ROSEN'S

Emergency Medicine
Concepts and Clinical Practice

10th Edition

ROSEN'S
Emergency Medicine
Concepts and Clinical Practice

Editor-in-Chief

Ron M. Walls, MD
Neskey Family Professor of Emergency Medicine
Department of Emergency Medicine
Harvard Medical School;
Chief Operating Officer
Mass General Brigham
Boston, Massachusetts

Senior Editors

Robert S. Hockberger, MD
Chair Emeritus
Emergency Medicine
Harbor-UCLA Medical Center
Torrance, California;
Emeritus Professor of Emergency Medicine
David Geffen School of Medicine at UCLA
Westwood, California

Marianne Gausche-Hill, MD
Medical Director
Los Angeles County EMS Agency;
Professor of Clinical Emergency Medicine
and Pediatrics
David Geffen School of Medicine at
University of California, Los Angeles
Los Angeles, California;
Clinical Faculty
Departments of Emergency Medicine and
Pediatrics
Harbor-UCLA Medical Center
Torrance, California

Timothy B. Erickson, MD,
FACEP, FACMT, FAACT
Department of Emergency Medicine
Brigham and Women's Hospital;
Chief, Division of Medical Toxicology
Mass General Brigham;
Associate Professor of Emergency
Medicine
Harvard Medical School
Boston, Massachusetts

Susan R. Wilcox, MD
Chief, Division of Critical Care
Department of Emergency Medicine
Massachusetts General Hospital;
Associate Professor of Emergency Medicine
Harvard Medical School
Associate Chief Medical Officer
Boston MedFlight
Boston, Massachusets

Editors

Katie Bakes, MD
Rocky Mountain Regional VA Medical
Center
Professor of Emergency Medicine and
Pediatrics
University of Colorado School of Medicine
Denver, Colorado

Calvin A. Brown III, MD
Department of Emergency Medicine
Brigham and Women's Hospital;
Associate Professor of Emergency
Medicine
Harvard Medical School
Boston, Massachusetts

David F.M. Brown, MD
MGH Trustees Endowed Professor
Department of Emergency Medicine
Harvard Medical School;
President
Massachusetts General Hospital
Boston, Massachusetts

Jonathan Davis, MD
Professor and Academic Chair
Department of Emergency Medicine
Georgetown University and MedStar Health
Washington, DC

Andy Jagoda, MD, FACEP
Professor and Chair Emeritus of
Emergency Medicine
Department of Emergency Medicine
Icahn School of Medicine at Mount Sinai
New York, New York

Amy H. Kaji, MD, PhD
Interim Chair
Department of Emergency Medicine
Harbor-UCLA Medical Center
Torrance, California;
Professor of Emergency Medicine
David Geffen School of Medicine at UCLA
Los Angeles, California;
Attending Physician
Department of Emergency Medicine
Long Beach Memorial Medical Center
Long Beach, California

León D. Sánchez, MD, MPH
Chief
Department of Emergency Medicine
Brigham and Women's Faulkner Hospital
Associate Professor of Emergency
Medicine
Harvard Medical School
Boston, Massachusetts

J. Adrian Tyndall, MD, MPH
Executive Vice President for Health Affairs
Professor and Dean
Morehouse School of Medicine
Atlanta, Georgia

Michael VanRooyen, MD, MPH
Chair
Department of Emergency Medicine
Brigham and Women's Hospital
Massachusetts General Hospital;
Enterprise Chief of Emergency Medicine
Mass General Brigham;
J. Stephen Bohan Professor of Emergency
Medicine
Harvard Medical School
Boston, Massachusetts

Content Editor—
Pharmacology

Bryan D. Hayes, PharmD, DABAT,
FAACT, FASHP
Clinical Pharmacy Manager
Emergency Medicine, Pediatric, and Overnight
Services
Massachusetts General Hospital;
Associate Professor
Department of Emergency Medicine
Division of Medical Toxicology
Interim Director
Graduate Pharmacy Education
Harvard Medical School;
Immediate Past-President
American Board of Applied Toxicology (ABAT)
Boston, Massachusetts

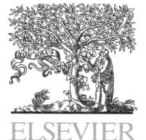

ELSEVIER

Elsevier
1600 John F. Kennedy Blvd.
Ste 1600
Philadelphia, PA 19103-2899

ROSEN'S EMERGENCY MEDICINE: CONCEPTS AND CLINICAL PRACTICE,
TENTH EDITION
VOLUME 1
VOLUME 2

ISBN: 978-0-323-75789-8
ISBN: 978-0-323-75847-5
ISBN: 978-0-323-75848-2

Senior Content Strategist: Kayla Wolfe
Content Development Specialist: Kristen Helm
Publishing Services Manager: Catherine Jackson
Senior Project Manager: Kate Mannix
Design Direction: Patrick Ferguson

Printed in India.

Last digit is the print number: 9 8 7 6 5 4 3 2

ACKNOWLEDGMENTS

Never has family meant so much. To my wife, Barb; my children, Andrew, Blake, and Alexa; and their spouses and children, thank you for reminding me why this work is so important. I was inspired and profoundly moved by the response of our specialty, and our colleagues across the healthcare spectrum, to this pandemic scourge. We embrace a brighter future, with a deep and unwavering look to the past, and with enormous gratitude. To Peter and John, thanks again, for all of it.

RMW

It has been both an honor and a pleasure to serve as an editor of this book for 10 editions, and I would like to express my appreciation to those who made this career-spanning journey for me both professionally fulfilling and personally rewarding. To Peter, John, and Ron for their vision and leadership as editors-in-chief, and for their friendship over the years, in good times and bad; to the 28 other leaders in our discipline who gave generously of their time and talent to serve as editors on different editions of the book; to the Elsevier staff (particularly Laura, Kathy, Stephanie, Kate, and Dee) for the support and encouragement they provided over the years; and to my wife Patty for bringing color, perspective, and broader meaning to my life.

RSH

I would like to thank my family for their continued understanding of my work to improve emergency care. My husband, David, and our three children, Katie, Jeremiah, and Sarah, provide the love, joy, and encouragement that makes participation on endeavors as important as this text worthwhile. Finally, I would like to thank my editor colleagues for their leadership and willingness to work through the pandemic to create a truly state-of-the-art textbook.

MGH

I would like to thank my incredible husband, Peter—I love you more each day—and our three amazing daughters, Sam, Jessie, and Avery—being your mom has been the joy of my life. I would also like to thank Denver Health's humanistic, incredibly talented, and brave Emergency Medicine residents—you are the hope for the future of medicine. And finally, I am deeply indebted to our patients, who allow us to witness their most vulnerable moments, and in doing so, offer us a chance to connect through our shared humanity.

KB

Thanks to my family for their understanding and support of all that pulls me away from time to time. Many thanks to Ron, Bob, Marianne, Tim, and Susan for the opportunity to work on this critical resource for our specialty. It has been an honor and a wonderful learning experience.

CAB

Forged during the scourge of the COVID-19 pandemic, this edition was for me a personal tribute to Peter Rosen, whose voice I can still hear and whose wisdom I still need. Looking forward to a brighter, kinder, safer, and more just future for all we serve, including those most dear to me: Deborah, Jacob, Sally, and Jaylin.

DFMB

With sincerest gratitude to Ron for the opportunity to contribute to this humbling body of work, to Bob, Marianne, Tim, and Susan for their sage wisdom and guidance throughout the process, and to Christine, Marisa, and Matthew—you are a source of perpetual strength, grounding, and encouragement that forever reminds me of the really important things in life.

JED

I extend my heartfelt thanks to Valerie, Camille, Isabelle, Celeste, Julian, and my parents, Robert and Gladys. I also give full credit to my mentors and colleagues in Emergency Medicine, Toxicology, Wilderness Medicine, and Global Humanitarian Health. Special thanks (with deep reverence) to the scientists who helped lay the foundation for us all: Paracelsus, Alice Hamilton, Rosalind Franklin, and Percy Lavon Julian.

TBE

To all the faculty, residents, and staff at the Mount Sinai Department of Emergency Medicine—their commitment to excellence in clinical care, teaching, and research inspires me every day. To Silvana, my wife and closest colleague, for her support and for keeping me focused on the important things in life. To Ron for being a mentor throughout my career; and to John and Peter, who live forever in our hearts and in the soul of our specialty.

ASJ

I am grateful to Ron, Bob, Marianne, Tim, and Susan for their incredible mentorship and patience with me, and to our Elsevier team for their editorial guidance. I also want to thank all the faculty, fellows, and residents at Harbor-UCLA Medical Center for inspiring me to always be the better teacher, learner, faculty member, and physician. Thank you!

AHK

To my wife Ami, thank you for your boundless patience. To all the residents I have played a role in training, I hope you have learned from me as much as I have from you.

LDS

I am grateful to my family who put up with late nights, early mornings and weekends, understanding this labor of love. To the authors for incredible work, and to my senior editors, Bob, Marianne, Tim, and Susan for their tremendous guidance. To Ron, for his incredible leadership and artful mentorship and for bringing me on. To the Elsevier team for first class support. To my late mother, Belle Patricia Tyndall, a teacher of English, who made this all possible for me.

JAT

With love and thanks to my wife, Julie, and my three wonderful kids, Izzy, Jack, and Alex, to my family, ever patient and ever supportive, and to my friends and mentors who continue to advance this critical field. This book is more important than ever as our specialty forms the front line of medicine and faces the most challenging clinical and social issues of our time. I remain inspired by all of the emergency providers everywhere who strive to provide expert care to every patient, every day; thank you. And especially to my daughter, Isabella VanRooyen, who is striving toward a career in medicine. May she be as fortunate as I was to find wonderful colleagues, inspiring mentors, and generous patients to lead her into a fulfilling career in a field that she loves.

MVR

I would like to thank Ron for the opportunity to work with this incomparable team of authors and coeditors. I have learned from each of you. I also want to thank my residents. Over the years, I have been fortunate to work with gifted EM residents who push me each day to be a better physician. Their asking the "why" behind the medicine, wanting to know the evidence, and insisting upon excellence from themselves have elevated my knowledge and practice. I am deeply indebted to you all.

SRW

Emily L. Aaronson, MD, MPH
Department of Emergency Medicine, Massachusetts General Hospital, Harvard Medical School, Boston, Massachusetts

Ethan E. Abbott, DO, MSCR, FACEP
Assistant Professor, T32 Research Fellow, Department of Emergency Medicine, Ichan School of Medicine at Mount Sinai, New York, New York

Gallane Abraham, MD
Assistant Professor, Department of Emergency Medicine, Associate Director, Geriatric Emergency Department, Icahn School of Medicine at Mount Sinai, New York, New York

Michael K. Abraham, MD, MS
Adjunct Assistant Professor, Department of Emergency Medicine, University of Maryland School of Medicine, Baltimore, Maryland; Chairman, Department of Emergency Medicine, Upper Chesapeake Health System, Bel Air, Maryland

Miguel Agrait-Gonzalez, MD, CAQ-SM
Assistant Professor, Department of Emergency Medicine, Ponce Health Sciences University, San Lucas Hospital, Ponce, Puerto Rico; Attending Physician, Emergency Medicine, Bayamon Medical Center, Bayamon, Puerto Rico

Saadia Akhtar, MD
Associate Dean for Graduate Medical Education and Residency Program Director, Department of Emergency Medicine, Mount Sinai Beth Israel, New York, New York

Steven E. Aks, DO
Director, The Toxikon Consortium, Department of Emergency Medicine, Cook County Health and Hospitals System; Professor of Emergency Medicine, Department of Emergency Medicine, Rush University, Chicago, Illinois

Patricia Ruth Atchinson, DO
Assistant Professor of Emergency Medicine and Medicine, Department of Emergency Medicine, Geisel School of Medicine, Dartmouth-Hitchcock Medical Center, Lebanon, New Hampshire

Marc Auerbach, MD, MSci, FAAP
Professor, Departments of Pediatrics and Emergency Medicine, Yale University School of Medicine, New Haven, Connecticut

Tom P. Aufderheide, MD, MS
Professor of Emergency Medicine, Department of Emergency Medicine, Medical College of Wisconsin, Milwaukee, Wisconsin

Katie Bakes, MD
Rocky Mountain Regional VA Medical Center, Professor of Emergency Medicine and Pediatrics, University of Colorado School of Medicine, Denver, Colorado

Laura L. Banks, DVM, MPH
Associate Professor of Emergency Medicine, University of New Mexico School of Medicine, Albuquerque, New Mexico

Aaron N. Barksdale, MD, FACEP
Associate Professor, Vice Chair of Research, Department of Emergency Medicine, University of Nebraska Medical Center, Omaha, Nebraska

Whitney Barrett, MD
Associate Professor, Department of Emergency Medicine, University of New Mexico School of Medicine, Albuquerque, New Mexico

Bruce M. Becker, MD, MPH
Professor, Departments of Emergency Medicine and Community Health, Warren Alpert School of Medicine at Brown University, Providence, Rhode Island

Zheng Ben Ma, MD, MHCM
Assistant Medical Director of Emergency Services, Memorial Hermann Hospital-Texas Medical Center; Assistant Professor of Emergency Medicine, UT Health McGovern Medical School, Houston, Texas

Kevin Biese, MD, MAT
Departments of Emergency Medicine and Internal Medicine, University of North Carolina at Chapel Hill, Chapel Hill, North Carolina

Michelle H. Biros, MD, MS
Professor, Department of Emergency Medicine, University of Minnesota Medical School, Minneapolis, Minnesota

Robert A. Bitterman, MD, JD, FACEP
President, Bitterman Health Law Consulting Group, Inc., Harbor Springs, Michigan

Thomas H. Blackwell, MD, FACEP, FAEMS
Professor of Emergency Medicine, University of South Carolina School of Medicine Greenville; Executive Director, Greenville County Emergency Medical Services, Greenville, South Carolina

Frederick C. Blum, MD
Professor, Department of Emergency Medicine, West Virginia University School of Medicine, Morgantown, West Virginia

Ira J. Blumen, MD, FACEP, FAMPA
Professor, Department of Medicine, Section of Emergency Medicine, University of Chicago; Program and Medical Director, University of Chicago Aeromedical Network (UCAN), University of Chicago Medicine, Chicago, Illinois

Edward B. Bolgiano, MD, FACEP, FACP
Assistant Professor, Department of Emergency Medicine, University of Maryland School of Medicine, Baltimore, Maryland

Michael C. Bond, MD
Associate Professor, Department of Emergency Medicine, University of Maryland School of Medicine, Baltimore, Maryland

Kelly Bookman, MD
Professor, Department of Emergency Medicine, University of Colorado, Denver, Colorado

Joelle Borhart, MD
Associate Professor, Department of Emergency Medicine, Georgetown University, Washington, DC

Brittany Boswell, MD
Fellow, Pediatric Emergency Medicine, University of Washington, Seattle Children's Hospital, Seattle, Washington

William J. Brady, MD
Professor, Departments of Medicine and Emergency Medicine, University of Virginia, Charlottesville, Virginia

Sabina A. Braithwaite, MD, MPH
Associate Professor and EMS Fellowship Director, Department of Emergency Medicine, Washington University, St. Louis, Missouri; Clinical Associate Professor, Department of Emergency Medicine, University of Kansas Medical Center, Kansas City, Kansas

Aaron Brody, MD, MPH, FACEP
Attending Physician, US Acute Care Solutions, Denver, Colorado

Calvin A. Brown III., MD
Department of Emergency Medicine, Brigham and Women's Hospital, Associate Professor of Emergency Medicine, Harvard Medical School, Boston, Massachusetts

David F.M. Brown, MD
MGH Trustees Endowed Professor, Department of Emergency Medicine, Harvard Medical School; President, Massachusetts General Hospital, Boston, Massachusetts

James E. Brown, MD, MMM
Professor and Chair, Department of Emergency Medicine, Wright State University Boonshoft School of Medicine, Dayton, Ohio

Jennie Alison Buchanan, MD, FACEP, FACMT
Staff Physician, Rocky Mountain Poison & Drug Safety; Department of Emergency Medicine, Denver Health & Hospital Authority; Associate Program Direct, Denver Health Residency in Emergency Medicine; Associate Professor, Department of Emergency Medicine, University of Colorado School of Medicine, Aurora, Colorado

Alice Kidder Bukhman, MD, MPH
Director of Clinical Operations, Brigham and Women's Faulkner Hospital; Instructor in Emergency Medicine, Harvard Medical School, Boston, Massachusetts

Jeffrey Bullard-Berent, MD
Professor of Emergency Medicine and Pediatrics, University of New Mexico, Albuquerque, New Mexico

E. Bradshaw Bunney, MD, FACEP
Professor, Residency Program Director, Vice Chair for Clinical Affairs, Associate CMO for GME, Department of Emergency Medicine, University of Illinois at Chicago, Chicago, Illinois

John H. Burton, MD
Chair, Professor of Emergency Medicine, Department of Emergency Medicine, Carilion Clinic, Roanoke, Virginia

Derya Caglar, MD
Associate Professor, Department of Pediatrics, University of Washington; Fellowship Director, Pediatric Emergency Medicine, Seattle Children's Hospital, Seattle, Washington

John D. Cahill, MD
Senior Attending in Emergency Medicine and Infectious Disease, Global Health Director, Department of Emergency Medicine, Mount Sinai Hospital, New York, New York; Senior Lecturer, International Health and Tropical Medicine, The Royal College of Surgeons, Dublin, Ireland

David J. Carlberg, MD
Assistant Professor of Emergency Medicine, Deparent of Emergency Medicine, Georgetown University School of Medicine; Associate Program Director, Program Director-Simulation and Safety Fellowship, Attending Physician, Department of Emergency Medicine, MedStar Georgetown University Hospital/MedStar Washington Hospital Center Emergency Medicine Residency, Washington, DC

Andrew K. Chang, MD, MS
Vincent P. Verdile, MD, '84 Endowed Chair for Emergency Medicine, Vice Chair for Research and Academic Affairs, Department of Emergency Medicine, Professor of Emergency Medicine, Albany Medical College; Attending Physician, Department of Emergency Medicine, Albany Medical Center, Albany, New York

Michael A. Chary, MD, PhD
Instructor, Department of Emergency Medicine, Cornell University, New York, New York

Paul Chen, MD, MBA
Director of Clinical Operations, Department of Emergency Medicine, Brigham and Women's Hospital; Instructor, Department of Emergency Medicine, Harvard Medical School, Boston, Massachusetts

Corrie E. Chumpitazi, MD, MS
Associate Professor, Department of Pediatrics, Baylor College of Medicine; Sedation Oversight Committee Co-Chair, Department of Pediatrics, Texas Children's Hospital, Houston, Texas

Stephen John Cico, MD, MEd
Assistant Dean for Graduate Medical Education, ACGME Designated Institutional Official (DIO), UCF-HCA Healthcare GME Consortium, Pediatric Emergency Medicine, University of Central Florida College of Medicine, Orlando, Florida

Ilene Claudius, MD
Associate Professor, Department of Emergency Medicine, David Geffen School of Medicine at University of California Los Angeles, Los Angeles, California; Physician Specialist, Department of Emergency Medicine, Harbor-UCLA Medical Center, Torrance, California

Wendy C. Coates, MD
Emeritus Professor of Emergency Medicine, Department of Emergency Medicine, David Geffen School of Medicine at University of California, Los Angeles, Los Angeles, California; Department of Emergency Medicine, Harbor-UCLA Medical Center, Torrance, California

Jon B. Cole, MD
Medical Director, Minnesota Poison Control System; Professor of Emergency Medicine, Department of Emergency Medicien, University of Minnesota Medical School, Hennepin Healthcare, Minneapolis, Minnesota

Christopher B. Colwell, MD
Professor and Vice Chair, Department of Emergency Medicine, University of California at San Francisco; Chief, Department of Emergency Medicine, Zuckerberg San Francisco General Hospital and Trauma Center, San Francisco, California

Theodore Corbin, MD, MPP
Department of Emergency Medicine, Rush University Medical Center, Chicago, Illinois

Robert Cooper, MD, MBA, MPH
Assistant Professor, Department of Emergency Medicine, Ohio State University College of Medicine; Medical Director, Ohio State University Health Plan, Columbus, Ohio

Brian Niall Corwell, MD
Assistant Professor, Departments of Emergency Medicine and Orthopaedics, University of Maryland School of Medicine, Baltimore, Maryland

Amelia M. Curtis, MD
Toxicology Fellow in Training, Department of Emergency Medicine, University of Massachusetts, Worcester, Massachusetts

Shawn D'Andrea, MD, MPH, FACEP
Affiliated Faculty, Harvard Humanitarian Initiative, Harvard University, Boston, Massachusetts

Daniel F. Danzl, MD
Professor and Emeritus Chair, Department of Emergency Medicine, University of Louisville, Louisville, Kentucky

Moira Davenport, MD
Attending Physician, Department of Emergency Medicine, Allegheny General Hospital, Pittsburgh, Pennsylvania

Alysa S. Davis, DO
Department of Emergency Medicine, Unity Point Health-Trinity, Rock Island, Illinois

Jonathan Davis, MD
Professor and Academic Chair, Department of Emergency Medicine, Georgetown University and MedStar Health, Washington, DC

Natalie L. Davis, MD, MMSc
Associate Professor, Department of Pediatrics, University of Maryland School of Medicine, Baltimore, Maryland

Mohamud R. Daya, MD, MSc
Professor, Department of Emergency Medicine, Oregon Health & Science University, Portland, Oregon

Lindsey M. DeGeorge, MD
Attending Physician, Department of Emergency Medicine, MedStar Southern Maryland Hospital, Clinton, Maryland

Robert W. Derlet, MD
Professor, Emergency Department, University of California, Davis School of Medicine, Sacramento, California

Valerie A. Dobiesz, MD, MPH
Department of Emergency Medicine, Brigham and Women's Hospital; Director of Internal Programs, STRATUS Center for Medical Simulation; Assistant Professor of Emergency Medicine, Harvard Medical School, Boston, Massachusetts

Alan A. Dupré, MD, FACEP, FAAEM
Assistant Professor, Department of Emergency Medicine, Wright State University/Wright-Patterson Air Force Base, Dayton, Ohio

Petra Duran-Gehring, MD, RDMS, FACEP
Associate Professor, Director of Emergency Ultrasound, Department of Emergency Medicine, University of Florida College of Medicine-Jacksonville, Jacksonville, Florida

Joshua S. Easter, MD, MSc
Associate Professor, Department of Emergency Medicine, University of Virginia, Charlottesville, Virginia

Christopher J. Edwards, PharmD, BCPS
Assistant Professor, University of Arizona College of Pharmacy, Tucson, Arizona

Wesley P. Eilbert, MD
Professor of Clinical Emergency Medicine, Department of Emergency Medicine, University of Illinois College of Medicine, Chicago, Illinois

Erick Eiting, MD, MPH, MMM
Associate Professor of Clinical Emergency Medicine, Department of Emergency Medicine, Icahn School of Medicine at Mount Sinai, New York, New York

Marie-Carmelle Elie-Turenne, MD, FACEP, FAAEM, FCCM
Professor and Chair, Department of Emergency Medicine, The University of Alabama at Birmingham School of Medicine, Birmingham, Alabama; Adjunct Professor, Department of Emergency Medicine, University of Florida, Gainesville, Florida

Timothy B. Erickson, MD, FACEP, FACMT, FAACT
Department of Emergency Medicine, Brigham and Women's Hospital; Chief, Division of Medical Toxicology, Mass General Brigham; Associate Professor of Emergency Medicine, Harvard Medical School, Boston, Massachusetts

Andrew J. Eyre, MD, MS-HPEd
Attending Physician, Assistant Residency Director, Department of Emergency Medicine, Brigham and Women's Hospital, Instructor in Emergency Medicine, Harvard Medical School, Boston, Massachusetts

Romeo Fairley, MD, MPH, FACEP
Assistant Professor, Director, Disaster Preparedness and Response, Director, Disaster Medicine Fellowship, Department of Emergency Medicine, University of Texas Health-San Antonio, San Antonio, Texas

Susan E. Farrell, MD, EdM
Director, OSCE Program and Associate Professor, Emergency Medicine, Program in Medical Education, Harvard Medical School; Director, Continuing and Professional Development, Center for Interprofessional Studies and Innovation, MGH Institute of Health Professions, Boston, Massachusetts

John J. Fath, MD, MPH, FACS, FCCM
Former Clinical Professor of Surgery, Wayne State University, Detroit, Michigan; Former Director of Trauma, Beaumont Hospital Dearborn, Dearborn, Michigan

Madonna Fernandez-Frackelton, MD
Program Director, Vice Chair of Medical Education, Department of Emergency Medicine, Harbor-UCLA Medical Center, Torrance, California; Professor of Medicine, David Geffen School of Medicine, University of California, Los Angeles, Los Angeles, California

John T. Finnell, MD, MSc
Professor of Clinical Emergency Medicine, Department of Emergency Medicine, Indiana University, Indianapolis, Indiana

Vanessa Franco, MD, PhD
Assistant Professor, Department of Emergency Medicine, University of California, Los Angeles, Los Angeles, California

Bradley W. Frazee, MD
Attending Physician, Department of Emergency Medicine, Alameda Health System-Highland Hospital, Oakland, California; Clinical Professor of Emergency Medicine, University of California San Francisco, San Francisco, California

Benjamin W. Friedman, MD, MS
Department of Emergency Medicine, Albert Einstein College of Medicine, Bronx, New York

Jeremiah D. Gaddy, EMT-P, MD
Assistant Professor, Department of Emergency Medicine, Wright State University, Dayton, Ohio

Michael Ganetsky, MD
Assistant Professor of Emergency Medicine, Harvard Medical School; Department of Emergency Medicine, Beth Israel Deaconess Medical Center, Boston, Massachusetts

Marianne Gausche-Hill, MD, FACEP, FAAP, FAEMS
Medical Director, Los Angeles County EMS Agency; Professor of Clinical Emergency Medicine and Pediatrics, David Geffen School of Medicine at University of California, Los Angeles, Los Angeles, California; Clinical Faculty, Departments of Emergency Medicine and Pediatrics, Harbor-UCLA Medical Center, Torrance, California

Joel M. Geiderman, MD
Professor and Co-Chairman, Department of Emergency Medicine, Ruth and Harry Roman Emergency Department, Cedars-Sinai Medical Center, Los Angeles, California

Carl A. Germann, MD, MHPE, FACEP
Associate Professor, Department of Emergency Medicine, Tufts University School of Medicine, Boston, Massachusetts; Attending Physician, Emergency Department, Maine Medical Center, Portland, Maine

George F. Glass III., MD
Assistant Professor, Department of Emergency Medicine, University of Virginia, Charlottesville, Virginia

Jonathan M. Glauser, MD, MBA, FACEP
Professor, Department of Emergency Medicine, Case Western Reserve University; Faculty, Emergency Medicine Residency, MetroHealth Medical Center, Cleveland, Ohio

Steven A. Godwin, MD, FACEP
Professor and Chair, Department of Emergency Medicine, Assistant Dean, Simulation Education, University of Florida COM-Jacksonville, Jacksonville, Florida

Scott A. Goldberg, MD, MPH
Director of Emergency Medical Services, Department of Emergency Medicine, Brigham and Women's Hospital; Assistant Professor of Emergency Medicine, Harvard Medical School, Boston, Massachusetts

Jeffrey M. Goodloe, MD, NRP, FACEP, FAEMS, LSSBB
Chief Medical Officer, Medical Controll Board, Emergency Medical Services System for Metropolitan Oklahoma City; Professor and EMS Section Chief, Department of Emergency Medicine, Oklahoma Cetner for Prehospital and Disaster Medicine, University of Oklahoma School of Community Medicine, Tulsa, Oklahoma

Diane L. Gorgas, MD
Professor, Vice Chair of Academic Affairs, Department of Emergency Medicine, Executive Director, Office of Global Health, The Ohio State University and Wexner Medical Center, Columbus, Ohio

Thomas J. Green, MD, MSc, Dip Sports Med (CASEM)
Clinical Assistant Professor, Department of Emergency Medicine, University of British Columbia, Royal Columbian Hospital, New Westminster, British Columbia, Canada

Shamai A. Grossman, MD, MS
Associate Professor of Medicine and Emergency Medicine, Vice Chair for Health Care Quality, Department of Emergency Medicine, Harvard Medical School, Harvard Medical Faculty Physicians, Beth Israel Deaconess Medical Center, Boston, Massachusetts

Kama Guluma, MD
Clinical Professor, Department of Emergency Medicine, University of California San Diego School of Medicine; Faculty Physician, Department of Emergency Medicine, University of California San Diego Health System, San Diego, California; Associate Dean of Admissions and Student Affairs, University of California San Diego School of Medicine, La Jolla, California

Joshua Guttman, MD, FRCPC, FAAEM, FACEP
Assistant Professor, Department of Emergency Medicine, Emory University School of Medicine, Atlanta, Georgia

Nathan L. Haas, MD
Clinical Assistant Professor, Department of Emergency Medicine, University of Michigan, Ann Arbor, Michigan

Elizabeth J. Haines, DO
Ronald O. Perelman Department of Emergency Medicine, New York University, New York

Christina Hajicharalambous, DO, MSEd, MS
Residency Director, Department of Emergency Medicine, Hackensack University Medical Center, Hackensack, New Jersey

Matthew M. Hall, MD
Department of Emergency Medicine, Providence Regional Medical Center, Evertt, Washington; Clinical Associate Professor, Elson S. Floyd College of Medicine, Washington State University, Pullman, Washington

Laurie Seidel Halmo, MD
Fellow, Rocky Mountain Poison and Drug Center, Denver Health and Hospital Authority, Denver, Colorado; Instructor Fellow, Pediatrics, University of Colorado School of Medicine, Aurora, Colorado

Bhakti Hansoti, MBChB, MPH, PhD
Associate Professor, Department of Emergency Medicine, Johns Hopkins School of Medicine and Department of International Health Bloomberg School of Public Health, Baltimore, Maryland

N. Stuart Harris, MD, MFA, FRCP Edin.
Chief, Division of Wilderness Medicine; Fellowship Director, MGH Wilderness Medicine Fellowship, Department of Emergency Medicine, Massachusetts General Hospital, Associate Professor of Emergency Medicine, Harvard Medical School, Boston, Massachusetts

Nicholas Harrison, MD, MSC
Assistant Professor of Emergency Medicine, Indiana University School of Medicine, Indianapolis, Indiana

Danielle Hart, MD
Program Director, Emergency Medicine Residency, Co-Fellowship Director, Medical Education & Simulation Fellowship, Department of Emergency Medicine, Hennepin County Medical Center, Minneapolis, Minnesota

Benjamin W. Hatten, MD, MPH
Assistant Professor, Section of Medical Toxicology, Department of Emergency Medicine, University of Colorado School of Medicine, Aurora, Colorado

Carlton E. Heine, MD, PhD, FACEP, FAWM
Associate Professor, Department of Medical Education and Clinical Sciences, Elson S. Floyd College of Medicine, Washington State University, Spokane, Washington

Jason D. Heiner, MD
Staff Physician, Emergency Medicine, University of Washington, Seattle, Washington

Megan C. Henn, MD
Assistant Professor of Emergency Medicine, Department of Emergency Medicine, Emory University, Atlanta, Georgia

H. Gene Hern Jr., MD, MS
Associate Clinical Professor of Emergency Medicine, University of California San Francisco, San Francisco, California; Vice Chairman of the Emergency Department, Alameda Health System, Oakland, California

Jamie M. Hess, MD
President, UW Medical Foundation, Associate Professor of Emergency Medicine, Director of Quality, Patient Safety, and Interprofessional Education, University of Wisconsin School of Medicine and Public Health, Madison, Wisconsin

Adam D. Hill, MD
Assistant Professor, Department of Emergency Medicine, Icahn School of Medicine at Mount Sinai, New York, New York

Nadine T. Himelfarb, MD
Assistant Professor of Emergency Medicine, Clinician Educator, Department of Emergency Medicine, Warren Alpert Medical School of Brown University, Providence, Rhode Island

Robert S. Hockberger, MD
Chair Emeritus, Emergency Medicine, Harbor-UCLA Medical Center, Torrance, California; Emeritus Professor of Emergency Medicine, David Geffen School of Medicine at UCLA, Westwood, California

Christopher Hogrefe, MD
Clinical Associate Professor, Department of Emergency Medicine, University of Iowa Hospitals and Clinics, University of Iowa Carver College of Medicine, Iowa City, Iowa; Assistant Team Physician, Chicago Cubs, Chicago, Illinois

Carolyn Kluwe Holland, MD, MEd, FACEP, FAAP
Clinical Associate Professor and Physician Director of Quality, Department of Emergency Medicine, Affiliate Clinical Associate Professor, Department of Pediatrics, Division Chief, Pediatric Emergency Medicine, Medical Director, UF Health Pediatric Emergency Department, University of Florida Health, Gainesville, Florida

James F. Holmes, MD, MPH
Professor and Executive Vice Chair, Department of Emergency Medicine, UC Davis School of Medicine, Sacramento, California

Jason A. Hoppe, DO
Associate Professor, Department of Emergency Medicine, Section of Pharmacology and Toxicology University of Colorado School of Medicine, Aurora, Colorado; Rocky Mountain Poison & Drug Safety, Denver Health & Hospital Authority, Denver, Colorado

Timothy Horeczko, MD, MSCR
Associate Professor of Clinical Emergency Medicine, David Geffen School of Medicine at University of California, Los Angeles, Los Angeles, California; Director of Pediatric Emergency Medicine Fellowship, Harbor-UCLA Medical Center, Torrance, California

Christopher Hoyte, MD
Rocky Mountain Poison Center, Medical Toxicology, Denver Health and Hospital Authority, University of Colorado School of Medicine, Denver, Colorado

Dennis Hsieh, MD, JD
Chief Medical Officer, Contra Costa Health Plan; Clinical Faculty, Harbor-UCLA Medical Center; Assistant Professor, David Geffen School of Medicine at University of California, Los Angeles, Los Angeles, California

Korin Hudson, MD
Associate Professor, Department of Emergency Medicine, MedStar Georgetown University Hospital, Washington, DC

Karl Huesgen, MD, MS
Associate Professor, Department of Emergency Medicine, University of Missouri, Columbia, Missouri

Ula Hwang, MD, MPH
Department of Emergency Medicine, Yale University School of Medicine, New Haven, Connecticut; Geriatric Research, Education, and Clinic Center, James J. Peters VA Medical Center, Bronx, New York

Kenneth V. Iserson, MD, MBA, FACEP, FAAEM, FIFEM
Professor Emeritus, Department of Emergency Medicine, University of Arizona, Tucson, Arizona

Janetta L. Iwanicki, MD
Scientific Director of Research, Medical Toxicology, Rocky Mountain Poison and Drug Center; Emergency Medicine Attending Physician, Department of Emergency Medicine, Denver Health and Hospital Authority, Denver, Colorado; Assistant Professor, Department of Emergency Medicine, University of Colorado School of Medicine, Aurora, Colorado

Andy Jagoda, MD, FACEP
Professor and Chair Emeritus of Emergency Medicine, Department of Emergency Medicine, Icahn School of Medicine at Mount Sinai, New York, New York, New York

Thea James, MD, MPH
Vice President of Mission, Associate Chief Medical Officer, Office of Chief Medical Officer, Boston Medical Center; Associate Professor of Emergency Medicine, Department of Emergency Medicine, Boston University School of Medicine, Boston, Massachusetts

Corlin Jewell, MD
Assistant Professor, Department of Emergency Medicine, University of Wisconsin School of Medicine and Public Health, Madison, Wisconsin

Nicholas J. Johnson, MD, FACEP, FCCM
Assistant Professor, Department of Emergency Medicine, Division of Pulmonary, Critical Care, and Sleep Medicine (Adjunct), University of Washington, Washington

Alan E. Jones, MD
Tenured Professor, Department of Emergency Medicine, University of Mississippi Medical Center, Jackson, Mississippi

Emily M. Jones, MD
Clinical Assistant Professor, Northwestern University Feinberg School of Medicine, Chicago, Illinois

Nicholas J. Jouriles, MD
Professor and Chair, Department of Emergency Medicine, Northeast Ohio Medical University, Rootstown, Ohio; Vice Chair, Faculty Development, Department of Emergency Medicine, Summa Health and US Acute Care Solutions, Akron, Ohio; Past President, American College of Emergency Physicians, Dallas, Texas

Christopher Kabrhel, MD, MPH
Director, Center for Vascular Emergencies, Department of Emergency Medicine, Massachusetts General Hospital; MGH Endowed Chair in Emergency Medicine, Professor of Emergency Medicine, Harvard Medical School, Boston, Massachusetts

Colin G. Kaide, MD
Professor of Emergency Medicine, Wexner Medical Center, The Ohio State University, Columbus, Ohio

Amy H. Kaji, MD, PhD
Interim Chair, Professor of Clinical Emergency Medicine, Harbor-UCLA Medical Center, Torrance, California; Professor of Emergency Medicine, David Geffen School of Medicine at UCLA, Los Angeles, California; Attending Physician, Department of Emergency Medicine, Long Beach Memorial Medical Center, Long Beach, California

Julius (Jay) A. Kaplan, MD, FACEP
Medical Director, Care Transformation, LCMC Health; Clinical Associate Professor and Academic Faculty, Department of Emergency Medicine, University Medical Center, LSU Health Sciences Center, New Orleans, Louisiana; Past President, American College of Emergency Physicians, Irving, Texas

Stephanie Kayden, MD, MPH
Deputy Chair and Brigham Distinguished Chair in Emergency Medicine, Department of Emergency Medicine, Brigham and Women's Hospital, Associate Professor of Emergency Medicine, Harvard Medical School, Boston, Massachusetts

Ryan D. Kearney, MD, MPH
Staff Physician, Summit Health, Bend, Oregon

Matthew P. Kelly, MD
Assistant Professor, Department of Emergency Medicine, University of Alabama, Birmingham, Birmingham, Alabama

Hyung T. Kim, MD
Associate Professor of Clinical Emergency Medicine, Department of Emergency Medicine, David Geffin School of Medicine, University of California, Los Angeles, Los Angeles, California

Sean M. Kivlehan, MD, MPH
Fellowship Director, Global Emergency Medicine, Department of Emergency Medicine, Brigham and Women's Hospital, Boston, Massachusetts

Kristi L. Koenig, MD, FACEP, FIFEM, FAEMS
Medical Director, San Diego County EMS Office, San Diego, California; Professor Emerita of Emergency Medicine and Public Health, University of California, Irvine, Irvine, California

Joshua M. Kosowsky, MD
Attending Physician, Department of Emergency Medicine, Brigham and Women's Hospital; Assistant Professor of Emergency Medicine, Harvard Medical School, Boston, Massachusetts

Christine E. Koval, MD
Section Head, Transplant Infectious Diseases, Associate Professor, Lerner College of Medicine of Case Western Reserve University; Department of Infectious Diseases, Transplant Center, Cleveland Clinic, Cleveland, Ohio

Alex Koyfman, MD
Assistant Professor, Attending Physician, Department of Emergency Medicine, University of Texas Southwestern Medical Center, Parkland Memorial Hospital, Dallas, Texas

Michael C. Kurz, MD, MS, FACEP, FAHA
Professor and Vice Chair for Research, Department of Emergency Medicine; Professor, Department of Surgery, Division of Acute Care Surgery, University of Alabama School of Medicine, Birmingham, Alabama

Michelle D. Lall, MD, MHS, FACEP
Associate Professor, Department of Emergency Medicine, Emory University, Atlanta, Georgia

Spenser C. Lang, MD
Assistant Professor, Department of Emergency Medicine, University of Cincinnati, Cincinnati, Ohio

Jeffrey E. Lee, MD
Associate Clinical Professor, Residency Program Director, Department of Ophthalmology, University of California San Diego School of Medicine, La Jolla, California; Chief of Ophthalmology, University of California San Diego Medical Center, University of California San Diego Health System, San Diego, California, San Diego, California

Charles Lei, MD
Assistant Professor of Emergency Medicine, Department of Emergency Medicine, Vanderbilt University Medical Center, Nashville, Tennessee

Michael D. Levine, MD
Associate Professor of Emergency Medicine, Department of Emergency Medicine, University of California, Los Angeles, Los Angeles, California

Matthew J. Levy, DO, MSc
Assistant Director of Special Operations, Department of Emergency Medicine, Johns Hopkins University School of Medicine, Baltimore, Maryland

Phillip D. Levy, MD, MPH, FACEP, FAHA, FACC
Professor of Emergency Medicine, Associate Vice President for Translational Science, Wayne State University, Detroit, Michigan

Christopher S. Lim, MD
Senior Physician, Department of Emergency Medicine. Kaiser Permanente San Jose Medical Center, San Jose, California

Daniel Lindberg, MD
Associate Professor, Departments of Emergency Medicine and Pediatrics, University of Colorado Anschutz Medical Campus; Children's Hospital Colorado, Denver, Colorado

Ari M. Lipsky, MD, PhD
Chair, Department of Emergency medicine, HaEmek Medical Center, Afula, Israel

J. Marc Liu, MD, MPH
Professor, Department of Emergency Medicine, Medical College of Wisconsin, Milwaukee, Wisconsin

Brit Long, MD
Physician, Department of Emergency Medicine, SAUSHEC, Brooke Army Medical Center, Texas

Wendy Macias-Konstantopoulos, MD, MPH
Associate Professor, Department of Emergency Medicine, Havard Medical School, Boston, Massachusetts

Carolina Barbosa Maciel, MD, MSCR
Assistant Professor of Neurology and Neurosurgery, Department of Neurology and Neurosurgery, University of Florida, Gainesville, Florida; Adjunct Assistant Professor of Neurology, Yale University School of Medicine, New Haven, Connecticut; Adjunct Assistant Professor of Neurology, University of Utah, Salt Lake City, Utah

Patrick J. Maher, MD, MS
Assistant Professor, Department of Emergency Medicine, Icahn School of Medicine at Mount Sinai, New York, New York

Gerald E. Maloney Jr., DO, MS
Associate Medical Director, Emergency Department, Louis Stokes Cleveland VA Medical Center; Associate Professor, Department of Emergency Medicine, Case Western Reserve University, Cleveland, Ohio

Patrick J. Maloney, MD
Clinical Faculty, University of South Carolina School of Medicine-Greenville, Greenville, South Carolina

Catherine Anna Marco, MD
Professor, Department of Emergency Medicine, Wright State University Boonshoft School of Medicine; Attending Physician, Department of Emergency Medicine, Miami Valley Hospital, Dayton, Ohio

Keith A. Marill, MD, MS
Department of Emergency Medicine, Massachusetts General Hospital; Associate Professor of Emergency Medicine, Harvard Medical School, Boston, Massachusetts

Joseph P. Martinez, MD
Associate Professor, Departments of Emergency Medicine and Medicine, University of Maryland School of Medicine, Baltimore, Maryland

Aaron G. Matlock, MD, MBA
Attending Physician, Department of Emergency Medicine, Brooke Army Medical Center, Joint Base San Antonio, Texas

Ryanne J. Mayersak, MS, MD
Assistant Professor, Associate Residency Program Director, Director of Residency Wellness, Department of Emergency Medicine, Oregon Health and Science University, Portland, Oregon

Larissa S. May, MD, MSPH
Professor, Department of Emergency Medicine, University of California, Davis, Sacramento, California

Nicole S. McCoin, MD
Chair, Department of Emergency Medicine, Ochsner Medical Center, Metairie, Louisiana

Michael T. McCurdy, MD
Clinical Professor, Departments of Medicine and Emergency Medicine, Division of Pulmonary & Critical Care, University of Maryland School of Medicine, Baltimore, Maryland; Chief, Department of Medicine and Division of Critical Care, Department of Medicine, University of Maryland St. Joseph Medical Center, Towson, Maryland

Jeffry McKinzie, MD
Assistant Professor, Departments of Emergency Medicine and Pediatrics, Vanderbilt University Medical Center, Nashville, Tennessee

Christopher W. Meaden, MD, MS
Assistant Professor, Department of Emergency Medicine. Rutgers New Jersey Medical School, Newark, New Jersey

Timothy J. Meehan, MD, MPH
Associate Professor of Emergency Medicine and Medical Toxicology, The University of Illinois at Chicago, UI Health, Chicago, Illinois

Niyati Mehta, MD
Assistant Professor, Department of Pediatric Neurology, Medical College of Wisconsin, Milwaukee, Wisconsin

William J. Meurer, MD, MS
Professor, Departments of Emergency Medicine and Neurology, University of Michigan, Ann Arbor, Michigan

Nathan W. Mick, MD
Vice Chair, Department of Emergency Medicine, Maine Medical Center, Portland, Maine; Associate Professor of Emergency Medicine, Tufts University School of Medicine, Boston, Massachusetts

Eli M. Miloslavsky, MD
Assistant Professor, Department of Medicine, Division of Rheumatology, Allergy, and Immunology, Massachusetts General Hospital, Harvard Medical School, Boston, Massachusetts

James R. Miner, MD
Professor and Chair, Department of Emergency Medicine, University of Minnesota; Chief, Department of Emergency Medicine, Hennepin County Medical Center, Minneapolis, Minnesota

Nicholas M. Mohr, MD, MS
Department of Emergency Medicine, University of Iowa Hospitals and Clinics, Iowa City, Iowa

Joel Moll, MD
Associate Professor, Vice Chair of Education, Residency Program Director, Medical Education Fellowship Director, Department of Emergency Medicine, Virginia Commonwealth University, Richmond, Virginia

Jessica Monas, MD
Assistant Professor, Consultant, Department of Emergency Medicine, Mayo Clinic, Phoenix, Arizona

Andrew A. Monte, MD, PhD
Associate Professor, Department of Emergency Medicine, Section of Pharmacology and Toxicology, University of Colorado School of Medicine, Aurora, Colorado; Rocky Mountain Poison & Drug Safety, Denver Health & Hospital Authority, Denver, Colorado

Martha M. Montgomery, MD, MS
Attending Physician, Department of Emergency Medicine, Highland Hospital-Alameda Health System, Oakland, California

Malia J. Moore, MD
Assistant Professor of Emergency Medicine, Indiana University School of Medicine, Indianapolis, Indiana

Gregory J. Moran, MD
Professor of Clinical Emergency Medicine, David Geffen School of Medicine at University of California Los Angeles, Los Angeles, California; Department of Emergency Medicine and Division of Infectious Disease, Olive View-UCLA Medical Center, Sylmar, California

Mark B. Mycyk, MD
Director, Toxicology Research, Department of Emergency Medicine, Cook County Health; Associate Professor, Department of Emergency Medicine, Rush Medical College, Chicago, Illinois

Jose V. Nable, MD, NRP
Associate Professor, Department of Emergency Medicine, Georgetown University School of Medicine; Attending Physician, Department of Emergency Medicine, MedStar Georgetown University Hospital, Washington, DC

Joshua Nagler, MD, MHPEd
Associate Division Chief, Fellowship Director, Division of Emergency Medicine, Boston's Children's Hospital; Associate Professor of Pediatrics and Emergency Medicine, Harvard Medical School, Boston, Massachusetts

Denise Nassisi, MD
Associate Professor, Department of Emergency Medicine, Icahn School of Medicine at Mount Sinai, New York, New York

Joshua B. Nathan, MD
Clinical Assistant Professor of Psychiatry and Behavioral Sciences, Department of Psychiatry and Behavioral Sciences, Rosalind Franklin University of Medicine and Science, Chicago, Illinois

Lewis S. Nelson, MD
Professor and Chair, Department of Emergency Medicine, Rutgers New Jersey Medical School, Newark, New Jersey

Michael E. Nelson, MD, MS
Attending Physician, Departments of Emergency Medicine, Toxicology, and Addiction Medicine, NorthShore University Health System, Evanston, Illinois; Attending Physician, Departments of Emergency Medicine, Toxicology, and Addiction Medicine, Cook County Hospital (Stroger), Chicago, Illinois

Kim Newton, MD
Clinical Associate Professor, Department of Emergency Medicine, Los Angeles County Medical Center, Keck School of Medicine at University of Southern California, Los Angeles, California

Thomas Nguyen, MD
Associate Professor, Department of Emergency Medicine, Mount Sinai Beth Israel, New York, New York

Adam M. Nicholson, MD
Assistant Professor, Department of Emergency Medicine, University of Wisconsin, Madison, Wisconsin

L. Connor Nickels, MD, RDMS
Ultrasound Director, Attending Physician, Department of Emergency Medicine, University of Florida, Gainesville, Florida

Jenna Karagianis Nikolaides, MD, MA
Assistant Professor of Emergency Medicine and Medical Toxicology, Department of Emergency Medicine, Assistant Professor of Addiction Medicine, Department of Psychiatry, Rush University Medical Center; Medical Toxicologist, Illinois Poison Center, Chicago, Illinois

Micah J. Nite, MD
Assistant Professor, Department of Emergency Medicine, Icahn School of Medicine at Mount Sinai, New York, New York

Michael Nitzberg, MD, FACEM, FAAEM, FACEP
Staff Specialist, Emergency Medicine, Illawarra Shoalhaven Local Health District, Wollongong Hospital, Wollongong, New South Wales, Australia

Marquita S. Norman, MD, MBA
Associate Professor, University of Texas Southwestern Medical Center, Dallas, Texas

Ashley Booth Norse, MD, FACEP
Associate Chair of Operations, Associate Professor, Department of Emergency Medicine, University of Florida COM-Jacksonville, Jacksonville, Florida

Richard M. Nowak, MD, MBA
Chair Emeritus, Department of Emergency Medicine, Henry Ford Health System; Clinical Professor, Department of Emergency Medicine, Wayne State Medical School, Detroit, Michigan; Clinical Professor, Department of Emergency Medicine, University of Michigan Medical School, Ann Arbor, Michigan

Adedamola A. Ogunniyi, MD
Associate Program Director, Department of Emergency Medicine, Harbor-UCLA Medical Center, Los Angeles Department of Health Services, Torrance, California; Assistant Clinical Professor, Department of Emergency Medicine, David Geffen School of Medicine at University of California, Los Angeles, Los Angeles, California

Daniel L. Overbeek, MD
Medical Toxicology Fellow, Departments of Emergency Medicine and Medical Toxicology, University of Rochester Medical Center, Rochester, New York

Patricia Padlipsky, MD, MS
Associate Clinical Professor of Pediatrics, David Geffen School of Medicine, University of California at Los Angeles, Los Angeles, California; Director, Pediatric Emergency Department, Harbor-UCLA Medical Center, Torrance, California

Jessica Palmer, MS, MD
Attending Physician, Department of Emergency Medicine, MedStar Georgetown University Hospital, Washington Hospital Center, Washington, DC

Linda Papa, MD, MSc
Director of Academic Clinical Research, Department of Emergency Medicine, Orlando Regional Medical Center; Adjunct Professor, Department of Emergency Medicine, University of Central Florida, Orlando, Florida; Adjunct Professor, Departments of Neurology and Neurosurgery, McGill University, Montreal, Quebec, Canada; Adjunct Professor, Department of Emergency Medicine, University of Florida, Gainesville, Florida

David A. Peak, MD
Associate Residency Director, Department of Emergency Medicine, Massachusetts General Hospital; Assistant Professor of Emergency Medicine, Harvard Medical School, Boston, Massachusetts

Ryan Anthony Pedigo, MD, NHPE
Associate Residency Program Director, Department of Emergency Medicine, Harbor-UCLA Medical Center, Torrance, California; Assistant Professor of Medicine, David Geffen School of Medicine at University of California, Los Angeles, Los Angeles, California

Jack Perkins Jr., MD
Department of Emergency Medicine, Virginia Tech, Roanoke, Virginia

James A. Pfaff, MD
Attending Physician, San Antonio Univformed Services Health Education Consortium (SAUSHEC), Emergency Medicine Residency, Brooke Army Medical Center, Joint Base San Antonio, Texas

Camiron L. Pfennig, MD, MHPE
Prisma Health-Upstate Department of Emergency Medicine, Emergency Medicine Residency Director, Associate Professor, University of South Carolina School of Medicine Greenville; Clemson University School of Health Research, Greenville, South Carolina

Michael P. Phelan, MD
Associate Professor, Lerner College of Medicine of Case Western Reserve University, Emergency Medicine Institute, Cleveland Clinic, Cleveland, Ohio

Ava E. Pierce, MD
Associate Chair of Diversity and Inclusion, Department of Emergency Medicine, University of Texas Southwestern Medical Center, Dallas, Texas

Melissa A. Platt, MD
Professor, Department of Emergency Medicine, University of Louisville, Louisville, Kentucky

Elizabeth P.D. Pontius, MD
Associate Professor of Emergency Medicine, Emergency Department, Georgetown University School of Medicine; Attending Physician, Emergency Department, Assistant Program Director, Emergency Medicine Residency, Georgetown/ MedStar Washington Hospital Center, Washington, DC

Trevor R. Pour, MD
Associate Residency Program Director, Department of Emergency Medicine, Mount Sinai Hospital, New York, New York

Kian Preston-Suni, MD, MPH
Assistant Chief, Department of Emergency Medicine, Greater Los Angeles VA Medical Center; Assistant Professor of Clinical Emergency Medicine, David Geffen School of Medicine at University of California, Los Angeles, Los Angeles, California

Timothy G. Price, MD
Professor, Department of Emergency Medicine, University of Louisville, Louisville, Kentucky

William B. Prince, MD
Clinical Assistant Professor of Pediatrics, Seattle Children's Hospital, University of Washington School of Medicine, Seattle, Washington

Marc Probst, MD, MS
Assistant Professor, Director of General Emergency Medicine Research, Department of Emergency Medicine, Columbia University Irving Medical Center, New York, New York

Michael Pulia, MD, MS
Assistant Professor, Director, Emergency Care for Infectious Diseases (ECID) Research Program, Department of Emergency Medicine, University of Wisconsin School of Medicine and Public Health, Madison, Wisconsin

Michael A. Puskarich, MD
Director of Research, Department of Emergency Medicine, Hennepin County Medical Center; Associate Professor of Emergency Medicine, Department of Emergency Medicine, University of Minnesota, Minneapolis, Minnesota

Tammie E. Quest, MD
Professor, Department of Emergency Medicine, Emory University School of Medicine, Decatur, Georgia; Division Chief, Palliative Medicine, Family and Preventive Medicine, Emory University, Atlanta, Georgia

Ali S. Raja, MD, MBA, MPH
Executive Vice Chair of Emergency Medicine, Mooney-Reed Endowed Chair, Massachusetts General Hospital; Professor of Emergency Medicine, Harvard Medical School Boston, Massachusetts

Neha P. Raukar, MD, MS, California QSM
Associate Professor, Department of Emergency Medicine, Mayo Clinic, Rochester, Minnesota

Robert F. Reardon, MD
Professor, Department of Emergency Medicine, University of Minnesota; Assistant Chief, Department of Emergency Medicine, Hennepin County Medical Center, Minneapolis, Minnesota

Kevin C. Reed, MD
Vice Chief, Department of Emergency Medicine, MedStar Georgetown University Hospital; Assistant Professor of Emergency Medicine, Georgetown University School of Medicine, Washington, DC

David B. Richards, MD, FACEP
Associate Professor, Department of Emergency Medicine, University of Colorado School of Medicine; Denver Health Medical Center, Denver, Colorado

Megan L. Rischall, MD
Faculty Physician, Department of Emergency Medicine, Hennepin County Medical Center; Assistant Professor, Department of Emergency Medicine, University of Minnesota Medical School, Minneapolis, Minnesota

Daniel W. Robinson, MD, MHPEc
Emergency Physician, Veteran's Affairs Puget Sound; Clinical Instructor, Departments of Emergency Medicine and Family Medicine, University of Washington, Seattle, Washington

Howard Rodenberg, MD, MPH
Physician Advisor, Clinical Documentation Integrity, Baptist Health, Jacksonville, Florida; Emergency Physician, Speaker, Consultant, and Blogger, University of Missouri-Kansas City School of Medicine, Kansas City, Missouri

Matthew A. Roginski, MD, MPH
Assistant Professor of Emergency Medicine and Medicine, Departments of Emergency Medicine and Medicine, Section of Pulmonary and Critical Care Medicine, Geisel School of Medicine, Dartmouth-Hitchcock Medical Center, Lebanon, New Hampshire

Chad E. Roline, MD
Emergency Medicine Physician, Emergency Physicians Professional Association, North Memorial Health Hospital and Maple Grove Hospital, Bloomington, Minnesota

Emily Rose, MD
Associate Professor of Clinical Emergency Medicine (Educational Scholar), Department of Emergency Medicine, LA County + USC Medical Center, Keck School of Medicine of the University of Southern California; Director for Pre-Health Undergraduate Studies, Medical Education, Keck School of Medicine of the University of Southern California, Los Angeles, California

Jeremy Rose, MD, MPH, FRCPC
Associate Professor, Department of Emergency Medicine, Icahn School of Medicine at Mount Sinai, New York, New York

Nicholas G.W. Rose, MD, PhD, FRCPC, Dip Sports Med (CASEM)
Clinical Assistant Professor, Department of Emergency Medicine, University of British Columbia, Vancouver General Hospital, Vancouver, British Columbia, Canada

Tony Rosen, MD, MPH
Assistant Professor of Emergency Medicine, Department of Emergency Medicine, Weill Cornell Medical College, NewYork-Presbyterian Hospital, New York, New York

Weston Ross, DO, MBA
Emergency Medicine Staff Physician, Bellevue Medical Center, Bellevue, Nebraska

C. Craig Rudy, MD
Attending Physician, Department of Emergency Medicine, Samaritan Health Services, Albany, Oregon

Anne-Michelle Ruha, MD
Chair, Medical Toxicology, Banner-University Medical Center Phoenix; Professor, Departments of Internal Medicine and Emergency Medicine, University of Arizona College of Medicine, Phoenix, Arizona

Megan M. Rybarczyk, MD, MPH
Assistant Professor of Clinical Emergency Medicine, Department of Emergency Medicine, Perelman School of Medicine at the University of Pennsylvania, Philadelphia, Pennsylvania

Carolyn Joy Sachs, MD, MPH
Clinical Professor, Emergency Department, David Geffen School of Medicine, University of California, Los Angeles; Chair, Domestic Violence Committee, UCLA Health Sciences, David Geffen School of Medicine at University of California, Los Angeles, Ronald Reagan-UCLA Medical Center, Los Angeles, California; Voluntary Medical Director, FNS Sexual Assault Examination Program, Long Beach, California

Matthew Salzberg, MD, MBA
Assistant Professor, Department of Emergency Medicine, University of Colorado Medical School; Assistant Medical Director, Department of Emergency Medicine, University of Colorado Anschutz Medical Center, Aurora, Colorado

León D. Sánchez, MD, MPH
Chief, Department of Emergency Medicine, Brigham and Women's Faulkner Hospital; Associate Professor of Emergency Medicine, Harvard Medical School, Boston, Massachusetts

Arthur B. Sanders, MD, MHA
Professor, Department of Emergency Medicine, University of Arizona College of Medicine Tucson, Tucson, Arizona

Christopher E. San Miguel, MD
Assistant Professor of Emergency Medicine, Wexner Medical Center, The Ohio State University, Columbus, Ohio

Richard J. Scarfone, MD
Associate Professor, Department of Pediatrics, Perelman School of Medicine at the University of Pennsylvania; Attending Physician, Division of Emergency Medicine, Medical Director, Emergency Preparedness, Division of Emergency Medicine, Program Director, Pediatric Emergency Medicine Fellowship, Children's Hospital of Philadelphia, Philadelphia, Pennsylvania

Andrew Schmidt, DO, MPH
Assistant Professor, Department of Emergency Medicine, University of Florida-Jacksonville, Jacksonville, Florida

Eric R. Schmitt, MD, MPH
Health Sciences Associate Clinical Professor of Emergency Medicine, Department of Emergency Medicine, University of California, San Francisco Fresno Medical Education Program; Attending Physician, Department of Emergency Medicine, Community Regional Medical Center, Fresno, California

Benjamin H. Schnapp, MD, MEd
Assistant Professor, Department of Emergency Medicine, University of Wisconsin School of Medicine and Public Health, Madison, Wisconsin

Benjamin Schoener, MD
Assistant Professor, Department of Emergency Medicine, Central Michigan University, Saginaw, Michigan

Carl H. Schultz, MD, FACEP
Professor Emeritus of Emergency Medicine and Public Health, University of California, Irvine, School of Medicine, Irvine, California; EMS Medical Director, Emergency Medical Services, Orange County Health Care Agency, Santa Ana, California

Raghu Seethala, MD
Department of Emergency Medicine, Brigham and Women's Hospital; Instructor of Emergency Medicine, Harvard Medical School, Boston, Massachusetts; Associate Visiting Professor, Department of Emergency Medicine, University of California San Francisco-Fresno, Fresno, California

Jeffrey A. Seiden, MD, MHA
Medical Director, Pediatric Emergency Medicine, CHOP at Virtua, Voorhees, New Jersey; Associate Professor of Clinical Pediatrics, Perelman School of Medicine at The University of Pennsylvania, Philadelphia, Pennsylvania

Todd A. Seigel, MD
Senior Physician, Emergency Medicine and Critical Care Medicine, Kaiser Permanente, Oakland Medical Center, Oakland, California; Clinical Assistant Professor, Department of Clinical Science, Permanente Bernard J. Tyson School of Medicine, Pasadena, California

Sarah Tolford Selby, DO
Assistant Professor, Department of Emergency Medicine, University of Colorado School of Medicine; Medical Director, Forensic Nursing Program, University of Colorado, Denver, Colorado

Wesley H. Self, MD, MPH
Vice President, Vanderbilt Institute for Clinical and Translational Research, Vice Chair, Department of Emergency Medicine, Vanderbilt University Medical Center, Nashville, Tennessee

Joseph Sexton, MD, FACEP
Emergency Physician, Lehigh Valley Health Network, Allentown, Pennsylvania

Huma Shaikh, MD
Assistant Professor, Department of Pediatrics, Baylor College of Medicine, Houston, Texas

Michael A. Shapiro, MD
Assistant Professor, Department of Psychiatry, University of Florida, Gainesville, Florida

Nathan I. Shapiro, MD, MPH
Professor of Emergency Medicine, Department of Emergency Medicine, Beth Israel Lahey Health, Harvard Medical School, Boston, Massachusetts

Eric Shappell, MD, MHPE
Assistant Professor, Department of Emergency Medicine, Massachusetts General Hospital, Harvard Medical School, Boston, Massachusetts

Dag Shapshak, MD
Associate Professor, Department of Emergency Medicine, University of Alabama, Birmingham, Birmingham, Alabama

Andrea C. Sharp, MD, MS
Assistant Professor, Department of Emergency Medicine, Mayo Clinic Florida, Jacksonville, Florida

Trent She, MD
Department of Emergency Medicine, Mount Sinai St. Luke's and West, New York, New York

Pranav Shetty, MD, MPH
Health Sciences Assistant Clinical Professor, Department of Emergency Medicine, EMS and Disaster Medicine Fellow, Harbor-UCLA Medical Center, Torrance, California

Sanjay N. Shewakramani, MD
Associate Professor, Department of Emergency Medicine, University of Cincinnati, Cincinnati, Ohio

Ashley Shreves, MD
Senior Physician, Department of Emergency Medicine, Ochsner Medical Center, New Orleans, Louisiana

Barry C. Simon, MD
Chairman, Department of Emergency Medicine, Alameda County Medical Center, Oakland, California; Professor, Department of Emergency Medicine, University of California, San Francisco, California

Leslie V. Simon, DO
Associate Professor, Emergency Medicine, Department of Emergency Medicine, Mayo Clinic Florida, Jacksonville, Florida

Manpreet Singh, MD, MBE
Assistant Professor in Emergency Medicine, Department of Emergency Medicine, Harbor-UCLA Medical Center, Torrance, California

Sonia Singh, MD, MPH, MBA
Fellow, Department of Emergency Medicine, UC Davis School of Medicine, Sacramento, California

Aaron B. Skolnik, MD
Assistant Professor, Department of Emergency Medicine, Consultant, Department of Critical Care Medicine, Mayo Clinic, Phoenix, Arizona

Corey M. Slovis, MD
Professor of Emergency Medicine and Medicine, Chairman Emeritus, Department of Emergency Medicine, Vanderbilt University Medical Center; Medical Director, Nashville Fire Department, Nashville International Airport, Nashville, Tennessee

Janet Smereck, MD
Associate Professor of Clinical Emergency Medicine, Department of Emergency Medicine, MedStar Georgetown University Hospital, Washington, DC

Clay Smith, MD
Associate Professor of Emergency Medicine, Internal Medicine, and Pediatrics, Department of Emergency Medicine, Vanderbilt University Medical Center, Nashville, Tennessee

Peter E. Sokolove, MD
Professor and Chair, Department of Emergency Medicine, University of California San Francisco School of Medicine, San Francisco, California

Philippa Soskin, MD, MPP
Assistant Professor, Department of Emergency Medicine, MedStar Georgetown University Hospital, Washington, DC

Jaron Soulek, MD
Associate Program Director, Department of Emergency Medicine, University of Oklahoma School of Community Medicine, Tulsa, Oklahoma

Lauren T. Southerland, MD
Associate Professor, Department of Emergency Medicine, The Ohio State University Wexner Medical Center, Columbus, Ohio

Brian L. Springer, MD, FACEP
Associate Professor, Department of Emergency Medicine, Wright State University, Dayton, Ohio

Bryan A. Stenson, MD
Clinical Fellow, Emergency Medicine, Beth Israel Deaconess Medical Center, Boston, Massachusetts

Hanni Stoklosa, MD, MPH
Department of Emergency Medicine, Brigham and Women's Hospital, Assistant Professor of Emergency Medicine, Harvard Medical School, Boston, Massachusetts; CEO, HEAL Trafficking

Christopher R. Tainter, MD, RDMS
Clinical Professor, Department of Anesthesiology, Division of Critical Care, University of California, San Diego, San Diego, California

Sukhjit S. Takhar, MD, SM
Attending Physician, Department of Emergency Medicine/Infectious Disease, Mills Peninsula Medical Center, Burlingame, California

Nelson Tang, MD, FACEP
Vice Chair of Operational Medicine, Department of Emergency Medicine, Johns Hopkins University School of Medicine, Baltimore, Maryland

Todd Andrew Taylor, MD
Associate Professor, Department of Emergency Medicine, Emory University, Atlanta, Georgia

Jillian L. Theobald, MD, PhD
Associate Professor, Department of Emergency Medicine, Medical College of Wisconsin; Associate Medical Director, Wisconsin Poison Center, Milwaukee, Wisconsin

Molly E.W. Thiessen, MD
Emergency Physician, Department of Emergency Medicine, Denver Health Medical Center, Denver, Colorado; Associate Professor, Department of Emergency Medicine, University of Colorado School of Medicine, Aurora, Colorado

Anita A. Thomas, MD, MPH
Assistant Professor, Pediatric Emergency Medicine, University of Washington, Seattle Children's Hospital, Seattle, Washington

Natasha Thomas, MD, MPH
Assistant Clinical Professor, Assistant Director, Adult Emergency Department, Director, Trauma Recovery Center, Department of Emergency Medicine, Harbor-UCLA Medical Center, Torrance, California

Holly Thompson, MD, FACEP, FAAEM
Associate Program Director, Department of Emergency Medicine, The Brooklyn Hospital Center, Brooklyn, New York

Trevonne M. Thompson, MD
Associate Professor/Director of Medical Toxicology, Department of Emergency Medicine, University of Illinois at Chicago, Chicago, Illinois

Joseph E. Thornton, MD, DFAPA
Adjunct Clinical Associate Professor, Department of Psychiatry, University of Florida College of Medicine, Gainesville, Florida

J. Adrian Tyndall, MD, MPH
Executive Vice President for Health Affairs, Professor and Dean, Morehouse School of Medicine, Atlanta, Georgia

Sam Torbati, MD
Co-Chair, Department of Emergency Medicine, Medical Director, Ruth and Harry Roman Emergency Department, Associate Professor, Emergency Medicine, Cedars Sinai Medical Center, Los Angeles, California

Michael VanRooyen, MD, MPH
Chair, Department of Emergency Medicine, Brigham and Women's Hospital, Massachusetts General Hospital; Enterprise Chief of Emergency Medicine, Mass General Brigham, J. Stephen Bohan Professor of Emergency Medicine, Harvard Medical School, Boston, Massachusetts

Meagan B. Verbillion, DO
Assistant Professor, Department of Emergency Medicine, Wright State University/Wright-Patterson Air Force Base, Dayton, Ohio

Taher T. Vohra, MD
Residency Program Director, Vice Chair of Education, Department of Emergency Medicine, Henry Ford Hospital; Clinical Associate Professor, Department of Emergency Medicine, Wayne State University School of Medicine, Detroit, Michigan

Leslie R. Vojta, MD, FACEP
Assistant Professor, Department of Military and Emergency Medicine, Uniformed Services University of the Health Sciences, Bethesda, Maryland

Christopher P. Waasdorp Jr., DO, FAWM, FAAEM
Assistant Professor of Emergency Medicine, Assistant Professor of Family & Community Medicine, Virginia Tech Carilion School of Medicine; Assistant Program Director of Wilderness Medicine Fellowship, Attending Physician, Physician Informaticist, Carilion Clinic, Roanoke, Virginia

David A. Wacker, MD, PhD
Assistant Professor, Division of Pulmonary, Allergy, Critical Care, and Sleep Medicine, Department of Internal Medicine, University of Minnesota Medical School, Minneapolis, Minnesota

Mary Jo Wagner, MD
Chief Academic Officer/DIO, GME, Central Michigan University Medical Education Partners; Professor, Department of Emergency Medicine, Central Michigan University College of Medicine, Saginaw, Michigan

Laura E. Walker, MD
Assistant Professor, Department of Emergency Medicine, Mayo Clinic Alix School of Medicine; Consultant, Department of Emergency Medicine, Mayo Clinic, Rochester, Minnesota

Joshua Wallenstein, MD, FACEP
Associate Professor, Department of Emergency Medicine, Emory University, Atlanta, Georgia

Ron M. Walls, MD
Neskey Family Professor of Emergency Medicine, Department of Emergency Medicine, Harvard Medical School; Chief Operating Officer, Mass General Brigham, Boston, Massachusetts

George Sam Wang, MD, FAAP, FAACT
Associate Professor of Pediatrics, Section of Emergency Medicine and Medical Toxicology, University of Colorado School of Medicine, Aurora, Colorado

Gabriel Wardi, MD, MPH
Assistant Clinical Professor, Department of Emergency Medicine, Division of Pulmonary, Critical Care, and Sleep Medicine, University of California, San Diego, San Diego, California

Matthew A. Waxman, MD, DTM&H
Clinical Professor of Emergency Medicine, David Geffen School of Medicine at University of California, Los Angeles, Los Angeles, California; Department of Emergency Medicine and Internal Medicine, Olive View-University of California Los Angeles Medical Center, Sylmar, California

Lori Weichenthal, MD, FACEP
Professor of Clinical Emergency Medicine, Department of Emergency Medicine, University of California San Francisco, Fresno, Fresno, California

Katherine Louise Welker, MD, MPH
Staff Physician, Emergency Department and Toxicology, Kaiser (Southern California Permanente Group), San Diego, California

Amanda L. Wessel, MD
Assistant Professor, Department of Emergency Medicine, Vanderbilt University Medical Center, Nashville, Tennessee

Benjamin White, MD
Department of Emergency Medicine, Massachusetts General Hospital; Associate Professor of Emergency Medicine, Harvard Medical School, Boston, Massachusetts

William White, MD
Fellow, Emergency Medicine, Harbor-UCLA Medical Center, Torrance, California

Susan R. Wilcox, MD
Chief, Division of Critical Care, Department of Emergency Medicine, Massachusetts General Hospital; Associate Professor of Emergency Medicine, Harvard Medical School; Associate Chief Medical Officer, Boston MedFlight, Boston, Massachusetts

Craig A. Williamson, MD, MS
Clinical Assistant Professor, Neurosurgery and Neurology, University of Michigan, Ann Arbor, Michigan

Allan B. Wolfson, MD, FACEP, FACP
Professor of Emergency Medicine, Vice Chair for Education, Department of Emergency Medicine, University of Pittsburgh, Pittsburgh, Pennsylvania

Andrea W. Wu, MD, MMM
Vice Chair of Clinical Operations, Department of Emergency Medicine, Harbor-UCLA Medical Center, Los Angeles Department of Health Services, Torrance, California; Associate Clinical Professor, Department of Emergency Medicine, David Geffen School of Medicine at University of California, Los Angeles, Los Angeles, California

Donald M. Yealy, MD
Professor and Chair, Department of Emergency Medicine, University of Pittsburgh, Pittsburgh, Pennsylvania

Henry W. Young II., MD
Assistant Professor, Assistant Program Director, Department of Emergency Medicine, University of Florida, Gainesville, Florida

Ken Zafren, MD
Department of Emergency Medicine, Stanford University Medical Center, Stanford, California; Department of Emergency Medicine, Alaska Native Medical Center, Anchorage, Alaska; International Commission for Mountain Emergency Medicine (ICAR MedCom), Zürich, Switzerland

Michael J. Zdradzinski, MD
Assistant Professor, Department of Emergency Medicine, Emory University School of Medicine, Atlanta, Georgia

Brian J. Zink, MD
Professor, Department of Emergency Medicine, Senior Associate Dean for Faculty and Faculty Development, University of Michigan Medical School, Ann Arbor, Michigan

Leslie S. Zun, MD, MBA
Professor of Emergency Medicine, Rosalind Franklin University of Medicine and Science, Chicago Medical School, Chicago, Illinois

PREFACE TO THE TENTH EDITION

We introduce this tenth edition of the most important textbook in our field with a deep humility, born of the uncertainty that has shaken our beliefs and our world community. Through the extraordinary challenges of 2020 through 2022 we learned anew the precious and inestimable joy of companionship—of family, friends, loved ones, and colleagues. We learned to rely on one another as never before, and we learned the strength of numbers, of teams, of collective effort to face down a daunting and unfamiliar foe. We learned about the indominable spirit that drives our specialty, and the unquestioning trust our patients place in us. And we affirmed, as never before, the power of science to lift us all up, to transform and respond, to solve and to cure, and to relentlessly breach the faulty logic of the deniers.

This edition of *Rosen's* was born in three labors. In the first, we set about to build a creative new editorial team, one that would make this current edition undeniably better, but also position us to expand the influential leadership position of this book as a source of truth for the next generation of learners and practitioners. We celebrated the contributions of editors departing and welcomed a new and diverse team to lead us into the future. Ron reprised his role as Editor-in-Chief. Tim and Susan joined Bob and Marianne as Senior Editors, Tim moving from his role of Associate Editor for the ninth edition, Susan stepping into the role directly from the solid foundation of her body of work in emergency medicine and critical care. We welcomed our outstanding returning Associate Editors, Katie Bakes, Andy Jagoda, Amy Kaji, and Mike VanRooyen, who generously agreed to again shoulder the enormous load as primary editors. We bolstered our team with new Associate Editors from leading academic centers: Calvin Brown III, David Brown, and Leòn Sanchez, from the Harvard Medical School affiliates Brigham and Women's Hospital and Massachusetts General Hospital; Adrian Tyndall, from the University of Florida; and Jonathan Davis, from Georgetown University. With our outstanding editorial team from Elsevier, we held detailed discussions about how to make the book better, more succinct, easier to access, and with more clear guidance for our readers. We brainstormed new topics and chapters, identified promising new authors, debated whether some existing topics should be consolidated or retired, and what content should be in the book versus available online only. Little did we know, when we held our planning meetings in Cambridge, MA, in June, 2019, that we would never again be together in one room until after the book was in print.

The second labor was, in reality, a pause. When the pandemic hit in full force in spring of 2020, we recognized that neither authors nor editors should be distracted from their complete commitment to caring for their teams, patients, and communities. From month to month, we gathered editors in virtual meetings to discuss the evolving situation, so we could collectively decide when it would be appropriate to turn our attention back to the important work of editing. These meetings kept us together as a team, reminded us of the long future ahead in a post-pandemic world, and also informed us about new information that was sorely needed, such as how to safely intubate patients with high infectivity, high morbidity respiratory disease, and the need to shift coronaviruses from a brief topic in a general chapter on viruses to a chapter all of its own. Through it all, we supported one another and a found common purpose.

The third labor was in bringing the book over the finish line when we resumed our task, reconnected with authors, and attacked the work with renewed energy. Fortunately, at the time of our pause, the book was well ahead of schedule, a tribute to the diligence of our authors and editors, which made the final steps less daunting than otherwise would have been the case. Our editorial team from Elsevier never missed a beat, always ready to help, support, cajole, remind, problem-solve, bolster, and cheer; often with a moment or two of humor, encouragement, and respite.

And we got there. Not just there, not just to a good place, not simply to the relief of finishing, but to the profound satisfaction of producing what we know, without the slightest doubt, represents yet another significant advance in the evolution of Peter Rosen's vision from almost 40 years ago. So, to you, the reader, we submit this, our finest work, born of one of our finest hours, and perhaps the finest hour of our specialty.

Ron M. Walls
Robert S. Hockberger
Marianne Gausche-Hill
Tim Erickson
Susan Wilcox

When we began planning for this ninth edition, we challenged ourselves to make substantial and meaningful improvements to a book that has become the trusted standard in our field. With broad and rapid changes occurring in health care and information sciences, we recognized that relevance is not an accidental or passive concept. To advance in relevance and consolidate the book's position as the defining reference in our specialty, we carefully and deliberately undertook bold changes that we know make the book at once fresh, directive, and current in a way we have never before dared.

First, we created a substantially enhanced role for our editors, one that would demand a great deal more of their time, creativity, and energy. This helped us build a substantially different team of editors, a perfectly balanced blend of those with great experience with prior editions and those who would bring new ideas and challenge our assumptions. Ron Walls was asked to serve as Editor-in-Chief, with Bob Hockberger in his long-standing role as senior editor. Marianne Gausche-Hill, a highly respected academic emergency physician with service as editor on four previous editions, stepped up to complete our senior editorial ranks. At the editor level, Dr. Andy Jagoda returns and is joined by six brilliant new editors drawn from academic programs from coast to coast—Drs. Katherine Bakes, Jill Baren, Timothy Erickson, Amy Kaji, Michael VanRooyen, and Richard Zane. This dynamic and innovative editorial team has dramatically redrawn our text's blueprint by preserving what has served our readers the best, such as well-written discussions of the pathophysiologic basis of illness and injury, while moving in entirely new directions in providing pithy, clear, and succinct recommendations for diagnosis and treatment.

We collectively determined that all references prior to 2010 have been sufficiently long in the public domain that they no longer warrant citation. The infrequent exception to this is for guidelines that were issued in 2007 or later and have not been reissued or supplanted since. Strict adherence to our referencing policy required authors to diligently provide well-researched and detailed updates to their chapter content, based on only the most recent and relevant medical literature. In cases in which the literature is controversial or unclear, we have used the combined experience and expertise of our authors and editors to present cogent analyses of diagnostic and treatment options, make specific recommendations, and give the reader clear indications of the preferred actions. This makes the book much more immediately relevant for emergency clinicians. We recognize that emergency medicine is practiced by specialist emergency physicians, other physicians, residents and other trainees, and a variety of nonphysician practitioners, so were careful to ensure that we are addressing all these groups with the same concise, highest quality information and recommendations.

We revisited page counts for every chapter, adjusting allocations where indicated, and added new chapters on several important topics. We focused anew on consistency and redundancy, enhancing the former and minimizing the latter. We moved some chapters to online access only, allowing us to add new topics of interest, such as drug therapy for older patients, and have provided a rich array of dynamic videos and images, especially in emergency ultrasound. We substantially expanded and reorganized the pediatric emergency medicine section, introducing dedicated pediatric chapters on airway management, procedural sedation, and drug therapy. We introduced significant new material on emergencies in the pregnant woman, the patient with cancer, and a variety of other highly important clinical conditions. And, in every possible case, we insisted on adherence to referencing and writing requirements, a focus on relevant directive information, and appropriate use of prose and illustrations to provide the perfect balance of depth, breadth, and ready accessibility.

We are enormously proud of the result, a different, more readable "Rosen," preserving the gravitas earned over 30 years as the most important book in our specialty while embracing the modern era of emergency medicine practice and research and an entirely new generation of learners and practitioners. For those who have owned prior editions, we appreciate your loyalty over so many years and hope to reward it with a significantly improved and useful companion for your continuing learning and practice of this great specialty. For our newer readers, welcome, and thank you for inspiring us to make significant changes to an iconic and timeless part of our academic heritage.

Ron M. Walls
Robert S. Hockberger
Marianne Gausche-Hill

HOW THIS MEDICAL TEXTBOOK SHOULD BE VIEWED BY THE PRACTICING CLINICIAN AND JUDICIAL SYSTEM

The editors and authors of this text strongly believe that because of the variations of human diseases, the unpredictability of pathologic conditions, and the functions, dysfunctions, and responses of the human body, the complex practice of medicine cannot be definitively explained or comprehensively dictated by any written document. Therefore, it is neither the purpose nor intent of our textbook to serve as the definitive source of truth regarding any medical condition, treatment plan, or clinical intervention. Specifically, our textbook is intended to educate and inform learners and practitioners, and is not to be used to rigorously define a standard of care that should be followed by all clinicians in all settings.

Our written word represents our best efforts to present the clinician with scientifically based and clinically sound information to provide reasonable and reliable clinical guidance. This science is interpreted by our authors and editors through the lenses of their own knowledge, years of clinical experience, teaching of others, and the study of adverse outcomes and human and system error. No textbook can fully account for the range of limited information, varying clinical clues, instincts, judgments, and responses that occur during the care of emergency and critical care patients. In fact, other experts might interpret the same evidence differently, based on their own experience and analysis of available information. No human being can possibly assimilate the entire depth and breadth of the treatments, procedures, and medical conditions described in this textbook—in fact, that is why this book and others exist. Finally, many of the described complications and adverse outcomes associated with implementing or withholding complex medical and surgical interventions may occur, even when the clinicians have used sound clinical judgment and made decisions and performed interventions according to the tenets of this and other standard medical references.

The editors and authors of *Rosen's Emergency Medicine: Concepts and Clinical Practice,* Tenth Edition

CONTENTS

83

Renal Failure

Allan B. Wolfson

KEY CONCEPTS

- The causes of acute kidney injury (AKI) can be classified as prerenal, post-renal, and intrinsic renal disorders. Abrupt cessation of glomerular filtration typically results in a rise of the serum creatinine level of 1 to 2 mg/dL per day.

- Management of AKI is directed first at potentially lethal complications such as hyperkalemia or volume overload and then at reversal of the underlying cause of renal dysfunction. It is important to avoid any further hemodynamic or toxic insults to the kidneys.

- Patients with acute or chronic kidney disease have a limited ability to handle fluid and solute loads and have altered metabolism of many drugs. Therefore, the patient's impaired renal function must be considered when fluid is administered or drugs are prescribed.

- The most rapidly lethal complication of acute and chronic kidney disease is hyperkalemia.

- The most common problems with vascular access devices used for hemodialysis are thrombosis, hemorrhage, and infection. Access infection often presents as fever without an obvious source and, if suspected, appropriate IV antibiotics should be administered presumptively while awaiting blood culture results.

- Peritoneal dialysis–associated peritonitis typically presents with cloudiness of the peritoneal dialysis effluent. The diagnosis is made by a positive Gram stain or finding of more than 100 WBC/mm³ in the effluent, with at least 50% polys. It is generally treated on an outpatient basis with intraperitoneal antibiotics self-administered by the patient.

- Chest pain in the dialysis patient should be presumed initially to be due to acute coronary syndrome, although other potentially serious causes may also be responsible. Serum troponin levels tend to be elevated in patients with poor renal function, but patients with myocardial infarction show the typical temporal pattern of rise and fall of troponin levels.

- Hypotension in patients with chronic kidney disease (CKD) may be caused by infection but may also be the result of rapid fluid removal during dialysis. This often responds readily to fluid administration. Pericardial tamponade is another cause of hypotension that should be considered for these patients.

- Altered mental status is most commonly due to causes similar to those seen in patients without renal disease but is sometimes the result of over-rapid shifts in intravascular fluid and solutes during dialysis, termed *disequilibrium syndrome*.

RENAL FAILURE

The evaluation of renal disease in the emergency department (ED) requires an approach that incorporates the urinalysis, serum and urine chemical determinations, and renal imaging studies. This approach assesses the degree of renal dysfunction and establishes the foundation for distinguishing acute kidney injury (AKI) from chronic kidney disease (CKD).

ACUTE KIDNEY INJURY

Foundations

The hallmark of AKI (formerly termed *acute renal failure* [ARF]) is progressive azotemia, which commonly is accompanied by a wide range of other disturbances, depending on the severity and duration of renal dysfunction. These include metabolic derangements (e.g., metabolic acidosis, hyperkalemia), disturbances of body fluid balance (particularly volume overload), and a variety of effects on almost every organ system (Box 83.1).

The causes of AKI are divided into those that decrease renal blood flow (prerenal), produce a renal parenchymal insult (intrarenal), or obstruct urine flow (obstructive, or postrenal). Identification of a prerenal or postrenal cause of AKI generally makes it possible to initiate specific corrective therapy; if these two broad categories of AKI can be excluded, an intrarenal cause is implicated. The renal parenchymal causes of AKI can be usefully subdivided into those primarily affecting the glomeruli, intrarenal vasculature, or renal interstitium. The term *acute tubular necrosis* denotes another broad category of intrinsic renal failure that cannot be attributed to a specific glomerular, vascular, or interstitial cause (Fig. 83.1).

Renal failure can lead to numerous other systemic and organ-specific effects. Uremia impairs host defenses, particularly leukocyte function, and infection is a significant cause of morbidity and mortality in AKI. Pericarditis, which has a prevalence of 10% to 20% in dialyzed patients with CKD, also may occur in patients with AKI. Urgent dialysis is indicated when there is associated pericardial effusion and tamponade. Neurologic abnormalities in AKI may be precipitated by electrolyte abnormalities, medications, or uremia. Anorexia, nausea, vomiting, gastritis, and pancreatitis also are associated with AKI and significant gastrointestinal (GI) hemorrhage is seen in about 10% of patients.

Impaired erythropoiesis, shortened red blood cell (RBC) survival, hemolysis, hemodilution, and GI blood loss all play a role in the normocytic normochromic anemia that usually accompanies AKI. Although mild thrombocytopenia may be present, it is the qualitative defect in platelet function thought to be caused by the effect of circulating uremic toxins that contributes to these patients' bleeding tendencies.

Clinical Features

When the presence of azotemia or renal failure has been discovered, the first consideration in the ED evaluation should be the possibility of potentially life-threatening complications (e.g., hyperkalemia, pulmonary edema). Assuming that these have been satisfactorily ruled out, the next step is to determine whether the condition represents AKI or is the result of preexisting renal disease. The clinical distinction

---

BOX 83.1 Clinical Features of Acute Kidney Injury

Cardiovascular
Pulmonary edema
Arrhythmia
Hypertension
Pericarditis
Pericardial effusion
Myocardial infarction
Pulmonary embolism

Metabolic
Hyponatremia
Hyperkalemia
Acidosis
Hypocalcemia
Hyperphosphatemia
Hypermagnesemia
Hyperuricemia

Neurologic
Asterixis
Neuromuscular irritability
Mental status changes
Somnolence
Coma
Seizures

Gastrointestinal
Nausea
Vomiting
Gastritis
Gastroduodenal ulcer
Gastrointestinal bleeding
Pancreatitis
Malnutrition

Hematologic
Anemia
Hemorrhagic diathesis

Infectious
Pneumonia
Septicemia
Urinary tract infection
Wound infection

---

between AKI and CKD often is difficult, especially if prior records and laboratory results are not available. The finding of small kidneys on abdominal imaging or bone changes of secondary hyperparathyroidism on hand films demonstrating abnormal calcifications suggests that the renal failure is chronic. Anemia, hypocalcemia, and hyperphosphatemia, however, should not be relied on to identify patients who have CKD because these abnormalities can develop rapidly in AKI.

In evaluating the patient with azotemia, the emergency clinician uses history, physical examination, and laboratory studies to seek clues to the cause and to identify signs and symptoms of uremia, volume overload, or other complications of renal failure. In attempting to identify the cause, the general strategy is to rule out prerenal and postrenal causes before considering the many intrinsic renal causes. First, potential sources of volume loss and causes of decreased cardiac output are sought in the history, and the patient should be questioned about lightheadedness, bleeding, GI fluid loss, abnormal polyuria, or symptoms of congestive heart failure (CHF). In men, a history of nocturia, frequency, hesitancy, or decreased urinary stream suggests prostatic obstruction. A history of lower tract symptoms or of abdominal or pelvic tumor in either gender is sought, as is a history of kidney stones or chronic urinary tract infection (UTI). A history of acute anuria, defined as the production of less than 100 mL of urine/ day, is most often the result of high-grade urinary tract obstruction, although it also may accompany severe volume depletion, severe acute glomerulonephritis, cortical necrosis, or bilateral renal vascular occlusion. Intermittent anuria, on the other hand, is characteristic of obstructive disease. Medication use and possible exposure to radiographic contrast agents or other exogenous toxins are other key components of the history. A history of hypertension, dark-colored urine, rash, fever, or arthritis suggests intrinsic renal disease or a multisystem disorder.

The physical examination focuses on signs of volume depletion, such as tachycardia and decreased skin turgor. Documented short-term changes in body weight also offer a valuable clue in assessing volume status, particularly in patients who are chronically ill. Volume overload

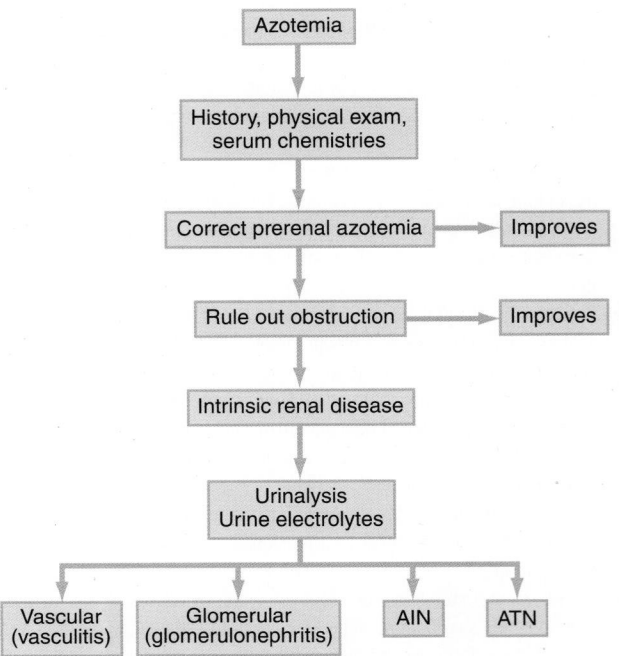

Fig. 83.1 Evaluation of azotemia. *AIN,* Acute interstitial nephritis; *ATN,* acute tubular necrosis.

is suggested by findings of jugular vein distention and the presence of rales or peripheral edema.

A distended bladder is percussible when it contains at least 150 mL of urine, and the dome is palpable abdominally when the bladder contains 500 mL. Ultrasonography can be used to detect bladder distention or postvoid residual volume if there is a question of urinary retention. A prostate examination in men and pelvic examination in women are also necessary components of the examination. The presence of rash, purpura, pallor, or petechiae on skin examination may be noted, as is arthritis, musculoskeletal tenderness, and findings suggestive of infection or malignancy.

Differential Diagnosis

The management of AKI requires a systematic approach to the potential underlying causes. Once prerenal and postrenal causes are considered, the diagnostic and management strategies focus on the intrarenal pathologies.

Prerenal Azotemia

Decreased renal perfusion that is sufficient to cause a decrease in the glomerular filtration rate (GFR) results in azotemia. The possible causes are grouped into entities causing intravascular volume depletion, volume redistribution, or decreased cardiac output (Box 83.2). Patients who have preexisting renal disease are particularly sensitive to the effects of diminished renal perfusion.

Prerenal azotemia is characterized by increased urine specific gravity, a blood urea nitrogen (BUN) to creatinine ratio generally between 10:1 and 20:1, urine sodium concentration less than 20 mEq/dL, and fractional excretion of sodium (FENa) less than 1%. The condition generally can be corrected readily by expanding extracellular fluid volume, augmenting cardiac output, or discontinuing vasodilating antihypertensive drugs. However, severe prolonged prerenal azotemia can result in acute tubular necrosis (ATN).

Patients who have CHF or cirrhosis form an important subset of those with prerenal azotemia. These patients often are sodium-overloaded and water-overloaded, yet the effective intra-arterial volume is decreased. Administration of diuretics has the potential to decrease intravascular volume further, resulting in decreased glomerular filtration and prerenal azotemia. For some patients with advanced CHF or hepatic disease, a state of chronic, stable, prerenal azotemia may be the best achievable compromise between symptomatic volume overload and severe renal hypoperfusion.

Glomerular perfusion also may be decreased in patients with normal intravascular volume and normal renal blood flow who take angiotensin-converting enzyme (ACE) inhibitors or, more commonly, prostaglandin inhibitors. All nonsteroidal antiinflammatory drugs (NSAIDs), including aspirin, inhibit prostaglandin synthesis. Renal vasodilator prostaglandins are critical in maintaining glomerular perfusion in patients with conditions such as CHF, chronic renal insufficiency, and cirrhosis, in which elevated circulating levels of renin and angiotensin II decrease renal blood flow and GFR. In this setting, a decrease in the production of vasodilator prostaglandins may result in acute intrarenal hemodynamic changes and a reversible decrease in renal function. This phenomenon also is seen with the selective cyclooxygenase-2 inhibitor class of NSAIDs. Other risk factors include advanced age, diuretic use, renovascular disease, and diabetes. This entity is distinct from other renal complications of NSAIDs such as interstitial nephritis and papillary necrosis.

Postrenal (Obstructive) Acute Kidney Injury

Obstruction is an eminently reversible cause of AKI and should be considered in every patient with newly discovered azotemia or worsening renal function. Obstruction may occur at any level of the urinary tract but usually is caused by prostatic hypertrophy or functional bladder neck obstruction (e.g., secondary to medication side effects or neurogenic bladder; Box 83.3). Intrarenal obstruction may result from the intratubular precipitation of uric acid crystals (e.g., with tumor lysis), oxalic acid (as in ethylene glycol ingestion), phosphates, myeloma proteins, methotrexate, sulfadiazine, acyclovir, or indinavir. Bilateral ureteral obstruction (or obstruction of the ureter of a solitary kidney) may be caused by retroperitoneal fibrosis, tumor, surgical complications (such as inadvertent ligation of the ureter), stones, or

---

BOX 83.2 Causes of Prerenal Azotemia

Volume Loss
Gastrointestinal—vomiting, diarrhea, nasogastric drainage
Renal—diuresis
Blood loss
Insensible losses
Third-space sequestration
Pancreatitis
Peritonitis
Trauma
Burns

Cardiac Causes
Myocardial infarction
Valvular disease
Cardiomyopathy
Decreased effective arterial volume
Antihypertensive medication
Nitrates

Neurogenic Causes
Sepsis
Anaphylaxis
Hypoalbuminemia
Nephrotic syndrome
Liver disease

BOX 83.3 Causes of Postrenal Renal Failure

Intrarenal and Ureteral Causes
Kidney stones
Sloughed papillas
Bilateral ureteral compression related to malignancy or benign gynecologic causes
Retroperitoneal fibrosis
Uric acid, oxalic acid, or phosphate crystal precipitation
Sulfonamide, methotrexate, acyclovir, or indinavir precipitation

Bladder
Kidney stone
Blood clot
Prostatic hypertrophy
Bladder carcinoma
Neurogenic bladder

Urethra
Phimosis
Stricture

blood clots. A sudden deterioration in renal function in the setting of diabetes mellitus, analgesic nephropathy, or sickle cell disease suggests papillary necrosis.

Intrinsic Acute Kidney Injury

Of the specific intrarenal disorders that cause AKI, glomerulonephritis, interstitial nephritis, and abnormalities of the intrarenal vasculature are amenable to specific therapy and are important to consider as possible causes. These entities are responsible for only 5% to 10% of cases of AKI in adult inpatients; most cases are caused by ATN. In adults in whom AKI develops outside the hospital, the incidence of glomerular, interstitial, and small vessel disease is much greater. In children, these entities account for approximately 50% of the cases of AKI (Box 83.4).

Acute Glomerulonephritis. This may represent a primary renal process or may be the manifestation of any of a wide range of other disease entities (see Box 83.4). Patients may have dark urine, hypertension, edema, or CHF (secondary to volume overload) or may be completely asymptomatic, in which case the diagnosis rests on an incidental finding on urinalysis. The hematuria associated with glomerular disease may be microscopic or gross and may be persistent or intermittent. Proteinuria, although often in the range of 500 mg/day to 3 g/day, is not uncommonly in the nephrotic range, defined as 3.5 g/day or more. The presence of hematuria, proteinuria, or red cell casts is highly suggestive of glomerulonephritis. Conversely, the absence of red cell casts, proteinuria, and hematuria essentially excludes glomerulonephritis as the cause of AKI.

The specific diagnosis of acute glomerulonephritis caused by primary renal disease often is ultimately made by renal biopsy. However, when glomerulonephritis is secondary to a systemic disease such as systemic lupus erythematosus, the clinical signs and symptoms and results of laboratory assessment aid considerably in narrowing the scope of the differential diagnosis. As a rule, extensive laboratory testing to identify the cause of acute glomerulonephritis is not indicated in the ED setting and is more appropriately performed as part of an inpatient evaluation.

Acute Interstitial Nephritis. Acute interstitial nephritis (AIN) is usually precipitated by drug exposure or by infection. Drug-induced AIN is poorly understood, but the absence of a clear relationship to the dose, and recurrence of the syndrome on rechallenge with the offending agent, suggests that an immunologic mechanism is responsible. The most commonly incriminated drugs are the penicillins, diuretics, and NSAIDs. AIN has been reported in association with bacterial, fungal, protozoan, and rickettsial infections.

Patients with AIN typically have rash, fever, eosinophilia, and eosinophiluria, but it is common for one or more of these cardinal signs to be absent. Pyuria, gross or microscopic hematuria, and mild proteinuria are observed in some cases. A definite diagnosis sometimes can be made only on renal biopsy. Treatment of AIN is directed at removing the presumed cause; infections should be treated and offending drugs discontinued. Renal function generally returns to baseline over several weeks, although chronic renal failure has been reported to occur.

Intrarenal Vascular Disease of the Kidney. This can be classified according to the size of the vessel that is affected. Disorders such as renal arterial thrombosis or embolism, which affect large blood vessels, must be bilateral—or affect a single functioning kidney—to produce AKI. Whether to attribute such cases of AKI to a prerenal or intrarenal vascular cause is a matter of semantics. The most common cause of thrombosis probably is trauma; thrombosis also may occur after angiography or may be secondary to aortic or renal arterial dissection. Renal atheroembolism is thought to occur commonly, at least on a microscopic level, after arteriography but it is an uncommon cause of AKI. Similarly, patients with chronic atrial fibrillation or infective endocarditis may experience embolization of the kidney but rarely develop AKI as a result. Renal arterial embolism can

---

BOX 83.4 Intrinsic Renal Diseases That Cause Acute Kidney Injury

Vascular Diseases
Large-Vessel Diseases
Renal artery thrombosis or stenosis
Renal vein thrombosis
Atheroembolic disease

Small- and Medium-Sized Vessel Diseases
Scleroderma
Malignant hypertension
Hemolytic uremic syndrome
Thrombotic thrombocytopenic purpura
HIV-associated microangiopathy

Glomerular Diseases
Systemic Diseases
Systemic lupus erythematosus
Infective endocarditis
Systemic vasculitis (e.g., periarteritis nodosa, Wegener granulomatosis)
Henoch-Schönlein purpura
HIV-associated nephropathy
Essential mixed cryoglobulinemia
Goodpasture syndrome

Primary Renal Diseases
Poststreptococcal glomerulonephritis

Other postinfectious glomerulonephritis
Rapidly progressive glomerulonephritis

Tubulointerstitial Diseases and Conditions
Drugs (many)
Toxins (e.g., heavy metals, ethylene glycol)
Infections
Multiple myeloma

Acute Tubular Necrosis
Ischemia
Shock
Sepsis
Severe prerenal azotemia

Nephrotoxins
Antibiotics
Radiographic contrast agents
Myoglobinuria
Hemoglobinuria

Other Diseases and Conditions
Severe liver disease
Allergic reactions
NSAIDs

HIV, Human immunodeficiency virus; *NSAIDs*, nonsteroidal antiinflammatory drugs.

cause acute renal infarction, generally manifested by sudden flank, back, chest, or upper abdominal pain. Urinary findings, including hematuria, are variable. The diagnosis usually is made by renal flow scanning or arteriography.

Several diseases that affect the smaller intrarenal vessels can cause AKI (see Box 83.4). Patients whose disease is severe enough to cause AKI also are generally found to have hypertension, microangiopathic hemolytic anemia, and other systemic and organ-specific manifestations. Infection with *Escherichia coli* O157:H7 has emerged as a major cause of hemolytic uremic syndrome, an important cause of AKI in children.

Patients with scleroderma (systemic sclerosis) may have so-called scleroderma renal crisis, characterized by malignant hypertension and rapidly progressive renal failure. Whereas vasculitis associated with glomerular capillary inflammation typically causes gross or microscopic hematuria and the formation of red cell casts, vascular involvement of the medium-sized vessels, such as that produced by scleroderma, often spares the preglomerular vessels and tends not to produce an active urine sediment. Extrarenal manifestations (e.g., rash, fever, arthritis, pulmonary symptoms) are usually evident.

For malignant hypertension, both as a separate entity and as a part of scleroderma renal crisis, appropriate treatment can produce remission of AKI. Patients with malignant hypertension have been reported to recover renal function after aggressive antihypertensive therapy, with temporary maintenance on dialysis if necessary. In patients with scleroderma renal crisis, specific therapy with ACE inhibitors has been shown to result in improvement in renal function in a significant proportion of cases.

Acute Tubular Necrosis. ATN refers to a generally reversible deterioration of kidney function associated with a variety of renal insults. Oliguria may or may not be a feature. The diagnosis is made after prerenal and postrenal causes of ARF and disorders of glomeruli, interstitium, and intrarenal vasculature have been excluded. In a few disorders, these discrete categories overlap. For example, AKI associated with multiple myeloma or ethylene glycol toxicity is associated with intrarenal obstruction and interstitial disease, as well as a probable direct toxic effect on the renal tubule itself.

The most common precipitant of ATN is renal ischemia occurring during surgery or after trauma and sepsis. The remainder of cases occur in the setting of medical illness, usually as a result of the administration of a nephrotoxic aminoglycoside antibiotic or in association with rhabdomyolysis. Multiple causes can be identified in some cases; in others, a definitive cause cannot be established.

Decreased renal perfusion results in a continuum of renal dysfunction that ranges from transient prerenal azotemia at one extreme to ATN at the other. Early during the period of renal ischemia, renal function can be restored completely by restoring renal blood flow but, at some point, continued hypoperfusion results in renal dysfunction unresponsive to volume repletion, and ATN supervenes. ATN may occur in the absence of frank hypotension; even modest renal ischemia may result in ATN in susceptible persons. Individual susceptibility to ATN may be related to the balance of prostaglandin-mediated vasopressor and vasodilatory influences on the renal vasculature.

Postischemic ATN can occur in the setting of volume loss from the GI tract (upper or lower), skin, or kidneys or can result from severe hemorrhage or major burns. Heat stroke commonly is associated with the development of ATN, which is thought to result from a combination of volume loss, hyperpyrexia, and rhabdomyolysis. Another cause of ATN is hyperglycemic hyperosmolar syndrome, which can be associated with loss of as much as 25% of total body water. ATN also is seen in the setting of cardiogenic shock, sepsis, and third spacing of fluids in pancreatitis and peritonitis.

ATN is common in postoperative patients, although not all cases can be attributed to intraoperative hypotension or hemorrhage. Concomitant sepsis, increased age, preexisting renal disease, and other comorbid conditions are associated with a worse outcome.

Recently, it has been noted that patients hospitalized for coronavirus disease 2019 (COVID-19) may develop AKI during the course of their illness, particularly when intensive care is required. The mechanism is likely to be multifactorial, including hypovolemia, cardiac dysfunction, exposure to nephrotoxins, and direct renal endothelial damage related to viremia, immune dysfunction, or hypercoagulability. Patients may initially present with proteinuria early in the course; AKI is felt to be a marker of the severity of disease. Treatment is supportive, with careful management of fluid balance and optimization of renal perfusion. More severe cases require hemodialysis or other forms of renal replacement therapy.[14]

Nephrotoxins constitute the other major cause of ATN. Among the most prominent of these are the endogenous pigments myoglobin and hemoglobin, associated with rhabdomyolysis (Box 83.5). Hypotension secondary to fluid loss into damaged muscle is thought to worsen the effects of myoglobinuria on the renal tubule, as does acidemia. Hemolysis, resulting in the release of hemoglobin into the circulation and hemoglobinuria, can cause ATN but usually only in the presence of coexisting dehydration, acidosis, or other causes of decreased renal perfusion. ATN may be associated with the hemolysis of as little as 100 mL of blood.

ATN associated with rhabdomyolysis is often oliguric; it is characterized by rapid increases in the serum creatinine, potassium, phosphorus, and uric acid levels. Creatine released from muscle is metabolized to creatinine, which may result in serum creatinine level increases of more than 2 mg/dL/day, in contrast to the increase of 0.5 to 1.0 mg/dL/day typically seen in other forms of AKI. The BUN/creatinine ratio often is *less* than 10 : 1. Intracellular potassium released from damaged muscle may raise the serum potassium level by 1 to 2 mEq/L in several hours. Likewise, phosphate released from muscle may cause dramatic increases in the serum phosphate level. Uric acid, produced by the metabolism of purines released from damaged muscle, may accumulate to levels high enough to cause acute uric acid nephropathy.

BOX 83.5   Causes of Pigment-Induced Acute Kidney Injury

Rhabdomyolysis and myoglobinuria
  Crush injury
  Compartment syndrome
  Electrical injury
  Myonecrosis from coma or immobilization
  Acute arterial occlusion
  Vigorous exertion
  Status epilepticus
  Hyperthermia/heat stress
  Metabolic myopathy
  Drugs/toxins
  Hypokalemia
  Hypophosphatemia
Hemoglobinuria
  Acute hemolysis
  Transfusion reaction
  Drugs/toxins
  Infections

G6PD, Glucose-6-phosphate dehydrogenase; *RBCs,* red blood cells.

Urine dipstick testing yields a positive result for heme in, at most, 50% of patients with rhabdomyolysis, because myoglobin is rapidly cleared from the serum and may therefore be undetectable in the urine at the time of presentation. Thus, a negative result on urine dipstick testing does not rule out the diagnosis. Serum creatine kinase (CK) is cleared much more slowly, so measurement of serum CK levels is a more sensitive test.

Antibiotics are commonly implicated in the development of ATN, with aminoglycosides being the most commonly associated. Higher doses and longer duration of therapy are associated with higher serum drug levels, leading to greater accumulation of drug in the renal parenchyma and a greater likelihood of nephrotoxicity. Increased age, impaired renal function, dehydration, and exposure to other nephrotoxins are additional risk factors. Once-daily administration of a somewhat higher dose is associated with less nephrotoxicity but has equal antimicrobial effectiveness.

Aminoglycoside-induced ATN typically has a gradual onset. Clinically significant renal dysfunction usually occurs only after several days and often after more than 1 week of therapy. However, renal failure can develop as late as 10 days after a drug has been discontinued, an observation that appears to be explained by the prolonged tissue half-life characteristic of these agents. Renal function returns to normal after an average of 6 weeks, but the condition occasionally progresses to permanent renal injury.

Radiographic contrast agents have long been considered a common cause of hospital-acquired renal insufficiency. AKI associated with these agents has been defined as an increase in serum creatinine level of 25% or an increase of 0.5 mg/dL over baseline, with a temporal relation to contrast medium administration and in the absence of other identifiable causes. Cases have been noted after any procedure involving intravascular administration of contrast material.

Radiocontrast-associated AKI presents on a spectrum ranging from asymptomatic nonoliguric renal insufficiency to severe renal failure requiring dialysis. Most cases are mild, however, likely due at least partially to the broad criteria by which the entity has been defined.[1-3] Typically, an increase in the serum creatinine level is noted within 3 days of exposure, with a return to normal levels within 10 to 14 days.

The most important risk factor for radiocontrast agent–induced AKI is preexisting renal insufficiency. Diabetes mellitus, multiple myeloma, age older than 60 years, and volume depletion are also associated with greater risk. Diabetic patients with a serum creatinine level less than 1.5 mg/dL appear to be at lower risk than those whose serum creatinine level is more than 1.5 mg/dL. Importantly, large doses and repeated doses of contrast material are associated with increased risk of ATN, particularly if a second study is performed within 72 hours of the first.

Volume depletion is an independent risk factor for contrast nephropathy, and aggressive volume expansion before contrast exposure appears to have a protective effect.[4] Modest volumes of intravenous normal saline (3 mL/kg over 1 hour, followed by 1.5 mL/kg/hr for 4 hours after contrast exposure) appear to be effective in decreasing the likelihood of nephrotoxicity. Sodium bicarbonate does not appear to offer an advantage over normal saline, and the weight of evidence does not favor a beneficial effect of administering oral N-acetylcysteine as part of the treatment regimen.[5]

Diagnostic Testing

Laboratory evaluation of renal dysfunction begins with a dipstick and microscopic urinalysis and measurement of urine output. BUN, serum creatinine, urine sodium, and FENa levels are determined to help evaluate renal function and provide clues about the cause of AKI. A complete blood count, serum electrolyte panel (expanded to include calcium, phosphorus, and magnesium determinations), electrocardiogram (ECG), and chest radiograph help establish the patient's baseline status and provide information about possible complications.

Urine Volume

Urine flow does not diminish until the GFR is sharply decreased; thus, urine volume is a poor indicator of renal dysfunction. Oliguria, defined as a urine volume of 100 to 400 mL/24 hr, may be seen with prerenal (blood flow–dependent), intrinsic (intrarenal), or postrenal (obstructive) causes of AKI. Although uncommon, alternating oliguria and anuria (the latter defined as less than 100 mL/24 hr), is a classic indicator of intermittent obstruction, which occurs as urine collects behind an obstructing stone or tumor and then is allowed to flow past as the obstructing material shifts position.

Urinalysis

The standard urinalysis consists of dipstick screening for heme pigment, protein, glucose, ketones, pH, leukocyte esterase, and nitrite and microscopic examination of a spun specimen of freshly voided urine and should be performed on all patients with AKI. Dipstick testing for heme and protein can provide important information related to renal function.

Heme. The dipstick detects free hemoglobin from lysed RBCs (or myoglobin) and the hemoglobin inside RBCs but is more sensitive to free hemoglobin. Although as few as three RBCs/high-power field (hpf) can be detected, on any given sample the dipstick may fail to identify 10% to 15% of patients who are otherwise found to have microscopic hematuria, typically defined as more than three RBCs/hpf. A positive result on dipstick testing should prompt microscopic examination of the urine. If red cells are seen, the diagnosis of hematuria is confirmed, though a level of two to three RBCs/hpf is commonly accepted as normal. If the dipstick result is positive but findings on microscopic examination are negative, pigmenturia (myoglobin or free hemoglobin) is suspected.

Protein. The dipstick test for protein, which uses the color change of tetrabromophenol blue, can detect protein at concentrations of 10 to 15 mg/dL but does not yield reliably positive results until the concentration is greater than 30 mg/dL. Moreover, the relation between color intensity and protein concentration is only approximate. The dipstick reagent is three to five times more sensitive to albumin than to globulins and immunoglobulin light chains (e.g., Bence Jones protein), an important limitation. False-positive results are caused by alkaline urine, hematuria, or prolonged immersion of the dipstick in the urine. False-negative results are seen with dilute urine. After dipstick testing has been completed, the sediment from a spun urine specimen is examined under the microscope.

Casts are formed from urinary Tamm-Horsfall protein—a product of the tubular epithelial cells that gels at low pH and high concentration and when mixed with albumin—or from red cells, tubular cells, or cellular debris in the urine. The composition of a cast reflects the contents of the tubule. Casts are classified according to their appearance or constituents (e.g., hyaline, red cell, white cell, granular, or fatty casts). Hyaline casts, those that are devoid of contents, are seen with dehydration, after exercise, or in association with glomerular proteinuria. Red cell casts indicate glomerular hematuria, as seen in glomerulonephritis; the presence of even a few red cell casts is significant. White cell casts imply the presence of renal parenchymal inflammation. Granular casts are composed of cellular remnants and debris. Fatty casts, like oval fat bodies, generally are associated with heavy proteinuria and nephrotic syndrome.

Microscopic examination of the urinary sediment can be helpful in establishing the cause of AKI. A sediment without formed elements or with only hyaline casts is characteristic of prerenal azotemia or obstruction. Red cell casts suggest glomerulonephritis or vasculitis. Fatty casts also suggest glomerular disease. In ATN, the urinary sediment commonly shows granular casts and renal tubular epithelial cells. Large numbers of polymorphonuclear leukocytes are observed in interstitial nephritis, papillary necrosis, and pyelonephritis. Eosinophil-containing casts, appreciated only after staining of the sediment, are typical of allergic interstitial nephritis. Uric acid crystals suggest uric acid nephropathy but are extremely nonspecific; oxalic acid or hippuric acid crystals may be seen in cases of ethylene glycol ingestion.

Serum and Urine Chemical Analysis

Creatinine and Blood Urea Nitrogen. The normal range for the serum creatinine level extends from 0.5 mg/dL in thin people to 1.5 mg/dL in muscular persons. Spurious elevations (up to 2 mg/dL) can be caused by acetoacetate, which cross-reacts with creatinine in some commonly used assays, and by certain medications (such as trimethoprim and cimetidine) that reversibly inhibit tubular creatinine secretion, causing a modest elevation of the serum creatinine despite a normal GFR. Serum creatinine concentration is a function of the amount of creatinine entering the blood from muscle, its volume of distribution, and its rate of excretion. Because the first two are usually constant, changes in the serum creatinine concentration generally reflect changes in GFR. The creatinine clearance is commonly estimated by the Cockcroft-Gault equation:

$$\text{Creatinine clearance (mL/min)} = ([140-\text{age}] \times \text{weight}) / (72 \times \text{serum creatinine}) (\times 0.85 \text{ if female})$$

Under steady-state conditions, if the GFR is halved, the serum creatinine doubles. Abrupt cessation of glomerular filtration causes the serum creatinine level to rise by 1 to 2 mg/dL per day. Thus, a daily increment of less than 1 mg/dL suggests that at least some renal function has been preserved. Rhabdomyolysis releases creatine into the plasma and may cause the serum creatinine level to increase by more than 2 mg/dL per day. The BUN level also rises with renal dysfunction but is also influenced by many extrarenal factors. Increased protein intake, GI bleeding, and the catabolic effects of fever, trauma, infection, and drugs such as tetracycline and corticosteroids all increase protein turnover and result in increased hepatic urea production and increased BUN levels. Conversely, the BUN level tends to be decreased in patients with liver failure or protein malnutrition.

When glomerular filtrate has been formed, renal urea clearance is largely a function of flow rate. Urea clearance is thus decreased in patients with prerenal azotemia or acute obstruction, despite preservation of tubular function. In such cases, the BUN/creatinine ratio usually is greater than the normal value of 10:1, whereas this ratio usually is not markedly increased in cases of uncomplicated intrinsic AKI.

Urine Sodium and Fractional Excretion of Sodium. Normally, urine sodium concentration parallels sodium intake. A low urine sodium concentration thus indicates not only intact tubular reabsorptive function but also the presence of a stimulus to conserve sodium. The urine sodium concentration, as well as the FENa, an additional measure of tubular sodium handling, helps distinguish between the two most common causes of AKI, prerenal azotemia and ATN.

Measurement of urinary indices can be helpful in oliguric patients. An oliguric patient with a urine sodium concentration less than 20 mEq/L and FENa less than 1% is likely to have prerenal azotemia, whereas a urine sodium concentration more than 40 mEq/L and FENa more than 1% suggest ATN. Values in patients with prerenal azotemia overlap somewhat with those in patients with nonoliguric ATN,

particularly if the renal injury is mild and some capability to retain sodium has been preserved. Thus, intermediate values for urine sodium concentration and FENa are of little help in differentiating between the two conditions. The administration of mannitol or a loop diuretic within the several hours preceding urine collection also may make interpretation of urine values difficult because the urinary sodium level will tend to be higher and the urine less concentrated, causing the results in prerenal azotemia to resemble those in intrinsic renal failure.

In glomerulonephritis, the urinary indices generally reflect intact tubular sodium handling, but the diagnosis is more accurately made by urine microscopy. In obstructive uropathy, the values of the urinary indices depend on the duration of obstruction and cannot be relied on to indicate the presence or absence of obstruction.

Renal Imaging

Renal imaging is often helpful in the evaluation of the patient with kidney dysfunction, particularly when obstruction is suspected. Computed tomography (CT) scanning provides an anatomic image of the urinary tract but does not provide an evaluation of renal function. The classic CT findings of obstruction are kidneys that are normal to large in size, and demonstration of hydronephrosis or hydroureter. Since contrast-enhanced CT subjects the kidneys of an already azotemic patient to the risk of an additional potential insult from the contrast agent, ultrasonography and noncontrast CT are much preferred for patients with preexisting renal insufficiency (Fig. 83.2).

Computed Tomography. Noncontrast CT may be useful in evaluating some azotemic patients. Hydronephrosis can be recognized without the use of contrast material. Often, dilated ureters can also be seen without contrast enhancement, and the level of obstruction can be determined. The cause of obstruction (e.g., bilateral stones, lymphoma, retroperitoneal hemorrhage, metastatic cancer, retroperitoneal fibrosis) often can also be delineated. Occasionally, bilateral ureteral obstruction produced by malignancy or retroperitoneal fibrosis may not cause detectable proximal dilation of the urinary tract. When noninvasive studies yield negative results, the diagnosis of obstruction can be made by retrograde pyelography or antegrade pyelography performed via a percutaneous nephrostomy.

Ultrasonography. Ultrasonography is a safe and reasonably reliable method for excluding obstruction as a cause of AKI. The normal kidney shows an echo-free renal parenchyma surrounding the echogenic central

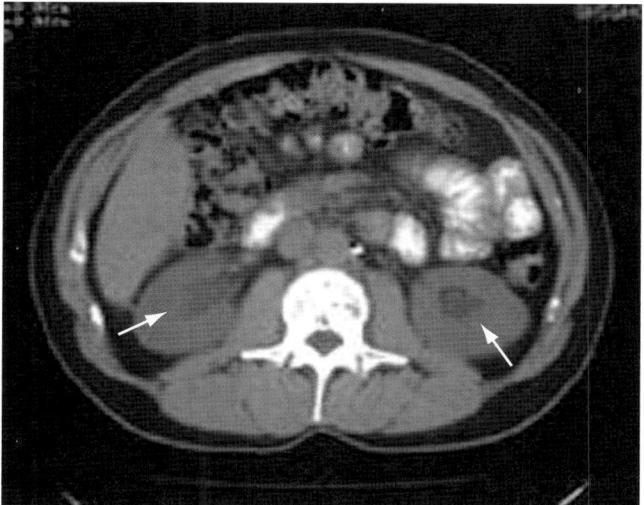

Fig. 83.2 CT scan of bilateral hydronephrotic kidneys without IV contrast medium.

urothelium of the renal pelvis and calices. The sonographic appearance of the kidney in obstruction is that of an enlarged, central, sonolucent area that spreads the normal central echo densities. A similar pattern may be produced by renal cysts, but without associated ureteral dilation. Dilation of the collecting system generally is apparent within 24 to 36 hours of the onset of obstruction, but obstruction may not be evident in patients who are evaluated early in the development of obstructive AKI.

Diagnosis

Prerenal azotemia is suspected in the setting of volume loss, volume redistribution, or decreased effective renal perfusion. It typically is associated with a normal urinalysis, high BUN/creatinine ratio, increased urine osmolality, urine sodium concentration less than 20 mEq/L, and FENa less than 1%. A rapid response to volume repletion also is characteristic.

Urethral or bladder neck obstruction is documented by the finding of significant amounts of residual urine in the bladder by catheterization or ultrasound examination after the patient has voided or attempted to void spontaneously. An important point is that the ability to void does not rule out obstruction. In fact, the urine volume in the presence of obstruction may range from zero to several liters per day. Flank pain is likewise an insensitive marker for obstruction. Urine indices and the BUN/creatinine ratio tend not to be helpful, although an increase in the latter is common in obstruction. A renal parenchymal disorder often can be diagnosed by its manifestations on microscopic urinalysis or by associated extrarenal manifestations (e.g., with multisystem disease) or clinical setting (e.g., recent exposure to a new medication). The absence of evidence of prerenal or postrenal causes in a patient with AKI may be taken as presumptive evidence of an intrarenal parenchymal process. Among these, the possibility of an acute or ongoing vascular insult should be kept in mind because timely intervention can be important in preserving ultimate renal function.

Management

ED management of AKI is directed at reversing decreases in GFR and urine output (if possible) while minimizing further hemodynamic and toxic insults, maintaining normal fluid and electrolyte balance, and managing other complications of AKI, as required. Because renal failure alters the metabolism and action of many drugs, often in ways that are not predictable, great care should be exercised in prescribing all medications. Easy access to online sources that provide guidelines for drug dosages in renal failure, and readily available consultation with a hospital pharmacist are of great help for this purpose.

After ensuring that the vital signs are adequate and the patient is in no immediate danger from volume or metabolic derangements, the next step is to correct prerenal and postrenal factors, if any are identified. Intravascular volume is repleted in hypovolemic patients and maintained in euvolemic patients by matching input to measured and insensible output. Inadequate cardiac output is augmented when possible. Postrenal or obstructive AKI is treated by restoration of normal urine outflow. Bladder outlet obstruction may be relieved by passage of a Foley catheter, whereas upper tract obstruction may require percutaneous nephrostomy.

Renal insufficiency secondary to NSAIDs generally is reversible after withdrawal of the causative agent. For patients who are at increased risk but require treatment with NSAIDs, a short-acting preparation (e.g., ibuprofen) should be prescribed and follow-up monitoring of renal function and the serum potassium level should begin within days rather than weeks. If renal function is unchanged after a short course of treatment, adverse effects from continuing therapy are unlikely, although other potential mechanisms for the development of renal dysfunction (e.g., interstitial nephritis) should be kept in mind.

Treatment of postrenal AKI consists of relief of the obstruction. In the absence of infection, full renal recovery is possible, even after 1 to 2 weeks of total obstruction, although the serum creatinine level may not return to baseline for several weeks. Because the onset of irreversible loss of renal function with obstruction appears to be gradual, a few days' delay in diagnosis generally is considered acceptable. Still, common sense dictates that obstructions should be detected and relieved promptly.

When prerenal and postrenal factors have been ruled out, the challenge is to identify the cause of intrinsic renal AKI, keeping in mind the multitude of known possible causes (see Box 83.4). The differential diagnosis can often be significantly narrowed by considering the clinical setting and physical and laboratory findings. The clinical picture is often most consistent with the broad category of ATN.

Patients who have oliguric AKI have a significantly higher mortality rate and much greater risk of complications than those who are not oliguric. The difference in prognosis may simply reflect a more severe renal insult in patients who are oliguric, however, and it is not clear that interventions aimed at converting oliguric to nonoliguric AKI have a beneficial effect on renal function or mortality. Nevertheless, because nonoliguric patients are easier to manage, an attempt to increase urine flow is warranted.

The use of loop diuretics or mannitol often is effective in increasing urine flow when intravascular volume deficits have been corrected. Furosemide has not been shown to shorten the clinical course or affect mortality. Mannitol appears to be most useful when given at the time of, or shortly after, the renal insult; the recommended adult dose is 12.5 to 25 g, intravenous (IV). If urine output does not increase, further doses may cause hyperosmolality and clinically significant intravascular volume overload in patients with impaired renal function. Dopamine also has been used in an effort to increase urine output, but it has not been proven effective.

Certain specific considerations apply to toxin-induced ATN. Pigment-induced ATN may be prevented by avoidance of hemolysis and muscle injury and correction of the factors (e.g., dehydration, acidemia) known to predispose patients with pigmenturia to the development of renal failure. When hemolysis or rhabdomyolysis has occurred, treatment is directed at eliminating the cause and preventing the development of renal failure.

Mannitol has been shown to prevent AKI in experimental models of myoglobinuria, presumably by inducing osmotic diuresis and decreasing intratubular deposition of pigment. Furosemide, on the other hand, has not consistently shown a beneficial effect. Other studies have suggested that myoglobin precipitates in an acidic urine but not in an alkaline urine. Thus, aggressive volume repletion, alkalinization, and mannitol infusion have traditionally been recommended after crush injuries to reduce the likelihood or severity of AKI. However, there is good evidence that aggressive volume resuscitation alone is equally effective. When AKI has occurred, management is similar to that for other forms of AKI, but early dialysis may be required to control rapidly developing hyperkalemia, hyperphosphatemia, and hyperuricemia.

Patients who have radiocontrast agent–induced ATN usually require only supportive therapy. A more significant aspect of ED management is identifying patients who are at risk when contrast studies are being considered. BUN and serum creatinine levels should be checked before contrast exposure in patient with risk factors, such as older age, diabetes, volume depletion, and underlying renal disease. Patients at risk should be volume-repleted (if not contraindicated) before undergoing the study, the administered dose of contrast agent should be kept as low as possible, and multiple exposures to contrast should be avoided, as should concomitant use of other nephrotoxins.[4]

In addition to general measures aimed at minimizing decreases in GFR and increasing urine output, an important component of the management of AKI is the prevention or control of systemic complications. Of particular significance in this regard are metabolic derangements (e.g., hyperkalemia, hypocalcemia, hyperphosphatemia, metabolic acidosis) and complications of volume overload (e.g., hypertension, CHF).

Hyperkalemia and Other Metabolic Derangements

Hyperkalemia. The most common metabolic cause of death in patients with AKI results from an inability to excrete endogenous and exogenous potassium loads. In oliguric patients, the serum potassium level typically increases by 0.3 to 0.5 mEq/L per day, but greater increases occur in catabolic, septic, or traumatized patients and in the presence of acidosis or exogenous potassium loads from diet or medication. This is of particular concern in patients with rhabdomyolysis and associated AKI.

Hyperkalemia results in serious disturbances in cardiac electrophysiology that may culminate in cardiac arrest. Calcium chloride is considered the second choice agent given its irritating effect when administered parentally. Hyperkalemia is essentially asymptomatic until major manifestations of cardiotoxicity appear. Accordingly, detection of hyperkalemia is a primary consideration in these patients. Electrocardiographic changes correlate only roughly with the serum potassium level. Mild hyperkalemia (serum potassium < 6.0 mEq/L) may be cautiously observed without specific treatment while all exogenous sources of potassium are eliminated. If the serum potassium level is greater than 6.5 mEq/L, and particularly if electrocardiographic changes are present, urgent intervention is necessary.

When cardiotoxicity must be reversed immediately (e.g., when there is hemodynamic compromise), IV calcium (10 mL of 10% calcium gluconate infused over 2 minutes, repeated after 5 minutes if necessary) is the treatment of choice. Calcium directly antagonizes the membrane effects of hyperkalemia. IV insulin, given with glucose to prevent hypoglycemia, temporarily shifts potassium to the intracellular space. The safety and efficacy of β-agonists in hyperkalemic patients have been well documented; like insulin, inhaled albuterol (in a dose of 10–20 mg for adult patients; for pediatric patients, a fixed dose should be given based on patient weight [<25 kg: 2.5 mg, 25 to 50 kg: 5 mg, >50 kg: 10 mg]) causes potassium to move into cells, thereby controlling hyperkalemia for 2 hours or more. Bicarbonate appears to be less effective in shifting potassium into cells than once thought. It should be used with caution in patients with renal failure because of its potential to cause volume overload and provoke hypocalcemic tetany or seizures. Sodium polystyrene sulfonate (Kayexalate), a potassium-binding ion exchange resin, has long been administered with sorbitol to promote elimination of potassium from the body, but it is no longer considered to be effective or free of adverse effects.[6] More recently, other nonabsorbable cation exchangers such as patiromer and sodium zirconium cyclosilicate have been used to control hyperkalemia in patients with renal failure, but they have not been evaluated in patients who present with acute hyperkalemia.[7]

Hypocalcemia. Hypocalcemia is a common feature of AKI that can develop rapidly after its onset. Vitamin D–dependent intestinal absorption of calcium is decreased in AKI because of decreased renal synthesis of 1,25-dihydroxyvitamin D. Another factor promoting hypocalcemia is the complexing of calcium with retained phosphate. Rhabdomyolysis-associated AKI, in particular, is often associated with the deposition of complexed calcium in muscle and other tissues. Asymptomatic hypocalcemia requires no immediate treatment, but subtle or frank tetany should be treated with IV calcium (10–20 mL of 10% calcium gluconate infused over several minutes).

Hyperphosphatemia. Hyperphosphatemia resulting from decreased renal elimination of phosphate is another common feature. The serum phosphorus level usually ranges from 6 to 8 mg/dL but may be much higher with rhabdomyolysis or in catabolic states. A calcium-phosphate product greater than 70 mg^2/dL^2 may result in metastatic soft tissue calcification. Hyperphosphatemia often is treated with oral calcium-based antacids that bind ingested phosphate in the gut.

Acids produced in normal metabolic processes accumulate in AKI and are buffered in part by serum bicarbonate, resulting in a decrease in the serum bicarbonate level and a high anion gap metabolic acidosis. Compensatory hyperventilation may be mistakenly attributed to primary cardiac failure or volume overload. The metabolic acidosis associated with AKI usually is mild, and treatment generally is not necessary if the serum bicarbonate level is greater than 10 mEq/L. Overzealous correction may result in hypokalemia, hypocalcemia, or volume overload.

Hypermagnesemia. This may complicate AKI when patients are given magnesium-containing antacids or laxatives. Thus, these products, as well as magnesium itself (e.g., when given for preeclampsia or for treatment of arrhythmia or wheezing), should be avoided in the setting of AKI.

Disturbances of Volume Regulation. These can be expected to occur in most patients with AKI. Some nonoliguric patients excrete enough salt and water to produce intravascular volume depletion if adequate fluid replacement is not provided. Volume depletion prolongs recovery from AKI. Much more commonly, AKI is complicated by volume overload because sodium and water excretion may be inadequate to match even modest intakes. Volume overload is largely responsible for the hypertension often seen in those with AKI and commonly leads to CHF and pulmonary edema. Iatrogenic volume overload is particularly common and can be prevented only by careful attention to fluid intake and output, with prudent estimates of insensible loss. Volume overload can be treated with diuretics or intravenous nitroglycerin while preparations are being made to initiate dialysis.

Disposition

Patients with new-onset severe AKI should be hospitalized. If nephrology consultation and dialysis facilities are not available, transfer to another institution is advisable once volume and metabolic abnormalities have been controlled and the patient is hemodynamically stable.

Decisions regarding dialysis generally are made by the nephrology consultant and take into account many factors, including laboratory test abnormalities and the presence or absence of signs and symptoms of uremia (e.g., nausea, vomiting, change in mental status). Many nephrologists choose to initiate dialysis when the BUN level exceeds 100 mg/dL or the serum creatinine level exceeds 10 mg/dL. Intractable volume overload and life-threatening hyperkalemia are the two most common indications for emergency dialysis.

CHRONIC KIDNEY DISEASE

Foundations

CKD denotes kidney damage or decreased renal function for 3 months or longer and is characterized by irreversible nephron loss and scarring. Chronic renal insufficiency, which denotes a condition in which the GFR has been moderately reduced but not to a degree sufficient to cause clear-cut clinical symptoms, has been replaced by an indication of the degree to which the GFR is reduced. End-stage renal disease, now termed *kidney failure,* describes a condition in which renal function has diminished to a low level and in which serious, life-threatening manifestations can be expected to occur without dialysis or transplantation. At this stage, the kidneys often are shrunken and diffusely scarred to such a degree that it may be impossible to make an etiologic diagnosis, even on pathologic examination.

The causes of CKD are numerous; their relative frequency depends primarily on the population studied. As with AKI, they can be conveniently classified as prerenal (vascular), intrinsic renal (glomerular and tubulointerstitial), or postrenal (obstructive; Box 83.6). Glomerular disease accounts for approximately one-third to half of the cases of CKD; in the United States, diabetic nephropathy forms the largest group of these. Hypertensive nephrosclerosis is another important cause, particularly among blacks, in whom it may be the cause of 25% or more of cases of CKD. Among children and adolescents, reflux nephropathy is the most common cause of CKD. Renal failure related to IV drug use or human immunodeficiency virus disease is a major consideration in some populations. Clues to other specific causes may be gained from elements of the history, physical examination, and laboratory and imaging studies. Although determining the underlying cause of CKD can permit the underlying disease to be treated and can lead to some improvement in renal function in some cases, this is the exception rather than the rule.

BOX 83.6   Major Causes of Chronic Kidney Disease

Vascular Causes
Renal arterial disease
Hypertensive nephrosclerosis

Glomerular Causes
Primary Glomerulopathies
Focal sclerosing glomerulonephritis (GN)
Membranoproliferative GN
Membranous GN
Crescentic GN
IgA nephropathy

Secondary Glomerulopathies
Diabetic nephropathy
Collagen vascular disease
Amyloidosis
Postinfectious
HIV nephropathy

Tubulointerstitial Causes
Nephrotoxins
Analgesic nephropathy
Hypercalcemia or nephrocalcinosis
Multiple myeloma
Reflux nephropathy
Sickle nephropathy
Chronic pyelonephritis
Tuberculosis

Obstructive Causes
Nephrolithiasis
Ureteral tuberculosis
Retroperitoneal fibrosis
Retroperitoneal tumor
Prostatic obstruction
Congenital abnormalities

Hereditary Causes
Polycystic kidney disease
Alport syndrome
Medullary cystic disease

HIV, Human immunodeficiency virus; *IgA*, immunoglobulin A.

Barring renal transplantation, CKD is an essentially irreversible condition generally characterized by a relentless decrease in renal function. The most common problems requiring emergent intervention are severe hyperkalemia and symptomatic volume overload. In the patient with CKD who has an acute problem, the focus should be on the identification and treatment of an intercurrent illness that has caused clinical decompensation, with the goal of returning the patient to a stable, chronically compensated status.

Pathophysiology

Progressive loss of renal function eventually results in a recognizable syndrome termed *uremia*. Clinical manifestations do not generally appear, however, until the GFR has been reduced to approximately 15% to 20% of normal. As the patient becomes unable to excrete an ingested salt or water load promptly, the external balance of sodium and water is affected; volume overload or hypernatremia or hyponatremia may result. Inability to concentrate the urine is an early manifestation of renal insufficiency and may be manifested as nocturia. Potassium homeostasis is likewise disrupted, and a relatively small potassium load may lead to dangerous hyperkalemia. The acid-base balance is affected because the kidney fails to clear the daily metabolic acid load owing to a decreased ability to excrete ammonium and phosphate; the result is a non–anion gap acidosis in the earlier stages of CKD and a superimposed anion gap acidosis as the GFR decreases further. Calcium and phosphate metabolism is affected as well; retention of phosphate and progressive loss of the kidney's capacity to synthesize 1,25-dihydroxycholecalciferol, the active form of vitamin D, lead to hypocalcemia, secondary hyperparathyroidism, and eventually the development of renal osteodystrophy.

Nitrogenous byproducts of protein catabolism retained in the blood are the presumed cause of many of the diverse abnormalities of organ function in renal failure. Most patients with CKD show decreased glucose tolerance, although it is rarely severe enough to require treatment unless the medical history includes established diabetes. In the latter case, insulin or other hypoglycemic therapy may need to be continued, but generally at a lower dosage than required before the onset of renal failure because the normal kidney has a major role in insulin degradation. Alterations in lipid metabolism result in elevated low-density lipoprotein levels and hypertriglyceridemia in many patients with CKD.

Clinical Features

Uremia has specific effects on a variety of organ systems. Many of these manifestations are relieved by dialysis, but others are not. A number have been attributed in some degree to the retention of nitrogenous wastes and to derangements in vitamin D and parathyroid hormone metabolism.

Cardiovascular System

The cardiovascular system is perhaps most dramatically affected in CKD. Many of the manifestations can be attributed to the effects of chronic volume overload, anemia, hyperlipidemia, alterations in calcium and phosphorus metabolism, and volume- and hormone-mediated hypertension. Pericarditis, with or without pericardial fluid accumulation, also is common in CKD, particularly among patients who have not undergone dialysis.[8]

Pulmonary Effects

Uremic pleuritis, with or without associated pleural fluid collections, may develop in some patients. So-called "uremic lung," often manifested radiographically by bat wing perihilar infiltrates, represents pulmonary edema and is almost always caused by volume overload or myocardial dysfunction. Noninflammatory pleural effusion caused by volume overload also is fairly common. Of special importance in the ED evaluation is that the radiographic appearance in pulmonary edema may at times be misleading, simulating an infectious lobar infiltrate or even assuming a nodular appearance in some cases.

Neurologic Features

Neurologic dysfunction is common in those with advanced uremia and may manifest as lethargy, somnolence, difficulty concentrating, or frank alteration in mental status. Seizures may occur, although causes other than uremia alone must be ruled out. Uremic encephalopathy commonly manifests with hiccups, asterixis, or myoclonic twitching. The latter should not be confused with tetany caused by hypocalcemia, which also is common in untreated CKD patients. In the peripheral nervous system, uremia often causes cramps and a distal sensorimotor neuropathy.

Gastrointestinal System

Anorexia and nausea are nearly constant features of uremia. These GI manifestations are caused by the accumulation of nitrogenous wastes that correlate roughly with the BUN level and may be relieved even in the undialyzed patient by introduction of a low-protein diet.

Dermatologic Features

The skin of patients with CKD has a characteristic yellowish tinge. Uremic frost, the result of the deposition of urea from evaporated sweat on the skin, is a classic finding that, like so-called uremic fetor, is seen only rarely now with the widespread use of dialysis (Fig. 83.3). Diffuse pruritus is often a major source of discomfort for the patient with CKD; in some cases, it may be caused by calcium deposition in the skin secondary to derangements in calcium metabolism.

The use of gadolinium-based contrast agents for magnetic resonance imaging has been associated with the development of nephrogenic systemic fibrosis, a potentially fatal disorder that occurs in patients with moderate-to-severe chronic kidney failure.

Musculoskeletal System

The complex disturbances of calcium and phosphate metabolism in CKD result in renal osteodystrophy, a clinical entity encompassing

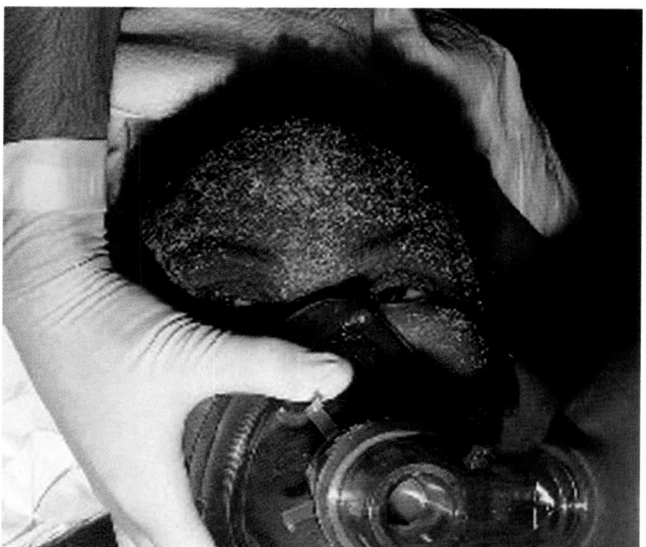

Fig. 83.3 Uremic frost. Note the fine white powder on the skin of this patient with kidney failure.

several overlapping varieties of bone disease that can cause bone pain or frank fractures. Patients with CKD generally are treated with long-term oral calcium and vitamin D in an effort to prevent secondary hyperparathyroidism and uremic osteodystrophy. Occasional patients will have a poor response to therapy and require parathyroidectomy. A specific type of arthritis caused by the deposition of calcium hydroxyapatite or calcium oxalate crystals in joints is seen in some patients, as are periarticular calcium deposition, spontaneous tendon rupture, myopathy, and carpal tunnel syndrome.

Immunologic Considerations

Uremic patients have long been noted to have an increased susceptibility to infection due to alteration of both humoral and cellular immunity. The relative importance of each in the pathogenesis of infection in renal failure is not completely clear, but defects in cellular immunity appear to be more significant clinically. Although patients with renal failure should be considered to be immunocompromised, most infections in patients with CKD are caused by common pathogens rather than opportunistic organisms.

Hematologic Effects

A pronounced normochromic normocytic anemia, with a hematocrit value commonly in the range of 18% to 25%, is nearly universal in those with untreated CKD, except among patients with polycystic disease. It is caused primarily by the kidneys' decreased production of erythropoietin, a hormone that stimulates red cell production by the bone marrow. Other contributing factors are increased red cell hemolysis, nutritional deficiencies, and increased bleeding secondary to platelet dysfunction.

Although the platelet number generally is normal in uremia, the bleeding time is prolonged because of defective platelet adhesiveness and activation. Numerous ecchymoses, seen in many patients with CKD, are a common manifestation.

Differential Diagnosis

Patients with CKD commonly present with nonspecific complaints that are often of insidious onset, such as generalized weakness, poor appetite, or deterioration of mental functioning. However, because CKD can affect all organ systems, a number of life-threatening conditions, including hyperkalemia and myocardial infarction, are in the differential, and a comprehensive evaluation is generally indicated.

In patients without an established diagnosis of CKD, the first consideration is to determine that the renal failure is chronic rather than acute. An explicit history to that effect, obtained from previous medical records or from the patient or family, provides the most straightforward and reliable confirmation, as does the presence of a dialysis access device on physical examination. If such a history is unavailable, the finding of bilaterally small kidneys, readily detected by plain abdominal radiography or ultrasonography, constitutes equally good evidence. However, the converse is not necessarily true—a finding of normal-sized or large kidneys does not rule out CKD. In such cases, additional diagnostic steps are required to establish the diagnosis. A convincing history of the long-standing presence of the presenting symptoms or of symptoms, such as nocturia, may be helpful in suggesting chronicity, as may a history of familial kidney disease, such as polycystic kidney disease or Alport syndrome.

Laboratory abnormalities such as anemia, acidosis, hyperuricemia, hypocalcemia, and hyperphosphatemia can occur in patients with acute kidney failure as early as 10 days after onset. Although urinary findings likewise tend not to be helpful, the presence of broad waxy casts on microscopic examination is suggestive of chronic disease, whereas the finding of an active sediment (e.g., red cell casts) is good evidence for an acute process.

Although as a rule chronic kidney failure is irreversible and slowly progressive, an essential component of the ED evaluation is to exclude the possibility of potentially reversible factors (in effect, ruling out "acute on chronic" renal failure) and to ensure that treatable causes of CKD—disorders that if treated might allow for some return of renal function—have not been overlooked. These potentially reversible factors and treatable causes of CKD are important to keep in mind because they represent the only potential opportunity to reverse the patient's disease rather than simply to manage its results (Box 83.7).

Primary among superimposed reversible factors are those that lead to decreased renal perfusion. Of these, the most common is volume depletion. Regardless of the initiating cause, the process is exacerbated by the diseased kidney's impaired ability to conserve sodium and concentrate the urine appropriately. Decreased renal perfusion caused by cardiac dysfunction of any cause is another extremely common and potentially reversible factor. An uncommonly encountered but important vascular cause of reversible deterioration of renal function is scleroderma renal crisis, a syndrome of accelerated hypertension and severe vasoconstriction in patients with underlying scleroderma that can be reversed by timely treatment with ACE inhibitors. Increased catabolism caused by infection, trauma, surgery, corticosteroids, or GI bleeding is another reversible factor that often is responsible for worsening azotemia and the development of uremic symptoms.

Drugs and toxins constitute another important group of reversible factors. Not only may these agents exacerbate renal insufficiency by causing intravascular volume depletion (diuretics), decreased renal perfusion (antihypertensive agents), or increased catabolism (tetracycline), they also can cause ATN (aminoglycosides, rhabdomyolysis), AIN (many drugs), or inhibition of renal prostaglandin synthesis (NSAIDs). Particularly noteworthy is the dramatic decrease in renal function produced when an ACE inhibitor is administered to a patient with renal insufficiency caused by bilateral renal artery stenosis or renal artery stenosis in a solitary kidney.

Postrenal reversible factors also are important because of their frequency, particularly obstructive disease in the older male patient and reflux nephropathy in the child. Papillary necrosis should remain a consideration in the diabetic patient and the patient with sickle cell disease. Stone disease, retroperitoneal fibrosis, and even rarer entities such as ureteral tuberculosis also should not be overlooked.

Finally, treatment of the underlying disorder that has caused the CKD can occasionally result in the return of some renal function, most notably in cases of myeloma kidney, some forms of secondary glomerulonephritis, and severe hypertensive disease. Although this consideration relates to long-term care and follow-up, it is appropriate that ED management address this issue to ensure that appropriate evaluation and disposition are arranged.

Diagnostic Testing

Diagnostic testing for CKD generally follows the principles outlined for AKI (see earlier section "Acute Kidney Injury: Diagnostic Testing"), though prerenal causes are of concern mostly as exacerbating factors in patients with CKD.

Management

CKD patients are susceptible to infection, bleeding, and the numerous other complications associated with renal failure, as well as those that may be associated with the underlying causative disorder. Moreover, these patients are more vulnerable to the effects of any intercurrent illness or trauma. Those who are maintained with chronic hemodialysis or peritoneal dialysis are subject to potential complications from the dialysis therapy itself.

Patients with CKD also are uniquely susceptible to iatrogenic illness. First, they are less able to handle fluid and solute loads than normal persons. Just as important, the presence of renal failure significantly alters the metabolism and action of many drugs, often in ways that are not predictable (Box 83.8). Thus, the dose and schedule of every agent administered, even those that are apparently innocuous, such as antacids, laxatives, antiemetics, or multivitamin preparations, should be carefully considered, and the hospital pharmacist or other dependable resource consulted. In general, consultation with the patient's nephrologist is recommended on completion of the initial ED evaluation because management and follow-up monitoring after the patient has left the ED are often complex.

In the United States, most patients with advancing CKD eventually will require dialysis, but several true emergencies may develop in the patient with CKD before chronic dialysis has been instituted. Specific diagnostic and therapeutic considerations apply to the management of these conditions, regardless of whether they occur in dialyzed or undialyzed patients.

Hyperkalemia

Potentially the most rapidly lethal complication of CKD is severe hyperkalemia. As a rule, this condition is clinically silent until it causes

---

BOX 83.7 Reversible Factors and Treatable Causes of Chronic Kidney Disease

Reversible Factors
Hypovolemia
Congestive heart failure
Pericardial tamponade
Severe hypertension
Catabolic state, protein loads
Nephrotoxic agents
Obstructive disease
Reflux disease

Treatable Causes
Renal artery stenosis
Malignant hypertension
Acute interstitial nephritis
Hypercalcemic nephropathy
Multiple myeloma
Vasculitis (e.g., systemic lupus erythematosus, Wegener granulomatosis, polyarteritis nodosa)
Obstructive nephropathy
Reflux nephropathy

BOX 83.8 Mechanisms of Drug Toxicity in Renal Failure

Excessive drug level
Impaired renal excretion of drug
Impaired renal excretion of active metabolite
Impaired hepatic metabolism
Increased sensitivity to drug
Changes in protein binding
Changes in volume of distribution
Changes in target organ sensitivity
Metabolic loads administered with drug
Misinterpretation of measured serum drug level (i.e., change in therapeutic range)

potentially life-threatening manifestations. Accordingly, hyperkalemia must be looked for in every patient with CKD. These patients can become severely hyperkalemic when required to handle even modest exogenous and endogenous potassium loads; moreover, even drugs that have only minimal effects on the serum potassium level in normal persons, such as β-blockers and ACE inhibitors, can cause hyperkalemia in these patients. There is concern that the use of succinylcholine in patients with CKD has the potential to cause rapid deterioration in patients who are already hyperkalemic, although this appears to be rare.

An ECG should be obtained whenever hyperkalemia is a possibility and, if signs of hyperkalemia are noted, appropriate therapy should be started immediately, even before laboratory confirmation of a high serum potassium level. Electrocardiographic changes may be completely absent, even when hyperkalemia is severe; thus, a normal ECG does not preclude the need for laboratory confirmation of a normal serum potassium level. A potassium level of 6 mEq/L should be considered potentially dangerous, even though many patients with CKD chronically tolerate levels somewhat above this threshold, without electrocardiographic changes. A patient with CKD who is in cardiac arrest should be assumed to be hyperkalemic and treated accordingly while the usual resuscitative measures are taken. See earlier ("Acute Kidney Injury: Management") and Table 83.1.

In patients who still retain some renal function, the most effective way to treat hyperkalemia in patients with CKI may be to administer an IV diuretic such as furosemide (if the patient is not hypovolemic) and to provide volume, if necessary. Large doses of diuretic may be necessary for a satisfactory diuresis to be induced. In light of the potential for ototoxicity with the use of loop-active diuretics, these drugs should be administered by slow infusion rather than by bolus and may be contraindicated in patients who also are receiving other potentially ototoxic agents. During the course of any of these therapeutic interventions, the electrocardiographic and serum potassium levels must be monitored frequently.

Pulmonary Edema

Perhaps the most common ED problem in patients with CKD is pulmonary edema secondary to volume overload. Surprisingly, the diagnosis is not always straightforward. A history of increasing dyspnea on exertion or paroxysmal nocturnal dyspnea may be suggestive, but the physical examination may not reveal the expected signs of CHF, and even chest radiography may be deceptive. Recent weight gain or a body weight considerably over dry weight (typically >5 pounds) is the most reliable clue and, in the absence of convincing evidence of another cause for dyspnea, volume overload should be assumed to be the cause.

Treatment of pulmonary edema in the patient with CKD is of necessity somewhat different from that in other patients. Arrangements for initiation of dialysis should be made as soon as possible because it is the most rapidly effective means to decrease intravascular volume in the absence of renal function. Other immediate measures should be instituted in the meantime. Although such measures may occasionally prove to be effective enough to avoid dialysis temporarily in patients who possess some residual renal function, it should nevertheless be anticipated that the response to even extremely aggressive medical therapy, short of dialysis, will be inadequate.

The CKD patient with pulmonary edema is placed in the sitting position, and high-flow oxygen is administered by mask. The use of continuous or bilevel positive airway pressure (CPAP or BiPAP) is a useful adjunct for patients with CKD, as it is for patients without renal failure. Sublingual nitroglycerin can be administered immediately and functions rapidly to reduce preload and afterload; an IV infusion beginning at 10 to 20 µg/min can be initiated promptly and titrated to effect. Diuretics are not expected to be helpful unless the patient has retained a significant level of renal function.

Infection

Because infection is a major contributor to morbidity and mortality among patients with CKD, the possibility of serious infection should be entertained, even when the expected classic findings are not all present. For example, bacteremia may manifest with fever alone, just as in other patients with impaired immunity. Patients with pneumonia may have only vague dyspnea or malaise, symptoms that may be attributed to volume overload or uremia. Thus, all diagnostic possibilities should

TABLE 83.1 Treatment of Hyperkalemia

Agent or Modality	Dose and Regimen	Onset/Duration of Action	Mechanism of Action	Comments
Calcium gluconate (10%)	10 mL IV (may repeat × 2 prn every 5–10 min)	1–5 min/≈1 hr	Antagonizes membrane effects of K	Monitoring of ECG required; do not mix with HCO_3^- *Beware*—hypercalcemia
Albuterol	10–20 mg (nebulized) by inhalation	30 min/2 hr or more	Intracellular movement of K	Relatively free of significant side effects; tachycardia
Glucose and insulin	10–20 units regular insulin/100 g glucose	30 min/while infusion continued	Intracellular movement of K	*Beware*—hyperglycemia, hypoglycemia Infused volume may be decreased by giving $D_{10}W$, $D_{20}W$, or $D_{50}W$
Sodium bicarbonate	150 mEq/L IV infusion (rate variable)	Approximately 10–15 min/1–2 hr	Possible intracellular movement of K	Most effective with organic acidosis
Dialysis	HD, PD	Minutes/while continued	Removal of K from blood	HD may remove 50 mEq/hr *Beware*—K rebound PD may remove 15 mEq/hr
IV diuretics (IV fluid if patient is hypovolemic)	Furosemide 40–80 mg IV	15 minutes/while diuresis continued (depending on renal function)	Urinary K excretion	Only in patients with some residual renal function

$D_{10}W$, 10% dextrose in water; $D_{20}W$, 20% dextrose in water; $D_{50}W$, 50% dextrose in water; *ECG*, electrocardiogram; *HD*, hemodialysis; *IV*, intravenous; *PD*, peritoneal dialysis; *PO*, orally.

be pursued, and empirical broad-spectrum antibiotic coverage often is advisable until infection has been ruled out in the hospital. Bacteremia resulting from vascular access infection is common in patients undergoing hemodialysis, as is peritonitis in patients undergoing peritoneal dialysis.

A UTI can occur even in patients with minimal urine output or those with long-standing renal failure. Urinary stasis is undoubtedly a predisposing factor. However, asymptomatic pyuria is common in these patients and is not necessarily indicative of infection. For patients with symptoms, urine culture is helpful in guiding treatment decisions. An upper UTI associated with a clinical picture typical of pyelonephritis or renal colic is unusual, but when seen it is often in patients with polycystic kidney disease and requires parenteral treatment. A clinical diagnosis can be made presumptively in the ED, but invasive measures sometimes are necessary to document infection and guide therapy. For infected cysts, lipid-soluble antibiotics (e.g., ciprofloxacin, trimethoprim-sulfamethoxazole) offer the best antibiotic penetration, although surgical intervention for these infections sometimes becomes necessary.

Dialysis

Dialysis can normalize fluid balance, correct electrolyte and other solute abnormalities, and remove uremic toxins or drugs from the circulation when the patient's kidneys are unable to do so. Dialysis also can reverse some uremic symptoms, but generally to a lesser degree, and permit better long-term control of hypertension, anemia, and renal osteodystrophy.

The two major dialysis modalities are hemodialysis and peritoneal dialysis. Each is based on a technique whereby the patient's blood comes into contact with a semipermeable membrane, on the other side of which is a specially constituted balanced physiologic solution. Water and solutes diffuse across the membrane by moving along concentration and osmotic gradients, effectively normalizing the blood's composition.

Hemodialysis. This requires special access to the patient's circulation, generally through a surgically created arteriovenous fistula or an implanted artificial graft or through a surgically placed tunneled catheter. The vascular access site must be treated with care because hemodialysis cannot be performed without it. Careless manipulation or puncture can cause bleeding, infection, or thrombosis, which may result in loss of the access. The involved arm should not be used for blood pressure determinations and a tourniquet should not be applied.

In general, blood is drawn and IV lines are established in other locations. In exceptional circumstances, if no other site is available and it is essential to obtain blood samples quickly, the fistula or graft may be used, but with precautions. A tourniquet is not applied, the area is cleansed scrupulously before the puncture, and extreme care is taken not to puncture the back wall of the access. After the puncture, firm but nonocclusive pressure is applied for at least 10 minutes. The presence of a thrill before and after the procedure is documented. Similar precautions are taken in the exceptional cases in which the fistula or graft must be used for IV access. If this is done, an automated infusion pump is essential to control the infusion rate into these relatively high-pressure blood vessels.

Peritoneal Dialysis. In peritoneal dialysis, the patient's peritoneum functions as the dialysis membrane. Dialysate is infused through a surgically implanted Silastic catheter (Tenckhoff catheter) that penetrates the lower abdominal wall. Fluid exchanges are generally performed several times daily, typically by the patient at home. As compared with hemodialysis, peritoneal dialysis offers the theoretical advantages of greater patient independence, avoidance of anticoagulation, and smoother control of volume and hypertension,

without the intermittent rapid shifts of solute typical of hemodialysis. Medications such as insulin and antibiotics can be administered via the intraperitoneal (IP) route, allowing smoother absorption and more stable blood levels. The main disadvantage of peritoneal dialysis is a significant incidence of bacterial peritonitis, which is usually readily treatable.

Indications for Dialysis. The decision to initiate chronic dialysis in the patient with CKD generally is made by the patient's nephrologist in the setting of a gradually decreasing GFR and progressive manifestations of renal failure. The absolute value of the BUN or serum creatinine level generally is used only as a rough guide to determine when chronic dialysis should be instituted. The provision of vascular or peritoneal access usually has been arranged weeks to months before the anticipated initiation of dialysis to allow the access site to mature and to minimize any mechanical complications of the procedure.

For patients who come to the ED with AKI, however, as well as for patients with CKD in whom acute problems have developed, the emergency clinician must be prepared to make the decision to arrange for emergent dialysis (Box 83.9). How urgently dialysis must be initiated depends not only on the severity and acuteness of the presenting problem, but also on the availability of technical facilities and trained dialysis personnel and the effectiveness of available temporizing measures for the problem at hand.

The most common problem requiring emergent dialysis, particularly in the patient with CKD, is pulmonary edema secondary to volume overload. In general, the inciting cause is over-ingestion of fluid and salt in excess of the patient's greatly diminished renal excretory capacity. Despite the effectiveness of temporizing measures, many of these patients require immediate dialysis—emergency hemodialysis or, in the case of the patient maintained on peritoneal dialysis, intensification of the usual dialysis regimen.

A related problem that may require emergent, or at least urgent, dialysis is malignant hypertension, particularly when associated with hypertensive encephalopathy or cardiovascular decompensation. Because hypertension in patients with renal failure is commonly volume-dependent, correction of volume overload, even if not apparent clinically, is a central component of therapy. Temporizing measures such as the administration of IV nitroglycerin often permit hypertension to be controlled sufficiently for dialysis to be delayed for several hours. However, in many cases, hypertension and associated symptoms are difficult to control until dialysis permits the volume overload to be corrected. Because blood pressure often is dramatically responsive to reduction of circulating volume, other antihypertensive agents with more prolonged effects should be withheld until after dialysis to avoid hypotension after circulating volume has been acutely reduced.

Severe hyperkalemia is another common indication for emergent or urgent dialysis, particularly in the patient with AKI who is hypercatabolic. In the patient with CKD, hyperkalemia usually is caused by excessive potassium intake, but endogenous causes such as hemolysis or rhabdomyolysis should also be kept in mind. The available temporizing measures can be used to control the serum potassium level, but dialysis remains the most effective means of removing potassium from

---

BOX 83.9 Indications for Emergency Dialysis

- Pulmonary edema
- Severe uncontrollable hypertension
- Hyperkalemia
- Other severe electrolyte or acid-base disturbances
- Some overdoses
- Pericarditis (possibly)

the body. For rapid control of the serum potassium level, hemodialysis leads to high clearance rates and is preferred to peritoneal dialysis.

Other severe electrolyte and acid-base disturbances, including diabetic ketoacidosis, may sometimes necessitate emergent dialysis. Occasional patients with renal failure and severe hypercalcemia uncontrollable by other modalities (e.g., patients with multiple myeloma causing both renal failure and hypercalcemia) may require dialysis. The occasional patient with renal failure in whom severe hypermagnesemia develops after inappropriate therapy or magnesium ingestion may require immediate dialysis to reverse life-threatening paralysis or cardiac dysrhythmia. Severe metabolic acidosis in the setting of renal failure is another indication for emergent dialysis, particularly if volume overload or hypocalcemia (with the risk of tetany and convulsions) precludes the administration of bicarbonate.

A related situation is one in which a patient with renal failure has taken an overdose or inadvertently been administered medication that is ordinarily cleared by the kidneys. If the agent is adequately dialyzable and its continued presence in the circulation poses a significant risk to the patient, immediate dialysis can be lifesaving. An example is the ingestion of methanol or ethylene glycol by a dialysis patient. Similarly, ill-advised use of magnesium-containing cathartics or phosphate-containing enemas by patients with CKD can lead to dangerous hypermagnesemia and hyperphosphatemia and may necessitate urgent dialysis.

The serum creatinine and BUN levels themselves are not considered definitive indications for dialysis. A creatinine level of 10 mg/dL or BUN level of 100 mg/dL often is used as a guideline for beginning chronic dialysis in the patient with progressive renal failure. In dialyzed patients, however, the serum creatinine level often is considerably greater than 10 mg/dL but is a reflection of total body muscle mass more than of the adequacy of dialysis. The BUN level is a somewhat better indicator; in well-dialyzed persons, it generally is in the range of 50 to 80 mg/dL and is more than 100 mg/dL in less well-dialyzed patients. Neither blood level, however, correlates more than roughly with uremic symptoms, even in undialyzed patients, or has any direct bearing on how urgently dialysis should be initiated.

The occurrence of uremic symptoms or signs such as nausea, vomiting, lethargy, or twitching indicates a need for dialysis but does not necessitate immediate initiation of dialysis unless symptoms are severe. Pericarditis, even in the absence of cardiac tamponade, often is considered an indication for urgent dialysis, but pericarditis can also occur in well-dialyzed CKD patients. In a previously undialyzed patient with progressive renal insufficiency, the appearance of pericarditis indicates that it is time to initiate dialysis, although not necessarily on an emergency basis.

COMPLICATIONS OF DIALYSIS

A number of complications can be manifested after dialysis has been initiated.

Hemodialysis

Vascular Access–Related Complications

The performance of hemodialysis depends on reliable vascular access, and it is the vascular access device that is responsible for the complications of dialysis that most often require evaluation in the ED setting. These problems must be attended to promptly to minimize the risk of losing the patient's dialysis lifeline.

Bleeding from the dialysis puncture site can occur hours after a hemodialysis treatment, either spontaneously or after inadvertent minor trauma to the site. Such bleeding can usually be stopped by applying firm pressure to the access site. Care should be taken not to

occlude and possibly cause thrombosis of the vessel by compressing it too vigorously, and the presence of a thrill immediately after the procedure should be documented in the chart. It may be necessary to keep the patient in the ED for a time to ensure that bleeding does not recur. Recurrent bleeding, especially from an aneurysm or a pseudoaneurysm, is best evaluated by a vascular surgeon.

Similarly, if the patient reports that the thrill in the access has been lost, a vascular surgeon is consulted immediately. Although thrombolytic agents are generally used, definitive treatment is usually surgical revision. The access device should not be forcefully manipulated or irrigated because rupture of the vessel or venous embolization may result.

Infection of the vascular access can result in persistent or recurrent bacteremia, as well as loss of the access. Infection appears to be a consequence of contamination at the time of puncture for dialysis, and most infections are caused by staphylococci typical of skin flora. Infections are more likely to occur in grafts than in native fistulas. The signs and symptoms of an access infection—redness, warmth, and tenderness over the site—often are obvious, but in many cases localizing findings are absent and the patient has only a fever or a history of recurrent episodes of fever and documented bacteremia. For this reason, it is common practice to obtain blood cultures for all patients on hemodialysis who have a fever without an obvious source of infection and to treat them presumptively for an abscess infection. A careful search for other sources of infection should be performed before an abscess infection is assumed to be the cause. Infections such as odontogenic abscess, extremity cellulitis (particularly in diabetics), and perirectal abscess can easily be missed.

Although some nephrologists prefer to admit all dialysis patients with fever to the hospital, management of these patients on an outpatient basis often is possible, provided that they otherwise feel well and do not appear to be septic and provided that they can care for themselves at home and return promptly if their condition worsens. This course is made possible by the fact that they can be loaded with IV antibiotics that dependably maintain adequate blood levels until the next scheduled dialysis treatment, at which time the culture and sensitivity test results can be checked and therapy adjusted accordingly. IV vancomycin, 1 to 1.5 g, given as a single loading dose, is the drug of choice in this case because most abscess infections are staphylococcal and because this drug is only minimally hemodialyzable and needs to be given only every 4 to 7 days in the chronic dialysis patient. If a gram-negative infection also is thought to be likely, as in a patient who has had recent episodes of gram-negative bacteremia, a loading dose of a second drug (e.g., a third-generation cephalosporin or aminoglycoside) also can be administered. Patients can be reloaded with these drugs at the end of their next hemodialysis session if culture results prove to be positive.

Non–Vascular Access–Related Complications of Dialysis

The hemodialysis procedure itself, which entails invasion of the vasculature, anticoagulation, and significant shifts of fluid and solutes, often is associated with acute complications such as hypotension, shortness of breath, chest pain, and neurologic abnormalities.

Hypotension. Hypotension that occurs after dialysis is usually the result of an acute reduction in circulating intravascular volume and failure of the patient's homeostatic mechanisms to compensate for it. Because hemodialysis is episodic, each treatment must remove the excess fluid that has accumulated over the period since the last dialysis (generally, 2–3 days), and patients often are relatively volume-overloaded at the beginning of each treatment. With rapid removal of extracellular fluid, there is inadequate time for transcellular fluid shifts to replace intravascular volume. Antihypertensive medications that are required when the patient is in a volume-expanded state, particularly β-blockers, can contribute to the hypotension when intravascular volume is normalized.

Most episodes of hypotension that occur during hemodialysis resolve spontaneously or can be readily managed by a decrease in blood flow rate or by infusion of small volumes of saline (to cause transient volume expansion) or hypertonic solutions (to reverse transient acute hypo-osmolality). Patients with significant hypotension who do not respond to these maneuvers often are brought to the ED for further evaluation. Patients on dialysis with persistent hypotension should be considered to be at risk for acute myocardial infarction, acute dysrhythmias, and sepsis (Box 83.10).

Acute blood loss is another consideration when a hemodialysis patient presents with hypotension, symptomatic angina, or CHF. Dialysis patients are commonly treated with epoetin or darbepoetin to prevent severe anemia; untreated patients typically have low baseline hemoglobin levels. Serum levels of clotting factors are normal in CKD, but patients are routinely anticoagulated for each hemodialysis treatment and, although transient thrombocytopenia may occur during the dialysis procedure, the qualitative platelet defect characteristic of renal failure is an important factor in bleeding that continues beyond the peridialytic period. This abnormality is only partially reversed by dialysis but can be corrected by the administration of desmopressin (DDAVP), which increases the release of factor VIII–von Willebrand factor polymers from vascular endothelium. DDAVP has been used successfully to normalize the bleeding time in preparation for surgery in patients with CKD.[9] Cryoprecipitate and conjugated estrogen both have been shown to produce similar effects for a longer period·

Overt bleeding from the GI tract, often caused by angiodysplasia or peptic ulcer disease, is common and can be dramatic. Occult hemorrhage in other locations, however, can present a diagnostic challenge because symptoms and signs of volume loss tend to be overshadowed by local manifestations of bleeding into a closed space. Spontaneous retroperitoneal or pleural hemorrhage may manifest with flank pain or with chest pain and shortness of breath, respectively.

Acute pulmonary embolism and acute air embolism are two less likely possibilities. The former, although it does occur occasionally in dialysis patients, is unusual. The latter, although reported occasionally in the past, has been all but eliminated by improved dialysis monitoring equipment and safety mechanisms.

Two additional entities in the differential diagnosis for hypotension are of particular importance in the patient with CKD—acute pericardial tamponade and severe, life-threatening hyperkalemia. Acute pericardial tamponade may be the result of sudden pericardial hemorrhage or sudden worsening of a formerly compensated pericardial effusion after acute correction of elevated preload. The clinical features of tamponade in the dialysis patient are similar to those in other populations, but the common preexistence of cardiomegaly may make the chest film difficult to interpret unless it shows the typical water bottle shape and a definite increase in heart size from previous examinations.

Similarly, an elevated central venous pressure is of little use in differentiating tamponade from underlying right-sided heart failure. Even the finding of pericardial fluid on bedside ultrasonographic examination, although suggestive, is not proof that tamponade is present, because many dialysis patients chronically have pericardial effusions that do not cause hemodynamic compromise. The ultrasonographic demonstration of right ventricular diastolic collapse is more specific. A definitive diagnosis of tamponade depends on the direct demonstration of equal pressures in the right and left atria on cardiac catheterization.

Emergency pericardiocentesis must occasionally be performed in the ED to relieve acute tamponade, but there often is enough time for the patient to be transported to the catheterization suite or operating room for safer and more definitive therapy in a controlled setting. If immediate pericardiocentesis is believed to be necessary, the emergency clinician should not hesitate to perform this potentially lifesaving procedure, despite the many potential complications and increased risk of bleeding in patients with CKD. Similarly, in the case of a dialysis patient who is in cardiac arrest, pericardiocentesis generally should be attempted if initial resuscitative efforts have not been successful.

Severe life-threatening hyperkalemia, although unusual in a dialyzed patient, can occur in the presence of underlying catabolic illness or with a prolonged period of hypotension and low flow. Patients who are hyperkalemic can have profoundly slow heart rates, particularly if they have been treated with β-blockers or calcium channel blockers. If a dialysis patient is in cardiac arrest, it should be assumed that hyperkalemia is present, and IV calcium should be given immediately.

Shortness of Breath. Shortness of breath in dialysis patients generally is caused by volume overload. In the patient who becomes short of breath while being dialyzed, however, other causes must be sought—primarily sudden cardiac failure, pericardial tamponade, pleural effusion, or pleural hemorrhage. Air embolism and anaphylactoid reactions are unusual causes. Pneumonia or underlying reactive airway disease may be responsible.

Chest Pain. Cardiovascular disease is a leading cause of death in patients with CKD, and most episodes of chest pain occurring during dialysis are likely to be ischemic in origin. Most dialysis patients have risk factors for coronary artery disease, related to CKD itself or to the underlying condition that led to renal failure, and many have well-documented coronary artery disease. CKD is commonly associated with hypertension, hyperlipidemia, carbohydrate intolerance, and disturbances of calcium and phosphorus metabolism. In addition, dialysis patients may be anemic, and many are chronically volume-overloaded. During hemodialysis, these underlying factors may be added to acute physiologic stresses such as transient hypotension and hypoxemia, which often are associated with the dialysis procedure, thereby increasing myocardial oxygen demand while decreasing oxygen delivery.

In evaluating presumed ischemic chest pain in a patient with CKD, reversible precipitants should be considered. It should be determined whether increasing anemia, poorly controlled hypertension, or uncorrected volume overload are factors, particularly when a patient whose angina has been stable begins to experience more frequent or more severe anginal episodes. Patients who repeatedly experience chest pain during dialysis are candidates for a complete cardiac evaluation. Dialysis patients who have repeated ED visits for chest pain should have a coordinated strategy developed by their nephrologist and cardiologist to set guidelines regarding further admissions.

The presence of renal failure and its associated electrolyte and acid-base disturbances does not obscure the usual electrocardiographic changes of angina or acute myocardial infarction. The pattern of change of serum cardiac enzyme levels with acute infarction also is not altered by CKD, although the baseline level of these enzymes may be higher than in the general population.[10-12] Troponin appears to perform best as a marker of infarction in patients with CKD.[10-12] Treatment of ischemic chest pain is the same as for other populations.

Among nonischemic causes of chest pain, pericarditis should always be a consideration, even in the well-dialyzed patient. The presentation is essentially the same as in nonrenal patients; fever, a friction rub, or atrial dysrhythmias may be associated findings. Signs of pericardial effusion or early tamponade should be sought by bedside ultrasonography. Indomethacin often is effective in relieving pain, but some patients eventually require further measures, such as pericardiocentesis with corticosteroid instillation or pericardial stripping. Patients with pericarditis may require more frequent or intensified dialysis because pericarditis is thought to be a marker for inadequate dialysis.[8]

Neurologic Dysfunction. Neurologic symptoms during or immediately after hemodialysis may be caused by disequilibrium syndrome, a constellation of symptoms and signs thought to result from rapid changes in body fluid composition and osmolality during hemodialysis. It usually occurs only in patients with high BUN levels who are just starting hemodialysis and does not occur with peritoneal dialysis. Typically, patients have headache, dizziness, nausea, vomiting, and muscle cramps, but in more severe cases features may include altered mental status, seizures, or coma. Symptoms resolve over several hours as fluid and solutes are redistributed across cell membranes.

Altered mental status in the CKD patient should not be attributed to disequilibrium syndrome unless other causes have been ruled out (Box 83.11), particularly when symptoms persist, fluctuate, or worsen during a reasonable period of observation. Likewise, when seizures occur during dialysis, they should not be attributed to disequilibrium syndrome without considering other potentially serious causes, even in patients who have had seizures in the past. Any new focal neurologic abnormality requires an immediate head CT scan to detect intracranial hemorrhage. Similarly, if fever or other evidence of infection is present, meningitis should be a serious consideration. Other considerations include hyperglycemia and hypoglycemia, especially in the diabetic patient, as well as electrolyte abnormalities, hypoxic states, hypotension, and other toxic or metabolic causes. The acute treatment of seizures in patients with CKD is essentially the same as for other populations.

Peritoneal Dialysis

As with hemodialysis, most of the complications of peritoneal dialysis are related to the dialysis access device, in this case the peritoneal catheter. In contrast to hemodialysis, however, the dialytic process in peritoneal dialysis occasions few immediate difficulties.

Peritonitis is the most common complication of peritoneal dialysis. Fortunately, it is generally much less severe than other types of peritonitis and can be treated readily on an outpatient basis, despite the

---

> **BOX 83.11** **Differential Diagnosis of Altered Mental Status in Dialysis Patients**
>
> **Structural Conditions**
> Cerebrovascular accident (particularly hemorrhage)
> Subdural hematoma
> Intracerebral abscess
> Brain tumor
>
> **Metabolic Conditions**
> Disequilibrium syndrome
> Uremia
> Drug effects
> Meningitis
> Hypertensive encephalopathy
> Hypotension
> Postictal state
> Hypernatremia or hyponatremia
> Hypercalcemia
> Hypermagnesemia
> Hypoglycemia
> Severe hyperglycemia
> Hypoxemia
> Dialysis dementia

---

continued presence of a foreign body—the Tenckhoff catheter—in the peritoneal cavity. Occasionally, when an episode of peritonitis responds poorly to antimicrobial therapy or when a patient has repeated episodes of peritonitis caused by the same organism, the catheter must be removed and the patient sustained with hemodialysis until the infection is completely cleared and a new catheter can be placed. Repeated infections carry the risk of permanently altering peritoneal permeability or effective surface area and necessitating a permanent switch to hemodialysis.

Peritonitis in patients who are on peritoneal dialysis is presumably caused by inadvertent bacterial contamination of the dialysate or tubing during an exchange or by extension of an infection of the exit site or subcutaneous tunnel into the peritoneal cavity. Most cases of peritonitis are caused by *Staphylococcus aureus* or *Staphylococcus epidermidis,* and most of the remainder (≈30%) by gram-negative enteric organisms.[13] Fungal infections are uncommon but generally are refractory to medical therapy and are often considered as an indication for catheter removal. Polymicrobial infection suggests direct contamination from the GI tract and mandates a search for the site of perforation or fistula, although such a source is identified in only a minority of cases. No organism is identified in approximately 10% to 20% of cases of peritoneal dialysis–associated peritonitis.

The diagnosis of peritonitis usually is made by the patient when a cloudy dialysis effluent is noted, corresponding with the appearance of white blood cells (WBCs) in the dialysate. Peritonitis is often accompanied by nonspecific abdominal pain, malaise, or fever. When a patient has fever or abdominal symptoms, even in the absence of cloudy fluid, it is advisable to consider peritonitis and check the fluid, because early peritonitis may manifest in an atypical manner. In more severe cases, peritonitis is accompanied by nausea, vomiting, severe pain, and hypotension, necessitating hospitalization and consideration of the possibility of acute surgical disease.

In the ED setting, the diagnosis of peritonitis is confirmed by the finding of more than 100 WBCs/mm^3 in the peritoneal fluid, with more than 50% neutrophils, or by a positive result on Gram stain. A sample of fluid is obtained for analysis. If a specialized dialysis nurse is available to obtain the fluid, this may be preferable. If not, the fluid is obtained through the use of sterile technique. Fluid is sent for cell count and differential, Gram staining, and culture, with the use of blood culture bottles.

Peritoneal dialysis–associated peritonitis is treated with an initial intraperitoneal (IP) loading dose of antibiotic, followed by a 10- to 14-day course of IP antibiotics self-administered by the patient on an outpatient basis. After the diagnosis has been confirmed, consultation with the patient's nephrologist or dialysis nurse specialist is indicated to determine antibiotic therapy and to plan for outpatient management and follow-up evaluation or, occasionally, if peritonitis is severe or outpatient management is precluded by psychosocial considerations, for hospitalization. A common treatment regimen is a loading dose of vancomycin, 15 to 30 mg/kg IP, followed by further IP doses every 4 to 7 days, plus ceftazidime or cefepime, 1 g IP, or gentamicin, 0.6 mg/kg IP. The last two regimens are given as a loading dose followed by maintenance doses administered IP once daily at the time of an exchange.[13] Heparin, 500 to 1000 units, may also be added to each liter of dialysate for the first few days of treatment to help reduce the formation of fibrin strands that may obstruct the catheter. Patients should be seen by the dialysis nurse in 24 to 48 hours for assessment of the response to therapy and adjustment of antibiotic therapy as necessary after review of the results of culture and sensitivity testing.

Catheter contamination or leaks from the catheter, tubing, or dialysate bag should be managed in the same fashion as for frank peritonitis. The site and cause of leakage are identified, and damaged elements are promptly replaced. Occasionally, with leakage of peritoneal fluid from around the catheter, surgical correction of the underlying problem will be necessary.

Patients who have severe abdominal pain, vomiting, ileus, chills or high fever, or hypotension require hospital admission and management. Likewise, patients with severe underlying illness and those who cannot reliably perform exchanges or administer antibiotics at home also require inpatient management. Dialysis exchanges are continued on the same schedule. The inpatient antibiotic regimen is essentially the same as for outpatients.

Perhaps the most serious potential pitfall in caring for the patient maintained on peritoneal dialysis with abdominal pain or other signs of peritonitis is to overlook other serious intra-abdominal conditions whose presentation may mimic that of peritonitis. Patients on peritoneal dialysis are at increased risk for abdominal wall or inguinal hernia because of chronically increased intra-abdominal pressures; previous abdominal surgery also places them at risk for hernia, as well as for obstruction secondary to adhesions. The manifestations of serious disorders unrelated to dialysis (e.g., acute appendicitis, diverticulitis, cholecystitis, acute pancreatitis, ischemic bowel, perforated viscus, or spontaneous bacterial peritonitis in patients with chronic liver disease) also may be attributed to ordinary peritoneal dialysis–associated peritonitis, with the potential for disastrous consequences. The accessibility of the peritoneal fluid for examination may prove to be helpful in documenting the presence of an inflammatory process, but it also has the potential to mislead ED investigation of its cause. A finding of brownish or fecal material in the peritoneal drainage should suggest a ruptured viscus until proven otherwise and immediate surgical consultation should be sought. Detection of a localized tenderness, palpable mass, or incarcerated hernia on physical examination can be extremely helpful in making the diagnosis. Plain abdominal radiography or abdominal CT may be useful for demonstrating the presence of ileus, but pneumoperitoneum may reflect only the introduction of air during a recent fluid exchange rather than a perforated viscus.

Infection of the catheter exit site or tunnel is another relatively common problem for which the patient on chronic peritoneal dialysis may seek care in the ED. These infections tend to be caused by typical skin flora and manifest with local signs of infection. Although not serious in themselves, exit site infections may lead to infection of the subcutaneous tunnel, which can cause repeated episodes of peritonitis and may ultimately necessitate removal of the catheter. Any visible exudate is cultured and Gram-stained and therapy with an oral antibiotic such as cephalexin or dicloxacillin is started, pending the results of culture and sensitivity testing. The patient is instructed to cleanse the site meticulously several times a day using povidone-iodine or peroxide solution.

Tunnel infections can be difficult to detect on physical examination and may be suspected only after the patient has several bouts of peritonitis caused by the same organism. As with other closed space infections, tunnel infections tend to be difficult to eradicate unless the tunnel is partially unroofed and drained.

Patients maintained on peritoneal dialysis also may come to the ED with positional or mechanical problems with the site, of which the most common is failure of the dialysate to drain completely at the time of an exchange. Occasionally this problem is caused simply by kinking or inadvertent clamping of the external catheter or tubing. More often, however, it is the result of catheter obstruction by fibrinous debris or kinking or migration of the catheter within the peritoneal cavity, often associated with constipation. Catheter position is best assessed by a CT scan of the abdomen. Specific intervention may be guided by a contrast catheterogram. Fibrinolytic agents have been used successfully to open occluded catheters, but surgical intervention for catheter replacement often is required. Severe metabolic disturbances are much less common among patients on peritoneal dialysis than patients on hemodialysis, because in the former group dialysis is being performed essentially continuously and the blood remains in near-equilibrium with the dialysate. However, significant disturbances do occasionally occur, usually in association with hypercatabolic states, major dietary indiscretions, or significant GI fluid loss. One derangement that occurs occasionally in diabetic patients undergoing peritoneal dialysis is a syndrome of severe hyperglycemia—sometimes even despite continuation of the usual insulin dose—that results from absorption of glucose from the hyperosmolar dialysate, with associated nonspecific symptoms of malaise, weakness, and headache. Although glucose levels may be as high as 1500 mg/dL in these patients, they cannot undergo an osmotic diuresis and remain clinically euvolemic. Correction of hyperglycemia must be undertaken carefully to avoid causing rapid osmolar and volume shifts.

The references for this chapter can be found online at ExpertConsult.com.

Sexually Transmitted Infections

Jeffry McKinzie

FOUNDATIONS

Sexually transmitted infections ((STIs) are a diverse group of conditions caused by more than 30 viral, bacterial, and parasitic organisms that are transmitted through sexual contact. Four of the pathogens that contribute most to the global incidence of STIs (chlamydia, gonorrhea, syphilis, and trichomoniasis) are curable, often with a single dose of an antibiotic.[1,2] More than 1 million newly acquired cases of these curable STIs occur worldwide each year.[3] Viral pathogens responsible for common STIs (herpes simplex virus, human papillomavirus, and HIV) cause chronic infection in which symptoms and progression of disease can be modified with appropriate antiviral therapy.

STIs are seen across all demographic, cultural, and socioeconomic strata, and all sexually active persons are at risk for acquiring them. Factors associated with higher risk for STIs reflect the importance of individual sexual practices and risk-taking behaviors (i.e., multiple sex partners, substance abuse, commercial sex workers, men who have sex with men, and unsafe sex practices), as well as various demographic and social determinants that influence health status (i.e., adolescents and young adults, minorities, and low socioeconomic status).

STIs are among the most common urogenital conditions encountered in the ED. The management of patients with STIs is particularly challenging for multiple reasons: (1) the clinical presentation is highly variable; (2) available diagnostic tests have limited sensitivity and results are usually delayed; (3) compliance with treatment, follow-up, and partner notification is often poor; and (4) misdiagnosis and suboptimal treatment can result in serious sequelae. In addition to the morbidity associated with individual STIs, many of these infections also increase the risk of human immunodeficiency virus (HIV) transmission and acquisition in both the infected person and their sexual partners. Thus, STIs have a significant impact on both individual and public health.

Patients with STIs frequently present with complaints related to the genitalia but may also present with a variety of nonspecific dermatologic, gastrointestinal, musculoskeletal, and systemic complaints. Because the signs and symptoms of many common STIs are often nonspecific, one must maintain a high level of awareness for these conditions and their associated complications. A thorough history, including sexual history, and focused physical examination facilitate appropriate diagnosis and treatment. The sexual history should include number and gender of sexual partners, types of sexual practices, use of barrier contraception (condoms), and past history of STIs. Obtaining an accurate sexual history may be difficult due to the sensitive nature of the subject, lack of established physician-patient rapport, and other constraints of the ED setting. Evaluation is facilitated by the use of a nonjudgmental approach, maintenance of patient privacy, and assurance of confidentiality.

The differential diagnosis for STIs is extensive, including many other infectious and noninfectious conditions (Table 84.1). Most STIs can be broadly categorized as conditions characterized by one of the following manifestations: genital ulcers, genital discharge, epithelial cell infections, and infestation by ectoparasites. Some STIs, such as syphilis, frequently have associated systemic symptoms in addition to their genitourinary manifestations. Other STIs, such as HIV, may have systemic manifestations in the absence of genitourinary signs and symptoms.

STIs frequently coexist. Diagnosis of one STI should prompt consideration of other coexisting infections, which may not be clinically apparent. Screening for other STIs, including HIV, should be considered, because early diagnosis and treatment benefits both the individual patient and the public health. Despite current recommendations from the Centers for Disease Control and Prevention (CDC) for routine HIV screening among patients age 13 to 64 years in all health care settings, systematic HIV testing is not routinely performed in most EDs. When available, rapid HIV testing should be considered. Patients should be counseled regarding the need for HIV testing if it is not performed in the ED.

Empirical antibiotic treatment designed to cover the most likely infecting organisms is recommended for patients with suspected STIs

TABLE 84.1   Differential Diagnosis of Common Sexually Transmitted Infection Syndromes

Genital Ulcers	Genital Discharge	Epithelial Cell Lesions	Ectoparasites
Genital herpes	Gonorrhea	Genital warts	Pubic lice
Primary syphilis	Chlamydia	Secondary syphilis	Scabies
Chancroid	Nongonococcal urethritis (NGU)	Molluscum contagiosum	Other lice (body, head)
Lymphogranuloma venereum	Pelvic inflammatory disease	Neoplasm	Other mites (chiggers)
Granuloma inguinale	Trichomoniasis	Nevi	Ticks
Trauma	Bacterial vaginosis	Skin tags	
Neoplasm	*Candida* vaginitis		
Behçet disease	Foreign body		
Abscess (draining)	Irritants/allergens		

to maximize eradication of disease in the individual patient and reduce the spread of infection to other susceptible persons. Empirical therapy is particularly important when there are concerns about the patient's ability to obtain appropriate follow-up care. Confirmatory diagnostic studies should still be considered, even when empirical therapy is provided. Microbiologic diagnosis confirms the appropriate choice of empirical therapy, provides guidance for potential changes in treatment, and facilitates reporting of specific STIs to public health authorities. Point-of-care rapid diagnostic testing may minimize the need for empirical antibiotic treatment by providing confirmatory test results before treatment decisions are made and prior to patient discharge from the ED. This reduces the unnecessary use of antibiotics with associated costs, side effects, and development of antimicrobial resistance.

The diagnosis of an STIs provides the physician with a "teachable moment" to educate the patient regarding important factors, including (1) nature of the infection and how it is transmitted; (2) compliance with prescribed therapy and recommended follow-up; (3) importance of preventive measures, including condom use and other safe sex practices; and (4) partner notification and treatment. Patients diagnosed with STIs should be counseled to abstain from sexual intercourse for at least 7 days after the patient and partner(s) complete treatment. Proper counseling helps to ensure the success of initial treatment and reduce the incidence of reinfection. When the diagnosis of an STI is suspected but not confirmed, the patient should be informed of the uncertainty of the diagnosis and the rationale for empirical treatment. The physician should be sensitive to the stress and anxiety that may ensue when discussing the diagnosis of an STI, particularly with a patient who assumes he or she is in a monogamous relationship. A respectful, nonjudgmental, and compassionate approach should be maintained.

The CDC recommends the use of expedited partner therapy (EPT) to ensure treatment in sexual partners of selected patients diagnosed with gonorrhea or chlamydia. With EPT, the clinician provides patient-delivered medication or prescriptions for sexual partners without personally evaluating them. The use of EPT in the ED is potentially problematic due to lack of knowledge regarding the partner's medical history, allergies, pregnancy status, and other factors. In addition, some states prohibit the prescribing or dispensing of medications to patients who have not been seen and are unknown to the provider. Updated information regarding the use of EPT and applicable state regulations is available online from the CDC website.[4] All patients diagnosed with an STI in the ED should be advised to notify their sexual partners to seek prompt evaluation and treatment.

An organized mechanism for follow-up of positive diagnostic test results is recommended when these results are not available until after the patient and physician have left the ED. Obtaining accurate contact information at the time of the initial visit is important in ensuring timely patient notification. Reporting requirements vary by state, but the following STIs must be reported in all 50 states: gonorrhea, chlamydia, syphilis, chancroid, and HIV. Reporting may be laboratory-based or provider-based, or both. The clinician should be familiar with applicable state reporting requirements and the reporting mechanism used at their hospital.

This chapter reviews the clinical features, diagnosis, and treatment of selected common STIs encountered in the ED setting. Readers are referred to the "Sexually Transmitted Infections Treatment Guidelines" published by the CDC for additional information regarding the diagnosis and treatment of these conditions, as well as other less common STIs.[5] Updates regarding changes in treatment guidelines are provided by the CDC in the *Morbidity and Mortality Weekly Report,* available at www.cdc.gov/mmwr.

DISORDERS CHARACTERIZED BY GENITAL ULCERS

Genital ulcers may be caused by several different STIs, as well as various other infectious and noninfectious conditions. Genital herpes is the most common ulcerating STI seen in the United States, followed by syphilis. Chancroid is an uncommon cause of genital ulcers in the United States, and other STIs that may be manifested by genital ulcers (lymphogranuloma venereum, granuloma inguinale) are rare. Although the history, clinical appearance of the ulcers, and other associated findings provide helpful clues in differentiating the various causes of genital ulcers, these features are not specific enough to provide a definitive diagnosis. Diagnostic studies such as darkfield microscopy, serology for syphilis, polymerase chain reaction (PCR), and viral culture should be considered to discriminate between the various etiologies and facilitate a definitive diagnosis, even when empirical therapy is initiated. Diagnostic testing is particularly important in patients that are unresponsive to previous empirical antibiotic therapy. Ulcerating STIs play an important role in facilitating the transmission and acquisition of HIV.

Herpes

Background and Importance

Genital herpes is a lifelong viral infection caused by one of two types of herpes simplex virus (HSV): HSV-1 or HSV-2. Sexual transmission occurs more commonly with HSV-2, but both types of HSV can be transmitted through sexual or nonsexual contact. Many cases of HSV are undiagnosed. HSV is often transmitted by persons who are unaware that they are infected, or who are asymptomatic at the time of transmission. HSV transmission occurs through viral contact with a break in the skin or intact mucous membranes. The average incubation

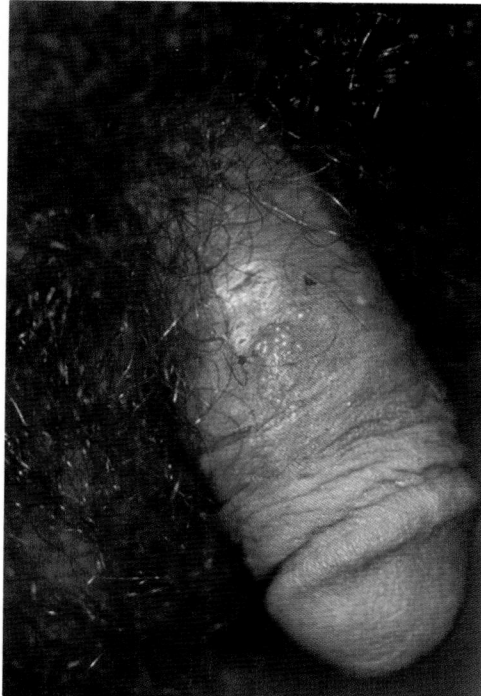

Fig. 84.1 Genital herpes lesions on the penile shaft.

period is 4 days but may range from 2 to 12 days. The virus ascends via sensory nerves to the dorsal root ganglia, where it becomes latent but may reactivate periodically. Herpes, like other ulcerating STIs, facilitates the transmission and acquisition of HIV. Herpes infection in pregnant women may result in transmission to the infant at the time of delivery, with devastating associated neonatal morbidity and mortality.

Clinical Features

Typical herpetic lesions begin as a cluster of small erythematous painful vesicles, which quickly ulcerate (Fig. 84.1). Lesions may occur anywhere the organism is inoculated, but they are typically seen on the skin of the external genitalia, perineum, and buttocks and on the mucous membranes of the vagina, rectum, and oropharynx. Primary infection occurs when a patient is infected with HSV-1 or HSV-2 with no preexisting antibodies to either type. The primary infection is usually more painful and symptomatic, with associated tender regional lymphadenopathy, fever, malaise, headache, and other systemic symptoms. Dysuria is common due to the proximity of the lesions to the urethra. The symptoms of untreated primary infection typically last from 2 to 4 weeks before resolving spontaneously.

Recurrent episodes of genital herpes tend to be less symptomatic and shorter in duration, with lesions occurring in the same distribution due to reactivation of latent HSV infection in the affected nerve roots. Recurrences are more frequent with infection caused by HSV-2 than with HSV-1. Recurrent outbreaks are often heralded by prodromal symptoms of itching, burning, and paresthesias prior to the development of skin or mucous membrane lesions. Reactivation of latent HSV may occur in response to a variety of stressors, including acute illness or injury, immunosuppression, psychological stress, and menses. Recurrences typically become less frequent and less severe over time. Extragenital complications of HSV infection include meningoencephalitis, transverse myelitis, hepatitis, pneumonitis, and disseminated infection. Asymptomatic viral shedding and transmission occurs even in the absence of visible lesions on the skin or mucous membranes.

Diagnostic Testing

The diagnosis of genital herpes is frequently made based upon clinical findings. Although the presence of typical skin or mucous membrane lesions is suggestive of herpes, the clinical diagnosis is both insensitive and nonspecific. A history of similar lesions in the same anatomic distribution supports the clinical diagnosis. HSV type-specific nucleic acid amplification tests (NAATs) are the diagnostic tests of choice, with the highest sensitivity and specificity in the presence of active lesions. Viral culture is also specific but less sensitive than NAATs. Darkfield microscopy and serologic testing for syphilis should be considered to help differentiate cases of syphilis. The utility of these diagnostic studies is limited in the ED because test results are delayed, but results may be helpful at the time of follow-up. Direct fluorescent antibody (DFA) and serology for HSV are available, but less commonly used in the ED setting. Cytologic testing (Tzanck preparation) is nonspecific and insensitive and should not be relied upon to make the diagnosis of HSV.

Management

Genital herpes is treated with the antiviral medications acyclovir, famciclovir, or valacyclovir. Antiviral therapy is not curative but has been shown to decrease the duration and severity of symptoms and the development of complicated HSV infection, particularly when started early during the primary infection. Prompt initiation of antiviral treatment is key to obtaining optimal clinical benefit. Although most studies have evaluated drug initiation within 72 hours of symptom onset, antiviral therapy may still be offered after this time frame in the presence of ongoing symptoms and the development of new lesions. Multiple regimens are available for treatment of primary and recurrent episodes of genital herpes with oral antiviral medications (Table 84.2). Oral antiviral therapy is generally well tolerated with few side effects. Suppressive therapy with daily antiviral use has been shown to decrease the frequency of recurrences while the medication is being taken, but it does not affect the frequency or severity of recurrences after the drug is discontinued. Topical antiviral therapy provides minimal clinical benefit and is not recommended.

Disposition

Most patients with genital herpes are managed as outpatients. Hospitalization for parenteral therapy with acyclovir is indicated for systemic complications of HSV infection, including meningoencephalitis, hepatitis, pneumonitis, and disseminated infection. Patients with genital herpes should be counseled that transmission may occur even in the absence of clinical symptoms. Condom use has been shown to reduce but not eliminate the incidence of HSV transmission. Discordant couples (i.e., those in which one partner is HSV+) should be advised to avoid sexual contact during active outbreaks, which is when viral transmission is highest. Condoms should be used during asymptomatic periods. Patients with genital herpes should also be counseled regarding the increased risk of acquisition and transmission of HIV in the presence of genital ulcers.

Syphilis

Background and Importance

Humans are the only known host for *Treponema pallidum,* the spirochete that causes syphilis. The incidence of syphilis has declined significantly since penicillin became widely available in 1945, but outbreaks still occur intermittently. After a progressive decline in the incidence of syphilis from 1990 to 2000, there has been an increase in recent years. More than 35,000 cases of primary and secondary syphilis were reported to the CDC in 2018.[6] The rates of primary and secondary syphilis are higher among those between 20 to 34 years old, minority groups, and men who have sex with men (MSM). It is more common in

TABLE 84.2 Treatment of Common Ulcerating Sexually Transmitted Infections[a]

Disease	Recommended Treatments
Herpes simplex	
Primary episode	Acyclovir 400 mg PO tid for 7 to 10 days *or*
	Valacyclovir 1000 mg PO bid for 7 to 10 days *or*
	Famciclovir 250 mg PO tid for 7 to 10 days
Recurrent episodes	Acyclovir 800 mg PO bid for 5 days *or*
	Acyclovir 800 mg PO tid for 2 days *or*
	Valacyclovir 500 mg PO bid for 3 days *or*
	Valacyclovir 1000 mg PO daily for 5 days *or*
	Famciclovir 125 mg PO bid for 5 days *or*
	Famciclovir 1000 mg PO bid for 1 day *or*
	Famciclovir 500 mg PO once, then 250 mg bid for 2 days
Syphilis[b]	
Primary, secondary, and early latent syphilis	Benzathine penicillin G 2.4 million units IM single dose
Neurosyphilis	Aqueous penicillin G 3 to 4 million units IV every 4 hours for 10 to 14 days
Chancroid	Ceftriaxone 250 mg IM single dose *or*
	Azithromycin 1000 mg PO single dose *or*
	Ciprofloxacin 500 mg PO bid for 3 days *or*
	Erythromycin 500 mg by mouth TID × 7 days

[a]Alternative treatment regimens for selected patients (including pregnancy, drug allergies) can be found at www.cdc.gov/std/treatment.
[b]Pregnant women with syphilis who are allergic to penicillin should be admitted for desensitization and treatment with penicillin.
IM, Intramuscular; *PO*, per os (by mouth).

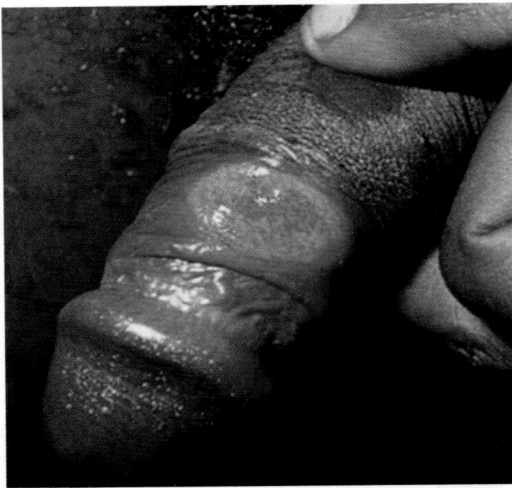

Fig. 84.2 Chancre of primary syphilis. (From: Morse S, Ballard RC, Holmes KK, et al, eds. *Atlas of Sexually Transmitted Diseases and AIDS*, ed 4. London: Saunders/Elsevier; 2010: Fig. 7.9, p 185.)

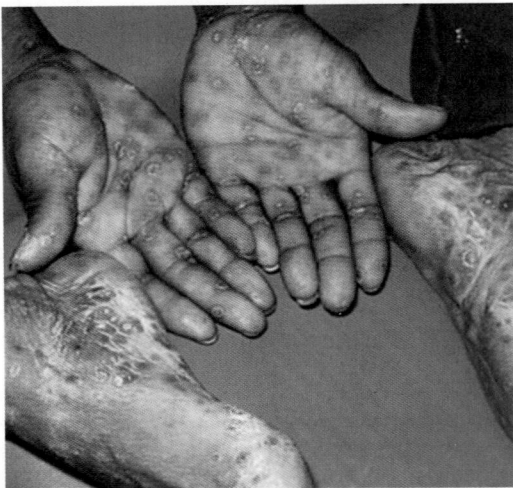

Fig. 84.3 Rash of secondary syphilis on palms and soles. (From: Morse S, Ballard RC, Holmes KK, et al, eds. *Atlas of Sexually Transmitted Diseases and AIDS*, ed 4. London: Saunders/Elsevier; 2010: Fig. 7.24, p 188.)

the western and southeastern United States compared to other regions of the country.

Clinical Features

Syphilis has been called "the great imitator," because its clinical manifestations are protean. The classification and staging of syphilis based upon clinical and serologic findings was updated in 2017.[7] The primary and secondary stages of syphilis are most commonly seen in the ED setting. Transmission occurs when the spirochetes gain access through disrupted epithelium of the skin or mucous membranes. The average incubation period is approximately 21 days but may range from 3 to 90 days.

Primary syphilis is initially manifested by the development of a painless papule at the site of inoculation. The lesion ulcerates, forming the chancre of primary syphilis (Fig. 84.2). The chancre is classically described as a relatively painless clean-based ulcer with well demarcated indurated edges, measuring approximately 1 to 2 cm in size. Nontender regional lymphadenopathy may be seen. Although the chancre often occurs in the genital or perianal area, it may occur at any site of inoculation, including the oropharynx, breasts, hands, and other sites. The chancre will heal spontaneously over the course of 3 to 6 weeks. Because the chancre is relatively painless, it may go unnoticed by the patient.

Secondary syphilis will develop in approximately 25% of patients with primary syphilis over a period of several weeks to months. Manifestations of secondary syphilis include rash, generalized lymphadenopathy, mucous membrane lesions, and systemic symptoms. The rash is diffuse, involving the face, trunk, and extremities, including the palms and soles.

The appearance of the rash is highly variable. Lesions may be macular, papular, scaly, or pustular in appearance (Fig. 84.3). Mucous patches are multiple shallow erosions of the oropharyngeal mucosa that are usually accompanied by other dermatologic and systemic manifestations of secondary syphilis. Condyloma lata, which resemble genital warts, are broad-based papular lesions that occur on the genitalia and perineum and typically have a moist surface appearance (Fig. 84.4). Lymphadenopathy is typically diffuse, rubbery, and nontender. Epitrochlear adenopathy is particularly suggestive of secondary syphilis. A nonspecific "moth-eaten" alopecia may be seen. Systemic manifestations include low-grade fever, anorexia, headache, malaise, myalgias, and weight loss. Symptoms of secondary syphilis will resolve without treatment, with subsequent progression to latent syphilis.

Patients infected with syphilis who exhibit no clinical manifestations of primary or secondary syphilis are classified as *early nonprimary, nonsecondary syphilis* if infection occurred within the past 12 months. *Unknown duration or late syphilis* includes those patients infected more than 12 months previously and those in whom time

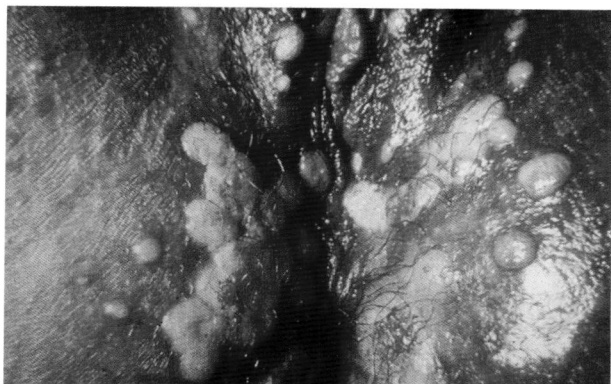

Fig. 84.4 Condyloma lata of secondary syphilis.

of infection is unknown.[8] Neurologic, ophthalmologic, and otologic manifestations can occur at any stage of syphilis. *Neurosyphilis* may be manifested by meningitis, dementia, tabes dorsalis, and general paresis. Patients with *ocular syphilis* may exhibit uveitis, optic neuropathy, and retinal vasculitis. Otic syphilis may cause sensorineural hearing loss, vertigo, and tinnitus.

Tertiary syphilis, which includes cardiovascular manifestations and gummatous disease, is uncommon in the United States. Aortitis, aortic aneurysm, and gummatous lesions of the skin, bones, and other organs may be seen. In patients with untreated syphilis, the estimated risk of eventual progression to tertiary syphilis ranges from 25% to 40%.

Congenital syphilis is transmitted perinatally to the fetus and has significant associated morbidity in infected children. Although relatively uncommon in the United States, congenital syphilis has increased in prevalence in recent years.

Diagnostic Testing

T. pallidum is fastidious and cannot be cultured in the laboratory. The diagnosis of syphilis can be confirmed with darkfield microscopy or by serologic testing. Visualization of the spirochete on darkfield examination of specimens obtained from a chancre or from the moist lesions of secondary syphilis provides an immediate diagnosis. Darkfield microscopy is particularly useful in primary syphilis when false-negative serology is common. The utility of darkfield microscopy is limited by the need for specialized laboratory equipment and appropriately trained personnel, which are lacking at many hospitals.

Serologic tests for syphilis include nonspecific nontreponemal tests and specific treponemal tests. Nontreponemal tests include the Venereal Disease Research Laboratory (VDRL) and the rapid plasma reagin (RPR). The VDRL and RPR provide quantitative measurements of nonspecific antibodies that are produced in response to *T. pallidum* infection. The titers correlate with disease activity, typically rising with active syphilis infection and declining after successful treatment. The sensitivity of nontreponemal tests is approximately 70% to 80% in primary syphilis but rises to nearly 100% in secondary syphilis. False-positive nontreponemal tests may be seen in a variety of conditions, including pregnancy, endocarditis, autoimmune disease, and other acute or chronic illnesses. A positive nontreponemal test should always be confirmed with a specific treponemal test. Specific treponemal tests include the *T. pallidum* enzyme immunoassay (TP-EIA), the fluorescent treponemal antibody absorption (FTA-ABS) and the microhemagglutination test for antibodies to *T. pallidum* (MHA-TP). These treponemal tests provide qualitative measurements of specific antitreponemal antibodies. Although these treponemal tests are highly specific for syphilis, they may remain positive for life even after successful treatment and cure.

The traditional testing algorithm begins with a nontreponemal test for screening purposes, because the quantitative titers serve as a better marker for acute infection. A specific treponemal test is used to confirm the diagnosis when the nontreponemal test is positive. An acceptable alternative testing algorithm begins with the specific treponemal test, which is then confirmed with the quantitative titers of the nontreponemal test. Both types of serologic testing are necessary for the proper diagnosis of syphilis.

Management

Penicillin is the cornerstone of treatment for syphilis, with *T. pallidum* remaining highly sensitive to penicillin. The dosage and preparation of penicillin and the length of treatment vary depending upon the stage of the disease and the associated clinical manifestations (see Table 84.2). A single dose of long-acting benzathine penicillin G (2.4 million units intramuscularly [IM]) is curative in the majority of cases of primary and secondary syphilis. Patients with significant penicillin allergy can be treated with doxycycline or tetracycline (preferred in late latent syphilis) for 2 weeks if no contraindication to these drugs exists. Ceftriaxone has antitreponemal activity, but the optimal dosage and duration of therapy have not been established. Azithromycin has some efficacy but is not recommended as a first-line therapy due to documented resistance and treatment failures. Penicillin remains the drug of choice for patients with neurosyphilis, congenital syphilis, and syphilis during pregnancy even in the presence of penicillin allergy, due to the known efficacy of penicillin and the absence of proven alternative therapies. Patients with these conditions should be admitted for desensitization and treatment with penicillin.

The Jarisch-Herxheimer reaction is an acute worsening of symptoms that may develop after antibiotic therapy is initiated for syphilis. The patient typically reports worsening malaise, myalgias, and fever within 24 hours of antibiotic treatment. The condition has traditionally been thought to be caused by the sudden lysis of spirochetes, but the mechanism is poorly understood. Treatment is supportive, including rest, hydration, and antipyretics. The symptoms resolve spontaneously. Anticipatory guidance regarding the appropriate management of this common self-limited reaction may prevent a return visit to the ED.

Disposition

Most cases of syphilis are treated on an outpatient basis. Hospitalization is recommended for patients with penicillin allergy who require desensitization prior to penicillin therapy, including pregnant women with syphilis and patients with neurosyphilis or congenital syphilis.

Chancroid

Background and Importance

Chancroid is an ulcerating STI caused by the gram-negative organism *Haemophilus ducreyi.* Chancroid is common in parts of the developing world but is rare in the United States, with only 3 cases reported in 2018. Like other ulcerating STIs, chancroid is a cofactor for the transmission and acquisition of HIV.

Clinical Features

After an incubation period of less than 1 week, a tender erythematous papule develops at the site of inoculation. The initial lesion rapidly ulcerates, and multiple painful ulcers subsequently develop (Fig. 84.5). The ulcers typically have an irregular, inflamed, and "dirty" appearance compared to the well circumscribed clean-based chancre of syphilis, and the smaller punched-out appearance of herpetic ulcers. Painful inguinal lymphadenopathy is common and may progress to bubo formation. A *bubo* is a large, painful, fluctuant unilateral inguinal lymph node, which may spontaneously rupture and drain purulent material.

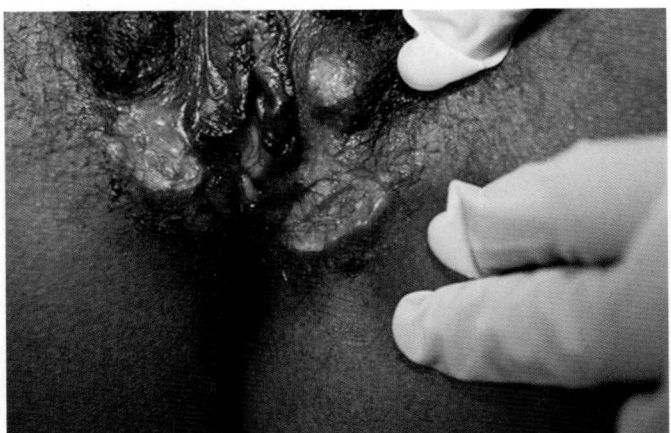

Fig. 84.5 Multiple vulvar ulcers due to chancroid. (From: Morse S, Ballard RC, Holmes KK, et al, eds. *Atlas of Sexually Transmitted Diseases and AIDS*, ed 4. London: Saunders/Elsevier; 2010: Fig. 8.14, p 219.)

Diagnostic Testing

Differential diagnosis of genital ulcers includes herpes and syphilis, both of which are more common than chancroid in the United States. Although the appearance of the ulcers may suggest the diagnosis of chancroid, the clinical diagnosis may be inaccurate. Darkfield microscopy and serologic testing are useful in identifying syphilis, whereas NAAT and viral culture can confirm HSV infection. Chancroid is usually a clinical diagnosis based upon the presence of typical painful genital ulcers and associated tender adenopathy. Culture provides definitive diagnosis but is difficult due to the fastidious nature of *H. ducreyi*, which requires special culture media. No FDA-approved NAAT is available in the U.S., but some clinical laboratories have developed their own NAAT and have performed the necessary Clinical Laboratory Improvement Amendment (CLIA) studies to allow for their use in the diagnosis of chancroid.

Management

Patients with chancroid are treated as outpatients. Single-dose therapy with azithromycin or ceftriaxone is recommended for suspected chancroid (see Table 84.2). Alternative treatment regimens include oral ciprofloxacin or erythromycin.

DISORDERS CHARACTERIZED BY GENITAL DISCHARGE

Foundations

Some STIs, including gonorrhea, chlamydia, trichomoniasis, and pelvic inflammatory disease (PID), are frequently characterized by the presence of genital discharge in absence of genital ulcers and lymphadenopathy. The differential diagnosis of genital discharge is broad, including infections that are not sexually transmitted and noninfectious conditions (see Table 84.1). For example, bacterial vaginosis and candidiasis are common conditions that are not considered to be sexually transmitted but are frequently found during the evaluation of a woman with vaginal discharge. Urethritis, cervicitis, and vaginitis caused by various organisms can present with associated genital discharge.

Infectious causes of urethritis are generally divided into two categories: gonococcal urethritis and nongonococcal urethritis (NGU). Urethritis occurs in men and women and may be asymptomatic, particularly in persons with NGU. When present, symptoms include dysuria, urethral pruritus, and urethral discharge. The absence of visible discharge does not exclude the diagnosis. A clinical diagnosis of urethritis can be made on the basis of any of the following findings in the setting of compatible symptoms: (1) mucoid, mucopurulent or purulent urethral discharge, (2) Gram stain of urethral discharge containing two or more white blood cells (WBCs) per oil immersion field, (3) first-void urine sediment containing 10 or more WBCs per high-power field, and (4) positive leukocyte esterase test on first-void urine. Diagnosis and management of specific causes of urethritis are discussed later.

Cervicitis is characterized by the presence of purulent or mucopurulent discharge from the endocervix and the presence of cervical friability. Many women with cervicitis are asymptomatic. The discharge may be visible in the endocervical canal or noted on an endocervical swab specimen. Cervical friability is demonstrated when endocervical bleeding is easily induced with gentle passage of a swab through the cervical os. Gonorrhea and chlamydia are common causes, but trichomonas and HSV may also cause cervicitis. Frequently, no organism is isolated despite the presence of clinical findings consistent with cervicitis. Women with cervicitis may complain of abnormal vaginal discharge, dyspareunia, and postcoital vaginal bleeding. Pelvic examination may demonstrate endocervical discharge and friability. These findings are insensitive, and the absence of these findings on history and examination do not exclude the diagnosis of cervicitis. Specific causes of cervicitis and their management are discussed later.

Gonorrhea

Background and Importance

Gonorrhea is the second most commonly reported STI in the United States, with more than 500,000 cases reported to the CDC annually. Humans are the only reservoir for the causative organism, *Neisseria gonorrhoeae*, a gram-negative intracellular diplococcus. The prevalence of gonorrhea varies widely, with higher rates of gonorrhea seen among adolescents and young adults, minorities, people with low socioeconomic status, those with a history of substance abuse, and those who engage in high-risk sexual behaviors.

Clinical Features

The signs and symptoms of gonorrhea vary depending upon the sex of the patient, the site of inoculation, and the local or systemic spread of the infection. The incubation period for gonorrhea typically ranges from 3 to 7 days. Most men with gonococcal urethritis become symptomatic within 1 to 2 weeks, prompting them to seek curative treatment. Patients complain of urethral discharge and dysuria. The discharge is usually copious and purulent, although the clinical appearance alone cannot differentiate gonococcal urethritis from NGU (see Fig. 84.6). Women with gonococcal cervicitis are often asymptomatic until ascending infection develops. Because many women remain asymptomatic for prolonged periods, a larger reservoir of untreated women exists. When present, symptoms of gonococcal cervicitis may include abnormal vaginal discharge, dyspareunia, and intermenstrual bleeding. Women with gonococcal cervicitis may also complain of dysuria due to associated urethritis.

Gonococcal proctitis may occur in men and women who engage in receptive anal intercourse and in women who are inoculated by infected vaginal secretions. Patients with gonococcal proctitis are often asymptomatic but may complain of rectal pain, tenesmus, rectal discharge, or bleeding. Anoscopy may reveal abnormal discharge and inflamed friable rectal mucosa.

Gonococcal pharyngitis is usually acquired from oral sexual exposure. Patients with pharyngitis are usually asymptomatic but may complain of sore throat. Tonsillar erythema and cervical lymphadenopathy may be present. Differentiating gonococcal pharyngitis from common

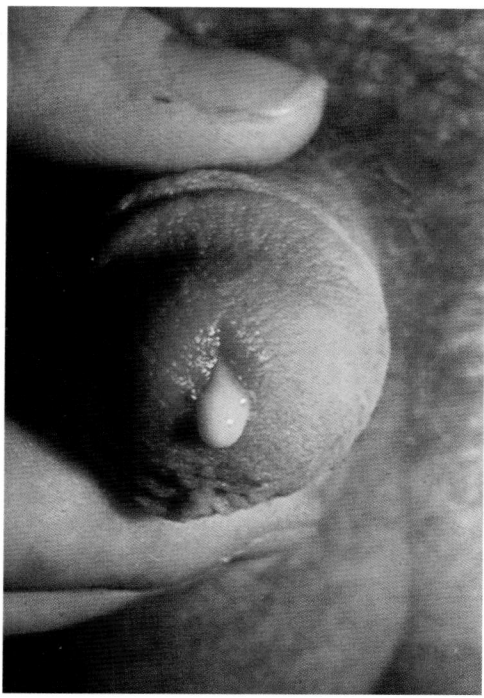

Fig. 84.6 Purulent urethral discharge due to gonococcal urethritis.

viral or bacterial forms of pharyngitis requires a careful history in patients presenting with symptoms of pharyngitis.

Gonococcal conjunctivitis was historically seen most often in infants born to infected mothers. Because infants are now routinely prophylaxed at birth, gonococcal conjunctivitis is now more common in adults who self-inoculate by rubbing the eye with contaminated fingers. Severe conjunctival injection with copious purulent discharge is typically seen. The infection can progress rapidly to corneal ulceration, perforation, and blindness if untreated.

Disseminated gonococcal infection (DGI) results from hematogenous spread of *N. gonorrhoeae*. DGI may occur in the absence of any signs or symptoms of the initial local infection. Characteristic clinical findings include rash, polyarthralgias, tenosynovitis, and septic arthritis. The rash usually consists of petechial or pustular lesions in an acral distribution on the distal extremities. The rash is sparse, with 2 to 10 skin lesions being typical and more than 40 lesions uncommon. Septic arthritis presents as a swollen, red, warm, and painful joint. One or more joints may be involved. The knees, wrists, and ankles are the most common sites. Rarer complications of DGI include hepatitis, meningitis, and myocarditis.

Diagnostic Testing

Nucleic acid amplification tests (NAATs) have replaced culture as the gold standard for the diagnosis of gonorrhea. These tests are widely available and have a higher sensitivity compared to culture. A wide variety of specimens can be used for NAATs, including first-void urine and swabs from the urethra, cervix, vagina, oropharynx, and rectum. Suitable specimens can be obtained by the examining clinician or provided by the patient.

Culture with selective Thayer Martin media is still useful in selected patients and has the advantage of allowing antimicrobial susceptibility testing. Isolation of *N. gonorrhoeae* from the blood, synovial fluid, or skin lesions establishes a definitive diagnosis of DGI, but sensitivity of these cultures is poor. The organism may be more readily identified from other sites (urethra, cervix, rectum, or pharynx) even in the absence of localized symptoms at these sites. When accompanied by the appropriate clinical presentation, identification of gonorrhea by NAATs or culture from any site is sufficient for a presumptive diagnosis of DGI. In symptomatic men, a Gram stain of urethral discharge that reveals gram-negative intracellular diplococci has a sensitivity and specificity approaching 100% for the diagnosis of gonorrhea. A positive Gram stain does not exclude coinfection with chlamydia or other organisms. Gram stain of genitourinary specimens in female patients is not recommended due to potential false-positive results caused by nonpathogenic *Neisseria* organisms that may be normal flora in the female reproductive tract.

Treatment

Recommended treatment options for gonorrhea have changed in recent years due to the increasing antimicrobial resistance of *N. gonorrhoeae*. Ceftriaxone remains the drug of choice for the treatment of gonorrhea. Single-dose therapy with an intramuscular injection of ceftriaxone 500 mg is recommended for gonococcal urethritis, cervicitis, proctitis, and pharyngitis in patients weighing <150 kg. The recommended single dose of ceftriaxone is increased to 1 g IM for patients weighing ≥150 kg (see Table 84.2). Concomitant single-dose therapy with azithromycin is no longer recommended for treatment of gonorrhea due to increasing antimicrobial resistance patterns. When chlamydial infection has not been excluded, antichlamydial therapy should also be administered (discussed later in this chapter). The use of oral cephalosporins or fluoroquinolones is also no longer recommended. DGI and gonococcal arthritis are treated with parenteral ceftriaxone 1 g daily. Several parenteral antibiotic regimens are available for treatment of severe or complicated PID (discussed later in this chapter).

Disposition

Uncomplicated gonococcal infections are treated on an outpatient basis. Hospitalization may be warranted for more severe cases of upper tract infection, such as PID or epididymo-orchitis. Admission and treatment with parenteral ceftriaxone is recommended for DGI, septic arthritis, and conjunctivitis.

Chlamydia

Background and Importance

Chlamydia is the most commonly reported STI in the United States, with more than 1.7 million cases reported to the CDC in 2018. *Chlamydia trachomatis,* an obligate intracellular organism, is the causative pathogen. Approximately 50% of men and 70% of women who are infected with chlamydia are asymptomatic. Adolescents and young adults 15 to 24 years old have the highest rate of chlamydia infection. The reported rate of chlamydia is twice as high among women compared to men, reflecting the higher number of women screened for this infection.

Clinical Features

Chlamydia infection is a common cause of NGU. When present, the urethral discharge associated with chlamydia is typically scant, mucoid, and less purulent than the discharge seen with gonorrhea. Dysuria is less pronounced and presentation is often delayed. Chlamydia cervicitis may present with mucopurulent cervical discharge or postcoital bleeding but is often asymptomatic. When untreated, chlamydia can progress to upper tract infection, including epididymitis and orchitis in men and PID in women. Patients with epididymitis and orchitis complain of unilateral scrotal pain and swelling, and they may also report symptoms of urethritis. Swelling and tenderness of the epididymis and testicle are usually present. Epididymitis is more common with chlamydia infection alone or combined gonorrhea and chlamydia infections, rather than with gonorrhea alone. Chlamydia frequently

TABLE 84.3   Treatment of Sexually Transmitted Infections Associated With Genital Discharge[a]

Disease	Recommended Treatments
Gonorrhea	
Urethritis, cervicitis, proctitis, pharyngitis	Ceftriaxone 500 mg[b] IM single dose
Chlamydia	
Urethritis, cervicitis, proctitis, pharyngitis	Doxycycline 100 mg PO bid for 7 days
Nongonococcal urethritis (NGU)	Doxycycline 100 mg PO bid for 7 days
Trichomoniasis	Men: Metronidazole 2 g PO single dose
	Women: Metronidazole 500 mg PO bid for 7 days

[a]Alternative treatment regimens for selected patients (including pregnancy, drug allergies) can be found at www.cdc.gov/std/treatment.
[b]For weight ≥150 kg, ceftriaxone 1 g IM single dose.
IM, Intramuscular; *PO,* per os (by mouth).

contributes to the development of PID, which may be indolent or clinically silent, but results in significant chronic sequelae.

Diagnostic Testing

Differentiation between chlamydial and gonococcal infection based solely upon history and physical examination is unreliable, and these infections frequently coexist. NAATs are the diagnostic test of choice, with sensitivity greater than 90% and specificity of 99% for the diagnosis of chlamydia. Concurrent testing for gonorrhea can be performed on the same NAATs specimen obtained from either genital or extragenital sites.

Management

The recommended treatment for chlamydia urethritis, cervicitis, pharyngitis or proctitis is doxycycline 100 mg PO bid for 7 days (Table 84.3). Single-dose azithromycin 1 g PO is no longer the preferred treatment for uncomplicated chlamydia infection, but remains an alternative treatment for use during pregnancy or when doxycycline is otherwise contraindicated. Levofloxacin may also be used in the nonpregant patient. Suspected upper genitourinary tract infection with chlamydia (i.e., epididymitis, PID) requires a longer course of antibiotic therapy ranging from 10 to 14 days (Table 84.4).

Empirical treatment for both gonorrhea and chlamydia is recommended when confirmatory test results are unavailable, because history and physical examination cannot reliably differentiate these conditions and coinfections often occur. Weight-based single-dose ceftriaxone IM plus doxycycline 100 mg PO bid for 7 days treats uncomplicated gonorrhea in addition to lower tract chlamydia infection.

Disposition

Most chlamydia infections are treated on an outpatient basis. Patients with severe upper tract infection and those with associated complications may require hospitalization for parenteral antibiotics. Indications for admission include suspected tubo-ovarian abscess, Fitz-Hugh-Curtis syndrome, patients with intractable vomiting, septic patients, those with peritonitis, prepubertal children, and women with an indwelling intrauterine device (IUD).

Nongonococcal Urethritis

NGU is most often caused by *Chlamydia trachomatis,* but may also be caused by *Trichomonas vaginalis, Mycoplasma genitalium,*

TABLE 84.4   Treatment of Complicated or Upper Genitourinary Tract Sexually Transmitted Infections[a]

Disease	Recommended Treatments
Disseminated gonorrhea	Ceftriaxone 1 g IV or IM every 24 hours
	Hospitalization and infectious disease (ID) consult recommended
Gonococcal conjunctivitis	Ceftriaxone 1 g IV or IM single dose[b]
	Consider hospitalization & ID consult
Epididymitis/orchitis	Ceftriaxone 500 mg[b] IM single dose *plus*
	Doxycycline 100 mg PO bid for 10 days[c]
	Or
	Ceftriaxone 500 mg[b] IM single dose *plus*
	Levofloxacin 500 mg PO every day for 10 days[d]
	Or
	Levofloxacin 500 mg PO every day for 10 days[e]
Pelvic inflammatory disease (PID)	
Inpatient	Cefotetan 2 g IV every 12 hours *plus*
	Doxycycline 100 mg PO or IV every 12 hours
	Or
	Cefoxitin 2 g IV every 6 hours *plus*
	Doxycycline 100 mg PO or IV every 12 hours
	Or
	Ceftriaxone 1 g IV every 24 hours *plus*
	Doxycycline 100 mg PO or IV every 12 hours *plus*
	Metronidazole 500 mg PO or IV every 12 hours
Outpatient	Ceftriaxone 500 mg[b] IM single dose *plus*
	Doxycycline 100 mg PO bid for 14 days
	± Metronidazole 500 mg PO bid for 14 days

[a]Alternative treatment regimens for selected patients (including pregnancy, drug allergies) can be found at www.cdc.gov/std/treatment.
[b]For weight ≥150 kg, ceftriaxone 1 g IM single dose.
[c]For suspected gonorrhea and/or chlamydia.
[d]For suspected gonorrhea and/or chlamydia *and* enteric organisms (i.e., men who practice insertive anal intercourse).
[e]For suspected enteric organisms.
IM, Intramuscular; *IV,* intravenous; *PO,* per os (by mouth).

other *Mycoplasma* species, *Ureaplasma* species, and other organisms. Patients with NGU are often asymptomatic. Symptoms, when present, are usually less prominent than those seen with gonococcal urethritis. Clinical features are not sufficiently specific to distinguish between gonococcal urethritis and NGU, and coinfection is common. NAATs have high sensitivity and specificity for chlamydia, gonorrhea, trichomoniasis and *M. genitalium* infection. Wet mount microscopy can identify cases of trichomoniasis, but is less sensitive than NAATs, which are now the gold standard. Diagnostic testing is not routinely performed for other causes of NGU. Recommended treatment for NGU is doxycycline 100 mg PO bid for 7 days. Additional empirical treatment with weight-based single-dose ceftriaxone IM is recommended when gonorrhea has not been ruled out with negative NAATs. Treatment of trichomoniasis is discussed separately.

Persistent or recurrent NGU may be caused by treatment failure or reinfection following successful treatment. Management of these patients should be guided by results of diagnostic testing for causative organisms, when possible. *M. genitalium* is increasingly recognized

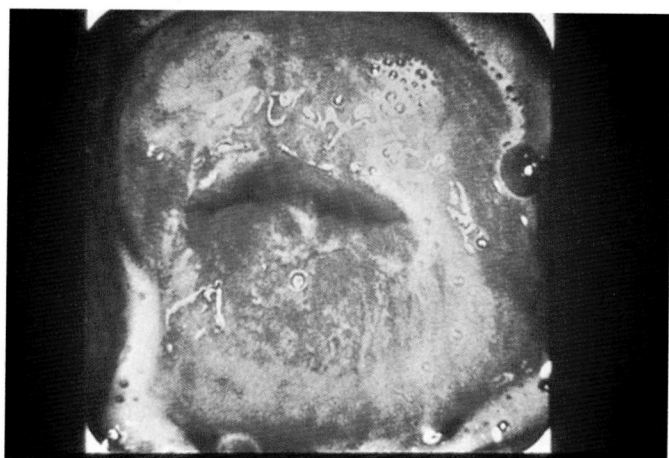

Fig. 84.7 Frothy vaginal discharge due to trichomoniasis. (From: Morse S, Ballard RC, Holmes KK, et al, eds. *Atlas of Sexually Transmitted Diseases and AIDS*, ed 4. London: Saunders/Elsevier; 2010: Fig. 5.23, p 140.)

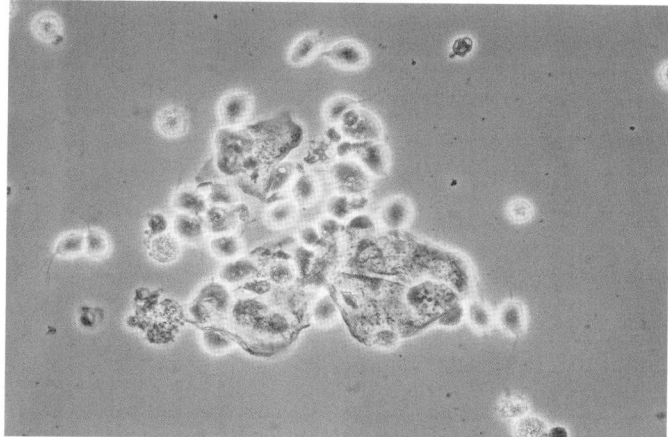

Fig. 84.8 *T. vaginalis* on a wet mount slide prep. (From Centers for Disease Control and Prevention [CDC]: Public Health Image Library [PHIL]. Image #14500. Available at phil.cdc.gov/phil/.)

as a cause of NGU that may be resistant to treatment with doxycycline alone. NAATs for *M. genitalium* should be obtained. The recommended two-stage treatment for confirmed *M. genitalium* infection is doxycycline 100 mg PO bid for 7 days, followed by moxifloxacin 400 mg PO once daily for 7 days. If antimicrobial resistance testing confirms sensitivity to macrolides, then azithromycin 1 g PO initial dose, followed by 500 mg PO once daily for 3 additional days may be considered as an alternative to moxifloxacin following the recommended 7 day course of doxycycline.

Trichomoniasis

Background and Importance

Trichomonas vaginalis is the flagellated protozoan organism responsible for trichomoniasis, the most common curable STI worldwide. Women are typically more symptomatic than men, but asymptomatic infection occurs in both sexes. Trichomoniasis usually causes mild disease, but significant morbidity can occur. Trichomoniasis has been associated with PID, preterm birth among pregnant women, prostatitis, epididymitis, and increased susceptibility to HIV acquisition.

Clinical Features

Trichomoniasis causes vaginitis in women. Common symptoms include vaginal discharge, pruritus, dysuria, urinary frequency, dyspareunia, and postcoital bleeding. The discharge is classically described as malodorous, frothy, and greenish yellow in color (Fig. 84.7). Pelvic examination may reveal erythema of the vaginal mucosa and vulva, in addition to the discharge. Punctate hemorrhages of the cervix ("strawberry cervix") are seen in up to 10% of cases. Trichomoniasis is often asymptomatic in men but may cause urethritis with associated dysuria and urethral discharge.

Diagnostic Testing

The diagnosis of trichomoniasis is often confirmed with microscopic examination of a saline wet mount slide, which reveals motile flagellated trichomonads and leukocytes (Fig. 84.8). The sensitivity of the wet mount slide is approximately 50% to 65%. Trichomonas may be seen incidentally on microscopic analysis of the urine sediment. NAATs are superior to microscopic examination, with reported sensitivity and specificity greater than 95% for some assays. Point-of-care antigen detection kits are now available. Culture is also confirmatory, but seldom used in the ED.

Management

Treatment of trichomoniasis is indicated in both symptomatic and asymptomatic men and nonpregnant women. Although single-dose metronidazole 2 g PO was previously recommended for treatment of trichomoniasis in men and women, studies have demonstrated increased efficacy using a multi-dose regimen of metronidazole in women. The recommended treatment in women is metronidazole 500 mg PO bid for 7 days. Metronidazole 2 g PO single dose is still recommended for treatment in men. (see Table 84.3). Tinidazole 2 g PO single dose is an acceptable treatment alternative in men and nonpregnant women, but should be avoided during pregnancy. Metronidazole is the recommended treatment for symptomatic trichomoniasis during pregnancy. The treatment of asymptomatic pregnant women with trichomoniasis is controversial, because there is conflicting data regarding the possible increased incidence of preterm labor in pregnant women treated with metronidazole.

Disposition

Trichomoniasis is treated on an outpatient basis. Patients should be counseled to avoid alcohol use for at least 24 hours after completion of metronidazole therapy and 72 hours after completion of tinidazole therapy, due to the occurrence of a disulfiram-like reaction following alcohol use.

Pelvic Inflammatory Disease

Background and Importance

PID is an ascending infection that begins at the level of the endocervix but progresses to the upper reproductive tract, causing endometritis, salpingitis, and peritonitis. *N. gonorrhoeae* and *Chlamydia trachomatis* have traditionally been implicated in the development of PID, but many women diagnosed with PID do not test positive for either of these organisms. Negative testing for gonorrhea and chlamydia from endocervical specimens does not reliably exclude them as a cause for upper tract infection. Polymicrobial involvement is common, with anaerobes, enteric organisms, vaginal flora, and other STIs often implicated in PID. An estimated 10% to 20% of women with gonorrhea or chlamydia may develop PID if they do not receive proper treatment. Other recognized complications of PID include chronic pelvic pain, infertility, and ectopic pregnancy.

Clinical Features

PID causes a spectrum of illness ranging from asymptomatic infection to severe illness with associated peritonitis and systemic toxicity. Lower abdominal pain is the most common presenting complaint. Other

TABLE 84.5 Diagnosis of Pelvic Inflammatory Disease[a]

Minimum Criteria	Additional Criteria[b]
Cervical motion tenderness *or*	Mucopurulent cervical discharge
Adnexal tenderness *or*	Cervical friability
Uterine tenderness	Oral temperature >101°F
	Elevated erythrocyte sedimentation rate
	Elevated C-reactive protein
	White blood cells (WBCs) on microscopy of vaginal secretions
	Laboratory confirmation of endocervical gonorrhea or chlamydia

[a]In a sexually active woman at risk for sexually transmitted infections (STIs) who presents with abdominal pain and no alternative diagnosis is identified, a presumptive diagnosis of pelvic inflammatory disease (PID) may be based upon the criteria listed in this table.
[b]Additional criteria increase specificity but decrease sensitivity for the diagnosis of PID.

symptoms include dyspareunia, abnormal vaginal discharge or bleeding, dysuria, and fever. Nausea, vomiting, diarrhea, and anorexia may be present, mimicking gastrointestinal conditions. Physical findings may include lower abdominal tenderness, cervical friability, mucopurulent discharge, cervical motion tenderness, and adnexal tenderness. Vital sign abnormalities, such as fever and tachycardia, may be seen.

Diagnostic Testing

PID is a clinical diagnosis. No single historical, physical, or laboratory finding or combination of findings is sufficiently sensitive or specific to make a definitive diagnosis of PID. Because PID causes significant morbidity, the CDC recommends a low threshold for the diagnosis and empirical treatment of PID. The diagnosis of PID should be considered and presumptive treatment initiated in any sexually active woman at risk for STIs who presents with lower abdominal or pelvic pain if no alternative diagnosis is identified and if one or more of the following findings are present on pelvic examination: (1) cervical motion tenderness, or (2) uterine tenderness, or (3) adnexal tenderness. These criteria have high sensitivity but low specificity for the diagnosis of PID. Because the use of these criteria will result in the over-diagnosis of PID, one should consider other possible diagnoses. The use of the additional criteria improves the specificity of the diagnosis of PID but decreases the diagnostic sensitivity (see Table 84.5).

NAATs for gonorrhea and chlamydia are recommended. A pregnancy test should always be obtained, because ectopic pregnancy and other pregnancy-related conditions may mimic PID. Computed tomography (CT) and pelvic ultrasonography may reveal findings supporting the diagnosis of PID, including evidence of swelling and inflammation within the endometrial cavity and fallopian tubes. Imaging studies are also helpful in ruling out other diagnoses, such as appendicitis, and for identifying complications of PID, such as tubo-ovarian abscess. Laparoscopy can confirm the diagnosis but is of limited utility due to its invasive nature, limited availability, and expense. In addition, laparoscopy may not identify mild cases of PID.

Management

Treatment should be initiated as soon as possible after the diagnosis is made and should not await the results of microbiologic testing or other delayed diagnostic studies. Delays in the initiation of antibiotic therapy contribute to the development of complications of PID. Multiple

inpatient and outpatient antibiotic regimens are available for the treatment of PID (see Table 84.4). The total duration of antibiotic therapy is 14 days. Antibiotic selection should include empirical coverage of gonorrhea and chlamydia. Anaerobic coverage with metronidazole was previously considered optional, but is now recommended in the routine outpatient treatment of PID. Recommended inpatient parenteral treatment regimens also include anaerobic coverage with metronidazole or cephalosporins. Supportive care measures include analgesics, antipyretics, and hydration. Sexual intercourse should be deferred until symptoms have resolved and antibiotic therapy has been completed by the patient and her partner.

Disposition

Most women with PID are treated as outpatients. Current recommendations no longer mandate hospitalization for adolescents or for HIV-positive patients with PID. Follow-up within 72 hours is recommended to ensure appropriate response to initial treatment. Women who meet any of the following criteria should be considered for inpatient treatment of PID:

- Surgical emergencies cannot be excluded (i.e., appendicitis)
- Pregnancy
- Tubo-ovarian abscess
- Severe illness, nausea and vomiting, or high fever
- Inability to follow or tolerate outpatient oral regimens
- Failure to respond to oral antibiotic therapy

In addition, to chronic pelvic pain, ectopic pregnancy, and infertility, other complications of PID are common. Tubo-ovarian abscess or pyosalpinx may be identified on pelvic ultrasound or CT. Perihepatitis, known as *Fitz-Hugh-Curtis syndrome,* is occasionally seen and may result in associated right upper quadrant abdominal pain.

Bacterial Vaginosis

Background and Importance

Bacterial vaginosis (BV) is the most common cause of abnormal vaginal discharge in the United States. Although BV is not considered to be an STI, it is often encountered during the evaluation of patients with an abnormal vaginal discharge. BV is due to an alteration in the vaginal flora with replacement of normal *Lactobacillus* species by a polymicrobial group of organisms, including *Gardnerella vaginalis*, anaerobes, and others.

Clinical Features and Diagnostic Testing

Many women with bacterial vaginosis are asymptomatic. Symptomatic women complain of a malodorous thin whitish vaginal discharge. A fishy odor is often reported and can be accentuated with the addition of 10% potassium hydroxide (KOH) solution to a wet mount slide at the time of pelvic examination (the "whiff test"). The pH of vaginal fluid is greater than 4.5. Microscopic examination of the wet mount slide reveals clue cells, which are vaginal epithelial cells with indistinct borders due to a coating of bacteria. Multiple available NAATs have high sensitivity and specificity for BV. Bacterial vaginosis is associated with an increased risk of PID and complications of pregnancy (premature rupture of membranes and preterm delivery). Bacterial vaginosis may also be a cofactor in the acquisition and transmission of other STIs, including HIV.

Management

Treatment is recommended for all symptomatic women with bacterial vaginosis, regardless of pregnancy status. The established benefit of therapy is the relief of vaginal symptoms. There is conflicting data regarding the efficacy of treatment in reducing the incidence of associated illnesses in pregnant and nonpregnant women. Treatment of bacterial vaginosis in asymptomatic women is not recommended.

Treatment of male sexual partners is of no benefit. Recommended treatment regimens for bacterial vaginosis include: (1) metronidazole 500 mg PO twice a day for 7 days, (2) metronidazole gel 0.75% 5 g intravaginally once a day for 5 days, and (3) clindamycin cream 2% 5 g intravaginally at bedtime for 7 days. Symptomatic pregnant women can be treated with the same oral or topical regimens recommended for nonpregnant women. The use of intravaginal *Lactobacillus* preparations and other probiotics are of no proven benefit in the restoration of normal vaginal flora or in the treatment of bacterial vaginosis.

Vulvovaginal Candidiasis

Background and Importance

Vulvovaginal candidiasis is usually caused by the yeast species *Candida albicans*. An estimated 75% of women will have at least one episode of candidiasis during their lifetime, and recurrent episodes are common. Like bacterial vaginosis, candidiasis is not considered to be an STI but is frequently encountered in the evaluation of patients with abnormal vaginal discharge.

Clinical Features and Diagnostic Testing

Common nonspecific symptoms include pruritus, abnormal discharge, dyspareunia, and external dysuria. Pelvic examination may reveal vulvar erythema and edema with satellite lesions, erythema of the vaginal mucosa, and a thick curdy whitish vaginal discharge. Microscopic examination of a wet mount slide may reveal the presence of budding yeast or pseudohyphae. Diagnosis is facilitated with the use of 10% KOH, which disrupts other cellular structures and facilitates visualization of fungal elements. Fungal culture is the diagnostic gold standard but is rarely performed.

Management

Multiple topical antifungal azole drugs are recommended for the treatment of vulvovaginal candidiasis, including clotrimazole, miconazole, butoconazole, terconazole, and tioconazole. Several topical agents are available over the counter. Fluconazole is the only oral antifungal agent approved by the FDA for treatment of candidiasis. A single dose of fluconazole 150 mg PO is highly effective in nonpregnant women but is contraindicated during pregnancy. A 7-day course of topical azoles is recommended during pregnancy. Single-dose and short-course therapy with azoles is associated with a cure rate of 80% to 90% in uncomplicated *Candida* vulvovaginitis. Male sexual partners may develop *Candida balanitis,* which typically responds to topical antifungal therapy. Treatment of asymptomatic sexual partners is of no proven benefit.

EPITHELIAL CELL INFECTIONS

Condyloma Acuminata (Genital Warts)

Background and Importance

Genital warts are caused by human papillomavirus (HPV). More than 40 types of HPV can infect humans, with the majority of HPV infections remaining asymptomatic or unrecognized. Clinically apparent warts occur in approximately 1% of cases. HPV types 6 and 11 cause most cases of visible genital warts and are considered non-oncogenic. HPV types 16 and 18 are responsible for most cases of cervical cancer and are also associated with vaginal, vulvar, anal, penile, and oropharyngeal cancers. The 9-valent vaccine currently available in the United States provides protection against the most common HPV types that cause cancer and visible genital warts. This vaccine is approved for use in women and men from 9 to 45 years of age, with the optimal timing of vaccine initiation prior to an individual's sexual debut.

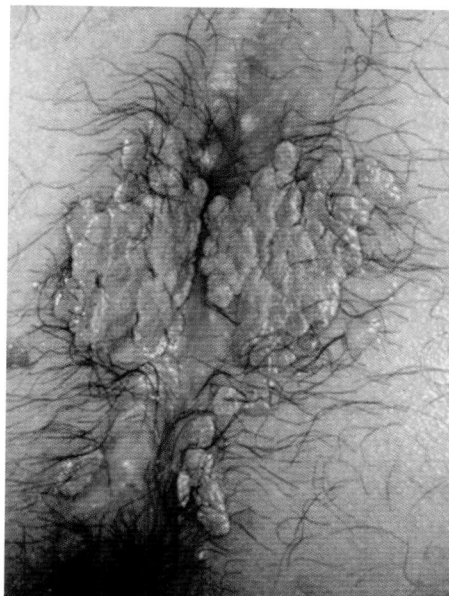

Fig. 84.9 Perianal condyloma acuminata. (From: Morse S, Ballard RC, Holmes KK, et al, eds. *Atlas of Sexually Transmitted Diseases and AIDS,* ed 4. London: Saunders/Elsevier; 2010: Fig. 11.10, p 294.)

Clinical Findings

Genital warts are typically manifested by small painless fleshy papular lesions on the skin or mucous membranes (Fig. 84.9). The slow-growing lesions gradually become more lobulated, pedunculated, or verrucous in appearance. Lesions may become friable and painful due to local irritation or secondary infection. Warts are typically found on the external genitalia, buttocks, and perineum, but they may occur anywhere the organism is inoculated.

Diagnostic Testing

A clinical diagnosis of genital warts is usually made by visual inspection. Differential diagnosis includes molluscum contagiosum, skin tags, nevi, neoplasm, and condyloma lata. Genital warts may have a moist appearance in intertriginous areas, but they do not usually have the denuded surface typically seen with condyloma lata in secondary syphilis. The duration of lesions and presence of associated symptoms are helpful features, because genital warts are often present for months or years but have no associated systemic symptoms. Darkfield microscopy and serology are useful in excluding a diagnosis of syphilis. Although not generally performed in the ED, biopsy can confirm the diagnosis and exclude neoplasm. The application of topical acetic acid to mucosal lesions to screen for HPV is nonspecific and is not recommended.

Management

All available treatments for HPV have significant failure rates. Treatment options include patient-applied regimens and provider-administered regimens. Patient-applied regimens include topical application of imiquimod cream, podofilox solution or gel, or sinecatechins ointment. The patient must be able to adequately visualize and reach the lesions to use these patient-applied agents. These modalities are preferable to some patients, because they can administer the treatment in the privacy of their own home. Provider-administered treatments include surgical excision, cryotherapy, or topical therapy with trichloroacetic acid (TCA) or bichloracetic acid (BCA). Podophyllin-based therapy is contraindicated during pregnancy due to possible teratogenic effects. The emergency clinician may elect to defer initiation of treatment for genital warts and refer the patient to a primary care provider or STI clinic, because the condition is not emergent and a prolonged course of treatment is usually required.

Molluscum Contagiosum

Molluscum contagiosum is a localized skin infection caused by a member of the pox virus family. The condition is common in childhood when it is usually acquired via nonsexual contact. It may be sexually acquired in adolescents and adults. Clinical appearance consists of one or more small 2- to 5-mm papules. The lesions have a waxy appearance, and central umbilication is common. Spontaneous resolution typically occurs within 6 to 12 months. Differential diagnosis may include genital warts, skin cancers, nevi, skin tags, and other benign skin lesions. Clinical diagnosis is made based upon the typical appearance of the lesions. No specific diagnostic testing or treatment is necessary in the ED. The patient can be referred to a primary care provider or dermatologist for curettage, cryotherapy, or treatment with topical agents for lesions that persist.

ECTOPARASITES

Pediculosis Pubis

Pediculosis pubis is a parasitic infestation caused by *Phthirus pubis,* the pubic louse. Although pubic lice are usually sexually transmitted, they can be transmitted via nonsexual contact with infected individuals or contact with infested fomites, such as linen or clothing. Symptoms include pruritus and mild discomfort at the site of the bites. Small erythematous maculopapular lesions with associated punctate bleeding may be seen. The lice are visible in the pubic hair or attached to the skin while feeding. The eggs (nits) are attached to the shaft of the pubic hairs. Diagnosis is confirmed by visual inspection.

Treatment includes topical permethrin 1% creams and rinses which are available over the counter. Permethrin should be applied to the affected area and washed off after 10 minutes. Alternative topical agents include pyrethrin shampoo and malathion. The patient should attempt to remove any visible nits, because topical treatment is not always ovicidal. Potentially infested linen and clothing should be washed in hot water with detergent. Repeat topical treatment can be applied in 1 to 2 weeks to kill any newly hatched lice. Resistance to pediculicides has been widely reported. An alternative topical agent or oral ivermectin may be used for treatment failures.

Scabies

Sarcoptes scabiei is the mite responsible for scabies. The organism is transmitted via direct person-to-person contact or exposure to infested linens and clothing. Although sexual transmission is common, many cases occur from nonsexual contact. The mite creates superficial burrows in the skin where eggs and excrement are deposited. Intense pruritus is caused by a hypersensitivity reaction to the foreign material in the skin. Careful inspection often reveals characteristic burrows in the skin. Excoriations, papules, and nodules are frequently seen. Commonly affected areas include the groin, genitalia, axilla, and interdigital web spaces of the hands. Diagnosis can be confirmed by microscopic examination of scrapings from characteristic skin lesions, which reveals the mites. Recommended treatments for scabies includes topical permethrin 5% cream, topical ivermectin 1% lotion or oral ivermectin. Permethrin is nontoxic and can be used safely in pregnancy and in patients of all ages. Linen and clothing should be washed in hot water with detergent.

The references for this chapter can be found online at ExpertConsult. com.

Urologic Disorders

Carl A. Germann

URINARY TRACT INFECTION IN ADULTS

Background

Urinary tract infections (UTI) occur when bacteria, often from the skin or rectum, ascend the urethra and infect the urinary tract. In the United States, the urinary tract is the most common source of infection of patients presenting in septic shock, with an associated mortality of 10% to 20%.

UTI describes an inflammatory response of the urothelium to microorganisms in the urinary tract, resulting in clinical symptoms that include dysuria, frequency, urgency, hematuria, and suprapubic or costovertebral angle discomfort. The diagnosis of a UTI requires the presence of urinary-specific symptoms or signs in a patient who has bacteriuria and no other identified source of infection. Bacteriuria is the presence of bacteria in the urine but is not considered to represent a UTI in the absence of clinical manifestations. Bacteriuria accompanied by symptoms should be treated, whereas bacteriuria in the absence of symptoms should be treated only in select patients (e.g., pregnant women, immunosuppressed patients).

UTIs are classified as lower (confined to the bladder) or upper (involving the ureters or kidneys) and as uncomplicated or complicated. An uncomplicated infection occurs in a nonpregnant individual with a structurally and functionally normal urinary tract. A complicated UTI is a heterogeneous term that may be associated with an underlying functional or structural abnormality, history of urinary instrumentation or organ transplantation, or systemic disease, such as renal insufficiency, diabetes, and immunodeficiency. UTIs in men are generally categorized as complicated given the higher incidence of associated urologic abnormalities. However, men can experience a UTI without an underlying structural or functional abnormality. Complicated UTIs often require a prolonged course of antibiotic therapy and a more in-depth approach to testing and anatomic evaluation.

The term *urethritis* refers to the inflammation of the urethra secondary to an infection or trauma. Frequently, urethritis may be a manifestation of a sexually transmitted infection (STI), such as gonococcal urethritis in *Neisseria gonorrhoeae* infection, but may occur in other clinical scenarios as well. *Cystitis* generally refers to inflammation of the bladder resulting in increased urinary frequency, urgency, dysuria, and suprapubic pain. The causes of cystitis can be separated into bacterial and nonbacterial (e.g., radiation) categories. *Acute pyelonephritis* is a UTI involving the renal parenchyma and collecting system, manifesting with the clinical syndrome of fever, chills, and flank pain. Management and disposition of patients with acute pyelonephritis depend on whether the infection is simple or complicated.

Anatomy and Physiology

In women, the urethra is short and opens close to the vulvar and perirectal areas. This contributes to the much higher incidence of UTI in women. The route of infection in men is also usually ascending, from the urethra to the prostate to the bladder and then to the kidney. Risk factors for cystitis and pyelonephritis include sexual intercourse, use of spermicides, previous UTI, new sex partner, and history of UTI in a first-degree female relative suggestive of possible inherited urethral anatomic pathology.

Pathophysiology

UTIs arise when urinary pathogens from the bowel or vagina colonize the periurethral mucosa and ascend through the urethra and into the collecting system. Infrequently, bacterial infection of the urinary tract arises from hematogenous or lymphatic sources. This is frequently the pathologic mechanism in debilitated and chronically ill patients who are immunosuppressed. Obstruction from any cause, with resultant stasis of urine, is a common contributor to infection. Urinary calculi may cause obstruction and increased susceptibility to the development of a UTI. Likewise, numerous abnormalities of the urinary tract may interfere with its innate ability to resist infection.

Subgroups of patients who are more susceptible than the normal population to UTIs include diabetics, pregnant women, elders, patients who are unable to empty their bladder completely, patients with indwelling urinary catheters, and those with immunodeficiency disorders. Lower UTIs are more common in aging men in the setting of prostatic enlargement or obstruction.

Escherichia coli is responsible for approximately three-quarters of cases of UTI in men and women.[1] Other less common bacteria that may be responsible for infection include *Staphylococcus saprophyticus* and other members of the Enterobacteriaceae family (*Klebsiella pneumonia* and *Proteus mirabilis*). Unusual microorganisms may be found in institutionalized or hospitalized populations. Such settings and conditions predispose the patient to alterations in the normal gastrointestinal (GI) flora, leading to complex UTIs. The uropathogens in these patients include more resistant strains of *Escherichia, Klebsiella, Proteus,* and *Enterobacter,* as well as *Pseudomonas, Enterococcus, Staphylococcus, Providencia, Serratia, Morganella, Citrobacter, Salmonella, Shigella,* and *Haemophilus* spp., *Mycobacterium tuberculosis,* and fungi.

Clinical Features

UTI is usually manifested as dysuria, with or without frequency, urgency, hematuria, or suprapubic discomfort. Symptoms of dysuria, frequency, hematuria, nocturia, and urgency all increase the probability of UTI, whereas vaginal discharge decreases the likelihood of UTI. The probability of cystitis is greater than 90% in women who have dysuria and frequency without vaginal discharge or irritation.

Symptoms of UTI in men may also represent storage or voiding disturbances that are common in aging men (e.g., prostatic enlargement). Commonly, men with lower UTIs have symptoms of urinary urgency, frequency, dysuria, hematuria, and suprapubic pain. If fever and chills are present in association with irritative symptoms and difficulty voiding, acute bacterial prostatitis should be strongly considered. A digital rectal examination of the prostate gland with attention to size, shape, and consistency can identify prostatic enlargement, inflammation, or cancer.

Clinical signs and symptoms suggestive of pyelonephritis include fever, chills, flank pain, costovertebral angle tenderness, and nausea or vomiting, with or without symptoms of cystitis. The presentation of UTI and pyelonephritis can be particularly challenging in those who are debilitated and elders because they may not be able to verbalize their symptoms and can present without fever; these patients may present with nonspecific complaints such as altered mental status, lethargy, abdominal pain, or generalized weakness.

Differential Diagnosis

Bacterial UTI is the most common cause of dysuria. Differential considerations include acute urethritis or acute vaginitis from STI, as well as mechanical trauma or irritation (Table 85.1). In the ED setting, UTI is often overdiagnosed and associated with missed STI diagnoses.[2] In general, if historical information includes contact with multiple sexual partners, recent change in sexual partners, or sexual partner with

TABLE 85.1 Clinical Differentiation of Major Causes of Dysuria

Cause	Clinical Features
Urinary tract infection	Internal dysuria
	Frequency, urgency, voiding small volumes
	Abrupt onset
	Suprapubic pain
	Often associated with diaphragm use
	Presence of pyuria
	Presence of hematuria (50% of patients)
Sexually transmitted disease	Internal dysuria
	Occasional history of frequency, urgency, voiding small volumes
	Gradual onset
	History of new or multiple sexual partners
	Vaginal discharge
Vaginitis	External dysuria
	Gradual onset
	Vaginal discharge
	Vaginal odor
	Pruritus

dysuria or discharge, *Chlamydia trachomatis* and *N. gonorrhoeae* infection should be strongly considered. Because the diagnosis of UTI is rarer in men, a high suspicion for an STI such as gonococcal or nongonococcal urethritis should be maintained. Trauma, calculi, chemical irritation, candidal infections, psychogenic disorders, neoplasm, and malformations or space-occupying lesions compressing the distal genitourinary tract can also cause dysuria.

Diagnostic Testing

Urinalysis and Urine Culture

A clean-catch, midstream specimen is the preferred type of urine sample for analysis. This is particularly important in woman in whom contamination from the perineum may result in a false-positive test result. However, even when the procedure is performed correctly, a specimen may be contaminated because the surrounding areas can be difficult to clean. A predominance of epithelial cells suggests that the specimen is contaminated. Sterile catheterization is the most accurate method of obtaining a urine specimen in women and may be the best solution for achieving a reliable urinalysis if the patient is unable to provide a clean-catch specimen or is actively menstruating. In men, the specimen is usually not affected by lack of cleansing or by the timing of specimen collection. Therefore, it is not appropriate to catheterize an adolescent or adult man for the purpose of collecting a urine specimen unless he is experiencing urinary retention.

Urine screening tests provide a quick and inexpensive diagnostic tool, with a goal of reliably predicting specimens that will provide positive or negative cultures. The most commonly used screening tests measure urinary leukocyte esterase and nitrite. Both can be detected by a color change on dipstick testing. Leukocyte esterase is an enzyme found in neutrophils, and nitrite is produced from nitrate reductase, present in gram-negative bacteria. Nitrite positivity is highly sensitive at 95% or greater. However, not all uropathogens, such as *S. saprophyticus* and *Enterococcus,* convert nitrate into nitrite. A urine dipstick test indicating the presence of nitrite and leukocyte esterase has a specificity of almost 100% for UTI. However, dipstick tests should be used with caution because they can be less sensitive than the microscopic examination of urine (urinalysis). Given the limited negative predictive value of urine dipstick testing, a UTI may be difficult to rule out, even when all features are negative.[3] However, when there is a low pretest probability of UTI, a negative dipstick result for leukocyte esterase and nitrites excludes infection.[4] When the history is strongly suggestive of a UTI and the dipstick is negative, we recommend that a urine culture be sent.

Urine microscopy is an adjunct to the dipstick and helps reduce the number of urine cultures performed. Although no accepted level of pyuria is diagnostic of UTI, careful quantitation with a hemocytometer chamber will find pyuria in nearly all cases of acute UTI caused by coliforms. Pyuria is defined as 10 or more WBCs/mm³. Microscopic examination of urine to identify bacteria remains the most reliable test for a diagnosis of UTI, but availability varies by institution.

The diagnosis of a UTI can be made only with clinical symptoms and the determination of bacteriuria; however, the diagnosis is confirmed with urine culture. A generally accepted definition of a positive culture is 10^5 or more colony-forming units (CFU)/mL. There is no absolute number of CFUs that is definitive for a UTI; the culture results alone are not diagnostic of infection and must be combined with symptoms suggestive of a UTI. The presence of 10^5 CFUs/mL of bacteria in a urine culture is associated with a 95% likelihood of infection, whereas 10^4 CFUs/mL is associated with a 50% likelihood of infection. The presence of bacteria on culture in the absence of clinical manifestations does not always indicate infection but may be due to patient colonization or contamination of the specimen.

The decision to perform a urine culture should be assessed for its relevance to patient care. Patients with frequency, dysuria, urgency, and suprapubic pain should be treated on the basis of symptoms, and a urine culture is not required to guide therapy. Patients with relapse or recurrent infections, complicated infection, or those in whom multidrug-resistant organisms are suspected based on previous microbiology or exposure to antibiotics should have a culture performed (Box 85.1).

An STI may mimic a UTI and, in sexually active patients, cultures for *C. trachomatis* and *N. gonorrhoeae* should be considered. Other causes of acute dysuria include infections with *Trichomonas vaginalis* and herpes simplex virus.

Imaging

Most patients with acute cystitis or pyelonephritis do not need emergency imaging of the urinary tract. Imaging is reserved for patients with a clinical suspicion for underlying structural abnormalities or complicating factors such as abscess, urolithiasis, or emphysematous pyelonephritis. Patients with pyelonephritis who have severe or worsening illness or persistent fever 48 to 72 hours after the initiation of appropriate antimicrobial treatment should undergo imaging to exclude renal stones, abscesses, or obstruction.

Ultrasonography is indicated to assess for potential urinary obstruction. Ultrasound is a sensitive tool for detecting postvoid residual bladder volume, intrarenal and perinephric abscess, and presence of hydroureter and hydronephrosis (Figs. 85.1 and 85.2). Ultrasound can also detect the presence of pyelonephritis and congenital anomalies. Regardless of patient age, this procedure is relatively inexpensive and avoids the hazards of contrast and radiation exposure. A suggestion of obstruction based on clinical suspicion or lack of response to medical therapy necessitates performance of an abdominal ultrasound or noncontrast CT scan.

A contrast CT scan of the abdomen is the most comprehensive test for assessing the kidneys, ureters, and bladder.[5] It has a high sensitivity for detecting abscess, obstruction, and acute inflammation. Imaging

BOX 85.1 Patient Groups for Whom Urine Culture Is Indicated

- Children
- Adult men
- Immunocompromised patients
- Patients with treatment failure (i.e., with persistent urinary symptoms despite recently completed course of antibiotics)
- Patients with duration of symptoms more than 4–6 days
- Older patients at risk for bacteremia
- Ill-appearing patients with signs and symptoms suggestive of pyelonephritis or bacteremia
- Pregnant women
- Patients with known chronic or recurrent renal infection
- Patients with known anatomic urologic abnormalities
- Patients in whom urinary tract obstruction is suspected (e.g., stones, benign prostatic hypertrophy)
- Patients with serious medical diseases, including diabetes mellitus, sickle cell anemia, cancer, and other debilitating diseases
- Patients with alcoholism or drug dependence
- Recently hospitalized patients
- Patients taking antibiotics
- Patients who recently have undergone urinary tract instrumentation (e.g., cystoscopy, catheterization)

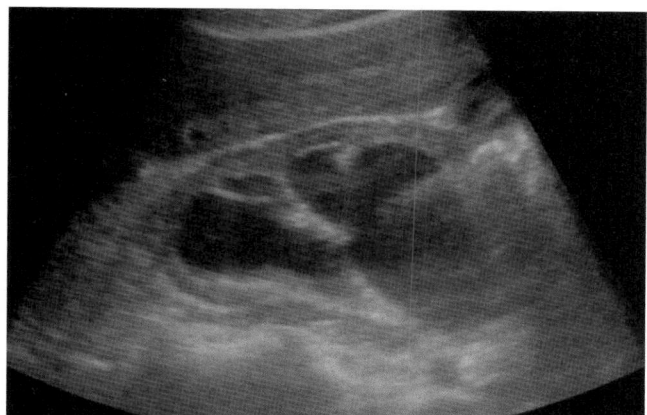

Fig. 85.1 Ultrasound Image Demonstrating Hydronephrosis With a Dilated Collecting System. (Courtesy Dr. Peter Croft.)

with an abdominal CT scan is recommended for those with pyelonephritis and known functional or anatomic abnormalities, recent instrumentation, immunosuppression, or concern for obstruction. Its disadvantages include radiation exposure, cost, and potential to induce contrast reactions.

Management

Simple Urinary Tract Infection

The options for treating uncomplicated lower UTI include single-dose therapy with fosfomycin, 5 days of nitrofurantoin, or 3 days of trimethoprim-sulfamethoxazole (Table 85.2). Fluoroquinolones such as ciprofloxacin or levofloxacin should not be used as first-line agents for empirical treatment of uncomplicated UTIs. Instead, they should be reserved for patients who have failed or have contraindications to first-line antibiotics. Fluoroquinolones achieve therapeutic levels in renal and prostate parenchyma and are indicated for complicated or more severe infections. However, they are not routinely used for

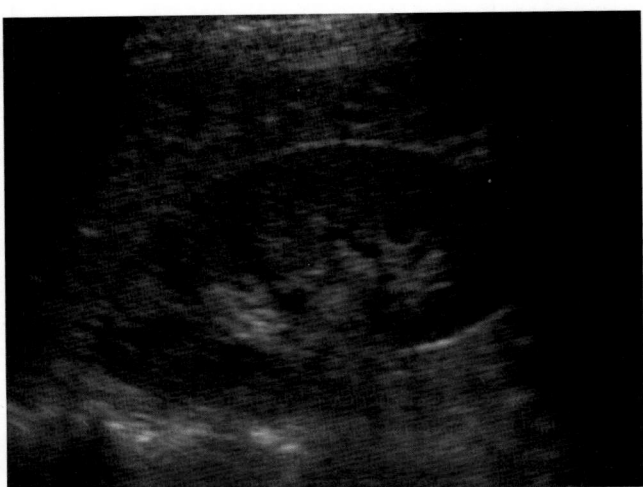

Fig. 85.2 Ultrasound Image Demonstrating a Normal Kidney. (Courtesy Dr. Peter Croft.)

TABLE 85.2 Antibiotic Options for Acute Uncomplicated Cystitis

Antimicrobial	Dose (Oral)	Duration	Common Side Effects
Trimethoprim-sulfamethoxazole	160/800 mg bid	3 days	Nausea, vomiting, anorexia, hypersensitivity reactions
Nitrofurantoin	100 mg bid	5 days	Gastrointestinal disturbance, headache, allergic reactions
Fosfomycin	3 g as a single dose		Diarrhea, nausea, headache, vaginitis, dizziness

uncomplicated cystitis due to adverse side-effect profiles and increasing resistance.

Antibiotics should be chosen with local resistance patterns in mind. The Infectious Disease Society of America (IDSA) recommends avoiding antimicrobial agents when local resistance exceeds 20%, emphasizing the need to be familiar with local outpatient resistance patterns. Although most hospitals monitor the resistance of organisms cultured in their microbiology laboratory, these data may reflect drug-exposed, hospital-acquired organisms more than community-acquired, outpatient-based illnesses. Thus, hospital antibiograms likely overestimate community resistance patterns.

Nitrofurantoin is a useful drug for the treatment of acute bacterial cystitis. It is inexpensive and maintains low serum and high urine levels. Nitrofurantoin is effective against *E. coli* but is inactive against other pathogens, such as *Proteus* and *Pseudomonas aeruginosa*. The rate of clearance is proportional to the creatinine clearance, and dose adjustments are necessary with renal impairment. The most common adverse effects of using nitrofurantoin are GI effects, including nausea, vomiting, and diarrhea.

Fosfomycin is an inhibitor of cell wall synthesis, structurally unrelated to any other antibiotic, and is active against most urinary tract pathogens, including multi-drug resistant gram-negative organisms. Fosfomycin is appealing for emergency department (ED) use because it can be given as a single dose for simple cystitis and does not require that a patient go to a pharmacy. However, we recommend the use of Fosfomycin only when other first-line therapies cannot be used because overuse might lead to an increased rate of resistance. Both nitrofurantoin and fosfomycin remain effective against extended-spectrum, β-lactamase–producing bacteria.[6]

A useful adjunctive therapy for UTIs in patients experiencing significant discomfort is phenazopyridine (Pyridium). It produces topical analgesia in the urinary tract and helps relieve dysuria. Patients should be cautioned that body secretions and excretions (e.g., tears, urine) will turn orange. This side effect can stain contact lenses and alarm unknowing patients.

The clinical presentations of UTIs and STIs can overlap. When coexisting vaginitis or pelvic inflammatory disease is suspected, empirical treatment should include the possibility of coinfection. In such cases, levofloxacin (500 mg/day for 7 days) has activity against common uropathogens as well as chlamydia and can be used with a single intramuscular dose of ceftriaxone (500 mg) for gonorrhea coverage.

Complex Urinary Tract Infection

Patients with mild to moderate pyelonephritis without complicating factors can be safely treated on an outpatient basis as long as the patient is able to eat and drink, has achieved adequate pain control, and has appropriate social support in the home. Given the risk for systemic illness, bacteremia, and progression to severe sepsis, medications must achieve therapeutic levels not only in the urine but also in the renal tissues and bloodstream. Therefore, fluoroquinolones are a first-line choice (Table 85.3). In areas in which the prevalence of resistance of fluoroquinolones is less than 10%, we recommend a 7-day course of ciprofloxacin for empirical outpatient treatment for uncomplicated pyelonephritis. In areas in which there is more than 10% fluoroquinolone resistance, the most recent IDSA guidelines recommend giving a long-acting parenteral antibiotic, such as 1 g ceftriaxone, followed by 10 to 14 days of an oral cephalosporin. Trimethoprim-sulfamethoxazole (TMP-SMX) for 10 to 14 days is an alternative treatment. Nitrofurantoin and fosfomycin do not achieve adequate blood and tissue levels and therefore are not effective for pyelonephritis.

A severe upper tract UTI necessitating hospitalization initially should be treated with parenteral antibiotics, such as cefepime, ceftriaxone, piperacillin-tazobactam, aztreonam, or a fluoroquinolone, with transition to oral therapy after the patient has been afebrile for 24 to 48 hours (Table 85.4). Oral therapy should be continued for 10 to 14 days. Follow-up urine cultures are recommended given the diverse flora and high rate of antimicrobial resistance.

In men, if there are no signs of toxicity, the patient can be treated on an outpatient basis with any of the urinary antibacterial agents (e.g., TMP-SMX, nitrofurantoin, fluoroquinolones) for 7 to 14 days. If concomitant prostatitis is suspected, TMP-SMX or a fluoroquinolone is recommended for 14 days. If evaluation demonstrates suspicion for prostate involvement, recurrent infection, or hematuria, the patient should be referred to a urologist for further evaluation. Patients with symptoms of prostatic enlargement can be treated with α-adrenergic receptor antagonists and/or 5-alpha-reductase inhibitor therapy (Table 85.5). Surgical treatment produces the most significant, long-term symptom improvement; it includes transurethral

TABLE 85.3 Antibiotic Options for Acute Uncomplicated Pyelonephritis

Antimicrobial	Dose (Oral)	Duration	Common Side Effects
Ciprofloxacin	500 mg bid	7 days	Gastrointestinal disturbance, headache, dizziness, tremors, restlessness, confusion, rash, *Candida* infections
Levofloxacin	750 mg once daily	5 days	Same as for ciprofloxacin
Trimethoprim-sulfamethoxazole	160/800 mg bid	10–14 days	Nausea, vomiting, anorexia, hypersensitivity reactions

TABLE 85.4 Antibiotic Options for Complicated Pyelonephritis

Antimicrobial	Dose (IV)	Common Side Effects
Cefepime	1–2 g every 8 h	Abdominal pain, muscle cramps, nausea, vomiting
Ceftriaxone	1 g every 24 h	Fever, cough, sore throat, fatigue
Piperacillin-tazobactam	3.375 g every 6 h	Diarrhea, nausea, vomiting, rash
Aztreonam	1 g every 8–12 h	Cough, abdominal pain, nausea, vomiting
Ciprofloxacin	400 mg every 12 h	GI disturbance, headache, dizziness, tremors, restlessness, confusion, rash, *Candida* infections
Levofloxacin	500 mg every 24 h	Same as for ciprofloxacin

TABLE 85.5 Medication Options for Prostatic Enlargement

Antimicrobial	Dose
Alpha-Adrenergic Receptor Antagonist	
Alfuzosin	10 mg once daily
Doxazosin	1 mg once daily
Tamsulosin	0.4 mg once daily
Terazosin	1 mg once daily or at bedtime
5-Alpha-Reductase Inhibitors	
Dutasteride	0.5 mg once daily
Finasteride	5 mg once daily

prostate resection, open prostatectomy, laser vaporization, transurethral microwave therapy, or needle ablation. Decisions regarding treatment options are based on the degree of obstruction and symptoms.

Disposition

Hospitalization is required in the presence of clinical toxicity (e.g., fever, tachycardia, hypotension, vomiting), inability to take oral medications, an immunocompromised state, third-trimester pregnancy, failure of oral outpatient therapy, urologic abnormalities, or patients with significant comorbid conditions, including heart failure and renal insufficiency. Patients who don't fall into these categories often benefit from short-term treatment in the ED or observation unit with IV hydration, pain and fever control, and the first dose of an IV fluoroquinolone. If these patients improve clinically, and can tolerate food and drink, they can be safely discharged home on a 10- to 14-day course of an oral fluoroquinolone, with close primary physician follow up. Urine culture with sensitivity testing and further diagnostic evaluation are not necessary in this patient population.

COMPLICATED URINARY TRACT INFECTION IN HIGH-RISK POPULATIONS

Pregnancy

UTI during pregnancy represents a special situation. Although the incidence of UTI in pregnancy is approximately the same as in nonpregnant women, pyelonephritis is more common during pregnancy. This is likely a result of the physiologic changes that occur within the urinary tract of pregnant women, which include ureteral and renal pelvis dilation. Factors associated with a higher risk of bacteriuria include a history of prior UTI, preexisting diabetes mellitus, increased parity, and low socioeconomic status.

Unlike bacteriuria in nonpregnant females, bacteriuria in pregnant women, even if they are asymptomatic, should be treated. Untreated bacteriuria in pregnancy is associated with premature labor, low birth weight, perinatal mortality, maternal anemia, and maternal pyelonephritis. Like nonpregnant women, *E. coli* is the most common uropathogen. The symptoms of UTI and pyelonephritis are also the same as in nonpregnant patients; however, urinary frequency and urgency may be symptoms of a normal pregnancy. Specimen collection and diagnostic strategies are also similar. A urine culture specimen should be obtained, along with a follow-up culture as a test of cure.

Options for empirical treatment for UTI include amoxicillin-clavulanate, cefpodoxime, nitrofurantoin, fosfomycin, and TMP-SMX (Table 85.6). The evidence regarding an association between the nitrofuran and sulfonamide classes of antibiotics and birth defects is mixed.[7] Previous American College of Obstetricians and Gynecologists (ACOG) recommendations were to avoid TMP-SMX and nitrofurantoin during the first trimester. Current recommendations state that it is appropriate to prescribing sulfonamides or nitrofurantoin in the first trimester when no other suitable alternative antibiotics are available.[7]

During the second and third trimesters, sulfonamides and nitrofurantoins may be used as first-line agents for the treatment of UTIs.[7] Fluoroquinolones should be avoided in pregnancy.

Hospital admission should be considered for patients in their last trimester, who appear ill, or who have evidence of pyelonephritis and would benefit from treatment with parenteral antibiotics and IV fluids. Parenteral regimens for the empirical treatment of pyelonephritis are similar to those for nonpregnant patients, except the use of fluoroquinolones, and include ceftriaxone, cefepime, aztreonam, and piperacillin-tazobactam (Table 85.7). Nitrofurantoin and fosfomycin do not achieve tissue levels adequate to treat pyelonephritis

TABLE 85.6 Antibiotic Options for Bacteriuria in Pregnancy

Antimicrobial	Dose (Oral)	Duration	Contraindications
Amoxicillin-clavulanate	500 mg tid	3–7 days	
Cefpodoxime	100 mg bid	5–7 days	
Nitrofurantoin	100 mg bid	5–7 days	First trimester and 38 weeks to delivery
Fosfomycin	3 g as a single dose		
Trimethoprim-sulfamethoxazole	160/800 mg bid	3 days	First trimester and term

TABLE 85.7 Parenteral Antibiotic Options for Pyelonephritis in Pregnancy

Antimicrobial	Dose (IV)
Ceftriaxone	1 g every 24 h
Cefepime	1 g every 8 h
Piperacillin-tazobactam	3.375 g every 6 h
Aztreonam	1 g every 8–12 hours

appropriately. Hospitalized pregnant patients who are afebrile for 48 hours can be discharged on oral antibiotics, directed by culture susceptibility results, to be completed in 10 to 14 days.

Indwelling and Temporary Urinary Catheters

Catheter-associated UTI (CAUTI) is defined as urine containing greater than 1000 CFU/ml of one or more bacterial species in a catheterized patient with suggestive symptoms, such as pelvic discomfort, flank pain, fever, rigors, malaise, altered mental status or lethargy with no other identified cause, costovertebral angle tenderness, or acute hematuria.

Screening for or treating asymptomatic bacteriuria in patients with indwelling catheters is not indicated. Antibiotic treatment results in the development of resistant microorganisms, whereas removal of the catheter leads to the spontaneous elimination of bacteria in many patients. Treatment of patients with a UTI in whom permanent removal of the catheter is contraindicated includes antibiotic therapy and urine culture and sensitivity. Replacement of the catheter and strong consideration for hospitalization is indicated in those who exhibit altered vital signs, systemic symptoms, or a toxic appearance.

Many patients with indwelling urinary catheters who present to the ED are older and not able to verbalize their symptoms or lack clinical signs of infection. Given that a catheter-associated UTI is a common cause of subsequent bacteremia and mortality, empirical antimicrobial therapy, in addition to replacement or removal of the catheter, is often appropriate in such patients. Urine culture with antibiotic sensitivity testing will help guide antibiotic therapy in this patient population. The most important risk factor for bacteriuria is the duration of catheterization. The most effective strategy for addressing CAUTIs is to prevent the infection from occurring by placing urinary catheters only when necessary and considering the use of intermittent catheterization and condom catheters, when appropriate.

PROSTATITIS

Background

Males with cystitis often have involvement of the prostate.[8] Prostatitis encompasses four distinct clinical processes—acute bacterial prostatitis, chronic bacterial prostatitis, chronic prostatitis–chronic pelvic pain syndrome, and asymptomatic inflammatory prostatitis.

Acute bacterial prostatitis generally affects men between the ages of 20 and 40 years, with a second peak in men older than 60 years. Acute prostatitis is caused by a bacterial infiltration that is usually precipitated by reflux of urine infected by *E. coli, Klebsiella, Enterobacter, Proteus,* or *Pseudomonas* spp.

Chronic bacterial prostatitis is a persistent bacterial infection of the prostate lasting more than 3 months. Approximately 10% of acute bacterial prostatitis cases develop into chronic bacterial prostatitis.[9] This can be caused by undertreated acute bacterial prostatitis or highly virulent strains. Like acute bacterial prostatitis, gram-negative bacteria are responsible for most cases of chronic prostatitis.

Whereas acute and chronic bacterial prostatitis have clear bacterial etiologies and are managed as infectious diseases, *chronic prostatitis/chronic pelvic pain syndrome (CP/CPPS)* is characterized by chronic pelvic pain and voiding symptoms in the absence of a clear bacterial etiology.[10] CPPS is defined as urologic pain in the pelvic region associated with urinary symptoms or sexual dysfunction lasting for at least 3 of the previous 6 months. Symptoms of chronic bacterial prostatitis may not differ from those of CP/CPPS. It is a heterogeneous condition with broad diagnostic criteria and uncertain cause, making it difficult to determine an effective treatment regimen reliably.

Asymptomatic inflammatory prostatitis is a painless inflammation of the prostate gland in the absence of infection. It is a common finding in men with benign prostatic hyperplasia and a diagnosis of exclusion in the ED.

Clinical Features

Patients with acute prostatitis often report UTI symptoms such as fever, chills, dysuria, urinary frequency or urgency, and/or perineal and low back pain. A rectal examination will reveal an exquisitely tender and swollen prostate gland in more than 90% of patients. There is no evidence that performing a rectal examination induces clinically significant bacteremia.

Clinical manifestations of chronic prostatitis vary widely, making recognition difficult. Most patients report some degree of voiding symptoms (e.g., frequency, urgency, dysuria), low back and perineal pain and, occasionally, myalgias. Fever and chills are uncommon except during an acute exacerbation of the chronic infection. Findings on the physical examination, including examination of the prostate, often are unremarkable. The diagnosis is based on history, physical examination, and positive urine culture.

Diagnostic Testing

Acute bacterial prostatitis is a clinical diagnosis. A urine Gram stain and culture are recommended to identify causative organisms and guide treatment. Blood cultures are recommended for patients with acute prostatitis and fever who have not yet received antibiotics.[8] Although acute bacterial prostatitis is usually caused by typical urinary pathogens, an STI such as chlamydia and gonorrhea should be

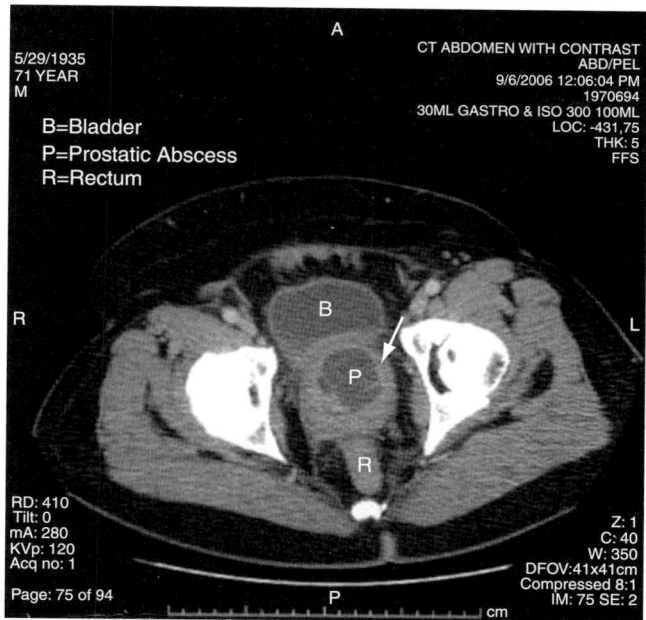

CT ABDOMEN WITH CONTRAST
ABD/PEL
9/6/2006 12:06:04 PM
1970694
30ML GASTRO & ISO 300 100ML
LOC: -431,75
THK: 5
FFS

5/29/1935
71 YEAR
M

B=Bladder
P=Prostatic Abscess
R=Rectum

RD: 410
Tilt: 0
mA: 280
KVp: 120
Acq no: 1
Page: 75 of 94

Z: 1
C: 40
W: 350
DFOV:41x41cm
Compressed 8:1
IM: 75 SE: 2

Fig. 85.3 Prostate Abscess. *B,* Bladder; *P,* prostate; *R,* rectum. (From Vandover JC, Patel N, Dalawari P. Prostatic abscess. *J Emerg Med.* 2011;40:e83–e85.)

TABLE 85.8 Oral and Parenteral Antibiotic Options for Prostatitis (4 to 6 Weeks' Duration)

Antimicrobial	Dose
Ciprofloxacin	400 mg every 12 h (IV)
Levofloxacin	500 mg every 24 h (IV)
Ceftriaxone	2 g every 24 h (IV)
Ciprofloxacin	500 mg every 12 h (PO)
Levofloxacin	500 mg once daily (PO)
Trimethoprim-sulfamethoxazole	160/800 mg bid (PO)

considered, especially in sexually active patients. Urethral swabs or first-voided urine, with subsequent culture or DNA amplification, should be obtained if a STI is suspected.

The most common complications of acute prostatitis are acute urinary retention (AUR) and prostatic abscess. Approximately 10% of men with acute prostatitis will have some urinary retention, which can be diagnosed using bedside ultrasound. Transrectal ultrasound or CT can detect prostatic abscess and should be considered in patients who fail to improve with antibiotics (Fig. 85.3).

Management

Outpatient therapy can be used if the patient is not systemically ill, can tolerate oral medications, and does not have urinary retention. General support measures for outpatients should include bed rest, analgesics, nonsteroidal antiinflammatory drugs (NSAIDs), hydration, and stool softeners. Alpha blocker therapy is also recommended for obstructive voiding symptoms related to prostatitis (see Table 85.5).

There is no consensus regarding an optimal treatment regimen, so regional patterns of antibiotic resistance should be considered. Few antimicrobial agents are able to penetrate the prostrate and achieve sufficient concentrations to eradicate infection. Fluoroquinolones, such as ciprofloxacin or levofloxacin, achieve the highest concentrations in the prostate and are the first-line agents in the treatment of bacterial prostatitis. Empirical parenteral antibiotics such as ciprofloxacin, levofloxacin, or ceftriaxone are recommended until fever and other symptoms have subsided. After improvement, oral antibiotics are recommended for at least 4 weeks (Table 85.8). Hospitalization for parenteral antibiotics is recommended for patients who appear systemically ill, cannot tolerate oral medications, or have urinary retention as determined by ultrasound or catheterization. Antibiotic options include ciprofloxacin 400 mg IV every 12 hours, levofloxacin 500 mg IV every 24 hours, or ceftriaxone 2 g IV every 24 hours. Following clinical improvement, the patient may be transitioned to an oral regimen, such as a fluoroquinolone. The duration of treatment should be a minimum of 2 weeks, although 4 to 6 weeks may be necessary.

The treatment of chronic bacterial prostatitis consists of antibiotics for 4 to 12 weeks. Of the researched treatments, α-adrenergic receptor blockers and antibiotics used alone or in combination result in the greatest improvement in symptoms (see Tables 85.5 and 85.8). Antiinflammatories may also be beneficial. Patients thought to have chronic prostatitis or CPPS should be referred to a urologist.

Treatment of prostatic abscess consists of broad-spectrum intravenous antibiotics (e.g., ciprofloxacin, 400 mg IV every 12 hours) and urologic consultation for perineal drainage or surgical debridement.

RENAL CALCULI

Background

Urolithiasis affects about 12% of the world population and occurs approximately twice as much in men than women.[11] Multiple pathogenic factors interact to cause the formation of renal calculi. Risk factors include older age, male gender, obesity, and family history (Box 85.2). Its incidence depends on geographic, ethnic, dietary, and genetic factors. Approximately 50% of patients will have a recurrence within 5 years.

Pathophysiology

Most ureteral calculi originate in the kidney and then pass into the collecting system. The chemical composition of urinary tract stones is the key factor for determining optimal management. Stones are generally composed of calcium, struvite, or uric acid. Most stones (75%) are composed of calcium oxalate, alone or in combination with calcium phosphate. The hyperexcretion of calcium is a major contributor to stone formation; its most common identified cause is hyperparathyroidism. Other medical conditions that lead to increased calcium levels include hypercalcemia of malignancy, sarcoidosis, and excessive calcium ingestion or increased absorption from the gut. The other major component of calcium stones, oxalate, is influenced by diet. Hyperoxaluria occurs in the presence of small bowel disease, bariatric surgery, Crohn disease, ulcerative colitis, and radiation enteritis.

Magnesium ammonium phosphate (struvite) stones account for approximately 15% of all renal calculi. Struvite stones occur almost exclusively in patients with UTIs and are sometimes referred to as infection stones. They form as a result of the presence of urea-splitting organisms, such as *Proteus, Providencia, Klebsiella, Pseudomonas,* and *Staphylococcus.* Patients with anatomic abnormalities that predispose them to recurrent UTIs are at increased risk of developing struvite stones. Most staghorn calculi—stones that fill the greater part of the collecting system—are composed of struvite.

Uric acid stones account for 10% of all stones in the United States. Approximately 15% of patients with symptomatic gout have uric acid calculi, and the incidence of uric acid stones increases with the use of uricosuric agents. In addition to hyperuricosuria, aciduria is

BOX 85.2   Risk Factors for Urolithiasis

Metabolic disease or disturbance
   Crohn disease
   Milk-alkali syndrome
   Primary hyperparathyroidism
   Hyperoxaluria
   Hyperuricosuria
   Sarcoidosis
   Recurrent UTI
   Renal tubular acidosis (type I)
   Gout
   Laxative abuse
Positive family history
   Hot arid climates (southeast United States)
   Male gender (white men affected more commonly than black men)
   Previous kidney stone
   Dehydration

UTI, urinary tract infection.

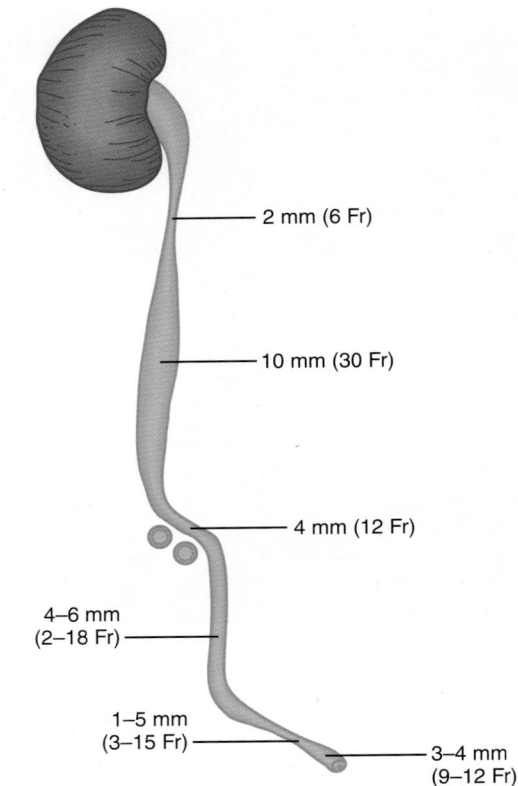

Fig. 85.4 Variations in Caliber of the Ureter. *Fr,* French catheter size. (Adapted from Eisendrath, Rolnick. Lich R Jr, et al. Childhood disorders and diseases. In: Harrison JH, Gittes RF., eds. *Campbell's Urology.* Vol. 1. 4th ed. Philadelphia: WB Saunders; 1978.)

considered necessary because the precipitation of uric acid is unlikely at a higher urine pH. A distinctive feature of uric acid stones is their radiolucency.

Impaction along the genitourinary tract is a serious complication of renal calculi and can cause several physiologic changes. Once obstruction occurs, a rapid redistribution of renal blood flow results in a decrease in the glomerular filtration rate (GFR). As glomerular and tubular function decrease, renal excretion shifts to the unaffected kidney. Obstruction also causes a rapid decrease in ureteral peristaltic activity. In the presence of infection, renal and ureteral function may be impaired. Complete obstruction of the ureters may lead to loss of renal function with an increased incidence of irreversible damage after 1 to 2 weeks. Partial obstruction is associated with a lower likelihood of renal injury but may still result in irreversible damage.

Although calculus size and location are important determinants of the degree of disease, the major cause of progressive renal damage is associated infection. The stone behaves as a foreign body and leads to stasis and obstruction, decreasing host resistance and increasing the incidence of infection. Subsequent infectious complications include pyelonephritis, perinephric abscess, and gram-negative bacterial sepsis.

The three primary predictors of stone passage without the need for surgical intervention are calculus size, location, and degree of patient pain. The most important factor that relates to passage of a calculus though the genitourinary tract is its size. Approximately 90% of stones smaller than 5 mm pass spontaneously within 4 weeks. This percentage decreases to 15% for stones 5 to 8 mm in size. Up to 95% of stones larger than 8 mm become impacted along the genitourinary tract, and lithotripsy or surgical removal is usually required. Surgical intervention can be performed on an outpatient basis, provided the patient is able to tolerate oral intake and has adequate pain control unless the stone is infected, renal damage is considerable, there are bilateral obstructing stones, or there is obstruction of a solitary or transplanted kidney. Spontaneous passage is more frequent with stones located below the midureter than those located above the midureter.

Renal calculi seldom cause complete obstruction. There are five sites along the ureter at which calculi are likely to become impacted (Fig. 85.4). First, a stone may lodge in the calyx of the kidney or

pass into the renal pelvis and become lodged at the ureteropelvic junction. Second, the relatively large renal pelvis (1 cm) narrows abruptly at its distal portion, where it is equal in diameter to its adjoining ureter (2 to 3 mm). The third region is near the pelvic brim, where the ureter arches over the iliac vessels posteriorly into the true pelvis. The most constricted area along the ureter, and a common location for impaction, is the ureterovesicular junction. This is the site at which the ureter enters the muscular coat of the bladder (intramural ureter). At the time of diagnosis, up to 75% of stones are located in the distal third of the ureter. Finally, calculi may become lodged in the vesical orifice.

Clinical Features

The onset of pain usually is abrupt, with a crescendo of extreme pain that begins in the flank, extends laterally around the abdomen, and radiates into the groin. Pain may radiate to the testicles in men and the labia majora in women. A constant, underlying dull ache in the flank is common between episodes of colic. The cause of colicky, severe flank pain is hyperperistalsis of the smooth muscle of the calyces, pelvis, and ureter, whereas the cause of a dull ache can be acute obstruction and renal capsular tension. GI symptoms of nausea and vomiting are common.

One-third of patients experience gross hematuria, with or without blood clots in the urine. Symptoms of urinary urgency and frequency often develop as the stone nears the bladder. A history of fever and chills strongly suggests superimposed infection; these cases should be regarded as true urologic emergencies.

BOX 85.3 Differential Diagnosis for Pain Associated With Urolithiasis

Urologic Disease
Upper Urinary Tract
Renal infarct
Renal parenchymal tumors
Urothelial tumors
Papillary necrosis
Pyelonephritis
Hemorrhage (blood clot)

Ureter
Urothelial tumors
Hemorrhage (blood clot)
Previous surgery (e.g., stricture)
Metastatic tumors

Lower Urinary Tract
Urothelial tumors
Urinary retention

Nonurologic Disease
Intra-abdominal
Peritonitis (especially appendicitis)
Biliary colic
Intestinal obstruction

Vascular
Abdominal aortic aneurysm
Superior mesenteric artery occlusion

Retroperitoneal
Retroperitoneal lymphadenopathy
Retroperitoneal fibrosis
Tumor

Gynecologic
Cervical cancer
Endometriosis
Ovarian vein syndrome

Musculoskeletal
Muscle strain or bony injury

A patient with renal colic often is in severe pain and paces or writhes in pain on the stretcher, unable to find a comfortable position. The abdomen should be auscultated and palpated in search of bruits and thrills over the abdominal aorta and iliac vessels because the clinical manifestations of aortic abdominal aneurysms (AAAs) may mimic those of renal colic. Patients commonly have intermittent pain that may nearly resolve between episodes of severe discomfort.

Differential Diagnosis

A number of clinical diseases can produce pain similar to that of renal colic (Box 85.3). Potentially serious or life-threatening alternate diagnoses include pulmonary embolism, ectopic pregnancy, biliary disease, bowel obstruction, incarcerated inguinal hernia, pancreatitis, appendicitis, AAA, renal vein thrombosis, and renal malignancies and infarction.

Diagnostic Testing

Urinalysis and Culture
Red blood cells (RBCs) generally are found in the urine of patients with urolithiasis. However, the absence of RBCs in the urine does not exclude the diagnosis. Up to 20% of patients with documented urolithiasis have no microscopic hematuria.[12] Furthermore, there is no correlation between the degree of obstruction and absence of hematuria.

Sterile pyuria can occur in the absence of infection as a result of ureteral inflammation, but the presence of a UTI should be investigated if other clinical signs of infection are present, such as fever and chills. A urinalysis with culture should be performed to look for pyuria and bacteriuria and to measure nitrite and leukocyte esterase levels when infection is suspected.

The kidney does not produce urine with a pH greater than 7.5 under normal conditions, so a urinary pH higher than 7.5 should raise suspicion for the presence of urea-splitting organisms such as *Proteus*. Renal tubular acidosis and ingestion of absorbable alkali also may increase the urinary pH and should be considered in the differential diagnosis. A pH less than 5 often is associated with the formation of uric acid calculi.

Other Laboratory Tests
Measurement of blood urea nitrogen (BUN) and serum creatinine levels is not routine but should be performed in patients who have a renal calculus with a solitary kidney, transplanted kidney, or history of renal insufficiency. On rare occasions, urolithiasis can present as acute renal failure resulting from obstruction of both ureters or the ureter of a solitary kidney. A slightly elevated white blood cell (WBC) count in patients with renal calculi may be the result of demargination from acute pain, but this is not a sensitive test and should be performed only in patients who are thought to be infected. A significantly elevated WBC count or left shift on the differential suggests active infection.

Imaging
Imaging is not needed in all patients with renal colic but should be performed when signs and symptoms are atypical and the diagnosis is in question, the patient has a solitary or transplanted kidney, or appears toxic, or high-grade obstruction is suspected.

Radiography of the Kidney, Ureter, and Bladder
As an initial imaging study, kidney, ureter, and bladder (KUB) radiography provides only presumptive evidence of calculi (<70% specificity), so it should be followed by a more definitive study or avoided altogether. It is of limited usefulness on its own except to monitor progression of a previously identified radiopaque stone in a stable patient.

Intravenous Pyelography
Intravenous pyelography is an accurate imaging modality to detect renal stones, but is seldom used now because CT scanning and ultrasonography have become first-line imaging modalities. It is very sensitive, capable of establishing the diagnosis of calculous disease in 96% of cases, and it can quantify the presence and severity of obstruction (Fig. 85.5A and B).

Computed Tomography
Non–contrast-enhanced helical (spiral) CT scanning is the standard imaging modality in the U.S. It is 95% sensitive and 98% specific for

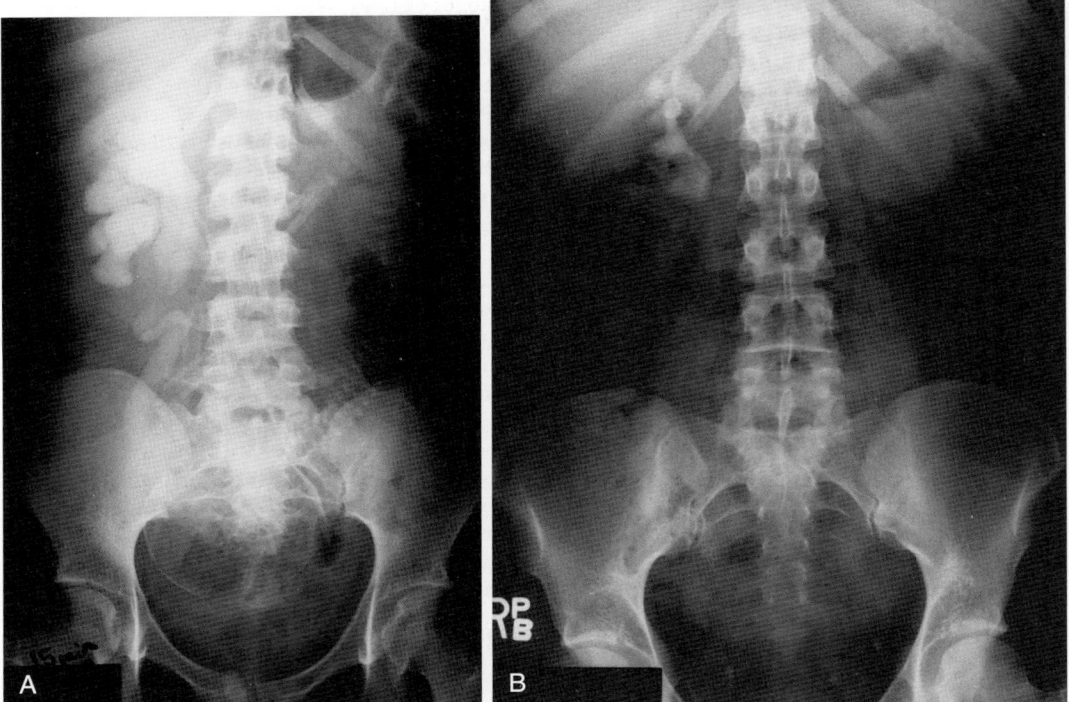

Fig. 85.5 (A) In a near-term pregnant woman with an obstructed left kidney, this intravenous pyelogram demonstrates a delayed nephrogram. (B) The right kidney has physiologic hydronephrosis from ureteral compression by the fetal head.

detecting ureteral calculi.[13] CT may detect calculi as small as 1 mm in diameter and provide direct visualization of complicating conditions such as hydroureter, hydronephrosis (Fig. 85.6), and ureteral edema. Some kidney stones, such as uric acid stones, may be radiolucent. CT is also superior to alternate imaging modalities in its ability to recognize other pathologies, such as malignancy, renal abscess, and AAA. Other advantages include lack of contrast exposure, short duration of testing, and ease of interpretation. For patients with a body mass index less than 30 kg/m², low radiation dose protocols can be used, with sensitivities and specificities still reported as more than 90%.[14] However, many patients with a history of nephrolithiasis and clinical picture consistent with renal colic do not require imaging. Patients with a history of nephrolithiasis who lack fever, a urinalysis showing infection, a solitary or transplanted kidney, suspicion for complicated urolithiasis, or diagnosis other than renal colic may forego CT imaging.[15]

Ultrasonography

Ultrasound, whether performed by a radiology technician or point of care in the ED, may provide diagnostic information to guide further evaluation and treatment. Performing an ultrasound as the initial imaging test often eliminates the need to obtain an abdominal and pelvic CT scan and decreases radiation exposure to the patient. Ultrasound has been found to be up to 100% sensitive and 90% specific for the diagnosis of ureteral obstruction in patients presenting with acute flank pain.[5] This has resulted in some guidelines to recommend it as the initial imaging modality for suspected obstructing ureterolithiasis and identification of hydronephrosis (Fig. 85.7).[16] Ultrasound may also guide clinical suspicion and need for further imaging in patients with less typical signs and symptoms of calculi. It is also the study of choice for ruling out hydronephrosis for pregnant and pediatric patients if obstructive urolithiasis is a concern.[17]

Ultrasound is less sensitive and specific than CT imaging for detecting stone size and location and has been found to be 54% sensitive and 91% specific for the diagnosis of urolithiasis.[18] For potential urological intervention, CT is generally performed given the accuracy for identification of stones and identification of other potential etiologies of flank pain.

Management

The first priority for a patient with a presumed diagnosis of kidney stone is adequate pain control. NSAIDs are first-line agents, but parenteral administration often is necessary because of nausea and vomiting. Ketorolac, 30 mg IV, or diclofenac, 75 mg intramuscularly (IM), provide rapid effective analgesia and decrease both ureteral spasm and renal capsular pressure by diminishing the GFR in the obstructed kidney. Accordingly, caution is advised with use of these agents in patients with underlying renal insufficiency or peptic ulcer disease. An IV narcotic such as fentanyl (1 to 2 µg/kg) is also very effective in providing rapid analgesia. The combination of NSAIDS and opiates may reduce length of stay in the ED. In the patient who is unable to tolerate oral fluids, IV fluids and an antiemetic such as ondansetron, 4 mg IV, should be given. There have been no definitive studies proving that high-volume fluid therapy in those with acute renal colic facilitates stone passage or improves outcomes.[19]

Concomitant infection with an obstructive stone and hydronephrosis constitutes a true urologic emergency and may warrant immediate urologic intervention for placement of ureteral stents or decompression of the renal pelvis by percutaneous nephrostomy.

Disposition

Indications for Admission

Hospitalization is recommended for patients who are severely dehydrated, are experiencing unrelenting pain or vomiting, or have an

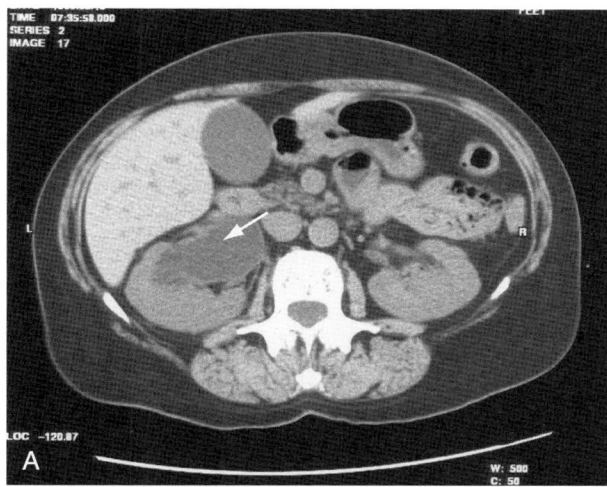
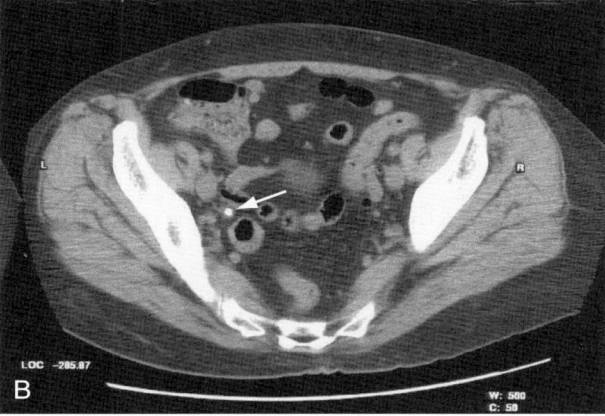

Fig. 85.6 CT Scans Obtained in a Patient With Renal Colic. (A) Right-sided hydronephrosis. (B) Right ureteral calculi.

underlying urinary infection (Box 85.4). Sepsis and renal damage are risks in the presence of obstruction and infection, so these patients require an emergent urologic consultation to evaluate the need for immediate operative intervention to provide drainage and relieve the obstruction. If signs of sepsis (e.g., tachycardia, fever, hypotension, shock) are present, parenteral antibiotics, such as ceftriaxone 1 g IV, should be given and fluid resuscitation carried out pending urologic evaluation.

Several interventional strategies are available to the urologist for the management of stones that do not pass spontaneously. Optimal therapy depends on the size, location, and composition of the stone. Ureteroscopy and extracorporeal shock wave lithotripsy (ESWL) are the two most commonly used techniques. Ureteroscopic removal of ureteral stones, compared to ESWL, achieves a greater stone-free state and lowers the need for retreatment.[20] Both treatment options have a low complication rate.[20] Percutaneous nephrolithotomy, which establishes a tract from the skin to the collecting system, is used for stones too large or hard for ECSWL or ureteroscopy by removing them directly from the renal pelvis.

Outpatient Management

Most patients with nephrolithiasis may be safely managed as outpatients. They should be instructed to return to the ED immediately for intractable or severe pain, persistent nausea and vomiting, fever or chills, or difficulty voiding. Spontaneous passage usually occurs within 4 weeks after the onset of symptoms. Patients with first-time

stones or those who have not had chemical analysis of their stones should strain all urine or simply void into a glass jar; the calculus should be visible at the bottom. The stone can be submitted to the follow-up urologist for analysis. If a stone has not been passed within 4 weeks, intervention is indicated, because the risk of complications such as ureteral stricture and renal function deterioration increase. The patient should be instructed to drink a moderate amount of fluids, take analgesics as needed for pain, and engage in activity as tolerated.

Medical expulsive therapy is a potentially useful treatment modality for the management of ureteral stones. α_1-Antagonists (e.g., tamsulosin, 0.4 mg PO daily) may facilitate stone expulsion and decrease the time to spontaneous stone passage by blocking ureteral smooth muscle contraction and improving antegrade stone movement.[21-23] Some studies have questioned the effectiveness of tamulosin,[24-26] while others have suggested, and current guidelines acknowledge, a therapeutic benefit for patients with larger distal stones (5 to 10 mm).[22,25,27,28]

BLADDER (VESICAL) CALCULUS

Background

Approximately 5% of calculi originate in the bladder. Bladder stones occur almost exclusively in older men, often as a complication of an infection of residual bladder urine with urea-splitting organisms or an indwelling catheter. Other disorders predisposing to the formation of bladder stones include bladder neck obstruction (usually secondary to prostatic hyperplasia), neurogenic bladder, vesical diverticula, damage from irradiation, and schistosomiasis.

Clinical Features

Bladder stones cause pain on voiding and hematuria. The patient may report a sudden interruption of the urinary stream, which strongly suggests a vesical stone that intermittently obstructs the bladder outlet. Frequency, urgency, and dysuria are described by up to 50% of patients, and UTIs are common.

The physical examination is rarely helpful; the rectal examination may reveal an enlarged prostate or prostatic malignancy. Poor sphincter tone may suggest a neurogenic bladder.

Diagnostic Testing

Urinalysis generally reveals pyuria, bacteriuria, and hematuria. Plain radiographs of the pelvis reveal a bladder stone in 50% of cases. Contrast scans may demonstrate obstructive changes in the upper tracts or bladder diverticula. Ultrasonography also is useful in the diagnosis of bladder stones.

Management

Surgery is currently the gold standard of care. Depending on the size of the stone, an endoscopic or open approach is used.

ACUTE SCROTAL PAIN

Background

The most common causes of acute scrotal pain are epididymitis and torsions of the testicle and testicular appendage (Table 85.9). Some are emergent surgical conditions such as Fournier gangrene and incarcerated hernias. Others require less invasive and time-dependent therapies, such as antibiotics for epididymitis and observation for benign masses or torsion of the appendix of the testes. Box 85.5 lists a number of other disorders that can present as scrotal swelling.

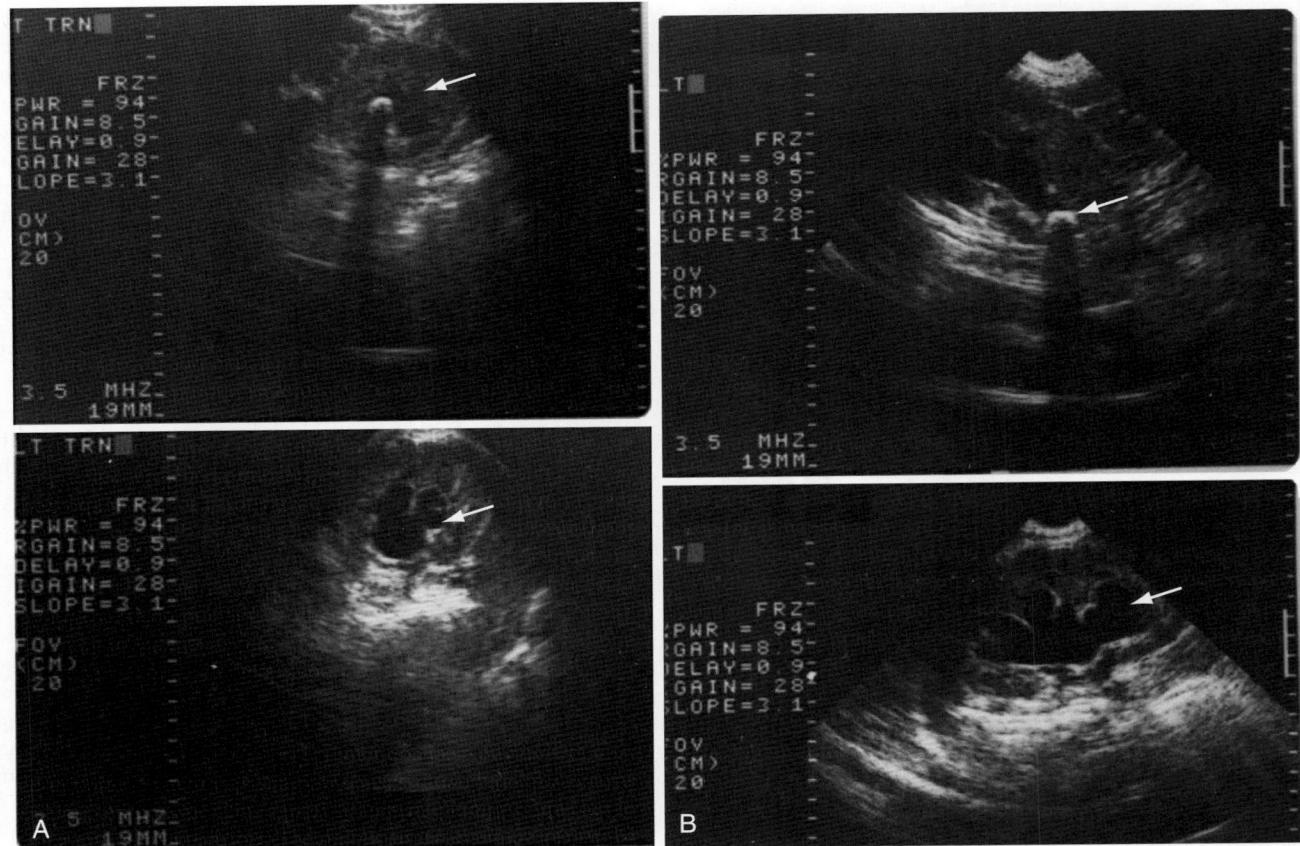

Fig. 85.7 (A) Ultrasound images of the kidney in a patient with renal colic. Hydronephrosis and a calcification with an acoustic shadow are visualized. (B) Ultrasound images of the kidney in a patient with renal colic. Short axis reveals a kidney stone and hydronephrosis.

BOX 85.4   Indications for Hospitalization of Patients With Urolithiasis

Absolute
Obstructing stone with signs of urinary infection
Intractable nausea or vomiting
Severe pain requiring parenteral analgesics
Urinary extravasation
Hypercalcemic crisis

Relative
Significant comorbid illness complicating outpatient management
High-grade obstruction
Leukocytosis
Solitary kidney or intrinsic renal disease
Psychosocial factors adversely affecting home management

Fig. 85.8 demonstrates the anatomy of the scrotum and testis. A normal scrotum is relatively symmetric, and both testicles are of equal mass and volume. The left testicle often is higher than the right because its blood flow empties into the large, low-pressure vena cava, whereas the right drains into the relatively smaller, high-pressure renal vein. A normal testis is found in the vertical axis with a slight forward tilt, and the epididymis is above the superior pole in the posterolateral position. The epididymis is located posterolateral to the testis and is normally nontender and soft. The cremasteric reflex is elicited by stroking or pinching the inner aspect of the thigh; more than 0.5 cm of elevation of the ipsilateral testicle is considered evidence of a normal reflex. This reflex normally is absent in 50% of male infants younger than 30 months.

SPECIFIC DISORDERS

Testicular Torsion

Background

The incidence of testicular torsion in males below 25 years old is approximately 1:4000.[29] Torsion can occur at any age, but has a bimodal age-incidence in the first year of life and at puberty during testicular growth (Fig 85.9). In neonatal torsion, extravaginal torsion usually occurs, with twisting of the entire cord including the tunica vaginalis. In older children and adults, intravaginal torsion (twisting of the cord within the tunica vaginalis) occurs and is commonly associated with a bell-clapper deformity.[30] A bell-clapper deformity is a congenitally abnormal fixation of the tunica vaginalis to the testicle that results in increased mobility of the testicle.

With torsion, abnormal testicular rotation of the spermatic cord results in obstruction of venous outflow, subsequent compromised arterial flow, and testicular ischemia. Testicular salvage hinges on the degree of torsion and duration of the ischemia. Testicular torsion in neonates has few known etiological factors, poor testicular viability, and rarely present to the ED.[31] Thus, the remainder of this discussion will focus on intravaginal torsion. Torsion that presents to the ED within 6 hours of the start of pain is associated with testicular salvage rates greater than 90%. After 6 hours of torsion, the rate of testicular

TABLE 85.9   Differentiation Among Common Causes of the Acute Scrotum

Parameter	Testicular Torsion	Appendix Torsion	Epididymitis
Age	<1 year, puberty	7–14 years	Adult
Onset	Hours	1–2 days	Days to weeks
Location of pain	Entire testicle	Upper pole	Epididymis
Testicle position	High-riding testicle Transverse alignment	Normal position Vertical alignment	Normal position Vertical alignment
Systemic symptoms	Nausea, vomiting	None	Possibly fever
Cremasteric reflex	No	Intact	Intact
Pyuria	Rare	No	Yes
Ultrasound findings	Diffusely hypoechoic Asymmetric testicles Normal or decreased flow Spermatic cord twist	Focally hypoechoic Symmetrical testicles Normal flow	Hypoechoic epididymis Symmetric testicles Increased flow
Treatment	Surgery	Supportive	Antibiotics; prepubescent—supportive only

Note: No single finding in patients with an acute scrotum can reliably differentiate torsion from other causative disorders. When torsion is a diagnostic possibility, prompt urology consultation and further testing are mandatory.

BOX 85.5   Causes of Acute Scrotal Swelling

Infant
Hernia
Hydrocele

Child
Hernia
Torsion
Epididymitis

Adolescent
Epididymitis
Torsion
Trauma

Adult
Epididymitis
Hernia
Trauma
Tumor
Torsion
Fournier gangrene

atrophy and orchiectomy increases rapidly. There is poor testicular viability if detorsion is delayed 24 hours or more.[29]

Clinical Features

Patients with testicular torsion typically report the sudden onset of rapidly escalating pain in the scrotum, lower abdomen, or inguinal area that awakens them from sleep or develops several hours after physical activity. While torsion can occur after trauma, it usually occurs without any specific preceding event. Patients with testicular torsion may describe similar pain in the past, caused by previous intermittent torsion in a predisposed testicle. Because torsion may present with abdominal pain and no scrotal pain, the scrotum should be examined in all patients presenting with abdominal pain.

The physical examination is more reliable than the history in determining the presence of testicular torsion. Patients with torsion frequently have a tender firm testicle that can be higher than the contralateral testicle owing to shortening of a twisted spermatic cord. Twisting also can leave the testicle in the transverse position and displace the epididymis from its usual location along the posterior aspect of the scrotum. Often, the patient's scrotum is so swollen and tender that a complete physical examination is impossible. The cremasteric reflex is usually absent in patients with torsion; however, its presence cannot be used to rule out torsion. The cremasteric reflex occurs when the ipsilateral testicle elevates after stroking the medial thigh. This reflex may be absent in normal patients as well as those with upper and lower motor neuron disorders or spinal cord trauma.[32]

Differential Diagnosis

There is no single historical or physical finding that reliably differentiates testicular torsion from other causes of acute scrotal pain (see Table 85.9).

Diagnostic Testing

Urinalysis

In patients in whom the history and physical findings strongly suggest torsion, emergent surgical consultation is warranted. If the diagnosis is equivocal, adjunctive tests should be performed to determine the cause of the pain. Although urinalysis results suggestive of infection are consistent with epididymitis, such findings also may be noted in patients with torsion and a concomitant UTI.

Imaging

Ultrasound is the diagnostic modality of choice for detecting torsion and has a sensitivity of 96% to 100% and specificity of 84% to 95%.[33] The torsed testicle is typically hypoechoic and enlarged (Fig. 85.10). False-negative findings occur when the testicle is examined early in the course of the disease, when blood flow is still present, and with intermittent torsion. Examination of the spermatic cord for twisting, instead of the testicle itself, has been shown to reduce the frequency of these false-negative results. Ultrasound is helpful when it demonstrates torsion in patients with equivocal findings on the history and physical examination, but it does not have sufficient sensitivity to rule out a diagnosis of torsion. A urologist should evaluate any patient in whom ultrasound findings are negative but history and physical

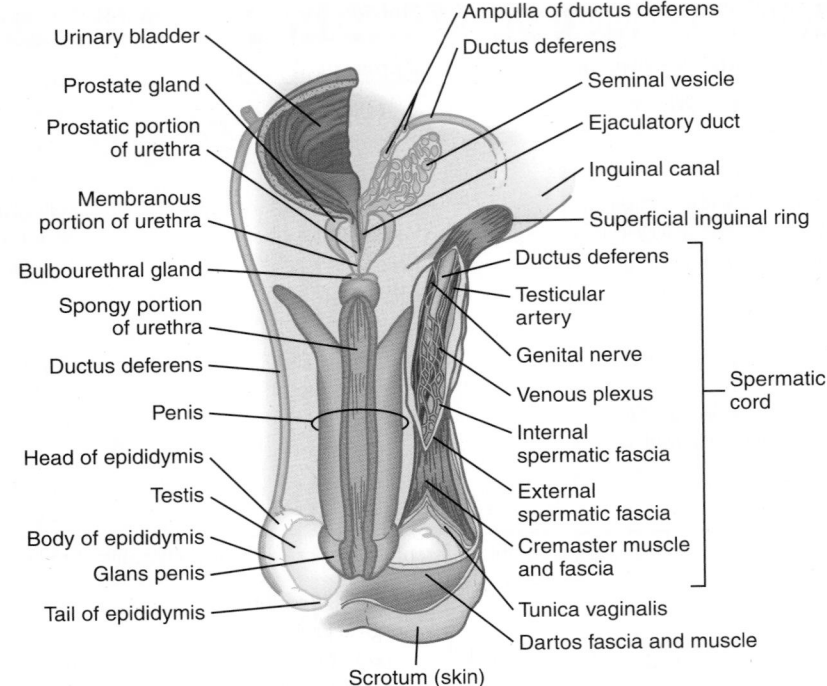

Fig. 85.8 Testes, Epididymis, Ductus Deferens, and Glands of the Male Reproductive System. (From Seeley RR, et al., eds. *Anatomy and Physiology.* New York: McGraw-Hill; 1985.)

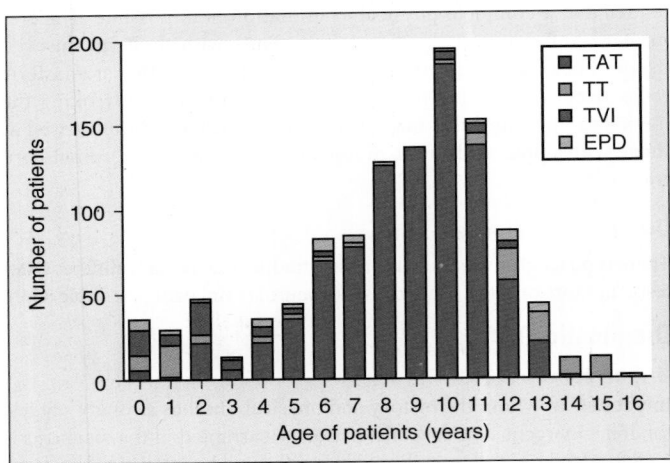

Fig. 85.9 Age distribution of boys with torsion of the appendix testis *(TAT)*, testicular torsion *(TT)*, tunica vaginalis inflammation *(TVI)*, and epididymitis *(EPD)*. (From Yang C, Song B, Liu X, et al. Acute scrotum in children: an 18-year retrospective study. *Pediatr Emerg Care.* 2011;27:270–274.)

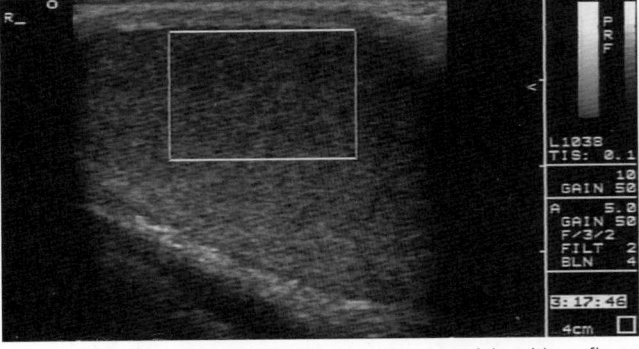

Fig. 85.10 Doppler ultrasound image showing a testicle with no flow as a result of torsion *(white box).* (From Blaivas M, Brannam L. Testicular ultrasound. *Emerg Med Clin North Am.* 2004;22:723–748.)

findings are suggestive of torsion. Moreover, an ultrasound examination should never delay evaluation by a urologist in a patient with probable torsion.

Ultrasound imaging for testicular torsion includes both grayscale and Doppler examination. Grayscale imaging can identify a spermatic cord twist, called a "whirlpool sign," above the testis. The parenchymal echotexture on ultrasound may help predict the viability of the testicle. Homogeneous echotexture portends extremely well for testicular viability. However, varying degrees of heterogeneous parenchymal echotexture may be seen in testicular torsion and significant heterogeneity indicates late torsion and testicular nonviability.[34–36] Grayscale

imaging can also identify other diagnoses such as inflammation due to epididymitis and scrotal masses.

The Doppler ultrasound appearance of the testicle depends on the degree of twisting of the spermatic cord. With 180 degrees or less of twisting of the cord, venous flow from the testicle ceases but arterial flow persists. This leads to edema of the testicle on ultrasound that can be misinterpreted as inconsistent with torsion. In contrast, with more than 180 degrees of twisting of the cord, arterial flow also ceases, leading to a lack of Doppler signal on ultrasound.

Doppler studies can be more difficult to interpret in younger boys because blood flow is physiologically low in the testicles of prepubertal boys. As many as 50% of boys younger than 8 years do not show intratesticular flow. This hypovascularity can result in false-positive diagnoses, which could potentially lead to unnecessary surgical exploration. Comparison with the contralateral testicle can help avoid this misdiagnosis; as in normal patients, blood flow to the two testicles will be similar.

Magnetic resonance imaging (MRI) and radionuclide scanning of the scrotum have also been used to diagnose testicular torsion but are time-consuming. They have largely been replaced by ultrasound.

Management

The first step in the management of suspected testicular torsion is immediate consultation with a urologist. The longer the spermatic cord remains twisted, the lower the likelihood of testicular salvage. In addition, early consultation allows the urologist to accompany the patient to ultrasound—if imaging is obtained—where images can be reviewed in real time with the radiologist. Analgesia is provided systemically or with a spermatic cord block.

If the urologist is not readily available, manual detorsion may improve testicular salvage and should be attempted (Fig. 85.11).[37] Relief should be felt when the operator rotates the affected testicle away from the midline, as if turning the pages of a book. If this maneuver is successful, patients should report immediate improvement of symptoms. If only partial relief of pain is noticed, an attempt should be made to untwist past 360 degrees because a higher degree of rotation may be present. If pain increases or there is no relief, consider reversing the direction of reduction because over one-third of patients may be torsed laterally.[36] Unfortunately, no independent predictors of the direction of torsion have been identified to guide decision-making on manual detorsion.[36] If manual detorsion is attempted, a spermatic cord block or systemic analgesics should be administered (see Fig. 85.11).

Evaluation by a urologist should never be delayed to perform manual detorsion or any other maneuver. Likewise, regardless of the outcome with manual detorsion, patients require prompt urological evaluation. A surgeon can confirm the reduction and stabilize the testes with orchiopexy. Even for symptoms lasting beyond 24 hours, testicular salvage is possible for incomplete torsion, and orchiopexy can help prevent recurrence. Removal of a necrotic testicle speeds recovery.

Disposition

Rapid diagnosis of testicular torsion is essential and should be followed by emergent surgical scrotal exploration and bilateral orchiopexy, if necessary. Loss of the testicle is usually a result of delay in seeking medical attention. However, many cases of failed testicular salvage have been attributed to misdiagnosis, which almost always leads to orchiectomy and represents a common source of litigation.

TORSION OF APPENDAGES OF THE TESTIS

Background

A normal scrotum has several vestigial appendages that can also twist and become ischemic, with resultant scrotal pain. This process is most common between 7 and 14 years of age, with a mean age of 10 years. In retrospective analyses, torsion of an appendage rivals epididymo-orchitis as the most common cause of the acute scrotum.

The appendix testis, a remnant of the paramesonephric duct, is present in 92% of patients. It is located on the superior aspect of the testicle, between the testis and epididymis (Fig. 85.12). This appendage is prone to torsion owing to its pedunculated shape. After several days of ischemia from torsion, it will undergo necrosis, with eventual reabsorption. Its loss does not permanently affect fertility or have any impact on surrounding structures.

Clinical Features

As with testicular torsion, patients with torsion of an appendage complain of scrotal pain but report milder symptoms, with a more gradual onset. They report nausea, vomiting, urinary symptoms, or previous episodes of similar pain less commonly than patients with testicular

torsion. They usually seek medical attention later than patients with testicular torsion, generally after 48 hours of symptoms.

On physical examination, twisting of the appendix testis leads to formation of a hard, tender, 2- to 3-mm nodule at the upper pole of the testicle. Unlike in testicular torsion, the entire testicle is not tender. The testicle also does not change in overall size, and the scrotum typically does not swell until late in the disease process. The cremasteric reflex typically is intact. On transillumination, the ischemic appendage may rarely be seen as a blue dot.

Diagnostic Testing

Urinalysis should not show evidence of infection. On ultrasound imaging, the appendix under torsion will appear hypoechoic. Color Doppler ultrasound can show decreased flow in normal and torsed appendages. With torsion of the appendix, a hypoechoic spherical nodule with a diameter more than 5 mm is present over the superior aspect of the testicle (Fig. 85.13).

Management and Disposition

If testicular torsion is ruled out, surgical excision of the appendix is rarely necessary. Treatment consists of scrotal support, ice packs, and NSAIDs. Resolution of symptoms can be expected within 7 to 10 days. Surgical excision is reserved for uncontrollable pain.

EPIDIDYMITIS

Background

Epididymitis is the most common intrascrotal inflammatory disease. Most cases occur in men between 18 and 35 years of age, but the disease can affect males at any age. It is uncommon in prepubertal males. If untreated, it can lead to orchitis, testicular abscess and, rarely, sepsis.

The epididymis is a tightly coiled tubular area along the posterior aspect of the testes, where sperm mature before their transit to the vas deferens. The epididymis becomes infected when organisms travel retrograde from the vas deferens. With infection, the ipsilateral testicle is also commonly involved, a condition referred to as epididymo-orchitis.

The common route of infection is local extension, mainly due to infections spreading from the urethra (sexually transmitted pathogens) or bladder (urinary pathogens). The particular organisms involved in the infection depend on the sexual activity of the patient. Although the literature classically describes men younger than 35 years who are prone to *C. trachomatis* and *N. gonorrhoeae* infections, all sexually active men, regardless of age, are at risk for epididymitis from these organisms. Acute epididymitis caused by sexually transmitted enteric organisms occurs in men who are the insertive partner during anal intercourse. Other rare causes of epididymitis include *M. tuberculosis*, *Treponema pallidum*, fungal infections, amiodarone use, and systemic inflammatory conditions such as Behçet syndrome.

In men older than 35 years, urinary tract pathogens become the predominant cause of epididymitis. Unlike younger patients, older men with epididymitis tend to have urinary tract abnormalities that predispose them to these infections. Over 50% of men older than 60 years with epididymitis have lower urinary tract obstruction. Older men also are more likely to have concomitant prostatitis, benign prostatic hypertrophy (BPH), immunosuppression, or systemic disease or have undergone recent genitourinary instrumentation, surgery, or catheterization.

Epididymitis in children is usually idiopathic, although children can also have congenital genitourinary anomalies that predispose them to recurrent infection. The most commonly associated abnormality is neurogenic bladder, which produces increased pressure during urination and reflux into the ejaculatory ducts. In infants, bacterial causes are more common.

MANUAL TESTICULAR DETORSION

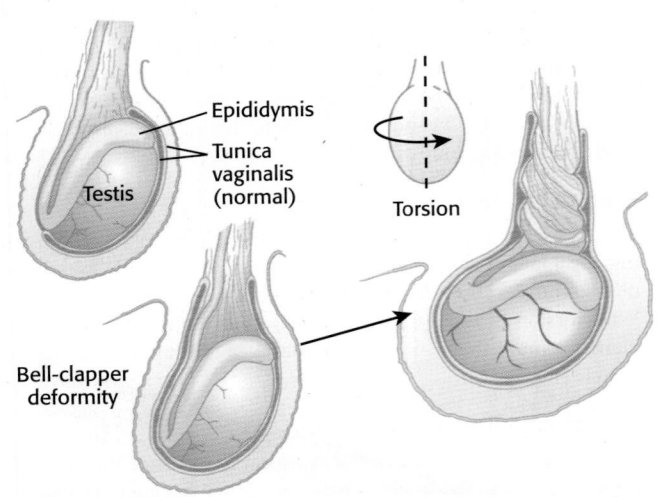

A. **Anatomy of testicular torsion**. Testicular torsion occurs when the testis twists within the tunica vaginalis. Patients with the bell clapper deformity (i.e. incomplete fusion of the tunica along the epididymis, which results in incomplete attachment of the testicle to the scrotum) are at higher risk.

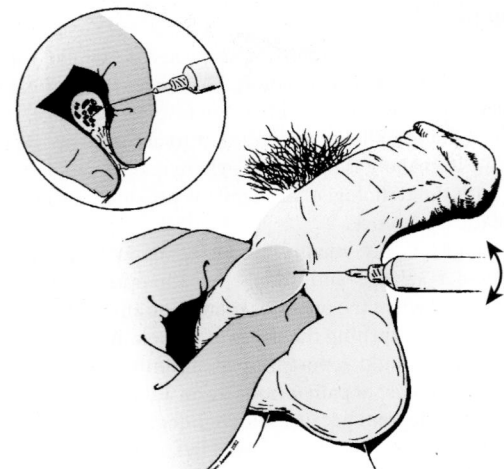

B. **Spermatic cord block**. Grasp the spermatic cord between your thumb and index finger. Use a 30-gauge needle to infiltrate the entire cross section of the spermatic cord and its surrounding rim with anesthetic. This will cause visual ballooning of the grasped segment of the cord. Gently massage this bulge to disperse the anesthetic. Usually about 10 mL is required.

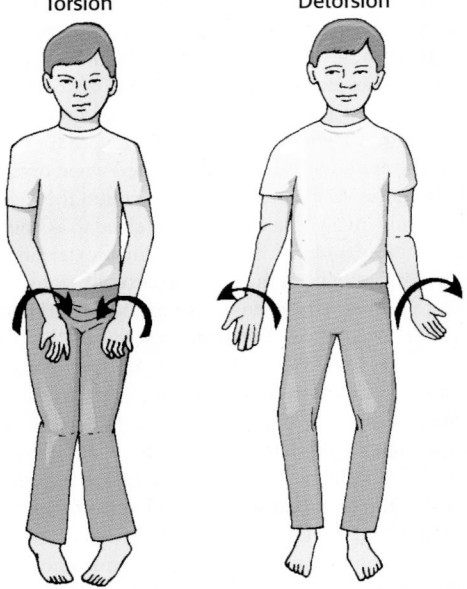

C. Testicular torsion more commonly occurs in a medial direction. Initially attempt detorsion by rotating the testis outward toward the thigh. This is most successful if attempted within the first few hours of torsion, before the onset of significant scrotal swelling. Intravenous narcotics (e.g. fentanyl) can be administered or a cord block performed before attempting detorsion.

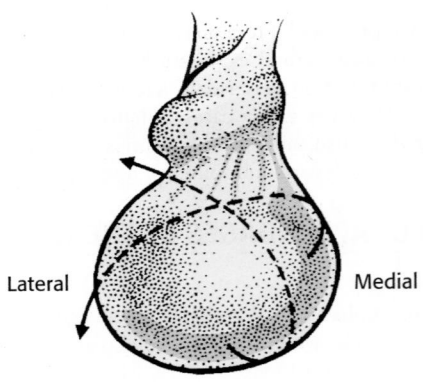

D. **Detorsion maneuver**. Detorsion of the testicle may require testicular rotation through two planes. To release the cremasteric muscle, rotate the testis in a caudal-to-cranial direction simultaneously with medial-to-lateral rotation. The right testis is shown.

Fig. 85.11 Manual Testicular Detorsion. (Adapted from Roberts J, Custalow CB, Thomsen TW, eds. *Roberts and Hedges' clinical procedures in emergency medicine*. 6th ed. St. Louis: Elsevier Health Sciences; 2014.)

Clinical Features

Patients with epididymitis experience scrotal pain of gradual onset, prompting them to present later in the clinical course than patients with torsion. Initially, this pain may reside in the lower abdomen or flank, caused by inflammation of the vas deferens. Fever is uncommon.

In the early stages of the disease, tenderness is localized to the epididymis but quickly spreads to the ipsilateral testicle. Later in the course, the scrotum can become edematous, erythematous, and extremely tender. The testis is located in the normal anatomic position, with an intact cremasteric reflex. Although Prehn sign—decrease in pain with

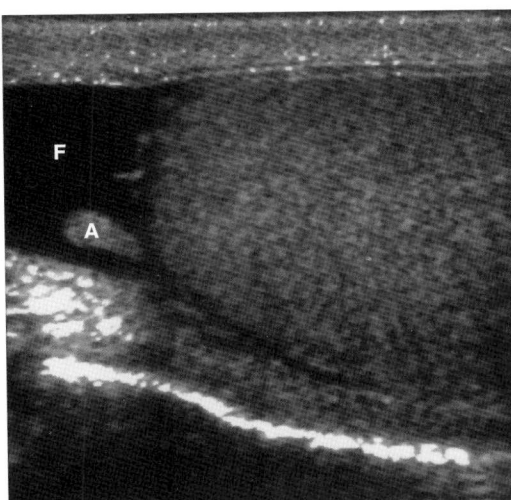

Fig. 85.12 Ultrasound image showing the testicular appendage (A) surrounded by a hydrocele (F). (From Blaivas M, Brannam L. Testicular ultrasound. *Emerg Med Clin North Am.* 2004;22:723–748.)

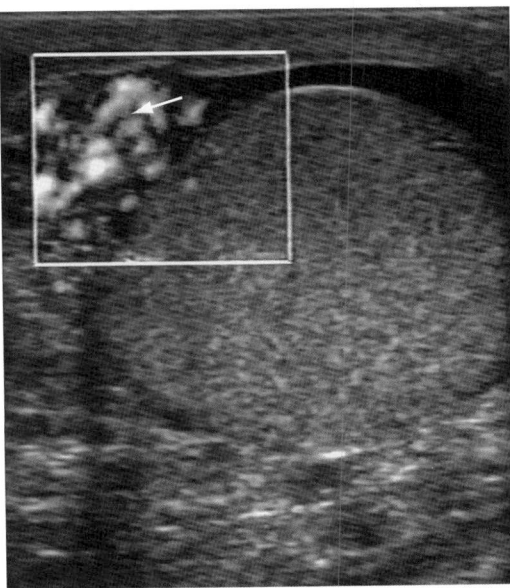

Fig. 85.14 Ultrasound of the testicle showing an enlarged epididymis and increased blood flow on Doppler ultrasound imaging (white box). (From Blaivas M, Brannam L. Testicular ultrasound. *Emerg Med Clin North Am.* 2004;22:723–748.)

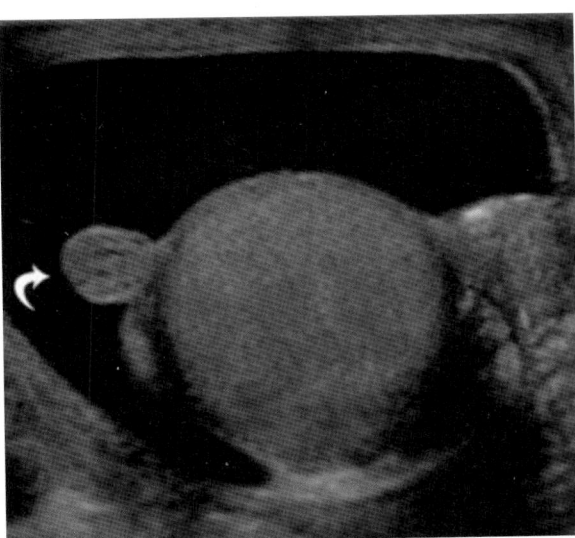

Fig. 85.13 Transverse ultrasound image shows a hyperechoic mass (curved arrow) with tiny central hypoechoic areas adjacent to the left testes and epididymis with a reactive hydrocele and mild scrotal wall thickening. (From Mirochnik B, Bhargava P, Dighe MK, Kanth N. Ultrasound evaluation of scrotal pathology. *Radiol Clin North Am.* 2012;50:317–332.)

Systemic leukocytosis may be present but is a nonspecific finding and does not differentiate epididymitis from torsion. In prepubertal children, urinalysis and urine culture rarely are positive. Nevertheless, in these patients, urine cultures should still be obtained to rule out bacterial infection because untreated bacterial infections may lead to long-term complications.

Because the history and physical examination features and laboratory results cannot reliably distinguish torsion from epididymitis or other diseases, equivocal presentation for epididymitis versus testicular torsion should be assessed using testicular ultrasound with Doppler. On ultrasound, an inflamed epididymis appears enlarged and hypoechoic (Fig. 85.14). However, a minority of patients with torsion have preserved flow that can appear similar to that of epididymitis; in these cases, the presence of a spermatic cord twist, indicative of torsion, should be sought.

Prepubertal children with recurrent epididymitis should undergo renal ultrasound and cystography to identify potential underlying urinary tract abnormalities. These are important to identify to reduce the risk of future inflammation.

Management

Empirical antibiotics are selected in accordance with the patient's risk for chlamydia and gonorrhea and/or enteric organisms (Table 85.10). Treatment goals include curing infection, preventing transmission, and reducing future complications such as infertility and chronic pain.

In patients with a suspected sexually acquired infection, ceftriaxone, 500 mg IM, should be given to treat possible *N. gonorrhoeae* infection. In conjunction, doxycycline, 100 mg PO twice a day for 10 to 14 days, should be started to treat *C. trachomatis* or *Ureaplasma urealyticum* infection.[38] Men with suspected or confirmed *N. gonorrhoeae* or *C. trachomatis* infection should be advised to abstain from sexual intercourse until they and their partners have been treated. Treatment of sexual partners should be arranged, even if the partner's culture demonstrates no growth.

In patients with infection by enteric organisms, levofloxacin, 500 mg PO once daily, or ofloxacin, 300 mg PO every 12 hours, is recommended. If the patient is high risk for STIs and enteric organisms,

elevation of the scrotum—has been touted as indicative of epididymitis, it has low sensitivity and specificity. Only 10% of patients with epididymitis from sexually transmitted organisms have symptoms of urethritis or a urethral discharge on examination. No single historical factor or physical finding has been shown to differentiate torsion from epididymitis reliably.

Diagnostic Testing

The diagnosis of epididymitis is typically made based on compatible physical examination findings and confirmed by laboratory testing. A urinalysis usually demonstrates evidence of pyuria. If patients are at risk for STI, a urethral swab or first-void urine sample should be tested for *C. trachomatis* and *N. gonorrhoeae*; a polymerase chain reaction (PCR) assay and other nucleic acid amplification tests have the greatest sensitivity and should be used, when available.

TABLE 85.10 Treatment of Epididymitis

Drug of Choice	Dose and Route
Presumed Sexually Acquired Epididymitis	
Ceftriaxone *plus*	500 mg IM once
Doxycycline	100 mg PO twice a day for 10 days
Presumed Enteric Epididymitis[a]	
Levofloxacin	500 mg PO daily for 10 days
Potential Sexually Acquired or Enteric Epididymitis[a]	
Ceftriaxone *plus*	500 mg IM once
Levofloxacin	500 mg PO daily for 10 days

[a]Adjust antibacterial therapy according to results of urine culture.
IM, Intramuscularly; *PO,* orally.

treatment should include ceftriaxone and fluoroquinolones (see Table 85.10). Despite the absence of evidence to support benefit, we also recommend bed rest, scrotal elevation, ice packs, and NSAIDs. Discomfort may not completely resolve until weeks after completing an antibiotic regimen.

Most cases of pediatric epididymitis are idiopathic, and antibiotics are not routinely recommended. Urine culture specimens should be obtained and antibiotic therapy should be initiated only if cultures reveal bacteria. Despite the absence of evidence to support benefit, we recommend that boys limit activity, elevate the scrotum with ice packs, and reduce inflammation with NSAIDs. In contrast, infants often have bacterial epididymitis and should be treated empirically with antibiotics pending urine culture results.

Disposition

Patients with systemic signs of toxicity (fever, chills, nausea, vomiting) usually have extension of the infection to involve the testicle, termed epididymo-orchitis. These patients often require hospitalization and treatment with parenteral antibiotics. Most well-appearing patients with uncomplicated epididymitis can be managed as outpatients. Urology referral should be arranged for those likely infected with enteric organisms. Signs and symptoms of epididymitis that do not subside within 3 days require reevaluation of the diagnosis and therapy.

ORCHITIS

Background

Orchitis is a rare acute infection of the testis. With the exception of viral diseases, genitourinary tract infections seldom primarily involve the testis. Orchitis often presents as a progression of epididymitis and may be caused by bacterial or viral infection. Bacterial causes are usually associated with epididymo-orchitis. The most common viral cause of orchitis is mumps. Orchitis due to mumps tends to arise several days after the onset of parotitis. Although vaccination has significantly reduced the incidence of mumps infection, sporadic outbreaks have occurred. Infections in vaccinated individuals are increasingly common, presumably resulting from vaccine failure or antigenic differences between the infecting and vaccine strains.

Owing to the testes' relatively high threshold of resistance to infection, bacterial orchitis usually results from local bacterial spread from the epididymis, frequently referred to as epididymo-orchitis. The most frequent bacterial pathogens are *N. gonorrhoeae, C. trachomatis, E. coli, Klebsiella,* and *P. aeruginosa.* These organisms tend to infect postpubertal males and men older than 50 years with BPH.

Clinical Features

A patient with mumps orchitis has testicular pain and swelling that commonly begins 4 to 6 days after the onset of parotitis, although it can develop in the absence of parotitis. The clinical course varies, with adults having more severe symptoms. Clinical resolution generally occurs in 4 to 5 days.

Patients with bacterial orchitis typically have fever and scrotal pain. They often have constitutional signs and symptoms, including nausea, vomiting, myalgias, and malaise. The disease may be bilateral in up to 30% of patients. The affected testicle and scrotum are swollen, tender, and erythematous.

Diagnostic Testing

As with all causes of scrotal pain, the first priority is to exclude testicular torsion. If the patient clearly has mumps orchitis based on the clinical presentation and a history of preceding parotitis, no other tests are necessary. For all other patients, urinalysis, urine culture, and ultrasound should be performed. On ultrasound, orchitis shows hypervascularity, commonly described as a testicular inferno. Blood tests are typically not helpful, because false-negative results are common with serologic testing, particularly in vaccinated individuals.

Management

In sexually active patients, ceftriaxone and doxycycline should be used to cover *N. gonorrhoeae* and *C. trachomatis.* In older patients, fluoroquinolones provide the best coverage of gram-negative organisms (see Table 85.10). Treatment of viral orchitis is supportive only. Although steroids may improve symptoms, they can reduce testosterone levels. All patients should receive local scrotal care as described for epididymitis. Patients with marked pain, high fever, or constitutional symptoms merit hospitalization and parenteral antibiotics.

TESTICULAR TUMORS

Background

Tumor of the testis is the most common malignancy in young men but accounts for only 1% of all cancers in men. These tumors are more common in infertile patients and patients with cryptorchidism. Approximately 95% of testicular tumors are germ cell tumors, with 50% of these being seminomas and the other 50% being mixed types, including teratomas, choriocarcinomas, and yolk sac tumors. The other 5% of testicular tumors are sex cord stromal tumors. The disease course will depend on the type of tumor present, as well as the age of the patient.

Clinical Features

Testicular cancer usually presents as a painless, unilateral scrotal mass or as an incidental ultrasound finding. However, scrotal pain may be the first symptom in up to 20% of cases. Unlike other painless scrotal masses, such as hydroceles and varicoceles, tumors cannot be separated from the underlying testicle. Palpable tumors are more likely to be malignant compared with tumors identified only with imaging.

Diagnostic Testing

All patients with a scrotal enlargement or palpable scrotal lesions on physical examination should undergo a scrotal ultrasound examination. This study can reveal a concomitant hydrocele or homogeneous hypoechoic lesion. Intratesticular tumors are typically hypervascular, with irregular branching vessels. Leydig cell tumors are unique, because they show hypervascularity around the lesion but no internal color Doppler flow. Although helpful for staging purposes, CT scans of the chest and abdomen are necessary in the ED only if the patient has complaints related to these parts of the body. Most paratesticular masses are benign lesions such as epididymal cysts, epididymitis, spermatoceles, hydroceles, or hernias.

Management and Disposition

Urgent referral to a urologist is indicated for patients with intratesticular masses. The radiosensitive nature of seminomas renders the combined treatment of orchiectomy and radiation therapy highly successful for early-stage disease. Testicular cancer has become one of the most curable solid neoplasms, with an expected 5-year survival rate over 95%.[39]

TESTICULAR TRAUMA

The most concerning injury associated with trauma is rupture of the testicle. Testicular rupture is characterized by tear of the tunica albuginea and extrusion of the seminiferous tubules. The presentation can range from a tender, large, blood-filled scrotum to minimal swelling, with mild pain of the testicle. If there is any concern for rupture, scrotal ultrasound is indicated. Disruption in the echogenic tunica albuginea is 100% sensitive and 65% specific for rupture. Early surgical intervention is associated with higher rates of testicular salvage. Hematomas can be intratesticular or extratesticular, with or without testicular rupture. Similar to rupture, rapid evacuation of an intratesticular hematoma will reduce the risk of necrosis. Extratesticular hemorrhage into the tunica vaginalis is termed a *hematocele* and is the most common finding after blunt scrotal injury. Surgical exploration with hematoma extraction is recommended for patients with large hematoceles to prevent testicular atrophy. Approximately 10% of patients with testicular trauma have associated torsion and require prompt identification and detorsion.

INGUINAL HERNIA, ACUTE HYDROCELE, VARICOCELE, AND SPERMATOCELE

Inguinal hernias, hydroceles, varicoceles, and spermatoceles are considerations in the differential diagnosis of an acute scrotal mass. These clinical entities are typically painless and readily identifiable on physical examination.

Most children with inguinal hernias will not have a palpable mass on examination but will report a history of intermittent bulge in the groin that appears with straining or crying. Less commonly, an inguinal mass is palpable and may extend into the scrotum. If this mass becomes incarcerated, it will be tender, and often the overlying skin will be edematous and erythematous. Children typically will develop irritability, vomiting, or abdominal distention. Incarcerated hernias should be reduced promptly to prevent bowel infarction from strangulation. Reduction can be accomplished by placing the patient in a Trendelenburg position and applying gentle pressure to expel the gas and stool in the bowel from the hernia. Pressure is then applied over the distal aspect of the hernia to reduce the bowel. If this technique fails, surgery is consulted. After reduction of an incarcerated hernia, children typically require hospitalization and delayed surgical repair.

Acute hydroceles typically are benign. They are caused by the accumulation of fluid between the two layers of the tunica vaginalis. They are painless, localized to the scrotum, and will transilluminate.

Varicoceles are enlarged spermatic cord veins that typically are painless or cause only minimal discomfort. On examination, they are often described as feeling similar to a bag of worms, just superior to the testicle, and decrease in size when the patient is supine. In contrast, a spermatocele is a sperm-containing cyst that is palpated as a nontender mass posterior to the testicle. Ultrasound is diagnostic of these conditions. No emergent treatment is necessary, but patients require outpatient urologic evaluation.

Regardless of the cause of the scrotal swelling, concomitant pathology is always a consideration. A careful evaluation for torsion, epididymitis, and tumors should be performed.

ACUTE URINARY RETENTION

Background

AUR is the sudden inability to pass urine voluntarily from the bladder. The lifetime risk of AUR increases with age, occurring in 10% of men in their 70s and in 33% of men in their 80s. AUR is usually caused by an obstructive lesion but also can be the presenting manifestation of other pathologic processes. AUR in women is much less common than in men; common causes in women include an atonic bladder, inflammation occurring postpartum or secondary to herpes, Bartholin abscess, acute urethritis, or vulvovaginitis. Causes in younger patients include obstruction, cystitis, and neurologic disturbances.

Physiology and Pathophysiology

Holding urine requires relaxation of the bladder detrusor muscle, through parasympathetic inhibition and β-adrenergic stimulation, and contraction of the bladder neck and internal sphincter, through α-adrenergic stimulation. Conversely, micturition requires a coordinated contraction of detrusor muscle, with the simultaneous relaxation of the urethral sphincter muscle. AUR results from a disruption of this coordinated physiology caused by an increased resistance to flow via mechanical (e.g., urethral stricture, clot retention) or dynamic means (e.g., increased α-adrenergic activity, prostatic inflammation) or decreased neurogenic control of the detrusor muscle (e.g., drugs inhibiting bladder contractility, diabetes cystopathy).

The most common cause of AUR seen in the ED is obstruction of the urinary tract distal to the bladder. In men, BPH is the most common precipitant. Enlargement of the prostate coupled with constriction of the prostatic urethra from heightened α-adrenergic tone obstructs urinary output. Strictures of the urethra after prior procedural trauma, infection, or radiation therapy can also lead to AUR. Other less common obstructive causes of AUR include prostate cancer, phimosis (inability to retract the foreskin over the glans penis), and paraphimosis (inability to reduce the foreskin over an edematous glans). In women, the most frequent obstructive causes are pelvic masses and prolapse of pelvic organs such as the bladder, rectum, or uterus. These structures cause AUR by compressing the urethra and obstructing urine flow. Finally, congenital posterior urethral valves are the most common source of AUR in children.

Infectious and inflammatory conditions can also cause AUR from urethral edema and obstruction, particularly in the setting of underlying prostatic disease. The most common infectious causative disorder is acute prostatitis, followed by urethritis and vulvovaginitis. In pediatric patients. UTIs can induce sufficient dysuria that the child refuses to void, with consequent urinary retention.

Pharmacologic agents associated with AUR include the anticholinergic and sympathomimetic agents. Anticholinergic agents inhibit detrusor muscle contraction, whereas sympathomimetic agents increase α-adrenergic tone in the prostate. NSAIDs and calcium channel blockers have also been known to increase the rate of AUR by inhibiting prostaglandin and calcium-mediated detrusor muscle contraction.

Neurogenic causes of AUR result from a cortical, spinal cord, or peripheral nerve deficit in the sensory or motor nerve supply of the detrusor muscle. Most neurologic causes of AUR are chronic conditions such as multiple sclerosis, Parkinson disease, neoplasms, and diabetic peripheral neuropathy. Other more acute neurologic conditions that should be diagnosed emergently as causative factors in the ED include spinal trauma, stroke, epidural abscess, and intervertebral disk herniation.

Clinical Features

Although the potential causes of AUR are many, the history and physical examination can considerably narrow the scope of the differential diagnosis (Table 85.11). Most patients with AUR report sudden pain and have a distended tender bladder. Patients with dementia or limited verbal ability may only present with restlessness and agitation. With lesions proximal to the bladder, patients typically note pain in the flank, whereas lesions distal to the bladder can produce pain radiating to the scrotum or labia. With acute obstruction, pain is often quite severe. Patients with slowly developing or chronic obstructions are typically older and report overflow incontinence and little to no pain.

When obstruction is the cause of AUR, the patient often will recall multiple previous episodes of urinary retention. In addition to this history, patients with BPH report frequency, urgency, hesitancy, nocturia, difficulty initiating the urinary stream, decreased force of the stream, sensation of incomplete voiding, and terminal dribbling. The prostate is enlarged, firm, and nonnodular. Normal findings on the prostate examination do not exclude BPH. Patients with prostate cancer can have similar symptoms, but these are more often accompanied by weight loss, bone pain, and other constitutional signs and symptoms. These patients generally will have an enlarged nodular prostate. Examination of the penis is important to identify phimosis or paraphimosis. In women with obstruction, pelvic pain and pressure are symptoms commonly associated with AUR. A prolapsed bladder, rectum, or uterus and enlarged ovaries or uterus can be identified on pelvic examination.

Patients with an infectious cause for their symptoms may complain of dysuria, frequency, urgency, hematuria, fever, chills, and low back pain. In acute prostatitis, these symptoms can be associated with penile discharge and a tender boggy prostate. Despite the obstruction, the patient may nevertheless be able to void small amounts of urine. In vulvovaginitis and urethritis, presenting complaints also may include discharge, pruritus, and vulvar skin findings.

Patients with a neurogenic cause for AUR may already have a history of neurologic disease that contributes to AUR. The examination should focus on any findings suggestive of acute neurologic deficit. Strength, sensation, and reflexes in the lower extremities should be examined because they have similar innervation to that of the bladder. The status of the bulbocavernosus reflex, anal reflex, sphincter tone, and perineal sensation should also be assessed.

Differential Diagnosis

The differential diagnosis for AUR is very broad and dependent on the patient's symptoms (Box 85.6). AUR presenting as lower abdominal pain may present similarly to small bowel obstruction, UTI, or prostatitis. Flank and back pain secondary to hydronephrosis can be confused with nephrolithiasis, pyelonephritis, and spinal pathology. Urinary symptoms of overflow incontinence and urinary hesitancy can be confused with UTI or spinal cord compression. Genital pain may present similarly to trauma, testicular torsion, or inguinal hernia.

TABLE 85.11   Presentation and Diagnosis of Acute Urinary Retention

Cause	History	Physical Examination Findings	Diagnosis[a]
Benign prostatic hypertrophy	Frequency, urgency, hesitancy Prior retention	Enlarged, firm prostate	UA
Prostate cancer	Frequency, urgency, hesitancy Previous retention Constitutional symptoms	Enlarged, firm prostate Nodular prostate	UA
Phimosis, paraphimosis	Penile pain	Nonretractable foreskin Edematous penis	Clinical only
Prostatitis	Dysuria, frequency, urgency Fever, chills	Warm, tender, boggy prostate Penile discharge	UA Urine culture
Urethritis, vulvovaginitis	Dysuria, frequency, urgency Itching	Discharge	UA Urine culture Urethral or cervical culture
Pelvic mass	Pelvic pain pressure	Prolapse of rectum, bladder, uterus	UA Ultrasound imaging, CT
Neurogenic bladder	Other neurologic complaints	Neurologic deficits	UA CT, MRI

[a]In the emergency department setting, each of these diagnoses is made primarily by the history and findings on the physical examination. Additional tests are needed as described.
CT, Computed tomography; MRI, magnetic resonance imaging; UA, urinalysis.

Diagnostic Testing

A urinalysis is recommended for AUR as it can reveal infection or the presence of hematuria from infection, tumor, or calculi. A basic chemistry panel for the assessment of renal function should be performed only when renal damage or hydronephrosis is a concern. There is no history, physical examination, or ultrasound finding that can reliably correlate with an acutely elevated creatinine level. It should be considered for patients with prolonged obstruction or preexisting renal insufficiency.

Additional studies are selectively indicated based on the history and physical examination to identify potentially serious or reversible causes, or when the diagnosis of AUR is unclear. With an equivocal history or physical examination, bedside ultrasound can confirm AUR.

BOX 85.6 Causes of Acute Urinary Retention in Adults

Obstructive
Benign prostatic hypertrophy
Prostatitis
Phimosis
Paraphimosis
Meatal stenosis
Tumor
Foreign body
Calculus
Stricture
Hematoma
Carcinoma

Infectious, Inflammatory
Urethritis (severe)
Urinary tract infection
Prostatitis
Severe vulvovaginitis
Genital herpes

Neurologic Causes
Motor Paralytic
Spinal shock
Spinal cord syndromes

Sensory Paralytic
Tabes dorsalis
Diabetes
Multiple sclerosis
Syringomyelia
Spinal cord syndromes
Herpes zoster

Drugs
Antihistamines
Anticholinergic agents
Antispasmodic agents
Tricyclic antidepressants
α-Adrenergic stimulators
Cold tablets
Ephedrine derivatives
Amphetamines

Psychogenic Problems
Psychodynamic stressors (e.g., lazy bladder syndrome)

Renal and bladder ultrasound studies provide visualization of an elevated postvoid residual, obstruction, hydronephrosis, or other cause of upper urinary tract disease. Pelvic ultrasound examination and CT scan evaluate for masses or malignancy causing obstruction. MRI of the spine detects disk herniation, cord compression, and cauda equina syndrome. Cystoscopy and retrograde cystourethrography can identify problems in the lower urinary tract and usually are performed as outpatient procedures. A prostate-specific antigen assay is not helpful in diagnosing or differentiating prostate cancer from other causes of AUR and should not be routinely performed.

Management

Treatment focuses on bladder decompression and identification of the underlying cause. Immediate placement of a 14 to 18 Fr Foley catheter should provide decompression of the bladder. If this fails, placement of an elbowed catheter (coudé catheter) with a cephalad orientation should be attempted to assist bypassing by any obstruction. If both these techniques prove to be unsuccessful, urologic consultation is indicated. If obstruction is believed to be caused by retained blood clots, a three-way catheter should be placed to allow for bladder irrigation. When immediate bladder decompression is required and a urologist is not available, major urethral trauma is present, or the patient has recently undergone urethral surgery, suprapubic bladder drainage should be performed.

Placement of a catheter has been reported to cause post-obstructive diuresis, hypotension, and hematuria. Such problems are believed to be related to rapid bladder decompression so, historically, gradual decompression has been recommended to prevent these complications. Neither has been proven to have any clinical significance. We recommend that all patients with AUR undergo rapid and complete decompression of the bladder.

Although the catheter is an inconvenience for the patient, and chronic use has been associated with UTIs, trauma, stones, and urethral strictures, early removal of the catheter is also associated with heightened risk for recurrence of AUR, which has been reported in up to 70% of cases. Leaving the catheter in place for 3 to 7 days decreases the incidence of recurrent retention.

Studies have suggested that administration of an α-adrenergic blocker, such as tamsulosin, at the time of catheter insertion in patients with BPH improves the likelihood of spontaneous voiding after catheter removal and may also improve the likelihood that a patient will not require ongoing catheter placement (see Table 85.5). While we recommend this approach, these medications are associated with an increased risk of orthostatic hypotension, particularly in older adults, so initiation of treatment should be coordinated with the patient's primary care physician. 5-Alpha-reductase inhibitors, another agent typically used for BPH, have not been shown to reduce the recurrence of AUR.

Prophylactic antibiotic therapy is not recommended for patients with AUR. Although bacteriuria often develops in patients with indwelling catheters, it typically is not clinically significant, and the use of prophylactic antibiotics only promotes resistance.

Definitive therapy often requires surgical correction of any underlying obstruction. This should not be performed emergently because early surgery is associated with increased morbidity.

Disposition

After bladder drainage, healthy and reliable patients can be safely discharged from the ED with an indwelling catheter and urology follow-up. Patients with concomitant infection, significant comorbid illnesses, impaired renal function, neurologic deficits, or complications from catheterization require further diagnosis and treatment and probably admission.

HEMATURIA

Background

Blood in the urine can be microscopic or gross. Although generally associated with a benign process, microscopic hematuria can reflect serious underlying pathology, such as a urothelial malignancy. Therefore, following ED assessment, patients with any degree of hematuria require outpatient follow-up. Less commonly, patients come to the ED complaining of gross blood in their urine. Compared to microscopic hematuria, gross blood in the urine is more likely to be a presenting symptom of an underlying malignancy. Regardless of age or visibility of blood in the urine, patients with hematuria require evaluation in the ED to rule out life-threatening diagnoses, such as malignancy and AAA.

Gross and microscopic hematuria can arise from anywhere along or near the urinary tract. In the upper and lower portions of the urinary tract, infection, trauma, and renal calculi are the most common causative disorders. Patients also can have more serious causes of hematuria, such as malignancy or vascular lesions (e.g., AAA), and these diagnoses should be excluded. Up to 5% of patients with asymptomatic microscopic hematuria and 30% to 40% of patients with gross hematuria are found to have a urinary tract malignancy. The risk of urologic malignancy is increased in patients older than 35 years, male gender, and those with a history of smoking.

Occasionally, hematuria also has been attributed to warfarin use, BPH, and exercise. Supratherapeutic anticoagulant therapy can lead to blood in the urine, but therapeutic anticoagulation does not typically produce spontaneous hematuria. Similarly, BPH can lead to increased vascularity of the prostate but does not increase the risk of hematuria. High-intensity exercise also can produce hematuria. This bleeding typically is transient and clinically inconsequential. Because warfarin use, BPH, and exercise do not directly cause persistent hematuria, patients with ongoing bleeding require further urologic evaluation.

Clinical Features

A careful history will often identify a benign cause for hematuria, such as menstruation, recent heavy exercise or urologic procedure, sexual activity, or use of agents that can produce red urine without blood (Box 85.7). Repeated episodes of bleeding during and after menstruation in women suggest endometriosis of the urinary tract. Patients may report frequency, urgency, and dysuria in the setting of infection. They may note flank pain with urolithiasis or pyelonephritis. Microscopic hematuria in the setting of a UTI should resolve after appropriate antibiotic treatment.

The physical examination may point toward the underlying cause. For example, hypertension occurs with glomerulosclerosis and, in the setting of peripheral edema, suggests nephrotic syndrome. An abdominal bruit may be caused by an arteriovenous fistula, whereas a palpable abdominal mass may represent an AAA. Flank pain and tenderness can arise with pyelonephritis or nephrolithiasis. The external genital examination can show evidence of trauma or a tumor and may reveal a rectal or vaginal source for the bleeding. A pelvic examination should be performed in women to identify a vaginal or uterine source of bleeding.

Diagnostic Testing

Microscopic hematuria is defined as the presence of three or more RBCs/high-power field (hpf) of urinary sediment. A clean-catch or catheterized urine specimen should be obtained in all patients with hematuria. Catheterization itself induces hematuria in approximately 15% of patients, but the amount of bleeding is inconsequential, rarely exceeding three RBCs/hpf. If available, bedside urine dipstick testing

---

BOX 85.7 Causes of Red-Colored Urine Without Hematuria

Phenazopyridine
Nitrofurantoin
Rifampin
Chloroquine
Hydroxychloroquine
Iodine
Bromide
Food coloring
Beets
Berries
Rhubarb

---

should be performed. A negative urine dipstick rules out the presence of hematuria and obviates the need for urine microscopy. If positive for blood, urine microscopy should be performed.

As little as 1 mL of whole blood in 1 L of urine can produce gross hematuria, turning the urine red. A number of other substances and reactions can turn the urine red, and centrifugation of the urine and microscopic analysis differentiate these false-positive results from true hematuria. After centrifugation, the red color persists only in the urine sediment with hematuria. By contrast, a red supernatant that contains no RBCs on microscopic analysis typically represents a benign condition (see Box 85.7).

Microscopy will reveal WBCs in addition to RBCs in the presence of infection. Proteinuria, cellular casts, and dysmorphic RBCs are seen with glomerular disease. Patients with these findings may also have cola-colored urine and should be referred to a nephrologist.

Management and Disposition

The combination of a careful history, physical examination, and laboratory studies should identify benign causes of microhematuria such as infection, menstruation, vigorous exercise, and trauma. According to the American Urological Association (AUA) Guideline on Asymptomatic Microhematuria, once benign causes have been ruled out, a prompt outpatient urologic evaluation should occur.[40] This evaluation generally consists of an assessment of renal function (BUN and creatinine levels, calculated GFR) and multiphasic CT urography, including sufficient phases to evaluate the renal parenchyma and urothelium of the upper tracts.

CT urography identifies hydronephrosis, urinary calculi, and renal and ureteral lesions. For patients with contraindications to contrasted CT, MR urography is an acceptable alternative imaging approach. Finally, the AUA guidelines recommend that cystoscopy be performed on all patients aged 35 years or older or those with risk factors for urinary tract malignancy, such as tobacco use, exposure to carcinogenic chemicals (e.g., aniline dye, benzidine, petroleum products), or history of chronic UTIs.[40] Risk factors for urinary tract malignancy in patients with microscopic hematuria are listed in Box 85.8. For persistent microhematuria following a negative evaluation, yearly urinalyses are recommended, with consideration for a repeat urologic examination every 3 to 5 years.

By contrast, patients with gross hematuria require a thorough evaluation before discharge from the ED. Renal function should be assessed to rule out the development of renal insufficiency. The patient should also undergo appropriate imaging tests, although clear consensus is lacking on the appropriate radiographic study. If the initial assessment fails to identify a benign cause for the hematuria, a CT scan with contrast or renal ultrasound study should be performed. CT scanning is

---

BOX 85.8 Risk Factors for Urinary Tract Malignancy

Age >35 years
Past or current cigarette smoking
Occupational exposure (chemicals or dyes)
Analgesic abuse
Chronic indwelling foreign body
Chronic urinary tract infection
Exposure to known carcinogenic or chemotherapeutic agent
Gross hematuria
Irritative voiding symptoms
Pelvic irradiation
Urologic disorder or disease

---

highly sensitive for stones, masses, and other diseases of the upper urinary tract. If contrast CT must be avoided owing to pregnancy, renal insufficiency, or history of anaphylaxis to contrast medium, ultrasound imaging is the modality of choice. Ultrasound is less sensitive than a CT scan for detecting stones, small masses, and traumatic causes of hematuria.

CT is the appropriate imaging modality for traumatic hematuria because its sensitivity and specificity exceed those of ultrasound. The exact level of hematuria that should trigger imaging is unclear, but it appears that patients without gross hematuria or evidence of coexisting abdominal or pelvic injuries are unlikely to have clinically significant injuries on CT.

The references for this chapter can be found online at ExpertConsult.com.

Gynecologic Disorders

Trevor R. Pour and Christina S. Hajicharalambous

KEY CONCEPTS

- Adnexal torsion is easily missed on initial presentation and should be considered in any patient with known risk factors, even if symptoms are subtle or atypical.
- Doppler ultrasound is the preferred initial imaging study for suspected adnexal torsion.
- An ultrasound examination may distinguish among the various types of ovarian cysts and identify associated complications, such as torsion, hemorrhage, and malignancy. Most ovarian cysts are simple follicular cysts that resolve without pharmacologic or surgical intervention.
- Abnormal uterine bleeding (AUB) has many structural, hormonal, and coagulopathic causes. Selected imaging and laboratory testing, based on a careful history and physical examination, can often lead to determination of the cause. Combined oral contraceptive pills can help to regulate the cycle and alleviate AUB.
- Emergency contraception is a safe, effective option to prevent an undesired pregnancy. Levonorgestrel and ulipristal are both effective oral medications and are associated with fewer side effects than the traditional combined contraceptive method. Intrauterine devices should also be considered for emergency contraception if a patient desires a long-term contraceptive option.

GYNECOLOGIC DISORDERS

Many women present to the emergency department (ED) with pelvic pain or vaginal bleeding. After the possibility of pregnancy-related diagnoses has been eliminated, the primary goal is to recognize the presence of conditions that warrant urgent intervention, such as adnexal torsion, versus those that can be managed as an outpatient, such as new postmenopausal uterine bleeding. Most patients also benefit from symptom relief and reassurance. This chapter specifically addresses the ED management of adnexal torsion, ovarian cysts, abnormal uterine bleeding (AUB), and emergency contraception. The general approach to vaginal bleeding is discussed in Chapter 30, complications of pregnancy are discussed in Chapter 173, and sexually transmitted disease is discussed in Chapter 84.

ADNEXAL TORSION

Foundations

The bilateral adnexal structures consist of the ovaries and fallopian tubes. Torsion accounts for approximately 3% of gynecologic emergencies and refers to the twisting of the ovary and/or fallopian tube on the axis between the utero-ovarian and infundibulopelvic ligaments. Although most commonly both structures are involved in this process, isolated ovarian torsion and, more rarely, isolated fallopian tube

torsion may occur. In the early phases of torsion, venous and lymphatic obstruction initially occur, followed subsequent congestion and edema of the adnexal structures, which then progress to ischemia and necrosis.

In addition to loss of tubal or ovarian function, torsion left untreated can progress further to hemorrhage, peritonitis, and infection. Because of the dual blood supply of the ovary from the uterine and ovarian arteries, total arterial obstruction is rare but can develop (Fig. 86.1).

Ovarian torsion can occur at any age but is most common in the reproductive years due to the regular development of a corpus luteal cyst during the menstrual cycle. Torsion may be a complication of pregnancy, more likely to occur in the first and early second trimesters.[1] A history of tubal ligation is a risk factor for ovarian torsion.[2] A predominance of torsion on the right side has been noted in approximately a 2:1 ratio to cases on the left, likely related to the stabilizing effect of the fixed sigmoid colon.

In premenarchal patients, torsion frequently occurs despite normal ovarian size, thought to be secondary to the excessive mobility of the adnexa due to relatively longer supporting ligaments and the smaller size of the uterus.[3,4]

Most cases of torsion in the postmenarchal population are associated with an enlarged ovary with a diameter greater than 5.0 cm as the result of a benign neoplasm or cysts, which can be the result of ovulation induction, hyperstimulation syndrome, or polycystic ovarian syndrome. Masses prone to developing adhesions and therefore restricting mobility of adnexal structures, such as malignant tumors, endometriomas, or tubo-ovarian abscesses, are less likely to develop torsion than benign lesions.

Clinical Features

Despite advances in imaging modalities, the definitive preoperative diagnosis rate of ectopic pregnancy approaches only 40%, making clinical assessment the primary driver of management decisions. The classic symptoms of ovarian torsion are severe, sharp, unilateral lower abdominal pain accompanied by nausea and vomiting; however, these elements are not consistently present in all cases.[5] The presence of known risk factors, such as an ovarian mass or recent assisted reproductive treatments, may suggest the diagnosis in postmenarchal patients.

Patients typically report pain lasting from several hours to days, sometimes with intermittent resolution likely owing to spontaneous detorsion. Rarely, patients report pain for weeks to months in duration, most likely due to intermittent or chronic torsion.[6] Nausea and vomiting are present in approximately 60% to 70% of cases. Fever is a an uncommonly reported finding, typically seen late in the course of disease and likely secondary to ischemia and necrosis of adnexal tissue.

Most patients will have unilateral tenderness on abdominal palpation, but peritoneal signs are rare, especially in early presentations. Only 50% of patients will have a palpable adnexal mass on pelvic

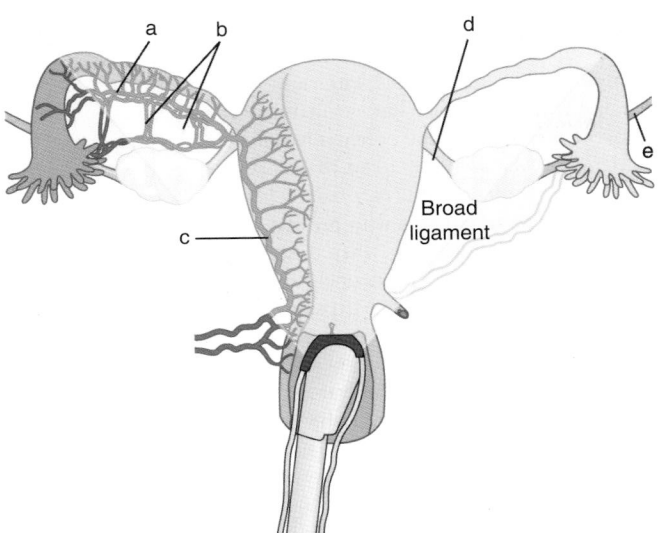

Fig. 86.1 Ovarian Blood Supply. *a*, Ovarian artery and vein. *b*, Branching arterioles supplying ovary. *c*, Uterine artery. *d*, Utero-ovarian ligament. *e*, Infundibulopelvic ligament. (From Andreotti RF, Shadinger L, Fleischer A. The sonographic diagnosis of ovarian torsion: pearls and pitfalls. *Ultrasound Clin.* 2007;2:155.)

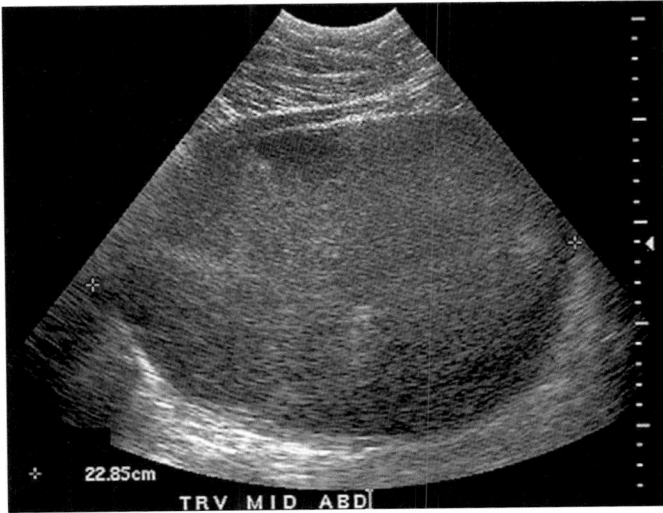

Fig. 86.2 Ovarian Torsion with a Large Pelvic Mass. This transabdominal image reveals a largely homogeneous 22.8-cm pelvic mass. (From Cicchiello LA, Hamper UM, Scoutt LM. Ultrasound evaluation of gynecologic causes of pelvic pain. *Obstet Gynecol Clin North Am.* 2011;38:85–114.)

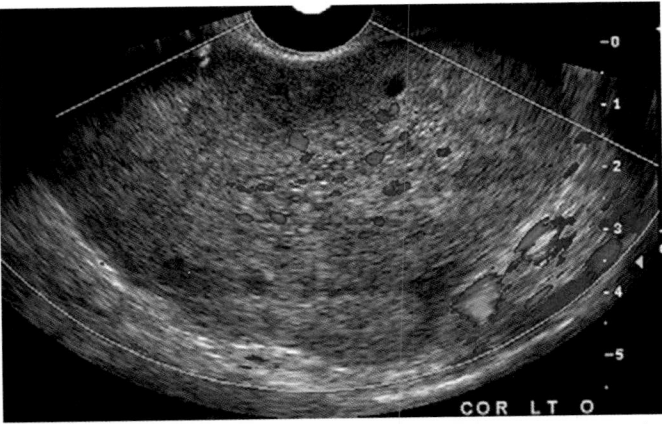

Fig. 86.3 Ovarian torsion with color Doppler image demonstrating venous and arterial flow. (From Cicchiello LA, Hamper UM, Scoutt LM. Ultrasound evaluation of gynecologic causes of pelvic pain. *Obstet Gynecol Clin North Am.* 2011;38:85–114.)

examination; a palpable mass is more common in adults than pediatric patients with torsion.[7] Predictive scoring systems for adnexal torsion—typically involving a combination of clinical elements and imaging or laboratory findings—have been developed but have not yet been shown to be generalizable to all populations and therefore cannot be recommended at this time.[8,9] Clinical signs of isolated tubal torsion are indistinguishable from those of ovarian or full adnexal torsion.[10]

Differential Diagnoses

The differential diagnosis of adnexal torsion includes appendicitis, ruptured ovarian cyst, cystitis or pyelonephritis, nephrolithiasis, pelvic inflammatory disease, uterine leiomyoma, diverticulitis, bowel obstruction, and ectopic pregnancy. A pregnancy test, physical examination, and imaging with ultrasound, computed tomography (CT), or magnetic resonance imaging (MRI), if necessary, can typically distinguish among these possibilities.

Diagnostic Testing

Laboratory Tests

No specific laboratory tests are routinely used in the diagnosis of adnexal torsion, although preoperative labs should be drawn on all patients suspected of torsion. A negative pregnancy test may exclude ectopic pregnancy from the differential, but importantly a positive test does not rule out adnexal torsion. Leukocytosis and elevated C-reactive protein (CRP) are occasionally associated with torsion but both are nonspecific and cannot be used as reliable predictors.

Small studies on serum interleukin-6 (IL-6) and D-dimer levels have revealed moderate sensitivity and specificity for detection of ovarian torsion, especially when coupled with findings suggestive of torsion on ultrasonography.[11,12] These tests in combination may eventually prove to be useful if early findings are confirmed by larger trials, but neither is considered a routine test at this time.

Imaging Tests

Ultrasonography. Ultrasound examination is the optimal initial imaging test in the evaluation of patients with pelvic pain highly suggestive of torsion, but findings can vary depending on timing and

duration of symptoms. Asymmetric enlargement of the ovary is the most common finding. Enlargement of an ovary with a heterogeneous stroma secondary to edema along with small, peripherally displaced follicles is the classic ultrasound appearance of torsion but is often absent, particularly in the setting of prolonged ischemia.[13] Ultrasound may also reveal a discrete ovarian mass, evidence of hemorrhage, or free pelvic fluid (Fig. 86.2). Hemorrhagic cysts and other nonneoplastic masses frequently are associated with torsion; these may appear fluid filled, exhibit a complex pattern with debris and septations, or be visualized as a solid mass. The characteristic appearance of torsion may be difficult to appreciate if the ovary is obscured by an associated mass. In isolated tubal torsion, tubal lesions such as hydrosalpinx or a tubo-ovarian abscess may be seen.

Doppler ultrasound findings are inconsistent in the definitive diagnosis of adnexal torsion. Up to 60% of surgically proven cases have ovarian blood flow on the preceding Doppler examination (Fig. 86.3).[14] These findings may vary depending on the time of the examination because torsion may occur intermittently, and clinical symptoms commonly precede arterial compromise. If a large adnexal mass is present, the examination may also be technically difficult to perform. Despite these limitations, the Doppler examination is still useful, as recognition of ovarian enlargement or masses, as well as detection of abnormal venous flow is particularly important in early cases of torsion (Fig. 86.4). Absence of arterial flow is highly specific for torsion, with a positive predictive value nearing 100%. Visualization of the twisting of the pedicle and coiled vessels is referred to as a "whirlpool sign" and has a 90% positive predictive value for torsion.[15]

Computed tomography. When alternative abdominal pathologies are strong considerations in the differential diagnosis of a patient's acute pelvic pain, abdominopelvic CT may be the best initial study, particularly in patients who have a presentation less typical for torsion. In ovarian torsion, CT findings include asymmetric ovarian enlargement or asymmetric adnexal enhancement following intravenous (IV) contrast, fallopian tube thickening, twisted vascular pedicle, fat stranding surrounding the affected adnexa, and uterine deviation to the affected side.[16] Pelvic free fluid can also be seen, especially in cases of hemorrhagic infarction.

Multiple studies show that patients with ultrasonographic or surgically confirmed torsion have evidence of at least one abnormal finding on CT. This suggests that a completely normal contrast-enhanced CT scan of the abdomen and pelvis—including the absence of ovarian enlargement or masses in addition to the aforementioned findings—may be sufficient to rule out ovarian torsion.[17] Negative CT imaging findings should be interpreted with caution when clinical suspicion is high, but with lower suspicion, normal-appearing pelvic structures on a CT scan is reassuring and potentially sufficient imaging.

Magnetic resonance imaging. MRI may also demonstrate findings consistent with torsion. It is particularly helpful when the diagnosis is unclear, such as in patients who present with intermittent pain over days, or for pregnant patients when the history is suggestive of torsion but ultrasound findings are inconclusive or equivocal and CT scans are not preferred. Findings on MRI suggestive of torsion are similar to those on CT (Box 86.1).

Laparoscopy. Given the frequency of equivocal findings on imaging studies, the lack of reliable clinical decision tools, the absence of a proven biomarker, and the variable clinical presentation, adnexal torsion is commonly a surgical diagnosis. Diagnostic laparoscopy is therefore indicated for patients in whom clinical suspicion is high despite negative imaging results. Laparoscopy also allows for the diagnosis of other unsuspected conditions, including appendicitis or tubo-ovarian abscess.[18]

Management and Disposition

Once the diagnosis of suspected torsion has been made, the patient should be taken to the operating room as soon as possible. The adnexal

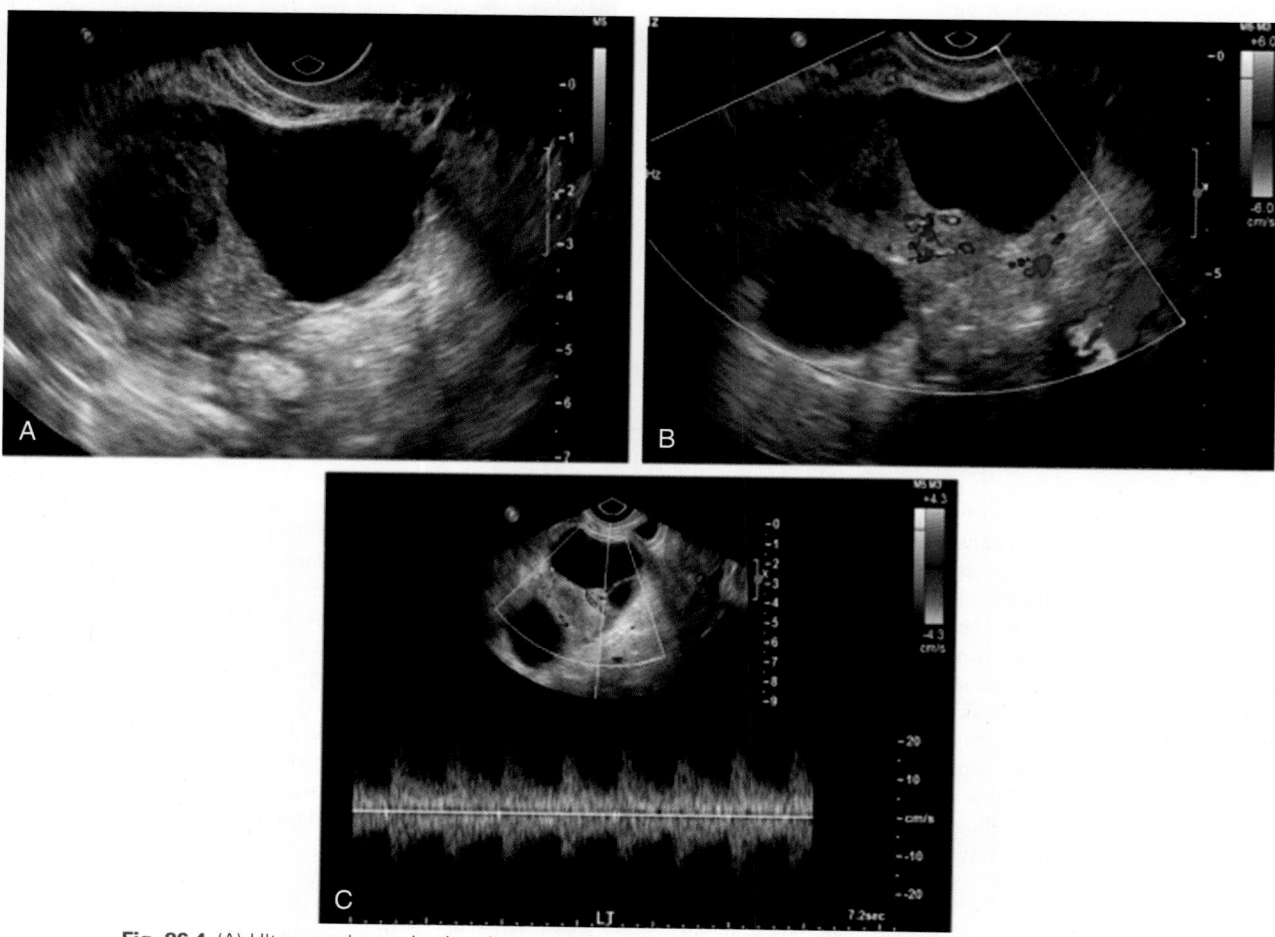

Fig. 86.4 (A) Ultrasound examination demonstrating a large associated hemorrhagic cyst. (B and C) Arterial Doppler signal without venous signal in a patient with surgically proven torsion. (From Andreotti RF, Shadinger L, Fleischer A. The sonographic diagnosis of ovarian torsion: pearls and pitfalls. *Ultrasound Clin.* 2007;2:155.)

structures often will recover, even if visibly ischemic or dusky in appearance at the time of surgery. Because of its dual blood supply and potential to recover function, attempts at ovarian salvage are warranted even if the diagnosis is delayed. This is particularly true in adolescent patients.

OVARIAN CYSTS AND MASSES

Foundations

Cysts are the most common cause of gynecologic masses. They occur at any stage of life but are most frequent in the reproductive years because of the cyclic changes of the ovary associated with menstruation (Fig. 86.5). Most ovarian cysts in premenopausal and postmenopausal women are benign and resolve without intervention, but on occasion they may be malignant or associated with complications such as hemorrhage or torsion.[19,20]

BOX 86.1 Imaging Characteristics of Adnexal Torsion

Ultrasonography
Enlargement of the ovary
Associated ovarian mass
Loss of enhancement
Edema
Free pelvic fluid
Loss of venous waveforms
Loss of arterial waveforms

Computed Tomography and Magnetic Resonance Imaging
Enlargement of the ovary
Associated ovarian mass
Thickening of the fallopian tube
Free pelvic fluid
Edema of the ovary
Deviation of the uterus to the affected side
Associated hemorrhage

The most common type of cyst is a simple follicular, or functional cyst, developing from a follicle that fails to rupture or regress, and is defined as pathologic when the diameter exceeds 3.0 cm. Follicular cysts are typically thin-walled and filled with clear fluid, whereas a corpus luteal cyst is often filled with hemorrhagic fluid. Several other types of cystic masses can occur in the ovary, including endometriomas (often called "chocolate cysts"), nonneoplastic lesions such as benign cystic teratoma or dermoid cyst, fibroma, cystadenoma, and various types of malignant neoplasms.[21]

Clinical Features

The most common presentation for patients with an ovarian cyst is pelvic pain. Rupture of a follicular cyst may produce transient pelvic pain, be associated with dyspareunia, or be asymptomatic. Because of the thin and fragile wall, a follicular cyst may rupture during sexual intercourse or during the pelvic examination. Follicular cysts are rarely associated with hemorrhage.

Presentation of a corpus luteal cyst may range from an asymptomatic mass to dull, chronic pelvic pain to severe pain associated with rupture. Rupture of a corpus luteal cyst is frequently associated with a significant degree of hemorrhage. As with a follicular cyst, rupture may follow a pelvic examination, sexual intercourse, exercise, or trauma. Rupture of a large or complex cyst may result in severe pain and peritoneal signs. Occasionally, a large cyst may be discovered on a routine pelvic examination as an asymptomatic mass, but this is uncommon.

Differential Diagnoses

Diagnostic considerations in the patient with symptomatic ovarian cysts and masses include other causes of pelvic pain that require urgent intervention, such as ectopic pregnancy, pelvic inflammatory disease, urinary tract infections, nephrolithiasis, appendicitis, and diverticulitis. Tumors or abscesses of the gastrointestinal tract may also mimic adnexal masses.

Diagnostic Testing

Laboratory Tests

The initial step in the evaluation of pelvic pain or a pelvic mass is to exclude pregnancy with a urine or serum β-human chorionic gonadotropin (β-hCG) test. A hematocrit may be valuable in the unstable

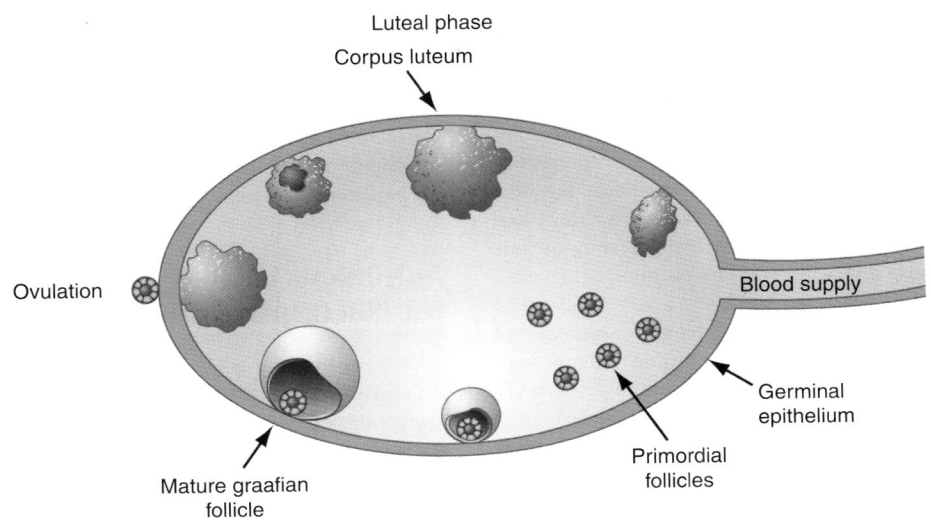

Fig. 86.5 Ovulatory cycle and maturation during the normal menstrual cycle. (From Lambert MJ, Villa M. Gynecologic ultrasound in emergency medicine. *Emerg Med Clin North Am.* 2004;22:683–696.)

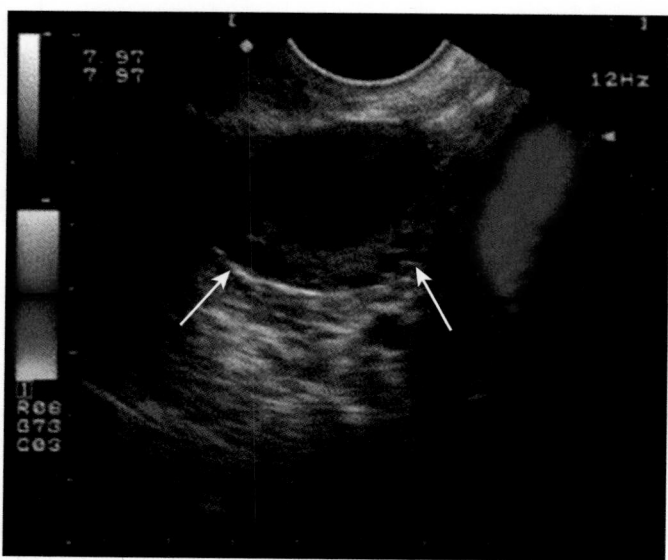

Fig. 86.6 Endovaginal ultrasound image of a normal ovary with a dominant follicle *(arrows)*. (From Lambert MJ, Villa M. Gynecologic ultrasound in emergency medicine. *Emerg Med Clin North Am.* 2004;22:683–696.)

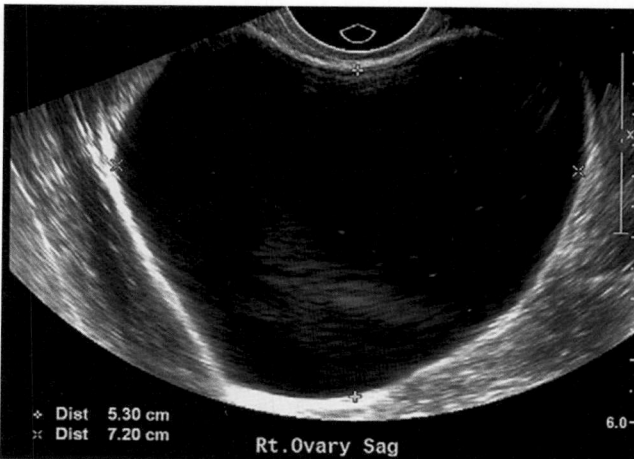

Fig. 86.7 Endovaginal ultrasound image of a follicular cyst, with smooth wall and posterior wall enhancement. (From Cicchiello LA, Hamper UM, Scoutt LM. Ultrasound evaluation of gynecologic causes of pelvic pain. *Obstet Gynecol Clin North Am.* 2011;38:85–114.)

patient as a marker of blood loss. The serum antigen CA-125 is elevated in 80% of women with epithelial ovarian cancer but can also be elevated by nonmalignant conditions such as endometriosis, pregnancy, and pelvic inflammatory disorder, limiting its usefulness in the emergency setting.

Imaging Tests

Ultrasonography. Ultrasonography is used to diagnose and characterize all ovarian pathologic processes and lesions, including cysts and masses. Approximately 90% of adnexal masses are adequately characterized by ultrasound imaging alone. Transabdominal and endovaginal examinations provide useful information. The transabdominal approach is performed with a full bladder as a sonographic window. It permits an overall view of the pelvis and will visualize large masses and pelvic free fluid. Use of the endovaginal probe, which should be performed with an empty bladder to reduce artifact, provides a detailed picture of the ovary. Follicles are part of the normal architecture of the ovary and are typically smaller than 1.0 cm in diameter, whereas the dominant follicle may measure up to 2.5 cm at the time of ovulation. Depending on the timing of the scan and degree of clot formation and lysis, hemorrhage may be seen; serial bedside abdominal ultrasound imaging can also serve as a rapid assessment tool to detect worsening hemoperitoneum in the setting of hemorrhagic cyst rupture. Fig. 86.6 demonstrates a normal ovary with a dominant follicle, Fig. 86.7 demonstrates a large cyst, and Fig. 86.8 demonstrates hemorrhage and free pelvic fluid. Ultrasound findings suggestive of malignancy include internal septations, solid elements within cystic structures, a thickened wall, and large amounts of ascites or free fluid.[22]

Computed tomography. When the differential diagnosis of unilateral pelvic pain is broad, particularly in the patient with symptoms or physical findings not solely confined to the pelvis, a CT scan may be a more appropriate initial imaging study. However, it is not recommended as the first line imaging study if an adnexal mass is of primary concern due to poor soft tissue discrimination.[23] However, once the diagnosis of potential malignancy has been made, ultrasound is insensitive for staging or follow-up imaging, and contrast-enhanced CT is indicated at that time. A CT scan can detect a cyst and associated complications, including torsion, as noted earlier in this chapter. CT

findings suggestive of malignancy are a cystic solid mass, necrosis in a solid lesion, complex or cystic lesion with thick, irregular walls, and the presence of ascites, peritoneal metastases, and lymphadenopathy.

Magnetic resonance imaging. MRI provides better soft tissue contrast than CT and has been shown in multiple studies to differentiate benign from malignant adnexal masses better than ultrasound. Its use is often limited by availability, cost, and duration of examination. MRI should be considered for pregnant patients or those with equivocal findings on ultrasound or CT.

Management and Disposition

Patients with a simple cyst, no evidence of additional pathology, and improvement in symptoms may be safely discharged with referral for outpatient gynecologic follow-up to ensure resolution. Most uncomplicated simple cysts will resolve without further intervention. Pain should be controlled with nonsteroidal antiinflammatory drugs (NSAIDs) as a first line approach and with oral opioids reserved only for severe cases. Oral contraceptives are not recommended for the routine management of ovarian cysts; despite being theorized to accelerate the regression of ovarian cysts, multiple randomized controlled trials have shown no difference in cyst resolution when compared to expectant management.

A complex cyst concerning for malignancy requires more urgent gynecologic intervention. Such patients may benefit from gynecologic consultation in the ED, particularly if reliable follow-up is unlikely or if the patient is particularly symptomatic.

ABNORMAL UTERINE BLEEDING IN THE NONPREGNANT PATIENT

Foundations

An understanding of the normal menstrual cycle is necessary to understand the potential causes of AUB (Fig. 86.9). The menstrual cycle starts on the first day of menses. During the first part of the menstrual cycle, the endometrium thickens under the influence of estrogen, and a dominant follicle develops in the ovary, releasing an ovum at the midpoint of the cycle. After ovulation, the luteal phase begins and is characterized by the production of progesterone from the corpus luteum. Progesterone matures the lining of the uterus and, if implantation does

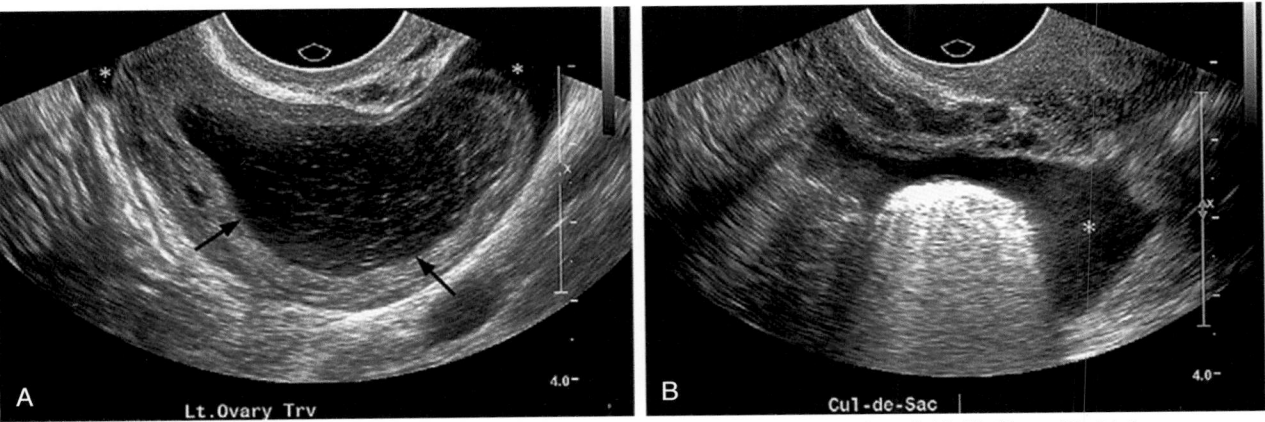

Fig. 86.8 Endovaginal ultrasound image of a hemorrhagic ovarian cyst with free fluid *(*)*. (From Cicchiello LA, Hamper UM, Scoutt LM. Ultrasound evaluation of gynecologic causes of pelvic pain. *Obstet Gynecol Clin North Am.* 2011;38:85–114.)

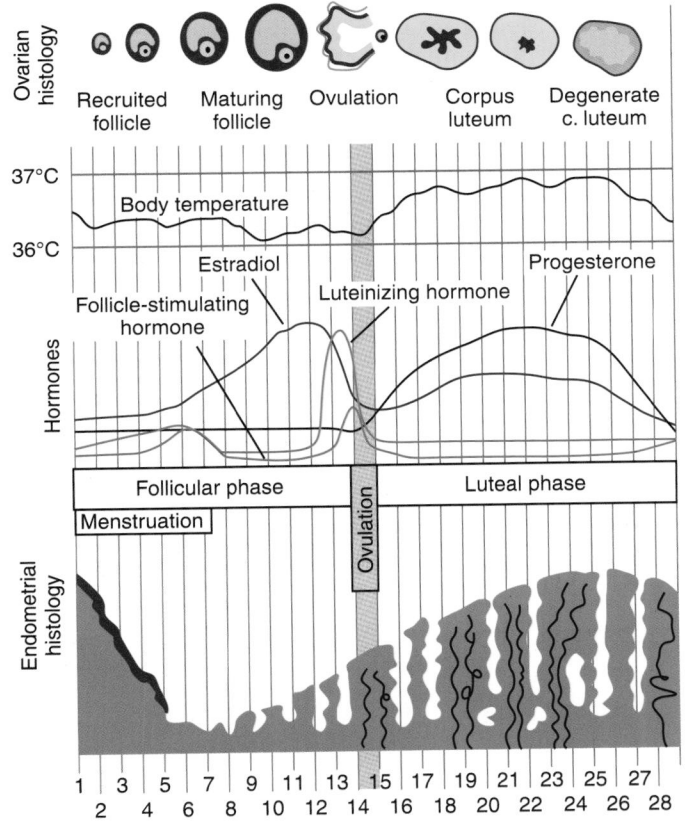

Fig. 86.9 Normal Menstrual Cycle.

BOX 86.2 PALM-COEIN Classification for Abnormal Uterine Bleeding (AUB)

PALM—Structural Causes
Polyp (AUB-P)
Adenomyosis (AUB-A)
Leiomyoma (AUB-L)
    Submucosal leiomyoma (AUB-LSM)
    Other leiomyoma (AUB-LO)
Malignancy and hyperplasia (AUB-M)

COEIN—Nonstructural Causes
Coagulopathy (AUB-C)
Ovulatory Dysfunction (AUB-O)
Endometrial (AUB-E)
Iatrogenic (AUB-I)
Not yet classified (AUB-N)

---

multiinstitutional investigation (Box 86.2).[24] The first four letters, PALM, represent structural causes for AUB—*p*olyp, *a*denomyosis, *l*eiomyoma, and *m*alignancy or hyperplasia, whereas the latter, COEIN, represent nonstructural causes—*c*oagulopathy, *o*vulatory dysfunction, *e*ndometrial, *i*atrogenic, and *n*ot yet classified. The term *dysfunctional uterine bleeding* is obsolete and should not be used.

Clinical Features

History

Many conditions cause AUB, defined as any change in the frequency, regularity, duration, or volume of bleeding. A systematic history and physical examination tailored to the patient's menstrual development will help narrow these possibilities. Vaginal bleeding in prepubertal patients can be concerning and may be the result of infection, trauma such as sexual abuse or a vaginal foreign body, or a structural lesion. Adolescents who develop heavy bleeding at the time of menarche may be presenting with their first sign of an inherited bleeding disorder. In the postmenopausal woman, any bleeding 12 months after the cessation of menses or unpredictable bleeding during hormone therapy is abnormal. The volume and frequency of bleeding, the duration of symptoms, and the relationship between bleeding and the patient's normal menstrual cycle should be established. A menstrual cycle shorter than 21 days in duration or more than 35 days apart, or flow for

not occur, the corpus luteum dies, accompanied by sharp drops in progesterone and estrogen levels. These changes typically are followed by menstruation. Menstrual bleeding is usually predictable, cyclic, and results from withdrawal of the effects of hormones on the endometrium, which occurs approximately 14 days after ovulation.

A revised system of terminology, PALM-COEIN, regarding AUB was created in 2011 by the International Federation of Gynecology and Obstetrics (FIGO) to standardize language and facilitate

less than 2 or more than 7 days, is classified as abnormal. A pattern of irregular bleeding between cycles or an abrupt change in the previous pattern of bleeding should also be determined.

Systemic conditions, such as liver or thyroid disease, may be associated with AUB. Endometrial cancer is associated with underlying diabetes mellitus, metabolic syndrome and obesity, anovulatory cycles, nulliparity, and age older than 55 years. Cervical dysplasia or other genital tract pathology may cause postcoital or irregular bleeding, and patients should routinely be questioned on risk factors for sexually transmitted infections. Prior history of cesarean section may contribute to iatrogenic AUB; studies have found that irregular scarring postoperatively leads to a higher prevalence of vaginal spotting.

Disruption along the hypothalamus-pituitary-ovarian pathway leading to anovulation is frequently the cause of AUB. Disruption of this pathway may be physiologic, such as during adolescence, perimenopause, or lactation. Pathologic causes include polycystic ovary syndrome (PCOS), hypothalamic dysfunction seen in anorexia nervosa, hyperprolactinemia, and primary pituitary disease.

Patients should be questioned about excessive bleeding or bruising or any family history of bleeding disorders because up to 20% of women presenting with heavy menstrual bleeding will have an underlying coagulopathy. Von Willebrand disease is the most common of these, seen in up to 13% of cases of AUB, and often first presents with heavy uterine bleeding since menarche.

Physical Examination

In the setting of acute, heavy bleeding, the initial physical examination should focus on signs of hypovolemia and anemia. PCOS is a common cause of AUB and suggested by the presence of obesity, acne, hirsutism, and acanthosis nigricans. The examination should include inspection of the thyroid, particularly for nodules, as well as a comprehensive skin examination for petechiae and ecchymosis. Other causes of bleeding include vaginal or cervical lesions, which may be visible on the vaginal speculum examination. A leiomyoma or fibroid uterus may be palpable on the bimanual examination.[25]

Differential Diagnoses

The differential diagnosis of AUB in the nonpregnant patient is extensive but may be narrowed by patient age. In adolescents, consider undiagnosed coagulopathy, pelvic infection, or hypothalamic-pituitary-ovarian axis dysregulation due to physiologic immaturity or PCOS. Young adults often have structural lesions such as polyps or leiomyomas, endometrial hyperplasia, or anovulation secondary to PCOS or the other conditions listed earlier. In patients older than 40 years but not yet postmenopausal, anovulatory bleeding due to perimenopause becomes more likely, as does endometrial carcinoma or hyperplasia and leiomyoma. Postmenopausal patients require an outpatient evaluation for malignancy.

Diagnostic Strategies

Laboratory Tests

A urine or serum pregnancy test is essential in evaluating a woman of reproductive age with vaginal bleeding. In a patient with excessive bleeding, hemodynamic instability, or clinical evidence of anemia (e.g., excessive fatigue, pale conjunctiva), a hemoglobin or hematocrit is indicated. If coagulopathy is suspected, platelet count, prothrombin and partial thromboplastin time should be measured. In the emergency setting, testing for von Willebrand disease and other specific coagulopathies can usually be deferred to outpatient follow-up. Sexually transmitted infections should be tested for in patients with risk factors or clinical signs of infection, particularly *Chlamydia trachomatis*. The presence of chlamydial antigens has been linked to AUB, likely due

to endometrial inflammation. Thyroid dysfunction, particularly hypothyroidism, is associated with AUB, and therefore screening to determine the thyroid-stimulating hormone serum level is recommended.

Imaging Tests

The decision to perform ultrasound imaging to evaluate AUB in the ED depends on the urgency to determine the cause of bleeding and the reliability of outpatient follow-up. Transvaginal ultrasonography (TVUS) may reveal a fibroid uterus, endometrial thickening, or a focal mass (Fig. 86.10). In postmenopausal patients with AUB, an endometrium measuring less than 4 to 5 mm of thickness on TVUS reliably excludes endometrial cancer. A thickened endometrium may indicate an underlying lesion or excess estrogen. For most nonpregnant patients with AUB, ultrasound findings do not immediately affect ED decision making. In patients who have reliable access to outpatient gynecologic services, imaging may be deferred until follow-up evaluation.

Management

The likely causative disorder coupled with the volume of bleeding and overall stability of the patient will guide ED management. Patients with uncontrolled bleeding and hemodynamic instability on presentation should receive standard resuscitation IV fluids and blood products, and surgical options should be considered, including urgent dilation and curettage, uterine artery embolization, endometrial ablation, or hysterectomy. Alternatively, conjugated equine estrogen may be administered at a dose of 25 mg given IV every 4 to 6 hours for 24 hours or until the bleeding stops. In emergent situations, intrauterine tamponade with a 26-French foley catheter instilled with 30 mL of saline can also be attempted.

In less emergent situations, oral medications can be considered for the treatment of AUB. Disruption of the hypothalamic-pituitary-ovarian axis from a variety of causes can result in bleeding related to ovulatory dysfunction (AUB-O). Restoring the balance of estrogen and progesterone with oral contraceptives will help many patients regulate the cycle, with reduction in or cessation of AUB. Combination oral contraceptive pills can help regulate the cycle and counteract the long-term effects of unopposed estrogen on the endometrium. We recommend a combination oral contraceptive with 35 µg of ethinyl estradiol or 20 mg or medroxyprogesterone three times daily for 1 week. Contraindications must be reviewed with the patient prior to prescribing

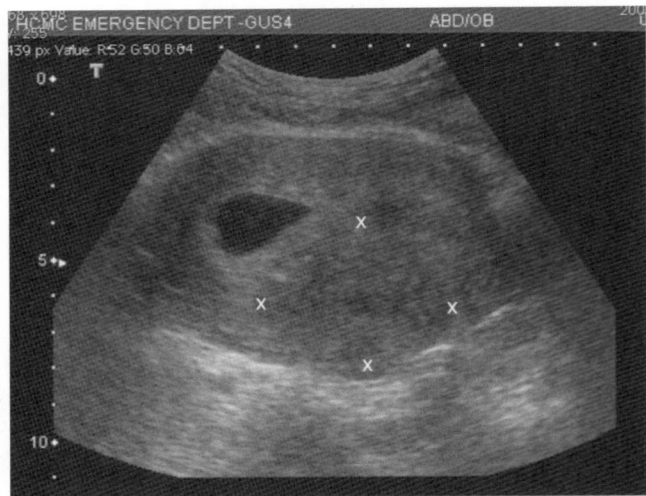

Fig. 86.10 Longitudinal view of the uterus with thickened endometrium. (Courtesy Dr. Robert Reardon, Hennepin County Medical Center, Minneapolis; with permission.)

these medications, specifically to determine a history of thromboembolic events, cigarette smoking, breast cancer, or liver disease. However, patients with contraindications to estrogen-progesterone combination treatment can also consider progestin-only treatment, given as 5 mg norethindrone orally three times daily for 1 week.[23] The levonorgestrel intrauterine device (IUD) is also a nonemergent option to treat AUB in patients who are interested in long-term contraception.[26]

Nonhormonal medications also have been shown to be effective in AUB. Tranexamic acid, an antifibrinolytic agent, may also be used for either emergent or outpatient management of bleeding. It can be administered IV at 10 mg/kg with a maximum dose of 600 mg, or orally at a dose of 1.3 g every 8 hours for 5 days. NSAIDs are generally safe and well tolerated and are effective for relief of associated cramping pelvic pain. They have also been shown to be more effective than placebo to reduce heavy menstrual bleeding, although less effective than either tranexamic acid or a hormonal IUD, with limited data to compare efficacy to oral contraceptives.[27,28] In patients with suspected bleeding disorders, specifically those with platelet dysfunction, NSAIDs should be used with caution.

Disposition

Most patients with pelvic pain from ovarian cysts or AUB without hemodynamic compromise may be managed with specific therapies to minimize symptoms and should be referred to a gynecologist for definitive management on an outpatient basis. Patients with severe, acute AUB and hemodynamic instability require urgent gynecologic consultation and hospitalization.

EMERGENCY CONTRACEPTION

Emergency contraception, more commonly known as the "morning after pill," consists of medical therapy to prevent pregnancy immediately following unprotected or inadequately protected sexual intercourse. At present, there are three oral formulations available: ulipristal acetate (a progesterone receptor modulator), levonorgestrel (a progestin), and combined oral contraceptives consisting of progestin and estrogen taken together and often referred to as the Yuzpe regimen. In addition to oral options, the copper IUD is extremely effective as emergency contraception and works through inhibition of sperm function, inhibition of fertilized egg transport, and likely inhibition of implantation.[29]

The most commonly used regimen, and the only formulation available without a prescription in the United States, consists of a single dose of 1.5 mg or two doses of 0.75 mg levonorgestrel spaced 12 hours apart. The one-time dose of 1.5 mg is simpler to use and is at least as effective as the two-dose regimen and is therefore recommended.[30] It is labeled for use for up to 72 hours following intercourse. Studies have indicated an association between higher patient body mass index (BMI) and decreased effectiveness of levonorgestrel, suggesting that perhaps an increased dose may be indicated in obese individuals. However, further study is necessary before this can be definitively recommended.[31]

Another regimen, a single tablet of 30 mg of ulipristal acetate, is available only with a prescription but has demonstrated effectiveness for up to 120 hours from intercourse, making it a preferred choice over levonorgestrel beyond the 72-hour window. Both forms of contraception—levonorgestrel and ulipristal—are maximally effective when used within 24 hours. Combined oral contraceptives, consisting of 100 µg of ethinyl estradiol and 0.5 to 1.0 mg of levonorgestrel, have largely fallen out of favor due to the simplicity and success of levonorgestrel alone.

Adverse effects of oral emergency contraception include nausea and headache, with the combined oral contraceptive regimen producing significantly higher rates of nausea than levonorgestrel or ulipristal alone. Irregular menstrual bleeding, which can occur within 1 week to 1 month after treatment, resolves without intervention.

The copper IUD is highly effective when placed within 5 days of intercourse and appears to be effective for as long as 10 days. It carries a 1/1000 risk of uterine perforation and is associated with uterine cramping but also provides ongoing contraceptive benefit. The major barrier to utilization for emergency contraception is the requirement to make a clinic appointment or visit with a qualified provider within the timeframe outlined earlier.[32]

Both levonorgestrel and ulipristal act to delay or inhibit ovulation, whereas the copper IUD prevents fertilization. As such, a common misconception is that emergency contraception is equivalent to medical abortion. None of the methods discussed involve the termination of a preexisting pregnancy, and emergency contraception has not been shown to have adverse effects on a developing fetus when taken during an established pregnancy. It is still possible for a patient who uses emergency contraception to get pregnant in the same menstrual cycle, so patients should be advised to use an alternative form of contraception and to undergo a pregnancy test if menstruation is delayed for more than 3 weeks. Patients who receive emergency contraception should be counseled regarding birth control and have a follow-up pregnancy test should they miss their next period.

The references for this chapter can be found online at ExpertConsult.com.

87

Stroke

Linda Papa and William J. Meurer

FOUNDATIONS

Background and Importance

Stroke is the fifth leading cause of death in the United States and a leading cause of long-term disability. It affects nearly 800,000 people per year. On average, someone has a stroke every 40 seconds, and someone dies of a stroke every 4 minutes.[1] Stroke patients have an in-hospital mortality rate of 5% to 10% for ischemic stroke and 40% to 60% for intracerebral hemorrhage (ICH).[2] Only 10% of stroke survivors will recover completely, 25% will recover with minor impairments, and 40% will have moderate to severe impairments, making stroke a leading cause of adult disability.

Stroke is any vascular injury that reduces cerebral blood flow (CBF) to a specific region of the brain, retina, or spinal cord, causing neurologic impairment. The onset of symptoms may be sudden or stuttering, often with transient or permanent loss of neurologic function. Approximately 87% of all strokes are ischemic in origin, caused by the occlusion of a cerebral vessel, and 13% are hemorrhagic strokes caused by the rupture of a blood vessel into the parenchyma of the brain (ICH) or into the subarachnoid space (subarachnoid hemorrhage [SAH]). Only ischemic stroke involving the brain and ICH are discussed in this chapter. SAH is discussed in Chapters 16 and 33.

Current acute interventional treatment regimens are designed to reverse or minimize brain damage. Strategies include blood pressure (BP) management, anticoagulation, thrombolytic therapy, catheter-based interventions, and surgery.[3]

Ischemic Stroke

About 600,000 "first-ever" ischemic strokes occur each year in the United States. These may result from either in situ thrombosis or embolic obstruction from a more proximal source, usually the heart. In more than one-third of these first-ever strokes, no clear cause is identified. Strokes of all subtypes are more common in Blacks and Hispanics versus non-Hispanic whites.[1]

Approximately one-third of all ischemic strokes are thrombotic in nature, caused by either large- or small-vessel occlusions. Common areas for large-vessel occlusions are cerebral vessel branch points, especially in the distribution of the internal carotid artery (ICA). Thrombosis usually results from clot formation in the area of an ulcerated atherosclerotic plaque that forms in the area of turbulent blood flow, such as a vessel bifurcation. A marked reduction in flow results when the stenosis occludes more than 90% of the blood vessel diameter. With further ulceration and thrombosis, platelets adhere to the region. A clot then either embolizes or occludes the artery.

Lacunae, or small-vessel strokes, involve small terminal sections of the vasculature and more commonly occur in patients with diabetes and hypertension. About 80% to 90% of patients experiencing lacunar strokes have hypertension. The subcortical areas of the cerebrum and brainstem often are involved. Infarcts here range in size from a few millimeters to 2 cm and are seen most commonly in the basal ganglia, thalamus, pons, and internal capsule. They may be caused by small emboli or by a process termed *lipohyalinosis,* which occurs in patients with hypertensive cerebral vasculopathy.

One-fourth of all ischemic strokes are cardioembolic in nature. Embolization of a mural thrombus in patients with atrial fibrillation is the most common mechanism, and patients with atrial fibrillation have an approximate fivefold increased risk for development of a stroke. Noncardiac sources of emboli most commonly include diseased portions of extracranial arteries, resulting in an artery-to-artery embolus. One common example is amaurosis fugax, in which emboli from a proximal carotid artery plaque embolizes to the ophthalmic artery, causing transient monocular blindness. Aortic atheromas represent another non-cardiac source of emboli.

Although stroke risk increases with age, approximately 3% to 4% of all strokes occur in patients 15 to 45 years old, and there have been trends observed showing the average age of first stroke is becoming younger.[1,4] Atherosclerosis is the most common cause in elders while causative disorders and conditions in younger patients often are uncommon and may be reversible. Pregnancy, the use of oral contraceptives, antiphospholipid antibodies (such as lupus anticoagulant and anticardiolipin antibodies), protein S and C deficiencies, sickle cell anemia, and polycythemia all predispose patients to sludging or thrombosis, thereby increasing the risk of stroke. Fibromuscular dysplasia of the cerebral vasculature also may lead to stroke, and in rare instances prolonged vasoconstriction from a migraine syndrome causes stroke. Recreational drugs such as cocaine and amphetamines are potent vasoconstrictors that have been associated with both ischemic and hemorrhagic stroke. Infectious processes, particularly varicella and recently fungal meningitis, can induce vasculopathies that lead to stroke as well or can induce longer-term inflammatory processes that ultimately cause a clinical stroke.

Carotid and vertebral dissections often are associated with trauma but may follow mild events such as sneezing. Dissections are the leading determined cause of stroke in the young and are slightly less common than idiopathic strokes. Carotid and vertebral dissections also are seen more frequently in people with underlying pathology of the vessel wall, such as in fibromuscular dysplasia and connective tissue disorders. Alteration in the vessel intima can lead to vessel stenosis, occlusion, or embolism. The patient may report a minor preceding event, such as spinal manipulation, strenuous exercise, yoga, coughing, or vomiting. Presenting manifestations may include headache, facial pain, visual changes, cranial nerve (CN) palsies, pain over the affected vessel, Horner syndrome, amaurosis fugax, SAH, or an ischemic stroke. The headache frequently is unilateral and may occur days before onset of the other neurologic symptoms. Dissections are typically diagnosed by noninvasive modalities, such as ultrasonography, magnetic resonance angiography (MRA), and computed tomography angiography (CTA).

Transient Ischemic Attack

A transient ischemic attack (TIA) was previously defined as a neurologic deficit that completely resolves within 24 hours; however, a portion of TIA cases have evidence of permanent brain ischemia on neuroimaging. Therefore, the American Heart Association (AHA) has adopted a tissue-based definition: "A transient episode of neurologic dysfunction caused by focal brain, spinal cord, or retinal ischemia, without acute infarction."

About 240,000 TIAs per year occur in the United States, with an incidence rate of 8 per 1000 person years. TIAs constitute an important warning sign for the future development of cerebral infarction. Approximately 10% of the patients who experience a TIA will sustain a stroke within 3 months of the sentinel event, and one-half of these occur within the first 2 days. High-grade carotid stenosis in the neck and cardioemboli are two key causes that contribute to early stroke following TIA. In addition, recurrence data is primarily derived from an era where MRI was much less commonly used; patients with DWI negative TIAs generally have a much lower risk of recurrence.[5,6]

Hemorrhagic Stroke

Spontaneous ICH causes 10% to 15% of all acute strokes, affecting approximately 65,000 patients per year. It carries a 30-day mortality rate of up to 50% with one-half of patients dying in the first 2 days. Among survivors, only one in five are living independently at 6 months.

The two major underlying causes of ICH are hypertensive vasculopathy (caused by long-standing hypertension) and cerebral amyloid~angiopathy (usually found in elder patients, which is the result of amyloid deposition in cerebral vessel walls). Hypertensive hemorrhage results from degenerative changes in the small penetrating arteries and arterioles, leading to lipohyalinosis of small, deep penetrating arteries. Such hemorrhages generally occur in the deep regions, including basal ganglia and thalamus. The most common sites for hypertensive hemorrhage are summarized in Box 87.1. ICH caused by amyloid angiopathy tends to be lobar in nature and to occur more commonly in older adults.

Other factors leading to ICH include underlying vascular malformations (i.e., arteriovenous malformations [AVMs] and aneurysms, drug intoxication [particularly sympathomimetics, such as cocaine], malignant hypertension, saccular aneurysms, blood dyscrasias, venous sinus thrombosis, hemorrhagic transformation of an ischemic stroke,

---

BOX 87.1   Most Common Sites for Hypertensive Intracranial Hemorrhage

Affected Area (Frequency)
Putamen (44%)
Thalamus (13%)
Cerebellum (9%)
Pons (9%)
Other cortical areas (25%)

Common Clinical Presentation
Contralateral motor/sensory loss
Limb pain, speech difficulty
Uncoordinated movements of trunk and limbs
Numbness, weakness, ataxia, dizziness
Numbness, weakness, language disturbances

---

moyamoya disease, and tumors). High-risk features for such secondary forms of ICH include lobar location, presence of intraventricular blood, and younger age.

Anatomy, Physiology, and Pathophysiology

The cerebral vasculature supplies the brain with a rich flow of blood that contains the critical supply of oxygen and glucose necessary for normal brain function. When a stroke occurs, there are immediate alterations in CBF and extensive changes in cellular homeostasis. The normal CBF is approximately 40 to 60 mL/100 g of brain per minute. When CBF drops below 15 to 18 mL/100 g of brain per minute, several physiologic changes occur. The brain loses electrical activity, becoming electrically "silent," although neuronal membrane integrity and function remain intact. Clinically, the areas of the brain maintaining electrical silence manifest a neurologic deficit, even though the brain cells are viable. When CBF is below 10 mL/100 g of brain per minute, membrane failure occurs, with a subsequent increase in the extracellular potassium and intracellular calcium and eventual cell death.

The ischemic penumbra is the area of the brain surrounding the primary injury, which is preserved by a tenuous supply of blood from collateral vessels. This border zone of neuronal tissue is the area of greatest interest to investigators for possible salvage in both ischemic and hemorrhagic stroke. In ischemic stroke, the duration of occlusion plays a critical role in neuronal survival.

In ICH, acute vessel rupture is most often caused by underlying small vessel disease and causes injury by several mechanisms. First, there is mass effect from the hematoma itself, followed by activation of the coagulation cascade, release of inflammatory cytokines, and blood-brain barrier (BBB) disruption. This leads to perihematomal edema formation and secondary brain injury. Finally, continued bleeding, or hematoma expansion, occurs in many patients—either continued bleeding from the primary source, or secondary bleeding at the periphery of the hemorrhage.

Blood is supplied to the brain by the anterior and posterior circulations. The anterior circulation originates from the carotid system and perfuses 80% of the brain, including the optic nerve, retina, and frontoparietal and anterior-temporal lobes. The first branch off the ICA is the ophthalmic artery, which supplies the optic nerve and retina. As a result, the sudden onset of painless monocular blindness (*amaurosis fugax*) identifies the stroke as involving the anterior circulation (specifically the ipsilateral carotid artery) at or below the level of the ophthalmic artery. The ICAs terminate by branching into the anterior and middle cerebral arteries (MCAs) at the circle of Willis.

The anterior cerebral artery supplies the basal and medial aspects of the cerebral hemispheres and extends to the anterior two-thirds of the parietal lobe. The MCA feeds the lenticulostriate branches that supply the putamen, part of the anterior limb of the internal capsule, the lentiform nucleus, and the external capsule. Main cortical branches of the MCA supply the lateral surfaces of the cerebral cortex from the anterior portion of the frontal lobe to the posterolateral occipital lobe.

Although the posterior circulation is smaller and usually supplies only 20% of the brain, it supplies the brainstem (which is critical for normal consciousness, movement, and sensation), cerebellum, thalamus, auditory and vestibular centers of the ear, medial temporal lobe, and visual occipital cortex. The posterior circulation is derived from the two vertebral arteries that ascend through the transverse processes of the cervical vertebrae. The vertebral arteries enter the cranium through the foramen magnum and supply the cerebellum by the posterior inferior cerebellar arteries. They join to form the basilar artery, which branches to form the posterior cerebral arteries. Some variants exist, importantly, the fetal origin posterior cerebral artery, which is where the posterior cerebral artery is actually fed by the anterior circulation.

The extent of injury in either an anterior or a posterior stroke depends on both the vessel involved and the presence of collateral blood flow distal to the vessel occlusion. A patient with adequate collateral blood flow from the contralateral hemisphere may have minimal clinical deficits despite a complete carotid occlusion. By contrast, a patient with poor collateral flow may have hemiplegia with the same lesion.

CLINICAL FEATURES

Ischemic Stroke

The signs and symptoms of an ischemic stroke may appear suddenly and without warning or may have a stuttering, insidious onset. Disruption of the flow to one of the major vascular limbs of the cerebral circulation will result in physiologic disruption to the anatomic area of the brain supplied by that blood vessel. Ischemic strokes involve either the anterior or posterior circulation strokes and the neurologic deficits are highly dependent on amount of collateral blood flow. In addition to the vascular supply involved, ischemic strokes can be further described by the temporal presentation of their neurologic deficits.

A "stroke in evolution" is one in which focal neurologic deficits worsen over the course of minutes or hours. Approximately 20% of anterior circulation strokes and 40% of posterior circulation strokes will show evidence of progression. Since a single low score on the National Institutes of Health Stroke Scale (NIHSS) may not be sufficient to determine t-PA eligibility, repeating the NIHSS and reassessing these patients is recommended. Anterior circulation strokes may progress within the first 24 hours, whereas posterior strokes may progress for up to 3 days. Propagation of thrombus is postulated as a likely mechanism for progression. With anterior circulation strokes (involving primarily the carotid, anterior, and MCAs), the clinical presentation rarely includes complete loss of consciousness unless the lesion occurs in the previously unaffected hemisphere of a patient who has experienced a previous contralateral stroke.

Occlusions in the anterior cerebral artery mainly affect frontal lobe function. The patient has altered mentation coupled with impaired judgment and insight, as well as the presence of primitive grasp and suck reflexes on physical examination. Bowel and bladder incontinence may be features of anterior cerebral artery stroke. Paralysis and hypesthesia of the lower limb opposite the side of the lesion are characteristic. Leg weakness is more pronounced than arm weakness in anterior cerebral distribution stroke. Apraxia or clumsiness in the patient's gait is often observed.

Marked motor and sensory disturbances are the hallmarks of occlusion of the MCA. They occur on the side of the body contralateral to the side of the lesion and usually are more pronounced in the arm and face than the leg. Such disturbances may involve only part of an extremity or the face but almost always are accompanied by numbness in the same region as that of the motor loss. Hemianopsia, or blindness in one-half of the visual field, occurs contralateral to the lesion. Agnosia, or the inability to recognize previously known subjects, is common, and aphasia may be present if the lesion occurs in the dominant hemisphere. Patients often have a gaze preference toward the affected hemisphere because of disruption of the cortical lateral gaze centers.

Aphasia, a disorder of language in which the patient articulates clearly but uses language inappropriately or comprehends it poorly, also is common in dominant-hemisphere stroke. Aphasia may be expressive, receptive, or a combination of both. *Wernicke aphasia* occurs when the patient is unable to process sensory input, such as speech, and thus fails to understand verbal communication (receptive aphasia). *Broca aphasia* refers to the inability to communicate verbally in an effective way, even though understanding may be intact (expressive aphasia). Aphasia should be distinguished from dysarthria, which is a motor deficit of the mouth and speech muscles; the dysarthric patient articulates poorly but understands words and word choices. Aphasia is important to recognize because it usually localizes a lesion to the dominant cerebral cortex (typically the left side) in the MCA distribution. *Aphasia* and *dysphasia* are terms that are used interchangeably but must be distinguished from *dysphagia,* which is difficulty in swallowing.

Chemoreceptor Trigger Zone for Emesis

Pathology in the vertebrobasilar system (i.e., posterior circulation strokes) can cause the widest variety of symptoms and as a result may be the most challenging to diagnose. The symptoms reflect CN deficits, cerebellar involvement, and involvement of neurosensory tracts. The brainstem also contains the reticular activating system, which is responsible for mediating consciousness, and the chemoreceptor trigger zone (CTZ) for emesis (commonly referred to as the "vomiting center"). Unlike those with anterior circulation strokes, patients with posterior circulation stroke can have loss of consciousness and frequently have nausea and vomiting. The posterior cerebral artery supplies portions of the parietal and occipital lobes, so vision and thought processing are impaired. Visual agnosia, the inability to recognize seen objects, is a common feature, as is alexia, the inability to understand the written word. A third CN palsy may occur, and the patient may experience homonymous hemianopsia. One of the more unique facets of this syndrome is that the patient may be unaware of any visual problem (visual neglect). Vertigo, syncope, diplopia, visual field defects, weakness, paralysis, dysarthria, dysphagia, spasticity, ataxia, or nystagmus may be associated with vertebrobasilar artery insufficiency. Posterior circulation strokes also demonstrate crossed deficits, such as motor deficits on one side of the body and sensory loss on the other. In anterior circulation strokes, by contrast, abnormalities are limited to one side of the body.

A focused neurologic examination should assess level of consciousness, speech, CN function, motor and sensory function, and cerebellar function. Level of consciousness and fluency of speech can be rapidly assessed in a dialogue with the patient to determine the presence of dysarthria or aphasia. The head should be evaluated for signs of trauma. Pupillary size and reactivity and extraocular movements provide important information about brainstem function, particularly CN III through CN VI; an abnormal third nerve function may be the

first sign of tentorial herniation. Gaze preference suggests brainstem or cortical involvement. Central facial nerve weakness from a stroke should be distinguished from the peripheral causes of CN VII weakness. With a peripheral lesion, the patient is unable to wrinkle the forehead. Assessment of facial sensation, eyebrow elevation and squinting, smiling symmetry, gross auditory acuity, gag reflex, shoulder elevation, sternocleidomastoid strength, and tongue protrusion complete the CN evaluation.

Motor and sensory testing is performed next. Muscle tone can be assessed by moving a relaxed limb. Proximal and distal muscle group strength is assessed against resistance. Pronator drift of the arm is a sensitive sign of motor weakness and can be tested simultaneously by having the patient sit with eyes closed and arms outstretched, with palms toward the ceiling for 10 seconds. Asymmetrical sensation to pain and light touch may be subtle and difficult to detect. Double simultaneous extinction evaluation tests for sensory neglect and can be performed by simultaneously touching the right and left limbs. The patient may feel both the right and left sides being touched individually but may not discern touch on one side when both are touched simultaneously. Similarly, the ability to discern a number gently scratched on a forearm, termed graphesthesia, is another readily performed test of cortical parietal lobe. These tests can help differentiate a pure motor deficit of a lacunar stroke from a sensorimotor MCA deficit.

Cerebellar testing and the assessment of reflexes and gait complete the neurological examination. Finger-to-nose and heel-to-shin evaluations are important tests of cerebellar functions. Asymmetry of the deep tendon reflexes or unilateral Babinski sign may be an early finding of corticospinal tract dysfunction. Gait testing is commonly omitted yet is a critical part of the neurologic examination when it can be safely performed. Observing routine ambulation and heel-to-toe walking can assess for subtle ataxia, weakness, or focal cerebellar lesions.

Several prehospital stroke scales have been created to assist emergency medical service (EMS) personnel with the rapid assessment of potential stroke patients. Many of these prehospital stroke scales have been prospectively validated for their accuracy in stroke detection. Two of the more commonly used scales include the Cincinnati Prehospital Stroke Scale (Fig. 87.1) and the Los Angeles Prehospital Stroke Screen (Fig. 87.2). Scales that can reliably identify patients with large vessel occlusion (LVO) who may benefit from preferential triage to a thrombectomy capable stroke center are being evaluated.[7] The Los Angeles Motor Score (LAMS) performed by paramedics in the field has potential for identifying individuals with LVOs.[8]

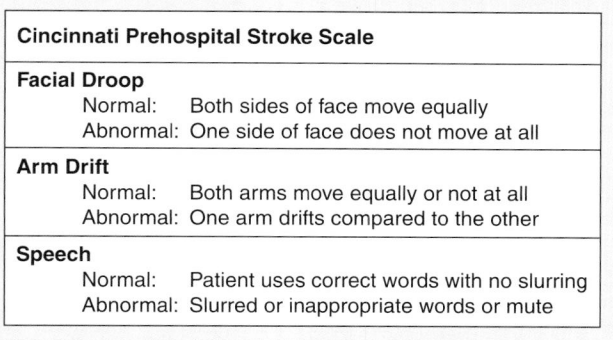

Cincinnati Prehospital Stroke Scale	
Facial Droop	
Normal:	Both sides of face move equally
Abnormal:	One side of face does not move at all
Arm Drift	
Normal:	Both arms move equally or not at all
Abnormal:	One arm drifts compared to the other
Speech	
Normal:	Patient uses correct words with no slurring
Abnormal:	Slurred or inappropriate words or mute

Fig. 87.1 Cincinnati Prehospital Stroke Scale. (Adapted from Kothari RU, Pancioli A, Liu T, et al. Cincinnati Prehospital Stroke Scale: reproducibility and validity. *Ann Emerg Med.* 1999;33[4]:373–378.)

The NIHSS is a useful and rapid tool for quantifying neurologic deficit in patients with stroke and can be used in determining treatment options (Table 87.1). NIHSS scores have been shown to be reproducible, valid, and correlate well with the amount of infarcted tissue on computed tomography (CT) scan. The baseline NIHSS score can identify patients who are appropriate candidates for fibrinolytic therapy, as well as those at increased risk for hemorrhage. It is, however, possible for patients to have disabling strokes with an NIHSS of zero (severe truncal ataxia). In addition, it has been used as a prognostic tool to predict outcome and is currently being used by certain stroke centers to stratify patients for entry into treatment trials.

Hemorrhagic Stroke

The classic presentation of ICH is the sudden onset of headache, vomiting, severely elevated BP, and focal neurologic deficits that progress

---

Los Angeles Prehospital Stroke Scale (LAPSS)

Patient name: _____
Rater name: _____
Date: _____

Screening criteria	Yes	No
4. Age over 45 years	___	___
5. No prior history of seizure disorder	___	___
6. New onset of neurologic symptoms in last 24 hours	___	___
7. Patient was ambulatory at baseline (prior to event)	___	___
8. Blood glucose between 60 and 400	___	___

9. Exam: *Look for obvious asymmetry*

	Normal	Right	Left
Facial smile / grimace:	☐	☐ Droop	☐ Droop
Grip:	☐	☐ Weak grip ☐ No grip	☐ Weak grip ☐ No grip
Arm weakness:	☐	☐ Drifts down ☐ Falls rapidly	☐ Drifts down ☐ Falls rapidly

Based on exam, patient has only unilateral (and not bilateral) weakness: Yes ☐ No ☐

10. If yes (or unknown) to all items above LAPSS screening criteria met: Yes ☐ No ☐

11. If LAPSS criteria for stroke met, call receiving hospital with "CODE STROKE," if not then return to the appropriate treatment protocol. (Note: The patient may still be experiencing a stroke if even if LAPSS criteria are not met.)

Provided by the internet stroke center — www.strokecenter.org

Fig. 87.2 Los Angeles Prehospital Stroke Screen. (Adapted from Kidwell CS, Starkman S, Eckstein M, et al. Identifying stroke in the field: prospective validation of the Los Angeles Prehospital Stroke Screen [LAPSS]. *Stroke.* 2000;31:71–76.)

TABLE 87.1 National Institutes of Health Stroke Scale Scoring Form

Item	Scoring Definitions	Score
1a. Level of consciousness (LOC)	0 = Alert and responsive 1 = Arousable to minor stimulation 2 = Arousable only to painful stimulation 3 = Reflex responses or unarousable	
1b. LOC-related questions: Ask patient's age and month. Must be exact.	0 = Both correct 1 = One correct (or dysarthria, intubated, foreign language) 2 = Neither correct	
1c. Commands: Open and close eyes, grip and release nonparetic hand. (Other one-step commands or mimic also acceptable.)	0 = Both correct (acceptable if impaired by weakness) 1 = One correct 2 = Neither correct	
2. Best gaze: Horizontal EOM by voluntary or doll's eye maneuver.	0 = Normal 1 = Partial gaze palsy; abnormal gaze in one or both eyes 2 = Forced eye deviation or total paresis that cannot be overcome by doll's eye maneuver	
3. Visual field: Use visual threat if necessary. If monocular, score field of good eye.	0 = No visual loss 1 = Partial hemianopsia, quadrantanopia, extinction 2 = Complete hemianopsia 3 = Bilateral hemianopsia or blindness	
4. Facial palsy: If patient is stuporous, check symmetry of grimace to pain.	0 = Normal 1 = Minor paralysis, flat NLF, asymmetrical smile 2 = Partial paralysis (lower face = UMN lesion) 3 = Complete paralysis (upper and lower face)	
5. Motor arm: Arms outstretched 90 degrees (sitting) or 45 degrees (supine) for 10 seconds. Encourage best effort. Indicate paretic limb in score box.	0 = No drift for 10 seconds 1 = Drift but does not hit bed 2 = Some antigravity effort, but cannot sustain 3 = No antigravity effort, but even minimal movement counts 4 = No movement at all X = Unable to assess owing to amputation, fusion, fracture, and so on	L or R
6. Motor leg: Raise leg to 30 degrees (from supine) for 5 seconds. Indicate paretic limb in score box.	0 = No drift for 5 seconds 1 = Drift but does not hit bed 2 = Some antigravity effort, but cannot sustain 3 = No antigravity effort, but even minimal movement counts 4 = No movement at all X = Unable to assess owing to amputation, fusion, fracture, and so on	L or R
7. Limb ataxia: Check finger-nose-finger, heel-shin position sense; and score only if out of proportion to paralysis.	0 = No ataxia (or aphasic, hemiplegic) 1 = Ataxia in upper or lower extremity 2 = Ataxia in upper *and* lower extremity X = Unable to assess owing to amputation, fusion, fracture, and so on	L or R
8. Sensory: Use safety pin. Check grimace or withdrawal if patient is stuporous. Score only stroke-related losses.	0 = Normal 1 = Mild-moderate unilateral loss but patient aware of touch (or aphasic, confused) 2 = Total loss, patient unaware of touch; coma, bilateral loss	
9. Best language: Describe cookie jar picture, name objects, read sentences. May use repeating, writing, stereognosis.	0 = Normal 1 = Mild-moderate aphasia (speech difficult to understand but partly comprehensible) 2 = Severe aphasia (almost no information exchanged) 3 = Mute, global aphasia, coma; no one-step commands	
10. Dysarthria: Read list of words.	0 = Normal 1 = Mild-moderate; slurred but intelligible 2 = Severe; unintelligible or mute X = Intubation or mechanical barrier	
11. Extinction or neglect: Simultaneously check bilateral visual fields and auditory sensation, touch in both hands and recognition of body parts looking for extinction or neglect.	0 = Normal, none detected (visual loss alone) 1 = Neglects or extinguishes to double simultaneous stimulation in any modality (visual, auditory, sensation, spatial, body parts) 2 = Profound neglect in more than one modality	

Android Free App: https://play.google.com/store/apps/details?id=com.myprograms.nihss
Apple Free App: https://itunes.apple.com/us/app/nih-stroke-scale-from-statcoder/id408788598?mt=8
Online NIHSS Calculator: www.mdcalc.com/nih-stroke-scale-score-nihss/
EOM, Extraocular movement; *L,* left; *LOC,* level of consciousness; *NLF,* nasolabial fold; *R,* right; *UMN,* upper motor neuron.
Modified from Massachusetts General Hospital Stroke Service. NIH stroke scale materials. Scoring form. Available at www2.massgeneral.org/stopstroke/pdfs/scoring_form.pdf.

over minutes. Similar to ischemic stroke, ICH is often associated with a motor and sensory deficit contralateral to the brain lesion. Almost 40% of patients will demonstrate significant growth in hemorrhage volume within the first few hours.

Although headache, vomiting, and coma are common, many patients do not have these findings, and the clinical presentation can be identical to that of patients with ischemic stroke; the two cannot be reliably differentiated in the absence of neuroimaging.

Ongoing assessment of airway and mental status is part of a comprehensive care plan since patients with ICH can precipitously deteriorate. Emergency airway management requires careful judgment: On the one hand, airway control can prevent aspiration, hypoxia, and hypercarbia; on the other, sedation and paralysis can make it difficult to follow serial neurologic exams, which can help monitor for hemorrhage expansion, elevated intracranial pressure (ICP), seizure activity, and brainstem herniation.

As with ischemic stroke, the neurologic examination localizes the region and extent of injury. Baseline NIHSS and Glasgow Coma Scale scores can be used to assess stroke severity, although the Glasgow Coma Score (GCS) may be more practical to follow for neurologic or mental status deterioration (Table 87.2). In addition, serial examinations can detect early changes that may suggest ongoing bleeding during the acute phase. The ICH score can also predict mortality (Table 87.3).

Baseline characteristics associated with unfavorable outcome for patients with ICH include a decreased level of consciousness on arrival, intraventricular hemorrhage, and large ICH volume, all of which can be assessed in the emergency department (ED) (Fig. 87.3). Prognostic studies of ICH have been biased by early care limitation; newer research suggests a number of patients with early care limitations could have acceptable outcomes. Based on the uncertainty, emergency clinicians are best served in avoiding specific predictions regarding chances of recovery shortly after ICH.[9]

DIFFERENTIAL DIAGNOSES

Ischemic Stroke

Extra-axial collections of blood secondary to trauma can mimic stroke. An epidural or subdural hematoma can cause an altered mental status, focal neurologic signs, and rapid progression to coma. Elders, who represent the age group at highest risk for stroke, can be victims of recurrent falls that lead to chronic subdural hematomas (particularly those on anticoagulation therapy). Carotid dissection may occur after neck trauma or sudden hyperextension and may be associated with focal neurologic signs and symptoms, as with an aortic dissection that extends into the carotid arteries.

Other structural lesions that may cause focal neurological findings include brain tumors and abscesses. Air embolism should be suspected in the setting of marked atmospheric pressure changes, such as in scuba diving or during medical procedures or injuries that may allow air into the vascular system. Seizure activity, altered mental status, and focal neurologic findings also may be manifestations of air embolism.

Metabolic abnormalities also can mimic stroke syndromes. Hypoglycemia often is responsible for an altered mental status and is a common cause of sustained focal neurologic symptoms that can persist for several days. Wernicke encephalopathy from thiamine deficiency causes ophthalmoplegia, ataxia, and confusion that can be mistaken for signs of cerebellar infarction.

Complex migraines may present with focal neurologic findings, with or without headache. A seizure followed by Todd postictal paralysis may mimic stroke. Bell or peripheral facial nerve palsy, labyrinthitis, vestibular neuronitis, peripheral nerve palsy, and demyelinating diseases may all mimic stroke. Ménière disease may be difficult to distinguish from a posterior circulation stroke or TIA. Dizziness, vertigo, hearing loss, and tinnitus in Ménière disease are common, whereas difficulties with vision or speech or other focal symptoms are less common.

Similar to stroke, giant cell arteritis is a disease of elder adults. It may cause severe headache, visual disturbances, and, rarely, aphasia and hemiparesis. Other symptoms include intermittent fever, malaise,

TABLE 87.3 Intracerebral Hemorrhage Score Predicting Mortality After Acute Intracerebral Hemorrhage

Feature	Points
Glasgow Coma Scale Score	
3–4	2
5–12	1
13–15	0
Intracerebral Hemorrhage Volume	
>30 mL	1
≤30 mL	0
Intraventricular Hemorrhage (Intraventricular Blood)	
Present	1
Absent	0
Intracerebral Hemorrhage Location	
Infratentorial	1
Supratentorial	0
Age	
≥80 years	1
<80 years	0
30-Day Mortalities for Total Intracerebral Hemorrhage Scores	
0 = 0%	
1 = 13%	
2 = 26%	
3 = 72%	
4 = 97%	
5 = 100%	
6 = Estimated to be 100%; no patients in the study fell into this category	

Adapted from Hemphill JC, Bonovich DC, Besmertis L, et al. The ICH Score. *Stroke.* 2001;32:891–897.

TABLE 87.2 Glasgow Coma Scale Score[a]

Eye Opening (E)	Verbal Response (V)	Motor Response (M)
4 = Spontaneous	5 = Normal conversation	6 = Normal
3 = To voice	4 = Disoriented conversation	5 = Localizes to pain
2 = To pain	3 = Words, but not coherent	4 = Withdraws to pain
1 = None	2 = No words; only sounds	3 = Decorticate posture
	1 = None	2 = Decerebrate posture
		1 = None

[a]Total score = E + V + M.
Shoestring Graphics: Glasgow coma score.
Available at www.ssgfx.com/CP2020/medtech/glossary/glasgow.htm.

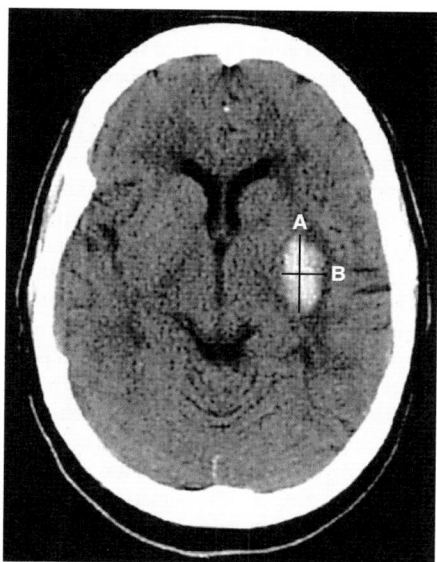

Fig. 87.3 The computed tomography (CT) slice with the largest area of hemorrhage is identified. The largest diameter of the hemorrhage on this slice is measured in centimeters *(line A)*. The largest diameter 90 degrees to A on the same slice is measured *(line B)*. C is the approximate number of 10-mm slices on which the intracerebral hemorrhage (ICH) was seen. (Many centers use 5-mm slices, in which case an adjustment can be made by dividing by 2.) The volume of the hemorrhage = A × B × C ÷ 2 (ABC/2).

jaw claudication, morning stiffness, and myalgias. The diagnosis should be suspected in patients with an elevated erythrocyte sedimentation rate (ESR) and is confirmed by temporal artery biopsy. Collagen vascular diseases such as polyarteritis nodosa, systemic lupus erythematous (SLE), and other types of vasculitis may cause stroke syndromes.

Cerebral venous sinus thrombosis (CVST) is another cause of focal neurologic symptoms that most commonly affects the superior sagittal sinus and lateral sinuses (see Chapter 89).[10] The diagnosis of CVST can be difficult because of the nonspecific nature of symptoms, as well as the variable time frame of symptom onset (from hours to weeks). Patients may have generalized headaches, nausea, vomiting, paresis, visual disturbances, depressed level of consciousness, seizures, or symptoms generally ascribed to psychiatric disorders (such as depression). Depending on the location of the thrombus, physical examination of the patient may reveal papilledema, proptosis, or palsies of CNs III, IV, and VI, as well as other focal neurologic signs. Risk factors for CVST include trauma, infectious processes, hypercoagulable states, low-flow states, compression of the venous sinus, dehydration, pregnancy, postpartum state, and certain drugs (such as androgens, designer amphetamines, and oral contraceptives).

Hemorrhagic Stroke

Differential diagnoses for ICH is similar to that for ischemic stroke; considerations include migraine, seizure, brain tumor, abscess, hypertensive encephalopathy, and head trauma. Hypertensive encephalopathy and migraine also can manifest with headache, nausea, and vomiting, although focal neurologic signs are less common in these entities. With hypertensive encephalopathy, patients usually exhibit marked elevation in BP and other evidence of end-organ injury, such as proteinuria, cardiomegaly, papilledema, and malignant hypertensive retinopathy. These patients usually improve with treatment of their hypertension. The posterior reversible encephalopathy syndrome

(PRES) is a subset of hypertensive encephalopathy presentations and has characteristic CT or magnetic resonance imaging (MRI) changes.

Once ICH is diagnosed on neuroimaging, it can be difficult to determine the underlying cause. Primary ICH typically manifests as a parenchymal hematoma with new onset neurologic symptoms. Patients with hemorrhagic transformation of an ischemic stroke may have recurrence or worsening of previously established neurological deficits. Patients with known underlying cancer, or perihematomal edema out of proportion to the hemorrhage, should be considered for hemorrhage into a metastatic lesion or primary tumor. Finally, patients with known underlying venous thromboembolic risk factors may have underlying CVST.

DIAGNOSTIC TESTING

Ischemic Stroke

Although clinical data can help establish the diagnosis and location of the stroke, confirmatory diagnostic tests are often required to establish the final cause or to eliminate other processes. The immediate evaluation includes cranial imaging, an electrocardiogram (ECG), and laboratory testing, particularly blood glucose determination.

An emergent noncontrast cranial CT of the head is the standard initial imaging technique for evaluating a patient with a potential stroke. However, it has limited sensitivity to assess strokes involving the posterior circulation, especially in the posterior fossa structures. It can quickly differentiate an ischemic stroke from ICH and other mass lesions. This information is crucial to the subsequent therapeutic decisions that need to be rapidly made. A CT scan can identify the vast majority of parenchymal hemorrhages larger than 1 cm in diameter and it has a high sensitivity for the detection of SAH. With most ischemic strokes, gross signs of infarction will not appear on routine CT scans for at least 6 to 12 hours, depending on the size of the infarct. However, subtle, early ischemic changes have been noted in up to 67% of noncontrast CT head scans within the first 3 hours. These early ischemic changes include the hyperdense artery sign (acute thrombus in a vessel), sulcal effacement, loss of the insular ribbon, loss of gray-white interface, mass effect, and acute hypodensity (Fig. 87.4).

In addition, CTA or MRA can be used to identify the presence of intravascular thrombosis, vasculature dissection, or stenosis. CTA can be used for the triage of patients who may be candidates for endovascular therapy to determine if there is an LVO. CTA can be obtained concurrently with head CT. Imaging with CTA can also be helpful to identify patients who might benefit from thrombectomy following t-PA administration. Vigilance should be taken to avoid delaying administration of thrombolytics as the thrombectomy trials with the largest treatment effects were predominantly populated with patients who had received t-PA promptly prior to thrombectomy.

Automated CT perfusion (CTP) has emerged as an additional methodology to identify patients who may benefit from reperfusion in extended time windows.[11–13] CTP is generally not helpful in the first 6 hours following stroke onset in that most of these patients will either qualify for t-PA on clinical grounds and for thrombectomy based on CTA findings. MRI has also been investigated to identify candidates for systemic thrombolysis with "wake up" strokes.[14] Advanced imaging should not delay the administration of t-PA.

The clinical importance of early ischemic CT findings with regard to fibrinolytic therapy within 3 hours of symptom onset is controversial, because the ability of treating clinicians to reproducibly identify these findings is poor and their clinical significance is questionable. Only acute hypodensity and mass effect have been shown to be associated with an increased risk of ICH after fibrinolysis (over that in treated patients without these findings). However, these findings do

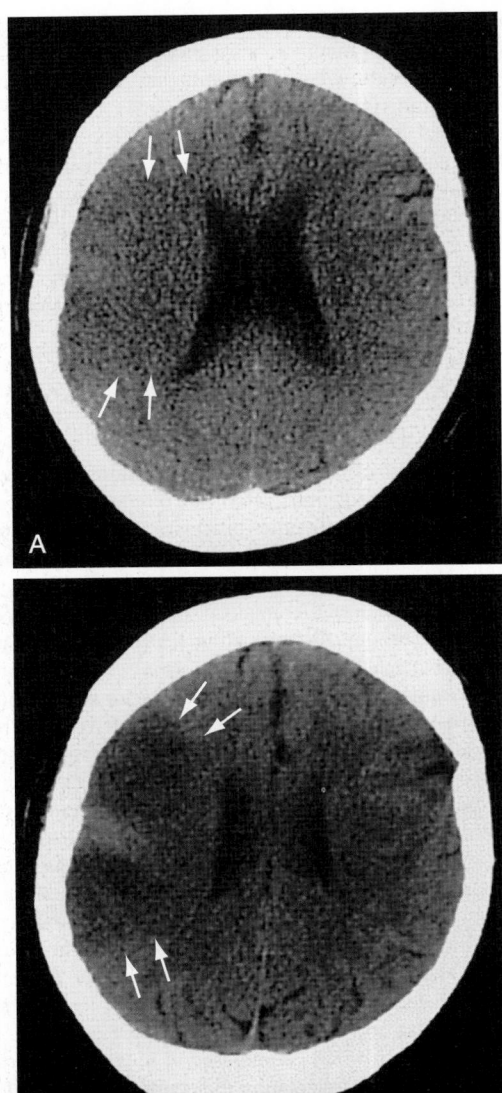

Fig. 87.4 (A) Computed tomography (CT) scan taken 2 hours and 50 minutes after a large right middle cerebral artery occlusion. There are subtle, ultra-early ischemic changes, including loss of the gray-white interface *(arrows)* and subtle evidence of sulcal effacement. (B) CT scan of same patient approximately 8 hours after symptom onset shows acute hypodensity *(arrows)* and more prominent sulcal effacement.

initial imaging modality of choice. The choice of initial cranial imaging modality is highly dependent on the speed with which these scans can be performed and interpreted at each individual center.

Diffusion-weighted imaging (DWI) and perfusion-weighted imaging (PWI) are MRI techniques that take minutes to perform and may allow differentiation between reversible and irreversible neuronal injury. Other potential imaging modalities include CTA and perfusion scans. In CTA, CT imaging is enhanced by an intravenous (IV) contrast agent to better define the vasculature of the brain. Areas of vascular stenosis and occlusion can be visualized with this technique. This information can then be used by interventionalists to determine whether a lesion is amenable to endovascular thrombectomy. Also requiring IV contrast, perfusion CT scans can reveal perfusion deficits within different regions of the brain. In addition, CTA and perfusion CT can differentiate reversible from irreversible ischemic insults.

An ECG is indicated in all patients with acute ischemic stroke; atrial fibrillation and acute myocardial infarction are associated with up to 60% of all cardioembolic strokes. The hematologic evaluation includes a complete blood and platelet count, prothrombin time (including international normalized ratio [INR]), partial thromboplastin time, troponin levels, and serum glucose measurement. Elevated blood viscosity, even when hematocrit levels are not polycythemic, can affect blood flow and prognosis. A platelet count can identify thrombocytosis or thrombocytopenia, which may precipitate a thrombosis or hemorrhage. Coagulation studies are especially helpful to guide management for patients in whom anticoagulation is being considered or for patients with an acute hemorrhagic stroke.

Other ancillary diagnostic tests to consider include an echocardiogram, carotid duplex scan, and angiogram. Some stroke centers are performing these studies as part of a TIA observation unit protocol to exclude a patent foramen ovale or valvular vegetation in those patients in whom a cardioembolic stroke is suspected. An echocardiogram should also be performed in patients with no obvious cause for their stroke.[3] Finally, conventional angiography can demonstrate stenosis or occlusion of both large and small blood vessels of the head and neck. It can detect subtle abnormalities, such as with dissection, that may not be demonstrated with noninvasive imaging techniques.

Transient Ischemic Attack

Patients with new-onset TIAs should receive an expedited evaluation and treatment owing to the substantial short-term risk of stroke and other adverse events. In 2016, a multi-national study reported a 2% stroke recurrence rate in the week following a presentation for TIA or minor stroke.[15] Emergency neuroimaging, vascular imaging (such as with a carotid Doppler study, MRA, or CTA), electrocardiography, and basic blood tests should be performed. A medically or surgically treatable cause for TIAs (e.g., high-grade carotid stenosis, mural thrombus) should be considered, which would require in-hospital treatment such as anticoagulation, stenting, or carotid endarterectomy.

Hemorrhagic Stroke

The hematologic evaluation for the patient with hemorrhagic stroke should be performed in the same manner as for the patient with ischemic stroke. Particular attention should be directed to uncovering the presence of a coagulopathy. A drug screen should be obtained to evaluate for use of sympathomimetics (such as cocaine) if substance abuse is suspected. Increased sympathetic outflow secondary to the hemorrhage may lead to an increase in dysrhythmias. Dysrhythmias also may signal impending brainstem compression from an expanding hemorrhage.

As in ischemic stroke, the cranial CT scan is the diagnostic test of choice to evaluate for an ICH. The noncontrast CT scan will reliably

not exclude patients from fibrinolytic therapy, which is associated with an improved neurological outcome. Patients with a hyperdense artery sign and acute hypodensity of one-third of the MCA distribution tend to have a poorer prognosis. Their outcomes, however, are still better with t-PA treatment than without fibrinolytic therapy.

MRI can visualize ischemic brain infarcts earlier and identify acute posterior circulation strokes more accurately than CT, and it is as effective as CT in identifying ICH. However, availability, proximity to the ED, difficulty in accessing critically ill patients, and image time limit the use of MRI in acute stroke. Advances in MRA technology have allowed a noninvasive method of demonstrating large-vessel occlusions of the anterior and posterior circulation, although small intracranial vascular occlusions may not be readily apparent. With the improvements in MRI and MRA speed and resolution, some stroke centers are replacing CT protocols with limited "stroke protocol" MRI or MRA as the

diagnose patients with clinically relevant acute ICH. Hemorrhages that are several days old may not be as apparent as acute hemorrhages and appear as isodense regions on CT imaging.

Also, as with ischemic stroke, advanced neuroimaging modalities are gaining favor in ICH. CTA produces high-quality images of the larger arterial vessels and can help exclude secondary causes, such as aneurysm, AVM, or fistula. Some patients with primary ICH show contrast extravasation on CTA, and such patients are at particularly high risk of ongoing bleeding and hematoma expansion. A venous phase can be added to this study (computed tomography venography [CTV]) to evaluate for CVST. An MRI can help detect underlying lesions (such as a brain tumor) and may offer better resolution for evaluating perihematomal edema. When available, MRA and magnetic resonance venography (MRV) can be used in place of CTA and CTV.

MANAGEMENT

Ischemic Stroke

With a focus on rapid recognition, evaluation, and treatment of stroke, many medical centers have streamlined care to meet recommended time goals (Table 87.4). This has led to the development of stroke protocols, critical pathways, and acute interventional stroke teams that may even be deployed in the field by EMS personnel before the patient arrives at the ED.

Prehospital Considerations: In the prehospital setting, the focus should be on ensuring central nervous system (CNS) oxygenation and perfusion, rapid identification, early hospital notification, and rapid transport. Although it is unusual for patients with ischemic stroke to be unresponsive on presentation, their ability to communicate may be altered by dysphasia. After an ischemic stroke, patients usually can maintain their airway unless the brainstem is affected or significant cerebral edema is compressing the opposite hemisphere. Patients with intact protective airway reflexes should receive oxygen if they are hypoxic (oxygen saturation less than 95%). Routine oxygen supplementation of normoxic stroke patients should be avoided.

A monitor and IV line should be established. Overhydration should be avoided to prevent cerebral edema. By contrast, dehydration may lead to decreased cerebral perfusion, and saline infusion should be given if dehydration is suspected. Dextrose-containing solutions should be avoided in normoglycemic patients suspected of having had a stroke because elevated blood glucose levels may worsen an ischemic deficit.

Prehospital personnel should rapidly ascertain the patient's blood sugar. Both hypo- and hyperglycemia can mimic acute stroke

presentations. Electrocardiographic monitoring is recommended to identify life-threatening arrhythmias and atrial fibrillation.[3]

Prehospital providers should document the exact time the patient was last seen to be neurologically normal and the level of neurologic functioning using one of the validated prehospital stroke scores. The level of consciousness, gross focal motor deficits, difficulty with speech, clumsiness, facial asymmetry, and any other focal deficits should be noted. Prehospital stroke scales assist in identifying patients who have had a stroke and who are potential candidates for fibrinolytic therapy. Early recognition, notification, and transport by EMS are associated with expedited delivery of fibrinolytic treatment and improved patient outcomes.

In the ED setting, the vital signs should be reassessed on an ongoing basis because patients may rapidly deteriorate even with subacute stroke. Some stroke patients are found at home 1 or 2 days after the event has occurred and may have concomitant illnesses, such as aspiration pneumonia, dehydration, hypothermia, rhabdomyolysis, or myocardial ischemia. Fever necessitates an evaluation to identify sources of infection, followed by prompt institution of treatment, including appropriate antibiotics. Even minor degrees of hyperthermia have been associated with increased neurologic injury. Oral medications, liquids, and food should be withheld until some form of swallowing assessment has been performed, given the risk of aspiration in patients with an acute stroke.

Blood Pressure Management

Current guidelines for the management of hypertension in patients with acute ischemic stroke recommend that antihypertensive treatment be reserved for those with markedly elevated BPs, unless fibrinolytic therapy is anticipated or specific medical indications are present. These medical indications include acute myocardial infarction, aortic dissection, hypertensive encephalopathy, and severe left ventricular heart failure. Oral or parenteral agents are withheld unless the patient's systolic pressure is greater than 220 mm Hg, diastolic pressure is greater than 120 mm Hg, or mean arterial pressure (MAP) is greater than 130 mm Hg (Box 87.2).

If thrombolytic therapy is indicated, stringent control of BP is indicated to reduce the potential for intracranial hemorrhage (see Box 87.2). Thrombolytic therapy is not recommended for patients whose systolic pressure is consistently higher than 185 mm Hg or whose diastolic pressure is 110 mm Hg at the time of treatment. Patients who have elevated BP and are otherwise eligible for treatment with IV thrombolytics should have their BP carefully lowered so that their systolic BP is less than 185 mm Hg and their diastolic BP is less than 110 mm Hg before IV fibrinolytic therapy is initiated. In patients for whom mechanical thrombectomy is planned and who have not received IV fibrinolytic therapy, it is reasonable to maintain BP ≤185/110 mm Hg before the procedure.[3] Simple measures can be used to lower the BP below this level: Recommended approaches include the use of IV labetalol 10 to 20 mg over 1 to 2 minutes; or continuous nicardipine 5 mg/h IV, titrate up by 2.5 mg/h every 5 to 15 minutes (maximum 15 mg/h); or clevidipine 1 to 2 mg/h IV, titrate by doubling the dose every 2 to 5 minutes (maximum 21 mg/h). Other agents such as hydralazine and enalaprilat can be used.[3] Once thrombolytic therapy has been initiated, hypertension should be treated aggressively and monitored closely for the first 24 hours after treatment.

Just as problematic as an elevated BP can be, low BP can be equally detrimental to patients with ischemic stroke. Hypotension and hypovolemia should be corrected to maintain systemic perfusion levels necessary to support organ function. Normally normotensive stroke patients with low BP or normally hypertensive stroke patients with low or even

TABLE 87.4 National Institute of Neurological Disorders and Stroke Recommended Stroke Evaluation Targets for Potential Thrombolytic Candidates	
Management Component	**Target Time Frame**
Door to doctor	10 min
Door to CT completion	25 min
Door to CT scan reading	45 min
Door to treatment	60 min
Access to neurologic expertise[a]	15 min
Access to neurosurgical expertise [a]	2 h

[a]By phone or in person.
CT, Computed tomography.

low-normal BP are given a fluid bolus to try to increase cerebral perfusion. This is especially important in patients in a dehydrated state. If initial fluid challenge is ineffective, the patient may require vasopressor therapy to gradually increase MAP and improve cerebral perfusion.

Temperature

Sources of hyperthermia (temperature >38°C) should be identified and treated, and antipyretic medications should be administered to lower temperature in hyperthermic patients with stroke.[3] For patients with stroke peak temperature in the first 24 hours less than 37°C and greater than 39°C is associated with an increased risk of in-hospital death compared with normothermia.[16] The benefit of treatment with induced hypothermia remains unclear. To date, studies of hypothermia in acute ischemic stroke show no benefit in functional outcome and suggest that induction of hypothermia increases the risk of infection, including pneumonia.[3]

BOX 87.2   Emergency Antihypertensive Therapy for Acute Ischemic Stroke

Indication That Patient Is Eligible for Treatment With Intravenous Recombinant Tissue Plasminogen Activator or Other Acute Reperfusion Intervention
Blood Pressure Level
Systolic >185 mm Hg or diastolic >110 mm Hg
  Labetalol 10–20 mg IV over 1–2 min; may repeat 1 time
  or
  Nicardipine infusion, 5 mg/h; titrate up by 2.5 mg/h at 5- to 15-min intervals, maximum dose 15 mg/h; when desired BP attained, reduce to 3 mg/h
  or
  Clevidipine 1 to 2 mg/h IV, titrate by doubling dose every 2 to 5 minutes (maximum 21 mg/h)
Other agents (e.g., hydralazine, enalaprilat) may be considered when appropriate.
If BP does not decline and remains >185/110 mm Hg, do not administer rtPA.

Management of Blood Pressure During and After Treatment With Recombinant Tissue Plasminogen Activator or Other Acute Reperfusion Intervention
Monitor BP every 15 min during treatment and then for another 2 h, then every 30 min for 6 h, and then every hour for 16 h.

Blood Pressure Level
Systolic 180–230 mm Hg or diastolic 105–120 mm Hg
  Labetalol 10 mg IV over 1–2 min; may repeat every 10–20 min; maximum dose of 300 mg
  or
  Labetalol 10 mg IV followed by an infusion at 2–8 mg/min
Systolic >230 mm Hg or diastolic 121–140 mm Hg
  Labetalol 10 mg IV over 1–2 min; may repeat every 10–20 min; maximum dose of 300 mg
  or
  Labetalol 10 mg IV followed by an infusion at 2–8 mg/min
  or
  Nicardipine infusion, 5 mg/h; titrate up to desired effect by increasing 2.5 mg/h every 5 minutes to maximum of 15 mg/h
If BP not controlled, consider sodium nitroprusside.

BP, Blood pressure; *IV,* intravenous; *rtPA,* recombinant tissue plasminogen activator.
Adapted from Jauch EC, Saver JL, Adams HP Jr, et al. Guidelines for the early management of adults with ischemic stroke: a guideline for healthcare professionals from the American Heart Association/ American Stroke Association. *Stroke* 2013;44(3):870–947.

Blood Glucose

Evidence indicates that persistent in-hospital hyperglycemia during the first 24 hours after stroke is associated with worse outcomes than normoglycemia, and thus we recommend treating hyperglycemia to achieve blood glucose levels in a range of 140 to 180 mg/dL and to closely monitor to prevent hypoglycemia. Hypoglycemia (blood glucose <60 mg/dL) should be treated with IV dextrose solution.

Reperfusion Therapy

The ultimate goal of reperfusion therapy for acute ischemic stroke is to improve outcome by reducing stroke-related disability and mortality. Restoring perfusion to ischemic areas of the brain that are not yet infarcted is critical to achieving this goal and is time dependent. There are two reperfusion strategies that have been extensively studied and proven effective: (1) IV thrombolytic therapy and (2) mechanical thrombectomy.

Thrombolytic Therapy

Agent and Dosage

Options for thrombolytic therapy that are proven effective include two types of recombinant tissue plasminogen activators (t-PA): IV alteplase and IV tenecteplase. Alteplase is the primary IV thrombolytic agent approved by the U.S. Food and Drug Administration (FDA) for treatment of patients with acute ischemic stroke within 3 hours of clearly defined symptom onset to restore blood flow to the regions of brain that are ischemic. Approval was initially based on the results of the National Institute of Neurological Disorders and Stroke (NINDS) trial. The dosage of alteplase is 0.9 mg/kg (maximum dose 90 mg) over 60 minutes with initial 10% of dose given as bolus over 1 minute. The ENCHANTED trial evaluated a low-dose alteplase (0.6 mg/kg IV) versus standard-dose alteplase (0.9 mg/kg IV) in 3300 patients (63% Asian) with acute ischemic stroke. Low-dose alteplase was noninferior to standard-dose alteplase with respect to death and disability at 90 days and there were significantly fewer symptomatic ICHs with low-dose alteplase.[17] Low-dose alteplase is the standard of care in Japan but current AHA/ASA guidelines still recommend 0.9 mg/Kg.

There is moderate- to high-quality evidence that IV tenecteplase 0.25 mg/kg (maximum 25 mg) given in a single bolus has similar rates of functional outcome, symptomatic ICH, and mortality at 90 days compared with alteplase.[18–20] The EXTEND-IA TNK trial (Tenecteplase Versus Alteplase Before Endovascular Therapy for Ischemic Stroke) randomized 202 patients with acute ischemic stroke within 4.5 hours of symptoms undergoing endovascular therapy to thrombolysis with tenecteplase versus alteplase.[21] Tenecteplase was associated with a higher incidence of reperfusion and better functional outcome compared with alteplase. Intracranial hemorrhage was similar between groups.[21] Tenecteplase can be used in place of alteplase in patients without contraindications for IV fibrinolysis who are also eligible to undergo mechanical thrombectomy.[3,21] From a practical standpoint, the bolus infusion of tenecteplase is easier to administer than a 1-hour infusion of alteplase.

The potential risks should be discussed with the patient when determining eligibility for thrombolysis and weighed against the anticipated benefits during decision making (Table 87.5).

Time Window

Within 3 hours of symptom onset: The safety and efficacy of alteplase treatment when administered within the first 3 hours after stroke onset are solidly supported by combined data from multiple RCTs[3,22] and confirmed by extensive community experience in many countries.[23] The eligibility criteria for IV thrombolytic therapy have evolved over time as its usefulness and true risks have become clearer (see eligibility criteria).

TABLE 87.5 2019 AHA/ASA Acute Stroke Management Guidelines for Alteplase Treatment in Acute Ischemic Stroke

A. Eligibility Recommendations for IV Alteplase in Patients With Acute Ischemic Stroke

Within 3 h	IV alteplase (0.9 mg/kg, maximum dose 90 mg over 60 min with initial 10% of dose given as bolus over 1 min) is recommended for selected patients who may be treated within 3 h of ischemic stroke symptom onset or patient last known well or at baseline state.
Within 3 h—Age	For otherwise medically eligible patients ≥18 years of age, IV alteplase administration within 3 h is equally recommended for patients ≤80 and >80 years of age.
Within 3 h—Severe stroke	For severe stroke, IV alteplase is indicated within 3 h from symptom onset of ischemic stroke. Despite increased risk of hemorrhagic transformation, there is still proven clinical benefit for patients with severe stroke symptoms.
Within 3 h—Mild disabling stroke	For otherwise eligible patients with mild but disabling stroke symptoms, IV alteplase is recommended for patients who can be treated within 3 hours of ischemic stroke symptom onset or patient last known well or at baseline state.
3–4.5 h	IV alteplase is also recommended for selected patients who can be treated within 3 and 4.5 h of ischemic stroke symptom onset or patient last known well.
3–4.5 h—Age	IV alteplase treatment in the 3- to 4.5-h time window is recommended for those patients ≤80 years of age, without a history of both diabetes mellitus and prior stroke, NIHSS score ≤25, not taking any oral anticoagulants, and without imaging evidence of ischemic injury involving more than one-third of the MCA territory.
Urgency	Treatment should be initiated as quickly as possible within the above-listed time frames because time to treatment is strongly associated with outcomes.
BP	IV alteplase is recommended in patients with BP <185/110 mm Hg and in those patients whose BP can be lowered safely to this level with antihypertensive agents, with the physician assessing the stability of the BP before starting IV alteplase.
Blood glucose	IV alteplase is recommended in otherwise eligible patients with initial glucose levels >50 mg/dL.
CT	IV alteplase administration is recommended in the setting of early ischemic changes on NCCT of mild to moderate extent (other than frank hypodensity).
Prior antiplatelet therapy	IV alteplase is recommended for patients taking antiplatelet drug monotherapy before stroke on the basis of evidence that the benefit of alteplase outweighs a possible small increased risk of sICH. IV alteplase is recommended for patients taking antiplatelet drug combination therapy (e.g., aspirin and clopidogrel) before stroke on the basis of evidence that the benefit of alteplase outweighs a probable increased risk of sICH.
End-stage renal disease	In patients with end-stage renal disease on hemodialysis and normal aPTT, IV alteplase is recommended. However, those with elevated aPTT may have elevated risk for hemorrhagic complications.

B. Exclusions for IV Alteplase in Patients With Acute Ischemic Stroke

0- to 3-h window—Mild nondisabling stroke	For otherwise eligible patients with mild nondisabling stroke (NIHSS score 0–5), IV alteplase is not recommended for patients who could be treated within 3 h of ischemic stroke symptom onset or patient last known well or at baseline state.
3- to 4.5-h window—Mild nondisabling stroke	For otherwise eligible patients with mild nondisabling stroke (NIHSS score 0–5), IV alteplase is not recommended for patients who could be treated within 3 and 4.5 h of ischemic stroke symptom onset or patient last known well or at baseline state.
CT	There remains insufficient evidence to identify a threshold of hypoattenuation severity or extent that affects treatment response to alteplase. However, administering IV alteplase to patients whose CT brain imaging exhibits extensive regions of clear hypoattenuation is not recommended. These patients have a poor prognosis despite IV alteplase, and severe hypoattenuation defined as obvious hypodensity represents irreversible injury.
ICH	IV alteplase should not be administered to a patient whose CT reveals an acute intracranial hemorrhage.
Ischemic stroke within 3 months	Use of IV alteplase in patients presenting with AIS who have had a prior ischemic stroke within 3 months may be harmful.
Severe head trauma within 3 months	In AIS patients with recent severe head trauma (within 3 months), IV alteplase is contraindicated.
Acute head trauma	Given the possibility of bleeding complications from the underlying severe head trauma, IV alteplase should not be administered in posttraumatic infarction that occurs during the acute in-hospital phase.
Intracranial/intraspinal surgery within 3 months	For patients with AIS and a history of intracranial/spinal surgery within the prior 3 months, IV alteplase is potentially harmful.
History of intracranial hemorrhage	IV alteplase administration in patients who have a history of intracranial hemorrhage is potentially harmful.
Subarachnoid hemorrhage	IV alteplase is contraindicated in patients presenting with symptoms and signs most consistent with an SAH.
GI malignancy or GI bleed within 21 days	Patients with a structural GI malignancy or recent bleeding event within 21 days of their stroke event should be considered high risk, and IV alteplase administration is potentially harmful.
Coagulopathy	The safety and efficacy of IV alteplase for acute stroke patients with platelets <100 000/mm3, INR >1.7, aPTT > 40 s, or PT >15 s are unknown, and IV alteplase should not be administered. (In patients without history of thrombocytopenia, treatment with IV alteplase can be initiated before availability of platelet count but should be discontinued if platelet count is <100,000/mm³. In patients without recent use of OACs or heparin, treatment with IV alteplase can be initiated before availability of coagulation test results but should be discontinued if INR is >1.7 or PT is abnormally elevated by local laboratory standards.)

(continued)

TABLE 87.5   2019 AHA/ASA Acute Stroke Management Guidelines for Alteplase Treatment in Acute Ischemic Stroke—cont'd.

LMWH	IV alteplase should not be administered to patients who have received a full treatment dose of LMWH within the previous 24 h.
Thrombin inhibitors or factor Xa inhibitors	The use of IV alteplase in patients taking direct thrombin inhibitors or direct factor Xa inhibitors has not been firmly established but may be harmful. IV alteplase should not be administered to patients taking direct thrombin inhibitors or direct factor Xa inhibitors unless laboratory tests such as aPTT, INR, platelet count, ecarin clotting time, thrombin time, or appropriate direct factor Xa activity assays are normal or the patient has not received a dose of these agents for >48 h (assuming normal renal metabolizing function). (Alteplase could be considered when appropriate laboratory tests such as aPTT, INR, ecarin clotting time, thrombin time, or direct factor Xa activity assays are normal or when the patient has not taken a dose of these ACs for >48 h and renal function is normal.)
Concomitant Abciximab	Abciximab should not be administered concurrently with IV alteplase.
Concomitant IV aspirin	IV aspirin should not be administered within 90 min after the start of IV alteplase.
Infective endocarditis	For patients with AIS and symptoms consistent with infective endocarditis, treatment with IV alteplase should not be administered because of the increased risk of intracranial hemorrhage.
Aortic arch dissection	IV alteplase in AIS known or suspected to be associated with aortic arch dissection is potentially harmful and should not be administered.
Intra-axial intracranial neoplasm	IV alteplase treatment for patients with AIS who harbor an intra-axial intracranial neoplasm is potentially harmful.

AIS, Acute ischemic stroke; *aPPT,* activated partial thromboplatin time; *CT,* computed tomography; *GI,* gastrointestinal; *ICH,* intracerebral hemorrhage; *INR,* international normalized ratio; *IV,* intravenous; *LMWH,* low molecular weight heparin; *MCA,* middle cerebral artery; *NCCT,* noncontrast computed tomography; *SAH,* subarachnoid hemorrhage; *sICH,* spontaneous intracerebral hemorrhage.

The benefit of IV alteplase is well established for adult patients with disabling stroke symptoms regardless of age and stroke severity.[24] Patients should receive IV thrombolytics without delay, if eligible, even if mechanical thrombectomy is being considered.

Three to 4.5 hours of symptom onset: Subsequent studies have demonstrated the usefulness of IV thrombolytics at 3 to 4.5 hours of ischemic stroke symptom onset or patient last known well or at baseline state. Treatment with IV alteplase initiated within 4.5 hours of stroke onset improves functional outcome at 3 to 6 months for patients across the age spectrum and severities of stroke.[24,25] However, the earlier that treatment is initiated, the greater the benefit, as the benefit decreases continuously over time from symptom onset. Faster IV thrombolysis delivery is associated with less disability at 3 months especially for door-to-needle time less than 30 minutes.[26] IV tenecteplase has been compared with alteplase up to 6 hours after stroke and appears to be similarly safe, but it is unclear whether it is as effective as or more effective than alteplase.[3]

In patients with acute ischemic stroke known or suspected to be associated with extracranial cervical arterial dissection, who are otherwise eligible for thrombolysis, it is reasonably safe to administer thrombolytics within 4.5 hours of symptom onset.[3] However, the usefulness and hemorrhagic risk of thrombolytics in acute ischemic stroke known or suspected to be associated with intracranial arterial dissection remain unknown and thrombolysis is not recommended.[3]

4.5 to 9 hours of symptom onset or unwitnessed onset or "wake-up" stroke: In patients with acute ischemic stroke who awake with stroke symptoms or have unclear time of onset greater than 4.5 hours from last known well or at baseline state, MRI to identify DWI-positive (diffusion weighted imaging) and FLAIR-negative (fluid-attenuated inversion recovery) lesions can be useful for selecting those who can benefit from IV alteplase administration within 4.5 hours of stroke symptom recognition (Fig. 87.5).[3] The WAKE-UP trial (Efficacy and Safety of MRI-based Thrombolysis in Wake-Up Stroke) randomized 503 patients who awoke with stroke (90%) or had unclear time of onset greater than 4.5 hours from last known well (10%) and were otherwise eligible for IV alteplase. Favorable outcome (mRS score of 0 to 1) at 90 days was achieved in significantly more patients in the IV alteplase

group versus the placebo group (53% vs. 42%). Mortality rate was not significantly higher in the alteplase group (4% vs. 1%) as was the rate of symptomatic intracranial hemorrhage (2% vs. 0.4%).[14]

The EXTEND trial (EXtending the time for Thrombolysis in Emergency Neurological Deficits) enrolled 225 adults who had hypoperfused but salvageable brain tissue on automated perfusion imaging (CT or MRI) and could be treated between 4.5 and 9 hours after the onset of ischemic stroke or awoke with stroke symptoms (9 hours from the midpoint of sleep) and randomly assigned them to IV alteplase or placebo. Favorable outcome (mRS score of 0 to 1) at 90 days was more likely for the IV alteplase group compared with the placebo group (35% vs. 30%); when adjusted for age and severity, there was no significant difference between alteplase and placebo in the unadjusted analysis. Symptomatic intracranial hemorrhage within 36 hours of treatment was higher with alteplase (6% vs. 1%) (*P* = .053) though mortality was not significantly higher with alteplase (12% vs. 9%).[11] Similarly, in the ECASS-4 trial, IV alteplase administered between 4.5 and 9 hours after the onset of symptoms in patients with salvageable tissue did not result in a significant benefit over placebo.[27]

Therefore, beyond 4.5 hours, the benefit of IV alteplase is not clear. The application of DWI-positive (diffusion-weighted imaging) and FLAIR-negative (fluid-attenuated inversion recovery) lesions on MRI to identify patients with a stroke onset time greater than 4.5 hours or an unknown stroke onset time who would benefit from IV alteplase, is promising.

Thrombolysis for Mild Disabling Versus Nondisabling Acute Ischemic Stroke

For otherwise eligible patients with *mild nondisabling* stroke symptoms (NIHSS score 0 to 5), IV alteplase is not recommended for patients who could be treated within 3 or 4.5 hours of ischemic stroke symptom onset or patient last known to be well or at baseline state.[3] The PRISMS trial (A Study of the Safety and Efficacy of Alteplase in Patients With Mild Stroke) evaluated IV alteplase in 313 patients with mild acute ischemic stroke within three hours of symptom onset (NIHSS score 0 to 5) whose acute neurological deficits were judged to not interfere with activities of daily living or prevent return to work (nondisabling).

Excluded

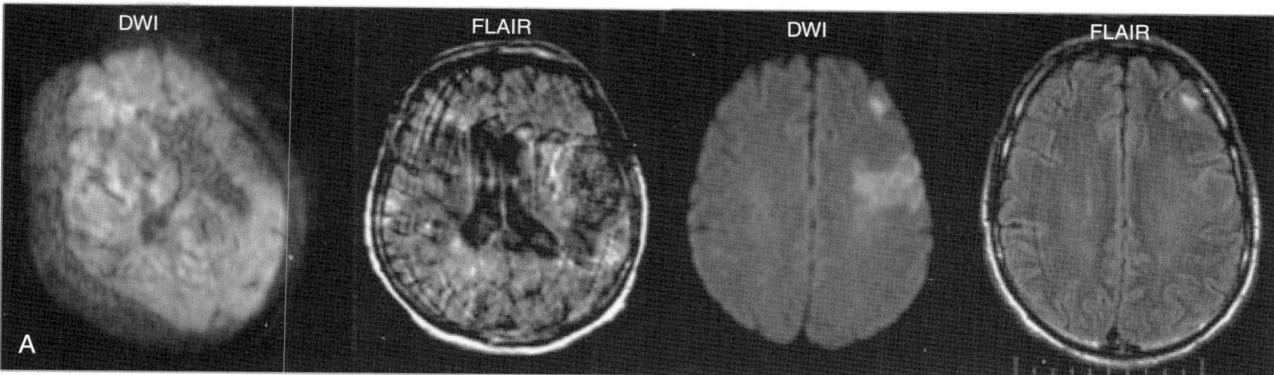

FLAIR-negative (DWI-FLAIR mismatch)

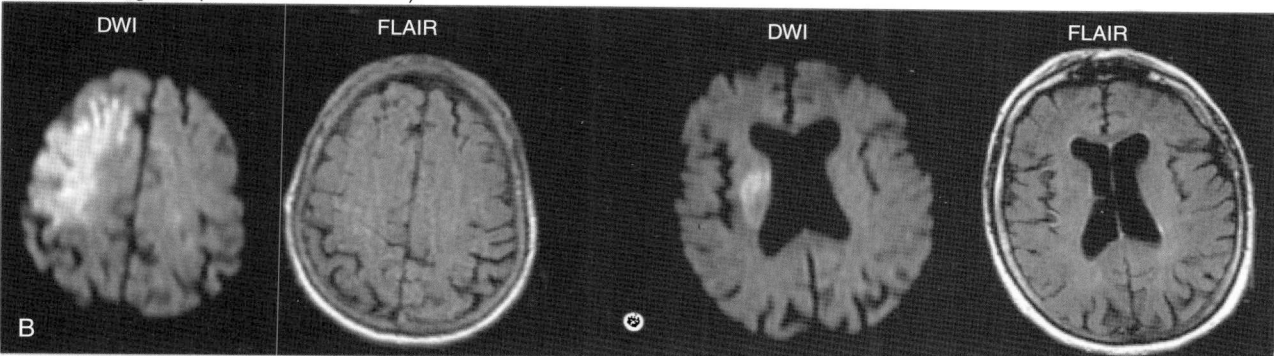

FLAIR-positive (no DWI-FLAIR mismatch)

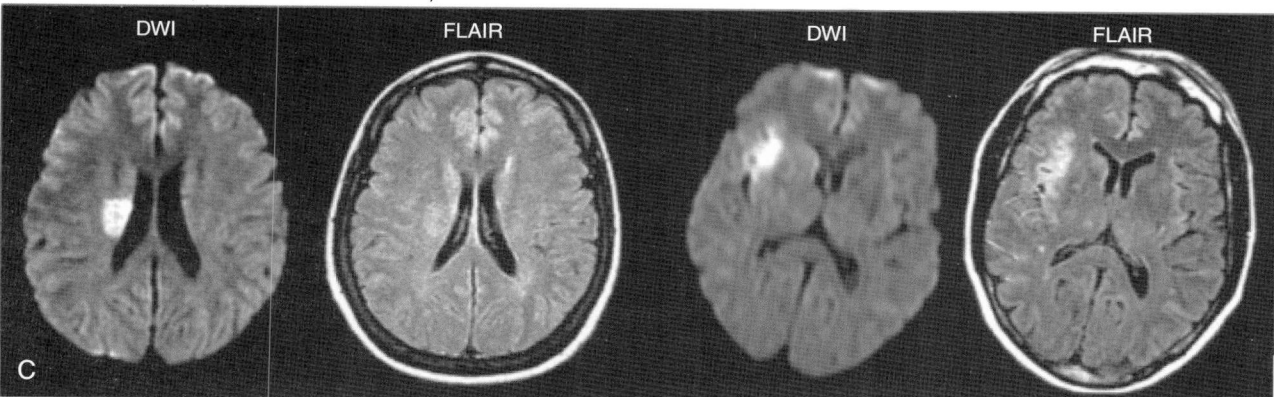

Fig. 87.5 Examples of DWI and FLAIR images. (A) Diffusion-weighted imaging (DWI) and fluid-attenuated inversion recovery (FLAIR) images excluded from the final analysis because of poor quality (left) or the presence of multiple acute and subacute ischemic lesions of different ages, precluding the attribution of symptom onset to one specific lesion (right). (B) Pairs of images showing acute ischemic lesions on DWI but not on FLAIR imaging (FLAIR-negative, DWI-FLAIR mismatch). (C) Pairs of images showing acute ischemic lesions on DWI together with a corresponding subtle (left) or obvious (right) parenchymal hyperintensity on FLAIR imaging (FLAIR-positive, no DWI-FLAIR mismatch). (Reprinted with permission from Elsevier. From Thomalla G, Cheng B, Ebinger M, et al. DWI-FLAIR mismatch for the identification of patients with acute ischaemic stroke within 4.5 h of symptom onset (PRE-FLAIR): a multicentre observational study. *Lancet Neurology*, 2011;10(11):981; Figure 2.)

There was no difference in the rate of a favorable functional outcome (mRS of 0 or 1) at 90 days for patients assigned to treatment with IV alteplase or to aspirin (78% vs. 82%).[28,29]

However, for otherwise eligible patients with *mild but disabling* stroke symptoms, IV alteplase is recommended for patients who can be treated within 3 hours and within 3 and 4.5 hours of ischemic stroke symptom onset or patient last known to be well or at baseline state (Powers et al., 2019).[30]

Thrombolysis in Patients on Anticoagulants Before the Stroke

Antiplatelet: IV alteplase is recommended for patients taking antiplatelet drug monotherapy before stroke on the basis of evidence that the benefit of alteplase outweighs a possible small increased risk of symptomatic ICH. Similarly, IV alteplase is recommended for patients taking antiplatelet drug combination therapy (e.g., aspirin and clopidogrel) before stroke on the basis of evidence that the benefit of alteplase outweighs a probable increased risk of ICH.

LMWH: IV alteplase should not be administered to patients who have received a full treatment dose of low molecular weight heparin (LMWH) within the previous 24 hours.

Factor IIa and Factor Xa Inhibitors: The use of IV alteplase in patients taking direct thrombin inhibitors or direct factor Xa inhibitors has not been firmly established but may be harmful. Therefore, IV alteplase should not be administered to patients taking direct thrombin inhibitors or direct factor Xa inhibitors unless laboratory tests such as activated partial thromboplastin time (aPTT), INR, platelet count, ecarin clotting time, thrombin time, or appropriate direct factor Xa activity assays are normal, or the patient has not received a dose of these agents for greater than 48 hours (assuming normal renal metabolizing function).[3]

Symptomatic Intracerebral Hemorrhage Following Thrombolysis

IV thrombolysis with tissue plasminogen activator after acute ischemic stroke carries a risk of symptomatic ICH with an incidence from 2% to 7%[31] with greatest risk in patients with the most severe strokes.[25] Asymptomatic ICH occurs more frequently and usually occurs within 36 hours after t-PA infusion and half of the events are diagnosed within 5 to 10 hours. Intracranial hemorrhage occurring after 36 hours is unlikely to be caused by thrombolysis. Classification of symptomatic ICH after thrombolytic therapy is based on two main factors: (1) radiographic appearance of the hemorrhage and (2) the presence of associated neurological deterioration.[31] Unfortunately, variability in the definition of clinical neurological deterioration has a dramatic impact on the reported incidence of ICH in different studies.

Radiographically, hemorrhage is graded as: (1) *petechial* hemorrhage along the infarcted tissue margin (HI1), (2) *confluent petechial* hemorrhage within the infarcted tissue (HI2), (3) *parenchymal* hematoma involving 30% or less of the infarcted tissue with slight mass effect (PH1), (4) *parenchymal* hematoma involving greater than 30% of the infarcted tissue with significant mass effect (PH2). Subtype PH2 is the most clinically significant as it carries a poor prognosis, approaching 50% mortality and significant morbidity in survivors. Subtypes HI1, HI2, and PH1 occur more frequently than PH2.[32]

In a systematic review and meta-analysis of 55 studies, older age, greater stroke severity, higher baseline glucose, hypertension, congestive heart failure, renal impairment, diabetes mellitus, ischemic heart disease, atrial fibrillation, baseline antiplatelet use, leukoaraiosis, and visible acute infarction on brain imaging were all associated with increased risk of symptomatic ICH (Box 87.3).[31] Several risk scores have been developed to predict the risk of ICH or prognosis for patients treated with IV thrombolysis.[33] They include the HAT score, DRAGON score, SEDAN score, Stroke-Thrombolytic Predictive Instrument, SPAN-100 index, and the SITS SICH risk score. The predictive ability of the risk scores varies with absolute risk for symptomatic ICH for SITS at 0.2% for a score of zero to 14% for a score of 10 or more. For SEDAN the risk has ranged from 1% for a score of zero to 28% for a score of five points. For HAT the symptomatic ICH rate has ranged from 3% to 14%. Validation studies are needed to confirm their utility before they can be instituted in clinical practice.

Current protocols include ICU monitoring for 24 hours with repeat neuroimaging if there is any neurological deterioration. Treatment of post-thrombolytic hemorrhage includes cardiovascular and respiratory support, BP management, neurological monitoring, prevention of hematoma expansion, control of elevated ICP, and seizure control. Treatment options for ICH related to IV thrombolytics include the administration of agents to reverse the effects of thrombolytic therapy and antithrombotic therapy but no specific agent has been shown

> ### BOX 87.3 Factors Associated With Increased Risk for Symptomatic Intracerebral Hemorrhage After Thrombolysis
>
> Older age
> Greater stroke severity
> Higher baseline glucose
> Hypertension
> Congestive heart failure
> Renal impairment
> Diabetes mellitus
> Ischemic heart disease
> Atrial fibrillation
> Baseline antiplatelet use
> Leukoaraiosis (periventricular white matter disease)
> Visible acute infarction on brain imaging
> Cerebral microbleeds

to be most effective.[31] These include antifibrinolytic agents (epsilon-aminocaproic acid and tranexamic acid), cryoprecipitate, fresh frozen plasma, platelets, prothrombin complex concentrate, and vitamin K. It's preferable to withhold the use of activated Factor VIIa (rFVIIa) until more studies establish its safety in this setting, given that it is associated with relatively high thrombosis rates.[31] Of these treatment options, we recommend cryoprecipitate. Once symptomatic ICH is diagnosed, consider immediately sending a fibrinogen level and empirically transfusing with 10 U cryoprecipitate intravenously over 10 to 30 minutes.[3] Additional cryoprecipitate may be needed to achieve a fibrinogen level of ≥150 mg/dL. Neurosurgical intervention may also be considered if clinically indicated.[31]

Cerebral Microbleeds

Cerebral microbleeds (CMBs) are small accumulations of blood products in brain tissue that are associated with cerebrovascular disease, dementia, and aging. They occur in the setting of impaired small vessel integrity due to hypertension or cerebral amyloid angiopathy.[34] In the setting of acute ischemic stroke, CMBs are considered markers of bleeding-prone cerebral vessel microangiopathies that increase the risk of ICH[35-37] along with poor 3- to 6-month functional outcome after administration of IV thrombolysis.[37-39] The risk of symptomatic ICH in patients with greater than 10 CMBs is significantly greater (30% to 47%) than in those without CMBs (1% to 4%).[35,36,38] Thus, the presence of CMBs increases the risk of ICH and the chances of poor outcomes after thrombolytics, but it is unclear whether these negative effects fully negate the benefit of thrombolytics.[37] Therefore, in patients who have previously had a high burden of CMBs (>10) demonstrated on MRI, the benefits of thrombolytic treatment are uncertain.[3]

Mechanical Thrombectomy

The recent trials demonstrating clear benefit of endovascular thrombectomy come after a decade of negative studies. The difference in results is due to a combination of improved devices, emphasis on early intervention, advanced imaging techniques and careful patient selection. These studies have conclusively demonstrated that patients with severe strokes and evidence of proximal LVOs have significantly better functional outcomes when treated with the new-generation devices. Mechanical thrombectomy is now indicated for patients with acute ischemic stroke with large artery occlusion in the anterior circulation who meet selected criteria and who present within 24 hours of last known to be well regardless of whether they receive IV alteplase for the same ischemic stroke event.

Timing

Shorter time to endovascular-reperfusion therapy is significantly associated with better outcomes.[40,41] In pooled patient-level data from five trials (MR CLEAN, ESCAPE, REVASCAT, SWIFT PRIME, and EXTEND-IA), shorter time from symptom onset to arterial puncture with mechanical thrombectomy was associated with lower degrees of disability at 3 months but the benefit became nonsignificant after 7 hours.[42] The majority of these patients also received thrombolytics. Among those who achieved substantial reperfusion each 1-hour delay to reperfusion was associated with a less favorable degree of disability and less functional independence, but no change in mortality.[42]

Zero to 6 hours of symptom onset: Guidelines from the AHA/American Stroke Association (ASA) recommend mechanical thrombectomy for adults with: (1) no significant prestroke disability (i.e., a mRS score of ≤1); (2) a causative occlusion of the ICA or the M1 segment of the MCA; (3) NIHSS score of ≥6; and (4) ASPECTS of ≥6 (associated with better functional outcome at 3 months). These guidelines are based on results from 6 recent randomized trials of mechanical thrombectomy using predominantly stent retriever devices (MR CLEAN, SWIFT PRIME, EXTEND-IA, ESCAPE, REVASCAT, THRACE).[3]

The benefits of thrombectomy are uncertain for patients with occlusion of the ICA or proximal MCA (M1), who have a prestroke mRS score greater than 1, or an NIHSS score less than 6, or a larger infarct core (i.e., ASPECTS score <6). Using pooled patient data, the direction of treatment effect for mechanical thrombectomy over standard care appears favorable in M2 occlusions but does not reach statistical significance.[43–45] Therefore, the benefits of thrombectomy for distal MCA occlusion, MCA segment 2 (M2) or MCA segment 3 (M3), are uncertain. Additionally, the benefits are uncertain in those with occlusion of the anterior cerebral arteries, vertebral arteries, basilar artery, or posterior cerebral arteries.

Pooled patient-level data showed that mechanical thrombectomy had a favorable effect over standard care in patients ≥70 years of age and ≥80 years of age.[43,44,46] However, the number of patients in these trials who were ≥90 years of age was very small. As with any treatment decision in an elderly patient, consideration of comorbidities and risks should factor into the decision-making for mechanical thrombectomy.

Six to 16 hours of symptom onset: In selected patients with acute ischemic stroke within 6 to 16 hours of last known normal who have LVO in the anterior circulation and meet other DAWN or DEFUSE 3 eligibility criteria, mechanical thrombectomy is recommended (without thrombolysis).[3]

The DAWN trial used clinical-core mismatch (a combination of NIHSS score and imaging findings on CT perfusion or diffusion-weighted MRI) as eligibility criteria to select patients with large anterior circulation vessel occlusion for treatment with mechanical thrombectomy between 6 and 24 hours from last known to be at their normal neurological baseline. This trial demonstrated an overall significant benefit in function outcome at 90 days in the treatment group (mRS score 0 to 2) of 49% versus 13%.[13] Only 12% with witnessed onset of symptoms. The DEFUSE 3 trial used perfusion-core mismatch and maximum core size as imaging criteria to select patients had large anterior circulation occlusion 6 to 16 hours from last seen well for mechanical thrombectomy (Fig. 87.6). This trial showed a significant benefit in functional outcome at 90 days in the treated group (mRS score 0 to 2) of 45% versus 17%.[12] Benefit was independently demonstrated for the subgroup of patients who met DAWN eligibility criteria and for the subgroup who did not. DAWN and DEFUSE 3 are the only RCTs showing benefit of mechanical thrombectomy greater than 6 hours from onset. Therefore, only the eligibility criteria from one or the other of these trials should be used for patient selection. Although future RCTs may demonstrate that additional eligibility criteria can be used to select patients who benefit from mechanical thrombectomy, at this time, the DAWN or DEFUSE 3 eligibility should be strictly adhered to in clinical practice.[3,12,13]

Sixteen to 24 hours of symptom onset: In selected patients with acute ischemia stroke within 16 to 24 hours of last known normal who have

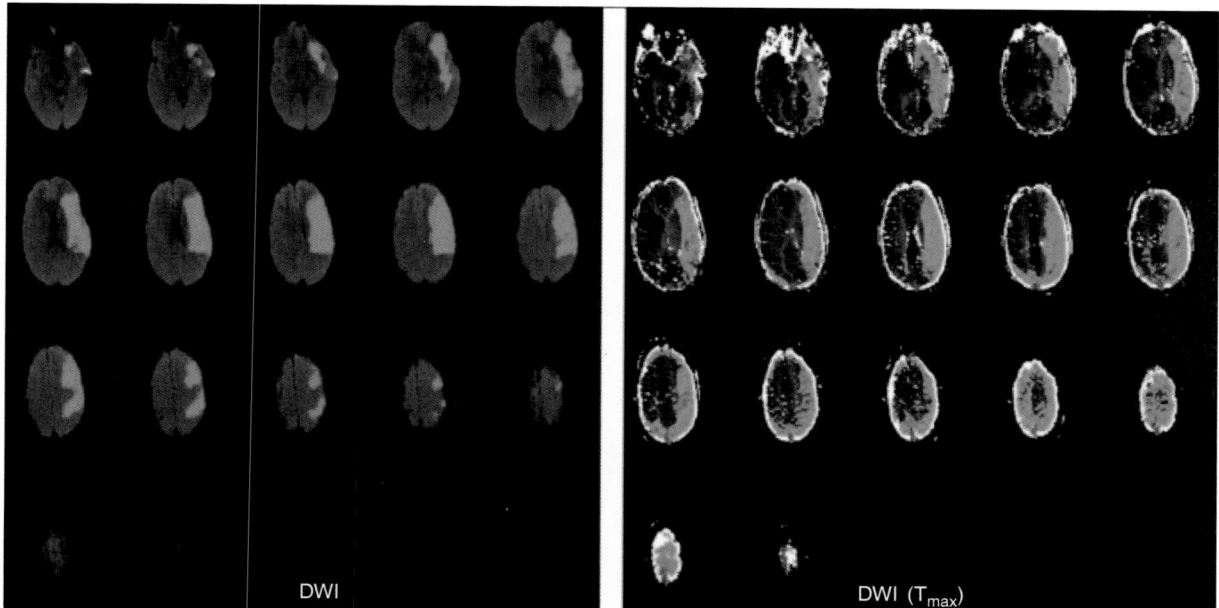

Fig. 87.6 Malignant penumbral profile unfavorable for treatment more than 3 h after stroke onset. MRI scan with DWI showing large established infarct core (*left*; 143 cm³) and perfusion-weighted imaging showing extremely large region of tissue at risk (*right*; 255 cm³). Although mismatch is present (ratio 1:8), and the patient presented within the treatment window, the large size of the already completed infarct in the dominant hemisphere shows reperfusion would probably be futile, because tissue loss sufficient to cause death or severe dependency has already occurred. DWI, diffusion-weighted imaging; Tmax, time-to-maximum of the residue function. (Images courtesy of Greg Albers, Stanford University, School of Medicine, CA, USA).

LVO in the anterior circulation and meet other DAWN eligibility criteria, mechanical thrombectomy is a reasonable approach.[3]

Mechanical Thrombectomy and Thrombolysis

Mechanical thrombectomy can be used in addition to treatment with IV thrombolytics. However, pretreatment with IV thrombolytics (if initiated within 4.5 hours of symptom onset) is not required prior to thrombectomy.[26] Mechanical thrombectomy treatment should be initiated as quickly as possible and should not be delayed to assess the response to IV alteplase.[3] A post hoc analyses of pooled data compared thrombectomy alone versus dual therapy (IV thrombolysis and thrombectomy) for LVO and concluded that dual therapy was associated with a higher likelihood of 3-month functional independence and lower odds of 3-month mortality. The two groups did not differ in functional improvement or symptomatic intracranial hemorrhage.[47] There are no randomized controlled trials of mechanical thrombectomy for posterior circulation LVOs.[48]

Intra-arterial fibrinolysis initiated within 6 hours of stroke onset in carefully selected patients who have contraindications to the use of IV alteplase might be considered, but the consequences are unknown and therefore not recommended. In this scenario, mechanical thrombectomy with stent retrievers is recommended over intraarterial fibrinolysis as first-line therapy.[3]

Spontaneous Intracerebral Hemorrhage (Hemorrhagic Stroke)

Evidence from clinical trials to guide management for spontaneous ICH has lagged behind that of ischemic stroke and aneurysmal SAH. Initial goals of treatment include preventing hemorrhage expansion (which occurs in about 20% to 30% of patients) and prevention of secondary brain injury via stabilization of airway, breathing, and circulation. Patients may require intubation and mechanical ventilation, anticoagulation reversal, BP control, interventions for elevated ICP, treatment for seizures, or neurosurgical hematoma evacuation.

Monitoring

Patients with spontaneous ICH are frequently medically and neurologically unstable, particularly within the first few days after onset and they can deteriorate from hematoma expansion (which most often occurs within the first few hours), elevations in ICP, hydrocephalus, seizures, and herniation. Admission to an intensive care unit or dedicated stroke unit is recommended as it is associated with a lower mortality rate.[2]

Blood Pressure Management

Two large phase III, multicenter, prospective randomized controlled trials (RCTs) have shown that early lowering of SBP to less than 140 mm Hg is safe without significant adversary effects. The INTERACT2 (Intensive Blood Pressure Reduction in Acute Cerebral Hemorrhage Trial 2) trial evaluated the efficacy of intensive BP lowering within 6 hours of spontaneous ICH in 2839 patients with systolic BP between 150 and 220 mm Hg. Patients were randomized to intensive BP lowering (target systolic BP less than140 mm Hg within 1 hour) versus standard treatment (target systolic BP <180 mm Hg). Intensive lowering of BP did not result in a significant reduction in death or severe disability but did improve functional outcomes at 90 days. In the ATACH 2 trial (Antihypertensive Treatment of Acute Cerebral Hemorrhage), IV nicardipine was administered within 3 hours of ICH in 1000 patients and the rate of death or disability was not different between subjects randomized to a target SBP of 110 to 139 mm Hg compared to a target of 140 to 179 mm Hg. The rate of renal adverse events within 7 days was significantly higher in the intensive-treatment group than in the standard-treatment group (9.0% vs. 4.0%).[49] A pooled analysis of

individual patient-level data from INTERACT2 and ATACH2 showed early and steady reduction in SBP (potentially down to 120 to 130 mm Hg) seemed to be safe and associated with favorable outcomes in patients with ICH that were mild to moderate in severity. However, a rapid and large reduction (≥60 mm Hg) within 1 hour of the initiation of treatment was associated with some harm.[50] Further analysis on the INTERACT2 data revealed that intensive BP lowering was beneficial across a wide range of baseline BPs (<160, 160 to 169, 170 to 179, 180 to 189, and ≥190 mm Hg) and that lowering SBP to 130 to 139 mm Hg was likely to be maximally beneficial.[51]

Therefore, for ICH patients presenting with SBP between 150 and 220 mm Hg and without contraindication to acute BP treatment, acute lowering of SBP to 140 mm Hg is safe and can be effective for improving functional outcome. For ICH patients presenting with SBP greater than 220 mm Hg, it may be reasonable to consider aggressive reduction of BP with a continuous IV infusion and frequent BP monitoring, but the target BP is less clear.[2] IV calcium channel blockers (e.g., nicardipine) and β-blockers (i.e., labetalol) are the treatments of choice for early BP reduction, given their short half-life and ease of titration. Nitrates should be avoided given their potential for cerebral vasodilation and elevated ICP.[52]

Reversal of Anticoagulation

All anticoagulants such as vitamin K antagonists (e.g., warfarin), antiplatelet medications (aspirin, clopidogrel, prasugrel, ticagrelor), and non–vitamin K antagonists known as direct oral anticoagulants (DOACs) such as Factor IIa (thrombin) inhibitors (e.g., dabigatran, argatroban and bivalirudin) or Factor Xa inhibitors (rivaroxaban, apixaban, edoxaban, betrixaban, darexaban) should be discontinued acutely and reversed immediately with appropriate agents.[53]

Patients taking vitamin K antagonists with INR ≥1.4 can be reversed with IV vitamin K and 3-factor or 4-factor prothrombin complex concentrate (PCC) or fresh frozen plasma administered intravenously.[53] Vitamin K 10 mg is administered slowly IV but its effects are delayed. 3-factor or 4-factor prothrombin complex concentrate is preferred over fresh-frozen plasma due to more rapid correction of INR, lower volume, and lower risk of infection and pulmonary edema.[53] PCC is an inactivated concentrate of factors II, IX, and X, with variable amounts of factor VII. Variation in factor VII concentrations in PCC has led to their classification as either 3- or 4-factor.[52]

Although direct thrombin inhibitors (Factor IIa inhibitors) have less risk of ICH than vitamin K antagonists, reversal is indicated if patients present within 3 to 5 half-lives of drug exposure.[52] Idarucizumab is a Fab fragment of a monoclonal antibody that binds to and inactivates dabigatran and 5 g is administered as two consecutive 2.5-g IV bolus injections.[54] If idarucizumab is not available or if other direct thrombin inhibitors have been ingested, clotting factor products such as prothrombin complex concentrates or fresh-frozen plasma can be used.[55] Dabigatran can also be reversed with hemodialysis. Idarucizumab should not be combined with other clotting factor products.

Patients requiring emergent reversal of Factor Xa inhibitors can be treated with Andexanet alfa or 4-factor prothrombin complex concentrates.[56] Andexanet alfa is a class-specific antidote targeted to competitively inhibit Factor Xa inhibitors.[57] The initial dose depends on the dose of the Factor Xa inhibitor and the interval since the last dose. Andexanet should not be combined with other clotting factor products.

There is inadequate evidence to support the routine use of platelet transfusion for ICH in patients taking preinjury antiplatelet medications.[58] Platelet transfusion should be considered for patients with aspirin- or adenosine diphosphate receptor (ADP) inhibitor-associated ICH who will undergo a neurosurgical procedure.[53] Desmopressin (ddAVP) (0.4 µg/kg IV single dose) can be considered in ICH associated with cyclooxygenase (COX) inhibitors or ADP receptor inhibitors.[53]

Hemostatic Agents

The TICH2 was an international double-blind randomized trial of 2325 patients with ICH comparing 2 g of tranexamic acid to placebo given within 8 hours of onset. Tranexamic acid did not affect functional status at 90 days compared to placebo, although potential benefits were seen with reductions in hematoma expansion, early death, and serious adverse events.[59]

Seizures

Patients with ICH have up to 16% risk of clinical seizures within 1 week, with the majority occurring at or near onset. There is no association between clinical seizures and neurological outcome or mortality.[52] Clinical seizures should be treated with anticonvulsants. Patients with a change in mental status who are found to have electrographic seizures on EEG should also be treated with anticonvulsants (e.g., levetiracetam 1000 to 1500 mg IV). Continuous EEG monitoring is probably indicated in ICH patients with depressed mental status that is out of proportion to the degree of brain injury. However, prophylactic antiseizure medication is not recommended.[2]

Prognosis

Factors that may affect outcome after ICH include hematoma volume and location, hematoma expansion, age, GCS score on presentation, intraventricular extension, and anticoagulant use. However, none of the existing ICH prediction models has proven reliable.[52] When health care providers initiate early do not resuscitate (DNR) orders, patients with otherwise equivalent prognoses are more likely to die. Therefore, current AHA/ASA guidelines recommend early and aggressive care for ICH patients and postponement of any new DNR orders until at least the second full day of treatment. Patients with pre-existing DNR orders are excluded from this recommendation.[2] However, DNR status should not limit appropriate medical and surgical interventions, unless explicitly indicated.

Increased Intracranial Pressure

In patients with supratentorial ICH with radiographic hydrocephalus, especially in patients with decreased level of consciousness, an external ventricular drain is advised. Patients with a GCS score of ≤8, those with clinical evidence of transtentorial herniation, or those with intraventricular hemorrhage or hydrocephalus should be considered for ICP monitoring and treatment. A CPP of 50 to 70 mm Hg is recommended.[2]

Mannitol and hypertonic saline (HTS 3% or 23.4%) are the first-line medical therapies for patients with symptomatic cerebral edema and elevated ICP. In an analysis of the INTERACT2 patients, there was no significant difference in outcome in mannitol and non–mannitol-treated patients so mannitol was safe, but did not improve outcome.[60] In a small retrospective study, treatment with 23.4% of HTS was associated with rapid reversal of transtentorial herniation and reduced ICP. Early continuous infusion of 3% of HTS for sodium goal of 145 to 155 mmol/L was associated with less cerebral edema and ICP elevations. A meta-analysis showed that HTS is slightly more effective than mannitol for the treatment of elevated ICP.[52]

Both hyperglycemia and hypoglycemia should be avoided. Corticosteroids should not be administered for treatment of elevated ICP. The risk of central fever is increased in patients with larger ICH and in those with IVH and negatively impacts outcome.[61] Sources of hyperthermia (temperature > 38°C) should be identified and treated, and antipyretic medications should be administered.[3]

Neurosurgical Intervention

Urgent neurosurgical consultation is recommended for assessment for hydrocephalus and the possible need for surgical decompression or hematoma evacuation.[62] Cerebellar ICH is considered a neurosurgical emergency. Patients with cerebellar hemorrhage who are deteriorating neurologically or who have brainstem compression or hydrocephalus from ventricular obstruction should undergo surgical removal of the hemorrhage as soon as possible.[2]

For most patients with supratentorial ICH the benefits of surgical evacuation of the hematoma are still under investigation. Open craniotomy hematoma evacuation has not been found to have any benefit in large randomized trials.[63] Current guidelines suggest that evacuation may be considered in patients with supratentorial ICH who exhibit neurological deterioration, coma, midline shift, or elevated ICP refractory to medical treatment.[2]

As an alternative to open surgical approaches, minimally invasive approaches to evacuate clots are being investigated. These approaches use small incisions and burr holes and insert either a catheter into the clot for drainage or a small tube into the clot for direct evacuation. A meta-analysis of five randomized trials and nine prospective studies in patients with supratentorial ICH found that minimally invasive approaches conferred a mortality benefit, as well as a lower rate of rebleeding and higher rate of good recovery.[64] The MISTIE III (Minimally Invasive Surgery Plus rt-PA for Intracerebral Hemorrhage Evacuation III) trial was an open-label blinded endpoint trial that randomized 506 patients to minimally invasive surgery (catheter evacuation followed by thrombolytic irrigation of the clot with alteplase) versus standard medical treatment. Eligible patients had a supratentorial ICH measuring ≥30 mL, NIHSS ≥6, good baseline status, a CT angiogram negative for an underlying lesion, and a repeat CT demonstrating clot volume stability for at least 6 hours. At one year, the number of patients with good functional outcome (mRS score of 0 to 3) was similar for the minimally invasive surgery group compared with the standard care group (45% vs. 41%). Mortality was lower in the minimally invasive surgery group (19% vs. 26%).[63]

The ENRICH (Early MiNimally-invasive Removal of ICH) is a multicenter randomized clinical trial of ICH patients aged 18 to 80 years with a GCS score of 5 to 14 and an intraparenchymal hemorrhage volume of 30 to 80 mL comparing standard medical management to early surgical hematoma evacuation within 24 hours using minimally invasive parafascicular surgery (MIPS). An initial single-arm surgical evaluation of this endoport system in 39 patients with primary IPH reported functional independence in 52% of patients at follow-up and no mortality.[65]

Intraventricular extension of the ICH (intraventricular hemorrhage or IVH) occurs in up to 45% of patients with ICH[52] and puts patients at risk for hydrocephalus, especially if the third and fourth ventricles are involved because the normal circulation of cerebrospinal fluid (CSF) can become interrupted. Such patients should be closely monitored with frequent neurological assessments. When neurologic deterioration occurs, an emergent CT scan should be done to exclude the development of hydrocephalus. Patients with neurologic deterioration in the setting of ventricular enlargement may be candidates for ventriculostomy and external ventricular drainage.[2] The CLEAR III trial (Clot Lysis: Evaluating Accelerated Resolution of Intraventricular Hemorrhage III) was a double-blinded, placebo-controlled trial conducted in 500 ICH patients with intraventricular hemorrhage obstructing the third or fourth ventricles. Patients were randomized to irrigation of the extraventricular drain with alteplase versus saline. Alteplase did not substantially improve functional outcomes at the mRS 3 cutoff compared with irrigation with saline.[66]

Decompressive craniectomy is a procedure that removes a portion of the skull bone enabling the brain to expand to decrease ICP. In small non-randomized studies decompressive craniectomy treatment for spontaneous supratentorial ICH showed lower rates of in-hospital mortality and better functional status compared with medically managed patients in certain populations.[67,68] The SWITCH trial (Swiss trial of decompressive craniectomy versus best medical treatment of spontaneous supratentorial ICH) is currently enrolling ICH patients between 18 and 75 years with hemorrhage into the basal ganglia or thalamus with a GCS 8 to 13, NIHSS ≥10 and ≤30, and volume of hematoma 30 to 100 mL.

TRANSIENT ISCHEMIC ATTACK

TIA is no longer defined by an arbitrary time of 24 hours. Patients with symptoms less than 24 hours can have representative ischemic lesions on diffusion-weighted or perfusion-weighted MRI, so TIA has moved from time-based to tissue-based definition. Patients with TIA or non-disabling strokes are at increased risk of recurrent stroke and should be evaluated and treated immediately in order to reduce the risk of subsequent stroke and to identify patients who may benefit from preventive therapy or from revascularization of large vessels.

Some centers have developed rapid outpatient TIA clinics to ensure an expedited evaluation within 24 hours of presentation. However, patients at higher risk for subsequent stroke should be hospitalized. Previous guidelines have used the ABCD2 score (i.e., ABCDD, for Age, BP, Clinical features, Duration of symptoms, and Diabetes) as a prognostic assessment tool designed to identify TIA patients at high risk of ischemic stroke and thus requiring admission (Table 87.6). More recent studies have found the score does not provide an accurate estimate of stroke risk.[69,70] Others have combined the ABCD2 score with imaging such as MRI and MRA (ABCD2-I and ABCD3-I)[6,71,72] to improve the short-term prediction of cerebral infarction but have yet to be validated.

Most patients without a contraindication will be started on antithrombotic therapy in the ED after consultation with a neurologist. Dual antiplatelet therapy with clopidogrel and aspirin is effective for secondary prevention after minor ischemic stroke or TIA.[73] Pooled analysis of two RCTs, POINT and CHANCE, showed that early and short-term clopidogrel-aspirin treatment was associated with a reduction in the risk of major ischemic events compared to aspirin alone. The benefit of dual antiplatelet therapy appeared to be confined to the first 21 days after minor ischemic stroke or high-risk TIA.[74] The risk for major hemorrhages in patients receiving either clopidogrel plus aspirin or aspirin alone after TIA was low. Nevertheless, treatment with clopidogrel plus aspirin increased the risk of major hemorrhages over aspirin alone from 0.2% to 0.9%.[75] In patients presenting with minor noncardioembolic ischemic stroke (NIHSS score ≤3) who did not receive IV alteplase, treatment with dual antiplatelet therapy (aspirin and clopidogrel) started within 24 hours after symptom onset and continued for 21 days is effective in reducing recurrent ischemic stroke for a period of up to 90 days from symptom onset.[3]

In patients with new onset atrial fibrillation, immediate anticoagulation should be considered, except those for whom the risks of bleeding exceed the benefits or those with a CHA2DS2-VASc score of 0 in men or 1 in women who have short paroxysms of AF that self-terminate (see Chapter 65 for suggested anticoagulants).

DISPOSITION

"Stroke center" definitions have been established, and there is a national certification process for primary stroke centers (PSCs) and comprehensive stroke centers (CSCs) in the United States. In broad terms, institutional certification as a PSC requires the establishment of a stroke infrastructure (i.e., a dedicated stroke team, stroke unit, patient care protocols, and support services, including CT/MRI scanning and laboratory testing availability), as well as institutional administrative support and specialty-qualified leadership. CSCs offer advanced imaging modalities, perform surgical and endovascular interventions, and maintain a core infrastructure, such as a stroke unit and stroke registry. The establishment of PSCs and CSCs is intended to improve outcomes for stroke patients by ensuring a high level of coordinated care. Early identification and transfer of patients with acute stroke to a PSCs or CSCs results in more favorable outcomes.

The most recent level of stroke classification for hospitals is the acute stroke-ready hospital (ASRH). These hospitals are typically smaller facilities with lower stroke patient volumes. An ASRH is capable of establishing the initial stroke diagnosis, as well as providing acute stabilization and treatment. The use of tele-technologies between the ASRH and PSC/CSC will likely serve a pivotal role in support of clinical care. After initial stabilization and treatment, stroke patients will frequently be transferred to PSC or CSC institutions. A systematic review of retrospective studies evaluating the safety and efficacy of IV alteplase delivered within 3 hours of symptom onset through telestroke networks concluded that there was no difference in mortality or functional independence at 3 months between telestroke-guided and stroke center–managed patients.[76]

Reducing the time interval from ED presentation to initial brain imaging can help to reduce the time to treatment initiation. Studies have shown that median or mean door-to-imaging times of ≤20 minutes can be achieved in a variety of different hospital settings.[77-79] The benefit of bypassing the closest hospital that offers thrombolytic therapy to transporting the patient directly to an institution that offers a higher level of stroke care (including mechanical thrombectomy) has not been established. However, it is reasonable to introduce prehospital procedures to identify patients who have a strong probability of LVO stroke and are eligible for thrombectomy and facilitate rapid transport of these patients to centers that perform mechanical thrombectomy.[3] Telestroke networks may also be reasonable for triaging patients with acute ischemic stroke who may be eligible for interfacility transfer in order to be considered for emergency mechanical thrombectomy.[76]

Patients with acute ischemic stroke may deteriorate over the first 24 hours and require close in-hospital monitoring. There is evidence suggesting a benefit from admission to a stroke-specific unit. Patients with large acute hemispheric strokes (associated with increased risk of herniation) or with significant posterior circulation-related changes and those treated with a fibrinolytic agent should be monitored in an ICU for at least 24 hours.

The references for this chapter can be found online at ExpertConsult.com.

TABLE 87.6 ABCD2 Score for Assessing Stroke Risk in Patients With a Transient Ischemic Attack	
Risk Factor	**Points**
Age >60 years old	1
Initial BP >140/90 mm Hg	1
Unilateral weakness	2
Speech Impairment	
Without weakness	1
Symptoms 10–59 min	1
Symptoms ≥60 min	2
History of diabetes	1
Result	
0–3 = Low risk (1% risk of stroke in 48 h)	
4–5 = Moderate risk (4.1% risk of stroke in 48 h)	
≥6 = High risk (8% risk of stroke in 48 h)	

BP, Blood pressure.

Seizure

Carolina Barbosa Maciel and Marie-Carmelle Elie-Turenne

KEY CONCEPTS

- Epilepsy is a neurologic condition associated with an intrinsically lower seizure threshold and a higher risk of recurrent seizures without a clear trigger.
- The characterization of seizure semiology, duration, and etiology is important for accurate classification of seizures and status epilepticus; these impact definitive treatment choices.
- There is no single test to confirm that a patient seized, and several seizure mimics, including convulsive syncope, exist. A postictal alteration in mental status makes a seizure five times more likely than syncope.
- Key factors in the evaluation of epilepsy patients who present with breakthrough seizures include: changes in anti-seizure regimen, compliance, the addition of new medications that may lower the seizure threshold or levels of antiseizure drugs, presence of common infections or metabolic derangements, and recent sleep habits.
- Although most seizures are self-limited, the management of patients with seizures involves a targeted search for underlying pathology, treatment of complications associated with convulsions, and the prevention of future episodes.
- Serious systemic complications of seizures and status epilepticus include cardiac arrest, arrhythmias, apnea, hypoxia, acute kidney injury, rhabdomyolysis, acidosis, and death. The prognosis of status epilepticus is directly related to the etiology of seizures.
- Primary seizure prophylaxis should only be given for 7 days following traumatic brain injury. The period is shorter, although less well-defined, in unsecured aneurysmal subarachnoid hemorrhage. Prolonged primary prophylaxis is not recommended because it has not been demonstrated to reduce long-term seizure risk. The duration of secondary seizure prophylaxis and the anti-seizure regimen in patients with acute brain injury who had a seizure during hospitalization should be individualized.
- Patients with a first-time seizure who have no known structural brain pathology, normal serum glucose and sodium levels, and normal neurologic examination can be discharged from the ED with appropriate outpatient follow-up.

- Emerging evidence supports the consideration of secondary seizure prophylaxis for first-time unprovoked seizures in selected patients. However, data are heterogeneous, and a thorough discussion with the patient and a specialist is advised before the initiation of anti-seizure drugs.
- Alcohol withdrawal syndrome can include seizures resulting from the cessation or reduction of alcohol consumption leading to an unopposed excitatory sympathomimetic response. Benzodiazepines are the drug of choice and should be supplemented by supportive measures, including electrolyte and thiamine supplementation. In pregnant patients, evaluations for new-onset seizures before 20 weeks should be the same as in nonpregnant patients. After 20 weeks, and up to 8 weeks postpartum, eclampsia is a major cause of seizures and should be included in the differential. IV magnesium remains first-line treatment for patients with eclamptic seizures and should not be delayed. Benzodiazepines and non-teratogenic antiseizure medications are reasonable alternatives in magnesium-refractory cases.
- Post-anoxic status epilepticus, including myoclonic status, frequently observed following cardiac arrest, was considered pathognomonic of poor neurologic outcome. However, in patients lacking factors with high predictive value for poor outcome post cardiac arrest, early antiseizure therapy can lead to improved outcomes.
- Therapeutic approaches to nonconvulsive status epilepticus are commonly extrapolated from convulsive generalized status epilepticus guidelines. However, the presumed etiology of seizures, extent of cortical area involved (focal versus diffuse or generalized), comorbidities, and response to therapy should be considered when selecting an antiseizure therapeutic algorithm.
- Immunomodulation remains the cornerstone of therapy for autoimmune epilepsies, in conjunction with antiseizure drugs. Transdisciplinary decision making is warranted before initiating immune-targeted therapy, which may include high-dose methylprednisolone, intravenous immunoglobulin, plasma exchange, rituximab, cyclophosphamide, and more recently, tocilizumab.

FOUNDATIONS

Background and Classification

Seizures are excessive excitatory neuronal activity associated with hypersynchrony of neighboring cells, resulting in sensory, motor, autonomic, or cognitive function alterations. *Convulsion* refers specifically to the motor manifestations of a seizure. The *ictal period* is the time during which a seizure or seizure-like activity occurs. A *postictal period* is an interval of transient neurologic dysfunction (commonly altered mental status or weakness) immediately following a seizure, generally lasting less than 1 hour. Longer ictal activity is associated with more prominent and prolonged postictal symptoms. When precipitating

factors can be identified, provoked seizures are termed *acute symptomatic seizures*. Conversely, *primary seizures* are unprovoked and have no acute inciting pathology. Epilepsy refers to a condition of recurrent unprovoked seizures.

The International League Against Epilepsy defines epilepsy as a disease in which the threshold for seizures is lower than the normal population reflected by meeting at least one of the following: (A) diagnosis of epilepsy syndrome (e.g., juvenile myoclonic epilepsy, Lennox-Gastault syndrome, benign rolandic epilepsy, infantile spasms); (B) two or more seizures occurring more than 24 hours apart without an identified trigger; (C) one unprovoked seizure coupled with a higher likelihood of recurrent seizures over the subsequent decade (similar to the recurrence risk for fulfilling criterion B, or ≥60% recurrence risk). For example, a patient who suffers head trauma might have a seizure in close proximity to the acute brain injury but would not be considered to have epilepsy unless unprovoked seizures recur remotely from the initial brain injury. Epilepsies are classified further according to seizure onset and semiology (focal with or without impairment of awareness, generalized or unknown onset; see Figure 14.1 in Chapter 14),[1] epilepsy syndrome (e.g., idiopathic generalized and self-limited focal epilepsies), and etiology (e.g., structural, genetic, infectious, metabolic, immune, or unknown).[2]

The majority of epilepsy syndromes have onset during childhood or adolescence. However, there have been reports of onset in early adulthood[2]; a thorough evaluation with a specialist is indicated in these cases. Breakthrough seizures in patients with epilepsy are commonly triggered by sleep deprivation, emotional or physical stress, and menses. Additionally, even slight adjustments in the antiseizure regimen or missing doses of medications may precipitate a recurrent seizure. A specific sensory stimulus, such as flashing lights or a specific smell, may also trigger seizures in epilepsies; these are still considered "unprovoked" when triggered by a process that would not cause a seizure in the patient that does not have epilepsy.

Medically refractory epilepsy (also known as "uncontrolled" or "drug-resistant") refers to patients who are unable to achieve or maintain seizure freedom despite 2 trials of adequately dosed antiseizure regimens. These patients continue to have seizures with a variable baseline frequency of occurrence. There are several definitions for seizure *clusters* reported in the literature: 3 or more seizures in 24 hours, 2 or more seizures in 24 hours, or 2 or more seizures in 6 hours.[3] The timely recognition of seizure clusters allows for prompt administration of seizure abortive measures (at home as instructed by the neurologist or epileptologist, in the pre-hospital, or in the hospital settings). Patients with medically refractory epilepsy presenting with seizure clusters are at a higher risk for status epilepticus.

Uncontrollable seizures, or status epilepticus, are seizures that have reached a prespecified duration according to specific seizure types (see Table 14.1 in Chapter 14) or recur with a frequency that does not allow a patient to return to the baseline neurologic status in between seizures.

Seizures may be provoked by a multitude of insults, such as acute brain injury (e.g., ischemic and hemorrhagic strokes, trauma, meningoencephalitis), toxins, and metabolic derangements. The main cause of status epilepticus and epilepsy in the elderly remains cerebrovascular disease. Patients with diabetes, higher stroke severity, cortical location of infarcts, and thromboembolic mechanisms are at the highest risk for experiencing seizures in the acute phase, with an incidence of up to 5% of all ischemic strokes in some series.[4,5] Nevertheless, the true incidence of seizures in the setting of stroke is difficult to ascertain because studies had variable methods of detection, use of primary seizure prophylaxis, and follow-up duration. Box 88.1 summarizes etiologies of seizures and status epilepticus according to the type of insult or neurologic process. Being familiar with common seizure triggers allows for identifying patients at higher risk for seizures and status epilepticus who may benefit from further diagnostic workup such as neuroimaging, EEG, or neurologic consultation.

When seizures are prolonged and the duration exceeds the respective threshold according to type (convulsive, nonconvulsive, or absence; see Table 14.1 in Chapter 14), they are termed *status epilepticus*. Overall, status epilepticus is associated with significant morbidity and mortality, particularly convulsive generalized status epilepticus. In the United States, reported status epilepticus incidence ranges from 10 to 40 persons per 100,000 annually. In a meta-analysis, the leading cause of status epilepticus globally was acute symptomatic (in close temporal relationship with a brain insult).[6] Overall case fatality rates were 15%; the highest case fatality rates were seen in low- and middle-income countries, refractory status epilepticus, and in the elderly population.

Several different scores exist to predict outcomes in status epilepticus. The Epidemiology based Mortality Score in Status Epilepticus (EMSE; Table 88.1) accounts for etiology of seizures, age, comorbidities, and EEG findings and performs well in predicting mortality and morbidity, but fails to predict responses to therapy satisfactorily.[7]

Anatomy, Physiology, and Pathophysiology

Neuronal cell membranes are stabilized by transmembrane electrochemical gradients and equilibrium among inhibitory neurotransmitters (e.g., GABA) and excitatory neurotransmitters (e.g., glutamate and acetylcholine). Seizures start when the equilibrium across the cell membrane is disrupted by an imbalance between these factors, leading to abnormal electrical discharge of cortical and subcortical neurons. The recruitment of neighboring neurons leads to spreading of this abnormal excitation. It may manifest clinically by propagating clonic activity in adjacent areas in the body following their corresponding topography in the brain (i.e., *Jacksonian March*, when focal motor seizure symptoms spread in a step-wise fashion). If there is involvement of large areas in both hemispheres, thalami, or deeper structures, and of the reticular activating system in the brainstem, impairment in consciousness ensues.

Physiologic mechanisms implicated in seizure termination involve reflex inhibition, hyperpolarization of neurons preventing their depolarization, and neuronal exhaustion, among others. Most drugs used to interrupt seizures act on $GABA_A$ subtype receptors, therefore enhancing inhibitory activity. However, with prolonged seizure activity, $GABA_A$ receptors are sequestered inside the cells and become unresponsive to GABA[8] (and GABA-ergic medications), whereas excitatory N-methyl-D-aspartate (NMDA) receptors may be upregulated. This perpetuates an excitatory state and leads to sustained seizure activity, explaining why timely treatment of seizures is of utmost importance.

CLINICAL FEATURES

In caring for patients who may have seized, the first step is to determine whether the event in question was truly a seizure. A common clinical scenario for the emergency clinician is the patient who presents with a history of having had a seizure-like episode, usually involving sudden loss of consciousness and some type of motor activity. Characterizing the episodes with particular attention to the predominant features at onset helps define the seizure type. In Chapter 14, Figure 14.1 depicts the revised expanded classification of seizure types according to their semiology at onset[1] and Table 14.1, the operational definition of status epilepticus according to time domains and seizure types.[9]

Once a seizure has met the criteria for status epilepticus, it can be further subdivided according to response to treatment: refractory status epilepticus when seizures persist despite 2 appropriately dosed antiseizure therapies, or super-refractory status epilepticus when seizures do not entirely resolve despite at least 24 hours of therapeutic coma with anesthetics (including propofol and benzodiazepines) or when seizures recur preventing tapering off anesthetics. Status epilepticus persisting for over 7 days despite appropriate management is termed prolonged and is associated with complications and longer hospital length-of-stay[10] (Table 88.2).

Recently revised definitions of clinical syndromes have been proposed for new-onset refractory status epilepticus (NORSE) and febrile infection-related epilepsy syndrome (FIRES).[10] NORSE includes patients without a known diagnosis of epilepsy or clear triggers (absent toxic exposure, metabolic derangements, or structural brain injury)

BOX 88.1 Etiologies of Seizures and Status Epilepticus According to Class of Insult/Pathology

Autoimmune
Acute disseminated encephalomyelitis
Antibody-mediated autoimmune and paraneuroplastic encephalitides
CREST, Goodpasture syndrome, and systemic lupus erythematosus
Multiple sclerosis
Rasmussen encephalitis
Thrombotic thrombocytopenic purpura

Cerebrovascular Disease
Acute ischemic stroke
Cavernous and arteriovenous malformations
Cerebral venous thrombosis
Intracerebral hemorrhage
Nontraumatic subarachnoid hemorrhage
Posterior reversible encephalopathy syndrome
Reversible cerebral vasoconstriction syndrome

Dementias
Alzheimer disease
Corticobasal degeneration
Frontotemporal dementia
Vascular dementia

Genetic Syndromes and Structural Anomalies
Focal cortical dysplasia
Hydrocephalus
Inherited metabolic diseases
Mitochondrial diseases
Polymicrogyria
Porphyria
Tuberous sclerosis complex
Wilson disease

Hypoxic-Ischemic Brain Injury
Cardiac arrest

Intracranial Tumor
Dysembryoplastic neuroepithelial tumor
Gangliogliomas
Gliomas
Lymphoma
Meningioma
Metastases
Primitive neuroectodermal tumor

Metabolic Derangements
Acidosis
Elevated blood urea nitrogen
Hyperammonemia
Hyperglycemia
Hypernatremia
Hypocalcemia
Hypoglycemia
Hypomagnesemia
Hyponatremia
Wernicke encephalopathy

Medications and Toxins
Alcohol intoxication and withdrawal
Alkylating agents
Baclofen intoxication and withdrawal
Benzodiazepine and barbiturate withdrawal
Beta-interferons
CAR-T (chimeric antigen receptor T cell therapy)
Carbapenems (imipenem in particular)
Cephalosporin (cefepime in particular)
Cyclosporine
Digoxin
Fentanyl
Heavy metals
Lidocaine
Metronidazole
Mexiletine
Theophylline
Tramadol
Tacrolimus
Subtherapeutic antiseizure drug levels

Systemic Disease
Acute and chronic renal failure
Cirrhosis

Trauma
Blunt or penetrating head injury (skull fracture)
Epidural hematoma
Subarachnoid hemorrhage
Subdural hematoma
Diffuse Axonal Injury

Although this list includes many recognized etiologies for epilepsy and acute symptomatic seizures, several entities were clustered into themes, and less common etiologies were omitted.

presenting with de novo refractory status epilepticus. FIRES is a subcategory of NORSE to specify the subset of patients with a clear prodrome of febrile illness for 24 hours up to 2 weeks prior to status epilepticus presentation; FIRES is common but not exclusive to the pediatric population. Box 88.2 summarizes other status epilepticus classifications according to their semiology, etiology, age, and EEG correlate.[9]

Classifications are important because they often dictate the aggressiveness of treatment. Not all types of status epilepticus warrant seizure suppression with third-tier therapy (therapeutic coma with anesthetics). An example is *epilepsia partialis continua* which, as the name implies, is characterized by continuous focal seizures that are notoriously refractory to antiseizure therapies. These patients learn how to live with ongoing focal clonic activity, and the therapeutic goal is shifted towards minimizing the side effects of medications. In this condition, seizures remain confined to a relatively small cortical region without spreading, which often leads to EEG recordings without epileptiform activity in most cases.

Seizures produce many secondary physiologic derangements that can result in poor outcomes. Epilepsy patients with poorly controlled generalized tonic-clonic seizures are at highest risk of sudden unexpected death in epilepsy (SUDEP), which exceeds the expected death rate in the general population by 24 times, primarily affecting young adults between 15 and 44 years of age.

The potential systemic complications of convulsive status are summarized in Table 88.3.[11,12] Sympathetic stimulation increases body temperature, heart rate, respiratory rate, serum glucose, and lactic acid.

The involvement of the insula, a highly epileptogenic area in which the cortical representation of the heart is also located, may be implicated in tachy- and bradyarrhythmias associated with ictal activity. Ictal asystole is a syndrome implicated in focal epilepsies, particularly of left temporal onset, female sex, and prior history of a heart condition. However, ictal asystole lasting longer than 30 seconds is associated with extra-temporal seizure focus and secondary generalized tonic-clonic seizures.[13]

Prominent autonomic dysregulation and apnea, possibly associated with spreading depolarization in the brainstem, and postictal diffuse suppression of cortical electrical activity have been implicated as potential mechanisms leading to SUDEP. With more prolonged convulsions, hypoglycemia, neurogenic pulmonary edema, skeletal muscle damage, and, rarely, frank rhabdomyolysis may ensue. A rise in the peripheral white blood cell count without an increase in bands is also often seen. Autonomic discharge and bulbar muscle involvement may result in urinary or fecal incontinence, vomiting, tongue biting, and potential airway impairment. Rarely, the force generated by the muscle contractions in these seizures can be strong enough to cause posterior shoulder dislocations or fractures.

TABLE 88.1 Epidemiology-Based Mortality Score in Status Epilepticus (EMSE)[34]

Age	Points	Comorbidity (Score Each Disease)	Points
>80	10	AIDS, metastatic solid tumor	60
71–80	8	Moderate to severe liver disease	30
61–70	7	Moderate to severe renal disease, any tumor (includes lymphoma and leukemia), hemiplegia, diabetes with end-organ damage	20
51–60	5		
41–50	3		
31–40	2	Peripheral vascular disease, connective tissue disease, diabetes, myocardial infarction, cerebrovascular disease, congestive heart failure, dementia, mild liver disease, peptic ulcer disease, chronic pulmonary disease	10
21–30	1		
Score one	_____	Score each disease	_____
EEG	Points	Etiology	Points
Spontaneous burst suppression	60	Anoxia	65
		Acute central nervous system infection	33
		Acute cerebrovascular disease	26
After status epilepticus ictal discharges	40	Metabolic disorders	22
		Metabolic, sodium imbalance	17
		Brain tumor	16
Lateralized periodic discharges (LPDs)	40	Cryptogenic	12
		Head trauma	12
		Drug overdose	11
Generalized periodic discharges (GPDs)	40	Alcohol abuse	10
		Hydrocephalus	8
		Remote cerebrovascular event or brain injury	7
No LPDs, GPDs, or ictal discharges	0	Multiple sclerosis	5
		Drug withdrawal, reduction, or poor compliance	2
		Central nervous system anomalies	2
Score only worst	_____	Score one	_____
Total Score = Sum of above scores			

Leitinger M, Holler Y, Kalss G, et al. Epidemiology-based mortality score in status epilepticus (EMSE). *Neurocrit Care.* 2015;22(2):273-282.

TABLE 88.2 Status Epilepticus Nomenclature According to Refractoriness and Duration[10]

Subtype of Status Epilepticus	Refractoriness to Treatment
Refractory (RSE)	Ongoing seizures despite first-line (benzodiazepine) and at least one second-line (appropriately selected parenteral antiseizure drug) therapies. Both first- and second-line therapies must have been adequately dosed to meet this criterion; status epilepticus may have any duration.
Super-Refractory (SRSE)	Ongoing seizures lasting over 24 hours from initiation of third-line therapy (therapeutic coma with anesthetics, regardless of which drug); status epilepticus may have any duration. This includes those that had a partial response at any point, but not completely subsided (recurred after or during attempts to wean anesthetics).
± Prolonged (qualifier for either types: refractory or super-refractory)	Status epilepticus lasting over 7 days despite adequate step-wise escalation of therapy: it may be refractory (no anesthetic trial introduced) or super-refractory (therapeutic trial with anesthetics included).

Hirsch LJ, Gaspard N, van Baalen A, et al. Proposed consensus definitions for new-onset refractory status epilepticus (NORSE), febrile infection-related epilepsy syndrome (FIRES), and related conditions. *Epilepsia.* 2018;59(4):739-744.

BOX 88.2 Status Epilepticus Subclassifications According to Semiology, Etiology, Age Group, and Electroencephalographic Correlate[35]

Semiology

Predominant motor features: convulsive status epilepticus (generalized, focal onset evolving to bilateral convulsive, unknown), myoclonic status epilepticus (with coma, without coma), focal motor status epilepticus (repeated focal motor, epilepsia partialis continua, adversive status, oculoclonic status, ictal paresis), tonic status epilepticus, hyperkinetic status epilepticus

Without prominent motor features (nonconvulsive status epilepticus): with coma, without coma (generalized: typical absence status, atypical absence status, myoclonic absence status; focal: without impairment of consciousness, aphasic status, with impaired consciousness; unknown focal versus generalized: autonomic status)

Etiology

Known or symptomatic: acute, remote, progressive, or status epilepticus in defined electroclinical syndromes

Unknown or cryptogenic

Age

Neonatal (0–30 days)

Infancy (1–24 months)

Childhood (>2–12 years)

Adolescence and adulthood (>12–59 years)

Elderly (+60 years)

Electroencephalographic Characteristics

Location: generalized, lateralized, bilateral independent, or multifocal

Pattern: periodic discharges, rhythmic delta activity, or spike-and-wave/sharp-and-wave

Morphology characterization of discharges according to sharpness, number of phases, amplitude and polarity

Time-related features of patterns according to prevalence, frequency, duration, onset, dynamics, daily burden

Modulation: spontaneous or stimulus-induced

Response to therapy

Leitinger M, Beniczky S, Rohracher A, et al. Salzburg Consensus Criteria for Non-Convulsive Status Epilepticus: approach to clinical application. *Epilepsy & Behavior : E&B.* 2015;49:158-163.

Clinical History

Identifying the circumstances surrounding the event, such as possible inciting factors and progression and duration of symptoms, provides important clues regarding whether the episode was a seizure and the likely etiology (a framework of cardinal features of seizures is provided in Chapter 14). The clinician should obtain any history of trauma (either before or during the seizure), alcohol intoxication or abuse, and pregnancy. Although febrile seizures are common in children (see separate discussion of seizures in pediatric patients in Chapter 169), hyperthermia alone as seizure etiology of adults is uncommon, and seizures in the setting of fever are highly suggestive of meningoencephalitis. Immunocompromised patients and those with recent neurosurgical instrumentation with or without hardware (e.g., shunt, drug delivery devices, spinal cord stimulator) are at particularly high risk for infection. Other red flags suggesting acute brain injury is thunderclap and severe headache preceding seizures or sudden neurologic deficits. New or recent changes in medication regimen, and history of comorbidities are also important in both patients with new-onset seizures and epilepsy because they assist in unveiling potential triggers: medications lowering seizure threshold, interacting with antiseizure regimen, or even leading to severe metabolic derangements such as hypoglycemia or hypocalcemia (Table 88.4).

In epilepsy patients, characterizing typical seizure semiology, typical seizure frequency, last known seizure, common precipitating factors, and neurologic baseline provides a meaningful comparison with the current presentation. Noncompliance with the antiseizure regimen is the most common cause for the ED presentation of recurrent seizures. Certain recreational drugs (e.g., cocaine, phencyclidine, ecstasy, and synthetic marijuana) are known to decrease the seizure threshold. Common causes of adult-onset focal seizures in low- and middle-income countries include neurocysticercosis (especially Central and South America) and malaria, both of which should be considered in travelers and immigrants. Finally, investigating potential precipitants (such as sleep deprivation, infection, or new medications, especially those that can lower the seizure threshold or affect antiseizure drug metabolism) is key to managing the patient with a known seizure disorder who has a typical event while on medications. Further details on key historical features are provided in Chapter 14; a stepwise approach to evaluating a patient with suspected seizures in the emergency department is displayed in Figure 14.2.

TABLE 88.3 Potential Systemic Complications Related to Seizures and Status Epilepticus[11,12]

Cardiac and Others	Heme/Musculoskeletal and tegmentum/ Gastrointestinal	Pulmonary	Renal/Acid-Base/ Metabolic	Prolonged Course Complications
Arrhythmias and conduction abnormalities	Dislocation	Airway obstruction	Acute renal failure	Critical illness myopathy or neuropathy
Cardiac arrest	Fracture	Apnea/ hypoventilation	Acidosis: lactic, respiratory	Deep vein thrombosis or pulmonary embolism
Cardiomyopathy	Hepatotoxicity and pancreatitis	Aspiration	Hyperglycemia	Gastrostomy
Cardiac necrosis	Leukocytosis/leukopenia/ thrombocytopenia	Hypoxia	Hyperkalemia	Infection
Hypertension	Rhabdomyolysis	Mucous plugging	Myoglobinuria	Tracheostomy
Thermodysregulation	Life-threatening rash	Pulmonary edema		Skin breakdown and poor wound healing
	Ileus and bowel ischemia			

Sutter R, Dittrich T, Semmlack S, Ruegg S, Marsch S, Kaplan PW. Acute systemic complications of convulsive status epilepticus: a systematic review. *Crit Care Med.* 2018;46(1):138-145; Legriel S, Bresson E, Deye N, et al. Cardiac arrest in patients managed for convulsive status epilepticus: characteristics, predictors, and outcome. *Crit Care Med.* 2018;46(8):e751-e760.

TABLE 88.4   Management of "Special Situations" Seizures in the Emergency Department

Clinical Situation	Agent of Choice	Dosage/Comment
Hyponatremia	Hypertonic (3%) saline	Adults: 100 mL 3% NaCl over 10 min; children: 2 to 5 mL/kg, up to 150 mL/dose 3% NaCl over 20 min
Hypocalcemia	Calcium chloride or gluconate	Sequential ampules until seizures stop
Tricyclic antidepressant overdose	Sodium bicarbonate	Administer 1 to 2 mEq/kg IV bolus; repeat as needed to maintain ECG QRS complex ≤ 100 msec
Salicylate overdose	Sodium bicarbonate; hemodialysis for severe cases	Administer 1 to 2 mEq/kg IV bolus; repeat as needed to maintain a blood pH of 7.4 to 7.5
Isoniazid overdose	Pyridoxine	5 g IV (adult) or 70 mg/kg (pediatric)
Cocaine intoxication	Benzodiazepines	As per idiopathic seizures
Lithium toxicity	Hemodialysis	
Alcohol-associated seizure	Lorazepam	0.05 to 0.10 mg/kg, or fixed doses of 2 to 4 mg for adults
MDMA	Benzodiazepines	Be aware of possible hyperthermia or hyponatremia
Eclampsia	Magnesium sulfate	IV loading dose of 4 to 6 g over 15 to 20 minutes, then 1 to 2 g/h infusion; monitor patients for hyporeflexia; alternatively, lorazepam (Ativan) 4 mg IV over 2 to 5 minutes or diazepam (Valium) 5 to 10 mg IV slowly can be used to terminate the seizure, after which magnesium sulfate is administered

Physical Examination

An accurate set of vital signs is the foundation of any physical examination and may direct the clinician to potential etiologies (e.g., fever suggesting meningoencephalitis, tachycardia and hypertension suggesting sympathomimetic intoxication) and indicate the existence of an ominous intracranial diagnosis (e.g., hypertension and bradycardia suggest herniation syndromes).

If the patient presents actively seizing, observe the specifics of the motor activity and pay close attention to focal findings and asymmetries such as dystonic posturing, clonic or tonic activity, eye deviation, or nystagmus. Apply gentle manual pressure to the limb in an attempt to suppress clonic activity: if suppressible, this suggests nonepileptic spells or movement disorders. Anecdotally, pupils are often reported to be dilated during or after a seizure; persistent mydriasis may reflect anticholinergic or sympathomimetic toxicity. Subtle automatisms, facial myoclonus, and nystagmus following convulsive activity suggest nonconvulsive status epilepticus.

A systematic neurologic exam should be performed including mental status. Postictal patients may be hyperreflexic, have an extensor plantar response, or have a focal motor deficit (e.g., Todd paralysis), all of which generally resolve within one hour of a seizure. Todd paralysis is associated with a high likelihood of an underlying structural cause for the seizure. If it does not quickly resolve, a new structural lesion should be suspected.

Seizures are often associated with injury, and the patient must be evaluated for both soft tissue and skeletal trauma. Head trauma and tongue lacerations are common. Seizure activity can also produce dislocations and fractures. Posterior shoulder dislocations are extremely rare but, when present, should prompt suspicion that a seizure has occurred. Seizure-induced fractures are rare but frequently missed; the humerus, thoracic spine, and femur are most commonly involved. Extremities should be inspected for signs of intravenous drug use and signs of systemic embolism and endocarditis, which may raise suspicion for intoxication, septic strokes or cerebral abscesses. Dysmorphic features and stigmata of neurocutaneous diseases help diagnose epilepsy syndromes, particularly in the pediatric population.

DIFFERENTIAL DIAGNOSIS

Common differential diagnoses to consider when evaluating for seizure are summarized in Chapter 14 and listed in Box 14.2. The history surrounding the circumstances of the event and precipitating factors help distinguish seizures from their mimics. However, as a general rule, no single clinical feature or diagnostic modality is 100% confirmatory of the diagnosis of seizures.

Commonly regarded features suggestive of seizures include postictal disorientation and amnesia, lateral tongue biting, cyanosis during the event, auras (e.g., déjà vu or jamais vu, which are focal nonconvulsive seizures), non-suppressible rhythmic limb shaking, and dystonic posturing. Conversely, diaphoresis, palpitations, nausea, and dizziness preceding seizures may suggest arrhythmias and transient cerebral hypoperfusion.

Convulsive syncope is characterized by some component of motor activity, most commonly involving tonic extension of the trunk or myoclonic jerks of the extremities, at times associated with bradycardia. As cerebral perfusion is restored, abnormal muscle activity ceases, and there is no postictal period; these events are usually not associated with tongue biting, but urinary incontinence may occur.

Nonepileptic spells, or psychogenic seizures/attacks, are paroxysmal events that may be misdiagnosed as a seizure or as status epilepticus. Psychogenic seizures are rarely caused by malingering but are more commonly a psychiatric disorder (e.g., a conversion disorder). Avoidance of eye contact with the examiner, asynchronous, stop-and-go clonic activity, forward pelvic thrusting, horizontal head movements, maintaining eyes closed during the spell, and relative short postictal confusion are findings consistent with nonepileptic spells. Spells lasting 5 minutes or longer were 24 times more likely to be nonepileptic than ictal in a video EEG study.[14] Approximately 10% of subjects in clinical trials of convulsive status epilepticus are ultimately diagnosed with nonepileptic spells. Given the characteristically long duration and overt convulsions in nonepileptic spells, these patients are more likely to receive higher cumulative doses of benzodiazepines, and up to 15% result in intubation and mechanical ventilation in the emergency department.[15] Lack of leukocytosis and metabolic acidosis despite prolonged events may also help differentiate nonepileptic spells from seizures. Video EEG monitoring capturing the spell and documenting an absence of an associated electrographic ictal pattern is required to establish the diagnosis of nonepileptic spells.

DIAGNOSTIC TESTING

A thorough history and physical examination primarily directs the evaluation and management and may obviate the need for extensive

BOX 88.3 Proposed Seizure Triggering Thresholds for Metabolic Derangements

Serum Glucose: <36 mg/dl (2.0 mm); >450 mg/dl (25 mM) associated with ketoacidosis
Serum Sodium: <115 mg/dl (<5 mm)
Serum Calcium: <5.0 mg/dl (<1.2 mm)
Serum Magnesium: <0.8 mg/dl (<0.3 mm)
Blood Urea Nitrogen: >100 mg/dl (>35.7 mM)
Serum Creatinine: >10.0 mg/dl (>884 μM)

diagnostic testing. Due to the challenges of obtaining an accurate history in an actively seizing or postictal patient, vigilance in seeking collateral information is warranted from witnesses,[16] relatives, paramedics, medical alert bracelets, old medical records, and medication lists or containers. These data will often provide critical elements in the patient assessment.

Laboratory Studies

If a patient with a new-onset seizure has no significant comorbid disease and a normal examination (including mental status), the likelihood of an electrolyte disorder is extremely low; thus, extensive metabolic testing in patients who have returned to a normal baseline after a first-time seizure is not indicated.[17] Patients with persistent alteration of mental status, those in status epilepticus, and those who have fever or new neurologic deficit require extensive diagnostic testing, including serum glucose, electrolytes (i.e., sodium, magnesium, calcium), urea nitrogen, creatinine, complete blood count, pregnancy tests in women of childbearing age, antiseizure drug levels, AST, ALT, and drugs-of-abuse screening. Box 88.3 lists proposed cutoff values for metabolic derangements lowering the seizure threshold. Blood alcohol level and toxicology screening should be considered in patients with first-time seizures, although there is no evidence that such testing changes outcomes. A positive drug-of-abuse screen does not prove causation, and the patient may still require further evaluation with EEG and neuroimaging. Seizure due to alcohol intoxication or withdrawal is a diagnosis of exclusion because alcoholics are at increased risk for electrolyte abnormalities and traumatic injuries. Chapter 14 summarizes key laboratory diagnostics in patients presenting with seizures.

Radiology

Neuroimaging is recommended in patients with a first-time seizure, though in select patients who have a normal examination, have returned to baseline, do not have headaches, and have access to follow-up care, imaging can be obtained as an outpatient. Patients with a history of epilepsy and who have returned to baseline do not need neuroimaging in the emergency department. Urgent neuroimaging is indicated in cases with status epilepticus, focal neurologic deficits, prominent headache, known or suspected trauma, history of malignancy or immunocompromised state, and use of systemic anticoagulation. Additionally, elderly patients and those with neurocutaneous syndromes are at higher risk for structural brain abnormalities. Box 14.1 summarizes factors that should prompt consideration for neuroimaging.

Computed tomography (CT) has the advantages of being widely available and requiring shorter imaging acquisition times. However, other modalities such as magnetic resonance imaging (MRI) and CT perfusion may provide additional information (see Chapter 14). Figure 88.1 depicts the typical diffusion restriction corresponding to a seizure focus in an MRI of a patient with refractory focal status epilepticus.

Special Procedures and Tests

Lumbar puncture is indicated in patients with fever, severe headache, persistent altered mental status, or immunocompromise, unless a clear alternative diagnosis is present. Obtaining an EEG is often logistically challenging in the ED, but can be of high yield for patients whose diagnosis is unclear or who remain altered. EEG assists in the diagnosis of both epilepsy and nonepileptic spells, the detection of nonconvulsive seizures, and status epilepticus in those with altered mental status. Moreover, EEG guides management in monitoring the duration and depth of therapeutic coma management in refractory status epilepticus.

MANAGEMENT

Stabilization and Empirical Therapy

The initial approach to a patient with seizures centers on the characterization of the nature of events (seizures versus not seizures and underlying etiology), implementing supportive measures, and identifying critical and emergent diagnoses, listed in Box 14.3 in Chapter 14. The timely administration of adequate doses of first-line therapy (i.e., lorazepam 0.1 mg/kg [max 4 mg/dose] or midazolam 0.2 mg/kg [max 10 mg/dose]) remains the cornerstone of empirical abortive seizure therapy.[18,19] In status epilepticus, the use of benzodiazepines as the first line of treatment and a higher cumulative dose of antiseizure medications were associated with quicker cessation of status epilepticus.[20] Approximately 1 in 3 patients with status epilepticus require endotracheal intubation.[21] Proposed algorithms for the initial assessment, support, and implementation of empiric therapy of seizures and status epilepticus are displayed in Figure 14.2 and Figure 14.3, and most commonly used agents in first-, second- and third-line therapies are included in Table 14.2.

Definitive Management

While the empirical therapy centers on benzodiazepines as first-line therapy for most seizures that warrant abortive drugs, certain underlying pathologies warrant specific treatments; these are summarized in Table 88.3 which also provides specific dose considerations.

SPECIAL CASES

Alcohol-Related Seizures

Alcohol-withdrawal seizures account for a substantial portion of alcohol-related seizures. Alcohol suppresses glutamate-mediated excitatory tone while enhancing the inhibitory GABA-ergic receptors; in chronic use, there is upregulation of excitatory receptors. The interruption of alcohol use leads to excess excitation and a sympathomimetic response characterized by tachycardia, hypertension, disorientation, agitation, and seizures (See Chapter 137).

While seizures are witnessed in the setting of withdrawal, clinical findings cannot predict who is likely to have a recurrent seizure in the ED. Signs of alcohol withdrawal (tachycardia, confusion, or tremors) do not necessarily correlate with the likelihood of seizures. Although withdrawal seizures are an important etiology, patients with a history of alcohol abuse and dependence have several other potential risk factors for seizures, including increased incidence of traumatic brain injury, hypomagnesemia related to malnutrition, hyponatremia and hyperammonemia as a consequence of decompensated cirrhosis, hypoxic-anoxic events (i.e., aspiration) and co-ingestion of other toxins. In over half of the cases, alcohol-related seizures occur as a result of concomitant factors, such as epilepsy, structural brain abnormalities, and recreational drugs.

A first-time "withdrawal" seizure must be evaluated as any first-time seizure. Other conditions must be ruled out by history, physical examination, and diagnostic testing, including electrolytes, glucose,

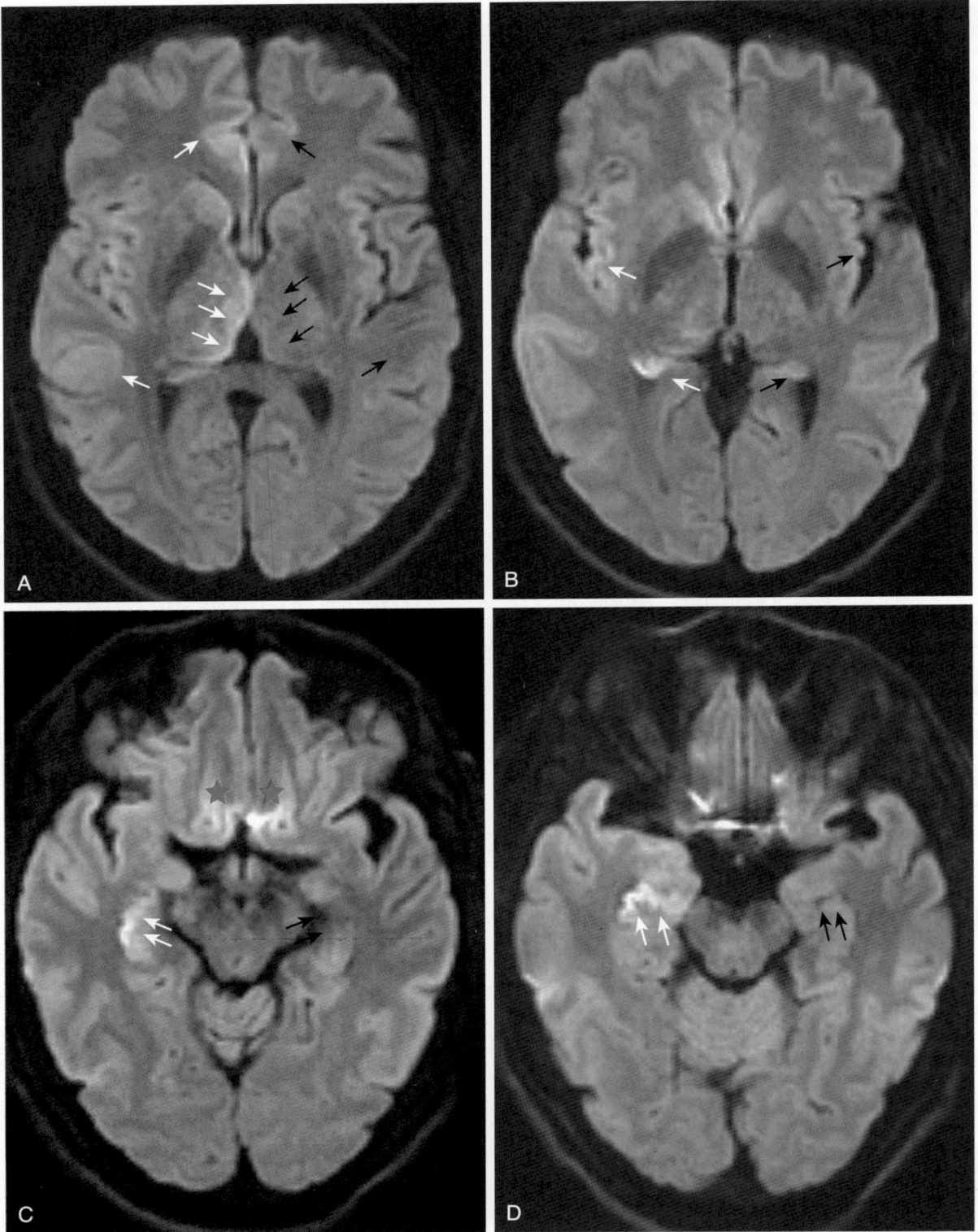

Fig. 88.1 Magnetic Resonance Imaging of Cortical Changes from Prolonged Seizures. Diffusion-weighted imaging (DWI) sequence of magnetic resonance imaging (MRI) of the brain of a 55-year-old woman with prolonged refractory status epilepticus from autoimmune etiology demonstrating restriction of diffusion (hyperintensities) in the areas of seizure involvement. From anterior to posterior, *white arrows* contrast the high signal in involved areas on the right hemisphere with the *black arrows* demarking spared areas in the contralateral left hemisphere. (A) Mesial frontal lobes, thalami, superior temporal cortex; (B) insular cortices and hippocampi; (C & D) hippocampi. *Red stars* depict artifactual symmetric hyperintensities in the inferior frontal lobes.

CT head, and lumbar puncture if indicated, particularly if fever is present. Testing results in an increased diagnostic yield in this population and is likely to affect management. After excluding other etiologies, the diagnosis of alcohol-withdrawal seizure is based on a history of recurrent events temporally related to ceasing or decreasing alcohol intake. Importantly, the presentation of alcohol withdrawal is frequently preceded by an illness or injury, leading to a decrease in alcohol consumption. A thorough history should include the precipitating reason for abstinence as well as a comprehensive assessment for concomitant illness if the cessation was not intentional. Alcohol-withdrawal seizures are usually generalized and occur between 6 and 48 hours after cessation of drinking. Judicious monitoring of these time intervals is warranted in scenarios where patients with a history of alcohol dependence are anticipated to have prolonged stays in the emergency department or are to be admitted.

Benzodiazepines are the treatment of choice in alcohol-withdrawal seizures, given the GABA-ergic pathway modulation, reducing the signs and symptoms of alcohol withdrawal and increasing the seizure threshold. All benzodiazepines appear to be equally efficacious in terminating an alcohol-withdrawal seizure; however, lorazepam is the only benzodiazepine that has been shown to decrease the incidence of seizure recurrence and decrease the need for hospitalization with a number needed to treat of 5 to prevent additional seizures in the subsequent 6 hours. Patients requiring 40 mg/h of diazepam equivalents are considered to have benzodiazepine-resistant alcohol withdrawal syndrome.[22] Adjunctive therapy such as phenobarbital[22] and ketamine (infusions ranging from 0.012 to 1.6 mg/kg/h) are potential alternatives

in such cases.[23] The placement of a definitive airway may be considered in refractory withdrawal seizures where repeated intravenous bolus or infusion dosing is anticipated to control symptoms.

Seizures Related to Other Toxins

Other toxins may lower the seizure threshold by disrupting the balance between excitatory and inhibitory neuronal transmission. Treatment is supportive and relies on the use of benzodiazepines as first-line therapy in most cases. Cases of toxin-induced refractory status epilepticus pose a particular challenge because the mechanism of status epilepticus may be different from status epilepticus with other causes. Some toxins (e.g., isoniazid) cause depletion of GABA neurotransmitter. Some of the typical antiseizure medications act by sensitizing the GABA receptor, making them less effective when GABA is depleted. In these cases, early administration of pyridoxine may be advantageous because it replenishes GABA in the brain. As with alcohol-induced seizures, phenytoin is ineffective for most drug-induced seizures. In some cases, such as in theophylline or tricyclic overdose, it may be harmful due to the increased risk of cardiac toxicity given the sodium channel antagonism of phenytoin and other antiseizure drugs (Fig. 88.2).

Post-Traumatic Seizures

Post-traumatic seizures are the hallmark of acute symptomatic seizures related to acute brain injury. Early post-traumatic seizures occur within the first week, with over 50% occurring within the first 24 hours. For primary seizure prophylaxis, antiseizure drugs may be initiated in the absence of seizures on presentation following acute brain injury

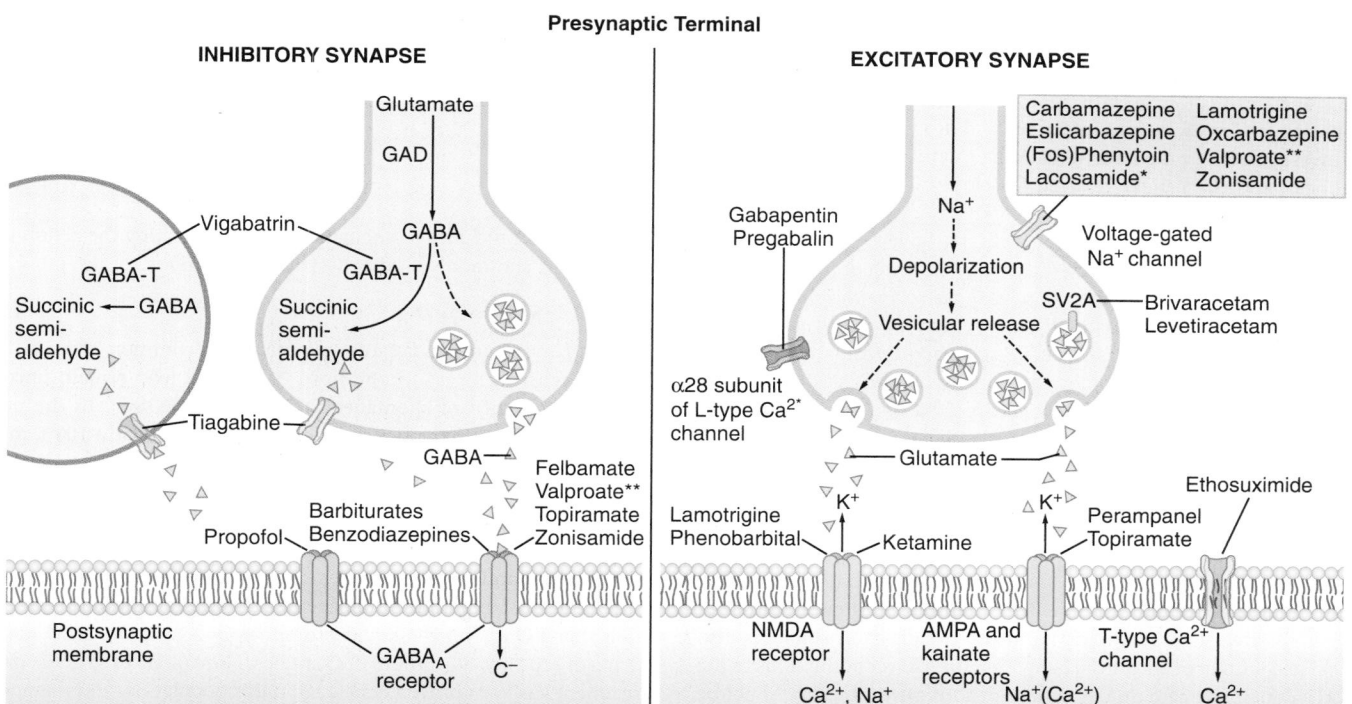

Fig. 88.2 Schematic Display Illustrating the Action Targets of Most Commonly Used Antiseizure Medications. *Lacosamide acts in Na+ channels by enhancing the slow inactivation of voltage-gated Na+ channels; other antiseizure drugs that target Na+ channels act by enhancing their fast inactivation. **Valproic acid (valproate) is considered a broad-spectrum antiseizure drug because it acts in both inhibitory and excitatory pathways. The enzyme GAD is responsible for catalyzing the decarboxylation of glutamate into GABA. *AMPA,* Alpha-amino-3-hydroxy-5-methyl-4-isoxazole propionic acid; *GABA,* gamma-aminobutyric acid; *GABA-T,* GABA transaminase; *GAD,* glutamic acid decarboxylase; *GAT1,* GABA transporter; *NMDA,* N-methyl-D-aspartate; *SV2A,* synaptic vesicle glycoprotein 2A. (Adapted from Morris M, Owusu K, Maciel CB. Status Epilepticus. In: Rabinstein A, ed. *Neurological Emergencies: A Practical Approach.* Vol 1. 1 ed. Springer: Switzerland; 2020:15 47.)

(e.g., traumatic brain injury, ischemic stroke, intracerebral hemorrhage, subarachnoid hemorrhage). Guidelines recommend 7 days in traumatic brain injury[24] and short-term therapy in subarachnoid hemorrhage. Although secondary prophylaxis helps reduce the risk of seizures during the subacute phase following traumatic brain injury, it fails to impact the risk of late seizures (or localization-related epilepsy).

Seizures in Pregnancy

Seizures in pregnancy are classified as one of three types: (1) those that occur in epileptic patients who are also pregnant, (2) new-onset seizures in pregnant patients, and (3) seizures that occur in the setting of eclampsia. Among patients with a history of seizure disorders, factors that may lower the seizure threshold in women who are pregnant include noncompliance, sleep deprivation, nausea and vomiting, or an increase in drug clearance resulting in subtherapeutic levels of antiseizure drugs—in particular, lamotrigine, phenytoin, carbamazepine, levetiracetam, and topiramate.[25] Additionally, pregnant patients with epilepsy commonly undergo adjustments in antiseizure regimens because several drugs are known for their teratogenic potential; these adjustments may lead to breakthrough seizures in otherwise well-controlled epilepsies. Overall, there is not an increased risk of status epilepticus during pregnancy.

Although few data guide the use of antiepileptic drugs for status epilepticus during pregnancy, the risks to the fetus from status epilepticus–related hypoxia and acidosis are greater than the potential teratogenicity of anticonvulsant medications. Therefore, patients who are actively seizing should be managed as the nonpregnant patient. In patients who are more than 24 weeks pregnant, fetal monitoring during and after a seizure should be arranged.

Pregnant patients with noneclamptic new-onset seizures should be worked up as any new-onset seizure patient, with a metabolic profile, EEG, and head CT scan with appropriate abdominal shielding. Precipitating etiologies, such as infections and drug toxicities, should also be investigated. If no source is identified, anticonvulsants should be withheld, and the patient referred for close follow-up. Cortical vein thrombosis should be on the differential for pregnant patients who present with headaches and focal seizures, given the relative prothrombotic state of pregnancy. Eclampsia is a major consideration in pregnant patients of at least 20 weeks' gestation who present with new-onset seizures. The pathophysiology may be due to disruption of cerebral autoregulation and resulting hyperperfusion and edema, similar to posterior reversible encephalopathy syndrome (PRES). Generalized seizures in pregnant women are typically preceded by preeclampsia, HELLP (hemolysis, elevated liver enzymes, low platelets), or hypertension.

Postpartum eclampsia represents 25% of eclamptic seizures, and importantly can occur up to 8 weeks after delivery without preceding preeclampsia or hypertension. Magnesium is the therapy of choice to treat acute eclamptic seizures and prevent a recurrence. It is more effective and has a better safety profile than phenytoin in preventing recurrence of convulsions and maternal death. Magnesium sulfate is also associated with benefits for the baby, including fewer admissions to the neonatal intensive care unit. Magnesium administration should not be delayed while awaiting definitive results when evaluating first-time seizures in a pregnant woman. An in-depth discussion of eclampsia can be found in Chapter 174.

First-Time Seizures

Adult patients with first-time unprovoked seizures may not have epilepsy, but should be informed that the risk of recurrence is highest in the subsequent 2 years, ranging from 21% to 45%,[26] especially in patients with prior brain insults such as trauma and stroke, those with epileptiform findings on EEG and abnormal neuroimaging, and nocturnal type of seizures. Starting secondary seizure prophylaxis reduces seizure recurrence in the initial 2 years; however, a careful risk-benefit assessment is warranted because there are conflicting data on the impact of antiseizure medicines on quality of life due to potential side effects.[26,27,28] Thus, starting an antiseizure regimen routinely in the emergency department is not recommended without input from a specialist and an individualized plan.

In children, the recurrence risk is much higher, particularly in those younger than 3 years.[29] One in three patients with newly diagnosed epilepsy remains untreated up to 3 years after diagnosis in the United States; this gap between diagnosis and adequate therapy may increase the risk of medical events and increase health care resource utilization.[30] Further, of those initiated in an antiseizure regimen, one-third discontinue treatment in the initial year.[31] The establishment of a reliable plan for follow-up care with a primary physician or neurologist is essential in patients with epilepsy.

Breakthrough Seizures

Patients with epilepsy presenting with breakthrough seizures should be evaluated for subtherapeutic levels whenever possible, as noncompliance and adjustments in regimens are common triggers. Table 88.5 includes reference levels for commonly used antiseizure drugs and suggested empiric reloading doses. A general formula for supplementing bolus of phenytoin is:

$$(\text{target total phenytoin level} - \text{current total corrected phenytoin level}) \times (\text{weight in Kg} \times 0.8).$$

A similar formula is available for valproic acid, and the volume of distribution is adjusted:

$$(\text{target total valproic acid level} - \text{current total valproic acid}) \times (\text{weight in Kg} \times 0.2).$$

Figure 88.2 includes a schematic display illustrating the action targets of most commonly used antiseizure medications.

Post-Anoxic Seizures

Post-anoxic seizures and status epilepticus are common after cardiac arrest, occurring in up to one-third of patients who remain unconscious after return of spontaneous circulation (ROSC). In the past, post-anoxic status epilepticus was associated with nearly 100% mortality, but immediate and aggressive seizure abortive measures may improve outcomes in select cases. Patients with a higher chance for recovery include those with the presence of brainstem reflexes, preserved median nerve somatosensory evoked potentials, and preserved EEG background reactivity to external stimuli.[32] In patients treated with targeted temperature management, seizures may occur at any time after ROSC, which should prompt early continuous EEG monitoring or repeated 30-minute EEG studies. No standardized antiseizure treatment has been proven beneficial in this population, and therapeutic algorithms are largely extrapolated from convulsive status epilepticus guidelines. Post-ROSC myoclonus may occur and requires EEG monitoring for an accurate diagnosis.

Nonconvulsive Status Epilepticus

The treatment of nonconvulsive status epilepticus should be individualized according to the risk of additional brain injury, extent of brain area involved by seizures, etiology of seizures, and comorbidities. No

TABLE 88.5   Loading Dose Route of Administration for Antiepileptic Drugs When Resuming Treatment in the Emergency Department

Drug	Loading Dose, Route, Therapeutic Range	Potential Adverse Effects
Carbamazepine	8 mg/kg oral suspension, single oral load Therapeutic level 4–12 µg/mL IV formulation recent; not widely available	Drowsiness, nausea, dizziness, nystagmus
Fosphenytoin	5–20 PE/kg depending on level IV at maximum rate of 150 PE/min; can also give IM Free level target ≈1.5 µg/mL; adjusted total level 15-20 µg/mL	Hypotension, bradycardia, nystagmus, dizziness, drowsiness
Gabapentin	900 mg/day oral at 300 mg tid for 3 days IV not available	Somnolence and fatigue, dizziness, myoclonus Uncommonly used as antiseizure regimen.
Lacosamide	200–400 mg IV or PO	Dizziness, somnolence, brady- or tachyarrhythmias
Levetiracetam	1000–2000 mg IV or PO	Somnolence or irritability. Usually well tolerated.
Oxcarbazepine	150–450 mg PO, single oral load IV formulation not available	Drowsiness, nausea, dizziness
Phenobarbital	15–20 mg/kg, IV or PO Therapeutic level 10–30 µg/mL	Drowsiness, sedation, hypotension
Phenytoin	5–20 mg/kg depending on level, IV or PO; if IV, infusion no faster than 50 mg/min Free level target ≈1.5 µg/mL; adjusted total level 15–20 µg/mL	Drowsiness, nausea, dizziness, nystagmus IV: Hypotension, bradyarrhythmias, extravasation injuries
Valproate	20–40 mg/kg depending on level, IV or PO Free level target 5–15 µg/mL; total level 50–100 µg/mL	Local irritation, thrombocytopenia, transaminitis, hyperammonemia

IM, Intramuscular; *IV*, intravenous; *PE*, phenytoin sodium equivalents; *PO*, by mouth
Medications were listed in alphabetic order; agent selection should be individualized.
Adapted from: Huff JS, Melnick ER, Tomaszewski CA, Thiessen ME, Jagoda AS, Fesmire FM. Clinical policy: critical issues in the evaluation and management of adult patients presenting to the emergency department with seizures. *Ann Emerg Med.* 2014;63(4):437-447.e415; and Morris M, Owusu K, Maciel CB. Status epilepticus. In: Rabinstein A, ed. *Neurological Emergencies: A Practical Approach.* Vol 1. 1 ed: Springer: Switzerland; 2020:15-47.

specific guidelines address nonconvulsive status epilepticus, and treatment algorithms are extrapolated from convulsive status epilepticus literature. Nonconvulsive seizures and epileptiform patterns bordering nonconvulsive status epilepticus are associated with metabolic crisis in the acutely injured brain. The threshold for starting third-tier medications (anesthetic coma) should be ascertained based on the perceived risk-benefit assessment for each patient. For example, an older patient with focal refractory nonconvulsive status epilepticus and sepsis is not the ideal candidate for pentobarbital or high-dose midazolam, because the morbidity associated with this treatment may surpass the evidence justifying its benefits.

Inflammation-Related Seizures

Inflammation-related seizures and status epilepticus comprise a heterogeneous group of epilepsies that may be triggered by an infection, tumor (i.e., paraneoplastic syndrome), or idiopathic autoimmune response. In paraneoplastic and autoimmune cases, seizures tend to be refractory to conventional antiseizure therapies, and the role of immunotherapy has been increasingly recognized. High-dose methylprednisolone, intravenous immunoglobulin, rituximab, plasma exchange, cyclophosphamide, and more recently tocilizumab, are potential rescue therapies that have been reported with variable degrees of success. Immunotherapy for seizures and status epilepticus requires coordination of care with multiple specialties for most cases, such as hematology, neurology, and rheumatology.

DISPOSITION

Patients with status epilepticus and those with critical diagnoses require admission for continued monitoring for complications and response to therapy. Admission to the intensive or neurocritical care unit, when available, is preferred in patients who require therapeutic coma with anesthetic agents. Disposition plans are less straightforward in other scenarios, including those presenting after a first-time seizure. The best predictor of seizure recurrence is the causative etiology combined with EEG findings. This information often requires modalities that are not routinely available in the ED, and there are few ED-based studies to direct disposition. At present, there is insufficient evidence to guide the decision pertaining to admission. We recommend this decision be tailored to the patient and shared decision making be employed, taking into consideration the patient's access to follow-up care and social risk factors (e.g., alcohol use disorder or lack of health insurance). Patients with comorbidities (including those older than 60 years old), known cardiovascular disease, history of cancer, or history of immunocompromise, should be considered for admission to the hospital. Patients with medically refractory epilepsies who live in assisted care facilities are often best served by being discharged back to the facility if they have returned to their baseline following breakthrough seizures.

Patients and their families or caregivers should be counseled on basic safety measures to prevent complications during seizures. For example, patients should be advised to avoid swimming or cycling following a seizure, at least until they have been reassessed by their neurologist and their antiepileptic therapy optimized if needed. The need for a "medical alert" bracelet or other medical condition identifier should be considered, and state-specific regulations should be followed. A crucial point for seizure patients is education against driving. Although evidence remains controversial on this issue, there is general agreement that uncontrolled epileptic patients who drive are at risk for a motor vehicle collision, with potential injury to themselves and others. For this reason, most states do not allow these patients to drive unless they have been seizure-free on medications for at least 6 months to 1 year. Although physicians are required to report patients with seizures to driving authorities in several states, mandatory reporting has not been proven to reduce the risk of motor vehicle crashes in patients with epilepsy.

Even a single seizure can induce an array of physical and psychosocial challenges that can affect the quality of life of the patient and caregivers. The psychological and social implications of the new diagnosis of a seizure disorder for the patient can be profound.

Fear of seizures and stigmatization are common; employability and insurability may be adversely affected. Emergency clinicians may consider coordination with social work and the referral of patients with seizures to counseling and community-based local epilepsy support groups.

The references for this chapter can be found online by accessing ExpertConsult.com.

89

Headache Disorders

Benjamin W. Friedman

KEY CONCEPTS

- The goals of headache evaluation in the ED are (1) to distinguish between benign primary headache disorders and potentially life-threatening secondary causes of headache and (2) to treat the headache pain effectively and rapidly without causing undue side effects.
- Patients with the following headache presentations are at risk for serious underlying disease: sudden explosive headache; new-onset headache after the age of 50 years; headache associated with papilledema, alteration in or loss of consciousness, or focal neurologic symptoms; subacute headache with increasing frequency or severity; headache associated with fever, cancer, or immunosuppression; and headache triggered by exertion, sexual activity, or Valsalva maneuver.
- The need for diagnostic studies is dictated by the suspected secondary cause of headache.
- Antidopaminergic agents, such as metoclopramide or prochlorperazine, are first-line therapy for migraine.

- Opioids are not first-line therapy for the primary headaches.
- Patients with migraine treated in the ED require a discharge "rescue plan" if the headache recurs.
- High-flow oxygen will terminate the majority of cluster headaches.
- The differential diagnosis of sudden severe headache includes subarachnoid hemorrhage, cerebral venous thrombosis, cervical artery dissection, and idiopathic intracranial hypertension.
- Cerebral venous thrombosis should be suspected in women who have a new type of headache and are pregnant or on birth control pills.
- Carotid artery dissection may cause headache, ptosis, and miosis.
- Patients with post-traumatic headache should only be imaged if they have high-risk features on the Canadian CT Head rule.

Headache is divided into primary and secondary disorders. *Primary headache disorders* include migraine, cluster, and tension-type headaches, and represent the majority of headaches seen in clinical emergency practice. *Secondary headache disorders* include a variety of organic illnesses in which head pain is a symptom of an identifiable, distinct pathologic process. To facilitate a standardized approach to headache management, the International Headache Society published a classification system and diagnostic criteria for headache disorders, cranial neuralgias, and facial pain.[1] This comprehensive and widely accepted system includes 14 major categories of headache disorders and uses specific operational diagnostic criteria to define each headache type (Box 89.1). Most patients presenting to an ED with headache have a benign process requiring only symptomatic treatment and referral. The challenge for the emergency clinician is to identify the very small subset of patients who have headache as a symptom of a serious or potentially life-threatening disease.

PRIMARY HEADACHE DISORDERS

Migraine Headache

Principles

Migraine is a common, chronic, sometimes incapacitating neurovascular disease characterized by recurrent attacks of severe headache, autonomic nervous system dysfunction, and, in some patients, an aura causing visual, sensory, motor, or other neurologic symptoms. It is a primary headache disorder with a genetic basis.

Migraine is a common disorder; attacks typically begin in the second decade of life and peak in prevalence in the fourth decade, affecting about 1 of 4 women and 1 of 12 men. There is no gender difference in the prevalence of migraine in children. After menopause, the prevalence of migraine among women decreases.

Historically, migraine headaches were considered to be vascular in origin. However, this hypothesis is no longer tenable as alterations in cerebral blood flow do not correlate with the various phases of the headache attack or vascular territories and do not explain features of an acute migraine, such as premonitory mood disturbances, nausea, and osmophobia (aversion to odors). Rather, vascular changes are now thought to be an epiphenomenon to what is a primary neurologic event. Abnormal trigeminal nerve and thalamic activity, possibly triggered by a sterile neuropeptide-induced inflammatory process, leads to activity and sensitization of higher order neurons in the brainstem and thalamus. Descending modulation is likely to be compromised as well. It is not yet known what initiates the pathophysiologic process that leads to a migraine attack. Migraine is commonly thought of in two major categories: (1) migraine without aura, which accounts for approximately 75% of all cases (Box 89.2); and (2) migraine with aura, which has specific reversible neurologic symptoms that precede the actual headache (Box 89.3). Cortical spreading depression, a neuroelectrical event characterized by a slow wave of depolarization, is the mechanism behind the symptom of migraine aura.

Clinical Features

Migraine is by definition a chronic and recurrent disease. The headache, characteristically, is unilateral, pulsating in quality, moderate to severe in intensity, and exacerbated by routine activities. The side of the headache can vary with individual attacks, and the headache may be bilateral in 40% of patients. The onset usually is gradual, and the attacks typically last 4 to 72 hours. Headache frequency is variable;

BOX 89.1 International Headache Society Classification of Headaches

Primary Headaches
1. Migraine
2. Tension-type headache
3. Cluster headache and trigeminal autonomic cephalalgias
4. Other primary headaches

Secondary Headaches
5. Headache attributed to trauma or injury to the head or neck
6. Headache attributed to cranial or cervical vascular disorder
7. Headache attributed to nonvascular intracranial disorder
8. Headache attributed to a substance or its withdrawal
9. Headache attributed to infection
10. Headache attributed to disorder of homeostasis
11. Headache or facial pain attributed to disorder of cranium, neck, eyes, ears, nose, sinuses, teeth, mouth, or other facial or cranial structures
12. Headache attributed to psychiatric disorder

Painful Cranial Neuropathies, Other Facial Pains, and Other Headaches
13. Cranial neuralgias and other facial pain
14. Other headache disorders

BOX 89.2 Migraine Without Aura Criteria

A. At least five attacks fulfilling criteria in B, C, D, and E
B. Attack lasts 4 to 72 hours (untreated or unsuccessfully treated)
C. Headache has at least two of the following characteristics:
   1. Unilateral location
   2. Pulsating quality
   3. Moderate to severe pain intensity
   4. Aggravation by or causing avoidance of routine physical activity (e.g., walking or climbing stairs)
D. During headache, at least one of the following:
   1. Nausea or vomiting (or both)
   2. Photophobia and phonophobia
E. Not attributable to another disorder

Reproduced with permission of International Headache Society, Headache Classification Committee of the International Headache Society (IHS). The International Classification of Headache Disorders, 3rd edition. *Cephalagia* 2018;38:1–211.

BOX 89.3 Migraine With Aura Criteria

A. At least two attacks that fulfill criterion B
B. Presence of at least three of the following four characteristics for a diagnosis of classic migraine:
   1. One or more fully reversible aura symptoms indicating focal cerebral cortical or brainstem dysfunction (or both)
   2. At least one aura symptom developing gradually over more than 4 minutes, or two or more symptoms occurring in succession
   3. No single aura symptom lasting longer than 60 minutes
   4. Headache beginning *during* aura or *afterward,* with a symptom-free interval of less than 60 minutes (also may begin *before* aura)
C. Exclusion of related organic diseases by means of an appropriate history, physical examination, and neurologic examination with appropriate diagnostic tests

Reproduced with permission of International Headache Society, Headache Classification Committee of the International Headache Society (IHS). The International Classification of Headache Disorder, 3rd edition. *Cephalagia* 2018;38:1–211.

those patients with more than 15 headache days per month are considered to have chronic migraine. Associated symptoms and signs include nausea, vomiting, anorexia, photophobia, phonophobia, osmophobia, blurred vision, lightheadedness, vertigo, muscle tenderness, and nasal congestion. Many patients have dramatic light and sound sensitivity and seek a dark, and quiet room. Some patients experience premonitory cognitive impairment during the days leading up to the acute attack producing forgetfulness, irritability, and depression.

The migraine aura consists of focal neurologic symptoms that usually precede the headache, though patients may experience aura without headache. By definition, the aura is fully reversible and typically lasts 10 to 20 minutes, although it may continue for as long as 1 hour. The most common aura is visual; features may include scintillating scotoma (bright rim around an area of visual loss), teichopsia (subjective visual image perceived with eyes open or closed), fortification spectra (zigzagged lines that slowly drift across the visual field), photopsias (poorly formed brief flashes or sparks of light), and blurred vision. Less common auras include somatosensory phenomena, such as tingling or numbness, motor disturbances, and cognitive or language disorders.

Retinal migraine is a rare syndrome consisting of recurrent attacks of monocular visual dysfunction, including positive features (such as scintillations) or negative features (such as blindness). As with aura, these symptoms are completely reversible.

Hemiplegic migraine is characterized by a motor aura consisting of hemiparesis or hemiplegia. The progression of the motor deficit is gradual and, in most cases, is accompanied by a visual, sensory, or speech disturbance. The neurologic symptoms last up to 60 minutes, followed by headache. Rarely, the motor deficit is persistent, resulting from a true stroke. A familial version of hemiplegic migraine is associated with genetic channelopathies.

Migraine with brainstem aura presents with an aura referable to the brainstem. Common neurologic findings include dysarthria, tinnitus, vertigo, diplopia, and altered level of consciousness.

Status migrainosus is a severe unremitting migraine headache that persists unabated for more than 72 hours.

Many factors can trigger migraine headaches in predisposed persons. Common precipitants include sleep deprivation, stress, hunger, hormonal changes, including menstruation, and use of certain drugs, including oral contraceptives and nitroglycerin. In addition, some patients report specific food sensitivities to chocolate, caffeine, and foods rich in tyramine, monosodium glutamate, and nitrates. Alcohol, specifically red or port wine, has also been implicated. In others, certain sensory stimuli, such as a strong glare or strong odors, loud noises, and weather changes, can trigger an attack.

Differential Diagnoses

Among patients without stereotypical recurrent headaches, migraine may be difficult to distinguish from secondary causes of headache, see Chapter 16 and Table 16.1. Headaches with an acute onset may have a cerebrovascular etiology. Headaches that have lingered for longer than several weeks may be due to an intracranial mass lesion or other causes of high cerebrospinal fluid (CSF) pressure. Headaches that occur in the setting of upper respiratory infections may be due to sinus inflammation. Medication overuse headache, which is a disorder characterized by worsening headache frequency in the setting of increased use of analgesic or migraine abortive medication, may coexist with migraine.

Diagnostic Testing

Neuroimaging is not necessary for patients with typical recurrent migraine headaches. Neuroimaging should be considered for older or immunocompromised patients with new-onset headaches, headaches associated with unexplained neurologic abnormalities, and new headaches with an abrupt onset. (Please see Chapter 16 for the diagnostic

TABLE 89.1 Selected Medications for Acute Migraine Attacks

Medication	Dosage and Route Administered	Comments
Oral Medication		
Ibuprofen	400 mg PO	Gastrointestinal upset
Naproxen sodium	500 mg PO	Gastrointestinal upset
Acetaminophen + metoclopramide	650 mg + 10 mg PO	Combination therapy has better efficacy than acetaminophen alone
Sumatriptan	50–100 mg PO	Use cautiously in patients with cardiovascular risk factors
Eletriptan	40 mg PO	Use cautiously in patients with cardiovascular risk factors
Ubrogepant	50–100 mg	May cause transaminitis
First-Line Parenteral Medication		
Prochlorperazine	10 mg IV	Sedation and dystonic reaction
Metoclopramide	10 mg IV	Dystonic reaction
Droperidol	2.5 mg IV	QT prolongation; dystonic reaction
Ketorolac	15 mg IV or 15 mg IM	Gastrointestinal upset; avoid this medication in elderly patients and in patients with renal insufficiency
Sumatriptan	6 mg SC	Chest pain, throat tightness, flushing Contraindicated with hypertension, coronary artery disease, peripheral vascular disease, and pregnancy Cannot be used within 24 hours of ergot use
Second-Line Parenteral medication:		
Dihydroergotamine (DHE)	1 mg IV or IM; may be repeated in 1 hour	Nausea (pretreat with antiemetic) Often causes chest pain Caution in inhibitors of enzyme CYP450 3A4
Magnesium sulfate	2 g IV	More efficacious in migraine with aura
Procedures		
Greater occipital nerve block	6 mL of bupivacaine 0.5% injected bilaterally	Can also target lesser occipital nerve
To Prevent Headache Recurrence After Emergency Department Discharge		
Dexamethasone	10 mg IV	Use cautiously in diabetics

IM, Intramuscular; *IV*, intravenous; *PO*, per os (by mouth); *SC*, subcutaneous.

algorithm.) Such patients have a higher likelihood of having a secondary cause of headache, such as an intracranial bleed or space-occupying lesion. Among patients with an acute migraine headache, laboratory testing should be limited to a pregnancy test for those who are to be treated with medications that may be teratogenic and electrolytes for those patients with marked nausea, anorexia, or vomiting sufficient to require intravenous (IV) fluid hydration.

Management

The pharmacologic treatment of migraine is divided into abortive therapies, which attempt to limit the intensity and duration of a given episode, and preventive therapies, which are intended to decrease the frequency and intensity of attacks. The goals of abortive therapy include rapid pain relief, minimization of headache recurrence and medication side effects, and restoration of the patient's ability to function.

There are several approaches to treatment of the acute headache episode, depending on the severity of the attack (Table 89.1).[2] The choice of agents depends on the patient's previous response to specific therapies, the existence of comorbid conditions, and the presence or absence of nausea or vomiting. Gastric stasis is common during acute migraine attacks and may limit the effectiveness of oral agents.

For mild to moderate attacks, simple analgesics such as acetaminophen or nonsteroidal antiinflammatory drugs (NSAIDs), such as ibuprofen or naproxen, are often effective. In the presence of nausea

or vomiting, administration of intravenous metoclopramide 20 to 30 minutes before the oral analgesic enhances the absorption and effectiveness of these medications. Appropriate doses for these and other oral medications are listed in Table 89.1.

For moderate to severe attacks, three classes of medications are recommended as initial parenteral therapy: the antiemetic dopamine antagonists, such as metoclopramide and prochlorperazine; migraine-specific agents, such as the triptans and dihydroergotamine (DHE); and parenteral nonsteroidal medications, such as ketorolac.

Dopamine antagonists, such as the neuroleptic prochlorperazine, and the antiemetic metoclopramide, are highly effective as monotherapy for acute migraine attacks. Because of their efficacy, safety, tolerability, and few contraindications, we recommend either of these agents as first-line therapy for acute migraine. Metoclopramide is a less potent antinauseant, and is less likely to induce drowsiness and sleep, which can be factored into the choice of agents, depending on the patient's circumstances. For this class of medication, the mechanism of action is not known, but migraine pathogenesis likely involves dopaminergic pathways. The most common side effects after parenteral administration include sedation and extrapyramidal symptoms, most notably akathisia, which can be treated with diphenhydramine, 25 to 50 mg IV, or midazolam, 2 mg IV.

Sumatriptan, the first-approved medication of the triptan class, a class of selective 5-HT (1B/1D) receptor agonists, is the most frequently used triptan in the ED, and is available for oral (50 to 100 mg)

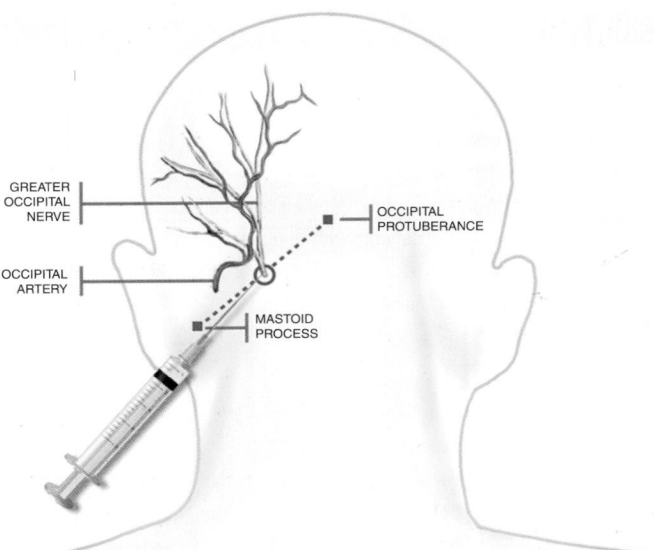

Fig. 89.1 Technique of Greater Occipital Nerve Block. The injector identified the appropriate location using landmarks on the patient's head. The medial landmark was the occipital protuberance. The lateral landmark was the mastoid process. Using these landmarks to form a line, the injector identified the correct location, which was one-third of the distance from the occipital protuberance along this line (two-thirds of the distance away from the mastoid process). The injector felt for pulsation of the occipital artery and attempted to elicit pain or paresthesia in the distribution of the GON by pressing slightly. The injector then used a fan technique, placing 1 mm of anesthetic at the correct spot, 1 mm slightly medial of the correct spot, and 1 mm slightly lateral to the correct spot.

and subcutaneous (6 mg) administration; the latter is more efficacious but also more likely to cause adverse effects. If the patient has experienced insufficient relief with sumatriptan previously, eletriptan 40 mg orally may be administered. Common side effects of triptans include tingling, flushing, warm or hot sensations, heaviness in the chest, and initial worsening of the underlying headache. Sumatriptan is contraindicated in patients with coronary artery disease and should not be used within hours of administration of an ergotamine-containing medication. Sumatriptan is classified as a category C drug for pregnancy, though there does not seem to be an increase in adverse pregnancy outcomes with its use. A smaller dose of subcutaneous sumatriptan may limit side effects.

DHE is often effective when prochlorperazine or metoclopramide have failed, and is administered intravenously in a dosage of 1 mg over 2 minutes; this can be repeated in 1 hour if pain control has not been achieved. Because DHE can cause nausea and vomiting, patients who have not already received an antiemetic, should be given metoclopramide 10 mg IV or prochlorperazine 10 mg IV at least 15 minutes before administration of DHE. Contraindications to use of DHE include pregnancy, breast-feeding, poorly controlled hypertension, coronary artery disease, and peripheral vascular disease. DHE should not be used if the patient has already taken any drug in the triptan class or if the patient is using macrolides or protease inhibitors.

Alternatively, greater occipital nerve block with bupivacaine 0.5% may be attempted among patients with symptoms refractory to first-line medications (Fig. 89.1).

Calcitonin gene related peptide (CGRP) receptor antagonists and monoclonal antibodies likely will play an increasing role in the management of migraine in the coming years as multiple placebo-controlled studies have demonstrated safety and efficacy. The relative efficacy and safety of these medications vis-à-vis the antidopaminergic antiemetics is still unknown. It is clear that CGRP is released during acute migraine attacks and contributes to migraine symptoms.

Opioid analgesics are nonspecific for migraine pain, and rarely, if ever, are indicated in the treatment of acute migraine. They have not been shown to be more effective than nonsteroidal antiinflammatory agents for treatment of migraine. Opioid requests by patients with "migraine" often represent misunderstanding of effective therapy based on past experience. We recommend that opioids not be used for treatment of migraine. Rare cases may exist where a neurologist who knows the particular patient's syndrome rationally validates the use of opioids. Opioids should not be administered on the basis of a "doctor's letter" or other document produced by the patient (see Chapter 151).

Status migrainosus can often be treated successfully using the various medications or combinations of the medications discussed in the previous paragraphs.

Recurrence of migraine within 24 hours of ED discharge occurs in two-thirds of patients who initially improve after treatment in the ED, regardless of medication administered or pain intensity at discharge. Patients should be discharged home with oral medication to treat the headache recurrence, such as naproxen 500 mg or sumatriptan 100 mg. Dexamethasone 10 mg IV decreases migraine recurrence after ED discharge and should be administered to all patients without contraindications.[2]

Preventive therapy is indicated for patients who have more than two or three functionally disabling headaches per month. Several classes of medications are used for migraine prevention, including beta-blockers, tricyclic antidepressants, antiepileptic drugs, and botulinum toxin. Patients who meet criteria for preventative therapy and are not on it, and those for whom preventative therapy has failed, should be referred to a primary care physician or neurologist for evaluation.

Disposition

Most patients who present to an ED for treatment of migraine can be treated and discharged after one or several doses of medication and IV fluids if required. Only rarely do patients with migraine require hospitalization. Patients requiring admission often have chronic migraine, with more than 15 days of migraine monthly, or concomitant *medication overuse headache*. Migraine patients admitted to the hospital receive IV fluids, frequent doses of parenteral migraine medication, and detoxification from medications contributing to the overuse headache.

Cluster Headache
Principles

Cluster headache is the only headache syndrome that is more common in men than in women. It typically occurs in young to middle-aged adults who smoke, almost always onsetting before the age of 50 years. The headaches tend to occur repeatedly during a defined time interval, hence the term *cluster*. Several attacks can occur in a single day, and a typical cluster period may last weeks to months. Several precipitating factors have been implicated, most notably the ingestion of alcohol. Stress and climate changes may also play a role in susceptible persons. As with migraine, abnormal activation of the trigeminal nerve contributes to headache nociception. Typically, secondary parasympathetic activation causes ipsilateral lacrimation and rhinorrhea, a characteristic of cluster headache syndrome.

Clinical Features

Cluster headaches occur suddenly with little warning, and multiple episodes can occur within a 24-hour period. Each headache lasts from 15 minutes up to 3 hours, with a mean duration of about two hours.

TABLE 89.2 Treatment of Cluster Headaches

Medication	Dosage and Route Administered	Comments
Acute Treatment		
First-Line		
Sumatriptan	6 mg SQ	
Oxygen	At least 6–12 L/ min	
Second-Line		
Octreotide	100 micrograms SQ	GI symptoms
Metoclopramide	10 mg IV	Dystonic reaction
Discharge Treatment		
Dexamethasone	10 mg IM or IV	Most efficacious dose unknown
Verapamil	240–480 mg/day PO in 2–4 divided doses	May cause constipation, use cautiously if BP or HR are low
Melatonin	10 mg qHS	Well tolerated

The headache typically begins with a unilateral sharp, stabbing pain in the eye, which may awaken the patient from sleep. The attacks occur exclusively in the territory of the trigeminal nerve. Unlike the patient with migraine, the patient with cluster headache presents agitated and anxious, rocking, rubbing the head, and pacing. The attack subsides rapidly, often leaving the patient exhausted.

Accompanying the headache are ipsilateral autonomic symptoms, such as ptosis, miosis, and forehead or facial sweating. The eye often is injected and tearing, and many patients have unilateral nasal congestion or rhinorrhea.

Differential Diagnoses

Other headache disorders that mimic cluster headache include carotid artery dissection, trigeminal neuralgia, and rare trigeminal autonomic cephalalgias, including paroxysmal hemicranias and short-lasting uniform neuralgiform headache attacks with conjunctival injection and tearing (SUNCT). Carotid artery dissection should be excluded as the diagnosis in patients who present with unilateral face or neck pain and Horner syndrome. With trigeminal neuralgia, the pain peaks within seconds, lasts only a few minutes, and can be provoked by specific trigger points on the face or oral mucosa. The less common trigeminal autonomic cephalalgias are manifested by brief unilateral headaches that recur dozens of times per day, often accompanied by the same unilateral eye and nasal symptoms as cluster.

Diagnostic Testing

Diagnostic testing is not indicated for patients with a well-established history of cluster headache. Cluster headache is a characteristic syndrome with specific onset, distribution, duration, and accompanying symptoms, so in patients younger than 50 years without a prior diagnosis, particularly if they have a previous pattern of similar attacks, the presumptive diagnosis can be made with confidence. Patients with a presentation more consistent with carotid artery dissection, particularly neck pain, Horner syndrome, or unilateral neurologic deficit, should undergo neurovascular imaging

Management

Treatment should focus both on relieving the acute headache and preventing the next headache in the cluster (Table 89.2). Because cluster headache is brief in duration, it may resolve before a patient presents to medical attention. For acute headache relief, high-flow oxygen is first-line therapy. It should be administered at rates of 15 liters/minute or greater through a non-rebreather mask until that headache has remitted completely. High-flow oxygen aborts the headache within 15 minutes in approximately 80% of patients. Subcutaneous sumatriptan, 6 mg, is also an effective therapy for acute cluster headache if the headache fails to resolve after 20 to 25 minutes of high-flow oxygen.[8] Larger doses do not confer additional benefit and may contribute to medication side effects. Antidopaminergic agents and NSAIDs can be used if the patient does not experience relief with oxygen and sumatriptan or if the patient has contraindications to the latter. As with migraine, opioid medications are not indicated for treatment of acute cluster headache, in part because of the evanescent nature of the headache symptoms.

Once the acute attack has been relieved, focus shifts to the ongoing "cluster" of headaches that likely will recur over hours to days. Corticosteroids have long been theorized to help break the cluster, although high-quality evidence is not available. Based on retrospective data, we recommend a 10-day prednisone taper, starting with 60 mg for at least two days. Verapamil, dosed at 120 mg three times a day, may decrease the frequency of attacks by the end of the first week of therapy and should be considered for patients without calcium channel blocker contraindications who are discharged from the ED.

Disposition

Patients with cluster headache usually do not require admission to the hospital. Because these headaches are likely to continue over the following days and weeks, the patient should be referred to a physician with expertise in headache management.

Tension-Type Headache
Principles

Tension-type headache is the most common recurrent headache disorder, with one year prevalence of 40% of the population in the United States, but it is an infrequent cause of ED visits. Women are affected slightly more frequently than men, and as with migraine, peak prevalence is in the fourth decade of life. These headaches typically do not cause substantial functional disability, and patients are able to continue with their normal daily activities. Autonomic symptoms, such as nasal congestion, nausea, or vomiting are absent. By definition, episodic tension-type headache lasts as little as 30 minutes and as long as 7 days.

The pathophysiology underlying tension-type headache is not yet clear. There is no consistent evidence that increased muscle activity is present. Physical examination will reveal tender areas of the scalp and neck with both tension and migraine headaches. Despite different epidemiologic profiles, a similar response to many therapeutics suggests that tension and migraine headaches may share pathophysiologic mechanisms.

Clinical Features

Patients typically complain of a tight, bandlike discomfort or pressure around the head that is nonpulsating and dull. They also may experience tightening of the neck muscles. A majority of patients do not seek medical assistance, because the headache usually is mild in intensity and not functionally disabling. On occasion, the discomfort can build up slowly and fluctuate in severity for several days. Unlike in migraine, the headache does not worsen with physical activity, and accompanying symptoms (such as nausea, vomiting, phonophobia, and photophobia) are unusual. Anxiety and depression may coexist with chronic tension headache, which by definition, occurs more than 15 days a month and can be daily and unremitting.

Differential Diagnoses

Tension headache is the least distinct of all of the primary headache disorders, and its diagnosis is based mainly on the absence of features that would suggest another headache diagnosis. The most common disorders mimicking tension headache are migraine, IIH, cervical spondylosis, sinus or eye disease, and intracranial masses. Subtle indolent infections (such as cryptococcal meningitis) should be considered in the immunocompromised.

Diagnostic Testing

Patients who present with a headache similar in quality to previous headaches do not require diagnostic evaluation in the ED. New-onset headache with features of tension-type headache requires evaluation in patients 50 years and older, as well as immunocompromised patients. This evaluation can take place in the outpatient setting, where a scheduled MRI offers more sensitivity for a range of pathologies than a noncontrast CT.

Management

Because the pain of tension-type headache is rarely severe or disabling, the emergency physician should try to understand why the patient with tension-type headache presented to the ED. For a majority of patients with tension headaches, simple analgesics, such as acetaminophen or an NSAID, are adequate for pain control. Opioids are never indicated and consideration of a need for any parenteral treatment, such as metoclopramide, should prompt serious concern that the diagnosis of tension headache is not correct. For chronic outpatient management, acupuncture has shown benefit for some patients. Despite muscle pain and tenderness in many of these patients, spinal manipulation therapy is unlikely to provide a benefit for most patients.

Disposition

Absent comorbidities, patients with tension-type headache do not require admission to the hospital. Chronic tension-type headache is difficult to manage; these patients often have underlying mental health or personal stress issues, and should be referred to clinicians who can evaluate them for these underlying issues and work with them over time.

SECONDARY HEADACHE DISORDERS

Subarachnoid Hemorrhage

Principles

SAH refers to extravasated blood in the subarachnoid space. (For discussion of other intracranial hemorrhages, please see Chapter 87.) Presence of the blood activates meningeal nociceptors, leading to headache and, in about one-third of cases, signs of meningismus. SAH accounts for up to 10% of all strokes and is the most common cause of sudden death from a stroke.

Approximately 80% of patients with nontraumatic SAH have ruptured saccular (berry) aneurysms, which are small (usually <15 mm diameter) aneurysms that usually form at or near the junction of major cerebral vessels, particularly within the circle of Willis. The remainder are in the posterior circulation, particularly the basilar artery and its ramifications. Approximately 25% of people with a berry aneurysm have more than one aneurysm, and most aneurysms do not rupture, but are found incidentally by cerebral imaging or by autopsy. Other etiologies requiring emergent treatment include arteriovenous malformations, cavernous angiomas, mycotic aneurysms, neoplasms, and CNS vasculitis. Perimesencephalic hemorrhage is a benign form of SAH, in which a localized hemorrhage occurs anterior to the midbrain, without extension, and with no vascular abnormalities on cerebral vascular imaging. These hemorrhages resolve spontaneously and do not require intervention. SAH may also be caused secondarily by an intraparenchymal hematoma that dissects its way into the subarachnoid space.

The risk for aneurysmal SAH increases with age; most cases occur between 40 and 60 years old. In children and adolescents, aneurysms are uncommon, and SAH usually is secondary to an arteriovenous malformation. It is estimated that 2% of the general population harbor a berry aneurysm, with the vast majority never rupturing. Risk of rupture appears to be related to the rate of growth of the aneurysm and increases with aneurysmal size. Other risk factors associated with SAH include hypertension, smoking, excessive alcohol consumption, and use of sympathomimetic drugs. Both genetic and familial associations of cerebral aneurysms have been identified, and there is association with several diseases, including autosomal dominant polycystic kidney disease, coarctation of the aorta, Marfan syndrome, and Ehlers-Danlos syndrome type IV.

Less than 1% of patients presenting to the ED with a primary complaint of headache have SAH, but the diagnosis is of great importance because of the morbidity and mortality associated with aneurysmal rupture. One-quarter of patients with SAH die before reaching the hospital. Median mortality in the United States is about one-third with approximately one-third of survivors having functional and cognitive deficits.

Clinical Features

The clinical presentation of SAH is often distinctive. Most patients present with a sudden, cataclysmic thunderclap headache, which often is described as the worst headache of one's life. The onset of headache may be associated with exertion, the Valsalva maneuver, or sexual intercourse, but the majority occur in the absence of strenuous physical activity. The headache of SAH classically peaks in intensity within seconds to minutes. Headaches that take longer than 60 minutes to peak in intensity are unlikely to be SAH. Associated signs and symptoms include syncope, nausea and vomiting, neck stiffness, photophobia, and seizures. The patient may experience sudden syncope as the initial manifestation, with headache occurring as the patient regains consciousness and increasing thereafter.

Physical findings depend on the extent of the SAH. Up to 20% have focal neurologic abnormalities. Patients may have isolated third or sixth nerve palsy or meningismus. Oculomotor (third) nerve compression secondary to an expanding posterior communicating artery aneurysm causes pupillary dilation. Approximately 50% of patients with a ruptured aneurysm are restless or have a fluctuating or altered level of consciousness. Up to one-third of patients recall an earlier, less severe episode of headache (sentinel headache) days to weeks before the diagnosis of subarachnoid hemorrhage.[3]

TABLE 89.3 Hunt and Hess Clinical Grading Scale for Cerebral Aneurysms and Subarachnoid Hemorrhage

Grade	Condition
0	Unruptured aneurysm
1	Asymptomatic or minimal headache and slight nuchal rigidity
2	Moderate or severe headache, nuchal rigidity, no neurologic deficit other than cranial nerve palsy
3	Drowsiness, confusion, or mild focal deficit
4	Stupor, moderate to severe hemiparesis
5	Deep coma, decerebrate posturing, moribund appearance

BOX 89.4 Ottawa Subarachnoid Clinical Decision Rule

Age ≥ 40 years
Neck pain or stiffness
Loss of consciousness
Onset during exertion
Thunderclap (instantly peaking) headache
Limited neck flexion on examination

(Absence of all of these features obviates the need for further diagnostic workup.)

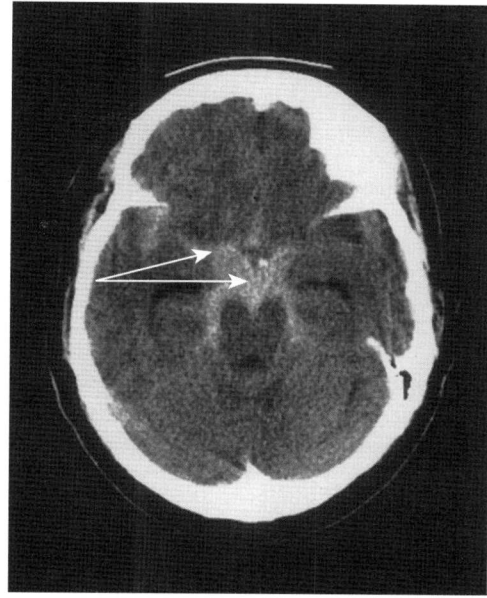

Fig. 89.2 Cerebral Aneurysm. Shown is a computed tomography (CT) scan of an aneurysmal subarachnoid hemorrhage (SAH) in a 55-year-old woman. Subarachnoid blood can be seen within the interpeduncular and ambient cisterns and the right sylvian fissure from a ruptured aneurysm at the junction of the right carotid artery and the posterior communicating artery. (From Brisman JL. Neurosurgery for cerebral aneurysm. Emedicine, updated Sep 23, 2010. Available at http://emedicine.medscape.com/article/252142-overview#a1.)

The patient's prognosis is related to neurologic status at hospital admission. The Hunt and Hess scale stratifies patients according to their clinical signs and symptoms at the time of presentation and is predictive of outcome (Table 89.3). Patients who present with a grade 1 or grade 2 hemorrhage tend to have a good prognosis. Patients with grade 4 or 5 hemorrhages tend to do poorly, presenting with an altered mental status, ranging from stupor to deep coma, together with focal neurologic signs and symptoms. Patients with grade 3 hemorrhage present with drowsiness or confusion and are at risk for rapid clinical deterioration.

Differential Diagnoses

Several clinical entities can mimic the abrupt onset headache associated with SAH. These include cervical artery dissection (CAD), cerebral venous thrombosis (CVT), reversible cerebral vasoconstriction syndrome, hemorrhagic or ischemic stroke, and primary headache disorders, including migraine and cluster headaches. CNS infections cause altered mental status and meningismus but can usually be distinguished by the presence of fever and much longer period of onset.

Diagnostic Testing

The Ottawa clinical decision rule can help risk stratify patients with possible SAH. In this rule, high (near 100%) sensitivity is achieved, but with low (less than 20%) specificity. Use of the rule may not improve accuracy compared to clinical gestalt, but a diagnosis of SAH is of sufficient gravity that high use of advanced imaging for diagnosing "positive" patients is justified (Box 89.4).

A non–contrast-enhanced head CT scan should be obtained emergently when SAH is suspected (Fig. 89.2). For acute hemorrhages less than 24 hours old, the sensitivity of third-generation multidetector row CT scanners in identifying hemorrhage is greater than 90%; however, sensitivity decreases to approximately 50% by the end of the first week, as blood is resorbed. The sensitivity of non–contrast-enhanced head CT performed within 6 hours of headache onset approaches 100%. For patients in whom CT has been performed more than 6 hours after headache onset, a normal non-contrast CT should be followed with subsequent diagnostic testing, which may include spinal fluid analysis or cerebrovascular imaging.[4] The choice of whether to perform LP or a subsequent imaging test depends upon patient preference, local availability, and what else is on the differential diagnosis. For example, if the physician is also concerned about meningitis or idiopathic intracranial hypertension, then an LP would be preferred; if the differential diagnosis includes other neurovascular etiologies such as cervical artery dissection or reversible cerebral vasoconstriction syndrome, then imaging is preferred. Options for cerebrovascular imaging include computed tomography angiography (CTA) or magnetic resonance angiography (MRA). The two-stage approach (non-contrast CT first followed by vascular imaging) is as sensitive as non-contrast CT followed by LP.

Interpretation of LP results can be challenging because up to one-third of spinal fluid analyses contain blood or blood degradation products. The presence of xanthochromia may help differentiate a traumatic LP from SAH. This yellowish pigmentation is secondary to the metabolism of hemoglobin to pigmented molecules of oxyhemoglobin and bilirubin, a process that can take up to 12 hours to occur. SAH cannot be ruled out if a substantial number of RBCs persist in tube 4; however, an RBC count of less than 100 in tube 4 indicates that aneurysmal SAH does not need to be pursued further. CSF xanthochromia in association with normal findings on the CT scan is suggestive of SAH. After the diagnosis is established, angiography should be performed to study the vascular anatomy and to identify the source of hemorrhage.

A normal non–contrast-enhanced head CT scan followed by a normal spinal fluid analysis definitively rules out SAH and does not need to be followed with angiography, even in patients at high risk of disease. However, this strategy does not rule out other causes of thunderclap headache that may be in the differential diagnosis, such as cervical artery dissection, cerebral venous sinus thrombosis, and reversible cerebral vasoconstrictor syndrome.

Up to 90% of patients with SAH have cardiac arrhythmias or electrocardiographic abnormalities suggestive of acute cardiac ischemia, which may lead to an erroneous primary cardiac diagnosis, especially when syncope has occurred. Typical electrocardiographic findings include ST-T wave changes, U waves, and QT prolongation.

Management

The management of SAH is aimed at treating acute medical and neurologic complications, preventing recurrent hemorrhage, and forestalling the ischemic complications of vasospasm. Because of an altered level of consciousness, patients with SAH of grade 3 or higher are at risk for respiratory depression and hypercapnia, which can lead to further increases in intracranial pressure (ICP); therefore, early endotracheal intubation should be considered in these patients, using a technique consistent with that used for patients with elevated intracranial pressure (see Chapter 1). Blood pressure should be closely monitored because of the risk of continued bleeding or recurrent hemorrhage. The typical treatment goal is a systolic blood pressure below 160 mm Hg or a mean arterial pressure (MAP) below 130 mm Hg. To achieve this, the physician should use intravenous nicardipine or labetalol. Care is required to maintain MAP above 95 mm Hg, though, because iatrogenic hypotension may cause more harm than elevated blood pressure. Nimodipine, a calcium channel blocker, should be started soon after a diagnosis of aneurysmal SAH is made to lessen the likelihood of poor outcome due to vasospasm, even if the patient's blood pressure is normal. Because nimodipine may cause transient hypotension in some patients, hemodynamic monitoring is required during its administration. The recommended dosage is 60 mg by mouth or nasogastric tube every 4 hours.

Corticosteroids have not been demonstrated to be of benefit. Opioids should be used for persistent headache, though modest doses of short-acting agents should be used to avoid interference with evaluations of neurologic status. Intravenous fentanyl, titrated in 50 microgram aliquots is an appropriate first-line agent. In patients who are nauseated or at risk for vomiting, antiemetics such as metoclopramide 10 mg IV or ondansetron 4 mg IV should be administered. Agitated patients require sedation. Short-acting opioids such as fentanyl 50 micrograms IV may achieve this goal. If not, short-acting benzodiazepines such as midazolam 1 mg IV may be added. All patients should be placed on bed rest in a quiet and dark environment. Clinically evident seizures should be treated with levetiracetam or fosphenytoin. Prophylactic anticonvulsant therapy is of unknown benefit, and we recommend leaving this to the discretion of the admitting consultant or in consultation with the receiving consultant when transfer to another center is planned. For definitive management, endovascular coil embolization is preferable to neurosurgical clipping, but this decision is based on size, location, and morphologic features of the aneurysm, as well as local expertise.

Disposition

Patients with ruptured aneurysms require monitoring of hemodynamics and neurological status in an intensive care setting. Patients requiring transfer to a higher level center for care should be managed in collaboration with the receiving center, including contingency plans for complications (e.g. seizures, decreasing level of consciousness) that might arise in transport.

Intracranial Neoplasm
Principles

Headache may be a presenting complaint among patients with brain tumors, though is less common in older patients, presumably because of age-related atrophy. Headache can be caused by primary neoplasms

---

BOX 89.5   Most Common Types of Intracranial Malignancy Causing Headache

Metastatic
  Breast
  Lung
  Gastrointestinal
  Melanoma
Meningioma
Glioblastoma
Primary CNS lymphoma
Pituitary adenoma

---

of the CNS, as well as by metastatic lesions (Box 89.5). The most common causes of metastasis are lung and breast carcinoma, followed by malignant melanoma and carcinomas of the gastrointestinal tract.

The headache of intracranial neoplasms can be caused by several mechanisms, including traction on pain-sensitive structures (such as meninges or larger cerebral vessels), or it may be a symptom of increased ICP or hydrocephalus. The pain patterns produced are highly variable, depending on the location and size of the mass and the structures involved. Rapidly growing tumors are more likely to be associated with headache.

Clinical Features

The location of the headache may be ipsilateral, contralateral or bilateral and does not predict tumor location. The patient may present with complaints of a worsening headache that has been present for weeks to months. The headache may have been present initially only on awakening (most likely in patients with increased ICP), gradually becoming continuous. The classic triad of brain tumor headache—sleep disturbances, severe pain, and nausea and vomiting—is seen in a minority of patients. If increased ICP is present, the headache often is bilateral and worsened by coughing, sneezing, bending, defecation, and sexual intercourse. Other presentations of intracranial neoplasms include seizures, personality changes, and cognitive difficulties.

Differential Diagnoses

A number of disease processes can mimic brain tumor headache. These include other space-occupying lesions, such as an abscess or an intra-axial or extra-axial brain hemorrhage; diseases associated with increased ICP, such as idiopathic intracranial hypertension; and a vasculitis, such as giant cell arteritis (GCA). Once malignant causes of headache have been excluded, many of these patients will be diagnosed with a chronic headache disorder, such as chronic migraine, chronic tension-type headache, or *new daily persistent headache*, which is a primary headache disorder, characterized by abrupt onset and unremitting course.

Diagnostic Testing

The diagnosis of brain tumor headache may be suspected from the history and neurologic examination. Early in the course, patients may present with headache and an intact neurologic examination, although the majority of intracranial neoplasms will eventually cause focal neurologic deficits. Neuroimaging with CT or MRI is the most efficient way to confirm the diagnosis and is appropriate for all patients with a new persistent headache, particularly those patients older than 50 years. Contrast enhancement on CT often improves the identification of the underlying mass lesion and helps differentiate it from other causes, including abscess, hematoma, and vascular malformation.

Choice of imaging modality depends on local availability and should be tailored to the differential diagnosis.

Management

The treatment of headache associated with brain tumors depends on the type of tumor, patient functional status, and stage of the disease. Management consists of urgent referral to specialty care and treatment of any acute complications, including increased ICP and seizures. For patients who present with symptoms suggestive of increased ICP (e.g., headache, nausea, vomiting, confusion, weakness), treatment with corticosteroids to treat associated edema often provides dramatic temporary relief of headache and other symptoms of increased ICP. Dexamethasone is most commonly used. The exact dose of steroids necessary for each patient varies in accordance with histologic features, size, and location of the tumor and the amount of edema present. An appropriate starting dosage in the ED is 10 mg IV, followed by 4 mg every 6 hours. NSAIDs are appropriate initial therapy.

Patients with seizures should receive levetiracetam or fosphenytoin. Empirical or prophylactic treatment with antiepileptic medication should be avoided as this does not delay or prevent the onset of seizure activity and may expose the patient to unnecessary complications and toxicity.

Disposition

Patients with brain tumor headache should be managed in consultation with the patient's primary health care team. Hospitalization versus discharge will depend upon the severity of the patient's presentation.

Giant Cell Arteritis
Principles

GCA is an inflammatory vasculopathy that occurs in medium and large arteries with well-developed wall layers and adventitial vasa vasorum. It typically involves the major branches of the aorta and has a predilection for the extracranial branches of the carotid artery (e.g., temporal and occipital arteries). It can involve the ophthalmic, vertebral, and distal subclavian arteries, as well as the thoracic aorta. GCA is often named *temporal arteritis* because it commonly affects the superficial temporal arteries.

The mean age at onset of GCA is 71 years old, and it is rare before 50 years old. Women are affected more commonly than men. Pathologically, the arteritis causes an inflammatory infiltrate in the arterial wall resulting in intimal hyperplasia and subsequent stenosis and occlusion, leading to a variety of ischemic complications. In the vast majority of cases, loss of vision is due to anterior ischemic optic neuropathy.

Clinical Features

Temporal arteritis is the most typical presentation of GCA and presents with a broad spectrum of clinical features attributable to both ischemia and systemic inflammation (Box 89.6). Headache is the most common initial manifestation and occurs in more than 70% of patients. The headache often is of 2 to 3 months' duration and can be continuous or intermittent; it can worsen at night or on exposure to cold. The pain may be described as sharp, throbbing, boring, or aching and usually is localized to the temporal region but may occur anywhere in the head. The physical examination may reveal tenderness over the scalp in the area of the temporal artery, with exacerbation of the pain by wearing a hat or resting the head on a pillow. Patients also can experience jaw claudication secondary to vascular insufficiency of the masseter and temporalis muscles. Systemic signs and symptoms are often present, including fever, anorexia, and weight loss. Approximately 40% of patients develop symptoms of polymyalgia rheumatica, pain in their large proximal joints, with symptoms referable to the neck, torso, and

---

BOX 89.6 Diagnostic Criteria for Giant Cell Arteritis (Require 3 of 5)

Age ≥ 50 years old

New headache type, particularly in association with visual loss or jaw claudication

Temporal artery tenderness or tenderness of other extracranial arteries

ESR ≥ 50 mm/h or CRP ≥ 10 mg/L

Positive imaging finding or temporal artery biopsy

---

lower back. The pain and stiffness are typically worse in the morning and lessen as the day goes on.

The most serious complication of GCA is permanent visual loss, which occurs in approximately 15% of patients. Amaurosis fugax (transient monocular blindness) can occur before permanent visual loss. Other complications include peripheral neuropathies, transient ischemic attacks, and stroke. The physical examination may reveal abnormalities of the temporal arteries best detected by light palpation just anterior and slightly superior to the tragus of the ear. Findings include tenderness, reduced or absent pulsations, erythema, and nodularity or swelling. Visual acuity, visual field testing, and thorough funduscopic examination should be followed over time. The presence of a relative afferent pupillary defect (Marcus-Gunn pupil) should increase the suspicion for GCA, although these patients usually will also have a visual loss or a visual field defect.

Differential Diagnoses

The systemic symptoms of GCA are nonspecific. Therefore, the differential diagnosis is quite broad and includes infections, malignancies, and other vasculitides. Takayasu arteritis can affect the aorta and its primary branches as well, but it affects younger patients and visual loss is uncommon. Polyarteritis nodosa, microscopic polyangiitis, and granulomatosis with polyangiitis (formerly known as *Wegener granulomatosis*) can rarely affect the temporal artery but have different histopathology and vascular involvement. Ischemic stroke can cause headache with visual loss or amaurosis fugax. Pituitary apoplexy classically presents with thunderclap headache and bitemporal visual field loss.

Diagnostic Testing

The diagnosis of GCA is based on the history and physical examination, laboratory and imaging studies, and biopsy of the temporal artery. The majority of patients will have elevations of both the C-reactive protein (CRP), and the erythrocyte sedimentation rate (ESR), usually to more than 50 mm/hr and often more than 100 mm/hr, as well as the presence of thrombocytosis and anemia. The sensitivity of an elevated ESR or an elevated CRP has been reported in the range of 85%, but their specificity is only 30%. However, very few patients with GCA have both a normal ESR and CRP at the time of diagnosis. Ultrasonography of the temporal arteries may reveal a periluminal hypoechoic halo representing vessel wall edema. MRI of the temporal arteries has similar test characteristics as ultrasonography. The decision about which test to order should be made in consolation with the interpreting radiologist. If these imaging studies are performed in the ED, they may confirm the diagnosis and obviate the need for biopsy. Temporal artery biopsy is an imperfect test and is not required for diagnosis if the diagnosis is apparent based on clinical, laboratory, and imaging results (see Box 89.6).[4]

Management

Patients who present with visual symptoms (such as amaurosis fugax or diplopia) must be treated emergently with glucocorticoids, because they are at risk for visual loss, which is typically permanent. Given the available evidence, we recommend methylprednisolone 1000 mg per day for 3 consecutive days to optimize immunosuppression and suppress tissue edema. For patients without visual symptoms, lower doses of steroids, in the range of 40 to 60 mg/day of prednisone should be used. Tocilizumab, a monoclonal antibody against the interleukin 6 receptor may be used in the outpatient setting to prevent relapse during corticosteroid tapering.[9]

Disposition

Patients with GCA should be managed in consultation with appropriate specialists, including neurology, ophthalmology, and rheumatology. They can be discharged if symptoms have resolved and rapid outpatient follow-up has been assured.

Carotid and Vertebral Artery Dissection

Principles

Approximately 2% of all ischemic strokes are caused by cervical artery dissection. In patients younger than 50 years old, cervical artery dissection is the most frequent cause of ischemic stroke and accounts for 10% to 25% of cases. These values likely underestimate the true incidence because patients with minimal symptoms are often not diagnosed. Although dissections may occur spontaneously, a careful history frequently identifies an association with sudden neck movement or trauma preceding the event. Reported mechanisms include neck torsion, chiropractic manipulation, coughing, minor falls, heavy lifting, various sports including basketball and volleyball, sexual intercourse, childbirth, and motor vehicle collisions. Early symptoms and signs may be subtle, and delays in diagnosis are common in the absence of neurologic findings. The median delay from symptom onset to diagnosis can be several days.

The pathologic lesion in cervical artery dissections is intramural hemorrhage within the media of the arterial wall. The hematoma can be localized or extend circumferentially along the length of the vessel, resulting in partial or complete occlusion. Damage to the intima results in platelet aggregation and thrombus formation further compromising vessel patency or causing distal embolization. The timing of these events is variable, and a patient may experience symptoms of cerebral ischemia days to years after dissection.

Clinical Features

The typical presentation of cervical artery dissection is the abrupt onset of pain in the head or neck, often in association with symptoms resulting from ischemic consequences of the dissection and emboli. Neurologic findings secondary to cerebral ischemia usually occur within the first few hours following the onset of the headache or neck pain. Although carotid dissection and vertebral artery dissection have many commonalities, their clinical presentations have some unique features.

Carotid Artery Dissection. The classic presentation of symptoms for carotid artery dissection includes (1) unilateral headache or neck pain, sometimes radiating to the ipsilateral eye; (2) ipsilateral ptosis and miosis (a partial Horner syndrome); and (3) either blindness, due to retinal ischemia, or contralateral motor deficits, caused by cerebral ischemia. However, this complete triad is only present in a minority of patients. The headache is often severe and throbbing but may be subacute and similar to previous headaches and may be associated with pulsatile tinnitus.

Acute severe retro-orbital pain in a previously healthy person with no history of cluster headaches is suggestive of carotid dissection. Patients with a carotid dissection are at risk of sustaining embolic cerebral ischemia. Warning symptoms include transient ischemic attacks, amaurosis fugax, episodic lightheadedness, and syncope. Spontaneous dissection of the carotid artery has a favorable prognosis and

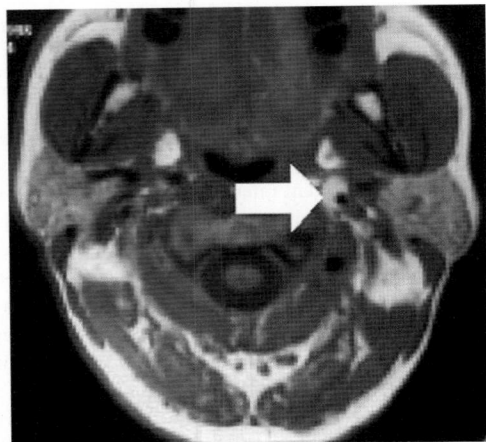

Fig. 89.3 Axial T1-weighted magnetic resonance image (MRI) demonstrating a crescent sign *(arrow)* in a patient with a left internal carotid artery dissection. (From Kidwell C. Dissection syndromes. Emedicine, updated Sep 19, 2011. Available at http://emedicine.medscape.com/article/1160482-overview.)

recurrence is uncommon. Factors associated with a worse prognosis include older age, occlusive disease on angiography, and stroke as the initial presenting symptom.

Vertebral Artery Dissection. Vertebral artery dissections are less common than carotid dissections. The classic presentation is that of a relatively young person with severe, unilateral posterior headache and a rapidly progressive neurologic deficit with symptoms of brainstem and cerebellar ischemia. Common findings include vertigo, severe vomiting, ataxia, diplopia, hemiparesis, unilateral facial weakness, and tinnitus. Stroke severity tends to be lower than that seen with carotid dissection. Spontaneous vertebral artery dissection appears to be relatively rare. Approximately 10% of patients who develop a vertebral dissection die during the acute phase, secondary to massive stroke. For patients who survive, the prognosis is usually good.

Differential Diagnoses

The differential diagnoses of unilateral headache and neck pain with or without Horner syndrome include migraine and cluster headache. Cluster headache in particular can present with ptosis. Cervical arterial dissection may present with an abrupt onset of severe headache, which may be confused with SAH or other vascular causes of headache. For patients who present with symptoms of cerebral ischemia, both ischemic and hemorrhagic stroke should be considered as possible etiologies. Conversely, cervical artery dissection should be considered in patients who present with acute stroke, particularly younger patients.

Diagnostic Testing

Identification of patients with dissection can be challenging, especially in the absence of cerebral ischemia. A non–contrast-enhanced head CT scan is often normal in uncomplicated dissection. Digital subtraction angiography remains the diagnostic gold standard, although several studies have found CTA and magnetic resonance angiography (MRA) to have sensitivities of approximately 95%, making them appropriate choices for initial screening. Cerebrovascular imaging of the head and neck should be considered in all patients in whom CAD is suspected and in young patients with stroke, because it is a more common cause of stroke in a younger population. Cerebrovascular imaging should be considered in unresponsive patients who may have basilar artery pathology. Figure 89.3 shows an example of carotid artery dissection on MRI.

Management

Cervical artery dissection patients with acute ischemic stroke are candidates for thrombolytic therapy or endovascular thrombectomy (see Chapter 87). Studies have shown these treatments to be safe with efficacy similar to stroke from other causes.

For patients with cervical artery dissection without acute ischemic stroke, the primary goal of treatment is the prevention of cerebral ischemic complications. Antiplatelet agents including aspirin, clopidogrel, or dipyridamole, and anticoagulation with unfractionated or low–molecular-weight heparin are comparably effective at preventing stroke, which is relatively uncommon.[5]

Disposition

Patients with cervical artery dissection should be admitted to the hospital for monitoring and further management.

Cerebral Venous Thrombosis
Principles

Thrombosis of the intracranial veins and sinuses is a rare disorder causing approximately 1% of all strokes. It typically presents with headache and disproportionately affects younger individuals without traditional cerebrovascular risk factors.

There are multiple causes for CVT, and risk factors are classically linked to the Virchow triad of blood stasis, blood vessel wall abnormalities, and a hypercoagulable state. Both genetic and acquired prothrombotic conditions have been associated with CVT. Inherited thrombophilias such as antithrombin III, protein C and protein S deficiencies, and factor V Leiden mutation are the most common genetic causes. Acquired causes for CVT include pregnancy and the puerperium, malignancy, head trauma, surgery, parameningeal infections, and exogenous hormones, such as oral contraceptives. Other causes include systemic inflammatory disorders, including vasculitis, inflammatory bowel disease and connective tissue disorders, and neurosurgical procedures.

Clinical Features

Clinical findings in CVT usually fall into two major categories, depending on the mechanism of neurologic dysfunction: (1) Those that are related to increased ICP due to impaired venous drainage, and (2) those related to focal brain injury from venous occlusion resulting in ischemia, infarction, or hemorrhage. Diffuse headache increasing in severity over days to weeks is the most common symptom experienced by patients with CVT and is often associated with increased ICP. Focal neurologic findings, when present, are related to the region of the brain that has been injured and bilateral brain involvement may occur. Seizures, both focal and generalized, frequently occur. Ocular findings associated with CVT include orbital pain, proptosis, chemosis, extraocular muscle paralysis, and papilledema.

Differential Diagnoses

The differential diagnoses of early CVT, when symptoms are limited to headache and papilledema, include brain tumor and idiopathic intracranial hypertension. Late presentations of CVT include altered sensorium, seizures, and focal neurologic deficits. At this point, the differential diagnosis includes ischemic and hemorrhagic stroke; intracranial infections, such as brain abscess, meningitis, and encephalitis; and systemic conditions, including sarcoidosis and systemic lupus erythematosus. With CVT, neurologic findings do not follow a typical arterial territory. CVT is a rare and often subtle diagnosis. To avoid missing the diagnosis, it should be considered for all patients with a new headache type who have thromboembolic risk factors or recent head or neck surgery.

Diagnostic Testing

Routine blood work including a complete blood count (CBC), chemistry panel, ESR, and clotting studies, including a prothrombin time (PT) and partial thromboplastin time (PTT), should be obtained in all patients with suspected CVT. These studies are helpful in determining the presence of an underlying hypercoagulable state, an infectious process, or an inflammatory disorder contributing to the development of CVT. A normal D-dimer can exclude this diagnosis among patients without thromboembolic risk factors or recent head or neck surgery who have a normal neurologic exam and the absence of papilledema.[6] The definitive diagnosis of CVT is based on neuroimaging of the area of thrombosis. This is best accomplished by a combination of MRI to visualize the thrombosed vessel and magnetic resonance venography (MRV) to detect nonvisualization of the same vessel. Non–contrast-enhanced CT by itself is an insensitive test, but it may reveal nonspecific late lesions, such as an infarct, hemorrhage, or edema. Occasionally, hyperdensity of a cortical vein or sinus may be seen. CTA and CTV may be used to visualize the cerebral venous system, especially in patients who have a contraindication to MRI.

Management

Patients with CVT should be anticoagulated to prevent propagation of the thrombosis and development of embolic complications. Treatment is adjusted dose unfractionated heparin or weight-based low–molecular-weight heparin in full anticoagulant doses, regardless of the presence of intracerebral hemorrhage. In patients whose clinical condition worsens despite anticoagulation, thrombolysis or thrombectomy may be considered in centers with expertise in interventional procedures. Seizures are treated with antiepileptic drugs such as phenytoin or levetiracetam.

The prognosis with CVT is based on the underlying etiology, the patient's condition at time of diagnosis, and the development of complications. The overall mortality is low compared with other types of strokes, but morbidity may be increased with delays in recognition and treatment.

Disposition

Patients with CVT require hospitalization, preferentially to a stroke unit, for systemic anticoagulation.

Idiopathic Intracranial Hypertension
Principles

Although this disease is sometimes called *pseudotumor cerebri,* the term *idiopathic intracranial hypertension (IIH)* best reflects current understanding of the pathophysiology and the fact that this disorder is not benign because permanent visual field loss can occur. Compared with other headache disorders, IIH is a relatively uncommon neurologic disease seen primarily in young, obese women of childbearing age. Several predisposing factors have been suggested, including antibiotics (most commonly tetracyclines), vitamin A and retinoids, and human growth hormone. The pathophysiologic mechanism of this disease is not understood, but it is often attributed to an imbalance between CSF production and reabsorption.

Clinical Features

Clinical and diagnostic criteria for IIH are listed in Box 89.7. The most prominent symptom is generalized headache, which may take the form of migraine or tension-type headache.[10] No specific localizing pattern has been documented, although in some patients the headache is worsened by eye movement. It may awaken the patient from sleep and is exacerbated by bending forward and the Valsalva maneuver, both of which impede cerebral venous return. Visual complaints are common, and patients may experience transient visual obscurations (TVOs), which are momentary blackouts of vision most likely due to temporary disruption of the microcirculation to the optic nerve head. They usually occur with postural changes and are not predictive of permanent visual loss. Patients may also complain of nausea, vomiting, dizziness, and pulsatile tinnitus. The physical examination will reveal papilledema, and visual field deficits or visual loss occurs in up to 50% of patients. Fortunately, in the majority of patients, visual defects are reversible with treatment. On occasion, a sixth nerve palsy is noted.[2]

Differential Diagnoses

The differential diagnoses of IIH include other causes of increased ICP in a patient presenting with headache. Important considerations include cerebral venous sinus thrombosis, mass lesions, obstructive hydrocephalus, and leptomeningeal infiltration by neoplastic or infectious processes.

Diagnostic Testing

Ultrasonographic measurement of the diameter of the optic nerve sheath, 3 mm behind the optic disc, is consistent with elevated intracranial pressure if greater than 5 mm. MRI with MRV or MRI with contrast is the preferred modality for diagnosing IIH. MRI should occur early in the workup of IIH because of its ability to detect not only mass lesions and hydrocephalus but also cerebral venous sinus thrombosis and other meningeal processes. If neuroimaging is normal, an LP should be performed in the lateral decubitus position to measure CSF opening pressure and to obtain CSF diagnostic studies. An opening pressure of 250 mm H_2O or more (normal is 70 to 180 mm H_2O) is necessary to make the diagnosis. Ophthalmology follow-up should be arranged for detailed visual field testing.

Management

Many patients present without visual field loss, and symptomatic therapy is all that is necessary. Historically, removal of a large enough amount of CSF (>20 mL) to decrease CSF pressure has been recommended to relieve headache. However, studies of patients with IIH reveal no association between CSF pressure and headache, and CSF is produced relatively quickly, which limits the duration of benefit.[10] Therefore, we believe treatment with NSAIDs such as ketorolac 15 mg IV or antidopaminergic medication such as metoclopramide 10 mg IV may allow the patient with an established diagnosis of IIH to avoid a therapeutic lumbar puncture. In patients with evidence of visual field loss, treatment with medications to lower ICP is indicated. Acetazolamide, starting at doses of 250 to 500 mg orally BID, can improve 6-month visual outcomes though it does not improve headache. If a

patient is not responsive to medications or has progressive symptoms, an optic nerve sheath decompression or CSF diversion procedure (e.g., lumboperitoneal or ventriculoperitoneal shunt) may be indicated.

Disposition

Once the headache has been controlled, patients with IIH can be discharged, assuming visual loss is not marked and has not progressed rapidly. Because visual loss can occur early or late in the course of IIH, outpatient follow-up with ophthalmology and neurology should be recommended.

Post–Dural Puncture Headache and Other Low CSF Pressure Headaches
Principles

Post–dural puncture headache (PDPH) is the most frequent cause of low CSF pressure headache seen in the emergency department, though spontaneous intracranial hypotension can also cause orthostatic headaches. The former is a recognized complication of dural puncture, whether performed for diagnostic or therapeutic purposes or accidentally, as a complication of epidural anesthesia, whereas the latter is caused by spinal CSF leak without localized trauma.

The pathophysiology of low CSF pressure headaches is not entirely clear. The most likely explanation is a persistent CSF leak that exceeds CSF production, resulting in CSF hypotension. If sufficient CSF is lost, the brain descends in the cranial vault when the patient assumes the upright position, leading to increased traction on the pain fibers. Thus the headache is characteristically positional and increases with the upright position and decreases with recumbency. The amount of time a patient remains recumbent after lumbar puncture does not affect the incidence of PDPH.

Equipment-related factors have been implicated as causes of PDPH, including the size or diameter of the spinal needle, the orientation of the bevel during the procedure, and the amount of fluid withdrawn. Smaller-diameter needles (e.g., 20- or 22-gauge cutting needle) cause less leakage, and it is postulated that insertion of the needle with the bevel up (i.e., bevel pointing up when the patient is in the lateral position) minimizes damage to the dural fibers. Use of noncutting needles (e.g., Whitaker or Sprotte) also has been shown to reduce the incidence of PDPH.

Clinical Features

The cardinal feature of PDPH is orthostatic or positional headache that is precipitated by the upright position and relieved when the patient lies down. About 90% occur within the first 72 hours after the LP and typically resolve within 1 week, though headaches may persistent for months. Associated signs and symptoms include neck stiffness, nausea, vomiting, auditory disturbances including tinnitus and hypoacusis, and photophobia.

Differential Diagnoses

For most patients, PDPH is a benign disorder. However, in patients who do not respond to standard treatment modalities, other secondary headache disorders must be considered. This is especially true in the postpartum period when CVT and preeclampsia are important considerations.

Diagnostic Testing

The diagnosis of PDPH is based on clinical features, with a headache occurring after an LP or epidural catheter placement, and most patients have a benign course that requires no diagnostic testing. Spontaneous CSF leaks present with orthostatic headaches, which are sometimes severe and should be considered in the absence of a recent LP. The diagnosis is made when low CSF pressures are found on LP, which should be considered in patients with orthostatic headaches who have not experienced recent dural puncture. In the postpartum period, CVT should be excluded with MRV.

Management

Most PDPHs resolve spontaneously within 5 to 7 days with bed rest, hydration, and analgesics. For persistent headaches not responding to over-the-counter analgesics, methylxanthine agents (such as caffeine 500 mg IV drip over 1 hour) and corticosteroids may be of benefit. For severe headaches that do not respond to these conservative measures, an epidural blood patch (EBP) should be used. This procedure involves the injection of 15 to 30 mL of autologous blood into the epidural space near the site of the original dural puncture resulting in a blood clot that seals off the dural hole.[7]

Disposition

The vast majority of patients with PDPH will have a benign course requiring only conservative treatment. These patients can be discharged home. For patients with persistent complaints, consultation with anesthesia or radiology for an EBP should be considered.

Post-Traumatic Headache
Principles

Headache is the most common symptom following a concussion or other traumatic brain injury (TBI). It is often part of a complex post-concussive syndrome that can include dizziness, fatigue, insomnia, irritability, memory loss, and difficulty with concentration. Persistent headache (>3 months) occurs in over 50% of patients who have suffered a TBI. Paradoxically, patients with milder injuries are more likely to report persistence of symptoms, as are patients with preexisting headache disorders. For the emergency clinician, management of post-traumatic headache (PTH) requires excluding life-threatening causes of headache and treating the headache, associated symptoms, and contributing factors (e.g., cervical strain, cranial neuropraxias). The pathophysiologic mechanism for the symptoms is unclear and may have both anatomic and functional components.

Clinical Features

By international criteria, PTH develops within 7 days of the injury or regaining consciousness. Acute PTH resolves within 3 months, whereas persistent PTH persists beyond 3 months. Patients in whom PTH develops after minor head injuries have normal findings on neurologic examination and routine neuroimaging studies. Many patients are more concerned about the cause of the headache than about the headache itself, underscoring the importance of patient education on the post-concussive syndrome.

PTH may assume a variety of characteristics, including the pulsating unilateral pain and associated features of migraine, the bland, squeezing pain of tension-type headache, or nonspecific headache often relating to the musculature of the neck.

Differential Diagnoses

In the acute setting, pathological causes of headache including intracranial hemorrhage, or skull or cervical fractures should be excluded. Cervical strain and subtle oculomotor nerve palsies are additional etiologies of PTH that should be considered. After the acute setting, it may be difficult to distinguish PTH from migraine or tension-type headache, a distinction that, as time passes, becomes less important.

Diagnostic Testing

In the acute setting following TBI, traumatic injuries to the brain, skull, and neck should be evaluated using available clinical decision rules (see Chapter 34). Patients who return to the ED with persistent symptoms after normal initial imaging should be reassured that follow-up imaging is not required, assuming the patient has a normal neurologic examination and is not using anticoagulants or antiplatelet medication. Neuroimaging is indicated in the setting of focal neurologic deficits or persistent altered mental status.

Management

We recommend that PTH be treated with the same armamentarium of medications used to treat acute primary headaches, specifically, antiemetic dopamine antagonists such as metoclopramide or prochlorperazine, and NSAIDs. Opioids should be avoided.

Disposition

Patients with PTH should be discharged home with appropriate outpatient follow-up. These patients should be informed that they may continue to suffer from headache and other symptoms over the subsequent weeks and should be provided with medication, advice about how to manage symptoms, and referrals to local physicians with relevant expertise.

Hypertensive Headache
Principles

There is uncertainty about whether elevated blood pressure can cause headache. Ambulatory blood pressure monitoring studies have not demonstrated an association, although these studies are limited by relatively modest blood pressure elevations during the study period. Nearly one-quarter of patients who present to an ED with headache have a systolic blood pressure above 150 mm Hg or diastolic blood pressure over 95 mm Hg. Patients who present with headache are more likely to have a markedly elevated blood pressure than patients with other chief complaints. However, the causal pathway, if one exists, is not apparent based on current evidence. In fact, both chronic hypertension and acute elevation in blood pressure have been linked to decreased pain sensitivity in animal and human models. International criteria attribute headache to elevated blood pressure when the pressure is greater than 180 mm Hg systolic or 120 mm Hg diastolic and when the headache resolves with resolution of the elevated blood pressure.

Clinical Features

The headache of severe hypertension is generally characterized as bilateral and throbbing. Early reports of a typical hypertensive headache come from patients with marked, untreated hypertension, who had early morning headaches that were of greatest intensity before the patient arose and typically resolved as the patient engaged in morning activities.

Differential Diagnoses

Based on population prevalence, the most likely diagnoses in patients with elevated blood pressure and headache are migraine or tension-type headache with concomitant hypertension.

Pre-eclampsia, a disorder characterized by elevated blood pressure and headache, should be considered in patients in the latter stages of pregnancy and the recent postpartum period. Posterior reversible encephalopathy syndrome (PRES) is characterized by white matter changes on diagnostic imaging. Malignant hypertension, including drug-induced hypertension, requires evidence of end-organ damage (Table 89.4).

Diagnostic Testing

In the absence of altered sensorium, focal neurologic deficits or visual deficits, a diagnostic evaluation is not indicated.

TABLE 89.4 **Pathological Processes That May Present With Headache and Elevated Blood Pressure**

Disease Process	Clinical Features	Diagnostic Criteria
Pre-eclampsia	Elevated blood pressure and proteinuria in the second half of pregnancy	Should be considered in all patients greater than 20 weeks pregnant with blood pressure > 140/90 mm Hg
Posterior reversible encephalopathy syndrome	Risk factors include immunosuppressant medication, chemotherapeutics, and underlying renal disease	Abnormal MRI imaging
Intracranial hemorrhage	Acute onset of focal neurologic deficits	Abnormal neuroimaging

Management

It is uncertain if strategies aimed at lowering the blood pressure acutely will alleviate the headache. We recommend use of antidopaminergic or nonsteroidal agents, with use of antihypertensive agents reserved for patients with evidence of end-organ damage. Blood pressure can be reassessed after the headache has improved. Oral antihypertensive therapy may be prescribed in the ED if timely outpatient follow-up cannot be assured (see Chapter 70).

Disposition

In the absence of objective neurologic symptoms, patients with hypertension and headache do not require admission to the hospital. Elevated blood pressure should be treated on an outpatient basis.

Reversible Cerebral Vasoconstriction Syndrome

Principles

Reversible cerebral vasoconstriction syndrome (RCVS) is a cerebral arteriopathy characterized by segmental areas of vasoconstriction within large- and medium-sized vessels. RCVS causes recurrent thunderclap headache in susceptible patients and may cause ischemic or hemorrhagic stroke. The prevalence of this presumably rare disorder is not known. RCVS is being reported with more frequency given the wide availability of noninvasive neurovascular imaging. Some data suggest that this disorder may cause the majority of thunderclap headaches.

Clinical Features

The headache of RCVS is characteristically a thunderclap headache, abrupt in onset, and severe. It is often throbbing and associated with nausea, vomiting, and photophobia. The headache may be provoked by use of vasoactive medications or substances such as recreational sympathomimetics or nasal decongestants.

Differential Diagnoses

The differential diagnoses for thunderclap headache include SAH and other hemorrhagic strokes, CVT, cervical artery dissection, and pituitary apoplexy. Unlike these other pathological diagnoses, RCVS is characterized by recurrent thunderclap headache within a discrete period of time. Thunderclap headache during sexual activity may occur pre- or post-orgasm and is classified as *primary headache associated with sexual activity* after other causes of thunderclap headaches have been excluded. Once that happens, a diagnosis of *primary thunderclap headache* is assigned.

Diagnostic Testing

Patients with the initial presentation of thunderclap headache should have a head CT and LP or neurovascular imaging performed to exclude SAH and other intracranial pathology. Repeat neurovascular imaging, or diagnostic angiography, should be pursued in patients with recurrent thunderclap headache if the diagnosis of RCVS was not confirmed by the initial imaging.

Management

There are no evidence-based treatment options available for RCVS. Goals of treatment include prevention of ischemic and hemorrhagic stroke and elimination of headache. To date, the natural history of this disorder is incompletely understood. Treatment with calcium channel blockers, such as nimodipine 30 to 60 mg PO q4h, has been described and we recommend that it be offered to patients with progressive or refractory symptoms.

Disposition

Patients with thunderclap headache who have received an appropriate diagnostic evaluation with neurovascular imaging in the ED may be discharged home with follow-up within a defined period. An inpatient workup is appropriate for patients with recurrent thunderclap headache, refractory pain, or for those with focal neurologic deficits.

The references for this chapter can be found online at ExpertConsult. com.

90

Delirium and Dementia

Gallane Abraham and Patrick J. Maher

OVERVIEW

Delirium and dementia are syndromes defined through impairment of specific cognitive domains including attention, social cognition, memory, language, perceptual-motor ability, and executive function. Both delirium and dementia affect cognition but in different ways and over different time courses. However, delirium can occur concomitantly in a patient with dementia, making the diagnosis challenging. Other nonspecific terms including *acute confusional state, encephalopathy,* and *organic brain syndrome* have been used to describe a number of abnormal cognitive states with often overlapping symptoms. These terms are frequently used synonymously with *delirium* to reflect an alteration of consciousness from presumptive underlying medical etiology. The *Diagnostic and Statistical Manual of Mental Disorders, Fifth Edition* (DSM-5) classifies these pathologies as *neurocognitive disorders,* although prior editions have used the heading *delirium, dementia, amnestic,* and *other cognitive disorders.*

Delirium is characterized by a fluctuating neurobehavioral disturbance typically progressing over a short period. It is a direct consequence of an acute systemic or central nervous system (CNS) stressor. Dementia, on the other hand, tends to follow a more gradual course, with evolution occurring over months to years. Although patients with dementia may exhibit confusion, unlike delirium, a disturbance in attention is usually absent and other acute medical abnormalities cannot explain the changes in cognition.

The evaluation of patients who present to the emergency department (ED) with a neurobehavioral disturbance is best conducted in accordance with the following basic guidelines:

1. The first step is to establish a safe and supportive environment to facilitate further diagnostic and therapeutic efforts. Verbal de-escalation and nonpharmacological means of treating agitation are preferred, but sedative adjuncts may be employed if needed.
2. The second step is to determine whether this state represents delirium or dementia by obtaining a careful history from the patient, family members, and caregivers. Screening tools for delirium and cognitive assessments for dementia can assist in the diagnosis. Clinical findings may be subtle, and distinguishing between these syndromes can be challenging, especially as acute delirium may be superimposed on chronic dementia.
3. The third step is to rapidly treat the underlying disorder in patients with delirium and to evaluate for causes of reversible dementia.

DELIRIUM

Background

Delirium is an acute or subacute state of cognitive dysfunction caused by an underlying physiologic condition.[1] Several key features are necessary for a diagnosis of delirium (Box 90.1). The hallmark finding in delirium is the disturbance in attention and awareness, manifested as an inability to focus attention and reduced orientation to the environment. Patients with delirium may show changes in several other cognitive domains including memory, language, and perception. Arousal and awareness may be normal or impaired. These disturbances tend to develop during a short time (hours to days), but in certain cases they may last weeks to months despite treatment of the underlying cause. Symptoms often have a fluctuating course over time, in distinction to the progressive changes of dementia. Deficiencies in attention may be manifested by reduced maintenance of attention, increased distractibility, or reductions in task processing speed. Memory impairments can manifest as reduced recall of recent information or repeating oneself in conversation. Either expressive or receptive language may be affected. Perceptual disturbances include hallucinations and delusions. The extent of cognitive derangement may range from mildly disturbed to grossly disorganized. The patient's sleep-wake cycle may be altered or reversed; agitation often is present during the night. The level of psychomotor activity in delirium can be specified as hyperactive, hypoactive, or a mixed level of activity. Hyperactive individuals demonstrate

BOX 90.1   Diagnostic Criteria for Delirium

Four Key Characteristics
- Disturbance in attention and awareness.
- The disturbance develops over a short time period, represents a change from baseline attention and awareness, and tends to fluctuate in severity during the day.
- There are additional disturbances in cognition, such as memory, disorientation, language, visual-spatial ability, or perception.
- The disturbances are not better explained by another preexisting, established, or evolving neurocognitive disorder and do not occur in context of a coma.

Adapted from American Psychiatric Association. *Diagnostic and Statistical Manual of Mental Disorders*, ed 5. Arlington, VA: American Psychiatric Association; 2013.

TABLE 90.1   Risk Factors for Delirium

Advanced age
Male gender
Visual or hearing impairment
Alcohol and drug use
Dementia
Hypertension
Heart failure
Previous delirium
Chronic respiratory disease
Chronic kidney disease
Heart failure
Sedative medications (e.g., benzodiazepines and opioids)
Malnutrition
Depression

emotional lability, agitation, and may refuse care; hypoactive individuals demonstrate sluggishness and lethargy; the mixed type describes either a normal level of psychomotor activity but with disturbance of attention and awareness, or individuals having fluctuations in activity levels. Although hyperactive delirium is the most easily recognizable presentation, hypoactive delirium is the most common form and carries the highest risk of mortality.

Delirium occurs frequently, particularly in older ED patients, and it is associated with increased morbidity and mortality, particularly when unrecognized.[2] Predisposing factors for delirium include comorbid illness, dementia, older age, male gender, medications, neurologic deficits, and psychiatric illness (Table 90.1). Drug intoxication and withdrawal (including ethanol) are the most common cause of delirium in the younger adult population. Within the older population, medication side effects are another common cause of delirium; drugs with anticholinergic properties are often implicated but many drug classes can act as a precipitant. Environmental exposures (e.g., heavy metals, insecticides, cyanide, carbon monoxide), herbal medications, and ingestion of psychoactive botanicals (e.g., nutmeg, foxglove, jimsonweed, psilocybin-containing mushrooms) are yet other causes of delirium to consider.

Delirium can be a prominent feature of any CNS or systemic infection, particularly in the very young, older patients, and immunocompromised patients. Many metabolic disorders put patients at risk for delirium, with hypoglycemia and hypoxia being the most common. Delirium is common in patients with strokes, but isolated delirium without other neurologic abnormality is not a common stroke presentation. CNS vasculitis and paraneoplastic syndromes are additional considerations.

Pathophysiology

At a cellular level, delirium is the result of a widespread alteration in cerebral metabolic activity, with secondary deregulation of neurotransmitter synthesis and metabolism. Both the cerebral cortex and the subcortical structures are affected, producing changes in arousal, alertness, attention, information processing, and the normal sleep-wake cycle.

Although the exact pathophysiologic process is not well understood, multiple neurotransmitters have been implicated in causing delirium.[3,4] Given the phenotypic heterogeneity of delirium, it is likely that a number of various neurophysiologic mechanisms underlie the clinical presentation in different patients. Delirium has classically been associated with a derangement of central cholinergic transmission. Cholinergic deficiency is most pronounced in patients experiencing delirium secondary to anticholinergic drugs. Increased glutamatergic activity and neuroinflammation are seen in hepatic encephalopathy, uremic encephalopathy, sepsis, and alcohol withdrawal. Some of the disturbances that occur in delirium are deficiencies of substrates for oxidative metabolism (e.g., glucose, oxygen); GABA-ergic deficit; imbalance of normal noradrenergic, serotoninergic, dopaminergic, and cholinergic tone; and disturbance of the neuroendocrine axis.

Drugs and exogenous toxins can produce delirium through direct effects on the CNS. Although the limbic system appears to be particularly vulnerable to the effects of drugs, the cerebral hemispheres and the brainstem also can be profoundly affected. Tricyclic antidepressants can cause delirium by cholinergic inhibition; sedative-hypnotics depress activity in the CNS, especially in the limbic system, thalamus, and hypothalamus. Narcotics affect CNS activity primarily by interacting with various opioid receptor sites. Psychedelic drugs may act via agonism at serotonin receptor sites. Phencyclidine (PCP) antagonizes the NMDA receptor and inhibits dopamine reuptake.

Hyperthermia and hypothermia can cause delirium due to changes in the cerebral metabolic rate. Patients suffering from heatstroke may have cerebral edema and degenerative neuronal changes leading to the development of oxidative stress and neuroinflammation. Normalizing the core temperature can reverse these changes. Delirium occurring at temperatures below 40°C is not usually caused solely by increased core temperature, and infection should be considered in cases not meeting the criteria for heatstroke.

Delirium caused by metabolic abnormalities, such as hyponatremia, hypernatremia, hyperosmolarity, hypercapnia, and hyperglycemic disorders, is associated with a variety of metabolic disturbances at the cellular level. Such disturbances may include impairments in energy supplies, changes in resting membrane potentials, in cellular morphology, and in the brain water volume.

Most patients with delirium have reduced cerebral metabolic activity. This reduction in cerebral metabolism is reflected by a slowing of background electrical activity on the electroencephalogram (EEG). Exceptions are hyperthermia, sedative-hypnotic withdrawal, delirium tremens, and certain drug-induced states, in which the cerebral metabolism is either normal or increased. In addition, patients experiencing delirium due to a postictal state or to nonconvulsive status epilepticus can show abnormal epileptiform discharges.

Clinical Features

Delirium can present as the first manifestation of underlying disease. The natural history of a patient's delirium can progress from apathy to marked agitation over hours (see Box 90.1). Nonspecific prodromal symptoms such as anxiety, restlessness, and insomnia may emerge in the hours to days before diagnosis.

Key aspects of cognitive impairment should become evident during a careful history and physical examination. Disturbance in attention is central to the diagnosis of delirium. The patient can be easily distractible or have difficulty remaining focused on a particular topic or interacting with a single person. Disorientation often accompanies the inattention but is not an invariable feature. The patient usually is disoriented with respect to time and occasionally to place; in extreme cases, disorientation to person also may be noted. Delirium, however, may be present in a patient who is completely oriented to person, place, and time. A mental status examination that consists solely of questions that assess orientation will not detect delirium in these instances.

The patient with delirium frequently has some degree of memory impairment, with the greatest impact on short-term memory. Thought processes and speech may be disorganized in patients with previously normal cognition. Disturbance in the sleep-wake cycle often occurs early in the course of delirium. Perceptual disturbances, including poorly formed delusions and hallucinations, are common. Delusions may involve a perception of harmful intent of others. Hallucinations are classically visual, but can also be auditory, tactile, gustatory, or olfactory. In addition, the delirious patient has a reduced capacity to modulate fine emotional expression and may demonstrate extreme emotional lability.

The cognitively impaired patient may provide an unreliable history. Valuable information often can be obtained from family, friends, in-home medical care providers, and paramedics. The baseline premorbid mental condition of the patient in relation to the current presentation should be established early in the examination. Specific inquiry should be made about the patient's current medical problems and previous medical history, including diabetes, hypertension, kidney or liver disease, immune status, and any neurologic or psychiatric problems. A detailed medication history, including the use of prescribed and over-the-counter medications, dietary supplements, and alcohol or other substances, is essential. Information about the home environment, medication bottles belonging to the patient or found near the patient, and the possibility of trauma can help clarify the underlying condition leading to the delirium.

The physical examination should begin with a careful assessment of vital signs. The delirious patient often exhibits autonomic nervous system abnormalities, including elevated or decreased pulse rate, blood pressure, respiratory rate, and temperature. The examination also includes assessment of the head for signs of trauma and the pupils for size, symmetry, and light reflex; evaluation of the neck for nuchal rigidity, bruits, and thyroid enlargement; assessment of the heart and lungs; evaluation of the abdomen for organomegaly and ascites;

and examination of the extremities for cyanosis. The skin should be carefully examined for rashes, petechiae, ecchymosis, splinter hemorrhages, and needle tracks.

The neurologic examination includes assessment of the cranial nerves, motor strength, sensation, reflexes, and presence of abnormal movements (e.g., ophthalmoplegia, tremor, asterixis, myoclonus). The reflexes are assessed for symmetry and presence of hyperreflexia or hyporeflexia. Signs that suggest either a metabolic or a structural neurologic problem are helpful but can be nonspecific. For example, asterixis is a hallmark of hepatic encephalopathy but can also be seen in uremia and hypercapnia. Likewise, focal neurologic signs typically associated with structural CNS lesions also can be present in metabolic abnormalities such as hypoglycemia, hyperglycemia, hepatic encephalopathy, uremia, and hypercalcemia. A specific constellation of physical and neurologic findings may suggest a diagnosis. One such example is the classic triad of Wernicke encephalopathy: ophthalmoplegia, ataxia, and confusion. Other examples would include the classic toxidromes found in the presence of sympathomimetic, anticholinergic, sedative/hypnotic, and opioid medications.

Standardized screening tools can facilitate recognizing delirium and avoid missing the diagnosis. Similar to the diagnostic algorithm in other conditions, a fast, sensitive screen may first be applied before proceeding with a longer, more specific test. The most recent guidelines for geriatric emergency care recommend the Delirium Triage Screen (DTS) followed by the brief Confusion Assessment Method (bCAM).[5] The DTS can be performed in less than one minute and is 98% sensitive for delirium. The bCAM, a modification of the full Confusion Assessment Method (CAM) often used during inpatient evaluations, is 84% sensitive and 96% specific for delirium in older emergency department patients. The bCAM uses four key features in screening for delirium: (1) acute onset and fluctuating course, (2) inattention, (3) disorganized thinking, and (4) altered level of consciousness. For a definitive diagnosis of delirium, the first two features, and one of the last two, must be present (Table 90.2).

In addition to the above recommended tools, there are several other delirium assessments in clinical use, but these instruments lack similar acceptance and utility within the ED setting. The Richmond Agitation-Sedation Scale (RASS) can be performed rapidly but has reduced sensitivity and specificity when used alone.[6] The Mini-Mental State Examination (MMSE) evaluates cognition in multiple domains, but it takes longer to perform and is best used for baseline assessments of dementia, rather than delirium. Other screening tools include the 4A's Test (4AT), the Nursing Delirium Symptom Checklist (Nu-DESC), and 3-Minute Diagnostic Assessment (3D-CAM), among others.[7]

TABLE 90.2 Common Emergency Department Assessments for Delirium and Dementia

Tests for Delirium	Item(S)	Application	Administered By	Time (Minutes)
Delirium Triage Screen (DTS)	2	Clinical, screening	Interviewer	1–2
Brief Confusion Assessment Method (bCAM)	4	Clinical, screening	Interviewer	1–2
TESTS FOR DEMENTIA	ITEM(S)	APPLICATION	ADMINISTERED BY	TIME (MINUTES)
Short Blessed Test (SBT)	6	Screening	Interviewer	5–10
Abbreviated Mental Test (AMT-4)	4	Clinical, screening	Interviewer	1–2
Brief Alzheimer's Screen	5	Clinical, screening	Interviewer	2–5
Clock drawing test	1	Clinical, screening	Patient	3
Mini-Mental State Examination (MMSE)	30	Clinical, screening	Interviewer	5–10

Differential Diagnosis

Considerations in the differential diagnosis for delirium include dementia and psychiatric disorders. Dementia, depression, mania, paranoia, and schizophrenia all may resemble delirium but can be distinguished using historical and clinical features such as onset, time course, fluctuating mental status, and inattention (Table 90.3). Unlike delirium, dementia and psychiatric disorders tend to be insidious processes that develop over months to years. Typically, the patient's vital signs are normal. In addition, cognitive impairment of dementia exhibits little fluctuation during hours or days and occurs primarily in elders. However, patients with dementia are more likely to develop delirium, and as such, the two may often coexist.

Diagnostic Studies

Because delirium results from an underlying medical disorder, a comprehensive evaluation looking for structural, metabolic, and infectious etiologies is indicated (Table 90.4). Despite these diagnostic evaluations, no cause may ultimately be found for many patients. Basic laboratory tests, such as serum electrolytes, have variable diagnostic yield. An elevated anion gap (>15 mEq/L) may indicate the presence of unmeasured anions, such as ketoacids in diabetic or alcoholic ketoacidosis; lactate in postictal states or associated with hypotension; sulfate in renal failure; and exogenous toxins, such as ethylene glycol, methanol, and salicylates.

In addition to a pulse oximetry measurement to screen for hypoxemia, blood gas analysis from an arterial or venous sample is warranted in patients at risk for respiratory failure with hypercarbia. Urinalysis and chest radiography may be obtained to exclude an occult infection, which is the most common cause of delirium in older patients.

An electrocardiogram and troponin may be obtained to assess for an acute coronary syndrome in patients at risk for heart disease, including older patients. Thyroid hormone testing may reveal hypothyroid or hyperthyroid state. Furthermore, additional laboratory studies outside the usual scope of the ED evaluation may be appropriate when the cause of delirium remains unknown or when suggested by the clinical history and exam. These additional studies may include vitamin B_{12} and folic acid assays in cases of possible malnutrition, rapid plasma reagin test to exclude neurosyphilis, measurement of serum antinuclear antibodies if lupus encephalitis is suspected, urinary porphobilinogen assay in acute porphyria, and screens for heavy metals in intentional or accidental ingestions.

Adverse prescription medication effects, including drug-drug interactions, are another common cause of delirium and may occur at therapeutic doses and levels. A comprehensive review of all medications should be performed, with testing for levels when indicated and available. Standard toxicology screens may have limited usefulness in the evaluation of patients with delirium, since both false-positive and false-negative results may occur, and early diagnostic closure based on these tests may result in an incorrect diagnosis.

Neuroimaging with a head computed tomography (CT) scan should be performed on patients with a history or signs of trauma (especially those taking anticoagulant medications), recent neurosurgical procedures or with implanted devices (e.g., cerebrospinal fluid shunt), or focal neurologic signs to detect structural lesions causing delirium. Advanced imaging may be indicated if there is suspicion for

TABLE 90.3 Comparison of Delirium and Dementia

	DELIRIUM	DEMENTIA
Onset	Acute	Gradual
Attention	Impaired	Normal
Level of consciousness	Fluctuates	Normal
Orientation	Variable	Impaired
Memory	Often impaired	Impaired
Hallucinations	Present	Usually absent
Language	Slowed, aphasia	Word finding difficulty

TABLE 90.4 Delirium Diagnostic Studies and Clinical Findings

Diagnostic Studies	Examples of Delirium Precipitants
Vital signs	Hypoxemia, hypotension/hypertension, hypothermia/hyperthermia, pain, fever
Fingerstick glucose	Hypoglycemia/hyperglycemia
Blood gas	Hypoxemia, hypercarbia, respiratory alkalosis, metabolic acidosis
CBC: Hemoglobin, leukocyte count with differential, platelet count, mean corpuscle volume	Anemia, occult infection, thrombocytopenic purpura, megaloblastic anemia, hyperviscosity from myelogenous leukemia, polycythemia
Serum electrolytes: Glucose, sodium, calcium, chloride, bicarbonate, BUN, creatinine, magnesium, phosphate, osmolality	Hypoglycemia/hyperglycemia, hyponatremia/hypernatremia, uremia, hypo-osmolar/hyperosmolar, anion gap acidosis
Urinalysis: Nitrites, leukocytes, ketones	Occult infection, proteinuria
Chest x-ray	Occult infection, pneumothorax
Drug levels	Digoxin, lithium, quinidine, salicylate, antiepileptics
Additional tests: Troponin, liver and thyroid function studies, ammonia, PT, PTT, INR, vitamin B_{12} and folic acid assays, rapid plasma reagin test, measurement of serum antinuclear antibodies, urinary porphobilinogen assay, screens for heavy metals, toxic screens of blood and urine, methanol, ethylene glycol, carbon monoxide, cyanide	Myocardial infarction, liver failure, hypothyroid/hyperthyroid, bleeding disorder, excess anticoagulation, vitamin B_{12} or folate deficiency, occult infections, vasculitis, acute porphyria, toxins
CT Head/MRI	Cerebrovascular accident, structural lesions, traumatic head injury
LP/CSF analysis	Meningitis, encephalitis, subarachnoid hemorrhage
EEG	Nonconvulsive status epilepticus, delirium

BUN, Blood urea nitrogen; *CBC*, complete blood count; *CSF*, cerebrospinal fluid; *CT*, computed tomography; *EEG*, electroencephalogram; *INR*, international normalized ratio; *LP*, lumbar puncture; *MRI*, magnetic resonance imaging; *PT*, prothrombin time; *PTT*, partial thromboplastin time.

early infarctions, small brainstem lesions, closed head injuries, sagittal venous sinus thrombosis, or small isodense subdural hematomas that may be missed on a CT scan. In addition, a small percentage of acute subarachnoid hemorrhages are not detected by head CT scan and require LP for diagnosis.

The role of magnetic resonance imaging (MRI) in the evaluation of the delirious patient has not been clearly established. MRI is superior to CT for detection of small intracerebral and brainstem lesions, small brain contusions, certain infectious and inflammatory encephalitides, and abnormalities of white matter (e.g., leukoencephalopathy). The posterior reversible encephalopathy syndrome (PRES) can present with confusion, visual changes, and headache in the setting of malignant hypertension, with MRI abnormalities often, but not exclusively, in the posterior cerebrum.

Cerebrospinal fluid (CSF) analysis is an essential part of the evaluation in selected patients with delirium. In patients with fever and cognitive dysfunction, a LP should be considered to rule out infectious, inflammatory or neoplastic etiologies particularly in cases of new headache, meningismus, seizures, community-living adults, recent neurosurgery, or when other testing has failed to identify an infectious source. This test is particularly important in children under age 5, older adults over age 65, and immunocompromised patients, who are less likely to show classic signs of meningitis. Patients with focal neurologic deficits, immunocompromised states, or evidence of increased intracranial pressure should undergo head CT before LP. Antibiotic therapy should not be delayed for the results of LP testing.

Although it is rarely practical in the ED setting, the EEG can be a valuable tool for ruling out nonconvulsive status epilepticus (NCSE) in the presence of delirium. Typical EEG findings in delirium from metabolic causes include nonspecific generalized slowing without epileptiform discharges. In critically ill inpatients with no alternative explanation for decreased level of consciousness, observational studies have shown up to one-third of patients had NCSE on EEG. This condition, even when diagnosed promptly, may be associated with poor patient outcomes in acutely ill patients when mental status abnormalities fail to resolve.

Management

Delirium is a medical emergency. The outcome depends on the cause, the patient's overall health status, and the timeliness of treatment. The hypoactive form of delirium tends to be more common in older adults and carries a worse overall prognosis, perhaps because it often goes unrecognized. Acute recognition and management of delirium in older patients is essential because delirium in this population is associated with increased risk of long-term institutionalization, development of dementia, and increased overall mortality.[2,8]

After recognition of delirium, patients should be screened quickly for readily treatable causes, such as hypoglycemia, hyperglycemia, hypoxia, hypercarbia, and opioid overdose. Acute intoxication due to medications or illicit substances requires prompt attention, and antidotes provided when available.

Initial management of agitation in hyperactive delirium should be accomplished with nonpharmacologic interventions such as verbal reassurance, assistance from family caregivers when present, and calming environment. When nonpharmacologic measures fail, or in the setting of immediate threat to the patient or staff, sedative medications may be administered through an intravenous or intramuscular route to prevent unsafe behavior and facilitate rapid clinical assessment and management.

Supportive care for all patients with delirium ideally includes an environment with adequate lighting and minimization of sensory overload; the patient should be placed in an area that can be easily observed

by staff, and use of stretcher side rails to prevent falls. Use of "sitters" may be necessary to provide continuous supervision on a 1:1 or 1:2 basis with the patient. The patient must be protected from self-harm or from injuring other patients or staff. In cases of hyperactive delirium, the patient may need to be initially physically restrained until pharmacologic control takes effect. Physical restraints should be viewed only as a temporizing action because they can increase agitation and the risk of injury to the patient. Death in restraint is a recognized phenomenon, occurring more frequently in patients restrained in nonsupine positions and with agitated delirium.

Following the initial evaluation, care should be directed towards conditions requiring immediate medical intervention. Patients with signs of acute meningitis or sepsis should rapidly receive antibiotics along with appropriate fluid resuscitation. Other conditions that may manifest as delirium and necessitate immediate intervention include severe hypothermia, hyperthermia, and CNS vascular conditions, including hypertensive encephalopathy, acute epidural or subdural hematoma, subarachnoid hemorrhage, and stroke. Patients with Wernicke encephalopathy require immediate treatment with 200 to 500 mg of intravenous (IV) thiamine, with titration of additional doses until the ophthalmoplegia resolves. Traditionally, glucose administration in patients with severe thiamine deficiency was deferred given concern for precipitating Wernicke encephalopathy, but evidence for this phenomenon occurring is poor.

The specific treatment of delirium tremens (and other alcohol withdrawal syndromes) involves the substitution of a long-acting drug that is cross-tolerant with the alcohol. Benzodiazepines are the agents of choice in treatment of delirium due to sedative withdrawal, but caution should be used with these medications in other conditions because they may worsen delirium severity. Treatment for delirium secondary to dehydration or electrolyte abnormality begins in the ED, but care is needed to prevent overcorrection in patients with sodium abnormalities because this can lead to permanent neurologic damage. In patients with hepatic or renal disease, inpatient treatment with medications for hepatic encephalopathy or dialysis for renal disease may be required before disturbances in cognition resolve.

Pharmacologic interventions are a cornerstone of behavioral management while the underlying medical condition that caused the delirium is being addressed. Antipsychotics and benzodiazepines have been used in the management of acute agitation in the undifferentiated patient with delirium (Table 90.5); opioids have no role.

Antipsychotic medications used to treat delirium include the typical antipsychotics, especially the butyrophenones including haloperidol and droperidol, and the newer atypical antipsychotic agents. Evidence for the superiority of any individual agent is limited, and no one drug is ideal for treatment of all cases. The typical antipsychotic, haloperidol, a potent dopamine-blocking medication with minimal anticholinergic and vasodilatory side effects, is recommended as monotherapy for controlling agitation in acute delirium on the basis of extensive clinical experience and best evidence base.[9] The main acute response to the drug is tranquilization. The incidence of extrapyramidal side effects in patients receiving IV haloperidol for management of delirium with agitation is relatively low, generally less than 10% of patients.

As with all the antipsychotics, haloperidol can prolong the QTc interval, more so when given intravenously, but this effect is clinically insignificant in most patients and does not require a pretreatment electrocardiogram. Caution is warranted with use of this agent in patients taking medications that prolong the QTc and in patients with acute coronary ischemia, uncompensated congestive heart failure, or hepatic dysfunction. Another agent in this class, droperidol, received a "black-box" warning from the US Food and Drug Administration (FDA) in 2001 for concerns of QTc prolongation. Although an effective therapy

TABLE 90.5   Medications for Agitation

Etiology	Agent	Dose	Notes
Acute undifferentiated agitation	Typical antipsychotics		
	• Haloperidol	0.5–1 mg IV or 1–2.5 mg IM	Maximum of 10–20 mg/day. Black-box warning of increased mortality in older patients with dementia-related psychosis.
	• Droperidol	2.5–5 mg IV or 5 mg IM Q30 minutes as needed	Maximum dose of 20 mg/day. Black-box warning for QT prolongation.
Parkinson dementia with agitation; acute undifferentiated agitation	Atypical antipsychotics		
	• Quetiapine	12.5–25 mg PO one to three times daily	Black-box warning of increased mortality in older patients with dementia-related psychosis.
	• Olanzapine	2.5–5 mg IM or IV every 2–4 hours	Maximum of 30 mg/day based on patient toleration. Black-box warning of increased mortality in older patients with dementia-related psychosis.
Agitation from acute intoxication or withdrawal syndromes; acute undifferentiated agitation	Benzodiazepines		
	• Lorazepam	0.5–1 mg IM or IV every 4–6 hours as needed	Maximum 4 mg per episode. Has additive CNS depressant effects with other medications.
	• Midazolam	2.5–5 mg IV or IM every 15 minutes as needed	Maximum 10 mg per episode. Has additive CNS depressant effects with other medications.

for agitation in many patients, this warning led to a reduction in the use of droperidol and research into its effects in comparison to other agents. Large observational studies of droperidol use in the emergency department have not supported this concern and we consider droperidol a viable option in the management of acute agitation.[10]

Dosing of haloperidol should be adjusted for the patient's level of agitation, age, weight, and response to treatment. In most patients, 2.5 to 5 mg intramuscularly or intravenously (adjusted according to weight and comorbidities) is well tolerated as an initial dose, and levels can be titrated as needed. For older patients, a lower initial dose of 0.5 to 1 mg is recommended. In highly agitated patients, combination therapy with haloperidol and lorazepam, 0.5 to 2 mg IV or IM, may be more effective than monotherapy with haloperidol. Combinations of sedatives with anticholinergics, such as diphenhydramine, is discouraged, given the likelihood of prolonging the delirium state.

The newer atypical antipsychotic agents (risperidone, olanzapine, ziprasidone, aripiprazole) may have similar efficacy but different side effect profiles, which may be desirable in some cases of acute agitation. The mechanism of action includes antagonism of alpha$_1$-adrenergic, serotonin, dopamine, and histamine receptors. These drugs can also block the reuptake of dopamine and serotonin. Olanzapine, since it has both IV and IM formulations, has received support in the literature as being a safe and effective treatment for acute agitation in the ED, with reduced need for additional sedation in comparison to haloperidol.[11-13] Because of the limited dopamine antagonism effect, atypical antipsychotics are preferred over haloperidol for patients with Parkinsonism and agitation, although benzodiazepines may be a better choice in this population given concerns about increased mortality with the use of atypical antipsychotics in Parkinson disease.[14]

Benzodiazepines are another means to effectively sedate patients with acute undifferentiated agitation, but they are especially useful in cases of substance intoxication or withdrawal syndromes. Lorazepam, with onset of sedation within 2 to 3 minutes, is the preferred agent for treatment of withdrawal symptoms. Midazolam has a similar onset of action to lorazepam, but shorter duration of effect, and may be preferable in some cases. Diazepam should be avoided as an agent for treatment of agitated behavior in most delirious patients because of its long half-life and risk of drug accumulation with repeated dosing. Both midazolam and diazepam have prolonged half-lives in hepatic and renal impairment.

The management of acute behavior change in elderly patients in the emergency department has been identified by national groups as an area requiring further research.[15] Based on the best available evidence, we recommend screening and treatment of readily reversible causes of delirium and initial nonpharmacologic management followed by a selection of pharmacologic agents based upon the etiology of delirium and patient comorbidities.[2] We recommend an antipsychotic (typical or atypical) be used as monotherapy for undifferentiated patients with agitated delirium, or benzodiazepines for patients suspected of having substance intoxication or withdrawal who require sedation. As an alternative, a combination of a low-dose antipsychotic plus benzodiazepine (e.g., haloperidol 5 mg plus lorazepam 2 mg IM) can be used in combative patients with immediate safety threats. The combination approach has been found to be superior to monotherapy in the control of undifferentiated acute agitation.[11,16]

Disposition

Patients with delirium secondary to acute drug intoxication may be discharged from the ED provided the process resolves during a short period of observation and the drug has no potentially serious delayed toxicity. For most patients with delirium from metabolic, infectious, or CNS processes, hospitalization is necessary for further diagnostic evaluation and treatment. The only readily reversible metabolic problem associated with delirium that can be completely managed in the ED is hypoglycemia.

For most patients with treatable medical illness who have delirium, the outcome is full recovery. Time for return to baseline function can be prolonged, particularly in older patients. In some patients, a persistent decline in their baseline level of functioning may occur despite resolution of the acute cognitive dysfunction. Delirium in older adults hospitalized without baseline dementia is associated with higher 1-year mortality rates, higher rates of institutionalization, and a greater risk for development of dementia. These long-term consequences can occur despite optimal supportive multidisciplinary care.

DEMENTIA

Principles

Background

Dementia is a gradual progressive cognitive decline in complex attention, executive function, learning and memory, language, perceptual motor function or social cognition that interferes with daily function and independence. Dementia may be a primary progressive irreversible neurodegenerative disease, a secondary potentially reversible non-neurodegenerative disease or a mixed dementia arising from multiple etiologies. The predominant dementia is Alzheimer dementia representing 60% to 80% of all cases; vascular dementia represents 20% of all cases, and dementia from multiple etiologies represents 20%.

Dementia is not a single disease entity but rather a highly variable clinical syndrome characterized by the gradual progressive deterioration of cognitive function. Prognosis depends on the underlying cause (Box 90.2). Dementia onset may be categorized as "presenile" when arising before age 65, or "senile" dementia otherwise. Severity is classified according to the degree of cognitive impairment. Mild dementia implies some impairment of work and social activities; however, the capacity for independent living remains intact. With moderate dementia, independent living is hazardous, and some degree of supervision is necessary. With severe dementia, continual supervision and often custodial care are needed.

Primary neurodegenerative dementias include Alzheimer disease, dementia with Lewy bodies, subcortical dementias involving the basal ganglia and thalamus (e.g., progressive supranuclear palsy, Huntington chorea, Parkinson disease), and dementia of the frontal lobe type, which includes Pick disease. Dementia with Lewy bodies, clinically manifested by persistent, well-formed visual hallucinations and prominent extrapyramidal movements, has been found to be the third most common type of dementia. With advanced aging, dementia may have mixed causes, with Alzheimer disease and vascular dementia frequently coexisting. A smaller percentage of dementias are attributable to causes such as anoxic encephalopathy, hepatolenticular degeneration, tumors, alcohol abuse, and slow virus infections.

Potentially reversible secondary non-neurodegenerative dementias are caused by adverse drug reactions, endocrinopathies, metabolic abnormalities, intracranial processes, and depression. The disorder may manifest clinically as acute or gradual progressive cognitive impairment that reverses once the underlying etiology is addressed and resolved. Drug-induced dementia occurs primarily in older adults and can be caused by various psychotropic drugs, antihypertensive medications, anticonvulsants, anticholinergics, and miscellaneous medications, such as L-dopa.[17] Dementia also may be caused by heavy

---

BOX 90.2   Causes of Dementia

Primary Degenerative Dementias
Alzheimer disease
Lewy bodies disease
Frontal lobe disease (Pick disease)

Subcortical Dementias
Parkinson disease
Huntington disease

Vascular Dementia
Multi-infarct dementia

Intracranial Processes
Space occupying lesions (tumor, subdural hematoma)
Hydrocephalus
CNS infections (i.e., HIV-1, neurosyphilis, chronic meningitis, encephalitis secondary to measles, John Cunningham (JC) virus, rubella, *Candida albicans*, Creutzfeldt-Jakob disease (CJD), and variant CJD subacute spongiform viral encephalopathies, or slow virus infections)
Repetitive head trauma

Endocrinopathies
Addison and Cushing diseases
Thyroid and parathyroid disease

Nutritional Deficiencies
Thiamine
Niacin
Folate
Vitamin B_{12}

Toxic Exposures
Heavy metals
Carbon monoxide
Carbon disulfide

Drugs
Psychotropics
Antihypertensives
Anticonvulsants
Anticholinergics

Depression
Pseudodementia

Adapted from American Psychiatric Association. *Diagnostic and Statistical Manual of Mental Disorders*, ed 5. Arlington, VA: American Psychiatric Association; 2013.

---

metals and other exogenous agents, such as carbon monoxide, carbon disulfide, and trichloroethylene.

Endocrinopathies and metabolic abnormalities that can cause secondary and potentially reversible dementia include hypothyroidism, hyperthyroidism, parathyroid disease, Addison disease, Cushing disease, and panhypopituitarism. Metabolic abnormalities such as nutritional deficiencies that cause dementia include thiamine deficiency (Wernicke syndrome), niacin deficiency (pellagra), vitamin B_{12} deficiency, and folate deficiency.

Intracranial processes, space-occupying lesions, and hydrocephalus may also cause dementia. Repetitive intracranial trauma resulting from contact sports can produce a chronic organic brain syndrome without evidence of hematoma or significant contusion (dementia pugilistica).

BOX 90.3   Diagnostic Criteria for Dementia

A. Cognitive decline from a previous level of performance in one or more cognitive domains: Complex attention, executive function, learning and memory, language, perceptual motor function, or social cognition.

B. The disorder has an insidious onset and gradual progression.

C. The deficits do not occur exclusively during the course of a delirium.

D. The cognitive deficits are not better explained by another mental disorder, such as major depression or schizophrenia.

Adapted from American Psychiatric Association. *Diagnostic and Statistical Manual of Mental Disorders*, ed 5. Arlington, VA: American Psychiatric Association; 2013.

Intracranial processes that may eventually lead to a chronic organic brain syndrome include infections with slow viruses, human immunodeficiency virus type 1 (HIV-1) infection, chronic meningitis (tubercular or fungal), brain abscess, and neurosyphilis. In addition to primary HIV-1 CNS infection, toxoplasmosis, cryptococcal meningitis, malignant disease, and infections due to herpesvirus, cytomegalovirus, varicella-zoster virus, and JC virus (progressive multifocal leukoencephalopathy) can cause progressive cognitive impairment in this compromised group of patients and must be excluded.

Worldwide, approximately 24.3 million persons suffer from dementia, and as the population ages, 4.6 million new cases are diagnosed yearly. The prevalence of dementia is approximately 10% in adults over 65 years old and 50% in adults over 85 years old. The incidence of dementia in the United States is expected to increase as life expectancy continues to increase, but rates may decline as risk factors are controlled in older adults.[18] ED-based studies of cognitive impairment report that up to 70% of older adults seen with cognitive impairment have undiagnosed dementia. Dementia is a strong predictor of mortality, which varies with age and subtype. Older adults with dementia have high rates of ED utilization, with greater numbers of comorbidities and higher rates of admission compared to those without dementia.[19]

DSM-5 criteria for the diagnosis of dementia are presented in Box 90.3. There must be cognitive impairment that interferes with independence in one of six domains: complex attention, executive function, learning and memory, language, perceptual-motor function, or social cognition. Several clinical features deserve emphasis. Impairment in memory must involve both short-term and long-term memory. The cognitive impairment commonly involves abstract thinking, judgment, and other higher cortical functions. The cognitive impairment must interfere with interpersonal relationships, work, and social activities. Although mild decline in intellectual functioning characterized as inability to learn and retain new information without impairment of daily functions can be part of the normal aging process, gross intellectual impairment of short- and long-term memory or confusion is not normal. Mild cognitive impairment is distinct from early dementia.

The goals of ED evaluation for suspected dementia are (1) to recognize the signs and symptoms of undiagnosed and potentially reversible forms of dementia, (2) to identify the manifestations of acute illness in the demented patient promptly, and (3) to assess the clinical findings in lieu of the patient's cognitive impairment and facilitate a safe disposition and expedited follow-up.

Pathophysiology

Alzheimer disease is the best-understood dementia and involves several characteristic anatomic, pathologic, and neurochemical changes. The predominant change is cortical atrophy most prominent in the temporal and hippocampal regions caused by progressive synaptic and neuronal loss in the cerebral gray matter. This atrophy generally is followed by loss of white matter (subcortical atrophy). The degree of neuronal loss correlates with symptomatic severity of Alzheimer dementia and is typically beyond the amount expected in normal aging. Not all patients with histopathologic features of Alzheimer disease will have extensive neuronal losses. There is no ischemic component to Alzheimer disease.

Histologic features characteristic of Alzheimer disease include extracellular deposition of β-amyloid protein and intracellular neurofibrillary tangles contributing to neuron loss. The abnormal processing of β-amyloid protein is likely central to the pathogenesis of Alzheimer disease. The neurofibrillary tangles are intraneuronal paired helical filaments composed of the abnormally phosphorylated protein tau, the structural protein involved in the regeneration of neurites. Senile plaques are extracellular lesions composed of the degenerating neuronal processes and abnormal β-amyloid protein. These plaques are extensively spread throughout the cerebral cortex and do not correlate with the severity of dementia. Other consistent neurohistopathologic changes in Alzheimer disease include granulovascular degeneration (membrane-bound bodies within vacuoles of hippocampal pyramidal cells containing small basophilic granules), Hirano bodies (eosinophilic rod-shaped bodies in hippocampal pyramidal cells composed of actin-associated protein aggregates), β-amyloid deposition in the small cortical blood vessels, and neuronal loss in the limbic area.

Many biochemical abnormalities have been described in patients with Alzheimer disease. A decrease in the neurotransmitter acetylcholine is characteristic. Levels of the enzyme choline acetyltransferase, which synthesizes acetylcholine in the brain, can be reduced to 20% of that in age-matched control subjects.

Risk factors for Alzheimer and vascular dementia range from potentially modifiable cardiometabolic and lifestyle factors to genetic factors. The Framingham Cardiovascular Risk Profile (FCRP) and Cardiovascular Risk Factors Aging and Dementia (CAIDE) risk score reflect the common risk factors of high cholesterol, high blood pressure, diabetes.[20] In addition, advancing age, gender, smoking, air pollution, depression, family history, low education level, and head trauma are associated risk factors for the development of cognitive impairment and dementia. The apolipoprotein E epsilon 4 allele on chromosome 19 has been associated with both familial and sporadic late-onset Alzheimer disease. Apolipoprotein E is responsible for transporting of the cholesterol and phospholipids necessary for dendritic and synaptic repair. There are several allelic variants, but those homozygous or heterozygous for the E4 variant have an increased risk for the development and expression of the disease. Abnormalities on chromosomes 1 and 14 also have been associated with Alzheimer disease.

The frontotemporal dementias are less prevalent than Alzheimer disease and are categorized by a frontal and temporal atrophy caused by cell death. The most common histologic finding in the frontotemporal dementias is the combination of prominent cell loss and gliosis in frontal and temporal regions of the cortex, termed *dementia lacking distinctive histology* (DLDH).

Approximately 15% to 20% of dementias are caused by multiple vascular insults to the CNS; the resulting deficit is termed *multi-infarct dementia*. The multiple infarcts typically involve the cerebral hemispheres and basal ganglia. Multi-infarct dementia often has an earlier age at onset than Alzheimer disease and occurs more often in adult men and patients with risk factors for atherosclerosis. Approximately 20% of dementias are mixed combinations of both ischemic cerebrovascular disease and Alzheimer dementia.

Inflammatory conditions of the CNS contribute to the development of dementia and can be caused by conventional viruses or fungal infections including subacute sclerosing panencephalitis from measles virus infection, progressive multifocal leukoencephalopathy from infection by the John Cunningham (JC) virus (a papovavirus), progressive rubella encephalitis, HIV disease, and *Candida albicans*.[20] The unconventional viral infections include kuru, Creutzfeldt-Jakob disease (CJD), and variant CJD (which appears to be linked to bovine spongiform encephalopathy, the pathologic process in "mad cow disease"). The infectious agents in these diseases are virus-like particles known as *prions*. A prion is a proteinaceous infectious particle with the apparent ability to start a chain reaction that changes the shape of benign protein molecules into abnormal, slowly destructive forms. These diseases cause a fine vacuolation of the nervous tissue and hence are referred to as *subacute spongiform viral encephalopathies*. With these diseases, months to years pass between infection and the appearance of clinical illness.

One of the most prevalent slow virus infections causing progressive dementia is HIV-1 infection. HIV may produce a primary neurotrophic disorder in addition to causing the immunologic compromise that permits other viruses to replicate and damage nervous tissue. HIV dementia or acquired immunodeficiency syndrome (AIDS) dementia complex occurs in approximately one-fourth of patients with AIDS. It is believed to be caused by the HIV-1 virus targeting the microglial cells and the macrophages, which may produce cytotoxic substances, such as tumor necrosis factor and interleukins. Pathologic changes occur mostly in the hippocampus and basal ganglia and include atrophy, ventricular dilation, and fibrosis.

Several of the potentially reversible causes of dementia also are associated with neuropathologic or neurochemical abnormalities. Normal-pressure hydrocephalus generally affects younger people; 50% of patients are younger than 60 years. Most of the conditions that cause hydrocephalus involve a defect in uptake of CSF by arachnoid villi, which results in gradual ventricular dilation.

Chronic, heavy ethanol consumption is associated with dementia. The neurotoxicity of ethanol appears to be independent of thiamine deficiency. Heavy chronic alcohol consumption causes cerebral cortical atrophy, but no single alcohol-related dementia syndrome exists.

Clinical Features

Family or friends often bring the patient to the ED because of a sudden worsening in mental status, a change in the patient's activities (e.g., refusal to eat), or a change in the ability of the caregiver to manage the patient. Presentations vary by the cause of the dementia and the stage of progression. Many older adults with dementia have a superimposed delirium on presentation.

The symptoms, signs, and progression of chronic cognitive impairment rarely are so diagnostic as to permit identification of the specific cause of the dementia. Alzheimer disease begins insidiously. Signs and symptoms of cognitive dysfunction may be present for months to years before the diagnosis is made. The earliest symptoms and signs of Alzheimer disease often are vague and nonspecific; patients manifest anxiety, depression, insomnia, frustration, and somatic complaints that often are more prominent than the memory loss. Patients often deny any cognitive deficits and change the subject of the conversation frequently rather than admit their increasing forgetfulness. Physicians often overlook the subtle signs of dementia in this phase of the disease. Family and close informants are often the source of a reliable history of cognitive and functional changes for patients with chronic cognitive impairment. Various tests of cognitive function can be used to improve the detection rate of subtle cases, document a change in level of cognition or assist in determination of competency (see Table 90.2).

Depression often is the initial manifestation of Alzheimer disease and is present in up to 40% of cases. Early in the illness, short-term memory is affected with forgetfulness of recent events, such as appointments and names of new acquaintances. Patients often repeat questions. The memory impairment may cause them to withdraw from social situations and recreational pursuits. Attempts to perform complex tasks may produce anxiety and confusion. The patient often has difficulty with interpersonal relationships. Affect may be shallow and labile, and minor events may trigger inappropriate laughter or tears. Compensation for early deficits includes excessive orderliness and avoidance of situations in which the defects may be observed. Patients in this early phase who are treated with antidepressants with anticholinergic properties may experience worsening of their symptoms. Sedative-hypnotics prescribed for anxiety also may accelerate cognitive dysfunction.

As dementia progresses, cognitive deficits are more obvious and should be readily apparent on a mental status examination. Problems with recent memory, impairment of remote memory, language deficits, and difficulty with spontaneous speech may be noted. With moderate severity of the disease, patients have difficulty naming objects (dysnomia). As many as 50% of patients have delusions, usually of the paranoid type. Atypical presentations of Alzheimer disease include aphasia, visual agnosia, right parietal lobe syndrome, focal neurologic findings, extrapyramidal signs, gait disturbances, and pure memory loss. In the final stage of dementia, patients exhibit marked cognitive impairment, apraxia, and personality changes. They often are bedridden and unable to perform the routine activities of daily living.

Because Pick disease dementia affects the frontal and temporal lobes, patients often have frontal lobe release signs, including dramatic behavioral changes of disinhibition and social inappropriateness. Basal ganglia degenerative disorders that have dementia as a prominent feature are Huntington chorea, Parkinson disease, and Wilson disease. One of several features that distinguish cortical from subcortical dementias is a prominent movement disorder, including posturing, ataxia, tremor, and chorea, that tends to occur early in the illness. Other features of these dementias include slowness of speech, hypotonia, and dysarthria, which can progress to mutism.

Patients with vascular dementia have a stepwise deterioration in memory and cognitive function with each cerebrovascular insult. The clinical presentation may follow one of two scenarios. In the more common scenario, the patient suffers several strokes that involve large volumes of cortical and subcortical structures in both hemispheres. The patient then exhibits dementia along with other neurologic disabilities (e.g., focal weakness, hyper-reflexia, extensor plantar response). In a second group of patients, the presentation is subtle. These patients characteristically are hypertensive and suffer multiple tiny infarcts (lacunae) that involve deep subcortical structures. There may be no focal neurologic residua except progressive dementia with psychomotor retardation. Antihypertensive management in older adults moderately reduces the incidence of dementia and Alzheimer disease for patients with hypertension.[21]

The clinical manifestations of slow virus CNS infections are protean. After an insidious onset of mental deterioration in subacute sclerosing panencephalitis, a rapid progression ensues that is associated with myoclonic jerks, incoordination, and ataxia. In progressive multifocal leukoencephalopathy, neurologic signs and symptoms reflect diffuse asymmetrical involvement of both cerebral hemispheres. Sporadic CJD, of unknown etiology, tends to affect older people, with a rate of disease of one case per million people per year. Among these patients, rapidly evolving dementia with myoclonus is characteristic. The hallmarks of the disorder are mental deterioration, multisystem neurologic signs, myoclonus, and typical electroencephalographic changes that evolve during months. Variant CJD affects younger patients (median age of 24 years) with key features that include early affective symptoms progressing to cognitive impairment and gait disturbances and ultimately leading to progressive neurologic deterioration. The incubation period appears to be in the range of 10 to 15 years, and most patients die within 14 months after the clinical onset of symptoms.

The classic triad of progressive dementia, ataxia, and urinary incontinence occurs in patients with normal-pressure hydrocephalus. Hydrocephalus secondary to previous head trauma or infection carries a more favorable prognosis than that for primary hydrocephalus.

In approximately 20% of reversible cases, dementia is secondary to an intracranial mass. Patients may exhibit focal or nonfocal neurologic signs. Of the reversible dementias, 10% to 15% are caused by medications or chemical intoxications, frequently compounding a history of heavy alcohol use. Older adults have increased susceptibility to the toxicities owing to polypharmacy and age-related changes in metabolism. The clinical presentation of a patient with a drug-related or toxin-related dementia may be indistinguishable from that of a patient with a primary degenerative process.

In addition, chronic traumatic encephalopathy (CTE) is a controversial diagnosis that is proposed to be caused by repetitive mild traumatic brain injuries though well-designed studies have not eliminated confounders that could contribute to the process.[22] It is characterized by progressive neurodegeneration, deposition of hyperphosphorylated tau (p-tau) as neurofibrillary tangles in a distinct pattern and may present as dementia and cognitive impairment. This form of encephalopathy is proposed to develop many years after trauma and progresses to dementia, gait and speech abnormalities, and Parkinsonism. It is unclear if CTE is unique to trauma and its symptomatology overlaps with other types of dementias.

Differential Diagnosis

Senescent Forgetfulness

Subacute or chronic cognitive decline may be caused by a dementing illness or can be a manifestation of senescent forgetfulness, delirium, or depression. Senescent forgetfulness is an almost inevitable reality of aging. Mild impairment of both short-term and long-term memory is usual. Unlike dementia, the cognitive disturbance in senescent forgetfulness does not interfere with work or customary social activity.

Delirium

In most cases, the distinction between delirium and dementia is obvious (see Table 90.3). The onset of symptoms, progression of signs and symptoms, perceptual disturbances, abnormalities on assessment of vital signs, and fluctuations in the level of consciousness are key distinguishing features. However, dementia is a risk factor for delirium, and it is more difficult to differentiate delirium when superimposed on a patient with dementia.

Depression

Depression in older adults may closely mimic dementia. Diagnosis of pseudodementia or depression masquerading as dementia can be difficult and may require therapeutic interventions to confirm the clinical diagnosis. Confounding the issue, depression often coexists with dementia; one study found that 40% of patients with dementia were depressed. Depression, anxiety, and apathy are common in the prodrome and course of Alzheimer disease. Several distinguishing features suggest that the problem is depression rather than dementia. The onset of cognitive changes in pseudodementia often can be pinpointed, and symptoms usually are of short duration before medical help is sought. The progression of symptoms is rapid, and the family usually is aware of the severity of the dysfunction. A history of psychiatric illness is common. Patients with pseudodementia usually complain of cognitive dysfunction and emphasize their failures and disabilities. The affective change often is pervasive, and the patient makes little effort to perform simple tasks. Loss of social skills usually occurs early in the illness, and patients communicate a strong sense of distress and inability to function. Intellectual functioning in pseudodementia often is difficult to

---

BOX 90.4   Elements of the Mental Status Examination in the Evaluation of Dementia

Routinely Observed
Appearance, behavior, and attitude
Mood and affect

Require Inquiry
Sensorium and intelligence: Cognitive impairment
Disorders of thought: Suicidal and homicidal ideation
Insight and judgment: Knowledge about illness
Disorder of perception: Hallucinations and delusions

---

assess because of lack of patient cooperation or inconsistent findings on neuropsychometric testing. Attention and concentration often are intact, but patients commonly give answers such as "I don't know" on tests of orientation, concentration, and memory. Memory losses for recent and remote events usually are equally severe, and variability in the performance of tasks with similar degrees of difficulty may be marked. Tasks of high capacity (e.g., testing of delayed memory with distraction) may be helpful in identifying the depressed patient.

Diagnostic Testing

The evaluation of the patient with suspected dementia includes a focused medical, psychiatric, and medication history plus a collateral history from family and friends. Physical examination should include a detailed neurologic examination with a mental status evaluation. Dementia often goes unrecognized in the patient who is alert, pleasant, and cooperative. A validated cognitive evaluation test can play a key role in the early identification of dementia in patients who have maintained social and conversational ability.

Cognitive Evaluation

A mental status examination should be performed in all patients suspected to have cognitive dysfunction. In the demented patient, mental status testing can uncover subtle forms of delirium. Assessment of orientation to person, place, and time are not sensitive enough to establish cognitive dysfunction. A cognitive assessment should include both psychiatric and neurologic components (Box 90.4).

Several standardized tools for rapid cognitive assessment have been successfully applied in the ED and can be performed in 7 to 10 minutes. Mini-mental status exam (MMSE) testing includes assessment of orientation, memory, attention, and concentration; several tests also incorporate assessments of constructional tasks, spatial discrimination, arithmetic ability, and writing. Memory assessment requires testing of the patient's ability to repeat short series of words or numbers (immediate recall), to learn new information (short-term memory), and to retrieve previously stored information (long-term memory). Constructional apraxia is assessed by having the patient perform tasks, such as drawing interlocking geometric figures or clock faces and connecting dots. Dysnomia (inability to name objects correctly) and dysgraphia (impaired writing ability) are two of the most sensitive indicators of delirium superimposed on dementia. Almost all acutely confused patients exhibit writing impairments, including spatial disorganization, misspelling, and tremor. Therefore, if patients screen positive for delirium the standardized tools cannot be used to assess for dementia.

No single bedside cognitive test that can be administered quickly is ideal. There are various tests of cognitive function, some of which have been tested in the ED (see Table 90.2). The MMSE developed by Folstein and colleagues has been validated more than any other test and is regarded as the reference standard for dementia diagnosis in most studies in the ED as well. For hospitalized patients, this test has a sensitivity of 87% and a specificity of 82% for detection of organic brain syndrome. Limitations of the MMSE include copyright protection, meaning that official tests must be ordered individually through its distributor although multiple free versions are available online, concerns about false positives in certain lower socioeconomic groups and non-English speakers, and length of the test in comparison to brief screening tools.

The MMSE consists of a short series of questions that test orientation, registration (memory), attention, calculation, recall, and language scored on a 30-point scale. The time for the test to be administered can be reduced to 5 minutes by elimination of the writing and drawing components with only a modest reduction in sensitivity. The registration section tests both immediate and short-term memory; the recall section also assesses short-term memory. The ability to recall two of three objects has 81% sensitivity and 74% specificity for exclusion of organic brain syndrome. Asking the patient to subtract "serial sevens" backward from 100 assesses attention, concentration, and arithmetic ability. This test is specific but not sensitive for absence of an organic brain syndrome; up to 40% of nondelirious, nondemented people fail to perform the tasks of this test correctly, reflecting limitations due to language ability and education. A total score of 23 or less is considered markedly abnormal and indicates an organic brain syndrome. Generally, patients with mild cognitive impairment have a score of 18 to 26 out of 30, those with moderate impairment have a score of 10 to 18, and those with severe impairment have a score of less than 10.

The most recent Geriatric Emergency Department Guidelines, endorsed by the American College of Emergency Physicians and the American Geriatrics Society, suggest the Short Blessed Test (SBT) for ED Dementia Screening. The SBT is a 6-item screening tool evaluating a combination of orientation, registration, and attention. SBT scores correlate well with full MMSE testing, can be performed in 5 to 10 minutes, and has high diagnostic accuracy. Other tests include the clock drawing test, Montreal Cognitive Assessment (MoCA), Abbreviated Mental Test (AMT-4), and Brief Alzheimer's Screen.[23] The clock drawing test is scored on a 6-point scale from no errors to no reasonable representation of a clock. MoCA testing includes assessment of visuospatial, language (naming), memory, attention, recall, and orientation domains of cognition, for a total of thirty possible points. Both the AMT-4 and Brief Alzheimer's Screens are shorter mental status exams validated in the ED as screening tools to prompt more comprehensive testing. The AMT-4 focuses on memory and orientation, and the Brief Alzheimer's Screen includes a spelling item.

The screening tests provide limited detection of mild cognitive impairment (without dementia) or early dementia. In addition, bedside tests of cognition represent cognitive functioning at only one point in time and can be influenced by the patient's level of education and general intelligence; therefore, further history and testing is recommended to establish the diagnosis in symptomatic patients.

Alzheimer disease is a clinical diagnosis typically made on probability; no routine available laboratory tests have been found to confirm the presence of the disorder. MRI scans, functional scans looking at regional blood flow or glucose metabolism, assays for specific biomarkers, and CSF analysis can increase the probability of the presence of the disease. The physical examination is rarely helpful in detecting treatable dementias because of the considerable clinical overlap with irreversible dementias.

Laboratory Tests and Imaging Studies

Data clearly supporting or refuting the ordering of "routine" laboratory studies for evaluation of dementia are lacking; however, several studies are recommended to exclude treatable causes (see Box 90.2). For symptomatic ED patients with suspected undiagnosed dementia, a baseline laboratory evaluation, including CBC, comprehensive metabolic panel, and urinalysis, is recommended. If neurosyphilis is clinically suspected based on risk factors such as HIV co-infection or possible sexual exposure, a serum fluorescent treponemal antibody absorption test should be performed in addition to a Venereal Disease Research Laboratory (VDRL) test because the serum VDRL assay may yield negative results in patients with tertiary syphilis. Rapid Plasma Reagin (RPR) accuracy may be inferior compared to the VDRL for neurosyphilis. The radiologic evaluation may include a non–contrast-enhanced head CT scan. The CT scan is used to diagnose or to exclude the presence of hydrocephalus or space-occupying lesions, and CT findings may support a vascular etiology.

Patients may require additional laboratory tests on follow-up evaluation; such tests may include determination of serum vitamin B_{12} and folate levels, thyroid function studies, erythrocyte sedimentation rate, fluorescent antinuclear antibody assay, measurement of urine corticosteroid levels, and, if indicated by history, urine screens for drugs and heavy metals. Selected patients, particularly those younger than 60 years of age, those with rapidly progressive symptoms or patients in whom confirmatory biomarker testing is desirable, should undergo a LP with CSF analysis. Neuroimaging with head CT or MRI is controversial but indicated in patients with acute onset or rapid deterioration of cognitive impairment to identify rapidly progressive dementia and cerebrovascular accidents. An MRI finding of medial temporal atrophy suggests Alzheimer disease but is not specific or sensitive for diagnosis of this disorder. Confirmatory options in certain patients, most typically performed in outpatients being evaluated for Alzheimer disease, would include formal neuropsychological testing, testing of visual evoked potentials, brainstem auditory evoked potentials, and somatosensory evoked potentials. The EEG rarely is helpful in establishing the diagnosis of senile dementia, although in CJD characteristic slowing and periodic complexes may be electroencephalographic features.

Management

Initial management focus is on accurate diagnosis, symptomatic treatment of behavioral and sleep changes, nonpharmacologic environmental and safety interventions, management of chronic comorbid medical conditions, and specific pharmacologic therapies. Accurate and rapid identification of reversible dementias and conditions that cause worsening of baseline dementia require early diagnosis and disease-specific management. Determination of reversible causes of dementia during the ED evaluation occasionally is possible based on the history (including medication history), physical examination, and head CT scan. Patients with acute changes in mental status or a relatively rapid onset of symptoms will require hospitalization for comprehensive evaluation. Patients presenting with recent gradual decline in cognitive function without an underlying acute medical condition may undergo further evaluation and management on an outpatient basis.

Pharmacotherapy approved by the FDA for the treatment of mild to moderate Alzheimer disease includes the cholinesterase inhibitors donepezil (Aricept), rivastigmine (Exelon), and galantamine (Razadyne). There are multiple randomized, placebo-controlled, large-scale clinical trials with these drugs establishing efficacy in improving cognitive functions and activities of daily living in patients with mild to moderate dementia. These drugs are not considered disease modifying, and there are limited data at present on the benefit of these drugs beyond 2 or 3 years (a significant number of patients discontinue medications because of side effects). The most common side effect of these agents is due to the cholinergic effects, including nausea, vomiting, and diarrhea.

Memantine (Namenda) is a disease-modifying agent that helps regulate the excitatory effects of glutamate by antagonizing the *N*-methyl-D-aspartate receptor. Whether this drug alters the underlying disease process is unclear, but short-term studies show improved cognition in patients with moderate and moderate to severe Alzheimer disease. There are conflicting studies on the effectiveness of other agents, such as gingko biloba, vitamin E, nonsteroidal agents, and statins. Estrogen replacement is not indicated for cognitive improvement or maintenance in women with Alzheimer disease and can be detrimental. Ultimately, the key to altering the course of the disease is halting neuron loss. In severe dementia, the goal of management is supportive care, and we recommend that initiation and maintenance of medical therapy be conducted by a patient's primary clinician or by a specialized clinic with a focus on dementia treatment.

Many therapies currently are under investigation for the modulation and early treatment of Alzheimer disease. These therapies include antibiotics (directed against *Chlamydophila pneumoniae*), secretase modulators to reduce serum β-amyloid levels, immunization to reduce amyloid plaque burden, chelators to promote dissolution of β-amyloid, nonsteroidal antiinflammatory medications, supplementation with omega-3 fatty acids, and testosterone. In addition, aerobic exercise, diet, cardiovascular and metabolic risk factor modification are recommended.

Increasing evidence suggests that certain nonpharmacologic measures, including behavioral methods and avoidance of environmental triggers, may be effective in reducing agitation and anxiety in patients with dementia. On occasion, medications are needed for behavioral symptoms of dementia. Affected patients typically do not improve with anxiolytics. Adverse effects offset the modest advantages in the efficacy of antipsychotic drugs for the treatment of psychosis, aggression, or agitation in many patients with Alzheimer disease, and these drugs should be avoided when possible. However, despite the lack of consensus in the indication for use and dosages in older demented patients, butyrophenones (such as, haloperidol, 1 to 2.5 mg IM) or atypical antipsychotic olanzapine (2.5 to 5 mg IM) have been found to be effective in the management of acute agitation.

Clozapine may be effective in treating psychosis associated with both Alzheimer- and Parkinson-type dementias. However, the FDA issued a black-box warning that the use of atypical antipsychotics to treat older patients with dementia-related psychosis was associated with an increased risk for death due to cardiovascular and infectious causes compared with placebo, thus the risks and benefits of using these drugs must be considered as part of a unified treatment strategy with the patient's outpatient clinicians, with the above shorter-acting agents used for acute agitation in the ED.

A clear treatment choice for agitation and psychosis in those with dementia has not been identified. The antipsychotics raise a concern for QT prolongation, extrapyramidal symptoms, sedation, and anticholinergic and drug-drug interaction; the benzodiazepines have a risk of falls, confusion, memory impairment, and oversedation. Regardless of intervention used, the lowest dose possible should be used and then titrated carefully to effect.

Agitation in patients with dementia may occasionally be due to unrecognized pain, depression or sleep disturbances. A trial of adequate pain management or selective serotonin reuptake inhibitors (SSRIs) (such as citalopram 20 mg PO) may be warranted. Selection of a SSRI should be based upon side effect profile and drug interactions, and the medication should be initiated only with a plan for follow-up assessments by a clinician capable of monitoring its effect. Sleep disturbances may be treated with temazepam (7.5 mg oral), though the half-life of temazepam is 8 to 10 hours, potentially placing patients at an increased risk for falls.

Disposition

Patients with dementia present to the ED because of an acute deterioration, behavioral change, or crisis due to family stress. A brief observation, acute inpatient medical or psychiatric hospitalization, nursing home stay, or other institutional stay (respite program) may stabilize the patient and give the family time to mobilize resources to resume the home care regimen. Social workers can play a vital role in attempting to facilitate continued management. A key to successful disposition planning is to use screening tools to assess the cognitive, functional, and psychosocial status of patients with delirium and dementia. Anticipating and addressing cognitive or functional barriers to compliance with discharge and transitional care planning is essential.

The references for this chapter can be found online at ExpertConsult.com.

91

Brain and Cranial Nerve Disorders

Joshua Wallenstein

KEY CONCEPTS

Multiple Sclerosis
- The clinical picture of multiple sclerosis (MS); is one of marked heterogeneity. The classic clinical syndrome consists of recurring episodes of neurologic symptoms that rapidly evolve over days and slowly resolve over weeks.
- Magnetic resonance imaging (MRI) is a high-yield diagnostic test for MS. When the emergency department (ED) MRI is an option, it should be considered as it may expedite follow up and initiation of treatment.
- MS relapse is treated with high-dose methylprednisolone, typically 1000 mg IV over a course of 3 to 5 days. There is emerging evidence supporting oral therapy as efficacious in the treatment of relapse.

Cerebral Venous Thrombosis
- Cerebral venous thrombosis (CVT) should be suspected in patients (particularly female patients under age 50) presenting with stroke symptoms without risk factors, unexplained new seizures or refractory headaches, or signs of intracranial hypertension.
- The combination of MRI and magnetic resonance venography (MRV) is considered the gold-standard for diagnosis of CVT, though contrast-enhanced computed tomography (CT) with venous phase imaging is an alternative.
- Primary treatment of CVT in the ED is anticoagulation with a weak recommendation for low molecular-weight heparin over unfractionated heparin. Neuro-interventional treatment may have a role in severe cases, and hospital transfer may be needed for advanced neurological care.

Trigeminal Neuralgia
- Trigeminal neuralgia (TN) is characterized by intermittent, unilateral, severe and sharp facial pain precipitated by innocuous sensory stimuli and not explained by other local causes.
- Secondary TN can be associated with MS and other cranial nerve disorders and neurologic conditions. A careful history and physical examination can help identify these causes though imaging may be needed.
- Sodium-channel blockers are first line therapy, either carbamazepine (200 to 400 mg/day, titrated up to 1200 mg/day) or oxcarbazepine (300 to 600 mg/day

in two divided doses, titrated up to 1800 mg/day); adverse side effects may lead to treatment failure. While secondary therapies are available, treatment failure with sodium-channel blockers is an indication for surgical referral.

Facial Nerve Paralysis
- The diagnostic dilemma related to facial nerve paralysis typically revolves around distinguishing Bell's palsy from other causes. While diagnostic imaging is not needed to make a diagnosis of Bell's palsy, it may be indicated in cases where the etiology of facial weakness is unclear.
- Patients at high risk for stroke and infection or with features atypical for Bell's palsy (particularly intact forehead movement or bilateral facial paralysis) should be considered for an alternate diagnosis and often require additional diagnostic testing.
- Corticosteroids improve the outcome in Bell's palsy and should be started as soon as possible to maximize their benefit. We recommend 5 days of prednisone, 60 mg, followed by a taper over 5 days.
- Adding antiviral therapy to corticosteroids confers little or no benefit and evidence supporting its use is very weak except in cases of Ramsay Hunt Syndrome.

Vestibular Schwannoma
- Vestibular schwannomas are a common cause of sensorineural hearing loss and may lead to other distressing neurological symptoms. The primary role of the emergency clinicians is referral for testing and treatment when the diagnosis is suspected or confirmed.

Diabetic Cranial Mononeuropathy
- The differential diagnosis for diabetic cranial mononeuropathy includes aneurysm and stroke; a careful history and physical examination can identify cases that require neuroimaging.
- Diabetic patients presenting with a CN III palsy with spared pupillary response and no other deficits in general do not require neuroimaging.

MULTIPLE SCLEROSIS

Foundations

MS is an inflammatory disease of the central nervous system (CNS) manifested by demyelination of discrete regions (plaques) with a relative sparing of axons. An environmental trigger superimposed on genetic susceptibility appears to be a likely etiology. One theory proposes that this trigger establishes autoreactive T cells in the CNS that after a long latency period become reactivated on subsequent exposure to a systemic trigger, such as a viral infection or superantigen. This sets off a complex immunologic cascade that leads to demyelination.

MS presents with highly variable symptoms, making the illness difficult to definitively diagnose on a patient's first presentation. Symptoms evolve over time with a broad range of severity. Women are more commonly affected than men, with a peak age of onset between 25 and 30 years. Management of MS continues to evolve, and early treatment with disease-modifying therapy results in improved outcomes.[1] The emergency clinician will encounter patients with established diagnoses presenting with acute exacerbations (relapse) and undiagnosed patients presenting with initial symptoms. While familiarity with treatment options for managing relapse is necessary, arguably the most important role for the clinician is to recognize symptoms of MS and expedite testing and referral.

TABLE 91.1 Clinical Features of Multiple Sclerosis

Function	Symptoms and Findings
Cranial nerves	Optic neuritis, diplopia, nystagmus, facial paresis, and pain
Motor	Weakness, spasticity, exaggerated deep-tendon reflexes
Sensory	Numbness, tingling, "pins and needles" paresthesia, coldness
Cerebellar	Gait imbalance, dysarthria, truncal ataxia.
Bladder, bowel and sexual dysfunction	Urinary incontinence, constipation, erectile dysfunction.
Cognition	Poor memory, distractibility, cognitive impairment

Clinical Features

The clinical picture in MS is one of marked heterogeneity. The classic clinical syndrome consists of recurring episodes of neurologic symptoms that rapidly evolve over days and slowly resolve over weeks. Variability occurs in age at onset, location of CNS lesions, frequency and severity of relapses, and degree and time course of progression. Four basic disease courses have been identified by the International Advisory Committee on Clinical Trials of MS. (2) The most common form is relapsing and remitting MS (RRMS, 85%), characterized by clearly defined attacks of new or increasing neurologic symptoms that are followed by periods of partial or complete recovery. The less common primary and secondary progressive MS syndromes are characterized by worsening neurologic function and accumulation of disability, either from symptom onset (primary), or after RRMS (secondary). The remaining course, radiologically isolated syndrome (RIS), has been used to classify those with radiographic abnormalities of MS who have no neurological symptoms or findings.

The clinical features of MS are divided into areas of specific CNS impairment and are described in Table 91.1: cranial nerves, motor pathways, sensory pathways, cerebellar pathways, bowel/bladder/sexual dysfunction, and cognition. While MS has no single pathognomonic finding, optic neuritis has a particularly strong association with the disease. Optic neuritis is a unilateral syndrome characterized by pain in the eye and a variable degree of visual loss primarily affecting the central vision. It is the most common cranial nerve dysfunction related to MS, and not infrequently the first presenting symptom for which patients will seek care. It is the initial presentation in about 20% of MS patients. One study found that 65% of patients who presented to an ED with a first episode of optic neuritis were diagnosed with MS within one year.[2] Other common cranial nerve symptoms include diplopia and nystagmus. The nystagmus may be severe enough to cause oscillopsia (a subjective oscillation of objects in the visual field). Cranial nerve impairment may also include impairment of facial sensation, which is relatively common. Unilateral facial paresis also may occur. In addition, the occurrence of trigeminal neuralgia in a young person may be an early sign of MS.

Motor pathways, specifically the corticospinal tract, are commonly involved. Paraparesis or paraplegia occurs with greater frequency than upper extremity lesions owing to the common occurrence of lesions in the motor tracts of the spinal cord. In patients with motor weakness, spasms of the legs and trunk may occur on attempts to stand from a seated position. This dysfunction is manifested on physical examination as spasticity that is typically worse in the legs than in the arms. The deep tendon reflexes are markedly exaggerated, and sustained clonus may be demonstrated. Although these symptoms may be bilateral, they are generally asymmetric. Sensory manifestations are a frequent initial feature of MS and will be present in nearly all patients at some point during the course of the disease. Sensory symptoms are commonly described as numbness, tingling, "pins and needles" paresthesias, coldness, or a sensation of swelling of the limbs or trunk.

Impairment of the cerebellar pathway may result in gait imbalance, difficulty with coordinated actions, and dysarthria. Physical examination reveals the typical features of cerebellar dysfunction, including dysmetria, dysdiadochokinesis (an impairment of rapid alternating movements), breakdown in the ability to perform complex movements, intention tremor in the limbs and head, truncal ataxia, and dysarthria. Impairment of bowel, bladder, and sexual function is also common with patients complaining of constipation, incontinence, and erectile dysfunction. Finally, cognitive impairments in MS are common, and may be underreported by patients, and underrecognized by care providers.

Differential Diagnoses

Given the marked heterogenicity of MS symptoms, the differential diagnosis is vast and includes central and peripheral nervous system disorders, ophthalmologic and neuropsychiatric disorders, and a large number of systemic and inflammatory/autoimmune disorders. Considerations will vary based on presenting symptoms, but may include ischemic and hemorrhagic stroke, CNS infection or malignancy, neuropathy, and rheumatologic conditions such as systemic lupus erythematosus. Several conditions can also present with radiographic features similar to MS. These include CNS tumors, spinal cord compression, vasculitides, Behçet disease, neuro-sarcoidosis, encephalomyelitis, HIV encephalopathy, Lyme disease, and vitamin B_{12} deficiency. The evolution of symptoms over time can be an important diagnostic finding in differentiating symptoms of MS from other conditions.

Diagnostic Testing

Patients previously diagnosed with MS presenting with acute exacerbations should be evaluated for an acute precipitating trigger, though most often one will not be found. The two most high-yield tests for diagnosing MS are a lumbar puncture (LP) and MRI of the brain and spinal cord. CT of the brain, with or without contrast, is not a useful test in evaluating MS but may be used to investigate other potential diagnoses. CSF analysis is abnormal in most cases of MS, but there is no definitive diagnostic biomarker and many of the more specialized CSF tests may not be done within the ED visit. Nevertheless, LP with CSF analysis can be useful in considering other causes of symptoms, and individual CSF proteins have been demonstrated to be biomarkers of disease activity and progression.[3]

The initial imaging test to aid in the diagnosis of MS is gadolinium-enhanced MRI of the brain and spinal cord. MRI is a sensitive test for the detection of lesions consistent with MS and also is useful to assess disease severity. Lesions usually are multiple and commonly are found in the periventricular white matter. Recent studies point to the important role of ED MRI in patients with suspected MS: In one study, concordance between signs of demyelination of ED-based MRI and later final diagnosis of demyelinating disorder was approximately 52%.[4] Given the importance of timely diagnosis and initiation of treatment, emergency clinicians should consider obtaining an MRI when feasible.

Management

Early treatment with disease-modifying therapies can lower relapse rates, reduce disability progression and improve survival. Management of MS in the ED typically entails treating MS relapse. Ongoing therapies, including disease-modifying therapies and management of MS-related complications are best made by a patient's neurologist or primary care physician.

Treatment with high-dose IV corticosteroids diminishes the duration of symptoms and is an accepted best practice to manage MS relapse; however, there is no agreed upon best dosing regimens or durations of therapy. A common treatment regimen is IV methylprednisolone, 500 to 1000 mg daily for 3 to 5 days with or without a tapering dose of oral steroids (whether there is any benefit to divided doses versus a single daily dose is unclear).

There is an emerging body of evidence supporting the use of high-dose oral prednisone alone (typically 500 to 1250 mg daily) in the treatment of MS relapse. A recent meta-analysis failed to demonstrate clear-cut differences in efficacy and safety outcomes between oral and IV strategies.[5] Outpatient oral prednisolone therapy may reduce health system and patient-borne expenses related to IV infusions, hospital stay, and lost work productivity, as well as minimize patient discomfort and improve patient satisfaction. The decision of oral versus IV therapy should ideally be made through shared decision-making and in consultation with the patient's MS specialist. Other potential therapies of acute exacerbation include repository corticotrophin injection, plasmapheresis, and intravenous immunoglobulin.

Disposition

Patients with a history of MS who seek treatment for relapse must first be evaluated to rule out a worrisome acute trigger, and admission may be required for an identified systemic illness, infection, or other acute condition which is thought to have triggered the MS relapse. While patients initiated on IV steroids therapy will generally require admission for continued treatment, initiation and discharge home with high-dose oral prednisolone therapy is safe and effective. In these cases, the clinician should consider safety at home related to any neurologic disability brought on by the relapse, as well as management of pain and other symptoms.

When a new diagnosis of MS is suspected clinically or based on imaging results, further testing and treatment evaluation can often be performed as an outpatient, again assuming adequate mobility, home safety, and symptom control. Current consensus on quality standards for MS patients suggests that patients with new symptoms be referred to a neurologist within 4 weeks if not sooner.[6] While often an achievable goal after ED discharge, hospital admission for advanced diagnostic testing and neurology consultation may be considered, particularly when access-to-care is a concern.

CEREBRAL VENOUS THROMBOSIS

Foundations

Cerebral venous thrombosis (CVT) accounts for 0.5% to 1.0% of all strokes, often occurring in otherwise healthy young adults, though any age can be affected. The mean age at presentation is about 40 years, with the majority of cases (80%) presenting before the age of 50 years. Women are three times more commonly affected than men. Risk factors include thrombophilias (protein C and S deficiencies, factor V Leiden mutation), pregnancy and the post-partum period, oral contraceptives, infections of the head and neck, cancer, chronic inflammatory states, head trauma, and recent lumbar puncture or neurosurgical procedures. At least one risk factor is identified in 85% of patients, and multiple risk factors are found in 50% of patients.

CVT is caused by systemic or local imbalances in thrombotic and thrombolytic pathways, leading to thrombus formation in cerebral

TABLE 91.2 Cavernous Venous Thrombosis Clinical Syndromes

Clinical Syndrome	Features
Intracranial hypertension	Persistent headache, decreased visual acuity, papilledema
Focal neurological deficits	Motor weakness, aphasia
Seizures	Focal, generalized, status epilepticus
Encephalopathy	Altered mental status, coma

dural sinuses or veins. As the flow of venous blood from the brain is impeded, an increase in venous and capillary pressure occurs. Anastomoses of the cerebral venous system can initially compensate for increases in pressure, but when this capacity is overwhelmed a disruption of the blood-barrier occurs, leading to a decrease in cerebral perfusion pressure. This in turn, can lead to cerebral edema, infarction, and hemorrhage.

Clinical Features

There are four major CVT syndromes, which overlap in presentation and are detailed in Table 91.2. The most common, isolated intracranial hypertension, typically presents with headache. Headache from CVT will often be described as localized, persistent or gradually worsening, though it may also be sudden, diffuse and severe, mimicking subarachnoid hemorrhage. Decreased visual acuity and papilledema may also result. Headache may worsen with transient increases in intracranial pressure (coughing, Valsalva). The second and third syndromes, focal neurologic deficits and seizures, are each found in approximately 30% to 40% of CVT cases. Motor weakness (which may be unilateral or bilateral) is the most common focal symptom, and aphasia may also be present. Sensory deficits are possible, though less common. Seizures may be focal or generalized and may present as status epilepticus. CVT should be considered in an at-risk patient presenting with both focal neurologic deficit and seizure. The final syndrome, encephalopathy, may present as altered mental status and confusion. This syndrome is less common and may be seen in more severe cases of thrombosis.

Differential Diagnoses

The differential diagnosis of CVT is vast owing to its highly variable clinical presentations. Depending on the clinical presentation, this may include the broad differential diagnoses of headache, papilledema, motor weakness, seizure, and altered mental status. It is vital to check for risk factors for CVT in considering this often easily overlooked diagnosis. Though only a subset of at-risk patients, women who are pregnant, postpartum, or on oral contraceptives should be considered for further testing when presenting with these symptoms in the absence of an identified cause.

Diagnostic Testing

Routine laboratory testing, including CSF analysis, may be helpful in considering alternative diagnoses of seizure, altered mental status, and other presenting symptoms, but generally have little value in the diagnosis of CVT. Studies evaluating the use of d-dimer in the evaluation of CVT have demonstrated its role; one recent study found that a normal d-dimer had a negative predictive value of 99% and concluded that the test may help guide further diagnostic testing.[7] The authors however noted a need for replication of this single-site study, and did not advocate relying solely on a negative d-dimer as exclusion in at-risk patients.

Imaging is the standard of care when CVT is suspected. The non-contrast head CT may demonstrate an elongated hyper-attenuating clot ("cord sign") but is more likely to show indirect signs of CVT such as sulcal effacement and decreased grey/white matter differentiation, or it may not demonstrate any abnormality. Although this is an appropriate initial test, it is inadequate to rule out CVT. CT venography or MR venography (MRV) are far more sensitive in demonstrating signs of CVT, and MRI in combination with MRV is generally considered the gold standard. Given the young age of many patients with suspected CVT, radiation exposure further supports the choice of MRI/MRV when available. That said, CT venography has a sensitivity and specificity of 75% to 100% depending on anatomic location of the clot, and recent guidelines suggest that CT venography can be used as a reliable alternative to MRV.[8]

Management

Current therapeutic consensus strongly recommends systemic anticoagulation to prevent further clot formation and to promote recanalization, even in patients with intracranial hemorrhage on initial imaging. There is some evidence to support the use of low-molecular-weight heparin (LMWH) over unfractionated heparin (UFH) based on improved outcomes with LMWH and lower hemorrhagic complications when compared to UFH. This recommendation does not apply to patients with contraindication to LMWH or in situations when rapid-reversal (such as surgical intervention) may be desired. The use of new oral anticoagulants such as rivaroxaban and dibigatran after initial heparin therapy has been evaluated, but there is insufficient evidence to support their use, particularly in the acute phase.

There is insufficient evidence to recommend the routine use of acetazolamide or steroids in the treatment of symptoms or signs thought to be related to increased intracranial pressure due to CVT. There is some evidence to recommend the short-term use of antiepileptic drugs in patient with supratentorial lesions who have had seizures as prophylaxis to prevent early recurrent seizures, but no evidence to support their long-term use. Finally, endovascular mechanical thrombectomy (EMT) may have a role in severe or refractory CVT and has been demonstrated to be an effective strategy with a reasonable safety profile.[9]

Disposition

All patients with confirmed or suspected CVT should be admitted to a unit capable of providing a high level of care with neurologic consultation. Considerations for hospital transfer include the need for and availability of neurocritical care with neurosurgical and/or interventional neuroradiology consultation.

CRANIAL NERVE DISORDERS

The cranial nerves are 12 paired nerves that emerge from the brainstem and primarily transmit information to and from structures in the head and neck, including sense organs and muscles controlling facial expression, eye movement, and mastication. Owing to these varied functions, cranial nerve disorders often lead to sense-organ dysfunction, as well as facial pain and motor weakness. Cranial nerve dysfunction can occur through multiple etiologies including compression, infection and inflammation, ischemia, and trauma (including injury resulting from surgery). Given the multiple diverse causes of cranial nerve dysfunction, there is no well-defined at-risk population, though cancer, immunocompromise, and microvascular disease certainly may be relevant risk factors for select patients.

Cranial nerve disorders can present either with sensory dysregulation, motor weakness, or as a mixed disorder. Many of these symptoms can also be related to inflammation of local facial structures as well as systemic infections, leading to a broad differential diagnosis. Table 91.3 describes the normal function and pathologic considerations for each cranial nerve.

Trigeminal Neuralgia (Cranial Nerve V)

Foundations

Trigeminal neuralgia (TN) is an often debilitating illness causing bouts of severe facial pain, often associated with chronic underlying pain. Triggers are usually innocuous sensory stimuli, and attacks can be unpredictable, leading to a marked disruption of normal daily activities. The term *tic douloureux*, often used synonymously with TN, describes the characteristic wince patients may exhibit with a pain paroxysm. TN is slightly more common in women than in men, and most frequently affects individuals over the age of 50 years.

Trigeminal neuralgia is an idiopathic disorder, though evidence points to vascular compression of the trigeminal nerve root in many cases. This compression may be caused by a tortuous arterial or venous loop in the posterior fossa, an arteriovenous malformation, or rarely a tumor.

Clinical Features

TN is defined by three or more attacks of unilateral facial pain occurring in one or more divisions of the TN that have at least three of the following four characteristics: recurring in paroxysmal attacks, severe intensity, electric shock-like or sharp/stabbing in quality, and precipitated by innocuous stimuli to the affected side of the face. The pain is commonly associated with physical triggers such as chewing and swallowing, facial hygiene (brushing, shaving, washing), and exposure to hot or cold temperature. Patients tend to experience the pain in clustered episodes that last a few seconds to several minutes. TN can be subclassified as TN with purely paroxysmal pain or with concomitant persistent pain, which can be seen in up to 50% of affected patients. TN most frequently affects the second and third trigeminal divisions with symptoms occurring slightly more commonly on the right side of the face. Bilateral TN is very rare and should raise suspicion for an alternate or underlying cause. Autonomic symptoms such as tearing and rhinorrhea may also occur during a pain episode.

TN can also be subclassified as idiopathic/classical, or as secondary TN caused by other neurological disease such as MS or cerebellopontine tumor. As such, patients may present with additional neurological symptoms or findings. Although there are no diagnostic physical examination findings of TN, special attention should be paid to alternate possible sources of facial pain, including the teeth, temporomandibular joints, sinuses, and ears. The skin of the face and scalp should be examined for the painful vesicular eruption of zoster. Though pain is not the dominant feature of other cranial nerve disorders, it can be an associated symptom and the cranial nerves should be carefully examined.

Differential Diagnoses

Other painful facial conditions that are considered in patients with facial pain include odontogenic infections, sinus disease, otitis media, acute glaucoma, temporomandibular joint disease, and herpes zoster. Although the temporal components of the pain in these conditions are not similar to the sudden onset, lancinating pain of TN, the distribution is similar and these diagnoses should be considered before anchoring on a diagnosis of trigeminal neuralgia. There is an association between TN and MS, and though not common, TN can be the first presenting symptom of MS, and this diagnosis should be considered in the presence of other unexplained neurologic findings.

TABLE 91.3 Cranial Nerve Function and Pathologies

Cranial Nerve	Clinical Function Relevant to Emergency Medicine	Pathologic Features	Possible Causes
CN I: Olfactory nerve	Sense of smell	Unilateral anosmia	Trauma: Skull fracture or shear injury interrupting olfactory fibers traversing the cribriform plate Tumor: Frontal lobe masses compressing the nerve
CN II: Optic nerve	Vision	Unilateral vision loss	Trauma: Traumatic optic neuropathy Tumor: Orbital compressive lesion Inflammatory: Optic neuritis (MS) Ischemic: Ischemic optic neuropathy
CN III: Oculomotor nerve	Extra oculomotor function via motor fibers to levator palpebrae, superior rectus, medial rectus, inferior rectus, inferior oblique muscles Pupillary constriction via parasympathetic fibers to constrictor pupillae and ciliary muscles	Ptosis caused by loss of levator palpebrae function Eye deviated laterally and down Diplopia Dilated, nonreactive pupil Loss of accommodation	Trauma: Herniation of the temporal lobe through the tentorial opening, causing compression and stretch injury to the nerve Ischemic: Especially in diabetes; microvascular ischemic injury to nerve causes extraocular muscle paralysis but usually is papillary sparing (often painful) Vascular: Intracranial aneurysms may press on the nerve, leading to dysfunction Myasthenia gravis can lead to atraumatic ocular muscle palsy
CN IV: Trochlear nerve	Motor supply to the superior oblique muscle	Inability to move eye downward and laterally Diplopia Patients tilt head toward unaffected eye to overcome inward rotation of affected eye	Trauma is the most common cause of nerve dysfunction
CN V: Trigeminal nerve	Motor supply to muscles of mastication and to tensor tympani Sensory to cornea, face, scalp, oral cavity (including tongue and teeth)	Partial facial anesthesia Episodic, lancinating facial pain associated with benign triggers, such as chewing, brushing teeth, light touch	Trauma: Facial bone fracture may injure one section, leading to area of facial anesthesia Tic douloureux
CN VI: Abducens nerve	Motor supply to the lateral rectus muscle	Inability to move affected eye laterally Diplopia on attempting lateral gaze	Tumor: Lesions in the cerebellopontine angle Any lesion, vascular or otherwise, in the cavernous sinus may compress nerve Elevated ICP: Because of its position and long intracranial length, increased ICP from any cause may lead to injury and dysfunction of the nerve
CN VII: Facial nerve	Motor supply to muscles of facial expression Parasympathetic stimulation of the lacrimal, submandibular, and sublingual glands Sensation to the ear canal and tympanic membrane	Hemifacial paresis: Lower motor neuron lesion leaves entire side of face paralyzed Upper motor neuron lesion leaves forehead musculature functioning Abnormal taste Sensory deficit around ear Intolerance to sudden loud noises	Lower motor neuron: Infection (viral): The likely cause of Bell's palsy Lyme disease: The most common cause of bilateral CN VII palsy in areas where Lyme disease is endemic Bacterial infection extending from otitis media Upper motor neuron: Stroke, tumor
CN VIII: Vestibulocochlear nerve	Hearing and balance	Unilateral hearing loss Tinnitus Vertigo, unsteadiness	Tumor: Acoustic neuroma Mimics Ménière disease, perilymphatic fistula

Continued

TABLE 91.3 Cranial Nerve Function and Pathologies—cont'd.

Cranial Nerve	Clinical Function Relevant to Emergency Medicine	Pathologic Features	Possible Causes
CN IX: Glossopharyngeal nerve	General sensation to posterior third of tongue Taste for posterior third of tongue Motor supply to the stylopharyngeus	Clinical pathology referable to the nerve in isolation is very rare Occasionally painful paroxysms beginning in the throat and radiating down the side of the neck in front of the ear but behind the mandible	Brainstem lesion Glossopharyngeal neuralgia
CN X: Vagus nerve	Motor to striated muscles and muscles of the pharynx, larynx, and tensor (veli) palatini Motor to smooth muscles and glands of the pharynx, larynx, thoracic and abdominal viscera Sensory from larynx, trachea, esophagus, thoracic and abdominal viscera	Unilateral loss of palatal elevation: Patients complain that on drinking liquids, the fluid refluxes through the nose Unilateral vocal cord paralysis: Hoarse voice	Brainstem lesion Injury to the recurrent laryngeal nerve during surgery
CN XI: Spinal accessory nerve	Motor supply to the sternocleidomastoid and trapezius muscles	Downward and lateral rotation of the scapula and shoulder drop	Trauma to the nerve
CN XII: Hypoglossal nerve	Motor supply to the intrinsic and extrinsic muscles of the tongue	Tongue deviations: Upper motor neuron lesion causes the tongue to deviate toward the opposite side Lower motor neuron lesion causes the tongue to deviate toward the side of the lesion, and the affected side atrophies over time	Stroke or tumor can cause upper motor neuron lesion Amyotrophic lateral sclerosis can cause bilateral lower motor neuron lesion with atrophy Metastatic disease to the skull base may involve the nerve

Diagnostic Testing

The diagnosis of TN is primarily based on history and physical as there are no definitive laboratory or imaging tests. Patients with normal findings on the head and neck examination and no neurologic deficits who have episodic, unilateral facial pain associated with nonpainful triggers are likely to have TN. The presence of a neurologic deficit should prompt suspicion of a structural lesion, such as aneurysm or tumor. Patients with a neurologic deficit require urgent imaging studies, typically MRI, to rule out a mass or vascular abnormality. As classical and secondary TN cannot be confidently separated based on history and exam, MRI of the brain and brainstem has been proposed as part of the early workup on TN,[10] though in the absence of a neurologic deficit there is no recommendation for imaging in the ED.

Management

The first-line treatment of TN is sodium channel blockers, either carbamazepine (200 to 400 mg/day, titrated up to 1200 mg/day) or oxcarbazepine (300 to 600 mg/day in two divided doses, titrated up to 1800 mg/day). Generally, sodium channel blockers are effective in most TN patients; however, high dosages are often necessary, leading to frequent adverse side effects including drowsiness, dizziness, tremor, and rash. Treatment failure is typically not due to drug inefficacy, but rather to side effects leading to treatment interruption or dosage reduction to ineffective levels. Oxcarbazepine may be preferred by patients due to its more favorable side effect profile, but its higher cost may put it out of reach for some. An ECG should be obtained prior to initiating therapy as both drugs are contraindicated in patients with atrioventricular block. A complete blood count and liver function studies are performed periodically to monitor for hematologic and hepatic side effects.

Combination treatment can be considered when carbamazepine or oxcarbazepine are not effective alone or not tolerated at higher dosages. Additional agents that have been used to treat TN include phenytoin, baclofen, lamotrigine, gabapentin, and levetiracetam. That said, guidelines recommend surgical consultation as a reasonable next step if sodium channel blockers prove ineffective. Microvascular decompression is the first-choice treatment for many patients, as it provides the longest duration of pain freedom compared to other surgical techniques. While major complications are rare, sensory loss and other mild or transient cranial dysfunction are more common. Stereotactic ("gamma knife") radiosurgery, is minimally invasive but less efficacious with more frequent minor complications.

Disposition

Patients with newly suspected trigeminal neuralgia should be referred for specialty evaluation and possible neuroimaging. In patients with established diagnoses presenting for management of symptoms, consultation with a neurologist can help in therapeutic decision making. Patients with an established diagnosis who present with uncontrolled pain refractory to maximum pharmacologic management may benefit from a neurosurgical referral.

Facial Nerve Paralysis (Cranial Nerve VII)

Foundations

The facial nerve (CN VII) has motor, sensory, and parasympathetic components. It controls facial musculature, sensation to portions of the external auditory meatus and taste to the anterior two-thirds of the tongue. It also controls salivary and lacrimal glands through its parasympathetic pathways. Facial nerve dysfunction can cause facial weakness and asymmetry, abnormalities of taste, as well as dry eyes and dry

TABLE 91.4 Clinical Features Associated With Causes of Facial Nerve Paralysis

Condition	Common Clinical Features
Bell's palsy	Abrupt onset of unilateral facial weakness involving forehead improving over weeks. May include mild to moderate pain, altered taste, hyperacusis, dry eye and mouth
Stroke	Forehead sparing facial weakness, other neurological deficits.
Neoplastic	Insidious onset, minimal improvement over time or recurrent episodes, other cranial neuropathies.
Ramsey-Hunt syndrome	Pronounced pain, vesicular eruptions, vestibulocochlear dysfunction
Lyme disease	Bilateral symptoms, rash, arthralgia, exposure to endemic area
Ear infection	Ear pain, fever, hearing loss

mouth. There are multiple etiologies of facial nerve dysfunction including stroke, compression or disruption from mass lesions and trauma, infection, and others. The most frequent cause of facial nerve paralysis, Bell's palsy, is incompletely understood, though the proposed mechanisms include viral infection and ischemia.

Facial weakness can be caused by lesions of the upper motor neurons in the contralateral motor cortex, or lower motor neurons in the ipsilateral facial nerve. The bilateral innervation of forehead musculature by upper motor neurons leads to a key distinguishing characteristic: upper motor neuron lesions spare the forehead while lower motor neuron lesions typically cause weakness affecting the entire ipsilateral face.

Facial nerve paralysis, while often transient, can be a devastating event for patients causing functional and esthetic issues, particularly when recovery is delayed or incomplete. The underlying etiology may impose additional morbidity and mortality, and there are a variety of etiologies with divergent treatment strategies that may be encountered. A careful history and physical exam (particularly of the face and neurologic system) are the primary diagnostic tools, with imaging indicated in select cases.

Clinical Features

The medical history in patients with facial paralysis focuses on the distribution, onset and timing of the paralysis, concentrating on forehead involvement (involved in peripheral disease and spared in central disease as the result of crossed innervation), rapidity of onset, and associated signs and symptoms. Common clinical features associated with causative conditions are described in Table 91.4.

Bell's palsy is characterized by an abrupt onset of a lower motor neuron paresis that typically develops over 72 hours and can progress over 1 to 7 days to complete paralysis. A prodromal viral-like illness is described by 60% of patients. Symptoms and signs frequently associated with the facial paresis include ear pain, perception of sensory change on the involved side of the face, decreased tearing, overflow of tears on the cheek, sound sensitivity (hyperacusis), and impaired taste.

To make the diagnosis of Bell's palsy, both the upper and lower facial muscles must be involved. If only lower face involvement can be appreciated, there should be a suspicion for a central lesion, such as a cerebral infarct or neoplasm. Other red flags that should prompt consideration of an alternative diagnosis include vestibular or hearing abnormalities (other than hyperacusis), severe pain, rash, an unwell appearing patient, and history of cancer or tick bite.

Ramsay-Hunt syndrome may present with paresis similar to Bell's palsy, but is also characterized by a herpetiform vesicular eruption, vestibulocochlear dysfunction, and marked pain. The vesicular eruption, which may follow the facial paralysis by a few days, may occur on the pinna, external auditory canal, tympanic membrane, soft palate, oral cavity, face, and neck as far down as the shoulder. The pain is considerably more severe than that associated with Bell's palsy, and it frequently is out of proportion to physical findings. In addition, outcomes are worse than with Bell's palsy, with a lower incidence of complete facial recovery and the possibility of sensorineural hearing loss.

Systemic symptoms or bilateral facial paresis should raise the possibility of Lyme disease or other systemic infection. Lyme disease is the most frequent vector-borne infection in the United States. It is caused by the spirochete *Borrelia burgdorferi* and is spread by the bite of *Ixodes* genus ticks. Neurologic manifestations can arise in any phase of the disease, and facial palsy accounts for up to 50% of the neurologic presentations. In regions in which Lyme disease is endemic, it is the leading cause of facial paralysis in children. Infectious mononucleosis can also cause bilateral facial paralysis.

Facial paralysis can be caused by acute bacterial infections of the middle ear, mastoid, or external auditory canal. While it is very rare for an uncomplicated ear infection to result in facial paralysis, this may be seen with malignant otitis externa. This disease entity is most commonly seen in immunocompromised patients and usually is caused by *Pseudomonas* infection.

Differential Diagnoses

In addition to the disorders previously discussed, paralysis of CN VII can be caused by disruption of the nerve as a result of trauma or surgical procedures. Neoplasia, either tumors of the facial nerve itself or tumors that compress the nerve, can also lead to facial nerve paralysis. The course is typically (though not always) of slower onset than Bell's palsy. Although very rare overall, a neoplastic cause should be suspected in patients who suffer from recurrent ipsilateral facial paralysis, significant pain, prolonged symptoms, or any other concomitant CN abnormality.

Diagnostic Testing

The diagnostic evaluation of acute facial nerve paresis is based on whether the clinical picture is suggestive of a disease process other than Bell's palsy, highlighting the importance of a focused history and physical examination. In the absence of atypical features or identifiable risk factors, routine laboratory testing and diagnostic imaging are not recommended.[11] The presence of a "central" seventh nerve paralysis (upper face sparing) should prompt imaging with CT or MRI, and consideration given to the possibility of an acute stroke or other hemispheric lesion. History or physical findings suggestive of a possible tumor require imaging to rule out a neoplasm. A history that poses potential exposure to Lyme warrants serologic evaluation for the disease.

Management

The primary medical therapy for Bell's palsy is corticosteroids. Multiple studies have demonstrated that corticosteroids reduce the incidence of post infection residual facial weakness. A recent meta-analysis calculated the number needed to treat (NNT) as 10 in order to prevent one person left with facial weakness.[12] Guidelines recommend a 10-day course of oral corticosteroids with at least 5 days of high dose (prednisolone 50 mg for 10 days or prednisone 60 mg for 5 days with a 5-day taper).[13] Early treatment improves outcomes and therapy should be started as soon as possible, ideally within 72 hours of symptom onset.

Reflecting on the theory that herpes simplex virus may be a cause of Bell's palsy, a number of studies have considered the use of antivirals, either alone or in combination with corticosteroids. One meta-analysis demonstrated that antivirals alone were less effective than corticosteroids alone, and that the addition of antiviral therapy to corticosteroid therapy added little to no benefit over steroids alone.[14]

The treatment of Ramsey-Hunt syndrome is similar to that of Bell's palsy; however, antiviral treatment (acyclovir 400 mg five times daily or valacyclovir 1000 mg TID) is recommended. Both prednisone and antiviral therapy should be continued for 7 to 10 days. Other infectious causes of facial nerve paralysis (Lyme disease, infectious mononucleosis, malignant otitis externa) should be treated with directed antimicrobial therapy; severe local infection (such as malignant otitis externa) may require surgical debridement.

Patient education regarding meticulous eye care is of key importance. Inability to close the eyelids combined with decreased lacrimation can lead to corneal abrasions, keratitis, and ulcers. Prophylactic eye care includes barrier precautions (protective glasses, eye patches) as well as artificial tears, ideally with a thicker protective ointment during sleep.

Disposition

Most patients who have a seventh CN paralysis will have a clinical diagnosis of Bell's palsy and may be discharged with referral for short-term follow-up. Patients with a possible hemispheric process, such as stroke or tumor, require further evaluation and often hospitalization. Patients thought to have Lyme disease require immediate initiation of antibiotic therapy. Patients should be counselled regarding their expected timeline for recovery. Although mild paresis typically recovers within 2 to 3 weeks, complete paralysis may take up to 6 to 12 months for recovery, and some patients may not fully recover all function.

Vestibular Schwannoma (Cranial Nerve VIII)

Foundations

Vestibular schwannomas (VS) are tumors of the vestibular nerve, that though histologically benign, can impact the quality of life through hearing loss, imbalance, and other symptoms. VS, also referred to as acoustic neuroma, account for 80% of all cerebellopontine angle tumors. The incidence has increased over recent decades, though this is likely related to increased frequency of neuroimaging for other causes and identification of VS as an incidental finding. The median age of onset is about 50 and hearing loss is almost always unilateral (bilateral disease occurs in approximately 5% of cases and generally associated with type 2 neurofibromatosis).

Vestibular schwannomas arise from the Schwann cells covering the vestibular branch of the CN VIII as it passes through the internal auditory canal. The tumor may compress the cochlear (acoustic) branch of the CN VIII, causing hearing loss, tinnitus, and disequilibrium. Continued growth of the tumor may result in compression of structures in the cerebellopontine angle, where CN V and CN VII may be compressed and damaged. Larger tumors may further encroach on the brainstem and, if large enough, may compress the fourth ventricle, ultimately resulting in signs of increased intracranial pressure (ICP).

Clinical Features

Asymmetrical sensorineural hearing loss is the hallmark of vestibular schwannoma. Up to 15% of patients with this tumor, however, will have normal results on audiometry. These patients typically have symptoms such as unilateral tinnitus, imbalance, headache, fullness in the ear, otalgia, and facial nerve weakness. Thus, patients with asymmetrical symptoms should be further evaluated for vestibular schwannoma even with normal findings on audiometry. Vestibular schwannomas

are extremely slow-growing tumors, averaging a 1-mm increase per year, although some do not grow at all. The median time from symptom onset to diagnosis is 12 months.

Differential Diagnoses

While symmetrical sensorineural hearing loss has numerous causes, asymmetrical sensorineural hearing loss has few causes other than VS. Ménière disease may present with asymmetrical findings, but it can be differentiated from VS in that the tinnitus of Ménière disease is usually intermittent, whereas that of VS is continuous. In addition, patients with Ménière disease typically describe true vertigo, whereas those with a VS are more likely to describe imbalance or disequilibrium. Meningiomas, the second most common cerebellopontine angle tumor, more frequently cause symptoms of facial palsy or trigeminal nerve abnormality. However, there can be some clinical similarity between the two tumor types.

Diagnostic Testing

In general, diagnostic testing for VS can be performed as an outpatient. When suspected, testing includes MRI and audiometry. MRI is extremely sensitive and has led to earlier diagnosis and a decrease in mean size at detection of vestibular schwannoma. CT lacks the necessary sensitivity in the posterior cranial fossa to reliably rule out the presence of VS. The smaller the tumor at the time of diagnosis, the more options there are for therapy and the better the prognosis.

Management

There are currently three main approaches for managing newly diagnosed VS: observation with active surveillance, surgical resection, and stereotactic radiation therapy. Observation may be appropriate for elderly patients with comorbidities, small tumor size, and absence of symptoms. Due to the continued growth of most tumors however, observation is often associated with progressive hearing loss. In appropriately selected patients, there is little difference in long-term quality-of-life based on surgical resection versus radiotherapy. In general, tumors larger than 3 cm are recommended for microsurgery because radiation poses a risk of brain stem compressions due to posttreatment edema. Smaller tumors may be treated with surgery or radiation.

Disposition

Patients with suspected acoustic neuroma should be referred for audiometry or MRI and evaluation by a specialist in either otolaryngology or neurosurgery.

Diabetic Cranial Mononeuropathy

Foundations

Cranial mononeuropathies are uncommon and are usually a complication of diabetes. They most often affect the extraocular muscles causing ophthalmoplegia. The oculomotor nerve (CN III) is most commonly affected, followed by the trochlear (CN IV) and abducens (CN VI) nerves. CN palsies occur in 1% of diabetics versus 0.1% of nondiabetics. They are more likely to occur in patients over the age of 50 years. The pathologic basis of diabetic mononeuropathy appears to be ischemia caused by occlusion of an intraneural nutrient artery serving the nerve. This occlusion leads to injury located primarily in the core fibers, whereas the peripheral nerve fibers are less affected because they also are supplied by collateral vessels. In the oculomotor nerve, the preservation of the circumferentially located parasympathetic fibers explains the pupillary sparing that usually is found in this condition.

The anatomy of the third CN is particularly important to consider. Centrally located motor fibers controlling extraocular movement are likely to be affected by vascular ischemic disease. Parasympathetic fibers associated with the pupillary light reflex run superficially within the nerve; while pupillary findings can result from microvascular ischemia, they should raise concern for compression of CN III from aneurysm in the posterior cerebral arteries.

Clinical Features

Diabetic cranial nerve palsy often results in diplopia, which may be worsened by the direction of gaze. Physical examination may demonstrate asymmetric positioning of the eyes at rest or with directional gaze. The physical manifestations of a CN III palsy include the inability to move the eye superiorly and medially (leading to the "down and out" position at rest), accompanied by ptosis. The pupillary light reflex usually is present. Although it is a less common finding, CN IV and CN VI may be affected. Patients with a CN IV palsy are unable to move the eye inferolaterally, and those with a CN VI palsy are unable to move the eye laterally. Because of the long intracranial course of CN VI, a patient with an isolated sixth nerve palsy should be evaluated for an intracranial lesion or increased ICP.

Differential Diagnoses

Diabetic mononeuropathy is generally a diagnosis of exclusion. Considerations in the differential diagnosis include trauma, tumor, vertebrobasilar ischemia, aneurysm, and brainstem hemorrhage. Unequal pupils or an abnormal pupillary light reflex should be considered a red flag for a more worrisome cause.

Diagnostic Testing

The key clinical dilemma in a diabetic patient presenting with new onset oculomotor neuropathy relates to the use of diagnostic imaging to rule out potentially life-threatening etiologies. There is no clear clinical consensus on neuroimaging, with a recent meta-analysis demonstrating discrepancies in practice between neurologists and ophthalmologists (with neurologists being more likely to use imaging).[15] It is generally accepted that pupillary involvement warrants evaluation for aneurysm with either MR or CT angiography. Similarly, if other CN are involved or there are other acute neurologic deficits, neuroimaging for stroke is warranted. While there is not a clear treatment recommendation for the ED provider, clinical history and physical examination are thought to be sufficient in the majority of cases, and there is no evidence that diagnostic imaging is required in the diabetic patient presenting an isolated CN III palsy with sparing of the pupillary light reflex and no other neurologic abnormalities.

Management

Treatment consists of patching the affected eye and administration of analgesics and antiplatelet therapy. The prognosis is good and the neuropathy generally resolves within 3 to 6 months.

Disposition

Assuming aneurysm and stroke have been excluded as causes of cranial mononeuropathy, patients may be discharged home. There is some evidence demonstrating that patients with diabetes diagnosed with a CN palsy have a higher risk of subsequent ischemic stroke.[16] While the evidence for this is limited, there is certainly no downside to using the clinical encounter to identify modifiable risk factors for stroke and encourage treatment compliance and outpatient follow up.

The references for this chapter can be found online at ExpertConsult.com.

92

Spinal Cord Disorders

Adam D. Hill and Micah J. Nite

KEY CONCEPTS

- Nontraumatic spinal cord disorders can be intrinsic or extrinsic, some of which require prompt diagnosis, advanced imaging, and specialist intervention to prevent or limit permanent neurologic dysfunction.
- The bulbocavernosus reflex is cord-mediated. Return of this reflex following a spinal injury marks the termination of spinal shock.
- Anterior cord syndrome is marked by symmetrical motor loss but intact proprioception and vibration sense.
- In patients with sudden severe back pain, consider spinal subarachnoid hemorrhage (SSAH) or spinal epidural hematoma (SEH), both of which are diagnosed using magnetic resonance imaging (MRI).
- Transverse myelitis is inflammation of the spinal cord often associated with a prior viral infection resulting in paraplegia and a defined sensory level impairment. MRI with contrast enhancement is the diagnostic modality of choice. Roughly one-third of patients have a good outcome.
- Cauda equina syndrome can be difficult to differentiate from conus medullaris lesions because both can result in bladder retention, fecal incontinence, leg weakness, and sensory loss in the perineum. Conus lesions are more typically bilateral, whereas cauda equina syndrome may be unilateral. Upper motor neuron findings are expected with conus lesions while cauda equina syndrome is associated with hypo- or areflexia.
- Central cord syndrome is often due to a hyperextension injury. Physical findings are represented with the mnemonic **MUD**: **M**otor deficits > sensory, **U**pper extremities > lower, **D**istal extremity findings > proximal.
- Brown-Séquard syndrome is due to a functional hemisection of the spine (frequently traumatic) resulting in ipsilateral loss of motor function, proprioception, and vibration with contralateral loss of pain and temperature sensation below the level of injury.
- The diagnostic imaging of choice in the majority of suspected spinal disorders is MRI with contrast.
- A syrinx is a cavitary lesion in the spinal cord that presents with a sensory disassociation predominately in the upper extremities. With progression, it can lead to upper extremity weakness and wasting. Symptom exacerbation with cough or Valsalva is typical.
- With compressive lesions of the spinal cord, neurologic status at the time of intervention and the duration of symptoms are directly related to outcome.
- Autonomic dysreflexia is a complication of spinal cord injury that can result in life-threatening hypertension. Hypertension may be the result of bladder distention, fecal impaction, pain, or infection. Treatment focuses on blood pressure management and the identification and treatment of inciting noxious stimuli.

FOUNDATIONS

This chapter focuses on nontraumatic processes affecting the spinal cord, both extrinsic and internal. The ultimate neurologic outcome of patients with many of these disorders depends on expeditious recognition and management in the emergency department (ED).

Anatomy

In adults, the spinal cord is approximately 40 cm long and extends from the foramen magnum, where it is continuous with the medulla oblongata, to the body of the first or second lumbar vertebra (L1 to L2). The spinal cord is covered in the same three meningeal layers as the brain: the pia mater (innermost), arachnoid mater (middle), and dura mater (outermost). Inferiorly, the cord tapers into the conus medullaris (L1), where several segmental levels are represented in a small area. The lumbar and sacral nerve roots form the cauda equina as they descend caudally in the thecal sac before exiting the spinal canal at the respective foramina. The filum terminale, a non-neural strand of fibrous tissue composed of pia whose function is to suspend the cord in the subarachnoid space, runs from the tip of the conus and inserts into the dura at the level of the second sacral vertebra (S2).

Two symmetrical enlargements of the spinal cord contain the segments that innervate the limbs. The first occurs at the junction of the cervical (C) and thoracic (T) vertebrae. The *cervical enlargement* (C5 to T1) gives rise to the brachial plexus and peripheral nerves of the upper extremity. The second area is located at the junction of the thoracic and lumbar (L) vertebrae. The *lumbar enlargement* (L2 to S3) gives rise to the lumbosacral plexus and peripheral nerves of the lower extremity. The space surrounding the cord at these particular levels is reduced leaving it more vulnerable to external compression. At each segmental level, anterior (ventral) and posterior (dorsal) roots arise from rootlets along the anterolateral and posterolateral cord surfaces. Anterior roots convey the outflow of the motor neurons in the anterior horn of the spinal cord while posterior roots contain neurons and fibers that convey sensory inflow.

The arterial supply of the spinal cord is derived primarily from two sources (Fig. 92.1). The single anterior spinal artery arises from the paired vertebral arteries at the base of the skull. It runs the entire length of the cord in the midline anterior median sulcus and supplies the anterior two-thirds of the spinal cord. Blood supply to the posterior third of the spinal cord is derived from the smaller paired posterior spinal arteries that arise from the vertebral arteries near the skull base and run bilaterally along the posterior cord. These three major spinal arteries receive segmental contributions from radicular arteries throughout their caudal projection, the largest being the artery of Adamkiewicz, which typically originates from the aorta between T8 and L4. The venous drainage of the cord largely parallels the arterial supply.

The internal anatomy of the spinal cord is divided into central gray matter, containing cell bodies and their processes, and surrounding white matter, where the ascending and descending myelinated fiber tracts are located. These white matter fiber tracts are organized into discrete bundles; the ascending tracts convey sensory information while the descending tracts convey the efferent motor impulses and visceral innervation.

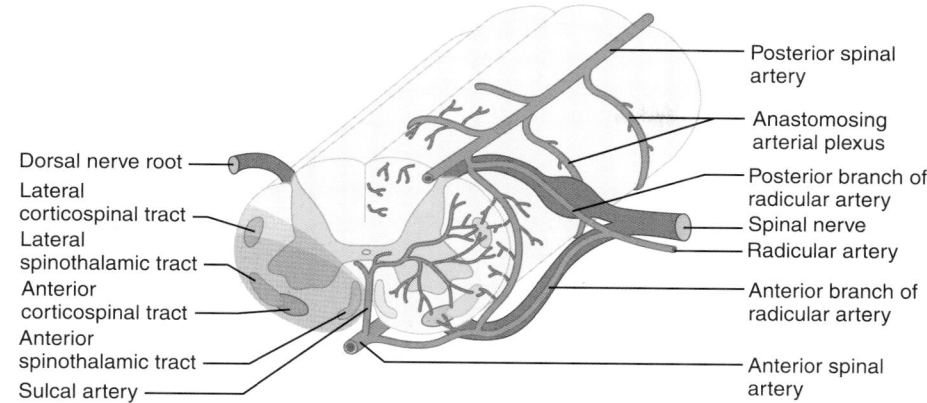

Fig. 92.1 Arterial blood supply to the spinal cord. The anterior spinal artery supplies blood to most of the anterior spinal cord, as well as the lateral column area of the cord (*darkly shaded area*). Some areas of the cord are supplied blood by both the anterior and posterior circulation (*light gray–shaded area*); there is variation among individuals. The anterior horn cells and lateral spinothalamic tracts rely on the anterior spinal artery for blood supply. (Modified from: Yang ML, Connolly AM. Other Motor Neuron Diseases of Childhood. In: Swaiman KF, Ashwal S, Ferriero DM, et al., eds. *Swaiman's Pediatric Neurology*, ed 6. Philadelphia: Elsevier; 2017.)

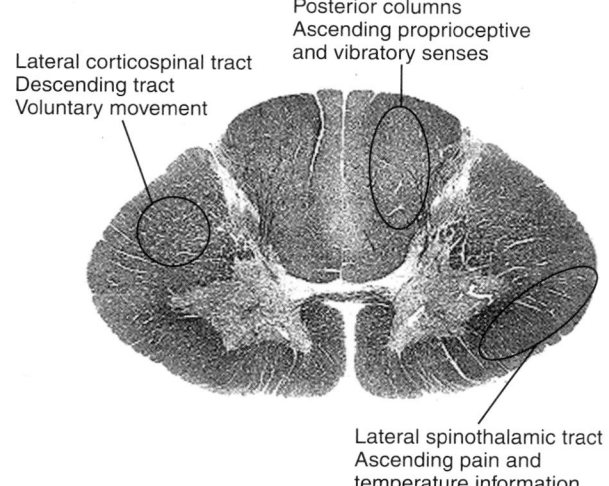

Fig. 92.2 Simplified spinal cord anatomy showing clinically essential motor and sensory tracts. (Photomicrograph courtesy John Sundsten, Digital Anatomist Project, University of Washington.)

For clinical purposes, neuroanatomy of the spinal cord may be greatly simplified, as depicted in Figure 92.2. Tracts are named starting with the point of origin followed by the destination; the spinothalamic tract, for example, arises in the spinal cord and travels to the thalamus. Major ascending sensory tracts are labeled on the right side of the figure, with descending motor tracts on the left. The posterior column (dorsal column) carries afferent ascending proprioceptive and vibratory information on the ipsilateral side of the cord from the area stimulated to the brain; crossing of these fibers occurs in the medulla resulting in contralateral cortical representation. Within the cord, the posterior column is arranged with the sacral fibers existing medially and the cervical fibers laterally. The lateral spinothalamic tract conveys afferent information about pain and temperature in a portion of the lateral column of white matter. The tract is arranged so that sacral fibers are located laterally and cervical fibers medially, a reversal from the posterior column arrangement. Crossing of fibers from this tract occurs near the level of entry of the spinal nerve resulting in

contralateral representation in the cord. This is why an isolated cord lesion affecting a spinothalamic tract results in decreased or absent pain and temperature perception below the level of injury on the opposite side of the body.

The major descending motor tract is represented in the lateral corticospinal tract, originating in the cortex of the brain and traveling to the spinal cord. Crossing of this tract occurs in the medulla, similar to the ascending posterior column, meaning that motor signals from one side of the brain ultimately descend down the opposite cord side and result in motion of the contralateral body. This tract is organized similar to the lateral spinothalamic, with sacral fibers located laterally and the cervical fibers medially. The cell bodies of the lower motor neurons (anterior horn cells) are in the ventral portion of the gray matter of the spinal cord.

Classification of Spinal Cord Syndromes

The anatomic organization of the spinal cord lends itself to a corresponding anatomic-pathophysiologic classification of cord dysfunction (Table 92.1). Any of the different cord syndromes may be the final clinical picture of a variety of pathologic processes. These syndromes do frequently exist in partial or incomplete forms, adding to the diagnostic challenge.

Complete (Transverse) Spinal Cord Syndrome

Complete spinal cord lesions may be manifested as either acute or subacute processes. It is defined as a total loss of sensory, autonomic, and voluntary motor innervation distal to the spinal cord level of injury. Neural responses mediated at the spinal level, such as deep tendon reflexes, may persist but may also be absent (early stages) or hyperreflexic (later stages). Autonomic dysfunction may be manifested acutely with hypotension (neurogenic shock) or priapism. The most common cause of a complete cord syndrome is trauma, though other etiologies are possible including infarction, hemorrhage, and extrinsic compression. In patients with complete syndromes that persist for more than 24 hours, functional recovery almost never occurs. Any evidence of preserved cord function below the level of injury denotes a partial rather than complete lesion. Signs such as persistent perineal sensation (sacral sparing), reflex rectal sphincter tone or voluntary rectal sphincter contraction, and even slight voluntary toe movement suggest a partial cord lesion, which carries a better prognosis than a complete lesion.

TABLE 92.1   Spinal Cord Syndromes

Syndrome	Sensory	Motor	Sphincter Involvement
Central cord syndrome	Variable	Upper extremity weakness, distal > proximal	Variable
Brown-Séquard syndrome	Ipsilateral position and vibration sense loss; Contralateral pain and temperature sensation loss	Motor loss ipsilateral to cord lesion	Variable
Anterior cord syndrome	Loss of pain and touch sensation; Vibration, position sense preserved	Motor loss or weakness below cord level	Variable
Transverse (complete) cord syndrome	Loss of sensation below level of cord injury	Loss of voluntary motor function below cord level	Sphincter control lost
Conus medullaris syndrome	Saddle anesthesia may be present; Sensory loss may range from patchy to complete transverse pattern	Weakness may be of upper motor neuron type; Bilateral	Sphincter control impaired
Cauda equina syndrome	Saddle anesthesia may be present; Sensory loss may range from patchy to complete transverse pattern	Weakness may be of lower motor neuron type; Unilateral	Sphincter control impaired

Spinal shock refers to the loss of muscle tone and reflexes with a complete cord syndrome during the acute phase of injury. It typically lasts less than 24 hours but has been reported to occasionally last days or weeks. A marker of spinal shock is loss of the bulbocavernosus reflex, which is a normal cord-mediated reflex that may be preserved in complete cord lesions. The bulbocavernosus reflex involves involuntary contraction of the anal sphincter in response to a squeeze of the glans penis, clitoris, or outward tug on a Foley catheter. Termination of the spinal shock phase of injury is heralded by the return of the bulbocavernosus reflex, with increased muscle tone and hyperreflexia following later.

Incomplete (Partial) Spinal Cord Lesions

Incomplete lesions are characterized by functional preservation of various portions of the spinal cord. Of the many possible incomplete lesions, most can be classified as one of three clinical syndromes based on functionality: (1) central cord syndrome, (2) Brown-Séquard syndrome, or (3) anterior cord syndrome.

Central Cord Syndrome. Central cord syndrome is the most common of the partial cord syndromes. Because of the anatomic organization of the spinal cord, a central cord injury is characterized by bilateral motor paresis. The upper extremities and distal muscle groups are affected to a greater degree than the lower extremities and proximal muscle groups. Sensory impairment and bladder dysfunction are variable features. At times, burning dysesthesias in the upper extremities may be the dominant clinical feature. The mnemonic "MUD" can aid in recall of these features: **M**otor greater than sensory, **U**pper greater than lower, **D**istal greater than proximal.

Central cord syndrome affects the central gray matter and the central portions of the corticospinal and spinothalamic tracts. It is most often caused by a hyperextension injury, frequently from falls or motor vehicle accidents. The postulated mechanism is squeezing of the cord anteriorly and posteriorly due to inward bulging of the dorsally located ligamentum flavum resulting in a contusion to the spinal cord which most affects the central cord. This injury often occurs in elders with degenerative arthritis and spinal stenosis in the cervical area but can affect patients with cervical canal narrowing of any etiology (i.e., disc protrusion, tumor, or congenital narrowing as in achondroplasia). The prognosis depends on the degree of injury at presentation as well as the patient's age, with advanced age predicting decreased functional outcome. In patients younger than 50 years old, more than 80% regain bladder continence and approximately 90% return to full ambulatory status; in patients older than 50 years, only 30% regain bladder function and approximately 50% regain the ability to ambulate.

Brown-Séquard Syndrome. Brown-Séquard syndrome is the result of an anatomic or functional hemisection of the spinal cord. Usually associated with penetrating injuries, Brown-Séquard syndrome also may be seen with compressive or intrinsic lesions. It has been reported in association with spinal cord tumors, spinal epidural hematomas, vascular malformations, cervical spondylosis, degenerative disc disease, herpes zoster myelitis, radiation injury, and as a complication of spinal instrumentation. In its pure form, it is characterized by ipsilateral loss of motor function, proprioception, and vibration sense with contralateral loss of pain and temperature sensation below the level of injury. Because fibers associated with the lateral spinothalamic tract ascend one or two spinal cord segments before crossing to the contralateral side, ipsilateral anesthesia (pain and temperature modalities) may be noted one or two segments above the lesion, although this observation is variable. Most patients with this syndrome incur only partial sensory and motor impairment, so the classic pattern is not always seen. Brown-Séquard syndrome carries the best prognosis of any of the incomplete spinal cord syndromes. Fully 80% to 90% of patients regain bowel and bladder function, 75% regain ambulatory status, and 70% become independent in their activities of daily living.

Anterior Cord Syndrome. Anterior cord syndrome is characterized by loss of motor function, pinprick, and light touch below the level of the lesion with preservation of the posterior column modalities, including position, vibration, and some touch. Although most reported cases of anterior spinal cord syndrome follow aortic surgery, it may also occur after severe hypotension, infection, myocardial infarction, vasospasm from drug reaction, and aortic angiography. Mechanically, the lesion may be caused by cervical hyperflexion resulting in a cord contusion or by protrusion of bone fragments or herniated cervical disc material into the canal. Rarely, it is produced by laceration or thrombosis of the anterior spinal artery or a major radicular vessel. Functional recovery varies, with most improvement occurring during the first 24 hours and little improvement thereafter. Although anterior cord lesions from ischemia usually are incomplete, patients without motor function at 30 days have little or no likelihood of regaining any motor function by 1 year. Only 10% to 20% of patients regain some muscle function, and even in this group there is little power or coordination.

Conus Medullaris and Cauda Equina Syndromes

The differentiation between conus medullaris and cauda equina lesions in clinical practice is difficult because the two disorders overlap in their clinical presentation. In addition, a combined lesion can mask clear clinical symptoms or signs of either an upper or a lower motor neuron type of injury.

Physical features of conus medullaris syndrome may involve disturbances of urination (usually from a denervated, spastic, autonomic bladder that manifests as overflow incontinence) and

sphincter impairment (decreased rectal tone) or erectile dysfunction. Sensory involvement may affect the sacral and coccygeal segments, resulting in saddle anesthesia. Pure lesions of the conus medullaris are rare. Upper motor neuron signs, such as increased motor tone and hyperreflexia, may be present, but their absence does not exclude the syndrome.

Conus medullaris syndrome can be caused by central disc herniation, neoplasm, trauma, or vascular insufficiency. Because the conus is such a small structure, with lumbar and sacral segments represented in a minimal area, a lesion will usually cause bilateral symptoms. This finding may help distinguish conus medullaris lesions from those in the cauda equina, which often are unilateral.

Cauda equina (Latin for "horse's tail") is the name given to the lumbar and sacral nerve roots that continue on within the dural sac distal to the conus medullaris. Not a true "cord syndrome" as the cord itself is unaffected, cauda equina syndrome represents dysfunction at the level of nerve roots. The anatomic clustering of nerve roots within the lumbar dural sac allows insult to multiple nerve roots to occur simultaneously.

Cauda equina syndrome is usually caused by the midline rupture of an intervertebral disc most commonly at the L4 to L5 level, but any compressive mass can cause it. As in conus medullaris syndrome, patients generally present with progressive symptoms of fecal or urinary incontinence, impotence, decreased rectal tone, distal motor weakness, and saddle anesthesia. Deep tendon reflexes may be reduced. All of these findings have low sensitivity but moderately good specificity in the diagnosis, with saddle anesthesia and bowel/bladder changes having a specificity range of 70% to 89%.[1] Of note, a complaint of low back pain may or may not be present.

CLINICAL FEATURES

History

Weakness, sensory abnormalities, and autonomic dysfunction are the cardinal manifestations of spinal cord dysfunction. The tempo and degree of impairment often reflect the disease process. Past medical history is vital because an underlying coagulopathy or other systemic process may be elicited. A history of cancer suggests the possibility of metastatic disease. Recent trauma raises the possibility of vertebral fracture or disc protrusion. The acuity of pain can help narrow the differential diagnosis as well, with sudden pain or dysfunction more likely to be a vascular catastrophe, and slower onset, midline pain in the setting of fever points toward an infectious source.

Physical Examination

The physical examination pertinent to spinal cord dysfunction involves testing in three areas: (1) motor function, (2) sensory function, and (3) reflexes. Each component is best tested with the anatomic organization of the spinal cord in mind to help determine the level of dysfunction. A detailed description of neurologic deficits and their correlating spinal level can be found in Chapter 35.

Motor Function

Testing of motor function encompasses examination of muscle bulk, tone, and strength. Muscle bulk is easily examined in large motor groups, such as the thigh, the calf, or the upper arm. Inspection of intrinsic hand muscles may also be helpful in determination of bulk; wasting may be evident as hollowed or recessed regions of the hand. Any decreased mass, asymmetry, or fasciculations should be noted. Tone is tested with repeated passive knee, elbow, or wrist flexion, or by rapid passive forearm pronation-supination, with the examiner assessing for abnormally increased or decreased resistance. Increased

TABLE 92.2   Grading of Neuromuscular Weakness

Grade	Physical Findings
0	No firing of the muscle is present.
1	The muscle fires but is unable to move the intended part.
2	The muscle is able to move the intended part with gravity eliminated.
3	The muscle is able to move the intended part against gravity.
4	The muscle is able to move the intended part but not at full strength.
5	Full muscle strength is present.

tone may indicate spasticity or an upper motor neuron lesion whereas decreased tone corresponds with lower motor neuron, motor end-plate, or muscle problems. Motor strength is then graded in the upper and the lower extremities. Motor grading for the neurologic examination is relatively straightforward; scored on a scale of 0 to 5, as shown in Table 92.2.

A rectal examination and the bulbocavernosus reflex (involuntary anal sphincter contraction in response to a squeeze of the glans penis or clitoris or a tugging on a Foley catheter) are performed to assess voluntary sphincter contraction and resting tone. Although not commonly thought of as a physical examination maneuver, a post-void residual (PVR) urine volume is useful to evaluate bladder function. A PVR of more than 100 to 200 mL in a patient without prior voiding difficulty suggests bladder dysfunction of a neurologic cause.

Sensory Function

Sensory testing requires a cooperative patient and an attentive examiner. Assessment of the patient's response to pinprick and light touch (contralateral spinothalamic tract) and proprioception (ipsilateral posterior column) in all four extremities is necessary. Testing of sacral dermatomes is indicated, as sparing suggests that a lesion may be incomplete. The sensory fibers from these dermatomes are more peripherally located in the ascending fiber bundles, thus, central or partial cord lesions may ablate sensation in the extremities yet allow some perception in the sacral area.

Reflexes

Deep tendon (muscle stretch) reflexes are graded on a scale of 0 to 4+, with 2 being normal. Hyperactive reflexes suggest upper motor neuron disease (affecting the neurons or their outflow from the brain or spinal cord) as do sustained clonus and Babinski sign. If present, hyperactive or abnormally brisk reflexes may be a key finding suggesting a myelopathy. However, absence of hyperreflexia does not exclude one. Reflexes may be diminished or absent when sensation is lost, when spinal shock is present, or in diseases of muscles or the neuromuscular junction. In acute cord injury, reflexes can be diminished in the acute phase, therefore, the bulbocavernosus reflex may be helpful in this assessment.

DIFFERENTIAL DIAGNOSES

The prime principle in management of spinal cord dysfunction is to consider and diagnose potentially treatable and time-sensitive conditions. The clinician should rule out any nonstructural cause of neurologic dysfunction (e.g., hypoglycemia, hypokalemia) early in the evaluation process. Once a true neurologic entity is suspected, the next step is to differentiate the location of the lesion (i.e., brain, spinal cord, nerve or motor end-plate). When the pathologic process is suspected to be spinal in origin, liberal use of specialist consultation and imaging is generally warranted. Spinal cord disorders may mimic many other disease processes, and neither the history nor physical examination can reliably enable a true diagnosis until appreciable neurologic dysfunction has developed.

The picture of a complete (transverse) spinal cord syndrome with paraplegia, sensory loss at a clear anatomic level, and sphincter dysfunction cannot be fully mimicked by other anatomic lesions; incomplete or evolving spinal cord syndromes, however, can. Ataxia, for example, is often a finding in cerebellar disease but has been reported as a rare, isolated finding in spinal cord compression.

In general, pathologic processes involving the spinal cord may be divided into those affecting the cord or its blood supply (e.g., demyelination, infection, or infarction) and ones that compress the cord. Of note, *myelitis* is a comprehensive term for spinal cord inflammation with dysfunction. The clinical presentation is often similar across the many etiologies of cord compression, but the tempo of the process may yield a different clinical picture. In chronic compression, muscle wasting and abnormal reflexes may be present, whereas both of these findings are likely to be lacking in acute compression.

DIAGNOSTIC TESTING

The purpose of diagnostic testing in patients suspected of having spinal cord dysfunction is to detect or exclude extrinsic compressive lesions or other potentially treatable entities. Conventional radiographs and computed tomography (CT) scans are essential in patients with trauma or suspected bony involvement by tumor or degenerative process because they better define bone and can show some soft tissue abnormalities. However, due to its ability to clearly define the spinal cord and the soft tissue structures around it, magnetic resonance imaging (MRI) is the preferred modality in assessing spinal cord disorders. It may also detect tissue damage patterns within the cord, such as hemorrhage and edema, as well as bone pathology. When utilized, MRI assessment of the entire spine should be considered because lesions can frequently occur at multiple levels.

MRI with gadolinium contrast enhancement is indicated when looking for pathology that affects the blood–central nervous system (CNS) barrier. Specific indications include primary or metastatic tumor, multiple sclerosis (MS), and spinal infections (i.e., spinal epidural abscess, discitis, and osteomyelitis). An example of the utility of gadolinium enhancement is seen in Figure 92.3. CT myelography is an option when MRI is unavailable or contraindicated, although it does not yield the same level of detail.

After imaging studies exclude compressive lesions or other masses affecting the spinal cord, the possibility of inflammatory or demyelinating disorders remains. In these cases, lumbar puncture with cerebrospinal fluid (CSF) analysis may be diagnostic.

MANAGEMENT

The treatment of many of the disease processes causing spinal cord dysfunction is nonspecific and based on limited evidence. Steroids have been used with many nontraumatic causes of cord compression, particularly spinal cord tumors, despite the lack of rigorous clinical studies supporting this practice. Radiation treatment is recommended for cord compression by tumor; surgical consultation for decompression may be considered, although the indications and timing for surgery are controversial.

Pre-gadolinium

Post-gadolinium

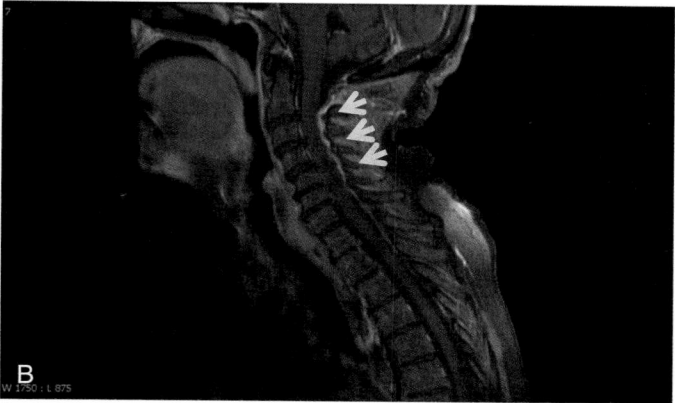

Fig. 92.3 90-year-old female with recent pyelonephritis presenting with severe neck pain. Pregadolinium sequence (A) compared with postgadolinium sequence (B) demonstrates posterior spinal epidural abscess (SEA) *(yellow arrowheads)*.

TABLE 92.3	Causes and Characteristics of Nontraumatic Spinal Cord Dysfunction		
Disease Process	**Symptoms/Examination Findings**	**Testing**	**Treatment**
Intrinsic Lesions			
Multiple Sclerosis	Symptoms include sensory, visual (optic neuritis), GI, fatigue, weakness, labile mood, hyperreflexia.	MRI, LP, consider biopsy	Steroids + disease-modifying medications
Transverse Myelitis	Paraplegia, transverse sensory impairment, and sphincter disturbance.	MRI	±Glucocorticoid therapy (etiology dependent)
Spinal Subarachnoid Hemorrhage	Usually have focal deficits on examination at level of bleed. May also complain of headache and/or demonstrate nuchal rigidity on exam.	MRI +/− LP	Anticoagulation reversal +/− clot evacuation
Syringomyelia	Headache with neck pain and sensory disturbances. Frequently demonstrate lower limb hyperreflexia with hand weakness and dissociative anesthesia.	MRI	Neurosurgical consultation vs. outpatient follow-up
HIV Myelopathy	Advanced HIV infection with weakness, gait disturbance, and sensory abnormalities.	Diagnosis of exclusion	Supportive therapy, HAART
Spinal Cord Infarction	Findings depend on location of infarction but anterior cord syndrome is most common.	Diagnosis of exclusion	Dependent on etiology
Surfer's Myelopathy	Back pain, paresis, and urinary retention.	MRI	Conservative therapy
Extrinsic Lesions			
Spinal Epidural Hematoma	Sudden severe radicular back pain usually presents prior to onset of deficits. Exam findings depend on location of hematoma.	MRI	Decompressive laminectomy
Spinal Epidural Abscess	Classically febrile with progressive neurological deficits. Back pain may be worse with percussion.	MRI	IV antibiotics ± surgery vs. needle decompression
Discitis	Children with back pain at level of lesion. Subacute presentation with fever but no neurologic deficits.	MRI	IV antibiotics
Neoplasm	Nighttime pain worse with lying flat. Deficits depend on location of lesion.	CT or MRI	Glucocorticoid therapy + radiation therapy or surgery

SPECIFIC DISEASE PROCESSES

Spinal cord disorders are grouped into lesions resulting from processes intrinsic to the cord or vasculature and lesions causing extrinsic compression (Table 92.3).

Intrinsic Cord Lesions

Multiple Sclerosis

Demyelination denotes a disease process with the prominent feature of partial or complete loss of the myelin surrounding the axons of the CNS. Multiple sclerosis (MS) is the most common example of such a process. The spinal cord is involved in as many as 90% of MS patients. In approximately 20% of patients, the spinal cord lesions will be the only area where plaques are identified. The pathophysiology, diagnosis, and management of MS is discussed in Chapter 94.

Transverse Myelitis

Foundations. *Acute transverse myelitis* (TM) refers to acute or subacute spinal cord dysfunction characterized by paraplegia, a transverse level of sensory impairment, and sphincter disturbance. It is often considered part of a heterogeneous group of inflammatory processes known as neuromyelitis opticum spectrum disorders (NMOSD).[2] TM affects the spinal cord by interrupting the ascending or descending pathways. The presentation may be mimicked by compressive lesions, trauma, infection, or malignant infiltration.

The pathogenesis of transverse myelitis is unknown, although it is noted to follow a viral infection in approximately 30% of patients and therefore often termed *postinfectious myelitis*. Other postulated etiologies include infectious, autoimmune, and idiopathic disorders. It can be seen with a wide variety of connective tissue diseases, such as lupus, Sjögren syndrome, antiphospholipid syndrome, and other mixed connective tissue diseases. More recent research points to the presence of anti-AQP4 antibodies, particularly in cases thought to be part of NMOSD.[3] No cause is identified in 30% of patients. Progression of symptoms is usually rapid, with 66% of the cases reaching maximal deficit by 24 hours. However, symptoms may progress over days to weeks. The thoracic cord region is affected in 60% to 70% of cases, with the cervical cord being rarely involved. When TM lesions span 3 or more spinal cord levels, it is termed *longitudinally extensive transverse myelitis* (LETM) and is considered a hallmark of NMOSD.[4]

Clinical Features. In addition to motor, sensory, and urinary disturbances, patients with acute transverse myelitis may complain of back pain as well as a low-grade fever, raising concern for SEA. As with MS, the examination may reveal weakness progressing to paresis, hypertonia, hyperreflexia, clonus, Babinski response, and anal sphincter dysfunction. A distinct sensory level deficit is usually present. Autonomic dysfunction may also be noted as hyper- or hypotension and tachy- or bradycardia.

Differential Diagnoses. Considerations in the differential diagnosis for transverse myelitis include MS, SEA, spinal epidural hematoma (SEH), primary or metastatic spinal neoplasm, spinal cord infarct, surfer's myelopathy, and vitamin B_4 deficiency.[3]

Diagnostic Strategies. MRI with gadolinium enhancement is the diagnostic modality of choice for suspected transverse myelitis (Fig. 92.4). In cases of diagnostic uncertainty, a lumbar puncture may be performed; however, the results of CSF studies are normal in 40% of cases, with only mildly elevated protein levels or pleocytosis in the remaining 60%. The most essential aspect of the evaluation is to eliminate a potentially treatable cause. If testing is available, serum can be sent to detect the presence of specific antibodies (e.g., antiphospholipid, anti-AQP4, ANA).

Management. Treatment is tailored to the suspected underlying etiology. There are no good studies supporting a role for steroids. The exception for this would be in the setting of NMOSD-related TM, where steroids and immunosuppressant agents are the current recommended treatment. Methylprednisolone 1 gram IV is commonly administered. Neurologic consultation is suggested and hospitalization is usually required.

The clinical course of acute transverse myelitis varies widely, ranging from complete recovery to death from progressive neurologic compromise. Most patients with idiopathic disease have at least partial recovery, which usually begins within 1 to 3 months. Maximal improvement usually is obtained within 3 to 6 months with 30% of patients having "good" recovery, 25% "fair" recovery, and 30% having a "poor" outcome; there is 15% mortality at 5 years.

Spinal Subarachnoid Hemorrhage

Foundations. Intraspinal hemorrhage is rare and may occur in the same anatomic locations as intracranial hemorrhages; epidural, subdural, subarachnoid, and intramedullary hemorrhages are all possible. Spinal subarachnoid hemorrhage (SSAH) is usually caused by

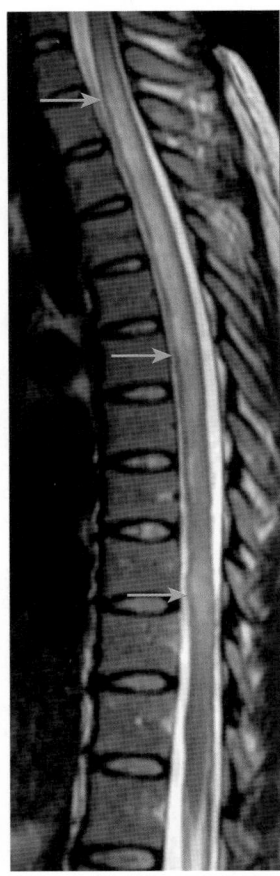

Fig. 92.4 Sagittal T2 MR shows a long segment of abnormal hyperintensity *(blue arrowheads)* and expansion of the visualized spinal cord, characteristic of transverse myelitis. (From: Merrow AC, Hariharan S. Transverse myelitis. In: Merrow AC, Hariharan S, eds. *Imaging in Pediatrics*, ed 1. Philadelphia: Elsevier; 2018.)

an arteriovenous malformation. Hemorrhage from tumors or cavernous angiomas and spontaneous hemorrhage secondary to anticoagulation therapy have also been reported. Diagnostic lumbar puncture is documented as a rare cause.[5] Bleeding may occur exclusively in the subarachnoid space or within the spinal cord tissue itself.

Clinical Features. Patients with SSAH present with excruciating back pain of a sudden and severe nature at the level of the hemorrhage. This pain may be in a radicular distribution or extend into the flank. Patients can complain of headache and exhibit cervical rigidity if the blood migrates into the intracranial subarachnoid space, simulating an intracranial subarachnoid hemorrhage. Variable neurologic deficits depend on the magnitude and anatomic location of the hemorrhage. These deficits typically include extremity numbness, weakness, and sphincter dysfunction. Nuchal rigidity or signs of meningeal irritation may also be present.

Differential Diagnoses. Considerations in the differential diagnosis include disc herniation, tumor, ischemia from aortic dissection, and anterior spinal artery thrombosis.

Diagnostic Testing. Because bone artifact may obscure the presence of blood in the spine, the diagnostic study of choice in patients with suspected SSAH is MRI without contrast. Lumbar puncture can help to confirm the presence of blood in the CSF. Angiography may be recommended if arteriovenous malformation is suspected. CT may be of benefit in detecting SSAH if MRI is not immediately available, but a negative CT does not definitively rule out the disease.[6]

Management. The treatment of spinal subarachnoid hemorrhage depends on the etiology of the hemorrhage. Neurosurgical referral is obtained for further evaluation and potential clot evacuation if compression is present. Reversal of anticoagulant medications should be considered in the proper clinical setting.

Syringomyelia

Foundations. Syringomyelia is the presence of a cavitary lesion within the tissue of the spinal cord. The word *syrinx* is derived from the Greek *surinx* for "pipe" or "channel." A syrinx is usually a chronic, progressive lesion with its specific location within the cord determining the constellation of neurologic findings. Ninety percent of patients with syringomyelia have a Chiari I malformation (projection of the cerebellar tonsils and medulla into the spinal canal) with nearly 5% of these patients requiring urgent surgical decompression due to acute neurologic deterioration.[7] This particular pathology, however, can be seen in almost all types of craniocervical junctional malformations.[8] Other etiologies of syringomyelia include spinal cord trauma (often months to years post-injury), compressive tumors, postinfectious (meningitis), and postinflammatory (transverse myelitis, MS).

Clinical Features. Headache and neck pain are the most common presenting complaints of patients with syringomyelia, followed by sensory disturbance, gait disorder, and lower cranial nerve dysfunction (CN IX–XII). Symptoms may be exacerbated by activities that increase intracranial pressure: sneeze, cough, or Valsalva maneuver. Patient-specific symptoms of syringomyelia develop and progress in accordance with the intracavitary pressure and anatomic location of the syrinx.

The most common features on physical examination are lower limb hyperreflexia, upper limb/hand weakness and muscle wasting, dissociated sensory loss, and gait abnormality. The classic pattern of sensory deficit involves a loss of pain and temperature sensation in the upper extremities with preservation of proprioception and light touch. This phenomenon is described as a "dissociative anesthesia" because of the discrepant loss of sensory modalities. This deficit often is described as being in a "capelike" distribution over the shoulders and arms. The anatomic basis for the neurologic features of a syrinx is the location near the central canal. Crossing fibers of the lateral spinothalamic tract carrying pain and temperature fibers are impaired while crude touch, position, and vibratory sensation from the posterior columns are unaffected. Sensory fibers from the lower limbs are similarly spared. Motor fibers from the corticospinal tract, when affected, will often result in upper extremity weakness due to the anatomic layout of the tract and the predominant cervical location of most syrinxes.

Differential Diagnoses. Considerations in the differential diagnosis for syrinx include intrinsic spinal tumor, demyelination, and trauma resulting in central cord syndrome.

Diagnostic Testing. Syringomyelia is best seen on MRI (Fig. 92.5). No other modality currently in widespread use is equivalent in diagnostic ability.

Management. When the diagnosis of syringomyelia is considered, emergent imaging in the ED may not be necessary if follow-up evaluation can be arranged; in approximately two-thirds of patients this condition is a slowly progressive process. If MRI studies are obtained and the diagnosis is made, referral to a neurosurgeon is indicated. Patients with acute neurologic deterioration, however, likely benefit from a more expedited evaluation, as urgent surgical decompression may be indicated in specific anatomic malformations (i.e., Chiari I malformations).

Human Immunodeficiency Virus Myelopathy

Human immunodeficiency virus (HIV) myelopathy typically occurs in patients with advanced HIV infection, often in conjunction with a

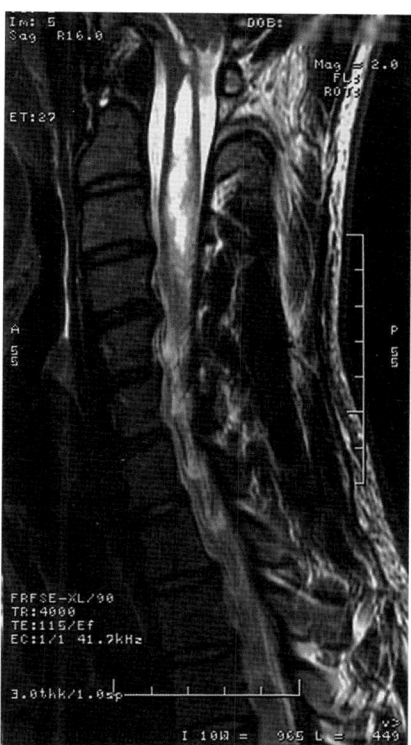

Fig. 92.5 T2-weighted magnetic resonance imaging of a patient with Chiari malformation and syringomyelia. (From: Batzdorf U. Syringomyelia. In: Shen FH, Samartzis D, Fessler RG, eds. *Textbook of the Cervical Spine*, ed 1. Maryland Heights: Saunders; 2015.)

very low CD4 count.[9] Weakness, gait disturbance, sphincter dysfunction, sensory abnormalities, and signs of spasticity are all features of this progressive process. Because diseases such as toxoplasmosis, lymphoma, varicella-zoster, and cytomegalovirus may produce a similar clinical picture in immunocompromised patients, HIV myelopathy is a diagnosis of exclusion. It more often affects the thoracic cord, so symptoms are frequently localized to the lower extremities. Treatment is primarily supportive, but improvement may be seen with utilization of highly active antiretroviral therapy (HAART).

Spinal Cord Infarction

Spinal cord infarction is extremely rare and considered a diagnosis of exclusion, but certain clinical clues may point to it. Aortic dissection, aortic surgery, and global ischemia are the most common causes. It can also occur as a complication of lupus or vasculitis or be cryptogenic. The clinical picture depends on the extent of infarct as well as the vascular territory affected (anterior versus posterior spinal artery). An anterior spinal cord syndrome is the most common clinical picture. Recovery is variable and etiology dependent.

Surfer's Myelopathy

Surfer's myelopathy is a recently described etiology of atraumatic cord dysfunction.[10] It is most often seen in novice or first-time surfers presenting with back pain, paresis, and urinary retention. Anesthesia or hyperesthesia may be present. The suggested mechanism is static hyperextension of the spine that occurs when lying prone on a surfboard with arms extended and head up for long periods of time, resulting in transient cord ischemia. Recovery is generally favorable but permanent paresis is possible. Awareness of this etiology is important, as it's symptoms mimic transverse myelitis.

Extrinsic Cord Lesions

Spinal Epidural Hematoma

Foundations. Spinal epidural hematoma (SEH) is a relatively rare condition where blood accumulates in the epidural space and can cause compression of the spinal cord. A hematoma may occur spontaneously but is more commonly traumatic or iatrogenic following lumbar puncture, epidural anesthesia, spinal surgery, and even acupuncture. SEH can occur at any level of the spine and can even extend to the cranium. It is more likely to occur in anticoagulated or thrombocytopenic patients such as those with liver disease or alcoholism. Spontaneous bleeding is rare but may arise from a spinal or dural arteriovenous malformation or a vertebral hemangioma. One-quarter of all cases are associated with anticoagulation therapy, including low-molecular-weight heparin and direct thrombin inhibitors.

Clinical Features. Patients usually present with sudden, severe, constant back pain. The pain is frequently radicular and may occur after a straining episode; it is often worsened by percussion over the spine and by maneuvers that increase intraspinal pressure (cough, sneeze, Valsalva).[11] Due to the severity of pain, patients are often in distress and seek care prior to the development of neurologic signs, which may actually lead to a delay in diagnosis. Neurologic deficits follow the onset of pain and may progress over a period of hours to days. Motor and sensory findings are variable because they depend on the level and size of the hematoma. Symptoms can include weakness, paralysis, loss of bowel or bladder function, and virtually any sensory deficit.

Differential Diagnoses. Considerations in the differential diagnosis include SEA, epidural neoplasm, acute disc herniation, and SSAH. SEH has even been known to mimic a stroke. This diagnosis should be considered in a patient presenting with a stroke syndrome who also has acute neck or back pain.

Diagnostic Testing. MRI with and without IV contrast is the diagnostic study of choice. CT myelography will frequently pick up the hematoma or show contrast medium in the subarachnoid space. The hematoma may initially be identified on CT due to its high density but is inferior to MRI in localizing and characterizing the lesion.

Management. In patients with SEH, recovery without surgery is rare. Neurosurgical consultation for emergent decompressive laminectomy is indicated as soon as the diagnosis is considered. Functional recovery is related both to the length of time the symptoms are present and to the initial neurologic status. Recovery after 72 hours of symptoms is rare but has been reported even without surgery, primarily in younger patients with rapidly improving symptoms. In the setting of anticoagulation therapy that is reversible, measures should be taken to do so.

Spinal Epidural Abscess

Foundations. Spinal epidural abscess (SEA) is an infectious process usually confined to the adipose tissue of the dorsal epidural space where there is a rich venous plexus. Abscesses that form in this space are limited by the bony confines of the spinal column. Damage to the spinal cord can be caused by direct compression on neural or vascular structures, but septic thrombophlebitis and vascular occlusion secondary to bacterial and inflammatory substances may also cause injury. Major risk factors for the development of SEA include underlying disease (immunosuppression, diabetes, chronic renal failure, alcoholism), spinal abnormality, recent spinal intervention (surgery, epidural analgesia), or local or systemic infection (skin and soft tissue infections, cystitis, sepsis, osteomyelitis, endocarditis, IV drug abuse), but the disease can be seen in individuals without any risk factors. The incidence of this disease is increasing, likely due to a higher rate of spinal instrumentation, an aging population, and higher prevalence of IV drug use. An acute or subacute presentation is most frequently seen in the ED, though some patients may develop a chronic form.

The thoracolumbar spine is the most frequent site of infection because the epidural space is larger and contains more adipose tissue. Infection typically extends over multiple vertebral segments but can also occur at noncontiguous locations. The dura mater limits the spread of an epidural infection, making subdural or intraspinal spread uncommon. Hematogenous spread to the epidural space from a discrete infection occurs in about half of the cases via the epidural space or the adjacent vertebra with subsequent extension into the epidural space. Local spread of bacteria occurs in another third of cases with the remainder having no clear source of infection identified.

Skin and soft tissue infections are the most frequently identified source of bacteria. *Staphylococcus aureus* is the most prevalent organism, cultured in nearly two-thirds of cases; the percentage of cases caused by MRSA has been increasing in recent years. Other frequently identified pathogens include gram-negative pathogens (*Escherichia coli, Pseudomonas aeruginosa*), *Streptococcus*, and coagulase-negative *Staphylococcus*. Anaerobic or fungal causes are rarely identified. *Mycobacterium tuberculosis* should be considered as a potential cause in the developing world. Multiple organisms are identified in 10% of cases.

Clinical Features. The clinical presentation of SEA begins with back pain localized to the level of the affected spine, often associated with tenderness to percussion. Symptoms usually progress over a few days but may extend for weeks. Radicular symptoms develop as the disease progresses to involve the nerve root radiating from the involved vertebrae. Without treatment, myelopathic signs will result, usually beginning with bowel and bladder disturbance. Weakness and sensory deficits develop, followed by paraplegia or quadriplegia. Once paralysis develops it quickly becomes irreversible within 24 to 48 hours. Bacteremia, either as a cause or as a result of SEA, may be present in over 50% of patients. Patients should be questioned about fevers, chills, or rigors, as they are present in up to 75% of cases. The classic triad of back pain, fever, and progressive neurologic deficits is rarely present and thus a delay in clinical diagnosis is common. In rare cases, SEA may also present as acute delirium.

Differential Diagnoses. SEA is frequently misdiagnosed on initial presentation, especially in a patient who is neurologically intact. In someone with infectious symptoms, more common causes such as cystitis, pneumonia, bacteremia, or osteomyelitis may be incorrectly diagnosed. Any compressive spinal lesion can mimic the neurologic manifestations of SEA.

Diagnostic Testing. MRI with IV contrast is the imaging modality of choice and should be performed emergently if the diagnosis of SEA is considered (see Fig. 92.3). CT myelography is also highly sensitive (>90%) in diagnosing SEA but MRI is more useful for surgical planning and differentiating a mass from an abscess.[12] Plain radiographs or noncontrast CT may show bony vertebral lysis but should not replace MRI.

A white blood cell (WBC) count is usually elevated and may support the diagnosis but is neither sensitive nor specific. The erythrocyte sedimentation rate (ESR) and C-reactive protein (CRP) tests, although not highly specific for epidural abscess, are virtually always elevated with this condition and have been studied as screening tests for SEA in certain "at-risk" populations.[12] Blood cultures are not beneficial in diagnosis but should be obtained as they may help to identify the causative organism. Lumbar puncture is relatively contraindicated with known or suspected SEA, because the procedure may further seed the infection. If performed, CSF findings are consistent with a parameningeal infection, showing protein elevation and increased inflammatory cells. The Gram stain is usually negative and CSF cultures are no more useful than blood cultures.

Management. Urgent surgical consultation for possible decompression is required for SEA. Antibiotics effective against the most common pathogens (particularly *S. aureus*) should be started empirically to cover gram-positive and gram-negative organisms: We recommend IV vancomycin (15 to 20 mg/kg IV every 8 to 12 hours) plus a third- or fourth-generation cephalosporin (e.g., ceftriaxone 2 g every 12 hours) or meropenem (2 g every 8 hours). If MSSA is a concern, nafcillin or oxacillin should be added. Cefepime (2 g every 8 hours) should be used in cases of known or suspected pseudomonas. CT-guided needle decompression is an option for drainage, particularly if the abscess is located posteriorly and the patient is a high-risk surgical candidate. Independent risk factors for failure of a nonoperative management plan include a motor deficit at the time of presentation, a pathologic or compression fracture, active malignancy, diabetes, and sensory changes.[13]

Outcome in SEA is related to the speed of diagnosis before the development of neurologic deficits. The primary indicator of final outcome is the patient's neurologic status just prior to the operating room. Even if treated, the disease can be fatal, and patients with neurologic changes rarely improve if surgical intervention is delayed more than 12 to 36 hours after onset of paralysis. Patients operated on before development of neurologic symptoms generally have good outcomes.

Discitis

Foundations. Discitis is an uncommon primary infection of the vertebral disc, specifically the nucleus pulposus, with secondary involvement of the cartilaginous end plate and vertebral body. Bacteria can spread to the disc by direct inoculation after surgical procedures, by local spread from infected tissue, or hematogenously. Children are more likely to develop primary infections of this space due to persistent vascular supply of the vertebral disc. Higher rates occur in immunocompromised patients and patients with systemic infections. The lumbar spine is the most common site of disease.

Clinical Features. Clinical presentation can be quite variable. In general, patients present with moderate to severe pain localized to the level of involvement and exacerbated by almost any movement of the spine. The hallmark of diagnosis, however, is a usual lack of neurologic deficits. In neonates or infants, cases are usually severe and present as sepsis with multiple infectious foci. In older children, symptom onset tends to be gradual; they may refuse to crawl, walk, or stand and demonstrate general irritability. Low-grade temperature elevations are noted in most patients. Radicular symptoms are present in 50% to 90% of cases. Because of the lack of neurologic deficits in the early stage, there is often a latent period (2 to 8 weeks) between the onset of back pain and the development of significant clinical findings on the physical examination. *S. aureus* is the most common pathogen, but gram-negative, fungal, and tuberculous infections have all been recognized. *Kingella kingae*, identified by PCR in a number of culture-negative cases of discitis, is an emerging pathogen in young children.[14]

Differential Diagnoses. Considerations in the differential diagnosis of discitis include vertebral osteomyelitis, spinal epidural abscess, neoplasm, and hematoma.

Diagnostic Testing. MRI with IV contrast is the radiographic study of choice for suspected discitis, because it not only enables diagnosis but also rules out paravertebral or epidural abscess. Plain radiographs usually are not helpful for early diagnosis of discitis, but destruction of the disc space is highly suggestive if present. Radiographic findings become abnormal after 2 to 4 weeks of disease. In addition to disc space narrowing, plain films may show irregular destruction of the vertebral body endplates. Aspiration of the affected disc for culture is generally

not performed. Laboratory studies often show an elevated ESR, but the WBC count is often normal and blood cultures are frequently negative.

Management. With timely diagnosis and treatment, outcome is usually very good and medical treatment with IV antibiotics that cover *Staphylococcus* and *Streptococcus* in accordance with local resistance patterns is usually curative. An antibiotic regimen similar to that recommended for the treatment of SEA is appropriate. Of note, *K. kingae* is covered by this treatment regimen. In a patient with a severe penicillin allergy or contraindication to a cephalosporin, meropenem (2 g IV) or aztreonam (2 g IV) may replace the cephalosporin. Finally, in patients with a vancomycin allergy or high resistance, linezolid (600 mg IV) is recommended. Surgery is generally not necessary.

Neoplasm

Foundations. Spinal cord tumors are classified according to their relationship to the dura and spinal cord (extradural, intradural extramedullary, and intradural intramedullary). Primary spinal cord tumors are generally benign but produce neurologic symptoms by compression, invasion, or destruction of myelinated tracts. The resulting neurologic symptoms are directly related to the growth rate and the location of the tumor. Overall, primary spinal cord tumors account for less than 10% of CNS tumors and only 1% of all cancers.

Most tumors affecting the spinal cord are metastatic in origin. Approximately 10% of patients with known cancer are diagnosed with a spinal metastasis at some point in the course of their disease; 5% to 10% of patients ultimately diagnosed with cancer first present with spinal metastases. Lung, breast, and prostate cancer represent the majority of the primary malignant neoplasms that subsequently develop spinal metastases, spreading both hematogenously and via direct extension. Intramedullary spinal cord metastases are rare. Multiple myeloma and lymphoma are generally more widespread at diagnosis but may also cause symptoms of cord compression. Most spinal lesions occur in the thoracic spine, but nearly 20% of patients with metastases will have lesions at multiple levels.[15]

Clinical Features. In nearly all patients with spinal neoplasm, the initial complaint is pain, either in the back at the level of the tumor or in a radicular distribution. Pain often is characterized as dull, constant, and aching and may worsen with recumbency (whereas pain from a herniated disc is classically improved when lying flat). Nighttime pain that is severe is characteristic of spinal neoplasm. Any action that increases intraspinal pressure may be associated with increased pain. Neurologic deficits vary by the location of the lesion. Metastatic spinal cord compression may present as a Brown-Séquard syndrome. Motor deficits are estimated to be found in almost half of patients at the time of initial diagnosis while sensory changes are less often reported. Besides a thorough neurologic examination, a search for possible primary sites of malignancy should be performed during the patient assessment.

Differential Diagnoses. Considerations in the differential diagnosis of spinal neoplasm include any of the compressive lesions (e.g., hematoma, infection, disc herniation). Tumors can also mimic intrinsic spinal cord lesions, such as transverse myelitis and cord infarction.

Diagnostic Testing. Patients presenting with new back pain (<6 weeks) and no risk factors or neurologic deficits on examination generally do not require imaging. If imaging is performed, plain radiographs are usually the initial modality in patients with minimal risk factors for or no previous diagnosis of cancer. The sensitivity and specificity of plain radiographs in detecting abnormalities consistent with malignancy are 60% and 95%, respectively.[15] In the presence of normal radiographs, an ESR measurement is helpful in that a cancer diagnosis is very unlikely in a patient with a normal ESR, normal radiographs, no clinical findings, and no or low risk for neoplasm. Patients with neurologic abnormalities, a history of cancer, and suspicious findings on plain films or elevated ESR are candidates for emergent MRI with IV contrast; in contrast-allergic patients, MRI without contrast is recommended.[13] CT myelography is an option if MRI is unavailable or the patient has contraindications.

Management. Acute compressive myelopathy from neoplasm constitutes an oncologic emergency. Immediate treatment is required to preserve function and prevent deterioration. With onset of paraplegia and incontinence, less than 5% of patients regain ambulatory status. Of patients who are ambulatory at the time of diagnosis, 60% will remain ambulatory. Spinal instability or neurologic deficits are indications for immediate surgical decompression. In patients with symptoms of cord compression, high-dose glucocorticoid therapy is recommended (i.e., 10 mg dexamethasone IV followed by 4 mg orally every 6 hours). Higher initial doses of dexamethasone have not been associated with better outcomes. Steroids are generally not initiated in patients with small lesions or in the presence of a normal neurologic examination.[16] Radiation therapy is frequently indicated in the treatment of spinal cord tumors and can be combined with surgical intervention, if indicated.

CHRONIC COMPLICATIONS OF SPINAL CORD INJURY

Autonomic Dysreflexia

Foundations

Autonomic dysreflexia (AD) is defined as the loss of coordination between heart rate and vascular tone in response to increased demand. It can be seen in spinal cord injury (SCI) due to a disruption of splanchnic innervation that occurs when the lesion is at or above the T6 level. Noxious stimuli below the injury level can result in an uninhibited sympathetic response causing vasoconstriction and resultant hypertension that is not overcome by compensatory parasympathetic activity (bradycardia and vasodilation) above the lesion. Over 50% of SCI patients suffer from AD with most developing symptoms within the first year post-injury. Common examples of noxious stimuli are bladder distention, bowel impaction, pain (even from sources as seemingly benign as in-grown toenails), pressure ulcers, tight clothing, and infection. AD will persist until the underlying cause is resolved.

Clinical Features

AD is defined as an elevation in systolic blood pressure 20 to 40 mm Hg or greater from baseline (15 to 20 mm Hg in pediatric population) or a systolic reading of 150 mm Hg or greater with symptoms in the absence of a known baseline; 88% of patients will present with severe headache and diaphoresis above the spinal level. Other possible symptoms include nasal congestion, blurred vision, anxiety, and nausea. There may be accompanying bradycardia due to the parasympathetic compensation but the absence of it does not rule out AD.

Management

Treatment centers on managing blood pressure while working to identify and treat the underlying cause. Assessing for bladder distention and, if present, relieving by catheterization or the flushing of an obstructed indwelling catheter may be necessary. Digital rectal exam will help assess for fecal impaction and a full skin examination will identify pressure ulcers, skin infections, or lesions. Removing tight clothing and sitting the patient upright if possible may help to engage hydrostatic redistribution.

Topical, oral, or IV anti-hypertensive medications may be indicated when an elevated blood pressure persists in order to prevent acute complications of severe hypertension. Application of 1 to 2 inches of 2% nitroglycerin paste to the skin above the spinal lesion is recommended to relax vascular smooth muscles and cause vasodilation. Likewise, IV nitroglycerin (5 mcg/minute increasing by 20 mcg/minute every 1 to 3 minutes to a maximum of 400 mcg/min) for severe cases is indicated. Beta blockers are avoided to prevent potential uninhibited alpha-adrenergic activity but not contraindicated. Oral anticholinergics and botulinum toxin injections into the bladder have been used to help manage neurogenic detrusor overactivity, the most common cause of bladder distention resulting in AD, but would be of little benefit in severe, acute cases in the ED.

Spasticity

More than 60% of SCI patients will develop spasticity to some degree, defined as a velocity-dependent increase in muscle tone (hyperexcitability). It is thought to be caused by disruption of descending inhibitory modulation of alpha-motor neurons. Care should be taken when evaluating spasticity because a sudden increase in patient or caregiver reported spasticity may be indicative of occult infection.

Treating spasticity is not only difficult but may not be beneficial as spasms and contractures can aid the patient or caregiver in transfer or other activities. Any suggested treatment should focus on functionality and often starts with physical therapy (stretching, braces) and progresses to include medications such as baclofen (5 mg PO 1 to 3 times daily, increasing by 5 mg per dose every 3 days up to 80 mg/day in divided doses), tizanidine (2 mg PO at bedtime, initially, increasing by 4 mg daily dose every 3 to 4 days up to 36 mg/day given in 3 to 4 doses), and benzodiazepines; unfortunately, these medications have little proven efficacy aside from tizanidine and are frequently limited by their sedative properties.

Infection

Pneumonia is a frequent complication of SCI with roughly 50% of SCI patients developing it during their acute hospital stay post-injury; it is often the ultimate cause of death in SCI patients. Pressure ulcers, frequently located over bony prominences, are an additional nidus of infection and a thorough skin exam should be performed on any SCI patient presenting with infectious signs or symptoms.

Urinary tract infections (UTIs) occur at an estimated rate of 2.5 episodes per patient per year and are the third leading cause of death among this population. This high rate is primarily due to patients with chronic indwelling catheters but also includes patients who void, have suprapubic catheters, or intermittently catheterize. In the latter group, it is thought that frequent catheterization not only introduces bacteria but the scheduled nature of the procedure allows for large volumes of urine to collect in the bladder prior to drainage, increasing the risk of infection. Symptomatic UTIs frequently present with fevers, foul-smelling urine, increased spasticity, or autonomic dysreflexia and should be treated with antibiotics. Asymptomatic bacteriuria, however, should not be treated as doing so has no effect on the frequency of symptomatic infections and risks increasing microbial resistance. An additional consideration in the management of symptomatic UTI is to consider a diagnosis of infected renal calculi in that up to 20% of SCI patients have hypercalciuria from altered bone metabolism which contributes to higher rates of nephrolithiasis.

The references for this chapter can be found online at ExpertConsult. com.

93

Peripheral Nerve Disorders

Ethan E. Abbott and E. Bradshaw Bunney

OVERVIEW

Principles

The nervous system is divided into central nervous system (CNS) and peripheral nervous system (PNS) components. The PNS is subdivided into 12 cranial and 31 spinal nerves. Disorders of the cranial nerves are discussed in Chapter 91. Because diseases of the neuromuscular junction and the myopathies are located distal to the neuron itself, they are also considered separately in Chapter 95. Radiculopathies, which are disorders of the roots of the PNS, are so commonly associated with musculoskeletal neck and back pain that they are mentioned only briefly here and are discussed in detail in Chapter 36.

Current estimates suggest that about 2.4% of the population suffers from peripheral neuropathy, rising to 8% for those over 50 years of age. Diabetes mellitus is a leading contributor.

The simplest approach to categorizing diseases of the PNS is to distinguish focal from nonfocal disease. In the PNS, the first broad category is the focal group, which is divided into those with evidence of single versus multiple lesions of peripheral nerves, known respectively as *simple mononeuropathies* and *multiple mononeuropathies* (or *mononeuropathy multiplex*). The second broad category, which constitutes the nonfocal group of peripheral neuropathies, contains the polyneuropathies. These tend to produce bilaterally symmetrical symptoms and signs, reflecting the widespread nature of the underlying pathologic processes.

The evaluation of PNS disease involves a goal-directed history and physical examination targeted at answering the three questions, each of which corresponds to a stratum of the algorithm presented in Figure 93.1:

1. Are the sensorimotor signs and symptoms symmetrical or asymmetrical?
2. Are the sensorimotor signs and symptoms distal or both proximal and distal?
3. Is the modality involved exclusively motor, sensory, or mixed sensorimotor?

By systematically combining responses to these questions, seven discrete categories of peripheral neuropathy are identified, each of which contains a finite set of possible diagnoses. Because pure motor or pure sensory findings tend to occur mainly in an asymmetrical, distal distribution, this is the only category in Figure 93.1 subdivided into pure motor and pure sensory abnormalities.

The spinal component of the PNS is shown schematically in Figure 93.2. The anterior and posterior nerve roots exit the spinal cord at each segmental level. Just distal to the dorsal root ganglion they converge to form a mixed (motor and sensory) spinal nerve, of which there are 31

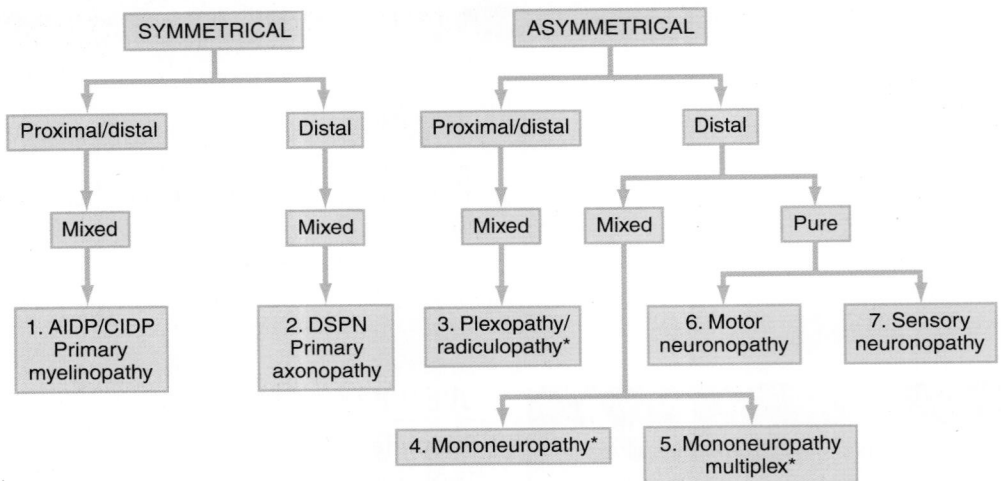

Fig. 93.1 An approach to peripheral neuropathy in the emergency department. *AIDP,* Acute inflammatory demyelinating polyneuropathy (Guillain-Barré syndrome); *CIDP,* chronic inflammatory demyelinating polyneuropathy; *DSPN,* distal symmetrical polyneuropathy. *A proximal distribution of sensorimotor findings may dominate the clinical picture in patterns 3, 4, and 5, depending on the location of the lesions.

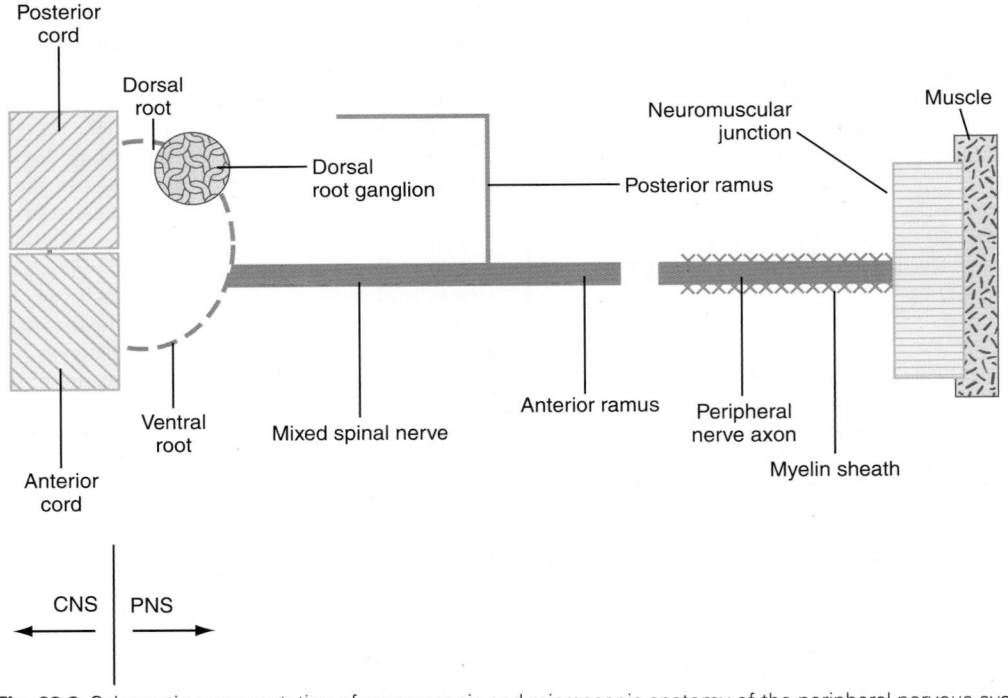

Fig. 93.2 Schematic representation of macroscopic and microscopic anatomy of the peripheral nervous system *(PNS)* and its interface with the central nervous system *(CNS)*. See the text for an explanation.

pairs: 8 cervical, 12 thoracic, 5 lumbar, 5 sacral, and 1 coccygeal. The spinal nerves immediately bifurcate into anterior (ventral) and posterior (dorsal) rami. The posterior ramus travels to the back. The anterior ramus innervates the anterolateral portion of the body and supplies all peripheral nerves for the upper and lower extremities through the brachial and lumbosacral plexus, respectively. Interweaving of fibers occurs within a plexus, producing a mixed sensorimotor innervation of peripheral nerves exiting the plexus.

In addition to the motor and sensory modalities of the PNS, the autonomic nervous system has a peripheral component. Anatomically and functionally, the autonomic nervous system is divided into two parts: (1) a sympathetic (thoracolumbar) component and (2) a parasympathetic (craniosacral) component. Autonomic dysfunction may cause systemic abnormalities, such as orthostasis, or local problems, such as atrophic, dry skin.

The PNS has three basic categories of pathology (see Fig. 93.2): (1) the myelinopathies, in which the primary site of involvement is limited to the myelin sheath surrounding the axon; (2) the axonopathies, in which the primary site of involvement is the axon, with or without secondary demyelination; and (3) the neuronopathies, in which the cell body of the neuron itself is the primary site of involvement, ultimately affecting the entire peripheral nerve. Although overlap occurs, each of

BOX 93.1 Causes of Acute, Emergent Weakness and Possible Respiratory Compromise

Autoimmune
  Demyelinating
  • Guillain-Barré syndrome (GBS)
  • Chronic inflammatory demyelinating polyneuropathy
  Myasthenia gravis
Toxic
  Botulism
  Buckthorn
  Seafood
  • Paralytic shellfish toxin
  • Tetrodotoxin (puffer fish, newts)
  Tick paralysis
  Metals
Arsenic
Thallium
Metabolic
  Dyskalemic syndromes
  • Acquired (especially with thyrotoxicosis)
  • Familial
  Hypophosphatemia
  Hypermagnesemia
  Porphyria
Infectious
  Poliomyelitis
  Diphtheria

Note: Although several of the disorders listed are myopathies (see Chapter 95) rather than peripheral neuropathies, they are combined here to emphasize the importance of identifying patients at risk for respiratory failure early in the course of their evaluation.

TABLE 93.1 Patterns and Prototypes of Peripheral Neuropathies

Type	Pattern Distribution	Prototypical Disease Modalities
1	Proximal and distal, symmetrical, sensorimotor polyneuropathy	GBS
	Proximal and distal	Symmetrical
	Motor > sensory	
2	Distal, symmetrical, sensorimotor polyneuropathy	Diabetic DSPN
	Distal	Symmetrical
	Sensory > motor	
3	Proximal and distal, asymmetrical, sensorimotor neuropathy	Brachial plexopathy
	Proximal and distal	Asymmetrical
	Sensory and motor	
4	Distal, asymmetrical, sensorimotor mononeuropathy	CTS (median mononeuropathy)
	Distal	Asymmetrical
	Sensory and motor	
5	Distal, asymmetrical, sensorimotor mononeuropathy multiplex	Vasculitic mononeuropathy multiplex
	Distal	Asymmetrical
	Sensory and motor	
6	Distal, asymmetrical, pure motor neuronopathy	ALS
	Distal	Asymmetrical
	Motor	
7	Distal, asymmetrical, pure sensory neuronopathy	Pyridoxine toxicity
	Distal	Asymmetrical
	Sensory	

ALS, Amyotrophic lateral sclerosis; *CTS*, carpal tunnel syndrome; *DSPN*, distal symmetrical polyneuropathy; *GBS*, Guillain-Barré syndrome.

these prototypes has a distinctive clinical presentation, electrophysiologic profile, and microscopic appearance.

Differential Diagnosis

The differential diagnosis for any patient presenting with sensory, motor, or sensorimotor complaints, particularly if they are localized to the extremities, should include a peripheral neuropathy. Within this group, patients with focal weakness are most concerning, because they are at greatest risk for respiratory compromise. Box 93.1 lists the causes of acute weakness that may affect respiration.

As soon as the emergent causes of weakness have been excluded, the individuals with focal weakness are next assessed to exclude CNS disease (e.g., stroke; see Chapter 87). After a CNS cause has been exonerated, the systematic evaluation of peripheral neuropathy is performed. The distinguishing features of each of the seven peripheral neuropathic patterns are described by distribution and modality and represented by a disease prototype (see Fig. 93.1; Table 93.1).

Diagnostic Testing

Testing in the evaluation of the patient with a suspected peripheral neuropathy is presented in Box 93.2. Electrophysiologic testing (nerve conduction studies [NCSs] and needle electromyography [EMG]) detects underlying pathologic abnormalities. Because neither test is readily available in the acute care setting, they are discussed only briefly here. Information gathered from these tests can be used to obtain objective information regarding the anatomic distribution of involvement (symmetrical versus asymmetrical and distal versus proximal and distal) and the modalities involved (sensory, motor, or mixed).

NCSs and EMG can also identify the level of the neuraxis affected by the disease process (i.e., root, plexus, or nerve). If the nerve is affected, electrophysiologic testing can help determine whether the lesion is mononeuropathic (either an isolated mononeuropathy or mononeuropathy multiplex) or polyneuropathic.

Finally, EMG and NCSs can distinguish axonal from myelin disease, further narrowing the differential diagnosis. Prognosis is determined by the nature of pathologic involvement of the PNS. Primary demyelination spares the axon and thus carries the best prognosis. The prognosis is worse in axonopathies because reestablishment of nerve function is dependent on the much slower process of axonal regeneration. Neuronopathies, which begin with primary destruction of the nerve cell body, produce pure motor or pure sensory syndromes. Eventually the entire nerve is affected, resulting in the worst prognosis of the three.

Antibody tests are commercially available that aim to aid in the diagnosis of peripheral neuropathies, especially those that are immune-mediated in etiology. However they are controversial, lack sensitivity and specificity, and may offer limited benefit beyond the focused neurologic examination and existing screening tests.

BOX 93.2   Ancillary Diagnostic Testing in Suspected Peripheral Neuropathy

Obtained in Most Patients

Complete blood count
Erythrocyte sedimentation rate
Glucose
Creatine kinase
Creatinine

Obtained in Some Patients Based on History

Human chorionic gonadotropin
Magnesium
Phosphate
Vitamin B_{12}
Hemoglobin A_{1c}
Serum protein electrophoresis with immune fixation electrophoresis
Venereal Disease Research Laboratory (VDRL) or rapid plasma reagin screen with fluorescent treponemal antibody absorption test, as appropriate
Thyroid function
Human immunodeficiency virus (HIV) titer
Lyme enzyme-linked immunosorbent assay and Western blot
Rheumatoid factor and antinuclear antibody
Blood, urine, hair, or nails for metal, depending on suspected chronicity of exposure
Specific serum antibodies to components of peripheral nervous system (PNS)
Cerebrospinal fluid (CSF) for cells, protein, Lyme titer
Electrodiagnostic testing
    Nerve conduction studies (NCS)
    Electromyography (EMG)
Neurodiagnostic imaging
    Magnetic resonance imaging (MRI)
    Computed tomography (CT)
    Sonography
Quantitative sensory testing
Nerve biopsy
    Sural
    Intraepidermal nerve fiber density

BOX 93.3   Demyelinating Polyneuropathies

Guillain-Barré syndrome (GBS)
    Acute inflammatory demyelinating polyradiculoneuropathy
    Acute motor axonal neuropathy
    Acute motor and sensory axonal neuropathy
    Miller Fisher syndrome
Chronic inflammatory demyelinating polyradiculoplexoneuropathy
Malignant disease
Human immunodeficiency virus (HIV) infection
Hepatitis B
Buckthorn
Diphtheria

Campylobacter jejuni infection is the most commonly associated etiology for GBS with a frequency reported in 25% to 50% of adult cases.[2] Cytomegalovirus, Epstein-Barr virus, and *Mycoplasma pneumonia* have also been associated with the subsequent development of GBS.

Clinical Features

The majority of patients with GBS seek treatment days to weeks after resolution of an upper respiratory or gastrointestinal illness; patients present with progressive, symmetrical distal (and usually to a lesser extent proximal) weakness. Symptom progression ranges from rapidly progressive to a more insidious course over days to weeks. Signs and symptoms are usually worse in the lower extremities and are associated with diminution or loss of deep tendon reflexes (DTRs) in the affected limbs, variable sensory findings, and sparing of the anal sphincter. The presence of distal paresthesias increases the likelihood of GBS as the diagnosis.

About half of patients with GBS have autonomic dysfunction, experience a peak of disease severity within a week of onset, have some form of cranial nerve involvement (usually cranial nerve VII), and suffer long-term sequelae of their illness.

Patients with neck or bulbar weakness are more likely to require mechanical ventilation than those patients without. Predicting outcomes among GBS patients can be challenging and several scoring systems are available to aid with prognosis in the inpatient setting. The Erasmus GBS outcome score (EGOS) is a validated prognostic scoring tool, performed at 14 days of admission, that utilizes three measures: age of onset of disease, the presence or absence of diarrhea, and then folds in another scoring system, the GBS disability score, to predict inability to ambulate independently at 6 months. A modified EGOS (mEGOS) utilizes Medical Research Council score (MRC) instead of the GBS disability score and can be used earlier, at one week of admission. There is no score to predict outcomes from the ED, however.

Diagnostic Testing

GBS is typically diagnosed on clinical findings, but additional testing with EMG is indicated when the diagnosis is uncertain. The most frequent finding of demyelination includes nerve conduction slowing with prolonged distal motor latency.

In addition to electrophysiologic testing, cerebrospinal fluid (CSF) analysis and respiratory function testing may aid in the diagnosis of GBS. CSF analysis is useful when it demonstrates the characteristic picture of markedly elevated protein with only a mild pleocytosis (albuminocytologic dissociation). In the clinical setting of suspected GBS, this finding is highly specific. Early in the disease, however, patients may have normal CSF values. One study noted only 50% of patients had elevated protein and mild pleocytosis in the first week of symptoms, rising to 75% in the third week. Consequently, normal CSF

SPECIFIC TYPES OF NEUROPATHIES

Type 1: Demyelinating Polyneuropathy (Guillain-Barré Syndrome)

Principles

The pattern of symmetrical weakness, usually worse distally, accompanied by variable sensory findings is characteristic of acute Guillain-Barré syndrome (GBS). It is a heterogeneous and unpredictable disorder, characterized by areflexic paralysis with albuminocytologic dissociation, with marked variation in latency between antecedent infection and symptom onset.

Mortality rates in Europe and North America are estimated between 3% and 7% and up to 20% of patients remain disabled after six months, unable to ambulate without assistance.[1]

The most common form of GBS is an acute inflammatory demyelinating polyneuropathy, representing 90% of the cases seen in the United States. Less common variants are acute motor axonal neuropathy, acute motor and sensory axonal neuropathy, and the Miller Fisher syndrome. Acute motor axonal neuropathy, which accounts for most of the remaining cases seen in the United States, afflicts those of Asian descent more often. Miller Fisher syndrome is a rare form of GBS characterized by the triad of ophthalmoplegia, ataxia, and areflexia (Box 93.3).

cannot be used to exclude GBS, though a lumbar puncture performed early in the disease process can help identify infectious or neoplastic causes that may present similarly to GBS. Because of the potential for a missed diagnosis, a lumbar puncture should be performed in the emergency department for patients in whom there is concern for GBS.

Individuals with suspected GBS should have their respiratory function tested, as they may present without overt signs of respiratory distress. A decrease in forced vital capacity (FVC) to less than 20 mL/kg is associated with pending respiratory failure and the need for intubation, whereas patients with an FVC of more than 40 mL/kg do not usually require intubation. Likewise, patients with a negative inspiratory force of less than 30 cm H_2O are more likely to require mechanical ventilation. Other tests, such as the forced expiratory volume in 1 second (FEV_1) and peak flow rate (PFR), can also be used to assess respiratory function, but there has been limited study of these modalities. A PFR of less than 250 L/min increased the likelihood of needing mechanical ventilation in a retrospective study of patients with GBS. Patients unable to perform these tests and those with less than 100% of predicted values should have a blood gas performed to assess for hypercapnia and an impending need for mechanical ventilation. However, hypercapnia may be a late sign of weakness, and therefore, the decision to intubate should be made considering the overall clinical picture.

Management

In practice, patients with symmetrical weakness of relatively acute onset, decreased or absent DTRs, and variable degrees of sensory loss are managed as if they have GBS or one of its variants. These patients are at risk for respiratory compromise, which develops in 20% of patients. Conversely, patients with predominantly sensory signs and symptoms are less likely to develop acute respiratory distress and have a more favorable prognosis.

The definitive treatments for GBS are plasma exchange or intravenous immune globulin (IVIG). Both of these treatments are supported by well-designed studies, although there are no studies comparing IVIG to placebo. Combination or sequential therapy confers no therapeutic advantage over either intervention alone. Plasma exchange is cumbersome and not available at many hospitals. IVIG is more readily available and is usually administered in a dose of 400 mg/kg per day for 5 days. However, IVIG is expensive, costing roughly double a standard course of plasma exchange.

Corticosteroids are not recommended; oral steroids have been shown to delay recovery, and intravenous steroids alone have no benefit. The combination of intravenous steroids and IVIG may hasten recovery but does not have an effect on long-term outcome and is not currently recommended.[3]

Disposition

Patients with suspected GBS should receive neurologic consultation and admission for respiratory monitoring and treatment with either plasma exchange or IVIG. Evidence of alveolar hypoventilation (elevated carbon dioxide [Pco_2]) in a patient with an unsecured airway requires an intensive care level of monitoring, as these patients may require intubation.

Type 2: Distal Symmetrical Polyneuropathy

Principles

Distal symmetrical polyneuropathy (DSPN) is the most common type of peripheral neuropathy. Diabetes, alcoholism, human immunodeficiency virus (HIV) disease, and toxic metabolic causes are the most frequent etiologies (Box 93.4). DSPN in diabetics, termed *diabetic polyneuropathy,* is the most common chronic complication of diabetes mellitus.

BOX 93.4 Distal Sensorimotor Polyneuropathies

Diabetes mellitus
Alcoholism
Neoplastic or paraneoplastic
Hereditary motor and sensory neuropathies (Charcot-Marie-Tooth)
Cryptogenic sensorimotor polyneuropathies
HIV infection
Toxins
  Organic or industrial agents
  • Acrylamide
  • Allyl chloride
  • Carbon disulfide
  • Ethylene oxide
  • Hexacarbons
  • Methyl bromide
  • Organophosphate-induced delayed polyneuropathy
  • Polychlorinated biphenyls
  • Trichloroethylene
  • Vacor
  Metals
  • Arsenic
  • Gold
  • Mercury (inorganic)
  • Thallium
  Therapeutic agents
  • Amiodarone
  • Antiretrovirals
  • Dapsone
  • Disulfiram
  • Isoniazid
  • Metronidazole
  • Nitrofurantoin
  • Paclitaxel (Taxol)
  • Phenytoin
  • Statins (HMG-CoA reductase inhibitors)
  • Thalidomide
  • Vinca alkaloids (vincristine, vinblastine)
Nutritional
  • Beriberi (thiamine or vitamin B_1)
  • Pellagra (niacin, B vitamins)
  • Pernicious anemia (vitamin B_{12})
  • Pyridoxine deficiency (vitamin B_6)
End-organ dysfunction
  • Acromegaly
  • Chronic pulmonary disease
  • Hypothyroidism
  • Renal failure (uremic neuropathy)
Paraproteinemias
  • Amyloidosis
  • Monoclonal gammopathy of unknown significance
  • Multiple myeloma
  • Waldenström macroglobulinemia
Porphyria

HIV, Human immunodeficiency virus; *HMG-CoA,* hydroxymethylglutaryl coenzyme A.

Although the association between alcoholism and peripheral neuropathy has been well established for centuries, demonstration of a direct neurotoxic effect of alcohol remains elusive. The preponderance of evidence from both observational studies in humans and experimental data from animal models suggests that the association between alcohol and peripheral neuropathy may be confounded by nutritional status (i.e., deficiency states might be the true underlying cause of alcoholic peripheral neuropathy).

With the widespread use of highly active and effective antiretroviral treatment, peripheral neuropathies have become the most common neurologic complication of HIV infection. The typical HIV neuropathy is a DSPN, estimated to affect up to 35% of the HIV population; the pathogenesis is currently unknown.

Clinical Findings

Most polyneuropathies are characterized by a pattern of distal, symmetrical sensorimotor findings, worse in the lower than in the upper extremities, with a stocking-glove distribution of sensory abnormalities that gradually diminishes as one moves proximally. Motor weakness and loss of DTRs, which lag behind the sensory features, follow a similar pattern of progression from distal to proximal. The diffuse, distal, symmetrical nature of this pattern is most consistent with a toxic-metabolic disease process that causes a length-dependent axonopathy.

Initial symptoms usually consist of "positive" sensory complaints (e.g., dysesthesias, such as tingling and burning) beginning on the plantar surfaces of both feet. At the early stages of a typical DSPN, there may be some asymmetry. At this juncture, it may be impossible to distinguish a focal neuropathic process such as a mononeuropathy from a polyneuropathy, although this location strongly favors a polyneuropathy. As the process advances, the plantar surfaces of both feet become dysesthetic before the dorsum of either foot is involved.

Weakness of dorsiflexion of the big toe is usually the first motor sign, followed by weakness of foot dorsiflexion, footdrop, loss of the Achilles reflex, and later a "steppage gait," in which footdrop causes the toes to point downward and scrape the ground while walking, requiring the patient to lift the leg higher than normal when walking.

Sensory loss continues to move proximally, and before it reaches the knees, the fingertips are usually involved. DTRs are progressively lost, as is proprioception. If loss of proprioception becomes severe, patients may develop sensory ataxia. As the neuropathy continues to progress, sensory abnormalities ultimately involve all modalities and extend to a diamond-shaped periumbilical area. Far-advanced disease may affect sensation over the skull vertex and facial midline structures. Atrophy and areflexia occur as weakness worsens. Severely impaired patients may be unable to ambulate or to grasp objects. These symptoms have an impact on the patient's quality of life, affecting not only physical functioning but also sleep and emotional and social functioning. Many of these patients display signs of depression or anxiety. Polyneuropathies can be difficult to diagnose and are best approached by the performance of electrodiagnostic studies for patients with a constellation of symptoms and signs suggesting a particular neuropathy.

Diabetic foot ulcers are a common and often late complication of diabetes, ranging from 2% to 10% of the population. Repetitive stress or unperceived minor trauma is the leading cause, likely from the associated polyneuropathy.

The clinical picture of alcoholic neuropathy is similar to that of diabetic DSPN. However, in alcoholism, severe myopathy and cerebellar degeneration often complicate the clinical picture. Autonomic skin changes with atrophy and hair loss accompany the sensorimotor abnormalities. Often, other systemic effects of alcoholism are so severe that the patient may not notice the neuropathic symptoms.

Differential Diagnosis

Box 93.4 lists the differential diagnoses of DSPN. On the basis of results from a case-control study, the statins have been added to the list of drugs that are implicated.

Diagnostic Testing

Electrodiagnostic studies are commonly employed in the evaluation of DSPN. This includes both NCSs and needle electromyelography. Screening laboratory tests should be considered for all patients who present with DSPN. The high yield tests in evaluating a DSPN include blood glucose, serum B12, and serum protein immunofixation electrophoresis. A complete blood count (CBC), comprehensive metabolic panel, hemoglobin A1c or oral glucose tolerance test, and thyroid-stimulating hormone (TSH) are recommended as part of the initial workup.

Management

In diabetic DSPN, the initial steps in management focus on tight glucose control and lifestyle modifications. Tight glucose control in type 1 diabetes is associated with a more profound reduction in the incidence of DSPN than is found among those with type 2 diabetes. If discomfort is severe, the etiology of the neuropathy seems likely to be diabetic, and referral is delayed, it may be necessary to provide the patient with some symptomatic relief. Because the treatment of neuropathic pain has traditionally been linked to etiology, the choice of pharmacologic agents is empirical with substantial practice variation. Nonsteroidal antiinflammatory drugs (NSAIDs) have little proven efficacy and a high potential for renal impairment; therefore they are not a first-line therapy. Pregabalin, duloxetine, and tapentadol have all received regulatory approval by the US Food and Drug Administration for the treatment of DSPN, with duloxetine and pregabalin considered first-line treatments.[4] Pregabalin has a mechanism of action similar to that of gabapentin and is dosed at 50 to 150 mg/day in divided doses. Duloxetine, a selective serotonin and norepinephrine reuptake inhibitor, is effective at a dose of 60 mg per day. Tapentadol ER, dosed at 50 mg twice daily, also provides pain relief in patients with diabetic neuropathy, however, given the risk of addiction with opioids, it is not considered a first-line agent.[5] Other evidence supports the use of tricyclic antidepressants, anticonvulsants, and the serotonin and norepinephrine reuptake inhibitor duloxetine. Imipramine or amitriptyline are started at a daily dose of 25 mg at bedtime (10 mg in the elderly) and titrated slowly up to a dose of 100 mg. Gabapentin 900 to 3600 mg per day in divided doses are also effective treatments. Tramadol, a centrally acting analgesic and mixed opioid, has been effective in several trials for the treatment of DSPN, but safety concerns regarding its abuse potential make it a less desirable option. Topical capsaicin provides relief in some patients, but the burning associated with its application has limited its use. Topical lidocaine patches, 5%, are yet another option.

We recommend pregabalin, duloxetine, or gabapentin at a low dose to manage the pain from DSPN; this is best done in consultation with the patient's primary physician who can then titrate to therapeutic effect on follow-up. In patients who have localized symptoms, who cannot tolerate the side effects or have the potential for adverse drug interactions, topical agents such as lidocaine patches or capsaicin cream can be offered. In addition to pain management as discussed earlier, all patients with suspected alcoholic DSPN should receive dietary supplements and referral for outpatient management.

There are no first-line agents for the treatment of HIV-associated neuropathy, and limited randomized controlled trials have not demonstrated any specific analgesic that is more effective over placebo.

Type 3: Asymmetric Proximal and Distal Peripheral Neuropathies (Radiculopathies and Plexopathies)

Radiculopathies and plexopathies often result from trauma (Box 93.5). In general, a plexopathy, whether brachial or lumbosacral, is identified by process of elimination (i.e., a pattern of sensorimotor and reflex

BOX 93.5 Asymmetrical Proximal and Distal Peripheral Neuropathies

Brachial Plexopathy
Open
   Direct plexus injury (knife or gunshot wound)
   Neurovascular (plexus ischemia)
   Iatrogenic (central line insertion)
Closed
   Traction injuries
     • "Stingers" (neck or shoulder injury resulting in transient brachial plexus injury)
     • Traction neurapraxia
     • Partial or complete nerve root avulsion
   Radiation
   Neoplastic
   Idiopathic brachial plexitis
   Thoracic outlet

Lumbosacral Plexopathies
Open
Closed
   Traction injuries
     • Pelvic double vertical shearing fracture
     • Posterior hip dislocation
     • Retroperitoneal hemorrhage
   Vasospastic (deep buttock injection)
   Neoplastic
   Radiation
   Idiopathic lumbosacral plexitis
   Infectious
     • Herpesvirus (sacrococcygeal)
     • Herpes simplex 2
     • Herpes zoster
     • Cytomegalovirus polyradiculopathy (HIV infection)

HIV, Human immunodeficiency virus.

abnormalities that fit neither a radicular nor an individual peripheral nerve distribution). Although this approach does not exclude a mononeuropathy multiplex on physical examination alone, a careful history should determine whether the patient is at risk for development of a mononeuropathy or plexopathy based on underlying disease

Most plexopathies are seen in young men after motor vehicle accidents, many of whom present for evaluation of radicular pain several months after the initial injury. Therapeutic intervention is often delayed to maximize the potential for spontaneous recovery. Several surgical repairs exist, including neurotization.

Radiation (actinic) plexopathy occurs after a variable period of latency following treatment, which may extend to 20 years or more. Almost all series include women who received radiation treatment for breast cancer. Among neoplastic causes, most originate from the lung or breast. Patients with probable neoplastic brachial plexopathy need imaging studies and may require immediate radiation therapy. Pain control is the focus of management.

Thoracic outlet syndrome (TOS) describes a constellation of symptoms caused by compression of the neurovascular bundle at the thoracic outlet. As our understanding of this condition has improved, treatment has evolved but remains controversial. Manifestations include both neurogenic and vascular (arterial or venous) TOS. It is estimated that over 90% of cases are neurogenic in origin; 3% to 5% are venous, and less than 1% are arterial.

Neurogenic TOS is caused by compression of the brachial plexus, presenting with upper extremity weakness, numbness, paresthesias, and pain in a nonradicular distribution. Symptoms are usually present during normal daily activities and sleep. Treatment is typically nonsurgical, involving education, activity modification, and physical therapy.

Vascular TOS can be either arterial or venous and is characterized by swelling of the upper extremity, pain, and a feeling of heaviness after exertion. Discoloration can also be seen. If arterial TOS is occurring, caused by compression of the subclavian artery, the typical findings of arterial insufficiency can be seen—pain, numbness, coolness, pallor. Treatment is typically surgical, involving decompression of the thoracic outlet.

Because of the complexity of plexopathies, the goal in the ED is to localize the probable pathologic process to the brachial or lumbosacral plexus. Depending on severity and suspected etiology, the patient should either be admitted or referred to a neurologist with experience in PNS disease.

Type 4: Isolated Mononeuropathies

The pattern of asymmetrical, sensorimotor, usually distal, peripheral neuropathy is characteristic of a mononeuropathy. Mononeuropathies are of two main types: isolated and multiple. The isolated mononeuropathies are discussed in this section; the multiple mononeuropathies, also termed mononeuropathy multiplex, are discussed in the next section as a Type 5 peripheral neuropathy.

Isolated mononeuropathies are usually caused by trauma, either blunt or penetrating (Box 93.6). If the trauma is blunt, the injury may be secondary to compression from an internal or external source. Entrapment neuropathies are a subset of compression neuropathies occurring at anatomic locations where nerves traverse potentially constricting compartments or tunnels. Isolated mononeuropathies may be acute, intermittent, or chronic and continuous. Antecedent peripheral neuropathy may be a risk factor for the development of compression neuropathy (so-called double-crush syndrome), particularly in diabetics.

Radial Mononeuropathy

Principles. The radial nerve arises from the C5 to T1 roots. After exiting the brachial plexus, it passes behind the proximal humerus in the spiral groove and takes a lateral (radial) course down the upper arm (Fig. 93.3). At about the level of the antecubital fossa, it bifurcates into the posterior interosseous (pure motor) and superficial radial (pure sensory) nerves.

The radial nerve controls extension of the fingers, thumb, wrist, and elbow (triceps). In contrast to the median and ulnar nerves, the radial nerve provides only *extrinsic* motor innervation to the hand (i.e., it does not supply motor fibers to any muscles that both originate and insert within the hand). In further contrast to the median and ulnar nerves, which supply most of the sensation to the hand, the radial nerve makes a contribution only to a cutaneous dorsal area overlying the first dorsal interosseus muscle, sometimes extending part of the way up the dorsa of the thumb, index, and long fingers.

Radial mononeuropathy caused by involvement at the level of the axilla is uncommon. When it occurs, it is usually associated with other upper extremity mononeuropathies or a brachial plexopathy. Although improper use of crutches may cause this syndrome, it usually occurs after an extended period of unconsciousness during which the arm is positioned in such a way that prolonged, deep compression is applied to the axilla. The most common are due to the so-called "Saturday night palsies," which is derived from the association of radial mononeuropathy with improper positioning of the arm during deep, commonly inebriated sleep. Consequently, the radial nerve is trapped for a prolonged period between the humeral shaft and some firm surface, causing

BOX 93.6   Isolated Mononeuropathies

Upper Extremity

Radial nerve
  Axilla
  Humerus
  Elbow (posterior interosseous neuropathy)
  Wrist (superficial cutaneous radial neuropathy)
Ulnar nerve
  Axilla
  Humerus
  Elbow
  Condylar groove
  Cubital tunnel
  Wrist (Guyon's canal)
  Hand
  • Superficial terminal ulnar neuropathy
  • Deep terminal ulnar neuropathy: proximal hypothenar; distal hypothenar
Median nerve
  Axilla
  Humerus (musculocutaneous mononeuropathy)
  Forearm
  • Anterior interosseus
  • Pronator syndrome
  Wrist (carpal tunnel)
  Hand (recurrent motor branch)
  Suprascapular mononeuropathy
  Axillary mononeuropathy

Lower Extremity

Sciatic nerve
Femoral nerve
  Iliacus compartment (proximal)
  Saphenous mononeuropathy (distal)
Lateral femoral cutaneous (meralgia paresthetica)
Peroneal nerve
  Common peroneal mononeuropathy (fibular head, popliteal fossa)
  Deep peroneal mononeuropathy (anterior compartment)
Tibial nerve
  Popliteal fossa (proximal)
  Tarsal tunnel (distal)
Sural nerve
  Popliteal fossa, calf (proximal)
  Fifth metatarsal base (distal)
Plantar nerve
  Distal to tarsal tunnel
  Interdigital neuropathies (Morton neuroma)
Obturator mononeuropathy

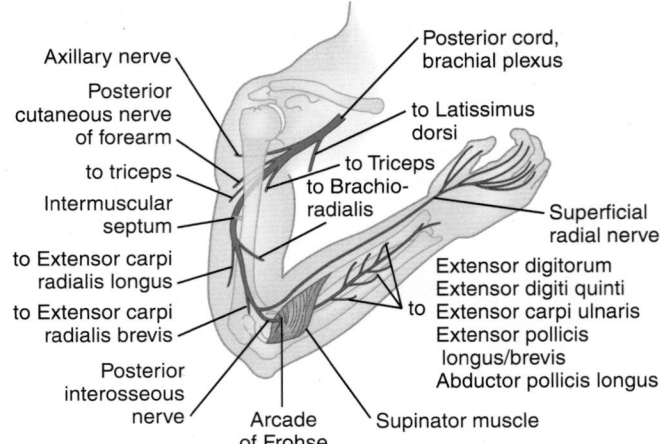

Fig. 93.3 Radial nerve, major branches, right arm, lateral view. (From Stewart JD. *Focal Peripheral Neuropathies*, ed 3. Philadelphia: Lippincott Williams & Wilkins; 2000.)

are characterized by wrist and finger drop and mild numbness over the skin of the first dorsal interosseus muscle. Depending on the level, degree, and duration of compression, some fascicles of the nerve may remain functional, resulting in a partial radial mononeuropathy. Thus the superficial radial nerve may remain intact, resulting in no loss of sensation, or loss of wrist and finger extension may be incomplete.

Because the finger drop of radial mononeuropathy places the hand at a mechanical disadvantage, examination of ulnar function by testing of the interossei may produce false-positive findings of weakness. To adjust for this, the examiner should ask the patient to place the palm on a horizontal supporting surface, such as a stretcher. With the fingers extended and no longer "dropped" at the metacarpophalangeal joints, interosseous strength can now be fairly tested. Failure to perform this maneuver may cause misdiagnosis of a simple radial mononeuropathy as a brachial plexopathy in an effort to explain what appears to be radial and partial ulnar nerve involvement.

About 90% of radial nerve palsies occurring during sleep, coma, or anesthesia recover fully, usually within 6 to 8 weeks. Evidence of denervation on EMG studies predicts a slower rate of recovery. Tourniquet injuries to the radial nerve usually recover spontaneously within 2 to 4 months. If axonal degeneration is seen on electrophysiologic testing, recovery may take longer, although virtually all radial mononeuropathies caused by tourniquets eventually resolve.

The radial nerve courses closely to the humerus, so it follows that about 22% of humeral shaft fractures are associated with radial nerve injury, with "wrist drop" the hallmark injury. Spontaneous resolution has been reported between 60% and 92%, so many authors suggest observation of these injuries is appropriate. In contrast, surgical intervention is needed to free the nerve from entrapment associated with complex fractures.

Diagnostic Testing. There exists no diagnostic test per se for this disease entity beyond the physical examination. EMG testing is employed to aid in predicting recovery times.

Management. While patients are waiting for spontaneous recovery to occur, the hand should be maintained in about 60 degrees of dorsiflexion. Although a simple dorsal plaster or fiberglass splint treats the wristdrop, atrophy and contractures can be minimized, and function of the hand can be improved if wide rubber bands anchored to the splint at a point proximal to the wrist are attached to individual fingers to provide passive dorsiflexion.

an external compression mononeuropathy. "Bridegroom's palsy" is another eponym for radial mononeuropathy, so named because the radial nerve may be compressed by the bride's head resting on the bridegroom's arm during sleep. Axillary radial mononeuropathy is distinguished from the more common humeral form by the finding of triceps involvement in addition to typical wrist and finger drop. Triceps involvement occurs because the innervation to the triceps is proximal to the point where the nerve is most vulnerable as it winds around the humeral shaft (see Fig. 93.3).

Clinical Findings. Because innervation of the wrist and finger extensors occurs distal to this area of the humeral shaft, findings

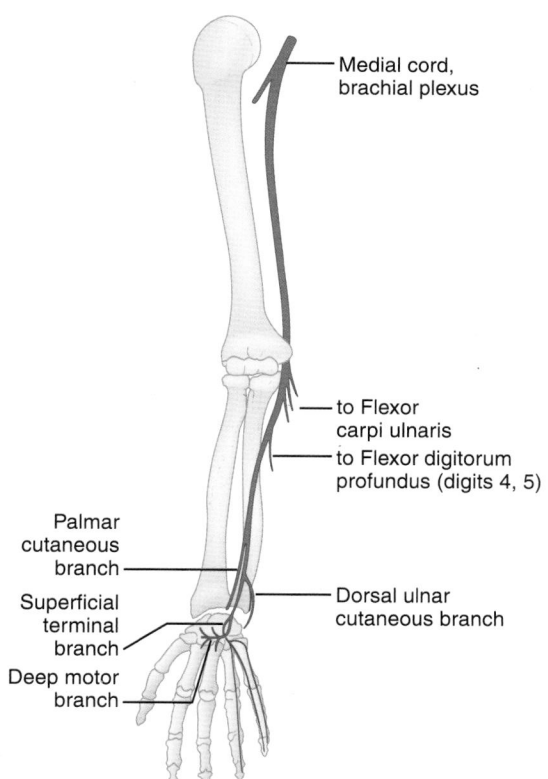

Fig. 93.4 Ulnar nerve, major branches, right arm, anterior view. (From Stewart JD. *Focal Peripheral Neuropathies*, ed 3. Philadelphia: Lippincott Williams & Wilkins; 2000.)

Ulnar Mononeuropathy

Principles and Clinical Findings. The ulnar nerve includes C7 to T1 roots and passes through the brachial plexus to descend medially, without branching, to the ulnar (medial) condylar groove at the elbow. It then enters the cubital canal, where it gives off branches to the ulnar wrist flexor and the deep flexors of the fourth and fifth digits.

Just proximal to the wrist, two important sensory branches leave the main trunk to supply cutaneous sensation to part of the hand (Fig. 93.4). These are the palmar and dorsal cutaneous branches, which do *not* pass through the Guyon canal. The palmar branch supplies sensation to the hypothenar eminence and the dorsal branch innervates the ulnar side of the dorsum of the hand, extending out nearly to the tip of the fifth and ulnar half of the fourth digit.

At the wrist, the nerve enters the Guyon canal (Fig. 93.5) between the pisiform and hook of the hamate, then bifurcates into the superficial terminal sensory branch and the deep motor branch.

The superficial sensory nerve supplies ulnar sensation to the palmar side of the fifth and half of the fourth digit (see Fig. 93.5). The deep motor nerve supplies the hypothenar muscles, then crosses to the radial side of the palm to innervate the ulnar intrinsics (all interossei and the ulnar lumbricals of the fourth and fifth digits), terminating in the first dorsal interosseus. The interossei abduct and adduct the fingers and are all innervated by the ulnar nerve. The lumbrical muscles flex the metacarpophalangeal joints and are evenly divided between the ulnar (fourth and fifth) and median (second and third) digits. The ulnar nerve can be thought of as the complement to the median nerve in the hand, because it supplies all of the muscles and all palmar sensation not innervated by the median nerve.

The ulnar nerve may be injured at two locations near the elbow: in the ulnar condylar groove and distally in the cubital canal. Because

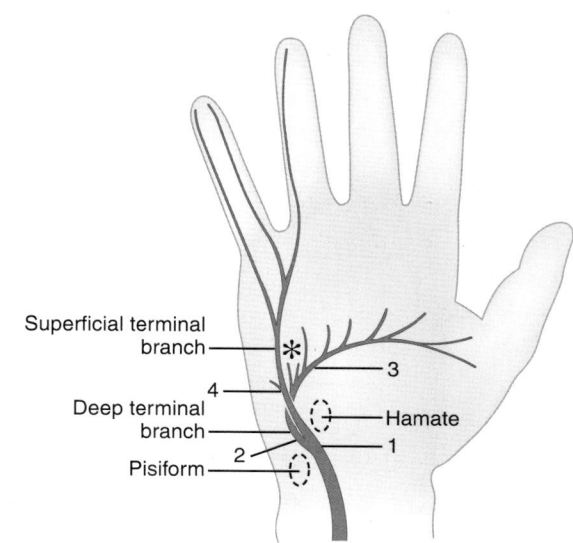

Fig. 93.5 Distal ulnar nerve and branches, right hand, palmar view. *Numbers* indicate four main sites of distal ulnar mononeuropathy in the wrist and hand. Asterisk *(*)* denotes hypothenar branches. (From Stewart JD. *Focal Peripheral Neuropathies*, ed 3. Philadelphia: Lippincott Williams & Wilkins; 2000.)

the condylar groove is shallow, the ulnar nerve runs superficially in this location and is vulnerable to injury, usually from external pressure or from a fracture or dislocation. The ulnar nerve has a propensity to develop a "tardy ulnar palsy," occurring years after a traumatic event. Many of these delayed ulnar mononeuropathies can be localized to the elbow on electrophysiologic testing.

Some ulnar mononeuropathies occur secondary to compression just proximal to entry into the cubital canal or are entrapped within the canal itself. Transient symptoms may occur during prolonged flexion or with repeated flexion and extension at the elbow.

Although it is difficult to distinguish a condylar from a cubital ulnar mononeuropathy, it is usually possible to localize the problem to the region of the elbow or the wrist. In addition to prior probability heavily favoring the elbow, the presence of sensory abnormalities in an ulnar distribution in the hand and fingers (i.e., usually including the fifth digit and "splitting" the fourth digit) strongly suggests that the lesion is at the level of the elbow rather than the wrist. The ulnar cutaneous innervation to the hand branches off from the main trunk proximal to the nerve entering the Guyon canal (see Figs. 93.4 and 93.5). Thus a lesion at the wrist should not produce sensory abnormalities, whereas one at the elbow would be expected to do so.

Compression of the ulnar nerve within the Guyon canal is rare. When it does occur, it affects all of the ulnar intrinsics (i.e., the two ulnar [fourth and fifth] lumbricals) and all the interossei. However, the ulnar extrinsics (i.e., the deep flexors of the fourth and fifth digits) are not affected, nor is the ulnar flexor of the wrist. The only sensory abnormalities are those in the distribution of the superficial terminal sensory branch, sparing other areas of ulnar innervation (see Fig. 93.5).

There are three ulnar mononeuropathies that occur distal to the Guyon canal in the hand. The two most common ones involve the deep terminal branch, either proximal or distal to the separation of the hypothenar branches (see Fig. 93.5). If the lesion is proximal, it produces weakness of all the ulnar-innervated muscles of the hand without sensory loss. If it is distal, the hypothenar ulnar intrinsics are spared, but the picture is otherwise similar. Usually, this occurs secondary to a laceration or repeated compression in the hand from use of certain tools, a cane, or the handle of a crutch.

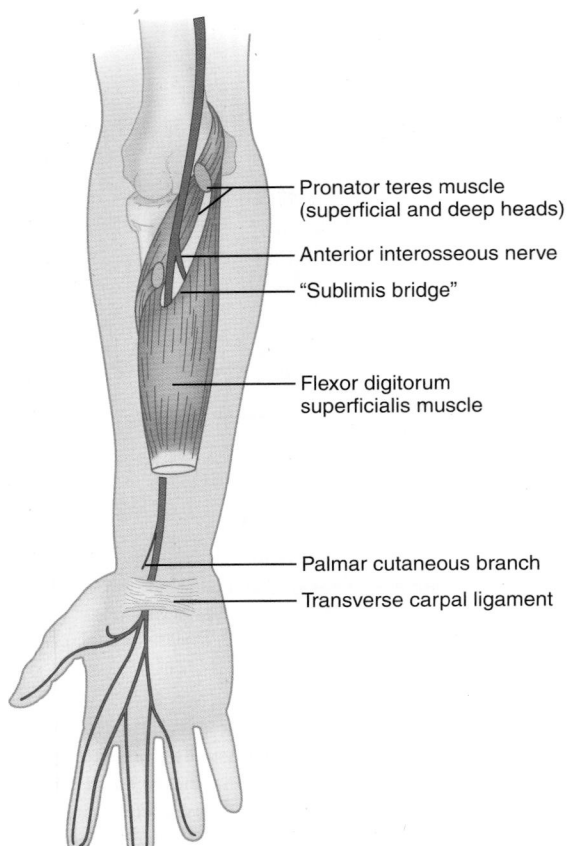

- Pronator teres muscle (superficial and deep heads)
- Anterior interosseous nerve
- "Sublimis bridge"
- Flexor digitorum superficialis muscle
- Palmar cutaneous branch
- Transverse carpal ligament

Fig. 93.6 Median nerve, major branches, right arm, anterior view. (From Stewart JD. *Focal Peripheral Neuropathies*, ed 3. Philadelphia: Lippincott Williams & Wilkins; 2000.)

Involvement of the superficial terminal branch (see Fig. 93.5) produces a pure sensory loss of the palmar surface of the fifth digit and ulnar half of the fourth digit caused by direct compression of this branch just distal to the Guyon canal. The dorsal surface of these two digits should have normal sensation except for the distal tips. This configuration of findings is due to the intact innervation provided by the dorsal and palmar cutaneous branches that enter the hand without passing through the Guyon canal (see Fig. 93.4).

Diagnostic Testing. There exists no true diagnostic entity for this disease process beyond the physical examination.

Management. Most ulnar mononeuropathies will spontaneously resolve. The evidence and options for nonoperative management are limited, but include splinting or padding, limiting flexion at the elbow, and activity modification. However, if muscle atrophy, particularly in the hypothenar area, is detected, surgery may be considered. There is no noted difference in outcomes between the two surgical options of simple decompression and decompression with transposition.

Median Mononeuropathy

Principles. The median nerve arises from the C5 to T1 spinal nerve roots and exits the brachial plexus through the lower trunk (Fig. 93.6). Median mononeuropathy is usually diagnosed as carpal tunnel syndrome (CTS), which is the most common of all entrapment neuropathies. The incidence of CTS is estimated at 1 in 1000 for the general population and a lifetime risk of 10%.[6] It is defined by the Academy of Orthopedic Surgeons as "a symptomatic compression neuropathy of the median nerve at the level of the wrist."

Clinical Findings. Although the patient may complain of bilateral symptoms, a careful history usually reveals that symptoms in one hand preceded those in the other. A common symptom of CTS is awakening at night and shaking the hand. Symptoms are often worsened by activity. For unclear reasons, the pain may spread as high as the arm or shoulder, although the paresthesias are generally confined to the fingers. Many patients initially state that their entire hand is involved, although this is not elicited by careful sensory examination. Patients may note, progressively over time, that their hands are clumsy or weak, and also note associated loss of fine motor function. The skin of the fingers innervated by the median nerve may be drier and rougher to the touch than the corresponding ulnar skin, depending on the duration of entrapment.

When motor involvement occurs in CTS, it is confined to the median intrinsics, which innervate the *l*umbricals (flexion of the metacarpophalangeal joints) and subserve thumb *o*pposition, *a*bduction, and *f*lexion, known as the *LOAF* muscles. However, the hallmark of CTS is sensory involvement, with motor abnormalities occurring later. The typical pattern of sensory innervation of the hand by the median, ulnar, and radial nerves shows marked individual variation. The most specific finding for CTS is splitting of the fourth digit (i.e., normal sensation of the ring finger on the ulnar palmar side with abnormal sensation on the median [radial] palmar side of the same finger). The most sensitive finding is abnormal sensation of the distal palmar tip of the index finger. If sensory findings are absent in the presence of motor findings consistent with median nerve involvement, it is highly unlikely that the patient has CTS, and an alternative diagnosis should be sought.

CTS appears to be associated with the conditions listed in Box 93.7. Of these, the two most common are diabetes mellitus and pregnancy.[7] CTS associated with systemic illness is commonly bilateral. CTS in pregnancy appears to be common, but the prevalence varies widely in the literature from 30% to 60%; resolution occurs among the majority of patients postpartum, but several studies have demonstrated that symptoms can persist for months to years among a subset of patients even after delivery.

Diagnostic Testing. The Tinel sign (percussion of the median nerve at the wrist) and Phalen sign (maximal palmar flexion at the wrist) are provocative tests to reproduce the sensory symptoms of CTS if neither sensory nor motor symptoms are evident on initial examination. Unfortunately, neither sign has adequate sensitivity or specificity to determine which patients should be referred for electrodiagnostic studies. Dropping of objects is indicative of severe CTS. The best way to examine patients for sensory findings is to touch the distal palmar tips very lightly, asking the patient whether the sensation feels "abnormal."

A nerve conduction study is an objective test that provides information on the physiologic health of the median nerve across the carpal tunnel and is the diagnostic gold standard. Magnetic resonance imaging (MRI) delineates the site of the nerve compression with a sensitivity of 96% but a specificity of 33% to 38%. Ultrasonography may be useful, particularly in patients with symptoms and a normal NCS. The most reliable ultrasonographic measurement is to obtain the cross-sectional area of the median nerve at the level of the pisiform. Thus, if all diagnostic studies in a symptomatic patient are normal, or if only the MRI result is abnormal, they should be repeated within three months if symptoms do not resolve. This recommendation is based on the theory that the CTS will progress over time to the point that an objective indicator, such as the NCS, will become positive.

Management. There are a variety of nonsurgical treatments, with splinting and steroid injections being the most common. A neutral wrist splint, typically worn at night during sleep, has commonly been used as the initial treatment. A Cochrane review found splinting more effective than no treatment in the short term, but the evidence that supported this conclusion was not robust.[8] A randomized trial comparing the effectiveness of night splinting versus a single corticosteroid injection found steroid injection benefit at six weeks, but at six months outcomes between the two treatment groups were the same.[9] We recommend providing patients with a splint to be worn during the night time hours and education regarding hand positioning or avoidance of repetitive activities that could lead to exacerbation of their symptoms. Oral NSAIDs can be offered, but there is no good quality supporting evidence.

Because of the possibility of a disabling "median hand" after inadvertent direct injection of the median nerve, we recommend that emergency clinicians defer the injection of the carpal tunnel with steroids to the consulting hand surgeon who can also obtain NCS and determine if splinting, injection, or surgical division of the transverse carpal ligament is indicated. Surgical treatment involves the division of the transverse carpal ligament, which reduces pressure on the median nerve by increasing the space in the carpal tunnel. This carpal tunnel "release" surgery can be performed open or endoscopically with no significant difference in outcomes noted.

Sciatic Mononeuropathy

Principles. The sciatic nerve includes L4 to S3 spinal nerve roots that pass through the lumbosacral plexus and divides into two terminal branches: the common peroneal and tibial nerves. The nerve exits the pelvis through the sciatic notch, passes behind the hip, and remains deep in the thigh until its terminal bifurcation in the proximal popliteal fossa (Fig. 93.7).

Lesions of the sciatic nerve occur with posterior hip dislocation or with virtually any form of penetrating or blunt trauma that causes formation of a buttock hematoma. Other causes include deep gluteal injection and prolonged supine immobilization on a firm surface. Because the sciatic nerve innervates the hamstrings and provides all sensorimotor function distal to the knee, a complete sciatic mononeuropathy is a devastating injury.

Clinical Findings. Ambulation is extremely difficult because of inability to flex the knee and a flail foot (i.e., neither flexion nor extension is possible at the ankle). Fortunately, many sciatic mononeuropathies are incomplete. For unknown reasons, a partial lesion typically involves only the trunk of the sciatic nerve, which subsequently becomes the common peroneal nerve, sometimes making the two difficult to distinguish from one another clinically.

Diagnostic Testing. This condition is mainly diagnosed by physical findings. If used, electrophysiologic studies show evidence of involvement of gluteal muscles or of any muscles innervated by the tibial nerve. This readily distinguishes a partial sciatic mononeuropathy from a lesion of the common peroneal nerve.

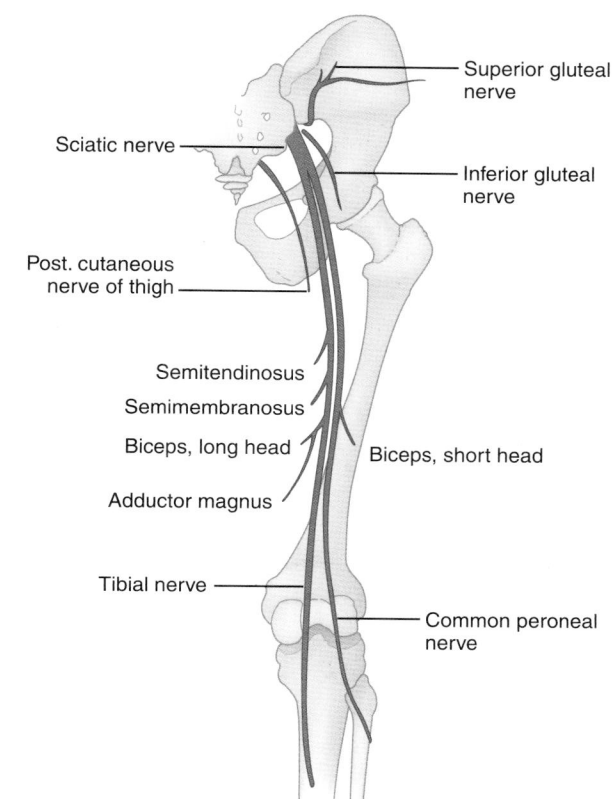

Fig. 93.7 Sciatic nerve, major branches, right leg, posterior view. (From Stewart JD. *Focal Peripheral Neuropathies,* ed 3. Philadelphia: Lippincott Williams & Wilkins; 2000.)

Management. Treatment of footdrop requires a posterior splint to maintain the ankle at 90 degrees until a brace can be obtained (see the Common Peroneal Mononeuropathy section).

Lateral Femoral Cutaneous Mononeuropathy

Principles. Lateral femoral cutaneous mononeuropathy (meralgia paresthetica) is a common syndrome believed to be caused by injury to this pure sensory nerve as it passes through or over the inguinal ligament, where it may become entrapped or kinked. Along with facial nerve neuropathy, meralgia paresthetica is one of the most commonly reported mononeuropathies associated with HIV infection. Risk factors include obesity, diabetes, pregnancy, and wearing tight-fitting clothing or belts. In addition, patients who have undergone surgical procedures of the hip and spine are also at risk for developing the syndrome.

Clinical Findings. Numbness and dysesthesia over the skin of the upper lateral thigh is typically found on physical examination.

Diagnostic Testing. There is no diagnostic test for this disease process beyond the physical examination.

Management. Resolution usually occurs spontaneously. In select patients, such as obese patients with BMI of 30 or greater, recommendations to avoid tight-fitting clothing or belts and/or to lose weight should be made. Ultrasound-guided nerve blocks utilizing corticosteroids and lidocaine are an option. Recurrence is possible and may require an inguinal ligament surgical release procedure.

Common Peroneal Mononeuropathy

Principles. The common peroneal nerve is a continuation of one trunk of the sciatic nerve. It is most vulnerable to injury where it winds around the fibular neck (Fig. 93.8). It then passes through the fibular

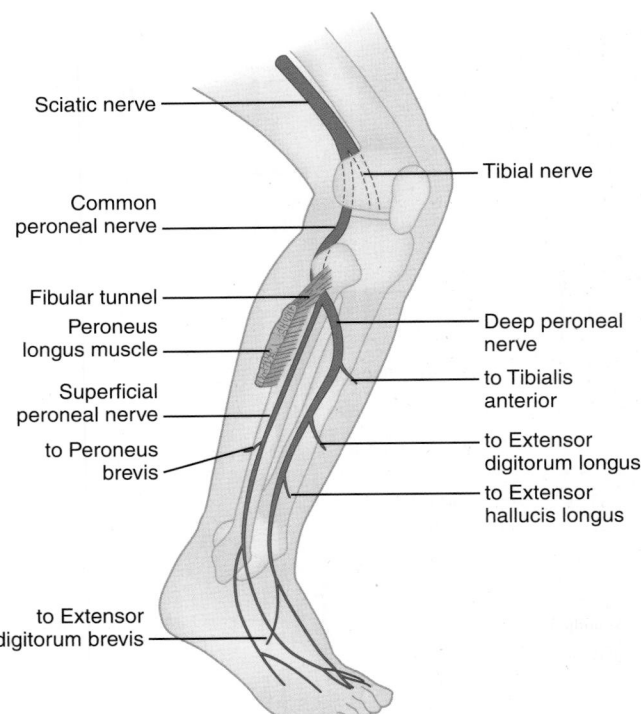

Fig. 93.8 Common peroneal nerve, major branches, right leg, antero-lateral view. (From Stewart JD. *Focal Peripheral Neuropathies*, ed 3. Philadelphia: Lippincott Williams & Wilkins; 2000.)

canal and bifurcates into its terminal branches, the superficial and deep peroneal nerves. The superficial peroneal nerve innervates the peroneal muscles (foot evertors) and supplies sensation to the lateral, distal lower leg and dorsum of the foot. The deep peroneal nerve traverses the anterior compartment and supplies innervation to the dorsiflexors of the foot and toes plus cutaneous sensation between the first and second toes.

Most common peroneal mononeuropathies are idiopathic and thought to be related to compression where the nerve is superficially located lateral to the fibular neck. Because this common neuropathy is often noted on awakening, it may be secondary to position during sleep. Leg crossing may also be a risk factor for development of this mononeuropathy.

Clinical Findings. The most striking feature of a complete common peroneal mononeuropathy is footdrop caused by weakness of foot dorsiflexion. At testing, the evertors of the foot are also weak, but the inverters, which are innervated by the tibial nerve, remain strong. This is the single most reliable clinical feature distinguishing sciatic from common peroneal mononeuropathy. Analogous to radial mononeuropathy in the upper extremity, sensory abnormalities in the leg and foot are inconsistent and easily overlooked in peroneal mononeuropathy.

Diagnostic Testing. Most patients with peroneal palsy recover. Those who do not should be studied electrophysiologically to ensure that the point of compression is not proximal to the fibular neck (i.e., in the popliteal fossa). If the point of peroneal injury appears to be in the region of, or distal to, the fibular neck on EMG, patients whose footdrop does not resolve should be considered candidates for exploration to determine whether the nerve is compressed within the fibular canal.

Management. Treatment of common peroneal palsy requires a posterior splint to maintain the ankle at 90 degrees until the nerve regenerates. This splinting prevents the foot from falling into sustained

---

BOX 93.8 Mononeuropathy Multiplex

Vasculitis
  Systemic vasculitis
  • Polyarteritis nodosa
  • Rheumatoid arthritis
  • Systemic lupus erythematosus
  • Sjögren syndrome (keratoconjunctivitis sicca)
  Nonsystemic vasculitis
Diabetes mellitus
Neoplastic
  Paraneoplastic
  Direct infiltration
Infectious
  Lyme disease
  HIV infection
Sarcoid
Toxic (lead)
Transient (polycythemia vera)
Cryoglobulinemia (hepatitis C)

HIV, Human immunodeficiency virus.

equinus (plantar flexion), which in turn allows the intermalleolar distance to narrow, effectively locking the talus out of the ankle mortise.

The treatment of isolated mononeuropathies depends on their etiology, location, and natural history of spontaneous recovery. All penetrating neuropathies should have surgical exploration and repair performed. Blunt trauma may cause a mononeuropathy indirectly by entrapment of a nerve within a fracture, hematoma, or compartment, requiring surgical intervention. Alternatively, nerves may be injured at a point where they are superficial, either by a single direct blow or by sustained pressure caused by immobility (pressure palsies). Most of these resolve spontaneously over time, depending on the severity of injury and length of the nerve. If entrapment can be confirmed by imaging or electrophysiologic studies, a release procedure is indicated. The mononeuropathies that do not require timely surgical exploration should be referred for further evaluation to confirm the location of the neuropathic lesion.

Type 5: Mononeuropathy Multiplex

Principles

Mononeuropathy multiplex is characterized by an asymmetrical, sensorimotor, usually distal pattern of peripheral neuropathy (Box 93.8). Common causes include vasculitis, diabetes, and Lyme disease.

Clinical Findings

As with isolated mononeuropathies, sensory abnormalities tend to be located in the same general anatomic region as the accompanying motor findings. Whether DTRs are affected depends on which nerves are involved. For example, if the process includes the femoral nerve, the patellar reflex is likely to be diminished or absent.

Lyme Disease. The PNS manifestations of Lyme disease are divided into early and late. The early PNS syndromes commonly include facial nerve involvement (rarely other cranial nerve palsies) and radiculoneuritis. Late PNS involvement occurs as a DSPN, mononeuropathy multiplex, or radiculoneuropathy. The most common neurologic abnormality in Lyme disease is unilateral or bilateral facial nerve palsy, usually occurring within a month of exposure. Patients may also complain of headache and constitutional symptoms. Early in the course of Lyme disease, severe neuritic pain may develop in a radicular distribution, often in or near the dermatome where the tick bite occurred. There may also be associated sensory changes, motor weakness, and decreased reflexes consistent with nerve root involvement.

Patients with chronic Lyme disease present with sensory symptoms, particularly distal paresthesias in the lower extremities. Less commonly, they develop a picture consistent with mononeuropathy multiplex or a radiculopathy, which is much less severe than the early radiculoneuritis of Lyme disease.

Diagnostic Testing

Vasculitis-related multiple mononeuropathy is diagnosed with a sural nerve biopsy.

The most useful diagnostic tests for patients with suspected Lyme disease are a serum enzyme-linked immunosorbent assay, Western blot, and CSF examination. CSF abnormalities suggestive of Lyme disease are a lymphocytic pleocytosis, elevated protein level, and normal glucose concentration. The CSF is almost always abnormal in early radiculitis, sometimes abnormal with isolated facial palsy, and typically normal in chronic Lyme disease.

Management

Facial nerve palsy in Lyme disease without CSF abnormalities may be treated with oral doxycycline 100 mg twice a day for 2 weeks. Intravenous (IV) ceftriaxone is the drug of choice for all other neurologic syndromes associated with Lyme disease. The adult dosage is 2 g/day, and the pediatric dosage is 50 to 75 mg/kg per day. The standard course of treatment with IV ceftriaxone is at least 2 weeks.

Type 6: Amyotrophic Lateral Sclerosis
Principles

Although *amyotrophic lateral sclerosis (ALS)* and *motor neuron disease (MND)* are often used synonymously, the latter represents a spectrum of diseases ranging from primary lateral sclerosis, in which degeneration is confined to upper motor neurons, to progressive muscle atrophy, in which only lower motor neurons are involved. ALS, which requires the presence of both upper and lower motor neuron findings, resides in the middle of this spectrum, representing the most common form of MND. The incidence of ALS is 1.5 to 2.5 per 100,000. Most develop symptoms in middle-adult life, with motor weakness in the extremities, spasticity, paralysis, and eventually death, typically within 3 to 5 years of symptom onset.

In ALS, the primary pathologic process in the PNS component of the disease is a neuronopathy of the anterior horn cell. Because this structure is located proximal to the point where motor and sensory fibers merge to form mixed spinal nerve roots, the signs and symptoms of MND are purely motor (see Fig. 93.2). In the CNS, there is a loss of Betz cells from the motor cortex with secondary degeneration of the corticospinal tracts.

Clinical Findings

Box 93.9 lists some representative upper, lower, and mixed motor signs. Patients typically demonstrate asymmetrical distal weakness without sensory findings. Positive motor phenomena in the form of fasciculations are found in almost all patients at diagnosis but are rarely an initial complaint. Although there is electrophysiologic evidence of autonomic involvement in ALS, this is generally subclinical.

Diagnostic Testing

All patients in whom this diagnosis is suspected should be referred for electrophysiologic confirmation against standardized criteria, with denervation combined with the physical findings typically confirming the diagnosis. Confirmation is particularly important because

> ### BOX 93.9 Objective Clinical Findings Consistent With Amyotrophic Lateral Sclerosis
>
> **Upper Motor Neuron Signs**
> Hyperreflexia
>   Sustained clonus, especially at ankle
>   Finger flexors and jaw jerk
> Spasticity, especially of gait
> Presence of Babinski sign
>
> **Lower Motor Neuron Signs**
> Positive motor phenomena
>   Fasciculations
>   Cramps
> Negative motor phenomena
>   Asymmetrical distal weakness
>   Atrophy
>
> **Combined Upper and Lower Motor Neuron Signs**
> Dysarthria
> Dysphagia
> Respiratory compromise

multifocal motor neuropathy, a rare disease that masquerades as ALS, responds dramatically to cyclophosphamide and immune globulin administration.

Management

Riluzole and edaravone are the only two drugs approved for treatment of ALS by the FDA. A systematic review found that riluzole increased median survival time by 2 to 3 months.[10] Edaravone, only recently approved for ALS in 2017, demonstrated a 33% decrease in ALS severity scores over six months and improved quality of life measures.[11] The development of a multidisciplinary team approach has had a much higher impact on overall quality of life for patients with ALS. This team includes ALS-focused neurologists, nurses, occupational therapy, and speech therapy amongst others. Patients presenting to the emergency department with undifferentiated or early signs of ALS can be challenging to diagnose and will benefit from prompt neurologic consultation to avoid a delay in diagnosis. Those with an established diagnosis of ALS and demonstrated disease progression are at high risk for aspiration pneumonia and respiratory compromise and may require admission to the hospital, which should be done with consideration for the patient's advanced directives and long-term goals of care.

Type 7: Sensory Neuronopathy (Ganglionopathy)
Principles

This category of peripheral neuropathy is characterized by a selective or predominant involvement of the dorsal root ganglion, producing a relatively pure sensory syndrome analogous to the pure motor syndrome of ALS.

Clinical Findings

Although all sensory modalities are affected, proprioception is profoundly altered, leading to sensory ataxia and loss of DTRs without weakness. The distribution is typically asymmetrical and distal at the outset, but depending on severity and extent of progression, it may become functionally symmetrical.

BOX 93.10   Sensory Neuronopathies (Ganglionopathies)

Herpes
    Herpes simplex 1 and 2
    Varicella-zoster (shingles)
Inflammatory sensory polyganglionopathy
Paraneoplastic
Primary biliary cirrhosis
Sjögren syndrome (keratoconjunctivitis sicca)
Toxin induced
    Pyridoxine (vitamin B_6) overdose
    Metals
      • Platinum (cisplatin)
      • Methyl mercury
Vitamin E deficiency

Diagnostic Testing

Sensory ganglionopathies can be confirmed by MRI of the spinal cord and surrounding areas, showing degeneration of central sensory projections that localize the disease process to the dorsal root ganglion. Some of the more common causes of this type of peripheral neuropathy are listed in Box 93.10.

Management

The management of sensory neuropathies is symptomatic in nature and best left to the patient's primary physician.

The references for this chapter can be found online at ExpertConsult.com.

94

Neuromuscular Disorders

Jeremy Rose, Trent She

FOUNDATIONS

Disorders of the neuromuscular unit result in clinical presentations that range from subtle symptoms to acute respiratory failure. In most cases, the pathophysiologic mechanisms and characteristics of these disorders are well understood, which permits an organized approach to diagnosis and treatment based on the distribution and severity of the neuromuscular system affected.

The neuromuscular unit has four components: the anterior horn cells of the spinal cord, the spinal and peripheral nerves, the neuromuscular junctions, and the muscles. The level of the pathologic process determines associated signs and symptoms (Fig. 94.1 and Table 94.1). *Myelopathies* involve the spinal cord; *radiculopathies* involve the nerve roots as they leave the spinal cord; *neuropathies* involve the peripheral nerves; and *myopathies* involve the muscle. The use of physical signs to differentiate these disorders is discussed in Chapter 9.

Neuropathies involve the axon or the myelin sheath of the nerve. Nerve conduction studies can differentiate the locations of involvement. As the conduction along the axon is disrupted, the subsequent delay in transmission first causes symptoms in the muscles controlled by longer nerve axons, resulting in ascending weakness. Progression of the destruction or axonal degeneration causes a slowly progressive course of symptoms.

The neuromuscular junction comprises the presynaptic membrane, the postsynaptic membrane, the synaptic cleft, and the neurotransmitter acetylcholine (ACh), which carries the signal across the cleft between the two membranes. The neuromuscular junction features postsynaptic nicotinic ACh receptors, distinct from muscarinic ACh receptors that effect autonomic nervous system functions. Disorders of these postsynaptic nicotinic receptors produce weakness. Postsynaptic ACh receptors are continually turned over at a rate that is related to the amount of stimulation. A disorder of transmission often leads to an increase in the density of ACh receptors. Myasthenia gravis is the archetype of neuromuscular diseases.

CLINICAL FEATURES

History

Initial history of patients with complaints of weakness focuses on the acuity of the process and the potential for airway compromise. A complaint of difficulty in breathing or swallowing indicates possible bulbar or respiratory muscle compromise with the potential for life-threatening deterioration. As with other neurologic diseases, the anatomic distribution of symptoms can be the key to diagnosis. Neuromuscular diseases are often progressive or intermittent in nature, so a detailed history of the chronology of symptoms is important. Specific historical features, such as diarrhea (botulism), tick exposure (tick neurotoxin–mediated paralysis), or recurrent episodes of weakness over time (hereditary hypokalemic paralysis) may be helpful. Factors elicited during the history help to guide further history taking, targeted physical examination, and testing, as the differential diagnosis forms and is narrowed by the historical information the patient provides.

Physical Examination

The clinician should first assess adequacy of airway protection and ventilation before a more generalized examination evaluates for the degree of weakness and the location of the lesion. The presence of swallowing and a strong cough suggest that the patient has sufficient protective and ventilatory reserve. The muscles used to lift the head off the bed may weaken before those of respiration and should be assessed. A patient who is not yet intubated but is complaining of shortness of breath or difficulty in breathing should have frequent measurements of forced vital capacity (FVC). Normal FVC ranges from 60 to 70 mL/kg; when the FVC reaches 15 mL/kg, ventilatory support is necessary. Maximal negative inspiratory force (NIF), also called a maximal inspiratory pressure (MIP), is an alternative to FVC. An NIF or MIP of less than 15 cm H_2O suggests the need for intubation. Neuromuscular disorders interfere with ventilation not oxygenation, so capnography is a better monitoring modality than pulse oximetry in these cases. Hypercarbia is a late finding and should be regarded as a sign of impending respiratory failure. A subnormal PCO_2 may also represent developing respiratory failure. As the patient's respiratory effort falls, tidal volume is reduced, and alveolar CO_2 is not exhaled sufficiently (hypopneic hypoventilation).

A systematic neurologic examination assesses the patient's mental status, cranial nerves, motor and sensory function, deep tendon reflexes, and coordination, including cerebellar function. The motor examination begins by determining whether the weakness is unilateral or bilateral and which muscle groups are involved. Key components of the examination include motor strength, muscle bulk, and presence of fasciculations. Box 94.1 provides the grading system used in motor strength assessment. Table 94.2 provides the findings used to distinguish upper motor neuron from lower motor neuron processes.

DIFFERENTIAL DIAGNOSIS

Myelopathies

Myelopathies are spinal cord disorders that are manifested with signs of upper motor neuron dysfunction, such as muscle weakness with increased spinal reflexes, including an extensor plantar reflex (Babinski sign). There may be bladder and bowel involvement. When sensory findings are present, they often define the level of the lesion. The presence of back pain suggests a compressive lesion, such as a herniated intervertebral disk, tumor, or epidural hematoma. Concomitant systemic signs, such as a fever, or a history of intravenous (IV) drug use, can suggest an epidural abscess. Increasing postprocedural pain, for example following lumbar puncture, epidural anesthesia, or spine surgery, warrants consideration of an epidural hematoma. Acute, painless spinal cord lesions include transverse myelitis and spinal cord infarction.

Motor Neuron Disease

The characteristic findings of motor neuron disease combine signs of both upper and lower motor neuron dysfunction, including hyperreflexia, muscle wasting, and fasciculations. Pain is not a component of the clinical picture. Amyotrophic lateral sclerosis (ALS; Lou Gehrig disease) is the archetypal motor neuron disease.

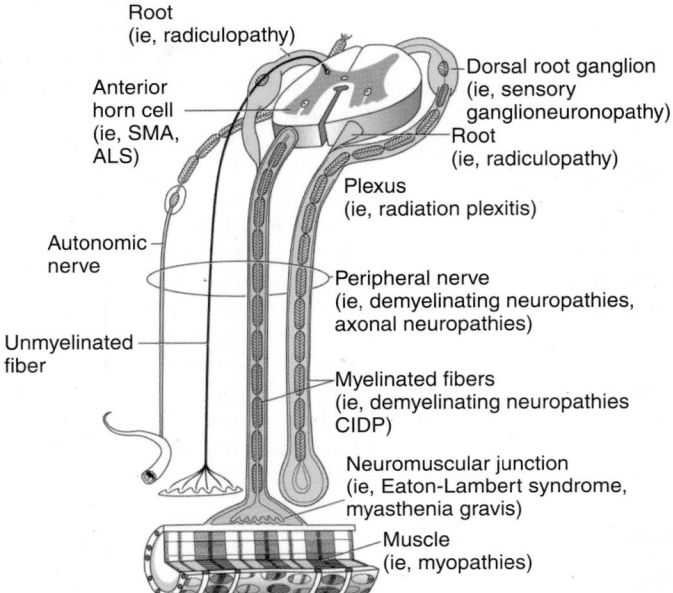

Fig. 94.1 The anatomic elements of the peripheral nervous system and related neurologic disorders. *ALS,* Amyotrophic lateral sclerosis; *CIDP,* chronic inflammatory demyelinating polyneuropathy; *SMA,* spinal muscular atrophy. (From Bertorini TE. Neuromuscular anatomy and function in neuromuscular case studies. In: *Neuromuscular Case Studies.* Philadelphia: Butterworth-Heinemann/Elsevier; 2008.)

BOX 94.1 **Grading Score for Motor Strength**
5 = Normal strength
4 = Weak but able to resist examiner
3 = Moves against gravity but unable to resist examiner
2 = Moves but unable to resist gravity
1 = Flicker but no movement
0 = No movement

TABLE 94.1 Clinical Characteristics of Neuromuscular Diseases

Disease	History	Strength	Deep Tendon Reflex	Sensation	Wasting
Myelopathy	Trauma, infection, cancer	Normal to decreased	Increased	Normal to decreased	No
Motor neuron disease (ALS)	Progressive difficulty swallowing, speaking, walking	Decreased	Increased	Normal	Yes
Neuropathy	Recent infection Ascending weakness	Normal or decreased Distal > proximal	Decreased	Decreased	Yes
Neuromuscular junction disease	Food (canned goods) Tick exposure Easy fatigability	Normal to fatigue	Normal	Normal	No
Myopathy	Thyroid disease Previous similar episodes	Decreased Proximal > distal	Normal	Normal	Yes

ALS, Amyotrophic lateral sclerosis.

TABLE 94.2	Distinguishing Upper Motor Neuron From Lower Motor Neuron Involvement				
Motor Neuron	Deep Tendon Reflex	Muscle Tone	Atrophy	Fasciculations	Babinski Response
Upper motor neuron	Increased	Increased	No[a]	No	Present
Lower motor neuron	Decreased	Decreased	Yes	Yes	Absent

[a]Not significant but can occur.

Poliomyelitis affects the anterior horn cells and results in lower motor neuron disease without sensory involvement. The weakness is often asymmetric. Patients initially have a clinical picture similar to that of viral meningitis with fever and neck stiffness. The cerebrospinal fluid (CSF) analysis resembles that of viral meningitis. Polio has been eradicated in many parts of the world but remains prevalent in areas of conflict where public health systems have eroded.[1] The United States has seen an increase in acute flaccid myelitis (AFM), a paralyzing illness affecting pediatric patients that is described as "polio-like." AFM appears to have a temporal relationship with enteroviruses D68 and A71, but it is unclear if these viruses are the cause of the syndrome.[2]

Neuropathies

Weakness from a neuropathy is often noted first in distal muscles and then progresses centrally. Decreased grip strength and foot drop are common initial presentations. The differential diagnosis includes Guillain-Barré syndrome, toxic neuropathies, diabetic neuropathy, and tick paralysis (which is caused by inhibition of both nerve conduction and function of the neuromuscular junction). Neuropathies are discussed in Chapter 93.

Diseases of the Neuromuscular Junction

Disorders of the neuromuscular junction cause motor fatigability. The initial depolarization at the nerve end plate stimulates a maximum number of ACh receptors on the muscle cell, producing a normal or nearly normal strength response. Repeated stimulation leads to diminishing motor strength, which is caused by one of three mechanisms: blockage of the receptors, as in myasthenia gravis, decrease in the amount of ACh released, as in botulism, or inactivation of ACh by irreversible binding, as in organophosphate poisoning.

A decrease in the release of ACh can cause a combination of nicotinic and muscarinic effects. The clinical manifestations of this are anticholinergic findings, such as dilated pupils, confusion, urinary retention, tachycardia, low-grade fever, and dry, flushed skin. In the case of Lambert-Eaton myasthenic syndrome, weakness is more pronounced at the beginning of muscle use and improves with repeated use as more ACh builds up in the synaptic cleft with each stimulation. Muscle tone is generally diminished and sensation is preserved in diseases of the neuromuscular junction.

Myopathies

Myopathies produce generalized, symmetric weakness. Reflexes are diminished, muscle tone is usually diminished, but sensation is preserved. Myopathies due to inflammatory disorders (polymyositis, dermatomyositis, polymyalgia rheumatica, and viral myositis) cause muscle pain and tenderness. Metabolic disorders affecting muscle strength (e.g., electrolyte and endocrine disorders) cause diffuse weakness without pain. Electrolyte alterations affecting muscular and cardiac function are discussed in Chapter 114.

DIAGNOSTIC TESTING

Serum electrolyte determination, with emphasis on potassium, calcium, and phosphorus concentrations, should be assessed in patients

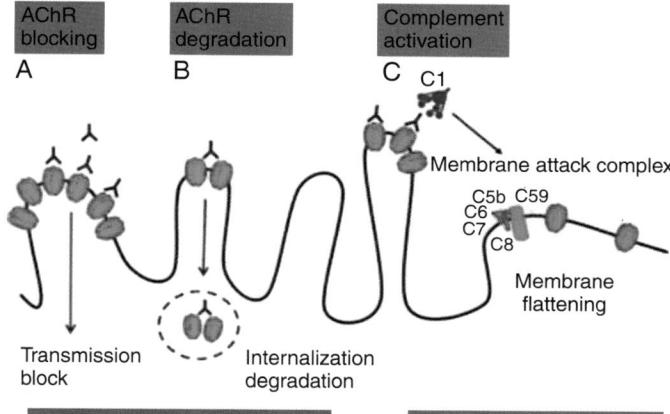

Fig. 94.2 Mechanisms of action of acetylcholine receptor *(AChR)* autoantibodies. Neuromuscular synapse in myasthenia gravis. AChR antibodies interfere with signal transduction by direct blocking of AChR (A), by cross-linking and increased degradation (B), or by immune-mediated destruction including complement activation (C). (From Sommer N, Tackenberg B, Hohlfeld R. The immunopathogenesis of myasthenia gravis. In Engel AG, ed. *Handbook of Clinical Neurology, volume 91, Neuromuscular Junction Disorders.* St Louis: Elsevier; 2008:169–212.)

with acute weakness. An electrocardiogram (ECG) may provide an earlier clue to potassium or calcium disturbance. Thyroid function tests are recommended in cases of suspected myopathies. A creatine kinase (CK) level assesses for muscle inflammation, and if CK is markedly elevated, serial renal function studies should be obtained to assess for developing acute kidney injury.

Magnetic resonance imaging (MRI) is the preferred imaging modality for suspected cases of acute myelopathy caused by a compressive lesion. CSF analysis is indicated when Guillain-Barré syndrome or transverse myelitis is suspected.

DISORDERS OF THE NEUROMUSCULAR JUNCTION

Myasthenia Gravis

Principles

The age at onset of myasthenia gravis is influenced by gender; women are most commonly affected between 20 and 40 years old and men between 50 and 70 years old. Although new cases of myasthenia gravis are occasionally diagnosed in the emergency department (ED), it is much more common for patients with established disease to present with exacerbations of their disorder, often caused by precipitating factors.

In most patients with myasthenia gravis, weakness and fatigue result from circulating autoantibodies against the nicotinic ACh receptor on the junctional folds of the postsynaptic membrane. The effects are the result of several pathologic processes: direct blocking of the receptor, complement mediated destruction of the folds, and internalization and degradation of the receptors (Fig. 94.2). With

BOX 94.2 Drugs That May Exacerbate Myasthenia Gravis

Cardiovascular
  Beta-blockers
  Calcium channel blockers
  Quinidine
  Lidocaine
  Procainamide
Antibiotics
  Aminoglycosides
  Tetracyclines
  Clindamycin
  Lincomycin
  Polymyxin B
  Tobramycin
  Fluoroquinolones
  Colistin
Other
  Phenytoin
  Neuromuscular blockers
  Corticosteroids
  Thyroid replacement

repeated stimulation, fewer and fewer receptor sites are available for ACh binding, and fatigue develops. Fatigability and muscle weakness are the hallmarks of myasthenia gravis. Muscarinic receptors are also affected but to a much lesser extent, so muscular weakness is the dominant presentation of myasthenia gravis. Ocular muscle weakness is the first sign of myasthenia gravis in up to 40% of patients, although 85% of patients eventually have ocular involvement. When ptosis is present, it is often worse toward the end of the day. New-onset diplopia also may signal development of myasthenia gravis. Respiratory failure is rarely the initial symptom of myasthenia gravis. Bulbar muscles may be involved myasthenia gravis, producing dysarthria or dysphagia.[3] Facial and extremity muscles may also be involved, producing some classic symptoms of myasthenia gravis (i.e., difficulty in combing hair or brushing teeth, weakness of the muscles in the posterior neck causing a "dropped-head appearance," and a limited ability to form a full smile due to weakness of lateral facial muscles).

The prognosis for patients with myasthenia gravis has markedly improved in recent years due to the demonstrated benefit of thymectomy and the approval of the drug eculizumab for refractory cases.[4] Nevertheless, stable disease can be pushed to crisis by commonly used drugs that are known to exacerbate myasthenia gravis (Box 94.2). Even topical medications, such as tobramycin eye drops, can cause an exacerbation.[5] Assessing drug-disease interactions is a particularly important step when prescribing to patients with myasthenia gravis, even if the disease is well controlled.

Myasthenic crisis. Myasthenic crisis is defined as respiratory failure requiring mechanical ventilation. It occurs in 15% to 20% of patients with myasthenia gravis, usually within the first 2 years of disease onset. Although it is potentially life threatening, the mortality from this complication of myasthenia gravis has declined dramatically with appropriate care in the ED and intensive care unit (ICU) and the use of plasma exchange or immunomodulatory therapy with intravenous immune globulin (IVIG).

Crises are most often precipitated by underlying infection, aspiration, and medication changes, such as stopping anticholinergic medications or initiating a new medication that precipitates weakness. Other precipitants can be surgery and pregnancy (see Box 94.2).

Lambert-Eaton syndrome. Lambert-Eaton myasthenic syndrome is a rare disorder. Almost 50% of cases are associated with small cell carcinoma of the lung. Autoantibodies cause inadequate release of ACh from nerve terminals, affecting both nicotinic and muscarinic receptors. With repeated stimulation, the amount of ACh in the synaptic cleft increases, leading to a progressive increase in strength with muscle use, an effect opposite of that seen with myasthenia gravis. The classic syndrome includes weakness that improves with use of muscles, particularly proximal hip and shoulder muscles; hyporeflexia; and autonomic dysfunction, most commonly seen as dry mouth. Management focuses on treatment of the underlying cancer, although IVIG may be useful.

Diagnostic Testing

The diagnosis of new-onset myasthenia gravis is based on history, clinical findings, and a combination of serologic testing and electromyographic testing. In rare cases, the diagnosis is further clarified through bedside testing with the ice bag test (or, historically, the edrophonium test). Serum testing for ACh receptor antibodies is positive in 80% to 90% of patients with myasthenia gravis, but results are not available in the ED. Myasthenia gravis can be associated with a thymoma as a paraneoplastic syndrome. Initial evaluation of patients with newly diagnosed myasthenia gravis includes a contrast-enhanced computed tomography (CT) scan to evaluate for presence of a thymoma or other anterior mediastinal masses.

The edrophonium (Tensilon) test has an unacceptable number of false-positives and false-negatives and can cause serious adverse reactions through enhanced muscarinic effects of ACh. The test is rarely, if ever, indicated, and we do not recommend it.

The ice bag test can be performed at the bedside for patients with suspected myasthenia gravis and ptosis, whose diagnosis is otherwise uncertain. Cooling decreases symptoms in myasthenia gravis and heating exacerbates symptoms, so placing an ice bag to the eyelids can reduce ptosis. The degree of ptosis is measured before and after application of an ice bag. The distance from the upper to the lower eyelid in the most severely affected eye is measured first. An ice pack is applied to the affected eye for approximately 2 minutes. An improvement in the amount of ptosis of at least 2 mm is considered positive. The pooled sensitivity and specificity of the ice bag test for detecting ocular myasthenia are 0.94 and 0.97, respectively.

Management

The initial step in managing the myasthenic patient in crisis is stabilization of the airway and supporting ventilation. Respiratory failure ensues from muscle weakness, not inadequate oxygenation; therefore supplemental oxygenation does not address the problem, and mechanical ventilation is indicated. Endotracheal intubation may be necessary, but biphasic positive airway pressure (BiPAP) support may be sufficient if the patient is otherwise able to protect their airway. Capnometry monitoring can be useful in detecting respiratory fatigue well in advance of oxyhemoglobin desaturation and obvious clinical findings of respiratory distress.

Pyridostigmine, thymectomy, immunosuppressant drugs, steroids, rituximab, and eculizumab are all used for maintenance management of myasthenia gravis in the outpatient setting. The mainstays of ED myasthenic crisis management are plasma exchange or IVIG.

Plasma exchange, performed as multiple exchanges over 1 to 2 weeks, is effective in up to 95% of patients in acute myasthenic crisis and is generally considered the first line treatment for patients with severe myasthenic crisis.[5] IVIG is also effective for myasthenic crisis, usually given as 2 g/kg in divided doses over several days. Given the rarity of this condition, we recommend consultation with a neurologist with expertise in neuromuscular disease to aid in decision making between plasma exchange and IVIG and the initiation of either of these interventions. Patients treated by either IVIG and plasma exchange should also receive high-dose oral glucocorticoids, such as prednisone, 60 mg daily, beginning as soon as possible. High-dose steroids can worsen weakness, so they should be given only as a complement to plasma exchange or IVIG therapy, in consultation with a neurologist.

Ambulatory treatment of myasthenia gravis is often initiated using oral pyridostigmine, an acetylcholinesterase inhibitor. If the patient is newly diagnosed, or the patient's increased weakness is a result of discontinuation or dosage reduction of pyridostigmine, initiating or reestablishing treatment with pyridostigmine (60 to 120 mg by mouth every 4 to 6 hours) will prolong the presence and activity of ACh in the synaptic cleft and improve symptoms. Initiation or reestablishment of pyridostigmine therapy should be done in consultation with the outpatient physician from whom the patient will receive ongoing ambulatory management. The most common side effects of pyridostigmine are those of excessive cholinergic stimulation, such as increased airway secretions and increased bowel motility. These side effects can be treated with glycopyrrolate (1 mg with each dose of pyridostigmine), which preferentially blocks muscarinic cholinergic receptors that are responsible for these symptoms.

Cholinergic crisis, caused by excessive ACh activity related to acetylcholinesterase inhibitor therapy, is rarely seen, particularly with close management of pyridostigmine dosing. It may occur when patients deliberately or inadvertently take pyridostigmine in excess of the recommended dose. Cholinergic crisis is manifest by excessive cholinergic activity, which may include bradycardia, diarrhea and abdominal cramping, increased secretions, and muscle weakness, which might mimic a myasthenic crisis (Table 94.3).

Disposition

The decision to admit or to discharge a patient with myasthenia gravis from the ED is based on the potential for neuromuscular deterioration. Patients requiring plasma exchange or IVIG often require admission to ensure response to therapy and close monitoring for respiratory

compromise. For some patients, a short stay in an observation unit under the care of a team comprising emergency medicine and neurology specialists will aid in evaluation of the patient's likelihood of successful outpatient treatment. Patients being admitted to the hospital should have an NIF or FVC measured to help determine the level of monitoring and care needed. These measurements need to be trended during the admission.

Botulism

Principles

Botulism is a toxin-mediated illness that can cause weakness leading to respiratory insufficiency. In 2017, the Centers for Disease Control and Prevention (CDC) reported 182 cases of botulism in the United States: 10% food-borne, 77% infant botulism, 10% wound botulism, and 3% unknown etiology.[6] *Clostridium botulinum* is an anaerobic, spore-forming bacterium. Three of eight known toxins produced by *C. botulinum* (types A, B, and E) cause human disease. Recent outbreaks have been traced to home canned peas in New York[7] and whale flipper in Alaska.[8]

Clinical Features

The botulinum toxin blocks both voluntary motor and autonomic functions. There is no pain or sensory deficit. The onset of symptoms is 6 to 48 hours after the ingestion of toxin. Symptoms of gastroenteritis may or may not be present. The classic feature of botulism is a descending, symmetric, flaccid paralysis. Cranial nerves and bulbar muscles are affected first, causing diplopia, dysarthria, and dysphagia, followed later by generalized weakness. Because the toxin decreases cholinergic output, anticholinergic signs may be present: constipation, urinary retention, dry skin and eyes, and increased temperature and dilated, nonreactive pupils. This can help to differentiate botulism toxicity from myasthenia gravis. Deep tendon reflexes are normal or diminished.

Infantile botulism results from the ingestion of *C. botulinum* spores that are able to germinate and produce toxin in the high pH of the gastrointestinal tract of infants. Botulism spores can survive in honey, so it is recommended that honey not be fed to infants. The clinical presentation includes constipation, poor feeding, lethargy, and weak cry; consequently, this diagnosis must be included in the differential diagnosis of the floppy infant.

Wound botulism is a rare presentation of botulism stemming from the colonization of a wound or other skin lesion by *C. botulinum* spores, which are then able to produce toxin that can travel through the bloodstream to cause systemic effects. Wound botulism is generally seen in IV drug users, classically in users of "black tar" heroin. In addition to causing the classic symptoms of botulism as described earlier, wound botulism tends to present with fever and lesser gastrointestinal manifestations.

Diagnostic Testing

The diagnosis of botulism is made by both clinical findings and exclusion of other processes. The toxin can be identified in serum and stool, but the assay is not commonly available in most hospitals and requires a prolonged turnaround time. If the suspected food source is available, it should also be tested for the toxin. Wound cultures should be sent in anaerobic transport medium for patients with suspected wound botulism.

Management

Treatment is initially focused on stabilization of the airway and supportive measures. In 2010, the CDC announced a new equine heptavalent

TABLE 94.3 Notable Differences Between Myasthenic Crisis and Cholinergic Crisis Pertaining to Myasthenia Gravis Patients

Myasthenic Crisis	Cholinergic Crisis
Generally minimal abdominal symptoms	Presence of abdominal pain, nausea and vomiting
Increased HR and BP	Decreased heart rate and blood pressure
Normal secretions	Increased secretions
Mydriasis	Miosis
Caused by undermedication of myasthenia gravis treatment	Caused by overmedication of myasthenia gravis treatment
Treat with cholinergic agent (edrophonoium)	Treat with anticholinergic agent (atropine)

botulinum antitoxin (HBAT) that is now the only antitoxin available in the United States for noninfant botulism.[9] For suspected cases and to obtain HBAT, clinicians should contact their state health departments. The CDC also maintains a 24-hour botulism duty officer at the CDC Emergency Operations Center (770-488-7100). An IV human-derived botulism immune globulin (BabyBIG) has been developed for treatment of infantile botulism and is available 24 hours/7 days through the California Department of Public Health Infant Botulism Treatment and Prevention Program on-call physician at 510-231-7600. Wound botulism patients should have emergent surgical consultation for débridement of the wound. Tetanus toxoid is administered unless previously received within the past 5 years. In addition, antibiotic coverage is recommended. Penicillin G 3 million units every 4 hours and metronidazole 500 mg every 8 hours intravenously provide effective coverage against *C. botulinum*. Aminoglycosides, tetracyclines, and polymixins are not recommended because they can potentially worsen neuromuscular blockade. The duration of treatment is generally 7 to 10 days but may need to be extended based on the severity of disease. We recommend infectious disease consultation for this rare disorder.

Disposition

All patients being treated for botulism need to be hospitalized, and most will be admitted to an ICU setting given the likelihood of progression of neuromuscular weakness. Infants and children will need to be transferred to the most appropriate neonatal intensive care unit (NICU) or pediatric intensive care unit (PICU) setting.

Tick Paralysis

Principles

This extraordinarily rare cause of an acute, ascending, flaccid paralysis is most often found in North America (Rocky Mountain region, US Pacific Northwest, and Southwestern Canada) and the east coast of Australia. Although the pathogenesis of tick paralysis is not fully understood, it is thought that a salivary neurotoxin is injected while the female tick feeds. The toxin functions like botulinum toxin to decrease the release of ACh from the presynaptic membrane of the neuromuscular junction.[10]

Clinical Features

Tick paralysis causes an acute, ascending, flaccid motor paralysis that can be confused with Guillain-Barré syndrome, botulism, and myasthenia gravis. Symptoms usually begin 1 to 2 days after the female tick has attached and begun to feed, although delays of up to 6 days have been reported. There may be associated ocular signs, such as fixed and dilated pupils, that can help to distinguish it from Guillain-Barré syndrome.

Management

The management is supportive care and tick removal. A tick can be removed by use of forceps to grasp it as closely as possible to the point of attachment. Care should be taken not to leave mouth parts in the patient's tissue. Injecting a small amount of lidocaine with epinephrine just below the tick facilitates removal by starving the animal of blood supply and encouraging it to release. Although symptoms may resolve rapidly after removal of the tick, supportive measures such as intubation should not be withheld pending resolution of symptoms. Although there is little new research on the topic, there are many reports of cases misdiagnosed as other causes of weakness (e.g., Guillain-Barré syndrome, acute inflammatory demyelinating polyneuropathy) until the offending tick was found and removed.

Disposition

These patients may begin to show improvement upon removal of the tick and may be able to be discharged from the ED. If symptoms are slow to resolve, the patient is admitted to an observation unit.

DISORDERS OF THE MUSCLES

Newly acquired weakness originating at the muscle level can be divided into two types: inflammatory and toxic-metabolic. Inflammatory disorders usually produce pain and tenderness, whereas metabolic disorders do not.

Inflammatory Disorders

Principles

The most common inflammatory myopathies are polymyositis and dermatomyositis. Polymyositis may be idiopathic in nature, occur secondary to infections (viral or bacterial), or be seen in conjunction with other disorders, such as sarcoidosis and hypereosinophilic syndromes. Inflammatory myopathies cause weakness, pain, and tenderness of the muscles involved.

Clinical Features

Dermatomyositis and polymyositis can occur at any age, although adults are more often affected than children. They can be associated with various malignant neoplasms, such as of the breast, ovary, lung, and gastrointestinal tract, and lymphoproliferative disorders. Proximal muscle weakness predominates and leads to complaints of difficulty in rising from a seated position or climbing stairs and weakness in lifting the arms over the head. There is often pain and tenderness in these proximal muscles as well. There is a decrease in reflexes proportionate to the decrease in strength. Fasciculations are not seen, and atrophy is a very late finding. Inclusion body myositis, another type inflammatory myositis, has a similar presentation to polymyositis but presents more gradually and with predominantly distal muscle weakness that extends to proximal muscle weakness with progression of disease.

Dermatomyositis is similar to polymyositis, but it is also associated with classic skin findings. These are more prominent in childhood but are also found in adults. They include a periorbital heliotrope rash and erythema and swelling of the extensor surfaces of joints. The heliotrope rash is usually photosensitive and may also involve the exposed areas of the chest and neck.

Diagnostic Testing

The diagnosis of an inflammatory myopathy requires exclusion of electrolyte abnormalities. Serum CK level is interpreted in light of the entire clinical picture; an elevated CK level does not establish the cause of weakness as a myopathy because some neuropathies can also produce an elevated CK level. Similarly, a normal CK level does not rule out a myopathy as the cause of weakness. Electromyography and muscle biopsy are used to confirm the diagnosis. Erythrocyte sedimentation rate (ESR) and C-reactive protein (CRP) are often normal or only mildly elevated, thus they have no role in diagnosis or prognosis. Aldolase and other specific myositis autoantibodies should be considered after consultation with a neurologist or rheumatologist.

Management

Inflammatory myositis syndromes are usually managed with oral prednisone in a dose of 1 to 2 mg/kg/day. When steroids prove ineffective and during acute exacerbations, cytotoxic drugs such as azathioprine (initial dose of 50 mg/day) and methotrexate (initial dose of 15 mg/week) are added. Fortunately, the degree of rhabdomyolysis seen with the inflammatory myopathies is not sufficient to cause renal impairment.

Disposition

The majority of these patients will likely be discharged, some following an observation period. Hospitalization should be considered for patients with comorbidities, elders, and those who do not improve with treatment in the ED or observation unit.

Metabolic Disorders

Acute, generalized muscle weakness is seen with a number of severe electrolyte abnormalities of any cause: hypokalemia, hyperkalemia, hypocalcemia, hypercalcemia, hypomagnesemia, and hypophosphatemia. (See Chapter 114.) Acute painless myopathies are also seen with endocrine disorders involving the thyroid, parathyroid, or adrenal glands (see Chapter 117).

There are several disorders referred to collectively as the *periodic paralyses,* which include periodic paralysis of the hyperkalemic and hypokalemic forms and thyrotoxic periodic paralysis, which is similar to hypokalemic periodic paralysis except that it is associated with hyperthyroidism.

Periodic Paralysis

Principles. Periodic paralysis of the hypokalemic and hyperkalemic forms is a rare hereditary disorder of ion channels resulting in intermittent attacks of flaccid extremity weakness, which can be mild to moderate or sufficiently severe that the patient goes to the ground and cannot get up. The hypokalemic form is more common. Periodic paralysis is most often associated with an inherited genetic mutation. Patients usually report a personal and family history of similar episodes. Thyrotoxic periodic paralysis is an acquired rather than inherited form of hypokalemic periodic paralysis.

The clinical picture of thyrotoxic periodic paralysis is almost identical to that of periodic paralysis, and indeed a small number of patients with hypokalemic periodic paralysis have hyperthyroidism. In thyrotoxic periodic paralysis, symptoms related to hyperthyroidism are often present at the same time the patient has weakness. The relation of the hyperthyroidism to hypokalemia is probably due to increased sodium-potassium adenosine triphosphatase (Na^+/K^+-ATPase) pump, which causes a rapid shift of potassium from the extracellular into the intracellular compartment. There is probably a genetic predisposition to this form of periodic paralysis, although it may be due to different genes in different patient populations.[11] Patients with a first episode of hypokalemic paralysis should undergo thyroid function testing.

Clinical features. Patients may suffer either isolated or recurrent episodes of flaccid paralysis. The lower limbs are involved more often than the upper, although both can be affected. Bulbar, ocular, and respiratory muscles are usually not involved. Onset is rapid often

following a high oral carbohydrate intake (with subsequent insulin rise) and a period of rest. This reflects the intracellular shift of potassium rather than the total body depletion of potassium. A typical complaint is acute weakness noted on waking in the morning after a large meal.

Diagnostic testing. The ECG may demonstrate signs of hyperkalemia or hypokalemia. ECG findings of hyperkalemia include peaked T waves, prolongation of the PR interval and QRS complex, loss of P waves, and finally a sinusoidal pattern and asystole in severe cases. ECG findings of hypokalemia include flattening and inversion of T waves, prolongation of the QT interval, presence of a U wave and ectopic beats, and ventricular arrhythmias in severe cases. An immediate serum potassium level should be obtained; in the hypokalemic form, the potassium level during an attack falls to values well below 3.0 mEq/L. Magnesium and glucose levels should also be measured.

Management. Many cases resolve spontaneously with supportive care alone. The mainstay of management is the treatment of the underlying electrolyte imbalance, with awareness that the changes in potassium concentration in patients with periodic paralysis are not due to depletion or excess of potassium but rather intracellular and extracellular shifts (i.e., in the hypokalemic state, the total body potassium is not reduced but has shifted intracellularly). Thus, in the repletion of potassium, caution is necessary to prevent overtreatment. For this reason, we recommend that IV potassium be given sparingly at one or two 10-mEq IV doses of potassium chloride, each over 1 hour. This can be done in parallel with 40-mEq oral potassium repletion and retesting of serum potassium levels. IV hydration helps to redistribute the body's potassium stores; magnesium supplementation is not necessary. In the hyperkalemic state, glucose, insulin, and albuterol may be used to promote intracellular shifting of potassium. Treatment of the hyperthyroid symptoms in thyrotoxic periodic paralysis, such as tachycardia, may help the paralysis as well. Counseling should also be provided to the patient to avoid triggers. These include avoidance of sudden, high-intensity exercise followed by resting, excessive dietary potassium, and alcohol.

Disposition. In the past, most cases of periodic paralysis required an inpatient stay, but most patients can be managed in less than 24 hours in an observation unit. Admission may be necessary for patients with their first episode of periodic paralysis in the context of thyrotoxicosis.

The references for this chapter can be found online at ExpertConsult. com.

95

Central Nervous System Infections

Benjamin H. Schnapp and Corlin Jewell

FOUNDATIONS

Background and Pathophysiology

The etiology of CNS infections continues to change as a result of new therapeutic interventions, vaccines, and the growing number of immunosuppressed patients. Despite advances, however, the morbidity and mortality from a CNS infection remains high; good outcomes can be maximized with early recognition and treatment.

The two most common CNS infections, *meningitis* and *encephalitis,* are delineated by the tissue that is infected. Meningitis refers to an infection of the meningeal layers lying between the bony covering of the CNS and the brain tissue. If the infection is present in the brain parenchyma itself, then it is termed encephalitis. However, these disease states are not mutually exclusive and exist on a continuum of *meningoencephalitis*. Generally, greater degrees of encephalitis portend a worse prognosis, as more tissue is involved.

Bacterial Meningitis

Bacterial meningitis has a high mortality rate despite treatment, with rates variable depending on the organism, time to appropriate treatment, and patient factors. *Streptococcus pneumoniae* remains the predominant pathogen in adult patients, accounting for over half of cases despite a recent decline in incidence.[1] Other common causes in adults include *Neisseria meningitidis, Haemophilus influenzae*, and *Listeria monocytogenes*. *N. meningitidis* is the predominant organism in children. *Listeria* is more commonly seen in elderly adults and infants. In the first six weeks of life, Group B streptococcus species as well as *Escherichia coli* also represent common causes of bacterial meningitis. Bacterial meningitis caused by *H. influenzae* was previously responsible for a much larger proportion of cases, but the incidence has declined sharply since the introduction of the vaccine for type B (HiB).

Meningococcal disease refers to meningitis caused by *N. meningitidis,* and is most common in younger individuals, particularly those living in very close proximity to others such as in military barracks or college dormitories. A, B, and C represent the major groups. Group B is particularly prevalent in Europe, while group C is commonly isolated in the United States. A conjugate vaccine containing serogroups A, C, Y, and W-135 has been developed, as well as a separate vaccine for serogroup B. These vaccines are highly effective in children, but have yet to be broadly distributed to developing countries.

The infection process in bacterial meningitis generally begins with nasopharyngeal colonization and invasion of the mucosa. The varying capsular properties of each organism protect the bacteria. Once bacteria cross the blood-brain barrier to enter the CSF, host defense mechanisms within the CSF are often ineffective. Bacteria then proliferate, which causes the body to signal for leukocytes to enter the CSF. Meningeal and subarachnoid space inflammation is associated with the release of cytokines into the CSF, inciting an inflammatory cascade that promotes increased permeability of the blood-brain barrier, cerebral vasculitis, edema, and increased intracranial pressure (ICP). A subsequent decrease in cerebral blood flow can then lead to cerebral hypoxia.

Meningeal infection may also occur in association with a dural leak secondary to neurosurgery or trauma to the CNS. Skin flora, including coagulase-negative staphylococcus species, *Staphylococcus aureus*, and *Cutibacterium acnes* are seen most commonly in this population, though infections caused by *Pseudomonas aeruginosa* also occur.

Mortality from bacterial meningitis is highest in patients with advanced presentations, serious underlying disease or advanced age. The fatality rate is highest with *Listeria* meningitis with a mortality rate up to 27%.[2] Overall, many survivors have some degree of residual neurologic deficit, with the highest rates found in those with pneumococcal meningitis.[3]

Meningitis from Lyme disease (*Borrelia burgdorferi*) presents similarly to other causes of bacterial meningitis, but can also cause other neurologic symptoms, including facial palsies and radiculopathies. Late Lyme infection, occurring in some cases years after initial infection, can cause encephalopathy which can manifest as migraines, psychosis, and somatoform disorders.

Viral Meningitis

Given the decrease in the incidence of bacterial meningitis, largely secondary to vaccination efforts, viral infections are now the most common cause of meningitis. Enteroviruses and herpesviruses are the most common causes,[4] often occurring in those with risk factors such as a suppressed immune system. The overall prognosis for the majority of cases of viral meningitis is excellent.

Viral Encephalitis

The same organisms responsible for viral meningitis may also be associated with encephalitis. A common mechanism of viral transmission is through the skin via insect vectors (e.g., Zika virus or West Nile virus), although clinical disease develops in only a small percentage of the people bitten. Tick-borne viral encephalitis is endemic to parts of Europe and Russia and is an important consideration for residents and recent travelers to those regions; a vaccine is available. Transmission of viral encephalitis often occurs by hematogenous spread from infections of the respiratory, gastrointestinal, or urogenital tracts. Other mechanisms include retrograde transmission along neuronal axons, as seen in the herpes virus, and direct invasion of the subarachnoid space after infection of the olfactory submucosa, as seen in rabies or herpes.

The outcomes in viral encephalitis, including permanent neurologic sequelae, are dependent on both the host and the infecting agent. Acyclovir treatment has reduced the mortality from HSV encephalitis from up to 70% down to 9%, but with 34% of surviving patients having moderate to severe neurologic disability.[5] Common complications include seizures, motor deficits, and impaired cognition. Encephalitis caused by Japanese encephalitis virus, Eastern equine virus, and St. Louis encephalitis virus is severe, with high mortality rates and high rates of neurologic sequelae among survivors. West Nile virus produces encephalitis in less than 1% of those infected but has resulted in 2000 deaths in the United States as of 2016.[6] Western equine virus and California encephalitis virus cause milder infections, and death is rare. Zika virus has been associated with the development of Guillain-Barré syndrome (GBS) as well as severe encephalitis in developing fetuses of infected mothers, resulting in devastating neurologic defects. It is not entirely clear if the virus also causes neuroinvasive disease in adults. Powassan virus, another tick-borne cause of CNS infection in North America, is known to cause severe encephalitis with a mortality of approximately 10% and a high rate of neurologic disability in survivors. CMV can also cause encephalitis, particularly in patients who are infected with HIV or are otherwise immunocompromised. Influenza virus, well-known for its respiratory effects, is another rare cause of high-mortality encephalitis in adults. Encephalitis secondary to measles and mumps has almost disappeared in the developed world due to widespread vaccination, but still can occur, particularly in those who are immunocompromised. Primary measles encephalitis is typically self-limited but carries a mortality of approximately 10% to 15%. Patients with this disease can go on to develop both subacute and chronic encephalitis (sometimes occurring years later) which is universally fatal.

Tuberculous Meningitis

Mycobacteria typically gain access to the CNS via hematogenous spread, and once present will begin to form granulomas. These can rupture, inciting an inflammatory response from the host. This can have the side effect of causing vasculitis and potentially a stroke. Tuberculous meningitis is also frequently complicated by hydrocephalus requiring neurosurgical intervention; in advanced disease, up to 25% of patients may require some neurosurgical procedure for obstruction (ventriculoperitoneal shunt or drainage). Tuberculous meningitis leads to severe disability or death in roughly half of the cases, and, as with bacterial meningitis, depends on the patient's age, comorbidities, time to diagnosis, and the progression of their disease.

Fungal Meningitis

CNS infections caused by fungal species are most commonly caused by *Cryptococcus* (typically *C. neoformans* and *C. gattii*) and have been increasing in recent years. Other common causes of fungal meningitis include *Aspergillus* species and *Coccidioides immitis*. Diabetic patients are at high risk of developing cerebral mucormycosis via direct invasion of the sinuses, and CNS invasion by *Histoplasma capsulatum* is also commonly seen in AIDS patients.

Over a million cases of fungal CNS infections are estimated to occur annually, likely via similar mechanisms as bacterial meningitis. Because these infections typically affect those with compromised immune systems, this increase is likely secondary to an increasing number of people living with iatrogenic chronic immunosuppression and HIV infection. Pulmonary exposure, followed by hematogenous spread, is the primary pathogenic mechanism in most cases of cryptococcal meningitis. Infection with *C. neoformans* is considered an acquired immunodeficiency syndrome (AIDS)-defining illness but can occur in those with immunocompromised states arising from other causes. Infection with *C. gatti* can occur even in immunocompetent patients. *Candida* species are also a major cause of fungal meningitis. These infections typically occur in those with candidemia or via the implantation of neurosurgical hardware (such as CNS shunts).

Common CNS complications of fungal meningitis include abscesses, increased ICP, neurologic deficits, seizures, bone invasion, fluid collections, and ocular abnormalities (seen in up to 40% of patients with cryptococcal meningitis). The mortality rate of fungal meningoencephalitis is usually around 20% to 30%, but may be up to 97% in untreated *Candida* meningitis, and varies with the severity of illness, timeliness of diagnosis, and administration of appropriate treatment.

Central Nervous System Abscess

CNS abscesses occur due to both local contiguous invasion as well as hematogenous spread from remote infections. They are also associated with intravenous (IV) drug use, neurologic surgery, and cranial trauma. In cases of contiguous spread, the location of the abscess within the brain is typically dictated by the source of invasive infection or the surgical procedure (Fig. 95.1). Brain abscesses secondary to otitis media are most often found within the temporal lobe or cerebellum, whereas cases arising from sinusitis usually result in abscesses in the frontal or temporal lobes. Hematogenous spread of microorganisms (most commonly from the pulmonary system) often results in multiple brain abscesses, although solitary lesions may also occur. Rarely, patients present without a clear source or the presence of risk factors. Antibiotic prophylaxis in the immunosuppressed, improved diagnostic imaging, and neurosurgical interventions have all contributed to more favorable outcomes.[7]

The spinal epidural space also represents a common site of CNS abscesses. Increasing numbers of spinal surgeries, immunosuppressed

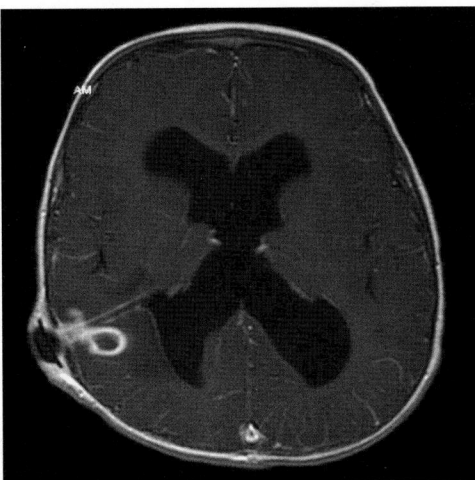

Fig. 95.1 A brain abscess which has developed adjacent to the site of a CSF shunt, as seen on MRI. CNS abscesses commonly develop adjacent to surgical sites, as this is one way bacteria can bypass the blood-brain barrier.

patients, and high rates of intravenous drug use are contributing factors to an increase in the incidence of these abscesses, which are associated with high rates of permanent neurologic morbidity. Infection typically enters the epidural space via the blood but can also arise from contiguous spread from nearby infections (e.g., psoas abscess, vertebral osteomyelitis).

CLINICAL FEATURES

Meningitis

The clinical picture of bacterial and viral meningitis is classically defined by fever, headache, photophobia, and nuchal rigidity. Unfortunately, subtle presentations lacking these classic features are common. In immunosuppressed or geriatric patients, alteration in mental status may be the only finding, and therefore requires a lower threshold for ruling out meningitis in these special populations. Clinical presentations in neonates may include a bulging fontanelle, but are often subtle, such as changes in behavior, decreased tone, or weakness as noticed by parents; consequently, guidelines universally recommend a lumbar puncture as part of the evaluation of a neonate with a suspected infection.

The physical findings in meningitis are variable depending on patient factors (e.g., age, comorbidities), pathogen, and time course of the disease (early vs. late). Two classic exam maneuvers, the Kernig sign (inability to straighten leg to a position of full knee extension when patient is lying supine with hip flexed to a right angle) and Brudzinski sign (attempts to flex the neck passively are accompanied by flexion of the hips), have a low sensitivity of less than 12%; however, they have a high specificity and strongly suggest meningitis if they are present (Table 95.1).[1]

Patients with suspected meningitis should first be examined for evidence of a structural lesion precipitating their symptoms, as these patients may require CT imaging to rule out other causes of their symptoms. Signs of mass lesions can include papilledema, decreased venous pulsations, new-onset seizures, abnormal level of consciousness, or focal neurologic deficits. An accurate fundoscopic exam can be challenging to obtain and bedside ultrasound offers an alternative tool for assessing intracranial pressure.[8] Patients without abnormal findings on neurologic examination may proceed to lumbar puncture without CT.[9]

Because meningitis can result from both contiguous and hematogenous spread, the physical examination should include a search for an inciting infection, such as a skin abscess, sinusitis, endocarditis, or osteomyelitis. Manifestations of endocarditis may be present, particularly in cases found to be due to S. aureus. Petechiae and cutaneous hemorrhages are widely reported with meningococcemia, typically on the extremities although they can occur anywhere on the body. Endotoxic shock with vascular collapse and DIC often develops in severe meningococcal disease, but shock may be present in the advanced stages of any bacterial meningitis. A finding of a systemic infection in a patient with signs of potential meningeal irritation should encourage rather than dissuade the clinician from considering the possibility of a concomitant CNS infection.

Cerebral venous thrombosis occurs in approximately 1% of patients with meningitis, likely due to coagulopathy induced by the robust CNS immune response; this rare complication can manifest as new-onset seizures, altered sensorium, and new focal neurologic deficits. Meningococcemia may cause Waterhouse-Friderichsen syndrome, or bilateral adrenal hemorrhage, often accompanied by other signs of severe systemic infection such as DIC and purpura.

The presentation of fungal meningitis can sometimes be subtle even in the healthy adult population. Headache, low-grade fever, malaise, and weight loss may be present but often to such a mild degree that CNS infection is not initially considered. Tuberculous meningitis, in contrast to other types of meningitis, can have a subacute or even chronic presentation, with symptoms developing months after onset of infection. Cases can be vague and nonspecific, including fever, weight loss, night sweats, and malaise, with or without headache and meningismus. In some cases, CNS involvement may be the only manifestation of tuberculosis, but CNS infection can also present alongside pulmonary tuberculosis or disseminated (miliary) infection.

Encephalitis

Encephalitis can occur from a viral, bacterial or fungal cause; it is not possible to definitively distinguish the etiology of the infection based on clinical features, although certain presentations can be suggestive. Viral encephalitis can occur secondary to primary viral invasion of the CNS, such as West Nile or rabies virus. Alternatively, it can be caused by reactivation of a previously dormant viral illness, such as varicella-zoster virus (VZV).

The diagnosis of encephalitis requires an alteration of consciousness or behavior without another known cause. Fever, headache, seizures, and disorientation can be present. The symptoms exhibited by the patient are representative of the affected area of the brain. For example, HSV has a predilection for the temporal lobes and therefore, patients with HSV encephalitis can present with psychosis, personality or behavior changes, or hallucinations, occasionally prompting an initial diagnosis of a psychiatric disorder. A thorough skin and mucosal examination may reveal the presence of herpetic lesions, as encephalitis can be associated with cutaneous outbreak in some cases. West Nile virus can result in neuroinvasive disease resulting in a wide range of symptoms, including muscle weakness, memory loss, behavioral changes, and difficulty concentrating. In cases of rabies encephalitis, patients also present with agitation, extreme hydrophobia, and muscular spasms.

Central Nervous System Abscess

The most common finding in patients with an intracranial abscess is headache. Findings seen consistently in other CNS infections, such as fever and altered mental status, may not be present. Most patients with intraparenchymal abscess have a subacute clinical course with symptoms progressing over 1 or more weeks. Just as with encephalitis, the

TABLE 95.1 Approximate Sensitivity, Specificity, Positive and Negative Likelihood Ratios of Clinical Findings and Examination Maneuvers for CSF Pleocytosis in Patients With Suspected Meningitis

	Sensitivity	Specificity	LR+	LR-
Headache	91%	16%	1.1	0.5
Fever	30%	58%	0.7	1.2
Jolt accentuation	21%	82%	1.2	1.0
Kernig sign	2%	97%	0.8	1.0
Brudzinski sign	2%	98%	1.0	1.0
Nuchal rigidity	13%	80%	0.6	1.1
Focal neurologic deficit	2%	96%	0.5	1.0
Vomiting	4%	85%	0.3	1.1
Rash	2%	96%	0.6	1.0
Physician suspicion	44%	40%	0.8	1.4

Adapted from Nakao JH, Jafri FN, Shah K, Newman DH. Jolt accentuation of headache and other clinical signs: poor predictors of meningitis in adults. *Am J Emerg Med.* 2014;32(1):24–28.

symptoms exhibited by patients depends on the site affected by the abscess. For example, those with abscesses near the frontal lobe may present with disinhibited behavior, and abscesses near the motor cortex may demonstrate focal weakness. Seizures occur in approximately 25% of patients. Abrupt neurologic deterioration and death can result from abscesses that rupture into the ventricular system.

Abscesses can also present in the epidural space in the spine, most commonly in the lumbar region.[10] However, multiple areas may be affected which can be discontiguous.[11] Like brain abscesses however, presentations can be nonspecific and mimic more benign causes of back pain. The most common presenting symptom of an abscess within the epidural space is midline pain, which is present in the majority of patients. Conversely, fever is only present in approximately half of cases, particularly early in the course. Complications of a spinal abscess primarily result from cord compression, including paralysis, motor and sensory deficits, and bowel and bladder dysfunction. These deficits may be permanent once they develop, even with prompt treatment, making prompt diagnosis critical to avoid serious morbidity.

CSF Shunt Infection

These infections typically manifest with signs of increased intracranial pressure and hydrocephalus such as headache, altered mental status, nausea, and vomiting. They most often occur within 6 months of shunt placement and are typically the result of skin flora being introduced into the CSF space.

DIFFERENTIAL DIAGNOSES

The diagnoses of acute, subacute, and chronic meningitis and the other potential pathologies that must be considered vary based on the time course of the presenting symptoms. *Acute meningitis* encompasses patients with clear signs and symptoms of meningitis who are evaluated within 24 hours of the onset of their symptoms. While other diagnoses can be considered during the initial evaluation, antibiotic therapy should be initiated as soon as possible in these patients to cover for the possibility of bacterial meningitis. In this group of patients with rapid onset of symptoms, the most important differential diagnostic

considerations are viral meningitis, acute subarachnoid hemorrhage (SAH), acute arterial dissection, and the noninfectious causes of meningitis including drugs, malignancy, or autoimmune conditions.

Distinguishing between viral and bacterial meningitis is described in the Diagnostic Testing section. Because subarachnoid blood is irritating to the meninges, it will cause neck pain similar to meningitis, but can be distinguished using CT imaging and LP. Generally, patients with SAH and cervical artery dissection will lack associated infectious symptoms and signs, such as a prodrome or fever.

In *subacute meningitis*, symptoms develop over a period of 1 to 7 days. Although this time course makes viral meningitis most likely, bacterial and fungal etiologies remain possible. Brain tumor, spinal abscess, infections outside the CNS such as osteomyelitis, and drug effects are potential diagnoses. Other considerations that may mimic subacute meningitis include CNS malignancy, intracranial hemorrhage, brain abscess and nonconvulsive status epilepticus. CNS abscess should be considered especially if fever is minimal or absent or if there are focal neurologic findings. Nonconvulsive status epilepticus is a consideration in patients with altered mental status, especially if there is a seizure history or a known structural brain lesion.

The spectrum of *chronic meningitis* includes the viral meningitides, as well as meningitis caused by tuberculosis, syphilis, and fungi. Symptoms have generally been present in this group for at least 1 week and generally have a prolonged, indolent course. The potential causes of culture-negative meningitis symptoms are broad and varied, including rheumatologic, neoplastic, and medication-induced symptoms. Generally, these atypical causes will present during the timeframe for *chronic meningitis* but may occasionally be seen with a *subacute* course.

Spinal epidural abscess should be suspected in patients with back pain accompanied by fever, back pain with neurologic deficits on exam, or relatively rapid onset atraumatic back pain, though patients may not always present with classic signs and symptoms. Patients with spinal surgery and instrumentation, IV drug abuse, and immunosuppression are at higher risk, and benefit from a lower threshold for testing. Epidural hematoma, osteomyelitis, discitis, aortic aneurysm rupture, aortic dissection, and pulmonary embolism are other considerations.

DIAGNOSTIC TESTING

Blood Testing

Currently, no test can substitute for cerebrospinal fluid analysis. The complete blood count (CBC) with differential is a nonspecific adjunct in the diagnostic evaluation of a patient suspected to have a CNS infection. However, a normal leukocyte count and differential does not rule out the diagnosis of a CNS infection.

Procalcitonin has been shown in multiple studies to have some value in the discrimination between bacterial and viral etiologies of meningitis. With an estimated sensitivity of 90% and specificity of 98% for bacterial infection, it may be useful as an adjunct when the clinical picture is unclear, but it is currently not considered definitive to rule out bacterial meningitis.[12] In addition, elevation in serum erythrocyte sedimentation rate (ESR) and C-reactive protein (CRP) are potentially useful but not diagnostic in the differentiation of bacterial and viral meningitis.[13]

A serum glucose level is needed to interpret the CSF glucose level. Although most patients do not require coagulation studies, patients who are taking warfarin should have their INR checked. Patients on direct oral anticoagulants can be checked for anti-Xa levels, if available, to assess for current anticoagulant activity. Coagulation status should be considered in patients on anticoagulants prior to attempting a lumbar puncture given the risk of bleeding complications.

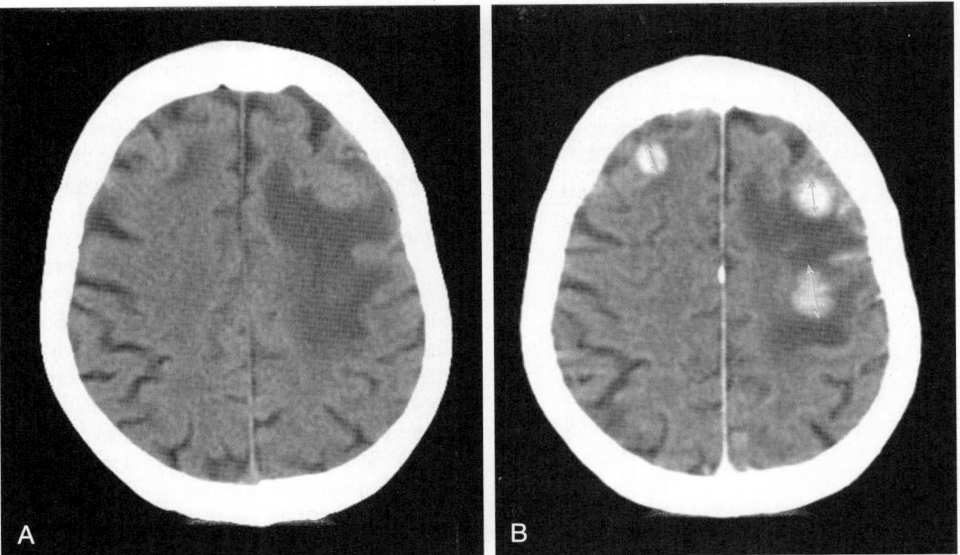

Fig. 95.2 CT image of multiple brain metastases with surrounding edema. When evaluating for CNS infection, findings such as this may suggest that LP is unnecessary or unwise.

Blood cultures should be obtained for all patients who are being evaluated for a CNS infection, ideally on arrival. However, they may still have benefit later in the patient's course even if antimicrobial therapy has already been administered, because pneumococcal and meningococcal infections may be identified in the blood of patients with these CNS infections.

Neuroimaging

A CT scan without contrast of the head or magnetic resonance imaging (MRI) scan of the brain is indicated in any patient with a suspected CNS infection in which an intracranial hemorrhage or mass lesion is suggested by history or examination. Contrast studies are more sensitive if a mass lesion is high on the differential (Fig. 95.2). A CT scan may show hypodense lesions in the temporal lobes in patients with HSV encephalitis, although an MRI scan reveals enhancement with greater sensitivity (Fig. 95.3). Neuroimaging should not delay antimicrobial therapy, which can be initiated prior to imaging, and LP should still be obtained expeditiously.

A contrast-enhanced cranial CT or MRI scan is diagnostic for a CNS abscess, though the MRI is more sensitive. Large lesions are generally visible on non–contrast-head CTs, although again, MRI is more sensitive and can show smaller lesions that may be mimicking meningitis or encephalitis. When evaluating for spinal abscess, CT imaging of the spine is insufficiently sensitive. MRI of the entire spine is the test of choice (Fig. 95.4), as lesions may be multiple and discontinuous, and can be difficult to localize by exam alone. In patients with contraindications to MRI, a CT myelogram of the spine is an alternative, although definitive testing is preferred if possible due to the high morbidity associated with missed spinal abscess. Transfer to an MRI-capable center may be appropriate if imaging is not available in a timely manner.

Bedside ultrasound of the optic nerve sheath diameter is a rapid and accurate way to evaluate for increased intracranial pressure. This is performed using a high-frequency probe placed over a closed eye. The optic nerve can be assessed in either longitudinal or transverse planes and measured 3 mm behind the globe of the eye;[14] the upper limit of normal for optic nerve sheath dilation is 5 mm (Fig. 95.5). A diameter greater than 5 mm suggests increased intracranial pressure but does not distinguish among potential causes.

Lumbar Puncture

A lumbar puncture (LP) for CSF analysis is indicated whenever meningitis or encephalitis is suspected unless the skin overlying the puncture site is infected or there is potential for brain herniation. In the majority of patients with suspected meningitis who have no focal neurologic findings (including no altered mental status), LP can be safely performed without delay and without preceding neuroimaging studies. Coagulation studies do not need to be routinely obtained prior to LP, but should be considered in those with personal or family history of coagulopathy, use of anticoagulation medications, organ failure, or evidence of DIC. A platelet count below 40,000 should also prompt consideration for delaying an LP. An INR greater than 1.4 in patients on warfarin is a relative contraindication to LP. The guidelines for DOACs depend on the agent being used; ideally these should be held at least 24 hours prior to an LP.[15] The need for a LP cannot be anticipated in most cases in the ED, however, and the emergent need for the procedure must be weighed against the increased risk of bleeding.

Herniation has been described in patients following LP, hence the recommendation to avoid a LP in patients with evidence of increased intracranial pressure. A recent study showed the risk of herniation to be only 0.1% in the first hour following LP, suggesting that some reported cases of herniation may be due to the infectious process itself.[9] Regardless, at the present time, we recommend that LP be avoided in those patients with the presence of papilledema, increased optic nerve sheath diameter on ultrasound, mass lesions on CT imaging or other signs of increased ICP. Early initiation of antimicrobial therapy should not be delayed pending LP for patients with high clinical suspicion for CNS infections. However, the CSF can be sterilized within as little as one hour post-antibiotics, so LPs should proceed as expeditiously as is feasible.

If the physician is unable to obtain CSF during the LP, consideration should be given to a prompt radiology-guided LP. If no LP can be performed, the blood cultures obtained on presentation may still be of assistance in identifying the causative microbe.

Opening Pressure

The normal upper limit of CSF pressure in an adult is 20 cm H_2O. The opening pressure is only valid for patients in the lateral recumbent position, because it may increase substantially when the patient is in

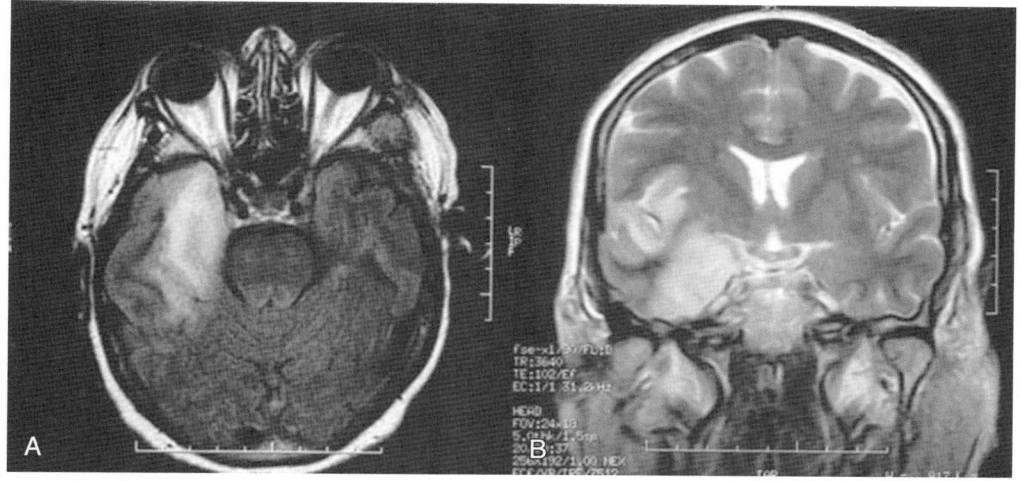

Fig. 95.3 Temporal lobe enhancement on brain MRI. This is a common imaging finding in patients with HSV encephalitis.

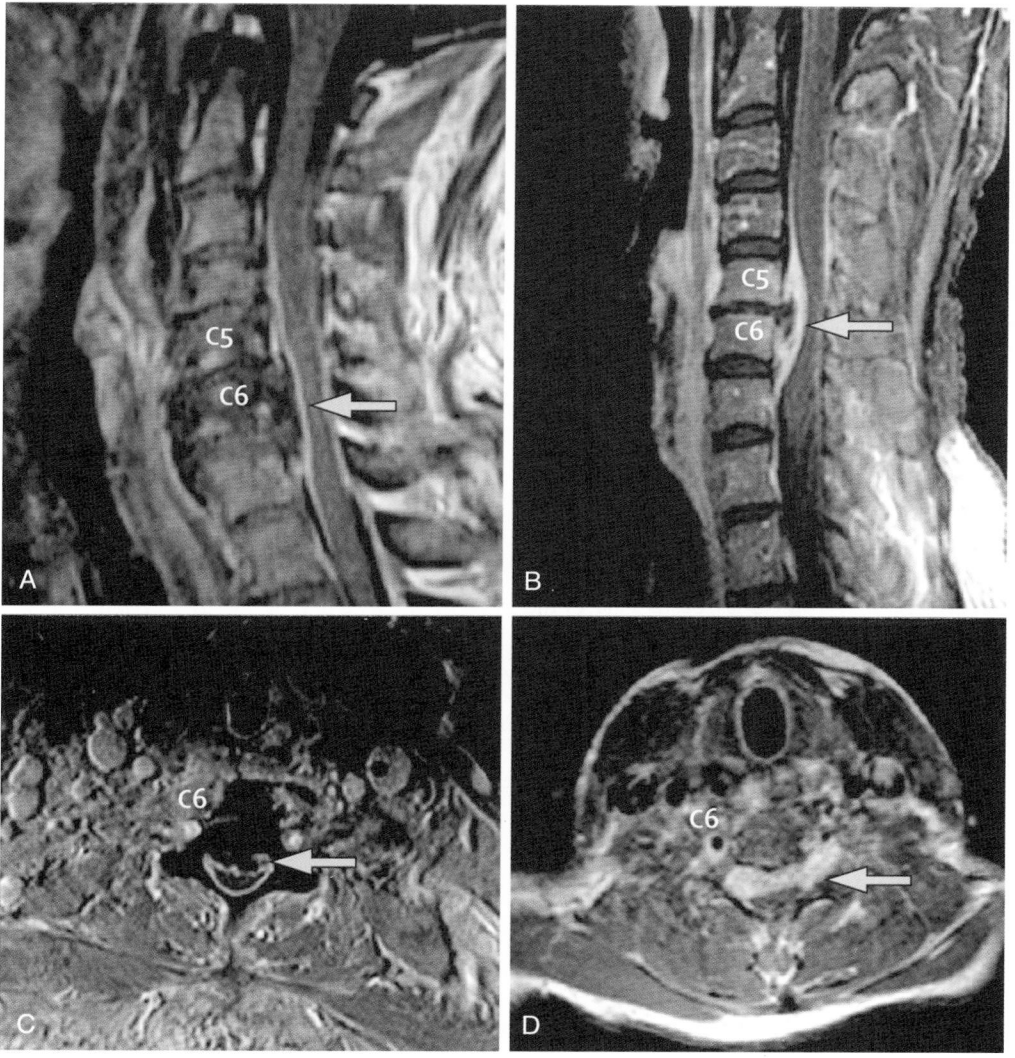

Fig. 95.4 Epidural abscess as seen on lumbar spine MRI. CT imaging may miss smaller spinal cord lesions such as these.

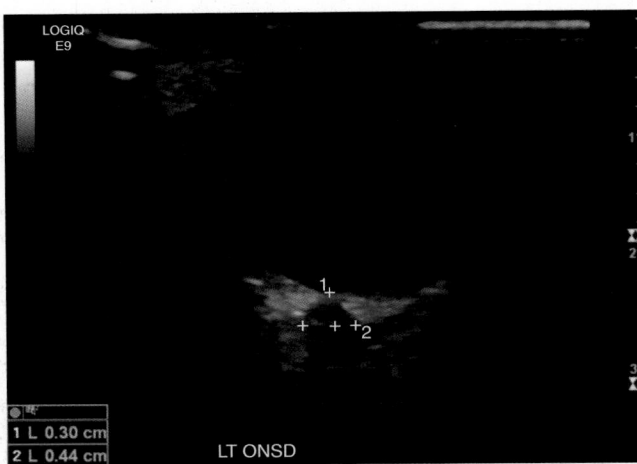

Fig. 95.5 The optic nerve sheath diameter using ultrasound is measured 3 mm behind the optic disc. This method can be used by the clinician at bedside to quickly assess patients for increased intracranial pressure.

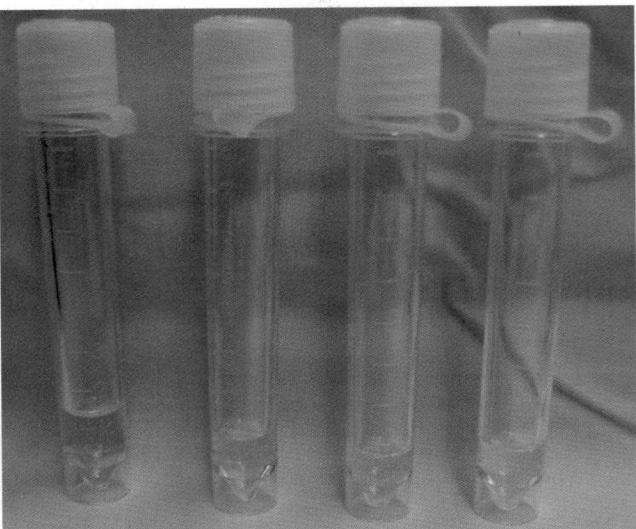

Fig. 95.6 CSF specimens after collection. The clear appearance, indistinguishable from water, is a normal finding; any degree of cloudiness can suggest CNS infection.

the sitting position. It may also be falsely elevated when the patient is tense, has marked muscle contraction, or is obese. The pressure is often elevated in bacterial, tuberculous, and fungal meningitides and a variety of noninfectious processes, and often normal in viral meningitis. There is little data however on the sensitivity and specificity of this marker. As such, obtaining an opening pressure when possible prior to collecting CSF provides an additional data point to support a viral or bacterial clinical picture but cannot be used in isolation. If CSF collection requires the patient to sit up for mechanical reasons or patient comfort, opening pressure may be safely omitted.

Cerebrospinal Spinal Fluid Analysis

When possible, at least three sterile tubes each containing 1 to 1.5 mL of CSF should be obtained and numbered in sequence. A fourth tube is desirable in case additional studies are later necessary. The fluid should then be sent to the laboratory for immediate analysis of turbidity, xanthochromia, glucose, protein, cell count and differential, Gram stain, and bacterial culture. When only a small amount of fluid can be obtained, the most important studies are the cell count with differential, the Gram stain, and culture. Depending on the clinical scenario and patient risk factors, such as HIV, immunosuppression, travel history, or exposures, additional testing can be valuable as well. These studies can include cryptococcal antigens, acid-fast bacilli stain, or the Venereal Disease Research Laboratory (VDRL) test for neurosyphilis. Ideally, a cell count should be performed on both the first and last tubes collected to help differentiate true CSF pleocytosis from contamination of the specimen by peripheral blood from a traumatic LP.

The CSF should be assessed immediately for turbidity or cloudiness by the person performing the LP. Normal CSF is completely clear, colorless, and indistinguishable from water (Fig. 95.6); any degree of turbidity is pathologic. Changes in CSF clarity can generally be seen when leukocyte counts are greater than 200 to 500 cells/mm³.

Cerebrospinal Spinal Fluid Cell Count

Normal adult CSF contains no more than 5 leukocytes/mm³ with at most one granulocyte (polymorphonuclear [PMN] leukocyte); the presence of more than one PMN or a total cell count of more than 5 cells/mm³ is evidence of CNS infection. The presence of any eosinophil in the CSF is abnormal; occasionally basophils may be seen in the absence of disease. The cell counts in bacterial meningitis often exceed

1000 cells/mm³ with a neutrophil predominance (Table 95.2). However, the initial CSF analysis exhibits lymphocytosis (lymphocyte count greater than 50%) in approximately 10% of cases of bacterial meningitis. In some cases of *L. monocytogenes* meningitis, CSF analysis shows a cell count of less than 1000 cells/mm³ with lymphocyte predominance but near-normal CSF glucose levels. In viral meningitis, encephalitis, tuberculous meningitis, or fungal meningitis, counts are typically less than 1000 cells/mm³ with lymphocyte predominance. However, early (within 48 hours) viral presentations may reveal neutrophils and be indistinguishable from presentations of bacterial meningitis. Treatment with antibiotics before the LP will decrease the yield of Gram stain and cultures but likely does not affect the CSF cell counts or total CSF protein in meningitis.

A traumatic LP is suggested by the presence of 10,000 or more red blood cells (RBCs)/mm³ or fewer RBCs in the final tube than in the initial tube. In the presence of a traumatic LP, the CSF white blood cell (WBC) pleocytosis can be estimated by subtracting one leukocyte for every 500 to 1000 RBCs.

Normal CSF cell counts, although reassuring, do not completely exclude bacterial meningitis, especially in immunocompromised patients. Lumbar puncture for brain abscess is unlikely to offer diagnostic yield except in cases of abscess rupture into the ventricular space. Although abnormalities can be seen, the CSF can also be entirely normal. Lumbar puncture is generally contraindicated in cases of spinal epidural abscess due to concern for seeding the infection.

Gram Stain

A Gram stain of a CSF specimen may identify the causative organism up to 75% of the time in cases of bacterial meningitis, however this is highly dependent on the concentration of the bacteria present. The yield is diminished to 40% to 60% when there has been prior treatment with antibiotics.[16] Gram-stain appearance of the CSF of a patient with *N. meningitidis* is shown in Figure 95.7.

Xanthochromia

Xanthochromia is the yellowish discoloration of the supernatant of centrifuged CSF specimens, detectable by visual inspection or spectrophotometry. Xanthochromia is an abnormal finding and is concerning

TABLE 95.2 Typical CSF Findings for Various Etiologies of Meningitis and Encephalitis

	Normal	Bacterial	Viral	Fungal/TB
Pressure (cm H$_2$0)	5–20	>30	Normal or increased	Increased
Protein (mg/dL)	18–45	Increased	Normal or increased	Normal or increased
Glucose	2/3 serum glucose	Decreased	Normal	Normal or decreased
Gram stain	Negative	60–90% positive	Negative	Negative
White blood cells	<5	Usually >1000	100–1000	50–500
WBC differential predominance	None	Neutrophils	Lymphocytes	Lymphocytes or monocytes

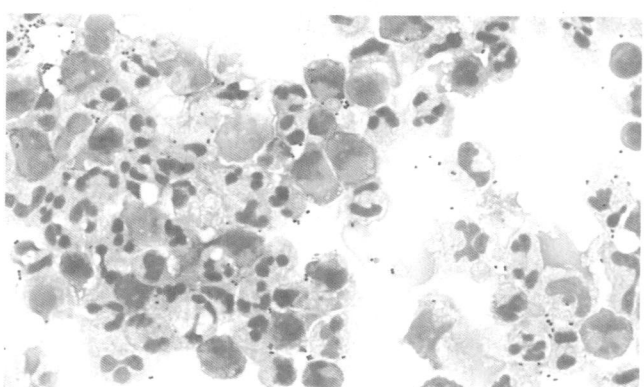

Fig. 95.7 The Gram stain appearance of a CSF sample infected with *N. meningitidis*, a gram-negative coccus. Magnification 1000x.

for SAH when detected. It results from the lysis of RBCs with the release of the breakdown pigments oxyhemoglobin, bilirubin, and methemoglobin into the CSF. This process takes hours to occur, though in patients presenting between 12 hours and 2 weeks of symptom onset, the sensitivity is close to 100% if analyzed using spectrophotometry. Visual inspection of the centrifuged specimen has been found to be much lower (47%). If a traumatic tap has introduced enough plasma to raise the CSF protein level to 150 mg/dL or more, blood pigments may cause xanthochromia. If the CSF protein level is less than 150 mg/dL, however, xanthochromia of a centrifuged CSF specimen almost always indicates that a SAH has occurred.

Glucose

The CSF glucose level is normally two-thirds of the serum glucose; when the serum glucose is within normal range, the CSF glucose is usually between 50 and 80 mg/dL. In the first 4 hours after food intake or parenteral glucose administration, however, the ratio is decreased, and the results are difficult to interpret with certainty. A CSF-to-serum glucose ratio of less than 0.5 in normoglycemic subjects is abnormal and may represent the impaired glucose transport mechanisms and increased CNS glucose use associated with bacterial meningitis. Mild decreases in the CSF glucose level may occur in viral, fungal, or tuberculous meningitis. However, bacterial meningitis should be presumed to be the cause of low CSF glucose until it is clearly excluded.

Protein

The normal CSF protein level in adults is typically below 45 mg/dL. An elevated CSF protein (higher than 100 mg/dL) commonly occurs with acute bacterial meningitis. When a traumatic LP has occurred, the CSF protein can be corrected for the presence of blood by subtracting 1 mg/dL of protein for each 1000 RBCs. Elevated CSF protein concentrations can result from any cause of meningitis, SAH, CNS vasculitis, syphilis,

viral encephalitis, neoplasms, and demyelination syndromes. HSV and VZV can have higher CSF protein values than are typically seen in viral CNS infection (>100 mg/dL).

Other Stains

Historically, an India ink staining of the CSF was performed to diagnose cryptococcal meningitis. Though it is a rapid means of diagnosis, it has poor sensitivity (as low as 30% in non-AIDS patients). Cryptococcal antigen testing is now the gold standard for investigating cryptococcal infection, with baseline serum and CSF antigen titers providing a good estimate of fungal burden and prognosis but not response to therapy. Latex agglutination and enzyme immunoassay techniques have high sensitivity for cryptococcus as well but are inferior to antigen testing. Acid-fast bacilli (AFB) staining has been used for diagnosis of tuberculous meningitis but has poor sensitivity (typically <60%).

Lactic Acid

The normal reference range for CSF lactate is between 0.88 to 2.7 mmol/L. Although nonspecific, elevations in CSF lactic acid concentrations are suspicious for bacterial meningitis, while normal lactate levels (<2.7 mmol/L) are usually seen in patients with viral causes of meningitis. Recent studies have shown CSF lactate to have excellent predictive value in differentiating bacterial from viral meningitis,[17] and CSF lactate may be useful as an adjunct in the workup of suspected meningitis. We recommend its use, when available, to aid in determining the cause of CNS infection.

Antigen Detection

Nucleic acid amplification tests such as PCR have sensitivities of 67% to 100% for *H. influenza,* 79% to 100% for *S. pneumoniae,* and 91% to 100% for *N. meningitides;* specificities are nearly 100% for all three organisms.[1] The value of antigen testing has been demonstrated in multiple studies in which acute bacterial meningitis was confirmed only by PCR.[1] The sensitivity of bacterial culture is much lower and varies considerably based on the specific causative microorganism; under ideal conditions, cultures may miss a third of organisms, and sensitivity can be even lower if the patient has been treated with antibiotics. PCR testing has been demonstrated to have a sensitivity of 70% despite antibiotic therapy up to 1 week following initiation of treatment.[18]

Antigen and antibody testing have particular utility in HSV encephalitis. Although enzyme-linked immunosorbent assays (ELISAs) can detect HSV antibody production, the appearance of antibodies in CSF occurs too late to aid in any therapeutic decision analysis. PCR amplification and the identification of HSV DNA have a sensitivity of 96% and a specificity of 99% early in the disease, such that brain biopsy is no longer needed to make this diagnosis. PCR testing is sensitive for other viral infections as well, including VZV and enterovirus, though identification of the exact virus usually does not affect management. Diagnosis of VZV encephalitis is further improved by testing for IgG and IgM antibodies in the CSF.

TABLE 95.3   Common Bacterial Pathogens and Initial Antibiotic Regimens for Suspected Bacterial Meningoencephalitis,[a] Listed by Age Group and Risk Factors

Patient Subgroup	Most Common Bacterial Pathogen	Most Common Intravenous Therapy
Neonates (up to 4 weeks)	*S. agalactiae, E. coli, L. monocytogenes, S. agalactiae,* gram-negative bacilli	Ampicillin (100 mg/kg/dose q8h for 0-7 days and 75 mg/kg/dose for 8-28 days) AND Cefotaxime (50 mg/kg every 8 hrs; may increase to 50 mg/kg q6h for 8-28 days)
Infants and children	*S. pneumoniae, N. meningiditis*	Ceftriaxone (100 mg/kg every day) OR Cefotaxime (75 mg/kg every 6 hrs)
Adults	*S. pneumoniae, N. meningiditis*	Ceftriaxone (2 g every 12 hrs) OR Cefotaxime (2 g q4–6h) AND Vancomycin (loading dose: 20–35 mg/kg actual body weight [not to exceed 3000 mg] or 20–25 mg/kg actual body weight not to exceed 3000 mg in patients with obesity, then 15–20 mg/kg actual body weight every 8–12 hrs)
Elderly	*S. pneumoniae, N. meningiditis, L. monocytogenes*	Ceftriaxone (2 g every 12 hrs) OR Cefotaxime (3 g every 6 hrs) AND Vancomycin (loading dose: 20–35 mg/kg actual body weight [not to exceed 3000 mg] or 20–25 mg/kg actual body weight not to exceed 3000 mg in patients with obesity, then 15–20 mg/kg actual body weight every 8–12 hrs) AND Ampicillin (2 g every 4 hrs)
Immunocompromised	*S. pneumoniae, N. meningiditis, H. influenzae*	Ceftriaxone (2 g every 12 hrs) OR Cefotaxime (3 g every 6 hrs) AND Vancomycin (loading dose: 20–35 mg/kg actual body weight [not to exceed 3000 mg] or 20–25 mg/kg actual body weight not to exceed 3000 mg in patients with obesity, then 15–20 mg/kg actual body weight every 8–12 hrs) AND Ampicillin (2 g every 4 hrs)
Suspected hospital-acquired organism	*S. aureus, S. epidermidis,* aerobic gram-negative bacilli	Vancomycin (15–20 mg/kg every 8 hrs) AND Cefepime (2 g every 8 hrs) OR Meropenem (2 g every 8 hrs)

Adapted from Dorsett M, Liang SY. Diagnosis and treatment of central nervous system infections in the emergency department. *Emerg Med Clin North Am.* 2016;34(4):917-942.[25]
[a]In addition to dexamethasone (adults 0.4 mg/kg IV, up to 10 mg; infants and children 0.15 mg/kg, up to 10 mg

PCR has improved the diagnosis of tuberculous meningitis as well and newer assays continue to show improved performance characteristics. One of the latest assays, Xpert Ultra, was recently shown to have a sensitivity of 95% (compared to previous assays and culture with a 45% sensitivity) and has been endorsed as the initial diagnostic test of choice by the World Health Organization.[19]

Bacterial Cultures

Bacterial cultures of CSF should be performed despite some organisms, such as mycobacterium, being difficult to culture. Although results of cultures will not be available in the ED, they can be helpful to the subsequent treatment team for guiding antimicrobial therapy if positive. Bacterial culture yields can be decreased in patients pretreated with antibiotics, depending on the timing of the antibiotics and the cultures. Although antigen testing holds promise, it alone cannot replace bacterial cultures at this time.

Additional Investigations

Other ancillary investigations such as echocardiography, body fluid cultures, chest X-ray, CT of the maxillary region, and urinalysis may be undertaken as necessary to evaluate suspected coexistent disease, such as a distant infection that may be seeding the CNS.

Characteristic EEG abnormalities have been associated with HSV type 1 encephalitis, including diffuse high-amplitude slow waves, temporal lobe spike-and-wave activity, and periodic lateralized epileptiform discharges, although these changes are not specific enough to make them diagnostic. More than half of patients with viral encephalitis may have an abnormal EEG, most commonly in patients with HSV; it is not routine however to obtain an EEG emergently in the ED and EEG is unlikely to acutely change management unless nonconvulsive status epilepticus is diagnosed.

MANAGEMENT

Initial management of the patient with suspected CNS infection focuses on ensuring CNS oxygenation and perfusion. In cases of severely elevated ICP, management is with endotracheal intubation, mannitol, hypertonic saline, and maintenance of eucapnia on the ventilator.

Bacterial Meningitis

Treatment of bacterial meningitis requires bactericidal antibiotics that penetrate the blood-brain barrier and achieve therapeutic CSF concentrations. Until the causative organism is identified, broadspectrum coverage of the most common pathogens is indicated (Table 95.3). Ceftriaxone (2 g every 12 hours) or cefotaxime (3 g every 6 hours) are the most commonly used agents, with vancomycin (15–20 mg/kg every 8 hours) added to cover potentially resistant organisms. In neonates, especially those with hyperbilirubinemia, ceftriaxone should be avoided, because it displaces bilirubin from albumin binding sites and can further increase bilirubin levels in the blood. Cefotaxime is instead recommended in this population. We recommend high-dose ampicillin (2 g every 4 hours) be added in adults over 50 years old and infants younger than 1 month old (100 mg/kg/dose q8h for 0–7 days and 75 mg/kg/dose for 8–28 days) because they are at risk for *Listeria*. If *Listeria* meningitis is suspected, gentamicin may also have a mortality benefit if added to ampicillin, though this should be used cautiously in patients with renal dysfunction.

Patients who have had a recent hospitalization, especially for surgery, may be at risk for hospital-acquired antibiotic-resistant organisms and may benefit from broader coverage with cefepime (2 g every 8 hours) instead of ceftriaxone. In patients allergic to cephalosporins, meropenem or chloramphenicol is recommended. Linezolid (600 mg every 12 hours) or moxifloxacin (400 mg once daily) with vancomycin can be used in cephalosporin-resistant strains of pneumococcus.

Treatment with corticosteroids (0.15 mg/kg up to 10 mg IV dexamethasone every 6 hours for 4 days) decreases mortality in patients with pneumococcal meningitis and decreases the incidence of hearing loss in patients with *H. influenzae* meningitis. Interestingly, this benefit has only been shown in high-income countries and not in low-income countries, likely secondary to better access to medications and specialist care in the former.[20] Though some data suggest benefit persists if started within 12 hours of antibiotic initiation, the first dose of steroids should be given with or 20 minutes before initiation of antibiotics in suspected adult bacterial meningitis. However, a recent large, prospective study showed an increased incidence of adverse outcomes related to dexamethasone in cases of *Listeria* CNS infections and therefore steroids should be discontinued if this organism is identified.[21]

Tuberculous Meningitis

Early antimicrobial intervention in acute tuberculous meningitis improves the patient's prognosis and a strong clinical suggestion of this disease is an appropriate indication to begin antituberculous therapy. A standard treatment regimen consists of 4-drug therapy with isoniazid (5 mg/kg once daily; max dose 300 mg), rifampin (20 to 30 mg/kg once daily; max dose 600 mg), pyrazinamide (<40 kg: 35 mg/kg/dose; 40 to 55 kg: 1000 mg daily; 56 to 75 kg: 1500 mg daily; 76 to 90 kg: 2000 mg daily), and ethambutol (<40 kg: 25 mg/kg/dose; 40 to 55 kg: 800 mg daily; 56 to 75 kg: 1200 mg daily; 76 to 90 kg: 1600 mg daily). Alternative dosing strategies exist that involve less-frequent dosing and can be considered with infectious disease consultation. Neurosurgical consultation may be required in cases of hydrocephalus or mass lesions. Corticosteroids have also been shown to decrease secondary complications, and we recommend an initial dose of 0.15 mg/kg of IV dexamethasone.

Fungal Meningitis

Because fungal meningitis most often has a prolonged course and can be difficult to diagnose in the ED, the initiation of antifungal treatment is rarely required in the ED unless clinical suspicion is high. Four agents are commonly used to treat fungal meningitis: amphotericin B, flucytosine, miconazole, and fluconazole. Of these, amphotericin B, either alone or in combination with flucytosine, is the most common regimen. Fluconazole can be used if flucytosine is not available and can be used as monotherapy if amphotericin B is not available, though it is associated with higher rates of treatment failure.

Viral Meningitis

The majority of viral meningitis cases have a short, relatively benign and self-limited course followed by a complete recovery. Acyclovir (10 mg/kg IV every 8 hours) is recommended in immunocompromised patients with HSV meningitis and should be considered based on the theoretical benefit in immunocompromised patients with VZV meningitis. Benefit has not been shown in HSV or VZV meningitis in immunocompetent patients. In these cases, as with most types of viral meningitis, care is mainly supportive, because no treatments have been shown to be effective for relieving symptoms, shortening the course of disease, or preventing disease progression.

Early cases of viral meningitis may be indistinguishable from bacterial meningitis, and diagnostic certainty may not be provided by initial CSF analysis. When doubt exists about the veracity of the diagnosis, it is reasonable to initiate workup and empiric antibiotics and admit the patient to the hospital.

Viral Encephalitis

In cases of suspected viral encephalitis, empiric IV acyclovir (10 mg/kg IV every 8 hours) is recommended as it targets both HSV and VZV,

two common causes of this disease. Patients with CMV encephalitis can be treated with ganciclovir (5 mg/kg every 12 hours), although this diagnosis is unlikely to be made in the ED. Otherwise, patients should largely be treated supportively.

Central Nervous System Abscess

The location, size, and number of abscesses influences the choice of medical management, surgical excision, or aspiration. Consideration of empiric antimicrobial therapy is ideally accomplished in consultation with neurosurgical providers, as it is reasonable to withhold antimicrobial therapy prior to aspiration or surgical excision if an urgent neurosurgical intervention is planned. If neurosurgery is delayed, however, we recommend initiating empiric treatment, as prolonged time without antibiotics has been associated with adverse outcomes.

Abscesses originating from sinus or ear infections are treated with cefotaxime (2 g IV every 4-6 hours) or ceftriaxone (2 g IV every 12 hours) plus metronidazole (500 mg IV every 6 to 8 hours). Abscesses related to trauma or neurosurgical procedures require vancomycin for *S. aureus* or methicillin-resistant *S. aureus* coverage. Patients at high risk for tuberculous, fungal, or parasitic abscess may also receive coverage for the suspected etiologic agent. Corticosteroids may mitigate superimposed cerebral edema and a recent meta-analysis did not show an increase in mortality with their use.[22] We therefore recommend 10 mg IV dexamethasone for CNS abscesses associated with cerebral edema.

Spinal epidural abscesses should also be managed with a combined medical and surgical approach. Neurosurgical consultation should be obtained as soon as possible to evaluate the need for emergent intervention, particularly if neurologic deficits are present. Additionally, we recommend empiric vancomycin (loading dose: 20 to 35 mg/kg actual body weight [not to exceed 3000 mg] or 20 to 25 mg/kg actual body weight not to exceed 3000 mg in patients with obesity, then 15 to 20 mg/kg actual body weight every 8 to 12 hrs) and ceftriaxone (2 g IV every 12 hours) for antimicrobial treatment. When atypical organisms such as *Pseudomonas* are present or suspected, broader coverage is recommended with a fourth-generation cephalosporin (e.g., cefepime 2 g IV every 8 hours).

CSF Shunt Infection

After obtaining neuroimaging (either CT or rapid MRI protocol), management generally includes neurosurgical consultation and empiric antibiotics directed at skin flora, including *S. aureus and Streptococcus* as well as MRSA and *Pseudomonas*. We recommend vancomycin (loading dose: 20 to 35 mg/kg actual body weight [not to exceed 3000 mg] or 20 to 25 mg/kg actual body weight not to exceed 3000 mg in patients with obesity, then 15 to 20 mg/kg actual body weight every 8 to 12 hrs) and an anti-pseudomonal beta-lactam, such as cefepime (2 g every 8 hours).

Chemoprophylaxis

The risk for developing meningococcal meningitis is increased 400 to 800 times in individuals with close contact with an infected person. Close contacts at risk include health care workers exposed to the patient's secretions (as might occur during endotracheal intubation or nasotracheal suctioning), those exposed for a prolonged period (e.g., spending more than 8 hours less than three feet away from the patient such as roommates, intimate partners, daycare attendants) or those exposed to an infected person's oral excretions. At risk contacts should be treated with four doses of oral rifampin (600 mg every 12 hours) or a single dose of oral ciprofloxacin (500 mg). Pregnant women can receive a single intramuscular (IM) dose of ceftriaxone (250 mg). In addition, close contacts should be advised to

TABLE 95.4   Recommended Population for Prophylaxis and Antibiotic Dosing Regimens, Listed by Exposure Type

	Population	Medication	Dose	Frequency
N. meningitidis	Close contacts (roommates, partners, daycare workers), health care workers exposed to secretions	Ciprofloxacin	500 mg	Once
		Rifampin	600 mg	Every 12 hours for 2 days
		Ceftriaxone	250 mg	Once (preferred in pregnancy)
H. influenzae	Immunocompromised children (including unvaccinated), contacts with unvaccinated children <4 years old	Rifampin	20 mg/kg	Daily for four days
All others (bacterial, viral, fungal)	All	None	None	None

watch for fever, sore throat, rash, or any symptoms of meningitis. If there are signs of active meningococcal disease, the close contact should be hospitalized for IV antibiotics as presented above, because rifampin is not recommended as therapy against invasive meningococcal disease.

Rifampin prophylaxis (20 mg/kg once daily; max dose 600 mg for four days) is currently recommended by the Centers for Disease Control (CDC) for contacts of patients with *H. influenzae* meningitis in households with members aged younger than 4 years who have not completed their vaccination schedule or immunocompromised children (<18 years old), regardless of their vaccination status. It is only recommended in childcare facilities caring for immunocompromised or unvaccinated children in instances where two confirmed cases have occurred. There is no current recommendation for chemoprophylaxis in pneumococcal meningitis. See Table 95.4 for a summary of the guidelines.

Immunoprophylaxis

Although vaccinations against pathogens implicated in CNS infection are not routinely administered in the ED, it is useful to be aware of currently available vaccinations so that patients and family members may be queried regarding their risk for vaccine-preventable diseases.

A quadrivalent meningococcal vaccine based on the polysaccharide capsule and conferring protection against group A, C, Y, and W-135 meningococci has been in routine use since it was approved in 1978. It is currently recommended for routine use in children and adolescents aged 11 to 21 years old. People living in close quarters with other individuals (e.g., college students, military recruits), travelers to endemic areas, as well as asplenic individuals are at increased risk of meningococcal disease and should receive the vaccine. Two vaccines targeting serogroup B also have been approved for use in the United States since 2014 but have yet to be routinely administered. The capsular polysaccharide vaccines used to immunize adults are not protective in children younger than 2 years old because of poor antibody response.

The development of a highly effective pneumococcal vaccine has been hampered by the large number of serotypes of the organism. Despite this, a single dose of the vaccine should be considered for elderly or debilitated patients, especially those with pulmonary disease, and for patients with impaired splenic function, splenectomy, or sickle cell anemia. Vaccination against pneumococcus is recommended in patients who have been treated for an episode of pneumococcal pneumonia to prevent recurrent infection. A heptavalent conjugated pneumococcal vaccine has also been developed and is recommended for universal childhood immunization by the ACIP.

A conjugate vaccine effective against Hib has been developed for use in the pediatric population and is recommended for all infants starting at 2 months.

DISPOSITION

With the exception of obvious presentations of viral meningitis, the majority of CNS infections require inpatient evaluation and treatment for IV antimicrobials, monitoring for acute decompensation, following of cultures, specialist input, and potential surgical intervention, depending on the infection. Because normal CSF cell counts do not completely exclude bacterial meningitis, patients with a high likelihood of meningitis require hospitalization with frequent reevaluation, antimicrobial therapy, and possible repeat LP.

Some patients with suspected viral meningitis should be considered for hospitalization. These include patients who are immunocompromised, patients with more severe disease or refractory symptoms, patients who are unable to tolerate oral intake, and those in whom the diagnosis is unclear.

The references for this chapter can be found online at ExpertConsult.com.

96

Thought Disorders

Matthew P. Kelly and Dag Shapshak

KEY CONCEPTS

- Thought disorder symptoms can be precipitated by psychiatric, underlying medical, and toxicologic etiologies.
- Diagnostic testing should be patient specific and based on the particular medical processes that the clinician feels may be causing or exacerbating the thought disorder, rather than panels of routine tests.
- Consider nonphysical interventions first when appropriate, but chemical sedation or physical restraints may become immediately necessary for patients who demonstrate life-threatening aggressive and dangerous behaviors.
- Appropriate disposition depends on the etiology of the underlying psychosis and response to treatment while addressing patient and community safety considerations. Psychiatric consultation is often required.

FOUNDATIONS

Background and Importance

Patients with a history of mental disorders have a higher rate of emergency department (ED) visits than the general population. Patients with at least one primary psychiatric visit to an ED are four times more likely to become frequent ED users compared to patients with none, and the severity of mental illness correlates with the frequency of ED utilization.[1] The rate of ED visits for patients with mental disorders has increased substantially over the last several years for both adults[2] and children.[3] Schizophrenia is among the top 10 most disabling and economically catastrophic medical disorders as ranked by the World Health Organization, and the global burden of disease continues to increase,[4] affecting almost 1% of the world's population. Slightly more men than women are affected and at a younger age. The modal age of onset is between 18 and 25 years for men and between 25 and 35 years for women.

Groups at high risk for developing schizophrenia include migrants, urban dwellers, people born in late winter to early spring, and those with advanced paternal age at conception. The mortality rate for patients with schizophrenia is 2.5 times that of the general population and continues to grow, especially in populations with low socioeconomic status. Patients diagnosed with schizophrenia have a mean life expectancy almost 15 years shorter than the general population and a 5% to 10% life-time risk of death by suicide.[5] Financial costs associated with schizophrenia are disproportionally high relative to other chronic mental and physical health conditions, reflecting both direct costs of care, and indirect costs of lost productivity, criminal justice involvement, social needs, and homelessness.

Pathophysiology

Although the etiology of schizophrenia is multifactorial, it has a substantial genetic component with approximately 80% of disease expression attributed to genetic factors. In addition to genetic factors, environmental and neurodevelopmental influences increase risk of the disease.[6] Such influences include perinatal stress and hypoxia, poor nutrition, infections, and vitamin D and zinc deficiencies. Newer research is showing that schizophrenia may be detectable at earlier stages of development, prior to the first psychotic episode, which may open the window for earlier interventions.[7]

Alterations in the dopaminergic, serotonergic, cholinergic, glutamatergic, and GABA-ergic pathways have been implicated in the pathophysiology of schizophrenia. Symptoms may be caused by cortical excitatory-inhibitory imbalance and subcortical dopamine dysregulation in the frontal, temporal, and mesostriatal brain regions.[8] Imaging and postmortem studies have revealed disturbed oligodendroglia-related processes, altered gene expression, disturbed myelination, and altered numbers of oligodendrocytes in the brains of patients with schizophrenia.[9] Genetic predisposition, coupled with early neurodevelopmental disturbances during postnatal brain maturation, are thought to trigger the onset of overt schizophrenia.

Patients often present to the ED via family, police, or EMS exhibiting symptoms of disorganized thought and behavior. They may express language, ideas, and behavior found to be inappropriate and disruptive to accepted patterns of social interaction. Whether the issue involves thought content (delusions), hallucinations or thought form (structure of thinking), the clinical impression is that of psychosis (detachment from reality and societal norms). Acutely psychotic patients raise concerns for the safety of themselves, those around them, and those attempting to care for them.

The emergency clinician's role is to prevent and control violent and disruptive behavior while simultaneously determining if the underlying etiology of the psychosis is functional versus organic in nature. Functional causes include schizophrenia and schizophrenia-like illness, mania, and mood disorder–associated psychosis. Organic causes can mimic a functional psychosis. Medication effects, substance abuse, and certain medical disorders must be excluded before symptoms of psychosis can be attributed to an underlying psychiatric illness.

CLINICAL FEATURES

Thought disorders broadly affect mental activity and can be associated with varying degrees of functional impairment. Schizophrenia is the most common thought disorder characterized by psychotic symptoms of hallucinations, delusions, and disorganized speech. The core psychopathology of schizophrenia and other thought disorders according to the *Diagnostic and Statistical Manual of Mental Disorders, Fifth Edition* (DSM-5) includes both negative and positive symptoms. Negative symptoms include decreased motivation, diminished expressiveness, cognitive deficits involving impaired executive functions, memory, and speed of mental processing.[10]

Positive symptoms of schizophrenia are the most easily identified and can be classified as delusions, hallucinations, and abnormal motor behavior in varying degrees of severity. Significant cognitive symptoms include disorganized speech, thought, and attention, which may impair the individual's ability to communicate. Hallucinations are the perception of a sensory process in the absence of an external source. They can be auditory, olfactory, visual, gustatory, or somatic in nature. The vast majority of patients with schizophrenia suffer with auditory hallucinations.

Patients with schizophrenia typically display disorganization of behavior and cognition. They use disjointed speech patterns that reflect poor organization of thought and lack of a coherent focus of ideas. Their speech patterns are tangential and circumstantial, causing the narrative to wander away from the initial topic of conversation. More severe thought disorders include derailment, neologisms (invented words), word salad (confused, incomprehensible language), and preservations (severely repetitive language). In debilitating cases, there may be no understandable content and speech is utterly incomprehensible.

A separate group of patients with a more extreme deficit in communication are those suffering from catatonia. Catatonia includes immobility, stupor, mutism, resistance to instructions, oppositionalism, echo phenomena, and withdrawal. Although classically associated with schizophrenia because of the profound communication and thought deficiencies, recent studies highlight a strong association of catatonia with mood and medical disorders with only a minority diagnosed with schizophrenia.[11] Treatment is with benzodiazepines.[12]

The development of schizophrenia involves three phases: premorbid, progressive, and residual phases. The premorbid phase is characterized by the development of negative symptoms with deterioration in personal, social, and intellectual functioning. The first indications of schizophrenia typically appear in the late teens and early twenties. Children who later develop schizophrenia may demonstrate social awkwardness, physical clumsiness, and lower IQs than peers and siblings. There may be years of subtle changes in behavior and declining function in school and interpersonal relationships. The progressive phase is often precipitated by a stressful life event precipitating the development of positive symptoms. The progressive phase is said to begin when the patient develops the classic characteristics of schizophrenia mentioned earlier. Patients can become agitated or exhibit a hypervigilant withdrawal state characterized by rocking, staring, violence, or bizarre behavior. It is during the progressive phase that the patient is most likely to be brought to the ED by family, friends, police, or concerned bystanders. The residual phase is characterized by persistence of progressive symptoms and disability. Impaired social and cognitive ability, poor hygiene, delusions, bizarre behavior, and social isolation, and homelessness can all occur. On average, functional outcome is poor and patients have varying levels of

BOX 96.1 Medical Disorders That May Cause Acute Psychosis

Metabolic Disorders
- Hypercalcemia
- Hypercarbia
- Hypoglycemia
- Hyponatremia
- Hypoxia

Inflammatory Disorders
- Sarcoidosis
- Anti-NMDAR encephalitis
- Systemic lupus erythematosus
- Temporal (giant cell) arteritis

Organ Failure
- Hepatic encephalopathy
- Uremia

Neurologic Disorders
- Alzheimer disease
- Cerebrovascular disease
- Encephalitis (including HIV infection)
- Encephalopathies
- Epilepsy
- Huntington disease
- Multiple sclerosis
- Neoplasms
- Normal-pressure hydrocephalus
- Parkinson disease
- Pick disease
- Wilson disease

Endocrine Disorders
- Addison disease
- Cushing disease
- Panhypopituitarism
- Parathyroid disease
- Postpartum psychosis
- Recurrent menstrual psychosis
- Sydenham chorea
- Thyroid disease

Deficiency States
- Niacin
- Thiamine
- Vitamin B_{12} and folate

HIV, Human immunodeficiency virus.

treatment resistance, especially in those with predominantly negative symptoms.[13]

DIFFERENTIAL DIAGNOSES

Medical Disorders

Numerous acute and chronic medical conditions can precipitate thought disorders and mimic acute psychosis (Box 96.1). Patients with underlying psychiatric diseases may develop medical conditions that can exacerbate behavioral symptoms and cloud the distinction between psychiatric and organic brain disease.

BOX 96.2 Pharmacologic Agents That May Cause Acute Psychosis

Antianxiety Agents
- Alprazolam
- Chlordiazepoxide
- Clonazepam
- Clorazepate
- Diazepam
- Ethchlorvynol

Antibiotics
- Isoniazid
- Rifampin

Anticonvulsants
- Ethosuximide
- Phenobarbital
- Phenytoin
- Primidone

Antidepressants
- Amitriptyline
- Doxepin
- Imipramine
- Protriptyline
- Trimipramine

Cardiovascular Drugs
- Captopril
- Digitalis
- Disopyramide
- Methyldopa
- Procainamide
- Propranolol
- Reserpine

Drugs of Abuse
- Alcohol
- Amphetamines
- Cannabis
- Cocaine
- Hallucinogens
- Opioids
- Phencyclidine
- Sedative-hypnotics

Miscellaneous Drugs
- Antihistamines
- Antineoplastics
- Bromides
- Cimetidine
- Corticosteroids
- Disulfiram
- Heavy metals

BOX 96.3 Diagnostic Criteria for Schizophrenia From *Diagnostic and Statistical Manual of Mental Disorders, Fifth Edition*

A. Two (or more) of the following, each present for a significant portion of time during a 1-month period (or less if successfully treated). At least one of these must be (1), (2), or (3):
   1. Delusions
   2. Hallucinations
   3. Disorganized speech (e.g., frequent derailment or incoherence)
   4. Grossly disorganized or catatonic behavior
   5. Negative symptoms (i.e., diminished emotional expression or avolition)

B. For a significant portion of the time since the onset of the disturbance, level of functioning in one or more major areas, such as work, interpersonal relations, or self-care, is markedly below the level achieved prior to the onset (or when the onset is in childhood or adolescence, there is failure to achieve expected level of interpersonal, academic, or occupational functioning).

C. Continuous signs of the disturbance persist for at least 6 months. This 6-month period must include at least 1 month of symptoms (or less if successfully treated) that meet Criterion A (i.e., active-phase symptoms) and may include periods of prodromal or residual symptoms. During these prodromal or residual periods, the signs of the disturbance may be manifested by only negative symptoms or by two or more symptoms listed in Criterion A present in an attenuated form (e.g., odd beliefs, unusual perceptual experiences).

D. Schizoaffective disorder and depressive or bipolar disorder with psychotic features have been ruled out because either (1) no major depressive or manic episodes have occurred concurrently with the active-phase symptoms, or (2) if mood episodes have occurred during active-phase symptoms, they have been present for a minority of the total duration of the active and residual periods of the illness.

E. The disturbance is not attributable to the physiological effects of a substance (e.g., a drug of abuse, a medication) or another medical condition.

F. If there is a history of autism spectrum disorder or a communication disorder of childhood onset, the additional diagnosis of schizophrenia is made only if prominent delusions or hallucinations, in addition to the other required symptoms of schizophrenia, are also present for at least 1 month (or less if successfully treated).

Primary medical conditions are more commonly associated with the new onset of symptoms, acute changes in mental status, recent fluctuations in behavioral symptoms, onset in fifth decade of life or later, the presence of nonauditory hallucinations, lethargy, abnormal vital signs, and poor performance on cognitive testing, particularly orientation to time, place, and person. The onset of psychotic symptoms after a patient has been admitted to a medical care setting is often caused by a medical disorder.

Primary psychiatric conditions are more commonly associated with auditory hallucinations, family history of psychosis, and insidious onset in the late teens to mid-twenties, stable vital signs, and normal orientation. Medical delirium is common in elders and special attention should be paid to patients who develop psychosis later in life.[14]

Patients intoxicated with drugs of abuse are often brought to the ED with bizarre or dangerous behavior. Street drugs such as cocaine, cannabinoids, kratom, amphetamines, bath salts, hallucinogens, and synthetic cannabinoids affect the serotonergic and dopaminergic pathways and can provoke psychotic reactions resembling a primary psychiatric condition, or can unmask latent schizophrenia.[15] Certain pharmacologic agents may also cause acute psychosis mimicking a thought disorder (Box 96.2).

Psychiatric Disorders

Once medical causes have been reasonably ruled out, it can be helpful to classify the type of functional psychosis the patient is exhibiting. The DSM-5 uses four classes of information to distinguish among the various types of psychosis: type of psychotic symptom, course of illness, consequences of illness, and exclusions. Each category can help distinguish schizophrenia from other psychiatric disorders that include psychosis among their symptoms. The DSM-5 definition of schizophrenia is included in Box 96.3.

A brief psychotic disorder involves the sudden onset of psychotic symptoms in response to major stress and lasts from several days up to one month. Peripartum psychosis is included under the diagnosis of brief psychotic disorder. Patients with schizophreniform disorder have similar symptoms to a brief psychotic disorder that lasts longer than one month but less than 6 months. Roughly one in three patients with schizophreniform disorder recover within 6 months; the others progress to develop clinical schizophrenia. Patients diagnosed with mood disorders may develop psychotic symptoms as part of their disease. If psychotic symptoms develop during periods of mood disturbances, the diagnosis of mood disorder with psychotic features applies. If symptoms consistent with schizophrenia persist for more than 2 weeks in the absence of prominent mood episode, the diagnosis of schizoaffective disorder is made. Patients with personality disorders may occasionally develop brief psychotic episodes, especially under duress. None of the aforementioned disturbances can be attributable to the effects of a substance or another medical condition.[16]

Delusional disorder is characterized by one or more delusions that are present for longer than one month, and the DSM-5 criteria for schizophrenia have not been met. Patients may believe famous people are in love with them (erotic type) or that they have extraordinary power or possess a special relationship with a deity or famous person (grandiose type). Other common delusions are sexual partners being unfaithful (jealous type), physical defect, or medical condition (somatic type). Function is not typically impaired, and behavior is often not bizarre separate from the impact of the delusions. Individuals may appear and behave normally when not actively discussing their delusions, but social, marital, work, and legal problems can result from the delusional beliefs.

DIAGNOSTIC TESTING

Diagnostic tests are indicated when a patient's clinical presentation cannot be explained by the history and physical examination alone. Often there is not enough information readily available to accurately ensure that the patient is suffering from a thought disorder alone. The potential medical causes of thought disorders are very broad; therefore, if a medical evaluation is indicated, testing should be patient specific and based on the particular medical processes that the clinician feels may be causing or exacerbating the thought disorder. The clinical judgment of the treating physician, rather than panels of routine tests, should be used to efficiently and appropriately guide diagnostic testing.

The evaluation of a "first-time" psychosis or thought disorder presentation in an emergency patient differs substantially from the evaluation of a patient with chronic disease who is experiencing recurrent symptoms. The evaluation for the first-time thought disorder patient may include a larger, more detailed laboratory and radiological evaluation. Complete blood counts, electrolyte panels, glucose levels, thyroid function, urine testing, vitamin B_{12}, and rapid plasma regain (RPR) testing are useful in certain clinical situations and should be ordered as appropriate for individual patients.

Neuroimaging for intracranial injury, vasculitis, demyelinating diseases, tumor, cerebrovascular disease, or abscess may be indicated based upon findings noted on the history and physical examination. A 2017 guideline from the American College of Emergency Physicians (ACEP) recommends the use of individual patient risk assessment to guide the ordering of brain imaging in the ED for patients presenting with new-onset psychosis without focal neurologic deficit.[17] The ACEP medical clearance guidelines are included in Box 96.4.

The new onset of primary thought disorders is rare in older adults. Medical illness often presents differently in elders, and a complete history and physical examination alone may not detect important medical presentations.[18] Geriatric medical assessment is more complex due to increased comorbidities, medication use, and variable baseline functional status with vague and nonspecific symptoms. Even for patients who have a previous psychiatric history or diagnoses, the presence of organic processes that may be exacerbating or contributing to the psychiatric decompensation should be considered. Most often, infections, electrolyte abnormalities, and medication side effects are the offending process. In one study, even after extensive ED testing was performed, a significant percentage of patients admitted to a geriatric psychiatric unit still required transfer out to a medical unit. The authors however concluded that further ED testing would not have prevented the transfers, which likely were related to the ongoing complex medical management issues rather than being related to missed opportunities for diagnosis in the ED.[18]

Ancillary testing beyond that required for medical clearance of psychiatric emergency patients rarely alters care, especially for patients with an established diagnosis of schizophrenia or other chronic thought

---

BOX 96.4 Summary of ACEP Medical Clearance Guidelines

Level B Recommendation

1. In adult ED patients with primary psychiatric complaints, diagnostic evaluation should be directed by the history and physical examination.
2. Routine laboratory testing of all patients is of low yield and need not be performed as part of the ED assessment.

Level C Recommendations Regarding UDS

1. Routine urine toxicologic screens for drugs of abuse in alert, awake, cooperative patients do not affect ED management and need not be performed as part of the ED assessment.
2. Urine toxicologic screens for drugs of abuse obtained in the ED for the use of the receiving psychiatric facility or service should not delay patient evaluation or transfer.

Level C Recommendations Regarding EtOH

1. The patient's cognitive abilities, rather than a specific blood alcohol level, should be the basis on which clinicians begin the psychiatric assessment.
2. Consider using a period of observation to determine if psychiatric symptoms resolve as the episode of intoxication resolves.

Data from: Lukens TW, Wolf SJ, Edlow JA, et al. Clinical policy: critical issues in the diagnosis and management of the adult psychiatric patient in the emergency department. *Ann Emergency Med.* 2006;47:79–99.

American College of Emergency Physicians Clinical Policies Subcommittee on Critical Issues, et al. Clinical policy: critical issues in the diagnosis and management of the adult psychiatric patient in the emergency department. *Ann Emerg Med.* 2017;69(4):480-498.

---

disorders. Policies that require panels of testing prior to psychiatric admission are costly and unnecessary.[19] One of the largest unnecessary costs is incurred with the routine use of urine drug screens, which have been found to rarely alter disposition for psychiatric patients from the ED, especially when combined with a good substance abuse history. Greater emphasis should be placed on identifying a clinical toxidrome and history of use when attempting to determine if drugs and medications are contributing to the symptoms of psychosis.

MANAGEMENT

Maintaining patient and staff safety are important when a patient presents with aggressive and unpredictable psychotic behavior. Risk factors for violence in patients with schizophrenia include extreme excitement, prior violence, auditory hallucinations, systematization of delusions, incoherence of speech, and long duration of illness. In contrast, traits such as substance abuse and antisocial episodes are not recognized as significant violence-associated factors. Strategies to control disruptive and violent behavior in psychosis and thought disorders include de-escalation techniques, chemical sedation, and physical restraints.

Although chemical and physical intervention can be appropriate when patients are demonstrating dangerous behavior, verbal de-escalation should be considered first. The clinician should demonstrate a calm, nonjudgmental demeanor while showing appropriate concern and avoiding excessive stimulation, posturing, and prolonged eye contact. The patient should be given an opportunity to express their concerns, as well as identify unmet needs that can be easily corrected (e.g., inadequate pain control, communication failures, or social concerns). If available, consider recruiting trusted others (e.g., family, friends, case managers) to help prevent further agitation.

TABLE 96.1 Common Drugs for Sedation

Drug	Usual Adult Dose	Adverse Events
Midazolam	2.5 to 5 mg IM (rapid onset)	Respiratory depression
Lorazepam	1 to 2 mg PO or IM	Oversedation
Diazepam	5 to 10 mg PO or IM (longer acting)	Hypotension
		Paradoxical excitation reaction in patients with organic brain disease
Haloperidol	5 to 10 mg PO or IM	Increased mortality risk in elderly dementia-related psychosis
Ziprasidone	10 to 20 mg PO or IM	
Olanzapine	5–10 mg PO or IM	
Loxapine	10 mg PO or INH	Caution in prolonged QT or history of neutropenia

IM, Intramuscular; INH, Inhaled; PO, per os (by mouth).

When verbal de-escalation is ineffective or inappropriate, physical restraint or use of seclusion may be necessary. Risk factors predicting the need for restraint or seclusion include referrals initiated by a third party, patients arriving to the ED in restraints, and clinician perception of the patient as severely disruptive, already exhibiting psychosis, or experiencing a manic episode.

Chemical restraint for psychomotor agitation is a common and necessary intervention. Speed of onset and reliability of delivery are two important factors to consider when selecting a route of administration of sedation in the behaviorally disturbed patient. Oral sedation is indicated when the patient can be safely verbally de-escalated, is not at imminent risk of harm to self, and agrees to take oral medications. When more expedient sedation is required, parenteral and inhaled routes have the advantage of immediate effect and titration of dosing. Inhaled loxapine has also been found to be a safe and effective alternative medication to reduce agitation with rapid onset[20,21] and reduces risks of needle sticks in an un-cooperative patient. The goal of titration in this setting is the induction of rousable sleep, not unconsciousness.

Benzodiazepines and antipsychotics are the two medications most commonly used for chemical restraint with the trend of moving towards use of second-generation antipsychotics.[22,23] Using a single agent or, for more disturbed patients, a combination of the two classes, can be considered. Common agents and dosages are listed in Table 96.1.

Combined with concurrent physical restraint and the risk of previously ingested intoxicants, there is significant risk for over-sedation and respiratory compromise. The combination of haloperidol and lorazepam can cause respiratory depression in patients, with a significant number experiencing a hypoxic event. As a result, we recommend the use of pulse oximetry or CO_2 monitoring in chemically restrained patients to detect early signs of respiratory depression. In addition to monitoring of airway and level of consciousness, sedated and restrained patients should have frequent behavioral monitoring. The use of physical restraints may cause excess pressure on the patient's neck, chest or abdomen, and requires ongoing direct visualization. Potentially hazardous articles and possessions should be removed from the patient's area. Restrained patients are known to forcibly remove Foley catheters without deflation of the balloon if their limbs are released prior to removal of the catheter, resulting in urethral injury.

DISPOSITION

Making an appropriate disposition for patients with decompensated thought disorders is often difficult in today's emergency medicine practice environment. Although institutional and community psychiatric resources vary widely by region, there appears to be a nationwide trend of diminishing psychiatric referral resources in the presence of rising numbers of psychiatric-related ED visits. The number of inpatient psychiatric beds nationwide has decreased, and many EDs "board" psychiatric patients for extended periods of time.

Appropriate disposition is based on the etiology of the underlying psychosis, response to treatment, consideration of patient and community safety, and the availability of an appropriate outpatient follow-up plan. Patients who are actively suicidal, dangerous to others, possess severe mental debilitation precluding self-care, or are having their first psychotic episode should be hospitalized.[17] The evaluation and disposition of potentially suicidal patients is discussed in Chapter 101. Psychiatric consultation can help confirm safety for discharge, help facilitate inpatient admission or transfer, and aid in developing an outpatient follow-up plan. Telemedicine is emerging as a technology that may ease the growing lack of adequate psychiatric resources for ED patients by facilitating urgent psychiatric consultation. Telemedicine can often be used safely and is not associated with significant differences in care when compared with face-to-face psychiatric evaluations.

Medication noncompliance is a common reason for a known schizophrenic to present to the ED with a decompensated psychotic episode. A patient whose psychosis stabilizes in the ED with medication can sometimes be safely discharged back into the community. Safe discharge planning can be accomplished provided that the patient has adequate ability to care for self and does not pose a risk of harm to self or others. Insight by the patient and judgment to adhere to an agreed course of action, including taking medication, is typically required. Patients with severe underlying psychiatric illnesses may have some degree of persistent mental disability even when optimally treated. For these patients, recruiting family or friends familiar with the patient can help establish that the patient is back to his or her baseline to ensure safety.

A safe transition to the community setting requires adequate social support, including follow-up with a mental health service. However, even when appropriately discharged, patients with a history of alcohol or drug dependence, dementias, psychotic disorders, autism, impulse control disorders, and personality disorders are at high risk for ED recidivism with repeat visits within 12 months. Uninsured status was also highly associated with repeat psychiatric admission and ED visits.[24]

The references for this chapter can be found online at ExpertConsult. com.

97

Mood Disorders

Leslie S. Zun and Joshua B. Nathan

KEY CONCEPTS

- Patients with apparent mood disorders should be evaluated for medical disorders, medication effects, or substance abuse or withdrawal because these conditions can mimic both depression and mania.
- Mood disorders should be suspected in patients with multiple, vague, nonspecific complaints and in patients who are frequent, heavy users of medical care.
- Patients with mood disorders should be assessed for their suicide potential.
- Pharmacologic treatment and linkage to care after discharge are important parts of managing mood disorders in the emergency setting.

FOUNDATIONS

Background and Importance

Mood is a subjective emotional state. It is normal human experience to have fluctuations in mood in response to occurrences in everyday life. A change in mood becomes a "mood disorder" when it significantly impairs functioning. In the emergency department (ED), patients with mood disorders often present grossly debilitated, with thoughts of suicide, homicide, or profound self-neglect. These patients frequently present in moments of emotional crisis, but this may not be their presenting complaint. Approximately one-fourth to one-third of ED patients screen positive for mood disorders.

The *Diagnostic and Statistical Manual of Mental Disorders, Fifth Edition* (DSM-5), divides mood disorders into two broad categories: depressive disorders and bipolar disorders.[1] Mood disorders may also be due to a general medical condition or substance-induced mood disorders. Because the specific pathophysiologic mechanisms of these disorders are not fully understood, they are categorized by groupings of symptoms that persist for defined lengths of time.

EPIDEMIOLOGY

The World Health Organization (WHO) ranks major depressive disorder as one of the most prevalent and disabling diseases in the world.[2] The 12-month prevalence for major depressive disorder is 5% and the lifetime prevalence is 13%. Patients with major depressive disorder frequently have other comorbid mental health issues, including anxiety disorders, personality disorders, and substance use disorders.

The lifetime prevalence of bipolar spectrum disorders is approximately 4%. Both severe depression and mania are serious and potentially life-threatening. Up to 80% of patients with bipolar disorder will exhibit suicidal behavior, and half will attempt suicide. Suicidal behavior can occur during all phases of bipolar disorder, but patients experiencing a depressed or a mixed episode are at higher risk, especially those with severe depressive symptoms and a sense of hopelessness.

Doctors, including residents and medical students, die by suicide at twice the rate of the general population, with 300 to 400 physicians dying by suicide every year. This also means doctors are in the highest risk profession for suicide. Unlike the general population, male and female physicians have equal rates of suicide attempts and suicide completion. While the high rate of suicide among physicians may seem counterintuitive, concerns about privacy, accessibility of services, and lack of time are commonly stated barriers to physicians seeking help. As a result, doctors fare worse with burnout, depression, and suicide than almost anyone else.[3]

Neuroanatomy

Neuroimaging studies of the brain suggest that abnormalities in certain areas and the interconnections between those areas may be involved mood disorders. A common magnetic resonance imaging (MRI) finding in patients with mood disorders, especially bipolar disorder, is an increased occurrence of subcortical hyperintensities in the periventricular areas, basal ganglia, and thalamus. High-resolution MRI demonstrates reduced volumes in the hippocampus, orbital cortex, and anterior cingulate. These findings are associated with more severe illness, bipolar disorder, and increased cortisol levels. Volume reduction in the hippocampus is associated with high illness chronicity.

The amygdala is a clustering of nuclei that process emotional stimuli, especially fear, anger, and sadness. Functional neuroimaging suggests that amygdala activity is increased when the subject is exposed to emotionally relevant stimuli. The amygdala has connections throughout the brain. A decreased amygdala volume has been associated with unipolar depression.

PATHOPHYSIOLOGY

The pathophysiology of the mood disorders is not well established, but much is known about the neurophysiology, genetics, and psychosocial aspects of the disorders.[4,5]

Neurophysiology

Antidepressants work by increasing the availability and activity of serotonin and norepinephrine at the synapse to stimulate the postsynaptic neuron. This is done by direct binding to the presynaptic and postsynaptic receptors, blocking reuptake of the neurotransmitter or inhibiting the enzymatic breakdown of the neurotransmitter. Because norepinephrine and serotonin systems traverse large portions of the brain, monoamine deficiency is hypothesized as a cause of depression. Depletion of oral tryptophan and tyrosine, amino acids essential for the production of serotonin and norepinephrine, respectively, can induce a depressive episode in subjects with a history of depression but not in healthy controls. Monoamine metabolite levels in cerebrospinal fluid, plasma, urine, and postmortem brains of patients with depression have not been reliably found to be deficient, indicating that there could be downstream effects involving second-messenger systems, such as cyclic adenosine monophosphate and phosphatidylinositol.

Other neurotransmitter systems may play a role in the development of depression. Decreased levels of both glutamate and γ-aminobutyric acid (GABA) have been found in the prefrontal cortex of depressed subjects. Intravenous (IV) ketamine, an *N*-methyl-D-aspartate (NMDA) antagonist, induces a rapid antidepressant effect and suggests a role for glutamate in the pathophysiologic process of depression. The brain relies on the actions of protective and regenerative cytokines, such as brain-derived neurotrophic factor (BDNF). All known antidepressants raise levels of BDNF and subsequently result in neurogenesis of certain brain regions, such as the hippocampus. Other theories include the melatonergic system and related abnormalities in circadian rhythm, decreased neurosteroid synthesis, impaired endogenous opioid functioning, monoamine-acetylcholine imbalance, inflammatory effects of cytokines, and dysfunction of specific brain structures and circuits.

The neurophysiology of bipolar disorder is less well understood than unipolar depression, in part because of the fluctuating mood states and the heterogeneity of the disorder. Bipolar disorder may in part arise from abnormalities in the connections within and between structures in the brain.[5] Specifically implicated are circuits interconnecting the amygdala, hypothalamus, striatum, and subdivisions of the frontal cortex, all of which are involved in both the generation and regulation of emotion.[6]

Endocrine System

Physiologic changes such as increased alertness, decreased appetite, increased heart rate, and activation of the hypothalamic-pituitary-adrenal (HPA) axis occur when a person is stressed. The HPA axis may play a role in depression, especially in cases of early childhood and chronic stress. Activation of the HPA axis releases corticotropin-releasing hormone (CRH) from the hypothalamus. Although not specific, patients with depression may have increased levels of free cortisol in the plasma, cerebrospinal fluid, and urine. Increased CRH has been demonstrated in cerebrospinal fluid, and increased levels of CRH messenger RNA and protein have been demonstrated in limbic brain regions. Although none of these measures is reliable as a diagnostic tool, successful treatment to remission has been shown to reverse some of these abnormalities, and antiinflammatory agents have demonstrated benefit in the treatment of depression in small controlled trials.[5]

Genetics

Genetic vulnerability to mood disorders has not been traced to a single gene. It is likely to be due to the additive effects of many genes and environmental influences on how these genes are expressed. Family, twin, and adoption studies provide evidence that major depressive disorder is a familial disorder but is less heritable than bipolar disorder. Bipolar disorder is one of the most heritable medical illnesses with a heritability of 80% to 85% and a monozygotic twin concordance of about 40%.

Psychosocial Factors

The etiology of most psychiatric problems, including mood disorders, involves complex interactions between both biologic and psychosocial factors.[1] The complex neural mechanism that regulates mood responds to and is modified by each person's experience, including events in early childhood, such as childhood sexual abuse, reward and punishment during growth and development, other lifetime trauma, marital problems, low social support, and various kinds of loss. Psychosocial theories of mood disorder form the basis for psychotherapy.

CLINICAL FEATURES

Major Depressive Disorder

Major depressive disorder is characterized by one or more major depressive episodes, as defined by DSM-5 criteria (Boxes 97.1 and 97.2).[1] A major depressive episode is characterized by disturbances in four major areas: mood, psychomotor activity, cognition, and vegetative function. The patient must have at least five symptoms for a minimum of 2 weeks and one of the five must be depressed mood or anhedonia (decreased interest or pleasure).[1]

Mood Disturbances

Patients in a depressed state often feel profoundly hopeless and helpless. There are many words and phrases that can be used to describe feeling depressed; some patients will not recognize that they are "depressed" but rather they may describe the feeling in some other manner. Someone feeling no emotion (profoundly depressed) may answer "no" when asked about depressed mood.

On the other hand, a person may meet criteria for a major depressive episode and not be experiencing a depressed mood. Depression can also be manifested as a decreased capacity to experience pleasure or interest in otherwise pleasurable activities. This loss of interest is known as *anhedonia*.

As noted previously, the patient must exhibit a depressed mood or anhedonia to meet DSM-5 criteria for a diagnosis of a major depressive episode.[1]

Disturbances in Psychomotor Activity

Physical activity in depression can be either increased or decreased. Psychomotor retardation is a significant slowing of physical activity. When suffering from psychomotor retardation, thinking and speaking can be slow, causing delayed responses to answers. Depressed patients often describe feeling fatigued with a general lack of energy and motivation. Conversely, patients may display psychomotor agitation, which can be manifested as fidgeting, pacing, hand-wringing, or restlessness.

Vegetative Disturbances

Vegetative symptoms include disturbances in three major areas: sleep, appetite, and sexual function. Depressed patients may complain of insomnia or hypersomnia. Insomnia may be manifested as difficulty in falling asleep, frequent awakenings throughout the night, or early-morning wakening. Depressed patients with hypersomnia may report sleeping 12 to 14 hours or more a day. Alterations in appetite and eating patterns can also occur, resulting in significant weight gain or loss during a short time. Loss of interest in sexual activity and impaired sexual functioning may also accompany depression, although this is not listed as a DSM-5 criterion.

Thought Process and Content

Depressed patients often describe impaired concentration and forgetfulness. Executive functioning can also be impaired. In severe cases, this results in a decreased ability to perform basic activities of daily living.

Thought content tends to be negatively biased, such as recurrent thoughts of guilt, failure, worthlessness, and self-criticism. Patients in a depressed episode are at increased risk for suicide. Suicidal thoughts may range from vague notions that life is not worth living (passive) to fully envisioned suicide plans with definitive intent to kill themselves (active). All depressed patients must be questioned about suicidal

BOX 97.1 Summary of *Diagnostic and Statistical Manual of Mental Disorders, Fifth Edition,* Criteria for a Major Depressive Episode

A. Five or more of the following symptoms have been present almost every day during the same 2-week period and represent a change from previous functioning; at least one of the symptoms is either (1) depressed mood or (2) loss of interest or pleasure. *Note:* Do not include symptoms caused by a general medical condition.
   1. Depressed mood (can be irritable mood in children and adolescents)
   2. Loss of interest or pleasure in activities
   3. Significant weight loss when not dieting or weight gain, or decrease or increase in appetite
   4. Insomnia or hypersomnia
   5. Psychomotor agitation or retardation
   6. Fatigue or loss of energy
   7. Feelings of worthlessness, or excessive or inappropriate guilt
   8. Diminished ability to think or concentrate, or indecisiveness
   9. Recurrent thoughts of death (not just fear of dying), recurrent suicidal ideation, or a suicide plan or attempt
B. Symptoms cause clinically significant distress or impairment in social, occupational, or other functioning.
C. Symptoms are not caused by direct physiologic effects of a substance (e.g., drug of abuse, medication) or a general medical condition (e.g., hypothyroidism).
D. Symptoms are not better explained by another mental health disorder.
E. There has never been a manic or hypomanic episode.

Modified from: American Psychiatric Association. *Diagnostic and Statistical Manual of Mental Disorders,* ed 5. Arlington, VA: American Psychiatric Association; 2013.

BOX 97.2 Mnemonics for the Symptoms of Depression and Mania

Mnemonic for the Symptoms of Depression
Sig E Caps
Sleep amount increased or decreased
Interest (anhedonia)
Guilt
Energy level decreased
Concentration decreased
Appetite increased or decreased
Psychomotor activity increased or decreased
Suicidal ideation

Mnemonic for the Symptoms of Mania
Dig Fast
Distractibility
Irritability
Grandiosity
Flight of ideas
Activity increased
Sleeplessness
Thoughtlessness (impulsivity, increased risk-taking)

thoughts. Because patients are not often forthcoming with their thoughts on suicide, a thorough review of risk factors and protective factors needs to form the basis of clinical decisions for providing the necessary level of care.

Patients with severe depression may have psychotic symptoms. The hallucinations and delusions that accompany depression are usually mood-congruent, meaning that the themes of the psychotic content are consistent with the depressed mood.

Masked Depression

Mood disorders may not be clear at presentation. The depressed patient may have only vague somatic symptoms. Common complaints include weakness, fatigue, headache, and abdominal pain with medical evaluations occurring in response. Patients may not be aware of their depression and are often heavy users of medical care. Over half of patients with major depressive disorder initially present with somatic symptoms only, which can mask a hidden depression. Clues that suggest a mood disturbance include the recent onset of a set of unusual behaviors, significant social disturbance, such as job loss, financial stress, and marital difficulties, and self-destructive behavior (e.g., substance abuse, sexual promiscuity).

Special Considerations

Children and Adolescents. Criteria for depression in children and adolescents are the same as for depression in adults. Depression in these age groups can, however, present differently. Prepubertal children are more likely to have somatic complaints, psychomotor agitation, and mood-congruent hallucinations and less likely to have disturbances in sleep and appetite. Some children are misdiagnosed as having attention deficit disorder, especially if symptoms involve poor concentration, listlessness, agitation, and withdrawal from daily activities.

Adolescents with depression may show increased irritability, oppositional behavior, and substance abuse. Other characteristics include social withdrawal, increased rejection sensitivity, and decline in school performance. Some adolescents may be first diagnosed with depression on receiving treatment for drug and alcohol problems.

Disruptive Mood Dysregulation Disorder. A newly described phenomenon for children who may have been previously diagnosed with depression or bipolar disorder is disruptive mood dysregulation disorder. Children and adolescents given this diagnosis display severe, recurrent outbursts that are out of proportion for the situation and are inconsistent with developmental level. The outbursts must occur three or more times a week, and the mood in between outbursts is irritable or angry most days. There are duration criteria of 12 months with no periods of three or more consecutive months not meeting criteria. Symptoms must occur prior to age 10.[1]

Geriatric Patients. Depression is more common in elders because of more frequent occurrences of loss, comorbid health issues, and loss of autonomy. The elderly have a tendency to report more somatic complaints when depressed. They are also more vulnerable to development of melancholic depression, which is characterized by early morning awakening, diurnal variation in mood, low self-esteem, and low mood reactivity. Older depressed patients can also present with symptoms involving memory loss, inattention, withdrawal from daily activities, and lapses in personal and social hygiene that suggest dementia rather than depression. When such symptoms are from depression, the condition is called *pseudodementia*. Serious depression in elders is a highly treatable, reversible condition.

Other Depressive Disorders

Peripartum Depression

Postpartum depression is a depressive disorder that occurs during pregnancy or within 4 weeks of delivery and would allow for the specifier "with peripartum onset." Symptoms of depression are common in the perinatal period. As noted in the DSM-5, between 3% and 6% of women will experience the onset of major depression during pregnancy or within the following weeks to months.[1] Similarly, but less severe, up to 65% of mothers report some depressed mood after childbirth, often called *postpartum blues.* Symptoms are generally mild and transient; although in 10% of mothers, it may lead to a full-fledged episode of major depression.

Postpartum mood episodes with psychotic features can be particularly dangerous. Infanticide is most often associated with command hallucinations to kill the infant or associated delusions. The risk for this is most closely related to a past history of postpartum episodes with psychosis, a history of depression or bipolar disorder, or a family history of bipolar disorder.

Persistent Depressive Disorder

Persistent depressive disorder is a new diagnosis that combines two former diagnoses: chronic major depressive disorder and dysthymic disorder. Specific criteria include the following: depressed mood most of the day, most days for at least 2 years; two or more of the following: poor appetite or overeating, insomnia or hypersomnia, low energy or fatigue, low self-esteem, poor concentration or difficulty making decisions, and feelings of hopelessness; never more than 2 months of the 2 years without symptoms; and must cause significant distress or impairment in functioning. Exclusion criteria include a history of hypomania or mania and a history of psychotic illness. Also, it cannot be due to a substance or medical condition.[1] There are multiple specifiers that can be applied to this diagnosis.

Premenstrual Dysphoric Disorder

Premenstrual dysphoric syndrome is a new diagnosis included in the DSM-5. At least five of the listed symptoms must be present in the final week before the onset of menses and start to improve within a few days after the onset of menses, and be absent or minimal in the week post menses. These symptoms must be present for most cycles over the preceding year. The onset can occur at any point after menarche. Risks for development include stress, history of interpersonal trauma, seasonal changes, and sociocultural aspects of female sexual behavior.

Seasonal Affective Disorder

Seasonal affective disorder is not a separate mood disorder, but rather, a specifier of major depressive disorder. An example of the use of a specifier is "major depressive disorder, recurrent, moderate, with seasonal pattern." This specifier can only be used with a recurrent major depressive disorder. The criteria for this include the following: a regular temporal relationship between the onset of a depressive episode and a particular time of year, full remissions at a specific time of year, two depressive episodes within 2 years that demonstrate a temporal relationship, no nonseasonal episodes within the same period, and substantially more seasonal depressive episodes than nonseasonal episodes over the person's lifetime.[1] Melatonin, a hormone secreted in the brain and produced at high levels in the dark, has been implicated in the etiology of this disorder. Phototherapy is an effective and safe treatment of seasonal depression. Light exposure to the eyes seems to be essential, but the exact mechanism of action is still unknown.

Bipolar Disorders

Bipolar disorder is a chronic, progressive illness with onset for men between their mid-teens and mid-twenties and for women between their mid-teens and mid-thirties. The illness involves extreme mood episodes associated with exacerbation of other symptoms and deterioration of function. Patients with bipolar disorder may require different forms and intensities of treatment at different stages of the illness. *Bipolar I disorder* includes at least one manic episode, and patients have typically had one or more major depressive episodes, although

a depressive episode is not necessary for diagnosis. *Bipolar II disorder* involves a hypomanic episode and at least one major depressive episode. A hypomanic episode includes the features of a manic episode without psychosis, marked impairment of function, or the need for hospitalization.[1]

Manic Episode

During a manic episode (see Boxes 97.2 and 97.3), the disturbance in mood must be severe enough to include psychosis, the need for hospitalization, or marked impairment in functioning. Bipolar disorders are much less common than major depressive disorder. The overall prevalence of a manic episode is about 2% in both women and men.

In many cases, manic patients are brought to the ED by someone else (e.g., family, police, or emergency medical services). Patients who are experiencing a manic episode may present with extreme mood lability; at time gregarious, humorous, and engaging, alternating suddenly with belligerence and irritability. Patients may display pressured speech, in which they keep talking, often rapidly and loudly without pauses between thoughts or sentences and are difficult to interrupt. The thought process in mania is characterized by illogical associations and flight of ideas. An inflated self-esteem and grandiose delusions may lead them to also be argumentative, impatient, and condescending. Grandiosity often centers on very broad dramatic or universal themes, such as religion or politics. The patient may describe a massive undertaking, such as "uniting the world's churches" or "solving world poverty." These severe symptoms are usually accompanied by a profound lack of insight. Despite obvious altered behavior, impaired judgment, and poor impulse control, the patient may insist that there is nothing wrong or blame problems on others.

BOX 97.3 Summary of *Diagnostic and Statistical Manual of Mental Disorders, Fifth Edition,* Criteria for a Manic Episode

A. Distinct period of abnormally and persistently elevated, expansive, or irritable mood, and abnormally and persistently increased goal-directed activity or energy lasting at least 1 week (or any duration if hospitalization is necessary).

B. During the period of mood disturbance and increased energy or activity, three or more of the following symptoms have persisted (four, if the mood is only irritable) and have been present to a significant degree:
  1. Inflated self-esteem or grandiosity
  2. Decreased need for sleep (e.g., feels rested after only 3 hours of sleep)
  3. More talkative than usual or pressure to keep talking
  4. Flight of ideas or subjective experience that thoughts are racing
  5. Distractibility (i.e., attention too easily drawn to unimportant or irrelevant external stimuli)
  6. Increase in goal-directed activity (either socially, at work or school, or sexually) or psychomotor agitation
  7. Excessive involvement in pleasurable activities that have a high potential for painful consequences (e.g., buying sprees, sexual indiscretions, foolish investments)

C. Mood disturbance is sufficiently severe to cause marked impairment in occupational functioning or social activities or to necessitate hospitalization to prevent harm to self or others, or psychotic features are present.

D. Symptoms are not caused by direct physiologic effects of a substance (e.g., drug of abuse, medication) or a general medical condition (e.g., hyperthyroidism).

Modified from: American Psychiatric Association. *Diagnostic and Statistical Manual of Mental Disorders,* ed 5. Arlington, VA: American Psychiatric Association; 2013.

Manic patients have decreased or no need for sleep and typically report being awake for days. They may be involved in a massive project (e.g., writing a novel), may completely disregard consequences of actions, may have difficulty with spending (e.g., credit cards revoked), and may engage in risky behavior (e.g., sexual liaisons with strangers, risky driving). Because the patient's abnormal thought process can make the history of present illness unreliable, whenever possible, a corroborating history should also be obtained from family or others who know of the patient's behavior.

Manic patients may present as trauma patients, injured by an action reflecting the patient's grandiosity (e.g., attempting to fly), impulsivity, or belligerence (e.g., fighting, resisting arrest). A manic episode may be punctuated by abrupt periods of tearfulness and profound depression, including suicidal ideation. When depressive and manic features occur concurrently in such a manner, the episode is termed *mixed* or *bipolar, mixed phase.*

Cyclothymic Disorder

Cyclothymic disorder is characterized by chronic mood swings that do not meet criteria for a hypomanic or depressive episode. The mood episodes must occur over at least 2 years, present for at least half the time, and the individual cannot be symptom-free for more than 2 months at a time.[1]

Mood Disorders Caused by a General Medical Condition

This diagnosis requires a prominent and persistent period of depressed mood or anhedonia that predominates the clinical picture, with evidence that the disturbance is the direct pathophysiological consequence of a medical condition, and not better explained by another mental disorder or occurring during the course of delirium.[1] Bipolar disorder requires a prominent and persistent period of abnormally elevated, expansive, or irritable mood; and abnormally increased activity or energy that predominates the clinical picture, with evidence of direct pathophysiological consequence of another medical condition, and it is not better explained by another mental disorder or occurs during the course of delirium.[1]

Certain medical illnesses have a well-known association with mood disorder. In Parkinson disease, electrical stimulation to a certain area of the substantia nigra alleviates symptoms of depression. Stimulation of an area only 2 mm away can cause acute reversible symptoms of depression, such as crying, not wanting to live, and hopelessness. Parkinson disease has a well-known association with depression, with up to 40% of patients demonstrating major depression.

Certain malignant neoplasms have a well-known association with depression, including pancreatic carcinoma, brain neoplasm, and disseminated malignant disease (e.g., lymphoma). Coronary artery disease, myocardial infarction, stroke, end-stage renal disease, acquired immunodeficiency syndrome, several endocrine diseases, and connective tissue disease are also associated with major depressive disorder. After a myocardial infarction, patients with depression have a 3.5-fold increase in cardiovascular mortality compared with nondepressed patients. The development of stroke, diabetes, and osteoporosis is more likely in patients with depression than in those who are not depressed.

Depression related to medical conditions may be different in some respects from primary depression and responds less favorably than primary depression to antidepressant medication. Treatment-resistant depression, defined as depression that has not responded to at least two adequate trials of medication, should prompt clinical investigation for a general medical condition causing the depressive episode.

Mood Disorders Caused by Medications or Other Substances

These are very similar to mood disorders caused by medical conditions, with the exception that the symptoms must develop during or soon after substance intoxication or withdrawal, or after exposure to a medication capable of producing the symptoms.[1]

Many medications are associated with symptoms of mood disorders. Multiple antihypertensives, anticonvulsants, and hormones have been associated with depressive symptoms, and certain antibiotics and steroids are associated with manic symptoms. Intoxication with or chronic heavy use of alcohol, sedatives, hypnotics, anxiolytics, narcotics, and other depressants can cause symptoms of a major depressive episode. Stimulants such as cocaine, phencyclidine, hallucinogens, and amphetamines can cause symptoms of a manic episode. Mood disorder symptoms can also develop during withdrawal. To qualify for this diagnosis, the symptoms must not occur exclusively during a course of delirium, must cause significant distress or impairment of functioning, and must develop within a month of either substance intoxication or withdrawal. When the mood disorder predates the period of substance abuse or lasts longer than 1 month after the period of abuse, the diagnosis may be an underlying mood disorder, such as a major depressive disorder or bipolar disorder, with a comorbid substance use disorder.

DIFFERENTIAL DIAGNOSES

Medical Disorders, Medications, and Substance Abuse or Withdrawal

Medical disorders, medications, and substance abuse or withdrawal can either cause or mimic mood disorders. The patient with symptoms and signs of depression may have an unrecognized malignant neoplasm or sedative intoxication. Differential diagnostic considerations for manic symptoms include stimulant abuse (e.g., cocaine, amphetamines), hallucinogen abuse, alcohol or sedative withdrawal, delirium, hyperthyroidism, and other medical conditions causing agitation. See the previous section for further information. Patients may be treated with antidepressant medication for a variety of disorders other than depression, such as anxiety, obsessive-compulsive disorder, posttraumatic stress disorder, pain syndromes, smoking cessation, and vasodepressor syncope.

Grief and Bereavement

Grief and bereavement are normal human reactions to the acute loss of another person, health, social position, or job. The period of mourning is characterized by sadness, diminished sense of well-being (somatic complaints), sleeplessness, and sadness triggered by thoughts of the loss. Normal grief, however, does not include loss of self-esteem, feelings of worthlessness, suicidal intent, psychomotor retardation, or occupational dysfunction. The duration of normal grief and bereavement differs among cultures and among individuals within cultures, but severe symptoms normally resolve within 6 to 12 months.

Adjustment Disorders

Adjustment disorders are behavioral or emotional disorders that occur in response to an identifiable stress or stressors, with marked distress that is out of proportion to the severity of the stressor. The emotional component can involve sadness, low self-esteem, suicidal behavior, hopelessness, helplessness, or other self-threatening behavior. Acute adjustment disorder occurs within 3 months of the stressor and does not last longer than 6 months.[1] The stressors are typically not as severe as those precipitating bereavement reactions, and the responses are often more maladaptive.

Borderline Personality Disorder

Borderline personality disorder is characterized by unstable personal relationships, unstable self-image, and self-destructive behaviors. The disorder may include chronic feelings of emptiness, which may be misdiagnosed as depression, or reactivity of mood, which may be mistaken for mania or hypomania. These patients typically live lives of crisis and constant conflict.

Dementia

Dementia can be confused with depression but is characterized by abnormal mental status, including abnormalities in tests of memory, calculation, and judgment (see Chapter 90).

Diagnostic Testing

History and physical examination should focus on determining if the patient has a mood disorder or the possibility that drug abuse, medications, or a general medical condition may be responsible for the patient's condition instead. It is essential to identify medical conditions that may exacerbate a psychiatric presentation. The psychiatric history should ask about current symptoms, precipitating events (e.g., job loss or relationship), past psychiatric and substance use history, history of self-harm or suicide attempts, and identification of support systems. Even if not suggested by the patient, careful questioning of suicidal thoughts is necessary. If possible, history should be confirmed by speaking with the patient's regular health care providers and interviewing family, friends, or eyewitnesses to the events that precipitated the ED visit. A tentative diagnosis can be established by use of DSM-5 criteria.

Laboratory tests to investigate medical conditions may be necessary based on the specifics of the clinical presentation, but no tests can confirm or exclude mood disorders. Patients with new symptoms compatible with mood disorders need a more extensive medical and psychiatric investigation than those with a known disorder.

MANAGEMENT

Patients presenting with mood disorder symptomology are frequently in crisis, often overwhelmed, and frankly scared. The ED is a chaotic, stimulating environment that may cause or exacerbate the patients' level of agitation. Creation of a safe and stable environment for the patient is a high priority. Individuals experiencing an acute manic episode may be disruptive, refuse medical evaluation, and make repeated attempts to leave the ED. The initial step in treating such a disruptive patient is to offer assistance in reducing the agitation, which may begin with verbal de-escalation.[7] One key is offering anxiolytic medication early in the patient's presentation. If de-escalation techniques and medication do not resolve the agitation, the patient may need to be placed in seclusion or restraints for his or her safety and that of others. This is a last resort after other de-escalation measures have failed. Chapter 185 discusses the use of seclusion and restraints in the ED. If a medical cause for agitation is found, treatment is aimed at the underlying cause (e.g., oxygen for hypoxic delirium). Often in the ED, treatment may need to begin prior to the cause of the agitation being fully recognized.[8,9] Figure 97.1 shows a simple algorithm for approaching the agitated patient.

Treatment of depression in the ED is more controversial. Selective serotonin reuptake inhibitors (SSRIs) and serotonin norepinephrine reuptake inhibitors (SNRIs) are the main treatments for depression. For the patient who is awaiting inpatient psychiatric placement, these medications can be initiated in consultation with the admitting service. Patients with mild to moderate depression, not requiring hospitalization, may be started on an SSRI as long as they have close follow-up arranged. SSRIs are known to have a myriad of side effects that can lead to premature discontinuation.[10] For the patients who are already on psychotropic medications but have discontinued them for a reason unrelated to adverse effects, it is reasonable to restart these medications in the ED.

A non-agitated manic patient may be able to inform the treatment team about what has worked well in the past. There are two medication choices for acute mania: antipsychotics and mood stabilizers.[11] All of the atypical, or second-generation, antipsychotics have been approved to treat acute mania as monotherapy or as an adjunctive therapy, except paliperidone and iloperidone. Lithium, valproic acid/divalproate, and carbamazepine are the most well-studied mood stabilizers. Lithium and carbamazepine need to be titrated, but valproic acid can be loaded in the ED at 20 to 30 mg/kg a day in a healthy person with normal liver function.

The atypical antipsychotic medicines, including ziprasidone, risperidone, olanzapine, aripiprazole, quetiapine, asenapine, and lurasidone, have a lower risk of acute side effects (such as acute dystonia) than conventional antipsychotic agents. Oral doses should be offered first, and several agents, including risperidone, olanzapine, and aripiprazole, are available in rapidly dissolving tablet form. Two are available as a short-acting intramuscular injection: ziprasidone (Geodon) and olanzapine (Zyprexa). Ziprasidone 10 mg every two hours or 20 mg every four hours is effective; however, its use is limited to 40 mg per 24 hours. Olanzapine 2.5 mg to 10 mg is effective, but is limited to 30 mg per 24 hours. Also, olanzapine is associated with postural hypotension so should not be used in combination with parenteral benzodiazepines because of the risk of cardiopulmonary depression. It is valuable to obtain psychiatric consultation during the initiation of agitation treatment, because these patients will generally require significant ED treatment or psychiatric hospitalization.

DISPOSITION

To determine the appropriate disposition for patients presenting with a mood disorder, a suicide risk assessment is required. The Substance Abuse and Mental Health Services Administration developed a practical tool referred to as the Suicide Assessment Five-Step Evaluation and Triage (SAFE-T).[12] Current suicidal thoughts, risk factors, and protective factors should be identified, as well as past suicidal thoughts, plans, or acts. Chapter 101 provides an in-depth discussion of suicide assessment. It is only after considering this information that an appropriate intervention can be determined. With the help of social workers or a mental health worker, many patients can be safely discharged home with close follow-up. Patients receiving initial treatment in the ED, without a proper handoff to outpatient care, are at an increased risk for return. If available, it is preferred that a social worker or mental health worker connect discharged patients with outside agencies and services, rather than providing patients with a referral list.

The references for this chapter can be found online at ExpertConsult.com.

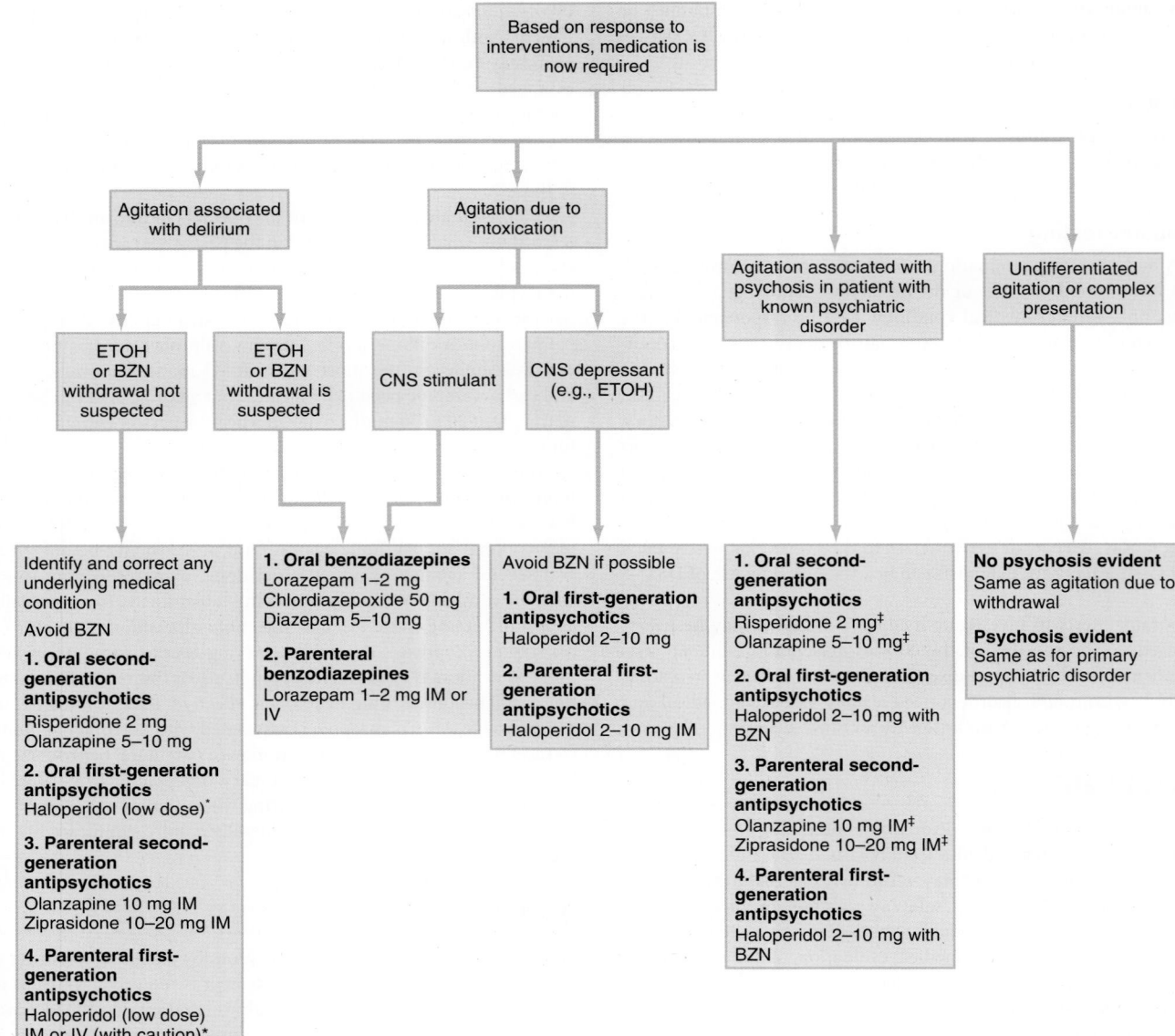

Fig. 97.1 Protocol for treatment of agitation. *BZN,* Benzodiazepine; *CNS,* central nervous system; *ETOH,* ethyl alcohol; *IM,* intramuscular; *IV,* intravenous. *See U.S. Food and Drug Administration (FDA) guidelines. ‡If an antipsychotic alone does not work sufficiently, add lorazepam 1 to 2 mg (oral or parenteral). (Redrawn from Wilson MP, Pepper D, Currier GW, et al. The psychopharmacology of agitation: consensus statement of the American Association for Emergency Psychiatry Project BETA Psychopharmacology Workgroup. *WJEM.* 2012;13[1]:26-34.)

98

Anxiety Disorders

Leslie S. Zun and Joshua B. Nathan

KEY CONCEPTS

- Patients who present with predominant symptoms of anxiety may be suffering from medical disorders, medication effects, or substance abuse or withdrawal.
- Anxiety may accompany the onset of serious medical disease, cause significant metabolic demands, and stress a marginally compensated organ system.
- Anxiety caused by non-psychiatric illness is usually suggested by the patient's physical examination findings but may require testing to further delineate the cause.
- Oral, intravenous, or intramuscular medication may be necessary for patients who are a significant threat to themselves or others and for anxious patients with significant medical illness.
- Limited benzodiazepine therapy may be helpful for select patients.

FOUNDATIONS

Background and Importance

Anxiety is a specific unpleasurable state of tension that forewarns the presence of danger, real or imagined, known or unrecognized, and is often verbalized as an intense feeling of worry. Anxiety is often a normal adaptation to life events or stressors, and in many circumstances, could be considered appropriate given the context and would represent a reasonable emotional response to a perceived threat or circumstance. Even extreme levels of anxiety could be considered appropriate given the level of perceived threat. An anxiety disorder, however, describes a condition in which a response to a given circumstance or threat becomes significantly disproportionate or uncontrollable, leading to the deterioration of performance and an inability to cope. As the level of dysfunction increases, the patient is much more likely to have a true anxiety disorder. Anxiety disorders are considered to be among the most prevalent of mental health behavioral and emotional disorders worldwide.

Acute anxiety is common in emergency department (ED) patients who have primary anxiety disorders, concomitant anxiety disorders, and crisis situations. Emergency physicians are frequently called upon to diagnosis and treat anxiety disorders in the ED and therefore need to be familiar with both the diagnostic criteria as well as the differential diagnoses and treatment modalities. The *Diagnostic and Statistical Manual of Mental Disorders, Fifth Edition* (DSM-5) criteria for anxiety disorders include general anxiety disorder, panic disorder, agoraphobia, and specific phobia. Obsessive-compulsive disorders (OCD), post-traumatic stress disorder (PTSD), and acute stress disorder, which have now been moved to their own category in the DSM-5, will also be discussed in this chapter.[1]

Epidemiology

The most recent available national statistics on past-one-year and lifetime prevalence of anxiety disorders amongst adults (age 18 or older) is derived from the National Comorbidity Study Replication (NCS-R) originating from the Harvard Medical School National Comorbidity Survey (NCS). Data updated as of 2007 reveals 19.1% past-year prevalence with a female predominance (23.4% versus 14.3%) and an overall lifetime prevalence of 31.1% among all adults in the United States (US).[2]

Many patients seeking primary health care have significant mood and anxiety symptoms, such as panic disorder, generalized anxiety disorders (GAD), and depression, but almost half of these symptomatic patients never receive appropriate treatment. Patients with chronic illness and those who make frequent medical visits have higher rates of anxiety and depression. The prevalence of anxiety disorders surpasses that of any other mental health disorder, including substance abuse. There is a close relationship between alcohol abuse and anxiety disorders.

Anxiety disorders in children and adolescents lead to anxiety disorders in adulthood, but anxiety disorders often go unrecognized and untreated in the pediatric population.[3] The same is true of geriatric patients with a prevalence rate of 1.2% to 15%. Except for generalized anxiety disorder and agoraphobia, anxiety disorders typically start earlier in life.[4]

The incidence of specific anxiety disorders varies: specific phobia is 7% to 9%, social anxiety is 7%, panic disorder is 3%, and GAD is 3%. The lifetime risk for post-traumatic stress disorder (PTSD) is about 9%, but the 12-month prevalence is approximately 4%. Substance or medication-induced anxiety and anxiety due to a medical condition have an unknown prevalence but may be relatively high in those seeking emergency medical care.

A different form of anxiety related to fear of suffering from an illness, now known as *illness anxiety disorder* (formerly hypochondriasis), may be as high as 8% in ambulatory medical populations.[2] In these cases, patients may disguise their anxiety, presenting with a physical complaint rather than bear the perceived stigma associated with psychiatric complaints. This is distinct from patients with a somatoform disorder.

Pathophysiology

There are many forms of anxiety disorders and the precise mechanisms underlying the development of anxiety have not been fully established. However, the serotonin, noradrenergic gamma-aminobutyric acid (GABA) and dopaminergic systems are the most studied neurotransmitter systems implicated in anxiety disorders[5] (see Box 98.1). It is hypothesized that low serotonin system activity and elevated

BOX 98.1 Neurotransmitters Involved in Anxiety Disorders

Neurotransmitter	Neuroanatomical Association and Mechanism
Serotonin	Amygdala. Periaqueductal gray matter increased in AD
Dopamine	Mesolimbic mesocortical and nigrostriatal cortex; evidence of role in AD
Norepinephrine and epinephrine	Autonomic nervous system directly correlated in AD
GABA	Inhibitory neurotransmitter decreased in AD

Adapted from: Hingray C, McGonigal A, Kotwas I, Micoulaud-Franchi JA. The relationship between epilepsy and anxiety disorders. *Curr Psychiatry Rep.* 2019 Apr 29;21(6):40. https://doi.org/10.1007/s11920-019-1029-9. PMID: 31037466. Vismara M, Girone N, Cirnigliaro G, et al. Peripheral biomarkers in DSM-5 anxiety disorders: an updated overview. *Brain Sci.* 2020;10(8):564. Published 2020 Aug 17. https://doi.org/10.3390/brainsci10080564.

BOX 98.2 Predictors of Anxiety Caused by an Underlying Medical Issue

Onset of anxiety symptoms after 35 years old
Lack of personal or family history of an anxiety disorder
Lack of childhood history of significant anxiety, phobias, or separation anxiety
Lack of avoidance behavior
Absence of significant life events generating or exacerbating the anxiety symptoms
Poor response to antianxiety agents

BOX 98.3 Characteristics of a Panic Attack

Abrupt surge of intense fear or discomfort that reaches a peak within minutes, in which four or more of the following occur:
Palpitations
Sweating
Trembling
Shortness of breath or feeling of being smothered
Feeling of choking
Chest pain or discomfort
Nausea or abdominal distress
Feeling dizzy or lightheaded
Chills or heat sensations
Paresthesias
Derealization or depersonalization
Fear of losing control or going "crazy"
Fear of dying

Adapted from: American Psychiatric Association. *Diagnostic and Statistical Manual of Mental Disorders*, ed 5. Arlington, VA: American Psychiatric Association; 2013.

noradrenergic system activity may play a role, and thus selective serotonin reuptake inhibitors (SSRIs) and serotonin norepinephrine reuptake inhibitors (SNRIs) are frequently used as treatment. There is also considerable comorbidity with depressive disorders, with evidence showing genetic and neurobiologic similarities, especially related to serotonin.

The well-established effectiveness of benzodiazepines in the treatment of anxiety has led to the study of the GABA system and its relationship to anxiety. GABA is the principal inhibitory neurotransmitter in the central nervous system, and benzodiazepines act on the GABA_A receptors. Studies have also focused on the role that corticosteroids may play in fear and anxiety. Steroids are thought to induce chemical changes in select neurons that strengthen or weaken certain neural pathways to affect behavior under stress.

Family research suggests that genetic factors play a role in anxiety, but the precise nature of the inherited vulnerability is unknown. Five major anxiety disorders (panic disorder, GAD, phobias, OCD, and PTSD) share genetic and environmental risk factors. Psychological and environmental factors also contribute to the generation of anxiety in biologically predisposed individuals.

CLINICAL FEATURES

Anxiety may be a manifestation of another medical disorder or an expression of an underlying psychiatric disorder. It may be difficult to make the distinction between anxiety as a symptom and anxiety as a syndrome in the ED. The physical symptoms of autonomic arousal (e.g., tachypnea, tachycardia, diaphoresis, lightheadedness) may be the only manifestations of anxiety. Classic panic disorder symptoms of chest pain, shortness of breath, and the sense of impending doom will often lead the patient to the ED, especially if it is the very first episode. Box 98.2 lists clinical predictors of anxiety caused by an underlying medical disorder. Patients may also exhibit anxiety associated with experiencing uncertainty about their illness and the potential implications of the illness. In addition, many patients seeking care in the ED may experience anxiety related to encountering internal and external dangers, such as assaults on body integrity in the form of uncomfortable procedures and forced intimacy with strangers.

Clinical manifestations of specific anxiety disorders are considerably different, warranting a review of each of the major types.

Panic Disorder

Panic disorder (PD) is a diagnosis of exclusion, even in patients with known psychiatric illness, because several mental illnesses cause panic attacks as a secondary manifestation. For a diagnosis of panic disorder, one must experience recurrent, unexpected panic attacks (Box 98.3), as well as either persistent concern of future attacks or a maladaptive behavioral change related to the attacks. As with other disorders, the disturbance should not be better explained by substance use, another medical condition, or another psychiatric illness.[2]

A panic attack, differentiated from panic disorder, is an abrupt fear or discomfort that reaches a peak within minutes and has associated physical and cognitive symptoms.[2] It may occur with any anxiety disorder or as part of another psychiatric or other medical disorder. A panic attack is not a diagnosis but rather an indication of an underlying disorder. The presence of panic attacks often influences the treatment and outcome of the primary illness. An attack can be replicated by intentional hyperventilation, which can be distinguished from medical hyperventilation by its irregularity and interruptions. When there is doubt, formal psychiatric evaluation is indicated, particularly before a potentially dangerous or addictive drug therapy is prescribed.

Generalized Anxiety Disorder

GAD is defined as excessive worry that occurs most days over a 6-month period involving several events or activities.[2] The anxiety must cause significant distress or impairment in functioning. GAD has been linked to overuse of medical services and often is not recognized, which leads to ineffective treatment.

BOX 98.4 Characteristics of Post-Traumatic Stress Disorder*

Exposure to actual or threatened death, serious injury, or sexual violence.
Presence of intrusion symptoms associated with the traumatic event.
Persistent avoidance of stimuli associated with the traumatic event.
Negative alterations in cognition and mood associated with the traumatic event.
Marked alterations in arousal and reactivity associated with the event.
Duration is greater than 1 month.
Disturbance causes clinically significant distress or impairment.
Disturbance is not attributable to the physiological effects of a substance or another medical condition.

* Specifiers include "with dissociative symptoms" and "with delayed expression."
Adapted from: American Psychiatric Association. *Diagnostic and Statistical Manual of Mental Disorders*, ed 5. Arlington, VA: American Psychiatric Association; 2013.

Post-Traumatic Stress Disorder

PTSD is caused by experiencing or witnessing a highly traumatic event. Those with PTSD manifest symptoms of re-experiencing the event, avoidance of triggers, changes in cognition and mood, and changes in arousal and reactivity (Box 98.4). Rates of PTSD are higher among military veterans and those whose occupation involves risk of traumatic exposure.[2] ED staff are also at risk for experiencing PTSD related to unusual traumatic events and unexpected deaths. Those suffering from PTSD may also be suffering from other disorders such as OCD, personality disorders, and substance use disorders, and may even exhibit suicidal ideations.

Specific Phobias

A phobia is an irrational fear that results in avoidance behavior. Phobia becomes a disorder when it interferes with day-to-day function in an individual's life. Social phobia, now termed *social anxiety disorder,* is characterized by clinically significant anxiety about one or more social situations in which the individual may be scrutinized.[2] This fear often leads to avoidance or other changes in behavior for such activities, such as public speaking, performing, visiting people, sitting in classrooms, attending social events using public showers or restrooms, or eating in public places.

Obsessive-Compulsive Disorder

OCD is characterized by recurrent, intrusive, unwanted thoughts (obsessions), such as fears of contamination, or compulsive behaviors or mental acts (compulsions) that a person feels compelled to perform, such as handwashing or counting. OCD is considered an anxiety disorder because (1) anxiety or tension is often associated with obsessions and resistance to compulsions, (2) anxiety or tension is often immediately relieved by yielding to compulsions, and (3) OCD often occurs in association with other anxiety disorders.[2] In summary, the obsessions and intrusive thoughts increase anxiety, and the compulsions and repetitive behaviors decrease anxiety but with significant disruption of one's life.

Hyperventilation Syndrome

Hyperventilation syndrome is a disorder characterized by intermittent episodes of increases in minute ventilation, together with feelings of doom and anxiety, associated with somatic symptoms such as dyspnea, chest pain, lightheadedness, perioral numbness and tingling, and muscle spasm of the hands and feet. Underlying conditions that may cause or contribute to this syndrome include primary psychological or neurologic dysfunction as well as cardiopulmonary etiologies. The diagnosis of hyperventilation syndrome may be challenging since there are no widely accepted diagnostic criteria. Patients presenting with new-onset hyperventilation require an extensive history, as well as physical examination and screening laboratories to rule out lethal etiologies. Patients with known hyperventilation syndrome from a psychological etiology can benefit from reassurance, breathing therapy, and low doses of benzodiazepines. A study of patients presenting to an ED with hyperventilation syndrome found 30% had previous episodes and more than 50% had a psychiatric comorbidity.[6]

Somatic Symptoms and Related Disorders

Although not necessarily categorized as anxiety disorders, this group of disorders has an undefined but established link to anxiety and depressive disorders and includes somatic symptom disorder, illness anxiety disorder (formerly hypochondriasis), conversion disorder (formerly functional neurological symptom disorder), and psychological factors affecting other medical conditions. With somatic disorders, the patient will complain about one or more physical symptoms, which cause impairment notwithstanding a negative evaluation. These symptoms are not intentionally feigned, as in the case of malingering or factitious disorder. A high utilization of medical services is correlated with these disorders, independent of comorbidity. Patients with somatoform disorders may seek as much psychiatric attention as do those with panic disorder.

DIFFERENTIAL DIAGNOSIS

It is important to differentiate the origin of anxiety to provide appropriate treatment. Many medical conditions mimic anxiety disorders, and up to 42% of patients initially thought to have anxiety disorders are later found to have a medical etiology.

Emergency clinicians should be able to distinguish between anxiety disorders and other medical illness (see Box 98.2) and, if necessary, treat both entities. Because anxiety states cause an increase in metabolic demands, they can cause a marginally compensated organ system to fail.

In patients who present with predominant symptoms of anxiety, even when the patients have known anxiety disorders, before considering which of the previously discussed DSM-5 anxiety-related diagnoses the patient might have, the clinician should first consider the possibility of medical and pharmacologic-related conditions associated with anxiety.

Patients with anxiety disorders may present with an apparently different medical disease, and many medical diseases are strongly associated with symptoms of anxiety. Several factors help distinguish an anxiety syndrome caused by an underlying medical issue from a primary anxiety disorder (see Box 98.2).

Anxiety may be the most obvious symptom of an underlying disease or condition, and therefore, the patient should be evaluated for exacerbation of known preexisting disease, as well as for the onset of new illness, because of the increased risk of acute medical exacerbation of chronic illness.

Anxiety disorder classifications in the DSM-5 include anxiety caused by another medical condition.[2] Post–myocardial infarction patients with anxiety have poorer outcomes than those without documented anxiety. Patients with respiratory diseases, such as asthma and chronic obstructive pulmonary disease, often have anxiety associated with long-standing illnesses. In addition, many of the medications used to treat these illnesses may induce anxiety. One of the most common medical causes of anxiety is alcohol and drug use from either intoxication or, more typically, withdrawal states.

Cardiac Diseases

Approximately 25% of patients with chest pain who present to the ED have panic disorder, which often goes undiagnosed, resulting in multiple visits and expensive cardiac evaluations. Symptoms of anxiety, like those of a myocardial infarction or angina pectoris, may include crushing chest pain, shortness of breath, nausea, palpitations, heavy perspiration, and a feeling of impending doom. The associated chest pain is usually described as atypical, and patients are generally female and younger. Because of the morbidity and mortality of cardiovascular disease, a patient warrants an appropriate cardiac evaluation when the differentiation between myocardial infarction and acute anxiety is unclear.

Cardiac dysrhythmias can also cause symptoms similar to a panic attack including palpitations, discomfort, dizziness, respiratory distress, and even syncope. Mitral valve prolapse syndrome can be associated with palpitations and panic attacks indistinguishable from a panic disorder. Benzodiazepines can be used to provide symptomatic relief to patients who experience chest pain due to anxiety.

Endocrine Diseases

The most common endocrinologic conditions associated with anxiety states are hypoparathyroidism, hyperthyroidism and hypothyroidism, hypoglycemia, pheochromocytoma, and hyperadrenocorticism. Anxiety is the predominant symptom in 20% of patients with hypoparathyroidism. Studies indicate a higher incidence of anxiety in the subset of patients with surgically removed parathyroid glands. Even though other symptoms may improve with supplementation, patients have been found to have significant depression, anxiety, somatization, and phobic anxiety, even after being given calcium and vitamin D.

Anxiety symptoms are seen in up to 40% of people with diabetes mellitus, and 14% of diabetic patients suffer from anxiety disorders.[7] There is evidence that people with diabetes mellitus and anxiety have worse glycemic control when anxiety is untreated.

Pheochromocytomas are rare tumors that produce elevated levels of catecholamine in the body. Pheochromocytoma attacks may manifest similar to panic attacks and can be precipitated by emotional stress. Elevated urinary catecholamine or plasma metanephrine levels confirm a pheochromocytoma.

Hyperthyroidism is one of the most frequently encountered endocrine diseases associated with anxiety. As with panic disorders, hyperthyroidism is associated with acute episodic anxiety. Thyrotoxicosis causes anxiety, palpitations, perspiration, hot skin, rapid pulse, active reflexes, diarrhea, weight loss, heat intolerance, proptosis, and lid lag. A substantial portion of patients continue to have psychiatric manifestations even after treatment.

Psychiatric presentations can be the first sign of hypothyroidism, occurring as the initial symptom in 2% to 12% of reported cases along with deficits of impaired recent memory and learning. The severity of anxiety disorders in hypothyroid states is related to the rapidity of thyroid hormone level changes and not to the absolute hormone levels. In general, checking serum thyroid-stimulating hormone and free thyroxine levels will suffice in the ED to establish the diagnosis of thyroid disease.

Respiratory Diseases

Most conditions causing airway compromise or impairment of gas exchange do not mimic psychiatric disorders. However, some conditions that cause hypoxemia or hypercarbia may lead to the development of significant anxiety. Up to a third of the patients with chronic obstructive pulmonary disease meet the criteria for anxiety disorder.

Patients who have severe asthma are twice as likely to have an anxiety disorder and almost five times as likely to have a phobia compared with nonasthmatics. Acute dyspnea from a pure panic attack with good air movement and normal lung sounds is easily differentiated from an asthma attack, but studies consistently show that anxiety disorders increase asthma morbidity and mortality.

Acute shortness of breath in any patient should not be immediately attributed to anxiety, especially because pulmonary embolism can present with only shortness of breath as the major symptom. Fortunately, pulmonary embolism can almost always be distinguished by history and physical examination, assessment of risk factors for thromboembolic disease, and laboratory testing (e.g., pulse oximetry, electrocardiography, chest radiography, and D-dimer assay) as indicated. The Multidimensional Dyspnea Profile tool uses the verbal subjective descriptors of feeling depressed, air hunger, and breathing concentration to help differentiate patients with pulmonary disease with and without panic disorder.[8]

Neurologic Disorders

Many neurologic conditions are associated with anxiety symptoms. For example, stress is one of the most common reported causes of seizures. Those who report stress as a trigger tend to have higher scores on anxiety tests, and the stress may be either acute or chronic.[12] Temporal lobe seizures, complex partial seizures, tumors, arteriovenous malformation, and cerebral ischemia or infarction have all been reported with panic attacks. Anxiety disorders also occur in the aftermath of traumatic brain injury (TBI). Approximately 23% of those who sustain a mild TBI are at risk for developing an anxiety disorder; this is frequently found in military personnel. In Huntington disease, anxiety is the most common prodromal symptom. Anxiety occurs in up to 40% of patients with Parkinson disease and up to 37% of patients with multiple sclerosis. Similarly, anxiety symptoms are common in moderate Alzheimer disease.

Drug Intoxication and Withdrawal States

Amphetamines, cocaine, and other sympathomimetic drugs are abused for their stimulant and mind-altering properties. Patients often present agitated and anxious, particularly when these drugs are taken in large doses and with prolonged use. Caffeine is a very commonly used stimulant, and studies suggest that about 400 mg/day is the threshold for toxicity in healthy adults (19 years or older), 100 mg/day in healthy adolescents (12-18 years old) and 2.5 mg/kg/day in healthy children (11 years old or younger). With the consumption of higher doses, caffeine intoxication may result, causing restlessness, nervousness, excitement, insomnia, diuresis, gastrointestinal disturbance, tachycardia, psychomotor agitation, as well as other unpleasant symptoms.[2] The acute symptoms of caffeine intoxication and GAD are almost identical.

Marijuana use may result in depersonalization that provokes severe anxiety, fearfulness, and symptoms of agoraphobia. Cannabis intoxication is associated with behavioral or psychological changes, such as anxiety, and physical signs, such as conjunctival injection, dry mouth, and tachycardia. Although marijuana use is sometimes associated with anxiety reduction, there is evidence to suggest that therapy for anxiety disorder using cannabis is limited with the potential harm out weighing the risk.[7]

Lysergic acid diethylamide (LSD), phencyclidine (PCP), and ecstasy (3,4-methylenedioxy-methamphetamine [MDMA]) are hallucinogens that can produce anxiety and paranoia from chronic use or "bad trips." Flashbacks affect some users of LSD; the person may experience the symptoms of anxiety and paranoia weeks or months after use.

Sedative, hypnotic, or anxiolytic drugs (e.g., benzodiazepines, barbiturates) are taken to relieve anxiety or sleeplessness, but their discontinuation can cause sedative withdrawal and rebound anxiety.[2] The severity of the withdrawal syndrome depends on the drug, dosage, duration of use, and speed of elimination. Symptoms include hyperalertness, motor tension, muscle aches, agitation, anxiety, insomnia, tremulousness, nausea, vomiting, convulsions, delirium, and even death.[2]

Although antidepressants are rarely abused, their abrupt cessation can cause a discontinuation syndrome, which may present as sensory and gastrointestinal-related symptoms, insomnia, lethargy, and extreme anxiety.[9]

Alcohol withdrawal can appear 6 to 12 hours after the last drink or significant reduction in consumption. Patients often have a detectable serum alcohol level at this time. Anxiety is one of the first and most prominent symptoms and is seen within 24 to 48 hours of the withdrawal state. Symptoms of anxiety, insomnia, and autonomic dysfunction can last up to 6 months following alcohol withdrawal.[2]

DIAGNOSTIC TESTING

The initial history and physical examination should focus on the presenting complaints to determine if the patient has an anxiety disorder or anxiety caused by drug abuse, medication use, or a general medical condition. The psychiatric history should, at minimum, include current symptoms, precipitating events and significant life stressors, past psychiatric and substance history, history of self-harm or suicide attempts, and identification of support systems. A thorough risk assessment for suicidality is key. Among ED patients, panic attacks have been found to be closely associated with suicidal ideation (43%) and intent (55%). Chapter 101 discusses suicide risk assessment.

A physical examination focused on any bodily area of complaint is necessary, even when there is no overt evidence of disease. Abnormal vital signs suggest an organic medical cause of the anxiety symptoms. Laboratory tests may be necessary based on the clinical presentation, but no tests can confirm or exclude anxiety disorders.[11] Patients with new symptoms require a more extensive medical and psychiatric investigation than those with a known disorder.

MANAGEMENT

The patient should be placed in a quiet area for evaluation. Some patients experience calm when they are removed from a chaotic ED environment. If that is not possible, reducing environmental stimulants, such as dimming lights, can be helpful. If the clinician encounters difficulty in calming the patient, supportive family members may help.

Pharmacologic Treatment

Use of oral, intravenous, or intramuscular medication may be necessary when an anxiety state results in the threat to safety for the patient or others. Medication may also be appropriate for the anxious patient experiencing a significant medical illness or undergoing a medical procedure. Low doses of benzodiazepines (e.g., lorazepam) in small increments can be helpful in alleviating the anxiety associated with substance withdrawal states. Midazolam reduces anxiety and increases amnesia for ED procedures.

SSRIs and SNRIs have become first-line treatment of most anxiety disorders because of their broad spectrum of efficacy and high tolerability by most patients. They have a low potential for dependence and are safer than older classes of antidepressants and anxiolytics. Improvement is usually seen in 4 to 6 weeks, but doses may have to be adjusted. Patients with known anxiety disorders may need a refill of their prescribed medication in the ED. Patients with new-onset anxiety may be started on an SSRI/SNRI in the ED in consultation with a psychiatrist or primary care physician who will see them in follow-up for a thorough evaluation of the type of anxiety and provide a long-term treatment plan. There is no difference in efficacy in drugs in the same class nor between SSRI and SNRI for all anxiety disorders except social anxiety disorders.[10]

Benzodiazepines can be prescribed for motivated patients with acute exogenous anxiety for time-limited stress. Benzodiazepines are an attractive alternative to the delayed response of an SSRI when an immediate reduction of symptoms is desired or a short-term treatment is needed. Benzodiazepines have a role in emergency medical treatment, but their use is questionable for long-term treatment. In most circumstances, benzodiazepines should be prescribed for a week or less. Patients may need to be prescribed several weeks of benzodiazepines until SSRIs/SNRIs take effect. Patients with a history of alcoholism or drug abuse, who are emotionally dependent, or who become anxious in response to normal stress are at greater risk of drug dependency and are not good candidates for this treatment. Hydroxyzine has also been used in select patients as an alternative to benzodiazepines for rapid anxiolytic effect, and are indicated for the treatment of anxiety.

Monoamine oxidase inhibitors and tricyclic antidepressants have been effective in treating anxiety but have been largely supplanted by SSRIs and SNRIs. Buspirone, a 5-hydroxytryptamine receptor 1A agonist, has been shown to work well for generalized anxiety disorders in some studies with few side effects but requires 1 to 3 weeks to become effective.[13]

Nonpharmacologic Therapy

Patients with associated agitation may need verbal de-escalation as first-line treatment prior to the use of medications. Supportive therapy can be used to calm patients and give them room to problem-solve. Emergency clinicians and staff can also use psychoeducation to normalize perception and to teach skills of coping such as breathing techniques. It is also particularly useful to educate the patient on the role that stimulants (e.g., caffeine) and depressants (e.g., alcohol) play in promoting anxiety.

There are multiple longer-term therapies that can be helpful for treating anxiety but are not applicable in the acute care setting. Psychotherapy may be helpful for individuals whose psychological makeup, coping style, interpersonal dynamics, and situational stressors contribute to their pathologic anxiety. The use of supportive, insight-oriented, or family therapy is helpful when these factors appear prominently in the patient's presentation. Cognitive-behavioral therapy helps the patient correct the cognitive misperceptions and overreactions that occur. Psychotherapy is as effective as medication in treating anxiety, but requires commitment from the patient. Meditation, biofeedback, and suggestive hypnosis may also have a role in long-term treatment.[13]

DISPOSITION

Patients receiving initial treatment in the ED without a proper referral to outpatient care are at an increased risk for return. If available, it is preferred that a social worker or mental health worker connect discharged patients with outside agencies and services, rather than providing patients with a referral list.

Most patients with an anxiety disorder can be safely discharged with close primary care physician or psychiatrist follow-up. Some who may have difficulty navigating the outpatient setting may benefit from a short stay in psychiatric observation or in a crisis stabilization unit even if suicide risk is low. Patients with an anxiety disorder associated with suicidal or homicidal ideation or with severe depression require urgent psychiatric attention and hospitalization.

The references for this chapter can be found online at ExpertConsult.com.

99

Somatic Symptoms and Related Disorders

Karl Huesgen and J. Adrian Tyndall

- Several conditions previously classified in the fourth edition of the Diagnostic and Statistical Manual of Mental Disorders (DSM-IV) as somatoform disorders are now classified under DSM-V as *Somatic Symptom and Related Disorders* (SSRD). These include somatic symptom disorder (SSD), illness anxiety disorder (IAD), and conversion disorder. They share a common feature of patients' maladaptive and inappropriate psychological response to somatic (bodily) symptoms.
- SSRD patients have approximately twice the rate of medical disease seen in the general population. It is unclear whether this is the consequence of more frequent health care use or whether an increased disease burden prompts these patients to have a greater concern for bodily sensations.
- *SSD* is characterized by disproportionate or persistent health-related thoughts, anxiety, and time and energy devoted to somatic (bodily) symptoms, resulting in disruption of daily life.
- Patients with *IAD,* formerly known as hypochondriasis, have excessive anxiety regarding the possibly having or acquiring a serious medical illness in the presence of minimal or absent somatic symptoms.
- *Conversion disorder*, also known as *functional neurologic symptom disorder*, is characterized by abnormal sensory or voluntary motor function that is found to be incompatible with known neurologic or medical conditions, and that causes significant distress or life impairment.
- The differential diagnoses for SSRD may be broadly divided between (a) psychiatric disorders that manifest somatic symptoms and (b) medical conditions with signs or symptoms that might be attributed to psychiatric disorders.
- A "positive review of systems" in an emergency department (ED) evaluation is similar to a high score on SSRD symptoms severity scales and thus may serve as an inadvertent screen for SSRD. Further research is needed to ascertain whether this is clinically reliable.
- ED care goals for patients with SSRD include establishment of rapport, building a therapeutic alliance, legitimizing the patient's distress, and enhancing the patient's ability to function despite the symptoms.
- Multiple care modalities are available for SSRD treatment. These are typically managed by the patient's primary care physician or psychiatrist.

FOUNDATIONS

Somatic symptom and related disorders (SSRD), formerly known as somatoform disorders, are described as the borderland between psychiatry and medicine and are responsible for some of the most challenging and the least understood patient encounters in the emergency department (ED). Individuals who suffer from these disorders must be identified and treated appropriately to avoid patient suffering, inappropriate resource use, and iatrogenic injuries.

Box 99.1 lists the disorders classified in the fifth edition of the Diagnostic and Statistical Manual of Mental Disorders (DSM-5) as SSRD. They include somatic symptom disorder (SSD), illness anxiety disorder (IAD, formerly known as hypochondriasis), conversion disorder, psychological factors affecting medical illness, and factitious disorder (discussed separately in Chapter 100). Body dysmorphic disorder (excessive concern for a perceived defect in physical features) is no longer included in this group.

Although prior versions of the DSM emphasized medically unexplained symptoms and their putative psychological causes, current descriptions of these disorders focus on patients' maladaptive and inappropriate cognitive and affective responses to somatic symptoms rather than the lack of explanation for them.[1,2] These disorders are thought to be mediated by abnormal sensory perception, processing, interpretation, attribution to pathologic causes, and subsequent hypervigilance toward further sensations.[3–7]

SSRD are common, with a prevalence of approximately 5% to 7% of the adult population, and are present in many patients with medically unexplained symptoms.[1,8] The defining features of these disorders, a maladaptive response to bodily sensations, cause patients to seek help for their illness through medical routes rather than psychiatric avenues. However, the SSRD are typically formally diagnosed only via structured psychiatric interview, and these disorders may take many years to diagnose even in longitudinal primary care settings.[9] The disorders are even more challenging to diagnose during a brief ED encounter prioritizing life-threatening illness.

Difficulty identifying the root cause of patients' distress may cause frustration for both patients and physicians. For example, patients with SSD may have excessive anxiety regarding nonpathologic sensations, whereas patients with IAD may be certain they have a serious medical condition despite contradictory evidence. Thus, after a negative ED work-up, the very nature of the patients' psychiatric condition may leave them feeling that their concerns have not been adequately addressed, prompting pursuit of extensive, expensive, and invasive medical evaluations. SSRD patients have approximately twice the rate of medical disease seen in the general population. It is unclear whether this is the consequence of more frequent health care use or whether an increased disease burden prompts these patients to have a greater concern for bodily sensations.[10]

Clinicians may also feel frustrated by encounters with patients with SSRD. Frequent ED use by patients with unrealistic expectations and subsequent frustrations may cause physicians to feel these encounters were suboptimal. These patients frequently exhibit an extensive "positive review of symptoms," which clinicians may feel obligated to evaluate. Even when clinicians suspect SSRD, they are often unwilling to ascribe patient concerns to psychiatric illness at the exclusion of rare but consequential medical diagnoses with nonspecific presentations. However, if the patients' concerns are recognized and addressed within

---

BOX 99.1 Somatic Symptom and Related Disorders

Somatic symptom and related disorders share a common feature of patients' maladaptive and inappropriate psychological response to somatic (bodily) symptoms

Somatic symptom disorder

Illness anxiety disorder

Conversion disorder (functional neurologic symptom disorder)

Psychological factors affecting other medical conditions

Factitious disorder

BOX 99.2 Differential Diagnosis of Somatic Symptom Disorder

Psychiatric Conditions	Medical Conditions
Depression disorders	Transient ischemic attack
Anxiety disorders	Multiple sclerosis
Obsessive-compulsive disorder	Systemic lupus erythematosus
Schizophrenia	Thyroid and parathyroid disorders
Personality disorders	Electrolyte disorders
Substance abuse disorders	Human immunodeficiency virus (HIV)
Malingering	Anti-NMDA receptor encephalitis

---

a patient-centered framework, clinicians may recognize that the "difficult patient" with a "positive review of systems" may have a psychiatric illness requiring further evaluation in an outpatient medical or psychiatric setting.

CLINICAL FEATURES

Patients with SSRD experience physical symptoms associated with significant distress and impairment that cannot be adequately explained by demonstrable physical pathology despite appropriate medical investigation. These disorders are most common in women of lower socioeconomic status in their 20s and 30s but may be present in any demographic group. Depressive and anxiety disorders are common comorbid conditions, as are nonpsychiatric medical diagnoses.[1]

Somatic Symptom Disorder

Patients with SSD have disproportionate or persistent health-related thoughts, anxiety, and time and energy devoted to somatic (bodily) symptoms, resulting in disruption of daily life. Previous editions of the DSM described a causal relationship between a patient's emotions and subsequent symptoms (termed somatization). The disorder criteria now focus upon the abnormal psychological response to bodily sensations rather than to a lack of medical explanation for symptoms.[1] Research indicates these patients have abnormal autonomic activity and reactivity, as well as measurably altered emotional processing and bodily awareness.[7] A subset of SSD patients includes patients for whom pain is the primary concern. Previously called pain disorder, this diagnosis is now termed *SSD with predominant pain*. For these patients, pain may represent normal bodily function in conjunction with spinal or higher-CNS sensitization from prior experience and genetic factors.[1,11] Of note, because the diagnosis of SSD depends upon the maladaptive psychological response to bodily sensations rather than the lack of medical explanation alone, the symptoms alone from fibromyalgia, irritable bowel syndrome, or multiple chemical sensitivities do not meet criteria for SSD.[1]

Illness Anxiety Disorder

Patients with IAD have minimal or absent somatic symptoms but present with excessive anxiety regarding possibly having or acquiring a serious medical illness. Formerly known as hypochondriasis, IAD is now the preferred nomenclature to avoid pejorative connotations. IAD persists despite repeatedly negative medical evaluations, and the anxiety associated with this condition can produce either excessive health-related behaviors or maladaptive health care avoidance, resulting in care-seeking and care-avoidant subtypes, respectively. Care-seeking subtypes are at risk for iatrogenic complications of excessive testing.[1]

Conversion Disorder

Patients with conversion disorder, now commonly referred to as *functional neurologic symptom disorder*, have altered sensory or voluntary motor function that is found to be incompatible with known neurologic or medical conditions and that causes the patient significant distress or life impairment. This disorder may have a variety of presentations, including seizure-like activity, focal weakness, memory disturbances, dysphonia, blindness, or alterations of any sensory system. Upon medical examination, however, no pathologic correlates are identified, and serial neurologic examinations often demonstrate inconsistent disability. For example, in the Hoover test, a supine patient may demonstrate normal hip extension (pushing down) with a "paralyzed" leg when asked to flex (lift) the contralateral hip. Similarly, patients may demonstrate inability to turn their head toward a "paralyzed" side but use the "paralyzed" sternocleidomastoid to turn from it. Coincident life stress is associated with but not essential for the diagnosis. The presence of *la belle indifference* (i.e., an inappropriate lack of concern regarding a seemingly profound disability) is also associated with but not specific to this disorder. Proven intentionality is not necessary for the diagnosis.[1]

Factitious Disorder

In contrast to conversion disorder, factitious disorder is characterized by purposefully deceptive falsification of disease signs or symptoms for the sole purpose of causing others to see the person with the disorder as ill. In the case of Munchausen by proxy, the person induces symptoms in another patient, typically a child.[1,12] These disorders are discussed in greater detail in Chapter 100.

Psychological Factors Affecting Medical Illness

Psychological factors affecting medical illness is a separate category included in SSRD due to the predominance of somatic symptoms and propensity to present in medical settings. This includes psychological factors that exacerbate or delay recovery from medical conditions, reduce adherence to medical treatment, or pose additional risk harm. Examples include anxiety-exacerbated asthma, or stress-induced Takotsubo cardiomyopathy.[1]

DIFFERENTIAL DIAGNOSES

Other psychiatric disorders may initially present with somatic symptoms, including major depressive disorder and anxiety disorders. The differential diagnoses for the SSRD may be broadly separated into two groups: psychiatric disorders that manifest somatic symptoms and medical conditions with signs or symptoms that might be attributed to psychiatric disorders (Box 99.2).[1,13] For example, psychiatric patients with panic disorder may present with complaints of palpitations and dyspnea, and patients with major depressive disorder might present with sleep disturbances. Alternatively, many medical diagnoses can have subtle or variable presentations which might be attributed to psychiatric disorders (e.g., hypothyroidism-induced fatigue attributed to depression, sensory loss due to multiple sclerosis, or behavioral disturbances secondary to anti-N-methyl-d-aspartate (NMDA) receptor encephalitis).[14]

DIAGNOSTIC TESTING

The very nature of SSRD often prompts repeated and extensive evaluations of patients' somatic complaints. Diagnostic testing for possible organic diagnoses should be based upon a physician's standard practice for evaluating a presenting medical complaint and not upon a patient's desire for additional testing to reassure them that an undiagnosed medical disorder is not present. Unnecessary testing may put patients at risk for diagnostic false-positives and iatrogenic injury. The exception to this rule is the patient with functional neurologic symptom disorder or conversion disorder. Neurologic disorders such as transient ischemic attacks, multiple sclerosis, and atypical migraine headaches may have subtle presentations. In these cases, it may require imaging studies and both neurologic and psychiatric consultations to avoid the misdiagnosis of a patient who requires intervention.

Specific SSRD diagnoses are suggested by the overall clinical picture rather than single discrete findings. For example, excessive anxiety despite a negative chest pain work-up would suggest SSD, or an inappropriate lack of concern regarding a hemiparesis would suggest conversion disorder. Diagnostic reliability for SSRD is improved with formal structured clinical interviews, typically in psychiatric or primary care settings.[15] Self-report questionnaires have shown promise in these settings.[16,17] Clinicians typically have neither the time nor the clinical training to perform structured clinical interviews for formal SSRD diagnosis; however, brief 2- to 3-minute self-report instruments (e.g., SSD-12) are available for outpatient screening of patients' symptom-related thoughts, feeling, and behaviors, although further research is needed regarding whether these are applicable to an emergency setting.[18,19] It is notable that tests of SSRD patients' symptoms severity (e.g., Patient Health Questionaire-15 [PHQ-15]) resemble a standard emergency medicine review of symptoms (e.g., has the patient had chest pain, shortness of breath, dizziness, nausea, headaches in the past month, and whether these symptoms bothered patient not at all, a little, or a lot). On this test, a score at greater than 10 indicates high risk for somatoform disorders.[20] Therefore a positive review of systems in a normal ED evaluation may serve as an inadvertent screen for SSRD.

If organic causes of patients' symptoms are not identified, psychiatric consultation or referral could be considered for formal SSRD diagnosis.

MANAGEMENT

The management of patients with SSRD is challenging. Whereas most patients trust their doctors' conclusions, SSRD produce an inherent conflict between the patient beliefs and physician reassurance. Even patients with insight into their disorder may harbor unshakable beliefs of physical illness despite evidence to the contrary. On the other hand, one must be aware of the possibility of an unexplained medical illness that can confound diagnosis and management. It is thus incumbent upon the physician to build rapport by demonstrating attention, empathy, and the desire to alleviate the patient's suffering. One should recognize and communicate understanding of the life impact of the patient's somatic and psychiatric symptoms. After building a therapeutic alliance, it may be helpful to discuss the patient's illness with them in terms of a chronic disease that can be mitigated but not fully alleviated. In this way, patients may focus on maximizing life function in spite of their disorder rather than eliminating the symptoms.[13] Naming the disorder itself may improve the therapeutic alliance.[21] Long-term treatment of SSRD typically involves the use of medications (e.g., SSRIs) with or without therapy (e.g., cognitive behavioral therapy) that is best managed by primary care physicians or psychiatrists. These treatments are not initiated by an emergency clinician but may be started by a psychiatric consultant.[22]

DISPOSITION

In the absence other factors necessitating medical or psychiatric admission, patients with SSRD may be discharged with outpatient primary care or psychiatric follow-up. They should be told that acute life-threatening diagnoses have been ruled out and that further testing and additional medications are not indicated at this time. Emphasize to the patient that even in the absence of a satisfactory explanation for their symptoms, psychiatric intervention may be useful in mitigating life impacts of their symptomatology.

The references for this chapter can be found online at ExpertConsult. com.

100

Factitious Disorders and Malingering

Henry W. Young II and Joseph E. Thornton

FOUNDATIONS

Patients may present to the emergency department (ED) with symptoms that are simulated or intentionally produced. The reasons that cause this behavior define two disorders: factitious disorders and malingering.

Factitious disorders are characterized by symptoms or signs that are intentionally produced or feigned by the patient in the absence of apparent external incentives.[1,2] These patients constitute up to 3% of general psychiatric referrals.[3] However, the prevalence of factitious disorders in emergency departments is thought to be higher because these patients rarely accept psychiatric treatment and are frequently undiagnosed.[2,4] These patients are often seen in other health care settings including infectious disease for fever of unknown origin, epilepsy clinics for psychogenic seizures, and nephrology clinics for renal stones.[3] Factitious disorders have been associated with costs up to $1 million per case.[3] Early diagnosis of factitious disorder can have a significant impact on the utilization of unnecessary investigations, treatments, and hospital admissions within a health care system.[3]

The *Diagnostic and Statistical Manual of Mental Disorders, Fifth Edition* (DSM-5) classifies factitious disorders into two types: factitious disorder imposed on self (FDIS) and factitious disorder imposed on another (FDIA).[1]

Munchausen syndrome, the most dramatic form of FDIS, was originally described in 1951.[8] This rare syndrome takes its name from Baron Karl F. von Munchausen (1720–1797), a revered German military officer and noted raconteur who had his embellished life stories stolen and parodied in a 1785 pamphlet.[4] While commonly discussed, the incidence of Munchausen syndrome is estimated to be approximately 0.5 to 2 per 100,000 children.[5] Other names used to describe FDIS include the "hospital hobo syndrome" (patients wander from hospital to hospital seeking admission), peregrinating (wandering) patients, hospital addict, polysurgical addiction, and hospital vagrant.[3,6]

Factitious disorder imposed on another (FDIA) involves the simulation or production of a factitious mental or physical disease in an individual by a caregiver. It was first described in 1977.[1] Due to the difficulty in identification, the prevalence of FDIA is not known.[5] This condition often involves a child and a mother. The condition excludes straightforward physical abuse or neglect and simple failure to thrive; mere lying to cover up physical abuse is not FDIA. The key discriminator is motive: the caregiver is making the child ill so that they can vicariously assume the sick role with all its benefits.[3] FDIA has a mortality rate of 6% to 30%.[6,7] Permanent disfigurement or permanent impairment of function can occur directly from induced disease or indirectly from invasive procedures, multiple medications, or major surgery. Other names applied to this condition include *Polle syndrome* (Polle was a child of Baron Munchausen who died mysteriously), *factitious disorder by proxy, pediatric condition falsification, Munchausen syndrome by proxy,* and *Meadow syndrome.*[3,7]

Malingering is the simulation of disease by the intentional production of false or grossly exaggerated physical or psychological symptoms, motivated by external incentives, such as avoidance of military responsibility, avoidance of work, obtaining financial compensation, evading criminal prosecution, obtaining medication, hospital admission (for the purpose of obtaining free room and board), or securing of better living conditions.[1] The most common goal among such "patients" presenting to the ED is to obtain medications, whereas in the office or clinic the gain is more commonly insurance payments or industrial injury settlements. The true incidence of malingering is difficult to gauge because of underreporting, but estimates include a 1% incidence among mental health patients in civilian clinical practice, and as high as 10% among inpatient psychiatric patients with suicidality.[8-10] In one review, 33% of patients assessed in a psychiatric emergency department were suspected of malingering.[8] Some clinicians are resistant to document malingering in a patients' chart due to concern for lack of reimbursement and legal liability.[8,9] The most likely conditions to be feigned are conditions that are difficult to exclude objectively, such as suicidal ideations, depression, mild head injury, fibromyalgia, chronic fatigue syndrome, and chronic pain.[3,7,11-13]

CLINICAL FEATURES

Factitious Disorders

Factitious Disorders Imposed on Self

The diagnosis of FDIS depends on specific criteria (Box 100.1).[1] With a factitious disorder, the production of symptoms and signs is compulsive; the patient is unable to refrain from the behavior even when its risks are known. The behavior is voluntary only in the sense that it is deliberate and purposeful (intentional) but not in the sense that the acts can be fully controlled. The underlying motivation for producing these deceptions, securing the sick role, is primarily unconscious.[1,2] Individuals who readily admit that they have produced their own injuries (e.g., self-mutilation) are not included in the category of factitious disorders. Presentations may be acute, in response to an identifiable recent psychosocial stress (termination of romantic relationship, threats to self-esteem), or a chronic life pattern, reflective of the way in which the person deals with life in general. The symptoms involved may be either psychological or physical.[3,5,7]

Psychological Symptoms. Individuals may intentionally produce or feign psychological (often psychotic) symptoms suggestive of a mental disorder. Stimulants may be used to induce restlessness or insomnia; hallucinogens, to create altered levels of consciousness; and hypnotics, to produce lethargy. This psychological factitious condition is less common than factitious disorders with physical symptoms and is almost always superimposed on a severe personality disorder.[1,3,5]

Physical Symptoms. The intentional production of physical symptoms may take the form of fabricating symptoms without signs (e.g., feigning abdominal pain), simulation of signs suggesting illness (e.g., fraudulent pyuria, induced anemia), self-inflicted conditions (e.g., the production of abscesses by injection of contaminated material under the skin), or genuine complications from the intentional misuse of medications (e.g., hypoglycemic agents).[3] These patients are predominantly unmarried women younger than 40 years old.[1] They typically accept their illness with few complaints and are generally well-educated, responsible workers or students with moral attitudes and otherwise conscientious behavior. A majority of individuals with factitious disorder are employed in health care settings, including laboratory technicians, nurses, and physicians. There is an increased rate of personality disorders and depression among individuals with factitious disorder.[2-5,7]

These patients are willing to undergo incredible hardship, limb amputation, organ loss, and even death to perpetuate the masquerade.[4] Although multiple hospitalizations often lead to iatrogenic physical conditions, such as postoperative pain syndromes and drug addictions, patients continue to seek hospitalization for its own sake. They typically have a fragile and fragmented self-image and are susceptible to psychotic and suicidal episodes.[3] Interactions with the health care system and relationships with caregivers provide the needed structure that stabilizes the patient's sense of self.[4] Some patients are driven by the conviction that they have a real but as yet undiscovered illness. Consequently, artificial symptoms are contrived to convince the physician to continue a search for the elusive disease process. Factitious illness behavior has also emerged on the internet. "Virtual support groups" offering person-to-person communications through chat rooms or websites have been perpetrated by individuals, under the pretense of illness or personal crisis, for the purpose of extracting attention or sympathy, acting out anger, or exercising control over others.[4]

Munchausen Syndrome. The uncommon patient with true Munchausen syndrome has a prolonged pattern of "medical imposture," usually years in duration. The diagnosis may be delayed several years.[12] The average age at presentation is 34 years, and the syndrome is most commonly found in women. Patients' entire adult lives may consist of trying to gain admission to hospitals and then resisting discharge. The majority of patients work in the health care field.[2,3,14] The quest for repeated hospitalizations often takes these patients to numerous and widespread cities and states.[6]

These individuals see themselves as important people, or at least related to such persons, and their life events are depicted as exceptional. They possess extensive knowledge of medical terminology. There is frequently a history of genuine disease, and the individual may exhibit objective physical findings.[4]

The symptoms presented are "limited only by the person's medical knowledge, sophistication, and imagination."[1] Common presentations are those that most reliably result in admission to the hospital, such as abdominal pain, self-injection of a foreign substance, feculent urine, bleeding disorders, hemoptysis, paroxysmal headaches, seizures, shortness of breath, asthma with respiratory failure, chronic pain, acute cardiovascular symptoms (e.g., chest pain, induced hypertension, and syncope), renal colic and spurious urolithiasis, fever of unknown origin, and profound hypoglycemia.[3] Some self-induced conditions are highly injurious or even lethal.[15]

The patient usually presents during evenings or on weekends so as to minimize accessibility to psychiatric consultants, personal physicians, and past medical records. In teaching institutions, these patients often present in July, shortly after the change in resident house officers. They relate their history in a precise, dramatic, even intriguing fashion, embellished with flourishes of pathologic lying and self-aggrandizement. *Pseudologia fantastica,* or pathologic lying, is a distinctive peculiarity of such patients. In a chronic, often lifelong behavior pattern, the patient typically takes a central and heroic role in these tales, which may function as a way to act out fantasy.[16] The history quickly becomes vague and inconsistent, however, when the patient is questioned in detail about medical contacts. Attempts to manage the complaint on an outpatient basis are adamantly resisted. Once admitted, the patient initially appeals to the physician's qualities of nurturance and omnipotence, lavishing praise on the caregivers. Behavior rapidly evolves, however, as the patient creates havoc on the ward by insisting on excessive attention while ignoring both hospital rules and the prescribed therapeutic regimen. When the hoax is uncovered and the patient confronted, fear of rejection may abruptly change into rage against the treating physician, closely followed by departure from the hospital against medical advice.

Factitious Disorder Imposed on Another

The diagnosis of FDIA depends on specific criteria (Box 100.2).[2] FDIA is also referred to as Munchausen by proxy or medical child abuse, or a subset of battered child syndrome.[4,7,17] The diagnostic term is applied to the perpetrator of an abuse of a child, which is a criminal event and in most states requires referral once suspected.[4,18,19] The presenting complaints typically evade definitive diagnosis and are refractory to conventional therapy for no apparent reason. They usually present with more than five symptoms, presented in a confused picture; they are unusual or serious and, by design, unverifiable. Gold standard diagnostic methods include a separation test and covert video surveillance.[3,19]

Simulated illness, faked by the caregiver without producing direct harm to the patient (e.g., the addition of blood to a urine specimen), is present in 25% of cases. Produced illness, which the caregiver actually inflicts on the patient (e.g., the injection of feces into an intravenous line), is found in 50% of cases. Both simulated and produced illnesses are found in 25% of cases.[4]

FDIA most commonly arises with factitious bleeding, seizures, central nervous system (CNS) depression, apnea, diarrhea, vomiting, fever, and rash. Reported techniques of simulation or production of disease include fever manipulations and administration of drugs or toxins (e.g., chronic arsenic poisoning, mercury poisoning, ipecac, warfarin, salt, imipramine, laxatives, or CNS depressants), or caustics applied to the skin.[4,17] Techniques of asphyxiation include (1) covering the mouth or nose with one or both hands, a cloth, or plastic film, and (2) inserting the fingers into the back of the mouth. In such instances, even struggling infants may sustain no cutaneous markings. Cases involving seizures are common and may involve third-party witnesses. On personal questioning, however, these witnesses frequently deny the occurrence of seizure activity.[4]

Perpetrator Characteristics. Ninety-eight percent of perpetrators are biological mothers who come from all socioeconomic groups.[7,17,18] Many have a background in health professions or social work, or a past history of psychiatric treatment, marital problems, or suicide attempts. Depression, anxiety, and somatization are common, but overt psychotic behavior by the mother is atypical.[7] Perpetrators of FDIA are skilled in manipulating health care workers and child protection services. They are pleasant, socially adept, cooperative, and appreciative of good medical care. They often display a peculiar eagerness to have invasive procedures performed on their child. They often prefer to stay in the hospital with their child, cultivate unusually close relationships with hospital staff, and thrive on staff attention. This affable relationship with the medical team rapidly changes to excessive anger and denial when the perpetrator is confronted with suspicions.[7,18]

Most of these mothers have had an abusive experience early in life, and they use the health care system as a means to satisfy personal nurturing demands.[7] They often cannot distinguish their needs from the child's and satisfy their own needs first. They derive a sense of purpose from the medical and nursing attention gained when their children are in the hospital. Alternatively, the behavior may enable the mothers to escape from their own physical or psychological illnesses, marital difficulties, or social problems.[4]

Victim Characteristics. Victims of FDIA are equally male and female children. The proper diagnosis for the victims of FDIA is the coding for confirmed or suspected child physical abuse (995.4) and the appropriate injury code.[1,4] The child or vulnerable adult may also suffer physical or psychological consequences of unnecessary medical procedures. The mean age at diagnosis is 40 months, and the mean duration from the onset of signs and symptoms to diagnosis is 15 months.[17,18] A known physical illness that explains part of the symptoms is common among these children.[13] Most have a history of significant failure to thrive and have been hospitalized in more than one institution. Delays in many areas of performance and learning, difficulty with family relationships, attention deficit disorder, or clinical depression may coexist. Some of these victims may have factitious disorder later in life or even PTSD.[4] Elders may also be victims of FDIA, although this is uncommon.[4]

Malingering

Malingering is frequently found in association with antisocial personality disorder and substance abuse.[20] On questioning, malingerers are vague about prior hospitalizations or treatments. The physicians who previously treated them are usually unavailable. At times, malingerers may be careless about their symptoms and abandon them when they believe no one is watching. Common sources for secondary gain include opiate drug administration, shelter among the homeless, financial gains or avoidance of incarceration.[8,13] Since pain is a subjective experience, providers may have little objective evidence to quantify the degree of pain an individual is having. Malingerers who pursue drugs may report an unusually large number of drug allergies to persuade the physician to prescribe their drug of choice or simply insist on a specific drug (e.g., meperidine [Demerol] or hydromorphone [Dilaudid]). Unfortunately, the internet offers a wide availability of quality medical advice on how to convincingly feign pain and disability. In other persons, the external incentive may be obscure.

In contrast to the person with factitious disorders, the malingerer prefers counterfeit mental illness, because it is objectively difficult to verify or to disprove. Suicidal ideation is the most common psychological presentation, followed by psychosis, depression, and withdrawal syndromes.[8]

Malingering should be strongly suspected with any combination of certain factors (Box 100.3).[1] A definitive diagnosis of malingering is rare and can be established only with the patient's confession. Because malingering could constitute criminal behavior, documentation of this diagnosis must be made with care. In the absence of proof of wrongdoing, it is best to assume that the patient is not a malingerer but rather a somatizer. Due to the possible implications for diagnosing a patient as a malingerer, it is most appropriate to document the individual's behaviors.[27]

The clinical interview is especially important in identifying an individual that is malingering, with additional care to identify atypical presentations. The health care provider should be mindful in phrasing their questions to avoid providing insight on the typical presentation and begin the interview with open-ended questions, first allowing the individual to recount their symptoms in their own words and then asking more specific questions. Also be aware that patients who malinger often have true illnesses such as substance abuse or paranoia.[16,20,21]

DIFFERENTIAL DIAGNOSES

The most important diagnoses to be excluded are genuine medical and psychiatric conditions that might account for the presenting symptoms. Patients with conversion disorder, somatic disorder, delusional disorder of somatic type, and borderline personality disorder can present with symptoms similar to FDIS. The differences can be subtle and psychiatric consultation or referral is indicated.

Patients with factitious disorders are distinguished from malingerers because their desired hospitalization or surgery seems to offer no secondary gain other than to play the sick role.[1] The clinical presentation of the majority of patients with factitious disorders, unlike those with Munchausen syndrome, is relatively subtle and convincing. The complaints are generally chronic in nature rather than emergent and precipitous, and there are no obvious associated behavioral aberrations. The chronicity of malingering is usually less than that associated with factitious disorder, and malingerers are more reluctant to accept expensive, possibly painful, or dangerous tests or surgery.[4,21]

It can be useful to consider factitious disorders along a continuum of malingering, which are symptoms consciously produced for obvious secondary gain; factitious disorders, which are symptoms which are intentionally produced without obvious secondary gain; and somatization disorders, which are symptoms unconsciously produced for unconscious psychological gain. In fact, even within a patient, clinical presentations may present along this continuum at different times.[5,22] Additionally, it is important to know that there is significant morbidity and occasionally mortality associated with this spectrum of disorders. When a clinician suspects that there may be a factitious component to the clinical presentation due to an unexpected clinical course, it is useful to continue to think of a comprehensive and systematic differential diagnosis, but instead of aggressive pursuit of a rare diagnosis, to consider with the patient what problems the patient is facing and how their symptoms impact those problems.[4] The clinician can then formulate a treatment plan that addresses the root cause of these somatic symptoms.

DIAGNOSTIC TESTING

Unnecessary tests, medications, and hospitalizations should be avoided in the absence of objective evidence of a medical or psychiatric disease, and patients should be referred for ongoing primary care.

Factitious Disorder

The initial diagnosis of FDIS is often delayed because the possibility of factitious disease is not considered, physicians may be unfamiliar with this problem, or the physician is concerned about the consequences of making a mistaken diagnosis of FDIS.[9,23] Diagnosis may be confounded by genuine medical illnesses predating and coexisting with a factitious disorder. For example, patients with factitious hypoglycemia may have a history of insulin-dependent diabetes mellitus, or factitious skin disorders may be preceded by true dermatologic diseases.[4] Identification of a factitious disorder is usually made when (1) the patient's account of symptoms is patently inconsistent, (2) the patient's symptoms are too consistent with textbook descriptions, (3) laboratory findings are inconsistent (e.g., low C-peptide in context of high insulin confirms exogenous administration of insulin), (4) the patient is accidentally[4] discovered in the act, (5) incriminating items are found, (6) a combination of the preceding, or (7) the diagnosis is made by a historical pattern of medical documentation and exclusion.[4,21]

There has been increasing recognition of factitious illness produced by children. These children, ranging in age from 8 to 18 years old, are typically "bland, flat and indifferent during their extensive medical interventions, depressed, socially isolated, and often obese."[4] Among the most common presentations are fever without clear etiology, diabetic ketoacidosis, purpura, and recurrent infections. The prognosis is good if identification and psychotherapeutic intervention can be carried out at a young age.[4,12]

Suspected FDIA requires a detailed description of the event or illness and a search for caregiver witnesses, who should be interviewed personally. Although it is essential to see the child when the symptoms

are present, the caretaker often makes this difficult.[7,11] Additional history of unusual illness in siblings and parents should be sought. Child victims who are verbal should be interviewed in private about foods, medicines, and their recollection of the symptoms or events. Prior medical records of the victim and, if possible, the siblings should be examined, although parents may impede such data-gathering.[5,11]

The major obstacle to early discovery of FDIA is its omission from the differential diagnosis. When it is considered, the diagnosis is generally made easily and quickly.[11] A suspected diagnosis may be confirmed through separation of the parent from the child or individual (with consequent cessation of symptoms), covert video surveillance during hospitalization, or toxicologic screens.[7] The caregiver may attempt to induce episodes surreptitiously while in the hospital.[7]

Malingering

There have been several tools designed to assist with the identification of malingerers. Two common tools are the Structured Interview of Reported Symptoms (SIRS) and the Miller Forensic Assessment of Symptoms Test (M-FAST). Although both tools have been assessed in a variety of populations, neither has been thoroughly assessed in the ED. The SIRS questionnaire has been well studied and validated, but its duration makes it less suitable for performance in an emergency setting. Although the M-FAST is considerably shorter, highly sensitive, and easy to interpret, there is inadequate data to recommend this tool for clinical use in the ED at this time.[10] Similarly, tests designed to assess malingered pain currently lack validity studies involving known populations with malingered pain and have not been found to reliably detect malingering pain.[24]

MANAGEMENT

The initial management of patients suspected of fabricating disease should include a caring, nonjudgmental attitude and a search for objective clinical evidence of treatable medical or psychiatric illness.

Factitious Disorders

Treatment options for factitious disorders depend on the patient's characteristics. Although it is challenging, management of common forms of factitious disorder can be more rewarding, especially with adolescents, than management of Munchausen syndrome.[5] The prognosis is more favorable for cases with an underlying depression than for those associated with borderline personalities.[5]

The best approach to patients with factitious disorder, other than Munchausen syndrome and FDIA, is controversial. Direct nonaccusatory confrontation has been advocated as "the foundation of effective management" when it is coupled with the assurance that an ongoing relationship with a physician will be provided. This may be the first step in the acceptance of outpatient therapy.[25]

Others point out that confrontation is ineffective in most patients and may even be counterproductive in that it threatens to undermine a needed psychological defense. Enforced recognition of external objective reality, while simultaneously disallowing the patient's subjective experience, may generate even more dysfunction directed at legitimizing and maintaining symptoms and may even place the patient at risk for escalation of symptoms.[9,25] Because emergency clinicians rarely, if ever, provide longitudinal care to patients with factitious disorders, we recommend referral for ongoing care, rather than direct confrontation in the ED.

Individuals with Munchausen syndrome typically demonstrate sociopathic traits or a borderline personality disorder and are demanding and manipulative, especially regarding analgesics. They can be difficult to treat. Early confrontation or limit-setting, especially regarding drug use, is recommended. Although Munchausen patients typically do not want to be examined extensively, a thorough physical examination should be performed to rule out physical disease.[12,24,25]

FDIA constitutes a form of child (or elder) abuse, and appropriate action to protect the victim, including notification of state social service agencies, should take immediate priority. If available, a pediatrician who has expertise in child abuse should assess the case.[5,11] When the diagnosis has been established and the parents have been confronted, psychiatric care should be made immediately available to the parents because escalation of symptoms, including repeat abuse, abuse of siblings, and even fatalities, have been reported.[26]

Malingering

Malingerers do not want to be treated. Because they are "gaming the system" for personal gain, they do not want an accurate identification of their behavior and appropriate intervention. The emergency clinician should maintain clinical neutrality, offering the reassurance that the symptoms and examination are not consistent with any serious disease.[25] If there is no medical issue necessitating admission, admission is not recommended for malingerers. Among patients found to be malingering, admission was more likely in those feigning suicidality or seeking housing or social services.[8]

Some authors have characterized patients' use of medical resources under false pretenses as criminal behavior, and several states have enacted legislation against the fraudulent acquisition of medical services with successful prosecution of such behavior.[9,27] Conversely, patients with malingering disorders can and do sue.[27] In dealing with such patients, it is advisable to involve hospital administration and risk management. Clandestine searches are inadvisable, and respect for the patient's confidentiality should be maintained.[25]

DISPOSITION

Patients suspected of having a factitious disorder should be referred for primary care follow-up, and if it is acceptable to the patient, psychiatric referral should also be arranged. Referral to other medical specialists or hospitalization should be avoided when possible.[8,25]

The manner of presentation and the unavailability of past medical history often allow patients with Munchausen syndrome to achieve hospital admission. If the patient is discharged from the ED, outpatient primary care follow-up and psychiatric referral should be offered, although both are likely to be refused.

Because perpetrators of FDIA typically induce symptomatic episodes soon after hospitalization, admission of the victims (children or elders) without taking appropriate precautions may actually place them at increased risk. Visits by the suspected perpetrator should be closely supervised, and no food, drink, or medicines should be brought in by the family.[5] Protective services should be notified. Out-of-home placement of children in established cases of FDIA is recommended, and the best outcomes are seen among children taken into long-term care at an early age without access to their mother.[5] Children allowed to return home have a high rate of repeated abuse.[5] After the removal of the index child, the subsequent abuse rate of previous siblings is as high as 50%.[5]

After courteous but assertive reassurance, suspected malingerers should be offered primary care follow-up if the symptoms do not resolve. These individuals may become threatening when they are either denied treatment or overtly confronted.

There is a risk for escalation by the patient when they do not receive the therapy or outcome that they desire. This escalation can include threats of harm to the staff and/or the patient. While prior studies suggest that threats of suicide in these circumstances are usually not acted upon, the risk should be assessed. If necessary, consider involving psychiatry for a safety evaluation.[25]

Because prior encounters involving malingering and factitious disorder are important to recognizing similar presentations in the future, it is important to record visits for factitious disorder and malingering in the electronic medical record in a manner that is easily located such as in the problem list or past medical history. Included with the diagnosis should be a narrative including subjective and objective events during that encounter that were used to identify this disorder. In doing so, it is possible to limit unnecessary testing in the future. The goal of inclusion of this information is not to encourage cognitive bias for future providers, but to inform them of features of prior encounters that were concerning. It is important that every new complaint and encounter is evaluated, and that all identified medical needs are addressed.[25]

Once a decision for discharge is made, there should be a discussion with the treatment team including the concern that the patient may not receive the notice of discharge positively. A plan should be made with the treatment team to prepare for possible escalation by the patient. Consider having security presence nearby, if needed. All prescription orders and necessary forms should be prepared and readied to be provided to the patient at the conclusion of the conversation. During the discussion with the patient, direct language and a neutral tone should be used. After the patient is discharged, a debrief should be conducted among the treatment team to identify opportunities to improve the process in the future.[25]

The references for this chapter can be found online at ExpertConsult.com.

101

Suicidal Behavior

Henry W. Young II and Michael A. Shapiro

KEY CONCEPTS

- Many suicidal individuals see a physician shortly before their death. An ED visit for suicidal thoughts or behaviors represents an opportunity for a critical intervention that may prevent a subsequent suicide.
- Suicidal thoughts or behaviors are often triggered by short-term crisis, and most survivors are grateful to be alive.
- An empathetic, patient-centered, collaborative approach that incorporates information from collateral sources (e.g., family) can optimize care.
- Suicide precautions in the ED include appropriate use of staff to monitor the patient to prevent attempts of self-harm while in the ED.
- Routine laboratory tests provide little value for most ED patients with self-harm behaviors. Evaluation should be directed to specific concerning signs or symptoms.
- Suicide risk changes over time, and estimation of imminent risk is not currently evidence-based.
- Brief risk assessment by the clinician can identify patients in need of a comprehensive evaluation and consultation with a mental health specialist.
- Patients at low risk of suicide may be discharged to a safe and supportive environment where access to firearms or risk of overdose or poisoning is minimized.
- Discharged patients should receive education and safety planning in the ED and be referred for early mental health follow-up.

FOUNDATIONS

Background and Importance

Emergency clinicians care for many patients with suicidal ideation and self-harm behaviors. Two facts are especially important to remember in the care of suicidal patients. First, many suicide attempts occur during an acute crisis, such as a personal loss or the exacerbation of an underlying psychiatric disorder. This acute crisis is usually time-limited and is often resolvable or treatable. Second, suicidal patients are usually ambivalent about dying and grateful for help. An empathetic, patient-centered, and evidence-based approach by emergency care providers offers the opportunity to save lives.

Medical literature contains numerous terms to describe different types and degrees of suicidal thoughts and behaviors. *Suicidal behavior* refers to any observable mental state or outward behavior related to ending one's life. *Suicidal ideation* refers to thoughts of killing oneself. *Suicidal intent* refers to the desire to proceed with suicide. A *suicidal plan* refers to a conceived specific method in which a person would attempt suicide, such as by firearm, hanging, poisoning/overdose, or cutting oneself. *Lethal means* refers to someone having accessibility to a method in which to carry out a suicidal plan, for example, having physical possession of a firearm.

A *suicide attempt* is a self-directed act with the intent to die. *Non-suicidal self-injury* (NSSI) is an intentional act of self-harm without the intent to die as a result of the behavior. Terms to avoid because of implicit value judgement of a derogatory nature include *committed* or *successful* suicide, *suicidal gesture, manipulative act,* and *suicide threat.*[1]

Epidemiology

Suicide was the tenth leading cause of death in the United States in 2017.[2] It is the second leading cause of death for people 10 to 34 years of age, the fourth leading cause among people 35 to 54 years of age, and the eighth leading cause among people 55 to 64 years of age.[3] There were more than one million suicide attempts and 47,000 suicide deaths in the United States in 2017, and rates continue to rise.[3,4] It is estimated that in 2017 there were almost 500,000 visits to emergency departments (EDs) nationally for intentional nonfatal injuries.[5,6]

Contrary to popular belief, the majority of individuals (54%) in the United States who die by suicide do not have a known mental illness at the time of death; these individuals are much more likely to be male (84%) and to die by firearm (55%).[4] Of the individuals who die with known mental health conditions, the majority are still male (69%) and more likely to die by firearm (41%) or suffocation (31%).[4] Although women make up a higher proportion of suicide attempts, men are more likely to die by suicide due to use of more lethal methods.[4]

The ED plays a critical role in acute stabilization and initiation of appropriate preventative efforts to reduce subsequent suicide mortality.[7,8] It is estimated that 1 in 5 suicide fatalities are seen in an ED in the month prior to their death, which suggests 9,000 suicide deaths each year could be reduced through improved ED suicide prevention efforts.[9] An empathic, patient-centered, and evidence-based approach offers the opportunity to save lives.

Risk Factors

Precipitating Factors

Many precipitating factors are associated with suicide attempts among individuals with and without mental illnesses. The most common precipitants to suicide are "dynamic" factors such as interpersonal relationship stressors (42%), recent crises (29%), problematic substance use (28%), physical health problems (22%), financial circumstances, (16%), criminal or legal issues (9%), and homelessness (4%).[4] The most important risk factor for suicide is a previous suicide attempt.

At Risk Populations

In addition, there are also several "static" factors associated with increased risk of suicide, including age, ethnicity/race, geography, employment, and other population characteristics.

In a national survey of high school students in the United States, in the previous year 17% had serious thoughts of suicide, 13% made a suicide plan, and 8% made a suicide attempt.[10] Unfortunately, only half of the youths with suicide-related behavior sought mental health care or support.[10] Similar to adults, girls are more likely to attempt suicide, whereas boys are more likely to die by suicide; however, the rates for girls has been climbing.[4] History of suicide attempt and of non-suicidal self-injury are particularly strong risk factors in this population.[10]

Suicide rates are also particularly high in the geriatric population, especially older white men, who account for over 80% of suicide deaths among elders.[11] Older adults are more likely to die from suicide attempts because of the use of more lethal methods, more advanced planning, and a lower likelihood of asking for help or of having warnings recognized by others. Depression is the strongest risk factor for suicide among elders, with a prevalence of up to 80% among older suicide decedents.[11] Additional important risk factors in elders include cognitive dysfunction, decreased functional ability, bereavement or other stressful life events, social isolation, and loneliness.[11]

Suicide rates are highest across the life span among non-Hispanic American Indian/Alaska Native and non-Hispanic White populations. Other Americans disproportionately impacted by suicide include veterans and other military personnel. Among military personnel, suicide risk is increased in males and those with psychiatric history, alcohol abuse, or previous deployment.[12]

Certain occupations also convey higher suicide risk, including the health professions and physicians. Worldwide, physicians have a suicide rate almost twice that of the general population and the highest suicide rate of any profession, with the highest rates in the United States.[13] Female physicians have a suicide rate 250% to 400% higher than females in other professions and, unlike the general population, female physicians may be at higher risk for suicide than male physicians.[13] Physicians may also not seek help for their mental health for reasons that may include busy professional schedules, the de-emphasis of professional support or avoiding risk of disclosure.

Gender and sexual minorities, particularly youth, bear a large burden as well, and experience increased suicidal ideation and at-risk behaviors compared to their non–sexual minority peers.[14]

Suicide rates vary geographically, with higher rates in rural communities and in areas with higher levels of firearm ownership.[15] The rate of suicide with firearms is almost twice as high among rural compared to urban residents.[15] Important risk factors for suicide in rural areas include social isolation, lack of access to health care, socioeconomic factors such as unemployment and poverty, and sociocultural factors like increased mental illness stigma that prevent help-seeking.[15] In addition, the risk of death by suicide in rural settings is compounded by a decreased likelihood of rapid life-saving intervention as well as reduced timely access to emergency medical services and trauma centers.[15]

Mental Illness

The presence of a mood disorder, especially major depressive disorder, is a strong independent risk factor for suicide. The most common mental disorders presenting to the ED with suicidal ideation are adjustment disorders, mood disorders, and personality disorders.[16] However, many other psychiatric disorders are associated with increased rates of suicide. Overall, the risk of suicide in patients with mental illness increases with the presence of prior attempts, recent psychiatric hospitalization, male gender, more severe symptoms, comorbid psychiatric disorders, use of alcohol or drugs, and family history of suicide. In

patients hospitalized for psychiatric disorders, the risk for suicide is greatest in the first month after discharge, and especially in the first week.[16]

Alcohol and Substance Abuse Disorders

Both chronic and acute alcohol abuse are associated with suicide.[17,18] Individuals with alcohol use disorder who die from suicide usually have multiple risk factors, including major depression, unemployment, medical illness, and interpersonal loss.[17] Acute alcohol use is associated with increased risk of suicide in both those with and without chronic alcohol abuse, and this risk persists for 24 to 48 hours, particularly after heavy drinking.[18] This effect is largest among younger adults and is more often associated with violent means of suicide (e.g., firearms or hanging).[18] Substance abuse is associated with increased frequency and lethality in suicide attempts, and illicit substances are often detected at the time of suicide.

Chronic Illness

Many chronic medical illnesses are associated with increased risk of suicide, particularly those that affect the central nervous system such as epilepsy,[19] or those with chronic pain or impairment in activities of daily living.[20] Infection with human immunodeficiency virus (HIV) or presence of the acquired immunodeficiency syndrome (AIDS) remains associated with increased risk of suicide, but specific risk factors may vary based on nationality, socioeconomic status, age, and comorbidity with mental illness.[21]

Pathophysiology

The etiology of a suicide attempt is a complex mix of social, genetic, and psychological factors, what psychiatrists would refer to as a "bio-psycho-social" model.[22] Several genetic and neurobiological factors have been proposed as contributors to suicide risk, including abnormalities in the serotonin transport system, the stress response systems (hypothalamic–pituitary–adrenal (HPA) axis and polyamine system), neuroinflammation, and lipid metabolism.[22] Psychological factors associated with the highest suicide risk are hopelessness and impulsivity.[23]

The social contributions to risk of suicide have perhaps the most immediate, temporal relationship with suicide attempts. Many of the most prevalent precipitating factors associated with suicide occur in the social domain, namely relationship problems, recent crises, financial problems, criminal or legal problems, and homelessness.[4] There is a growing body of evidence suggesting that adverse childhood experiences are strong risk factors for future suicide that affect individuals on biological, psychological, and social levels.[22,24,25]

Methods of Suicide

Firearms account for half of all deaths from suicide for patients with and without mental illness,[4] as this is the most lethal method with little to no opportunity for the individual to experience regret or ask for help. There is a well-established relationship between the presence of a firearm in the home and higher rates of suicide.[26,27]

The next most lethal method is hanging or suffocation (25%), followed by poisoning or overdose (16%).[4] Overdose and poisoning attempts are relatively common, and account for over two-thirds of ED visits for suicide attempt or self-harm.[28] Intentional overdose is particularly common among adolescents; 63% of all overdoses for patients ages 13 to 19 years were intentional.[28] These attempts are less frequently lethal due to delayed lethality from absorption, ability for the individual to express regret and ask for help, and opportunities for emergent treatment once help is obtained. Death by suicide from overdose is most commonly due to opioids, although it is often difficult in public health records to distinguish death by suicide from deaths due to unintentional overdose, abuse, or misuse.[29] Children and adolescents use whatever is readily available, such as commonly used over-the-counter medications like acetaminophen and ibuprofen, which can be quite lethal or lead to severe complications.[30]

CLINICAL FEATURES

Initial Recognition and Screening

Due to stigma and fear of repercussions, patients who present to the ED following a traumatic event may not disclose the cause of their injury was a suicide attempt. The potential for suicide should be considered in patients who present with unintentional overdose or accidental gunshot wounds, lacerated wrists, automobile crashes, or falls from heights. Patients who are not overtly suicidal but who exhibit one or more of these high-risk presentations require assessment in an empathic but direct manner using a "graduated" approach. Rapport can first be established during a general medical and psychiatric history, with an evaluation of the patient's home, work, and social situation, followed by specific questions about recent psychosocial stressors, signs and symptoms of depression, and the presence of suicidal thoughts. Such questioning does not cause a person to consider suicide who has not already been considering it. This approach can be described as *indicated screening* of those with acute risk factors.[31]

A more systematic screening approach would be *selective screening* of all patients in high-risk groups, such as those with chronic risk factors for suicide including prior suicide attempts or mental illness.[32] *Universal screening* for suicidal risk involves questioning all patients about suicidal thoughts or behaviors.[32] Universal screening is supported by evidence suggesting that approximately 10% of all ED patients have recent suicidal ideation or behaviors, and 40% of suicide victims have visited an ED within the prior year.[33] For ideal functioning, any screening program can be integrated into available electronic medical records and work flow to optimize efficiency, increase provider uptake, and maximize impact.[34,35]

History and Physical Examination

The history includes details about the patient's suicidal thoughts (including onset and frequency), plans (including method, intent to act, and access to lethal means), and behaviors (including prior or recent attempts, as well as aborted or interrupted attempts). Other important points include prior medical and psychiatric conditions, prior outpatient or inpatient psychiatric care, current medications, and current drug or alcohol use (including recent use). The history also assesses for symptoms suggestive of concomitant medical illness. Intoxication does not preclude taking an initial history, but it is important to repeat interviews when patients are sober to ensure accuracy.

The physical examination assesses for evidence of drug ingestion, trauma, or associated medical illness, as well as evidence of self-harm behavior such as cutting. Roughly 10% of individuals presenting to the ED for suicidal ideation have an associated injury.[6] An evaluation of the patient's cognitive status, vital signs, pupils, skin, and nervous system are helpful in detecting organic conditions, particularly toxidromes associated with common ingestions (see Chapter 135).

The clinician should identify medical conditions requiring immediate treatment in the ED or acute or chronic conditions that may require less urgent but timely intervention, and note incidental findings requiring further outpatient management or conditions that may affect psychiatric care.

DIFFERENTIAL DIAGNOSES

Normal Colloquialisms and Expressions of Suffering

People in nonclinical settings may use colloquialisms such as "I could die!" to express exasperation or suffering that may be misinterpreted in clinical settings.[36] Individuals who have suffered with chronic illnesses or pain may vocalize statements akin to a "wish to hasten death," which could have many meanings aside from an intent to end one's life.[4] Such statements may serve to communicate feelings, thoughts, or wishes about suffering, relief, help, and concerns about the illness or dying process. These thoughts and statements typically have a theme of suffering and loss of control.[4] It is important to carefully ascertain the presence of true suicidal ideations in these circumstances.

Malingering

Malingering is not a psychiatric illness; it is the intentional fabrication of symptoms, such as that of a mental illness, or even a claim, exaggeration, or feigning of suicidality for the purpose of obtaining an external gain.[37] There are no indicated treatments for malingering and no role for hospitalization. Studies have suggested that up to 10% of patients admitted to psychiatric hospitals have fabricated or exaggerated suicidal ideation to gain hospital admission. Suicidal ideation is the most frequently malingered psychiatric symptom, likely because of its subjective nature and the implicit additional leverage associated with the risk of mortality if unaddressed.

Non-Suicidal Self-Injury

The term *non-suicidal self-injury* (NSSI) refers to "the direct, deliberate destruction of one's own body tissue in the absence of intent to die," such as cutting or burning oneself.[38] There is conflicting evidence regarding whether NSSI and suicidal behavior are diagnostically distinct or exist on a spectrum of self-harm behavior. There is, however, sufficient evidence to suggest that NSSI is a risk factor for future suicide attempts.[38] There are cases where NSSI may have potentially lethal consequences, even if the intent was not suicide, so it is critical to consider both lethality and intent when performing a safety assessment.

Unintentional Injury or Ingestion

Over three-quarters of all overdoses are classified as unintentional, including most cases in children ages 5 years and younger.[28] In almost a quarter of single-substance overdoses that involved pharmaceutical substances, the reason for exposure was intentional, compared to only 4% when the exposure involved a nonpharmaceutical substance. The ingestion of multiple drugs is more reflective of an intentional overdose, and generally leads to more serious and potentially lethal complications.[28]

Substance Intoxication, Abuse, or Misuse

Patients may make suicidal statements while intoxicated or when presenting with an injury that may be a result of a suicide attempt. Patients may also make suicidal statements or inflict self-harm while intoxicated, then deny suicidal ideation later. An electronic medical record study in the United Kingdom showed that patients who presented as an emergency due to any alcohol-related cause had a three-times higher risk of future suicide; and when they were admitted to the hospital, the risk was 22-fold higher in women and 5-fold higher in men. When the diagnosis was "toxic effects of alcohol or poisoning through alcohol," the risk was 30-fold higher for women and 18-fold higher for men, a risk even higher than for those with a previous mental health disorder.[39]

Suicide attempts using illicit drugs are relatively uncommon. Overdose with an illicit drug or a prescription pain medication may be lethal and intentional, but not with death as a desired outcome.

Opioids are the most frequent cause of fatal overdoses today, yet many of these are likely not suicides, but rather abuse, misuse, or the development of tolerance leading to high-dose use and fatal overdoses.[28]

Suicidal Obsessions or Preoccupations

Suicidal ideation must be differentiated from having "thoughts of suicide" or "thinking of hurting oneself," without the desire, intent, or plan to pursue an act of ending one's life. Such thoughts may represent obsessions, such as occur in obsessive-compulsive disorder (OCD), or the ruminations or preservative thinking that occurs in autism spectrum disorder (ASD).[40,41] It is important to note that individuals with OCD and ASD can experience frank suicidal ideation as well. To make the differentiation, it is helpful to clarify whether the patient prefers death over life, or harbors a desire, intent, or plan to end his or her life.

DIAGNOSTIC TESTING

Emergency clinicians are often asked to provide "medical clearance" for patients with psychiatric emergencies. However, this term substantially undervalues the importance of a focused medical assessment of patients who may have active acute or chronic conditions, to determine stability and appropriateness for treatment in a psychiatric setting.[42] Obtaining an adequate patient history and physical examination is essential in the focused medical assessment.

Mandatory nontargeted diagnostic testing of all suicidal patients is not necessary and has not demonstrated any clinical benefit, particularly in younger patients.[42,43] Less than 1% of suicidal patients have their disposition changed through use of testing believed to be unnecessary by the emergency clinician.[43] Targeted diagnostic testing should be based on clinical indications, including the new onset of psychiatric symptoms in those with no known past psychiatric history.[42,43] There is little evidence to show that screening urine drug testing alters management or disposition of the psychiatric patient in the ED.[42,43] However comorbid substance use is an important factor in subsequent treatment, and receiving psychiatric facilities may request this study, as it is a time-sensitive study and may affect the direction of further mental health treatment.[42,43] Local practices vary and some mental health facilities may require routine baseline testing. EDs and local receiving psychiatric facilities should create guidelines to clarify minimal testing required for medical clearance.

MANAGEMENT

Overview

Care of potentially suicidal patients requires an empathetic and patient-centered approach. Patients feel more comfortable discussing personal issues when health care personnel are friendly, nonjudgmental, and supportive.[44] Providers can improve the ED experience by explaining to patients what to expect from the evaluation, stating the estimated length of wait for evaluation and disposition, and focusing initially on basic comforts.[44] The use of a patient-centered approach can also enhance patient satisfaction and the likelihood of outpatient follow-up.[44] Attitudes towards suicide prevention are highly correlated with effective suicide prevention skills of emergency medical service providers.[44,45,46] Personal beliefs or inadequate training of clinical providers, or lack of time or personnel to provide appropriate psychiatric evaluation, can result in inadequate patient assessment and adversely impact outcomes.

The priority in management is immediate medical stabilization and treatment of injuries, poisonings, or overdose. Following stabilization, a focused medical assessment should be performed to identify and treat associated medical conditions that may underlie a patient's altered mental status or suicidal behavior. Hospitalization for significant injury, poisoning, or other acute medical problems is imperative so that medical problems can be treated as patients remain under constant observation for suicide risk and later receive appropriate psychiatric evaluation.

Suicide Precautions

Protocols for managing potentially suicidal individuals focus on patient safety and the prevention of self-harm. While the practice of constant physical observation by ED personnel of all patients exhibiting suicidal behavior may be considered essential, alternative means of monitoring through careful patient selection and use of technology may be similarly effective.[44,47,48] The effectiveness of electronic bracelets and other forms of virtual monitoring are currently being evaluated.[48]

As part of standard procedure, patients being evaluated for suicidal behavior are searched during the initial assessment for possible weapons, medications, and other possessions that might be used to inflict injury (e.g., belts, neckties, and long shoelaces),[44] and are evaluated in an area cleared of all potentially harmful objects, including medications, instruments, and glass objects.[44,47] Use of restraints is rarely necessary. Mechanical and chemical restraint use is most commonly employed for patients who are agitated or physically aggressive, but such measures are a last resort because they can be traumatic, impair rapport, exacerbate an underlying psychiatric condition, or impair early psychiatric evaluation.[44]

Pharmacologic Treatment

Prescription psychiatric medications are commonly used to treat depression and other underlying psychiatric disorders, but they are generally not effective for acute suicidality and may take weeks to become effective.[49]

Children, adolescents, and young adults may have increased suicidal thoughts or attempts soon after the initiation of antidepressant medications.[50] Although current studies do not support a direct causation between antidepressant medication and suicidality in youth, clinicians should recognize the time period around initiation of antidepressant therapy as one requiring heightened scrutiny for suicidal thoughts or behaviors.[51]

There are no generally accepted or evidence-based protocols for drug treatment of suicidal ideation in the ED. However, ketamine and its enantiomer, esketamine, have demonstrated promise as a potential acute treatment for suicidal ideations.[52-56] Ketamine at sub-anesthetic doses has been used in several studies for treatment-resistant depression, and such studies show that ketamine encompasses a specific and rapid suppression of suicidal ideation.[52,53,54] Meta-analyses have revealed single-dose intravenous (IV) infusion of ketamine to be associated with reduction of suicidality within as little as 40 minutes and lasting as long as 3 days to 2 weeks.[52-54] The intranasal form of esketamine was approved by the United States Food and Drug Administration for treatment-resistant depression in 2019, but patients must be monitored by a health care provider in a doctor's office, clinic, or hospital for at least 2 hours following administration due to risk of sedation and dissociation.[55]

Ketamine's application is not straightforward, as repetitive doses are required due to the short duration of action.[52-54] Additionally, use may be hindered by the drug's potential for abuse, dependence, and dissociative effects.[55] Despite increasing evidence showing the suicide-mitigating effect of ketamine, the underlying neurobiology is poorly understood, and a preliminary study suggests that the antidepressant effects of ketamine may actually be due to its action at opioid receptors.[56] We do not recommend the routine use of ketamine for this purpose in the ED in the absence of psychiatric consultation.

Risk Assessment

Analogous to the evaluation of chest pain and other physical complaints, the emergency clinician's role in managing potentially suicidal patients lies in assessing suicide risk, providing brief interventions, and facilitating consultation with specialists as indicated.[57]

Suicide risk assessment should be performed when the patient is sober, although intoxicated patients who endorse suicidal thoughts may still be at risk, even if they disavow these feelings when sober.[58] Risk assessment includes collateral information from a family member or friend who can provide additional background information and discuss whether there are sufficient resources available to support a safe discharge if considered.[59] Such contacts are most appropriately made with the consent of the patient, if possible, but can occur without consent in cases when disclosure of protected health information is required to prevent or mitigate an imminent, serious safety threat to an individual or the public.[59]

Assessing hopelessness, desperation, and a wish or intent to die are also important predictors of future suicide.[60-62] Assessment of risk of the lethality of a plan for death by suicide is paramount even though patients with strong suicidal ideations without a plan may still remain at high risk.[60] Patients who initially hide or conceal their suicide attempt may also be at higher risk of death.[60-63]

A practical, stepwise approach to suicide risk assessment (see Fig. 101.1) consists of both brief and comprehensive steps. *Brief risk assessment* typically involves a short set of questions to assess suicide risk and help determine the most appropriate actionable steps.[64,65] An example is the short version of the Columbia-Suicide Severity Rating Scale (C-SSRS; see Fig 101.2), which is available for free in English and Spanish with suggested cut-points for referral and consultation.[66] The C-SSRS can be modified for use by clinicians in a variety of settings, including the ED. It is a quick 6-item questionnaire that helps triage patients as acutely low, medium, or high risk for suicide and allows for individual EDs, hospitals, or hospital systems to use the

tool appropriately within their system depending on what resources are available.

A *comprehensive* or *formal risk assessment* involves more-detailed questions about a patient's various suicide risk and protective factors and is most often performed by a mental health consultant.[65] In cases where psychiatric consultation is not possible, the clinician can complete a comprehensive suicide risk assessment assisted by a validated tool such as the Suicide Assessment Five-step Evaluation and Triage (SAFE-T; see Fig. 101.3) tool. The SAFE-T is available as a pocket card or smartphone application. It guides one in assessing a patient's risk, the presence of protective factors and the specifics of suicidal thoughts or plans, and then combines these factors to estimate a level of suicide risk.[67]

The Ask Suicide-Screening Questions (ASQ) Toolkit is a free combined brief and comprehensive risk assessment developed by the National Institute for Mental Health (NIMH) and the Substance Abuse and Mental Health Services Association (SAMHSA) specifically for youth at risk for suicide.[32,68]

Ultimately, suicide risk assessment remains a matter of clinical judgment with tools such as the C-SSRS and SAFE-T to inform, reinforce, and justify the provider's decision making.[65]

Documentation

Documentation of the evaluation of potentially suicidal patients is important because of the variable nature of suicide risk, low compliance rates of follow-up with outpatient care, and the difficulty of predicting imminent risk. It is especially important when patients are either hospitalized involuntarily or discharged. If a patient requires involuntary hospitalization, providers should document why the patient is a danger to self or others. If the patient is discharged, appropriate documentation includes the decision making as to why the patient was considered to be at low risk of imminent self-harm, referencing access to potentially lethal methods of suicide, information from collateral sources, and the follow-up plan.[69] Use of standardized electronic health record templates may prove useful in ensuring sufficient system-wide documentation of suicide assessment and decision making.[70]

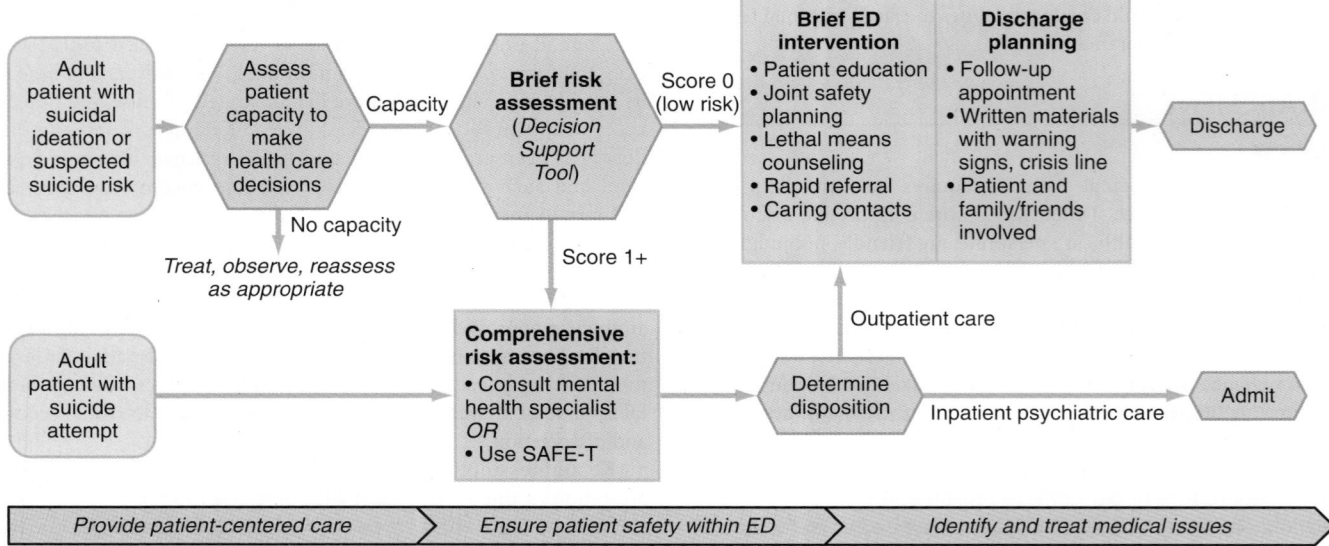

Fig. 101.1 Framework for using the decision support tool and emergency department (ED)-based suicide prevention interventions. (Adapted from: Capoccia L, Labre M. *Caring for Adult Patients With Suicide Risk: A Consensus-Based Guide for Emergency Departments*. Waltham, MA: Education Development Center, Inc., Suicide Resource Prevention Center; 2015.)

Columbia-suicide severity rating scale
*screen with triage points for **emergency department***

Ask questions that are bolded and <u>underlined</u>.	Past month	
Ask questions 1 and 2	YES	NO
1) ***Have you wished you were dead or wished you could go to sleep and not wake up?***		
2) ***Have you actually had any thoughts of killing yourself?***		
If YES to 2, ask questions 3, 4, 5, and 6. If NO to 2, go directly to question 6.		
3) ***Have you been thinking about how you might do this?*** E.g. *"I thought about taking an overdose but I never made a specific plan as to when where or how I would actually do it….and I would never go through with it."*		
4) ***Have you had these thoughts and had some intention of acting on them?*** As opposed to *"I have the thoughts but I definitely will not do anything about them."*		
5) ***Have you started to work out or worked out the details of how to kill yourself?*** ***Do you intend to carry out this plan?***		
6) ***Have you ever done anything, started to do anything, or prepared to do anything*** ***to end your life?*** Examples: Collected pills, obtained a gun, gave away valuables, wrote a will or suicide note, took out pills but didn't swallow any, held a gun but changed your mind or it was grabbed from your hand, went to the roof but didn't jump; or actually took pills, tried to shoot yourself, cut yourself, tried to hang yourself, etc.	**Lifetime**	
If YES, ask: *Was this within the past three months?*	**Past 3 months**	

Item 1 behavioral health referral at discharge
Item 2 behavioral health referral at discharge
Item 3 behavioral health consult (psychiatric nurse/social worker) and consider patient safety precautions
Item 4 immediate notification of physician and/or behavioral health and patient safety precautions
Item 5 immediate notification of physician and/or behavioral health and patient safety precautions
Item 6 over 3 months ago: Behavioral health consult (psychiatric nurse/social worker) and consider patient safety precautions
Item 6 3 months ago or less: Immediate notification of physician and/or behavioral health and patient safety precautions

Fig. 101.2 Columbia-Suicide Severity Rating Scale Triage and Risk Identification Tool from The Columbia Lighthouse Project. (From: Posner K, et al. The Columbia-Suicide Severity Rating Scale: initial validity and internal consistency findings from three multisite studies with adolescents and adults. *Am J Psychiatry.* 2011 Dec;168(12):1266-1277. PMID: 22193671. Available at https://cssrs.columbia.edu/the-columbia-scale-c-ssrs/risk-identification/.)

DISPOSITION

Determining the most appropriate disposition for the potentially suicidal patient involves integrating information about the precipitating crisis and event, the patient's current emotional state and prior mental health history, and the presence or absence of a safe and supportive environment. Addressing the crisis that precipitated a suicide attempt can substantially diminish the risk of suicide. Emergency psychiatric evaluation and psychiatric hospitalization are often strongly considered to ensure this crisis can be resolved.

Psychiatric Hospitalization

Voluntary hospitalization is preferable to involuntary hospitalization.[71] The efficacy of hospitalization as a long-term preventive measure is controversial and is not proved to prevent future suicide.[72-74] Still, hospitalization remains a primary intervention when patients are

deemed acutely suicidal as a means to provide a safe environment for close monitoring where medical or somatic therapies can be started, positive coping skills can be taught and reinforced, and social supports can be mobilized.[75] Depending upon outpatient resource availability, other options may include partial hospitalization programs, intensive outpatient programs, and assertive community treatment.

Statutes regulating involuntary hospitalization, otherwise known as civil commitment, differ between states and regions. Most states have emergency involuntary commitment provisions that typically require that a patient both have a mental illness and pose a threat to self or others.[76] The length of emergency commitments varies by state, from 72 hours to 15 days.[76-79] In some states, patients who agree to hospitalization may still need involuntary commitment documentation completed for transport to a receiving psychiatric facility; this provides the legal basis for holding patients if they change their mind during transportation.

1. Identify risk factors

- **Suicidal behavior**: prior suicide attempts or self-injurious behavior
- **Current/past psychiatric disorders**: especially mood disorders, psychotic disorders, alcohol/substance abuse, ADHD, TBI, PTSD, Cluster B personality disorders, conduct disorders (antisocial behavior, aggression, impulsivity)
- **Key symptoms**: anhedonia, impulsivity, hopelessness, anxiety/panic, insomnia, command hallucinations
- **Family history**: of suicide, attempts, or Axis 1 psychiatric disorders requiring hospitalization
- **Precipitants/Stressors/Interpersonal**: triggering events leading to humiliation, shame or despair (e.g., loss of relationship, financial or health status—real or anticipated); ongoing medical illness (esp. CNS disorders, pain); intoxication; family turmoil/chaos; history of physical or sexual abuse; social isolation
- **Change in treatment**: discharge from psychiatric hospital, provider or treatment change
- **Access to firearms**

2. Identify protective factors

- **Internal**: ability to cope with stress, religious beliefs, frustration tolerance
- **External**: responsibility to children/pets, positive therapeutic relationships, social supports

3. Conduct suicide inquiry

- **Ideation**: frequency, intensity, duration–in last 48 hours, past month, and worst ever
- **Plan**: timing, location, lethality, availability, preparatory acts
- **Behaviors**: past attempts, aborted attempts, rehearsals (tying noose, loading gun), vs. non-suicidal self-injurious actions
- **Intent**: extent to which the patient (1) expects to carry out the plan and (2) believes the plan/act to be lethal vs. self-injurious
- **Explore** ambivalence: reasons to die vs. reasons to live

4. Determine risk level & intervention

- **Assessment** of risk level is based on clinical judgment, after completing steps 1–3

Low risk	Moderate risk	High risk
• Denial of suicidal thoughts, plan, intent • No or mild sadness or anger; no psychosis • No or 1 recent attempt with low lethality • No or limited substance use • Good support, accepting of help, hopeful for future	• Suicidal ideation, plan, intent, or attempt • Moderate depression, anger, hopelessness • Frequent ideation or threats; low lethality • Substance abuse • Moderate support, unwilling to accept help • Access to lethal means	• Frequent, intense, enduring ideation • Specific plans • High intent (e.g., attempt with high lethality) • Impaired self-control, severe dysphoria, hopelessness, worthlessness • Poor corroborative history • Many risk factors, refusing help

5. Document

- Risk level and rationale; treatment plan to address/reduce current risk (e.g., setting, medication, psychotherapy, ECT, contact with significant others, consultation); firearm instructions, if relevant; follow-up plan
- For youths, treatment plan should include roles for parent/guardian

Fig. 101.3 Suicide assessment five-step evaluation and triage. (Modified from: Davidson CL, Olson-Madden JH, Betz ME, et al. Emergency department identification, assessment, and management of the suicidal patient. In: Koslow SH, Ruiz P, Nemeroff CB, eds. *A Concise Guide to Understanding Suicide*. Cambridge, UK: Cambridge University Press; 2014: 244–255; Suicide Assessment Five-Step Evaluation and Triage [SAFE-T]. Substance Abuse and Mental Health Services Administration. Available at http://store.samhsa.gov/product/Suicide-Assessment-Five-Step-Evaluation-and-Triage-SAFE-T-/SMA09-4432; and Substance Abuse and Mental Health Services Administration [SAMHSA]. Suicide safe: the suicide prevention app for health care providers, free from SAMHSA. Available at http://store.samhsa.gov/apps/suicidesafe/.)

Patients may lack capacity to refuse hospitalization but maintain the capacity to accept or refuse other treatments, such as management of medical conditions and administration of medications for pain or agitation.[80]

Discharge

Some patients who report suicidal thoughts can be safely managed as outpatients if the risk of subsequent suicide is judged to be acceptably low. Although the emergency clinician can make this determination in many cases, evaluation by a mental health professional can be useful if the safety of outpatient management is in doubt. The patient can be discharged to a stable and supportive home environment with a willing friend or family member, and without access to guns or lethal medications. The discharge planning process ideally includes (1) brief patient education, (2) joint safety planning, (3) lethal means restriction counseling, (4) referral for outpatient care, and (5) provision of "caring contacts."[77,81-83]

Brief Patient Education

Brief patient education for suicide prevention includes the use of verbal and written information and "teach back" techniques whereby the patient explains the information back to the provider.[81] Information can include a personalized list of risk and protective factors, home care and follow-up instructions, and warning signs that would trigger a call for help. The educational process engages the patient in an empathetic and respectful manner and can, with patient consent, include family members or close friends.[81] Educational materials are available from a number of national organizations.

Joint Safety Planning

In joint safety planning, a provider works with a patient to develop a plan regarding what to do if symptoms worsen.[77,81] The plan should be in the patient's own words and easy to understand, and it includes warning signs, a list of coping strategies, and resources such as hotlines or contact information for trusted family or friends (specify "adults" in the case of suicidal children or adolescents). The National Suicide Prevention Hotline (1-800-273-TALK [8255]) and/or text line (741-741) is a helpful resource for all discharged patients; in late 2019 the Federal Communications Commission (FCC) approved using 988 as a three-digit suicide prevention hotline number.[84] Importantly, safety planning is not the same as a "contract for safety" or "no suicide contract." Such "contracts" not only lack evidence of effectiveness but may deter patients from being truthful in disclosing future episodes of suicidality.[83] These contracts may create a false sense of security regarding safety and should not be used.

Lethal Means Restriction Counseling

Counseling about lethal means restriction—one of only two suicide prevention approaches with a strong empirical foundation—is another valuable resource.[84-85] Many suicidal crises are acute and short-lived and are impulsive (sometimes with only minutes or seconds between the decision to act and the attempt). The method chosen may be the one most readily available, and the lethality of the chosen method affects the likelihood of mortality. Numerous studies have shown a consistent association between firearm access and death by suicide, even after controlling for other risk factors, with a strong correlation amongst males.[26,86-87] Safe gun-storage practices—namely keeping firearms locked, unloaded, and separate from ammunition—can mitigate the risk of suicide. At a population level, firearms regulations such as waiting periods and training requirements are associated with reduced rates of firearm-related suicide.[87,88]

ED counseling about lethal means safety can affect patient behavior, and lethal means counseling for suicidal patients is supported by multiple physician organizations and listed as a best practice for suicide prevention.[89] Clinicians should counsel potentially suicidal patients and their families to remove guns temporarily from the home for storage off-site in an appropriate location, or to use gun locks or cabinets to which the patient has no access.[90]

Referral for Outpatient Care

Suicide risk remains high shortly after discharge from the ED, so it is important to arrange short-term outpatient care, ideally within 72 hours of discharge.[89] Evidence-based outpatient treatment can reduce future suicide risk, and emergency clinicians play a key role in linking patients to care.[89] A significant number of discharged ED patients do not keep their follow-up appointments, but compliance with follow-up may be increased by making a specific appointment for patients. Employing the support of family or friends helps ensure that the patient keeps the follow-up appointment. In addition, it may be helpful to provide physician contact information or to provide a list of community mental health resources. With the patient's consent, the physician can send visit information to the patient's primary care provider or outpatient referral provider to enhance continuity of care.

Caring Contacts

Other promising interventions for discharged patients include caring contacts, or brief communications from the ED after discharge.[91,92] These empirically supported interventions take a variety of forms, including text messages, emails, phone calls, and postcards, and they may be unidirectional or bidirectional. An automated system, supported by the electronic health record, can facilitate the process, or the contacts can be made by a clinical or nonclinical ED staff member. Such continued contacts have been shown to improve follow-up to outpatient appointments and lower suicide risk.[92]

ADDITIONAL ETHICAL CONSIDERATIONS

Do-Not-Resuscitate Orders

The presence of a do-not-resuscitate (DNR) order in a patient with a suicide attempt raises ethical and legal dilemmas.[93] Policies vary among states, and there are unfortunately no definitive guidelines for emergency care providers.[81] When possible, consultation with an ethics consultant or committee or legal representation from the hospital can be helpful, but in emergent time-sensitive conditions it is preferred to err on the side of resuscitation.

The principle of beneficence dictates that treatment be pursued when a suicidal patient may not be capable of making decisions about his or her own welfare. Because DNR orders and palliative care generally apply to progressive terminal illnesses and do not exclude or limit all other care, it is necessary to treat self-inflicted conditions even in the presence of a DNR order.[89] Treatment does not have to be indefinite and can be discontinued later following appropriate consultation with ethics and legal experts. Institutions have a responsibility to examine these issues proactively and pursue policies that address how to respond to patients with a DNR order who attempt suicide.[93] Such policies need to address specific state laws regarding prehospital DNR orders.

Physician-Assisted Dying

As of 2018, five states and the District of Columbia have passed legislation legalizing assisted dying, with other jurisdictions considering such legislation.[94] Physician-assisted dying refers to patients who voluntarily and orally ingest medications that are prescribed to them only after they pass a series of safeguards. Such safeguards typically include (1) having a prognosis of fewer than 6 months, confirmed by two physicians: (2), retaining medical decision-making capacity: and (3) making multiple requests separated by time to allow adequate reflection and reconsideration. Although EMS and ED involvement may be rare (approximately 1% of cases in Oregon), when they do occur, they require rapid decision making, often with limited information and challenging emotions.[42] As more states allow physician-assisted dying, it is expected that more such cases will come to clinical attention in the ED. It is appropriate to involve palliative care and ethics consultations in such cases with supporting institutional protocols in place that achieve consensus on recommendations for action.[94] The legal authorization of physician-assisted dying intent draws a sharp distinction in these cases from an impulsive suicide attempt, and ED providers must be prepared to adapt to new state laws and their application in medicine.

The references for this chapter can be found online at ExpertConsult. com.

102

Arthritis

Korin Hudson, Miguel Agrait-Gonzalez

GENERAL APPROACH TO ARTHRITIS

Foundations

Background

Arthritis and its related conditions were among the earliest diseases described. Ancient cultures including the Romans, Greeks, and Egyptians all referenced conditions such as gout and rheumatoid arthritis (RA), while Hippocrates and others contributed to the further description and classification. In modern times, arthritis has become a common cause of disability in the United States and around the world. More than 20% of adults in the United States carry the diagnosis of arthritis, leading to millions of prescriptions, procedures, and profound activity limitations.[1] Patients with arthritis may present to the emergency department (ED) for a variety of reasons. First among these is pain related to their primary condition; however, complications related to systemic illness are also common in patients with autoimmune or inflammatory conditions. Furthermore, the medications and treatments used to manage these conditions may themselves have side effects which lead patients to seek emergency care.

Pathophysiology

Arthritis typically occurs in synovial or diarthrotic (moving) joints. These joints are made up of two ends of subchondral bone, each covered with articular cartilage and surrounded by a fibrous capsule (Fig. 102.1). This capsule is supported by ligaments, tendons, and muscle. The capsule is lined with a thin synovial membrane and contains synovial fluid, a viscous, lubricating substance which allows near frictionless movement of the joint. The bones of the joint are lined by a specific form of hyaline cartilage known as articular cartilage, which allows load bearing and contributes to the friction-free movement of the joint when combined with synovial fluid. Numerous conditions and specific processes will lead to degradation of these tissues and ultimately to degeneration and arthritis.

Clinical Features and Differential Diagnosis

When evaluating a patient with a complaint of joint pain, it is important to use a systematic approach and consider several key factors (Box 102.1).

It is also helpful to think of arthritis in three broad categories: degenerative/osteoarthritis (OA) including posttraumatic arthritis, infectious or septic arthritis, and inflammatory arthritis. Table 102.1 and Fig. 102.2 outline the differential diagnosis and decision pathways that may be used when evaluating patients with an acutely painful joint.

History

The acutely painful joint or joints is usually the primary complaint for the patient presenting with arthritis. The patient's age, as well as the timing of symptoms, specific location and description of pain, presence of associated symptoms, and factors that aggravate or alleviate symptoms, can provide clues to the etiology. Once the history and characteristics of the pain have been reviewed, further classifying the problem as monoarticular or polyarticular is of great importance. In cases of polyarticular arthritis, care should be taken to assess for the presence of symmetric versus asymmetric symptoms. These specific characteristics can be used when creating a differential diagnosis, as detailed in Table 102.1.

OA or degenerative joint disease is a clinical finding expected in the older population and is uncommon in younger patients except in the setting of previous traumatic injuries or prior surgeries or in patients

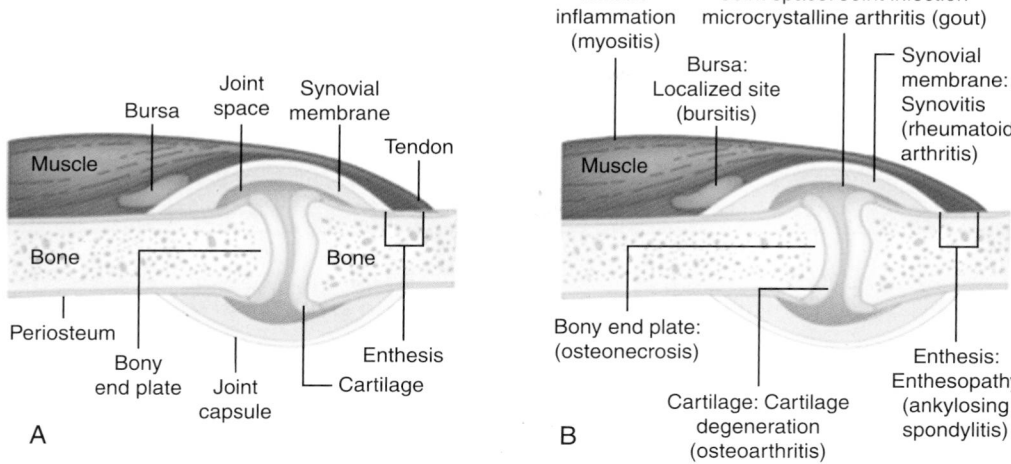

Fig. 102.1 Panel A: Example of a diarthrotic joint; Panel B: Sites of periarticular and articular disease and pain. (Redrawn from Goldman L, Ausiello DA, editors: *Cecil Medicine*, ed 23, Philadelphia, 2008, Saunders/Elsevier.)

BOX 102.1 Clinical Factors to Consider in the Evaluation of Joint Pain

Age
Single vs. multiple joint(s)
Time course:
- Acute (hours to <7 days)
- Subacute (7 days to 2–3 weeks)
- Chronic/progressive (>3 weeks to months)

History of acute or remote trauma to the joint
Associated systemic symptoms
Description and specific location of pain
Aggravating and alleviating factors

---

with certain comorbidities such as diabetes or obesity. OA will often present with pain in and around the joint, which worsens with activity. This pain is often accompanied by swelling, warmth, and discomfort to palpation diffusely around the joint. The most commonly affected joint in patients presenting to the ED will be the knee, but the shoulder, fingers, low back, or other joints may also be affected. In general, true arthritis pain will be more poorly localized in and around the joint. When the patient's pain is well localized and easily reproduced by palpation, common mimics such as bursitis or tendinitis should be considered.

Inflammatory or rheumatologic joint pain classically presents with symmetric and bilateral distribution with a predilection for the small joints of the hands. Inflammatory arthritides are more common in females and are usually diagnosed at an earlier age than degenerative arthritis. In general, the pain associated with inflammatory arthritis is worse in the morning and is associated with significant joint stiffness which improves with activity throughout the day. It is important to query the patient regarding the presence of systemic symptoms, because inflammatory conditions are often associated with symptoms distant from the affected joint. Many of the most common systemic symptoms are listed in Table 102.2. In addition, a careful medication history is important because many drugs can cause joint pain that mimics inflammatory arthritis. Certain viral conditions can also mimic inflammatory arthropathies and are discussed separately.

Acute monoarticular arthritis should always raise concern for the possibility of infectious arthritis, often referred to as septic arthritis, which is the most important condition to consider in the patient who presents to the ED with acute joint pain. There is significant morbidity and mortality associated with any delay in diagnosis of a septic joint. Therefore it is important to ask the patient about rapid progression of symptoms, associated skin changes, presence of fever, and any recent procedures or breaks in the skin that may have led to infection in the joint. Unfortunately, there are no adequately sensitive or specific findings either on history or physical examination that can safely rule out the possibility of a septic joint without a joint aspiration and analysis of joint fluid.

Physical Examination

General examination. The initial examination should focus on the affected joint or joints and should also assess for systemic or distant findings which may provide clues to the underlying problem. Vital signs, specifically presence of fever or tachycardia, should be noted because they may indicate infection, although most patients with confirmed septic arthritis will be afebrile on presentation.[2] The examination should begin with evaluation of general appearance, patient's position of comfort, and an assessment of ambulatory gait. A focused physical examination follows, directed by the patient's history and complaints.

Joint examination. The examination of the painful joint is performed in a systematic manner following the general principle of inspection, palpation, range of motion (ROM), neurovascular evaluation, special tests, and imaging when appropriate. Although the general examination is the same for all joints, each joint has different aspects to its exam and will be discussed independently. See Table 102.3.

Inspection. Begin the examination by watching the patient move in the exam room. Gait can provide important clues to discomfort and disability because pain, swelling, or weakness can all affect ambulation. The extent to which an affected joint is used and positions of comfort can also provide valuable information. Paired joints are compared, assessing each for deformity, skin integrity, erythema, swelling, ecchymosis, effusion, previous surgical scars, or rashes. Findings can suggest inflammation, infection, trauma, or prior surgery.

Palpation. When palpating, begin with an assessment of joint warmth. Large joints, such as the knee, should feel cool to the touch

TABLE 102.1   Differential Diagnosis of Arthritis

Monoarticular	Polyarticular: Symmetric	Polyarticular: Asymmetric
Septic arthritis	Rheumatoid arthritis	Gonococcal arthritis
Gout	Psoriatic arthritis	Lyme arthritis
Pseudogout	Polymyalgia rheumatica	Acute rheumatic fever
Osteoarthritis	Enteric arthritis	Reactive arthritis
Trauma, hemarthrosis	Ankylosing spondylitis	Viral arthritides

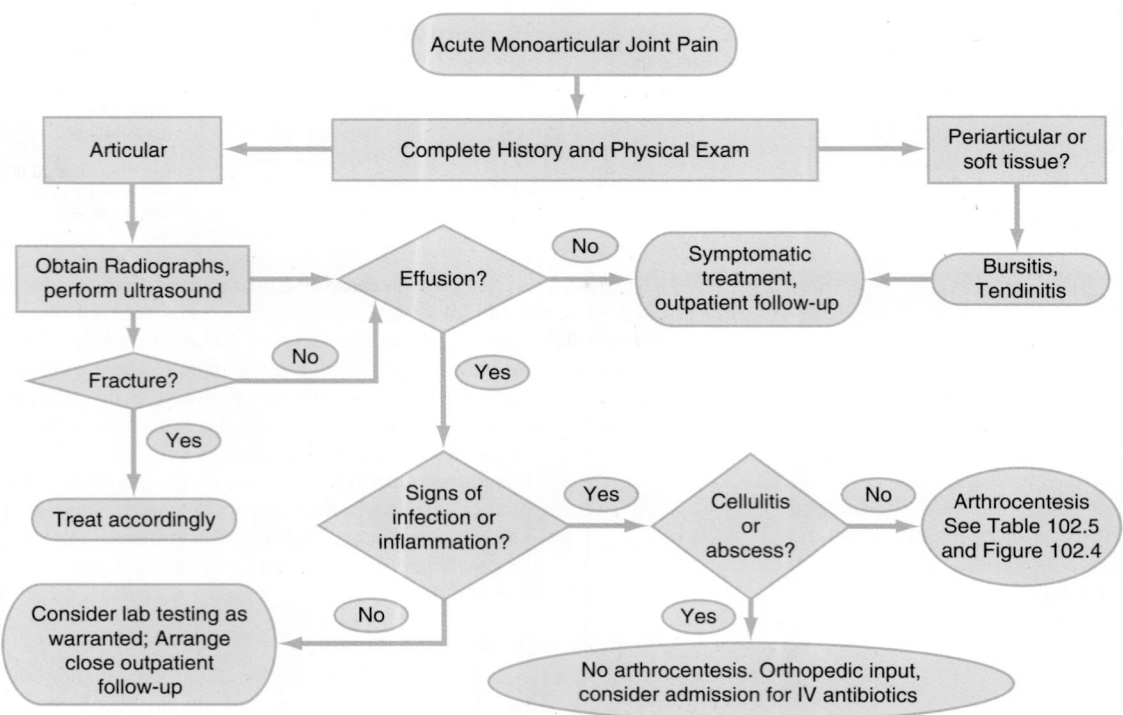

Fig. 102.2 Algorithm for Acute Monoarticular Joint Pain.

TABLE 102.2   Associated Systemic Findings for Common Arthritides

Condition	Findings
Rheumatoid arthritis	C-spine instability, pericarditis, pulmonary nodules, anemia
Psoriatic arthritis	Cutaneous plaques (most commonly on elbows, knees), inflammatory bowel disease
Ankylosing spondylitis	Uveitis/Iritis, cardiac abnormalities, aortic regurgitation, inflammatory bowel disease
Reactive arthritis	Conjunctivitis, genital/urethral discharge, oral ulcerations
Lyme disease	Erythema chronicum migrans, cardiac conduction abnormalities, Bell palsy
Gout	Tophi (usually nontender collections of uric acid crystals found most commonly in the subcutaneous tissue near affected joints)
Acute rheumatic fever	Erythema marginatum, chorea, carditis, subcutaneous nodules

or similar in temperature to the tissue proximal and distal to the joint. If a joint is found to be warm to the touch, this finding is suggestive of an inflammatory process or joint effusion. When a joint is hot to the touch, an infectious etiology should be considered.

Systematic palpation of the joint space and surrounding structures is performed with particular attention to areas of significant focal tenderness. Evaluate bony landmarks, ligamentous attachments, tendinous insertions, and nearby bursae. Identifying pain as articular (from the joint itself) or periarticular (due to proximate extra-articular structures) is important in determining diagnosis and management.

Range of motion. Both active and passive ROM should be assessed and compared with the unaffected extremity whenever possible. Active ROM refers to the patient moving the affected joint through its ROM, whereas passive ROM is performed by the physician without effort by the patient. Joints should be evaluated through their full ROM, which may be in multiple planes depending on the affected area. Pain with only active ROM or pain that is much worse with active ROM suggests a periarticular cause such as tendinopathy or bursitis, whereas pain with both active and passive ROM is more indicative of a true articular cause. Restricted or limited active and passive ROM due to severe pain suggests an inflammatory or infectious etiology.

TABLE 102.3 Components of a Comprehensive Joint Examination

Joint	Inspection	Palpation	Range of Motion (with normal ROM)	Neurovascular	Special Tests
Shoulder	Deformity Swelling Erythema Ecchymosis Muscle washing	Bony: SC joint, AC joint, scapular spine, grater tuberosity of humerus Soft tissue: subacromial space/bursa, biceps tendon	Forward flexion: 180° Extension: 35–45° Abduction: 180° IR and ER: 90° (both with arm adducted at side with elbow flexed and with arm adducted to 90°)	Neuro: Axillary nerve (deltoid sensation), radial, median, and ulnar nerves distally Vascular: radial and ulnar arteries at wrist	Numerous eponymic tests of variable clinical significance. No tests specifically for arthritis. Neer, Hawkins, O'Brien all evaluate RTC or labral pathology
Elbow	Deformity Specific location of pain (e.g., olecranon vs. radial head) Erythema Bruising Tophi (uric acid depositions)	Bony: olecranon, radial head, medial and lateral epicondyles of humerus Soft tissue: triceps tendon, distal biceps tendon	Supination and pronation Flexion: 150° Extension: 0°[a]	Neuro: Median, radial, ulnar nerves distally in forearm, wrist, and hand Vascular: radial and ulnar arteries at wrist	Valgus and varus stress at extension and slight flexion Resisted supination and resisted pronation
Wrist/Hand	Deformity Erythema Ulnar deviation Symmetric vs. asymmetric findings	Distal radius, scaphoid, anatomic snuffbox, ulnar styloid, CMC joint, TFCC, carpal tunnel, metacarpals	Wrist: Extension: 70° Flexion 80° Radial/ulnar deviation: 20° Supination 75°–90° Pronation: 90° Fingers/Thumb: Flexion, extension, abduction, adduction	Neuro: Radial, ulnar, median nerves, grip strength Vascular: radial and ulnar arteries at wrist, capillary refill in digits	Tinnel at carpal tunnel Finkelstein/Eichoff for De Quervain tenosynovitis
Hip	Observe gait Leg positioning at rest Shortening compared to contralateral leg	Bony: Greater trochanter, ischial tuberosity, pubic symphysis, iliac spine Soft tissue: proximal hamstring tendon, proximal quadriceps, inferior abdominal walls	Flexion: 90°–110° (Hyper)extension: 30° Abduction: 40° Adduction: 20° External rotation: 50° Internal rotation: 40° (performed with patient supine and hip flexed to 90° or by passive "log roll" with leg extended)[b]	Neuro: Evaluate strength and sensation in the foot to identify subtle muscle weakness or sensation deficits, patellar and Achilles ankle reflex Vascular: Dorsalis pedis in foot, posterior tibialis in ankle	FABER: Flexion, ABduction, External Rotation FADIR: Flexion, ADduction, Internal Rotation Log roll with internal and external rotation
Knee	Observe gait Swelling Erythema Fullness Calf or lower leg swelling	Bony: Patella, fibular head, distal femur, posterior patellar faces Soft tissue: peripatellar area, quad tendon, popliteal fossa, joint space, hamstring tendons, MCL, LCL Palpate for fluid in suprapatellar pouch	Flexion to 135° Extension to 0°	Neuro: Leg extension and flexion strength, patellar reflex Test strength more distally to find subtle weakness Vascular: Dorsalis pedis in foot, posterior tibialis in ankle	Lachman/anterior drawer Varus/valgus stress McMurray
Ankle/Foot	Swelling Erythema Bruising Arches	Bony: 5th metatarsal base, 1st MTP, medial and lateral malleoli, calcaneus, Lisfranc joint Soft tissue: Tibialis anterior tendon, Achilles insertion and tendon	Dorsiflexion: 20° Plantar flexion: 40° Inversion: 30° Eversion: 20° Toe flexion, extension	Neuro: Inversion (L4) Eversion (S1) Great toe extension strength (L5) Vascular: Dorsalis pedis in foot, posterior tibialis in ankle, capillary refill in toes	Anterior drawer Talar tilt Thompson test (Achilles)

[a]Limitation in terminal extension suggests joint effusion.
[b]Limited or painful IR suggestive of hip joint pathology
AC, Acromioclavicular; *CMC*, carpometacarpal; *ER*, external rotation; *IR*, internal rotation; *LCL*, lateral collateral ligament; *MCL*, medial collateral ligament; *MCP*, metacarpophalangeal; *MTP*, metatarsophalangeal; *SC*, sternoclavicular; *TFCC*, triangular fibrocartilage complex.

Neurovascular evaluation. Strength and sensation should be assessed in the affected joint, as well as the joints directly above and below the painful area. Strength is best assessed by testing small muscle groups whenever possible, because this allows the clinician to find subtle strength differences which may be missed when evaluating only large muscle groups (e.g., evaluate L4 with ankle inversion or L5 using great toe extension rather than testing leg extension). Distal pulses should be palpated and compared with the unaffected side. In the setting of severe peripheral vascular disease or difficult to palpate pulses, doppler or ultrasound may be useful in assessing peripheral arterial flow.

Diagnostic Testing

Radiographic Tests

Plain radiographs. Plain radiographs or X-rays (XR) are useful in determining possible etiologies of acute arthritis. Although they are more helpful in patients who have long-standing disease and therefore more obvious radiographic findings, even in the acute setting, radiographs may guide therapy by demonstrating soft tissue swelling, foreign bodies, or fractures. Whenever possible, weight-bearing images (Fig. 102.3) should be considered for lower extremity joints

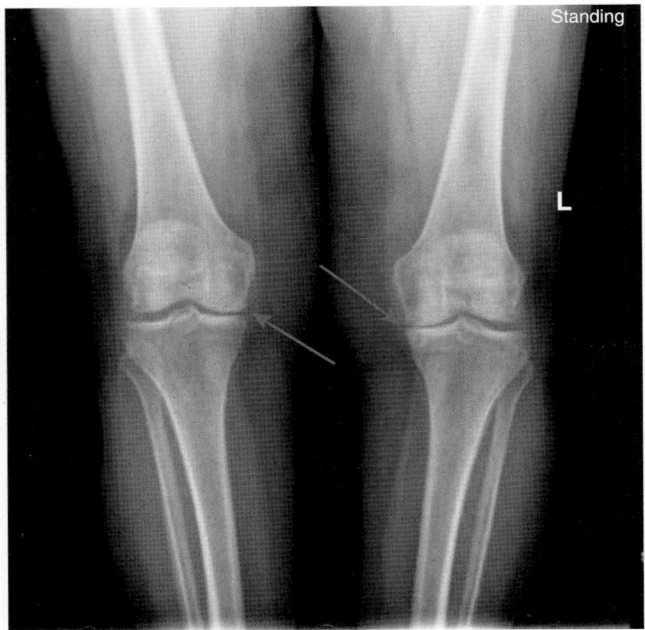

Fig. 102.3 Knee X-ray shows osteoarthritis with narrowing of the medial compartment bilaterally *(arrows)* on this weight-bearing radiograph.

because they may provide information such as presence of joint space narrowing or significant degenerative changes (Table 102.4). XR has limited utility in the evaluation for joint effusion.

Ultrasound. Bedside ultrasound may be used to complement the physical examination in cases of acute joint pain. The simple evaluation for joint effusion is safe, noninvasive, and easily learned by even novice ultrasound users. Evaluation of, and comparison with, the unaffected side allows direct, real-time visualization of the joint and surrounding areas, providing more expeditious diagnosis and disposition. Determining whether an effusion is present, as compared with a soft tissue abnormality such as an abscess or cellulitis without effusion, will inform the treatment course. Ultrasound may also be used to visualize the largest pocket of fluid in an effusion to help plan for and perform an arthrocentesis. Likewise, the use of bedside ultrasound has also been shown to decrease the incidence of nondiagnostic or "dry" joint taps. In rheumatologic illness, ultrasound has proved useful in determining active disease as well as the need for additional treatment modalities.

Computed Tomography and Magnetic Resonance Imaging. Advanced imaging modalities may add to the evaluation by showing the presence or absence of osteomyelitis, joint effusions, abscesses or other fluid collections, occult fractures, foreign bodies, and ligament or tendon injuries. Magnetic resonance imaging (MRI) is expensive, time-consuming, and generally not used in the ED for nonemergent indications. MRI should be considered when indicated to evaluate for specific conditions. For example, if the clinical suspicion for osteomyelitis is high, MRI is the diagnostic modality of choice. Computed tomography (CT) imaging can be useful if there are suspected fractures that were not visualized on XR, although the use of ionizing radiation should be minimized when feasible. In general, neither MRI nor CT should be used to guide the decision regarding performance of an arthrocentesis in the ED because the decision should be based on clinical findings and concern for infection. CT and MRI may show an effusion but will not be able to specify whether the effusion is infected or not.

Laboratory Testing

Aside from arthrocentesis and joint fluid analysis, specific laboratory tests lack adequate sensitivity or specificity to reliably exclude a septic joint. A serum white blood cell (WBC) count, erythrocyte sedimentation rate (ESR), or C-reactive protein (CRP) may be helpful, although it cannot be used to rule out an infectious cause and thus should not be used in isolation to guide ED decision making. An ESR level greater than 30 mm/h or CRP level of greater than 1.5 mg/mL has a sensitivity of greater than 90%, although it is poorly specific for septic arthritis, with specificities of approximately 20%.[2] Serum uric acid, although commonly ordered and elevated in patients with gouty arthropathies, provides little additional value in helping with diagnosis and patient

TABLE 102.4	Common Radiographic Findings in Arthritis
Arthritis	**Findings**
Acute arthritis (gout, pseudogout, septic)	Soft-tissue swelling
Late septic arthritis (>7–8 days)	Subchondral bone destructions, periosteal reaction, loss of joint space
Late pseudogout (knee, hip, radiocarpal, MCP)	Linear calcification in joint, asymmetric joint space narrowing
Degenerative arthritis (AC, CMC, MTP, DIP, knee, hip, c-spine, lumbosacral spine)	Asymmetric joint space narrowing (more pronounced on weight-bearing views), sclerosis of juxta-articular bone, bone spurs and cysts, minimal to no osteoporosis
Late rheumatoid arthritis (wrist MCP, PIP, MTP, 1st IP foot, atlantoaxial, glenohumeral)	Symmetric joint space narrowing, osteoporosis of periarticular bone marginal erosions

AC, Acromioclavicular; *CMC,* carpometacarpal; *DIP,* distal interphalangeal; *IP,* interphalangeal; *MCP,* metacarpophalangeal; *MTP,* metatarsophalangeal; *PIP,* proximal interphalangeal.

TABLE 102.5 Arthrocentesis Techniques by Joint

Joint	Patient Positioning	Landmarks	Needle trajectory	Ultrasound
Shoulder	Seated with arm flexed resting on thigh with hand supinated Or Lateral decubitus with affected arm internally rotated	Palpate posterolateral edge of acromion Coracoid process	Insert inferior to posterior acromial edge guided toward coracoid process	Performed in-plane: Probe on posterior aspect of acromion (parallel to floor if seated), needle from lateral to medial into joint
Elbow	Arm flexed and pronated Use supination and pronation to find radial head	Palpate lateral epicondyle of humerus and then anterior to it, palpate radial head. "Soft spot" between the two is joint space	Insert into soft spot just anterior to lateral epicondyle	Place probe on tip of lateral epicondyle and find radial head. Probe will be parallel to arm. Guide needled out of plane into joint space
Wrist	Wrist pronated resting on a towel in slight flexion	Lister's tubercle on dorsal radius and extensor pollicis longus tendon located radial to tubercle	Insert needled just ulnar to tendon and just distal to Lister's tubercle	Out of plane approach: Probe long to radius visualizing both radius and scaphoid. Joint space is between.
Hip	Supine in stretcher with leg neutral or slight external rotation if using US Internal rotation if performing without US	Greater trochanter (if not using US)	Insert needle superior to trochanter, horizontal and parallel to the stretcher. Aspirate throughout. Redirect slightly cephalad if bone encountered[a]	Low frequency curvilinear probe used for in-plane approach Find femoral head and neck, guide needled from distal to proximal (side to side on screen) to touch bone at femoral head-neck junction[b,c]
Knee	Supine with knee flexed ~20°	Lateral edge of superior half of patella	Lateral to medial guided to area just posterior to patella	Probe positioned transverse just superior to patella with quad tendon in short axis. Fluid will be inferior to tendon, superior to femur. Guide needle in plane from lateral to medial
Ankle	Supine with plantarflexed foot	Tibialis anterior tendon and anterior edge of medial malleolus	Insert between tibialis anterior and medial malleolus aiming directly posterior	Slight out of plane approach lateral to medial BELOW tibialis anterior tendon into joint space. Tibialis anterior tendon will be in long axis at top of screen
MTP	Supine or sitting with neutral foot, slight flexion of the affected toe	Distal metatarsal head, extensor tendon, and base of first phalanx	Insert dorsally medial to the extensor tendon	Out of plane. Probe is parallel to toe (short to joint), needle will be inserted from medial aspect of foot/toe into joint

[a]Not recommended.
[b]Preferred approach.
[c]Find and mark arteries to avoid in needle path.

disposition from the ED. Many patients with known gout and gouty arthritis have normal uric acid levels and many patients with elevated uric acid levels do not have gout. We therefore do not recommend the routine use of serum uric acid levels in the evaluation of acute arthritis in the ED setting.

Arthrocentesis and Synovial Fluid Analysis

Arthrocentesis. Joint fluid aspiration with synovial fluid analysis is the most important modality used to diagnose the cause of an acutely painful joint. Whenever possible, the procedure should be done with the aid of ultrasound which has demonstrated greater success rates in both aspiration and therapeutic injection when compared with palpation-guided techniques.[3] Arthrocentesis methods for various joints are discussed in Table 102.5.

Indications and contraindications. Indications for urgent arthrocentesis include (1) to obtain joint fluid for analysis for possible infection or crystals, (2) to drain a large hemarthrosis secondary to trauma or injury, (3) to inject medication into the joint, and, less frequently, (4) to evaluate a laceration for possible extension into the joint. Arthrocentesis should be considered for any patient with a newly swollen and painful joint in the absence of trauma.

Contraindications to the procedure are relative and should be discussed with the patient. It is generally accepted practice that arthrocentesis should not be performed if the needle must be inserted through an area of cellulitis or infected skin overlying a joint. Coagulopathy is a relative contraindication, although these procedures have been performed successfully with a less than 0.5% complication rate even in patients with therapeutic international normalized ratio (INR) levels. We recommend performing arthrocentesis in patients with suspected septic arthritis even if currently on therapeutic anticoagulation. A prosthetic joint should only be aspirated after discussion with the operating surgeon, and, in general, patients with prosthetic joints should have neither joint aspiration nor intra-articular injections until the case is discussed with an orthopedist. However, if orthopedic consultant is not available and suspicion for a septic joint remains high, arthrocentesis can be performed by the ED clinician.[4]

Complications. Patients should be counseled about the potential risks of the procedure, the most serious of which include inoculation of infection or bleeding, either into the joint or externally. Less serious complications include pain, allergic reaction to medication, or adverse outcomes when instilling corticosteroids or local anesthetics into the joint space. It is possible that the

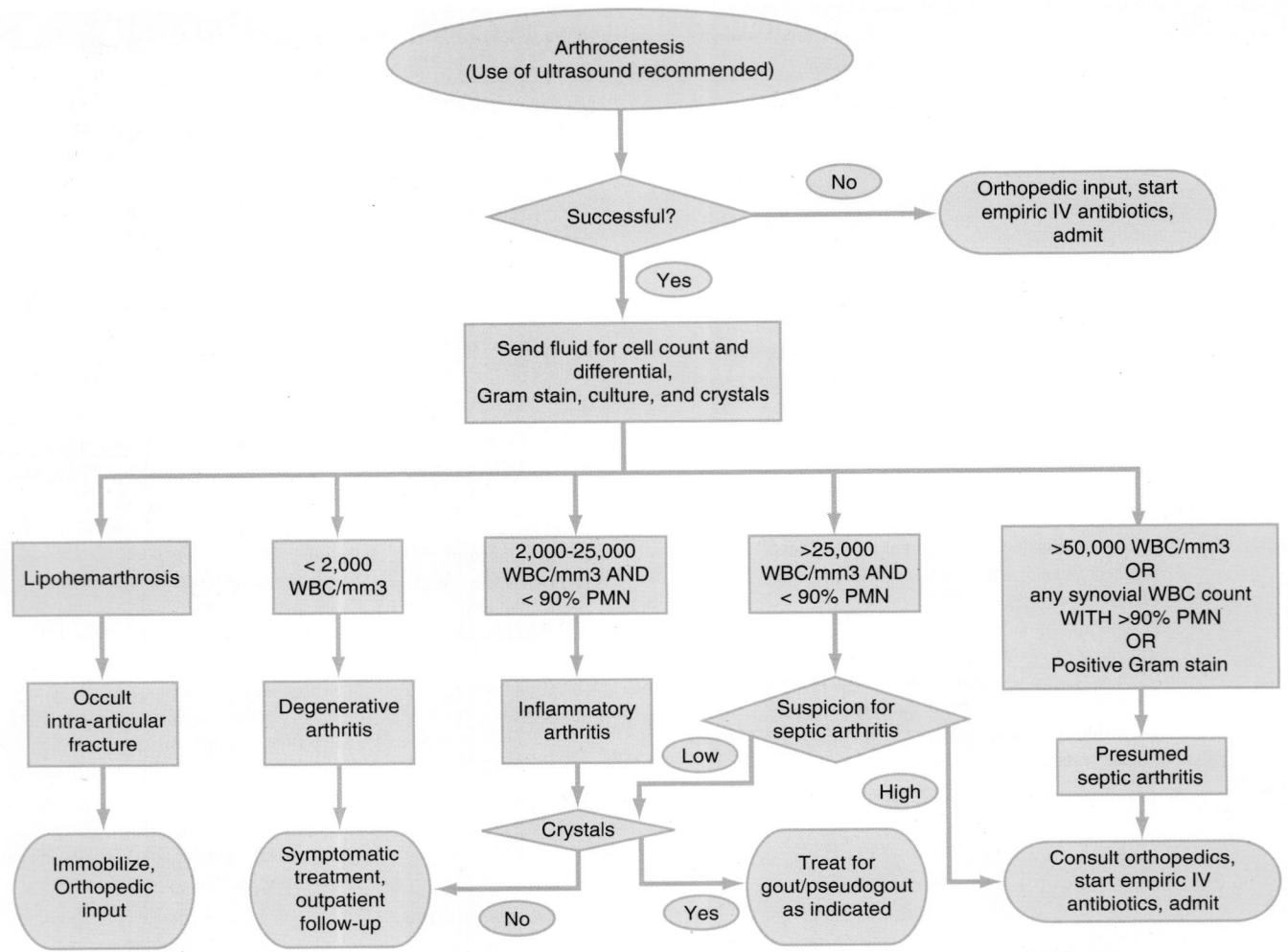

Fig. 102.4 Algorithm for Arthrocentesis for Suspected Septic Joint. *PMN,* Polymorphonuclear; *WBC,* white blood cell.

TABLE 102.6	Key Findings in Joint Fluid Analysis Among Various Causes of Arthritis			
	Degenerative	**Inflammatory**	**Septic/Infectious**	**Hemorrhagic**
Color/appearance	Clear to yellow	Yellow	Cloudy/turbid, may be dark or purulent	Bloody, may contain fat droplets
Viscosity	Thick, stringy	Variable	Variable, usually thin	Variable
Synovial WBC count	<2,000/mm³ <25,000/mm³ (+LR 0.32)	2,000–50,000/mm³	>25,000 (+LR 3.2) >50,000 (+LR 4.7) >100,000 (+LR 13.2)	<2,000/mm³
Synovial PMN%	Variable	Variable, generally <90%	>90%	<25%
Gram stain	Negative	Negative	Positive in 50%–60% of confirmed cases	Negative

LR, Likelihood ratio; *PMN,* polymorphonuclear neutrophil; *WBC,* white blood cell.

aspiration attempt may be unsuccessful, although if ultrasound is used, the fluid can generally be visualized to maximize the chance for success.

Synovial fluid examination. Analysis of the joint fluid obtained via arthrocentesis is a critical step in determining the cause of acute arthritis. Examination should be based on the general appearance of the fluid, color, fluid WBC count, crystal analysis, Gram stain, and ultimately on bacterial fluid culture (Fig. 102.4 and Table 102.6).

General appearance. Visual inspection of the fluid upon aspiration can aid in diagnosis, although no findings are diagnostic without microscopic fluid analysis. Normal fluid is mostly clear and colorless

but develops increased viscosity and a more intense yellow color with increased inflammation. Turbid, opaque, or grossly purulent fluid is more suggestive of acute infectious process. A hemarthrosis suggests internal derangement of the joint, including occult fracture or ligamentous injury. A lipohemarthrosis, identified by fat droplets in the aspirate, suggests a fracture, classically seen in a knee arthrocentesis with an occult tibial plateau fracture.

White blood cell count. The synovial WBC count is helpful in distinguishing different causes of arthritis. Although the number of WBCs is generally used to determine the cause of the effusion, there is significant overlap in accepted values among causes of arthritis and the absolute numbers can be misleading. Classically, septic arthritis presents with greater than 50,000/mm³ WBC in the synovial fluid, but it has been repeatedly shown that early, or partially treated, septic arthritis may present with significantly lower absolute numbers of WBCs. Nonetheless, the likelihood for septic arthritis increases along with the absolute number of WBCs. The relative number of neutrophils (polymorphonuclear [PMN] cells) is also used to diagnose septic arthritis with levels greater than 90% generally accepted to be associated with infection. No absolute number should be used to diagnose or exclude the presence of a septic joint when the clinical suspicion is high.

In inflammatory arthritis, WBC counts tend to be lower than in septic arthritis, in the range of 25K to 50K/mm³. However, there may be significant overlap between inflammatory and septic arthritis, and there are instances where patients with RA or gout may have synovial fluid WBC counts well above 50,000/mm³. We recommend that any synovial sample with a WBC count greater than 50,000/mm³ be treated as presumptive septic arthritis until further information confirms another etiology.[5]

Prosthetic joints have significantly lower thresholds for diagnosis, and a WBC count greater than 1100/mm³ should be considered diagnostic of infection.

Lactate and C-reactive protein. Much like synovial WBC count and pleocytosis, increasing lactate and CRP levels in the synovial fluid correlate with an increased likelihood of infection. However, these tests have not been shown to be significantly better than the synovial WBC count or PMN pleocytosis for predicting infection.[6] Due to the associated cost and unlikely additional benefit, we do not recommend the routine use of these tests in the evaluation of possible septic arthritis in the ED.

Crystal evaluation. Analysis under light microscopy to evaluate for monosodium urate or calcium pyrophosphate is used to diagnose gout or pseudogout, respectively. Monosodium urate crystals seen in gout are needle-shaped and negatively birefringent, whereas calcium pyrophosphate crystals seen in pseudogout are rhomboid-shaped and positively birefringent. Importantly, the presence of crystals does not rule out the possibility of infection and in fact, gout is a risk factor for septic arthritis due to chronic joint damage predisposing to hematogenous spread of bacteria into the joint.

Gram stain and culture. A positive Gram stain is diagnostic of septic arthritis though is only found in 30% to 50% of confirmed infections. A negative Gram stain does not exclude the possibility of a septic joint and thus should not be used in isolation to exclude infection. Gonococcal (GC) infections in particular are difficult to identify in synovial fluid and their diagnosis may depend on cultures of genital discharge or oral lesions taken at the same time. Whenever GC septic arthritis is suspected, we recommend obtaining samples from mucosal or skin lesions, as well as urine for nucleic acid amplification testing (NAAT) or Gram stain and culture.

A positive synovial fluid culture is the gold standard for the diagnosis of septic arthritis, but the results are not immediately available in the ED setting. For patients who are discharged, a mechanism should be in place for the follow-up of culture results with the patient. Blood cultures are recommended if septic arthritis is strongly suspected, because they may be positive in up to 50% of septic arthritis cases and may aid in identifying the causative organism if synovial cultures are negative.

Management

The mainstays of treatment of acute arthritis are antiinflammatory medications and, in the case of septic arthritis, antibiotics. The management of specific causes of acute arthritis are discussed in subsequent sections of the chapter.

Disposition

The ultimate disposition of the ED patient with acute arthropathy will depend on clinical findings. Although most patients with acute exacerbations of chronic conditions can be managed with oral medications in the outpatient setting, the challenge for the emergency clinician remains in identifying patients who are at risk for rapid deterioration, progressive disease, or permanent joint disability. When septic arthritis is suspected, hospital admission, parenteral antibiotic therapy, and orthopedic input remain prudent. Patients with known or suspected rheumatologic conditions can typically be followed on an outpatient basis. Patients with other noninfectious causes of joint pain can often be treated with analgesics or antiinflammatory medications until seen in follow-up by a primary care physician.

ACUTE MONOARTICULAR JOINT PAIN

Acute joint pain, when confined to a single joint and particularly if associated with erythema, warmth, or systemic infectious symptoms, should prompt urgent evaluation for a septic joint. However, acute trauma and inflammatory conditions of the periarticular tissues can also cause monoarticular joint pain. Therefore conditions such as bursitis, tendonitis, synovitis, and sprains or other trauma should also be considered.

Nongonococcal Bacterial Septic Arthritis

Foundations

The incidence of septic arthritis is approximately 6 per 100,000 population per year in industrialized countries. This number increases to 30 to 60 per 100,000 population per year in patients with underlying disease or prosthetic joints. Young children and elders are at greater risk, as are patients with immune compromise, diabetes, and history of hemodialysis or IV drug use. Patients with prosthetic joints or those who have had recent intra-articular steroid injections are at particular risk. The presence of chronic joint inflammation such as RA or gout is also a significant risk factor for joint infection, particularly as many of these patients are on chronic immunosuppression. Exacerbations of crystal arthropathies can coexist with infectious arthritis, and the presence of crystals should not be used to eliminate the possibility of septic arthritis. Box 102.2 lists factors that increase the risk of septic arthritis.

The most common method of joint space inoculation is by hematogenous spread although direct inoculation from local injury or infection in surrounding tissues may also occur. Once the joint space is inoculated, there is little defense against rapid bacterial proliferation. This unchecked bacterial growth and the associated inflammatory cascade typically leads to severe pain, synovial proliferation, neovascularization, and extensive

---

BOX 102.2 Factors Increasing Risk of Septic Arthritis

Age >80
Diabetes
Rheumatoid arthritis
Gout/pseudogout
Recent joint surgery
Hip or knee prosthesis
Skin infection
Prosthesis PLUS skin infection
Intravenous drug abuse
Endocarditis
Human immunodeficiency virus (HIV) disease

TABLE 102.7	Common Pathogens in Septic Arthritis
Group	**Organisms**
Neonates and infants	*Staphylococcus aureus*, group B *Streptococcus*
Children	*S. aureus*, group A *Streptococcus*, *Streptococcus pneumonia*, *Kingella Kingae*, Lyme
Adolescents and young adults	*Neisseria gonorrhea*, *S. aureus*
Older adults	*S. aureus*, *Streptococcus*, gram-negative rods
Sickle cell anemia	*S. pneumonia*, *Salmonella* (although more commonly causes osteomyelitis)
Intravenous drug use	Pseudomonas, *S. aureus*, gram-negative rods
Prosthetic joint	Coagulase-negative *Staphylococcus*, *S. aureus*, gram-negative rods, *Streptococcus* species

TABLE 102.8	Empiric Antibiotics for Suspected Septic Arthritics Intravenous
Gram Stain Results	**Antibiotic Regimen (IV Dosing)**
Unavailable or negative Gram stain	Vancomycin loading dose: 20 to 35 mg/kg actual body weight (not to exceed 3000 mg) or 20 to 25 mg/kg actual body weight (not to exceed 3000 mg) in patients with obesity, then 15 to 20 mg/kg actual body weight every 8 to 12 hrs IV WITH IV cephalosporin (ceftriaxone 2 g, cefepime 2 g, ceftazidime 2 g) OR aztreonam 2 g IV OR daptomycin 6 mg/kg IV WITH IV cephalosporin OR linezolid 600 mg IV WITH IV cephalosporin
Gram-positive cocci	Vancomycin loading dose: 20 to 35 mg/kg actual body weight (not to exceed 3000 mg) or 20 to 25 mg/kg actual body weight (not to exceed 3000 mg) in patients with obesity, then 15 to 20 mg/kg actual body weight every 8 to 12 hrs IV OR daptomycin 6 mg/kg IV OR linezolid 600 mg IV
Gram-negative bacilli	Ceftriaxone 2 g IV OR aztreonam 2 g IV
Gram-negative diplococci	Ceftriaxone 2 g IV, can consider adding azithromycin 1000 mg orally (PO) for chlamydia coverage

damage of the articular cartilage if not quickly identified and appropriately treated.

The most common bacterial causes of non-GC septic arthritis include gram-positive organisms such as methicillin-resistant or methicillin-sensitive *Staphylococcus aureus* and *Streptococcus* species, which are found in almost 80% of culture-confirmed infections. Anaerobes and mycobacteria are less common causes. Likewise, *Haemophilus* and pneumococcal species are less common in the postvaccine era. *Neisseria gonorrhoeae* accounts for less than 20% of monoarticular arthritis and more frequently presents as polyarticular arthritis. Certain patient populations are more likely to develop specific infections as discussed in Table 102.7.

Prosthetic joint infections deserve specific mention, with these infections classically being described as either early, defined as occurring within a month of surgery, or late. Late infections develop via hematogenous spread or by organisms introduced into the joint space during surgery, which may not become clinically evident for up to a year later. Arthrocentesis should be performed in discussion with, or optimally by, an orthopedic surgeon when feasible. In the prosthetic joint, a synovial WBC count of more than 1,100/mm^3 or PMNs greater than 60% are both sensitive and specific for joint infection. In the setting of a prosthetic joint, the host immune response and antibiotic delivery to the joint space are both impaired, and thus the management of infection can be complex.

Clinical Features and Differential Diagnosis

Patients with septic arthritis will often present with fever, joint pain, and effusion, most often in a large joint such as the knee. Fever response may be blunted in elders or those who have a suppressed immune system. At particular risk are patients with autoimmune arthritis, overwhelming sepsis, or meningococcal infections. Up to 20% of patients with septic arthritis may present with polyarticular involvement. Physical examination findings, such as decreased ROM, joint tenderness, or erythema, have inadequate sensitivity and specificity for determination of septic arthritis.

Diagnostic testing. Laboratory testing, including a serum WBC, ESR, and CRP, is commonly performed although often is of limited utility. Elevated values only slightly increase the likelihood of septic arthritis, and normal values do not exclude the condition. Likewise, radiographs are of limited utility in diagnosing a septic joint but may occasionally identify alternative diagnoses. Although plain radiographs may help to identify osteomyelitis, the bony changes associated with septic arthritis are a late finding. CT or MRI may be useful in identifying early changes associated with septic arthritis or may help to assess joints that are difficult to evaluate clinically, including joints that are challenging to aspirate.

The gold standard test for the patient with acute monoarticular arthritis remains joint aspiration and synovial fluid analysis. Elevated synovial fluid WBC count, increased proportion of PMNs, and elevated synovial fluid lactate all increase the likelihood of septic arthritis. A fluid Gram stain and aerobic and anaerobic cultures should be performed. Synovial fluid should also be evaluated for characteristic crystals of gout or pseudogout.

Management

Early identification and treatment of septic arthritis is crucial. Delays in definitive care can lead to increased morbidity and mortality. Hospitalization for intravenous (IV) antimicrobial therapy is appropriate. Empiric antibiotic therapy should be directed at organisms found on Gram stain, or alternatively, broad-spectrum therapy is appropriate and can be tailored once speciation and sensitivity results are available. Table 102.8 details recommended antibiotic therapy for suspected septic arthritis.

Depending upon the specific joints involved, either surgical drainage or repeated joint aspirations are often required. Early coordination with an orthopedic surgeon is critical in the management of infection in prosthetic joints. Antibiotics are often continued for several weeks and infectious disease input may be helpful in selecting the most appropriate antibiotic regimen.

CHRONIC MONOARTICULAR ARTHRITIS

Osteoarthritis

Foundations

OA or degenerative joint disease is the most common form of arthritis among adults and is more common in obese patients and elders. Changes in load on the joint, due to excess weight or trauma, combined with biochemical and genetic factors, lead to changes in cytokine signaling and thus alterations in composition of the extracellular matrix. This ultimately leads to overgrowth of subchondral bone, degradation of the articular cartilage, and inflammation of the synovium.

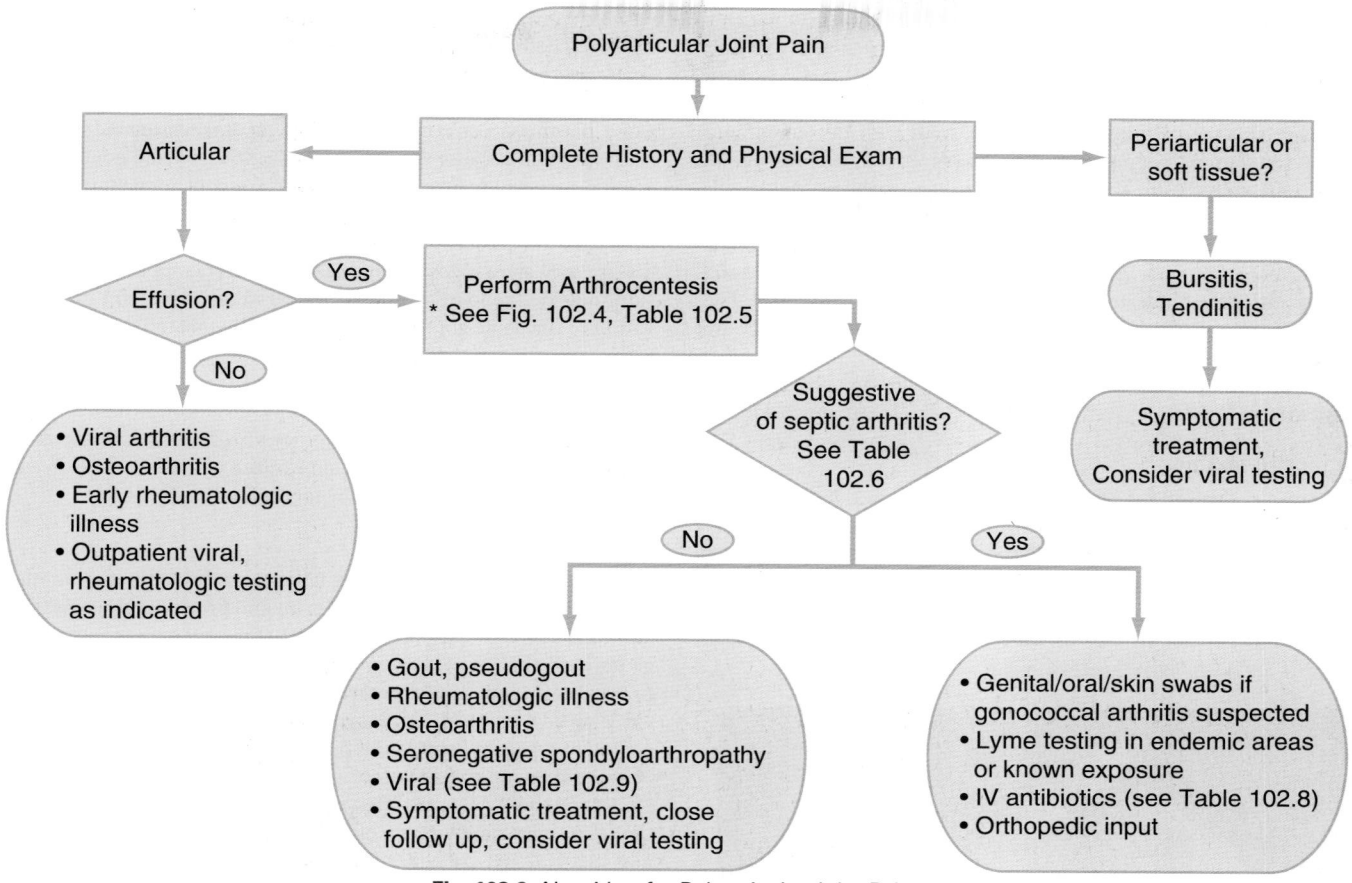

Fig. 102.6 Algorithm for Polyarticular Joint Pain.

common form of joint infection in the young, sexually active population. Hematogenous dissemination of the initial mucosal infection occurs in less than 3% of cases overall and is thought to play a major role in the pathogenesis of GC arthritis. The risk of dissemination is higher in immunocompromised patients, women (particularly during pregnancy), IV drug users, and patients with multiple sexual partners. The time from initial infection to presentation with arthritis symptoms may be 1 to 3 months.

Clinical Features

Although GC arthritis may present in a single joint, it often manifests as an oligoarthritis, affecting two to four joints simultaneously, often in the wrist, knee, or ankle. The effusions associated with this condition may be modest compared with other infections. Diffuse, migratory arthralgias and fever are also common. Simultaneous skin findings, also resulting from hematogenous spread, may also be present with small painless, nonpruritic lesions that may be papular, pustular, or vasculitic.

Management

The diagnosis of GC arthritis can be particularly challenging because cultures of blood and synovial fluid may be negative, although diagnostic yield is greatly improved when polymerase chain reaction (PCR) testing is performed. When GC infections are suspected, all possible sites should be tested, including blood, synovial fluid, oropharynx, genitalia, and any suspect skin lesions. When the diagnosis is made, hospitalization is advised, and treatment should be initiated with ceftriaxone 2 g IV or intramuscular (IM) every 24 hours. Antibiotic

sensitivity results will assist the transition to appropriate oral antibiotics. Simultaneous treatment for chlamydia is advised with azithromycin 1 g PO, as is testing for other sexually transmitted infections. Repeated arthrocentesis is rarely required, and when diagnosed and treated promptly, residual joint damage is rare.

Gout

Foundations

Acute gout occurs in approximately 4% of adults in the United States, impacting approximately 5% of adult males and 3% of adult females. Gout is more prevalent among older adults.[15] Risk factors include obesity, hypertension, diabetes, and use of thiazide diuretics or cyclosporin. Acute gout attacks may be precipitated by a purine-rich diet including meats, beer, legumes, and seafood, especially shellfish or anchovies. Uric acid is a normal by-product of purine metabolism, and hyperuricemia results from its undersecretion by the kidney or, less commonly, from overproduction caused by inborn errors in metabolism. Acute attacks result from inflammation that occurs when uric acid crystals precipitate from supersaturated extracellular fluid. During an acute attack, these crystals are ingested by PMN cells, resulting in release of cytokines and an inflammatory reaction of the synovium. Asymptomatic hyperuricemia may exist for years, and the absolute serum uric acid level does not correlate well with the risk or frequency of acute attacks.

Clinical Features

Gouty attacks occur most commonly in the first metatarsophalangeal (MTP) joint, causing the condition termed podagra. The knee, ankle, tarsal joints, and hand are also frequently affected. Usually patients experience an acute flair in a single joint, but up to 20% of patients have polyarticular involvement or associated bursitis, tenosynovitis, and skin changes that can resemble cellulitis (Fig. 102.7). Onset of pain is sudden, and the pain may be exquisite, both with movement and while at rest. Systemic symptoms, including fever, may be present and should raise concern for the possibility of septic arthritis. Acute episodes of gout are self-limited, usually with peak symptoms within 1 to 2 days and resolution within a week. If left untreated, attacks may become more frequent, involve more joints, and may have lasting sequelae including bony erosion and tophi, which are gritty, chalk-like nodules composed of deposits of monosodium urate crystals which are generally painless. These are most commonly found in the subcutaneous tissue, although they may also be found in bursae, joint space, or soft tissues.

Diagnostic Testing

Diagnostic evaluation for gout includes arthrocentesis and evaluation of joint fluid particularly in patients who are having their first episode of gout. Patients who have an established history of gout and are otherwise well appearing without other risk factors for septic arthritis may be treated without a joint aspiration. The acute gouty joint will have synovial fluid crystals visible that appear negatively birefringent when

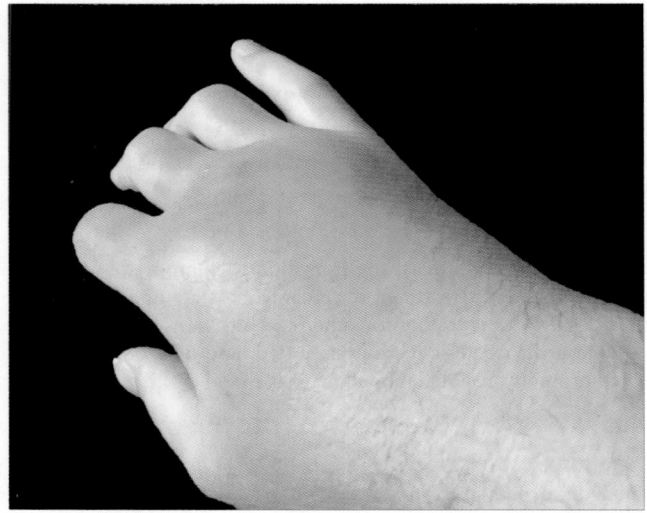

Fig. 102.7 Patient with confirmed gout in the second metacarpophalangeal joint mimicking hand cellulitis.

viewed with a polarizing microscope. Serum laboratory tests are largely unhelpful because gouty attacks can occur in patients with normal uric acid levels, and some patients may have elevated uric acid levels without signs or symptoms of clinical disease. Serum WBC count may be elevated, but this is also a nonspecific finding. It is reasonable to evaluate renal function because there is an association between gout and renal insufficiency and many of the treatments for gout are nephrotoxic.

Plain radiographs of the acutely affected joint may show only the associated soft-tissue swelling. However, patients with long-standing disease may show signs of asymmetric, sclerotic-appearing bony erosions outside the joint capsule. Ultrasound may be useful in the evaluation of the acute gouty joint: The crystalline material reflects sound waves, revealing an irregular, hyperechoic signal along the surface of the articular cartilage, sometimes referred to as the "double contour sign"—one representing the crystals and the second the hyperechoic bony surface below. Chronic tophi may also be visible on ultrasound and are described as having the appearance of "wet clumps of sugar" with a heterogenous center and hypoechoic rim (Fig. 102.8).

Management

The management of gout is divided into therapies to treat acute attacks and those aimed at long-term treatment and prophylaxis against future attacks. Patients often present to the ED for symptoms related to an acute exacerbation. Contrary to previous guidelines, long-standing prophylactic medications, such as allopurinol, febuxostat, or probenecid, may be continued—although they should not be initiated—in the setting of an acute gout flare.[16] The mainstays for ED management of acute gout include NSAIDs, corticosteroids, or colchicine.

Although NSAIDs are often considered first line, there is little evidence to suggest superiority of one drug over another, or even to suggest that NSAIDs are better than other pharmacologic options. When started promptly after the onset of symptoms, relief typically occurs within 24 hours, and the NSAID should be continued for at least another 24 hours after symptom resolution. Indomethacin, naproxen, and ibuprofen are all reasonable choices. NSAIDs should be avoided in patients with a history of peptic ulcer disease, GI bleeding, renal insufficiency, or other known contraindications.

Colchicine acts by inhibiting the formation of microtubules, thereby inhibiting the inflammatory response to the presence of crystals in the synovium and has been shown to be effective for the treatment of gout. However, it is contraindicated in patients with renal or hepatic insufficiency, can cause GI distress in many patients, and has a narrow therapeutic window making it potentially lethal in overdose. Because it shares similar contraindications to NSAIDs as well as a similar efficacy, we recommend traditional NSAIDs over colchicine for acute symptom management.

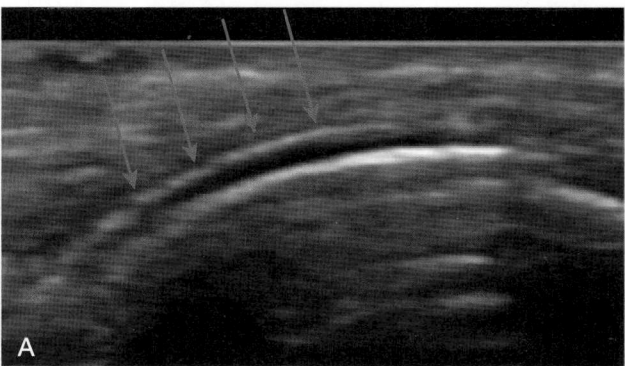
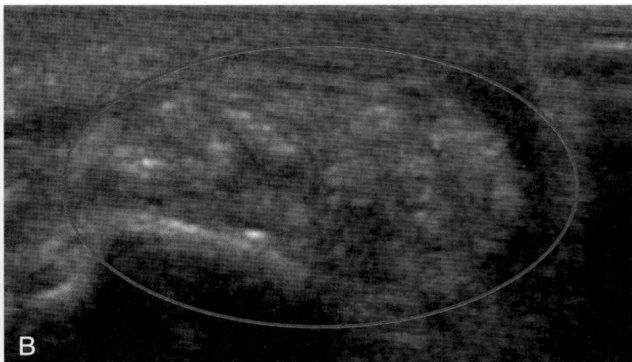

Fig. 102.8 Ultrasound Appearance of Gout. (A) Double contour sign showing gout in a metatarsal phalangeal joint. (B) Tophus seen on ultrasound showing "clump of sugar" appearance.

Steroids, whether oral or intra-articular, can also be beneficial in an acute gout attack. Intra-articular steroids may be most effective but should not be used in any patient with possible septic arthritis, and their use may be impractical in patients with small joint disease or when multiple joints are involved. Oral steroids, such as prednisone 40 mg daily for 5 to 7 days or a tapered pack of solumedrol, may also be effective.

Combination therapy, such as intra-articular steroid injection combined with colchicine or NSAIDs, is a reasonable option, particularly for patients with debilitating symptoms and those who have required such treatment previously. Oral corticosteroids with simultaneous NSAID use are not recommended due to the risk of GI side effects. Other treatment options include a short course of opioid analgesics, regional anesthetic blocks, or short-term cessation of diuretic therapy. Nonpharmacologic treatments such as ice, elevation, oral hydration, or avoidance of known triggers may also be helpful.

Pseudogout

Foundations

Calcium pyrophosphate deposition disease (CPPD), also known as pseudogout, is caused by deposits of calcium complex crystals on the articular surfaces. These deposits are evident on plain radiographs as chondrocalcinosis. The precipitation of these crystals leads to an inflammatory synovitis. Although the pathophysiology of the condition is not well understood, it is most commonly seen in elders and those with prior trauma or recent joint surgery. There is also an association with hemochromatosis, amyloidosis, hypothyroidism, and hyperparathyroidism. This condition is most often asymptomatic, but when acute inflammation occurs, the resulting condition is known as pseudogout.

Clinical Features

The acute presentation of pseudogout is similar to gout, although patients with pseudogout tend to be older and the knee is the most commonly affected joint. A warm and swollen joint that is acutely tender is typical, and it may be difficult to differentiate between the two conditions based on history and physical examination findings alone. However, compared with gout, acute pseudogout attacks may take longer to reach maximum symptom intensity and symptoms may persist for up to 2 to 3 months despite therapy.

Many patients with CPPD crystal deposition follow a chronic, progressive course of articular degeneration known as pseudo-OA. This may manifest in multiple joints, often involving the knees, wrists, metacarpophalangeal (MCP) joints, hips, shoulders, spine, elbows, or ankles. Approximately half of these patients will experience acute attacks of pseudogout superimposed on their chronic symptoms, whereas the remainder may present with signs and symptoms more consistent with classical OA.

Diagnostic Testing

Diagnostic testing for pseudogout is similar to that for gout. Plain radiographs may demonstrate chondrocalcinosis within the articular cartilage or in the joint capsule, although these radiographic findings may be present in less than half of cases. Given the association with systemic disease, laboratory testing may be warranted in select cases, including serum electrolytes, alkaline phosphatase, thyroid studies, or iron studies. Joint fluid analysis reveals weakly positive birefringent crystals that are rhomboid-shaped. As with gout, the symptoms may mimic septic arthritis, and it is important to note that crystals and acute infection may be present simultaneously.

Management

Asymptomatic CPPD does not require acute treatment unless it is directed at the underlying conditions (e.g., hypercalcemia due to hyperparathyroidism). When considering acute exacerbations of pseudogout, there are no specific pharmacologic agents that directly target the deposition of calcium crystals, and available anticrystal agents have not yet been proved to be effective in humans. In small studies, methotrexate, interleukin-1 (IL-1) inhibitors, and anti–tumor necrosis factor (TNF) alpha agents show promise in decreasing the frequency and severity of acute attacks, particularly in periarticular disease. Thus treatment is typically initiated using antiinflammatory medications. NSAIDs remain a mainstay of therapy, although they may be contraindicated in some older adults or those with comorbidities. Steroids, either systemic or intra-articular, can provide rapid symptomatic relief. Much like for gout, colchicine can be effective for acute exacerbations through its effect on PMNs; however, its narrow therapeutic window limits its utility.

Lyme Disease

Foundations

The spirochete *Borrelia burgdorferi* causes the infection responsible for Lyme disease, one of the most common vector-borne diseases in the Western Hemisphere. Transmitted by the *Ixodes* tick, the CDC estimates nearly 300,000 cases of Lyme disease per year in the United States.[17]

Clinical Features

Lyme disease presents as an unfolding pattern of symptoms which develop over weeks to months following infection. The early symptoms occur within weeks or months after a tick bite and may include rash as well as migratory myalgias or arthralgias without evidence of discrete arthritis. However, arthritis is the hallmark of the late stage of disease, and when untreated, approximately half of patients develop asymmetric arthritis within 6 months of initial infection. Lyme disease typically affects the large joints, in particular the knees, and if left untreated may cause intermittent episodes that persist for years. The arthritis associated with Lyme disease appears to be an autoimmune effect rather than a direct result of the spirochete infection. Early antibiotic therapy reduces the incidence of subsequent joint involvement.

Diagnostic Testing

The history of a tick bite, particularly in Lyme-endemic areas, or the classic erythema migrans rash may aid the clinician in making the diagnosis. However, many patients may not recall either the tick exposure or the resulting rash. The patient presenting with acute Lyme arthritis will typically have large joint effusions but may not have other systemic symptoms such as fever. Joint aspirate will reveal an inflammatory pattern with a predominance of PMNs. Although *B. burgdorferi* is difficult to culture from the synovial fluid, PCR testing may provide more accurate results when performed prior to the initiation of antibiotic therapy. Synovial fluid analysis and culture should be used to help exclude other etiologies, including septic arthritis. Lyme serologies (IgM and IgG) may be helpful in the outpatient setting but are of little utility in the ED. Routine lab testing is otherwise unhelpful.

Management

Prophylaxis against Lyme disease is not typically recommended unless an engorged *Ixodes* tick is found attached to a patient for greater than 24 to 36 hours in a Lyme-endemic area. In such cases, a single dose of doxycycline 200 mg PO (4.4 mg/kg in children) is recommended for prophylaxis. In the acute phase of disease, when patients present with rash, myalgias, or arthralgias, the treatment is doxycycline 100 mg PO twice daily for 10 days. Lyme arthritis is treated with a 28-day course of doxycycline 100 mg PO twice daily. Amoxicillin 50 mg/kg/day divided every 8 hours (max 500 mg per dose) may be substituted for doxycycline in children, pregnant women, or the setting of tetracycline allergy. IV therapy, typically with a second- or third-generation cephalosporin (e.g., ceftriaxone 2 g IV daily), is reserved for patients with moderate or severe, persistent arthritis despite adequate oral antibiotic therapy. A small subset of patients may experience ongoing symptoms even after appropriate therapy, but a more prolonged course of antibiotics is unlikely to be beneficial.[18]

Acute Rheumatic Fever

Foundations

Acute rheumatic fever (ARF) is a complex systemic disease triggered by a hyperimmune response that follows pharyngitis due to group A streptococcal infection. The cellular and humoral response to the infection affects joints as well as cardiac tissue. The incidence of ARF has declined in recent years due to several factors including improved hygiene, increased antibiotic use, and mutations in prevalent group A *Streptococcus* strains. The worldwide incidence may be as high as 20 per 100,000, but in the United States and other developed nations the incidence is less than 2 per 100,000. In certain indigenous populations, including Australia and New Zealand, the incidence among children aged 5 to 14 years is significantly higher.

Clinical Features

The diagnosis of ARF is based on the Jones Criteria and the presence of two major criteria and one or more of the minor criteria (Table 102.10). Laboratory evidence of antecedent group A streptococcal infection is also required. Arthritis occurs in up to 75% of patients with ARF and presents as a migratory polyarthritis typically affecting the large joints and lasting 2 to 3 days per joint. Joints may appear inflamed and patients often display pain out of proportion to the apparent severity of the arthritis.

Diagnostic Testing

The value of laboratory testing for ARF is limited in the ED setting. Evaluation of synovial fluid reveals a sterile, inflammatory pattern. If suspected, obtain formal two-dimensional (2D) echo and Doppler imaging to evaluate for cardiac involvement.

Management

Recommended treatment of ARF includes IM benzathine penicillin 1.2 million units or a 10-day course of oral penicillin (penicillin V 500

TABLE 102.10   Jones Criteria for Rheumatic Fever

Major Criteria	Minor Criteria
Joint pain (polyarthritis)	Arthralgia
Carditis (echo/Doppler used to diagnose)	Fever
	Elevated erythrocyte sedimentation rate (ESR)
Subcutaneous nodules	(>60 mm) or C-reactive protein (CRP)
Erythema marginatum	(>3.0 mg/dL)
Sydenham chorea	Prolonged PR interval

Two major criteria or one major with two minor criteria required for diagnosis. Also requires either elevated streptococcal antibody titer or positive throat culture/rapid streptococcus test.

mg PO 3 times daily for 10 days or amoxicillin 500 mg PO twice daily for 10 days). Oral clarithromycin 250 mg PO twice daily for 10 days may be used in penicillin-allergic patients. High-dose NSAIDs, such as oral aspirin 50 to 100 mg/kg/day divided into four daily doses may be used to treat arthritis and fever but do not have an effect on the cardiac sequelae. Small studies have suggested that oral or IM corticosteroids such as hydrocortisone 1 to 2 mg/kg/day PO slowly tapered over 2 to 4 weeks may be better than aspirin in patients with cardiac involvement. Recurrence may occur at a rate of 8% to 10% within 5 years; and monthly antibiotic prophylaxis with oral or IM penicillin for at least 5 years, or until adulthood, is recommended.

CHRONIC POLYARTHRITIS

Rheumatoid Arthritis

Foundations

Although RA is typically a chronic condition with insidious onset and progression, approximately 20% of patients with RA present with acute exacerbations. With a worldwide prevalence of approximately 1%, incidence peaks between the ages of 35 and 50 years, and the condition is approximately 3 times more common in women. It is characterized by immune complexes that stimulate PMN cells to produce and release enzymes that lead to joint destruction. Over time, the number of synovial cells dramatically increases, leading to progressive release of inflammatory substances and progressive joint damage.

Clinical Features

At the time of initial diagnosis, patients may report weeks or months of fatigue, weakness, malaise, and joint pain, with or without associated fevers or weight loss. Over time, joint pain, swelling, and inflammation may progress often starting symmetrically in the proximal interphalangeal (PIP) and MCP joints of the hands, associated with stiffness that is worse in the morning. Over time, patients with RA may develop persistent symmetric polyarthritis of hands and feet, progressive articular deterioration with characteristic deformities including ulnar deviation, swan neck, and boutonniere deformities of the hands (Figs. 102.9 and 102.10). Patients may also have associated tenosynovitis and signs of extra-articular disease, including constitutional symptoms and difficulty performing activities of daily living. During an acute exacerbation, patients may present with only warm, swollen, or tender joints, which may be difficult to differentiate from other arthritides.

Diagnostic Testing

In the emergency setting, the evaluation of a patient with known or suspected RA should be directed at identifying other possible causes of acute arthritis, particularly septic arthritis. An elevated ESR and CRP may be seen in patients with either acute or chronic disease and remain nonspecific findings. Early radiographic findings are similarly nonspecific and include soft-tissue swelling or joint-space narrowing; subluxation or other bony deformities are late findings (see Fig 102.10). Synovial fluid analysis tends to reveal a nonspecific inflammatory pattern, although it may be useful in excluding crystal arthropathy or acute infection in selected patients.

Management

Care of patients with RA includes both pharmacologic and nonpharmacologic therapies. Pharmacologic options include NSAIDs, both biologic and nonbiologic disease-modifying antirheumatologic drugs (DMARDs), immunosuppressants, and corticosteroids. In acute exacerbations, relative rest and antiinflammatory medications are appropriate, including NSAIDs or low-dose systemic corticosteroids. Short-term use of additional analgesic medication may also be required.

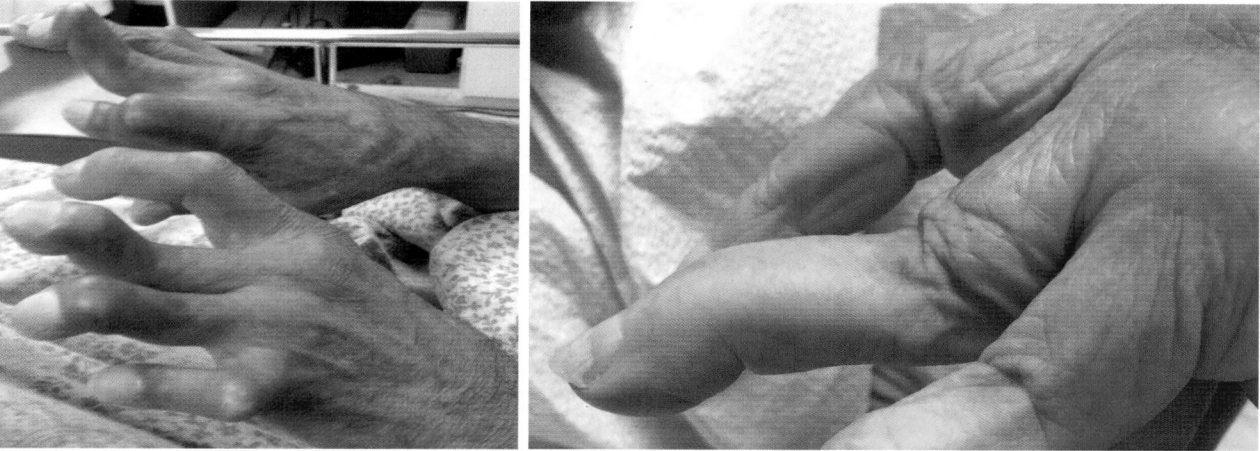

Fig. 102.9 Example of severe deformities including swan neck deformity of multiple digits in poorly controlled rheumatoid arthritis.

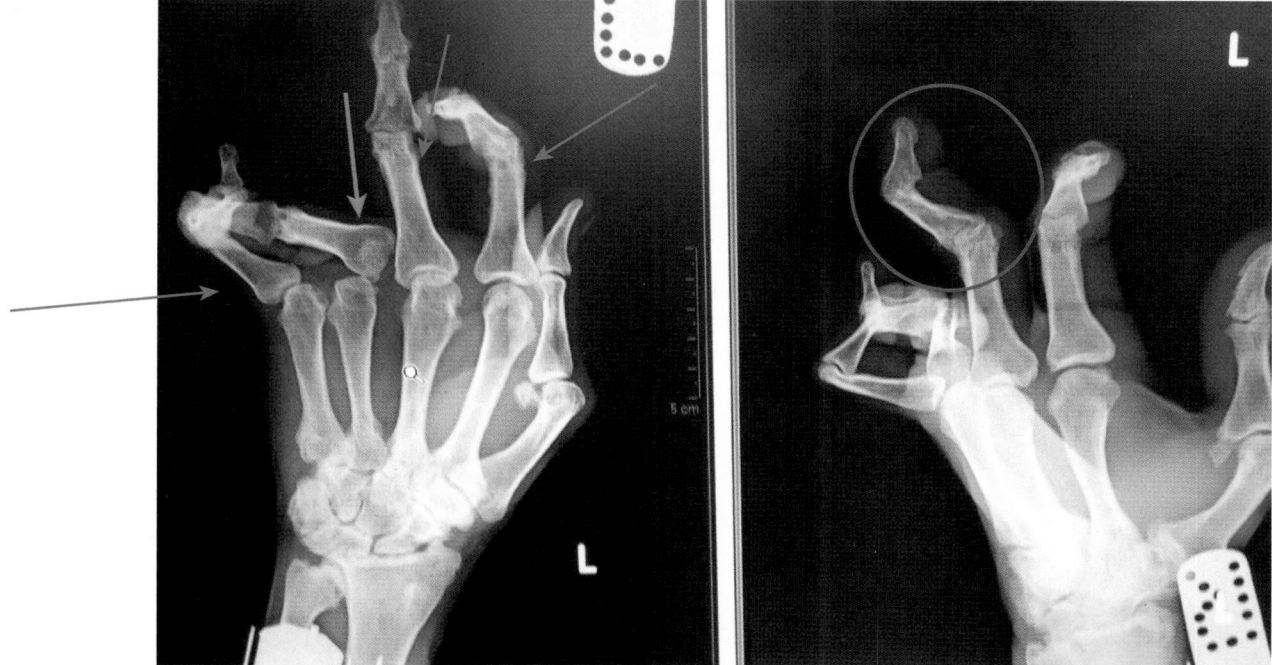

Fig. 102.10 X-ray demonstrating severe deformities associated with long-standing untreated rheumatoid arthritis. Note profound ulnar deviation *(small arrows)*, joint subluxations *(large arrow)*, and swan neck deformity *(circle)*.

Studies have shown that biologic agents may be the most effective option in patients who have failed other treatments as well as in patients who have not yet been started on any chronic maintenance therapy for their RA. Early initiation of biologic or nonbiologic DMARDs has become routine as they can lead to remission of symptoms as well as limit progression of disease. Nonpharmacologic interventions are generally directed at long-term mitigation of symptoms and include interventions such as exercise, diet, stress reduction, cryotherapy, physical therapy, massage, or surgery including synovectomy, arthroplasty, or arthrodesis.

Seronegative Spondyloarthropathies
Foundations
The seronegative spondyloarthropathies are a broad category of conditions that share the clinical features of sacroiliac joint involvement and inflammatory arthropathy affecting multiple distal/peripheral joints with pathologic changes seen at the entheses (ligament and tendon insertion sites, see Fig. 102.1). Rheumatoid factor is typically absent, and HLA-B27 may be positive. The most common of these conditions include ankylosing spondylitis (AS), reactive arthritis, psoriatic

arthritis, and arthropathy associated with inflammatory bowel disease, so-called enteropathic arthritis.

Ankylosing Spondylitis

Clinical features. Patients with AS are more likely to be male and younger (younger than 40 years of age) and often report chronic back pain with insidious onset. This may be associated with radiographic evidence of sacroiliitis or the characteristic "bamboo spine," as well as extra-articular disease, most commonly uveitis. Urethritis and vasculitis may also occur, including potentially life-threatening disease affecting the aortic root. Up to 30% of patients may have associated enthesopathies such as plantar fasciitis or Achilles tendinopathy.

Management. Acute therapies are directed at managing pain and reducing inflammation. Therefore analgesics and antiinflammatory medications are appropriate. Biologic or nonbiologic DMARD therapy will be appropriate for chronic management and to prevent disease progression.

Reactive Arthritis (Formerly Termed Reiter Syndrome)

Clinical features. Reactive arthritis, formerly termed Reiter syndrome, generally occurs in patients 20 to 40 years of age following infection with *Chlamydia, Salmonella, Shigella, Yersinia,* or *Campylobacter* species, with symptoms of arthritis presenting 2 to 6 weeks after an episode of dysentery, or cervicitis/urethritis in the case of *Chlamydia* species. The condition presents with asymmetric polyarticular pain, often affecting joints of the lower extremities. Associated conjunctivitis, uveitis, or oral ulcers may also be seen.

Diagnostic testing. In reactive arthritis, synovial fluid demonstrates an inflammatory pattern. The joint fluid is sterile, although antigen testing for *Chlamydia, Salmonella,* or *Yersinia* may be positive. Radiographs may reveal abnormalities at tendon insertion sites.

Management. Patients with reactive arthritis respond well to antiinflammatory treatment with NSAIDs. Antibiotics may be appropriate in patients with *Chlamydia* but have not been shown to improve the clinical course in patients with reactive arthritis following dysentery.

Psoriatic Arthritis

Psoriatic arthropathy may occur in 20% of patients with psoriasis, causing a range of clinical presentations such as asymmetric oligoarthropathy, symmetric polyarthropathy, spondylitis, distal interphalangeal (DIP) joint involvement—in distinction from other rheumatoid conditions that tend to affect the PIP or MCP joints—or arthritis mutilans, a particularly severe condition in which there is evidence of bone resorption with associated collapse of the soft tissue. First-line treatment is with NSAIDs, and local corticosteroid injections may also be considered. There is little evidence for systemic steroid use, and DMARDs are often initiated early.

Enteropathic Arthritis

Up to 40% of patients with inflammatory bowel disease will experience musculoskeletal manifestations. This may present as an acute, asymmetric, migratory, inflammatory polyarthritis, commonly affecting the knees. The acute exacerbations of joint pain often accompany acute flares of GI symptoms. Although NSAIDs are first-line treatment for joint pain, they may exacerbate GI symptoms. Sulfasalazine and intra-articular corticosteroid injections are alternatives for symptom management.

Other conditions such as fibromyalgia, polymyalgia rheumatica, and scleroderma may also have characteristic musculoskeletal pain and joint stiffness. These conditions tend to cause more widespread pain, rarely present with acute arthropathy or joint effusions, and do not represent a true arthritis.

The references for this chapter can be found online at ExpertConsult. com.

103

Tendinopathy and Bursitis

Christopher Hogrefe and Emily M. Jones

KEY CONCEPTS

Tendinopathy

- Mechanical overload and repetitive microtrauma are key underlying mechanisms in the development of tendinopathy. Patients most often present with a history of progressively worsening localized pain after repetitive work- or sports-related activities.
- Tendinopathy may also be associated with nonmechanical causes, including systemic manifestations of diseases, infectious etiologies, and the use of fluoroquinolones or statins.
- Most patients with tendinopathy can initially be treated with conservative measures, such as activity modification/protection, icing, medications (e.g., short-term use of nonsteroidal antiinflammatory drugs [NSAIDs] or nitroglycerin patches for certain tendinopathies), bracing/splinting, ergonomic modifications, and graduated exercises.
- Overuse syndromes can take at least 6 to 12 weeks to heal. Advise patients accordingly and provide appropriate referral for follow-up to a musculoskeletal specialist (e.g., a sports medicine, orthopedic, or physical medicine and rehabilitation specialist).
- Emergent imaging may be indicated in the ED when fracture or a condition such as calcific tendinopathy is suspected. The use of point-of-care ultrasound to evaluate tendinopathy can help to identify tendon disruption/rupture.

- Operative treatment may be indicated for selected cases of tendon injury that require primary repair (e.g., rupture of the Achilles tendon) or that have failed to respond to conservative treatment (e.g., rotator cuff tendinopathy).

Bursitis

- Consider the possibility of an infectious cause in all cases of acute bursitis.
- The definitive diagnosis of bursitis is made by aspiration of the bursa and evaluation of the fluid.
- Septic bursitis is most commonly caused by *Staphylococcus aureus*.
- Nonseptic bursitis may be traumatic, rheumatologic (e.g., gout and pseudogout), or idiopathic in nature. It is prudent to consider other conditions, such as septic arthritis, osteomyelitis, or an underlying fracture, in the differential diagnosis of bursitis.
- The management of bursitis includes treatment with appropriate medication (antibiotics for septic bursitis, NSAIDs for nonseptic bursitis), rest, application of ice, compression, elevation, and prompt referral for appropriate follow-up. Hospitalization should be considered for severe local infections, for patients who are immunosuppressed, and in the presence of systemic toxicity.

TENDINOPATHY

Foundations

Background and Importance

Tendons are collagenous, dynamic structures that connect muscle to bone. They transmit forces originating in muscles to bone by stiffening, thereby enabling joint motion. *Tendinopathy* is an umbrella term that also encompasses tendinitis and tendinosis. The diagnosis of *tendinitis,* a commonly used term implying "inflammation of the tendon," has long been associated with numerous overuse injuries. Many practitioners now advocate use of the term *tendinosis* as a more accurate reflection of the pathologic process, representing a degenerative process without evidence of inflammation. To date, reliable, well-conducted epidemiologic studies have not been performed for most tendinopathies; however, histopathologic analysis often reveals degenerative tendon pathology with few inflammatory cells. This chapter will utilize the term *tendinopathy,* referring to a painful, impaired tendon that encompasses the various pathologic processes.

Approximately 30% of all musculoskeletal evaluations performed in the emergency department (ED) or urgent care settings are attributed to tendinopathy, and the incidence is rising. A contributing factor is the increasing level of daily participation in athletics and fitness-related activities, up 3.6% across a recent 12-year period.[1] Nearly half of all sports participants will be injured at some point, with up to 50% of injuries involving tendinopathy. For instance, with approximately 1.5% of the population running on a daily basis the number of affected runners accumulates quickly.[1] One study found that over one year, 27% of novice runners, 32% of long distance runners, and 52% of marathon participants sustained injuries with the majority related to overuse.[2] In another investigation, 70% of professional and 25% of youth basketball injuries were due to tendinopathy.[3]

Exercise is not the only culprit precipitating tendinopathy, however. Occupational exposures are a prominent cause of tendinopathy, resulting from lower demand, highly repetitive tasks (contrasted with higher demand, explosive sporting activities). Professions that involve repetitive motion, localized contact stress, awkward positions, vibrations, or forceful exertion are more likely to result in overuse injury such as tendinopathy. Shoulder tendinopathies are particularly common in the workplace, representing up to 13.6% of all musculoskeletal complaints regardless of one's occupation.[4] The nature of such work is further

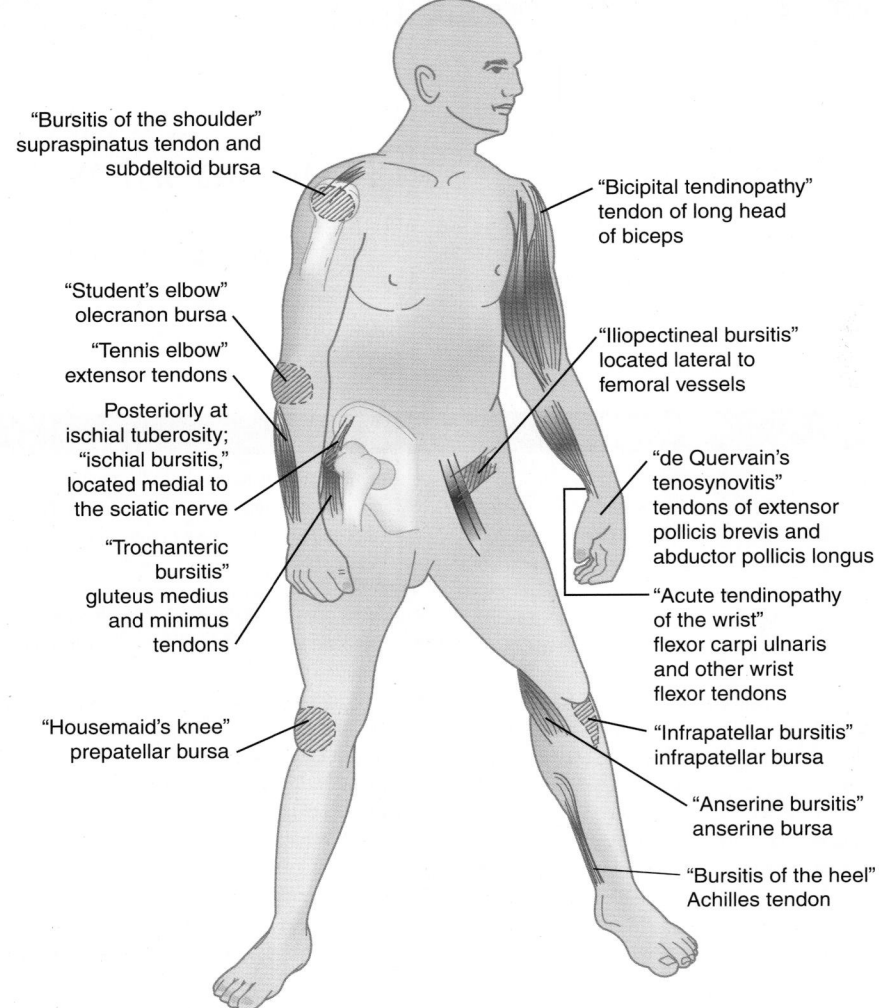

"Bursitis of the shoulder"
supraspinatus tendon and
subdeltoid bursa

"Bicipital tendinopathy"
tendon of long head
of biceps

"Student's elbow"
olecranon bursa

"Tennis elbow"
extensor tendons

Posteriorly at
ischial tuberosity;
"ischial bursitis,"
located medial to
the sciatic nerve

"Trochanteric
bursitis"
gluteus medius
and minimus
tendons

"Housemaid's knee"
prepatellar bursa

"Iliopectineal bursitis"
located lateral to
femoral vessels

"de Quervain's
tenosynovitis"
tendons of extensor
pollicis brevis and
abductor pollicis longus

"Acute tendinopathy
of the wrist"
flexor carpi ulnaris
and other wrist
flexor tendons

"Infrapatellar bursitis"
infrapatellar bursa

"Anserine bursitis"
anserine bursa

"Bursitis of the heel"
Achilles tendon

Fig. 103.1 Location of common sites for tendinopathy or bursitis. (Modified from Branch WT. *Office Practice of Medicine*, ed 2. Philadelphia: Saunders; 1987.)

compounded by longevity; those working 25 to 35 years are 7.1 times more likely to develop tendinopathy. The economic end result is staggering, with an estimate of nearly $800 billion in health care costs over a 3-year span attributed to these conditions.[5] Furthermore, for all non-fatal injuries in the United States (U.S.), tendinopathies account for the fifth most days away from work, totaling on average 14 days (with only fracture-related injuries accounting for more lost days of work).[6] Ergonomic and medical intervention programs may reduce the incidence of work-related injuries and decrease their socioeconomic impact.

Aside from the acute pain and functional limitations, tendinopathies often become chronic (i.e., greater than 3 months in duration) and can be disabling. Patients may experience symptoms for extended periods despite appropriate therapy and recurrence is common, affecting 49% of athletes with patellar tendinopathy.[7] Meanwhile, 40% to 50% of patients with rotator cuff tendinopathy exhibit symptoms at 6 to 12 months.[8]

Mechanical overload and repetitive microtrauma to the musculotendinous unit are thought to be the major precipitating causes of most tendinopathies. While the affected tendon is primarily under tensile overload, compression of the tendon occurs as well (e.g., fiber bundles contacting each other or friction/shearing against bone). Broadly, there are intrinsic and extrinsic factors that modify the pathophysiologic state of the tendon. Intrinsic factors such as age, gender, blood type O, adiposity, tobacco use, malalignment, joint laxity, muscle weakness, and imbalance can result in excessively high or frequent mechanical loads during normal activity. Extrinsic factors such as ergonomics, equipment changes, abnormal movements, excessive duration of activity, increased frequency or intensity of activity, and environmental conditions can also contribute to the development of tendinopathy.

Other potential contributing etiologies include excessive protein intake, systemic disease (e.g., coronary artery disease, diabetes mellitus, and gout), or medication use. An increased incidence of tendinopathy and tendon rupture, particularly of the Achilles tendon, has been attributed to fluoroquinolone antibiotics. This risk appears greatest within the first month of use, in those over age 60 years, in patients receiving corticosteroid treatment (4.68-fold increase for all tendons and 14.72-fold increase for Achilles tendon rupture), and in those with renal disease.[9] Statins have been implicated as contributing to tendinopathy as well (2% incidence), although simvastatin is thought to actually decrease this risk.[10] Overall, most tendinopathies are multifactorial in origin. Several of the common areas affected by tendinopathy are shown in Fig. 103.1.

Under optimal conditions, such as appropriately graduated athletic training, the musculotendinous units adapt to tension overload. This results from the ability of bone to increase its load-bearing capacity combined with an increase in size and strength generated by the hypertrophy of existing muscle fibers. An enhancement of tendon and ligament strength occurs through an increase in collagen content, collagen cross-linking, and mucopolysaccharide content. Unfortunately, many athletes may not allow sufficient time for this adaptive process to occur. For example, a soccer player may increase the number of games played, the duration of time per game played, participation intensity, or any combination of these factors with haste, restricting the cellular changes required to adapt to the increased stress. Poor running technique, suboptimal playing surfaces, environmental conditions, or improper equipment (particularly footwear) may also contribute to the development of an overuse syndrome.

Pathophysiology

The pathophysiologic mechanism of tendon healing has mainly been described in the context of acute injury (e.g., rupture), and correlation to the healing process in tendinopathy remains under investigation. Acutely injured tendons go through several stages in the healing process, starting with the hemorrhagic phase as blood accumulates and clots at the site of injury. The inflammatory stage then follows as neutrophils and macrophages initiate phagocytosis, removing the existing necrotic material. Healing then progresses to the proliferative phase where extrinsic cells (e.g., tendon sheath, fascia, periosteum) and intrinsic cells migrate and proliferate at the injured tendon.[11] At this point, type III collagen is synthesized, which tends to be thinner and possesses less tensile strength than the tendon's original type I collagen. The process then advances to the formative stage, which can last upwards of 2 months. In this stage, collagen fibers mature and orient themselves to handle tension forces. Finally, the remodeling phase features a shift toward the normalization of the ratio between type I and type III collagen followed by the reintroduction of physiologic load into the tendon.[11] It may take up to 12 weeks for the tendon to regain its former strength. As the healing process ensues, unrestricted activity is generally avoided. However, atrophy associated with immobilization should also be avoided as the strength in healing tendons and ligaments increases more rapidly when controlled forces are applied. Consequently, optimal loading is now advocated as a means of advancing from rest to a balanced, incremental rehabilitation program. Such rehabilitation focuses on flexibility forces, core strengthening, eccentric strength training, and a measured return to resistive exercises so long as pain is minimal. Most patients with overuse tendinopathies fully recover within 3 to 6 months.

Clinical Features

General Tendinopathy

The history of the patient presenting with a tendinopathy can vary, although certain clinical features are characteristic. Recent repetitive stress may be reported due to work activities, changes in the workplace environment, or alterations in sport or recreational activities. It is important to ask patients to consider the weeks to months preceding the onset of symptoms to identify a potential inciting event or change (e.g., workplace ergonomics, protective footwear, new sports equipment). Occasionally, no cause is identified for a mechanical overload. A history of fluoroquinolone therapy, statin use, infectious disease, or other systemic illness (e.g., coronary artery disease, diabetes mellitus, gout) should also be obtained as initial presentations of rheumatologic disorders or infections, such as those from *Mycobacterium,* have been described.

Nonradiating, increasing pain at the site of the affected tendon is the most common presenting symptom of tendinopathy. The discomfort is frequently described as more severe following periods of rest. Unlike

BOX 103.1 Differential Diagnosis for Tendinopathy

Tendon rupture
Ligamentous injury
Inflammatory arthritis (e.g., rheumatoid)
Fractures (e.g., avulsion, stress)
Tumors
Tenosynovitis
Osteochondrosis (e.g., Osgood-Schlatter disease)
Bursitis
Septic arthritis
Osteoarthritis
Foreign bodies
Rhabdomyolysis
Osteomyelitis
Nerve entrapment syndromes
Tendon sheath infections (e.g., pyogenic)

the discomfort of morning stiffness associated with arthritis, the pain of tendinopathy may resolve after initial movement only to be manifested as a throbbing pain after the cessation of exercise. Individuals may report similar prior episodes, whereas continued episodes may be accompanied by increased pain severity. Consequently, it may be helpful to inquire about a related previous diagnosis, how it was made, and which treatments (if any) were effective in resolving the prior episode.

When evaluating a patient suspected to have tendinopathy, a thorough, directed musculoskeletal examination offers valuable diagnostic information. Edema, swelling, erythema, atrophy, deformity, asymmetry, or visible signs of trauma may be identified. Palpate the tendon, noting warmth or crepitus (particularly with movement), or tenderness over the tendon, especially when localized and reproducing the patient's pain. Although tendon palpation can be sensitive for reproducing tendinopathy-related symptoms, it is nonspecific in determining the affected structure. Check for underlying bone tenderness and consider the differential diagnoses listed in Box 103.1. Motor function (particularly passive and active range of motion), strength (and evidence of weakness or pain), and joint involvement/stability should be noted.

In narrowing the diagnosis, it is important to determine whether the source of pain is articular (within the joint capsule) or periarticular (around the joint capsule). Arthritis typically produces generalized joint pain, warmth, swelling, and diffuse tenderness. The discomfort of arthritis increases with both passive and active motion of the joint. Conversely, the pain of a tendinopathy tends to be more localized. Tenderness and swelling do not occur uniformly across the joint, and pain may be produced only with certain movements, particularly with resisted active contraction or passive stretching of the affected muscles or tendons. Mechanical hyperalgesia (i.e., increased pain with passive and active range of motion) may reduce the specificity of the commonly used clinical tests discussed later in this chapter.

Specific Tendinopathies

Shoulder. Tendinopathies of the shoulder joint include impingement syndrome (which includes subacromial bursitis or rotator cuff tendinopathy), bicipital tendinopathy, calcific tendinopathy, and adhesive capsulitis (frozen shoulder syndrome).

Impingement Syndrome and Rotator Cuff Tendinopathies. The shoulder joint is predisposed to soft tissue injury because of its extensive range of motion and unique anatomic structure (Fig. 103.2). Although inherently unstable, the muscles of the rotator cuff (supraspinatus,

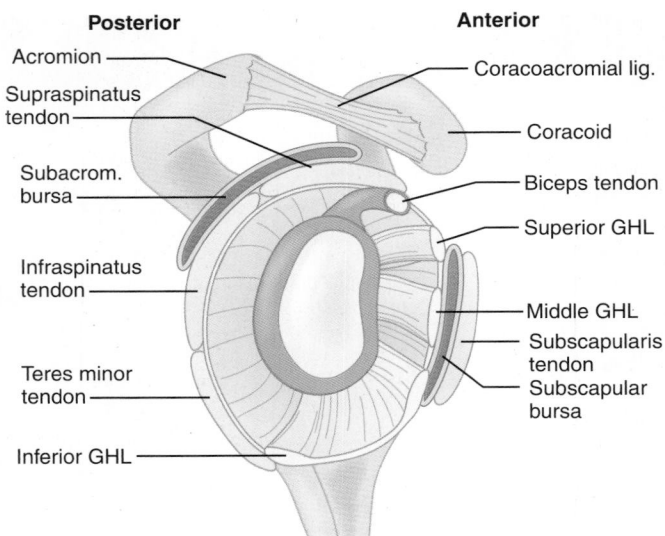

Fig. 103.2 Anatomy of the shoulder rotator cuff and supporting ligaments. *GHL,* Glenohumeral.

infraspinatus, teres minor, and subscapularis) and the glenohumeral ligaments (GHL) stabilize the joint. The muscles of the rotator cuff originate from the scapula and their tendinous insertions are found on the fibrous capsule of the glenohumeral joint after traversing through the subacromial space. The presence of the subacromial bursa serves to ensure fluidity of movement though may become inflamed as a part of an impingement syndrome.[12] Impingement of the tendons occurs because of their position interposed between the humeral head and the acromion. The functional arc of the elevated shoulder is forward and in the anterior plane. As a result of this position, the greater tuberosity of the humerus may compress (impinge) the tendons of the rotator cuff (usually the supraspinatus) against the undersurface of the anterior third of the acromion. Additionally, the long head of the biceps may be involved in impingement syndrome due to its location between the supraspinatus and subscapularis tendons in the rotator interval. This compressive component may combine with tensile loads on the rotator cuff to predispose patients to a chronic tendinopathy. Development of this tendinopathy may be the result of overuse of the extremity that leads to microtrauma of the tendinous fibers, individual anatomic differences (congenital or from the process of aging, such as osteophytic changes), or both. Other entities that may coexist and complicate an impingement syndrome include subacromial bursitis, bicipital tendinopathy, or calcific tendinopathy.

Ninety-five percent of rotator cuff tears are associated with impingement, exclusive of tears due to a one-time traumatic event. Three progressive stages of impingement syndrome as a result of overuse have been described. The first stage is frequently seen in athletes younger than 25 years of age who participate in sports that require repetitive overhead motions of the shoulder (e.g., swimming, volleyball, baseball). The pain is usually described as a dull ache over the anterolateral shoulder, extending from the shoulder to the middle upper arm, often occurring after an activity involving flexion and abduction of the arm. Point tenderness may be elicited over the greater tuberosity without the presence of weakness or loss of motion. This condition is generally believed to be reversible with appropriate treatment. In the second stage, as mechanical trauma continues, fibrosis and thickening of the tendon and subacromial bursa can occur. This generally affects patients between 25 and 40 years of age. The pain becomes constant and may worsen at night. Active motion may be limited by pain and any activity

involving overhead movement can exacerbate the symptoms. Passive range of motion is generally preserved and on physical examination the pain is more diffuse and intense. The third stage resembles the second stage but may also involve a prolonged history of shoulder problems. At this point, the range of motion of the shoulder is usually decreased owing to either disuse or a partial rotator cuff tear. On pathologic examination, tendon degeneration may be present. Partial-thickness tears may occur or extend with stress or minor trauma. Complete tears of the rotator cuff, biceps tendon rupture, or osteophytic bone changes are sometimes seen.

Specific physical examination maneuvers can exacerbate the symptoms of shoulder impingement and suggest a diagnosis of rotator cuff tendinopathy. Because the supraspinatus tendon is most often involved, the *empty can test* (describing the position of the arm and hand as one empties an aluminum can, also referred to as the *Jobe sign*) is helpful in assessing the supraspinatus tendon via resistance testing. With the arm abducted at 90° in the scapular plane (30° anterior to the coronal plane), the arm is internally rotated with the thumb pointed downward. The examiner places a downward force on the distal upper extremity and the patient is instructed to resist the examiner and to keep the arm parallel to the floor (Fig. 103.3A). Weakness or pain is considered a positive finding. When assessing for supraspinatus tendinopathy, the empty can test has a sensitivity of 62% with a specificity of 54%. If the patient is unable to resist the force of the examiner, a supraspinatus tear should be suspected.

Another sign of rotator cuff tendinopathy is elicited by the *Neer test,* which suggests mechanical impingement due to a decrease of the subacromial space. The examiner forward flexes the arm to 180°, which causes impingement of the greater tuberosity of the humerus against the anterior and inferior edge of the acromion. A positive result elicits pain produced at the end range of the arc. Studies assessing the utility of this test report significant variability, with sensitivities ranging from 75% to 86% and specificities from 48% to 49%.

The *Hawkins-Kennedy test,* also indicative of mechanical shoulder impingement, is performed by forcibly internally rotating the proximal humerus while the shoulder is forward flexed to 90° and the elbow flexed to 90°. Pain with this maneuver constitutes a positive finding. Again, there is fluctuation in the literature regarding this test's sensitivity (75% to 82%) and specificity (44% to 48%).

A complete rotator cuff tear can be evaluated via the *drop arm test,* in which the arm is passively abducted at 90° and the patient is asked to slowly maintain control of the arm while adducting it (i.e., returning the arm to one's side) (Fig. 103.3B). If the arm drops to the side, a significant rotator cuff tear should be considered. Previous studies suggest that this test is 74% sensitive, although more recent literature reported a 10% sensitivity for full-thickness supraspinatus tears. The specificity is much better, cited as 98%. The *shrug sign* is exhibited when a patient with acute macrotrauma to the rotator cuff is asked to abduct the arm at 90° and appears to be giving a shrug with that side. This movement stems from the rotator cuff's inability to assist in abducting the arm. While such a finding may be secondary to other shoulder pathology (e.g., glenohumeral osteoarthritis or adhesive capsulitis), a positive result may suggest rotator cuff pathology.

Bicipital Tendinopathy. The tendon of the long head of the biceps, given its passage between the supraspinatus and subscapularis tendons in the anterior shoulder, can be associated with impingement syndrome. Patients with bicipital tendinopathy may describe pain in the anterior shoulder radiating to the elbow. Discomfort may occur when the individual rolls onto the shoulder at night, attempts to reach into a pocket, or turns a door handle. Focal tenderness may be provoked via direct palpation of the groove between the greater and lesser tuberosities of the anterior humerus. While the sensitivity (57%

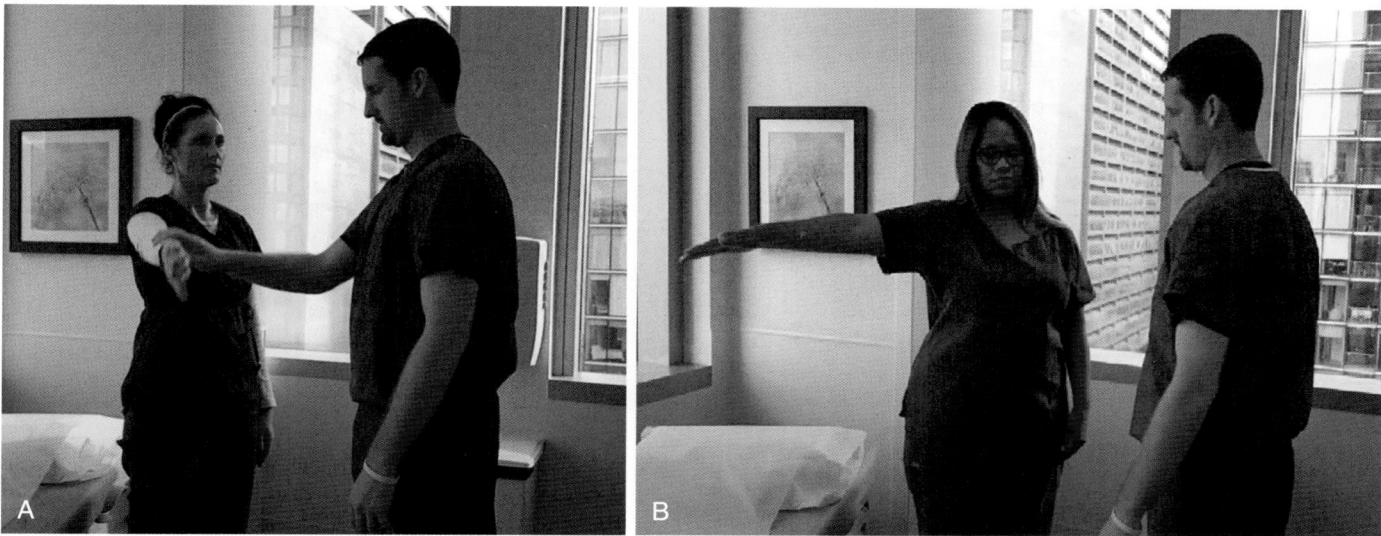

Fig. 103.3 Illustrations of the proper positioning for (A) *empty can test* and (B) *drop arm test* when assessing for rotator cuff tendinopathy or a rotator cuff tear.

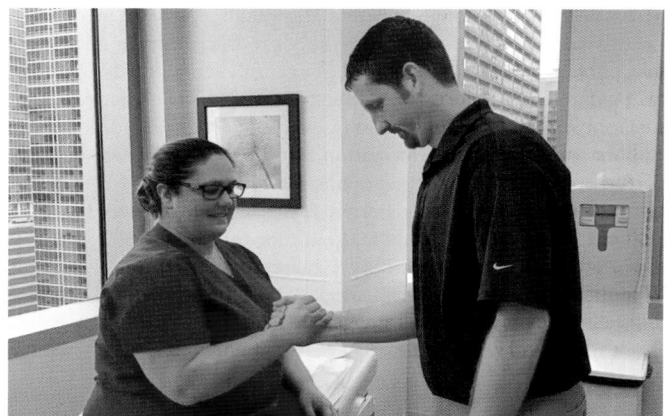

Fig. 103.4 A depiction of the *Yergason test* in the evaluation of biceps tendinopathy, which entails resisting a patient's supination.

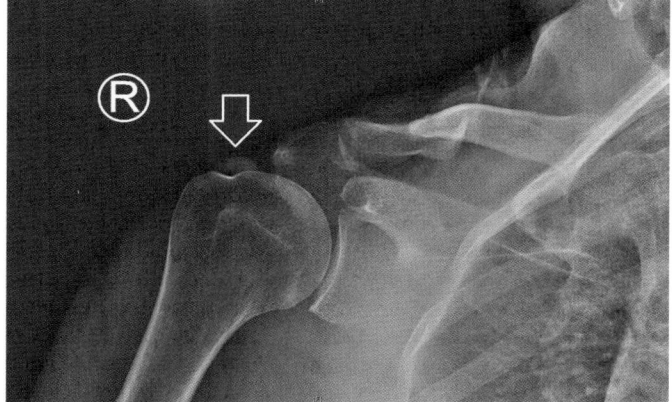

Fig. 103.5 Plain films of the right shoulder revealing a prominent calcium deposit in the supraspinatus tendon resulting in acute pain and decreased range of motion secondary to calcific tendinopathy.

to 85%) and specificity (49% to 72%) of this finding suggest that the test has utility, the accuracy of a clinician in directly palpating the long head of the biceps tendon has been questioned.[13] This accuracy can be further enhanced with the use of ultrasound.[14] The *Yergason sign* can also assist in the diagnosis of bicipital tendinopathy. This test is performed by having the patient flex the elbow to 90° with the arm against the body and the provider resisting the individual's forearm supination (Fig. 103.4). Pain in the area of the proximal tendon is considered a positive finding and indicative of biceps tendinopathy. Although the sensitivity is low (37%), the specificity (83%) and positive likelihood ratio (2.20) of this test are stronger.[15]

Another physical examination tool in the diagnosis of bicipital tendinopathy is *Speed's test*. With the elbow extended, the forearm supinated (i.e., palm facing upward), and the shoulder adducted at 60°, the patient is instructed to resist forward flexion of the shoulder. Pain in the area of the bicipital groove is indicative of a positive finding. Although Speed's test may be suggestive of glenohumeral labral pathology as well, meta-analyses suggest that it is more sensitive (61% to 83%) for bicipital tendinopathy with similar specificity (33% to 71%).[13,15]

Calcific Tendinopathy. Calcific tendinopathy is an acutely or chronically painful condition associated with the deposition of

calcium crystals in or around tendons. Although it can impact any tendon, the condition appears to be more prevalent in the rotator cuff. The underlying cause is still debated though has been attributed to tissue hypoxia and degeneration due to overuse. More common in females, studies have shown an association with diabetes mellitus, thyroid disorders, and nephrolithiasis along with a potential genetic predisposition. While it can affect any of the rotator cuff tendons, it seems to have a predilection for the supraspinatus, up to 80% of the time. The symptoms are similar to those of an impingement syndrome and the condition generally affects individuals between the ages of 30 and 60 years. Calcium deposition occurs over time and then undergoes spontaneous resorption. This resorptive phase is thought to contribute to the observed pain, though the severity of the symptoms is not correlated with the size of the deposit. Pain is believed to be in response to the local chemical pathologic disorder or direct mechanical irritation. On physical examination, there may be specific tenderness over the greater tuberosity as well as symptoms consistent with impingement. Plain film radiographs may show calcification in or around the rotator cuff tendons (Fig. 103.5). The presence of calcium in the tendon does not necessarily confirm the origin of the pain because

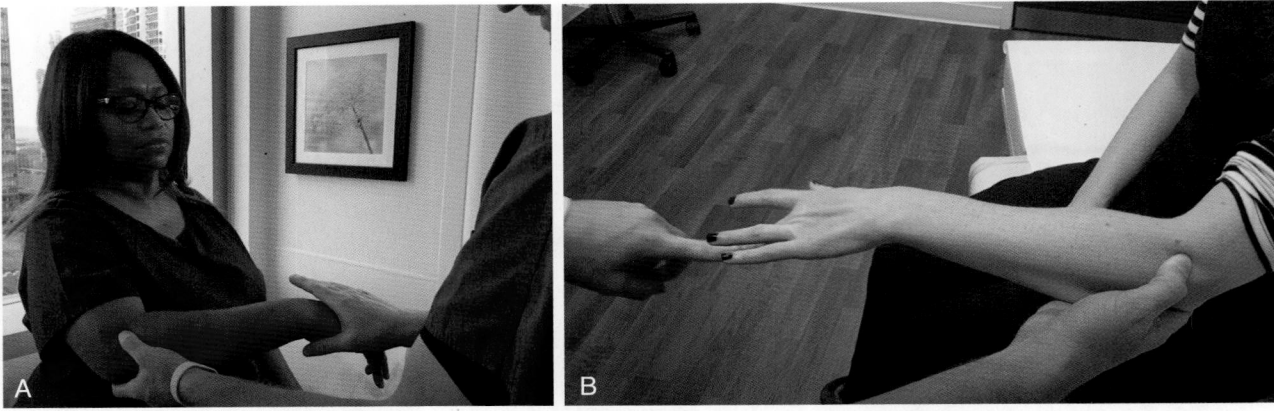

Fig. 103.6 When evaluating for lateral epicondylitis, (A) *Cozen's test* and (B) *Maudsley's test* may aid in confirming the diagnosis.

asymptomatic patients may demonstrate evidence of calcification on a routine radiograph. Ultrasound has proven useful in both the diagnosis and treatment (i.e., percutaneous needle lavage) of calcific tendinopathy.

Elbow. Increasingly, athletes of all ages and skill levels are participating in sports involving overhead arm motions. Consequently, the incidence of elbow injuries is rising. Such maladies also result from everyday life, including household chores and workplace exposures. From an anatomic and functional perspective, the extensors and supinators of the wrist attach to the lateral elbow, and the flexors and pronators attach medially.

Lateral Epicondylitis. Lateral epicondylitis ("tennis elbow") is a painful elbow condition that occurs at the insertion of the common extensor tendon (extensor carpi radialis brevis) onto the lateral epicondyle of the humerus. Although it occurs in many tennis players, epidemiologic studies suggest that less than 5% of patients with such a syndrome actually play tennis. Activities such as turning screws, using a wrench, and repetitive work on an assembly line have also been implicated. In fact, the prevalence of lateral epicondylitis in the workforce approaches 14.5%.[16] Symptoms often begin as a dull ache along the lateral aspect of the elbow. The discomfort can be exacerbated by activities that involve extension or supination of the wrist, such as grasping and twisting. *Cozen's test* is performed by grasping the patient's forearm with the one hand while resisting the patient's wrist extension (on the affected side) with the other hand. A positive finding includes the reproduction of pain at the lateral epicondyle and is associated with a sensitivity of 74%.[17] Studies have demonstrated poor specificity for this test.

Active extension of the middle finger (third digit) against resistance with the elbow in extension, or *Maudsley's test,* can also reproduce the pain over the lateral epicondyle at the insertion of the extensor carpi radialis brevis. Additionally, patients will typically note tenderness to palpation just distal to the lateral epicondyle, over the origin of the extensor carpi radialis brevis. With a sensitivity of 54%, its clinical utility in isolation is limited and it also offers poor specificity for this malady.[17] Illustrations of *Cozen's* and *Maudsley's tests* can be found in Figure 103.6.

Radiographs can be beneficial in cases of atypical or prolonged symptoms to rule out other pathologic conditions. Approximately 20% of patients demonstrate tendon calcification or a reactive exostosis at the tip of the epicondyle. The differential diagnosis of lateral epicondylitis includes fractures, posterior interosseus nerve entrapment (motor aspect of the radial nerve in the forearm), plica lesions, synovitis, chondromalacia, or adolescent osteochondral defects.

Medial Epicondylitis. Less common than its lateral counterpart, medial epicondylitis ("pitcher's elbow" or "golfer's elbow") can result from microtrauma at the site of the insertion of the flexor carpi radialis on the medial epicondyle. It is important to differentiate medial epicondylitis from other causes of medial elbow pain, including a medial ulnar collateral ligament injury. As a result of repetitive valgus stress placed on the joint, microtrauma and valgus instability at the ligament can also occur leading to disruption of the medial ulnar collateral ligament. Subsequently, abnormal stress is placed on the articular surfaces, which may lead to degenerative changes and osteophyte formation. Another diagnostic possibility worth considering is stress reactions/fractures. In the case of medial epicondylitis, patients will generally report tenderness over the flexor pronator origin slightly distal and anterior to the medial epicondyle. The pain of medial epicondylitis can be reproduced with resisted wrist flexion or resisted forearm pronation and may result in decreased grip strength. One should also evaluate for concomitant injuries elsewhere in the ipsilateral arm, which may be present in up to 84% of work-related injuries.

Wrist

de Quervain's Tenosynovitis. The wrist and hand include several tendons that pass through thick, fibrous retinacular tunnels. These help to prevent subluxation of the tendons and serve as a pulley system. Overuse syndromes are thought to result from changes of the synovial lining between these tendons and the retinaculum. de Quervain's tenosynovitis involves the synovial lining of the abductor pollicis longus and extensor pollicis brevis tendons. Although the term *tenosynovitis* suggests inflammation of the tendon sheath, it has been noted that there are many potential forms of tenosynovitis. Classic acute inflammatory changes that are characteristic of tenosynovitis may be related to systemic manifestations of disease (e.g., rheumatoid arthritis or gout). Tenosynovitis related to de Quervain's syndrome is referred to by some clinicians as *stenosing tenosynovitis.* The pathologic process of de Quervain's tenosynovitis does not generally involve inflammation but instead likely thickening of the extensor retinaculum covering the first dorsal compartment of the wrist combined with fibrous tissue depositions and increased vascularity in this region. It has been suggested that de Quervain's disease is a result of intrinsic degenerative mechanisms rather than extrinsic inflammatory ones.

The patient's history may consist of chronic, repetitive trauma or otherwise uncommon repetitive efforts, such as firmly grasping an object and moving the hand radially. However, studies have not found a causal relationship between this condition and specific occupational risk factors.[18] Direct trauma, such as a direct blow or fall,

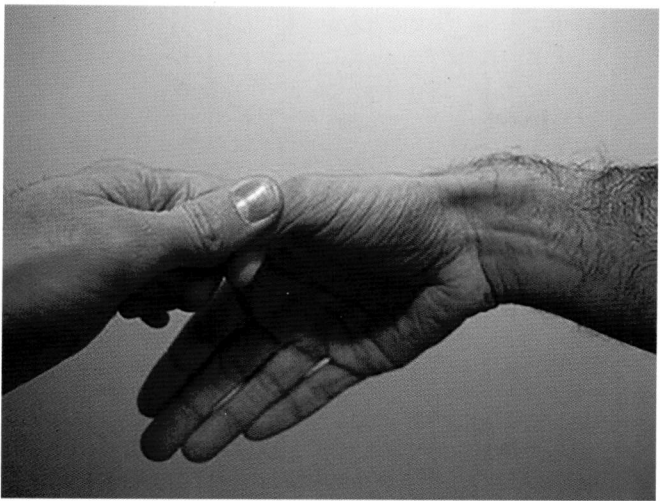

Fig. 103.7 *Finkelstein's test* can be useful in identifying de Quervain's tenosynovitis. The provider should then deviate the wrist toward the ulna. Note the position of the thumb. The patient should not enclose the thumb in a fist, which constitutes *Eichhoff's test.*

has occasionally been implicated. Yet, in most cases of de Quervain's tenosynovitis the onset is gradual. The discomfort of de Quervain's tenosynovitis is typically localized over the radial styloid process. Radiation of pain proximally to the forearm or distally down the thumb has been described. The pain is generally constant but may be exacerbated by movements that include grasping, abduction of the thumb, or ulnar deviation of the wrist.

On physical examination, swelling (sometimes subtle) may be appreciated over the radial styloid. Crepitus may be palpated over the abductor pollicis longus and extensor pollicis brevis tendons with flexion and extension of the thumb. An increase in the tensile load (passive stretching or active contraction) of these tendons increases pain. The *Finkelstein's test* is the most pathognomonic physical sign of de Quervain's tenosynovitis. While the provider holds the thumb in a neutral position, the patient deviates the wrist toward the ulna (Fig. 103.7). Pain is elicited near the radial styloid, which is also the point of tenderness, reflecting a positive finding. This test is often confused with the *Eichhoff's test*, which entails the patient placing the affected thumb in the palm, making a fist, and then deviating the wrist toward the ulna. Finkelstein's test is preferred when assessing for de Quervain's tenosynovitis given its specificity of 100% (compared with 89% for Eichhoff's test).[19]

Radiographs are characteristically normal. The pertinent differential diagnosis includes scaphoid fracture (tenderness in the anatomic snuffbox or at the scaphoid tubercle) and osteoarthritis of the carpometacarpal joint (pain precipitated by longitudinal traction and compression involving that joint). It should be noted that Finkelstein's test can produce pain at the carpometacarpal joint, potentially reducing its specificity. Rarely, infections such as tuberculosis or disseminated gonococcal infections can manifest as tenosynovitis as well.

Knee

Patellar Tendinopathy. Patellar tendinopathy ("jumper's knee") commonly occurs in sports featuring a prominent jumping component, although it can also occur as the result of other sporting activities or occupations. Patients report pain at the inferior pole of the patella. The discomfort may abate with activity in the early stages of this tendinopathy but later progresses to the point of discomfort with both exercise and rest. When the quadriceps musculature is relaxed with the knee flexed at 30°, tenderness may be localized to the deep surface of the proximal attachment of the patellar tendon at the inferior pole of

the patella. It should be noted that healthy active athletes sometimes have tenderness in this location on physical examination.

The differential diagnosis for patellar tendinopathy includes patellofemoral syndrome, which arises from imbalances in the forces that control patellar tracking during knee flexion and extension. Patients usually complain of anterior knee pain, described as "behind" or "around" the patella, which is classically worse with ascending or descending stairs or upon rising from a seated position. Occasionally, there is tenderness of the medial or lateral retinacula or facets.

Imaging with ultrasonography or magnetic resonance imaging (MRI) may reflect tendon degeneration, irregularity, or calcifications within the tendon. However, these findings should serve as an adjunct to the distinctive history and physical examination findings. It should be noted that some asymptomatic "jumping" athletes may have imaging findings similar to those of symptomatic individuals; thus, prognosis and outcomes are not predicted by imaging findings alone.

Ankle

Achilles Tendinopathy. Achilles tendinopathy is a common overuse syndrome that historically was thought to affect male athletes more frequently than their female counterparts, although that is currently subject to debate.[20] The Achilles tendon arises from the medial and lateral heads of the gastrocnemius muscle and the deep layers of the soleus muscle, inserting on the calcaneal tuberosity. Its major function is plantar flexion of the foot. The strongest and largest tendon in the body, it can withstand tensile loads more than 12 times the body's weight during running.

The Achilles tendon is vulnerable to injury from either trauma or overuse. A tendinopathy can also develop as a result of systemic disease (e.g., diabetes mellitus, renal disease, ankylosing spondylitis, reactive arthritis [previously known as Reiter's syndrome], gout, or pseudogout). The use of fluoroquinolones and statins have been associated with Achilles tendinopathy. Additionally, moderate alcohol use (7 to 13 units per week for men or 4 to 6 units per week for women) may predispose to this condition. The same association was not found for heavy alcohol use.[20]

The occurrence of Achilles tendinopathy is highest among individuals who participate in middle- and long-distance running, track and field, tennis, badminton, basketball, volleyball, or soccer. Some studies have noted a 5.2% incidence of Achilles tendinopathy in all runners and a 7.4% incidence in marathon runners.[21] Most cases of Achilles tendinopathy are thought to be multifactorial in origin. Anatomically, the vascular supply to the tendon creates a watershed area approximately 2 to 6 cm above the calcaneal insertion. This is responsible for the clinical symptoms and pathologic disruption commonly seen at this site. Otherwise, body mechanics and environmental factors (e.g., uneven terrain) may apply valgus or varus stress to the tendon. Activity technique (e.g., running form) and equipment (e.g., type of shoes) can also contribute to the development of tendinopathy.

The patient's history provides most of the information necessary to make the diagnosis. Pain, a cardinal symptom of Achilles tendinopathy, is often the impetus for an individual to seek medical evaluation. Some have argued that a patient's symptoms reflect the degree of tendon pathology, which has been validated in MRI studies assessing abnormal signal within the Achilles tendon. However, studies focusing on other changes associated with Achilles tendinopathy, such as neovascularization, have not shown a correlation with pain severity.[22] Regardless, as with many tendinopathies, pain after strenuous activity is reported in the early phase, whereas pain in the later phase occurs both during activity and at rest. Once an individual reaches this point, work and sporting activities are often limited by symptoms.

On physical examination, inspect the contour of the muscle-tendon unit while also assessing for swelling and erythema. In acute Achilles tendinopathy, the tendon may be diffusely swollen and reveal tenderness to palpation, usually most prominent over the middle third. Typically, in such patients the area of swelling and tenderness does not move with dorsiflexion of the ankle joint. On palpation, warmth, crepitus, or palpable tendon nodules or defects may be noted. Examination for ankle instability and biomechanical faults (e.g., excessive ankle supination or pronation) should be entertained.

Achilles Tendon Rupture. Although rupture of the Achilles tendon most often occurs when it is preceded by tendon damage, it is possible for untrained athletes to apply excessive force and rupture the tendon in the absence of prior changes of tendinopathy. Partial and complete rupture may occur, most commonly in men between 30 to 40 years of age. Complete rupture is more common in the middle-aged recreational athlete. Historically, the patient may note a "pop" followed by acute weakness and an inability to continue with activity. Patients may report feeling as though they were "struck" in the posterior ankle.

On physical examination, a defect in the tendon can sometimes be palpated. If enough time has elapsed to allow hematoma formation, bogginess may be noted over the injured area. The ability to plantar flex the foot does not rule out a complete rupture of the Achilles tendon. There are multiple plantar flexors of the foot and toes. Muscles such as the tibialis posterior, flexor digitorum longus, flexor hallucis longus, peroneus brevis, and peroneus longus can remain functional and therefore disguise a complete rupture given the persistent ability to plantar flex the foot.

Several observations can aid in the diagnosis of an Achilles tendon rupture by placing the patient in the prone position. Assess for decreased resting plantar flexion compared to the contralateral side, which is normally 20° to 30°. The *Thompson (Simmonds') test* can also be performed to evaluate for a complete rupture. With the patient prone and feet hanging over the edge of the bed, the examiner squeezes the calf muscles at their widest point and looks for passive plantar flexion. The absence of plantar flexion is considered a positive finding, indicative of a complete tear of the Achilles tendon. The presence of induced plantar flexion does not, however, eliminate the possibility of a partial tear of the Achilles tendon. Overall, the diagnosis of an Achilles tendon rupture can be made with 2 or more of the following findings on physical examination: palpable defect 2 cm to 6 cm proximal to its insertion, positive Thompson test, increased passive ankle dorsiflexion, and decreased plantar flexion strength. The absence of the first three of these findings has a negative predictive value of 100%, effectively ruling out the diagnosis of an Achilles tendon rupture.

Differential Diagnoses

The differential diagnoses of tendinopathy are listed in Box 103.1.

Diagnostic Testing

The diagnosis of tendinopathy is typically made on clinical grounds. While plain radiographs may be helpful in identifying calcific tendinopathy and in excluding bony abnormalities, ultrasonography has been recommended by some practitioners as the modality of choice for the evaluation of pathologic tendon conditions. Ultrasonography can be especially useful when other conditions, such as gouty arthritis, obscure the findings of concomitant tendinopathy. Emergency clinicians are proficient in identifying tendon injuries with point-of-care ultrasound, operating with 100% sensitivity and 95% specificity in such contexts. In cases of acute or chronic tendinopathy, one or more of the following features may be visualized: loss of the fibrillar echotexture, focal tendon thickening (Fig. 103.8), diffuse thickening, focal hypoechoic areas, extended hypoechogenicity, irregular and ill-defined borders, microruptures, intratendinous calcifications, or

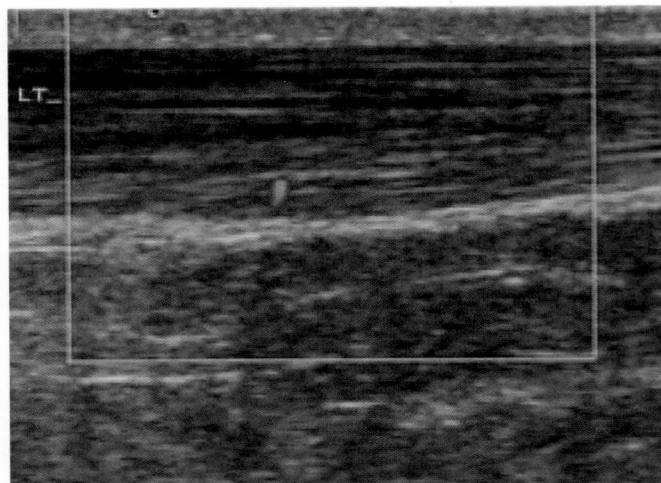

Fig. 103.8 A longitudinal view of the Achilles tendon showing focal thickening with peritendinous fluid.

peritendinous inflammatory edema. Hypoechoic areas surrounding tendons are consistent with surrounding soft tissue inflammation. Tendon tears, both partial and complete, can also be delineated by ultrasonography.

MRI has been utilized to visualize pathologic conditions of the tendon. It provides high intrinsic tissue contrast, which permits the distinction between normal tendons and abnormal tendons as well as high spatial resolution that facilitates the identification of detailed anatomic structures. MRI has superb resolution of the soft tissue structures and can aid in the diagnosis of a variety of tendon disorders. Although the accuracy in identifying clinically relevant tendinopathy appears to be good (70%), perhaps counterintuitively, the sensitivity of MRI in these patients has been found to be as low as 50%. Additionally, cost, availability, the need to have the patient remain still during the examination, and the loss of the dynamic component compared with ultrasound examination remain relative disadvantages.

Management
General Tendinopathy

The management of tendinopathy is summarized in Box 103.2. Cryotherapy (cold treatments, 20 minutes at a time every several hours, for the first 24 to 48 hours) may be beneficial in reducing pain. However, there are no high-quality studies supporting its use to resolve the underlying tendinopathy or to increase load tolerance of the tendon. The role of NSAIDs in treating tendinopathy remains controversial. They can provide short-term analgesic benefits in some patients, although the efficacy is variable. The mechanism of their benefit remains unclear though likely relates to the progressive nature of the condition and associated inflammation of surrounding tissues. However, studies have shown that NSAIDs can impair long-term tendon healing. Thus, emergency clinicians should use their clinical judgement when considering NSAIDs for the treatment of tendinopathy, with a preference for a short course (e.g., one week) when prescribed.

Additional treatment modalities include graduated range-of-motion exercises. Aside from ruptures, complete rest is relatively contraindicated due to the subsequent loss of muscle power, decrease in mechanical properties of the tendon, and effect on the kinetic chain. Although pain may be immediately reduced with rest, it will increase again when the tendon is loaded due to the aforementioned physiologic sequelae. Unless the provider has in-depth

BOX 103.2 Components of Tendinopathy Management[8]

Identify the cause of discomfort
Eliminate the sources of the primary tendinopathy
Institute treatment modalities
- Analgesic medications (e.g., NSAIDs)
- Protection
- Relative rest
- Optimal loading (e.g., ergonomic alterations)
- Application of ice, compression, and elevation as necessary

Educate patients regarding the underlying mechanical causes
Modify patient behavior to minimize or eliminate sources of continuing irritation (e.g., biofeedback, coaching)
Enhance the patient's diet (e.g., add vitamin D sources)
Refer patients for appropriate follow-up care and early rehabilitation.

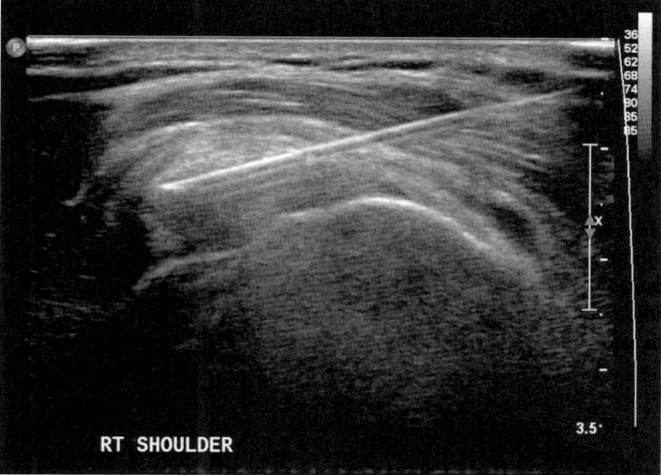

Fig. 103.9 Ultrasound-guided aspiration of a calcific deposit from the supraspinatus tendon causing calcific tendinopathy.

knowledge regarding the optimal rehabilitation regimen for a given tendinopathy (e.g., graduated eccentrics integrated with concentric exercises), it is prudent to avoid making specific recommendations. Instead, refer the patient to physical therapy, sports medicine, or an orthopedic specialist.

Corticosteroid injections have been utilized for short-term pain relief in the setting of tendinopathy. However, they likely have detrimental effects on both tendon pain and function for up to one year. Intratendinous corticosteroid injections should be avoided, particularly in the Achilles and patellar tendons, due to their potential for subsequent rupture. There are certain conditions that warrant consideration of peritendinous corticosteroid injections (i.e., de Quervain's tenosynovitis). Of interest, systemic corticosteroids may have a different impact on the healing process when administered after the early inflammatory stage of tendinopathy (e.g., post-injury day 5). A study in animal models assessing Achilles tendon injuries found that a five-day course of systemic dexamethasone starting at post-injury day 5 resulted in greater peak force, increased (beneficial) tendon stiffness, and decreased tendon thickness when compared to placebo.[23] While sufficient supporting evidence in humans has not yet been widely reported, this is an area of clinically relevant research to monitor moving forward.

The use of nitroglycerin patches has been shown to be effective in the treatment of certain tendinopathies. Questions remain as to whether their efficacy is due to an analgesic effect or promoting healing of the affected tendon. Medial and lateral epicondylitis, noninsertional Achilles tendinopathy, and rotator cuff tendinopathy typically respond well to this intervention.[24] However, no significant benefit in patellar tendinopathy has been reliably supported by the literature. Overall, chronic tendinopathies seem to respond better to nitroglycerin compared with acute injuries. Patients prescribed this treatment should be aware of the potential side effects, which include headaches and contact dermatitis. The use of nitroglycerin patches for tendinopathy remains off-label and is more likely to be prescribed by a musculoskeletal specialist.

Platelet-rich plasma (PRP) injections, a process by which a patient's platelets are concentrated in a centrifuge and then injected into the affected tendon, are utilized by some specialists in the management of tendinopathy. The literature on the efficacy of this intervention is widely variable. There is some support for this modality, although it is not definitively beneficial. It can be safely asserted that PRP should not be utilized as a first-line treatment and is most efficacious when administered under ultrasound guidance.[25,26] Accordingly, while some patients may reach this point in the treatment

algorithm of tendinopathies, it is not advocated for use in the ED setting at this time.

Specific Tendinopathies

Impingement Syndrome and Rotator Cuff Tendinopathies. The treatment of rotator cuff tendinopathies and impingement syndrome follows the treatment of tendinopathy in general. Emphasis is placed on physical rehabilitation and graduated strengthening exercises. A significant proportion of patients will improve with conservative management; otherwise, surgical intervention (e.g., acromioplasty, debridement, or repair) may be considered.[27]

Calcific Tendinopathy. The initial treatment of calcific tendinopathy is mainly conservative and consists of analgesia and brief immobilization (e.g., a shoulder sling for rotator cuff calcific tendinopathy) because prolonged immobilization may result in decreased range of motion. Both extracorporeal shock wave therapy (akin to that which is used for nephrolithiasis) and ultrasound-guided needle lavage and aspiration (Fig. 103.9) are effective treatments for this condition. The latter option has been shown to result in improved pain and functional outcomes compared to extracorporeal shock wave therapy or corticosteroid injection.[28] A small percentage of patients who do not respond to these interventions may need surgery. Follow-up care from the ED is important because calcific tendinopathy has been described as the most well-known cause of reactive cuff failure.

Lateral and Medial Epicondylitis. In up to 95% of patients, epicondylitis will improve with time and conservative therapy. Initial efforts include making the patient more comfortable with the standard principles of protection, compression, medications (e.g., NSAIDs for significant pain), biomechanical or ergonomic adjustments, and physical therapy modalities. *Relative rest* is appropriate and implies the avoidance of overuse as opposed to the absence of activity. Activities that aggravate pain should be eliminated and an attempt to protect the tendon through strategies such as a reduction in playing time or intensity should be entertained. The use of a counterforce brace should be recommended in order to control force loads and improve performance technique. This intervention has been shown to significantly reduce the frequency and severity of epicondylitis-related pain in the short term (i.e., 2 to 12 weeks) as well as improve elbow function at 26 weeks.[29] Corticosteroid injections remain a commonly employed treatment despite ample evidence that they are ineffective. At 4 to 6 weeks, patients may note a reduction in pain. However, at

26 weeks, outcomes (e.g., pain and function) were worse in those who received a corticosteroid injection compared to those who received a saline injection or no treatment.[30] In fact, corticosteroid injections may serve to increase the risk of nonoperative treatment failure.[31] Consequently, corticosteroid injections should be avoided in the ED while follow-up with a musculoskeletal specialist is pursued.

de Quervain's Tenosynovitis. The initial treatment of de Quervain's tenosynovitis consists of immobilization with a thumb spica splint, antiinflammatory medications, and prompt referral. Corticosteroid injections have been shown to be a beneficial treatment of de Quervain's disease, and failure to respond may be due to anatomic variation or poor technique (Fig. 103.10). Studies have shown this

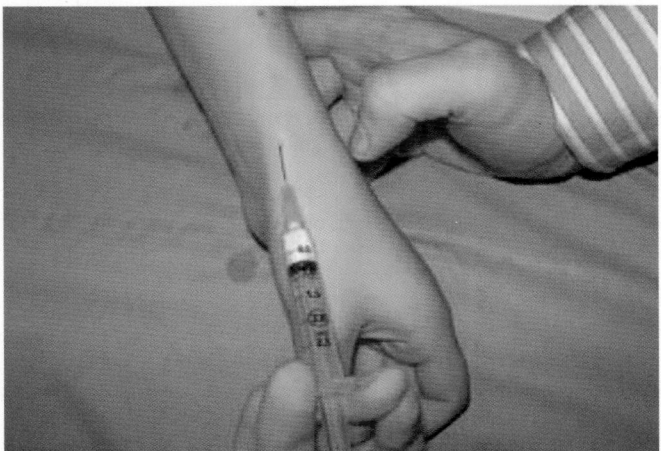

Fig. 103.10 The proper needle placement for a corticosteroid injection to address de Quervain's tenosynovitis.

intervention to be effective in resolving the associated pain 52% of the time.[32] A mixture of 20 mg of methylprednisolone acetate or triamcinolone combined with 1 mL to 2 mL of lidocaine or bupivacaine is appropriate for this injection. The associated benefit may be further enhanced when combined with a thumb spica splint or similar orthosis.[33] Surgical decompression of the first dorsal compartment may be indicated if these treatments fail.

Achilles Tendinopathy and Rupture. In addition to routine conservative treatment, patients with Achilles tendinopathy should be referred for orthopedic evaluation and correction of limb malalignment with the use of orthotics or heel lifts. Eccentric loading exercises (Fig. 103.11) and low-energy shock wave therapy are typically effective therapies for Achilles tendinopathy.

The management of Achilles tendon rupture may be either operative or nonoperative, depending on patient circumstances. In the ED, acute Achilles tendon ruptures should be treated with a posterior lower leg splint featuring the ankle placed in approximately 20° of equinus (i.e., plantar flexion). If this is not feasible for any reason, a walking boot with 2 inches of heel lift can suffice. This management brings the affected ends of the ruptured tendon closer to reapproximation, decreasing the amount of remodeling necessary to reconstitute the tendon. The individual should remain nonweightbearing until consultation by a musculoskeletal specialist is completed. Some authors contend that complete ruptures in active athletes should be treated surgically in most cases. And while scenarios differ, the outcomes for the nonoperative and operative management of Achilles tendon ruptures are similar, leaving both as viable options for many patients.[34]

Disposition

Most patients with tendinopathy are safely discharged home with proper instructions, relative rest of the tendon, analgesia, and appropriate follow-up care. Exceptions include elders and disabled patients

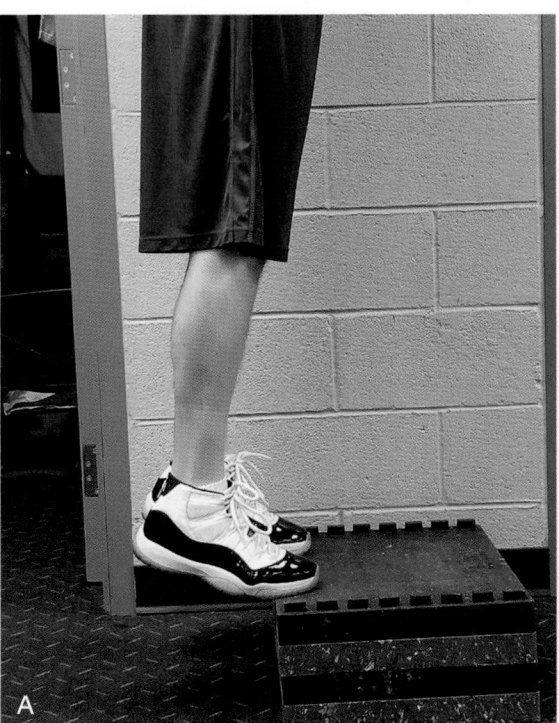
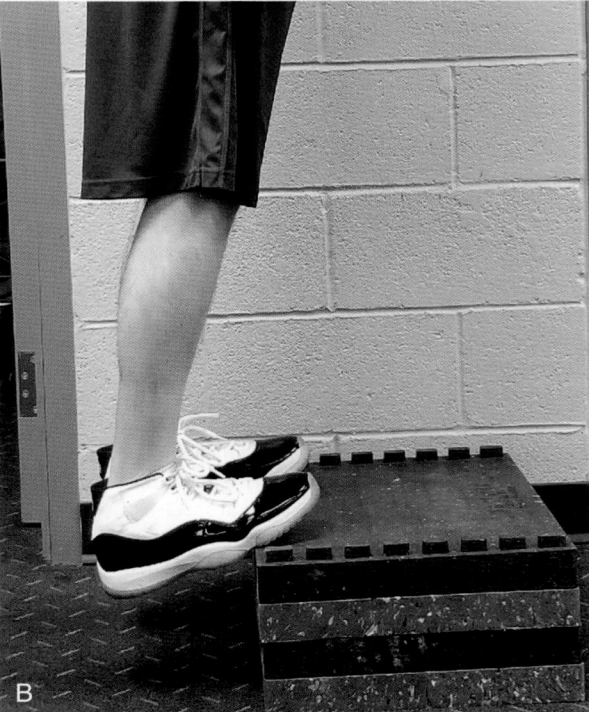

Fig. 103.11 Demonstration of eccentric Achilles tendon rehabilitation exercises, emphasizing bilateral toe raises (A). One should then lower the heel below neutral (B).

who may be unable to perform activities of daily living due to the tendinopathy. Although appropriate rest and analgesia provide symptomatic relief, underlying causes should be considered and addressed in follow-up.

BURSITIS

Foundations

A *bursa* is a closed sac lined by synovial membrane, which occurs in areas of friction between two layers of tissue. It permits fluid movement of soft tissue over areas of potential impingement (e.g., subacromial bursa) or friction (e.g., olecranon and prepatellar bursae). There are more than 150 bursae throughout the body. They develop after birth, most likely as a result of pressure or friction from movement. Superficial bursitis most commonly occurs in the olecranon and prepatellar bursae, which are located on the extensor surface of the elbow and knee, respectively.

Bursitis is most often due to trauma (acute direct trauma to or prolonged pressure on the bursa), systemic inflammation (from disorders such as gout, pseudogout, rheumatoid or psoriatic arthritis), or infection (most commonly due to *Staphylococcus aureus*). However, there are cases of idiopathic bursitis as well. Septic bursitis is most commonly due to spread from a nearby cellulitis, direct inoculation from trauma, or as a result of aspiration or injection.

Clinical Features

Olecranon and Prepatellar Bursitis

About one-third of patients with olecranon or prepatellar bursitis are found to have septic bursitis. Distinguishing septic from nonseptic bursitis can be difficult because clinical information and diagnostic data can be similar. Patients with septic bursitis generally present earlier in their clinical course and tend to have more pain, tenderness, erythema, and warmth compared to those with nonseptic bursitis. While septic and nonseptic bursitis are both frequently caused by trauma, septic bursitis is almost always preceded by some kind of trauma, including minor and repetitive microtrauma. Other predisposing factors include chronic illness (e.g., diabetes mellitus or alcohol abuse), chronic skin conditions (e.g., atopic dermatitis), and previous noninfectious inflammation of the bursae (e.g., rheumatoid arthritis or gout). It is also more common in people whose occupation results in repetitive knee or elbow trauma.

The olecranon bursa, found on the extensor surface of the elbow, is the only bursa of the elbow joint and is easily traumatized, which can result in inflammation, pain, and swelling. Infection can also occur from local trauma (e.g., puncture wounds or lacerations), but may also present without any preceding history of trauma. Hematogenous bacterial seeding is rare due to the limited vascular supply to the bursal tissue.

On physical examination, localized swelling and fluctuance are usually present over the bursa. There may or may not be evidence of trauma. Tenderness and warmth are typical in most patients with septic bursitis. Erythema with overlying cellulitis is also common in septic bursitis, and a fever can suggest infection, although this is inconsistent and reported to be present in 20% to 77% of patients. Tenderness, erythema, and warmth can also be seen in patients with purely inflammatory causes of bursitis, though the frequency and severity of these findings are less and patients with septic bursitis usually present earlier in their clinical course.

Passive range of motion should not produce noteworthy pain except for full flexion, at which point there may be discomfort as the inflamed bursa is compressed. Evidence of significantly diminished range of motion, generalized joint swelling, or other signs and symptoms of joint involvement (e.g., joint pain, warmth, effusion) should raise concern for septic arthritis. Although the olecranon and prepatellar bursae generally do not communicate with the joint space, septic arthritis should be considered in the differential diagnosis, especially if trauma is involved and the integrity of the underlying joint is disrupted. Arthrocentesis to assess for septic arthritis should be considered in these cases.

Subacromial Bursitis

The subacromial bursa lies between the rotator cuff tendons and the undersurface of the acromion, the acromioclavicular joint, and the deltoid muscle. Subacromial bursitis is thought to be nearly synonymous with supraspinatus tendinopathy and may be involved in the stages of rotator cuff impingement. Pain and tenderness to palpation, localized to the lateral aspect of the shoulder, in addition to signs of impingement may be noted on physical examination *(Neer test or Hawkins-Kennedy test)*. Septic subacromial bursitis is rare, but a few cases have been reported in the literature.[35]

Trochanteric Bursitis

The trochanteric bursa has both deep and superficial components. The deep bursa is located between the greater trochanter and the tensor fasciae latae; the superficial bursa is located between the greater trochanter and the skin. Trochanteric bursitis is more common in middle-aged women, who usually report acute or chronic pain over the bursal area as well as the lateral thigh. Lying on the hip and walking may exacerbate the pain. It can also occur as a complication of rheumatoid arthritis. On examination, the pain of superficial bursitis may be reproduced by direct palpation and hip adduction while the pain of deep trochanteric bursitis may be reproduced with hip abduction. The hip joint itself usually has normal examination findings. Septic trochanteric bursitis is rare but has been described.

Ischiogluteal Bursitis

The ischiogluteal bursa is located adjacent to the ischial tuberosity and overlies the sciatic and posterior femoral cutaneous nerves. Inflammation, known as *weaver's bottom,* is described as pain over the center of the buttocks with radiation down the back of the leg. It can be caused by prolonged sitting, running, repetitive jumping, or kicking. Sitting on a hard surface exacerbates the pain, and palpation over the ischial tuberosity causes discomfort.

Iliopsoas Bursitis

The iliopsoas bursa has been shown to be the largest bursa in the body. It lies between the iliopsoas tendon and the lesser trochanter. The pain of iliopsoas bursitis usually manifests as anterior hip pain that can radiate down the medial thigh to the knee and is exacerbated by hip extension.

Pes Anserine Bursitis

The anserine bursa lies deep to the three tendons (sartorius, gracilis, and semitendinosus) that form the pes anserinus ("foot of the goose") and superficial to the medial collateral ligament of the knee. Patients with anserine bursitis usually complain of medial knee pain approximately 2 or 3 cm distal to the joint line. There is usually tenderness to palpation in this area and occasionally swelling. Risk factors for pes anserine bursitis include osteoarthritis of the knee, diabetes mellitus, and possibly obesity.[36]

Differential Diagnoses

Conditions that mimic bursitis include underlying fracture, osteomyelitis, septic or inflammatory joint arthritis, and cellulitis. Radiography and bone scan or MRI may be necessary to evaluate for these alternative conditions. Box 103.3 lists the differential diagnoses for atraumatic, nonseptic bursitis.

Diagnostic Testing

When there are signs of acute inflammation, aspiration of the bursa should be considered to exclude the presence of infection or crystal-induced disease. Bursal aspiration is performed with sterile technique utilizing an 18- to 20-gauge needle. A lateral approach to the aspiration of any bursa, when feasible, has been recommended to lower the risk of iatrogenic sinus tract formation, although the relation between the two is unclear. A distal approach can also be used when the olecranon bursa is aspirated. In cases of septic bursitis, the aspirate usually appears purulent though can occasionally appear serosanguinous or straw-colored. In the case of nonseptic bursitis, the aspirate varies from bloody to straw-colored. The bursal fluid is typically evaluated for white blood cell count with differential, crystal analysis, Gram stain, appropriate cultures and sensitivities, and glucose level. Peripheral blood is typically sent for complete blood cell count with differential, C-reactive protein, erythrocyte sedimentation rate, and glucose. A bursal fluid to serum glucose ratio of less than 50% was initially thought to be diagnostic of septic bursitis, though recent studies have shown this comparison to be unreliable.

The identification of organisms on either Gram stain or culture is diagnostic for septic bursitis. There are no definitive guidelines regarding the use of WBC count to distinguish between septic and nonseptic bursitis. A bursal fluid WBC count higher than $1000/\mu L^3$ is almost always seen, and a value greater than $5000/\mu L^3$ suggests bursal fluid infection, even in the presence of a negative Gram stain. However, counts can be much lower in septic bursitis or above this threshold in nonseptic cases. Culture is the definitive test though will not be available during the initial evaluation. *S. aureus* is by far the most common organism in bursal infection, followed by streptococcal and other staphylococcal species, remaining unchanged in the last several decades. Because most cases of septic bursitis occur in the olecranon or prepatellar bursae, the diagnosis is made clinically in conjunction with aspiration. MRI can be used to aid in the diagnosis of inflammation or infection of deep bursae. Ultrasonography has also been used as a modality for aspiration of deep bursae.

Management

Septic Bursitis

Large-scale clinical prospective trials are lacking, thus the optimal treatment of septic bursitis remains unclear. Debate persists regarding the use of outpatient (oral) or inpatient (intravenous [IV]) antibiotics,

duration of therapy, role of needle aspiration or incision and drainage, and the need for operative intervention.

Patients who have bursal inflammation with suspicion (clinical or laboratory) of infection should be treated with appropriate antibiotics. Empirical therapy (including coverage for *S. aureus* and streptococcal species) is indicated until definitive culture results are available. A recent study on septic bursitis revealed the incidence of methicillin-resistant *S. aureus* (MRSA) as a causative pathogen to be around 17%.[37] It is more common in the United States compared to Europe, and MRSA was found to be the most common cause of community-onset adult septic bursitis in one case series from an ED population. Therefore, empirical coverage for this organism in septic bursitis should be considered. A trial of oral antibiotic therapy (up to 14 days) and treatment on an outpatient basis in the patient with uncomplicated septic bursitis and no underlying disease is reasonable. We recommend oral dicloxacillin (500 mg PO four times daily), trimethoprim/sulfamethoxazole (160 mg/800 mg strength, one to two tablets PO twice daily), or oral clindamycin (300 mg PO four times a day) for penicillin-allergic patients, as first-line therapy. However, failure in up to 50% of cases has been reported for outpatient treatment of septic bursitis. One of the largest observational studies on the successful outpatient treatment of septic bursitis showed an admission rate of only 1 of 118 patients, though all patients in this study received sequential IV antibiotics for approximately 4 days at an outpatient clinic followed by a course of oral antibiotic therapy. Consequently, treatment in an observation unit or inpatient setting with IV antibiotics is a consideration for patients with significant symptoms, overlying cellulitis, or those unlikely to receive close follow-up. For such patients, we recommend IV vancomycin (loading dose: 20 to 35 mg/kg actual body weight [not to exceed 3000 mg] or 20 to 25 mg/kg actual body weight [not to exceed 3000 mg] in patients with obesity, then 15 to 20 mg/kg actual body weight every 8 to 12 hours) as initial empirical treatment.

Needle aspiration is a technique commonly used for the diagnosis and management of septic bursae. Successful treatment of septic bursitis can typically be achieved in patients receiving oral antibiotics on an outpatient basis following initial needle aspiration. One study showed no difference between patients who received aspiration and those who did not, though patients who had more severe disease were also more likely to be selected for drainage. These patients were also initially treated with parenteral antibiotics. Furthermore, the diagnosis of septic bursitis was confirmed by culture in only 26% of patients, potentially underestimating the importance of bursal drainage in individuals with true septic bursitis. As needle aspiration is utilized in the diagnosis of septic bursitis, initial drainage at the same time seems reasonable. Those with a purulent aspirate may require repeated aspiration at 1- to 3-day intervals if the effusion persists. In all cases, appropriate follow-up to assess response to therapy should be arranged. Warm soaks and wound care are also indicated. Surgical incision and drainage or bursectomy may become necessary in severe, recurrent, or refractory cases.

Nonseptic Bursitis

Most cases of nonseptic bursitis improve with conservative therapy, although complete recovery can take many months. Initial treatment typically consists of NSAIDs, compression to prevent recurrent fluid accumulation, and occasionally aspiration of the bursa to relieve pain and increase range of motion. Systemic causes of bursitis (e.g., crystalline disease) should be treated as indicated. Avoidance of local trauma is important for treatment and successful prevention of bursitis. Recurrent olecranon bursitis may be caused by underlying anatomic disorders, such as bone spurs.

Bursal injection with a combination of local anesthetics and steroids at the time of diagnostic aspiration is often therapeutically beneficial for inflammatory bursitis of deeper areas, such as the subacromial, pes anserine, medial collateral ligament, or trochanteric bursae. Injections into superficial bursae have been used as a treatment modality, but multiple complications have been described, including skin atrophy over the bursa, persistent pain, development of septic bursitis, bleeding, postinjection flare as a result of release of microcrystals, and tendon rupture. However, a systematic review of the treatment of olecranon bursitis found that patients who received a corticosteroid injection were no more likely to develop an infection or persistent pain than those who did not. A recent randomized trial comparing compression and NSAIDs versus aspiration alone versus aspiration and steroid injection showed no appreciable differences between groups in treatment success rates.[38] At this point in time, we recommend starting with noninjection treatment (e.g., compression, NSAIDs, and possible aspiration) for suspected inflammatory bursitis of superficial bursae.

Disposition

Patients without underlying medical problems who present with uncomplicated septic bursitis can usually be discharged with appropriate oral antibiotics. Those with underlying diseases (e.g., immunocompromise, leukopenia, diabetes mellitus) or those with systemic toxicity or signs of severe bursal infection (e.g., purulent drainage) are candidates for IV antibiotics and inpatient therapy. Patients with a purulent aspirate or persistent infection may require serial aspirations. Close follow-up is necessary to ensure an appropriate response to therapy. Patients with presumed nonseptic bursitis require close follow-up as well.

The references for this chapter can be found online at ExpertConsult.com.

104

Musculoskeletal Back Pain

Susan E. Farrell and Zheng Ben Ma

- Most patients presenting to the emergency department (ED) with back pain have uncomplicated musculoskeletal pain that is self-resolving with conservative therapy and does not require imaging.
- Indications for emergent imaging include "red flags" such as an acute neurologic deficit, bowel or bladder dysfunction, or saddle anesthesia.
- Risk factors for compressive myelopathy include immunocompromised patients with a history of malignancy, injection drug use, fever, chronic steroid or anticoagulant use.
- Back pain due to metastatic disease is more common than primary tumors in the spine, and thoracic metastases are more common than lumbar metastases.
- Epidural abscess or hematoma, cauda equina syndrome (CES), spinal malignancy with compressive symptoms, and spinal osteomyelitis are all indications for emergent surgical consultation or transfer to a center where surgical spine consultation is available.
- Empirical parenteral antibiotics active against staphylococci, streptococci, and gram-negative bacilli should be administered for suspected epidural abscess. Specific antibiotics should be directed against the known pathogen if the culture or Gram stain of the aspirate is positive.
- Corticosteroids given as a single dose in the ED (10 mg dexamethasone) or as a 15-day tapering course after discharge (prednisone 60 mg, 40 mg, 20 mg daily for 5 days each) may improve functional ability but does not improve nerve root pain secondary to disc herniation.

FOUNDATIONS

Background

Back pain is one of the most common patient complaints encountered in emergency departments (EDs). Most cases of musculoskeletal back pain are related to physical motion of the vertebrae, intervertebral discs, or musculature of the back; however, a precise pathoanatomic etiology and diagnosis is identified in only 10% of cases.[1] As a result, the symptom of back pain can present the emergency clinician with a challenging diagnostic dilemma. Although most cases of acute or acute-on-chronic back pain are due to uncomplicated musculoskeletal causes, certain types of back pain are true emergencies requiring timely diagnosis and intervention. It is critical to distinguish between the large number of benign presentations of self-limited pain versus less common, high-morbidity causes of back pain that require immediate intervention.

Epidemiology

Back pain occurs in children and adults, females and males, with a lifetime prevalence in adults of 60% to 80%.[2] Total direct health care costs and indirect economic expenses associated with back pain are estimated to be in the tens of billions of dollars annually in the United States.[1-2] Risk factors associated with the development of back pain are numerous and include repetitive lifting and twisting movements, prolonged static (seated) postures, obesity, smoking, and psychosocial factors, such as anxiety and depression.[3]

Anatomy and Physiology

The spine consists of seven cervical, twelve thoracic, five lumbar, and five fused sacral and coccygeal vertebrae. The vertebrae articulate with each other superiorly and inferiorly at bilateral facet joints, creating four facet joints at each vertebral level. The thoracic vertebral bodies also have bilateral rib facets, which articulate with twelve pairs of ribs. Each vertebral body has bilateral transverse processes and a spinous process. Between the spinous process and the transverse processes are the lamina, and between the transverse processes and the posterior aspect of the vertebral body are the pedicles. Together, the pedicles and lamina form the neural arch, which, along with the posterior aspect of the vertebral body, forms the confines of the vertebral canal that contains the spinal cord and nerve roots. At each level, there are intervertebral (neural) foramina, where the spinal nerves exit.

Between the vertebral bodies are the intervertebral discs, which provide elasticity and stability to the spine. Each disc is comprised of the outer annulus fibrosis, a ring of fibrous tissue, and the collagenous inner nucleus pulposus. The spinal column is connected and stabilized by a network of spinal ligaments including anterior longitudinal ligament (ALL), the posterior longitudinal ligament (PLL), and the ligamentum flavum.

The spinal cord runs superiorly from the foramen magnum, inferiorly to the L1 to L2 interspace, but may extend as low as L3, where it then divides into the cauda equina. The cord is surrounded by three membranes: the tough dura mater, and the delicate arachnoid and pia mater (referred to as the leptomeninges). Cerebrospinal fluid bathes the spinal cord between the arachnoid and pia mater. The epidural space, between the bony vertebral canal and the dura, contains connective tissue padding and the spinal venous plexus. The dural sac ends between S1 and S3. The dura also protects the spinal nerve roots as the nerves exit the spine at each level, just below the correspondingly numbered vertebral body. The movements of the spine are governed by four groups of muscles: posterior extensor muscles of the back; forward flexors of the abdominal wall and the psoas and iliacus; lateral flexors, consisting of the quadratus lumborum, assisted by abdominal wall muscles; and rotators, which are a combination of the extensors and lateral flexors used with unilateral movements.

Pathophysiology

Nonspecific or Uncomplicated Back Pain

In as many as 90% of patients with back pain, no pathologic cause for the symptom can be identified.[1] Research indicates that in many instances of nonspecific pain, factors that increase spinal loading pressure such as obesity and musculoskeletal dysfunction, also reduce spinal stability. Static postures that reduce lateral flexor flexibility and restrict hamstring range of motion contribute to reduced core muscle strength and inadequate support of the spinal column. Weakened core muscles, including those of the anterior abdominal wall, threaten the stability of the remaining muscular and ligamentous spinal support structures, placing patients at risk for activity-related strain.[3] Patients with nonspecific muscular back pain typically have localized pain without radicular symptoms.

Nerve Root Syndromes

Nerve root syndromes comprise a heterogenous group of disease processes that can present with similar clinical symptoms and signs. These syndromes result when there is compression or irritation of a nerve root, causing pain or paresthesias that often radiate into an extremity. Nerve root irritation may occur as the result of muscle tightness or intervertebral disc herniation; however, it can also be caused by pathologies that require urgent diagnosis and management. Therefore, nerve root syndromes should be carefully evaluated to avoid misdiagnoses of etiologies that require emergent intervention. There are multiple possible etiologies for nerve root syndromes. Three major etiologies are discussed in detail here.

With age, intervertebral discs desiccate and degenerate and the nucleus pulposus can herniate through the annulus fibrosis, compressing the nerve root at the neural foramen. Conversely, the annulus fibrosis itself can tear without a true herniation of the nucleus pulposus, also resulting in nerve root irritation. Herniations tend to occur at the L4 to L5 and L5 to S1 levels. This is because most flexion and extension of the spine occurs at the lumbosacral joint and to a lesser degree at L4 to L5, and the supporting PLL is relatively weak at this level of the spine. Although most disc herniations are posterolateral, causing unilateral symptoms, intervertebral discs sometimes herniate centrally, at the level of the cauda equina, causing severe compression of multiple nerve roots, resulting in cauda equina syndrome (CES), as discussed in the following.

Nerve root compression can also be caused by spinal stenosis. Aging causes intervertebral disc space narrowing and deterioration of spine joints. Osteophytes can form at the facet joints, and the ligamentum flavum calcifies over time. These degenerative changes can narrow both the neural foramina and the central canal, causing nerve root compression from osteophytes and increased intrathecal pressure in the narrowed canal. The subsequent pain is often bilateral, unlike that caused by disc herniation. Spinal stenosis also results in leg pain that is typically worse while walking and relieved with forward flexion (thus reducing pressure on the nerve root). This historical information is referred to as the *pseudoclaudication sign.*

Epidural space occupying lesions can also cause compression to nerve roots or to the cauda equina. Spinal epidural abscesses or hematomas causing nerve compression are true emergencies. Spinal epidural abscesses can result from hematogenous spread of bacteria (often staphylococcal species), in the setting of injection drug use, or from direct inoculation after epidural steroid injection or spinal surgery. Epidural hematomas can result from instrumentation of the epidural space or spinal surgery, although they can also develop spontaneously or following trauma in anticoagulated patients. Regardless of the cause, epidural space lesions causing nerve root compression requires emergent imaging and consultation.

Skeletal Causes of Back Pain

Common bony causes of back pain include fractures, infection, and malignancy.

Fractures may occur in any part of the spine secondary to trauma (see Chapter 35). Although a significant amount of force is required to fracture the bones of a normal spine, patients with osteopenia can incur bony fractures with minor trauma. Age-related osteopenia can result in vertebral compression fractures, causing sudden acute back pain with or without trauma. Spontaneous compression fractures occur most commonly within the thoracic or lumbar vertebral bodies. Vertebral fractures may cause radicular symptoms, depending on the location of the injury and impingement on the spinal canal or nerve roots.

Osteomyelitis of the spine is generally caused by hematogenous spread and seeding of the bone by bacteria, resulting in inflammation of the bone and periosteum, and subsequent pain. Injection drug use, spinal surgery, and tuberculosis of the spine (Pott disease), can all cause vertebral osteomyelitis.

Cancer of the vertebral bones is due to primary or metastatic lesions. Primary tumors, such as Ewing sarcoma, multiple myeloma, and osteosarcoma, are less common and usually occur in patients younger than 30 years old, often involving the posterior vertebral elements. Metastatic tumors typically involve the vertebral body and are most common in the thoracic spine, but multiple levels can be affected. Lung and breast cancers make up over 50% of metastatic spinal lesions. Lymphoma, melanoma, cancers of the gastrointestinal (GI) tract, prostate, and kidney, and multiple myeloma may also present as metastatic spinal lesions.

Skeletal back pain can also be caused by nontraumatic congenital or acquired abnormalities of the spine. Spondylolisthesis, or slippage of one vertebral body on another, results from degenerative changes but can also occur after trauma. Retrolisthesis occurs with the posterior slippage of one vertebral body on another. Facet arthropathy is an age-related degenerative cause of skeletal back pain. Inflammatory arthropathies, such as ankylosing spondylitis, rheumatoid and osteoarthritis, can cause similar spinal changes, including pathologic fractures.

CLINICAL FEATURES

History

A thorough history and a directed physical examination is essential in evaluating patients with back pain. Although nonspecific uncomplicated back pain is common, it is critical that emergency clinicians elicit historical information that indicates a higher risk of compressive myelopathy, including history of cancer, unexpected weight loss, trauma, chronic steroid use, anticoagulation, fever, an impaired immune system, injection drug use, or spinal surgery. It is important to assess for "red flag" findings that require emergent evaluation and intervention, such as bowel or bladder dysfunction, saddle anesthesia, and acute neurologic deficits such as bilateral extremity weakness. Important historical data concerning the pain includes: the onset, location, character, severity, duration and radiation of the pain (such as to the abdomen, chest or extremities).

Aggravating and alleviating factors are also important to elicit. Pain that is exacerbated by coughing, sneezing, or bearing down with bowel movements, all of which increase intrathecal pressure, may be associated with a radicular or spinal cause. Pain that is worse with walking or prolonged standing, particularly if relieved by bending forward, suggests spinal stenosis. Pain associated with stiffness that is worse in the mornings and improves through the day suggests a rheumatic etiology. In contrast, pain that is improved with rest is more likely to be muscular or skeletal in nature.

Prior history of back pain, medical or surgical history, and any traumatic events should be documented. Any history of malignancy, or systemic symptoms such as fever, chills, or malaise may indicate metastatic or infectious causes. A history of spinal procedures or surgery should be elicited. Medications such as anticoagulants (associated with epidural hematoma) or chronic corticosteroids (associated with osteopenia) should be reviewed. A family history of autoimmune inflammatory diseases or malignancy may be contributory.

The patient should be asked about any neurologic findings that indicate serious pathology of the spine or nerve roots. These symptoms include sensations of numbness or paresthesias, pain in other locations of the spine, bowel or bladder dysfunction, or weakness in the extremities.

Physical Examination

A directed physical examination with the patient undressed is important in evaluating patients with back pain. The examination should include inspection, observation of the patient's normal movements, palpation, strength and sensory testing, specific maneuvers to assess for serious pathology, and an assessment of deep tendon reflexes. Inspect the overlying skin for erythema, warmth, or areas of swelling, noting any evidence of prior spine surgery or scoliosis. Observe the patient's general appearance including the presence of jaundice, rashes or contusions, and the patient's degree of discomfort. Observe the patient's gait and balance while ambulating. Because core and postural muscle dysfunction contributes to back pain through muscle inflexibility and tightness, range of motion should be tested in several planes.[3] Assess range of motion through flexion and extension at the waist, lateral flexion, and rotation. Palpate the spine to identify areas of maximal tenderness or the presence of muscle spasm.

Perform thorough neurologic testing for strength and sensation. Strength testing of the lower extremities is best done with the patient standing. Instruct the patient to flex both hips and knees, assuming a partial sitting or squatting position. Ask the patient to lift one leg briefly, then the other. Assess heel and toe walking (while holding the examiner's hands). Performing this activity requires full plantar and dorsiflexion strength, because the entire body weight is carried on a single extremity. If the patient is unable to comply with this approach to strength testing because of pain, this assessment can be performed with the patient reclining, although it is less reliable. Sensory testing is done with the patient reclining or sitting. Testing should include both upper and lower extremities, since some conditions, such as spinal stenosis, may occur at multiple spinal levels, including the cervical spine.

Straight leg and contralateral straight leg raise maneuvers are important in identifying radicular pain. The straight leg raise test is more sensitive but less specific than the contralateral straight leg raise test for the diagnosis of radiculopathy due to disc herniation.[4] The straight leg raise test is performed as follows:
- Position the patient supine with legs passively extended, without engaging the quadricep muscles. (This can be determined by noting that the patella can move freely side to side.)
- Raise each leg, flexing at the hip with the knee in extension.
- A positive test is elicited when pain is reproduced, radiating from the back to a point *below* the knee of the raised leg at 30 to 40 degrees of elevation. A positive result predicts lumbosacral radiculopathy with a high sensitivity though a relatively low specificity.[5]

Because L5 or S1 discs are implicated in the majority of disc herniations, a negative straight leg raise test is reassuring in ruling out disc pathology. Of note, radiation of pain from the back to the area of the posterior knee or above is a nonspecific finding and of less clinical value.

The contralateral straight leg raise test is performed in an identical manner. A positive test is elicited when pain is reproduced that radiates below the knee of the *contralateral* leg (the leg that is not being raised). Converse to the standard straight leg raise test, the sensitivity of the contralateral test for disc herniation is low, but the specificity is high. A positive contralateral straight leg raise test strongly suggests disc pathology at the L5 or S1 levels. In summary, if the straight leg raise test is positive, a positive contralateral straight leg raise test can

be considered confirmatory of the presence of disc impingement. If the straight leg raise test is negative, but the contralateral straight leg raise is positive, disc herniation or impingement is still highly likely.

Further assessment can provide additional information. Assess the patellar and Achilles deep tendon reflexes, and the plantar reflex. Hyperreflexia, clonus, or a Babinski sign (positive plantar reflex) suggests upper motor neuron pathology, such as a cord impingement. Perineal sensation and anal sphincter tone should be assessed in patients with bilateral symptoms or findings, gait disturbance, severe pain, complaints consistent with saddle anesthesia, or bowel or bladder dysfunction. The cauda equina syndrome is a spinal cord compression below the termination at the conus medullaris (L1–L2) and loss of function of the lumbar plexus. The S3, S4, and S5 dermatomal nerves innervate the "saddle" region and compression causes numbness or tingling to the perineum, anus, and genitalia. Decreased rectal muscle tone may cause loss of bowel function. Bladder dysfunction due to an inability to urinate generally presents as overflow incontinence as a result of urinary retention.

Finally, because pain from abdominal or pelvic pathology often radiates to the back, a thorough abdominal examination, including an assessment of costovertebral angle tenderness and, when indicated, a prostate or gynecologic examination should be performed to exonerate non-musculoskeletal causes of low back pain.

DIFFERENTIAL DIAGNOSES

Table 104.1 lists various causes of low back pain and historical findings that are suggestive of specific etiologies. In constructing the differential

TABLE 104.1   Historical Clues to the Cause of Low Back Pain

Questions for Patient	Potential Diagnosis
Does the back pain radiate down past the knees?	Radiculopathy and possible herniated disk
Is the pain worse with walking and better with bending forward and sitting?	Spinal stenosis
Do you have morning back stiffness that improves with exercise?	Ankylosing spondylitis
Are you older than 50 years old?	Osteoporotic fracture, spinal malignancy
Has there been any recent history of blunt trauma?	Fracture
Do you take long-term corticosteroids?	Fracture, spinal infection
Do you have a history of cancer?	Spinal metastatic malignancy
Does your pain persist at rest?	Spinal malignancy, spinal infection
Has there been persistent pain for longer than 6 weeks?	Spinal malignancy
Has there been unexplained weight loss?	Spinal malignancy
Is the pain worse at night?	Spinal malignancy, spinal infection
Are you immunocompromised?	Spinal infection
Have you had fevers or chills?	Spinal infection
Do you have pain, weakness, or numbness in both legs?	CES
Do you have bladder or bowel control problems?	CES

CES, Cauda equina syndrome.

diagnoses of musculoskeletal back pain, the emergency clinician should incorporate key findings of the history and physical examination to assess the likelihood of common, nonspecific uncomplicated back pain, while determining the presence of serious findings that are associated with specific pathoanatomic etiologies that require urgent evaluation and intervention (Table 104.2).

Other nonmuscular life-threatening pathologies which cause back pain should be considered. As an example, patients with vascular disease can present with seemingly innocuous back pain, but this may be an early warning symptom of an abdominal aortic aneurysm or thoracic aortic dissection. Gastrointestinal, pelvic, and genitourinary causes of back pain should also be assessed and excluded.

DIAGNOSTIC TESTING

Most patients presenting with back pain have nonspecific uncomplicated musculoskeletal back pain that does not require diagnostic testing. When clinical suspicion exists for a concerning etiology, or red flags are noted on either history or physical examination, diagnostic testing is warranted to identify causes of back pain that require urgent or emergent intervention.

Laboratory Testing

Laboratory testing is generally not indicated for low back pain and when performed is often adjunctive to specific diagnostic imaging. An abnormal white blood cell count (WBC), erythrocyte sedimentation rate (ESR) or C-reactive protein (CRP) may suggest an infectious or inflammatory etiology. For example, while the presence of an elevated ESR is not specific, it should increase the suspicion of spinal epidural abscess, osteomyelitis, or discitis. Marked elevations in the ESR and CRP are often due to infection, but noninfectious disorders such as malignancy, chronic or inflammatory disease, trauma, and tissue ischemia should also be considered. The presence of elevated inflammatory markers should prompt diagnostic imaging.

Coagulation testing is indicated for patients on long-term warfarin; however, the value of coagulation studies has diminished with the increasing prevalence of direct oral anticoagulant (DOAC) use. If coagulation studies are abnormal in the setting of low back pain, epidural or retroperitoneal bleeding should be explored. Urinalysis, and urine pregnancy testing in female patients, can be useful in establishing nonmusculoskeletal causes of back pain, such as nephrolithiasis, pyelonephritis or pelvic etiologies.

Imaging Studies

The vast majority of patients with self-limited, nonspecific back pain do not require emergent diagnostic imaging.[6] Routine imaging for low back pain is not associated with improved patient outcomes and

abnormalities, if found, are often incidental and not necessarily the cause of the presenting symptoms.[7] Therefore, emergent imaging in the setting of acute back pain should be reserved for patients with suspected diagnoses that would necessitate emergent intervention. Signs, symptoms, and historical features that should lead the clinician to consider imaging studies are provided in Box 104.1.

Point-of-Care Ultrasound

Bladder dysfunction as a result of cauda equina syndrome can be evaluated by post-void ultrasonographic measurement of bladder volume. A completely normal bladder should have about 20 mL of residual urine after voiding. In adults, 100 mL of residual urine is considered to be an abnormal level; in children, a residual urine volume in excess of 10 per cent of bladder capacity is also considered abnormal.

Plain Radiographs

Clinicians may obtain plain radiographs when there is concern for spontaneous compression fractures in patients with osteopenia and nontraumatic back pain. The sensitivity of plain radiographs is inadequate to safely exclude traumatic injuries, whether in elderly patients with minor trauma, in patients with major trauma, or in presentations that are suggestive of pathoanatomic etiologies. In these scenarios, more accurate, advanced diagnostic imaging should be performed.

Computed Tomography

Computed tomography (CT) is superior to plain radiographs in delineating the nature and extent of acute fractures. As compared to MRI, CT also has superior sensitivity in detecting cortical bone abnormalities and is preferable to MRI for the evaluation of acute bony injuries. Therefore, when there is a high pretest probability of vertebral fracture, CT imaging is warranted. In a multitrauma patient undergoing CT scans of the head, neck, chest, abdomen, and pelvis (or whole-body CT "pan-scans"), CT images can be reconstructed to facilitate the evaluation of the spine.

Magnetic Resonance Imaging

Magnetic resonance imaging (MRI) is the test of choice for evaluating the spinal cord and surrounding structures, including the canal, intervertebral discs, soft-tissue ligaments, and the epidural space. MRI defines the bony anatomy but is more sensitive and specific than CT in defining soft tissues and neural structures, such as the conus medullaris and spinal nerve roots within the canal and neural foramina. MRI can delineate epidural hematoma or abscess, herniated disc, ligamentous

TABLE 104.2 Physical Findings Corresponding to Herniated Disc Location

Level	Pain Location	Motor Loss	Sensory Loss	Reflex Loss
L3	Front of leg	Hip flexion and knee extension	Anterior thigh, medial calf	Loss of patellar
L4	Front of leg	Leg extension at knee	Around knee	Loss of patellar
L5	Side of leg	Foot dorsiflexion	Web of big toe	None
S1	Back of leg	Foot plantar flexion	Lateral foot	Loss of Achilles

BOX 104.1 Possible Indications for Advanced Imaging in the Setting of Back Pain

History
History of malignancy or unexplained weight loss
Fever with localized back pain
Immunocompromised status
History of injection drug use or bacteremia
History of anticoagulant use
Trauma of high force relative to patient
History of recent spinal procedure or surgery

Physical Examination
New weakness of extremities
Sensory level or saddle anesthesia
Abnormal reflexes, including positive Babinski sign
Urinary retention or incontinence with post-void residual volume >100 mL
Sphincter dysfunction: loss of sphincter tone or bowel incontinence

injury, and spinal stenosis, and it is the test of choice for diagnosing osteomyelitis. MRI is also the imaging study of choice in evaluating spinal infection and malignancy. Emergent MRI is indicated for suspected CES, epidural hemorrhage, or back pain accompanied by new neurologic findings in oncology patients. MRI is superior to plain radiographs or CT when determining the acuity or chronicity of a fracture. Contrast administration provides little additional information to MRI imaging except in the evaluation of possible intraspinal infection or metastasis.

When imaging to evaluate spinal cord lesions, it is important to clarify the possible level of the lesion. A thorough neurologic examination that includes the upper extremities may be used to exclude the need for cervical spine imaging. However, it is important to remember that spinal processes, such as malignancy or stenosis, can occur simultaneously in several levels, and the region of pain may not always correspond to the lesion causing a neurologic deficit, requiring imaging of the spine above or below the suspected affected area.

Computed Tomography Myelogram

Myelography is rarely performed in the emergency department setting and is generally indicated for patients who require advanced imaging but are unable to undergo MRI. Emergency clinicians should discuss the indications with their consulting radiologist and spine specialist before ordering this diagnostic study.

MANAGEMENT

Figure 104.1 presents a detailed algorithmic approach to ED management of patients with low back pain based on physical or ancillary test findings.

Nonspecific or Uncomplicated Back Pain

Emergency department management of acute or exacerbations of chronic back pain consists of supportive care, including patient reassurance and education and symptomatic relief. Current management guidelines for the treatment of patients with acute nonspecific back pain include attention to patient self-care and behavior modification, physical activity, and oral and topical analgesia.[8,9] Patients whose evaluations do not reveal red flags in history or physical examination should be given reassurance about the likely recovery from muscular back pain. Patients should be given advice and education about an early return to normal activities as tolerated, while avoiding heavy lifting or repetitive strenuous twisting movements. Physical activity, whether gentle exercise therapy or postural rehabilitation, has been shown to ease pain and facilitate recovery in both acute and chronic back pain. This approach also offers additional benefits of improving disability and mental health in those with nonspecific lower back pain.[8-11] Furthermore, those who use exercise to facilitate recovery are predicted to have better functional outcomes over time than those who do not exercise or use bedrest to help recovery.[11]

Topical therapies are a reasonable initial approach alone or in combination with pharmacologic treatment to offer symptomatic relief in uncomplicated back pain. Application of heat has been weakly recommended for short-term improvements in pain.[11,12] Topical capsicum or its derivative capsaicin has also demonstrated some relief in neuropathic pain, including neuropathic back pain due to lumbosacral radiculopathies.[13,14] Alternatively, transdermal application of lidocaine, whether in medicated gels, ointments, or more often in patches or plaster, has also gained increasingly widespread use. Despite the popularity of these topical agents, relatively little high-quality evidence exists for their definitive recommended use in low back pain.[11] Nonetheless, its

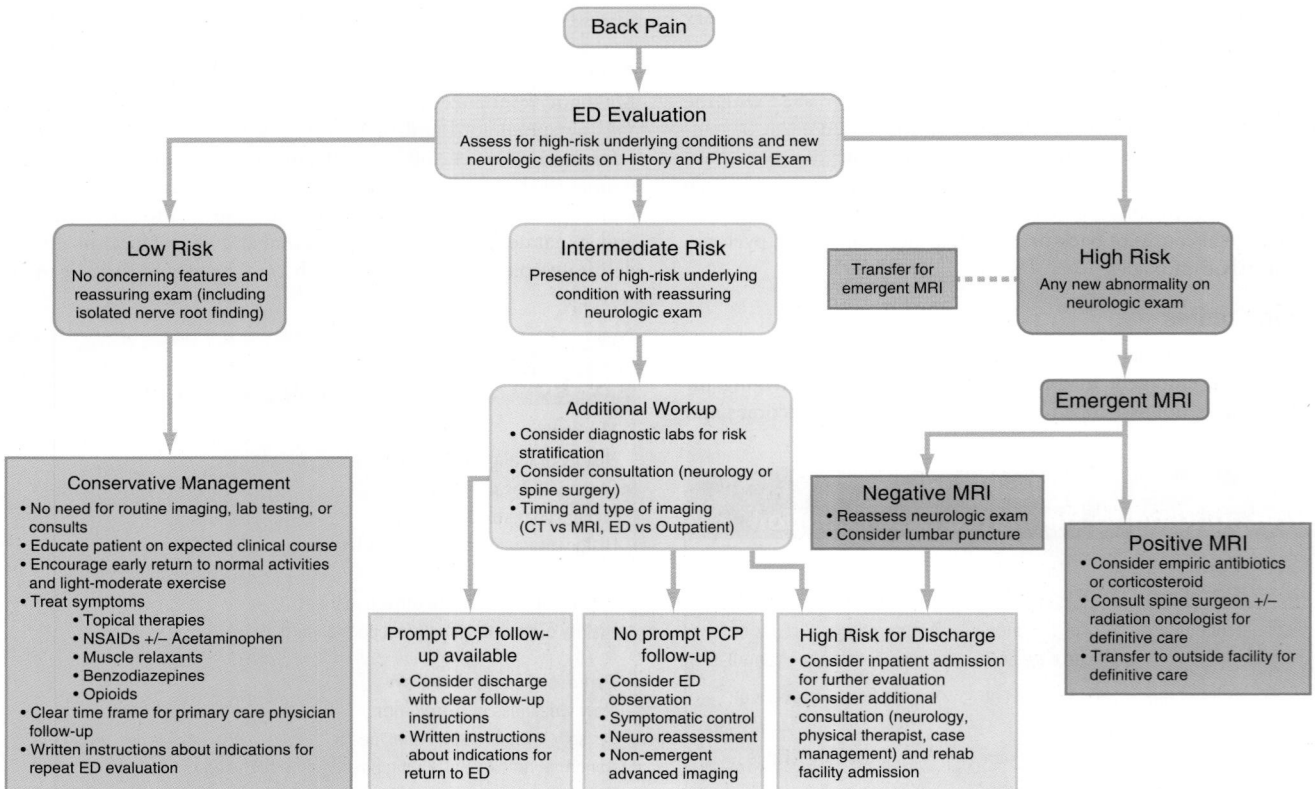

Fig. 104.1 Algorithmic approach to emergency department (ED) management of low back pain. *MRI*, Magnetic resonance imaging; *NSAID*, nonsteroidal antiinflammatory drug; *PCP*, primary care physician.

low incidence of serious adverse effects confers a clinical benefit, particularly among the elderly and medically complex.[15]

We recommend oral analgesia consisting of nonsteroidal antiinflammatory drugs (NSAIDs) alternating with or without acetaminophen. A very short course of opioid therapy may be warranted for the treatment of severe acute back pain that limits the patient's normal activity.[16] However, the use of opioid pain medications in treatment of back pain should be cautiously limited.[11-12,16] Combination therapy with NSAIDs and opioids, as compared to NSAIDs alone, does not appear to improve functional outcomes or pain at one-week follow-up.[17] A benzodiazepine may be considered to supplement analgesia when the patient has failed an NSAID regimen or when the pain is causing substantial anxiety or sleep disturbance. However, the available evidence has not demonstrated substantial effects in pain, function, or long-term outcomes.[18,19]

Early return to work, with or without activity restrictions, is associated with better long-term outcomes. Physical therapy, spinal manipulation, and multimodal rehabilitation including acupuncture have not been consistently demonstrated to be superior therapies to the above recommendations.[11,18] Approximately 10% of patients develop long-term chronic pain, often because of contributing psychosocial factors, such as anxiety or depression. Chronic back pain is more likely to develop in patients with psychiatric disorders, obesity, poor overall health status, and nonorganic signs. Development is not associated with demographic variables, prior episodes of back pain, or chronic baseline pain.[20]

In summary, nonspecific uncomplicated etiologies will account for the vast majority of patients who present to the emergency department for back pain. For these patients, the emergency clinician should focus treatment on supportive care including moderate careful exercise, low-risk topical therapies, and educating the patient regarding the self-limited nature of the disease. In those who require pharmacologic therapy, nonsteroidal antiinflammatories and acetaminophen are considered first-line. Abbreviated courses of opioids and benzodiazepines are reserved for those who have failed initial

therapy after consideration of the individual's benefits and risks. There is no role for invasive procedures, such as lumbar epidural injections, or certain classes of medications, such as anticonvulsants or antidepressants, for treatment of back pain in the emergency department.

Disc Herniation and Nerve Root Pain

Herniated disks and nerve root pain (often caused by intervertebral disc disease) without neurologic deficits on examination are initially managed similarly to nonspecific uncomplicated back pain. Signs and symptoms that indicate the need for advanced imaging and emergent spine service consultation include acute bowel or bladder dysfunction, new localized motor weakness or progressive leg weakness, and acute worsening of symptoms or findings in patients with known herniated discs and chronic back problems.

Although oral steroids do not have proven efficacy in general acute back pain, there is evidence that a subset of patients with nerve root pain and acute radiculopathy benefit from a single pulse dose of 6 to 10 mg of IV dexamethasone in the ED.[21] Alternatively, a 15-day course of a tapering dose of prednisone (60 mg, 40 mg, 20 mg daily for 5 days each) improves functional ability, but not pain.[20]

Epidural Abscess and Spinal Osteomyelitis

An epidural abscess is a surgical emergency. Emergent spine surgery consultation should be obtained at the treating hospital, or if unavailable, the patient should be transferred to a facility equipped for emergent spine surgery. Empiric antibiotics should be administered to cover suspected pathogens, usually Staphylococcus, Streptococcus, and gram-negative organisms. Vancomycin should be included to treat methicillin-resistant Staphylococcus aureus (MRSA) infection and pseudomonal coverage should be considered if hematogenous spread is suspected, particularly in immunocompromised patients with diabetes or sickle cell disease. As summarized in Box 104.2, appropriate empiric parenteral antibiotic regimens include:

BOX 104.2 Antibiotic Recommendations for Epidural Abscess and Spinal Osteomyelitis

Recommended Empiric Antibiotics Spinal and Epidural Infections	Regimen	Coverage
Epidural abscess	Vancomycin (loading dose: 20–35 mg/kg actual body weight [not to exceed 3000 mg] or 20–25 mg/kg actual body weight [not to exceed 3000 mg] in patients with obesity, then 15–20 mg/kg actual body weight every 8–12 hours)	Methicillin-resistant Staphylococcus aureus (MRSA), methicillin-sensitive Staphylococcus aureus (MSSA), and Streptococcus species
	PLUS	Anaerobic species
	Metronidazole (500 mg IV every 6 hours)	Methicillin-sensitive Staphylococcus aureus (MSSA), Streptococcus species, and gram-negative species
	PLUS	Preferred for additional coverage of Pseudomonas peruginosa
	Cefotaxime (2 g IV every 4 hours) OR Ceftriaxone (2 g IV every 12 hours) OR Ceftazidime (2 g IV every 8 hours)	
Spinal osteomyelitis	Inpatient Treatment: Nafcillin (2 g every 4 hours) OR Vancomycin (30–60 mg/kg IV per day in two equally divided doses adjusted for renal function)	Methicillin-sensitive Staphylococcus aureus (MSSA) Methicillin-resistant Staphylococcus aureus (MRSA)
	Outpatient Treatment: Ciprofloxacin (750 mg PO two times a day) OR Trimethoprim-sulfamethoxazole (1–2 DS twice a day)	Aerobic gram-negative organisms including Pseudomonas aeruginosa and Salmonella species Second-line for aerobic gram-negative organisms

- Vancomycin (30 to 60 mg/kg IV per day in two equally divided doses adjusted for renal function) for empirical coverage of MRSA

plus

- Metronidazole (500 mg IV every 8 hours)

plus

- Either cefotaxime (2 g IV every 6 hours), ceftriaxone (2 g IV every 12 hours), or ceftazidime (2 g IV every 8 hours); ceftazidime is preferable when *Pseudomonas aeruginosa* is considered a possible or likely pathogen.

Spinal osteomyelitis is treated with antibiotics (with similar broad-spectrum coverage to that of epidural abscess) in conjunction with spine surgery consultation. Surgical intervention may be less emergent than in the case of epidural abscess as long as there is no compression on the spinal cord or a purulent fluid collection. Whenever possible, antibiotic therapy should be delayed in stable patients until tissue cultures can be obtained. If tissue culture is not obtainable and in advance of tissue culture results, broad-spectrum empiric therapy should be administered (see Box 104.2). These empiric antibiotics commonly include:

- Inpatient treatment:
  - Nafcillin (2 g every 4 hours) for methicillin-sensitive *Staphylococcus aureus* (MSSA) coverage *or*
  - Vancomycin (30 to 60 mg/kg IV per day in two equally divided doses adjusted for renal function) for empirical coverage of MRSA *or*
  - Cefepime (2 g IV every 8 hours) for gram-negative and *Pseudomonas* coverage
- Outpatient treatment:
  - Ciprofloxacin (750 mg by mouth BID) *or*
  - Trimethoprim-sulfamethoxazole (1 double-strength tablet twice daily)

Epidural Hematoma

An epidural hematoma is a surgical emergency. Emergent spine surgery consultation should be obtained at the treating hospital, or if unavailable, the patient should be transferred to a facility equipped for emergent spine surgery. Patients who are anticoagulated should have their anticoagulation reversed as described in Chapter 111.

Cauda Equina Syndrome

CES, when suspected, requires rapid confirmation by emergent MRI and emergent surgical decompression. Whenever possible, spine surgery consultation should be obtained in parallel with imaging to facilitate definitive treatment. Although prompt surgery provides the best opportunity for a good outcome, some patients may not recover function after decompressive surgery. In consultation with the spine specialist, surgical intervention may be deferred in patients with long-standing or chronic symptoms of CES. Emergent administration of intravenous corticosteroids should also be determined by the treating spine surgeon.

Malignancy

Patients who are diagnosed with a compressive malignant lesion of the spine or spinal cord may benefit from emergent corticosteroids to reduce the severity of any mass effect. Once this diagnosis is made, patients with neurologic deficits should receive a single dose of 10 mg intravenous dexamethasone in the ED.[22] The ameliorative effects of corticosteroids are transient, however, and prompt consultation with spine surgery and radiation oncology specialists is imperative to consider surgical decompression or directed radiation therapy.

Fracture

The management of acute traumatic spinal fractures is extensively discussed in Chapter 35.

DISPOSITION

Most patients presenting to the ED with acute back pain will be discharged with symptomatic treatment and an appropriate outpatient follow-up plan. As mentioned previously, patient reassurance and education about muscular back pain, in conjunction with oral and topical analgesics, are foundations of care. Patients with back pain thought to be secondary to a herniated disc with no neurologic findings should have prompt follow-up with a primary care physician or a spine surgeon.

Patients with suspected radiculopathy should be given clear return precautions, including the development of weakness, inability to stand or ambulate, saddle anesthesia, or bowel or bladder dysfunction. Patients who require emergent surgical intervention for spinal epidural abscess, compressive neoplasm, osteomyelitis, fracture, or other compressive spine lesions should be emergently transferred to the care of a spine surgeon, which may involve transfer to a tertiary or quaternary care center.

Patient transfer may be necessary if emergent spine surgery is not present at the treating facility or if emergent MRI is not available to image patients with suspected emergent infectious or compressive pathologies. Patients believed to have an epidural abscess or osteomyelitis should receive empiric parenteral antibiotics prior to transfer. Patients with findings consistent with CES or other compressive lesions due to malignancy should receive parenteral steroids prior to transfer if ordered by the receiving physician or the onsite consultant.

The references for this chapter can be found online at ExpertConsult. com.

105

Systemic Lupus Erythematosus and the Vasculitides

Eric Shappell and Eli M. Miloslavsky

SYSTEMIC LUPUS ERYTHEMATOSUS

KEY CONCEPTS

- Systemic lupus erythematosus (SLE) is a chronic autoimmune disorder that can affect any organ system. A general approach to determine whether SLE is the cause of a nonspecific or single-organ symptom is to search for evidence of other organ involvement or systemic inflammation, which is expected in SLE-mediated presentations.
- Patients with SLE are at significantly higher risk of coronary artery or thromboembolic disease, which should prompt more thorough evaluation for these etiologies even in otherwise low-risk patients, such as young women.
- SLE itself, as well as its treatment, may lead to immunosuppression; thus, it is important to remain vigilant for the possibility of infection in patients with SLE.
- Glucocorticoids are the mainstay for the initial management of the majority of conditions that are associated with increased SLE disease activity, including musculoskeletal, cutaneous, renal, pleural, or pericardial disease.
- Antiphospholipid antibody syndrome (APS) is common in patients with SLE and carries with it an increased risk of venous and arterial thromboembolic disease.
- Rheumatology input may be helpful in diagnostic, management, or disposition decisions for select patients with SLE.

FOUNDATIONS

Background and Importance

Systemic lupus erythematosus (SLE) is a chronic autoimmune disorder with complex pathophysiology that can affect nearly any organ system in the body. The prevalence of SLE varies by age, gender, geography, and race. Women are the most commonly affected group worldwide, representing approximately 90% of cases. The disease is more common in young people with more than two-thirds of cases diagnosed before the age of 50. In the United States, the prevalence of SLE is higher in African, Asian, and Hispanic Americans compared to Caucasians.

Patients with SLE have an increased risk of mortality (2.6-fold) as compared to the general population.[1] Morbidity and mortality for patients with SLE derive from four processes: (1) organ damage secondary to disease-mediated inflammation (e.g., nephritis, cerebritis, coronary artery disease), (2) hypercoagulability (e.g., stroke, pulmonary embolism), (3) complications of treatment (e.g., infection related to immunosuppression), and (4) increased risk of cardiovascular events. Care for the patient with SLE in the emergency department (ED) hinges on the recognition and treatment of these processes.

Etiology and Pathophysiology

The etiology of SLE is complex and incompletely understood. It appears to be related to multiple factors; genetics, hormones, and environmental factors such as smoking have all been implicated to varying degrees. With women representing 90% of SLE cases, a strong role for estrogen in disease development has been well supported in large cohort studies. The disease also has a strong genetic link, with high rates of monozygotic twin concordance.

The pathophysiology of SLE is mediated by the creation of autoantibodies with a multitude of downstream impacts. These effects include the formation and deposition of immune complexes leading to inflammation and tissue destruction (largely via complement activation) as well as autoantibodies directly targeting cell surface antigens and phospholipids, which may lead to tissue cell death, hemolysis, and hypercoagulability. The pathophysiologic mechanism of SLE may differ for each organ system. The organ systems involved in any given patient's disease may be different and relate to antigen expression in those tissues, among other factors.

CLINICAL FEATURES

Overview

SLE activity follows a relapsing and remitting pattern: acute episodes of increased disease activity ("flares") are separated by periods of stable disease or relative quiescence. The frequency and severity of flares can vary significantly between patients and over time, as can the baseline level of disease activity. While SLE is a chronic condition, it is not necessarily progressive. Whether additional organs become involved and the degree to which previously involved organs are affected is variable.

Recognition of SLE-mediated morbidity can be challenging, as SLE can affect nearly any organ system in the body, and many symptoms of the disease lack specificity. In general, ED presentations for SLE are related to one or more of the following: (1) flares of increased SLE disease activity (e.g., nephritis, arthritis), (2) SLE-mediated hypercoagulability (e.g., stroke, pulmonary embolism), and (3) complications of treatment for SLE (e.g., opportunistic infection due to immunosuppression).

Even with good medication adherence, patients with SLE are prone to flares. SLE flares are typified by worsening physical symptoms from increased organ inflammation and destruction. Flares commonly involve organ systems previously affected by SLE, though new organ systems may also become affected. As a systemic disease, worsening symptoms in one organ system are often associated with evidence of systemic inflammation and, commonly, evidence of disease activity in other organs.

As a general approach, when evaluating whether a symptom is due to SLE, providers should look for other SLE manifestations and biomarkers that can point to active disease, such as those in the Systemic Lupus International Collaborating Clinics (SLICC) Criteria for Systemic Lupus Erythematosus (Table 105.1). Single-organ symptoms without systemic inflammation should prompt consideration of

TABLE 105.1 Systemic Lupus International Collaborating Clinics Criteria for Systemic Lupus Erythematosus[a]

Criteria	Description
Clinical Criteria	
Acute cutaneous lupus	May include acute cutaneous lupus (lupus malar rash, bullous lupus, toxic epidermal necrolysis variant of SLE, maculopapular lupus rash, photosensitive lupus rash) or subacute cutaneous lupus
Chronic cutaneous lupus	Classic discoid rash, generalized hypertrophic (verrucous) lupus, lupus panniculitis, mucosal lupus, others
Oral ulcers	Palate (buccal, tongue) or nasal ulcers
Non-scarring alopecia	Diffuse thinning or hair fragility
Synovitis	Involving two or more joints (swelling, effusion, or tenderness and ≥30 minutes of morning stiffness)
Serositis	Pleural (pleuritis, effusion, rub) or pericardial (pericarditis, effusion, rub)
Renal disorder	500 mg protein/24 h or red blood cell casts
Neurologic disorder	Seizures, psychosis, mononeuritis multiplex, myelitis, peripheral and cranial neuropathies, acute confusional state
Hemolytic anemia	
Leukopenia	<4000/mm^3 at least once
Thrombocytopenia	<100,000/mm^3 at least once
Immunological Criteria	
Anti-nuclear antibody	Any level above the laboratory reference range
Anti-dsDNA	Level above the laboratory reference range (or twofold the reference range if tested by ELISA)
Anti-Sm	Presence of antibody to Sm nuclear antigen
aPL antibody	As determined by a positive test for lupus anticoagulant or anti-2-glycoprotein, false-positive result for rapid plasma regain, medium- or high-titer anticardiolipin antibody level
Low complement	May include C3, C4, or CH50
Direct Coombs test	In the absence of hemolytic anemia

[a]Fulfillment of at least four criteria, with at least one clinical and one laboratory criterion, is required to establish the diagnosis of systemic lupus erythematosus.

aPL, Antiphospholipid; *ds*, double-stranded; *ELISA*, enzyme-linked immunosorbent assay; *SLE*, systemic lupus erythematosus; *Sm*, Smith.

pathology other than SLE. It is important to identify when overall disease activity is increased as this signals the need to initiate or escalate systemic therapy. In many cases, patients themselves are able to provide direction about the predictable course of their exacerbations and can be helpful in decision-making for therapy and disposition.

Specific Symptoms

Fever

Fever in a patient with SLE can be related to systemic disease activity, infection (including opportunistic infection related to immunosuppression), or pathology unrelated to SLE. Recurrent fevers without evidence of infection may be the presenting symptom that leads to an initial diagnosis of SLE. Similarly, patients with diagnosed SLE may present with fever as a symptom attributable to a disease flare. Before attributing fever to SLE disease activity, however, care should be taken to exclude acute infection. This is particularly important for patients taking immunosuppressive medications. Most infections in SLE are caused by typical organisms. However, largely because of the immunomodulating therapies that are the cornerstone of SLE management, opportunistic diseases are possible; *Pneumocystis (carinii) jiroveci* pneumonia, cryptococcal meningitis, *Listeria* infection, and herpes zoster have all been described.

Cardiopulmonary Presentations

There is a broad range of cardiac and pulmonary pathology associated with SLE that may present with chest pain or shortness of breath. Given the lengthy differential for this spectrum of presentations and the significant degree of overlapping symptoms for the varied underlying disease processes, an anatomic approach may be useful when working through the differential.

Coronary Artery Disease. As with other systemic inflammatory conditions, there is a significantly increased risk of coronary artery disease (CAD) in patients with SLE. While SLE is associated with higher incidences of traditional risk factors such as hypertension and hypercholesterolemia, the increased risk of CAD persists even after controlling for these factors.[4] Thus, whereas there are many considerations for the cause of chest pain in patients with SLE, acute coronary syndromes (ACS) should be considered highly in these cases, including in patients who would otherwise be deemed low risk (e.g., young women). Coronary disease should also be considered in patients with SLE presenting with atypical symptoms of ACS, such as shortness of breath, epigastric pain, or fatigue.

Pericardial and Myocardial Disease. Pericarditis and effusions of the pericardium occur commonly in patients with SLE and are among the classification criteria for the disease (see Table 105.1). An estimated 25% of patients with SLE will experience symptomatic pericarditis during the course of their lives, and pericardial effusion (often asymptomatic) occurs even more frequently. In patients with pericarditis, dyspnea and chest pain that is sharp, pleuritic, and positional (improved with leaning forward) are classic features of the disease. Auscultation may reveal a friction rub. Electrocardiography may reveal classic findings of diffuse ST elevation and PR depression (Fig. 105.1); however, patients with pericarditis may also have normal or nonspecific ECG findings. Given the increased risk of CAD in patients with SLE, obtaining cardiac biomarkers in patients with ST elevation that would otherwise be diagnosed as pericarditis is generally encouraged. If there is diagnostic uncertainty as to whether ST elevation is related to pericarditis or an ST elevation myocardial infarction (STEMI), urgent cardiology consultation for consideration of cardiac catheterization is warranted. There are no specific signs of pericarditis on echocardiography. Visualization of pericardial effusion is supportive of the diagnosis of pericarditis; however, this finding may also be present in patients with SLE that do not have symptomatic pericarditis. Echocardiography is also useful to assess for associated cardiac tamponade, which is a rare but life-threatening complication of SLE. The presentation and diagnosis of cardiac tamponade are the same for patients with SLE as the general population. SLE myocarditis may present with chest discomfort and symptoms of heart failure, though acute symptomatic presentations are rare.

Valvular Disease. SLE is associated with a type of noninfectious endocarditis known as *Libman-Sacks endocarditis* (Fig. 105.2). Mitral valve disease is most common, though other valves may also be affected. While the lesions formed on heart valves in this condition are more often associated with embolization than valvular dysfunction, some patients may develop valvular insufficiency that may present with shortness of breath, fatigue, or, in rare severe cases, pulmonary edema.

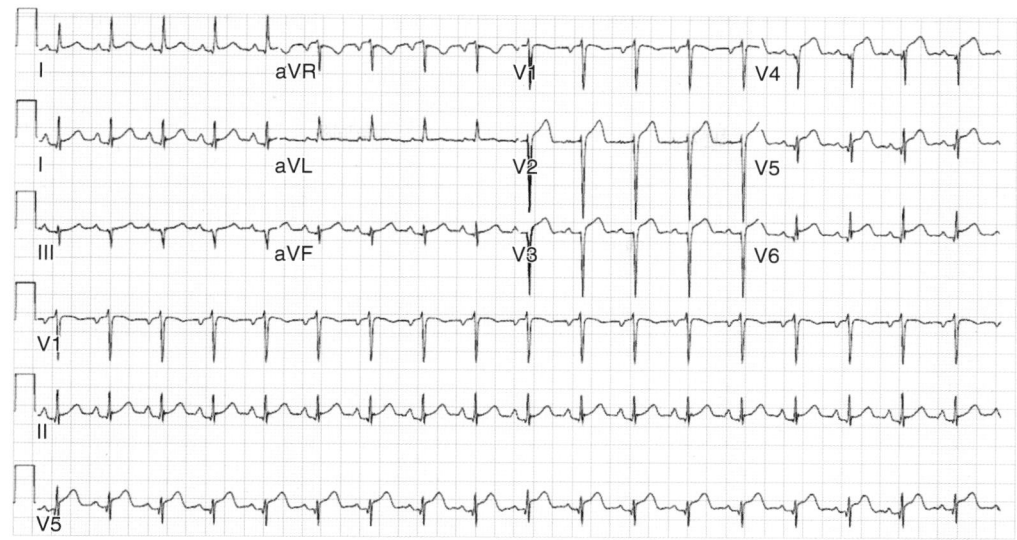

Fig. 105.1 Electrocardiogram of a 38-year-old woman with systemic lupus erythematosus (SLE) who presented to the emergency department (ED) with seizures and had chest pain while in the ED. Note diffuse ST elevation (with the absence of any reciprocal changes) and PR depression (particularly evident in lead II). Q waves anteriorly are related to prior myocardial infarct.

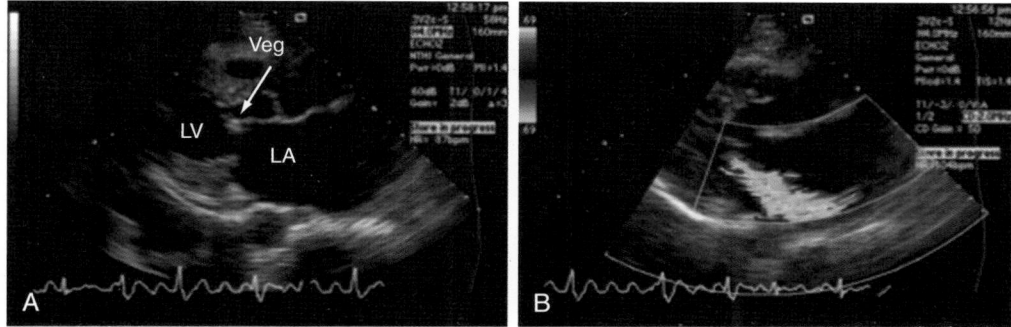

Fig. 105.2 Noninfectious endocarditis, known as a *Libman-Sacks lesion*, in a 56-year-old woman with systemic lupus erythematosus (SLE), a heart murmur, and dyspnea on exertion. (A) A parasternal long-axis view of the heart; a vegetation *(Veg)* is identified *(arrow)* on the mitral valve. (B) When color flow is superimposed on the valve, moderate to severe mitral regurgitation can be seen as a color jet entering the left atrium during systole. *LA,* Left atrium; *LV,* left ventricle. (Courtesy Martin Goldman, MD, Mount Sinai School of Medicine.)

Pulmonary Vascular Disease. Due to disease-associated hypercoagulability, deep venous thrombosis (DVT) and pulmonary embolism (PE) are more frequent in patients with SLE when compared to the general population. The degree of hypercoagulability in patients with concomitant **antiphospholipid syndrome** (APS) is even higher. Outside of the context of increased thromboembolic risk lowering the threshold for further testing, the evaluation for thrombosis and embolism in a patient with SLE does not differ from that of patients in the general population.

Though uncommon, patients with SLE may also develop pulmonary hypertension, which can present with shortness of breath, chest discomfort, and fatigue. Evaluation, in this case, may reveal a history of pathology known to lead to pulmonary hypertension (e.g., chronic thromboembolism, interstitial lung disease), physical exam findings of right heart failure, or evidence of right ventricular hypertrophy on electrocardiography or echocardiography. A definitive diagnosis is made via right heart catheterization.

Pleural Disease. Pleuritis is the most common respiratory condition occurring in SLE. Characterized by pleuritic chest pain with or without a pleural effusion or pleural rub, it has symptoms that overlap with those of other more serious conditions. A diagnosis of pleuritis should be arrived at only after other causes of pleuritic chest pain (e.g., PE) have been excluded.

Parenchymal Disease. Diseases of the lung parenchyma associated with SLE include infectious pneumonia, acute and chronic pneumonitis, interstitial lung disease, and, rarely, diffuse alveolar hemorrhage (DAH). The symptoms associated with infectious pneumonia, pneumonitis, and DAH have significant overlap; each of these entities may present with fever, cough, shortness of breath, and hemoptysis, and chest radiography may reveal nonspecific opacifications. Differentiating between these entities is difficult in the ED setting and may require further evaluation with bronchoscopy for bronchoalveolar lavage.

Mechanical Respiratory Disease. Shrinking lung syndrome is a rare condition associated with SLE that is characterized by symptoms of shortness of breath and pleurisy with low lung volumes and a restrictive pattern on pulmonary function testing. Patients may also have the elevation of one or both hemidiaphragms and pleural effusions. The etiology of this syndrome is unclear but appears to involve some degree of restriction of chest wall expansion with or without diaphragmatic dysfunction.

Renal Disease

Renal disease is a common complication of SLE occurring in approximately one-half of patients.[5,6] Renal disease related to SLE may cause a nephrotic-type disease, primarily characterized by significant proteinuria or nephritic disease with hematuria and increased creatinine concentration. Diagnosis based on clinical criteria alone is not possible as many patients with renal impairment are asymptomatic. Patients that do have symptoms may report hematuria, foamy urine, generalized edema, or an elevated blood pressure from baseline. Given the high prevalence and morbidity of renal disease and its tendency to carry few if any symptoms, a screening urinalysis and basic metabolic panel are prudent in all but the most straightforward presentations concerning SLE-mediated disease. Renal biopsy is indicated for all patients with new-onset lupus nephritis and can be considered in those with relapsing or refractory disease.

Gastrointestinal Presentations

The most common gastrointestinal (GI) manifestation of SLE is oral ulceration. Esophageal dysmotility and reflux are also more common in patients with SLE and may present with dysphagia or pain in the epigastric region or chest. In patients with SLE, most causes of abdominal symptoms (e.g., pain, nausea, diarrhea, constipation) are the same as in the general population. Accordingly, the ED evaluation should be largely similar for each of the two groups. Special considerations for patients with SLE, however, include an increased risk of pancreatitis due to medications, mesenteric vasculitis (also known as lupus enteritis), peritonitis due to serositis, or the side effects of medications including chronic NSAIDs (e.g., peptic ulcer disease), glucocorticoids (e.g., peptic ulcer disease, perforation, infection), or immunosuppressive agents (infection).

Patients taking glucocorticoids or other immunosuppressive medications may also have masking of traditional symptoms, so a lower threshold for further testing (e.g., computed tomography [CT] imaging) should be used for this population.

Dermatologic Presentations

The most characteristic cutaneous manifestation of SLE is the malar rash. The rash has a "butterfly" distribution of raised erythema over the bridge of the nose and malar eminences while sparing the chin, forehead, and nasal-labial folds (Fig. 105.3). This sparing of the nasal-labial folds can help distinguish the classic malar rash from mimics such as rosacea or seborrheic dermatitis. Other common skin findings in patients with SLE include discoid lupus erythematosus (DLE) and subacute cutaneous lupus erythematosus (SCLE). Each of these skin findings can present years before systemic manifestations of SLE occur, and while the characteristic malar rash is highly specific for SLE, DLE and SCLE more commonly present in isolation, without progression to SLE. DLE lesions are circular and raised, scaly lesions that may be commonly found on the face, scalp, and ears, often in association with pigment change, alopecia, and scarring (Fig. 105.4). SCLE lesions are annular with an erythematous border, scaling, and central clearing. At times, these areas may coalesce to form more complex linear patterns of erythema. These lesions can be triggered by sunlight and are most commonly found in sun-exposed areas of the upper extremities, torso, and neck. The face is not usually affected by SCLE.

Musculoskeletal Presentations

Arthritis commonly afflicts those with SLE, and increasing severity of joint pain may be a marker of increasing disease activity or an SLE flare. Arthritis or arthralgias are typically symmetrical and nonerosive (unlike rheumatoid arthritis, which is erosive) and always involve multiple joints. Arthritis most commonly presents in the hands (metacarpophalangeal and proximal interphalangeal joints), wrists, feet, and knees but may be manifested in any joint. While swelling may be present, often, the joint pain of lupus presents with arthralgia alone. Uncommonly, septic arthritis may complicate SLE. An isolated swollen joint is not typical of SLE and should prompt consideration for infectious arthritis. If septic arthritis is suspected, diagnostic arthrocentesis is recommended.

Myalgias are common in SLE and may be an early marker of increasing disease activity for some patients. It should be kept in mind that fibromyalgia may also coexist with SLE and chronic myalgia not associated with other disease activity or elevated inflammatory markers may point to this diagnosis. While generalized muscle pain is sometimes seen, muscle weakness is uncharacteristic. If muscle weakness is present, an underlying myositis or myopathy, potentially related to steroid or hydroxychloroquine use, should be considered. Musculoskeletal chest pain, related to underlying pectoral, intercostal muscle,

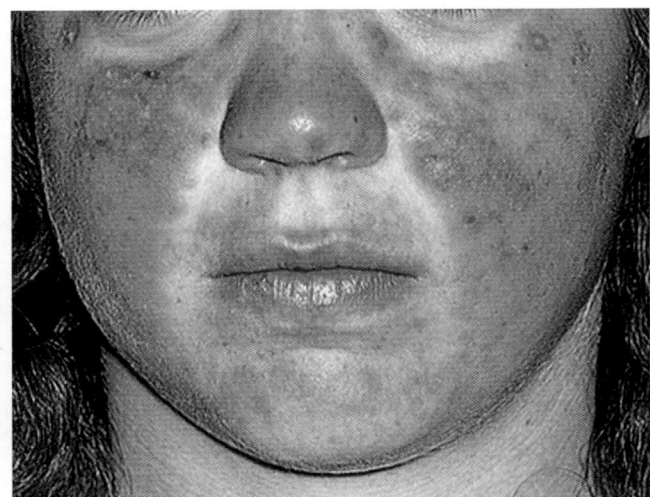

Fig. 105.3 The Malar or Butterfly Rash Is the Hallmark of Systemic Lupus Erythematosus (SLE). (From Habif TP. *Clinical Dermatology.* 5th ed. New York: Mosby; 2009:592–606.)

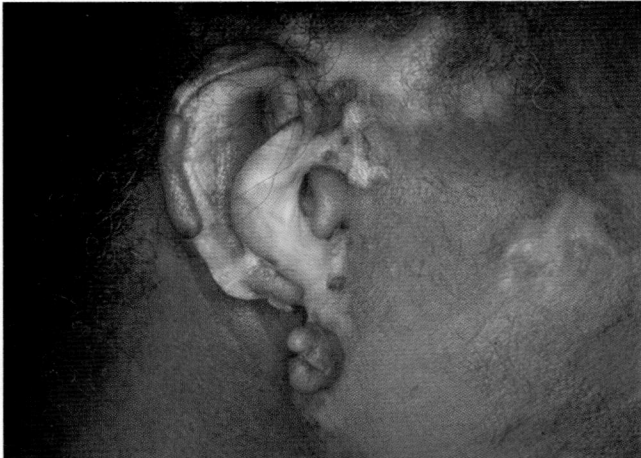

Fig. 105.4 Right Ear of a Patient Suffering From Chronic Discoid Lupus. Note pigment change and tissue destruction. (Courtesy Professor Gregory Raugi, University of Washington.)

or costochondral joint inflammation may also occur and should be treated the same as in patients without SLE. Similar to pleuritis, the threat of a more malicious underlying cause of the pain should prompt the clinician first to seek other causes before arriving at this more benign diagnosis.

Hematologic Disease

Anemia, present in up to 50% of patients with SLE, may present with a chief complaint of dyspnea or weakness. Iron deficiency anemia, anemia of chronic disease, autoimmune hemolytic anemia, or medication-induced bone marrow suppression can all contribute to anemia in a patient with SLE. SLE also shares a strong association with APS, which is associated with a significantly increased risk of thromboembolic disease.

Complications Due To Medications

Chronic NSAID use for the musculoskeletal consequences of SLE may contribute to peptic ulcer disease, especially if they are coadministered with glucocorticoids. Chronic glucocorticoids are associated with an increased risk of multiple conditions including CAD, osteoporosis, avascular necrosis, psychosis, hyperglycemia, hypertension, and weight gain, among many others. Therapy with antimalarials, such as hydroxychloroquine, is common and generally well tolerated; however, retinopathy has been associated with prolonged use. Medications that interfere with DNA synthesis such as cyclophosphamide, methotrexate, mycophenolate mofetil, and azathioprine suppress the immune response, leaving patients vulnerable to both conventional and opportunistic infections. These medications are also frequent causes of cytopenias and liver function test elevations. Cyclophosphamide is one of the most potent immunosuppressants and particular care should be given to assessing for infection in patients receiving this agent. Biologic agents such as rituximab and belimumab are also associated with an increased risk of infection or cytopenias.

DIFFERENTIAL DIAGNOSIS

In keeping with its highly varied presentations and permutations of disease activity, a number of other diseases may be confused with SLE before diagnosis. These include infection, thrombotic thrombocytopenic purpura (TTP), APS, vasculitis, rheumatoid arthritis, mixed connective tissue disease, undifferentiated connective tissue disease, Sjögren syndrome, fibromyalgia, and drug-induced lupus, among others. In the ED setting, the priority should be identifying severe illness with an acute threat to organ function or risk of death. Mild, subacute, and nonspecific disease processes generally do not require definitive diagnosis in the ED setting if not associated with evidence of near-term risk to organ function. Chief complaint-driven considerations for acute presentations of SLE are listed in Table 105.2.

DIAGNOSTIC TESTING

Patients carrying a diagnosis of SLE presenting with symptoms concerning SLE-related pathology will typically require evaluation for evidence of systemic disease activity in addition to symptom-specific testing. In general, patients will not undergo testing for an initial diagnosis of SLE in the ED.

The general approach to assessing whether a symptom is caused by overall SLE disease activity is to look for signs and symptoms of the disease in other organs or systemically. For example, a patient presenting with pleurisy, arthralgias, and fever that has laboratory testing consistent with increased disease activity and chest radiography that is negative for evidence of infection may be diagnosed with a lupus flare. A patient with isolated pleurisy in the absence of other symptoms,

laboratory tests, or imaging studies consistent with active SLE, however, is less likely to be suffering from an SLE flare and therefore warrants further evaluation for non-SLE pathology.

Symptom-specific testing will be the same for patients with and without SLE, with the caveat that certain testing thresholds may be lowered for patients with SLE given the increased risks associated with this disease and its treatment (e.g., cardiovascular disease, thromboembolic disease, infection).

Laboratory Tests

While patients will not typically undergo laboratory testing for an initial diagnosis of SLE in the ED, special circumstances such as low resource settings, poor outpatient follow-up, or severe illness requiring expedited diagnosis may prompt emergency physicians to begin this evaluation.

TABLE 105.2 **Common or Specific Differential Considerations for Patients With Systemic Lupus Erythematosus Based on Common Presentations, Comorbidities, or Complications**

Chief Complaint	Condition
Altered Mental Status	Neuropsychiatric lupus Medication effect (e.g., steroid psychosis) Seizure Infection
Fever	Infection Increased disease activity (SLE flare)
Chest pain	Acute coronary syndrome Pulmonary embolism Pericarditis/pericardial effusion Pleuritis/pleural effusion Musculoskeletal chest wall pain (diagnosis of exclusion)
Shortness of breath	Acute coronary syndrome Pulmonary embolism Pulmonary hypertension/right heart failure Pneumonia Pericarditis/pericardial effusion Pleuritis/pleural effusion Interstitial lung disease Shrinking lung syndrome Anemia
Abdominal pain	Pancreatitis Peptic ulcer disease Pseudo-obstruction Lupus enteritis
Leg swelling	Deep venous thrombosis Nephrotic syndrome Renal failure Heart failure (left- or right-sided)
Pruritic or painful rash	Discoid SLE Drug reaction Sun exposure
Arthritis	Increased disease activity (SLE flare) Osteoarthritis Septic arthritis

SLE, Systemic lupus erythematosus.

For patients carrying a diagnosis of SLE with all but the most trivial presentations of potential SLE-mediated disease, laboratory studies are indicated to assess for increased disease activity as the etiology of the patient's symptoms.

Initial Diagnosis

The diagnosis of SLE can be difficult. The broad, heterogeneous, waxing and waning nature of the disease, lack of specificity of many presenting symptoms, multitude of diseases with overlapping symptoms, and lack of uniform diagnostic criteria all contribute to this difficulty. While classification criteria for SLE have been published by the European League Against Rheumatism/American College of Rheumatology and Systemic Lupus Collaborating Clinics, these are not set forth as diagnostic criteria.[7,8] However, clinicians may find these criteria helpful in remembering salient elements for the evaluation of a patient with possible SLE, including relevant laboratory studies. Laboratory testing relevant to SLE diagnosis includes a complete blood count to assess for leukopenia, lymphopenia, and thrombocytopenia; hemolysis testing if anemia is present; complement levels; urinalysis for hematuria, proteinuria, and casts; and immunologic assays including anti-nuclear antibody (ANA), anti-double-stranded DNA (dsDNA) antibody, anti-Smith (Sm) antibody, and aPL antibodies. The Ro, La, and ribonucleoprotein (RNP) antibodies may also be seen in lupus but are less specific for SLE and are also associated with Sjögren's and mixed connective tissue disease, respectively. A positive ANA is present in nearly all patients with SLE but is also present in more than 10% of the general population. The ANA titer is important to consider as the majority of patients with SLE have high-titer ANAs. In general, the temptation to pursue a new diagnosis of SLE in the ED should be avoided due to the lack of uniform diagnostic criteria, reliance on laboratory investigations that are uncommonly carried out in the ED, and rarity that a diagnosis made emergently will significantly change patient outcomes.

Disease Activity

Routine laboratory tests with correlation to increased SLE disease activity include a complete blood count (leukopenia, anemia, thrombocytopenia), basic metabolic panel (creatinine elevation), erythrocyte sedimentation rate (ESR, elevated), and urinalysis (hematuria, proteinuria). Patients found to have new or worsening anemia should be evaluated for hemolysis, which is associated with increased SLE disease activity. This evaluation may include a direct Coombs test, peripheral blood smear, LDH, and haptoglobin. It should be noted that the ESR is not always elevated in active disease; therefore, patients with compelling symptoms without an alternative explanation can be diagnosed with SLE flare despite normal inflammatory markers. C-reactive protein (CRP) is frequently normal in active lupus. Therefore, an elevated CRP should prompt strong consideration of infection. Other more specialized laboratory markers of SLE disease activity include low complement levels (C3, C4) and elevated anti-dsDNA.

Evaluation for Infection

Leukocytosis may suggest infection in some cases; however, it has poor specificity. This finding may be even less useful in SLE patients taking glucocorticoids, as these medications are associated with baseline leukocytosis. Leukopenia may also suggest infection in some cases; however, this is also a sign of active SLE and therefore cannot be relied upon as a marker specific for infection in patients with SLE. Immature cells (e.g., band cells) on a differential are relatively specific for infection and are not routinely associated with SLE disease activity. CRP may also be a useful marker as it can be normal despite increased disease activity in SLE but typically rises in the case of infection. ESR is nonspecific and will rise in both cases of infection and SLE flares.

Imaging Studies

While SLE is also associated with a wide variety of other pathology routinely diagnosed on imaging studies (e.g., stroke, pneumonia, PE), the imaging studies of choice for these entities do not differ between patients with and without SLE. Lupus cerebritis, a blanket term for organic SLE-related CNS pathology with neuropsychiatric manifestations and no alternate diagnosis, is typically evaluated with magnetic resonance imaging (MRI) of the brain in addition to lumbar puncture. MRI of the brain in patients with lupus cerebritis may be normal or reveal nonspecific findings such as hyperintense white matter lesions, and should assist in excluding alternate diagnoses (e.g., stroke).

MANAGEMENT

Emergent Stabilization

Emergent stabilization of patients with SLE does not differ from that of patients without the disease. Management of life-threatening presentations associated with SLE such as myocardial infarction, stroke, PE, seizure, and infection should all proceed as usual. For patients with SLE in refractory shock, stress dose glucocorticoids (hydrocortisone 100 mg IV q8h) should be considered given the high incidence of chronic steroid therapy and related adrenal suppression in this population. Advanced SLE therapies (e.g., immunosuppressive agents, plasma exchange) can be coordinated with the appropriate consulting services (e.g., rheumatology, nephrology) for patients with a critical illness.

General Systemic Disease Activity

Nearly all manifestations of active SLE are managed with the introduction or escalation of immunomodulatory therapy.

Patients Diagnosed With Systemic Lupus Erythematosus

For patients that carry a diagnosis of SLE and evidence of active disease, treatment and disposition will be guided by the severity of symptoms. Mild to moderate disease with manifestations such as joint pain, serositis, or cutaneous disease typically respond to prednisone 15 to 20 mg PO daily or NSAIDs in the case of joint pain and serositis. For pericardial and pleural effusions in the absence of hemodynamic compromise or respiratory distress, respectively, drainage in the ED setting is rarely required. For patients with severe disease and end-organ dysfunction (e.g., seizures, transverse myelitis, cardiac tamponade, nephritis), either pulse glucocorticoids (e.g., methylprednisolone 1 g/day IV) or prednisone 1 mg/kg/day PO and admission are generally appropriate. If worsening renal dysfunction is discovered, admission should be considered for hydration, escalation of therapy, and consideration of renal biopsy to help classify the disease and guide treatment. In each of the presented scenarios, management and disposition decisions can be made in consultation with a patient's rheumatologist, if available.

Patients Not Diagnosed With Systemic Lupus Erythematosus

For patients who do not carry a diagnosis of SLE and who have only mild evidence of disease (e.g., rash, arthralgias, uncomplicated pleurisy), symptomatic treatment and referral to a rheumatologist or primary care physician are appropriate provided that end-organ disease such as nephritis has been considered. In patients with evidence of severe systemic SLE-related disease (e.g., seizures, transverse myelitis, cardiac tamponade), empiric pulsed glucocorticoids should be considered while a formal diagnosis of SLE is pending.

Specific Presentations

Infection

Management of infection in patients with SLE includes appropriate antimicrobial coverage based on the suspected source, prior culture data (as available), and the patient's degree of immunosuppression, as well as source control. Patients on chronic steroid therapy with refractory hypotension associated with infection should typically be treated with stress dose glucocorticoids (e.g., hydrocortisone 100 mg IV every 8 hours). Generally, nonglucocorticoid immunosuppression should be stopped while infection is treated, with the exception of hydroxychloroquine, which has not been associated with an increased risk of infection.

Musculoskeletal Pain

Much of the pain associated with SLE is related to inflammation that is amenable to treatment with NSAIDs or low-dose glucocorticoids. Ibuprofen 600–800 mg three times daily a day or naproxen 500 mg orally twice daily is useful for conditions such as pericarditis, pleuritis, arthralgias, myalgias, and fever. It is important to distinguish inflammatory joint pain from fibromyalgia, which does not typically respond to NSAIDs or glucocorticoids. Use of NSAIDs in patients with chronic kidney disease or a history of peptic ulcer disease is discouraged. In such patients, acetaminophen is used for mild to moderate pain. Adjunctive therapies such as lidocaine patches and heating or cooling packs may also be useful in controlling musculoskeletal pain related to SLE. The use of opioid medications is discouraged in the management of chronic rheumatologic diseases, including SLE.

Cutaneous Manifestations

In cases of isolated cutaneous findings, treatment with topical corticosteroids is preferable to systemic therapy. Topical therapy may be initiated with a medium potency steroid such as triamcinolone 1% cream to the affected area. In cases in which higher potency topical corticosteroids are necessary, preparation of 0.05% betamethasone dipropionate applied once daily to the affected area for 2 weeks is appropriate. Moderate to severe cases may be treated with topical calcineurin inhibitors or systemic therapy in consultation with the patient's internist, dermatologist, or rheumatologist. In nearly all cases of SLE, avoidance of sun exposure is advisable and will help minimize cutaneous disease.

SPECIAL CONSIDERATIONS

Antiphospholipid Syndrome
Foundations

Present in approximately 15% of patients with SLE, APS is considered when patients both have a clinical history of thrombosis and test positive for one or more antiphospholipid (aPL) antibodies. These antibodies include those corresponding to anticardiolipin, lupus anticoagulant, and β_2-glycoprotein I. The thrombotic risk profile varies based on which antibody or combination of antibodies are present. In addition to its role as a strong risk factor for both venous and arterial thrombosis, the presence of APS in SLE has been shown to be an independent predictor of more severe disease. Whether it is present in the context of SLE or independently, APS is an important cause of morbidity and mortality due to thrombosis.

Clinical Features

APS may present with a number of clinical features (Box 105.1), typically related to thrombosis or thromboembolism. A small subset of those with APS may present with multiple thrombotic sites or multiorgan failure due to microvascular thrombosis. Catastrophic APS (CAPS) is diagnosed when three or more sites or organs are affected.[9,10]

Diagnostic Testing

Similar to the workup for other hypercoagulable conditions, diagnostic testing for APS is unlikely to be indicated in the ED setting. Assays detecting the presence of aPL antibodies (anticardiolipin, lupus

anticoagulant, and β_2-glycoprotein I), at two timepoints 12 weeks apart, are necessary for the laboratory component of the diagnosis of APS. Two additional laboratory findings that are supportive of APS (though not diagnostic) are a spuriously elevated PTT in the setting of a normal PT/INR, due to interference of the coagulation study by aPL antibodies, or a falsely positive Venereal Disease Research Laboratory (VDRL) assay to test for syphilis, as the antigen in the VDRL test contains cardiolipin.

Management

For acute thrombotic events, anticoagulation with heparin (unfractionated or low–molecular-weight) is generally indicated. After an initial thrombotic event, anticoagulation with a low–molecular-weight heparin or vitamin K antagonists such as warfarin is recommended indefinitely. Direct oral anticoagulants carry an increased risk of thrombosis compared to vitamin K antagonists and therefore are not recommended for first-line treatment. For patients with catastrophic APS, in addition to anticoagulation and glucocorticoids, intravenous immune globulin (IVIG), immunosuppressive agents, and plasma exchange may all be indicated. Arrangement of these therapies can be considered in discussion with the relevant consultants (e.g., rheumatology, hematology, nephrology). Despite treatment, mortality for catastrophic APS approaches 50%.

Drug-Induced Lupus

Drug-induced lupus is an SLE-like, self-resolving illness characterized by arthralgias, myalgias, rash, and serositis. It may be brought on by as many as 80 different medications, including hydralazine, isoniazid, and tumor-necrosis factor (TNF) alpha inhibitors. Notably, the malar rash and major organ involvement are rare in this condition. In drug-induced lupus, antibodies against the body's own histone proteins are common and purported to be a major mechanism of disease. Although the list of potentially implicated medications is long, those agents with the most evidence for causing drug-induced lupus are summarized in Box 105.2. The diagnosis is typically clinical and confirmed by resolution of symptoms with the withdrawal of the offending medication. In addition to cessation of the culprit drug, NSAIDs or glucocorticoids may be prescribed for control of symptoms in the interim.

DISPOSITION

Disposition for the patient with SLE will vary significantly by clinical presentation. For patients with mild presentations, such as increased musculoskeletal symptom burden, uncomplicated pleurisy, or cutaneous disease, discharge with symptomatic care, return precautions, and follow-up is usually appropriate. However, patients with more acute pathology, poor insight into their disease, significant comorbidities, or weak home support may require hospitalization.

Disorders characteristic of moderate SLE flares (e.g., nephritis, pneumonitis), thrombotic events, or infectious complications in the setting of immunosuppression usually require admission for initiation or escalation of systemic therapy (e.g., glucocorticoids, anticoagulation, antibiotics) and monitoring for response to treatment. Select

---

BOX 105.1 Common Clinical Features of the Antiphospholipid Syndrome

Venous thrombosis
Arterial thrombosis (including stroke or transient ischemic attack)
Recurrent miscarriage
Livedo reticularis (rash)
Thrombocytopenia

patients with milder forms of illness may still be appropriate for discharge, particularly if in collaboration with the patient's rheumatologist. Admission to the intensive care unit should be considered for those who, despite initial resuscitation, suffer persistent severe circulatory or respiratory derangement.

Finally, the complexity of SLE is challenging for physicians not specialized in its many nuances and intricate pathophysiologic changes. General reasons for rheumatologic consultation or referral of patients with SLE are presented in Box 105.3.

BOX 105.2 Selected Drugs Definitively Implicated in Causing Drug-Induced Lupus

TNF alpha inhibitors
Procainamide
Hydralazine
Methyldopa
Chlorpromazine
Isoniazid
Quinidine
Minocycline

BOX 105.3 Considerations for Rheumatologic Consultation or Referral for Patients With Systemic Lupus Erythematosus

To establish a new diagnosis
To assess disease activity and severity
To provide general disease management
To manage uncontrolled disease
To manage organ involvement or life-threatening disease
To manage or prevent treatment toxicities
Special circumstances: Antiphospholipid syndrome (APS), pregnancy, surgery

Modified from Guidelines for referral and management of systemic lupus erythematosus in adults. American College of Rheumatology Ad Hoc Committee on Systemic Lupus Erythematosus Guidelines. *Arthritis Rheumatol.* 1999;42:1785–1796.

VASCULITIS

KEY CONCEPTS

- Giant cell arteritis should be considered in patients with new onset headache, visual changes, or jaw claudication combined with elevated inflammatory markers. Large-vessel vasculitides also affect the aorta and the great vessels leading to stenosis, claudication, and aneurysm formation.
- Small- and medium-vessel vasculitis syndromes should be considered in the presence of constitutional symptoms, glomerulonephritis, diffuse alveolar hemorrhage, mononeuritis multiplex, or cutaneous vasculitis.
- Many patients with established vasculitis are receiving high-intensity immunosuppression, making them vulnerable to opportunistic infections and sepsis.

FOUNDATIONS

The vasculitides are a heterogeneous group of disorders characterized by inflammation of blood vessel walls. Arteries and veins of all sizes can be affected to varying degrees. Presentations can range from benign and self-limited to serious and life-threatening. Diagnosis can be challenging, as early vasculitis syndromes are nonspecific and can mimic infectious, inflammatory, or neoplastic conditions. Approximately 1 in 2000 adults are affected by some form of vasculitis, with a higher incidence in adults in their sixth to eight decades of life.

Most vasculitis syndromes are idiopathic, although infection, medications, or recreational drugs can be causative. The pathophysiology of vasculitic conditions is complex and heterogenous; however, two overarching mechanisms play a role. Inflammation in blood vessel walls results in wall damage and necrosis, leading to stenosis, occlusion, and subsequent end-organ ischemia. In addition, a number of symptoms such as fever, fatigue, and joint pain are caused by a generalized systemic inflammatory process. Serologic testing, imaging, and biopsy all have a role in the diagnostic workup that at times can begin in the ED setting. In addition, empiric treatment is sometimes necessary to avoid end-organ damage.

Early recognition of vasculitis is critical, as these conditions can lead to irreversible end-organ damage and, if untreated, have a high mortality rate. While vasculitis can affect almost any organ system, the recognition of cardinal features that are common across multiple vasculitic conditions is critical to diagnosis. Constitutional symptoms such as fever, night sweats, weight loss, joint pain, and fatigue are common to all vasculitic syndromes. However, other manifestations vary considerably by the size of the blood vessel involved; therefore, large-vessel vasculitides differ markedly in their presentation from medium- and small-vessel vasculitides, which have overlapping features.[11] Table 105.3 summarizes the common and unique features of different vasculitides.

LARGE-VESSEL VASCULITIS

Large-vessel vasculitis involves the aorta and its immediate branches and is generally caused by giant cell arteritis (GCA) and Takayasu arteritis (TAK). These two vasculitides have a similar distribution of large-vessel involvement but differ in two important respects. GCA typically presents with cranial symptoms caused by involvement of the branches of the external carotid artery and affects patients older than 50 years of age. TAK in contrast does not have the same cranial features and generally affects younger patients.

Giant Cell Arteritis

Background

GCA, also known as temporal arteritis, is a systemic vasculitis that affects the aorta and its branches as well as the branches of the external carotid artery, which are medium and small arteries.[12] The disease typically occurs in patients over 50 with the highest incidence in the eighth decade of life. It is the most common vasculitis in older patients. Women are affected more commonly than men. GCA is most common in patients of Scandinavian descent, and the disease is relatively rare in black patients. The most feared complication of GCA is irreversible vision loss, occurring in up to one-third of patients. Early treatment can help prevent this complication, and thus the diagnosis is an important consideration in patients older than 50 years old presenting with any combination of constitutional symptoms, headache, visual changes, jaw claudication, or symptoms of polymyalgia rheumatica,

TABLE 105.3 Common and Unique Features of Vasculitides

Vasculitis	Common Clinical Features	Unique Clinical Features
LARGE-VESSEL VASCULITIS		
Takayasu arteritis	Aortitis	Carotidynia
Giant cell arteritis	Vasculitis of great vessels Diminished pulses Claudication	Headache, visual changes, jaw claudication, scalp tenderness, polymyalgia rheumatica
MEDIUM-VESSEL VASCULITIS		
Polyarteritis nodosa	Mononeuritis multiplex Mesenteric ischemia	Cutaneous ulcers, nodules, renal infarcts, testicular involvement Does not cause glomerulonephritis or lung involvement
SMALL-VESSEL VASCULITIS		
ANCA-Associated Vasculitis		
Granulomatosis with polyangiitis	Glomerulonephritis Diffuse alveolar hemorrhage	Granulomatous manifestations such as destructive sinusitis, nasal crusting, pulmonary nodules, retroorbital mass
Microscopic polyangiitis	Mononeuritis multiplex	Similar to GPA but without granulomatous manifestations
Eosinophilic granulomatosis with polyangiitis	Mesenteric ischemia Purpura	Eosinophilia, asthma, nasal polyps, cardiac involvement
Immune Complex Mediated Vasculitis		
Cryoglobulinemic vasculitis	Glomerulonephritis Palpable purpura	Associated with hepatitis B and C, lupus, Sjögren syndrome
IgA vasculitis	Mononeuritis multiplex GI involvement	Rare in the absence of skin lesions Does not typically cause mononeuritis multiplex or pulmonary involvement Intussusception is unique

which is characterized by the subacute onset of symmetric shoulder and pelvic girdle pain and prominent morning stiffness.

Clinical Features

GCA symptoms typically develop over weeks. Headache, the most common presenting symptom, occurs in three-quarters of patients with GCA. Although it is classically described as temporal, the headache of GCA can occur in any location. The most salient historical feature is that the headache is new or markedly different from prior headaches. Temporal artery tenderness or other abnormalities on examination increase the probability of GCA but are not sensitive for the diagnosis. Constitutional symptoms are present in more than half the patients. Visual symptoms are also common and importantly can herald visual loss. GCA can present with a variety of visual symptoms; however, the presence of unexplained amaurosis fugax or double vision should raise particular concern in the appropriate clinical setting. Jaw claudication is a particularly important symptom because, when present, it is the most specific GCA feature. Importantly, jaw claudication should be distinguished from temporomandibular joint (TMJ) disorder, which is much more common. Jaw claudication only occurs with chewing, resolves completely with rest, and tends to be reproducible over time. In contrast to TMJ disorder, it does not occur with mouth opening or other specific motions of the jaw not associated with chewing. Scalp tenderness occurs in up to a third of patients and is typically described as superficial discomfort with pressure such as lying on a pillow. Finally, polymyalgia rheumatica (PMR), which manifests as the subacute onset of symmetric shoulder and pelvic girdle pain and prominent morning stiffness, is present in nearly half of GCA patients and represents another important clue to the diagnosis. It should be

kept in mind that PMR is relatively common and, in up to 90% of cases, exists without GCA.

The large-vessel manifestations of GCA are similar to those of TAK. Involvement of the subclavian, axillary, or iliac arteries can lead to extremity claudication. Aortitis can lead to aneurysm formation and rupture. Thoracic aortic aneurysms are up to 17 times more likely to occur in patients with GCA compared with age-matched controls, and abdominal aortic aneurysm formation is twice as common. Involvement of vertebral-basilar arteries can lead to posterior circulation stroke. Other intracranial circulation is typically spared.

Diagnostic Testing

Inflammatory markers (ESR and CRP) should be evaluated when GCA is suspected. Normal inflammatory markers argue strongly against GCA, as more than 95% of patients have elevated markers at diagnosis. Temporal artery biopsy is the gold standard for diagnosis with sensitivity ranging from approximately 50% to 90%. Therefore, the diagnosis should be suspected even with a negative biopsy if suggestive clinical features are present in the setting of markedly elevated inflammatory markers without an alternative explanation. Increasingly, temporal artery ultrasound is being used in centers with experienced operators prior to biopsy. Demonstration of the halo sign around involved vessels is specific and can potentially eliminate the need for a biopsy. However, in patients with moderate to high suspicion of the disease and a negative ultrasound, biopsy should be pursued. Ophthalmologic evaluation is indicated for patients with acute visual symptoms. Fundoscopic examination can detect arteritic ischemic optic neuropathy, which is highly suggestive of GCA. The role of large-vessel imaging with CTA, MRA, or PET-CT is evolving.

Management

Patients with a moderate to high suspicion for GCA and no contraindication should be treated empirically with glucocorticoids, while simultaneously undergoing the diagnostic workup, to prevent visual loss. A typical initial regimen is oral prednisone 1 mg/kg. For patients with severe visual symptoms such as double vision or amaurosis fugax, admission for intravenous glucocorticoids (typically methylprednisolone 1 g daily for 3 days) can be considered. Tocilizumab (an IL-6 inhibitor) has recently been approved for the treatment of GCA in combination with glucocorticoids.[13] Initiation of tocilizumab should be made in consultation with rheumatology.

Takayasu Arteritis

Background

TAK is a systemic large-vessel vasculitis of unknown etiology.[14] It is eight times more common in women and is most prevalent in Asia, although it occurs worldwide. TAK typically affects a much younger population than GCA, with most patients diagnosed before the age of 40.

Clinical Features

TAK affects a similar distribution of arteries as GCA with the aorta and its branches being typically involved. However, in contrast to GCA, TAK typically presents with symptoms of more advanced vascular occlusion. This may be due to the absence of cranial symptoms as a heralding feature which leads to earlier diagnosis in GCA. The most common presenting symptoms include claudication (most commonly of the upper extremity, 35%), reduced or absent pulse (25%), hypertension (20%), or asymmetrical arm blood pressures (15%). Internal carotid artery involvement commonly causes carotidynia, lightheadedness, or headaches in approximately 20% of patients. In contrast to GCA, other cranial symptoms such as visual changes, scalp tenderness, and jaw claudication are absent. Aortitis can lead to aneurysm formation and aortic insufficiency. Constitutional symptoms are common in the early phase of the disease but are frequently absent in the stenotic phase when the disease is often diagnosed.

Diagnostic Testing

The diagnosis is made on the basis of clinical assessment and diagnostic imaging. Patients who present with symptoms of large-vessel occlusive disease (bruit, absent pulse, claudication) are candidates for imaging of the aorta and its major branches with CTA, MRA, or PET-CT.[15] Inflammatory markers are elevated in approximately 70% of patients with active disease. It should be noted that large-vessel vasculitis on imaging must be distinguished from atherosclerotic disease and noninflammatory vasculopathies, such as fibromuscular dysplasia or Ehlers Danlos syndrome, among others. Vasculitis typically causes long smooth stenoses and vessel wall thickening. In contrast, noncalcified atherosclerotic lesions cause focal stenoses. Noninflammatory vasculopathies generally cause beading, dissection, and aneurysm formation, rather than stenotic lesions and vessel wall thickening.

Management

TAK is managed with glucocorticoids in combination with steroid-sparing agents such as methotrexate, tumor-necrosis alpha inhibitors, or IL-6 inhibitors. Glucocorticoids are typically started at 60 mg and tapered over 6 to 12 months. Choice of steroid-sparing agent should be discussed with rheumatology. Surgical revascularization is reserved for patients with refractory stenotic lesions whose inflammatory disease is well controlled.

SMALL AND MEDIUM VESSEL VASCULITIS

Background

Small-vessel vasculitides as a group are the most common vasculitis syndromes. Polyarteritis nodosa, the only medium-vessel vasculitis affecting adults, is relatively rare but shares some common features with small-vessel diseases. Therefore, we will consider small- and medium-vessel vasculitis together.

Clinical Features

While each vasculitis causes multiple manifestations, it is important to recognize that there are common features shared by most small-vessel vasculitides which should alert the provider to consider this set of conditions. Specifically, the presence of DAH, glomerulonephritis, mononeuritis multiplex, mesenteric ischemia not due to atherosclerosis, or palpable purpura should prompt consideration of a small- or medium-vessel vasculitis. Joint pain and constitutional symptoms are also common to all forms of vasculitis.

DAH typically manifests with dyspnea and hemoptysis. Respiratory symptoms and signs of impaired gas exchange may develop before a drop in the hemoglobin level, which may be seen in cases of severe or persistent bleeding. It should be noted that hemoptysis is absent in approximately one-third of patients with DAH. CT imaging typically reveals diffuse ground-glass or consolidative opacities that must be differentiated from pulmonary edema or infection. The diagnosis is made on bronchoscopy with serial bronchoalveolar lavages returning increasingly bloody fluid. It should be noted that infection can also cause DAH.

Glomerulonephritis is typically asymptomatic although rarely patients will notice macroscopic hematuria. The key to diagnosis is an active urinary sediment with proteinuria and hematuria with red blood cell casts and dysmorphic RBCs. Pulmonary-renal syndrome, with both DAH and glomerulonephritis, is a classic presentation of small-vessel systemic vasculitis and anti-glomerular basement membrane (anti-GBM) disease.

While vasculitis can cause any type of peripheral neuropathy, the most common is mononeuritis multiplex, which is uncommon in other diseases. This condition generally affects large sensorimotor nerves in an asymmetric distribution. Patients may present with a combination of foot or wrist drop associated with sensory deficits, or less commonly cranial neuropathy occurring in an asymmetric manner over time.

Gastrointestinal manifestations are less common and can be nonspecific. However, symptoms of chronic mesenteric ischemia in the setting of elevated inflammatory markers or other systemic features without an alternative explanation, such as atherosclerotic disease, should prompt consideration of a small- or medium-vessel vasculitis.

The most common cutaneous manifestation of vasculitis is palpable purpura. Palpable purpura typically involves the lower extremities, is nonblanching, and is not painful or pruritic. A biopsy may be needed to distinguish the lesions of vasculitis from other causes of purpura.

Differential Diagnosis

A useful approach to vasculitis is to first recognize the common features of small- and medium-vessel vasculitis. Second, when evaluating patients with suspected vasculitis, it is important to confirm the scope of the disease by evaluating organs that may be asymptomatic such as the lung and kidneys. Finally, because these vasculitic features should prompt a workup for vasculitis but do not differentiate well between the various types of small- and medium-vessel vasculitis, it is important to focus on the differentiating features of each vasculitic condition to make a specific diagnosis. The differentiating features include clinical symptoms, laboratory testing, and biopsy results.

Small-vessel vasculitides can be broadly divided into antineutrophil cytoplasmic antibody (ANCA)-associated vasculitis and vasculitis caused primarily by immune-complex deposition. There are three ANCA-associated vasculitides: granulomatosis with polyangiitis (GPA, formerly Wegener granulomatosis), microscopic polyangiitis (MPA), and eosinophilic granulomatosis with polyangiitis (EGPA, formerly Churg-Strauss syndrome).[16] Immune complex vasculitides include cryoglobulinemic vasculitis, IgA vasculitis (IgAV, formerly Henoch–Schonlein purpura), drug-induced vasculitis, and connective tissue disease-associated vasculitis. Anti-GBM (Goodpasture disease) is not a true vasculitis but should be considered in the setting of either glomerulonephritis or pulmonary hemorrhage. Polyarteritis nodosa (PAN) is a medium-vessel vasculitis that shares some features with small-vessel diseases.

Specific Disorders

ANCA-Associated Vasculitis

Granulomatosis With Polyangiitis. GPA is a granulomatous vasculitis affecting small- and medium-sized vessels. It affects individuals in their fifth and sixth decade of life most commonly and has a slight male predominance. In addition to the vasculitic manifestations such as glomerulonephritis, DAH, mononeuritis multiplex, and palpable purpura, GPA is unique in that it causes "granulomatous" manifestations, mainly sinusitis and mass lesions. Sinusitis is one of the most common manifestations of GPA. The presence of significant nasal crusting may alert the physician to the presence of an inflammatory process because crusting is typically absent in allergic and bacterial sinusitis. Bony destruction and nasal septal perforation are other distinguishing features that may be present. In addition, GPA can cause pulmonary nodules (Fig. 105.5), bronchial lesions, retroorbital mass, or subglottic stenosis. Sensorineural hearing loss or otitis media can also be seen. Limited GPA is a well-recognized subset of disease and can present only with chronic sinusitis or other granulomatous features without vasculitic features.

The presence of ANCA in the appropriate clinical setting is highly suggestive of the diagnosis. It should be noted that when renal involvement is present, ANCA sensitivity is approximately 90% but drops to approximately 60% in nonsevere diseases without renal involvement. GPA is typically associated with proteinase 3 (PR3)-ANCA (c-ANCA immunofluorescence pattern). If the diagnosis is uncertain, biopsy of the affected organ should be performed. Pathology generally demonstrates vasculitis without significant immune complex deposition. Granulomatous inflammation may also be present.

Treatment of GPA requires the combination of glucocorticoids and another immunosuppressant (typically rituximab or cyclophosphamide).[17] In patients with glomerulonephritis or pulmonary hemorrhage, pulse dose glucocorticoids (methylprednisolone 1 g IV for 3 days) are often used. Plasma exchange has been used previously in severe cases, but recent studies have questioned the utility of this modality, except when ANCA-associated vasculitis occurs with anti-GBM disease.

Microscopic Polyangiitis. MPA is a non-granulomatous vasculitis affecting small- and medium-sized vessels. MPA most commonly affects patients in their sixth and seventh decades and has a relatively equal sex distribution. It shares the same vasculitic features as GPA but lacks the "granulomatous" manifestations. Therefore, sinusitis and mass lesions are not seen in MPA, and the most common presenting features include glomerulonephritis, pulmonary hemorrhage, mononeuritis multiplex, and palpable purpura. Diagnosis relies on the presence of myeloperoxidase (MPO)-ANCA (p-ANCA immunofluorescence pattern) that is present in approximately 70% of patients. If ANCA is negative or the diagnosis is uncertain, biopsy typically demonstrates findings of vasculitis lacking both immune complex deposition and granulomatous inflammation. Treatment is identical to that of GPA with a combination of glucocorticoids and rituximab or cyclophosphamide.

Eosinophilic Granulomatosis With Polyangiitis. EGPA is an eosinophilic vasculitis of small and medium vessels.[18] Mean age of the diagnosis is in the fourth and fifth decade with men and women equally affected. While it shares vasculitic features with GPA and MPA, it has a number of unique features related to the eosinophilic infiltration of organs. Over 90% of patients develop asthma as one of the first manifestations, typically preceding vasculitic features. The asthma is often severe, requiring treatment with agents such as prednisone. Migratory ground-glass opacities on CT chest imaging are common and may help differentiate EGPA from severe asthma. Allergic rhinitis and nasal polyps are also frequent. Eosinophilic myocarditis, which can present with arrhythmia or heart failure, is another unique feature, present in 10% to 20% of patients. Notably, cardiac involvement has been suggested to account for nearly half of the deaths due to EGPA.

All patients with EGPA have prominent peripheral eosinophilia, typically above 1000 cells/μL, which is not a feature of other vasculitides. It should be kept in mind that treatment with glucocorticoids markedly

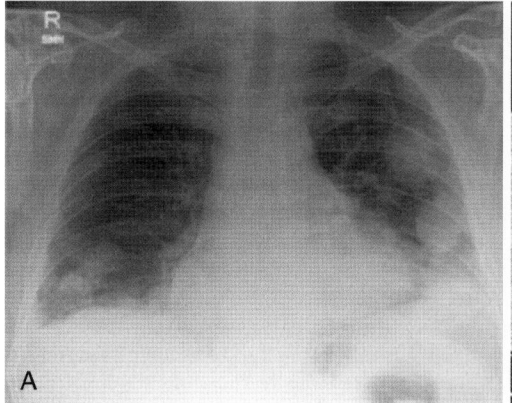
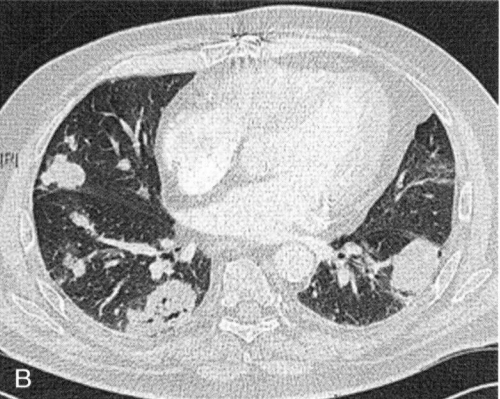

Fig. 105.5 (A) Multiple intrapulmonary nodules on a chest radiograph of a patient with granulomatosis with polyangiitis (GPA, formerly Wegener granulomatosis). (B) Pulmonary nodules seen on computed tomography (CT) imaging. (From Adam A, Dixon AK. *Grainger & Allison's Diagnostic Radiology*. 5th ed. Philadelphia: Churchill Livingstone; 2008.)

reduces peripheral eosinophilia; therefore, it may be absent in patients already receiving glucocorticoids. Differentiating EGPA from severe atopic disease or hypereosinophilic syndrome can be challenging. Generally, atopic disease lacks end-organ involvement outside of the lung, while hypereosinophilic syndromes lack asthma and vasculitic features. The diagnosis relies on the presence of MPO-ANCA, which is only seen in 50% of patients, or eosinophilic vasculitis on biopsy. Treatment of EGPA is dictated by disease severity. Severe vasculitic manifestations are generally treated similarly to GPA and MPA with a combination of pulse intravenous glucocorticoids and rituximab or cyclophosphamide. Patients without severe vasculitis may be treated with glucocorticoids alone or in combination with mepolizumab (anti-IL-5), methotrexate, azathioprine, or mycophenolate mofetil.

Anti-Glomerular Basement Membrane Disease (Goodpasture Disease)

Anti-GBM disease is caused by disruption of the basement membrane by circulating anti-GBM antibodies causing glomerulonephritis with or without alveolar hemorrhage.[19] The disease can affect individuals of all ages, with white patients more commonly affected. The incidence is bimodal; one peak occurs in 20- to 30-year-old men, and a second in 50- to 70-year-olds of both sexes. Because it is not a vasculitis per se, other vasculitic features are generally absent. The diagnosis is made by the presence of anti-GBM antibodies and demonstration of crescentic glomerulonephritis with linear staining along the basement membrane on immunofluorescence. Treatment requires the addition of plasma exchange to a combination of prednisone and cyclophosphamide. Of note, ANCA-associated vasculitis and anti-GBM disease can coexist; treatment of this syndrome is similar to that of anti-GBM disease alone.

Immune Complex Mediated Vasculitis

IgA Vasculitis. IgAV, formerly known as Henoch-Schonlein purpura, is a small- and medium-vessel vasculitis that is characterized by IgA deposition in vessel walls.[20] It is more common in children than adults at an approximately 3:1 ratio. IgAV has a strong association with infection, with 50% of cases occurring after an upper respiratory tract illness. It can also occur as a manifestation of a drug reaction. In contrast to other vasculitides, it does not typically involve the lung or the peripheral nervous system. The three organ systems typically affected are the skin, kidneys, and gastrointestinal tract. Joint pain and constitutional symptoms are also frequent. Skin manifestations, most commonly palpable purpura, are present in essentially all adults and the majority of children as the initial manifestation (Fig. 105.6). This is in contrast to other systemic vasculitides, where any of the manifestations can be the presenting feature. Gastrointestinal symptoms are nonspecific; intussusception is the most common finding, in contrast to other vasculitides where mesenteric ischemia tends to be the most common gastrointestinal presentation. Renal involvement manifests as hematuria most commonly but can be more severe with nephritic syndrome, particularly in adults, who have a worse renal prognosis. In children, the diagnosis is commonly made clinically, as it is much more common than other vasculitides. The diagnosis in adults typically requires a biopsy. Biopsy of an affected organ will demonstrate IgA deposition in vessel walls. IgAV is typically a self-limited illness. NSAIDs (e.g., naproxen 500 mg BID or ibuprofen 800 mg TID) can be helpful for fever and joint pain. Treatment with glucocorticoids should be considered in patients with severe renal or gastrointestinal manifestations. Similar to other vasculitides, prednisone should be started at 1 mg/kg or pulse intravenous dosing 1 g/day for 3 days in cases of severe end-organ involvement.

Cryoglobulinemic Vasculitis. Cryoglobulinemic vasculitis is characterized by a primarily small-vessel vasculitis in association

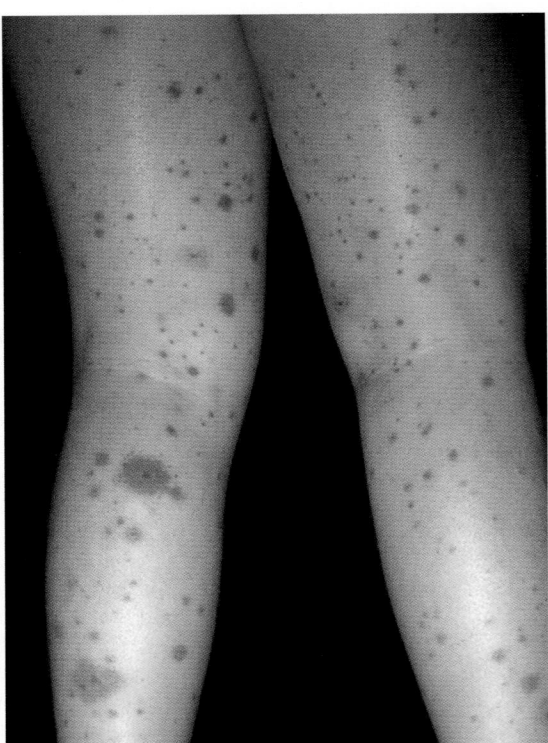

Fig. 105.6 Purpuric Lesions Associated with IgA Vasculitis, Some of Which Have Coalesced and Undergone Central Necrosis. (From Habif TP. *Clinical Dermatology.* 5th ed. New York: Mosby; 2009.)

with cryoglobulins in the peripheral blood, which are proteins that precipitate at temperatures below 37°C.[21] There are three types of cryoglobulins. Type I is typically associated with Waldenstrom macroglobulinemia and causes a hyperviscosity syndrome rather than a vasculitis. In contrast, types II and III cause vasculitis and are associated with chronic hepatitis C infection, malignancy, or autoimmune diseases (SLE, Sjögren's). Cryoglobulinemia can also be idiopathic. Cryoglobulinemic vasculitis generally causes vasculitic features such as glomerulonephritis, mononeuritis multiplex. palpable purpura, nonspecific myalgias, and arthralgias, or weakness are particularly common, while DAH is relatively uncommon. Diagnosis is made by demonstrating the presence of cryoglobulins in the bloodstream. Biopsy of an affected organ can be helpful if the diagnosis remains uncertain. Treatment includes immunosuppression if end-organ involvement is present, similarly to other vasculitides, and treating the precipitating illness (e.g., HCV).

Polyarteritis Nodosa

Polyarteritis nodosa is a necrotizing vasculitis primarily affecting medium-sized arteries.[22] It affects patients in their fifth and sixth decade of life and has a slight male predominance. A small percentage of cases are associated with hepatitis B infection. In contrast to the small-vessel vasculitides, it does not typically involve the lung and does not cause glomerulonephritis, as both of these manifestations are due to small-vessel involvement. The renal manifestations of PAN are typically reno-vascular hypertension or renal infarcts. Similarly, cutaneous features of PAN are typically ulcers or nodules rather than palpable purpura. However, similarly to the small-vessel vasculitides, PAN can cause mononeuritis multiplex, mesenteric ischemia, joint pain, or constitutional symptoms. A unique manifestation is testicular involvement. There are no antibodies associated with PAN. Diagnosis is made by either biopsy of the involved organ demonstrating a medium-vessel vasculitis or abdominal imaging demonstrating characteristic microaneurysms in the splanchnic vasculature. Treatment includes glucocorticoids and another immunosuppressant, most commonly cyclophosphamide. Glucocorticoid dosing is similar to other vasculitides with pulse dosing for severe end-organ involvement and prednisone 1 mg/kg for less severe end-organ involvement.

Other Vasculitides

Behçet Disease. Behçet disease (BD) is a vasculitis that affects all blood vessel sizes and is characterized by the presence of recurrent oral aphthous ulcers.[23] It affects populations living along the Silk Road most commonly, such as Turkey, Saudi Arabia, Iraq, Iran, and China, but can occur in any part of the world. In contrast to other vasculitides, the typical manifestations of vasculitis such as glomerulonephritis, DAH, mesenteric ischemia, peripheral neuropathy, or palpable purpura are rare. The most common manifestations include inflammatory eye disease such as uveitis, genital ulcers, and various skin manifestations including erythema nodosum (Fig. 105.7), among others. Gastrointestinal manifestations mimic those of Crohn's disease. Importantly, because BD can involve large vessels, it can cause aneurysmal arterial lesions with resultant rupture as well as DVT, including Budd-Chiari syndrome or cavernous sinus thrombosis. Uniquely, BD can also cause central nervous system disease, with a predilection for the brainstem.

Diagnosis is made on clinical grounds. BD should be considered in patients with recurrent oral ulcers (Fig. 105.8) and the presence of genital ulcers, inflammatory eye disease, or other systemic features. In the evaluation for BD, it is important to exclude other causes of oral and genital ulceration, in particular, herpes simplex virus infection. Treatment is guided by disease severity. Mucocutaneous manifestations are generally treated with colchicine. Internal organ involvement requires glucocorticoids 1 mg/kg or pulse dosing in severe end-organ involvement. Another immunosuppressant such as azathioprine, cyclophosphamide, or TNF alpha inhibitors should be considered with end-organ involvement in consultation with rheumatology. Notably, DVT associated with BD generally requires treatment with immunosuppression, which has been shown to decrease the rate of recurrence. Anticoagulation should be considered on an individualized basis.

Cutaneous Vasculitis. Cutaneous small-vessel vasculitis (CSVV) is the most common single-organ vasculitis.[24] It has been previously known as hypersensitivity vasculitis or leukocytoclastic vasculitis, among others. CSVV can occur as a manifestation of a drug reaction or be idiopathic. It is only distinguished clinically from the systemic vasculitides such as ANCA-associated vasculitis, IgAV, and cryoglobulinemia due to the absence of other systemic symptoms, negative serology, and absence of IgA deposition on skin biopsy. Diagnosis is made on tissue biopsy with histology generally demonstrating leukocytoclastic vasculitis. It is critical to exclude systemic involvement; therefore, a urinalysis should be obtained in patients with CSVV to investigate for glomerulonephritis. Treatment may include topical corticosteroids, NSAIDs (e.g., naproxen 500 mg BID or ibuprofen 800 mg TID), colchicine (0.6 mg BID), dapsone (50 mg daily: dapsone requires lab monitoring and should be started in

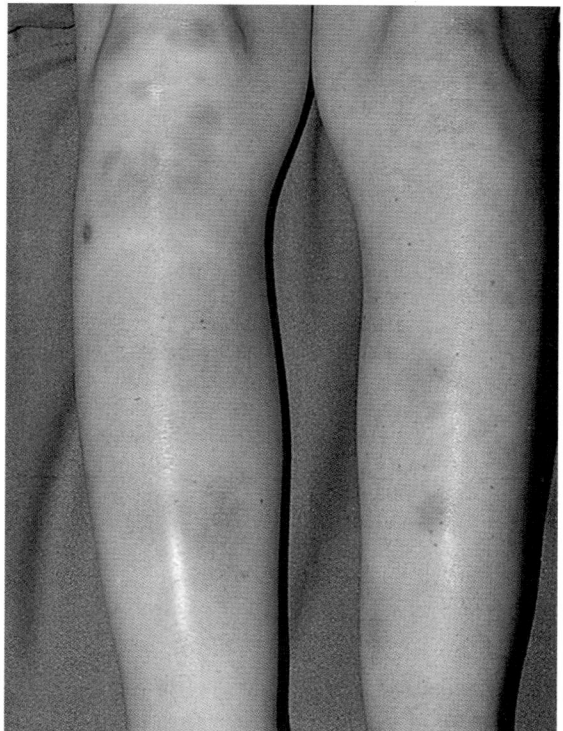

Fig. 105.7 Tender Subcutaneous Nodules Associated With Erythema Nodosum. (From Kliegman R. *Nelson Textbook of Pediatrics.* 18th ed. Philadelphia: WB Saunders; 2007.)

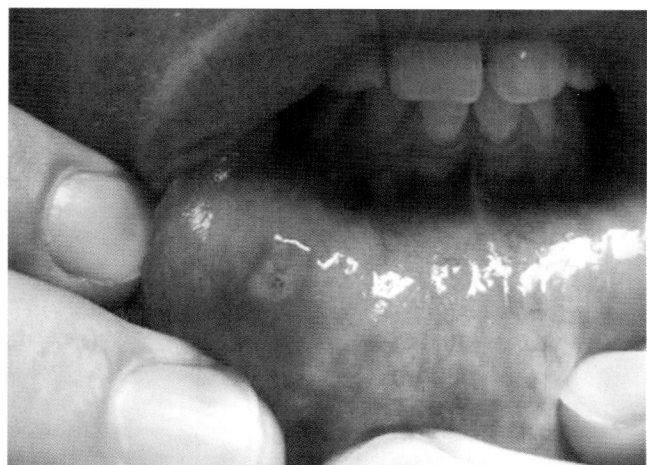

Fig. 105.8 Oral Aphthae Associated With Behçet Disease. (From Firestein GS. *Kelley's Textbook of Rheumatology.* 8th ed. Philadelphia: WB Saunders; 2008.)

consultation with dermatology or rheumatology), or glucocorticoids (ranging from 20 to 60 mg daily depending on severity), among others.

The references for this chapter can be found online at Expert-Consult.com.

106

Allergy, Anaphylaxis, and Angioedema

Aaron N. Barksdale and Weston Ross

ALLERGY

FOUNDATIONS

Background and Terminology

The prevalence of allergic disease has significantly increased over the past several decades, particularly in developed societies. It is currently estimated that 30% of the worldwide population suffer from some component of allergy, including 5% to 8% with food allergies. This has contributed to increased financial burdens on our health care systems and morbidity in affected individuals.[1-4] This is largely attributed to changes in lifestyle, diet, antibiotic use, smaller families, and the "hygiene hypothesis," which centers around decreased microbial exposure in developed countries.[1,3]

The human immune system comprises cellular and humoral components working together in a highly complex and coordinated fashion to achieve the primary goal of protecting the human host from potentially harmful offenders. The immune system, however, can overreact to otherwise harmless agents, producing an inappropriate response that may be harmful to the host, thereby giving rise to allergy or allergic diseases. These hypersensitivity reactions are manifested in clinical symptoms ranging from nuisance-level to fatal. For practical purposes, the term *allergy* is used in this chapter to refer to mast cell–mediated hypersensitivity reactions. For most allergic diseases to occur, predisposed individuals require exposure to allergens through *sensitization*. Substances that elicit an allergic reaction are referred to as *allergens*, and those that elicit an antibody response are termed *antigens*.

On the allergic continuum, there are several important allergic syndromes (Fig. 106.1). *Urticaria* (wheels, hives) is a common allergic reaction to foods, drugs, temperature changes, or physical stimuli. It is clinically characterized by a raised central swelling of variable size with surrounding reflex erythema, combined with an itching or burning sensation, with the skin typically returning to its baseline appearance within 30 minutes to 24 hours.[5]

Angioedema is characterized by sudden swelling of the subcutaneous or mucous membranes and tends to be more painful than pruritic. In general, it is slower to resolve compared to urticaria, and if the tongue or larynx is involved, it can result in airway compromise.[5] Angioedema can occur through one of two different mechanisms. Allergic (histaminergic) angioedema occurs in response to exposure to foods, drugs, or physical stimuli. Nonallergic (non-histaminergic) angioedema may be hereditary (termed hereditary angioedema [HAE]) or medication-induced (e.g., angiotensin-converting enzyme [ACE] inhibitor angioedema).

At the other extreme of this allergic continuum is *anaphylaxis*, a life-threatening systemic reaction, characterized by acute onset and multiorgan involvement.[6-8] It is a type I hypersensitivity reaction (allergic), mediated by immunoglobulin E (IgE). In its most common form, anaphylaxis is precipitated by exposure to allergens in previously sensitized individuals (immunologic). Previously, the term *anaphylactoid reaction* referred to a syndrome clinically similar to anaphylaxis that is not mediated by IgE (non-immunologic). Its clinical presentation and treatment are identical to that of anaphylaxis. Non-IgE (non-immunologic) reactions appear to result from direct degranulation of mast cells (and basophils) and may follow a single, first-time exposure to certain inciting agents (e.g., NSAIDs, monoclonal antibodies, local anesthetics, chemotherapeutic drugs). The World Allergy Organization (WAO) guidelines use the term *anaphylaxis* to refer to both IgE- and

Allergic rhinitis　　　Contact dermatitis　　　Urticaria (hives)　　　Anaphylaxis

Mild　　　　　　　　　　　　　　　　　　　　　　　　　　　　**Severe**

Allergic conjunctivitis　　　Atopic dermatitis (eczema)　　　Angioedema

Fig. 106.1 Severity Spectrum of Allergic Disease.

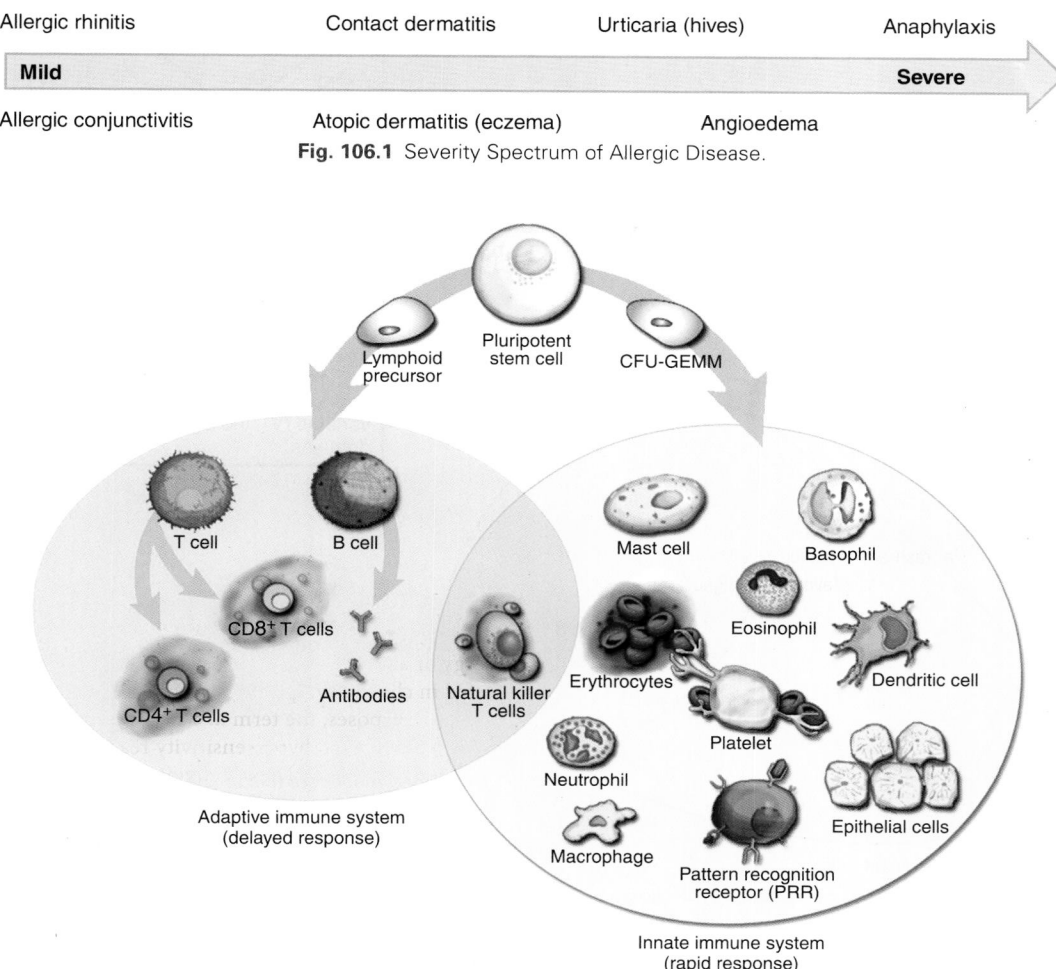

Fig. 106.2 Developmental Pathways of the Immune and Hematopoietic Systems. *CFU-GEMM,* Colony-forming unit for granulocyte, erythroid, myeloid, and megakaryocyte.

non-IgE-mediated reactions, obviating the need for the term *anaphylactoid reaction,* although this term is still often used.[6,9]

Pathophysiology

Immunologic responses to *antigens* are coordinated by two systems: the *innate* immune system, and the more recently evolved *adaptive* immune system (Fig. 106.2). The innate immune system is considered the first line of defense and is characterized by its nonspecific but rapid responses to offending agents or microbes. Its effector components include resident cells (epithelial cells, mast cells, macrophages, dendritic cells, antimicrobial proteins), infiltrative cells (natural killer cells, neutrophils, monocytes, dendritic cells), and various proteins (antimicrobial peptides, complements, cytokines, and the pathogenic pattern recognition receptor [PRR] system). The innate system responds to danger signals rapidly and nonspecifically, whereas the adaptive immune system takes time for antigen-specific cells (B and T cells) to amplify through a process known as *clonal expansion* to mount a specific immune response. The T and B lymphocytes are capable of recognizing a myriad of antigens through a vast library of antibodies and receptors (up to 10^{15}).[1,3,4]

The adaptive and innate immune systems originate from the common pluripotential hematopoietic stem cells. When the host encounters a foreign antigen, the cellular components of the adaptive immune system interact with the cellular and protein components of the innate immune system to mount a coordinated defense aimed at neutralization of the antigen.

Mast cells, basophils, and their mediators are the central effectors in allergy and anaphylaxis. Exposure of a genetically predisposed individual to an allergen leads to the synthesis and release of allergen-specific IgE by plasma cells into the circulation. Fixation of this allergen-specific IgE to surface receptors on mast cells completes the process known as *sensitization.* These IgE-bearing mast cells usually reside in the mucosal surfaces, submucosal tissue (around venules), and cutaneous surfaces, where they are capable of becoming activated on reexposure to a specific allergen. Cross-linking of the mast cell receptors by a specific multivalent allergen sets off a cascade of conformational and biochemical events, causing the degranulation of preformed mediators, subsequent generation and release of arachidonic acid metabolites, elaboration of cytokines and chemokines, and activation of the cellular components by the innate and adaptive systems. This series of events ultimately leads to the clinical syndromes of allergy and anaphylaxis (Fig 106.3).[1,3,4]

Classification of Reactions

The term *allergy* is commonly used to describe clinical illnesses produced by excessive immune responses by a normal immune system to otherwise innocuous allergens. The classic Coombs and Gell

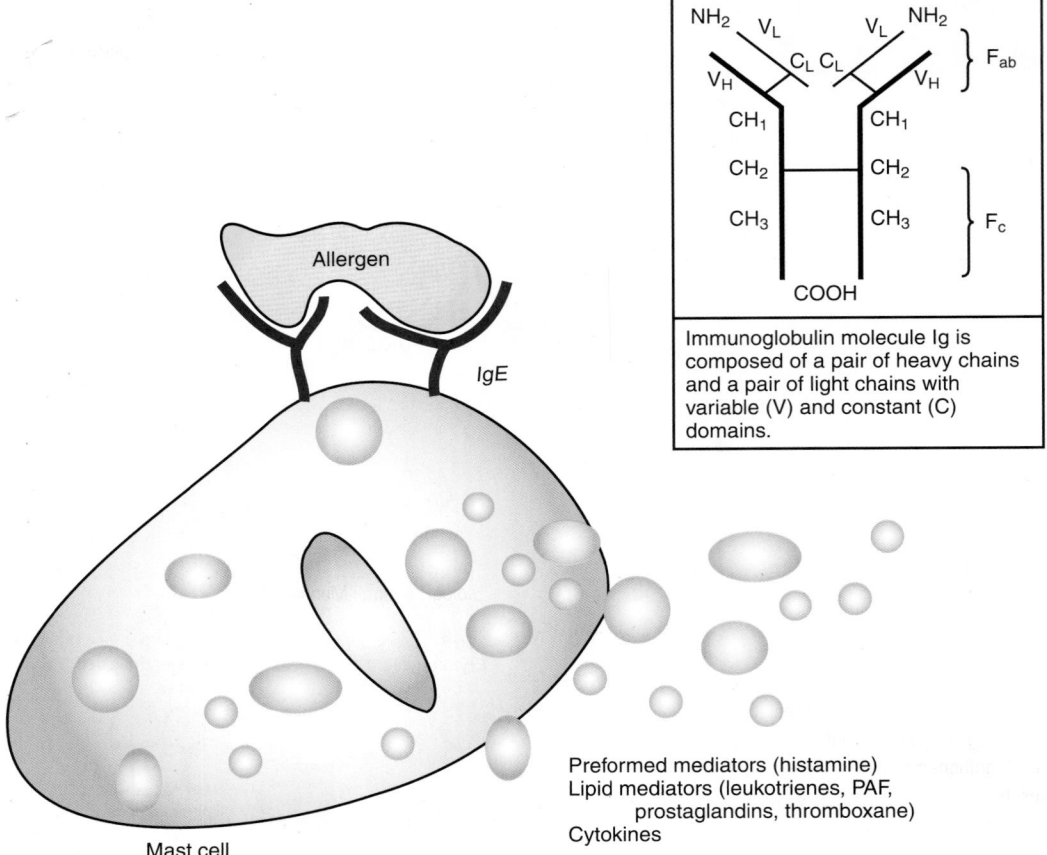

Immunoglobulin molecule Ig is composed of a pair of heavy chains and a pair of light chains with variable (V) and constant (C) domains.

Fig. 106.3 Activation of mast cells with degranulation of mast cell mediators by antigen cross-linking of adjacent immunoglobulin E *(IgE)* on the cell surface. *PAF,* Platelet-activating factor.

BOX 106.1 Gell and Coombs Classification of Immune Reactions

Type I: Immediate Hypersensitivity

Binding of multivalent antigens to IgE on the surface of mast cells and basophils leads to degranulation of mediators. In previously sensitized individuals, the reaction develops quickly (minutes). This type of hypersensitivity reaction is seen in allergic diseases (e.g., hay fever, allergic asthma, urticaria, angioedema, and anaphylaxis). *Non-immunologic* (previously termed anaphylactoid) *reaction* refers to the direct release of preformed mediators of mast cells independent of IgE.

Type II: Cytotoxic Antibody Reaction

Antibody (IgM, IgG) binding of membrane-bound antigens leads to cytotoxicity and cell lysis of cells through the complement or mononuclear cell system (macrophages, neutrophils, and eosinophils). This type of reaction is seen in transfusion reaction and Rh incompatibility.

Type III: Immune Complex–Mediated Reaction

Binding of antibody (IgM, IgG) to antigens forms soluble immune complexes, which are deposited on vessel walls, causing a local inflammatory reaction (Arthus reaction) leading to inflammation and tissue injury. This type of reaction is seen in systemic lupus erythematosus and serum sickness (after antithymocyte globulin administration).

Type IV: Cell-Mediated Delayed Hypersensitivity

Sensitized lymphocytes (T$_H$1 cells) recognize the antigen, recruit additional lymphocytes and mononuclear cells to the site, and start the inflammatory reaction. No antibodies are involved. This type of reaction is seen in contact dermatitis, erythema multiforme, Stevens-Johnson syndrome, and toxic epidermal necrolysis.

IgE, Immunoglobulin E; *IgG,* immunoglobulin G; *IgM,* immunoglobulin M; *T$_H$1,* type 1 helper.

---

classification can be adapted to categorize these hypersensitivity reactions (Box 106.1).

Type I reactions (immediate hypersensitivity) are IgE mediated and account for most allergic and anaphylactic reactions. Exposure to sensitizing allergens causes mediators from mast cells and basophils to be released through both IgE-dependent and IgE-independent (direct mast cell degranulation) mechanisms. Rhinitis caused by ragweed pollen and anaphylaxis caused by foods are examples of the IgE-dependent mechanism.

ANAPHYLAXIS

FOUNDATIONS

Epidemiology and Risk Factors

The prevalence of anaphylaxis and related hospital admissions has increased over the past two decades. The incidence is difficult to determine, but anaphylaxis is estimated to occur in roughly 2% of the

BOX 106.2 **Risk Factors for Anaphylaxis and Increased Anaphylaxis Severity and Mortality**

Risk Factors for Having Anaphylaxis
Age and sex
    Pregnant women, infants, teenagers, elderly
Route of administration
    Parenteral > oral
Higher social economic status
Time of the year
    Summer and fall (the outdoor seasons)
    History of atopy
    Emotional stress
    Acute infection
    Physical exertion
    History of mastocytosis
Risk Factors for Increased Anaphylaxis Severity and Mortality
Extremes of age
    Very young (under-recognition)
    Elderly (decreased physiologic reserves)
Comorbid conditions
    Cardiovascular disease (heart failure, ischemic heart disease, hypertension)
    Pulmonary disease (asthma, obstructive airway disease)
Others
    Concurrent use of anti-hypertensive agents, specifically beta-blockers and angiotensin-converting enzyme (ACE) inhibitors
    Concurrent use of cognition-impairing drugs (e.g., alcohol, recreational drugs, sedatives, tranquilizers)
    Recent anaphylaxis episode
    Upright posture at the onset of symptoms

BOX 106.3 **Etiologic Agents Causing Anaphylaxis by Immunologic Mechanisms**

Immunologic Mechanisms (IgE-Dependent)
Foods: Peanut, tree nut, milk, egg, shellfish, soybean, cow milk, mammalian meats (after sensitization to alpha-gal protein following tick bite)
Medications: Antibiotics, NSAIDs, chemotherapeutic agents, immunomodulators
Insect stings: *Hymenoptera* venoms, fire ant stings
Natural rubber latex
Hormones: Insulin, methylprednisolone, parathormone, estradiol, progesterone, corticotropin
Local anesthetics: Mostly ester family (procaine, tetracaine, benzocaine)
RCM
Occupational allergens: Enzymes, animal protein, plant protein
Aeroallergens: Pollen, dust, spores, pet dander

Immunologic Mechanisms (Ige-Independent)
RCM
NSAIDs
Dextrans
Biologic agents: Monoclonal antibodies, immunomodulators

Non-Immunologic Mechanisms (Direct Mast Cell Activations)
Physical factors: Exercise, cold, heat, sunlight
Ethanol
Medications: Some opioids
Idiopathic (no apparent trigger)

IgE, Immunoglobulin E; *NSAID,* nonsteroidal antiinflammatory drug; *RCM,* radiocontrast media.

worldwide population and as high as 5% in the United States.[6–8,10] While fatal anaphylaxis is rare, representing less than 1% of cases, there is evidence that medication-induced fatalities are increasing in North America and that food-induced fatalities are increasing in Australia.[11]

The severity of anaphylaxis varies between different age groups depending on the specific trigger and cofactors, but in general, pregnant women, infants, teenagers, and elders have been shown to have an increased incidence of anaphylaxis.[6] Additional risk factors include atopy (genetic predisposition to develop allergic disease), peanut and tree nut allergy, emotional stress, seasonal occurrence in summer to fall months, higher socioeconomic status, premenstrual age, and the presence of acute infection. Severe anaphylaxis has been associated with poorly controlled asthma, history of mastocytosis, heavy physical exertion, exposure to a trigger during the concomitant use of certain medications (ACE inhibitors, beta-blockers, and nonsteroidal antiinflammatory drugs [NSAIDs]), history of a previous anaphylactic reaction, delayed epinephrine administration, and upright position at the onset of symptoms (Box 106.2).[6,8,10,12,13]

In general, the more rapid an anaphylaxis reaction occurs after an exposure, the more likely it is to be severe and potentially fatal. The dose, frequency, duration, and route of administration of a drug can also affect the tendency to develop an anaphylactic reaction (e.g., the parenteral route is more likely to lead to an anaphylactic reaction than the oral route).[6,7,10] One interesting aspect of drug-related anaphylaxis is the constancy of administration. An anaphylactic reaction may not occur in an otherwise susceptible patient as long as a drug is administered at regular intervals. The same patient, however, may experience an anaphylactic reaction if the drug is resumed after an interruption of therapy.

ACE-inhibitor use can cause an accumulation of kinins and bradykinin and thus can exacerbate the angioedema component of anaphylaxis. Beta-adrenergic blockers may oppose the actions of adrenergic agents used in anaphylaxis treatment. Recent evidence suggests that taking an ACE inhibitor or a beta-blocker increases the risk of severe anaphylaxis (and even more so when taken concurrently) but does not necessarily increase the incidence of initial anaphylactic reactions.[6,14]

Common Triggers for Anaphylaxis

Virtually any agent that is capable of activating mast cells or basophils can potentially precipitate an anaphylactic reaction. However, in up to 60% of adults and 10% of children, an inciting agent cannot be identified, which is classified as *idiopathic anaphylaxis.*[15] When a trigger can be determined, foods, insect stings, and medications are the most common causes. Box 106.3 lists many of the common agents by their proposed immunologic mechanism.[6,9,10,12]

Foods

Food allergens are the most common identifiable agents and represent up to a third of reported anaphylactic cases. The incidence has significantly increased over the past decade, especially among children. Symptoms typically occur within 5 to 30 minutes of ingestion with fatalities reported within 30 minutes of exposure, though in some cases onset can be significantly delayed. In particular, reactions to mammalian foods (e.g., beef and pork) can be delayed 3 to 6 hours following exposure; recent research strongly suggests sensitization to the alpha-gal protein following a tick bite in this circumstance.[16–19] The most commonly implicated foods include peanuts, shellfish, tree nuts, fish, soy, cow's milk, and eggs. Fatal outcomes have been more commonly reported in adolescents and young adults, as well as those with a history of asthma, tree nut or peanut allergy, anaphylactic cases presenting without skin manifestations, or when epinephrine administration was delayed.[6,9–11] The majority of reactions occur after ingestion, but may also occur following inhalation of food particles or even after skin contact with vomit containing the instigating agent. In the setting of a known allergy, it may be difficult to avoid certain allergens, as their identity may be obscured during processing (e.g., consuming wine contaminated with *Hymenoptera* venom).

Drugs

Medications represent the second most frequent cause of anaphylactic reactions but are the most common trigger in adult subjects and result in the highest incidence of fatalities across all age groups. NSAIDs, antibiotics (specifically beta lactams), and neuromuscular blocking agents (NMBAs) are the most commonly reported triggers, but over the past decade, there has been a significant rise in chemotherapeutic or immunomodulator agent–related reactions.[6,10,20,21] Fatal drug-induced anaphylaxis has been associated with hypertension, obesity, male gender, beta-blocker use, and old age.[6,10,11]

Penicillin is the most common antibiotic cause of anaphylaxis. Although many report a history of penicillin allergy, studies have shown that less than 10% of individuals with a reported history of penicillin are truly allergic via skin testing. These individuals are often mislabeled as penicillin allergic at some point, or their allergy senesces after years of avoidance. Parenterally administered penicillin is responsible for the majority of anaphylactic reactions.[20,21]

Cephalosporins share the β-lactam ring structure and side chains of the penicillins, but allergic cross-reactivity appears to be low, in 1% to 8% of patients. Patients who have experienced urticaria or anaphylactic reactions after taking penicillin are more likely to have an adverse reaction to cephalosporins, but even in this setting, the risk of an anaphylactic reaction is low. There have been rare reports of cross-reactivity to aztreonam and carbapenems in penicillin-allergic patients, but these antibiotics should not be withheld when clinically indicated.[6,21]

NSAIDs are the most common trigger of drug-induced anaphylaxis and are believed to occur through interruption of the arachidonic acid metabolism, a non-IgE (non-immunologic) mediated process. The incidence of anaphylaxis to NSAIDs varies widely, and these reactions appear to be drug specific and without cross-reactivity to other NSAIDs. Aspirin exacerbated respiratory distress (AERD) and NSAID-induced respiratory distress syndromes are unique in individuals with a history of asthma or allergic rhinitis and are not considered anaphylactic reactions.[6,9,20,21]

Insect Stings

Anaphylactic reactions occur in up to 3% of adults and 1% of children who suffer an insect sting. The majority are associated with hymenoptera venoms (wasps, bees, ants, and sawflies) and fire ant stings. These reactions typically require a sensitizing exposure, but there have been numerous reports of anaphylactic reactions following first known stings or bites. Increased risk of fatal venom anaphylaxis has been associated with middle-aged white males, preexisting cardiovascular disease, and upright posture at the time of exposure.[9–11]

Natural Rubber Latex

Natural rubber latex (NRL) allergy is the result of sensitivity to the proteins or chemicals contained in the latex products. This sensitivity reaction can be delayed (type IV) contact dermatitis or an immediate hypersensitivity (type I) reaction (see Box 106.1). In addition to rubber gloves, NRL can be found in an array of other medical supplies, including endotracheal tubes, blood pressure cuffs, stethoscope

> **BOX 106.4   A Standard Treatment Protocol for Patients With a History of Radiocontrast-Induced Anaphylaxis**
>
> Prednisone 50 mg by mouth given 13, 7, and 1 h before the procedure
> Diphenhydramine 50 mg PO given 1 hour before the procedure
> Consider ephedrine 25 mg by mouth given 1 hour before the procedure
> Consider an H_2 antagonist, such as famotidine 20 mg by mouth given 3 h before the procedure

tubing, airway masks, tourniquets, and catheters. In the United States, most health care settings have incorporated the use of non-NRL gloves and products, but in many countries, it is still a common anaphylactic trigger.[6] NRL can also found in balloons, condoms, pacifiers, sports equipment, and toys.

Radiocontrast Media

Approximately 38 million computerized tomography (CT) scans, and 17 million magnetic resonance imaging (MRI) examinations using radiocontrast media (RCM) are performed in the United States annually.[22] CT scans use iodinated contrast media (ICM). ICM reactions can be divided into two types based on timing: immediate reactions occur within the first hour of administration, and delayed reactions occur from 1 hour to several days after administration. Anaphylactic reactions to ICM are largely idiosyncratic and occur within minutes of infusion. Delayed reactions are generally mild to moderate and typically limited to the integumentary system manifesting as maculopapular rash, urticaria, and angioedema. Delayed reactions rarely escalate to the levels of toxic epidermal necrolysis or Stevens-Johnson syndrome. The pathophysiologic mechanism of anaphylactic reactions to ICM is unknown, but it is believed to be non-immunologic (non-IgE). Risk factors for an anaphylactic reaction include a previous adverse reaction to ICM, a history of atopy or allergic disease, asthma, and certain medications including ACE inhibitors, β-blockers, or proton pump inhibitors.[23] A history of allergy to fish or shellfish is not a contraindication to the use of the currently available ICM, nor does it increase the risk of an adverse reaction to ICM. Clinically, the risk for severe adverse reaction to ICM is less than 1%. The death rate from ICM reactions is estimated at 1 per 170,000 administrations and accounts for 27% of drug-induced anaphylactic fatalities.[22,23] Protocols using pretest administration of antihistamines and/or glucocorticoids have been developed to minimize the risks of serious allergic reactions in patients who have had a previous adverse reaction to ICM (Box 106.4). However, there is currently little evidence to support the use of these agents to prevent anaphylaxis in patients receiving low or iso-osmolar RCM for emergently needed tests. We do not recommend delaying necessary tests for ED patients requiring emergent imaging with RCM to administer these medications as a prophylactic measure.[8]

Gadolinium-based contrast agents (GBCAs) are another type of RCM used in MRI. There is no cross-reactivity in allergies to ICM and GBCA, as they are unique structurally. Risk factors for reactions to GBCA include a history of asthma, food allergies, allergies to medications, and female gender. Reactions to GBCA are exceedingly rare, with an incidence of 0.004% to 0.01%, and typically occur within minutes of administration.[23] Like ICM, the pathophysiology of these reactions is poorly understood. Finally, adverse reactions to RCM are not related to iodine and these individuals should not be labeled as having an "iodine allergy."[8]

Exercise-Induced Anaphylaxis

Exercise-induced anaphylaxis (EIA) is a clinical syndrome in which anaphylactic-like reactions occur in relation to physical exertion.

TABLE 106.1 Mediators in Anaphylaxis and Their Physiologic Actions and Clinical Manifestations

Mediators	Physiologic Activity	Clinical Manifestation
Histamine, leukotrienes, thromboxane, prostaglandins, platelet-activating factor, nitric oxide	Vascular permeability, vasodilation, smooth muscle spasm, mucous gland secretion, nociceptor stimulation, myocardial depression	Generalized urticaria and angioedema, pruritus, wheezing, bronchoconstriction, rhinorrhea and bronchorrhea, coryza, conjunctivitis, syncope, tachycardia, hypotension, shock, abdominal pain, nausea, vomiting, diarrhea
Tryptase, carboxypeptidase, chymase, cathepsin G	Activation of the complement system, chemoattraction, activation, and degranulation of mast cells	Anaphylaxis response is amplified by recruitment and activation of the complement system and further degranulation of mast cell mediators
TNF-α, cytokines, chemokines, eosinophil chemotactic factors	Induction of anti-platelet-activating factor production, control migration of eosinophils and other inflammatory cells	May be responsible for the intensity, protracted symptoms, and multiphasic reaction of anaphylaxis

TNF-α, Tumor necrosis factor alpha.

There are two subtypes: Exercise-induced anaphylaxis (EIA), and food-dependent exercise-induced anaphylaxis (FDEIA). EIA can be dependent on other various cofactors including alcohol, environmental temperatures, pollen levels, medications such as NSAIDs (especially aspirin), or endogenous progesterone during female menstrual cycles. EIA can occur with varying levels of exertion or types of activity. While it is more commonly seen with moderate to intense physical activity, it has also been described during less strenuous activities like walking and raking leaves. Reactions can occur inconsistently with physical activities, thus increasing the difficulty of diagnosis. FDEIA only occurs if specific foods have been ingested prior to initiating exercise that would otherwise not cause symptoms without associated physical exertion. Wheat has been identified as the most common food to cause FDEIA. Avoidance of the offending food agent minimizes the risk of symptom development. Ingestion of triggering food 4 to 6 hours, or NSAIDs up to 24 hours, prior to physical activity may precipitate a reaction in susceptible individuals.[9,24-26]

Patients should be instructed to discontinue exercise at the first sign of symptoms, as continued activity can lead to clinical deterioration. Patients with suspected EIA should be prescribed epinephrine autoinjectors. They should be counseled to avoid exercising alone and preferably only exercise with a partner who is aware of their condition and able to administer an epinephrine autoinjector if necessary.[9,24]

Idiopathic Anaphylaxis

Thirty percent to 60% of adults, and up to 10% of children, have no identifiable trigger for an anaphylactic episode. The diagnosis of idiopathic anaphylaxis is often made after evaluation and testing by an allergist. In an attempt to prevent recurrent episodes, these patients may be treated with daily prophylactic medications, such as oral antihistamines with or without oral corticosteroids. A newer treatment option is omalizumab, which has been shown to reduce episodes of idiopathic anaphylactic reactions.[15] The prevalence of idiopathic anaphylaxis is unknown and difficult to estimate. Newly identifiable causes of anaphylaxis, such as alpha-gal, and other allergens have reframed prior idiopathic anaphylaxis diagnoses in some individuals.[27]

Pathophysiology

Anaphylaxis is the result of a variable intracellular signaling process, and severity depends on the specific allergen, route of exposure, and amount of effector cell activation. Mast cells and basophils appear to be the primary effector cells, but research has demonstrated other blood cell and platelet involvement as well.[28] Numerous mediators released by mast cells and basophils exert overlapping physiologic effects on target organs and tissues, making it difficult to ascribe specific clinical manifestations to any single mediator. Histamine and typtase are the two most abundant, with histamine serving as the predominant contributor to immediate hypersensitivity and inflammation.[28-30] Table 106.1 lists the primary mediators in anaphylaxis and their physiologic actions and associated clinical manifestations.

CLINICAL FEATURES

Anaphylactic reactions vary in duration and severity but typically are rapid in onset with most occurring within 2 hours of allergen exposure. Clinical presentations depend on the degree of hypersensitivity, the quantity, route, and rate of antigen exposure, as well as the target organ sensitivity and responsiveness. Presentations include a combination of clinical characteristics, affecting an array of organ systems including the skin (80% to 90%), respiratory tract (70% to 80%), gastrointestinal tract (25% to 30%), cardiovascular (30% to 50%), or the central nervous system (20% to 30%).[9,12,13,20] The National Institute of Allergy and Infectious Diseases/Food Allergy and Anaphylaxis Network (NIAID/FAAN) and WAO adopted specific diagnostic guidelines to help clinicians recognize and develop consistency in the diagnosis of anaphylaxis (Box 106.5). The criteria were initially validated with a sensitivity and specificity of 97% and 82%, respectively. A subsequent prospective validation study demonstrated a sensitivity and specificity of 95% and 71%, respectively.[31,32]

The majority of anaphylactic reactions (80% to 90%) involve the skin. This may present as isolated warmth and tingling, generalized flushing, pruritus, diffuse urticarial eruption, or any combination of these findings. Nasal congestion, sneezing, ocular itching, or tearing are also common. Patients presenting with angioedema complain of swelling and a burning sensation in the affected area. Respiratory symptoms (70% to 80%) are not always as severe as stridor or audible wheeze and may consist of cough, sense of chest tightness, subjective dyspnea, or throat tightness.[9,12,13] Hypotension or dysrhythmias may be manifested as lightheadedness or syncope. Seizure activity due to decreased cerebral perfusion is infrequently seen. Gastrointestinal symptoms are more common in elders or when triggered by a food allergen. This may include crampy abdominal pain, associated nausea and vomiting, diarrhea, or tenesmus.[9,12] Anaphylactic reactions vary a great deal from one individual to another and even among different episodes in the same individual. It should be noted that hypotension or shock are rarely presenting features in infants and children, and remain much more common in adults.[9,33] A summary of the clinical

BOX 106.5   Clinical Criteria for Diagnosis of Anaphylaxis

Anaphylaxis is highly likely when any one of the following three criteria is fulfilled:

1. Sudden onset of an illness (minutes to several hours) with involvement of the skin, mucosal tissue, or both (e.g., generalized hives, itching or flushing, swollen lips-tongue-uvula) and at least one of the following:
   a. Respiratory compromise (e.g., shortness of breath, wheeze, cough stridor, hypoxemia)
   b. Reduced BP or associated symptoms of end-organ dysfunction (e.g., hypotonia [collapse], syncope, incontinence)
2. Two or more of the following occurring rapidly (minutes to several hours) after exposure to a likely allergen or other triggers for that patient:
   a. Involvement of the skin-mucosal tissue (e.g., generalized hives, itch-flush, swollen lips-tongue-uvula)
   b. Sudden respiratory compromise (e.g., shortness of breath, wheeze, cough, stridor, hypoxemia)
   c. Sudden reduced BP or symptoms of end-organ dysfunction (e.g., hypotonia [collapse], syncope, incontinence)
   d. Sudden gastrointestinal symptoms (e.g., crampy abdominal pain, vomiting)
3. Reduced BP after exposure to known allergen for that patient (minutes to several hours):
   a. Infants and children: Low systolic BP (age specific) or greater than 30% decrease in systolic BP*
   b. Adults: Systolic BP of <90 mm Hg or greater than 30% decrease from that person's baseline

* Low systolic blood pressure for children is defined as <70 mm Hg from 1 month to 1 year old, <70 mm Hg + (2 × age) from 1 to 10 years old, and <90 mm Hg from 11 to 17 years old.
Modified from Simons ER, Ardusso LRF, Bilò MB, et al. 2012 Update: World Allergy Organization Guidelines for the assessment and management of anaphylaxis. *Curr Opin Allergy Clin Immunol.* 2012:12:389–399.
BP, Blood pressure.

manifestations of anaphylaxis, along with related pathophysiologic changes, is presented in Table 106.2.

DIFFERENTIAL DIAGNOSES

The diagnosis of anaphylaxis is readily apparent in a patient presenting with acute rash, respiratory difficulty, and hypotension after allergen exposure. Common anaphylaxis mimics include syncope, panic attack, or acute asthma exacerbation. A history of asthma is commonly seen in patients experiencing anaphylaxis.[6,9] Flush syndromes may occur related to certain ingestions such as scrombroidosis, sulfites, or monosodium glutamate (MSG) but typically lack the hypotension, urticaria, or airway involvement that may be seen with anaphylaxis. Vasovagal syncope often presents with bradycardia, hypotension, and pallor, rather than the tachycardia, urticaria, and respiratory distress more commonly associated with anaphylaxis.[9,12] Differential diagnostic considerations for suspected anaphylaxis are found in Box 106.6.

DIAGNOSTIC TESTING

Anaphylaxis is primarily a clinical diagnosis. Box 106.5 lists the NIAID/FAAN and WAO diagnostic criteria for anaphylaxis. Elevated serum histamine levels acquired within 1 hour and tryptase levels (specifically in hymenoptera venom-induced anaphylaxis) within 3 hours of the onset of symptoms have been shown to correlate with

anaphylaxis. In addition, there is now a commercially available serum-specific test for IgE anti-alpha-gal to help identify sensitivity to mammalian meats following tick exposure. These laboratory tests are rarely helpful in the acute setting as they take time to perform. In addition, tryptase levels may not be elevated in food-induced anaphylaxis.[6,9] Diagnostic studies should be aimed at excluding other emergency conditions that could potentially be confused with anaphylaxis (Box 106.6).

MANAGEMENT

Overview

Prompt recognition and initiation of the appropriate interventions remain key in avoiding adverse outcomes. Treatment delays, even by a few minutes, could potentially lead to hypoxia, circulatory collapse, and even death.[10]

Epinephrine should be immediately administered in the distal and lateral thigh once anaphylaxis is identified, followed by a quick effort to remove any triggering agent (e.g., insect stinger and infusing medication). Initial interventions should include continuous cardiac and pulse oximetry monitoring, intravenous (IV) access, and supplemental oxygen.[6,9,12] Most of the morbidity and mortality associated with anaphylaxis is caused by acute respiratory failure or cardiovascular collapse. Therefore, the next steps in management should focus on the triad of repeat epinephrine administration as necessary, maintenance of airway patency, and expansion of intravascular volume. Antihistamines (H₁ and H₂ blockers) and corticosteroids are commonly given for anaphylaxis, but there is no objective evidence that they improve the overall outcome and should not be considered first-line medications.[6,9,12] Box 106.7 summarizes the recommended treatment algorithm in anaphylaxis.

Positioning

Hypotensive patients should be placed in the supine position with their lower extremities elevated. If they are experiencing airway difficulties or vomiting, allow the patients to place themselves in a comfortable position and attempt to elevate their legs if possible. Pregnant women should be placed in the left lateral decubitus position to prevent vena cava compression and to promote the venous return of blood to the heart.[9,12]

Epinephrine

Epinephrine is the sole first-line medication and should be given immediately whenever anaphylaxis is suspected. Delay in administering epinephrine has been associated with increased ED length of stay, hospitalization, hypoxic encephalopathy, and death. Conversely, there is a strong correlation between early epinephrine administration and decreased hospitalization or fatality.[34,35] Despite NIAID/FAAN guidelines for diagnosis and treatment of anaphylaxis being established in 2006, studies have shown that only about 30% of patients receive epinephrine in the prehospital setting, and only 50% to 70% of those ultimately diagnosed with anaphylaxis receive epinephrine in the ED.[16,33–36]

The dose of aqueous epinephrine is 0.3 to 0.5 mg of 1 mg/mL intramuscularly (IM) for adults, and 0.01 mg/kg of 1:1000 concentration IM for pediatric patients. It can be repeated every 5 to 10 minutes, as up to 30% will require more than one dose and should optimally be administered IM in the lateral, distal thigh (vastus lateralis). This provides more rapid peak plasma concentrations (8 minutes) when compared to the previously suggested subcutaneous route (34 minutes). Subcutaneous or inhalation administration of epinephrine is no longer routinely recommended.[9,12,34,37]

TABLE 106.2   Clinical Manifestations of Anaphylaxis and Related Pathophysiologic Changes

Organ System	Reaction	Symptoms	Signs	Pathophysiologic Changes
Respiratory tract				
Upper	Rhinitis	Nasal congestion	Nasal mucosal edema	Increased vascular permeability
		Nasal itching	Rhinorrhea	Vasodilation
		Sneezing		Stimulation of nerve endings
	Laryngeal edema	Dyspnea	Laryngeal stridor	As above, plus increased exocrine gland secretions
		Hoarseness	Supraglottic and glottic edema	
		Throat tightness		
		Hypersalivation		
Lower	Bronchospasm	Cough	Cough	As above, plus bronchiole smooth muscle contraction
		Wheezing	Wheeze, rhonchi	
		Retrosternal tightness	Tachypnea	
		Dyspnea	Respiratory distress	
			Cyanosis	
Cardiovascular system	Circulatory collapse	Lightheadedness	Tachycardia	Increased vascular permeability
		Generalized weakness	Hypotension	Vasodilation
		Syncope	Shock	Loss of vasomotor tone
		Ischemic chest pain		Increased venous capacitance
	Dysrhythmias	As above, plus palpitations	ECG changes:	Decreased cardiac output
			Tachycardia	Decreased mediator-induced myocardial suppression
			Nonspecific and ischemic ST-T wave changes	Decreased effective plasma volume
			Right ventricular strain	Decreased preload
			Premature atrial and ventricular contractions	Decreased afterload
			Nodal rhythm	Hypoxia and ischemia
			Atrial fibrillation	Dysrhythmias
				Iatrogenic effects of drugs used in treatment
				Preexisting heart disease
	Cardiac arrest		Pulseless	
			ECG changes:	
			Ventricular fibrillation	
			Asystole	
Skin	Urticaria	Pruritus	Urticaria	Increased vascular permeability
		Tingling and warmth	Diffuse erythema	Vasodilation
		Flushing		
		Hives		
	Angioedema	Nonpruritic extremity, periorbital, and perioral swelling	Nonpitting edema, frequently asymmetrical	Increased vascular permeability
Eye	Conjunctivitis	Ocular itching	Conjunctival inflammation	Stimulation of nerve endings
		Increased lacrimation		
		Red eye		
Gastrointestinal tract		Dysphagia	Nonspecific	Increased secretion of mucus
		Cramping, abdominal pain		Gastrointestinal smooth muscle contraction
		Nausea and vomiting		
		Diarrhea (rarely bloody)		
		Tenesmus		
Miscellaneous central nervous system		Apprehension	Anxiety	Secondary to cerebral hypoxia and hypoperfusion
		Sense of impending doom	Seizures (rarely)	Vasodilation
		Headache	Coma (late)	
		Confusion		
Hematologic	Fibrinolysis and disseminated intravascular coagulation	Abnormal bleeding and bruising	Mucous membrane bleeding, disseminated intravascular coagulation	Mediator recruitment and activation
			Increased uterine tone	Uterine smooth muscle contraction
			Vaginal bleeding	Bladder smooth muscle contraction
Genitourinary		Pelvic pain	Urinary incontinence	
		Urinary incontinence		

ECG, Electrocardiographic.

BOX 106.6   Differential Diagnosis of Anaphylaxis

Acute generalized urticaria
Asthma exacerbation
Myocardial infarction
Pulmonary embolus
Syncope
Adverse cutaneous drug reaction
Anxiety/panic attacks

Flush Syndrome
Flushing associated with food
Alcohol
MSG
Sulfites
Scombroidosis
Carcinoid tumor
Peri-menopause
Thyrotoxicosis

Basophilic leukemia
Mastocytosis (systemic mastocytosis and urticaria pigmentosa)
Vasointestinal peptide tumors

Shock Syndromes
Septic shock
Hypovolemic shock
Cardiogenic shock
Distributive shock

Miscellaneous
Hypoglycemia
Acquired and HAE
ACE-inhibitor-associated angioedema
Red man syndrome (Vancomycin)
Neurologic disorders (seizure, stroke, autonomic epilepsy)
Vocal cord dysfunction syndrome
Pheochromocytoma

ACE, Angiotensin-converting enzyme; *HAE,* hereditary angioedema; *MSG,* monosodium glutamate.

BOX 106.7   Treatment Algorithm for Anaphylaxis

Emergency Measures (Taken Simultaneously)
Remove any triggering agent.
Place the patient in the supine position.
Begin cardiac monitoring, pulse oximetry, and blood pressure monitoring.
Begin supplemental oxygen if indicated.
Establish large-bore IV lines (e.g., 16 or 18 gauge preferred).
Ensure a patent airway.
Be prepared for endotracheal intubation with or without rapid sequence intubation.
Be prepared to use an adjunct airway technique (e.g., awake fiberoptic intubation, surgical airway).
Start a rapid infusion of isotonic crystalloid (normal saline):
  Adults: 1000 mL IV in the first 5 min in the adult (several liters of normal saline may be required), titrated to response
  Pediatrics: 20–30 mL/kg IV increments

Anaphylaxis Treatment Medications
First-Line Agent
Epinephrine is the first-line medication and should be given immediately at the first suspicion of an anaphylactic reaction.
  Adult: 0.3–0.5 mg IM (1 mg/mL concentration) in anterolateral thigh every 5–10 minutes as necessary
  Pediatric: 0.01 mg/kg IM (1:1000 concentration) in anterolateral thigh every 5–10 minutes as necessary
Alternatively, epinephrine (EpiPen, 0.3 mL; or EpiPen Jr, 0.15 mL) can be administered into the anterolateral thigh

Second-Line Agents (Should Not Precede the Administration of Epinephrine)
Antihistamines
Diphenhydramine:
  Adults: 50 mg IV or 50 mg oral
  Pediatric: 1 mg/kg IV or oral
Famotidine:
  Adult: 40 mg IV (40 mg oral)
  Pediatric: 0.5 mg/kg IV or oral

Aerosolized Beta-Agonists (if Bronchospasm Is Present)
Adult:
  Albuterol: 2.5 mg, diluted to 3 mL of normal saline; may be repeated as needed or continuous
  Ipratropium: 0.5 mg in 3 mL of normal saline; may be repeated as necessary
Pediatric:
  Albuterol: 2.5 mg, diluted to 3 mL of normal saline; may be repeated as needed or continuous
  Ipratropium: 0.25 mg in 3 mL of normal saline; may be repeated as necessary

Glucocorticoids (No Benefit in the Acute Management)
Methylprednisolone:
  Adult: 125–250 mg IV
  Pediatric: 1–2 mg/kg IV
Prednisone/prednisolone:
  Adult: 40–60 mg oral
  Pediatrics: 1–2 mg/kg oral

Refractory Hypotension
Consider continuous IV epinephrine drip (dilute 1 mg (1 mg/mL concentration) in 1000 mL of normal saline or D_5W to yield a concentration of 1 μg/mL)
Adults: 1–10 μg/min IV (titrated to desired effect)
Pediatrics: 0.1–1.5 μg/kg/min IV (titrated to desired effect)

Other Adjunctive Vasopressors to Consider
Dopamine: 5–20 μg/kg/min continuous IV infusion (titrated to the desired effect)
Norepinephrine: 0.05–0.5 μg/kg/min (titrated to desired effect)
Phenylephrine: 1–5 μg/kg/min (titrated to desired effect)
Vasopressin: 0.01–0.4 units/min (titrated between 0.01–0.04 units/min)

Patients Receiving Beta-Blockade
Glucagon: 1–5 mg IV over 5 min, followed by 5–15 μg/min continuous IV infusion

D_5W, 5% dextrose in water; *IM,* intramuscular; *IV,* intravenous.

For patients who remain hypotensive after multiple doses of IM epinephrine and adequate volume expansion aimed at increasing blood pressure, IV epinephrine should be considered. IV epinephrine increases the risks of cardiac dysrhythmias, thus requiring cautious cardiac and hemodynamic monitoring. Dilution and slow administration are recommended to reduce untoward effects.[12,38] In adults, we suggest preparing a concentration of 1.0 µg/mL and initially infusing at a rate of 1 µg/min. The rate should be increased until hemodynamic stability is achieved, or a maximum dose of 10 µg/min. This can be prepared by mixing 1 mg (1 mL) of 1:1000 concentration of epinephrine with 1000 mL of 5% dextrose in water or normal saline; this provides an infusion of 1 mL/min equaling 1 µg/minute. In children and infants, an infusion rate of 0.1 µg/kg/min is advised, increasing in increments of 0.1 µg/kg/min to a maximum of 1.5 µg/kg/min.[37] Central venous access is encouraged when administering IV epinephrine because of the risk of tissue necrosis from extravasation.

Epinephrine derives its therapeutic value from its combined alpha-adrenergic and beta-adrenergic actions that work directly to improve the most commonly observed clinical features.

Alpha$_1$-adrenergic stimulation increases vasoconstriction, increases peripheral vascular resistance, and decreases mucosal edema. Through beta$_1$-adrenergic stimulation, inotropic and chronotropic cardiac activity is enhanced. Beta$_2$-adrenergic stimulation also provides stabilization of mast cells and basophils, and it induces bronchodilation. These combined effects result in decreased mediator release from mast cells and basophils, which improves bronchospasm, decreases mucosal edema and swelling, and reverses systemic hypotension.[12,34]

Epinephrine can produce a number of undesirable side effects, though there is no absolute contraindication in the setting of anaphylaxis. Common side effects include palpitations, anxiety, tremor, pallor, dizziness, or headache. There is a common misconception that epinephrine should be avoided in patients with a history of cardiovascular disease due to the concern of inducing life-threatening arrhythmias and other adverse cardiovascular events. These events are rare, and the majority are associated with improper dosing or administration. The benefits of the early administration of epinephrine in anaphylaxis far outweigh the risks.[34,36,37]

Airway

Patients in respiratory distress and receiving multiple doses of epinephrine should be placed on supplemental oxygen and prepared for possible advanced airway management. Patients with bronchospasm may benefit from bronchodilators, but this should not preclude the administration of epinephrine. Upper airway obstruction from laryngeal angioedema can progress rapidly, so preparations for a difficult airway should be made early. This may include an awake intubation with assistance fiberoptic laryngoscopy or the equipment to convert to a surgical airway procedure if needed.[6,9,12]

Volume Expansion

Along with airway assessment, fluid resuscitation should be initiated. For adults, infuse 1 to 2 L of normal saline rapidly through large-bore (e.g., 16-gauge) IV lines. Pediatric patients should be given boluses in 20 to 30 mL/kg increments. When IV access cannot be established, intraosseous catheter placement is an alternative. The assistance of an infusion pump or pressure bag should be considered when administering fluids in this manner. Large volumes of normal saline (2 to 7 L) may be required to reverse the effects of fluid extravasation into the extravascular space and the circulatory collapse sometimes seen in anaphylaxis. Patients with heart or renal failure should be monitored closely for signs of volume overload.[6,9,12]

Antihistamines

H$_1$ and H$_2$-antihistamines should never be used as the sole or initial treatment in anaphylaxis. They may be considered as second- or third-line treatments and can be helpful in relieving cutaneous symptoms, such as urticaria, pruritus, flushing, eye, or nasal symptoms.[6,12,34] See Box 106.7 for suggested dosing.

Glucocorticoids

While glucocorticoids are frequently administered, they have no immediate effect on the management of anaphylaxis and thus should be considered a second- or third-line intervention. Their onset of action typically takes several hours. In theory, they may provide benefit by preventing protracted symptoms or a biphasic reaction, but there is no strong evidence to support their use for those purposes.[8,39–41] With these limitations in mind, glucocorticoids are an optional adjunct in the treatment of anaphylaxis but should never precede the administration of epinephrine. See Box 106.7 for suggested dosing.

Patients Receiving Beta-Blockade

Glucagon, with positive inotropic and chronotropic cardiac effects mediated independently of alpha and beta receptors, may be helpful in patients with anaphylactic reactions who are receiving beta-blockers and fail to respond to epinephrine or other standard treatments. The initial IV dose is 1 to 5 mg for adults or 20 to 30 µg/kg (maximum dose 1 mg) for children and may be followed by an infusion of 5 to 15 µg/min. Nausea and vomiting are common side effects, so the clinician should be prepared to administer an antiemetic when indicated.[9,12]

DISPOSITION

Up to 20% of patients with anaphylaxis may experience a biphasic reaction defined as a reoccurrence of anaphylactic symptoms without re-exposure to the triggering agent. Most of these reactions occur within 8 hours but have been reported as far out as 72 hours.[8] The majority respond to the appropriate treatment, and recent literature suggests that clinically important biphasic reactions and fatalities are actually much rarer than previously reported.[41,42] Many clinicians administer corticosteroids in hopes of preventing a biphasic reaction, but recent studies have failed to show significant effect.[8,39,40] Patients at increased risk for biphasic reactions include those presenting with hypotension, wide pulse pressure, unknown trigger, greater than 1 dose of epinephrine, cutaneous signs and symptoms, prior anaphylaxis, and delayed epinephrine administration.[8,43,44]

Consensus guidelines suggest that patients who respond to initial treatments and experience complete resolution of symptoms can generally be discharged home after an observation period of 4 to 6 hours. Recent literature suggested a 95% NPV of a biphasic reaction in those observed for 1 hour and 97.3% after 6 hours of observation. Therefore, we suggest a minimum of 1 hour of asymptomatic observation and 6 hours or longer in those with increased risk of biphasic reactions (as previously mentioned).[8,45] Hospitalization should be strongly considered for patients who present with protracted anaphylaxis, hypotension, or airway involvement; receive more than two doses of IM epinephrine; or have poor outpatient social support, or inability to acquire an auto-injectable epinephrine device.[8,9]

Prior to discharge, the clinician should take an active role in educating the patient or caretakers about their allergy and anaphylaxis. It is also important to explain and demonstrate how to use the auto-injectable epinephrine device. Patients should be encouraged to develop an individualized anaphylaxis emergency action plan and to consider acquiring a medical identification device (e.g., bracelet, wallet

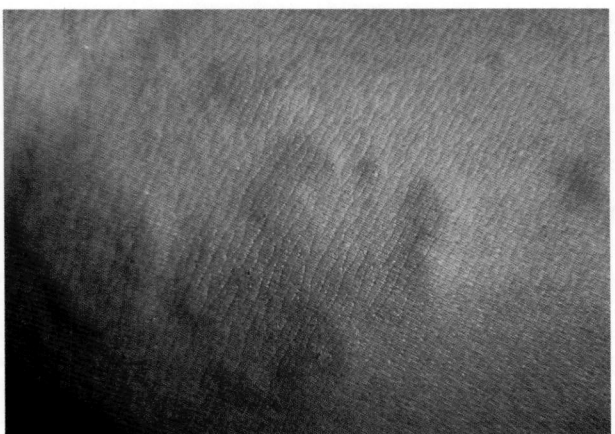

Fig. 106.4 Acute Urticaria. (©2001–2003, Johns Hopkins University School of Medicine. http://dermatlas.med.jhmi.edu/derm.)

card). Emphasis should be placed on timely follow-up, preferably with an allergist-immunologist.[9,34,46]

URTICARIA AND ANGIOEDEMA

PATHOPHYSIOLOGY AND CLINICAL FEATURES

Urticaria is commonly encountered in the ED. It is estimated that 25% of the population will experience an episode of urticaria in their lifetime. Urticaria is characterized by the presence of wheals (hives), angioedema, or both. It should be distinguished from other conditions, such as autoinflammatory syndromes or other causes of non-histaminergic angioedema. Urticaria appears as papules or wheals that consist of central swelling with surrounding reflex erythema and is associated with itching or a burning type sensation (Fig. 106.4).[5] These lesions are a result of mediators (predominately histamine) released from mast cells. They tend to occur on the extremities and are usually transient, with skin often returning to its normal appearance within 24 hours. Urticaria can be classified based on its duration, with acute urticaria lasting less than 6 weeks and chronic episodes lasting longer than 6 weeks. There are also several types of inducible urticaria including cold contact, delayed pressure, heat contact, solar, aquagenic, or cholinergic.[5]

Angioedema is characterized by edema of the subcutaneous or sub-mucosal tissues, commonly involving the face, mouth, lips, tongue, extremities, or genitalia. It is a result of abrupt vasodilation and increased vascular permeability, allowing fluid to move from the vascular to the interstitial space. As the swelling is located in the deeper layers of the skin, the appearance is often normal in color and patients often complain of pain or a pressure sensation, rather than an itch. Of particular concern is when the tongue, posterior pharynx, or larynx is involved, which could progress to airway obstruction and compromise. Angioedema can be mediated by an allergic mechanism in response to exposure to foods, drugs, or physical stimuli or by a nonallergic mechanism such as HAE, acquired angioedema, or ACE-inhibitor-induced angioedema.[47]

Non-histaminergic (nonallergic) angioedema is typically a result of elevated bradykinin levels. This classification includes four subtypes: Hereditary angioedema (HAE) with or without C1 esterase inhibitor deficiency, acquired C1 esterase inhibitor deficiency (ACID), ACE-inhibitor-induced, and idiopathic angioedema. HAE is an autosomal dominant condition, with an estimated frequency of 1:50,000 globally.[48] The median age at which patients develop symptoms is 12 years.[47]

ACID onset usually occurs later in life and may be associated with an underlying lymphoproliferative disorder such as lymphoma, or benign monoclonal gammopathy.[47,49] ACID is a rare condition with limited epidemiologic data. Other than familial history and age of onset, HAE and ACID are clinically indistinguishable. HAE with C1 inhibitor deficiency and ACID share the same mechanism: The lack of C1 inhibitor causes activation of the kallikrein-kinin system, increasing the consumption of kininogen, resulting in increased production of brady-kinin. In the case of ACE-inhibitor-induced angioedema, bradykinin levels accumulate due to the inhibition of the angiotensin-converting enzyme, which is one of two main enzymes responsible for the breakdown of bradykinin. Bradykinin binds the bradykinin 2 receptor (β2), inducing vasodilation and vascular permeability, ultimately resulting in angioedema.[49–51]

Recent literature suggests that in the United States, non-histaminergic angioedema is responsible for approximately 110,000 ED visits annually, with 30% resulting from ACE-inhibitor-induced angioedema. ACE-inhibitor-induced angioedema has an overall incidence of 0.3% to 0.7% and is 3 to 4 times more likely in African Americans, and women are at a 50% higher risk than men. ACE-inhibitor-induced angioedema has a predilection for the face, often involving the lips, eyelids, tongue, larynx, or pharynx. The highest incidence occurs in the first month of therapy but has also been reported to occur years after initiation of therapy.[49–51]

DIAGNOSTIC TESTING

Similar to anaphylaxis, angioedema is a clinical diagnosis. Laboratory tests are not helpful in the acute setting. If a hypersensitivity reaction is suspected, a detailed history should focus on identifying any recent exposures to foods, drugs, physical stimuli, infection (especially viral hepatitis), occupational elements, or insect stings. Patients should also be questioned about prior history of similar symptoms as well as any family history of non-histaminergic angioedema.

MANAGEMENT

Angioedema With Urticaria

Angioedema that occurs in conjunction with urticaria is typically histaminergic (allergic) in nature. In cases that do not meet the criteria for anaphylaxis, antihistamines are considered the first-line treatment. Second-generation H_1-antihistamines, such as cetirizine, loratadine, and fexofenadine, are the preferred agents, and up to fourfold the conventional dose may be considered. Because 15% of dermal histamine receptors are H_2, the addition of an oral H_2-antihistamine may also be beneficial. A short course of oral corticosteroids (e.g., prednisone) may be considered as a second-line therapy.[5] In patients with severe symptoms and no cardiac risk factors, epinephrine should be given (anaphylactic dosing). In an effort to prevent reoccurrence, patients should be educated to avoid exposure to potential triggering agents.

Angioedema Without Urticaria

Acute attacks of non-histaminergic (bradykinin-related) angioedema do not typically respond to treatment with epinephrine, antihistamines, or steroids. In patients presenting with airway-threatening angioedema and no prior history, we suggest initially administering epinephrine and antihistamines at anaphylactic doses. In situations requiring intubation, awake fiberoptic intubation when available is the preferred method and paralytics should be utilized with caution. The clinician must be prepared to rapidly work through a difficult airway algorithm using alternative measures (e.g., fiberoptic laryngoscopy, surgical airway), as discussed in Chapter 1. When available, early

TABLE 106.3 Treatment Options for Hereditary Angioedema

Drug	Age Approved Use	Mechanism of Action	Dose/Route	Median Time to Symptom Relief
Berinert	Adult and pediatric patients	C1-INH protein replacement, human	20 units/kg IV	48 min
Ruconest	Adults and pediatric patients >11 years of age	C1-INH protein replacement, recombinant	50 units/kg IV (max 4200 units IV)	90 min
Ecallantide	Adults and pediatric patients >12 years of age	Plasma-Kallikrein inhibitor	30 mg SC	67 min
Icatibant	Adult patients >18 years of age	Bradykinin-2 receptor antagonist	30 mg SC	2 h

C1-INH, C1 esterase inhibitor; *IV,* intravenous; *SC,* subcutaneous.
Modified from Bernstein JA, Cremonesi P, Hoffmann TK, et al. Angioedema in the emergency department: a practical guide to differential diagnosis and management. *Int J Emerg Med.* 2017;10(15):1–11.

mobilization of ENT, anesthesiology, or another emergency physician colleague may be beneficial. In cases with suspected laryngeal or supraglottic angioedema, evaluation with nasopharyngoscopy may assist in formulating treatment plans, interventions, and disposition.

Fresh frozen plasma (FFP), which contains a C1 inhibitor, has been reported to be effective in acute attacks; however, there are rare reports of exacerbation of the angioedema by FFP. The FDA has approved four medications for use in the United States for patients with acute HAE (see Table 106.3).[49]

For ACE-inhibitor-induced angioedema, treatment is mainly supportive. Theoretically, the medications described for the treatment of HAE would be effective in ACE-inhibitor-induced angioedema, but none are FDA-approved for use at this time. There are multiple case reports of FFP being used with success in the treatment of ACE-inhibitor angioedema. Early treatment (within several hours of symptom onset) may be necessary to be successful.[52] Initial studies looking at ecallantide and icatibant have yielded mixed results, and there is no strong recommendation for their use at the time of this publication. We suggest administering one of these agents if available at your institution and the patient is showing signs of progressing airway involvement.[53–56]

Special Considerations

Thrombolytic induced angioedema is a well-recognized, yet rare complication following administration of recombinant tissue plasminogen activator (tPA). While usually transient in nature, it can be rapidly progressive and potentially life-threatening. The reported incidence is 1% to %5.[49] It is classically described as asymmetric orolingual angioedema. Increased risk is associated with ACE-inhibitor use. The mechanism of angioedema development is thought to be multifactorial. Also, tPA can increase bradykinin levels through its production of plasmin, which can also activate the complement cascade, triggering mast cell degranulation and histamine release. Recommended treatment includes antihistamines and corticosteroids. There are reports of successful treatment with epinephrine, although blood pressure control is a potential concern.[57,58]

DISPOSITION

There is a lack of data to provide concrete guidelines for disposition. Most will agree that patients who experience a complete resolution of angioedema or have only extra-oral facial involvement can be discharged home after a period of observation in the ED. Individuals suspected of HAE or ACID should be referred to an allergist, as further evaluation and potential preventative medications may be warranted. We suggest hospitalization for patients with persistent angioedema of the sublingual area, tongue, soft palate, pharynx, or larynx.

The references for this chapter can be found online at ExpertConsult.com.

107

Dermatologic Presentations

Catherine Anna Marco

- Accurate descriptions of dermatologic lesions are essential for diagnosis and management. Primary and secondary lesions are described in Tables 107.1 and 107.2.
- Systemic illnesses with cutaneous findings include systemic infections, autoimmune or connective tissue disorders, malignancies, diabetes mellitus, endocrine disorders, and immunodeficiency states.
- Cutaneous signs of systemic disease include pruritus, urticaria, erythema multiforme, erythema nodosum, pyoderma gangrenosum, or others.
- Most skin and soft tissue infections should be treated with antibiotics to cover methicillin-resistant *Staphylococcus aureus*.
- Cutaneous abscesses are treated with incision and drainage plus antibiotics.
- Tinea capitis requires 4–8 weeks of systemic antifungal treatment.
- Onychomycosis requires long-term systemic treatment.
- Allergic reactions are treated with antihistamines and discontinuation of exposure to the allergen. Nonsedating antihistamines are the preferred agents to control pruritus and histamine-mediated rashes because they allow patients to remain active.
- Suspected infestations should be diagnosed clinically and treated expeditiously, even without definitive proof of the infestation.
- Medication reactions are common and may result from any agent, typically within 4–28 days after use.
- Rashes that are associated with mucosal lesions, blisters, or desquamating skin are often caused by significant soft tissue infections, drug eruptions, or immune disorders.
- Patients with Stevens-Johnson syndrome or toxic epidermal necrolysis require inpatient treatment, preferably in a burn unit.
- Clinicians should be familiar with one or two topical steroid preparations of low, medium, and high potency, and their appropriate therapeutic use.
- The majority of patients with dermatologic complaints are managed as outpatients. Indications for hospitalization include significant fluid and electrolyte abnormalities, disordered thermoregulation, systemic infection or other underlying disorder requiring inpatient management, and inability to care for self or maintain appropriate oral intake.

OVERVIEW

Foundations

Background and Importance

Diseases of the skin and subcutaneous tissue account for over 5 million emergency department (ED) visits annually, approximately 3.5% of all ED visits.[1] Dermatologic conditions often have a significant impact on quality of life.[2] Common diagnoses among ED patients include infections, inflammatory conditions, allergic reactions, or drug reactions.

Anatomy, Physiology, and Pathophysiology

The skin is composed of three layers: the epidermis, dermis, and subcutaneous layer (Fig. 107.1). The epidermis is a thin layer of stratified squamous epithelium, consisting mainly of keratinocytes, which progress through stages of differentiation as they migrate from the basal to the superficial layer. These layers are the stratum basale (base of the epithelium), stratum spinosum, stratum granulosum, stratum lucidum, and stratum corneum (superficial layer). The epidermis also includes other cells, such as melanocytes and Langerhans cells. Melanocytes produce melanin, which functions to add pigment to the skin and also to absorb ultraviolet radiation. Langerhans cells are a component of the immune system and function to ingest and process foreign antigens. The epidermis lacks direct blood supply and is dependent on the dermis for nutrients by diffusion through the dermal-epidermal junction. This junction is the site of immunologic injury resulting in separation of these layers, which appears as bullae.

The dermis consists of connective tissue, blood vessels, lymphatic vessels, nerve endings, and immune cells. The main function of the dermis is to support the epidermis and contribute to the protective functions of the skin. Fibroblasts produce procollagen and elastic fibers used to form the connective tissues that give support and elasticity to the skin. Sweat glands and the network of blood vessels in the dermis assist with thermoregulation.

The subcutaneous layer is composed of connective tissue and adipose tissue, functions to cushion the overlying skin, and contains lymph and neurovascular structures.

The skin serves several important physiologic functions. It serves as a barrier between the internal and external environment. The skin protects from external toxic and infectious materials, and assures homeostatic balance of fluids and electrolytes. The skin serves an integral role in temperature homeostasis through its barrier function, sweating mechanism, and blood vessel dilation or constriction; it functions in the absorption of ultraviolet radiation and production of vitamin D; sensory nerve endings in skin serve important functions of sensation; and finally, certain cells within the skin serve important immunologic functions, including Langerhans cells, lymphocytes, mast cells, and keratinocytes.

Clinical Features and Differential Diagnoses

A step-by-step approach to evaluating an unknown rash is listed in Box 107.1.

Important historical factors include the time of onset, duration of symptoms, and exposure to potential allergens, such as foods, medications, soaps, pets, or jewelry. Information about changes over time should be sought, including whether the rash has progressed, improved, or waxed and waned. Associated pain, pruritus, fever, sexual history, occupation, and hobbies should be identified. Relevant past medical history includes medical conditions, skin conditions,

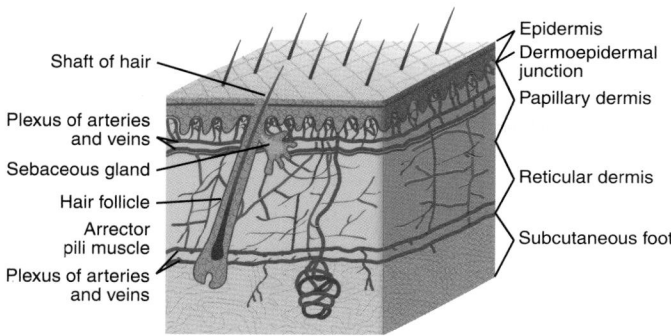

Fig. 107.1 Skin Anatomy.

Shaft of hair
Plexus of arteries and veins
Sebaceous gland
Hair follicle
Arrector pili muscle
Plexus of arteries and veins

Epidermis
Dermoepidermal junction
Papillary dermis
Reticular dermis
Subcutaneous foot

BOX 107.1 Approach to Management of the Unknown Rash

1. Time of onset
2. Historical features
3. Medical history
4. Primary lesion
5. Secondary lesions
6. Distribution of the lesions
7. Systemic illness
8. Diagnostic tests
9. Category of rash
   a. Infectious
   b. Immune
   c. Vascular
   d. Allergic
   e. Malignancy
10. Treatment

TABLE 107.1 Primary Lesions

Lesion	Description	Size
Macule	Flat circumscribed pigmented area	<0.5 cm in diameter
Patch	Flat circumscribed pigmented area	>0.5 cm in diameter
Papule	Elevated, solid, palpable lesion, variable color	<0.5 cm in diameter
Plaque	Elevated, solid, palpable lesion, variable color	>0.5 cm in diameter
Nodule	Solid, palpable, subcutaneous lesion	<0.5 cm in diameter
Abscess	Erythematous, fluctuant, tender, fluid-filled nodule	Any
Tumor	Solid, palpable, subcutaneous lesion	>0.5 cm in diameter
Vesicle	Elevated, thin walled, circumscribed, clear fluid-filled lesion	<0.5 cm in diameter
Bulla	Elevated, thin walled, circumscribed, clear fluid-filled lesion	>0.5 cm in diameter
Pustule	Elevated, circumscribed, purulent fluid-filled lesion	Any
Petechiae	Flat, erythematous or violaceous non-blanching lesions	<0.5 cm in diameter
Purpura	Erythematous or violaceous non-blanching lesions, may be palpable	>0.5 cm in diameter

TABLE 107.2 Secondary Lesions

Secondary Lesion	Description
Scale	Thickened area of keratinized epithelium
Crust	Dried area of plasma proteins, resulting from inflammation
Fissures	Deep cracks in skin surfaces, extending into dermis
Erosions	Disruption of surface epithelium, usually linear, traumatic
Ulcer	Deep erosion extending into dermis
Scar	Dense collection of collagen, a result of healing after trauma or procedures
Excoriation	Linear erosions typically secondary to scratching or rubbing
Infections	Bacterial, viral, fungal, or protozoal infection, caused by breaks in dermal-epidermal junction, often erythematous
Hyperpigmentation	Increase in melanin containing epidermal cells
Lichenification	Abnormally dense layer of keratinized epidermal cells

medications, illicit drug use, allergies, recent travel, sunlight exposure, and family history.

The physical examination is essential to identifying the diagnosis. The examination should be performed with adequate lighting. Primary and secondary lesions, as well as characteristics and patterns of lesions, should be identified. Lesions may be palpated wearing gloves to identify texture, blanching, or sloughing characteristics. Nikolsky sign may be tested, and when positive, gentle rubbing of the skin results in sloughing of the top layer of the epidermis. For patients with systemic complaints, a thorough visual examination from head to soles of feet should be performed, including skin, mucosa, and genitalia.

Identification and description of lesions is essential. Lesions may be classified as primary or secondary lesions. Primary lesions arise directly from the disease process. Secondary lesions result from factors such as scratching, treatment, healing, or complicating infections. Primary and secondary lesions and descriptions are listed in Tables 107.1 and 107.2. The significance of distribution of lesions is outlined in Table 107.3.

Diagnostic Testing

Laboratory testing is unnecessary for most patients with a rash. Specific tests for clinically suspected diseases may be indicated, such as a blood test for secondary syphilis, heterophile antibody (Monospot) for mononucleosis, or throat swab for rapid testing and culture of group A streptococcus for scarlet fever. Adjunctive skin tests may be considered, including potassium hydroxide (KOH) prep, Tzanck smear, gram stain, erythrocyte sedimentation rate (ESR), or biopsy. For the patient with severe systemic illness, a complete blood count, blood cultures,

lumbar puncture studies, electrolytes, blood urea nitrogen (BUN), creatinine, glucose, and liver function tests may be considered. Ultrasound may be helpful in identifying features such as fluid collection, blood flow, septations, inflammation, and to determine the extent of soft tissue lesions.[3]

Management

The treatment of specific dermatologic conditions is addressed in the following sections of this chapter covering infectious, allergic, inflammatory, autoimmune, and malignant disorders. More detailed discussions of the systemic manifestations and overall management of many

TABLE 107.3   Distribution and Patterns of Selected Disease States

Dermatologic Diagnosis	Distribution and Patterns of Lesions
Atopic dermatitis, infantile	Face, scalp, flexor surfaces of extremities
Atopic eczema, adult	Face, neck, flexor surfaces of extremities
Dermatomyositis	Dorsal MCP joints, periorbital area
Disseminated gonorrhea	Distal extremities, near joints
Erythema nodosum	Anterior shins, ulnar surfaces
Herpes zoster infection	Dermatomal distribution, common on trunk
Lichen planus	Wrists, ankles, flexor surfaces
Nummular eczema	Distal extremities
Neurotic excoriations	Extremities, face, upper back, neck
Pityriasis rosea	Trunk, extremities, "Christmas tree" pattern
Porphyria cutanea tarda	Sun-exposed areas, hands, forearms, feet
Psoriasis	Extensor surfaces of extremities, sacral area
Rosacea	Face, neck
Sarcoidosis	Face, extremities, back
Seborrheic dermatitis	Chest, nasolabial folds
Secondary syphilis	Torso, palms, soles
Systemic lupus erythematosus	Nose and cheeks, head and neck, photosensitivity, alopecia
Tinea versicolor	Upper back and chest

MCP, Metacarpophalangeal.

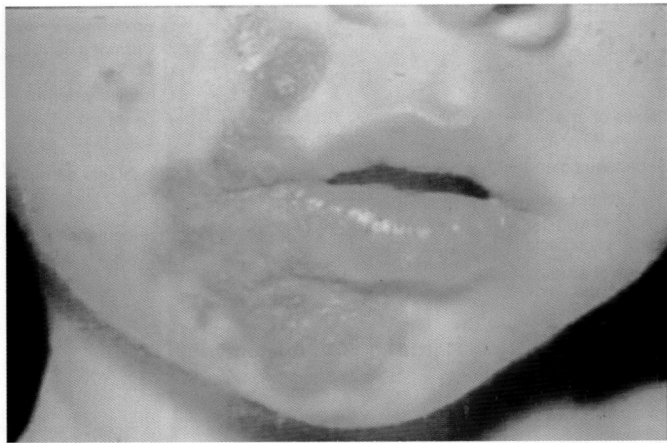

Fig. 107.2 Impetigo. (Courtesy Jonathan Singer, MD.)

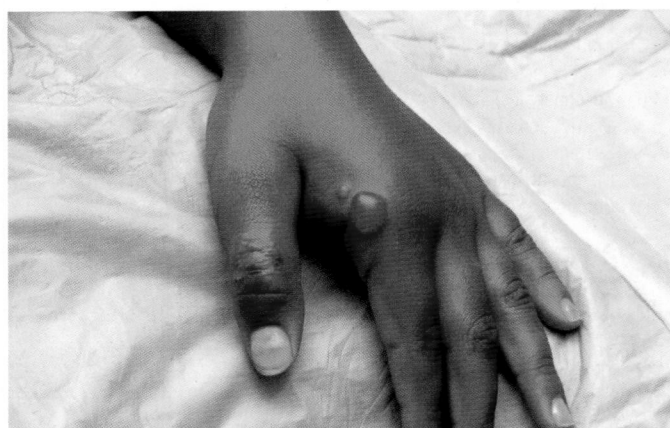

Fig. 107.3 Bullous Impetigo. (Courtesy David Effron, MD.)

of the conditions can be found elsewhere in this textbook. Soft tissue, bacterial, viral, tick-borne, and sexually transmitted infections are covered in Chapters 126, 118, 122, 123, and 84, respectively. Urticaria is discussed in Chapter 106.

Disposition

Most patients with dermatologic complaints are managed as outpatients. Indications for hospitalization include significant fluid and electrolyte abnormalities, disordered thermoregulation, systemic infection, underlying disorders requiring inpatient management, and inability to care for self or maintain appropriate oral intake. Dermatologic outpatient follow-up or inpatient consultation may be appropriate.

INFECTIOUS DISORDERS

Bacterial Infections

Impetigo

Impetigo is typically caused by *Staphylococcus aureus* or β-hemolytic *Streptococcus.* Pediatric patients are commonly affected. Streptococcal impetigo (ecthyma) is found most often on the face and other exposed areas. The eruption often begins as a single pustule and later progresses to multiple lesions, often with a golden yellow crust (Fig. 107.2). Lesions may be pruritic but usually are not painful. Regional lymphadenopathy is commonly present. Lesions are contagious among infants and young children and less so in older children and adults. Postpyodermal acute glomerulonephritis is a recognized complication of streptococcal impetigo.

Staphylococcal impetigo is differentiated from streptococcal impetigo in that it is more superficial, and there is little surrounding erythema. Other diagnostic considerations include herpes simplex virus (HSV) or inflammatory fungal infections. Methicillin-resistant

Streptococcus aureus (MRSA) impetigo is increasingly common. Bullous impetigo is caused by the toxin released by staphylococcus. It is seen primarily in infants and young children. The initial skin lesions are thin-walled, 1- to 2-cm bullae (Fig. 107.3). When these rupture, they leave a thin serous crust and collarette-like remnant of the blister roof at the rim of the crust. The face, neck, and extremities are most often affected. The differential diagnosis includes contact dermatitis, HSV infection, superficial fungal infections, and pemphigus vulgaris.

Empirical therapy should be instituted with oral or topical antibiotics. Topical therapy is initiated with bacitracin, mupirocin, retapamulin, minocycline, or ozenoxacin.[4-7] Oral antibiotics are indicated for severe or multiple lesions. Oral therapies include an agent active against *S. aureus,* such as dicloxacillin or cephalexin. If MRSA is suspected, doxycycline, clindamycin, or trimethoprim-sulfamethoxazole (TMP-SMX) is recommended. Therapy for bullous impetigo consists of a systemic oral antibiotic, such as dicloxacillin, erythromycin, or azithromycin. Even without treatment, impetigo generally resolves within 3 to 6 weeks (see Chapter 126).

Folliculitis

Folliculitis is an inflammation in the hair follicle, usually caused by *S. aureus.* It appears as pustules with a central hair. The lesions are commonly on the buttocks and thighs, in the beard or scalp, and may cause mild discomfort. The differential diagnosis includes acne, keratosis pilaris, or fungal infection. Gram-negative folliculitis with

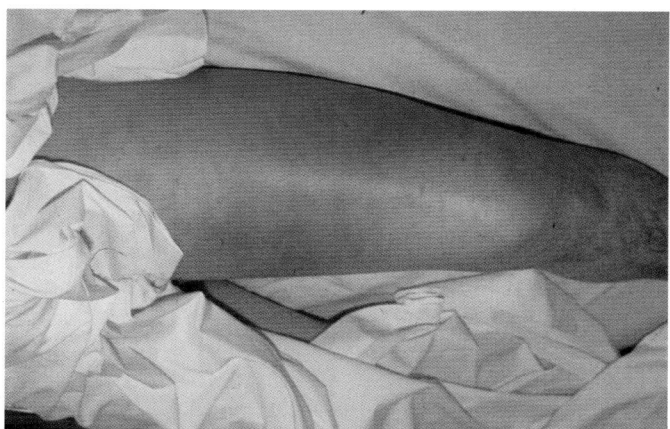

Fig. 107.4 Cellulitis. (Courtesy Jonathan Singer, MD.)

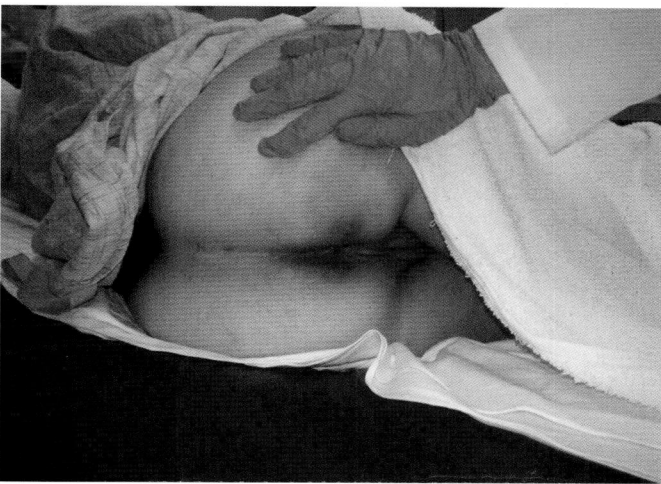

Fig. 107.5 Methicillin-Resistant *Staphylococcus aureus* (MRSA) Abscess With Cellulitis.

Pseudomonas aeruginosa can occur after exposure to infected hot tubs and swimming pools, or in individuals taking antibiotics for acne.

Local treatment with an antiseptic cleanser such as povidone-iodine or chlorhexidine every day or every other day for several weeks is usually adequate. For patients with extensive involvement, a course of systemic oral antibiotics may be added, such as doxycycline or dicloxacillin (see Chapter 126).

Cellulitis

Cellulitis presents with localized erythema, swelling, and pain of the soft tissues (Fig. 107.4). Erysipelas is a streptococcal infection of the skin and subcutaneous tissue and typically has an erythematous appearance with a well demarcated border, often with fever, malaise, or myalgias. Cellulitis may be a cause of sepsis. Ultrasound may be helpful in differentiating from abscess.

Mild cases of cellulitis may be treated with an oral antibiotic, such as a cephalosporin, dicloxacillin, or clindamycin. Moderate cases requiring IV therapy should be treated with a penicillin, ceftriaxone, cefazolin, or clindamycin. Severe cases should be treated with IV vancomycin plus piperacillin/tazobactam. Chapter 126 provides detailed management recommendations.

Abscess

Abscesses are accumulations of pus within body tissues. *Furuncles* are skin abscesses caused by staphylococcal infection involving hair follicles and surrounding tissue. They may present with localized soft tissue swelling, erythema, and fluctuance (Fig. 107.5). Ultrasound may be helpful in differentiating abscess, which appears as a fluid-filled cavity from cellulitis, which appears as cobblestoning, with fine reticular (net-like) areas of hypoechoic stranding.[8-10]

Carbuncles are large abscesses that develop in the thick, inelastic skin of the back of the neck, back, or thighs and usually involve multiple hair follicles. They may produce severe pain and fever. Septicemia may be a complication.

Abscesses should be treated with incision and drainage. Recent literature suggests higher cure rate for antibiotic treatment with TMP-SMX in addition to incision and drainage.[11-15] TMP-SMX and clindamycin have demonstrated efficacy in cure rates following incision and drainage.[16] Moderate or severe abscesses should ideally have culture and sensitivity performed. If IV antibiotics are indicated, agents may include vancomycin, daptomycin, linezolid, telavancin, or ceftaroline. Chapter 126 provides detailed management recommendations.

Hidradenitis suppurativa affects the apocrine sweat glands. Recurrent abscess formation in the axillae and groin resembles localized furunculosis. The condition tends to be recurrent and may be resistant to therapy. Ultrasound will help differentiate abscesses from vascular or lymphoid structures. Hidradenitis suppurativa may be treated with drainage of abscesses if they are fluctuant, painful, and large. Antistaphylococcal antibiotics are useful if they are administered early and for a prolonged period. Begin treatment for mild disease with topical clindamycin for 3 months. In patients with more severe or nonresponsive disease, oral clindamycin combined with rifampin for 3 to 6 months is indicated. Antiandrogen therapy may be considered if antibiotics fail to produce improvement. Recurrent cases should be referred for surgical management.

Methicillin-Resistant *Staphylococcus aureus* (MRSA)

The incidence of community-associated MRSA has risen steadily since the first report in 1993. In many major cities in the United States, MRSA is now the most common pathogen cultured from ED patients presenting with skin and soft tissue infections. Hospital-acquired MRSA isolates can survive on a variety of inanimate surfaces, sometimes for weeks. Pets (including dogs and cats), livestock, and birds have been identified as MRSA carriers; their role in MRSA transmission to humans is unclear.

MRSA infections are most often manifested as skin and soft tissue suppuration, such as an abscess, furuncle, or cellulitis. Lesions frequently exhibit central necrosis and are often confused with spider bites by patients. Clinical features cannot distinguish with certainty skin and soft tissue infections caused by MRSA from those caused by methicillin-susceptible *S. aureus*. Although rare, MRSA infection can present as necrotizing fasciitis. Recurrences of MRSA cellulitis are common. Contagion among the close household contacts of patients as well as correctional facility, school, or sports team contacts is well recognized.

Local resistance patterns should guide therapy. Agents typically effective against MRSA include TMP-SMX, clindamycin, minocycline, or doxycycline. Cephalosporins and macrolides are typically ineffective against MRSA. Fluoroquinolones should be avoided as *S. aureus* resistance develops readily.

Patients with large abscesses, abscesses in high-risk locations, fever, signs of systemic infection, young age, or immunodeficiency should be considered for inpatient treatment. Vancomycin is considered the parenteral drug of choice for patients with invasive *S. aureus* infection, although clinical failures have been reported. It is reasonable to combine vancomycin with another effective

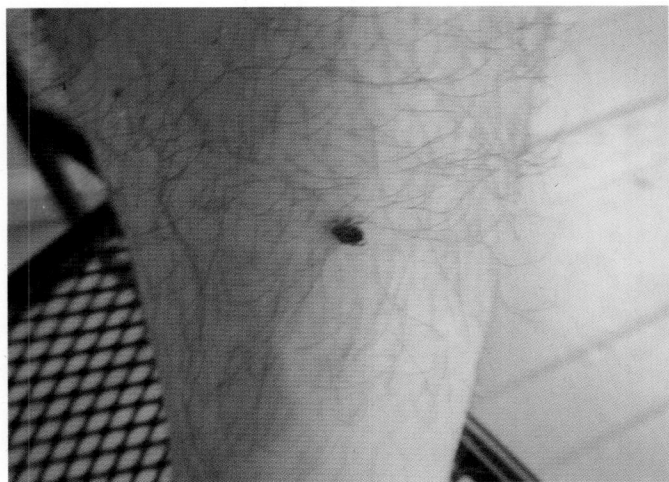

Fig. 107.6 Tick.

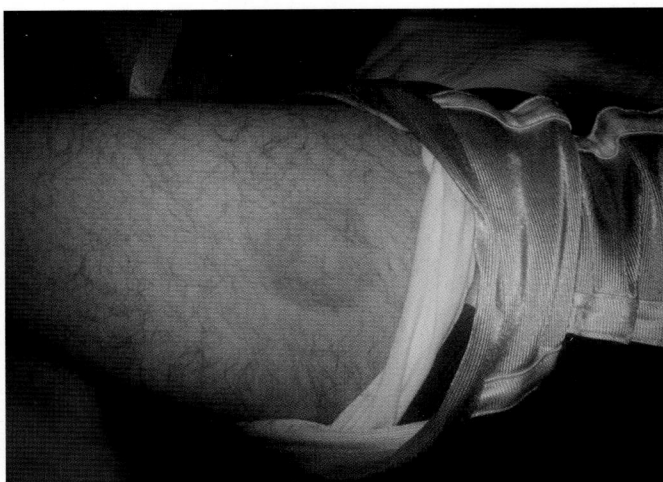

Fig. 107.7 Erythema Migrans.

anti-staphylococcal agent as many antibiotics have better bactericidal activity. In severely ill patients, carbapenems such as meropenem, panipenem, and ertapenem are recommended, because they are active against MRSA and synergistic with vancomycin. Other effective parenteral agents may include clindamycin, linezolid, daptomycin, tigecycline, or telavancin. Chapter 126 provides detailed management recommendations.

Although decolonization strategies have been recommended by some, neither the indications for their use nor their effectiveness in reducing the risk of recurrences has been established. Common antiseptics appear to retain reasonable activity against MRSA, although the results of studies are somewhat conflicting. Good personal hygiene, including appropriate handwashing techniques, separation of infected patients, and routine cleaning of shared equipment, remain essential to limiting MRSA spread.

Erythema Migrans

Lyme disease is caused by the organism *Borrelia burgdorferi* and is transmitted by the deer tick bite (Fig. 107.6). Most cases occur in the spring and early summer. Endemic areas in the U.S. include the Northeast, Midwest, West, and scattered other areas. Although 36 to 48 hours of tick attachment is necessary to transmit disease, less than 33% of patients recall a tick bite. The incubation period is 3 to 30 days.

Clinical presentations include three disease stages. Stage I occurs early and is manifested by malaise, headache, fever, lymphadenopathy, and arthralgias. Stage I typically resolves in 4 weeks. Erythema migrans occurs in 60% to 80% of cases and manifests as erythematous annular, non-scaling lesion with central clearing (Fig. 107.7). Stage II presents with secondary annular lesions, fever, lymphadenopathy, neurologic manifestations, or cardiac conduction abnormalities that may last weeks to months. Stage III manifests as chronic arthritis, dermatitis, or central nervous system (CNS) disease.

Diagnostic tests may include a nonspecific elevated ESR and serologic tests, which are helpful in establishing the definitive diagnosis but are not typically available acutely. Serologic testing includes a two-tiered serologic analysis consisting of an enzyme-linked immunoassay or immunofluorescence assay, followed by reflexive immunoblotting.[17]

Management should include appropriate antibiotic administration. The antibiotic regimen may include doxycycline or amoxicillin, for 10 to 21 days, or as alternates, cefuroxime, clarithromycin, erythromycin, or azithromycin.[18,19] Chapter 123 provides detailed management recommendations.

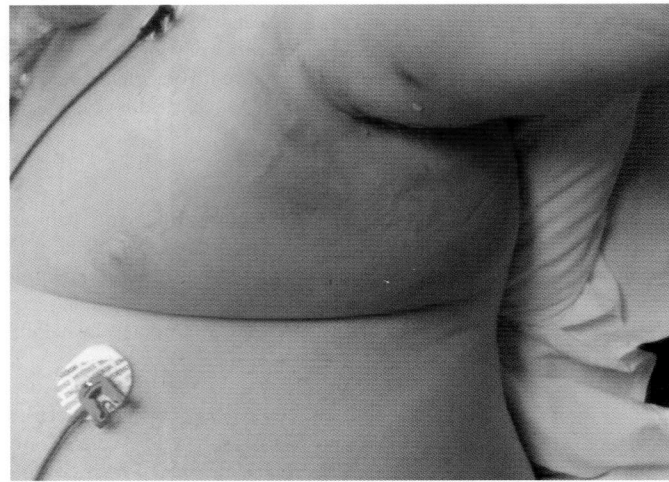

Fig. 107.8 Necrotizing Fasciitis.

Necrotizing Fasciitis

Necrotizing fasciitis should be considered with skin and soft tissue infection with signs of systemic toxicity, or severe infection (Figs. 107.8, 107.9, and 107.10). The etiology is often polymicrobial (mixed aerobic/anaerobic microbes) or monomicrobial (group A streptococci, community-acquired MRSA). Radiographic tests may demonstrate soft tissue air. Prompt surgical consultation is indicated.

Empirical antibiotic treatment should be instituted with broad coverage, such as vancomycin or linezolid plus one of the following: piperacillin-tazobactam, carbapenem, or a combination of ceftriaxone and metronidazole. Chapter 126 provides detailed management recommendations.

Meningococcal Infection

Meningococcal infection is caused by the organism *Neisseria meningitides*, typically transmitted by respiratory secretions. Meningococcal disease may manifest as one of three syndromes: meningitis, bacteremia, or pneumonia. Meningococcal disease typically affects healthy children and adolescents, and it may result in significant morbidity and mortality. Infection is fatal in approximately 10% of cases.

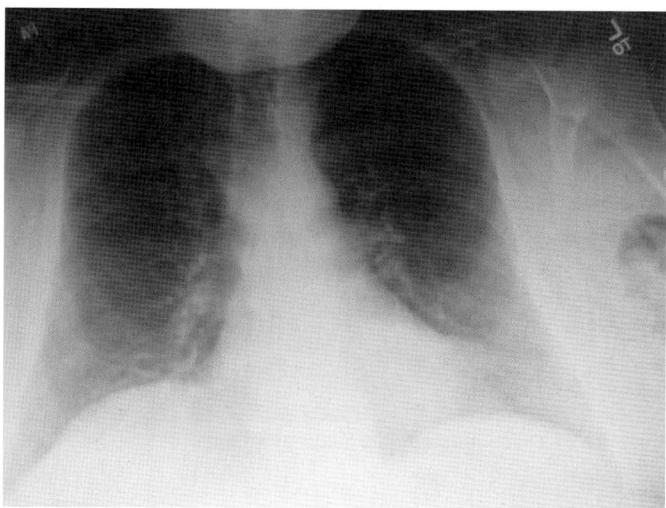

Fig. 107.9 Necrotizing Fasciitis. Note air in subcutaneous tissues.

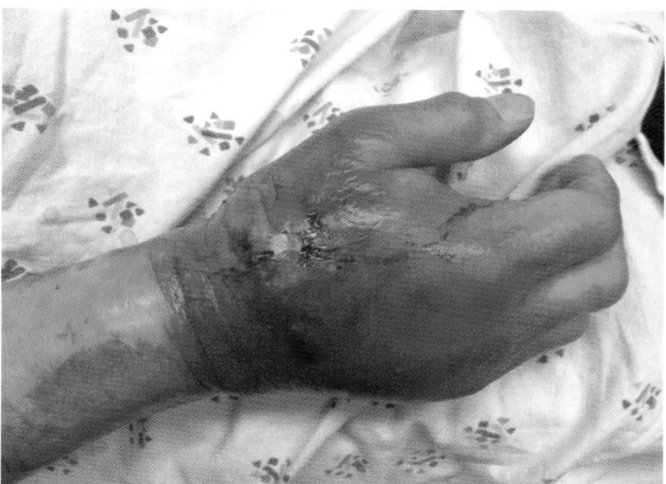

Fig. 107.10 Necrotizing Fasciitis.

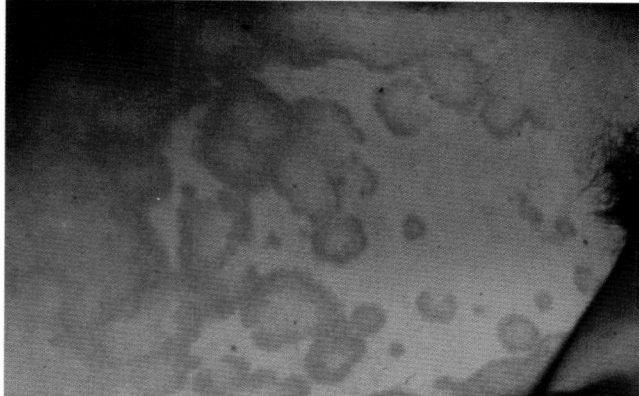

Fig. 107.11 Erythema Marginatum Associated With Rheumatic Fever. (Courtesy David Effron, MD.)

a rough sandpaper-like texture due to a multitude of tiny papules. The pharynx is typically injected, and there may be erythematous lesions or petechiae on the palate. After the resolution of symptoms, desquamation of the involved areas may occur. Erythema marginatum may be seen in 10% of cases and presents with annular erythematous lesions that may be transient and reappear over days, weeks, or months (Fig. 107.11).

Complications include the development of a streptococcal infection of lymph nodes, tonsils, middle ear, or respiratory tract. Late complications include rheumatic fever or glomerulonephritis.

Treatment should be initiated with oral penicillin VK (children <27 kg: 250 mg twice daily or three times daily for 10 days; adolescents and adults: 250 mg four times daily or 500 mg twice daily for 10 days) or IM benzathine penicillin (given as Bicillin C-R (<27 kg: 600,000 units as a one-time dose; ≥27 kg: 1,200,000 units as a one time dose). In patients allergic to penicillin, treatment may be initiated with erythromycin, other macrolides, or a cephalosporin.

Syphilis

Syphilis is the third most common sexually transmitted infection in the United States (following chlamydia and gonorrhea) and is transmitted by direct contact with an infectious lesion. The incidence of reported cases has risen steadily since 2001. The causative organism is the spirochete *Treponema pallidum*. After an incubation period of 10 to 90 days, the primary lesion appears, which lasts 3 to 12 weeks and heals spontaneously. If untreated, in 6 weeks to 6 months after exposure, the secondary stage may be manifest. These lesions also heal spontaneously in 2 to 6 weeks as the disease enters the latent phase. Tertiary syphilis or latent syphilis may occur in months to years after untreated secondary syphilis.

The chancre is the dermatologic manifestation of primary syphilis. Chancres usually appear as single lesions but may be multiple. They appear at the site of spirochete inoculation, usually the mucous membranes of the mouth or genitalia. The chancre begins as a papule and characteristically develops into an ulcer approximately 1 cm in diameter with a central base and raised borders (Fig. 107.12). The chancre is typically painless unless it is secondarily infected, and it may be accompanied by painless lymphadenopathy. Many patients do not recall the primary chancre.

The secondary stage usually follows the primary stage by 6 weeks or more. There are a number of cutaneous manifestations of secondary syphilis. Lesions may be erythematous or pink macules or papules, usually with a generalized symmetric distribution. Secondary syphilis should be considered in the differential diagnosis of any maculopapular

Clinical presentation may include fever, malaise, arthralgias, nausea, and vomiting. Cutaneous findings of macules, papules, vesicles, or petechiae and purpura may be present.

Ten percent of cases may present with Waterhouse-Friderichsen syndrome characterized by shock with intracutaneous hemorrhage.

The diagnosis should be suspected clinically and treated promptly. Confirmatory tests may include blood cultures, cerebrospinal fluid (CSF) cultures, or skin scrapings.

Empirical therapy should be instituted with agents, such as a third-generation cephalosporin (e.g., ceftriaxone or cefotaxime) plus vancomycin. Alternative antibiotics may include penicillin G, chloramphenicol, a fluoroquinolone, or aztreonam. Dexamethasone should also be considered for suspected or proven meningitis.[20,21] Immunization against meningococcal infection is recommended for groups at increased risk for infection, including adolescents. Chapter 118 provides detailed management recommendations.

Scarlet Fever

Scarlet fever results from group A strep infection. The illness presents with fever, chills, malaise, and sore throat, followed within 12 to 48 hours by a distinctive rash that begins on the chest and spreads rapidly, usually within 24 hours. Circumoral pallor may be noted. The skin has

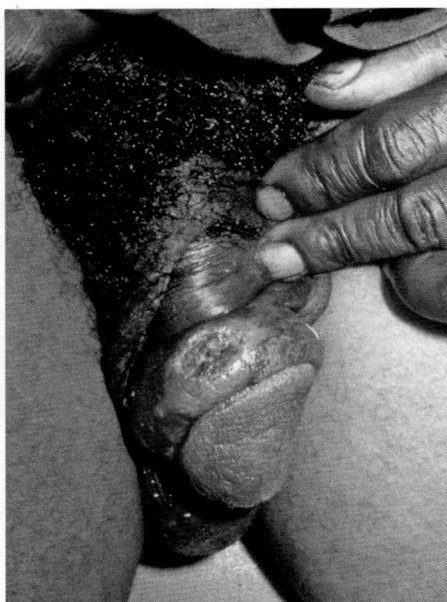

Fig. 107.12 Primary Syphilis (Courtesy David Effron, MD.)

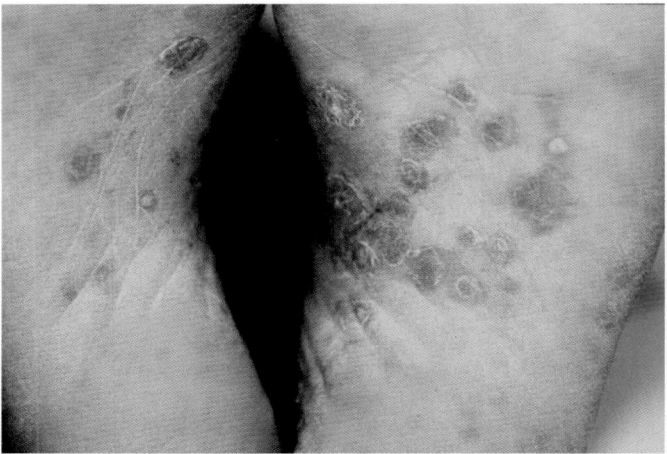

Fig. 107.13 Secondary Syphilis. (Courtesy David Effron, MD.)

rash. Pigmented macules and papules may appear on the palms and soles (Fig. 107.13). Generalized lymphadenopathy and malaise accompany the skin lesions. Moist, flat, verrucous condyloma latum may appear in the genital area. These lesions are highly contagious.

The diagnosis of primary or secondary syphilis should be made in the ED based on clinical presentation. Definitive diagnosis is made by the identification of spirochetes with darkfield microscopy and by serologic testing. The result of the Venereal Disease Research Laboratory (VDRL) test, the most commonly used diagnostic nontreponemal serologic test, is positive in approximately three-fourths of patients with primary syphilis but may be negative early in the course of the disease. The VDRL test result is positive in cases of secondary syphilis. Rapid plasma reagin (RPR) is an alternative nontreponemal test. The most specific and sensitive serologic test is the fluorescent treponemal antibody absorption (FTA-ABS) test.

Current guidelines for syphilis treatment, including in penicillin allergic individuals, are available at www.cdc.gov.[22] Treatment should be initiated in the ED based on clinical diagnosis. Primary and secondary syphilis is treated with benzathine penicillin G in a dose of 2.4

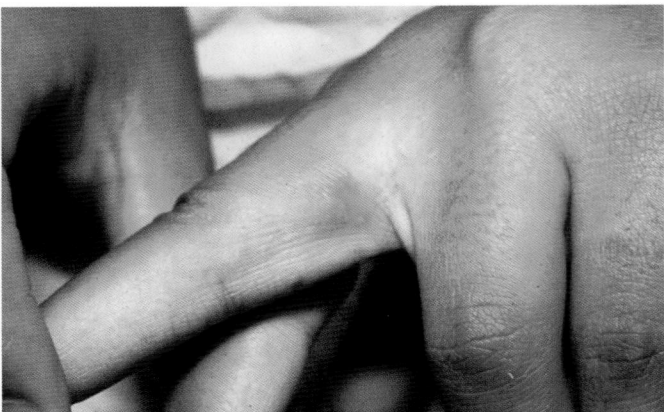

Fig. 107.14 Disseminated Gonococcal Infection. (Courtesy David Effron, MD.)

million units IM.[23] Pregnant women should be treated with the regimen appropriate for their disease state. Doxycycline or azithromycin are alternatives in patients with penicillin allergy. Patients with early latent syphilis are treated the same as patients with primary disease, whereas late latent syphilis and tertiary syphilis are treated with benzathine penicillin G, three doses of 2.4 million units IM at weekly intervals for a total of 7.2 million units. Treatment of neurosyphilis requires infusion of aqueous crystalline penicillin, 3 to 4 million units IV every 4 hours for 10 to 14 days. Following antibiotic therapy, patients may experience a *Jarisch-Herxheimer reaction,* with symptoms of fever, headache, and myalgia.

Disseminated Gonococcal Infection

Gonococcal infections are the second most common notifiable condition in the U.S., following *Chlamydia trachomatis* infections.[24] The incidence of reported gonococcal infection has risen consistently since 2009. Disseminated gonococcal infection (DGI) occurs in less than 2% of patients with gonorrhea, affecting women primarily. Symptoms typically include fever and migratory asymmetric polyarthralgias, tenosynovitis, or skin lesions. The lesions have a predilection for periarticular regions of the distal extremities. The lesions typically begin as erythematous or hemorrhagic papules that evolve into pustules and vesicles with an erythematous halo (Fig. 107.14). They may be tender and may have a gray necrotic or hemorrhagic center. Healing with crust formation usually occurs within 4 or 5 days, although recurrent crops of lesions may appear even after antibiotics have been started. Rare complications may include perihepatitis, endocarditis, or meningitis.

The organism may be cultured from the cutaneous lesions. A more reliable diagnostic technique is immunofluorescent antibody staining of direct smears from pustules.

Treatment should be initiated with ceftriaxone, 1 g IV q 24 hours, and treatment for chlamydia with doxycycline 100 mg bid for 7 days. Alternatives include cefotaxime or ceftizoxime, plus doxycycline. Patients allergic to β-lactam antibiotics or those with severe penicillin allergies may be treated with spectinomycin. Ciprofloxacin and ofloxacin are not recommended owing to increasing resistance patterns. Hospitalization is recommended for patients with DGI. Chapter 84 provides detailed management recommendations.

Staphylococcal Scalded Skin Syndrome

Staphylococcal scalded skin syndrome (SSSS) typically occurs in children 6 years old or younger. It is caused by an infection with phage group 2 exotoxin-producing staphylococci. The illness begins with erythema and crusting around the mouth. The erythema then spreads down the body, followed by bulla formation and desquamation. Mucous membranes are typically spared. After desquamation occurs, the lesions dry up quickly, with clinical resolution in 3 to 7 days.

Treatment should be initiated promptly with intravenous antibiotics, such as nafcillin, oxacillin, or vancomycin. For patients allergic to penicillin, alternatives may include clarithromycin or cefuroxime.[25] Chapter 126 provides detailed management recommendations.

Toxic Shock Syndrome

Toxic shock syndrome (TSS) is an acute febrile illness characterized by a diffuse desquamating erythroderma. Clinical presentation may include high fever, hypotension, constitutional symptoms, multiorgan involvement, and rash. The syndrome gained notoriety in the early 1980s because of association with tampon use. However, it is also well known in men and children. Its appearance has often been linked to exotoxin-producing *S. aureus*. Approximately 50% of cases are associated with menstruation. Other cases occur in the postoperative setting, or related to burns, postpartum infection, osteomyelitis, arthritis, empyema, fasciitis, septic abortion, pharyngitis, peritonsillar abscess, sinusitis, or subcutaneous abscess.[26]

TSS is typically caused by *Staphylococcus aureus* or *Streptococcus pyogenes*. It has been reported in previously healthy patients, immunocompromised patients, and elders. Fatigue, localized pain, and nonspecific symptoms herald the onset of this disease, followed by septic shock and multisystem organ failure.

Diagnosis of TSS requires the presence of (1) temperature of at least 38.9°C; (2) hypotension, with a systolic blood pressure of 90 mm Hg or less; (3) rash; and (4) involvement of at least three organ systems. Systemic involvement may include the gastrointestinal tract, muscular system, or CNS and laboratory evidence of renal, hepatic, or hematologic dysfunction. Headache, myalgias, arthralgias, alteration of consciousness, nausea, vomiting, or diarrhea may be present.

The rash is typically a diffuse, blanching, macular erythroderma. Accompanying nonexudative mucous membrane inflammation is common. Pharyngitis, sometimes accompanied by a "strawberry tongue," conjunctivitis, or vaginitis, may be seen. As a general rule, the rash fades within 3 days of its appearance. This is followed by a full-thickness desquamation, most commonly involving the hands and feet.

Initial treatment of TSS consists of IV fluid replacement, ventilatory support, pressor agents, antibiotics covering *S. aureus* (including MRSA) and *S. pyogenes*. Initial empirical antibiotic regimens may include clindamycin, vancomycin, linezolid, imipenem, meropenem, ticarcillin-clavulanate, or piperacillin-tazobactam. Chapter 126 provides detailed management recommendations.

Rocky Mountain Spotted Fever

Rocky Mountain spotted fever is caused by *Rickettsia rickettsii*, an organism harbored by a variety of ticks. The organism is transmitted to humans through tick saliva at the time of a tick bite, or when the tick is crushed while in contact with the host. Many patients do not report tick exposure. Although originally described in the Rocky Mountain region, this disease occurs in other areas of North, South, and Central America. Most reported cases are from the southeastern United States.

The onset of the illness is usually abrupt, with headache, nausea and vomiting, myalgias, chills, and fever. On occasion, the onset is more gradual, with progressive anorexia, malaise, and fever. The disease may last 3 weeks and may be severe with prominent involvement of the CNS, cardiac, pulmonary, gastrointestinal, and renal systems, disseminated intravascular coagulation, or shock.

The rash develops on the second to sixth day. It begins with erythematous macules that blanch on pressure, appearing first on the wrists and ankles. These macules spread up the extremities and to

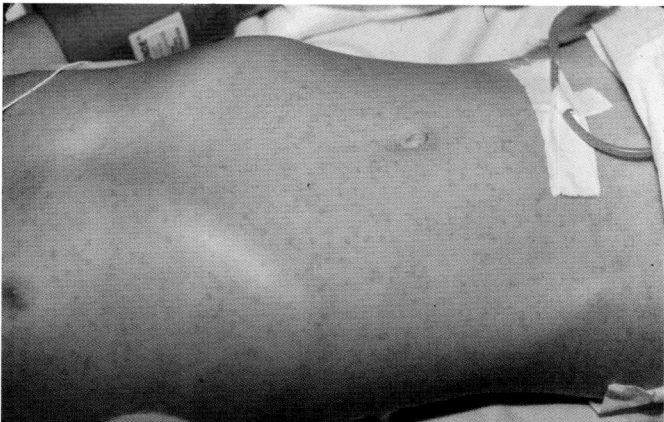

Fig. 107.15 Rocky Mountain Spotted Fever. (Courtesy Jonathan Singer, MD.)

the trunk and face. They may become petechial or hemorrhagic (Fig. 107.15). Lesions on the palms and soles are characteristic. Increased capillary fragility and splenomegaly may be present.

The diagnosis of Rocky Mountain spotted fever should be made based on clinical presentation in the ED. Definitive testing is not available in the ED and may include the Weil-Felix reaction and more specific immunofluorescent procedures.

Treatment should be initiated promptly based on a clinical diagnosis (see Chapter 126). Failure to administer antibiotics in a timely fashion dramatically increases morbidity and mortality. Treatment should be initiated with doxycycline.[27] Chloramphenicol may be used for patients allergic to tetracyclines, or in children younger than 9 years old. Sulfa drugs should be avoided, as they may exacerbate the illness. Rickettsiae are routinely resistant to penicillins, cephalosporins, aminoglycosides, and erythromycin. Ehrlichiosis may be difficult to differentiate from Rocky Mountain spotted fever clinically, though it is also reliably treated with doxycycline.

Viral Infections

Herpes Simplex Virus

Two known variants of HSV routinely cause human infection: HSV-1 and HSV-2. HSV-1 primarily affects nongenital sites, whereas lesions caused by HSV-2 are found predominantly in the genital area and are transmitted primarily by sexual contact. There is significant variation in viral type and anatomic site of infection.

The characteristic presentation is painful, grouped vesicles on an erythematous base (Fig. 107.16). The lesions are usually localized in a clustered, nondermatomal distribution. The skin distribution may become more generalized in patients with atopic dermatitis or other dermatoses. Adults with HSV infection should avoid contact with children with atopic dermatitis, especially in the first 3 to 5 days of infection.

The mouth is the most common site of HSV-1 infections. Children are affected more commonly than adults. Small clusters of vesicles appear but are soon denuded, leaving irregularly shaped, crusted erosions. The severity of gingivostomatitis varies from the presence of small ulcers to extensive ulceration of the mouth, tongue, and gums accompanied by fever and cervical lymphadenopathy (Fig. 107.17). The infection may be so severe that oral fluid intake is difficult, and dehydration may result. Healing typically occurs in 7 to 14 days unless a secondary bacterial infection occurs.

Herpetic whitlow is a herpes infection of the hand, typically affecting the distal phalanx (Fig. 107.18). It may be caused by HSV-1 (60%) or HSV-2 (40%).

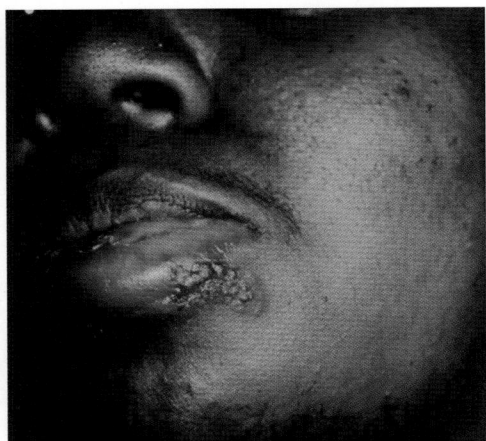

Fig. 107.16 Herpes Simplex Virus 1 (HSV-1) Infection. (Courtesy David Effron, MD.)

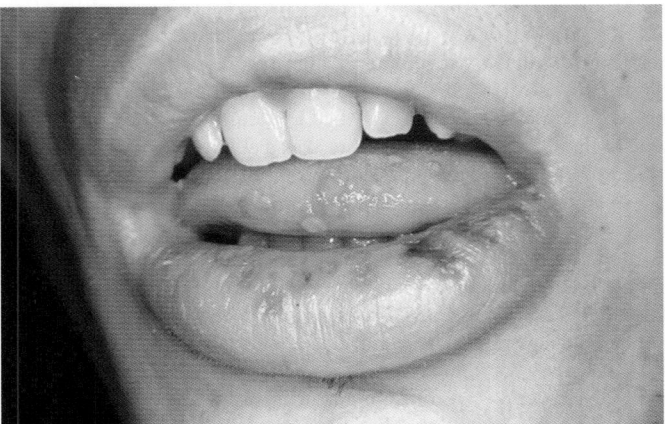

Fig. 107.17 Herpes Simplex. (Courtesy Centers for Disease Control and Prevention [CDC] Public Health Image Library, Robert E. Sumpter.)

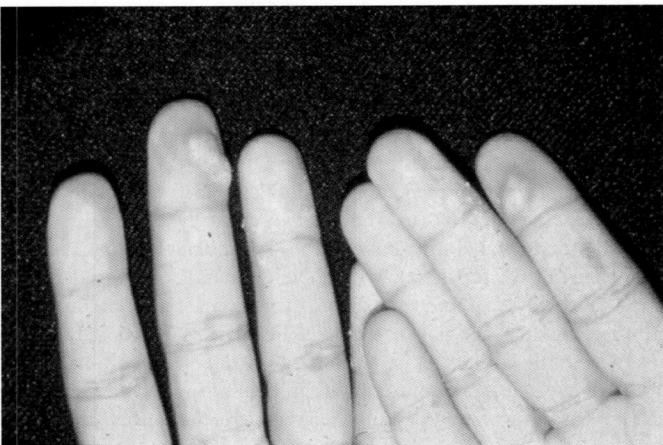

Fig. 107.18 Herpetic Whitlow. (Courtesy Jonathan Singer, MD.)

HSV-2 infections in men present with either single or multiple vesicles or erosions on the penile shaft or glans penis. Fever, malaise, and regional adenopathy may be present. A prodrome of local pain and hyperesthesia may precede the appearance of the cutaneous lesions. The vesicles erode after several days, become crusted, and heal in 10 to 14 days. Infections in women involve the introitus, cervix, or vagina.

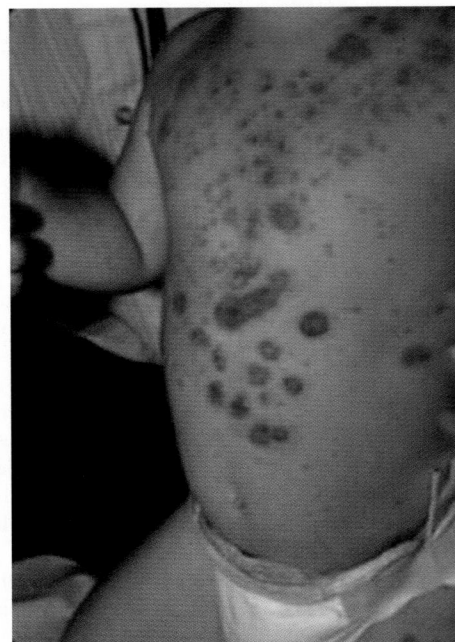

Fig. 107.19 Varicella Zoster. (Courtesy Jonathan Singer, MD.)

Vesicles may be grouped or confluent, and may be denuded, leaving erosions and ulcerations. Herpetic cervicitis or vaginitis may be the cause of pelvic pain, dysuria, or vaginal discharge. Recurrence is common, and recurrent episodes tend to be less severe.

Recommended treatment for a first clinical episode of genital herpes is with acyclovir, famciclovir, or valacyclovir. These agents reduce the duration of viral shedding, accelerate healing, and shorten the duration of symptoms, but they do not prevent recurrent episodes. Prophylactic administration of acyclovir may be effective in ameliorating the severity of recurrent genital herpes.

IV therapy should be considered for immunocompromised patients. A mucocutaneous herpes infection in such patients is potentially fatal, as it has a propensity for generalization and dissemination to the internal organs.

Any vesicular eruption on skin or mucous membranes in a neonate should prompt concern for HSV infection, as there is a high likelihood of dissemination in this group. Unless an alternative diagnosis is established, testing of the vesicle fluid for HSV and acyclovir therapy are indicated.

Supportive care and pain control are important components of treatment. Systemic analgesics or topical anesthetic agents may be useful. Education of the patient about the prevention or spread of the disease during sexual contact and the birth process is imperative. Chapter 119 provides detailed management recommendations.

Varicella-Zoster Virus

Varicella. Varicella, or chickenpox, is an infection caused by the varicella-zoster virus. After an incubation period of 14 to 21 days, the illness begins with a low-grade fever, headache, and malaise. The exanthem coincides with these symptoms in children and follows them by several days in adults.

The skin lesions rapidly progress from macules to papules to vesicles to crusting, sometimes within 6 to 8 hours. The vesicle of varicella is 2 or 3 mm in diameter and surrounded by an erythematous border (Fig. 107.19). An unusual form of varicella has larger bullae. The drying of the vesicle begins centrally, producing umbilication. The dried scabs typically disappear in 5 to 20 days.

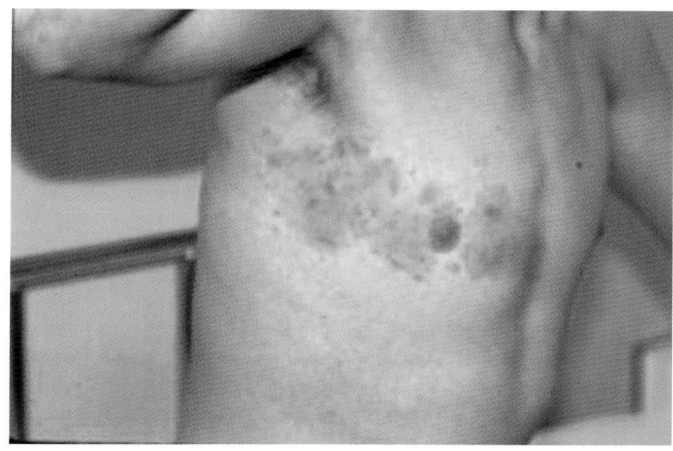

Fig. 107.20 Herpes Zoster. (Courtesy David Effron, MD.)

Lesions appear in crops on the trunk, where they are seen in the highest concentration, and on the scalp, face, or extremities. The hallmark of varicella is the appearance of lesions in all three stages of development in one region of the body. Extensive eruptions are often associated with a high and prolonged fever.

Complications include encephalitis or meningitis, pneumonia, secondary staphylococcal or streptococcal cellulitis, thrombocytopenia, arthritis, hepatitis, or glomerulonephritis. Varicella pneumonia occurs more commonly in adults than in children.

The illness is typically self-limited, and treatment is symptomatic. Salicylates should be avoided to minimize the risk of subsequent Reye syndrome. Oral acyclovir may be effective if it can be started within 24 hours of development of rash for patients with chronic respiratory or skin disease. Chapter 119 provides detailed management recommendations.

The disease has the potential to be contagious until all vesicles are crusted and dried, thus infected persons should be kept at home until this stage is reached. Isolation of infected patients is often futile as the disease may be transmitted before the diagnosis is clinically evident.

Varicella zoster immune globulin (VariZIG) is indicated for administration to high-risk individuals within 10 days (ideally within 4 days) of varicella zoster virus exposure.[28]

The varicella vaccine is a live attenuated virus; it is highly efficacious and very safe. A single dose is effective in children between the ages of 1 and 13 years. For older children, two doses separated by 4 to 8 weeks are recommended. In addition, the incidence of zoster occurring after vaccination appears to be lower than that of naturally acquired disease.

Herpes zoster. Herpes zoster, or "shingles," is an infection caused by the varicella-zoster virus. It occurs in individuals who have previously had chickenpox and is caused by reactivation of the latent virus from the dorsal root ganglion. At risk populations include female sex, Caucasian race, family history, or comorbidities including autoimmune diseases, asthma, diabetes mellitus, or chronic obstructive pulmonary disease.[29] Dermatomal pain may precede the eruption by 1 to 10 days and is variable in intensity; it may be described as sharp, dull, or burning in quality. The typical rash consists of grouped vesicles on an erythematous base involving one or several adjacent dermatomes. The thorax is involved in most cases, and the trigeminal distribution is the next most commonly involved region.

The vesicles initially appear clear and then become cloudy and progress to scab and crust formation. This process takes 10 to 12 days, and the crusts fall off in 2 or 3 weeks (Fig. 107.20). Herpes zoster has a peak incidence in patients 50 to 70 years old and is unusual in children. Complications may include CNS involvement, ocular infection, stroke,

meningoencephalitis, myelitis, peripheral neuropathy, or myocardial infarction.[30] Ocular complications occur in 20% to 70% of cases involving the ophthalmic division of the trigeminal nerve. The severity varies from mild conjunctivitis to panophthalmitis, which threatens vision. Corneal dendritic lesions may be visible on fluorescein examination. Eye involvement may produce anterior uveitis, secondary glaucoma, optic neuritis, or corneal scarring. There is a close correlation between vesicles located at the tip of the nose and eye involvement (Hutchinson sign).

Herpes zoster generally tends to be more severe in immunosuppressed patients, especially those with acquired immunodeficiency syndrome (AIDS), Hodgkin disease, or other lymphomas. Individuals with immunosuppression or stress are at higher risk for disseminated herpes zoster infection.[31]

Herpes zoster infection is a clinical diagnosis, and treatment should be initiated based on clinical findings. If the diagnosis is in question, definitive diagnosis may be made by VZV DNA PCR or skin biopsy.

Antiviral medications are usually indicated, especially within 48 hours of onset of rash, to decrease the duration of symptoms and associated pain (see Chapter 119). Antiviral therapy may be initiated with first-line therapy with acyclovir, famciclovir, or valacyclovir. Intravenous acyclovir is indicated for treatment of disseminated HZV infection. Supportive care is important for pain and pruritus control. Burow's solution compresses (over-the-counter solution of aluminum triacetate) may be applied to hasten drying of lesions. Steroids have not been shown to reduce the incidence of postherpetic neuralgia.

IV administration of acyclovir may be of benefit in the treatment of severe ocular herpes zoster. Treatment includes mydriasis and the application of topical corticosteroids at the direction of an ophthalmologist. Eye involvement caused by herpes zoster does not appear to be exacerbated by corticosteroids, which differs from herpes simplex conjunctivitis.

Postherpetic neuralgia may occur in 15% of patients and is more common in the elderly. Treatments may include opioids, topical capsaicin, topical lidocaine, topical or oral gabapentin, or tricyclic antidepressants.[32-34] The varicella vaccine has been shown to reduce the incidence and severity of herpes zoster virus infection and is recommended for patients 60 years old and older.[35-37]

Viral Exanthems

An exanthem is defined as a skin eruption that occurs as a symptom of a general disease. In the pediatric population, an estimated 72% of cases of fever and rash are caused by viruses. Approximately 30 enteroviruses, predominantly the coxsackievirus and echovirus groups, and four types of adenoviruses are known to produce exanthems (Fig. 107.21). Most viral exanthems are maculopapular, although scarlatiniform, erythematous, vesicular, or petechial rashes are occasionally seen. The eruptions are variable in their extent, are typically nonpruritic, and do not desquamate. Oropharyngeal lesions may be present.

The classic viral exanthems are rubeola (measles), rubella (German measles), herpesvirus 6 (roseola), parvovirus B19 (erythema infectiosum or fifth disease), and the enteroviruses (echovirus and coxsackievirus).

Roseola infantum. Roseola infantum, otherwise known as *exanthem subitum* or *sixth disease,* is a benign illness caused by human herpesvirus 6 and human herpesvirus 7 and is typically spread by saliva. It is characterized by fever and a skin eruption. Ninety-five percent of cases are seen in children 6 months to 3 years old. The fever typically has an abrupt onset, with temperature rising rapidly to 39°C to 41°C, and is present consistently or intermittently for 3 or 4 days, at which time the temperature drops to normal. The rash typically appears with fever defervescence. The lesions are discrete pink or rose-colored macules

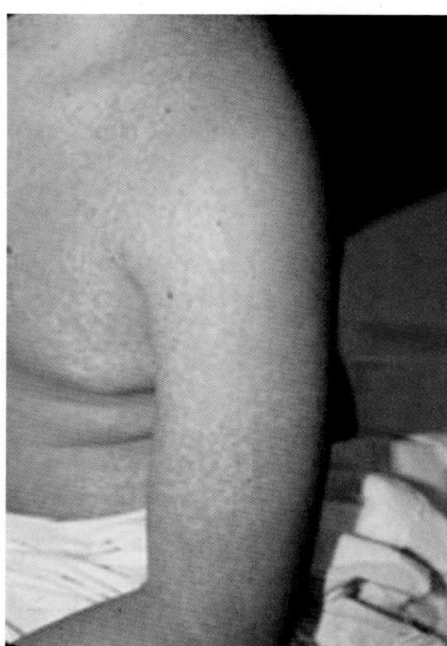

Fig. 107.21 Enterovirus. (Courtesy Jonathan Singer, MD.)

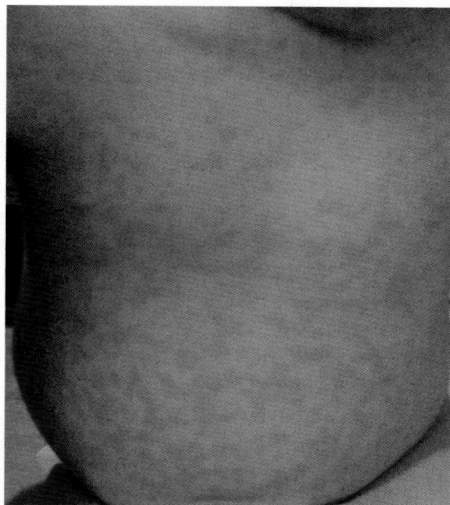

Fig. 107.22 Roseola.

or maculopapules, 2 or 3 mm in diameter, that blanch on pressure and rarely coalesce (Fig. 107.22). The trunk is involved initially, with the eruption typically spreading to the neck and extremities. The rash clears in 1 or 2 days.

Despite the presence of a high fever, the infant usually appears well. A febrile seizure may occur. Encephalitis is a very rare complication of the disease. The prognosis is excellent, and no treatment is necessary.

Measles. Measles, or rubeola, is a highly contagious viral illness spread by contact with infectious droplets, with an incubation period of 10 to 14 days. Although measles was declared eradicated in the US in 2000, the incidence has risen since that time.[38] Measles is most likely to infect unvaccinated individuals. Patients are considered to be contagious from 5 days prior to onset of symptoms until 5 to 6 days after the onset of dermatologic involvement.

Symptoms begin with fever and malaise. Symptoms include the "three C's": cough, coryza, and conjunctivitis. On the second day of

the illness, Koplik spots, which are pathognomonic of the disease, may appear on the buccal mucosa as small, irregular, bright red spots with bluish white centers. Beginning opposite the molars, Koplik spots may spread to involve a variable extent of the oropharynx.

The cutaneous eruption of measles typically begins on the third to fifth day of the illness. Maculopapular erythematous lesions involve the forehead and upper neck and spread to involve the face, trunk, arms, and finally the legs and feet. Koplik spots begin to disappear coincident with the appearance of the rash. By the third day of its presence, the rash begins to fade, doing so in the order of its appearance, and the fever subsides.

Complications may include otitis media, encephalitis, or pneumonitis. Otitis media is the most common complication. Encephalitis or pneumonia may be life-threatening.

Treatment is primarily supportive and should include antipyretics, hydration, and treatment of pruritus (see Chapter 119). Vitamin A should be administered to hospitalized patients at the time of diagnosis and repeated the second day, to help prevent eye damage and blindness.[39] If bacterial invasion occurs with otitis media or pneumonia, antibiotics are indicated. Isolation of infected children is of limited value as exposure usually occurs before the appearance of the rash. Infection typically confers lifelong immunity. Postexposure prophylaxis may be administered with the measles virus vaccine or human immunoglobulin.

Rubella. Rubella, or German measles, is a viral illness characterized by fever, skin eruption, and generalized lymphadenopathy. It is spread by droplet contact, and peak incidence is in the winter and early spring. The incubation period is typically 14 to 21 days, and the rash heralds the onset of the illness in children. The maximum time of communicability is in the few days before and 5 to 7 days after the onset of the rash. Infants with congenital rubella may shed virus for more than 1 year. In adults, a 1- to 6-day prodrome of headache, malaise, sore throat, coryza, and low-grade fever precedes the rash. These symptoms generally disappear within 24 hours after the appearance of the skin eruption.

The rash of pink to red maculopapules appears first on the face and spreads rapidly to the neck, trunk, and extremities. Those on the trunk may coalesce, but lesions on the extremities typically do not. The rash remains for 1 to 5 days, and often disappears at the end of 3 days. Although clearing may be accompanied by fine desquamation, this sign is usually absent.

The major complications of rubella include encephalitis, arthritis, or thrombocytopenia. Rubella during pregnancy may result in congenital defects. No treatment is required in most cases of rubella. Antipyretics may be administered to treat headache, arthralgias, and painful lymphadenopathy.

Erythema infectiosum. Erythema infectiosum, or "fifth disease," is caused by parvovirus B19 infection and typically affects pediatric patients. It is characterized by mild systemic symptoms, fever in 10% to 15% of patients, and a characteristic rash. Arthralgia and arthritis occur commonly in adults but rarely in children. The rash is intensely red on the face and gives a "slapped-cheek" appearance with circumoral pallor. A reticular (netlike) maculopapular eruption, which may be noted on the arms, moves caudally to the trunk, buttocks, and thighs. The rash may recur with changes in temperature and exposure to sunlight. The incubation period is usually between 4 and 14 days. The infection is benign and management is supportive.

Fungal Infections

Fungal infections may affect the skin, scalp, or mucous membranes. The dermatophytoses are superficial fungal infections that are limited to the skin. Dermatophytes generally grow best in warm, moist environments,

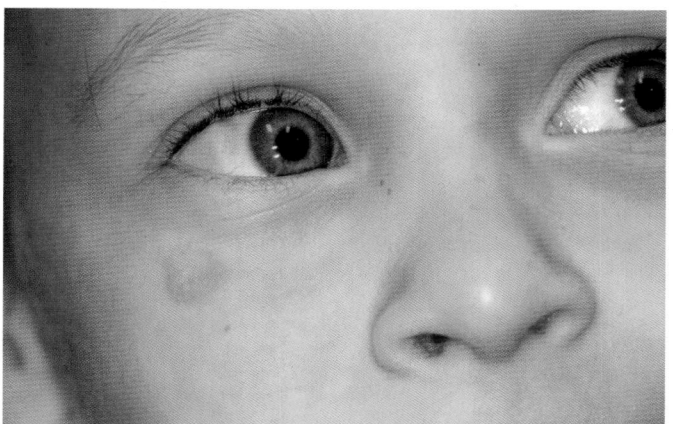

Fig. 107.23 Tinea Corporis. (Courtesy David Effron, MD.)

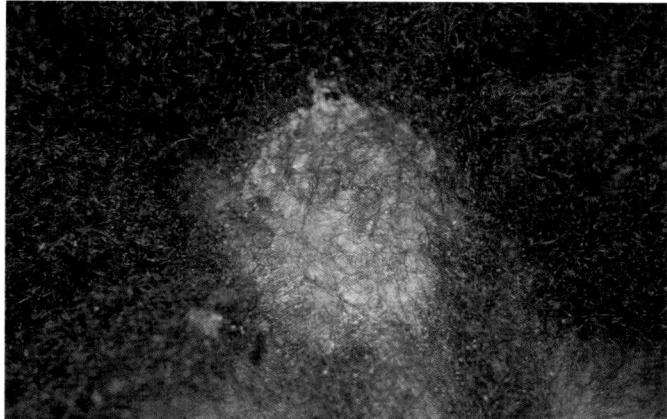

Fig. 107.24 Kerion of Tinea Capitis. (Courtesy David Effron, MD.)

and grow only in the keratin or outer layer of the skin, nails, or hair. Any potential dermatophyte infection can be examined under the microscope in a KOH preparation if available. The specimen is examined for the characteristic branching hyphae of the dermatophytes or the short, thick hyphae and clustered spores of tinea versicolor.

Tinea Corporis

Tinea refers to superficial dermatophytic infection of the skin, hair, or nails, usually by the *Trichophyton* organism. Tinea corporis, commonly referred to as "ringworm" infection, presents as a sharply marginated, annular lesion with raised or vesicular margins and central clearing (Fig. 107.23). Lesions may be single or multiple. Other related forms of tinea may be seen, including tinea cruris involving the groin, tinea manuum affecting the hands, and tinea pedis of the feet.

The differential diagnosis of tinea corporis includes erythema migrans (associated with Lyme disease, with annular lesions with central clearing without scale), granuloma annulare (idiopathic skin condition that causes raised annual lesions without scale), psoriasis (erythematous plaques with silvery scale), cellulitis (erythema without central clearing or scale), or erythrasma (superficial bacterial infection that presents with hyperpigmented patches).

Infections of the body, groin, or extremities usually respond to topical antifungal agents, such as clotrimazole, miconazole, tolnaftate, terbinafine, or naftifine. Two or three daily applications of the cream form of any of these preparations result in healing of most superficial lesions in 1 to 3 weeks.

Tinea Capitis

Tinea capitis is a fungal infection of the scalp, and it is the most common cutaneous fungal infection in children. Common organisms include *Microsporum* and *Trichophyton* species. Although it is often seen in pediatric patients 6 to 10 years old, tinea capitis may also occur in adults. Nosocomial transmission of dermatophyte infections, such as *Trichophyton tonsurans,* has also been reported. Alopecia may be seen, typically with thickened, scaly scalp. Broken hairs resembling black dots near the scalp may be seen. Hair loss is the result of hyphae growing within the hair shaft, rendering it fragile, so that the hair strands break off 1 to 2 mm from the scalp. The disease may be transmitted by close child-to-child contact, or contact with household pets, hats, combs, barber's shears, or similar items. Complications may include kerion formation, lymphadenitis, bacterial cellulitis or abscess, or scarring alopecia.

The differential diagnosis of tinea capitis includes alopecia areata (alopecia without scalp changes), atopic dermatitis (patches of thickened skin with scale), nummular eczema (eczema in small circular patterns), bacterial infection (such as cellulitis or abscess), psoriasis (erythematous patches with silvery scale), seborrheic dermatitis (pruritic yellow or white patches), or trichotillomania (hair pulling).

The diagnosis is made based on clinical presentation. If in question, a fungal culture specimen may be obtained.

Systemic therapy is required for tinea capitis, due to fungal invasion of the hair follicles. Treatment should be with a systemic antifungal agent, such as terbinafine (<25 kg: 125 mg/day PO for 6 weeks; 25 to 35 kg: 187.5 mg/day PO for 6 weeks; >35 kg: 250 mg/day PO for 6 weeks). Alternatives include itraconazole, fluconazole, or griseofulvin.[40] Therapy should be given for 4 to 8 weeks. Topical treatments such as selenium sulfide, ketoconazole, or ciclopirox shampoo in addition to systemic antifungal therapy may increase cure rates.[41] Patients should be referred for outpatient follow-up with primary care or dermatology within 4 weeks. Family members should be evaluated for possible infection.

Kerion

A kerion is a fungal infection affecting hair follicles that is characterized by intense inflammation, and a boggy, erythematous mass, typically affecting the scalp (Fig. 107.24). The lesion may contain frank pus. It usually affects the scalp and is more common in children and in African Americans. Local alopecia and scarring can result. Lymphadenopathy may be present. Accurate differentiation of a kerion with or without superinfection can be challenging. Wood's lamp examination can be helpful in confirming the diagnosis.

Kerions are treated the same as tinea capitis, with systemic antifungal agents for 6 to 8 weeks. If bacterial superinfection exists, an antibiotic is added. Antibiotic options include oral cephalexin, dicloxacillin, or clindamycin. Clindamycin is recommended when community-acquired MRSA is a concern. Surgical drainage of kerions is rarely helpful and should be avoided.

Tinea Pedis

Tinea pedis, commonly referred to as *athlete's foot,* presents with scaling, maceration, vesiculation, and fissuring between the toes and on the plantar surface of the foot. Common etiologies include *Trichophyton rubrum, Trichophyton interdigitale,* and *Epidermophyton floccosum.* Secondary bacterial infection may occur. The vesicular pustular form of tinea pedis should be considered when vesicles and pustules on the instep are noted. Interdigital lesions may cause minimal symptoms and serve as a portal of entry for bacterial cellulitis. The differential diagnosis includes contact dermatitis, and dyshidrotic eczema which usually presents as pruritic vesicles on the lateral aspects of fingers. A KOH preparation is helpful to differentiate among these processes.

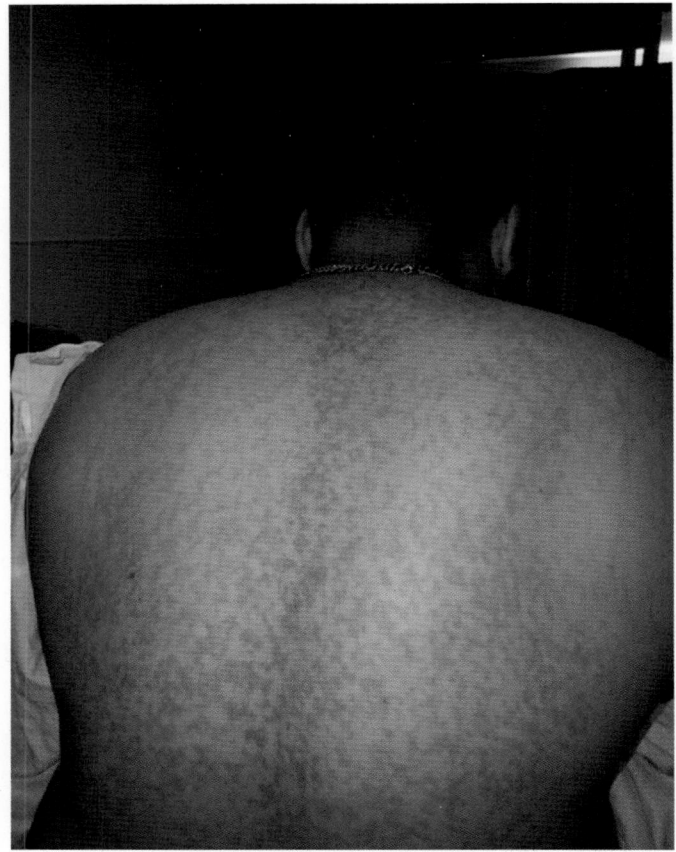

Fig. 107.25 Tinea Versicolor.

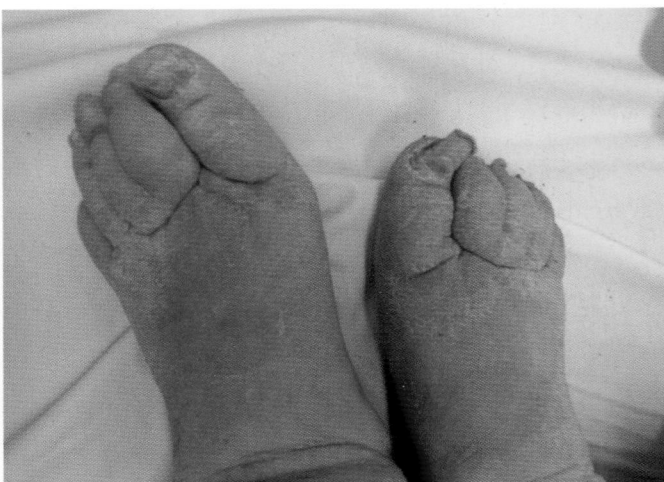

Fig. 107.26 Onychomycosis.

Treatment options include topical antifungal agents, such as terbinafine 1% cream, applied BID for 1 to 2 weeks. Alternatives include miconazole cream, powder, or spray, and clotrimazole cream, solution, or ointment. For severe disease or if topical treatment has failed, systemic therapy may be instituted with terbinafine, fluconazole, or griseofulvin.

Tinea Versicolor

Tinea versicolor, or pityriasis versicolor, is a superficial fungal infection caused by genus *Malassezia*. Superficial hypopigmented or hyperpigmented patches occur mainly on the chest and trunk, but may extend to the head and limbs. As the name implies, lesions can be a variety of colors, including pink, tan, or white. The disease may be associated with pruritus. On examination, a fine subtle scale is noted that may appear hypopigmented (Fig. 107.25). Pale yellow or orange fluorescence under Wood's light may be seen. The differential diagnosis includes vitiligo and seborrheic dermatitis. A KOH preparation reveals short hyphae mixed with spores ("chopped spaghetti and meatballs").

Tinea versicolor may be treated with topical antifungal agents, such as 2.5% selenium sulfide shampoo, applied daily for 1 weeks. Alternative therapies include imidazole creams, and ketoconazole cream or foam. For topical treatment failures, systemic therapy may be indicated, such as fluconazole, as a single 150- to 300-mg weekly dose for 2 to 4 weeks. Recurrence is common. Pigmentation may not return to normal for months.

Tinea Unguium (Onychomycosis)

Tinea unguium may be caused by dermatophytes, candida, or other fungal species. Paronychia or untreated tinea pedis may be predisposing factors. Onychomycosis presents with toenails or fingernails that are thickened, opaque, cracked, or destroyed. Subungual debris is present, and the nail may contain yellowish longitudinal streaks (Fig. 107.26). The nail of the great toe is most commonly involved. Differential diagnosis includes tinea pedis, psoriasis, or warts.

Topical therapy of the nails may be initiated if less than 25% of the nail bed is involved, but often may not result in cure due to poor penetration into the nail keratin.[42] Fingernails typically respond more rapidly to therapy than toenails. Involvement of one or two nails may be treated with topical antifungal agents. More extensive infection or risk factors (including advanced age, diabetes, immunosuppression, or widespread infection) requires systemic therapy with an antifungal agent, such as terbinafine (250 mg PO daily for 6 weeks [fingernail]) or 12 weeks [toenail]) or itraconazole (200 mg bid for 1 week, repeated q4wk for 2 mo [fingernail] or 200 mg/day PO for 12 weeks [toenail]).[43] Third-line agents may include griseofulvin or ketoconazole, which require prolonged courses, with high relapse rates and numerous side effects. Treatment failures or relapses are common, and they may be attributed to poor patient compliance, low bioavailability, lack of drug penetration into the nail, drug resistance, or drug interactions. Additional therapies may include surgical removal of the nail, photodynamic therapy, or laser therapy.

Candidiasis

Infection by *Candida albicans* may occur in patients of all ages. Many conditions predispose to infection, including diabetes mellitus, HIV infection, pregnancy, obesity, smoking, malnutrition, malignancy, or treatment with corticosteroids, antibiotics, or immunosuppressive agents.

Oral candidiasis. Oral candidiasis ("thrush") is the most common clinical expressions of *Candida* infection. It is common in newborns with one-third being affected by the first week of life, and also in elder persons, immunosuppressed individuals, or persons wearing dentures. It appears as patches of white or gray friable material covering an erythematous base on the buccal mucosa, gingiva, tongue, palate, or tonsils. Fissures or crust at the corners of the mouth may be present. The differential diagnosis of oral candidiasis includes lichen planus (which unlike *C. albicans* is not easily scraped off), or hairy leukoplakia (villous white patches on the lateral tongue). Oral mucous membrane infection with *C. albicans* is an AIDS-defining illness. If the patient does not use dentures and has not taken antibiotics recently, underlying immunosuppression should be considered.

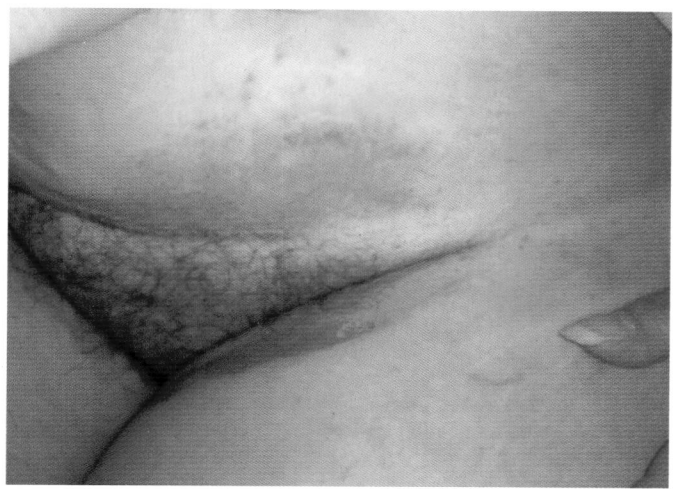

Fig. 107.27 Candida Intertrigo.

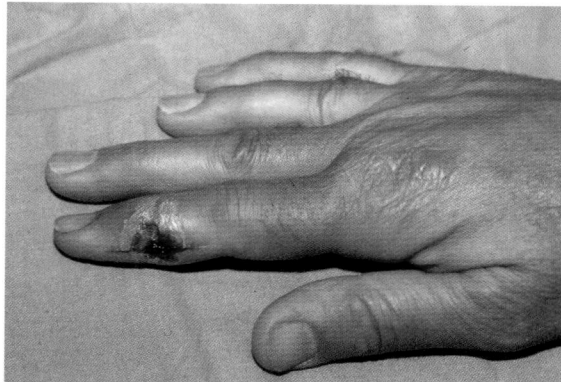

Fig. 107.28 Sporotrichosis. (Courtesy David Effron, MD)

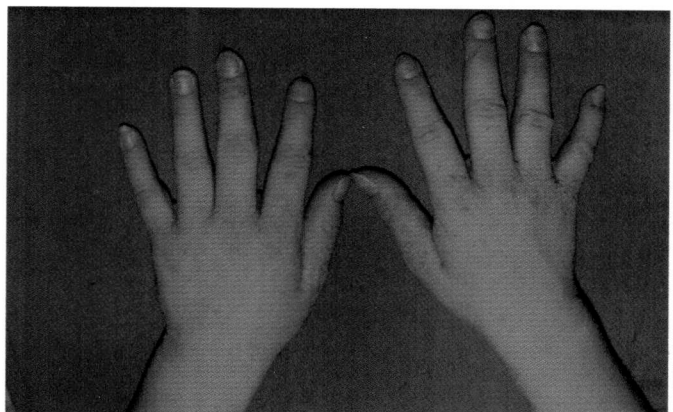

Fig. 107.29 Scabies. (Courtesy David Effron, MD.)

Treatment of oral candidiasis includes topical antifungal agents, such as clotrimazole troches five times daily, or oral nystatin suspension four times daily, or nystatin pastilles four times daily. Treatment is continued for 5 to 7 days after the lesions disappear. For esophageal candidiasis, systemic antifungal therapy is typically required, with oral fluconazole, IV fluconazole, or IV amphotericin B. Chapter 121 provides detailed management recommendations.

Cutaneous candidiasis. Cutaneous candidiasis affects intertriginous areas, including the interdigital web spaces, groin, axilla, and intergluteal or inframammary folds. Lesions appear as moist, bright red macules rimmed with a collarette of scale, with small satellite papules or pustules just peripheral to the main body of the rash (Fig. 107.27). These satellite lesions are typical indicators of a *Candida* infection. Intertriginous lesions are prone to bacterial superinfection.

The differential diagnosis of cutaneous candidiasis includes contact dermatitis, tinea cruris, intertrigo, herpes simplex such as herpetic whitlow, and folliculitis. Candidiasis, however, is less sharply demarcated than tinea cruris and brighter red than intertrigo. A KOH preparation of a specimen taken from a pustule and roof of the lesion will reveal hyphae and pseudohyphae.

Intertriginous lesions should be treated with topical imidazole creams, such as clotrimazole, 1% cream BID for 4 weeks. Alternative topical therapies include miconazole, ketoconazole, or sulconazole. Extensive infection may be treated with fluconazole (100 mg PO daily for 2 weeks) or itraconazole (100 mg PO daily for 2 weeks). The area should be kept dry.

Vulvovaginal candidiasis. Vaginal candidiasis accounts for 20% to 25% of vaginitis. It has been estimated that 75% of women will experience vaginal candidiasis at least once. Predisposing factors include diabetes, pregnancy, immunosuppression, or hormone replacement therapy. Pruritus is a common presenting complaint. Other symptoms may include dyspareunia, dysuria, or vaginal burning. Differential diagnosis includes sexually transmitted infection, bacterial vaginosis, or urinary tract infection. A KOH preparation will reveal hyphae and budding yeast forms.

Treatment should be initiated with over-the-counter intravaginal imidazoles, such as clotrimazole or miconazole, or a single 150-mg dose of oral fluconazole.

Sporotrichosis. Sporotrichosis, caused by a variety of *Sporothrix* species, is a fungal infection that may be transmitted by contact with soil, or by zoonotic transmission from animals such as snakes, birds, or cats. Most cases present with lymphocutaneous findings, such as papules, nodules, or ulcerations (Fig. 107.28). Rarely, systemic involvement may be seen with joint, pulmonary, or neurologic complications. Definitive diagnosis may be made with serologic testing. Treatment should be initiated with an oral antifungal agent such as itraconazole, 200 mg PO daily until 2 weeks after lesions have resolved, usually 3 to 6 months. Alternative oral agents include terbinafine, or intravenous amphotericin B in the setting of systemic sporotrichosis or treatment failure.[44] Dermatologic follow-up is essential to ensure adequate resolution.

Infestations

Scabies

Scabies is a skin infestation caused by the penetration of the parasitic mite *Sarcoptes scabiei-var hominis* into the epidermis. It is an infestation of worldwide impact; over 100 million persons are affected annually. It occurs more commonly in winter months. It is transmitted mostly through close personal contacts. It may also be spread by exposure to fomites, as the scabies mite can live off the human skin for 3 days. The average number of mites harbored by a host is usually less than 20. Scabies presents with intense pruritus and rash, which usually develop after 1 to 8 weeks following exposure. The pruritus is typically worst at night. Clinical findings include small (<5 mm) papules or pustules, often with excoriations due to scratching. Burrows are uncommonly seen. Classically scabies affects several skin sites, including interdigital folds of the upper extremities and abdomen, genitalia, breasts, buttocks, or subungual skin of fingers (Figs. 107.29 and 107.30).[45] Scabies in infants and young children often

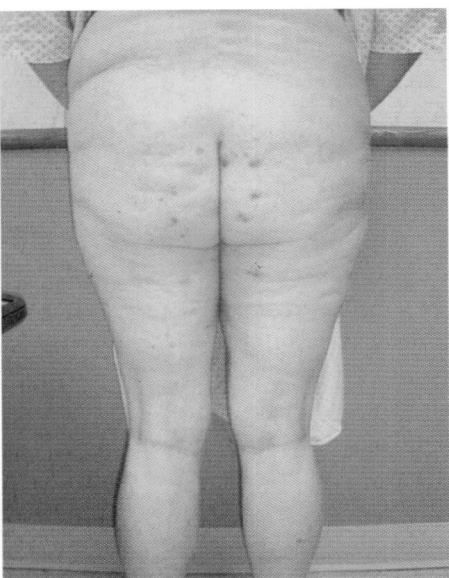

Fig. 107.30 Scabies.

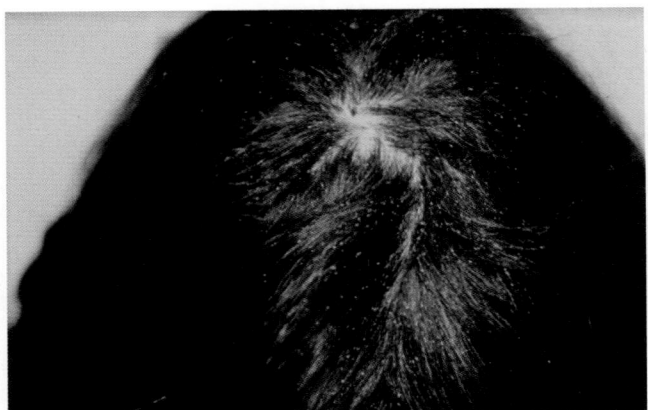

Fig. 107.31 Nits as Seen in Head Lice. (Courtesy David Effron, MD.)

may present with generalized involvement of the skin, including the face, scalp, palms, and soles. In infants, the most common presenting lesions are papules and vesicopustules.

In *crusted scabies* (previously known as *Norwegian scabies*), hyperkeratotic plaques develop diffusely, often on the palmar and plantar regions, with thickening and dystrophy of the toenails and fingernails. Crusted scabies is highly contagious, as a host may harbor thousands or millions of mites. Individuals with immunosuppression, including human immunodeficiency virus infection, elders, and patients with dementia or neuropathy are at risk of developing crusted scabies.[46,47]

Scabies is a clinical diagnosis that is based primarily on the history and examination. The definitive diagnosis is made by the microscopic identification of the scabies mites, eggs, or fecal pellets (*Scybala*). As these techniques may be impractical in the ED, treatment should be instituted based on a clinical suspicion of the diagnosis.

The differential diagnosis of scabies includes pityriasis rosea (symmetric maculopapular rash), papular urticaria, secondary syphilis (symmetric maculopapular rash), folliculitis, contact dermatitis, atopic dermatitis, seborrhea, dermatitis herpetiformis (autoimmune blistering disorder associated with celiac disease), lichen planus (pruritic violaceous polygonal lesions on the extremities), and psoriasis (erythematous patches with silvery scale).

Scabies should be treated with topical permethrin 5% cream or oral ivermectin.[48,49] Permethrin cream should be applied from the neck down, covering all areas of the body including under the nails, in the umbilicus, around the nipples, and genitals. Face and scalp should be treated in affected infants and young children. Preferably, it should be applied prior to bedtime, left on overnight, and then washed off 8 to 12 hours later. It is vital to treat not only the patient but family members and close contacts as well. A second treatment should be administered in 1 to 2 weeks. Alternative therapy may be initiated with oral ivermectin, although the cure rate may be lower than permethrin.[50] For heavily infested or immunocompromised patients, it is recommended that ivermectin be given once a week for 2 to 3 weeks. Lindane, a previously utilized agent, is not recommended, due to potential neurotoxicity as well as resistance. Emollients and antihistamines may provide symptomatic relief of pruritus.[51]

Equally important in the treatment is the decontamination of clothing, bed linens, and towels by washing them in hot water and hot machine drying. Items that cannot be washed or dry-cleaned can be decontaminated by sealing the items in an airtight container for at least 72 hours.

Pediculosis

Pediculosis may affect the scalp hair (pediculosis capitis, caused by the mite *Pediculus humanus capitis*), body (pediculosis corporis, caused by *Pediculus humanus corporis*), or genitalia (pubic lice, caused by *Pthirus pubis*). Infestation is typically associated with significant pruritus. Lesions may be erythematous macules, papules, or wheals.

Pediculosis capitis is the most common form of lice infestation in the United States and is frequently seen in children 3 to 12 years old. An estimated 10% to 40% of school children in the United States have been infected with pediculosis capitis. It can be transmitted by sharing hairbrushes, combs, or hats, and through contact with infested furniture, clothing, or linens. Lice can live on fomites for up to 4 days. Hygiene and hair length are unrelated to infection. Incidence is greatest during autumn. Scalp, occipital, or postauricular pruritus are common in patients with pediculosis capitis. Neck and auricular erythema, papules, vesicles, or lymphadenopathy may be seen.

Pediculosis corporis can present with intense pruritus and erythematous macules or wheals. Pediculosis corporis typically occurs in patients with poor hygiene or living in crowded conditions.

Pediculosis pubic ("crabs") is a sexually transmitted disease and is most commonly seen among young adults. Other concurrent sexually transmitted diseases should also be considered.

The differential diagnosis includes conditions such as tinea capitis, seborrheic dermatitis, atopic dermatitis, eczema, scabies, folliculitis, or contact dermatitis.

The diagnosis of pediculosis is made by identification of lice or nits on the hair shaft (Fig. 107.31). Nits (eggs), which appear as white dots or grains, are more easily identified than the louse itself. Nits fluoresce with the Wood's lamp. Examination with a louse comb improves the diagnostic accuracy and is faster than direct visualization.

Therapy for pediculosis should be initiated with a pediculicide, such as pyrethrin shampoo or permethrin 1% lotion, with retreatment on day 9.[52,53] Spinosad 0.9% suspension (Natroba) is a newer agent with demonstrated pediculicidal efficacy. Spinosad 0.9% is approved for use in patients older than 4 years of age and is also effective against permethrin-resistant populations of lice. Spinosad is ovicidal, killing both nits and lice; thus extensive nit combing is not necessary. However, the cost may be prohibitive. Oral ivermectin has a high cure rate and may be used as alternate therapy (200 mcg/kg PO once).[54] Other treatments may be considered, including malathion, albendazole or thiabendazole, benzyl alcohol lotion, or levamisole. Lindane, an older therapy, should be avoided, because of neurotoxicity and poor pediculicidal activity. Over-the-counter products have variable success rates, in part due to resistance. Nits should be removed with a special fine-toothed comb. The environment should also be treated. Hats, hairbrushes and combs, and linens as well as clothing should be treated. Items should be boiled or washed and dried at high temperatures. Floors and furniture should be vacuumed. Family members should be examined and treated if infested. Sexual partners of patients with pediculosis pubis should be treated. The American Academy of Pediatrics recommends that children do not miss school simply because of head lice.

Bed Bugs

Bed bugs *(Cimex lectularius)* appear brown and are approximately 5 to 6 mm in length. Bed bugs may be potential vectors for many fungi, viruses, and bacteria, including MRSA and vancomycin-resistant *Enterococcus faecium*, although disease transmission to humans has not been documented.[55] Bed bugs are found not only in linens, but on furniture, luggage, and in walls, baseboards, and buildings, including hotels, hospitals, or apartments.[56,57] They often feed on humans at night with a painless bite.

Clinical presentation may appear as erythematous welts, macules, papules, urticaria, purpura, vesicles, or bullae, with intense pruritus. The distribution is often over uncovered areas, such as arms, legs, or shoulders. Lesions resolve spontaneously in 1 to 2 weeks.

Symptomatic treatment should be undertaken with antihistamines and topical corticosteroids. If there is suspicion for scabies, empiric treatment should be initiated with permethrin 5% cream, ivermectin, or crotamiton. Eradication from the environment is challenging, due in part to increasing resistance to insecticides. Eradication methods may include insecticides, heat, steam, freezing, or vacuuming. The hazards of widespread insecticide use, including potential for malignancy or CNS adverse effects, have created a dilemma of eradication.

ALLERGIC REACTIONS

Contact Dermatitis

Contact dermatitis is an inflammatory reaction of the skin to a chemical, physical, or biologic agent, which acts as an irritant or allergic sensitizer. Allergic contact dermatitis is a form of delayed hypersensitivity mediated by lymphocytes sensitized by the contact of the allergen to the skin. It is less common than irritant contact dermatitis. Caustics, industrial solvents, or detergents are common causes of irritant dermatitis. Clothing, jewelry, soaps, cosmetics, latex, plants, and medications contain allergens that commonly cause allergic contact dermatitis. The most common allergens include rubber compounds; plants of the *Toxicodendron* species, including poison ivy, oak, and sumac; nickel, often used in jewelry alloys; paraphenylenediamine, an ingredient in hair dyes and industrial chemicals; and ethylenediamine, a stabilizer in topical medications.

The primary lesions of contact dermatitis are papules, vesicles, or bullae on an erythematous base. Streaky, linear, intensely pruritic lesions are characteristic. A pattern in the dermatologic region in contact with the allergen is typical (Fig. 107.32). Eruptions associated with contact dermatitis can appear as soon as several hours after the exposure or may be delayed for days.

Treatment of contact dermatitis includes avoidance of the irritant or allergen, and treatment of the resulting inflammation. Low-potency topical steroid creams may be applied to inflamed areas around orifices, and medium-potency creams can be used elsewhere, for example triamcinolone 1% cream bid for 1 week, or other options

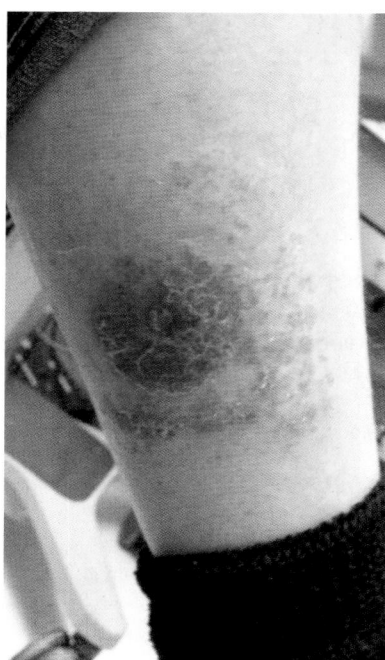

Fig. 107.32 Neomycin Allergy. (Courtesy Joanna Marco, MD.)

as listed in Table 107.4). Topical steroids are ineffectual on blistered areas. Oozing or vesiculated lesions should be treated with cool wet compresses of Domeboro or Burow's solutions (aluminum acetate). Topical baths, available over the counter, may also be comforting. Systemic antihistamines, such as hydroxyzine and diphenhydramine, may help control pruritus; nonsedating antihistamines are preferred for use during the day. If present, secondary bacterial infection should also be treated.

Urticaria

Urticaria may occur in isolation or as part of a systemic anaphylactic reaction. Approximately 15% to 20% of the population experiences urticaria during their lifetime. Acute urticaria is seen in both sexes. Chronic urticaria is more common in women in their 40s and 50s. Half of all patients with chronic urticaria have the disease for 5 years or more.

Various mediators, including histamine, bradykinin, kallikrein, and acetylcholine, are thought to play a role in urticaria production. Urticaria may be initiated by immunologic or nonimmunologic mechanisms. Nonimmunologic urticaria may be produced by degranulation of mast cells, which may be caused by foods and drugs, including aspirin and narcotics.

Almost any medication may produce urticaria, although penicillin and aspirin are the most common. Traces of penicillin may be present in dairy products, as well as in other medications. The mechanism of production of urticaria by aspirin is unclear, but is probably nonimmunologic, and the effects of aspirin may persist for weeks after ingestion. Substances that can cause urticaria by contact with the skin include foods, textiles, animal dander and saliva, plants, topical medications, chemicals, or cosmetics. Food allergies, such as seafood, tree nuts, peanuts, or eggs, may result in urticaria. In addition, foods such as lobster or strawberries can release histamine through a nonimmunologic mechanism.

Infection is a common cause of urticaria. Viral infections that produce urticaria include rhinovirus, rotavirus, hepatitis, mononucleosis, and coxsackievirus infections. Occult infections with *Candida,* the dermatophytes, bacteria, viruses, or parasites may also cause urticaria.

TABLE 107.4 Potency of Topical Steroids

Brand Name	Generic name	Brand Name	Generic name
Class 1: Superpotent		Synalar ointment, 0.025%	Fluocinolone acetonide
Clobex lotion, spray, or shampoo, 0.05%	Clobetasol propionate	Westcort ointment, 0.2%	Hydrocortisone valerate
Cormax solution, 0.05%	Clobetasol propionate		
Diprolene ointment, 0.05%	Betamethasone dipropionate	**Class 5: Lower Midstrength**	
Olux E foam, 0.05%	Clobetasol propionate	Cordran cream, lotion, or tape, 0.05%	Flurandrenolide
Olux foam, 0.05%	Clobetasol propionate	Cutivate cream or lotion, 0.05%	Fluticasone propionate
Temovate cream, 0.05%	Clobetasol propionate	Dermatop cream, ointment, 0.1%	Prednicarbate
Ultravate cream or ointment, 0.05%	Halobetasol propionate	Desonate gel, 0.05%	Desonide
Vanos cream, 0.1%	Fluocinonide	Locoid cream, lotion, ointment, or solution, 0.1%	Hydrocortisone butyrate
		Pandel cream, 0.1%	Hydrocortisone probutate
Class 2: Potent		Synalar cream, 0.03%, 0.025%	Fluocinolone acetonide
ApexiCon E ointment, 0.05%	Diflorasone diacetate	Westcort cream, 0.2%	Hydrocortisone valerate
Diprolene cream AF, 0.05%	Betamethasone dipropionate		
Halog ointment, solution, or cream, 0.1%	Halcinonide	**Class 6: Mild**	
Lidex cream, gel, or ointment, 0.05%	Fluocinonide	Aclovate cream or ointment, 0.05%	Alclometasone dipropionate
Psorcon ointment, 0.05%	Diflorasone diacetate	Capex shampoo, 0.01%	Fluocinolone acetonide
Topicort cream, spray, or ointment, 0.25%	Desoximetasone	Derma-Smoothe/FS oil, 0.01%	Fluocinolone acetonide
Topicort gel, 0.05%	Desoximetasone	DesOwen lotion, 0.05%	Desonide
		Synalar cream or solution, 0.01%	Fluocinolone acetonide
Class 3: Upper Midstrength		Verdeso foam, 0.05%	Desonide
Cutivate ointment, 0.005%	Fluticasone propionate		
Elocon ointment, 0.1%	Mometasone furoate	**Class 7: Least Potent**	
Lidex-E cream, 0.05%	Fluocinonide	Aquanil HC, 1%	Hydrocortisone
Luxiq foam, 0.12%	Betamethasone valerate	Cortaid cream, spray, or ointment, 1%	Hydrocortisone
		Hytone cream, 1%, 2.5%; lotion, 2%	Hydrocortisone
Class 4: Midstrength		MiCort-HC cream, 2.5%	Hydrocortisone
Cordran ointment, 0.05%	Flurandrenolide	Nutracort cream, 2.5%	Hydrocortisone
Elocon cream, lotion, solution, 0.1%	Mometasone furoate		
Kenalog cream, 0.1%, or spray, 0.2 mg/2 second spray	Triamcinolone acetonide		

Synacort cream, 1% Modified with permission from National Psoriasis Foundation: Topical steroids potency chart. Available at www.psoriasis.org/page.aspx?pid=469.

Inhalation of pollens, mold, animal dander, dust, plant products, or aerosols may produce urticaria. Respiratory symptoms may accompany the dermatosis, and a seasonal pattern of occurrence may be present. Stings and bites of insects, arthropods, or various marine animals may also produce an urticarial eruption.

Systemic diseases such as systemic lupus erythematosus, lymphoma, carcinoma, hyperthyroidism, rheumatic fever, or juvenile rheumatoid arthritis may induce an urticarial eruption.

Physical agents may produce urticaria. Dermatographism is present when firm stroking of the skin produces an urticarial wheal within 30 minutes and is the most common form of physical urticaria. Pressure urticaria is distinct from dermatographism in that the onset of urticaria is delayed by 4 to 8 hours after the application of physical pressure.

Cold urticaria may be either familial or, more commonly, acquired. Cold urticaria may also be associated with underlying illness, such as cryoglobulinemia, cryofibrinogenemia, syphilis, or connective tissue disease. Antihistamines taken 30 to 60 minutes before cold exposure may be helpful. Cholinergic urticaria is induced by exercise, heat, or emotional stress. It may be associated with pruritus, nausea, abdominal pain, or headache. The lesions of cholinergic urticaria are wheals, 1 to 3 mm in diameter, surrounded by extensive erythematous flares and, occasionally, satellite wheals. Nonsedating antihistamines are generally used to treat cholinergic urticaria.

Heat is a rare cause of hives. Solar urticaria, also uncommon, is confined to sun-exposed areas of skin and clears rapidly when the light stimulus is removed. Extensive sun exposure may cause wheezing, dizziness, or syncope in a susceptible individual. Sunscreens have not been proven to be effective for the prevention of solar urticaria. Phototherapy may be used in an attempt to induce tolerance.

Urticaria appears as edematous plaques with pale centers and red borders and is easily recognizable (Fig. 107.33). Individual hives are typically transient, lasting less than 24 hours, although new lesions may continuously develop, which represents localized dermal edema produced by transvascular fluid extravasation.

The differential diagnosis of urticaria includes drug eruption, exanthems, erythema multiforme, erythema marginatum, and juvenile rheumatoid arthritis.

Treatment of urticaria involves the removal of the inciting factor, when applicable, and the administration of antihistamines or other antipruritics. Hydroxyzine can treat pruritus for symptomatic relief. For chronic urticaria, long-term therapy with antihistamines may be needed. Nonsedating antihistamines are preferred. Cetirizine, fexofenadine, or loratadine can be used. An H_2 blocker may be added.

Steroids may be a useful adjunctive therapy. Patients with moderate or severe urticaria may benefit from prednisone or dexamethasone. Patients with recurrent urticaria may benefit from longer courses of

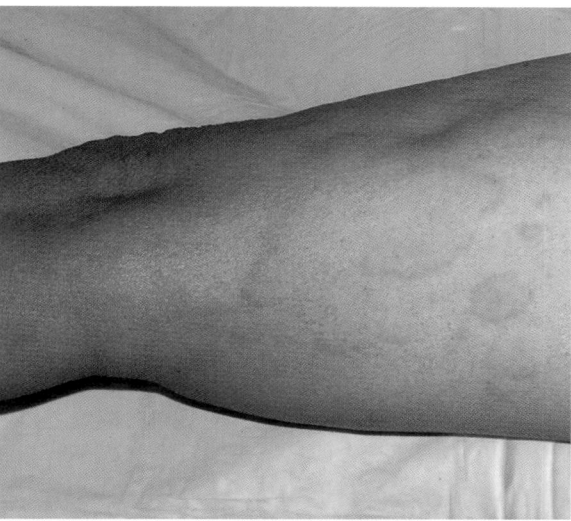

Fig. 107.33 Urticaria. (Courtesy David Effron, MD.)

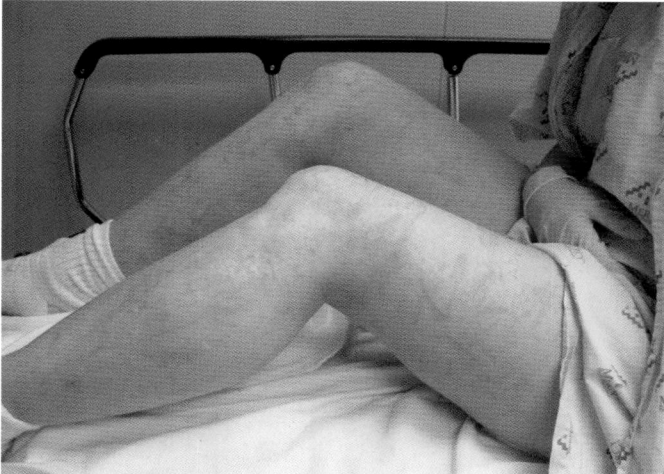

Fig. 107.34 Toxicodendron (Poison Ivy).

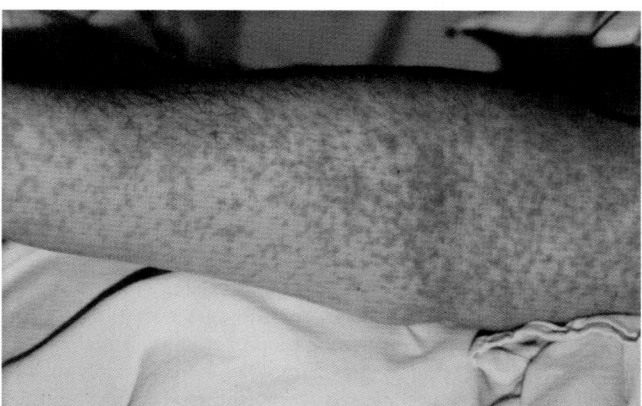

Fig. 107.35 Morbilliform Drug Eruption. (Courtesy David Effron, MD.)

oral steroids (14 to 21 days with a taper). Chronic administration of steroids is not recommended.

Patients with chronic urticaria may be treated with a prescription for a combination of an H_1 and H_2 antihistamine.

Poison Ivy

Exposure to *Toxicodendron* species may cause vesicular or bullous eruptions. Oozing, crusting, scaling, and fissuring may be found, with lichenification in chronic lesions. The distribution of the eruption depends on the specific contact and may be localized, asymmetric, linear, unilateral, or disseminated (Fig. 107.34). Mucous membranes are usually spared unless they are directly exposed to the inciting agent. Sensitization to poison ivy may result in sensitization to other plants in this family, including cashew, mango, lacquer, and ginkgo trees, thus patients may present with a dermatologic reaction to these exposures as well.

In addition to treatment regimens for contact dermatitis, a course of systemic corticosteroids may be indicated to treat *Toxicodendron*-associated dermatitis. Patients should be counseled to wash all clothes or items that might have contacted the plant as the irritant plant oil can remain on inanimate objects. Once the offending agent is reliably removed from the skin and clothes, ongoing outbreak is attributable to the initial contact, not spread from the serous fluid from the bullae. The patient is not contagious to others unless there is direct contact with the plant oil in those who are sensitized.

DRUG REACTIONS

Reactions to medications are common and are estimated to occur in 1% to 5% of patients. Cutaneous reactions are the most common type of reaction. Immediate reactions, occurring within 1 hour, may include urticaria, anaphylaxis, or angioedema.[58] Delayed hypersensitivity reactions often appear within 4 to 28 days after the drug is taken. Many medications have the potential to produce a drug reaction. Patients at higher risk of drug reactions include those with immunodeficiency, certain infections, or genetic predisposition. The most common eruptions are a morbilliform rash (Fig. 107.35), urticaria, or fixed drug eruption. More severe reactions may include vasculitis, erythema nodosum, angioedema, anaphylaxis, Stevens-Johnson syndrome, toxic epidermal necrolysis, blistering dermatoses, drug-induced lupus, lichenoid drug eruptions, psoriasiform drug eruptions, drug-induced neutrophilic dermatoses (i.e., Sweet's

syndrome, erythema nodosum, and pyoderma gangrenosum), and cutaneous lymphoma-like drug reactions.

Treatment of drug eruptions includes discontinuation of the inciting agent.[59] Most cutaneous drug reactions fade within 1 week of discontinuation. Antihistamines, H_2-antagonists, and topical or systemic steroids may be indicated for symptomatic treatment.

Toxic Epidermal Necrolysis

Stevens-Johnson syndrome and toxic epidermal necrolysis are considered a continuous spectrum of the same disease, an immune-complex–mediated hypersensitivity reaction. Stevens-Johnson syndrome is considered a minor form of toxic epidermal necrolysis with less than 10% body surface area (BSA) involved. Toxic epidermal necrolysis includes patients with more than 30% BSA involved. There is overlap with patients with 10% to 30% BSA involved.[60] The main feature of non–staphylococcal-induced toxic epidermal necrolysis, or Lyell's disease, is the separation of large sheets of epidermis from underlying dermis. Toxic epidermal necrolysis may be caused by medications, infection, malignancy, or idiopathic (30% to 50% of cases). Medications that can cause toxic epidermal necrolysis include sulfa drugs, nonsteroidal antiinflammatory drugs (NSAIDs), penicillin, aspirin, barbiturates, phenytoin, carbamazepine, or allopurinol.

Mortality may be up to 30% with toxic epidermal necrolysis. Risk factors for poor prognosis include age older than 40 years, underlying malignancy, heart rate greater than 120 beats/min, initial percentage

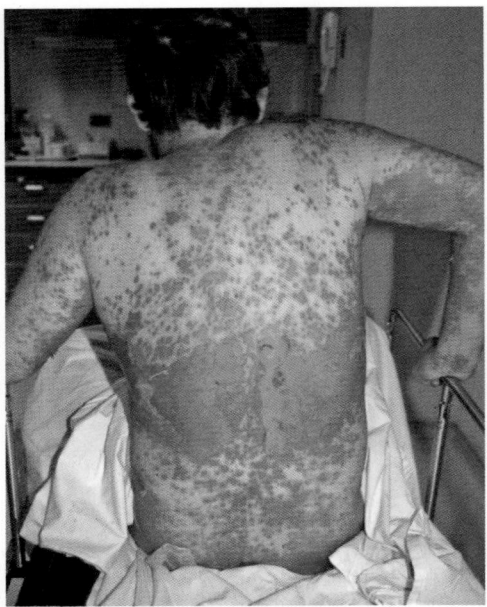

Fig. 107.36 Toxic Epidermal Necrolysis. (Courtesy David Effron, MD.)

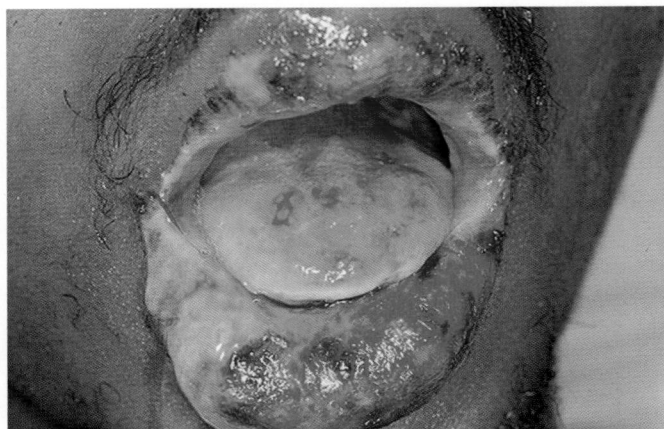

Fig. 107.37 Toxic Epidermal Necrolysis. (Courtesy David Effron, MD.)

INFLAMMATORY CONDITIONS

Atopic Dermatitis

Atopic dermatitis is a common dermatologic condition often referred to as *eczema* or *chronic dermatitis*. Atopic dermatitis is the cutaneous manifestation of an atopic state, and it is associated with allergic diseases, such as asthma and allergic rhinitis. Patients with atopic dermatitis are known to have abnormalities of both humeral and cell-mediated immunity. The exact mechanism is unclear, but eosinophil, mast cell, and lymphocyte activation triggered by increased production of interleukin-4 by specific T helper cells seems to be involved. The course of atopic dermatitis includes remissions and exacerbations. More than 90% of patients have the onset of atopic dermatitis before 5 years of age.

Atopic dermatitis is an inflammatory skin condition. Diagnostic criteria include itchy skin plus three or more of the following: generalized dry skin in the past year, history of asthma or hay fever, onset of rash before 2 years old, and flexural dermatitis.

Skin lesions generally appear as inflammatory thickened, papular, or papulovesicular lesions. The skin is typically dry and may be scaly, but in the acute phase, it may also be vesicular, weeping, or oozing. In the chronic stage, lesions are thickened and lichenified.

The distribution of lesions varies with the age. In infants, inflammatory exudative plaques are seen on the cheeks, on the extensor surfaces, or in the diaper area. Older children and adults have lesions in the antecubital and popliteal flexion areas, neck, face, or upper chest. Infantile atopic dermatitis usually begins in the fourth to sixth month of life and improves by the third to fifth year of life. The childhood form occurs between 3 and 6 years of age, and it resolves spontaneously or continues into the adult form.

Intense pruritus is a hallmark of atopic dermatitis. During flares, patients may present with complaints of intense itching and failure of routine treatments to control their symptoms. Patients may also present with secondary infections. The itching may be focal or generalized, is worse during the winter, and is triggered by increased body temperature or emotional stress. It may be particularly challenging at night. Excoriations may be prominent, and secondary bacterial infection of excoriated lesions is common. Repeated scratching and rubbing produce lichenification, a condition of hyperpigmentation, thickening of the skin, and accentuation of skin furrows. Lichenification is a common feature of chronic atopic dermatitis.

Treatment should be aimed at control of inflammation, dryness, and itching. Topical emollients and topical corticosteroids are the cornerstone of therapy.

of epidermal detachment more than 10%, BUN level more than 10 mmol/L, serum glucose level more than 252 mg/dL, and bicarbonate level less than 20 mmol/L.

Toxic epidermal necrolysis commonly begins with prodromal symptoms, such as fever, malaise, rhinitis, sore throat, or myalgias. These are followed by the abrupt development of a macular rash that may appear as target lesions. The extremities are commonly involved, although any area may be affected. The exanthem becomes confluent, and dermal-epidermal dissociation ensues; Nikolsky sign (denudation with shear stress) is present, and the skin is commonly painful to the touch (Fig. 107.36). Mucous membrane involvement may occur with erythema, blistering, sloughing, or necrosis (Fig. 107.37). Involvement of the conjunctivae and cornea may lead to permanent scarring and blindness. Systemic involvement may occur, with renal, gastrointestinal, or respiratory tract lesions, resulting in hematuria, diarrhea, bronchitis, or pneumonia. Morbidity and mortality are often related to infection and dehydration.

The treatment of Stevens-Johnson syndrome and toxic epidermal necrolysis includes discontinuation of the offending agent and supportive care, including hydration, prevention of secondary infection, pain control, and wound management.[61,62] This is usually best accomplished in a center with burn care expertise. Treatment may also include systemic steroids, intravenous immune globulin (IVIG), or cyclosporin A.[61] Plasmapheresis may be considered in consultation with a specialist with experience in treating these serious skin disorders.[63]

DRESS syndrome. Drug reaction with eosinophilia and systemic symptoms (DRESS syndrome) is a severe drug reaction characterized by a morbilliform skin eruption, fever, lymphadenopathy, hematologic abnormalities (eosinophilia, atypical lymphocytosis), and internal organ involvement (hepatic, renal, pulmonary, cardiac, gastrointestinal, neurologic, or endocrine abnormalities).[64,65] Mortality may be as high as 10%. Common inciting medications include anticonvulsants, antibiotics, or allopurinol. Onset may be 2 to 8 weeks after beginning the medication. Treatment includes withdrawal of the inciting agent and treatment with systemic steroids.

Skin dryness is treated with topical emollients, such as oils, ointments, lotions, and creams. In some cases, emollients are as effective as topical steroids.[66] The choice of agent should be based on patient preference and may be applied several times daily. Pruritis may be treated with topical emollients and systemic antihistamines.

Approximately 80% of patients have improvement of symptoms with topical steroid treatment. When the dermatitis is severe, the application of a fluorinated corticosteroid ointment (such as betamethasone valerate) is recommended (Table 107.4). Fluorinated corticosteroids should not be used on the face, as they can produce cutaneous atrophy. Milder corticosteroid preparations, such as 0.025% triamcinolone ointment, may be used on the face or intertriginous areas. Patients with severe disease may require systemic steroids. Other treatment modalities include calcineurin inhibitors, topical phosphodiesterase inhibitors, or UV radiation.[67]

Patients with atopic dermatitis are susceptible to infection and colonization by a variety of organisms because of their defective skin barrier functions and local skin immunodeficiency. Widespread disseminated viral infections, such as eczema molluscum (molluscum contagiosum in the setting of eczema), eczema herpeticum (herpes virus infection in the setting of eczema), or recurrent staphylococcal pustulosis may complicate atopic dermatitis.

Inpatient admission is a consideration in rare cases, for those patients who have generalized erythema and exfoliation (erythroderma) or intractable itching with skin breakdown and heightened risk for severe secondary bacterial or viral skin infections.

Pityriasis Rosea

Pityriasis rosea is a mild skin eruption predominantly found in children and young adults. The etiology is unknown, although viral, bacterial, and fungal etiologies have been suggested. Patients aged 10 to 35 years are commonly affected. Clinical presentation includes multiple pink or pigmented oval papules or plaques 1 to 2 cm in diameter on the trunk and proximal extremities. A history may reveal an initial larger patch ("herald patch") that precedes the widespread eruption (Figs. 107.38 and 107.39). Mild scaling may be present. The lesions are parallel to the ribs, forming a Christmas tree–like distribution on the trunk and extremities. Oral lesions are rare. In children, papular or vesicular variants of the disease may occur. The eruption is usually asymptomatic, although pruritus may be present. The differential diagnosis includes tinea corporis (erythematous lesions with scale and central clearing), guttate psoriasis (small psoriatic lesions over trunk and proximal extremities), lichen planus (pruritic violaceous polygonal

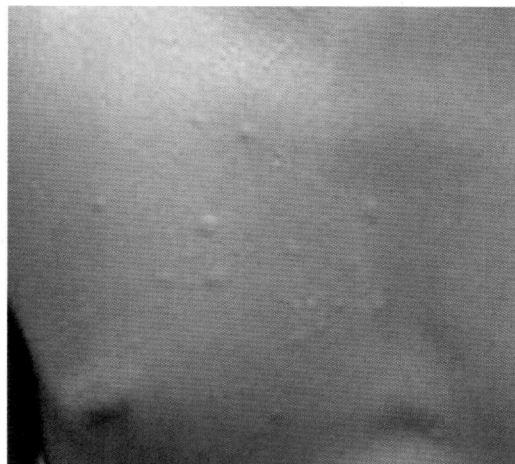

Fig. 107.39 Pityriasis Rosea.

lesions), drug eruption, Lyme disease, or secondary syphilis (erythematous maculopapular lesions).

Pityriasis rosea is self-limited, resolving in 8 to 12 weeks. Recurrences are rare. Treatment should include supportive care, including alleviation of pruritus. Topical zinc oxide or calamine lotion are useful for pruritus. Typically steroids are not indicated. If the disease is severe or widespread (e.g., vesicular pityriasis rosea), topical or oral steroids may be used (Table 107.4). No restriction of activity or isolation is indicated.

Kawasaki Disease

Kawasaki disease (mucocutaneous lymph node syndrome) is one of the most common vasculitides of childhood. The peak age is between 1 and 2 years old. The disease is very uncommon in children older than 14 years old or in adults. It is more common in boys. Although cases of Kawasaki disease have been reported in children of all ethnic origins, the highest incidence is among children of Asian descent. The disease typically occurs in winter and spring and is usually self-limiting, resolving spontaneously without treatment within 2 to 4 weeks. However, 15% to 20% of patients will develop complications, such as damage to coronary arteries, leading to myocardial infarction and heart failure. Kawasaki disease is the leading cause of pediatric acquired heart disease in the U.S.

Clinical features are characterized by three phases. The acute febrile period (phase I) is manifested by the abrupt onset of fever, lasting approximately 12 days. During phase I, cutaneous findings include erythematous lesions on the palms and soles. Within 2 days, the blotchy, erythematous, macular lesions spread to the extremities and trunk. Nonexudative injected conjunctivae, seen in approximately 90% of patients, may be present for 1 to 3 weeks. Diffuse oropharyngeal erythema with a "strawberry" tongue appearance is often present. Symptoms of diarrhea, arthritis, or photophobia may be present. In the subacute phase (phase II), desquamation, thrombocytosis, arthritis, arthralgias, or carditis may be present. This phase may last 30 days. There is a high risk for sudden death during this phase of the illness if it has gone untreated. During the convalescent phase (phase III), which occurs within 8 to 10 weeks after the onset of the illness, most signs of the illness have resolved. Coronary aneurysms present in 25% of cases and may be diagnosed by echocardiography or coronary angiography.

For epidemiologic surveillance, the Centers for Disease Control and Prevention (CDC) defines a case of Kawasaki disease as illness in

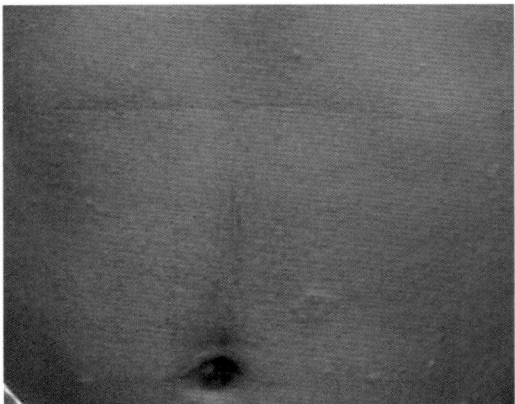

Fig. 107.38 Herald Patch of Pityriasis Rosea.

a patient with fever of 5 or more days duration, and the presence of at least four of the following five clinical signs[68]

- Rash
- Cervical lymphadenopathy (at least 1.5 cm in diameter)
- Bilateral conjunctival injection
- Oral mucosal changes
- Peripheral extremity changes.

The diagnosis is made based on clinical findings. Laboratory tests that support the diagnosis include elevated liver function tests, leukocytosis, thrombocytosis, and an elevated C-reactive protein (CRP). The ESR is elevated during phase II and returns to normal in phase III. Pyuria may be seen on urinalysis. Electrocardiography (ECG) may show PR and QT prolongation or acute ST/T wave changes.

Management of Kawasaki disease includes hospital admission, and treatment with high-dose IVIG and aspirin during hospitalization.[69] Treatment with IVIG within the first 10 days of illness reduces the incidence of coronary artery aneurysms fivefold, compared with children not treated with IVIG. Early cardiology evaluation is important to identify and treat possible coronary artery involvement.

Erythema Multiforme

Erythema multiforme is considered to be a hypersensitivity reaction. Potential etiologies include drug reaction; HSV infection or other viral infections; fungal diseases, such as dermatophytosis, histoplasmosis, or coccidioidomycosis; and bacterial infections, especially streptococcal infections or tuberculosis. Collagen vascular disorders have been known to precipitate erythema multiforme, including rheumatoid arthritis, systemic lupus erythematosus, dermatomyositis, or periarteritis nodosa. Pregnancy and various malignant neoplasms have also been associated with erythema multiforme. The etiology is unknown in approximately 50% of cases. The differential diagnosis includes urticaria, scalded skin syndrome, pemphigus, and pemphigoid or viral exanthems.

Erythema multiforme is an acute, usually self-limited disease. It is characterized by skin lesions that are erythematous or violaceous macules, papules, vesicles, or bullae. Their distribution is often symmetric, most commonly involving the soles and palms, the backs of the hands or feet, and the extensor surfaces of the extremities. The presence of lesions of the palms and soles is particularly characteristic. The target lesion with three zones of color is the hallmark of erythema multiforme (Fig. 107.40).

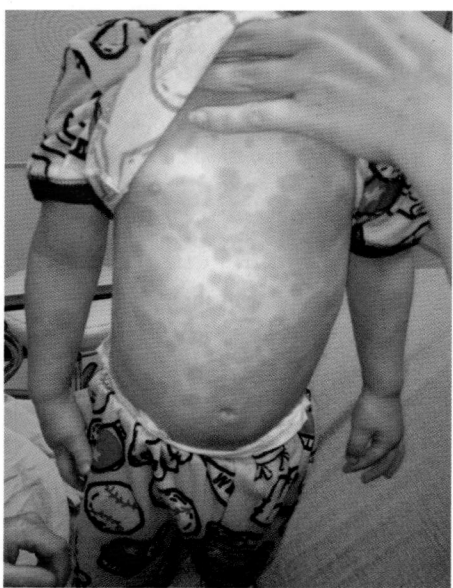

Fig. 107.40 Erythema Multiforme.

Treatment should include treatment of the underlying cause. Mild forms with no systemic symptoms, lesions limited to extremities, and no mucous membrane involvement typically resolve spontaneously in 2 or 3 weeks. Patients with lesions on the trunk or patients who are immunocompromised, especially those with multiple lesions, should receive a course of systemic steroids for 14 to 21 days with a taper and urgent dermatology referral.

Erythema Nodosum

Erythema nodosum is an inflammatory reaction of the dermis and adipose tissue that presents with painful, palpable erythematous or violaceous subcutaneous nodules. These painful nodules occur most commonly over the anterior tibia but may also be seen on the arms or body (Fig. 107.41). Fever and arthralgia of the ankles or knees may precede the rash. As the lesions evolve, they may turn yellow-purple and resemble bruises. Women are affected more often than men, with the highest incidence in the third to fifth decades of life.

A number of diseases are associated with erythema nodosum; these include drug reactions, sarcoidosis, coccidioidomycosis, histoplasmosis, tuberculosis, ulcerative colitis, regional enteritis, pregnancy, malignancy, or infections. Approximately 50% of erythema nodosum cases are idiopathic.[70]

Management includes treatment of the underlying etiology. Chest radiography may be considered to exclude findings characteristic of sarcoidosis, tuberculosis, or pulmonary fungal infection. Bed rest, elevation of the legs, and elastic stockings reduce pain and edema. Aspirin or other NSAIDs may provide pain relief. Erythema nodosum is a self-limited process that usually resolves in 3 to 8 weeks. Patients

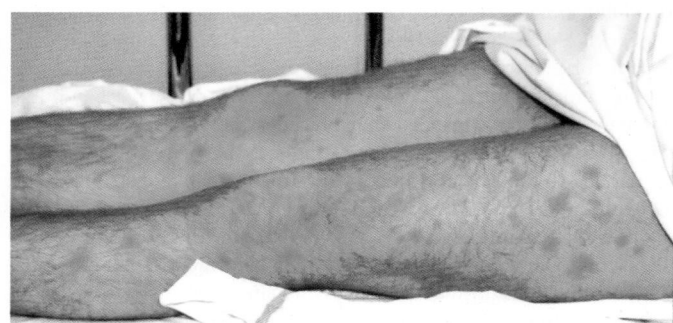

Fig. 107.41 Erythema Nodosum. (Courtesy David Effron, MD.)

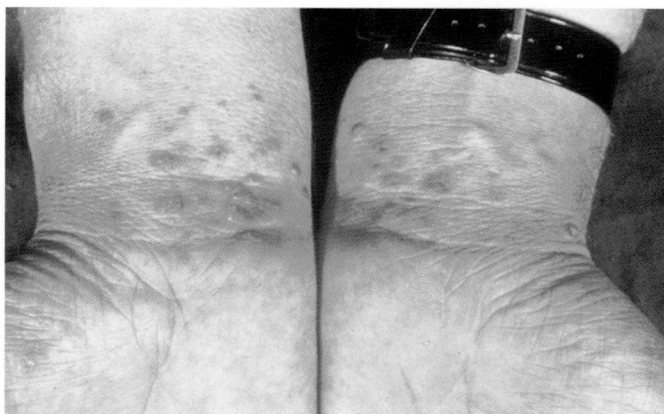

Fig. 107.42 Lichen Planus. (Courtesy Centers for Disease Control and Prevention [CDC] Public Health Image Library, Susan Lindsley.)

with severe pain may be treated with potassium iodide daily for 3 or 4 weeks.[71]

Lichen Planus

Lichen planus (LP) is an autoimmune condition that results in inflammation. LP typically presents with lesions that are flat-topped violaceous papules with pruritus (also known as the five "Ps": purple, planar, polygonal, pruritic, papules). Lesions typically appear on the wrists and ankles (Fig. 107.42). The lesions may occur in an area of trauma (Koebner phenomenon). Other areas may be affected, such as oral mucosa, anogenital region, scalp, or other areas.

Medium- to high-potency topical steroids are the treatment of choice (Table 107.4). Pruritus may be treated with systemic agents, such as diphenhydramine or hydroxyzine. Systemic steroids may be indicated if greater than 15% BSA is involved, or for topical treatment failures. Alternate therapies include topical calcineurin inhibitors, methotrexate, topical or systemic retinoids, or phototherapy.[72,73]

AUTOIMMUNE DISORDERS

Bullous Pemphigoid

Bullous pemphigoid is an autoimmune blistering disorder that most commonly affects geriatric patients. Clinical manifestations are often pruritus and generalized blistering of the skin (Fig. 107.43). Nikolsky sign is negative. It often has a waxing and waning clinical course. It has been associated with numerous systemic conditions, including malignancy, diabetes, stroke, Parkinson disease, or cardiovascular disease.

Topical steroids may be prescribed as initial therapy.[74] For example, clobetasol propionate cream, 0.05% may be applied BID for 1 to 3 weeks. Systemic steroids or doxycycline may be necessary to treat widespread lesions. Patients with topical treatment failure may be treated with a systemic agent, such as doxycycline (100 mg BID for 1 to 3 weeks) or prednisone (40 mg daily for 1 to 3 weeks).

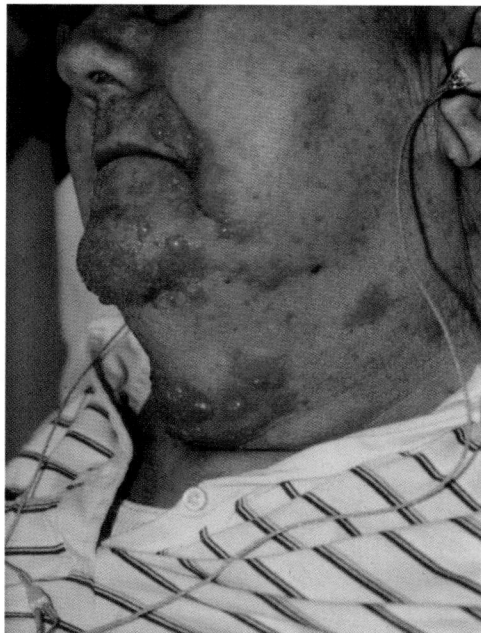

Fig. 107.43 Bullous Pemphigus. (Courtesy David Effron, MD.)

Pemphigus Vulgaris

Pemphigus vulgaris is an uncommon but important dermatologic disorder to identify. The mortality rate before the use of steroids was approximately 95%. The current mortality rate is 10% to 15%, with appropriate treatment. Pemphigus is a bullous disease, affecting both sexes equally, and is most common in patients 40 to 60 years old. The disease is mostly prevalent in people of Jewish, Mediterranean, or south Asian descent.

The typical skin lesions are small, flaccid bullae that break easily, forming superficial erosions and crusted ulcerations. Any area of the body may be involved. Nikolsky sign is positive and characteristic of the disease.

Many patients also have oral lesions (50% to 60%). The oral lesions typically antedate the cutaneous lesions by several months. The most common site is in the mouth, especially the gums and vermilion borders of the lips. Oral lesions are bullous but commonly break, leaving painful, denuded areas of superficial ulceration.

Pain control and local wound care are essential components of therapy. Treatment with oral glucocorticoids should be instituted. Other treatments may include immunosuppressive agents, intravenous immunoglobulins, immunoadsorption, or rituximab.[75] Morbidity and mortality may ensue, related to an uncontrolled spread of the disease, secondary infection, dehydration, side effects of steroid therapy, or thromboembolism.

CUTANEOUS MALIGNANCIES

The most common cutaneous malignancies are basal cell carcinoma, squamous cell carcinoma, and melanoma.[76]

Basal cell carcinoma is the most common skin cancer in the United States.[77] Basal cell carcinomas are commonly seen in patients with fair skin, sun exposure, outdoor occupation, and older age. Clinical presentation is typically on sun exposed areas, commonly on the head or neck. Clinical presentations include nodular, superficial, and morphea-form subtypes. The typical nodular appearance is a pearly papule with well-defined borders and telangiectasias. Suspicious lesions should be referred to a dermatologist for biopsy and management.

Squamous cell carcinoma is the second most common skin cancer in the United States. It is more common in men than in women. The risk of developing squamous cell carcinoma of the skin is increased with advancing age and sun exposure. Squamous cell carcinomas are typically found in sun-exposed areas, most commonly on the head or neck. The appearance is typically an irregular growth with erythema, induration, inflammation, crusting, or oozing. Suspicious lesions should be referred to a dermatologist for biopsy.

Melanoma is less common, and accounts for only 4% to 5% of skin cancers. However, it is responsible for most deaths from cutaneous malignancies. Risk factors include fair skin, dysplastic nevi, multiple (>50) nevi, prior history of melanoma, family history of melanoma, immunocompromised state, or xeroderma pigmentosum (an inherited condition resulting in UV light sensitivity). Melanoma may occur in any area of the skin, though tends to appear more often on lower extremities in women, and on the head, neck, or trunk in men. The typical appearance is an asymmetric lesion with irregular pigmentation, border, and texture, and diameter greater than 6 mm or increasing in size. Suspicious lesions should be referred to a dermatologist for biopsy.

Kaposi sarcoma appears more often in patients with underlying immunosuppression. Clinically, it presents with painless, raised, brown-black or purple papules and nodules that do not blanch. Common sites are the face, chest, genitals, and oral cavity, but widespread

TABLE 107.5 Cutaneous Signs of Systemic Disease

Anatomic Site	Sign	Systemic Disease
Generalized	Urticaria	Drug reaction
		SLE
		Infection
	Pruritus	Anemia
		Renal disease
		Cholestasis
		Polycythemia
		Lymphoma
		Malignancies
		Thyroid disease
Head and neck	Xanthelasma	Hyperlipidemia
	Spider nevi	Liver disease
		Hyperthyroidism
	Malar erythema	SLE
	Photosensitive rash	SLE
		Porphyria
	Alopecia	Thyroid disease
		Drugs
		Anemia
		Malnutrition
		SLE
		Fungal infection
	Heliotrope discoloration and eyelid edema	Dermatomyositis
Hands	Gottron papules	Dermatomyositis
		Internal malignancy
	Raynaud phenomenon	Normal
		Connective tissue diseases
	Clubbing	Normal
		Internal malignancy
		Cyanotic cardiac disease
		IBD
		Lung disease
	Erythema multiforme	Drugs
		Infections
	Palmar erythema	Normal
		Liver disease
		Pregnancy
		Rheumatoid arthritis
		SLE
Legs	Erythema nodosum	Strep infection
		Drugs
		Pregnancy
		Tuberculosis
		Sarcoidosis
		IBD
	Pyoderma gangrenosum	IBD
		Hepatitis
		Rheumatoid arthritis
		Malignancy
	Pretibial myxedema	Hypothyroidism
		Hyperthyroidism
	Necrobiosis lipoidica	Diabetes mellitus

IBD, Inflammatory bowel disease; *SLE*, systemic lupus erythematosus.

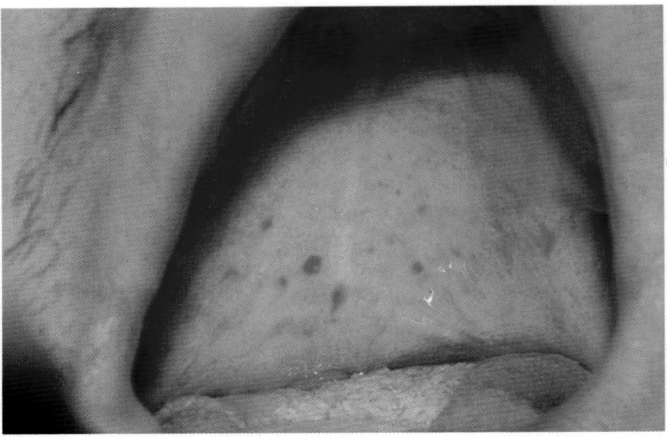

Fig. 107.44 Palatal petechiae secondary to thrombocytopenia in a patient with acute myelogenous leukemia (AML). (Courtesy Jason R. Pickett, MD.)

dissemination involving internal organs may occur. Because cutaneous Kaposi sarcoma is not generally associated with morbidity or mortality, therapy is indicated only for extensive, painful, or cosmetically disfiguring lesions.

Although the ED does not provide definitive management for cutaneous malignancies, recognition of possible malignant lesions may facilitate prompt and expeditious referral for definitive management. Any lesion with irregular pigmentation, irregular borders or texture, easy bleeding, or recent change in lesion should be referred to a dermatologist.

SKIN CONDITIONS ASSOCIATED WITH SYSTEMIC DISEASE

Systemic illness should be considered with generalized dermatologic presentations. Systemic illness should be suspected in patients with systemic symptoms, such as fever, fatigue, weight loss or gain, weakness, immunosuppression, or other generalized symptoms. Systemic illnesses with cutaneous findings may include systemic infections, autoimmune or connective tissue disorders, malignancies, diabetes mellitus, endocrine disorders, or immunodeficiency states (Table 107.5).

Cutaneous lesions most directly indicative of an internal malignant disease arise from the extension of the tumor to the skin, or by hematogenous or lymphatic metastasis. The neoplasms that most commonly produce cutaneous extension are lymphomas, leukemias, and carcinomas of the breast, gastrointestinal tract, lung, ovary, prostate, uterus, or bladder. Skin metastases generally signify a poor prognosis.

Pruritus may be a sign of systemic disease, such as liver disease, renal disease, endocrine disorder, rheumatologic disorder, malignancy, or neurodegenerative disease.[78] Malignancies associated with pruritus include Hodgkin disease, leukemia, adenocarcinoma or squamous cell carcinoma of various organs, carcinoid syndrome, multiple myeloma, or polycythemia vera. Pruritis may be present years before the underlying malignant disease is identified. It may be intractable and associated with urticaria, erythroderma, excoriation, or lichenification.

Purpura may be a manifestation of acute granulocytic and monocytic leukemia, myeloma, lymphoma, or polycythemia vera. Purpura is caused by vascular abnormalities, thrombocytopenia, or other coagulation defects. A variety of diseases and conditions may be the underlying cause, and the treatment should be directed toward this cause whenever possible. Thrombocytopenic and nonthrombocytopenic forms are differentiated by the platelet count.

Petechiae are manifestations of intradermal hemorrhage. Petechiae may be associated with thrombocytopenia, allergic reactions, endocarditis, Rocky Mountain spotted fever, viral hepatitis, infections, trauma, or malignancy (Fig. 107.44).[79]

Generalized erythroderma may indicate systemic condition, such as drug reaction, SSSS, erythema multiforme, toxic epidermal necrolysis, malignancy, exacerbation of underlying skin condition, or collagen vascular disorder.[80]

The references for this chapter can be found online at ExpertConsult. com.

108

Blood and Blood Components

Christopher E. San Miguel and Colin G. Kaide

KEY CONCEPTS

- Red blood cell transfusion is indicated only to increase oxygen delivery at the tissue level.
- One unit of packed red blood cells (PRBCs) can be expected to raise an adult's hemoglobin level by 1 g/dL. A similar increase is expected in children following the transfusion of 10 mL/kg of PRBCs.
- Controlled trials have supported newer, restrictive, red cell transfusion strategies. Pending further trials, a transfusion trigger of a hemoglobin level below 7 to 8 g/dL is appropriate for most stable hospitalized patients.
- Platelet transfusions are typically used prophylactically for counts less than 10 K/μL in adults without bleeding. For patients undergoing central venous catheter placement, a level of 20 K/μL is recommended. Patients undergoing lumbar puncture and non-neuroaxial surgery should be prophylactically transfused to a level of 50 K/μL.
- Prospective and retrospective reports have suggested a benefit to massive transfusion protocols, with most advocating a 1 : 1 : 1 ratio of fresh frozen plasma (FFP) to platelets to PRBCs.
- When available, low-titer whole blood is safe and effective for transfusion and provides a physiologic mix of blood products.
- When available, prothrombin complex concentrate (PCC) should be given over FFP for reversal of vitamin K antagonism in the setting of a life-threatening bleeding. When PCC is not available, FFP can be used for this purpose, but is considered a second-line therapy.
- Transfusion reactions can vary from minor symptoms to fatal systemic reactions. If any transfusion reaction is suspected, the transfusion should be stopped while the cause and extent of the reaction is investigated.
- An intravascular hemolytic transfusion reaction is usually the result of ABO incompatibility and typically results in immediate symptoms that can include fever, chills, headache, nausea, vomiting, sensation of chest restriction, severe joint or low back pain, burning sensation at the site of the infusion, and feeling of impending doom. Treatment involves stopping the transfusion, fluid resuscitation, and monitoring for the development of renal failure and disseminated intravascular coagulation (DIC).
- Transfusion-related acute lung injury (TRALI) is now the leading cause of reported transfusion-related mortality. Treatment involves stopping the transfusion and providing supportive respiratory care, which may include noninvasive positive-pressure ventilation (NIPPV) or intubation and mechanical ventilation.
- Improved techniques for selecting and testing blood donors has dramatically reduced the risk of viral transmission of disease by transfusion.

FOUNDATIONS

Background and Importance

The modern blood transfusion era began with identification of the ABO red cell antigen system in the early 1900s. The subsequent discovery that adding citrate enabled the storage of anticoagulated blood led to the establishment of the first blood banks in the United States in the 1930s, and blood banking expanded rapidly after World War II. In subsequent decades, transfusion research focused primarily on critical issues such as developing component therapy, prolonging the storage life of blood products, and reducing the risk of transfusion reactions and transfusion-related infections. In 2015, approximately 11.4 million red blood cell units, 2.7 million plasma units, and 2 million platelet units were transfused in US acute care hospitals.[1]

Anatomy, Physiology, and Pathophysiology

Sound transfusion decision making is informed by a thorough working knowledge of the underlying physiology and pathophysiology, as well as familiarity with the key clinical trials that support up-to-date, evidence-based guidelines. This knowledge facilitates the effective ordering and interpretation of laboratory tests, delivery of blood products, and management of common or serious complications.

Blood Banking

Red blood cell (RBC) storage methods aim to ensure viability of at least 75% of the cells 24 hours after infusion. Blood collection bags contain an anticoagulant that ensures a shelf life of 35 days and a hematocrit of 70% to 80% for packed RBCs (PRBCs). Additive solutions provide additional nutrients and extend maximum storage to 42 days.

A number of biochemical and structural changes have been documented to occur during red cell storage, including loss of deformability, leakage of potassium, irreversible membrane changes, and biochemical alterations that have the potential to affect the ability of RBCs to unload oxygen in the microcirculation.[2] These changes worsen with increased storage duration and have been collectively referred to as the storage lesion. A number of observational studies and a few randomized prospective trials have reported conflicting results as to whether these changes are clinically relevant. The most recent four, large randomized trials have found no statistically significant difference in patient outcomes based on the age of the transfused blood product. Due to methodological limitations however, these results are not yet universally considered definitive.[3]

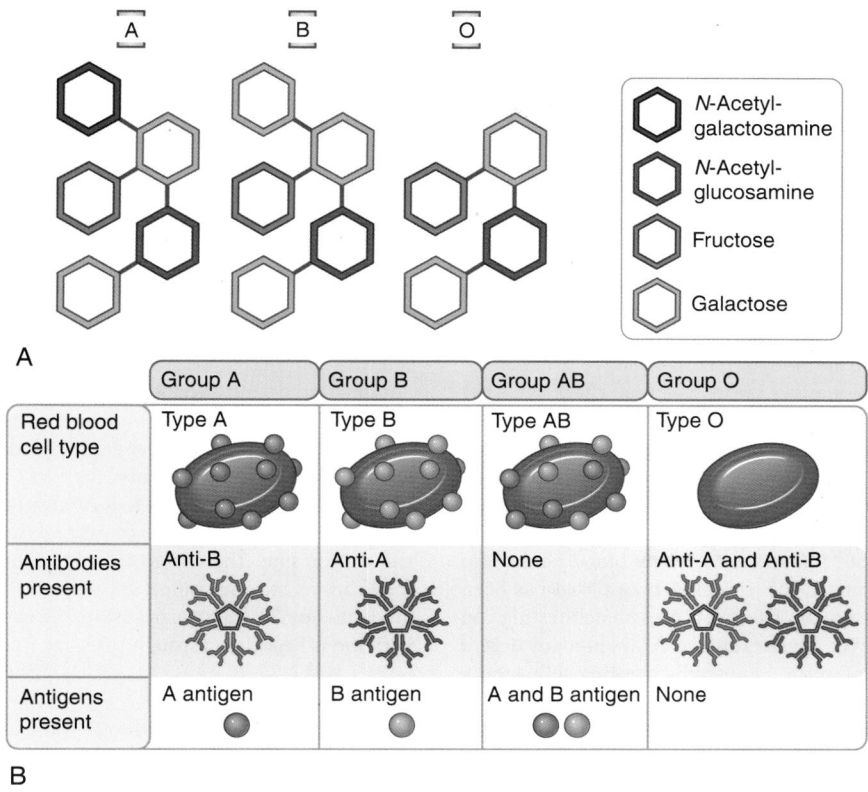

Fig. 108.1 Overview of red blood cell ABO grouping. (From: Abbas AK, Lichtman AH, Pillai S, eds. Transplantation immunology. In: *Cellular and Molecular Immunology*, 9th ed. Philadelphia: Elsevier; 2018.)

Blood Typing

Blood typing refers to the process by which blood is categorized by the antigens expressed on the red blood cells and the antibodies contained in the serum. There are currently over 30 known blood type systems, with the most important systems being the ABO and Rh systems. Kell, Duffy, and Kidd are examples of other blood type systems which generally have less of an impact on clinical practice.

Within the ABO system, there are type A and type B antigens. Red blood cells can express either, both, or neither of these antigens on their cell membranes. Throughout the first year of life, antibodies are formed against whichever antigens are not expressed on an individual's red blood cells. Type O blood, for instance, describes red blood cells that express neither type A nor type B antigens and thus is associated with anti-A and anti-B antibodies in the serum (Fig. 108.1). This seemingly spontaneous production of antibodies is theorized to be triggered by natural exposure to similar antigens in food, bacteria, or the environment and is unique to the ABO blood type system. Conversely, if type A, B, or both antigens are expressed on an individual's red blood cells (as is the case for type A, type B, and type AB blood respectively), the immune system recognizes these naturally occurring antigens as self-antigens and antibodies are not produced. Antibodies against antigens from other blood type systems can certainly be formed, but they generally require an exposure to red blood cells that express those antigens, for instance through blood transfusions or pregnancy. The "natural" production of ABO antibodies combined with the fact that ABO antigens and antibodies cause agglutination and hemolysis when mixed, means that patients can suffer from severe or even fatal transfusion reactions the first time they receive a PRBC transfusion from an ABO incompatible donor.

The second most clinically important blood type system is the Rh system. There are numerous known antigens in this system, but the D antigen is the most immunogenic. When a blood type is described as positive or negative (as in AB+), the report is referring to the presence or absence of the RhD antigen. Unlike in the ABO system, the mixing of Rh antigens and antibodies from a single transfusion is unlikely to result in a severe hemolytic reaction. This blood type system is most clinically relevant in the setting of pregnancy (or potential future pregnancies). If through a previous blood transfusion or pregnancy, an RhD negative mother has been exposed to RhD and subsequently developed anti-RhD antibodies, these antibodies can cross the placenta and into the fetal circulation. If the fetus is RhD positive, prolonged mixture of antigen and antibody can result in hemolytic disease of the newborn. Therefore, unstable hemorrhaging female patients who are not post-menopausal should receive O– blood, while male patients and postmenopausal female patients can receive O+ blood. Of note, hemolytic disease of the newborn is not seen with an ABO incompatible mother and fetus, as the vast majority of anti-ABO antibodies are IgM, which do not cross the placenta.

Type and Screen. An individual blood type and screen test includes ABO grouping, Rh typing, and antibody screen for unexpected, non-ABO/Rh antibodies. ABO grouping tests patient red cells with anti-A and anti-B serum and also with A and B red cells. Rh typing is accomplished by adding a commercial anti-D reagent to patient RBCs. To complete the antibody screen, the patient's serum is combined with commercially prepared mixtures of red cells expressing clinically significant antigens. The incidence of unexpected antibodies in the general population is low (<1%–2%), but a positive screen prompts further compatibility testing. In ideal circumstances, type-specific, yet uncrossmatched, blood can generally be made available within 15 minutes of receiving a sample of the patient's blood.

Type and Crossmatch. When a unit of blood is ordered for transfusion, a crossmatch follows the initial type and screen. In an ideal situation, blood identical to the patient's own ABO and Rh group is utilized. Local blood supplies, however, might dictate that a nonidentical but compatible unit be used. Patients with blood group AB are known as universal recipients—they can receive packed red blood cells from any of the ABO groups, given their lack of anti-A and anti-B antibodies. Type O is commonly referred to as the universal donor of packed red blood cells, given the lack of A and B antigens.

A crossmatch procedure involves mixing the recipient's serum with donor RBCs and observing for agglutination as a final compatibility test before transfusion. If the antibody screen is negative, an abbreviated crossmatch at room temperature serves as a final check for ABO incompatibility. An antibody screen and abbreviated crossmatch requires at least 45 to 60 minutes to complete. If the antibody screen is positive, a complete crossmatch is generally required before transfusion. This requires the mixture of donor RBCs and recipient serum be incubated to 37°C (98.6°F) with the addition of antihuman globulin (Coombs reagent) to promote agglutination. Many blood banks also substitute a computer crossmatch for patients whose blood has been tested at least twice in their system. Complete crossmatch testing can take up to several hours, or even days, leading to delays in many urgent or emergent situations. If complete compatibility testing following a positive antibody screen would substantially delay transfusion of blood products to a critically ill patient, the emergency clinician may choose to bypass this step. Direct communication with the blood bank will facilitate determination of the best course of action.

Titer Testing for Whole Blood Donation. Although patients with type O blood are considered to be universal donors of packed red cells (PRBCs), whole blood from type O donors contains plasma and therefore may contain a concentration of anti-A and anti-B antibodies that can cause destruction of the recipient's type A or B RBCs. A strategy to mitigate this issue is either to transfuse only type-specific whole blood or to test donors or, more commonly, donor blood in advance to identify those with a "low titer" for anti-A and anti-B antibodies. Donors with a titer less than 256 saline dilution (immediate spin method) are designated low titer O universal whole blood (LTOWB) donors. A recent study showed LTOWB does not cause hemolysis when used in resuscitation of non–group O civilian trauma patients when up to 4 units are given.[4] LTOWB may be fresh (fresh whole blood, FWB) or stored (stored whole blood, SWB).

The use of LTOWB was standard practice in wartime settings for decades. In civilian practice in the United States, however, it has generally been unavailable and rarely used, comprising less than 1% of transfusions. More recently, interest in the use of whole blood has been growing, including the use of banked and fresh warm whole blood, despite the associated logistic hurdles.[5] In wartime settings, individuals designated as low-titer could be called upon to donate FWB acutely if needed. In the civilian setting, SWB is used on an as needed basis.

MANAGEMENT

Decision Making

Considerations in patient selection for blood product transfusion in the emergency care setting include the cause of the deficit, severity of symptoms, likelihood of ongoing hemorrhage, tissue oxygen requirements, and the patient's ability to compensate for decreased oxygen-carrying capacity. These considerations are influenced by the patient's age, underlying medical conditions, and hemodynamic stability. Clinical evaluation, including appearance (pallor, diaphoresis), mentation,

heart rate, blood pressure, and nature of the bleeding (active, controlled, uncontrolled), as well as laboratory evaluation all inform transfusion decision making.

Pharmacology

PRBCs are administered through a filter and an intravenous (IV) line or intraosseous (IO) line, along with normal saline. No other in-line solutions should be utilized, unless approved for this purpose. For example, combining calcium containing fluids, such as lactated Ringers solution, with PRBCs can cause clotting in the line as the calcium binds with the citrate which is added to the PRBCs to act as an anticoagulant. Of note, this concern for clotting was mostly established in laboratory studies, and over the last 20 years there is anesthesiology literature that suggests that this clotting is not seen in clinical practice given the rapidity of administration and the PRBC to lactated Ringers ratios used. Nonetheless, no large study has demonstrated the safety of this practice, and therefore it is not routinely recommended. Dextrose containing fluids should also be avoided because the PRBCs may take up the dextrose, which causes osmotic shifts that can lead to cell lysis. Likewise, medications should not be added or pushed through the blood component transfusion line. There is growing literature demonstrating that some medications may be compatible with PRBC administration, and local guidelines or clinical pharmacist input is prudent if medication administration is necessary through the same line as a PRBC transfusion.

Devices and Techniques

Urgent or emergent transfusion requires flow rates faster than gravity can provide. An administration set with an in-line pump that is squeezed by hand is the simplest method to speed infusion. Pressure bags and rapid infusion devices are commercially available for clinical scenarios that require infusion of units of PRBCs within a matter a minutes. With high-pressure infusion, large-bore catheters are recommended so that hemolysis is prevented, however the literature supporting this recommendation is sparse.

Whole Blood

Reports on the successful use of FWB in military field hospitals have been published. In civilian practice in the United States, however, it has generally been unavailable and rarely used. The military experience with using whole blood dates back to World War I where type-specific, crossmatched blood was used in combat. This was almost 25 years before Rh typing was developed.[5] The use of citrate phosphate dextrose (CPD) or citrate phosphate double dextrose (CP2D) can allow for safe preservation of SWB for 21 days at 1°C to 6°C. The use of citrate phosphate dextrose adenine (CPDA-1) at 1°C to 6°C can increase storage time to 35 days. Owing to time dependent degradation of clotting factors and platelets, whole blood older than 2 weeks may require the addition of fresher whole blood or supplemental platelets to avoid contributing to coagulopathy.[5]

When PRBCs, plasma, and platelet transfusions in the 1 : 1 : 1 ratio are used, the mixture is significantly more diluted than when SWB is transfused. Average hematocrit and platelet count in 1 : 1 : 1 mixtures were 29% and 90 K/μl, respectively, when compared to 35% to 38% and 150 to 200 K/μl with SWB. Coagulation factors were also higher in SWB transfusions.

Current studies show that the use of SWB results in outcomes at least as good as component (RBC + plasma + platelet) therapy in hemorrhaging patients. We recommend the use of whole blood when available. Although the shelf-life of whole blood is shorter than component therapy, it can still be cost-effective owing to the higher cost of separating blood into components. The argument for using SWB early in the resuscitation process can be summarized as follows:[4,6-9]

- SWB provides a physiologic balance of blood components that are simultaneously transfused.
- A smaller volume of anticoagulant/preservative solution is transfused with SWB.
- Platelet function in SWB may be significantly enhanced compared to component therapy.
- Higher levels of hemostatic factors are delivered with SWB.
- Fibrinogen delivery is higher when utilizing SWB, as FFP does not deliver significant amounts of fibrinogen.
- Hemolytic transfusion reaction rate in SWB is low (about 1 : 120,000), therefore transfusions are generally safe and confer fewer donor exposures compared with component therapy, such as 1 : 1 : 1 protocols.
- Administration of all components together in one unit can improve the time to complete a transfusion.
- Errors associated with transfusion of type-specific blood can be minimized.

One potential complication from the lack of Rh typing in LTOWB, is the possibility of isoimmunization causing hemolytic disease of the newborn. Premenopausal women who receive LTOWB are potential candidates for anti-D immunoglobulin (Rhogam) and consultation with obstetrics.[9]

Autotransfusion may also be used in the emergency setting in the event of severe chest trauma. A large retrospective trial showed it to be both safe and effective. Autotransfusion is the process of giving a patient back his or her own blood that has been collected from an uncontaminated active bleeding site. This is most frequently done using blood from the thorax after trauma. This strategy has numerous advantages—immediate availability, blood compatibility, elimination of donor to patient disease transmission, lower risk of circulatory overload, and fewer direct complications related to the transfusion itself, such as hyperkalemia, hypothermia, hypocalcemia, or metabolic acidosis. It is also more acceptable to patients whose religious convictions prohibit non-autologous transfusions. It is impractical in some settings owing to a relatively limited number of appropriate trauma patients, specific training required to operate the equipment, and time required for equipment setup.

Packed Red Blood Cells

PRBCs are indicated only to improve oxygen delivery to tissues at the microvascular level and thus improve intracellular oxygen consumption, yet definitive demonstration of the efficacy of red cells for this purpose (or improved clinical outcomes) has proven elusive. A definitive randomized prospective study in which RBCs are withheld completely from one treatment group is unlikely to be conducted given ethical considerations.

In 2016, the AABB (formerly, the American Association of Blood Banks), published a clinical practice guideline regarding red blood cell transfusion after reviewing trials published between 1950 and May 2016. This review found strong support for using a restrictive transfusion strategy and a hemoglobin treatment threshold of 7 g/dL for most stable hospitalized patients. In those patients undergoing orthopedic surgery, cardiac surgery, or with preexisting cardiovascular disease, they recommend a hemoglobin treatment threshold of 8 g/dL. Of note, these recommendations are less universal to patients with a history of acute coronary syndrome, severe thrombocytopenia, or chronic transfusion–dependent anemia.[10]

For many patients, the decision to transfuse RBCs requires clinical judgment. The appropriate trigger for patients with active hemorrhage, for example, is not well-established, despite numerous trials.[11] With increasing support for permissive hypotension treatment strategies, clinicians must balance adequate tissue perfusion and hemostasis. We recommend transfusion with ongoing signs of inadequate perfusion, such as elevated serum lactate level, altered mental status, or decreased urinary output. Transfusions may be stopped once a patient has a stable blood pressure, even if hypotensive, combined with signs of adequate perfusion without overt ongoing hemorrhage. Of note, the hemoglobin level in acute hemorrhage can be misleading and should not exclusively be used to guide acute management. Because the hemoglobin level is a concentration, and individuals bleed whole blood and not just red cells, it takes time for fluid to shift into the intravascular space and cause the hemoglobin level to drop. Unfortunately, the amount of time required for this equilibration to occur has not been clearly established. A recent study of trauma patients demonstrated that a hemoglobin level of 11.8 g/dL or below on arrival to the hospital was only 88% sensitive for predicting significant hemorrhage.[12]

Special Preparations of PRBCs

Washed RBCs. PRBCs can be washed to remove residual plasma and any remaining leukocytes, platelets, microaggregates, plasma proteins, and free hemoglobin. Washing reduces the titer of anti-A and anti-B antibodies, thereby permitting safer transfusion of type O PRBCs into non–type O recipients. Washed cells are used in patients who have had recurrent allergic reactions to transfusion, as most of these reactions are a response to donor proteins in the plasma. Patients with IGA deficiency from circulating anti-IGA antibodies can react to IGA in the donor plasma and may also benefit from washed cells. Washing takes about an hour and reduces the viability of the unit to 24 hours.

Leukocyte-Reduced RBCs. A typical unit of whole blood or packed red cells can contain from 1 to 3 billion white blood cells (WBC), which can cause a variety of problems in the recipient including febrile (non-hemolytic) reactions, immune sensitization, or transmission of disease. Non-leukocyte-reduced products can be a major source of viral transmission, including human T-lymphotropic virus 1 and 2, Epstein-Barr virus (EBV), and cytomegalovirus (CMV). Additionally, increased rates of bacterial contamination and postoperative or vascular line infections have been associated with the use of non-leukocyte-reduced products.

By passing the blood through a leukocyte filter, the number of WBCs can be reduced by 99.99%. This can lead to a significant reduction in complications in vulnerable populations. Leukoreduction is not effective enough, however, to prevent transfusion-associated graft-versus-host disease (TA-GvHD), thus blood transfused to susceptible patients must be irradiated. Leukocyte-reduced red cell products are now used for more than 95% of patients in the United States.

Irradiated RBCs. Blood products can be irradiated to reduce the risk for TA-GvHD in susceptible patients, which occurs in about 1 per 1 million transfusions but is associated with 90% mortality.[13] Irradiation can be performed either directly before transfusion on an individual unit or batches of irradiated PRBCs may be maintained in locations for use in the care of immunosuppressed patients. Irradiation destroys donor lymphocytes. This prevents WBCs in donor blood from recognizing the host's cells as foreign and attacking them, potentially leading to severe illness or death. Susceptible patients are those who are unable to mount an immune response to the donor lymphocytes. Although there is some variation in the literature as to who should receive irradiated PRBCs, generally the categories center on those who are immunocompromised or who have a close human leukocyte antigen (HLA) match to the donor, as occurs in the case of a directed donation. The latter group may not be able to recognize the donor cells as foreign. As a result of irradiation, post-transfusion red cell recovery is decreased and the rate of intracellular potassium release increases. PRBCs irradiated within 14 days of collection expire 28 days after

TABLE 108.1   Indications for Special Preparations of PRBCs

Special Preparation	Process	Use
Irradiated PRBCs	Irradiation of the donor blood destroys WBCs thereby decreasing the risk of transfusion-associated graft-versus-host disease.	• Neonatal or intrauterine transfusion • Hematologic malignancy • Stem cell transplant patients or donors within a week prior to cell harvesting • Hodgkin lymphoma • Directed donations from family members (biological) • Congenital cellular immune deficiency • Transfusions from HLA-matched donors • Patients treated with antithymocyte globulin or chemotherapy with purine analogs (e.g., fludarabine, bendamustine, etc.)
Washed PRBCs[14]	PRBCs are washed with saline to remove residual plasma and protein. Reduces allergic reactions to foreign proteins.	• History of severe allergic transfusion reactions • IgA-deficiency • Paroxysmal nocturnal hemoglobinuria
Leukocyte Reduced PRBCs	PRBCs are filtered to remove 99.99% of the leukocytes	• Patients undergoing chemotherapy • Multiparous females • Patients receiving multiple transfusions
CMV Negative PRBCs[15]	CMV testing is performed on units of PRBCs	• Seronegative patients who are currently pregnant • Fetal or intrauterine transfusion • Solid organ, stem cell, or bone marrow transplant recipients who are CMV negative

collection, and PRBCs irradiated more than 14 days after collection expire either 5 days after irradiation or at the original expiration date, whichever comes first.

CMV Negative Blood. Because CMV is endemic worldwide and seropositivity rates in the United States are reported at 30% to 97%, most donated blood is CMV positive. Even after an acute infection with CMV is cleared, it remains present in leukocytes. CMV testing can identify units of PRBCs that are free of the virus and safe to transfuse in at-risk populations. Leukocyte-reduced PRBCs are typically an acceptable alternative if CMV negative products are not available. Indications for CMV negative PRBCs and other special preparations are summarized in Table 108.1.

Fresh Frozen Plasma

A unit of fresh frozen plasma (FFP) contains all the clotting factors and typically has a volume of 200 to 250 mL. It must be ABO compatible and is administered through blood tubing. Triggers for FFP are not clearly defined; indications for FFP are based primarily on observational trials and expert opinion. The following indications seem reasonable based on current evidence: massive hemorrhage, as a component of a plasma exchange procedure, emergency reversal of a vitamin K antagonist in the presence of clinically significant hemorrhage or in the treatment of ace inhibitor–induced angioedema. It is worth noting, however, that the therapeutic effect is difficult to predict, and the international normalized ratio (INR) level of FFP itself is around 1.5, thus FFP can't lower an INR level below 1.5. A large volume of FFP is needed to reverse coagulopathy caused by vitamin K antagonism (at least 10 mL/kg, and perhaps as much as 30 mL/kg), which can place patients at risk for volume overload. This, in part, justifies the recommendation for prothrombin complex concentrate (PCC) over FFP when available for reversal of vitamin K antagonism in the setting of life-threatening bleeding.

Evidence from retrospective trials has supported increased use of FFP in patients anticipated to require more than 10 units of PRBCs (massive transfusion). This should not be generalized to all patients receiving a transfusion, however, as limited benefit and increased complications have been observed in patients with mild or moderate active blood loss who receive FFP.

Likewise, limited available evidence has failed to support the use of FFP in patients with an elevated INR before invasive procedures such as central line placement or lumbar puncture. The INR level itself often proves to be a poor predictor of risk for clinical bleeding. If a specific factor deficiency is identified, as in hemophilia, targeted factor replacement, if available, is preferred over FFP.

The use of FFP has also recently been described in the treatment of ace inhibitor–induced angioedema, as FFP contains c1-inhibitor and kininase II enzymes. Case reports and series suggest that the administration of 2 units of FFP may lead to significant reduction of edema within 2 to 4 hours.[16]

Platelets

The decision to transfuse platelets is multifactorial. The underlying cause of the thrombocytopenia and the age of the patient are just two factors that greatly affect transfusion recommendations. In 2015, the AABB published a clinical practice guideline concerning the general transfusion of platelets. They recommended, in most cases, transfusing adults below 10 K/μL given the risk of spontaneous hemorrhage. For patients undergoing central venous catheter placement, consideration of transfusion is recommended below 20 K/μL. Patients undergoing lumbar puncture and non-neuroaxial surgery should be considered for transfusion below 50 K/μL.[17]

Other than in the setting of massive transfusion, pediatric platelet transfusion should be discussed with a hematologist. Children with immune thrombocytopenic purpura (ITP) and no signs of active bleeding can often be managed without transfusion, even at levels below 10 K/μL.[18] If thrombotic thrombocytopenic purpura (TTP) is suspected as the cause of thrombocytopenia, platelet transfusion should be avoided. Platelet transfusion in this case may serve to exacerbate the underlying problem by adding platelet substrate for unbalanced thrombotic reactions within the vasculature. Administration of platelets in TTP is associated with increased arterial thrombosis and mortality.[19] Similarly, platelet administration is not routinely recommended in heparin-induced thrombocytopenia (HIT), though it may be beneficial in patients with significant active bleeding.[20]

Crossmatching is generally unnecessary for platelet transfusions, but Rh-negative, premenopausal women should be transfused with Rh-negative platelets because there may be enough red cells in the platelet concentrate to cause Rh sensitization. The use of leukocyte-reduced platelets has been shown to reduce the risk of HLA sensitization and is therefore beneficial in patients receiving frequent platelet transfusions. Once sensitization has occurred and patients have developed immune-mediated platelet refractoriness, various management strategies may be considered in consultation with a hematologist, including HLA-based donor selection or platelet crossmatching.

Cryoprecipitate

Cryoprecipitate is prepared from single-donor plasma by gradually thawing rapidly frozen plasma. The result of this process is the precipitation of fibrinogen, factor VIII, factor XIII, von Willebrand factor, and fibronectin. Per AABB standards, each unit (5–20 ml) of cryoprecipitate should contain at least 150 mg of fibrinogen and 80 IU of factor VIII. Because cryoprecipitate is a plasma product, ABO compatibility is necessary. Like FFP, cryoprecipitate has similar risks for both allergic and febrile reactions. It has also been associated with the development of TRALI.

Cryoprecipitate is indicated for patients with fibrinogen deficiency, congenital afibrinogenemia, or dysfibrinogenemia. Clinically, low fibrinogen levels are most often encountered in the setting of massive hemorrhage and DIC. Although not recommended as a primary treatment, cryoprecipitate can also be given to patients with hemophilia A or von Willebrand disease when recombinant factor VIII preparations are not readily available. As cryoprecipitate does not contain factor IX, it is of no value in the treatment of factor IX deficiency (hemophilia B).

Prothrombin Complex Concentrate

Both three- and four-factor PCC products are now FDA-approved in the United States, with four-factor products containing all the vitamin K–dependent clotting factors (factor II, VII, IX, and X), whereas three-factor products lack any significant amounts of factor VII. Guidelines published by the American College of Chest Physicians recommend that PCC be used for the reversal of an elevated INR level in patients with life-threatening bleeding or intracranial hemorrhage, and available evidence has shown that a more rapid normalization of the INR in these patients occurs with the administration of PCC rather than FFP. Studies comparing three- and four-factor PCCs in patients with serious warfarin-associated bleeding have found that the four-factor product is more reliable in reducing the INR to below 1.5 within 1 hour, and we recommend its use, when available.[21,22]

OUTCOMES

Safety and Effectiveness

In an average adult, 1 unit (≈450 mL) of PRBCs increases the hemoglobin level by about 1 g/dL or the hematocrit by about 3%. A similar increase in pediatric patients is observed with administration of 10 mL/kg of PRBCs. Most transfusions are given over 60 to 90 minutes. Owing to an increased risk of bacterial growth when PRBCs are exposed to room temperature, transfusion of a single unit should not last longer than 4 hours. Unused blood should be returned promptly to the blood bank. Any units unrefrigerated for more than 30 minutes should be discarded.

One unit of activity for any coagulation factor is equal to the clotting activity found in 1 mL of FFP. Appropriate dosing of FFP has not been well grounded in evidence from clinical trials. In massive transfusion,

many centers now incorporate FFP in proportion with red cells and platelets. For other indications, it seems reasonable to start with an infusion of 10 to 30 mL/kg, recognizing that results will be variable and follow-up laboratory and clinical assessment is necessary to guide further management.

Platelets are often given to adults in a dose of 6 units of platelet concentrate ("six-pack" of platelets) and in children at a dose of 1 unit per 10 kg of body weight, an amount expected to raise the platelet count by about 40 to 60 K/μl in adults or children. Administering additional platelets does not generally improve hemorrhage outcomes.[17] The AABB recommends giving either a six-pack or three-pack of platelets. Alternatively, a single apheresis unit (derived from a single donor) provides roughly the same amount of platelets as a six-pack. The advantage of apheresis platelets is that they expose the recipient to the plasma proteins of only one donor as opposed to 6 donors in a pooled unit. This, in turn, decreases the risk of allergic reactions.

Cryoprecipitate is used to correct significant hypofibrinogenemia (<100 mg/dL). A typical adult dose of around 10 bags of cryoprecipitate raises the fibrinogen level by up to 1 g/L (100 mg/dL). Cryoprecipitate can also be used in cases of post-tPA (tissue plasminogen activator) bleeding. A consensus on dosing has not been reached, though many sources recommend between 10 and 12 bags.[23]

PCC dosing is based upon the concentration of factor IX, which varies between different specific formulations. Some products also have variable dosing based upon the pretreatment INR. Consequently, emergency clinicians should consult their local protocols and pharmacists to ensure proper dosing of PCC. We also recommend that all patients with life-threatening warfarin-associated hemorrhage also receive 10 mg of vitamin K by slow IV infusion, administered at 1 mg/min or slower.

Massive Transfusion Protocols

Massive transfusion was traditionally defined as the administration of more than 10 units of PRBCs over 24 hours, but a more practical and efficacious application of the concept is the transfusion of 3 units of PRBCs over an hour or the use of 4 components over 30 minutes. The concept of utilizing a massive transfusion protocol (MTP) that called for the use of plasma and platelets along with PRBCs was born from the understanding that acute blood loss involves more than just the loss of red cells. Physiologically it makes sense to replace all components of blood after more than a few units of PRBCs have been transfused. Although protocols for MTP are variable and often predicated on institutional protocol, most now use a ratio of 1 : 1 : 1 (PRBCs : FFP : platelets) when transfusion needs exceed 3 units of PRBCs. When large and ongoing blood loss is anticipated, the initiation of a MTP should be considered.

A systematic review concluded that the available evidence could not support any definite recommendations regarding specific ratios of blood components in massive transfusion.[24] A large, multicenter randomized clinical trial compared the use in massively transfused trauma patients of a 2 : 1 : 1 ratio (PRBCs : FFP : platelets) with a 1 : 1 : 1 ratio and found no difference in mortality at 24 hours or 30 days, although fewer patients in the 1 : 1 : 1 group died of exsanguination at 24 hours.[25] Until evidence supports otherwise, we recommend a 1 : 1 : 1 ratio of blood products when a MTP is initiated.

The use of thromboelastography (TEG) or rotational thromboelastometry (ROTEM) has been studied as a way to better predict which blood components may be helpful in normalizing coagulation. While TEG/ROTEM does alter transfusion patterns, a 2015 systematic review was unable to show that TEG/ROTEM was superior to standard coagulation studies, such as prothrombin time ratio and/or the INR.[26] A subsequent study in trauma patients compared goal-directed transfusion

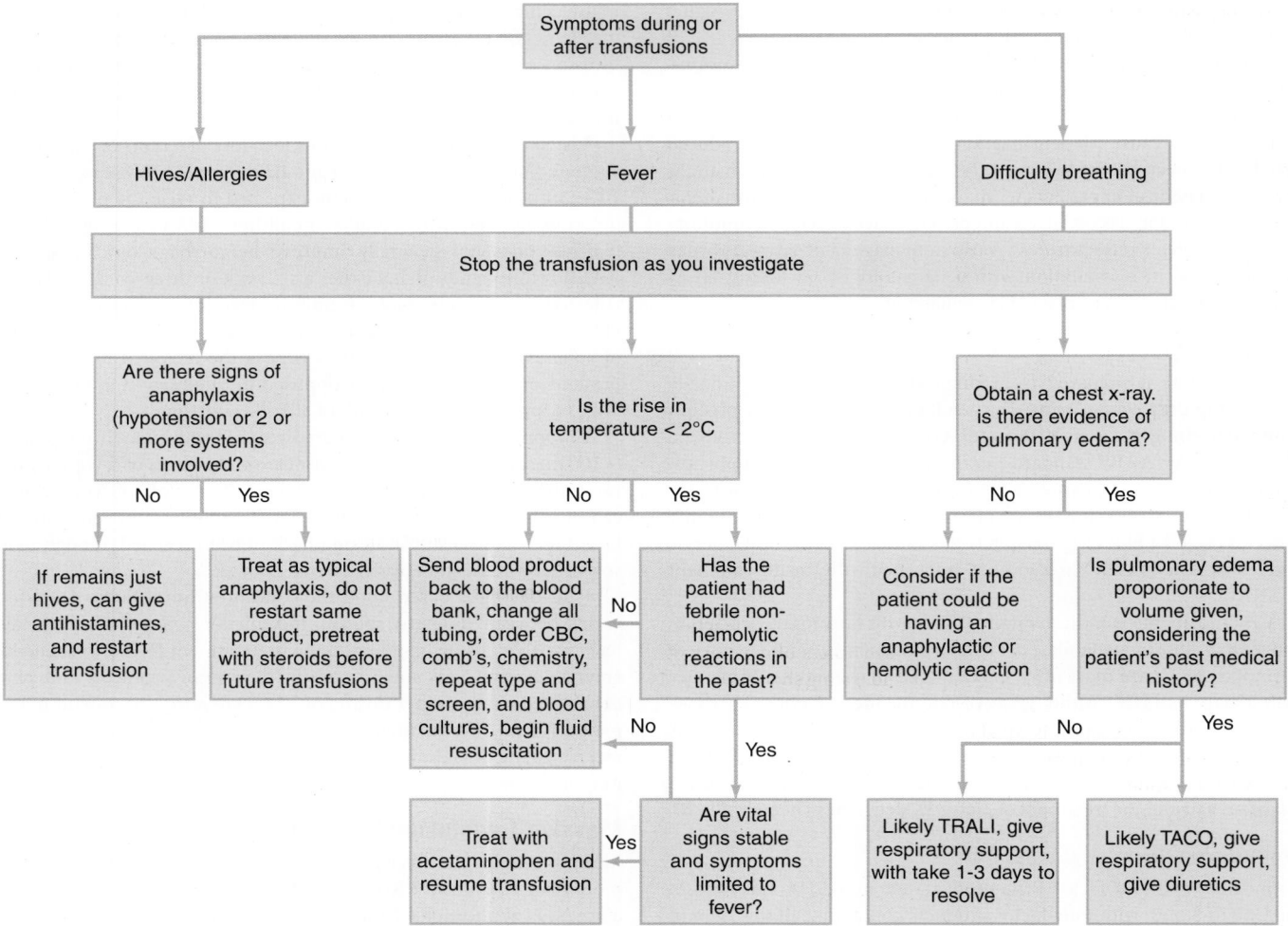

Fig. 108.2 Algorithm for treatment of transfusion reactions.

based on TEG to transfusion based on conventional coagulation parameters. In this study, the risk of death was higher in the conventional coagulation group.[27] While promising, further study is needed to clarify the role of routine TEG/ROTEM in trauma care.

Complications of massive transfusion are well-understood and many can be managed anticipatorily. Hypothermia is common and can reduce clotting factor activity. Warmed IV fluids, blood warmers, and warming lights or blankets are often needed. Frequent laboratory testing will identify electrolyte disturbances, including low magnesium and calcium levels and low or high potassium levels, which are generally treated in a standard fashion. Acidosis is a common finding with massive hemorrhage and can also be caused by hypoperfusion with or without contributions from transfused blood. Citrate from banked blood is metabolized in the liver to bicarbonate, which can result in metabolic alkalosis at times. With rapid infusion or reduced hepatic function, however, this pathway can be overwhelmed and the net effect of infusing large amounts of citrate can be worsening metabolic acidosis. A rational response to metabolic acidosis is to optimize oxygen delivery and ventilation. The benefit of administering sodium bicarbonate in this setting remains unproven and, as such, is not routinely recommended.

Complications and Adverse Effects of Nonmassive RBC Transfusion

Transfusion reactions are complications developing during or after transfusion of whole blood or individual blood components. Reactions can range from mild to life-threatening, with most acute reactions classified as mild and with upwards of 90% occurring rapidly after transfusion initiation. Delayed reactions tend to occur days to weeks after the transfusion is completed. See Figure 108.2 for a generalized and algorithmic approach to managing transfusion reactions.

Acute Transfusion Reactions

Minor Allergic. The most common manifestation of a minor allergic transfusion reaction is urticaria. In some cases, however, wheezing and angioedema can also be observed. Minor allergic reactions develop in 1% to 3% of transfusions and are generally attributed to an allergic, antibody-mediated response to donor plasma proteins. If a patient develops allergy symptoms, the transfusion should be stopped. The reaction can be treated like any other allergic reactions using antihistamines and steroids. If the reaction remains mild and is limited to the skin, the transfusion can be resumed after symptomatic treatment.

Anaphylactic. The reported incidence of transfusion-associated anaphylaxis is 1 in 20,000 to 50,000 transfusions, with most cases being idiopathic in nature. There are case reports of patients with IgA deficiency and anti-IgA antibodies developing anaphylactic reactions to IgA in donor blood, but this is not generalizable to most cases of transfusion-related anaphylaxis.

The presentation is similar to anaphylactic reactions from other causes and may include hypotension, angioedema, dyspnea, bronchospasm, or laryngospasm. The symptoms are typically rapid in onset and begin within seconds to minutes of transfusion initiation. The transfusion should be stopped immediately, with symptoms treated in the same way as other forms of anaphylaxis. If a transfusion is still required, pretreatment with steroids and antihistamines 30 to 60 minutes before the transfusion is prudent, and the patient should be given a new transfusion product, rather than restarting the original product. In addition, transfusion of washed cellular products may further decrease risk.

Febrile (Nonhemolytic) Transfusion Reaction. A febrile, nonhemolytic transfusion reaction (FNHTR) is defined as a temperature elevation of 1°C (1.8°F) or higher that occurs with transfusion and for which no other medical explanation is identified. It is often associated with rigors and chills. Reactions are believed to result from both recipient anti-leukocyte antibodies that react with donor WBCs and from cytokines released during a storage lesion (damage to and loss of some RBCs over time during storage) of the transfused unit, the latter of which increases with the duration of blood storage.[28] The use of leuko-reduction has been shown to decrease the risk of FNHTR by around 50% for RBCs and up to 93% for platelets.

If a febrile reaction occurs in a first-time transfusion, it should be treated as an acute hemolytic reaction until proven otherwise. Similarly, any vital sign instability, rise in temperature greater than 2°C, or symptoms other than fever and chills should prompt the reaction to be treated as an acute hemolytic reaction, regardless of a history of FNHTR. The transfusion should be stopped, and testing should be done to prove the reaction is non-hemolytic (see the next section for details). When a hemolytic reaction is ruled out and the event is considered to be a simple FNHTR, treatment with acetaminophen is appropriate and the unit in question should be discarded with a fresh unit transfused in its place. Many institutions routinely utilize leukocyte-reduced blood, however if this is not the case, leukocyte-reduced blood may decrease the likelihood of a recurrent reaction. If the original unit was already leukocyte-reduced, switching to a different unit may also decrease the chance of another reaction.

Pretreatment, or treatment for symptoms, with antipyretics is appropriate for patients with recurrent reactions. If a patient has a history of FNHTR, no vital sign instability, no symptoms other than fever and chills, and the rise in temperature is less than 2°C, the transfusion may be continued as normal. Antihistamines are usually not helpful in either treatment or prophylaxis for FNHTR. Patients with severe chills and rigors may also benefit from other analgesics in addition to acetaminophen, such as ibuprofen or an opiate medication. The now infrequently used opiate pain medication meperidine has been recommended for the prevention and treatment of rigors at the dose of 0.5 to 0.75 mg/kg over 4 minutes. When meperidine is not available, other opiates such as hydromorphone (0.015 mg/kg IV) or fentanyl (0.5 to 0.75 mcg/kg IV) can be used.

Acute Hemolytic Transfusion Reaction. Intravascular hemolytic transfusion reaction is the most serious transfusion reaction. It generally results from ABO incompatibility, usually caused by a clerical or laboratory error. The incidence of acute hemolytic transfusion reactions ranges from 2 to 8 per 100,000 units transfused with a fatality rate of 1 per 100,000 units transfused. When incompatible blood is given, the impact may range widely from asymptomatic to death. While mortality from hemolytic reactions increases in proportion to the amount of blood transfused, as little as 30 ml can be fatal.

In an ABO incompatibility, the recipient's serum has preformed antibodies directed against the donor RBCs. The donor cells will begin to hemolyze within seconds or minutes. In most cases, donor blood is agglutinated (clumped and stuck together) and then hemolyzed. Vasoactive substances released by responding macrophages may cause fever, chills, hypotension, and shock.

BOX 108.1 Laboratory Abnormalities in Acute Hemolytic Transfusion Reactions

- Decrease in hemoglobin or hematocrit
- Hemoglobinemia
- Hemoglobinuria
- Increased serum lactate dehydrogenase (LDH)
- Increased serum indirect bilirubin
- Decreased serum haptoglobin
- Evidence of DIC, including: prolonged PT, PTT, decreased fibrinogen level, increased D-dimer
- Schistocytes or spherocytes on peripheral smear

BOX 108.2 The National Healthcare Safety Network Hemovigilance Surveillance Protocol Definition of TRALI

- No evidence of acute lung injury before transfusion, AND
- Acute lung injury onset during or within 6 hours of cessation of transfusion, AND
- Hypoxemia defined as either $Pao_2/Fi o_2$ less than or equal to 300 mm Hg or oxygen saturation less than 90% on room air, AND
- Radiographic evidence of bilateral infiltrates, AND
- No evidence of left atrial hypertension (i.e., circulatory overload).

(Adapted from Centers for Disease Control and Prevention (CDC). National Healthcare Safety Network Biovigilance Component Hemovigilance Module Surveillance Protocol. Available at: https://www.cdc.gov/nhsn/pdfs/biovigilance/bv-hv-protocol-current.pdf. Accessed May 10 2021.)

The onset of symptoms is usually immediate but can take up to 24 hours to fully manifest. Fevers and rigors are an early indication of an AHTR. Patients may also complain of headache, nausea, vomiting, sensation of chest restriction, severe joint or low back pain, burning sensation at the site of the infusion, or a feeling of impending doom.

Treatment includes immediate cessation of the transfusion, replacement of all blood administration tubing, and initiation of vigorous crystalloid fluid therapy. The use of vasopressors or diuretics may also be considered in order to maintain a urine output of 1 to 2 mL/kg/hr. Blood and urine specimens, as well as the remainder of the transfusion and blood tubing, should be sent for laboratory testing. The diagnosis can be confirmed by detection of free hemoglobin in blood or urine and a positive result of Coombs test on posttransfusion, but not pretransfusion, specimens. See Box 108.1 for associated laboratory abnormalities in AHTR.

Recipient blood should be sent for a direct antiglobulin test (DAT), plasma-free hemoglobin level, CBC, chemistry, haptoglobin, LDH, bilirubin, PT/PTT, D-dimer, fibrinogen, and a repeat type and crossmatch. Urine should be tested for free hemoglobin. In cases of severe intravascular hemolysis, the urine and/or plasma can become pink or dark brown in color from the free hemoglobin. Dialysis is occasionally required for either severe hyperkalemia as a direct result of the hemolysis or renal failure as a result of DIC.

Transfusion-Related Acute Lung Injury. TRALI refers to noncardiogenic pulmonary edema occurring during or shortly after the transfusion of virtually any blood products. See Box 108.2 for the definition and diagnostic criteria of TRALI. Although TRALI has been traditionally associated more with platelet and plasma transfusion, the increased use of PRBCs relative to other components seems to have

TABLE 108.2   Acute Transfusion Reactions

Condition	Notes	Clinical Findings	Laboratory Findings
TACO	Proportional to volume transfused. Onset 6–12 hours after transfusion started.	Evidence of volume overload with dyspnea, edema, rales, tachycardia, hypertension	Elevated BNP level, pulmonary edema on chest x-ray
TRALI	Not associated with volume of transfusion	Hypotension, fever, hypoxia	pulmonary edema on chest x-ray
Anaphylaxis	Not associated with volume of transfusion	Hypotension, tachycardia, urticaria, wheezing	None specific
Hemolysis	Not necessarily associated with volume transfused though generally worse with increased amounts of incompatible blood	Fever, chills, hypotension, bleeding (DIC), back pain, discoloration of urine	Evidence of hemolysis (increased LDH, decreased haptoglobin, schistocytes) Evidence of DIC (prolonged PT/PTT, low platelets, decreased fibrinogen, elevated D-dimer, schistocytes)
FNHTR	Associated with fever	Fever	None specific, lack of evidence of hemolysis

TACO, Transfusion-associated circulatory overload; *TRALI*, transfusion-related acute lung injury; *FNHTR*, febrile non-hemolytic transfusion reaction; *DIC*, disseminated intravascular coagulation.

balanced the risk as similar across different blood products. Owing to strategies designed to mitigate TRALI, the incidence has decreased significantly in recent years. Nonfatal TRALI occurs in about 1 in 60,000 transfusions, but it still accounts for 29% of transfusion-related deaths.

A proposed mechanism for the development of TRALI includes a reaction between transfused antibodies and leukocytes in the recipient, as well as the effects of biologically active factors that accumulate in stored blood, including cytokines and lipids. Another proposed mechanism involves the alloimmunization of plasma from female donors. During a prior pregnancy the donor may have produced IgG antibodies against the paternally inherited antigens in the fetus. These antibodies can persist and be transfused into the recipient contributing to the TRALI reaction. This issue seems to become relevant when high-volume plasma transfusion is used. The ultimate effect is an increase in pulmonary capillary permeability leading to leakage of high protein fluid into the alveoli. Clinical effects can include noncardiogenic pulmonary edema, with dyspnea, hypoxemia, or bilateral infiltrates on the chest radiograph. Fever, hypotension, and transient leukopenia may also be seen.

If TRALI is suspected, the transfusion should be stopped, and the blood bank notified. Respiratory support should be provided, which may include noninvasive positive-pressure ventilation (NIPPV) or intubation and mechanical ventilation. It is safe to continue transfusion of blood products from a different donor. Complete resolution is usually seen within 48 to 96 hours. The overall prognosis is better than would be expected with many other causes of acute lung injury, with a reported mortality rate of 6% in one series. One strategy suggested for reducing TRALI has been to use only male donors for plasma to avoid allotypic leukocyte antibodies or to screen for these antibodies and exclude donors when the antibodies are found.

Transfusion Associated Circulatory Overload. Transfusion associated circulatory overload (TACO) is volume overload after transfusion that is proportional to the volume transfused. Smaller volume transfusions, such as cryoprecipitate, are less likely to produce an overload state than FFP or PRBCs. Risk factors for developing TACO include preexisting heart disease (e.g., CHF), significant renal insufficiency, and extremes of age. A recent animal model suggested a two-hit hypothesis for the development of TACO. The first hit is volume incompliance and the second hit is the composition of the fluid given (PRBCs versus crystalloid solutions). A preexisting volume incompliance (myocardial infarction [MI] or acute kidney injury) confers a significant and clinically relevant difference in left ventricular end-diastolic pressure (LVEDP), heart rate, and blood pressure in

animals receiving PRBCs (the second hit) as opposed to equal volumes of lactated Ringers solution. This difference was not noted in animals without the first hit in whom equal volumes of PRBCs and lactated Ringers solution were given.[30] This appears to explain similar findings in humans with heart and kidney disease.

TACO appears to develop in about 1% of transfused patients, however this number may underestimate the true incidence since many cases spontaneously resolve with diuresis.[31] There is no specific test or single criteria to definitively diagnose TACO. It should be considered in patients who develop shortness of breath, hypertension, tachycardia, and other signs of volume overload. It is also important to distinguish TACO from immune-mediated conditions such as TRALI, allergic reactions or other conditions causing shortness of breath (e.g., pulmonary embolism, MI). Some clinical clues to help differentiate TACO from other causes can be seen in Table 108.2.

Management of TACO is similar to other causes of volume overload. The transfusion (if ongoing) should be stopped. Diuretics should be given. Theoretically, nitroglycerine would have similar effect in TACO as in any other volume overload situation and can be started at 50 to 100 mcg/min IV and titrated to effect. NIPPV can be initiated early to improve oxygenation and the work of breathing. If the patient develops intractable symptoms, intubation and mechanical ventilation may be required. In future transfusions, the rate of transfusion may be slowed, and prophylactic diuretics can be given to decrease the risk of another episode of TACO.

Infectious Complications of Transfusions

Though rare, transmission of infectious diseases is the transfusion-related complication most feared by the lay public. Transmission of a wide variety of infectious diseases has been reported, but modern screening methods, of both donors and the blood itself, have sharply reduced the frequency of transmission. The risks of transmission of viral infections such as HIV, hepatitis B, and hepatitis C are all well below 1 in a million. Concerns for bacterial infections prompted the practice of completing transfusions within 4 hours and returning unused blood products to the blood bank only if they have been unrefrigerated for less than 30 minutes.

In a recent study, bacterial culture positive transfusion reactions (BCPTRs) were defined as a positive bacterial culture result from the transfused blood product, from the recipient, or from both the blood product and the recipient. A septic transfusion reaction (STR) was further distinguished as a BCPTR that met definitive CDC hemovigilance criteria with absolute "imputability" and matching culture results from both the donor unit and the patient's blood culture.[32] Over an 8-year period the study recorded 688,514 transfusions (52%, PRBCs, 23% apheresis platelets, 18% plasma, and 8% cryoprecipitate) and identified a total of 15 BCPTRs (0.002%). Further, only half of these met the more strict STR definition. A majority of the infectious cases resulted from platelet transfusions.[32]

Although a relatively rare occurrence, STR should be at least considered in any patient who develops a fever during a transfusion when it does not improve after cessation of the transfusion and the use of antipyretics.[33] The AABB developed criteria for consideration of STR which included a temperature of 38°C or higher and a 1°C rise above pretransfusion temperature in conjunction with associated symptoms such as rigors, nausea/vomiting, dyspnea, hypotension, or shock. They also used isolated hypotension or shock (and/or cardiovascular collapse) irrespective of fever as reasons to investigate for STR.

The Biomedical Excellence for Safer Transfusion (BEST) Collaborative found an increased sensitivity for detecting an STR with modification of the AABB criteria to include isolated high fever (>39°C) and a greater than 1°C rise above pretransfusion temperature irrespective of the presence of associated symptoms. In addition, they used predefined vital sign criteria to indicate hypotension (SBP < 90 mm Hg/DBP < 60 mm Hg or a 15% decrease from baseline) and tachycardia (HR > 100 or a 15% increase from pretransfusion baseline). Finally, they took into account the use of pretransfusion use of antipyretics which could blunt fever response.[34]

When an STR is suspected the transfusion should be paused and a culture of the transfusion unit and a blood culture from the patient are indicated.

Delayed Transfusion Reactions

Delayed Hemolytic Transfusion Reaction. A delayed hemolytic transfusion reaction (DHTR) typically occurs 3 to 10 days following transfusion with blood that initially appeared to be compatible. This can result from a non–ABO-mediated immune response, usually caused by an anamnestic response in a patient previously sensitized to red cell minor antigens through transfusion, pregnancy, or transplantation. Decreased survival of transfused red cells develops as a result of extravascular hemolysis. A related phenomenon termed delayed serologic transfusion reaction (DSTR) can develop when anamnestic antibodies are detected but there is no evidence of hemolysis. Together DSTR and DHTR occur in about 1 in 1500 transfusions, with the former occurring about four times more frequently than the latter.

Clinical effects can include fever, anemia, or jaundice. Symptoms are usually mild, though rarely significant complications such as oliguria or DIC can occur. Hemoglobinemia and hemoglobinuria are generally absent. Treatment is primarily supportive and the blood bank should be notified.

Transfusion-Associated Graft-versus-Host Disease. This rare but typically fatal complication results when transfused lymphocytes proliferate and attack a recipient who is incapable of mounting an immune response to the transfused cells.

Cell-mediated immunodeficiency places patients at risk, as does having an HLA type that is similar (sharing some but not all of the HLA antigens) between donor and recipient (most often seen among first-degree relatives).

Symptoms begin 3 to 30 days after transfusion and include fever, erythematous skin rash, diarrhea, elevated liver enzyme levels, and pancytopenia. Mortality is greater than 95%.

Efforts are directed at prevention through the use of gamma irradiation of cellular components, which renders the donor lymphocytes incapable of proliferating. The use of leukocyte-reduced components is not sufficient to prevent TA-GvHD. This condition should be kept in mind when transfusion is being considered for high-risk patients, including:

- Congenital immunodeficiency
- Hematologic malignancy (Hodgkin disease)
- Stem cell transplantation
- Treatment with purine analogues (e.g., fludarabine)
- Directed donor products from a close relative

Discussion with a hematologist is prudent when deciding whether to use irradiated cellular components in these high-risk groups.

Treatment is palliative and aims to restore the recipient's immune function. It is largely unsuccessful.[35]

Post-transfusion Purpura. Rarely, profound thrombocytopenia can develop 1 to 3 weeks after a transfusion associated with an antibody response to a platelet antigen. Eventually, this low-affinity antibody is eliminated, and the thrombocytopenia resolves spontaneously. Patients at risk for bleeding or with active hemorrhage are considered for treatment with high-dose immune globulin, plasmapheresis, or platelet transfusion.

The references for this chapter can be found online at ExpertConsult. com.

109

Anemia and Polycythemia

Meagan B. Verbillion and Alan A. Dupré

KEY CONCEPTS

- Anemia is caused by three basic mechanisms: loss of red blood cells (RBCs) through bleeding, destruction of RBCs, or decrease in production of RBCs.
- RBC indices along with a peripheral blood smear can help determine the mechanism of anemia.
- Anemia in the elderly often occurs as an exacerbation of pre-existing comorbid diseases.
- Anemia of uncertain etiology should be thoroughly evaluated. If the patient has no adverse hemodynamic consequences, the evaluation can proceed on an outpatient basis or management initiated in an observation setting until the patient is stable.
- Patients with sickle cell disease should be considered to have an acute pain crisis and treated appropriately until proven otherwise.
- Acute chest syndrome is one of the most common causes of death in sickle cell disease and presents with fever, dyspnea, cough, and a new infiltrate on chest radiograph.
- Transfusion therapy is most useful in sickle cell disease associated with acute stroke, acute chest syndrome, or splenic sequestration.
- Primary polycythemia vera is treated with serial phlebotomy to a goal hematocrit of less than 45%.

ANEMIA

Foundations

Background and Importance

Anemia affects a third of the global population and accounted for the primary hospital discharge diagnosis in approximately 188,000 emergency department (ED) visits in 2014 as reported by the Centers for Disease Control (CDC).[1] Anemia is an absolute decrease in the number of circulating red blood cells (RBCs). The diagnosis is made when laboratory measurements fall below accepted normal values (Table 109.1).

Anemia is divided into two broad categories: emergent, having immediate life-threatening complications, and typically secondary to acute blood loss; and non-emergent, with less imminent danger to the patient and many times can be further evaluated on an outpatient basis. Factors other than the absolute number of circulating RBCs may place the patient in one category or another (e.g., rate of onset and underlying hemodynamic reserve of the patient). Both groups necessitate a sound diagnostic approach, though emergent anemia may require immediate supportive therapy concomitant with or in advance of the definitive diagnosis. Although patients with non-emergent anemia are usually referred to a specialist, the urgency of consultation depends predominantly on the patient's hemodynamic tolerance of the anemia.

Anatomy, Physiology, and Pathophysiology

Understanding anemia starts with the structure and function of the RBC. RBCs are primarily composed of hemoglobin, which has a quaternary structure containing 4 heme polypeptide subunits bound to an iron molecule that is contained in the center of a porphyrin ring. The major function of the RBC is oxygen transport from the lung to the tissue, and carbon dioxide transport in the reverse direction. Oxygen transport is influenced by the amount of hemoglobin and its oxygen affinity, as well as blood flow. An alteration in any of these major components usually results in compensatory changes in the other two. For example, a decrease in hemoglobin is compensated for by both inotropic and chronotropic cardiac changes that result in increased blood flow and decreased hemoglobin affinity at the tissue level, thereby allowing more oxygen release. Due to disease severity or underlying pathologic conditions, these compensatory responses may fail, resulting in tissue hypoxia and cell death.

Anemia stimulates the compensatory mechanism of erythropoiesis controlled by the hormone erythropoietin, which is a glycoprotein produced in the kidney (90%) and liver (10%). It regulates the production of RBCs by controlling differentiation of committed erythroid stem cells and is stimulated by tissue hypoxia or products of RBC destruction during hemolysis. Elevated in many types of anemia, erythropoietin enhances the growth and differentiation of erythroid progenitors.

Bone marrow contains pluripotent stem cells that can differentiate into erythroid, myeloid, megakaryocytic, or lymphoid progenitors. When the late normoblast extrudes its nucleus, it still contains a ribosomal network, which identifies the reticulocyte. The reticulocyte retains its ribosomal network for approximately 4 days, 3 days of which are spent in bone marrow and 1 day in the peripheral circulation. The RBC matures as the reticulocyte loses its ribosomal network and becomes an erythrocyte which circulates for 110 to 120 days in the peripheral circulation. Erythrocytes are anucleate, flexible, biconcave discs. The erythrocyte is scavenged and removed by macrophages that detect senescent signals. Under steady-state conditions, RBC mass remains constant as an equal number of reticulocytes replace the destroyed, senescent erythrocytes.[2]

The most common cause of emergent anemia is acute blood loss. Common sites of blood loss in the trauma patient include pleural, peritoneal, pelvic, long bone (e.g., thigh), and retroperitoneal spaces. In non-traumatic circumstances, especially in patients receiving anticoagulants, the gastrointestinal tract, retroperitoneal space, uterus, or adnexa need to be considered. Certain hemolytic conditions, such as disseminated intravascular coagulopathy (DIC), can also cause rapid intravascular destruction of RBCs leading to emergent anemia (Box 109.1).

Non-emergent anemias can be subdivided into microcytic, normocytic, and macrocytic based on the mean corpuscular volume (MCV), which measures size and volume of the RBC. Microcytic anemias are caused by low iron production, gene mutations, toxins (e.g., lead poisoning), or defective heme synthesis. Normocytic anemias can be caused by primary or secondary bone marrow failure and can

TABLE 109.1 Hemogram Normal Values

Age	Hemoglobin (g/dL)	Hematocrit (%)	Red Blood Cell Count (×10⁶)
3 Months	10.4–12.2	30–36	3.4–4.0
3–7 years	11.7–13.5	34–40	4.4–5.0
Adult man	14.0–18.0	40–52	4.4–5.9
Adult woman	12.0–16.0	35–47	3.8–5.2

BOX 109.1 Causes of Rapid Intravascular Red Blood Cell Destruction

Mechanical hemolysis associated with disseminated intravascular coagulation
Massive burns
Toxins (e.g., some poisonous venoms: brown recluse spider, cobra)
Infections such as malaria or *Clostridium* sepsis
Severe glucose-6-phosphate dehydrogenase (G6PD) deficiency with exposure to oxidant stress
ABO incompatibility transfusion reaction
Cold agglutinin hemolysis (e.g., *Mycoplasma* organisms, infectious mononucleosis)
Paroxysmal nocturnal hemoglobinuria exacerbated by transfusion
Immune complex hemolysis (e.g., quinidine)

be further subdivided into hemolytic and non-hemolytic. Anemia of chronic disease is the most common non-hemolytic anemia, caused by an inflammatory response to underlying disease states. Hemolytic anemias are either intrinsic or extrinsic in nature. Intrinsic hemolytic anemias are typically caused by underlying genetic mutations or enzyme deficiencies (e.g., sickle cell disease) that lead to abnormal RBC production. Extrinsic hemolytic anemias result from defects outside of the RBC (e.g., DIC). Macrocytic anemias are caused primarily by nutritional deficiencies such as folate or vitamin B_{12}, as well as various disease states (e.g., alcoholism) that retard the maturation of the RBC.

Clinical Features

The clinical manifestation of anemia depends on how rapidly the hematocrit falls and on the patient's ability to compensate for the loss. Clinical signs and symptoms of acute blood loss include tachycardia, hypotension, orthostasis, lightheadedness, dyspnea, pallor, or tachypnea. Complaints of thirst, altered mental status, or decreased urine output may also be present. The patient's age, concomitant illness, and underlying comorbidities can tremendously influence the presenting clinical findings. Children and young adults may tolerate significant blood loss with largely unaltered vital signs, preceding a precipitant hypotensive episode. Elderly patients commonly have underlying disease states that compromise their ability to compensate for blood loss, which can lead to the earlier vital sign alterations and a higher potential for rapid clinical deterioration.[3] Pertinent elements of the history and physical examination of patients with acute anemia are listed in Box 109.2.

In contrast, nonemergent anemias are usually seen in ambulatory patients complaining of fatigue and weakness, irritability, headache, postural dizziness, angina, decreased exercise tolerance, shortness of breath, or decreased libido. The history and physical examination is typically paramount in helping to identify the cause of anemia (Box 109.3). The rate of loss of hemoglobin also dictates symptom onset. When anemia is slow in onset, the patient may compensate well until the hemoglobin is very low, at which point symptoms worsen or vital sign changes occur. Most of these patients do not need immediate stabilization and can be further evaluated in the outpatient setting.

BOX 109.2 History and Physical Examination for Clinically Severe Anemia

History
General
Out-of-hospital status, therapy, response to therapy
Bleeding diathesis
Previous blood transfusion
Underlying diseases, including allergies
Current medications, especially those causing platelet inhibition
Trauma: Nature and Time of Injury, Blood Loss at Scene
Nontrauma
Skin: Petechiae, ecchymoses
Gastrointestinal: Hematemesis, hematochezia, melena, peptic ulcer
Genitourinary: Last menstruation, menorrhagia, metrorrhagia, hematuria

Physical Examination
Vital Signs Measured Serially
Blood pressure, pulse, respiratory rate, oxygen saturation
Level and content of consciousness
Skin: pallor, diaphoresis, jaundice, cyanosis, purpura, ecchymoses, petechiae
Cardiovascular: Murmurs, S_3, S_4, quality of femoral and carotid pulses
Abdomen: Hepatosplenomegaly, pain, guarding, rebound on palpation, stool hemoglobin testing

BOX 109.3 History and Physical Examination for Nonemergent Anemia

History
Symptoms of Anemia
Chest pain, decreased exercise tolerance, dyspnea
Weakness, fatigue, dizziness, syncope

Bleeding Diathesis
Bleeding after trauma, injections, tooth extractions
Spontaneous bleeding, such as epistaxis, menorrhagia
Spontaneous purpura and petechiae

Sites of Blood Loss
Respiratory: Epistaxis, hemoptysis
Gastrointestinal: Hematemesis, hematochezia, melena
Genitourinary: Abnormal menses, pregnancies, hematuria
Skin: Petechiae, ecchymoses
Intermittent jaundice, dark urine
Dietary history: Vegetarianism, poor nutrition
Drug use and toxin exposure, including alcohol
Racial background, family history
Underlying disease
    Uremia, liver disease, hypothyroidism
    Chronic disease states, such as cancer, rheumatic or renal disease
    Previous surgery

Physical Examination
Skin: Pallor, Purpura, petechiae, angiomas, ulcerations
Eye: Conjunctival jaundice, pallor
Oral: tongue atrophy, papillary soreness
Cardiopulmonary: Heart size, murmurs, extra cardiac sounds, rales indicating pulmonary edema
Abdomen: Hepatomegaly, splenomegaly, ascites, masses
Lymph nodes
    Neurologic: Altered positions or vibratory sense, ataxia, peripheral neuritis
    Rectal and pelvic: masses

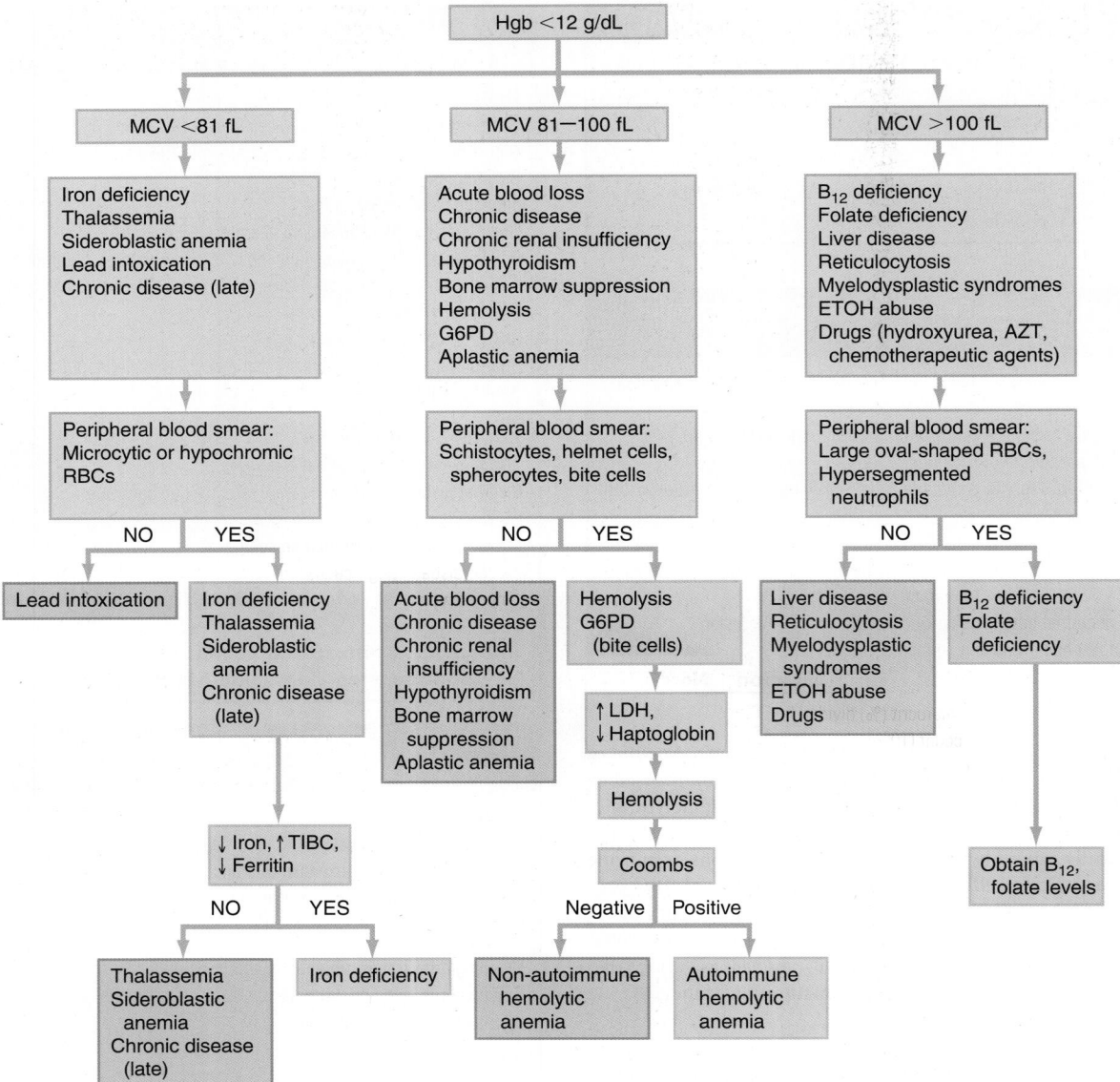

Fig. 109.1 Algorithm for the Evaluation of Anemia. *AZT,* Azathioprine; *ETOH,* ethanol; *fL,* femtoliter; *G6PD,* glucose-6-phosphate dehydrogenase; *Hgb,* hemoglobin; *LDH,* lactate dehydrogenase; *MCV,* mean corpuscular volume; *RBCs,* red blood cells; *TIBC,* total iron-binding capacity.

Differential Diagnoses

The differential diagnosis of anemia is facilitated by classification of the anemia into one of three groups: decreased RBC production, increased RBC destruction, and blood loss. A complementary approach uses RBC morphology and indices. Fig. 109.1 presents an algorithm for the evaluation of anemia.

Diagnostic Testing

In a patient suspected of acute blood loss, the following initial laboratory tests may be helpful, depending on clinical circumstances:
- Complete blood count and peripheral smear
- Blood sample for type and crossmatch
- Prothrombin time and international normalized ratio
- Partial thromboplastin time
- Serum electrolyte levels
- Glucose level (particularly if the patient has altered consciousness)

- Creatinine level
- Urinalysis for free hemoglobin

Obtaining a hemoglobin and hematocrit in the emergency department (ED) is useful for determining a baseline even though it may not be reflective of the true degree of blood loss for many hours. Depending on severity, a blood sample should be sent for type and crossmatch.

The initial laboratory evaluation for a patient with non-emergent anemia also includes a complete blood count with leukocyte differential, reticulocyte count, peripheral smear (Fig. 109.2), as well as RBC indices, including MCV, mean corpuscular hemoglobin (MCH), and mean corpuscular hemoglobin concentration (MCHC). RBC indices are useful in classifying anemias caused by a production deficit (Table 109.2). MCV is a measure of RBC size and volume; decreases or increases reflect microcytosis and macrocytosis, respectively. MCH incorporates both RBC size and hemoglobin concentration. It is influenced by both and is rarely helpful in the ED setting. The MCHC index

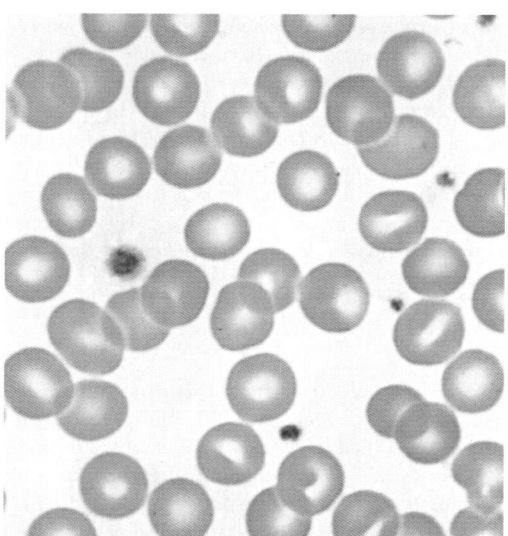

Fig. 109.2 Normal Smear. (From Hoffbrand AV, Pettite JE. *Color Atlas of Clinical Hematology.* 3rd ed. London: Mosby; 2000:22.)

TABLE 109.2 Calculation of Red Blood Cell Indices and Normal Values

Index	Formula for Calculation	Normal
Mean corpuscular volume	Hematocrit (%) divided by RBC count ($10^6/\mu L$)	81–100 fL
Mean corpuscular hemoglobin	Hemoglobin (g/dL) divided by RBC count ($10^6/\mu L$)	26–34 pg
Mean corpuscular hemoglobin concentration	Hemoglobin (g/dL) divided by hematocrit (%)	31%–36%

fL, Femtoliter; *RBC,* red blood cell; *pg,* picograms.

is a measure of the concentration of hemoglobin. Low values represent hypochromia, whereas high values are noted in patients with decreased cell membrane relative to cell volume, such as in the case of spherocytosis. An additional index is the RBC distribution width (RDW), a measure of RBC homogenicity. RDW is automatically calculated as the standard deviation of MCV divided by MCV multiplied by 100. A normal RDW is 13.5 ± 1.5%. The RDW is elevated in anemias caused by nutritional deficiencies; however, it is not specific for any abnormality.

Measurements of coagulation status, serum electrolytes, glucose, blood urea nitrogen, and creatinine are useful in the diagnosis of underlying disease processes that may relate to the patient's anemia. When the cause of anemia is unknown and the patient requires transfusion, consider ordering folate, vitamin B12, iron, total iron-binding capacity (TIBC), reticulocytes, and direct antiglobulin (Coombs test) pretreatment. Post-transfusion, these levels will be unreliable and could mask an underlying diagnosis.

Management
Stabilization of emergent anemia commonly runs in parallel with assessment. If the signs and symptoms suggest potential life-threatening conditions, multiple large bore intravenous lines are placed in preparation for resuscitation and transfusion.

Disposition
Criteria for the admission of patients with non-emergent anemia are shown in Box 109.4.

ANEMIAS DUE TO DECREASED RED BLOOD CELL PRODUCTION

Foundations
Anemias caused by decreased RBC production are insidious in onset and are associated with a decreased reticulocyte count. A subclassification by indices of anemias caused by decreased RBC production is listed in Box 109.5. RBC indices and a peripheral smear are useful in securing the diagnosis, although a definitive diagnosis may require more extensive outpatient work up including a bone marrow examination. Replacement of iron, vitamin B12, or folate by the emergency clinician without proof of cause is generally unnecessary and not routinely recommended.

Hypochromic microcytic anemias are subdivided into deficiencies of the three building blocks of hemoglobin: iron (iron deficiency anemia; Fig. 109.3), globin (thalassemia), and porphyrin (sideroblastic anemia and lead poisoning). Anemia of chronic disease, a secondary iron abnormality, is also included on the differential and can be microcytic or normocytic.[2]

Iron Deficiency Anemia
Foundations
Iron deficiency is a frequent cause of chronic anemia seen in the ED. It is the most common cause of anemia globally.[4] It is defined by microcytic,

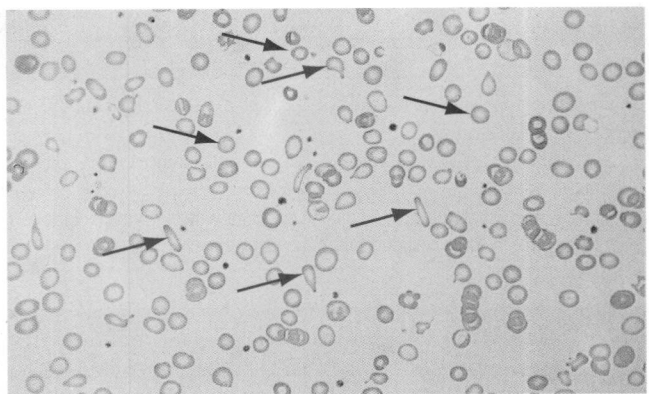

Fig. 109.3 Iron Deficiency Anemia With Hypochromic, Microcytic Cells and Poikilocytes (Abnormally Shaped Cells). (From Hoffbrand AV, Pettite JE. *Color Atlas of Clinical Hematology.* 3rd ed. London: Mosby; 2000:44.)

hypochromic RBC. Iron deficiency can either be absolute or functional. Absolute iron deficiency reflects low or exhausted total body iron stores, while functional iron deficiency is caused by inadequate iron supply to the bone marrow.[5] Iron is a critical component needed for effective erythropoiesis, and also essential for mitochondrial function, DNA synthesis, and cellular enzymatic reactions. Dietary iron is absorbed in the duodenum, thus nutritional deficiency or malabsorption syndromes can be a cause of iron deficiency anemia.[2] Occult blood loss should always be excluded in the setting of iron deficiency anemia. This is common in older patients, especially with gastrointestinal blood loss, as well as in menstruating women. Changes in RBC size, number, and hemoglobin content occur only after bone marrow and cytochrome iron stores are depleted; therefore, a patient may have early symptoms of iron deficiency (e.g., fatigue) without anemia. These non-hematologic symptoms are the result of impaired muscle-tissue oxidative capacity and decreased activity of iron-containing enzymes in the setting of iron deficiency.

Clinical Features

Most anemias secondary to iron deficiency are non-emergent in nature. The symptoms related to anemia are secondary to the body's ability to adapt to the low hemoglobin levels over time, and the eventual inability of the tissues to receive adequate oxygen for metabolic demands.

Diagnostic Testing

The diagnosis is made by laboratory evaluation of the fasting level of serum iron, serum ferritin, and TIBC. The laboratory interpretation and pitfalls are outlined in Table 109.3. A concentrated search for occult blood loss remains an important component of the evaluation.

Management

Therapy consists of oral iron replacement. A cost-effective form is ferrous sulfate. The dosage is 325 mg PO for adults (65 mg of elemental iron) three times daily, or 2 mg/kg/day of elemental iron orally for children.[5] This medication is generally well tolerated, although it may cause nausea, vomiting, or constipation. Ascorbic acid can improve the bioavailability of iron and is recommended in conjunction with iron replacement, although it can increase the frequency of side effects. Patients should be warned that iron frequently leads to black stools, and that bleeding from the digestive tract can also be manifested as black stool. In patients with poor oral tolerance or absorption, parenteral iron therapy may be necessary. Parenteral iron replenishes iron stores more effectively than oral replacement in CKD, inflammatory bowel disease, and in the post-partum period.[5,6]

The patient may experience a sense of improvement in as few as 24 hours after initiating replacement therapy. Reticulocytosis appears during a 3- to 4-day period in children, but may take more than 1 week in adults, with complete repletion of iron stores in approximately 3 to 6 months.[4] The hemoglobin concentration rises on a similar schedule. Failures of iron replacement therapy can occur due to a variety of causes, including patient noncompliance with iron supplementation, insufficient replacement, incorrect diagnosis, or presence of an additional process complicating the iron deficiency, such as anemia of chronic disease.

Thalassemia

Foundations

The hemoglobin molecule is present as two-paired globin chains. Each type of hemoglobin is made up of different globins. Normal adult hemoglobin (HbA) is made up of two alpha chains and two beta chains ($\alpha_2\beta_2$). HbA2 is a variant of hemoglobin A that contains two alpha and two delta chains ($\alpha_2\delta_2$). Fetal hemoglobin (HbF) contains two alpha and two gamma chains ($\alpha_2\gamma_2$). A separate autosomal gene controls each globin chain.

Pathophysiology

Thalassemia is a genetic autosomal recessive disorder reflected by the decreased synthesis of and abnormal structure of globin chains. Deletions in these globin genes result in an absence or decreased function of the messenger RNA that codes for particular globins. The various globins (α, β, δ, and γ) may be affected by a number of genetic combinations. Decreased globin production in thalassemia precipitates the formation of reactive oxygen species leading to apoptosis of erythroblasts, decreased hemoglobin synthesis, and ineffective erythropoiesis, leading to hemolytic anemia.[7] Beta thalassemia is associated with reduced or absent beta-globin synthesis and an excess of alpha-globins, leading to the formation of alpha-globin tetramers. Alpha thalassemia results in an excess of β-globins and the formation of β-globin tetramers termed *hemoglobin H*. The abnormal formation of hemoglobin at various concentrations results in complications, including red cell membrane breakage and hemolysis. A common method of classification is by phenotype. Beta thalassemias are broken down into silent (carrier), minor, intermedia, and major variants. Alpha thalassemias include silent (carrier), alpha thalassemia trait, HbH, and Hb Barts. This historical classification method is now being replaced by a simpler system: transfusion-dependent thalassemia (TDT) or non-transfusion-dependent thalassemia (NTDT), with patients often shifting clinically between the two categories depending on their transfusion needs. NTDT includes thalassemia minor, mild HbE, HbH disease, and alpha-thalassemia trait. Despite its name, NTDT treatments can range from no transfusion requirement to intermittent transfusions required. Transfusion is also offered to some NTDT patients to prevent or manage disease complications. TDT includes thalassemia major, severe HbE/Beta-thalassemia, and Hb Barts hydrops. Hb Barts is almost always fatal at birth. TDT, as reflected in its name, typically requires regular, lifelong transfusions for survival, usually starting before the age of 2 years.[7]

CLINICAL FEATURES

Homozygous β-chain thalassemia (thalassemia major or Cooley anemia) occurs predominantly in Mediterranean populations. It is one of the most common single-gene disorders, resulting in no functional beta chains. The disease is characterized by severe anemia, hepatosplenomegaly, jaundice, abnormal development, and premature death. Symptoms are typically evident by the age of 2 years. Patients are transfusion dependent and die as a result of iron deposition in tissues, particularly in the myocardium, or infection.

TABLE 109.3 Diagnostic Tests for Iron Deficiency Anemia

Test	Normal	Iron Deficiency	Interpretation
Fasting serum iron	60–180 µg/dL	<60 µg/dL	Diurnal variation (draw in morning); increased by hepatitis, hemochromatosis, hemolytic anemia, or aplastic anemia; decreased in infection
Total iron-binding capacity	250–400 µg/dL	>400 µg/dL	Increased in late pregnancy or hepatitis; decreased in infection
Percentage of saturation (serum iron) of total iron-binding capacity	15%–45%	<15%	
Serum ferritin	10–10,000 mg/mL	<10 mg/mL	Reflects iron stores; may increase as an acute-phase reactant in infection
Bone marrow stainable iron	Hemosiderin granules in reticuloendothelial cells	Absent	Standard for assessment of iron stores

Heterozygous β-chain thalassemia (thalassemia minor or intermedia) results in some functional beta chains and is manifested as a mild to moderate anemia. Thalassemia minor patients are typically asymptomatic and rarely, if ever, require transfusion. Thalassemia intermedia patients usually have a moderate anemia and require occasional transfusions. Heterozygous beta thalassemia is most prevalent in Asia, the Middle East, and Mediterranean countries. This widespread distribution is attributed to a natural selection toward heterozygote carriers, as this offers protection against falciparum malaria.[7] This same protection is also offered in sickle cell trait carriers.

Alpha-thalassemia varies in spectrum from an asymptomatic carrier state to prenatal death. Four gene loci are responsible, and disease severity increases as the number of gene deletions increase. The tolerated forms are more commonly seen in Asians and African Americans. One missing gene results in a silent carrier state while two missing genes, commonly referred to as alpha thalassemia trait, results in a minor anemia. Three missing genes, also called hemoglobin H disease, can lead to a mild to moderate anemia, but most affected lead normal lives. Four defective genes result in Hb Barts, which causes hydrops fetalis and fetal death.[8]

Diagnostic Testing

Thalassemia is a microcytic, hypochromic anemia. Hypochromia, target cells, and basophilic stippling are noted on the peripheral smear. The MCV is commonly lower than seen with iron deficiency, and serum iron levels are typically normal. The diagnosis is made with hemoglobin electrophoresis and genetic testing. Screening for carriers is performed by measurement of RBC indices and estimation of the HbA_2 concentration. Prenatal diagnosis can be made by analysis of fetal blood or by fetal DNA obtained by chorionic villus sampling.[7]

Management

Usually, no treatment is necessary for silent carriers, beta thalassemia minor, and alpha thalassemia trait. Therapy for the remaining types of thalassemia consists of blood transfusions, where the goals of transfusion therapy include correction of anemia, suppression of ineffective erythropoiesis, and inhibition of increased gastrointestinal iron absorption. TDT requires transfusions every 2 to 5 weeks to maintain a pre-transfusion hemoglobin between 9 and 10.5g/dL. Transfusion is usually started when patients are young to ensure normal growth and physical activity capacity. Recurrent transfusion does increase risk of blood-borne infection, alloimmunization, and iron overload, the latter of which may lead to multi-organ dysfunction and is a common cause of death. Guidelines for transfusion are not well established in patients with NTDT, but transfusion should be considered during times of significant stress such as pregnancy, surgery, or infection, or when

hemoglobin levels are low. More frequent transfusion may be used in children with NTDT if they develop signs of growth failure or reduced exercise tolerance.

Transfusion therapy improves long-term survival in patients with TDT when combined with iron chelation therapy. Iron chelation therapy can also reduce systemic and hepatic iron burden in NTDT, but it is not effective in all patients. Deferoxamine can be administered parenterally or subcutaneously. It was the first commercially available chelator. Its demanding treatment regimen, however, often leads to poor adherence. Dosages are weight based, with treatments required for 8 to 12 hours, 5 to 7 nights per week.[7] Two oral chelators are available, deferiprone and deferasirox. Deferiprone is administered two or three times daily, and deferasirox is a once-daily medication.[9,10]

Hydroxyurea, a cytotoxic anti-metabolite that induces fetal hemoglobin, is also used in some cases of NTDT. Hydroxyurea is hypothesized to improve chronic anemia and reduce the need for transfusion by reducing alpha and beta chain imbalance through the production of fetal hemoglobin. It is well tolerated by patients and has no major long-term adverse effects. Commonly reported side effects included mild transaminitis, nausea or vomiting, and transient bone marrow suppression. It is associated with a decrease in the need for recurrent transfusions. In patients with mild NTDT, it can raise baseline Hb by at least 1 g/dL and in some patients with severe NTDT (>3 transfusions per year) it can lead to a complete cessation of transfusion requirement.[11]

Splenectomy is considered in some patients and can improve hemoglobin concentration, decreasing the need for recurrent transfusions. Hematopoietic stem cell transplantation (HSCT) is another therapy in use and is potentially curative in patients with TDT with disease-free survival rates greater than 80% at 2 years. It is, however, only appropriate for a subset of patients due to age restrictions and the need for sibling donor compatibility. HSCT carries with it a 5% to 10% risk of mortality, as well as potential permanent fertility impairment.[7]

Gene therapy and gene editing are becoming more promising as possible future treatment modalities for thalassemia; data from clinical trials is in progress.

Sideroblastic Anemia

Foundations

Sideroblastic anemia involves a defect in porphyrin synthesis and can be congenital, idiopathic, or acquired. The resultant impaired hemoglobin production causes excess iron to be deposited in the mitochondria of the RBC precursor as well as increased serum iron, ferritin, and transferrin saturation levels. The defective heme synthesis results in ineffective erythropoiesis, mild to moderate anemia, and a dimorphic peripheral smear with hypochromic microcytes along with normal and macrocytic cells, as well as characteristic ringed sideroblasts.[12] A ringed sideroblast is an erythroid precursor with a minimum of five siderotic granules covering the nucleus after Prussian blue staining.[13]

Clinical Features

Congenital sideroblastic anemia is a relatively rare disease resulting from iron metabolism related gene mutations.[14] The most common congenital cause is X-linked sideroblastic anemia (XLSA) which occurs secondary to missense substitutions in 5′-Aminolevulinste Synthase 2 (ALAS2) genes.[13] Idiopathic sideroblastic anemia is a common type of refractory anemia in elderly patients. Pallor and splenomegaly may be noted, and iron staining of the peripheral smear may demonstrate iron-containing inclusion bodies in RBCs. Idiopathic sideroblastic anemia is considered a pre-leukemic state, with acute myelogenous leukemia developing in approximately 5% of patients.

Differential Diagnoses

Acquired causes of sideroblastic anemia include drugs, alcoholism, copper deficiency, lead poisoning, zinc toxicity, myelodysplastic syndrome, or myeloproliferative disorders. Chloramphenicol, isoniazid, linezolid, and penicillamine are known causes of drug-induced sideroblastic anemia.[13] Lead poisoning, one reversible cause of sideroblastic anemia, may be suggested by basophilic stippling on the peripheral smear and the presence of metaphyseal lead lines on imaging. Elevated blood lead levels are diagnostic. Alcohol abuse may also result in disordered heme synthesis, which can be corrected by alcohol cessation or by parenteral pyridoxal phosphate (active form of vitamin B6) in cases of continued abuse. Oral pyridoxine (vitamin B6) may be ineffective because of impaired conversion to the active form in alcoholic patients.

Management

Management varies based on underlying cause. Most congenital or acquired sideroblastic anemia is treated with pyridoxine (vitamin B_6) and responds to treatment with 100 mg PO three times a day. Although a trial of treatment with pyridoxine is advised, most patients remain anemic and will require transfusion. If long-term transfusion therapy is necessary, iron overload will need to be managed and usually responds well to chelation therapy. Stem cell transplantation can be curative in some patients with congenital or myelodysplastic sideroblastic anemias.[13,14]

Anemia of Chronic Disease

Foundations. Anemia of chronic disease (ACD) is secondary to reduced erythropoiesis and reduced RBC survival time in the peripheral circulation in chronic inflammatory states, which result in decreased iron release from macrophages secondary to increased cytokines and hepcidin. It is a multifactorial, acquired disorder of iron homeostasis. Common causes include malignancy, arthritis, renal insufficiency, chronic heart failure, chronic obstructive lung disease, or chronic infections (e.g., tuberculosis or osteomyelitis).[2] ACD is commonly found in older adults and is associated with increased morbidity and mortality, largely due to the effects of anemia on comorbid disease processes and the underlying etiology of the ACD.[3]

Clinical Features

Symptoms are usually those related to the underlying disease and not from the anemia itself.

Diagnostic Testing

Anemia of chronic disease is common and typically normochromic, normocytic, though can be microcytic. It is characterized by low serum iron levels, low TIBC, and normal or elevated ferritin levels.[3] Bone marrow is typically normal, but staining reveals an abnormality

TABLE 109.4   Clinicopathologic Correlation of Manifestations of Megaloblastic Anemia

Clinical Features	Pathologic Condition
Lemon yellow skin	Combination of pallor with low-grade icterus from ineffective erythropoiesis
Petechiae, mucosal bleeding	Thrombocytopenia
Infection	Leukopenia
Fatigue, dyspnea, orthostasis	Anemia
Sore mouth or tongue	Megaloblastosis of mucosal surfaces
Diarrhea and weight loss	Malabsorption from mucosal surface change
Paresthesias and ataxia	Related to myelin abnormality in vitamin B_{12} deficiency only

in the mobilization of iron from reticuloendothelial cells. This anemia can be differentiated from iron deficiency by TIBC, ferritin, bone marrow examination, and non-responsiveness to a trial of iron therapy. A complete search for occult blood loss is prudent during evaluation. It should be recognized that true iron deficiency may also be superimposed on anemia of chronic disease.

Management

Acute or emergent therapy is not usually required, as the hemoglobin and hematocrit is typically modest. Treatment should be directed at the underlying cause.

Macrocytic and Megaloblastic Anemias

Foundations

Macrocytic anemia is the hematologic manifestation of a total-body alteration in DNA synthesis caused primarily by vitamin B_{12} or folic acid deficiency, which appears clinically in tissues with rapid cell turnover, including hematopoietic cells or those of mucosal surfaces, particularly in the gastrointestinal tract. This deficiency is characterized by ineffective erythropoiesis and pancytopenia. Vitamin B_{12} and folate deficiencies have different developmental histories, but the clinical result is similar. Differentiation of folate and vitamin B_{12} deficiencies usually depends on laboratory measurements.

Clinical Features

Macrocytic anemias can be divided into megaloblastic and nonmegaloblastic categories. Megaloblastic macrocytic anemia is the most common cause of macrocytic anemia and pancytopenia. Table 109.4 lists a number of the problems associated with megaloblastic anemia and their underlying pathologic states. Nonmegaloblastic macrocytic anemia is caused by disease states such as alcoholism, liver dysfunction, hypothyroidism, myelodysplastic syndromes, and certain drugs (e.g., hydroxyurea, methotrexate, zidovudine, valproic acid).[15] Like other causes of anemia, easy fatigability is the most common symptom reported in patients with macrocytic anemia. Additional symptoms include anorexia, dyspnea on exertion, palpitations, oral ulcers, or weight loss.[16] A unique feature of vitamin B_{12} deficiency is its neurologic involvement. Patients may have paresthesias of their hands or feet, decreased proprioception, or decreased vibratory sense; weakness and spasticity of the lower extremities with altered reflexes; and variable mental changes, such as depression, paranoid ideation, irritability, or forgetfulness. The neurologic manifestations of folic acid deficiency overlap with those of vitamin B_{12} deficiency, but the neuropsychiatric manifestations (e.g., depression and forgetfulness) predominate in folic acid deficiency. A devastating consequence of vitamin B_{12} deficiency

BOX 109.6 Causes of Folate Deficiency

Inadequate dietary intake
  Poor diet or overcooked or processed food diet
  Alcoholism
Inadequate uptake
  Malabsorption with sprue and other chronic upper intestinal tract disorders, drugs such as phenytoin and barbiturates, or blind loop syndrome
Inadequate use
  Metabolic block caused by drugs, such as methotrexate or trimethoprim
  Enzymatic deficiency, congenital or acquired
Increased requirement
  Pregnancy
  Increased red blood cell (RBC) turnover: Ineffective erythropoiesis, hemolytic anemia, chronic blood loss
  Malignant disease: Lymphoproliferative disorders
Increased excretion or destruction or dialysis

BOX 109.7 Causes of Vitamin B$_{12}$ Deficiency

Inadequate dietary intake
  Total vegetarianism: No eggs, milk, or cheese
  Chronic alcoholism (rare)
Inadequate absorption
  Absent, inadequate, or abnormal intrinsic factor, as seen in patients with pernicious anemia and gastrectomy; in pernicious, autoimmune antibodies act against gastric parietal cells and intrinsic factor
  Abnormal ileum, as can occur in sprue and inflammatory bowel disease
Inadequate use
  Enzyme deficiency
  Abnormal vitamin B$_{12}$–binding protein
Increased requirement by increased body metabolism
Increased excretion or destruction

is the development of subacute combined degeneration of the spinal cord resulting from loss of myelin in the dorsal and lateral columns. The syndrome has a gradual and uniform onset of progressive weakness, spastic paresis, ataxia, and loss of proprioception. Vitamin B$_{12}$ deficiency can also cause elevated homocysteine levels which can lead to thrombosis.[15,16]

Differential Diagnoses

Folic acid, absorbed in the upper jejunum, is commonly found in green vegetables, cereals, and fruit. It may be destroyed completely by cooking. The recommended daily intake is approximately 240 µg/day in adults and 400 µg/day if pregnant or lactating. The body stores 6 to 20 mg.[15] Therefore, a 2- to 4-month body store is available for consumption before megaloblastic changes occur. Causes of folate deficiency are listed in Box 109.6. Most patients with folate deficiency have either an inadequate dietary intake, such as alcoholic patients, or increased use, as in pregnancy.

Vitamin B$_{12}$ is found in foods of animal origin and is absorbed in the terminal ileum after binding to intrinsic factor, which is a glycoprotein secreted by gastric parietal cells. Once absorbed, B$_{12}$ acts as a coenzyme to produce methionine from homocysteine which assists in folic acid conversion to its active form. Therefore, a deficiency in B$_{12}$ can also contribute to folic acid deficiency. The adult requirement of vitamin B$_{12}$ is 1 or 3 µg/day, with a body store of 5 mg. Therefore, megaloblastic changes and clinical problems may take 5 to 10 years to develop after cessation of vitamin B$_{12}$ uptake. The various causes of vitamin B$_{12}$ deficiency are listed in Box 109.7. The most common cause is chronic malabsorption resulting from pernicious anemia.[15]

Megaloblastic anemia that is not responsive to folate or vitamin B$_{12}$ is commonly related to antimetabolites used in chemotherapy or rare inherited disorders of DNA synthesis.

Liver disease, often associated with alcoholism, is the most common cause of non-megaloblastic macrocytic anemia. However, alcoholism can also cause concomitant megaloblastic anemia secondary to poor dietary intake. Thyroid hormone stimulates erythropoietin; thus hypothyroidism is commonly associated with nonmegaloblastic macrocytic anemia as well as normocytic anemia. Drugs can also cause macrocytosis and anemia. Commonly implicated agents include antiretrovirals, phenytoin, chemotherapeutic agents, valproic acid, or azathioprine. Macrocytic target cells may be seen on the peripheral smear in conjunction with this disorder.[15]

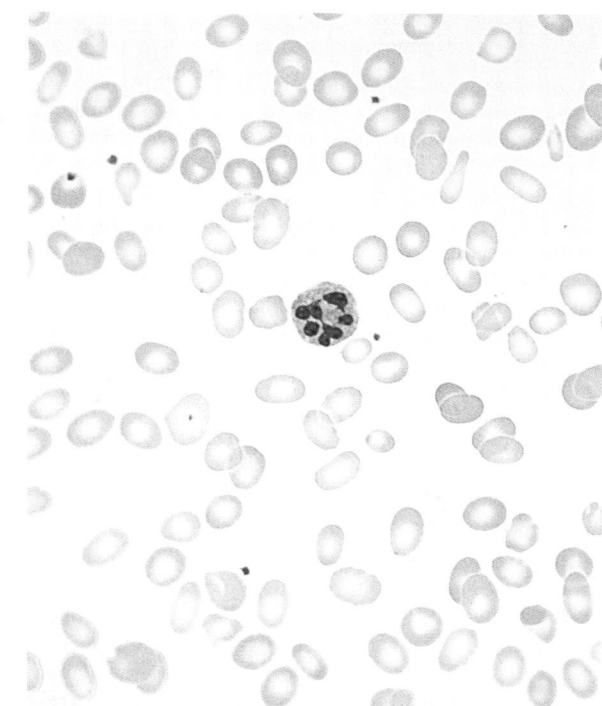

Fig. 109.4 Megaloblastic Anemia With Macrocytic Red Cells and Hypersegmented Polymorphonuclear Neutrophils. (From Hoffbrand AV, Pettite JE. *Color Atlas of Clinical Hematology.* 3rd ed. London: Mosby; 2000:61.)

Diagnostic Testing

Macrocytic anemia is suggested when the MCV is greater than 100 fL, but other criteria need to be met for megaloblastosis to be considered the cause of the macrocytic anemia. On the peripheral smear, large oval red cells (macro-ovalocytes), anisocytosis, hypersegmented polymorphonuclear neutrophils, as well as an elevated serum LDH level are diagnostic (Fig. 109.4). A bone marrow aspirate may reveal morphologic changes consistent with megaloblastic erythropoiesis. Other useful laboratory tests include vitamin B$_{12}$, folate level, and homocysteine levels. Laboratory techniques, values, and interpretations are listed in Table 109.5.

Management

As one form of deficiency may cause gastrointestinal absorption changes that beget other deficiencies, the clinician may need to initiate

TABLE 109.5   Serum Tests for Diagnosis and Differentiation of Megaloblastic Anemia

Test	Technique	Value	Interpretation
Vitamin B$_{12}$	Microbiologic or radioisotope	Normal: 300–900 μg/L Deficient: <200 μg/L	Vitamin B$_{12}$ level is usually normal in folate deficiency.
Folate	Microbiologic or radioisotope	Deficient: <3 μg/L	Vitamin B$_{12}$ deficiency may elevate folate levels by blocking transfer of serum folate to RBCs; hemolysis may elevate folate levels.
Lactate dehydrogenase	Spectrophotometric	Normal: 95–200 IU Megaloblastic anemia: 4–50 times normal	Normal in other macrocytic anemias; elevated two to four times normal in hemolytic anemias

RBC, Red blood cell.

therapy before the final diagnosis is made. However, it is important to obtain baseline laboratory specimens.

The usual dosage for patients with megaloblastic anemia secondary to folate deficiency is 1 mg of oral folic acid per day, and it is recommended to follow RBC folate levels to determine effectiveness as well as improvement in clinical symptoms. Parenteral administration is generally unnecessary as most cases are due to dietary deficiency.[15] In contrast, malabsorption is the most common cause of vitamin B$_{12}$ deficiency, and parenteral therapy is initiated at 1000 mcg IM daily for 7 to 10 days, then monthly 1000 mcg IM injections. Weekly 1000 mcg IM doses for 4 weeks in between daily and monthly injections may be considered. If neurologic symptoms are present, therapy is initiated at 1 mg IM every other day for up to three weeks, followed by 1 mg IM weekly for up to twelve weeks. Thereafter, monthly 1 mg IM doses are necessary as needed to maintain B$_{12}$ levels if the underlying cause of deficiency is not treatable. The response is often dramatic with levels of RBC, WBC, and platelets returning to normal within 4 weeks. During hematopoietic recovery, an iron deficiency may develop and should be treated in the usual manner.[15] We do not recommend vitamin B$_{12}$ or folate supplements in patients with undiagnosed anemia. Unfortunately, the routine injection of vitamin B$_{12}$ in the elderly is still a common practice.

Normochromic and Normocytic Anemias

Foundations

A hematologic parameter that can aid in the diagnosis of normocytic anemia associated with hypoproduction is the reticulocyte count, which reflects new RBC bone marrow production. Reticulocytes are released from bone marrow every 1 to 3 days and contain residual RNA that can be detected by supravital staining. With an average MCV of 160 fL, sufficient numbers of reticulocytes can increase the overall MCV of the total erythrocyte count. The reticulocyte count is expressed as a percentage of the total RBC population and needs to be related ("corrected") to the RBC count of the patient. The corrected reticulocyte count is equal to the measured percentage of reticulocytes multiplied by the patient's hematocrit (%), divided by the patient's normal hematocrit for age and gender.[17] The normal range is 1% to 3%.

Normocytic anemias may be classified as hemolytic or nonhemolytic. Nonhemolytic anemias are typically caused by chronic disease states or bone marrow failure, that is, decreased RBC production. Hemolytic anemia is defined by the premature destruction of RBCs.

Clinical Features

Non-hemolytic normocytic anemias include anemia of chronic disease, hypoendocrinism, aplastic anemia, and myelodysplastic or myeloproliferative syndromes.

Anemia of chronic disease may have microcytic or normocytic indices, and is associated with chronic inflammation (e.g., rheumatoid arthritis, chronic infections, or malignancy). The anemia of chronic renal failure is thought to be caused by a number of factors including

BOX 109.8   Aplastic Anemia Caused by Drugs or Chemicals

- Chloramphenicol
- Phenylbutazone
- Anticonvulsants
- Insecticides
- Solvents
- Solvents
- Sulfonamides
- Gold
- Benzene

decreased erythropoietin production, hemolysis, suppression by dialyzable factors, and increased blood loss caused by platelet abnormalities. Correction is with erythropoietin replacement therapy, as necessary.

Hypoendocrinism caused by hypothyroidism, hypoadrenalism, or hypopituitarism results in a hypometabolic state in which the bone marrow responds poorly to erythropoietin, and erythropoietin levels may be low resulting in normocytic normochromic anemia.

Aplastic anemia results from destruction of myeloid stem cells leading to pancytopenia. It is suspected in anemic patients with normal indices, a low reticulocyte count, neutropenia, thrombocytopenia, or a history of exposure to certain drugs or chemicals (Box 109.8) which is the cause in 50% of cases. Autoimmune disease, viral hepatitis, radiation exposure, viral illness (Parvovirus B19, HIV, Epstein-Barr virus), and pregnancy have also been associated with aplastic anemia. Infection with Parvovirus B19 can precipitate an aplastic crisis in sickle cell patients and can lead to severe anemia requiring emergent transfusion. Patients can present with symptoms of anemia, however more commonly they present with infections secondary to neutropenia or mucosal bleeding from the accompanying thrombocytopenia. Diagnosis is suspected based on CBC findings, and can be confirmed with bone marrow evaluation. Treatment involves removal of any known causative factor as well as supportive care measures with avoidance of aspirin, effective oral hygiene, and pharmacologic suppression of menses if necessary. Transfusions of RBC or platelets are given in life-threatening circumstances. Bone marrow or peripheral blood stem cell transplantation from a histocompatible sibling can prove to be curative. In patients not amenable to transplantation, immunosuppression with antithymocyte globulin, antilymphocyte globulin, or other cytotoxic chemotherapy may be used. The disease has a wide range of severity, and the overall 5-year survival rate is 30% to 40%. Even with supportive therapy, severe aplastic anemia may prove fatal in up to 80% of patients.

Myelodysplastic syndromes are a class of hematopoietic stem cell disorders that are characterized by cytopenia, myelodysplasia, and ineffective hematopoiesis. It is caused by an accumulation of oncogenic mutations and is associated with an increased risk of progression to leukemic states. It is the cause of anemia in up to 5% of elderly patients. Laboratory evaluation can present with normocytic anemia, thrombocytopenia, and neutropenia. A definitive diagnosis is made by bone marrow examination with evidence of dysplastic cell lines and blast cells.

Treatment is selected based on MDS subtype and age and can range from supportive care to allogeneic hematopoietic stem cell transplantation.[15]

Myeloproliferative neoplasms, specifically primary myelofibrosis, results in primary bone marrow fibrosis and splenomegaly due to extramedullary hematopoiesis, that may ultimately transform to an acute leukemia. The diagnosis is made by bone marrow examination. Treatment is supportive, although a splenectomy or alkylating agents may help treat complications of extramedullary blood cell production, such as hepatosplenomegaly.[18]

Diagnostic Testing

Diagnostic testing in nonhemolytic normocytic anemias consists of a CBC with differential, and additional testing based on presumed underlying cause.

Management

Treatment is based on underlying cause, and in the ED is directed at resuscitation in the event of life-threatening anemia and appropriate admission or outpatient referrals.

Increased Red Blood Cell Destruction

Foundations

Hemolytic anemias are caused by premature RBC destruction. In the appropriate clinical context, this can be defined by evidence of anemia with elevated LDH and decreased Haptoglobin on laboratory evaluation. They can be acute or chronic, with acute hemolytic anemias requiring prompt intervention and management. There are multiple classification systems for describing hemolytic anemias based on Coombs test reactivity, intrinsic versus extrinsic defects, intravascular versus extravascular hemolysis, and congenital or acquired forms.

Pathophysiology

Defined by a shortened life span of the erythrocyte, acute hemolytic anemias can be devastating and require rapid diagnosis and intervention (see Box 109.1). Fortunately, they are relatively rare in comparison to the chronic hemolytic conditions. Chronic disorders may be related to primary blood disorders (e.g., sickle cell anemia) or may be a result of other disease states (e.g., chronic renal failure). These disorders may be manifested as acute hemolytic anemia if the tenuous balance between RBC production and destruction is upset. If the patient can be simultaneously demonstrated to have a normal hematocrit and reticulocyte count, differentiation between acquired and inherited hemolytic anemia is particularly challenging.

Clinical Features

The clinical signs and symptoms of hemolytic anemia are, in general, caused by either intravascular or extravascular processes, and this division assists in the differential diagnostic approach. Emergency physicians should consider hemolysis as a cause of anemia in patients presenting with the typical symptoms of anemia in addition to new-onset jaundice, hematuria, fever, hepatosplenomegaly, abdominal or back pain, or altered mental status.[17,19] A thorough past medical and family history is also critical in the evaluation of hemolytic anemias.

Intravascular hemolysis presents acutely and dramatically due to an acute decrease in oxygen-carrying capacity as the hemolytic process releases free hemoglobin into circulation. Free hemoglobin initially binds to haptoglobin and hemopexin. This complex is transported to the liver, conjugated to bilirubin, then excreted. Once the degree of hemolysis overwhelms the ability of the binding and transport system, free hemoglobin will start to appear in the bloodstream and urine leading to hemoglobinemia and hemoglobinuria, respectively.[17] Jaundice occurs due to excessive bilirubin production, and

> ### BOX 109.9 Classification of Hemolytic Anemia
>
> **Intrinsic**
> *Enzyme defect*: Pyruvate kinase deficiency, G6PD deficiency
> *Membrane abnormality*: Spherocytosis, Paroxysmal nocturnal hemoglobinuria
> *Hemoglobin abnormality*: Hemoglobinopathies, Thalassemias (anemias)
>
> **Extrinsic**
> *Immunologic*: Alloantibodies, autoantibodies
> *Mechanical*: Microangiopathic hemolytic anemia, prosthetic heart valve disease
> *Environmental*: Drugs, toxins, infections, thermal
> *Abnormal sequestrations*

hemoglobin complexes can cause acute renal failure due to plugging of the microtubules.

The clinical appearance of intravascular hemolysis may vary from mild chronic anemia to severe acute anemia requiring emergent intervention. Mild anemia is commonly caused by mechanical hemolysis from prosthetic valves, or from chronic diseases such as paroxysmal nocturnal hemoglobinuria. Acute severe anemia can be seen with ABO incompatibility, autoimmune hemolytic anemias, infections, DIC, or toxins.

Extravascular hemolysis usually causes mild to moderate anemia, intermittent jaundice, and enlargement of the spleen. It occurs when RBCs are prematurely removed by macrophages in the liver, spleen, or bone marrow due to an abnormality in their shape or the binding of an antibody.[17] Hereditary spherocytosis, glucose-6-phosphate dehydrogenase deficiency (G6PD), sickle cell disease, and some autoimmune hemolytic anemias represent the most common causes of extravascular hemolysis. The signs and symptoms vary with the severity and chronicity of the hemolysis. Splenic blood flow slows as RBCs travel in the sinusoids close to the reticuloendothelial system, which is uniquely designed for removal of older or damaged cells. Once disassembled in the reticuloendothelial cell, hemoglobin is recycled and ultimately converted to bilirubin and subsequently conjugated by the liver. Primary splenic overactivity, antibody-mediated changes, or RBC membrane abnormalities may cause this normal splenic function to increase to a pathologic degree.

Differential Diagnoses

Hemolytic anemias may be classified as (1) congenital or acquired, (2) Coombs positive or Coombs negative, or (3) caused by processes intrinsic or extrinsic to the cell membrane, and the latter classification provides a useful differential diagnosis of hemolysis (Box 109.9).

Intrinsic enzyme defects. Of the membrane-sustaining energy production of the erythrocyte, 85% to 90% is through the anaerobic glycolytic pathway. At least eight known enzyme deficiencies are associated with this pathway. The most common is pyruvate kinase deficiency, which is manifested with hemolytic jaundice that is usually diagnosed in infancy.

The remaining 10% to 15% of RBC glycolysis occurs by way of the hexose monophosphate shunt. This bypass mechanism occurs in the early stages of the glycolytic pathway and generates reduced nicotinamide adenine dinucleotide phosphate (NADPH), which is important in maintaining reduced glutathione. Glutathione is essential in the protection of hemoglobin from oxidant injury. A deficiency of the first enzyme in this pathway, G6PD, is X linked and most common in African Americans or those of Mediterranean descent.[19] G6PD has a wide range of severity which is dependent on the degree of deficiency and the ability of the body to overcome oxidant stress. Clinical symptoms present when oxidative hemolysis occurs typically as an acute hemolytic episode that may be both intravascular and extravascular. It occurs 24 to 48 hours after the ingestion of an oxidant drug (Box 109.10) or after acute infections, such as viral hepatitis. The anemia induced by oxidant drugs is dose related. The oxidant creates forms of activated oxygen, such as peroxide, that either denature the hemoglobin or destroy cell membranes. The former process produces Heinz bodies, which are clumps of denatured hemoglobin found in RBCs that are removed by the spleen. The diagnosis is made by enzymatic screening for G6PD, but this test cannot be performed immediately after the hemolytic episode. A 3-week delay avoids a false-negative result caused by a predominance of young cells. Treatment includes supportive care and discontinuation of oxidant drugs.[19]

Intrinsic Membrane Abnormality

These abnormalities are manifested in a number of ways. An altered shape is the main feature of autosomal dominant hereditary spherocytosis. It is caused by mutations in genes encoding the cytoskeleton of the RBC membrane resulting in spherically shaped, rigid RBCs that are susceptible to premature destruction by the spleen.[20] Clinical sequelae range from compensated asymptomatic anemia to severe life-threatening acquired aplastic crises. The diagnosis is made by reviewing the family history, RBC indices (increased MCHC and RDW), blood smear, and osmotic fragility testing. Treatment is supportive in mild cases. Splenectomy is the treatment of choice for patients with severe disease requiring therapeutic intervention, and usually results in disappearance of anemia with a median increase in hemoglobin by 3g/dL.[20] Due to the complications associated with splenectomy, if possible, it is delayed until the age of 6 years or older.

Paroxysmal nocturnal hemoglobinemia is a stem cell defect causing abnormal erythrocyte, neutrophil, and platelet sensitivity to complement. It is most often seen clinically as chronic hemolysis, hemosiderinuria, leukopenia, and thrombocytopenia. The peripheral smear is normal, and the direct Coombs test result is negative. Its major complication is thrombosis, with a predilection for the hepatic vein. Normal activation of complement with the use of sucrose or acid hemolysis (the Ham test) is diagnostic. Treatment is with supportive care and Eculizumab, a complement inhibitor that has been shown to improve RBC indices and clinical symptoms.[21] Transfusion can be life-threatening in patients with this disease as RBC lysis is caused by donor complement. Thus, only washed packed cells should be utilized. Treatment varies based on disease severity.

Intrinsic Hemoglobin Abnormality

More than 350 types of abnormal hemoglobin have been documented. Problems that may be seen include unstable hemoglobins that appear as Heinz body–positive anemia, M hemoglobins that fix iron in its ferric or methemoglobin state, or hemoglobins with increased oxygen affinity that result in tissue hypoxia and erythrocytosis.

Extrinsic Alloantibodies

Alloantibodies are formed in response to foreign RBC antigens. In the case of the ABO system, these antibodies are preformed and ABO incompatibility resulting in donor cell destruction by the recipient's alloantibodies can be life-threatening. These immunoglobulin M (IgM) antibodies can act as a hemolysin, both agglutinating RBCs, fixing complement, and consequently causing intravascular hemolysis.

The Rh system is another set of antigens on the RBC. Individuals do not have antibodies that correspond to antigens in the Rh system unless they have been sensitized by previous exposure to antigens that they lack. The antibodies produced are IgG in nature, and they accelerate extravascular destruction of RBCs by the spleen and liver. Most autoimmune antibodies are directed toward antigens in the Rh system.

Extrinsic Autoantibodies

Evaluation of autoimmune hemolytic anemia (AIHA) is as complex as its origin, caused by autoantibody-mediated destruction against RBC surface antigens. Autoimmune hemolytic anemias are acquired disorders, with 40% to 50% remaining idiopathic. The remainder are associated with a number of diseases (Box 109.11). A sub-classification of autoimmune hemolytic anemias is based on the optimal temperature at which the antibody reacts with the RBC membrane. Therefore, there are warm-reacting (>37°C) and cold-reacting (<37°C) antibodies. The direct antiglobulin test (DAT) or Coombs test is useful in revealing cells coated with antibody or complement and can aid in diagnosis. A positive DAT alone, however, does not define AIHA and must be supported by clinical context and evidence of hemolysis on laboratory evaluation.[22] AIHA can have a varied presentation from compensated hemolysis with mild anemia and no symptoms to severe symptomatic anemia requiring immediate intervention. Splenomegaly, pallor, or jaundice are common exam findings.

Warm-reacting antibodies are characterized by a higher incidence in younger patients, predominance in women, variable complement fixation, and positive direct antiglobulin test result for IgG. IgG binds to either Rh proteins or glycophorins A-D. IgG-coated RBCs are then removed by reticuloendothelial macrophages and sequestered in the spleen for extravascular destruction. Warm agglutinins are common in

BOX 109.12 Drugs Associated With Immune Hemolytic Anemia

Hapten and drug absorption mechanisms: Penicillin, Cephalosporin, Tetracycline, Hydrocortisone, Oxaliplatin, Tolbutamide

Immune complex mechanism: Metformin, quinine, quinidine, amphotericin b, thiopental, diclofenac, doxepin, probenecid

Autoantibody mechanism: Cephalosporins, methyldopa, mefenamic acid, fludarabine, procainamide, diclofenac

Non-immunologic protein adsorption: Cephalosporins, carboplatin, cisplatin, oxaliplatin

Miscellaneous drug: insecticides, chlorpromazine, acetaminophen, ibuprofen, thiazides, omeprazole, erythromycin, streptomycin

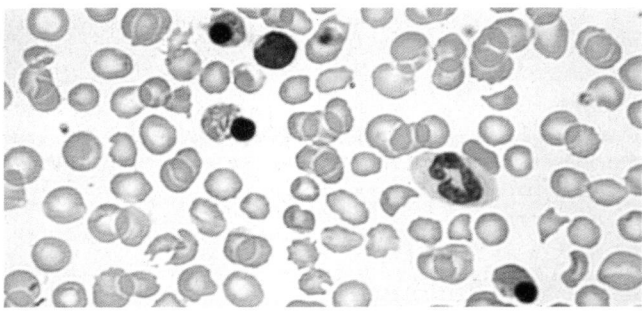

Fig. 109.5 Schizocytes (Fragmented Cell and Nucleated Red Cells). (From Hoffbrand AV, Pettite JE. *Color Atlas of Clinical Hematology.* 3rd ed. London: Mosby; 2000, p 115.)

systemic lupus erythematosus, common variable immunodeficiency, myasthenia gravis, autoimmune hepatitis, myelodysplastic syndromes, or lymphoma. First-line treatment is supportive with management of the underlying condition, in conjunction with glucocorticoids and rituximab. Second- or third-line treatments include intravenous immunoglobulin (IVIG), plasma exchange, hematopoietic stem cell transplantation, azathioprine, cyclosporine, or mycophenolate. Transfusion of blood products should be used in severe cases as needed. Splenectomy is an alternative treatment option for some patients, and up to 40% achieve complete remission post-operatively.[19,22] Disease course can be relapsing and remitting.

Cold-reacting antibodies, or cold agglutinins, are seen predominantly in men and older patients and with IgM complement fixation. IgM antibodies react with surface antigens at low temperatures and cause intravascular or extravascular hemolysis due to complement fixation and activation upon rewarming. Due to the high density of IgM-antigen complexes on RBC, RBC aggregates can be seen on peripheral blood smear. They may also be found in patients with infectious mononucleosis, *Mycoplasma* infection, or lymphoma. The DAT result is positive for complement. Treatment is largely supportive with folic acid and vitamin B_{12} supplementation if deficient, avoidance of triggers, and underlying disease control.[19,22] Blood transfusions should be utilized when anemia is severe. Thrombosis is a common complication of cold agglutinin disease due to agglutinating RBCs, thus thromboprophylaxis should be considered in patients with acute exacerbations or for chronic disease in high-risk situations (i.e., immobilization, long-flights, etc.).

Drug-induced hemolytic anemia may be difficult to diagnose. It is helpful to recognize the drugs most often associated with this Coombs-positive phenomenon, and realize that the result of this test is sometimes positive only in the drug's presence. Removal of the offending agent is the mainstay of treatment. Common drugs are listed in Box 109.12.[19,22]

Extrinsic Mechanical Causes

Hemolysis may be caused by trauma to RBCs. The peripheral smear may demonstrate schistocytes or fragmented cells (Fig. 109.5). Microangiopathic hemolytic anemia, cardiac trauma, and exercise-induced hemoglobinemia are the most commonly encountered forms of traumatic hemolysis.

Microangiopathic hemolytic anemia is a form of microcirculatory fragmentation by threads of fibrin deposited in the arterioles. An underlying disease may be found in renal lesions, such as malignant hypertension or preeclampsia, vasculitis, thrombotic thrombocytopenic purpura, disseminated intravascular coagulation, or vascular anomalies. Signs and symptoms are those of intravascular hemolysis and thrombosis; treatment is supportive and directed at the underlying cause.[17]

Cardiac trauma to RBCs results from increased turbulence. This may be found in patients with prosthetic valves, arteriovenous fistula, aortic stenosis, or other left-sided heart lesions. Surgical correction may be necessary. Supportive therapy with iron is usually required.

March hemoglobinemia is a form of trauma caused by breaking of intravascular RBCs by repetitive pounding. Soldiers, marathon runners, or anyone with repetitive striking against a hard surface may incur this problem. Reassurance and a change in the patient's pattern of activity are the recommended therapies.

Environmental Causes

Hemolysis may be seen in cases of severe burns, freshwater drowning, or hyperthermia. Toxic causes of hemolysis have been documented to be of animal origin, such as brown recluse spider or some venomous snake bites; vegetable origin, such as castor beans or certain mushrooms; and of mineral origin, such as copper. Certain infections are associated with hemolytic states, including malaria, *Bartonella* infection, or *Clostridium* sepsis.

Abnormal Sequestration

Hypersplenism may be caused by any disease that enlarges the spleen or stimulates the reticuloendothelial system. An unfortunate cycle can be established in which the enlarged spleen traps more blood components and grows larger. It is usually apparent clinically as splenomegaly with pancytopenia and marrow hyperactivity. Therapy for symptomatic or severe disease is splenectomy. Adults usually tolerate splenectomy well, though children should be approached conservatively because the risk of postsplenectomy life-threatening sepsis is increased significantly.

Diagnostic Testing

Once hemolysis is suspected, the history and laboratory testing have diagnostic precedence over physical examination. Important historical and physical examination points are listed in Box 109.13. Important diagnostic tests for hemolysis are included in Box 109.14, and the interpretations of the laboratory evaluation of hemolytic anemias is included in Table 109.6. Reticulocyte count should be obtained to evaluate bone marrow response. An elevated reticulocyte count indicates the bone marrow's attempt to increase RBC production and is usually seen in hemolytic anemias due to premature destruction of RBCs.[17] Examination of spun whole blood demonstrates clear serum in myoglobinemia, pink serum with free hemoglobin in the setting of intravascular hemolysis, and yellow serum from increased bilirubin production in the case of extravascular hemolysis. The blood smear is often more diagnostic than bone marrow examination. The typical cell seen in intravascular hemolysis is the schistocyte (see Fig. 109.5). The classic cell of extravascular hemolysis is the spherocyte. It may be seen in congenital spherocytosis, but more commonly indicates splenic activity against an antibody-coated RBC membrane. An increase in macrocytes reflects the presence of younger cells associated with reticulocytosis. The specific diagnosis may be made by a blood smear, as with sickled cells in sickle cell disease or Heinz bodies in G6PD deficiency.

Haptoglobin binds free hemoglobin on a molecule-for-molecule basis. Its absence implies saturation and degradation after binding with hemoglobin and is an early finding in hemolysis. A haptoglobin of less than 25mg/dL is 95% specific for hemolysis.[22] Haptoglobin is decreased in hepatic failure and increases as an acute-phase reactant. After haptoglobin is bound, hemoglobin binds with hemopexin, transferrin, and albumin before circulating in its free form. Plasma free hemoglobin levels are determined in suspected cases of intravascular hemolysis. The result is considered positive if the level is greater than 40 to 50 mg/dL. Hemoglobin is excreted by the kidney and may appear as a smoky red pigment that is orthotoluidine positive with no associated RBCs. Prussian blue–staining granules of hemosiderin may be found intracellularly in renal tubule cells excreted in urine during chronic hemolytic states.

LDH is released when the RBC is broken down peripherally or in the marrow. It is elevated in hemolytic, thalassemic, sideroblastic, or megaloblastic anemias but may also be seen in cases of uremia, heart failure, polycythemia vera, or erythroleukemia.

In extravascular hemolysis, bilirubin is often delivered to the liver faster than the conjugating mechanism can handle it, leading to an indirect or unconjugated hyperbilirubinemia. Normal total levels are less than 1.5 mg/dL, with an indirect component less than 0.5 mg/dL. Indirect bilirubin may rise as high as 4 or 5 mg/dL even with normal liver function. Higher levels connote some degree of underlying hepatic insufficiency.[17]

The DAT (Coombs) test detects antibody or complement on human RBC membranes by adding a polyspecific antihuman globulin reagent which will detect IgG, IgA, IgM, and complement. It is used in the evaluation of AIHA. The reaction causes an agglutination of RBCs that

TABLE 109.6 Laboratory Evaluation of Hemolytic Anemias

Extravascular Destruction	Lactate Dehydrogenase	Haptoglobin	Reticulocyte Count	Coombs Test	Peripheral Smear
Congenital Red Blood Cell Defects					
Enzyme defects (e.g., G6PD)	↑	↓	↑	Negative	"Bite" cells
Hemoglobinopathies (sickle cell disease)	↑	↓	↑	Negative	Sickle cells
Membrane defects (e.g., hereditary spherocytosis)	↑	↓	↑	Negative	Spherocytes
Acquired Red Blood Cell Defects					
Autoimmune hemolytic anemia	↑	↓	↑	Positive	Spherocytes
Liver disease	↑	↓	↑	Negative	Spur cells
Infections (e.g., malaria)	↑	↓	↑	Negative	RBCs with inclusions
Toxins (e.g., nitrates, dapsone, aniline dyes)	↑	↓	↑	Negative	Spherocytes
Hypersplenism	↑	↓	↑	Negative	Howell-Jolly bodies
Intravascular Destruction					
Microangiopathic hemolytic anemia (e.g., DIC, TTP, HUS)	↑	↓	↑	Negative	Schistocytes, helmet cells
Transfusion reactions	↑	↓	↑	Positive	Schistocytes, helmet cells
Sepsis	↑	↓	↑	Negative	RBC "ghost" cells, schistocytes, helmet cells
Paroxysmal nocturnal hemoglobinuria	↑	↓	↑	Negative	Schistocytes, helmet cells
Heat injury	↑	↓	↑	Negative	Schistocytes, helmet cells

DIC, Disseminated intravascular coagulation; *G6PD,* glucose-6-phosphate dehydrogenase; *HUS,* hemolytic uremia syndrome; *RBC,* red blood cell; *TTP,* thrombotic thrombocytopenic purpura.

is graded 0 to 4. Agglutinating properties depend on the size of the immunoglobulin. It can have false negative results if the RBC-bound antibodies are below the threshold of the test or in the presence of low affinity autoantibodies. A false positive DAT can occur after administration of intravenous immunoglobulins or Rh immunoglobulins. It is also important to recognize that a positive DAT can occur without AIHA and can be present in patients that have been recently transfused or have delayed hemolytic transfusion reactions.[22] The indirect test measures antibody titers in serum (cold agglutinin autoimmune hemolytic anemia). The indirect antiglobulin test (IAT) assumes that IgG or C3 is in the serum and tests for serum antibody activity against RBCs. Test RBCs are first mixed with patient serum, washed, and then incubated with polyspecific antihuman globulin reagent. Agglutination will occur if serum antibodies directed toward RBCs are present. Positive tests for immunologic markers do not correlate agglutination activity with the severity of hemolysis.[22]

Management. In patients with newly diagnosed reticulocytopenia or severe hemolytic anemia, the emergency clinician may need to institute rapid transfusion therapy. Compatible blood may be almost impossible to find as the antibody can react with almost all donors. The most compatible donor cells in terms of the ABO and Rh systems should be transfused with the knowledge that they will be no more compatible than the patient's own blood cells. If emergency blood transfusion is required, type-specific or type O blood (Rh-positive for men; Rh-negative for women of childbearing age) is indicated, as well as prednisone or its equivalent in a dose of 1 mg/kg to assist with slowing the rate of hemolysis. During transfusion, patients should be closely monitored for signs of hemolytic transfusion reactions. Death commonly results from uncontrolled hemolysis, infection, the underlying primary disorder, or pulmonary embolism.[17]

Sickle Cell Disease

Foundations

Sickle cell disease is an inherited autosomal recessive mutation that produces an abnormal hemoglobin known as HbS. It affects approximately 100,000 people in the United States, and an estimated 2 million Americans carry the sickle cell trait.[23,24] It is predominantly found in the African American population, however up to 10% of patients with various sickling disorders are not ethnically African American, includes people of Mediterranean, Indian, or Middle Eastern descent.[23,25]

The globin in hemoglobin is made up of two pairs of identical polypeptide globin chains. Each person has two non–sex-linked gene foci for β-globin chains, one from each parent. Six different types of hemoglobin from varying globin chain combinations are expressed: three embryonic hemoglobins, HbA (α2β2), HbA2 (α2δ2), and HbF (α2γ2, fetal hemoglobin). Embryonic hemoglobins are expressed only in utero, and after 6 months of age, HbA typically accounts for more than 95% of hemoglobin. The sickle syndromes result from mutations in the β-globin gene. Instead of HbA (α2β2), an abnormal hemoglobin, HbS, is produced. Embryonic and fetal hemoglobin do not contain β-globin; thus, there are no clinical manifestations in early infancy. As production declines, and normal HbA (α2β2) decreases, symptoms develop.

HbS is formed when an abnormal allele at the gene loci for the hemoglobin beta chain produces altered messenger RNA, which in turn results in replacement of glutamic acid by valine at the sixth position from the N-terminal end of the beta chain. When subjected to deoxygenation or various stressors, the RBC sickles and becomes a rigid, adhesive cell that is less deformable and prone to lysis. Sickled cells increase the viscosity and sludging tendency of blood, and ultimately undergo sequestration in the spleen and liver.[25,26] The clinical complex of vaso-occlusive events, chronic hemolysis, thrombosis, and organ injury is derived from this pathologic process.

In sickle cell trait (HbAS), the patient is heterozygous and only one parent contributes the abnormal S allele. In each cell, approximately 40% of the hemoglobin is HbS. Patients usually have a benign and asymptomatic clinical course. Sickle cell disease (HbSS) is homozygous, more than 85% of the hemoglobin is HbS, and it is associated with severe disease.[25] Because a parent may contribute alleles other than S, a wide number of variants can exist. Patients with HbSS are also subject to other causes of anemia such as iron deficiency, G6PD, or megaloblastic anemias. Two clinically important S variants are sickle cell–β-thalassemia and sickle cell–hemoglobin C disease.

The diagnosis is usually made after newborn sickle cell screening via hemoglobin electrophoresis. Most individuals with sickle cell trait are asymptomatic but can present with spontaneous hematuria, renal papillary necrosis, splenic infarction, pulmonary embolism, traumatic hyphema, exertional rhabdomyolysis, or exertional sudden death. In stark contrast to sickle cell disease, which is associated with increased maternal mortality and stillbirth, recent literature suggests that pregnancy in women with sickle cell trait is not associated with an increased risk of adverse events.[27]

Clinical Features

Sickle cell disease is characterized by two major clinical features, hemolysis and acute vaso-occlusive events. The hallmark manifestation of sickle cell disease and the most common reason for ED visits is painful vaso-occlusive crises.[25] Potential precipitating factors include antecedent infection, cold exposure, or stress such as trauma. A painful crisis is believed to have its origin in tissue ischemia which furthers irreversible sickling of cells, leading to increased viscosity, sludging, and microvascular obstruction. Sludging and vascular blockage cause stasis, deoxygenation, and local acidosis, which promotes continued sickling. Pain is caused by activation of nociceptors as inflammatory mediators are released in response to vascular damage. The pain is commonly deep and aching, and is most often found in the abdomen, chest, back, or extremities.[25,26,28] The disease may mimic an acute abdomen, pulmonary embolus, renal colic, or other painful condition. A directed history that relates this pain pattern to previous sickling episodes, a careful repeated physical examination, and specific organ-related laboratory tests can be used to differentiate "uncomplicated" crises from another serious pathologic condition. Children may be seen more often with skeletal crises, especially in the hips and lower extremities, leading to bone deformities. In these cases, osteomyelitis, avascular necrosis, and bone infarct needs to be differentiated. Acute pain crisis is treated with analgesia, including opioids and nonsteroidal anti-inflammatories, and intravenous hydration. Pain control adjuvants should be considered and include sedatives, anxiolytics, or antihistamines. If pain control is able to be achieved in the ED, patients can typically be discharged on an oral pain control regimen, otherwise, hospitalization may be required for further management.[23,28]

Neurologic complications include transient ischemic attack, cerebral infarction, intracranial hemorrhage, spinal cord infarction, or vestibular and hearing problems. Patients presenting with the sudden onset of acute neurologic abnormalities should be presumed to have a stroke until proven otherwise, typically necessitating prompt imaging. Risk factors for CVA in sickle cell patients include low hemoglobin level, history of acute chest syndrome, or history of hypertension.[23,25] Transcranial Doppler (TCD) is useful in children to identify those at highest risk of developing stroke by measuring the maximum time-averaged mean velocity of blood flow in the intracranial arteries.[25,28] TCD combined with brain MRI can be used in adults to assess stroke risk. The use of regular blood transfusions can reduce the risk of cerebrovascular events in selected patients. In the setting of an acute stroke, exchange transfusion is often recommended with the goal of hemoglobin S of less than 30% and a total hemoglobin level of 10 g/dL.[23,25] Tissue plasminogen activator (tPA) should be considered in adult sickle cell disease patients with acute non-hemorrhagic strokes, although extreme caution is advised due to increased risk of intracranial hemorrhage.[23]

Acute chest syndrome is the most common pulmonary condition associated with sickle cell disease, and one of the most common causes of death.[23,25] Patients with acute chest syndrome often have fever, cough, hypoxia, chest pain, dyspnea, or new infiltrates on chest radiograph. The pathophysiologic mechanism of the syndrome is not well understood and is postulated to be related to pulmonary microvascular sludging, infarction of pulmonary parenchyma, and bone marrow fat embolization from infarcted bone. Macrovascular pulmonary embolism and infection may also have a pathogenic role. Acute chest syndrome is commonly associated with infection, including *Mycoplasma* or *Chlamydia* species. The differential includes pneumonia, pulmonary embolism, congestive heart failure, fat embolism, or adult respiratory distress syndrome. Management consists of hydration, analgesia, maintenance of adequate oxygenation and ventilation, and empiric antibiotics with a parenteral cephalosporin, such as ceftriaxone 1 to 2g (50 mg/kg) IV daily, and a macrolide, such as azithromycin 500 mg (10 mg/kg) IV daily.[23,25] Exchange blood transfusions should be considered in patients with multi-lobe involvement, persistent or worsening hypoxemia, neurologic abnormalities, or multi-organ failure.[28] However, there are no randomized controlled studies demonstrating an improvement in outcome with exchange transfusions. Acute chest syndrome can rapidly progress to acute respiratory distress syndrome due to pulmonary sequestration or infarct, and typically requires mechanical ventilation. Long-term complications include pulmonary fibrosis, pulmonary hypertension, and cor pulmonale.[23]

Sickle cell disease is a chronic hemolytic state, often with reasonably compensated hematocrit values in the 20% to 30% range and elevated reticulocyte counts. This compensated balance may be disrupted by iron deficiency or, more commonly, by folate deficiency. A potentially life-threatening aplastic crisis may be seen as a result of suppression of erythropoiesis by an acute post-infectious condition (e.g., Parvovirus B19) or folate deficiency. Aplastic crisis is suspected when the hemoglobin level falls 2 g/dL or more from previous stable levels and the reticulocyte count is low (<2%).

Children may have an acute splenic sequestration syndrome or can develop splenic auto-infarction. This commonly occurs between 10 and 27 months of age. Acute splenic sequestration syndrome involves acute splenic enlargement from increased intrasplenic sickling and obstruction. Rapid sequestration results in a rapidly falling RBC count and circulatory collapse.[28] A Hb drop by greater than 4 g/dL is associated with 35% mortality in the pediatric population.[23] Emergency management is aimed at restoring circulating blood volume with transfusion. Splenectomy is curative, although asplenia results in an increased risk of infection with encapsulated organisms such as *Streptococcus pneumoniae* or *Haemophilus influenzae*. Autosplenectomy occurs as a result of occlusion of the splenic artery, leading to infarction and functional asplenia.[23,25]

Bacterial infections are common due to functional asplenia, and may result in life threatening pneumonia, sepsis, or meningitis, especially in infancy or childhood. Pneumococcal vaccination has dramatically reduced the incidence of invasive pneumococcal disease in sickle cell patients and is a mainstay of preventative therapy, in addition to *H. influenza* type b and meningococcal vaccination series. Prophylactic daily antibiotics, with either amoxicillin or penicillin, are usually required for all children 2 months to 5 years old with functional asplenia.[23,25] A WBC count, blood cultures, urine cultures, and a chest radiograph should be considered in the evaluation of a febrile patient

TABLE 109.7   Organ Damage Seen in Sickle Cell Disease

Organ or System	Injury
Skin	Stasis ulcer
Central nervous system	Cerebrovascular accident
Eye	Retinal hemorrhage, retinopathy
Cardiac	Congestive heart failure
Pulmonary	Intrapulmonary shunting, pulmonary hypertension, embolism, infarct, infection
Vascular	Occlusive phenomenon at any site
Liver	Hepatic infarct, hepatitis resulting from transfusion, hepatic sequestration, intrahepatic cholestasis
Gallbladder	Increased incidence of bilirubin gallstones caused by hemolysis
Spleen	Acute sequestration
Urinary	Hyposthenuria, hematuria, glomerulosclerosis, end-stage renal disease
Genital	Decreased fertility, impotence, priapism
Skeletal	Bone infarcts, osteomyelitis, aseptic necrosis
Placenta	Insufficiency with fetal wastage
Leukocytes	Relative immunodeficiency
Erythrocytes	Chronic hemolysis

with sickle cell disease. Early institution of appropriate antibiotics, such as ceftriaxone 1 to 2 g IV or IM with consideration for vancomycin 15 mg/kg IV, is necessary in patients with a discernible source of infection or sepsis. An increased incidence of *Salmonella* osteomyelitis occurs in sickle cell patients and should be considered in the differential. The origin of immunologic deficiency in sickle cell disease is believed to be multifactorial, involving functional asplenia leading to increased infection risk with encapsulated organisms, poorly migrating neutrophils, and decreased opsonin production.

Major, chronic organ damage in patients with sickle cell anemia is common (Table 109.7). Severe, life threatening multi-organ failure can also occur acutely due to sudden vaso-occlusion in the lungs, liver, or kidneys presenting as abrupt hemodynamic compromise.[23] Acute chest syndrome, sepsis, and multiorgan failure are the leading causes of death in HbSS.

Differential Diagnoses

Sickle cell–β-thalassemia disease is seen most commonly in those of Mediterranean descent. The severity of the disease is related to the concentration of HbS in RBCs, and the decrease in MCHC. It should be considered in a patient with a low MCV and a positive response on sickle preparation. The peripheral smear demonstrates a combination of sickled cells and normocytic target cells. It is generally a milder form than homozygous HbSS, though can also be severe.

HbSC accounts for 30% of the sickle cell disease in the United States and United Kingdom. HbSC results from co-inheritance of HbS and HbC beta globin gene mutations. HbC defect occurs due to a glutamic acid to lysine mutation at position six on the beta chain. Patients with HbSC disease have higher mean Hb and lower absolute reticulocyte counts. RBC lifespan is twice that of HbSS. Anemia in HbSC is mild, and both target cells and sickle cells are seen on peripheral smear. It is considered to be a milder variant, though may be associated with all of the typical HbSS complications as well as an increased incidence of retinopathy.[29]

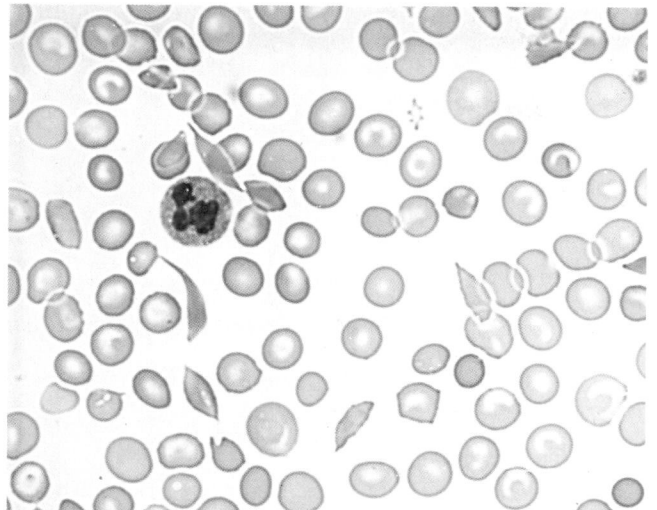

Fig. 109.6 Sickle Cells. (From Hoffbrand AV, Pettite JE. *Color Atlas of Clinical Hematology.* 3rd ed. London: Mosby; 2000:103.)

Diagnostic Testing

The initial diagnosis of sickle cell disease is usually performed via hemoglobin electrophoresis in the neonatal period as a screening test in at risk populations, or at the onset of symptoms. Patients with known or suspected sickle cell disease presenting to the ED should have a complete blood count with differential performed and compared with those of previous visits. A reticulocyte count is recommended whenever the patient's hemoglobin level has decreased by 2 g/dL from baseline. In sickle cell disease, the typical absolute reticulocyte count is three or four times the upper limit of normal. A reticulocyte count 3% or lower than the patient's usual value may suggest an aplastic crisis. A reticulocyte count greater than 12%, particularly if it is accompanied by numerous nucleated RBCs, may indicate rapid hemolysis. Unfortunately, no test is available that detects whether a patient is in a crisis, and the diagnosis is based largely on clinical presentation. In undiagnosed cases, the peripheral smear may show sickled cells (Fig. 109.6), but the definitive diagnosis of sickle cell disease is confirmed by hemoglobin electrophoresis.

Management

Current therapies, including rest, adequate nutrition, hydration, oxygenation, analgesia, transfusion, and therapy for infection, are directed toward symptomatic relief and attempts to interrupt the cycle of deoxygenated sickling and intravascular sludging. Although the use of supplemental oxygen may have some theoretical advantages, it has not been shown to reduce opioid use or hospitalization in patients that are not hypoxic.

Analgesia is a major benefit and essential early therapy for acute sickle cell vaso-occlusive crises. Many emergency clinicians caring for large populations of sickle cell patients have developed protocols to establish better physician-patient rapport, and to lessen the potential for narcotic addiction or manipulation. The following is a protocol for severe pain in adults and children weighing more than 50 kg: patients are evaluated, treated with oxygen and hydration, and given intravenous morphine sulfate, 5 to 10 mg every 2 to 4 hours, or intravenous hydromorphone, 1.5 mg every 3 to 4 hours. For children weighing less than 50 kg, intravenous bolus doses of morphine sulfate, 0.1 to 0.15 mg/kg, can be given every 2 to 4 hours, or intravenous hydromorphone, 0.015 to 0.020 mg/kg, can be given every 3 to 4 hours. At 4 to 6 hours, the patient is allowed to decide whether pain is appropriately controlled. Outpatient therapy includes 4 to 6 days of an effective oral analgesic. A 40-mg dose of oral morphine sulfate or equivalent is given 1 or 2 hours prior to discharge.[23] A major disadvantage of protocols has been a tendency to treat patients reflexively, rather than carefully considering the potential acute complications of sickle cell disease. A variety of analgesics (nonsteroidal anti-inflammatory drugs, mixed opioid agonist-antagonists, and opioids), dosages, and timing intervals may be selected. As many sickle cell disease patients can have varying degrees of hepatic or renal dysfunction, acetaminophen and nonsteroidal anti-inflammatory drugs should be used with caution. The most important aspect of pain management is a consistent, thorough, and attentive approach that offers true pain relief and helps mitigate potential under treatment.

The antisickling agent hydroxyurea reduces pain crises, the need for blood transfusions, and has reduced mortality.[28] The beneficial effects of hydroxyurea include the induction of fetal hemoglobin and mild myelosuppression. Hydroxyurea can reduce the incidence of acute painful crisis, with the potential to ameliorate chronic organ damage and prolonged survival.[26] However, the effects of hydroxyurea can take weeks to be appreciated, and it is not routinely recommended for acute episodes. Dosing of hydroxyurea should be titrated up to the maximum tolerated dose, usually ranging from 20 to 25 mg/kg/day PO.[26]

RBC transfusion is a mainstay in treatment, and more than 90% of adults with sickle cell disease have received at least one transfusion in their lifetime. Transfusion can be given acutely for severe acute exacerbation of chronic anemia with evidence of hypoxia or hypoperfusion, acute organ damage, or preoperatively as a prophylactic measure.[25] Acute chest syndrome, stroke, aplastic crisis, or acute splenic sequestration represent conditions that typically necessitate acute exchange transfusion, and the decision to initiate should be made in consultation with a hematologist. Chronic transfusions are indicated as stroke prevention in selected patients, or in those with progressive multisystem organ failure. The overall goal of transfusion therapy for symptomatic anemia is a hemoglobin level no higher than 10 g/dL, and a target HbS < 30%. Asymptomatic patients should not be transfused, regardless of hemoglobin value.

Alloimmunization, delayed hemolytic reactions, infection transmission, or iron overload are a few of the devastating complications that can result from long-term transfusion, thus transfusion needs should be carefully considered. Iron overload is treated in the usual manner with oral iron chelation therapy with deferiprone or deferasirox.[23,25]

Priapism is a painful complication of sickle cell disease that may lead to impotence. First-line therapy for priapism is aspiration of blood from the corpus cavernosum and irrigation with an α-adrenergic agent (e.g., phenylephrine). Urologic surgical management is typically reserved for patients who fail aspiration and irrigation.[23,28]

Stem cell transplantation offers the only current cure for sickle cell disease, and is associated with survival rates greater than 90% if the transplant comes from an HLA-matched, disease-free sibling. Due to the restrictive criteria for transplantation, as well as long-term conditioning regimen toxicities and transplant-related mortality, there is limited use of this modality and it remains unclear which patients will benefit most.[25]

Other agents and experimental therapies are showing promise and may have a future role in treatment, including steroids, statins, heme-oxygenase, Hb affinity modulators, antioxidants, and gene therapy.[24,28]

Disposition

If pain can be controlled, patients with painful crises can often be discharged with analgesics. Hospitalization may be warranted if pain cannot be adequately controlled. Hospitalization is also typically recommended in patients with acute chest syndrome, acute infections,

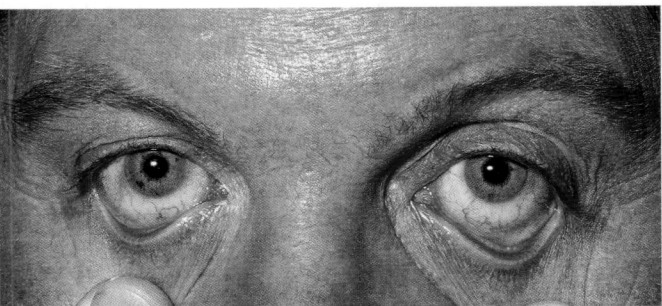

Fig. 109.7 Polycythemia Vera. Facial plethora and conjunctival suffusion in a 40-year-old woman (hemoglobin, 19.5 g/dL). (From Hoffbrand AV, Pettite JE. *Color Atlas of Clinical Hematology*. 3rd ed. London: Mosby; 2000:248.)

acute osteomyelitis, acute stroke, or other complications or disease states requiring further inpatient intervention.

POLYCYTHEMIA

Foundations

Polycythemia is a term commonly used for erythrocytosis (i.e., increased number of RBCs). This disorder is seen occasionally in EM, though rarely requires emergency intervention. An elevated RBC count, usually greater than the hematocrit, defines the disorder. It results in a low MCV, usually related to low serum iron and iron stores.

The major complications of polycythemia are related to the increase in blood viscosity associated with increased RBC numbers. As the hematocrit rises past 60%, viscosity increases in an almost exponential manner, resulting in reduced tissue flow, thrombosis, and hemorrhage.

Clinical Features

Symptoms may range from mild headaches to a fulminant syndrome of hypervolemia (vertigo, dizziness, blurred vision, or headache), hyperviscosity (arterial or venous thrombosis), and platelet dysfunction (epistaxis, spontaneous bruising, or gastrointestinal bleeding).[30]

On examination, the skin and mucous membranes may manifest plethora, engorgement, and venous congestion (Fig. 109.7). Other findings include venous congestion of the optic fundus, splenomegaly, or signs of congestive heart failure.[30] Investigation for uterine, central nervous system, renal, or hepatic tumors should be sought, as such tumors may result in secondary polycythemia.

Differential Diagnosis

Erythrocytosis can be absolute or relative (Box 109.15), and polycythemia is typically classified as primary, secondary, or apparent. Apparent polycythemia is a decrease in plasma volume, and RBC volume does not exceed the upper limit of normal. This is typically seen in the dehydrated patient and is consistent with volume contraction. Treatment is with hydration.

Primary polycythemia vera (PV) is a chronic myeloproliferative neoplasm caused by JAK2 mutations found predominantly in middle-aged or older patients. Initial symptoms are nonspecific and include headache, weakness, dizziness, excessive sweating, plethora, or pruritus after a hot water exposure.[31] The most serious complications include thrombotic episodes (cerebrovascular accident, myocardial infarction, or deep venous thrombosis), bleeding, and risk of leukemic or fibrotic transformation. Primary PV involves all cell lines—hematopoietic stem, erythroid, granulocytic, and megakaryocytic, and presents with elevated hemoglobin and RBC mass, thrombocytosis, and leukocytosis. The diagnostic criteria used by the World Health Organization and revised in 2016 are listed in Box 109.16.[31]

BOX 109.15 Causes of Absolute and Relative Polycythemia

Absolute Erythrocytosis
Right-to-left shunt
Pulmonary disease
Carboxyhemoglobinemia
High-altitude acclimatization
High affinity hemoglobins
Sleep apnea syndrome
Renal disease: focal sclerosing glomerulonephritis, renal transplantation
Tumors: hepatoma, adrenal tumors, meningioma, pheochromocytoma, hemangioblastoma
Drugs: Androgenic steroids, Recombinant erythropoietin
Polycythemia vera

Relative Erythrocytosis
Loss of fluid from vascular space: emesis, diarrhea, diuretics, burns, hypoalbuminemia
Chronic plasma volume contraction: hypoxia, hypertension, tobacco use, ethanol abuse

---

BOX 109.16 Diagnostic Criteria for Polycythemia Vera[a]

Major Criteria
1. Hemoglobin >16.5 g/dL in men or >16 g/dL in women or hematocrit >49% in men or >48% in women or increased red blood cell mass
2. Bone marrow tri-lineage proliferation with pleomorphic mature megakaryocytes
3. Presence of JAK2 mutation

Minor Criterion
Subnormal serum erythropoietin level

[a] Diagnosis of polycythemia vera requires all three major criteria or two major criteria and minor criterion.

The mainstay of therapy is phlebotomy to a hematocrit of less than 45% to assist in preventing thrombosis. The reduced hematocrit improves some symptoms, though neither leukocytes nor platelet counts are decreased.[30,31] In addition to phlebotomy, once-daily low-dose aspirin (40 to 100 mg PO) is recommended to prevent thrombosis. In patients with high-risk disease (history of thrombosis or >60 years of age), the addition of hydroxyurea is recommended at a dose of 500 mg PO twice daily. If there has been a prior history of arterial thrombosis, aspirin may be dosed twice daily. Venous thrombosis is typically treated with systemic anti-coagulation. In patients intolerant or resistant to hydroxyurea, interferon, busulfan, or ruxolitinib can be considered.[31] Complications necessitating additional therapy include hyperuricemia, refractory increased RBC mass, severe pruritus, excessive splenomegaly, or symptomatic thrombocytosis. Additional therapies may include paroxetine, transexamic acid, pipobroman, allopurinol, low-dose thalidomide, or prednisone. Splenectomy may be warranted in the setting of severe splenomegaly.[30] The natural history of the disease is protracted with survival less than but comparable to the general population. The most common causes of death include thrombosis, or worsening disease resulting from transformation to myelofibrosis or acute leukemia.[32]

Diagnostic Testing

Secondary polycythemia is classified according to appropriate erythropoietin response to abnormal tissue oxygen levels. This group of disorders may be excluded by normal measured arterial oxygen saturation. Also, inappropriate autonomous erythropoietin production is considered, which can be assessed with an erythropoietin assay. Because of a strong association with renal pathologic conditions and malignancies, computed tomography should be considered to evaluate a patient with a suspected inappropriate erythropoietin response. Patients with secondary polycythemia infrequently have central nervous system symptoms or splenomegaly. As erythropoietin stimulates only the red cell pathway, WBC and platelet counts should be unchanged.

Management

The emergency treatment of symptomatic polycythemia is phlebotomy. A commonly employed approach is to remove approximately 500 mL of blood and replace it with a comparable amount of saline. Hemodynamic compromise should be averted if this procedure is performed slowly. In true emergencies, 1 to 1.5 L of blood may be removed during a 24-hour period. The initial goal is to lower the hematocrit toward 60%; the ultimate goal is a level less than 45%.

Disposition

Selected patients with known polycythemia may be managed by serial outpatient phlebotomies. Newly diagnosed or symptomatic patients should be considered for admission for further diagnostic evaluation.

The references for this chapter can be found online at ExpertConsult. com.

110

White Blood Cell Disorders

Brian L. Springer and Alan A. Dupré

FOUNDATIONS

Background and Importance

The white blood cell (WBC) and accompanying differential count are among the most common laboratory tests ordered in the emergency department (ED) setting. Unfortunately, the WBC count has not proved to be a highly sensitive or specific test, and the absence of leukocytosis does not exclude the presence of significant infection or disease. Acute infection remains the most common nonmalignant cause of leukocytosis. In evaluation of the bacterial infectious potential in febrile children and adults, the WBC and differential counts have demonstrated limited usefulness as stand-alone biomarkers. Other tests, such as procalcitonin and C-reactive protein (CRP), may have more predictive value.[1,2] Thus, the WBC count should be viewed as having limited screening value in the acute care setting. However, when combined with history and physical examination findings, the WBC and differential counts can be of utility in helping determine the presence of acute infection or other processes.[1,3]

Anatomy and Physiology

The WBC (leukocyte) series can be divided into three basic cell types: granulocytes (neutrophils, eosinophils, and basophils), monocytes (nongranulated cells that mature into macrophages), and lymphocytes. WBCs reach their site of action through the circulation. The rate at which new cells enter the circulation is usually in equilibrium with the rate of loss in tissues. The granulocytic series is primarily involved in phagocytic activity. Its origin is the pluripotential stem cells located in the bone marrow. A subset of these cells differentiates and matures into the phagocytic cell lines, which include neutrophils, basophils, and eosinophils. Nongranulated phagocytic monocytes also develop from this same lineage. Granulocytes originate, mature, and are stored in the bone marrow, with a lifespan of days once released into the peripheral circulation. The postmitotic storage pool for neutrophils, which represents 15 to 20 times the circulating population, contains metamyelocytes, band neutrophils, and mature neutrophils (polymorphonuclear neutrophils). The pool can be drawn on as a ready reserve during rapid consumption of granulocytes. Circulating neutrophils are subdivided equally into the circulating neutrophil pool and the marginal pool, consisting of mature cells adherent to the blood vessel walls. During times of physiological stress, the marginal pool can rapidly enter the circulating pool and cause a substantial increase, even doubling, of the WBC count with neutrophilic predominance. This typically resolves within 24 to 48 hours; persistent elevation may be an indicator of leukemia or other malignancy. These patients should be referred to a primary care physician or hematologist for further evaluation.

The lymphocytic series matures in lymphoid tissues located in the bone marrow, thymus, spleen, lymph nodes, or elsewhere. They are involved in the immune response against foreign substances. There are two morphologically indistinguishable lymphocyte cell types: B cells (humoral immunity) and T cells (cellular immunity). Because lymphocytes can freely leave and return to the circulation, the storage pools are less well defined. Only a relatively small number of total body lymphocytes are in circulation at any point in time.

One unique problem in WBC disorders is the wide variability in normal values and the multiple factors influencing them. WBC counts are generally performed automatically by electrical impedance or optical diffraction techniques. Although differential counts are commonly performed by direct examination of 100 to 500 cells with the oil immersion lens of the microscope, automated techniques are becoming more popular. Normal values for the WBC count are listed in Table 110.1. The "normal" count is age dependent and may be shifted upward by exercise, female gender, smoking, or pregnancy. Similarly, certain ethnic populations such as Blacks have a lower total WBC count and neutrophil, with a higher percentage of monocytes and lymphocytes.[4] Laboratory errors may be due to improper sample preparation, nucleated red blood cells (RBCs), or platelet clumping. The blood smear differential count may also be influenced by small sample size, improper cell identification, and age group (children). Differential ranges are listed in Table 110.2. One common yet easily corrected error in laboratory analysis is reporting of results in terms of the percentage of cell types. Absolute counts for each cell type are more accurate and useful in assessing the risk for infection.

Pathophysiology

Alterations in cell counts are due to changes in production, the marginal pool, or the rate of tissue destruction. The differential diagnosis of increased or decreased WBC counts can be organized by processes impacting production, destruction, loss, or sequestration. Decreased production is caused by suppression of the bone marrow secondary to chemotherapy, radiation therapy, or viral infections. Beta-lactam antibiotics, rheumatoid arthritis, and other autoimmune diseases can destroy neutrophils and reduce the WBC count. Overwhelming bacterial infections can deplete the supply of WBCs faster than the bone marrow can increase production, resulting in net loss. Finally, sequestration may occur secondary to ischemic reperfusion injury, major trauma, or other tissue insults.

Given the spectrum of anticipated values, WBC count determinations should be interpreted in the context of the overall clinical picture. A careful history and physical examination, absolute cell counts, and review of the peripheral smear differential counts are valuable in determining the origins of quantitative WBC disorders.

Leukocytosis, or elevation in WBC count, is most frequently caused by increases in the neutrophil or lymphocyte cell lines. Neutrophilic leukocytosis (neutrophilia) is defined as an absolute neutrophil count greater than 7500 cells/mm³ and is commonly associated with infection

or inflammation (Box 110.1). This is manifested as a "left shift" in the differential count and represents movement of immature neutrophils from the postmitotic pool into the circulation. Because infection or inflammation is also associated with heightened peripheral neutrophil destruction, the proportion of immature (band) to mature neutrophils may increase beyond the baseline ratio of 1 band to 10 mature neutrophils.

WBC counts can also increase through demargination of neutrophils from the vessel walls, which often occurs in response to physiologic stress, endogenous or administered epinephrine, and exercise.[5,6]

Leukopenia is a broad definition that indicates any reduction in the circulating WBCs. The term *leukopenia* is often used interchangeably with *neutropenia*, which specifically refers to a reduction of the neutrophil cell line. Neutropenia is the most clinically significant leukopenia.

By definition, adult neutropenia is defined as an abnormally low absolute neutrophil count (ANC), calculated by multiplying the WBC count by the combined percentage of segmented and band neutrophils. An ANC below 1500 cells/mm³ is considered mild neutropenia, less than 1000 cells/mm³ is moderate, and less than 500

TABLE 110.1 Normal Ranges for the Blood Leukocyte Count (cells/mm³)[a]

Age	Average	95% Range (Average Value ±2 Standard Deviation)
1 week	12,200	5000–21,000
6 months	11,900	6000–17,500
12 months	11,400	6000–17,500
4 years	9100	5500–15,500
8 years	8300	4500–13,500
Adults	7400	4500–11,000

[a]Normal leukocyte count varies with ethnicity, age, gender, smoking, pregnancy, and aerobic exercise.
Modified from: Lanzkowsky P, Lipton JM, Fish JD. *Lanzkowsky's Manual of Pediatric Hematology and Oncology*. Sixth ed. London: Academic Press; 2016.

BOX 110.1 Common Causes of Leukocytosis

Leukocytosis
Primary
Myeloproliferative disorders: Chronic myeloid leukemia (CML), polycythemia vera
Hereditary neutrophilia
Familial myeloproliferative disease
Chronic idiopathic neutrophilia
Leukemoid reaction

Secondary
Infection
Tissue necrosis: Cancer, burns, infarctions
Metabolic disorders: Diabetic ketoacidosis, thyrotoxicosis, uremia
Non-hematologic malignant disease
Physiologic stress: Exercise, pain, surgery, hypoxia, seizures, trauma
Drugs: Epinephrine, corticosteroids, lithium, cocaine
Laboratory error: Automated counters, platelet clumping, precipitated cryoglobulin

Lymphocytosis
Viral infection: Mononucleosis, rubeola, rubella, varicella, toxoplasmosis
Lymphoproliferative: Acute or chronic lymphocytic leukemia (ALL, CLL)
Immunologic response: Immunization, autoimmune diseases, graft rejection

TABLE 110.2 Normal Percentages for the Leukocyte Differential Count in Blood[a]

Age	Segmented Neutrophils	Lymphocytes	Monocytes	Eosinophils
1 week	45% (5500)	41% (5000)	9% (1100)	4% (500)
6 months	32% (3800)	61% (7300)	5% (600)	3% (300)
12 months	31% (3500)	61% (7000)	5% (600)	3% (300)
4 years	42% (3800)	50% (4500)	5% (500)	3% (300)
8 years	53% (4400)	39% (3300)	4% (400)	2% (200)
Adult	59% (4400)	34% (2500)	4% (300)	3% (200)

[a]Numbers in parentheses indicate the average number of cells per cubic millimeter.
Modified from: Lanzkowsky P, Lipton JM, Fish JD. *Lanzkowsky's Manual of Pediatric Hematology and Oncology*. Sixth ed. London: Academic Press; 2016.

cells/mm³ is severe. Severe neutropenia is a well-known risk factor for increased susceptibility to bacterial infection.

Clinical Features

WBC disorders often present with clinical features characteristic of the underlying cause of the WBC disorder (e.g., characteristics of inciting infection in the setting of leukocytosis). The exception is hyperleukocytosis (WBC >100,000/mm³) which can result in leukostasis, a syndrome characterized by metabolic abnormalities, coagulopathy, and multiorgan failure.[7] Although any organ system may be affected, symptoms most often arise from involvement of the cerebral, pulmonary, or renal microvasculature. Central nervous system (CNS) signs and symptoms may include headache, confusion, lethargy, dizziness, blurred vision, ataxia, papilledema, and retinal or intracranial hemorrhage. Pulmonary signs and symptoms may include dyspnea, tachypnea, hypoxia, pulmonary infiltrates, or respiratory failure. Mechanical obstruction of the capillaries also commonly results in peripheral vascular occlusion, acute renal failure, or myocardial infarction.

Differential Diagnoses

Leukocytosis can be caused by primary WBC disorders, including myeloproliferative disorders, hereditary leukocytosis, congenital anomalies, or a leukemoid reaction, which is a pronounced leukocytosis associated with acute inflammation or infection that may be mistaken for leukemia. Secondary forms of leukocytosis are more common. Box 110.1 lists common causes of primary or secondary leukocytosis, as well as lymphocytosis.

Diagnostic Testing

A complete blood count (CBC) often identifies the WBC disorder. Coexisting anemia, thrombocytopenia, or thrombocytosis may also have diagnostic significance. For example, the presence of pancytopenia may indicate aplastic anemia and bone marrow failure due to bone marrow neoplastic disease, toxins, chemotherapy or radiation therapy, or an autoimmune disorder. Additional laboratory tests that may aid in the evaluation of a WBC disorder include a peripheral blood smear, sedimentation rate, or CRP. Peripheral blood smears allow the clinician to examine the cells and identify abnormal cell morphology. Elevation of the ESR or CRP may indicate occult infection and guide the emergency physician to initiate antimicrobial treatment. In the setting of hyperleukocytosis, a chest radiograph or neurologic imaging are often indicated, particularly if pulmonary or CNS signs or symptoms are present, respectively.

Automated hematology counters are increasingly able to quantify the number of immature granulocytes (IG) in the peripheral blood stream. IG measurements include granulocyte precursors other than band neutrophils. Elevation of IG may have a role in identifying patients with severe sepsis and other diseases associated with systemic inflammatory response syndrome.[8]

Management

The management of most WBC disorders is related to the underlying disease process. Hyperleukocytosis, however, is a hematologic emergency and efforts should be made to lower the WBC as rapidly as possible. Reduction in the WBC can be achieved with chemotherapy, often hydroxyurea, or leukapheresis. Rapid reduction with chemotherapy may induce the tumor lysis syndrome. Decisions regarding chemotherapy and leukapheresis should be made with a hematologist. Because the presence of pulmonary or CNS clinical features resulting from hyperleukocytosis is associated with a high mortality rate, leukapheresis is often the therapeutic modality of choice.[9]

Disposition

As WBC disorders are most commonly associated with an underlying disease process, patient disposition is dependent on the type and severity of the underlying cause.

SPECIFIC DISORDERS

Chronic Myeloid Leukemia

Foundations

Chronic myeloid leukemia (CML) accounts for approximately 10% to 15% of newly diagnosed adult leukemia, making it the least common of the major leukemias. The vast majority of cases arise from a genetic translocation, resulting in an aberration known as the Philadelphia chromosome. The initiating factor that triggers this somatic mutation remains unknown, but the mutation is found only in affected cells and is not inherited. The resulting peripheral blood smear in the chronic phase is characterized by myeloid cells in all stages of differentiation demonstrating a leukocytosis with immature myelocytes, metamyelocytes, band cells, and mature polymorphonuclear leukocytes (Fig. 110.1). Risk increases with age, with the median age of diagnosis between 57 and 60 years, with a slight male predominance. Overall, rates of diagnosis have remained stable over the last several decades.[10]

Clinical Features

Clinical staging of CML reflects progression through three phases in the absence of effective treatment: chronic, accelerated, and blastic. Symptom onset during the chronic phase tends to be insidious, with up to 50% of patients remaining asymptomatic at the time of diagnosis. Eventually, the abundance of immature cells begins to crowd out and impair the function of normal white and red blood cells, as well as platelets and other elements of the circulatory system. The most common presenting features in those who are symptomatic include GI features such as abdominal pain, decreased appetite, nausea, or early satiety resulting from hepatomegaly and splenomegaly. Significant left upper quadrant pain may result from splenic infarction. Hypermetabolism associated with the disease can result in fatigue, weight loss, diaphoresis, or low-grade fevers. Patients in the accelerated or blastic phase often present with abnormal bleeding and bruising, petechiae, bone pain, or fever. Fever in the late stages often results from opportunistic infection. Hyperleukocytosis and hyperviscosity are uncommon, and the more mature granulocytes seen in CML are less likely to result in leukostasis.

Late problems in the natural history of CML involve progressive loss of cell differentiation or response to therapy. The term *blastic crisis* represents the sudden appearance of an acute form of leukemia, which is rare and associated with poor outcomes.[11] The condition may occur in lymphoid or myeloid forms. Presenting signs and symptoms of blastic crisis are related to leukostasis and bone marrow infiltration and include anemia, abnormal bleeding due to thrombocytopenia, dyspnea, or neurologic symptoms. Prognosis remains poor despite intensive supportive treatment with chemotherapeutic agents.

Differential Diagnoses

The differential diagnoses include a leukemoid reaction or lymphocytic leukocytosis, including CLL or ALL. The initial presentation may be similar to that of CLL or ALL, though patients tend to be older, with WBC counts greater than 50,000 cells/mm³ in CML. A leukemoid reaction is a nonleukemic reactive leukocytosis that resembles CML. It may be triggered by infection, including *Clostridium difficile* disease, nonhematopoietic neoplasm, or bleeding.[12]

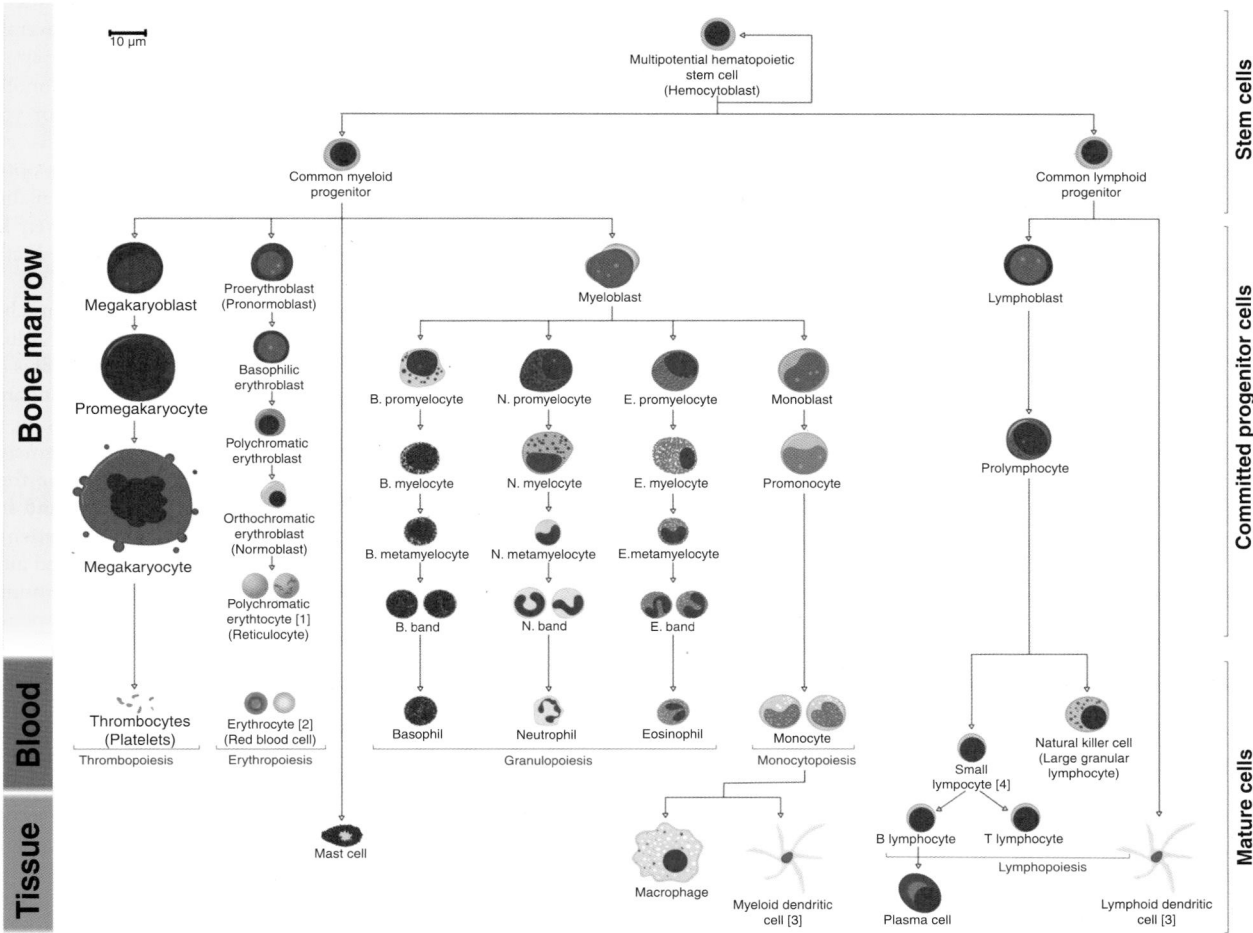

Fig. 110.1 Hematopoiesis, including myeloid and lymphoid cells in all stages of differentiation. Note immature myelocytes, metamyelocytes, band cells, as well as mature polymorphonuclear leukocytes present on the blood smear of patients with chronic myeloid leukemia. (From https://commons.wikimedia.org/wiki/Category:Mikael_Häggström/Medical_diagrams#/media/File:Hematopoiesis_(human)_diagram_en.svg.)

Diagnostic Testing

Associated laboratory abnormalities include a decreased leukocyte alkaline phosphatase and increased vitamin B_{12} levels, neither of which are associated with leukemoid reactions.

Management

Treatment for CML has evolved over the last several years to include the use of tyrosine kinase inhibitors (TKIs) that target the proteins that result from the Philadelphia chromosome genetic anomaly. Overall, survival has improved to the point where life expectancy nears that of the general population.[13] Patients in the accelerated phase may also respond to TKIs, although longer-term response to therapy tends to be limited. Patients in the blast phase may respond to chemotherapy agents targeted towards ALL, although long-term response is rare and palliative therapy may be indicated. Stem cell transplant, once a hallmark of treatment for CML, is rarely performed in the era of TKIs, though may be considered in young patients and in the setting of an accelerated or blast phase, or nonresponse to TKIs.

The need for urgent therapy in CML is usually related to hyperuricemia and renal injury, or severe anemia and subsequent angina or heart failure. Given the comparatively more mature, "less sticky" cells seen in CML, hyperleukocytosis rarely occurs unless WBC counts

exceed 500,000 cells/mm^3. A higher cell count may cause leukostasis and result in deafness, visual impairment, pulmonary ventilation-perfusion abnormalities, or priapism. Treatment includes hydration, leukapheresis, allopurinol to prevent severe hyperuricemia, and specific chemotherapy. Given the risk of increased blood viscosity, red blood cell transfusion should be reserved for symptomatic anemia.[9]

Disposition

Asymptomatic patients should be promptly referred to an oncologist. Patients requiring urgent treatment for symptomatic anemia, leukostasis, or blast crisis will require hospitalization for emergent treatment, guided by oncology consultation.

Lymphocytic Leukocytosis

Foundations

The definition of lymphocytic leukocytosis (lymphocytosis) varies by age: greater than 9000 cells/mm^3 for ages 1 to 6 years, greater than 7000 cells/mm^3 for ages 7 to 16 years, and greater than 5000 cells/mm^3 for adults. It is seen in a variety of disorders, primarily infections or lymphoproliferative disease. The terms *acute* or *chronic* are currently utilized to describe the cell maturity, rapidity of onset, and aggressiveness of therapy. Chronic lymphocytic leukemia (CLL) is the most common type of leukemia seen in individuals aged 50 years or older, and the most common leukemia seen in Western countries. The median age of diagnosis is 72 years. It is primarily a B-cell disorder, initiated by genomic alterations that impair apoptosis of clonal B cells. The disease is characterized by an accumulation of mature B lymphocytes in the peripheral circulation, bone marrow, lymph nodes, and spleen. The risk of developing CLL increases with age.[14]

Acute lymphocytic leukemia (ALL) is the most common cancer diagnosed in children. Like CLL, it is a clonal disease of the bone marrow, in this case characterized by proliferation of B-cell or T-cell precursors that ultimately crowd out and impair the development of other normal marrow elements. This results in anemia, neutropenia, and thrombocytopenia. Lymphoblasts outside the marrow result in lymphadenopathy, splenomegaly, or hepatomegaly. In pediatric ALL, an acquired or inborn genetic mutation creates susceptibility to the disease. It is theorized that a subsequent infection, toxin exposure, or other immune insult triggers further mutations that activates the disease process.[15] ALL is less common in older adults. The etiology of ALL in adults is less well understood and is related to genetic alterations that result in proliferation of lymphocyte precursors.[16]

Clinical Features

CLL is associated with a heterogenous presentation and clinical course. Patients are most often diagnosed after incidental findings such as an abnormal WBC count, enlarged lymph nodes, a palpable spleen, or an enlarged liver. Lymphadenopathy is common and seen in more than half of CLL patients at diagnosis, while splenomegaly is found in almost half. The most common symptoms are reflective of lymphocytic proliferation affecting other bone marrow cell lines and include fatigue and malaise, weight loss, decreased appetite, or decreased exercise tolerance. Signs include pallor, petechia, purpura, or other abnormal bleeding. Increased susceptibility to infection may be seen. The majority of patients follow an indolent clinical course, requiring either no treatment or delayed treatment once the disease becomes symptomatic. Rarely, patients experience aggressive early disease necessitating treatment and associated with recurrent relapses. The majority of patients have survival rates of 5 to 10 years, with increasing survival attributable to improvements in immunotherapy and chemotherapy.[17]

Although the symptoms commonly associated with ALL are nonspecific, persistence of symptoms may prompt further evaluation, particularly in the nonemergency setting. The potential for leukostasis increases in ALL when the blast count rises above 50,000 cells/mm³.

Diagnostic Testing

The CBC may demonstrate a preponderance of B lymphocytes, with an absolute lymphocyte count greater than 5000 cells/mm³ in adults. The diagnosis of CLL is confirmed when these B cells are determined to be monoclonal, either through flow cytometry or molecular assays.[18]

Abnormalities in ALL include anemia or thrombocytopenia. The WBC count may be normal, low or elevated, though the WBC differential will typically show diminished neutrophils at the expense of an increased percentage of lymphocytes. Definitive diagnosis is made through bone marrow aspiration and biopsy demonstrating proliferation of lymphoblasts. Immune and genetic testing help identify the disease subtype and specific cytogenetic-molecular abnormalities that may guide targeted therapy in order to improve survival.[19]

Management

Patients with CLL require treatment once they become significantly symptomatic. Progressive anemia or thrombocytopenia,

symptomatic splenomegaly or lymphadenopathy, or rapid increase in lymphocytosis are indications for initiating treatment. Several treatment options exist, with multiple regimens of chemotherapy agents and monoclonal antibodies that may either be used as monotherapy or in various combinations. In patients aged 65 years or younger, combination chemoimmunotherapy is used and may have curative potential. Allogenic stem cell transplantation remains an option for high-risk patients, but is used less with the current availability of novel agents.[20] Hyperleukocytosis and leukostasis are rarely seen as complications of CLL, but when present warrant leuko-reduction via leukapheresis.

Multiagent chemotherapy regimens are effective in children, with complete remission seen in over 90% of patients. Adult ALL has a much poorer prognosis, with complete remission rates of only 20% to 40%. This is largely driven by intolerance to standard-dose chemotherapy regimens and high rates of myelosuppression-related complications and mortality.[16] The additions of tyrosine kinase inhibitors, monoclonal antibodies, and targeted immune therapies as treatment options appear to be improving remission and survival rates and are better tolerated by the elderly.[21] Adult patients who respond to initial chemotherapy were traditionally offered allogenic bone marrow transplant, though novel targeted and immune therapies lead to questions regarding the necessity of transplantation. Patient age, comorbidities, disease subtype, and genetics, as well as response to therapy all factor into decision making regarding transplant therapy.[22]

Leukopenia

Foundations

Leukopenia is a broad definition that indicates any reduction in the circulating WBCs. The term *leukopenia* is often used interchangeably with *neutropenia*, which specifically refers to a reduction of the neutrophil cell line. Neutropenia is the most clinically significant leukopenia.

By definition, adult neutropenia is defined as an abnormally low absolute neutrophil count (ANC), calculated by multiplying the WBC count by the combined percentage of segmented and band neutrophils. An ANC below 1500 cells/mm³ is considered mild neutropenia, less than 1000 cells/mm³ is moderate, and less than 500 cells/mm³ is severe. Severe neutropenia is a well-known risk factor for increased susceptibility to bacterial infection.

Neutropenia may be caused by decreased production, impaired maturation, movement of circulating neutrophils into marginal or tissue pools, increased destruction, or artificially by laboratory error (Table 110.3). Neutropenia increases susceptibility to overwhelming infection. Infectious disease or drug-mediated reactions commonly cause neutropenia in adults. Common infectious etiologies include HIV, EBV, hepatitis, parasitic infections such as malaria, or bacterial sepsis.[23] Medications may cause an immune-mediated neutropenia by forming immune complexes or inducing antibody formation that destroys granulocytes, or by direct cytotoxic effects on the marrow stem cells or neutrophil precursors. Among cancer patients of all ages, treatment-associated neutropenia secondary to cytotoxic chemotherapy is the most common dose-limiting complication.[24] In children, the most common cause of acquired neutropenia is viral infection, followed by medications and autoimmune neutropenia. In healthy children, neutropenia typically resolves in step with resolution of viremia.

Clinical Features. Signs and symptoms of neutropenia are nonspecific and may include fatigue, sweats, or weight loss. Due to the body's inability to mount a substantial inflammatory or purulent response, symptoms of serious bacterial infection in neutropenic patients may be minimal or absent. The clinician should ask patients

TABLE 110.3 Linkage of Leukopenia to Phases of Neutrophil Maturation

Mechanism	Example
Proliferation in bone marrow	Aplastic anemia, leukemia, cancer chemotherapy (cyclophosphamide, azathioprine, methotrexate, chlorambucil) Drugs: Phenothiazines, phenylbutazone, indomethacin, propylthiouracil, phenytoin, cimetidine, semisynthetic penicillins, sulfonamides Infection: Viral, tuberculosis, sepsis
Maturation in bone marrow	Folate or vitamin B_{12} deficiency, chronic idiopathic neutropenia Starvation
Distribution	Hypersplenism: Sarcoidosis, portal hypertension, malaria
Increased use	Infection: Viral most common (mononucleosis, rubella, rubeola), *Rickettsia* organisms, overwhelming bacterial infection Autoimmune disease: Systemic lupus erythematosus, AIDS, Felty syndrome
Laboratory error	Leukocyte clumping, long delay in performing test

AIDS, Acquired immunodeficiency syndrome.

found to be neutropenic about their medication list, a personal or family history of neutropenia, as well as recent suspected infections or other illnesses. The physical examination is directed toward sites of infection, lymphadenopathy, hepatosplenomegaly, or underlying disease.

Diagnostic Testing and Management. Neutropenic fever, defined as a single oral temperature greater than or equal to 101°F (38.3°C) in a neutropenic patient, or greater than or equal to 100.4°F (38°C) for at least an hour, may herald a life-threatening infection and should prompt the initiation of a rapid workup and commonly the administration of broad-spectrum antibiotics. Neutropenic fever is common in those receiving chemotherapy, with up to 80% of patients developing it at least once during the course of treatment.[25] The evaluation should focus on identifying any infectious agents, with particular attention to common locations, such as the lungs, urine, or bloodstream. As such, consideration of chest radiography, urinalysis, and cultures of blood and urine remain prudent.

Disposition

The disposition for febrile neutropenic patients is evolving, and carefully selected patients may be eligible for discharge following ED evaluation. Although it remains the norm, inpatient treatment incurs significant costs and resource utilization, along with exposing the neutropenic patient to nosocomial pathogens. Select patients without significant comorbidities or signs of sepsis, and with reliable follow-up plans, may be considered for outpatient therapy. Disposition decisions should be made in conjunction with the patient's oncologist.[26] Septic patients will require hospitalization and neutropenic isolation precautions. Asymptomatic patients with incidental neutropenia can generally be referred for follow-up, which may include further investigation depending on repeat ANC or clinical course. Patients with a clear reversible source or without significant clinical findings and mild to moderate levels of neutropenia may have outpatient follow-up arranged, preferably after discussion with their physician.

The references for this chapter can be found online at ExpertConsult. com.

111

Disorders of Hemostasis

Jeremiah D. Gaddy and Alan A. Dupré

KEY CONCEPTS

- Although hemostatic disorders are confirmed through laboratory testing, a careful history and thorough physical examination may provide clues to the diagnosis.
- The use of antithrombotic agents remains widespread, whereas diseases such as hemophilia or disseminated intravascular coagulation (DIC) are encountered infrequently in the emergency department (ED) setting.
- Critical thrombocytopenia increases the risk of bleeding, particularly with trauma or invasive procedures. Platelet dysfunction may occur with platelet levels outside of or within the normal range. Aspirin therapy or renal disease, for instance, can cause platelet dysfunction in the setting of a normal platelet count.
- Patients with suspected new diagnosis of immune thrombocytopenic purpura (ITP) should typically be admitted for further management; glucocorticoid therapy is the mainstay of treatment.
- In patients with possible heparin-induced thrombocytopenia (HIT), clinical scoring systems are helpful in risk stratifying the possibility of HIT, prompting early cessation of heparin, alternative anticoagulation, and hematology consultation. Spontaneous HIT should be considered in patients following major surgery (typically an orthopedic procedure), or with recent serious infection.
- Thrombotic thrombocytopenic purpura (TTP) should be suspected if both thrombocytopenia and microangiopathic hemolytic anemia (MAHA) are identified. Early treatment includes plasma exchange therapy.
- Platelet transfusion is rarely indicated unless platelet counts are below 10,000/mm^3 or severe life-threatening bleeding occurs. Platelet transfusion should be avoided in the setting of thrombotic microangiopathies, such as TTP, hemolytic uremic syndrome (HUS), the "hemolysis, elevated liver function tests, and low platelets" (HELLP) syndrome complicating pregnancy, or HIT.
- Hemophiliacs are often highly informed about their disease. It is imperative that prompt intervention with replacement therapy occurs early when bleeding or the potential for bleeding is suspected. As a general rule, 1 U/kg of factor VIII will increase the circulating factor VIII level by 2%.
- Hemophilia with inhibitors creates a challenge for emergency resuscitation, and a treatment option is recombinant Factor VIIa.

FOUNDATIONS

Hemostasis is a dynamic process that is geared to preventing blood from escaping the boundaries of the vessel. This complex process occurs in phases: maintenance of vessel integrity, formation of a platelet plug, propagation of the coagulation cascade, subsequent clot development, followed by fibrinolysis and clot disintegration. Often the steps of platelet plug formation (primary hemostasis) and the coagulation process (secondary hemostasis) are utilized interchangeably, though the processes are distinctly unique yet collaborative. Common hemostatic abnormalities are acquired and result from iatrogenic causes such as medications (e.g., aspirin, warfarin, or direct thrombin inhibitor), from disease (e.g., hepatic insufficiency), and less frequently from congenital abnormalities. Disorders of hemostasis may result in hemorrhage. Identification and expeditious treatment of the underlying cause remains paramount.

Anatomy and Physiology

Vascular integrity is maintained by a lining of overlapping endothelial cells supported by a basement membrane, connective tissue, and smooth muscle. These cells are important in maintaining a barrier to macromolecules, secreting clot-preventing substances and, when injured, in contributing to the metabolic response and local vasoconstriction. The endothelium regulates clot formation by secreting substances such as tissue factor pathway inhibitor (TFPI) and heparin sulfate, preventing propagation of the coagulation pathway, as well as prostacyclin and nitric oxide, which prevent platelet aggregation and act as vasodilators. The endothelium also expresses CD39 (cluster of differentiation 39), which degrades adenosine triphosphate (ATP) and adenosine diphosphate (ADP) to adenosine monophosphate (AMP), a potent antiplatelet and antithrombotic, and adenosine, a potent locally acting platelet inhibitor that prevents platelet plug formation[1] (Fig. 111.1A). When the endothelium's physical barrier has been compromised, exposed von Willebrand factor (vWF) links to platelet glycoprotein Ib (gpIb) receptors allowing platelet adhesion to the intravascular surface. Normal inhibitory mechanisms are disrupted through damage to the endothelial cells, allowing ATP and ADP to interact with receptors to amplify platelet activation (Fig. 111.1B).

Platelets have multiple roles in hemostasis. They are complex cytoplasmic fragments released from bone marrow megakaryocytes largely regulated by thrombopoietin. After initial exposure to damaged endothelium, platelets display glycoproteins to aid in adhesion and aggregation, such as gpIb and gpIIa/IIIb. Platelets also contain lysosomes, microtubules, and granules, among other components. Granules contain over 300 metabolically active substances, including platelet factor 4, additional adhesive and aggregation glycoproteins, coagulation factors, and fibrinolytic inhibitors. Each participates in the process of coagulation and contributes to overall wound healing through the mediation of inflammation, immune response, and infection control. Platelet activity is summarized in Box 111.1. Any step in the platelet pathway may be absent, altered, or inhibited by inherited or acquired disorders. The coagulation cascade forms fibrin, and cross-linked fibrin serves to reinforce the initial platelet plug.

The coagulation pathway is a complex system of checks and balances that results in controlled formation of a fibrin clot. Coagulation factors are summarized in Box 111.2, and a simplified coagulation pathway is

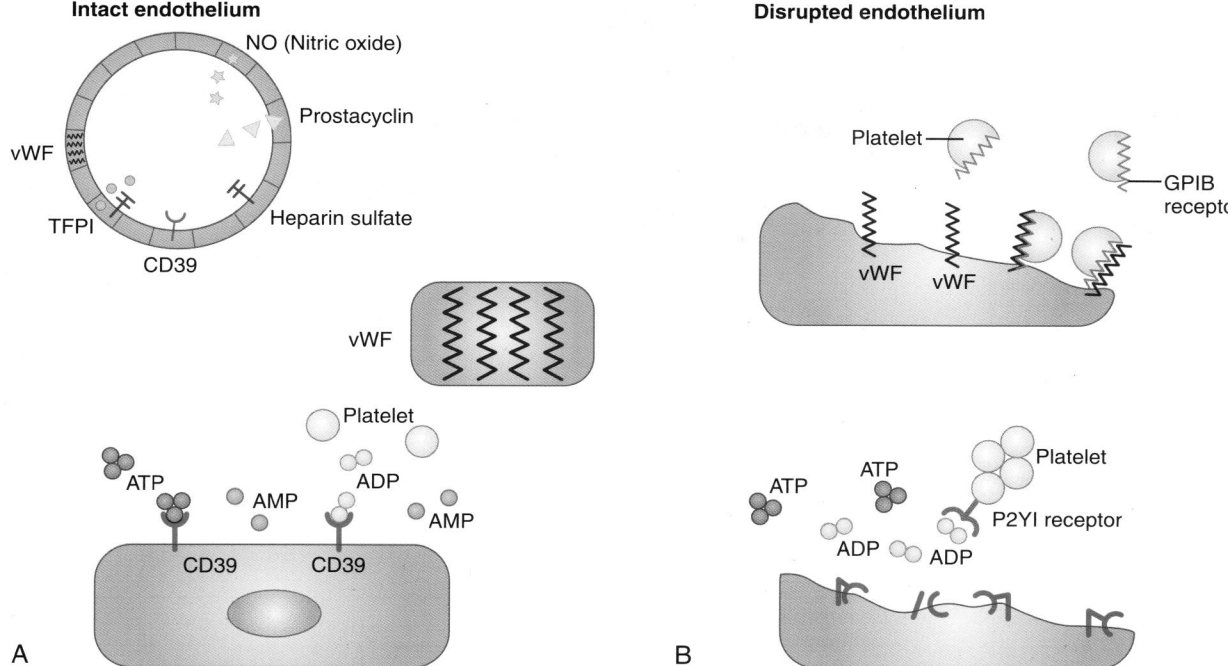

Fig. 111.1 (A) The endothelium regulates clot formation through expression of a number of substances including: CD39 (cluster of differentiation 39), which degrades adenosine triphosphate (ATP) and adenosine diphosphate (ADP) to adenosine monophosphate (AMP), a potent antiplatelet and antithrombotic, and adenosine, a potent locally acting platelet inhibitor that prevents platelet plug formation. (B) When the endothelium is injured the exposed von Willebrand factor (vWF) links to platelet glycoprotein Ib (gpIb) receptors allowing platelet adhesion to the intravascular surface and allowing ATP and ADP to interact with receptors to amplify platelet activation.

BOX 111.1 Role of Platelets in Hemostasis

1. Adhesion to subendothelial connective tissue: Collagen, basement membrane, and noncollagenous microfibrils; serum factor VIII and von Willebrand factor (vWF) permit this function; adhesion creates the initial bleeding arrest plug
2. Release of adenosine diphosphate, the primary mediator and amplifier of aggregation; release of thromboxane A, another aggregator and potent vasoconstrictor; release of calcium, serotonin, epinephrine, and trace thrombin
3. Platelet aggregation over the area of endothelial injury
4. Stabilization of the hemostatic plug by interaction with the coagulation system:
   - Platelet factor 3, a phospholipid that helps accelerate certain steps in the coagulation system
   - Platelet factor 4, a protein that neutralizes heparin
   - Pathway initiation and acceleration by thrombin production
   - Secretion of active forms of coagulation proteins
5. Stimulation of limiting reactions of platelet activity

BOX 111.2 Coagulation Factors

Factor I. Fibrinogen
Factor II. Prothrombin
Factor III. Tissue thromboplastin
Factor IV. Calcium
Factor V. Labile factor (proaccelerin)
Factor VI. Not assigned
Factor VII. Proconvertin
Factor VIII. Antihemophilic A factor
Factor IX. Antihemophilic B factor (plasma thromboplastin component, Christmas factor)
Factor X. Stuart-Prower factor
Factor XI. Plasma thromboplastin antecedent
Factor XII. Hageman factor (contact factor)
Factor XIII. Fibrin-stabilizing factor

presented in Figure 111.2. The clotting cascade is traditionally depicted as consisting of intrinsic and extrinsic pathways. A more modern approach is to view the extrinsic pathway as the initiation phase with exposed tissue factor at the site of vessel injury, and the intrinsic pathway as a parallel and amplification pathway. Both pathways converge to activate factor X, which then converts prothrombin to thrombin. Tissue factor is a critical cofactor that is required for activation of factor VII. Because of limited amounts of tissue factor and rapid inactivation by TFPI, the extrinsic pathway initiates the clot process, though sustained generation of thrombin and clot formation is dependent on the intrinsic pathway through activation of factor IX by activated factor VII. Once coagulation is initiated, controls are necessary to prevent overzealous local or generalized thrombosis (Box 111.3).

Pathophysiology

Hemostasis is dependent on normal functioning and integration of the vasculature, platelets, and coagulation pathway. The most commonly encountered disorder of hemostasis is antithrombotic drug administration, including use of antiplatelet or anticoagulant medications. Disorders of hemostasis may also be congenital, or secondary to disease states that affect the various steps of the hemostatic pathway

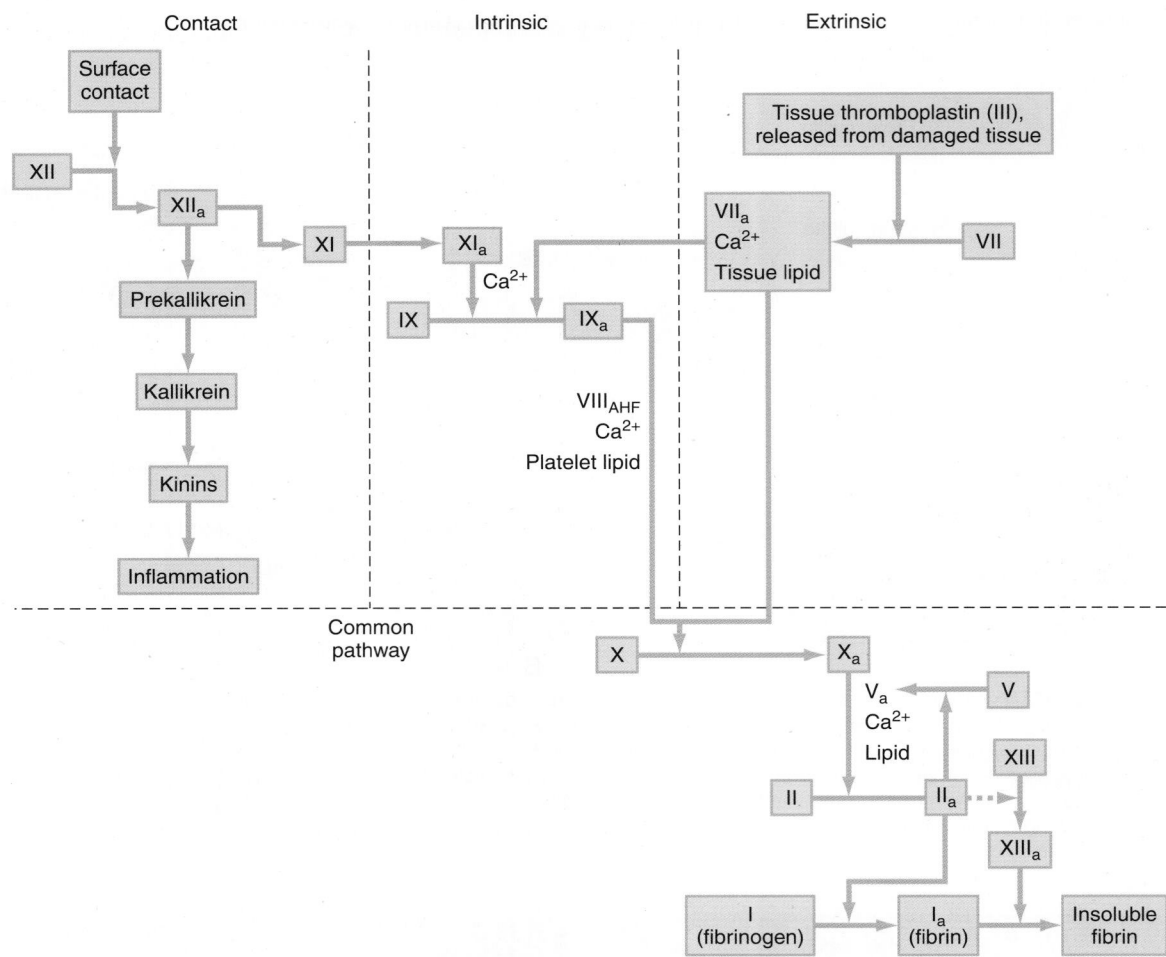

Fig. 111.2 Coagulation pathway.

BOX 111.3   Normal Controls of Coagulation

Removal and dilution of activated clotting factors through blood flow, which also mechanically opposes growth of the hemostatic plug

Alteration of platelet activity by endothelium-generated nitric oxide and prostacyclin

Removal of activated coagulation components by the reticuloendothelial system

Regulation of the clotting cascade by antithrombin III, protein C, protein S, and tissue factor pathway inhibitor (TFPI)

Activation of the fibrinolytic system

---

such as malignancy or hepatic dysfunction. Due to the interconnectedness between the endothelium and platelets, vascular disorders may share similar historical or examination features with platelet disorders. Despite some overlap, disorders of hemostasis are frequently grouped into vascular disorders (often with a component of platelet dysfunction), platelet disorders, and coagulation disorders.

CLINICAL FEATURES

Disorders of hemostasis may become evident through hemorrhage that is out of proportion to what would otherwise be anticipated, excessive ecchymosis, or the presence of a petechial or purpuric rash. Hemostatic

disorders may complicate any medical or traumatic problem, and platelet disorders or coagulopathy can rapidly develop in critically ill patients. Patients that fail to respond to usual hemostatic measures should be considered to have a potential bleeding disorder. When a bleeding disorder is diagnosed or suggested, the assessment initially includes stabilization, which may necessitate intravenous fluids, transfusion of red blood cells (RBC), or other blood component or factor replacement. In the setting of a known disorder, clinical complications associated with the underlying pathophysiologic condition must be considered. If the disorder is unknown, a rapid differential diagnosis should be pursued.

Key components of the history and physical examination are presented in Box 111.4. The history alone may in some cases be useful in differentiating between platelet and coagulation factor disorders.

Platelet disorders are usually manifested as acquired petechiae, purpura, or mucosal bleeding, and are more common in women. Platelet abnormalities can be caused by congenital disorders, though most are related to acquired conditions. The bleeding source is usually a capillary with resultant cutaneous and mucosal petechiae or ecchymosis. Epistaxis, menorrhagia, and gastrointestinal bleeding are common initial symptoms. The bleeding is generally mild and may occur immediately after surgery or dental extractions. The presence of petechiae or purpura may be noted on examination, and superficial ecchymoses may develop around venipuncture sites. The purpura associated with platelet disorders is typically asymptomatic and not palpable. This is

BOX 111.4 Clinical Evaluation of a Bleeding Patient

History
Nature of bleeding
  Petechiae
  Purpura
  Ecchymosis
  Significant bleeding episodes
Sites of bleeding
  Skin
  Mucosa: Oral or nasal
  Muscle
  Gastrointestinal
  Genitourinary
  Joints
Patterns of bleeding
  Recent onset or lifelong
  Frequency and severity
  Spontaneous or following injury
Challenges to hemostasis
  Dental extraction
  Operative or other invasive procedures
  Medications
Associated diseases
  Uremia: most commonly associated with platelet dysfunction
  Liver disease: most commonly associated with coagulation factor deficits
  Infection: could be associated with either platelet or coagulation deficits
  Malignant neoplasm: could be associated with either platelet or coagulation deficits
Previous transfusion history
Family history

Physical Examination
Vital signs
Skin: Nature of bleeding, signs of liver disease, petechial, purpura and distribution of skin abnormalities.
Mucosa: Oral or nasal, epistaxis
Lymphadenopathy
Abdomen: Liver size and shape, splenomegaly
Joints: Signs of previous bleeding (limited joint movement, pain mimicking osteoarthritis)
Other sites of blood loss: Pelvic, rectal, urinary tract, intramuscular or deep soft tissue

BOX 111.5 Features of Coagulation Disorders That Differentiate From Platelet Disorders

The bleeding source is often an intramuscular or deep soft tissue hematoma from small arterioles.
The congenital form of the disease occurs predominantly in men, often via sex-linked inheritance.
Bleeding may occur after surgery or trauma but may be delayed in onset up to 72 hours.
Epistaxis, menorrhagia, and gastrointestinal sources of bleeding are rare, whereas hematuria or hemarthrosis are common in severe cases.
The bleeding time is normal except in patients with von Willebrand disease (vWD).

BOX 111.6 Differential Diagnosis of Platelet Disorders

Decreased Platelet Count (Thrombocytopenia)
Decreased production
  Decreased megakaryocytes secondary to drugs, toxins, or infection
  Normal megakaryocytes with megaloblastic hematopoiesis or hereditary origin
  Platelet pooling and splenic sequestration
Increased destruction
  Immunologic
    • Related to collagen vascular disease, lymphoma, leukemia
    • Drug related
    • Infection
    • Post-transfusion
    • Immune thrombocytopenia
  Mechanical
    • Disseminated intravascular coagulation (DIC)
    • Thrombotic thrombocytopenic purpura (TTP)
    • Hemolytic-uremic syndrome (HUS)
    • Hemolysis elevated liver function tests & low platelets (HELLP) syndrome related to pregnancy
  Vasculitis
Dilutional secondary to massive blood transfusion

Platelet Dysfunction (Thrombocytopathy)
Adhesion defects such as von Willebrand disease (vWD)
Release defects: Acquired or drug related
Aggregation defects, such as in thrombasthenia

Elevated Platelet Count (Thrombocytosis)
Autonomous (primary thrombocythemia)
Reactive (secondary thrombocythemia)
Iron deficiency
Infection or inflammation
Trauma
Nonhematologic malignant disease
Post-splenectomy
Rebound from alcohol, cytotoxic drug therapy, folate or vitamin B_{12} deficiency

in contrast to purpura associated with vasculitis, which can burn or itch and is palpable. Vascular disorders such as vasculitis are associated with signs and symptoms similar to those of thrombocytopenic states. Inherited vascular disorders are rare, and acquired forms are usually associated with connective tissue changes or endothelial damage.

Coagulation issues may be congenital in nature, characterized by delayed deep muscle or joint bleeding, and occur more often in men. Clinically significant coagulation disorders have a number of characteristic features that help differentiate them from platelet disorders (Box 111.5).

DIFFERENTIAL DIAGNOSIS

The differential of platelet disorders is listed in Box 111.6. The differential of vascular disorders is listed in Box 111.7. The differential for coagulation disorders is listed in Box 111.8.

DIAGNOSTIC TESTING

A definitive diagnosis is dependent on laboratory evaluation. Tests pertinent to the ED setting are discussed in the following sections and are listed in Box 111.9.

BOX 111.7 Differential Diagnosis of Vascular Disorders

Inherited
Disorders of connective tissue
  Pseudoxanthoma elasticum
  Ehlers-Danlos syndrome
  Osteogenesis imperfecta
Disorders of blood vessels
  Hemorrhagic telangiectasia

Acquired
Scurvy (vitamin C deficiency)
Simple or senile purpura
Purpura secondary to steroid use
Vascular damage
  Infection (meningococcemia)
  Hemolytic-uremic syndrome (HUS)
  Hypoxemia
  Thrombotic thrombocytopenic purpura (TTP)
  Dysproteinemic purpura

BOX 111.8 Differential Diagnosis of Coagulation Disorders

Inherited
Von Willebrand disease
Hemophilia A (factor VIII) or hemophilia B (factor IX)
Factor XIII, factor XI, factor X, factor VII, factor V or factor II deficiency
Afibrinogenemia/hypofibrinogenemia

Acquired
Medication
Snake bite (venom-induced consumptive coagulopathy)
Liver disease
Disseminated intravascular coagulation (DIC)
Autoimmune disorders (including autoantibodies towards factors such as fibrinogen)
Acquired factor inhibitors, from treatment of congenital disorder such as hemophilia, or malignancy

BOX 111.9 Diagnostic Hemostasis Tests

Complete blood count and smear (EDTA—purple top)
Platelet count (EDTA—purple top)
Bleeding time
Prothrombin time/International normalized ratio (PT/INR; citrate—blue top)
Partial thromboplastin time (PTT; citrate—blue top)
Other coagulation studies: Fibrinogen level, anti-factor Xa assay, thrombin time, clot solubility, factor levels, inhibitor screens
As necessary: Serum electrolyte levels; serum glucose, BUN, and creatinine concentrations; type and crossmatch

BUN, Blood urea nitrogen; *EDTA,* ethylenediaminetetraacetic acid.

Complete Blood Count and Blood Smear

The complete blood count can, in some cases, assess the degree of anemia associated with a bleeding episode. Reductions in hemoglobin and hematocrit often lag behind the actual loss of RBCs in acute hemorrhage owing to the time necessary for equilibration. The peripheral blood smear may demonstrate schistocytes or fragmented RBCs in microangiopathic hemolytic anemias, such as TTP or DIC. Teardrop-shaped or nucleated RBCs may reflect myelophthisic disease where hematopoietic bone marrow is infiltrated and replaced by fibrosis, tumors, or granulomas. Characteristic white blood cell morphologies are seen with thrombocytopenia associated with infectious mononucleosis (e.g., increased WBC cytoplasm and nucleoli in the nuclei), folate or vitamin B_{12} deficiency (e.g., hypersegmented neutrophils), or leukemia (e.g., immature WBCs, hairy cell lymphocytes, and myeloblasts with Auer rods).

Platelet Count

The platelet count may be estimated from the peripheral blood smear. Normally, one platelet is present per 10 to 20 RBCs. Often, the count is automated with a normal reference range of 150,000 to 400,000/mm³. Thrombocytopenia is defined as a platelet count of less than 100,000/mm³. With normal platelet function, the bleeding time with platelet counts below 100,000/mm³ increases in direct relation to the level of thrombocytopenia. Levels below 20,000/mm³ may be associated with serious spontaneous hemorrhage. However, the platelet count provides no information regarding platelet function.

Bleeding Time and Platelet Function Assay

Historically, bleeding time was considered the best test to determine both vascular integrity and platelet function. A normal bleeding time is 8 minutes. A bleeding time of 8 to 10 minutes is borderline, and a bleeding time longer than 10 minutes is considered abnormal. However, bleeding time is insensitive in identifying medication-related platelet dysfunction, Von Willebrand disease (vWD), or in predicting surgical bleeding. Many institutions have replaced the traditional bleeding time with a platelet function analyzer instrument, which is more convenient, with improved clinical value. The platelet function assay has been found to be highly sensitive in detecting moderate to severe vWD, medication-related platelet dysfunction, or severe platelet function disorders. Although less sensitive to mild disease, the platelet function assay is useful in detecting platelet pathology relevant to the emergency clinician. Given the pervasiveness of drug-induced platelet dysfunction, it is critical to inquire about the use of medications, particularly aspirin and other antiplatelet medications (e.g., clopidogrel). Platelet function testing is independent of the coagulation pathways.

Prothrombin Time

The PT tests the factors of the extrinsic and common coagulation pathways. The patient's anticoagulated plasma is combined with calcium and tissue factor protein. Sensitivity to factor deficiencies depends on the source of the tissue factor. The PT is capable of detecting deficiencies in fibrinogen, prothrombin (factor II), factor V, factor VII, and factor X. Results are reported in seconds or as the prothrombin ratio. To generate the prothrombin ratio, the time in seconds of the sample is given over the time of a normal control, for example, 12.5/11.5. Results are also usually reported as the international normalized ratio (INR), which compensates for differences in sensitivity of various thromboplastin reagents to the effects of warfarin by calculating the prothrombin ratio raised to the power of an international sensitivity index for specific thromboplastin reagents. The test is helpful in monitoring the use of coumarin anticoagulants, and the time may be prolonged in patients with liver disease or other abnormalities of vitamin K–sensitive factors.

If all other test results are normal with an abnormal prothrombin time, the elevated PT reflects an extrinsic pathway abnormality mediated through deficiency of factor VII. The hereditary form, congenital proconvertin deficiency, is caused by a rare autosomal recessive gene on chromosome 13. The acquired form is commonly seen and may be a result of vitamin K deficiency, warfarin use, or liver disease. Given factor VII's short half-life (3 to 5 hours), it is typically the first to manifest a deficiency when its active form is underproduced. The PT is a sensitive gauge of hepatic function and the efficacy of warfarin administration. It is recommended with routine warfarin therapy that the INR level is maintained between 2.0 and 3.0, except in the setting of cardiac valvular disease, in which the target INR level is usually in the 2.5 to 3.5 range.

Partial Thromboplastin Time

The PTT tests the components of the intrinsic and common pathways, essentially all factors but factor VII and factor XIII. In this test, a phospholipid source and a contact-activating agent (kaolin) are added to anticoagulated citrate plasma. After an incubation period that allows factor XII to become activated, calcium is added and the clotting time is recorded. A normal control sample is run simultaneously. Normal ranges may vary by laboratory. The average time is 25 to 29 seconds. The sensitivity of the test varies from factor to factor, though factor levels less than 40% are typically required before the PTT is prolonged. The test may be altered by clotting factor inhibitors of external origin (e.g., heparin) or internal origin (e.g., anti–factor VIII antibody). Spurious high values may occur in the setting of heightened plasma turbidity. The activated PTT is most sensitive to abnormalities in the sequence of the coagulation cascade preceding activation of factor X.

Two groups of inherited disorders manifest as an isolated elevation in the PTT. The first group involves deficiencies of the contact factors, including factor XII (Hageman factor), prekallikrein (Fletcher factor), and high-molecular-weight kininogen. They may cause a relatively benign disorder in which the PTT is elevated but the patient has no bleeding diathesis. These deficiencies exist as isolated laboratory abnormalities, and thus they should not be invoked as a cause of the patient's bleeding problem. They may be specifically assayed when a precise diagnosis is necessary. The second group causes significant bleeding problems resulting from deficiencies of factors within the intrinsic coagulation system. They are the most common inherited abnormalities of the clotting system. Deficiencies of factors VIII, IX, and XI account for 99% of inherited bleeding disorders. Patients with active life-threatening bleeding who are thought to have a congenital bleeding disorder can be supported with fresh frozen plasma, 15 mL/kg, while additional information is being obtained and initial diagnostic studies are being performed.

In a patient with a prolonged PTT and a lifelong history of bleeding, the most important test is an assay of factor VIII and factor IX. This test measures the ability of the patient's plasma to correct the prolonged PTT of plasma deficient in a given factor. This ability is compared with that of normal plasma, and the result is given as a percentage of normal. These tests measure the procoagulant activity of the factor, although they do not discriminate between diminished activity resulting from abnormal factor VIII versus lower levels of normal factor VIII. Factor VIII deficiency is found in both hemophilia A and vWD, and factor IX deficiency is found in hemophilia B.

Anti-Xa Assay

The anti-Xa assay is a chromogenic assay that may be available to emergency clinicians for monitoring of unfractionated and low-molecular-weight heparin levels, or drug quantification of direct factor Xa inhibitors such as rivaroxaban and apixaban. When monitoring heparin levels, the test should ideally be performed 3 to 4 hours after medication administration for peak level monitoring. Because this test is not subject to the same variability as the PTT, it has become an attractive alternative as costs of the assay have declined in recent years. The test is

considered the reference standard for measurement of in vivo heparin activity, and presently represents the only reliable means of quantifying rivaroxaban and apixaban drug levels.

Fibrinogen

Fibrinogen is the final coagulation substrate, and its level reflects the balance between production and consumption. It may be decreased by low production, as in severe liver disease, or by overconsumption, as in DIC. Low levels or altered function increase the PT, PTT, and thrombin clotting time. Because fibrinogen is an acute-phase reactant, certain conditions, including malignant disease, sepsis, inflammation, or pregnancy, may impact fibrinogen levels.

Thrombin Time

Measurement of the thrombin clotting time bypasses measurement of the intrinsic and extrinsic pathways by directly analyzing conversion of soluble fibrinogen to insoluble fibrin. It is a useful screening test for both qualitative and quantitative abnormalities of fibrinogen and inhibitors, such as heparin and fibrin split products. The test is also an available means to measure drug activity of direct thrombin inhibitors, such as dabigatran.

Clot Solubility

The result of clot solubility testing may be the only abnormality in disorders involving factor XIII deficiency, which has a role in cross-linking fibrin to stabilize the fibrin clot. A washed clot is incubated in acetic acid or urea. If the fibrin clot is not properly cross-linked by factor XIII, it dissolves.

Factor Level Assays

Factor levels are determined either by bioassay, in which the ability of the sample of plasma to normalize controlled substrate-deficient plasma is evaluated, or by immunologic assay. Inhibitor screening tests reveal antibodies in plasma that prolong the normal plasma clotting time when mixed. Inhibitors may play a disruptive role in disease states such as hemophilia or when associated with certain malignancies.

MANAGEMENT

Thrombocytopenia

Thrombocytopenia can be grouped into two main causes: decreased production or increased destruction. Most experts agree that thrombocytopenia is defined as a platelet count of less than 100,000 micro/mm^3. Thrombocytopenia from decreased bone marrow production is usually caused by the effects of chemotherapeutic drugs, myelophthisic disease, or direct bone marrow effects of agents, such as alcohol or thiazides. Splenic sequestration is a rare cause of thrombocytopenia seen primarily with hypersplenism resulting from malignant hematologic disease, portal hypertension, or disorders involving increased splenic red blood cell (RBC) destruction, such as hereditary spherocytosis, autoimmune hemolytic anemia, or sickle cell disease.

Most platelet disorders are not treated by platelet transfusion, as its efficacy is questionable and alloimmunization may occur. Platelet transfusions are commonly indicated for primary bone marrow disorders (e.g., aplastic anemia or acute leukemia). Assessment of the risk for spontaneous bleeding due to thrombocytopenia is an imprecise science. In contrast to disorders with primary bone marrow involvement, less mature platelets associated with peripheral consumption or sequestration generally have more robust functionality and thus patients are less prone to spontaneous hemorrhage. An estimate of platelet functionality is combined with the platelet count for a more accurate prediction of primary hemostasis potential. At counts higher than 50,000/

BOX 111.10 **Immune Thrombocytopenia Chronicity**

Newly diagnosed: Up to 3 months since diagnosis
Persistent: 3 to 12 months since diagnosis
Chronic: Over 12 months since diagnosis

mm^3, hemorrhage attributed to platelet deficiency is unlikely. At counts below $40,000/mm^3$ to $50,000/mm^3$, a variable degree of risk exists, particularly in the setting of trauma, gastric ulcers, or invasive procedures. Spontaneous bleeding in the absence of surgery, trauma, or other risk factors is more likely when platelet counts reach below $10,000/mm^3$, thus prophylactic platelet infusions should typically be reserved for this degree of thrombocytopenia; however, this threshold may be lower in stable pediatric patients but should initiate hematology consultation.[2] Patients requiring urgent central venous access or lumbar puncture may require platelet transfusion if the count is less than $20,000/mm^3$ or $50,000/mm^3$, respectively.[2] Although literature is sparse, platelet transfusion is generally recommended for patients requiring neurosurgical or invasive ophthalmologic intervention if counts are less than 80,000 to $100,000/mm^3$.[2]

Immune Thrombocytopenia

Immune thrombocytopenia (ITP) is a broad acquired condition that results from autoantibodies against platelet antigens. ITP includes the diseases previously termed idiopathic thrombocytopenic purpura and autoimmune thrombocytopenic purpura. ITP is further broken down into separate categories: primary ITP; secondary ITP, typically resulting from pathogens, disease states, or malignancy; and drug-induced thrombocytopenia (DITP).

Primary ITP is an acquired autoimmune thrombocytopenia that has no apparent trigger or associated condition, and can result in both increased destruction as well as decreased platelet production. Severe ITP is characterized by a platelet count of less than 20,000 micro/mm^3. ITP is further characterized as newly diagnosed, persistent, or chronic (Box 111.10). The acute form of ITP is seen most often in children aged 2 to 6 years old. A viral prodrome commonly occurs within 3 weeks preceding its onset. The platelet count decreases, usually to less than $20,000/mm^3$. The course is self-limited, with a greater than 90% rate of spontaneous remission. Morbidity and mortality rates are low, although full recovery may take several weeks. The chronic form of ITP is primarily an adult disease found three times more often in women. The onset of chronic ITP is insidious, generally without a prodrome, and is manifested as easy bruising, prolonged menses, and mucosal bleeding. Petechiae or purpura are common, with platelet counts typically between $30,000/mm^3$ and $100,000/mm^3$.

Secondary ITP results from various infectious or other chronic disease states. Autoimmune disease, particularly systemic lupus erythematosus and rheumatoid arthritis, may cause an antiplatelet antibody-related thrombocytopenia. Similar associations have been noted with leukemia and lymphoma, particularly lymphocytic lymphoma. Postinfectious immune thrombocytopenia is usually associated with viral diseases, such as HIV, hepatitis (HBV or HCV), Epstein-Barr virus (EBV), rubella, rubeola, or varicella.

DITP is caused by drug-dependent platelet antibodies, which is a distinct mechanism from drugs that cause direct bone marrow suppression. Numerous drugs have been associated with DITP, and the resulting thrombocytopenia is expected to resolve after discontinuation of the offending drug. Owing to its relatively high frequency of use, heparin is an important cause of drug-induced thrombocytopenia in hospitalized patients.

ITP treatment is often supportive, with treatment recommendations distinguished between adult and pediatric patients. Corticosteroids are recommended for newly diagnosed adult patients with platelet counts of less than $30,000/mm^3$ who are asymptomatic or have only minor mucocutaneous bleeding. Dexamethasone, 40 mg PO or IV daily for 4 days, is the preferred glucocorticoid. Admission for further diagnostic evaluation may be considered for newly diagnosed adult patients with platelet counts of less than $20,000\ mm^3$.[3] IVIG in addition to corticosteroids should be considered for patients with platelet counts of less than $10,000\ mm^3$, significant bleeding, or when a more rapid increase in platelet count is necessary, such as the need for surgery or invasive procedure. Use of glucocorticoids with IVIG can be associated with a more sustained response than with IVIG alone.[3] If IVIG is indicated, a one-time dose of 1 g/kg should be given. A thrombopoietin receptor agonist (TPO-RA), such as eltrombopag, should be considered for life threatening bleeding in the setting of inadequate response to corticosteroids, IVIG, and platelet transfusion. Because eltrombopag takes days to weeks to normalize platelets, this will rarely be given in the emergency department and discussion with a hematologist would be prudent. Plasmapheresis and recombinant factor VIIa are no longer recommended.[4] Splenectomy is often considered a last resort for ITP that is refractory to medical management.[3]

Pediatric patients with newly diagnosed ITP and only mild bleeding (skin manifestations) can typically be managed without medication, even when platelet counts are less than $20,000\ mm^3$.[3] Though the overall platelet count is low, a relatively high fraction of newly minted platelets with robust functionality is seen in the circulation, thus patients remain at relatively low risk for significant spontaneous hemorrhage. Admission should be considered when there is uncertainty regarding the diagnosis or lack of close follow-up. Prednisone, IVIG, or anti-D immunoglobulin are available options for pediatric patients with newly diagnosed ITP.[3] As with adult patients, IVIG can be considered if there is a need for a more rapid correction of the platelet count. Treatment options should be discussed with the child's pediatrician or a pediatric hematologist.

Drug-Induced Thrombocytopenia

A number of drugs have been associated with thrombocytopenia of immunologic origin. Quinine and quinidine are common offenders that affect platelets through an "innocent bystander" mechanism. The platelet is coated with a drug-antibody complex, complement is fixed, and intravascular platelet lysis occurs. Beta lactams, quinolones, digoxin, sulfonamides, phenytoin, and aspirin may also be associated with thrombocytopenia, usually within 24 hours of use. Clinical trials with platelet glycoprotein IIb/IIIa antagonists show an increased risk for associated thrombocytopenia, independent of heparin therapy.[5] The platelet count may fall below $10,000/mm^3$ and be complicated by serious bleeding. Laboratory testing may confirm the presence of antibody, especially with the use of quinine and quinidine.

DITP is difficult to discern from ITP, especially during the initial evaluation by the emergency clinician. In DITP, the platelet count should improve within the first 1-2 days of cessation of the offending drug, and return to normal range within a week. In the setting of active bleeding with thrombocytopenia of unclear cause, corticosteroids, IVIG, and possibly platelet transfusion in selected patients are all considerations.

Heparin-Induced Thrombocytopenia. Heparin-induced thrombocytopenia (HIT) is a serious immune-mediated process associated with unfractionated heparin (UFH) and other forms of heparin such as low-molecular-weight heparin (LMWH). Heparin is thought to pair with platelet factor 4 (PF4), a procoagulant substance found in platelet granules. This paired complex results in rapid generation of

TABLE 111.1 4Ts Scoring System

4Ts	2 points	1 point	0 point
Thrombocytopenia	Platelet count fall >50% and platelet nadir ≥ 20	Platelet count fall 30–50% or platelet nadir 10–19	Platelet count fall < 30% or platelet nadir < 10
Timing of Platelet Count Fall	Clear onset between days 5–10 or platelet fall ≤ 1 day (prior heparin exposure within 30 days)	Consistent with days 5–10 fall, but not clear; onset after day 10; or fall ≤ 1 day (prior heparin exposure 30–100 days ago)	Platelet count fall < 4 days without recent exposure
Thrombosis or Sequelae	New thrombosis (confirmed) or skin necrosis; acute systemic reaction post-intravenous unfractionated heparin (UFH) bolus	Progressive or recurrent thrombosis; Non-necrotizing (erythematous) skin lesions; Suspected thrombosis (not proven)	None
Other Causes of Thrombocytopenia	None Apparent	Possible	Definite

TABLE 111.2 4Ts Point Risk Stratification

Total Points	Probability
<3 points	Low probability
4–5 points	Intermediate probability
6–8 points	High probability

antibodies, which coat platelets resulting in thrombocytopenia. The antibodies generated also activate platelets, thus creating a potential hypercoagulable state. Approximately 33% to 50% of patients with HIT will develop HIT with thrombosis (HITT).[6] A HIT-like reaction may also occur in the absence of exposure to heparin.

The overall risk for HIT ranges from 0.1% to 7.0% in patients receiving heparin.[6] The risk of HIT is related to drug and dosage factors, including duration of exposure (risk greatest following 5 days of heparin therapy), heparin type (UFH carries higher risk than LMWH), or dosage (greatest risk with higher doses). In addition, female patients are at twice the risk, and surgical or trauma patients have a higher risk for HIT than medical patients. Delayed HIT occurs a median of 14 days following the initiation of heparin, though may occur up to 40 days out.

The 4Ts Score for HIT is aimed at differentiating patients with HIT from those with alternative causes of thrombocytopenia (Tables 111.1 and 111.2).[6,7] Patients are stratified into low, intermediate or high risk based on degree of thrombocytopenia, timing of onset, presence of thrombosis, and other possible etiologies for the thrombocytopenia. For patients with intermediate or high risk for HIT based on 4Ts Score, heparin should be stopped and an immunoassay ordered. Most anti-PF4-heparin enzyme immunoassays have excellent negative predictive value, thus an unremarkable result effectively rules out HIT.[6] If the immunoassay is positive, a more specific functional test, such as a serotonin release assay, a heparin-induced platelet aggregation assay, or a solid-phase immunoassay, is indicated to confirm the diagnosis.

Current treatment recommendation for HIT is geared primarily toward management of thrombotic complications. If HIT is clinically suspected, immediate cessation of heparin is paramount. Vitamin K antagonists have been shown to increase thrombosis risk and potential for limb loss by decreasing the level of the endogenous anticoagulant protein C upon initiation.[6] Treatments for HIT include non-heparin anticoagulants, such as argatroban, bivalirudin, danaparoid, fondaparinux, or a direct oral anticoagulant (DOAC).[6] Argatroban has US Food and Drug Administration (FDA) approval for HIT, has quick onset of action, and has the most evidence supporting its use

and thus is the most widely utilized anticoagulant for the treatment of HIT. Danaparoid is an alternative available outside of the United States. Recently there has been evidence supporting the safety and efficacy of DOACs for HIT or HITT. Rivaroxaban is the most well studied though favorable results have been shown with apixaban and dabigatran as well.[8] Current recommendations suggest that argatroban or bivalirudin may be preferred in the setting of increased bleeding risk, critical illness, or the need for urgent procedures.[6] For patients with normal hepatic function and who are not critically ill, the initial dose of argatroban is 2 mcg/kg/min IV. An aPTT should be drawn after 2 hours with goal to be 1.5 to 3 times the baseline aPTT. For patients with compromised hepatic function (bilirubin >1.5 mg/dL), cardiac surgery, anasarca, or who are critically ill, the recommended dosage range is 0.5 to 1.2 mcg/kg/min IV with the same aPTT. In addition to anticoagulation, evidence is increasing regarding the utility of IVIG for severe HIT.[9,10]

Post-Transfusion Purpura

Post-transfusion purpura (PTP), also known as post-transfusion thrombocytopenia, is a rare disorder that causes a precipitous fall in platelets approximately one week following transfusion. It is frequently linked to human platelet antigen 1 (HPA1) on platelets, although other antigens have also been implicated. When an HPA1 antigen–negative patient receives a platelet transfusion, the platelets with attached HPA1 antibodies provoke an anamnestic response, though the actual mechanism of platelet destruction is uncertain. Patients are usually middle-aged women with a history of prior pregnancy, during which they may have been previously sensitized to the HPA1 antigen. The platelet count often falls precipitously below 10,000/mm³, with a significant associated risk of major bleeding.

High-dose IVIG, 1g/kg IV, is considered the first-line treatment for patients with severe thrombocytopenia or major bleeding. Glucocorticoids may be given with IVIG. Plasma exchange therapy is no longer considered a preferred therapy. Transfused platelets are often rapidly destroyed, thus platelet transfusion is generally not recommended except in the setting of severe thrombocytopenia and life-threatening bleeding, preferably with HPA1-negative blood products.

Thrombotic Microangiopathy

Thrombotic microangiopathies (TMA) represent a group of disorders that are characterized by their clinical presentation of microangiopathic hemolytic anemia (MAHA) and thrombocytopenia, and confirmed by histopathology or other specific tests. Microvascular thrombosis leads to abnormalities in the vessel wall of arterioles or capillaries, leading to consumption of platelets and destruction of RBCs. Presence or severity of clinical symptoms guide treatment decisions. There are many systemic disease states that have characteristics similar to TMA, and

TABLE 111.3   Plasmic Score

Criteria	Response	
Platelet count < 30 × 10⁹/L	No (0 point)	Yes (1 point)
Hemolysis (Reticulocyte count > 2.5%, haptoglobin undetectable, or indirect bilirubin > 2.0 mg/dL)	No (0 point)	Yes (1 point)
Active cancer or treated for cancer within the past year	No (1 point)	Yes (0 point)
History of solid organ or stem cell transplant	No (1 point)	Yes (0 point)
MCV < 9.0 × 10⁻¹⁴ L (<90 fL)	No (0 point)	Yes (1 point)
INR < 1.5	No (0 point)	Yes (1 point)
Creatinine < 2.0 mg/dL	No (0 point)	Yes (1 point)

TABLE 111.4   Plasmic Risk Stratification

Total Score	Risk
0–4 points	Low risk. Consider alternative diagnosis
5 points	Intermediate risk. Consult hematology and consider plasma exchange
6–7 points	High risk. Consult hematology and immediate plasma exchange

treatment is focused on the underlying disease. The most common primary TMA disorders include thrombotic thrombocytopenic purpura (TTP) and hemolytic-uremic syndrome (HUS).

Thrombotic Thrombocytopenic Purpura. TTP is most often acquired and results from autoantibodies to ADAMTS13, an endothelial protein that cleaves large vWF multimers. Large vWF multimers increase adhesiveness to platelets, and large VWF-platelet aggregates can form microthrombi inducing tissue ischemia, platelet consumption, and MAHA.[11] TTP is rarely inherited, including disorders such as Upshaw-Schulman syndrome. HUS shares some similarities to TTP, and is generally associated with less central nervous system and more renal involvement than TTP. The first acute episode of TTP often occurs during adulthood (approximately 90%), and occurs twice as frequently in women.[12] HUS, on the other hand, frequently occurs in children, often after a gastrointestinal illness. TTP is classically, though not always, seen as a constellation of thrombocytopenia, MAHA (schistocytes seen on blood smear), and fluctuating neurologic symptoms such as mental clouding or confusion. It may be associated with cardiac (25% of the time) or mesenteric ischemia (35%), resulting in abdominal pain or diarrhea. Acute renal manifestations consist mainly of proteinuria or hematuria and rarely acute renal failure.[12] This is in contrast to HUS, where acute kidney injury is common. For patients with thrombocytopenia and MAHA, the PLASMIC score should be utilized in hospitalized patients to identify candidates for early initiation of treatment with plasma exchange (Tables 111.3 and 111.4).[13] The differential diagnosis for TTP includes HUS or other TMA syndromes associated with sepsis, malignancy, or pregnancy (HELLP).

Prior to the availability of plasma exchange, TTP followed a progressive and often fatal course, with a 90% mortality rate within a few months of diagnosis. Therapeutic plasma exchange is now the standard treatment, often with accompanying glucocorticoids.[11] Typical glucocorticoid dosage for patients without neurologic deficits or cardiac ischemia is prednisone 1 mg/kg PO daily. If patient is considered to be in severe condition, 1 g methylprednisolone intravenously for 3 days may be considered. If TTP is suspected, hematologist involvement is essential prior to initiation of therapies. Addition of rituximab may be considered in patients who are refractory to standard treatment, though its use in the acute phase of TTP is still debated. Additionally, caplacizumab (11 mg IV initial dose, followed by 11 mg subcutaneously daily for 10 days) may also be advantageous to add to the standard treatment of plasma exchange and immunosuppression.[11] With the exception of life-threatening bleeding, platelet transfusion is avoided, as platelets may cause additional thrombi in the microcirculation. Current trials are assessing the effectiveness of N-acetylcysteine, recombinant ADAMTS13, or an inhibitor of VWF-glycoprotein Ib binding.

Dilutional Thrombocytopenia

Dilutional thrombocytopenia as a complication of massive transfusion, exchange transfusion, or fluid resuscitation. Current guidelines for 1 : 1 : 1 ratio of fresh frozen plasma (FFP), platelets, and RBCs may assist in alleviating dilutional thrombocytopenia in the setting of massive transfusion.

Hereditary Thrombocytopenia and Thrombocytopathy

Hereditary thrombocytopathy and thrombocytopenic syndromes are not as rare as once thought. It has been suggested that as many as 1 in 7 patients initially diagnosed with ITP have a hereditary thrombocytopenic syndrome.[14] This may in part explain the variable success rates in the treatment of ITP. A detailed history is important, as patients diagnosed with thrombocytopathy may have at least one family member who has been treated with splenectomy for presumed ITP. Inherited thrombocytopenias are often characterized by platelet size (large, normal, or small). A blood smear is helpful in evaluating platelet size and granules. Further evaluation with light transmission aggregometry or specific tests may also be necessary.

Thrombocytopathy. Knowledge of abnormal platelet function as a clinical disorder has grown rapidly in recent years, with identified disorders of platelet adhesion, aggregation, or granule secretion.

Adhesion Defects. Bernard-Soulier Syndrome (BSS) results from an abnormality in the platelet gpIb complex, which allows platelet adhesion to vWF and thus the subendothelium.

Aggregation Defects. Glanzmann thrombasthenia (GT) is a rare autosomal-recessive disorder that results from a defect in the integrin complex glycoprotein IIb/IIIa. This protein complex is important for platelet aggregation via fibrinogen. The glycoprotein IIb/IIIa complex is the site of action for particular antiplatelet agents utilized, often employed during percutaneous coronary intervention procedures.

Secretory Defects. Secretory defects comprise two pathologic groups: defective platelet granule formation or defective secretory machinery. These include "storage pool" syndromes with decreased amounts of adenosine diphosphate, calcium, and serotonin. Congenital disorders such as Hermansky-Pudlak syndrome will often be associated with other systemic features including immune or pigmentation defects. Other secretory defects may be acquired, such as in association with systemic lupus erythematosus, alcoholism, or lymphoma. Various medications may induce secretory issues. Aspirin blocks the enzyme cyclooxygenase, which participates in thromboxane A_2 formation. Decreased release of thromboxane A_2 results in diminished platelet aggregation and reduced local vasoconstriction.

Despite the advances in the diagnosis of inherited platelet disorders, little progress has been made in targeted therapies for specific platelet disorders. There has been an increase in use of tranexamic acid (TXA) for mucocutaneous bleeding, menorrhagia, or epistaxis. Patients with severe thrombocytopenia and bleeding may benefit from platelet transfusion, though this recommendation is limited to severe bleeding due to the risk of developing antibodies or platelet alloimmunization. Platelet transfusions should preferably include human leukocyte antigen (HLA) matching and leukocyte depletion. Desmopressin has traditionally been utilized for the theoretical benefit of increasing factor VIII and VWF in patients with a diagnosed thrombocytopathy, but with only equivocal success in BSS, no evidence for benefit in GT, and variable response rates in secretory disorders.

Thrombocytosis

Thrombocytosis is defined as a platelet count of greater than 600,000/mm³ (Box 111.6). It is frequently secondary to infection or iron deficiency, and in these circumstances, thrombocytosis is generally not associated with other platelet-related complications. Primary (or autonomous) thrombocytosis may lead to thrombosis or bleeding, resulting from high numbers of dysfunctional platelets. Primary thrombocytosis is associated with polycythemia vera, myelofibrosis, and chronic myelogenous leukemia, or Kawasaki disease in children. Primary thrombocytosis requires a thorough hematologic evaluation.

Coagulation Disorders

Hemophilia A

Hemophilia A is caused by a deficiency of factor VIII. Most cases are sex-linked recessive in nature, as the disease is carried on the X chromosome. The prevalence of hemophilia A is approximately 17 cases per 100,000 males, with approximately 1,125,000 affected worldwide.[15] Approximately 13,500 people in the United States have hemophilia A.[16] The severity of hemophilia is categorized by factor VIII activity level. Severe hemophilia is less than 1% of normal factor activity, moderate is 1% to 5%, and mild is 5% to 40%. Approximately 42% of cases are considered severe.[16] The more severe, the more likely the patient will need replacement factor VIII. Patients with severe hemophilia require more replacement therapy and have an increased risk to develop alloantibodies, termed inhibitors, that may serve to inactivate factor VIII and may therefore limit replacement therapy. Recombinant DNA technology currently supplies most factor utilized for replacement therapy, though there is evidence that plasma-derived factor VIII has reduced immunogenicity and is associated with a lower incidence of inhibitor development.[17] Emicizumab is a recombinant immunoglobulin that substitutes for part of the function of activated factor VIII and is utilized for prophylactic treatment. It works by bridging activated factor IX and factor X to restore the function of missing activated factor VIII that is necessary for effective hemostasis. Factor VIII typically circulates in low concentrations in plasma bound to vWF. Given this close relationship, a diagnosis of vWD may present with similar symptoms.

Hemophilia is seen as a disorder of secondary hemostasis with a characteristic pattern of bleeding. Bleeding can occur anywhere, though deep muscles, joints, the urinary tract, and intracranial sites are the most common. Recurrent hemarthrosis and progressive joint destruction are major causes of morbidity. Intracranial hemorrhage (ICH) is a major cause of death in all age groups, and studies indicate probabilities for ICH of 1 in 50,000 to 1 in 140,000 male patients.[18] Mortality from ICH remains around 20% in hemophiliacs.[19] Mucosal bleeding, such as epistaxis, oral bleeding, or menorrhagia, remain rare unless associated with comorbid vWD or platelet dysfunction, such as occurs with aspirin use. Gastrointestinal bleeding is rare unless peptic ulcer disease is present. Trauma is a common initiator of bleeding irrespective of perceived severity and the bleeding may be delayed for days or weeks following initial injury. As such, a careful history of distant or seemingly negligible trauma should be included.

Comprehensive management of hemophilia involves a team effort including physicians, specialized nursing, physical therapy, social work, as well as the patient and their caregivers. ED management of hemophilia is best accomplished with advanced planning, including

---

BOX 111.11 Indications for Factor Replacement in Hemophilia

Suspected bleeding into a joint or muscle

Any significant injury to the head, neck, mouth or eyes

Any new or unusual headache, particularly following trauma even if seemingly minor

Severe pain or swelling at any location

All wounds that require surgical closure (sutures, staples), wound adhesive, or Steri-Strip placement

History of blunt trauma that might result in bleeding

Prior to any invasive procedure or surgery

Suspicion of uncontrolled GI bleeding leading to anemia or signs or symptoms of hypovolemia

Acute fractures, dislocations or sprains

Suspicion of uncontrolled heavy menstrual bleeding, leading to anemia or signs or symptoms of hypovolemia

---

protocols for the administration of factor VIII developed in collaboration with a hematologist. Emergency clinicians should have rapid access to relevant information, including primary care physician, hematologist, diagnosis, factor VIII activity level, blood type, antihemophilic factor antibodies (inhibitor) status, and date of last hospitalization.

The severity of hemophilia, with last known factor level, as well as inhibitor status, must be considered with any bleeding in a patient with hemophilia. Many patients are well versed in their disease and often come prepared with their own treatment. The emergency clinician should institute early therapy for patients in whom bleeding is suspected. It is advisable to engage the patient's hematologist, if able, prior to initiating therapy.

Treatment decisions should be based on the *suspicion* of a bleeding related complication (Box 111.11).[20] Factor replacement therapy may need to be administered prior to diagnostic studies, particularly if ICH is suspected.

Replacement typically includes recombinant-derived factor VIII, or alternatively the patient's usual product of choice. Plasma-derived concentrate is a suitable alternative in an emergency situation. Cryoprecipitate or fresh frozen plasma are no longer generally recommended unless faced with life-threatening bleeding without alternatives.

Desmopressin can be used for patients with documented mild hemophilia A without inhibitors who are experiencing bleeding that is not life or limb threatening. Desmopressin raises factor VIII by three to six times baseline levels. This therapy should be reserved for situations when there is history of a prior favorable hemostatic response.[20] With suspicion for more significant bleeding, treatment follows as for other forms of hemophilia A.

As a general rule, 1 U/kg of factor VIII will increase the circulating factor VIII level by 2%. If the patient has a known recent factor level, this may be utilized into the calculation. In emergent therapy, however, the present factor VIII level is presumed as zero. Factor VIII activity goals are typically 40% to 50% for minor bleeding or trauma, and 80% to 100% for serious or life-threatening bleeding or trauma. Table 111.5 provides guidelines for treatment in patients without inhibitors.[21] Because the half-life of factor VIII is 8 to 12 hours, the desired level is maintained by giving half of the initial dose every 8 to 12 hours.

The response to therapy can be monitored by clinical improvement, a decreasing PTT, and, optimally, serial factor VIII activity levels. Of note, aPTT-based assays including clot-based FVIII activity assays should not be performed if patients are on emicizumab as it will artifactually shorten aPTT and elevate FVIII activity.[22] The lack of a response to factor VIII administration should raise suspicion for the presence of

TABLE 111.5 Recommended Factor VIII Therapy and Dosing for Complications Associated With Hemophilia

Type of Bleeding	Initial Dosage	Comment
Skin		
Abrasion	None	Treat with local pressure and topical tranexamic acid
Superficial laceration	Usually none; if closure is needed then then 25 U/kg	Local pressure and tranexamic acid may benefit; watch 4 hours after suturing; reexamine in 24 hours
Deep laceration	25 U/kg	May need hospitalization for observation; repeated dose may be necessary for suture removal
Superficial muscle hematoma	25 U/kg	May be complicated by local pressure on nerves or vessels; monitor for compartment syndrome
Deep muscle hematoma (e.g., iliopsoas)	50 U/kg	May be complicated by local pressure on nerves or vessels; monitor for compartment syndrome if in an extremity
Epistaxis		
Spontaneous	Usually none; but if persistent, consider 25 U/kg	Uncommon; consider platelet inhibition; treat in usual manner and consider tranexamic acid application
Traumatic	25 U/kg to 50 U/kg	Trauma-related bleeding can be significant. Consider 50 U/kg given head trauma and possible development of ICH.
Oral		
Mucosa or tongue bites or other similar minor injuries	Usually none; treat with 25 U/kg if bleeding persists	Saliva is rich in fibrinolytic activity; oral ε-aminocaproic acid (Amicar) may be given as 5 g (or 100 mg/kg) during the first hour, then 1 g per hour for 8 hours or until bleeding is controlled to block fibrinolysis; oral tranexamic acid may also be used (25 mg/kg) PO every 6 to 8 hrs, check for contraindications (patients receiving PCC or high risk of thrombosis); hospitalize patients with severe bleeding
Traumatic oral lesion (laceration) or dental extraction	25 U/kg to 50 U/kg	Saliva is rich in fibrinolytic activity; oral ε-aminocaproic acid (Amicar) may be given as 5 g (100 mg/kg) during the first hour, then 1 g per hour for 8 hours or until bleeding is controlled to block fibrinolysis; oral tranexamic acid may also be used (25 mg/kg) PO every 6 to 8 hrs, check contraindications (patients receiving PCC or high risk of thrombosis); hospitalize patients with severe bleeding
Hemarthrosis		
Early or moderate	25 U/kg	Treat at earliest symptom (pain); knee, elbow, ankle more common
Late hemarthrosis or nonresponsive to earlier treatment	40 U/kg	Arthrocentesis rarely necessary, immobilization is a critical component of therapy
Hematuria	25 U/kg	Painless hematuria should be treated with bed rest and hydration. With persistent hematuria, an anatomic cause should be excluded. Antifibrinolytics are not recommended as they prevent lysis of clots in the ureter causing serious obstructive uropathy.
Major/Life-Threatening Bleeding	50 U/kg	Administer on the suspicion of a major or life threatening bleed.

inhibitors. Up to 20% of patients develop IgG inhibitor antibodies, and usually have a severe deficiency necessitating multiple factor VIII infusions. The treatment may be complex, thus discussion with a hematologist or hospitalization may be necessary. A variety of therapies have been considered, and current treatments of choice include bypassing agents or immune tolerance induction.[23] In the emergency care setting, generally the safest immediate action is to administer recombinant factor VIIa at a dose of 90 mcg/kg IV. For patients not currently on emicizumab, an additional consideration is activated prothrombin complex concentrate at a dose of 75 to 100 units/kg IV.[20]

Hemophilia B (Christmas Disease)

Hemophilia B is a deficiency of factor IX activity. Its genetic pattern and clinical findings are indistinguishable from those of hemophilia A, but its incidence is only a fifth that of hemophilia A. Factor IX is

a vitamin K–dependent glycoprotein. Its deficiency is diagnosed by a factor IX assay, usually after the factor VIII assay is found to be normal.

Clinical presentations and treatment strategies associated with hemophilia A also generally apply to hemophilia B, including those for patients who have developed inhibitors. The replacement factor therapy is similar to that for hemophilia A, with use of a recombinant factor IX preparation. Plasma-derived concentrate is a suitable alternative in an emergency situation when recombinant factor IX is unavailable. Fresh frozen plasma is not routinely recommended for hemophilia B treatment, and cryoprecipitate does not contain factor IX. Given the comparatively longer half-life of factor IX, the maintenance factor dosing schedule is every 24 hours. When bleeding is severe, the appropriate dose of factor IX is 100 to 140 units/kg IV, which should result in a factor level of 80% to 100%. For hemophilia B with inhibitors, the safest immediate action is recombinant factor VIIa at a dose of 90 mcg/

kg IV. For those not currently on emicizumab, an additional consideration is activated prothrombin complex concentrate at a dose of at 75 to 100 units/kg IV.[20] As with hemophilia A, a hematologist should be included in the decision making as soon as is feasible.

von Willebrand Disease

Von Willebrand disease is the most common hereditary bleeding disorder, with an estimated prevalence of 1%. Quantitative or qualitative deficits in vWF are associated with clinical findings. Platelet adhering properties or factor VIII activity may be altered in vWD.

Manifestations of vWD are usually milder and less debilitating than those of hemophilia. The factor VIII activity level is in the 6% to 50% range. Bleeding sites are predominantly mucosal or cutaneous. Hemarthroses are rare, and menorrhagia and gastrointestinal bleeding are common.

Desmopressin, 0.3 mcg/kg IV, is of benefit in patients with mild to moderately severe vWD. Desmopressin is the preferred treatment for patients with mild to moderately severe disease, given its low risk profile and low cost. Adjunctive antifibrinolytic agents, such as tranexamic acid, have also shown benefit in vWD. In extreme circumstances, fresh frozen plasma or cryoprecipitate may be utilized. Severe vWD, with very low or absent vWF levels, is rare (1–5%) and presents early in life.

In patients with severe vWD, or in those with mild to moderately severe vWD who do not respond to desmopressin, replacement therapy with factor VIII in the form of lyophilized concentrate of factor VIII/vWF at a dose of 50 IU/kg is indicated. A unique response to the transfusion of plasma components in patients with vWD is the stimulation of a progressive increase in factor VIII activity that lasts 12 to 40 hours. After the initial dose, fewer units are necessary, and longer dosage schedules may be followed by clinical or laboratory response.

Miscellaneous Coagulation Disorders

A number of other disorders may be caused by deficiencies in the coagulation pathway. An altered level, or abnormal function, of fibrinogen may occur, leading to an abnormal thrombin time. The inherited forms are rare, and acquired forms are associated with fibrin-blocking substances or hypofibrinogenemia, which are found most often in the setting of DIC, or dysfibrinogenemia associated with macroglobulinemia, multiple myeloma, or hepatoma.

Rare inherited deficiencies may occur with other components of the common pathway (factors II, V, and X). Acquired forms are far more common and typically relate to vitamin K deficiency or warfarin use (decreased factor II, VII, IX, and X activity), hepatic insufficiency (potentially all factors except factor VIII), or massive transfusion of stored blood (low in factors V and VIII).

Medication-Induced Anticoagulation

The use of oral anticoagulants for conditions such as atrial fibrillation or venous thromboembolic disease continues to rise. Oral anticoagulation includes vitamin K antagonists such as warfarin, as well as the increasingly utilized direct-acting oral anticoagulants (DOACs). The first to gain FDA approval, dabigatran, is a direct thrombin inhibitor. Other common DOACs include rivaroxaban and apixaban, which are selective factor Xa inhibitors. Patients with impaired renal or liver function may experience excessive anticoagulation in the setting of DOAC use. Excessive anticoagulation related to warfarin occurs from a number of causes, including interactions between warfarin and other drugs or foods, or accompanying conditions that may interfere with its absorption or metabolism. Patients may present to the ED for concerns regarding supratherapeutic dosing of anticoagulants or for hemorrhage.

> **BOX 111.12 Critical Sites for Hemorrhage in Anticoagulated Patients**
>
> Intracranial
> Intraocular
> Spinal
> Pericardial tamponade
> Airway (including posterior epistaxis)
> Thorax
> Intra-abdominal bleeding
> Retroperitoneal hematoma
> Intramuscular
> Intra-articular

Bleeding related to heparin therapy is less of an issue in the ED setting, though still can occur (e.g., patient coming from a dialysis center). In addition to discontinuation of heparin, protamine sulfate can urgently reverse the effects of heparin. The full neutralizing effect of UFH is achieved with 1 mg of protamine for every 100 units of heparin. Protamine can also be utilized in an attempt to reverse the effects of LMWH, though in a less predictable or complete fashion as occurs with UFH. This is an off-label use and should be considered in life-threatening bleeding and, if possible, discussed with a hematologist. In this setting, the dose of protamine is 0.5 to 1 mg for every 1 mg of LMWH depending on timing of last administration; if ≤8 hr, use 1 mg, if >8 hr, use 0.5 mg. Administration of protamine should not exceed more than 50 mg over 10 minutes, as more rapid injection may result in adverse effects including hypotension.

In the setting of over-anticoagulation or hemorrhage related to DOAC use, management has shifted with the more recent development of drug-specific reversal agents. Careful consideration of the risk of thromboembolic events weighed with the benefits of bleeding cessation must be taken into account. If bleeding occurs in critical sites (Box 111.12) or is associated with hemodynamic compromise, then reversal should be strongly considered.[24] For dabigatran, the FDA-approved reversal agent idarucizumab, 5 g IV, can be administered. If idarucizumab is unavailable, consider activated prothrombin complex concentrate (aPCC) at a dose of 50 units/kg IV. 4F-PCC has been studied in vitro, and healthy volunteer studies but not prospectively with dabigatran-associated bleeding at this time. If aPCC is unavailable, then 4F-PCC is a reasonable alternative.[24] 4F-PCC (K-centra) includes factors II, VII, IX and X along with protein C and S whereas aPCC such as Factor Eight Inhibitor Bypass Agent (FEIBA) has inactive factors II, IX, X, and activated VII. In addition, dialysis may be considered for dabigatran, as approximately 57% of the drug is removed with 4 hours of dialysis. Caution needs to be exercised in dialysis catheter placement, however. For apixaban or rivaroxaban, the FDA-approved reversal agent for use in life-threatening bleeds is andexanet alfa.[25] An alternative to andexanet alfa is 4F-PCC at a dose of 25 to 50 units/kg IV, or a fixed dose of 2000 units IV. aPCC has been studied in vitro, and healthy volunteer studies but not prospectively with oral factor Xa–associated bleeding at this time.[26] If no andexanet alfa or 4F-PCC is unavailable, then aPCC is a reasonable alternative for life-threatening bleeding. For other DOACs, such as edoxaban or betrixaban, off-label use of andexanet alfa is a possible intervention, or use of 4F-PCC at a dose 50 units/kg or fixed dose of 2000 units IV.

Management of excessive anticoagulation from warfarin depends on the degree of elevation of the INR and whether there is accompanying bleeding (Table 111.16). If the INR is below 4.5 and not accompanied with bleeding, treatment consists of withholding additional warfarin. If the INR level is between 4.5 and 10 without bleeding, we recommend holding additional warfarin doses for 1 to 2 doses. There

TABLE 111.6   Treatment for Supratherapeutic INR

INR Level/Bleeding	Recommendation
Major, life-threatening bleeding	Cessation of warfarin
	Vitamin K 10 mg (IV over 30 minutes)
Any INR	4F-PCC (KCENTRA) (See dosage in Table 111.7)
INR > 10, active bleeding	Cessation of warfarin
	Vitamin K 10 mg (IV over 30 minutes)
	4F-PCC (KCENTRA) 50 U/KG, maximum dose 5000 units.
INR > 10, no bleeding	Cessation of warfarin
	Vitamin K 5 mg oral
INR 4.5 < 10, no bleeding	Cessation of warfarin
	If higher risk of bleeding or lower chance of thromboembolism, consider vitamin K 2.5 mg oral
INR < 4.5, no bleeding	Cessation of warfarin

TABLE 111.7   4F-PCC Dosage for Warfarin Reversal in Major Bleeding

Baseline INR Level	4F-PCC Dosage
INR 2 < 4	25 U/KG, maximum dose 2500 units
INR 4 < 6	35 U/KG, maximum dose 3500 units
INR > 6	50 U/KG, maximum dose 5000 units

are differing opinions on whether or not a small dose of 1.0 to 2.5 mg of oral vitamin K is indicated. It appears reasonable to give to those patients with a higher chance of bleeding or lower risk of thromboembolism vitamin K.[27,28] Treatment for patients presenting with an INR level above 10 but not bleeding includes holding warfarin and treating with 5 mg of oral vitamin K. Patients presenting with an elevated INR and active bleeding require cessation of warfarin, 10 mg of vitamin K IV, plus the administration of 4F-PCC or fresh frozen plasma (Table 111.17).[24,27] Vitamin K can be administered orally, intravenously, or subcutaneously. Oral dosing is superior to other routes of administration, and subcutaneous dosing is the least desirable method of administration owing to erratic serum level. Intravenous vitamin K given should be administered as a slow infusion over 20 to 30 minutes rather than a rapid bolus injection.

Disseminated Intravascular Coagulation

DIC is a relatively common acquired coagulopathy reflecting dysregulated coagulation and fibrinolytic pathways. Hemostasis is normally achieved by a fine balance between procoagulants and inhibitors, and thrombus formation and lysis. This balance may be disturbed by multiple pathologic processes, most often encountered in the critical care setting, resulting in DIC. The abnormal clotting sequence observed in DIC is shown in Box 111.13. Its ubiquitous nature, multiple origins, and potentially devastating sequelae, combined with potentially effective treatment modalities, make early diagnosis critical.

The clinical consequences include the potential for a life-threatening combination of bleeding from loss of platelets and clotting factors, fibrinolysis, and fibrin degradation product interference; small-vessel obstruction and tissue ischemia from fibrin deposition; and RBC injury and anemia from microvascular hemolysis. The condition should be

BOX 111.13   Disseminated Intravascular Coagulation Abnormal Clotting Sequence

Platelets and coagulation factors are consumed, especially fibrinogen and factors V, VIII, and XIII.

Thrombin is formed, and it overwhelms its inhibitor system and acts to accelerate the coagulation process and directly activate fibrinogen.

Fibrin is deposited in small vessels in multiple organs.

The fibrinolytic system by means of plasmin may lyse fibrin and impair thrombin formation.

Fibrin degradation products are released and affect platelet function and inhibit fibrin polymerization.

Coagulation inhibition levels (e.g., antithrombin III, protein C, and tissue factor pathway inhibitor) are decreased.

considered in any patient in whom purpura, a bleeding tendency, and signs of organ injury, particularly of the central nervous system or kidney, develop. This is further confounded clinically by the variable acuteness and intensity of intravascular clotting, the effectiveness of fibrinolysis, and other systemic manifestations of the precipitating disease. The clinical diagnosis of DIC is confirmed by laboratory testing (Table 111.8).

Severe liver disease or primary fibrinolysis may be confused with DIC. Liver disease of this severity is usually manifested by clinical jaundice and splenomegaly. Primary fibrinolysis is a rare disorder that affects fibrinogen and fibrin, though generally preserves other coagulation components (platelets, factor V, and factor VIII) in the low-normal range. Additional laboratory tests can be used to confirm the diagnosis of primary fibrinolysis in conjunction with a hematologist.

When planning therapy, it is critical to factor that DIC is secondary to a serious underlying pathologic process. Once the underlying diagnosis is confirmed, the initial treatment is focused on reversal of the triggering mechanism. Many episodes of DIC are self-limited, such as in a transfusion reaction, or compensated, such as in association with a tumor mass, and do not require specific intervention other than general supportive care.

If the patient demonstrates active bleeding, a significant risk of bleeding and requires an invasive procedure, arterial or venous thromboembolism, skin necrosis, or acral ischemia, specific management of DIC is warranted. In these cases of severe hemorrhagic or thromboembolic complications, in addition to treatment of the precipitating condition, specific management is based on which of the two major pathologic components of DIC predominates the clinical picture. In the setting of active bleeding, replacement therapy with platelets, fresh frozen plasma, and cryoprecipitate is recommended. Replacement therapy is instituted simultaneously with attempts to manage the primary inciting condition. The goal is to avoid depletion of clotting factors. Selective replacement therapy can be based on both laboratory and clinical response. Slowing of bleeding, a decrease in fibrin degradation products, and a rise in platelet count and fibrinogen level are useful monitors. Normalization of clotting times occurs later in the course, thus is of less value in initial monitoring.

Heparin can be selectively utilized in the treatment of DIC when fibrin deposition and thrombosis predominate the pathologic picture. Certain disease states are associated more with fibrin deposition, in which case heparin therapy should be considered. Examples include purpura fulminans, retained nonviable fetus before delivery, giant hemangioma, or acute promyelocytic leukemia. Conversely, heparin is

TABLE 111.8 Laboratory Diagnosis of Disseminated Intravascular Coagulation

Test	Finding	Pathophysiology
Peripheral smear	Low platelets, schistocytes, RBC fragments	RBC fragmentation on fibrin strands; schistocytes not always seen
Platelet count	Low (usually < 100,000/mm^3)	Consumed in clotting
Prothrombin time (PT)	Prolonged	Factors II and IV (calcium) consumed
Partial thromboplastin time (PTT)	Prolonged	Factors II, V, and VIII consumed
Thrombin time	Prolonged	Factor II consumed, decreased fibrinogen levels from the consumptive process of DIC (actual fibrinogen levels are variable as discussed below), and in vivo fibrinolysis leads to prolonged thrombin time even when fibrinogen levels are normal
Fibrinogen level	Low	Factor II consumed; may be difficult to interpret because it is an acute-phase reactant
Fibrin degradation products (including D-dimer)	Negligible to elevated	Dependent on the amount of secondary fibrinolysis
Serum creatinine or urinalysis	May be abnormal	Functional assessment of the kidney, as it is commonly impacted by microvascular fibrin deposition

RBC, Red blood cell.

generally of little benefit in the setting of meningococcemia, abruptio placentae, severe liver disease, or trauma. LMWH may also be utilized as an alternative to UFH. Continuous monitoring of the clinical response, heparin activity levels, and bleeding status is essential.

Other therapeutic agents have been evaluated, including antithrombin III, PCC, recombinant factor VIIa, and activated protein C, though none has demonstrated an improved outcome in DIC.

The goals of emergency care for patients with DIC include early recognition and close monitoring, focus on mitigation of the precipitating condition when possible, identifying potential life-threatening complications, and only rarely initiation of blood product or anticoagulation therapy.

DISPOSITION

Patients with bleeding disorders of unknown cause or of a significant degree should be considered for admission for further evaluation. Transfer may be necessary, particularly if hematologic expertise is not readily available. Owing to the potential for delayed bleeding in hemophiliacs, long-distance transports may be especially hazardous. Early notification and appropriate primary care or hematologic follow-up is prudent for other patients.

The references for this chapter can be found online at ExpertConsult. com.

112

Oncologic Emergencies

David A. Wacker and Michael T. McCurdy

FOUNDATIONS

As improved therapies prolong the lives of cancer patients, the prevalence of oncologic emergencies continues to increase. However, nonspecific clinical features misattributed to the underlying cancer complicate their diagnosis. In this chapter, we review febrile neutropenia, metastatic spinal cord compression (MSCC), malignant pericardial disease, hypercalcemia of malignancy, tumor lysis syndrome (TLS), leukostasis, superior vena cava (SVC) syndrome, and complications of cancer immunotherapies including monoclonal antibodies, T-lymphocyte checkpoint inhibition, and adoptive cell transfer therapy.

KEY CONCEPTS

- Patients whose absolute neutrophil count is or is expected to soon be 500 cells/mm³ or lower are considered severely neutropenic. A single temperature of 38.3°C or sustained temperature of 38.0°C for 1 to 2 hours or longer is considered fever.
- Any neutropenic patient with fever or with infectious signs or symptoms (even in the absence of fever) should be evaluated for an infectious source, including drawing of blood cultures, and started on empirical antibiotics. Those with high-risk features (e.g., prolonged or profound neutropenia, pneumonia, hypotension, abdominal pain, neurologic changes, Multinational Association for Supportive Care in Cancer (MASCC) score < 21) should be started on an antipseudomonal beta-lactam (e.g., cefepime, piperacillin-tazobactam, antipseudomonal carbapenem). Those with low-risk features may be appropriate for oral antibiotics. Empirical gram-positive bacterial, antifungal, and antiviral coverage is unnecessary unless the clinical situation dictates otherwise.
- Neutropenic patients with fever should generally be hospitalized, including all high-risk patients. Select low-risk patients may be managed as outpatients.

FEBRILE NEUTROPENIA

Foundations

Whether due to underlying malignancy or as a cytotoxic effect of chemotherapeutics, cancer patients regularly experience depleted levels of circulating neutrophils. Risk of infection rises when a patient's absolute neutrophil count (ANC) drops below 1000 cells/mm³. However, the increase in risk is most marked in patients with ANC less than 500 cells/mm³. Historically, ANC of 1000 to 1500 cells/mm³ has been considered mild, 500 to 1000 cells/mm³ moderate, and less than 500 cells/mm³ severe. Current guidelines do not emphasize these gradations, and neutropenia is defined as an ANC less than 500 cells/mm³ or an ANC expected to drop below this threshold within 48 hours.[1,2] The

ANC is calculated from a complete blood count (CBC) with differential count by the following formula:

$$\frac{([\% \text{ granulocytes}] + [\% \text{ bands}]) \times [\text{total WBC count}]}{100}$$

Neutropenic patients are particularly susceptible to infection, even from their own existing microbial flora, and such infection carries significant mortality risk. Twenty to thirty percent of patients with neutropenic fever require hospitalization, and of those patients, about 10% will not survive to discharge.[1] Most commonly, neutropenic fever is caused by pneumonia, anorectal lesion, skin infection, pharyngitis, or urinary tract infection. However, because local inflammatory responses are dampened by the absence of granulocytes, the only sign of infection may be fever, defined as a single temperature 38.3°C or greater or a sustained temperature of 38.0°C or greater for 1 hour or more. However, fever is not a requisite for infection; any neutropenic patient with signs or symptoms of infection should be treated as having neutropenic fever, whether actually febrile or not. In fact, suppressed temperature on presentation (<36.5°C) may portend higher mortality than fever or normothermia.

Clinical Features

Due to underlying immunosuppression, neutropenic patients often do not manifest infectious signs or symptoms beyond fever, making a thorough history and physical examination crucial. The interview should include a standard infectious review of systems, questioning for presence of diarrhea, nausea or vomiting, headache, neck stiffness, rashes, dysuria, cough, dyspnea, and pain at any location, including the abdomen, chest, joints, throat, sinuses, and ears.[2] Specific note should be made of indwelling venous catheters, because these increase the risk of bacteremia and skin infection.[1] To evaluate for perianal infection, the perineal region should be examined and inquiry made about pain with defecation. Although there is no hard evidence, expert opinion suggests against digital rectal examination to avoid compromise of the barrier between blood and rectal flora. Due to the chemosensitivity of the rapidly dividing epithelial cells of the mouth, mucositis is a common adverse effect of chemotherapy and provides a portal for oral flora into the bloodstream. This can be evaluated by examination and inquiry about oral pain.

Differential Diagnoses

Causes of fever in cancer patients are diverse and include infection, venous thrombus or embolus, adverse effect of chemotherapy or other medication, and direct effect of tumor burden. A clear source of infection is identified in only about one-third of neutropenic fever cases. Nonetheless, because of the potentially life-threatening effects of an infection in this population, all febrile neutropenic patients should receive empirical antibiotics and a full evaluation for an infectious source.

1500

Diagnostic Testing

Neutropenic patients with fever should have at least two sets of blood cultures drawn before administration of antibiotics. Both may be drawn peripherally in patients without preexisting central access. In patients with a preexisting central line, one of the two blood cultures should be obtained peripherally, whereas other cultures should be simultaneously drawn off each lumen of the central catheter. Bacterial growth in the catheter-drawn samples greater than 2 hours prior to the peripheral samples may suggest a catheter-associated infection. Patients with neutropenic fever should also have a CBC with differential count performed to assess severity of neutropenia, as well as urinalysis, urine culture, chemistries, and renal and hepatic function tests. Serum lactate should be measured if sepsis is suspected. Additional cultures may be sent according to the clinical presentation (e.g., sputum culture if productive cough, stool culture, and testing for *Clostridium difficile* if diarrhea or abdominal pain).[1,2]

Initial imaging usually consists of chest x-ray, although this is often low-yield in the absence of specific respiratory symptoms.[3] If fever persists for 72 hours without identified source, empirical computed tomography (CT) scan of the chest and sinuses, and bronchoalveolar lavage may be considered to evaluate for occult fungal infection. Patients with a history of invasive aspergillosis, and those with profound or prolonged neutropenia are at higher risk of fungal pneumonia, and consideration should be given to pulmonary imaging if there is little clinical response within the first day of therapy.[1] Similarly, directed CT scans may be performed sooner in the setting of appropriate clinical signs (e.g., chest CT for a patient with coughing and bronchial breath sounds, but a clear chest x-ray, abdominal CT for a patient with unexplained abdominal tenderness).

As nucleotide sequencing becomes more reliable, assays employing this technique for pathogen identification[4-7] are being aggressively developed. Although these assays provide a useful adjunct, and may direct antibiotic therapy prior to culture growth, they are not yet sufficiently developed to stand in lieu of conventional diagnostics, and a full set of cultures should always be obtained.

Management

Febrile neutropenic patients should receive antibiotics prior to confirmation of an infectious source. Recommendations for specific regimens are based on risk of clinical decompensation. According to the Infectious Disease Society of America (IDSA), high-risk features include an expected duration of neutropenia greater than 7 days, expected nadir ANC less than 100 cells/mm³, hypotension, pneumonia, new-onset abdominal pain, neurologic changes, or existence of other significant medical comorbidities. A current or prior infection with a resistant organism and treatment at a center with a high prevalence of resistant organisms should also be viewed as high risk. Alternatively, several scoring systems exist to assess risk of deterioration in neutropenic fever. The Multinational Association for Supportive Care in Cancer (MASCC) risk index identifies low-risk patients based on clinical features (Table 112.1). Patients scoring at least 21 points are considered low-risk, because nearly 90% of cases have uncomplicated resolution of their fever within 5 days. Similarly, the Clinical Index of Stable Febrile Neutropenia (CISNE) index (Table 112.2) has been validated to indicate patients with low (score 0), intermediate (score 1–2), and high (score ≥ 3) risk of clinical deterioration.[8-11]

High-risk patients should receive a parenteral broad-spectrum antibiotic regimen. Local antibiograms should be considered when choosing specific agents, but guidelines recommend monotherapy using a broad-spectrum beta-lactam with antipseudomonal coverage, such as ceftazidime, cefepime, piperacillin-tazobactam, or antipseudomonal carbapenem.[1,2] Among head-to-head studies of these agents

TABLE 112.1 Clinical Features and Corresponding Point Values for the Multinational Association of Supportive Care in Cancer (MASCC) Risk Index[a]

Clinical Feature	Point Value
Age < 60 years	2
Onset of fever while outpatient	3
Overall moderate symptom burden	3
Absence of dehydration	3
No prior fungal infections or solid tumor type	4
No history of chronic obstructive pulmonary disease	4
Absence of hypotension	5
Asymptomatic or overall mild symptom burden	5

[a]A score of ≥ 21 suggests low risk of complication and likely resolution of fever within 5 days.

TABLE 112.2 Clinical Features and Corresponding Point Values for the Clinical Index of Stable Febrile Neutropenia (CISNE)[a]

Clinical Feature	Point Value
Eastern Cooperative Oncology Group Performance status ≥ 2	2
Stress-induced hyperglycemia	2
Chronic obstructive pulmonary disease	1
Chronic cardiovascular disease	1
Mucositis of grade ≥ 2	1
Monocyte count < 200 per μL	1

[a]A score of zero indicates low risk of clinical deterioration prior to resolution of the episode of neutropenic fever.

in neutropenic patients, all have shown good effectiveness and none has consistently out-performed the others.[12-14] For patients with signs of sepsis or septic shock, double coverage for gram-negative bacteria with a fluoroquinolone or aminoglycoside in addition to beta-lactam therapy should be considered;[15] however, a meta-analysis of studies comparing beta-lactam monotherapy with combination beta-lactam/aminoglycoside therapy showed that patients receiving aminoglycoside had no survival benefit and were more likely to suffer adverse events, including nephrotoxicity and fungal superinfection. We therefore recommend antipseudomonal beta-lactam monotherapy for patients with neutropenia and fever but without signs of sepsis and septic shock. Regimens meeting these criteria for patients with normal renal function include piperacillin-tazobactam 4.5 g IV q6 hours or cefepime 2 g IV q8 hours; dosing adjustments must be made for patients with renal impairment. Further empirical antibiotics administered will depend on clinical presentation and consultation with oncology or infectious disease consultants.

Despite increasing rates of bacteremia with gram-positive organisms in cancer patients,[16,17] randomized controlled studies and meta-analyses have failed to demonstrate a survival benefit to immediate empirical gram-positive–specific coverage[18] and have previously suggested increased rates of adverse effects. Empirical gram-positive–specific therapy, such as with intravenous vancomycin or other glycopeptides, is not recommended except in cases of suspected cellulitis, catheter-associated infection, or pneumonia, or in the case of clinical instability. Similarly, randomized controlled trials have not shown a benefit in immediate, empirical antifungal therapy, and guidelines suggest against empirical antifungal agents, unless there is specific concern for a fungal source. Recent guidelines do suggest, however, that evaluation for fungal pneumonia with high-resolution chest CT scan, serum beta-galactomannan assay, and consideration of bronchoscopy with lavage is beneficial in patients with prolonged or profound neutropenia.[1] In cases requiring empirical antifungal coverage, echinocandins (e.g., micafungin 100 mg IV q24 hrs) compare well with other agents both in terms of effectiveness and safety profile.[19,20]

Neutropenic patients with community-acquired pneumonia should be covered for atypical pathogens and possibly pneumocystis pneumonia (PCP). For atypical pathogens we recommend either levofloxacin 750 mg IV q24 hrs or azithromycin 500 mg IV q24 hrs and doxycycline 100 mg q12 hrs (levofloxacin dose must be adjusted for impaired renal function). For PCP coverage, the preferred regimen is trimethoprim-sulfamethoxazole (TMP-SMX) at 15 to 20 mg of TMP per kilogram of patient's total body weight per day IV, divided into 3 or 4 doses per day (e.g., 5 mg/kg IV q6 hrs will result in a 20 mg/kg/day dose). TMP-SMX dosing must be adjusted for impaired renal function. For patients with gastrointestinal symptoms, one randomized controlled trial suggests improved 28-day survival with cefepime/metronidazole combination therapy when compared to piperacillin-tazobactam monotherapy. We recommend cefepime 2 g IV q8 hrs and metronidazole 500 mg PO q8 hrs (cefepime dose must be adjusted to renal function). Patients with a vesicular rash or other evidence of herpes infections should receive empirical acyclovir; an initial regimen of 5-10 mg/kg IV every 8 hrs is appropriate for severe cases. In the case of renal impairment, acyclovir dosing must be adjusted.

Although no specific timing of antibiotic administration is recommended in the current IDSA guidelines, evidence is mounting that delays in initiation of antibiotic therapy are correlated with worsened outcomes.[21,22] We therefore recommend that high-risk patients receive antibiotic therapy as soon as possible after obtaining blood cultures. Many process improvement efforts have been shown to reduce time to antibiotics in the ED setting, including implementation of neutropenic fever order sets and a dedicated neutropenic fever response team,[23] elevation of patients with neutropenic fever in the triage queue,[24] and establishment of a protocol for initiation of antibiotics by the bedside nurse in appropriate patients.[25]

Observational studies and a meta-analysis have demonstrated that low-risk patients may be treated with an enteral regimen, usually amoxicillin/clavulanate (875 mg PO q12 hrs) and a fluoroquinolone (e.g., ciprofloxacin 500 mg PO q12 hrs). Both amoxicillin/clavulanate and levofloxacin doses must be adjusted in the case of impaired renal clearance. Alternatively, low-risk patients may be started empirically on parenteral broad-spectrum therapy as outlined previously with transition to an enteral regimen after 24 to 48 hours if no complications arise.[26,27]

Disposition

Regardless of risk category, the majority of febrile neutropenic patients will be hospitalized for observation and initial treatment,[28,29] ideally to a unit specialized for oncology patients. Hemodynamically unstable patients and those with a deteriorating course should be admitted to an intensive care unit (ICU). A small fraction of patients may be safely treated with enteral antibiotics in the outpatient setting.[30,31] These patients should (1) meet the low-risk criteria of a MASCC score of 21 or less; (2) have no evidence of pneumonia, line infection, cellulitis, or organ failure; (3) have reliable daily follow-up with their oncologist; (4) demonstrate clinical stability during observation in the ED for 4 hours or longer; (5) carry low suspicion of infection with a drug-resistant organism.[26,27] Prior to discharge, an initial dose of parenteral

antibiotics should be given in the ED, reliable follow-up and access to the outpatient antibiotic regimen must be ensured, and discharge should be coordinated with the patient's oncologist.[26,27]

METASTATIC SPINAL CORD COMPRESSION

KEY CONCEPTS

- Vertebral metastasis and spinal cord compression should be considered in any cancer patient, particularly those who have back pain, peripheral strength or sensory loss, or bowel or bladder dysfunction.
- MRI of the spine is the preferred diagnostic test when evaluating spinal cord compression. CT of the spine with myelography may be performed if MRI is contraindicated or unavailable. Plain films are not sufficiently sensitive to rule out spinal cord compression.
- Intravenous corticosteroids (dexamethasone 10 mg bolus) should be given to any patient with neurologic deficits from known or suspected MSCC. Consideration should be given to emergent surgical and radiotherapeutic intervention if compatible with goals of care.

Foundations

Malignancy-related compromise of the spinal cord most commonly occurs from an extradural neoplasm that has metastasized to the vertebral column. The lesion then typically expands locally from the marrow space through a vertebral vein foramen to invade the spinal canal. Although the resulting cord injury is termed *metastatic spinal cord compression (MSCC)*, direct nerve compression by tumor is uncommon. Cord injury is more commonly caused by occlusion of the epidural venous plexus, leading to breakdown of the blood-cord barrier and vasogenic edema. If untreated, tumor expansion eventually leads to arterial obstruction, causing cord ischemia and infarct. Less commonly, direct compression of the cord over time may lead to demyelination and axonal injury.

The most common tumors causing MSCC are prostate, breast, and lung cancer, each accounting for about 15% to 20% of total cases. Renal cell cancer, non-Hodgkin lymphoma, and multiple myeloma each account for an additional 5% to 10% of all cases. Most cases of MSCC affect the thoracic spine (60%), with the lumbosacral and cervical spine each making up 25% and 15% of cases, respectively. Twenty to forty percent of patients with MSCC have multiple loci of spinal metastasis.

Clinical Features

Back pain, weakness, sensory loss, and autonomic function loss are the most frequent presenting symptoms of MSCC. Back pain occurs in more than 95% of patients with MSCC and is the most common initial symptom.[32] Extremity weakness occurs in up to 75% and generally (but not always) precedes sensory loss. Patients with MSCC may also present with autonomic nerve dysfunction, including loss of bowel or bladder function, but it is a late finding and rarely presents in isolation.

Differential Diagnoses

In addition to MSCC, patients with back pain with or without neurologic symptoms should be considered for nonmalignant musculoskeletal etiologies (e.g., muscle strain, ligamentous sprain, pathologic fracture, disc displacement, radicular stenosis, vertebral osteoarthritis) and paraspinal or vertebral infections (e.g., paraspinal abscess, vertebral osteomyelitis, discitis). In patients with known malignancy, new back pain and neurologic deficits (motor, sensory, or autonomic) carry high specificity for MSCC,[32] and this diagnosis should be presumed

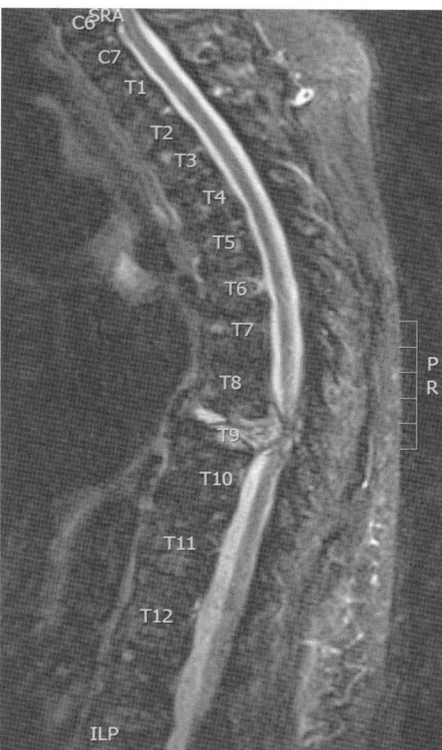

Fig. 112.1 Magnetic resonance imaging (MRI) short tau inversion recovery (STIR) image of T9 vertebral malignancy with pathologic fracture causing spinal cord compression in a patient with multiple myeloma. Vertebral numbering as marked. (Photo courtesy of the Department of Radiology, University of Maryland School of Medicine and Department of Internal Medicine, University of Maryland School of Medicine.)

and investigated. In patients without known cancer, however, new back pain is the heralding symptom of cancer in 20% of cases of MSCC, which commonly takes up to two months from original presentation to diagnose.

Diagnostic Testing

A thorough physical examination should be performed, including palpation of the entire spine, as well as testing of strength, sensation, deep tendon reflexes, and rectal tone. The diagnosis is confirmed by imaging, for which magnetic resonance imaging (MRI) has become the gold standard[32] with sensitivity of 93% and specificity of 97% (Fig. 112.1). Even in patients in whom MSCC has been established by another modality, MRI should still be performed when possible, because its added resolution changes treatment strategy in approximately 50% of cases. Because multiple separate lesions can occur simultaneously, both the thoracic and lumbar spine should be imaged in any patient with MSCC. Although the incidence of a second lesion in the cervical spine is much lower, this segment should also be included when possible.

If MRI is unavailable or contraindicated (e.g., patients with incompatible pacemakers), CT scan of the spine is the next most informative study. If vertebral metastasis is seen on initial scans, presence of cord compression can be assessed by CT myelography, in which contrast is introduced into the subarachnoid space.[32] Sensitivity of this technique rivals that of MRI, but MRI offers similar information noninvasively. Thus, CT myelography is reserved for those rare patients in whom MRI is contraindicated yet radiographic confirmation of cord compression as the cause of symptoms is required prior to intervention. Plain radiographs, positron emission tomography (PET) scans, and radionuclide

scans may demonstrate vertebral metastasis, but sensitivity is limited. Furthermore, these techniques provide no information about the state of the spinal cord itself or the precise location of suspected compression. These studies are therefore insufficient to rule out MSCC.[32]

Management

Treatment of MSCC in the ED entails administration of corticosteroids and initiation of definitive treatment with surgery, radiation therapy, or both.[33,34] Corticosteroids provide the most immediately available therapy for cord compression; unlike surgery or radiation, their administration does not require significant logistical planning or knowledge of the exact anatomic location of tumor. Early steroid administration has been shown to improve ambulation rates at 3- and 6-month intervals, and patients receiving corticosteroids have improved long-term pain scores. Current guidelines suggest a 10 mg intravenous bolus of dexamethasone followed by 16 mg orally per day in divided doses for any patient with neurologic deficits believed secondary to MSCC.[34] Patients with severe deficiencies, such as paraplegia, may receive a higher dose of 100 mg intravenous dexamethasone, followed by 96 mg orally per day in divided doses. Steroids are generally unnecessary in patients with vertebral metastases on imaging but without neurologic deficits.

Corticosteroids temporize vasogenic cord edema, but cord damage will ensue without definitive correction with radiation therapy, surgery, or both. For patients who can tolerate surgery and have goals of care in line with surgery, a combination of surgical decompression followed by radiation therapy provides better long-term rates of continence, ambulation, and survival than radiation therapy alone, and combined management is recommended in the most recent guidelines.[34,35] Surgical intervention is especially important in patients with spinal instability or cord compression by bony fragments.[35] Although surgery carries a high complication rate,[36] development of mini-open approaches[37,38] and use of postoperative stereotactic body radiation therapy to limit the degree of necessary resection[35] show promise to reduce complication rates and shorten recovery times. For patients unable to tolerate surgery or with incompatible goals of care, radiation alone may be pursued. Conventional fractionated radiotherapy has previously been the standard of care and continues to be an important modality for radiation therapy. Stereotactic body radiation therapy (SBRT), which employs advanced tumor mapping and beam-focusing techniques to allow safe delivery of significantly higher bolus doses of radiation to tumor cells without collateral injury to nearby tissues, is rapidly developing a central role in the management of MSCC. This is particularly true for patients with tumor histology known to be insensitive to fractionated radiotherapy, and for those with tumor in an area that has already received a maximum allowable radiation dose.[39] Neurointerventional radiology technologies such as injection of cement into spinal column fractures, or intra-arterial tumor embolization and other ablative techniques also show promise for patients whose goals of care are incompatible with major surgery.[35]

Although some recovery of lost neurologic function is possible after decompression, often the greater impact of treatment is prevention of further damage. In fact, neurologic status at initiation of treatment is the strongest indicator of functional outcome, and every effort should be made to expedite appropriate therapy to prevent further neurologic decline. No direct evidence exists to guide the exact timing of treatment, but most experts recommend definitive treatment within 24 hours whenever possible.[32]

Disposition

Following corticosteroid administration, patients with neurologic deficits (i.e., motor, sensory, or autonomic) should be hospitalized for definitive therapy. Asymptomatic patients with incidentally noted vertebral metastasis may be managed as outpatients, provided they have reliable follow-up. Given the complexity intrinsic to management of MSCC, a multidisciplinary approach involving oncology, radiation oncology, and neurosurgery should be employed regardless of disposition.[40]

MALIGNANT PERICARDIAL DISEASE

KEY CONCEPTS

- No clinical sign or symptom is entirely sensitive for cardiac tamponade, but echocardiographic findings of a large pericardial effusion (anechoic circumferential stripe around the heart) and right atrial or ventricular collapse during diastole, combined with clinical findings of shock are highly suggestive.
- If compatible with goals of care, pericardial effusion causing tamponade should be emergently drained. Intravenous fluid or inotrope administration may be trialed as a temporizing measure, but these therapies are unreliable and should not delay definitive management.

Foundations

Pericardial manifestations of malignant disease, including pericarditis, pericardial neoplasm (usually metastatic), and pericardial effusion affect greater than 10% of cancer patients and cause about 25% of all effusive pericardial disease in the developed world.[41] Approximately two-thirds of malignancy-associated pericardial disease is clinically insignificant. However, in the remaining one-third of cases, hemodynamic compromise, organ failure, or death occurs.

Neoplastic disease is believed to cause pericardial effusion when lymphatic flow, which normally drains fluid from the pericardium, becomes obstructed or reversed by congestion in proximal malignant lymph nodes. An effusion develops both by obstruction of fluid outflow, and by metastatic spread to the pericardial lining, leading to a nonphysiologic increase in pericardial fluid production. The most common culprits in this process are lung, breast, and hematologic tumors, as well as melanoma.[41] Effusions not directly caused by malignancy may also develop in cancer patients secondary to hypoalbuminemia or as an adverse effect of radiation or chemotherapy.

Although the pericardial sac has the elastic potential for gradual expansion to greater than 1 L, it is poorly distensible in short (i.e., hours to days) time frames, and rapid accumulation of even a few hundred milliliters of fluid may precipitate cardiac tamponade. This life-threatening condition occurs when intrapericardial pressures rise to match or surpass those of the atria and then ventricles, reducing or eliminating cardiac output and leading to shock.

Clinical Features

The classic presenting symptoms of pericardial disease are dyspnea and chest pain. Weakness and fatigue are often associated, and large, slowly accumulating effusions may result in mass effect on nearby structures, causing nausea, early satiety, cough, hiccups, hoarseness, or dysphagia. Cardiac tamponade presents with shock, but other classic stigmata of the disease are unreliable. Pulsus paradoxus, defined as a 10 mm Hg systolic blood pressure gradient between inspiration and expiration in the respiratory cycle, is the most sensitive sign, present in about 80% of cases. Kussmaul sign (paradoxically increased jugular venous pressure [JVP] with inspiration) and Beck triad (hypotension, elevated JVP, and muffled heart sounds) are seen in less than half of cases. Hypotension may not even be a presenting symptom, particularly in patients with underlying hypertension.

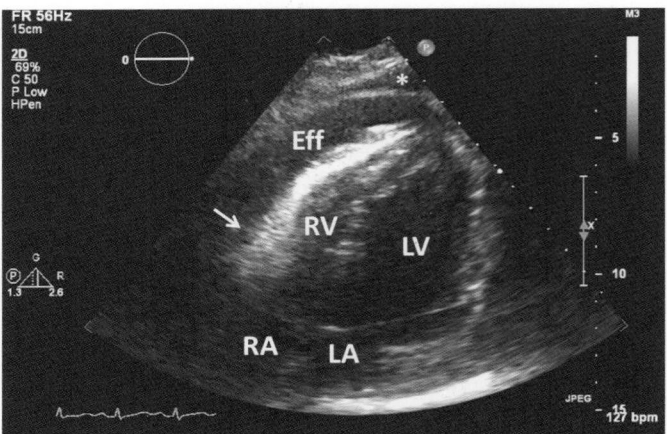

Fig. 112.2 Four-chamber apical view demonstrating pericardial effusion *(Eff)* with tamponade physiology in a patient with breast cancer. Buckling of the right ventricle wall is marked by a *white arrow*. Left ventricle *(LV)*, left atrium *(LA)*, right ventricle *(RV)*, and right atrium *(RA)* are all as marked. Incidentally noted pleural effusion is marked with an asterisk *(*)*. (Photo courtesy of the Division of Cardiology, Department of Internal Medicine, University of Maryland School of Medicine.)

Differential Diagnosis

Because of its nonspecific presentation, the differential diagnosis for malignant pericardial effusion is broad. Considerations should include acute coronary syndrome, acute heart failure or valve failure, pulmonary embolism, pleural effusion, pneumonia, and pneumothorax.

Diagnostic Testing

Evaluation for a patient with suspected malignant pericardial effusion should include chest radiography, electrocardiogram (ECG), and transthoracic echo (TTE). Electrocardiographic manifestations may include nonspecific ST or T changes, or low amplitude QRS voltage. Electrical alternans (alternating high and low QRS amplitudes) is only seen in 10% of cases. An enlarged cardiac silhouette on chest x-ray may suggest a large effusion. Echocardiography, which approaches 100% sensitivity and specificity for pericardial effusion, can also identify characteristics of tamponade physiology, such as cardiac chamber collapse and abnormal tissue imaging markers (e.g., tricuspid valve annular plane systolic excursion).[42] Emergency clinicians, who are trained in basic bedside cardiac ultrasound, can reliably identify pericardial effusion and should perform the initial examination to hasten diagnosis (Fig. 112.2).

Management

Malignant pericardial effusion generally serves as evidence of advanced cancer, and therapies should be tailored to match each patient's goals of care. If aggressive therapy is desired, cardiac tamponade is a medical emergency and warrants immediate drainage, ideally under real-time ultrasonographic guidance (Fig. 112.3). Ultrasound-guided drainage by the intercostal approach results in fewer complications and higher success rates than blind drainage by the subxiphoid approach. If ultrasound is unavailable, a subxiphoid approach should be employed by inserting the needle at a 15-degree angle to horizontal between the xyphoid process and left costal margin. After clearing the rib cage, the needle should be leveled and advanced toward the left shoulder until return of fluid is achieved. Temporizing measures such as inotropes (e.g., epinephrine in hypotensive patients, dobutamine in normotensive patients) or intravenous fluids may be attempted, but, despite

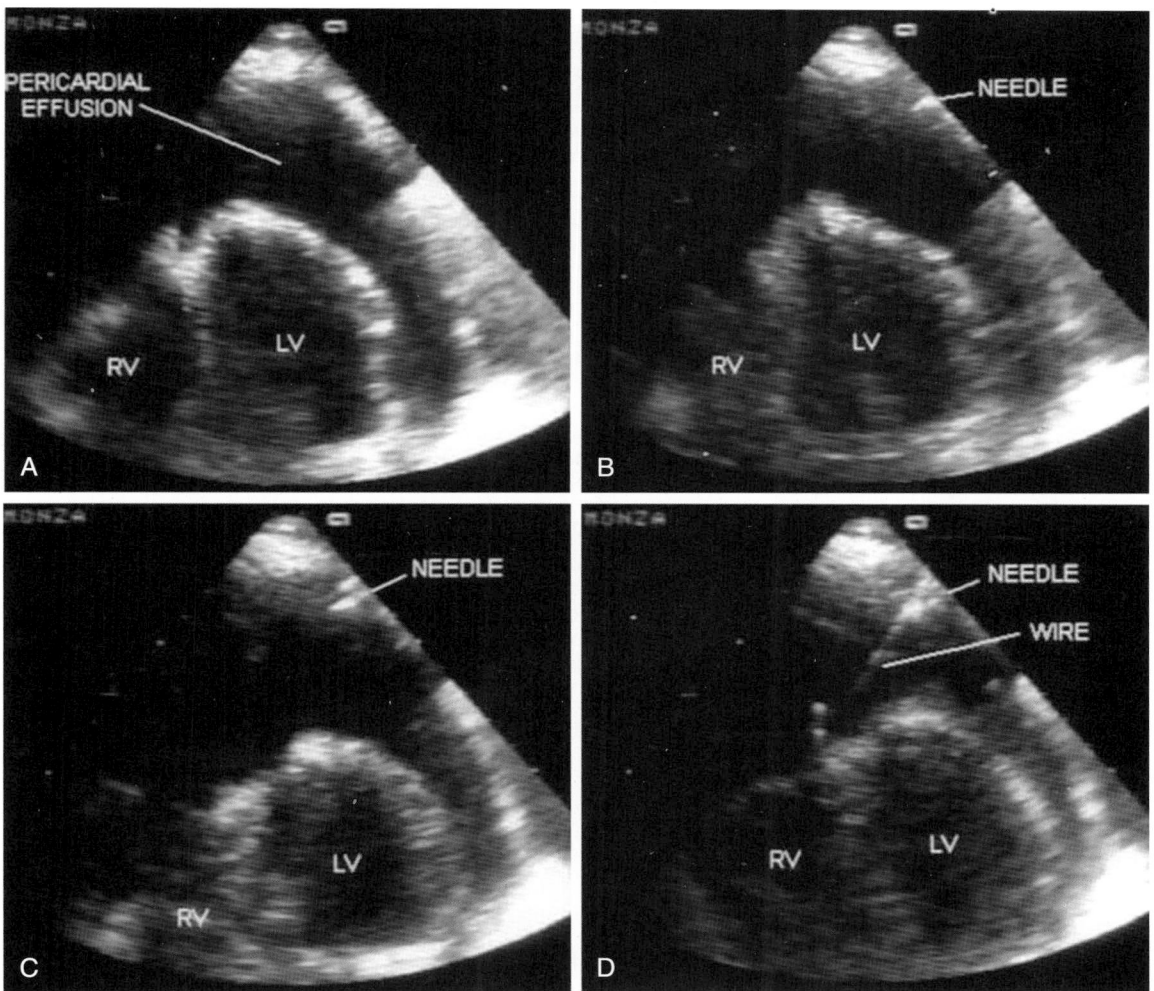

Fig. 112.3 Ultrasound-guided drainage of pericardial effusion. (A) A four-chamber apical view reveals a large pericardial effusion. (B and C) Under ultrasound guidance, a needle is advanced through an intercostal space and to the pericardial sack. (D) Upon reaching the pericardial sack fluid can be drained directly, or a wire advanced for drain placement by Seldinger technique. *LV*, Left ventricle; *RV*, right ventricle. (Reproduced from: Maggiolini S, et al. Echocardiography-guided pericardiocentesis with probe-mounted needle: report of 53 cases. *J Am Soc Echocardiogr.* 2001;14:821-824, with permission.)

early successes in trials on anesthetized animal models, these measures have not demonstrated reproducible benefit in humans and should not be viewed as a substitute for timely drainage.

Effusion without tamponade can be managed nonemergently. Fluid sampling for cytology and tumor marker analysis can help confirm etiology of effusion. This also allows intrapericardial chemotherapy or injection of sclerosing agents in a more controlled fashion. Malignant effusions tend to recur, so a long-term evacuation strategy by way of percutaneous drain,[43] surgical window,[44] or percutaneous balloon pericardiotomy[45] should be considered.

Disposition

Disposition depends on the hemodynamic effect of the pericardial effusion. Patients without tamponade or with a low likelihood of tamponade in the near future (i.e., slow evolution of symptoms) can be managed nonemergently as an outpatient. Those with tamponade or rapid development of effusion should undergo pericardiocentesis and be hospitalized to monitor for fluid reaccumulation.

HYPERCALCEMIA

KEY CONCEPTS

- Calcium levels in hypercalcemic patients should be assessed by measuring ionized calcium concentration, rather than total calcium concentration.
- First-line management of hypercalcemia includes intravenous fluids (1–2 L crystalloid bolus followed by 200–250 mL/hr), and loop diuretics only for volume management, as well as bisphosphonate therapy (pamidronate 90 mg or zoledronate 4 mg, intravenously). Calcitonin is faster acting than bisphosphonates, but tachyphylaxis may develop; consider calcitonin in hypercalcemic patients with active cardiac or neurologic symptoms (e.g., dysrhythmias, seizures).

FOUNDATIONS

Serum calcium regulation is achieved by parathyroid hormone (PTH) and calcitriol (the activated form of vitamin D), which both increase serum calcium level, and to a lesser extent by calcitonin, which

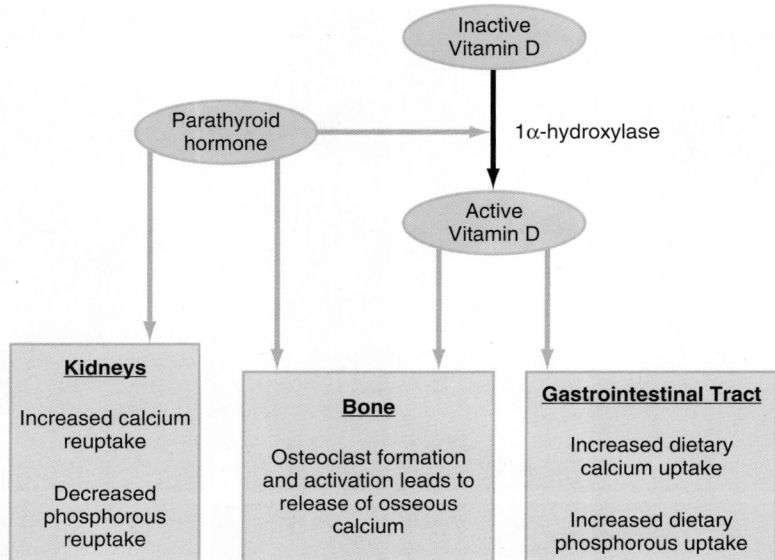

Fig. 112.4 Schematic representation of normal calcium homeostasis. Signaling molecules are represented by *circles*, targets of each signaling molecule and effects on the target are represented by *green arrows* and *boxes*. Activation of vitamin D by 1α-hydroxylase is represented by a *black arrow.*

decreases it (Fig. 112.4). Approximately a third of cancer patients will experience dysregulation of calcium homeostasis, usually caused by one or more of the following: (1) synthesis of the PTH analog PTH-related protein (PTHrP), (2) overproduction of calcitriol, (3) bone osteolysis due to direct spread of tumor, or, (4) less commonly, ectopic production of PTH.[46] In most cases, malignancy-associated hypercalcemia signifies advanced disease, with median survival of less than two months.[47-49]

Synthesis of PTHrP, classically called *humoral hypercalcemia*, causes about 80% of cases of malignancy-associated hypercalcemia, and is usually associated with squamous cancers, such as head and neck, lung, esophageal, cervical, ovarian, and endometrial carcinomas. Calcitriol overproduction is usually seen in Hodgkin and non-Hodgkin lymphomas, in which secreted cytokines inappropriately activate the vitamin D–activating enzyme 1α-hydroxylase in macrophages. Bony metastasis can cause local cytokine-induced osteolysis and, if extensive, can lead to hypercalcemia. Ectopic PTH production is a rare feature of malignancies, mainly limited to case reports. Primary hyperparathyroidism occurring coincidentally with cancer is much more common.[46]

Clinical Features

Presenting symptoms often include weakness, lethargy, confusion, abdominal pain, nausea, vomiting, constipation, polyuria, polydipsia, and kidney injury. Signs of dehydration may also be present. Manifestations depend not only on the absolute value of serum calcium but also on the patient's age and comorbidities and the rate of increase of serum calcium.[46] Acute hypercalcemia most commonly presents with neurologic abnormalities and acute kidney injury, as well as cardiac dysrhythmias if severe. Nephrolithiasis and nephrocalcinosis occur more commonly with chronic hypercalcemia, and they are infrequent manifestations of malignancy-associated hypercalcemia. Physical examination findings are often nonspecific. Electrocardiogram findings may initially exhibit QT interval shortening, progressing to dysrhythmias and heart block as hypercalcemia worsens.[50]

Differential Diagnoses

Because of its nonspecific presentation, the differential diagnosis for malignancy-associated hypercalcemia is quite broad. Consideration should be given to infection with systemic manifestations, direct neurologic injury (e.g., cerebrovascular accident or central nervous system [CNS] infection), or other metabolic derangements (e.g., hyper- or hyponatremia, acidemia, or TLS).

Diagnostic Testing

Accurate measurement of the free serum calcium level is the most important step in the evaluation of malignancy-associated hypercalcemia. Measurements of total serum calcium, which are often included in basic metabolic panels, include a large fraction of physiologically inert calcium, which is bound to albumin and other serum proteins. Approximations of the bound fraction of serum calcium can be made using serum albumin measurements, but factors affecting the avidity of calcium for serum proteins, such as pH and the presence of medications that compete for binding sites, as well as abnormal concentrations of non-albumin proteins, may lead to inaccuracies in this calculation. It is therefore recommended that free or ionized levels of calcium be obtained for any patient with suspected malignancy-associated hypercalcemia.

Testing for additional metabolic abnormalities including serum levels of sodium, potassium, bicarbonate, chloride, magnesium, and phosphorous should be performed, as should an assessment of kidney function with blood urea nitrogen and creatinine.[46] A brief review of reversible factors exacerbating hypercalcemia such as thiazide diuretic use or exogenous calcium supplementation may be helpful. Further testing to determine the etiology of malignancy-associated hypercalcemia (PTH, PTHrP, and calcitriol levels, as well as skeletal survey for bone metastasis) may eventually be undertaken but is generally unnecessary in the ED, because initial therapy is not etiology-specific.

Management

Severe hypercalcemia, especially if rapidly developing, will lead to death if untreated. First-line treatment for malignancy-associated hypercalcemia is intravenous fluid. Hypercalcemia impairs renal resorption of water and sodium, leading to hypovolemia. Hypovolemia further limits the kidneys' ability to eliminate calcium, creating a feedback loop that propagates hypercalcemia and hypovolemia. To break this loop, euvolemia must be restored, generally by administration of intravenous fluid. An initial bolus of 1 to 2 liters of crystalloid followed by 200 to 250 mL/hr has been recommended.[46] We recommend that patients with acute oliguria or anuria be vigorously volume challenged, because poor urine output may simply be a product of hypovolemia. However, if urine output does not improve, as may be the case with heart or kidney failure, resulting hypervolemia should be treated with a combination of diuresis, dialysis, and positive-pressure ventilation. Historically, loop diuretics have been used even for euvolemic patients in an attempt to force calciuresis; however, this has led to high complication rates and the calciuretic effect is minimal.[46] We therefore recommend the use of loop diuretics only for volume overload. Thiazide diuretics enhance distal tubule calcium resorption and should be avoided in hypercalcemic patients. Hypercalcemic patients with baseline oliguria or anuria may require dialysis.

Bisphosphonates are the primary pharmacologic treatment for hypercalcemia. Analogs of pyrophosphate, which is produced in bone catabolism, bisphosphonates inhibit bone turnover by reducing osteoclast function and directly stabilizing hydroxyapatite crystals. Typical regimens consist of single doses of either 90 mg of pamidronate given over 2 to 4 hours, or 4 mg of zoledronate given over 15 to 30 minutes.[46] Both should be given intravenously, because oral availability may be limited. An average reduction of serum calcium concentration of 3 to 4 mg/dL can be expected with either regimen, but maximum effect may not be seen for 7 to 10 days. Bisphosphonates can cause an acute phase reaction in up to one-third of cases, consisting of fever, myalgia, arthralgia, and headache, usually within 36 hours. Such side effects can be managed with antipyretics and antihistamines. Bisphosphonates have also been associated with renal dysfunction and jaw osteonecrosis.

Although effective, bisphosphonates require days to lower serum calcium levels. Calcitonin has a quicker onset (12 to 24 hours) and may be useful for manifestations of hypercalcemia requiring immediate reduction of serum calcium level, such as dysrhythmias.[46] The effects of calcitonin are short-lived due to tachyphylaxis, so definitive therapy with bisphosphonates should be simultaneously given. Calcitonin should be given subcutaneously or intramuscularly 4 to 8 units/kg every 6 hours, which typically reduces the serum calcium level by 1 to 2 mg/dL.

Other pharmacologic therapies include denosumab, a human monoclonal antibody inhibiting the RANK ligand that has been used in patients with bisphosphonate-resistant hypercalcemia, as well as plicamycin (mithramycin) and gallium nitrate. Denosumab is not significantly more effective nor faster-acting than bisphosphonates but is more expensive, thus it is generally used second-line in cases of bisphosphonate failure. It may be the preferred agent in patients with renal dysfunction and CrCl <30 mL/min. Plicamycin and gallium nitrate have both fallen out of favor due to long administration times and unfavorable adverse effect profiles; we generally recommend against their use. Hemodialysis can quickly reduce serum calcium levels and should be considered in patients who are dialysis-dependent, recalcitrant to other therapies, or have life-threatening manifestations of hypercalcemia.[51,52] Regardless of other therapies, treatment of the underlying malignancy should be immediately pursued if this is compatible with goals of care, because this is the only way to reverse the underlying cause of hypercalcemia and generally does not increase serum calcium levels.

Disposition

Patients with severe hypercalcemia (>14.0 mg/dL) or an acutely increasing calcium level should be admitted to a monitored bed. Patients with a stable serum calcium concentration less than 14 mg/dL, and close, reliable follow-up may be managed on an outpatient basis in consultation with the their oncologist or primary care doctor.

TUMOR LYSIS SYNDROME

KEY CONCEPTS

- TLS is manifested by the combination of hyperkalemia, hyperuricemia, hyperphosphatemia, and hypocalcemia, often accompanied by acute renal failure.
- Patients with TLS should have their potassium, phosphate, calcium, and uric acid levels, as well as renal indices monitored closely. Intravenous fluids should be administered, as well as therapies to reverse hyperkalemia. Hyperuricemia may be prevented with allopurinol or treated with rasburicase. Calcium should only be repleted in patients with cardiac or neurologic manifestations of hypocalcemia.

Foundations

TLS occurs when destruction of malignant cells occurs so rapidly that the body's mechanisms for regulating the unwanted products of this destruction are overwhelmed. Such cell lysis releases intracellular contents, causing hyperuricemia, hyperkalemia, hyperphosphatemia, and hypocalcemia. Acute kidney injury, caused by crystal deposits of uric acid or calcium-phosphate in the renal tubules or by crystal-independent mechanisms of damage by uric acid, often accompanies TLS, further compounding the patient's ability to regulate serum electrolyte levels and eliminate products of cellular destruction. Not infrequently, kidney injury can occur to the point that renal dialysis is required.[53] TLS is most likely to occur in patients with tumors that are high-burden, rapidly growing, and highly chemosensitive, such as Burkitt lymphoma or acute lymphoblastic leukemia (ALL). TLS occurs less commonly in rapidly growing solid tumors, such as breast, testicular, and small cell lung cancers; overall the types of malignancies with potential for TLS is growing as more effective and fast-acting chemotherapeutics are developed.[54,55] Patient factors predisposing to TLS include preexisting renal failure, hypovolemia, and hyperuricemia.

Clinical Features

Although spontaneous TLS is possible, patients undergoing cytotoxic therapy are particularly at risk for TLS. Symptoms result from metabolic derangements or kidney failure and include nausea, vomiting, lethargy, confusion, edema, seizure, myalgias, and tetany; dysrhythmias may result in cardiac arrest. Release of immunoactive proteins such as cytokines from lysed cells may cause sepsis-like symptoms. Due to the immunocompromised state of these individuals, an infectious source should be presumed in patients with septic symptoms and empiric antibiotics should be administered. Electrocardiographic changes may include QT interval prolongation due to hypocalcemia and P-wave flattening, PR and QRS interval prolongation, and T-wave peaking due to hyperkalemia.

Differential Diagnoses

Differential diagnosis for patients with TLS varies with presenting symptoms. For those with nonspecific symptoms such as fatigue or myalgia, consideration should be given to other metabolic derangements such as malignancy-associated hypercalcemia, or systemic manifestations of an infectious source. Patients presenting with cardiac dysrhythmia should be considered for acute coronary syndrome, pulmonary embolism, other sources of metabolic derangements, and other causes of myocardial irritation. Seizure and other neurologic symptoms may suggest cerebrovascular accident, CNS infection or metastasis, or other metabolic abnormalities.

Diagnostic Testing

Evaluation begins with measurement of serum potassium, phosphate, ionized calcium, urea nitrogen, creatinine, uric acid, and lactate dehydrogenase (LDH). For patients who have received rasburicase, uric acid specimens should be sent on ice to prevent artificially low results.[56] If the patient is presenting with sepsis-like symptoms, investigation for a source including cultures and appropriate imaging should be undertaken. Renal imaging (e.g., ultrasound) to rule out obstructive pathology as well as urinalysis and measurement of fractional excretion of sodium (FE_{Na}) should be performed for patients presenting with acute kidney injury. Further evaluation may be indicated by specific presenting symptoms, such as head imaging for patients presenting with seizure, or abdominal imaging for patients with nausea and vomiting.

Management

Intravenous fluids to promote renal clearance of unwanted metabolites should be the initial therapy for TLS; volumes of 3 L/m^2/day are suggested, or as high as 5 to 6 L daily.[56] Acutely oliguric or anuric patients should be similarly fluid challenged because these may be the result of hypovolemia, but plans should be made for diuresis or renal replacement therapy if urine output does not improve or hypervolemia ensues. Patients with oliguria or anuria at baseline may require initial management with renal replacement therapy. Although previously recommended, treatment guidelines no longer support alkalinization of the urine, because this may instigate worse metabolic derangements, including phosphate nephropathy and xanthine crystal nephropathy.[56]

Hydration provides the primary therapy for hyperphosphatemia but limiting dietary phosphate intake and eliminating phosphate-containing supplements are also indicated. Hypocalcemia is a direct result of free calcium precipitating with excess phosphate to form the insoluble, nephrotoxic compound calcium phosphate. The extent of calcium phosphate formation is directly related to the product of serum calcium and phosphate concentrations. Products greater than 55 suggest a worsened long-term risk of calcium phosphate deposition in the viscera, although short-term outcomes are not well studied. To minimize the risk of calcium phosphate nephropathy, asymptomatic patients should go without calcium repletion. Patients with cardiac (e.g., dysrhythmia, heart blocks) or neurologic (e.g., seizure, coma) manifestations of hypocalcemia should receive intravenous calcium repletion.

Management of hyperkalemia is the same as that from any other etiology. Intravenous calcium given as a bolus can transiently (less than 1 hour) stabilize the myocardium of patients with existing or an imminent dysrhythmia (e.g., QRS widening). Efforts can then be made to shift potassium intracellularly via administration of insulin, bicarbonate, and beta-agonists. Ultimately, potassium must be removed from the body by the gastrointestinal tract with administration of potassium binders, by the kidneys with hydration and possibly loop diuretics, or by dialysis.

Uric acid is a metabolite in the degradation pathway of nucleic acids. Hyperuricemia from massive release of free nucleic acids can cause nephropathy both directly and by crystal formation in the renal tubules. In addition to hydration, hyperuricemia can be managed pharmacologically by administration of allopurinol, febuxostat or rasburicase.[56] Allopurinol, an analog of the uric acid precursor hypoxanthine, competitively inhibits enzymatic conversion of xanthine to uric acid. Although this decreases uric acid production, it does not eliminate uric acid already present in the body, and it leads to buildup of xanthine, which itself has limited solubility and potential to cause nephropathy. Febuxostat functions similarly to allopurinol, though its inhibition of the xanthine oxidase enzyme is noncompetitive. Febuxostat has been shown to be noninferior to allopurinol for prevention of tumor lysis syndrome,[57,58] however due to its high cost relative to allopurinol[59] it should only be used in patients who can't tolerate allopurinol (e.g., allopurinol allergy). Rasburicase, a recombinant form of the enzyme urate oxidase, eliminates uric acid directly by converting it into the more soluble metabolite allantoin. It is usually given as a single, intravenous dose. Significant reduction in uric acid levels within 1 day have been observed with weight-based doses of 0.05 to 0.15 mg/kg, and with fixed doses of 3 to 6 mg, with a single 6 mg dose for adults or 0.15 mg/kg dose for children reliably demonstrating effective reduction of uric acid levels.[60-62] Those with glucose-6-phosphate dehydrogenase (G6PD) deficiency should not receive rasburicase, because hydrogen peroxide is a byproduct of its activity and this may trigger hemolytic crisis. Methemoglobinemia may also result from rasburicase administration.[56]

Disposition

The Cairo-Bishop definition of TLS, a systematic classification of lab abnormalities and clinical manifestations of TLS, divides patients with only laboratory manifestations of TLS (laboratory TLS, or LTLS) from those with clinical manifestations of TLS (clinical TLS, or CTLS), such as kidney injury, dysrhythmia, or seizure. Patients with clinical TLS consisting of dysrhythmia or seizure should be admitted to an ICU; those with kidney injury may be admitted to a standard telemetry bed, but ICU care should be considered because mortality in patients with kidney injury and TLS increases relative to that with TLS alone. Patients with laboratory TLS only may be admitted to a monitored bed for observation and treatment.

LEUKOSTASIS

KEY CONCEPTS

- Leukostasis arises due to congestion of blood vessels by excessive numbers of leukocytes. This most often occurs in the lungs and CNS, and the resulting clinical picture may be difficult to differentiate from other diseases that afflict cancer patients (e.g., pneumonia, pulmonary embolism, CNS hemorrhage).
- Intravenous fluids should be administered in the ED to reduce blood viscosity, and red blood cell transfusions should generally be avoided. Therapies to lower the WBC count should be performed in consultation with an oncologist, and may include leukapheresis, administration of hydroxyurea, or initiation of chemotherapy.

Foundations

Leukostasis arises when the white blood cell (WBC) count is sufficiently high to cause vascular congestion, leading to organ dysfunction, typically in the lungs[63] or CNS. No single threshold exists for leukostasis to occur, and different types of leukemia cells cause leukostasis at widely variable cell counts. Patients with chronic lymphocytic leukemia (CLL) may tolerate WBC counts greater than 500,000 cells/µL, whereas patients with acute myeloid leukemia (AML) may develop leukostasis with WBC counts less than 100,000 cells/µL.

Two mechanisms are believed to drive leukostasis. First, blast cells are larger and less deformable than normal WBCs. As the number of blast cells in the blood increases, blood viscosity increases. Second, because certain cell types are more prone to causing leukostasis than others with similar size and physical characteristics, intrinsic features of leukemic cells, such as cytokine-induced activation of endothelial adhesion mechanisms, may also contribute.[64]

Clinical Features

Pulmonary leukostasis presents as dyspnea, tachypnea, and hypoxemia. Auscultation of pulmonary leukostasis may mimic lung infection with crackles or rhonchi, and bilateral opacities are often seen on imaging.[63] CNS leukostasis may present with confusion, audio or visual abnormalities, headache, ataxia, or coma. Intracranial hemorrhage may be seen on head imaging. Other clinical manifestations may include retinal hemorrhage, myocardial infarction, acute limb ischemia, priapism, renal vein thrombosis, and renal infarction.

Differential Diagnoses

Diagnosis of leukostasis is challenging because symptoms of leukostasis are similar to those of other problems common to leukemia patients. Pulmonary leukostasis presents with similar history, physical examination findings, and imaging as pneumonia or pulmonary edema. Patients with CNS leukostasis may present with nonspecific alteration of mental status, similar to that seen in metabolic derangement, medication side effect, or systemic manifestation of infection. Intracranial hemorrhage seen on head imaging may be related to leukostasis itself or may result from thrombocytopenia or disseminated intravascular coagulopathy (DIC), both of which often accompany hyperleukocytosis.

Diagnostic Testing

The gold standard diagnostic test for leukostasis is the presence of leukocyte-clogged blood vessels on tissue pathology. Because this is rarely available, the diagnosis must often be inferred and empirically treated based on knowledge of leukocyte count, cancer type, and clinical picture. A CBC with peripheral smear should be sent from the ED. Further evaluation is indicated to determine cancer type (if not known), including cytology and immunostaining, although results are not actionable in the ED. Symptom-specific imaging should be performed, such as chest plain films or CT for respiratory problems, and head CT or MRI for neurologic symptoms. Normal imaging findings do not exclude leukostasis, however.[63] If sent, blood gases should be processed immediately, because metabolically active leukocytes will continue to consume oxygen in the phlebotomized sample, resulting in falsely low oxygen levels.

Management

ED management of leukostasis centers on reduction of blood viscosity. Intravenous fluids should be administered to dilute the blood as much as possible. Although patients with hyperleukocytosis are often anemic, transfusion of red blood cells should be avoided in asymptomatic patients, because erythrocytes exacerbate blood viscosity. Platelets and plasma may be given as needed because these components make little or no contribution to blood viscosity.

The definitive treatment for hyperleukocytosis is reduction of leukocyte count, either by physically removing excess cells using leukapheresis or by destroying excess cells pharmacologically. Leukapheresis involves continuous removal of fractions of the patient's blood, selective extraction of leukocytes from the fractions, and return of the remaining product to the patient. Leukapheresis can reduce leukocyte count by 20% to 50% in only a few hours, but insertion of a central large-bore catheter is necessary, and leukapheresis requires specialized equipment not available at all institutions. Studies of outcomes with and without leukapheresis are small and nonrandomized, and none have shown a long-term survival benefit (>90-day survival) from the therapy. Results are conflicting as to short-term survival benefits of leukapheresis (7 to 30 days),[65,66] and expert opinion regarding use of leukapheresis for this application remains mixed overall.[67] Hydroxyurea, an inhibitor of deoxyribonucleotide synthesis, can pharmacologically

reduce leukocyte burden by similar margins over 24 to 48 hours, and in studies has inconsistently shown a reduction in in-hospital mortality when used prior to induction chemotherapy.[68] Chemotherapy induction, which should only be initiated in consultation with an oncologist, can also quickly reduce leukocyte counts, but the patient should be monitored for signs of TLS.[67] Given the paucity of evidence supporting a single approach to leukoreduction, treatment varies significantly between hospitals, and should be guided by local experts. Due to the difficulty of clinically distinguishing leukostasis from other serious pathologies, treatments for other diagnoses may be simultaneously initiated. Such concomitant therapy (e.g., antibiotics) is particularly important for suspected pneumonia, because patients with hyperleukocytosis may be functionally neutropenic.

Disposition

Patents with leukostasis require hospitalization for monitoring, hydration, and leukocyte-reducing therapy. Asymptomatic patients with leukocytosis also warrant hospitalization if they have a blast count greater than 20,000 cells/μL, have a tumor type of AML, or have a new leukemia of unknown type. Patients with asymptomatic hyperleukocytosis who do not meet these criteria may be discharged with close, reliable follow-up, but this decision should be made in conjunction with the patient's oncologist.

SUPERIOR VENA CAVA SYNDROME

> **KEY CONCEPTS**
>
> - SVC syndrome occurs due to either external (e.g., tumor) or internal (e.g., thrombus) obstruction of the SVC.
> - ED management of SVC syndrome is largely supportive. The head of the bed should be elevated, and supplemental oxygen provided if needed. If the cause of SVC syndrome is determined to be thrombus, anticoagulation may be initiated if not contraindicated.
> - SVC syndrome is life-threatening only in the rare case of cerebral edema, hemodynamic collapse, or tracheal compromise. With the exception of these situations, definitive anti-cancer treatment should be postponed in order to allow for tissue diagnosis of the underlying mass if not already known.

Foundations

The superior vena cava (SVC) spans the final stretch of venous return from the upper body, spanning from the juncture of the brachiocephalic veins to the heart. The SVC is thin-walled, and blood pressures in the SVC are relatively low (≈2 to 8 mm Hg), making it particularly susceptible to external compression. When SVC flow is compromised, its internal pressure can reach 20 to 40 mm Hg, potentially resulting in symptoms or cardiac decompensation. Such clinical deterioration constitutes SVC syndrome.[69] Malignancy is the cause for more than 60% of total cases. Lung cancer and lymphoma cause over 90% of cases of malignancy-induced SVC syndrome. SVC syndrome due to an intraluminal mass, such as thrombosis, is increasing in prevalence. Cancer patients are at high risk for thrombosis due to their hypercoagulable state and indwelling venous catheters in the SVC.[69]

Clinical Features

Patients with SVC syndrome most commonly present with upper extremity, chest, or face edema or erythema, but dyspnea, dysphagia, chest pain, or cough may also be present. Physical examination

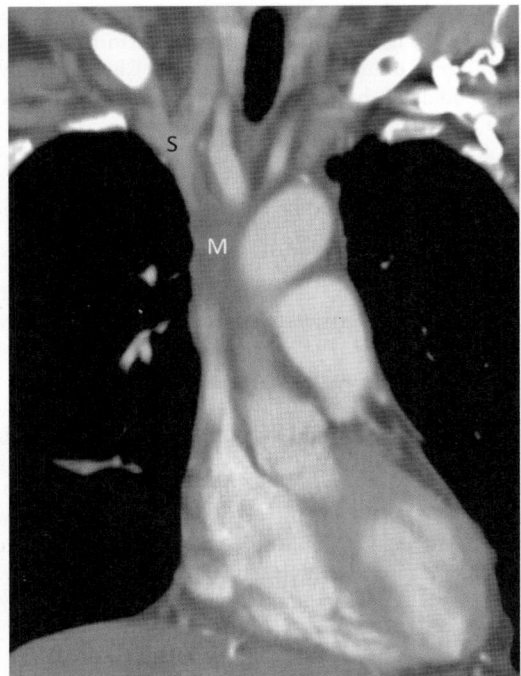

Fig. 112.5 Computed tomography (CT) scan of the chest with intravenous contrast demonstrating superior vena cava (SVC) compromise due to external mass in a patient with primary lung malignancy. *S*, SVC; *M*, intrathoracic mass. (Photo courtesy of the Department of Radiology, University of Maryland School of Medicine.)

findings often reflect elevated venous return pressures, including jugular venous distention (JVD) and edema, flushing, or cyanosis of the face, arms, and upper trunk. Distention of the SVC and compression of other nearby structures may cause vocal cord paralysis, blurred vision, and Horner syndrome.[69] Pleural effusion may be apparent on chest films or bedside sonography.[70] Overall, the type and severity of symptoms greatly depend on the acuity of SVC compression; patients with a slowly developing obstruction develop collaterals, which enable asymptomatic high-grade compression.

Differential Diagnoses

Edema and flushing isolated to the upper body is highly suspicious for SVC syndrome, particularly in a patient with known lung cancer or lymphoma. Other considerations include cellulitis or deep tissue infection (e.g., Ludwig angina), thoracic inlet syndrome, or obstruction of other deep veins (e.g., occlusive deep venous thrombosis in an internal jugular vein or subclavian vein). Other symptoms such as JVD, dyspnea, or cough are less specific and may suggest congestive heart failure, pneumonia, pericardial tamponade, or pulmonary embolism.

Diagnostic Testing

Thoracic imaging, and contrast-enhanced CT in particular, is the most important and commonly employed diagnostic modality for SVC syndrome (Fig. 112.5), but MRI is a viable alternative. In confirmed cases of SVC syndrome, a tissue diagnosis of the offending mass should be made prior to initiation of treatment.[69] This may be obtainable by sputum cytology, or by invasive means, such as bronchoscopy, lymph node biopsy, mediastinoscopy, or thoracotomy. Radiographically guided minimally invasive biopsy techniques performed by interventional radiologists have increasingly been employed for patients with SVC syndrome.[70] Moderate sedation or general anesthesia may be used safely to enable these procedures, however, in cases involving tracheal

compromise, an airway should be emergently and carefully (e.g., awake fiberoptic intubation) established prior to anesthesia induction.

Management

In the ED, management of SVC syndrome is largely conservative. Elevating the head of bed to promote gravitational drainage of the upper body and administration of supplemental oxygen, when appropriate, may provide significant symptomatic relief. For patients with SVC syndrome due to obstructing thrombus, anticoagulation with or without thrombolytics should be initiated. Diuretics or steroids have historically been administered and in some practices continue to be used[70]; however, they have no proven benefit, may simply provoke complications, and we do not recommend them.

Although the symptoms of SVC syndrome are unpleasant, risk to life occurs only with the rare and extreme complications of airway obstruction, cerebral edema or hemodynamic compromise. Definitive treatment of malignant SVC syndrome can often be safely delayed until biopsy specimens are obtained because of the rare need for emergent therapy and the increasing ability to tailor anti-cancer therapy based on exact tissue diagnosis. Once a histologic diagnosis is made, the ideal combination of chemotherapy, radiation, and surgery, if indicated, is guided by specialty consultation.

In cases requiring emergent resolution of SVC syndrome, the initial steps in the ED are aimed at achieving basic medical stabilization (e.g., intubation and mechanical ventilation, hemodynamic optimization). Thereafter, endovascular stenting of SVC may be employed for rapid and effective reduction of SVC pressures.[69] Although no large randomized controlled trials have been performed, in smaller observational studies endovascular stenting for SVC syndrome has been safe and effective[71] and resulted in rapid symptomatic relief.[72] Stenting carries the additional advantages that a tissue diagnosis isn't required prior to implementation, and that stent placement doesn't interfere with later plans for radiation or chemotherapy.[69] Endovascular stenting may also be considered nonemergently in cases of failure of or contraindication to conventional therapies (e.g., radiation or chemotherapy).[69] Open surgical bypass or replacement of the SVC can be performed but is reserved for the most extreme cases, because less invasive measures are often successful.

Disposition

Although SVC syndrome is seldom life-threatening, symptomatic relief first requires diagnosis and treatment tailored to the underlying etiology. Hospitalization generally expedites this evaluation. Patients with hemodynamic compromise, cerebral edema, or tracheal compromise should be admitted to an ICU following initial stabilization.[70]

MONOCLONAL ANTIBODY THERAPIES AND COMPLICATIONS

KEY CONCEPTS

- Monoclonal antibody therapies function through various mechanisms using a range of targets. This leads to a diverse collection of known complications including infection and organ dysfunction.
- Identifying and treating infections, including opportunistic infections, is the most important element of management for the emergency physician in treating a patient with suspected complications of monoclonal antibody therapy.

Foundations

As the molecular foundations of cancer are further explored, it has become increasingly feasible to target therapeutics against

TABLE 112.3 Properties and Complications of Anti-neoplastic Monoclonal Antibody Therapies

	Target/Mechanism	Indication	Notable complications
Alemtuzumab	CD52/ADCC and CDC	CLL	Cytopenias, infusion reactions, opportunistic infections including PCP (black box warnings)
Bevacizumab	VEGF-A/direct inhibition	Glioblastoma, cancers of colon, lung, and renal cell	Bowel perforation, wound healing complications, bleeding complications (black box warnings)
Blinatumomab	CD19/BiTE	ALL	CRS, neurotoxicity (black box warnings)
Brentuximab	CD30/cytotoxic agent delivery	HL, ALCL	PML (black box warning)
Cetuximab	EGFR/direct inhibition	Cancers of colon, lung, head/neck	Anaphylactic reaction in those with alpha-gal antibodies
Ibritumomab tiuxetan	CD20/radioisotope delivery	B-cell NHL	Infusion reactions, cutaneous reactions, persistent cytopenias (black box warnings)
Inotuzumab ozogamicin	CD22/cytotoxic agent delivery	B-cell ALL	Hepatotoxicity, hepatic veno-occlusive disease (black box warnings)
Ofatumumab	CD20/ADCC and CDC	CLL, NHL	PML, hepatitis B reactivation
Panitumumab	EGFR/direct inhibition	Colon cancer	Dermatologic toxicities (black box warning), ocular keratitis
Pertuzumab	HER2/direct inhibition	Breast cancer	Embryo-fetal toxicity (black box warning), cytopenias
Rituximab	CD20/ADCC and CDC	NHL, HL, CLL	Severe infusion reactions, TLS, severe mucocutaneous reactions, PML (black box warnings)
Trastuzumab	HER2/direct inhibition, ADCC and CDC	Breast cancer	Cardiomyopathies, infusion reactions, pulmonary toxicity (black box warnings)

ADCC, antibody-dependent cell-mediated cytotoxicity; *ALCL*, anaplastic large cell lymphoma; *ALL*, acute lymphoblastic leukemia; *Alpha gal*, galactose-α-1,3-galactose; *BiTE*, bispecific T-cell engager; *CLL*, chronic lymphocytic leukemia; *CRS*, cytokine release syndrome; EGFR, epidermal growth factor receptor; *HER2*, receptor tyrosine-protein kinase erbB-2; *HL*, Hodgkin lymphoma; *NHL*, non-Hodgkin lymphoma; *PCP*, *Pneumocystis jirovecii* pneumonia; *PML*, progressive multifocal leukoencephalopathy; *TLS*, tumor lysis syndrome; *VEGF-A*, vascular endothelial growth factor A.

tumor-specific molecules. While this specificity can be achieved by small molecules such as tyrosine kinase inhibitors, the natural targeting abilities of antibodies lend themselves well to efficient development of new therapies, and this has led to steady expansion of the repertoire of anti-neoplastic monoclonal antibodies.

Monoclonal antibody therapies have been engineered to work by various mechanisms. In their simplest form, non-conjugated antibodies bind to tumor-associated targets, marking tumor cells for killing by antibody-dependent cell-mediated cytotoxicity (ADCC) and complement-dependent cytotoxicity (CDC). Monoclonal antibodies tethered to cytotoxic payloads such as radioisotopes (e.g., ibritumomab) or cytotoxic medications (e.g., brentuximab) have increased the killing power of these therapeutics. Monoclonal antibodies tethered to the cytotoxic T cell–specific protein CD3, called bispecific T-cell engagers (BiTEs), are designed to amplify the efficiency of ADCC (e.g., blinatumomab). Monoclonal antibodies may also be designed to target and inhibit growth receptors on the tumor cell surface (e.g., trastuzumab) in addition to promoting cell destruction by ADCC and CDC. A list of common monoclonal antibodies along with their mechanisms of action and complications is given in Table 112.3.

Clinical Features

Because of the wide range of targets and mechanisms of action they employ, the complications of monoclonal antibody therapies are

diverse, vary between therapies, and are too numerous to list here. A broad outline of the clinical features of common complications is provided in the following sections; additionally, Table 112.3 lists therapy-specific complications including black box warnings. Due to their immunomodulatory nature, patients receiving monoclonal antibody therapies are particularly susceptible to infectious complications. Clinical features will vary depending on the nature of infection, but may include fever, rigors, fatigue, malaise, and leukocytosis. Opportunistic infections have been noted (especially with use of alemtuzumab), so the emergency physician should be wary of features such as a vesicular rash which may represent reactivation of a herpetic virus, respiratory symptoms which may represent *Pneumocystis jirovecii* pneumonia (PCP) or activation of tuberculosis, or jaundice and liver function abnormalities which may represent reactivation of viral hepatitis. Monoclonal antibody therapies can also cause cytokine release syndrome (blinatumomab especially[73]) which may have presenting features very similar to infection and sepsis.

Infusion reactions can occur with all monoclonal antibody therapies but are especially common to rituximab, cetuximab, alemtuzumab, ibritumomab tiuxetan, and trastuzumab. These reactions typically occur during or shortly after infusion. Clinical features may be similar to a type I hypersensitivity reaction (anaphylaxis) or may be nonspecific. These can include rash, tachycardia, dyspnea, and hypotension.

Dysfunction of particular organ systems may also occur with monoclonal antibody therapies. Several adverse pulmonary events have been known to occur over a broad time frame, ranging from acute respiratory distress syndrome (ARDS) occurring within hours after an infusion, to organizing pneumonia developing weeks to months after completion of therapy. Various cardiac complications have been reported, including sudden cardiac death (cetuximab especially), and cardiomyopathy (trastuzumab especially). A broad range of neurologic symptoms may also occur, including progressive multifocal leukoencephalopathy (PML). Hepatotoxicity believed due to veno-occlusive disease has also been noted with inotuzumab.[74] As with all cancer therapeutics, rapid killing of cancer cells may lead to tumor lysis syndrome.

Differential Diagnoses

The differential diagnosis for patients with complications of monoclonal antibody therapies varies widely depending on presentation. Patients presenting with fever and symptoms of sepsis should be considered to have an infection until proven otherwise, though cytokine release syndrome and some infusion reactions can have a similar presentation. Opportunistic infection must also be considered. Patients with symptoms of heart or respiratory failure (e.g., dyspnea, chest pain, edema) may have primary toxicity from their therapy, but may also have pneumonia, pericardial disease, or acute coronary syndrome. For patients with neurotoxicity, other central nervous system insults such as cerebrovascular accident and meningitis should be considered.

Diagnostic Testing

Diagnostic testing must be guided by the patient's clinical picture. Patients with symptoms consistent with infection or sepsis should undergo blood and urine culturing, chest x-ray, and other workup as guided by presentation (e.g., sputum culture for productive cough). Those with symptoms of cardiac or pulmonary dysfunction should have cardiac biomarkers, electrocardiogram, chest x-ray, and echocardiogram performed. Patients with neurologic symptoms should undergo brain imaging.

Management

Aside from prompt recognition and treatment of infections, treatments for complications of monoclonal antibody therapies are largely supportive. Mild cases of cytokine release syndrome may be treated with antipyretics, and mild infusion reactions may respond to histamine blockers. However, both of these conditions may require hemodynamic support (e.g., IV fluids, vasopressors) in more severe cases. For patients experiencing infusion reactions, management with epinephrine IM and close airway monitoring should commence if there is any question of anaphylaxis. Cardiomyopathies may be managed with inotropic agents and diuresis. Pulmonary complications should be managed with appropriate respiratory support (including mechanical ventilation if needed), and corticosteroids may be considered once infectious etiology has been ruled out.

Disposition

Disposition of patients with complications of monoclonal antibody therapy depends largely on the clinical picture and severity of symptoms and should be determined in conjunction with the patient's oncologist.

T-LYMPHOCYTE CHECKPOINT INHIBITOR THERAPIES AND COMPLICATIONS

KEY CONCEPTS

- Because it involves reduction of immune self-tolerance, T-lymphocyte checkpoint inhibition therapy is marked by a wide variety of complications
- For symptoms severe enough to affect quality of life, systemic corticosteroids may be initiated. This should be done in consultation with an oncologist.

Foundations

Many cancer cells carry surface markers which are unique to tumor cells and not found on normal cells (e.g., due to mutations or fusion proteins).[75] Although these tumor-specific antigens (TSAs) can be recognized and attacked by host T cells, many are sufficiently similar to host antigens that they are protected by the same mechanisms that protect host cells from autoimmune attack, known collectively as self-tolerance.[76] The goal of T-lymphocyte checkpoint inhibitor therapy is to reduce T-cell self-tolerance, thereby allowing a T-cell immune response against TSA-bearing cancer cells.

Self-tolerance is achieved by several mechanisms, including a series of protein interactions known as checkpoints which are designed to prevent mature T cells in the peripheral tissues from attacking self-antigen bearing cells. By inhibiting these checkpoints, T-lymphocyte checkpoint inhibitor therapy enables a more vigorous antitumor immune response. Current therapies achieve this through antibody-driven inhibition of two such checkpoint pathways: the CTLA-4 pathway and the PD-1 pathway. Therapeutic antibodies targeting the PD-1 pathway exist both for PD-1 itself and its ligand PD-L1. The CTLA-4 pathway is targeted via the CTLA-4 protein (Table 112.4).[76]

Clinical Features

Inhibiting the mechanisms of the immune system that maintain self-tolerance imparts a steep price in the form of diverse complications across all organ systems. Clinical features of these complications as well as approximate rates of incidence are summarized in Table 112.5. Perhaps the most feared of these are hypophysitis, an immune-mediated pituitary disease which can cause shock due to glucocorticoid deficiency, and colitis, which can be life-threatening.[77] Additionally, patients undergoing checkpoint inhibitor therapy are susceptible to all of the other complications listed in this chapter, such as tumor lysis syndrome.[78]

TABLE 112.4   Molecular Targets for T-lymphocyte Checkpoint Inhibition Therapy, FDA-Approved Inhibitors, and Overall Complication Rates by Target

Molecular Target	Approved Inhibitors	Overall Complication Incidence
CTLA-4	Ipilimumab	60–85%[85]
PD-1	Nivolumab, Pembrolizumab	16–37%[85]
PD-L1	Atezolizumab, Avelumab, Durvalumab	12–24%[85]

TABLE 112.5 Immune-Related Adverse Events, Presenting Symptoms, Differential Diagnoses, and Initial Workup, Listed by Organ System

Organ System	Immune-Related Adverse Event and Approximate Incidence Rate (CR = case reports only)	Clinical Features	Differential Diagnosis	Diagnostic Testing
Cardiac	Pericardial effusion (CR[86-88])	See above section on Malignant Pericardial Disease.		
	Myocarditis (CR[89])	Dyspnea, fatigue, pulmonary edema[89]	ACS, pneumonia	CXR, ECG, echocardiogram
Endocrine	Hypophysitis (≈5% for all therapies; greater with anti-CTLA-4 therapy [up to 17%] than anti-PD-1 or anti-PD-L1[90])	Anorexia, fatigue, headache, nausea, diplopia, confusion, temperature intolerance, subjective fever and chills. Average onset 6–12 weeks after starting therapy.	Infection/sepsis, adrenal crisis, cerebral metastases[90]	Visual field testing; brain MRI (evaluate for pituitary stalk enlargement); pituitary function testing (e.g., thyrotrophin, gonadotrophin, and corticotrophin levels)[90]
	Thyroid dysfunction (≈10% for anti-PD-1 and anti-PD-L1 therapy; >50% for anti-CTLA-4 therapy[90])	Thyroiditis (thyroid gland pain/induration), fatigue, temperature intolerance	Hypophysitis, infection/sepsis	Thyroid function testing, antithyroglobulin and anti-thyroperoxidase antibody testing, corticotropin testing (rule out hypophysitis)
Gastrointestinal	Colitis (0–2% with anti-PD-1 therapy; 5–10% with anti-CTLA-4 therapy[90])	Abdominal pain, fever, diarrhea, hematochezia, constitutional symptoms. Average onset 6–7 weeks after therapy initiation.[90]	Infection/sepsis, bowel ischemia, cytomegalovirus colitis, *Clostridium difficile* infection, IBD, other intra-abdominal pathology[90]	CT imaging of abdomen/pelvis, testing for stool pathogens (e.g., *C. difficile* toxin), endoscopic examination of colon (e.g., colonoscopy, flexible sigmoidoscopy)[90]
	Diarrhea (12–14% with anti-PD-1 therapy; 30–35% with anti-CTLA-4 therapy[90])	Diarrhea only	Colitis, GI infection, bowel ischemia, cytomegalovirus colitis, *Clostridium difficile* infection, IBD, other intra-abdominal pathology	CT imaging of abdomen/pelvis, testing for stool pathogens (e.g., *C. difficile* toxin)
	Hepatotoxicity (5–10% for all therapies)[90]	Elevated transaminases; in severe cases abdominal pain, jaundice, coagulopathy, liver synthetic function loss	Infectious hepatitis, hepatic metastases	Liver function testing, testing of liver synthetic functions (e.g., albumin, coagulation studies), hepatic imaging (e.g., ultrasound)
Hematologic	Neutropenia (1% for anti-PD-L1 therapy[91])	Largely asymptomatic; may present with fever/infection	Neutropenia due to alternative cause (e.g., chemotherapy, primary malignancy)	Complete blood count with manual differential; workup for neutropenic fever (see separate section above) if symptoms dictate
	Anemia (10% for anti-PD-L1 therapy[91])	Largely asymptomatic; severe cases may present with fatigue or dyspnea	Anemia due to alternative cause (e.g., chemotherapy, primary malignancy, blood loss), autoimmune hemolytic anemia (incidence of 0.5% with anti-PD-1/PD-L1 therapy[92])	Complete blood count with manual differential, evaluation for hemolysis (e.g., lactate dehydrogenase, serum haptoglobin, bilirubin levels), iron studies, evaluation for sources of blood loss (e.g., inquire about history of melanotic or bloody stools)
	Immune thrombocytopenia (<0.5% for anti-PD-1/PD-L1 therapy[92])	Often asymptomatic; may present with bleeding-related complications (e.g., excessive bruising)	Immune thrombocytopenic purpura, thrombotic thrombocytopenic purpura, disseminated intravascular coagulation	Complete blood count with manual differential, evaluation for hemolysis (e.g., lactate dehydrogenase, serum haptoglobin, bilirubin levels), coagulation testing

Continued

TABLE 112.5   Immune-Related Adverse Events, Presenting Symptoms, Differential Diagnoses, and Initial Workup, Listed by Organ System—cont'd.

Organ System	Immune-Related Adverse Event and Approximate Incidence Rate (CR = case reports only)	Clinical Features	Differential Diagnosis	Diagnostic Testing
Integumentary	Skin toxicity (up to 25% with anti-CTLA-4 therapy[89])	Rash, pruritis, vitiligo. Onset usually within a few weeks of starting treatment, but can be delayed.[89]	Contact dermatitis, viral rashes, vasculitis[89]	Skin biopsy is usually feasible and yields definitive diagnosis.[89]
	Intraoral lesions (<10% for all therapies[93])	Mucositis, xerostomia, lichenoid tongue lesions[93]	Intraoral infection (e.g., herpes simplex, hand foot and mouth disease), mucositis from an alternative cause (e.g., chemotherapy)	Testing for intraoral infection (e.g., herpes serologies), consider biopsy of lesion if diagnosis is unclear
Neurologic	Myasthenia gravis (CR[89])	Weakness, ptosis, diplopia, dysarthria	Cerebrovascular accident, brain metastases, paraneoplastic syndrome, metastatic spinal cord compression	Brain imaging (CT or MRI), consideration of LP, electromyography can be helpful but often not needed in ED[89]
	Guillain-Barré syndrome (CR[89])	Weakness usually developing centrally from the extremities. Loss or attenuation of peripheral reflexes.	Cerebrovascular accident, brain metastases, paraneoplastic syndrome, metastatic spinal cord compression	Brain imaging (CT or MRI), consideration of LP, electromyography can be helpful but often not needed in ED[89]
Pulmonary	Pneumonitis (2–5% for anti-PD-1 therapy[90])	Dyspnea, hypoxemia, cough. Usual onset ≈3 months after initiation of therapy, but can occur as long as years later.[90]	Disease progression or pseudoprogression, infection, pulmonary embolus, exacerbation of coexisting lung disease[90]	Chest imaging (CXR or ideally high-resolution CT scan). Testing for underlying lung infection (sputum culture, urine legionella antigen, consideration of testing for PCP if immunocompromised, flu test if seasonally appropriate)
Renal	Acute kidney injury (≈2% for all therapies[94])	May be asymptomatic. In severe cases volume overload, uremia, acidosis, electrolyte disturbances.	AKI due to alternative cause such as sepsis, dehydration, or malignant obstruction of genitourinary tract	Measurement of serum creatinine, blood urea nitrogen, pH, and electrolytes. Renal imaging (e.g., ultrasound) to exclude obstruction. Fraction of excreted sodium testing (FENa).
Rheumatologic	Vasculitis (CR, most frequently large vessel and nervous system vasculitides[95])	Fever, fatigue, rash, numbness, weakness	Infection, paraneoplastic polyarteritis nodosa, leukocytoclastic vasculitis due to melanoma or other cancers, worsening metastatic disease, new onset of primary vasculitis[95]	Difficult to definitively diagnose from the ED; often requires biopsy of blood vessel or affected tissue[95]
	Myalgias and Arthralgias (2–12% for all therapies[89])	Morning stiffness, synovitis, proximal weakness[89]	New onset of primary rheumatologic disease (e.g., rheumatoid arthritis), drug-induced lupus or myositis	Testing for rheumatologic markers (e.g., rheumatoid factor, anti-nuclear antibody) to rule out new onset rheumatologic disease

ACS, Acute coronary syndrome; *CR,* incidence limited to case reports; *CXR,* chest x-ray; *ECG,* electrocardiogram; *LP,* lumbar puncture; *PCP, Pneumocystis jirovecii* pneumonia.

Differential Diagnoses

Differential diagnoses vary based on the presenting symptoms. Differentials for each complication are listed in Table 112.5.

Diagnostic Testing

Diagnostic testing varies based on the presenting symptoms. Diagnostic strategies for each complication are listed in Table 112.5.

Management

Management strategies for complications of checkpoint inhibitor therapy are laid out based on the severity of the complication. Scales to judge the grade of each type of complication have been developed[79] but are beyond the scope of this text. In general, symptoms that negatively impact daily life and are recalcitrant to targeted management (e.g., oral analgesics for myalgia, or topical prednisone for rash) are considered grade 3, and warrant initiation of prednisone 1 to 2 mg/kg/d or methylprednisolone IV 1 to 2 mg/kg/d.[79] This is particularly true of suspected hypophysitis with hemodynamic instability, for which methylprednisolone 1 to 2 mg/kg/d intravenous should immediately be initiated. Whenever possible, steroids should be initiated in consultation with an oncologist. For severe colitis, initial reports suggest that infliximab may be helpful in steroid-recalcitrant cases.[77]

Disposition

Disposition will vary based on specific complication and severity and may range from discharge with close oncology follow-up to ICU admission. Whenever possible, disposition decisions should be made in consultation with the patient's oncologist.

ADOPTIVE CELL TRANSFER THERAPIES AND COMPLICATIONS

KEY CONCEPTS

- Adoptive cell transfer therapy (CAR T-cell therapy) involves using the patient's own T-cells to attack tumor cells. Cytokine release syndrome (CRS) and immune effector cell–associated neurotoxicity syndrome (ICANS) are the most common and serious complications of this treatment.
- Expressive aphasia is a very specific and early sign of ICANS. Presence of this finding should increase clinical suspicion for ICANS, though its absence should not be used to exclude the diagnosis.
- Tocilizumab (anti-IL-6 receptor antibody) and corticosteroids may be used to treat severe CRS. ICANS is typically only responsive to corticosteroids. Because of the effects these treatments may have on the underlying antineoplastic therapy, they should only be administered in collaboration with oncology.

Foundations

Adoptive cell transfer therapies, often referred to as chimeric antigen receptor (CAR) T-cell therapies, employ the patient's own T cells, reprogrammed to attack cancer cells. Following harvest of the patient's T cells via leukapheresis or other methods, the cells are genetically modified by insertion (e.g., by lentivirus) of a chimeric antigen receptor (CAR) protein expression cassette. The CAR protein subsequently expressed by the cells is a combination of a recognition domain for a tumor-specific antigen, and an effector domain that activates the T cells to armed effector status and triggers clonal expansion when the tumor antigen is bound. Following genetic modification, the altered T cells are expanded in vitro and then transfused back to the patient.[80]

As of August 1, 2020, two FDA-approved CAR-T therapies exist: tisagenlecleucel and axicabtagene ciloleucel. Both are designed to recognize CD-19, a B cell–specific surface marker which is often overexpressed on B cell lymphoma and leukemia cells.[80]

Clinical Features

As with other immunotherapies, reprogramming the immune system comes at the cost of severe adverse effects. In the case of CAR T-cell therapy, cytokine release syndrome (CRS), and immune effector cell–associated neurotoxicity syndrome (ICANS) are particularly prevalent.[81] CRS, in which uncontrolled cytokine release leads to a potentially life-threatening inflammatory syndrome, occurs in nearly 60% of patients receiving CAR T-cell therapy.[82] Severe CRS, causing end-organ dysfunction or requiring multiple pressors to achieve hemodynamic stability, occurs in up to 25% of patients.[82,83] CRS may appear clinically similar to infection or sepsis, as symptoms include fever, malaise, myalgias, fatigue, and rash. In severe cases, hypotension, respiratory failure, and end-organ dysfunction will develop.[81] Median time from CAR T-cell therapy to onset of CRS is 3 days.[82] ICANS, in which the central nervous system undergoes immune cell–mediated damage, occurs in up to 50% of patients receiving CAR T-cell therapy.[84] Clinical features range from confusion, headache, aphasia, tremor, behavioral changes, peripheral numbness, and weakness to grand mal seizures and cerebral edema.[84] Expressive aphasia is a very specific and early sign of ICANS in at least one study, and may help differentiate ICANS from other etiologies of neurologic insult, though the absence of this finding should not be used to exclude the diagnosis.[81] Median onset of ICANS is four to seven days after CAR T-cell therapy.[84] Interestingly, while ICANS is considered a distinct entity from CRS, severe cases of ICANS are rarely seen in the absence of accompanying or preceding CRS.[84]

Differential Diagnoses

Patients presenting with symptoms of CRS should be considered to have an infection and sepsis until proven otherwise. This is especially important because lympho-depleting chemotherapy is often given prior to CAR T-cell infusion, thus imparting some degree of immunocompromise.[80] The symptoms of ICANS overlap with other CNS injuries such as cerebrovascular accident, infectious meningoencephalitis, or CNS metastasis.

Diagnostic Testing

Patients suspected to have cytokine release syndrome should undergo thorough testing for an underlying infectious source of symptoms (see earlier section on neutropenic fever). Patients with symptoms of ICANS should undergo CNS imaging by CT or MRI and consideration should be given to lumbar puncture and electroencephalography as symptoms dictate. Although brain imaging studies may be normal in ICANS, MRI imaging may show T2 hyperintensities in the white matter and thalami,[84] and appropriate imaging may be used to exclude other diagnoses. Cerebrospinal fluid of patients with ICANS may have elevated levels of protein and leukocytes,[84] so infection-specific cultures and diagnostics may be needed to rule out infectious meningitis.

Management

Due to their propensities for CRS and ICANS, FDA approval of CAR T-cell therapies to date has been contingent on provision of specific risk evaluation and mitigation strategies (REMS) for grading and management of these conditions. Due to the complexities involved, CAR T-cell therapy patients should be treated at a facility approved to administer these therapies, and the patient's oncologists should be involved in all management decisions.

Low-grade CRS (fever, malaise, and constitutional symptoms, but otherwise normal vital signs and organ function) may be treated symptomatically. For patients with more severe CRS, REMS protocols vary somewhat but generally involve escalating to therapy with the anti-IL-6 receptor antibody tocilizumab, followed by corticosteroids in the most severe cases or if there is no response to tocilizumab. Supportive therapies such as intravenous fluids, vasopressors, and respiratory support should be provided. Similarly, patients with low-grade ICANS (symptoms not affecting activities of daily life) may be treated symptomatically. Those with more severe manifestations generally receive corticosteroids, as tocilizumab generally has minimal effect on ICANS.[81] In all cases, decisions to give corticosteroids should be made in conjunction with the patient's treating oncologist because this may have a detrimental effect on the antitumor effects of CAR T-cell therapy.[80]

Disposition

Disposition decisions should be made in consultation with the patient's oncologist, but most if not all patients with suspected complications of CAR T-cell therapy should be admitted to the hospital. Because of the specialized nature of these relatively new therapies, whenever possible the patient should be transferred to the center where they received CAR T-cell therapy, or another center experienced in these treatments.

The references for this chapter can be found online at ExpertConsult. com.

113

Acid-Base Disorders

Nicole S. McCoin and Wesley H. Self

KEY CONCEPTS

- Metabolic acidoses are classified into wide anion gap and normal anion gap acidoses, based on basic metabolic panel (BMP) values. A wide anion gap metabolic acidosis is present when the gap exceeds 15 mmol/L.
- Common causes of a wide anion gap metabolic acidosis are summarized with the mnemonic MUDPILES (Methanol, Uremia, DKA, Paraldehyde, Polyethylene glycol, or Paracetamol (Acetaminophen), Iron, Lactate, Ethylene Glycol, Salicylates).
- When a wide anion gap metabolic acidosis is identified on the BMP, the potential underlying causes can be determined through analysis of the delta gap and the osmolar gap.
- Common causes of a normal anion gap acidosis are summarized with the mnemonic HARDUP (Hyperalimentation/Hospital-acquired administration of saline, Acid infusion, Addison's disease, Carbonic Anhydrase Inhibitors, Renal Tubular Acidosis, Diarrhea, Ureterosigmoidostomy, and Pancreatic drainage/fistula.)
- The optimal use of sodium bicarbonate therapy for metabolic acidosis is not clear and is the subject of ongoing research. A common strategy is to use sodium bicarbonate to increase pH above 7.10 in severe metabolic acidosis or above 7.20 for patients with severe metabolic acidosis and acute kidney injury.
- Metabolic alkalosis is associated with decreased circulating volume. GI-based chloride losses can be corrected with the administration of sodium chloride–containing intravenous fluids.
- Metabolic alkalosis caused by impaired renal excretion of sodium chloride that does not respond to intravenous fluids.
- Respiratory acidosis or alkalosis relates to carbon dioxide (CO_2) clearance, and thus is dependent on minute ventilation. Respiratory acidoses are caused by etiologies that decrease the ability of the body to rid itself of CO_2, such as primary lung disease, chest wall disorders, and entities that decrease respiratory drive.
- Respiratory alkalosis results from disorders that increase CO_2 clearance such as hyperventilation and salicylate toxicity. Values from the blood gas are used primarily to identify the presence of respiratory acid-base disorders.

FOUNDATIONS

The body's homeostatic mechanisms must keep acid-base balance under tight control. Acid-base disturbances can be life-threatening, with severe acid-base disorders leading to cellular compromise and death within hours due to alterations in hydrogen bonds, protein structures, and enzyme function.

The pH of the blood summarizes the systemic acid-base balance. pH is the negative logarithm of hydrogen-ion concentration (H^+) and has a normal range of 7.35 to 7.45. This normal pH is maintained by the kidneys' regulation of plasma bicarbonate (HCO_3^-) and the lungs' regulation of the partial pressure of arterial carbon dioxide ($Paco_2$). The relationship of [HCO_3^-] and $Paco_2$ to pH is described by the Henderson-Hasselbach equation: $pH = pK + log_{10}$ ([HCO_3^-]/[0.03 × $Paco_2$]), where pK denotes the acid dissociation constant, [HCO_3^-] is measured in millimoles per liter (mmol/L), and $Paco_2$ is measured in millimeters of mercury (mm Hg).

The terms *acidemia* and *alkalemia* describe the summary acid-base state, or the pH of the blood, while the terms *acidosis* and *alkalosis* describe discrete conditions. Blood pH less than 7.35 defines acidemia, while a pH greater than 7.45 defines alkalemia. An acidosis is an acid-base disturbance that increases [H^+] and lowers the pH. An alkalosis is an acid-base disturbance that decreases [H^+] and increases the pH. Multiple acidoses and alkaloses may be present at the same time; in these situations, pH describes the balance among all the acid-base disturbances.

The "metabolic system" includes cellular production and renal excretion of acids and bases. The respiratory system ventilates acid, in the form of carbon dioxide, out of the body through the lungs. The metabolic system and respiratory system are tightly coordinated to maintain acid-base hemostasis. Metabolic acid-base disorders are caused by abnormalities of cellular function, altered renal excretion of acids and bases, and exogenous gain or loss of acids and bases through the gastrointestinal tract. In clinical medicine, the principal test to evaluate for metabolic acid-base disturbances is plasma bicarbonate concentration ([HCO_3^-]). When a primary metabolic acid-base disturbance develops, the respiratory system compensates through increased or

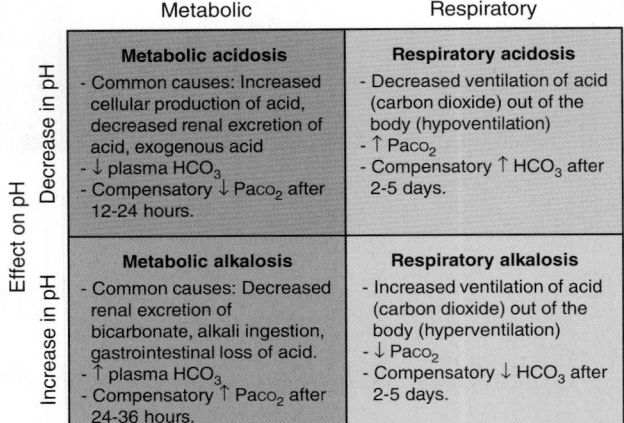

Fig. 113.1 Classification of the four major categories of acid-base disorders.

decreased ventilation of carbon dioxide to maintain acid-base hemostasis. Respiratory compensation typically takes 12 to 24 hours for a metabolic acidosis and 24 to 36 hours for a metabolic alkalosis.[1]

Respiratory acid-base disorders are caused by abnormalities in ventilating carbon dioxide out of the body through the lungs. In clinical medicine, a common method of evaluating ventilation is by measuring the partial pressure of carbon dioxide in arterial blood ($Paco_2$). After a primary respiratory acid-base disturbance develops, the metabolic system compensates by altering the excretion of acid in the kidneys to maintain acid-base hemostasis. Metabolic compensation typically takes between 2 and 5 days after a respiratory acidosis or alkalosis develops.[1]

Acid-base disorders are categorized by their pathophysiologic mechanism (metabolic or respiratory) and effect on pH (acidosis or alkalosis). Hence, the four broad categories of acid-base disorders are metabolic acidosis, metabolic alkalosis, respiratory acidosis, and respiratory alkalosis (Fig. 113.1). A simple acid-base disturbance describes a physiologic state with a single acid-base disorder with or without compensation. A mixed-acid base disturbance describes a state with more than one primary acid-disorder, each with or without compensation.

This chapter provides an overview of the identification and classification of acid-base disorders in emergency medicine. Specific acid-base disorders are discussed in detail in other disease-focused chapters.

CLINICAL FEATURES

A variety of patient presentations may prompt a clinician to search for acid-base disorders. This typically occurs in one of the three following scenarios in the emergency department:

1. The patient presents with undifferentiated signs and symptoms and is ill-appearing with vital sign abnormalities, respiratory distress, or altered mental status.
2. The patient presents with signs, symptoms or chronic medical conditions known to potentially cause acid-base abnormalities, such as toxic ingestions, vomiting, diarrhea, pregnancy, diabetes mellitus, chronic kidney disease, chronic liver disease, chronic lung disease, or neuromuscular disease.
3. The patient is well-appearing and does not have an overt clinical presentation consistent with an acid-base disorder, but laboratory studies demonstrate an acid-base abnormality.

Once an acid-base abnormality is suspected, the clinician should initiate targeted diagnostic testing to identify the type of acid-base disorder present and its underlying cause.

DIFFERENTIAL DIAGNOSIS AND DIAGNOSTIC TESTING

The initial phase of evaluating most patients with acid-base disorders is interpretation of laboratory data. These data can assist the clinician in classifying the type of acid-base disorder(s) present: metabolic acidosis, metabolic alkalosis, respiratory acidosis, or respiratory alkalosis. Once the class of acid-base disorder is identified, the clinician can develop a differential diagnosis for the cause of the disorder.

Diagnostic Testing

Acid-base disorders can be characterized by the pH, $Paco_2$, and HCO_3 concentration. Hence, interpretation of the basic metabolic panel (BMP) and blood gas is essential. Blood gas measurements can be obtained from either an arterial sample (arterial blood gas, ABG) or a venous sample (venous blood gas, VBG). Respiratory and acid-base physiology were classically described using ABG values, and ABG measurements provide a direct evaluation of oxygenation status as opposed to VBGs. However, obtaining an ABG requires arterial puncture, which is painful for patients, time-consuming for clinicians, and higher risk than venous blood sampling.

A VBG can be obtained from a routine venous blood draw with other laboratory studies and is a reasonable screening test in many settings. In the following sections, we provide a detailed discussion using ABG values; many of these concepts also apply to VBG values with the following considerations. On average, pH on a VBG is about 0.03 less than a concurrent ABG pH. The relationship between venous Pco_2 ($Pvco_2$) and $Paco_2$ is more variable, with $Pvco_2$ about 5 to 9 mm Hg higher than concurrent $Paco_2$ for many patients. $Pvco_2$ less than 45 mm Hg has nearly 100% negative predictive value for ruling out hypercapnia (defined as $Paco_2 > 50$ mm Hg). Pvo_2 does not correlate with Pao_2 and cannot be used to guide management decisions about oxygen supplementation. However, oxygenation can be adequately measured noninvasively in most patients with pulse oximetry providing saturation of peripheral oxygen (Spo_2) values. Hence, the combination of a VBG and Spo_2 is a useful screen for acid-base disturbances and hypoxemia in most patients. Patients with a complex acid-base disorder or severe respiratory illness often benefit from an ABG in addition to the initial screen with a VBG and Spo_2.

Goals for the clinician include identifying whether an acid-base disorder is present, and if so, determining the primary disturbance. Once the primary disturbance has been identified, simple formulas can be used to understand if an appropriate compensatory response has occurred and if another primary acid-base order is also present. Compensatory processes adjust the pH toward normal, but usually not completely to normal and never beyond normal.

Several methods for identifying, classifying, and understanding acid-base disorders have been described, including the physiologic, physiochemical (also known as the Stewart method), and base-excess approaches. A simplified method for acid-base classification that incorporates concepts from each approach can be rapidly applied by clinicians at the bedside and is described in detail below. This method involves a five-step approach that primarily focuses on the interpretation of the BMP to evaluate for metabolic acid-base disturbances and a three-step approach that primarily focuses on the interpretation of the ABG to evaluate for respiratory acid-base disturbances.

Basic Metabolic Panel Interpretation

The BMP is the primary test to evaluate for metabolic acid-base disturbances and includes plasma concentrations for the following: sodium (Na), chloride (Cl), potassium (K), bicarbonate (HCO_3), blood urea nitrogen (BUN), creatinine (Cr), and glucose. Normal ranges for

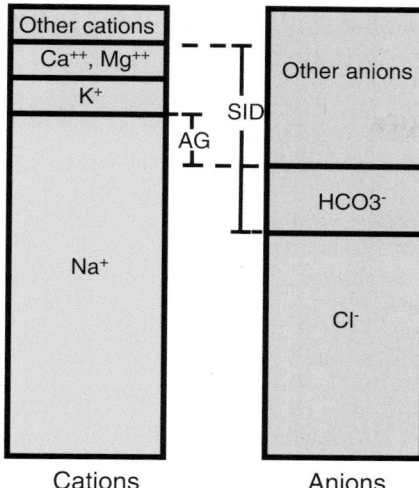

Fig. 113.2 Schematic representation of the anion gap (AG) and strong ion difference (SID). Human plasma is maintained at electroneutrality (no net charge). Thus, the sum of cations in plasma is equivalent to the sum of the anions. Calculation of the anion gap and strong ion difference can help identify the relative contribution of different cations and anions to plasma composition. An increase in anion gap indicates an increase in the contribution of "other anions," such as lactate in lactic acidosis or ketone bodies in diabetic ketoacidosis. A relative increase in chloride concentration compared to the strong cations (Na^+, K^+, Ca^{++}, Mg^{++}), such as occurs during saline infusion, leads to an increase in "other cations," including H^+, and a decrease in the SID.

laboratory tests vary, and clinicians should be familiar with the normal ranges in their institutions. Specific thresholds are shown below for illustrative purposes.

Five-Step Acid-Base Approach to the BMP

BMP Step 1. Check for Abnormal Values. Evaluate the BMP for any abnormalities. A low HCO_3 concentration (for example, <22 mmol/L) identifies a metabolic acidosis, whereas a high HCO_3 concentration (for example, >29 mmol/L) identifies a metabolic alkalosis.

BMP Step 2. Check the Anion Gap. The anion gap (AG) is calculated with the formula: $AG = [Na^+] - ([Cl^-] + [HCO_3^-])$. The anion gap is used to evaluate for the presence of a wide anion gap metabolic acidosis. A wide anion gap metabolic acidosis is present if the anion gap is elevated, regardless of values for HCO_3 and pH. The anion gap is normally between 9.0 and 15.0 mmol/L, and thresholds to signify a wide anion gap vary between 10 and 15 mmol/L due to differences in laboratory technique.[1] For illustrative purposes, a threshold of 15 mmol/L is used to define a wide anion gap in this chapter.

Plasma is electrically neutral. Hence, the sum of positive ion charges is equal to the sum of negative ion charges, as detailed in the equation: $[Na^+] + [K^+] + [Ca^{2+}] + [Mg^{2+}] + [H^+] +$ unmeasured cations $= [Cl^-] + [HCO_3^-] + [CO_3^{2-}] + [OH^-] +$ albumin + phosphate + sulfate + lactate + unmeasured anions. Clinical laboratories only routinely measure plasma concentrations of the major ions, resulting in some cations and anions being "unmeasured." A greater proportion of cation charge is typically measured than the anion charge, resulting in the concept of an "anion gap"—that is, the difference between measured cations and anions (Fig. 113.2). The calculation for the anion gap accounts for the most plentiful measured cation (Na^+) and the two most plentiful measured anions (Cl^- and $HCO3^-$).

Accumulation of "unmeasured anions"—that is, any anion other than chloride and bicarbonate—results in a wide anion gap metabolic acidosis. An acidosis in which the decrease in $[HCO3^-]$ is accompanied by an increase in $[Cl^-]$ of approximately the same magnitude results in a normal anion gap acidosis, also known as hyperchloremic metabolic acidosis.

BMP Step 3. If a Metabolic Acidosis is Present, Apply the Rule of 15. The rule of 15 is used to evaluate for concomitant respiratory acid-base disturbances in addition to a metabolic acidosis. According to the rule of 15, in an isolated metabolic acidosis, $HCO_3 + 15$ should equal the $Paco_2$ (±2 mm Hg) and the two digits of the pH following the decimal (±0.02). If measured $Paco_2$ equals the predicted value, simple respiratory compensation for a primary metabolic acidosis exists. If measured $Paco_2$ is less than the predicted value, there is a superimposed primary respiratory alkalosis on top of metabolic acidosis. If the $Paco_2$ is higher than the predicted value, a superimposed primary respiratory acidosis is present.

The rule of 15 has an important caveat. When HCO_3 falls below 10 mmol/L, the rule of 15 loses validity because HCO_3 and $Paco_2$ have a nonlinear relationship. In cases with HCO_3 between 5 mmol/L and 10 mmol/L, the expected $Paco_2$ is about 15 mm Hg and the expected pH is about 7.15 (this is known as the corollary to the rule of 15). Alternatively, in these cases with HCO_3^- less than 10 mmol/L, Winters equation can be used to calculate a more precise expected $Paco_2$: expected $Paco_2 = [HCO_3^-] * 1.5 + 8 \pm 2$. There are examples of the interpretation of the BMP using anion gap calculations and the rule of 15 available at the end of this chapter on ExpertConsult.com

BMP Step 4. If a Wide Anion Gap Metabolic Acidosis Is Present (Anion Gap ≥15), Check the Delta Gap. Calculation of the delta gap is used to identify additional metabolic acid-base disturbances superimposed on a wide anion gap metabolic acidosis. The delta gap explores the difference between the calculated anion gap and 15 mmol/L, which is the upper limit of normal for the anion gap, as well as the change in measured bicarbonate level from 24 mmol/L, which is the upper limit of normal for the bicarbonate level. In an isolated wide anion gap metabolic acidosis, each incremental increase in the anion gap is matched by an incremental decrease in HCO_3 of approximately the same magnitude. For example, each 1 mmol/L increase in the anion gap above 15 mmol/L is expected to be accompanied by a 1 mmol/L drop in HCO_3 below 24 mmol/L. A measured bicarbonate concentration higher than predicted by the delta gap calculation indicates a concomitant metabolic alkalosis. A measured bicarbonate concentration lower than predicted by the delta gap calculation indicates a concomitant normal anion gap metabolic acidosis. There are examples of delta gap calculations available at the end of this chapter on ExpertConsult.com

BMP Step 5. If a Wide Anion Gap Metabolic Acidosis Is Present (Anion Gap ≥15), But the Cause Is Not Evident, Check the Osmolar Gap. The osmolar gap is used to screen for the presence of abnormal particles dissolved in the blood. In the evaluation of acid-base disorders, calculation of the osmolar gap is commonly used to screen for the possibility of toxic alcohol ingestion as a cause for an unexplained wide anion gap metabolic acidosis.

Osmolality is a direct measure of the number of separate particles (solute) dissolved in a unit of water (solvent) within the blood. Calculated osmolarity is a calculated value of the expected number of osmotically active solutes in blood based on measured concentrations of the most common solutes. In normal physiologic states, the major solutes are sodium, the counter anions to sodium (e.g., chloride, bicarbonate, others), glucose, and urea. In patients who have been drinking ethanol, ethanol concentration (ETOH) is easily measured and is also a major contributor. Thus, the calculated osmolarity is calculated with the equation:

$$\text{calculated osmolarity} = (2 * Na) + (\text{glucose}/18) + (BUN/2.8) + (ETOH/3.7)$$

In this equation, Na is measured in mmol/L, and glucose, BUN, and ETOH are measured in mg/dL. Units for osmolarity are mOsm/kg of water; the equation above has built-in constants that convert mg/dL to mmol/L.

Osmolality can be measured in clinical laboratories. The measured osmolality includes the solutes in the calculated osmolarity equation and other solutes in the blood not included in the equation. The difference between measured osmolality and calculated osmolarity is the osmolar gap:

$$\text{Osmolar gap} = \text{(measured osmolality)} - \text{(calculated osmolarity)}$$

$$= \text{(Measured osmolality)} - [(2*Na) + (glucose/18) + (BUN/2.8) + (ETOH/3.7)]$$

A normal osmolar gap is 10 mOsm/kg or less. A wide osmolar gap (>10 mOsm/kg) indicates accumulation of a significant volume of solute not included in the osmolarity equation (that is, a significant volume of "unanticipated" osmotically active solutes). In the setting of a wide anion gap metabolic acidosis, a wide osmolar gap may indicate the presence of toxic alcohols, such as methanol or ethylene glycol. However, it is important to note that a normal osmolar gap does not eliminate the possibility of a toxic alcohol poisoning, because the osmolar gap decreases as toxic alcohols are metabolized. Additionally, the calculation assumes a normal baseline osmolality, which is not always true. When an elevated osmolar gap is caused exclusively by a toxic alcohol, the plasma concentration of methanol or ethylene glycol can be estimated from the osmolar gap. To estimate the concentration of methanol in mg/dL, multiply the osmolar gap by 3. To estimate the concentration of ethylene glycol in mg/dL, multiply the osmolar gap by 6. There is an example of the osmolar gap calculation in Box 113.1.

Blood Gas Interpretation

Blood gases are the primary tests to evaluate for respiratory acid-base disturbances and include measurements for pH, the partial pressure of carbon dioxide (PCO_2) and the partial pressure of oxygen (PO_2).

Three-Step Acid-Base Approach to the ABG

ABG Step 1. Determine if the Patient Is Acidemic or Alkalemic. Evaluate the pH. A pH less than 7.35 indicates acidemia; pH greater than 7.45 indicates alkalemia. pH is a summary measure that describes the overall balance of acid-base status. A pH in the normal range (7.35 to 7.45) may indicate no acid-base disturbance is present, a disturbance is present with compensation resulting in pH within the normal range, or multiple disturbances are present that, when combined, result in a pH in the normal range.

ABG Step 2. Determine if a Predominant Respiratory or Metabolic Acid-Base Disturbance Is Present. Evaluate $PaCO_2$ and place it into context with the pH. In predominant respiratory acid-base disturbances, the change in $PaCO_2$ is in the opposite direction of the change in pH. Using $PaCO_2$ of 40 mm Hg and pH of 7.40 as idealized normal values, a $PaCO_2$ greater than 40 with a pH less than 7.40 indicates a predominant respiratory acidosis. In predominant metabolic acid-base disturbances, the change in $PaCO_2$ and pH are in the same direction. For example, a $PaCO_2$ less than 40 mm Hg with a pH less than 7.40 indicates a predominant metabolic acidosis. There are two examples illustrating the use of ABG to determine the predominant respiratory or metabolic acid-base disturbance available at the end of this chapter on ExpertConsult.com.

ABG Step 3. If a Predominant Respiratory Acid-Base Disturbance Is Present, Determine If There Is a Concurrent Metabolic Disturbance. Compare the magnitude of changes in $PaCO_2$ and pH. In a pure respiratory disturbance, a 10 mm Hg change in $PaCO_2$ results in approximately a 0.08 change in pH in the opposite direction. If this delta-$PaCO_2$: delta-pH ratio of 10:0.08

BOX 113.1   Identifying Acid-Base Disturbances With the Five-Step Focused Algorithm for Interpreting a Basic Metabolic Panel (BMP)

Clinical Concern: Acute Antifreeze (Ethylene Glycol) Ingestion
Laboratory Data
Na = 140 mmol/L
Cl = 100 mmol/L
HCO_3 = 8 mmol/L
BUN = 30 mg/dL
Cr = 2.5 mg/dL
Glucose = 80 mg/dL
ETOH = 240 mg/dL
$PaCO_2$ = 17 mmHg
pH = 7.13
Measured Osmolality: 425 mOsm/kg

1. *Check the numbers*: Na = 140 mmol/L; Cl = 100 mmol/L; HCO_3 = 8 mmol/L; BUN = 30 mg/dL; Cr = 2.5 mg/dL; Glucose = 80 mg/dL. A low bicarbonate indicates a metabolic acidosis.
2. *Calculate the anion gap*: AG = 140 − (100 + 8) = 32. A high anion gap indicates wide anion gap metabolic acidosis.
3. *Apply the rule of 15*: HCO_3 is below 10 mmol/L. According to the corollary to the rule of 15, simple respiratory compensation would lead to a $PaCO_2$ of approximately 15 mm Hg (±2), which is consistent with the patient's measured $PaCO_2$ of 17 mm Hg. The patient's acid-base status is consistent with a primary metabolic acidosis with respiratory compensation without an additional primary respiratory acid-base disturbance.
4. *Calculate the delta gap*: Change in AG = measured AG − 15 = 32 − 15 = 17. Change in HCO_3 = 24 − measured HCO_3 = 24 − 8 = 16. The predicted change in bicarbonate concentration is 17 mmol/L, and the measured change is very similar at 16 mmol/L; this indicates the metabolic acid-base state is fully accounted for by a wide anion gap metabolic acidosis.
5. *Calculate the osmolar gap*: Calculated osmolarity = (2*Na) + (Glucose/18) + (BUN/2.8) + (ETOH/ 3.7) = (2*140) + (80/18) + (30/2.8) + (240/3.7) = 360 mOsm/kg. Osmol gap = (measured osmolality) − (calculated osmolarity) = 425 mOsm/kg − 360 mOsm/kg = 65 mOsm/kg. An osmolar gap >10 mOsm/kg indicates accumulation of a significant volume of abnormal solute in the blood. In the setting of suspected ethylene glycol ingestion, the wide osmolar gap is presumed to be due to ethylene glycol until plasma ethylene glycol concentration results are available. The estimated ethylene glycol concentration = (osmolar gap) * 6 = 65 * 6 = 390 mg/dL.

---

is not present, a concurrent metabolic disturbance is present along with the primary respiratory disturbance. The predicted pH assuming an isolated respiratory disturbance can be calculated with the equation:

$$\text{predicted pH} = \text{normal pH} + [(\text{normal } PaCO_2 - \text{measured } PaCO_2)/10*0.08]$$

$$= 7.40 + [(40 - \text{measured } PaCO_2)/10*0.08]$$

If the measured pH is higher than predicted for the magnitude of $PaCO_2$ change, a metabolic alkalosis is also present. If the pH is lower than expected for the magnitude of $PaCO_2$ change, a metabolic acidosis is also present. An example highlighting the three steps in the use of the ABG to determine which acid-base disorders exist both as primary and concomitant/compensatory processes is noted in Box 113.2. Another example of this three-step approach can be found at the end of this chapter on ExpertConsult.com.

BOX 113.2 Identifying Acid-Base Disturbances With the Three-Step Focused Algorithm for Interpreting an Arterial Blood Gas (ABG)

Clinical Concern: Salicylate Toxicity

Laboratory Data

ABG: pH = 7.47/$Paco_2$ = 25 mm Hg/Pao_2 = 180 mm Hg

Determine if the patient is acidemic or alkalemic. The patient's pH is 7.47, indicating alkalemia.

Determine if a predominant respiratory or metabolic acid-base disturbance is present. The patient's $Paco_2$ is low at 25 mm Hg and pH is high at 7.47. This is consistent with a respiratory alkalosis.

Determine if there is concurrent metabolic disturbance. Change in $Paco_2$ = 40 – measured $Paco_2$ = 40 – 25 = 15. Assuming a pure respiratory alkalosis with no metabolic acid-base disturbance, predicted pH = 7.40 + [(40 – 25) / 10 * 0.08] = 7.40 + 0.12 = 7.52. The measured pH of 7.47 is lower than the predicted pH of 7.52, indicating a concurrent metabolic acidosis.

BOX 113.3 Causes of Metabolic Acidosis, Divided into Wide Anion Gap and Normal Anion Gap Metabolic Acidosis

Wide Anion Gap Metabolic Acidosis—Mnemonic: MUDPILES

Methanol
Uremia
Diabetic ketoacidosis/alcoholic ketoacidosis
Paraldehyde/**P**olyethylene glycol/**P**aracetamol (acetaminophen)
Iron
Lactic acidosis
Ethylene glycol
Salicylates

Normal Anion Gap Metabolic Acidosis—Mnemonic: HARDUP

Hyperalimentation/**H**ospital-acquired administration of saline
Acid infusion/**A**ddison disease / Carbonic **A**nhydrase Inhibitors
Renal tubular acidosis (RTA)
Diarrhea
Ureterosigmoidostomy (and ileal diversion)
Pancreatic drainage/fistula

Differential Diagnosis of Acid-Base Disorders

Each of the four acid-base disorders—metabolic acidosis, metabolic alkalosis, respiratory acidosis, and respiratory alkalosis—have multiple potential causes.

Metabolic Acidosis

As previously described, the metabolic acidoses are classified based on anion gap. Accumulation of "unmeasured" anions results in a wide anion gap metabolic acidosis. A decline in bicarbonate with a concomitant increase in chloride results in a normal anion gap metabolic acidosis.

Wide Anion Gap Metabolic Acidosis. An elevated anion gap using the threshold of 15 mmol/L, regardless of the value of the pH or [HCO3−], indicates that a wide anion gap metabolic acidosis is present. The mnemonic MUDPILES can be used to recall common causes of a wide anion gap metabolic acidosis (Box 113.3). Lactic acidosis is the most common cause of a wide anion gap metabolic acidosis, accounting for approximately half of the cases. Other important causes include ketoacidosis (e.g., diabetic ketoacidosis) and toxic alcohol poisoning (e.g., methanol and ethylene glycol). A normal anion gap does not eliminate the possibility of lactic acidosis, ketoacidosis, or toxic alcohol poisoning, and these acids should be directly measured when clinical concern is high despite a normal anion gap.

Normal Anion Gap Metabolic Acidosis. The mnemonic HARDUP (see Box 113.3) can be used to recall the causes of a normal anion gap metabolic acidosis, which is also called hyperchloremic metabolic acidosis. Common causes of normal anion gap metabolic acidosis include renal tubular acidosis (failure of the kidney to properly excrete acid), diarrhea (gastrointestinal loss of bicarbonate), and saline infusion (hyperchloremia leading to the retention of acid to maintain electroneutrality).

Metabolic Alkalosis

Metabolic alkalosis can be caused by an increase in alkali or impaired renal excretion of bicarbonate. The differential for metabolic alkalosis can be divided into chloride-responsive and chloride-unresponsive conditions.

Chloride-Responsive Metabolic Alkalosis. When the circulating volume is decreased, the renin-angiotensin-aldosterone system is activated, and the kidneys reabsorb filtered sodium, bicarbonate,

BOX 113.4 Causes of Metabolic Alkalosis, Divided into Chloride-Responsive and Chloride-Unresponsive Metabolic Alkalosis

Chloride-Responsive Metabolic Alkalosis
Nasogastric suction
Vomiting
Chloride-wasting diarrhea
Villous adenoma
Persistent diuretic use

Chloride-Unresponsive Metabolic Alkalosis
Primary hyperaldosteronism
Secondary hyperaldosteronism (Bartter syndrome, Gitelman syndrome, congestive heart failure, liver failure, chronic renal failure)
Steroids
Cushing disease
Severe hypercalcemia
Severe hypomagnesemia
Bicarbonate ingestion
Licorice overdose (glycyrrhizic acid)

and chloride. This leads to metabolic alkalosis through retention of bicarbonate and decreased concentration of urine chloride (spot urine chloride concentration < 25 mmol/L). When sodium chloride–containing fluids are administered, circulating volume increases, and the metabolic alkalosis is corrected. Causes of chloride-responsive metabolic alkalosis are listed in Box 113.4.

Chloride-Unresponsive Metabolic Alkalosis. Causes of metabolic alkalosis that cannot be corrected with infusion of sodium chloride containing fluids are called chloride-unresponsive metabolic alkaloses (see Box 113.2). A common mechanism is hyperaldosteronism, which causes inappropriate renal excretion of H+ and Cl− and a spot urine chloride concentration greater than 40 mmol/L.

BOX 113.5　Causes of Respiratory Acidosis Based on Pathophysiologic Mechanism

Respiratory Disease (Lungs and Airways)
Airway obstruction
Obstructive pulmonary diseases (e.g., chronic obstructive pulmonary disease)
Pneumothorax
Pulmonary effusion
Pulmonary edema
Pneumonia
Mechanical ventilation (iatrogenic hypoventilation)

Chest Wall Disease
Chest wall trauma (e.g., flail chest)
Obesity hypoventilation syndrome

Respiratory Muscle Weakness
Myopathies (e.g., muscular dystrophy)
Neuropathies (e.g., Guillain-Barré)
Electrolyte abnormalities (e.g., hypokalemia, hypophosphatemia)

Decreased Respiratory Drive
Brain space-occupying lesion (e.g., intracranial mass, intracranial hemorrhage)
Drugs/toxins (e.g., sedative-hypnotics, narcotics)

BOX 113.6　Causes of Respiratory Alkalosis Based on Pathophysiologic Mechanism

Respiratory
Conditions that cause hypoxemia (e.g., pulmonary embolus)
Mechanical ventilation (iatrogenic hyperventilation)

Gastrointestinal
Hepatic encephalopathy
Neurologic
Brain lesion

Genitourinary
Pregnancy

Psychiatric
Anxiety

Toxic-Metabolic
Drugs (e.g., salicylates, catecholamines, progesterone)
Hyperthyroidism

Infectious
Fever
Sepsis

Miscellaneous
Pain

Respiratory Acidosis

Failure to adequately ventilate carbon dioxide out of the body results in increased $PaCO_2$ and respiratory acidosis. Mechanisms of respiratory acidosis include hypoventilation leading to hypercapnic respiratory failure and increased production of carbon dioxide overwhelming mild to moderately impaired pulmonary function. Common causes of hypercapnic respiratory failure and respiratory acidosis include primary lung disease, chest wall disease, respiratory muscle weakness, and decreased respiratory drive from central nervous system disease or toxins. Specific causes of respiratory acidosis within these categories are listed in Box 113.5.

Respiratory Alkalosis

Respiratory alkalosis occurs when increased minute ventilation (hyperventilation) leads to decreased $PaCO_2$. In the emergency department, anxiety-related hyperventilation is a common cause of respiratory alkalosis, but other medical illnesses, including salicylate toxicity, can also present with respiratory alkalosis (Box 113.6). Of note, respiratory alkalosis results in increased binding of calcium to albumin, thereby decreasing free serum calcium. Many of the classic symptoms of acute respiratory alkalosis are caused by hypocalcemia—lip and extremity paresthesia, carpal pedal spasm, muscle cramps, syncope. These symptoms quickly resolve as pH declines and free calcium concentrations return to normal.

MANAGEMENT

The management of acid-base disorders focuses on treating the specific cause of an acid-base derangement (e.g., treating diabetic ketoacidosis, managing an overdose, providing ventilatory support). Detailed discussions on the management of specific causes of acid-base disorders are included in other disease-focused chapters. Here, we discuss general principles of managing acid-base disorders.

Intravenous Fluids

Intravenous fluid administration is a common method of both causing and treating acid-base disorders. Thus, understanding the typical clinical effects of common intravenous fluid formulations is key to acid-base management. Although many intravenous fluid formulations are available, intravenous fluid use in the ED is dominated by crystalloid solutions. Three of the commonly used crystalloids are saline (0.9% sodium chloride, "normal saline"), lactated Ringers (also known as Hartmann solution), and Plasma-Lyte (Table 113.1).

One liter of saline is composed of 9 g of sodium chloride diluted in water to a total volume of 1000 ml; therefore, the mass concentration of saline is 9 g/1000 ml = 0.009 or 0.9%. The misnomer "normal saline" likely stems from in vitro red blood cell studies in the 1880s that were incorrectly interpreted as showing human blood is 0.9% salt; the actual concentration is approximately 0.6%. Saline contains 154 mmol/L of both sodium and chloride, which is supraphysiologic compared with human plasma (see Table 113.1). Thus, saline is not "normal" or physiologic. In the early 20th century, saline was adopted as a preferred intravenous fluid for patient care. The rationale behind the adoption of saline over other fluids more similar in composition to human plasma is unclear but may have been related to the ease and low cost of producing saline at the time.

The effect of intravenous crystalloid composition on acid-base status is described by the physiochemical (Stewart) model of acid-base. A key determinant of acid-base status, or the concentration of H^+ in plasma, is the relative concentrations of strong cations (Na^+, K^+, Ca^{++}, and Mg^{++}) and strong anions (Cl^-). As the concentration of strong anions increases relative to strong cations, the concentration of H^+, a weak unmeasured cation, increases to maintain electroneutrality. Thus, a relative increase in Cl^- compared with the strong cations results in acidosis.

The "strong ion difference" is a summary measure of the relative concentration of strong cations and strong anions (see Fig. 113.2). In human plasma and crystalloid solutions, the strong ion difference is approximated by the equation:

TABLE 113.1 Composition of Human Plasma and Commonly Used Intravenous Crystalloid Solutions

	Human Plasma	Saline	BALANCED CRYSTALLOIDS	
			Lactated Ringer	Plasma-Lyte
Sodium (mmol/L)	135–145	154	130	140
Potassium (mmol/L)	4.5–5.0	0	4	5
Chloride (mmol/L)	94–111	154	109	98
Calcium (mmol/L)	2.2–2.6	0	2.7	0
Magnesium (mmol/L)	0.8–1.0	0	0	1.5
Bicarbonate (mmol/L)	23–27	0	0	0
Lactate (mmol/L)	1–2	0	28	0
Acetate (mmol/L)	0	0	0	27
Gluconate (mmol/L)	0	0	0	23
pH	7.35–7.45	5.0	6.5	7.4
Osmolarity (mOsm/L)	291	308	273	294
Strong ion difference (mmol/L)	≈42	0	28	50

$$\text{Strong ion difference} = [Na^+] + [K^+] + [Ca^{++}] + [Mg^{++}] - [Cl^-]$$

Decreases in the strong ion difference indicate that unmeasured weak cations contribute more of the cation charge. At a physiologic pH of 7.40, infusion of intravenous fluids that have a strong ion difference of about 24 mmol/L has no effect on pH. Infusion of intravenous fluids with a strong ion difference of less than 24 mmol/L results in an increase in [H+] and acidosis, while fluids with a strong ion difference of greater than 24 mmol/L lead to a reduction in [H+] and alkalosis.

With a composition of 154 mmol/L of sodium and chloride, saline has a strong ion difference of 0. Therefore, infusing saline into human plasma results in a relative increase in chloride concentration compared with the strong cations, a decrease in the strong ion difference, and acidosis. Through these mechanisms, saline administration leads to a normal anion gap hyperchloremic metabolic acidosis.

"Balanced crystalloids" are crystalloids that more closely match the composition of human plasma than saline in terms of electrolyte concentrations. An idealized balanced crystalloid would contain the same electrolytes and concentrations as human plasma. However, bicarbonate-containing solutions are difficult to store in plastic containers for prolonged periods. Hence, balanced crystalloids are developed with alternative anions that serve as substitutes for bicarbonate. Historically, the primary balanced crystalloid was lactated Ringers (chloride concentration = 109 mmol/L; strong ion difference = 28 mmol/L), which is modeled after a fluid Dr. Sydney Ringer developed in the late 19th century. The primary anion in lactated Ringers is lactate, which is metabolized to bicarbonate after infusion. In terms of effects on acid-base, lactated Ringers is considered a neutral fluid that does not induce either acidosis or alkalosis.

The balanced crystalloid Plasma-Lyte (chloride concentration = 98 mmol/L) was developed with the anions acetate and gluconate and concentrations of sodium, potassium, and chloride that closely match human plasma (see Table 113.1). The calculated strong ion difference of Plasma-Lyte is 50 mmol/L, but the effective strong ion difference is

likely lower because gluconate does not fully metabolize into bicarbonate. The expected effect of Plasma-Lyte on acid-base status is a mild alkalinizing effect.

Saline infusion has been known to cause hyperchloremic metabolic acidosis since the early 20th century. While physiology studies have consistently suggested that saline-associated hyperchloremic metabolic acidosis may have negative effects on renal and immune function, the clinical consequences of saline infusion in human studies have only recently begun to emerge. The administration of balanced crystalloids instead of saline in volumes typically used in clinical medicine, including in the emergency department, reduces the number of patients who experience hyperchloremia and metabolic acidosis.[2,3] Additionally, recent data suggest balanced crystalloids lead to better patient outcomes than saline, including a survival benefit in sepsis.[2-4]

Although current data do not provide definitive evidence for scenarios in which clinicians should use balanced crystalloids instead of saline, it is reasonable to preferentially use a balanced crystalloid, such as lactated Ringers or Plasma-Lyte, in patients with hyperchloremia, metabolic acidosis, renal dysfunction, sepsis, and those receiving a large volume of fluid. Potential adverse effects of balanced crystalloids include the induction of metabolic alkalosis (especially with Plasma-Lyte), low tonicity potentially increasing intracranial pressure (especially with lactated Ringers), and hyponatremia (especially with lactated Ringers).

Sodium Bicarbonate Therapy

Although bicarbonate-containing solutions cannot be conveniently stored for prolonged periods, they can be mixed for immediate use. An isotonic sodium bicarbonate solution can be prepared by adding 150 mmol sodium bicarbonate, or three 50-ml ampules of 8.4% sodium bicarbonate, to one liter of D5W. This fluid can then be infused intravenously and has a strong alkalinizing effect. The addition of sodium bicarbonate to 0.9% sodium chloride (saline) should be avoided due to the hypertonicity and high sodium concentration of this mixture.

Intravenous sodium bicarbonate therapy is recommended for the treatment of some specific poisonings, such as sodium channel blocking toxicants and salicylates, but its role in the routine treatment of severe metabolic acidosis is controversial. Identifying and reversing the underlying cause of metabolic acidosis is the primary therapy. It remains unclear whether using sodium bicarbonate to increase pH while addressing the primary cause of acidosis provides benefit. Proponents of bicarbonate therapy in this setting note that acidosis can result in decreased myocardial contractility, systemic vasodilation, and decreased responsiveness to catecholamines. Opponents note potential harms of intravenous sodium bicarbonate therapy, including a paradoxical increase in CNS acidosis (bicarbonate does not readily cross the blood-brain barrier, and decreased drive for hyperventilation leads to increased CO_2 both systemically and in the CNS), hypernatremia, hypocalcemia, hypokalemia, increased lactate production, and fluid overload.

Historically, many clinicians have argued against bicarbonate therapy for metabolic acidosis due to its potential harms and no demonstrated clinical benefit. In a recent clinical trial of adults with metabolic acidosis (pH 7.20 or less), plasma bicarbonate concentration 20 mmol/L or less, and arterial lactate concentration 2.0 mmol/L or greater, sodium bicarbonate therapy demonstrated no effect on survival among all patients but was associated with a survival benefit among patients who presented with acute kidney injury.[5] Trial exclusions included diabetic ketoacidosis, respiratory acidosis, and severe chronic kidney disease.

While no evidence-based algorithms exist, a common and reasonable practice is to use intravenous sodium bicarbonate therapy for metabolic acidosis with a pH less than 7.10 with the goals of increasing pH above 7.10 and plasma bicarbonate concentration above 10 mmol/L. For patients with concomitant acute kidney injury, we recommend use of sodium bicarbonate therapy for a pH less than 7.20.[5] Based on current understanding, bicarbonate therapy is thought to be more beneficial for acidoses caused by loss of bicarbonate (e.g., diarrhea) or impairment of acid excretion (e.g., renal failure) than those caused by endogenous acid production (e.g., lactic acidosis, ketoacidosis).

DISPOSITION

Disposition of patients with acid-base disorders is based on treatment needs for the underlying etiology as well as the severity of the acid-base disorder. Most of the causes of acute acid-base disorders benefit from hospital admission because hours to days of monitoring and therapy are often needed to reverse the disorder. In some instances, a patient may be fully treated in the emergency department for a mild acid-base disorder or etiology that can be rapidly remedied. In these cases, repeat laboratory testing before discharge is often useful to assure that the acid-base disorder has been appropriately addressed.

ACKNOWLEDGEMENTS

We would like to recognize Corey M. Slovis, MD for helping develop many of the concepts presented in this chapter.

The references for this chapter can be found online at ExpertConsult. com.

114

Electrolyte Disorders

Camiron L. Pfennig and Corey M. Slovis

KEY CONCEPTS

- Electrolyte abnormalities are common in emergency medicine and can vary greatly in importance, severity, and symptoms. Asymptomatic electrolyte abnormalities can be gradually corrected, whereas those causing alterations in consciousness or life-threatening dysrhythmias require immediate therapy to avoid permanent sequelae or death. In some cases, therapy for life-threatening electrolyte disorders may precede laboratory confirmation.
- Asymptomatic electrolyte abnormalities can usually be corrected slowly, but those that cause profound mental status changes or life-threatening arrhythmias require immediate correction to avoid cardiac arrest or seizures.
- IV calcium should be used only for hyperkalemic emergencies, defined as the following: widening QRS; sine wave; bradycardias and cardiac arrest believed to be due to hyperkalemia; or rapidly evolving electrocardiographic changes, from normal to development of tall peaked T waves and loss of the P wave. Acute, rapid rises in serum potassium concentration are rare but may be seen in tumor lysis syndrome, rhabdomyolysis, or massive hemolysis.
- After the critical decision about administration of calcium has been made, a beta$_2$-agonist, insulin and glucose, normal saline, and bicarbonate (if the patient is acidotic) can be given to shift potassium intracellularly.
- When treating hypokalemia, the physician should also replace magnesium sulfate, in addition to potassium, or the patient will excrete most of the infused potassium in the urine.
- Low serum potassium levels reflect a substantial total potassium deficit; correction of large deficits can require several days.
- Hypertonic saline should be reserved for severely hyponatremic patients (typically in the 100 to 110 mEq/L range) who present with coma, seizures, or focal neurologic deficits. Central pontine myelinolysis can occur if serum sodium concentration is raised rapidly by more than 8 mEq/day.

HYPERKALEMIA

Foundations

Hyperkalemia, defined as a serum potassium level greater than 5.0 mEq/L, is the most dangerous acute electrolyte abnormality, potentially leading to life-threatening arrhythmias and death. Although hyperkalemia may have vague and varied symptoms, it is usually totally asymptomatic and can present with cardiac arrest as its first "symptom." Serum potassium concentration is normally between 3.5 and 5.0 mEq/L and is tightly regulated by the kidneys. Hyperkalemia usually develops from impaired renal excretion or intracellular release; however, in advanced chronic kidney disease or end-stage renal disease, dietary intake of potassium may be a significant factor in its development. Risk factors for hyperkalemia include impaired potassium excretion, such as dehydration and renal failure, as well as medications that cause potassium retention. Evaluation of the 12-lead electrocardiogram (ECG) of patients at risk for this electrolyte disturbance guides

management decisions. Hyperkalemia can be rapidly progressive, requiring lifesaving interventions at the earliest suspicion of toxicity.

Hyperkalemia causes cardiotoxicity by increasing the resting membrane potential of the cardiac myocyte, causing "membrane excitability," and conversely, sluggish depolarization, as well as decreased duration of repolarization. At very high levels, potassium causes the depolarization threshold to rise, leading to overall depressed cardiac function. Nearly any cardiac arrhythmia can be seen with hyperkalemia, including heart blocks, bradydysrhythmias, pseudoinfarction, ST-segment elevation, Brugada pattern, and the classic "sine wave" pattern.[1] As hyperkalemia advances, the end result is cardiac arrest, usually from deterioration into ventricular fibrillation, pulseless electrical activity, or asystole. A serum potassium level of 10.0 mEq/L is usually fatal, but decompensation and death can occur at any level above 7 to 8 mEq/L.

Clinical Features

Hyperkalemia is a difficult diagnosis to make on clinical grounds alone. Hyperkalemia is classified as mild (K 5.5 to 6.0), moderate (K 6.1 to 6.9) or severe (K >7.0). Patients with mild to moderate hyperkalemia are often identified during routine blood sampling for an unrelated condition. Patients with moderate to severe hyperkalemia may have gastrointestinal effects, such as nausea, vomiting, and diarrhea, which are often associated with their underlying disease. Patients with severe hyperkalemia may present with neuromuscular findings, including muscle cramps, generalized weakness, paresthesias, tetany, and focal or global paralysis. The signs and symptoms of progressive muscle weakness, paresthesias, dyspnea, and depressed deep tendon reflexes are neither sensitive nor specific, nor do they appear reliably with a particular serum potassium level. Patients with severe hyperkalemia may present with hemodynamic instability and cardiac arrhythmias requiring immediate intervention.

Differential Diagnosis

The most common cause of hyperkalemia is spurious elevation due to hemolysis during or after the blood draw. Thus, an ECG should be used to assess for true hyperkalemia while another sample is analyzed. Box 114.1 organizes the most common causes of hyperkalemia. The presence of one of these conditions may be the lone historical clue in hyperkalemia. Physicians should not rely solely on an ECG to determine the presence or absence of hyperkalemia in an otherwise stable patient.[2]

Diagnostic Testing

The ECG is helpful in making the diagnosis of hyperkalemia and can be used in unstable patients to initiate treatment (Figs. 114.1 to 114.3). Classic electrocardiographic changes—the peaked T wave, flattened p wave with prolonged PR interval or a totally absent P wave, wide QRS, and sine wave pattern, portending imminent cardiac arrest—have been well described as appearing sequentially with rising serum potassium levels. Peaked T waves usually appear as serum potassium levels exceed 5.5 to 6.5 mEq/L; P wave disappearance and PR prolongation are common with levels above 6.5 to 7.5 mEq/L; and levels above 7.0 to 8.0 mEq/L can result in QRS prolongation. Although these changes may occur in only half the patients, recognition of these patterns is vital to rapid diagnosis and initiation of lifesaving treatment. A serum potassium level above 5.0 mEq/L is diagnostic of hyperkalemia, but the value itself does not always predict electrocardiographic changes or the degree of cardiotoxicity. Furthermore, stable patients who are otherwise unlikely to have elevated potassium should not be presumptively treated for hyperkalemia based on subtle electrocardiographic changes alone. In addition, hyperkalemia may present as an atropine-resistant bradycardia, with or without apparent heart block.[1]

Management

Patients with suspected or known hyperkalemia should have intravenous (IV) access and continuous cardiac monitoring. Treatment of hyperkalemia should be directed by the clinical scenario combined with the ECG and laboratory potassium value, and consists of three main steps: (1) stabilization of the cardiac membrane, (2) shifting of potassium into the cells, and (3) removal of potassium from the body. A variety of treatment options are considered for the acute management of hyperkalemia, including calcium, insulin, beta$_2$-adrenergic agonists, sodium bicarbonate, resins, and dialysis (Table 114.1).

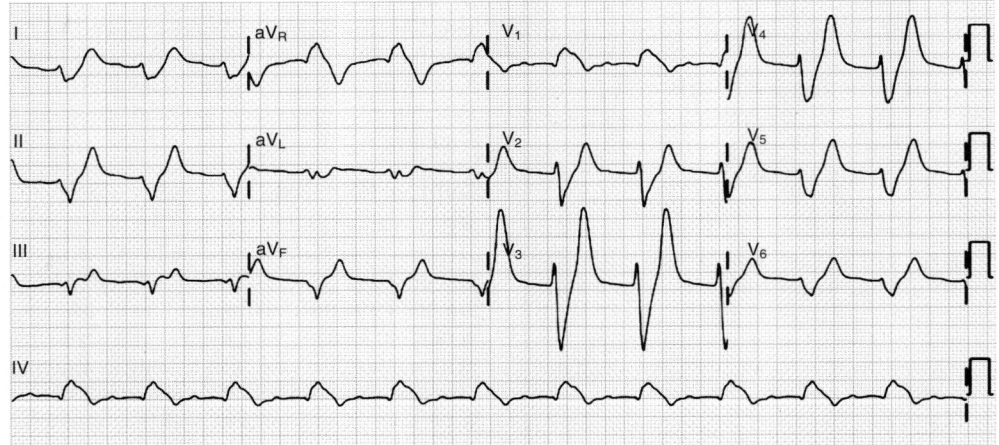

Fig. 114.1 Hyperkalemia with QRS widening merging into T wave, absent P wave.

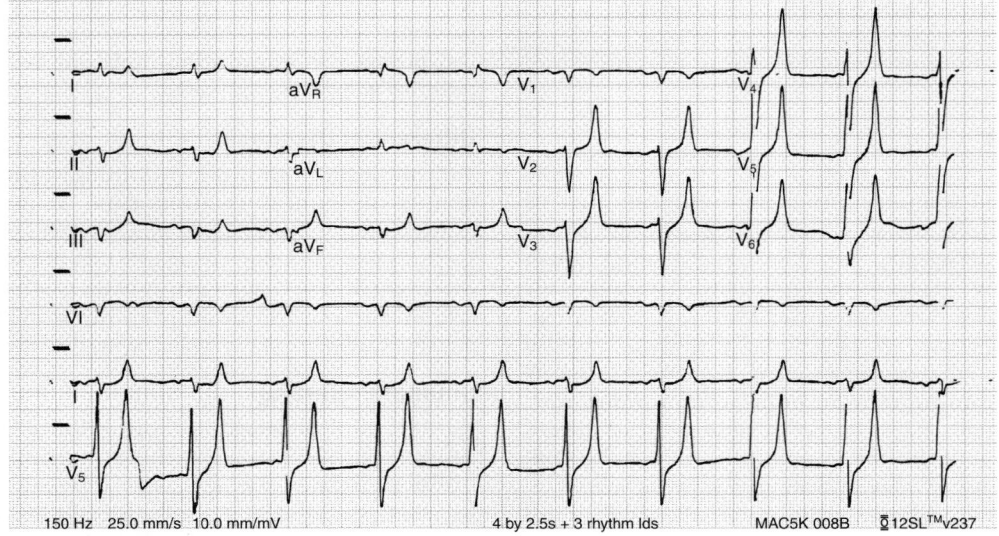

Fig. 114.2 Hyperkalemia in the same patient as in Figure 114.1 after potassium-lowering therapy has begun. Tall peaked T waves, decreased P wave.

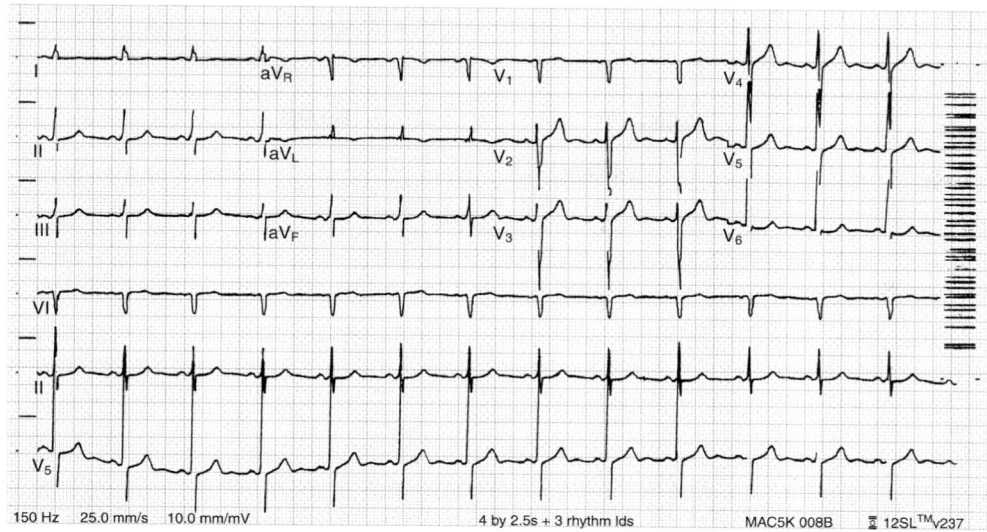

Fig. 114.3 The same patient as in Figures 114.1 and 114.2 after dialysis. The electrocardiogram (ECG) is now normal.

TABLE 114.1	Treatment of Hyperkalemia	
Treatment	**Medication**	**Features**
Stabilize cardiac membrane	Calcium chloride 1 g or calcium gluconate IV 2 g	For wide QRS, restores the electrical gradient; does not decrease serum potassium Onset within minutes; lasts 30 to 60 minutes
Shift potassium into cells	Regular insulin, 10 units, IV push, combined with 100 mL of 50% dextrose, IV push; 5 units IV insulin if renal dysfunction to avoid hypolgycemia High-dose nebulized albuterol by face mask (10 to 15 mg by continuous inhalation) Bicarbonate 50 to 100 mL Normal saline 100 to 250 mL	Insulin: Onset <15 minutes; maximum effect 30 to 60 minutes ($\approx$0.6 mEq/L decrease) Nebulized albuterol: Onset <15 minutes (0.5 to 1 mEq/L decrease) If severely acidotic In conjunction with nephrologist if dialysis dependent
Remove potassium from the body	Hemodialysis Normal saline and furosemide Ion exchange resin	Emergently in cardiac arrest, urgently in renal failure; may delay if renal function is normal In patients with rhabdomyolysis or tumor lysis syndrome with intact urine output, not effective acutely

IV, Intravenous.

IV calcium stabilizes the cardiac membrane by restoring the electrical gradient. Calcium increases the depolarization threshold and the calcium gradient across the cardiac membrane, quieting myocyte excitability and increasing cardiac conduction speed, thus narrowing the QRS. Calcium does not decrease serum potassium levels, and its effect is rapid (within 1 to 3 minutes), but transient (30 to 60 minutes or less). The dose is one ampule, or 10 mL of 10% calcium chloride solution. Calcium chloride is preferably administered through a central venous line due to the risk of tissue necrosis should it extravasate at the injection site. More than 10 mL of calcium gluconate will often be required, because it contains only one-third the calcium contained in calcium chloride. Calcium gluconate is preferred in pediatric cases, as well as in patients with less emergent (i.e., more chronic) hyperkalemic patients, when a slow infusion is desired or when only a smaller peripheral vein is available for administration.

Beta$_2$-agonists, insulin, saline, and potentially sodium bicarbonate shift potassium intracellularly. Insulin is the most reliable agent to move potassium into cells, but beta$_2$-adrenergic receptor agonists also

provide benefit in some patients. Insulin, given IV in combination with glucose to prevent hypoglycemia, also shifts potassium into cells by stimulation of the sodium-potassium adenosine triphosphatase (Na$^+$, K$^+$-ATPase) pump. The onset of action is less than 15 minutes, and the effect is maximal between 30 and 60 minutes, with a maximal drop of 0.6 mEq/L on average. Clinicians should follow glucose levels closely for hours post-therapy with glucose and insulin.

Nebulized albuterol is effective in shifting potassium into cells by stimulation of the Na$^+$, K$^+$-ATPase pump. Nebulized albuterol begins to take measurable effect after 15 minutes and lowers the serum potassium level by 0.5 to 1 mEq/L, depending on the dose. The effective dose is at least four times higher than that typically used for bronchodilation. The combination of nebulized albuterol and insulin with glucose appears to be additive, lowering serum potassium, on average, by 1.2 mEq/L.

Saline infusions also stimulate the Na$^+$, K$^+$-ATPase pump; only a few hundred milliliters are required for beneficial effects. Saline infusions should be given judiciously in anuric patients and in consultation with a nephrologist. Sodium bicarbonate is effective in hyperkalemic patients who are acidotic and has no benefit when used for hyperkalemia in non-acidotic patients. Sodium bicarbonate buffers hydrogen ions extracellularly while shifting potassium intracellularly, but it should be used in combination with other treatment options and reserved for patients with confirmed acidosis.[3]

Hemodialysis effectively and reliably decreases serum potassium levels by at least 1 mEq/L in the first hour and another 1 mEq/L during the next 2 hours. It is the only reliable method of potassium removal that has been experimentally studied and should be instituted early to treat life-threatening hyperkalemia in patients with renal failure. In patients with intact renal function, medical management alone is usually sufficient, even in extreme cases, and hemodialysis may not be necessary unless multiple medical modalities fail. There are no randomized trials addressing the use of diuretics (e.g., furosemide) in the emergent management of hyperkalemia. In cases such as rhabdomyolysis or tumor lysis syndrome, it may be appropriate to use a normal saline infusion supplemented by furosemide to enhance diuresis and urinary potassium excretion. Sodium polystyrene sulfonate (Kayexalate), does not decrease the serum potassium level within the first 4 hours of treatment, is not effective in the acute management of hyperkalemia, and may cause serious adverse gastrointestinal effects.[4]

Control of hyperkalemia in patients with chronic kidney disease and in those with heart failure continues to be difficult. However, two oral medications, patiromer and sodium zirconium cyclosilicate, have shown clinical promise in ongoing trials to lower serum potassium levels.[5,6] Zirconium is a highly selective cation exchanger that entraps potassium in the intestinal tract in exchange for sodium and hydrogen. Hypokalemia is often seen in association with hypomagnesemia, and patients with low serum potassium levels should be assumed to be hypomagnesemic also.

HYPOKALEMIA

Foundations

Hypokalemia is the most common electrolyte abnormality encountered in clinical practice. More than 20% of hospitalized patients and up to 40% of outpatients on thiazide diuretics have potassium values less than 3.5 mEq/L.[7] Moderate hypokalemia is a serum level of 2.5 to 3 mEq/L; severe hypokalemia is defined as a level less than 2.5 mEq/L. Although hypokalemia is usually asymptomatic, due to potassium's effect on the heart and muscle, very low levels can result in severe cardiac dysrhythmias or rhabdomyolysis, respectively.[8,9] Hypokalemia is often seen in association with hypomagnesemia, and patients with low serum potassium levels should be assumed to be hypomagnesemic as well.[10]

Clinical Features

Hypokalemia is usually asymptomatic but can present with nonspecific complaints, primarily weakness and muscle pain.[7] Although short periods of mild potassium depletion are typically well-tolerated in healthy individuals, severe potassium depletion can result in serious cardiovascular instability, neurologic dysfunction, glucose intolerance, gastrointestinal symptoms, and renal failure, as well as affect the acid-base balance in the body. The likelihood of symptoms appears to correlate with the rapidity of the decrease in serum potassium.

In patients without underlying heart disease, abnormalities in cardiac conduction are extremely unusual, even when the serum potassium concentration is below 3.0 mEq/L. Paresthesias, depressed deep tendon reflexes, fasciculations, muscle weakness, and confusion can occur when the serum potassium level is less than 2.5 mEq/L. However, in patients with cardiac ischemia or heart failure, even mild to moderate hypokalemia increases the likelihood of cardiac arrhythmias secondary to potassium's effect on the action potential. Hypokalemia is an independent risk factor contributing to reduced survival of cardiac

---

BOX 114.2   Five Most Common Causes of Hypokalemia

- Renal losses: Diuretic use, drugs, steroid use, metabolic acidosis, hyperaldosteronism, renal tubular acidosis, diabetic ketoacidosis (DKA), alcohol consumption
- Increased nonrenal losses: Sweating, diarrhea, vomiting, laxative use
- Decreased intake: Ethanol, malnutrition
- Intracellular shift: Hyperventilation, metabolic alkalosis, drugs
- Endocrine: Cushing disease, Bartter syndrome, insulin therapy

---

patients and increased incidence of arrhythmic death. Based on available evidence, serum potassium concentrations should be maintained above 4.5 mEq/L in patients having an acute myocardial infarction. Hypokalemic patients can demonstrate first- and second-degree heart block, atrial fibrillation, ventricular fibrillation, and asystole. Life-threatening cardiac arrhythmias are managed by restoration of serum potassium levels into the normal range. Thyrotoxic periodic paralysis is a rare disorder characterized by acute hypokalemia and muscle weakness. It is usually seen in patients of Asian descent and is potentially fatal when involvement includes respiratory muscles.[8]

Differential Diagnosis

The five most common causes of hypokalemia are renal losses, increased nonrenal losses, decreased potassium intake, intracellular shift, and endocrine etiologies (Box 114.2). Increased excretion of potassium, especially coupled with poor intake, is the most common cause of hypokalemia, and patients receiving diuretics represent the single most common patient group encountered in clinical practice. Thiazide diuretics are more likely than loop or osmotic diuretics to cause hypokalemia, but both the thiazide and loop diuretics block chloride-associated sodium and increase delivery of sodium to the collecting tubules. Hypokalemia is a common adverse effect of treatment with diuretics and may cause fatal arrhythmias and increase the risk of digitalis toxicity.[9] In addition to diuretics, other drugs and disorders can cause significant renal potassium losses, including hyperaldosteronism, steroid excess, metabolic acidosis, DKA, renal tubular acidosis, and alcohol consumption. When given in large doses, penicillin and its synthetic derivatives promote renal potassium excretion by increasing sodium delivery to the distal nephron. Individuals with secondary hyperaldosteronism, whether due to congestive heart failure (CHF), hepatic insufficiency, or nephrotic syndrome, may also exhibit hypokalemia. Patients with renal tubular acidosis can become hypokalemic, because a defect in the distal tubule leads to increased potassium excretion.

Administration of insulin may reduce serum potassium because of insulin's ability to stimulate the Na^+, K^+-ATPase pump and move potassium intracellularly; hypokalemia can be a dangerous complication with intentional overdoses of insulin or during treatment of DKA. Although most patients with DKA present with high-normal or mildly elevated serum potassium levels, patients are usually 2 to 3 mEq/kg deficient in total body potassium. To avoid hypokalemic arrhythmias or cardiac arrest from hypokalemia, a potassium infusion should be started once significant hyperkalemia has been ruled out and intact renal function confirmed.

Hypokalemia can also occur from gastrointestinal and dermal losses. In diarrheal states, large quantities of potassium can be lost in the stool, with consequent secondary hyperaldosteronism. Large doses of laxatives and repeated enemas also cause excessive potassium loss in the stool. Although hypokalemia is often seen after protracted vomiting or nasogastric suctions, only 5 to 10 mEq/L of potassium is lost in gastric fluid. Hypokalemia in this setting is secondary to metabolic alkalosis, chloride losses, and hyperaldosteronism. On occasion, excessive

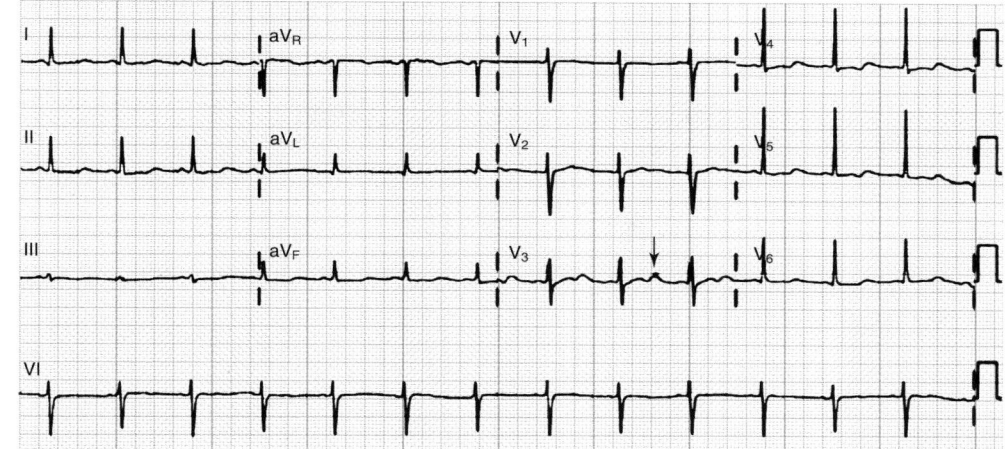

Fig. 114.4 Hypokalemic electrocardiographic changes, including flattened T wave, prolonged QT interval, nonspecific ST changes, and prominent U wave *(arrow)*.

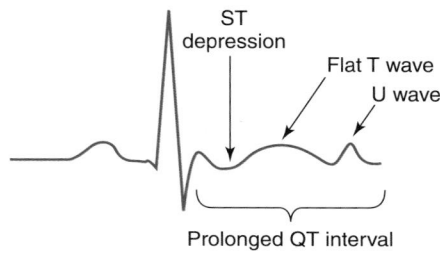

Hypokalemia

Fig. 114.5 Electrocardiographic changes in hypokalemia.

sweating can lead to hypokalemia from potassium losses through the skin. Patients with extensive burns can also suffer from hypokalemia because of significant skin losses. Dietary potassium deficiency should be considered in the severely malnourished patient or chronic alcoholic. Poor potassium intake combined with increased nonrenal losses can result in severe hypokalemia.

Hypokalemia can also result from an acute shift of potassium from the extracellular compartment into cells, most commonly in patients with metabolic alkalosis or hyperventilation, and in patients taking medications such as beta-agonists or decongestants. Stimulation of beta-receptors can lead to hypokalemia, especially in patients using repetitive and high doses of beta-agonists for chronic obstructive pulmonary disease or asthma. A standard dose of nebulized albuterol reduces serum potassium by 0.2 to 0.4 mEq/L, and a second dose taken within 1 hour can reduce it by almost 1 mEq/L. Patients with starvation or near-starvation may develop hypokalemia when fed, because insulin secretion and increased cellular uptake can cause an acute exaggerated intracellular migration of potassium.

Diagnostic Testing

Hypokalemia is rarely diagnosed on clinical presentation alone and is typically made by measurement of the serum potassium concentration during routine laboratory studies. If there is any suspicion for hypokalemia or a patient presents with generalized weakness, palpitations, or arrhythmias, an ECG should be obtained. Just as tall-peaked T waves are characteristic of hyperkalemia, flattened T waves can be seen in hypokalemia. Hypokalemia may produce U waves, which are small deflections after the T wave (Figs. 114.4 and 114.5). Hypokalemia may also cause a dangerously prolonged QT interval. Although there is no threshold of QT prolongation at which torsades de pointes is certain to occur, once the QT interval becomes longer than 500 milliseconds, the

risk of torsades de pointes increases twofold to threefold.[9] Hypokalemia is also notorious for causing nonspecific ST and T wave changes. In addition, prolonged potassium depletion of even a modest proportion can provoke or exacerbate kidney injury or hypertension. A severe degree of hypokalemia with paralysis is a potentially life-threatening medical emergency and may be seen as levels drop below 2.0 mEq/L.

Management

Because potassium is an intracellular cation; a low serum potassium level almost always reflects a significant total body potassium deficit; each 0.3 mEq potassium drop below normal correlates with an approximately 100 mEq total body deficit. In the absence of nausea or vomiting as the cause of hypokalemia, patients with mild or moderate hypokalemia may only need oral potassium replacement therapy. Oral replacement is available in liquid, powder, and tablet form. Potassium chloride is the most commonly used supplementation, and 40 to 60 mEq orally every 2 to 4 hours is typically well tolerated. If the cause of hypokalemia is not clear, or the hypokalemia is severe and associated with profound weakness, obtain a spot urine potassium level before starting therapy to assess whether the patient's kidneys are inappropriately wasting potassium from a renal or endocrine cause. Although a 24-hour serum is more accurate, a urinary potassium above 13 mEq/L per gram of creatinine is indicative of inappropriate renal potassium loses.[7] Treatment of hypokalemia is essential in multiple populations of patients. Hypokalemia is arrhythmogenic, especially in the settings of acute myocardial infarction, high catecholamine states, and hypertrophied or dilated ventricles. Hypokalemia is an important independent risk factor for morbidity and mortality in patients with heart failure, requiring serum potassium levels to between 4.0 and 5.0 mEq/L in this population.

If IV infusion is necessary, potassium chloride can be safely given at a rate of 10 to 20 mEq/hr. In the rare instance when IV repletion is planned at more than 20 mEq/hr, such as for levels below 2.0 mEq/L or QT interval greater than 500 milliseconds, the patient should have continuous cardiac monitoring and central line access established.

Hypokalemia is associated with hypomagnesemia, and the severity of the hypokalemia correlates with a similar degree of hypomagnesemia. Magnesium replacement should usually accompany potassium repletion.[10] Unless the patient receives at least 0.5 g/hr of magnesium sulfate along with potassium replacement, potassium will not move intracellularly and the patient will lose potassium through excretion. Correction of large potassium deficits may require several days, with simultaneous oral and IV replacement.

Disposition

Patients with mild hypokalemia, above 3.5 mEq/dl without any ECG changes can usually be discharged home with very close outpatient follow-up for a potassium recheck in a week. Hypokalemia due to diuretic therapy requires either increased potassium intake, the addition of a potassium sparing agent or switching the patient to a combined thiazide and potassium sparing diuretic.

Once the patient is discharged, if increased potassium intake is desired, then oral potassium repletion is best accomplished by encouraging the ingestion of potassium and magnesium-rich foods such as potatoes, avocado, black beans, tomatoes, and bananas.

Patients in whom the underlying cause of their hypokalemia cannot be successfully treated such as refractory nausea and vomiting require admission. Patients cannot be discharged until their potassium level is above 3.0 mEq/dl, they can tolerate food and liquids, and they have a QT interval of less than 500 msec.

HYPERNATREMIA

Foundations

Hypernatremia is defined as a serum sodium concentration above 145 mEq/L. It is rarely seen in previously healthy patients and usually portends a poor prognosis. Most hypernatremic patients have either an impaired sense of thirst or no access to water: elders, infants, patients with mental impairment, and those who are intubated and paralyzed are at highest risk for this disorder. Hypernatremia can be divided into three physiologic pairings: (1) hypernatremia with dehydration and low total body sodium, (2) hypernatremia with low total body water and normal total body sodium, and (3) hypernatremia with increased total body sodium (Box 114.3). Diabetes insipidus, an insufficient production of (or lack of response to) antidiuretic hormone, can lead to life-threatening hypernatremia (Box 114.4).

Clinical Features

Patients often have multiple causes of severe hypernatremia. Hypernatremia in adults is almost exclusively due to a free water deficit and should be considered in any patient presenting with altered mental status, as well as in bed-ridden patients with no access to water. Patients with impaired antidiuretic hormone function may complain of polyuria or polydipsia. Others may have obvious causes of extrarenal fluid losses, while some may have no complaints at all.

Diagnostic Testing

In addition to routine serum chemistries, serum osmolarity and urine sodium concentration and osmolality should be obtained. The degree of hypernatremia almost always equals the total body water (TBW) deficit in adults. The patient's TBW deficit can be estimated by the formula

$$\text{TBW deficit} = \text{TBW} \times (\text{serum Na}^+ - 140)/140$$

A patient's TBW is calculated by multiplying the patient's body weight in kilograms times 0.6. However, because of differences in the percentages of body fat, based on the age and sex of the patient, it is more accurate to use the correction factors listed in Table 114.2.

Management

The treatment of hypernatremia has three interdependent goals: first, to quickly correct underlying shock, hypoperfusion, or significant hypovolemia with normal saline; second, to treat the underlying cause of hypernatremia, such as fever, vomiting, or diabetes insipidus; and third, to carefully lower the serum sodium level, usually by replacement of the body's total water deficit.[11,12] Until hypoperfusion and

---

BOX 114.3 Three Types of Hypernatremia

Hypernatremia With Dehydration and Low Total Body Sodium
Heatstroke
Increased insensible losses: Burns, sweating
Gastrointestinal loss: Diarrhea, protracted vomiting, continuous gastrointestinal suction
Osmotic diuresis: Glucose, mannitol, enteral feeding

Hypernatremia With Low Total Body Water and Normal Total Body Sodium
Diabetes insipidus
Neurogenic
Elderly with "reset" osmostat
Hypothalamic dysfunction
Suprasellar or infrasellar tumors
Renal disease
Drugs (amphotericin, phenytoin, lithium, aminoglycosides, methoxyflurane)
Sickle cell disease

Hypernatremia With Increased Total Body Sodium
Salt tablet ingestion
Salt water ingestion
Saline infusions
Saline enemas
IV sodium bicarbonate
Poorly diluted interval feedings
Primary hyperaldosteronism
Hemodialysis
Cushing syndrome
Conn syndrome

IV, Intravenous.

BOX 114.4 More Common Causes of Diabetes Insipidus

Central
Idiopathic
Familial disease
Cancer
Hypoxic encephalopathy
Infiltrative disorders
Post supraventricular tachycardia
Anorexia nervosa

Nephrogenic
Chronic renal insufficiency
Polycystic kidney disease
Lithium toxicity
Hypercalcemia
Hypokalemia
Tubulointerstitial disease
Hereditary
Sickle cell disease

---

hypovolemia are corrected, homeostatic mechanisms for sodium balance promote sodium resorption to maintain intravascular volume, even at the expense of the serum sodium concentration.

The rate of correction in hypernatremia is extremely important to minimize morbidity and mortality. Both too quick and too slow

TABLE 114.2	**Calculation of Body Water**
Population	Total Body Water
Children and adult men	Body weight (kg) × 0.6
Adult women	Body weight (kg) × 0.5
Elderly men	Body weight (kg) × 0.5
Elderly women	Body weight (kg) × 0.45

correction speeds are associated with an increased risk of death, regardless of the initial sodium level.[11,12] In adult patients who develop hypernatremia over a short time due to sodium loading, "rapid correction" at a rate of at least 1 mEq/hr decrease in serum sodium appears relatively safe.[11,12] However, most adult patients develop hypernatremia over days to weeks. In this group of patients, serum sodium concentration should be corrected slowly, at no more than 0.5 mEq/hr or 10 to 12 mEq/day.

Normal saline should be started for volume replacement until the patient is hemodynamically stable, and then changed to half-normal saline at 100 mL/hr once vital signs have normalized. The treatment of central diabetes insipidus with desmopressin (DDAVP) is an effective means of improving polyuria and hypernatremia; initial doses in the acute setting range from 1 to 2 μg.

Disposition

The disposition is based on the patient's underlying etiology and severity of the hypernatremia. Almost all hypernatremic patients require hospitalization due to their dehydrated status and underlying comorbidities. Most of the time these patients have a free water deficit with a low chance of dangerous overcorrection. In mild cases, increasing water intake at home can restore the proper sodium balance.

HYPONATREMIA

Foundations

Hyponatremia, defined as serum sodium concentration of less than 135 mEq/L, is the second most common electrolyte abnormality encountered in clinical practice and can be a marker of underlying disease. The most common causes of severe hyponatremia in adults are therapy with thiazides, the postoperative state, the syndrome of inappropriate secretion of antidiuretic hormone (SIADH), psychogenic polydipsia, exercise-associated hyponatremia, and unintentional water intoxication. Gastrointestinal fluid loss, ingestion of overly dilute formula, accidental ingestion of excessive water, and receipt of multiple tap water enemas are the main causes of severe hyponatremia in infants and children. Most patients presenting to the emergency department (ED) with hyponatremia are asymptomatic and do not require emergent therapy. If symptoms are present, they are typically based on the degree of hyponatremia and how acutely the hyponatremia developed. Symptoms range from headache, nausea, and vomiting to confusion, seizures, and coma. There are two groups of hyponatremic patients that require treatment with either normal saline or hypertonic saline: (1) severe but asymptomatic hyponatremia with a sodium level of 110 mEq/L or less and (2) acute symptomatic hyponatremia with a sodium level below 120 mEq/L.

Central nervous system (CNS) damage due to hyponatremia may be caused by cerebral edema and increased intracranial pressure, by osmotic fluid shifts during overly aggressive treatment, or by both. When neurons are subjected to a hyponatremic environment, they become depleted of sodium and potassium in an attempt to limit their own osmolarity to prevent intracellular fluid shifts that would lead to cerebral edema. If fluid therapy raises extracellular sodium levels too quickly, fluids shift out of neurons and can cause diffuse demyelination.

BOX 114.5 Causes of Hyponatremia

Pseudohyponatremia
Hyperlipidemia
Hyperproteinemia (multiple myeloma, macroglobulinemia)

Dilutional
Hyperglycemia

Hypovolemic Hyponatremia: Decreased Total Body Water and Sodium, With a Relatively Greater Decrease in Sodium
Body fluid losses: Sweating, vomiting, diarrhea, gastrointestinal suction
Third spacing: Bowel obstruction, burns, pancreatitis, rhabdomyolysis
Renal causes: Diuretics, mineralocorticoid deficiency, osmotic diuresis, renal tubular acidosis, salt-wasting nephropathies

Hypervolemic Hyponatremia: Increased Total Body Sodium With a Relatively Greater Increase in Total Body Water
Heart failure
Chronic renal failure
Hepatic failure or cirrhosis

Euvolemic Hyponatremia: Increased Total Body Water With Nearly Normal Total Body Sodium
SIADH
Drugs causing SIADH (diuretics, barbiturates, carbamazepine, chlorpropamide, clofibrate, opioids, tolbutamide, vincristine)
Psychogenic polydipsia
Beer potomania
Hypothyroidism
Adrenal insufficiency
MDMA (ecstasy)
Accidental or intentional water intoxication

MDMA, N-methyl-3,4-methylenedioxyamphetamine; *SIADH*, syndrome of inappropriate secretion of antidiuretic hormone.

This can result in a flaccid paralysis and death due to central pontine myelinolysis, a syndrome more accurately labeled as the osmotic demyelinating syndrome (ODS).[13,14]

Causes of hyponatremia fall into four general categories: pseudohyponatremia, hyponatremia with dehydration and decreased extracellular volume, hyponatremia with increased extracellular volume, and euvolemic hyponatremia with increased TBW (Box 114.5).

Pseudohyponatremia

Pseudohyponatremia is a falsely low sodium reading caused by the presence of other osmolar particles in the serum. The phenomenon of pseudohyponatremia is explained by the increased percentage of large molecular particles that do not contribute to plasma osmolality relative to sodium. Severe hypertriglyceridemia and hyperproteinemia are two common causes of this condition. Blood draw or laboratory error should also be considered as a possible cause of hyponatremia, especially if the blood sample was drawn near an infusion site using 5% dextrose in water (D_5W) when a very abnormal sodium level is reported in an otherwise healthy patient.

Hyperglycemia is sometimes considered a cause of pseudohyponatremia; however, it causes a dilutional hyponatremia by pulling water into the vascular space through osmosis. In true pseudohyponatremia, serum osmolality is normal and no shifts of water occur. Two different formulas based on the degree of a patient's hyperglycemia are currently used to correct serum sodium levels. The most recommended formula advocates for the addition of 1.6 mEq/L to the measured sodium for every 100 mg/dL of glucose above 100. However, another acceptable formula recommends using this 1.6 mEq/dl only for the first 400 mg rise in glucose and then using 2.4 mEqs for each additional 100 mg/dl rise in glucose. Either formula is acceptable to use, the key concept being that as glucose levels rise significantly, a "normal" and not as lowered serum sodium is distinctly abnormal.

Hypovolemic Hyponatremia

Hypovolemic hyponatremia, or hyponatremia with dehydration, occurs when there is decreased extracellular volume combined with an even greater loss of sodium. Hyponatremia secondary to body fluid losses should be differentiated from that due to renal losses. Hyponatremia with dehydration due to body fluid losses includes sweating, vomiting, diarrhea, and gastrointestinal suction. Hypovolemic hyponatremia is also seen with "third spacing" in bowel obstruction, burns, and intra-abdominal sepsis. Hypovolemic hyponatremia due to renal causes includes diuretic use, mineralocorticoid deficiency, renal tubular acidosis, and salt-wasting nephropathy. Hypovolemic hyponatremia can be further exacerbated when fluid losses are replaced with hypotonic saline.

Hypervolemic Hyponatremia

Hypervolemic hyponatremia, or hyponatremia with increased extracellular volume, occurs when sodium and water are retained, but water retention exceeds sodium retention. Most of these patients present with edema. Hyponatremia with increased total body sodium occurs in patients with heart failure, chronic renal failure, and hepatic failure.[14,15] The fluid retention in these states is secondary to renal hypoperfusion, resulting in increased aldosterone secretion and a decrease in free water excretion.

Euvolemic Hyponatremia

The final category of hyponatremia is one in which patients are euvolemic but have increased TBW. Causes of this type of hyponatremia include SIADH, psychogenic polydipsia, beer potomania, hypothyroidism, diuretic use in patients with mild CHF, and accidental or intentional water intoxication. Euvolemic hyponatremia has also been described in patients after the use of the recreational drug N-methyl-3,4-methylenedioxyamphetamine (MDMA; or ecstasy). MDMA-induced hyponatremia is multifactorial and related to increased free water intake to avoid dehydration and rhabdomyolysis, along with the tendency to be very active while using the drug, leading to sweating and antidiuretic hormone secretion.[14] For similar reasons, there are extensive case reports of significant exercise-associated hyponatremia in endurance athletes.

SIADH is an important cause of hyponatremia that occurs when antidiuretic hormone is secreted independent of the body's need to conserve water. The process results from excess antidiuretic hormone production that increases TBW, causing the serum sodium to decrease. Patients with SIADH inappropriately concentrate their urine, despite a low serum osmolality and normal circulating blood volume. Despite excess TBW, they have no signs of edema, ascites, or heart failure, because most of the increased water is intracellular rather than intravascular. The three most common causes of SIADH are (1) pulmonary lung masses and infections, (2) CNS disorders, and (3) drugs (Box 114.6). Lung cancers (especially small cell cancer), pneumonia, and tuberculosis can lead to SIADH. CNS infections, masses, and psychosis can also cause SIADH. A large number of medications are associated with SIADH, the most common of which are thiazide diuretics, narcotics, lithium, oral hypoglycemics, barbiturates, and antineoplastics. The

---

BOX 114.6   Three Most Common Causes of Syndrome of Inappropriate Secretion of Antidiuretic Hormone

Lung Masses
Cancer (especially small cell)
Pneumonia
Tuberculosis
Abscess

Central Nervous System Disorders
Infection (meningitis, brain abscess)
Mass (subdural, postoperative, cerebrovascular accident)
Psychosis (with psychogenic polydipsia)

Drugs
Thiazide diuretics
Narcotics
Oral hypoglycemic agents
Barbiturates
Antineoplastics

---

mainstay of treatment of most patients with SIADH and other causes of euvolemic hyponatremia is free water restriction.

Clinical Features

The signs and symptoms of hyponatremia worsen as sodium levels decline and also correlate with how rapid hyponatremia develops. Nonspecific signs of hyponatremia include anorexia, nausea, vomiting, and generalized weakness. Acutely hyponatremic patients whose sodium level drops below 120 mEq/L over 24 to 48 hours may present with severe neurologic findings, including confusion, seizures, coma, and brainstem herniation. Determination of the hydration status of the patient may help establish the etiology of the hyponatremia and direct subsequent treatment. *Hypovolemic* hyponatremia is more likely in the patient with diminished skin turgor, increased capillary refill, dry mucous membranes, and orthostasis, whereas the patient with jugular venous distention, peripheral edema, or pulmonary congestion is much more likely to have *hypervolemic* hyponatremia. Patients with SIADH have no edema and normal skin turgor. Of note, in geriatric patients, the risk of hyponatremia doubles for those presenting with large-bone fractures.

Diagnostic Testing

A spot urinary sodium or urinary chloride level can help determine if hyponatremia is renal in origin (Table 114.3). Patients with hypovolemic hyponatremia due to nonrenal causes typically have a low urinary sodium or chloride level (<20 mEq/L), because they try to retain solute. Patients with hypovolemic hyponatremia due to renal causes have elevated urine sodium and chloride levels (>20 mEq/L) because their kidneys cannot retain sodium or chloride. Patients with euvolemic hyponatremia typically have a urinary sodium concentration more than 20 mEq/L secondary to volume expansion caused by water retention. Patients with psychogenic polydipsia who are ingesting large quantities of water have dilute urine with low quantities of urinary sodium. Patients with hypervolemic hyponatremia secondary to CHF or cirrhosis have urine sodium levels of less than 20 mEq/L because of renal hypoperfusion, whereas those with renal causes of hypervolemic hyponatremia or with SIADH have sodium levels more than 20 mEq/L, because their kidneys do not retain sodium. In interpreting serum sodium levels, consider the possibility of sampling error if the

TABLE 114.3 Spot Urine Interpretation

	Hypovolemic Hyponatremia	Hypovolemic Hyponatremia	Euvolemic Hyponatremia	Euvolemic Hyponatremia	Hypervolemic Hyponatremia	Hypervolemic Hyponatremia
Underlying etiologies	Nonrenal causes	Renal causes	SIADH, endocrinopathies	Psychogenic polydipsia	Edematous disorders: e.g., CHF, cirrhosis	Renal failure
Urinary sodium	<20 mEq/L	>20 mEq/L	>20 mEq/L	<20 mEq/L	<20 mEq/L	>20 mEq/L
Mechanism	Extrarenal solute loss	Renal solute loss	Volume expansion	Normal renal response to excess volume and sodium retention	Renal hypoperfusion	Renal solute loss

CHF, Congestive heart failure; SIADH, syndrome of inappropriate antidiuretic hormone secretion.

TABLE 114.4 Characteristics of Infusates

Infusate	Infusate Sodium (Mmol/L)	Extracellular Fluid Distribution (%)
3% Hypertonic saline	513	100
0.9% Normal saline solution	154	100
Lactated Ringers solution	130	97
Half-normal saline solution	77	73
0.2% Sodium chloride + D_5W	34	55
D_5W	0	45

D_5W, 5% dextrose in water.

reported value does not seem consistent with the patient's presentation and confirm that a diuretic such as furosemide, which will increase urinary sodium losses, has not been recently administered. Consider adrenal insufficiency when a dehydrated patient has both hyponatremia and hyperkalemia.

Of note, in geriatric patients, the risk of hyponatremia doubles for those presenting with large-bone fractures.

Management

Treatment of hyponatremia is guided by the patient's clinical presentation, severity of symptoms, estimated duration of illness, fluid status, and underlying cause of the sodium disturbance. Typically, sodium should be corrected during a time course of 48 to 72 hours. The neurologic changes, including flaccid paralysis, dysarthria, dysphagia, and hypotension, associated with overly rapid sodium correction are referred to as *osmotic demyelinating syndrome (ODS)*, previously termed *central pontine myelinolysis*. Most ODS cases occur in the alcoholic, malnourished, and geriatric population, although this devastating side effect can occur in young, healthy patients as well. If a patient develops symptoms of ODS during therapy, all sodium-containing fluids should be stopped and D_5W administered immediately to temporarily lower sodium values. Most patients presenting to the ED with hyponatremia are stable and require no emergent therapy. However, patients who have serum sodium levels of significantly less than 120 mEq/L and those who have acute alterations in mental status, seizures, or new focal findings due to hyponatremia need immediate intervention. Table 114.4 presents the sodium concentration of various infusates, and the following equation is helpful to estimate the effect of 1 liter of any infusate on serum sodium:

$$\text{Change in serum Na}^+ - \text{serum Na}^+/\text{TBW} + 1$$

There is no consensus regarding the optimal treatment of symptomatic hyponatremia. However, there is agreement that correction

should occur at a sufficient pace and magnitude to reverse the manifestations of hypotonicity but not be so rapid as to pose a risk for development of ODS.[13,14] For relatively asymptomatic patients with sodium values of 115 to 135 mEq/L, free water restriction is typically the most important treatment.

In more severe cases when the sodium value is 120 mEq/L or less and the patient has alterations in mental status, has focal findings, or is seizing, 3% hypertonic saline (513 mEq/L of sodium) is indicated.[15,16] Correction of hyponatremia by 4 to 6 mEq/L within 6 hours, with bolus infusions of 3% saline if necessary, is sufficient to manage the most severe manifestations of hyponatremia. Initially, 100 mL of 3% hypertonic saline should be infused over 10 minutes. If a second bolus is required, an additional 100 mL of the 3% solution may be administered during the next 50 minutes. To minimize the likelihood of ODS, it is essential that symptomatic patients with severe hyponatremia have serum sodium levels raised slowly. Previous guidelines endorsed the safety of raising the serum sodium by up to 10 to 12 mEq within the first 24 hours. However, in patients believed to have been hyponatremic for more than 48 hours, severe hyponatremia should be corrected by no more than 8 mEq in the first 24 hours.[13]

Potassium deficits should be replaced aggressively in the treatment of hyponatremic patients with a sodium disorder. If patients are retaining volume and diuresis is not adequate, furosemide can be used; D_5W is infused if the sodium level is rising too quickly.[16] Patients may be able to make full neurologic recoveries from ODS with the reinduction of hyponatremia in these extreme cases. Demeclocycline in a dosage of 600 to 1200 mg daily is effective in patients with refractory hyponatremia.

Hypovolemic Hyponatremia

Treatment of hypovolemic hyponatremia begins with rehydration. Hypotensive, dehydrated patients should be volume resuscitated with normal saline. Once the patient is hemodynamically stable, the infusion rate should be slowed. Typically, normal saline is started at 500 to 1000 mL/hr until the blood pressure is stable and then slowed to 200 mL/hr with frequent sodium checks. If the sodium value is below 120 mEq/L, the sodium concentration should be allowed to rise by less than an average of 0.5 mEq/hr or about 8 mEq/day until about 120 mEq.[13,15,16] The underlying cause of hyponatremia should be identified and treated.

Hypervolemic Hyponatremia

Normal saline and hypertonic saline can cause pulmonary edema in the hypervolemic hyponatremic patient. Restriction of fluid and sodium is the preferred treatment, although loop diuretics can be used in severe cases. Hemodialysis is an alternative in patients with renal impairment and should be considered for significantly hyponatremic renal failure patients with volume overload. Patients with CHF benefit from diuretics that increase water excretion and cause vasodilation to improve cardiac output.[17] In patients with liver failure, albumin is a consideration, along with diuretics and possibly paracentesis to improve the underlying pathologic process. Water restriction may make the largest impact on the long-term care of these patients.

Euvolemic Hyponatremia

The mainstay of treatment of euvolemic hyponatremia is free water restriction, as hypo-osmolality in SIADH results from a relative abundance of water in the intracellular and extracellular spaces, maintained by a reduced ability to excrete water. However, water restriction is insufficient to treat acute severe hyponatremia and is not recommended as a sole intervention for patients requiring more rapid correction based on clinical presentation. The only definitive treatment of SIADH is elimination of its underlying cause. Most cases of SIADH caused by malignant disease resolve with effective antineoplastic therapy; most due to medication resolve promptly when the offending agent is discontinued.

In patients with SIADH, normal saline may cause the serum sodium concentration to fall even more as free water is retained and hypertonic urine is excreted. If a patient is symptomatic because of a rapid decrease in serum sodium concentration, treatment with hypertonic saline is recommended. Rapid correction of hyponatremia may occur during hemodialysis. To minimize the risks of ODS, hemodialysis is reserved for patients with documented renal failure under close monitoring. Vaptans, which are oral agents that inhibit the effects of vasopressin, have been studied for treatment of patients with hyponatremia due to SIADH but need further evaluation before becoming standard of care.[15,16]

Disposition

Patients that are altered or lethargic with hyponatremia should be admitted to the ICU. Other hyponatremic patients that should be admitted to the ICU include patients on a hypertonic saline infusion and those who received a hypertonic saline bolus. In addition, nephrology should be consulted for patients with symptomatic hyponatremia or rapidly rising sodium to discuss the use of desmopressin or vaptans. Patients who have returned to neurologic baseline with stable sodium trended over 4 to 6 hours may be admitted to a monitored floor bed. Patients may be discharged once their sodium is approaching 130 mEq/L, their underlying cause has been identified and either corrected or more aggressively treated. Patients who have developed hyponatremia acutely (such as the endurance athlete) who present asymptomatically or with mild symptoms may be considered for discharge from the ED with close outpatient follow-up and a lab recheck.

HYPERCALCEMIA

Foundations

Hypercalcemia is usually defined as a serum calcium level above 10.5 mg/dL; normal levels are usually defined as between 9 and 10.5 mg/dL. Hypercalcemia is considered mild if the total serum calcium level is between 10.5 and 12 mg/dL; levels higher than 14 mg/dL can be life-threatening. Hypercalcemic crisis typically evolves from preexisting mild hypercalcemia, which develops into an acute severe hypercalcemic emergency.

Clinical Features

The clinical presentation of hypercalcemia is often vague and nonspecific. Symptoms include nonfocal abdominal pain, constipation, fatigue, body aches, anorexia, polydipsia, polyuria, nausea, and vomiting. Symptom severity depends on the degree of hypercalcemia, the rapidity of onset, and the patient's baseline neurologic and renal function. Neuropsychiatric disturbances include anxiety, depression, and hallucinations. The CNS manifestations that often predominate in more severe cases include lethargy, altered mental status, seizures, and coma. Death due to hypercalcemia is usually related to complications caused by coma, dehydration, or electrolyte disturbances. Cardiac conduction abnormalities may occur; bradydysrhythmias are the most common. Severe hypercalcemia (>14 mg/dL) has also been associated with sinus arrest, atrioventricular block, atrial fibrillation, and ventricular tachycardia.

Differential Diagnosis

There are five major causes of hypercalcemia (Box 114.7). Hyperparathyroidism is the most common cause of hypercalcemia in outpatients, whereas malignancy is the most common cause in hospitalized patients; together, these two etiologies account for the majority of hypercalcemia cases.[18] Mild hypercalcemia, in an otherwise normal person, may be due to thiazide diuretics in the setting of minimal dehydration. Other less common causes of elevated calcium concentration should be considered after malignant disease and parathyroid disease are ruled out. Malignancy-associated hypercalcemia occurs in up to 40% of all patients with advanced cancer and generally conveys a poor prognosis.[19] Other causes of hypercalcemia include granulomatous disease, such as sarcoidosis and tuberculosis; medications and pharmacologic agents; and a number of diverse conditions, such as rhabdomyolysis and prolonged immobilization.

BOX 114.7   Five Most Common Causes of Hypercalcemia

Malignant Disease
Ectopic secretions of parathyroid hormone, multiple myeloma, cancer metastatic to bone
   Most common: Breast, lung, hematologic, kidney, prostate

Endocrine
Hyperparathyroidism, multiple endocrine neoplasias, hyperthyroidism, pheochromocytoma, adrenal insufficiency

Granulomatous Disease
Sarcoidosis, tuberculosis, histoplasmosis, berylliosis, coccidioidomycosis

Pharmacologic Agents
Vitamins A and D, thiazide diuretics, estrogens, milk-alkali syndrome

Miscellaneous
Dehydration, prolonged immobilization, iatrogenic, rhabdomyolysis, familial, laboratory error

Diagnostic Testing

The diagnostic evaluation of a patient with suspected hypercalcemia begins with obtaining electrolyte and renal function tests and an ECG. Calcium is measured by determination of either a total serum calcium level or an ionized calcium level. Ionized calcium is the active form of the total calcium level. Ionized calcium is more accurate in the diagnosis and treatment of hypocalcemia but does need to be routinely evaluated in hypercalcemia. The serum total calcium level represents both bound and unbound calcium and, thus, should be corrected based on the albumin concentration. A correction of the total serum calcium is made by adjusting for deviations in the serum albumin level. The adjustment is accomplished by adding or subtracting 0.08 mg/dL to the measured total serum calcium for every 1.0 g/L of albumin below or above 4 g/L albumin, respectively.

A short QT interval can be seen in hypercalcemia and is considered a classic finding. However, although the incidence and duration of QT shortening appear to be correlated with the degree of hypercalcemia, it is not a reliable finding and is not routinely seen in most patients (Fig. 114.6). ST segment elevation may be the least well documented but most consistent electrocardiographic finding, making hypercalcemia a potential cause of ST segment elevation caused by conditions other than myocardial infarction.[20,21] Some hypercalcemic patients may have U waves in the precordial leads despite normokalemia, while others may have an Osborn wave despite normothermia.[22] In severe cases of hypercalcemia, sinus bradycardia, high-degree atrioventricular block, and ventricular fibrillation may also be seen.

Management

Patients in hypercalcemic crisis are usually dehydrated, often obtunded, and also predisposed to arrhythmias as a result of concomitant electrolyte disturbances; thus, they require IV access with a normal saline infusion and close monitoring. Normal saline inhibits proximal tubule reabsorption of calcium and corrects the patient's volume depletion. Normal saline should be infused "wide open" until blood pressure and perfusion are normalized. After the initial bolus, the saline infusion should be adjusted to a rate of approximately 200 to 300 mL/hr, depending on the patient's age, renal function, cardiac and other comorbid diseases, to establish adequate urine output (2 L/day). Although the administration of higher volumes of saline may further augment calcium excretion, it is much more likely to increase morbidity and mortality from volume overload, pulmonary edema, and myocardial ischemia. The routine use of furosemide in the management of hypercalcemia is no longer recommended.[18] Furosemide was once thought to block the distal reabsorption of calcium, thus complementing saline's proximal tubule effects. However, furosemide has not been shown to have significant calcium reabsorption blocking effects. The use of furosemide should be reserved for augmenting saline diuresis to avoid volume overload during the treatment of hypercalcemia. If a loop diuretic is given to patients who are not yet volume replete, not only can the patient's hemodynamics and renal status deteriorate, but hypercalcemia may worsen. Once calcium excretion by saline infusion has begun, other electrolyte values should be carefully monitored, with particular attention to serum potassium levels.

Osteoclast-inhibiting therapies for severe hypercalcemia are generally considered in consultation with the patient's primary physician or oncologist. Drugs that inhibit osteoclast-mediated bone resorption include the bisphosphonates, mithramycin, calcitonin, and glucocorticoids. IV bisphosphonates are the most extensively studied and most efficacious agents for the treatment of malignancy-associated hypercalcemia. Their calcium-lowering effect is achieved predominantly by inhibition of osteoclast function and survival. Zoledronic acid is the bisphosphonate of choice in hypercalcemia of malignancy. The infusion takes 15 minutes; zoledronic acid may be more effective than other bisphosphonates at keeping the calcium level down over time. The use of IV bisphosphonates is restricted to the treatment of acute hypercalcemia associated with serum calcium concentrations above 15 mg/dL and rapid deterioration of CNS, cardiac, gastrointestinal, and renal function. Denosumab for the management of hypercalcemia of malignancy provides a new option for the management of patients with persistent hypercalcemia despite bisphosphonates.[23] In the rare case in which a patient has a life-threatening hypercalcemic arrhythmia or heart block, hemodialysis should be considered. In cases of hypercalcemic crisis resulting from primary hyperparathyroidism, urgent parathyroidectomy is potentially curative. Hematology, oncology, and palliative care specialists should be involved early in the care of the patient with hypercalcemia associated with malignancy to assure the appropriate targeted therapies. Isolated mild hypercalcemia rarely requires urgent treatment; however, an outpatient hypercalcemia

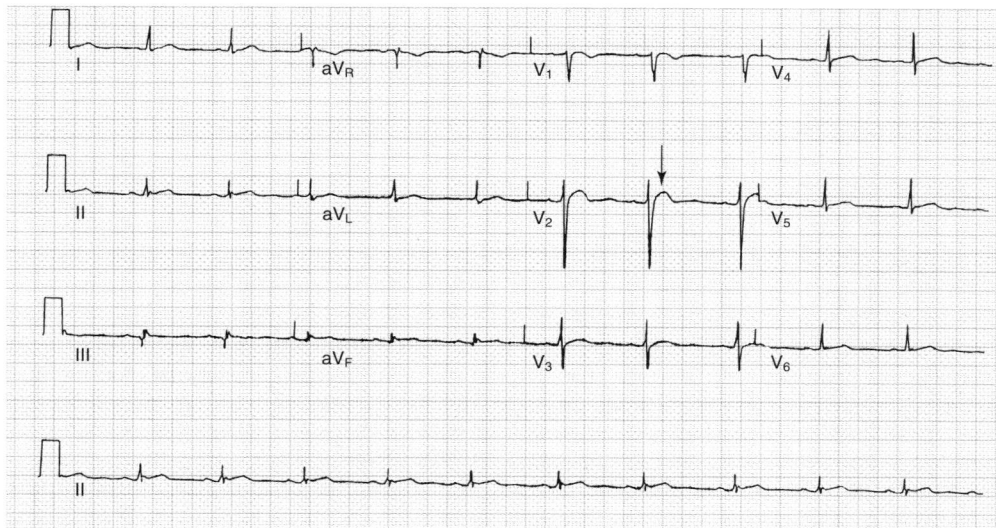

Fig. 114.6 Short QT interval *(arrow)* in a patient with multiple myeloma and a calcium level of 14.2 mg/dL. (Courtesy Dr. Barton Campbell.)

evaluation should be discussed at discharge, because many will ultimately be diagnosed with hyperparathyroidism.

Disposition

Patients with altered mental status or arrhythmias from hypercalcemia should be admitted to the intensive care unit for close monitoring, management of electrolytes, and frequent laboratory testing. In patients with symptomatic hypercalcemia, medical floor admission may be necessary for continuous fluid resuscitation and electrolyte monitoring. Patients with mild to moderate hypercalcemia may be discharged home with instructions to avoid dehydration and high calcium diets. In patients with known malignancy or suspicion for malignancy, disposition planning should be coordinated with the oncology team.

HYPOCALCEMIA

Foundations

Calcium regulation is critical for normal cell function, neural transmission, membrane stability, bone structure, blood coagulation, and intracellular signaling. Total body calcium is controlled by a feedback system in which parathyroid hormone induces the bone and the kidneys to increase serum calcium levels. Vitamin D facilitates intestinal calcium absorption. Conversely, elevated calcium levels normally inhibit parathyroid hormone release.

Clinical Features

Although there are many clinical manifestations of hypocalcemia, neuromuscular and cardiovascular findings predominate. Severity of symptoms is related to not only the absolute calcium level, but also the rate calcium rise. The patient may complain of muscle cramping, perioral or finger paresthesias, shortness of breath secondary to bronchospasm, and tetanic contractions. Symptomatic hypocalcemia may result in cardiovascular collapse, hypotension, and dysrhythmias. More severe hypocalcemia can lead to cardiovascular collapse, hypotension, syncope, dysrhythmias, CHF, angina, hypotension, and QT prolongation. Patients with a calcium level lower than 8.95 mg/dL have a 2.3-fold higher risk of sudden cardiac activity than those with calcium levels higher than 9.55 mg/dL.[24]

Chronic hypocalcemia may manifest with cataracts, poor dentition, dry skin, coarse hair, and pruritus. Chvostek sign may be present: when the examiner taps the facial nerve, facial or eye muscle twitching will be elicited. Trousseau sign may also be present; when the examiner inflates the blood pressure cuff to 20 mm Hg above the systolic blood pressure for 3 minutes, carpal spasms will be induced because of the increased excitability caused by local ulnar and median nerve ischemia. Trousseau sign is relatively specific for hypocalcemia, whereas Chvostek test is less diagnostic.

Differential Diagnosis

There are multiple causes of hypocalcemia, of which hypoalbuminemia is the most common (Box 114.8). Because calcium is bound to albumin and other serum proteins, hypoalbuminemia will cause a fall in the measured serum calcium by about 0.8 mg/dL for every 1 g/dL reduction in serum albumin. The active form of calcium is ionized calcium, which is not affected by changes in albumin.

Hypoparathyroidism is a common cause of hypocalcemia and often develops after surgery for head and neck cancers; it occurs in 1% to 2% of patients after total thyroidectomy. Patients with vitamin D deficiency, including those with malabsorption syndromes, liver disease, malnutrition, and very little sunlight exposure, are at high risk for development of hypocalcemia. Derangements in magnesium and phosphate can also lead to hypocalcemia. Hyperphosphatemic

---

> **BOX 114.8 Most Common Causes of Hypocalcemia**
>
> Hypoalbuminemia
> Hypoparathyroidism: inherited, postsurgical, autoimmune, infiltrative
> Vitamin D deficiency and vitamin D resistance: Malabsorption syndrome, liver disease, malnutrition, sepsis, anticonvulsants, lack of sunlight exposure
> Chronic renal failure
> Hyperphosphatemia
> Hypomagnesemia
> Respiratory alkalosis
> Severe pancreatitis
> Drugs: Bisphosphonates, phenytoin, phosphate, calcitonin
> Tumor lysis syndrome
> Rhabdomyolysis

> **BOX 114.9 Five Most Common Symptomatic Causes of Hypocalcemia Seen in the Emergency Department**
>
> - Hyperventilation: Anxiety, sympathomimetics
> - Ethanol abuse, chronic malnutrition: Hypoalbuminemia
> - Massive blood transfusion
> - Toxins: Hydrofluoric acid, ethylene glycol
> - Severe pancreatitis

patients often have hypocalcemia because of phosphate's affinity to bind calcium, whereas hypomagnesemia causes end-organ resistance to parathyroid hormone and inhibits the hypocalcemic feedback loop. Patients with sepsis demonstrate hypocalcemia usually associated with hypoalbuminemia.

The most common causes of symptomatic hypocalcemia are massive blood transfusions, toxins, pancreatitis, tumor lysis syndrome, and chronic malnutrition (Box 114.9). Patients receiving massive blood transfusions are at risk for development of hypocalcemia because of citrate toxicity.[25] Rapid blood transfusions and radiocontrast dyes containing citrate infusions should be monitored closely in patients with hepatic failure, CHF, or other low-output states to avoid hypocalcemia. Trauma patients that have sustained blood loss are at risk of hypocalcemia and those that require blood transfusions are at even higher risk of profound hypocalcemia.[26]

Hypocalcemia in acute pancreatitis is caused primarily by precipitation of calcium soaps in the abdominal cavity, but glucagon-stimulated calcitonin release and decreased parathyroid hormone secretion may play a role. Toxic exposures to hydrofluoric acid and ethylene glycol can cause profound hypocalcemia secondary to their abilities to complex and chelate with calcium. Patients being treated for malignant neoplasms are at risk for development of tumor lysis syndrome and multiple secondary electrolyte abnormalities. Hypocalcemia has been attributed to the precipitation of calcium phosphate salts. Finally, one should expect to encounter hypocalcemia in malnourished patients and chronic alcoholics who present to the ED, especially alcoholics with hyperventilation due to alcohol withdrawal.

Diagnostic Testing

Most cases of hypocalcemia are discovered by clinical suspicion followed by appropriate laboratory testing. A serum calcium level less than 8.5 mg/dL or an ionized calcium level less than 2.0 mEq/L is considered diagnostic. Total serum calcium is approximately 50% free (ionized) and 50% bound, primarily to albumin; thus the serum level should be "corrected" when hypoalbuminemia exists. The ionized calcium level, which is not affected by the albumin level, is more accurate. It is best to perform the whole blood ionized calcium determination rapidly to avoid changes in chelation and pH. In select cases, a parathyroid hormone level may be sent to assist the admitting or consulting physician. Electrocardiography and cardiac monitoring are recommended in suspected hypocalcemia patients to evaluate the QT interval and to provide continuous monitoring for potential dysrhythmias. The most common ECG finding in hypocalcemia is QT prolongation as a result of ST segment lengthening and can mimic acute myocardial infarct with J point elevation, absence of ST segment, and shortening of the QTc interval.[27,28]

Management

Most asymptomatic patients and those with mild symptoms can be treated with oral calcium supplementation, such as calcium carbonate. IV calcium is administered, either as calcium chloride or calcium gluconate, to patients with moderate to severe symptoms; 100 to 300 mg of elemental calcium given over 5 to 30 minutes will raise the ionized calcium level 0.5 to 1.5 mEq. Calcium chloride contains 272 mg of elemental calcium but can be caustic to veins, so it should be given via central venous access unless patients are critically ill without central access. Calcium gluconate contains 92 mg of elemental calcium. Although this is one-third the amount contained in calcium chloride, it is safer to administer and can be given peripherally. Most patients requiring IV calcium should be admitted to the hospital for monitoring and treatment of nausea, vomiting, hypertension, and bradycardia. Patients taking digoxin have increased cardiac sensitivity to fluctuations in serum calcium, so IV calcium administration should be accompanied by continuous electrocardiographic monitoring. Hypocalcemia is an independent predictor of all-cause mortality in heart failure and chronic kidney disease patients and these patients should be monitored very carefully.[29]

Disposition

Hypocalcemic patients need to be admitted to a monitored bed if ongoing calcium repletion is necessary due to the risk of bradycardia and hypertension. Other patients may be discharged home with internal medicine follow-up and the consideration of outpatient evaluation by an endocrinologist.

HYPERMAGNESEMIA

Foundations

Hypermagnesemia is a relatively rare electrolyte abnormality defined as a serum magnesium concentration above 2.2 mg/dL. Hypermagnesemia is usually iatrogenic and seen in patients who cannot optimally regulate magnesium excretion (e.g., renal insufficiency), especially as their magnesium load increases.

In patients with normal renal function, large amounts of magnesium can be excreted daily in the stool and urine. However, in patients with impaired renal function, hypermagnesemia can be seen even with therapeutic doses of magnesium-containing products. An adult dose of 10 ounces of laxative syrup results in consumption of approximately 2.0 g of elemental magnesium per single dose. A healthy adult can excrete more than 6.0 g of magnesium daily, but renally impaired patients may not be able to tolerate small doses of laxative syrup. In patients with constipation, retention of magnesium-based laxatives can serve as a reservoir for continuous magnesium absorption.[30] Thus, a patient with renal insufficiency should be cautious and minimize the use of magnesium citrate for treatment of constipation.

TABLE 114.5 Clinical Effects of Hypermagnesemia

Effect	Level (Mg/Dl)
Decreased deep tendon reflexes	4 to 5
Hypotension	5 to 7
Respiratory insufficiency	10
Heart block	10 to 15
Cardiac arrest	10 to 24

Decreased gastrointestinal elimination and increased gastrointestinal absorption of magnesium due to intestinal hypomotility can also result in toxicity. Hypermagnesemia can be seen with bowel obstruction, colitis, gastric dilation, and use of medications that decrease motility, including narcotics and anticholinergics. Other less common causes of hypermagnesemia include adrenal insufficiency, hyperparathyroidism, hypothyroidism, lithium therapy, rhabdomyolysis, and tumor lysis syndrome.

Clinical Features

Clinical manifestations of hypermagnesemia are concentration dependent, and typically symptoms begin to develop around magnesium levels of 4 mg/dL (Table 114.5). Hypermagnesemia is easily overlooked because of its nonspecific symptoms. Patients with mild hypermagnesemia (less than 7 mg/ dL) may present with headache flushing, nausea, vomiting, and weakness. As the magnesium level rises (7 mg/ dL to 12 mg/dL), the patient may also be confused, constipated, and found to have diminished deep tendon reflexes. When serum magnesium levels rise above 7 mg/dL, patients can have signs and symptoms of hypotension, respiratory insufficiency, and heart block. Severe hypermagnesemia (greater than 12 mg/dL) presents as progressive loss of neuromuscular, respiratory, and cardiovascular functions and can lead to coma and cardiorespiratory arrest. Magnesium acts as a calcium channel blocker and also blocks potassium channels needed for repolarization. As magnesium levels rise, hypotension and electrocardiographic changes, including QRS widening and QT and PR prolongation, begin to occur. In addition, hypermagnesemia can interfere with blood clotting by interfering with clotting time and platelet adhesiveness. Finally, hypermagnesemia causes suppression of parathyroid hormone secretion and can be associated with hypocalcemia. If a patient taking oral magnesium, especially an elderly patient, presents with clinical symptoms including altered mental status, hypotension, bradycardia, and respiratory failure, hypermagnesemia must be included in the differential.

Differential Diagnosis

Hypermagnesemia is most commonly seen in patients receiving parenteral treatment for pre-eclampsia or eclampsia, cardiac arrhythmias, or asthma exacerbations. In addition, hypermagnesemia is also seen in people utilizing laxatives and antacids, patients receiving cathartics for drug overdoses, and patients undergoing bowel preparations prior to colonoscopies. Even though most patients at risk for hypermagnesemia have underlying renal impairment, hypermagnesemia has been reported in patients with normal renal function, especially in elders.[31] Box 114.10 lists the most common causes of increased serum magnesium levels.

Diagnostic Testing

Measured plasma magnesium levels often do not reflect total magnesium content, making it difficult to correlate symptoms to specific magnesium levels consistently. Although there is some question of the role of measuring ionized magnesium in patients with hypomagnesemia, only total body magnesium needs to be followed in hypermagnesemic patients.

Management

Management of hypermagnesemia is dictated by the neuromuscular, cardiovascular, and CNS changes that occur. Most stable or asymptomatic hypermagnesemic patients can be treated with cessation of their magnesium therapy. As symptoms become more pronounced, IV isotonic fluids are administered to dilute the extracellular magnesium. Diuretics (furosemide 1 mg/kg) can be used to promote excretion of magnesium in patients with normal kidney function and reverse mild symptoms.

In patients with higher levels of serum magnesium or more severe symptoms, renal consultation should be initiated immediately to arrange for dialysis with magnesium-free dialysate. A dialysis session of 3 to 4 hours can reduce the magnesium level up to 50%. IV calcium therapy to reverse magnesium toxicity should be reserved for patients with life-threatening symptoms while dialysis is being arranged. Calcium directly antagonizes the neuromuscular and cardiovascular effects of magnesium and is recommended in hypotensive patients with respiratory depression and cardiac instability. In treating life-threatening hypermagnesemia, initially administer 1 g calcium chloride or 2 g calcium gluconate and repeat as needed. When needed, a continuous infusion at 2 to 4 mg/kg/hr can be administered while dialysis is being arranged. Most stable or asymptomatic hypermagnesemia patients can be treated with cessation of their magnesium therapy and discharged home with close outpatient follow-up. However, patients with higher levels of serum magnesium or more severe symptoms, should be admitted to a telemetry bed with ICU level of care discussed with the inpatient team. Unfortunately, severe hypermagnesemia often ends in death despite robust attempts to lower serum magnesium levels.

Disposition

Most stable or asymptomatic hypermagnesemia patients can be treated with cessation of their magnesium therapy and discharged home with close outpatient follow-up. However, patients with higher levels of serum magnesium or severe symptoms should be admitted to a telemetry bed with ICU level of care discussed with the inpatient team. Unfortunately, severe hypermagnesemia often ends in death despite robust attempts to lower serum magnesium levels.

HYPOMAGNESEMIA

Foundations

Hypomagnesemia is a common electrolyte abnormality that often goes undetected. Normal serum magnesium levels range from 1.5 to 3.0 mEq/L. Symptoms of hypomagnesemia typically begin to be manifested at serum levels below 1.2 mEq/L, although symptoms are often not well correlated with the patient's serum level. This is because most of the body's magnesium is intracellular, and thus a single blood sample with a low serum magnesium level may not accurately reflect total body magnesium or the extent of true hypomagnesemia. The incidence of hypomagnesemia is estimated to be 2% in the general population. In hospitalized patients, the risk is highest for patient requiring ICU level care.[32]

Magnesium exists in three states: (1) ionized magnesium, (2) protein bound, and (3) complexed to serum anions. Even though studies show the importance of measuring ionized calcium, most research shows that ionized magnesium can be inferred from total magnesium. Currently, the clinical role of measurement of ionized magnesium is unclear, and measurement of ionized magnesium is not standard practice in the ED; there may be a role for measurement of ionized magnesium in the intensive care setting.[33,34]

Clinical Features

Determination of the clinical consequences of isolated hypomagnesemia is often confounded by coexisting hypokalemia, hypocalcemia, or hyponatremia. However, many signs and symptoms are reported to correlate with hypomagnesemia, including muscle cramping, diffuse weakness, palpitations, vertigo, ataxia, depression, and seizures. Women with an adequate intake of magnesium are less likely to be affected by preeclampsia. The clinical manifestations most likely seen in the ED involve the neuromuscular and cardiovascular systems. Patients may present with hyperactive deep tendon reflexes, muscle cramps, Trousseau and Chvostek signs, and dysarthria and dysphagia from esophageal dysmotility. Cardiac conduction abnormalities secondary to magnesium depletion, and often coexisting hypokalemia, can result in PR and QT interval prolongation. Dysrhythmias including atrial fibrillation, multifocal atrial tachycardia, premature ventricular complexes, ventricular tachycardia, torsades de pointes, and ventricular fibrillation are the most common cardiovascular manifestations of hypomagnesemia.

Differential Diagnosis

There are many causes of hypomagnesemia (Box 114.11). The following sections describe the five most common ED presentations of hypomagnesemia.

Patients Maintained on Diuretics

Patients using either loop or thiazide diuretics are at increased risk for hypomagnesemia. Both types of diuretics can inhibit magnesium reabsorption. Conversely, potassium-sparing diuretics are also magnesium sparing, because they enhance magnesium reabsorption and decrease magnesium excretion. The degree of hypomagnesemia induced by the loop and thiazide diuretics is generally mild, in part because the associated volume contraction will tend to increase proximal sodium, water, and magnesium reabsorption.

Malnourished and Alcoholic Patients

Healthy patients consume enough magnesium in green vegetables, legumes, fruits, shellfish, fresh meat, and cocoa on a regular basis to maintain normal total body magnesium stores. However, hypomagnesemia is common in patients with chronic protein-calorie malnutrition because of an associated lack of essential minerals and vitamins including magnesium. This is especially true in chronic alcoholics who may not eat foods rich in magnesium. Magnesium losses are further increased in chronic alcoholics because of alcohol's diuretic effects may combine with episodes of pancreatitis and diarrhea.

Hypomagnesemia may also be seen in patients with malabsorption disorders (celiac sprue and short bowel syndrome), patients with increased magnesium excretion (chronic diarrhea or inflammatory bowel conditions), and patients with severe body dysmorphic disorders.

Patients With Hypokalemia

Both potassium and magnesium are critical to help stabilize the membrane potential, to decrease cell excitability, and for function of the Na+, K+-ATPase pump. Approximately 50% of patients with hypokalemia also have concomitant magnesium deficiency. Increasing degrees of hypokalemia are correlated with an increasing likelihood of a magnesium deficit. Hypokalemic patients who are refractory to potassium replacement are likely to also be hypomagnesemic.

Patients With Acute Coronary Artery Disease and Ventricular Arrhythmias

There appears to be a relationship between low serum magnesium levels and the subsequent development of coronary heart disease likely because low magnesium intake is associated with higher incidence of diabetes, hypertension, and metabolic syndrome.[35] Patients who have had a myocardial infarction are more likely than controls to be hypomagnesemic.[36] Patients with acute myocardial infarction who have mild hypomagnesemia appear to have a twofold to threefold increase in the frequency of ventricular arrhythmias in the first 24 hours compared with those with normal magnesium levels

There is controversy about whether magnesium should be administered empirically after acute myocardial infarction. At present, magnesium supplementation is recommended only for those acute coronary syndrome patients who have evidence of hypokalemia, prolonged QT, or known hypomagnesemia. However, Yuksel et al. found that the serum magnesium level is an independent predictor for electrocardiographic no-reflow in patients with STEMI who underwent PCI. In addition, it was demonstrated that initial Mg level is an independent predictor for long-term mortality in patients with STEMI who underwent PCI.[37]

Dysrhythmia is the most common cardiovascular manifestation of hypomagnesemia. Magnesium affects the duration of phase 2 of the action potential, and hypomagnesemia can prolong the QT interval. Magnesium also has effects on phase 4, the resting membrane potential, where it keeps the cell more negative by stimulating the sodium-potassium pump. The exact mechanism underlying a possible association between hypomagnesemia and arrhythmias is unknown. Arrhythmias are likely to be due to concurrent hypokalemia, hypomagnesemia, or both, resulting in a prolonged QT interval and increases in spontaneous depolarization.

Patients Receiving Specific Medications

In addition to diuretics, many nephrotoxic drugs, including aminoglycosides, amphotericin B, cisplatin, digoxin, and pentamidine, can produce magnesium wasting. Solid organ transplant patients maintained on calcineurin inhibitors including tacrolimus and cyclosporine are at risk for hypomagnesemia.[38] Long-term use of proton pump inhibitors, especially when combined with diuretics, may be associated with decreased intestinal absorption of magnesium.[39,40]

Diagnostic Testing

Clinical manifestations of hypomagnesemia begin at serum levels below 1.2 mEq/L, but symptoms do not always correlate with the total serum magnesium level. Because most of the total body magnesium is intracellular, the magnesium level alone does not guide therapy. The possibility of hypomagnesemia is considered in patients with depression, malnourishment, significant or refractory hypokalemia, and ventricular arrhythmias. Electrocardiographic findings in hypomagnesemia are nonspecific and may be caused by both the hypomagnesemia and concomitant hypokalemia. Hypomagnesemia should be suspected whenever electrocardiographic findings of hypokalemia are noted, including PR and QT interval prolongation, ST segment depression, flattening and widening of the T waves, loss of voltage, and U waves.

Management

The route of magnesium repletion varies with the severity of the clinical manifestations. Patients at risk of magnesium deficiency or with symptoms consistent with hypomagnesemia should be considered for treatment even with serum magnesium levels within normal range.[41] Parenteral magnesium is recommended for life-threatening conditions. In patients with normal renal function, 1 to 2 g of IV magnesium sulfate is an appropriate loading dose. A stable patient with hypomagnesemia can be treated with a loading dose of 1 to 2 g IV of magnesium sulfate during 10 to 60 minutes, followed by a maintenance dose of 0.5 to 1 g/hr until symptoms have resolved. The administration of 1 g of IV magnesium increases the serum magnesium concentration by 0.15 mEq/L within 18 to 30 hours.[42] Patients in cardiac arrest should receive a bolus of 1 to 2 g magnesium sulfate by IV push.

Magnesium administration is strongly encouraged for patients receiving IV potassium repletion. A dose of 0.5 g/hr is safe in patients who are well hydrated and have normal renal function. There are potential adverse effects to rapid magnesium replacement at more than 1 to 2 g/hr, including decreased deep tendon reflexes, respiratory depression, and heart block. Magnesium gluconate oral supplementation can be given if the patient is only mildly hypomagnesemic and asymptomatic. Oral absorption is variable, but most commonly magnesium oxide 400 mg twice daily can be administered to patients with adequate renal function.

Disposition

Patients with cardiac arrhythmias from hypomagnesemia should be admitted to a telemetry bed or critical unit in collaboration with cardiology. Other symptomatic patients may also need to be admitted to a monitored bed for parenteral magnesium. Asymptomatic patients can often be managed with supplements and strict follow-up instructions. When preparing any patient with hypomagnesemia for discharge, physicians can encourage lifestyle changes, including adequate magnesium intake that may benefit blood pressure control, promote weight loss, and improve chronic disease risk.

HYPERPHOSPHATEMIA

Foundations

Hyperphosphatemia is defined as a serum level above 2.5 mg/dL, but it is usually clinically significant only when levels are greater than 5 mg/dL. Although rare in the general population, hyperphosphatemia is extremely common in patients with renal insufficiency or renal failure. Almost all patients with renal failure experience hyperphosphatemia at some time during the course of their disease. Phosphate is a potential biomarker to predict mortality and disease severity in patients receiving dialysis.[43] Even in patients without renal failure, patients in the ICU with altered phosphate levels have increased morbidity and mortality.[44]

Clinical Features

Patients with hyperphosphatemia may present with multiple complaints related to electrolyte abnormalities, particularly hypocalcemia. Hyperphosphatemia causes hypocalcemia by precipitating calcium out of the blood and decreasing vitamin D production. It is this secondary hypocalcemia that can cause muscle cramping, tetany, and seizures. Chronic hyperphosphatemia can also lead to metastatic calcifications in joints, tissues, and arteries.

Differential Diagnosis

Hyperphosphatemia can occur via four major pathways: (1) decreased phosphate excretion, (2) excessive phosphate intake, (3) increased renal tubular reabsorption, and (4) shift of phosphate from intracellular to extracellular space. In addition, physicians should be aware of spurious elevations in phosphate (Box 114.12).[45]

Decreased excretion of phosphate combined with excessive intake is the most common mechanism for the development of hyperphosphatemia. Excessive phosphate intake alone is an uncommon cause of hyperphosphatemia in patients with normal renal function. When patients have glomerular filtration rates below 30 mL/min, the kidneys do not excrete the full amount of ingested phosphate to maintain homeostasis.[46] Exogenous phosphate, including IV or oral phosphate administration and phosphate enemas and laxatives can cause a large burden on the kidneys if they do not have normal baseline function. In 2014, the U.S. Food and Drug Administration (FDA) made a drug safety announcement after identifying over 50 cases of adverse events warning against utilizing a single dose of sodium phosphate larger than recommended or taking more than one dose in a day, especially in patients also taking medications that act on renal function.[47]

BOX 114.12   Five Most Common Causes of Hyperphosphatemia

Decreased Phosphate Excretion
Acute and chronic renal failure

Increased Renal Tubular Reabsorption
Hypoparathyroidism
Thyrotoxicosis
Excess vitamin D administration

Excessive Phosphate Intake
Phosphate enemas or laxatives
IV or oral phosphate administration

Shift of Phosphate From Intracellular to Extracellular Space
DKA
Tumor lysis
Rhabdomyolysis

Spurious Hyperphosphatemia
Paraproteinemia
Hyperbilirubinemia
Hemolysis
Hyperlipidemia

DKA, Diabetic ketoacidosis; *IV,* intravenous.

Hypoparathyroidism, vitamin D intoxication, and thyrotoxicosis increase renal phosphate reabsorption and may cause elevated phosphate levels. Hyperphosphatemia may also occur when there is a large shift of phosphate from the intracellular to the extracellular space and the kidneys' ability to excrete phosphate is overwhelmed. This cause of hyperphosphatemia is seen in rhabdomyolysis, tumor lysis syndrome, and DKA. Hyperphosphatemia can be a spurious finding in cases of hyperproteinemia, such as multiple myeloma, hyperlipidemia, hemolysis, or hyperbilirubinemia.

Diagnostic Testing

The diagnostic evaluation of a patient with suspected hyperphosphatemia begins with obtaining electrolyte and renal function tests with hyperphosphatemia defined as a serum level above 2.5 mg/dL. A low serum calcium level along with a high phosphate level is seen in patients with hypoparathyroidism, pseudohypoparathyroidism, and renal failure. The addition of the BUN and creatinine assist with narrowing down the differential to renal failure. Patients with hyperphosphatemia from renal failure are more likely to have elevated PTH levels when compared to those with hyperphosphatemia from hypoparathyroidism where low levels of PTH are expected.

Imaging studies are not typically indicated in the initial evaluation of hyperphosphatemia in the ED setting. However, some patients may need renal imaging studies and long-bone studies when admitted to differentiate the etiology of the hyperphosphatemia further.

Management

One of the most critical steps in management of hyperphosphatemia is the treatment of underlying causes while reducing the phosphate load in the body either by promoting urinary excretion or hemodialysis. Dietary restriction alone may suffice for control of hyperphosphatemia in persons with mild renal insufficiency, but it is inadequate for control in those with overt renal failure. Because most patients presenting with severe hyperphosphatemia also have hypocalcemia, treatment focuses on the correction of both.

In patients with normal renal function, phosphate excretion can be increased by saline infusion coupled with loop diuretics. Hyperphosphatemia usually resolves in 6 to 12 hours in patients with normal renal function. In patients with hyperphosphatemia with renal failure, hemodialysis or peritoneal dialysis should be considered early in the management. Currently, phosphate control is initiated only when hyperphosphatemia occurs, but it may be beneficial to intervene earlier in patients with chronic kidney disease. The optimal method for controlling serum phosphate in patients undergoing dialysis is unknown and may involve combinations of dietary modification, phosphate binders, and enhancement of phosphate clearance through longer dialysis sessions.[48]

Disposition

Often, hyperphosphatemic patients need to be admitted to reverse the underlying etiology of their electrolyte abnormality. All patients that require hemodialysis need to be admitted to a monitored bed on a phosphate-restricted diet. Patients should also be admitted to a monitored be if they require ongoing volume resuscitation with diuresis.

HYPOPHOSPHATEMIA

Foundations

Hypophosphatemia is defined as mild (2 to 2.5 mg/dL), moderate (1 to 2 mg/dL), or severe (<1 mg/dL). Mild to moderately severe hypophosphatemia is usually asymptomatic and, like hypomagnesemia, often goes unrecognized. Although most patients remain asymptomatic,

BOX 114.13 Clinical Manifestations of Hypophosphatemia

Central Nervous System
Irritability
Confusion
Paresthesias
Depression
Dysarthria
Seizure
Coma

Cardiovascular
Cardiomyopathy
Depressed myocardial contractility
Arrhythmias

Respiratory
Acute respiratory failure
Depressed myocardial contractility

Gastrointestinal
Ileus, dysphagia

Hematologic
Depressed levels of 2,3-diphosphoglycerate and adenosine triphosphate
Leukocyte dysfunction
Hemolysis
Platelet dysfunction

Renal
Acute tubular necrosis
Metabolic acidosis
Hypercalcemia

Endocrine
Insulin resistance
Hyperparathyroidism

BOX 114.14 Five Most Common Causes of Hypophosphatemia in the Emergency Department

Decreased Intake or Increased Absorptive States
Chronic alcoholism
Home parenteral nutrition
AIDS
Chemotherapy
Vomiting
Malabsorption syndromes
Secretory diarrhea
Vitamin D deficiency

Hyperventilatory States
Sepsis
Alcohol withdrawal
Salicylate poisoning
Neuroleptic malignant syndrome
Panic attacks
DKA
Hepatic coma

Hormonal and Endocrine Effects
Insulin loading
Glucose loading
Exogenous epinephrine
Hyperparathyroidism

Medications
Diuretics
Chronic antacid ingestion
Steroids
Phosphate binders
Xanthine derivatives
Beta2-agonists
Iron[49]

Disease States
Trauma
Severe thermal burns
Acute renal failure
Gout
Cannabinoid hyperemesis syndrome[50]

AIDS, Acquired immunodeficiency syndrome; *DKA*, diabetic ketoacidosis.

severe hypophosphatemia may result in potentially life-threatening complications. Major clinical sequelae usually occur only in severe hypophosphatemia. Symptoms of hypophosphatemia typically begin to be manifested at serum levels below 1.0 mg/dL.

Clinical Features

Mild to moderate hypophosphatemia is usually asymptomatic, but major clinical manifestations can occur with severe hypophosphatemia. Because phosphate is an essential component to adenosine triphosphate, hypophosphatemia can affect a variety of organ systems and a wide variety of symptoms (Box 114.13). Patients with hypophosphatemia may present with nonspecific complaints including joint pain, myalgias, irritability, and depression. Severe hypophosphatemia can be manifested as seizures, arrhythmias, cardiomyopathy, insulin resistance, acute tubular necrosis, rhabdomyolysis, and acute respiratory failure.

Differential Diagnosis

Hypophosphatemia is must commonly induced by one of the three causes: (1) Increased phosphate excretion, (2) inadequate phosphate intake, or (3) a shift in phosphate stores. Acute hypophosphatemia is most commonly due to a rapid intracellular shift. Hyperventilation, glucose, insulin, volume expansion, and resolving acidosis can lead to hypophosphatemia by rapid intracellular shift. The many causes of hypophosphatemia include decreased phosphate intake or increased absorptive states, hyperventilatory states, hormonal and endocrine effects, medications, and disease states (Box 114.14). The ED patients most likely to have hypophosphatemia are those who are malnourished with alcohol withdrawal, acute hyperventilation, or sepsis and patients with DKA or alcohol ketoacidosis in whom reintroduction of insulin and glucose causes phosphate uptake into cells.

Diagnostic Testing

The diagnostic evaluation of a patient with suspected hypophosphatemia begins with obtaining electrolyte and renal function tests with hypophosphatemia defined as a serum level below 2.5 mg/dL. Often, the etiology of hypophosphatemia can be determined by the history. However, if the etiology is unclear, the patient may need to have a renal phosphate excretion measured or calculated upon admission. Imaging in hyperphosphatemia is rarely indicated unless there are confounding cardiac, neurologic, or respiratory factors.

Management

We recommend patients with phosphate levels below 2.0 mg/dL be given phosphate repletion; patients with levels below 1.0 mg/dL necessitate treatment. Because hypophosphatemia is often coupled with hypokalemia, patients with hypophosphatemia often require potassium repletion as well. Oral phosphorous, 250 to 500 mg twice daily, can be given to stable or asymptomatic patients. IV preparations are available as sodium phosphate (Na_2PO_4 and $NaPO_4$) or potassium phosphate (K_2PO_4 and KPO_4), and rate of infusion and choice of initial dosage should be based on severity of hypophosphatemia and presence of symptoms.

If the serum phosphorus concentration is less than 1.5 mg/dL (0.48 mmol/L), 1.3 mmol/kg of elemental phosphorous (up to a maximum of 100 mmol) can be given in three or four divided doses in a 24-hour period. For routine replacement, give 0.5 mL/hr K_2PO_4; this may be increased to 1 mL/hr in severely symptomatic patients. Each milliliter of K_2PO_4 contains 3 mmol of phosphorus and 4.4 mEq of potassium.

Typical replacement therapy provides approximately 1 g of phosphorus per day. Patients should be monitored for the development of hypocalcemia, hyperkalemia, and hyperphosphatemia while IV phosphate is administered, especially in patients with renal insufficiency. Patients with DKA are initially hypophosphatemic. However, no studies have shown significant benefit to routine phosphate therapy in DKA. Risks of routine treatment with phosphate include hyperphosphatemia, renal failure, hypocalcemia, and hypomagnesemia. In patients with severe malnutrition or significant hypophosphatemia, replacement can be considered, but more than 60 mmol/day should not be administered without reason.

Disposition

Mild asymptomatic hypophosphatemia can be treated with oral phosphate while patients with severe or symptomatic hypophosphatemia should be treated with IV phosphate therapy and admitted for monitoring and subsequent serum electrolyte testing. In general, all symptomatic patients need treatment with phosphate. The outlook for patients depends on the primary condition causing the hypophosphatemia.

The references for this chapter can be found online at ExpertConsult.com.

115

Diabetes Mellitus and Disorders of Glucose Homeostasis

Gerald E. Maloney Jr. and Jonathan M. Glauser

KEY CONCEPTS

- The diagnosis of diabetes can be determined by one or more of four methods—random plasma glucose level above 200 mg/dL, fasting plasma glucose concentration above 126 mg/dL, 2-hour, 75-g post-load oral glucose tolerance test (OGTT) > 200 mg/dL, or HbA_{1c} value above 6.5%.
- Diabetic ketoacidosis (DKA) is diagnosed by the presence of hyperglycemia, anion gap metabolic acidosis, and elevated ketoacid levels.
- The essential treatment of DKA includes administration of insulin, correction of dehydration, correction of potassium level, correction of acidosis, and treatment of the underlying cause.
- The use of sodium bicarbonate to correct acidosis in DKA has not demonstrated any benefit and may be associated with worse outcomes.
- A hyperglycemic hyperosmolar state is usually seen in older adults with multiple comorbid conditions and is distinguished from DKA by the absence of ketoacidosis. In addition to fluid resuscitation and correction of hyperglycemia, treatment should address the underlying cause of the state, which includes infection, myocardial infarction, and cerebrovascular accident.
- Diabetic peripheral neuropathy is common and has multiple treatment options, including gabapentin, pregabalin, and duloxetine.
- Diabetic foot ulcers and other diabetic soft-tissue infections (e.g., gas gangrene, Fournier's gangrene) are frequently polymicrobial and require broad-spectrum antibiotic therapy covering gram-positives, gram-negatives, and anaerobes.
- Hypoglycemia may be associated with significant morbidity and mortality. When the diagnosis is suggested and, if possible, confirmed by laboratory evaluation, therapy should be initiated immediately.
- Hypoglycemia caused by sulfonylurea oral hypoglycemic agents may be prolonged. Patients should be observed for an extended period or hospitalized.

DIABETES MELLITUS

Diabetes Mellitus Foundations

Background and Importance

Diabetes mellitus is the most common endocrine disease. It comprises a heterogeneous group of hyperglycemic disorders characterized by a high serum glucose concentration and disturbances of carbohydrate and lipid metabolism. Acute complications include hypoglycemia and hyperglycemia, diabetic ketoacidosis (DKA), and hyperglycemic hyperosmolar state (HHS). Long-term complications affect multiple organ systems through involvement of the microvasculature and include retinopathy, nephropathy, neuropathy, and angiopathy. As a result, complications such as coronary and cerebral vascular disease, blindness, chronic kidney disease, complicated infections, and amputations occur with a much higher incidence in patients with diabetes than in patients without. Diabetes is ranked as one of the five major chronic diseases that account for a significant proportion of our health care spending. Several trials have shown to varying degrees that tight glucose control can reduce the risk of death and severe microvascular complications. Patients with diabetes mellitus incur emergency department (ED) costs three times higher than those of nondiabetic patients and are admitted to the hospital four times more often.[1,2]

Epidemiology

The most recent data (2015) estimate that some 30 million people, or 9.4% of all Americans and 13% of adults older than 20 years have diabetes.[1] The incidence of diabetes in those younger than 20 approaches as high as 45/100,000 by the teenage years. The type of diabetes depends on age; most of those younger than 10 years have type 1, whereas type 2 predominates among the 10- to 19-year-olds.[2] Additionally, 33% of the total US population is thought to have prediabetes.

Type 1 is less common than type 2. The peak age at onset of type 1 diabetes is 10 to 14 years, and approximately 1 of every 600 schoolchildren has this disease. In the United States, the prevalence of type 1 is approximately 0.26% by the age of 20 years, and the lifetime prevalence approaches 0.4%. The annual incidence among persons from birth to 16 years of age in the United States is 12 to 14 per 1 million population. The incidence is age-dependent, increasing from near-absence during infancy to a peak occurrence at puberty and another small peak at midlife.[1,2]

The morbidity of diabetes is related primarily to its vascular complications. A mortality rate of 36.8% has been attributed to cardiovascular causes, 17.5% to cerebrovascular causes, 15.5% to diabetic comas, and 12.5% to renal failure.

Anatomy, Physiology, and Pathophysiology

Normal Physiology. Because plasma glucose is the predominant metabolic fuel used by the central nervous system (CNS), maintenance of the plasma glucose concentration is critical to survival. The CNS cannot synthesize glucose, store more than a few minutes' supply, or concentrate glucose from the circulation. Brief hypoglycemia can cause profound CNS dysfunction, and prolonged severe hypoglycemia may cause cellular death. Glucose regulatory systems have evolved to prevent and correct hypoglycemia.

The plasma glucose concentration is normally maintained within a relatively narrow range, between 60 and 150 mg/dL, despite wide variations in glucose levels after meals and exercise. Glucose is derived from three sources—intestinal absorption from the diet, the breakdown of glycogen (glycogenolysis), and the formation of glucose from precursors (gluconeogenesis), including lactate, pyruvate, amino acids, and glycerol. After glucose ingestion, the plasma glucose concentration increases as a result of glucose absorption. Endogenous glucose production is suppressed, and the plasma glucose level rapidly declines in response to insulin to a level below the baseline.

Insulin. Insulin receptors on the beta cells of the pancreas sense elevations in the blood glucose concentration and trigger insulin release. For incompletely understood reasons, glucose taken orally results in more insulin release than parenteral glucose. Certain amino acids induce insulin release and even cause hypoglycemia in some patients. Sulfonylurea oral hypoglycemic agents work, in part, by stimulating the release of insulin from the pancreas.

The number of receptors determines the sensitivity of the specific tissue to circulating insulin. The number and sensitivity of receptors are also the primary factors affecting the long-term efficacy of the sulfonylurea oral hypoglycemic agents. Receptor sites are increased in glucocorticoid deficiency and may be relatively decreased in obese patients.

Under normal circumstances, insulin is rapidly degraded through the liver and kidneys. The half-life of insulin is 3 to 10 minutes. Whereas insulin is the major anabolic hormone implicated in diabetes, glucagon is the major catabolic hormone in disorders of glucose homeostasis.

Although most tissues have the enzyme systems required to synthesize and hydrolyze glycogen, only the liver and kidneys have glucose-6-phosphatase, the enzyme necessary to release glucose into the circulation. The liver is essentially the sole source of endogenous glucose production. Renal gluconeogenesis and glucose release contribute substantially to the systemic glucose pool only during prolonged starvation.

Glucose Regulatory Mechanisms. Maintenance of the normal plasma glucose concentration requires precise matching of glucose use with endogenous glucose production and dietary glucose intake. The regulatory mechanisms that maintain systemic glucose balance involve hormonal, neurohumoral, and autoregulatory factors. Glucose regulatory hormones include insulin, glucagon, epinephrine, cortisol, and growth hormone. Insulin is the main glucose-lowering hormone. Insulin suppresses endogenous glucose production and stimulates glucose use. Insulin is secreted from the beta cells of the pancreatic islets into the hepatic portal circulation and has important actions on the liver and peripheral tissues. Insulin stimulates glucose uptake and storage, and it is used by other insulin-sensitive tissues, such as fat and muscle.

Counterregulatory hormones include glucagon, epinephrine, norepinephrine, growth hormone, and cortisol. When glucose is not transported intracellularly because of a lack of food intake or lack of insulin, the body perceives a fasting state and releases glucagon, attempting to provide the glucose necessary for brain function. Glucagon is released in response to hypoglycemia as well as to stress, trauma, infection, exercise, and starvation. It increases hepatic glucose production within minutes, although transiently.

Epinephrine both stimulates hepatic glucose production and limits glucose use through direct and indirect actions mediated by α-adrenergic and β-adrenergic mechanisms. Epinephrine also acts directly to increase hepatic glycogenolysis and gluconeogenesis. It acts within minutes and produces a transient increase in glucose production but continues to support glucose production at approximately basal levels thereafter. Norepinephrine exerts hyperglycemic actions by mechanisms similar to those of epinephrine, except that norepinephrine is released from axon terminals of sympathetic postganglionic neurons.

Cortisol is released in response to stress, and it increases blood glucose by both increasing hepatic gluconeogenesis and inhibiting skeletal muscle uptake of glucose. These mechanisms contribute to the hyperglycemia seen during physiologic stress or illness.

Pathophysiology. Type 1 diabetes results from a chronic autoimmune process that usually exists in a preclinical state for years. The classic manifestations of type 1 diabetes—hyperglycemia and ketoacidosis—occur late in the disease, an overt sign of beta-cell destruction. The most striking feature of long-standing type 1 diabetes is the nearly total lack of insulin-secreting beta cells and insulin, with the preservation of glucagon-secreting alpha cells, somatostatin-secreting delta cells, and pancreatic polypeptide–secreting cells.[3]

Although the exact cause of diabetes remains unclear, research has provided some clues. Studies of the pathogenesis of diabetes mellitus have demonstrated that the cause of the disordered glucose homeostasis varies from individual to individual. This cause may determine the presentation in each patient. Individual patients are currently not studied for the source of their disease, except on an experimental basis. The goals of ongoing research are to identify who is susceptible to the development of diabetes, prevent diabetic emergencies and sequelae, and prevent expression of the disease.

Types of Diabetes

The American Diabetes Association (ADA) defines four major types of diabetes mellitus: type 1 diabetes mellitus, type 2 diabetes mellitus, gestational diabetes, and diabetes due to secondary disease processes or drugs.[1,4] Additionally, the diagnostic criteria of prediabetes was established for patients with glucose levels above the normal fasting range of 110 mg/dL but less than 126 mg/dL; this category has received much attention for the targeting of focused interventions to reduce progression to diabetes mellitus.[1] The 1997 National Diabetes Data Group discontinued the use of the terms *insulin-dependent diabetes mellitus* and *non-insulin-dependent diabetes mellitus* because they were confusing and clinically inaccurate. The most recent update to the standards of care for diabetes was published in January 2021.[1] The diagnostic criteria for the diagnosis of diabetes were changed in 2010 from the previous standards of elevated fasting glucose concentration and an abnormal result on the 2-hour oral glucose tolerance test (OGTT) to use of the hemoglobin A_{1c} (HbA_{1c}) value as the preferred confirmatory test.[4] A HbA_{1c} value above 6.5% is diagnostic of diabetes. However, the fasting plasma glucose concentration and 2-hour OGTT are still considered valid screening tests for diabetes, as is the presence of a random glucose measurement of more than 200 mg/dL in a non-fasting patient with symptoms of diabetes. Use of the fasting plasma glucose concentration may help identify patients at risk for diabetes when the glucose concentration is elevated but does not meet the threshold for the diagnosis of diabetes.

Type 1 Diabetes Mellitus. Type 1 diabetes is characterized by an abrupt failure of insulin production with a tendency to ketosis, even in the basal state. Parenteral insulin is required to sustain life. From 85% to 90% of patients with type 1 diabetes demonstrate evidence of one or more autoantibodies implicated in the cell-mediated autoimmune destruction of the beta cells of the pancreas. The autoimmune destruction has multiple genetic predispositions and may be related to undefined environmental insults.

Type 2 Diabetes Mellitus. Patients with type 2 diabetes may remain asymptomatic for long periods and show low, normal, or elevated levels of insulin. Ketosis is rare in type 2 disease. Patients frequently have hypertriglyceridemia and a high incidence of obesity. No association exists with viral infections, islet cell autoantibodies, or human leukocyte antigen (HLA) expression. Hyperinsulinemia may be related to peripheral tissue resistance to insulin because of defects in the insulin receptor. Defects in muscle glycogen synthesis have an important role in insulin resistance.

Gestational Diabetes. Gestational diabetes mellitus is characterized by an abnormal OGTT result that occurs during pregnancy and reverts to normal during the postpartum period or remains abnormal. The clinical pathogenesis is thought to be similar to that of type 2. The clinical presentation is usually nonketotic hyperglycemia during pregnancy. Screening is performed around the 24th to 28th week with a 75-g oral glucose load in a woman with no prior history of diabetes.[4]

Diabetes of Other Causes. Myriad causes of diabetes have been identified, including chronic pancreatitis, cystic fibrosis, genetic defects in the beta cell or in insulin receptors, and chemical-induced (e.g., Vacor; statins; chemotherapeutic, antipsychotic, or antiretroviral medications). The management of diabetes due to these conditions is cause-specific and depends on whether the underlying pathophysiologic process more closely resembles type 1 or 2 diabetes.[3]

Prediabetes. Impaired glucose tolerance (IGT) has been replaced by the term *prediabetes* to identify individuals at high risk for the development of diabetes.[4] The pathogenesis of prediabetes is thought to be related to insulin resistance. This group is composed of persons whose plasma glucose levels are between normal and diabetic; they are at increased risk for diabetes and cardiovascular disease. Prediabetes encompasses patients with both impaired fasting glucose (110 to 125 mg/dL) or IGT (level of 140 to 199 mg/dL after a 75 g oral glucose load). Presentations of prediabetes include nonketotic hyperglycemia, insulin resistance, hyperinsulinism, and often obesity. Prediabetes is not associated with the same degree of complications of diabetes mellitus, and many of these patients have normal glucose tolerance. However, each year, about 1% to 5% of patients with prediabetes will develop diabetes mellitus.[4]

Diabetes Mellitus Clinical Features

Type 1

The patient with type 1 diabetes is usually lean, younger than 40 years at diagnosis, and prone to ketosis. Plasma insulin levels are absent to low; plasma glucagon levels are high but suppressible with insulin, and patients require insulin therapy to treat their symptoms. The onset of symptoms may be abrupt, with polydipsia, polyuria, polyphagia, and weight loss developing rapidly. In some cases, the disease is heralded by ketoacidosis. Myriad problems related to type 1 diabetes may prompt an ED visit, including acute metabolic complications, such as DKA, and late complications, such as cardiovascular or circulatory abnormalities, retinopathy, nephropathy, neuropathy, foot ulcers, severe infections, and various skin lesions.

Type 2

The patient with type 2 diabetes is usually middle-aged or older and overweight, with normal to high insulin levels. Insulin levels are lower than would be predicted for glucose levels, however, leading to a relative insulin deficiency. Type 2 patients demonstrate impaired insulin function related to poor insulin production, failure of insulin to reach the site of action, or failure of an end-organ response to insulin. Although most adult patients with type 2 are obese, 20% are not.

Symptoms in type 2 diabetes tend to begin more gradually than in type 1. The diagnosis of type 2 is often made by the discovery of an elevated blood glucose level on routine laboratory examination. Hyperglycemia may be controlled by dietary therapy, oral hypoglycemic agents, or insulin administration. Decompensation of the disease usually leads to HHS rather than to ketoacidosis.

Diabetes Mellitus Differential Diagnosis

The differential diagnosis for diabetes includes hyperglycemia due to physiologic stress, catecholamine release, or certain toxins. Calcium channel blocker overdose has been known to cause insulin resistance and thus present with both significant hyperglycemia and metabolic acidosis. The rodenticide PNU (vacor), which destroys the pancreatic islet cells,

can induce a diabetes-like state. Patients with prediabetes may exhibit frank hyperglycemia with a large carbohydrate load or physiologic stress.

Diabetes Mellitus Diagnostic Testing

Serum Glucose Level

The diagnosis of diabetes can be established in one or more of four ways—random plasma glucose level above 200 mg/dL, fasting plasma glucose concentration above 126 mg/dL, 2-hour, 75-g postload OGTT higher than 200 mg/dL, or HbA_{1c} value above 6.5%.[4] In the absence of hyperglycemia with metabolic decompensation, these criteria should be confirmed by repeated testing on a different day. Confirmation can be made by the same test or two different tests (e.g., fasting plasma glucose and HbA_{1c}). A fasting value above 150 mg/dL is likely to distinguish diabetic from nondiabetic patients more accurately. Formal OGTTs are unnecessary except during pregnancy or in patients who are thought to have diabetes, but who do not meet the criteria for a particular classification. The World Health Organization and ADA have provided protocols for performing the OGTT.[4]

Glycosylated Hemoglobin

Measurement of glycosylated hemoglobin (HbA_{1c}) is one of the most important ways to assess the level of glucose control. An elevated serum glucose level binds progressively and irreversibly to the amino-terminal valine of the hemoglobin β chain. The HbA_{1c} measurement provides insight into the quality of glycemic control over time. Given the long half-life of red blood cells, the percentage of HbA_{1c} is an index of glucose concentration of the preceding 6 to 8 weeks, with normal values approximately 4% to 6% of total hemoglobin, depending on the assay used. Levels in patients with poorly controlled disease may reach 10% to 12%. The ADA has recommended at least biannual measurements of HbA_{1c} for the follow-up of all types of diabetes. The ADA currently sets an HbA_{1c} value of less than 7% as a treatment goal. Different medical societies have advocated for patient-specific A_{1c} goals, particularly in the elderly, who are more prone to adverse effects from hypoglycemia resulting from attempts at tight glucose control.[5,6] For functionally independent older adults, the HbA_{1c} goal is 7% to 7.5%, and 7% to 8% is recommended for functionally dependent, frail patients, or patients with dementia.[5]

Urine Glucose Level

Urine glucose measurement methods are of two types, reagent tests and dipstick tests. The reagent tests (e.g., Clinitest) are copper reduction tests. The reagent tests are rarely used because they are difficult to perform, and the test material is toxic for ingestion or dermal exposure. Dipstick tests generally use glucose oxidase, which may also be affected by different substances. Dipsticks are inexpensive and convenient but may vary in their sensitivity and strength of reaction to a given concentration of glucose. Dipstick interpretation can vary significantly, depending on the observer and type of lighting. Both falsely high and falsely low urine glucose readings can also occur. With the plus system, 1+, 2+, 3+, and 4+ have different implications about urine glucose concentrations, depending on the brand of the dipstick. The use of reflectance colorimeters to read dipsticks increases accuracy.

Urine Ketone Level

Urine ketone dipsticks use the nitroprusside reaction, which test for acetoacetate but does not measure β-hydroxybutyrate. Although the usual ratio of acetoacetate to β-hydroxybutyrate in DKA is 1:2.8, it may be as high as 1:30, and in which case, the urine dipstick does not reflect the true level of ketosis. When ketones are in the form of β-hydroxybutyrate, the urine ketone dipstick may infrequently yield a negative reaction in patients with significant ketosis.

Dipstick Blood Glucose Level

Dipsticks for testing the blood glucose level are clearly more accurate than urine dipsticks as a means of monitoring blood glucose concentration, but they also may be inaccurate. Hematocrits below 30% or above 55% cause inaccurately high or low readings, respectively, and a number of the strips specifically disclaim accuracy when used for neonates. The sensitivity of dipsticks to a variety of factors varies with the particular brand. The largest errors are in the hyperglycemic range. Dipstick readings rarely err more than 30 mg/dL when the actual concentration is below 90 mg/dL. Although specific glucose concentrations may not be accurately represented, blood glucose dipsticks are useful for estimating the general range of the glucose value. Reflectance meters increase the accuracy of the dipstick blood glucose level determination. The use of glucometers has supplanted the use of dipsticks in most clinical settings and tends to be fairly accurate, except, again, at the extremes of glucose levels (<30 or >600 mg/dL). If maximum accuracy is desired, a laboratory blood glucose level should be determined.

Diabetes Mellitus Management

Management of Hyperglycemia

Patients often present to the ED with typical diabetic symptoms, such as polyuria, polydipsia, and polyphagia. Many have serum glucose concentrations above 200 mg/dL but are not ketotic. Patients with newly diagnosed hyperglycemia with normal electrolyte values may be treated with intravenous (IV) hydration alone or with insulin, often reducing the glucose concentration to 150 mg/dL. In reliable patients whose initial glucose concentration is greater than 400 mg/dL, initiation of oral hypoglycemic therapy may be appropriate, with lifestyle modification and coordination with a clinician who will provide longitudinal care. An HbA$_{1c}$ value should be obtained before initiation of therapy to confirm a diagnosis of diabetes and to establish a baseline.

Detailed descriptions of oral hypoglycemics are provided below, but considerations for ED initiation in acute hyperglycemia are listed here. Initial therapy for type 2 diabetes generally includes metformin at a dose of 500 mg daily or twice daily depending on immediate or extended-release formulation. The extended-release formulation may be better tolerated in terms of GI side effects. Sulfonylurea therapy may be considered as well, with glyburide (2.5 to 5 mg once daily) or glipizide (5 mg once daily).[5-7] Patients with kidney disease may have complications from the use of a sulfonylurea or metformin and will likely need insulin therapy with or without a glucagon-like peptide-1 receptor agonist. Patients with heart failure or less severe renal disease might benefit from a sodium/glucose cotransporter-2 inhibitor (SGLT-2).[8-10] Recent studies have shown a mortality benefit to canagliflozin and empagliflozin. If possible, diabetic testing supplies should be given and patients should be taught how to test blood glucose prior to discharge. No target blood glucose level needs to be achieved for safe discharge; observational studies showed no difference in short-term outcomes whether a specific glucose target was achieved or not. Follow-up should be stressed and warning signs of hypoglycemia discussed.

Management of Diabetes Mellitus

Although emergency clinicians do not routinely provide longitudinal care for diabetic patients, these patients frequently present to the ED, and it is helpful to understand fundamental management principles of this important disease. The basic concepts of the diabetic diet remain unchanged, although many studies emphasize foods and medications that alter glucose absorption. Various high-fiber diets have improved glycemic control. The number of supplements or low–glycemic index snacks has risen in the last decade. Exercise continues to be a cornerstone of diabetes management, although care must be taken to balance it with appropriate calorie intake and medication use.

Oral Hypoglycemic Agents. Goals of diabetic management include lowering the hemoglobin A$_{1c}$ to less than 7% and maintenance of the fasting blood sugar level to within 90 to 130 mg/dL. When started on monotherapy, after 3 years, approximately 50% of patients need a second drug. There have been an increasing number of oral agents for hyperglycemia available in recent years. (Table 115.1) Some of these have serious side effects, requiring the emergency clinician to be familiar with these drugs. If these effects are expected to be prolonged, the patient may require observation. Categories of oral agents may be divided into those that increase the insulin supply, including sulfonylureas, secretagogues, and insulin itself. Medications that decrease insulin resistance include the biguanides and thiazolidinediones; drugs that reduce the rate of glucose absorption include α-glucosidase inhibitors. Metformin is generally used as the first-line agent for oral therapy. If the goal of lower HbA$_{1c}$ levels is not achieved, the addition of a sulfonylurea or pioglitazone should be considered.[8]

Biguanides. The ADA and European Association for the Study of Diabetes have recommended lifestyle changes, including weight control, at the time of diabetes diagnosis. Metformin (a biguanide) is the initial drug of choice because it does not induce weight gain, has low cost and good tolerability, and does not induce hypoglycemia. However, it lowers blood glucose by only about 100 mg/dL and lowers HbA$_{1c}$ by approximately 1.5%. Newly diagnosed diabetics frequently require additional agents to control their serum glucose and to lower their HbA1c levels.[8]

Metformin is renally excreted and should not be used with a glomerular filtration rate (GFR) < 30. The Food and Drug Administration (FDA) also recommends not starting metformin in patients with a GFR of 30 to 45, though increased rates of adverse events were not noted in this group.[8] Metabolic and lactic acidosis are a concern with biguanides. Historically, holding metformin after IV contrast and rechecking renal function before restarting has been advocated. However, evidence has failed to show the necessity of this approach for most patients. Patients with existing kidney disease, or those with dehydration or hypoperfusion, should probably have metformin held after IV contrast. There is no clear evidence to support holding metformin

TABLE 115.1	Common Oral Diabetic Medications	
Medication	**Function**	**Details**
Biguanides (metformin)	Decrease hepatic glycogenolysis	500–1000 mg daily or bid
Sulfonylureas (glipizide, glimepiride)	Stimulate pancreatic insulin release	2.5–5 mg daily or bid
Thiazolidinediones (pioglitazone, rosiglitazone)	Insulin sensitizers, decrease hepatic gluconeogenesis	Increased risk of adverse cardiac events
Meglitinides (repaglinide, nateglinide)	Stimulate postprandial insulin release	Take with meals only
Dipeptidyl peptidase 4 inhibitors (sitagliptin)	Decrease insulin degradation and gluconeogenesis	Once daily; can be found in multiple combination medications
α-Glucosidase inhibitors (acarbose, miglitol)	Delay breakdown of carbohydrates in the intestines	Major side effect is diarrhea

routinely for all patients. Metformin must be used with caution in patients with hypoxemia, pregnancy, heart failure, liver compromise, and alcohol abuse. These patients may be at increased risk for developing lactic acidosis, associated with a 50% mortality rate.[11]

Sulfonylureas. Developed in the 1940s, sulfonylureas have historically been a mainstay of oral diabetes treatment. These drugs increase insulin secretion by interacting with potassium channels in the beta cell membrane. This class of drugs is especially useful for patients with early-onset, type 2 diabetes mellitus, and fasting blood glucose levels less than 300 mg/dL. This class of drugs is contraindicated in patients with a known allergy to sulfa agents. Examples of sulfonylureas include glipizide (Glucotrol, Glucotrol XL), glimepiride (Amaryl), gliclazide (Diamicron), chlorpropamide (Diabinese), and glyburide (DiaBeta, Glynase PresTab, Micronase). The risk of hypoglycemia is greater in older adults and in those with impaired renal and hepatic function. This class of medication is also associated with weight gain. They generally lower the glucose level by 20%, and HbA_{1c} levels by 1% to 2%. Glipizide is shorter acting and therefore less likely than the other sulfonylureas to induce prolonged hypoglycemia. However, for all sulfonylureas, there have been several case reports of delayed onset of hypoglycemia from 12 to 21 hours after ingestion, leading to general recommendations to observe the patient for a 24-hour period. In addition to providing glucose, hypoglycemia due to sulfonylureas may be treated with octreotide, although the data supporting this recommendation is limited.

Thiazolidinediones. Thiazolidinediones reduce insulin resistance and are especially useful in patients who require large amounts of insulin and still lack adequate glucose control. They have been associated with hepatotoxicity and require liver function monitoring for at least 1 year after initiation. Due to its hepatotoxic effects, troglitazone has been removed from the market; pioglitazone (Actos) and rosiglitazone (Avandia) remain approved for monotherapy. Cardiovascular risks, including myocardial infarction, may be higher with rosiglitazone. These agents may also be associated with weight gain, fluid retention, and heart failure. They increase insulin sensitivity and may be expected to reduce the HbA_{1c} value by 0.5 to 1.4 points. They are contraindicated for patients with New York Heart Association class III or IV heart failure.[12]

α-Glucosidase Inhibitors. The *α-glucosidase inhibitors* delay intestinal monosaccharide absorption and prevent complex carbohydrate breakdown; these agents include acarbose (Precose and generic) and miglitol (Glyset). They must be titrated to minimize gastrointestinal (GI) side effects and should not be used in patients with certain GI disorders. Liver function must be monitored because of dose-dependent hepatotoxicity. The *α-glucosidase inhibitor* should be taken with meals because they delay the absorption of glucose. Side effects include abdominal pain, diarrhea, and flatulence from unabsorbed carbohydrates. They lower the $HgbA_{1c}$ by 0.5 to 0.8 points.

Meglitinides. The nonsulfonylurea secretagogues, the meglitinides, are similar to the sulfonylureas in action and mechanism. They bind to adenosine triphosphate (ATP)–sensitive potassium channels of beta cells to increase insulin secretion. They have a rapid onset of action and should be taken before a meal, involve less risk of hypoglycemia, and are suitable for patients allergic to sulfa medications. The specific agents available are nateglinide (Starlix) and repaglinide (Prandin). These may be better for patients with impaired renal function due to their hepatic metabolism. Similar to the management of refractory hypoglycemia with sulfonylureas, hypoglycemia due to meglitinides may be treated with octreotide by bolus or infusion.

Glucagon-Like Peptide Analogs and Agonists. Glucagon-like peptide (GLP-1) analogs and agonists stimulate the release of insulin from pancreatic cells. Exenatide (Byetta) is US FDA–approved for twice-daily subcutaneous injection in patients with type 2 diabetes who have not achieved satisfactory control with metformin, a sulfonylurea, pioglitazone, or lifestyle modifications. It lowers serum glucagon concentrations and slows gastric emptying. These agents should be used with caution if gastroparesis is a concern. Exenatide lowers HbA_{1c} by 1 to 1.5 points, even when administered once weekly.

GLP itself has a half-life of only a few minutes. The GLP agonists bind to the GLP receptor on the pancreas and have a much longer half-life. This class also includes the subcutaneously administered medications Liraglutide (Victoza), semaglutide (Ozempic), and lixisenatide. Recently, an oral version of semaglutide (Rybelsus) was approved by the FDA for once daily use. GLP-1 receptor antagonists have the following potential adverse effects: nausea, vomiting, diarrhea, renal impairment, pancreatitis, and thyroid carcinoma, with a warning against use if there is a personal or family history of medullary thyroid cancer. They have been associated with weight loss and may decrease hospitalization for heart failure.[9,10,13] Clinical experience with their toxicology is limited, but there have been episodes of hypoglycemia reported. Observation recommendations for hypoglycemia are not established, but, given the long half-life of the medications, we recommend a period of at least 24 hours.

Dipeptidyl Peptidase-4 Inhibitors. Dipeptidyl peptidase-4 (DPP-4) inhibitors include sitagliptin (Januvia), saxagliptin (Onglyza), and linagliptin (Tradjenta). DPP-4 degrades endogenous GLP; by preventing this degradation, the DPP-4 inhibitors prolong the half-life of GLP and increase insulin secretion. These are generally used as second- or third-line agents. Sitagliptin is FDA approved as monotherapy, but it is also available in combination with other oral hypoglycemic medications. Patients with chronic kidney disease may be at risk for hypoglycemia and should be treated symptomatically. DPP-4 inhibitors inhibit glucagon release and delay gastric emptying, and they are associated with a possible risk of pancreatitis.[10] Agents in the DPP-4 inhibitor class have not been associated with weight gain. They may be expected to produce a decrease in the HbA_{1c} of 0.4 to 0.8 points.

Amylin Analog. Pramlintide, administered three times daily before meals, is an amylinomimetic agent, or amylin analog, and decreases gastric emptying and glucagon secretion. It has been approved for use in patients with types 1 and 2 diabetes and may promote weight loss.

Sodium-Glucose Cotransporter 2 Inhibitors. Dapagliflozin (Farxiga), canagliflozin (Invokana), and empagliflozin (Jardiance) are sodium-glucose cotransporter 2 (SGLT2) inhibitors. Canagliflozin and empagliflozin have been FDA approved for cardiovascular risk reduction in patients with type 2 diabetes and established cardiovascular disease.[14] SGLT2 is a protein that transports filtered glucose from the proximal renal tubule into tubular epithelial cells, enhancing urinary excretion levels of glucose.[9] The typical threshold for urinary glucose excretion is typically a plasma glucose level of ~180 mg/dL the SGLT2 inhibitors decrease this threshold to ~40 mg/dL, markedly increasing urinary glucose excretion. They may also lower blood pressure and induce some degree of weight loss, possibly due to the loss of calories from glycosuria.[9]

SGLT2 inhibitors have been shown to reduce hospitalization for heart failure in people with diabetes, may reduce cardiovascular events, reduce albuminuria, and slow the progression of nephropathy.[9,10] Adverse events include hypotension, volume depletion, urinary and genital mycotic infections, and diabetic ketoacidosis, including normoglycemic DKA.

Insulin. Certain principles apply to all insulins, such as their ability to enhance gluconeogenesis and lipogenesis and suppress glycogenolysis. Human insulins are available today as regular insulin and neutral protamine hagedorn (NPH). Regular insulin, used in the treatment of DKA, has an onset of action within 30 to 60 minutes and is typically dosed 30 to 45 minutes before a meal. Its duration of action is approximately 4 to 12 hours. The longer-acting NPH insulin (e.g., Humulin, Novolin) is typically dosed 4 to 6 hours before a meal. It has a 12- to 24-hour duration of action and is administered two or three times daily. Regular and NPH insulin may be combined to reduce the number of daily injections.

The development of insulin analogs, with modification of the terminal end of the A or B chain of the insulin molecule, has resulted in rapid-acting and long-acting formulations. The rapid-acting insulins currently on the market are glulisine, insulin lispro (Humalog), and insulin aspart (NovoLog). Their onset of action is approximately 10 to 30 minutes, and their duration is 3 to 5 hours. They are typically administered 5 to 20 minutes before a meal. Ultrafast-acting insulin analogs reduce postprandial glucose fluctuations and abnormalities.[12] The intent is to match insulin absorption and action to food-related rises in the plasma glucose level.[5] These basal insulin analogs may enable the time of administration of the insulin to vary widely.[12]

Long-acting insulin analogs are detemir (Levemir), deglutec, and glargine (Lantus); their onset of action is 3 to 4 hours, and their duration of action approaches 24 hours, similar to that of NPH. Insulin deglutec has a half-life of 25 hours, with a duration of action of 42 hours. Insulin glargine and detemir, being long-acting but without a peak response, more closely mimic continuous pump infusion. Advances in basal insulin formulations have resulted in products with longer durations of activity, less inter-patient variability in plasma concentration, and "flatter," more predictable pharmacokinetic properties, including a lower frequency of severe hypoglycemia.[15]

Although treatment for type 2 diabetes has traditionally started with oral agents, analog insulin therapy has been recently advocated as initial therapy for type 2 diabetes. Type 2 diabetes is associated with a decline of beta-cell function over time, and early intensive insulin therapy has been suggested to rest the beta cells and possibly preserve their function. Emergency clinicians may, therefore, see patients who were started on insulin therapy early after their diagnosis. Starting patients on 10 units/ day of glargine, or detemir, 0.1 to 0.2 units/kg once daily in the evening or 10 units once or twice daily,[13,15] with 6 units of insulin aspart at mealtime, has been used as primary treatment for type 2 diabetes.[12] Basal insulin titration algorithms from numerous societies and colleges have recommended initial starting dosages of 10 units/day, titrating upward by 1 to 3 units every 1 to 3 days, with a target HbA_{1c} level below 6.5% to 7%.[16]

While many emergency clinicians are more comfortable starting patients on oral hypoglycemic agents to manage type 2 diabetes, on occasion, patients may be started on insulin from the ED. This approach involves the development of an outpatient protocol and follow-up with a specialty consultant, such as an endocrinologist. Glargine, detemir, or NPH insulin may be initiated at 0.1 to 0.2 units/kg, or roughly 10 units/ day, with follow-up within 3 to 4 days for dose adjustment.

Pancreas Transplantation. Solid organ pancreas transplantation has become more common; several centers have performed combined pancreas and kidney transplants in those with end-stage kidney disease due to diabetic nephropathy. Transplantation ameliorates many secondary complications of diabetes, such as nephropathy, neuropathy, gastroparesis, retinopathy, and microvascular changes. The percentage of grafts functioning after 1 year and 1-year survival rate of patients is greater than 75% in selected medical centers. However, rejection, post-transplantation pancreatitis, and graft thrombosis, as well as other vascular and immunosuppression problems, continue to plague transplant recipients.

New Trends in Diabetes Management. Changes in the therapy of diabetes have recently included greater use of human insulin, which has prevented some of the adverse reactions to beef and pork products.[12] Unfortunately, some patients demonstrate sensitivity reactions, even to human insulin.

The initiation of immunosuppressive therapy at the initial diagnosis of type 1 diabetes can prolong the patient's ability to secrete insulin.

This beneficial effect, whether achieved by azathioprine or cyclosporine, is not usually sustainable.[16] The potential side effects of immunosuppressive agents have precluded large trials in patients early in their disease.

Glycemic control now involves improved technology and more widespread individual monitoring of daily insulin dosage adjustments. Tight glycemic control limits the progression of microvascular disease, including neuropathy, renal disease, and certain types of retinopathy. However, those achieving tight control are more likely than other diabetic patients to experience hypoglycemic episodes.

Emergency clinicians and out-of-hospital care providers often encounter patients with insulin pumps.[17] Many types of insulin pumps are available, each with a pump mechanism, reservoir for insulin, tubing, and indwelling subcutaneous needles. They are attached, usually with tape, to the patient's body and administer insulin at a regular adjustable rate. Most pumps also allow the patient to administer additional boluses of insulin, as necessary. These pumps support tight glycemic control and are preferred by some patients. However, insulin pumps are associated with a variety of problems, including hypoglycemia. More recently, a wearable, automated bionic bihormonal pancreas has been noted to improve mean glycemic levels with less frequent hypoglycemic episodes among adults with type 1 diabetes mellitus. A consensus conference of the American Association of Clinical Endocrinologists and American College of Endocrinology supported the use of continuous glucose monitoring (CGM) for use in type I diabetes in reducing hypoglycemia, improving glucose control, and possibly reducing health care costs.[18] Real-time CGM provides users with updated glucose readings every 5 minutes.[19] The bionic pancreas receives data from a continuous glucose monitor to control subcutaneous delivery of insulin and glucagon.[19]

Because glucose rotates the polarization of light waves, new fiberoptic technology has been developed to determine the blood glucose level noninvasively.[19] This technique may be applied to the insulin pumps of the future. Ultrafast-acting insulins and biosimilar insulins may also be available in the near future. An inhaled insulin (Afrezza) has recently been released but has been associated with coughing and may exacerbate symptoms of reactive airway disease.

The pharmacologic treatment of diabetes continues to improve, with newer agents offering the promise of improving glycemic control for longer periods, with fewer glycemic fluctuations, less weight gain, and less hypoglycemia. New insulin analogs, such as deglutec and U-500, improve glycemic control without contributing to hypoglycemia.[18] The U500 insulin is much more concentrated, and errors in dosing are more frequent when using this product, however. Other new areas of research have included agents that increase the urinary excretion of glucose or increase hepatic gluconeogenesis.

LATE COMPLICATIONS OF DIABETES

Late complications of diabetes develop approximately 15 to 20 years after the onset of overt hyperglycemia, resulting in significant morbidity and mortality. The Diabetes Control and Complications Trial (DCCT) has shown that tight glycemic control significantly reduces the risk of microvascular disease, such as microalbuminuria (the earliest sign of nephropathy), neuropathy, and retinopathy, but at the expense of greatly increasing the risk of recurrent hypoglycemia.[2]

Vascular Complications

Diabetes is associated with an increased risk for atherosclerosis and thromboembolic complications, a major cause of morbidity and premature death. The cause of accelerated atherosclerosis is unknown, although it is probably related to oxidated low-density lipoprotein, and increased platelet activity. Atherosclerotic lesions are widespread, causing symptoms in many organ systems. Coronary artery disease and stroke are common. Diabetic patients have an increased incidence of so-called silent myocardial infarction, complicated myocardial infarctions, and congestive heart failure. Peripheral vascular disease is noted clinically by claudication, nonhealing ulcers, gangrene, and impotence. In addition, standard treadmill stress tests have a decreased sensitivity in the detection of coronary artery disease in diabetics. For this reason, exercise or pharmacologic stress echocardiography or a nuclear medicine imaging study should be considered when a provocative test is needed to evaluate the diabetic patient for acute coronary syndrome.[1]

Diabetic Nephropathy

Renal disease is a leading cause of death and disability in diabetic patients. Approximately 50% of cases of end-stage renal disease in the United States are caused by diabetic nephropathy. The appearance of microalbuminuria correlates with the presence of coronary artery disease and retinopathy. Azotemia generally does not begin until 10 to 15 years after the diagnosis of diabetes. The progression of renal disease is accelerated by hypertension. Meticulous control of diabetes can reverse microalbuminuria and may slow the progression of nephropathy. Blood pressure should be aggressively managed; angiotensin-converting enzyme inhibitors are effective in controlling hypertension and lowering microalbuminuria. Chronic hemodialysis and renal transplantation are unfortunate endpoints for many diabetic patients with renal disease.

Retinopathy

Diabetes is a leading cause of adult blindness in the United States. Approximately 11% to 18% of all diabetic patients have treatable diabetic retinopathy, ranging from mild to severe, and manifested in many forms. The severity of diabetic retinopathy is clearly related to the quality of glycemic control. Background retinopathy is found in most patients with prolonged diabetes and is characterized by microaneurysms, small vessel obstruction, cotton wool spots, soft or hard exudates, and macular ischemia. Proliferative retinopathy defines an entity of new vessel formation and scarring, as well as associated vitreal hemorrhage and retinal detachment. The diabetic patient may present with complaints ranging from the acute blurring of vision to sudden unilateral or even bilateral blindness. Less often, diabetic patients have more gradual vision loss caused by the common senile cataract (or snowflake cataract), which may disappear as the hyperglycemia is corrected. Diabetic patients with retinopathy should be referred to an ophthalmologist. Even in those with normal vision, ophthalmologic procedures may limit visual loss or prevent crises such as neovascular glaucoma.

Neuropathy

Autonomic and peripheral neuropathies are well-known complications of diabetes. The prevalence of peripheral neuropathy ranges from 15% to 60%. The cause of the neuropathy is not clearly understood, but studies have suggested several factors in its development, including the effects of diabetic vascular disease on the vasa nervorum. Neurologic manifestations of diabetes may regress with improved glycemic control.

Several distinct types of neuropathy have been recognized in diabetes.[20] Peripheral symmetric neuropathy is a slowly progressive, primary sensory disorder manifested bilaterally with anesthesia, hyperesthesia, or pain. The pain is often severe and worse at night. It affects the upper and lower extremities, although the lower extremities and distal most sections of the involved nerves are most often affected. There may be a motor deficit as well. The pain may be very difficult to control; opioid analgesics have been used, but nonopioid medications such as gabapentin, pregabalin, and amitriptyline are preferred. Nortriptyline has

been used, but the effects seem to dissipate after about 3 months of use. Pregabalin seems to hold the most promise when used at higher dosages (up to 600 mg/day). Duloxetine at a dosage of 60 mg/day is also effective. Both pregabalin and duloxetine achieve significant pain control in at least 50% of patients. Gabapentin, 300 mg tid, has some efficacy, achieving significant pain relief in about one-third of patients; amitriptyline 25 mg daily demonstrates similar results, though if there is no improvement after 5 to 7 days, any further efficacy is unlikely. N-methyl-D-aspartate receptor (NMDAR) antagonists such as memantine and dextromethorphan have shown promise in reducing pain and hyperalgesia in diabetic neuropathy.[21] A reasonable approach for the emergency clinician is the initiation of duloxetine or pregabalin, with the understanding that it may take several days for a peak effect to be reached.[20]

Mononeuropathy, or mononeuropathy multiplex, affects motor and sensory nerves, generally one nerve at a time. The onset is rapid, with wasting and tenderness of the involved muscles. There may be a sudden onset of wrist drop, foot drop, or paralysis of cranial nerves III, IV, and VI. Diabetic mononeuropathies may be most bothersome at night and generally resolve in a few months. Diabetic truncal mononeuropathy occurs rapidly in a radicular distribution. In contrast to other mononeuropathies, it is primarily, if not exclusively sensory. If it causes pain, it may mimic that of a myocardial infarction or acute abdominal inflammation. Whereas diabetic mononeuropathy is often the first indication of diabetes, truncal mononeuropathy is more often found in known diabetic patients. Management is similar to other diabetic neuropathies, with the exception of CN III palsy, which is usually expectant management.

Autonomic neuropathy occurs in many forms. Neuropathy of the GI tract, with resultant gastroparesis, is manifested by difficulty in swallowing, delayed gastric emptying, constipation, or nocturnal diarrhea. Impotence and bladder dysfunction or paralysis may occur. Orthostatic hypotension, syncope, and even cardiac arrest have resulted from autonomic neuropathy. Diabetic diarrhea responds to diphenoxylate and atropine, loperamide, or clonidine. There are small case series that also describe success using 5HT3 receptor antagonists successfully as well. Orthostatic hypotension is treated by sleeping with the head of the bed elevated, avoidance of sudden standing or sitting, and use of full-length elastic stockings. For gastroparesis, metoclopramide is recommended for its prokinetic and antiemetic properties, though caution must be taken with prolonged use due to the risk of tardive dyskinesia. Many patients with gastroparesis present with abdominal pain; opioids are not recommended for this group due to the risk of worsening dysmotility of the GI tract. In patients with acute presentations of pain and vomiting due to gastroparesis, intravenous haloperidol has shown effectiveness in a few small trials.

The Diabetic Foot

Approximately 20% of hospitalizations in diabetic patients are related to foot problems.[17] Sensory neuropathy, ischemia, and infection are the principal contributors to diabetic foot disease. Loss of sensation leads to pressure necrosis from poorly fitting footwear and small wounds going unnoticed. The most common cause of injury is pressure on plantar bone prominences. All neuropathic foot ulcers should be assessed for infection, devitalized tissue débrided, and radiographs obtained to evaluate for the presence of foreign bodies, soft tissue gas, or bone abnormalities (see Chapter 126).[19]

Not all ulcers are infected. Infection is suggested by local inflammation or crepitation. Conversely, some uninflamed ulcers are associated with underlying osteomyelitis. Most mild infections are caused by gram-positive cocci, such as *Staphylococcus aureus* or streptococci, and may be treated with oral antibiotics with activity against gram-positive

TABLE 115.2	Common Serious Infections in Diabetics and Their Antimicrobial Therapy
Infectious Condition	**Antimicrobial Therapy**
Diabetic foot infection	Mild—consider trimethoprim-sulfamethoxazole, 800/160 bid or clindamycin 300 mg q6h Moderate to severe—piperacillin-tazobactam (Zosyn), 3.375 g IV q6h and vancomycin, 15 mg/kg IV q12h
Malignant otitis externa	Oral—ciprofloxacin, 500 mg PO bid for 10–14 days IV—ceftazidime, 2 g IV q8h ± gentamicin, 2 mg/kg IV q8h
Mucormycosis	Amphotericin B, 1–1.5 mg/kg/day Posaconazole, 400 mg bid
Mucocutaneous candidiasis	Ketoconazole, 200 mg PO daily; may need several weeks of therapy
Nonclostridial gas gangrene (including Fournier's)	Clindamycin, 600 mg q6h + third-generation cephalosporin + vancomycin, 15 mg/kg q12h

organisms, such as trimethoprim-sulfamethoxazole, 800/160 mg bid, a first-generation cephalosporin such as cephalexin, 500 mg qid, or clindamycin, 300 mg qid. A strict non-weight-bearing regimen, meticulous wound care, and daily follow-up are also vitally important to wound healing. This approach may not be possible when patients do not have adequate home support or do not have ready access to follow-up care.

Deeper, limb-threatening infections—as evidenced by full-thickness ulceration, cellulitis more than 2 cm in diameter, with or without lymphangitis, bone or joint involvement, or systemic toxicity—are usually polymicrobial in origin and caused by aerobic gram-positive cocci, gram-negative bacilli, and anaerobes (see Chapter 125, Bone and Joint Infections). These patients require hospitalization and, after culture, broad-spectrum IV empirical antimicrobial therapy (Table 115.2). Additional measures include strict non-weight-bearing status, tight glycemic control, early surgical intervention for débridement, and meticulous wound care. Occult osteomyelitis should be considered in all cases of neuropathic ulceration.[19] Hyperbaric oxygen has been shown to have some efficacy in treating complicated infections, especially with anaerobic organisms. Up to one-third of patients eventually undergo amputation.

Infections

Diabetic patients are more susceptible to complications of infections because of their inability to limit microbial invasion with effective polymorphonuclear leukocytes and lymphocytes. They have an increased incidence of extremity infections and pyelonephritis compared with the general population. In addition, they are particularly susceptible to certain other infections, such as tuberculosis, mucocutaneous candidiasis, intertrigo, mucormycosis, soft tissue infections, nonclostridial gas gangrene, Fournier's gangrene, osteomyelitis, and malignant *Pseudomonas* otitis externa (see Table 115.2). Glycemic control, and hospitalization are usually required.

Cutaneous Manifestations

Dermal hypersensitivity is manifested by pruritic erythematous indurations that occur at insulin injection sites. The declining prevalence of this condition has paralleled the improved purification of insulin. Similarly, insulin lipoatrophy is subcutaneous depressions at injection sites and seems to be a result of insulin impurities. Although lipoatrophy is more common than dermal hypersensitivity, its prevalence has also declined sharply because of improved insulin preparations. Insulin lipohypertrophy is manifested by raised areas of subcutaneous fat deposits at insulin injection sites. These lesions generally reflect the failure of the patient to rotate injection sites adequately. They resolve spontaneously over months if insulin injection is avoided in the affected areas and sites are properly rotated.

Insulin pumps are often associated with localized skin problems, usually a reaction to the tape securing the tubing and needles. On occasion, sensitivity to the catheters is seen. Skin infections at the site of injection are the most common complication of insulin pumps. A few patients have been noted to have hard nodules at the injection site. The cause of these nodules is uncertain.

Diabetic patients who use oral hypoglycemic agents may have rashes associated with these medications. After consumption of ethanol, approximately 38% of type 2 patients taking chlorpropamide exhibit a flush consisting of redness of the face and neck and a sense of warmness or burning. Patients may demonstrate urticaria in response to insulin and oral hypoglycemics.

Skin Conditions

Diabetic skin conditions include fungal infections, acanthosis nigricans, necrobiosis lipoidica diabeticorum, xanthoma diabeticorum, bullosis diabeticorum, and diabetic dermopathy.

Acanthosis Nigricans. This is characterized by a velvety, brown-black thickening of the keratin layer, most often in the flexor surfaces. It is the cutaneous marker for a group of endocrine disorders with insulin resistance.

Necrobiosis Lipoidica Diabeticorum. This begins as erythematous papular or nodular lesions, usually in the pretibial area but in other areas as well. The early lesions may contain telangiectasias. These lesions spread and frequently form a single pigmented area of atrophic skin, often with a yellow and sometimes ulcerated center and an erythematous margin. A history of previous trauma is sometimes found.

Xanthoma Diabeticorum. These lesions are evidence of the hyperlipidemia associated with diabetes, similar to the xanthoma found in nondiabetic hyperlipidemic patients. Xanthomas have an erythematous base and a yellowish hue.

Bullosis Diabeticorum. This is a rare occurrence. Bullae are usually filled with a clear fluid and are most often found on the extremities, especially the feet. The fluid is occasionally slightly hemorrhagic. The bullae usually heal spontaneously without scarring.

Diabetic Dermopathy. Also known as skin spots, this is the most common skin finding in diabetes. It arises as discrete, depressed, and brownish lesions generally less than 15 mm in diameter and found in the pretibial area.

Impetigo or Intertrigo. Resistant, aggressive impetigo or intertrigo may suggest diabetes.

Diabetes Disposition

The decision to admit or discharge a diabetic patient depends on multiple factors. Primary considerations include the severity of illness,

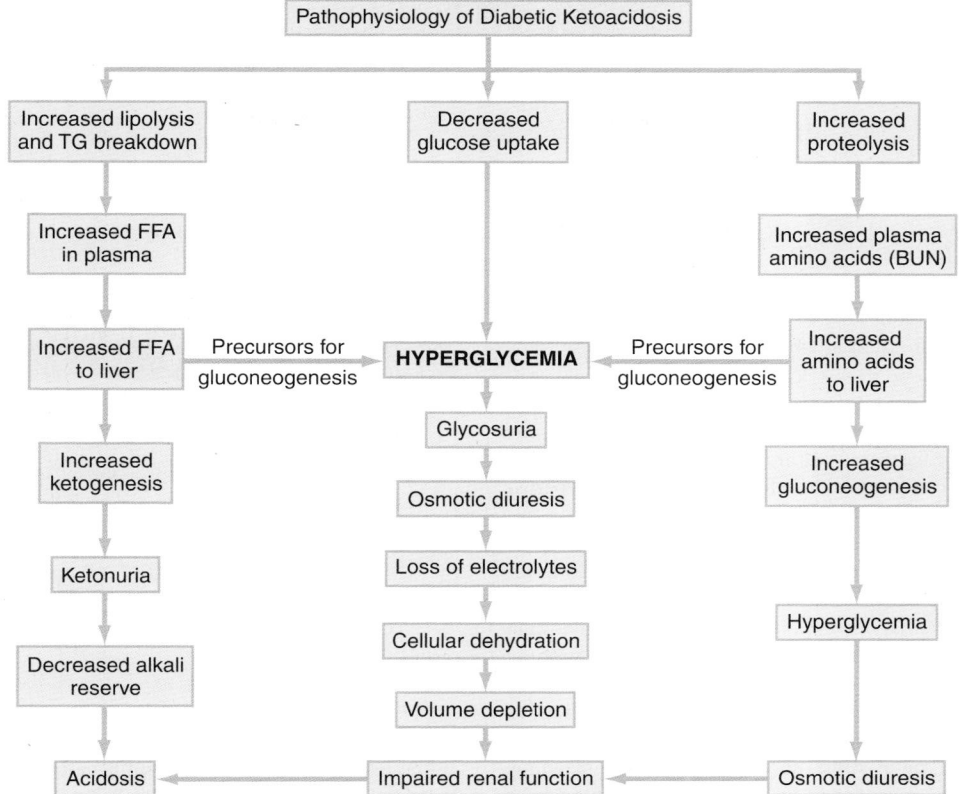

Fig. 115.1 Syndrome of Diabetic Ketoacidosis. *BUN,* Blood urea nitrogen; *FFA,* free fatty acids; *TG,* total glucose concentration.

whether this is a new diagnosis (where teaching, obtaining supplies, diabetic lifestyle education, and possibly insulin titration are needed) or an established diagnosis. Issues such as the ability to obtain medications and diabetic supplies and the ability to manage diabetes at home (particularly as relates to the measurement of blood glucose and insulin administration, which may be difficult in the elderly or those with low vision) are additional factors. Even in the absence of other complicating factors, such as DKA or infection, admission may be necessary for both achieving glycemic control and developing an appropriate outpatient plan for diabetes management. The elderly, socioeconomically disadvantaged populations, uninsured persons, and those with mental illness are at particular risk. Recent significant price increases for insulin have compelled many people with diabetes to forgo this part of their therapy. The mortality and morbidity rate from diabetes is also substantially higher in chronically underserved populations, such as African Americans; the rates of death, kidney disease, and amputations are all much higher in African-Americans as compared to Caucasians. African Americans have more than twice the incidence of diabetes compared to Caucasians (11.8 vs. 5.7) and are 2.3 times more likely to die from the disease as Caucasians.

DIABETIC KETOACIDOSIS

Foundations

Pathophysiology

DKA is a syndrome in which insulin deficiency and glucagon excess combine to produce a hyperglycemic, dehydrated, acidotic patient with profound electrolyte imbalances. All derangements producing DKA are interrelated and based on insulin deficiency (Fig. 115.1). DKA may be caused by the cessation of insulin intake or by physical or emotional stress, despite continued insulin therapy. The effects of insulin deficiency may be mimicked in peripheral tissues by a lack of insulin receptors or insulin sensitivity at receptor or post-receptor sites. When the hyperglycemia becomes sufficiently marked, the renal threshold is surpassed, and glucose is excreted in the urine. The hyperosmolarity produced by hyperglycemia and the dehydration are the most important determinants of the patient's mental status.[16]

Glucose in the renal tubules draws water, sodium, potassium, magnesium, calcium, phosphorus, and other ions from the circulation into the urine. This osmotic diuresis, combined with poor intake and vomiting, produces the profound dehydration and electrolyte imbalance associated with DKA (Table 115.3). Exocrine pancreatic dysfunction closely parallels endocrine beta-cell dysfunction, producing malabsorption that further limits the body's intake of fluid and exacerbates electrolyte loss.

In 95% of patients with DKA, the total sodium level is normal or low. Potassium, magnesium, and phosphorus deficits are also usually marked. As a result of acidosis and dehydration, however, the initially reported serum values for these electrolytes are often higher than actual body stores.

The cells, unable to receive fuel substances from the circulation, act as they do in starvation from other causes. They decrease amino acid uptake and accelerate proteolysis so that large amounts of amino acids are released to the liver and converted to two-carbon fragments.

Adipose tissue in the patient with DKA fails to clear the circulation of lipids. Insulin deficiency results in the activation of a hormone-sensitive lipase that increases circulating free fatty acid (FFA) levels. Long-chain FFAs, now circulating in abundance as a result of insulin deficiency, are partially oxidized and converted in the liver to acetoacetate and β-hydroxybutyrate. Despite the increased pathologic

TABLE 115.3   Average Fluid and Electrolyte Deficits in Severe Diabetic Ketoacidosis[a]

Weight	Water (mL/kg)	Sodium (mEq/L)	Potassium (mEq/L)	Chloride (mEq/L)	Phosphorus (mEq/L)
≤10 kg	100–120	8–10	5–7	6–8	3
10–20 kg	80–100	8–10	5–7	6–8	3
≥20 kg	70–80	8–10	5–7	6–8	3

[a]Per kilogram of body weight.

production of ketones, the body acts as it does in any form of starvation to decrease the peripheral tissue's use of ketones as fuel. The combination of increased ketone production with decreased ketone use leads to ketoacidosis.

Acidosis plays a prominent role in the clinical presentation of DKA. The acidotic patient attempts to increase lung ventilation to rid the body of excess acid with Kussmaul breathing. Bicarbonate is consumed in the process. Acidosis compounds the effects of ketosis and hyperosmolality to depress mental status directly.

Acidemia is not invariably present, even with significant ketoacidosis. Ketoalkalosis has been reported in diabetic patients vomiting for several days and in some with severe dehydration and hyperventilation. The finding of alkalemia, however, should prompt consideration of alcoholic ketoacidosis, in which alkalemia is much more common.

DKA most commonly occurs in patients with type 1 diabetes and is associated with inadequate administration of insulin, infection, or myocardial infarction. DKA can also occur in type 2 diabetics and may be associated with any type of stress, such as sepsis or GI bleeding. Approximately 25% of all episodes of DKA occur in patients whose diabetes was previously undiagnosed.

Clinical Features

Clinically, most patients with DKA complain of a recent history of polydipsia, polyuria, polyphagia, visual blurring, weakness, weight loss, nausea, vomiting, and abdominal pain. Approximately 50% of these patients, especially children, report abdominal pain. In children, this pain is usually idiopathic and probably caused by gastric distention or stretching of the liver capsule; it resolves as the metabolic abnormalities are corrected. In adults, however, abdominal pain more often signifies actual abdominal disease that may be triggering the DKA.

Physical examination may or may not demonstrate a depressed sensorium. Typical findings include tachypnea with Kussmaul breathing, tachycardia, frank hypotension or orthostatic blood pressure changes, odor of acetone on the breath, and signs of dehydration. An elevated temperature is rarely caused by DKA itself and suggests an inciting infection.

Differential Diagnosis

Alcoholics, especially those who have recently abstained from drinking, with Kussmaul's breathing, fruity odor to the breath, and acidemic blood gas values may have alcoholic ketoacidosis. These patients may be euglycemic or hypoglycemic, and a large part of their acidosis is often caused by the unmeasured β-hydroxybutyric acid. Alcoholic ketoacidosis accounts for approximately 20% of all cases of ketoacidosis. Ketoacidosis can also develop with fasting, commonly in the third trimester of pregnancy and in nursing mothers who do not eat.

The differential diagnosis for DKA is broad and includes any entity that may cause elevated anion gap acidosis, ketosis, or both. The presence of DKA should not exclude investigation for other causes of anion gap metabolic acidosis, such as sepsis, poisoning, or lactic acidosis, because physiologic stress from one of these other causes can precipitate DKA.

TABLE 115.4   Typical Laboratory Values in Diabetic Ketoacidosis and Hyperglycemic Hyperosmolar State

	DKA	HHS
Glucose (mg/dL)	>350	>700
Sodium (mEq/L)	Low 130s	140s
Potassium (mEq/L)	≈4.5–6.0	≈5
Bicarbonate (mEq/L)	<10	>15
Blood urea nitrogen (mg/dL)	25–50	>50
Serum ketones	Present	Absent

DKA, Diabetic ketoacidosis; *HHS,* hyperglycemic hyperosmolar state.

Diagnostic Testing

Initial tests allow preliminary confirmation of the diagnosis and initiation of therapy (Table 115.4).[22] Subsequent tests are carried out to determine more precisely the degree of dehydration, acidosis, and electrolyte imbalance and reveal the precipitant of DKA.

Laboratory studies should include serum glucose, electrolyte, and venous blood pH. Although serum ketoacid levels are frequently measured, they are not necessary to diagnose DKA and may be elevated in non-DKA states (e.g., starvation ketosis from inadequate utilization of glucose stores) or dehydration. If determination of the pH is the sole concern, venous blood gas samples correlate well with arterial pH and are preferable as they are less invasive and have a lower complication rate than arterial sampling. If there is concern about the degree of respiratory compensation and better assessment of ventilation is required, then arterial samples should be obtained.

Blood gas measurement usually reveals a low pH, with the aforementioned rare exception of a concomitant alkalemia, resulting in a pseudo-normalization of the pH. Metabolic acidosis with an anion gap is primarily the result of elevated plasma levels of acetoacetate and β-hydroxybutyrate, although lactate, FFAs, phosphates, volume depletion, and several medications may also contribute. Rarely, a well-hydrated patient with DKA may have a pure hyperchloremic acidosis with no anion gap if they have been aggressively rehydrated with normal saline. Again, although rare, there have been case reports of a normal anion gap in a patient with DKA. This can occur with vomiting sufficient to cause a concomitant metabolic alkalosis, resulting in pH and bicarbonate levels in the normal range.[22]

Knowledge of the relationship between the rise in anion gap (delta AG) and the fall in bicarbonate (delta HCO_3), or delta gap (delta AG-delta HCO_3), can delineate the existence of a mixed acid-base disorder. A delta gap greater than + 6 indicates a concomitant metabolic alkalosis, and a delta gap less than -6 indicates a concomitant hyperchloremic metabolic acidosis. Winter's formula (expected $Paco_2 = [1.5 \times$ serum $HCO_3^-] + [8 \pm 2]$) can be applied to determine if there is appropriate respiratory compensation or the presence of multiple acid-base disorders.

The glucose level is usually elevated above 350 mg/dL; however, euglycemic DKA (blood glucose level ≤ 300 mg/dL) has been reported in up to 18% of patients. The incidence of euglycemic DKA may be higher in patients treated with SGLT2 inhibitors.

If an immediate potassium level is not available through point-of-care testing or blood gas analysis, an electrocardiogram can reveal signs of hyperkalemia or hypokalemia. Initial serum potassium levels are typically normal or high in DKA due to intracellular potassium shifting out of cells in exchange for elevated serum hydrogen ions. However, as potassium is lost in the urine, the total body potassium usually declines by several hundred milliequivalents. This, in combination with the insulin doses administered in DKA, can result in life-threatening hypokalemia. A basic metabolic panel should be obtained to evaluate for an anion gap, potassium and glucose levels, and renal function. Because magnesium deficits are common in DKA, we recommend determining these levels as well. Urinalysis, in addition to the presence of ketones, may also help confirm a urinary tract infection as a precipitant of DKA. Whether to obtain blood or urine cultures should be determined by the clinical picture.

The serum sodium level is often misleading in DKA. It is often low in the presence of significant dehydration because it is strongly affected by hyperglycemia, hypertriglyceridemia, salt-poor fluid intake, increased GI and renal losses, and insensible loss. When hyperglycemia is marked, water flows from the cells into the vessels to decrease the osmolar gradient, thereby creating dilutional hyponatremia. Elevated lipid levels cause pseudohyponatremia by decreasing the fraction of serum that is water. Newer autoanalyzers remove triglycerides before the assay is performed, thus eliminating this artifact. The true value of the sodium level may be approximated by adding 1.6 mEq/L to the sodium value on the laboratory report for every 100-mg/dL glucose above the norm. Thus, if the laboratory reports a serum sodium level of 130 mEq/L and blood glucose level of 700 mEq/L, the corrected total serum sodium level is 139.6 mEq/L.

Acidosis and the hyperosmolarity induced by hyperglycemia shift potassium, magnesium, and phosphorus from the intracellular to extracellular space. Dehydration results in hemoconcentration, which contributes to normal or high initial serum potassium, magnesium, and phosphorus readings in DKA, even with profound total body deficits. The effect of acidosis on the serum potassium level determination can be corrected by subtracting 0.6 mEq/L from the laboratory potassium level for every 0.1-decrease in pH noted in the blood gas analysis. Thus, if the potassium level is reported as 5 mEq/L and the pH is 6.94, the corrected potassium value is 2 mEq/L, representing severe hypokalemia. As insulin is administered and the hydrogen ion concentration decreases, the patient needs considerable potassium replacement. The ADA algorithm for potassium repletion is helpful in guiding the management of potassium derangements. No conversion factor has been developed for the estimation of true magnesium levels, although initial values may be high.

All laboratory determinations must be interpreted with caution. Serum creatinine level determinations made by the autoanalyzer may be falsely elevated. Leukocytosis more closely reflects the degree of ketosis than the presence of infection. Only the elevation of band neutrophils has been demonstrated to indicate the presence of infection, with a sensitivity of 100% and specificity of 80% from a single retrospective study. Historically, the diagnosis of pancreatitis in a patient with DKA could be confounded by the elevation of amylase levels in DKA. Given the strength of the current literature demonstrating greater specificity of lipase for the diagnosis of pancreatitis, lipase (which must be three times the upper limit of normal to meet diagnostic criteria for pancreatitis) should be the blood test of choice if pancreatitis is a concern.

BOX 115.1 Summary of Treatment of Diabetic Ketoacidosis

Identify diabetic ketoacidosis—serum glucose, electrolyte, and ketone levels and arterial blood gas analysis; also obtain complete blood count with differential, urinalysis, chest radiograph, and electrocardiogram, if indicated.
Rehydrate.
- 1–2 L NS IV during 1–3 h
- Children—20 mL/kg NS during the first hour
- Correct electrolyte abnormalities.
- Sodium—correct with the administration of NS or 0.45% NS.
- Potassium—ensure adequate renal function. Add 20–40 mEq KCl to each liter (when serum potassium <5.5 mEq/L) of fluid until ketoacidosis is corrected and potassium is normalized. (Do not give insulin until potassium 3.3 mEq/L or greater.)
- Phosphorus—usually unnecessary to replenish.
- Magnesium—correct with 1–2 g $MgSO_4$. Serum magnesium levels may not correlate with body stores.
Supplement insulin.
- Insulin replacement—0.1 unit/kg/h regular insulin IV
- Change IV solution to D_5W/0.45% NS when glucose concentration is ≤300 mg/dL.
Correct acidosis.
- Administer IV fluids and insulin.
Search for and correct underlying precipitant.
Monitor progress and keep meticulous flow sheets.
- Vital signs
- Fluid intake and urine output
- Serum glucose, K^+, Cl^-, HCO_3^-, CO_2, pH
- Amount of insulin administered
Admit to hospital or intensive care unit.
Consider outpatient therapy in children with a reliable caregiver
and
- Initial pH ≥ 7.35
- Initial HCO_3^- ≥ 20 mEq/L
- Can tolerate oral fluids
- Resolution of symptoms after treatment in the emergency department
- No underlying precipitant requiring hospitalization

NS, Normal saline.

Management

When possible, intubation should be avoided in the patient with DKA. Patients often have tremendous respiratory drive, and matching this minute ventilation with the ventilator can be challenging. The comatose DKA patient, especially if vomiting, requires intubation however. Once the patient is intubated, maintenance of hyperventilation prevents worsening acidosis. The patient in hypovolemic shock requires aggressive fluid resuscitation with isotonic crystalloids before vasopressors are used, and clinicians should consider other possible causes of shock (e.g., sepsis or myocardial dysfunction secondary to myocardial infarction). Bedside ultrasonography may be of benefit in excluding other causes of hypotension and evaluating the volume status of an individual patient. Although it is not routinely used in the ED setting, in cases in which the volume status is difficult to ascertain because of complex underlying physiologic derangements (e.g., congestive heart failure, renal failure), the rapid ultrasound for shock and hypotension examination (see Chapter e5) or invasive hemodynamic monitoring may guide fluid therapy.

When hyperglycemia, ketosis, and acidosis have been established, fluid, electrolyte, and insulin therapy should be initiated (Box 115.1).

Intravenous Fluids

The severely dehydrated adult patient is likely to have a fluid deficit of 3 to 5 L. No uniformly accepted formula exists for the administration of fluid in this disorder. If the patient is in hypovolemic shock, the isotonic crystalloid solution should be given as rapidly as possible in the adult or in boluses of 20 mL/kg in the child until a systolic pressure of 80 mm Hg is obtained. There is no consensus regarding the ideal fluid to use; concerns have been raised using large amounts of normal saline exacerbating metabolic acidosis. At least one small trial has studied the use of a balanced crystalloid solution (Plasmalyte) in DKA, with reports of more rapid restoration of normal physiologic parameters.[18]

In the adult who has marked dehydration in the absence of clinical shock or heart failure, 1 L of fluid may be administered in the first hour. In general, 2 L of fluid resuscitation during the first 1 to 3 hours is followed by a slower infusion of a hypotonic solution, such as 0.45% normal saline solution. DKA patients without extreme volume depletion may be successfully treated with a lower volume of IV fluid replacement. An initial bolus of 20 mL/kg during the first hour is the usual fluid resuscitation therapy for a child. The fluid rate should be adjusted according to age, cardiac status, and degree of dehydration to achieve a urine output of 1 to 2 mL/kg/h.

Fluid resuscitation alone may help lower hyperglycemia. Because a low level of circulating insulin may be present, increased perfusion may transport insulin to previously unreached receptor sites. In addition, a large volume of glucose may be cleared by the kidneys in response to improved renal perfusion. The mean plasma glucose concentration has been noted to drop by 18% after the administration of saline solution without insulin.[18]

Acidosis also decreases after fluid infusion because increased perfusion improves tissue oxygenation and diminishes lactate formation while increasing lactate clearance. Increased renal perfusion promotes renal hydrogen ion loss, and the improved action of insulin in the better-hydrated patient inhibits ketogenesis. Although fluid administration decreases the serum glucose concentration and improves acidosis, the underlying deficiency in DKA requires administration of insulin for the correction of ketoacidosis.

Potassium

Potassium replacement is invariably needed in DKA. The initial potassium level is often normal or high, despite a large deficit because of severe acidosis. Potassium levels often plummet with correction of acidosis and administration of insulin. Once potassium levels reach 5.0 to 5.5 mEq/L and the patient is making urine, potassium should be administered while monitoring renal function (Table 115.5).[18] In patients with relatively lower serum potassium concentration at presentation (3.3 to 5.0 mEq/L), hypokalemia may become life-threatening when insulin therapy is administered; therefore, IV administration of potassium in concentrations of 20 to 40 mEq/L should be given with insulin administration. In patients with hypokalemia (<3.3 mEq/L),

insulin should only be initiated once potassium has been replaced to achieve levels of 3.3 mEq/L or higher. The primary rationale for such conservative recommendations regarding potassium administration is that serum levels do not correlate with total body stores in the DKA patient, and the potassium level can drop more rapidly than anticipated with insulin administration.

It was once believed that there was always a phosphorus deficit in DKA. However, there is no significant evidence to support this practice, and only isolated case reports have supported concerns about clinically significant hypophosphatemia in DKA. If the measured serum phosphorus level is low, it should be replaced with potassium phosphate.

Insulin

DKA cannot be reversed without insulin, and insulin therapy should be initiated as soon as the potassium level is determined to be adequate or potassium has been repleted. No randomized trials have compared insulin with placebo or other therapies for DKA. However, the mortality from DKA was 90% in historical controls before the development of exogenous insulin and 50% after insulin was introduced. With appropriate supportive therapy, mortality has reached the current levels of less than 10%.[11]

Although the dosing of insulin infusions has been established, an IV bolus before the infusion is no longer recommended. More recently, in selected patients with mild DKA, the subcutaneous or intramuscular administration of insulin has been proven safe and effective as IV administration of insulin. In selected cases with good outpatient follow-up, treatment of DKA with intermittent bolus dosing of regular insulin by the subcutaneous or intramuscular route without admission has also been shown to be safe. Such a strategy requires a well-hydrated, mildly acidemic patient, well versed in disease management, who has excellent outpatient follow-up. Poor perfusion may hamper the absorption of intramuscular or subcutaneous insulin, resulting in erratic absorption, making IV infusion the route of choice in sicker DKA patients.[5] The current initial therapy of choice, as recommended by the ADA, is regular insulin infused at 0.1 units/kg/h up to 5 to 10 units/h, mixed with IV fluids.

Children with DKA pose additional management challenges. Whereas the general principles of fluid and electrolyte repletion in concert with insulin therapy remain the same, controversy exists about the dosing and administration of fluids and insulin because of concerns related to the risk of inducing cerebral edema in children with DKA. Despite concerns about this complication, it remains rare, with an overall incidence of 1% in pediatric DKA patients. Virtually all current evidence supporting the contention that higher doses of insulin and aggressive fluid resuscitation contribute to the development of cerebral edema has come from retrospective reviews and small case studies. A recently completed large prospective study of 1255 pediatric DKA patients showed a similar risk of cerebral edema irrespective of restrictive or permissive fluid resuscitation.[15] Similarly, retrospective reviews of a large number of children with DKA did not show any significant difference in the development of cerebral edema based on insulin infusion rates. The degree of acidosis or uremia seem to be the best individual predictors of cerebral edema, as opposed to any specific fluid or insulin regimen, and earlier concerns about fluid resuscitation causing cerebral edema may have been the result of sicker patients getting more fluids (e.g., confounding by indication, since sicker patients are more likely to develop cerebral edema). Cerebral edema has a significant mortality rate, and patients should be carefully monitored and receive mannitol at the earliest suspicion of cerebral edema.

Because the half-life of IV regular insulin is 3 to 10 minutes, insulin should be administered IV by infusion rather than repeated bolus. When the blood glucose concentration has dropped to 250 to 300 mg/dL,

TABLE 115.5 **American Diabetes Association Recommendations for Potassium and Phosphorus Repletion**	
Potassium <3.3 mEQ/L	Replete to >3.3 mEq/L before starting insulin
Potassium 3.3–5.5 mEQ/L	Supplement potassium to maintain these levels while starting insulin
Potassium >5.5 mEQ/L	Do not start potassium supplementation until <5.5 mEq/L
Phosphorous <1.0 mEQ/L	Initiate supplementation with potassium phosphate

adding dextrose to the IV fluids reduces the risk of iatrogenic hypoglycemia and rapid shifts in osmolarity. In patients with euglycemic DKA, dextrose should be added to the IV fluids at the start of insulin therapy.

Insulin resistance rarely occurs in diabetic patients and requires an increase in dosage for a satisfactory response. Resistance may be caused by obesity or accelerated insulin degradation.

Magnesium

Magnesium deficiency is a common problem in patients with DKA without renal disease. Both the initial pathophysiologic process and therapy for DKA induce profound magnesium diuresis. Magnesium deficiency may exacerbate vomiting and mental changes, promote recalcitrant hypokalemia and hypocalcemia, or induce fatal cardiac dysrhythmia. If there is a concern for hypomagnesemia, we recommend adding magnesium to the IV fluids, with the typical adult patient requiring 1 to 3 g for repletion.

Sodium Bicarbonate

In the past, sodium bicarbonate was recommended for severely acidemic patients (pH < 7.0). However, research has demonstrated worse outcomes for patients receiving bicarbonate, including exacerbation of electrolyte deficits such as hypokalemia, delaying clearing of ketosis, paradoxical worsening of cerebrospinal fluid (CSF) acidosis due to suppression of respiratory compensations, and preferential permeability of the blood-brain barrier to CO_2. Unless needed to stave off impending cardiac arrest in a severely acidemic patient, we do not recommend routine bicarbonate administration. If a severely acidemic patient requires endotracheal intubation, the use of a bolus of bicarbonate in the immediate pre-intubation period may reduce the risk of cardiovascular collapse from a precipitous decline in pH after induction during rapid-sequence intubation; this recommendation is based on expert opinion as opposed to any specific clinical trials.[18]

Complications

The precipitating causes of DKA may have associated morbidity and mortality rates equal to or worse than those of DKA itself. These include iatrogenic causes, infection, and myocardial infarction. Morbidity in DKA is largely iatrogenic—hypokalemia from inadequate potassium replacement, hypoglycemia from inadequate glucose monitoring, failure to replenish glucose in IV solutions when the serum glucose concentration drops below 250 to 300 mg/dL, alkalosis from overaggressive bicarbonate replacement, and pulmonary edema from overaggressive hydration.

The mortality in treated DKA is approximately 5% to 7%. The primary causes of death remain infection, especially pneumonia, arterial thromboses, and shock. The decrease in the mortality rate over the last several decades has demonstrated the importance of appropriate therapy. Cerebral edema remains a rare but important cause of morbidity and mortality in children with DKA.

Cerebral edema should be considered when the patient in DKA becomes altered or lapses into a coma after the reversal of acidosis. Cerebral edema generally occurs 6 to 10 hours after the initiation of therapy, often without warning signs, and the associated mortality rate is 90%.[15] Cerebral edema is less common in adults or children older than 5 years and appears to be most strongly associated with severity of illness (acidemia and azotemia), although subclinical cerebral edema in children is probably common. Furthermore, subclinical cerebral edema may precede or follow the onset of therapy, raising the question of whether it is caused by therapy or is simply a manifestation of the basic pathophysiologic mechanisms of DKA. The treatment of cerebral edema is largely supportive. No large clinical trials have identified effective treatment, although some authors recommend mannitol. Steroids have not been shown to be effective.

Diabetic Ketoacidosis Disposition

Most patients with DKA require hospital admission, often to the intensive care unit. The use of observation units to manage uncomplicated DKA in selected patients has been shown to be effective (see Chapter e6). All pregnant diabetic patients in DKA require admission and consultation with an endocrinologist and obstetrician specializing in the care of high-risk pregnancies. Some children (initial pH ≥ 7.35; bicarbonate ≥ 20 mEq/L) who can tolerate oral fluids after 3 or 4 hours of treatment may be discharged home with a reliable caregiver. Patients who have mild DKA may be treated as an outpatient if the patient or parent can understand discharge instructions and are able to return, underlying causes do not require inpatient therapy, and close follow-up is confirmed.

HYPERGLYCEMIC HYPEROSMOLAR STATE

Foundations

HHS represents a syndrome of acute diabetic decompensation characterized by marked hyperglycemia, hyperosmolarity, dehydration, and decreased mental function that may progress to frank coma. The terminology has changed recently from the former term *hyperglycemic hyperosmolar nonketotic coma* because some patients have mild degrees of ketosis, and coma is not universally present.[4,18] Ketoacidosis is generally minimal or absent, although metabolic acidosis from another source, such as lactic acidosis from sepsis or uremia from acute renal failure, may be present. Focal neurologic signs may be present, or there may be a global encephalopathy. DKA and HHS may occur together.

Pathophysiology

As with DKA, the pathophysiologic mechanisms of HHS vary with the particular patient. Because most patients with HHS are older adults, decreased renal clearance of glucose produced by the decline of renal function with age often contributes to the illness. Decreased insulin action results in glycogenolysis, gluconeogenesis, and decreased peripheral uptake of glucose. The hyperglycemia pulls fluid from the intracellular into the extracellular space, transiently maintaining adequate perfusion. Soon, however, this fluid is lost in a profound osmotic diuresis, limited finally by hypotension, decreased renal perfusion, and a subsequent drop in the GFR. The urine is extremely hypotonic, with a urine sodium concentration between 50 and 70 mEq/L, compared with 140 mEq/L in extracellular fluid. This hypotonic diuresis produces profound dehydration, leading to hyperglycemia, hypernatremia, and associated hypertonicity. Often, the patient is unable to take in adequate fluids because of stroke, Alzheimer disease, or other diseases, greatly exacerbating the dehydration.

The reason for the absence of ketoacidosis in HHS is unknown. FFA levels are lower than in DKA, thus limiting the substrates needed to form ketones. The most likely reason for the blunted counterregulatory hormone release and lack of ketosis seems to be the continued secretion of tiny amounts of insulin that block ketogenesis.

HHS is a syndrome of severe dehydration that results from a sustained hyperglycemic diuresis in which the patient is unable to drink sufficient fluids to offset the urinary losses. The full-blown syndrome does not usually occur until volume depletion has progressed to the point of decreased urine output.

HHS is most common in geriatric patients with type 2 diabetes but has been reported in children with type 1 diabetes. HHS may occur in patients who do not have diabetes, especially after burns, parenteral hyperalimentation, peritoneal dialysis, or hemodialysis.

Clinical Features

The prodrome of HHS is significantly longer than that of DKA. Clinically, extreme dehydration, hyperosmolarity, volume depletion, and CNS findings predominate. If they are awake, patients may complain of fever, thirst, polyuria, or oliguria. Approximately 20% of patients have no known history of type 2 diabetes. The most common associated diseases are chronic renal insufficiency, GI bleeding, gram-negative pneumonia, and gram-negative sepsis. Approximately 85% of patients have underlying renal or cardiac impairment as a predisposing factor. Arterial and venous thromboses are common and often complicate the picture.

The patient often exhibits orthostatic hypotension or frank hypotension, tachycardia, and fever, with signs of marked dehydration. The depression of the sensorium correlates directly with the degree and rate of development of hyperosmolarity. Some patients have a normal mental status. Neurologic issues are common in HHS. Although a decreased level of consciousness is the most common neurologic finding, seizures, stroke syndromes, and movement disorders have been reported in various case series. Whether HHS is the cause or result of these disorders is unclear, and there is no current evidence to recommend the prophylactic use of antiepileptics or antithrombotic agents in HHS patients.

Differential Diagnoses

The differential diagnosis of HHS is identical to that of DKA (Table 115.6). In addition, diabetic patients receiving chlorpropamide are subject to water intoxication with dilutional hyponatremia, which may be manifested as coma without acidosis that is clinically indistinguishable from HHS. The patient with HHS who has a sharply depressed sensorium may not be initially distinguishable from the patient with profound hypoglycemia. When the blood glucose concentration cannot be rapidly checked, the immediate administration of one ampule of $D_{50}W$ minimally worsens HHS and may be lifesaving for patients with hypoglycemia.

Diagnostic Testing

Laboratory findings usually reveal a blood glucose level above 600 mg/dL and serum osmolarity above 350 mOsm/L. The blood urea nitrogen concentration is invariably elevated. Although patients with HHS do not have ketoacidosis caused by diabetes, they may have a metabolic acidosis secondary to some combination of lactic acidosis, starvation ketosis, and retention of inorganic acids attributable to renal hypoperfusion.

The patient with HHS typically has a more profound electrolyte imbalance than the patient with DKA. Levels of potassium, magnesium, and phosphorus may seem initially high, even in the presence of a marked total deficit. In the absence of acidemia, however, the discrepancy between the initial electrolyte reading and body stores is less than that of DKA. Initial serum sodium readings are inaccurate because of hyperglycemia.

Management

The fluid, electrolyte, and insulin regimens for the initial resuscitation in HHS are subject to the same controversies as the therapies for DKA (see Box 115.1). There have been varying recommendations about which IV fluids to administer, generally based on calculations of water deficits. There have been no well-done randomized trials comparing isotonic versus hypotonic fluid resuscitation; isotonic crystalloid is recommended in the volume-depleted patient. Cerebral edema has been noted in isolated case reports in adults, especially with glucose levels above 700 mg/dL. An association between IV fluid resuscitation and cerebral edema has not been shown in the literature; previous reports of this association may be due to the confounder that sicker patients often receive more aggressive fluid resuscitation.

Intravenous Fluids

For patients in hypovolemic shock, an initial IV fluid infusion is given as rapidly as possible. Glucose should be added to resuscitation fluids when the blood glucose level drops below 300 mg/dL. Because many HHS patients are older adults with coexisting diseases, such as congestive heart failure and renal failure, noninvasive or invasive forms of hemodynamic monitoring may be required to guide fluid administration when there is clinical suspicion of pulmonary edema or volume overload.

Electrolytes

Measurement of serum electrolyte levels should be used to guide replacement in the HHS patient. In particular, because acidosis is generally less, potassium levels more accurately reflect total body stores than they do in DKA.

Insulin

The pathophysiologic mechanisms of HHS are different from those of DKA, and there is usually enough basal insulin function to prevent frank ketoacidosis. Therefore, a continuous IV insulin infusion is not required in these patients, as with DKA. However, there are times when

---

TABLE 115.6 Features Distinguishing Diabetic Ketoacidosis Versus Hyperglycemic Hyperosmolar State

DKA	HHS
• Typically type 1 diabetic patients	• Typically type 2 diabetic patients
• Metabolic acidosis present	• Usually do not have metabolic acidosis as a result of glucose abnormality
• Blood sugars typically >250 mg/dL, though occasionally can be lower (euglycemic DKA)	• Sugars typically markedly high (>500 mg/dL)
• May have infection, trauma, myocardial ischemia as underlying triggers, or may be due to inadequate insulin administration	• Infection most common underlying cause, but may have other etiologies (dehydration, ischemic event, etc.)
• Associated with significant fluid deficits	• Associated with significant fluid deficits
• Insulin and fluids required to correct	• While insulin and fluids may be given, treatment is directed at an underlying cause
• Occurs across the age spectrum (toddler to geriatric)	• Typically seen in geriatric population

DKA, Diabetic ketoacidosis; *HHS*, hyperglycemic hyperosmolar state.

the use of an IV insulin infusion may help lower the glucose concentration in a more controlled fashion, particularly in patients with very high glucose levels (>700 mg/dL) or those who are severely hypoperfused, in whom intramuscular or subcutaneous insulin absorption may be erratic. If an IV insulin infusion is used, it should be a rate similar to that for DKA (0.1 unit/kg/h).

Other Considerations

A search for the underlying precipitant of HHS should be pursued. Response to therapy should be followed in the manner described for patients in DKA. Phenytoin (Dilantin) is contraindicated for the seizures of HHS because it is often ineffective and may impair endogenous insulin release.[5] Admitted patients should be given low-dose subcutaneous heparin to lessen the risk of thrombosis, which is increased by the volume depletion, hyperviscosity, hypotension, and inactivity associated with HHS.

Acute Complications

Reasons for high morbidity and mortality rates are not always clear, but many patients with HHS are older adults who have underlying cardiac and renal disease. Pediatric HHS differs from adult HHS in that children have a much higher incidence of fatal cerebral edema. Other causes of morbidity and mortality are similar to those described for DKA. The mortality rate of treated HHS patients has been 40% to 70% in the past but now ranges from 8% to 25%.[1,22]

Hyperglycemic Hyperosmolar State Disposition

In general, patients with HHS require hospitalization for IV hydration, glucose control, and evaluation of precipitating and complicating conditions.

DIABETES IN PREGNANCY

Before the discovery of insulin in 1922, diabetes in pregnancy was associated with a fetal death rate of 60% to 72% and maternal morbidity of approximately 30%.[7] In 1977, a linear relationship between glycemic control and perinatal mortality was discovered. Strict metabolic control is now a goal in all diabetic pregnancies.[6]

Pregnant patients are at particular risk from DKA due to the impact on both maternal and fetal health. For a variety of reasons, pregnant women are predisposed to glucose intolerance and excess ketone production. Although uncommon, DKA may reduce fetal oxygen delivery and cause perinatal asphyxia. Severe ketoacidosis is associated with a 50% to 90% fetal mortality rate due to hypoperfusion of the placenta.[18] Cognitive deficits in the offspring have been associated with maternal ketonuria from any cause. Hypoglycemia is common in pregnancy, in part because of intensive insulin treatment to maintain euglycemia. The effects of hypoglycemia on the fetus are unclear.

HYPOGLYCEMIA

Foundations

Hypoglycemia is a common problem in patients with type 1 diabetes, especially if tight glycemic control is practiced; it is the most dangerous, acute complication of diabetes. The estimated incidence of hypoglycemia in diabetic patients is 9 to 120 episodes/100 patient-years. As significant efforts continue to keep fasting and postprandial glucose concentrations within the normal range, the incidence of hypoglycemia may increase. The most common cause of coma associated with diabetes is an excess of administered insulin with respect to glucose intake.[22] Severe hypoglycemia is usually associated with blood glucose levels below 40 to 50 mg/dL and impaired cognitive function.

Protection against hypoglycemia is normally provided by the cessation of insulin release and mobilization of counterregulatory hormones, which increase hepatic glucose production and decrease glucose use. Diabetic patients using insulin are vulnerable to hypoglycemia because of insulin excess and failure of the counterregulatory system.

Hypoglycemia has many causes, such as missing a meal (decreased intake), increased energy output (exercise), and increased insulin dosage. It can also occur in the absence of any precipitant. Oral hypoglycemic agents have also been implicated in causing hypoglycemia, both when taken therapeutically and as an agent of overdose.

Hypoglycemia without warning symptoms, or hypoglycemia unawareness, is a dangerous complication of type 1 diabetes and is probably caused by previous exposure to low blood glucose concentrations because even a single hypoglycemic episode can reduce neurohumoral counterregulatory responses to subsequent episodes. Other factors associated with recurrent hypoglycemic attacks include overaggressive or intensified insulin therapy, longer history of diabetes, autonomic neuropathy, and decreased epinephrine secretion or sensitivity.

The Somogyi phenomenon is a common problem associated with iatrogenic hypoglycemia in type 1 diabetic patients. Excessive insulin dosing results in an unrecognized hypoglycemic episode that usually occurs in the early morning while the patient is sleeping. The counterregulatory hormone response produces rebound hyperglycemia, evident when the patient awakens. Often, the patient and physician interpret this hyperglycemia as an indication to increase the insulin dosage, which exacerbates the problem. Instead, the insulin dosage should be lowered or the timing changed.

Clinical Features

Symptomatic hypoglycemia occurs in most adults below a blood glucose level of 40 to 50 mg/dL. The rate at which the glucose level decreases, however, and the patient's age, gender, size, overall health, and previous hypoglycemic reactions contribute to symptom development. Signs and symptoms of hypoglycemia are caused by excessive secretion of epinephrine and CNS dysfunction; these include sweating, nervousness, tremor, tachycardia, hunger, and neurologic symptoms, ranging from bizarre behavior and confusion to seizures and coma. In patients with hypoglycemia unawareness, the prodrome to marked hypoglycemia may be minimal or absent, and these individuals may rapidly become unarousable. They may have a seizure or show focal neurologic signs, which resolve with glucose administration.

Differential Diagnoses

Hypoglycemia in the nondiabetic patient may be classified as postprandial or fasting. The most common cause of postprandial hypoglycemia is alimentary hyperinsulinism, such as that seen in patients who have undergone gastrectomy, gastrojejunostomy, pyloroplasty, or vagotomy. Fasting hypoglycemia is caused when there is an imbalance between glucose production and use. The causes of inadequate glucose production include hormone deficiencies, enzyme defects, substrate deficiencies, severe liver disease, and drugs. Causes of overuse of glucose include the presence of an insulinoma, exogenous insulin, sulfonylureas, drugs, endotoxic shock, extrapancreatic tumors, and a variety of enzyme deficiencies.

Diagnostic Testing

The cardinal laboratory test for hypoglycemia determines the blood glucose concentration. It should be performed, if possible, before therapy is begun. As noted, POC fingerstick testing helpful in permitting rapid, reasonably accurate blood glucose level estimates before therapy.

Laboratory testing should address any suggested cause of the hypoglycemia, such as ethanol, other drug ingestion, sepsis, or acute kidney injury causing decreased clearance of medications. If factitious hypoglycemia is suggested, testing for insulin antibodies or low levels of C peptide may be helpful. A patient who is surreptitiously administering exogenous insulin will have normal to low levels of C peptide and markedly elevated insulin levels.

Management

In alert patients with mild symptoms, oral consumption of sugar-containing foods or beverages is often adequate. In other patients, after blood is drawn for glucose determination, one to three ampules of $D_{50}W$ is administered IV while the patient's airway, breathing, and circulation are assessed and maintained. Augmentation of the blood glucose level by administration of an ampule of $D_{50}W$ may range from less than 40 mg/dL to more than 350 mg/dL. If alcohol use disorder is suggested, we recommend that thiamine be administered as well. In children younger than 8 years, providers should use $D_{25}W$ or $D_{10}W$. $D_{25}W$ may be prepared by diluting $D_{50}W$ 1:1 with sterile water. The dose is 0.5 to 1 g/kg body weight or 2 to 4 mL/kg when using $D_{25}W$. With recent shortages of $D_{50}W$, many emergency medical services (EMS) agencies and some hospitals have moved to the use of $D_{10}W$, giving boluses of up to 250 mL to achieve a similar glucose load to an ampule of $D_{50}W$.

If IV access cannot be rapidly obtained, 1 to 2 mg of glucagon may be given intramuscularly or subcutaneously. The onset of action is 10 to 20 minutes, and a peak response occurs in 30 to 60 minutes. It may be repeated as needed. Glucagon may also be administered IV; 1 mg has an effect similar to that of one ampule of $D_{50}W$. Glucagon is ineffective in causes of hypoglycemia resulting from absent glycogen, notably alcohol-induced hypoglycemia.

Families of type 1 diabetic patients are often taught to administer glucagon intramuscularly at home. Of the families so instructed, only 9% to 42% inject the glucagon when indicated. Intranasal glucagon has not been widely used. All patients with severe hypoglycemic reactions require aspiration and seizure precautions. Although the response to IV administration of glucose is generally rapid, older patients may require several days for complete recovery.

Treatment of hypoglycemia secondary to oral hypoglycemic agents depends on the agent. Metformin and the thiazolidinediones rarely cause significant hypoglycemia, whereas sulfonylureas, which are insulin secretagogues, can cause hypoglycemia. Sulfonylurea oral hypoglycemic agents pose particular problems because the hypoglycemia they induce tends to be prolonged and severe. Patients with an overdose of sulfonylurea hypoglycemic agents should be observed for a period of 24 hours if hypoglycemia recurs in the ED after management of the initial episode. Patients at risk for hypoglycemia from oral sulfonylureas include patients with impaired renal function, pediatric patients, and patients who are naïve to hypoglycemic agents. Although symptoms may occur after an overdose, several case reports in patients (e.g., with renal failure and pediatric patients) have described refractory hypoglycemia after ingestion of a single pill. One case series of pediatric patients presenting with sulfonylurea ingestion who were initially euglycemic demonstrated an average time to hypoglycemia of 8 hours.[22] However, in some patients, the onset of symptoms was delayed for up to 18 hours. As a result, we recommend 24 hours of observation for patients with known or suspected ingestion of hypoglycemic agents.

A patient with hypoglycemia from sulfonylureas, in addition to standard glucose replacement, frequently requires treatment with an agent to inhibit further insulin release, such as octreotide, a somatostatin analog. Several case series have described the use of octreotide in adult and pediatric patients suffering from sulfonylurea-induced hypoglycemia, frequently reporting successful results, with a significant decrease in the number of episodes of recurrent hypoglycemia. A randomized clinical trial has concluded that patients receiving octreotide had a decreased glucose supplementation requirement.[22] No single set protocol for use has been described; however, typical adult doses have ranged from 50 to 100 μg IV or subcutaneously every 12 hours, with pediatric dosages of 0.1 μg/kg IV or subcutaneously. Although experience thus far with octreotide has been positive, it does not obviate the need for prolonged observation and serial glucose level measurements.

Disposition

Type 1 diabetic patients with brief episodes of hypoglycemia uncomplicated by other conditions may be discharged from the ED if a cause of the hypoglycemia can be identified and corrected by instruction or medication. All patients should be given a meal before discharge to ensure their ability to tolerate oral feedings and to begin to replenish glycogen stores in glycogen-deficient patients. Patients who are discharged should receive short-term follow-up for ongoing evaluation. Patients with hypoglycemia caused by long-acting sulfonylurea medications should be observed in the hospital if they have recurrent hypoglycemia after a period of observation in the ED. Other agents, such as metformin, do not typically produce hypoglycemia, although they may have other issues, such as lactic acidosis, that may require admission.

The determination of inpatient (and if inpatient, type of bed, and monitoring required) versus outpatient evaluation of hypoglycemia in a nondiabetic patient should be based on the suggested cause and nature of the episode (i.e., factors such as severity, persistence, and recurrence).

The references for this chapter can be found online at ExpertConsult. com.

Rhabdomyolysis

Brit Long and Alex Koyfman

FOUNDATIONS

Background and Importance

Rhabdomyolysis is the result of damage to striated muscle, leading to release of creatine kinase, aspartate transaminase, lactate dehydrogenase, aldolase, the heme pigment myoglobin, and electrolytes. Patients most commonly present with diffuse muscle pain, weakness, and dark urine, which is caused by renal excretion of myoglobin pigment. Although most cases follow a benign course, patients with severe disease may experience renal failure, electrolyte derangements, compartment syndrome, or disseminated intravascular coagulation.

Anatomy, Physiology, and Pathophysiology

Skeletal muscle is 80% water and 20% protein, accounting for about half of the total body protein stores. Muscle cells require a significant amount of ATP and oxygen for appropriate cellular function, both at rest and with activity. Myoglobin delivers and releases oxygen to active skeletal muscle. Potassium, sodium, and calcium are strictly regulated by ATP-dependent cellular pumps, including sodium-potassium–adenosine triphosphatase (Na^+,K^+-ATPase) and an active calcium exchanger

(Ca^{2+}-ATPase pump) (Fig. 116.1). Under normal physiologic conditions, the concentration of free ionized calcium in the extracellular space is approximately 10,000 times greater than that in the intracellular space. Because extracellular calcium functions as an intracellular regulator and results in a sizeable electrochemical force on Ca^{2+}, even minor changes in the permeability of the plasma membrane to calcium will produce significant fluctuations in the cytosolic concentration, with potentially unfavorable consequences for the integrity of the cell.

Rhabdomyolysis involves four pathophysiologic processes (Fig. 116.2):

1. Impairment of the muscle's production or use of ATP at the cellular level. ATP concentrations within the cell fall; energy-dependent mechanisms falter, including Na^+,K^+-ATPase pumps, leading to disruption of chemical gradients, sarcolemma and cell membrane compromise, and cell destruction.
2. Disruption in the delivery of oxygen, glucose, and other nutrients to skeletal muscle.
3. Increased metabolic demands beyond the ability of the organism to deliver oxygen and nutrients.
4. Direct myocyte damage.

The pathogenesis of rhabdomyolysis follows a final common pathway—increased cytoplasmic calcium concentration from cell membrane damage and ATP depletion. Calcium activates proteases, phospholipases, and other proteolytic enzymes, which result in further ATP depletion, direct intracellular toxicity, and increased cellular membrane permeability. Increased intracellular calcium causes skeletal myocyte destruction and the release of toxic components into the extracellular and vascular spaces. Damage to adjacent capillaries causes local edema, increased local pressures, and tissue ischemia, resulting in further damage and energy depletion. Leukocytes adhere to damaged tissue and release radical oxygen species and enzymes that result in further cell damage. Ischemic etiologies of rhabdomyolysis may include reperfusion injury to myocytes.

Table 116.1 lists the various risk factors and causes of rhabdomyolysis.[1-4]

CLINICAL FEATURES

Rhabdomyolysis presents with a wide range of signs and symptoms. Patients may be asymptomatic or seriously ill with evidence of life-threatening complications, such as acute renal failure, disseminated intravascular coagulation, and dysrhythmias. In most patients, rhabdomyolysis presents in a mild form. Diagnosis in patients with a traumatic etiology is typically straightforward, but the diagnosis is often more challenging when rhabdomyolysis results from nontraumatic etiologies, or the patient is not able to provide a reliable history or cooperate with physical examination.

The classic presentation is localized muscle pain, stiffness, swelling, and tenderness, combined with dark-colored urine. However, this combination of factors is found together in less than 10% of patients. Localized muscle pain is the most common symptom (80%), followed by localized muscle weakness and swelling. The thighs are most commonly involved, followed by the calves and back. Other symptoms may include fever, palpitations, tachycardia, nausea and vomiting, agitation, focal sensory deficits, pain with passive range of motion, skin changes, and decreased urine output. The finding of dark urine depends on the severity of the injury and the patient's muscle mass, urine concentration, and baseline renal function. The absence of visibly dark urine does not exclude the diagnosis of rhabdomyolysis.

Children are more diagnostically challenging. Most pediatric patients with rhabdomyolysis experience muscle pain, but fewer than

5% present with dark urine. Children also more commonly present with symptoms suggestive of a viral syndrome.

A focused history provides important information regarding the symptoms of rhabdomyolysis, risk factors for the disease (see Table 116.1), prior history of the condition, or a family history consistent with rhabdomyolysis (due to inherited myopathies), which is associated with recurrent episodes of rhabdomyolysis. Other important historical points include changes in urine output and color, oral intake, and medication or illicit substance use. In patients with severe trauma or altered mental status, history from first responders, witnesses, or family members can assist.

Complications

Early Complications

Compartment Syndrome. Most skeletal muscles are encased in compartments formed by bones, fascia, and other structures. The massive influx of calcium and sodium in rhabdomyolysis leads to the accumulation of large amounts of extracellular fluid in myocytes, causing local edema and raised pressure within the compartments. Note that rhabdomyolysis can therefore be the cause and result of compartment syndrome.[5]

Electrolyte Disorders and Acidosis. Potassium released from damaged muscle may lead to hyperkalemia. Over 98% of the body's potassium is found in the intracellular space, and 60% to 70% of the total cellular mass of the human body consists of skeletal muscle. Therefore, damage to as little as 100 g of muscle may increase the serum

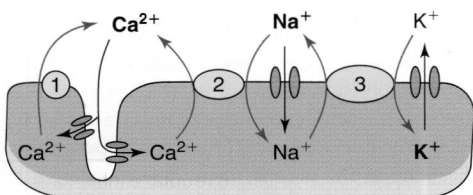

1 = ATP-dependent Ca^{2+} pump
2 = Na^+-Ca^{2+} exchanger (3:1)
3 = Na^+, K^+-ATPase pump (3:2)

Fig. 116.1 Normal Membrane Ionic Pump Function of Skeletal Muscle Cell. When the ATP supply is impaired, the intracellular sodium concentration increases, reversing the function of the Na^+-Ca^{2+} exchanger, with a subsequent increase in the intracellular calcium level.

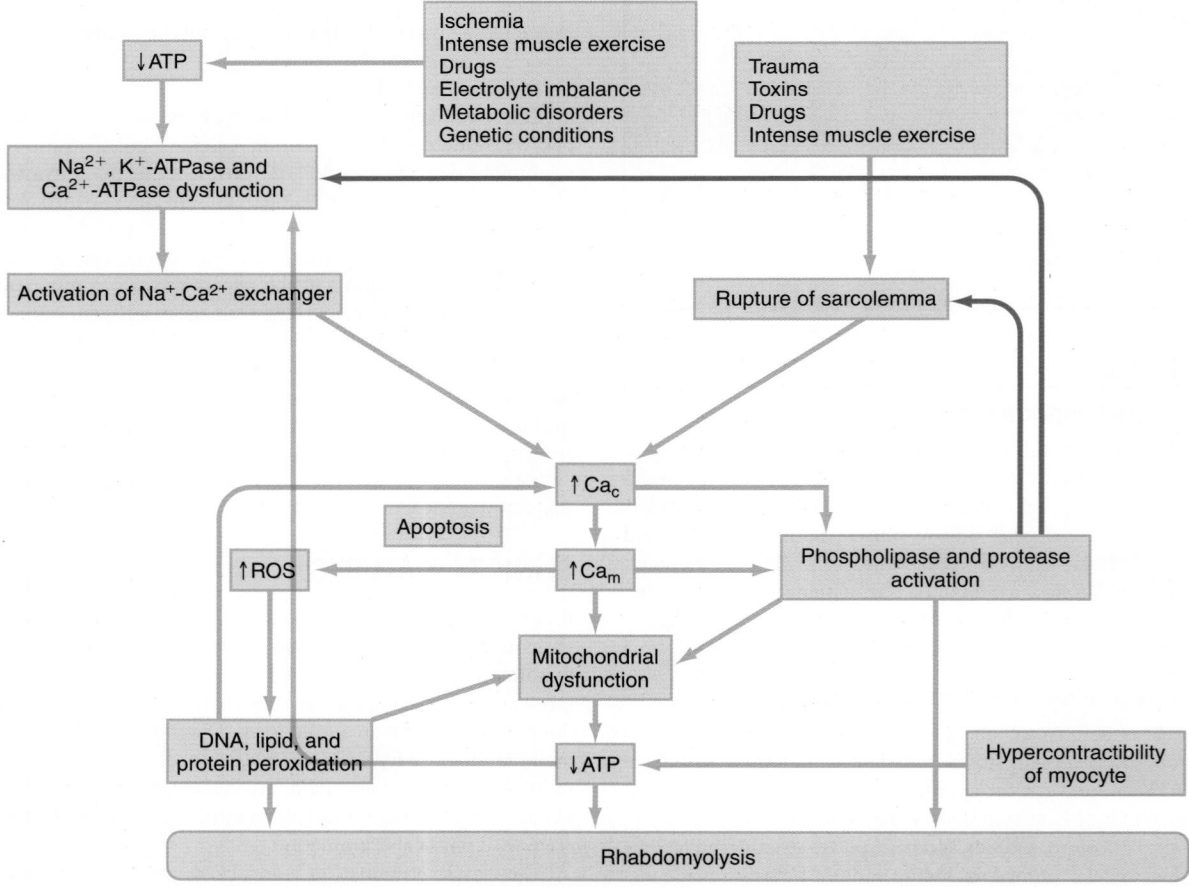

Fig. 116.2 Pathophysiology of rhabdomyolysis. Ca_c, cytosolic [Ca]; Ca_m, mitochondrial [Ca].

TABLE 116.1   Risk Factors and Etiologies of Rhabdomyolysis[1-4]

Exertion	Intense exercise, seizure, status asthmaticus, sickle cell crisis, alcohol withdrawal
Trauma or compression	Motor vehicle accidents, prolonged immobilization, crush syndrome, electrical injury, burns
Extreme changes in body temperature	Hyperthermia, hypothermia, serotonin syndrome, malignant hyperthermia, neuroleptic malignant syndrome
Electrolyte alterations	Hypokalemia, hypophosphatemia, hypocalcemia, hyponatremia, hypernatremia, hyperglycemia
Muscle ischemia/hypoxia	Arterial occlusion due to embolus, thrombus, or during vascular surgery
Infections	Sepsis, *Salmonella*, *Streptococcus pyogenes*, *Staphylococcus aureus*, *Clostridium* species, *Legionella*, influenza, coxsackie, Epstein-Barr virus, herpes virus, HIV
Drugs/toxins	Statins, anti-lipid agents (ezetimibe, clofibrate, gemfibrozil), proton pump inhibitors, psychiatric medications (SSRIs, SNRIs, TCAs, benzodiazepines, barbiturates, phenothiazines, lithium), alcohol, cocaine, opiates, amphetamines, LSD, phencyclidine, synthetic cannabinoids, bath salts, antihistamines, propofol, arsenic, carbon monoxide, azathioprine, quinidine, salicylates, succinylcholine, thiazides, vasopressin, pentamidine, terbutaline, theophylline
Endocrine	Thyroid abnormalities, hyperaldosteronism
Autoimmune	Dermatomyositis, polymyositis
Genetic	Krebs cycle disorders, G6PD deficiency, lipid metabolism disorders, mitochondrial chain disorders, muscular dystrophies
Foodborne	Ingestion of burbot, eel, pike, crayfish, buffalo fish, and other fish/crustacean species

HIV, Human immunodeficiency virus; *SSRI*, selective serotonin reuptake inhibitors; *SNRI*, serotonin norepinephrine reuptake inhibitors; *TCA*, tricyclic antidepressants; *LSD*, lysergic acid diethylamide; *G6PD*, glucose-6-phosphate dehydrogenase.
Data from Nguyen KA, Li L, Lu D, et al. A comprehensive review and meta-analysis of risk factors for statin-induced myopathy. *Eur J Clin Pharmacol.* 2018;74(9):1099-1109; Mousavi SR, Vahabzadeh M, Mahdizadeh A, et al. Rhabdomyolysis in 114 patients with acute poisonings. *J Res Med Sci.* 2015;20:239-243; Durand D, Delgado LL, de la Parra-Pellot DM, et al. Psychosis and severe rhabdomyolysis associated with synthetic cannabinoid use. *Clin Schizophr Relat Psychoses.* 2015;8:205-208; Fadila MF, Wool KJ. Rhabdomyolysis secondary to influenza a infection: a case report and review of the literature. *N Am J Med Sci.* 2015;7:122-124.

potassium by 1.0 mEq/L. Acidemia contributes to hyperkalemia and can be exacerbated by oliguria.

Rhabdomyolysis-related fluid sequestration or myoglobin-induced kidney injury reduces the kidney's ability to excrete acid. Metabolic acidosis is also caused by the release of organic acids (e.g., lactic acid, uric acid, and sulfur-containing proteins).

The disruption of muscle cells releases phosphoric components into circulation, and when massive, this can lead to hyperphosphatemia and ectopic calcification, typically depositing in necrotic tissue. In case of rhabdomyolysis with severe, extensive muscle damage, calcium phosphate crystal deposition in damaged muscle can lead to early-phase hypocalcemia, with potentially fatal dysrhythmias. This is rare and reported only in case reports. Hyperkalemia coupled with hypocalcemia predisposes patients to malignant dysrhythmias. Furthermore, excessively high phosphate levels shut down the 1α-hydroxylase enzyme of the kidneys, decreasing production of the active form of vitamin D, further contributing to early hypocalcemia. Late in the course of rhabdomyolysis, calcium initially deposited in the cytoplasm of necrotic muscle cells can reenter the plasma, resulting in late hypercalcemia.

Hypovolemia. In rhabdomyolysis, fluid moves from intravascular compartments into damaged muscle. In cases of massive muscle crush or electrical injury, this fluid shift may exceed 15 liters, causing profound intravascular volume depletion.

Hepatic laboratory abnormalities. Reversible elevations in aspartate transaminase (AST) levels may occur with rhabdomyolysis, possibly caused by myocyte release of proteases. The level of AST elevation is correlated with the severity of CK elevation in patients with rhabdomyolysis.[6] However, AST elevations may also be of skeletal muscle origin. Preexisting hepatic dysfunction may potentiate statin-induced rhabdomyolysis.[2] Rhabdomyolysis is not typically associated with abnormalities of other liver function tests or synthetic function such as alanine aminotransferase, prothrombin time, and albumin.

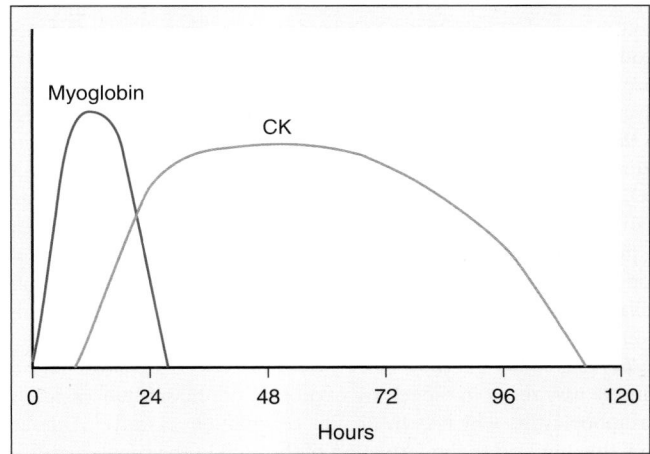

Fig. 116.3 Variations of Myoglobin and Creatine Kinase (CK) Levels During the Course of Rhabdomyolysis. Myoglobin is the first enzyme that increases but, because of its rapid clearance from the plasma, it returns to normal levels within the first 24 hours after the onset of symptoms. The CK level increases a few hours later than myoglobin, reaches its peak value within the first 24 hours, and remains at these levels for 3 days. CK is considered to be a more useful marker for the diagnosis and assessment of the severity of muscle injury because of its delayed clearance from the plasma.

Late Complications

Myoglobin-Induced Acute Kidney Injury. Experimental evidence suggests that myoglobinuric acute renal failure is caused by myoglobin cast formation in the distal convoluted tubules, the direct cytotoxic action of myoglobin on the epithelial cells of the proximal convoluted tubules, and ischemia from intrarenal vasoconstriction (Fig. 116.3).

Myoglobin concentrates along the renal tubules and precipitates in acidic urine with uric acid to form obstructive casts. This is enhanced by volume depletion and renal vasoconstriction, which reduce blood flow and the glomerular filtration rate (GFR), promoting the accumulation of necrotic epithelial cells into tubular casts. Tubule obstruction occurs at the level of the distal tubule, whereas direct cytotoxicity occurs mainly in the proximal tubules. There remains some controversy about the exact mechanism of renal dysfunction in rhabdomyolysis; some experts believe that casts and tubular obstruction are not the cause, but rather the consequence, of poor tubular clearance.

When the concentration of myoglobin filtered at the glomerulus exceeds normal levels, tubular cells at the proximal convoluted tubule increase their resorptive capacity to limit the excretion of myoglobin into the urine, protecting the kidney from its nephrotoxic effects. At a urine pH of 5.6 or lower, myoglobin, an iron-containing heme protein, dissociates into free iron (Fe), ferrihemate (Fe-heme complex), and globin inside the proximal tubular epithelial cell. Oxidation of ferrous oxide in the Fe-heme complex in combination with free iron reaction with H_2O_2 produces free radicals which may result in nephrotoxicity. Free iron may also act as a free radical, although its role in rhabdomyolysis-induced renal injury is unclear. Myoglobin itself has been shown to exhibit peroxidase-like enzyme activity. Ferrihemate causes direct nephrotoxic effects along with the resultant increased oxidative stress within the tubular epithelial cell. More recent evidence has argued against free iron's role in oxidative stress–induced renal injury, instead emphasizing the role of ferrihemate-induced lipid peroxidation in cell injury.

Fluid shifts and renal dysfunction lead to activation of the renin-angiotensin-aldosterone system and production of vasoconstricting molecules such as endothelin 1 and vasopressin. There is also decreased production of vasodilatory prostaglandins. Nitric oxide (NO), a potent vasodilator agent, assists with the maintenance of renal blood flow. Myoglobin released from damaged muscle may act as a NO scavenger in the renal microcirculation, itself reduced by NO buffering against oxidant injury. When increased myoglobin concentrations overcome NO, the kidney is deprived of the ability to autoregulate blood flow and maintain adequate perfusion. Thus, myoglobin is free to cause damage in proximal tubular epithelial cells, specifically under acidotic conditions. Other locally stimulated vascular mediators, including thromboxane A_2, tumor necrosis factor alpha, and F_2-isoprostanes, also reduce renal blood flow and cause oxidant injury.

Disseminated Intravascular Coagulation. Extensive muscle damage may result in the release of prothrombotic substances, mainly thromboplastin, which activate the coagulation cascade. Although rare, this can lead to the formation of thrombi in the capillary tufts of the glomeruli and disseminated intravascular coagulation.

DIFFERENTIAL DIAGNOSIS

The differential diagnosis of rhabdomyolysis includes conditions that may present with influenza-like symptoms, myalgias, extremity pain, or urinary changes. Such conditions include heatstroke, sepsis, infective endocarditis, myocarditis, spinal epidural abscess, pyomyositis, toxic ingestion or carbon monoxide exposure, thyroid abnormalities, compartment syndrome, vascular injury, and orthopedic injuries.

Red or dark urine can be seen with hemoglobinuria, urolithiasis, porphyria, ingestion of specific foods (blackberries, beets, rhubarb, food coloring) and numerous medications, including laxatives, rifampin, doxorubicin, chloroquine, hydroxocobalamin, and deferoxamine.

Notably, many of the conditions that mimic rhabdomyolysis can also cause rhabdomyolysis (e.g., heatstroke, bacterial or viral infection, and toxic ingestions).

DIAGNOSTIC TESTING

Serum Creatine Kinase

The definitive diagnosis of rhabdomyolysis is made by serologic testing for creatine kinase (CK). CK functions as an energy reservoir for ATP: creatine + ATP = creatine kinase + ADP (adenosine diphosphate). CK has a half-life of 1.5 days; it increases in the first 12 hours after injury, peaks during the first three days, and normalizes at approximately five days. A CK level five times the upper limit of normal (≈1000 U/L), without an alternative cause, confirms the diagnosis.

Serum and Urine Myoglobin

Myoglobin is a dark-red protein composed of globin and a molecule of heme. It supplies oxygen to skeletal and cardiac muscle in times of need and is renally excreted. It is initially filtered at the glomerulus and reabsorbed in the tubules, where it is broken down into its component parts, globin and heme. As with all other low-molecular-weight proteins, a small amount is excreted in the urine. The normal concentration of myoglobin in the urine is less than 10 μg/L. A normal serum concentration of myoglobin is less than 100 μg/L.

During rhabdomyolysis, myoglobin released by damaged muscle is increasingly filtered at the glomerulus. This leads to an initial increased resorptive capacity by glomerular and tubular epithelial cells, developed presumably as a protective response to increased filtered myoglobin. When serum myoglobin concentrations exceed 0.3 mg/L and the renal threshold of 1.0 mg/dL is met, this resorptive capacity is overwhelmed, and excess myoglobin appears in the urine. This myoglobin is detected by urine dipstick as positive for blood with microscopic urine analysis showing few, or no RBCs (Table 116.2).

In the past, the diagnosis of rhabdomyolysis was made by measuring serum myoglobin; however, myoglobin has a serum half-life of 1 to 3 hours, is completely absent after 24 hours, and normal levels depend upon the patient's muscle mass. These factors make serum myoglobin an unreliable diagnostic test. This is also true of urine myoglobin levels, which depend on the degree of muscle injury, volume status of the patient, and urinary flow rate. A well-hydrated patient with normal renal function can rapidly clear myoglobin from the body. The absence of plasma or urine myoglobin does not rule out rhabdomyolysis (Fig. 116.4).

Urine Dipstick and Urinalysis

Myoglobinuria causes a false-positive result for blood in urine dipstick testing. The drawback of this test is its inability to distinguish among heme compounds. In myoglobinuria, microscopic analysis will show few if any red blood cells, thereby distinguishing between hemoglobin and hemoglobin-rich red blood cells (from hemolysis or hematuria). Myoglobinuria, in combination with an elevated plasma CK level, confirms rhabdomyolysis. At plasma concentrations above 100 to 300 mg/L, macroscopic myoglobinuria manifests as tea-colored urine.

The urine dipstick test or urinalysis result is generally acidic in rhabdomyolysis, which plays a role in cast and uric acid crystal formation and pathologic myoglobin metabolism in tubular epithelial cells. Proteinuria may be noted because of the detection of the globin component of myoglobin. Urine sediment will show myoglobin casts and dead epithelial cells (see Table 116.2).

Other Laboratory Findings

Common electrolyte disturbances in patients with rhabdomyolysis include hyperkalemia, hyperphosphatemia, and early hypocalcemia followed by late hypercalcemia. Late hypercalcemia is postulated to be due to the mobilization of calcium that was initially sequestered in damaged muscle.

TABLE 116.2 Causes and Microscopic Features of Red and Brown Urine

Cause	Results for Blood in Urine[a]	Sediment[b]	Supernatant
Hematuria	+++	Red	Yellow
Myoglobinuria	+++	Normal	Red to brown
Hemoglobinuria	+++	Normal	Red to brown
Porphyria	–	Normal	Red
Bile pigments	–	Normal	Brown
Food and drugs[c]	–	Normal	Red to brown

[a]Urine tested with dipstick test.

[b]Normal refers to white or yellow color.

[c]Food and drugs that can cause red urine include beets, blackberries, rhubarb, food coloring, fava beans, phenolphthalein, rifampin, doxorubicin, deferoxamine, chloroquine, ibuprofen, and methyldopa. Those that cause brown urine include levodopa, metronidazole, nitrofurantoin, iron sorbitol, chloroquine, and methyldopa.

Adapted from Bosch X, Poch E, Grau JM. Rhabdomyolysis and acute kidney injury. *N Engl J Med.* 2009;361:62-79.

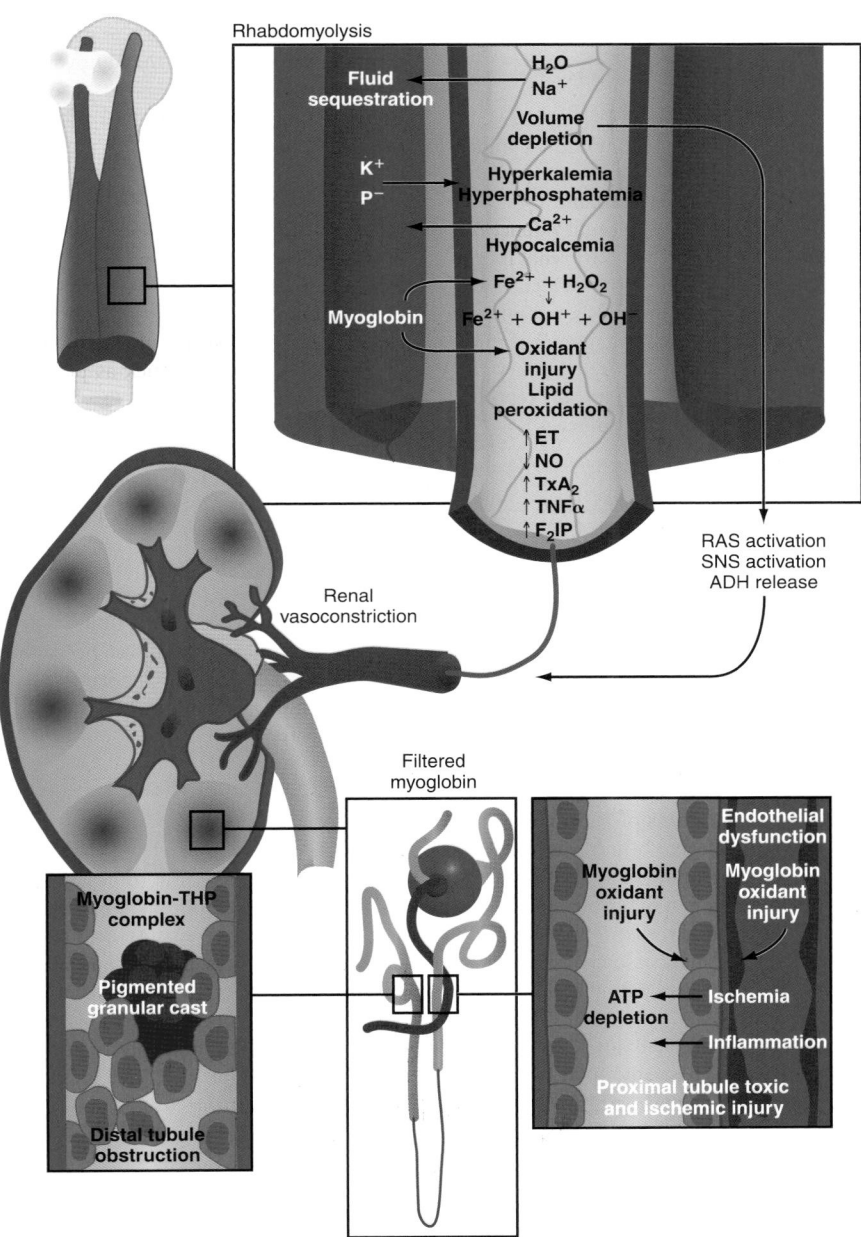

Fig. 116.4 Pathophysiologic Mechanisms in Rhabdomyolysis-Induced Acute Kidney Injury. *ADH,* Antidiuretic hormone; *ATP,* adenosine triphosphate; *ET,* endothelin; F_2IP, F_2-isoprostanes; *NO,* nitric oxide; *RAS,* renin-angiotensin system; *SNS,* sympathetic nervous system; *THP,* Tamm-Horsfall protein; *TNFα,* tumor necrosis factor alpha; TxA_2, thromboxane A_2. (Adapted from: Bosch X, Poch E, Grau JM. Rhabdomyolysis and acute kidney injury. *N Engl J Med.* 2009;361:62-72.)

Hyperuricemia from the release of muscle nucleic acids is especially common in patients with large muscle mass, as is elevation in serum lactate dehydrogenase (LDH). Metabolic acidosis typically occurs from the generation of organic acids from damaged muscle—namely, lactate and uric acid. Hypoalbuminemia and anemia result from capillary damage and release into the extracellular space.

Both blood urea nitrogen (BUN) and creatinine (Cr) concentrations increase, but with a characteristic decrease in the BUN/Cr ratio due to large amounts of creatinine released into the serum from damaged muscle. A normal BUN/Cr ratio is 10:1; in rhabdomyolysis, it can be 5:1 or even less. In severe cases with significant muscle necrosis and electrolyte abnormalities, disseminated intravascular coagulation (DIC) can ensue with bleeding or thrombosis and abnormal coagulation panel, thrombocytopenia, low fibrinogen, elevated D-dimer, and fragmented RBCs, triggered by the released thromboplastin from damaged tissue.

Prognostic Tests in Rhabdomyolysis

Although CK levels may correlate with the risk of developing acute kidney injury in patients with rhabdomyolysis due to traumatic injury, such as crush injury, the degree of CK level elevation is not a reliable predictor of acute kidney injury, need for dialysis, or death.[7,8]

However, patients with an estimated glomerular filtration rate (eGFR) of more than 60 mL/min/1.73 m^2 appear to have low risk for acute kidney injury or death. Based on the cumulative evidence, CK should be used as a diagnostic marker for rhabdomyolysis, but not as a prognostic indicator of acute renal injury.[9] Once the diagnosis of rhabdomyolysis is made, the eGFR can be used to predict renal injury and help determine the need for admission. The eGFR is typically reported routinely on basic metabolic panels that include creatinine.

MANAGEMENT

Management of rhabdomyolysis focuses on treatment of the cause, prevention of renal failure, and management of life- or limb-threatening complications.

Fluid Replacement

Volume expansion is critical to avoiding myoglobin-induced acute renal failure in those who are hypovolemic.[10] Fluid expansion increases renal blood flow, glomerular filtration, and urine production, while reducing the risk of renal injury. Patients with rhabdomyolysis can present with severe dehydration due to fluid sequestration in the affected skeletal muscles. Several case series, mostly from victims of natural disasters with crush injury, have shown that some degree of intravascular volume contraction is a prerequisite for developing acute renal failure. Because acute renal failure appears to develop in hypovolemic patients with a longer delay to supportive therapy, fluid resuscitation should be instituted as early as possible.[11] Victims of mass casualty events often have prolonged extrication times, so fluid resuscitation should begin before complete extrication, when possible.

Fluid resuscitation should generally be initiated at CK levels more than five times the upper limit of normal (typically, 1000 IU/L) and should be continued until levels trend down and drop below this level. Fluid boluses are recommended in patients with hypovolemia or crush injury. In euvolemic or hypervolemic patients, over-resuscitation may be harmful. In general, titration to a urinary output of 2 to 3 mL/kg/hr or more and patient euvolemia are reasonable targets for adults.[3]

Balanced crystalloids such as plasmalyte or lactated Ringers solution are recommended for initial resuscitation, though there are no studies demonstrating improved outcomes with balanced fluids in rhabdomyolysis compared to normal saline. Normal saline contains supraphysiologic concentrations of chloride ions. Massive infusion of normal saline leads to a disproportionate increase in serum chloride concentrations, inducing an iatrogenic metabolic (hyperchloremic) acidosis that may exacerbate myoglobin precipitation, tubular obstruction, and risk of hyperkalemia-related complications.

Urine alkalinization, achieved through addition of sodium bicarbonate to IV fluids, is no longer recommended. Animal data suggested potential value for alkalinization, based on: (1) decreased renal myoglobin precipitation; (2) decreased reduction-oxidation (redox) cycling of myoglobin and lipid peroxidation, and thus tubule injury; and (3) decreased myoglobin-induced renal vasoconstriction.

However, the clinical benefits of alkalinization over IV hydration were never established, and sodium bicarbonate therapy has not been proven superior to normal saline diuresis at increasing urine pH, or more importantly, improving patient outcomes such as mortality and renal failure.

We do not recommend the use of sodium bicarbonate to induce urinary alkalinization in rhabdomyolysis because there is no evidence of improved outcomes with its use. However, isotonic bicarbonate infusion may be considered for those with non-anion gap metabolic acidosis or uremic acidosis.

Mannitol and Other Diuretics

In human studies, the addition of mannitol has not demonstrated benefit over fluid expansion alone, and no randomized controlled trials have shown any beneficial effect. Accordingly, we do not recommend the use of mannitol in the treatment of rhabdomyolysis. Animal studies demonstrated that the bulk of mannitol's effect is attributable simply to its osmotic diuretic action, but large accumulated doses of mannitol may be detrimental by causing renal vasoconstriction and tubular toxicity, a condition known as osmotic nephrosis, as well as exacerbating hypovolemia.

There also is no evidence to support the use of loop diuretics or carbonic anhydrase inhibitor diuretics in the treatment of rhabdomyolysis.

Experimental Therapies

Antioxidants such as glutathione and vitamin E analogues have shown promise in experimental animal models of myoglobin-induced oxidant injury and may have a future role in management. Grape seed proanthocyanidin extract has been shown to have renoprotective effects in animal models. The xanthine oxidase inhibitor, allopurinol, is being studied as a prophylactic agent in those at risk for exertional rhabdomyolysis.[12]

Renal Replacement Therapy

Renal replacement therapy (RRT) is needed in up to 20% of patients with acute kidney injury from rhabdomyolysis. As with other causes of acute renal failure, the indications for emergent RRT remain (1) uncorrectable metabolic acidosis, (2) life-threatening hyperkalemia and other electrolyte disturbances despite medical management, and (3) manifestations of uremia, and anuria or oliguria, despite volume expansion in patients with complications related to fluid overload. The current literature does not demonstrate a mortality benefit with RRT in the setting of rhabdomyolysis, but in those with a previously mentioned indication for RRT, RRT is associated with more rapid removal of myoglobin and improvement in electrolyte, BUN, and creatinine levels. RRT should be continued until the indication for it is corrected and the patient has improved.

DISPOSITION

The majority of patients with rhabdomyolysis require hospitalization for fluid resuscitation and close monitoring of renal function. Discharge with close outpatient follow-up or observation stays can be considered in select, milder cases. Patients with a known etiology, mild symptoms, normal vital signs, normal renal function and electrolytes, and reliable follow-up may be discharged. Hemodynamically unstable patients or those requiring RRT should be considered for ICU admission, whereas those who do not meet these criteria or are not appropriate for outpatient management should be admitted to the hospital floor.

Prognosis

Rhabdomyolysis has an excellent prognosis when recognized and treated early. The majority of cases follow a benign course and resolve without complications. With the exception of hyperkalemia-related death or the rare complication of DIC, which typically occurs in patients with extensive muscle damage or crush injury, acute kidney injury is the most serious complication of rhabdomyolysis. Most patients who have acute renal failure will recover full renal function with fluid rehydration to euvolemia. Mortality data for patients with renal failure vary widely according to the study population, underlying etiology, presence of multiple causative agents, and comorbidities with no clear data; however, long-term survival among patients with rhabdomyolysis and acute renal injury tends to be very good when timely management is provided.

The references for this chapter can be found online at ExpertConsult. com.

117

Thyroid and Adrenal Disorders

Molly E.W. Thiessen

KEY CONCEPTS

Hyperthyroidism

- Hyperthyroidism induces a hypermetabolic state and increases β-adrenergic activity. The resulting clinical manifestations range from vague constitutional symptoms to more organ-specific symptoms (see Box 117.1).
- Hyperthyroidism in elders may be asymptomatic or may manifest with subtle nonspecific symptoms such as weight loss, shortness of breath, and/or dementia.
- The laboratory test of choice for suspected hyperthyroidism is the thyroid stimulating hormone (TSH) concentration with free T_4 and T_3 levels.
- Thyroid storm is a life-threatening thyrotoxic crisis that often presents with fever, extreme tachycardia, and/or altered sensorium. It requires prompt recognition and therapy, as well as identification and treatment of any precipitating cause, such as infection.
- The order of medication administration in thyroid storm is critical. Iodine can precipitate thyroid storm and must be given a minimum of 1 hour after thionamide therapy (PTU or methimazole). As such, the typical order is beta blocker (propranolol), PTU or methimazole, and then iodine (SSKI, Lugol solution).

Hypothyroidism

- Hypothyroidism results from lack of stimulation of the thyroid gland (central or secondary hypothyroidism) or intrinsic gland dysfunction limiting hormone production (primary hypothyroidism).
- Signs and symptoms of hypothyroidism range from asymptomatic to overt organ failure, which can lead to death (see Box 117.5).
- Determination of an elevated TSH level is the most sensitive and single best screening test to confirm the diagnosis of primary hypothyroidism.
- Replacement with levothyroxine (T_4) remains the treatment of choice and resolves physical and psychological signs and symptoms in most patients.
- Myxedema coma is a life-threatening event that presents with altered mental status and hypothermia, along with a concomitant precipitating event (see

Box 117.6). It usually occurs in patients with untreated or undertreated hypothyroidism. Treatment with thyroid hormone replacement must be initiated, often based solely on clinical findings.

Adrenal Excess States

- Adrenal excess states run the spectrum from Cushing syndrome, to primary and secondary hyperadrenalism, to pheochromocytoma.
- Symptoms of adrenal excess will vary, depending on the etiology, with chronic, nonspecific symptoms that arise from Cushing syndrome (generalized weakness, fatigue, menstrual irregularities, and weight gain), to simple refractory hypertension with hyperaldosteronism, to acute, refractory hypertension and hyperadrenergic symptoms with pheochromocytoma.
- Diagnosis of hyperaldosteronism is typically clinical, and confirmed by laboratory testing and imaging studies, depending on the etiology. In most cases, acute stabilization of the presenting complaint is paramount, and definitive diagnosis will occur outside the ED. Any adrenal incidentaloma discovered on imaging obtained in the ED, especially in the setting of hypertension, should prompt further evaluation for adrenal excess.

Adrenal Insufficiency

- Clinical manifestations of secondary adrenal insufficiency are often vague and nonspecific, including fatigue, weakness, dizziness, nausea, vomiting, and other nonspecific GI symptoms. Patients with primary adrenal insufficiency characteristically have more pronounced clinical manifestations and skin hyperpigmentation.
- The ACTH stimulation test and measurements of cortisol levels is the most convenient method and is considered the criterion standard to make the diagnosis.
- Refractory hypotension in the acutely ill patient may be the only clue to adrenal insufficiency and is readily treated with IV administration of glucocorticoids (hydrocortisone, 100 mg).

HYPERTHYROIDISM

Foundations

Background and Importance

Hyperthyroidism is a condition caused by overproduction and increased circulation of thyroid hormone. The disorder runs the spectrum from subclinical hyperthyroidism to thyrotoxicosis and thyroid storm, a life-threatening disorder. Thyrotoxicosis is a hypermetabolic condition that results from elevated levels of thyroid hormones—triiodothyronine (T_3) and thyroxine (T_4). This can occur from hormone overproduction, increased thyroid hormone release from an injured gland, or exogenous thyroid hormone. For the purpose of this discussion, the terms *hyperthyroidism* and *thyrotoxicosis* are used interchangeably.

Anatomy, Physiology, and Pathophysiology

The normal adult thyroid gland is a highly vascular bilobar organ overlying the anterior trachea (Fig. 117.1). The thyroid's function is to secrete two iodinated hormones, T_3 and T_4. Only about 20% of circulating T_3 is directly secreted by the thyroid; the remainder is produced by peripheral conversion of T_4 to the more biologically active T_3. The thyroid is the only endocrine gland that stores large quantities of hormone.

Hormone production is regulated by a negative feedback loop involving the hypothalamic-pituitary-thyroid axis (Fig. 117.2). As the serum levels of T_4 and T_3 fall, the hypothalamus releases the tripeptide thyrotropin-releasing hormone (TRH), which in turn stimulates the anterior pituitary gland's release of the polypeptide thyroid-stimulating hormone (TSH) from its thyrotroph cells. TSH then binds to epithelial

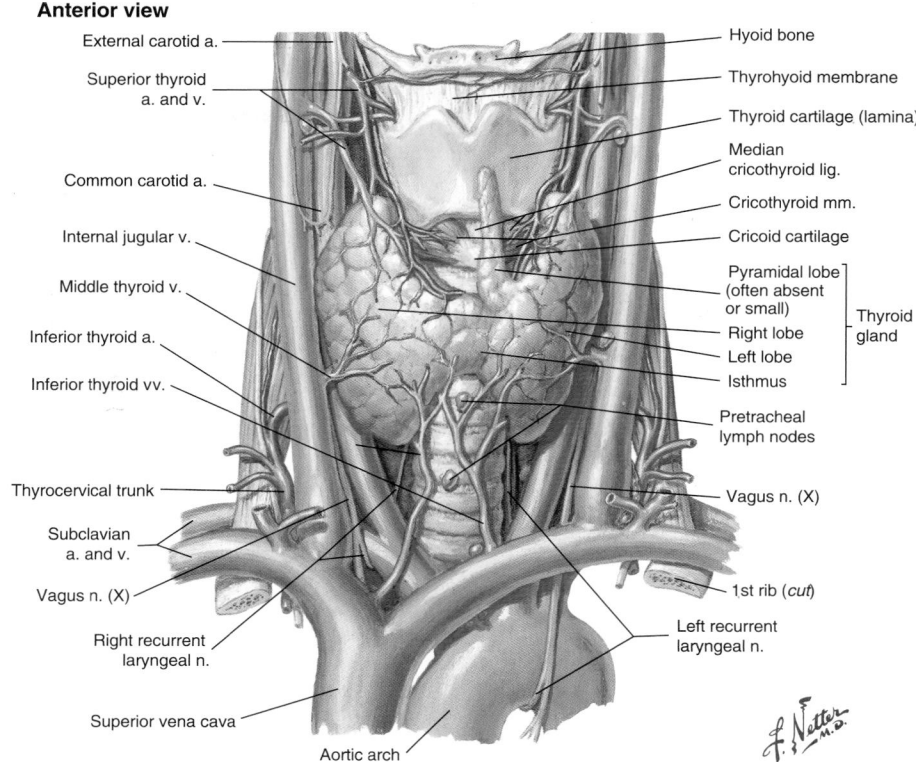

Fig. 117.1 Anatomy of the thyroid gland and related structures. (Netter illustration from www.netterimages. com. Copyright Elsevier. All rights reserved.)

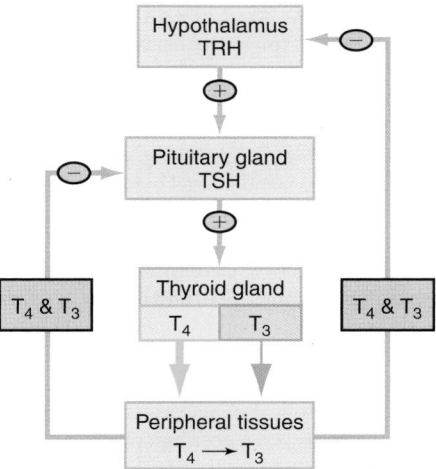

Fig. 117.2 Negative feedback loop of thyroid hormone regulation—hypothalamic-pituitary-thyroid axis. Thyroid hormone production is regulated by the hypothalamus and pituitary gland. Hypothalamic thyrotropin-releasing hormone (TRH) stimulates pituitary thyrotropin (TSH) synthesis and secretion. In turn, TSH stimulates the production and release of thyroxine (T_4) triiodothyronine (T_3) from the thyroid gland. Once released, T_4 and T_3 exert a negative feedback mechanism on the production of TRH and TSH. T_4 is converted to T_3 in the peripheral tissues.

cells on the thyroid gland, stimulating follicular cells to synthesize and secrete the thyroid hormones T_4 and T_3. TRH release may also result from exercise, stress, malnutrition, hypoglycemia, and sleep.

The function of thyroid hormone is to influence the metabolism of cells by increasing their basal metabolic rate. It has a role in protein synthesis and functions together with other hormones necessary for normal growth and development. T_3 and T_4 increase the expression and sensitivity of β-adrenergic receptors, increasing the response to endogenous catecholamines.

T_4 is a prohormone with only mild intrinsic activity; its deiodination produces T_3, the biologically active hormone. More than 99.5% of thyroid hormones are protein-bound in the serum to thyroxine-binding globulin (TBG) and other proteins, rendering them metabolically inactive. As a result, only free T_4 and free T_3 are clinically relevant.

Although iodide is a necessary substrate for thyroid hormone production, excess iodide can have two opposing effects. In the Wolff-Chaikoff effect, excess iodine inhibits the release of thyroid hormone from the gland by blocking iodide trapping and thyroglobulin iodination. This inhibition is transient, typically lasting only a matter of days. An iodine load can induce hyperthyroidism (Jod-Basedow effect) in some patients with multinodular goiter and occult Graves disease.

Clinical Features

History and Physical Examination

Hyperthyroidism induces a hypermetabolic state and increases β-adrenergic activity. The resulting clinical manifestations range from vague constitutional symptoms to more organ-specific symptoms (Box 117.1). Altered mental status and coma typify thyroid storm, the most severe manifestation of disease.

Hyperthyroidism in older adults often manifests in more subtle ways, often asymptomatic or with nonspecific symptoms of weight loss, shortness of breath, and/or dementia. Elders are more prone to cardiac manifestations of hyperthyroidism and may present with atrial fibrillation.[1] Elders who smoke or have higher circulating thyroid hormone levels appear to have more severe symptoms. Thyrotoxic periodic paralysis is a rare manifestation that presents as a sudden and

BOX 117.1   Symptoms of Thyrotoxicosis

Constitutional: Weight loss despite hyperphagia, fatigue, generalized weakness
Hypermetabolic: Heat intolerance, cold preference, excessive perspiration
Cardiorespiratory: Palpitations, dyspnea, dyspnea on exertion, chest pains, poor exercise tolerance
Gastrointestinal: Nausea, vomiting, diarrhea, dysphagia
Neuropsychiatric: Anxiety, restlessness, hyperkinesis, emotional lability, confusion, insomnia, poor attention
Neuromuscular: Myopathy, myalgias, tremor, proximal muscle weakness (difficulty getting out of a chair or combing hair)
Ophthalmologic: Tearing, irritation, wind sensitivity, diplopia, foreign body sensation
Thyroid gland: Neck fullness, dysphagia, dysphonia
Dermatologic: Flushed feeling, hair loss, pretibial swelling
Reproductive: Oligomenorrhea, amenorrhea, menometrorrhagia, decreased libido, gynecomastia, erectile dysfunction, infertility

BOX 117.2   Physical Findings in Thyrotoxicosis

Vital signs: Tachycardia, widened pulse pressure, bounding pulses, fever
Cardiac: Hyperdynamic precordium, systolic flow murmur, prominent heart sounds, systolic rub (Means-Lerman scratch), tricuspid regurgitation, atrial fibrillation, evidence of heart failure
Ophthalmologic: Widened palpebral fissures (stare), lid lag, globe lag, conjunctival injection, periorbital edema, proptosis, limitation of superior gaze
Neurologic: Fine tremor, hyperreflexia, proximal muscle weakness
Psychiatric: Fidgety, emotionally labile, poor concentration
Dermatologic: Warm, moist, smooth skin; rosy cheeks, blushing face; fine brittle hair; alopecia, flushed facies; palmar erythema; hyperpigmented pretibial plaques, nodules, or induration that is nonpitting; onycholysis (Plummer nails, separation of the distal portion of the fingernail from the nail bed)
Neck: Diffuse symmetric thyroid enlargement, sometimes with a bruit and palpable thrill; thyroid with multiple irregular nodules or a prominent single nodule; tracheal deviation, venous prominence with arm elevation (Pemberton sign)

profound muscle weakness progressing to flaccid paralysis, similar to familial hypokalemic periodic paralysis.

Ophthalmopathy is a classic finding in Graves disease. Patients subsequently present with eyelid edema, hyperemia, conjunctival hyperemia, and chemosis. Graves ophthalmopathy is also associated with restrictive extraocular myopathy, and exophthalmos. As the disease progresses, patients may experience restriction of their upward gaze from infiltration of the inferior rectus muscle and visual loss from optic nerve involvement (compression by inflamed, enlarged orbital contents). Increased activity at the sympathetic innervation of the eyelids leads to widening of the palpebral fissures, resulting in the characteristic stare and lid lag of thyrotoxicosis.

Physical examination findings of hyperthyroidism depend largely on age (Box 117.2). Younger patients typically present with signs of sympathetic stimulation, whereas older adults often lack the same adrenergic response and present with weight loss and fatigue, more consistent with apathetic hyperthyroidism.[1] In Graves disease, patients uncommonly have classic pretibial myxedema, which are confluent, painless, reddish raised nodules and plaques over the pretibial area and dorsum of the feet, often described as orange skin. Hyperpigmentation

and induration are present, but pitting is absent. Pretibial myxedema is often associated with Graves ophthalmopathy.

Tachycardia is the most common cardiac finding. Other findings include a widened pulse pressure, bounding peripheral pulses and, rarely, a friction rub heard along the left sternal border (Means-Lerman scratch). Atrial fibrillation is more common in elders, especially those over 65 years of age. Dilated cardiomyopathy may develop as a complication of a high cardiac output state. Patients can also develop primary pulmonary hypertension, as well as increased chamber size and poor right ventricular function.[2]

Most hyperthyroid patients have an enlarged thyroid gland, especially in toxic multinodular goiter or Graves disease, although many elders with Graves disease have nonpalpable thyroids. Retrosternal enlargement can occur, making detection difficult while causing the obstructive symptoms discussed earlier. Facial and neck vein engorgement can be elicited when arms are elevated above the head (known as the Pemberton sign). The absence of thyroid enlargement should suggest exogenous (factitious) thyroiditis as well as ectopic thyroid hormone production, such as a hydatidiform mole or struma ovarii, an ovarian tumor composed of some thyroid tissue.

Thyroid Storm

Thyroid storm is a rare, life-threatening form of severe thyrotoxicosis, with multiorgan dysfunction and significantly higher mortality rates than thyrotoxicosis without storm.[3] Although it can occur as the result of unrecognized or undertreated thyrotoxicosis, more often, it is an acute reaction to surgery, trauma, infection, iodine load or parturition in patients with preexisting hyperthyroidism. Other precipitants include acute myocardial infarction, pulmonary embolism, hyperemesis gravidarum, preeclampsia, and diabetic ketoacidosis. Untreated, mortality approaches 100%, but prompt recognition and therapy have lowered mortality to 10% to 30%.[3,4] Death in thyroid storm is caused by multiorgan dysfunction, congestive heart failure, respiratory failure, arrhythmias, disseminated intravascular coagulation, hypoxic brain insult, or sepsis.

The typical clinical manifestations of thyroid storm include marked pyrexia (104°–106°F [40°–41°C]), extreme tachycardia (often out of proportion to level of fever), and altered mental status. These findings, coupled with the clinical picture of a patient with hyperthyroidism, lid lag, stare, goiter, ophthalmopathy, and tremor, should alert the emergency clinician to the diagnosis. Cardiovascular collapse can result in congestive heart failure, hypotension, and cardiac arrhythmias. Hypotension can also result from volume depletion secondary to nausea, vomiting, and diarrhea. Abdominal pain is common; hepatic failure with cholestatic jaundice is less common but carries a poor prognosis. Thyroid storm is a clinical diagnosis, and no validated diagnostic criteria yet exist. However, a scoring system developed by Burch and Wartofsky in 1993 is repeatedly cited and utilized by practicing endocrinologists. Although the test characteristics (e.g., sensitivity and specificity) have not been published, it may help distinguish among thyrotoxicosis, impending thyroid storm, and frank thyroid storm (Table 117.1).[5]

Differential Diagnoses

The differential diagnosis for the thyrotoxic patient is broad. An anxious patient may be interpreted to be manic or experiencing a panic attack. The hyperadrenergic state may be confused with that seen in patients with sympathomimetic intoxication, suffering from anticholinergic crisis, or experiencing withdrawal from alcohol or sedative-hypnotics. The hyperpyrexia and altered mental status seen in thyroid storm may mimic other hyperthermic disorders such as heatstroke, neuroleptic malignant syndrome, serotonin syndrome, bacterial

TABLE 117.1   Diagnostic Criteria for Thyroid Storm

Criteria	Score[a]
Fever (°F)	
99–99.9	5
100–100.9	10
101–101.9	15
102–102.9	20
103–103.9	25
≥104	30
Tachycardia (beats/min)	
90–109	5
110–119	10
120–129	15
130–139	20
≥140	25
Mental Status	
Normal	0
Mild agitation	10
Delirium, psychosis	
Extreme lethargy	20
Coma, seizures	30
Congestive Heart Failure	
Absent	0
Mild (edema)	5
Moderate (rales)	10
Pulmonary edema	15
Atrial fibrillation	10
Gastrointestinal and Hepatic Symptoms	
None	0
Nausea, vomiting	10
Diarrhea, abdominal pain	
Unexplained jaundice	20
Precipitating Event	
None	0
Present	10

[a]Tally the maximum score from each category. A score of 45 or higher suggests thyroid storm, or impending storm, and a score below 25 is unlikely to represent thyroid storm.

TABLE 117.2   Thyroid Function Test Interpretation

Tsh	Free T$_4$	Free T$_3$	Disease
Normal	Normal	Normal	None
Low	High	High	Hyperthyroidism
Low	Normal	Normal	Subclinical hyperthyroidism
Low	Normal	High	T$_3$ toxicosis
Low	High	Normal	Thyroiditis, T$_4$ ingestion, hyperthyroidism in older adults or those with comorbid illness
Low	Low	Low	Euthyroid sick syndrome; central hypothyroidism
High	Normal	Normal	Subclinical hypothyroidism; recovery from euthyroid sick syndrome

T$_3$, Triiodothyronine; *T$_4$*, thyroxine; *TSH*, thyroid-stimulating hormone.

Severe systemic illness depresses TSH production, leading to low levels of TSH, free T$_3$, and free T$_4$.

Elevation of free T$_4$ and free T$_3$ levels in conjunction with TSH suppression is diagnostic of thyrotoxicosis. Because nearly all T$_3$ and T$_4$ is bound to TBG, assays measuring total T$_3$ or T$_4$ are influenced by changes in TBG; they are therefore unreliable and should not be used. Subclinical hyperthyroidism is likely if TSH is suppressed and the free T$_4$ level is normal. T$_3$ toxicosis occurs in about 5% of patients with thyrotoxicosis. These patients have an elevated free T$_3$ level and a normal free T$_4$ level. When the reverse pattern is present—normal free T$_3$ level and elevated free T$_4$ level—the differential includes thyroiditis, exogenous levothyroxine ingestion, and hyperthyroidism in elders, often with suppressed T$_4$ to T$_3$ conversion due to comorbid illness (Table 117.2). Since Graves is caused by autoantibodies to the TSH receptor, the presence of thyroid receptor antibodies in the serum can help distinguish it from other causes. Additionally, a radioiodine scan can help discern Graves from exogenous intake or hyperthyroidism due to struma ovarii. A magnetic resonance imaging (MRI) test of the brain and an ultrasound of the thyroid may help differentiate whether excess levels of thyroid hormone are emanating from either the pituitary or the thyroid gland.

Many thyrotoxic patients have hyperglycemia. This is likely to be the result of increased glycogenolysis and catecholamine-mediated antagonism of insulin. Mild hypercalcemia can be seen, is related to hormone-mediated bone resorption, and is associated with osteoporosis and increased fracture risk. Other frequent laboratory abnormalities include abnormal liver function tests, leukocytosis, mild anemia, and low serum cholesterol levels.

In thyroiditis, the diagnostic evaluation is more difficult. An exquisitely tender gland and elevated erythrocyte sedimentation rate (ESR) or C-reactive protein make the diagnosis of subacute thyroiditis likely. The other forms of thyroiditis lack these findings.

Factitious thyrotoxicosis can often be diagnosed by history. Laboratory testing will demonstrate low thyroglobulin levels and a low T$_3$/T$_4$ ratio (<20 ng/microgram).[5] Furthermore, radioactive iodine uptake is depressed in thyroiditis and factitious thyrotoxicosis but increased in hyperthyroidism.

Management

Management of thyrotoxicosis is based on etiology and symptom severity. For those with mild symptoms, outpatient referral and management are appropriate. Patients with moderate to severe symptoms are best managed in the emergency department (ED) setting. Treatment is divided into supportive, symptomatic, and thyroid-directed therapy.

meningitis, and sepsis. Elders with apathetic hyperthyroidism may be mistakenly diagnosed with psychiatric illness.

Diagnostic Testing

The initial diagnosis of thyrotoxicosis is based on the clinical picture and confirmed with laboratory values. Measurement of the serum TSH level is the most sensitive test for hyperthyroidism. In thyrotoxicosis, the serum TSH concentration is depressed or undetectable (<0.01 µU/mL in third-generation assays), and a normal TSH level excludes hyperthyroidism. Accuracy of the TSH determination is improved when the free T$_4$ test is added. Assessment of thyroid function during acute nonthyroidal illness is difficult, especially in critically ill patients.

BOX 117.3 Management of Thyrotoxicosis

β-Adrenergic Blockade
Propranolol 60–80 mg PO every 4 hours
or
Metoprolol, 25–50 mg PO every 6 hrs
If IV route is required, propranolol, 0.5–1.0 mg IV slow push test dose, then repeat 1–2 mg every 15 min as tolerated to desired effect, then 1–2 mg every 3 hr
or
Esmolol, 50–100 µg/kg/min infusion
Strict contraindication to beta blocker—reserpine 2.5–5 mg IM every 4 hr

Inhibition of Thyroid Hormone Synthesis
Propylthiouracil, 500–1000 mg loading dose, then 250 mg every 4 hr
or
Methimazole, 60–80 mg/day in divided doses
Preferred route, PO or nasogastric (NG); alternative route: PR (in rectum), enema prepared by pharmacy; same dose for all routes

Inhibition of Thyroid Hormone Release
Saturated solution of potassium iodide (SSKI, 50 mg iodide/drop), 1–2 drops PO or PR tid
or
Lugol solution (8 mg iodide/drop), 5–7 drops PO or PR tid
or
Sodium iodide, dosing as per Endocrinology recommendations
or
If allergic to iodine, lithium carbonate, 300 mg PO or NG qid

Administration of Corticosteroids
Inhibit T_4 to T_3 conversion; treat relative adrenal insufficiency.
Hydrocortisone, 300 mg IV, followed by 100 mg tid
or
Dexamethasone, 2–4 mg IV qid

Diagnosis and Treatment of Underlying Precipitant
Consider empirical antibiotics if critical.

Supportive Measures
Volume resuscitation and replacement of glycogen stores with D_5/0.9 NS (dose varies, depending on volume status and CHF)
Acetaminophen
Cooling blanket, fans, ice packs, ice lavage

Miscellaneous
Lorazepam or diazepam as anxiolytic and to decrease central sympathetic outflow
Cholestyramine (blocks enterohepatic recirculation of thyroid hormone), 1–4 g PO twice daily for severe or refractory thyrotoxicosis

CHF, Congestive heart failure; *D_5W/0.9 NS*, 5% dextrose in 0.9% normal saline; *IV*, intravenously; *NG*, by nasogastric tube; *PO*, by mouth; *PR*, by rectum; *T_3*, triiodothyronine; *T_4*, thyroxine.

Specific dosages of the drugs discussed in the following sections can be found in Box 117.3. The order of medication administration in thyroid storm is critical. Iodine can precipitate thyroid storm and must be given a minimum of 1 hour after thionamide therapy (PTU or methimazole). As such, the typical order is beta blocker (propranolol), propylthiouracil (PTU), or methimazole, and then iodine (saturated solution of potassium iodide [SSKI], Lugol solution). In addition, it is important to identify and treat the precipitating cause of thyroid storm.

Supportive Treatment

Supportive therapy for thyroid storm patients should include management of hyperthermia with cooling and acetaminophen. Aspirin should be avoided in thyrotoxic patients because it decreases the protein binding of T_4 and T_3. Agitation is controlled with benzodiazepines. Fluid resuscitation is needed to compensate for insensible and gastrointestinal (GI) losses; dextrose-containing solutions are helpful because glycogen stores are often depleted. Electrolyte replacement is guided by laboratory values.

Symptomatic Treatment

Symptomatic treatment consists primarily of beta blockade to diminish the adrenergic response. Propranolol is the beta blocker of choice because it has the added benefit of blocking conversion of T_4 to T_3; its nonselective effects also improve tremor, weakness, hyperpyrexia, restlessness, irritability, and emotional lability. The onset of action after oral dosing is about 1 hour.

For more rapid beta blockade, propranolol can be administered intravenously (IV). A short-acting agent such as esmolol may be used when concerns about beta blockade exist, due to underlying asthma or COPD, or pulmonary edema from heart failure. In asthmatics, a β_1-selective drug such as esmolol or metoprolol may be considered.

If beta blockers are contraindicated, reserpine, 2.5 to 5 mg intramuscularly (IM) every 4 hours, is also an option. Patients should be closely monitored for hypotension, regardless of the agent used, because thyrotoxicosis can lower systemic vascular resistance and cause congestive heart failure. Patients who develop clinically significant heart failure should be treated with the usual medications for heart failure, including diuretics and angiotensin-converting enzyme inhibitors. Atrial fibrillation is often refractory to rate control until antithyroid therapy is instituted.

Thyroid-Directed Treatment

Thyroid-directed therapy has three goals: reduce thyroid hormone production, prevent thyroid hormone release, and block peripheral conversion of T_4 to T_3. In conjunction with this treatment, an additional goal is the avoidance of therapeutic interventions that may worsen thyrotoxicosis. As such, certain drugs should be avoided in the thyrotoxic patient. Amiodarone and iodinated contrast material both contain iodine and can increase thyroid hormone production. Aspirin can increase free thyroid hormone concentrations through its effect on protein binding. Pseudoephedrine, ketamine, and albuterol increase sympathetic tone and can exacerbate the adrenergic effects of thyrotoxicosis; when indicated, they should be used cautiously.

Reducing Thyroid Hormone Production. Thionamides inhibit oxidation and organic binding of iodine to thyroglobulin, thereby blocking the synthesis of thyroid hormone. PTU or methimazole can be used. PTU has the additional effect of impairing the conversion of T_4 to T_3; methimazole has a longer duration of action. Both PTU and methimazole may be given by nasogastric tube or rectum as needed. PTU is preferred in the first trimester of pregnancy, and methimazole is preferred in the second and third trimesters. Methimazole is available in IV form outside the United States, but its use is not recommended by the most recent American Thyroid Association guidelines.[6]

Side effects of thionamide therapy vary from mild to life-threatening. These can range from urticarial, rash, arthralgia, GI upset, to agranulocytosis, hepatotoxicity and vasculitis.

Inhibiting Thyroid Hormone Release. Inorganic iodine blocks the release of stored thyroid hormone. Because an iodine load can increase the synthesis of thyroid hormone, these agents should not be administered until 1 hour after the initiation of PTU or methimazole therapy. Traditionally, oral iodine in the form of potassium iodide (SSKI), or Lugol solution, is administered. Like the thionamides, these agents may be given via nasogastric tube or retention enema, as needed. Lithium may be considered an alternative therapy for iodine-allergic patients. Lithium is also the agent of choice for iodine-induced hyperthyroidism, which is usually the result of the administration of amiodarone or iodinated contrast material.

Inhibiting Conversion of T_4 to T_3. Corticosteroids are capable of inhibiting the peripheral conversion of T_4 to T_3 and blocking the release of hormone from the thyroid gland. When steroids are used in conjunction with PTU and iodide, the concentration of T_3 can return to normal within 48 hours. Hydrocortisone may be administered, and dexamethasone is an alternative.

Miscellaneous Therapies

Cholestyramine, an anion exchange resin, interrupts the enterohepatic recirculation of thyroid hormone by binding it in the bowel lumen. Because it may help to decrease the level of circulating hormone more rapidly, its use is recommended for severe or refractory thyroid storm. Although it has been shown to result in a more rapid decline in hormone levels compared with thionamides alone, it requires weeks of therapy and, as such, is reserved for outpatient management.[7] Plasmapheresis has been used in thyroid storm as an attempt to remove circulating thyroid hormone.[5,8] Extracorporeal membrane oxygenation (ECMO) has been recently described as successful in supporting patients with severe thyroid storm and "rapid clinical deterioration."[9] Neither radioactive iodine nor surgery plays a role in the management of thyroid storm or thyrotoxicosis until a sustained euthyroid state has been established because these interventions can precipitate thyroid storm.

First-line treatment of subacute thyroiditis is the use of nonsteroidal antiinflammatory drugs (NSAIDs). Corticosteroids are used in refractory cases. Symptomatic patients are treated with beta blockers. Management of drug-induced hyperthyroidism depends on the inciting agent. In the case of AIT-1, treatment typically consists of stopping amiodarone and initiating antithyroid therapy. AIT-2 is managed with corticosteroids, and the decision to stop amiodarone is made on a case-by-case basis.[10] Management of drug-induced hyperthyroidism related to lithium involves stopping lithium. When related to immunomodulator therapy, discontinuation of the offending drug is not always mandatory.[11] Treatment is based on the determination of the type of reaction present; Box 117.4).

Identification and Treatment of the Precipitating Event

Thyroid storm is often precipitated by a physiologic stressor, such as infection, myocardial ischemia, pulmonary embolism, and stroke. Management of thyroid storm with PTU, followed by iodine, beta blockers, corticosteroids, fluid resuscitation, rapid cooling, and treatment of the precipitating illness, can resolve acute thyroid storm within 24 hours.

Disposition

The disposition of patients with hyperthyroidism is guided by symptom severity, with intensive care unit (ICU) admission for patients in thyroid storm. Patients with mild thyrotoxicosis controlled with a first-line medication who are otherwise stable can be managed as outpatients. Admission to the hospital may be appropriate for patients who require more than beta blockers for symptom control or whose symptoms persist despite therapy. Patients with rapid atrial fibrillation should be admitted to a monitored setting. Patients managed as outpatients can be sent to a primary care physician or referred to an endocrinologist. Lack of insurance and other socioeconomic factors have been linked to higher admission rates in patients with thyrotoxicosis.[12]

Note: Many subtypes and varying etiologies of hyperthyroidism have been identified. Table 117.3 provides descriptions of cases distinguished from the above general description.

BOX 117.4 Thyrotoxicosis and Thyroid Storm Special Situations

Congestive Heart Failure
If rate-related, high-output failure:
  Beta blockade is first-line therapy (dose as in Box 117.3)
  ACEI, digoxin, diuretics as needed
If depressed ejection fraction:
  Avoid beta blocker or one-quarter dose
  ACEI if blood pressure adequate
  Digoxin and furosemide as needed
If pulmonary hypertension:
  Oxygen
  Sildenafil

Atrial Fibrillation
Beta blocker preferred for rate control (dose as in Box 117.3)
Calcium channel blockers prone to hypotension; diltiazem, 10-mg test dose.
  Avoid verapamil.
Digoxin less effective but may be tried
Amiodarone should be avoided because of iodine load
Refractory to conversion to sinus rhythm unless euthyroid first

Thyroiditis (Subacute)
NSAIDs for inflammation and pain control
Prednisone, 40 mg/day, if refractory to NSAIDs
Beta blockade to control thyrotoxic symptoms
No role for PTU, methimazole, or iodides

Factitious Thyrotoxicosis
Beta blockade for thyrotoxic symptoms
Cholestyramine to block absorption of ingested thyroid hormone
No role for PTU, methimazole, or iodides

ACEI, Angiotensin-converting enzyme inhibitor; *NSAIDs*, nonsteroidal antiinflammatory drugs; *PTU*, propylthiouracil.

HYPOTHYROIDISM

Foundations

Background and Importance
Hypothyroidism is a condition in which the thyroid gland fails to produce or secrete sufficient circulating thyroid hormone to meet the needs of the peripheral tissues. The condition results from lack of stimulation of the thyroid gland (central or secondary hypothyroidism) or intrinsic gland dysfunction limiting hormone production (primary hypothyroidism). Hypothyroidism is the most common functional disorder of the thyroid gland.

Thyroid disorders are the second most common endocrine condition after diabetes mellitus. Higher incidence rates are found in women than in men, which is attributed to the higher prevalence of autoimmune disease found in women in general. In the United States (US), 1% to 2% of women are affected by hypothyroidism. Subclinical hypothyroidism affects 4% to 10% of the population. The incidence of subclinical hypothyroidism in pregnancy is 5% to 8%.[13] There is no specific race or ethnic predilection, but older age groups are at a higher risk for the development of hypothyroidism.

Pathophysiology
Intrinsic gland failure accounts for up to 99% of all cases of hypothyroidism. Factors that may result in primary hypothyroidism include autoimmune disorders, infiltrative disorders, congenital thyroid dysfunction, pregnancy, radiotherapy, medications, infection, surgery,

TABLE 117.3   Hyperthyroidism Summary

	Background and Importance	Pathophysiology	Clinical Features	Diagnostic Testing	Management
Graves Disease	Most common form of hyperthyroidism in the United States Strong genetic association, with frequent occurrence in the setting of other autoimmune disorders[1] Some environmental causes, such as smoking	Autoantibodies bind to the TSH receptor and stimulate thyroid hormone production and release. Infiltration of the inferior rectus muscles Increased activity at the sympathetic innervation of the eyelids	Enlarged thyroid gland • May be absent in the elderly Ophthalmopathy • eyelid edema • hyperemia • conjunctival hyperemia • chemosis • restrictive extraocular myopathy • exophthalmos • restriction of upward gaze • visual loss secondary to optic nerve compression • widening palpebral fissure • lid lag Pretibial Myxedema • confluent, painless, reddish raised nodules and plaques over the pretibial area and dorsum of the feet, often described as "orange skin" • hyperpigmented • indurated • nonpitting	Thyroid receptor antibody positive Radioiodide uptake increased	Patients should first be treated to stabilize their acute thyrotoxic symptoms. Patients can then be referred for: • radioactive iodine therapy • OR long-term antithyroid drug administration • OR thyroidectomy
Toxic Multinodular Goiter	Second leading cause of hyperthyroidism in the United States More common in women >50 years old	Multiple autonomously functioning nodules	Enlarged, palpable thyroid gland Milder, more gradual in onset than Graves disease May present acutely when iodine replacement is given to iodine-deficient patients.	A ^{123}I or ^{99m}Tc pertechnetate scan	Patients should first be treated to stabilize their acute thyrotoxic symptoms. Patients can then be referred for: • radioactive iodine therapy • OR thyroidectomy Treatment with antithyroid drugs may be appropriate on occasion, when specific contraindications to the above exist
Toxic Adenoma	Typically affects the same population as toxic multinodular goiter, but is less common	Single hyperfunctioning nodule within the thyroid	Typical hyperthyroid signs and symptoms	A ^{123}I or ^{99m}Tc pertechnetate scan	Patients should first be treated to stabilize their acute thyrotoxic symptoms. Patients can then be referred for: • radioactive iodine therapy • OR thyroidectomy Treatment with antithyroid drugs may be appropriate on occasion, when specific contraindications to the above exist

Thyroiditis	Hashimoto thyroiditis is most common form in the United States	Any inflammatory process that results in thyroid gland inflammation can lead to thyroiditis: • autoimmune • drug-induced • infectious • traumatic Inflammation leads to follicular cell breakdown, with resultant release of preformed thyroid hormone, resulting in thyrotoxicosis Hashimoto is the result of thyroid antibodies and lymphocytic infiltration of the thyroid gland.	Exquisitely tender thyroid gland Hashimoto patients may have transient thyrotoxicosis, followed by painless goiter and hypothyroidism secondary to the destruction of thyroid tissue.	Elevated ESR and CRP Radioiodide uptake depressed	NSAIDS Corticosteroids for refractory cases
Postpartum Thyroiditis	5% of pregnant women will develop this. 70% recurrence rate in subsequent pregnancies Some women will have permanent hypothyroidism.	Autoimmune etiology, presents as the immune system returns to its normal function following pregnancy. Triphasic course: (1) thyrotoxicosis, 2 to 6 months postpartum, although this phase may be asymptomatic; (2) a hypothyroid state lasting 2 to 3 months; and (3) a euthyroid state by the end of the first postpartum year.	20% to 30% may have only thyrotoxicosis 40% may have only hypothyroidism	Diagnostic Triad: • Lack of previous history of thyroid disorder • Abnormal TSH concentration during the first postpartum year • Absence of TSH receptor antibodies or a toxic nodule	Supportive treatment Beta blockers are recommended to control pulse and other symptoms Atenolol is contraindicated in breastfeeding because of excretion in breast milk; propranolol and metoprolol are preferred.
Subacute Thyroiditis	de Quervain thyroiditis Most common in women, ages 40–60	Thought to be caused by a viral infection of the thyroid	Viral prodrome • fever • fatigue • myalgias • pharyngitis Anterior neck pain, may radiate to ears/jaw/throat Exquisitely tender thyroid, may be enlarged About 50% of patients have mild, typical symptoms lasting 3 to 6 weeks. About one-third of patients will then have hypothyroidism for up to 6 months, followed by a return to a euthyroid state 5–15% of patients will have persistent hypothyroidism.	Clinical suspicion based on history and physical exam TSH low Free T4 *may* be elevated relative to T3 Elevation of ESR, CRP May also see mild leukocytosis and anemia Radioactive iodine uptake is low	Initial treatment with beta-adrenergic blocking agents and NSAIDs. • May substitute corticosteroids for NSAIDs if moderate to severe thyrotoxic symptoms at presentation or failure to respond to initial interventions

Continued

TABLE 117.3   Hyperthyroidism Summary—cont'd.

	Background and Importance	Pathophysiology	Clinical Features	Diagnostic Testing	Management
Painless Thyroiditis	"Silent thyroiditis" Common cause of post-partum thyroiditis Also seen in nonpregnant women and men	Likely autoimmune Medication related • lithium • cytokine therapy	Similar to subacute thyroiditis, but typically without viral prodrome, neck pain or inflammatory response Small, nontender goiter Mild symptoms Triphasic course	ESR, CRP normal No leukocytosis Anti-thyroid peroxidase antibodies present in 50% of patients Low radioactive iodine uptake in thyrotoxic phase Typical lab findings for thyrotoxicosis in this phase (low TSH and high free T4)	Beta-adrenergic blocking agents Corticosteroids for severe cases
Acute Suppurative Thyroiditis	Rare Life-threatening	Infection of the thyroid gland • bacterial • parasitic (rare) • mycobacterial (rare) • fungal (rare)In adults, most often secondary to hematogenous spread or iatrogenic In children and adolescents, can be secondary to pyriform sinus fistula	Fever Anterior neck pain Neck swelling and induration Neck erythema Dysphonia Dysphagia Patients may be euthyroid.	Ultrasound or CT may demonstrate inflammation, destruction of the thyroid, and/or abscess formation; these findings may be absent early in the course of the disease.	Beta-adrenergic blocking agents for tachycardia Antibiotics and/or surgical drainage Definitive treatment of pyriform sinus fistula, when present.
Drug Induced Thyroiditis	Amiodarone Lithium Immunomodulators • immune checkpoint inhibitors • tyrosine kinase inhibitors	Drug induced, related to specific drugs Amiodarone • Contains a large amount of iodine, and has a significant effect on thyroid function. • type-1 amiodarone induced thyroiditis (AIT) • iodine content of amiodarone unmasks subclinical Graves disease or goiters • type-2 AIT • direct destructive effect on thyroid cells, resulting in the release of preformed hormone[2] Immunomodulators • direct destructive effect on thyroid cells Lithium • more commonly causes hypothyroidism • exact mechanism unknown, theories include: • Increased iodide retention and stores in the thyroid resulting in increased thyroid hormone production • Autoimmune mechanism • Direct toxic effect.[3]	Exacerbation of the tachyarrhythmia for which the patient is being treated or heart failure. Immunomodulators • initial hyperthyroid phase (typically within a few weeks, but can present years later), followed by hypothyroidism[4]	Typical lab findings for thyrotoxicosis (low TSH and high free T4)	Treatment depends on the inciting agent and type of reaction Amiodarone AIT-1 • stop amiodarone • Antithyroid therapy AIT-2 • corticosteroids • may or may not stop amiodarone Lithium • stop lithium Immunomodulators • inciting agent may or may not be stopped, depending on the type of reaction

Factitious Thyroiditis	Exogenous thyroid ingestion • intentional • nutritional supplements, particularly those marketed for weight loss.[5] • accidental	Thyroid enlargement not present on physical exam	Low thyroglobulin levels Low T3/T4 ratio (<20 ng/microgram) Radioactive iodine uptake is depressed	Cessation of offending agent
Subclinical Hyperthyroidism	Risk factor for cardiovascular morbidity and mortality, as evidenced by coronary artery disease, acute coronary events and atrial fibrillation Patients older than 65 years at higher risk	Subclinical hyperthyroidism with suppressed TSH and variable levels of functional thyroid hormone in the body Over time, some patients may remit and some will progress to full hyperthyroidism.	Patients are clinically euthyroid, but there is association with cardiovascular disease, osteoporosis, and changes in mood and cognition	Low TSH • lower TSH imparts higher risk Normal free T4 and T3	Treatment is recommended in patients over 65 with TSH <0.1 mU/L over time, IF They are asymptomatic but have risk factors for cardiovascular disease, osteoporosis, or are postmenopausal women not on estrogens or bisphosphonates OR They are symptomatic

Unless otherwise specifically noted, information in this table summarizes that presented in: Ross DS, Burch HB, Cooper DS, et al. 2016 American Thyroid Association Guidelines for Diagnosis and Management of Hyperthyroidism and Other Causes of Thyrotoxicosis. *Thyroid.* 2016;26(10):1343-1421.

6 Ross DS, Burch HB, Cooper DS, et al. 2016 American Thyroid Association Guidelines for Diagnosis and Management of Hyperthyroidism and Other Causes of Thyrotoxicosis. *Thyroid.* 2016;26(10):1343-1421.

[1]Ferrari SM, Fallahi P, Ruffilli I, et al. The association of other autoimmune diseases in patients with Graves' disease (with or without ophthalmopathy): Review of the literature and report of a large series. *Autoimmun Rev.* 2019;18(3):287-292.

[2]Bartalena L, Bogazzi F, Chiovato L, Hubalewska-Dydejczyk A, Links TP, Vanderpump M. 2018 European Thyroid Association (ETA) Guidelines for the Management of Amiodarone-Associated Thyroid Dysfunction. *Eur Thyroid J.* 2018;7(2):55-66.

[3]Galindo RJ, Hurtado CR, Pasquel FJ, Garcia Tome R, Peng L, Umpierrez GE. National trends in incidence, mortality, and clinical outcomes of patients hospitalized for thyrotoxicosis with and without thyroid storm in the United States, 2004-2013. *Thyroid.* 2019;29(1):36-43.

[4]Ono Y, Ono S, Yasunaga H, Matsui H, Fushimi K, Tanaka Y. Factors associated with mortality of thyroid storm: analysis using a national inpatient database in Japan. *Medicine (Baltimore).* 2016;95(7):e2848.

[5]Satoh T, Isozaki O, Suzuki A, et al. 2016 Guidelines for the management of thyroid storm from The Japan Thyroid Association and Japan Endocrine Society (First edition). *Endocr J.* 2016;63(12):1025-1064.

inadequate dietary iodine intake, thyroid medication noncompliance, and previous treatment of thyrotoxicosis. Worldwide, iodine deficiency is the most common cause of hypothyroidism; however, in iodine-replete regions, the primary cause is autoimmune. Hypothyroidism may also be associated with other autoimmune diseases, most commonly diabetes mellitus.

Central causes of hypothyroidism are rare and result from hypothalamic dysfunction in the secretion of TRH or pituitary dysfunction in the secretion of TSH. Pituitary adenoma is the most common cause of central hypothyroidism. Other causes include pituitary hemorrhage (Sheehan syndrome), pituitary infiltrative processes, brain injury, and space-occupying mass. Sheehan syndrome is a result of postpartum pituitary hemorrhage that leads to pituitary ischemia and necrosis. Patients often have lactation failure, amenorrhea, adrenal insufficiency, and central hypothyroidism.

Clinical Features

History and Physical Examination

Signs and symptoms of hypothyroidism range from asymptomatic to overt organ failure, which may lead to death. Patients with early hypothyroidism often present with vague complaints. As a result, thyroid dysfunction should be considered in patients with generalized arthralgias, infertility or menstrual changes, depression, and hypercholesterolemia. Typical symptoms develop insidiously and progress with the disease (Box 117.5). Patients with subclinical hypothyroidism may present with varying nonspecific signs and symptoms similar to those of patients with overt hypothyroidism, but less pronounced. Patients with Hashimoto thyroiditis present typically with an insidiously developed goiter and hypothyroidism.

The thyroid plays a fundamental role in maintaining cardiovascular homeostasis in physiologic and pathologic states; it influences cardiac contractility, heart rate, diastolic function, and systemic vascular resistance. Increased peripheral vascular resistance and low cardiac output have been suggested to be additional links between hypothyroidism and impaired blood pressure regulation and resultant hypertension. Antihypertensive medications are usually ineffective in noneuthyroid individuals. The accelerated atherosclerosis in hypothyroidism is ascribed to dyslipidemia, diastolic hypertension, and impaired endothelial function. These cardiovascular findings are linked to overt and subclinical hypothyroidism.

Overt hypothyroidism leads to significant neuropsychiatric impairments of mood and cognition. Subclinical hypothyroidism may cause subtle deficits in memory and cognition.

Pulmonary abnormalities in hypothyroidism are primarily related to hypoventilation and hypercapnia; up to 65% of patients with pulmonary hypertension have concomitant thyroid dysfunction. Although the exact relationship is unknown, pulmonary artery pressures normalize after treatment of thyroid disease.

In pregnancy, hypothyroidism may be manifested typically, but it is often subtle and difficult to distinguish from normal changes in pregnancy.

In children, hypothyroidism may affect growth, development, and cognitive ability. Declining growth velocity noticed during several years might be the first clue to evaluate for thyroid disorders. T_4 replacement will induce a rapid growth spurt, although predicted bone maturation size might not be achieved. In adults, thyroid hormone functions to regulate and maintain bone mass; patients with hypothyroidism are at increased risk for fracture, although the underlying mechanism resulting in this association is unclear.

Myxedema Coma

Myxedema coma is a life-threatening event, presenting with altered mental status, hypothermia, and a concomitant precipitating event.[14] Precipitating events are listed in Box 117.6. Diagnosis must often be

---

BOX 117.5 Symptoms and Signs of Hypothyroidism

Vital Signs
Systolic blood pressure, normal or low
Diastolic blood pressure, normal or elevated
Slow pulse to sinus bradycardia
Respirations, normal or slow, shallow
Temperature, normal, but prone to hypothermia with stress

Hypometabolic Complaints
Cold intolerance
Fatigue
Weight gain, but decreased appetite

Cutaneous
Coarse, brittle hair
Alopecia
Dry skin, decreased perspiration
Pallor, cool hands and feet
Coarse, rough skin
Yellow tinge from carotenemia
Thin, brittle nails
Lateral thinning of the eyebrows

Neurologic
Slow mentation and speech
Impaired concentrating ability and attention span
Lethargy
Decreased short-term memory
Agitation, psychosis
Seizures
Ataxia, dysmetria
Mononeuropathy
  Carpal tunnel syndrome
  Sensorineural hearing loss
Peripheral neuropathy, paresthesias

Muscular
Proximal myopathy
Pseudohypertrophy
Delayed relaxation of reflexes (hung up or pseudomyotonic)

Cardiac
Decreased exercise capacity
Dyspnea on exertion
Sinus bradycardia
Long QT with increased ventricular arrhythmia
Chest pain, accelerated coronary disease
Diastolic heart failure (delayed ventricular relaxation)
Pericardial effusion (asymptomatic)
Peripheral edema

Respiratory
Dyspnea on exertion
Obstructive sleep apnea
Primary pulmonary hypertension

Gastrointestinal
Constipation
Ileus
Gastric atrophy

Reproductive
Oligomenorrhea and amenorrhea
Menorrhagia
Decreased fertility
Early abortions
Decreased libido
Erectile dysfunction

Rheumatic
Polyarthralgias
Joint effusions
Acute gout or pseudogout

Head, Ear, Eyes, Nose, and Throat
Hoarseness
Deep husky voice
Macroglossia
Hearing loss
Periorbital swelling
Broad nose
Swollen lips
Goiter

---

made on the basis of clinical findings (Box 117.7), and can be difficult because not all patients will present with all 3 elements described mentioned previously. Treatment of myxedema coma requires potentially toxic doses of thyroid hormone and can precipitate thyroid storm. Mortality rates are high, up to nearly 30%, even with optimum therapy. Higher mortality is seen in hospitalized patients who require steroids, mechanical ventilation, or exogenous catecholamines.[4] Without treatment, the mortality approaches 100%.

Differential Diagnoses

Differential considerations include other causes of the common clinical presentations of hypothyroidism, such as congestive heart failure,

BOX 117.6 Myxedema Coma: Aggravating or Precipitating Factors

Infection, sepsis (especially pneumonia)
Exposure to cold
Cerebrovascular accident
Drug effect
  Altered sensorium: sedative-hypnotics, narcotics, anesthesia, neuroleptics
  Decreased T_4 and T_3 release: amiodarone, lithium, iodides
  Enhanced elimination of T_4 and T_3: phenytoin, rifampin
  Inadequate thyroid hormone replacement: noncompliance; interference with absorption (iron, calcium, cholestyramine)
Myocardial infarction
Gastrointestinal bleeding
Trauma, burns
Congestive heart failure
Hypoxia
Hypercapnia
Hyponatremia
Hypoglycemia
Hypercalcemia
Diabetic ketoacidosis

T_3, Triiodothyronine; T_4, thyroxine.

TABLE 117.4 Myxedema Coma Scoring Tool

Criterion	Score
GCS 0-10	4
GCS 11-13	3
GCS 14	2
GCS 15	0
TSH > 30 mU/L	2
TSH 15-30 mU/L	1
Low FT4 (<0.6 ng/dL)	1
Hypothermia (<95 degrees F)	1
Bradycardia (<60 beats/minute)	1
Precipitating Event	1

For total scores 8–10, myxedema coma is most likely and proceeding with treatment is recommended; for total scores 5–7, myxedema coma is likely, and treatment is recommended if there are no other likely diagnoses; for total scores <5, myxedema coma is unlikely and clinicians should consider other diagnoses.
Adapted from: Chiong YV, Bammerlin E, Mariash CN. Development of an objective tool for the diagnosis of myxedema coma. *Transl Res.* 2015;166(3):233-243.

BOX 117.7 Recognition of Myxedema Coma

Patient profile—older woman in the winter
Known hypothyroidism; thyroidectomy scar
Hypothermia—temperature usually <95.9°F (36°C); <90°F (32°C) is poor prognostic sign; as low as 75°F (24°C) reported; nearly normal in presence of infection
Altered mental status—lethargy and confusion to stupor and coma, agitation, psychosis, and seizures (myxedema madness)
Hypotension—refractory to volume resuscitation and pressors unless thyroid hormone administered
Slow, shallow respirations with hypercapnia and hypoxia; high risk of respiratory failure
Bradycardia (sinus), long QT and ventricular arrhythmias
Myxedema facies—puffy eyelids and lips, large tongue, broad nose
Evidence of severe chronic hypothyroidism—skin, hair, reflexes, bradykinesis, voice
Acute precipitating illness (e.g., pneumonia)
Drug toxicity (e.g., sedative, narcotic, neuroleptic)
Hyponatremia

pulmonary edema, depression, encephalopathy, hypothermia, systemic infection, and shock.

Diagnostic Testing

Determination of an elevated TSH level is the most sensitive and single best screening test to confirm the diagnosis of primary hypothyroidism. An elevated TSH level with a low T_4 level is indicative of primary hypothyroidism. Central hypothyroidism is associated with a low or normal TSH level, with a low T_4 level. An increased TSH concentration with a normal T_4 level represents subclinical hypothyroidism.

If the TSH level is normal but the T_4 level is low, hypothyroxinemia exists; patients are often asymptomatic but can experience pathologic effects. A useful confirmatory test is the presence of thyroid antibodies (antithyroglobulin, antimicrosomal). They may help determine the cause of hypothyroidism or may serve to predict a future occurrence. Other laboratory findings may include mild anemia, hypercholesterolemia, elevated hepatic enzyme levels, elevated prolactin level, and hyponatremia. Blood glucose levels may be normal to low.

The electrocardiogram is nonspecific in hypothyroidism. It might reveal sinus bradycardia with low-voltage complexes and nonspecific ST-T wave changes.

The presence of myxedema coma carries a high mortality, and inappropriate treatment can cause thyroid storm, so appropriate identification is essential. A recent scoring system was proposed that indicates the risk of myxedema coma and recommended treatments (Table 117.4). While this scoring system requires wider validation, the elements listed are helpful in guiding the clinician to the diagnosis.[14]

Management

Hypothyroidism
Replacement with levothyroxine (T_4) remains the treatment of choice and resolves most physical and psychological signs and symptoms of hypothyroidism in most patients. Synthetic levothyroxine is a levo isomer of thyroxine and has activity identical to that of the endogenous hormone. Approximately 70% to 80% is absorbed from the GI tract, predominantly in the small intestine. T_4 levels peak approximately 4 hours after ingestion. The T_3 concentration rises more slowly because it depends on conversion from T_4. Dose optimization is guided by monitoring of serum TSH levels and symptoms.

Levothyroxine is the drug of choice for patients with subclinical hypothyroidism and a serum TSH concentration above 10 mIU/L and for symptomatic patients with a serum TSH concentration between 5.1 and 10.0 mIU/L. The usual daily dosage is between 50 and 75 μg. The TSH concentration guides thyroid hormone dosing, and should be checked every 6 to 8 weeks after initiation of treatment until TSH levels normalize. It is recommended that levothyroxine be taken at bedtime or 60 minutes before breakfast to improve absorption.[15]

Studies comparing combination therapy of levothyroxine (T_4) and T_3 (liothyronine) with levothyroxine monotherapy included variable combinations and dosages, and have not established a significant benefit for the vast majority of patients. The most recent American Thyroid

BOX 117.8   Treatment of Myxedema Coma

Protect airway, ventilatory support; monitor for alkalosis

Fluid resuscitation

0.9 NS or D_5/0.9 NS if hypoglycemia

Watch for unmasking of CHF

Thyroid hormone replacement

T4 200–400 µg IV (give lower doses to patients who are smaller, have coronary artery disease or a history of arrhythmia) loading dose

Subsequent daily replacement of 1.6 µg/kg body weight PO, give 75% of this dose if given IV

Hydrocortisone—100 mg IV every 8 hrs

Hyponatremia

Consider fluid restriction.

Avoid hypotonic fluids; use only 0.9 NS or D_5/0.9 NS.

If <120 mEq/L, consider 3% saline, 50- to 100-mL boluses.

Passive rewarming

Regular blankets; prevent heat loss

If heating blankets are considered, pretreat with IV fluids and monitor blood pressure closely.

Avoid mechanical stimulation.

Treatment of any precipitating illness, with special attention to infectious causes

CHF, Congestive heart failure; D_5/0.9 NS, 5% dextrose in 0.9% normal saline; IV, intravenous; PO, by mouth; T_3, triiodothyronine; T_4, thyroxine.

Association guidelines do not recommend combination therapy for routine treatment.[15]

Myxedema Coma

The cornerstone for the treatment of myxedema coma is rapid replacement of IV thyroid hormone (Box 117.8). An initial loading dose of 200 to 400 µg IV should be given, using lower doses in patients who are smaller, older, or have a history of coronary artery disease or arrhythmia. Subsequent daily replacement dose is 1.6 µg/kg body weight, decreasing the dose to 75% of the IV dose. In very ill patients, liothyronine administration can be considered in addition to levothyroxine therapy, with extreme caution because elevated levels of T3 in the serum are associated with increased mortality. Stress doses of an IV glucocorticoid are recommended due to possible concomitant adrenal insufficiency. Hydrocortisone, 100 mg IV, is the drug of choice because it has mineralocorticoid and glucocorticoid effects.

Hypotension may respond to crystalloid infusion, but vasopressors are occasionally required. In patients with initially refractory hypotension, the mere replacement of thyroid hormone may have a beneficial effect on improvement of blood pressure. Passive rewarming with blankets and removal from the cold are generally sufficient until the administered thyroid hormone takes effect.

Hyponatremia may occur and is associated with increased mortality. As with other causes of hyponatremia, hypertonic saline should be administered for severe cases of altered mental status or seizures and then corrected more slowly to avoid osmotic demyelination syndrome. The metabolism of sedatives, narcotics, and anesthetics may be slowed, prolonging their effects; lower dosages should be considered.

Disposition

Most patients with hypothyroidism may be treated on an outpatient basis. Patients with severe hypothyroidism or patients with myxedema coma require inpatient care, often in an ICU setting.

Note: There are varying etiologies of hypothyroidism, each with unique aspects of their pathophysiology, diagnosis, and management. These are summarized in Table 117.5.

ADRENAL EXCESS STATES

Foundations

Background and Importance

Adrenal excess states can arise from a variety of causes, including Cushing syndrome, primary and secondary hyperaldosteronism, and pheochromocytoma. Regardless of the etiology, these all result in an excess of adrenal function, which can result in various symptoms that will prompt a patient to present to the ED. In particular, adrenal excess states are to be considered in any patient with resistant hypertension.[16] Left untreated, the long-term metabolic and cardiovascular effects of these diseases can be devastating.

Cushing Syndrome

Pathophysiology

Cushing syndrome results from excessive exposure to cortisol. The most common cause of this syndrome is long-term exogenous steroid administration. Endogenous Cushing syndrome is caused by excessive release of cortisol internally, usually from a corticotropin (ACTH) released from the pituitary (Cushing disease), or cortisol secretion from primary adrenal lesions (adrenal adenoma or carcinoma or adrenal hyperplasia of the adrenal cortex), or ectopic production of a corticotropin-releasing hormone (CRH) by a nonpituitary or other neuroendocrine tumor.[17,18]

Clinical Features

Because of systemic excess in cortisol, patients with Cushing syndrome will present with a variety of nonspecific symptoms given the broad downstream effects of the glucocorticoid exposure. Patients may experience multiple nonspecific symptoms, including psychiatric symptoms, generalized weakness, fatigue, menstrual irregularities and weight gain. Physical examination may reveal obesity, hirsutism, abdominal striae, an increase in adipose distribution on the back and above the clavicles (the classic "buffalo hump") and thin skin.[16,18] According to Nieman and colleagues, easy bruising, facial plethora, proximal muscle weakness and abdominal striae are the physical findings most associated with Cushing syndrome.[18] Cushing syndrome has also been linked to hypertension, diabetes, central obesity, and osteoporosis.[17]

Differential Diagnoses

Because of symptoms that are similar across the spectrum of etiologies of adrenal excess states, the differential diagnosis spans the same gamut. Resistant hypertension and glucose disorders can also be seen in hyperaldosteronism and pheochromocytoma. It can be difficult to distinguish simple obesity and metabolic syndrome from Cushing syndrome.[19] There is also significant overlap in the presenting symptoms of simple depression. Menstrual irregularities can also be associated with a variety of other etiologies, in addition to Cushing syndrome.[18]

Diagnostic Testing

The diagnostic workup of patients with suspected endogenous Cushing syndrome is complex and usually performed in the outpatient setting. Patients who should be referred for evaluation include individuals with an incidentaloma consistent with adrenal adenoma on imaging; patients who have presentations that would not be typical for their age, such as hypertension or osteoporosis at a young age; and patients with multiple clinical findings that would suggest Cushing syndrome.[18]

TABLE 117.5 Hypothyroidism Etiologies

	Background and Importance	Pathophysiology	Clinical Features	Diagnostic Testing	Management
Primary	Most common etiology of hypothyroidism[1]	Results from thyroid hormone deficiency	Typical symptoms span the spectrum from hypothyroidism to myxedema coma	An elevated TSH level with a low T_4 level indicates primary hypothyroidism.	Levothyroxine replacement
Autoimmune	Hashimoto thyroiditis, also known as chronic autoimmune lymphocytic thyroiditis. One of the most common organ-specific autoimmune diseases. Most common cause of primary hypothyroidism in iodine-replete areas of the world	Infiltration of the thyroid gland by lymphocytic inflammatory cells results in destruction and eventual fibrous replacement of the gland's follicular tissue and subsequent functional hypothyroidism.	Patients typically present with an insidiously developed goiter and hypothyroidism.	Elevated TSH Low T_4	Levothyroxine replacement
Infiltrative disorders[1]	Rare cause of primary hypothyroidism	Infectious Malignant Autoimmune Inflammatory	Patients will present with typical hypothyroid symptoms	Elevated TSH Low T_4	Levothyroxine replacement
Congenital thyroid dysfunction	Most preventable cause of intellectual disability	Most commonly caused by thyroid dysgenesis, resulting in decreased production of T_4. Some infants have minimal thyroid tissue but it is insufficient to sustain normal thyroid hormone production. Cognitive deficit is directly related to the amount of delay in diagnosis and treatment	Typically discovered on newborn screening tests	Elevated TSH Low T_4	Levothyroxine replacement
Pregnancy-related hypothyroidism		Thyroxine binding globulin (RBG) and Total T_4 increase and peak by 16 weeks and stay elevated throughout pregnancy.[2] Human chorionic gonadotropin (hCG) and TSH have identical subunits, which then both stimulate the release of T_4 and T_3, resulting in a decreased level of TSH throughout pregnancy. Increased peripheral metabolism of thyroid hormone occurs primarily in the second and third trimesters	In pregnancy, hypothyroidism may be manifested typically, but it is often subtle and difficult to distinguish from normal changes in pregnancy. Other obstetric complications of hypothyroidism include miscarriage, anemia, abruptio placentae, postpartum hemorrhage, low birth weight, and neonatal respiratory distress[2]	TSH will be altered, interpret based on local trimester-specific TSH ranges[3]	Women with preexisting hypothyroidism will generally require increased doses of replacement hormone in pregnancy. At this time, the evidence is not sufficient to recommend universal screening for thyroid function and subsequent treatment in pregnant women without overt symptoms or risk factors for hypothyroidism.[2]
Medication related	Lithium. Lithium causes overt hypothyroidism in 14–17% of patients, and subclinical hypothyroidism in 19–35% of patients.	Lithium inhibits release of T_4 and T_3. Lithium may increase autoimmunity to the thyroid if it was preexisting.	Typical hypothyroid signs and symptoms	Elevated TSH Low T_4	Lithium: Treatment with exogenous thyroid hormone is effective, and lithium therapy need not be discontinued.

Continued

TABLE 117.5   Hypothyroidism Etiologies—cont'd

Background and Importance	Pathophysiology	Clinical Features	Diagnostic Testing	Management
Amiodarone[4] • Anti-thyroid peroxidase autoantibodies and female gender are linked with an increased risk of amiodarone induced hypothyroidism (AIH) • Increased incidence in iodine replete areas	Amiodarone is a class III antiarrhythmic medication Chemical structure similar to that of T_4 Contains large amounts of iodine. Inhibits the peripheral conversion of T_4 to T_3 Directly cytotoxic to the thyroid Blocks thyroid hormone entry into cells Decreases T_3 receptor binding	Typical hypothyroid signs and symptoms	Elevated TSH Low T_4	If amiodarone therapy must be continued for arrhythmia control, patients with AIH may be successfully treated with exogenous thyroid hormone replacement and amiodarone use may continue.[4] Patients should be screened with a TSH prior to starting amiodarone.[5]
Inadequate dietary intake	Uncommon in developed nations, but still a major concern in areas where the iodine content in the water is low.	Goiter	Elevated TSH Low T_4	Dietary iodine supplementation
	Insufficient dietary iodine intake leads to reduced T4 and T3 production, with compensatory increase in TSH concentration and gland cell proliferation, goiter.			
Prior hyperthyroid treatment	Thyroid known to be functionally absent based on prior anti-thyroid treatment	Typical hypothyroid signs and symptoms	Elevated TSH Low T_4	Levothyroxine replacement
Surgically removed	Thyroid known to be surgically absent based on prior anti-thyroid treatment	Typical hypothyroid signs and symptoms	Elevated TSH Low T_4	Levothyroxine replacement
Nonthyroidal Illness Syndrome (NTSI)[6-8] Previously known as euthyroid sick syndrome Transient form of central hypothyroidism that occurs in critically ill patients	Its molecular basis remains unclear, but its presence in critically ill patients predicts adverse outcomes and mortality.[6-8] In acute phases, this is likely related to changes in binding and uptake of thyroid hormone by cells, as well as decreased conversion of T_4 to T_3. In chronic phases, likely results from dysregulation of the hypothalamic-pituitary-thyroid axis in the setting of critical illness	Typical hypothyroid signs and symptoms in the setting of critical illness	Initially low T_3, followed by decrease in T_4 and TSH as illness progresses.	At this time, there is no evidence that treatment of patients with NTIS improves outcomes.

[1]Chaker L, Bianco AC, Jonklaas J, Peeters RP. Hypothyroidism. *Lancet.* 2017;390(10101):1550-1562.
[2]Alexander EK, Pearce EN, Brent GA, et al. 2017 Guidelines of the American Thyroid Association for the Diagnosis and Management of Thyroid Disease During Pregnancy and the Postpartum. *Thyroid.* 2017;27(3):315-389.
[3]Jonklaas J, Bianco AC, Bauer AJ, et al. Guidelines for the treatment of hypothyroidism: prepared by the American Thyroid Association Task Force on Thyroid Hormone Replacement. *Thyroid.* 2014;24(12):1670-1751.
[4]Bartalena L, Bogazzi F, Chiovato L, Hubalewska-Dydejczyk A, Links TP, Vanderpump M. 2018 European Thyroid Association (ETA) Guidelines for the management of amiodarone-associated thyroid dysfunction. *Eur Thyroid J.* 2018;7(2):55-66.
[5]Kinoshita S, Hosomi K, Yokoyama S, Takada M. Time-to-onset analysis of amiodarone-associated thyroid dysfunction. *J Clin Pharm Ther.* 2020 Feb;45(1):65-71.
[6]Gutch M, Kumar S, Gupta KK. Prognostic value of thyroid profile in critical care condition. *Indian J Endocrinol Metab.* 2018;22(3):387-391.
[7]Kothiwale VA, Patil P, Gaur S. Correlation of thyroid hormone profile with the Acute Physiology and Chronic Health Evaluation II Score as a prognostic marker in patients with sepsis in the intensive care unit. *J Assoc Physicians India.* 2018;66(7):59-62.
[8]Padhi R, Kabi S, Panda BN, Jagati S. Prognostic significance of nonthyroidal illness syndrome in critically ill adult patients with sepsis. *Int J Crit Illn Inj Sci.* 2018;8(3):165-172.

Diagnosis begins with urine free cortisol, late night salivary cortisol and/or a dexamethasone suppression test, and additional imaging studies as indicated.[18] Given that these tests typically occur outside of the ED, these patients should be referred to a primary physician for definitive testing, or have workup by an inpatient team when admission is indicated.

Management

Management in the ED is directed towards treating the manifestation of Cushing syndrome that prompted the current presentation. Acute control of hypertension and glucose disorders is as per routine clinical practice. Definitive management of the underlying causes follows appropriate diagnosis via the methods described above and requires surgical resection of responsible lesions.[18]

Disposition

The need for hospitalization of patients who present with extremes of the disorders associated with Cushing syndrome (uncontrolled hypertension, glucose disorders, fractures) is determined by usual practices for these presentations. Most patients with chronic Cushing syndrome and milder symptoms can be discharged and referred for further workup as outpatients.

Hyperaldosteronism

Pathophysiology

Hyperaldosteronism is the result of excessive aldosterone production. Aldosterone acts on the kidneys, regulating sodium absorption, potassium excretion, and subsequently, hydrogen excretion. In primary hyperaldosteronism, excessive aldosterone is produced by the adrenal glands, independent of the signals from the renin-angiotensin system and sodium administration.[20,21] It is the most common cause of secondary hypertension and is significantly linked to cases of refractory hypertension.[21] Because aldosterone has toxic effects on vascular structures, it can result in cardiovascular disease and stroke, in addition to hypertension.[16] Primary hyperaldosteronism is caused by an intrinsic abnormality of the adrenal glands, such as hyperplasia or malignancy. Secondary hyperaldosteronism is caused by increased action of renin on the adrenal glands, as seen in states of renal hypoperfusion, but has the same downstream effects.

Clinical Features

Patients with hyperaldosteronism most commonly present with hypertension and its associated symptoms, as it is significantly linked with refractory hypertension. Patients may also present with a variety of other cardiovascular events, such as atrial arrhythmias, heart failure, and strokes. Primary aldosteronism is associated with the metabolic syndrome of obesity, high-density lipoprotein cholesterol and hypertriglyceridemia, and hyperglycemia. Laboratory workup may also demonstrate hypokalemia.[22]

Differential Diagnoses

Hyperaldosteronism can mimic any disease that presents with hypertension and/or disorders of potassium regulation. Its differential diagnosis includes essential hypertension, other adrenal disorders, thyroid dysfunction, and diabetes.

Diagnostic Testing

The most recent Endocrine Society clinical practice guideline recommends referral for testing for any patient with hypertension that is not controlled with three or more medications, or any patient requiring four or more medications, any patients with hypertension and hypokalemia, sleep apnea, family history of early onset hypertension or

stroke, or a family history of primary aldosteronism. In the ED, significant hypertension and any incidentaloma on the adrenal should also be referred for further evaluation.[23] Workup (inpatient or outpatient) entails measurements of the plasma renin activity or plasma renin concentration and plasma aldosterone concentration, as well the plasma aldosterone/renin ratio. If the renin concentration or renin activity are suppressed, and the aldosterone level is inappropriately high, then further confirmatory testing with laboratory studies and imaging are indicated.[23]

Management

Presentations of acute cardiovascular events, refractory hypertension or severe electrolyte derangements are managed acutely in the ED according to usual practice. Further workup and treatment for underlying primary aldosteronism is initiated once the patient has been stabilized.

Disposition

Patients with severe, acute cardiovascular events or electrolyte derangements should be admitted to the hospital according to usual practice. Patients who are stable or improving and are otherwise appropriate for discharge based on their presenting symptoms and diagnosis can be discharged home with referral for further workup as described previously.

Pheochromocytoma and Paraganglioma

Pathophysiology

Emanating from adrenal medullary chromaffin cells, pheochromocytomas are rare catecholamine–secreting neuroendocrine tumors, whereas paragangliomas are catecholamine–secreting tumors arising from the thoracic and abdominal parasympathetic ganglia.[24] The excess catecholamine states result in significant downstream systemic effects, both based on the action of norepinephrine and epinephrine as vasopressors. There is also evidence that patients with pheochromocytomas and paragangliomas have increased circulating steroids, due to the interaction between the adrenal cortex and the medulla.[25] The tumors can be benign or associated with malignancy, especially in patients who are younger and have larger tumors.[26] Certain medications can potentiate the effects of catecholamines and result in an acute exacerbation of underlying pheochromocytoma. These include dopamine receptor antagonists, beta-blockers, sympathomimetics, opioid analgesics, norepinephrine reuptake inhibitors, serotonin reuptake inhibitors, monoamine oxidase inhibitors, corticosteroids, peptides, and neuromuscular blocking agents.[24]

Clinical Features

Clinical features of pheochromocytoma and paraganglioma are characteristic of catecholamine excess. Classic symptoms include paroxysms of hypertension, diaphoresis, palpitations, headache, abdominal pain, nausea, vomiting, and weight loss. In extreme cases, patients may present with hypertensive crisis.[27] With increasing use of CT and MRI imaging, a larger proportion of patients are diagnosed after a tumor is discovered incidentally (e.g., "incidentaloma").

Differential Diagnoses

Because catecholamine excess mimics any hyperadrenergic state, the differential diagnosis includes sympathomimetic toxicity, withdrawal syndromes, hyperthyroidism, serotonin syndrome, neuroleptic malignant syndrome, and presentations of typical untreated or refractory hypertension and underlying arrhythmias.

Diagnostic Testing

Definitive testing for pheochromocytoma and paraganglioma entails establishing a biochemical diagnosis via plasma free metanephrines or urinary fractionated metanephrines. Once the diagnosis is apparent via these tests, CT imaging of the thorax, abdomen, and pelvis with contrast is recommended. MRI is reserved for patients with metastatic disease, neck and skull base lesions, or other contraindications to CT.[24] Given the significant overlap in presentation and symptomatology with multiple diseases as listed previously, providers must maintain a high index of suspicion in certain patient populations. Testing for pheochromocytoma and paraganglioma is indicated for any patient with the signs and symptoms listed previously, especially if they are paroxysmal, symptoms like this that are precipitated by the medications listed previously, or a personal or family history of pheochromocytoma, paraganglioma, multiple endocrine neoplasia type 2 (MEN2), or Von Hippel-Lindau (VHL) disease. Any patient with an adrenal incidentaloma should also be referred, regardless of symptoms.[24]

Management

Acute management of pheochromocytoma and paraganglioma focus on controlling the catecholamine surge effects. The first-line treatment is typically alpha-adrenergic blockade, such as phenoxybenzamine (final dose typically between 20–100 mg daily) or doxazosin. If resultant tachycardia ensues, providers may add calcium channel blockers or beta-adrenergic blockers. Of note, in patients with pheochromocytoma and catecholamine excess, beta-adrenergic receptor blockade in isolation can result in hypertensive crisis because of unopposed alpha-adrenergic receptor stimulation. Beta-adrenergic blockade should only be performed following alpha-adrenergic blockade in these patients. Use of calcium channel blockers alone is not recommended as initial treatment, but can be used in patients with very mild hypertension or undesirable alpha-adrenergic receptor blocker side effects.[24] Surgical removal of the offending pheochromocytoma or paraganglioma is the definitive treatment, and is typically delayed until the hyperadrenergic state is adequately controlled.

Disposition

Patients who present in hypertensive crisis or other extreme presentation who are not controlled with initial doses of the medications listed above should be admitted for continued treatment and monitoring. Patients who are stable can be discharged for continued workup and referral as outpatients.

ADRENAL INSUFFICIENCY

Foundations

Background and Importance

Adrenal insufficiency is the failure of the adrenal glands to function appropriately, and is a potentially life-threatening disease. Acute manifestations of disease may result in severe, refractory hypotension. Secondary adrenal insufficiency is more common than primary adrenal insufficiency. Its most common cause is exogenous corticosteroid administration.

Anatomy and Physiology

The adrenal glands are responsible for the release of the hormone aldosterone, corticosteroids, and catecholamines. They are paired structures that sit in the retroperitoneum, one atop each kidney. The adrenal gland has two distinct structures—the outer adrenal cortex, comprised anatomically of the zona glomerulosa, and the medulla, comprised anatomically of the zona fasciculata and reticularis. The medulla acts in concert with the central nervous system to produce and secrete epinephrine and norepinephrine in response to sympathetic stimulation.

It also secretes the mineralocorticoid cortisol from the zona fasciculata and androgens from the zona reticularis. The outer cortex, which includes the zona glomerulosa, secretes the mineralocorticoid aldosterone.

ACTH, produced and secreted by the anterior pituitary, stimulates the adrenal cortex to synthesize and produce cortisol, which regulates carbohydrate, protein, and lipid metabolism, and aldosterone, which regulates fluid and electrolyte balance through sodium and potassium homeostasis. Cortisol is the primary glucocorticoid in humans, accounting for approximately 95% of all glucocorticoid activity.

Pathophysiology

Primary adrenal insufficiency, or Addison disease, is the failure of the adrenal gland to produce cortisol, aldosterone, or both, with an intact hypothalamic-pituitary-adrenal (HPA) axis (Fig. 117.3). Its most common cause in adults is autoimmune destruction of the adrenal gland. It can also be caused by infectious diseases and certain medications.[16] Adrenal insufficiency may occur alone, with other autoimmune diseases.

In primary disease, the HPA axis remains intact. Primary adrenal insufficiency is characterized by absent or low cortisol with high levels of circulating ACTH because of reduced negative feedback effects on the anterior pituitary. The increased ACTH concentration results in secretion of other hormones with similar chemical structure. One classic feature exemplifying this relationship is ACTH stimulation of melanocyte-stimulating hormone, which causes melanocytes to form a black pigment and the characteristic skin hyperpigmentation seen in those with primary adrenal insufficiency.

Secondary adrenal insufficiency is a result of impaired stimulation of the adrenals from the disruption of normal secretion of ACTH by the pituitary (see Fig. 117.3). It is characterized by a low plasma cortisol level, with low circulating ACTH levels.

Tertiary adrenal insufficiency is caused by hypothalamic disease. There is a decrease in release of corticotropin-releasing hormone, resulting in minimal ACTH and cortisol production. Aldosterone, sex hormone, and catecholamine synthesis are normal; the most common cause is long-term exogenous steroid administration.

Adrenal insufficiency may be further characterized as acute or chronic (Box 117.9). The most common cause of acute adrenal insufficiency is the exogenous administration of glucocorticoids, which results in suppression of the HPA axis. Although the time for HPA axis recovery after exogenous suppression is highly variable, adrenal insufficiency should be anticipated to occur in patients who receive corticosteroid therapy for prolonged periods, typically more than several weeks.

Adrenal crisis is usually seen in patients with Addison disease because of mineralocorticoid deficiency but can also present in patients with secondary or tertiary adrenal insufficiency who undergo severe physiologic stress, or exogenous steroid withdrawal (after suppression of the HPA axis). These stressors deplete cortisol stores and impair the ability to mount a normal stress response.

Clinical Features

The clinical manifestations of chronic adrenal insufficiency are nonspecific, as seen in Box 117.10. Primary and secondary adrenal insufficiency result in hyponatremia from different mechanisms—aldosterone deficiency and sodium wasting in primary adrenal insufficiency and a low cortisol level and free water retention in secondary adrenal insufficiency.

Primary adrenal insufficiency characteristically has more pronounced clinical manifestations than secondary adrenal insufficiency. Patients have symptoms related to a deficiency of glucocorticoids,

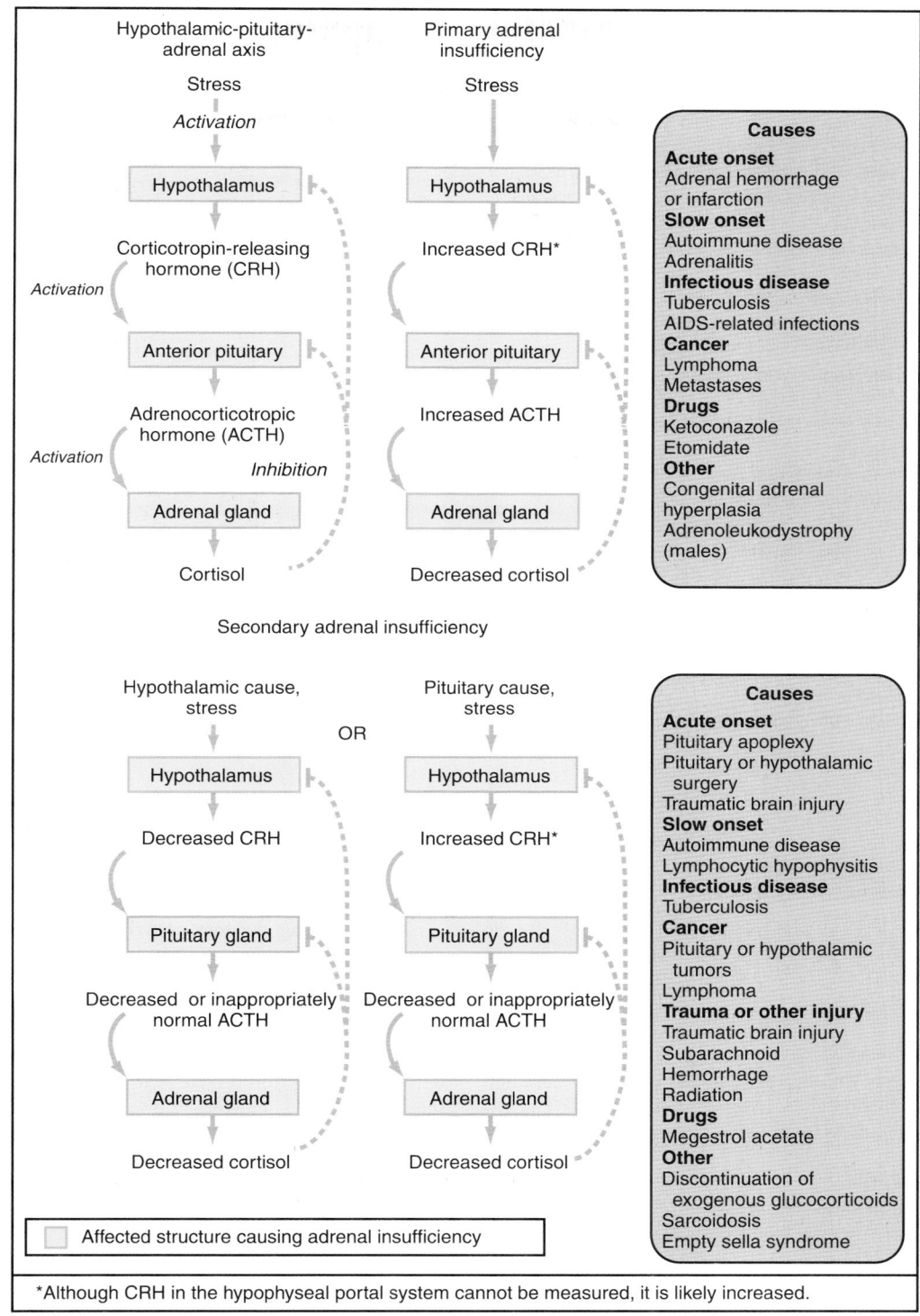

Fig. 117.3 Hypothalamic-pituitary-adrenal axis and causes of primary and secondary adrenal insufficiency. (Adapted from: Wallace I, Cunningham S, Lindsay J. The diagnosis and investigation of adrenal insufficiency in adults. *Ann Clin Biochem*. 2009;46[Pt 5]:351-367.)

mineralocorticoids, and androgens. Primary adrenal insufficiency more commonly presents with skin hyperpigmentation, particularly in areas exposed to the sun or subject to friction or pressure, salt craving, hyperkalemia, and acidosis. These patients may show signs of sodium and volume depletion (e.g., orthostatic hypotension and tachycardia). In secondary adrenal insufficiency, patients more often present with pale skin, loss of axillary and pubic hair, decreased libido, and impotence. Glucocorticoid deficiency and low ACTH concentrations may result in hypotension and hyponatremia with normal potassium levels.

BOX 117.9   Causes of Adrenal Insufficiency

Primary Adrenal Insufficiency
Chronic
Autoimmune adrenalitis (Addison disease): isolated or polyglandular deficiency, human immunodeficiency virus (HIV) infection (direct involvement or disseminated cytomegalovirus, *Mycobacterium avium-intracellulare*, tuberculosis, cryptococcosis, histoplasmosis, blastomycosis, toxoplasmosis, *Pneumocystis* pneumonia)
Tuberculosis and disseminated infections as seen with HIV
Metastatic cancer (breast, lung)
Infiltrative (sarcoid, hemochromatosis, amyloid)
Congenital (adrenal hypoplasia, adrenoleukodystrophy, ACTH resistance)
Bilateral adrenalectomy
Drug toxicity (e.g., etomidate, ketoconazole, rifampicin)

Acute
Adrenal hemorrhage
    Meningococcemia and other sepsis
    Anticoagulation (heparins and warfarin)
    Anticardiolipin antibody syndrome
    Trauma

Secondary Adrenal Failure
Chronic
Pituitary tumor (primary or metastatic)
Pituitary surgery or irradiation
Chronic steroid use with functional deficiency
Infiltrative (sarcoid, eosinophilic granuloma, tuberculosis)
Traumatic brain injury
Postpartum pituitary necrosis (Sheehan syndrome)
Empty sella syndrome

Acute
Pituitary apoplexy (hemorrhage into a pituitary tumor)
Postpartum pituitary necrosis (Sheehan syndrome)
Traumatic brain injury
Relative adrenal insufficiency (sepsis, hepatic failure, severe acute pancreatitis, trauma)

ACTH, Adrenocorticotropic hormone.

BOX 117.10   Clinical Features of Adrenal Insufficiency

General
Weakness, fatigue
Anorexia
Gastrointestinal symptoms
Weight loss
Hyponatremia
Blood pressure ≤ 110/70 mm Hg
Fevers (mild)
Depression, apathy
Myalgia, arthralgias
Auricular calcifications

Primary
Hyperpigmentation
Salt craving
Orthostasis, syncope
Vitiligo
Hyperkalemia
Hyperchloremia and acidosis
Hypoglycemia

Secondary
Hyperkalemia
Hyperpigmentation
Hypoglycemia
Orthostasis, hypotension
Amenorrhea
Axillary and pubic hair loss
Decreased libido

Crisis
Refractory hypotension

Adrenal crisis presents with hypotension and shock that does not respond to fluid resuscitation and pressors. Patients may have many other nonspecific symptoms, as listed above, but shock is the hallmark.

Differential Diagnoses

Because of the vague and nonspecific symptoms, the differential diagnosis of hypoadrenalism is extensive. The wasting associated with chronic adrenal insufficiency resembles that of anorexia nervosa or an occult carcinoma. The generalized weakness, fatigue, and myalgias can be confused with chronic fatigue syndrome, polymyalgia rheumatica, myopathy, hypothyroidism, or influenza syndromes.

Lack of recognition of acute adrenal crisis with refractory hypotension can result in evaluations for sepsis, GI bleeding, myocardial ischemia, or anaphylaxis. Abdominal pain in crisis may be clinically indistinguishable from an acute abdomen, especially if precipitated by adrenal hemorrhage. The headache and visual field cuts in pituitary apoplexy may resemble those of a hemorrhagic stroke. Finally, the constellation of symptoms seen in acute adrenal insufficiency—weakness, malaise, fatigue, nausea, dizziness, and arthralgias—is also present in steroid withdrawal syndrome. Because both can occur with the

cessation of chronic glucocorticoid administration, history is critical to distinguish between the two disease processes.

Diagnostic Testing

Although there are many tests available to confirm the diagnosis of adrenal insufficiency, they require a significant amount of time or serial testing. For this reason, if there is suspicion of adrenal crisis, treatment should be initiated immediately, prior to confirmatory tests.

Mild to moderate hyponatremia, with levels typically above 120 mEq/L, are seen in primary adrenal insufficiency. Aldosterone deficiency leads to sodium wasting, and decreased cortisol levels lead to increased antidiuretic hormone, resulting in increased water absorption. Hyperkalemia may be seen in primary adrenal insufficiency secondary to a low circulating aldosterone concentration, but is not seen in secondary causes when aldosterone is not affected.

In stable patients, cortisol measurement is the mainstay for an accurate diagnosis. Measurement of the cortisol level in the ACTH stimulation test is the standard method. Random basal serum cortisol concentrations are of limited value for assessment of HPA axis reserve. In most emergent presentations, these tests are reserved for inpatient workup after initial ED stabilization.

Management

Patients with adrenal insufficiency require hormone replacement to correct a lack of circulating glucocorticoid and mineralocorticoid. Treatment of adrenal crisis should begin as soon as possible and prior to diagnostic testing when crisis is suspected. The first-line treatment is hydrocortisone, 100 mg IV, with IV fluids, pressor support and glucose administration, as indicated (Box 117.11). An alternative is dexamethasone (4-mg IV bolus); in contrast to hydrocortisone, it does not interfere with serum cortisol assays.

Chronic management of adrenal insufficiency includes hydrocortisone (30 mg total daily in split doses; two-thirds of the daily dose is usually given in the morning and one-third in the late afternoon) and fludrocortisone, (50 to 200 µg/day) for mineralocorticoid replacement. In the setting of fever, infection, or other illness, these doses should be increased.

Whereas definitive treatment of secondary adrenal insufficiency is directed at replacement of missing hormone (ACTH or CRH) at the level of the hypothalamus or pituitary, in the ED setting, simple steroid hormone replacement is administered. Steroid tapering is necessary when gradual downregulation of the HPA axis has been provoked by exogenous glucocorticoids. There is no universally recommended method for steroid tapering.

Disposition

Severely ill patients should have the underlying disease process identified and treated; an ICU setting is indicated due to the high mortality rate. Most patients with mild symptoms of hypoadrenalism may be discharged for outpatient evaluation and treatment.

The references for this chapter can be found online at ExpertConsult. com.

BOX 117.11 Treatment of Hypoadrenalism

Maintenance
Hydrocortisone, 15–25 mg, divided into 2 or 3 doses daily
Fludrocortisone, 50–100 µg/day

Maintenance During Minor Illness
Hydrocortisone, double typical daily dosages
Fludrocortisone, 50–200 µg daily

Coverage During Procedural Stress
Hydrocortisone, 100 mg IV

Adrenal Crisis or Relative Adrenal Insufficiency of Critical Illness
Dexamethasone, 4 mg IV bolus
or
Hydrocortisone, 100 mg IV bolus, followed by additional dosing of 200 mg/24 hrs as bolus divided every 6 hrs or infusion if critically ill or major stress
0.9 NS, 2–3 L in the first few hours
Switch to D$_5$/NS if hypoglycemia
Treat precipitating illness

D$_5$/NS, 5% dextrose in normal saline; *0.9 NS,* 0.9% normal saline.

118

Bacteria

Manpreet Singh and Madonna Fernández-Frackelton

KEY CONCEPTS

- All septic patients should be treated with antibiotics as soon as possible, even before a definitive diagnosis is made. Patients with pneumococcemia, meningococcemia, and aggressive soft tissue infections can decompensate rapidly.
- The source of sepsis should be identified as soon as possible, and surgical causes should be addressed. A surgeon should be consulted as soon as possible for patients with sepsis and a débridable source of infection.
- Immunity to diphtheria, tetanus, and pertussis wanes significantly in adults. Pertussis should be considered a cause of persistent cough in adults. A tetanus vaccination history should always be obtained from patients with trauma or infection. When there is doubt about the history, the age-appropriate vaccine according to CDC guidelines should be administered.
- Consider botulism in the differential diagnosis for the infant with failure to thrive, constipation, or decreased muscle tone and for the patient who injects drugs with neurologic symptoms.

DIPHTHERIA

Foundations

Background and Importance

In the fifth century BCE, Hippocrates first described what was likely diphtheria, characterized by sore throat, membrane formation, and death from suffocation. In 1821, Pierre Bretonneau named the condition *diphtherite* (Greek for leather), describing the characteristic pharyngeal membrane. In 1890, von Behring and Kitasato created the first diphtheria antitoxin (DAT) and 1 year later administered the first dose of antitoxin to a human with diphtheria. Immunization dramatically decreased the incidence of diphtheria in the United States from 206,000 cases in 1921 with 15,520 deaths to only 2 cases between 2004 and 2017.[1,2]

Humans are the only known reservoir for *Cornybacterium diphtheriae*. Spread is person-to-person through respiratory droplets or by direct contact with secretions, skin lesion exudates, or rarely fomites or food. Transmission is associated with crowded living conditions. Individuals may spread the disease when they are actively ill, in the convalescent stage, or as asymptomatic carriers.[1,3,4]

Immunization against diphtheria is highly effective (Fig. 118.1). Before widespread immunization in the United States, the incidence of diphtheria exceeded 100 cases per 100,000 population, and the disease predominantly affected children. Most people acquired natural immunity to diphtheria by age 15, and recurrent exposure to toxigenic strains of the bacteria acted as a booster. Because childhood immunization nearly eliminates toxigenic strains in a population, adult immunity wanes, so more adults in industrialized nations are susceptible to diphtheria. By the 1980s the Centers for Disease Control and Prevention (CDC) reported 0 to 5 cases per year nationwide. Currently, sporadic cases occur primarily in inadequately immunized adolescents and adults.[2] Even in industrialized nations with high childhood vaccination rates, more than 50% of adults older than 40 years old lack protective antibodies. Recent reemergence due to disruption of national vaccination programs has led to outbreaks in Yemen and Venezuela, with a recent death in Spain from a traveling passenger from that region.

Anatomy, Physiology, and Pathophysiology

Diphtheria is caused by *C. diphtheriae*, an unencapsulated, nonmotile, gram-positive bacillus named for its shape (*korynee*, for "club") and its characteristic clinical presentation (*diphtheria*, for "leather," describing the leathery pharyngeal membrane).[1]

Infection with *C. diphtheriae* can occur at various sites of the respiratory tract or the skin. Respiratory diphtheria includes faucial (pharyngeal or tonsillar), nasal, and laryngeal (tracheobronchial) types, named for the primary location of infection. Cutaneous diphtheria can occur as a primary skin infection or as a secondary infection of a preexisting wound.[1,3]

Toxigenic strains of *C. diphtheriae* bacterium are lysogenized with the bacteriophage and produce an exotoxin that inhibits cellular protein synthesis. The diphtheritic membrane, composed of leukocytes, erythrocytes, fibrin, epithelial cells, and bacteria, results from necrosis caused by local effects of the exotoxin. Initially, the pharynx appears erythematous, but as necrosis occurs, grayish white patches appear and eventually coalesce. The membrane causes surrounding edema and cervical adenitis. The initial grayish white, filmy appearance changes to a thick, grayish black membrane with sharply defined borders. This membrane adheres to the underlying tissue, and bleeding occurs if removal is attempted.[1]

Circulating exotoxin causes the systemic symptoms of diphtheria, most profoundly affecting the nervous system, heart, and kidneys.[1,3] The degree of local and systemic toxicity depends on the location and extent of membrane formation. Pharyngeal diphtheria has the greatest toxicity and cutaneous diphtheria the least. As the exotoxin disrupts cellular protein synthesis, it causes peripheral neuropathy manifested

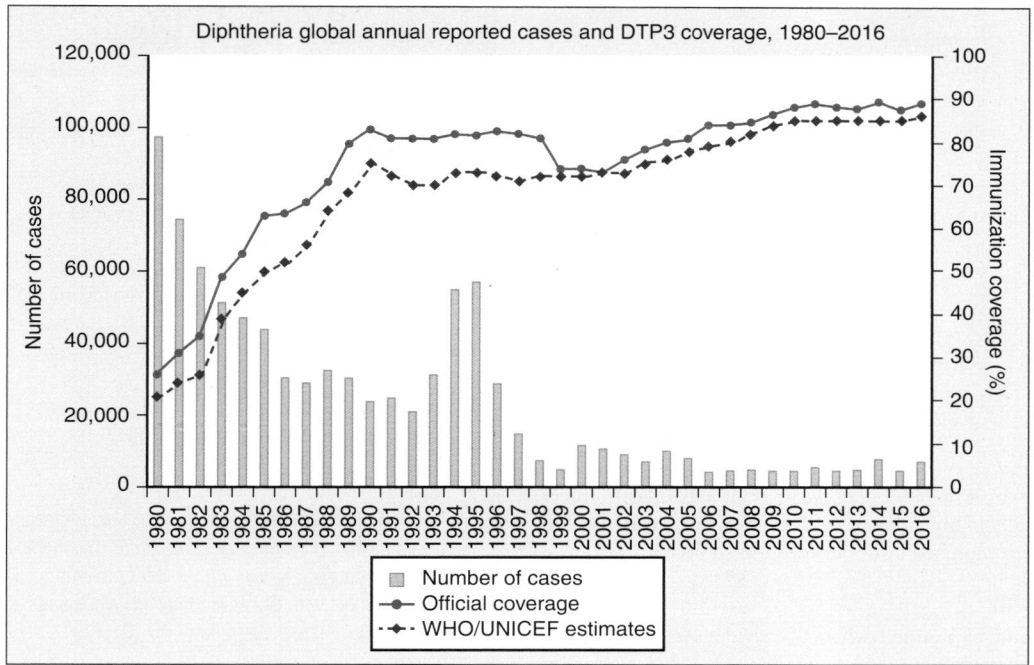

Fig. 118.1 Global annual reported cases of diphtheria compared with percentage of immunization coverage from 1980 to 2016. *DTP3,* Third dose of diphtheria-tetanus-pertussis vaccine; *UNICEF,* United Nations Children's Fund; *WHO,* World Health Organization. (From: World Health Organization, 2016 Global Summary. Geneva: WHO; 2016. World Health Organization: Immunization, vaccines and biologicals: diphtheria. Available at: www.who.int/immunization/monitoring_surveillance/burden/diphtheria/en/.)

by muscle weakness. About 5% of patients with respiratory infection develop polyneuritis; 75% of patients with severe disease have some form of neuropathy.[5] The muscles of the palate are usually affected first. Other cranial nerves, peripheral nerves, and the spinal cord may be affected. Degenerative lesions develop in dorsal root and ventral horn ganglia of the spinal cord and in cranial nerve nuclei. Cortical cells are spared. Proximal muscle groups are affected first. In severe cases, paralysis may develop in the first few days of illness. Paralysis typically does not last more than 10 days, but may last up to 3 months. Complete recovery over a longer time is the rule.[1]

The exotoxin directly damages myocardial cells. Cardiac dysfunction may appear 1 to 2 weeks after the onset of illness, but may arise earlier in severe cases. Electrocardiographic (ECG) changes suggestive of myocarditis occur in up to two-thirds of patients, but clinical manifestations of myocarditis occur in only 10% to 25% of cases.

Clinical Features

The average incubation period of respiratory tract diphtheria is 2 to 4 days (range 1–8 days). Signs and symptoms are indistinguishable from other upper respiratory tract infections, with low-grade fever and sore throat as the most frequent presenting complaints. Weakness, dysphagia, headache, voice changes, and loss of appetite are also common. Cough, shortness of breath, nasal discharge, and neck edema occur in less than 10% of patients. Cervical adenopathy occurs in approximately one-third of patients, and a membrane is observed in more than half of patients.

In patients with faucial diphtheria, the extent of the membrane parallels clinical toxicity. If the membrane is limited to the tonsils, disease may be mild; if it covers the entire pharynx, the onset of illness is usually abrupt and severe. Cervical lymphadenopathy and infiltration of neck tissues may be so extensive that the patient has a "bull-neck" appearance. Patients with this form of malignant diphtheria usually

have high fever, severe muscle weakness, vomiting, diarrhea, restlessness, and delirium. Respiratory tract obstruction or cardiac failure from myocarditis can result in death.

Nasal diphtheria presents with serous or serosanguineous nasal discharge, and these patients do not usually have constitutional symptoms. A membrane may be visible. Treatment is important to prevent a persistent carrier state. Laryngeal diphtheria may begin in the larynx or spread downward. Respiratory tract edema with subsequent upper airway obstruction may develop. In cutaneous diphtheria, patients typically do not develop systemic toxicity. The skin characteristically has an ulcer with a grayish membrane; however, wounds from which *C. diphtheriae* is cultured are clinically indistinguishable from other chronic skin conditions.[1]

The most serious complications of diphtheria are airway obstruction, congestive heart failure, cardiac conduction disturbances, and muscle paralysis. Overall mortality is less than 3% but rises to 7% in patients with myocarditis and 26% in patients with the malignant form of the disease with neck swelling.[5] Although invasive disease is rare, endocarditis, mycotic aneurysms, osteomyelitis, and septic arthritis have all been described in immunocompromised hosts.[1]

Differential Diagnosis

It may be difficult to differentiate respiratory diphtheria from many other respiratory conditions, especially in the early phase of infection (Box 118.1). In general, the diphtheritic membrane is darker, grayer, more fibrous, and more firmly attached to the underlying tissues than in other conditions that have a membrane-like appearance. Acute necrotizing ulcerative gingivitis (ANUG) frequently involves the gingivae, which are unaffected in diphtheria. Acute bacterial epiglottitis has a more rapid onset than diphtheria, and laryngoscopy reveals an erythematous, edematous epiglottis without membrane formation.[1] Cutaneous diphtheria is difficult to differentiate from other acute and

BOX 118.1 Differential Diagnosis of Respiratory Diphtheria

Streptococcal pharyngitis
Viral pharyngitis (Epstein-Barr virus, adenovirus, herpes simplex)
Tonsillitis
Gonococcal pharyngitis
Acute necrotizing ulcerative gingivitis (ANUG)
Acute epiglottitis
Mononucleosis
Laryngitis
Bronchitis
Tracheitis
Candida albicans (thrush)
Rhinitis

BOX 118.2 Check List for Assessing a Patient With Suspected Diphtheria

Suspect Case
- Pharyngitis, nasopharyngitis, tonsillitis, laryngitis, tracheitis (or any combination of these), absent or low-grade fever
- Grayish adherent pseudo-membrane present
- Membrane bleeds, if manipulated or dislodged

Probable Case
Suspect case above, plus one or more of the following:
- Stridor
- Bull-neck (cervical edema)
- Toxic circulatory collapse
- Acute renal insufficiency
- Submucosal or subcutaneous petechiae
- Myocarditis
- Death
- Recent return (<2 weeks) from travel to area with endemic diphtheria
- Recent contact (<2 weeks) with confirmed diphtheria case or carrier
- Recent contact (<2 weeks) with visitor from area with endemic diphtheria
- Recent contact with dairy or farm animals or domestic pets
- Immunization status: Up-to-date- any DTaP/DT/Tdap/Td shot within past 10 years?

Laboratory Confirmed Case
- Positive culture of *Corynebacterium diphtheriae* (or *Corynebacterium ulcerans*) and
  - Positive Elek test *or*
  - PCR for tox gene (positive for subunit A and B)

DT, Diphtheria-tetanus; *DTaP,* diphtheria, tetanus, and acellular pertussis; *PCR,* polymerase chain reaction; *Td,* diphtheria-tetanus; *Tdap,* tetanus, diphtheria, activated pertussis.
Available at: www.cdc.gov/diphtheria/downloads/dip-cklist-diag.pdf.

chronic ulcerative skin lesions. *C. diphtheriae* can secondarily infect these lesions, especially in high-risk patients such as those with alcohol use disorder and unimmunized or underimmunized people.

Diagnostic Testing

The laboratory should be notified when *C. diphtheriae* is suspected, because routine cultures do not identify the organism. Throat or nasopharyngeal swabs should be obtained for respiratory diphtheria, and if present, membranous material should be examined. Samples should be obtained from skin lesions in cutaneous infections. Specimens should be collected before antibiotic therapy is initiated and transported to the laboratory for rapid inoculation onto tellurite selective culture medium.[1,3] Definitive identification is made using a combination of colony morphology, microscopic appearance, and fermentation reactions.[1] *C. diphtheriae* isolates should be tested for toxin production. The Elek test for toxin A is available at the CDC. Polymerase chain reaction (PCR), which is more reliable but not as readily available commercially, can detect the toxin structural gene. Newer methods that rapidly detect the toxin by mass spectrometry are not readily available but may be used in the future.[6] A positive culture for group A beta-hemolytic streptococcus does not exclude diphtheria, as up to 30% of patients with diphtheria test positive for streptococcal coinfection or carrier state.

Leukocytosis, mild thrombocytopenia, and proteinuria are common but neither sensitive nor specific for diphtheria. Changes on ECG are nonspecific and include ST-T wave changes, varying degrees of atrioventricular block, and dysrhythmias.[1] The ECG may be normal in the presence of myocarditis (see Chapter 68). An echocardiogram may show dilated or hypertrophic cardiomyopathy. Cardiac enzymes may be elevated; serum troponin levels correlate with the severity of myocarditis.

Management

Patients with evidence of diphtheria should be placed in respiratory isolation and treated presumptively for *C. diphtheriae*. The goals of therapy are to protect the airway, limit toxin effects, and stop future toxin production by terminating bacterial growth. Although airway obstruction from diphtheria is rare in the United States, the management is identical to that of other forms of airway obstruction. Early intubation should be considered for patients with laryngeal involvement. Patients may be dehydrated from fever and decreased oral intake related to dysphagia or neurologic impairment. In the course of resuscitation, the patient should be assessed for fluid responsiveness, as the toxin's effect on the myocardium may result in heart failure[1] (see Chapter 3).

Equine serum diphtheria anti-toxin (DAT) should be administered if the diagnosis of respiratory diphtheria is deemed probable (Box 118.2) and before laboratory confirmation.[1,7] DAT is currently not licensed by the U.S. Food and Drug Administration (FDA) for use in the United States, and several countries do not currently hold DAT stockpiles.[8] The CDC can be contacted at 770-488-7100 to distribute DAT to physicians as an investigational new drug. The size and location of the membrane, duration of illness, and patient's overall degree of toxicity determine the DAT dose. Patients with probable or confirmed respiratory diphtheria are eligible to receive DAT (20,000 to 40,000 units for pharyngeal or laryngeal involvement of 2 days' duration; 40,000 to 60,000 units for nasopharyngeal lesions; 80,000 to 100,000 units for systemic disease of 3 days' duration or more or for diffuse neck swelling).[7] After conjunctival or intradermal sensitivity skin testing, the antitoxin is administered intravenously (IV). If the patient exhibits sensitivity to the antitoxin, desensitization should be performed. Active immunization against diphtheria should also be initiated because clinical infection may not confer immunity.

After DAT, antibiotics are initiated to prevent growth and spread of the organism but are no substitute for the antitoxin. Erythromycin 40 mg/kg/day (maximum of 2 g) intravenously or orally in divided doses is the preferred treatment. Procaine penicillin G 300,000 units/day q12h intramuscularly (IM) for those weighing 10 kg or less, and 600,000 units/day in q12h for those weighing more than 10 kg is an acceptable alternative.[1,3] Treatment failures are more common with penicillin than with erythromycin. Azithromycin and clarithromycin have activity similar to erythromycin in vitro and may result in better compliance. These agents have not been adequately tested in clinical disease. Daily oral therapy may be substituted when the patient can swallow. Negative cultures should be documented after treatment.

Myocarditis and neuritis are treated with supportive care and monitoring. Patients with ECG changes consistent with myocarditis have three to four times the mortality rate of those with normal ECGs. The mortality rate for patients with left bundle branch block and atrioventricular block is 60% to 90%. Serial ECGs are recommended, and survivors may have permanent conduction abnormalities. No data support the use of steroids.

Cutaneous lesions should be débrided of necrotic tissue and cleansed vigorously. A course of antibiotics is recommended, but DAT for cutaneous lesions is of questionable value. We recommend 20,000 to 40,000 units of antitoxin, but few data support its use in this setting.[1,7]

Carriers of *C. diphtheriae* should receive oral penicillin G or erythromycin for 7 days or IM benzathine penicillin (600,000 units for those weighing less than 30 kg and 1,200,000 units for those weighing more than 30 kg). Active immunization should also be provided to unimmunized and partially immunized carriers. After 2 weeks of therapy, cultures should be obtained; if positive, erythromycin therapy should be given for 10 additional days.[1]

Individuals who have been in close contact with infected patients should have cultures taken and be kept under surveillance for 7 days. Previously immunized close contacts should receive a booster of diphtheria toxoid if the last booster was more than 5 years earlier. The vaccine should be diphtheria, tetanus, and acellular pertussis (DTaP) or diphtheria-tetanus (DT or Td) as appropriate for age. Close unimmunized contacts or those whose immunization status is unknown should receive the same antimicrobial therapy as carriers (previously described), have culture specimens taken before and after therapy, and have active immunization initiated. Close contacts who cannot be kept under surveillance should receive IM benzathine penicillin to ensure compliance and a Td booster (appropriate for age and immunization history). DAT is not recommended for this group because of the risk of horse serum allergy.[7]

A universal primary immunization program with regular boosters every 10 years is the most effective method for controlling diphtheria. Emergency clinicians should routinely administer age-appropriate tetanus and diphtheria toxoids as part of wound management.

Disposition

All patients with possible pharyngeal diphtheria should be isolated, admitted, and monitored for arrhythmias. A cardiologist should be consulted for patients with evidence of myocarditis. The CDC should be contacted for all suspected or proven cases of diphtheria.

PERTUSSIS

Foundations

Background and Importance

Pertussis is an acute respiratory disease first described in 1578 when an epidemic swept through Paris. *Pertussis* means "violent cough." It is also called *whooping cough* because the severe episodes of coughing are followed by forceful inspiration, which creates a characteristic "whoop" sound. Bordet and Gengou identified the causative organism in 1900. Pertussis was a major cause of mortality among infants and children in the United States in the prevaccination era. A vaccine was developed in the 1940s, but pertussis remains a significant cause of morbidity and mortality worldwide.[9]

Pertussis is a highly contagious respiratory illness transmitted by aerosolized droplets. It can occur at any age but is predominantly a pediatric and adolescent illness. Infection rates are greater than 80% in adults exposed more than 12 years after completing a vaccination series and up to 90% in susceptible individuals with household exposure. Half of the cases in the United States occur from June through September. The average incubation period is 7 to 10 days (range less than 1 week to 3 weeks). Neither vaccination nor prior infection confers lifelong immunity.

Pertussis is prevalent worldwide. The World Health Organization (WHO) estimated over 24.1 million cases in 2017 with 160,700 annual deaths.[10] In the United States, annual pertussis rates declined sharply after the introduction of the vaccine, reaching a nadir of 1010 cases in 1976. There has been a steady increase since, with 11,647 cases reported in 2003 and more than 28,000 cases in 2014 (Fig. 118.2A and B).[11] The incidence is highest in infants who have not received the entire vaccine series (see Fig. 118.2C). Waning immunity in the adult population and increased reporting may be contributing factors, but the emergence of the antivaccination movement is a leading factor.

A 1991 report found a possible relationship between the vaccine and acute encephalopathy. Although there appears to be no relationship between the vaccine and long-term neurologic complications, the report resulted in a decline in the use of the whole-cell pertussis vaccine. The acellular pertussis vaccine has been approved in the United States since 1991 for persons 15 months to 64 years and since 1997 for infants.

Anatomy, Physiology, and Pathophysiology

Pertussis is caused by organisms of the *Bordetella* genus, which are small, aerobic, gram-negative coccobacilli. *Bordetella pertussis* and *Bordetella parapertussis* are responsible for human disease. The organisms are fastidious and require a medium containing charcoal, blood, or starch, and an optimal temperature of 95° to 98.6°F (35° to 37°C) to grow. *Bordetella bronchiseptica*, a flagellated, motile organism, causes illness in animals, including kennel cough, and may rarely cause respiratory infection in immunocompromised humans.[12] *Bordetella* adheres preferentially to ciliated respiratory epithelial cells, but does not invade beyond the submucosa and is seldom recovered in the bloodstream. It elaborates several toxins that act locally and systemically, including pertussis toxin, dermonecrotic toxin, adenylate cyclase toxin, and tracheal cytotoxin. Local tissue damage consists of inflammatory changes in the respiratory mucosa. Secondary pneumonia and otitis media may occur. Systemic effects of pertussis toxin include sensitization to the lethal effects of histamine and increased excretion of insulin. This hyperinsulinemia can cause hypoglycemia, particularly in young infants potentially leading to seizures.[9]

Clinical Features

Pertussis has three clinical stages: the catarrhal phase, paroxysmal phase, and convalescent phase. The *catarrhal* or *prodromal phase* begins after an incubation period of approximately 7 to 10 days and lasts approximately 1 to 2 weeks. Infectivity is greatest during the catarrhal phase, when the disease is clinically indistinguishable from other upper respiratory tract infections. Signs and symptoms include rhinorrhea, low-grade fever, malaise, and conjunctival injection. A dry cough usually begins at the end of the catarrhal phase.[9,12]

The *paroxysmal phase* begins as fever subsides. Cough increases and lasts 1 to 6 weeks, but may persist for up to 10 weeks. Paroxysms of staccato coughing occur an average of 15 times per day and are followed by a sudden, forceful inhalation that produces the characteristic "whoop." One-third of adults with pertussis develop this whoop, and it is rare in young infants, who may present with apneic episodes and

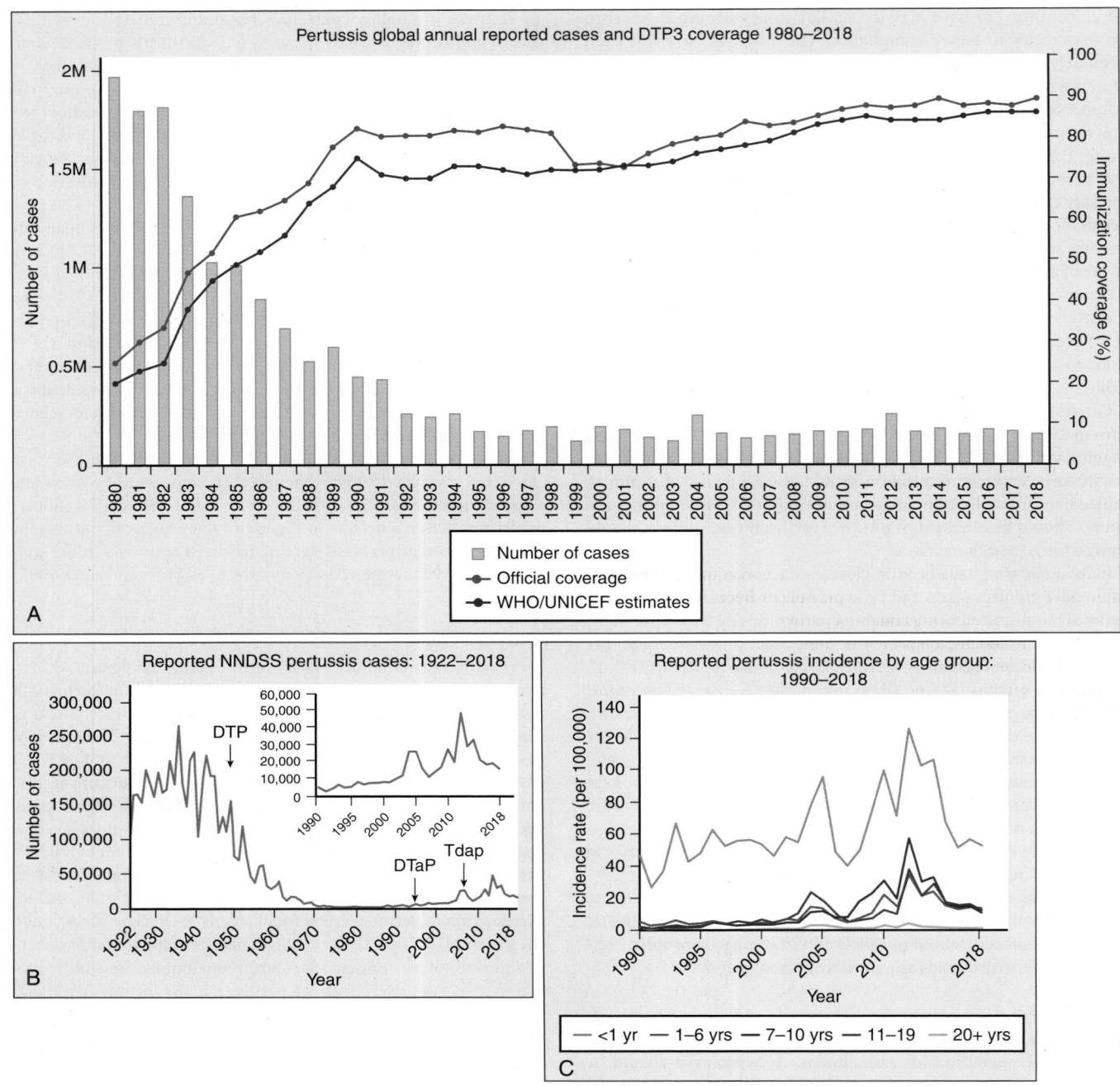

Fig. 118.2 (A) Global annual reported cases of pertussis compared with percentage of immunization coverage. (B) Incidence of reported pertussis cases in the United States by year. (C) Pertussis incidence in the United States by age, Centers of Disease Control and Prevention 2018. *DTaP,* Diphtheria, tetanus, and acellular pertussis; *DTP3,* Third dose of diphtheria-tetanus-pertussis vaccine; *NNDSS,* National Notifiable Diseases Surveillance System; *Tdap,* tetanus, diphtheria, activated pertussis; *UNICEF,* United Nations Children's Fund; *WHO,* World Health Organization. (A, From: World Health Organization. WHO/IVB database 2018; 194 WHO states. Available at www.who.int/immunization/monitoring_surveillance/burden/vpd/surveillance_type/passive/pertussis/en/. B and C, From: Centers for Disease Control and Prevention: National Notifiable Diseases Surveillance System: Pertussis (whooping cough). Available at: www.cdc.gov/pertussis/surv-reporting.html.)

no other symptoms. Paroxysms may be spontaneous, occur more frequently at night, or be precipitated by noise or cold. During the paroxysm, the patient may exhibit cyanosis, diaphoresis, tongue protrusion, salivation, and lacrimation. Post-tussive vomiting, syncope, and apnea may occur. Infants may be exhausted after a typical paroxysm. Between episodes of coughing, patients do not appear acutely ill.[9,12]

In the *convalescent phase* a residual cough may last weeks to months. Paroxysms of coughing may be triggered by unrelated respiratory infection or by exposure to a respiratory irritant. This recurrence of coughing does not represent recurrence of pertussis infection.

Atypical presentations can occur in young and preterm infants. Fever is usually absent in uncomplicated neonatal pertussis. Tachypnea,

---

BOX 118.3   Pertussis Complications

Periorbital edema
Subconjunctival hemorrhage
Petechiae
Epistaxis
Hemoptysis
Subcutaneous emphysema
Pneumothorax
Pneumomediastinum
Diaphragmatic rupture
Umbilical and inguinal hernias
Rectal prolapse

BOX 118.4   Pertussis Case Definition

Clinical Case
Cough and illness for more than 2 weeks with no apparent other cause *plus* one of the following:
- Paroxysms of coughing
- Inspiratory "whoop"
- Post-tussive emesis

Probable Case
All of the following:
- Meets clinical case definition
- Not laboratory confirmed (Only PCR and culture are considered laboratory confirmation.)
- Not epidemiologically linked to a laboratory confirmed case

Confirmed Case
One of the following:
- Acute cough illness of any duration with a positive culture for *Bordetella pertussis*
- A case that meets the clinical case definition and is confirmed by PCR for *B. pertussis*
- A case that meets the clinical case definition and is epidemiologically linked directly to a case confirmed by either culture or PCR

PCR, Polymerase chain reaction.

---

apnea, and cyanotic and bradycardic episodes may be the predominant symptoms.[13] Older children and adults who have partial protection from vaccination or previous illness may have a long-lasting intractable dry cough that is frequently misdiagnosed as bronchitis. Post-tussive vomiting in adults is highly suggestive of pertussis.[9,14]

Physical findings are nonspecific. Tachypnea is variably present and may be related to the degree of pulmonary involvement. Low-grade fever, conjunctival injection, and rhinorrhea are common during the catarrhal phase. Fever during other stages of illness suggests secondary infection. Petechiae above the nipple line, subconjunctival hemorrhages, pneumothorax, and epistaxis may occur because of increased intrathoracic pressure during coughing paroxysms.[9,12] Chest examination may reveal rhonchi; the presence of rales suggests pneumonia.

Complications of pertussis are listed in Box 118.3. Secondary pulmonary infection may result from decreased respiratory clearance cause by the *Bordetella* organism and its toxins on bronchial and lung mucosa. Bacterial or viral pneumonia superinfection complicating pertussis is a leading cause of death, especially in infants and young children. Aspiration of gastric contents and respiratory secretions may occur during paroxysm of coughing, whooping, and vomiting. A fever during the paroxysmal phase should alert the physician to a possible superinfection.[9,10,12]

Seizures and encephalopathy occur in approximately 1% of patients but are more common in infants. This may be due to hypoxia, hypoglycemia, cerebral petechiae, toxin effect, or secondary infection by neurotropic viruses or bacteria. Central nervous system (CNS) hemorrhages may occur from increased cerebrovascular pressures during paroxysm of coughing. Sudden increases in intrathoracic and intraabdominal pressures can result in other complications.[9,12] Bradycardia, hypotension, and cardiac arrest can occur in neonates and young infants with pertussis. Severe pulmonary hypertension has been recognized in this age group and can lead to systemic hypotension, hypoxia, and increased mortality.[13] Intensive care monitoring is recommended for these patients, regardless of how well they appear on admission.

Differential Diagnoses

The differential diagnosis includes acute viral upper respiratory tract infection, pneumonia, bronchiolitis, cystic fibrosis, tuberculosis, exacerbation of chronic obstructive pulmonary disease, and foreign body aspiration. The marked leukocytosis may suggest leukemia.

Diagnostic Testing

Pertussis should be considered in patients with cough lasting longer than 2 weeks with paroxysms, whoops, or post-tussive emesis, regardless of previous vaccination status.[13] Up to 27% of adults in the United States with a prolonged cough have serologic evidence of pertussis.

Ancillary studies are of limited value in the emergency department (ED). During the late catarrhal and early paroxysmal phases, a marked leukocytosis and a characteristic lymphocytosis are often present. A white blood cell (WBC) count of greater than 20,000/mL is common in pediatric patients.[12] Adults with pertussis frequently do not have the characteristic leukocytosis and lymphocytosis, and some infants and immunocompromised hosts may not mount this response. The chest radiograph (CXR) may show peribronchial thickening, atelectasis, or pulmonary consolidation.

Laboratory confirmation is important for epidemiologic purposes. Nasopharyngeal aspirate or swab (synthetic, non-cotton) should be obtained for culture and PCR, if both are available; sputum and throat swabs are inadequate because ciliated respiratory epithelial cells are required.[12] The *Bordetella* organism is fastidious, and isolation requires a medium impregnated with antibiotics to reduce overgrowth of competing bacteria. Colonies of *B. pertussis* take 3 to 7 days to appear. Pertussis cultures are 30% to 50% sensitive, and this drops to less than 3% three weeks after the onset of cough. Direct fluorescent antibody techniques are useful as a rapid screening test for pertussis but are variably specific and should not be relied upon as laboratory confirmation of *B. pertussis*. Adults generally come to medical attention late in the disease when cultures are rarely positive. PCR is more likely to identify the organism during the first 3 weeks of illness, but it has a high false-positive rate for various reasons, including asymptomatic carriers, recent vaccination, or contamination. Serologic testing is often performed as well. Most laboratories use enzyme-linked immunosorbent assay, which rises 2 to 3 weeks after infection or primary immunization. Paired serologic tests showing a twofold increase are considered positive, but they are reported as "probable" cases by the CDC unless performed at the CDC or the Massachusetts state laboratory. See Box 118.4 for the case definition.

Management

Acute Treatment

Treatment of pertussis is supportive and includes oxygen, frequent suctioning, appropriate hydration, parenteral nutrition as needed, and avoidance of respiratory irritants. Patients with suggested pertussis and associated pneumonia, hypoxia, CNS complications, or those experiencing severe paroxysms should be hospitalized. Children younger than 1 year old should also be admitted, because they are not yet fully immunized and have the greatest risk for morbidity and mortality. Neonates with pertussis should be admitted to a neonatal intensive care unit (NICU) because apnea and significant cardiac complications can occur without warning.[9,12]

Antibiotic treatment does not reduce the severity or duration of illness at any phase. The goal of antibiotic therapy is to decrease infectivity and carriage.[14] The CDC recommends macrolides; erythromycin, clarithromycin, and azithromycin are preferred for pertussis in persons 1 month of age and older. Erythromycin estolate ester 40 to 50 mg/kg/day (maximum of 2 g/day) has previously been recommended for four divided doses for 14 days, but a 7-day course of erythromycin estolate ester at 1 g/day is just as effective at eradicating *B. pertussis* with better compliance. Azithromycin 10 mg/kg/day for 5 days is recommended in infants younger than 1-year-old because of an association between oral erythromycin and infantile hypertrophic pyloric stenosis (IHPS). Alternative treatments include azithromycin (10 mg/kg on day 1, followed by 5 mg/kg on days 2 to 5) or clarithromycin (15 mg/kg/day; maximum of 1 g/day in two divided doses). Trimethoprim-sulfamethoxazole (8 mg/kg/day of trimethoprim) is an alternative for macrolide-allergic patients two months of age or older, but efficacy is unproven. Patients should be considered infectious for 3 weeks after the onset of the paroxysmal phase or until at least 5 days after antibiotics are started.[9] Droplet isolation is recommended during this period.

Corticosteroids, especially in young critically ill infants, may reduce the severity and course of illness, but effectiveness has not been established. Inhaled beta$_2$-adrenergic agonists do not reduce the frequency or severity of paroxysmal coughing episodes but may help patients with reactive airway disease. Past trials with pertussis immune globulin are limited and do not show benefit. Standard cough suppressants and antihistamines are ineffective.[15]

Postexposure prophylaxis with an appropriate macrolide is recommended for those at high risk for developing severe pertussis, including household contacts of a pertussis case, infants and women in their third trimester of pregnancy, persons with preexisting health conditions that may be exacerbated by a pertussis infection, and close contact with any of the above-listed people. This includes but is not limited to those who work in NICUs, childcare settings, and maternity wards. Women in their third trimester of pregnancy may be a source of pertussis to their newborn infant.[16]

Vaccination

Whole-cell and acellular pertussis vaccines are distributed in combination with diphtheria and tetanus toxoids as DPT and DTaP, respectively. The whole-cell vaccine is 70% to 90% effective at preventing serious pertussis infection. Pediatric recipients have fever, irritability, behavioral changes, and local discomfort at the site of inoculation. Moderately severe reactions are uncommon but include temperature above 104°F (40°C), persistent, high-pitched crying, and seizures. Severe neurologic complications (prolonged seizures and encephalopathy) occur rarely but led to decreased use of the whole-cell form of the vaccine and the development of DTaP.[17]

The acellular pertussis vaccines contain inactivated pertussis toxin and one or more other bacterial components; they are less effective than the whole-cell vaccine but have fewer reported adverse reactions.[18,19] DTaP has replaced DPT for childhood immunizations in the United States and is approved for children ages 6 weeks to 6 years old.[12,] Current American Academy of Pediatrics (AAP) guidelines state that acellular pertussis vaccinations are as safe as whole-cell vaccines, but new data suggest the latter provide a better, longer-lasting serologic response. There has also been a correlation between acellular vaccination and food allergies. Further studies are needed to guide future recommendations.

Pertussis immunity wanes 5 to 10 years after immunization and 15 years after natural infection, resulting in an increased incidence in people older than 15 years. Tetanus, diphtheria, acellular pertussis (Tdap) (with reduced diphtheria toxoid and pertussis antigens) is indicated as a booster vaccine in persons 11 to 18 years old. It is safe and effective in adults, including pregnant women and those over 65 years of age. Persons older than 65 years old who have never received Tdap and anticipate close contact with infants younger than 12 months old should receive a single dose of Tdap, regardless of interval since last Td vaccination. A live attenuated nasal vaccine has completed phase one trials in humans showing greater than 99.9 nasopharyngeal colonization and is undergoing further clinical development.[20]

TETANUS

Foundations

Background and Importance

Tetanus is a toxin-mediated disease characterized by severe uncontrolled skeletal muscle spasms. Respiratory muscle involvement leads to hypoventilation, hypoxia, and death. Dramatic descriptions of this disease date to ancient Egypt, when physicians recognized a frequent relationship between tissue injury and subsequent fatal spasm.[21] Prophylactic injection of tetanus antitoxin provided passive immunity to wounded soldiers during World War I. In 1924, an effective vaccine was developed, and large-scale testing during World War II indicated that the tetanus toxoid confers a high degree of protection against disease.[22] Despite the availability of an effective vaccine, tetanus remains endemic worldwide. It is more common in warm, damp climates and relatively rare in cold regions. The global annual incidence of reported cases of tetanus has declined with the introduction of vaccination programs (Fig. 118.3A). The WHO reported 15,103 cases of tetanus in 2018 but estimates that thousands of unreported cases occur annually resulting in approximately 34,000 neonatal deaths. Most of these cases occur in countries with low immunization rates.[23]

Since the introduction of vaccination programs in the United States, the incidence of tetanus has steadily declined from 4 cases per million population in the 1940s to fewer than 0.01 cases per million population in 2010 (see Fig. 118.3B).[24] The highest incidence occurs in people older than 65 years old (0.23 case per million population). Half of cases occur in injection drug users. The overall case fatality rate is 18% but approaches 50% in patients over 70 years old (Fig. 118.4). Cases have been reported in fully vaccinated patients, but no deaths occurred.[24]

Tetanus classically occurs as a result of a deep penetrating wound. A history of injury is present in more than 70% of patients, but the injury may be trivial. The remainder may have another identifiable condition or no apparent source.[21] The most common portals of entry are puncture wounds, lacerations, and abrasions. Tetanus has also been reported in association with chronic skin ulcers, abscesses, otitis media, foreign bodies, corneal abrasions, childbirth, and dental procedures. Postoperative tetanus has been reported in patients who have undergone intestinal operations and abortions. In these cases, the source of bacteria is probably endogenous because up to 10% of humans harbor *Clostridium tetani* in the colon. Inadequate primary immunization and waning immunity continue to be the primary risk factors for tetanus in the United States. As tetanus vaccination of children has improved, older people have accounted for an increasing percentage of reported cases.

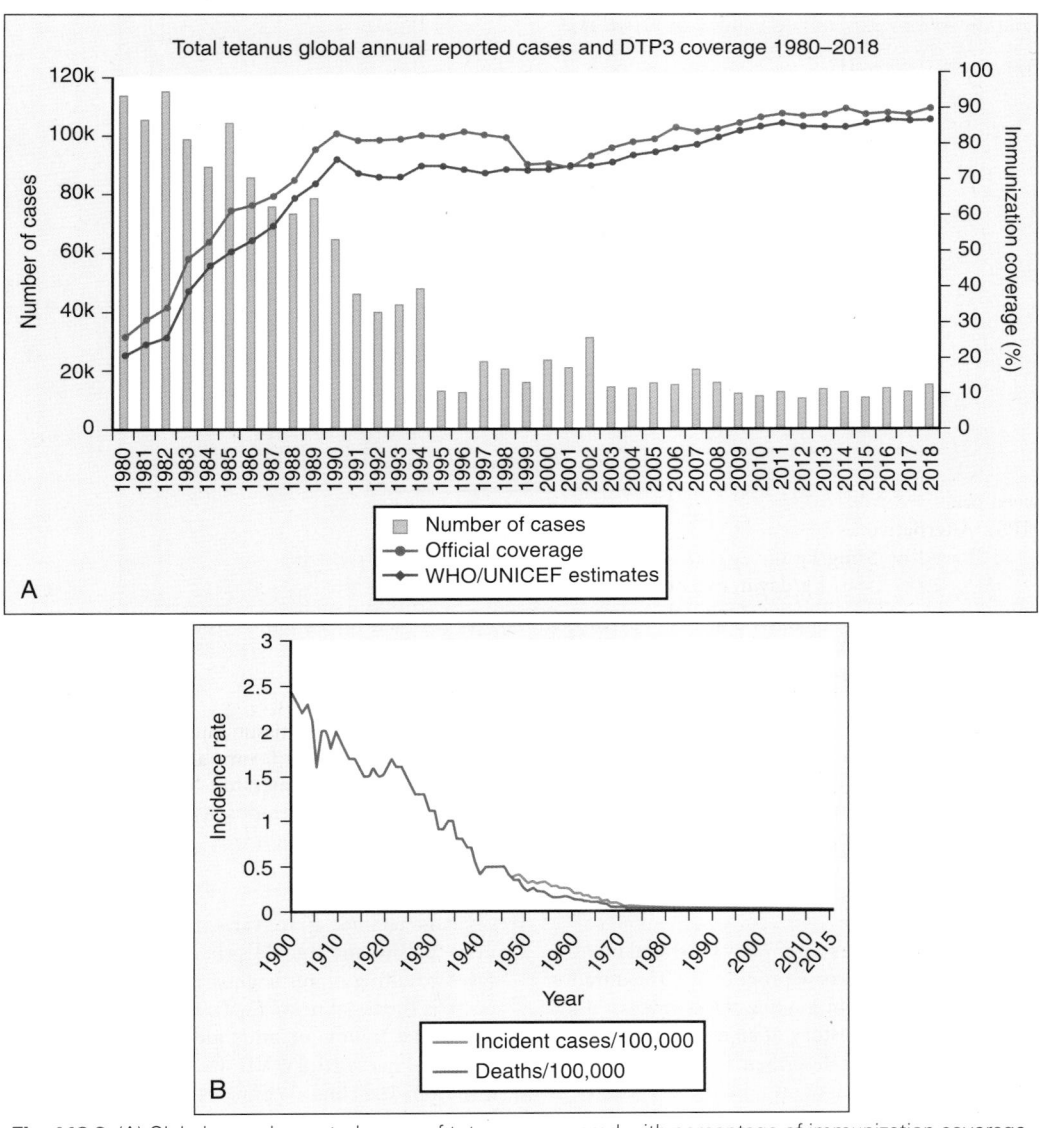

Fig. 118.3 (A) Global annual reported cases of tetanus compared with percentage of immunization coverage. (B) Incidence of reported tetanus cases in the United States by year. *DTP3*, third dose of diphtheria-tetanus-pertussis vaccine; *UNICEF*, United Nations Children's Fund; *WHO*, World Health Organization. (A, From: World Health Organization. Immunization, vaccines and biologicals: tetanus. Available at: https://www.cdc.gov/vaccines/pubs/surv-manual/chpt16-tetanus.html. B, From: Centers for Disease Control and Prevention National Notifiable Diseases Surveillance System. Available at: https://www.cdc.gov/vaccines/pubs/surv-manual/chpt16-tetanus.html.)

Anatomy, Physiology, and Pathophysiology

C. tetani is a spore-forming, motile, rod-shaped, obligate anaerobic bacillus. It stains gram-positive in fresh culture but has a variable staining pattern in culture and tissue samples. *C. tetani* is ubiquitous in soil and dust and is also found in the feces of animals and humans. Spores are resistant to heating and chemical disinfectants and can survive in the soil for months to years. When introduced into a wound, spores may not germinate for weeks because of unfavorable tissue conditions. When injury favors anaerobic growth, the spores germinate into mature bacilli, which form a single spherical terminal endospore to produce a characteristic drumstick appearance. Only these mature bacilli produce the tetanus toxin that causes clinical disease.[21]

C. tetani is a noninvasive organism. The development of clinical disease requires a portal of entry and tissue conditions that promote germination and growth in a susceptible host. Tetanus-prone wounds have damaged or devitalized tissue, foreign bodies, or other bacteria. Under these conditions, *C. tetani* produces the neurotoxin that causes clinical illness. Germination and replication of *C. tetani* can occur without clinical signs of wound infection.

C. tetani produces the neurotoxin tetanospasmin at the site of tissue injury. Tetanospasmin binds the motor nerve ending and moves by retrograde axonal transport and trans-synaptic spread to the CNS. It binds preferentially to inhibitory (GABAergic and glycinergic) neurons and blocks the presynaptic release of these neurotransmitters. Interneurons afferent to alpha motor neurons are affected first. Without inhibitory control, the motor neurons undergo sustained excitatory discharge, resulting in the muscle spasm characteristic of tetanus.[25] Tetanospasmin may also affect preganglionic sympathetic neurons and

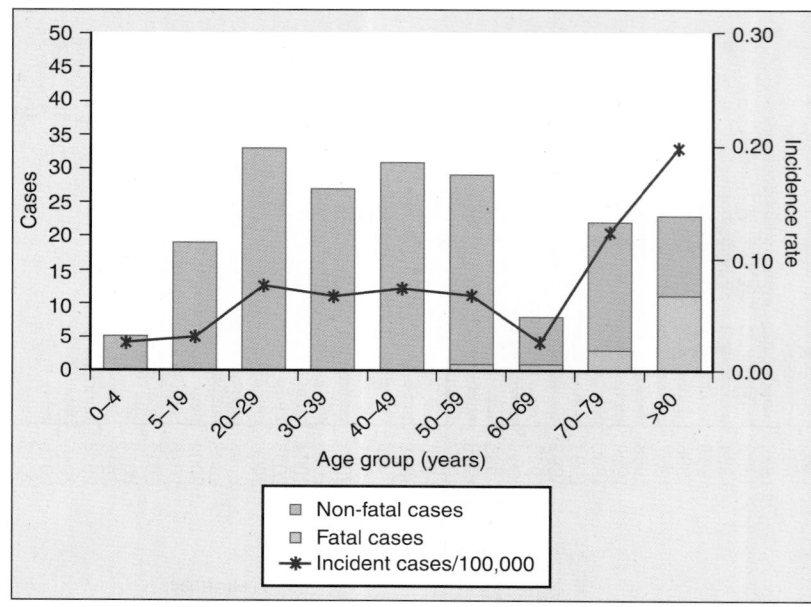

Fig. 118.4 Incidence of and mortality from tetanus by age group in the United States, 2009 to 2015. (Centers for Disease Control and Prevention. Manual for the surveillance of vaccine-preventable diseases. Available at: www.cdc.gov/vaccines/pubs/surv-manual/chpt16-tetanus.html.)

parasympathetic centers, resulting in autonomic nervous system dysfunction. The clinical manifestations include dysrhythmias and wide fluctuations in blood pressure and heart rate. The binding of tetanospasmin at the synapse is irreversible; recovery occurs only when a new axonal terminal is produced.[21]

Clinical Features

The incubation period for tetanus ranges from 1 day to several months. Shorter incubation periods portend a worse prognosis.[21] The duration of the incubation period is not useful in making the diagnosis of tetanus because many patients have no history of an antecedent wound. Four types of clinical tetanus have been described.

Generalized Tetanus

Generalized tetanus, the most common form of the disease, results in spasms of agonist and antagonist muscle groups throughout the body. The classic presenting symptom is trismus or "lockjaw," caused by masseter muscle spasm, and is present in 50% to 75% of patients. As the other facial muscles become involved, a characteristic sardonic smile (risus sardonicus) appears. Other early symptoms include irritability, weakness, myalgias, muscle cramps, dysphagia, hydrophobia, and drooling. As the disease progresses, generalized uncontrollable muscle spasms occur spontaneously or as a result of minor stimuli, such as touch or noise. Spasms can cause vertebral and long-bone fractures and tendon rupture. Opisthotonos is prolonged tonic contraction that resembles decorticate posturing. Spasms of laryngeal and respiratory muscles can cause ventilatory failure and death. Autonomic dysfunction is the major cause of death in patients who survive the acute phase and is manifested by tachycardia, hypertension, hyperpyrexia, cardiac dysrhythmias, and diaphoresis. The illness progresses over 2 weeks. If the patient survives, recovery is complete after 4 weeks or more. Throughout this illness, patients remain completely lucid unless they are chemically sedated.[21]

Localized Tetanus

Localized tetanus is a form of the disease characterized by persistent muscle spasms close to the site of injury. Symptoms may be mild or severe, but mortality is lower than with generalized tetanus. Local tetanus may progress to generalized disease. This form of illness may reflect partial immunity to tetanospasmin and may be present for weeks to months before resolution.[21]

Cephalic Tetanus

Cephalic tetanus, a rare variant of localized tetanus, results in cranial nerve palsies and muscle spasms. Palsies precede the spasm in many cases, resulting in misdiagnosis. The most commonly involved cranial nerve is the facial nerve (VII), mimicking Bell palsy. Most cases occur after facial trauma or otitis media. Patients have trismus and palsies of cranial nerve III, IV, VII, IX, X, or XII ipsilateral to the site of local infection. The clinical course is variable. In one-third of cases, resolution of symptoms is complete. The remainder progress to generalized tetanus with an overall mortality rate of 15% to 30%.[18,21]

Neonatal Tetanus

Neonatal tetanus is generalized tetanus of the newborn and occurs almost exclusively in countries where maternal immunization is inadequate and contaminated material is used to cut and dress umbilical cords. Symptoms begin during the first week of life and include irritability and poor feeding. Mortality approaches 100% because of the high toxin load for body weight and inadequate medical support. Even with limited resources, mortality can be reduced to less than 50% with medication and experienced medical personnel.

Complications

Acute respiratory failure results from respiratory muscle spasms or laryngospasms and airway obstruction. If patients survive the acute onset of illness and have adequate ventilatory support, autonomic dysfunction becomes the leading cause of death. Autonomic instability occurs several days after the onset of generalized spasms. Disinhibition of the sympathetic nervous system predominates and causes dysrhythmias, hypertension, myocarditis, and pulmonary edema. Dysrhythmias and myocardial infarction are the most common fatal events during this phase.

Forceful tetanic muscle spasms can cause vertebral subluxations and fractures, long-bone fractures, and shoulder and temporomandibular joint dislocations. Rhabdomyolysis occasionally occurs and can cause acute renal failure. Renal failure may also result from dehydration and sympathetic nervous system hyperactivity.

Secondary infection may occur in the initial inoculating wound or as a complication from invasive treatment modalities, such as mechanical ventilation. Hyperthermia may also result from muscle spasms and sympathetic hyperactivity. Prolonged immobility can lead to deep venous thrombosis and pulmonary embolism. Gastrointestinal complications include peptic ulcers, ileus, intestinal perforation, and constipation. The syndrome of inappropriate secretion of antidiuretic hormone occurs in a small number of patients. Hemolysis has also been reported.

Mortality is a function of the previous immunization status, incubation period, severity and rapidity of onset of illness, comorbid disease, age, and sophistication of medical treatment available. With appropriate intensive care treatment, older patients may fare as well as their middle-aged counterparts. Long-term physical complications in survivors are rare. The most common persistent problem is psychological trauma related to the disease and its treatment.[21]

Differential Diagnoses

Strychnine poisoning is the only clinical condition that truly mimics generalized tetanus. Strychnine, like tetanospasmin, antagonizes glycine release, but unlike tetanospasmin, it has no effect on GABA release. Patients have opisthotonos while remaining alert. The annual incidences of tetanus and strychnine poisoning are similar in the United States, and serum and urine tests for strychnine should be performed when tetanus is considered.

In patients who present with diffuse generalized spasms, the diagnosis is unlikely to be missed, but ideally the disease should be considered and diagnosed in the early stages to minimize complications and decrease mortality. Some conditions with clinical similarities to tetanus are listed in Box 118.5. Trismus is most commonly caused by intraoral infections. These can be excluded with careful history and physical examination. Mandibular dislocation can be ruled out with appropriate radiographs of the mandible and temporomandibular joints. Dystonic reactions can be differentiated from tetanus by medication history and symptoms alleviated by benztropine or diphenhydramine. Patients with encephalitis usually exhibit an altered mental status. Meningitis can be excluded by examination of the cerebrospinal fluid (CSF). Rabies should be considered when there are symptoms of brainstem dysfunction, including dysphagia and respiratory muscle dysfunction. A history of exposure to secretions of an infected animal is the most helpful historical point. In addition, rabies does not cause trismus.

Cephalic tetanus is especially difficult to diagnose when the cranial nerve palsy precedes trismus. The differential diagnosis of cephalic tetanus includes Bell palsy, botulism, cranial nerve palsies, and facial cellulitis with facial nerve compression and ophthalmoplegia.

Diagnostic Testing

The diagnosis of tetanus should be made on clinical grounds. Wound cultures are of little value and are positive in only one-third of cases. A positive culture does not indicate whether the bacterium is a toxin-producing strain. There are no laboratory tests to confirm or to exclude the diagnosis of tetanus. Lumbar puncture may be indicated to exclude meningitis in the neonate when the diagnosis of tetanus is uncertain. A computed tomography (CT) scan helps assess for intracranial disease. A serum calcium level is helpful to exclude hypocalcemia. Electromyography may be useful if the diagnosis of cephalic or localized tetanus is in doubt.

BOX 118.5 Differential Diagnosis of Tetanus

Acute abdomen
Black widow spider bite
Dental abscess/infection
Dislocated mandible
Dystonic reaction
Encephalitis
Head trauma
Hyperventilation syndrome
Hypocalcemia
Meningitis
Peritonsillar abscess
Progressive fluctuating muscle rigidity (stiff-man syndrome)
Psychogenic
Rabies
Sepsis
Status epilepticus
Strychnine poisoning
Subarachnoid hemorrhage
Temporomandibular joint syndrome

The spatula test involves touching the oropharynx with a tongue blade. With a negative test, the patient gags and expels the tongue blade. With a positive test, the patient has reflex masseter muscle spasm and bites the spatula. This test is 94% sensitive and 100% specific for tetanus.

Management

The four treatment strategies for patients with tetanus should be undertaken simultaneously: supportive care, elimination of unbound tetanospasmin, prevention of further toxin production, and active immunization.[22]

Supportive Care

Supportive care begins with controlling muscle spasms. Reflex spasms result from stimulation of the patient caused by any movement or loud noises. Unnecessary stimulation should be avoided. Benzodiazepines are the mainstay of symptomatic therapy. These drugs are GABA agonists and indirectly antagonize many of the effects of tetanospasmin, but they do not affect the glycine release inhibition by tetanospasmin. Diazepam is the most extensively studied, but lorazepam and midazolam are equally effective. Diazepam has a rapid onset of action, wide safety margin, and can be given orally, rectally, or IV. It is inexpensive and available in most parts of the world. Its long cumulative half-life and active metabolites can cause prolonged sedation and respiratory depression. The IV formulations of diazepam and lorazepam contain propylene glycol, which, at high doses, can produce lactic acidosis. Gastrointestinal delivery of these agents is limited by motility problems associated with tetanus. Midazolam has a short half-life and does not contain propylene glycol; it should be given by continuous infusion and is cost-prohibitive in many areas of the world. Propofol infusion is effective and expensive, but patients may not tolerate the lipid vehicle. Neuroleptics, barbiturates, and intrathecal baclofen have no advantage over benzodiazepines. Dantrolene is a direct muscle relaxant without CNS activity. It has been reported as an adjunctive agent for muscle spasms and may decrease the need for mechanical ventilation.[19] Magnesium sulfate infusion has been advocated as both adjuvant and first-line therapy for tetanus, with recent data showing effectiveness as first-line therapy to control spasms and muscle rigidity in mild-to-moderate tetanus.[26]

If spasms cannot be controlled with these regimens or airway compromise develops, the patient should receive neuromuscular blockade and mechanical ventilation. Succinylcholine should not be the first-line neuromuscular blockade because there is a risk of severe hyperkalemia resulting from its use in any neuromuscular disease. This effect does not begin until about 4 days after the onset of disease. Long-acting nondepolarizing agents are preferred. Vecuronium and rocuronium are shorter acting and lack significant cardiovascular side effects but require continuous infusion. Adequate sedation should be provided, and neuromuscular blockade should be withheld daily to assess the patient's status. All intubated patients should be considered for early tracheostomy to decrease reflex spasms caused by the endotracheal tube.

Autonomic instability requires monitoring and treatment. Sympathetic hyperactivity can be treated with combined alpha- and beta-adrenergic antagonists, such as labetalol and propranolol. The use of beta-antagonists alone can lead to unopposed alpha-activity, resulting in severe hypertension. If beta-antagonists are necessary, a short-acting agent such as esmolol should be used. Clonidine has variable success at modulation of sympathetic outflow in these cases. Morphine and magnesium sulfate infusions as well as spinal anesthesia and intrathecal baclofen have been shown to improve autonomic dysfunction.[21] Diuretics should be avoided for blood pressure control as volume depletion can worsen autonomic instability. Bradydysrhythmia should be treated with temporary pacing. Atropine and sympathomimetic drugs should be used with caution because the autonomic instability is essentially due to catecholamine excess.

Elimination of Unbound Toxin and Active Immunization. Passive immunization with human tetanus immune globulin (HTIG) and active immunization with Td should be initiated as soon as possible in all patients with suspected tetanus. HTIG neutralizes circulating toxin and reduces mortality. It does not neutralize toxin already present in the nervous system, nor does it treat any existing symptoms. HTIG should be administered at a site separate from the Td; 500 units is as effective as higher doses. Adult and pediatric doses are the same. Administration of a portion of the HTIG proximal to the site of inoculation is often recommended but has not been studied. The preparation of HTIG available in the United States is not licensed for intrathecal administration, which is of questionable benefit.[21]

Prevention of Further Toxin Production. Toxin production is eliminated by treatment of the *C. tetani* infection. Wound débridement and antibiotic administration can cause transient release of tetanospasmin, so these measures should be delayed until after the HTIG is administered. Metronidazole (500 mg orally or IV every 6 hours) is the antibiotic of choice for *C. tetani*. Table 118.1 lists pediatric doses of metronidazole based on age and weight.

Penicillin has good in vitro and in vivo activity against *C. tetani*, but it also has GABA antagonistic activity and may potentiate the effects of tetanospasmin. Metronidazole has better penetration into devitalized tissue and abscesses than penicillin and is superior in terms of recovery time and effect on mortality. Macrolides, doxycycline, chloramphenicol, and tetracycline are effective alternatives in metronidazole-allergic patients.[21]

Vaccination

Tetanus toxoid is an inactivated form of tetanospasmin. Vaccination confers protective antibody levels in nearly 100% of people who receive three doses. Immunity wanes between 5 and 10 years after completion of the series. In high-risk patients such as older patients, injection drug users, and immunocompromised patients, immunity wanes more quickly, and the response to the vaccine is slower.

Adults with uncertain primary immunization status should receive a primary series of three tetanus toxoid doses, followed by booster doses

TABLE 118.1 Pediatric Doses of Metronidazole Based on Age and Weight

Weight and Age	Dosage
Neonates <1200 g and 0 to 7 days	7.5 mg/kg IV or orally every 24 hours
Neonates <1200 g and 8 to 28 days	7.5 mg/kg IV or orally every 12 hours
Neonates >1200 g and 0 to 7 days	7.5 mg/kg IV or orally every 12 hours
Neonates >1200 g and 8 to 28 days	25 to 30 mg/kg/day IV or orally every 12 hours
Infants and children	30 mg/kg/day IV divided every 6 hours, maximum 4 g/day

IV, Intravenous.

every 10 years. Age-specific guidelines for tetanus prophylaxis have been developed by the Advisory Committee on Immunization Practices (ACIP) and published by the CDC (Tables 118.2 and 118.3). Tetanus vaccination should be updated for all patients who present for wound management. Those younger than 7 years old should receive diphtheria-tetanus or DTaP. Patients 7 years old or older should receive Tdap.

HTIG prophylaxis (250 units IM) is recommended for unimmunized and underimmunized patients with high-risk wounds (>6 hours old, >1 cm deep, contaminated, stellate, denervated, ischemic, infected). When tetanus toxoid and HTIG are given concurrently, separate injection sites should be used. The only contraindication to tetanus and diphtheria toxoids is a history of a neurologic or severe hypersensitivity reaction to a previous dose. The most common side effects of tetanus vaccine are minor: local swelling, pain, erythema, pruritus, fever, nausea, vomiting, malaise, and nonspecific rash. Local reactions do not preclude future use of toxoid. Serious anaphylactic reactions are rare. If a patient who requires toxoid gives a history suggestive of a neurologic or severe anaphylactic reaction, HTIG should be administered alone to protect the patient from development of tetanus as a result of the present injury. HTIG does not confer active immunity, and such patients should be referred to an allergist for measurement of antibody levels, antitoxin desensitization, and immunization. No evidence exists that tetanus and diphtheria toxoids are teratogenic and HTIG is not contraindicated in pregnancy. For inadequately immunized patients of any age, referral should be made to ensure that the patient receives the remainder of the immunizations required.

BOTULISM

Foundations

Background and Importance

Botulism is a rare life-threatening paralytic illness caused by neurotoxins produced by *Clostridium botulinum*. The disease occurs in one of five forms: food-borne botulism, infant botulism, wound botulism, unclassified botulism, and inadvertent botulism.[27] Since the approval of botulinum toxins A and B by the FDA for cosmetic and therapeutic uses in the United States, cases of iatrogenic botulism have been reported.[28]

The term *botulism* comes from the Latin *botulus*, meaning "sausage," because of an association noted between sausage ingestion and the paralytic illness. Botulism first received attention in the United States during World War I when women were encouraged to preserve fruits and vegetables. The recommended heating methods for home canning did not destroy spores, leading to epidemics of botulism. Wound botulism was first described in 1943, the CDC began surveillance of this form of the disease in 1950. Infant botulism, now the most common form of the illness, was first described in 1976.

TABLE 118.2 Routine Diphtheria, Tetanus, and Pertussis Vaccination Schedule for Children and Adults—United States

Dose	Customary Age	Age/Interval	Product
Primary 1	2 months old	6 weeks or older	DTaP
Primary 2	4 months old	4 to 8 weeks after first dose[b]	DTaP
Primary 3	6 months old	4 to 8 weeks after second dose[b]	DTaP
Primary 4	15 to 18 months old	6 to 12 months after third dose[b]	DTaP
Booster	4 to 6 years old, not needed if fourth vaccination administered after birthday[a]		DTaP
Additional booster	11 to 18 years old		Tdap
Adult booster	>18 years old All pregnant women	Every 10 years	Tdap or Td[c]

[a]If primary immunizations are started after the age of 6 years, the series should begin and continue with Tdap.
[b]Prolonging the interval does not require restarting of the series.
[c]Td should be given to adult patients who have previously received Tdap. Tdap can be given regardless of interval since Td.
DTaP, Diphtheria, tetanus, and acellular pertussis; *Td,* diphtheria-tetanus; *Tdap,* tetanus, diphtheria, activated pertussis.
Modified from: Recommended childhood immunization schedule—United States, 2020. Available at www.cdc.gov/vaccines/schedules/hcp/imz/child-adolescent.html and *MMWR.* 2019;68(5):112.

TABLE 118.3 Summary Guide to Tetanus Prophylaxis in Routine Wound Management

History of Absorbed Tetanus Toxoid (Doses)	CLEAN MINOR WOUNDS		ALL OTHER WOUNDS[a]	
	Tdap[b] or Td	TIG	Tdap[b] or Td	TIG
Unknown or less than three	Yes	No	Yes	Yes
Three or more[c]	No[d]	No	No[e]	No

[a]Such as, but not limited to, wounds contaminated with dirt, feces, soil, and saliva; puncture wounds; avulsions; and wounds resulting from missiles, crushing, burns, and frostbite.
[b]For children younger than 7 years old, DTaP is preferred. For persons older than 7 years old, Tdap is preferred to tetanus toxoid alone. Td is preferable in adults who have previously received one dose of Tdap.
[c]If only three doses of fluid toxoid have been received, a fourth dose of toxoid, preferably an adsorbed toxoid, should be given.
[d]Yes, if greater than 10 years old since last dose.
[e]Yes, if greater than 5 years old since last dose. (More frequent boosters are not needed and can accentuate side effects.)
HTIG, Human tetanus immune globulin; *Td,* diphtheria-tetanus; *Tdap,* tetanus, diphtheria, activated pertussis.
Modified from: Centers of Disease Control and Prevention. Pink Book. National enteric disease surveillance: botulism annual summary in 2017. Available at: www.cdc.gov/vaccines/pubs/surv-manual/chpt16-tetanus.html.

A total of 182 confirmed cases of botulism were reported to the CDC in 2017, a decrease from 205 cases in 2016. Of these, 77% were infant botulism, 10% were food-borne botulism, 10% were wound botulism, two cases were iatrogenic, and one was suspected adult intestinal colonization.[29] Despite the ubiquitous nature of botulinum spores and the variety of possible routes of toxin entry, the incidence of disease is low.

Typical food-borne botulism results from the ingestion of preformed heat-labile toxin rather than from the ingestion of spores or live bacteria. Food-borne botulism usually results from exposure to home-canned foods that are inadequately preserved and undercooked; large outbreaks occasionally occur after the ingestion of contaminated food at restaurants or from commercial sources. A variety of preserved foods have been implicated, and botulism has also been reported to result from ingestion of improperly prepared and stored fresh foods.

Infant botulism occurs in children younger than 1 year old with a peak incidence between the ages of 6 weeks and 6 months. In contrast to food-borne botulism in adults, infant botulism is caused by the ingestion of spores with in vivo production of toxin. Honey and to a lesser extent corn syrup have been implicated as sources of *C. botulinum* spores in infant botulism. Soil and vacuum cleaner dust have also been implicated, but the source of ingestion remains unknown in most cases. Types A and B botulinum toxins have been responsible for almost all infant cases. There appears to be no relationship between infant botulism and sudden infant death syndrome.

Wound botulism once accounted for approximately one botulism case per year, but the increased use of black tar heroin has resulted in a dramatic increase in cases. Most cases occur in California among injection drug users, with two confirmed cases in Los Angeles county associated with heroin injection. Toxin type A is the most frequent causative agent.[29,30]

Unclassified or adult infectious botulism is a rare illness that is analogous to infant botulism. The *Clostridium* bacterium produces toxin in vivo. Patients with compromised gastric acidity, disturbances of gastrointestinal motility, or abnormal gastrointestinal bacterial flora may be susceptible to in vivo production of botulinum toxin.

Inadvertent botulism is an iatrogenic form of the disease that occurs in patients who have been treated with botulinum toxin injections for dystonia and other movement disorders and for cosmetic purposes. Inadvertent generalized weakness as well as unintentional focal weakness may be seen.[31]

The potential exists for botulinum toxin to be used as a biologic weapon. It is highly potent and easy to produce. The Aum Shinrikyo, responsible for the 1995 sarin gas attack on the Tokyo subway, produced and dispersed aerosolized botulinum toxin in Japan on at least three occasions between 1990 and 1995. In 1995, Iraq admitted to the United Nations that it had produced 19,000 L of concentrated botulinum toxin and loaded approximately 10,000 L into warheads. These 19,000 L are not fully accounted for and constitute three times the amount needed to kill the entire human population by inhalation.

Anatomy, Physiology, and Pathophysiology

C. botulinum is an anaerobic, gram-positive, rod-shaped organism. It forms spores that germinate under certain environmental conditions. It produces a potent exotoxin that is responsible for the disease. Each strain of *C. botulinum* produces a specific toxin type—A through G. Only types A, B, E, and F produce disease in humans.[32] Botulinum toxins are the most potent known biologic compounds. Doses as small as 0.09 to 0.15 μg IV or 0.7 to 0.9 μg inhaled can cause death in a 70-kg human.[33] Heating at 185°F (85°C) for 5 minutes destroys any botulism toxin, and heating of toxin-contaminated food just before ingestion prevents food-borne botulism. Conversely, spores are highly heat resistant and can survive a temperature of 212°F (100°C) for several hours.

Food-borne botulism results from ingestion of food that contains preformed toxin. Toxin-contaminated food may have a normal appearance and taste or exhibit signs of spoilage. Because of the potency, one bite can expose a person to enough toxin to cause illness. Digestive enzymes do not destroy preformed toxin.

Infant and adult infectious botulism results from in vivo bacterial elaboration of toxin in the gastrointestinal tract. Achlorhydria and recent antibiotic use predispose the gastrointestinal tract to colonization with *C. botulinum*. Wound botulism results from in vivo bacterial elaboration of toxin in a wound. Inadvertent or iatrogenic botulism results from injection of preformed toxin for medical purposes.[32] Primate studies indicate that aerosolized botulinum toxin can also be absorbed systemically through the respiratory tract.[33]

The botulinum neurotoxin is similar in structure and function to the tetanospasmin toxin produced by *C. tetani*, but the clinical effects differ dramatically. Tetanospasmin targets inhibitory interneurons in the CNS, causing generalized muscle spasm, whereas botulinum toxin targets peripheral neuromuscular junctions and autonomic synapses, causing flaccid paralysis. When botulinum toxin is absorbed, it circulates until it reaches the neurons. The toxin binds to the presynaptic nerve membrane, becomes internalized, and inhibits the release of acetylcholine predominantly at the cholinergic synapses of the cranial nerves, autonomic nerves, and neuromuscular junction. Clinically, this is manifested by cranial nerve palsies, parasympathetic blockade, and descending flaccid paralysis. Once affected with type A toxin, the nerve is permanently damaged, and recovery requires axonal regeneration and the formation of new synapses, which may take several months. Recovery after type F toxin is substantially faster.[27]

Clinical Features

Food-borne botulism is the prototype for understanding the clinical signs and symptoms of all forms of botulism. Symptoms begin 6 hours to 8 days after the ingestion of toxin-containing food. A shorter incubation period is associated with a more severe form of illness. Early symptoms include weakness, malaise, lightheadedness, nausea, vomiting, and constipation. These symptoms are generally not severe and occur in fewer than half of the patients.

Neurologic symptoms may begin immediately or be delayed for several days. The cranial nerves are first affected. Patients experience diplopia, blurred vision, dysphonia, dysphagia, dysarthria, and vertigo. Next, a symmetrical descending muscle weakness occurs, involving the upper and lower extremities and the muscles of respiration. Blockade of the cholinergic fibers of the autonomic nervous system leads to a variety of symptoms. Decreased salivation causes a dry mouth, which may be so severe that the patient complains of a painful tongue and sore throat. Ileus and urinary retention may occur.

The patient with botulism is usually alert and afebrile unless a secondary infection is present. Postural hypotension may be present. Ocular signs include ptosis, extraocular palsies, and markedly dilated and fixed pupils; the absence of ocular abnormalities does not exclude the diagnosis. The oropharynx may be erythematous, with dry mucous membranes. The gag reflex is depressed or absent. Muscle weakness is usually present and varies from mild to severe. Neck muscles are often weak. Upper extremity muscles are affected more than those of the lower extremity, and proximal muscles are weaker than distal muscles. Deep tendon reflexes may be normal, symmetrically decreased, or absent. The sensory examination is normal. The abdomen may be distended with hypoactive or absent bowel sounds. Bladder distention may be apparent on examination. Respirations may be tachypneic and shallow or normal. In advanced illness, signs of respiratory failure may be present. Atypical presentations of food-borne botulism have been reported, and certain serotypes produce distinct variations in the pattern of symptoms. Type A disease may be more severe and is more commonly associated with bulbar findings and upper extremity weakness. Type A and type B disease may rarely cause a decreased level of consciousness. Type E is associated with a greater incidence of gastrointestinal symptoms.[27]

The presentation of *infant botulism* is different from that of food-borne botulism. Constipation is a common presenting complaint, followed by several days to weeks of poor feeding, weak cry, loss of head control, and hypotonia. Patients have decreased muscle tone and depressed deep tendon reflexes. Cranial nerve involvement causes alterations in facial expression, ptosis, and extraocular palsies. Respiratory failure occurs in 50% of patients. Fever is absent unless a secondary infection is present.[34]

Wound botulism has notable differences from food-borne botulism. The incubation period is longer, from 4 to 14 days, because the toxin must be produced within the wound after the spores have germinated. If the wound is infected, the patient may be febrile. Gastrointestinal symptoms are absent in wound botulism. Recurrent episodes are well described.[30]

The clinical presentation of *unclassified (adult infectious) botulism* is similar to food-borne botulism, although the mortality rate is significantly greater. Recovery from botulism is slow, and survivors are hospitalized for several weeks to months.

Complications from botulism include respiratory failure and problems associated with prolonged intensive care management. Aspiration of oral secretions and gastric contents because of loss of protective airway reflexes can occur. In the past 50 years, the overall mortality rate has decreased from 50% to less than 1% with modern intensive care. Mortality rates are higher in wound botulism patients (15% to 17%) and lower in infant botulism patients (<1%). For those who recover, muscle strength and endurance may not return to normal for up to 1 year, and persistent psychological problems are common.[29]

Differential Diagnoses

The differential diagnosis of *adult botulism* includes a wide variety of illnesses. The first presenting case is often misdiagnosed because early symptoms suggest pharyngitis or gastroenteritis, both of which can affect several members of a single household. Only after one or more cases progress to classic botulism is the diagnosis usually suggested.

Botulism should be differentiated from other illnesses that cause paralysis. In Guillain-Barré syndrome, weakness usually starts distally and ascends, paresthesias may be present, and the CSF protein level may be elevated. Tick paralysis is an ascending paralysis, which is notable for a lack of bulbar involvement and the presence of a tick. In myasthenia gravis, eye signs are also prominent, but pupillary response is preserved, no autonomic symptoms are present, and weakness responds to the administration of edrophonium or ice applied to the affected muscle group. Of note, minimal improvement in weakness after the administration of edrophonium has been reported in botulism.[35] Poliomyelitis causes fever, asymmetrical neurologic signs, and CSF abnormalities. Diphtheria can be distinguished by the prolonged interval between pharyngitis and neurologic symptoms. Eaton-Lambert syndrome does not usually involve bulbar muscles. Strokes of the brainstem have an acute onset and asymmetrical, neuroanatomically localizing signs and symptoms.

Certain toxins should be considered in the differential diagnosis of botulism. Anticholinergics (atropine, belladonna, jimson weed) cause pupillary dilation and dry, red mucous membranes but also cause delirium. Organophosphate insecticides cause hyperthermia and altered mental status. Dystonic reactions are self-limited and respond to diphenhydramine or benztropine. Neuromuscular blockade from the administration of aminoglycosides is distinguished by medication history. Heavy metal poisoning produces changes in mental status. Magnesium toxicity may mimic botulism, but history and serum magnesium levels distinguish these entities. In paralytic shellfish poisoning, paresthesias are prominent, a history of shellfish ingestion is present, and recovery occurs within 24 hours.

Infant botulism has a broader differential diagnosis. Common illnesses that can mimic infant botulism include sepsis, viral illnesses, dehydration, encephalitis, meningitis, and failure to thrive. Neurologic illnesses such as Guillain-Barré syndrome, myasthenia gravis, and poliomyelitis should also be considered.[34] Hypothyroidism, hypoglycemia, diphtheria, and toxin exposures are all part of the differential diagnosis, as are less common conditions such as inborn errors of metabolism, congenital muscular dystrophy, and cerebral degenerative diseases.

Diagnostic Testing

Botulism is a clinical diagnosis that should be considered in any patient who presents with the constellation of gastrointestinal, autonomic, and cranial nerve dysfunction. Bilateral cranial nerve involvement and the progression of neurologic findings should increase clinical suspicion. Routine laboratory studies are of no value in the diagnosis. If a lumbar puncture is performed, the CSF may show only a slight elevation of protein.[32]

The diagnosis is confirmed by detecting botulinum toxin or *C. botulinum* in gastric contents, stool, or wound of the patient, botulinum toxin in the patient's blood, or toxin or organisms in the suspected food source. Local health departments and the CDC should be notified for instruction on the handling of specimens. Ideally, the specimens should be obtained before administering antitoxin, but treatment should not await laboratory confirmation. Serial measurements of the patient's vital capacity are helpful in recognizing deteriorating ventilatory function.[27]

Electromyography (EMG) can detect abnormalities consistent with the diagnosis of botulism and may be useful in differentiating botulism from other paralytic illnesses. The EMG signature of botulism is decreased amplitude of the compound muscle action potential in response to a supramaximal stimulus and facilitation of the muscle action potential with repetitive nerve stimulation. Not all motor units are affected, and normal test results do not exclude the diagnosis.

Management

The treatment of botulism consists of supportive care and specific treatment with antitoxin and other medications to block the effects of the toxin. All patients with suspected botulism should be admitted to an intensive care unit (ICU) because respiratory failure may develop rapidly. A decrease in vital capacity to less than 30% of predicted or less than 12 mL/kg is an appropriate criterion for intubation. Ileus should be treated with nasogastric suction and urinary retention with an indwelling urinary catheter. The autonomic dysfunction of botulism is much less severe than that of tetanus and rarely requires intervention.

Saline enemas and cathartics have been recommended to cleanse the gastrointestinal tract of residual toxin, but no evidence supports these treatments. Cathartics should not be given in the presence of ileus. Magnesium-containing cathartics should be avoided because elevated serum magnesium levels can exacerbate muscle weakness. Special care should be taken with use of gastrointestinal clearance in infants with botulism. Because the source of toxin is outside the gastrointestinal tract in wound botulism, bowel decontamination is not indicated.

Equine antitoxin contains antibodies to toxin types A, B, and E. It should be administered as soon as possible after appropriate laboratory specimens have been obtained. It neutralizes circulating toxin but does not affect bound toxin. Early administration prevents illness progression, decreases hospital length of stay, prevents respiratory failure, and shortens the duration of respiratory failure in patients with severe disease. Antitoxin can be obtained from the CDC or state health department. After skin testing for hypersensitivity, one 10-mL vial should be given IV. The serum half-life is 5 to 8 days. Contrary to the information in the package insert, only one vial of antitoxin is required. Repeated doses are unnecessary and increase the risk of hypersensitivity reactions, which occur in approximately 9% of patients.[29]

Infant botulism is treated with human botulism immune globulin (BabyBIG), which is pooled plasma from immunized adults with high titers of antibodies to toxins A and B.[35] BabyBIG shortens hospital length of stay by a mean of 3.1 weeks and mechanical ventilation by a mean of 1.7 weeks. It can be obtained by calling the Infant Botulism Treatment and Prevention Program (IBTPP) on-call physician at 510-231-7600 (24/7/365).[34,35]

Antibiotics are not currently recommended for food-borne botulism and may increase cell lysis and promote toxin release. Because the source of toxin is in vivo production within an infected wound, débridement and antibiotic administration should be considered only after antitoxin has been administered. Otherwise, the use of antibiotics should be limited to treatment of secondary infections that may develop. Antibiotic treatment of both infant and wound botulism has no proven benefit. If antibiotics are used for any reason in a botulism patient, attempts should be made to avoid the aminoglycosides and tetracyclines because they can impair neuron calcium entry and worsen the effects of botulinum toxin.[27] Guanidine hydrochloride may enhance acetylcholine release from terminal nerve fibers and has been recommended as an experimental component of botulism therapy.[35]

Disposition

All patients with possible botulism should be admitted to an ICU because respiratory failure may develop rapidly and insidiously. An infectious disease specialist should be consulted for management issues. The CDC should be called for assistance in any case of suggested botulism. The CDC can be reached by calling 404-639-3311 (days) and 404-639-2540 (nights, weekends, and holidays). State and local health departments may also be helpful in investigating and preventing major epidemics. Area emergency departments should be alerted so that clinicains can be aware of possible subsequent cases.

PNEUMOCOCCEMIA

Foundations

Background

Streptococcus pneumoniae is a significant cause of morbidity and mortality worldwide. Pneumococcemia is defined as the presence of *S. pneumoniae* in the blood. The clinical presentation ranges from a mild illness to a fulminant, life-threatening, systemic syndrome. *S. pneumoniae* also causes myriad localized infections, including otitis media, pneumonia, meningitis, and, less commonly, endocarditis, septic arthritis, and peritonitis.[31,36]

S. pneumoniae was discovered in 1881 by Sternberg in the United States and simultaneously by Pasteur in France. The first pneumococcal vaccine was licensed for use in the United States in 1977, and today there are two forms available: one for infants younger than 2 years old and individuals with impaired host defenses, and one for otherwise healthy individuals older than 2 years old.[37-40] *S. pneumoniae* remains a substantial cause of serious illness despite the availability of antibiotics and vaccines. Infection appears sporadically in normal individuals and in patients with impaired host defenses. Most cases of pneumococcal infections are community acquired, with a peak incidence in winter. Invasive pneumococcal disease (IPD) is defined as isolation of *S. pneumoniae* from a normally sterile site (blood, pleural fluid, CSF). Pneumococcemia occurs in less than 2% of all hospitalized patients with community-acquired pneumonia, but up to 7.3% of those admitted to the ICU, 11.5% of those with multilobar infiltrates, 15% of those with a temperature 104°F (40°C) or higher or 95°F (35°C) or lower, 20% of those with a systolic blood pressure below 90 mm Hg, and 22% of those with HIV. Other sources include the meninges (8%) and the sinuses or middle ear (4%).

Bacteremia is primary in 18% of adults but is much higher in children. People at higher risk for pneumococcemia include those with chronic respiratory or cardiovascular disease, chronic alcohol abusers, patients with cirrhosis, diabetes mellitus, or an absent or functionally impaired spleen (postsplenectomy or sickle cell disease), those receiving immunosuppressive therapy, those with chronic renal failure, nephrotic syndrome, organ transplantation, lymphoma, Hodgkin disease, multiple myeloma, and acquired immunodeficiency syndrome (AIDS).[39] Pneumococcus is spread from person to person by close contact, and crowded living conditions are associated with epidemics. The mortality rate from pneumococcemia is 10% to 20% for young adults and much higher for older patients, those with underlying disease, and those with localized infections, such as meningitis.[40-41] The case fatality rate is significantly lower for children.

Anatomy, Physiology, and Pathophysiology

Pneumococcemia is caused by *S. pneumoniae*, an encapsulated, gram-positive, facultative anaerobic coccus. Antigenic differences in the polysaccharide capsule separate *S. pneumoniae* into 90 serotypes.[31] In the United States, seven serotypes account for most of invasive disease in children younger than 6 years old and 50% of invasive disease in people older than 6 years old. Worldwide, 10 capsular types account for two-thirds of invasive disease while in western industrialized nations, seven capsular types account for two-thirds of invasive disease.

S. pneumoniae enters the blood by one of two routes: (1) It begins as a pulmonary infection that spreads to mediastinal lymph nodes, the thoracic duct, and into the circulation; (2) it colonizes or causes infection in the upper respiratory tract and spreads to the subarachnoid space through the arachnoid villi to the venous sinus and into the blood (with or without meningeal involvement).

S. pneumoniae bacteremia causes a clinical picture that ranges from a minor febrile illness to life-threatening septic shock. Multiple virulence factors contribute to adherence to tissues, inhibition of phagocytosis, activation of complement, and stimulation of cytokines.[31] Host defenses rely heavily upon antibody and complement production, and people who have impaired humoral immunity are more susceptible to IPD. In patients with pneumococcal infections, antibodies specific to the capsule serotype develop within several days of onset of infection. This response occurs approximately 30 days after a patient receives the pneumococcal vaccine. Patients who demonstrate substantial host resistance are able to develop active immunity, and some children can spontaneously clear culture-proven pneumococcemia.

Clinical Features

The clinical presentation of pneumococcemia ranges from mild illness to fulminant disease, progressing to death within several hours. Occult bacteremia begins as a febrile illness in which the only direct indication of pneumococcemia is a positive blood culture (often at 24 to 48 hours). Sepsis is indicated by 2 or more systemic inflammatory response syndrome (SIRS) criteria or the quick SOFA (qSOFA) assessment[42] (see Chapter 127). Patients may present with lethargy, signs of poor tissue perfusion, cyanosis, and hypoventilation or hyperventilation. Either occult bacteremia or sepsis can occur in conjunction with a localized infection.

Symptoms include fever, chills, cough, shortness of breath, headache, and rash. The clinical presentation of pneumococcemia is similar to that of other common febrile illnesses. Although signs of focal infection, such as pneumonia, may be present, often the only indication of pneumococcemia is fever or other signs of bacterial toxicity. Most adult patients have fever or hypothermia. Cough, rigors, pleuritic pain, and gastrointestinal symptoms occur in about one-third of adult patients. Fever (temperature >101.3°F [38.5°C]) occurs in 90% of younger patients but in less than 60% of those older than 65 years old. Patients with signs of sepsis have an increased risk for a fulminant course with rapid deterioration. Physical examination findings vary with the site of primary infection. A focal primary source of infection is more common in adults than in children. Clinicians should evaluate for signs of otitis media, sinusitis, and meningitis. Pneumococcemia is considered primary in 18% of adults and 30% of children, so lack of localized infection as a source does not rule out IPD.

Cardiovascular collapse can occur with fulminant pneumococcal sepsis. Patients who develop severe illness from pneumococcemia may have end-organ damage from inadequate perfusion, disseminated intravascular coagulation (DIC), septic emboli, respiratory failure, meningitis, gastrointestinal bleeding, hepatic coma, renal failure, and myocardial infarction.

Pneumococcemia occasionally results in hematogenous seeding, causing peritonitis, arthritis, endocarditis, meningitis, and cellulitis. Adults and children with functional or anatomic asplenia may have fulminant pneumococcemia, or *overwhelming postsplenectomy infection (OPSI)*, characterized by septic shock, adrenal hemorrhage, and DIC. Although the incidence of OPSI is unknown, studies demonstrate that it is substantial and that the risk for it does not decrease over time after splenectomy. Most invasive pneumococcal infections occur in the first 2 years postsplenectomy, and about two-thirds occur between 5 and 20 years. OPSI may arise with symptoms indistinguishable from those of common viral illnesses.[43,44] The 100-fold increased incidence of pneumococcal bacteremia and meningitis in children with sickle cell disease is likely primarily due to splenic dysfunction, but complement abnormalities may also play a role.[45]

Differential Diagnoses

Pneumococcemia is challenging to distinguish from other causes of febrile illness. The presence of fever and shock, with or without a characteristic rash, suggests the possibility of sepsis caused by *Haemophilus influenzae, Neisseria meningitidis,* and other streptococcus types. The presence of confirmed pneumococcemia does not exclude other diagnoses, such as influenza.

Diagnostic Testing

The only test specific for pneumococcemia is a blood culture that grows *S. pneumoniae.* Ancillary testing should include a complete blood count with differential, blood and urine cultures, electrolyte values, glucose concentration, serum creatinine level, serum lactate, and blood urea nitrogen level. A CXR may demonstrate pneumonia. The results of sputum Gram stain, culture, and sensitivity testing may help direct later inpatient care. Sputum specimens should be collected before antimicrobial therapy is instituted if possible; however, therapy should not be delayed to obtain sputum. Antigen testing of urine for pneumococcal polysaccharide is up to 100% sensitive in IPD.[45]

If the patient appears toxic or has signs of respiratory compromise, an arterial blood gas, serum lactate, and coagulation profile should be obtained. If signs of meningitis or alterations in mental status are present, a lumbar puncture should be performed. Gram stain of the buffy coat may be positive in cases of overwhelming pneumococcal sepsis. The WBC count is usually elevated. A normal or low WBC count is suggestive of more serious disease, as are hypoxemia and hypercarbia. Increased mortality occurs in patients with serum creatinine levels higher than 2.0 mg/dL, bilirubin levels higher than 1.5 mg/dL, and albumin levels below 2.5 g/dL.

Management

Acute Treatment

Management of pneumococcemia consists of stabilization of life-threatening conditions, eradication of the infection, and treatment of predisposing or coexisting conditions. All septic patients should be managed with sepsis-directed therapy (see Chapter 127).[46,47] The decision to initiate antibiotic therapy is often made with limited objective data, which include the clinical findings, age of the patient, underlying conditions, and preliminary laboratory studies. Prompt initiation of antibiotics is essential to reduce the morbidity and mortality of pneumococcal infection, and should begin in the ED. To simplify selection of a treatment strategy, patients can be divided into two groups:

1. Bacteremia or sepsis suggested by clinical findings; organism not identified: Patients in this group are given antibiotics based on the most likely organism, patient's age, immune status, presence of coexisting disorders, and local patterns of antibiotic resistance. The antibiotic regimen is altered after identification of the organism and its sensitivities.

2. *S. pneumoniae* growth is reported from blood cultures (usually 1 to 2 days prior): The treatment regimen for occult bacteremia is guided by the patient's age, history, physical examination, general appearance, and ancillary test results. The antibiotic selected on initial visit may be sufficient to treat pneumococcal bacteremia subsequently identified by the laboratory. The patient should be reevaluated promptly. Repeated blood culture should be obtained if the patient has not been taking an antibiotic. For well-appearing children, a 7- to 10-day course of an appropriate oral antibiotic is reasonable. The decision to admit a child is based on the findings at the time of reevaluation.

Adult patients with laboratory-proven pneumococcemia may be treated with penicillin G if susceptibility has been documented: 2 to 4 million units IV every 4 hours if local penicillin resistance patterns are still low. Meningitis is treated with 4 million units of penicillin G every 4 hours. In children, the dosage for meningitis is 250,000 units/kg per 24 hours in divided doses every 4 hours IV up to a maximum of 20 million units.

S. pneumoniae susceptibility to penicillin in the United States continues to decline.[48] Unless penicillin susceptibility has been documented, treatment should begin with ceftriaxone (1 to 2 g IV every 12 to 24 hours; 50 to 100 mg/kg/day in children) or cefepime (1 to 2 g IV every 8 to 24 hours; 50 mg/kg every 8 hours in children). When meningitis is suspected, higher doses should be given. In areas where ceftriaxone resistance has emerged, vancomycin (weight-based loading dose 20 mg/kg, maintenance dose based on renal function in children) should be administered.

Ceftriaxone is commonly administered to children with suggested occult bacteremia treated as outpatients while blood, urine, and CSF culture results are pending. Ceftriaxone (initial dose of 50 to 100 mg/kg IM or IV, followed by daily dosage of 100 mg/kg in divided doses every 12 hours, up to a maximum of 4 g) and cefotaxime (200 mg/kg/day in divided doses every 6 hours IV, up to a maximum of 12 g) are excellent antibiotics for *N. meningitidis* and *H. influenzae.* Alternative initial treatment of pneumococcemia in penicillin- or cephalosporin-allergic patients includes vancomycin, imipenem, and chloramphenicol.

Patients with pneumococcemia may not respond to treatment for the first 24 to 48 hours of therapy. This may be attributed to the normal course of the disease, an incorrect diagnosis, the underlying illness, or an antibiotic regimen that does not treat the infection sufficiently.

Vaccination

Pneumococcal vaccine is effective in preventing infection; the 23-valent vaccine contains the purified polysaccharide antigens of the serotypes that cause 70% to 88% of pneumococcemia infections in the United States. Although it is only 60% to 70% effective at preventing invasive disease, it is safe, inexpensive, and of substantial value for well-defined groups at risk.[37,39] The 23-valent pneumococcal vaccine has limited immunogenicity in children younger than 2 years. The heptavalent conjugate vaccine PCV7, licensed in 2000, linked the polysaccharide to proteins, resulting in an improved immunogenic response in children younger than 2 years old.[49] This vaccine significantly decreased IPD caused by the included serotypes, but an increase in disease caused by non-vaccine serotypes prompted the development of a 13-valent conjugate vaccine. PCV13 was licensed in the United States in 2010 and has replaced PCV7.[37] Recommendations for the use of the PVC13 and 23-valent (PPSV23) vaccines are given in Tables 118.4, 118.5, and 118.6.[50,51]

Approximately 50% of IPD in children with comorbidities is caused by serotypes not included in either the 13-valent or 23-valent vaccine.[52] Other preventive measures for pneumococcemia include passive immunization with immunoglobulins for patients with congenital or acquired immunodeficiency diseases and daily antibiotic prophylaxis for children with functional or anatomic asplenia.[53]

Disposition

Toxic-appearing patients of any age should be treated with antibiotics and admitted to the hospital. Patients with underlying or coexisting conditions and those with an unclear course of illness should also be admitted or observed. Children who are afebrile and appear well on initial examination are unlikely to have serious sequelae. The decision to treat a febrile child with antibiotics on an outpatient basis is based on clinical findings, vaccination history, medical history, the ability of the parents to follow the discharge instructions, and availability of timely follow-up.

MENINGOCOCCEMIA

Foundations

Background

Few clinical situations in emergency medicine produce greater concern than meningococcal infection. Virtually all emergency clinicians

TABLE 118.4   Centers for Disease Control and Prevention Recommendations for the Use of the PVC13 and PPSV23 in Adults

| | | PCV13 | PPSV23[a] | |
| | | Recommended | Recommended | Revaccination at 5 Years After First Dose |
Risk Group	Underlying Medical Condition			
Immunocompetent persons	Chronic heart disease[b]		✓	
	Chronic lung disease[c]		✓	
	Diabetes mellitus		✓	
	CSF leaks	✓	✓	
	Cochlear implants	✓	✓	
	Alcoholism		✓	
	Chronic liver disease		✓	
	Cigarette smoking		✓	
Persons with functional or anatomic asplenia	Sickle cell disease/other hemoglobinopathies	✓	✓	✓
	Congenital or acquired asplenia	✓	✓	✓
Immunocompromised persons	Congenital or acquired immunodeficiencies[d]	✓	✓	✓
	HIV infection	✓	✓	✓
	Chronic renal failure	✓	✓	✓
	Nephrotic syndrome	✓	✓	✓
	Leukemia	✓	✓	✓
	Lymphoma	✓	✓	✓
	Hodgkin disease	✓	✓	✓
	Generalized malignancy	✓	✓	✓
	Iatrogenic immunosuppression[e]	✓	✓	✓
	Solid organ transplant	✓	✓	✓
	Multiple myeloma	✓	✓	✓

[a]All adults 65 years old or older should receive a dose of PPSV23, regardless of previous history of vaccination with pneumococcal vaccine.
[b]Including congestive heart failure and cardiomyopathies.
[c]Including chronic obstructive pulmonary disease, emphysema, and asthma.
[d]Includes B- (humoral) or T-lymphocyte deficiency, complement deficiencies (particularly C1, C2, C3, and C4 deficiencies), and phagocytic disorders (excluding chronic granulomatous disease).
[e]Diseases requiring treatment with immunosuppressive drugs, including long-term systemic corticosteroids and radiation therapy.
CSF, Cerebrospinal fluid; *HIV,* human immunodeficiency virus.

TABLE 118.5   Centers for Disease Control and Prevention Recommendations for the Use of the PCV13 Vaccine Among Infants and Children Who Have Not Received Previous Doses of PCV7 or PCV13, by Age at First Dose

Age At First Dose	Primary PCV13 Series[a]	PCV13 Booster Dose[b]
2 to 6 months old	3 doses	1 dose at age 12 to 15 months old
7 to 11 months old	2 doses	1 dose at age 12 to 15 months old
12 to 23 months old	2 doses	—
24 to 59 months old (healthy children)	1 dose	—
24 to 71 months old (children with certain chronic diseases or immunocompromising conditions	2 doses	—

[a]Minimum interval between doses is 8 weeks except for children vaccinated at age <12 months old for whom minimum interval between doses is 4 weeks. Minimum age for administration of first dose is 6 weeks old.
[b]Given at least 8 weeks after the previous dose.
Advisory Committee on Immunization Practices (ACIP), United States, 2019.

practicing before the meningitis vaccine have had a patient who appeared relatively well on initial presentation, only to be moribund with fulminant infection a few hours later. Vieusseux initially described "Epidemic cerebrospinal fever" in 1805, and Weichselbaum identified the causative bacterial agent in 1887. The introduction of sulfonamide therapy in 1937 dramatically improved outcomes. Sulfonamide prophylaxis was also effective at eradication of the carrier state and was used to prevent epidemics that occurred in military barracks. In the 1940s, sulfonamide resistance began to emerge. In 1963 an outbreak of resistant meningococcal disease occurred in the United States, which

TABLE 118.6 Underlying Medical Conditions That Are Indications for Pneumococcal Vaccination Among Children, by Risk Group

Risk Group	Condition
Immunocompetent children	Chronic heart disease[a]
	Chronic lung disease[b]
	Diabetes mellitus
	CSF leaks
	Cochlear implant
Children with functional or anatomic asplenia	Sickle cell disease and other hemoglobinopathies
	Congenital or acquired asplenia, or splenic dysfunction
Children with immunocompromising conditions	HIV infection
	Chronic renal failure and nephrotic syndrome
	Diseases associated with treatment with immunosuppressive drugs or radiation therapy, including malignant neoplasms, leukemias, lymphomas, and Hodgkin disease; or solid organ transplantation
	Congenital immunodeficiency[c]

[a]Particularly cyanotic congenital heart disease and cardiac failure.
[b]Including asthma if treated with prolonged high-dose oral corticosteroids.
[c]Includes B- (humoral) or T-lymphocyte deficiency; complement deficiencies, particularly C1, C2, C3, and C4 deficiency; and phagocytic disorders (excluding chronic granulomatous disease).
CSF, Cerebrospinal fluid; HIV, human immunodeficiency virus.
Advisory Committee on Immunization Practices (ACIP), United States, 2010.

spurred efforts to develop a vaccine. Subsequent worldwide resistance has resulted in continued efforts to develop safe and effective vaccines.[53]

Humans are the only reservoir for N. meningitidis. In 2013, 564 cases of meningococcal disease were reported in the United States. Active Bacterial Core surveillance by the CDC reports an incidence of 0.14 per 100,000 population, a marked decrease since the licensing of the first conjugated meningococcal vaccine in 2005 (Fig. 118.5). Of the more than 13 serogroups, groups A, B, C, Y, and W-135 cause most infections. Most cases occur sporadically, with occasional outbreaks, notably on college campuses in dormitories or other crowded living situations. More than half of the cases in infants are caused by serogroup B, for which there is no effective vaccine. Serogroups C, Y, and W-135 cause 75% of meningococcal disease in patients older than 11 years old.[54]

The incidence of meningococcal disease peaks in the winter. Superimposed on this annual variation are cyclic peaks of disease every 5 to 15 years. Approximately every 10 years, massive outbreaks of serogroup A occur in sub-Saharan Africa (the "meningitis belt"). The last outbreak was in 2013 with over 9000 cases and close to 900 deaths.[55] During nonepidemic periods, children younger than 5 years old have the highest incidence of infection. During epidemics, the incidence increases among children aged 5 to 9 years, an observation that may be of value in predicting the beginning of an epidemic. Crowded living conditions increase the risk for spread of meningococcal disease. The incidence of disease and the carrier state are several times higher among military recruits in the first few weeks of service than in the general public. This is also true of first-year college students, particularly those living in dormitories. Other risk factors for development of invasive meningococcal disease include close contact with an infected patient,

complement deficiency, properdin deficiency, asplenia, chronic alcohol abuse, active and passive smoking, corticosteroid use, and recent respiratory illness. The mortality rate of meningococcemia is 40% in the United States. Septicemia without meningitis carries a much higher mortality rate (up to 70%) than meningitis alone (less than 10%).[53,54,56]

Anatomy, Physiology, and Pathophysiology

Meningococcal disease is caused by N. meningitidis, a fastidious, aerobic, gram-negative diplococcus. N. meningitidis is an encapsulated organism classified into at least 13 serogroups based on the capsular polysaccharides.[53] N. meningitidis is an obligate human pathogen. It attaches to nonciliated epithelial cells in the nasopharynx. It may remain on the epithelial surface, causing an asymptomatic carrier state or producing mild upper respiratory tract infection symptoms. The carrier state acts as an immunizing process. In certain patients, the bacteria enter the bloodstream and cause localized infection, bacteremia, sepsis, or fulminant infection. Multiple host and microorganism characteristics determine whether clinical disease develops, but the presence of bactericidal antibodies is protective. Complement deficiency plays a role in a host's inability to fight this infection. The capsule is required for N. meningitidis to adhere to epithelium, but only unencapsulated meningococci enter epithelial cells; capsular biosynthesis has been shown to stop as the bacteria enter the epithelial cell.[53] The release of lipo-oligosaccharide (LOS) and endotoxin by autolysis of the N. meningitidis cell is the initial event in the development of meningococcal sepsis. LOS stimulates a massive host mediator response.

All of the major pathophysiologic events of meningococcal sepsis are caused by the host's inflammatory response to the organism causing functional and histologic damage to the microvasculature, resulting in increased vascular permeability, pathologic vasoconstriction and vasodilation, loss of thromboresistance, DIC, and profound myocardial dysfunction.[53]

Clinical Features

Presentation of meningococcemia ranges from a mild febrile illness to fulminant disease progressing to death within hours. Most patients have fever on presentation. Other complaints include headache, irritability, lethargy, myalgias, emesis, diarrhea, cough, and rhinorrhea. Anywhere from 27% to 77% of patients present with the classic hemorrhagic skin lesions.[53] These patients can rapidly progress to purpura fulminans, with hypotension, adrenal hemorrhage, and multiorgan failure. The following categories detail the five patterns of presentation.

Occult Bacteremia

This is a febrile illness in which the only direct indication of meningococcemia is a positive blood culture. In its mildest form, meningococcal bacteremia cannot clinically be distinguished from more benign febrile illnesses. Initial diagnoses include common childhood infections, such as otitis media, acute viral upper respiratory infections, and gastroenteritis. For some patients the illness resolves after treatment with an oral regimen of antibiotics; others experience spontaneous resolution without antibiotic treatment. N. meningitidis accounts for less than 1% of occult bacteremia cases, but these patients are much more likely to develop meningitis (up to 58%) than are those with S. pneumoniae. Despite the total absence of clinical clues to meningococcal infection at initial presentation, some untreated patients subsequently deteriorate rapidly.

Meningococcal Meningitis

Patients with meningococcal meningitis present similarly to those with meningitis of other causes, with headache, photophobia, vomiting, fever, and signs of meningeal inflammation. This classic triad of fever,

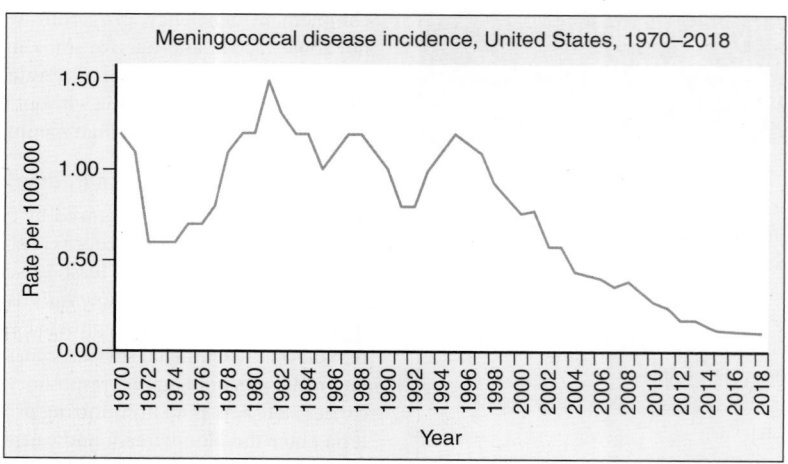

Fig. 118.5 Meningococcal disease incidence by year in the United States from 1970 to 2018. (Centers for Disease Control and Prevention. Manual for the surveillance of vaccine-preventable diseases. Available at: https://www.cdc.gov/meningococcal/surveillance/index.html)

neck stiffness, and altered mental status is present in less than 30% of patients.[57] Infants and small children may present with fever, irritability, and vomiting as the only complaints. More than half of patients with meningococcal meningitis have rash on presentation, and 20% present with seizures. Onset of symptoms is less abrupt (usually during 24 hours), and the prognosis is better for patients with meningococcal meningitis than for patients with meningococcemia without clinical signs of meningitis.

Meningococcal Septicemia

Patients with meningococcal septicemia present with lethargy, poor tissue perfusion, cyanosis, and hypoventilation or hyperventilation. Hemorrhagic skin lesions are present in 28% to 77% of patients, but a macular or maculopapular rash may occur and be mistaken for a variety of viral exanthems. Petechiae generally appear on the extremities and under pressure points, such as the elastic bands of socks and underwear. They may progress to involve almost any body surface, including the mucosa and sclera, but typically spare the palms, soles, and head. Macular lesions may progress to purpura and ecchymoses in fulminant meningococcemia.

Purpura fulminans, the most advanced form of meningococcal septicemia, occurs most often in children and is usually associated with DIC. This condition is characterized by rapidly spreading ecchymoses and gangrene of the extremities. Mucosal and gastrointestinal bleeding as well as oozing from IV sites may occur. Clinical signs of meningitis and CSF pleocytosis may not be present, even when diplococci are isolated from the CSF, likely because the systemic progression of the disease is so rapid that it precludes a host meningeal inflammatory response to the organism in the CSF. Shock can result from distributive shock, intravascular volume loss, and heart failure, probably related to myocarditis. Renal failure, coma, and bilateral adrenal hemorrhage often occur.[53]

Fever and a Nonblanching Rash

Up to 30% of patients present without signs of meningitis or septicemia. They are typically admitted for fever and a nonblanching rash and no other specific findings. If left untreated, meningitis or fulminant septicemia and shock can develop.[50,56]

Chronic Meningococcemia

This syndrome is characterized by fever, rash, and arthritis in conjunction with a positive blood culture for *N. meningitidis.* Headache and upper respiratory symptoms are often present. This is the rarest form of meningococcal disease, accounting for less than 2% of cases. It may progress to meningitis, endocarditis, or fulminant meningococcemia regardless of treatment.

Complications

Circulatory collapse is a common complication of meningococcemia and the most common cause of death. Many of the inflammatory mediators released during sepsis cause peripheral vasodilation, capillary leak, and myocardial dysfunction. Acidosis, hypoglycemia, hypokalemia, hypocalcemia, hypophosphatemia, and hypoxia also contribute to myocardial dysfunction, which may become unresponsive to inotropic medications.

Acute respiratory failure occurs from capillary leak, DIC, and large volume requirements in the setting of decreased cardiac function. Patients frequently require mechanical ventilation. Renal failure is common due to impaired renal perfusion. If meningitis accompanies meningococcemia, focal neurologic deficits and seizures may occur but are less common than with pneumococcal meningitis. Long-term neurologic sequelae include hearing loss, visual deficits, neurodevelopmental impairment, cranial nerve palsies, and hemi- and quadriparesis. Purpura fulminans may result in skin lesions and loss of digits or limbs from gangrene. Purulent or immune complex arthritis and pericarditis with tamponade may also occur.

Poor prognostic indicators include seizures, hypothermia, hyperpyrexia, total peripheral WBC count of less than 500/mm³, platelet count of less than 100,000/mm³, metabolic acidosis (pH <7.30), development of purpura fulminans, onset of petechiae within 12 hours of admission, absence of meningitis, presence of shock, low sedimentation rate, and extremes of age. In one study, all patients who developed organ system failure had one or more of the following at the time of initial presentation: circulatory insufficiency (hypotension or shock), peripheral WBC count of less than 10,000 cells/mm³, or a coagulopathy.[51]

Differential Diagnoses

It is difficult to distinguish the clinical signs of meningococcemia from bacteremia caused by *S. pneumoniae,* other streptococcal groups, *H. influenzae,* and *Neisseria gonorrhoeae.* A hemorrhagic rash is more commonly associated with meningococcal disease. The differential diagnosis of meningococcemia also includes viral exanthems, Rocky Mountain spotted fever, typhus, typhoid fever, endocarditis, vasculitis syndromes (polyarteritis nodosa and Henoch-Schönlein purpura), toxic shock syndrome (TSS), acute rheumatic fever, dengue fever, drug reactions, idiopathic thrombocytopenic purpura, and thrombotic thrombocytopenic purpura.

Diagnostic Testing

The tentative diagnosis of meningococcemia is based on clinical findings and confirmed by the isolation of *N. meningitidis* from blood cultures or any other usually sterile site, such as CSF or synovial, pleural, or pericardial fluid. Ideally, blood culture specimens should be obtained before the administration of antibiotics unless this delays the patient's treatment. Blood cultures are positive in approximately 50% to 80% of cases. A lumbar puncture should be performed in stable patients without evidence of DIC. The CSF shows either gram-negative diplococci on Gram stain or a positive culture in about 46% to 94% of cases. Even patients without clinical signs of meningitis frequently have the organism grown from the CSF. Gram stain of petechial scrapings may show gram-negative diplococci in up to two-thirds of cases, and the organism can rarely be seen in the peripheral blood buffy coat. Highly specific antigen tests for CSF are available but have a high false-negative rate. PCR of the buffy coat or CSF is more sensitive and specific than any of the preceding tests and is not affected by prior antibiotic therapy.[53,54]

Ancillary laboratory tests are of little value in establishing a specific diagnosis of meningococcal sepsis but may be useful in ruling out other disease, determining prognosis, and monitoring complications. The WBC count may be high, low, or normal, but a bandemia is typically present. The symptoms and signs of CNS infection may be nonspecific in the infant and child younger than 2 years old. If meningitis is present, the CSF opening pressure is usually elevated, the protein level is increased, and the glucose concentration is decreased. Pleocytosis is usually present, with a predominance of polymorphonuclear leukocytes. Gram-negative diplococci may be seen on microscopy. Early in the disease or with fulminant disease, the CSF may be free of inflammatory cells. Serologic evidence of DIC is frequently present.[54,55] A CXR is useful in evaluation for pneumonia and acute respiratory distress syndrome. An echocardiogram helps assess for myocardial dysfunction and pericardial effusion. Serum lactate may help direct therapy.

Management

Acute Treatment

Morbidity and mortality in meningococcemia are reduced with prompt recognition and intravenous antibiotic therapy. Patients can be divided into two general groups:

1. Bacteremia or sepsis suggested by clinical findings; no organism identified: Patients should receive empirical antibiotics based on factors that include the most likely organism, patient's age and immune status, presence of coexisting disorders, and local patterns of antibiotic resistance. A narrower-spectrum agent is selected after identification of the organism and its sensitivities.
2. *N. meningitidis* growth is reported from prior blood cultures: Treatment for occult bacteremia is guided by the patient's age, history, physical examination, general appearance, and ancillary test results. The antibiotic selected at the time of the initial visit may be sufficient to treat the meningococcal bacteremia subsequently identified by the laboratory. The decision to hospitalize the patient is based on the findings at the time of reevaluation and the risk of sequelae. We recommend repeating blood cultures, considering lumbar puncture, and admitting the patient to the hospital until results of repeated cultures are obtained.

The standard antibiotic regimen for laboratory-proven meningococcemia is penicillin G (4 million units every 4 hours IV for adults) and penicillin (250,000 to 300,000 units/kg/day in divided doses every 4 hours IV for children, up to a maximum of 20 million units). Penicillin resistance in *N. meningitidis* remains low in the United States but has been reported in Spain and the United Kingdom.[53]

Although appropriate first-line therapy, penicillin is rarely given as the initial agent in patients with suspected meningococcal sepsis or meningitis. Ceftriaxone (100 mg/kg IV, followed by daily dosage of 100 mg/kg in divided doses every 12 hours, up to a maximum of 4 g) and cefotaxime (100 mg/kg/day IV in divided doses every 6 hours, up to a maximum of 12 g) are appropriate initial antibiotics as well. The cephalosporins are safe and have rapid onset of action and excellent coverage for *S. pneumoniae* and *H. influenzae*. Chloramphenicol (100 mg/kg/day divided every 6 hours to a maximum of 4 g/day) should be considered in penicillin- and cephalosporin-allergic patients. IM ceftriaxone is occasionally administered to children with suspected bacteremia treated as outpatients while culture results are pending. Several reports have demonstrated the efficacy of ceftriaxone (80 to 100 mg/kg IV) in a single daily dose; however, twice-daily dosing remains the standard recommendation at this time. Ceftriaxone-treated patients have more rapid sterilization of the CSF and a lower incidence of hearing loss than conventionally treated patients.

Patients with fulminant meningococcemia often require airway management, IV fluid resuscitation, and vasopressor support. Fluid requirements may be high. In the setting of frequent myocardial dysfunction, intensive cardiovascular monitoring is required. Electrolyte and acid-base abnormalities should be corrected. If the patient is oliguric or anuric, hemodialysis may be necessary to correct these abnormalities. Fresh frozen plasma should be considered for patients with bleeding complications.

The role of steroids in the treatment of meningococcemia without meningitis is controversial. Although corticosteroids were once widely recommended to treat the adrenal insufficiency associated with fulminant meningococcemia, recent studies demonstrate that adrenal function is not impaired in all patients. If patients have persistent shock despite vigorous fluid resuscitation and vasopressor therapy, glucocorticoid therapy and adrenal function testing should be considered as this subgroup of patients may benefit.[57]

The use of corticosteroids in patients with bacterial meningitis is currently recommended for adults and children. Corticosteroid administration before antibiotic administration decreases long-term neurologic sequelae in adults and children. There is also a mild decrease in mortality. In neonates, there are limited data of low quality that suggest steroids decrease morbidity from hearing loss and may decrease mortality. Although these benefits are not seen in patients with meningococcal meningitis, the organism is typically not identified when steroids are initiated. Dexamethasone (0.4 to 0.6 mg/kg/day every 6 hours for 4 days) should be given to patients with bacterial meningitis. The first dose should be given before the first dose of antibiotics if possible.[58,59] Plasmapheresis, blood exchange, and extracorporeal membrane oxygenation have been described, but data are limited.

Antibiotic Prophylaxis and Vaccination

Close patient contacts (household, nursery schools, daycare centers, military recruits, college dormitories, teammates) should receive antibiotic prophylaxis. Intimate contacts and health care workers with intimate exposure (e.g., mouth-to-mouth resuscitation, intubation, or suctioning) should receive rifampin, 10 mg/kg (up to 600 mg) orally every 12 hours for four doses. The dose for neonates is 5 mg/kg. Patients should be warned that rifampin discolors the urine and secretions; contact lenses should be removed to avoid permanent staining.

IM ceftriaxone (125 mg for children younger than 15 years old and 250 mg for those older than 12 years old) is an effective alternative for pregnant women and for people in whom compliance with an oral regimen cannot be ensured. Ciprofloxacin (500 mg orally) is another alternative for adults.[56]

Meningococcal vaccine should be considered an adjunct to prophylaxis in epidemics and for close contacts in sporadic cases if one of the serotypes contained in the vaccine is identified as the causative agent. The currently available vaccines are quadrivalent vaccines for serogroups A, C, Y, and W-135. No vaccine is licensed for group B, a serogroup that causes a significant portion of meningococcal infection in the United States, but trials are currently underway.[60] The conjugate vaccines (MCV4: Menactra and Menveo) produce a superior immune response compared to the polysaccharide vaccine (MPSV4: Menomune). Routine vaccination with MPSV4 is not recommended and should be limited to patients over 55 years old, or when MCV4 is unavailable. Routine vaccination with MCV4 is recommended for persons 11 or 12 years old with a booster at 16 years old. Vaccination is also recommended for those at increased risk of meningococcal disease, including microbiologists who are routinely working with *N. meningitides*, military recruits, children with functional or anatomic asplenia, and people traveling to endemic areas of the world, such as sub-Saharan Africa.[54]

Disposition

All patients with possible or confirmed meningococcemia should be placed in respiratory isolation and hospitalized, preferably in an ICU, because they can decompensate rapidly and without warning. A possible exception is the well-appearing child who has culture-proven *N. meningitidis* and has been taking appropriate antibiotics as an outpatient. This child should have a lumbar puncture performed to determine CSF involvement if one was not performed at the initial evaluation. Antibiotics should be continued on an inpatient basis, but an ICU may not be necessary if the child appears well.

TOXIC SHOCK SYNDROME

Foundations

Background and Importance

Toxic shock syndrome (TSS) is a toxin-mediated systemic inflammatory response syndrome that was first described in 1978 in a series of seven children 8 to 17 years old who had high fever, rash, headache, confusion, conjunctival injection, edema, vomiting, diarrhea, renal failure, hepatic dysfunction, DIC, and shock. *S. aureus* was cultured from various body sites but not from the blood in five of the seven cases. The disease gained notoriety in the early 1980s when many cases were reported in association with tampon use in young, healthy menstruating women. The term *toxic shock syndrome* was coined to describe the constellation of signs and symptoms. Investigators noted positive vaginal cultures for *S. aureus,* recurrence of illness during subsequent menses, and the value of antistaphylococcal antibiotics in preventing recurrences. Nonmenstrual cases were also recognized in both men and women due to a variety of predisposing conditions, and a case definition was published in 1982 (Box 118.6).[61-64]

In the late 1980s, several reports described group A streptococcus infection (*S. pyogenes*) associated with shock and multisystem organ failure. This is called *streptococcal toxic shock syndrome* because it shares many features with staphylococcal TSS. Box 118.7 shows the case definition for streptococcal TSS.[65]

The peak incidence of TSS occurred in 1980, when 890 cases were reported, 91% of which were associated with tampon use. Since then, the reduction in cases of the menstrual form of TSS has followed an

---

BOX 118.6　Case Definition of Toxic Shock Syndrome (Revised)

Clinical Case Definition

Fever: Temperature >102°F (38.9°C)

Rash: Diffuse macular erythroderma

Desquamation 1 to 2 weeks after onset of illness, particularly of palms and soles

Hypotension: Systolic blood pressure <90 mm Hg for adults or below fifth percentile by age for children younger than 16 years old, orthostatic drop in diastolic blood pressure >15 mm Hg from lying to sitting, orthostatic syncope, or orthostatic dizziness

Multisystem involvement—*three* or more of the following:

　Gastrointestinal: Vomiting or diarrhea at onset of illness

　Muscular: Severe myalgia or creatine kinase level at least twice the upper limit of normal for laboratory

　Mucous membrane: Vaginal, oropharyngeal, or conjunctival hyperemia

　Renal: BUN or creatinine at least twice the upper limit of normal for laboratory or urinary sediment with pyuria (>5 leukocytes/high-power field) in the absence of urinary tract infection

　Hepatic: Total bilirubin, AST, and ALT at least twice the upper limit of normal for laboratory

　Hematologic: Platelets <100,000/mm³

　CNS: Disorientation or alterations in consciousness without focal neurologic signs when fever and hypotension are absent

Laboratory Criteria for Diagnosis

Negative results on the following tests, if obtained:

Blood, throat, or CSF cultures (blood culture may be positive for *Staphylococcus aureus*)

Rise in titer to Rocky Mountain spotted fever, leptospirosis, or rubeola

Case Classification

Probable: A case that meets the laboratory criteria and in which four of the five clinical findings are present

Confirmed: A case that meets the laboratory criteria and in which all five of the clinical findings are present, including desquamation, unless the patient dies before desquamation occurs

---

ALT, Alanine transaminase; *AST,* aspartate transaminase; *BUN,* blood urea nitrogen; *CNS,* central nervous system; *CSF,* cerebrospinal fluid.

---

active effort to decrease the absorbency of tampons and to change their composition. Menstruation remains the most common setting for TSS, but nonmenstrual TSS accounts for just under half of the reported cases. TSS has also been reported in association with barrier contraceptives and childbirth. Nonmenstrual TSS occurs in people of all ages and both sexes. The CDC reported an average of about 300 cases a year between 2010 and 2015, with a steady increase in the incidence of streptococcal TSS and a decrease in the incidence of staphylococcal TSS. The age and sex distribution reflects the association with menses. Streptococcal TSS accounts for two-thirds of the cases.[63]

Nonmenstrual staphylococcal TSS is associated with superinfection of various skin lesions, including burns, surgical sites, dialysis catheters, and lung (influenza-associated). It may also occur in association with staphylococcal respiratory infections or even with colonization by a toxigenic strain of the organism, without an obvious infectious source. Streptococcal TSS is classically associated with more severe soft tissue infections, such as necrotizing fasciitis and myositis, as well as with pneumonia, peritonitis, myometritis, and osteomyelitis.

The mortality rate from staphylococcal TSS has declined since the disease was first described. The case fatality rate in 1980 was 10% and is

BOX 118.7 Case Definition of Streptococcal Toxic Shock Syndrome

Clinical Case Definition

Hypotension: Systolic blood pressure ≤90 mm Hg for adults or below fifth percentile by age for children younger than 16 years old

Multisystem involvement—*two* or more of the following:

Renal: Creatinine >2 mg/dL (177 μmol/L) for adults or more than twice the upper limit of normal for age or more than twofold elevation above baseline for patients with preexisting renal disease

Hematologic: Platelets <100,000/mm³ or DIC, defined as prolonged clotting times, low fibrinogen level, and the presence of fibrin degradation products

Hepatic: Total bilirubin, AST, and ALT at least twice the upper limit of normal for laboratory, or a twofold increase in patients with preexisting liver disease

Acute respiratory distress syndrome: Defined by acute onset of pulmonary infiltrates and hypoxemia in the absence of cardiac failure or by evidence of diffuse capillary leak manifested by acute onset of generalized edema, or pleural or peritoneal effusions with hypoalbuminemia

Generalized erythematous maculopapular rash that may desquamate

Soft tissue necrosis, including necrotizing fasciitis, myositis, or gangrene

Laboratory Criteria for Diagnosis

Isolation of group A streptococcus

Case Classification

Probable: A case that meets the clinical case definition in the absence of another identified cause of the illness and with isolation of group A streptococcus from a nonsterile site

Confirmed: A case that meets the clinical case definition and with isolation of group A streptococcus from a normally sterile site (e.g., CSF or joint, pleural, or pericardial fluid)

ALT, Alanine transaminase; *AST,* aspartate transaminase; *CSF,* cerebrospinal fluid; *DIC,* disseminated intravascular coagulation.

BOX 118.8 Risk Factors for Toxic Shock Syndrome

Use of superabsorbent tampons

Postoperative wound infections

Postpartum period

Nasal packing

Cancer

Common bacterial infections

Ethanol abuse

Infection with influenza A virus

Infection with varicella virus

Diabetes mellitus

Human immunodeficiency virus (HIV) infection

Chronic cardiac disease

Chronic pulmonary disease

Nonsteroidal antiinflammatory drug (NSAID) use (may mask symptoms rather than be a risk factor)

an invasive organism and circulating group A streptococcus organisms induce the production of TNF-α and other cytokines by mononuclear cells.[64]

Clinical Features

The clinical presentations of streptococcal TSS and staphylococcal TSS are similar. The primary difference is that an identifiable infectious source is virtually always present with streptococcal TSS, and colonization alone may be the source in staphylococcal TSS.

TSS should be considered in patients who present with fever, rash, hypotension, and evidence of end-organ damage, such as respiratory failure or altered mental status. Patients may have a prodromal illness with fever, chills, nausea, vomiting, watery diarrhea, headache, myalgias, and pharyngitis, which can last 2 to 3 days before progression to frank sepsis and organ dysfunction. Other patients may become abruptly symptomatic within hours. Rapid progression is more typical of streptococcal TSS. Patients may complain of pain at a site of infection more often with streptococcal TSS. Risk factors for TSS are listed in Box 118.8.

The fever is usually high and abrupt in onset, although patients may have hypothermia. The classic rash is a nonpruritic, diffuse, blanching, macular erythroderma. It develops in the first few days of the illness and may be faint, evanescent, and mistaken for the flush associated with a fever. It is usually diffuse but may be localized to the trunk, extremities, or perineum. After about a week, fine flaky desquamation occurs on the face, trunk, and extremities, followed by full-thickness peeling of the palms, soles, and fingers. This classic rash progression is much more common in staphylococcal TSS and is present in less than 10% of patients with streptococcal TSS. Patients with streptococcal TSS may have a scarlet fever–like rash, petechiae, or maculopapular lesions. Mucosal involvement may also occur, including conjunctival and scleral hemorrhages, "strawberry tongue," and mucosal ulceration.

Altered mental status such as confusion, somnolence, agitation, and combativeness are present in 55% of patients with streptococcal TSS and in even more patients with staphylococcal TSS. Other findings on physical examination include pharyngeal and conjunctival erythema and peripheral edema. Vaginal mucosal erythema and purulent vaginal discharge may be present in menstrual TSS but are not required make the diagnosis. As multiple organ systems become involved, a wide constellation of signs and symptoms may be seen. Gastrointestinal involvement is manifested by vomiting, diarrhea, and severe abdominal pain. Hepatomegaly may be present. Acute respiratory distress syndrome

now 5%. Streptococcal TSS remains a highly fatal disease, with a mortality rate of 30% to 70%.

Anatomy, Physiology, and Pathophysiology

Staphylococcal TSS is caused by colonization or infection with toxigenic strains of *S. aureus,* which produce toxic shock syndrome toxin 1 (TSST-1). *S. aureus* is present in virtually all cases of both forms of the illness. Because the organism is often not invasive, the blood cultures are often negative. Streptococcal TSS is caused by invasive infection with toxigenic strains of group A streptococcus.[61,62,64]

The effects of various exotoxins produced by *S. aureus* and group A streptococcus cause the shock and multiorgan dysfunction associated with TSS. *S. aureus* produces TSST-1 and enterotoxin B. TSST-1 is identified in more than 90% of menstrual cases and 60% of nonmenstrual cases. Other toxins may play a role in nonmenstrual TSS. Antibodies to these toxins are protective against disease. Group A streptococcus produces streptococcal pyrogenic exotoxins A and B. These exotoxins are absorbed into the bloodstream through inflamed or traumatized mucous membranes or from areas of focal infection. Absorbed toxins act as superantigens, inducing mononuclear cells to synthesize and to release cytokines, tumor necrosis factor alpha (TNF-α), and interleukins at a rate and magnitude many fold greater than with the normal antigen presentation, which begin the cascade of systemic vasculitis and the multisystem manifestations of the disease. Host immune factors are important in the pathogenesis of TSS. Group A streptococcus is

(ARDS) develops in more than half of patients and is manifested by rales on pulmonary examination and hypoxia (see Chapter 2). Comparisons between staphylococcal and streptococcal TSS are presented in Table 118.7.

Complications of TSS include shock, gangrene, DIC, and a constellation of neuropsychiatric symptoms. Renal failure occurs in 80% of patients but is irreversible in only 10%. Less common findings in staphylococcal TSS include rhabdomyolysis, seizures, pancreatitis, pericarditis, and cardiomyopathy. Women with the menstrual form of TSS may experience recurrent episodes; recurrences of the nonmenstrual form are rare. Complication rates are higher with streptococcal TSS. Rhabdomyolysis occurs in up to 63% of patients with streptococcal TSS and is usually related to the underlying soft tissue infections.

Differential Diagnoses

The differential diagnosis of TSS includes any septic illness with exanthems. Other diseases to consider include heatstroke, cellulitis, Kawasaki disease, staphylococcal scalded skin syndrome, scarlet fever, drug reactions such as Stevens-Johnson syndrome, toxic epidermal necrolysis (TEN), Rocky Mountain spotted fever, clostridial gas gangrene, leptospirosis, meningococcemia, gram-negative sepsis, atypical measles, and viral illnesses.

Kawasaki disease occurs almost exclusively in children, usually does not progress to shock, lacks multisystem involvement, is manifested with a protracted fever, and is associated with thrombocytosis later in its course.[65] Staphylococcal scalded skin syndrome presents with a desquamating rash acutely, whereas the desquamation of TSS occurs in the convalescent phase. Staphylococcal scalded skin syndrome does not progress to shock, is not associated with multisystem illness, and lacks mucous membrane involvement. Scarlet fever differs in its clinical course by lack of shock and multisystem involvement, positive cultures for group A streptococcus, and a rise in the convalescent titer. Stevens-Johnson syndrome usually occurs after drug administration, has characteristic mucous membrane lesions, and lacks desquamation. TEN may be challenging to distinguish from TSS; TEN patients are typically febrile, are in shock, and can progress to multisystem failure. The desquamation of TEN occurs early in the course of the disease, and it usually occurs after administration of a drug.[66] Rocky Mountain spotted fever occurs after a tick bite, has a distinctive rash, and is associated with a severe headache without an altered mental status or hypotension. Leptospirosis occurs in endemic areas and may be distinguished by positive serologic studies and cultures. Petechiae and purpura occurring anywhere on the skin characterize the rash of meningococcemia.

Diagnostic Testing

Diagnosis of TSS does not require a positive culture for *S. aureus,* but isolation of *Streptococcus* organisms is a criterion. The case definitions (see Boxes 118.6 and 118.7) are useful, but they are neither specific nor foolproof. Suspecting the disease is key rather than meeting all CDC criteria for diagnosis.

No specific laboratory changes are associated with TSS, but many abnormalities are common. Leukocytosis or leukopenia with bandemia is common, and myelocytes and metamyelocytes may be seen. Elevated creatinine levels and hemoglobinuria occur in most patients. Renal dysfunction occurs before hypotension in half of the patients. Hypoalbuminemia (85%) and life-threatening hypocalcemia (79%) are prominent initially and persist throughout the disease. Other abnormalities include anemia, thrombocytopenia, prolonged prothrombin and activated partial thromboplastin times, hyper-bilirubinemia, elevated transaminase levels, severe metabolic acidosis, and sterile pyuria. Creatine phosphokinase (CPK)

TABLE 118.7 Comparison of Staphylococcal and Streptococcal Toxic Shock Syndrome

Feature	Staphylococcal	Streptococcal
Age	Primarily 15 to 35 years old	Primarily 20 to 50 years old
Sex	Greatest in women	Either
Severe pain	Rare	Common
Hypotension	100%	100%
Erythroderma rash	Very common	Less common
Renal failure	Common	Common
Bacteremia	Low	60%
Tissue necrosis	Rare	Common
Predisposing factors	Tampons, packing, NSAID use?	Cuts, burns, bruises, varicella, NSAID use?
Thrombocytopenia	Common	Common
Mortality rate	<3%	30% to 70%

NSAID, Nonsteroidal antiinflammatory drug.

levels may be elevated in patients with necrotizing fasciitis and myonecrosis.[64]

Blood cultures are positive for bacteria in 60% of cases associated with group A streptococcus but are rarely positive in staphylococcal TSS. Gram stains and cultures from wounds may identify the organism. Culture of the cervix or vagina is positive in 90% of menstrual cases of TSS, even in the absence of local infection.

A CXR may reveal bilateral heterogeneous opacities, consistent with ARDS, or a pulmonary source of the organism. Plain radiographs of any infected skin or soft tissue site typically show only soft tissue swelling but may reveal a retained foreign body or air in the soft tissue. A lack of air in the soft tissue does not rule out a necrotizing soft tissue infection.

An ECG may reveal evidence of ischemia, arrhythmias, and varying degrees of atrioventricular block associated with sepsis. A blood gas analysis may indicate metabolic acidosis secondary to hypotension or hypoxia. A lumbar puncture should be performed in febrile patients with altered mental status to evaluate for meningitis. It is prudent to wait for the results of a coagulation profile before the lumbar puncture is performed because these patients may have DIC at presentation. The CSF is normal in patients with TSS.

Management

Patients with TSS should receive fluid resuscitation with crystalloids due to severe volume depletion and third spacing from capillary leaking. Supplemental oxygen should be administered to treat an Spo_2 less than 95%, and mechanical ventilation with low tidal volumes may be necessary in patients with ARDS. The source of bacteria, such as tampons, nasal packs, and other foreign bodies, should be removed. Prompt surgical consultation should be obtained to débride wounds. If specimens are sent for culture, the laboratory should be informed of the suspected diagnosis. Patients who do not respond to fluid resuscitation require vasopressors, such as norepinephrine, vasopressin, and epinephrine (see Chapter 3).

Antibiotics should be initiated early in the treatment of TSS because the clinical presentation of the disease is similar whether the source is staphylococcal or streptococcal. For septic patients without an identified organism, broad-spectrum antibiotics should be administered. Although the penicillinase-resistant penicillins (nafcillin, oxacillin) have been widely used in TSS treatment, we recommend clindamycin as a first-line agent. Clindamycin is a potent suppressor of bacterial toxin synthesis; it also facilitates phagocytosis of streptococci by inhibiting M protein synthesis, decreases monocyte synthesis of cytokines, and has a more prolonged post-antibiotic effect than the β-lactams. The dose is 900 mg IV every 8 hours. (The pediatric dose is 20-40 mg/kg/day divided every 6 to 8 hours.)[64] Linezolid in combination with clindamycin may be better than either agent alone based on isolated case reports.

Patients who do not respond to appropriate fluid resuscitation, antibiotics, and vasopressors should be considered for intravenous immune globulin (IVIG) treatment, especially if pulmonary edema develops and mechanical ventilation is required. Pooled immune globulin has high titers for antibodies to TSST-1 and other exotoxins, and significant improvement has been reported with its use in streptococcal TSS. Because the data in staphylococcal TSS are inconclusive, and the mortality is relatively low, immunotherapy should be reserved for life-threatening cases. If used, the recommended dose is 1 to 2 g/kg on day 1 administered intravenously during several hours, followed by 400 to 500 mg/kg/day for up to 5 days.[61]

Hemodialysis or hemoperfusion may be necessary because more than half of streptococcal TSS patients develop renal failure. Both modalities may reduce concentrations of circulating toxins, and a study in Sweden demonstrated the lowest mortality rate ever recorded for strep TSS.[64]

The value of corticosteroids in TSS is unresolved. They are not currently recommended to treat staphylococcal or streptococcal TSS, but should be given to patients thought to have adrenal insufficiency related to underlying disease or chronic steroid use.

Disposition

All patients thought to have TSS should be admitted to an ICU. Prompt surgical consultation should be obtained for patients with a wound source.

The references for this chapter can be found online at ExpertConsult. com.

119

Viruses

Raghu Seethala, Sukhjit S. Takhar, Jeffrey Bullard-Berent, and Laura L. Banks

KEY CONCEPTS

- Recent outbreaks of vaccine-preventable childhood infections have occurred secondary to unvaccinated individuals and travel to areas where disease is still endemic. Emergency clinicians should recognize the possibility of these once rare diseases.
- Herpes simplex encephalitis is fatal if untreated. Clinicians should suspect this diagnosis when evaluating severely ill patients for suspected meningitis or encephalitis and promptly institute empirical therapy with IV acyclovir while awaiting diagnostic results.
- Primary varicella can be dangerous in select populations, including older children, adults, and pregnant patients. These patients require treatment with acyclovir.
- Zoster patients should be treated with acyclovir if they present within 72 hours of symptoms onset or if they are immunocompromised regardless of duration of illness. Disseminated zoster should be treated with IV acyclovir.
- In healthy patients with influenza infection, the duration of illness can be shortened by almost 1 day if antiviral treatment is administered within 48 hours of symptom onset. Hospitalized patients with influenza infection should be treated with antiviral medication regardless of duration of symptoms, because it may decrease mortality and influenza complications.
- Rabies has the highest case fatality rate of any recognized infectious disease.
- Almost 60,000 deaths per year worldwide are caused by dog-mediated human rabies, and this burden falls disproportionately on children and the poor in rural areas.
- Globally, human rabies results from bites by infected dogs. In North America human rabies results predominantly from wildlife exposures (bat, raccoon, and skunks).
- Treatment is rarely effective once symptoms of human rabies occur.
- Rabies postexposure prophylaxis (PEP) given strictly according to the World Health Organization (WHO) or US Centers for Disease Prevention and Control (CDC) guidelines is extremely effective. Discussion with public health officials is recommended to guide decisions regarding when PEP should be considered. The CDC clinician information line is 877-554-4625 or 800-CDC-INFO.
- Many emerging viral infections, including SARS-CoV2 and Ebola, should be considered in febrile patients. It is important to identify patients at risk by determining travel history and exposure history to individuals with confirmed infection. Once a patient is deemed at risk, the patient should be promptly isolated according to established guidelines while further investigation occurs. It is also important to immediately inform the hospital infection control program and public health agencies.

FOUNDATIONS

The vast majority of viral infections, such as the common cold, are minor and self-limiting. However, some are highly pathogenic, contagious, and have the potential to cause devastating illness. In addition to centuries-old infections such as chicken pox, there are also newer infections such as avian influenza, Middle East respiratory syndrome (MERS), enterovirus D68 (EV-D68), as well as SARS-CoV2 (see Chapter 120). With increasing international travel, emergency clinicians should be familiar with emerging infections spreading beyond their endemic origins. In addition to recognizing symptoms and knowing the treatment for these infections, emergency clinicians should be familiar with isolation and reporting practices vital to preventing global pandemics.

Advances in molecular biology have increased our knowledge of these infections, improved our diagnostic ability, and allowed more treatment options. Viruses are classified according to the type and structure of nucleic acid, capsid, and presence or absence of an envelope (Table 119.1). In practice, it is useful to group viruses based on clinical syndromes. This chapter reviews select viral illnesses with high morbidity and mortality, those with specific treatments, and those with major public health consequences. The chapter begins by reviewing several preventable diseases reemerging because of decreasing immunization rates caused by unfounded fears of complications or side effects.

VACCINE-PREVENTABLE INFECTIONS OF CHILDHOOD

Childhood immunization is among the most important public health measures globally. Immunizations save 2 to 3 million children per year from serious illness, disability, and death. However, there has been a troubling trend of people in industrialized nations refusing routine immunizations. These groups advocate for nonmedical exemptions from mandated school-entry vaccines in developed nations, and routine immunizations have been rejected by some over questions of safety and the lack of perceived threat for serious vaccine-preventable diseases.[1] The emergency clinicians may therefore play a significant role in educating parents on the safety and efficacy of childhood immunizations. The United States (US) Advisory Committee on Immunization Practices (ACIP), the American Academy of Pediatrics (AAP), and the American Academy of Family Physicians recommend a specific childhood immunization schedule each year. Table 119.2 summarizes the currently available viral vaccines and recommended schedule.

Mumps

Mumps is an RNA virus that is a member of the *Paramyxoviridae* family. It causes a febrile illness with swelling and tenderness of the parotid gland. Since the advent of the mumps vaccine in 1967, there has been a 99% decrease in mumps in the United States. Despite the vaccine, recent outbreaks in industrialized nations, even in vaccinated individuals, raised concerns about resurgence of mumps.[2]

Mumps is spread via infected respiratory secretions that enter a susceptible respiratory tract. The incubation period is typically 16 to 18

TABLE 119.1   Classification of Viruses

DNA Viruses

Poxviridae	Variola	Smallpox
	Orf	Contagious pustular dermatitis
Herpesviridae	HSV-1, HSV-2	Mucocutaneous ulcers, herpes encephalitis
	Cytomegalovirus	Pneumonitis in immunocompromised patients
	VZV	Chickenpox, shingles
	HHV-6	Roseola infantum
	EBV	Mononucleosis
	Kaposi sarcoma herpesvirus	Kaposi sarcoma
Adenoviridae	Adenovirus (50+ species)	Upper respiratory tract infections, diarrhea
Papillomaviridae	Papillomavirus (80+ species)	Warts (e.g., plantar, genital)
Polyomaviridae	JC virus	PML
Hepadnaviridae	Hepatitis B	Hepatitis
Parvoviridae	Parvovirus B19	Aplastic anemia

RNA Viruses

Reoviridae	Colorado tick fever	Fever and rash
	Rotavirus	Gastroenteritis
Togaviridae	Eastern equine encephalitis	Epidemic encephalitis
	Rubella	German measles
Flaviviridae	Yellow fever	Hemorrhagic fever
	Dengue	Dengue hemorrhagic fever
	Zika	Fever, rash, arthralgias
	West Nile virus	West Nile encephalitis
	Hepacivirus, hepatitis C	Chronic hepatitis
Coronaviridae	Coronavirus	Upper respiratory tract infections
	SARS-CoV	SARS
	MERS-CoV	MERS
	SARS-CoV-2	COVID-19
Paramyxoviridae	Respiratory syncytial virus	Bronchiolitis
	Measles	Measles (rubeola), SSPE
	Parainfluenza	Croup
Rhabdoviridae	Rabies	Rabies
Filoviridae	Ebola	Hemorrhagic fever
Orthomyxoviridae	Influenza A, B	Influenza
Bunyaviridae	La Crosse	Encephalitis
	Hanta	Hemorrhagic fevers, ARDS
Arenaviridae	Lassa	Hemorrhagic fever
	Lymphocytic choriomeningitis virus	Meningoencephalitis
Retroviridae	HIV	AIDS
Picornaviridae	Poliovirus	Polio
	Coxsackie B	Myocarditis
	Hepatitis A	Enteric hepatitis
	Rhinovirus (115+ species)	Upper respiratory infections
Caliciviridae	Norwalk virus	Gastroenteritis
Unclassified viruses	Hepatitis E	Enteric hepatitis

AIDS, Acquired immunodeficiency syndrome; *ARDS,* acute respiratory distress syndrome; *COVID-19,* coronavirus disease 2019; *EBV,* Epstein-Barr virus; *HHV,* human herpesvirus; *HIV,* human immunodeficiency virus; *HSV,* herpes simplex virus; *MERS-CoV,* Middle East respiratory syndrome coronavirus; *PML,* progressive multifocal leukoencephalopathy; *SARS-CoV,* severe acute respiratory syndrome–coronavirus; *SSPE,* subacute sclerosing panencephalitis; *VZV,* varicella-zoster virus.

TABLE 119.2   Viral Vaccines

Virus	Vaccine	Type	Indication	Recommended Schedule
Smallpox	Vaccinia	Live	For persons at risk or for emergency responders	Once, before anticipated risk of exposure
Polio	Oral polio vaccine (Sabin)	Live	During outbreaks Unvaccinated travelers	Inactivated polio vaccine preferred in almost all cases
	Inactivated polio vaccine (Salk)	Inactivated	All children	At 2, 4, 6–18 months, and at 4–6 years
Measles	Measles, mumps, rubella (MMR)	Live	All normal children	At 12–15 months and 4–6 years
Mumps	MMR	Live	All normal children	Same as for measles
Rubella	MMR	Live	All normal children	Same as for measles
Hepatitis A	HAV vaccine	Inactivated	Persons at risk (e.g., travelers, persons living in areas of high prevalence)	Two doses, 6 months apart. Ideally should be given one month prior to travel. Immune globulin should be given if travel is imminent
Hepatitis B	HBV vaccine	Inactivated or recombinant	All children	At birth, 1–2 months, and 6–18 months
			Persons at risk of exposure (e.g., health care workers)	Hepatitis B immune globulin (HBIG) should be given in addition in case of high-risk exposure
Influenza A and B	Influenza vaccine	Inactivated	In 2010, CDC expanded recommendation for annual influenza vaccination to include all persons aged 6 months and older	One dose yearly in the fall or winter
	Intranasal vaccine	Live, cold adapted	As above, for persons 2–49 years of age. Avoid if pregnant, immunosuppressed, young children with asthma, allergic to eggs	As above
Rabies	Human diploid cell vaccine (HDCV)	Inactivated	Postexposure prophylaxis or for preexposure prophylaxis in high-risk individuals	Postexposure: HDCV or PCEC 1.0 mL IM in the deltoid region on days 0, 3, 7, and 14. Rabies immune globulin (RIG) 20 IU/kg should be administered around the wound site, as possible, with the remainder given IM at an anatomically distant site. Preexposure: HDCV or PCEC 1.0 mL IM in the deltoid region on days 0, 7, 21, and 28.
	Purified chick embryo cell (PCEC)	Inactivated	Postexposure prophylaxis or for preexposure prophylaxis in high-risk individuals	As above
Yellow fever	17D virus strain	Live	Persons 9 months to 59 years of age traveling to endemic areas. Contraindicated in children younger than 6 months of age, precaution in age 6–8 months and 60 years or older	Boosters every 10 years
Rotavirus	RV1	Live	All healthy children	2 dose series, at 2 months and 4 months of age
	RV5	Live	All healthy children	3 dose series, at 2, 4, and 6 months of age
Varicella	Varicella	Live	All healthy children	At 12–15 months and 4–6 years
			At-risk adults (those without evidence of immunity and high risk for exposure or transmission)	Persons older than 13 years should receive two doses 4–8 weeks apart
Zoster	Zoster	Live	Anyone 60 years of age and older, contraindicated in severe immunodeficiency	A single one time dose in adults aged 60 years or older

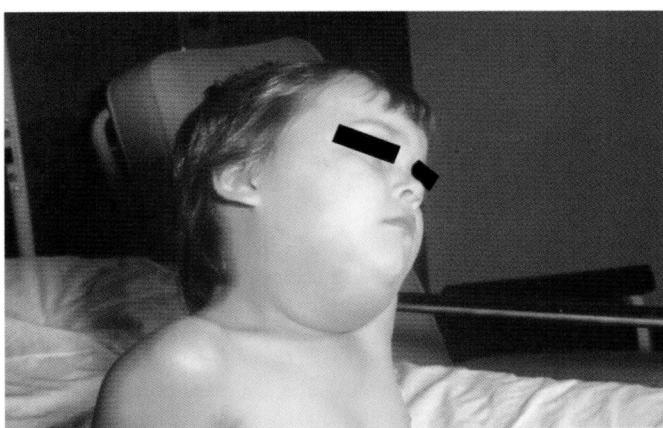

Fig. 119.1 Mumps infection demonstrating parotitis. (Courtesy of CDC website: http://phil.cdc.gov/phil/details.asp?pid=130)

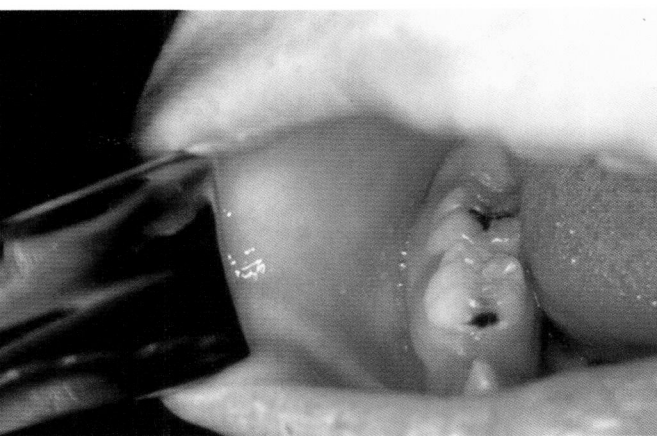

Fig. 119.2 Koplik spots. (Courtesy of CDC website: http://phil.cdc.gov/phil/details.asp?pid=6111.)

days, ranging from 12 to 25 days. Infected patients are most contagious 1 to 2 days before onset of disease but can be contagious as early as 7 days before symptoms and up to 9 days after symptoms start.

Clinical Features

Parotitis, either unilateral or bilateral, is the hallmark of this infection, occurring in over 95% of symptomatic patients (Fig. 119.1). Other salivary glands are not commonly affected. Symptoms usually begin with fever, malaise, and headache, but about one-third of mumps infections are asymptomatic. Up to 30% of mumps infections cause orchitis, which usually occurs 1 week after the onset of parotitis and is more commonly seen in older patients. Orchitis is usually unilateral but can occur in both testes in up to one-third of the cases. There is a high incidence of cerebrospinal fluid (CSF) pleocytosis in patients with mumps, but less than 10% have symptomatic meningitis, and less than 1% have encephalitis. The mortality from mumps is very low, and the majority of morbidity and mortality associated with mumps occurs in cases complicated by encephalitis.

Differential Diagnosis

During an outbreak, mumps can be easy to diagnose. Other viral infections that can cause parotitis (Epstein-Barr virus [EBV], parainfluenza, influenza A virus, coxsackievirus, adenovirus, parvovirus B19, lymphocytic choriomeningitis virus, and human immunodeficiency virus [HIV]), bacterial infections, facial cellulitis, and tumor are all other diagnoses that should be considered.

Diagnostic Testing

Mumps can be confirmed by detection of viral RNA, via reverse transcription polymerase chain reaction (RT-PCR), detection of the virus itself from clinical specimens, or detection of antibodies (immunoglobulin M [IgM] or a fourfold rise in immunoglobulin G [IgG] between acute and convalescent serum specimen). This entails collecting a buccal or oral swab specimen for virus isolation and blood sample for serologic testing. Collecting samples early improves yield as virus isolation greatly diminishes after the first week of symptoms.

Management and Disposition

The mainstay of treatment is supportive care with antipyretics and analgesics. There is no specific antiviral treatment. Most cases have a benign, self-resolving course and do not require admission to the hospital. In the hospital setting, these patients should have droplet precautions observed. Patients should be isolated for 5 days after the onset of parotid swelling. Individuals with close contact with the infected patient should receive vaccinations if not immunized.

Measles (Rubeola)

Measles is an RNA virus thought to be the most contagious infection known to humans. It was a common childhood illness, causing 3 to 4 million cases per year in the United States the 1960s, but the number of cases has dramatically decreased since the advent of the measles vaccine. Despite introduction of the measles vaccine in the 1960s, measles remains common in developing countries, mostly in parts of Africa and Asia. Global health initiatives aimed at eliminating measles focus on reaching and maintaining over 95% coverage with two doses of measles-containing vaccination. Progress has been made toward measles elimination; the World Health Organization (WHO) reported that from 2000 to 2018, the annual measles incidence decreased by 66% and measles-related deaths decreased by 73%.[3]

Measles still occurs in the United States and other developed nations, mostly among unvaccinated or incompletely vaccinated individuals who have exposures to individuals infected from an endemic region. In 2011, France had a measles outbreak with nearly 15,000 cases. A recent outbreak in New York City was linked to an unvaccinated child returning home from Israel with measles with over 600 cases occurring.[4]

Clinical Features

The incubation period for measles is 7 to 21 days. The first symptoms manifest during the prodromal phase, which lasts approximately 3 days. During this phase patients have fever, malaise, and the classically taught three Cs (cough, coryza, and conjunctivitis). Koplik spots, small raised bluish white spots on the buccal mucosa, often opposite the lower first and second molars, or the roof of mouth (Fig. 119.2), are pathognomonic for the diagnosis and can be seen during the prodromal phase. The patient will then develop the typical rash; a nonpruritic maculopapular rash beginning on the head and face and spreading down the entire body over the next 2 to 3 days (Fig. 119.3). Patients are contagious 4 days before and 4 days after the onset of the rash.

Complications of measles include otitis media, laryngitis, tracheobronchitis, bronchiolitis, pneumonitis, severe diarrhea, and acute encephalitis. The virus itself can also cause pneumonia. Bacterial superinfection can also occur. The populations that are at high risk for severe disease or complications include children younger than 5 years old, adults older than 20 years old, pregnant women, and the immunocompromised.

Subacute sclerosing panencephalitis (SSPE) is a rare but fatal complication of measles. SSPE is a slow progressive infection of the central nervous systems (CNS) that results from a prior measles infection. It is

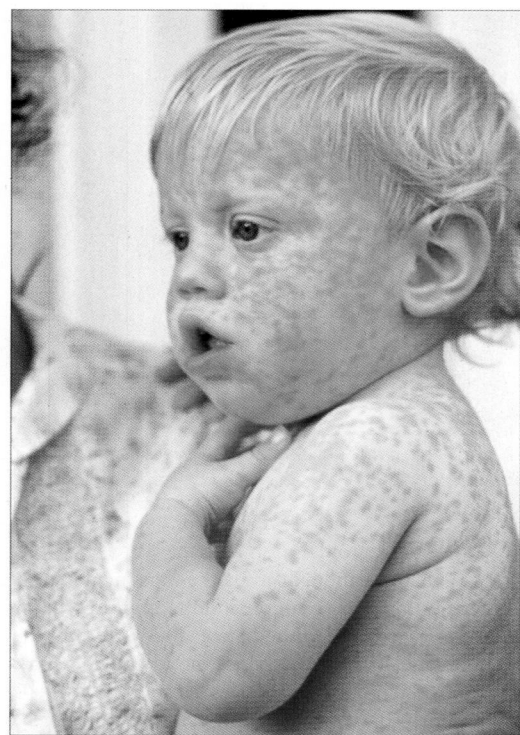

Figure 119.3 Typical rash associated with measles infection. (Kremer JR, Muller CP. Measles in Europe—there is room for improvement. *Lancet.* 2009;373(9661):356-358.)

thought to be due to continual measles infection of the CNS. The mean time of onset of SSPE is 7 years after measles infection. Symptoms include behavior change, decreased intellect, ataxia, and myoclonic seizures followed by progressive neurologic deterioration and death. Since the development of measles vaccine, this disease has almost disappeared in the United States.

Differential Diagnosis

Measles can be mistaken for other acute respiratory viral illnesses with rash or even noninfectious illnesses that present with fever and rash. Other diagnoses to consider include rubella, roseola, dengue, Kawasaki disease, and drug rash. Measles should be considered in patients that have traveled to endemic regions and return with fever and rash.

Diagnostic Testing

The diagnosis was usually made clinically by visualizing both Koplik spots and the characteristic rash along with cough, coryza, and conjunctivitis. However, the disease is not common in the developed world, and it may be mistaken for other illnesses. Clinicians suspecting a diagnosis of measles should contact local health departments. They can help instruct practitioners to obtain the necessary samples for diagnosis and surveillance. The most common methods of confirmation are serologic testing for measles-specific IgM antibody and detection of measles RNA from a nasopharyngeal specimen, blood, or urine by RT-PCR.

Management

The mainstay of treatment is supportive care. Bacterial superinfection should be treated appropriately. Postexposure prophylaxis is important in individuals who do not have evidence of measles immunity and have a measles exposure, because it can provide protection or lessen the severity of disease. Postexposure prophylaxis consists of either

the measles, mumps, and rubella (MMR) vaccine within 72 hours, or immunoglobulin within 6 days. Healthy infants should receive 0.25 mL/kg of immunoglobulin intramuscularly, and immunocompromised children should be given 0.5 mL/kg intramuscularly, up to 15 mL. Children and malnourished patients who are hospitalized with severe measles may benefit from vitamin A.

Disposition

Patients with measles require admission to the hospital based on the severity of illness. Uncomplicated measles patients should be treated at home to prevent spread of the disease. It is important, however, to observe appropriate isolation precautions in the hospital setting. All suspected cases of measles should be evaluated with airborne isolation precautions in place. Infected individuals should have airborne isolation for 4 days after they develop the rash, and those who are immunocompromised should remain on airborne precautions until complete recovery.

Rubella (German Measles)

Rubella is a single-stranded RNA virus that is a member of the *Togaviridae* family. Since the wide-scale implementation of the vaccine, cases have dropped by greater than 99%. As a result, rubella is no longer endemic in the United States. The virus is spread via contact with respiratory droplets. In pregnant patients, the virus spreads to the placenta with subsequent infection of fetal organs.

Clinical Features

Acquired rubella is a mild febrile illness associated with a diffuse maculopapular rash, malaise, headache, and arthritis. Encephalitis and thrombocytopenia are rare complications. Rubella is generally a mild disease, but consequences in pregnant patients can be devastating. It can cause miscarriage, intrauterine death, premature delivery, or congenital rubella syndrome. Congenital rubella syndrome is characterized by severe birth defects, including hearing impairment, cataracts, retinopathy, developmental delay, microcephaly, and a variety of congenital heart defects.

Differential Diagnosis

The diagnosis of rubella on a clinical basis can be difficult because of the overlap with many other illnesses. Diseases that share common features include measles, roseola, erythema infectiosum (fifth disease), toxoplasmosis, and scarlet fever.

Diagnostic Testing

The diagnosis of rubella can be made by virus detection or serologic testing. The most common method is detection of IgM antibodies or fourfold increase in IgG antibody titer between acute and convalescent specimen. Virus culture and RT-PCR can also be isolated from blood or the nasopharynx.

Management and Disposition

There is no specific antiviral treatment for rubella. The management centers on symptom control with antipyretics and analgesics. The course of this disease is short and benign. These patients can generally be treated at home but should be educated about the risks to pregnant women.

VIRAL INFECTIONS WITH VESICULAR RASH

Herpes Simplex

Herpes simplex virus type 1 (HSV-1) and herpes simplex virus type 2 (HSV-2) are double-stranded DNA viruses of the *Herpesviridae* family. Herpes simplex infections primarily involve the skin or mucosal

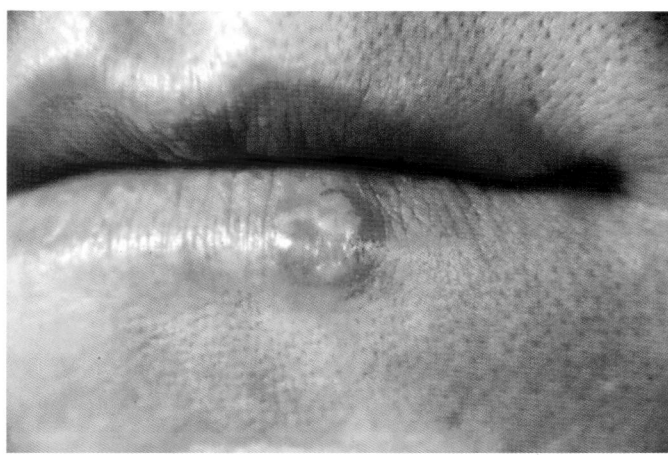

Fig. 119.4 Herpes labialis. (Courtesy of CDC website: http://phil.cdc.gov/phil/details.asp?pid=1573.)

surfaces with occasional severe involvement of organs. Herpes simplex virus (HSV) infections range in acuity from asymptomatic to life-threatening. HSV-1 typically causes orofacial infections but can affect liver, lung, eye, genitalia, and the CNS. HSV-2 typically causes genital herpes but can also affect the other systems as well. HSV infections are common; the seroprevalence of HSV-1 has been reported to be 57.7% in persons aged 14 to 49 years old in the United States, and the seroprevalence of HSV-2 has been reported to be 17.0% in the same population.

Initial HSV-1 infection usually occurs in childhood. HSV gains entry via breaks in the skin or mucosal surfaces. Viral replication is then initiated in epidermal and dermal cells. The infection then spreads to the nervous system, where it lays latent in the sensory nerve ganglia. Any stressor such as acute illness, emotional stress, trauma, intense sunlight, or fever can trigger reactivation of the virus. Recurrence rates are high for herpes infections. HSV-2 infections usually are acquired in adolescence or adulthood through sexual contact. Neonatal HSV-2 infections occur during childbirth via contact with the infected mother's birth canal.

Clinical Features

Oral Infection. The first episode of HSV-1 infections usually occurs early in life and manifests as a gingivostomatitis and pharyngitis. Symptoms include fever, malaise, and vesicular lesions anywhere in the mouth or oropharynx. Infections typically last between 10 to 14 days. Reactivation is usually much less severe and occurs as herpes labialis, small vesicles at the vermilion border of the lip (Fig. 119.4). These vesicles usually crust over within 48 hours.

Genital Herpes. This infection is characterized by painful vesicles and ulcers on the external genitalia. The first infection is usually the most severe and can be accompanied by systemic symptoms like fever, headache, malaise, and myalgias. It is also common to have dysuria and tender inguinal lymphadenopathy. Infections can also spread to the perianal and rectal region as well.

Central Nervous System Infection. HSV-1 is a common cause of infectious encephalitis; it causes necrotizing hemorrhagic encephalitis, typically involving the temporal lobes. Herpes simplex encephalitis is characterized by acute onset of symptoms, including fever, headache, altered mental status, seizures, and focal neurologic deficits resulting from frontal and temporal lobe necrosis. If left untreated, mortality is greater than 70%. HSV-2 can cause meningitis in over 25% of patients with primary infection, more commonly in women. In contrast to HSV encephalitis, HSV meningitis has a benign course. Neonatal HSV

encephalitis is caused by HSV-2 acquired during vaginal delivery of an infected mother.

Other Infections. Herpes can cause a variety of cutaneous manifestations. They typically present with the classic painful grouped vesicles on an erythematous base on the affected area. Herpetic whitlow refers to these vesicles occurring on the finger. Herpes gladiatorum is a skin infection that can arise anywhere on the body and is associated with contact sports. Herpes can also cause ocular infections, including keratitis, conjunctivitis, and acute retinal necrosis. Immunocompromised patients are at risk for rare infections like HSV pneumonitis, esophagitis, or hepatitis.

Differential Diagnosis

When suspecting orofacial HSV infection, considerations include other diseases with vesicles and ulcers, such as aphthous ulcers, coxsackievirus infections (herpangina and hand-foot-and-mouth disease), infectious mononucleosis, Stevens-Johnson syndrome, or Behçet disease. The differential diagnosis for genital herpes infection should include other sexually transmitted infections with ulcers and vesicles, such as syphilis or chancroid or noninfectious diseases like Behçet disease. HSV encephalitis can be difficult to distinguish from other acute CNS emergencies like bacterial meningitis, brain abscess, other viral encephalitides, brain tumor, or stroke.

Diagnostic Testing

Frequently, clinicians diagnose oral or genital HSV infections clinically, given the classic appearance of the vesicles and ulcers. However, because of the risk of transmission and the impact of this diagnosis on a patient, testing should be performed if possible. Definitive diagnosis can be made by viral culture, direct fluorescent antibody (DFA), or polymerase chain reaction (PCR) from vesicles, ulcers, or mucocutaneous sites. PCR is more sensitive than viral culture. Tzanck smear has a low sensitivity and specificity and is mainly of historical interest. Serology can differentiate between acute infection and reactivation.

The diagnosis of HSV encephalitis is made by PCR from the CSF. The routine laboratory tests sent after a lumbar puncture (LP) to assess for bacterial meningitis do not adequately assess for HSV encephalitis. Classically, CSF analysis shows an elevated white blood cell (WBC) count, with lymphocyte predominance. Depending on the degree of brain necrosis, an elevated red blood cell (RBC) count can also be seen. Although it is rare, CSF results can be normal in HSV encephalitis, particularly in immunocompromised individuals.[5] This underscores the importance of waiting for PCR results before considering discontinuation of treatment in suspected cases of HSV encephalitis. In cases of negative CSF PCR with a high suspicion of HSV encephalitis, especially those with who present early in their illness, we recommend continuing empirical treatment and resending CSF PCR in 72 hours. Neuroimaging with computed tomography (CT) or magnetic resonance imaging (MRI) can be highly suggestive of HSV encephalitis, but imaging can be negative early in the course of illness (Fig. 119.5).

Management

Antiviral agents are the mainstay of treatment. The treatment dose and duration for herpes simplex depends on the clinical syndrome that is present. Acyclovir, valacyclovir, and famciclovir are the commonly used antiviral drugs with activity against HSV. These drugs are nucleoside analogues that work by inhibiting viral DNA synthesis. Acyclovir is the only agent that is available in an intravenous (IV) formulation.

Herpes gingivostomatitis or labialis: First episodes are treated with oral acyclovir 200 mg five times a day (alternative regimen: 400 mg three times a day), valacyclovir 1 g twice daily, or famciclovir 250 mg three times a day for 7 days. Recurrent infections are treated with

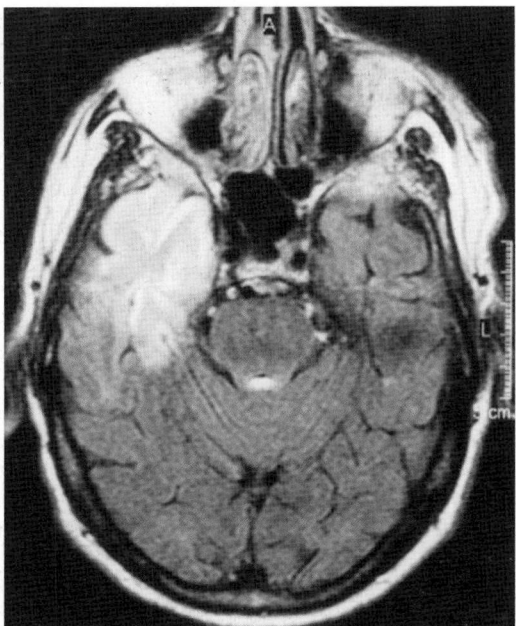

Fig. 119.5 T-2 weighted MRI with gadolinium demonstrating temporal lobe enhancement secondary to HSV-1 encephalitis. (Martin K, Franco-Paredes C. Herpes encephalitis. *Lancet.* 2002;360(9342):1286.)

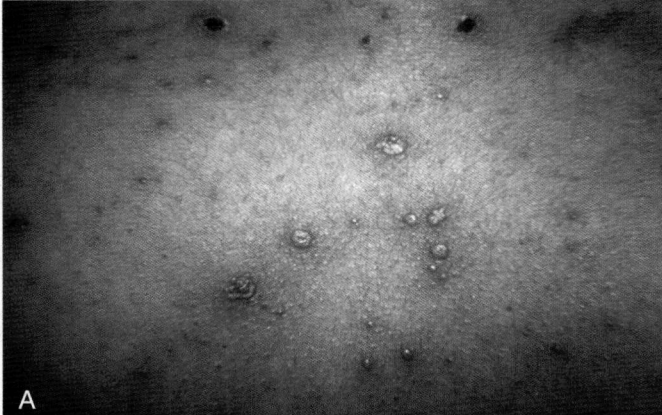

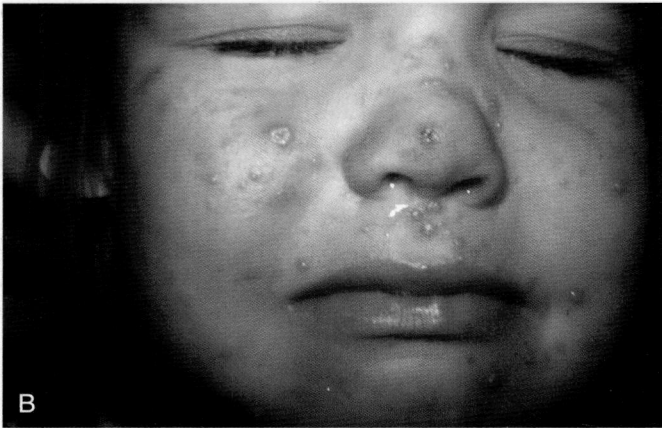

Fig. 119.6 (A and B) Varicella infection demonstrating the typical rash with lesions in different stages of healing. (Courtesy of CDC website: http://phil.cdc.gov/phil/details.asp?pid=10484   http://phil.cdc.gov/phil/details.asp?pid=10486.)

acyclovir 400 mg five times a day for 5 days, valacyclovir 2 g twice daily for 1 day, or famciclovir 1500 mg as a single dose.

Genital herpes: First episodes are treated with oral acyclovir 200 mg five times a day (alternative regimen: 400 mg three times a day), valacyclovir 1 g twice daily, or famciclovir 250 mg three times a day for 7 to 10 days. A shorter course is usually adequate for treatment of recurrence. For suppression of recurrent episodes, acyclovir 400 to 800 mg twice daily or valacyclovir 500 mg daily can be used.

Herpetic whitlow and other mucocutaneous manifestations: Administer acyclovir 200 mg five times a day or 400 mg three times a day for 5 days.

Herpes keratitis: Administer acyclovir 400 mg five times a day or valacyclovir 500 mg three times a day. Topical antiviral therapy with trifluridine, acyclovir, or ganciclovir are all equally effective.[6]

HSV encephalitis: Administer IV acyclovir 10 mg/kg every 8 hours for 14 to 21 days. Given the high mortality associated with this condition, antiviral therapy should be started as soon as the diagnosis is suspected.

Disposition

The majority of herpes infections can be treated with oral antiviral therapy on an outpatient basis. Patients who are immunocompromised and have severe mucocutaneous disease or disseminated disease benefit from inpatient admission with IV acyclovir treatment. All patients with suspected encephalitis should be admitted for empirical treatment and diagnostic testing. Intensive care unit (ICU) admission may be necessary depending on the severity of neurologic symptoms. For HSV encephalitis patients, we recommend early involvement of infectious disease consultants to help guide treatment and neurology for management of cerebral edema and severe neurologic symptoms.

Varicella-Zoster Virus

The varicella-zoster virus (VZV) is another double-stranded DNA virus that is a member of the *Herpesviridae* family. VZV causes two common infections: varicella (chicken pox) and zoster (shingles). Transmission

occurs via the respiratory tract through respiratory droplets and also by direct contact with virus present in the fluid-filled vesicles. VZV initially infects the nasopharynx and spreads to the lymphoid tissue. The virus is present in vesicles that develop on the skin and then infects the nerve endings in the skin and migrates to the dorsal ganglia where it lays latent.

Primary infection of VZV occurs as varicella (chicken pox). Varicella is highly contagious and historically occurred year round with a predilection for winter and spring months. Prior to the development of the varicella vaccine in 1995, most people would develop this infection in childhood. After widespread uptake of the vaccine, the incidence of varicella has decreased by 90%, with a subsequent decline in mortality. Zoster (shingles) is a result of reactivation of the latent virus. Risk factors for developing shingles include older age and immunosuppression.

Clinical Features

Varicella. Chicken pox is a febrile illness characterized by malaise and rash. The rash begins first on the scalp and face and then spreads to the trunk and extremities. The lesions start as maculopapular, and progress to fluid-filled vesicles that eventually crust over and form scabs (Fig. 119.6). The lesions occur as crops at various stages of development. Patients are contagious until all lesions are scabbed over, which can typically take 1 to 2 weeks.

This disease typically has a benign course, although adults have a more severe course than children. The most common complication is a secondary bacterial infection of the skin lesions. VZV has been

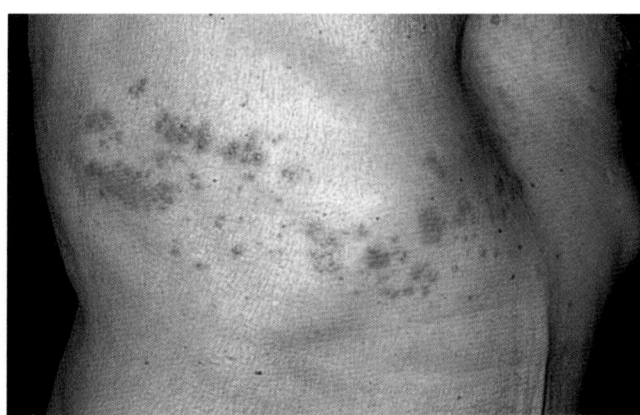
Fig. 119.7 Herpes zoster infection.

associated with invasive group A streptococcal infections and necrotizing fasciitis.[7] Immunocompromised patients are at risk for disseminated disease and visceral organ involvement. Pregnant patients are also at risk for severe disease. Varicella pneumonia accounts for most of the morbidity related to this disease. Neurologic complications are rare but can include encephalitis, aseptic meningitis, transverse myelitis, and Reye syndrome. Although exceedingly rare, it is important to recognize the association of aspirin use with Reye syndrome, a progressive encephalopathy with acute liver injury. Thus aspirin and other salicylates should be avoided in varicella treatment, especially in children.

Zoster. Herpes zoster typically causes a vesicular rash with an erythematous base that occurs unilaterally in a single dermatome (Fig. 119.7). The rash is often painful and preceded by paresthesias or hypesthesia. In immunocompetent individuals, the rash crusts in 7 to 10 days, and at that time patients are no longer contagious. Post-herpetic neuralgia, defined as pain that persists for more than 90 days, is the feared complication. Risk factors for post-herpetic neuralgia include older age and severity of pain at onset.[8]

Herpes zoster ophthalmicus is viral reactivation within the trigeminal nerve ganglion. Ocular involvement occurs in over 50% of these cases. The Hutchinson sign, a vesicle on the tip of the nose, is associated with ocular involvement. Herpes zoster oticus (Ramsay Hunt syndrome) is characterized by facial nerve palsy, pain, and vesicular rash on the ear and in the auditory canal. Disseminated zoster involving multiple dermatomes can occur in immunocompromised patients.

Differential Diagnosis

Classic varicella is distinctive, but the other major diagnoses to consider are other febrile illnesses with rashes like disseminated HSV infection, coxsackievirus infection, measles, or rickettsialpox. Prior to eradication, smallpox was a consideration, presenting with lesions in the same stage of development. The rash of zoster is also usually very characteristic. Other diagnoses to consider include herpes simplex infection or contact dermatitis.

Diagnostic Testing

The majority of chickenpox and shingles diagnosis is made clinically. Confirmatory diagnosis can be made through viral culture, DFA, or PCR testing of the vesicle fluid.

Management

Varicella. The management is mainly supportive care with antipyretics and antihistamines to decrease the pruritus caused by the skin lesions. Salicylates should be avoided in children because of the association with Reye syndrome. Antiviral therapy with acyclovir has been shown to decrease the duration of fever and total number of lesions in healthy children. It does not reduce the number of varicella-related complications, however. Therefore, we typically do not recommend treatment of otherwise healthy children with varicella. We recommend treating high-risk groups with acyclovir, including those older than 12 years old, pregnant patients, persons with chronic cutaneous or pulmonary disorders, persons on long-term salicylate therapy, persons on aerosolized corticosteroids, and immunocompromised patients. The treatment should be initiated within 24 hours after the rash appears for the most benefit. The dose of acyclovir for VZV treatment is higher than that of HSV, 800 mg orally four times a day for 5 days. If the patient is immunocompromised and has severe disease, IV acyclovir should be administered.

Zoster. The goals of treatment for zoster are to treat the viral infection and control the pain that occurs with the rash. Uncomplicated zoster in the immunocompetent host can be treated with the following regimens for 1 week: acyclovir 800 mg five times a day, famciclovir 500 mg three times a day, or valacyclovir 1 g three times a day. Antiviral treatment should be initiated within 72 hours of the onset of rash because the efficacy beyond 72 hours is unclear. Immunocompromised patients should be treated regardless of time of onset of rash. Zoster involving more than one dermatome or disseminated zoster should be treated with IV acyclovir. The disease is often painful enough to require opioid agents. Currently, there are no treatments that have reliably shown a reduction in the occurrence of post-herpetic neuralgia. Antiviral treatment has shown mixed results and is likely not useful in preventing post-herpetic neuralgia.[9] Corticosteroids have been studied extensively, but a recent review did not support their use in preventing post-herpetic neuralgia.[10]

Disposition

Most patients with varicella and zoster can be treated at home. Patients with varicella are highly contagious and should be instructed to avoid people who have not been fully vaccinated or never had the disease, immunocompromised persons, or pregnant individuals until all of their lesions have crusted over. Immunocompromised patients, patients with disseminated zoster, or patients with complications require admission to the hospital.

In general, patients with varicella should be under contact and airborne precautions until all of the lesions have crusted over. An immunocompetent localized zoster patient only requires standard precautions, whereas an immunocompromised or disseminated zoster patient is treated like a patient with varicella, requiring contact and airborne precautions.

VIRAL INFECTIONS CAUSING NONSPECIFIC FEBRILE ILLNESS

Epstein-Barr Virus

EBV is a member of the *Herpesviridae* family. It is classically known for causing infectious mononucleosis. It is also associated with several types of cancer, including Burkitt lymphoma, nasopharyngeal carcinoma, Hodgkin disease, and B cell lymphoma. EBV is ubiquitous, with most individuals testing positive for antibodies by adulthood. One British study demonstrated that 70% of 0- to 5-year-olds had antibodies to EBV, whereas 95% of 20- to 25-year-olds tested positive.[11] EBV is spread via salivary secretions. The virus infects the oropharynx and then spreads through the bloodstream and infects B lymphocytes resulting in proliferation of infected B lymphocytes and T lymphocytes, leading to enlargement of lymphoid tissue.

Clinical Features

EBV infection in young children is usually asymptomatic or presents as mild pharyngitis. Adolescents and young adults tend to have the classic infectious mononucleosis (fever, exudative pharyngitis, lymphadenopathy, myalgias, and fatigue). Splenomegaly is common, seen in up to 50% of cases. Hepatomegaly and jaundice occur less than 10% of the time. The symptom duration is typically 1 to 3 weeks, with some cases having malaise and fatigue for several months. Splenic rupture is rare, occurring in less than 0.5% of patients. It should be suspected in patients with left upper quadrant pain and is more common during the first 3 weeks of illness. Airway obstruction occurs in less than 5% of children with mononucleosis and is one of the common causes of hospital admission. Rare neurologic complications include encephalitis, aseptic meningitis, transverse myelitis, Guillain-Barré syndrome, retrobulbar neuritis, and peripheral neuropathies. Patients treated with amoxicillin or ampicillin for presumed streptococcal pharyngitis may develop a nonallergic maculopapular rash.

Differential Diagnosis

EBV causes 90% of infectious mononucleosis; the remaining 10% is caused by cytomegalovirus (CMV). Acute HIV infection, streptococcal pharyngitis, toxoplasmosis, and other viral pharyngitis causes should be considered in potential mononucleosis patients.

Diagnostic Testing

It is difficult to diagnose mononucleosis based on history and physical examination alone. Laboratory data can help confirm the diagnosis. Historically, the heterophile antibody test (monospot) has been the test of confirmation for primary EBV infection. The test has a sensitivity ranging from 63% to 84% and specificity ranging from 84% to 100%. The test is often not positive in younger children. The WBC count typically demonstrates lymphocyte predominance with many atypical lymphocytes. A lymphocyte count less than 4×10^9/L in adults is highly predictive of a negative monospot test. Health care providers can test for antibodies to EBV viral capsid and nuclear antigen if other testing is equivocal.

Management

Infectious mononucleosis typically has a self-limiting course. The treatment is supportive care with rest, antipyretics, and analgesia. Glucocorticoids have been used to decrease severity of symptoms, but there is insufficient evidence to support this practice. Antiviral treatment with acyclovir does not reduce the clinical symptoms of the disease. It is important to advise patients to avoid contact sports for at least 3 weeks to avoid the feared complication of splenic rupture. Abdominal ultrasound for assessment of spleen size may have a role in determining when it is safe to return to sports.[12]

Disposition

The majority of patients can be treated at home. Admission is necessary for airway obstruction and in patients with significant complications, such as splenic rupture.

Cytomegalovirus

CMV is a double-stranded DNA virus that belongs to the *Herpesviridae* family. Depending on geographic location, the seroprevalence ranges from 66% to 90%.[13] The spectrum of illness caused by CMV ranges from asymptomatic to severe disseminated disease in the immunocompromised patient. CMV is particularly harmful in pregnant patients because it can lead to congenital infection, causing profound neurologic defects and permanent hearing loss. CMV is present in breast milk, saliva, feces, urine, semen, cervical secretions, and blood. The virus spreads via prolonged exposure to these body fluids. After primary infection, CMV establishes a lifelong latent infection.

Clinical Features

The primary CMV infection is subclinical in most individuals. Some immunocompetent adults develop a mononucleosis-like syndrome. The illness can last from 2 to 6 weeks and is characterized by fever, fatigue, malaise, myalgia, and headache. Unlike EBV mononucleosis, exudative pharyngitis and lymphadenopathy are less common. Although it is rare, CMV can cause severe disease in the immunocompetent individual. CMV colitis and CNS infection (meningitis, encephalitis, transverse myelitis) are the most frequent forms of severe CMV infection in the immunocompetent host. Up to one-third of critically ill immunocompetent patients have evidence of CMV reactivation.

The majority of newborns who are infected with congenital CMV appear healthy or normal at birth. Common problems caused by congenital CMV infection include premature birth, intrauterine growth retardation, microcephaly, seizures, thrombocytopenia, hepatosplenomegaly, or pneumonitis. Sequelae of congenital CMV infection can present up to 2 years after birth. Frequent complications that occur are hearing loss, neurologic impairment, and ocular disturbances.

CMV can cause life-threatening disease in immunocompromised patients. CMV infection occurs in over 40% of solid organ transplant patients during the first 3 months when immunosuppressive therapy is the strongest. Transplant patients that are CMV seronegative and receive a CMV seropositive donor are at highest risk. HIV patients with CD4 count less than 100/μL are at high risk of CMV infection as well. In the immunocompromised host, CMV manifests initially as fever, malaise, and myalgias. The infection can then progress to cause leukopenia, pneumonia, esophagitis/gastritis, hepatitis, colitis, encephalitis, polyradiculopathy, and retinitis. CMV retinitis is the most common cause of blindness in patients with AIDS.

Differential Diagnosis

It is difficult to make the diagnosis of CMV infection solely on a clinical basis. Infectious mononucleosis caused by EBV presents very similarly. In the perinatal phase, infants with apparent infections should be evaluated for the other common congenital infections: toxoplasmosis, rubella, herpes simplex, syphilis, VZV, and parvovirus B19. Because the CMV infection can cause a wide array of disease in the immunocompromised host, the differential diagnosis should be broad and include other viral pathogens, bacterial infections, *Pneumocystis* infection, and fungal infections.

Diagnostic Testing

Making the diagnosis of CMV is unlikely in the ED. Confirmation of this diagnosis centers on either virus isolation, serologic testing, or histopathology. Common methods involve PCR, viral culture, or antibody testing. The WBC count may show lymphocyte predominance with more than 10% atypical lymphocytes, much like EBV infections.

Management

For the most part, CMV infection in the immunocompetent host only requires symptomatic care for the mononucleosis-like syndrome. The treatment recommendations for critically ill immunocompetent patients with CMV infection are less clear.[14] Immunocompromised patients with CMV infection are treated more aggressively. Antiviral treatment is necessary in sight and life-threatening infections.

Ganciclovir is an IV agent that is used to treat CMV infections. The treatment for CMV retinitis is induction therapy: 5 mg/kg/dose every 12 hours for 14 to 21 days followed by 5 mg/kg/dose once daily maintenance therapy for a prolonged course. Fever, diarrhea, and thrombocytopenia are common adverse reactions. Valganciclovir is an oral prodrug that is metabolized to ganciclovir. The treatment regimen is induction: 900 mg twice daily for 21 days followed by maintenance of 900 mg once daily. Foscarnet and cidofovir are IV agents used to treat CMV resistant to ganciclovir, and both can also be used to treat HSV resistant to acyclovir. The primary limiting toxicity of these drugs is renal toxicity.

Disposition

Most immunocompetent patients with CMV infection can be managed at home. In contrast, immunocompromised patients with CMV infection will usually require admission to the hospital, and depending on the extent of end-organ damage, may require ICU admission.

Enteroviruses

Enteroviruses are a group of single-stranded RNA viruses that can multiply within the gastrointestinal tract. Most infections are asymptomatic or mild undifferentiated illnesses. Despite their name, their major manifestation is not gastroenteritis. There are many enteroviruses; common ones include poliovirus, coxsackievirus A and B, echovirus, and enterovirus. These viruses are found globally and are transmitted via the fecal-oral route. Vaccination exists for poliovirus; in the United States and other industrialized nations, the disease has been declared eradicated.

Clinical Features

Most of the infections caused by enteroviruses are asymptomatic or self-limiting febrile illnesses. More of the severe infections are discussed in the following sections.

Poliovirus. The poliovirus causes a nonspecific febrile illness with malaise, myalgias, headache, and sore throat. The most feared presentation of the poliovirus infection is paralytic poliomyelitis. This manifests as aseptic meningitis followed by back, neck, and muscle pain and then the development of motor weakness. The paralysis is usually asymmetrical and affects proximal muscles more. Usually some recovery of motor function occurs months later, but approximately two-thirds of patients have some form of permanent weakness.

Non-Polio Enteroviruses. Most enterovirus infections are subclinical, but they can also cause a variety of symptoms and syndromes. Enteroviruses account for most causes of viral meningitis and encephalitis. Enteroviruses commonly cause pericarditis and myocarditis, particularly coxsackievirus B. Symptoms usually include chest pain, fever, dyspnea, and can progress to severe heart failure. Enteroviruses are a common cause of viral exanthems as well. Herpangina is caused by coxsackievirus A and presents with fever, sore throat, odynophagia, and vesiculopapular lesions on the cheeks and soft palate (Fig. 119.8). Hand-foot-and-mouth disease is caused by coxsackievirus A or enterovirus 71 and commonly manifests as fever and malaise, followed by vesicles in the mouth, and vesicles on the hands and feet (Fig. 119.9). Pleurodynia is a painful illness characterized by fever and spasms of the chest wall and abdomen that occur in paroxysms.

In 2014, there was an outbreak across the United States of EV-D68.[15] The virus affected mostly children and was severe in children with asthma. Typically EV-D68 causes mild respiratory illness, rhinorrhea, sneezing, cough, and myalgias but occasionally causes severe disease with wheezing and respiratory distress. There has also been an association with flaccid paralysis with anterior myelitis with EV-D68 infection.[16]

Differential Diagnosis

Clinicians should consider other diagnoses depending on the specific symptoms and syndrome caused by enterovirus infection. For the

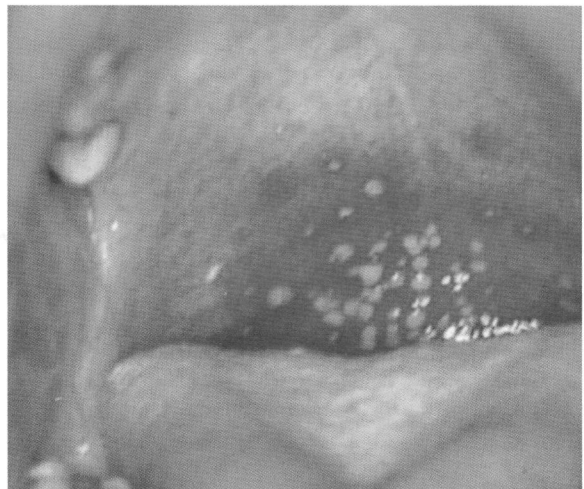

Fig. 119.8 Herpangina. (Originally from: Cohen J, Powderly WG. *Infectious Diseases*, ed 2. St. Louis: Mosby; 2004. Also found in: Bennett, JE. *Mandell, Douglas, and Bennett's Principles and Practice of Infectious Diseases*, ed 8. Philadelphia: Elsevier; 2015.)

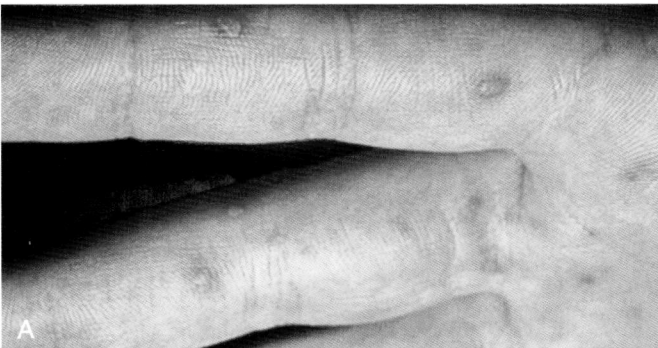

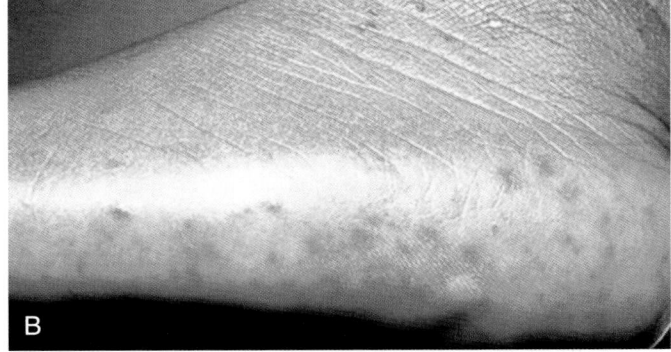

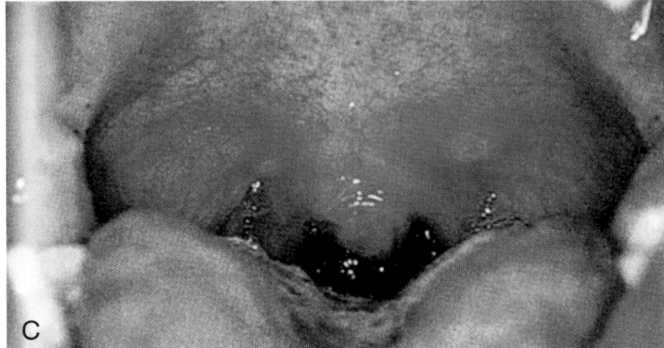

Fig. 119.9 Hand-foot-and-mouth disease. (From: Cohen BA. *Pediatric Dermatology*, ed 4. Philadelphia: Elsevier; 2013: 110.)

diseases with skin and oropharyngeal lesions, herpes simplex, aphthous stomatitis, mononucleosis, and bacterial pharyngitis should be considered. The diseases with primary neurologic manifestation present similarly to bacterial meningitis and other causes of viral meningitis or encephalitis, including herpes simplex encephalitis. Myopericarditis can present similar to pulmonary embolism, myocardial infarction, or pneumonia (see Chapter 68).

Diagnostic Testing

Diagnosis is confirmed by viral culture, serology, or PCR. Samples can be sent from nasopharynx or oropharynx via swabs or washings, CSF, serum, stool, or pericardial fluid. Other diagnostic testing should be tailored toward the symptoms, such as ECG, chest x-ray, and cardiac biomarkers for evaluation of myopericarditis. Lumbar puncture should be performed for meningitis or encephalitis evaluation.

Management

The treatment is primarily symptomatic, because currently, there are no recommended specific antiviral therapies for enteroviruses. Hand-foot-and-mouth disease can cause severe dehydration, because children refuse to eat secondary to the painful lesions in the mouth. This illness is typically treated with analgesia and encouragement of oral intake. Topical analgesia with diphenhydramine, aluminum hydroxide, and magnesium hydroxide can be used. Viscous lidocaine and topical benzocaine should be avoided in young children because of the risk of systemic toxicity and questionable efficacy. If there is concern for meningitis, empirical therapy for bacterial meningitis and herpes simplex encephalitis should be instituted while awaiting culture and PCR results because both of the aforementioned diseases have significantly higher morbidity and mortality with delayed treatment.

Disposition

The majority of enteroviruses cause a benign disease, and patients can be treated at home and expect no sequelae. Depending on the severity of symptoms, some patients may require hospitalization for dehydration, severe respiratory illness, or neurologic infection. Viral myocarditis can cause severe heart failure and dysrhythmias requiring hospitalization and ICU care. The outcome after viral myocarditis can be variable and range from return of normal heart function to severe cardiomyopathy requiring heart transplantation (see Chapters 66 and 67).

VIRUSES ASSOCIATED WITH RESPIRATORY INFECTIONS

Influenza

Influenza is an RNA virus from the *Orthomyxoviridae* family that causes acute respiratory symptoms. This virus is highly contagious and is transmitted through large-particle respiratory droplets. Transmission usually requires close contact between individuals less than 1 meter apart. Epidemics and outbreaks occur almost annually, with the peak influenza activity usually occurring in the winter months in the United States. Influenza occasionally causes devastating pandemics. During the 1918 influenza pandemic, approximately 50 to 100 million people were killed across the globe. The most recent pandemic occurred in 2009, when a new strain of H1N1 influenza emerged, killing over 284,000 globally.

There are three major types of influenza: A, B, and C. The majority of human infections are caused by influenza A and B. Influenza can be further subdivided based on the two major surface glycoproteins present, hemagglutinin (H) and neuraminidase (N). Influenza A is

BOX 119.1 Conditions that Increase Risk for Severe Influenza and Influenza-Related Complications

Age less than 2 years
Age 65 years and older
Chronic pulmonary disorders, including asthma
Chronic cardiovascular disorders except hypertension alone
Chronic renal insufficiency
Chronic hepatic disorders
Chronic hematological conditions including sickle cell disease
Metabolic and endocrine disorders including diabetes mellitus
Neurologic disorders including disorders of the brain, spinal cord, peripheral nerve, and muscle, such as cerebral palsy, seizure disorders, stroke, intellectual disability (mental retardation), moderate to severe developmental delay, muscular dystrophy, or spinal cord injury
Immunosuppression, including that caused by medications or by HIV infection
Pregnancy or postpartum state (within 2 weeks after delivery)
Ethnicity belonging to American Indians/Alaska Natives
Morbid obesity (i.e., body mass index is equal to or greater than 40)
Residency in nursing homes and other chronic care facilities

Adapted from Grohskopf LA, Sokolow LZ, Broder KR, et al. Prevention and control of seasonal influenza with vaccines: recommendations of the Advisory Committee on Immunization Practices—United States, 2017–18 influenza season. *MMWR Recomm Rep* 2017;66:1–20.

responsible for most of the severe epidemics and pandemics because of its ability of surface antigens to undergo periodic changes. This is known as *antigenic drift* when the changes are minor and *antigenic shift* when the changes are major.

Clinical Features

Influenza typically presents as fever with constitutional (headache, malaise, and myalgias) and respiratory symptoms (cough, sore throat, rhinitis). These symptoms typically last for 3 to 7 days. Individuals are usually contagious 1 day prior to symptom onset and up to 1 week after. The majority of influenza is a benign self-limited disease, but some patients are at risk for severe influenza and influenza-related complications (Box 119.1). The common influenza-related complications are bacterial pneumonia (typically due to *Staphylococcus aureus*), sinusitis, and otitis media. Influenza can also assert its pathogenic effects by exacerbating underlying cardiopulmonary and other chronic health conditions. Occasionally influenza itself can cause a rapidly progressing pneumonia that leads to acute respiratory distress syndrome (ARDS).

Differential Diagnosis

The differential diagnosis is broad, because many different infectious diseases can present with similar symptoms. Other respiratory viruses like RSV, rhinovirus, or coronavirus can have a similar presentation. Additionally, bacterial infections, like pneumonia and meningitis, can present similarly.

Diagnostic Testing

Influenza can be diagnosed clinically based on signs and symptoms, especially during influenza season, but the accuracy of clinical diagnosis in the absence of supportive tests is not high because influenza shares common features with many viral and bacterial infections. Clinical diagnosis alone is poor, with a sensitivity less than 50% and a specificity near 70%.[17]

There are several diagnostic tests available to emergency clinicians. Rapid influenza diagnostic tests are based on immunochromatographic assays that detect specific influenza antigens, yielding results in less than 30 minutes. The sensitivity of these tests can vary from 50% to 65%, with specificities above 95%.[18] Molecular assays, such as RT-PCR or rapid antigen tests, are far more sensitive than traditional rapid influenza tests. RT-PCR is the most sensitive test and, if available, is preferred. However, rapid molecular tests have sensitivity and specificity that approach RT-PCR, and results can be back in less than 20 minutes. Rapid molecular tests have sensitivities of over 90%.

Management

The management of influenza centers on symptom control with antipyretics, analgesics, and hydration. Several antiviral agents are available to treat influenza, but some controversy surrounds treatment with these agents.

Neuraminidase Inhibitors. Oseltamivir, zanamivir, and peramivir are the currently available neuraminidase inhibitors. They work by inhibiting the release of viral progeny from infected cells. These drugs are active against both influenza A and B.

Oseltamivir is available orally as a capsule or suspension. The treatment dose in adults and children weighing more than 40 kg is 75 mg twice daily for 5 days. For children younger than 1 year old, the dose is 3 mg/kg twice daily. For children 1 year or older, the dose varies by weight: for those weighing less than or equal to 15 kg the dose is 30 mg twice daily, for those weighing more than 15 to 23 kg it is 45 mg twice daily, and for those weighing more than 23 to 40 kg it is 60 mg twice daily. The dosing does require adjustment in renally impaired individuals based on creatinine clearance. The main side effects reported have been nausea and vomiting.

Zanamivir is available as an aerosol powder and is administered via inhalation through a specialized inhaler. It is approved for use in patients 7 years old and older. The treatment dose is two inhalations twice daily for 5 days. It is not recommended in patients with underlying asthma and chronic obstructive pulmonary disease (COPD), because it can cause bronchospasm. Peramivir is the first IV neuraminidase inhibitor available for treatment in influenza patients. The treatment dose is 600 mg IV administered once as a single dose.

Adamantane Antivirals. Amantadine and rimantadine are the currently available adamantane antivirals. They prevent or greatly reduce the uncoating of the viral RNA of influenza A after attachment and endocytosis by host cells. They have no activity against influenza B. In the past, they have been used for prophylaxis and treatment for influenza A. In recent years, the circulating influenza strains have demonstrated greater than 90% resistance to these drugs. They are not recommended for use for influenza treatment.

Other Antivirals. Baloxavir is a novel antiviral that gained US Food and Drug Administration (FDA) approval to treat influenza A and B in patients 12 years of age and older in 2018. Its unique mechanism of action is inhibition of influenza cap-dependent endonuclease. Studies have demonstrated similar efficacy to oseltamivir.[19] The treatment is a single oral dose based on weight. For 40 kg to less than 80 kg, it is 40 mg as a single dose within 48 hours of the onset of influenza symptoms. For 80 kg or greater, it is 80 mg as a single dose within 48 hours of the onset of influenza symptoms.

The controversy surrounding the use of antivirals for treatment of influenza, specifically neuraminidase inhibitors (NIs) has centered on its modest effect with treatment. The most recent Cochrane review found that oseltamivir reduced symptom duration by 16.8 hours in those treated within 48 hours of symptom onset but did not affect hospitalization or reduce severe influenza complications.[20] However, another recent meta-analysis found that treatment with oseltamivir was associated with accelerated symptom improvement, reduced risk in lower respiratory tract complications, and decreased admission to hospital.[21] Investigations have also found that treatment of hospitalized patients with NIs is associated with reduced hospital length of stay and mortality.[22,23] The greatest benefit is in very early treatment, but some studies have demonstrated benefit up to 5 days after symptoms onset in hospitalized patients.[24] The Infectious Diseases Society of America (IDSA) recommendations are to treat all patients as early as possible who are hospitalized, have severe progressive illness regardless of duration, or are at high risk for influenza-related complications.[25]

Disposition

The majority of patients with influenza are discharged home with symptomatic treatment instructions, although this depends on the specific virulence of the circulating strain of the season. Patients with severe influenza require admission. These patients usually have accompanying cardiopulmonary comorbidities. A small number of influenza patients will require ICU admission because of primary influenza or acute exacerbation of an underlying illness. Influenza can cause rapidly progressive ARDS with refractory hypoxemic respiratory failure. These patients with rapidly progressive ARDS may benefit from transfer to centers that perform extracorporeal membrane oxygenation (ECMO). During the 2009 H1N1 pandemic, some centers had success with managing ARDS patients on ECMO.

Coronavirus

Coronaviruses are single-stranded RNA viruses that typically cause respiratory illness. They are covered in detail in Chapter 120.

Rhinovirus

Human rhinovirus is the most common cause of the common cold. Infections peak in the fall and spring but can occur all year. The infection is spread via infected respiratory secretions and direct contact with infected patients. The virus can remain contagious on surfaces for several hours. Hand-to-face inoculation is likely one of the predominant mechanisms of spread, underscoring the importance of frequent handwashing to decrease transmission.

Clinical Features

Symptoms of rhinovirus infection are usually limited to the nose, nasopharynx, and pharynx. The common symptoms that occur are sore throat, nasal congestion, low-grade fever, sneezing, and cough. Less commonly in children, rhinovirus can cause lower respiratory tract infections like pneumonia and tracheobronchitis.

Differential Diagnosis

Other viruses that cause respiratory illness, such as coronaviruses, respiratory syncytial virus (RSV), parainfluenza viruses, influenza viruses, adenoviruses, and enteroviruses, can produce clinical syndromes similar to those produced by the rhinoviruses.

Diagnostic Testing

Definitive diagnostic testing is usually not necessary for rhinovirus. Viral panels do exist that use nucleic acid testing to detect rhinovirus.[26] Samples are typically taken from nose, nasopharynx, or oropharynx.

Management and Disposition

The cornerstone of treatment is symptomatic relief with analgesics and antipyretics. Cough medicines should be avoided in children younger than 6 years old. This infection has a benign course and can be treated at home.

Adenovirus

Adenoviruses are double-stranded DNA viruses consisting of 7 species (A–G) and greater than 100 types. They commonly cause upper respiratory tract infections, gastrointestinal symptoms, and conjunctivitis. Infection is spread via respiratory droplets and close contact. Outbreaks have been reported in crowded settings such as military personnel undergoing training and students living in dormitory style housing. In 2018 to 2019 there was a multistate outbreak on 5 college campuses, resulting in 168 infections, 11 hospitalizations, and 2 deaths.[27]

Clinical Features

The most common presentation of adenovirus is as a URI with sore throat, cough, and fever. Gastroenteritis and conjunctivitis are also common manifestations. Other syndromes less frequently caused by adenoviruses include hemorrhagic cystitis, urethritis, infantile diarrhea, myocarditis, encephalitis, and meningoencephalitis. In infants and immunocompromised patients, particularly hematopoietic stem cell transplant and solid organ transplant patients, adenovirus can cause severe life-threatening illness.

Differential Diagnosis

Other pathogens causing similar atypical pneumonia syndromes include influenza and parainfluenza viruses and *Mycoplasma pneumoniae*. Diarrheal syndromes may be similar to those caused by rotaviruses.

Diagnostic Testing

Because adenovirus mostly causes a benign self-limiting disease, routine diagnostic testing is unnecessary. If testing is required, qualitative or quantitative PCR from serum, tissue, or body fluid is the most diagnostic method.

Management and Disposition

The majority of these infections require only symptomatic treatment. There is no specific antiviral therapy that is routinely recommended. There have been reports of using cidofovir in immunocompromised patients with life-threatening adenovirus infection, but this is not routinely recommended. The majority of these patients will be treated at home. The most severe cases may require admission.

Parainfluenza

Parainfluenza is a single-stranded RNA virus that belongs to the *Paramyxoviridae* family. This infection is usually acquired in childhood. In the United States, parainfluenza infections have been reported to account for up to a quarter of respiratory disease in children. In adults, the burden of illness caused by parainfluenza is much less. Parainfluenza is transmitted by close contact via infected respiratory secretions. There are four types, each with its own clinical presentation.

Clinical Features

Parainfluenza type 1 is the most common cause of croup. Parainfluenza type 2 is also associated with croup but causes less morbidity. Croup symptoms usually worsen at night and are characterized by a barky cough. Typically patients have a fever and URI symptoms 1 to 2 days before the cough. Tachypnea and hoarse voice are common as well. In severe cases, stridor at rest may be present. Parainfluenza type 1 and 2 also cause lower respiratory tract infections in children. Parainfluenza type 3 more often causes bronchitis, bronchiolitis, and pneumonia. Parainfluenza type 4 is less common

and causes a mild respiratory illness. In adults and older children, parainfluenza infections are mild and present as a simple URI.

Differential Diagnosis

Adenoviruses, rhinoviruses, influenza viruses, RSV, echoviruses, coxsackieviruses, and coronaviruses all can cause similar URI symptoms. If the primary presentation is croup, it is important to differentiate this from epiglottitis as a potential diagnosis.

Diagnostic Testing

Diagnosis is made from viral culture, rapid antigen test, or nucleic acid testing, either rapid testing or RT-PCR. Specimens are usually obtained from nasal swabs, throat swabs, or nasopharyngeal washings.

Management

There is no specific antiviral treatment for parainfluenza infection. The treatment is mainly symptomatic. For mild and moderate croup, a single dose of oral dexamethasone (0.15–0.6 mg/kg, maximum dose 20 mg) or oral prednisolone (1 mg/kg) can be given.[28] For severe croup, nebulized racemic epinephrine should be administered in addition to oral or intramuscular dexamethasone (0.6 mg/kg, maximum dose 20 mg). Glucocorticoids improve symptoms, reduce rates of return visits, admissions, and readmissions.[29]

Respiratory Syncytial Virus

RSV is an RNA virus that belongs to the *Paramyxoviridae* family. RSV causes significant morbidity in children. It is an important cause of death in young children in the low- and middle-income countries. In the United States, RSV is associated with approximately 20% of hospitalizations and 18% of ED visits in children younger than 5 years old. RSV is also a significant cause of respiratory illness in older patients, affecting 3% to 10% of the population over age 65 each year. RSV is spread via contact with infected individuals, by exposure to respiratory secretions and fomites.

Clinical Features

RSV causes a range of respiratory disease. The illness is most severe in infants, causing pneumonia and bronchiolitis. Newborns with RSV can present with apnea. Symptoms usually begin with nasal congestion, rhinorrhea, low-grade fever, and cough. Then 1 to 2 days after symptom onset, patients develop wheezing and increased respiratory effort. Symptoms can last up to 2 weeks. In adults and older children, RSV usually causes a benign URI typically lasting less than 5 days. Geriatric patients, immunosuppressed patients, and adults with chronic medical problems can develop severe lower respiratory tract disease.

Differential Diagnosis

The clinical presentation caused by RSV infections is similar to other upper and lower respiratory tract pathogens, including rhinovirus, parainfluenza, influenza, enteroviruses, coronaviruses, and bacterial causes of pneumonia. It is important to consider noninfectious causes of hypoxemia in infants, such as foreign body aspiration and asthma.

Diagnostic Testing

The common methods of diagnosis include viral culture, molecular assays, and rapid antigen detection tests. Specimens are typically obtained from nasopharyngeal swabs or washings. Other routine diagnostic testing is generally unnecessary and should be symptom targeted.

Management

The mainstay of treatment is supportive care. Beta-agonist bronchodilators are not recommended by the most recent guidelines published by the AAP.[30] The authors agree that routine inhaled bronchodilators should not be used for RSV bronchiolitis given the lack of evidence of improved outcomes. However, it is reasonable to administer a trial of inhaled albuterol for severe disease, because most of these patients were excluded from studies and some of the patients may actually have viral-induced asthma exacerbation. Corticosteroids have not been shown to provide any benefit. Supplemental oxygen should be provided for pulse oximetry less than 90%. Nebulized hypertonic saline can be used as an inpatient, but currently data do not support use in the ED. For severe cases, nasal continuous positive airway pressure (CPAP) can be trialed to avoid intubation. It is also important to treat dehydration associated with the disease with IV or nasogastric fluids if the patient cannot maintain oral intake. For prevention of RSV infection in high-risk patients, the AAP recommends the use of palivizumab, a monoclonal anti-RSV antibody preparation, during the first year of life for infants with hemodynamically significant heart disease or chronic lung disease of prematurity defined as preterm infants younger than 32 weeks' gestation who require more than 21% oxygen for at least the first 28 days of life.

Disposition

Healthy adults and older children have a short disease course that is mild and can be treated at home. The majority of infants with RSV may also be treated at home but may have prolonged illness. Infants younger than 1 year old that visit the ED for bronchiolitis have a median duration of symptoms of 15 days, and over one-third of them have a subsequent unscheduled medical visit. Approximately 1% to 3% of infants with RSV require hospitalization for hypoxemia, respiratory distress, or dehydration. Approximately 15% of geriatric patients requiring ICU care with an acute cardiopulmonary diagnosis are diagnosed with RSV infection.

VIRUSES ASSOCIATED WITH DIARRHEAL ILLNESS

Norovirus and Rotavirus

Norovirus is a member of the *Caliciviridae* family and is the most common cause of nonbacterial gastroenteritis. It is highly infectious because only a few particles are necessary to transmit the disease. Norovirus is spread through direct transmission from person to person via the fecal-oral route. Transmission can also occur through contaminated water, food, and surfaces. Because of its structure as a nonenveloped RNA virus, norovirus is very stable in the environment and is resistant to most disinfectants, including alcohol hand wash. Outbreaks of norovirus occur in areas where people are in proximity, including long-term care facilities, restaurants, hospitals, schools, and cruise ships. ED visits for norovirus peak in the winter months.

Rotaviruses are double-stranded RNA viruses that belong to the *Reoviridae* family. These viruses are ubiquitous, and by 5 years old most children have been exposed to them. They are the leading cause of severe gastroenteritis in children. The introduction of rotavirus vaccine in industrialized countries has dramatically decreased encounters for this disease.[31,32]

Clinical Features

Norovirus. The disease causes a severe gastroenteritis, with vomiting, diarrhea, and abdominal cramping. In infants and children, vomiting is the primary symptom, whereas adults more commonly have diarrhea. The gastrointestinal symptoms can be accompanied by fever, headache, and myalgias as well. The diarrhea is typically nonbloody, watery, and profuse. The acute illness usually lasts for half a day to 3 days.

Rotavirus. The illness manifests as sudden onset of nausea, vomiting, and profuse watery diarrhea, with fever, headache, and myalgias. The disease course is usually 3 to 7 days. The spectrum of disease can range from asymptomatic to severe and fatal dehydration.

Differential Diagnosis

Other causes of viral gastroenteritis include adenovirus, enterovirus, and certain coronaviruses. *Clostridioides difficile* infection and some bacterial gastroenteritis can present similarly.

Diagnostic Testing

Norovirus diagnosis can be confirmed by PCR of stool or vomit specimen. Rapid antigen detection test, enzyme-linked immunosorbent assay (ELISA), and PCR of stool specimen are the methods of diagnosis for rotavirus.

Management

There is no specific treatment for these viral gastrointestinal infections. Management centers on ensuring that patients are adequately hydrated and correcting significant electrolyte derangements. Most patients can be treated with oral rehydration alone. Patients with severe dehydration warrant IV rehydration. Meticulous attention to standard precautions and hand hygiene is important to prevent spread of these diseases.

Disposition

The majority of patients can be managed at home with oral therapy. Very young patients or patients with chronic illness may be at risk for more severe disease and benefit from IV therapy and monitoring. Depending on the severity of illness, these patients could be managed in an observation unit or may require inpatient admission.

VIRAL INFECTIONS WITH NEUROLOGIC MANIFESTATIONS

Rabies

The natural history and clinical course of rabies disease is complex. After a bite from a rabid animal, the risk of developing clinical disease is unknown and depends on viral inoculation or migration into nerve tissue. The risk of death following untreated clinical disease, however, is almost 100%, and the risk of developing clinical disease following proper treatment approaches 0%.[33] Rabies remains a huge public health problem worldwide, particularly affecting vulnerable populations in poor and rural areas (Fig. 119.10). Human rabies disproportionately affects children, with an estimated 40% of rabid bites occurring in those 15 years of age and younger.[34]

Emergency medicine clinicians should be prepared to evaluate bites and other exposures for the risk of rabies inoculation as well as diagnose or rule out rabies disease in patients presenting with neurologic symptoms. The diagnosis of rabies requires a thorough medical history, noting the course of illness, and multiple laboratory tests. Likewise, the management of animal bites requires appropriate wound care, risk analysis in conjunction with local or state public health authorities, patient and physician decision making regarding the need for and timing of postexposure treatment, and appropriate bite reporting to animal control or public health authorities.[35]

The signs of rabies in all species of animals are extremely variable and cannot be used alone to determine the likelihood of rabies. Additionally, the incubation period for rabies (i.e., the time between when a human or animal is bitten by a rabid animal and the development of clinical signs) is highly variable, ranging from days to months or rarely years in both humans and animals.[36] For these reasons, thorough risk assessment based on environmental, historical, and clinical conditions is essential for every animal bite and exposure.

Epidemiology

All mammals are physiologically capable of becoming infected with rabies and transmitting the virus to humans, but globally the domestic

Rabies, countries or areas at risk

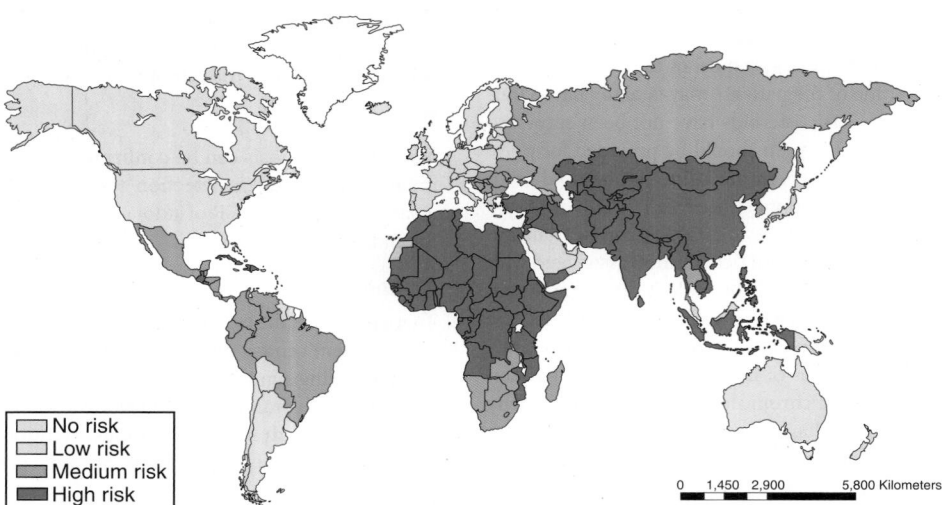

No risk
Low risk
Medium risk
High risk

In countries of categories 1, 2 and 3, contacts with suspect rabid animals including bats should be followed by rabies post-exposure prophylaxis.

No risk: no risk at all.
Low risk: pre-exposure immunization recommended for people likely to have contact with bats.
Medium risk: pre-exposure immunization recommended for travellers and other people for whom contact with bats and other wildlife is likely.
High risk: pre-exposure immunization recommended for travellers and other people for whom contact with domestic animals particularly dogs and other rabies vectors is likely.

Fig. 119.10 Rabies—countries or areas at risk. (Courtesy of World Health Organization (WHO).)

dog is the highest-risk species for rabies exposure.[37] In many countries, endemic dog rabies still occurs, and the cycle of dog-to-dog transmission spills into the human population. The global burden of human rabies from dogs is high, with an estimated 59,000 deaths and the equivalent of over $8.5 billion (US) in economic losses from premature death and postexposure treatment.[38] Although the United States was declared free of endemic canine rabies in 2007, travelers to countries where canine rabies is endemic can be exposed to rabies and subsequently express symptoms after returning to the United States. Since 2003, all fatal cases of canine-attributed human rabies in the United States have been acquired outside the continental United States.[39]

In the United States, certain wildlife species are high-risk for human exposure. This risk is due to shared habitats, interactions between humans and wildlife, and human proximity to locations of endemic rabies in certain species, including the bat, raccoon, skunk, and fox. Small rodents such as squirrels, hamsters, guinea pigs, chipmunks, rats, and rabbits are almost never found to be infected and have not been known to transmit rabies to humans.[39]

Other modes of transmission are rare but exist. Human rabies disease has been caused via organ transplantation and aerosolization (in laboratories or high-concentration environments such as caves).[40,41] Other than through organ transplantation, person-to-person transmission of rabies has not been reported.

Pathophysiology

Rabies is caused by an RNA virus from the genus lyssavirus, in the family Rhabdoviridae. The rabies virus (RABV) is responsible for most human and animal rabies cases worldwide, but other lyssavirus have been implicated. RABV is found extensively throughout the world in terrestrial carnivores, but non-RABV lyssavirus is rarely encountered in nonflying carnivores.[37,42]

Bites through the dermis allow the virus to enter tissues and initiate infection. The virus spreads from muscle tissue to the peripheral nervous system via the neuromuscular junction and then travels to the spinal cord and brain. Host cell machinery is usurped, and rapid replication occurs, resulting in clinically apparent disease. Infection of the brain is followed quickly by peripheral viral dissemination. For the reservoir species, transmission to the salivary glands proceeds through the parasympathetic and sympathetic nervous systems. The associated aggressive behavior and hypersalivation promotes transmission to new hosts.[43,44]

Clinical Features

Two forms of clinical rabies are described, encephalitic and paralytic. The encephalitic form predominates and represents approximately 80% of all human rabies presentations.[45] It is believed that the burden of infection is in the brain in the encephalitic form, whereas the burden is in the spinal cord in the paralytic form. The initial symptoms of rabies infection are vague and may be confused with other flu-like illnesses. Presenting symptoms of rabies include headache, malaise, pharyngitis, and weakness which are followed by or concomitant with pruritus and paresthesia at the site of inoculation. Fever, tachycardia, and tachypnea foretell the acute behavioral changes characteristic of rabies: agitation, aerophagia, hydrophobia, seizures, and coma.[36] The image of a patient in the final stages of rabies delirium with agitation and foaming of the mouth is aptly described by the genus name lyssavirus, named for Lyssa, a Greek goddess of rage, fury, madness, and frenzy (Fig. 119.11). Infection in the central and peripheral nervous systems leads to multiorgan failure.

Encephalitic Rabies. Encephalitic rabies progresses rapidly over days, and the presenting signs and symptoms are supplanted rapidly by diffuse neurologic involvement. A brief period of anxiety, confusion, insomnia, and cerebellar dysfunction are soon replaced by frank delirium, hallucinations, and the clinically defining behavioral changes: hydrophobia, aerophobia, aggressive behavior, and seizures. These are the clinical symptoms most associated with rabies infection,

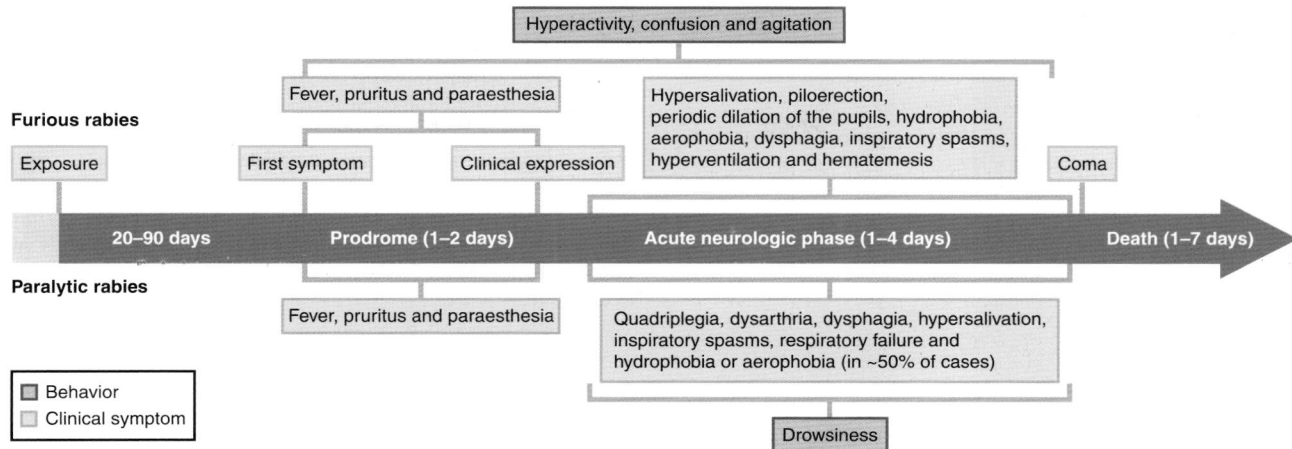

Fig. 119.11 Spectrum of clinical rabies. (From: Fooks AR, Cliquet F, Finke S, et al. Rabies. *Nat Rev Dis Primers.* 2017;3:17091.)

and these portend death.[45] In the final stage of encephalitic rabies, the patient has difficulty swallowing from involuntary muscle spasms of the pharynx, and hypersalivation occurs. If offered water, the patient may develop pharyngeal spasm with resultant gagging. Patients are unable to handle salivary secretions, leading to characteristic drooling and foaming of the mouth. The findings of hydrophobia with resultant gagging and hypersalivation are so characteristic of rabies infection that in many developing countries, water is offered to the patient as a diagnostic test. Coma and death follow rapidly, usually within 5 days of presentation.[36]

Paralytic Rabies. Paralytic rabies accounts for approximately 20% of human rabies infections. The presenting symptoms are similar to encephalitic rabies and include headache, weakness, and malaise. Muscle weakness and paresthesia occur at the site of the bite and, over days to weeks, an acute flaccid paralysis ensues. Unlike the encephalitic form, the patient does not develop agitation, hypersalivation, or hydrophobia. Rather, muscle weakness occurs over days to weeks, and the progression to coma and death takes longer than in the encephalitic form.[45] The paralytic form develops more often in patients who have been bitten by rabid bats than dogs and those who have had incomplete PEP, without a clear explanation. Exposed patients receiving the nerve cell–derived vaccine that is still used in a few countries are also at greater risk of developing the paralytic form.

Differential Diagnoses

The prodromal phase of rabies presents similarly to many common infections including mononucleosis, bacteremia, and meningitis. In its early stages, rabies may appear similar to other infectious encephalitis including herpes simplex, cerebral malaria, and West Nile infections. Noninfectious toxic or metabolic encephalopathies, including serotonin syndrome, alcohol withdrawal, organophosphate poisoning, elapid or scorpion envenomation, may mimic early rabies. On rare occasion, psychiatric disease, such as schizophrenia and conversion disorders, may resemble rabies.[46,47] Tetanus, dystonia, and strychnine poisoning all present with muscular rigidity which may appear similar to rabies. Once aerophagia, hydrophobia, or dysphagia appear, however, the diagnosis of rabies becomes clear.

The early presentation of paralytic rabies may mimic Guillain-Barré syndrome, but is distinguished by the onset of encephalitis, asymmetry of limb involvement, persistent fever, bladder incontinence, and intact sensory function. Percussion myoedema is the mounding of muscle at the site of percussion and is characteristic of rabies.[33] It is best elicited on the chest, deltoid, and thigh (Box 119.2).

BOX 119.2 Rabies Rigidity/Paralysis: Differential Diagnosis

Muscular Rigidity
Tetanus
Dystonia
Strychnine poisoning

Paralysis
Guillain-Barré
Acute flaccid paralysis
Envenomation
Hypokalemia

In atypical presentations of encephalitic rabies or paralytic rabies, the diagnosis may not be clear and may delay institution of appropriate public health and infection control measures. As improved antemortem techniques arise, more timely diagnosis will provide more opportunity for appropriate prophylaxis to family members, and more timely discussions with patient and family regarding prognosis.[42]

Diagnostic Evaluation and Testing

The diagnosis of human rabies requires clinical acumen, understanding of local capabilities of treatment, and public health issues in the community.[36] The emergency clinician must consider rabies in two scenarios: possible exposure to rabies and the diagnosis of clinical rabies. The decision to initiate postexposure prophylaxis requires understanding of the type of exposure and the local vector demographics. Because the risk assessment of the exposure is intricately tied to its management, this topic is addressed in the management section.

Clinical cases of human rabies are categorized as suspected, probable, or confirmed. A suspected case is one that is compatible with clinical findings, probable cases have a reliable history of contact suspected, probably or confirmed rabid animal as well as suspected clinical findings, and confirmed case definition indicates laboratory confirmation.[36] The WHO definition of confirmed rabies requires at least one of the laboratory criteria in Box 119.3.

Typical laboratory tests are rarely helpful in the diagnosis of rabies. Complete blood count often demonstrates a leukocytosis, and cerebrospinal fluid findings include lymphocytic pleocytosis with elevated protein and normal glucose. Neither of these studies and their findings are specific for rabies. MRI imaging may demonstrate T2 signals

BOX 119.3 Laboratory Criteria Used to Confirm Rabies

- Presence of viral antigens in samples (e.g., brain tissue, skin);
- Isolation of virus from samples in cell culture or in laboratory animals;
- Presence of viral-specific antibodies in the cerebrospinal fluid or serum of an unvaccinated person; and/or
- Presence of viral nucleic acids in samples (e.g., brain tissue, skin, saliva, concentrated urine).

The WHO definition of rabies requires at least one of the criteria to be met.[35]

in the hippocampus, hypothalamus, and brainstem, but is not clearly diagnostic.[33]

Effective antemortem testing remains elusive, particularly in endemic regions with limited laboratory capability. Patients with suspected rabies who have not been vaccinated may not have rabies antibodies in serum or CSF until obvious clinical signs are apparent, but positive titers are then diagnostic. Patients who have received rabies vaccine or rabies immunoglobulin (RIG) have serum titers of rabies antibody but require subsequent testing in 7 days to assess if titers are rising. Various forms of molecular methods-reverse transcription (RT) and polymerase chain reaction (PCR) assays have demonstrated high sensitivity for RABV in dog brain tissue. In humans, real-time PCR testing of cerebral spinal fluid, nuchal skin, and saliva using the TaqMan probes has demonstrated excellent sensitivity and specificity.[48] Consultation with local public health authorities to determine which tissues should be sampled and how to obtain and transport safely is paramount.[35]

Postmortem testing of fresh brain samples remains the gold standard for the diagnosis of rabies in all animal species. The WHO and World Organization for Animal Health (OIE) recommend fluorescent antibody testing (FAT) of brain smears or touch impressions.[49] FAT provides sensitive and specific results within a few hours. The best results are obtained with fresh brain tissue, but saline-washed tissue preserved in 50% glycerol saline also works well.

The direct rapid immunohistochemical test (dRIT) was developed in 2006 at the CDC. The dRIT assay is an immunohistochemical diagnostic assay that utilizes polyclonal or monoclonal antibody that is directly labeled, and is performed after a touch impression of brain tissues. A streptavidin reagent catalyzes the formation of a colored precipitate when bound to the rabies virus, making it visible with simple light microscopy. dRIT provides results in 1 hour, does not require expensive fluorescent-labeled antibodies, and has been field-tested in endemic areas with 100% sensitivity and specificity when compared to FAT.[50] The use of dRIT allows regions with limited resources to obtain important incidence data, as well as the possibility of carrying out more informed postexposure prophylaxis. However, one significant drawback of dRIT is that the reagents used for the test are only available through the CDC.

Management

The treatment of rabies exposure and rabies disease is divided into preexposure (PreP) recommendations in high-risk groups, animal bite or exposure assessment, wound care, postexposure prophylaxis, and treatment of human rabies (Fig. 119.12).

Preexposure Prophylaxis. Pasteur described the first rabies vaccine in 1885.[51,52] Nerve tissue–derived vaccines similar to Pasteur's were used worldwide until the 1940s, when they were replaced by cell culture–derived vaccines (CCVs) that were safer and more immunogenic. The nerve cell–derived vaccines contain myelin basic protein, which may

cause a severe immune response resulting in devastating neurologic adverse reactions. Despite warnings from WHO, some countries continue to manufacture and use nerve tissue–derived vaccines.[36]

All US-licensed rabies vaccines are inactivated cell culture vaccines that can be administered to immunocompromised individuals. Patients with immunosuppressive disorders and those taking corticosteroids, immunosuppressive agents, or antimalarials may have a reduced response to the vaccine, necessitating a 5-dose regimen. In this setting, serologic testing for neutralizing rabies antibody may be considered 4 weeks after the last vaccine dose to determine if a booster is necessary.[36]

Adverse reactions to rabies vaccines include local reactions, mild systemic reactions, and immediate hypersensitivity reactions. Typical local reactions include pain, swelling, redness, and induration at the injection site.[52] These symptoms are reported by 60% to 85% of recipients of the human diploid cell vaccine (HDCV) and by 11% to 57% of recipients of the purified chick embryo vaccine (PCEV). From 6.8% to 55.6% and up to 31% of recipients of HDCV and PCEV, respectively, have reported systemic reactions, including gastrointestinal symptoms, headache, dizziness, and fever. Immediate hypersensitivity occurs in 1.2% of previously unimmunized HDCV recipients and in up to 6% of those previously immunized receiving HDCV as a booster. No deaths have been reported from recipients of the human diploid cell vaccine or purified chick embryo cell vaccine.[53]

Preexposure vaccine (PrEP) is recommended for travelers to endemic areas and those in high-risk professions (e.g., veterinarians, laboratory staff handling the virus). The PrEP regimen recommended by the WHO and CDC are not currently aligned, with WHO recommending a 2-dose strategy and CDC recommending a 3-dose regimen.[36,52]

Intramuscular or intradermal administration of vaccine is recommended.[36,52] In the United States, the CDC recommends the intramuscular route only. The intradermal method, common in many countries, uses less total vaccine in multidose vials and is thus less expensive while still being highly efficacious.[54] While some recommend preexposure prophylaxis for children younger than 15 years old in endemic areas, due to this group being responsible for approximately 50% of rabies deaths,[33,55] the current 3-dose PrEP regimen is cost-prohibitive in endemic areas, even with the lower-cost intradermal method. A PrEP regimen that induces immunity with a single injection is needed.[36]

Numerous serologic studies have provided evidence of robust production of neutralizing antibody in response to cell culture–derived vaccines. Following the use of WHO-approved vaccines, 100% of healthy individuals were found to have a significant antibody response. No individuals with circulating neutralizing antibody levels above 0.5 IU/mL have ever contracted rabies.

Animal Bite Risk Assessment. An animal bite or potential rabies exposure is a medical urgency, not an emergency. In the emergency department, PEP is either administered at the time of presentation after consultation with public health authorities or is postponed until the rabies risk of the biting animal is determined (Table 119.3). Discharge instructions for patients with postponed PEP should reflect the on-going nature of the risk assessment. Because of periodic national shortages of vaccine and immune globulin used in PEP, clinicians should consult with local or state public health authorities and complete a risk assessment before administering internal stocks of PEP supplies.

Bats are responsible for the greatest number of rabies exposures in the United States.[38] Because of the difficulty in identifying the very small bite wounds created by bats, the CDC classifies all bats found indoors with a person who was asleep or incapacitated, or a bat found near an unattended child or an adult who cannot reliably attest to their

Decision tree for potential rabies exposure

Exposure = Confirmed or possible animal saliva or CNS tissue in contact with human broken skin or mucous membrane, or bat in a room with a child or sleeping/incapacitated adult

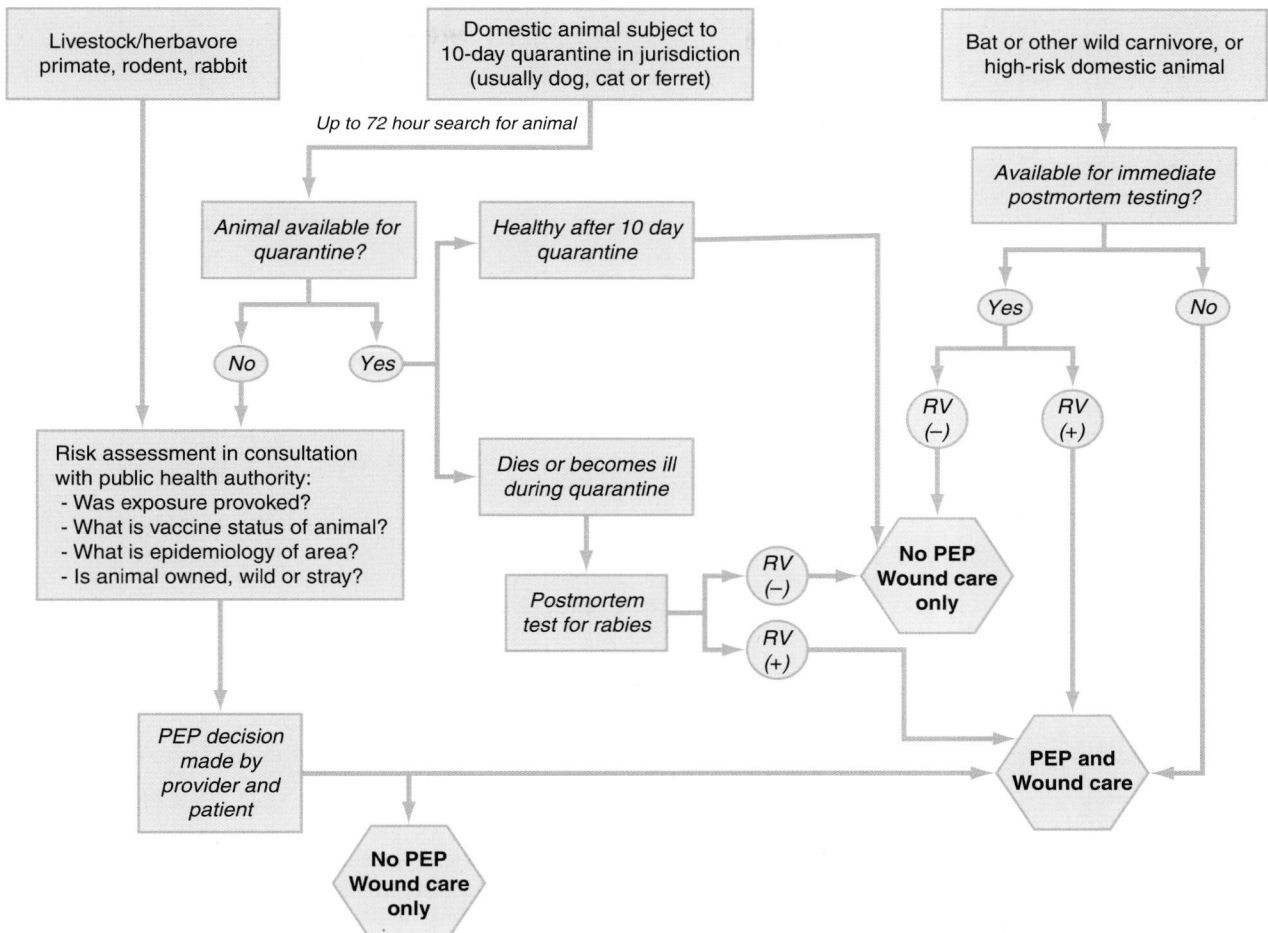

Fig. 119.12 Decision tree for potential rabies exposures.

physical contact with the bat, as an exposure. PEP is recommended under these conditions unless the bat is available for immediate testing and tests negative. In the United States, PEP always includes four doses of rabies vaccine and rabies immunoglobulin.[56]

Bites and exposure require a thorough history including geographic location where, when, and what type of exposure occurred (species, bite, scratch). Outside of the United States, WHO categorizes exposures in areas enzootic for rabies into three categories.[36] Category I includes touching or feeding animals, licks on intact skin, and contact of intact skin with secretions or excretions of a rabid animal or human. These are not regarded as significant exposures, and postexposure prophylaxis is not required. Category II includes nibbling of uncovered skin, minor scratches, or abrasions without bleeding. If these are caused by a bat, treat as category III. Vaccine should be injected as soon as possible, but RIG is not recommended for Category II. Category III includes single or multiple transdermal bites or scratches, licks on broken skin, contamination of mucous membrane with saliva from licks, and indoor exposure to bats. Category III contact requires full rabies prophylaxis including vaccine and rabies immunoglobulin.

Within the United States, most jurisdictions (state or local) require rabies vaccination of dogs and cats, and some require vaccination of pet ferrets. In addition, some livestock owners choose to vaccinate

their animals against rabies. These variations in vaccination implementation result in different postexposure treatment recommendations among state public health officials for humans bitten by domestic animals. Each state and territory maintains a contact phone number for consultation for potential rabies exposure. The list of contacts is available from the U.S. Centers for Disease Control and Prevention at www.cdc.gov/rabies or by calling the CDC's information line, 877-554-4625 or 800-CDC-INFO, 24 hours/day, 7 days/week. In addition to seeking consultation for PEP, in some jurisdictions, emergency medicine clinicians must comply with mandated reporting of PEP administration to public health authorities. Clinicians should be familiar with their local regulations. Clinicians are also mandatory reporters of animal bites to animal control authorities in many states and local jurisdictions. This bite reporting initiates the process of animal location and testing or quarantine.[35,54] These PEP and bite reporting requirements are not generally waived for people bitten by their own animals.

The only species for which the shedding period has been scientifically determined are the domestic dog, cat, and ferret. A 10-day quarantine, based on the viral shedding period, is used in lieu of postmortem testing to determine the rabies risk of domestic animals in geographic areas with high rates of vaccination. Quarantine establishes that if a dog, cat, or ferret is alive on the tenth day after biting

TABLE 119.3 Assessment of Rabies Exposure

Exposure	Rationale	Action/Timing
Bite by a wild terrestrial mammal other than small rodent or lagomorph	Rabies is abundant in wildlife and cross-species transmission occurs. Many small rodents and lagomorphs paralyze and die before salivary excretion of virus occurs.	Animal will be sacrificed and submit head to public health authorities to test brain for rabies. Urgent PEP pending test results[a] If animal unavailable for testing, prepare for PEP and consult public health authorities for risk assessment.
Unprovoked bite by a pet (dog, cat, or ferret)	Pet vaccination is imperfect. Cross-species transmission occurs. Incubation periods are well-defined.	Report to animal control authorities as required. Observation for 10 d[b,c] Urgent PEP if animal is determined to have rabies
Unprovoked bite by a domestic mammal (horse, cow, or other pet)	Vaccinations exist for horses, cattle, and sheep, but efficacy and incubation period are poorly defined.	Report the incident to the local public health department. The animal may be sacrificed and the head submitted for testing.[b] Urgent PEP pending test results.
Dog or cat brings fresh prey to their master.	Without direct bite by the prey, there is no human exposure. The dog or cat is exposed.	Refer the pet to a veterinarian for assessment and treatment.
Dog or cat brings dead, desiccated prey to their master.	Virus is rapidly inactivated by desiccation or sunlight—no exposure.	No action
Physical contact with a bat	Bat bites are hard to appreciate or find by examination. Most American deaths from bat rabies have no known exposure, so known exposure confers very high odds for death from rabies.	Animal will be sacrificed and submit for testing. If positive or if animal cannot be tested, urgent PEP
Bat seen in the same room as a responsible child (>6 y) or adult	Physical contact can be reliably excluded—no exposure	No action
Bat seen in the same room as a young child (<7 y),[d] sleeping, intoxicated or cognitively impaired person	Eight percent of bats found indoors are rabid. Physical contact CANNOT be reliably excluded—exposure occurred	Animal will be sacrificed and submit for testing. If positive or if animal cannot be tested, urgent PEP
Bat found in a room that was previously occupied or seen in a hallway or room adjacent to persons who cannot report physical contact with a bat.	Risk of undetected contact is substantially lower—no exposure	No action

WHO Expert Consultation on Rabies, third report: WHO Technical Series Report No. 1012. Geneva; 2018. ISBN 978-92-4-121021-8.

a human, it did not have virus *in its saliva* on the day of the bite.[57] All other species that potentially expose a human to rabies, including domestic-wild animal hybrids, must be evaluated on a case-by-case basis without quarantine.

Wound Care. All mammal bites require meticulous wound care, and if rabies prophylaxis is considered the initial wound care is critical. Rabies virus is very sensitive to sunlight, soap, and drying. When performed within 3 hours of inoculation, scrubbing and flushing with benzalkonium chloride, 20% soap solution, or Ivory soap is nearly 100% protective. Wounds from high-risk animals should be scrubbed with soap, water, and a virucidal agent (e.g., povidone-iodine) and then flushed with saline or water.[33] As with other mammalian bites, bacterial infection, cosmetic results, and tetanus prophylaxis need to be considered, but any indicated wound closure should be sutured loosely with delayed scar revision as needed. The bite location is a significant determinant of disease potential. Wounds to the face are at highest risk, as well as other highly vascular areas, including the head, neck, genitals, and hands.

Postexposure Prophylaxis. PEP is almost 100% effective when administered according to CDC or WHO guidelines. Treatment failures usually occur when local wound care is not complete, immunoglobulin is not given, or nerve cell–derived vaccine is used. No postexposure prophylaxis failures have occurred in the United States, but scattered reports worldwide do occur. These are typically associated with variance from the WHO PEP protocol.

Once the decision to initiate PEP has been made, it should be started immediately. Currently, WHO describes 6 different protocols using 2 different routes for postexposure treatment of unimmunized individuals, 4 intradermal and 2 intramuscular to accommodate clinical care settings and preferences in different countries.[36] In the United States, the CDC recommends the intramuscular route only and 4 vaccinations over 14 days[56] (Table 119.4). Both the CDC and WHO recommend an intramuscular dose of 1.0 mL/injection, and an intradermal dose of 0.1 mL. Effective intradermal injections must form a bleb at the site. Two vaccines are currently available in the United States, RabAvert (Novartis, Chiron Behring GmbH) and Imovax (Sanofi Pasteur).

The CDC Advisory Committee on Immunization Practices (ACIP) recommends the 4-dose vaccine schedule for postexposure prophylaxis in previously unvaccinated individuals.[58] This regimen should start as soon as possible after the exposure, day 0, and should then be followed by repeated doses on days 3, 7, and 14. The dose is 1 mL of vaccine administered intramuscularly. The deltoid is the preferred site for adults; the anterolateral thigh is the preferred site in children. There is a diminished immunologic response to gluteal injection of vaccine, so this site should be avoided. The intradermal vaccination regimes recommended by the WHO are shorter in duration, but require may require two ID injections at each visit.[59]

In addition to vaccination, in the United States, once a decision to start PEP is made, rabies immunoglobulin (RIG) should be given promptly in patients not previously vaccinated. WHO only

TABLE 119.4 Postexposure Vaccination Comparison of WHO and CDC Protocols

Vaccine Regimen	Protocol Organization	Number of Vaccinations per Clinic Visit (Days 0, 3, 7, 14, 21, 28)	Route
If no previous rabies vaccinations:			
1 week, 2 sites	WHO	2-2-2-0-0	Intradermal
2 week, 1 site	WHO	1-1-1-1-0	Intramuscular
3 weeks, 1 site	WHO	2-0-1-0-1	Intramuscular
1 month, 2 sites	WHO	2-2-2-0-2	Alternative Intradermal
1 month, 4 sites	WHO	4-0-2-0-1	Alternative Intradermal
1 week, 4 sites	WHO	4-4-4-0-0	Alternative Intradermal
2 weeks, 1 site	CDC	1-1-1-1-0	Intramuscular
If previously vaccinated: 1 day, 4 sites	WHO	4-0-0-0-0	Intradermal
If previously vaccinated:3 day, 2 sites	CDC	1-1-0-0-0	Intramuscular

Center for Disease Control and Prevention: Rabies Post Exposure Prophylaxis https://www.cdc.gov/rabies/medical_care/index.html. O'Brien KL, Nolan T, on behalf of the SAGE WG on Rabies. The WHO position on rabies immunization—2018 updates. *Vaccine.* 2019;37(Suppl 1): A85-A87. PMC [article]PMCID:PMC6863036. PMID:30342901DOI:10.1016/j.vaccine.2018.10.014.

recommends RIG for Category III wounds, which differs from US practice. RIG may be derived from equine or human sources (human rabies immunoglobulin). RIG inhibits viral spread during the interval when antibodies are produced in response to the rabies vaccine.[33] Human rabies immunoglobulin produced by Grifols (HyperRAB) is available, but equine immunoglobulin[60] or monoclonal antibodies to rabies may be necessary for passive immunization if human RIG is not available.[36] Human rabies immunoglobulin, 20 IU/kg, should be administered soon after the bite occurs and not more than 7 days after the first dose of rabies vaccine. As much RIG is injected into and around the wound site as the patient will tolerate, with the remainder injected intramuscularly at a distance from the vaccine administration site.

Adverse reactions to human RIG are common, but these are primarily local reactions. Pain, induration, swelling, and erythema have been reported in 30% to 100% of injections. Headache is the most common systemic reaction to HRIG occurring in more than 50% of recipients. No deaths have been reported from human RIG.

Postexposure vaccination for previously vaccinated individuals requires wound care and a 2-dose intramuscular vaccination (days 0 and 3) or 4-dose intradermal vaccination (all on day 0). RIG is not needed in previously vaccinated individuals who have received ACIP- or WHO-approved PrEP or PEP or other vaccinations with documented rabies virus–neutralizing antibody response.[56]

Outside the United States, RIG is in short supply, and some countries do not use WHO-approved vaccines.[61] Exposed travelers from these areas may require further vaccination on return to their native country, and it is imperative that providers clarify what patients have actually received in the originating country.

Management

Reversal of the disease process in rabies remains elusive. RABVs ability to evade neuro and humoral immune responses and cross the blood-brain barrier without causing axonal apoptosis, is not completely understood, but it results in neuronal dysfunction rather than neuronal death. Without a clear understanding of the pathogenesis of this disease, targeting treatment is difficult.

Regardless of new developments, management remains focused on palliative care. Because the vast majority of human rabies occurs in low-income and rural areas, one must be cognizant of the local medical capabilities, and the local culture. Care focuses on comfort through sedation, analgesia, and rehydration in a calm, draft-free environment.

The patient and family require support during the death process in a culturally sensitive manner. In resource-poor areas, the decision to initiate aggressive intensive care therapy should consider these factors: rabies vaccination prior to onset of disease, young age, rabies in previously healthy and immunocompetent individuals, initiation of treatment when neurologic signs are mild, New World bat variant rabies virus, and early detection of neutralizing anti–rabies virus antibodies in the serum and cerebrospinal fluid.[36]

Aggressive critical care management is rarely successful. In recent years, India reported survival in 6 individuals with aggressive therapy, but all suffered severe neurologic impairment.[62,63] Fifteen well-documented cases of survival with better cognitive outcomes were reported, but in all of these cases the patients had receive at least one preexposure vaccination.[45] The heralded Milwaukee Protocol, successful in treatment of a 15-year-old in Wisconsin in 2004, has not been replicated in spite of numerous attempts and should be abandoned.[64] Clinical trials for new protocols are limited. Thus, even in the ICU setting, sedation and analgesia with benzodiazepines, ketamine, haloperidol, and opiates remain the mainstay of therapy.

Disposition

Unfortunately, the survival of patients with rabies remains dismal and the disposition should focus on supportive therapy. Newer therapies may provide hope for patients in the future, but for now, prevention of canine rabies remains the single most important treatment for rabies and the best hope for eradication.

Arboviruses

Arboviruses are a group of viruses that are transmitted via arthropod vectors, generally mosquitoes and ticks. Encephalitis is a common manifestation of arboviral infection. Most of these viruses are primarily transmitted from the arthropod vector to another animal, and humans are only incidentally infected. The arboviral viruses that cause encephalitides belong to the following families: *Flaviviridae, Togaviridae, Bunyaviridae,* and *Reoviridae.*

St. Louis encephalitis virus, West Nile virus (WNV), Powassan virus, and Japanese encephalitis virus belong to the *Flaviviridae* family. Most of these viruses are maintained in a natural cycle of bird-mosquito-bird transmission. Given the mosquito vector, in North America and other temperate climates, these infections have a higher incidence in the summer months. WNV was popularized at the turn of the 20th century because of its first-time appearance in the western hemisphere. WNV emerged in New York City in 1999 and since then has spread to the Pacific coast, as far south as Argentina, and as far north as Canada. Now WNV is the leading cause of domestically acquired arboviral infection in the United States.[65] Powassan virus is maintained in a natural cycle of ticks to rodents. In Asia, Japanese encephalitis virus is the most prevalent cause of viral encephalitis with the greatest morbidity as well.

La Crosse virus and California encephalitis virus belong to the *Bunyaviridae* family. According to reports from the CDC, La Crosse virus is the most common cause of encephalitis among children in the United States.[65] Eastern equine encephalitis (EEE) virus, Western equine encephalitis virus, and Venezuelan equine encephalitis virus belong to the *Togaviridae* family and cause infections in certain parts of North and South America.

Clinical Features

Arboviral infections cause a wide range of presentations, including subclinical disease, nonspecific febrile illness, hemorrhagic fever, meningitis, acute flaccid paralysis, and severe encephalitis. Typically encephalitis patients begin with a nonspecific febrile illness accompanied by malaise, sore throat, and respiratory symptoms. Headache, photophobia, meningismus, lethargy, somnolence, and altered mental status will then follow. Severe disease can manifest as paralysis, coma, and seizures. Depending on the virus, it can be common for patients that recover to have some neurologic sequelae.

West Nile Virus. The majority of people who become infected with WNV are asymptomatic. The most common presentation of symptomatic WNV is West Nile fever, a self-limiting illness characterized by fever, headache, malaise, and myalgias. Patients can also experience gastrointestinal symptoms. Between a quarter to half of the patients can also have an accompanying maculopapular rash on the chest, back, and arms. It is estimated that around 1% of WNV causes neuroinvasive disease. The neuroinvasive disease manifests as meningitis, encephalitis, or flaccid paralysis. WNV neuroinvasive disease carries with it a 10% mortality rate. Age and immunosuppression have been identified as a risk factor for more severe neuroinvasive disease and mortality for WNV infections.[66]

Eastern Equine Encephalitis Virus. EEE virus is the most dangerous of the viruses that cause equine encephalitides. It occurs along the Gulf and Atlantic coast with predominance in the late summer months. The usual manifestation is fever, chills, headache, and myalgias lasting 1 to 2 weeks, typically followed by resolution. A small portion of patients will go on to develop encephalitis with headache, nausea, vomiting, altered mental status, and focal neurologic deficits. Approximately 2% to 6% of infected patients develop rapidly deteriorating severe encephalitis that results in coma. EEE virus infection that results in encephalitis is associated with 30% mortality.

St. Louis Encephalitis Virus. The majority of infections are asymptomatic, but as patients get older the rate of symptomatic infections increases dramatically. The incubation period varies from 4 to 21 days. Symptomatic disease presents as fever, myalgias, and headaches. Patients older than 60 frequently present with encephalitis, with mental status ranging from lethargy to coma. Acute flaccid paralysis occurs in approximately 6% of patients with encephalitis.

Powasson Virus. The infection usually presents as fever with neurologic complaints including headache, confusion, weakness, paralysis, lethargy, or even seizures. The mortality rate is near 10%, and survivors are often left with long-term neurologic impairment.

Differential Diagnosis

The diagnosis of arboviral encephalitis is difficult based on clinical presentation alone. It shares many features with other arboviral infections, other viral causes of encephalitis, bacterial meningitis, HSV encephalitis, leptospirosis, Lyme disease, and brain abscess.

Diagnostic Testing

The primary method of diagnosis is CSF analysis for serologic markers or PCR. WNV encephalitis is diagnosed by detecting IgM antibody in CSF. Viral culture is not commonly used for these diagnoses. There is often a broad differential diagnosis when evaluating these patients, so it is crucial to elicit travel and potential exposure history to narrow the differential diagnosis. When performing a lumbar puncture, it can be helpful to obtain an extra tube or vial of CSF to put on hold. This extra CSF sample is useful because testing for arboviral infections is often sent after the initial evaluation, assessing for more common etiologies of neurologic infection, such as bacterial meningitis or HSV encephalitis, is completed. CSF demonstrates an elevated WBC count with lymphocyte predominance. Early during a WNV infection there may be a neutrophil predominance. Ancillary testing with CT or MRI may be indicated, depending on the severity of neurologic symptoms.

Management

The treatment for these entities remains largely symptomatic. There is no specific antiviral therapy or immunoglobulin treatment with proven benefit. In patients that develop cerebral edema, the therapies focus on preventing secondary brain injury and treatment of cerebral edema by maintaining adequate cerebral perfusion pressure, treating seizures, and avoiding hypoxemia, high fever, and hypoglycemia or hyperglycemia (see Chapter 4).

Disposition

Patients with neurologic symptoms should be admitted to the hospital. These patients often require neurology and infectious disease specialists to consult in their care. Arboviral infections are reportable diseases. Long-term outcomes for these patients can vary. Full recovery can usually be expected in patients with WNV meningitis. WNV encephalitis patients often have residual effects, with over half of them reporting some type of persistent symptoms (fatigue, muscle aches, decreased activity, memory difficulty, concentration difficulty) beyond 6 months.[67]

Other Arboviral Infections

Dengue Virus

Dengue is the most common virus in the *Flaviviridae* family to cause human infection. It can be found all over the world, with most infections occurring in Southeast Asia, the Western Pacific, and Central and South America. It is one of the most important causes of fever in the returned traveler. It is transmitted via the mosquito vector, *Aedes aegypti* and *Aedes albopictus,* and humans are the natural host.

Clinical Features. Dengue can cause a wide spectrum of disease. Many infected individuals with dengue are asymptomatic. Dengue fever is a self-limited illness characterized by fever, headache, retro-orbital pain, severe myalgias, and arthralgias. Symptoms can last up to 1 week. Dengue hemorrhagic fever (DHF), a more severe syndrome, occurs when the following four criteria are present: (1) increased vascular permeability (pleural effusion, ascites, hemoconcentration), (2) thrombocytopenia, (3) fever lasting 2 to 7 days, and (4) hemorrhagic tendency or spontaneous bleeding. Dengue shock syndrome (DSS), the most severe presentation of dengue infection, is present when DHF occurs with circulatory shock.

Differential Diagnosis. Other diagnoses to consider in suspected dengue patients include Zika, malaria, chikungunya, rickettsial infections, leptospirosis, and other viral hemorrhagic fevers, including Ebola, Marburg, yellow fever, or bunyaviruses. It is also important to consider the diagnosis of measles in a returned febrile traveler with a rash, because many countries that have endemic dengue also have endemic measles.

Diagnostic Testing. The diagnosis can be made via serologic testing with IgM assay, antigen testing of the viral antigen nonstructural protein 1 (NS1), or viral RNA detection with RT-PCR. Early in the course the IgM is often negative. Other laboratory findings that may be present with dengue infection include leukopenia, thrombocytopenia, elevated hematocrit (due to hemoconcentration from fluid loss), and abnormal liver function tests. In DHF, coagulopathy can be present.

Management. There are no specific antiviral agents that treat dengue. The treatment is mainly supportive. Dengue fever is usually a self-limited illness and can be treated with rest, antipyretics, analgesics, and fluid replacement therapy. Nonsteroidal antiinflammatory drugs and aspirin should be avoided given the bleeding tendencies associated with these medications. Patients with DHF and DSS require close monitoring, IV fluid replacement therapy, and organ support as indicated. Hemorrhagic sequelae are treated with blood product transfusions as needed. Steroid therapy for severe dengue has been evaluated in several low-quality studies, but the evidence to date is inconclusive, and steroid treatment cannot be recommended at this time. The control of epidemics revolves around reducing the mosquito vector population and preventing humans from being bitten by mosquitoes.

Disposition. Depending on the severity of illness, patients with dengue fever can be treated as outpatients, but some may require admission for rehydration therapy. Patients with DHF will require admission to the hospital for monitoring and IV fluid resuscitation, and patients with DSS will require admission to the ICU.

Zika Virus. Zika virus is an arbovirus in the *Flaviviridae* family that is transmitted to humans via the *Aedes* species mosquitos. Although transmission is predominantly from mosquitos, there have been reports of perinatal, in utero, sexual, and blood product transfusion–related transmission as well. In 2016 there was a large uptake in cases reported in the United States. Over 5000 cases of Zika virus were reported, with most travelers returning from Zika endemic regions.[68] Over 200 cases were reported from local transmission within the United States. Although the case fatality is low, Zika virus infection during pregnancy has been linked to severe congenital anomalies including microcephaly and other neurologic defects. This has led to the CDC issuing travel advisories to avoid Zika endemic regions for pregnant women, women planning on pregnancy, men with a pregnant partner, or men with a partner planning pregnancy.

Clinical Features. The majority of patients infected with Zika virus are asymptomatic. For those who do develop symptoms, the clinical manifestations include maculopapular rash, fever, nonpurulent conjunctivitis, headache, retro-orbital pain, myalgias, arthralgias, and vomiting. The most commonly reported symptom is an erythematous maculopapular rash (Fig. 119.13).[69] The course of the disease is typically mild with resolution within 2 weeks. Although rare, Zika infection has been associated with a variety of neurologic complications, including Guillain-Barré syndrome, meningoencephalitis, and myelitis.[70,71]

Differential Diagnosis. Other diseases with fever, rash, myalgias, and travel history should be considered, including dengue, chikungunya, malaria, rickettsial infections, leptospirosis, measles, rubella, and meningococcal disease.

Diagnostic Testing. The diagnosis of Zika virus infection can be made with RT-PCR or serology. In nonpregnant symptomatic patients with symptoms for less than 7 days, serum RT-PCR is the preferred method for diagnosis. If symptoms are present for more than 7 days, then serology is the preferred method. In pregnant symptomatic patients, RT-PCR and IgM antibody testing on a serum specimen and RT-PCR on a urine specimen are recommended.[72] It is important to

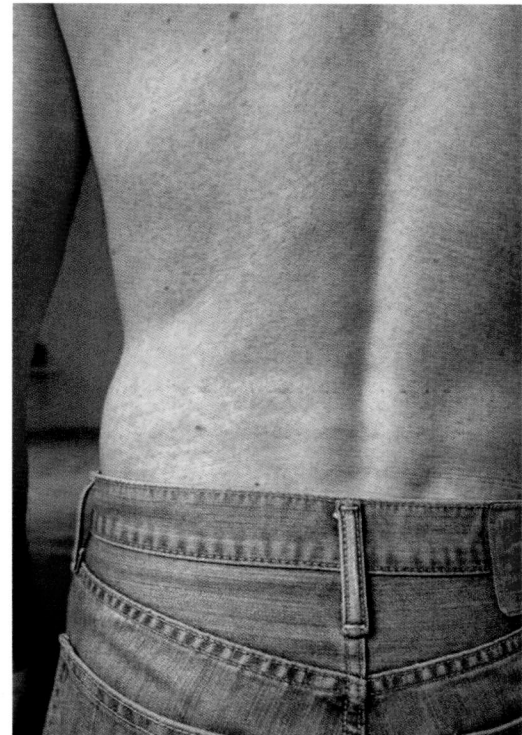

Fig. 119.13 Typical rash associated with Zika virus. (Courtesy of CDC website: https://phil.cdc.gov/Details.aspx?pid=21385)

test for dengue as well, as there is significant overlap in symptoms. Obtaining a CBC in severely symptomatic patients can be useful because significant thrombocytopenia has been reported in Zika infections.[73]

Management and Disposition. Similar to other flavivirus infections, treatment largely consists of symptom management and supportive care. Antipyretics, analgesics, and hydration are the cornerstone of management. Acetaminophen is the agent of choice. If there is concern for severe thrombocytopenia or dengue infection, aspirin and NSAIDs should be avoided. Most of these patients can be discharged, and treatment can continue at home. Pregnant patients should have definite follow-up with their OB/GYN providers, given the risk of fetal anomalies. Typically, this follow-up will entail psychosocial support as well

Chikungunya Virus. Chikungunya is an arbovirus in the *Alphaviridae* family that was originally endemic to West Africa. Since early this millennium, the infection has spread broadly, responsible for multiple outbreaks in Asia, Europe, and the Indian subcontinent. In 2013, local transmission was identified in the Americas for the first time. The vectors are the same as dengue, the *Aedes aegypti* and *Aedes albopictus* mosquitoes.

Clinical Features. Chikungunya causes a self-limiting disease very similar to dengue. Fever, myalgias, and polyarthralgias are the hallmark of this disease. The joint pain can be so severe that ambulation is impaired. Symptoms typically last for 7 to 10 days. More than half of infected individuals develop a maculopapular rash several days after fever onset. Risk factors for severe disease with higher mortality include age older than 65, diabetes, and underlying cardiopulmonary disorders.

Differential Diagnosis. Other febrile illnesses with rash, myalgias, and arthralgias should be considered, including dengue, Zika, malaria, African tick bite fever, leptospirosis, measles, rubella, relapsing fever,

EBV, and meningococcal disease. Noninfectious disorders such as adult-onset Still disease and other rheumatologic disorders should also be considered.

Diagnostic Testing. The diagnosis can be confirmed via enzyme-linked immunosorbent assay (ELISA) testing for antibodies, RT-PCR for detecting viral RNA, or viral culture. Lab abnormalities associated with acute infection include abnormal liver function tests, thrombocytopenia, and lymphopenia.

Management and Disposition. Treatment is mainly supportive. Antipyretics, antiinflammatory agents, and analgesics play an important role in symptom control. IV fluids may be necessary, depending on disease severity. Prevention of disease centers on reducing mosquito exposure. Most patients can be treated at home. Patients that present with severe disease may require admission for IV hydration and observation until they are stable.

VIRAL HEMORRHAGIC FEVERS

Yellow Fever Virus

Yellow fever virus is an arbovirus in the *Flaviviridae* family that can cause a viral hemorrhagic fever. Prior to the discovery of its mosquito vector transmission, there were multiple yellow fever epidemics in Africa, Europe, and the Americas. The vector is the *Aedes* or *Haemagogus* mosquito. Vector control and development of a vaccine have significantly reduced the burden of this disease over the past several decades. Currently yellow fever occurs in tropical regions of Africa and South America.

Clinical Features

The incubation period is between 3 to 6 days. Patients present with an acute febrile illness accompanied by chills, malaise, headache, myalgias, nausea, and dizziness. Patients can have a much lower heart rate than expected in reference to the high fever that is present. This acute febrile phase of the illness can last between 3 to 6 days. Patients then experience a short period of remission, lasting up to 24 hours; some patients recover completely, whereas others go on to have a more severe recurrence of illness with fever, vomiting, jaundice, acute liver injury, acute renal failure, and hemorrhagic manifestations. The hallmark feature of yellow fever is jaundice with hemorrhagic fever. The mortality of patients with hepatorenal involvement ranges from 20 to 50%.

Differential Diagnosis

One must consider other febrile illnesses that occur in these endemic areas, including leptospirosis, relapsing fever, viral hepatitis, malaria, and other viral hemorrhagic fevers, including dengue.

Diagnostic Testing

Laboratory diagnosis is usually made by detecting IgM and neutralizing antibodies in the serum. There are a number of laboratory abnormalities that occur in this illness, including elevated aspartate transaminase (AST), alanine transaminase (ALT), and direct bilirubin. Patients with severe disease also have hematologic labs consistent with disseminated intravascular coagulation (DIC).

Management

There are no specific antiviral treatments for yellow fever. The treatment is supportive. Fluids, antipyretics, and analgesia are the main symptomatic treatments. Given the risk of hemorrhagic fever, aspirin and nonsteroidal antiinflammatory drugs should generally be avoided. If severe disease with shock develops, patients may require IV fluid resuscitation, blood product resuscitation, vasopressors, mechanical ventilation, and renal replacement therapy.

Because there is no specific treatment for yellow fever, much attention has been placed on prevention. Personal protection measures to avoid mosquito bites and vector control at the community level are important in preventing disease. The live-virus vaccine is recommended for individuals 9 months old and older who live in or are traveling to endemic areas. Many countries where yellow fever is endemic require a certificate of vaccination for entry.

Disposition

Depending on the severity of illness, patients can be treated at home or may require admission to the hospital. Severe illness may require ICU admission given the high mortality associated with severe forms of yellow fever.

Ebola

Ebola virus is an RNA virus that belongs to the *Filoviridae* family. Ebola virus disease (EVD) causes severe viral hemorrhagic fever. Ebola was first described in 1976 in Sudan and what is now the Democratic Republic of the Congo (Zaire at that time). Since then, there have been several outbreaks occurring in rural areas in Africa. The 2014 to 2016 Ebola outbreak in West Africa was the most severe in history. It began March 2014 in Guinea and then spread to Sierra Leone and Liberia. Nigeria, Senegal, and Mali have also been affected. At the close of this outbreak, 28,652 cases were identified, and 11,325 lives were claimed.[74] Prior to this outbreak, the largest recorded outbreak had resulted in fewer than 300 deaths. This outbreak also resulted in the first cases of Ebola acquired outside of Africa. A nurse assistant in Spain acquired the disease after caring for an Ebola patient transported from Sierra Leone to Spain. Subsequently, two nurses contracted Ebola in the United States after caring for an Ebola patient who contracted the virus in Liberia.[75]

The mortality rate for Ebola infections ranges from 25% to 90%. Transmission of the virus occurs by direct contact of infected tissue or infected bodily fluids, including blood, saliva, vomit, feces, or semen. Individuals are not contagious until they show symptoms. The usual incubation time is 5 to 7 days but can range from 2 to 21 days.

Clinical Features

The initial symptoms include high fever, headache, myalgias, malaise, sore throat, and profuse vomiting and diarrhea. After 5 to 7 days, patients can progress to develop the hemorrhagic manifestations, which include spontaneous bleeding, ecchymosis, and petechia. It is also common for patients to not develop any hemorrhagic complications.[76] An erythematous maculopapular rash can occur during that time that eventually desquamates. Patients can become hypovolemic and develop severe metabolic derangements secondary to fluid losses via the gastrointestinal tract. Eventually patients advance to shock and multiorgan failure.

Differential Diagnosis

The symptoms of Ebola are initially nonspecific and overlap with other diseases. Other more common infections from the endemic regions include malaria, typhoid fever, other viral hemorrhagic fevers (i.e., Marburg, bunyaviruses), meningococcemia, leptospirosis, or other bacterial illnesses.

Diagnostic Testing

Testing should only be conducted for patients that meet clinical criteria of having exposure history *and* signs or symptoms of EVD. The hospital should also have a protocol for handling lab specimens of potential EVD patients. The risk of acquiring EVD through lab testing is low but not zero. RT-PCR assay using a plasma specimen is currently the main method of Ebola diagnosis. A rapid antigen point-of-care test with a turnaround time of 15 minutes has been developed with good sensitivity and specificity as compared to RT-PCR.[77] Laboratory findings that can accompany Ebola infection include thrombocytopenia, anemia, coagulopathy, transaminitis, elevated creatinine, hypocalcemia, and hypokalemia. All patients should have testing for malaria performed with thin and thick smear of the blood. Malaria is much more likely than Ebola in the endemic population and returned travelers. Coinfection is also common; in one study of Ebola patients in Guinea, 11% of the patients had concomitant malaria infection.[76]

Management

When managing a suspected EVD case, the important guiding principles are to treat the patient and prevent the spread of the infection. The CDC has developed practical algorithms for evaluating suspected EVD cases in United States EDs (www.cdc.gov/vhf/ebola/pdf/ed-algorithm-management-patients-possible-ebola.pdf). The basic tenets are to identify, isolate, and inform.

The main therapy for Ebola victims is supportive care. Patients are empirically managed with malaria treatment, broad-spectrum antibiotics, and antipyretics. They also require rehydration therapy, preferably with IV fluid and electrolyte repletion. Additionally, many EVD patients require support for organ failure, including renal replacement therapy, mechanical ventilation, vasopressors, or blood product administration.

Currently there are no clinically proven medical therapies against EVD. A number of therapies have been investigated, including monoclonal antibodies against Ebola viral antigens, convalescent plasma, and nucleotide analogue antiviral drugs. Unfortunately, many of these therapies have not shown clinical efficacy in studies.[78,79] The most promising therapies to date are a single monoclonal antibody, MAb114, and a triple monoclonal antibody, REGN-EB3.[80] Although specific therapies against Ebola are currently limited, a landmark breakthrough for the public health response was reached in 2019 when the FDA approved the first vaccine for prevention of EVD.[81]

Disposition

It is paramount that providers caring for potential EVD patients be familiar with proper isolation practices. The CDC stresses that health care providers should receive extensive training and demonstrate competency in Ebola-related infection control procedures, specifically in putting on and removing the PPE. Many hospitals have developed internal guidelines, but the CDC website is a useful resource and gives comprehensive guidance regarding how to deal with potential EVD patients in the United States health care setting (www.cdc.gov/vhf/ebola/healthcare-us/index.html).

The CDC has also developed a strategy to help hospitals prepare for suspected EVD cases (www.cdc.gov/vhf/ebola/pdf/preparing-hospitals-ebola.pdf). There is a tiered system categorized by frontline health care facilities, Ebola assessment hospitals, and then Ebola treatment centers. All hospitals should have and follow infection control protocols, ensure that staff is trained and competent in safe PPE practices, and have a system to manage waste disposal, cleaning, and disinfection. Patients with suspected EVD are admitted to hospital isolation rooms, and many of them will need ICU care. The mortality of EBV is high, but patients are likely to have much better outcomes than previously reported with access to medical facilities with ICUs. Of note, the Ebola patients treated in Europe and the United States had a mortality rate of 18.5%, much lower than reported in endemic regions.[82]

Marburg

Marburg virus is an RNA virus that belongs to the *Filoviridae* family. It is an important cause of viral hemorrhagic fever in central Africa.

Marburg cases have occurred in Uganda, Zimbabwe, the Democratic Republic of the Congo, Kenya, and Angola. Cases have been reported outside Africa, including Germany, the former Yugoslavia, Netherlands, and the United States, all with confirmed exposure to an African source. The virus was described first in 1967 after an outbreak occurred in Marburg, Germany, when laboratory personnel working with African Green monkeys developed fever and hemorrhagic shock. Direct transmission occurs with contact with blood, secretions, or solid organs of infected individuals. It is currently thought that the natural host of the Marburg virus is the African fruit bat. The incubation period is 3 to 9 days. The disease carries a similar fatality rate to Ebola, with case fatality rate ranging from 24% to 88%.

Clinical Features

Marburg and Ebola virus cause a very similar clinical syndrome. Marburg virus illness initially causes fever, headache, malaise, and myalgias. After the third to fifth day, severe abdominal pain, cramping, vomiting, and diarrhea occurs. Around the same time, a maculopapular rash may develop. Half of the patients will also develop hemorrhagic manifestations during this time. Hematemesis, diarrhea, oropharyngeal bleeding, and bleeding from venipuncture sites can all occur. Death usually occurs because of acute blood loss and septic shock.

Differential Diagnosis

The differential diagnosis of Marburg infection is very similar to that of Ebola infection in that the symptoms are initially nonspecific and overlap with other diseases. Other more common infections from the endemic regions include malaria, typhoid fever, other viral hemorrhagic fevers (i.e., Marburg, bunyaviruses), meningococcemia, leptospirosis, or other bacterial illnesses.

Diagnostic Testing

Diagnosis requires laboratory testing, because the clinical features overlap with many other viral hemorrhagic fevers. Diagnosis can be made via RT-PCR, ELISA, antigen detection tests, serum neutralization tests, and viral culture.

Management

The priorities of managing a suspected Marburg hemorrhagic fever (MHF) case are similar to a suspected EVD case. Early recognition is key for controlling the spread of this infection. It is important to consider this disease in potential patients by assessing the patient for travel history to countries with endemic MHF or contact with someone who has had MHF within the past 3 weeks and then assessing if symptoms consistent with MHF are present. Patients identified at risk by the screening process should be isolated to a private room with private bathroom. Public health authorities and hospital infection control personnel should be immediately informed. Please refer to the Ebola section of this chapter for further details.

There is no specific treatment for MHF. The treatment is mainly supportive and directed at the patient's symptoms. Patients initially require large fluid volume resuscitation and antipyretics. Patients who develop end-organ failure need advanced therapies, such as vasopressors, mechanical ventilation, and renal replacement therapy. Patients with hemorrhagic manifestations also require blood product resuscitation with packed red blood cells (PRBCs) and fresh frozen plasma.

Disposition

Patients with MHF require hospital admission, and many will require ICU admission. It is important to observe strict isolation practices and ensure that staff use PPE when caring for the patient. When appropriate, patients should be transferred to specialized treatment centers that are prepared for and designated to care for patients with viral hemorrhagic fevers.

Lassa Fever

Lassa virus is an *Arenavirus* that is endemic to West Africa. Its reservoir is the African rodent *Mastomys natalensis*. Humans contract the disease by exposure to urine or feces of *Mastomys natalensis*. Human-to-human transmission can occur via contact with blood or bodily secretions from infected humans. The incubation period is usually around 10 days, but can range from 3 to 21 days. Unlike Ebola and Marburg, the majority of Lassa infections are asymptomatic. The case fatality rate is less than 2%.

Clinical Features

When patients are symptomatic with Lassa fever, symptoms usually begin with gradual onset of fever and malaise. Headache, myalgias, sore throat, cough, chest pain, abdominal pain, nausea, vomiting, and diarrhea can all occur after a few days. Patients can also develop facial edema, pleural effusion, myocarditis, and encephalitis. Less than 20% of symptomatic patients progress to develop hemorrhagic manifestations. Patients that do go on to have full-blown hemorrhagic fever have a much higher mortality rate. Third-trimester pregnancy is associated with more severe disease with higher mortality as well.

Differential Diagnosis

The differential diagnosis is broad and includes that of other viral hemorrhagic fevers.

Diagnostic Testing

Diagnosis on clinical grounds alone is difficult, because Lassa fever shares features with many other diseases. Diagnosis can be made via RT-PCR, ELISA, antigen detection tests, and viral culture.

Management

Ribavirin has been shown to decrease overall mortality. The greatest effect occurs when treatment is initiated early within the first 6 days after fever onset. The remainder of treatment is supportive care with volume resuscitation, antipyretics, and blood product administration if hemorrhagic disease occurs. As with other viral hemorrhagic fevers, organ failure support with mechanical ventilation, vasopressors, and dialysis may also be needed. Although high-quality evidence does not exist, guidelines do recommend ribavirin as postexposure prophylaxis for definitive high-risk exposures.[83] Prevention of Lassa fever at the community level centers on good hygiene and rodent control.

Disposition

Symptomatic patients with Lassa fever require hospital admission. The same principles of the other viral hemorrhagic fevers of prompt recognition, identification, isolation, and informing authorities apply to Lassa fever as well. Please refer to the sections in this chapter on Ebola and Marburg for more details.

The references for this chapter can be found online at ExpertConsult.com.

120

Coronaviruses

Raghu Seethala and Sukhjit S. Takhar

KEY CONCEPTS

- Coronaviruses infect humans and animals and have the ability for recombination, generating novel viruses.
- Most human coronaviruses cause mild disease. Three coronaviruses, severe acute respiratory syndrome (SARS) associated virus, Middle East respiratory syndrome (MERS), and severe acute respiratory syndrome coronavirus 2 (SARS-CoV-2), have caused severe disease in humans.
- The hallmark presentation of severe disease in coronavirus patients is respiratory failure, usually manifesting as acute respiratory distress syndrome (ARDS).
- Public health measures, including social distancing, wearing face masks, limiting social gatherings, and vaccinations, remain integral to controlling the COVID-19 pandemic.
- The vast majority of children have a benign disease course. However, a small number may develop a severe hyperinflammatory illness called multisystem inflammatory syndrome in children (MIS-C).
- Treatment for COVID-19 is rapidly evolving with the available data. Management of nonsevere illness is largely supportive and can occur at home. Treatment of moderate to severe disease occurs in the hospital and focuses on supporting oxygenation and ventilation. These patients may benefit from antiviral and corticosteroid therapies. At this point, the remainder of therapeutics remain mostly investigational.

FOUNDATIONS

Coronaviruses (CoVs) are pathogens that cause a variety of human and veterinary diseases. Seven members of the coronavirus family infect humans, and three lethal CoVs have crossed species barriers over the last twenty years as the causative agents of severe acute respiratory syndrome (SARS), Middle East respiratory syndrome (MERS), and coronavirus disease 2019 (COVID-19). Two (SARS-CoV and MERS-CoV) have caused dangerous epidemics. Severe acute respiratory syndrome coronavirus 2 (SARS-CoV-2), the cause of COVID-19, was identified as the causative pathogen in a cluster of unusual pneumonia cases in Wuhan, China, in late 2019, leading to a worldwide pandemic with profound social, economic, and political consequences.[1] As of late December 2020, it has infected over 77 million and killed over 1,700,000 people globally with continued rapid spread.[2] Advances in molecular biology have increased our knowledge of these infections and have contributed to the massive scale-up of testing, development, and distribution of vaccines at an unprecedented pace. At the time of this chapter's writing, several SARS-CoV-2 vaccines are being distributed in a massive worldwide campaign.

Severe acute respiratory syndrome–coronavirus (SARS-CoV), resulting in SARS, is a virulent coronavirus that first appeared in China in November 2002. SARS affected at least 8098 individuals in 29 countries across Asia, Europe, and North and South America. Most of the cases were from China and Hong Kong, with a mortality rate near 10%. As the last reported case of SARS occurred in 2003, SARS will be discussed only briefly in this chapter.

In 2012, another novel coronavirus, *Middle East respiratory syndrome–coronavirus (MERS-CoV)*, emerged, causing international concern. The majority of cases have been reported from Saudi Arabia and the United Arab Emirates, but cases have been reported in the United States, Europe, and Asia. All reported cases have been associated with direct or indirect exposure to travel or residence in the following countries: Saudi Arabia, the United Arab Emirates, Qatar, Jordan, Oman, Kuwait, Yemen, Lebanon, and Iran. MERS is still circulating in the animal population in the Middle East, causing intermittent, sporadic cases and community clusters.[3]

Coronaviruses (CoVs) are large and spherical, enveloped positive-sense RNA viruses. The virus has four major structural proteins: membrane protein (M), envelope protein (E), nucleocapsid protein (N), and the spike protein (S) (Fig. 120.1). The spike protein gives the virus its characteristic look, binds with human cells, and is also the target of novel vaccines.

SARS-CoV-2, SARS-CoV, and MERS-CoV typically cause severe disease, whereas the other human coronaviruses (HCoVs)—HKU1, NL63, OC43, and 229E—are associated with mild illness. HCoVs cause about 15% of all colds (Table 120.1).

SARS-CoV-2 is under the genus beta-coronavirus, which includes a diverse group isolated from bats. Natural selection rather than laboratory manipulation is almost certainly the origin of SARS-CoV-2.[4] Potentially, this pathogen arose from genetic reassortment. The sizeable genetic composition, along with the possibility of reassortment, increases the probability of novel coronaviruses emerging.

Transmission

Knowledge of the transmission of SARS-CoV-2 continues to evolve. Person-to-person transmission occurs primarily during close contact with an individual infected with SARS-CoV-2 via respiratory droplets. These respiratory droplets, produced by sneezing, coughing, or even talking, can land on mucous membranes, starting the infective process. Transmission is much less likely to occur through contact with contaminated surfaces. The evidence that SARS-CoV-2 is spreading via aerosols in the community is mixed, and droplet transmission is likely much more important than the aerosol route. Transmission is highly overdispersed—80% of secondary infections arose from 8.9% of index cases.[5] Nasal viral concentration is usually highest in early and presymptomatic disease, and patients are most infectious during this time. Asymptomatic and presymptomatic spread of the virus has contributed to the difficulty in controlling outbreaks; asymptomatic or

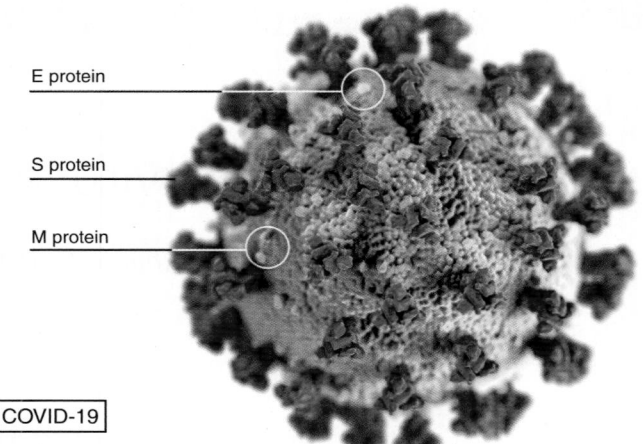

Fig. 120.1 Illustration of morphology exhibited by coronaviruses. Spikes are the S protein. (Courtesy of CDC website: https://phil.cdc.gov/Details.aspx?pid=23313.)

TABLE 120.1   Coronaviruses

Virus	Representative Disease	Clinical Features
SARS-CoV	SARS	Fevers, malaise, myalgias, chills, rigors, cough, dyspnea, tachypnea, pleuritic pain, ARDS
MERS-CoV	MERS	Fever, cough, dyspnea, sore throat, myalgias, GI symptoms, ARDS
SARS-CoV-2	COVID-19	Cough, fevers, chills, dyspnea, headaches, myalgias, diarrhea, nausea, anosmia, ageusia, ARDS
NL63, OC43, HKU1,229E	"Common cold"	Sore throat, rhinorrhea, nasal congestion, cough

presymptomatic individuals may cause as many as 50% of cases.[6-8] The duration of infectious viral shedding is unclear. Prolonged detection of viral RNA by PCR has been observed but does not necessarily mean that patients are infectious.[5] Patients are rarely contagious 10 days after symptom onset. However, those who are immune-compromised and those with severe disease can be contagious for much longer.[9] SARS-CoV-2 RNA has been detected in stool, blood, semen, and ocular secretions, but transmission via these routes is unlikely.

In health care settings, respiratory (either droplet or airborne) and contact precautions are recommended for COVID-19 patient contacts, with surgical or N95 mask, eye protection, gown, and gloves. Aerosolization can occur during certain procedures such as intubation or noninvasive ventilation. An N95 mask, powered air-purifying respirator (PAPR), or equivalent respirator, is recommended for aerosolizing procedures.

Emergency departments should screen patients with symptoms suggestive of COVID-19 so appropriate precautions can be quickly initiated. Because of the risk of asymptomatic spread during the pandemic, all persons entering medical facilities (both patients and visitors) should be masked. Persons in waiting areas and lines should be situated to maintain an adequate distance of 2 meters or more from each other. Health care workers should also be masked in the workplace to decrease the risk of asymptomatic spread to co-workers during the pandemic. In most health care settings, severe restrictions have been placed on patient visitors and accompanying family members.

MERS virus has a high mortality rate and shares many features with SARS-CoV. The mode of transmission has not been elucidated fully, but the most likely route is via direct droplet transmission. There have been case reports of transmission in the health care setting via a less than 10-minute encounter, maintaining 3 feet distance, but without any personal protective equipment (PPE). On the other hand, investigations have also revealed minimal transmission among close contacts at home, indicating that the viral load is higher in those who are more ill and in the hospital. In MERS and SARS, patients become more infectious as the illness progresses through the initial phase as viral replication increases. This contrasts with the early replication and infectivity of SARS-CoV-2, which makes the eradication of COVID-19 much more difficult.

CLINICAL FEATURES

Coronavirus Disease 2019

The incubation period for SARS-CoV-2 is up to 14 days from the time of exposure with a median of 4 to 5 days.[10] Patients present with a spectrum of illness, from minimally symptomatic, to a nonspecific influenza-like illness, with some developing a severe form requiring mechanical ventilation. Initial reports from China show 81% of individuals had mild or moderate disease, 14% had severe disease, and 5% were critical.[11] The most common presenting symptoms for patients who require medical care are cough, fevers or chills, and shortness of breath. Headaches, myalgias, diarrhea, and nausea also commonly occur. Anosmia and ageusia are also often reported.

Patients often worsen as the illness progresses, with a median time to dyspnea of 5 days after initial symptoms and acute respiratory distress syndrome (ARDS) occurring a few days after this.[12] Severe disease can occur in anyone, with the highest risk of fatal outcomes in people aged 65 years or older and those living in a nursing home or long-term care facility. Others at higher risk include those with comorbid conditions such as hypertension, cardiovascular disease, diabetes, chronic respiratory disease, cancers, renal disease, and obesity.[12] The COVID-19 pandemic has highlighted the disparities along several social determinants of health, including race, ethnicity, and socioeconomic status. Thrombotic complications are described in COVID-19 patients, leading to acute kidney injury, stroke, deep vein thrombosis, and pulmonary embolism.

Multisystem Inflammatory Syndrome in Children

Most children with COVID-19 infection have mild symptoms. Clinicians in the United Kingdom reported previously healthy children who presented with cardiovascular shock, fever, and hyper inflammation, which was later called multisystem inflammatory syndrome in children (MIS-C) (Box 120.1).[13] MIS-C has been reported to occur weeks after initial COVID-19 infection. MIS-C is also frequently associated with some degree of cardiac dysfunction. Cases of multisystem inflammatory syndromes have been reported in adults as well (MIS-A).[14] Features of MIS-C and MIS-A include cardiac dysfunction, abdominal pain, significantly elevated inflammatory markers, including C-reactive protein (CRP), D-dimer, ferritin, and interleukin-6. MIS-A is distinguished from severe COVID-19 by having minimal respiratory symptoms, hypoxemia, or radiographic abnormalities.

Severe Acute Respiratory Syndrome and Middle East Respiratory Syndrome

SARS and MERS both initially cause high fevers, malaise, myalgias, chills, and rigors. As with COVID-19, initial symptoms can be followed by cough, shortness of breath, tachypnea, and pleuritic pain. The reported incubation time for MERS-CoV is between 2 to 14 days, with a median incubation of 7 days.[3] MERS can rapidly deteriorate to acute respiratory failure. Close to half of the patients evaluated in the hospital setting will require ICU admission. Similar to COVID-19, age, diabetes mellitus, and other chronic health problems are risk factors for poor prognosis.

Sore throat and fever were less commonly manifested in SARS, and diarrhea can occur later in the course of the disease. About one-third of patients will have improvement in symptoms after the initial febrile illness. Approximately 20% to 30% go on to require mechanical ventilation secondary to hypoxemia. Severe respiratory failure, sepsis, and multiorgan failure are the common causes of death in these patients. Risk factors for mortality include age older than 60 years old, the presence of diabetes mellitus, and heart disease.

DIFFERENTIAL DIAGNOSES

The less severe, more common coronaviruses have similar presentations to the other benign upper respiratory tract infections like rhinovirus, adenovirus, parainfluenza, and other viral causes of upper respiratory infection (URI). For SARS, MERS, and COVID-19, other diagnoses to consider include bacterial pneumonia, influenza, other viral pneumonias, or other causes of ARDS.

DIAGNOSTIC TESTING

Coronavirus Disease 2019

The most common test for the diagnosis of COVID-19 is the reverse transcriptase-polymerase chain reaction (RT-PCR) test of nasopharyngeal (NP), mid-turbinate, or anterior nasal swabs.[15] The true sensitivity and specificity of available tests is difficult to establish in the absence of

> **BOX 120.1 Case Definition of Multisystem Inflammatory Syndrome in Children (MIS-C)**
>
> Age less than 21 years
> Evidence of infection with SARS-CoV-2
> Fever for at least 24 hours
> Laboratory evidence of inflammation
> Multisystem organ system inflammation or dysfunction
> Serious illness requiring hospitalization
> No alternative plausible diagnosis

From Centers for Disease Control and Prevention (CDC). MIS, multisystem inflammatory syndrome. "Information for Healthcare Providers about Multisystem Inflammatory Syndrome in Children (MIS-C)." 2020. https://www.cdc.gov/mis/mis-c/hcp/index.html?CDC_AA_refVal=https%3A%2F%2Fwww.cdc.gov%2Fmis%2Fhcp%2Findex.html. Accessed Sept 21, 2021.

an established gold standard. Testing of induced sputum samples may be more sensitive than NP swab, but collection carries risk of aerosolization.[16] RT-PCR tests can remain positive for weeks after infection but may not indicate an ongoing risk of transmission as it can detect noninfectious viral RNA fragments. Semi-quantitative methods in RT-PCR, which can identify the cycle threshold (CT), may prove useful in identifying who may be contagious, those with a low CT count being infectious. Antigen testing may be an alternative—though being less sensitive, it may be adequate in those who are contagious. Additionally, newer technology such as CRISPR may allow for widespread and cheaper testing.[17]

Serologic testing with IgM and IgG enzyme-linked immunosorbent assay (ELISA) can help determine community prevalence. (Refer to Table 120.2 to compare the various diagnostic tests.) IgM and IgG typically become detectable several days to a few weeks after symptom onset and are often negative when patients are evaluated during acute illness. Currently available tests have a range of sensitivity and specificity. There is a risk of a high proportion of false-positive tests when performed on a low-prevalence population. It is not known how long antibody levels remain detectable, and the level of immunity conferred by detectable antibodies is also unknown. The CDC does not recommend any change in personal protective equipment (PPE) use for health care workers who test positive for SARS-CoV-2 antibody.

Laboratory findings of hospitalized individuals commonly include lymphopenia, elevated levels of C-reactive protein, D-dimer, LDH, IL-6, and ferritin. There is a correlation between inflammatory marker elevation and progression to more serious illness, although the strength of associations and individual test thresholds are still being determined. Chest radiographs often show patchy bilateral infiltrates with a peripheral and basilar predominance (Figs. 120.2 and 120.3), and ground-glass opacifications in a peripheral and subpleural distribution are typically found on CT (Fig. 120.4). Lung point-of-care ultrasound has characteristic findings, including B-lines, pleural thickening, pleural irregularities, and focal consolidation (Fig. 120.5). Some early studies have demonstrated the ability of ultrasound in the ED to risk stratify the severity of illness for COVID-19 patients.[18]

Multisystem Inflammatory Syndrome in Children

As mentioned previously, patients with MIS-C have severely elevated inflammatory markers. Diagnostic testing involves measuring the degree of inflammation and assessing the severity of cardiac involvement. If MIS-C is suspected, clinicians should measure C-reactive protein (CRP), erythrocyte sedimentation rate (ESR), fibrinogen, procalcitonin, D-dimer, ferritin, lactic acid dehydrogenase (LDH), and interleukin 6 (IL-6). Troponin, B-type natriuretic peptide (BNP) or NT-proBNP, electrocardiogram, and echocardiogram assess the severity of cardiac involvement.

TABLE 120.2 Diagnostic Testing for SARS-CoV-2

Test Type	Use	Type of Specimen	Comments
Nucleic acid amplification tests (NAATs) (including RT-PCR)	Diagnosis of current infection	Respiratory tract specimens (e.g., nasopharyngeal, oropharyngeal, nasal mid turbinate, anterior nasal, saliva)	Highly sensitive and specific. Often positive for weeks after initial diagnosis
Antigen tests	Diagnosis of current infection	Respiratory tract specimens	Less sensitive than NAAT. Potentially useful to identify those who are contagious.
Serology (antibody testing)	Diagnosis of prior infection	Blood	Potentially useful in the diagnosis of Multisystem inflammatory syndrome in children (MIS-C). Unclear if positive test means they are immune.

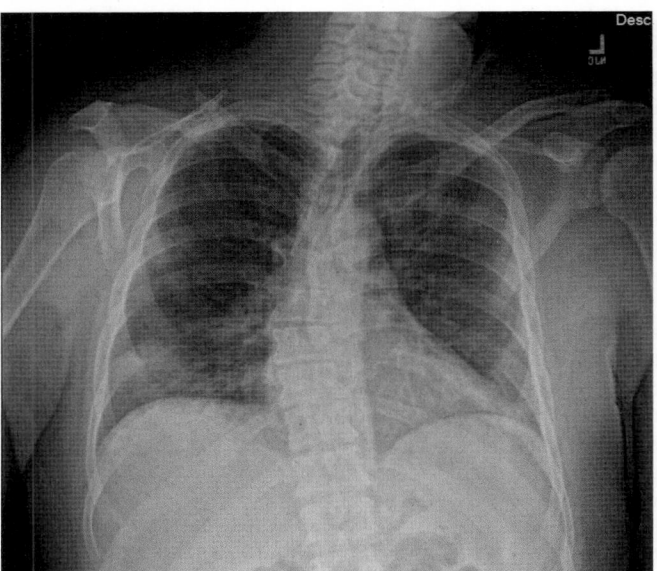

Fig. 120.2 Chest x-ray in mild disease demonstrating multifocal patchy bilateral airspace opacities.

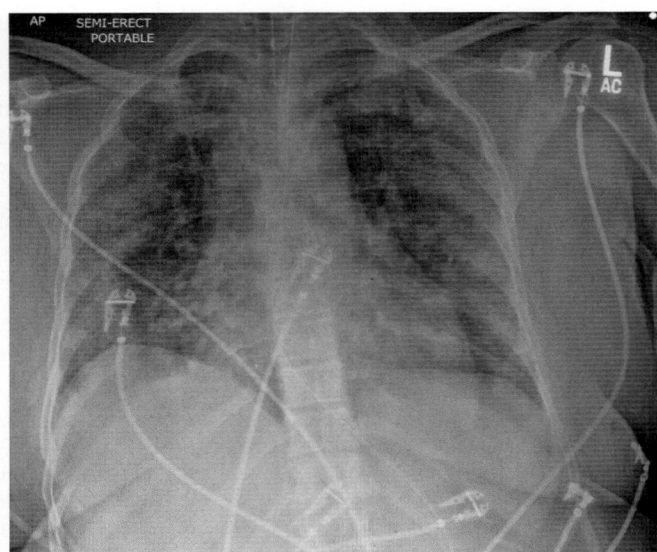

Fig. 120.3 Chest x-ray in severe disease demonstrating ground-glass opacities throughout the lungs, with the more coalescent opacities in the mid and lower zone subpleural regions.

Severe Acute Respiratory Syndrome and Middle East Respiratory Syndrome

The diagnosis of MERS can be also be confirmed by RT-PCR from upper or lower respiratory tract samples. MERS patients tend to have leukopenia, lymphocytopenia, and elevated transaminases as well. Over 80% of MERS patients have abnormalities on chest x-ray ranging from subtle findings to extensive bilateral infiltrates. SARS is thought to have been eradicated, but RT-PCR can be used to make the diagnosis.

MANAGEMENT

Coronavirus Disease 2019

Evidence on the management of COVID-19 is evolving, but treatment is largely supportive. The ED management of COVID-19 focuses on early identification, isolation, and risk stratification to decide which patients require further treatment and hospitalization. For patients that do not require hospitalization, management centers on symptom control and is similar to other nonspecific febrile viral illnesses (rest, hydration, antipyretics, and analgesics). The most important therapeutic interventions are supporting oxygenation and ventilation. At the time of this writing, only corticosteroids have been shown to decrease mortality. Some antiviral agents are thought to decrease hospital length of stay, although the data for this finding are mixed.

Oxygenation and Ventilation

Hypoxemia requiring supplemental oxygen or other ventilatory support is the most common reason for hospitalization. Patients should be given supplemental oxygen to target oxygen saturations of 92% to 96% as with other disease processes. There should be stepwise escalation to achieve this goal, starting with 1 to 6 L/min of oxygen via nasal cannula. If this support is not sufficient, oxygen therapy should be escalated to an Oxymizer or venturi mask. Patients with hypoxemic respiratory failure despite these measures should be tried on high-flow nasal cannula (HFNC).

Another therapeutic maneuver that has shown some promise is "awake proning" or "self-proning." This is the action of placing the non-intubated patient in the prone position. Proning increases oxygenation by improving ventilation-perfusion matching and increasing the recruitment of lung. This is typically done in moderate to severe ARDS patients who are intubated, but early on during the pandemic, multiple reports described an improvement in oxygenation with proning non-intubated patients with COVID-19 respiratory failure.[19] However, it is not clear that self-proning prevents the need for intubation.

Intubation and Mechanical Ventilation

Patients with COVID-19 may have rapid progression to respiratory failure, and these patients often meet criteria for ARDS. One study reported that approximately 12% of patients admitted to the hospital for COVID-19 required mechanical ventilation.[20] Intubation is an aerosol-generating procedure that can put the intubating clinician and other staff at increased risk. It is important to approach this procedure with caution. Guiding principles for intubation of a COVID-19 patient include reducing aerosolization of virus particles, maximizing the first attempt success rate, and reducing health care workers' exposure.[21] Intubations should be performed in a closed room, ideally a negative-pressure room, if available. All staff in the room should be protected with an N95 respirator, eye protection, gowns, and gloves. We recommend the use of high-dose neuromuscular blockade, with rocuronium 1.5 mg/kg or succinylcholine 2 mg/kg to reduce the risk of slow-onset or incomplete relaxation.[21] We also recommend videolaryngoscopy as a first-line approach to the airway, to maximize first-pass success and maintain distance between the intubating clinician and the patient.[21]

Because these patients typically meet moderate to severe ARDS criteria, postintubation management is similar to typical ARDS management. We recommend lung-protective ventilation with low tidal volumes (4–6 mL/kg/ideal body weight) targeting plateau pressures less than 30 cm H_2O (see Chapter 2). These patients usually require a moderate amount of PEEP. To tolerate these settings, these patients may need large doses of sedatives and analgesics.

Therapeutics

Medical treatments for COVID-19 are aimed at inhibiting viral replication, mitigating the inflammatory cascade, and augmenting immunity with antibodies to SARS-CoV-2. Patients may have sepsis, and treatment for bacterial pneumonia is also reasonable. Early optimism about various treatments has typically faded once results from trials have become available; these include lopinavir/ritonavir, hydroxychloroquine, with or without azithromycin, and interferons.[22-24]

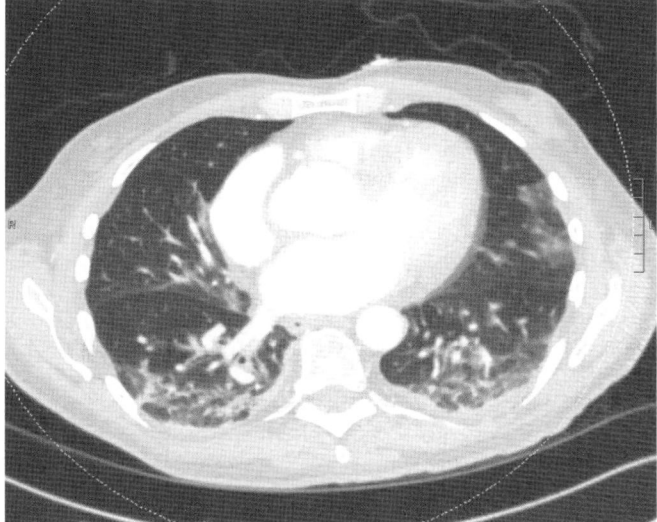

Fig. 120.4 CT scan demonstrating bilateral peripheral and peribronchovascular ground-glass opacities.

Most of the following treatments are primarily given to inpatients and are usually not administered in the ED. Symptoms can be treated with acetaminophen or NSAIDs as needed.

Antivirals. Remdesivir, an adenosine nucleotide analog active against a wide variety of RNA viruses including SARS-CoV-2, shows some promise in early studies and has gained FDA authorization for treatment of SARS-CoV-2. It may be more effective when started early in the course of infection.[25] The dose of remdesivir is 200 mg intravenously on day one and 100 mg a day for an additional 4 days days, depending on severity. The greatest benefits of remdesivir appear to be in hospitalized patients requiring low-flow supplemental oxygen and within 10 days of symptom onset.[25] A shorter course of 3-day remdesivir may be used for patients who are positive, largely symptomatic, but at high risk of developing severe disease. Results of ongoing trials continue to inform the role of remdesivir. However, due to the viral dynamics, we suspect that the benefit of remdesivir in hospitalized patients will be minimal, much like giving oseltamivir in those with later presentations of influenza.

Convalescent Serum and Monoclonal Antibodies. Convalescent serum has been used for over a century for viral infections and even bacterial infections. Studies are underway for pooled and concentrated antibodies specific for COVID-19, and for monoclonal antibodies that target SARS CoV-2. Serum obtained from people who have recovered from COVID-19 appears to be safe but likely will not prove to be effective. A monoclonal antibody targeting the spike protein recently obtained emergency use authorization for treatment of mild

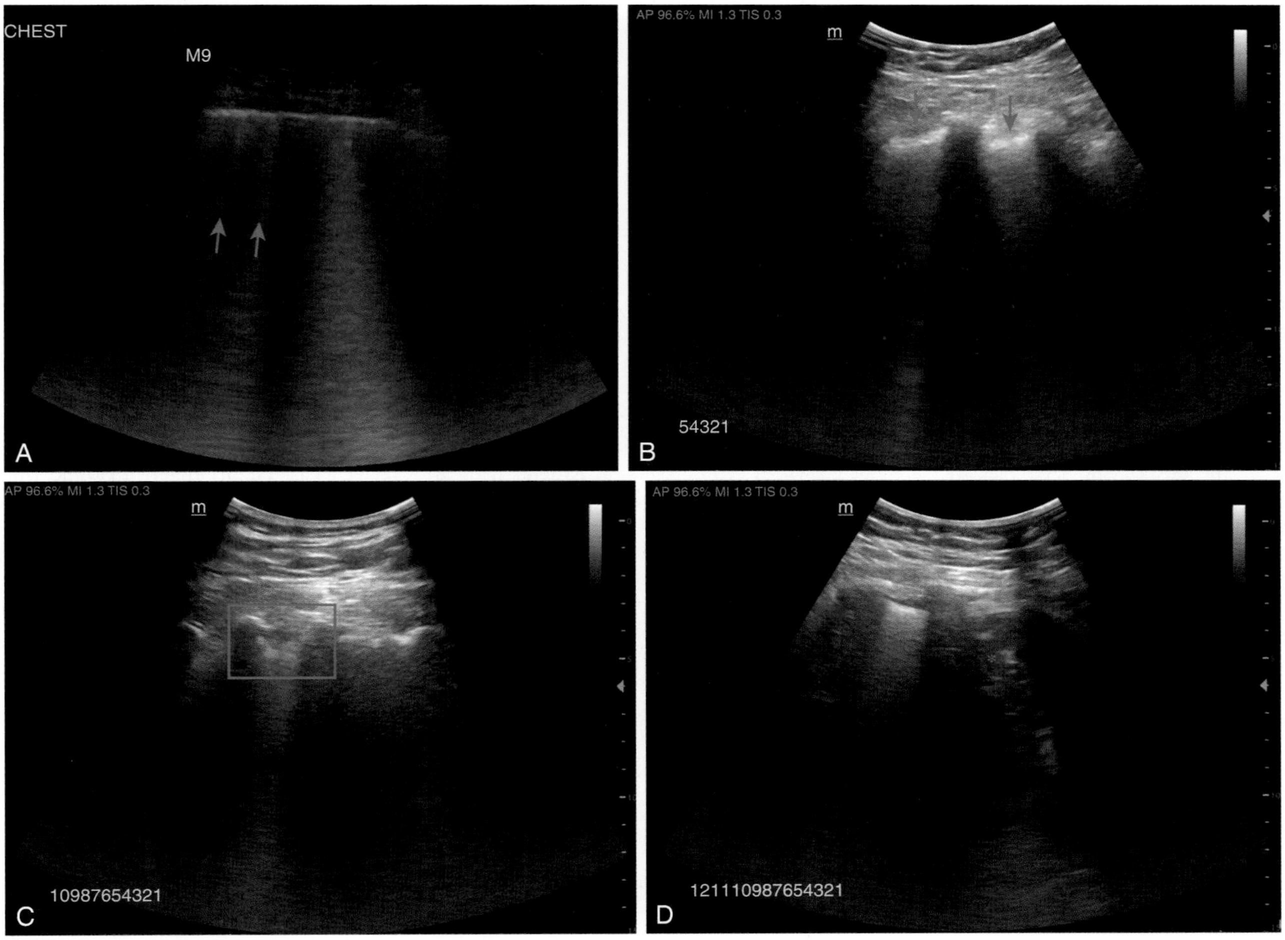

Fig. 120.5 Lung ultrasound demonstrating typical findings in COVID-19. (A) Isolated B-lines (*red arrow*). (B) Confluent B-lines (*red arrow*). (C) Irregular and thickened pleura (*red box*). (D) Subpleural consolidation (*red star*).

to moderate COVID-19.[26] Monoclonal antibodies are being evaluated for those early in their course and emergency departments may be a site where they are infused. We are hoping for a safe, oral medication for COVID-19, but at this time, there are no approved medications. Attempts at treatment with hydroxychloroquine, azithromycin, ivermectin, and zinc showed initial promise in small, uncontrolled studies but were found to be ineffective in more robust investigations.

Immunomodulatory Drugs Including Corticosteroids. Cytokine storm may trigger severe COVID-19 morbidity. Monoclonal antibodies targeting IL-6 and other components of the inflammatory cascade have been attempted as treatments, but preliminary data suggest they are not useful. In June 2020, data from the RECOVERY trial in England suggested that dexamethasone 6 mg daily orally or intravenously for up to 10 days is beneficial in patients with severe COVID-19, defined as those with oxygen saturations of less than 94% on room air and those who require supplemental oxygen, mechanical ventilation, or ECMO.[27-29] These data were the first to show any mortality benefit in treatments for patients hospitalized with COVID-19. Recently, hydrocortisone and other steroids have also been shown to improve mortality in critically ill patients, indicating a class effect.[30,31]

Several IL-6 pathway inhibitors are being studied in patients with severe COVID-19. Trials at this time have not shown a benefit of either tocilizumab, sarilumab, nor siltuximab, contrasting with observational studies.

Anticoagulation. Patients with COVID-19 are at risk for thrombotic complications, and those exhibiting evidence of thrombotic complications should undergo appropriate imaging and occasionally receive empirical anticoagulation. However, studies of empirical anticoagulation for COVID-19 patients without evidence of thrombosis have not shown better outcomes than DVT prophylaxis alone.[32] DVT prophylaxis with low-molecular-weight heparin does not have to be started in the ED, but should be initiated within 48 hours of admission. We do not recommend routine therapeutic anticoagulation in admitted patients without another indication. We also do not recommend anticoagulation in those who are discharged.

Prevention and Vaccination

Over one hundred first-generation COVID-19 vaccines are being developed, and several vaccines have been successfully brought to market, with aggressive roll out campaigns in the United States and Europe in December 2020. However, a SARS-CoV-2 vaccine is unlikely to lead to sterilizing immunity. The virus has a short incubation period and does not have a viremic phase, unlike measles. A variety of vaccine approaches are being used, either via a protein- or gene-based approach. The mRNA and DNA vaccines are not grown in cell cultures or eggs, which consumes time, making them theoretically easier to develop quickly. These genetic platforms have positive results but need to be refrigerated at −80°F.[33] This need for refrigeration presents a challenge to global scalability and a significant barrier to extending availability to low- and middle-income countries.

At this time, public health measures, such as physical distancing, wearing a mask, hand hygiene, and limiting gathering size, remain the most important factors in decreasing transmission. The best measures to control human coronaviruses rely on a strong public health system along with rapid diagnosis and isolating those who are infected.

Multisystem Inflammatory Syndrome in Children

The mainstay of treatment is supportive care and attenuating the inflammatory response. Patients typically require fluid therapy. More severe cases may require vasopressors, inotropes, mechanical ventilation, and in cases of refractory cardiogenic shock, ECMO. Patients are treated with immunomodulatory therapies such as IVIG, glucocorticoids, or interleukin antagonists.

Middle East Respiratory Syndrome

Obtaining an accurate travel history in febrile patients with an unknown respiratory illness, with a negative MERS-CoV-2 PCR, is key to early identification of MERS cases. Nosocomial outbreak was a critical component of the 2003 SARS outbreak as well as MERS outbreaks.

There is no specific antiviral treatment for MERS. The mainstay of treatment is supportive care. For the benign URI, nothing more than rest, antipyretics, and analgesics are needed. However, patients with MERS may require more invasive supportive measures. The diagnosis of MERS will not be immediately apparent, so patients should be treated initially with antibiotics covering community-acquired or health care–associated pneumonia. If mechanical ventilation is required, they should be ventilated with a lung-protective strategy with low tidal volumes to limit additional lung injury.

Prevention of transmission is an essential component of MERS management. This involves early identification of cases and prompt isolation of suspected cases. Obtaining an accurate travel history in all febrile patients with a respiratory illness is key to early identification of MERS cases. CDC guidelines on infection control measures for these infections can be found at www.cdc.gov/sars/infection/index.html and www.cdc.gov/coronavirus/mers/infection-prevention-control.html.

DISPOSITION

Most patients with coronaviruses can be treated at home. Those with moderate to severe COVID-19 will require hospitalization. Patients who have hypoxemia with an oxygen saturation of less than 94% on room air and those requiring oxygen or ventilatory support are classified as severe disease and require hospitalization. Children with suspected MIS-C should be admitted. All patients who are discharged should be counseled on infection control practices and self-isolation. Return precautions should be given. Patients should be counseled to return for dyspnea and confusion. If possible, we recommend providing patients who are discharged with a pulse-oximeter and clear instructions for use and interpretation.

Patients with MERS have a case fatality rate of 35% and will likely require admission to the hospital and ICU, depending on the severity of illness. Patients with suspected MERS should be isolated with contact precautions and airborne isolation, as are those with COVID-19. The hospital infection control team and department of public health should be notified immediately for patients under investigation for MERS.

The references for this chapter can be found online at ExpertConsult. com.

HIV

Bhakti Hansoti

FOUNDATIONS

Background and Importance

Acquired immunodeficiency syndrome (AIDS) is a pandemic caused by the human immunodeficiency virus (HIV). HIV has caused tremendous human suffering and has had an immeasurable impact on demographics, cultures, economics, and politics in most societies around the globe. There are an estimated 37.9 million people living with HIV infection worldwide, and approximately 770,000 deaths annually.[1] Significant strides have been made in areas of prevention and treatment. Since 2010 the number of new HIV infections has decreased by 16%, and the number of AIDS-related deaths by 33%.[1,2] Decline in the incidence of new cases of HIV infection and AIDS-related deaths is mostly due to the widespread use of highly active antiretroviral therapy (ART) and the treatment as prevention paradigm, resulting in a decline in the overall HIV incidence worldwide. Recent advances in HIV management have focused on the scale-up of preventative strategies such as preexposure prophylaxis (PreP), universal ART, and even same-day initiation (SDI). However, there is no cure for HIV and significant treatment gaps in at-risk populations have resulted in an increase in global HIV prevalence. Therefore, a significant number of patients in the ED may present with HIV coinfection, as well as ART-related or AIDS-related complications (Figs. 121.1 and 121.2).

Pathophysiology

HIV, a retrovirus from the lentivirus subfamily, is the cause of AIDS. There are two main subtypes of HIV, HIV-1 and HIV-2. Worldwide, the predominant virus is HIV-1. HIV-1 accounts for around 95% of all infections worldwide. HIV-2 is estimated to be more than 55% genetically distinct from HIV-1. The relatively uncommon HIV-2 virus is concentrated in West Africa but has been seen in other countries with links to West Africa. It is less infectious and progresses more slowly than HIV-1, resulting in fewer deaths. HIV-1 can be further divided into four groups; group M is the strain responsible for the global HIV epidemic and can be further divided into nine genetically distinct subtypes. The individual characteristics of each of the subtypes are beyond the scope of emergency medicine, but clinicians should be aware that most ART is largely tested on populations with subtype B, and tests used to diagnose HIV may not be sensitive to all subtypes. This is a concern in places where diverse subtypes are prevalent.

The mature HIV virion is a spherical structure with an outer envelope and inner core (Fig. 121.3). The core contains two copies of the RNA genome, enzymes (reverse transcriptase and integrase), and regulatory proteins. Surrounding the core is the viral membrane, containing the glycoproteins responsible for the attachment and entry of the virus into a CD4+ cell. In a multistep process, the HIV virion invades the host cell and integrates its genetic material into the host's chromosome (Fig. 121.4). The infection begins with the binding of the virus to the CD4+ host cell. The virus enters the cell by fusing its envelope with the target cell membrane. After internalization, reverse transcriptase forms viral DNA from the original RNA. The viral enzyme integrase then transports the newly formed viral DNA into the nucleus, where it integrates with human chromosomal DNA. Viral polyproteins and RNA are formed, and new infectious viral particles are created. This cycle continues with HIV infecting more CD4+ cells. Major targets of ART include reverse transcriptase, protease, integrase, and the CCR5 coreceptor.

The hallmark of HIV infection is CD4+ T cell destruction, leading to a deficient cell-mediated arm of the immune system. Humoral immunity is also impaired through B cell proliferation and the production of abnormal antibodies, making HIV-infected individuals more vulnerable to infections by encapsulated bacteria. HIV infection also leads to chronic immune activation. Ongoing viremia, along with pro-inflammatory cytokines, B cell proliferation, and hypergammaglobulinemia leads to a chronic inflammatory state that contributes to cardiovascular disease, cancer, and other chronic diseases in HIV-infected individuals.[2] Increased immune activation persists, even in patients with immune reconstitution on antiretroviral therapy.

HIV has been isolated from a wide range of body fluids, including semen, vaginal secretions, lymphocytes, cell-free plasma, cerebrospinal fluid (CSF), tears, saliva, urine, and breast milk.[3] However, only semen,

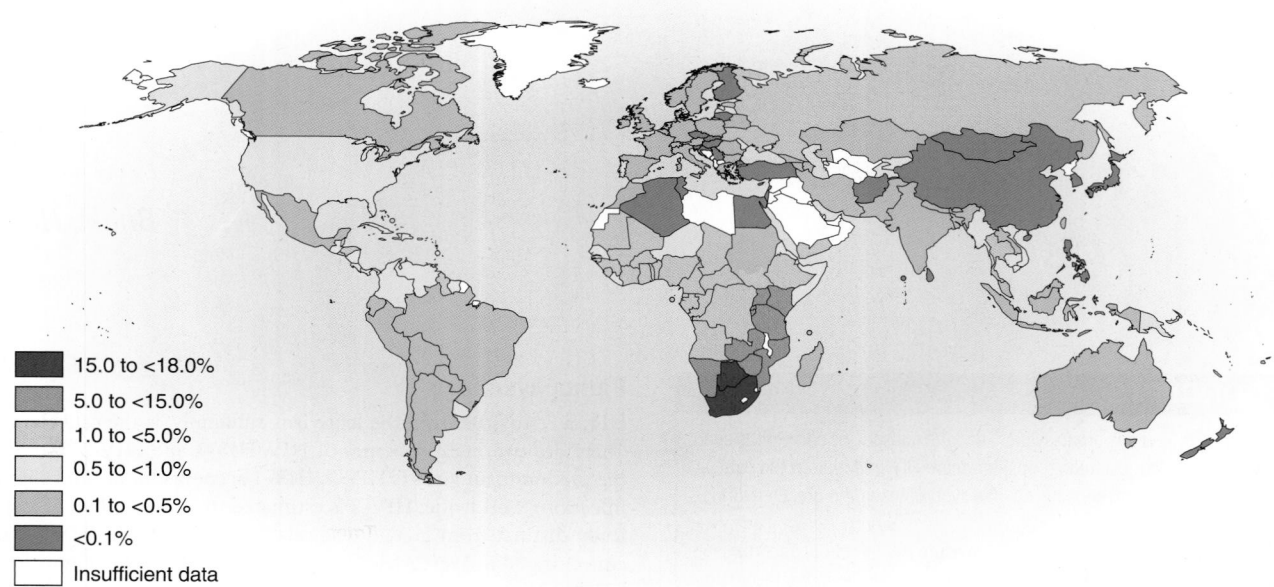

15.0 to <18.0%
5.0 to <15.0%
1.0 to <5.0%
0.5 to <1.0%
0.1 to <0.5%
<0.1%
Insufficient data

Fig. 121.1 Human immunodeficiency virus prevalence by country. (From Bennett JE, et al, eds. *Mandell, Douglas, and Bennett's Principles and Practice of Infectious Diseases*, ed 8. Philadelphia: Elsevier/Churchill Livingstone; 2015.)

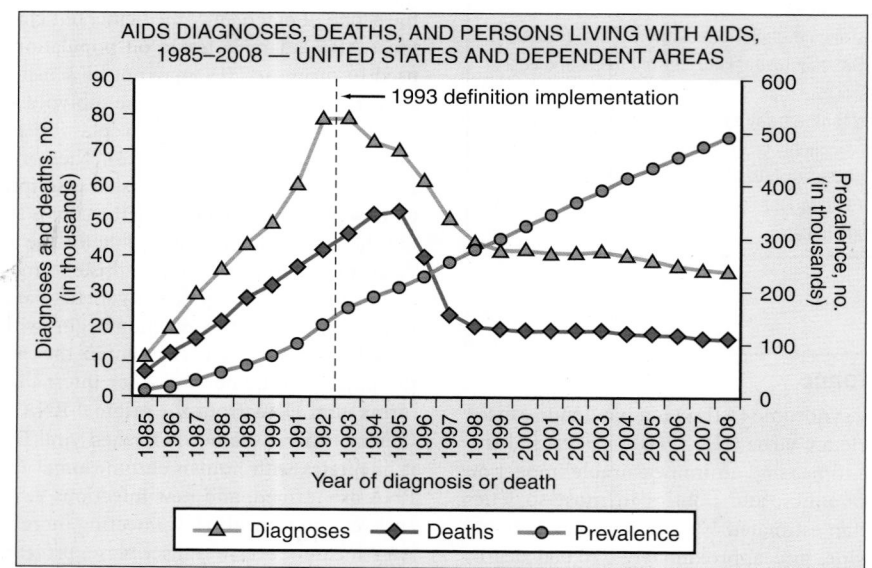

Fig. 121.2 AIDS diagnoses, deaths, and persons living with AIDS—United States. (From: Centers for Disease Control and Prevention. AIDS surveillance—trends [1985–2009]. www.cdc.gov/hiv/topics/surveillance/resources/slides/trends/index.htm.)

blood, vaginal secretions, and breast milk are significantly infectious. For transmission to occur, these fluids must come into contact with damaged tissue or with a mucous membrane or be directly injected into the bloodstream. After transmission, the virus replicates in the mucosal surface or lymphoid tissue at the site of entry in lymphocytes and macrophages. If enough cells are infected, the virus spreads to draining lymph nodes and infection is established, usually within 48 to 72 hours.

Means of transmission of HIV and the demographic distribution of the virus vary from country to country. Unprotected heterosexual intercourse with subsequent transmission of HIV to newborns and breast-fed babies (mother-to-child transmission) is the dominant mode of transmission worldwide, accounting for about 85% of all HIV infections. The main pattern of transmission in the higher-income countries of North America and western and central Europe is in men who have sex with men (MSM) and direct injection into the bloodstream in patients with intravenous drug use (IVDU).

The risk of transmission varies by modality. The average risk of HIV infection after a needlestick or cut exposure to HIV-infected blood is

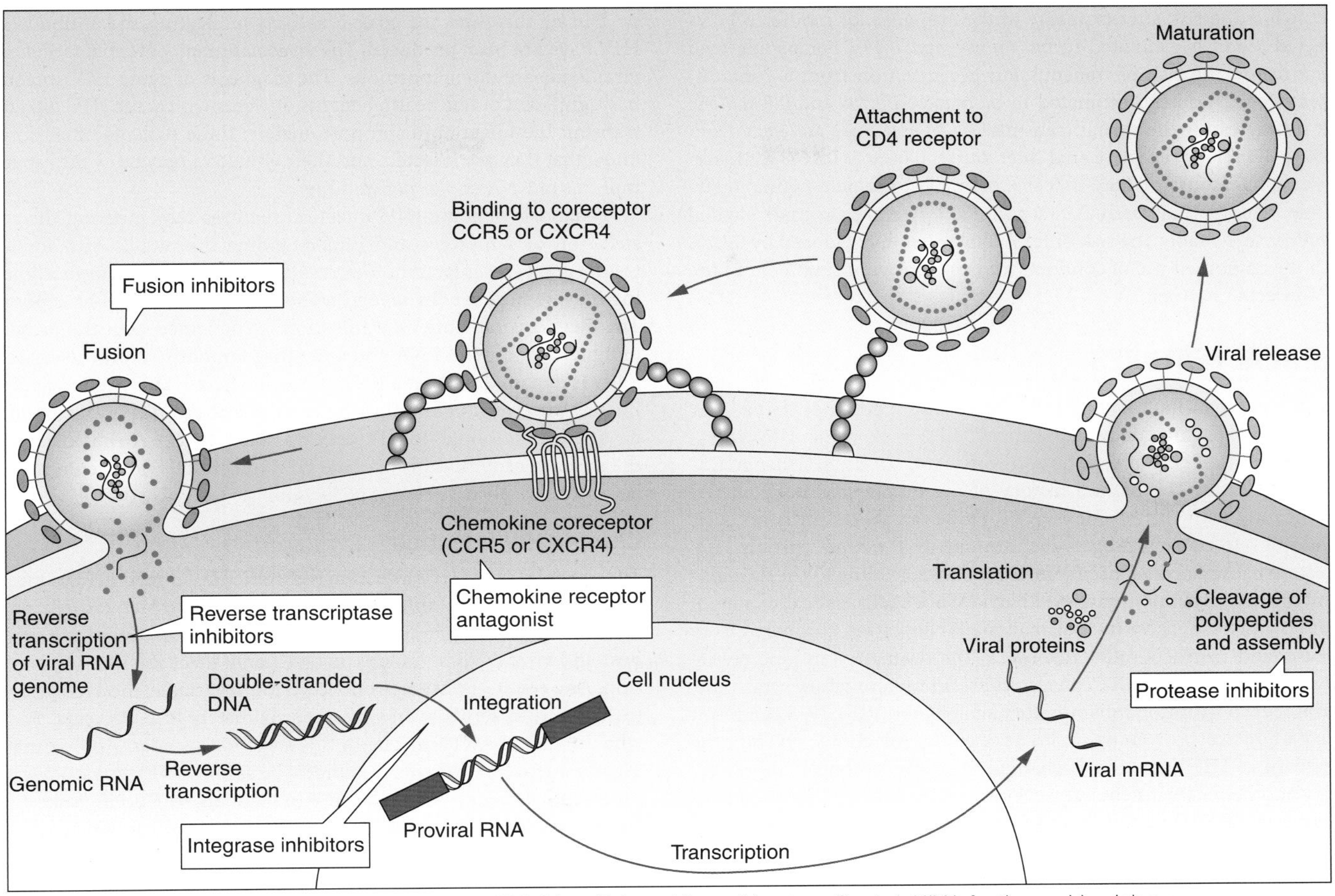

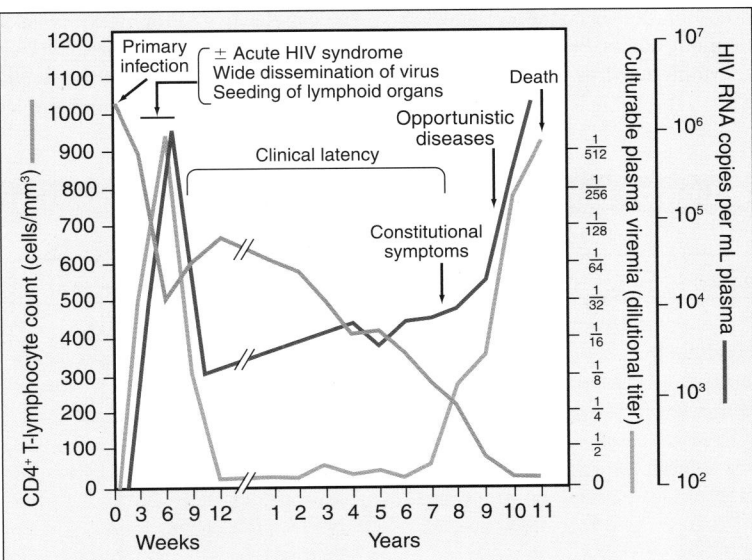

Fig. 121.3 Replicative cycle of the HIV virion. (Adapted from: Maartens G, et al. HIV infection: epidemiology, pathogenesis, treatment, and prevention. *Lancet.* 2014;384:258-271.)

Fig. 121.4 Natural history of HIV infection in the absence of therapy in a hypothetical patient. (Adapted from: Fauci AS, et al. Immunopathogenic mechanisms of HIV infection. *Ann Intern Med.* 1996;124:654-663.)

0.3% while the risk after exposure of the eye, nose, or mouth to HIV-infected blood is estimated to be, on average, 0.1%. For people who inject drugs, the risk of transmission per injection from a contaminated needle has been estimated to be between 0.7% and 0.8%.[3] The risk estimates for the sexual transmission of HIV, per act, vary from 0.5% to 3.38% for receptive anal intercourse; 0.06% to 0.16% for insertive anal intercourse; 0.08% to 0.19% for male-to-female vaginal intercourse; and approximately 0.05% to 0.1% for female-to-male vaginal intercourse. Notably, the risk of HIV transmission is reduced by 99.2% with the combined use of condoms and antiretroviral treatment of the HIV-infected partner.

CLINICAL FEATURES

The clinical manifestations of HIV infection are varied. Patients may present to the emergency department (ED) with acute HIV infection, medication side effects, opportunistic infections, or other AIDS-related illnesses. The natural history of the disease has been altered significantly with the advent of ART. However, there still is no cure. In addition to causing progressive immune dysfunction, chronic HIV infection causes a constant inflammatory state, leading to the development of numerous manifestations that have not been classically thought of as HIV disease. These include malignant neoplasms, coronary artery disease, and neurocognitive disorders. The dramatic immune recovery seen with modern ART can also cause an inflammatory syndrome, immune reconstitution inflammatory syndrome (IRIS). IRIS can result in a paradoxical worsening of any preexisting infections. Overall, the spectrum of HIV infection is changing because of longer life expectancy and better treatment. However, many patients still have undiagnosed HIV infection and can present with acute HIV infection.

Acute HIV Infection

Acute HIV infection, also referred to as primary HIV infection, describes the earliest stage of infection with the HIV virus. Patients present with symptoms consistent with an acute, self-limited viral infection, including fever, fatigue, sore throat, pharyngitis, lymphadenopathy, muscle aches, diarrhea, and a rash. They can occur within a few days of exposure or up to 6 weeks after, and usually last about 14 days. Acute HIV infection can be complicated by encephalitis, Guillain-Barré syndrome, and mononeuritis. CD4+ counts also transiently drop, occasionally to the level at which opportunistic infections can occur. Among others, *Pneumocystis jiroveci* pneumonia (PCP), toxoplasmosis, cytomegalovirus (CMV) infection, and thrush may occur in this stage.

During this time, the virus is actively replicating and antibodies to HIV have not been produced. The virus has many potential targets and viral loads are often enormous. The diagnosis of acute HIV infection has significant public health benefits. Patients with acute HIV infection transmit the infection disproportionately; these patients often do not know that they are infected, and their viral load may be in the range of millions of RNA copies per milliliter.

Diagnosis of acute HIV infection requires remembering the constellation of symptoms and understanding the pitfalls of laboratory testing for early infection. The results of routine HIV antibody testing may be negative for several weeks or even months after exposure. The diagnosis of acute HIV infection is confirmed with the presence of high titers of viral RNA and a negative antibody screen. Assay reactivity is dynamic; a plasma RNA test will detect HIV infection approximately one week before the ability to detect the p24 antigen and 12 days before antibodies to HIV develop (Table 121.1). A viral load test in the absence of symptoms of acute HIV infection is not recommended because false-positive results occur, and the test is costly.

Chronic HIV Infection

The second stage of HIV infection is chronic HIV infection (also known as asymptomatic HIV infection or clinical latency). Many patients have few or no clinical manifestations of HIV infection. There are several host and viral factors that are involved and affect the rate of progression. As a result, the asymptomatic period is variable; the average onset to AIDS from seroconversion is approximately 8 to 10 years. People who are taking ARTs may be in this stage for decades. Approximately 5% of patients are long-term nonprogressors (LTNP), sometimes also called elite noncontrollers; they are individuals who do not take ARTs and still maintain CD4 counts in the normal range indefinitely.

AIDS

AIDS is the final and most severe stage of HIV infection. Due to a severely immunocompromised state (CD4+ count <200 cells/μL), the body is unable to fight off opportunistic infections, which for diagnostic purposes are reported as AIDS-defining conditions (Box 121.1). The types and frequency of opportunistic infections are more severe as the CD4+ count continues to deteriorate. Some infections are so common in patients with AIDS that primary prophylaxis is indicated and is cost-effective.[4] Prophylaxis is started for PCP when CD4+ counts are less than 200 cells/μL, for toxoplasmosis when CD4+ counts are less than 100 cells/μL and, for *Mycobacterium avium* complex (MAC) infection when CD4+ counts are less than 50 cells/μL (Table 121.2).

TABLE 121.1   HIV Testing by Laboratory Stage

Stage	LABORATORY MARKER				HIV Stage
	RNA	p24 Antigen	Third-Generation Antibody (EIA)	Western Blot	
1	+	–	–	–	Acute HIV infection
2	+++	+	–	–	Acute HIV infection
3	+++	+/–	+	–	Seroconversion
4	+++	+/–	+	Intermediate	Seroconversion
5	++	+/–	+	+	Seroconversion
6	+–+++	+/–	+	+	Chronic HIV infection (all Western blot bands are positive, older antibody tests react)

EIA, Enzyme immunoassay.
Adapted from: Fiebig EW, et al. Dynamics of HIV viremia and antibody seroconversion in plasma donors: implications for diagnosis and staging of primary HIV infection. *AIDS.* 2003;17:1871-1879.

BOX 121.1   AIDS-Defining Conditions

Bacterial infections, multiple or recurrent
Candidiasis of bronchi, trachea, or lungs
Candidiasis of esophagus
Cervical cancer, invasive
Coccidioidomycosis, disseminated or extrapulmonary
Cryptococcosis, extrapulmonary
Cryptosporidiosis, chronic intestinal (>1 mo duration)
Cytomegalovirus disease (other than liver, spleen, or nodes), onset at age >1 mo
Cytomegalovirus retinitis (with loss of vision)
Encephalopathy, HIV related
Herpes simplex: chronic ulcers (>1 mo duration) or bronchitis, pneumonitis, or esophagitis (onset at age >1 mo)
Histoplasmosis, disseminated or extrapulmonary
Isosporiasis, chronic intestinal (>1 mo duration)
Lymphoma, Burkitt (or equivalent term)
Kaposi sarcoma
Lymphoma, immunoblastic (or equivalent term)
Lymphoma, primary, of brain
Mycobacterium avium complex or *Mycobacterium kansasii,* disseminated or extrapulmonary
Mycobacterium tuberculosis of any site, pulmonary, disseminated, or extrapulmonary
Mycobacterium, other species or unidentified species, disseminated or extrapulmonary
Pneumocystis jiroveci pneumonia
Pneumonia, recurrent
Progressive multifocal leukoencephalopathy
Salmonella septicemia, recurrent
Toxoplasmosis of brain, onset at age >1 mo
Wasting syndrome attributed to HIV

Furthermore, isoniazid preventative therapy is given to all patients with a positive tuberculin skin test (TST) to prevent latent TB.

Clinical Manifestations by Organ System

Manifestations of HIV infection vary greatly, depending on the patient's immune status and whether the patient is receiving ART. Some of the clinical manifestations are secondary to severe immunocompromise state and secondary opportunistic infections, and others are due to the proinflammatory pathology of the disease process.

Cardiac Manifestations

Patients with advanced HIV infection can have a constellation of cardiac manifestations, including pericarditis, myocarditis, cardiomyopathy, pulmonary vascular disease, pulmonary hypertension, valvular disease, and neoplastic involvement of the heart. Purulent pericarditis and cardiac tamponade are potentially lethal clinical manifestations of cardiovascular disease in patients with AIDS; *Mycobacterium tuberculosis* is often the causative organism, especially in low-resource countries.

The success of ART has led to prolonged survival in patients with HIV. Cardiovascular disease is now the major cause of morbidity and mortality. HIV-infected patients have a 50% increased risk of acute coronary syndrome compared to the general population, after adjustment for risk factors. Patients receiving ART also suffer from a number of metabolic abnormalities (e.g., hyperglycemia, hyperlipidemia, lipodystrophy) and accelerated atherosclerosis, which increases their cardiovascular risk profile. Protease inhibitors, particularly ritonavir in higher doses, are strongly associated with dyslipidemia. Non-nucleoside reverse transcriptase inhibitors (NNRTIs) are associated with increases in low-density lipoprotein cholesterol and total cholesterol but also a significant increase in high-density lipoprotein cholesterol. Discontinuing ART has been shown to result in systemic inflammation, coagulation cascade activation, an increase in biomarkers associated with endothelial activation, and increased risk of major

TABLE 121.2   Prophylaxis to Prevent First Episode of Selected Opportunistic Infections

Pathogen	Indication	First-Choice Therapy	Alternative
Pneumocystis jiroveci pneumonia (PCP)	• CD4+ < 200 cells/μL or oropharyngeal candidiasis • CD4+ < 14% or history of AIDS-defining illness • CD4+ > 200 cells/μL but <250 cells/μL if monitoring is not possible every 1–3 mo	TMP-SMZ	TMP-SMZ Dapsone Dapsone + pyrimethamine + leucovorin Aerosolized pentamidine Atovaquone Atovaquone + pyrimethamine + leucovorin
Toxoplasma gondii encephalitis	• *Toxoplasma* IgG–positive patients with CD4+ count < 100 cells/μL • Seronegative patients receiving PCP prophylaxis not active against toxoplasmosis should have *Toxoplasma* serology retested if CD4+ count declines to < 100 cells/μL • Initiate prophylaxis if seroconversion occurs.	TMP-SMZ	TMP-SMZ Dapsone + pyrimethamine + leucovorin Dapsone + pyrimethamine + leucovorin Atovaquone ± pyrimethamine + leucovorin
Disseminated *Mycobacterium avium* complex (MAC) disease	• CD4+ count < 50 cells/μL (after active MAC infection is ruled out)	Azithromycin or Clarithromycin	Rifabutin (adjust dose on basis of ART interactions); rule out active TB before rifabutin is started.

ART, Antiretroviral therapy; *TB,* tuberculosis; *TMP-SMZ,* trimethoprim-sulfamethoxazole.
Adapted from: Kaplan JE, et al. Guidelines for prevention and treatment of opportunistic infections in HIV-infected adults and adolescents: recommendations from CDC, the National Institutes of Health, and the HIV Medicine Association of the Infectious Diseases Society of America. www.cdc.gov/mmwr/preview/mmwrhtml/rr5804a1.htm.

cardiovascular events. Studies have also shown that the virus alone is associated with dyslipidemia, endothelial damage, inflammation, and hypercoagulability.

Pulmonary Manifestations

Noninfectious and infectious pulmonary diseases are more common in those with HIV infection compared to uninfected individuals. Although the incidence is greatly reduced in the era of ART, pulmonary manifestations of Kaposi sarcoma and non-Hodgkin lymphoma can occur. HIV-infected patients also appear to be at increased risk for lung cancer, emphysema, cryptogenic organizing pneumonia, sarcoidosis, drug hypersensitivity, primary effusion lymphoma, foreign body granulomatosis, and lymphocytic interstitial pneumonitis.

The most frequent respiratory infections in people with HIV infection are upper respiratory tract infections and acute bronchitis. The incidence of lower respiratory tract infections increases as CD4+ counts decline. Potential causes of lower respiratory tract infections include viruses (influenza, respiratory syncytial, parainfluenza), bacteria, and fungi (*P. jiroveci*; Table 121.3). Bacterial pneumonia is more frequent in people infected with HIV than in uninfected persons (most commonly caused by *Streptococcus pneumoniae*). In patients with a CD4+ count below 200 cells/μL, the prevalence of pneumocystis pneumonia (PCP) increases. The clinical presentation of PCP is characterized by the gradual onset of fever (79% to 100% of cases), cough (95%), and progressive dyspnea (95%). The cough is nonproductive, although sputum production does not exclude this diagnosis, and patients can be coinfected with bacterial pneumonia. Some patients, especially those taking nonsystemic prophylaxis (e.g., aerosolized pentamidine), may have extrapulmonary manifestations of PCP, such as hepatosplenomegaly,

skin lesions, and ocular lesions. The most common associated laboratory abnormalities are a CD4+ count below 200 cells/μL and elevated lactate dehydrogenase level. Although chest radiographs can be normal, they usually show diffuse, bilateral, interstitial, or alveolar infiltrates (Fig. 121.5). High-resolution computed tomography (CT) has a high sensitivity for PCP and often reveals ground glass or cystic lesions (Fig. 121.6). The definitive diagnosis is made by isolation of the organism, commonly from respiratory specimens obtained by sputum induction, bronchoalveolar lavage, or endotracheal aspiration. Trimethoprim-sulfamethoxazole (TMP-SMZ) is also the preferred treatment of PCP; the route is dependent on the severity of the disease. There are a number of other possible regimens for those who are intolerant (Table 121.4). Patients with severe (partial pressure of oxygen 70 mm Hg or less or an alveolar-arterial oxygen gradient 35 mm Hg or

TABLE 121.3 Differential Diagnosis of Respiratory Infections in HIV-Infected Patients by CD4+ Count

CD4+ Count and Stage	Differential Diagnosis
Present at any stage	Acute bronchitis
	Bacterial pneumonia
	Tuberculosis
>500 cells/μL	Bacterial pneumonia[a]
Early HIV infection	PCP[a]
	HHV-8–related Kaposi sarcoma
200–500 cells/μL	Bacterial pneumonia[a]
	PCP[a]
<200 cells/μL	Bacterial pneumonia[a] (consider bacteremia)
AIDS	PCP[a]
	Histoplasma capsulatum or *Coccidioides immitis* pneumonia
	Cryptococcus neoformans pneumonia
	Extrapulmonary or disseminated tuberculosis[a]
≤50 cells/μL	Bacterial pneumonia[a]
Advanced HIV infection	PCP[a]
	Toxoplasma gondii pneumonia
	Pulmonary Kaposi sarcoma
	Histoplasma capsulatum or *Coccidioides immitis* pneumonia
	Mycobacterium avium complex pneumonia

HHV-8, Human herpesvirus 8; *PCP*, *Pneumocystis jiroveci* pneumonia.
[a]Occurs more frequently as immune function declines.

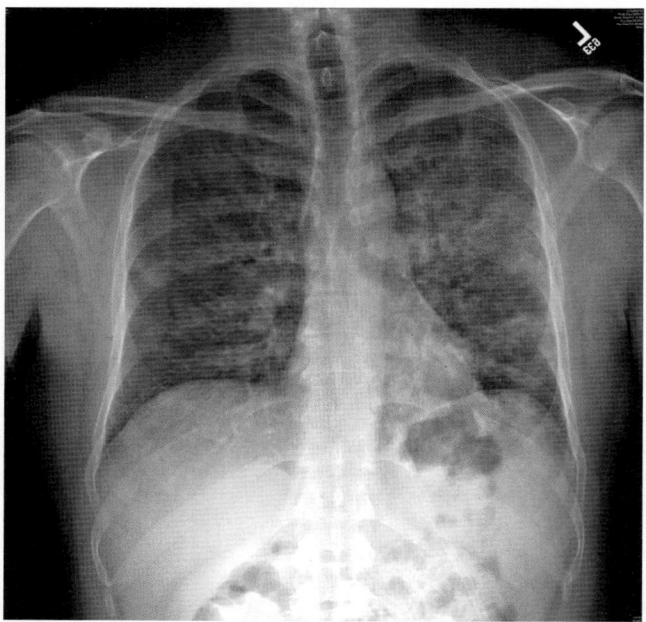

Fig. 121.5 Chest radiograph of *Pneumocystis* pneumonia. (From Mocroft A, et al: Decline in the AIDS and death rates in the EuroSIDA study: an observational study. Lancet 362:22–29, 2003.)

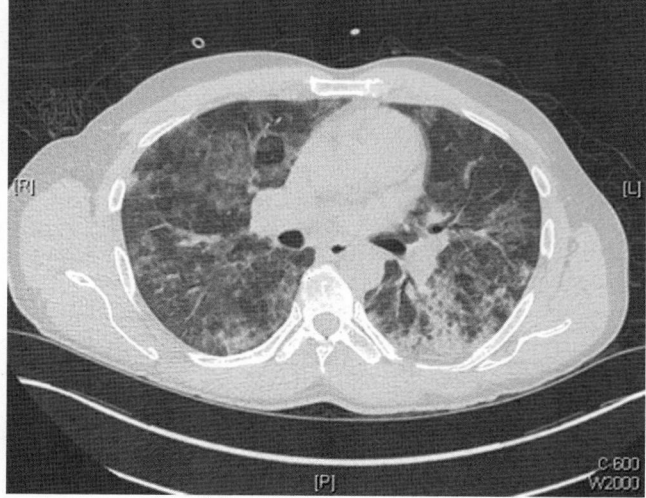

Fig. 121.6 Chest computed tomography scan of *Pneumocystis* pneumonia.

greater) PCP receive significant benefit from concurrent corticosteroid treatment and should receive a 21-day prednisone taper in addition to antibiotic therapy.

Pulmonary TB is so commonly found as a coinfection in HIV-positive patients that patients are recommended to take isoniazid preventative therapy (IPT). Patients with early HIV infection and TB have presentations similar to those of individuals without HIV infection; they often have classic symptoms of pulmonary TB, such as fever, cough, weight loss, malaise, and night sweats, with plain films showing upper lobe cavitations. In patients with advanced disease, atypical radiographic findings are more common, such as pulmonary infiltrates without preference for the upper lung fields. Patients with advanced HIV infection and severe immunosuppression may also present with extrapulmonary and disseminated TB. All patients with a clinical suspicion of TB should be placed in respiratory isolation. In addition to

plain films and sputum samples, evaluation of extrapulmonary disease includes specimens of suspected areas of involvement (e.g., CSF, lymph nodes, pleural fluid, pericardial fluid, blood, urine). The treatment of TB in people with HIV infection is complicated, and drug interactions between ART and anti-TB therapy are severe and common. After initiation of anti-TB therapy, the patient requires close monitoring for assessment of adequate treatment response and for observation of signs of IRIS, a complication more common in patients with CD4+ counts below 200 cells/μL.

Diagnostic evaluation of patients with HIV infection who present with respiratory complaints should be based on their HIV disease stage, as well as their clinical presentation (Table 121.5). Specific algorithms are difficult because of geographic differences in epidemiology. The evaluation includes pulse oximetry, chest radiography, and complete blood count. Additional tests may include arterial blood gas analysis to determine the need for corticosteroids in patients with PCP, levels of serum lactate dehydrogenase (elevated in PCP), 1,3-β-D-glucan (elevated in PCP), serum cryptococcal antigen, urine *Histoplasma capsulatum* antigen, and sputum studies (including Gram staining, acid-fast bacillus, and staining for *P. jiroveci*) if available. Blood cultures should be obtained before antibiotic therapy initiation. A thorough search for the pathogen is recommended in patients with HIV infection.

Oropharyngeal and Gastrointestinal Manifestations

HIV-infected patients with GI symptoms may present with common abdominal diseases or may have opportunistic infections, malignant neoplasms, or medication side effects. Patients receiving ART may suffer treatment-related adverse gastrointestinal events, including pancreatitis, hepatic steatosis, lactic acidosis, and drug-induced hepatotoxicity. Furthermore, a number of patients with HIV infection have concomitant hepatitis B virus (HBV) or hepatitis C virus (HCV) infection and may also have GI manifestations from these causes as well. Although improvements have been noted, end-stage liver disease remains a common cause of mortality in HIV-infected patients.

Patients with primary HIV infection often present with thrush (secondary to candida is most often the first manifestation of HIV

TABLE 121.4 Treatment of *Pneumocystis jiroveci* Pneumonia in Patients with HIV Infection

Severity of Illness	Preferred Therapy	Alternative Therapy
Moderate to severe	TMP-SMZ, IV; switch to oral administration after clinical improvement 21-day therapy	Pentamidine *or* Primaquine + clindamycin
Mild to moderate	TMP-SMZ	Dapsone + trimethoprim *or* Primaquine + clindamycin *or* Atovaquone

TMP-SMZ, Trimethoprim-sulfamethoxazole.
US Department of Health and Human Services. Guidelines for prevention and treatment of opportunistic infections in HIV-infected adults and adolescents. www.aidsinfo.nih.gov.

TABLE 121.5 Pulmonary Manifestations of Disease in HIV-Infected Patients

Disease	Presentation	Diagnostic Evaluation	Treatment
Bacterial pneumonia	Acute onset (<1 wk) Cough Purulent sputum Fevers, chills, rigors	Elevated white blood cell count Chest radiograph—unilateral focal consolidation CD4+ count variable	Antibiotic therapy targeting *Streptococcus pneumoniae* and *Haemophilus influenzae* Also cover atypical bacterial pathogens
Pneumocystis jiroveci pneumonia (PCP)	Gradual onset (>2 wk) Nonproductive cough Dyspnea Fever	Exercise-induced hypoxia Elevated serum lactate dehydrogenase level Chest radiograph—bilateral reticular or interstitial pattern Computed tomography scan—ground glass opacity (56%) CD4+ < 200 cells/μL	Trimethoprim-sulfamethoxazole for 21 days If Pao2 < 70 mm Hg at room air or alveolar-arterial oxygen gradient > 35 mm Hg, give prednisone; taper over 21 days.
Mycobacterium tuberculosis infection (TB)	Gradual onset (>2 wk) Cough Fever Night sweats Weight loss Lymphadenopathy	Chest radiograph—alveolar pattern (±cavitation), miliary pattern, nodules, adenopathy, effusions CD4+ count variable	Determine antituberculosis therapy with infectious disease consultant. Consider possibility of drug resistance. Multiple drug interactions exist between TB medications and antiretroviral therapy.
Kaposi sarcoma	Gradual onset (>2–4 wk) Cough Dyspnea Fever	Chest radiograph—bilateral perihilar nodules, opacities, effusions, adenopathy CD4+ < 200 cells/μL	Cryotherapy, radiation therapy Infrared coagulation Sclerosing agents, intralesional vinblastine Systemic chemotherapy

infection), pharyngitis, and severe aphthous ulcers. Less commonly, oral hairy leukoplakia, caused by Epstein-Barr virus (EBV), is manifested as raised white lesions on the side of the tongue. Unlike in thrush, the lesions cannot be scraped off and are not responsive to topical antifungal agents. Kaposi sarcoma, which can occur in the mouth, is usually found on the palate.

Patients with CD4+ counts below 100 cells/µl are particularly prone to esophagitis, presenting with dysphagia or odynophagia. The most common cause of esophagitis in patients with HIV infection is *Candida*, followed by herpes simplex virus, CMV, and deep aphthous ulcers. Diagnosis can be confirmed by endoscopic biopsy. Given the invasive nature of the testing, most patients are empirically treated by a 5- to 7-day course of fluconazole. However, the decision to start treatment is usually made in conjunction with the patient's infectious disease physician.

Gastroesophageal reflux is another common complaint, and treatment is with antacids. However, atazanavir requires an acidic environment to aid in absorption, and thus close monitoring is required post-treatment initiation.

Abdominal pain, diarrhea, cramping, and fever may be due to bacterial enteritis affecting the small or large bowel; causative organisms include *Clostridium difficile, Salmonella, Shigella, Campylobacter,* and *Yersinia* spp. Patients with advanced immunosuppression can have chronic diarrhea, often from opportunistic infections with *Cryptosporidium, Isospora,* and microsporidia. CMV is known to cause large bowel enteritis and generally occurs in severely immunosuppressed hosts with CD4+ counts below 50 cells/µL. In developing countries, extrapulmonary TB should also be on the differential for abdominal disease in HIV-positive patients. The evaluation for diarrhea involves laboratory stool studies (ova and parasite, *C. difficile* toxin, bacterial culture, modified acid-fast staining) and, occasionally, colonoscopy. For patients with mild to moderate symptoms, this can be arranged as an outpatient. For patients with severe cases, dehydration, or electrolyte abnormalities, these should be performed as an inpatient. Treatment is often supportive, maintaining hydration; symptoms often persist until immune reconstitution.

Rarely, malignancies such as Kaposi sarcoma or lymphoma, have been known to result in massive GI bleeding and bowel obstruction. Disseminated opportunistic infections such as MAC and *Bartonella* may cause secondary liver failure. AIDS-related cholangiopathy, biliary obstruction from infection-associated strictures of the biliary tract, is seen with severe immunosuppression.

Central Nervous System Manifestations

Common neurologic complications of HIV infection include aseptic meningitis, cryptococcal meningitis, toxoplasmosis, primary central nervous system (CNS) lymphoma, and progressive multifocal leukoencephalopathy. Patients present with a constellation of findings, including headaches, possible focal neurologic deficits, altered mental status, and fever.

HIV itself is a neurotropic virus, and patients with an acute infection can present with aseptic meningitis with complaints of fever, headaches, and meningismus. There usually is lymphocyte-predominant, moderate pleocytosis in the CSF. *Cryptococcus neoformans* is the most common cause of meningitis in patients with AIDS. It usually affects patients who are profoundly immunosuppressed, with CD4+ counts below 100 cells/µL. The disease is subacute, and patients present with fevers, malaise, and headache. Later in the course, because of increased intracranial pressure, patients experience vomiting and altered mental status. *Cryptococcus* often does not cause a significant inflammatory response, and meningeal signs are frequently absent. A lumbar puncture is diagnostic, demonstrating elevated opening pressures (70% with

pressures > 200 mm Hg), presence of cryptococcal antigen (CRAG), and low white blood cell count in the CSF (typically, <50/µL). Serum CRAG testing is readily available, sensitive, and especially useful in resource-poor settings. If the serum CRAG is negative, it will not likely be positive in the CSF and not the cause of cryptococcal meningitis. Poor prognostic factors for cryptococcal meningitis are altered mental status, absence of CSF pleocytosis, CSF antigen titers greater than 1:1024, and a positive serum fungal culture. These signs are indicative of a high organism burden, elevated CSF pressure, and lack of an inflammatory response. If left untreated, cryptococcal meningoencephalitis is fatal. Therapy involves three phases: induction, consolidation, and maintenance. Two weeks of amphotericin B and flucytosine is the recommended initial treatment. Fluconazole is used for the consolidation phase and is continued until immune reconstitution (CD4+ count > 100 cell/µL for more than one year). Elevated intracranial pressure is treated with repeated lumbar punctures; occasionally, a lumbar drain is needed. Cryptococcal meningitis immune reconstitution syndrome, a clinical deterioration in the setting of cryptococcal disease after the reversal of immune deficiency, can cause rapid clinical deterioration. A multicenter randomized trial has shown improved survival when ART is started five weeks after antifungal treatment compared to 1 to 2 weeks in those with risk factors.

Severely immunocompromised hosts (CD4+ count < 200 cells/µL) are likely to have opportunistic infections or AIDS-associated tumors (Table 121.6). In developed countries, common causes of mass effect are toxoplasmosis and EBV-related primary CNS lymphoma; in developing countries, the cause is more likely to be tuberculomas. Toxoplasmosis is caused by reactivation of latent infection by the parasite *Toxoplasma gondii.* Most infected patients have a CD4+ count below 100 cells/µL. Patients present with signs of increased intracranial pressure, such as headaches, confusion, lethargy, and seizures. Lesions are typically multiple and ring-enhancing on CT. Although the definitive diagnosis is made after a brain biopsy, patients who are serologically positive for toxoplasmosis are usually treated empirically with pyrimethamine and sulfadiazine, keeping in mind that toxoplasmosis is much less common in patients who have been receiving TMP-SMZ prophylaxis for PCP. Most patients will show radiographic improvement in 2 weeks; response to treatment obviates the need for a brain biopsy (Fig. 121.7).

Primary CNS lymphoma often looks identical to toxoplasmosis on magnetic resonance imaging (MRI) or CT scans. It also occurs with profound immunosuppression (CD4+ count < 50 cells/µL). EBV is the cause of primary CNS lymphoma, and a polymerase chain reaction (PCR) analysis of the CSF, looking for the virus, has become an integral step in the evaluation of mass lesions. Treatment involves ART and chemotherapy.

Progressive multifocal leukoencephalopathy, caused by the JC virus, is characterized by demyelinating lesions in the CNS. The diagnosis is suggested by nonenhancing, hypodense lesions on CT or MRI, with a CSF PCR assay positive for the JC virus. Advanced imaging with positron emission tomography, MRI, and single-photon emission CT can help differentiate among toxoplasmosis, lymphoma, and progressive multifocal leukoencephalopathy.

The gold standard for the diagnosis of CNS mass lesions remains brain biopsy. Corticosteroid therapy can cause false-negative results on brain biopsies in patients with lymphoma, and therefore the use of corticosteroids should be limited to patients with life-threatening mass lesions.

Renal Manifestations

The two main categories of HIV-related kidney disease are HIV-associated nephropathy (HIVAN) and HIV immune complex kidney

TABLE 121.6 Differential of Focal Central Nervous System Lesions in Patients With HIV Infection

	Common Clinical Presentation	Imaging and Diagnostic Testing
Toxoplasma encephalitis	Fever Headache Altered mental status Focal neurologic findings Seizure Evolves during days to weeks	Ring enhancing (≈90% of the time) CNS lesions Frequent edema and mass effect Toxoplasma antibodies (reflects past exposure) CD4+ often <100 cells/μL PCR detection of *Toxoplasma gondii*
Primary CNS lymphoma (PCNSL)	Confusion Lethargy Memory loss Hemiparesis Aphasia Seizure Fever Night sweats Weight loss Evolves during months	CNS lesion or lesions (may have mass effect) Solitary lesions are often large (>4 cm) Some ring enhancement may occur but less regular PCR assay for Epstein-Barr virus (associated with PCNSL)
Progressive multifocal leukoencephalopathy (PML)	Progressive focal neurologic deficits (during months) Hemiparesis Visual field defects Ataxia Aphasia Cognitive impairment	Multifocal areas of demyelination primarily involving white matter Less frequent mass effect or ring-enhancing PCR assay for DNA of JC virus (causes PML)
HIV encephalopathy	Memory and psychomotor speed impairment Depressive symptoms Movement disorders	Multiple hyperintense signals in T2-weighted images Often symmetrical; not well demarcated
Cytomegalovirus encephalitis	Delirium Confusion Focal neurologic abnormalities	Magnetic resonance imaging shows multifocal scattered micronodules and ventriculoencephalitis. CD4+ < 50 cells/μL
Brain abscess	Focal neurologic deficit Headache Bacteremia or craniofacial infection	Often concomitant evidence of disseminated infection
Tuberculoma	Focal neurologic deficit Headache Tuberculosis infection	Single or multiple mass lesions Can be manifested as focal lesion or meningeal infection

CNS, Central nervous system; *PCR*, polymerase chain reaction.

disease. HIVAN is a form of focal glomerulosclerosis that usually occurs in untreated individuals of African descent. Proteinuria, often severe, and an elevated creatinine concentration occur. Some patients recover renal function with ART, but many progress to end-stage renal disease and require dialysis. Transplantation is now widely accepted for patients with stable HIV infection.

ART can also affect the kidney. Indinavir, although less commonly used in industrialized countries, is associated with renal calculi. Tenofovir can cause acute renal failure, a Fanconi-like syndrome, and nephrogenic diabetes insipidus. Medications used to treat opportunistic infections can cause acute renal failure; amphotericin, pentamidine, and foscarnet are especially notorious.

Rheumatologic and Orthopedic Manifestations

HIV-infected patients are susceptible to the same types of orthopedic injuries and musculoskeletal disorders as patients without HIV infection. However, a few conditions specific to HIV infection are worth mentioning. Disseminated TB is more common in HIV-infected patients and can present with septic arthritis, spondylitis, osteomyelitis,

and bursitis. Risk factors include injection drug use and hemophilia. The most common causative organism involved is *Staphylococcus aureus*. Disseminated gonococcus causing septic arthritis is another possibility, especially in sexually active individuals. In late-stage AIDS, bacillary angiomatosis secondary to *Bartonella henselae* and *Bartonella quintana* can cause disseminated disease affecting the skin, lymph nodes, liver, and CNS and can also cause long-bone osteomyelitis.

Fractures of the hip, spine, and wrist are more common in HIV-infected individuals because they have lower bone mineral density than that of age-matched controls. Osteonecrosis, especially of the femoral head, is common. Predisposing factors include corticosteroid use, ethanol abuse, and hypertriglyceridemia.

HIV-related polymyositis can occur at any stage of infection. These patients may have proximal muscle weakness, myalgias, and fatigue. Medications, especially nucleotide reverse transcriptase inhibitors (NRTIs), such as azidothymidine (AZT), can be toxic to the mitochondria and are common causes of polymyositis. Myopathies, spondylarthritis, pyomyositis, and HIV-associated arthritis are also common musculoskeletal problems. Reactive arthritis and other seronegative

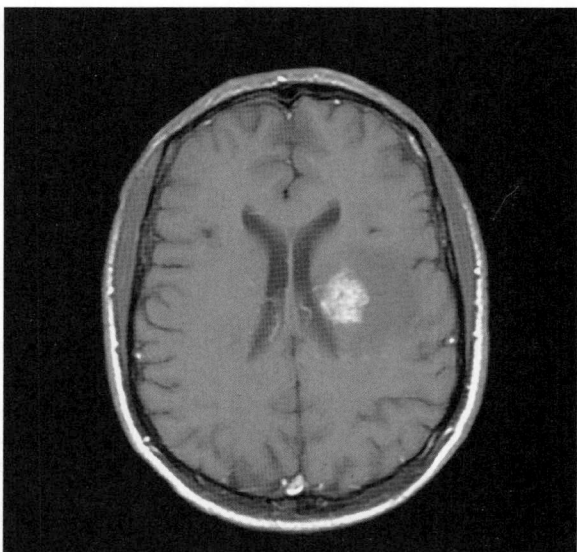

Fig. 121.7 Brain magnetic resonance image of a 38-year-old man with AIDS and *Toxoplasma* encephalitis. (From: Mandell GL, et al, ed. *Mandell, Douglas, and Bennett's Principles and Practice of Infectious Diseases*, ed 7. Philadelphia: Elsevier/Churchill Livingstone; 2010.)

arthropathies are common, although it is unclear if these are because of sexual activity, generalized immune suppression, or the inflammatory response from the virus itself.

Hematologic Manifestations

HIV infection is known to cause anemia, thrombocytopenia, and leukopenia. While anemia and leukopenia occur in later stages of HIV infection, thrombocytopenia can occur at any stage. Anemia and leukopenia are often secondary to medication-associated (AZT, TMP-SMZ, and ganciclovir) bone marrow toxicity. Thrombocytopenia is often immune-related, presenting as a disease process similar to idiopathic thrombocytopenic purpura; the treatment is ART. Thrombotic thrombocytopenic purpura is also well described in HIV-infected patients and tends to occur at later stages of the disease. Lastly, systemic fungal infections and mycobacterial disease such as disseminated MAC disease can infect the bone marrow and decrease all three cell lines, as can nutritional deficiencies, such as folate and vitamin B_{12}, which are also common.

AIDS-related lymphoma (Hodgkin and non-Hodgkin) occurs more frequently in patients with advanced HIV infection. Most non-Hodgkin's lymphomas are of B cell origin and tend to be more aggressive in HIV-infected than in noninfected patients. CNS lymphomas and Burkitt's lymphoma are almost always associated with EBV, and primary effusion lymphoma is associated with human herpesvirus 8. The treatment involves standard chemotherapy and ART.

Cutaneous Manifestations

Dermatologic manifestations of HIV infection are extremely common, occurring throughout the course of HIV infection. Some skin findings are manifested early in the disease; others, found later, can be suggestive of profound immunosuppression (Box 121.2). Skin problems increase as HIV infection progresses. Recognition of HIV-related dermatologic conditions can lead to early diagnosis and can help the emergency clinician gauge the patient's immune status (Box 121.3).

Acute HIV infection often is manifested with a generalized maculopapular or morbilliform rash shortly after the onset of fevers. Oral ulcers, lesions on the palms and soles, and mucosal lesions can all be present. Aside from HIV itself, a variety of viruses can involve the skin.

BOX 121.2 Dermatologic and Mucocutaneous Manifestations of WHO Stage 4 HIV Disease

Chronic herpes simplex virus ulcers
Extrapulmonary tuberculosis
Kaposi sarcoma
Extrapulmonary cryptococcosis
Disseminated mycosis
Atypical disseminated leishmaniasis
Disseminated nontuberculous mycobacterial infection
Extrapulmonary cryptococcosis including meningitis

WHO, World Health Organization.

BOX 121.3 Cutaneous Findings Highly Suggestive of HIV Disease

Any WHO criteria for stage 4 HIV disease
Facial molluscum in an adult
Proximal subungual onychomycosis
Herpes zoster scarring
Oral hairy leukoplakia
Bacillary angiomatosis
Widespread dermatophytosis
Severe seborrheic dermatitis

WHO, World Health Organization.

Herpes simplex virus infections are often more severe and recur frequently. Chronic ulcerating herpes simplex occurs later in the disease course and is an AIDS-defining opportunistic infection. Other common viral diseases include molluscum contagiosum, human papillomavirus infection, and oral hairy leukoplakia.

Kaposi sarcoma, a vascular neoplasm, is the most common AIDS-related malignant disease in the United States, and the skin is the most commonly involved organ. Lesions are violaceous patches, nodules, or plaques (Fig. 121.8). Bacillary angiomatosis is manifested with lesions that resemble those of Kaposi sarcoma.

Disseminated fungal infections are often signs of severe immunosuppression, and patients can present with skin manifestations. Disseminated cryptococcosis can be manifested with centrally umbilicated skin lesions resembling those of molluscum contagiosum. Other fungi (e.g., *Histoplasma capsulatum, Coccidioides immitis, Blastomyces dermatitidis, Penicillium marneffei*) can cause cutaneous disease and are a significant cause of morbidity and mortality.

Noninfectious skin disorders are common. Seborrheic dermatitis, characterized by greasy, scaly patches that are often located on the nasolabial folds, eyebrows, and scalp, affects up to 80% of patients with AIDS. Cutaneous drug reactions occur with increased frequency and severity, such as toxic epidermal necrolysis. Often, the reaction is from sulfa-containing drugs. Abacavir can cause a hypersensitivity reaction that can be fatal if not recognized.

DIFFERENTIAL DIAGNOSES

Initial Evaluation

HIV-infected patients are at risk for some of the same infections and medical problems as noninfected patients, but they are more vulnerable to opportunistic and unusual infections. Knowledge of the $CD4^+$ count, along with the patient's clinical presentation, is critical in ED management. Before ART, patients were primarily hospitalized for

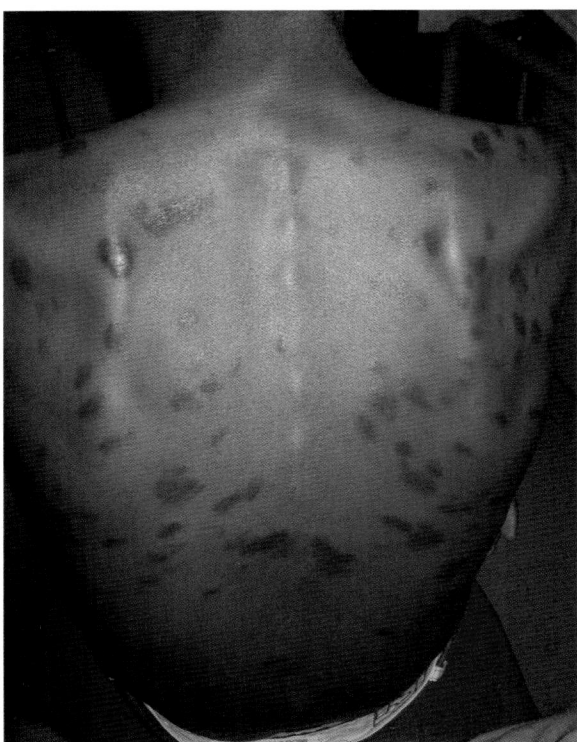

Fig. 121.8 Kaposi sarcoma lesions.

opportunistic infections. Patients with HIV infection are now dying of diseases that were not traditionally considered diseases of AIDS, such as heart disease, liver failure, and non–AIDS-related cancers.

The current CD4$^+$ count is a marker of the degree of immunosuppression and is critical background information for the interpretation of signs and symptoms. However, many ED patients have undiagnosed HIV infection or are medication noncompliant and may present with acute HIV infection, incidental HIV infection, or in later stages of the disease. Diagnostic clinical patterns are key to making an accurate diagnosis as to the stage of the disease. In lieu of a CD4$^+$ count, the total lymphocyte count may provide a rough approximation; a count between 1000 and 2000 cells/μL appears to be a reasonable surrogate of significant immunosuppression. Acute illness decreases peripheral lymphocyte counts and thus limits the value of the peripheral lymphocyte count as a diagnostic aid in an acute setting. However, an ED study has shown that patients with a peripheral lymphocyte count below 950 cells/μL are highly likely to have AIDS.

The possibility of HIV infection in patients presenting to the ED must be considered on a case by case basis. HIV infection should be considered in any patient who presents with unusual or recurrent serious infections without another explanation, especially patients with risk factors for HIV infection, such as IV drug users (IVDUs) and high-risk sexual practices. Although the opportunistic infections associated with AIDS can occur in the absence of HIV infection, they usually develop in patients with some form of immunosuppression. HIV infection should also be considered in younger patients who develop conditions that typically do not occur until later in life, such as herpes zoster.

Diagnostic Testing

HIV Testing
The diagnosis of HIV infection involves the detection of specific antibodies or viral antigens (see Table 121.1). Laboratory detection of HIV infection is a two-step process. The first step is a screening test; if the result is positive, a confirmatory test is performed.

The balance between public health and patient confidentiality has been an issue surrounding HIV testing and reporting. Most states and hospitals have developed policies related to these concerns. Regardless, testing should be done in a confidential manner, with appropriate follow-up and counseling.

With improved testing capabilities as well as efforts to diagnose existing cases of HIV infection in underserved populations, some experts have recommended routine screening tests. The advantages of testing in the ED include increased detection of HIV infection in difficult-to-reach populations and earlier diagnosis of HIV infection, allowing earlier ART implementation and therefore decreased viral transmission.

In 2006, the CDC published revised recommendations for HIV testing in health care settings, including hospital EDs.[5] This report recommended the use of diagnostic HIV testing and opt-out HIV screening in routine clinical care. Routine screening is recommended for 13- to 64-year-old patients, all patients who require TB treatment, those seeking treatment for sexually transmitted infections, and all pregnant women. Repeat annual screening is recommended for people at high risk. Recommendations specify that consent should be obtained for HIV testing, pretest information should be shared with patients, and those responsible for the patient's care should be notified verbally of the planned testing. The recommendations also call for reducing barriers to HIV testing. In April 2013, the U.S. Preventive Services Task Force issued similar recommendations.[3] Screening tests can include self-testing or provider-initiated testing. In emergency departments, given the resource constraints, there is a trend towards opt-out testing where the consent process is truncated and performed during triage. Testing can be in the form of a rapid point of care test, such as the INSTI©, or an oral test such as the Oraquick©. Local institutional availability and strategies for implementing testing in the ED will vary. Most rapid tests and self-tests are antibody tests; thus, it is recommended that patients with an initial negative test should retest at three months and, in the meantime, implement transmission reduction strategies such as condoms. The window period for a fourth-generation (antigen/antibody) test is still about four weeks.

MANAGEMENT

The care of the HIV-infected patient in the emergency department has evolved significantly, as has the management of HIV worldwide. In addition to the management of acute HIV infection, HIV-associated complications, and ART side effects, the modern ED physician may also be tasked with providing preexposure prophylaxis (PrEP), postexposure prophylaxis, ART initiation, and linkage to care.

The clinical management of acute HIV infection is supportive. Management of opportunistic infections in the ED should be guided by the presumptive causative organism and may require consultation with Infectious Diseases.

Side effects of antiretroviral medications are extremely common. Protease inhibitors are notorious for GI side effects; most cause nausea and diarrhea. The NRTIs are mitochondrial toxic and can cause pancreatitis and hepatitis. Nevirapine, an NNRTI, can cause hepatic necrosis. Atazanavir causes Gilbert-like syndrome. Efavirenz is commonly associated with self-limited neuropsychiatric problems

Preexposure Prophylaxis
The CDC guidelines for preexposure for the prevention of HIV infection in the United States were updated in 2017. Daily oral PrEP with the fixed-dose combination of tenofovir disoproxil fumarate (TDF)

300 mg and emtricitabine (FTC) 200 mg is safe and effective in reducing the risk of sexual HIV acquisition in adults. It is recommended for patients with a substantial risk of HIV infection and for patients with HIV-positive partners. Currently, the data on the efficacy and safety of PrEP for adolescents are insufficient. Acute and chronic HIV infection must be excluded by symptom history and HIV testing immediately before PrEP is prescribed. Patients should be counseled that HIV infection should be assessed at least every three months, and renal function should be assessed at baseline and monitored every six months while on PrEP. Furthermore, when PrEP is prescribed, clinicians should provide access, directly or by facilitated referral, to proven effective risk-reduction services. Because high medication adherence is critical to PrEP efficacy but was not uniformly achieved by trial participants, patients should be encouraged and enabled to use PrEP in combination with other effective prevention methods.

Postexposure Prophylaxis

Postexposure prophylaxis (PEP) using ART significantly decreases the risk of transmission. Potentially infectious body fluids include CSF and synovial, pleural, peritoneal, pericardial, and amniotic fluids. Unless they contain blood, the following fluids are not considered infectious for HIV: vomitus, feces, nasal secretions, saliva, sputum, sweat, tears, and urine. Low-risk injuries are those involving solid needles (e.g., suture needles), those that are superficial, and those involving a low-risk source patient or body fluid. High-risk injuries include those involving hollow bore needles with visible blood and percutaneous injury from a needle that was in an artery or vein of the source patient. Unless a mucocutaneous exposure involves large volumes of blood from a source patient with a plasma HIV viral load more than 1500 copies/µL, mucocutaneous exposures are considered to be low risk.

The US Public Health Services updated guidelines on managing occupational exposures to HIV are as follows: (1) PEP is initiated when occupational exposures to HIV occur; (2) the HIV status of the exposure source patient should be determined, if possible, to guide need for HIV PEP; (3) PEP medication regimens should be started as soon as possible after occupational exposure to HIV, and they should be continued for a 4-week duration; (4) PEP medication regimens should contain 3 (or more) antiretroviral drugs for all occupational exposures to HIV; (5) expert consultation is recommended for occupational exposures to HIV, especially in cases of delayed exposure report, pregnancy or breastfeeding status of exposed individual, known or suspected resistance of source virus, underlying medical illness in the exposed individual, and unclear source (e.g., needle in sharps disposal container or laundry); (6) close follow-up for exposed personnel should be provided that includes counseling, baseline, and follow-up HIV testing, and monitoring for drug toxicity; follow-up appointments should begin within 72 hours of an HIV exposure.[6] Most institutions have specific guidelines that specify treatment regimens and follow-up plan through occupational health.

In addition to PEP, the initial response to exposure is immediate cleansing of the exposed or injured site; soap and water can be used for intact skin, and viricidal antiseptic agents, such as alcohol-based hand hygiene agents, can be used for small punctures and wounds. Mucosal surfaces and eyes should be flushed with copious amounts of water. Efforts should be made to document clinical information about the source patient, including risk factors and previous test results for HIV, HBV, and HCV, as well as to provide a description of the exposure and the time it occurred.

In situations where local expertise is unavailable, the Clinician Consultation Center (PEPline) can be contacted at 888-448-4911 for rapid, expert guidance in managing health care worker exposures to HIV and hepatitis B and C, including recommendations on when and how to initiate PEP through an online Quick Guide.[7]

Some patients may present after possible exposure to HIV/AIDS with concern about the potential of transmission. Possible means of exposure include sexual contact, injection drug use, and exposure to body fluids through broken skin or mucous membranes. The CDC recommends PEP for persons presenting within 72 hours after an exposure to a source known to be HIV-positive if contact of body fluid contaminated with blood (including semen, vaginal secretions, rectal secretions, and breast milk) was made with the vagina, rectum, eye, mouth or other mucous membranes, or nonintact skin or by percutaneous injection. Efforts should be made to determine the current HIV status of the source.

All persons offered PEP should be prescribed a 28-day course of a 3-drug antiretroviral regimen. The preferred regimen for otherwise healthy adults and adolescents is tenofovir disoproxil fumarate (tenofovir DF or TDF) (300 mg) with emtricitabine (200 mg) once daily plus raltegravir (RAL) 400 mg twice daily or dolutegravir (DTG) 50 mg daily.[4] RAL is preferred if the woman is pregnant. A modification of this regimen is recommended for children, persons with decreased renal function, and pregnant women.

Whereas most seroconversions will occur in the first three months after the exposure, these patients should be checked for HIV at six weeks, 12 weeks, and six months. The PEPline is also available to provide advice (see earlier). In addition, all persons evaluated for possible nPEP should be provided any indicated prevention, treatment, or supportive care for other exposure-associated health risks and conditions (e.g., bacterial sexually transmitted infections, traumatic injuries, hepatitis B virus, and hepatitis C virus infection, or pregnancy). Persons who report behaviors or situations that place them at risk for frequently recurring HIV exposures (e.g., injection drug use, or sex without condoms) or who report receipt of 1 course or less of nPEP in the past year should be provided risk-reduction counseling and intervention services, including consideration of preexposure prophylaxis

ART Initiation and Linkage to Care

Immediate antiretroviral therapy (ART) refers to starting HIV treatment as soon as possible after the diagnosis of HIV infection, preferably on the first clinic visit (and even on the same day the HIV diagnosis is made). This strategy also is known as "rapid ART," "same-day ART," and "treatment upon diagnosis." Immediate ART initiation may bring earlier benefits in personal health and reductions in the risk of further transmission of HIV. For persons with acute infection, immediate ART may limit the HIV viral reservoir. In pilot studies in the United States and in randomized controlled trials in resource-limited settings, rapid ART initiation has been shown to reduce time to linkage to care and viral load suppression.[8,9]

As such, same-day initiation (SDI), has not only been piloted but is the standard of care at numerous institutions in the United States. Local institutional guidelines must be followed. To support this practice, the ED clinician should identify patients suitable for ART initiation, provide counseling, complete baseline laboratory testing, and prescribe a blister pack with a locally recommended treatment regimen. ART is started before the results of baseline testing (including HIV RNA, CD4 count, genotype, HLA-B*5701, and creatinine) are available. Thus, the ART regimens must be potent and effective in the setting of high viral load and/or transmitted NRTI resistance. The preferred recommended regimens are dolutegravir (Tivicay) + TAF/FTC (Descovy) or darunavir (Prezista) + booster (ritonavir or cobicistat) + TAF/FTC.[10]

ART initiation will be successful only if closely tied to linkage to care. Patients will need additional HIV-related education, information regarding the importance of medication adherence, counseling about preventing HIV transmission, and encouragement about living healthy lives with HIV. Most institutions will have a partnership with their local infectious disease clinic. It is recommended that patients have a phone call scheduled within 2 to 3 days of the index visit, and a clinic follow-up appointment at 1 to 2 weeks.

DISPOSITION

The widespread use of ART among HIV-positive individuals has dramatically changed the course of the disease; individuals often have sustained and lasting immune reconstitution and live relatively normal lives. Knowledge of their immune status is critical for disposition and treatment; patients with a normal or near-normal CD4$^+$ count should be treated like non–HIV-infected patients. Drug interactions are common. Patients with AIDS, unlike immunocompetent patients, often suffer from multiple, simultaneous underlying pathologic processes, making evaluation and treatment decisions even more difficult; a unifying diagnosis is not the norm. These patients are at greater risk of morbidity and mortality from common disease entities, as well as from complications of HIV/AIDS. Emergency clinicians who approach these patients with background knowledge of the potential manifestations of HIV/AIDS will be poised to deliver the best emergent care.

The references for this chapter can be found online at ExpertConsult.com.

122

Parasites

John D. Cahill and Bruce M.Becker

KEY CONCEPTS

- Parasitic diseases may manifest with almost any constellation of signs and symptoms.
- The combination of presenting signs and symptoms and a history of recent travel to specific geographic regions can lead to early diagnosis and the initiation of pharmacotherapy, decreasing morbidity and mortality and increasing the probability of eradication of the infection.
- Parasitic coinfections are particularly common in patients with HIV infection and AIDS. A travel history is essential because the clinical presentation may be atypical, morbidity and mortality are more severe, and treatment is often prolonged.
- Acute malaria should be suspected in patients with irregular high fevers associated with headache, abdominal pain, or respiratory symptoms. Falciparum malaria, which has a unique morphology easily identifiable on the peripheral blood smear, is the predominant species of malaria that causes coma and death. *P. falciparum* is the most highly resistant to chemotherapy, demanding close observation and clinical follow-up of patients. Patients who are clinically ill or who are suspected of having falciparum malaria should be hospitalized.
- Cysticercosis should be considered in the differential diagnosis of the patient with new-onset seizures, especially in patients who have been living in Central and South America.
- Giardiasis should be suspected in patients with diarrhea who have recently been camping or drinking unfiltered mountain spring water. Patients may have tolerated several weeks of severe bloating, flatulence, eructation, and weight loss without fever before seeking medical attention.
- *Trypanosoma cruzi* infection results in Chagas disease, most notable for the development of acute and chronic myocarditis. Cardiomyopathy can be severe, at times even necessitating heart transplant.

FOUNDATIONS

Parasitic infections are caused by a diverse group of eukaryotic organisms distributed across the globe, although the highest prevalence of these infections is found in tropical regions. Box 122.1 outlines the taxonomy of human parasites. Protozoal agents are unicellular, while the helminths are multicellular. These infectious organisms demonstrate complex life cycles that often include intermediate stages that target (human) hosts, along with stages of development in which they live freely in the environment. The modes of transmission to humans may include insect bites, the consumption of raw or undercooked and "infected" meat or seafood, the ingestion of water or food contaminated by human feces, or skin exposure to water or soil containing parasites at the infectious stage of development. The spectrum of clinical parasitic disease can vary from acute, life-threatening infection to chronic, progressive illness. Other infections may present with acute illness that can recover without sequalae and some cause asymptomatic infections that may manifest years later or never.

An understanding of parasitology has become increasingly crucial for emergency clinicians. In the last few decades, there has been a dramatic increase in immigration across the globe, including regions where parasitic infections are highly endemic. There has also been an increase in business and adventure travel to tropical regions, bringing immunologically naïve and vulnerable hosts to sites rich in parasitic disease. Patients with human immunodeficiency virus (HIV) infection or acquired immunodeficiency syndrome (AIDS) who travel to or emigrate from countries where parasitic illnesses are endemic are at higher risk of infection with these illnesses. In addition, there continues to be an increase in the prevalence of endemic parasitic diseases in many rural areas of the southeastern and southwestern United States, and in some parts of Europe. Climate change has been extending the habitat of what were previously known as tropical parasites and vectors to previously temperate regions. Thus, a growing population of patients with parasitic illness now present to emergency departments, requiring the emergency clinician to consider these unusual but important diseases.

Many parasitic infections follow an indolent course or present with nonspecific symptoms, posing a challenge to diagnosis especially in the ED setting. While correct diagnosis and pharmacologic treatment of parasitic infections usually leads to a rapid and complete recovery, delayed treatment or mismanagement of parasitic diseases can have severe long-term consequences. To diagnose parasitic infection, the emergency clinician must obtain a thorough travel history, including questions summarized in Box 122.2, perform a detailed physical examination, and order appropriate laboratory studies. This information must be integrated with an understanding of the basic life cycles of parasites, incubation periods between inoculation and clinical presentation, and intersecting geography of the organism and host. Physicians must have the ability to recognize both the classical and atypical presentations of particular parasitic infections and institute appropriate therapy (Table 122.1).

Parasitic illness should be considered in the differential diagnosis of patients who have spent time in areas of the world with endemic parasitic illnesses (Table 122.2). For patients who have recently immigrated to the United States, the emergency clinician should elicit additional information specific to the country of origin, also summarized in Box 122.2. The incubation period for the development of symptoms for parasitic diseases ranges from days (falciparum malaria) to months (vivax malaria) to years (filariasis).

Parasite biochemical pathways are generally different from those of their human host, permitting selective metabolic interference by using relatively small doses of chemotherapeutic agents. New and more effective antiparasitic agents continue to be developed. The list of

BOX 122.1 List of Conditions and Taxonomy

Protozoa
Apicomplexan/Coccidia
- Malaria
- Babesia
- Cryptosporidia
- Cyclospora
- Cystoisospora
- Sarcocystis
- Toxoplasma

Amoebae
- Entamoeba histolytica
- Naegleria fowleri
- Acanthamoeba spp.
- Balamuthia mandrillaris

Flagellates
- Leishmania
- Trypanosoma cruzi
- Trypanosoma brucei
- Giardia lamblia
- Trichomonas vaginalis

Ciliates
- Balantidium coli

Helminths
Nematodes
- Hookworm (Necator/Ancyclostoma)
- Trichuris
- Ascaris
- Enterobius
- Filaria (Wuchereria/Brugia/Onchocerca/Loa loa/Mansonella)

- Strongyloides
- Capillaria
- Anisakiasis
- Dracunculiasis
- Trichinella

Trematodes
- Schistosoma
- Fasciola spp.
- Paragonimus
- Clonorchis
- Opisthorchis
- Fasciolopsis/Echinostoma

Cestodes
- Taenia solium
- Taenia saginata
- Diphyllobothrium latum, D. pacificum
- Hymenolepis nana/diminuta
- Echinococcus granulosus, E. multilocularis
- Spirometra (sparganosis)—eyes, brain, other
- Sparganum (proliferative sparganosis)

Zoonotic Helminths
- Baylisascaris
- Angiostrongylus costaricensis, cantonensis
- Gnathostomiasis
- Toxocara
- Hookworm (Ancylostoma caninum, A. braziliense, Uncinaria)

BOX 122.2 Comprehensive Travel History for Evaluation of Parasitic Disease in the Emergency Department

Questions for All Patients
- What were the exact dates of travel?
- What countries did the patient visit?
- How much time was spent in each country?
- What was the patient doing in the country, and where was he or she living?
- Was the patient a tourist, an adventure traveler, or a worker?
- Did the patient stay in cities or rural villages?
- Was the patient sleeping in hotels or tents?
- Did the patient engage in protected or unprotected sexual intercourse?
- What did the patient eat and drink?
- What were the patient's activities (e.g., swimming in fresh water leads to schistosomiasis)?
- Did the patient receive prophylactic immunizations before travel?
- Did the patient take malaria chemoprophylaxis and comply with the regimen?
- Did the patient use mosquito repellent and netting?
- Does the patient have underlying chronic medical problems?
- What medications does the patient take?
- When did symptoms start, and what has been the chronology of symptoms, particularly fever and diarrhea?

Questions for Patients Who Are Recent Immigrants to the United States
- When did the patient arrive, and from where?
- What acute and chronic illnesses did the patient have previously while living in the country of origin?
- What treatment did the patient receive there?
- If a refugee or immigrant, what countries did the patient pass through, and what were the living conditions (especially relevant for persons who have lived in numerous refugee camps)?
- What was the season during the patient's stay or travel in the countries (e.g., monsoon vs. dry)?
- What animal exposures and bites has the patient experienced?
- Has the patient had exposure to fresh water in work or recreational activities?

drugs used to treat parasitic infestations is long and varied. Table 122.3 includes recommended agents. The newer antiparasitic drugs tend to be less toxic and more efficacious. In many cases, single-dose treatment can eradicate an entire parasite burden, thus supporting effective public health initiatives that include mass treatment programs for populations with a large burden of infection in endemic areas.

MALARIA

Background and Importance

More than 41% of the world's population lives in malarial areas where plasmodia are endemic (e.g., parts of Africa, Asia, Oceania, Central America, and South America). The World Health Organization (WHO) has estimated that in 2013, malaria was responsible for 198 million clinical episodes and 500,000 deaths. Most of these deaths were the result of infection with *Plasmodium falciparum*.[1] Immigrants and returning travelers presenting with malarial symptoms warrant particular consideration as acute falciparum malaria, if left untreated, carries a high mortality. Although it is classically associated with cyclical fevers, malaria presents various symptoms, including headache and diarrhea. Fever is common but not universal at initial presentation. When fever is present,

it is often continuous early in the course of illness. Some studies in low endemicity areas have suggested that the presence of fever or headache has a sensitivity greater than 95%. In recent years there has been an increase in the diagnosis of falciparum malaria in travelers returning to the United States; the most common region from which these travelers return is West Africa. Patients who have had a longer duration of travel and neglected to take prophylactic medications or who failed to adhere to prescribed regimens are at the greatest risk.

Most people contract malaria after being bitten by an infected vector mosquito in an endemic region. Other mechanisms of transmission have been reported, including blood transfusions, injection drug use with contaminated syringes, maternal-fetal perinatal transmission, transmission from infected organs after transplantation (worsened by immunosuppression), and what has been described as "airport malaria." This occurs when the infected mosquito is transported from the endemic region and released at the airport when the plane arrives, surviving long enough to transmit the parasite to a human host and then dying without establishing itself in its new location.

Pathophysiology

Malaria is caused by one of five species of the protozoan parasite *Plasmodium*: *P. falciparum*, *P. vivax*, *P. ovale*, *P. malariae*, and *P. knowlesi*. Of these species, *P. falciparum* poses the greatest risk of

TABLE 122.1   Drug Classes and Modes of Action of Agents Used for Treatment of Parasitic Diseases

Type of Drug	Examples[a]	Useful in the Treatment of:	Likely Target in the Parasite	Proposed Effects on Targets
Anthelmintic	Thiabendazole Mebendazole Albendazole	*Ascaris, Enterobius,* hookworm, *Strongyloides, Trichuris,* hydatid disease (long-term therapy)	Tubulin polymerization	Blocks cellular structural integrity and egg production; secondary effects on mitochondrial fumarate reductase and glucose uptake
	Ivermectin (Stromectol)	Many nematodes of humans (except hookworms) Filariasis Onchocerciasis	GABA-sensitive neuromuscular interface	Flaccidity or contraction (tight-binding drug effective at low dose)
Trematodicide	Praziquantel (Biltricide)	Schistosomes Most other flukes, such as *Clonorchis, Paragonimus, Fasciolopsis* (many tapeworms of humans)	Surface structure Carbohydrate metabolism	Vacuolization and surface disruption followed by immune attacks by the host; contraction of the muscles due to flooding of calcium through a permeable tegument; initial increase of glucose metabolism followed by shutdown
Antiprotozoal	Metronidazole (Flagyl) Tinidazole Niridazole	Amebiasis Balantidiasis Giardiasis *Schistosoma haematobium*	Molecular electron transport systems Acetylcholine recycling systems	Failure to sustain energy-producing systems Binds to acetylcholinesterase, inactivating normal neuromuscular function
Antimalarial	Chloroquine phosphate (Aralen)	Many species of susceptible malaria	Parasite digestive vacuole hemoglobinase	Local pH is changed so enzyme becomes inoperative
	Mefloquine	Many species of susceptible malaria		
	Proguanil-atovaquone	Many species of susceptible malaria	Mitochondrial electron transport prevents the normal function of the apicoplast	Works on erythrocytic and hepatic stages
	Doxycycline	Many species of susceptible malaria		Kills *Plasmodium falciparum*

[a]Some drugs may be available only from the CDC Drug Service, Centers for Disease Control and Prevention, Atlanta, GA 30333; telephone: 404-639-3670 (nights, weekends, and holidays: 404-639-2888).

GABA, γ-aminobutyric acid.

TABLE 122.2   Parasites Causing Human Disease: Geographic Location and Portal of Entry

Parasite	Geographic Distribution	Common Infective Stage and Portal of Entry
Protozoa Apicomplexan Amoeba Flagellate Ciliate		
Entamoeba histolytica	Especially prevalent in warm climates	Cyst via mouth
Balantidium coli	Warm climates	Cyst via mouth
Giardia lamblia	Found throughout temperate and warm climates	Cyst via mouth
Trichomonas vaginalis	United States	Trophozoite via vulva or urethra
Leishmania tropica	Mediterranean area to western India	Bite of sandfly introducing promastigote via skin, leading to visceral disease
Leishmania infantum	Southern Europe and Mediterranean	Bite of sandfly introducing promastigote via skin, leading to visceral disease
Leishmania donovani	China, India, Africa, Mediterranean area, continental Latin America	Bite of sandfly introducing promastigote via skin, leading to visceral disease
Leishmania chagasi	South America	Bite of sandfly introducing promastigote via skin, leading to visceral disease
Leishmania braziliensis	South America and Central America	Bite of sandfly introducing promastigote via skin, leading to cutaneous or mucocutaneous disease
Leishmania major, L. tropica	Africa and Asia	Bite of sandfly introducing promastigote via skin, leading to cutaneous disease

TABLE 122.2 Parasites Causing Human Disease: Geographic Location and Portal of Entry—cont'd.

Parasite	Geographic Distribution	Common Infective Stage and Portal of Entry
Leishmania mexicana, L. amazonensis, L. guyanensis, L. costaricensis	Central and South America	Bite of sandfly introducing promastigote via skin, leading to cutaneous disease
Trypanosoma brucei gambiense	West and Central Africa	Trypanosome via skin from bite of the tsetse fly
Trypanosoma brucei rhodesiense	Central and East Africa	Trypanosome via skin from bite of the tsetse fly
Trypanosoma cruzi	Continental Latin America	Trypanosome via skin from reduviid bug
Plasmodium vivax	Warm and cooler climates	Sporozoite via skin from *Anopheles* mosquito
Plasmodium ovale	Warm and cooler climates	Sporozoite via skin from *Anopheles* mosquito
Plasmodium malariae	Warm climates	Sporozoite via skin from *Anopheles* mosquito
Plasmodium knowlesi	Warm and cooler climates	Sporozoite via skin from *Anopheles* mosquito
Plasmodium falciparum	Warm climates	Sporozoite via skin from *Anopheles* mosquito
Babesia microti		
Cryptosporidium parvum		
Cyclospora cayetanensis		
Cystoisospora belli		
Toxoplasma gondii		
Sarcocystis hominis		
Naegleria fowleri		
Acanthamoeba spp.		
Balamuthia mandrillaris		
Nematodes		
Trichinella spiralis	Cooler and temperate climates	Encysted larva in pork or bear via mouth
Trichuris trichiura	Warm, moist climates	Embryonated egg via mouth
Strongyloides stercoralis	Warm, moist climates	Filariform larva via skin
Necator americanus	Common in warm climates	Filariform larva via skin
Ancylostoma duodenale	Common in warm climates	Filariform larva via skin
Enterobius vermicularis	Common in the United States	Embryonated egg via mouth
Ascaris lumbricoides	Global distribution; common in the United States	Embryonated egg via mouth
Wuchereria bancrofti	Prevalent in warm climates	Filariform larva via skin from bite of *Anopheles* or *Culex* mosquito
Brugia malayi	Asia	Filariform larva via skin from bite of *Anopheles* or *Culex* mosquito
Onchocerca volvulus	Tropical Africa, Mexico, Central America, and northern South America	Filariform larva via skin from bite of the blackfly
Loa loa	Tropical West Africa	Filariform larva via skin from bite of the *Chrysops* fly
Dracunculus medinensis	Increasingly rare	Ingestion of larva by copepod via mouth
Capillaria philippinensis		
Anisakis simplex		
Baylisascaris procyonis		
Angiostrongylus cantonensis		
Gnathostoma spinigerum/binucleatum		
Toxocara canis		
Ancylostoma braziliense		
Cestodes		
Taenia saginata	Global distribution; uncommon in the United States	Cysticercus in beef via mouth
Taenia solium	South America, Central America, Mexico, East Africa, India, China, Indonesia	
• Adult worm		Cysticercus in pork via mouth
• Cysticercus stage		Eggs in human infections via mouth
Echinococcus granulosus	Mediterranean, Russian Federation and neighboring countries, China, Central Asia, North and East Africa, and South America	Eggs from canines via fecal-oral transmission
Echinococcus multilocularis	Central Europe, northern Asia, Alaska	Eggs from foxes, dogs, and cats via fecal-oral transmission
Hymenolepis nana	Warm climates	Eggs in human infections via mouth

Continued

TABLE 122.2   Parasites Causing Human Disease: Geographic Location and Portal of Entry—cont'd.

Parasite	Geographic Distribution	Common Infective Stage and Portal of Entry
Hymenolepis diminuta	Warm climates	Larva in arthropod host via mouth
Diphyllobothrium latum *Diphyllobothrium pacificum* *Spirometra spp.* *Sparganum proliferum*	US Great Lakes region and Alaska, Scandinavia, Russia, Japan, Pacific Coast of South America, and Uganda	*Sparganum* larva in fish flesh via mouth
Trematodes		
Fasciola hepatica	Sheep-raising countries	Larva on vegetation via mouth
Fasciolopsis buski	Asia	Larva on water nuts
Clonorchis sinensis	Asia	Larva encysted in freshwater fish
Opisthorchis felineus	Europe, Asia	Larva encysted in freshwater fish
Opisthorchis viverrini	Thailand	Larva encysted in freshwater fish
Paragonimus westermani	Primarily Asia; also South America and Africa	Larva encysted in crabs or crayfish via mouth
Schistosoma japonicum	China, Southeast Asia, Philippines	Cercarial larva in water via skin
Schistosoma mansoni	Africa, Latin America, Middle East, Caribbean	Cercarial larva in water via skin
Schistosoma haematobium *Echinostoma hortense*	Africa, Middle East	Cercarial larva in water via skin

Adapted from: Beaver PC, Jung RC, Eddie Wayne Cupp EW. *Clinical Parasitology*, ed 9. Philadelphia: Lea & Febiger; 1984.

TABLE 122.3   Drug Regimens for Treatment of Parasitic Infections

Infection	Drug[a]	DOSAGE Adults	Children
Amebiasis (*Entamoeba histolytica*)			
Asymptomatic			
	DRUG OF CHOICE		
	• Iodoquinol	650 mg tid × 20 days	30 mg/kg/day in 3 doses × 20 days
	ALTERNATIVES		
	• Diloxanide furoate *or*	500 mg tid × 10 days	25–35 mg/kg/day in 3 doses × 7 days
	• Paromomycin	25–30 mg/kg/day in 3 doses × 7 days	25–30 mg/kg/day in 3 doses × 7 days
Mild to Moderate Intestinal Disease			
	DRUG OF CHOICE		
	• Metronidazole *followed by* • Paromomycin or iodoquinol	750 mg tid × 10 days	35–50 mg/kg/day in 3 doses × 10 days
	ALTERNATIVES		
	• Tinidazole *followed by* • Paromomycin or iodoquinol	2 g/day × 3 days	50 mg/kg (max, 2 g) qd × 3 days
Severe Intestinal Disease, Hepatic Abscess Drainage of liver abscess			
	DRUG OF CHOICE		
	• Metronidazole *followed by* • Paromomycin or iodoquinol	750 mg IV or PO tid × 10 days	35–50 mg/kg/day in 3 doses × 10 days
	ALTERNATIVES		
	• Tinidazole *followed by* • Paromomycin or iodoquinol	2 g/day × 5 days	50 mg/kg or 60 mg/kg (max, 2 g) qd × 3 days
Amebic meningoencephalitis, primary (*Naegleria* spp.)	DRUG OF CHOICE • Amphotericin B	1 mg/kg/day IV, uncertain duration	1 mg/kg/day IV, uncertain duration
Anisakiasis (*Anisakis*)			
Treatment of choice	Surgical or endoscopic removal		

TABLE 122.3   Drug Regimens for Treatment of Parasitic Infections—cont'd.

Infection	Drug[a]	DOSAGE	
		Adults	**Children**
Ascariasis (*Ascaris lumbricoides*)			
Roundworm	DRUGS OF CHOICE		
	• Mebendazole	100 mg bid × 3 days	100 mg bid × 3 days
	• Albendazole	400 mg × 1 dose	>6 yr, same dose as for adult
	• Nitazoxanide	500 mg bid × 3 days	200 mg bid × 3 days
	• Ivermectin	150–200 µg/kg for 1 dose; should be avoided in pregnant women	Should be avoided in young children
Balantidiasis (*Balantidium coli*)			
	DRUG OF CHOICE		
	• Tetracycline	500 mg qid × 10 days	40 mg/kg/day in 4 doses × 10 days (max, 2 g/day)
	ALTERNATIVES	650 mg tid × 20 days	40 mg/kg/day in 3 doses × 20 days
	• Iodoquinol		
	• Metronidazole	750 mg tid × 5 days	35–50 mg/kg/day in 3 doses × 5 days
Cutaneous Larva Migrans			
Creeping eruption	DRUG OF CHOICE		
	• Ivermectin	200 µg/kg once daily × 1 or 2 days	
Dracunculus medinensis			
Guinea worm; worm also needs to be extracted	DRUG OF CHOICE		
	• Metronidazole	750 mg tid × 5–10 days	25 mg/kg/day (max, 750 mg/day) in 2 doses × 10 days
	ALTERNATIVE		
	• Thiabendazole	50–75 mg/day bid × 3 days	50–75 mg/kg/day in 2 doses × 3 days
Enterobius vermicularis			
Pinworm	DRUGS OF CHOICE		
	• Albendazole	Single dose of 400 mg; repeat after 2 wk	11 mg/kg once (max, 1 g); repeat after 2 wk
	• Mebendazole	Single dose of 100 mg; repeat after 2 wk	Single dose of 100 mg; repeat after 2 wk
Filariasis (*Wuchereria bancrofti, Brugia malayi*)			
	DRUG OF CHOICE		
	• Diethylcarbamazine	Day 1: 50 mg PO Day 2: 50 mg tid Day 3: 100 mg tid Days 4–21: 6 mg/kg/day in 3 doses	Day 1: 1 mg/kg PO Day 2: 1 mg/kg tid Day 3: 1–2 mg/kg tid Days 4–21: 6 mg/kg/day in 3 doses
Loa loa	DRUG OF CHOICE		
	• Diethylcarbamazine	Day 1: 50 mg PO Day 2: 50 mg tid Day 3: 100 mg tid Days 4–21: 9 mg/kg/day in 3 doses	Day 1: 1 mg/kg PO Day 2: 1 mg/kg tid Day 3: 1–2 mg/kg tid Days 4–21: 6 mg/kg/day in 3 doses
Onchocerca volvulus	DRUG OF CHOICE		
	• Ivermectin	150 µg/kg PO once, repeated every 3–12 mo	150 µg/kg PO once, repeated every 3–12 mo
Hermaphroditic Fluke			
Clonorchis sinensis (Chinese liver fluke)	DRUG OF CHOICE		
	• Praziquantel	25 mg/kg/day in 4–6 doses × 1 day	25 mg/kg/day in 4–6 doses × 1 day
Fasciola hepatica (sheep liver fluke)	DRUG OF CHOICE	30–50 mg/kg on alternate days × 10–15 doses	30–50 mg/kg on alternate days × 10–15 doses
	• Bithionol		

Continued

TABLE 122.3   Drug Regimens for Treatment of Parasitic Infections—cont'd.

Infection	Drug[a]	DOSAGE	
		Adults	**Children**
Fasciolopsis buski (intestinal fluke)	DRUG OF CHOICE		
	• Praziquantel	25 mg/kg/day in 4 to 6 doses × 1 day	25 mg/kg/day in 4 to 6 doses × 1 day
Opisthorchis felineu	DRUG OF CHOICE		
	• Praziquantel	25 mg/kg/day in 4 to 6 doses × 1 day	25 mg/kg/day in 4 to 6 doses × 1 day
Paragonimus westermani (lung fluke)	DRUG OF CHOICE		
	• Praziquantel	25 mg/kg/day in 4 to 6 doses × 2 days	25 mg/kg/day in 4 to 6 doses × 2 days
	ALTERNATIVE	30–50 mg/kg on alternate days × 10–15 doses	30–50 mg/kg on alternate days × 10–15 doses
	• Bithionol		
Giardiasis (*Giardia lamblia*)	DRUG OF CHOICE		
	• Metronidazole	250 mg tid × 5 to 7 days	15 mg/kg/day in 3 doses × 5 to 7 days
	ALTERNATIVES		
	• Nitazoxanide *or*	500 mg bid × 3 days	200 mg PO bid × 3 days (>4 yr)
	• Tinidazole	2 g as a single dose	50 mg/kg as a single dose
Hookworm Infection (*Ancylostoma duodenale, Necator americanus*)			
	DRUGS OF CHOICE		
	• Albendazole *or*	400 mg × one dose	
	• Mebendazole *or*	500 mg × one dose	500 mg × one dose
	• Pyrantel pamoate	11 mg/kg (max, 1 g) × 3 days	11 mg/kg (max, 1 g) × 3 days
LEISHMANIASIS			
Leishmania braziliensis, Leishmania mexicana, Leishmania tropica, Leishmania donovani (kala-azar, black fever)	DRUGS OF CHOICE		
	• Miltefosine *or*	Not indicated in those ≤12 yr	2.5 mg/kg/day PO × 28 days
	• Stibogluconate sodium	20 mg/kg/day IV or IM × 20–28 days	20 mg/kg/day IV or IM × 20–28 days
	ALTERNATIVE		
	• Amphotericin B	0.25–1 mg/kg by slow infusion daily or every 2 days for 8 wk	0.25–1 mg/kg by slow infusion daily or every 2 days for 8 wk
Malaria, Treatment of (*Plasmodium falciparum, P. ovale, P. vivax, P. malariae*) **All Plasmodium *Species* (Except Chloroquine-Resistant P. falciparum)**			
Oral	DRUG OF CHOICE		
	Chloroquine phosphate	600 mg base (1 g), then 300 mg base (500 mg) 6 hr later, then 300 mg base (500 mg) at 24 and 48 hr	10 mg base/kg (max, 600 mg base), then 5 mg base/kg 6 hr later, then 5 mg base/kg at 24 and 48 hr
Parenteral	DRUGS OF CHOICE		
	• Quinine dihydrochloride *or*	20 mg/kg loading dose in 10 mg/kg 5% dextrose during 4 hr, followed by 10 mg/kg during 2–4 hr q8h (max, 1800 mg/day) until oral therapy can be started	Same as adult dose
	• Quinidine gluconate *or*	10 mg/kg loading dose (max, 600 mg) in normal saline slowly during 1–2 hr, followed by continuous infusion of 0.02 mg/kg/min for 3 days max	Same as adult dose
	• Artesunate for treatment failure or adverse reactions from quinidine or quinine (available from the CDC)		
	ALTERNATIVE		
	• Chloroquine hydrochloride	200 mg base (250 mg) IM q6h if oral therapy cannot be started	0.83 mg base/kg/hr × 30 hr continuous infusion or 3.5 mg base/kg q6h IM or SC

TABLE 122.3 Drug Regimens for Treatment of Parasitic Infections—cont'd.

Infection	Drug[a]	DOSAGE	
		Adults	Children
Chloroquine-Resistant P. falciparum			
Oral	DRUGS OF CHOICE		
	• Quinine sulfate *plus*	650 mg tid × 3 days	25 mg/kg/day in 3 doses × 3–7 days
	• Doxycycline *or*	100 mg bid × 7 days	
	• Clindamycin	900 mg tid × 3–5 days	20–40 mg/kg/day in 3 doses × 3–5 days
	ALTERNATIVES		
	• Mefloquine	1250 mg once	25 mg/kg once (<45 kg)
	• Atovaquone-proguanil	1000/400 mg qd × 3 days	
	• Artemether-lumefantrine	4 tabs bid × 3 days	
Parenteral	DRUGS OF CHOICE		
	• Quinine dihydrochloride *or*	Same as above	Same as above
	• Quinidine gluconate *or*	Same as above	Same as above
	• Artesunate	Same as above	Same as above
Prevention of relapses—*P. vivax* and *P. ovale* only	DRUG OF CHOICE		
	• Primaquine phosphate	15 mg base (26.3 mg)/day × 14 days or 45 mg base (79 mg)/wk × 8 wk	0.3 mg base/kg/day × 14 days
Malaria, Prevention of			
	DRUG OF CHOICE		
	• Chloroquine phosphate	300 mg base (500 mg salt) PO, once/wk beginning 1 wk before and continuing for 4 wk after last exposure	5 mg/kg base (8.3 mg/kg salt) once/wk, up to adult dose of 300 mg base, same schedule as for adults
Chloroquine-resistant areas	DRUGS OF CHOICE		
	• Mefloquine *or*	250-mg tablet PO once/wk × 4 wk, then every other wk, continuing for 4 wk after last exposure	Same schedule as for adults with the following dosing guidelines: 15–19 kg, ¼ tablet; 20–30 kg, ½ tablet; 31–45 kg, ¾ tablet; >45 kg, 1 tablet
	• Atovaquone-proguanil *or*	250/100 mg qd 1 day before travel, each day in endemic region, and for 1 week afterward	
	• Doxycycline	100 mg daily during exposure and for 4 wk afterward	>8 yr: 2 mg/kg/day PO, up to 100 mg/day
Schistosomiasis			
Schistosoma haematobium	DRUG OF CHOICE		
	• Praziquantel	40 mg/kg/day in 4–6 doses × 1 day	20 mg/kg/day in 4–6 doses × 1 day
Schistosoma japonicum	DRUG OF CHOICE		
	• Praziquantel	40 mg/kg/day in 4–6 doses × 1 day	20 mg kg/day in 4–6 doses × 1 day
Schistosoma mansoni	DRUG OF CHOICE		
	• Praziquantel	60 mg/kg/day in 4–6 doses × 1 day	20 mg/kg/day in 4–6 doses × 1 day
	ALTERNATIVE		
	• Oxamniquine	15 mg/kg once	20 mg/kg/day in 2 doses × 1 day
Schistosoma mekongi	DRUG OF CHOICE		
	• Praziquantel	60 mg/kg/day in 4–6 doses × 1 day	20 mg/kg/day in 4–6 doses × 1 day
Strongyloidiasis (*Strongyloides stercoralis*)	DRUGS OF CHOICE		
	• Ivermectin *or*	200 μg/kg/day × 1–2 days	200 μg/kg/day × 1 or 2 days
	• Thiabendazole	50 mg/kg/day in 2 doses (max, 3 g/day) × 2 days	50 mg/kg/day in 2 doses (max, 3 g/day) × 2 days

Continued

TABLE 122.3   Drug Regimens for Treatment of Parasitic Infections—cont'd.

| Infection | Drug[a] | DOSAGE | |
		Adults	Children
Tapeworm Infection			
Adult (Intestinal Stage)			
Diphyllobothrium latum (fish), *Taenia saginata* (beef), *Taenia solium* (pork), *Dipylidium caninum* (dog)	DRUG OF CHOICE Praziquantel	5–10 mg/kg once	5–10 mg/kg once
Hymenolepis nana (dwarf tapeworm)	DRUG OF CHOICE • Praziquantel	25 mg/kg once	25 mg/kg once
Tapeworm Infection, Larval (Tissue) Stage			
Echinococcus granulosus (hydatid cysts)	DRUG OF CHOICE • Albendazole	400 mg bid × 28 days, repeated as necessary	15 mg/kg/day × 28 days, repeated as necessary
Echinococcus multilocularis— treatment of choice	Surgical excision		
Cysticercus cellulosae (cysticercosis)	DRUG OF CHOICE • Praziquantel ALTERNATIVE • Surgery	50 mg/kg/day in 3 doses × 15 days	50 mg/kg/day in 3 doses × 15 days
Trichinosis (*Trichinella spiralis*)	DRUGS OF CHOICE • Steroids for severe symptoms *plus* • Mebendazole	200–400 mg tid × 3 days, then 400–500 mg tid × 10 days	Same as adult dose
Trichomoniasis (*Trichomonas vaginalis*)	DRUG OF CHOICE • Metronidazole	2 g once or 250 mg tid or 375 mg bid PO × 7 days	15 mg/kg/day PO in 3 doses × 7 days
Trichuriasis (*Trichuris trichiura*, Whipworm)	DRUGS OF CHOICE • Mebendazole *or* • Albendazole	100 mg bid × 3 days 400 mg once	100 mg bid × 3 days 400 mg once
Trypanosomiasis			
Trypanosoma cruzi (South American trypanosomiasis, Chagas disease)	DRUG OF CHOICE • Nifurtimox	10–15 mg/kg/day PO in 4 doses × 120 days	1–10 yr: 15–20 mg/kg/day in 4 doses × 90 days 11–16 yr: 12.5–15 mg/kg/day in 4 doses × 90 days
	Alternative • Benznidazole	5–7 mg/kg/day × 30–120 days	Same as adult dose
Trypanosoma brucei gambiense, Trypanosoma brucei rhodesiense (African trypanosomiasis, sleeping sickness), hemolymphatic stage	DRUG OF CHOICE • Suramin	100–200 mg (test dose) IV, then 1 g IV on days 1, 3, 7, 14, and 21 Weight based: 2 mg/kg test dose followed by 10–15 mg/kg/day on days 1, 3, 7, 14, and 21	20 mg/kg on days 1, 3, 7, 14, and 21
	ALTERNATIVE • Pentamidine isethionate	4 mg/kg/day IM × 10 days	4 mg/kg/day IM × 10 days

TABLE 122.3 Drug Regimens for Treatment of Parasitic Infections—cont'd.

Infection	Drug[a]	DOSAGE	
		Adults	**Children**
Late disease with central nervous system involvement	DRUG OF CHOICE		
	• Melarsoprol (Trypanosoma brucei rhodesiense)	2–3.6 mg/kg/day IV × 3 days; after 1 wk, 3.6 mg/kg/day IV × 3 days; repeat again after 10–21 days	18–25 mg/kg total during 1 mo; initial dose of 0.36 mg/kg IV, increasing gradually to max, 3.6 mg/kg at intervals of 1–5 days for total of 9 or 10 doses
	ALTERNATIVES (*T. b. gambiense* only)		
	• Tryparsamide	One injection of 30 mg/kg (max, 2 g) IV every 5 days to total of 12 injections; course may be repeated after 1 mo	Unknown
	• Eflornithine *plus*	400 mg/kg/day in 4 doses × 14 days injections; course may be repeated after 1 mo	Same as adult dose
	• Suramin	One injection of 10 mg/kg IV every 5 days to total of 12 injections; course may be repeated after 1 mo	Unknown
Visceral Larva Migrans Toxocariasis	DRUG OF CHOICE		
	• Diethylcarbamazine	6 mg/kg/day in 3 doses × 7–10 days	6 mg/kg/day in 3 doses × 7–10 days
	ALTERNATIVES		
	• Mebendazole *or*	100–200 mg bid × 5 days	Same as adult dose
	• Albendazole	400 mg bid × 3–5 days	400 mg bid × 3–5 days

[a]Some drugs may be available only from the CDC Drug Service, Centers for Disease Control and Prevention, Atlanta; telephone, 404-639-3670 (nights, weekends, and holidays: 404-639-2888).
CDC, Centers for Disease Control and Prevention; *max,* Maximum.
Adapted from: Drugs for parasite infections. *Med Lett Drugs Ther.* 1995;37:99-108.

severe disease and death to the infected host. The female Anopheles mosquito is the arthropod vector that transmits malaria. The female ingests plasmodial gametocytes from ingesting a blood meal from an infected source. The gametocytes reproduce in the gut of the mosquito, transitioning to their sporozoite phase and migrating to the salivary glands in preparation for transmission. The plasmodia parasites enter the bloodstream of their next human host from the salivary glands of the female *Anopheles* mosquito during her blood meal. The sporozoites are trophic for human liver parenchymal cells; in hepatocytes, they undergo multiple replication rounds to form liver (extraerythrocytic) schizonts. The hepatocytes rupture, usually within 2 to 10 days after infection, releasing merozoites into the bloodstream. The merozoites invade red blood cells (RBCs), transforming into trophozoites and feeding on the hemoglobin in RBCs. Trophozoites mature into erythrocytic schizonts, which divide asexually into additional merozoites. Eventually, the erythrocyte undergoes lysis, releasing merozoites capable of infecting additional red blood cells. Although some merozoites are destroyed by the host's immune system, many enter new erythrocytes. As this cycle repeats itself, there is amplification of the number of infected erythrocytes. After several repetitions of the erythrocytic cycle, the process changes, and male or female macrogametocytes develop instead of merozoites. These gametes ingested by the mosquito, subsequently complete the reproductive cycle by fusion, which is accomplished sexually within the gut of a new female *Anopheles* mosquito after she feeds on the infected human.

Infection with *P. vivax* or *P. ovale* can manifest a dormant stage in human hepatocytes; this stage is known as the hypnozoite.

Hypnozoites are metabolically inactive and thus less susceptible to standard pharmacologic therapies. Hypnozoites can eventually release merozoites into the blood stream weeks to months or even years after initial infection, initiating relapse in the host unless specific treatment for the hypnozoite stage was anticipated by the clinician treating the patient. Recrudescent infection occurs when primary blood stages of any species of *Plasmodium* are immunologically or pharmacologically controlled without being fully eradicated and the liver phase persists, thus leading to latent multiplication at a higher rate. This may occur later due to immune suppression or overlying acute illness. *P. malariae* can sometimes cause an initial asymptomatic infection, and clinical symptoms develop years or decades later.

Initial parasite replication cycles are asynchronous, as multiple liver schizonts may rupture and release merozoites into the bloodstream. The host immune response to these parasites can lead to cytokine production with fever and rigors, malaise, headache, and myalgia, in addition to a variety of other symptoms. Over time, cycles of parasite reproduction become synchronized, with 24-hour (*P. knowlesi*), 48-hour (*P. falciparum, P. vivax, P. ovale*), or 72-hour (*P. malariae*) intervals of fever. Erythrocytes parasitized by *P. falciparum* express the parasitic protein PfEMP1, which binds to several host endothelial proteins, leading to cytoadhesion. RBC adherence to the endothelium leads to stasis of blood flow and microvascular occlusion, which can cause hypoperfusion of end organs. End-organ hypoperfusion in the brain can led to seizure, coma, and cerebral edema, which can be fatal. Hypoperfusion of other organs may lead to lactic acidosis or renal failure. Cytoadherence of parasitized RBCs may also result in low measured levels of parasitemia or even false-negative blood smears due to sequestration of infected erythrocytes in capillary beds.

Clinical Features

Patients presenting with a fever or acute illness who have returned from travel in a region endemic for malaria should be evaluated for the possibility of malaria. Other signs and symptoms including anemia, headache, nausea, chills, lethargy, abdominal pain, and upper respiratory complaints should also be considered as manifestations of malaria.

P. falciparum is the malarial species most morbid to humans; it infects a larger percentage of the host's RBCs and is trophic for neural tissue leading to cerebral edema, seizures, encephalopathy, hypoglycemia (especially in children), metabolic acidosis, severe anemia, high-output cardiac failure, renal failure, pulmonary edema, disseminated intravascular coagulation, and death. In chronic malarial infection, increased cellularity from the host's exuberant immune response may lead to hepatosplenomegaly. Within the liver, parasites and malarial pigment distend the Kupffer cells. Parasitized RBCs also adhere to the sinusoidal system of the spleen, reducing its immunologic effectiveness. Anemia results from acute and chronic hemolysis. Hemoglobinuria caused by severe hemolysis leading to renal failure, known as blackwater fever, may occur in patients with chronic or acute falciparum malaria.

Signs of severe malaria requiring immediate IV antimalarial treatment include prostration, altered mental status (Glasgow coma scale <11), more than two generalized seizures, severe anemia (hemoglobin < 7 g/dL), acute renal failure (creatinine > 3 mg/dL or blood urea > 20 mmol/L), hyperbilirubinemia or clinical jaundice (total bilirubin > 3 mg/dL), respiratory distress or pulmonary edema, shock, hypoglycemia (glucose < 40 mg/dL), spontaneous bleeding or DIC, acidosis (bicarbonate < 15 mmol/L or lactate > 5 mmol/L), hemoglobinuria, and greater than 2% parasitemia on blood smear (i.e., more than 2% of the patient's RBCs contain malarial schizonts).

Cerebral malaria is a life-threatening complication of *P. falciparum* infection. Parasitized RBCs express malarial cell surface glycoproteins called knobs which adhere to capillary walls, resulting in sludging in the cerebral microvasculature. Impaired circulation leads to localized ischemia, capillary leakage, and petechial hemorrhages. Clinical manifestations of cerebral malaria include fever, altered mental status including obtundation and coma, and, not uncommonly, seizures. A careful history, rapid diagnosis, and immediate initiation of therapy are essential to prevent severe morbidity and death.

Differential Diagnosis

The emergency medicine clinician will most successfully diagnose parasitic infections by correlating historical features, such as exposure and travel history, with presenting symptoms that may be more non-specific, including fever, anemia, peripheral edema, visual impairment, skin complaints, and symptoms related to the pulmonary, cardiovascular, and gastrointestinal (GI) systems. Other diagnostic considerations in at-risk travelers returning with febrile illness include more common conditions such as viral infections such as influenza or viral respiratory infections, and bacterial infections such as infectious diarrhea, urinary tract infections, and pneumonia. Cerebral malaria may manifest with confusion and mental status changes and should be differentiated from meningitis and encephalitis.

Malarial infection is often associated with anemia, particularly in children younger than 5 years. Anemia may develop quickly, from massive hemolysis in acute infection, or may have a more insidious onset, developing over months. Mature merozoites lyse parasitized RBCs. Uninfected RBCs undergo immune destruction from cell surface antibodies produced in response to parasite-associated changes in RBC

surface proteins. This process of destruction is abetted by increased reticuloendothelial activity. The inhibition of erythropoietin secretion blunts the reticulocyte response in infected persons. Concomitant iron deficiency contributes to the severity of the anemia.

Diagnostic Testing

Microscopic examination of thick and thin blood films remains the gold standard for the diagnosis of malaria. Peripheral blood smears are stained with Giemsa or Wright stain and examined with ordinary light microscopy. The morphology of the intraerythrocytic schizonts allows the experienced clinician to determine the plasmodial species. In particular, *P. falciparum* has a very specific morphology, and the diagnosis can be made in a simply equipped laboratory. Even if the parasite is not visualized in the smear, treatment of malaria is indicated if the disease is suspected. The US Food and Drug Administration (FDA) has approved the use of an antigen-based rapid diagnostic test to screen patients. The Alere BinaxNOW kit provides qualitative testing for all four species and is available for approximately $5 per test. The test is not as sensitive as microscopy, which should still be performed for all patients with positive antigen test results to determine the species and severity of parasitemia.

Management

Untreated falciparum malaria can lead to coma and death; early treatment reduces morbidity and mortality. In the past, chloroquine phosphate was the treatment of choice for acute uncomplicated attacks of malaria. Resistance to chloroquine has been steadily increasing, and the drug is now recommended only in regions of known chloroquine sensitivity—Haiti, Dominican Republic, Central America north of the Panama Canal, and limited regions of the Middle East. For uncomplicated malarial infections in patients from chloroquine-resistant regions, oral quinine is given with doxycycline or clindamycin. Another suitable alternative combination is proguanil-atovaquone.

For severe *P. falciparum* infection or in patients unable to tolerate oral medication, intravenous (IV) artesunate is the recommended first-line treatment. It is available only as an expanded-access investigational new drug and must be obtained via request from the CDC (call CDC Malaria Hotline at 770-488-7788, Monday-Friday, 9 a.m. to 5 p.m. EST; at other hours call 770-488-7100). The artemisinin agents are excellent antimalarials and are available as enteral and parenteral preparations. They have a rapid onset of action and are well tolerated. An oral agent known as artemether-lumefantrine (Coartem) is now available for uncomplicated malaria, though other artemisinins are not approved for use in the United States.

Although not currently available in the United States, IV quinine or quinidine is another option for treatment of severe cases. Rapid infusion of IV quinine can cause profound hypoglycemia, as well as hyponatremia and coma vigil, a neurologic impairment due to high rates of parasite destruction. Patients should not receive IV quinine without cardiac monitoring.

Primaquine is used to eliminate the hepatic phases of *P. ovale* and *P. vivax* to prevent disease relapse. Primaquine therapy is contraindicated in patients with glucose-6-phosphate dehydrogenase (G6PD) enzyme deficiency because it can precipitate severe hemolysis.

Cerebral malaria is treated with IV quinine, quinidine, or artemisinin (as available), and supportive care, including mechanical ventilation for comatose patients and patients with noncardiogenic pulmonary edema, antiepileptics, and correction of acidosis and hypoglycemia. Hypoglycemia results from the high-grade falciparum parasitemia, as the protozoan is metabolically active, and the patient is often anorectic from the disease process or the quinine infusion and may be malnourished at baseline. The mortality rate is high, especially in children, but neurologic sequelae are rare if the patient recovers. Corticosteroids, including dexamethasone, provide no benefit and can worsen outcomes. A second antimalarial, such as doxycycline or clindamycin, should always be administered in conjunction with artemisinin or quinine in these cases.

BABESIOSIS

Background and Importance

Babesiosis is a malaria-like illness that is becoming increasingly prevalent in the Northeastern United States (*Babesia microti*), northwestern United States (*Babesia gibsoni*), and Europe (*Babesia divergens*). Babesiosis is particularly endemic to Long Island, Cape Cod, Martha's Vineyard, Nantucket, and Block Island. Babesiosis must be suspected, along with ehrlichiosis/anaplasmosis and Lyme disease, in patients who live or have traveled in these regions who present with flu-like illness (see Chapter 123). *Babesia* is a protozoan, similar in structure and life cycle to plasmodia. It is transmitted by the deer tick *Ixodes dammini*, which also is the vector of Lyme disease, ehrlichiosis, and anaplasmosis. Several cases of babesiosis have been correlated with transfusions with infected blood.

Clinical Features

Patients with babesiosis experience fatigue, anorexia, malaise, and emotional lability, with myalgia, chills, high spiking fevers, sweats, headache, and dark urine. Other manifestations include hepatosplenomegaly, anemia, thrombocytopenia, leukopenia, elevated liver enzyme levels (particularly the transaminases), and signs of hemolysis, with hyperbilirubinemia and decreased haptoglobin. In an otherwise healthy person, the disease may remit spontaneously. In asplenic, older, and immunocompromised patients, especially patients with AIDS and those taking corticosteroids, up to 85% of RBCs may contain organisms and infections may be fatal with vascular collapse and a septic shock-like presentation due to massive hemolysis, jaundice, renal failure, disseminated intravascular coagulation, hypotension, and adult respiratory distress syndrome (ARDS).

Diagnostic Testing

Diagnosis is based on clinical suspicion, multiple thin and thick blood smears (*Babesia* organisms resemble plasmodia in blood smears), and serologic testing (convalescent titers may not be positive for several weeks after infection).

Management

The treatment of choice consists of atovaquone (750 mg BID orally) plus azithromycin (500–1000 mg once followed by 250 mg once daily orally) or, for severe illness, quinine (650 mg TID orally) plus clindamycin (1.2 g bid IV or 600 mg TID). Patients infected with *B. divergens* tend to be sicker and require more supportive care. Coinfection with *Borrelia burgdorferi*, the agent of Lyme disease, results in a more severe and prolonged illness.

SCHISTOSOMIASIS AND KATAYAMA FEVER

Background and Importance

The acute phase of schistosomiasis infection causes Katayama fever. Schistosomiasis is a trematode infection acquired through skin contact with freshwater habitats of snail species that are the intermediate host for the parasite. Motile cercariae are released from the snail and penetrate the skin of a person wading in the water. In the human host, the cercariae mature into schistosomulae, which migrate through the bloodstream to the host's lungs, and, subsequently, to the venous plexi of the gastrointestinal or genitourinary organs where they mature into adult worms and begin laying eggs. One to three months after the host is exposed to the parasite during the migration and early egg-production phases of infection, patients who have experienced prior infection develop nocturnal fever, diaphoresis, cough, wheezing, myalgia, headache, or abdominal pain. Infected patients may report brief exposures to fresh water in endemic areas.

Diagnostic Testing

Diagnosis depends upon positive schistosome serology and appropriate exposure history, correlated with the detection of eggs in urine or stool. Initial serology and egg examination may be falsely negative at the time of initial presentation and should be repeated at three-month intervals. Lab tests often reveal eosinophilia. Radiographs may reveal diffuse pulmonary infiltrates or nodules.

Management

Treatment should be initiated based on clinical suspicion because initial testing may provide false-positive results. In returning travelers with isolated exposure and low infectious burden, the most concerning result of untreated schistosomiasis is the embolization of schistosome eggs to small venules in the central nervous system creating intense inflammation, fibrosis, and tissue destruction manifesting as transverse myelitis or central nervous system lesions. Treatment consists of praziquantel in single dose or three-day course, as well as corticosteroids to reduce the severity of the inflammatory reaction.

CYSTICERCOSIS

Background and Importance

Cysticercosis is caused by the larval form of *Taenia solium*, a tapeworm, which is neurotrophic and endemic in many tropical areas. Ingestion of undercooked pork containing *T. solium* cysterici leads to tapeworm infection in the human intestine. Human cysticercosis is acquired via the fecal-oral route through accidental ingestion of stool containing eggs shed by the adult tapeworm. Autoinfection may occur when an individual unknowingly infected with a tapeworm fails to practice adequate hand hygiene, and household infection may occur through contamination of the environment, or of food and water sources. Once the egg is ingested, it hatches in the small intestine, releasing a larva that penetrates the gut wall and migrates throughout the host's body with particular trophism for the CNS, muscle, and soft tissue. The larvae encyst, and the ensuing local inflammation and fibrosis create a nidus for seizure activity in the brain. Neurocysticercosis is the leading cause of acquired epilepsy worldwide.

Clinical Features

In the brain, a *T. solium* larva forms an expanding cyst that induces an intense immunologic reaction, including inflammation, edema, fibrosis, and, ultimately, calcification. Cysts may be single or multiple. Neurologic abnormalities develop when neural tissue cannot accommodate the enlarging cyst. Seizure activity is often the first indication of cysticercosis, which should be considered in the differential diagnosis of new-onset seizures in adults. Racemose cysticercosis occurs when cysterici lodge in the cerebral ventricles or subarachnoid space, leading to hydrocephalus, cranial nerve deficits, vasculitis, and stroke.

Diagnostic Testing

The diagnosis of cysticercosis can be made by pairing the finding of characteristic cysts with scolices on noncontrast cranial computed tomography (CT) or magnetic resonance imaging (MRI) with positive serology for *T. solium*. Stool may reveal eggs of *T. solium* if the patient has a living worm in their gut. Brain lesions can mimic a CNS abscess, metastatic malignant disease, or primary tumor such as glioblastoma multiforme.

Management

Treatment of neurocysticercosis consists of a 10- to 14-day course of albendazole 400 mg BID alone, or albendazole with praziquantel 50 to 100 mg/kg/day, divided q8hr, depending on the number of cysts present. Consultation with an infectious disease specialist is appropriate. Corticosteroids and antiepileptics are important adjunct medications during therapy, because CNS cysts can release highly antigenic inflammatory material as they die and necrose. We recommend dexamethasone 10 mg and levetiracetam 1000 mg for most adult patients. Neurosurgical consultation is warranted for ventricular or subarachnoid cysts, or in the presence of hydrocephalus, elevated ICP, or mass effect.

AFRICAN TRYPANOSOMIASIS

Background and Importance

African sleeping sickness is caused by *Trypanosoma brucei gambiense* and *Trypanosoma brucei rhodesiense*. This infection is endemic in limited areas of West and East Africa. Several recent cases have been reported in travelers who have returned from safari in East Africa. The motile organisms are transmitted by the bite of the *Glossina* (tsetse) fly, which introduces the infective form of the trypanosome into the host's blood. A small lesion or boil may develop and persist for several days. The flagellated organism travels throughout the bloodstream, invading the lymph nodes and spleen.

Clinical Features

The patient generally is febrile, and a maculopapular rash can often be seen. Once the parasite invades the CNS, cerebral inflammation causes severe headache. The Winterbottom sign, which is posterior cervical lymphadenopathy, usually is apparent at the time of initial presentation. Patients may display altered mental status, psychiatric symptoms, and eventually, extreme sleepiness and lethargy. Coma and death from starvation and trypanotoxins are inevitable in untreated patients.

Diagnostic Testing

An appropriate exposure history and characteristic symptoms should prompt the clinician to obtain diagnostic studies. The diagnosis is established when trypanosomes are found in peripheral blood, CSF, or lymph node and bone marrow aspirates. The presence of parasites in the CSF indicates advanced progression of the disease.

Management

Suramin sodium, given as 100 to 200 mg IV for a test dose, then 1 g IV on days 1, 3, 7, 14, 21, is the treatment of choice for early infection with *T. b. rhodesiense*. Pentamidine isethionate 4 mg/kg IM a day is the preferred treatment for early *T. b. gambiense* infection. Melarsoprol is used in CNS disease from *T. b. rhodesiense*; eflornithine is used in combination with nifurtimox in CNS disease from *T. b. gambiense* infection.

TOXOPLASMOSIS

Background and Importance

Toxoplasma gondii is a zoonotic protozoan that is estimated to infect one-third of the human population globally; however, clinically significant infection is rare, and is most often seen in congenitally acquired infection or in immunocompromised individuals, particularly those with HIV. CNS disease includes cerebral mass lesions, encephalitis, and chorioretinitis. Infections rarely occur in immunocompetent individuals.[3]

Clinical Features

Toxoplasma oocysts are infectious forms in the intestines of the usual host, members of the cat family. Oocysts shed in cat feces often contaminate food and water ingested by other mammals, leading to the formation of cysts in a variety of tissues. Humans generally become infected by one of two routes: ingestion of oocysts through environmental contamination in proximity to cats, or ingestion of raw or undercooked meat harboring tissue cysts. Upon ingestion of cysts, tachyzoites are released and disseminated through the blood or lymphatics, leading to an acute phase of infection. Acute infection manifests as fever, malaise, headache, myalgia, and lymphadenopathy, and can cause posterior uveitis in immunocompetent patients. Eventually, the host's immune system controls the acute infection, but cysts in tissues persist, supporting dormant infections. In immunocompromised hosts, the cysts release bradyzoites initiating reactivation. CNS toxoplasmosis has been a significant cause of morbidity and mortality in patients with advanced AIDS.

Diagnostic Testing

Serologic testing identifying IgM (acutely) or serially rising IgG levels support the diagnosis. The general population worldwide has a large prevalence of seropositivity with IgG titers, thus one positive titer does not suggest infection. PCR performed on body fluids or specific tissues is highly specific for infection and has a sensitivity of 70% to 95%. The classical finding in immunocompromised patients with CNS disease is a ring-enhancing lesion on contrast-enhanced CT.

Management

Therapeutic options include pyrimethamine 50 to 75 mg a day with sulfadiazine 1 to 1.5 gm QID or clindamycin 450 mg q6 to 8 hours. Pyrimethamine is a folate antagonist, so folic acid is often given with prolonged courses.

EOSINOPHILIC MENINGITIS

A number of helminths, including those that typically complete their life cycles in animal hosts, only infecting humans incidentally, can migrate to the brain and cause severe disease, including meningitis and intracerebral hemorrhage.

Angiostrongylus cantonensis, the rat lung worm, typically infects rats, and has snail species as intermediate hosts. Larvae may infect humans, either through ingestion of undercooked snail, which may be part of dietary practice in some cultures, or as has been reported in teens responding to a prank or dare, or through ingestion of vegetables that have been contaminated by snail slime. In infected humans, larvae migrate to the brain causing headaches, vomiting, and altered mental status. *Baylisascaris procyonis* is an intestinal roundworm found in racoons. Raccoon "latrines," sites of frequent raccoon urination and defecation, are often teeming with *B. procyonis* eggs. Geophagia or hand contamination and subsequent ingestion, especially among young children, can lead to significant human infection, with tropism for the brain and eye leading to severe neurologic sequelae and death.

Gnathostoma spinigerum is a roundworm that incidentally infects humans consuming raw or undercooked freshwater fish, including ceviche. Most cases occur in Southeast Asia and Latin America, initially manifesting as a migratory inflammatory swelling of the skin with subcutaneous hemorrhages. Migration to the brain and spinal cord causes eosinophilic meningitis, coma, cranial nerve deficit, and massive subarachnoid hemorrhage from erosion into cerebral arterioles. Cases of

CNS involvement with *Trichella spiralis* have been reported and are associated with cerebral edema and CNS vasculitis. *Toxocara canis* can also cause CNS disease. *Paragonimus westermani* occasionally causes eosinophilic meningitis or focal neurologic findings that demonstrate a classic cluster of ring-enhancing lesions on contrast-enhanced CT, with a "soap bubble" appearance.

Eosinophilic meningitis is diagnosed by CSF pleocytosis (>10 WBC/hpf) with at least 10% eosinophils, though up to 50% eosinophils may be seen. CT or MRI findings may suggest a particular helminthic infection, but serologic testing will be confirmatory. Treatment consists of appropriate antihelminthic therapy and corticosteroids. Albendazole is used for *Angiostrongylus, Baylisascaris, Gnathostoma,* and *Toxocara*. Ivermectin, in weight-based dosing, is an alternative for *Gnathostoma*. Praziquantel treats *Paragonimus* whereas mebendazole 100 mg PO q12hr or thiabendazole 500 mg PO are the drugs of choice for *Trichella*. The clinician should obtain neurosurgical consultation if there is evidence of mass or hemorrhage.

PARASITES ASSOCIATED WITH FEVER

Other parasitic illnesses that commonly present with fever include visceral leishmaniasis, and toxoplasmosis. Fascioliasis and amoebic liver abscess also generally present with fever.

Leishmaniasis

Leishmaniasis is spread to humans by the sandfly and is found in the Middle East, India, East Africa, Brazil, and along the Mediterranean coast. Although leishmaniasis can involve the skin (cutaneous) and mucosa (mucosal), fever is seen only in visceral leishmaniasis in immunocompetent persons. Patients present with massive hepatosplenomegaly, neutropenia, and weight loss.

Amebic Abscess

Amebic abscess of the brain or meningoencephalitis is a rare complication of infection with *E. histolytica* after ingestion of amebic cysts. Spread of amebae to the brain or meninges from the colonized large bowel wall is rare but should be considered in any patient with amebiasis and neurologic signs or symptoms. The diagnosis may be made by microscopic identification of trophozoites (motile amebae) in CSF; however, biopsy of affected tissue is more specific. CNS amebiasis is treated with IV metronidazole but may require neurosurgical intervention.

Naegleria fowleri, Acanthamoeba spp., and *Balamuthia mandrillaris* are free-living freshwater amoebae that infect patients swimming and diving in ponds and lakes. These organisms invade the CNS through the olfactory neuroepithelium or compromised corneal epithelium that has been violated by abrasion or contact lens wear, often resulting in devastating amebic meningoencephalitis. Cases of *Balamuthia* amoebic encephalitis are often preceded by skin lesions or rhinitis. Due to the rarity of the condition, there is little data on the efficacy of different therapeutic agents, but a pharmacologic regimen of five drugs is generally recommended. Therapeutic options include amphotericin B, miltefosine, fluconazole or miconazole, rifampin, azithromycin, flucytosine, and sulfadiazine. Treatment is initiated when motile amoebae are identified in CSF.

Strongyloides

Strongyloides stercoralis infection is a common disease in the tropics. The worm enters through the host's skin and migrates to their small bowel. Infection with *Strongyloides* is more clinically significant in immunosuppressed patients, particularly transplant patients or those with autoimmune disease who are treated with high-dose corticosteroids. Patients will manifest larval dissemination, with subsequent encephalitis and pyogenic meningitis. *Strongyloides* infection is treated with thiabendazole or albendazole. Ivermectin has recently been found to be as effective with fewer side effects, and we recommend this as a first-line agent.

WHIPWORM AND HOOKWORM

Infestation by the whipworm *Trichuris trichiura,* and especially by the two human hookworms *Necator americanus* and *Ancylostoma duodenale,* is a major cause of iron deficiency anemia worldwide. Adult worms penetrate intestinal mucosa and feed using mouthparts consisting of hooks or biting plates, causing significant luminal blood loss. Eggs are shed in the feces and mature in the soil, hatching to release a rhabditiform larva that subsequently develops into the infective filariform larva. These larvae penetrate the human skin, usually through the feet. In trichuriasis, anemia is seen only with massive parasite infestation. Ova from the whipworm are ingested through food and water contaminated with feces. Diagnosis of these infections requires identification of characteristic ova in the stool. As with most helminthic infections, peripheral eosinophilia is common. Mebendazole or albendazole effectively controls trichuriasis and hookworm infections in adults and children. Anemic patients should be further worked up and receive iron supplementation.

TAPEWORM

Infection with the fish tapeworm, *Diphyllobothrium latum,* is associated with pernicious anemia. This tapeworm competes with the human host, absorbing vitamin B_{12} from the host's intestine. Infection is acquired when the host ingests raw freshwater fish that contains the plerocercoid larvae in its muscle fiber. The larva develops in the human small intestine into an adult tapeworm that can grow to be longer than 15 meters and can live up to 20 years. The diagnosis is made by identification of the ova in the feces. Praziquantel is the drug of choice for adults and children.

PARASITES ASSOCIATED WITH CUTANEOUS MANIFESTATIONS

Elephantiasis

Elephantiasis, a manifestation of lymphatic filariasis, is the development of massive peripheral edema, with distention and thickening of the overlying epidermis, which acquires the appearance and texture of elephant skin. Elephantiasis is caused by infection with the filarial worm *Wuchereria bancrofti* or *Brugia malayi*. The infection is confined to humans and is widely distributed in the equatorial regions of the world, including Africa, Asia, South America, and Oceania. More than 90% of all infections are found in Asia, where the disease has reached epidemic proportions. Even in endemic regions in which most residents are infected, the disease is rare among travelers. Infected mosquitoes introduce larvae into the bloodstream of the human host during a blood meal. After infecting the host, the worms migrate into the lymphatic system and mature into coiled gravid adults. The adult worm triggers a robust inflammatory reaction in the lymphatic vessels, particularly in the lower extremities and genitalia. The macrophages, lymphocytes, plasma cells, giant cells, and eosinophils migrate to the inflamed and fibrotic lymphatic vessels, which becomes erythematous, edematous, and tender, suggesting the diagnosis of filariasis.

Chronic manifestations of filariasis include fibrosis of a lymphatic vessel containing a dead or calcified worm. Subsequent mechanical blockage of the lymphatic system leads inevitably to severe lower extremity and genital edema accompanied by thickening of the skin. Recurrent cellulitis is common in these patients; prevention of super-infection requires meticulous skin care.

Diethylcarbamazine 50 mg orally rapidly clears the microfilariae from the peripheral blood and slowly sterilizes the gravid female nematode. Combined therapy with diethylcarbamazine and albendazole, or ivermectin and albendazole, may be more effective. Treatment with doxycycline eradicates *Wolbachia,* a symbiotic bacterium of the filarial parasite, increasing rates of eradication of the adult worm. Established elephantiasis of the scrotum can be successfully treated surgically. Chronic lymphatic obstruction of the limbs rarely responds to operative intervention.

Cutaneous Leishmaniasis

Cutaneous leishmaniasis is one of the most important causes of painless, chronic, ulcerating skin lesions globally. *Leishmania braziliensis* and *Leishmania mexicana* are responsible for New World leishmaniasis; *Leishmania tropica* and *Leishmania major* commonly cause Old World leishmaniasis. During a blood meal, a female sandfly of the species *Phlebotomus* or *Lutzomyia* transmits the promastigotes, which are then ingested by host macrophages and survive in their amastigote form in the skin.

Skin papules and nodules are seen early in the course of infection at the insect bite site. A raised lesion also can appear, which subsequently develops painless central ulceration and a raised border. Lymphocyte and macrophage invasions of the epidermis and dermis cause the induration that occurs at the ulcer border. Secondary bacterial infection of these ulcers increases the risk of associated scarring. *L. braziliensis braziliensis* (subspecies of *L. braziliensis*) can lead to spread of parasites from the primary lesion to the mucocutaneous skin borders (i.e., in tissues of the nose and mouth). Mutilation of the face occurs after massive tissue and nasal cartilage destruction. The soft palate, larynx, and trachea also can be involved, compromising the airway. Disseminated cutaneous leishmaniasis (*L. mexicana amazonensis* in South America and *L. tropica aethiopica* in Ethiopia) is characterized by diffuse nodules and papules resembling those of lepromatous leprosy (Fig. 122.1). Persons with this manifestation of leishmaniasis are thought to have a defect in their cell-mediated immune response.

Definitive diagnosis of leishmaniasis is made by direct visualization of the parasite with light microscopy. Diagnosis can also be made by an indirect fluorescent antibody test. Results of intradermal skin testing with parasite antigen often are negative during the acute stages of the disease.

Many forms of cutaneous leishmaniasis, especially *L. tropica* and *L. mexicana* infection, are self-limited and require no treatment unless the wounds become secondarily infected. Treatment options for advanced disease include sodium stibogluconate, meglumine antimonate, amphotericin B, miltefosine, fluconazole, and paromomycin. These treatments are rarely initiated in the ED setting.

Cutaneous Larva Migrans

Cutaneous larva migrans (CLM), the creeping eruption, occurs in the host's epidermis when the skin is penetrated by *Ancylostoma braziliense* (dog or cat hookworm) larvae. Exposure usually occurs after the host walks barefooted or lies directly on beaches or other warm soil contaminated by animal feces. The diagnosis is visual with a characteristic meandering erythematous track on the skin surface caused by larval migration. Visceral larva migrans occurs in young children after the ingestion of soil containing ova from the dog ascarid *Toxocara canis.* Thiabendazole, ivermectin, or albendazole may be used for treatment of cutaneous larva migrans, and antipruritics give symptomatic

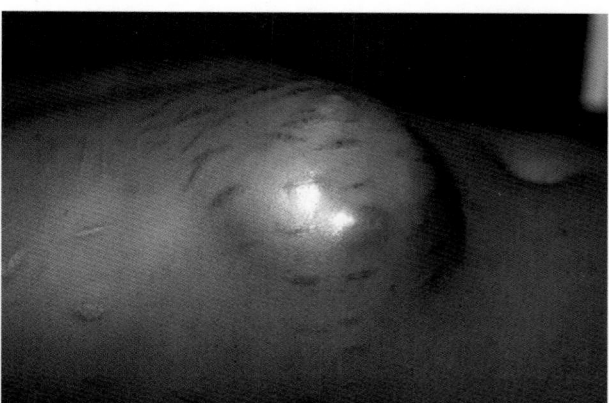

Fig. 122.1 Cutaneous leishmaniasis.

relief. Diethylcarbamazine treats visceral larva migrans. An alternative is thiabendazole.[2]

Swimmer's Itch (Cercarial Dermatitis)

Swimmer's itch is a dermatitis that occurs when skin is penetrated by a schistosome that is trophic for avians and nonhuman mammals while the patient usually was swimming in northern US freshwater lakes. The infection spontaneously resolves when the human host's immune system destroys the schistosome. A similar dermatitis also can occur after infection with schistosome species that are trophic for humans. Treatment is symptomatic.

Strongyloides

Strongyloides can cause a transient pruritic rash known as larva currens that may appear and then disappear within hours. *Taenia solium* can cause cysts in the soft tissues and muscles. These cysts often are an incidental finding. Onchocerciasis (from *Onchocerca volvulus*), common in West Africa and parts of South America, can cause severe pruritus and nodules overlying bony protuberances.

Dracunculus medinensis

Dracunculus medinensis, the fiery serpent, commonly referred to as Guinea-worm disease (GWD), is a parasite known since antiquity, which was once widely distributed in Africa and the Middle East. As the worm develops, it migrates to the subcutaneous tissues of the leg, where a painful blister forms; when the overlying skin is compromised, the worm emerges to release eggs into water. GWD has been eradicated and is currently primarily of interest for the success of this worldwide campaign, which has brought case numbers worldwide down from over 3 million in the 1980s to fewer than 100 per year over the last five years. While public health experts expect that GWD will be the first parasitic disease to be globally eradicated, COVID-19 has interrupted treatment programs and threatened years of progress.

PARASITES ASSOCIATED WITH OCULAR MANIFESTATIONS

Many different worms migrate to or through the eye, causing inflammation, tissue destruction, and blindness.

Onchocerciasis

Onchocerciasis is a major cause of blindness in the world; 95% of cases occur in Africa. The parasite is found only in humans and is transmitted by the bite of the *Simulium* fly. These flies live near rivers—hence, the common name of the disease, river blindness. Microfilariae of *O.*

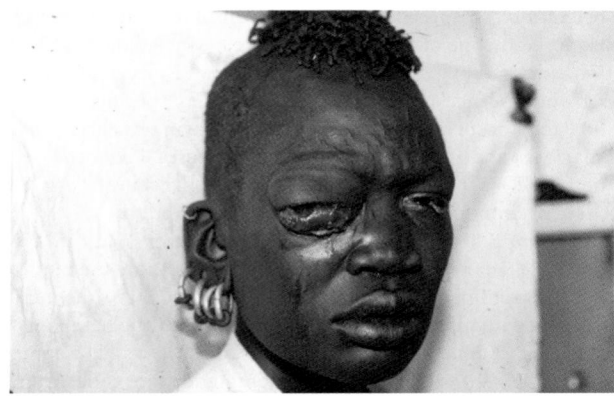

Fig. 122.2 Patient with onchocerciasis (river blindness).

volvulus are released by adult nematodes, which coil in subcutaneous nodules in the infected host; the microfilariae then migrate through the dermis and epidermis. The presence of adult worms stimulates a brisk immune response, including the infiltration of lymphocytes, macrophages, plasma cells, and eosinophils.

The skin becomes chronically edematous and pruritic; it then atrophies, resulting in loose, thin folds of skin, known as lizard skin. River blindness is more likely to develop in patients with nodules close to the eyes. When the microfilaria dies during its migration in the eye, the immunologic response to parasitic antigens leads to sclerosing keratitis, which is the major cause of ocular destruction and subsequent blindness (Fig. 122.2). Posterior ocular disease can also occur, leading to subretinal fibrosis.

Onchocerciasis is diagnosed by identifying characteristic microfilariae in skin snipped from the patient. Ivermectin is the therapeutic drug of choice. Surgical excision of the subcutaneous nodules is recommended when they are located on the head.

Loiasis

Loiasis is confined to forest areas in West and Central Africa. Transmission of *Loa loa* occurs through the bite of flies of the genus *Chrysops*. The disease is caused by migration of the adult worm in the subcutaneous tissue. The edema initially associated with migration of the worm is called a Calabar swelling. The adult worm occasionally migrates through the subconjunctival tissues of the eye and can be surgically excised from the conjunctiva. Although it is upsetting to the patient, the disease is generally fairly benign. The adult worm releases sheathed microfilariae into the peripheral bloodstream during the daytime.

Microfilariae can be detected in a thick blood smear, securing the diagnosis of loiasis. The treatment of choice for *L. loa* infection is diethylcarbamazine. Albendazole is also effective. Corticosteroids or antihistamines should be used to supplement specific chemotherapy because of the intense allergic reaction when the dead adult worms and microfilariae disintegrate. Heavy infections require plasmapheresis before administering antihelminthic treatment to avoid encephalitis precipitated by dying microfilaria.

Toxocara canis (Dog Roundworm)

Toxocara canis (dog roundworm) has a trophism for the host's eyes. Toxocariasis is a roundworm infection found in urban dogs. Humans ingest eggs by the fecal-oral route. The larvae migrate and often enter the retina, where they become trapped. They stimulate an immune response that culminates in granuloma formation. These granulomas can impair vision and sometimes are mistaken for retinal tumors. There is no means of direct diagnosis except tissue biopsy. Although serologic tests are available, results may be unreliable. Infection is treated with albendazole and steroids; larvae visible in the retina can be destroyed with a laser.

PARASITES ASSOCIATED WITH PULMONARY MANIFESTATIONS

A number of parasitic infections may be associated with pulmonary symptoms, although the presence of pulmonary findings may not be sufficient to differentiate between various forms of parasitic diseases. Patients with *P. falciparum* malaria initially may seek treatment for fever and cough, further necessitating the consideration of malaria in travelers with apparent respiratory symptoms. Early in the course of treatment for severe malaria, noncardiogenic pulmonary edema or ARDS may develop, necessitating mechanical ventilation with positive end-expiratory pressure.

E. histolytica can cause sympathetic pleural effusions, pulmonary or pleural involvement by direct extension or rupture of an amebic liver abscess, or direct hematogenous seeding of the lungs, leading to considerable additional morbidity and mortality among patients with underlying amebic infection.

Löffler syndrome, characterized by persistent and nonproductive cough, substernal chest pain, wheezing, rales, pulmonary infiltrates on the chest radiograph, and marked eosinophilia, often is seen when larvae from the roundworm *Ascaris lumbricoides,* the hookworms *N. americanus* and *A. duodenale,* and the threadworm *Strongyloides stercoralis* transit the lungs as part of their developmental cycles. *Ascaris* larvae penetrate the small intestinal wall to gain entry into the small venules of the GI tract and then migrate to the lungs. *Strongyloides* and hookworm filariform larvae penetrate through the skin of the feet, entering small cutaneous venules before migrating to the lungs. The pulmonary infiltrates and symptoms are transient, resolving within 2 weeks. Diagnosis depends on the discovery of larvae in sputum or gastric aspirates. Negative stool examinations initially are nondiagnostic because eggs do not appear in the stool for at least one month after initial infection.

Tropical pulmonary eosinophilia is a syndrome that can result from the patient's immune response to the microfilariae of *W. bancrofti* and *B. malayi*. Affected patients present with malaise, weight loss, new-onset nocturnal wheezing and asthma, shortness of breath, and chest discomfort. Chest radiographs may show nodular or interstitial infiltrates, consolidations, or cavitation, but are sometimes normal. Untreated infection may result in obstructive or restrictive lung disease. Patients have marked eosinophilia and elevations of serum immunoglobulin E levels. Serologic testing demonstrates antibodies to filaria, and microfilaria can be seen on nocturnal blood smears. Young men are more commonly affected.

Paragonimus westermani and echinococcal species are trophic for the lungs in their human hosts. *P. westermani* eggs are shed in stool, hatch in fresh water, and, as miracidia, infect a snail intermediary. After further development, cercariae are released from the snail, penetrating and encysting in freshwater crabs or crayfish. If the human host consumes raw or undercooked shellfish, the metacercariae excyst within the host's duodenum, penetrating the duodenal wall into the abdominal cavity. The larvae migrate from the peritoneal cavity through the diaphragm into the pleural cavity, finally migrating to the lungs, where they cause hemorrhage, necrosis, and a granulomatous response. Early in the process, patients may have infiltrates and eosinophilia; later disease is marked by bronchiectasis, chronic bronchitis, fever, hemoptysis, and cachexia. Pulmonary nodules and cysts may cavitate. Many of these patients may have a positive result on purified protein derivative (PPD) testing, and their symptoms and chest radiographic findings may mimic those of tuberculosis. Sputum often is blood-streaked and flecked with dark brown particles containing ova. Radiography, stool examination, and immune testing of sputum and blood are all helpful in making the diagnosis, and finding ova in sputum is diagnostic. Praziquantel is the therapeutic agent of choice.

E. granulosus causes pulmonary hydatid cyst disease; the host often remains asymptomatic until a cyst grows large enough to cause a mass effect or becomes superinfected. Pulmonary hydatid cysts also may be associated with cough, expectoration of cyst contents, chest pain, and/or hemoptysis. A thoracic CT scan may show a unilocular lung cyst; on a plain radiograph, a cyst with detached germinal membrane is said to resemble a water lily, a pathognomonic finding. Lung cysts can be treated with careful surgical excision or pharmacotherapy, depending on size.

PARASITIC DISEASES WITH CARDIOVASCULAR MANIFESTATIONS

Chagas Disease

Trypanosoma cruzi infection often leads to acute and chronic myocarditis. *T. cruzi* is endemic in South and Central America and causes Chagas disease. The vector is the reduviid bug (kissing bug) that inhabits the walls and roofs of thatched dwellings built adjacent to forests. Urban transmigration has expanded the epidemiologic scope of Chagas disease, which was previously a disease of rural populations. The disease is not seen commonly in travelers. The reduviid bug's bite is no longer the only source of *T. cruzi* infection; transfusion with blood containing live trypanosomes from infected hosts has been a growing source of infection. Oral transmission also has been reported through consumption of infected fruit.

The reduviid bug bites the patient, often around the eye, and excretes feces containing the trypomastigote of *T. cruzi*. The trypomastigote enters the inflamed bite wound or other mucosal or conjunctival surfaces, causing a local swelling called a chagoma. The Romaña sign (painless unilateral periorbital edema) is pathognomonic but rarely seen. The trypomastigote migrates to trophic tissues, including smooth muscle, cardiac muscle, and autonomic ganglia in the heart, esophagus, and colon, causing local inflammation and tissue destruction.

Acute infection is heralded by fever, facial and dependent extremity edema, hepatosplenomegaly, lymphadenopathy, malaise, lymphocytosis on peripheral blood smear, and elevated liver transaminase levels. At this stage, fatal left ventricular dysfunction and dysrhythmias are uncommon. Early illness lasts 1 to 2 months and resolves spontaneously, resulting in a latency known as the indeterminate phase, which can persist throughout the patient's lifetime.

In approximately 25% of cases, the infection progresses to chronic Chagas disease, principally with cardiomyopathy and GI pathology. Amastigotes invade cardiac muscle and the cardiac conduction system, causing chronic inflammation, mononuclear cell infiltration, and fibrosis. Involvement of the conduction system may lead to atrial bradydysrhythmias, right and left bundle branch blocks, complete heart block, and ventricular dysrhythmias, including ventricular fibrillation (see Chapter 65). Fibrosis and scarring from cardiac muscle infection leads to the development of right and left ventricular dysfunction and dilated cardiomyopathy. Mural thrombi are common, and the first indication of long-standing asymptomatic infection may be thromboembolic disease, such as stroke, pulmonary embolism, or peripheral arterial embolism. Heart failure is generally rapidly progressive and fatal within months unless treated with pharmacologic intervention and transplantation[4] (see Chapter 67).

Acute Chagas disease can be diagnosed by the presence of motile trypomastigotes in anticoagulated blood specimens. The organism also can be cultured in special liquid media. Chronic Chagas disease can be diagnosed by one of several serologic tests, including complement fixation, enzyme-linked immunosorbent assay (ELISA), and indirect immunofluorescence testing. The assays are nonspecific, and cross-reaction may occur in the presence of underlying malaria, syphilis, leishmaniasis, and some collagen vascular diseases. Polymerase chain reaction (PCR) is the gold standard for diagnosing acute or congenital infection, or immunosuppression-induced reactivation.

Nifurtimox 8 to 10 mg/kg/day orally divided every 6 to 8 hours and benznidazole 5 to 7 mg/kg/day orally every 12 hours are used for treatment of *T. cruzi* infection. Cure rates rarely exceed 50%. The duration of treatment with nifurtimox is prolonged, and the drug has many serious side effects. Benznidazole has fewer side effects, is FDA approved in children ages 2 to 12, and is now recommended for indeterminate-phase treatment. Nifurtimox is available under investigational protocols from the CDC. (It can be obtained by calling 404-639-2888).

Late complications of chronic diseases are modulated by autoimmune activity and do not respond to antiparasitic pharmacotherapy. Chronic Chagas disease of the heart, esophagus, or colon is treated symptomatically. Automated implantable cardioverter-defibrillators decrease the incidence of sudden death in infected patients. Patients receiving immunosuppressive therapy to prevent rejection after cardiac transplantation have developed recurrent disease in the transplanted myocardium.

PARASITIC DISEASES WITH GASTROINTESTINAL MANIFESTATIONS

Diarrhea

Diarrhea is one of the most common symptoms motivating travelers to seek medical attention. Diarrhea also is the leading cause of death in children younger than 5 years in developing countries and a major source of morbidity for older children and adults. Most diarrheal disease is viral or bacterial; however, some clinically significant diarrheal disease is caused by parasites.

Cryptosporidium and Cyclospora

Cryptosporidium parvum and *Cyclospora cayetanensis* are foodborne and waterborne coccidians that cause watery diarrhea. Both are particularly significant causes of morbidity in malnourished children and patients with AIDS. Cryptosporidial oocysts can be seen in stool when an acid-fast stain is used. ELISA and immunofluorescent assays of stool also are available for this organism. Paromomycin 25 to 30 mg/kg/day in 3 doses decreases diarrheal frequency in patients with AIDS with cryptosporidial infections; without treatment, patients have prolonged, disabling symptoms. Severe infections in immunocompetent patients can be treated with nitazoxanide 500 mg twice daily. *Cyclospora* oocysts can be detected in stool samples with a Ziehl-Neelsen stain. Trimethoprim-sulfamethoxazole treats this infection.

Entamoeba histolytica

E. histolytica causes an invasive or inflammatory diarrhea. Patients complain of fever, tenesmus, abdominal pain, and watery stool containing blood and mucus. Untreated disease can progress to widespread colitis and perforation of the bowel wall, with peritonitis and death. Stool examination reveals mobile trophozoites containing ingested RBCs. Cysts noted on stool studies do not necessarily reflect active infection because there are nonpathogenic ameba species occasionally found in the bowel of healthy adults. However, nonpathogenic entamoeba do not contain host RBCs. Immune assays of stool can now differentiate between *E. histolytica* and these nonpathogenic ameba species. Serologic tests may be useful for an infected patient from a nonendemic region, but patients will not have a positive test result for one month after initial infection. Metronidazole 750 mg every 8 hours is the drug of choice for treatment of amebiasis.

Entamoeba histolytica can also cause hepatic abscesses. The patient presents with high fevers, elevated white blood cell counts, right upper quadrant pain, weight loss, anorexia, but no jaundice. Affected patients typically do not have amebic dysentery and do not shed *Entamoeba* in their stool, but results of serologic studies are almost always positive. These patients are treated with metronidazole or tinidazole 2 g/day and a luminal amebicide, such as iodoquinol 650 mg three times a day or paromomycin. Drainage of the abscess is not indicated but will yield a viscous liquid often described "anchovy paste."

Balantidium coli

Balantidium coli is another protozoan that can cause invasive diarrhea. The usual hosts are pigs. It has tropism for the terminal ileum, sometimes causing a clinical picture suggestive of appendicitis. It can also infect the colon, causing abdominal pain, fever, diarrhea, and occasionally colonic perforation. Tetracycline, metronidazole, and iodoquinol are active against *B. coli*.

Giardia lamblia

Giardia lamblia can cause persistent diarrhea, abdominal bloating, cramps, flatulence, and significant weight loss. The organism is ingested and reproduces exponentially in the small bowel. In severe infection, the entire jejunum becomes covered with organisms, and the patient has malabsorption with steatorrhea. The organisms are rarely seen in fresh stool preparations because they quickly break down and become indiscernible. Accordingly, an antigen test often is used to confirm the diagnosis. *Giardia* has many animal reservoirs, including the beaver—thus the lay term, "beaver fever." Campers who drink unfiltered, "pure" mountain spring water in the United States commonly contract *Giardia* infection. Men who have sex with men are also at high risk from a fecal-oral route of transmission. Metronidazole, tinidazole, or nitazoxanide treats the disease.

S. stercoralis, Capillaria philippinensis, T. trichiura, and *Schistosoma* infections can cause diarrhea. Hyperinfection or dissemination of *Strongyloides* can cause persistent diarrhea, weight loss, and abdominal pain. *Trichuris* causes diarrhea when the parasite load in the intestine is high. Schistosomiasis can cause a chronic granulomatous colitis, which may resemble inflammatory bowel disease, or an acute, bloody, febrile colitis associated with Katayama fever in the immunologically naïve patient.

In chronic schistosomiasis, worm pairs in patients' mesenteric and portal venous systems lay eggs that become ensnared in the liver, causing intense local inflammation, scarring, and classic "pipestem" cirrhosis, with periportal fibrosis. Clinical manifestations in these patients include portal hypertension, ascites, and esophageal varices (Figs. 122.3 and 122.4). Upper GI bleeding is not as common as in patients with alcoholic cirrhosis; however, many patients are infected with schistosomiasis in endemic regions, so variceal bleeding is an important cause of GI hemorrhage in these populations.

Echinococcosis

Echinococcus granulosus is a tapeworm capable of causing disease in a number of organs, most commonly the liver, lung, bone, and CNS. The *Echinococcal* life cycle usually occurs outside of humans, with dogs and other canid species harboring the adult tapeworm in their intestinal tract. Sheep and other grazing animals ingest eggs shed in the stool of dogs in pastural areas. In the sheep, eggs hatch, penetrate the intestine, and migrate to other tissues where they form cysts. The life cycle is

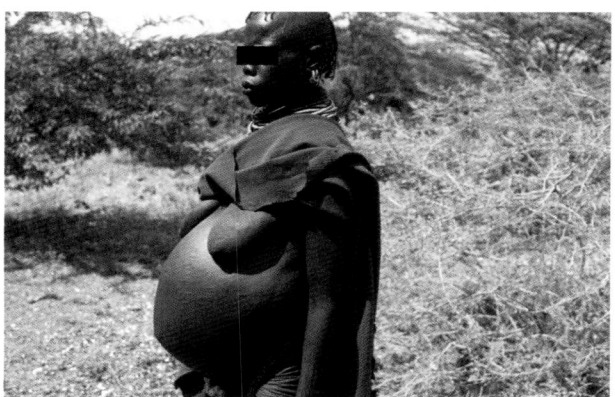

Fig. 122.3 Pipestem cirrhosis with extensive ascites in a patient with chronic schistosomiasis.

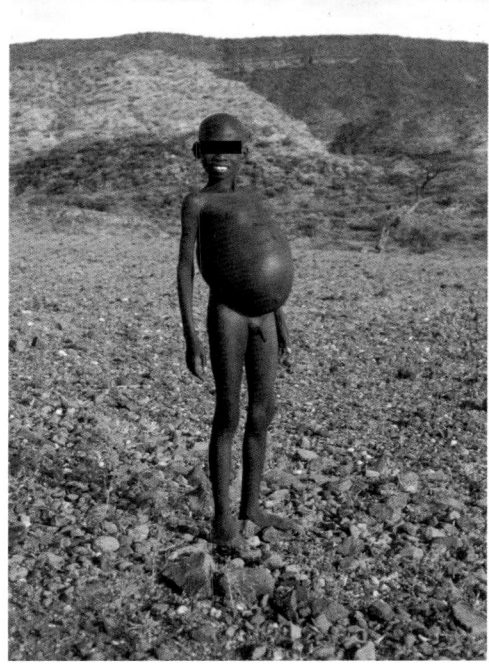

Fig. 122.4 Extensive ascites in a child, which may be from schistosomiasis or kala-azar (leishmaniasis).

completed when infected viscera of sheep are consumed by dogs. This usually occurs when sheep are slaughtered for food, and the discarded offal is fed to dogs. Humans become incidental end hosts when they ingest eggs from an environment (often food or water) contaminated by the feces of infected dogs.

In humans, infection results in the liberation of the embryonic oncosphere into the small intestine. *Echinococcal* larva then penetrate the intestinal wall and migrate to many organs, where they form enlarging hydatid cysts. Hydatid cysts are loculated structures containing a germinal epithelium, which produces the multiple infectious protoscoleces (heads) of the adult worm, as well as daughter cysts. The liver is the target organ in more than two-thirds of cases, with 20% occurring in the lungs, 6% in the spleen, and 2% or fewer in the heart, kidney, and brain.[5] Hydatid cysts typically grow slowly at a rate of 1 to 10 mm per year. The host immune response leads to a fibrous capsule around the cyst.

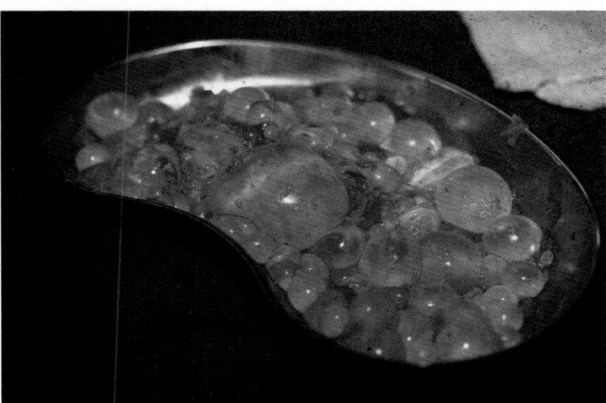

Fig. 122.5 Hydatid cysts removed surgically.

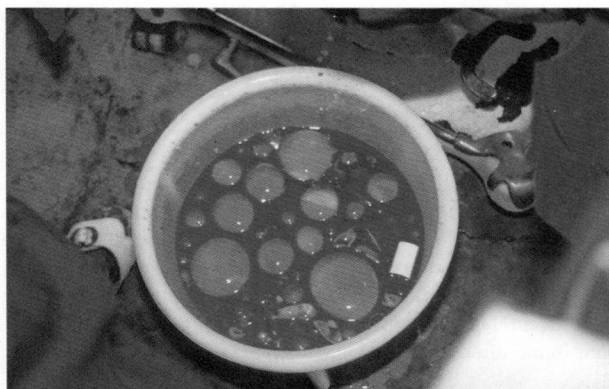

Fig. 122.6 Additional hydatid cysts removed surgically.

Over time, the metabolically active germinal layer can separate from the acellular laminar layer leading to cessation of growth and eventual involution and calcification. Hydatid cysts, especially larger ones, can rupture spontaneously or from direct trauma spilling cyst contents and initiating the proliferation of daughter cysts. This spilling and proliferation can lead to a disastrous seeding of the peritoneum or pleural space with metastatic growth which is very difficult to treat (so-called "white cancer") as well as the possibility of secondary bacterial infection of the ruptured cyst cavity, bronchopleural fistula, and anaphylactoid reactions to parasite antigens. When a pulmonary cyst ruptures, it may lead to the expectoration of salty cyst fluid, a phenomenon known as "hydatid vomica." *Echinococcus multilocularis,* the cause of human alveolar echinococcosis, is a related parasite found in the northern hemisphere, with relatively high incidence in China, Siberia, and central Europe. Like hydatid echinococcosis, *E. multilocularis* has a canid definitive host (foxes, coyotes, domestic dogs). Its intermediate host is a number of rodent species. When humans are incidentally infected, they develop proliferative multiloculated liver cysts that can resemble hepatic neoplasms.

The diagnosis of hydatid cyst disease is suggested by the appearance and localization of the cyst on ultrasound examination or CT scan. The Gharbi classification scheme describes ultrasonographic stages of hydatid cyst development and involution, which is important for determining treatment modality. Serologic evaluation of serum or cerebrospinal fluid (CSF) may help confirm the diagnosis. Simple aspiration of the cyst should not be attempted because of the risk of seeding the host's body with metastatic cysts.

Treatment options include albendazole, praziquantel, and surgical resection. PAIR (puncture, aspiration, instillation, re-aspiration) is a procedure that can be used on larger hydatid liver cysts and uses instillation of 95% alcohol to inactivate the germinal layer of an active cyst. Resection of the cyst may cause an anaphylactoid reaction if there is spillage of hydatid sand, which contains parasite antigenic proteins (Figs. 122.5 and 122.6). Treatment of alveolar hydatid disease is primarily with albendazole.

Fascioliasis, caused by the liver fluke *Fasciola hepatica,* is endemic on all continents except Antarctica and has been found in over 50 countries, especially where sheep or cattle are reared. Infection begins with ingestion of the metacercariae often found in watercress. Within 6 weeks, patients exhibit right upper quadrant abdominal pain, fever, nausea and vomiting, jaundice, tender enlarged liver, and elevated transaminase levels. This syndrome can mimic viral hepatitis; however, eosinophilia and urticaria are often present. Imaging studies, including CT, show the tracks of burrowing flukes. Serologic testing establishes

the diagnosis; the patient's stool may not contain eggs for several months after ingestion.

Several parasites have been identified in the pathologic examination of appendices of patients diagnosed with tropical appendicitis. These infections have included enterobiasis, amebiasis, ascariasis, trichuriasis, and taeniasis.

A. lumbricoides (roundworm) can cause significant persistent or recurrent abdominal pain in adults and partial intestinal obstruction in children with significant worm loads. Antihelminthics and conservative supportive therapy usually eliminate this infestation, thereby avoiding surgical intervention. Clinicians diagnose ascariasis by identifying eggs in the stool. Patients with large worm loads may excrete adult worms, especially after therapy is started. Severe intestinal amebiasis can be complicated by colonic perforation and peritonitis.

Angiostrongylus costaricensis, a species of rat lung worm, is common in Central America. Infected children may appear clinically to have Meckel diverticulum or acute appendicitis. Manifestations of the infection include nausea, vomiting, fever, abdominal pain localized to the right lower quadrant, and a tender mass. Surgical exploration may uncover abscesses, obstruction, or intestinal infarction. Anisakiasis is characterized by severe abdominal pain that occurs within hours of ingestion of raw fish (sushi and sashimi primarily). It is caused by *Anisakis simplex,* a nematode that burrows into the wall of the stomach or intestine. Treatment requires endoscopic removal of the worm.

Jaundice may result from hemolysis secondary to direct infection of RBCs with *Plasmodium* or *Babesia* or from biliary obstruction with pigmented stones. *Ascaris* can cause biliary colic, pyogenic cholangitis, pancreatitis, or liver abscess. Dead worms can be the nidus for gallstone formation. Biliary imaging and endoscopic retrograde cholangiopancreatography show worms in the biliary tree. Mechanical removal by endoscopy combined with antihelminthic therapy is curative. *Clonorchis sinensis* and *F. hepatica* are trophic for the biliary tree. Infection with these worms may be asymptomatic for years before eventually precipitating cholecystitis, cholangitis, or cholangiocarcinoma.

Enterobius vermicularis

Enterobius vermicularis, or pinworm, causes pruritus ani, a syndrome of intense perianal itching occurring primarily in children. Autoinfection is common, because children (and adults) scratch the pruritic anal area and then bite their nails or put their fingers in their mouth. The worm has a worldwide distribution. Diagnosis is clinical and is confirmed by finding the small adult worms wriggling the anal verge. Eggs are rarely seen in the stool but can be visualized by the tape test—transparent tape touched to the perianal region collects eggs, which can be seen with light microscopy. Albendazole or mebendazole is the drug of choice.

PARASITIC COINFECTIONS IN PATIENTS WITH HIV INFECTION AND AIDS

HIV infection is prevalent in developing countries. Heterosexual transmission and perinatal transmission are common; children and young adults of both sexes are primarily infected. Patients presenting to the ED may be coinfected with HIV and any other infectious agent, including all the parasites discussed in this chapter. HIV coinfection may worsen the symptoms and outcome, alter the presentation, increase the virulence, or assist the infective process.

AIDS causes abnormalities in almost every aspect of a host's immune response to infection; cell-mediated immunity, which is important in combating parasitic infection, is most affected. The diagnosis and response to therapy of many parasitic infections are monitored serologically. HIV infection interferes with this response, rendering many of these tests unreliable. Therapies that are extremely effective in the normal host may be ineffective in a patient with HIV infection. Pharmacologic agents may have to be given for long periods or the duration of the patient's life.

Specific Parasitic Coinfections

Malaria is not an opportunistic infection in patients with AIDS; however, many patients, especially children, with recurrent malaria and anemia from hemolysis have required transfusions from blood supplies not screened for HIV and have become infected. In regions where malaria is endemic, it is a common practice to treat most febrile patients with antimalarials. Some antimalarials are sulfonamides. Patients with AIDS have more severe allergic reactions to drugs, especially sulfonamides. Fever alone is not predictive of malaria in patients with AIDS; therefore, diagnosis should precede therapy.

Patients with HIV infection are at greater risk for severe clinical manifestations of babesiosis.

Visceral leishmaniasis is usually disseminated and often fatal in patients with AIDS. Latent leishmanial infections may be reactivated, and a prolonged febrile illness in an HIV-positive patient with a lifetime history of travel in leishmaniasis-endemic areas of the world should prompt consideration of this coinfection. Cutaneous infection also may become disseminated in these patients. Several clinical trials are examining the role of chemoprophylaxis for leishmaniasis in HIV-positive persons who live in endemic regions.

Chagas disease in the indeterminate phase can be reactivated in patients infected with HIV. These patients frequently have CNS involvement, with meningoencephalitis and severe myocarditis. Single-drug therapy may be insufficient because benznidazole penetration into the CSF is minimal. *T. gondii* infection is well recognized throughout the world as a common opportunistic infection for patients with AIDS, with a particular trophism for the CNS.

The coccidial organisms *Isospora belli, C. parvum,* and *C. cayetanensis* have been associated with prolonged diarrhea in patients with AIDS. These organisms cause difficult to treat infections and are almost impossible to eradicate in patients with AIDS. The diarrhea is extremely debilitating and can be as profuse as that seen in cholera. *E. histolytica* has a high prevalence among men who practice unprotected anal intercourse; however, invasive amebiasis is not an opportunistic infection associated with HIV infection.

Schistosomiasis may enhance the pathogenesis of HIV infection and is more difficult to treat and eradicate in patients who are HIV positive. Despite initial concerns, *S. stercoralis* infection does not appear to manifest more frequently as hyperinfection and disseminated disease in HIV-positive patients. In patients at risk for HIV infection and parasitic illness, it is essential to consider coinfection in the differential diagnosis. While many HIV-positive patients in industrialized countries are taking suppressive medication (HAART) and have fairly normal immune function, many patients who emigrate from developing countries may not have access to testing or HAART and thus may be HIV positive with active AIDS and parasitic coinfection.

The references for this chapter can be found online at ExpertConsult. com.

123

Tickborne Illnesses

Edward B. Bolgiano and Joseph Sexton

KEY CONCEPTS

- Tickborne illnesses frequently are misdiagnosed as common viral or bacterial infections. Diagnosis can be facilitated by considering tickborne illnesses in patients who recently have been in endemic areas and routinely asking for a history of recent tick or insect bites in patients with febrile illnesses.
- Lyme disease should be suspected in patients who present with signs of a viral illness, monarticular arthritis, meningitis, multiple neurologic abnormalities, or heart block. Diagnosis can be confirmed with serologic testing of acute and convalescent serum samples.
- Normal physiologic changes from tick bites should not be confused with erythema migrans.
- Relapsing fever should be suspected in patients who present with recurrent viral-like illness associated with high fever. The diagnosis can be confirmed by identifying spirochetes on a blood smear obtained during a period of rising temperature.
- Ulceroglandular tularemia should be suspected in patients with slow-healing extremity ulcers associated with large lesions of regional adenopathy (buboes). The diagnosis can be confirmed with serologic testing.
- Rocky Mountain spotted fever should be considered in patients who present with an unexplained febrile illness, even in the absence of a rash or known tick exposure. Delayed diagnosis and late initiation of specific antirickettsial therapy may lead to a fatal outcome. Treatment never should be delayed pending laboratory diagnosis.

OVERVIEW

Ticks are hematophagous parasites of humans and animals, distributed worldwide. They transmit rickettsial, bacterial, spirochetal, viral, and protozoal diseases and cause disease employing their own toxins (Table 123.1). As vectors of human disease, ticks rank second in importance only to mosquitoes. Although it is generally understood that people who travel during the summer months may return from endemic areas with tickborne disease, increasing reports of infection acquired within urban areas emphasize the need to consider tickborne illness even in the absence of a history of travel to high-risk areas. In addition, tularemia and Q fever are now considered by the Centers for Disease Control and Prevention (CDC) to be significant threats during biologic warfare, adding to the importance of research on ticks and tickborne diseases.

Reports on ticks, their feeding habits, and their possible relation to disease can be found from early human history. Tickborne illness was first recognized on the North American continent by Native Americans. The causative association of the tick vector with Rocky Mountain spotted fever (RMSF) was noted by missionaries and early settlers, who named the affliction tick fever, and physicians in Idaho and Montana recorded the classic clinical descriptions of the disease in 1899.

The majority of tickborne diseases in the United States occur east of the Mississippi River (Fig. 123.1). The reported cases of these diseases have nearly doubled since 2008, led by Lyme disease, the ehrlichioses, and the Rocky Mountain or other spotted fever rickettsioses (Table 123.2).

Identification of Ticks

Ticks are arthropods but not insects. They have eight legs instead of six and generally two fusing body parts—a capitulum (head) and opisthosoma (abdomen)—instead of three. Identification of an arthropod as a tick is not difficult (Figs. 123.2 and 123.3), but speciation requires a trained acarologist. However, tick identification has limited importance in clinical decision making. Color, which varies seasonally, and size, which varies by amount of blood ingested at the time of presentation, are unreliable criteria for identification purposes.

Physiology of Tick Feeding

An understanding of the physiology of feeding in arthropods is helpful when assessing the risks of disease transmission. Blood-sucking (hematophagic) arthropods are divided into two groups according to their method of acquiring blood. The solenophagic feeders insert their mouthparts directly into capillaries to obtain blood. Telmophagic feeders insert their mouthparts indiscriminately, lyse tissue along with capillaries, and feed on the resultant pool of blood, extracellular fluid, and tissue. Ticks and deer flies, for example, are telmophagic feeders, whereas mosquitoes are mostly solenophagic.

Argasid ticks (soft-bodied ticks) are short, rapid feeders with preformed distensible endocuticles. They therefore need to feed for only minutes to hours to acquire a full meal. As a result, they tend to be found in nests and burrows where their hosts visit frequently. The soft tick genus *Ornithodoros* is the vector for relapsing fever. Ixodid ticks (hard-bodied ticks) include the genera *Ixodes, Dermacentor, Amblyomma,* and *Rhipicephalus,* which are those responsible for the remainder of human tickborne diseases in the United States discussed in this chapter.

Two mechanisms prevent many species of tick from being removed from the skin—the barbed hypostome, or a calcified mouth-piece that anchors the tick to the skin, and a cement-like salivary secretion from the base of the hypostome, composed of lipoproteins and glycoproteins. This allows ixodid ticks to remain attached for as long as 2 weeks. Because argasids are much faster feeders, they secrete no cement substance.

During a bite, trauma and salivary gland products can cause local inflammation, hyperemia, edema, hemorrhage, and skin thickening. Hard and soft ticks produce a histolytic secretion injected during feeding that liquefies tissue, which is then sucked into the gut. Eventually, the secretion breaks down the walls of the dermal blood vessels and the released blood is ingested. To prevent hemostasis, the saliva contains

TABLE 123.1 Tickborne Illnesses

Type	Disease	Pathogen	Arthropod Vector	Geographic Distribution
Bacterial (including spirochetal)	Lyme disease	*Borrelia burgdorferi*	*Ixodes scapularis*	Northeastern United States
			Ixodes pacificus	Upper Midwestern United States
			Ixodes ricinus	Pacific Coast Europe
	Tularemia	*Francisella tularensis*	*Ixodes scapularis* *Amblyomma americanum* *Dermacentor variabilis*	Southwest central United States
Rickettsial	Rocky Mountain spotted fever	*Rickettsia rickettsii*	*Dermacentor andersoni* *Dermacentor variabilis* *Rhipicephalus sanguineus*	Predominantly southeastern United States Arizona
	Q fever	*Coxiella burnetii*	*Dermacentor andersoni*	Worldwide
	Human monocytic ehrlichiosis	*Ehrlichia chaffeensis*	*Amblyomma americanum*	South central and southeastern United States
	Human granulocytic anaplasmosis	*Anaplasma phagocytophilum*	*Ixodes scapularis* *Ixodes pacificus*	New England and north central United States Northern California
Parasitic (protozoal)	Babesiosis	*Babesia microti*	*Ixodes scapularis*	Coastal New England
Viral[a]	Colorado tick fever	Orbivirus	*Dermacentor andersoni*	Mountain areas of western United States and Canada
Miscellaneous	Tick paralysis	Ixobotoxin	*Dermacentor andersoni* *Dermacentor variabilis* *Amblyomma americanum* *Ixodes scapularis* *Ixodes pacificus* *Ixodes holocyclus*	Worldwide

[a]Many other viruses are transmitted to humans by ticks. In the United States, only Colorado tick fever occurs with any significant frequency.

a thrombokinase inhibitor, apyrase, which prevents platelet aggregation by depleting adenosine diphosphate, prostaglandin E_2, and prostacyclin (prostaglandin I_2) to prevent vasoconstriction, and cytolysins. *Ixodes scapularis* also secretes a carboxypeptidase that destroys other inflammatory mediators, such as anaphylatoxins and bradykinin, as well as anti–complement C3 factor. These other mediators normally would cause further inflammation, which would enhance hemostasis. The neurotoxins responsible for tick paralysis also are found in tick saliva. All infectious agents and excretory liquids from some argasids are transmitted through this saliva. Transmission of a disease from *Ixodes* ticks is unlikely if the tick is not yet engorged with blood at the time of removal.

The local physiologic changes associated with tick feeding produce the characteristic 1- to 4-mm erythematous mark typically seen on the skin after a tick bite. This is a common finding from most bloodsucking arthropods. The mark should not be confused with certain rashes associated with disease progression—for example, erythema migrans. Informing patients of this difference may be reassuring.

LYME DISEASE

Lyme disease, the most common vector-borne disease in the United States, is a tickborne illness caused by six species in the spirochete family Borreliaceae. In North America, infection is caused primarily by *Borrelia burgdorferi*. The recognition of Lyme disease began in 1975, when health officials at the Connecticut State Department of Health and physicians at Yale University were alerted by two skeptical mothers to an unusually large number of cases of apparent juvenile rheumatoid arthritis occurring in their small coastal community of Old Lyme, Connecticut. Investigation led to the description of a new entity called Lyme arthritis. The causative agent of Lyme disease was isolated in 1982.

Lyme disease occurs worldwide and has been reported on every continent except Antarctica. It now accounts for more than 95% of all reported cases of US vector-borne illness. The incidence of Lyme disease is unknown because many cases go unreported. Lyme disease occurs in people of all ages but is more common in children younger than 15 years and in adults 30 to 60 years of age. Persons at greatest risk live or vacation in endemic areas. In the United States, three distinct endemic foci are recognized—the northeastern coastal, Mid-Atlantic, and north central states. Twelve states (Connecticut, Maine, Maryland, Massachusetts, Minnesota, New Hampshire, New Jersey, New York, Pennsylvania, Vermont, Washington, and Wisconsin) account for 92% of US cases reported (Fig. 123.4).[1]

The principal tick vectors are *I. scapularis* in the Northeast and Midwest and *Ixodes pacificus* in the West. The *I. scapularis* population density depends on that of its preferred hosts, the white-footed field mouse, *Peromyscus leucopus,* for the larval and nymphal forms, and the white-tailed deer, *Odocoileus virginianus,* for the adult form. The white-footed mouse readily becomes infected after being bitten by infected ticks and remains highly infectious for periods that approach its life span, thereby providing an important reservoir for *B. burgdorferi*. Adult *I. scapularis* ticks feed primarily on deer, which are key hosts in the tick life cycle and in whose fur the adult tick may survive the winter. The repopulation

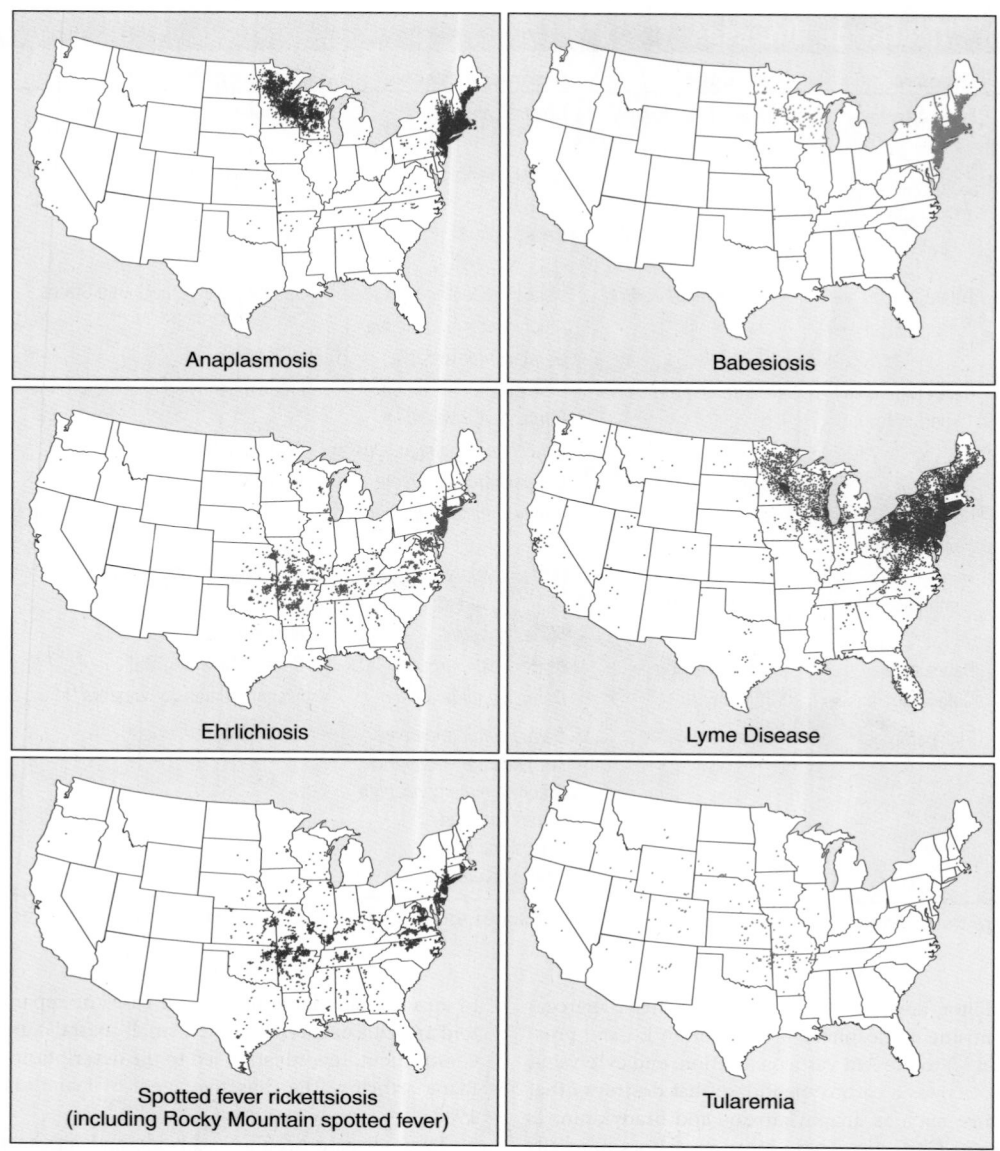

Fig. 123.1 Selected tickborne diseases reported to CDC, United States, 2016. (From: Centers for Disease Control and Prevention (CDC). Tickborne diseases of the United States: Overview of tickborne diseases. Available at: http://www.cdc.gov/ticks/tickbornediseases/overview.html. Accessed May 11 2021.)

TABLE 123.2   Tickborne Disease Surveillance Data Summary

Reported Tickborne Diseases, US	2016	2017	2018
Lyme disease (confirmed and probable)	36,429	42,743	33,666
Anaplasmosis/ehrlichiosis	5,750	7,718	6,123
Spotted fever rickettsiosis	4,269	6,248	5,544
Babesiosis	1,910	2,368	2,160
Tularemia	230	239	229
Powassan virus	22	33	21
Total	48,610	59,349	47,743

From: Centers for Disease Control and Prevention. Ticks: tickborne disease surveillance data summary. https://www.cdc.gov/ticks/data-summary/index.html.

of several areas in the United States by white-tailed deer preceded the recent emergence of Lyme disease in those regions.

Although all stages of the tick may feed on humans, the nymph is primarily responsible for transmitting Lyme disease. It is not surprising that more than two-thirds of patients with Lyme disease do not recall a tick bite, given the small size (1–2 mm) of nymphs (Fig. 123.5). The nymph feeds in the spring and summer, correlating with a peak incidence of early Lyme disease between May and August. In addition, recreational and occupational exposure is greatest during this time. Later manifestations of Lyme disease may appear throughout the year.

The spirochete *Borrelia burgdorferi* persists and multiplies in the midgut of its tick vector, *I. scapularis*. Transmission of the spirochete to humans occurs during feeding, generally about 2 days after attachment. The mechanism of transmission probably is inoculation with infectious saliva or with tick gut fluids periodically regurgitated during the feeding process.

After an incubation period that lasts several days to weeks, spiro-chetemia develops, and *Borrelia* organisms may migrate outward in the blood or lymph to virtually any site in the body. The spirochete appears to be tropic for synovial tissue, skin, and cells of the nervous system, but the mechanism of this tropism is not yet understood. Infection by the spirochete itself accounts for early clinical manifesta-tions. It remains unclear whether late disease manifestations require the continued presence of viable spirochetes or whether an ongo-ing host immune response to initial infection is sufficient to cause some late disease effects, but persistent live spirochetes are likely responsible for most later manifestations of the disease. The variable severity of Lyme disease may in part result from genetic variations in the human immune system. For example, patients with chronic Lyme arthritis have an increased frequency of human leukocyte anti-gen (HLA) specificity, in particular for HLA-DR4 and, less often, for HLA-DR2.

Clinical Features

Lyme disease, a multisystem disorder, can be classified into three stages—early localized, early disseminated, and late disease. Virtually any clinical feature may occur alone or recur at intervals, and some patients who had no early symptoms may have late symptoms. The disorder usually begins with a rash and associated constitutional signs and symptoms, suggesting a viral syndrome (early Lyme disease). Neu-rologic, joint, or cardiac manifestations may emerge weeks to months later (early disseminated Lyme disease), and chronic arthritic and neurologic abnormalities may appear weeks to years later (late Lyme disease). The time course for the clinical features of untreated Lyme disease is illustrated in Fig. 123.6.

Early Lyme Disease

Ticks may attach to human hosts at the initial point of contact, gen-erally around ankle level, or move about until they encounter an

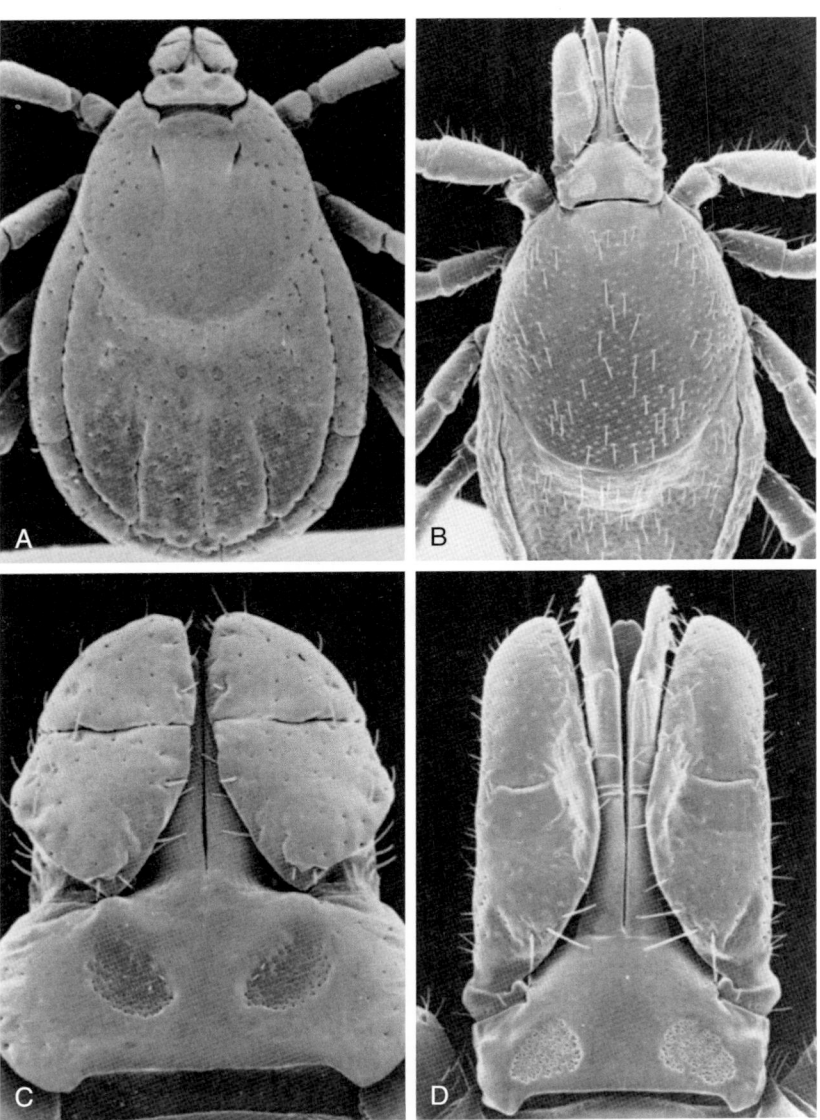

Fig. 123.2 Scanning electron micrographs of two tick species. (A) Dorsal view of adult female, *Dermacentor variabilis*. (B) Dorsal view of adult female, *Ixodes scapularis*. (C) Dorsal close-up view of *D. variabilis* head. (D) Dorsal close-up view of *I. scapularis* head. (Courtesy Dr. J. E. Keirans, Georgia Southern University, States-boro, Georgia.)

obstruction. The groin, popliteal fossae, gluteal folds, axillary folds, and earlobes are common sites of attachment. With transmission of *B. burgdorferi* through a tick bite, the initial site of infection is the skin at the site of the bite. After an incubation period of approximately 1 week (range, 1–36 days), the spirochetes cause a gradually spreading localized infection in the skin and a resultant skin lesion, erythema migrans.

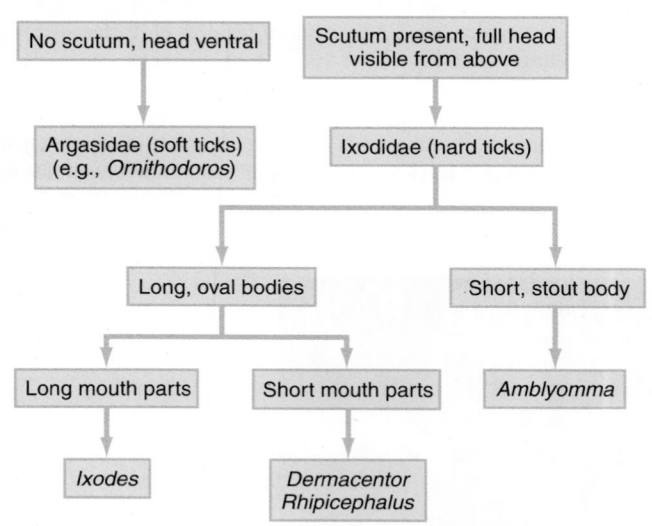

KEY TO IDENTIFICATION OF IXODIDAE AND ARGASIDAE TICKS

Fig. 123.3 Identification scheme for Ixodidae and Argasidae genera, the two primary disease-transmitting families of ticks.

Erythema migrans (EM) is the most characteristic clinical manifestation of Lyme disease and is recognized in 90% or more of patients. EM may go unnoticed if the entire skin surface is not examined. The characteristic rash begins at the site of the tick bite with an erythematous papule or macule. The lesion expands gradually (1–2 cm/day, a rate of expansion slower than cellulitis). The patch of erythema may be confluent or may have bands of normal-appearing skin. Central clearing may occur but is not an invariable feature. The lesion borders usually are flat but may be raised. The lesions generally are sharply demarcated and blanch with pressure. Most lesions are oval or round, but triangular and elongated patches may occur. In patients presenting 1 to 7 days after the appearance of lesions, the average lesion size is approximately 8 by 10 cm (range, 2 by 3 cm to 25 by 25 cm). In some cases, the center of some early lesions becomes red and indurated or vesicular and necrotic. The lesion is warm to the touch and may be described by the patient as nontender to minimally tender (Figs. 123.7 and 123.8).

Hematogenous spread of viable spirochetes (not additional tick bites) may result in one or more secondary lesions. These secondary lesions are smaller, migrate less, and typically spare the palms and soles. In all, 10% to 15% of patients have more than 20 such lesions; on rare occasions, they may number more than 100. Blistering and mucosal involvement do not occur. The primary and secondary skin lesions generally fade after approximately 28 days (range, 1 week to 14 months) without treatment and within several days of antibiotic therapy. Recurrent lesions may develop in patients who do not receive antibiotic therapy but not in those who receive appropriate antibiotics.

Constitutional signs and symptoms commonly appear in early Lyme disease (Table 123.3). Malaise, fatigue, and lethargy are most common (seen in ≈80% of patients) and may be severe. Fever typically is low grade and intermittent. Lymphadenopathy usually is regional in

Reported cases of Lyme Disease—United States, 2018

Each dot represents one case of Lyme disease and is placed randomly in the patient's county of residence. The presence of a dot in a state does not necessarily mean that Lyme disease was aquired in that state. People travel between states, and the place of residence is sometimes different from the place the patient became infected. Many high incidence states have modified surveillance practices. Contact your state health department for more information.

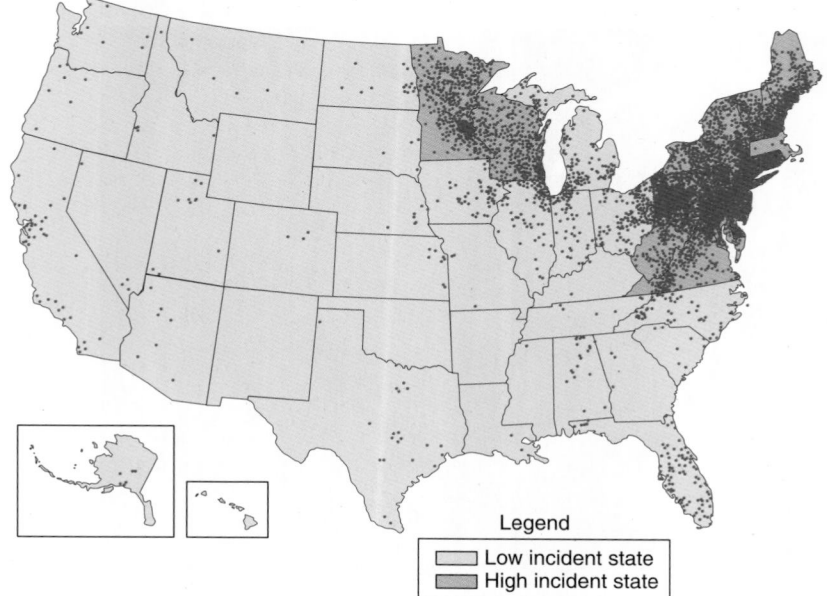

Legend
Low incident state
High incident state

Fig. 123.4 Reported cases of Lyme disease cases by county in the United States in 2018. The number of confirmed cases totaled 23,558. (Adapted from: Centers for Disease Control and Prevention: Lyme disease maps. https://www.cdc.gov/lyme/stats/maps.html.)

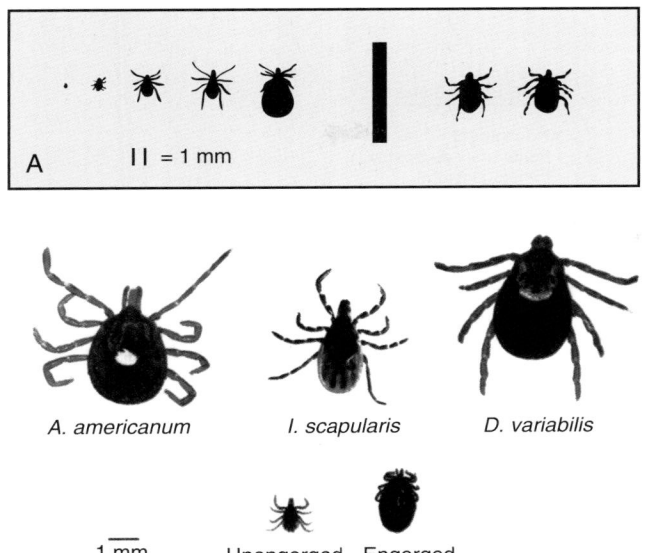

Fig. 123.5 (A) *Left to right,* Larva, nymph, adult male, adult female, and engorged adult female *Ixodes* ticks and adult male and female *Dermacentor* ticks; actual size. (B) Adult female *Amblyomma americanum* (Lone Star tick), adult female and nymphal *Ixodes scapularis* (deer tick), and adult female *Dermacentor variabilis* (dog tick). (From: Hayes EB, Piesman J, How can we prevent Lyme disease? *N Engl J Med.* 2003;348:2424-2430.)

the distribution of EM or may be generalized; splenomegaly may occur. Musculoskeletal complaints, such as arthralgias and myalgias, are common, and the discomfort typically is short-lived and migratory, sometimes lasting only hours in one location. Frank arthritis may occur at this stage but is rare.

Clinical manifestations of meningeal irritation are frequently seen. Headache, the most common symptom, usually is intermittent and localized. Nausea, vomiting, and photophobia occasionally accompany the headache. Kernig and Brudzinski signs typically are absent, and neck stiffness usually is noted only on extreme forward flexion. At this stage, the neurologic examination and cerebrospinal fluid (CSF) assessment usually yield normal findings.

Signs and symptoms of hepatitis, including anorexia, abdominal pain, right upper quadrant tenderness, nausea, and vomiting, may be present. Mild pharyngitis also may be present, but other upper respiratory symptoms, such as rhinorrhea, do not occur. Although the systemic symptoms of early Lyme disease often are described as flulike, that term can be misleading because clinically significant cough usually does not occur. Conjunctivitis develops in approximately 10% of patients.

The incidence of Lyme disease without EM appears to be approximately 10%. Because of the variety of nonspecific signs and symptoms at this stage, in the absence of the characteristic rash or history of tick bite, early Lyme disease may be easily confused with a viral or collagen vascular disease. The intermittent and rapidly changing nature of the early signs and symptoms of Lyme disease may be a helpful distinguishing feature, especially in a patient from an endemic area. In untreated disease, early symptoms usually last for several weeks but may persist for months.

Acute Disseminated Infection

Shortly after disease onset, hematogenous spread can cause various systemic signs and symptoms and result in secondary sites of infection. Organ systems commonly affected are the nervous system, heart, and

joints. Less commonly, the eyes, liver, skeletal muscle, subcutaneous tissue, and spleen are infected.

Neurologic Manifestations. A relatively symptom-free interval usually occurs between early and disseminated infection; however, neurologic signs and symptoms may be the presenting manifestations of Lyme disease or may overlap with early or late manifestations. Beginning at an average of 4 weeks (range, 0–10 weeks) after the onset of erythema migrans, neurologic involvement occurs in approximately 15% of untreated patients.

The most common neurologic manifestation of Lyme disease is a fluctuating meningoencephalitis, with superimposed symptoms of cranial neuropathy, peripheral neuropathy, or radiculopathy. A triad of lymphocytic meningitis, cranial neuropathies (usually Bell palsy), and radiculoneuritis (motor or sensory or both) has been described, but each entity may occur alone. Headache of variable intensity usually is present; other signs and symptoms of a mild meningoencephalitis may be noted, including lethargy or irritability, sleep disturbances, poor concentration, and memory loss. At this point, the disease often is misdiagnosed as viral meningitis. As in early disease, Kernig and Brudzinski signs are absent and computed tomography (CT) findings are normal. Unlike in early disease, however, findings on CSF examination often are abnormal, with a lymphocytic pleocytosis and moderately elevated protein level. CSF glucose concentration usually is normal. Intrathecal *B. burgdorferi* antibody (usually immunoglobulin G [IgG] or IgA) is present in 80% to 90% of patients. CSF polymerase chain reaction (PCR) assay results are positive in less than 50% of patients, probably reflecting the low number of organisms usually present in spinal fluid. Routine testing of CSF by PCR assay is not recommended.

Cranial neuropathies are common, occurring in approximately 50% of patients with Lyme meningitis; the seventh nerve is usually involved. Other cranial nerves are affected less often. Bell palsy is bilateral in approximately one-third of patients. Its duration usually is weeks to months, and the condition generally resolves spontaneously without treatment.

Peripheral nervous system manifestations also may occur in early disseminated Lyme disease. The spinal root and plexus and peripheral nerves may be involved in the form of thoracic sensory radiculitis, brachial plexitis, mononeuritis, and motor and sensory radiculoneuritis in the extremities. Patients may complain of weakness, pain, or dysesthesia. Examination may reveal loss of reflexes. Involvement of the extremities usually is asymmetrical, but cervical and thoracic dermatomes may be affected. Radiculoneuritis can mimic a mechanical radiculopathy (such as sciatica) and should be considered in endemic areas in patients without an apparent mechanical cause. Other rare neurologic abnormalities described in association with Lyme disease include chorea, transverse myelitis, ataxia, and pseudotumor cerebri. Cerebral vasculitis associated with Lyme disease also has been reported.

Cardiac Manifestations. Cardiac involvement in Lyme disease is uncommon, with an estimated incidence in untreated patients ranging from 4% to 10%. Carditis occurs during the early disseminated phase of the disease. The average time from initial illness to the development of carditis typically is 3 to 5 weeks (range, 4 days to 7 months). Direct myocardial invasion has been demonstrated with endomyocardial biopsy. Electrophysiologic testing has demonstrated widespread involvement of the conduction system.

The most common cardiac manifestation of Lyme disease is atrioventricular (AV) block, although conduction defects may involve any level of the conducting system.[2] Myopericarditis, tachydysrhythmias including atrial fibrillation,[3] and ventricular impairment occur less often. In a review of 105 reported cases of Lyme carditis, 49% of cases were third-degree, 16% were second-degree, and 12% were first-degree AV block. The degree of AV block seen in a specific patient may fluctuate rapidly.

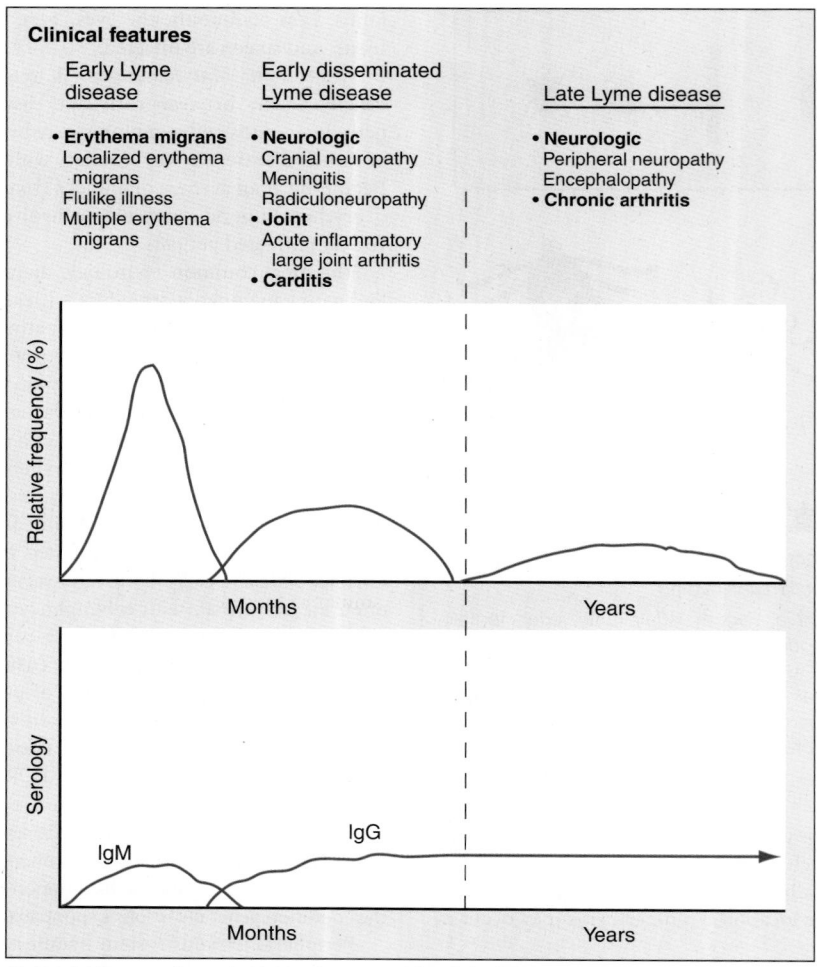

Fig. 123.6 Natural history of serologic response, with clinical features, in untreated Lyme disease. *IgG,* Immunoglobulin G; *IgM,* immunoglobulin M. (Adapted from: Rahn DW. Natural history of Lyme disease. In Rahn DW, Evans J, eds. *Lyme Disease.* Philadelphia: American College of Physicians; 1998, pp 35-48.)

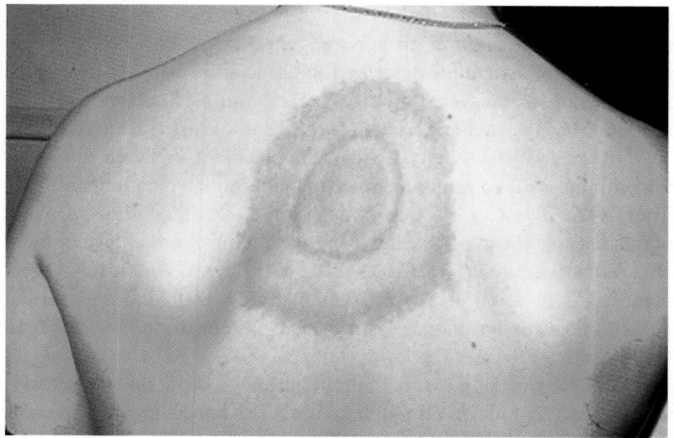

Fig. 123.7 Lyme disease usually begins with a slowly expanding skin lesion, erythema migrans, which occurs at the site of the tick bite. The classic bull's-eye or target lesion has partial central clearing, a bright red outer border, and a target center. (From: Bhate C, Schwartz RA. Lyme disease. Part I. Advances and perspectives. *J Am Acad Dermatol.* 2011;64:619-636.)

A commonly observed feature of AV block in patients with Lyme carditis is its gradual resolution, resembling that occurring after an acute inferior wall myocardial infarction and presumably related to the resolution of inflammation. Assessment of the level of the AV block is important to determine the prognosis of a patient with Lyme carditis. In most cases, the block appears to be at or above the AV node; therefore, the prognosis is favorable. However, infranodal AV block does occur and may be characterized by slow escape rhythms of wide QRS pattern, asystole, or fluctuating left and right bundle branch block. Other electrocardiographic findings include nonspecific ST and T wave abnormalities and intraventricular conduction delay.

Patients with high-degree AV block usually are symptomatic. Symptoms include lightheadedness, palpitations, syncope, chest pain, and dyspnea on exertion. The physical examination may reveal flow murmurs and murmurs of mild mitral regurgitation, pericardial friction rub, or evidence of congestive heart failure. Associated left ventricular dysfunction may be present and has been documented by two-dimensional echocardiography and radionuclide studies; in most reported cases, it has been mild and transient. Sudden cardiac death attributable to Lyme disease has also been reported.

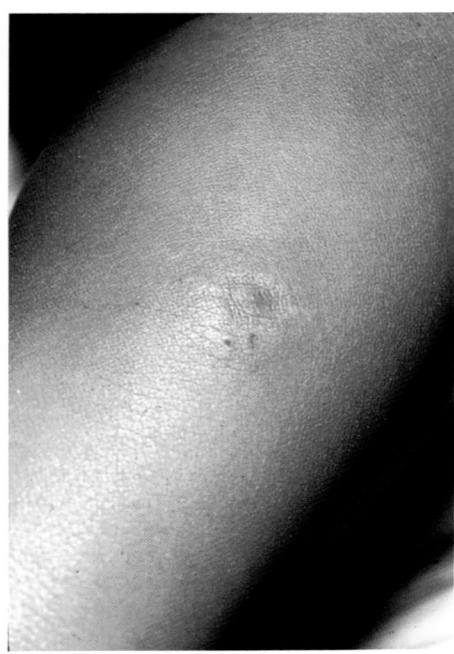

Fig. 123.8 Early erythema migrans on the lower leg. The erythematous nodular appearance could lead to misdiagnosis as a spider bite or MRSA cellulitis. (From: Bhate C, Schwartz RA. Lyme disease. Part I. Advances and perspectives. *J Am Acad Dermatol.* 2011;64:619-636.)

TABLE 123.3 Early Clinical Manifestations of Lyme Disease

Manifestation	No. of Patients (%)
Signs	
Erythema chronicum migrans[a]	314 (100)
Multiple annular lesions	150 (48)
Lymphadenopathy	
Regional	128 (41)
Generalized	63 (20)
Pain on neck flexion	52 (17)
Malar rash	41 (13)
Erythematous throat	38 (12)
Conjunctivitis	35 (11)
Symptoms	
Malaise, fatigue, lethargy	251 (80)
Headache	200 (64)
Fever and chills	185 (59)
Stiff neck	151 (48)
Arthralgias	150 (48)
Myalgias	135 (43)
Backache	81 (26)
Anorexia	73 (23)
Sore throat	53 (17)
Nausea	53 (17)
Dysesthesia	35 (11)
Vomiting	32 (10)

[a]Required for inclusion in this study.
From: Steere AC, Bartenhagen NH, Craft JE, et al. The early clinical manifestations of Lyme disease. *Ann Intern Med.* 1983;99:76-82.

Arthritis. Although it is generally considered a sign of late Lyme disease, acute arthritis may begin during the acute disseminated stage. Monarticular or oligoarticular arthritis, primarily affecting large joints, especially the knee, may develop weeks to months after the onset of initial illness. In an early study of the natural history of Lyme arthritis, approximately 50% of untreated patients experienced one episode or multiple intermittent attacks of arthritis. Acute arthritis typically is monarticular, with involvement of only one knee. The shoulder, elbow, temporomandibular joint, ankle, wrist, hip, and small joints of the hands and feet are involved less commonly. Episodes of arthritis typically are brief (lasting weeks to months) and are separated by variable periods of remission.

Arthrocentesis generally is nondiagnostic, yielding an inflammatory synovial fluid with a mean white blood cell count of approximately 25,000 cells/µL (75% polymorphonuclear leukocytes). Higher white blood cell counts have been reported, simulating septic arthritis. The synovial glucose concentration usually is normal, and protein levels are variable, ranging from 3 to 8 g/dL. Cultures of the fluid rarely identify the causative spirochete. The complement level generally is greater than one-third that of serum. Synovial biopsy reveals hypertrophy, vascular proliferation, and a mononuclear cell infiltrate. Findings, therefore, are similar to those in rheumatoid arthritis, except that rheumatoid factor and antinuclear antibody assays yield a negative result in Lyme arthritis. Radiography may reveal nonspecific abnormalities such as juxtaarticular osteoporosis, cartilage loss, cortical or marginal bone erosions, and joint effusions.

Ophthalmic Manifestations. Ocular involvement also may be seen in early disseminated disease; manifestations include conjunctivitis, keratitis, choroiditis, retinal detachment, optic neuritis, and blindness. These findings also may be seen in late disease.

Late Lyme Disease

The chronic phase of Lyme disease is characterized by arthritic and, less commonly, neurologic symptoms. Over time, the pattern of episodic inflammation in early disease transitions to a more indolent persistent inflammation. The term *chronic* (or *late*) *Lyme disease* describes continuous inflammation in an organ system for more than 1 year.

A pattern of exacerbation and remission of arthritis may extend for several years, with a gradual tendency toward less frequent and less severe occurrences. The spontaneous long-term remission rate approximates 10% to 20% annually in untreated patients. However, patients commonly have episodes of periarticular involvement, arthralgias, or fatigue interspersed between attacks of frank arthritis. During the second or third year of illness, attacks of joint swelling sometimes become longer in duration, lasting months rather than weeks. Chronic arthritis eventually develops in approximately 10% of patients.

Late neurologic complications include a wide variety of abnormalities of the central and peripheral nervous systems and fatigue syndromes. Diagnosis may be difficult because of the large number of other neurologic conditions that Lyme disease may imitate and because late neurologic symptoms may be the first symptoms of the disease. The manifestations of chronic neuroborreliosis (the neurologic manifestations of Lyme disease) usually appear months to years after the onset of infection.

The most common late neurologic manifestation of Lyme disease is a chronic encephalopathy manifested as a mild to moderately severe impairment of memory and learning. Hypersomnolence and mild psychiatric disturbances (depression, irritability, paranoia) also may develop.[4]

Peripheral nervous system manifestations often are seen in late disease, with involvement of cranial nerves, spinal roots, spinal plexuses, and peripheral nerves. A predominantly sensory polyradiculoneuropathy that is manifested as radicular pain or distal paresthesia is common. Significant overlap occurs with early symptoms. Less commonly, a demyelinating condition resembling multiple sclerosis may appear in late disease. Symptoms are variable and, as in multiple sclerosis, may undergo exacerbations and remissions. CT and magnetic resonance imaging (MRI) may reveal multiple white matter lesions.

Chronic inflammation also may occur in the skin, causing a seldom-recognized late cutaneous manifestation of Lyme disease, acrodermatitis chronica atrophicans. This condition usually involves the skin of distal extremities at the site of a tick bite. It is characterized in its initial stages by an edematous infiltration, which progresses to an atrophic lesion resembling localized scleroderma in its more established form. B. burgdorferi has been demonstrated in the skin of patients with acrodermatitis chronica atrophicans and positive findings on serologic studies.

Differential Diagnoses

The diagnosis of Lyme disease should be considered based on clinical and epidemiologic features. Identification of the disorder often is difficult, however, especially in the early stage. Although Lyme disease manifests in many ways, each stage has characteristic clinical findings that narrow the differential diagnosis. Early Lyme disease (EM and associated constitutional symptoms) may be easily confused with various other diseases, especially if the characteristic rash of EM is absent. A common clinical presentation is an influenza-like illness with headache, nausea, fever, chills, myalgias, arthralgias, stiff neck, and anorexia, occurring during the summer months. Even in endemic areas during the summer months, most patients with such symptoms do not have Lyme disease. When headache and stiff neck are the predominant symptoms, the principal diagnostic distinction to be made is between Lyme disease and the enteroviral diseases (and other causes of aseptic meningitis). The enteroviral diseases also have their peak incidence during the summer months; however, diarrhea, commonly associated with enteroviral infection, is not a feature of Lyme disease. Abdominal pain, anorexia, and nausea suggest hepatitis, sore throat, adenopathy, and fatigue suggest mononucleosis, and myalgias and arthralgias suggest connective tissue diseases. In many areas where Lyme disease is endemic, Ixodes ticks can be infected simultaneously with B. burgdorferi, Anaplasma phagocytophilum, and Babesia microti. Coinfection with more than one of these agents can occur.[5]

The rash of EM is characteristic of but not pathognomonic for Lyme disease. Some patients are not aware of having had such a rash and, in others, its appearance is atypical. An EM skin lesion is frequently misdiagnosed as a spider bite or community-acquired methicillin-resistant Staphylococcus aureus (MRSA) cellulitis, resulting in treatment with ineffective antibiotics. Other cutaneous entities in the differential diagnosis for EM include fungal infection, plant dermatitis, and fixed drug eruptions. Secondary lesions may be confused with the target lesions of erythema multiforme, which generally are smaller and nonexpanding. Erythema multiforme also may involve the mucous membranes, palms, and soles; EM does not. The presence of a malar rash in association with Lyme disease suggests systemic lupus erythematosus. Erythema nodosum generally causes more painful induration than EM and has a predilection for the extensor surfaces of the legs. Erythema marginatum of acute rheumatic fever also is in the differential diagnosis for EM; the Lyme disease rash differs in comprising generally fewer, larger, less evanescent lesions that migrate more slowly. Atypical EM manifesting as an urticarial rash may suggest hepatitis B infection or serum sickness. Lyme disease should be considered in a patient with an atypical rash accompanied by a viral syndrome or meningitis-like illness, especially during the months of peak incidence.

Acute rheumatic fever, coronary artery disease, or viral myocarditis may be suggested by the cardiac manifestations of Lyme disease. The carditis of Lyme disease, like the carditis of rheumatic fever, may follow pharyngitis and migratory polyarthritis. Erythema marginatum usually occurs with the onset of arthritis, in contrast with EM, which usually precedes the carditis. Although some patients with Lyme disease may satisfy the clinical aspects of the Jones criteria for acute rheumatic fever, they lack evidence of a preceding streptococcal infection; in addition, valvular involvement is not a prominent feature of Lyme carditis.

The differential diagnosis of the neurologic manifestations caused by Lyme disease is extensive. Considerations include aseptic meningitis, herpes simplex encephalitis, Bell palsy of other causes, radiculopathy due to mechanical causes, multiple sclerosis, Guillain-Barré syndrome, dementia, primary psychosis, cerebral vasculitis, and brain tumor. Neurologic symptoms often occur in the absence of any epidemiologic clues or preceding clinical symptoms suggestive of Lyme disease, making the diagnosis particularly challenging.

Lyme arthritis may mimic other immune-mediated disorders. The arthritis of Lyme disease generally is asymmetric, oligoarticular, and episodic. In contrast to patients with rheumatoid arthritis, those with Lyme arthritis rarely have symmetric polyarthritis, morning stiffness, a positive result on rheumatoid factor assay, or subcutaneous nodules. Lyme arthritis is commonly mistaken for seronegative rheumatoid arthritis; however, Lyme arthritis is most similar to the spondyloarthropathies, particularly reactive arthritis. Lyme disease and reactive arthritis both commonly cause huge knee effusions but, in Lyme disease, absence of the extra-articular features of reactive arthritis (conjunctivitis, urethritis or cervicitis, balanitis, keratosis blennorrhagica) at the time of the onset of arthritis helps distinguish it from reactive arthritis. In children, Lyme arthritis may mimic juvenile rheumatoid arthritis, but joint involvement in Lyme disease usually occurs in short intermittent attacks, and iridocyclitis typically is absent. Rheumatoid factor titers will be negative in juvenile rheumatoid arthritis and Lyme disease. The diseases resemble one another closely enough to have been confused at the time of the initial description of Lyme disease. Other diseases in the differential diagnosis for Lyme arthritis include acute gouty arthritis, septic arthritis, gonococcal arthritis, rheumatic fever, polymyalgia rheumatica, and temporomandibular joint syndrome.

Diagnostic Testing

Results of routine laboratory studies are nonspecific, and such studies generally are not helpful in the diagnosis of Lyme disease. Abnormalities may include an elevated erythrocyte sedimentation rate, mild anemia, total white blood cell count in the normal range with a decreased absolute lymphocyte count, microhematuria, proteinuria, and mildly elevated hepatic transaminases. Cultures of blood, tissue, and body fluids (including CSF and synovial fluid) for B. burgdorferi and direct visualization techniques are difficult to perform properly and have such a low yield that they are not clinically useful.

Serologic testing measuring the host's antibody response (for IgG and IgM) to B. burgdorferi is the most useful means of confirming a clinical diagnosis of Lyme disease, but is not without limitations. Results of serologic tests should be interpreted within the context of symptoms, considering the presumed stage of Lyme disease. These tests should be regarded only as adjuncts in the diagnostic process. Limitations of the tests' performance and the interpretation of their findings often result in diagnostic confusion. False-negative and, especially, false-positive results are common. The antibody response to B. burgdorferi develops slowly. The peak of IgM titers appears between 3 and 6 weeks after the onset of illness. Earlier in the course of the illness, IgM titers may be negative. IgM antibody usually returns to nondiagnostic levels 4 to 6 weeks after the peak, but elevations may persist. IgG antibody may be detectable 2 months after exposure and peaks at approximately 12 months. Early antibiotic therapy may blunt or even abolish the antibody response.

A two-tier strategy is recommended for serologic testing—a sensitive enzyme immunoassay (EIA) followed by a Western blot (immunoblot). Positive or equivocal EIA results should be followed by a Western blot. If the EIA is negative, no further testing is necessary. Several Lyme disease serologic assays have recently been cleared by the Food and Drug Administration (FDA) allowing use of an EIA rather than Western blot as the second test in a Lyme disease testing algorithm.[6] IgM and IgG immunoblots should be obtained if early disease is suspected. If late disease is suspected, IgG Western blot alone should be obtained. Criteria for positive Western immunoblotting (requiring the presence of bands at particular locations) have been adopted by the CDC.

About one-third of patients with early localized Lyme disease (erythema migrans) are seropositive at the time of presentation by the two-tier method. Patients with skin lesions typical of EM do not require confirmatory serologic testing, and the rash itself is sufficient for the diagnosis to be made. If the cause of the rash is uncertain, acute and convalescent phase serologic testing may be considered, with the convalescent sample drawn 2 to 4 weeks after the acute sample. In contrast to early localized disease, most patients with early disseminated Lyme disease or late Lyme disease are seropositive.

IgG (and occasionally IgM) antibody may persist for several years after adequate treatment and symptom resolution. Persistent seropositivity is not diagnostic of ongoing infection. Even an IgM response cannot be interpreted as a demonstration of recent infection or reinfection unless the appropriate clinical characteristics are present. IgG antibody that developed after natural infection does not always confer immunity against future infection by *B. burgdorferi*. Patients who are treated for EM may become reinfected; patients with Lyme arthritis, however, usually have high antibody titers to many spirochetal proteins and seem not to become reinfected. Thus, the expanded immune response of late disease appears to be protective against reinfection, at least in most patients, whereas the immature immune response of early disease does not.

False-positive enzyme-linked immunosorbent assay (ELISA) results are common. Serologic cross-reactivity can occur between *B. burgdorferi* and other spirochetes, most notably *Treponema pallidum*. False-positive results for Lyme disease also can occur with relapsing fever, gingivitis, leptospirosis, enteroviral and other viral illnesses, rickettsial diseases, autoimmune diseases, malaria, and subacute bacterial endocarditis. In addition, it is estimated that up to 5% of the normal population will test positive for Lyme disease by ELISA. Bayes theorem states that if the pretest likelihood of the disease is low, the positive predictive value is low: a positive test result is more likely to be a false-positive result. For this reason, screening serologic tests are not indicated in the absence of objective clinical evidence of Lyme disease.

Patients suspected of having acute Lyme neuroborreliosis should be evaluated with serologic tests and routine CSF examination, including cell counts and differential, protein, glucose, Gram stain, and culture. Most patients with neuroborreliosis have positive results on serum serologic testing, thereby making additional laboratory confirmation with CSF serology unnecessary. The PCR assay has low sensitivity when performed on CSF and is not routinely recommended. However, the PCR assay is superior to culture for detecting *B. burgdorferi* in synovial fluid and has a sensitivity of 73% and specificity of 99% in untreated Lyme arthritis.

Management

Prompt treatment of early disease can shorten the duration of symptoms and prevent progression to later stages of disease. Most manifestations of Lyme disease can be treated successfully with oral antibiotic therapy, with the exception of neurologic abnormalities, which usually require intravenous (IV) therapy. Treatment of Lyme disease is summarized in Table 123.4.

Early Disease

Prompt antibiotic therapy is essential in early Lyme disease because it generally shortens the duration of the rash and associated symptoms and, more importantly, prevents later illness in most patients. Some patients with severe early disease, however, progress to later stages, despite appropriate antibiotic regimens.

The drug of choice for men, nonpregnant and nonlactating women, and children older than 8 years is doxycycline, 100 mg bid for 3 weeks. An advantage of doxycycline is that it also is effective for the treatment of human granulocytic anaplasmosis, which is transmitted by the same tick that transmits Lyme disease. Pregnant or lactating women and children younger than 8 years should receive amoxicillin, 500 mg three times daily orally (20 to 40 mg/kg/day in three doses for children). Cefuroxime axetil has been shown to be as effective as doxycycline and may be used in children of any age, but cephalexin is ineffective in Lyme disease.

Macrolide antibiotics are not recommended as first-line agents for therapy for early Lyme disease. They should be reserved for patients who cannot tolerate doxycycline, amoxicillin, and cefuroxime axetil. Macrolide regimens for adults include azithromycin, 500 mg orally daily for 7 to 10 days, erythromycin, 500 mg orally qid for 14 to 21 days, and clarithromycin, 500 mg orally bid for 14 to 21 days.

A Jarisch-Herxheimer type of reaction may occur in the first 24 hours of antibiotic treatment, consisting of fever, chills, myalgias, headache, tachycardia, increased respiratory rate, and mild leukocytosis. Defervescence usually takes place within 12 to 24 hours. The pathogenesis of this reaction is controversial, but it probably is caused by the killing of spirochetes, with the release of pyrogens. The Jarisch-Herxheimer reaction occurs more commonly with penicillin and doxycycline than with erythromycin, probably because of their superior spirocheticidal activity.

Early Disseminated Infection

Neurologic Disease. For patients with relatively mild symptoms (e.g., solitary facial nerve palsy with normal findings on CSF examination), doxycycline or amoxicillin can be used in the same dosage as for early disease, but the duration of therapy should be extended to 28 days. The use of prednisone for facial nerve palsy from Lyme disease has been suggested but is not currently recommended.

Parenteral antibiotic therapy is required for patients with other objective neurologic abnormalities (e.g., meningitis or encephalitis, peripheral neuropathies, cranial neuritis other than facial nerve palsy) or evidence of the spirochete in the CSF. Ceftriaxone, 2 g/day IV for 14 days (75 to 100 mg/kg/day for pediatric patients), or penicillin G, 18 to 24 million units every 4 hours daily IV for 10 to 14 days, may be used. Ceftriaxone may be more effective than penicillin, and many experts recommend longer courses (e.g., up to 4 weeks). In cases of penicillin or cephalosporin allergy, oral doxycycline may be used for 28 days.

Cardiac Disease. Patients with mild cardiac conduction system involvement, such as a first-degree AV block with a PR interval less than 0.30 second, and no other significant symptoms usually can be treated safely on an outpatient basis with oral doxycycline or amoxicillin for 21 to 30 days.[7] Patients with higher degrees of AV block, including first-degree block with a PR interval of more than 0.30 second or evidence of global ventricular impairment, should be hospitalized for cardiac monitoring and treatment with parenteral antibiotics. Penicillin G, 18 to 24 million units IV in 4 divided doses, or ceftriaxone, 2 g daily for 21 days (50 to 80 mg/kg/day for children), may be used.

TABLE 123.4   Treatment of Lyme Disease

Syndrome and Manifestation	Drug	Adult Dosage	Pediatric Dosage[a]
Early Lyme disease	Doxycycline[b]	100 mg PO bid for 21 days	
	or		
	Amoxicillin	500 mg PO tid for 21 days	50 mg/kg/day tid
	ALTERNATIVE		
	Cefuroxime axetil	500 mg PO bid for 21 days	15 mg/kg/day bid (max dose of 250 mg bid)
	or		
	Erythromycin (less effective than doxycycline or amoxicillin)	500 mg PO qid for 14–21 days	
Neurologic disease			
• Facial nerve paralysis	With an isolated deficit, oral regimens for early disease, used for at least 28 days, may suffice. For a deficit associated with other neurologic manifestations, intravenous therapy is warranted (see below).		
• Lyme meningitis	Ceftriaxone	2 g IV by single dose for 14–28 days	75–100 mg/kg/day IV
	Penicillin G	20 million units daily in divided doses for 10–14 days	300,000 units/kg/day IV
	ALTERNATIVE		
	Chloramphenicol	1 g IV qid for 10–21 days	
Cardiac disease			
• Mild	Doxycycline[b]	100 mg PO bid	
	or		
	Amoxicillin	500 mg PO tid	50 mg/kg/day tid
• More severe	Ceftriaxone	2 g IV daily by single dose for 14–21 days	75–100 mg/kg/day IV
	or		
	Penicillin G	20 million units daily in divided doses every 4 hours for 14–21 days	300,000 units/kg/day IV
Arthritis	ORAL		
	Doxycycline[b]	100 mg PO bid for 30 days	
	or		
	Amoxicillin	500 mg PO tid for 30 days	50 mg/kg/day divided tid
	PARENTERAL		
	Ceftriaxone	2 g IV by single dose for 14–21 days	75–100 mg/kg/day IV
	or		
	Penicillin G	20 million units daily in divided doses for 14–21 days	300,000 units/kg/day IV

[a]Pediatric dosage should not exceed adult dosage.
[b]Tetracycline, 250 to 500 mg PO qid, may be substituted for doxycycline. Neither doxycycline nor any other tetracycline should be used for children younger than 8 years or for pregnant or lactating women.
[c]Regimens for radiculoneuropathy, peripheral neuropathy, and encephalitis are the same as those for meningitis.
[d]Oral regimens are reserved for mild cardiac involvement (see text).
Adapted from: New drugs for allergic conjunctivitis. *Med Lett Drugs Ther.* 2000;42:39-40; and Wormser GP, Dattwyler RJ, Shapiro ED, et al. The clinical assessment, treatment, and prevention of Lyme disease, human granulocytic anaplasmosis, and babesiosis: clinical practice guidelines by the Infectious Diseases Society of America. *Clin Infect Dis.* 2006;43:1089-1134.

The benefit of the adjuvant use of aspirin or prednisone in the treatment of Lyme carditis is uncertain and not currently recommended. Temporary cardiac pacing may be necessary in patients who have severe heart block with hemodynamic instability. The block generally resolves entirely with antibiotic treatment, so the recognition of Lyme carditis in young patients with unexplained heart block is critical for avoidance of unnecessary permanent pacemaker implantation.

Late Infection

Arthritis. In established Lyme arthritis, the response to antibiotic therapy may be delayed for several weeks or months. An oral regimen for 30 days, such as doxycycline, 100 mg orally bid, or amoxicillin, 500 mg tid, usually are effective and, for reasons of cost and convenience, may be selected as first-line therapy given on an outpatient basis before parenteral antibiotic therapy is considered. Persistent or recurrent joint swelling after recommended courses of antibiotic therapy can be treated with another 4-week course of oral antibiotics or with a 2- to 4-week course of IV ceftriaxone. A small percentage of patients with Lyme arthritis, particularly those with HLA-DR4 specificity or antibody reactivity with OspA, may have persistent joint inflammation, despite treatment with oral or IV antibiotics. Such patients often do not respond to any antibiotic therapy and may require arthroscopic synovectomy.

Neurologic Disease. Patients with late neurologic disease affecting the central or peripheral nervous system should be treated with ceftriaxone (2 g once daily IV for 2 to 4 weeks). Alternative parenteral therapy may include cefotaxime (2 g IV three times a day) or penicillin G (18–24 million units IV daily, given in divided doses every 4 hours). Response to treatment is usually slow and may be incomplete.

Lyme Disease and Pregnancy

Similar to the spirochetal agents of syphilis and relapsing fever, *B. burgdorferi* can be passed transplacentally. In rare cases, Lyme disease acquired during pregnancy may lead to infection of the fetus and possibly to stillbirth, but adverse effects on the fetus have not been documented conclusively. Counseling about the termination of a pregnancy because of maternal Lyme disease is unwarranted.

Lyme disease contracted during pregnancy can be treated and cured. Treatment of pregnant patients can be identical to that of nonpregnant patients with the same disease manifestations, except that doxycycline should be avoided. Most women give birth to normal infants despite documented Lyme borreliosis during their pregnancies.

Vaccination

No vaccine against Lyme disease is currently available in the United States. The LYMErix vaccine (SmithKline Pharmaceuticals, Philadelphia), initially licensed in 1999, was withdrawn from the market in 2002. The vaccine, directed against the outer surface protein A of *B. burgdorferi* (OspA), was apparently safe but required repeated doses for optimal protection. Ongoing questions about its safety and cost-effectiveness dampened demand for the vaccine.

A history of vaccination with the previously licensed vaccine should not change the approach to management. Because protective immunity produced by the vaccine is short-lived, it is unlikely that previous vaccination will provide any residual protective effect. Vaccination may cause a persistently positive ELISA result but a negative Western blot result.

Prophylaxis and Asymptomatic Tick Bites

A well-designed trial found that a dose of doxycycline given within 72 hours after a bite by a deer tick (*I. scapularis*) effectively prevented Lyme disease. A single 200-mg dose of doxycycline therefore should be considered for adult patients and children 8 years of age and older (4 mg/kg, up to a maximum dose of 200 mg) when all the following criteria are met: (1) the tick is an adult or nymphal *I. scapularis*; (2) the tick has been attached for 36 hours or more, as indicated by certainty of the time of exposure or degree of engorgement; (3) prophylaxis can be started within 72 hours after tick removal; (4) the local rate of infection of these ticks with *B. burgdorferi* is 20% or greater; and (5) doxycycline is not contraindicated. *B. burgdorferi* infects 20% or more of ticks in highly endemic areas such as New England, parts of the Mid-Atlantic region, and parts of Minnesota and Wisconsin. Most other areas of the United States do not have infection rates high enough to warrant prophylaxis.

The efficacy of single-dose doxycycline in patients who present more than 72 hours after removing a tick is unknown. In children, the dosing and efficacy of prophylactic treatment have not been evaluated. The effectiveness of doxycycline for preventing other infections transmitted by *I. scapularis* ticks (e.g., babesiosis, human granulocytic anaplasmosis) is unknown and should not be assumed. Other antimicrobial agents effective for treating Lyme disease (e.g., amoxicillin) and even other regimens of doxycycline (e.g., 100 mg bid) have unknown efficacy for Lyme disease prophylaxis. Anyone who has been bitten by a tick should be instructed to seek medical evaluation if symptoms of tickborne illness develop.

SOUTHERN TICK-ASSOCIATED RASH ILLNESS

A rash similar to erythema migrans (EM) has been described in humans following bites of the lone star tick, *Amblyomma americanum*, found from central Texas and Oklahoma eastward across the southern states and along the Atlantic coast as far north as Maine. The rash may be accompanied by fatigue, fever, headache, muscle and joint pains. This condition has been named southern tick-associated rash illness (STARI).[8] The cause of STARI is not known.

STARI is diagnosed based on symptoms, geographic location, and possibility of tick bite. Because the cause of STARI is unknown, no diagnostic blood tests are available.

It is not known whether antibiotic treatment is necessary or beneficial for patients with STARI. Because STARI resembles early Lyme disease, patients are often treated with oral antibiotics.

RELAPSING FEVER

Relapsing fever is caused by bacteria of the *Borrelia* species, order Spirochaetales. Human *Borrelia* infections occur worldwide, and all are associated with arthropod vectors. The epidemic (louseborne) form of relapsing fever is caused solely by *Borrelia recurrentis* and is found mostly in Africa, where mortality rates can reach 70% with outbreaks. The endemic form, tickborne relapsing fever (TBRF), is caused by a group of closely related *Borrelia* species, their names derived from the species names of *Ornithodoros* tick vectors that carry them. The more common species in North America are *Borrelia hermsii*, *Borrelia turicatae*, and *Borrelia parkeri*. *B. burgdorferi* has been recognized as the causative agent of the third and most recently described borrelial disease, Lyme disease.

TBRF is maintained in an animal reservoir consisting primarily of wild rodents, including squirrels, mice, rats, chipmunks, and rabbits. It is found predominantly at altitudes of 2000 to 7000 feet in coniferous forest habitats. The tick vectors are argasids (soft ticks) belonging to several species of the genus *Ornithodoros*, which routinely reside in the nests and burrows of their mammalian hosts. Ticks acquire the infection by feeding on a spirochetemic rodent. The borreliae remain viable in the ticks for several years and can be passed transovarially to the next generation. In addition, soft ticks—unlike hard ticks—can survive up to 10 years, making removal of all infested nests imperative.[9] Two unique characteristics make this genus a significant reservoir and vector. These soft ticks feed for brief periods (15–20 minutes), usually at night, and their painless bite generally is unnoticed by the sleeping victim. Transmission occurs by injection of infected saliva through the bite site or intact skin. Less common modes of transmission (e.g., venipuncture equipment in injection drug users) have been reported.

In the United States, TBRF occurs primarily in the western Mountain and Pacific states, including Montana, Wyoming, Nevada, Colorado, California, and Washington. Between 1990 and 2011, the CDC received 504 reports of TBRF. The groups most commonly affected were males and people between the ages of 10 to 14 and 40 to 44 years. Of all reported cases, 70% were collectively from California, Washington, and Colorado. Most cases involved visitors to those states. Although TBRF is not nationally reportable, it was reported in 12 states in 2011.[4] Outbreaks have been reported among groups of persons sleeping overnight in hunting cabins inhabited by wild rodents. In Texas, most cases were reported in the winter months among people who had been exploring caves.

Clinical Features

In TBRF, the initial febrile episode lasts 3 days. This is followed by an asymptomatic period of variable duration, usually, approximately 7 days. During this time, patients generally feel better and may return to their usual daily activity levels under the assumption that they have recovered from another viral illness. Relapse then occurs, with symptoms that mimic those of the original illness. With TBRF, this cycle repeats itself three to five times. Each successive relapse usually is less severe. Relapse is caused by the spirochete's unique ability to undergo antigenic variation within the body of the infected host. Each successive antigenic variation is cleared from the bloodstream by specific host antibodies, and a characteristic relapsing febrile course results.

Clinical illness is manifested in two classic stages as each fever episode resolves. The first stage is called the chill phase (high fevers with reported temperatures of up to 106.7°F (41.5°C), mental status changes, tachycardia, and tachypnea), lasting approximately 30 minutes, followed by a flush phase (rapid temperature decrease, sweats, and hypotension), which can be confused with a Jarisch-Herxheimer reaction.[5]

After a postbite incubation period of 4 to 18 days, during which time the host concentration of spirochetes increases, fever of abrupt onset occurs, often accompanied by shaking chills, headache, arthralgias, myalgias, nausea, and vomiting. On occasion, a pruritic eschar may be noted at the site of the tick bite, but this usually is absent by the onset of clinical symptoms. Consequently, the nonspecific nature of the clinical presentation may lead to misdiagnosis of the disease as a viral illness. The patient's temperature is high, and generalized muscle weakness and lethargy are common. Hepatomegaly, splenomegaly, and jaundice are sometimes seen. Neurologic involvement is less common but can be manifested as delirium, nuchal rigidity, peripheral neuropathy, or pupillary abnormalities. Uveitis, iritis, and other cranial neuropathies can present acutely or, rarely, as long-term sequelae. A macular or petechial rash, more apparent on the trunk than on the extremities, may be present. There is evidence that febrile illness caused by relapsing fever might cause *Plasmodium vivax* malaria relapse.

Severe cases of TBRF resulting in acute respiratory distress syndrome (ARDS) in California and Nevada near the Lake Tahoe area and in the state of Washington prompted a comprehensive epidemiologic investigation of cases in those areas during a 10-year period. This study showed that ARDS may be more common than was previously suspected. Reported occurrence rates for Jarisch-Herxheimer reaction varied between 6% and 21%, 16% for hypoxia, 8% for elevated liver function test values, and 6% for ARDS; 46% of patients with TBRF required hospitalization.

Differential Diagnoses

On initial presentation, the differential diagnosis is extensive; however, it narrows with the occurrence of relapse. A history of possible soft tick exposure together with recurrent fever should suggest the diagnosis. Other conditions that initially may be considered include malaria, typhus, dengue, yellow fever, Colorado tick fever, and tularemia. Careful examination of blood smears, together with clinical data and other laboratory tests, aid in making the correct diagnosis.

A recently discovered Borrelia species, phylogenetically related to those responsible for relapsing fever, is now known to cause a new tickborne illness called Borrelia miyamotoi disease (BMD). It has been found in the Upper Midwest, mid-Atlantic, and Northeast states and tends to occur in late summer months as opposed to Lyme disease, which tends to occur in midsummer. Caused by the spirochete of the same name, BMD resembles Lyme disease and human granulocytic anaplasmosis (HGA), but the vectors consist of several species of the hard tick genus Ixodes. Headache, fever, and myalgias are the most common symptoms and tend to be more severe than those associated with Lyme or HGA. Diagnosis can be made using blood PCR samples and antibody titers. Giemsa-stained acute blood smears may reveal spirochetemia. Lab tests often show leukopenia, thrombocytopenia, and elevated liver enzymes. Both amoxicillin and doxycycline are effective treatments.[10,11]

Diagnostic Testing

In contrast to other spirochetal diseases, the definitive diagnosis of relapsing fever depends on the demonstration of spirochetes in peripheral blood smears during a febrile episode. In most cases, spirochetes are readily visible on a routine blood smear prepared with Wright or Giemsa stain. Thick or thin blood smears, such as those prepared for malaria evaluation, also are satisfactory. The organisms are seen within the plasma spaces between blood cells or may overlie the blood cells. Several organisms per high-power field typically are visible in smears from febrile patients with relapsing fever. Blood specimens for the smears should be obtained as the temperature curve increases. Repeated samples may be required before a positive result is observed because sensitivity approaches only 70%.

Spirochetes also may be visible in wet mounts with the use of phase contrast microscopy. Culture, although it is the most sensitive diagnostic method available, requires a special medium, does not yield rapid results, and therefore is not commonly performed. Genus-specific PCR testing has been used successfully and may be higher in sensitivity than serology or blood smear, especially in the acute phase of disease. Serologic testing is available through public and private health facilities but is not useful for immediate diagnosis. Nonspecific laboratory findings may include mildly increased bilirubin and liver function levels, thrombocytopenia, and an elevated erythrocyte sedimentation rate.[5]

Management

Relapsing fever is effectively treated with tetracycline or erythromycin. Tetracycline should be avoided in children younger than 8 years and in pregnant women. Tetracycline or erythromycin should be given in an oral dose of 500 mg four times daily for 10 days. Other treatment regimens have been recommended, including doxycycline and chloramphenicol. Treatment with penicillin G has been associated with an increased rate of relapse. Success with ceftriaxone has been reported in a patient with relapsing fever who did not respond to penicillin. Prophylaxis with doxycycline for TBRF in exposed subjects in high-risk infested areas is effective.

As many as one-third of patients experience a Jarisch-Herxheimer type of reaction during treatment with antibiotics. The reaction can be severe, especially with louseborne relapsing fever, and has been associated with high levels of cytokine intermediaries and endogenous opioids, and accelerated phagocytosis of spirochetes.[12] Approximately 4 hours after antibiotic treatment, and coinciding with the clearance of spirochetes from the blood, the patient usually experiences an increase in temperature and severe rigors, accompanied by a drop in the leukocyte and platelet counts and onset of hypotension. Anticipation of this reaction is crucial because volume expansion with saline solution may be required to maintain the blood pressure; the reaction can be more threatening than the disease itself.

The prognosis is good for treated patients with relapsing fever; approximately 95% achieve complete recovery. Poor prognostic signs include the presence of jaundice, high spirochete counts in the blood, and hypotension. Transplacental transmission can occur in infected pregnant women. Spontaneous abortions occur in nearly 50% of cases in pregnant women. Death is rare in TBRF and is limited to infants and older adults.

TULAREMIA

Tularemia was first characterized in 1837 by Soken, who described a febrile illness with generalized lymphadenopathy in people who had eaten infected rabbit meat. In 1912, McCoy first isolated *Bacterium tularense,* now known as *Francisella tularensis,* from rodents in Tulare County, California, giving rise to the name of the disease.

Tularemia occurs worldwide and is endemic between 30 and 71 degrees north latitude. The incidence of tularemia is low. There were between 180 and 314 yearly reported cases of tularemia in the United

States between 2014 and 2018, and it is a nationally notifiable disease.[13] Tularemia has been seen in every state except Hawaii but is most common in the southwest central region. During this period, most cases have come collectively from Missouri, Oklahoma, South Dakota, Colorado, Kansas, and Arkansas. It is more common in men than in women. Persons at increased risk for infection include hunters, trappers, butchers, agricultural workers, campers, sheep herders, mink farmers, and laboratory workers.

Ticks, lagomorphs (hares, rabbits), and rodents (mice, rats) are believed to be the most important sources of transmission to humans; however, the organism has been recovered from animals of more than 100 species. Significant epidemics have been linked to contact with a variety of them, including domestic cats. In 2002, a large number of commercially distributed prairie dogs from Texas died of tularemia.

The ticks most commonly involved in transmission of tularemia in the United States are from the hard tick family Ixodidae, specifically the Lone Star tick (*A. americanum*) and the dog tick (*D. variabilis*), both of which have been associated with other tickborne illnesses. Ticks were responsible for approximately half of tularemia cases in the United States between 2004 and 2014.[14] Whereas mosquitoes are major vectors in many European countries, horse fly and deer fly bites have been implicated in endemic situations in the United States. In 2007, an outbreak in Utah was associated with deer fly bites.

While transmission to humans most commonly occurs through tick bites or handling of infected animals, it also can occur with ingestion of infected food or water, inhalation of dust or water aerosol, and insect bites. Nonimmune laboratory workers who work with *F. tularensis* can acquire the disease. Person to person transmission is rare. Tularemia has a bimodal prevalence in the United States; an increased incidence in May to August is associated with tickborne transmission, and a December to January peak is associated with hunting and skinning of infected mammals (primarily rabbits). *F. tularensis* has been found to coexist in reservoir populations harboring the agent responsible for Lyme disease. Eleven cases of pneumonic tularemia, found to be from aerosolization of contaminated vegetation clippings, were discovered in Martha's Vineyard, Massachusetts. Outside the United States, tularemia has been confirmed in hundreds of cases in Kosovo through rodent contamination of food. Sweden has reported a high number of cases, usually associated with aquatic environments and mosquitoes.[15]

Tularemia is manifested in different ways, depending on the portal of entry of the organism. The primary route of infection by *F. tularensis* is through the skin. Entry can occur through hair follicles or small cuts and abrasions that may be contaminated by exposure to an infected animal; tick exposure can also introduce the bacteria. Because the bacterium has not been isolated from the salivary glands of ticks, it is thought that they transmit the organism through their feces. Scratching after a tick bite introduces the infected feces into the skin. Inhalation or ingestion of the organism or transmission through the conjunctivae also can cause infection. The incubation period is approximately 2 to 6 days, depending on the size of the inoculum.

After penetration of the skin or epithelial membrane, the organism usually spreads to the regional lymph nodes. An erythematous tender papule develops at the primary infection site, followed by inflammation and skin ulceration. The regional nodes enlarge, necrose, and may rupture. The necrotic, purulent, painful lymph node is termed a *bubo*. In the ulceroglandular form of the infection, the organism may not spread farther than the regional lymph nodes. If the inoculum is sufficiently large or host defenses are inadequate, bacteremia ensues, with dissemination to phagocytic cells of the reticuloendothelial system.

Pulmonary tularemia may result from inhalation of small-particle aerosols containing *F. tularensis* or from hematogenous dissemination. Small areas of localized pneumonitis are most commonly seen,

although chest radiographic findings are nonspecific; lobar consolidation or abscess formation is rare. Oculoglandular tularemia occurs when the conjunctiva becomes infected from contact with material from an ulcer or contaminated finger. Typhoidal tularemia follows the systemic spread of *F. tularensis* from the oropharynx and probably the gastrointestinal tract when a large inoculum is swallowed.

Clinical Features

Presentations

Tularemia has six clinical presentations, depending on whether disease is localized to an entry site and its regional lymph nodes—ulceroglandular, glandular, oculoglandular, and oropharyngeal forms—or is more invasive and generalized—typhoidal and pulmonary forms. Ulceroglandular and glandular are the most common manifestations of tickborne tularemia.

Ulceroglandular Tularemia. This accounts for approximately 80% of cases. Typically, a skin lesion on an extremity at the site of primary inoculation begins as an erythematous papule, which then ulcerates 2 to 3 days later. The ulcer is slow to heal and often is still present when the subsequent regional lymphadenopathy and fever develop. The distribution of the regional adenopathy reflects the primary entry site; patients with tickborne tularemia usually have inguinal or femoral adenopathy, whereas those who acquire rabbit-associated tularemia have axillary or epitrochlear nodal involvement. Generalized lymphadenopathy also may be seen. On occasion, nodes suppurate and drain.

Glandular Tularemia. This is the second most common form. It is characterized by the development of lymphadenopathy (usually cervical) without an associated skin ulcer.

Oculoglandular Tularemia. This is seen in less than 2% of cases. It is characterized by unilateral conjunctivitis, with regional adenopathy involving preauricular lymph nodes.

Oropharyngeal Tularemia. This is manifested as severe exudative pharyngitis, with associated cervical lymphadenitis. It has been known to cause acute glaucoma.

Typhoidal Tularemia. This is a systemic form of the disease in which no obvious entry site can be found; it occurs in approximately 10% of cases. Only 10 to 50 organisms are required to induce disease; incubation time is 2 to 10 days. Symptoms and signs may include fever, chills, constipation or diarrhea, abdominal pain, and weight loss. A 30% to 60% case fatality rate is associated with untreated typhoidal tularemia.[16]

Pulmonary Tularemia. This has symptoms similar to those of other bacterial pneumonias—fever and chills, cough (usually nonproductive), substernal burning, dyspnea, malaise, and prostration. It may result from direct inhalation of aerosolized organisms or bacteremic spread from another site.

Other Considerations

Uncommon complications of tularemia include pericarditis, meningitis, endocarditis, peritonitis, appendicitis, perisplenitis, and osteomyelitis. Guillain-Barré syndrome associated with tularemia also has been reported.

Tularemia is one of the most widely studied diseases with respect to potential biologic warfare. The United States developed an aerosolized form in the 1950s, and the Japanese allegedly contaminated prisoners with the disease in the 1930s. It was removed from the national list of notifiable diseases in 1995 but then was reinstated in view of the heightened biologic weapons threat. It is classified by the CDC as one of the six category A critical biologic diseases.[7,13] An aerosolized form of the bacterium would be the most likely delivery mechanism used in biologic warfare. With the release of aerosolized particles, disease would be manifested clinically as acute fever, progressive pneumonia, pleuritis, and hilar lymphadenopathy, beginning as early as 3 to 5 days after delivery. The mortality rate for untreated tularemia in general ranges from 5% to 30%, but the rate for the pulmonary form can reach 60%. With appropriate antibiotic treatment, death is rare (mortality rate < 1%). Only approximately 55% of emergency departments (EDs) have been adequately educated on the recognition of and preparedness for tularemia.

Diagnostic Testing

The diagnosis of tularemia is based on clinical findings and serologic testing. Antibody titers begin to rise approximately 7 to 10 days after exposure and peak in 3 to 4 weeks. In a patient with a clinical presentation suggesting tularemia, an antibody titer of 1:160 or higher in a single specimen is diagnostic. Confirmatory evidence is provided by a fourfold or greater rise in titer in a second sample obtained 2 weeks later. Unfortunately, titers of IgG and IgM can continue to be high for up to 10 years, and cell-mediated immunity can be maintained for up to 25 years. Rapid testing with PCR assay is available, and point of care analysis using an immunochromatographic approach has proven useful in testing water sources.

As for most infectious organisms, culture is the gold standard for diagnosis; however, aspiration of affected lymph nodes for culture is not routinely recommended because of the associated risk to laboratory personnel. If tularemia is suspected, the laboratory should be alerted so that appropriate precautions can be taken in specimen handling and enriched culture medium can be used. The risk of tularemia transmission lies in the danger of any handling that might produce aerosols or droplets.

Management

Isolation of patients with tularemia is not required because it is not transmitted from person to person. Streptomycin is the drug of choice for the treatment of all forms of tularemia but is not widely available. When given intramuscularly in a dose of 10 mg/kg (pediatric: 30 to 40 mg/kg/day) bid, streptomycin usually produces symptomatic improvement and resolution of fever in 1 to 2 days. After the third treatment day, half of the dose is given for a total course of 7 to 14 days. With this regimen, relapses are unusual.

Gentamicin is effective for treatment, especially in children (3 to 5 mg/kg/day for 10 to 14 days) and is more readily available than streptomycin. Tetracycline and chloramphenicol are also effective; however, the risk of relapse is greater than that associated with the aminoglycosides. Imipenem-cilastatin, an antibiotic without nephrotoxicity, has been used successfully to treat pulmonary tularemia in a patient with acute renal failure. Ceftriaxone is not effective against *F. tularensis* infections. Prophylaxis for possible exposure requires doxycycline, 100 mg bid for 14 days. Doxycycline or ciprofloxacin prophylaxis is recommended for a large biologic attack.

Ulcers and tender lymph nodes usually heal within 7 to 10 days; however, enlarged nodes occasionally develop into fluctuant sterile buboes, requiring incision and drainage after completion of the course of antibiotics. The unique ability of *F. tularensis* to attenuate host inflammatory responses has been emerging as a basis for research investigating the use of immunomodulatory agents or antibodies for adjunctive treatment. There continues to be no approved vaccine for tularemia. Because of recent interest in biologic warfare, however, research on tularemia vaccines has resurged.

ROCKY MOUNTAIN SPOTTED FEVER

Rocky Mountain spotted fever (RMSF) is an acute, febrile, systemic tickborne illness caused by *Rickettsia rickettsii*. The genus *Rickettsia*

is divided into the spotted fever group and typhus group. *R. rickettsii* is considered the typical representative of the spotted fever group. Twenty-six species have been described.

RMSF is found in North, South, and Central America and is a nationally reportable disease. All cases are to be registered with the respective state department. As of 2010, reported cases of RMSF are categorized in the broader name of spotted fever rickettsiosis (Box 123.1).[16] The number of reported cases in the United States more than tripled between 2000 and 2007, especially in suburban areas.[17] The increase during this period was thought to be due to more widespread use of ELISA. Use of the assay has also resulted in a significantly lower

---

BOX 123.1   Diagnostic Criteria for Spotted Fever Rickettsiosis (*Rickettsia* spp.)

- Clinical criteria
  - Any reported fever and one or more of the following: rash, eschar, headache, myalgia, anemia, thrombocytopenia, or hepatic transaminase level elevation
- Laboratory-confirmed
  - Serologic evidence of a fourfold change in immunoglobulin G (IgG)–specific antibody titer reactive with *Rickettsia rickettsii* or other spotted fever group antigen by indirect immunofluorescence assay (IFA) between paired serum specimens (one taken in the first week of illness and a second 2 to 4 weeks later) *or*
  - Detection of *R. rickettsii* or other spotted fever group DNA in a clinical specimen via amplification of a specific target by PCR assay, *or*
  - Demonstration of spotted fever group antigen in a biopsy or autopsy specimen by immunohistochemistry (IHC), *or*
  - Isolation of *R. rickettsii* or other spotted fever group *Rickettsia* from a clinical specimen in cell culture
- Laboratory-supportive
  - Has serologic evidence of elevated IgG or immunoglobulin M (IgM) antibody reactive with *R. rickettsii* or other spotted fever group antigen by IFA, enzyme-linked immunosorbent assay (ELISA),[a] dot ELISA, or latex agglutination
- Exposure
  - Exposure is defined as having been in a potential tick habitat within the 14 days preceding the onset of symptoms. The patient's occupation should be recorded if relevant to exposure. A history of a tick bite is not required.
- Case classification
  - Suspected: A case with laboratory evidence of past or present infection but no clinical information available (e.g., laboratory report)
  - Probable: A clinically compatible case (meets clinical evidence criteria) that has supportive laboratory results
  - Confirmed: A clinically compatible case (meets clinical evidence criteria) that is laboratory-confirmed

[a] NOTE: Current commercially available ELISA tests are not quantitative, cannot be used to evaluate changes in antibody titer, and hence are not useful for serologic confirmation. IgM tests are not strongly supported for use in the serodiagnosis of acute disease because the response might not be specific for the agent (resulting in false-positives) and the IgM response might be persistent. Complement fixation (CF) tests and older test methods are neither readily available nor commonly used. CDC uses in-house IFA IgG testing (cutoff ≥ 1:64), preferring simultaneous testing of paired specimens, and does not use IgM results for routine diagnostic testing.

From: Centers for Disease Control and Prevention. National Notifiable Diseases Surveillance System: Spotted fever rickettsiosis (*Rickettsia* spp.) 2010 case definition. www.cdc.gov/NNDSS/script/casedef.aspx?CondYrID=853&DatePub=2010-01-01.

case fatality rate, which could be related to the high cross-reactivity of serologic tests with more benign rickettsioses. Higher awareness and more aggressive empirical treatment of RMSF might also have contributed to the decreased fatality rate. In 2016, there were 4,269 reported spotted fever cases in the United States, which included all spotted fever rickettsioses, not just RMSF, in accordance with the surveillance changes mentioned.[18] Another rare rickettsiosis that emerged in North America in 2004 was caused by *Rickettsia parkeri*, transmitted through the Gulf Coast tick, *Amblyomma maculatum*. It is distinguished from RMSF by sometimes causing eschars or a vesicular rash.

RMSF ranges in clinical severity from mild or even subclinical illness to fulminant disease, with vascular collapse and death within several days of onset. It is the only rickettsiosis still associated with significant mortality, causing approximately 40 deaths in the United States each year, with a mortality rate ranging from 3% to 5%, despite appropriate treatment. Before tetracycline and chloramphenicol were available, death occurred in as many as 30% of cases in the 1930s. The highest mortality rates occur in patients between the ages 5 and 9 years or older than 70 years, among Native Americans, and among immunosuppressed patients. In the South Atlantic United States, mortality reaches 9% in patients older than 70 years. The median time between onset of illness and death is 9.5 days, whereas death occurs in hospitalized patients in a median time of 3 days.

The recorded history of RMSF suggests that the disease was present at least before the European settlement of western North America among inhabitants of wooded Rocky Mountain regions. Early terms used to name the disease included *tick fever* and *black measles*. In 1899, RMSF was described as "an acute, endemic, noncontagious but probably infectious, febrile disease, characterized by a continuous moderately high fever, severe arthritic and muscle pains, and a profuse petechial or purpuric eruption in the skin, appearing first on the ankles, wrists, and forehead, but rapidly spreading to all parts of the body."

Although RMSF was first described in Montana and Idaho, it is now relatively rare in the Rocky Mountain states. Endemic in all 48 contiguous states except Maine, the disease continues to be most prevalent in the southeastern United States. RMSF has been reported in Canada, Central America, Mexico, and South America but never outside the Western Hemisphere. Recently, RMSF has become increasingly common in certain areas of Arizona, with 21 fatalities reported between 2003 and 2016. In 1987, four cases of RMSF were reported among residents of the Bronx in New York City; none of the affected persons had recently traveled to an area known for endemic disease, raising the possibility that other urban foci of RMSF may exist.

RMSF also tends to be focally endemic, with clustering of cases within a larger endemic area that may correspond to islands of infected ticks. These areas, ecologically distinct from surrounding areas, may be ideally suited to ticks; they usually consist of wild open fields, deciduous forests with thick ground cover and poor water drainage, or uncultivated areas. Geographic clusters of severe disease have been reported. In areas with frequent occurrence of RMSF (Oklahoma, North and South Carolina, Tennessee, Pennsylvania, Missouri, Arkansas, Arizona), an infectivity rate of 2% to 15% of the tick population has been reported. North Carolina and Oklahoma carry the highest incidence rates (35% of all cases) for RMSF.

R. rickettsii organisms are obligate intracellular bacteria with tropism for human endothelial cells. They often occur in pairs and possess a cell wall similar in structure and chemical composition to that of gram-negative bacteria. *R. rickettsii* contain RNA and DNA and, in contrast with other rickettsial organisms, can invade the nucleus as well as the cytoplasm.

The American dog tick, *Dermacentor variabilis*, and the Rocky Mountain wood tick, *Dermacentor andersoni*, have been the vectors responsible for human RMSF cases in the United States to date. However, the common brown dog tick, *Rhipicephalus sanguineus*, has emerged as a third vector. *R. sanguineus* has been the main RMSF vector in Mexico, Central America, and the southwestern United States. *Amblyomma imitator*, in the genus of the Lone Star tick, has been implicated as yet another vector because *R. rickettsii* has been found in its eggs.

Ticks feed on virtually any available warm-blooded animal and human; the occurrence of *R. rickettsii* in the United States does not depend on the presence of any given order of mammal. Domestic dogs infected with *R. rickettsii* can demonstrate clinical illness similar to that seen in humans. Although dogs do not play an important role in the amplification cycle of RMSF, they can serve as a conduit for infected ticks, carrying them into close contact with pet owners. Dogs may serve as sentinels for RMSF in humans. A high prevalence of rickettsial antibodies in stray dogs in Arizona was thought to be a major factor in the 70 cases and 8 deaths from RMSF reported there between 2003 and 2008. The deadliest spotted fever, Brazilian spotted fever, is also caused by *R. rickettsia*. The capybara, a common mammal in Brazil, appears to be the main reservoir through the vector tick *Amblyomma cajennense*.

Communication between physicians and veterinarians is important when cases of zoonotic diseases are detected. Humans serve only as accidental participants in the cycle of infection. A retrospective study has revealed that none of 10 recipients of blood products found to be from donors with confirmed or probable RMSF contracted the disease.[15]

Pathophysiology

After introduction of *R. rickettsii* into the host by the tick vector, the organisms invade and multiply in the vascular endothelial cells. They then enter deeper areas of the vessel walls and infect vascular smooth muscle. Rickettsial organisms move from cell to cell by actin-based motility. Damage to endothelial cells not only exposes subendothelium but also releases tissue plasminogen activator and von Willebrand factor, thereby causing microhemorrhage, microthrombus formation, and increased vascular permeability. In addition, antibody forms, with antigen activating the complement system (type III immune response), and a cellular response is recruited.

These widespread vascular lesions form the basis for most of the clinical features associated with RMSF. Hypotension, edema, and increased extravascular fluid space result from the increased small-vessel permeability. The early rash results from the vasculitis and associated changes in permeability; later petechial and hemorrhagic lesions are secondary to the vasculitis and thrombocytopenia. Microinfarcts and focal lesions develop in various organs, including the brain, heart, lungs, kidneys, adrenal glands, liver, and spleen. Rickettsial encephalitis and diffuse microinfarcts are usual features of central nervous system involvement. An interstitial pneumonitis caused by direct lung invasion by the organism may occur, and ARDS can ensue. Acute renal failure and hypovolemic shock, the primary causes of death, can occur as early as the second week of illness.

Clinical Features

Children from 5 to 9 years of age are the most common victims of RMSF. Two-thirds of all cases are in children younger than 15 years. More than 90% present with a fever and rash. A history of tick bite or presence in possible tick-infested areas is elicited in 60% to 70% of all patients with RMSF, although only 49% of the pediatric population reports a bite. The incubation period ranges from 2 to 14 days, with a mean of 7 days. A short incubation period may indicate a more severe infection. Factors that bring a higher risk of death include delayed onset of rash, glucose-6-phosphate dehydrogenase deficiency, hepatomegaly,

TABLE 123.5 Symptoms and Signs of Rocky Mountain Spotted Fever[a]

Symptom or Sign	FREQUENCY DURING ILLNESS (%)	
	Any Time	First 3 Days
Fever (temperature of 37.8°–38.9°C [100°–102°F])	99	73
Headache, mild to moderate	91	71
Fever (≥102°F [38.9°C])	90	63
Any rash	88	49
Myalgia, mild to moderate	83	57
Rash, maculopapular	82	46
Rash, palms and soles	74	28
Triad of fever, rash, history of tick exposure	67	3
Nausea and vomiting	60	38
Headache, severe	57	40
Abdominal pain	52	30
Rash, petechial and hemorrhagic	49	13
Myalgia, severe	47	25
Conjunctivitis	30	13
Lymphadenopathy	27	13
Stupor	26	6
Diarrhea	19	9
Edema	18	3
Ataxia	18	7
Meningismus	18	5

[a]In 262 patients.
From: Helmick CG, Bernard KW, D'Angelo LJ. Rocky Mountain spotted fever: clinical, laboratory, and epidemiological features of 262 cases. *J Infect Dis*. 1984;150:480-488.

neurologic deficits, renal insufficiency, increased period between symptoms and antibiotic treatment, and lack of tick bite history.

Onset of symptoms usually is abrupt but may be gradual in approximately one-third of patients. Early symptoms are nonspecific and similar to those of many acute infectious diseases, making early diagnosis difficult. Typical patients experience sudden onset of fever, severe headache, myalgias, prostration, nausea, and vomiting. Tenderness may be noted in large muscle groups (Table 123.5). As many as 80% of patients may have gastrointestinal symptoms secondary to myositis of the abdominal wall. Fever (temperature usually > 102°F [39°C]) is nearly always present during the first 2 to 3 days of illness and may precede other signs by 1 week or more. On occasion, the onset of illness is mild, with lethargy, headache, anorexia, and low-grade fever; these patients may remain ambulatory. Although the triad of fever, rash, and tick exposure traditionally was seen in only approximately 3% to 18% of cases, more recent data have shown that it is found in up to 45% of children with the disease. An extreme complication of RMSF is gangrene, which probably is induced by small-vessel occlusion.

Cutaneous Manifestations

Vasculitis secondary to rickettsial invasion of vascular endothelial cells causes the rash commonly associated with RMSF; however, the rash reportedly is absent in 4% to 16% of laboratory-confirmed cases, referred to as Rocky Mountain spotless fever. In addition, the rash may go unnoticed in dark-skinned patients. It usually appears on the third to fifth febrile day but can emerge as early as the second and as late as the sixth day. The initial lesions generally are restricted to the ankles and wrists, sometimes spreading to the palms and soles. The rash then spreads centripetally to the forearms, arms, legs, thighs, and trunk. The face can be involved, although it is usually spared. Despite the common belief that the palms and soles are critical for diagnosis, they are not consistently involved; rash on the palms and soles is reported in approximately 50% of cases. Involvement of the scrotum or vulva can be an evasive clue for RMSF. The rash of RMSF typically begins as 1- to 5-mm blanchable pink to bright red discrete macules that may be pruritic. At this initial stage, the lesions fade when pressure is applied and are not palpable. A warm compress applied to the area enhances the rash.

After 6 to 12 hours, the rash spreads centripetally. After 2 to 3 days, the rash becomes maculopapular and changes to a deeper red; at this stage, skin changes can be appreciated on light palpation. By approximately the fourth day, the rash becomes petechial and no longer fades with applied pressure. Applying tourniquets for several minutes or taking the blood pressure may cause additional petechiae to form distal to the site of occlusion (Rumpel-Leede phenomenon). The lesions occasionally coalesce to form large ecchymotic areas that may slough and form indolent ulcers (Fig. 123.9).

Prompt institution of specific therapy can cause the initial nonfixed lesions to disappear rapidly, unlike the later fixed lesions. Patients who have had the typical rash may exhibit brownish discolorations at the site during the convalescent period.

Cardiopulmonary Manifestations

Echocardiographic evidence of decreased left ventricular contractility secondary to myocarditis is commonly seen and often is detectable even before clinical signs of RMSF appear. Clinical manifestations of left ventricular dysfunction are uncommon, however, and hypotension and pulmonary edema, when present, usually have noncardiogenic causes. Chest radiographs may demonstrate cardiac enlargement. Electrocardiographic changes include low-voltage, nonspecific ST-T changes, first-degree AV block, dysrhythmias (e.g., sinus and nodal tachycardia, paroxysmal atrial tachycardia, atrial fibrillation), and left ventricular hypertrophy. Most cardiac abnormalities are transient, but persistent echocardiographic changes have been described. Decreased systolic function, elevated serum cardiac markers, no finding of vascular lesions, and a fourfold rise in antibody titers are consistent with myocarditis from RMSF.

Interstitial pneumonitis and increased pulmonary capillary permeability may result from infection of the pulmonary capillaries with rickettsiae. Nonproductive cough and dyspnea secondary to pneumonitis are sometimes seen on presentation. Chest radiographic abnormalities are identified in approximately 25% of patients. These abnormalities include interstitial infiltrates, patchy alveolar infiltrates, pleural effusions, and cardiomegaly with pulmonary edema. Pulmonary consolidation is rare. In severe cases, progression to noncardiogenic pulmonary edema and ARDS may occur.

Neurologic Manifestations

Neurologic manifestations of RMSF range from mild headache and lethargy to seizures and coma. Acute disseminated encephalomyelitis has been described. Headache, generally severe, is common, occurring in 50% to 90% of cases. Meningismus is present in 16% to 29% of patients. The CSF may be normal or show a slight protein elevation and pleocytosis of lymphocytes and polymorphonuclear cells (usually 8 to 35 cells/mL). The CSF glucose level and opening pressure usually are normal. Resolution of eosinophilic meningitis during RMSF after appropriate antibiotic treatment has been reported. Less than 40% of patients have a positive CSF finding.

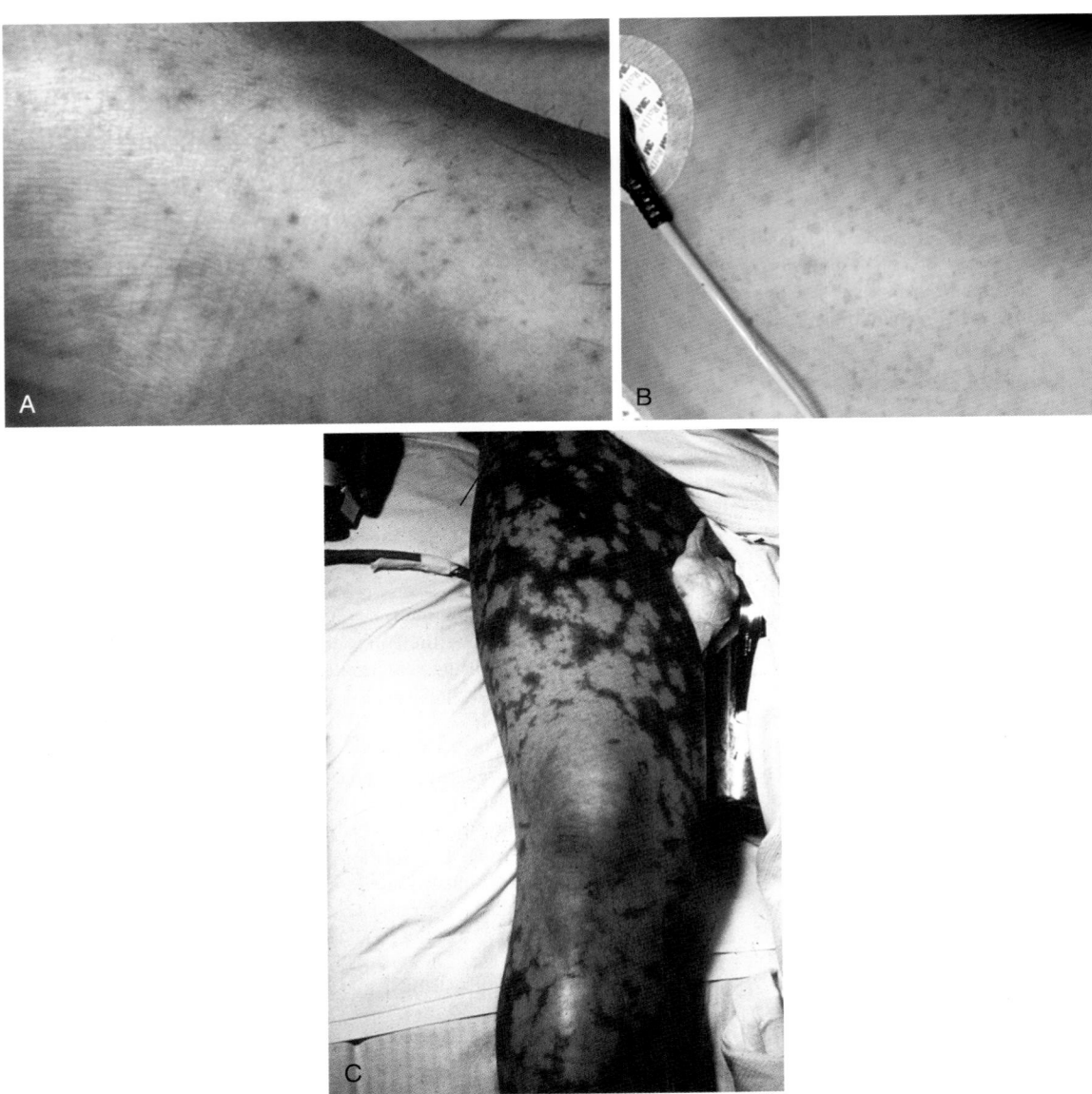

Fig. 123.9 Progression of rash of Rocky Mountain spotted fever. (A) Early, 2–4 days : Macular, maculopapular; small, flat, pink or red macules, usually on the wrists, forearms, and ankles. (B) Mid-stage, 5–7 days: Maculopapular, early petechia; progresses to maculopapular with petechiae, spreading centripetally to trunk. May involve palms and soles. (C) Late-stage, 7–9 days: Petechial, purpuric, necrosis; larger red to purple spots (petechiae) are considered a sign of progression to severe disease. These become diffuse, coalescing to form purpura. Areas of necrosis may occur. (A, From McGinley-Smith DE, Tsao SS. Dermatoses from ticks. *J Am Acad Dermatol.* 2003;49:363-392; B, From Centers for Disease Control and Prevention. RMSF training module: clinical diagnosis and treatment for healthcare providers [continuing education]. Accessed at: https://www.cdc.gov/rmsf/resources/module.html; Courtesy of Gerardo Álvarez; C, Courtesy Dr. Theodore Woodward.)

Cerebral thrombovasculitis may cause focal neurologic deficits, which usually are transient. Seizures can occur, especially during the acute phase of the illness. Generalized cerebral dysfunction ranging from lethargy to coma can occur secondary to systemic toxicity (e.g., fever, hypotension, hyponatremia) or vasculitic lesions involving the central nervous system. Coma is a late finding in patients with severe disease and is seen in less than 10% of cases. Some reports have described patients who remain alert but are amnesic for their illness after recovery. Other reported neurologic manifestations include transient deafness, tremor, rigidity, athetoid movements, paralysis, ataxia, opisthotonos, aphasia, and blindness. In general, neurologic signs abate without residual deficits, and permanent neurologic deficits are rare. Behavioral disturbances and learning disabilities have been reported after recovery from RMSF-associated coma in children.

Differential Diagnoses

Delayed diagnosis or misdiagnosis is the principal reason for the historically significant mortality associated with RMSF. Clinical diagnosis is difficult, especially early in the course of the illness, because of its nonspecific presentation. For avoidable deaths to be prevented, a diagnosis of RMSF should be considered in any patient with an unexplained febrile illness, with or without a rash and headache, even in the absence of a history of tick bite or travel to an area known to be endemic for the disease. The emergency clinician should remember to ask routinely about recent tick bites, especially when assessing children with unexplained febrile illness, because parents do not always spontaneously provide this important information. An atypical presentation or manifestation of RMSF also should be considered during the differential diagnosis, including the following: (1) absence of a rash (Rocky Mountain spotless fever) or late appearance of a rash; (2) predominant gastrointestinal features or abdominal pain suggestive of an acute condition in the abdomen; (3) cough and pulmonary congestion suggestive of pneumonitis; and (4) meningismus suggestive of viral meningitis. A presumptive diagnosis is advised, with the initiation of specific therapy, well before specific confirmatory laboratory values are available.

A wide variety of other infections with similar exanthems can be confused with RMSF.[19] The most common include meningococcal infection, measles (rubeola) and atypical measles, gonococcemia, infectious mononucleosis, toxic shock syndrome, and enteroviral infections. Less common diseases include dengue fever, leptospirosis, murine typhus, and epidemic typhus. *R. parkeri* rickettsiosis should be considered.

Diagnostic Testing

Most immediately available laboratory tests provide little help in the diagnosis of RMSF. Early in the course of the illness, the diagnosis is based primarily on the history and physical exam, so epidemiologic features should be correlated with clinical signs and symptoms. The initial presentation of RMSF is similar to that of many acute febrile infectious diseases, and almost invariably a therapeutic decision must be made on clinical grounds alone, without the luxury of confirmatory laboratory evidence. Abnormalities such as thrombocytopenia, hyponatremia, and acute renal failure may be detected by routine laboratory tests, but they are nonspecific and unhelpful diagnostically. Up to 30% of patients present with anemia. A definitive diagnosis of RMSF requires positive results on one or more of several tests—skin biopsy, serologic study, or direct isolation and identification of the organism (see Box 123.1).

Skin Biopsy

Identification by immunofluorescent assay (IFA) and immunoperoxidase staining of *R. rickettsii* in biopsy specimens of the rash from patients with suspected RMSF are the best rapid diagnostic tests currently available. In experienced laboratories, the diagnosis of RMSF can be confirmed as soon as 4 hours after the specimen is obtained. The organisms can be detected as early as day 3 of clinical illness and as late as day 10. Unfortunately, this technique can be used only when a rash is visible for accurate localization of the biopsy site. Biopsy specimens generally are obtained with a 3-mm punch in the center of the skin lesion. Immunofluorescent demonstration of rickettsiae in frozen sections of skin biopsy specimens has a sensitivity of 70%. Results of immunohistochemical staining of tissues at autopsy were positive in all fatal cases in one study, whereas IFA results were negative in most cases. Failure to obtain a biopsy specimen of a rickettsial cutaneous lesion or failure to obtain sections through its center is associated with false-negative results. Treatment with anti-rickettsial drugs for 24 hours does not appreciably alter the sensitivity of the test; however, after 48 hours, rickettsiae are substantially reduced in number. Detection of rickettsial DNA in a skin biopsy specimen by PCR assay is available through the CDC, some state health departments, and other clinical laboratories.

Serologic Studies

Rickettsial infection can be confirmed by demonstration of an antibody rise in paired sera. Even with the most sensitive serologic tests, however, elevations in antibody titers do not occur until approximately 5 to 7 days after the onset of initial symptoms. Especially given the need to start treatment when RMSF is suspected, serodiagnosis is retrospective. It is achieved by comparing acute serum, which typically yields negative findings, with convalescent serum, which yields positive results for antibodies. The indirect IFA generally is considered to be the reference standard for RMSF diagnosis and is the test currently used by the CDC and most state public health laboratories. It has a high specificity and sensitivity (94%). IFA can be used to detect IgG or IgM antibodies. An RMSF latex agglutination test with results in less than 24 hours is available in selected laboratories.[15]

A prior study has shown a 12% seroprevalence, with antibody titers of 1:64 or higher, in the pediatric population in the southeastern and south central regions of the United States. Accordingly, clinical correlation with titers in these regions is critical.

Convalescent-stage blood samples are best obtained 2 to 3 weeks after the onset of clinical illness. Antibiotic therapy does not affect the time of appearance of antibodies or titers if initiated several days after the onset of illness. However, if antibiotic therapy is started earlier in the course of the illness, the rise in titers can be delayed for 4 weeks or more. Under these circumstances, antibody titers should be tested again at 4 to 6 weeks after the onset of illness.

Nested PCR testing with a turnaround time between 1 and 2 days has been used but is not specific for individual rickettsial species. Real-time PCR assays that can be completed in 1 hour and are 100% specific for RMSF have been developed but are not readily available.

Isolation of Organism

For most pathogenic infections, the standard diagnostic criterion is isolation and identification of the causative organism from the patient's blood or tissues. This is seldom attempted in rickettsioses, however, because the isolation procedures are time-consuming, expensive, and hazardous to laboratory personnel. In addition, primary isolation of rickettsiae by inoculation in the yolk sac of a chick embryo usually fails because of the small number of organisms in the patient's blood.

Management

Treatment of RMSF consists of antibiotic therapy, supportive care, and possibly steroids. An understanding of the underlying pathophysiologic changes and appreciation of the systemic complications that can occur in the patient afflicted with RMSF are necessary for the formulation of a balanced therapeutic regimen. The course of the disease can be complicated by electrolyte imbalances, renal failure, circulatory collapse, and coma. Although these complications are often absent in the mildly ill patient, for whom antibiotic therapy alone usually suffices, they should be anticipated in the seriously ill patient, especially if the patient is first seen late in the disease course.

The most important factor contributing to the persistent case fatality rate of 5% is the delayed administration of specific antibiotic therapy. Without appropriate treatment, the fatality rate rises to 25%. For a select group of early-stage, mildly ill patients, outpatient therapy with oral antibiotics can be successful if the patient is reliable and close follow-up observation is arranged. More severely ill patients in whom the diagnosis is uncertain should be hospitalized for the administration of IV antibiotics.

As part of an effort to improve physician awareness and timely treatment for RMSF, the CDC offers a free online training module that includes a rash comparison tool and case-based exercises.[20]

Supportive Care

Major complications of RMSF, such as shock, congestive heart failure, disseminated intravascular coagulation, and ARDS, should be

TABLE 123.6 Antibiotic Therapy for Rocky Mountain Spotted Fever[a]

Patient	Doxycycline[b] (Oral or IV)	Chloramphenicol[c] (Oral or IV)
Adult	100 mg bid; consider initial loading dose of 200 mg IV for seriously ill patients	50–75 mg/kg/day, divided q6h
Child (<45 kg)	2.2 mg/kg PO q12h	50–75 mg/kg/day, divided q6h

[a]Continue treatment at least 3 days after fever subsides or until unequivocal clinical improvement is seen; minimum course, 7 to 14 days.
[b]Doxycycline should not be given to pregnant women.
[c]Chloramphenicol should not be given to patients with thrombocytopenia; maximum of 1 g/day for children.
From: Centers for Disease Control and Prevention, Division of Vector-Borne Diseases, National Center for Emerging and Zoonotic Infectious Diseases: Rocky Mountain spotted fever, www.cdc.gov/rmsf/symptoms/index.html#treatment; and Cunha BA. Clinical features of Rocky Mountain spotted fever. *Lancet Infect Dis*. 2008;8:143-144.

anticipated and standard supportive measures instituted when appropriate. Circulatory collapse is common in patients with severe illness and is a major contributor to morbidity and mortality in RMSF. Hypotension unresponsive to fluid administration may require the use of vasopressors. In the critically ill patient with widespread vasculitis, however, a delicate balance exists between maintaining effective circulating volume and excessive leakage of fluids into the tissues, including the lungs and brain. Under these circumstances, the excessive administration of IV fluids can be deleterious. Isolation of the patient is unnecessary unless the diagnosis is still uncertain and other highly communicable illnesses, such as meningococcemia and measles, have not been excluded.

Antibiotics

Antibiotic therapy is most effective when initiated during the early stages of disease, coincident with the initial appearance of the rash. Although data from randomized clinical trials about antibiotic selection for RMSF are lacking, doxycycline is still widely regarded as the therapeutic agent of choice for most patients, including children.[21] Chloramphenicol should be considered only for patients in whom tetracyclines have caused significant adverse events and for pregnant women, except for those who are near term. The recommended doses of doxycycline and chloramphenicol are summarized in Table 123.6.

The American Academy of Pediatrics and CDC recommend doxycycline as the agent of choice for treatment of RMSF in children of all ages. The risk of cosmetically perceptible tooth staining appears to be minimal for a single course of treatment and is subordinate to the potential lethality of this illness.[22]

The effectiveness of therapy depends on the duration of therapy and interval between the onset of illness and the initiation of therapy. Treatment should begin as early as possible and continue for 7 to 10 days or until the patient is afebrile for 2 to 5 days. Response to treatment, as manifested by decreasing fever and subsiding rash, generally occurs 36 to 48 hours after antibiotic therapy is begun. Resistance to chloramphenicol or tetracyclines has not been reported. Penicillin, erythromycin, cephalosporins, aminoglycosides, clindamycin, and sulfonamides are ineffective against RMSF. In fact, empirical use of these agents for presumed bacterial infections could permit progression of the illness.

Symptom overlap between early meningococcal infection and RMSF frequently leads to both diagnoses being considered simultaneously. After blood and CSF culture specimens are obtained, empirical antibiotic coverage with ceftriaxone plus doxycycline should be administered.

On occasion, secondary bacterial infection from the RMSF rash may occur. Although sulfonamides have become a mainstay for the empirical treatment of MRSA skin infections, the use of these agents should be avoided in RMSF patients because their mechanism of inhibiting *p*-aminobenzoic acid may worsen the primary RMSF infection. The role of the new quinolones as potential replacements for doxycycline and chloramphenicol in the treatment of RMSF is as yet unproved. At present, no vaccine is available for RMSF.

Corticosteroids

The use of steroids in RMSF is controversial and is not routinely recommended. However, along with concomitant specific antibiotic therapy, short-term, high-dose steroid therapy should be considered for severe cases of RMSF complicated by extensive vasculitis, encephalitis, and cerebral edema, although there are no robust data to support this recommendation.

Q FEVER

Q fever, or "query fever," was first described in 1937 in Australia as an occupational disease of abattoir workers and dairy farmers. Cattle, sheep, goats, and ticks are the primary reservoirs of the causative rickettsiae, *Coxiella burnetii*, but many other species may be infected. The disease is now endemic worldwide, although it is rare in Scandinavian countries. The southern area of the Netherlands experienced a serious outbreak and reported more than 4000 cases since 2007 and 500 cases, with 11 deaths, in 2010 alone. France and Australia have significantly more cases than the United States. Africa presently is hyperendemic with Q fever. In the United States, the Midwest and California have had the highest incidences of Q fever. More than 30 cases have been seen in US military personnel deployed in Iraq and Afghanistan. Approximately 80% of cases of Q fever occur in males.[23]

Pathophysiology

C. burnetii is an obligate intracellular gram-negative coccobacillus bacterium, with multiple strains having been identified. Although most Q fever infections are transmitted by particle inhalation, tick transmission does occur. Besides being a vector of the disease, extremely high levels of *C. burnetii* in the feces of infected ticks are found on ruminant animals on which they feed. The Rocky Mountain wood tick, *D. andersoni*, is the main tick vector in the United States, although the bacterium has been isolated in more than 40 hard tick and 14 soft tick species.

Q fever historically has been characterized as either an acute or chronic presentation, although the exact definitions and criteria are controversial, with some authors suggesting phases of infection, akin to tuberculosis.[24] The most common foci of infection are endocarditis, vascular infections, osteoarticular infections, or lymphadenitis. Both the type of bacterial strain and patient risk factors play a role in the course of illness.[24] It is extremely infectious for humans and animals; a single inhaled organism is likely sufficient to initiate infection. The Q fever rickettsiae are extremely resistant to desiccation, physical and chemical agents, and can survive for long periods in an inanimate environment. Consequently, it is classified as a category B biologic warfare agent by the CDC and has been a nationally notifiable disease since 1999.[25] The organism's infectivity and estimated casualty rate have been judged to be comparable with those of anthrax. Humans most commonly are infected by inhalation of aerosolized particles from contaminated environments. Patients with Q fever rarely recall a history of tick bite.

Clinical Features

The incubation period of Q fever ranges from 14 to 39 days, with an average of 20 days. Up to 60% of initial infections are asymptomatic. The acute form of the disease includes clinical manifestations such as severe retrobulbar headache, fever with temperatures to 40°C (104°F) or higher, shaking chills, general malaise, myalgia, and chest pain. Although Q fever is widely regarded as primarily a respiratory disease, the reported incidence of pulmonary involvement varies, ranging from 0% to 90%. The reasons for this reported variation are unclear, but explanations include geographic strain variation, plasmids that may regulate virulence, and source, route, and dose of the agent. Mild hepatic involvement is common. Osteomyelitis in children, acute renal failure, and lymphocytic meningitis secondary to *C. burnetii* have been described.

Rarely, Q fever may present as a "chronic infection," occurring in less than 5% of cases, with or without an antecedent acute episode. Clinical syndromes that historically have been labeled as a chronic form of the disease include granulomatous hepatitis and culture-negative endocarditis. Endocarditis has been documented in up to 68% of patients with chronic Q fever; the mortality rate for this group approaches 25%. Most patients with Q fever in whom endocarditis develops have a history of valvular heart disease, particularly affecting the aortic valve. These patients should be especially cognizant of the potential hazards of Q fever infection and should be restricted from certain at-risk occupational settings. Patients with aneurysms and vascular grafts also are at risk.

Human fetal demise and deaths have been attributed to *C. burnetii* infection. Persons infected with human immunodeficiency virus (HIV) are at increased risk for Q fever.

Diagnostic Testing

The diagnosis of Q fever should be suspected in any patient with a severe febrile illness without an obvious cause, especially someone who has had recent contact with sheep, cattle, goats, or animal byproducts. Few patients with this disease recall a tick bite. Because of the laboratory hazards associated with the cultivation of Q fever rickettsiae, isolation of *C. burnetii* is not recommended for routine diagnosis. Rather, serologic studies such as IFA, PCR, and ELISA are the preferred diagnostic tests, but the results are not identifiable until 2 to 3 weeks after the onset of illness.

C. burnetii displays an antigenic phase variation. In patients with acute Q fever, phase II antibodies dominate the humoral immune response and are detectable by the second week of illness, whereas phase I antibodies are prominent only in patients with chronic (persistent) Q fever. Confirmation of a Q fever case requires (1) a fourfold increase in IgG titers between acute and convalescent samples or the presence of IgM phase II antibodies, (2) a positive PCR test result, (3) the culture of *C. burnetii* from a clinical specimen, or (4) the positive immunostaining of the organism in tissue. Measurement of IgA and IgG together has been useful in the diagnosis of endocarditis. The finding of granulomatous changes on bone marrow biopsy can be characteristic of Q fever in patients with osteomyelitis.

Management

Uncomplicated acute Q fever is treated with doxycycline (200 mg once daily for 2–3 weeks). Acute disease with concomitant valvular heart disease is treated with doxycycline (200 mg once daily) plus hydroxychloroquine (600 mg once daily) for 1 year. Fluoroquinolones have also been successful in this situation. Patients with persistent infections should be continued on the same regimen for 1.5 to 3 years. Combination therapy with doxycycline and hydroxychloroquine is effective for treatment of endocarditis in HIV-infected patients. Strong evidence

has recommended combination therapy for endocarditis for 18 and 24 months in patients with native valves and prosthetic valves, respectively, with evidence of persistent infection. Cotrimoxazole is the recommended alternative treatment. Some macrolides and rifampin may also be effective. Treatment of pregnant women with Q fever with long-term cotrimoxazole, although not always curative, has been shown to decrease complications to the fetus.

In mass casualty situations, prophylaxis is recommended by treating with 5 to 7 days of doxycycline. Most acute Q fever infections resolve without treatment, but the risk of persistent infection makes treatment advisable. The mortality rate is less than 1% in untreated patients and lower still in those treated with antibiotics. The prognosis is worse in patients with protracted illness and hepatic involvement or endocarditis. Inactivated whole-cell vaccines for Q fever have proven to be effective for as long as 5 years. Vaccination can afford considerable protection to slaughterhouse and dairy workers and others at risk. Information on the handling of suspected or confirmed exposure to *C. burnetii* or bioterrorist threats can be found on the CDC website.

EHRLICHIOSES

There are currently two major forms of human ehrlichiosis in the United States—human monocytic ehrlichiosis (HME) and human granulocytic anaplasmosis (HGA), caused by the bacteria *Ehrlichia chaffeensis* and *Anaplasma phagocytophilum*, respectively. In 2001, restructuring of the *Ehrlichia* phylogenetic branches placed the previously known bacteria of human granulocytic ehrlichiosis into the genus *Anaplasma*—hence, the revised name. Both genera, *Ehrlichia* and *Anaplasma*, are now considered to be in the tribe Ehrlichieae, family Anaplasmataceae, but are still collectively referred to as being in the group of diseases called ehrlichioses. A total of seven different species are now thought to be possible human pathogens.[26] HME was discovered in 1986 and HGA (previously human granulocytic ehrlichiosis) in 1994. Both have been identified as emerging diseases by the CDC and are nationally notifiable diseases, reportable through the appropriate state departments.

More than 1650 cases of *E. chaffeensis* were reported in the United States between 2016 and 2017 (Fig. 123.10).[27] Dramatic increases in seroprevalence rates in both diseases during the past decade suggest that these diseases have previously been highly underdiagnosed, underreported, or both. Misclassification from failure to confirm *Anaplasma* serologically likely has led to underreporting of this disease.

Both diseases peak around June through August. High-risk populations are similar to those at high risk for Lyme disease, including those living in endemic areas or having frequent contact with wildlife or rural wooded areas. HME has been reported predominantly in the south-central and southeastern United States; HGA mostly is found in the upper Midwest, New England, parts of the Mid-Atlantic states, northern California, and many parts of Europe.

Pathophysiology

The causative agents in the ehrlichioses are gram-negative, obligate, intracellular, rickettsia-like coccobacilli. Transmitted from the midgut and salivary glands of their tick vectors, these organisms reside in specific circulating leukocytes in human and other mammalian hosts. Reservoirs include the white-tailed deer and white-footed mouse. *Ehrlichia canis* is the common pathogenic species in dogs. The species *Ehrlichia equina* has been isolated in California elk. HME, transmitted by the Lone Star tick, *A. americanum*, is most often caused by the organism *E. chaffeensis* (named for Fort Chaffee, Arkansas), which invades monocytes. *Ehrlichia ewingii* and *Ehrlichia muris* are also now known to be definite causative organisms.[28] *E. chaffeensis* has been isolated

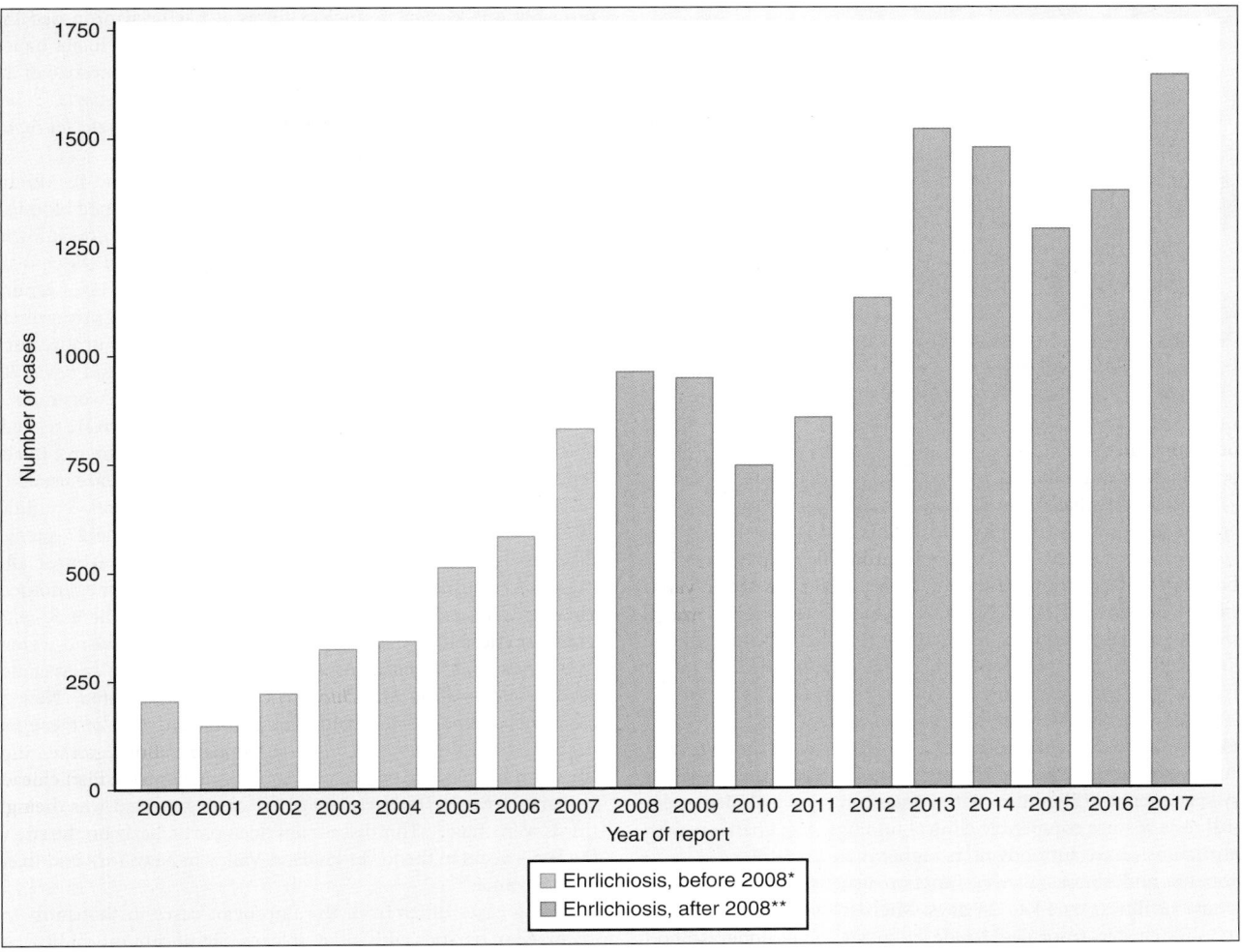

Fig. 123.10 More than 1650 cases of *Ehrlichia chaffeensis* were reported in the United States between 2016 and 2017.

from *I. pacificus* ticks in California. As of 2017, Missouri, Arkansas, New York, and Virginia are responsible for over half of reported HME cases.[27] *A. phagocytophilum* invades neutrophils (granulocytes), causing HGA and, in the United States, is transmitted by the black-legged tick, *I. scapularis*, and its West Coast counterpart, the western black-legged tick, *I. pacificus*. Deer, elk, and wild rodents are the main reservoirs for *Anaplasma*. Both ticks also are the vectors for Lyme disease. *A. phagocytophilum* has been detected in significant numbers in various *Ixodes* human tick species in mainland Portugal, Italy, and Japan.

Clinical Features

The clinical presentations of HME and HGA are similar and, for management, it is not necessary to differentiate between the two illnesses. The average time to onset of symptoms (for HME) from tick discovery is 9 days but ranges from 0 to 34 days. More than 90% of patients with HME report a history of tick bite or tick exposure. Ehrlichiosis characteristically is manifested with abrupt onset of fever, headache, myalgia, and shaking chills. Other, less frequent manifestations include nausea, vomiting, diarrhea, abdominal pain, cough, and confusion. Leukopenia, thrombocytopenia, and elevated liver function test values can be seen in 50% to 90% of patients.

Rashes occur in approximately one-third of patients with HME but in only 2% to 11% of those with HGA. In a small series of pediatric patients (average age, 7.4 years) with HME, a rash rate of 67% was found. Most of these patients suffered permanent cognitive or other neurologic damage.

Ehrlichiosis (HME) also has been associated with optic neuritis. ARDS, meningitis, pancarditis, renal failure, and disseminated intravascular coagulation have been associated with both ehrlichioses. Case fatality rates vary between studies but range from 0.5% to 3% for both diseases, with HGA usually reported as the lower of the two. Historically, data support only a 0.2% concurrence of lumbar puncture–proven meningitis or encephalitis with patients diagnosed with HGA who have a headache and/or stiff neck.[28] Approximately 45% of patients with HGA require hospitalization, although almost all recover without residual problems. HME has been associated with hemophagocytic lymphohistiocytosis.

Diagnostic Testing

For HME and HGA, the initial diagnosis is based largely on clinical presentation. With most tests, the diagnosis will be retrospective; results are rarely available immediately. The most common mode of diagnosis is confirmation of acute and convalescent antibodies with IFA. Enzyme immunoassay and confirmatory tests with Western blot have been developed but are not readily available. They provide only positive or negative results without titers. PCR testing for DNA fragments, although also not as readily available in most institutions, probably is most reliable in the acute phase of illness (at 1 week after onset of symptoms). Diagnostic serologic testing is available at the CDC through state health departments.

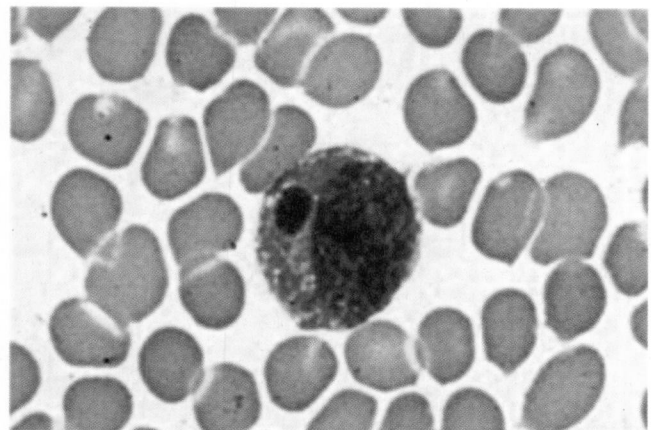

Fig. 123.11 Morulae detected in a monocyte on a peripheral blood smear associated with *Ehrlichia chaffeensis* infection (Wright stain; ×1000). (From: Centers for Disease Control and Prevention. Ehrlichiosis: symptoms, diagnosis, and treatment. www.cdc.gov/Ehrlichiosis/symptoms/index.html.)

Laboratory criteria required in the CDC's 2008 case definition to establish the presence of HME or HGA include detection of *E. chaffeensis* or *A. phagocytophilum*, respectively, through the use of the following diagnostic tests: (1) fourfold change in antibody titer to the organism antigen by IFA in paired serum samples; (2) positive result on PCR assay and confirmation of organism-specific DNA; (3) identification of morulae in leukocytes and a positive titer to the organism antigen; (4) immunostaining of the organism's antigen in a biopsy or autopsy specimen; or (5) culture of the organism from a clinical specimen. All tests require compatible clinical findings. Most patients with acute ehrlichiosis have antibody titers higher than 1:160.[29]

Cytopenia and abnormal liver function usually resolve after the acute phase of illness by 14 to 28 days. Microscopic identification of mulberry-like clusters (morulae) inside leukocytes on peripheral blood smears is helpful (Fig. 123.11). This finding, however, usually disappears after the first week of illness with HGA,[28] especially if the patient has been treated with doxycycline. Cultures take up to 2 weeks to grow the organisms.

Management

Doxycycline (100 mg bid; 2.2 mg/kg body weight bid for children weighing < 45 kg) and tetracycline regimens for 7 to 14 days are curative. Most patients respond rapidly after treatment is begun, and fever subsides within 24 to 48 hours. Tooth staining from doxycycline is no longer considered a concern for children and should not be a reason to withhold therapy. Rifampin is an effective alternative in children with human ehrlichiosis. Data supporting the use of chloramphenicol are inconclusive. The same ticks that transmit HGA (*Ixodes* spp.) also are responsible for Lyme disease and babesiosis. Each disease entity requires a full diagnostic evaluation because amoxicillin treats Lyme disease but not HGA or babesiosis, and doxycycline alone does not treat babesiosis. Failure of fever to resolve beyond 6 or 7 days of treatment of a suspected tickborne disease should heighten suspicion for another disease organism. There are no vaccines presently available for either of the ehrlichioses.

BABESIOSIS

Babesiosis is a tickborne, malaria-like, acute febrile illness caused by intraerythrocytic protozoal parasites of the genus *Babesia*. Babesiosis has long been recognized as an important veterinary disease and probably was known in ancient times; it has been proposed that the fifth plague described in the book of Exodus was likely babesiosis. The species almost solely causing the disease is the protozoan *Babesia microti*, which is transmitted via the tick *Ixodes scapularis*. *B. microti*'s main reservoirs are the white-footed mouse, *Peromyscus leucopus*, and the white-tailed deer, *Odocoileus virginianus*.

The first human cases of babesiosis were reported in Montana in 1904. Investigators seeking the cause of RMSF examined blood smears from local inhabitants and described parasitic forms now known to be characteristic of *Babesia*. Since the late 1950s, several widely scattered cases (mostly in Europe) of human babesiosis have been reported in splenectomized persons. *Babesia divergens*, a species primarily infecting cattle, is the most common agent reported in Europe, but other species have been implicated as well, including *Babesia bovis*, *Babesia equi*, and a single case of *Babesia caucasia* infection. Two strains, WA1, related to a canine pathogen, *Babesia gibsoni*, and MO1, related to *B. divergens*, also have been found to cause disease in humans. In all these reported cases, the course was fulminant and the disease usually fatal.

In 2011, babesiosis became a nationally reportable condition. In 2013, 1762 cases of babesiosis were identified by the 27 states mandated to report. This count reached 2358 in 2017. Almost all these cases were caused by *Babesia microti*, a rodent parasite, and occurred in the coastal regions of southern New England, where *B. microti* is endemic. New Jersey and the eastern part of Long Island were found to be endemic with babesiosis. Ninety-five percent of cases came from seven states—Connecticut, Massachusetts, Minnesota, New Jersey, New York, Rhode Island, and Wisconsin—and 85% of these patients presented with symptoms in June through August, coinciding with the nymphal feeding period and time of maximal human exposure in endemic areas.[30] The average age for cases reported was 62 and two-thirds were male.[31] This disease has been particularly on the rise within the last 8 years in the lower Hudson Valley in New York and in eastern Pennsylvania.[32]

These cases differ from the European cases in that most (≈80%) occurred in persons with intact spleens. Significant morbidity has been low in the United States, despite lack of specific therapy. Asplenic persons, older adults, and otherwise immunosuppressed patients usually have more severe disease.

Pathophysiology

B. microti is associated with mice and deer rather than with cattle. The ecology of *B. microti* is similar to that of *B. burgdorferi*, the causative agent of Lyme disease, with the same major vector, *I. scapularis*, and the same mammalian reservoirs—predominantly the white-footed mouse, which hosts the larval and nymphal stages of the tick, and the white-tailed deer, which hosts the adult ticks.

Human babesiosis results from accidental human intrusion on the natural cycle of infection. The nymphal form of the *Ixodes* tick most commonly transmits the disease to humans, although babesiosis also can be transmitted by the adult tick. *I. scapularis* nymphs measure only 1 to 2 mm long and thus are easily overlooked by the patient (see Fig. 123.5). In more than 50% of all cases of babesiosis, patients cannot recall tick exposure. Babesiosis acquired through blood transfusion has been well documented.

Clinical Features

Babesiosis has an incubation period of 1 to 4 weeks after tick exposure. A nonspecific influenza-like illness, with fever, chills, headache, fatigue, and anorexia, is characteristic. Less common manifestations are nausea, diaphoresis, depression, photophobia, myalgias, arthralgias, dark urine, emotional lability, and hyperesthesias. Unlike in Lyme disease, rash is not a feature of this illness; however, erythema figuratum, a widespread exanthem with well-established annular lesions, has been associated with septic babesiosis. The physical examination usually reveals normal findings, except for fever, which typically is present, and splenomegaly, which occurs in some patients. Meningeal signs are absent. More severe disease occurs in splenectomized patients; hypotension, severe hemolytic anemia, hemoglobinuria, jaundice, renal insufficiency, ARDS, and disseminated intravascular coagulation can be seen in these cases. Some patients with babesiosis are only mildly ill, and asymptomatic infection also may occur, as demonstrated by serologic surveys in endemic areas. The diagnosis of babesiosis should be considered in any febrile patient from an endemic area during the tick season and should be part of the differential diagnosis for posttransfusion infections. Mortality rates for hospitalized patients historically range from 6% to 9%, and up to 21% in immunocompromised patients.

Diagnostic Testing

The diagnosis may be established through microscopy, antibody detection through IFA staining, or PCR assay. Microscopic examination is done with thick and thin Giemsa-stained blood smears. Characteristic intraerythrocytic forms (piriform, ring, tetrad) may be present. Babesiosis has been known to be misdiagnosed as malaria. Malaria may be excluded by the absence of intracellular pigment granules, schizonts, and gametocytes. The presence of parasites in budding tetrad formation, resembling a Maltese cross, is more suggestive of babesiosis. Contrary to what is commonly taught, this finding is uncommon. Because parasitemia may vary, serial smears over the course of several days may be necessary in suspected cases. An immunohistochemical assay has been developed that further allows easier microscopic differentiation between babesiosis and malarial organisms.

The diagnosis can be confirmed by serologic studies. IFA antibody to *B. microti* is available through the CDC, and titers usually rise to 1 : 1024 or greater within the first few weeks of illness. IgM–indirect IFA is sensitive and specific in acute babesiosis. Serologic tests for Lyme disease, which shares a common tick vector with babesiosis, also should be performed; concurrent Lyme disease has been reported in up to 50% of cases of babesiosis. ELISA and IFA sensitivities rise significantly after 5 days of illness, whereas PCR is more useful in the earlier days of sampling.

Parasitemia observed at 1 to 4 weeks after inoculation of blood from infected patients into gerbils or hamsters supports the diagnosis. Other nonspecific laboratory findings include mild to moderate hemolytic anemia, which is present in most patients, and resultant mild elevations in bilirubin and serum lactate dehydrogenase levels.

Management

Patients who have not undergone splenectomy generally recover without specific therapy, although prolonged malaise and fatigue are common. In patients with severe disease and those who have had splenectomies, the combination of clindamycin (1.2 g bid IV or 600 mg tid orally) plus quinine (650 mg tid orally) has been shown to be effective and is the treatment of choice. An alternative regimen that may be better tolerated, especially by children and infants, consists of atovaquone (750 mg bid orally) plus azithromycin (500–1000 mg once followed by 250 mg once daily orally); up to 25% of patients may have an adverse effect from quinine. Pediatric doses need to be adjusted accordingly. Therapy should be continued for a minimum of 7 to 10 days. Development of resistance during treatment with azithromycin-atovaquone in immunocompromised patients has been described.

Other antimalarial drugs, such as chloroquine and quinacrine, are not effective. Fulminantly ill patients with marked degrees of parasitemia and hemolysis have benefited from exchange transfusion or apheresis.[33] Effective live vaccines have been developed for bovine babesiosis but have not been developed yet for human disease.[34]

COLORADO TICK FEVER

Endemic to the Rocky Mountain area, Colorado tick fever is an acute, tickborne viral infection characterized by headache, back pain, biphasic febrile course, and leukopenia. The causative agent of Colorado tick fever is a small RNA virus of the genus *Coltivirus,* family Reoviridae. It is one of more than 500 viruses in the heterogeneous group of arthropod-borne viruses (arboviruses). Colorado tick fever has a sharply defined endemic zone encompassing mountainous and highland areas, from an altitude of approximately 4000 to more than 10,000 feet, in the Canadian provinces of British Columbia and Alberta and in at least 11 western states (California, Colorado, Idaho, Montana, Nevada, New Mexico, Oregon, South Dakota, Utah, Washington, and Wyoming). The largest number of cases has been reported in Colorado. The distribution of the virus coincides with that of its principal tick vector, *D. andersoni,* the Rocky Mountain wood tick. Although RMSF is transmitted by the same vector, that disease is far less common in Colorado. The cases of RMSF are outnumbered at least 20-fold by cases of Colorado tick fever.

Pathophysiology

The Colorado tick fever virus has been isolated from at least eight species of ticks, but *D. andersoni* is the only proven vector for humans. The tick is a significant reservoir for the virus because trans-stadial transmission (from larva to nymph to adult) occurs, and the tick remains infected and infectious for life, up to 3 years. The primary vertebrate host species for Colorado tick fever virus maintenance are the chipmunk, *Tamias minimus,* and golden-mantled ground squirrel, *Spermophilus lateralis;* many other vertebrate hosts have been identified as well, including a species of porcupine in Colorado in Rocky Mountain National Park. Larval and nymphal stages of *D. andersoni* ticks are responsible for the transmission of Colorado tick fever virus among rodents, and overwintering of the virus is accomplished by nymphal and adult *D. andersoni.* Only adult ticks transmit Colorado tick fever virus to humans.

The CDC indicates that there were 83 cases reported between 2002 and 2012 in the United States. The actual incidence undoubtedly is much higher because many cases are diagnosed as nonspecific viral illness, and other cases may be mild or entirely subclinical. Human susceptibility to Colorado tick fever is universal, but it occurs most commonly in young men, reflecting greater occupational and recreational tick exposure. This disease is not notifiable nationally, but is in some states.

Clinical Features

After an incubation period of approximately 3 to 5 days (range, 0–14 days), a moderate to severe influenza-like illness occurs abruptly, with signs and symptoms similar to those in early-stage RMSF. Fever, chills, headache, retrobulbar pain, myalgia, lethargy, anorexia, and nausea are common; vomiting and abdominal pain are reported occasionally. Early physical findings are nonspecific. A macular or maculopapular rash has been reported in 5% to 12% of patients but, unlike the rash of RMSF, the rash of Colorado tick fever is not a prominent feature of the illness.

A distinct feature of the illness is a biphasic course that occurs in approximately 50% of patients, causing a characteristic saddleback fever curve. Initial symptoms resolve after 2 to 3 days, and the patient feels relatively well for 1 or 2 days, after which the fever, headache, and myalgias return. The second phase may be more intense than the first phase and generally lasts 2 to 4 days. There may even be a third febrile period. Alternatively, a single prolonged febrile illness may occur. Recovery from Colorado tick fever usually occurs within 2 weeks, but convalescence can be prolonged, especially in patients older than 30 years.

Colorado tick fever is a self-limited disease, and virtually all patients recover without sequelae. Reports of severe complications, such as meningoencephalitis and hemorrhagic diathesis, have been limited to children. Only a few fatal cases have been recorded.

Diagnostic Testing

The peripheral leukocyte count often is depressed during the acute phase of illness to as low as 1000/μL, with a relative lymphocytosis. Transient thrombocytopenia can accompany the leukopenia and, less often, a mild anemia can occur. These hematologic abnormalities normalize during convalescence, but persistence of the virus in red blood cells causes a prolonged viremia, even when clinical recovery is complete. Transfusion-acquired infection has been reported and is caused by this persistent viremia in asymptomatic blood donors.

The diagnosis of Colorado tick fever can be confirmed by serologic testing (IFA, neutralizing antibody, complement fixation, enzyme immunoassay) of acute and convalescent samples, but serologic study is of little help early because of the slow rise of titers. The most rapid confirmation of Colorado tick fever, with corresponding elimination of concern about possible RMSF, is provided by direct immunofluorescent staining of virus in red blood cells in peripheral blood smears. RT-PCR testing is available for more rapid diagnosis. ELISA has shown promising sensitivity in detection of the Colorado tick fever virus.

Management

The treatment of Colorado tick fever is supportive only. Although not commonly a fatal disease, up to 30% of patients require hospitalization. If RMSF remains a diagnostic possibility, initial treatment with tetracycline or chloramphenicol and a period of observation are necessary until the diagnosis of RMSF can be ruled out.

OTHER TICKBORNE VIRUSES

In addition to the virus responsible for Colorado tick fever, at least 40 viral species have been transmitted to humans by ticks and caused illness, approximately 25 of them in the United States. Tickborne viruses are found predominantly in the RNA virus families. Historically, the most severe cases involved the tickborne encephalitis virus and Crimean-Congo hemorrhagic fever virus, but these have not been reported in the United States. A few tickborne viral illnesses have received notable press in the United States because of their mortality rates—the Heartland virus, a phlebovirus (family Bunyaviridae); the Bourbon virus, a thogotovirus (family Orthomyxoviridae); and Powassan virus (POWV). Recently, the exotic tick *Haemaphysalis longicornis* has been identified in several East Coast states in the United States. This tick is responsible for severe hemorrhagic fever in China and Japan and, so far, two cases in the United States have been confirmed.[35]

Eight cases of Heartland virus (RNA) disease were found among residents of Tennessee and Missouri as of March 2014. Four patients were hospitalized, and there was one death. All cases presented with leukopenia, thrombocytopenia, and fever. The Bourbon virus, named after the county of its discovery, caused the death of a man in Kansas. POWV, named after Powassan, Ontario, where a young boy died from this flavivirus, is transmitted by several *Ixodes* tick species, including *I. scapularis*. It can cause a severe encephalitis and up to 50% of subjects acquire permanent neurologic deficits.[36] Presentations and laboratory results of these new viral syndromes resembled those of other

tickborne illnesses and were treated with antibiotics empirically and unsuccessfully. Other neurologic symptoms and encephalitis have been well-described with tickborne viral illnesses. As with most viral illnesses, treatment remains mostly supportive. The emergence and discovery of these newer tickborne diseases suggests that they have been underreported.[19,37]

TICK PARALYSIS

Tick paralysis occurs when an adult female tick attaches to a host and releases a neurotoxin that can produce cerebellar dysfunction or an ascending paralysis. Tick paralysis was recognized as early as the beginning of the 19th century. Hovell, while traveling through Australia, wrote in 1824 of "the small insect called the tick, which buries itself in the flesh, and would in the end destroy either human or beast if not removed in time."

Tick paralysis has been reported worldwide, but most cases occur in the southeastern and northwestern regions of the United States, western Canada, and Australia. Cases have been reported to occur in clusters; 43 species of ticks have been found to cause tick paralysis in humans, other mammals, or birds. Most cases in North America and Canada are caused by *D. andersoni* (Rocky Mountain wood tick) and *D. variabilis* (American dog tick). Species responsible for paralysis cases that also are associated with other tickborne diseases include *A. americanum* (Lone Star tick), *I. scapularis* (black-legged tick), and *I. pacificus* (western black-legged tick); in Australia, *Ixodes holocyclus* is primarily associated with this disorder. Family Argasidae ticks (soft ticks) also have been implicated. Tick paralysis usually occurs in the spring and summer months and most reported cases are in children, primarily girls, probably because ticks are more easily concealed in longer hair. Among adults, however, more men than women acquire the disease.

Pathophysiology

Tick paralysis is thought to be caused by a toxin secreted from the salivary glands of the tick during a blood meal. The toxin, ixobotoxin, affects sodium flux across axonal membranes without affecting the neuromuscular junction itself. The mechanism of action of the toxin is poorly understood, but it appears to produce a conduction block in the peripheral branches of motor fibers, resulting in a failure of release of acetylcholine at the neuromuscular junction. Electrophysiologic studies have confirmed a rapid reversal of significant impairment of motor nerve terminal function after tick removal, indicating that the disturbance is not a result of a neuromuscular junction defect. Possible central sites of action of the toxin have been postulated to explain cases in which the clinical picture is dominated by cerebellar dysfunction.

Clinical Features

The onset of symptoms usually occurs 4 to 7 days after the tick attaches. Initial manifestations include restlessness and irritability, followed by ascending flaccid paralysis, acute ataxia, or both. Deep tendon reflexes are almost invariably lost. These signs and symptoms can progress rapidly during a few days to bulbar involvement, respiratory paralysis, and ultimately death if the tick is not detected and removed.

The ascending nature of tick paralysis has been noted in most descriptions; however, ataxia and associated cerebellar abnormalities in the absence of muscle weakness may be seen. Thus, tick paralysis may sometimes be manifested as so-called tick ataxia. Isolated facial paralysis has been reported in patients with ticks embedded behind the ear. Fever, other systemic symptoms, and sensory deficits are unusual. Concomitant infection with Colorado tick fever has been reported.

Differential Diagnoses

Tick paralysis should be considered in the differential diagnosis for any patient thought to have Guillain-Barré syndrome, Eaton-Lambert syndrome, myasthenia gravis, poliomyelitis, botulism, diphtheritic polyneuropathy, or any disease with an acute onset of ascending flaccid paralysis or acute ataxia. Ocular findings, such as decreased convergence, unresponsive dilated pupils, and nystagmus (horizontal and vertical), seen early in tick paralysis can help distinguish this disease from Guillain-Barré syndrome.

Diagnostic Testing

No diagnostic tests to confirm tick paralysis are available other than the combination of the clinical scenario, presence of a tick, and improvement after its removal. The Tensilon test yields a negative result in patients with this condition, and CSF is normal.

Management

Treatment in the United States consists simply of removing the tick; improvement generally is seen within a few hours and complete recovery within 48 hours. Supportive care, including mechanical ventilation, may be necessary. The mortality rate is approximately 10%; nearly all patients who die are children. The recommended procedure for the removal of any tick, including ticks causing tick paralysis, is summarized in Box 123.2. Traditional methods, such as burning, forceful removal, and application of petroleum, viscous lidocaine, or gasoline, are not consistently successful and do not guarantee removal of mouthparts, where the salivary glands and toxin may remain. Retained mouthparts also may cause infection.

Tick paralysis in Australia is often more devastating than in the United States. Symptoms and signs of illness caused by the Australian tick, *I. holocyclus,* do not resolve and often worsen after tick removal. Hyperimmune serum is available in Australia and often is needed because symptoms may worsen up to 48 hours after removal.

TICK BITE PROPHYLAXIS WITH INSECT REPELLENTS

Insect repellents have long been used to prevent mosquito bites. With recent increased public awareness of and concern about tickborne illness, especially Lyme disease, skin and clothing repellents are now also being marketed for tick protection. Three active ingredients in repellents have been shown to be effective against blood-sucking arthropods, including ticks—*N,N*-diethyl-*m*-toluamide (DEET), picaridin in

---

BOX 123.2 Recommended Method for Tick Removal

1. Remove an embedded tick by grasping it with blunt forceps or tweezers as close to the point of attachment as possible.
2. Do not use bare fingers to remove ticks from animals or humans; when tweezers are unavailable, fingers should be shielded with a tissue, paper towel, or rubber glove.
3. Apply gentle, steady, upward traction with the forceps; do not twist or jerk the tick. Avoid squeezing or crushing the tick.
4. Do not handle the tick with bare hands. After removal of the tick, thoroughly disinfect the bite site and wash hands with soap and water.
5. Dispose of ticks by placing them in a container of alcohol or flushing them down the toilet.

Adapted from: Needham GR. Evaluation of five popular methods for tick removal. *Pediatrics.* 1985;75:997-1002.

KBR 3023 (known as Bayrepel, Hepidanin, and Autan Repel outside the United States), and *p*-menthane-3,8-diol (PMD) in oil of lemon eucalyptus. The most effective and most studied is DEET. Formulation percentages of DEET vary widely, ranging from 4.75% to 23.8%, giving 1.5 to 5 hours of protection, respectively.[38] A long-acting 35% DEET formulation (US Army Extended Duration Topical Insect/Arthropod Repellent [EDTIAR]), available in the United States as Ultrathon (3M), provides protection for 6 to 12 hours. Picaridin is as effective as the 35% DEET formulation. Despite some earlier concerns, toxic and allergic reactions to DEET have been uncommon, and serious adverse effects are rare. Used as directed, concentrations up to 50% appear to be safe, even in young children, although toxic encephalopathy rarely can occur. Use for infants younger than 2 months is not recommended.

Permethrin is actually a contact insecticide rather than a repellent. It can be used as a clothing spray for protection against ticks. Applied to the clothing as an aerosol, it is nonstaining, nearly odorless, and resistant to degradation by light, heat, or immersion in water. Permethrin is toxic to the nervous system of insects, but in mammals it is poorly absorbed and rapidly inactivated. Reported adverse effects have been limited to the skin and are uncommon.

Topical DEET and clothing impregnated with permethrin are effective in field trials when each is used alone. Wearing protective clothing treated with permethrin in addition to the use of DEET on exposed skin provides the greatest degree of protection against tick bites.

The references for this chapter can be found online at ExpertConsult. com.

Tuberculosis

Peter E. Sokolove and Robert W. Derlet

FOUNDATIONS

Background and Importance

The emergency department (ED) serves as the front line of contact for many persons with untreated tuberculosis (TB) in the United States. Undiagnosed patients, incompletely treated patients, or those with active disease who develop complications may first seek medical care in EDs. For this reason, emergency clinicians must fully understand the complexities of the disease, including the multiple presentations of undiagnosed disease, complications, and initial therapeutic options.

TB is currently the world's second leading infectious cause of death, and one-third of the world's population has been infected by TB. Each year, more than 8 million people acquire active TB infection globally, and over 1.5 million die of the disease. In the United States, close to 10,000 new cases of TB are diagnosed each year, and 65% of these cases are in patients from endemic countries.[1] The largest numbers of people with TB originate from Eastern Europe, Africa, and Asia. Ongoing challenges of the 21st century include increasing occurrence of TB in institutional living settings, increasing rates of poverty, and substance use disorders. Being undomiciled and urban crowding also have contributed to the spread of TB in the United States and globally.

The HIV/AIDS epidemic has increased the incidence of TB in the United States. The pandemic of HIV-related TB also increased TB cases among non–HIV-infected people owing to the higher numbers of source cases in the community. The rate of clinical TB among patients who are HIV-infected and have a positive TB skin test is higher the cohort of non–HIV-infected patients.

Pathophysiology

One microorganism, *Mycobacterium tuberculosis* (MTB), causes human TB in nearly all cases. Humans constitute the sole known reservoir for MTB. Two other pathogenic mycobacteria, *Mycobacterium bovis* and *Mycobacterium africanum* have, on rare occasions, been implicated in causing TB. *M. bovis* is transmitted by drinking milk from diseased cows, which is rare in industrialized nations. *M. africanum* also is a rare cause of human TB in rural Africa.

MTB is an intracellular, aerobic, nonmotile, non–spore-forming bacillus with a waxy lipid coat. This coating makes MTB resistant to decolorization with acid alcohol after staining—hence, the term *acid-fast bacillus* (AFB). MTB grows slowly. Its generation time is 15 to 20 hours, compared with less than 1 hour for some common bacteria, and cultures take 4 to 6 weeks to grow on standard solid media. MTB produces neither endotoxins nor exotoxins. Its cell components are immunoreactive: some are immunosuppressive, and others are the agents of granuloma formation, macrophage activation, host toxicity, and modification of the immune response.

Transmission

TB is transmitted with rare exception by the respiratory route, including droplet spread and true aerosolization into microparticles. Patients with active disease expel MTB in liquid droplets during coughing, sneezing, and vocalizing. A single cough or 5 minutes of talking can produce 3000 infectious droplets, and sneezing can produce an even higher number. The droplets rapidly evaporate, and the desiccated bacilli circulate airborne for prolonged periods. These infective particles, or droplet nuclei, measure 1 to 5 μm in diameter, contain one to three tubercle bacilli and, when inhaled, can travel to the distal alveoli. Transmission by nonrespiratory routes, such as direct inoculation, occurs primarily among health care workers.

The susceptible host may become infected when only a few of the droplet nuclei are inhaled. Fomites are not important in the transmission of the disease, and patients' rooms, eating utensils, and bedding do not require special decontamination procedures. Because the infectious droplet nuclei are airborne, exchange of contaminated air is the most important environmental control. In addition, MTB is susceptible to ultraviolet radiation, so transmission rarely occurs outdoors because of the dilution of infectious particles and exposure to ultraviolet radiation.

The risk for TB transmission increases when source patients have airway and cavitary disease. Infectivity correlates with the number of organisms seen on sputum smear, extent of pulmonary disease, and frequency of coughing. Currently, there is no clear epidemiologic evidence to define a patient's contagiousness once they have started effective therapy. Most patients who initially had AFB-negative sputum smears are noncontagious after 2 weeks of chemotherapy. In contrast, patients who initially were smear-positive may still have viable

MTB detectable in their posttreatment sputum cultures after 2 weeks of treatment. Patients with extensive disease may still have AFB detectable on their post-treatment sputum smears; these two groups should be considered contagious. The Centers for Disease Control and Prevention (CDC) has published guidelines requiring the presence of three negative smears on different days as the criteria for removal of a patient from respiratory isolation, but debate about this recommendation is ongoing.

Extrapulmonary TB also may be infectious, but only if it is in the oral cavity or open skin lesion. Transmission of MTB to health care workers caring for patients with skin ulcers and draining tuberculous abscesses has been reported. Irrigation of the abscess may aerosolize the bacilli, forming infectious droplet nuclei.

Pathogenesis

When infectious droplet nuclei are inhaled, the airflow through the bronchial tree tends to deposit them in the midlung zone on the respiratory surface of the alveoli. The deposition launches a complex series of immunologic events. The pathogenesis of TB is divided into four stages.

Stage 1

The first stage begins when an alveolar macrophage phagocytoses the recently inhaled bacillus. A macrophage from a resistant host can immediately destroy a less virulent bacillus. In these cases, no tuberculous infection develops, and the process ends. If a virulent bacillus can overcome a macrophage's microbicidal capability, the infection may progress to the next stage.

Stage 2

When the alveolar macrophage is unable to destroy the inhaled tubercle bacilli, the bacilli replicate until the macrophage lyses. Circulating monocytes are attracted to the site of infection by the released bacilli, cellular debris, and various chemotactic factors. The monocytes differentiate into macrophages and ingest the free bacilli. Initially, these new macrophages are not activated and cannot destroy or inhibit the mycobacteria. The bacilli multiply logarithmically within macrophages and accumulate at the primary focus of infection, called a tubercle. The infected macrophages also may be transported through lymphatics to regional lymph nodes, from which they can reach the bloodstream, with subsequent spread. During this lymphohematogenous dissemination, the pathogens tend to distribute preferentially to lymph nodes, kidney, epiphyses of long bones, vertebral bodies, meningeal areas, and apical posterior areas of the lungs.

Stage 3

The third stage of TB begins 2 to 3 weeks after the initial infection, with development of the immune response that terminates the unimpeded growth of MTB. Cell-mediated immunity occurs through CD4+ helper T cells. These T cells secrete cytokines that attract and activate monocyte-macrophages. Once activated, the macrophages, containing previously ingested mycobacteria and their progeny, kill the bacilli. Mild fever and malaise may develop in association with the immune response at 4 to 6 weeks, but the primary infection is generally insignificant clinically. Eventually, in the immunocompetent host with strong cell-mediated immunity, the caseous center inspissates (thickens) while the primary lesion is effectively walled off by epithelioid cells and is arrested. This sequence of events, from stage 1 to stage 3, represents the pathogenesis of primary TB in the immunocompetent patient. In most cases, primary TB is subclinical and self-limited. Clinically active TB develops in 8% to 10% of otherwise healthy persons. By contrast, in persons also infected with HIV, progression to acute primary TB occurs at a rate of 37% within 6 months.

Stage 4

The final stage usually occurs months to decades after an apparent recovery from the initial infection. TB may progress to stage 4 even in immunocompetent persons. Usually, host factors lead to decreased resistance and reactivation of dormant foci of MTB. Reactivation of dormant foci is responsible for the major clinical manifestations of TB. Exogenous reinfection of patients with well-documented previous TB infection causes clinical disease indistinguishable from that of reactivation TB. Because it may be incorrect to label all late-onset cases as reactivation disease, the preferred term is *postprimary TB*. Postprimary TB is active or chronic disease in a patient previously infected. In the United States and other developed countries, reactivation is thought to be the primary mechanism of postprimary TB. The primary walled-off tubercle eventually may erode through the bronchial wall and drains its contents, forming a cavity. The liquefied caseous material, teeming with mycobacteria, enters other parts of the lung and outside environment. The spilling of this liquefied material within the lung may produce a caseous bronchopneumonia.

CLINICAL FEATURES

Patients with TB may present with a primary infection or, more commonly, reactivation of an old infection. TB should be included in the differential diagnosis of common presenting complaints, such as isolated fever, chronic weakness, weight loss, failure to thrive, and night sweats.

Clinically significant pulmonary TB often is indolent, and signs and symptoms are absent or minimal until the disease advances. The constitutional symptoms of anorexia, weight loss, fatigue, irritability, malaise, weakness, headache, chills and, most commonly, fever can be caused by many other diseases. The fever usually develops in the afternoon; defervescence occurs during sleep, leading to the classic night sweats of TB.

Cough is the most common symptom of pulmonary TB patients presenting to the ED. It may initially be a dry nonproductive cough or, less commonly mucopurulent in nature. Hemoptysis, caused by caseous sloughing or endobronchial erosion, usually is minor but often indicates extensive lung involvement. Many otherwise asymptomatic MTB patients present for medical attention because they are alarmed by an episode of sudden hemoptysis. Patients also may complain of pleuritic chest pain, caused by parenchymal inflammation adjacent to the pleural surface. Dyspnea with chest pain may indicate a spontaneous pneumothorax. Shortness of breath from parenchymal lung involvement is unusual, however, and, if present, indicates extensive parenchymal disease or tracheobronchial obstruction.

The clinical manifestations of TB in patients presenting to the ED may be especially challenging. In one study, only one-third of ED patients with active pulmonary TB had pulmonary chief complaints. Any vague systemic disorder or fever of unknown cause may represent TB. Atypical presentations are particularly common in infants, older adults, and immunocompromised persons. In infants and young children, the development of large hilar lymph nodes is common. Pulmonary TB should be considered in older adults with chronic cough and failure to thrive. Young adults often show the adult pattern of apical pulmonary disease, including cavity formation, suggesting reactivation. Because of reduced immunocompetence, older adults typically have disease manifestations similar to those in young children.

Clinical manifestations of TB in patients coinfected with HIV are even more subtle and nonspecific, especially because these patients are vulnerable to opportunistic infections and neoplasms that can cause the same constitutional symptoms as TB. A synergy between MTB and HIV leads to a greatly increased viral load. Active TB with HIV coinfection has been associated with an increased risk for opportunistic infections and death. Patients with advanced HIV infection commonly have extrapulmonary involvement (seen in 30%) as well as combined pulmonary and extrapulmonary TB (in 32%).

Risk Factors

All ED patients who have been coughing should be screened for the presence of TB risk factors (Box 124.1). Individuals from endemic countries and those living with persons who recently emigrated from endemic areas are at risk, as are patients with unexplained weight loss or cachexia. One of the most important risk factors is HIV/AIDS with CD4[+] levels below 500 cells/μL.[10] Overseas, coinfection with HIV and TB is common and results in an increased TB mortality rate. Risks for acquiring TB may also be stratified by age. Because infants and toddlers have poorly developed cell-mediated immunity, they have a much higher incidence of TB than adults. Patients on immunosuppressant medications such as steroids or antiarthritic immunosuppressant agents are at increased risk. Patients with a history of purified protein derivative (PPD) conversion should be asked about the presence of immunosuppressive medical conditions, which are associated with an increased risk for the development of active postprimary disease through reactivation. Household contacts also have increased risk of TB infection. Health care providers should ask patients with a history of active TB about all antituberculosis medications previously or currently taken and about compliance. Failure to improve after 2 months with an appropriate regimen may signal nonadherence to therapy or the presence of a resistant strain.

Physical Examination

A wasted patient with a cachexic appearance is a hallmark of advanced disease. The patient may show signs of dyspnea or tachypnea. The mental status examination may show subtle abnormalities. Examination of the chest can reveal abnormalities, but is unlikely to establish the extent of disease. Over areas of infiltration, rales may be heard when the patient breathes in after a short cough (posttussive rales), and bronchial breath sounds may be present over areas of lung consolidation. Distant, hollow breath sounds (amphoric breath sounds) may be heard over cavities. Most physical findings are a result of complications of TB or from the extrapulmonary forms of the disease (see section on "Extrapulmonary Tuberculosis").

Complications of Pulmonic Tuberculosis

Hemoptysis

Minor hemoptysis is a common complication of acute infection. The destruction of lung parenchyma leads to the rupture of blood vessels. TB also may cause massive hemoptysis. An uncommon complication is the erosion of a tuberculous lesion or cavity into a pulmonary artery, leading to pseudoaneurysm formation (Rasmussen aneurysm), with potentially fatal hemoptysis. Alternatively, superinfection of cavities by invasive organisms or tumor development in the scarred lung may cause erosion of bronchial or pulmonary vessels, with resultant major hemorrhage. Affected patients often require emergency surgical resection or selective embolization.

Pneumothorax

Spontaneous pneumothorax is uncommon (affecting <5% of patients with severe cavitary disease) but may occur when a tuberculous cavity ruptures and creates a bronchopleural fistula or when a bleb ruptures into the pleural space (Fig. 124.1). If treatment with tube thoracostomy and suction is delayed, progressive infection and fibrosis of the pleura can lead to air trapping in the pleural space.

Pleural Effusion

Pleural extrapulmonary TB may occur early after primary infection with MTB and is manifested as pleurisy with effusion. More rarely, it may occur late in postprimary cavitary disease and arise as an empyema. Tuberculous pleural involvement often causes no symptoms and resolves spontaneously; however, a 65% relapse rate has been reported in untreated patients, with development of active pulmonary or extrapulmonary TB within 5 years. The diagnosis usually is confirmed by microscopic and chemical examination of pleural fluid or pleural biopsy tissue. White blood cell counts usually range from 500 to 2500 cells/mL. The fluid is an exudate with protein usually exceeding 50% of the serum protein, and the glucose concentration may be normal to low. Because there are few bacilli, AFB smears rarely are positive, and cultures grow MTB for only 25% to 30% of patients known to have the disease. Pleural biopsy can confirm the diagnosis in most patients.

Empyema

An empyema, characterized by extensive, progressive parenchymal disease and cavitation, may develop in patients with TB. Although it is rare, empyema is more common late in the course of the disease in debilitated patients. Rupture of a cavity into the pleural space usually is catastrophic and often is associated with bronchopleural fistula

---

BOX 124.1   Population Groups with Increased Risk for Tuberculosis

Close contacts of known case
Persons with HIV infection
From Eastern Europe, Asia, Africa, Latin America
Medically underserved, low-income populations
Older adults
Residents of long-term care facilities (e.g., nursing homes, correctional facilities)
Injection drug users
Undomiciled
Persons who have occupational exposure

HIV, Human immunodeficiency virus.

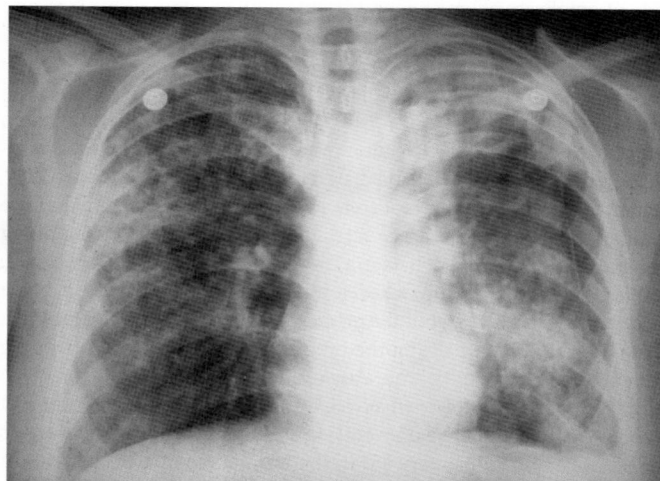

Fig. 124.1 Chest radiograph demonstrating cavitary tuberculosis with left-sided pneumothorax. The underlying cause of the pneumothorax was later determined to be a bronchopleural fistula. (Courtesy Dr. John Pearce.)

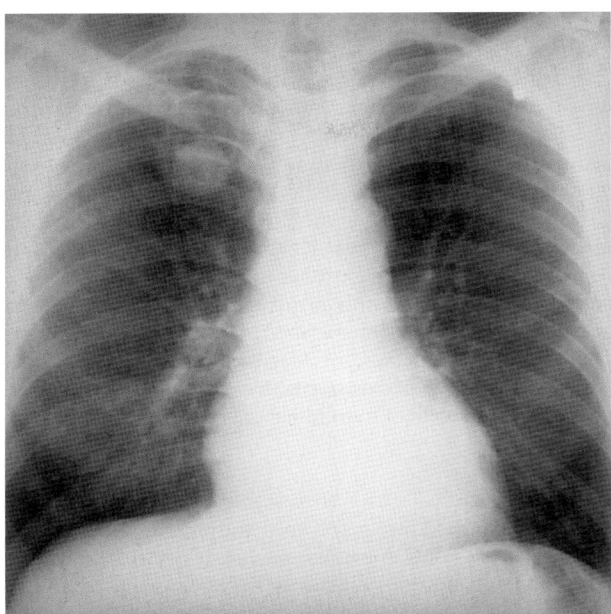

Fig. 124.2 Chest radiograph showing superinfection of healed tuberculous cavity. An aspergilloma can be seen in the right upper lung. (Courtesy Dr. John Pearce.)

formation. An untreated empyema can result in spontaneous pleurocutaneous fistula formation, presence of a chest wall mass on the radiograph, or rib and vertebral destruction.

Airway Tuberculosis

When a cavity drains its highly infectious material into the bronchial tree, the airways not only spread the infection but also develop endobronchial TB. Bronchiectasis commonly complicates endobronchial TB. Bronchial stenosis may result from extensive damage caused by endobronchial TB or from direct extension of infection by tuberculous adenitis or lymphatic dissemination to the airway. Tuberculous bronchostenosis may appear radiographically as persistent segmental or lobar collapse, lobar hyperinflation, and obstructive pneumonia. Tracheal and laryngeal TB are less common than endobronchial TB. Laryngeal disease is the most infectious form; it results from the proximal extension of lower airway disease, pooling of infected secretions in the posterior larynx, or hematogenous dissemination to the anterior larynx. Patients with laryngeal TB also usually have active pulmonary disease.

Superinfection with Fungi

Extensive TB infection often heals with open cavities and areas of bronchiectasis. Superinfection may occur with a wide variety of organisms, including *Aspergillus fumigatus*. The characteristic finding on chest radiographs is the aspergilloma or so-called fungus ball (Fig. 124.2). Aspergillomas are of particular clinical significance because they may cause massive and fatal hemoptysis.

Primary Tuberculous Pericarditis

Primary tuberculous pericarditis usually results from direct extension of infection from the tracheobronchial tree, mediastinal or hilar lymph nodes, sternum, or spine. Pericardial involvement also may result from hematogenous spread secondary to acute miliary TB or from another focus elsewhere in the body. TB is the leading cause of pericarditis among HIV-infected patients in the United States. The predominant

symptoms are cough, chest pain, and dyspnea, and the most common signs are cardiomegaly, audible rub, fever, and tachycardia. Complications of pericardial TB include pericardial effusion, constrictive pericarditis, myocarditis, and cardiac tamponade. Cardiac tamponade may result from the accumulation of pericardial fluid or rupture of enlarging lymph nodes into the pericardium. Emergency echocardiography reliably confirms the presence of pericardial fluid.

DIFFERENTIAL DIAGNOSES

Pulmonary Tuberculosis

Bacterial Pneumonia

Segmental or lobar infiltrates on chest radiographs in bacterial pneumonia may easily be confused with those seen in TB, especially primary disease. Compared with TB, however, bacterial pneumonias usually arise with more profound symptoms of systemic toxicity, more acute onset, and elevated white blood cell count. In pulmonary TB, there is no prompt response to antibiotics, as often seen in bacterial pneumonia.

Fungal and Nontuberculous Mycobacterial Infections

Histoplasmosis, coccidioidomycosis and blastomycosis, as well as nontuberculous mycobacterial infections—mainly with *Mycobacterium avium* complex and *Mycobacterium kansasii*—may be radiologically indistinguishable from TB. The incidence of these infections is influenced by geographic location; therefore the ED physician must take into account travel history and local epidemiologic risks. Nontuberculous mycobacterial infection usually involves chronic pulmonary infection in HIV-infected patients. Immunocompetent persons also may become infected with MTB, especially patients with chronic lung disease, such as cystic fibrosis. Other important risk factors include work in the mining industry, warm climate, advancing age, and male sex.

Pneumonias in Patients with HIV Infection

Bacterial pneumonias including upper lobe *Pneumocystis* pneumonia (due to *Pneumocystis jiroveci*) and, rarely, *Nocardia* and *Rhodococcus* infections may mimic TB in patients with HIV infection.

Cavitary Lesions

Lung abscess or cavitating pneumonia caused by *Klebsiella pneumoniae*, *Staphylococcus aureus,* or aspiration may appear similar to cavitary TB on chest radiographs. In older patients, especially smokers, bronchogenic carcinoma may mimic TB. This is particularly true of squamous cell carcinoma, which tends to cavitate. Because cancer may cause a focus of TB to spread, the two diseases may be present simultaneously. Other causes of nontuberculous cavitary lesions include *M. avium* complex infection in HIV-negative patients, pulmonary infarction secondary to pulmonary embolus, Wegener granulomatosis, and upper lobe bullous disease secondary to emphysema or neurofibromatosis.

Mediastinal Lymphadenopathy

The main considerations in the differential diagnosis for adenopathy include lymphoma and sarcoidosis. In sarcoidosis, lymphadenopathy usually is bilateral, symmetrical, and asymptomatic. Lymphadenopathy tends to be unilateral in TB; if it is bilateral, it is asymmetrical and associated with parenchymal lung disease. Lymphoma tends to involve bulky mediastinal lymphadenopathy.

Extrapulmonary Tuberculosis

Tuberculous infection involving multiple sites is usually seen in populations of patients less capable of containing MTB infection, such as infants, older adults, and immunocompromised persons.

Extrapulmonary TB may occur in multiple sites, with decreasing relative frequencies in lymphatic, pleural, bone or joint, genitourinary, meningeal, peritoneal, and other sites. The lymph nodes are the most common site of extrapulmonary TB for otherwise normal and HIV-infected patients. Involvement of the meninges is more common in young children than in other age groups (present in ≈4% of children with TB), and the incidence of TB in the remainder of the extrapulmonary sites increases with age. Less commonly involved locations for extrapulmonary TB include the skin, heart, pericardium, thyroid gland, mastoid cells, sclerae, and adrenal glands.

Lymphadenitis

Tuberculous lymphadenitis (scrofula) is the most common form of extrapulmonary TB. Scrofula is most commonly seen in young women but is also seen in children. The patient usually has an enlarging, painless, red, firm mass in the region of one or more lymph nodes, most commonly in the anterior or posterior cervical chain or supraclavicular fossa. Early on, the nodes are discrete rubbery masses that are freely mobile and the overlying skin is normal. Eventually, the nodes may become matted and harder and the overlying skin inflamed. Fluctuance as well as an abscess or sinus tract may be present if a node erodes through the skin. Systemic signs and symptoms are uncommon, except in HIV-positive patients, in whom lymphadenitis usually is generalized. Pulmonary infection is present in a minority of cases. Considerations in the differential diagnosis include lymphoma, metastatic cancer, fungal disease, cat-scratch disease, sarcoid, toxoplasmosis, reactive adenitis, and bacterial adenitis.

The diagnosis of scrofula usually is made by fine-needle aspiration of an affected lymph node. Although AFB smears are positive in only approximately 20% of cases, granulomatous inflammation may be obvious. Overall, fine-needle aspiration has a sensitivity of 77% and specificity of 93% for TB infection. First-line treatment of scrofula consists of antituberculosis drugs, but surgical excision may be performed when medical therapy has failed or if the diagnosis is unclear. Incision and drainage should not be done because permanent sinuses and prolonged drainage can result.

Bone and Joint Infection

Bone and joint TB remains a disease of older children and young adults in developing countries, and it is increasingly a disease of adults in developed countries. Skeletal TB presumably develops from reactivation of dormant tubercles originally seeded during stage 2 of the primary infection or, in the case of spinal TB, from contiguous spread from paravertebral lymph nodes to the vertebrae. In general, spinal TB (Pott disease) accounts for 50% to 70% of the reported cases; the hip or knee is involved in 15% to 20% of cases, and the ankle, elbow, wrists, shoulders, and other bones and joints account for 15% to 20% of cases. Approximately 50% of patients have a previous history or concurrent case of pulmonary TB, but the chest radiograph is normal in appearance in up to 50% of cases.

Patients with Pott disease may simply complain of back pain or stiffness. Early changes of spinal TB can be difficult to detect on plain radiographs and include loss of the so-called white stripe of the vertebral endplate subsequent to destruction of subchondral bone. Thus, computed tomography (CT) and magnetic resonance imaging (MRI) should be used when the disease is suspected. Paraspinal cold abscesses develop in 50% or more of cases, with occasional formation of sinus tracts. The abscess can spread the infection up and down the spine, sometimes sparing vertebral bodies along its course, forming the so-called skip lesions. These skip lesions can easily be missed in imaging of the spine for Pott disease. The main complication of Pott disease is spinal cord compression.

Renal Disease

The kidney is highly vascularized, and hematogenous dissemination to that organ can occur. After the typical tuberculous lesions develop within the parenchyma, infection can spread into the calyces, renal pelvis, ureters, and bladder. As a result, tuberculous granulomas, scarring, and obstruction can occur anywhere along the urinary tract. Advanced renal disease and destruction may occur before the diagnosis is made. The urinalysis often reveals pyuria, hematuria, and albuminuria. Sterile pyuria is a classic finding in renal TB but, in many cases with this finding, cultures will be positive for other urinary pathogens. The finding of pyuria in an acidic urine with no organisms isolated should increase clinical suspicion for TB. Complications of renal TB include nephrolithiasis, ureteral obstruction or reflux, recurrent bacterial infections, hypertension, papillary necrosis, renal insufficiency, autonephrectomy and, rarely, development of transitional cell cancer.

Genital Disease

Male genital TB is usually associated with coexistent renal TB. Spread of infection from the kidney may involve the prostate, seminal vesicles, epididymides, and testes. A painless or slightly painful scrotal mass is a typical finding, and the patient may have symptoms of prostatitis, epididymitis, or orchitis. Epididymal or prostatic calcifications may be clues to the diagnosis. TB involvement of the seminal vesicles may lead to infertility.

In women, genital TB disease usually begins with a hematogenous focus in the fallopian tubes. The infection then spreads to the endometrium (in 50% of cases), ovaries (30%), cervix (5%–15%), and vagina (1%). Clinical manifestations may include abdominal or pelvic pain, ascites, infertility, menstrual irregularities and, rarely, vaginal discharge. An ulcerating mass may be present on the cervix. Genital TB may be confused with ovarian or endometrial cancer, Meigs syndrome, vulvar or vaginal ulcer, pelvic abscess, cervicitis, or cervical carcinoma. Sexual transmission of TB by persons with active genital TB has been described.

Multisystem Disease

The term *acute disseminated tuberculosis* refers to active hematogenous spread of MTB to several organs in the body. The term *miliary tuberculosis* was first used to describe the pathologic lesions, which resemble small millet seeds. This is now used as a clinical term referring to the massive dissemination that leads to systemic illness. Miliary TB occurs when the host is unable to contain a recently acquired or dormant TB infection. In the past, miliary TB occurred mainly in young children after primary infection; today, it is more common in older adults and in persons infected with HIV. Miliary TB often is a subtle disease associated with alcohol use disorder, cirrhosis, neoplasm, pregnancy, collagen vascular disease, or use of corticosteroids or immunosuppressive medications. A presumptive diagnosis can be made rapidly if chest radiographs show a miliary infiltrate (Fig. 124.3). Unfortunately, the classic miliary pattern is absent on radiographs in approximately 50% of cases. Routine laboratory tests generally are not helpful. Hyponatremia from the syndrome of inappropriate secretion of antidiuretic hormone (SIADH) is common and often is associated with meningitis. Cultures of sputum, urine, draining lesions, and blood should be sent to the infectious disease laboratory.

Mortality rates for miliary TB are higher than for the other forms of TB, with one case series reporting a rate of 21%. The high mortality rate often is caused by delay in treatment, which should be initiated immediately on the basis of clinical suspicion and not delayed until confirmation of the diagnosis. A fulminant form of miliary TB may cause acute respiratory distress syndrome (ARDS) and disseminated intravascular coagulation (DIC).

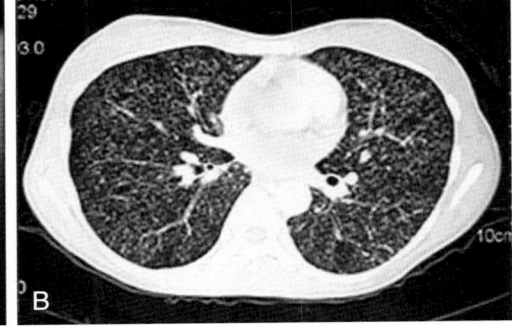

Fig. 124.3 Chest radiograph (A) and computed tomography scan (B) demonstrate a miliary pattern. (Reprinted with permission from: Golden MP, Vikram HR. Extrapulmonary tuberculosis: an overview. *Am Fam Physician.* 2005;72:1761. Copyright 2005, American Academy of Family Physicians. All rights reserved.)

Central Nervous System Disease

Approximately 6% of all cases of extrapulmonary TB involve the central nervous system (CNS), and CNS involvement remains a grave consequence of tuberculous infection. The peak incidence of CNS TB occurs in newborns to 4-year-old children.

Tuberculous meningitis usually results from the rupture of a subependymal tubercle into the subarachnoid space rather than from direct hematogenous seeding of the CNS. When it is a complication of miliary TB, meningitis usually develops within several weeks of infection. In children, it is an early postprimary TB event, usually appearing within 6 months. Tuberculous cerebral involvement is most marked at the base of the brain, and vasculitis of local arteries and veins may lead to aneurysm formation, thrombosis, and focal hemorrhagic infarction. The vessels to the basal ganglia are usually involved, leading to formation of lacunar infarcts or deficits associated with movement disorders. Involvement of other vessels, such as the middle cerebral artery, may lead to hemiparesis or hemiplegia. Tuberculous meningitis begins with a prodrome of malaise, intermittent headache, and low-grade fever. In 2 to 3 weeks, a protracted headache develops. Vomiting, confusion, meningismus and focal neurologic signs, and coma may follow. Nuchal rigidity may be absent. Diplopia resulting from basilar exudate is present in up to 70% of patients. Hyponatremia may be present because SIADH is common. The cerebrospinal fluid (CSF) white blood cell count varies widely, from 0 to 1500 cells/mL, with a predominance of lymphocytes when WBCs are present; however, polymorphonuclear cells may predominate early in the course of the disease. The CSF protein concentration usually is elevated, and the CSF glucose concentration typically is low. The classic triad of neuroradiologic findings in patients with TB meningitis consists of basal meningeal enhancement, hydrocephalus, and cerebral or brainstem infarction. CT or MRI also may reveal rounded lesions typical of evolving parenchymal tuberculomas (Fig. 124.4).

Gastrointestinal Disease

The most common clinical manifestations of gastrointestinal TB are abdominal pain, fever, weight loss, anorexia, nausea, vomiting, and diarrhea. Gastrointestinal TB infection usually is secondary to hematogenous or lymphatic spread but also may result from swallowed bronchial secretions or direct spread from local sites, such as lymph nodes or fallopian tubes. TB may occur in any gastrointestinal location from the mouth to the anus, but lesions proximal to the terminal ileum are rare. The ileocecal area is the most common site of involvement, producing signs and symptoms of pain, anorexia, diarrhea, obstruction, hemorrhage and, often, a palpable mass. The

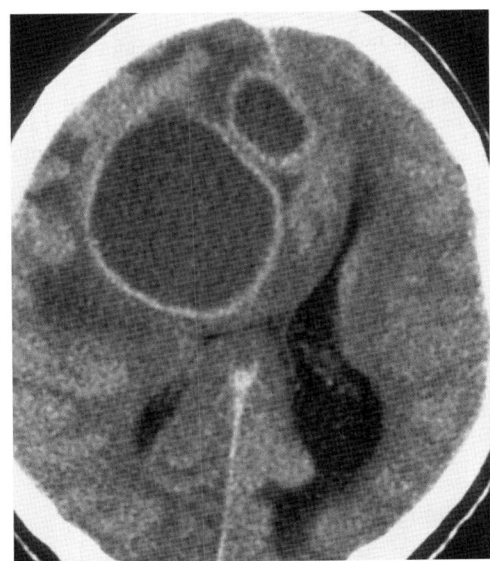

Fig. 124.4 Head CT scan demonstrating tuberculomas in a patient with AIDS.

nonspecificity of these findings, as well as of those on the physical examination, may lead to the misdiagnosis of gastrointestinal TB as an acute abdomen, appendicitis, intestinal obstruction, or cancer. The clinical manifestations of anal TB include fissures, fistulae, and perirectal abscesses.

Tuberculous peritonitis may develop from local spread of MTB infection from a tuberculous lymph node, intestinal focus, or infected fallopian tube. In addition, peritonitis can develop from seeding of the peritoneum in miliary TB or from the reactivation of a latent focus. The patient with tuberculous peritonitis commonly has pain and abdominal swelling associated with fever, anorexia, and weight loss. Diagnosis may be confounded by the similarity of this disease to alcoholic hepatitis and by the fact that this disease often coexists with other disorders, especially cirrhosis with ascites. Paracentesis is thus essential. The peritoneal fluid is exudative, with a cell count of 500 to 2000 cells/mL. Lymphocytes usually predominate, with rare exceptions early in the process, when polymorphonuclear leukocytes may predominate. AFB smears of the fluid have a low diagnostic yield. Peritoneal biopsy often is necessary to confirm the diagnosis. Treatment is the same as for pulmonary TB, with a 6-month therapeutic regimen.

DIAGNOSTIC TESTING

Laboratory Tests

Routine laboratory studies generally are not useful in suggesting or establishing the diagnosis of TB in the ED. Normochromic normocytic anemia, elevated erythrocyte sedimentation rate, elevated C-reactive protein (CRP) and serum globulin levels, hyponatremia, and hypercalcemia can occur in active pulmonary TB, but these findings are nonspecific.

White Cell Stimulation Tests

The patient's blood can be tested for sensitivity of its T cells to tuberculin antigens. These tests are called interferon-gamma (IFN-γ) release assays (IGRAs). The QuantiFERON-TB Gold (Quest Diagnostics) and T-Spot (Oxford Immunotec) tests are the most widely available IGRAs. They use an enzyme-linked immunosorbent assay (ELISA) to measure the amount of IFN-γ released in response to PPD. IFN-γ is a cytokine associated with cell-mediated immunity. Determination of IFN-γ levels also can be used as a diagnostic test for tuberculous pleural effusions, ascites, and pericardial effusions. Clinical studies have reported sensitivity ranges from 90% to 100%. TB infection can be rapidly confirmed in an individual in 2 days, compared with several weeks for a traditional culture. However, a normal study does not completely exclude TB; therefore, cultures should be sent when a person thought to have TB has a negative QuantiFERON-TB Gold test result.

Serology

Although ELISAs have been developed for several MTB serum antigens, in practice no serodiagnostic approach to the diagnosis of TB currently is in widespread clinical use in the United States. Other countries have discouraged the use of serology. Limitations of the ELISA include inadequate accuracy and reproducibility, inability to distinguish active from latent infection, poor discrimination between MTB and other mycobacteria, and relative cost.

Diagnostic Imaging

Plain radiography of the chest is the most useful study for a presumptive diagnosis of pulmonary TB. The availability of chest CT scans in most EDs has enhanced the sensitivity of detecting classic TB in the ED. A normal appearance on the chest radiograph has a high negative predictive value and is therefore useful in screening ED patients for active pulmonary TB. However, the low false-negative rate among immunocompetent adults increases significantly in HIV-positive patients. Therefore, depending on the clinical circumstances, the absence of specific abnormalities on the chest radiograph does not always exclude active TB, especially in patients with concomitant endobronchial disease and HIV infection.

Primary Tuberculosis

Chest radiographic manifestations of primary disease in adults often are not recognized as TB. Primary tuberculous infiltrates can occur in any lobe. In any age group, a pneumonic infiltrate with enlarged hilar or mediastinal nodes should strongly suggest the diagnosis. The infiltrate usually is homogeneous and most commonly involves a single lobe. Thus, primary TB may appear radiographically identical to a bacterial pneumonia, with associated lymphadenopathy, if present, being the only distinguishing feature.

Lymphadenopathy is considered the radiologic hallmark of primary TB in children but is seen less commonly in adults. When present, adenopathy usually is unilateral and associated with parenchymal infiltrate (Fig. 124.5). It may occur bilaterally or, less commonly, may be an isolated finding on chest radiography. Other

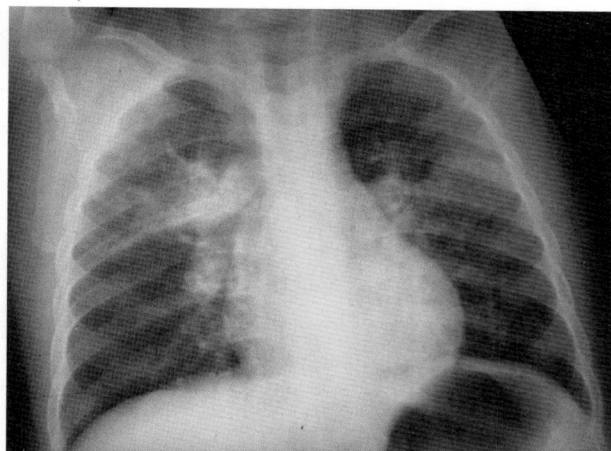

Fig. 124.5 Chest radiographic findings in a child with primary tuberculosis. Note the active Ghon focus, with associated hilar adenopathy and presence of bilateral infiltrates. (Courtesy Dr. John Pearce.)

primary TB chest radiographic findings include a moderate to large pleural effusion, which often is an isolated finding whose prevalence increases with age, and miliary TB characterized by the presence of innumerable, 1- to 3-mm noncalcified nodules dispersed throughout both lungs with mild basilar predominance. When the healed primary focus is visible on the chest radiograph as a calcified scar, it is known as the Ghon focus. Calcified secondary foci of infection in the lung apex are known as Simon foci. A Ghon focus associated with calcified hilar nodes is called a Ranke complex. A right-sided predominance in the distribution of the Ghon foci and Ranke complexes is well recognized and probably reflects the likelihood that an airborne infection will affect the right lung. Calcification seen on the chest radiograph indicates healing, but viable bacilli may still exist in a partially calcified lesion.

Postprimary Tuberculosis

Postprimary TB typically appears as an upper lung infiltrate or consolidation, with or without cavitation. The lesion may be small or extensive and usually is located in the apical or posterior segment of the upper lobe but may appear in the superior segment of the lower lobe. Postprimary disease also occurs in the lower lung. In addition, bronchogenic spread can occur, leading to the involvement of multiple lobes (Fig. 124.6). Patients with bilateral upper lobe disease are extremely likely to have TB. The other important recognizable characteristics of postprimary disease are fibrosis and cavitation. These lesions are not purely exudative in that they are associated with a fibrotic pattern of nodules and a few fine, linear densities. Fibroproductive lesions often are irregular and angular in contour, have strands extending toward the hilum, and demonstrate calcification of one or more nodules and distortion of vascular and mediastinal structures. Severe fibrosis with upper lobe volume loss may eventually lead to retraction of the interlobar fissure and upward displacement of the hilum. The chest radiographic appearance at this stage has been variably referred to as "old scarring," "no active disease," or "fibrotic, apparently well-healed TB." Cavitation should alert one to the potential for high infectivity of the patient and associated complications, such as bronchogenic spread of TB (see Fig. 124.4). The walls of the cavities initially are thick and rough and become thinner and smoother with healing. Chest radiographs of patients with pulmonary TB and HIV infection may be atypical in approximately one-third of cases. Patients with late HIV infection more often demonstrate

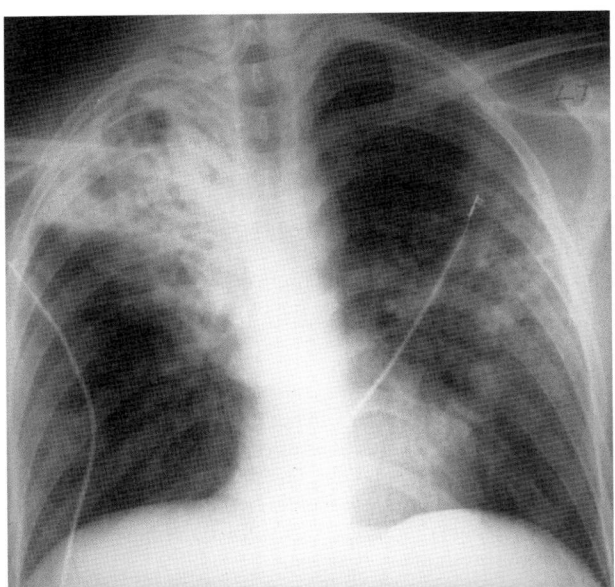

Fig. 124.6 Chest radiograph showing evidence of right upper lobe cavitary disease. Also note the left-sided infiltrate, secondary to endobronchial spread.

mediastinal adenopathy or atypical infiltrates and less often have cavitation. Severe immunosuppression has been reported to be associated with a miliary pattern of disease on chest radiographs.

Microbiologic Testing

Sputum Studies

If the clinical or chest radiographic findings suggest the diagnosis of pulmonary TB, mycobacteriologic studies of the patient's sputum should be ordered. A positive smear supports a presumptive diagnosis, and the number of bacilli seen correlates with infectivity. For patients who are not producing sputum, nebulized induction of sputum is the method of choice for the collection of samples. Induction of sputum with nebulization may increase the risk of TB transmission to health care workers and should be performed only in specially ventilated rooms, preferably not in the ED. When the sputum is not diagnostic in adults, fiberoptic bronchoscopy with bronchial washings, bronchoalveolar lavage, brushings, or transbronchial biopsy may be necessary for the laboratory diagnosis of TB.

Direct Microscopy. Direct microscopic examination of a stained sputum specimen for AFB (i.e., an AFB smear) is the most rapid laboratory test widely available to support a presumptive diagnosis of TB and results usually are available from hospital laboratories within 24 hours. Negative findings on an AFB smear, however, do not rule out active pulmonary TB because microscopy is relatively insensitive when performed on samples with small numbers of bacilli. At least 5000 bacilli/mL of sputum must be present for a positive result by microscopy. Overall, AFB smears have a sensitivity of 20% to 80% and a specificity of 90% to 100%. Despite limitations, microscopy remains an essential diagnostic test because of its ease of performance, low cost, rapid turnaround time, and reasonable diagnostic yield.

Nucleic Acid Amplification Tests. Nucleic acid amplification (NAA) tests are performed on sputum and take only 24 to 48 hours to yield results. Their overall positive predictive value is about 95%. In some cases, patients with positive TB sputum smears have had negative NAA test results because of inhibitors that may prevent amplification. This has been a rapidly growing field in TB diagnostics, although most

EDs do not yet have bedside capabilities. The best role of NAA is to aid emergency clinicians in decision making for patients thought to have active TB. It should not be ordered routinely when the clinical suspicion for TB is low.

Culture. Sputum culture is more sensitive than microscopy for the detection of MTB and is still considered the gold standard diagnostic modality. Liquid culture can detect 10 to 100 bacilli/mL, compared with 5000 to 10,000 bacilli/mL for an AFB smear. When the presence of mycobacteria is established, the specific identification of MTB may be accomplished by subjecting the initial mycobacteria to various isolation techniques. These include the detection of pigmentation on solid culture media, various biochemical tests, high-performance liquid chromatography, and nucleic acid probes. A presumptive diagnosis of TB based on a positive sputum smear usually is confirmed by isolation of MTB by culture. Traditional culture methods using solid media require 3 to 8 weeks for colony formation. The development of liquid culture systems has shortened the detection time to 7 to 14 days.

Tuberculin Skin Test

Although newer serologic diagnostic tests have become widely used in most US hospitals, the tuberculin skin test continues to be the diagnostic workhorse for the detection of exposure to MTB. The tuberculin test is based on the principle that MTB infection induces sensitivity to certain antigens of the bacillus. These antigens are contained in the tuberculin preparation called PPD. In a person infected with TB, the PPD test result usually turns positive 3 to 8 weeks after the infection, when the immune response is developed. The standard 0.1-mL dose used in skin testing contains 5 tuberculin units (TU). A properly placed needle should leave a blanched distinct wheal 6 to 10 mm in diameter. If the tuberculin dose is incorrectly administered, the test may be repeated immediately at a site several centimeters away. Test results are read 48 to 72 hours after administration of PPD. The largest diameter of palpable induration is measured and recorded in millimeters; erythema by itself is not measured. The precise measurement that denotes a positive test result depends on the patient's other clinical factors. The current CDC guidelines use 15 mm of induration as a positive test response for people without TB risk factors. Persons with previous TB immunization (see later, "Vaccines for *Mycobacterium tuberculosis*") may have a positive PPD result even though they are not infected with TB. However, a significant reaction to PPD and a long time interval between bacilli Calmette-Guérin (BCG) vaccination and the current skin test make it more likely that the reaction is due to MTB infection. Because the BCG vaccine is imperfect in protecting against MTB infection, and because most vaccinated persons come from areas of high TB prevalence, the CDC recommends that tuberculin skin test results be interpreted without regard to BCG vaccination status.

MANAGEMENT

Initial Management in the Emergency Department

Hemoptysis

The most emergent presentation of pulmonary TB is massive hemoptysis, defined as loss of at least 600 mL of blood in 24 hours. Exsanguination rarely occurs, and the major morbidity is due to asphyxiation from aspirated blood. Secure the airway with a large-diameter (8-mm) endotracheal tube that can accommodate a fiberoptic bronchoscope. The patient is positioned with the bleeding lung in a dependent position, and one should consider selective main bronchus intubation to allow ventilation of the unaffected lung and minimize the spread of blood from the affected lung. Emergency consultation for bronchoscopy, surgical resection, or angiography with selective embolization is required. Patients thought to have active pulmonary TB should be immediately placed in respiratory isolation.

Fever or Wasting

Patients with fever and wasting generally should be admitted for an in-hospital evaluation. Patients should be placed in respiratory isolation until the diagnosis of TB has been excluded.

History of Tuberculosis, Therapy Discontinued

In patients with vague symptoms and a history of TB, consider reactivation. Given the numerous considerations in resuming therapy, we recommend consulting a local TB health officer or an infectious diseases specialist.

Antituberculosis Medications

Three basic therapeutic principles govern the treatment of TB: (1) any treatment regimen must contain multiple drugs to which the MTB organism is susceptible; (2) the therapeutic agents must be taken regularly; and (3) therapy must continue for a sufficient period. In clinical practice, the last principle is the most problematic. The most up-to-date recommendations for the treatment of TB are available from the CDC through online publications or at the CDC website. Medications used to treat MTB generally are divided into first-line and second-line agents. Of these, 10 have been approved by the US Food and Drug Administration (FDA) for the treatment of MTB. The most commonly used first-line agents are isoniazid (INH), rifampin (RIF), pyrazinamide (PZA), and ethambutol (EMB).

First-Line Agents

INH demonstrates extremely potent early bactericidal activity and can rapidly decrease the patient's infectiousness. A small risk of hepatitis (<3%) occurs with long-term treatment. Supplemental pyridoxine is recommended for these patients. RIF also demonstrates strong early bactericidal activity. This agent causes orange discoloration of body fluids, including urine, tears, sweat, and sputum. PZA works against organisms contained in the acid environment of the macrophage. The chief side effect is hepatotoxicity, but this risk is very low at daily doses of 25 mg/kg or less. Polyarthralgias occur commonly (up to 40% of patients) but usually respond to nonsteroidal antiinflammatory drugs or aspirin. EMB is a first-line agent that helps prevent the emergence of RIF resistance during TB treatment. Retrobulbar neuritis can occur, resulting in decreased visual acuity to the point of blindness.

Second-Line Agents

Streptomycin must be given parenterally and has a peak of action 1 hour after the intramuscular dose is given. The chief side effects of this potentially teratogenic agent are ototoxicity and nephrotoxicity. Amikacin, kanamycin, and capreomycin also are injectable agents used for drug-resistant TB. As with streptomycin, ototoxicity and neurotoxicity are their major adverse effects. TB strains resistant to streptomycin usually are sensitive to amikacin and kanamycin, and resistance to these last two drugs usually is linked. Cycloserine, ethionamide, and p-aminosalicylic acid (PAS) are oral agents used for the treatment of patients with drug-resistant TB when the strain is presumed or known to be sensitive to these agents. The main adverse effect of cycloserine is psychosis or seizures, which occur in 3% to 16% of patients. Ethionamide is similar to INH in structure and toxicity. Major adverse effects of PAS include gastrointestinal distress (most common), hypothyroidism, and hepatitis. Fluoroquinolones have played a more recent role in the treatment of TB. They are less effective than the first-line agents and are used mainly in the treatment of drug-resistant disease.

Corticosteroids

Corticosteroids may prevent constriction in tuberculous pericarditis and decrease the neurologic sequelae in all stages of tuberculous meningitis, especially if they are given early in the disease. The CDC strongly recommends corticosteroids for MTB pericardial or CNS infections. Corticosteroids may provide some benefit to children with bronchial obstruction caused by enlarged lymph nodes. In addition, in patients with pulmonary TB, prednisone, 20 to 60 mg/day may benefit those who continue to experience temperature spiking and lose weight, despite a good bacteriologic response to appropriate antituberculosis therapy. In cases of miliary TB, 60 mg of prednisone should be added to the treatment regimen.

Initial Therapy

Emergency clinicians generally will not initiate treatment prior to consulting public health and infectious diseases specialists. To be successful, treatment must be continuous, ongoing, and monitored closely. A one-time dose of medications is fruitless in a patient who could be lost to follow-up. In some locations, this will require hospital admission with appropriate respiratory isolation.

Initial administration of anti-TB drugs in the ED is appropriate and necessary in certain circumstances, such as TB sepsis or miliary TB, critically ill HIV patients with TB, or life-threatening conditions. The CDC website should be reviewed for the most up-to-date treatment guidelines.[2,3] The goals of therapy are to rapidly kill large numbers of bacilli (bactericidal activity), prevent emergence of drug resistance, and prevent relapse by elimination of dormant or slowly dividing bacilli (sterilizing activity). In-person or telephone consultation with an infectious diseases specialist is critical, and they may recommend regimens that include INH, RIF, PZA, and/or EMB.[7]

Adequate treatment of active TB in patients coinfected with HIV is critical. It has been observed that immune activation from TB enhances systemic and local HIV replication and may accelerate the natural progression of HIV infection. Active TB in HIV-infected patients has been associated with increased risk for opportunistic infections and death. TB treatment alone leads to a reduction in viral load in these patients. Current recommendations for the initial treatment of MTB in HIV-infected patients are the same as those for patients who are not HIV-infected, with exceptions for complex drug interactions.[10] For example, significant drug interactions between rifamycins used for TB and antiretroviral drugs (protease inhibitors and nonnucleoside reverse transcriptase inhibitors [NNRTIs]) used for HIV infection complicate the treatment of patients with active TB who are coinfected with HIV. For treatment of MTB in patients who are taking protease inhibitors, rifabutin can be used instead of the other rifamycins. When TB treatment is initiated in HIV-positive patients, a paradoxical reaction to medical therapy may develop in some cases. The reaction is manifested with the development of fever, new or enlarging lymph nodes, or worsening of radiographic disease. Severe paradoxical reactions may be managed with a 2-week tapering course of prednisone or methylprednisolone.

Drug-Resistant Tuberculosis

Two types of drug-resistant MTB have emerged as a result of spontaneous mutations. Multidrug-resistant TB (MDR-TB) is defined as TB in which the mycobacteria are resistant to two or more first-line antituberculosis agents.[8] Extensively drug-resistant TB (XDR-TB) is TB characterized by resistance to first-line and at least three second-line drugs. Patients at high risk for MDR-TB and XDR-TB include those with HIV, those who have been treated in the past for TB, and those who live or lived in certain high-risk countries.

BOX 124.2 Risk Factors for Drug-Resistant *Mycobacterium tuberculosis* Infection

Previous unsuccessful antituberculosis treatment
Failure to respond or adhere to a treatment regimen
Human immunodeficiency virus infection
Injection drug abuse
Close contact with source cases
Recent immigration from area with a high prevalence of drug resistance
Cavitary lung disease
Undomiciled
Imprisonment
Drug malabsorption due to gastrectomy or ileal bypass surgery

Multidrug-Resistant Tuberculosis

The World Health Organization (WHO) has estimated the worldwide number of MDR-TB cases at close to one-half million persons. Airborne transmission of MDR-TB is a threat to those who come in contact with infected individuals, including family members, contacts in crowded living situations, and health care personnel. The spread of primary drug resistance is faster when HIV infection is highly prevalent in a population. Because initial TB infection in HIV-infected patients progresses rapidly to active disease, newly infected persons can quickly become source cases for further transmission of the resistant bacilli. In reports on hospital outbreaks of MDR-TB, more than 90% of patients had coinfection with HIV, and case fatality rates were as high as 70% to 90%. However, patients without HIV infection demonstrate excellent clinical responses when treated for MDR-TB.

For the identification of potential cases, health care workers should know the prevalence of drug resistance in their community and the risk factors for drug resistance (Box 124.2). Rapid identification and prompt isolation of these patients, along with other control measures, can reduce the nosocomial transmission of MDR-TB to patients and health care workers. Failure to control drug resistance may lead to wide dissemination of MDR-TB and to a public health crisis that physicians may confront without effective medications.

Treatment of drug-resistant TB can be challenging and requires familiarity with second-line agents. For MDR-TB, specialist consultation is essential. A general principle that applies in such cases is to use at least three drugs to which the organism is susceptible and that have not been used previously. In general, one of these medications should be an injectable agent. TB infection with strains that are resistant only to INH can be managed with shorter courses of RIF, PZA, and EMB.

Extensively Drug-Resistant Tuberculosis

XDR-TB was first recognized in patients coinfected with AIDS in South Africa in 2005 and is a major threat in Africa, Asia, and areas of the former Soviet Union. XDR-TB is found in 10% of patients presenting with MDR-TB. The strain has virulence similar to that of MTB, and disease does not progress faster in the absence of antibiotics. As resistance to so many antibiotics has developed, however, this strain has become a major threat, especially in patients with AIDS. Most alarming is a report that as many as 33% of patients with TB coinfected with HIV and MDR-TB had the XDR-TB strain. Mortality rates for this population of patients are high, because few alternative drugs exist. The CDC has reported cases in in the United States and has isolated patients as soon as they are identified. EDs could become a major focus for spread of this disease because of overcrowding, initial lack of recognition, and long wait times, exposing other patients to XDR-TB. Reports from Africa have shown that XDR-TB also can be transmitted directly to

health care workers. Of great concern is the potential for transmission of the disease within the ED by a previously undiagnosed patient with XDR-TB, who presents for treatment of TB-related symptoms or an unrelated condition.

Vaccines for *Mycobacterium tuberculosis*

The BCG vaccine has been used since 1921, but its overall efficacy, duration of protective immunity, and optimal age for administration are debated. Nonetheless, 100 million children receive BCG vaccine each year outside the United States (US). In developing countries, BCG is credited with reducing the incidence of the most severe forms of pediatric TB and death, and some hospitals overseas require that staff have a BCG vaccination as a requirement for work. In the United States, BCG is rarely recommended because of the belief that it may undermine the epidemiologic and diagnostic value of PPD skin testing. BCG use in children is common in some countries. Tuberculin skin tests in patients given previous BCG vaccination usually demonstrate less than 10 mm of induration. Thus, previous BCG vaccination status should be ignored in the interpretation of skin test results. Institutional outbreaks of TB and the emergence of MDR-TB have been sparking reassessment of the BCG issue in the United States. Reports of BCG vaccine efficacy range from 0% to 80%. A meta-analysis of international data reported the efficacy of BCG vaccine to be approximately 50%. This is consistent with an American study conducted over 60 years in a Native American population which showed a 50% reduction in the development of TB in persons receiving BCG vaccine.

BCG vaccine is currently recommended in the United States only for tuberculin-negative infants and children who cannot take INH and have ongoing exposure to a persistently untreated or inadequately treated patient with active TB, who are continuously exposed to persons with INH- and RIF-resistant TB, or who belong to groups with rates of new MTB infection exceeding 1% per year. WHO recommends that all infants in developing countries receive the vaccine.[6]

BCG vaccine is strongly contraindicated in persons with HIV infection or another immunosuppressive disease.

New vaccines against MTB are being researched, including those using attenuated strains of the MTB complex, recombinant mycobacteria, subunit proteins, and DNA vaccines. Vaccines are also under development for treatment of occult TB. A recent trial tested an adjuvanted recombinant protein vaccine, M72/AS01, in adults with a positive interferon-gama release assay, but without evidence of clinical disease.[4] Conducted in 3 African countries, a nearly 50% reduction in progression to active clinical disease was found in those receiving the vaccine.

DISPOSITION

Acutely ill or older patients may require hospitalization during the first few days of treatment because adverse reactions to TB chemotherapy are common and may occasionally be life-threatening. In addition, severely ill patients may require parenteral drug administration. Patients with TB have a high rate of HIV coinfection, and the comorbid illnesses associated with HIV infection, complex synergy between MTB and HIV, and potentially harmful drug interactions between the antiretroviral agents and rifamycins may favor inpatient treatment for the initial management of these complicated cases.

Hospital admission also is indicated for patients with active or suspected MDR-TB. These patients commonly require observation during initiation of therapy because of the complexity of the treatment regimens, toxicity of the drugs, and need for close monitoring to ensure adherence to treatment and isolation measures. Finally, social issues such as being undomiciled, presence of infants or immunocompromised persons in the household, substance abuse, and inability for self-care may necessitate hospitalization. The recalcitrant patient constitutes a potential threat to public health, and legal measures for involuntary hospitalization may be required.

Patients who are otherwise well but have suspected TB may be eligible for outpatient treatment in consultation with local county health officials, who agree to assume responsibility for ongoing care of the patient and investigate contacts for possible exposure to TB.

PREVENTION OF TRANSMISSION IN THE EMERGENCY DEPARTMENT

EDs often care for patients at increased risk for active pulmonary TB, such as those who are undomiciled, from endemic areas, recently incarcerated, or chronically ill. Accordingly, ED personnel can be at high risk for occupational TB infection. Increased hospital occupancy and ED crowding can lead to extended waiting periods for ED beds and hospital beds. Some EDs may lack an adequate number of TB isolation rooms.

Early Identification

For the most effective minimization of infectious exposures among health care workers and other patients, ideally, all patients with active pulmonary TB would be placed in respiratory isolation when they initially present. The CDC has recommended screening for TB at triage. Triage screening protocols can detect patients with more classic presentations of TB, but reported protocols are only moderately sensitive and somewhat cumbersome. Immediate respiratory isolation should be considered for patients with high-risk chief complaints, such as the HIV-positive patient with cough, the person with hemoptysis, or the patient with a history of TB presenting with cough or fever. The best guideline is to initiate respiratory isolation as soon as TB is considered a possible diagnosis. Masks should be placed on these patients before chest radiography is performed.

Isolation and Environmental Control

In addition to triage screening, the use of proper isolation facilities and environmental control measures can help prevent TB exposures. Airflow in the ED plays a central role, and inadequate ventilation has been a contributing factor in many nosocomial outbreaks of TB. Ideally, there should be single-pass airflow from waiting rooms to outside the facility. Within the ED, air should flow from clean areas to less clean areas, rather than vice versa. For EDs that frequently see patients with TB, at least one true respiratory isolation room should be available. The CDC recommends that respiratory isolation rooms have at least 12 air changes per hour and have negative pressure (air flows into the room from other ED areas). Other engineering approaches to TB infection control include the use of high-efficiency particulate air (HEPA) filters and upper room ultraviolet light irradiation.

Personal Respiratory Protection

ED personnel should be familiar with the appropriate use of respiratory protection against TB. Surgical masks (e.g., string tie masks) should be placed on potentially contagious patients to decrease the release of infectious droplets into the air. Air can leak around such masks, however, so they may not adequately prevent health care workers from inhaling infectious droplet nuclei. Thus, surgical masks are used only for source control, not for health care worker protection. More advanced personal respiratory protection devices include N95 particulate respirators. HEPA-filtered masks can also be used for health care worker respiratory protection; these masks were used more extensively before development of the N95 masks.

Preventive Therapy After Inadvertent Exposure

Health care workers who are exposed to patients with active pulmonary TB require referral to their primary care physicians or employee health services for follow-up testing and treatment. Tuberculin skin testing or IGRA blood testing usually is performed within days following exposure to establish whether the health care worker was previously infected with MTB. If the baseline test result is negative, a follow-up is performed 3 months later to determine whether conversion has occurred. The CDC has developed guidelines for the treatment of exposed personnel, which can be found on the CDC website.[9]

The references for this chapter can be found online at ExpertConsult.com.

125

Bone and Joint Infections

Neha P. Raukar and Brian J. Zink

KEY CONCEPTS

- Skeletal infection should be considered in the differential diagnosis of all patients who present with bone or joint pain.
- Laboratory evaluation is of little value in the diagnosis of bone and joint infections, with the exception of the ESR and CRP level, which are elevated in approximately 90% of cases of bone and joint infections.
- Joint aspiration is the definitive diagnostic procedure, and intraoperative synovial culture is the only reliable joint fluid test for establishing a diagnosis. When limited fluid is available, it should be sent for a cell count.
- With suspected septic arthritis, joint fluid and blood culture specimens are obtained before IV antibiotics are administered. With suspected osteomyelitis, blood culture specimens are obtained, and IV antibiotics are administered while plans are made for further imaging studies, surgical aspiration, or resection of bone.
- The most important aspect of antibiotic treatment of suspected bone and joint infections is to provide potent bactericidal activity against *S. aureus* with additional empirical antibiotic coverage aimed at suspected organisms on the basis of age, risk factors, and regional variability.

FOUNDATIONS

Background and Importance

Historically, bone and joint infections (BJIs) have been described in grim terms. *Aids to Surgery*, written in 1919, noted that "acute infective osteomyelitis … is a very fatal disease." With septic arthritis, "the patient becomes exhausted from toxaemia or pyemia," and "ankylosis is the usual most favourable termination." Advances in diagnostic methods, antibiotic therapy, and surgical techniques have resulted in better patient outcomes; however, new challenges are arising. The emergence of resistant bacteria endangers the efficacy of antibiotics, and antibiotic choices need to be informed by resistance patterns. Furthermore, there are increasing subsets of patients with reduced host immunity. This combination results in greater complexity in the management of BJIs than was previously encountered. The management focuses on prompt diagnosis, initiation of treatment, and avoidance of the complications and morbidity associated with bone or joint infections.

The overall occurrence of BJIs has remained constant during the past 4 decades.[1] In hospitalized patients in the United States, the incidence is approximately 1%. Osteomyelitis in children younger than 13 years occurs in 1 in 5000, whereas the incidence of septic arthritis ranges from 5.5 to 12/100,000 individuals.[1] In contrast to global patterns, socioeconomic factors or race do not affect the incidence of BJI in the United States. Both bone and joint infections show a bimodal age distribution, occurring most commonly in people younger than 20 years or older than 50 years. In children, BJIs usually occur in previously healthy individuals, with boys having a slightly increased susceptibility to bone infections. In adults, there are several known risk factors that lead to a higher risk of BJIs.

Orthopedic infections can be classified according to the site of involvement and include osseous (osteomyelitis), articular (septic, pyogenic, or suppurative arthritis), bursal (septic bursitis), subcutaneous (cellulitis or abscess), muscular (infectious myositis or abscess), and tendinous (infectious tendinitis or tenosynovitis) infections. The term *osteomyelitis* literally means inflammation of the marrow of the bone, but it is colloquially used to refer to infection in any part of the bone.

Infectious processes can also be categorized by their onset and are generally designated as acute, subacute, or chronic. An acute infection is one that is diagnosed within 2 weeks after disease onset, a subacute infection is one diagnosed after one to several months, and chronic infections after a few months. Periprosthetic infections follow a similar nomenclature, using time of onset after surgery. Chronic osteomyelitis is also used to define a bone infection that fails to respond to a normal course of antibiotic therapy.

For the emergency clinician, the most practical way to classify osteomyelitis is as hematogenous, which is more common, or contiguous, which is further subdivided based on the presence or absence of vascular insufficiency. This method of classification assists in the interpretation of diagnostic imaging examinations and helps guide management, including antibiotic therapy and surgical intervention.

Anatomy, Physiology, and Pathophysiology

Histologically, bone is composed of compact and trabecular tissue. Compact bone forms the shaft of long bones and also covers the epiphysis. Trabecular or spongy bone is found within the epiphysis and makes up irregular bones. Compact bone is dense and without cavities and consists of longitudinally running Haversian systems, which contain Haversian canals that house vasculature and nerves. Spongy bone, conversely, consists of a bony lattice, the trabeculae, which is located within the medullary cavity and contains marrow, making it more metabolically active. The central Haversian canals in spongy bone run parallel to the long axis of the bone and contain the blood supply and reticular connective tissue for the Haversian system.

The gross structure of long bones is divided into several sections. The diaphysis is the shaft of the bone and contains the compact cortical bone with an overlying periosteum and a medullary canal containing marrow. The metaphysis is the junctional region between the epiphysis and diaphysis. The metaphysis contains abundant trabecular bone, but the cortical bone thins here relative to the diaphysis. Finally, the epiphysis is the area at either end of a long bone and is made up of abundant trabecular bone and a thin shell of cortical bone (Fig. 125.1). In the skeletally mature individual, the epiphysis of most bones is involved in articulation and, instead of being covered by a periosteum, is covered with a thin layer of articulating cartilage. This cartilage is composed of a thin layer of secretory cells that sits on a loose fibrous stroma and allows frictionless movement of the bones.

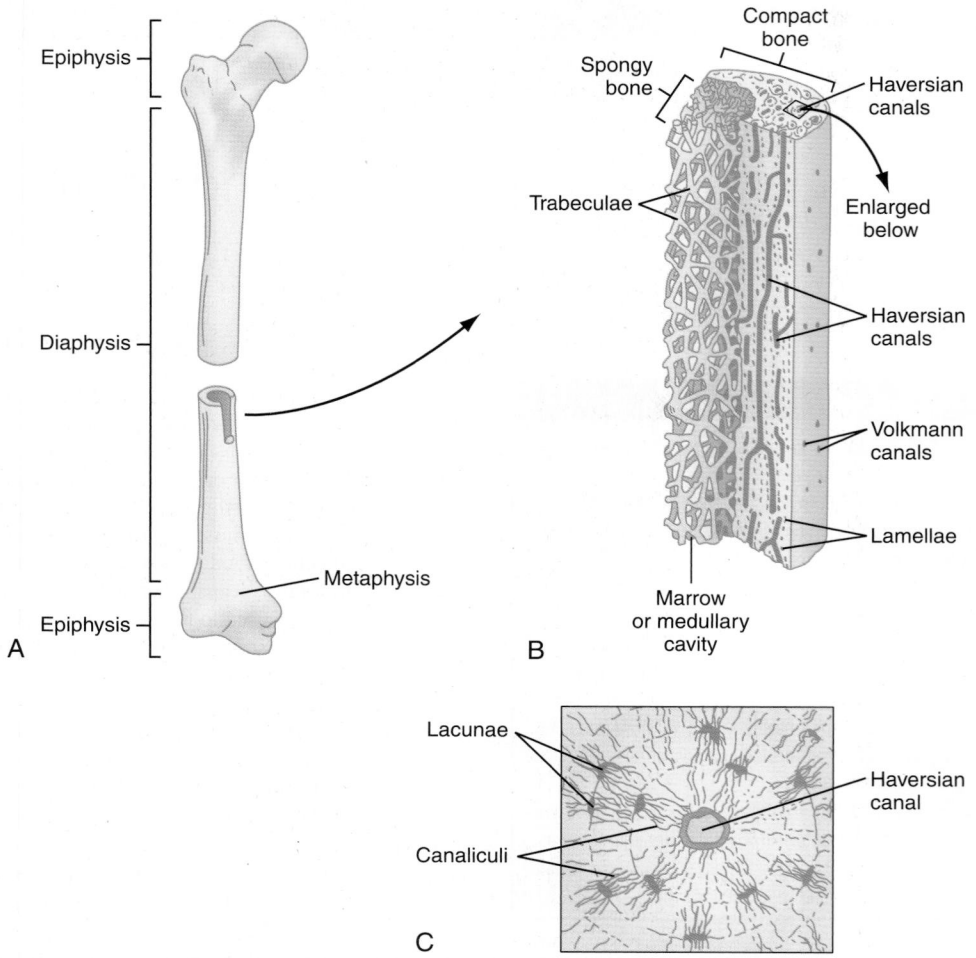

Fig. 125.1 Schematic drawing of long bone. (A) Regions of long bone. (B) Cross-sectional structure of long bone. (C) Microscopic structure.

Joints are enclosed by a synovial capsule. This layer of dense fibrous connective tissue offers structural integrity and is lined with synovial cells that secrete synovial fluid. This forms a sleeve around the articulating bones to which it is attached. The synovial membrane of the shoulder, hip, and knee joints extends beyond the epiphysis and attaches to the metaphysis allowing bacteria to spread directly from the metaphysis into the joint.

Osteomyelitis is an infection of the bone and medullary cavity. Bone is typically resistant to infection unless it is subjected to trauma, disruption of blood flow that deprives the bone of normal host immunity, a large inoculum of blood-borne or external microorganisms, or a foreign body. Hematogenous inoculation usually starts in the metaphysis, given the slow flow of blood in the sinusoidal blood vessels. Acute inflammatory cells migrate to the area, causing edema, vascular congestion, and small vessel thrombosis, which then leads to an increase in the intraosseous pressure compromising blood flow to the bone. The significantly reduced blood supply to this necrotic bone tissue makes bacterial infection difficult to eradicate with medication alone and, frequently, chronic osteomyelitis requires a combination of surgical debridement and antibiotic therapy. Eventually, lack of blood supply to the medullary canal and periosteum leads to areas of necrotic bone termed *sequestra*. Bony tissue attempts to compensate for the tensile stresses caused by infection by creating new bone around the areas of necrosis. This new bone deposition is called an involucrum.

The normal development of blood flow patterns at the metaphyseal-epiphyseal junction helps to explain the pathologic features of hematogenous osteomyelitis seen in the different age groups. In neonates and infants, osteomyelitis readily advances from the metaphysis to the epiphysis and adjacent joint space, leading to septic arthritis. After the first year of life, the infection usually spreads laterally through Volkmann canals, breaks through the cortex, and lifts the periosteum to form a subperiosteal abscess. In the adult, after the epiphyseal plate ossifies, anastomoses form between the metaphyseal and epiphyseal blood vessels and infection can once again spread from the metaphysis to the epiphysis and eventually into the synovium and joint space. In addition, because the periosteum becomes firmly attached to the underlying bone in adults, this limits subperiosteal abscess formation.

Bacteria congregate in a highly structured community, the biofilm, which plays an important role in the pathogenesis of septic arthritis and osteomyelitis. Within the biofilm, the bacteria are at varying stages of metabolism—some are active, some are slow-growing, and some are dormant. Antibiotics target metabolically active bacteria, such as those in the single cell state (planktonic state), and bacteria in other stages in the biofilm community are more resistant to the effects of antibiotics. Furthermore, Gram staining only identifies planktonic bacteria, which helps explain why Gram stains of aspirated synovial fluid in a suspected septic joint are often negative; therefore, a definitive diagnosis is made only by culture of the synovial fluid aspirate or synovial tissue. Biofilm formation also explains why optimal treatment of a septic joint, especially of prosthetic joints, involves complete surgical débridement.

Hematogenous spread of bacteria causes almost all cases of osteomyelitis in children and in the subset of adults who have vertebral osteomyelitis. In the appendicular skeleton of adults, such as in the foot, hand, skull, maxilla, and mandible, osteomyelitis usually occurs by spread of the pathogens from a contiguous source of infection or direct implantation. Head and neck osteomyelitis is usually caused by sinus disease and odontogenic infection.

Infections from direct implantation of bacteria are caused by deep puncture wounds, such as by an animal bite, and tend to occur in the hands and feet. Although cats account for only 10% of animal bites, significant infection results from 20% to 50% of cat bites versus only 5% of dog bites because of the morphology of feline teeth. Most human bite injuries are related to fistfights and contamination of the metacarpophalangeal joints and metacarpals, with infection due to oral flora. Direct implantation of pathogens is also common with open fractures and surgical instrumentation.

Septic arthritis is usually a consequence of hematogenous spread unless there is direct injection of bacteria into the joint. The lack of a basement membrane makes the highly vascular synovium vulnerable to bacterial seeding. Infection occurs first in the synovium, spreads into joint fluid, and finally affects the articular cartilage. Bacterial enzymes and toxins directly damage cartilage. The synovial membrane responds to infection by increasing synovial fluid production, resulting in a large joint effusion. In response to infection, synovial cells and polymorphonuclear leukocytes release lysosomal enzymes, which irreversibly degrade articular cartilage, creating a painful joint with limited range of motion. This is amplified by the damage produced by bacterial enzymes and toxins. Even a small bacterial load in the joint space elicits profound and persistent inflammatory and immune responses. Bacteria can be cleared from the joint, resulting in a sterile-appearing inflammatory response. In addition, other structures that are enclosed within or adjacent to the synovium, such as bursae, tendons, and bone, may also become damaged in those with septic arthritis.[2]

Causes and Microbiology

Typically, hematogenous osteomyelitis or septic arthritis is caused by a single strain of bacterium, with gram-positive organisms being responsible for most infections. Even though gram-negative organisms account for 43% of cases of community-acquired bacteremia, they result in only about 10% of septic arthritis cases. Trauma predisposes patients to osteomyelitis by environmental pathogens. Patients who are wounded or sustain open fractures in fresh water are susceptible to

infections with the gram-negative bacillus *Aeromonas hydrophila*. People who are bitten by animals, particularly dogs and cats, are at risk for the development of osteomyelitis from *Pasteurella multocida*. Osteomyelitis caused from human bites is most common in the hand and involves human oral flora, such as *Streptococcus anginosus*, *Fusobacterium nucleatum*, and *Eikenella* spp. In the population of injection drug users, *Staphylococcus aureus* is the most likely cause of infection, followed by *Pseudomonas* spp. *Pseudomonas aeruginosa* is also an important cause of osteomyelitis in puncture wounds, postsurgical wounds, and patients with sickle cell anemia.

Certain underlying disease states predispose a patient to BJI. These conditions include diabetes mellitus, sickle cell disease, HIV, alcohol use disorder, injection drug use, chronic corticosteroid use, preexisting joint disease (especially rheumatoid arthritis), and other immunosuppressed states. Postsurgical patients are also susceptible to BJIs, especially those who have implanted prosthetic devices.

Although most BJIs are bacterial, other pathogens include viruses, fungi, and parasites. The microbiology of osteomyelitis and septic arthritis is a function of several host and environmental factors. A patient's living environment also has some role in determining the incidence of BJIs. For example, people living in crowded conditions where tuberculosis is prevalent are at increased risk for tubercular BJIs, whereas older patients in hospitals and institutions may be more susceptible to infections with gram-negative bacteria. A summary of the organisms that cause osteomyelitis and septic arthritis is presented in Tables 125.1 and 125.2.

When considering the offending organism, *S. aureus* is the leading cause of osteomyelitis in all age groups except neonates. In neonates, group B streptococci, *Escherichia coli* and other gram-negative coliforms, and *Staphylococcus epidermidis* are the most common pathogens responsible for BJIs. Since the introduction of the vaccine, *Haemophilus influenzae* type b, once a common cause of septic arthritis and osteomyelitis in children younger than 2 years, has essentially disappeared as a pathogen in vaccinated children but cases of septic arthritis are being reported from other serotypes of *H. influenzae*. Another gram-negative coccobacillus in the Neisseriaceae family, *Kingella kingae* has been encountered with increasing frequency.[3] *K. kingae* can be part of the normal flora of the nasopharynx and can be spread hematogenously to bones and joints. It is a fastidious organism and may be mistaken for *Haemophilus* or *Neisseria* spp. and often requires PCR for diagnosis.[4] In older adults and patients with diabetes, gram-negative bacteria account for a higher percentage of cases of bone and joint infections.

P. aeruginosa has been reported as a cause of cervical spine osteomyelitis in injection drug users and lumbar spine osteomyelitis in patients

TABLE 125.1 Microbiology of Bacterial Septic Arthritis as Related to Age of the Patient

Organism	Child (%)[a]	Young Adult Engaging in High-Risk Sexual Behavior (%)	Adult (%)	Older Adult (%)
Staphylococcus aureus	10–20	15–20	60–0	45–65
Streptococcus species	5–10	1–5	15–20	10–15
Gram-negative bacterium	1–5	Rare	10–5	15–35
Haemophilus influenza	Rare[b]	Rare[b]	Rare[b]	Rare[b]
Neisseria gonorrhoeae	1–5	60–80	1–5	Rare

[a]Ages 6 months to 5 years.
[b]With widespread immunization.
Reprinted with permission from: Esterhai JL Jr, Rao N. The epidemiology of musculoskeletal infections. In: Cierny G 3rd, McLaren AC, Wongworawat MD, eds. *Orthopaedic Knowledge Update: Musculoskeletal Infection*. Rosemont, IL: American Academy of Orthopaedic Surgeons; 2009.

TABLE 125.2   Microbiology and Initial (Empirical) Antibiotic Treatment of Bone and Joint Infection

Age Group	OSTEOMYELITIS Common Organisms	Antibiotic Regimen	SEPTIC ARTHRITIS Common Organisms	Antibiotic Regimen
Neonate to <3 mo	Staphylococcus aureus Group B streptococcus Enterobacteriaceae Gram-negative rods	Ceph 3 PRP + gentamicin Consider vancomycin instead of PRP for MRSA.	S. aureus Group B streptococcus Enterobacteriaceae	PRP + Ceph 3 Alt—PRP + APAG Consider vancomycin instead of PRP for MRSA.
3 mo–14 yr	S. aureus Group A streptococcus Haemophilus influenzae	PRP + Ceph 3 Alt: vancomycin + Ceph 3, chloramphenicol PRP or Ceph 3 with allergy to penicillin or clindamycin with allergy to penicillin + Ceph 3	S. aureus Group A streptococcus Streptococcus pneumoniae H. influenzae	PRP + Ceph 3 Alt—vancomycin + Ceph 3
14 yr–adult	S. aureus	PRP Alt—vancomycin	S. aureus Streptococcal spp. Enterobacteriaceae	PRP or Ceph 3 Alt—vancomycin + Ceph 3 or penicillin + aminoglycoside or Ceph 3
Infection Subsets				
Sexually active adolescents or adults with acute arthritis			Neisseria gonorrhoeae[a]	Ceph 3 Alt—spectinomycin or penicillin if sensitive
Chronic osteomyelitis and diabetic foot infections	S. aureus Enterobacteriaceae Anaerobic bacteria	PRP + FLQ + metronidazole Alt—PRP + Ceph 3 + clindamycin		
Infected orthopedic joint prosthesis	Staphylococcus aureus Staphylococcus epidermidis Pseudomonas aeruginosa	Vancomycin + FLQ Alt—imipenem	S. aureus S. epidermidis P. aeruginosa	Vancomycin + FLQ Alt—PRP + APAG
Sickle cell disease	Staphylococcus aureus Salmonella sp.	PRP + Ceph 3 Alt—FLQ	S. aureus Salmonella spp.	PRP + Ceph 3 Alt—FLQ
Injection drug abuse	Staphylococcus aureus Pseudomonas aeruginosa Enterobacteriaceae	Ceph 3 + aminoglycoside Alt—Ceph 3	P. aeruginosa S. aureus Enterobacteriaceae	PRP + APAG or FLQ Alt—vancomycin + FLQ
Plantar puncture wound	Pseudomonas aeruginosa	AP Ceph Alt—FLQ	P. aeruginosa	AP Ceph Alt—FLQ
Human or animal bites	Eikenella corrodens Pasteurella multocida	Penicillin ± AC Alt—Ceph 3, TS	E. corrodens P. multocida	Penicillin ± AC Alt—Ceph 3, TS

Alt, Alternative antibiotics; APAG, antipseudomonal aminoglycoside; AP Ceph, antipseudomonal cephalosporin (ceftazidime or cefepime); Ceph 3, third-generation cephalosporin (e.g., ceftriaxone, cefotaxime, cefamandole, ceftizoxime, ceftazidime, cefazolin, moxalactam); FLQ, fluoroquinolone; MRSA, methicillin-resistant S. aureus; PRP, penicillinase-resistant penicillin (oxacillin, nafcillin, methicillin, amoxicillin-clavulanate [AC]); TS, trimethoprim-sulfamethoxazole.
[a]Concurrent treatment of Chlamydia trachomatis infection should be given to patients with suspected N. gonorrhoeae septic arthritis.

with chronic urinary catheters. Pseudomonas colonizes the rubber and plastic inserts in footwear and is therefore seen in soft tissue infections and osteomyelitis of the foot after a puncture wound through footwear.

Methicillin-resistant S. aureus (MRSA), methicillin-resistant S. epidermidis, and vancomycin-resistant enterococci (VRE) pose significant microbiologic problems. In fact, MRSA has become the most prevalent cause of acute hematogenous osteomyelitis in pediatric patients.[5] Traditional therapies, including vancomycin and clindamycin, remain effective for the treatment of much of pediatric AHO. Multiresistant enterococci pose the greatest potential danger in that bacteriocidal antibiotic regimens are limited.

The rise in injection opioid use in the United States since 2000 has also resulted in a rise in invasive bacterial infections, including

osteomyelitis. One study found that those who inject heroin were 16 times more likely to develop MRSA than those who did not inject drugs.[6]

Diabetic foot osteomyelitis, posttraumatic osteomyelitis, and chronic septic arthritis or osteomyelitis are often polymicrobial. Anaerobic bacteria can complicate polymicrobial infections and may be present more often than is commonly identified because standard culture techniques may be inadequate to identify them. Anaerobic bacteria are reportedly discovered in up to 40% of cases of chronic osteomyelitis.

Mycobacterium tuberculosis may infect bones and joints, usually in the axial skeleton. The two most common forms of skeletal infection are vertebral osteomyelitis (Pott disease), in which the spine is affected in 50% of cases, and tubercular arthritis, which manifests as a chronic, low-grade inflammatory process that resembles rheumatoid arthritis more than acute septic arthritis.

Patients with human immunodeficiency virus (HIV) infection and AIDS are predisposed to various common and opportunistic pathogens. Although *S. aureus* is still the most likely cause of bone and joint infections in patients with AIDS, fungal and other atypical organisms should be considered. One unusual but particularly characteristic form of osteomyelitis in HIV-positive patients is bacillary angiomatosis. This infection is caused by a gram-negative, rickettsia-like organism that frequently causes osteolytic bone lesions.

OSTEOMYELITIS

Clinical Features

History and Physical Examination

The symptoms and signs of osteomyelitis in adults vary. Patients with osteomyelitis often present with fever, rigors, and may even appear toxic. Systemic complaints of headache, fatigue, malaise, and anorexia are inconsistently reported and are less likely with chronic osteomyelitis. In children with lower extremity osteomyelitis, a sudden limp or inability to bear weight, localized warmth, swelling, and erythema may be reported. A careful review of the patient's past medical history should be performed to identify risk factors that may predispose to bone infection.

The predominant physical exam finding of osteomyelitis is point tenderness over the infected segment. Palpable warmth and soft tissue swelling with erythema may be present, but these findings are variable. In chronic osteomyelitis, the involucrum or sequestrum (fragments of necrotic bone separated from healthy bone) may be palpated, and sinus tracts that fistulize to the skin may be noted. A sympathetic effusion in the adjacent joint may develop in patients with osteomyelitis, even when the joint is not infected.

Complications

In addition to the development of chronic osteomyelitis, complications of acute osteomyelitis include bacteremia and sepsis. Depending on the location of osteomyelitis, local extension of an invasive suppurative process can lead to septic arthritis, brain abscess, meningitis, spinal cord compression, pneumonia, and empyema. In children, osteomyelitis damages the developing skeleton. If the infection involves the epiphysis, permanent growth alterations can occur, resulting in a shorter or deformed extremity on the affected side. Pathologic fractures may occur through sites of osteomyelitis.

Clinical Subsets of Osteomyelitis

Osteomyelitis in Children. Osteomyelitis in children tends to be acute, usually arising from hematogenous seeding of bone, and can often be treated with antibiotics alone. Acute hematogenous osteomyelitis (AHO) is seen in children as young as 3 months and as old as 16 years. *S. aureus* is the most common infecting organism in children of all ages, except neonates (see Tables 125.1 and 125.2) with MRSA being most common in AHO. As noted, *H. influenzae* is no longer a common cause of AHO.

AHO has a well-established male preponderance (male-female ratio of 2 : 1 to 3 : 1) and involves long bones approximately 80% of the time. The site of infection is usually the distal metaphysis because of its increased vascularity, but up to 30% of AHO occurs in other parts of the bone. Children with AHO may have fever, chills, vomiting, dehydration, and malaise, but they usually do not appear toxic. Most children have characteristic pain, limited use of the limb, and are point tender. The diagnostic evaluation for AHO is shown in Fig. 125.2. Blood cultures are positive for the bacterial cause of osteomyelitis in about 40%

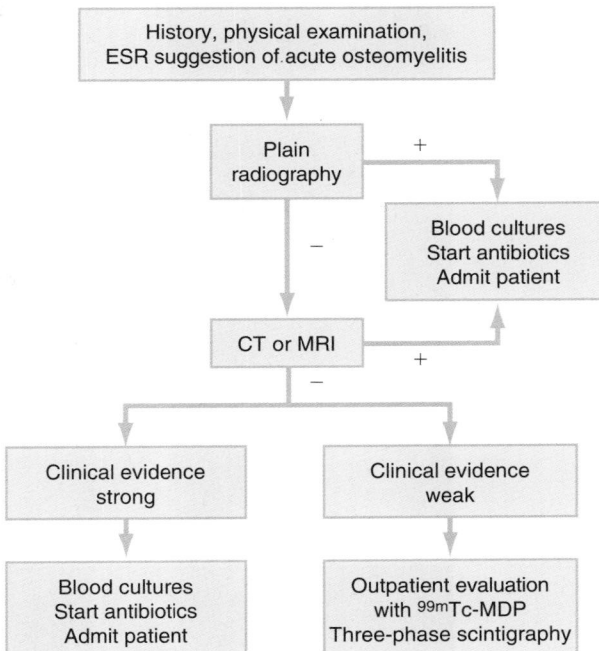

Fig. 125.2 Algorithm for the use of imaging studies in the emergency department diagnosis of osteomyelitis. *CT*, Computed tomography; *ESR*, erythrocyte sedimentation rate; *MRI*, magnetic resonance imaging; *^{99m}Tc-MDP*, technetium Tc-99m–labeled methylene diphosphonate.

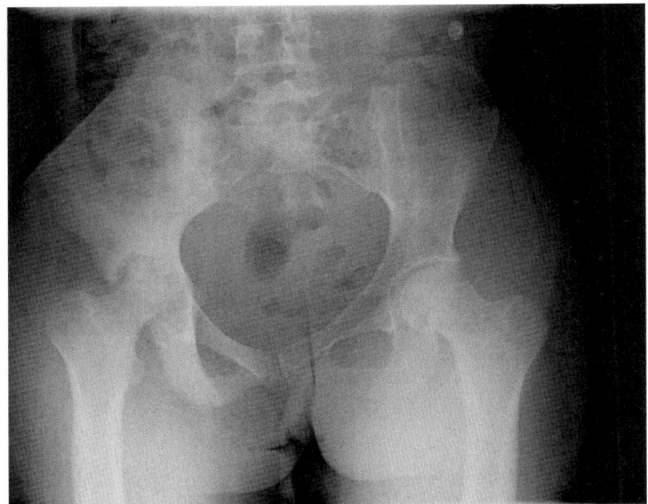

Fig. 125.3 Radiograph of chronic osteomyelitis. Diffuse sclerosis of the right hemipelvis includes the ischium and iliac bone, with extension to the right sacroiliac joint. The right acetabulum demonstrates whittling of the femoral head and neck, with marked loss of bone stock. Abutting the right symphysis pubis is increased cortical lucency suggestive of subchondral cystic changes. (Courtesy Dr. Peter Evangelista, Department of Diagnostic Imaging, Rhode Island Hospital, Brown University, Providence, RI.)

of pediatric patients[7] with AHO while tissue cultures are positive 86% of the time. A positive blood culture and physical examination consistent with osteomyelitis may be sufficient to diagnose AHO. Figs. 125.3 and 125.4 show typical radiographs of AHO.

Neonatal osteomyelitis is more commonly seen after an abnormal pregnancy or delivery and often accompanies other acute illnesses

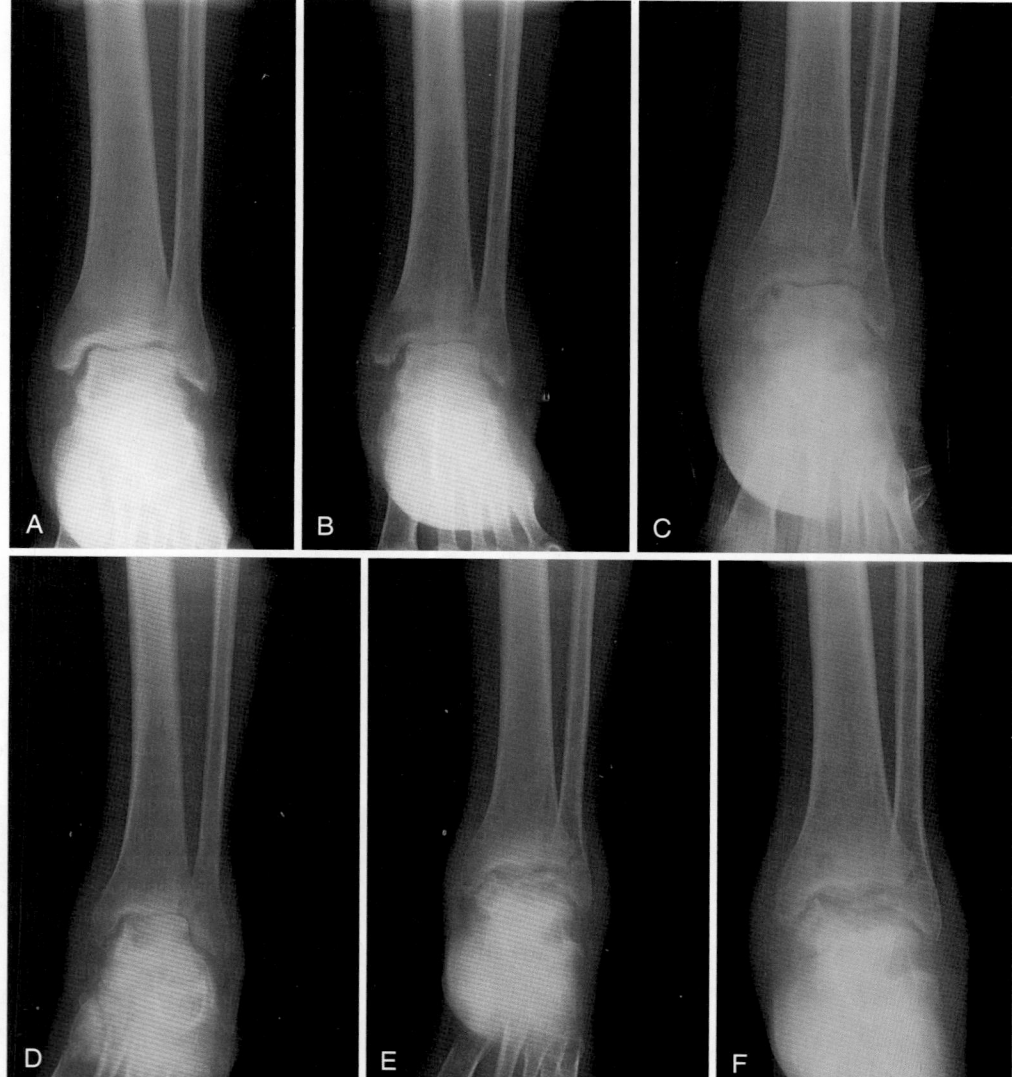

Fig. 125.4 Radiographic progression of acute osteomyelitis. (A) Soft tissue swelling at the medial and lateral aspects of the ankle, with a moderately sized effusion (August 2, 2006). (B) Large ankle effusion with extensive soft tissue swelling. There is complete loss of the tibiotalar joint space and widening of the medial joint space, suggesting chondrolysis. There are lucent areas in the distal tibia and fibula, suggestive of hyperemia, and the talus is diffusely sclerotic (September 11, 2006). (C) Increased erosion of the medial aspect of the talar dome, with increased joint effusion (October 12, 2006). (D) Talar bone destruction with demineralization involving all the osseous structures. There is also a small joint effusion (January 2, 2007). (E) Avascular necrosis of the talus and destruction of the articular surfaces of the tibia and talus is present, consistent with chronic osteomyelitis. There is diffuse osteopenia and loose bodies within the joint (April 19, 2007). (F) There is continued irregularity of the articular surface of the tibia and collapse of the talus. Loose bodies are still present within the joint, and there is a persistent joint effusion and soft tissue swelling (June 14, 2007). (Courtesy Dr. Thomas Egglin, Department of Diagnostic Imaging, Rhode Island Hospital, Brown University, Providence, RI.)

but is difficult to diagnose because of a paucity of systemic findings. Multiple sites of bone involvement are found in approximately 50% of reported cases. Because of the unique vascular anatomy of the neonate, septic arthritis often accompanies osteomyelitis. Osteomyelitis of the flat bones, such as the facial bones, is more common among neonates than any other age group. Group B streptococcus is the leading causative bacterium in neonatal osteomyelitis, but staphylococcal species are still common. As with adults, plain radiographs are a good initial test because abnormalities are identified within days of development of neonatal osteomyelitis, and radiographs are usually abnormal when the

disease is suspected. In the presence of a normal radiograph, the next step for the emergency clinician who suspects neonatal osteomyelitis is magnetic resonance imaging (MRI) in consultation with the orthopedic surgical service.

Two less common forms of osteomyelitis, subacute osteomyelitis and chronic recurrent multifocal osteomyelitis (CRMO), can occur in children, particularly older children (6–10 years) and adolescents. Subacute osteomyelitis refers to a form of the disease in which clinical symptoms and signs are slow to appear, and radiographs show small areas of osteomyelitis, usually in the metaphysis of long bones. Cultures of blood and bone are negative more than 50% of the time but usually implicate staphylococcal species when they are positive.

CRMO is characterized by small foci of infection at various sites in the skeleton. The disease is defined by multiple episodes of indolent infection. Diagnosis is made by radiography because culture of the bone sites is almost always negative. This disease may be associated with certain psoriatic subtypes.

Vertebral Osteomyelitis. Vertebral osteomyelitis usually affects older adults and is increasing in frequency as the population ages and has more chronic medical diseases. Risk factors in older adults include intravenous (IV) access devices, indwelling lines, and asymptomatic urinary infections, whereas in younger individuals risk factors include injection drug abuse. The spine is particularly susceptible to bacterial infection because the venous system surrounding vertebral bodies is valveless, permitting two-way flow of blood, and has transverse and longitudinal anastomoses. This anatomy allows bacteria to readily spread to adjacent vertebral bodies. Vertebral osteomyelitis usually results from hematogenous seeding, direct inoculation at the time of spinal surgery, or contiguous spread from an adjacent infection. A clear source of bacterial hematogenous seeding with positive blood cultures occurs in approximately 40% of cases of vertebral osteomyelitis. *S. aureus* (including MRSA) is the most common offending agent, followed by aerobic gram-negative rods from urinary or gastrointestinal sources.

Vertebral infections occur in the lumbar (58%), thoracic (30%), and cervical (11%) spine. Only 10% of patients with vertebral osteomyelitis appear septic or toxic; most patients present with insidious symptoms, leading to delays in diagnosis of up to 4 months. Back pain, seen in roughly 90% of patients, is the most common presenting symptom, and physical examination often reveals tenderness over the spinous process. Neurologic deficits are reported in less than 40% of patients with vertebral osteomyelitis and often coincide with a concomitant epidural abscess. Up to 60% of patients with these abscesses present without fever or leukocytosis. On laboratory testing, the erythrocyte sedimentation rate (ESR) and C-reactive protein (CRP) level are elevated in 98% and 100% of cases, respectively. Blood culture specimens should be obtained before antibiotic treatment is initiated. Rapid diagnosis and treatment of this medical emergency start with the initiation of empiric antibiotics, immediate imaging, and early orthopedic (or spine service) involvement. Diagnostic delay is an independent risk factor for an unfavorable outcome.

Similar to osteomyelitis in other parts of the body, findings on plain radiographs are not seen until at least the second week of vertebral infection and are nonspecific. MRI has largely replaced bone scintigraphy for imaging in suspected vertebral osteomyelitis. Although computed tomography (CT) is good for defining bone destruction and is often used to assist needle aspiration of the lesion, MRI can identify an epidural abscess and rule out other noninfectious vertebral conditions. MRI has a sensitivity of 90% for vertebral osteomyelitis, with T2-weighted images most valuable in establishing the diagnosis. When suspected, an MRI of the complete spine, with and without contrast, is the imaging study of choice.

Cervical spine osteomyelitis can cause a retropharyngeal abscess, whereas lumbar spine osteomyelitis may be complicated by a psoas muscle abscess. Vertebral osteomyelitis can cause spinal cord ischemia if the vertebral infection causes septic thrombosis or compression of local blood vessels. When osteomyelitis affects the thoracic spine, infection can spread to the chest. Paraspinal abscesses, reactive pleural effusions, and empyema have been reported as complications of vertebral osteomyelitis and may mislead the emergency clinician. The most dreaded complication of vertebral osteomyelitis is the spread of infection into the spinal canal, development of an epidural abscess, and progression of the infection to cause spinal cord injury and permanent

paralysis. Fortunately, this occurs in less than 15% of cases of vertebral osteomyelitis, and risk factors for this include older adults, those with cervical spine osteomyelitis, and those with serious underlying diseases (e.g., rheumatoid arthritis, diabetes mellitus).

Patients who present with a clinical picture consistent with vertebral osteomyelitis require rapid diagnostic confirmation to avoid progression and spinal cord compression. The diagnosis is suspected in patients who have recently undergone a spinal procedure or injection and have focal severe pain that is not relieved by rest. It can also result from hematogenous spread, making diagnosis elusive. The diagnostic procedure of choice for vertebral osteomyelitis is a spinal MRI with contrast, and needle biopsy may be indicated to identify the causative organism.

Patients with vertebral osteomyelitis initially require IV antibiotic therapy and can usually be successfully treated with antibiotics alone. Surgery may be required when there is spinal cord compression, for abscess drainage or débridement, for correction of the progressive anatomic deformity, and if the infection recurs after adequate treatment.

Diskitis is a variant of vertebral osteomyelitis. The disk is an avascular structure that depends on nutrient diffusion from adjacent blood vessels from the vertebral body and endplates. The avascular disk creates a rich environment for the bacteria to flourish. Due to the vascular anatomy, diskitis often coexists with vertebral osteomyelitis in adults while isolated diskitis is more common in children. The patient often complains of back pain and may refuse to walk. MRI demonstrates the anatomy of diskitis, whereas CT is used to guide aspiration. Cultures of the disk from needle aspiration are reported to be positive for bacteria 30% to 60% of the time, usually for *S. aureus*. The disease typically resolves with nonoperative treatment.

Posttraumatic Osteomyelitis. Posttraumatic osteomyelitis is a form of osteomyelitis that results from open fractures, burns, bites, puncture wounds, and surgery and invasive procedures. Open fractures are typically graded according to the Gustillo classification, which takes into account wound length and amount of soft tissue damage; this helps guide antibiotic treatment. Overall, the rate of osteomyelitis in open long-bone fractures is reported to be around 0.05%.[8] The fracture site may be contaminated directly from the environment or iatrogenically secondary to emergency procedures or surgery. When there is damage to soft tissues, a necrotic nidus of infection is created, and the bacteria can spread to bone. Polymicrobial infection is more common in this scenario. The imaging of posttraumatic osteomyelitis is complicated by changes induced by surgery and new bone formation in the fracture; therefore, the optimal imaging modalities are MRI and CT.

The intraoperative implantation of prosthetic devices increases the chance of infection. The rate of prosthetic joint infection is 0.5% to 1% for hips,[9] 0.5% to 2% for knees, and less than 1% for shoulder replacements. Osteomyelitis due to direct inoculation associated with joint arthroplasty and implantation of prosthetic devices typically becomes evident about 12 weeks after surgery. These patients generally do not report relief of their pain after surgery. Patients who have symptoms of infection more than 12 weeks after surgery and who have postoperative improvement of their pain are considered to have a hematogenous source of infection. Techniques to retain implanted prosthetic devices in the setting of an acute infection after total joint arthroplasty are evolving. Débridement and irrigation with prosthetic retention followed by antibiotic therapy is the treatment of choice in infections following total knee arthroplasty.[9,10] Postsurgical osteomyelitis should be considered in the postoperative patient with a painful joint. The prevalence of infection after total knee or hip arthroplasty is estimated to be approximately 1% to 2%, with infections within 3 months of injury likely the result of surgical contamination, and those that occur longer than 3 months postoperatively due to hematogenous seeding.

S. aureus and *S. epidermidis* account for 75% of postsurgical and prosthesis-related cases of osteomyelitis. Radiographs are often normal but may show subtle signs of bone resorption and loosening of the prosthetic components. It is difficult to distinguish mechanical from infectious loosening, so joint aspiration, synovial fluid analysis, and bone biopsy—all performed in a sterile operative setting—are undertaken to establish a diagnosis. Other imaging techniques such as CT and MRI are used but may be difficult to interpret because of scatter from the metallic components and postsurgical changes.

Puncture wounds to the feet have approximately a 2% incidence of development of osteomyelitis. The causative organism is usually *S. aureus* or beta-hemolytic streptococcus. *P. aeruginosa* is commonly associated with plantar wounds that occur while a person is wearing rubber-soled shoes. Invasive procedures that produce puncture wounds, such as venipuncture for central lines, intraosseous devices for intravascular access, and fetal scalp monitoring, may introduce infection that can lead to osteomyelitis. Proper antiseptic skin cleansing and avoiding punctures through infected skin will reduce the chance of contiguous bone infection.

Diabetic Foot Osteomyelitis. Diabetic foot infections lead to osteomyelitis 20% of the time, while diabetic ulcers have underlying osteomyelitis 15% of the time. This rate increases in ulcers greater in size than 2 cm². The pathologic changes induced by long-standing diabetes mellitus, such as compromised vascularity, encourage the development of osteomyelitis. Over 60% of patients report polyneuropathy, leading to repetitive trauma and subsequent foot ulcers. Once the skin has been violated and infected, the altered host defenses of diabetic patients make it easier for infection to occur and spread. Hyperglycemia resulting from the infection allows bacteria to proliferate, impairs leukocyte function, and results in defective chemotaxis, abnormal phagocytosis, decreased bactericidal function, defective antibody synthesis, and decreased complement levels, all of which impair healing and exacerbate osteomyelitis. The infection typically starts in the periosteum, spreads to the cortex, and eventually disrupts medullary bone.

Local findings in diabetic foot infections include swelling, erythema, and sometimes pain. Indolent ulcers and frank cellulitis are seen in more than 50% of cases. Laboratory testing cannot definitively diagnose osteomyelitis, though an ESR over 70 mm/h is associated with an 11-fold greater risk. Surgical biopsy of the bone is the only reliable way for the bacteriologic diagnosis to be made. The probe-to-bone (PTB) test can be performed by exploring the wound for palpable bone with a sterile blunt metal probe. The pretest probability plays a significant role in using PTB to diagnose osteomyelitis and the PTB result should be interpreted with the results of clinical, laboratory, and imaging findings.

Diabetic osteomyelitis is often chronic, so radiographic changes are often notable. Osteopenia, periosteal thickening, cortical erosions, new bone formation, and mottled lytic lesions are typical, and air may be present in the soft tissues. Bone biopsy for diabetic foot osteomyelitis has a reported sensitivity of 94%. Diabetic foot osteomyelitis is usually polymicrobial and often includes gram-negative bacteria. *S. aureus* is the most common pathogen; other organisms include streptococci, Enterobacteriaceae, and anaerobes. Surgical treatment with amputation had been the mainstay of treatment; however, a 10-week antibiotic treatment regimen, including IV administration followed by oral antibiotics, can be successful in select patients.[11]

Osteomyelitis in Sickle Cell Disease. Patients with sickle cell disease (SCD) are at increased risk for hematogenous infection, including osteomyelitis, often due to reduced or absent splenic function. In children, the difference in the vasculature of immature bone increases susceptibility to osteomyelitis. In contrast to AHO in non–sickle cell patients, AHO in children with sickle cell disease usually affects the diaphysis instead of the metaphysis. Also, although *S. aureus* is the most common bacterium in children without sickle cell disease, *Salmonella* spp. is the most common infecting organism in patients with SCD.[9,12] Reasons for this are not completely understood, although it has been postulated that microinfarcts in the bowel allow *Salmonella* bacteremia to seed the bloodstream and lead to hematogenous osteomyelitis.

The differentiation of bone infection from bone infarction and vaso-occlusive crisis in sickle cell patients is a challenge. Vaso-occlusive pain is typically consistent and far more common than either infarcts or infection. Fever, toxic appearance, and elevated ESR are more commonly associated with osteomyelitis than with bone infarction. Plain radiographs are not helpful in distinguishing between the entities, but MRI has been proving useful in differentiating between bone infarction and infection. Another approach is to note the response to conservative therapy; bone infarctions usually improve within 24 to 48 hours, whereas bone infections worsen. Empiric antibiotic treatment of osteomyelitis in the sickle cell patient should include coverage against *S. aureus, Salmonella,* as well as other gram-negative bacteria with vancomycin and ciprofloxacin.

Chronic Osteomyelitis. Most chronic bone infections occur as a complication of posttraumatic infection, surgical procedures, or diabetic foot infections. The inflammatory response to infection triggers bone resorption and cartilage destruction and ultimately leads to bone death (see Fig. 125.3). The necrotic bone provides an inanimate surface to which microorganisms adhere. Clinical signs that the infection has become chronic include the formation of sequestra and presence of draining tracts or fistulas. Chronic infection is almost always polymicrobial and commonly involves anaerobes. Because sinus tract culture is not a reliable method to predict which bacteria are active in the underlying bone infection, direct biopsy of bone is the only option for the accurate diagnosis of most cases of chronic osteomyelitis. Chronically established infections can be remarkably persistent or evolve even in the face of prolonged antibiotic therapy; therefore, treatment commonly involves surgery.

Differential Diagnoses

Many processes involving bone may masquerade as osteomyelitis. Bone tumors, such as osteoid osteomas and chondroblastomas, metastatic bone tumors, and lymphoma may produce local pain and radiographic changes consistent with osteomyelitis, such as small, round, radiolucent lesions. Ewing sarcoma is a tumor of bone marrow in children that can be mistaken for osteomyelitis. Finally, occult fractures, such as buckle fractures in children, present with point tenderness that may be mistaken for osteomyelitis.

Diagnostic Testing

Laboratory Tests

Initial evaluation in the emergency department (ED) often involves laboratory and radiographic evaluation, but the gold standard to confirm diagnosis is bone biopsy and culture, which also helps guide treatment. Laboratory data are not specific and can only suggest the diagnosis of osteomyelitis. In acute osteomyelitis, the white blood cell (WBC) count can be elevated—typical values range from normal to 15,000/mm³—whereas in chronic osteomyelitis the WBC count is often normal.

The ESR, a nonspecific measure of inflammation, is more helpful than the WBC count. The ESR is a relatively sensitive marker for infection, and many series have reported elevated ESR and CRP values in patients who have confirmed osteomyelitis. An elevated ESR in the presence of pertinent physical findings should lead one to suspect osteomyelitis, but a normal or slightly elevated ESR does not eliminate the diagnosis. Other inflammatory conditions, such as cellulitis, can

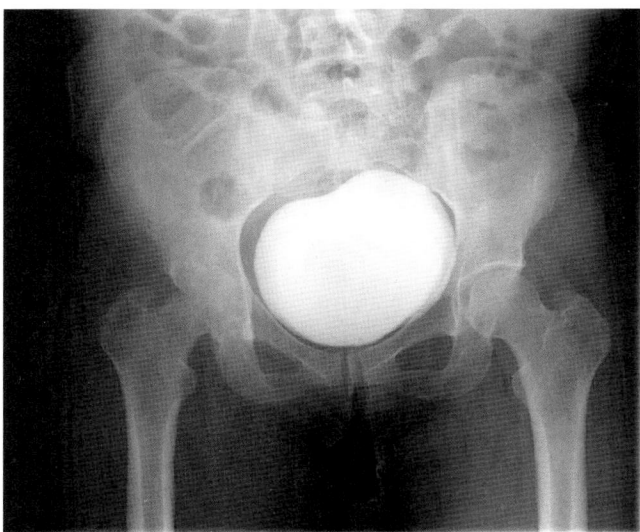

Fig. 125.5 Radiograph of right hemipelvis and proximal femur demonstrate permeative moth-eaten changes, with resultant femoroacetabular joint space narrowing consistent with osteomyelitis. (Courtesy Dr. Peter Evangelista, Department of Diagnostic Imaging, Rhode Island Hospital, Brown University, Providence, RI.)

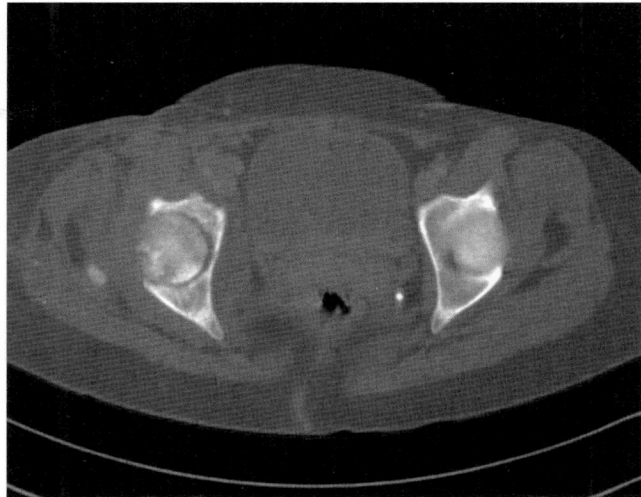

Fig. 125.6 CT scan of osteomyelitis. There is a diffuse moth-eaten appearance involving the right hemipelvis and right femoral head, with abundant periosteal reaction. (Courtesy Dr. Peter Evangelista, Department of Diagnostic Imaging, Rhode Island Hospital, Brown University, Providence, RI.)

cause an elevated ESR, although the degree of elevation of the ESR is often higher with osteomyelitis. In evaluating a diabetic foot infection, an ESR greater than 70 mm/hr predicts the presence of an underlying bone infection.

The CRP level, another nonspecific marker of inflammation, increases within the first 24 hours of infection, peaks within approximately 48 hours, and is usually normal within 1 week of therapy. The CRP level may be a better early indicator of disease, but the ESR is most valuable in following response to treatment. Typically, the ESR falls steadily as osteomyelitis resolves and increases should it recur. However, it is common to see elevations in one and not the other parameter, especially when there is development of a concurrent illness or the infection has progressed so that the ESR rises and stays elevated while the CRP rises and falls. In children, an elevated ESR or CRP level is seen in all cases of osteoarticular infection; sensitivity of the use of both the ESR and CRP value is 98%, but a leukocytosis is reportedly seen in only 35% of cases.

Diagnostic Imaging

Conventional Radiography. Conventional radiography is the initial modality of choice to evaluate osseous changes and, in most cases, will be the only imaging technique used to aid in the diagnosis of osteomyelitis.

Conventional radiography is readily available, relatively inexpensive, and useful in the differentiation of infection from trauma and tumors. The characteristic findings of early osteomyelitis on the plain radiograph are lucent lytic areas of cortical bone destruction (see Fig. 125.4). However, lucency is not detected on radiographs until approximately 50% of bone mineral is lost, which often takes up to 2 weeks from the onset of infection. Although these findings are often difficult to identify on plain radiographs, soft tissue edema, distorted fascial planes, and altered fat interfaces may be present within 3 to 5 days from the onset of infection and can serve as a clue to osteomyelitis in the underlying bone. A periosteal reaction, hypertrophy or elevation of the periosteum, and presence of an involucrum can also be seen, especially in children, given their thinner periosteum (Fig. 125.5). In advanced disease, the lytic lesions are surrounded by dense sclerotic bone, and

sequestra may be noted. By 28 days from the onset of osteomyelitis, 90% of the plain radiographs are abnormal.

Radionuclide Bone Scanning. Radionuclide skeletal scintigraphy (bone scanning) is more sensitive than plain radiography for the early diagnosis of osteomyelitis, and is especially useful in the presence of prosthetics or other hardware. Radionuclide scans can detect osteomyelitis within 48 to 72 hours after the onset of infection. A radioactive tracer is injected into the bloodstream and given time to bind or accumulate in body tissues, after which a camera is used to determine released radioactivity. An image is created that is evaluated for an increase or decrease in expected uptake of the radionuclide. Given the radiation burden associated with this modality, however, in the past 3 decades, there has been a movement away from skeletal scintigraphy to MRI to diagnose osteomyelitis. The amount of time this study requires makes this less than ideal in the emergency department.

Computed Tomography. Even though MRI is the best imaging modality to diagnose osteomyelitis because it can identify early changes in the bone, when it is not available, or is contraindicated, CT is a useful alternative. The bony cortex is seen particularly well on CT, and involucrum and sequestrum formation are easily identified. CT is generally used to detect and define areas of possible infection in bones that are difficult to visualize on plain radiographs, such as the sternum, vertebrae, pelvic bones, and calcaneus. On CT scan, osteomyelitis appears as lucent areas (Fig. 125.6), and gas may be seen in bony abscess cavities. The limitation of CT for the early diagnosis of osteomyelitis is the same as that for plain radiography, in that the disease must be present for more than 1 week for changes to be apparent. When required, the CT scan can guide the surgeon in débridement of infected bone and in choosing a site for diagnostic biopsy. However, the rate of a positive culture even with a CT guided bone biopsy is low and infrequently changes the course of the patient's care,[13] therefore, antibiotics should not be withheld while waiting for this procedure.

Magnetic Resonance Imaging. The use of bone scans and CT for the evaluation of osseous anatomy has been decreasing as the availability and image quality of MRI improves while its cost decreases. MRI findings are often evident before other modalities detect an abnormality with earlier detection of bone marrow involvement and medullary or cortical destruction, periosteal reaction, edema, soft tissue extension, joint

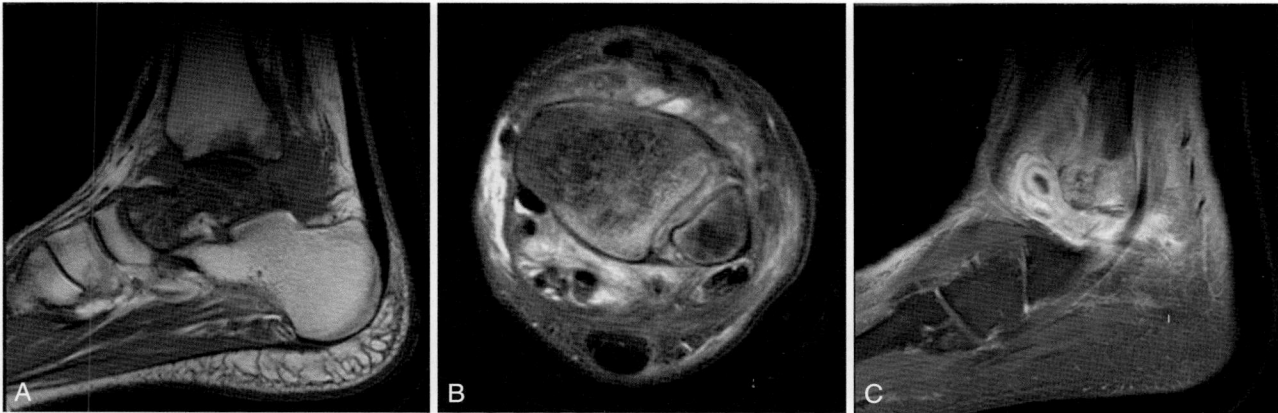

Fig. 125.7 MRI scan of osteomyelitis. (A) Sagittal T1 image shows decreased signal within the talus, suggesting osteomyelitis. (B) Axial T2 image demonstrating increased signal throughout the talus and distal fibula consistent with osteomyelitis (fat-suppressed image). (C) Sagittal T1 image after the administration of gadolinium demonstrates a small focus of nonenhancing fluid just anterior to the distal fibula, suggestive of an abscess. (Courtesy Dr. Thomas Egglin, Department of Diagnostic Imaging, Rhode Island Hospital, Brown University, Providence, RI.)

effusion, articular damage, and complications of osteomyelitis, such as abscess formation. Whereas the presence of ferromagnetic material is a contraindication to the use of MRI, most materials used in orthopedic surgery, such as titanium and chrome cobalt, do not interfere with this imaging modality. Metal may cause distortion of the signal in the area adjacent to a joint prosthesis, but this does not exclude MRI in this group of patients. Osteomyelitis produces a diminished intensity of the normal marrow signal on T1-weighted images and a normal or increased signal on T2-weighted images (Fig. 125.7). These findings, however, are not specific to osteomyelitis; the differential diagnoses for the MRI findings in acute osteomyelitis are trauma, noninfectious inflammatory and metabolic lesions, and cancer. In cases in which a surgical procedure will be done to obtain a microbiologic diagnosis or is needed to treat osteomyelitis, MRI has obvious advantages over other modalities in detailing the anatomy for the surgeon.

The administration of gadolinium as a contrast agent enhances the interface between normal and abnormal marrow, helps distinguish devitalized bone from normally perfused bone, helps identify sinus tracts, and helps differentiate between an abscess and a phlegmon. Gadolinium becomes localized in areas of increased vascularity and blood flow and also helps distinguish soft tissue infections, such as abscesses and cellulitis from osteomyelitis (Fig. 125.8). Contrast improves the specificity of the images on MRI and if there are no contraindications, gadolinium should be used.

Microbiologic Diagnosis

The most definitive way to diagnose osteomyelitis is to obtain infected bone by needle aspiration or surgical resection. This also helps guide antimicrobial therapy. Cultures from draining fistulas or sinus tracts are not an acceptable substitute because these cultured organisms often differ from those in the underlying infected bone. Because osteomyelitis may be polymicrobial or due to unusual microorganisms, especially in immunocompromised patients, cultures for fungal and anaerobic organisms should be included.

Particularly in cases of hematogenous osteomyelitis, cultures of blood, urine, cerebrospinal fluid, when necessary, and pus from other sites of infection can help identify the infecting bacteria. Blood cultures in patients with acute untreated osteomyelitis are positive for the offending bacteria approximately 50% of the time, while in chronic osteomyelitis, blood cultures are almost always negative.

The emergency clinician's diagnostic approach in suspected osteomyelitis is presented as an algorithm in Fig. 125.2. A few key points should be considered with use of this algorithm:

- Radiographs lag behind the clinical picture.
- In infants and children, the amount of radiation exposure with imaging techniques must be considered.
- If the clinical presentation strongly suggests osteomyelitis, a lengthy diagnostic evaluation should not delay empirical treatment. Culture specimens of blood, urine, and other appropriate sites should be obtained and antibiotic treatment started.
- Early osteomyelitis is best identified on MRI with contrast. Other imaging modalities are useful later in the disease course and play an important role, especially when MRI is unavailable or contraindicated, and in concert with other clinical and laboratory findings.

Management

The goal of therapy is to contain the infection before bone necrosis occurs because cure rates fall dramatically once this happens. Medical management with antibiotics is usually sufficient for asymptomatic osteomyelitis that is coincidentally discovered during the evaluation of a patient with fever, weight loss, or bacteremia, hematogenous infection caused by sensitive microbacteria or fungi, or hematogenous vertebral osteomyelitis caused by sensitive pathogens.

For all other types of osteomyelitis, including contiguous focus osteomyelitis, diabetic foot infections, posttraumatic osteomyelitis, and implant-related infection, definitive care is frequently surgical. In these cases, a discussion with an infectious disease or orthopedic surgery specialist, depending on the scenario and available services, is appropriate to plan surgical and medical therapy.

The ideal antibiotic in the treatment of osteomyelitis should be able to penetrate through the bone or the synovial membrane. While most antibiotics fulfill these criteria, penicillin and metronidazole do not penetrate bone as well as other antibiotic classes.[14] Penicillin is reserved for bone contaminated with soil to cover *Corynebacterium* which causes gas gangrene, and penicillin with gentamycin and metronidazole is reserved for bone infections that are contaminated with fecal content. Effective antibiotics should also be bactericidal against the offending bacteria, such as beta-hemolytic streptococci and staphylococci (including MRSA), have low toxicity, be chemically stable at the site of infection, and be relatively inexpensive. The low pH of infected

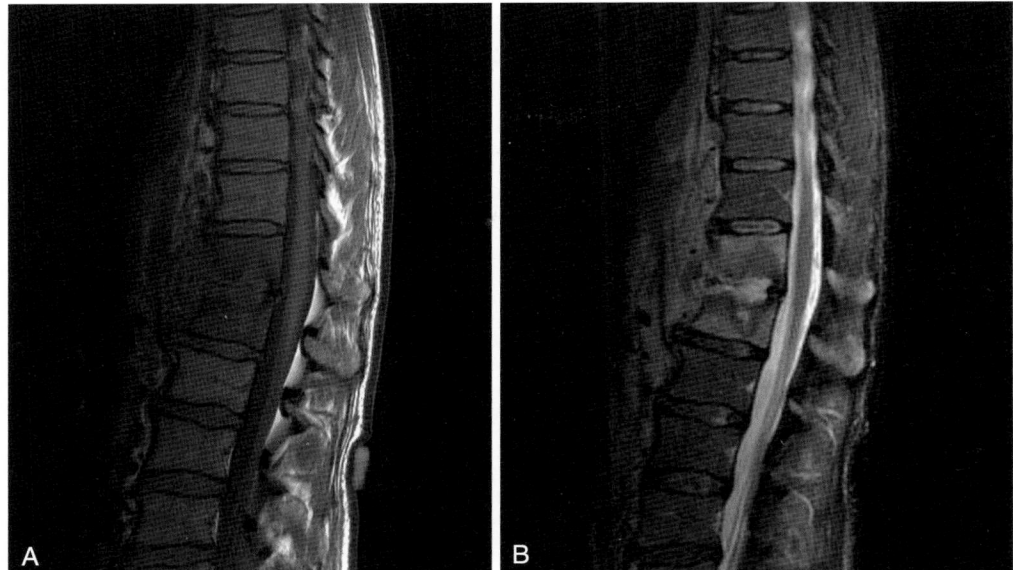

Fig. 125.8 MRI scan of osteomyelitis. (A) There is diffuse, abnormal, decreased T1 signal increase. (B) There is an increased STIR signal through the T12 and L1 vertebral bodies, with loss of the normal disk space and enhancement of these vertebral bodies consistent with osteomyelitis and diskitis. (Courtesy Dr. Peter Evangelista, Department of Diagnostic Imaging, Rhode Island Hospital, Brown University, Providence, RI.)

bone limits the bactericidal action of some antibiotics, particularly the aminoglycosides. Cephalosporins are stable in this environment.

In the ED, the first treatment priority is adequate coverage of *Staphylococcus* spp. with a penicillinase-resistant penicillin, such as oxacillin or nafcillin, or first-generation cephalosporin. In patients with a penicillin allergy, vancomycin is an acceptable alternative. Vancomycin is an often first-line antibiotic when MRSA is considered to be the causative organism. Retrospective studies have demonstrated higher relapse rates after vancomycin compared with those after a β-lactam for non-MRSA bone infections and in those with methicillin-sensitive *S. aureus* (MSSA), so vancomycin should be reserved for those patients with an actual type I penicillin allergy or in whom MRSA is strongly suggested.

Nonenterococcal streptococci are usually sensitive to antibiotics used to combat staphylococci. Gram-negative bacteria, including Enterobacteriaceae, *E. coli, Proteus mirabilis,* and *Serratia marcescens,* are rare causes of osteomyelitis. Third-generation cephalosporins, aminoglycosides, imipenem-cilastatin, and ampicillin are the usual choices for broad gram-negative coverage if this is identified on prior or current cultures. Beyond this initial broad-spectrum therapy, treatment for gram-negative anaerobic bacteria, *Pseudomonas,* and fungal organisms should be based on existing risk factors.

Antibiotics should be dosed to ensure a serum level eight times greater than its minimum inhibitory concentration. Table 125.2 lists common treatment regimens for the variety of bacteria that cause osteomyelitis. The standard recommendation is parenteral antibiotics for 4 to 6 weeks, then transition to an oral course of antibiotics.

Treatment of chronic osteomyelitis is a difficult surgical problem. A variety of adjunctive therapies have been investigated, such as installation of antibiotic-containing beads into infected bone and hyperbaric oxygen therapy.[15,16]

Prevention of posttraumatic osteomyelitis as can occur with an open fracture depends on reducing the concentration of bacteria on exposed bone. The proper management of open fractures in the field is to cut away surrounding clothing, pour sterile saline or water over the exposed bone, and cover the wound with moist sterile gauze bandages or a sterile sheet. Only in the case of severe vascular compromise to the distal limb should an open fracture site be manipulated or realigned because of the danger of introducing bacteria deeper into the wound. Wound surface cultures in the ED setting are not reliable in predicting future pathogens in bone infections and should not be performed. Even a single dose of antibiotics dramatically reduces the bacterial load and should be routinely administered in the emergency department.

Disposition

Patients with osteomyelitis are admitted for IV antibiotic treatment and some will also need operative débridement. After steady-state serum antibiotic levels have been achieved, patients can receive outpatient IV or oral antibiotic therapy.

SEPTIC ARTHRITIS

Foundations

Septic arthritis is an orthopedic emergency, and the incidence appears to be increasing. Even with prompt recognition and appropriate care, septic arthritis leads to a loss of function in 25% to 50% of patients. In the United States, the incidence of septic arthritis in native joints ranges from 2 to 10/100,000 and, in the subset of patients with rheumatoid arthritis, the incidence jumps to 30 to 70/100,000.

Septic arthritis usually results from hematogenous migration of bacteria into a joint and is often a monoarticular process. Like osteomyelitis, septic arthritis may also result from the spread from a contiguous focus of infection, direct inoculation from trauma, or iatrogenically after joint aspiration or injection. The synovial membrane extends beyond the epiphysis and attaches to the metaphysis in the knee, hip, and shoulder joints, allowing bacteria to spread easily from the metaphysis of the femur or humerus into the joint. This explains why septic arthritis may occur concomitantly with osteomyelitis, with infection spreading from bone to joint, and osteomyelitis may also be the result of septic arthritis with infection spreading from joint to bone. The most commonly isolated organism is *S. aureus.* Polyarticular involvement is present in less than 10% of pediatric cases and less than 20% of adult cases.[17] An adjacent infection, such as osteomyelitis and intramuscular abscesses can also occur. A reactive arthritis, which is more common than bacterial arthritis, is a sterile secondary inflammation of a joint, with no identifiable infecting microorganisms in the synovial fluid. Commonly, reactive arthritis occurs after a systemic viral infection but can also develop after a group A streptococcal infection.

Clinical Features

History and Physical Examination

Septic arthritis is usually more acute in onset than osteomyelitis. The predominant symptom of septic arthritis is joint pain, exacerbated with range of motion. The lower extremity is more commonly affected in all populations. In adults, the knee is the site of septic arthritis 50% of the time, followed by the hip (25%) and shoulder (15%). Immunosuppressed patients, especially those receiving corticosteroids, may have septic arthritis with minimal joint pain. It is important in obtaining the patient's history to identify underlying joint disease, such as osteoarthritis, gout, rheumatoid arthritis, or joint surgery or a past medical history for chronic systemic disease, immunodeficiency, prolonged steroid use, or history of injection drug use. In these patients, a careful history may help differentiate chronic joint pain from the acute pain associated with septic arthritis.

On presentation, more than 80% of children and 40% of adults with septic arthritis have a fever; constitutional symptoms such as weakness, malaise, anorexia, nausea, and diffuse myalgias are inconsistently reported. If the hip is infected, the patient may present with referred pain to the thigh or knee. Many children who have septic arthritis will not use the involved limb.

On physical examination, tachycardia and hypotension may indicate a generalized septic process. In the neonate or infant, there may be a so-called pseudoparalysis of the affected limb. This can be mistaken for a neurologic problem; however, an isolated true paralysis is far less common than septic arthritis. The inability of a child to bear weight on a lower extremity or to move any joint spontaneously should be considered a sign of septic arthritis and should be investigated.

In the older child and adult, signs may be more localized. The extremity will usually be held in the position of greatest comfort, which is slight flexion. Palpation of the septic joint will cause exquisite pain, and any maneuver that stretches the synovium, such as flexion and extension, will cause severe pain. The cardinal signs of inflammation—swelling, erythema, and warmth—are commonly found in the infected joint. Joint pain is 80% to 100% sensitive for septic arthritis, and tenderness is 100% sensitive. Periarticular processes such as bursitis, tendinitis, and cellulitis may produce erythema, warmth, and tenderness, but a thorough physical exam can help differentiate from septic arthritis. Palpation of the joint line and maneuvers that stretch the synovium and joint are usually not painful in cellulitis. Periarticular processes also do not commonly produce an effusion. In general, the triad of fever (seen in 45% to 60% of cases), pain (seen in 75% of cases), and impaired range of motion suggests septic arthritis. One caveat with the physical examination is that an increasing number of patients have been receiving chronic immunosuppressive drugs; in these patients, the classic history and examination findings are significantly less dramatic than in their immunocompetent counterparts.

Complications

Septic arthritis leads to two types of serious complications, those involving the joint itself and those that are systemic. The introduction of bacteria into a joint triggers a profound immune response that leads to destruction of the articular cartilage. Bacteria, host synovial cells, chondrocytes, neutrophils, and macrophages all release enzymes and inflammatory chemicals such as collagenase, elastase, hyaluronidase, lipase, and lipoproteinase, which are destructive to the joint. Damaged articular cartilage has limited repair capacity, and a common result of articular cartilage destruction is arthritis or ankylosis, which results in a stiff and immobile joint.

Children are at great risk for epiphyseal damage if the infection extends through subchondral bone. This can progress to growth impairment and limb length discrepancy.

Other tissues adjacent to the joint can be invaded, leading to suppurative destruction of bursae, tendons, ligaments, or muscles. Sinus tracts may lead the infection out through the skin. In the hip, the pressure and edema of a septic synovial effusion can occlude the tenuous blood supply to the femoral head, resulting in avascular necrosis, especially in neonates.

The hematogenous spread of bacteria from an infected joint can produce sepsis, septic shock, and death. Seeding of other sites with bacteria is also a possibility, though less common, and this can produce endocarditis, pneumonia, and systemic sepsis.[18]

Clinical Subsets of Septic Arthritis

Bites. The human mouth is a polymicrobial environment comprised of aerobic organisms, such as *Staphylococcus*, oral gram-negative rods, such as *Eikenella corrodens*, and anaerobes, such as *Fusobacterium*, making bone and joint infections caused by human bites difficult to treat. Similarly, animal bites also lead to a polymicrobial infection, with *Pasteurella multocida* an important additional organism seen in cat bites. Antibiotics should be empirically started, but treatment may also require drainage and débridement.

Infants and Children. Septic arthritis is more common in children than in adults, and the incidence of septic arthritis is twice that of osteomyelitis in children. Two-thirds of pediatric cases occur in children younger than 2 years, and boys are affected twice as often as girls. The offending agent in septic arthritis varies with age. In the post–*H. influenzae* vaccine era, overall, *S. aureus* (methicillin-sensitive more than methicillin-resistant) is the most common infecting organism in all pediatric and adult age groups, followed by group A streptococci and *Streptococcus pneumoniae*. In neonates, group B streptococci, *S. aureus,* and gram-negative enteric bacilli are usual pathogens. *Candida albicans* should also be considered in neonates and premature infants. *K. kingae* has been emerging as an important cause of septic arthritis and osteomyelitis in children younger than 2 years and often appears concurrent or shortly after an oropharyngeal infection. Prior trauma or skin infection may be more common with staphylococcal septic arthritis.

In the pediatric population, the hip and knee have equal rates of infection, with each accounting for about one-third of infections. Patients may have concurrent osteomyelitis, and this diagnosis impacts management.[17,19,20]

Laboratory work, including complete blood count and determination of the ESR and CRP level, are part of the routine evaluation of the limping child but, individually, do not have adequate sensitivity or specificity to rule in or rule out the diagnosis. The Kocher criteria of fever (temperature ≥38.5°C [101°F]), non–weight-bearing on the affected side, ESR greater than 40 mm/hr, and peripheral blood WBC count more than 12,000 cells/mm³ (Table 125.3), can be used to help identify children with septic arthritis of the hip and when combined with the CRP, can help determine which patients require arthrocentesis and orthopedic consultation. When all 5 markers are negative, patients were found to have less than a 1% chance of having septic arthritis.

A synovial fluid analysis should be performed if there is any suspicion for septic arthritis. Even when cultures of synovial fluid and blood are tested, a causative organism is not discovered in up to 30% of cases of septic arthritis in children. Prior antibiotic treatment in children decreases the yield on synovial fluid cultures from 80% to 38%.

TABLE 125.3 Kocher Criteria

No. of Kocher Criteria Met	Likelihood of Septic Arthritis of the Hip
1	3
2	40
3	93
4	99

Gonococcal Septic Arthritis. In the United States, *N. gonorrhoeae* is the most common cause of septic arthritis in sexually active patients. A person with gonorrhea of the urethra, cervix, rectum, or pharynx has a 1% to 3% chance to develop disseminated gonococcal infection (DGI). More than 75% of cases of DGI occur in women, possibly because of their increased risk of asymptomatic infection. DGI is common during pregnancy or after menstruation, when the alkaline vaginal environment makes the organism more resistant to host defenses in the bloodstream and therefore more likely to disseminate. Septic arthritis develops in approximately 40% of patients with DGI.

The classic triad of gonococcal bacteremia is migratory polyarthritis, tenosynovitis, and dermatitis. Asymmetric polyarthralgia, which may be migratory, is the most common presenting complaint, occurring in two-thirds of cases; 25% of patients have monoarthralgia. Polyarthralgia is usually asymmetric and most frequently involves the knee, although the elbow, wrist, metacarpophalangeal, and ankle joints are also affected. The sacroiliac and sternoclavicular joints may be involved, although these sites are far less common. The patient will present with classic signs of a septic joint, including a joint effusion, warmth, tenderness, decreased range of motion, and marked erythema. There is usually no clear progression of DGI and polyarthralgias to purulent monarticular arthritis, and many patients are afflicted with dermatitis and tenosynovitis without the development of true arthritis. Some strains of *N. gonorrhoeae* that produce DGI favor the development of tenosynovitis and dermatitis, whereas others favor the development of purulent arthritis.

Hemorrhagic pustules on the skin, scattered, painless, nonpruritic, small (0.5- to 0.75-cm) papules distributed below the neck that can involve the palms and the soles, are seen in 41% of cases. These papules can turn into pustules on a broad erythematous base with a necrotic or hemorrhagic center. There are usually fewer than 50 lesions, distinguishing DGI from the rash of meningococcus.

The diagnosis of gonococcal arthritis is difficult. In patients who present with localized purulent arthritis, *N. gonorrhoeae* will be isolated in only about 50% (range of 25% to 75%) of synovial fluid specimens.

In septic arthritis due to gonorrhea, the synovial fluid WBC count is often less than 50,000 cells/mm³, Gram stains of aspirated joint fluid are positive for bacteria only 25% of the time, and cultures of the joint fluid are negative in approximately 50% of cases. This may be due to poor culture techniques or because a suppurative reactive process can occur in the joint in DGI, even when bacteria are no longer present. When gonococcal arthritis is suspected, cultures for *N. gonorrhoeae* should be obtained from mucosal surfaces, because these may be the only places where bacteria are readily recovered. Cultures of the genital tract, pharynx, or rectum will be positive in 80% of cases of gonococcal arthritis. Nucleic acid amplification testing of either urine specimens in both men and women or vaginal swabs in women is preferred, if available. This has a sensitivity over 75% and should be performed if gonococcal arthritis is considered.

Gonococcal septic arthritis responds rapidly to antibiotic treatment and, unlike other types of bacterial arthritis, rarely causes permanent damage to the joint. Patients with gonococcal septic arthritis require hospital admission, with antibiotic coverage against the likely pathogens until laboratory results are available. With the rise in fluoroquinolone-resistant gonorrhea, the recommended treatment of gonococcal arthritis is a third-generation cephalosporin, such as ceftriaxone, ceftizoxime, or cefotaxime. Patients are given the first dose via the IV route or intramuscularly in the ED and admitted until culture results are available. A presumptive diagnosis of gonococcal arthritis, or disseminated gonorrhea, is best treated with inpatient therapy involving intravenous administration of 1 gm of ceftriaxone every 24 hours.

Lyme Arthritis. Lyme disease, the most common tickborne disease in the United States, is caused by infection with a spirochete, *Borrelia burgdorferi*. Transmitted by the *Ixodes* tick, it is an important cause of arthritis in endemic areas, and its incidence has been increasing. Lyme disease has been reported in all 50 states, but endemic areas, including Maryland, Massachusetts, Minnesota, New Jersey, New York, Pennsylvania, Wisconsin, Connecticut, Delaware, and Rhode Island, account for 93% of all cases annually. There is a bimodal age distribution in children aged 5 to 9 years and adults aged 55 to 59 years. Children infected by *B. burgdorferi* are more likely than adults to have arthritis as the initial manifestation of the disease. Although it is important to determine a history of a tick bite, up to 30% of people do not remember being bitten.

Arthritis, which is the most distinguishing feature of late-stage Lyme disease, develops in up to 60% of untreated Lyme patients and is manifested months after disease onset. After infection, spirochetes are disseminated and invade synovial joints, resulting in a profound immune response, similar to that seen in bacterial arthritis. Patients with Lyme arthritis present with migratory polyarthralgia that also involves bursae and tendons. This typically evolves into a monarticular process and usually involves single large joints. More than 90% of patients report knee inflammation, but other affected joints include the wrist, elbow, ankle, and hip.

The rash is often overlooked by patients and is generally not present in patients when they present with arthritis. However, fever is noted in up to 50% of all children who have Lyme arthritis. Clinically, the arthritis is similar to other inflammatory processes of the joint and includes warmth, erythema, swelling, and pain on motion of the joints; however, the effusion is usually large and out of proportion to the patient's complaints. The effusion also generally recurs after aspiration, even when the joint is appropriately treated.

The most widely used test for the diagnosis of Lyme disease is the serum antibody titer, including enzyme-linked immunosorbent assay (ELISA) and Western blot testing, but serum testing does not differentiate between acute and past infections. Synovial fluid analysis is not helpful in distinguishing Lyme arthritis and cultures are typically negative, but it usually reveals an inflammatory process with WBC counts that have been reported to have a very wide range, from 500 to 98,000 cells/μL. Arthrocentesis cannot differentiate between bacterial and Lyme arthritis because serologic analysis is similar. Testing of synovial fluid with ELISA or Western blot methods for Lyme disease is not recommended because no consensus exists on how to interpret these data. Lyme arthritis can be successfully treated with oral doxycycline, amoxicillin, or cefuroxime for 30 days. If this is unsuccessful, patients can be re-treated with the same oral regimen for another 30 days, or the antibiotic can be changed to IV ceftriaxone for 14 to 30 days.

Fortunately, Lyme arthritis has an excellent prognosis. Up to 95% of children remain asymptomatic after a single course of antibiotics; adults may show an increased incidence of persistent joint swelling months to years after the initial infection, even after appropriate antibiotics.

Periprosthetic Joint Infections. Infections occurring after joint replacement are a challenging and dangerous complication of arthroplasty, with rates reported to be 0.5 to 2% for knee replacements, 0.5 to 1% for hip replacements, and less than 1% for shoulder replacements. The prosthesis and cement are foreign bodies and are ideal sites for bacterial colonization. The most common infectious agents are *S. epidermidis* (40% of cases), *S. aureus,* methicillin-sensitive and methicillin-resistant (20%), and streptococcal species (20%). Risk factors for periprosthetic joint infections have been identified and include rheumatologic disease, preoperative anemia, coagulopathy, diabetes, depression, and low socioeconomic status. The American Academy of Orthopaedic Surgeons clinical practice guideline summary recommends that patients who present to the ED should initially be stratified to high or low probability for a periprosthetic joint infection. As with many diagnostic maneuvers performed in the ED, a pretest probability helps guide the evaluation.

On history and physical examination, the patient will complain of pain that is constant and present at rest, along with impaired function of the joint secondary to loosening of the hardware. Radiographs may also reveal movement of the prosthesis, bone erosion, new subperiosteal bone growth widening, or more than a 2-mm lucency at the bone-cement interface. The laboratory data should include an ESR and CRP level; if both test results are negative, a periprosthetic infection is unlikely (negative likelihood ratio, 0–0.06); when both test results are positive, a periprosthetic infection must be considered (likelihood ratio, 4.3–12.1). However, many inflammatory processes can result in an elevation of the ESR and CRP level, and these are not specific tests. The use of either test alone is less reliable, and no definitive conclusion can be drawn with just one result. In patients with an elevated ESR or CRP level in whom a prosthetic joint infection is suspected, consultation with the patient's orthopedic surgeon about the decision to perform joint aspiration in the ED and the selection and timing of antibiotics in suspected periprosthetic joint infection is advisable.

A synovial WBC count more than 1100 cells/mm^3 with more than 64% neutrophils is a sensitive and specific marker for periprosthetic joint infection in a patient with an elevated ESR (>30 mm/hr) and CRP level (>10 mg/L). Because of the difficulty in isolating infectious organisms from the prosthetic joint, even if done intraoperatively, in stable patients, antibiotics should not be started until after culture specimens are obtained.

Patients With Existing Joint Disease. Patients with underlying joint disease, especially rheumatoid arthritis or a crystal arthropathy, are at increased risk for septic arthritis. If septic arthritis is suspected, laboratory and radiographic evaluation are of lower yield in patients with these conditions compared to those without joint pathology. To reduce mortality, antibiotics are started immediately after synovial fluid is sent for testing. In patients with a crystal arthropathy, neutrophil invasion secondary to septic arthritis also leads to increased precipitation and release of crystals. Therefore, the emergency clinician who discovers crystals on joint fluid aspiration should not abandon the search for an infectious agent.

Atypical Joints. Septic arthritis can be particularly difficult to diagnose and treat if it occurs in fibrocartilaginous joints, such as the sternoclavicular, acromioclavicular, sacroiliac, or symphysis pubis. Septic arthritis of the axial skeleton, especially of the sternoclavicular joint, is commonly seen in injection drug users, with *Pseudomonas* a common infecting agent. In patients who are not injection drug users, the most common bacterial causes are *S. aureus* and *S. epidermidis.* The presentation is usually pain and point tenderness over the involved joint. Fever and an elevated ESR are commonly reported, although they are not always present because of the often suppressed immune status

of the patient. As with other cases of septic arthritis and osteomyelitis, MRI with contrast is the preferred imaging modality and is helpful in the diagnosis of septic arthritis in the fibrocartilaginous joints.

Differential Diagnoses

Many disease processes can be confused with septic arthritis. Toxic or transient synovitis, an inflammatory process common in children, especially after an upper respiratory infection, can be confused with septic arthritis. It occurs in the 3-month to 6-year age range, usually affects the hip, and is a self-limited disease, with no long-term morbidity. Children with transient synovitis have less pain with passive joint motion than patients with septic arthritis; they do not usually have a fever or appear ill but tend to favor the unaffected leg, as in septic arthritis. The diagnostic evaluation typically reveals a normal WBC count and ESR and no radiographic abnormalities.

Metaphyseal osteomyelitis may mimic septic arthritis because the adjacent joint may develop an effusion, and the two infections can be concurrent. Juvenile rheumatoid arthritis is usually more gradual in onset and produces polyarticular arthritis in children younger than 16 years but may be manifested as a monoarticular process that mimics septic arthritis.

Other diseases of the hip in children that are included in the differential diagnoses are Legg-Calvé-Perthes disease (avascular necrosis of the femoral head) and slipped capital femoral epiphysis; however, these processes are not as acutely disabling as septic arthritis. Rheumatic fever commonly presents with a migrating polyarthritis and may mimic gonococcal bacteremia. Patients with Lyme arthritis are not as debilitated as those with septic arthritis. In endemic areas, serum antibody titers for Lyme should be obtained early in the evaluation of the patient with an effusion.

In the adult, osteoarthritis, gout, and pseudogout may produce findings on joint examination similar to the findings of septic arthritis. Other arthropathies, such as psoriatic arthritis, arthritis associated with inflammatory bowel disease, ankylosing spondylitis, crystal-induced arthritis, and drug-induced arthritis should also be considered in the differential diagnosis of septic arthritis. Collectively, these are known as the seronegative spondyloarthropathies. Trauma to the joint can produce synovitis and hemarthrosis, which may be mistaken for septic arthritis. In a patient with hemophilia, hemarthrosis causes joint inflammation and destruction, and there may be superimposed infection.

Reactive arthritis has traditionally been considered to be a sterile inflammatory response to a distant infection. However, antigens from the infectious trigger are often present in the joint. Several viral and bacterial microorganisms can produce reactive arthritis. The most recognized syndrome is poststreptococcal reactive arthritis. Some other common organisms that cause reactive arthritis are *Chlamydia, Salmonella, Shigella, B. burgdorferi* (Lyme disease), *Yersinia,* human T-lymphotropic virus type 1, rubella virus, hepatitis B virus, adenoviruses, parvovirus, and Epstein-Barr virus. Reactive arthritis can usually be distinguished from septic arthritis because it tends to involve multiple joints in a migratory pattern, the inflammatory process is less severe with reactive arthritis, there is less effusion, the joint is not as hot or tender as it is with septic arthritis, and joint fluid cell counts are usually below 50,000 cells/mm^3.

Diagnostic Testing

Serum and Urine Tests

Blood tests are not consistently helpful in making a diagnosis of septic arthritis. Serum leukocytosis is nonspecific and nonsensitive for diagnosis of septic arthritis. Traditionally, a serum WBC count more than 10,000 cells/mm^3 may suggest a systemic illness but is present in only 50% of patients with septic arthritis, and many sterile inflammatory processes create a similar leukocytosis. The ESR is elevated in approximately 90% of cases and, along with the CRP level, can be used to help diagnose the infection and track resolution. When low thresholds are used in the ED, the sensitivity of ESR is reported to be 98%, with a cutoff of 10 mm/hr or more, and the sensitivity of CRP is 92%, with a threshold of 20 mg/L or more. A sensitivity of 96% for an ESR higher than 30 mm/hr has been demonstrated. A procalcitonin level more than 0.5 ng/mL is another possible serum marker for septic arthritis, but is also nonspecific and is often not readily available in the ED.[21] Synovial presepsin is another potential biomarker that seems to be both specific and sensitive in septic arthritis but needs to be tested further.[22]

Two sets of blood culture specimens should be obtained; however, blood cultures reveal the infecting organism in the minority of cases of both osteomyelitis and septic arthritis.[7,23] Cultures of infectious foci, such as the throat, cervix, and urine, may demonstrate the bacteria responsible for septic arthritis. Synovial leukocyte esterase has been studied as a possible new indicator for a septic arthritis; it is especially sensitive and specific in prosthetic joints, with initial studies showing a high sensitivity and specificity.[24]

Joint Fluid Analysis

The diagnosis of septic arthritis requires joint fluid for culture and analysis. The knee joint is the most likely to be infected and is the easiest to aspirate. Aspiration of other joints, such as the hip, often requires interventional radiology or orthopedic surgical consultation. When violating the joint capsule, aseptic technique should always be practiced. This has resulted in reducing the risk of introducing infection into a joint during intraarticular aspiration or injection, reported to be between 1 in 2000 to 1 in 15,000 injections,

Because joint fluid analysis is not performed as often as other diagnostic tests in the ED, a joint fluid protocol is useful to ensure that all necessary tests are prepared and ordered properly. To increase the bacterial yield from joint fluid, blood culture bottles should be inoculated with joint fluid immediately after joint aspiration. This allows some bacteria, which would normally die before being inoculated on culture media in the laboratory, to survive and grow in the blood culture bottle (brain-heart infusion broth). The sample should include special media to test for fastidious organisms such as *N. gonorrhoeae*. Anaerobic and fungal organisms should be cultured in patients with risk factors for these infections.

When only a small volume of synovial fluid is recovered from a joint aspiration, the single most important test is a cell count. If extra fluid is available after a cell count is obtained, other tests should be performed, including Gram stain and culture, crystal analysis, and joint fluid glucose level. The definitive test to determine bacterial arthritis is synovial culture. Tissue cultures from the operating room are more useful than fluid for identifying the offending organism and its susceptibility, but administration of antibiotics should not be delayed for these results.

Even with an adequate joint fluid sample, proper culture techniques, and the presence of fastidious organisms, synovial Gram staining results in clinically suspected septic arthritis are negative 45% to 71% of the time, likely due to the planktonic state of the bacteria in the joint. A positive result of Gram staining can be used to guide antibiotic treatment; however, empirical treatment should not be delayed if the result is negative.

Traditionally, a synovial fluid leukocyte count of more than 50,000 cells/mm³ with a predominance of polymorphonuclear leukocytes was used to define septic arthritis, but other processes can produce similar cell counts. Up to 30% of patients with septic arthritis have been documented to have counts well below 50,000 cells/mm³.

Many studies have not supported the idea that a specific range of elevation of the synovial fluid leukocyte count can be reliably used to

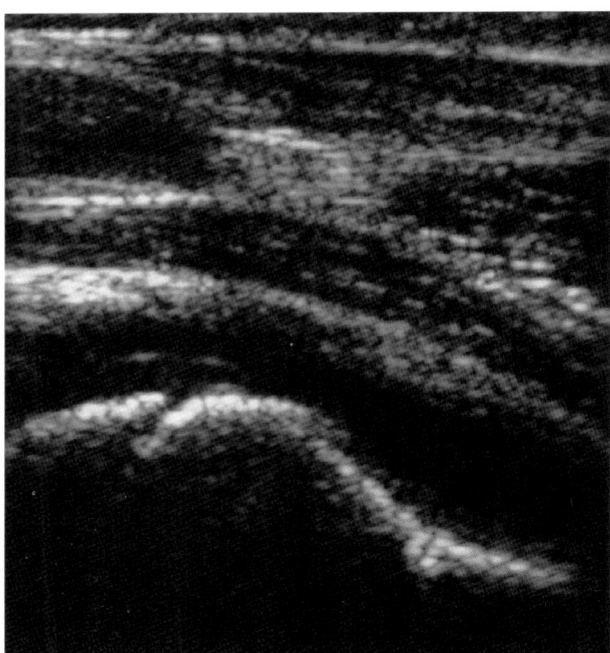

Fig. 125.9 Ultrasound image of the right hip in an 8-year-old girl with septic arthritis. A significant joint effusion can be seen just superior to the round contour of the femoral head. Joint aspiration revealed purulent fluid, with a white blood cell count of 71,000/mm³.

diagnose septic arthritis. One large study found that a synovial fluid WBC count higher than 17,500 cells/mm³ has a sensitivity of 83% and specificity of 67% for septic arthritis. The positive likelihood ratio at this level was 2.5, with a negative likelihood ratio of 0.25. A synovial fluid leukocyte differential count with at least 90% neutrophils suggests septic arthritis, with a likelihood ratio of 3.4; a count of less than 90% decreases the likelihood ratio. There is mounting evidence that one cannot rely solely on the synovial fluid leukocyte count to exclude or include the diagnosis of septic arthritis; this value should be used with the clinical, radiographic, and laboratory findings to help guide therapy as Gram staining and culture results become available.

The examination of synovial fluid under polarizing microscopy for the presence of crystals may be useful in the differentiation of inflammatory from noninflammatory joint disease but is not helpful in identifying infection in this population because the two often coexist. The identification of crystals does not rule out an infectious cause of the joint pain.

Imaging

Plain radiography is not an effective tool for the early evaluation of septic arthritis but may detect surrounding osteomyelitis. In most joints, the small areas of attachment of the synovial membrane to bone are devoid of cartilage. These so-called bare areas at the margins of the joint appear as lucencies or erosions early in the course of septic arthritis. Bone beneath the articular cartilage may start to erode 1 to 3 weeks into the disease. Air in the joint may be a sign of infection with gas-forming organisms but may be the result of a previous joint aspiration. In patients with existing joint disease, radiographs provide minimal assistance in the diagnosis of septic arthritis.

For joints that are not visualized, other than a physical examination, a variety of modalities are available to help detect a joint effusion, which under the right circumstances could suggest septic arthritis. Ultrasonography is a useful modality to help detect a joint effusion and assist in joint aspiration, particularly of the hip[25] (Fig. 125.9). CT and MRI provide detailed anatomic images of the joint, and MRI can also help

TABLE 125.4 Guidelines for Choice of Empirical Antibiotic Based on Gram Staining Results

Gram Stain or Clinical Condition	Probable Organism	Preferred Antibiotics	Alternative Antibiotics
Gram-positive cocci	Staphylococcus aureus Streptococci	Nafcillin or cefazolin	Clindamycin Trimethoprim-sulfamethoxazole Vancomycin
Gram-negative cocci or negative stain Healthy, sexually active patient	Neisseria gonorrhoeae	Ceftriaxone	Doxycycline
Gram-negative bacilli	Pseudomonas aeruginosa Enterobacteriaceae	Piperacillin ± gentamicin	Fourth-generation cephalosporin
Gram-positive bacilli	Propionibacterium acnes	Penicillin G	Nafcillin Vancomycin

Reprinted with permission from: Rao N, Esterhai JL Jr. Septic arthritis. In: Cierny G 3rd, McLaren AC, Wongworawat MD, eds. *Orthopaedic Knowledge Update: Musculoskeletal Infection.* Rosemont, IL: American Academy of Orthopaedic Surgeons; 2009.

determine if septic arthritis is complicated by concurrent osteomyelitis. CT and MRI can identify joint fluid but not necessarily an effusion, because a volumetric analysis cannot be done to assess the amount of fluid. In adult patients with an antalgic gait and painful internal and external rotation of the hip, MRI findings of bone marrow edema led to a diagnosis of septic arthritis only 6% of the time.

Skeletal scintigraphy (bone scanning) has been used in the diagnosis of septic arthritis, but its use has been decreasing. The main advantage of skeletal scintigraphy is for the detection of septic arthritis earlier than with other imaging techniques. In septic arthritis, scintigraphy shows symmetrical areas of increased uptake on both sides of the joint. In a three-phase ^{99m}Tc scan, all three phases will be hot with septic arthritis. In general, skeletal scintigraphy is used only when there is enough uncertainty about the diagnosis to warrant further investigation. However, in joints where aspiration is easier, skeletal scintigraphy has little role in diagnosis.

Management

Septic arthritis is an orthopedic emergency and, once synovial fluid is obtained, empirical antibiotics should be promptly administered based on Gram stain results, when possible (Table 125.4). Whereas many joint infections require surgical joint irrigation and débridement, there are a few cases in which medical management will suffice, such as gonococcal septic arthritis and Lyme arthritis.

Unlike most other infectious emergencies encountered in the ED, when time to antibiotic administration decreases morbidity and mortality, definitive management for most cases of septic arthritis requires surgical intervention and a prolonged course of antibiotics. Therefore, it is more important to obtain synovial fluid for Gram staining and culture than to start antibiotics, because this will guide appropriate long-term antibiotic treatment. In the hemodynamically stable patient in whom septic arthritis is a strong consideration, antibiotics should be held until blood and synovial fluid cultures are obtained.

The selection of antibiotics for the treatment of septic arthritis is outlined in Table 125.2. In most cases, because the emergency clinician does not know the identity of the causative organism, treatment should be tailored to the most likely causative agents based on the patient's age, history, and immune status, as well as results from the gram stain.

In general, if the initial Gram stain of synovial fluid demonstrates gram-positive cocci, empirical treatment starts with vancomycin whereas empirical treatment of gram-negative bacilli starts with a cephalosporin. In cases where pseudomonas is suspected, the antibiotic regimen should consist of two antipseudomonal agents such as ceftazidime with ciprofloxacin or gentamycin. Empirical antibiotic choices when the initial Gram stain is negative but there is still a high index of suspicion for a septic joint typically start with vancomycin.

S. aureus accounts for 44% of cases and remains the predominant pathogen for all age groups. Unless gonococcal arthritis, the most common cause of arthritis in young adults, is confirmed, the antibiotic selected should be bactericidal against *S. aureus*. Empirical antibiotics active against MRSA should be considered but should be based on the prevalence of this pathogen in the community. Group B streptococci have emerged as invasive pathogens in older adults, especially those with diabetes mellitus, cirrhosis, and neurologic disease. Penicillin- and fluoroquinolone-resistant strains of gonorrhea have become more prevalent, and a third-generation cephalosporin is the best choice for gonococcal arthritis. In older adults, gram-negative septic arthritis is more common, and agents such as the third-generation cephalosporins and aminoglycosides are added to the antistaphylococcal regimen. Establishment of good bactericidal serum levels of antibiotics will ensure that the levels in joint fluid are also bactericidal. In pediatrics, the use of dexamethasone to accelerate clinical improvement is no longer recommended.[26]

Disposition

Any patient thought to have septic arthritis requires joint aspiration. Patients for whom septic arthritis is considered to be the diagnosis should be given an initial parenteral dose of antibiotics after joint aspiration in the ED and admitted for culture results and continued management. If the joint fluid aspirate is not consistent with septic arthritis and clinical findings are equivocal, the patient can be discharged and reevaluated in 24 hours. In immunosuppressed patients, patients with preexisting joint disease, and patients with a joint replacement, septic arthritis can be difficult to detect. A conservative approach with in-hospital observation and treatment should be considered if there is any possibility of septic arthritis in these patients.

The prognosis for the patient with septic arthritis is favorable in most cases. From 50% to 75% of afflicted patients can expect to recover completely and achieve full painless range of motion of the joint. About one-third of patients have complications such as decreased mobility or ankylosis, pain on joint movement, chronic infection, or overwhelming sepsis and death. The patients most likely to do poorly include those who have had a delay in diagnosis and treatment, patients with underlying joint disease (especially rheumatoid arthritis), those with polyarticular septic arthritis, and those who have positive blood cultures. Despite many advances in diagnosis and treatment, the overall morbidity for patients with septic arthritis has not decreased in the last 3 decades. A general rule is that if the diagnosis of septic arthritis is made and treatment is initiated within 1 week of the onset of symptoms, the outcome is almost always favorable. Diagnosis and rapid treatment of septic arthritis have proven to be most elusive in two groups of patients, infants and people with existing joint disease. In infants and children, early symptoms can be nonspecific and difficult to assess; consequently, children with septic arthritis, especially of the hip, who experience a delay in diagnosis and treatment have a disappointingly high rate of complications. In patients with existing joint disease, septic arthritis may be mistaken for an acute exacerbation of the underlying disease process, so emergency clinicians must remain vigilant in their pursuit of the correct diagnosis.

The references for this chapter can be found online at ExpertConsult.com.

126

Skin and Soft Tissue Infections

Michael Pulia and Larissa S. May

KEY CONCEPTS

- Bacterial skin infections such as cellulitis and abscess are common and are rarely life-threatening.
- Necrotizing infection is suggested by pain out of proportion to physical findings, crepitance, gas seen on imaging studies, or clinical instability. Suspected necrotizing infection should be managed with prompt broad-spectrum antibiotics and surgical consultation.
- Emergency clinicians should be familiar with toxic shock syndrome and Rocky Mountain spotted fever, which are rare, life-threatening, systemic infections with skin manifestations.
- Antibiotics reduce treatment failure after surgical drainage of uncomplicated abscesses.
- Current recommendations for the treatment of uncomplicated cellulitis suggest selection of an agent effective against streptococci and methicillin-sensitive *Staphylococcus aureus* (MSSA) (e.g., cephalexin at maximal doses). The addition of community-associated methicillin-resistant *Staphylococcus aureus* (CA-MRSA) coverage does not improve outcomes for uncomplicated cellulitis.
- Clindamycin is no longer recommended for routine treatment of purulent SSTIs due to increasing rates of both MSSA and CA-MRSA resistance.
- White blood cell count should not be routinely measured in patients with uncomplicated skin infections.
- Blood cultures are not necessary to evaluate skin infections, except in cases of sepsis, necrotizing infections, immunocompromised hosts, and multifocal infections suggesting hematogenous seeding.
- Mimics such as venous stasis dermatitis are often misdiagnosed as cellulitis. These conditions are termed *pseudocellulitis* and novel tools are being developed that may assist clinicians improve diagnostic accuracy (e.g., ALT-70 and surface thermal imaging).

FOUNDATIONS

Background and Importance

Skin and soft tissue infections (SSTIs) exist on a clinical spectrum from common and typically mild bacterial infections, such as cellulitis and abscess, to relatively rare conditions with high mortality, such as necrotizing fasciitis and toxic shock syndrome. As a group, SSTIs are the third most common type of infection treated in the emergency department (ED), accounting for approximately 2.5% of all encounters.[1] The epidemiology of skin infections remained relatively stable over the past decade since the emergence of community-associated methicillin-resistant *Staphylococcus aureus* (CA-MRSA) as the predominant cause of purulent SSTIs in the early 2000s.

Anatomy and Physiology

The skin is the largest organ in the body and accounts for about 15% of total body weight. It has three layers, the hypodermis, dermis, and epidermis (Fig. 126.1). Hair is present throughout the body except on glabrous skin, which is the heavily keratinized skin found on the palms, soles, and parts of the genitals.

The skin has a rich supply of blood vessels, lymphatics, and nerves, although the epidermis is entirely avascular and relies on the dermis for nourishment. The main cell type in the epidermis is the keratinocyte, which has a cytoskeleton composed of keratin filaments, which are proteins. Also living in the epidermis is the Langerhans cell, a motile, macrophage-like, antigen-presenting member of the immune system that originates in the bone marrow. Melanocytes in the epidermis produce melanin.

The epidermis contains the pilosebaceous follicles and sweat glands, known collectively as epidermal appendages. The combination of the hair apparatus and sebaceous gland is known as a pilosebaceous follicle. The epidermal appendages are important as sites of infection because they provide a break in the otherwise continuous protective layer of keratinocytes and create a potential space for bacterial replication. There are two types, sweat glands and follicles. Sweat glands take three forms—eccrine, apocrine, and apoeccrine.

The dermal-epidermal junction is a complex basement membrane whose disruption results in vesicles and bullae. The dermis consists of cells, fibers, and ground substance, which is an acellular material composed of glycoproteins and other macromolecules. The hypodermis, or subcutaneous tissue, is composed largely of adipocytes. The lymphatic system drains interstitial fluid, and its disruption leads to interstitial fluid accumulation and edema.

Pathophysiology

The source of a skin infection may not always be evident. Skin infections may arise from nonvisible breaks in the protective epidermal layer or more obvious portals of entry such as injections, abrasions or lacerations. Hematogenous seeding from another infected site is a less common source. Venous blood and lymph drain from the orbits and skin around them into the cavernous sinuses; thus, bacterial infections in this area can lead to central nervous system infection.

CLINICAL FEATURES

Overview

Most skin infections present with redness (erythema), warmth, and induration. Erythema, caused by microvascular dilation due to the immune response, can present differently depending upon the patient's pigmentation. Thus, emergency clinicians should familiarize themselves with pathology on different skin types. Confluent erythema is typical of most skin infections; discrete macules and morbilliform (measles-like) eruptions are not typical. Induration means hardening and is a common finding with many inflammatory lesions of the skin. Skin that is indurated from cellulitis may become engorged with interstitial fluid and

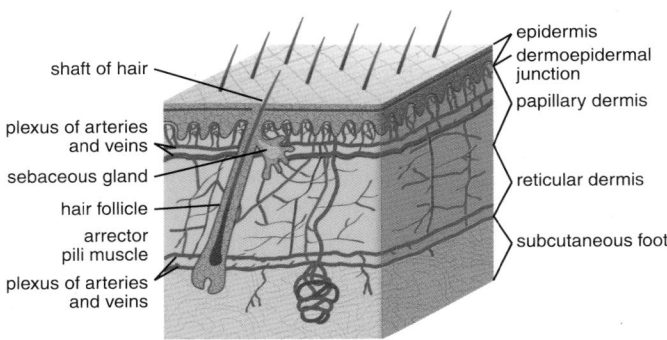

Fig. 126.1 Anatomy of the skin. (From Amirlak B: Skin anatomy. Available at http://emedicine.medscape.com/article/1294744-overview#a1.)

take on the texture of an orange peel due to dimpling where the skin is anchored by hair follicles. This classic finding is known by the French phrase *peau d'orange*. Fluctuance describes a fluid collection palpated on examination. "Pointing" or "coming to a head" conveys a sense of imminent rupture. Crepitance describes skin that feels crackly when palpated and suggests gas is present in the soft tissues.

Many skin infections have characteristic appearances. Well-demarcated erythema with a raised border, particularly on the face, is typical of erysipelas, a streptococcal cellulitis. Linear erythema tracking distally to proximally along a vascular pathway suggests lymphangitis or phlebitis. This usually represents the action of cytokines combating the infection, although proximal spread of the infection is a possibility. Vesicles suggest contact dermatitis, herpes simplex, varicella-zoster, or impetigo. Pruritic serpiginous (snakelike) lesions that are not particularly tender suggest an intracutaneous parasite, such as scabies (hands, intertriginous areas), hookworm larvae (feet or buttocks), or strongyloidiasis. Parasitic nematodes (e.g., Guinea worm) and insects (e.g., botfly) should be considered in the setting of a nodule after exposure to fresh water or insects in developing countries.

Other systemic infections may present with significant skin manifestations. Less common color changes associated with infection stem from small hemorrhages, vasculitis, or septic emboli. Janeway lesions are painless red, purple, or brown spots, usually seen on the hands or feet, due to septic emboli from infective endocarditis. Painless discolorations of the palms and soles may indicate secondary syphilis or Rocky Mountain spotted fever. Petechiae and purpura can indicate overwhelming bacterial infection, as with meningococcemia. When the diagnosis of infection is not clear, vasculitides such as Kawasaki syndrome in children and granulomatosis with polyangiitis should be considered. Intracutaneous pustules on the palms or soles of the feet are often due to a form of psoriasis called palmoplantar pustulosis, which can be uncomfortable for the patient, but is benign.

Fever is present in approximately 20% of patients with abscesses and 50% of patients with cellulitis presenting to the ED. Febrile skin infections are more common in children; in adults, fever may indicate a more serious infection. Skin infections can suggest underlying systemic illness. For example, a young man who presents with balanitis may have diabetes as the underlying problem. Disseminated varicella (other than the primary episode of chickenpox) suggests an immunocompromised state.

CELLULITIS

Clinical Features

Cellulitis is an inflammatory condition of skin and subcutaneous tissue caused by bacterial infection. Cellulitis may be purulent or nonpurulent

and may occur in the setting of wounds, foreign bodies, or impaired perfusion. Purulent cellulitis drains freely, in contrast to abscesses, which are walled off by fibrous tissue and epidermis. CA-MRSA is the leading cause of purulent skin and soft tissue infections in ED patients but is not a common cause of nonpurulent cellulitis.

The cardinal feature of cellulitis is inflammation with increased local blood flow. Pain may be variable, but most patients without neuropathy have some degree of tenderness. The inflammation of cellulitis is typically confluent, although it may be patchy. The borders are typically poorly defined and irregular. Linear or circular lesions should prompt a search for other underlying causes, such as contact dermatitis or Lyme disease. In some cases of cellulitis, there are streaks of inflammation extending proximally from the main area of inflammation along vascular tracts. This finding is known as lymphangitis and is commonly seen with cellulitis due to streptococci and bite wound–associated *Pasteurella multocida*.

When localized edema becomes severe, epidermal layers can separate, leading to vesicles or bullae. This can make it challenging to distinguish cellulitis from other infectious and noninfectious causes of dermatitis. When the border of an area of cellulitis becomes well-demarcated, raised, and palpable, the term *erysipelas* is used. This form of cellulitis is most often caused by *Streptococcus pyogenes*. The bacterial causes of cellulitis vary according to body site, comorbidities, and environmental exposures (Table 126.1).

Diabetic Foot Infections

Diabetic foot infections are the most common cause of hospitalization for patients with diabetes, and an infected wound precedes two-thirds of lower extremity amputations in patients with diabetes. Neuropathy, vascular insufficiency, and hyperglycemia are important factors in the development of diabetic ulcers and foot infections. Although early antibiotic therapy is important in diabetic infections, to avoid antibiotic overuse, uninfected ulcers should not be treated with antibiotics. In addition to antibiotics, diabetic foot infections require careful wound care and, in some cases débridement, revascularization, or amputation.

The most likely organisms in an acute diabetic foot infection are *S. aureus* and streptococci. Chronic wounds are more likely to be polymicrobial with gram-positive and gram-negative organisms, as well as anaerobes. Chronic wounds that have previously been treated with antimicrobials are more likely to involve multidrug-resistant organisms. *Pseudomonas* is uncommon, although is more likely to occur in patients with diabetes than those without. Deep tissue specimens for aerobic and anaerobic culture or bone samples should be obtained at the time of débridement if deep tissue infection or osteomyelitis is suspected. Organisms cultured from superficial swabs are not reliable for identifying pathogens responsible for deeper infection. Osteomyelitis should be considered a potential complication of any deep or extensive ulcer, especially one that is chronic or overlies a bony prominence.

Bite Wounds

A high proportion of cat bites become infected and presumptive antibiotic treatment is appropriate in the absence of signs of infection. The typical agent is *Pasteurella multocida*. Human bites also become infected frequently (≈25%) with polymicrobial (mixed aerobic and anaerobic) being the predominant pattern. Typical pathogens included oral flora (e.g. *Eikenella*, *Fusobacterium*, group A *Streptococcus*) and skin flora (e.g., *S. aureus*). Dog bites become infected infrequently (≈16%) and do not require routine antibiotic prophylaxis.[2] However, certain circumstances warrant prophylaxis, including those on the hands, face, genitals, or areas with poor perfusion, or in immunocompromised patients.

TABLE 126.1 Skin Infections: Bacteriology and First-Line Antibiotic Therapy

Anatomic Variant or Predisposition	Likely Bacterial Cause	First-Line Therapy (Nontoxic and Immunocompetent)[a]
Uncomplicated cutaneous abscess	CA-MRSA	Incision and drainage, consider antibiotics
Nonpurulent bacterial skin infections	Various *Streptococcus* spp., *Staphylococcus aureus*	Cephalexin or clindamycin; adjunctive measures
Purulent cellulitis and wound infections	CA-MRSA, *Streptococcus* spp.	TMP-SMX or doxycycline monotherapy; adjunctive measures
Diabetic foot infection	Mixed gram-positive, gram-negative, and anaerobes	Amoxicillin–clavulanic acid plus trimethoprim-sulfamethoxazole; avoid antibiotics for uninfected ulcers.
Any cat bite or infected dog bite	*Pasteurella multocida*, others	Amoxicillin–clavulanic acid
Human bite (treat presumptively)	Oral anaerobes, others	Amoxicillin–clavulanic acid
Erythema migrans	*Borrelia burgdorferi* (Lyme disease)	Doxycycline
Puncture wound through sole of shoe (treat presumptively)	*Pseudomonas aeruginosa*	Levofloxacin
Buccal cellulitis	*Haemophilus influenzae* type b (vaccine serotype)	Ceftriaxone or ampicillin-sulbactam
Balanitis	*Candida albicans* or group A streptococcus	Fluconazole plus penicillin or amoxicillin; consider diabetes
Liposuction	*Peptostreptococcus* (anaerobe), group A streptococcus	Ampicillin–clavulanic acid ± trimethoprim-sulfamethoxazole
Saltwater exposure	*Vibrio vulnificus*	Doxycycline
Freshwater exposure	*Aeromonas* species	Ciprofloxacin
Butcher, clam handler, veterinarian	*Erysipelothrix rhusiopathiae*	Amoxicillin
Black necrotic eschar with raised border and severe surrounding edema	*Bacillus anthracis* (anthrax)	Ciprofloxacin

[a]For life- or limb-threatening infections, use IV equivalents and add vancomycin.
CA-MRSA, Community-associated methicillin-resistant Staphylococcus aureus.

Water-Borne Infections

Exposure and travel history are important considerations in the evaluation of skin and soft tissue infections. *Vibrio* spp., in particular *Vibrio vulnificus*, are associated with exposure to seawater and can cause severe soft tissue infections and sepsis. Patients with liver disease, such as cirrhosis, are particularly at risk. Infection occurs from contamination of open wounds by seawater or shellfish and rarely by hematogenous spread from the ingestion of contaminated seafood, such as raw oysters. *Edwardsiella tarda* is a rare cause of wound infection after seawater exposure; it has been implicated in serious soft tissue infections, including myonecrosis, particularly in patients with liver disease. *Erysipelothrix rhusiopathiae* is usually associated with a localized erysipeloid eruption with minor trauma, often on the hands of seafood workers.

Aeromonas myonecrosis is associated with exposure to fresh water by penetrating trauma or exposure to aquatic animals. It causes rapidly progressive suppurative infections that often require surgical drainage. *Mycobacterium marinum* causes so-called fish tank granuloma. It typically is manifested weeks after exposure as a papule or nodule that may ulcerate and drain serosanguineous fluid. Multiple nodular lesions may develop along the lymphatics.

Differential Diagnosis

Consideration of potential mimics (i.e., pseudocellulitis) is critical when assessing potential cellulitis because the misdiagnosis rate may be as high as 30% in the ED. Common examples of pseudocellulitis include venous stasis dermatitis, burns, viral infections, fixed drug eruptions, lymphedema, venous thrombosis, gout, and contact dermatitis.[3,4] Venous stasis dermatitis in particular may appear similar to cellulitis. It is typically located above the ankle and is often (but not always) circumferential. Persistent erythema despite elevating the affected limb suggests cellulitis. Cellulitis is rarely bilateral and alternative diagnosis should strongly be considered with this presentation. Symmetric venous stasis dermatitis in the afebrile patient should not be confused with cellulitis. The ALT-70 (asymmetry, leukocytosis, tachycardia, age ≥70 years) scoring system has recently been proposed to help differentiate cellulitis from pseudocellulitis but requires further validation before utilization in clinical practice.[5,6] When any dermatologic presentation is accompanied by fever or lymphangitis, co-occurring cellulitis should be considered. Cellulitis must always be distinguished from more severe necrotizing infections, as discussed later.

Lyme disease causes a rash known as erythema chronicum migrans which can mimic cellulitis. It a bright red, round lesion, usually larger than 5 cm, with central clearing that gives a targetoid appearance. It occurs in only 80% of cases of Lyme disease. When the rash is observed in an endemic area, Lyme disease can be diagnosed and treated without further testing. Lyme disease is transmitted by the deer tick, *Ixodes scapularis*, and attachment of the tick for at least 24 hours is necessary for infection. Noninfectious, localized bite reactions from insects, arthropods, and hymenoptera can be mistaken for cellulitis despite their rapid development. In contrast, cellulitis typically develops over a period of days. The time course should be considered before initiation of antibiotics.

Diagnostic Testing

Wound Cultures

For nonpurulent cellulitis, needle aspiration, superficial swabs, and skin biopsy are unlikely to reveal the cause and are not recommended for typical cases. These can be considered in complex cases involving purulent cellulitis, immunocompromised patients, immersion injuries, surgical wound infections, or animal bites.[2]

Blood Cultures

Blood cultures are not indicated in patients with uncomplicated cellulitis. They are recommended in cases involving immunocompromised patients or those with systemic infection (e.g., sepsis). In the past, blood cultures were recommended for facial cellulitis, due to concern over *Haemophilus influenzae* bacteremia. However, the relevant strain (type b) is now covered by childhood vaccination, leading to a revision of this recommendation.

Radiographic Studies

Radiographic studies are not part of the standard diagnostic process for cellulitis but should be utilized in certain clinical scenarios. When a foreign body is suspected, plain radiographs are obtained, although they occasionally miss small or radiolucent foreign bodies. Ultrasonography can detect many foreign bodies. The location and extraction of foreign bodies can be challenging, however, and emergency clinicians must use their judgment in deciding when to use plain films, ultrasound, or both.

If necrotizing infection is suspected, plain radiographs or computed tomography (CT) may reveal soft tissue gas or inflammation along fascial planes, but cannot rule out necrotizing infection. Ultrasound examination is useful for differentiating abscess from cellulitis, as discussed later.

Plain radiographs are used to evaluate for evidence of osteomyelitis for chronic skin infections, especially in patients with diabetes, peripheral vascular disease, and secondarily infected nonhealing ulcers. Plain films are not definitive, and magnetic resonance imaging (MRI) has higher sensitivity for detecting osteomyelitis. CT with intravenous contrast is helpful when there is concern that a skin infection is an extension of a deeper infection (e.g., post-surgery).

Surface Thermal Imaging

Specialized cameras capable of measuring skin surface temperature have been proposed as a means to help differentiate cellulitis from pseudocellulitis by replacing the subjective assessment of tissue temperature through touch with quantitative data. In a recent study, temperature gradients between affected and unaffected limbs were observed to be significantly greater for cellulitis cases as compared to pseudocellulitis.[7] The use of surface temperature gradients in the diagnosis of cellulitis will require further validation before use in routine practice.

Management

Fig. 126.2 is a universal treatment algorithm for skin and soft tissue infections. The algorithm assumes no prior treatment as previously treated infections failing therapy generally require broader spectrum antibiotic coverage and customized management decisions. Table 126.2 summarizes the most commonly used antibiotics for skin and soft tissue infections. As *Streptococcus* spp. and *Staphylococcus aureus* are the predominant organisms causing cellulitis, first-line therapy is cephalexin 500 mg, four times daily for at least 5 days, or an equivalent oral β-lactam (e.g., penicillin VK, dicloxacillin). Trials examining the addition of CA-MRSA coverage for uncomplicated, nonpurulent cellulitis found no reduction in treatment failure and is not recommended.[8,9] CA-MRSA coverage should be added for all cases of purulent cellulitis and cases of treatment failure. The most common strain of CA-MRSA is highly susceptible to trimethoprim-sulfamethoxazole (TMP-SMX), making this the first-line empiric therapy. Critically ill patients (e.g., severe sepsis/shock) with suspected skin infection source should receive broad-spectrum empiric antibiotics, vancomycin plus piperacillin/tazobactam, and the emergency clinician should assess for a necrotizing soft tissue infection. Vancomycin is the recommended parenteral agent for MRSA.[2]

Two long-acting, broad-spectrum antibiotics, oritavancin and dalbavancin, recently have been approved for skin and soft tissue infections. These novel lipoglycopeptides cover all major cellulitis pathogens, including MRSA, and have extremely long half-lives. This results in oritavancin requiring only a single IV infusion for an entire treatment course and dalbavancin using a single IV infusion per week regimen. Clinical experience with these agents is limited but they have been proposed as a cost-effective alternative to hospital admission for complicated skin and soft tissue infections without an absolute need for admission (e.g., sepsis) or when concerns exist about medication compliance.[10-12] Due to the cost and logistical concerns (i.e., infusion time, follow-up plan) associated with these agents, we recommend using them only as part of an established ED pathway developed in partnership with pharmacy and infectious diseases.

We recommend amoxicillin–clavulanic acid for 3 to 5 days as a prophylactic regimen for high-risk bite wounds (i.e., cat or human source, puncture wound, immunocompromised patient, wounds to the hands/face, or penetrating the periosteum/joint capsule.) It is also the first-line agent for infected bite wounds. Doxycycline and moxifloxacin are second-line alternatives.[2] For severe infections, ampicillin-sulbactam is the first-line IV agent.

Patients allergic to penicillin may safely take cephalosporins in most cases due to limited cross-reactivity.[13] For patients with a cephalosporin or life-threatening penicillin allergy (e.g., anaphylaxis), clindamycin is the first-line alternative.

Although adjunctive measures are commonly recommended in the treatment of cellulitis. Extremity cellulitis responds dramatically to compression and elevation. Patients with cellulitis complicating venous stasis or lymphedema should be educated about the importance of compression with elastic socks, sleeves, or wraps. This is helpful for the acute infection and to prevent future episodes. Nonsteroidal antiinflammatory drugs (NSAIDs; e.g., ibuprofen) are helpful for pain control in the absence of contraindications.

Table. 126.1 summarizes the common skin and soft tissue infections, including causative organisms and first-line treatment. Recommendations in the table assume no treatment failure, necrotizing infection, or systemic illness. Cases involving these scenarios require broader-spectrum antibiotic coverage and customized management decisions.

Disposition

Immunocompetent patients with cellulitis who can take oral medications and adjunctive measures can be managed as outpatients. Hospitalization is generally required for patients with systemic symptoms (i.e., fever), immunosuppression, diabetic foot infections, infected lymphedema, or large, multifocal cellulitis. In severe cases, such as sepsis, broad-spectrum IV antibiotics are initiated in the ED prior to admission. ED infusion of novel lipoglycopeptides may represent an alternative option to admission for patients without an absolute indication for hospitalization.

ABSCESS

Clinical Features

An abscess begins when bacteria multiply beneath the epidermis. Neutrophils are drawn to the site of infection, and various cytokines combine with bacterial toxins to promote the development of purulence. A furuncle, or boil, is an abscess of the hair follicle. A carbuncle comprises multiple furuncles with loculations and connecting sinuses, often with multiple sites of drainage. Carbuncles are more likely to occur on the back of the neck and are more prevalent in diabetics.

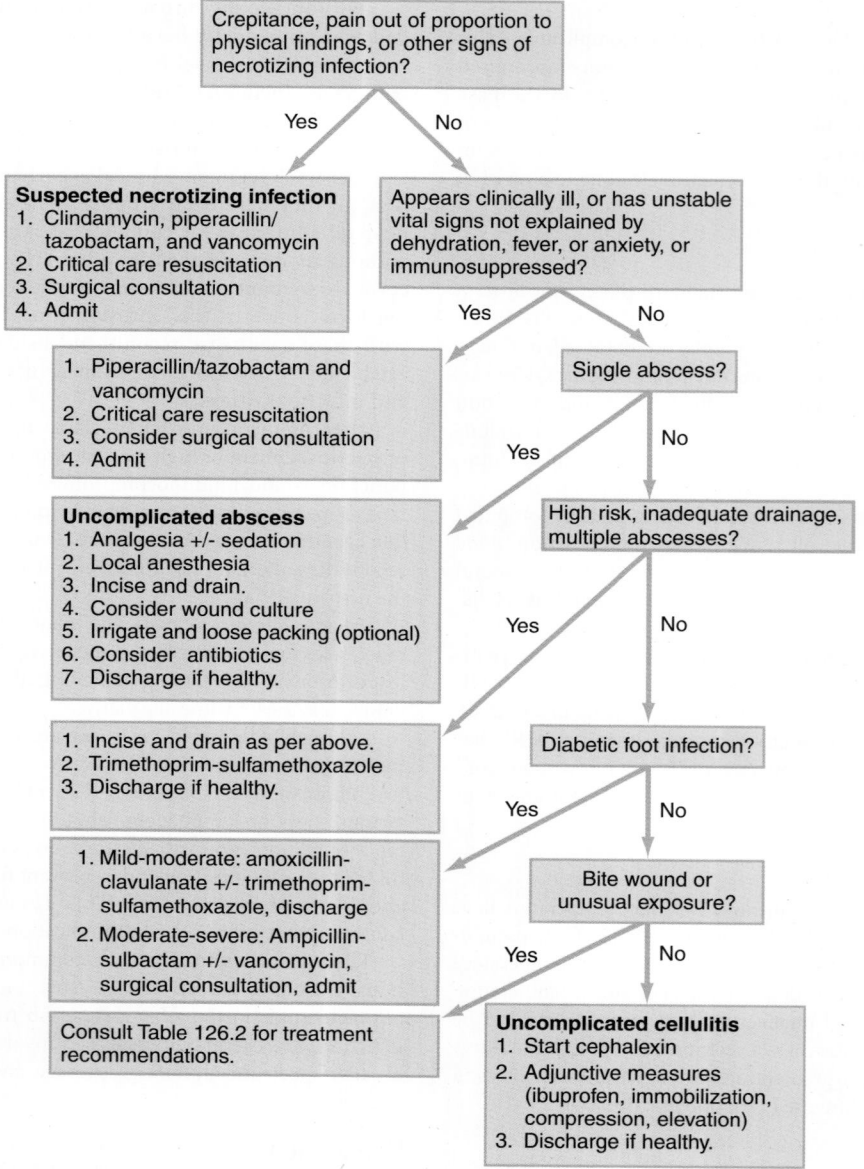

Fig. 126.2 Universal algorithm for skin and soft tissue infections, assuming no prior treatment.

In cutaneous abscesses, the overlying epidermis often prevents drainage and a painful, warm, and erythematous mass is usually seen. Skin abscesses rarely lead to systemic illness and most will eventually rupture through the epidermis and drain spontaneously. Historically, abscesses were caused by MSSA or mixed flora, but today CA-MRSA accounts for the majority of cases in the United States. Whirlpool baths at nail salons have been implicated in mycobacterial furunculosis.

Bartholin gland abscess is caused by an obstructed Bartholin duct. Bartholin gland is located at the upper part of the lower third of the labium majus, and its duct opens onto the mucosa in this area medially but externally to the labium minus. Bacteria cultured are usually a mixture of aerobic and anaerobic flora from the vagina. *Chlamydia trachomatis* or *Neisseria gonorrhoeae* is isolated approximately 10% of the time.

A pilonidal abscess is an abscess at the superior aspect of the gluteal cleft between the buttocks. Because they result from an infected pilonidal cyst, these abscesses are typically recurrent. Acute treatment is the same as for other cutaneous abscesses but patients should be referred for surgical excision of the cyst in recurrent cases.

A stitch abscess is a collection of pus around a suture. Stitch abscesses are generally caused by an inflammatory response in the suture tract and sterile. However, deeper wound infection can be confused with a stitch abscess.

Differential Diagnosis and Diagnostic Testing

The differentiation of abscess from cellulitis can be challenging. Bedside ultrasound examination with a high-frequency linear probe is the best option, improving diagnostic accuracy and management.[14] Abscesses are seen as hypoechoic areas with posterior acoustic enhancement. The hypoechoic areas are pus and may be heterogeneous, with some bright signals (Fig. 126.3A). Cellulitis is seen as a uniformly hyperechoic area or as hyperechoic areas separated by curvilinear hypoechoic areas (see Fig. 126.3B). This appearance is known as cobblestoning and results from interstitial edema.

TABLE 126.2   First-Line Oral Antibiotics for Skin and Soft Tissue Infection

Drug	Mechanism of Action	Pediatric Dose (Mg/Kg; Adult Dose Is Max)	Adult Dose (Mg)	Frequency (Doses/Day)	Special Instructions	Strep	MSSA	MRSA	Anaerobes
Cephalexin	Cell wall synthesis, bactericidal	12.5 qid	500 (max dose 2000 per day)	4		+	+	−	−
Dicloxacillin	Cell wall synthesis, bactericidal	10	250–500	4	Empty stomach	+	+	−	−
Amoxicillin	Cell wall synthesis, bactericidal	15	500	3		+	+	−	±
Amoxicillin–clavulanic acid	Cell wall synthesis, bactericidal	25 bid[a]	875 or 2000 for extended release formulation[a]	2		+	+	−	+
Clindamycin	Ribosome, bacteriostatic	10	300–450	3		+	+	±	±
Trimethoprim-sulfamethoxazole	DNA synthesis (folate metabolism), bacteriostatic	10[b]	160[b]	2	Warfarin interaction, avoid with glucose-6-phosphate dehydrogenase or folate deficiency	−	+	+	±
Doxycycline	Ribosome, bacteriostatic	2.2[c]	100	2	Empty stomach, sun sensitivity	±	+	+	−

[a]Dose by amoxicillin component.
[b]Dose by trimethoprim.
[c]Only for ≥ 8 years old.
MRSA, methicillin-resistant *S. aureus*; *MSSA*, methicillin-sensitive *S. aureus*.

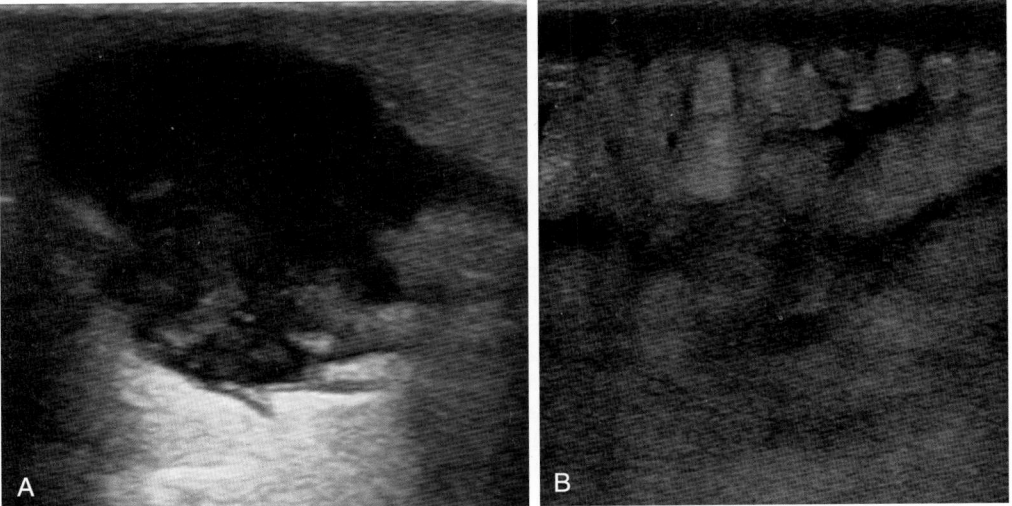

Fig. 126.3 Ultrasound examination to distinguish abscess from cellulitis. (A) Abscess visualized with 8-MHz linear probe demonstrating dark areas (pus) with posterior acoustic enhancement. (B) Cellulitis visualized with 8-MHz linear probe demonstrating cobblestoning. (Courtesy Dr. Mark W. Byrne, Department of Emergency Medicine, Brigham and Women's Hospital, Boston.)

Necrotizing fasciitis is always a consideration, although it is extremely rare relative to cellulitis. Fistula should be considered when perianal, perirectal, or perivaginal infections are evaluated, and the mucosa should be examined digitally. When perirectal abscess recurs, a deep abscess may be the source, and external examination may be unreliable. In this case, CT scanning should be performed.

The epidermoid cyst represents another diagnostic challenge. These lesions, formerly known as sebaceous cysts, are benign cystic tumors resulting from the pathologic accumulation of keratinaceous material. Patients report a long history of a cutaneous mass, often intermittently painful. These lesions become inflamed periodically and sometimes rupture spontaneously. With rupture, they drain a pearly white or yellowish, glistening, waxy material. Pus, which appears dull and viscous rather than waxy, may indicate an infected epidermoid cyst. Isolated mild inflammation of an epidermoid cyst does not contraindicate primary excision, although primary excision is more difficult during an episode of inflammation. A brief course of antibiotics and NSAIDs with delayed excision is also an option.

Vascular aneurysms and enlarged lymph nodes can be misdiagnosed as abscesses. Ultrasound examination is helpful to distinguish the pathology, and a color Doppler study should be used to investigate perivascular abscesses. When there is doubt, needle aspiration should be used to confirm the presence of pus and absence of blood.

Inflamed cutaneous nodules and cystic masses in returning travelers and immigrants from developing countries present special diagnostic challenges. Typical staphylococcal abscesses are most common, but parasitic causes, such as dracunculiasis and myiasis, should be considered.

Management

The primary treatment of abscess is surgical drainage. Needle aspiration alone has not been found to be an adequate alternative to incision and blunt dissection.

Abscess incision and drainage is a nonsterile procedure, but the operator and all environmental fomites should be protected from contamination and transmission of infectious material. The main challenge is to attain adequate analgesia. Injection of local anesthetics into the skin overlying an abscess is difficult because the skin is usually edematous and tense. Also, superficial anesthesia is often inadequate for blunt dissection. An alternative is to administer procedural sedation. Another excellent option is regional anesthesia with a nerve block. Oral analgesia plus a ring block may also provide adequate anesthesia and analgesia. The following medications are safe together and have additive effects: ibuprofen, acetaminophen, oxycodone, and low-dose diazepam. The ring block is performed with a 25-gauge needle (3.5-inch spinal needle for large areas) to inject bupivacaine in a ring around the abscess, with as few punctures through the skin surface as possible and with care taken that the injection not spread bacteria from infected to healthy tissue. At least 20 minutes should be allowed for this to take effect.

Once anesthesia has been attained, incision and drainage of an abscess involves four steps—incision, blunt dissection to disrupt loculations, irrigation, and packing. The skin is prepared with povidone-iodine, although this is a nonsterile procedure and expensive sterile gloves are not needed. A single incision across the abscess is made, but there is little evidence to guide us in determining how large to make the incision. Incisions parallel to cutaneous tension lines will leave smaller scars. A small clamp is used to probe the cavity and disrupt loculations by opening the clamp through the loculations. Blunt dissection rarely risks injury to vessels and nerves, but the initial sharp incision should be made with such structures in mind. The drained cavity can be irrigated to break loculations further, although there is no evidence to support the practice. Traditionally, the abscess is then packed and left to heal without closure; however, packing may increase pain and the evidence to support this practice is lacking. The loop technique, which involves placing a tied sterile rubber tube through the central incision and a secondary lateral incision, allows continuous drainage and has been proposed as a less painful alternative to traditional packing.[15,16] There is insufficient evidence to institute routine use of loop drainage or primary closure of abscesses immediately after incision and drainage, although these can be considered on a case by case basis.

Bartholin abscesses are drained from the mucosal rather than from the cutaneous surface. The Word catheter is a device used to keep the surgical wound from closing (Fig. 126.4) because the abscess will recur if the wound is allowed to close. A very small incision (≈3 mm) is made, and the cavity is drained. The catheter is inserted and inflated with about 4 mL of water or saline. The catheter should be left in place for 4 to 6 weeks so that a sinus tract will have time to form. Sitz baths may help keep the area clean and draining. Marsupialization is used in recurrent cases to prevent further recurrences and is usually deferred

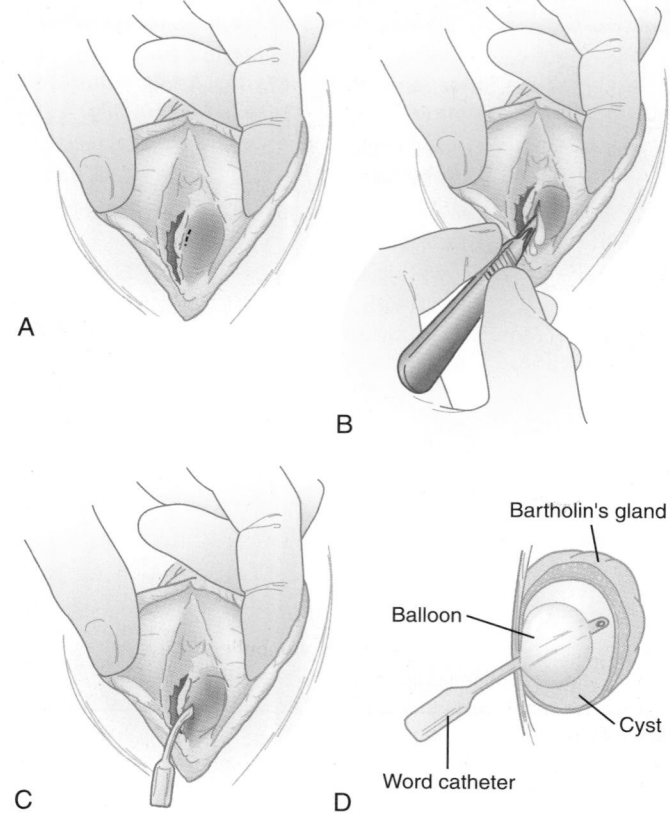

Fig. 126.4 (A–D) Drainage of Bartholin abscess and use of a Word catheter.

until the acute inflammation has subsided. A large incision is made, and the interior of the abscess is then sutured to the surrounding mucosa so that the abscess is sutured open.

The optimal approach to adjunct antibiotics following an adequate incision and drainage of abscesses is a matter of ongoing controversy.[17,18] Two recent, large randomized controlled trials focused on uncomplicated abscesses demonstrated a reduction in treatment failure (including recurrent abscesses) with antibiotic therapy. However, the numbers needed to treat ranged from 7 to 26 depending on how treatment failure was defined. A majority of patients in the control groups had clinical cure without antibiotics (70% to 90%).[19,20] Subgroup analysis of one trial demonstrated that patients with history of MRSA, MRSA as the causative organism, or fever derived the most benefit from antibiotic therapy.[21] Expert consensus suggests antibiotic decisions following incision and drainage for uncomplicated abscesses include an individualized patient risk/benefit assessment and shared decision making.[17,18] Routine antibiotics are recommended in patients with limited access to follow-up care and in severe or complicated cases, including: multiple sites of infection, associated cellulitis, systemic illness, associated comorbidities or immunosuppression, extremes of age, abscess in an area difficult to drain (e.g., face, hand, genitalia), septic phlebitis, and poor response to incision and drainage alone (see Fig. 126.2).

Universal wound cultures for uncomplicated abscesses are not recommended but they should be considered in cases of recurrent infections, treatment failure, or when considering treating with more than one antibiotic to facilitate tailoring of therapy. Although not widely implemented, rapid (≈90 minute) MSSA/MRSA polymerase chain reaction assays are available and can assist in tailoring of therapy to a single agent when providers are considering dual antibiotic coverage.[22]

Disposition

Patients can be discharged to home after incision and drainage of an uncomplicated abscess. It is traditional to schedule one or more visits for wound checks, but many patients can remove the packing themselves after 2 to 4 days and be instructed to return for reevaluation only in cases of persistent or worsening pain or other symptoms indicative of treatment failure. Admission can be considered for severe or complicated cases as defined previously.

IMPETIGO

Impetigo is a common superficial skin infection that is most prevalent in children aged 2 to 5 years, but it can occur at any age. It is communicable, spread by person to person transmission, autoinoculation, and fomites. It may be manifested as an infection of previously intact skin or may infect skin that has been damaged from minor trauma or atopic dermatitis.

Impetigo rarely progresses to systemic illness. However, most cases of poststreptococcal glomerulonephritis are believed to be caused by impetigo and not pharyngitis. Its onset is usually 10 days after the onset of impetigo but may occur up to 5 weeks later.

Clinical Features and Management

The two main forms of impetigo are nonbullous and bullous. Nonbullous impetigo, or impetigo contagiosa, is the most common. It was believed for many years that group A streptococci were the primary cause of this disorder, but studies have subsequently shown that most cases are due to *S. aureus*. Approximately one-third of cases have *S. pyogenes* isolated, usually in combination with *S. aureus*. The lesions begin as thin-walled vesicles that progress to pustules; subsequent rupture results in the characteristic so-called honey crusted lesions, typically found on the face or extremities. Associated lymphadenopathy is common.

Bullous impetigo is caused by *S. aureus,* including CA-MRSA. The bacteria produce an epidermolytic toxin that causes separation of the dermal-epidermal junction, resulting in bullae. The lesions in bullous impetigo are fewer and larger (0.5–3 cm) but rupture less readily than the vesicles of the nonbullous form. After rupture, the bullae leave a thin brown crust.

Ecthyma, or deep impetigo, is a less common ulcerative form of impetigo that extends through the epidermis into the dermis. It is manifested as ulcers with a punched-out appearance, with raised reddened margins covered with thick crust. It has a predilection for the lower extremities. Unlike impetigo, ecthyma can result in cutaneous scarring. Impetigo can be confused with contact dermatitis, varicella, herpes simplex, bullous pemphigoid, and Stevens-Johnson syndrome. It does not affect mucous membranes.

Nonbullous impetigo should be treated with topical mupirocin, which is active against most MRSA strains; however, extensive disease or multiple lesions should be treated with oral agents effective against MRSA. Bullous impetigo should be treated with systemic antibiotics active against MRSA and streptococcus (e.g., cephalexin plus trimethoprim-sulfamethoxazole). Ecthyma should also be treated with oral antibiotics, but it is rarely caused by CA-MRSA. Therefore, we recommend 7 days of either cephalexin or dicloxacillin as first-line treatment.

FOLLICULITIS

Folliculitis is a superficial inflammation of the hair follicle that is limited to the epidermis. It has many causes, including eosinophilic and drug-related factors, but it is usually an infection due to *S. aureus*.

Clinical Features and Management

Folliculitis is diagnosed clinically by its characteristic appearance of a small (2–5 mm), raised, erythematous, painful, tender lesion(s) that is typically pruritic. It can affect any hair-bearing area of the skin and is often associated with shaving. Folliculitis barbae involves the shaved beard area of the face or shaved scalp. Hot tub folliculitis is a pruritic condition caused by *Pseudomonas aeruginosa* that develops within 48 hours of bathing in a contaminated hot tub or swimming pool or from use of contaminated sponges. The rash consists of larger pustules and may have well-demarcated margins, typically involving the area of skin that was under the bathing suit. Candidal folliculitis occurs primarily in immunosuppressed patients and in individuals treated with broad-spectrum antibiotics. Eosinophilic folliculitis is a noninfectious recurrent disorder of unknown cause. It is more likely to occur in immunocompromised patients and is considered an AIDS-defining illness.

Folliculitis usually resolves on its own but can be treated with warm compresses or topical mupirocin. Multiple sites or a large cluster can warrant systemic antibiotics, although no randomized trials have been conducted on the efficacy of this treatment. Shaving of the involved area should be avoided. Hot tub folliculitis usually resolves on its own without specific treatment, but antihistamines and ciprofloxacin are treatment options. Fungal folliculitis is treated with topical antifungal agents. AIDS-associated folliculitis may be eosinophilic or fungal and may be treated with isotretinoin topically or systemic antifungals, respectively.

ACNE VULGARIS AND HIDRADENITIS SUPPURATIVA (ACNE INVERSA)

Acne vulgaris is a common cutaneous disorder involving the face, neck, or proximal upper extremities. It has an increased prevalence in adolescence with a male predominance. The exact pathogenic mechanism of acne is unknown but it is thought to originate in the sebaceous glands via androgen-mediated increased production of sebum and subsequent overgrowth of bacteria. An immune response then results in the formation of inflammatory papules, pustules, and nodules. Hidradenitis suppurativa (acne inversa) is an exquisitely painful condition usually seen in the axilla. It may also occur in other apocrine gland–bearing skin, including the perineum, breasts, and inner thighs. It is about three times more common in females than in males. There is some familial predisposition. The typical onset is between puberty and 40 years. It is currently believed to be an acneiform disorder that begins with follicular occlusion, rather than infection of the sweat glands. This has led to suggestions that the term *hidradenitis suppurativa,* which means suppurative inflammation of the sweat glands, be replaced with the term *acne inversa,* which implies an origin of follicular obstruction. The pathophysiologic mechanism remains incompletely understood and is likely to be a complex interaction of hormonal, environmental, and genetic factors.

Clinical Features and Management

Acne vulgaris manifests as papules, pustules, and nodules of varying severity. It is not typically associated with cellulitis or abscess formation. Acne fulminans is a rare complication involving large nodular lesions with associated ulcerations that can have systemic manifestations. Additional known complications include folliculitis, scarring, hyperpigmentation, and adverse psychosocial effects. The clinical course of hidradenitis varies from intermittent isolated inflamed nodules to recurrent draining cysts and sinuses that can progress to a chronic and debilitating condition that is difficult to treat. Recurrences can lead to scarring, sinus tract formation, and disfigurement. This is a debilitating disease, and patients suffer not only from pain but also from social stigma due to the odor that may accompany the lesions and may suffer reactive depression.

Recommended therapies for acne vulgaris include oral doxycycline, topical clindamycin, or topical retinoids. Acne fulminans is managed with systemic steroids initially followed by isotretinoin, and dermatology consultation is recommended.

For hidradenitis, incision of painful nondraining lesions can be considered for symptomatic relief although it is uncertain whether this accelerates healing. Systemic antibiotics are usually prescribed for symptomatic lesions and should cover CA-MRSA. Perianal and vulvar manifestations of Crohn disease can mimic hidradenitis and should be considered as part of the differential for lesions in these areas. Perianal and vulvar hidradenitis lesions should be treated more broadly with agents active against CA-MRSA, gram-negative organisms, and anaerobes. Amoxicillin–clavulanic acid plus trimethoprim-sulfamethoxazole is recommended in this scenario.

The optimal approach to long-term management of hidradenitis is unclear. Options include immunomodulators (e.g., steroids, cyclosporine), hormones, and en bloc resection. All patients should be instructed to stop smoking and keep the affected area(s) clean and dry. Pain control is essential. Patients rarely show signs of systemic illness and thus can be discharged and referred to a plastic surgeon or dermatologist.

NECROTIZING SKIN AND SOFT TISSUE INFECTIONS

Clinical Features

Necrotizing infections progress rapidly, cause extensive tissue destruction, and can be fatal despite prompt treatment. Clinical manifestations that suggest a necrotizing infection are signs of systemic toxicity, including abnormal vital signs, severe pain or pain out of proportion to physical findings, altered mental status, rapidly advancing infection, crepitus, hemorrhage, sloughing, and blistering. Some patients appear well at presentation, and overlying skin may not be involved initially. Extensive tissue destruction occurs eventually; the mortality rate is 20%.

Risk factors include diabetes, vascular insufficiency, and immunosuppression, although healthy people are vulnerable. Inciting events include penetrating trauma, recent surgery, varicella infection, injection drug use, burns, and childbirth.

Typical bacterial isolates include group A beta-streptococci, *S. aureus*, including CA-MRSA, enterococci, Enterobacteriaceae, and the anaerobes *Bacteroides* and *Clostridium*. Most cases are polymicrobial. The classification schemes historically used for necrotizing infections are less important than optimizing early identification and pursuing prompt surgical treatment.

Necrotizing fasciitis is an aggressive infection of subcutaneous tissues that spreads rapidly along fascial planes. In the operating room, the fasciae are inflamed, and tissue layers separate friably. It is caused by direct extension from a skin lesion in 80% of cases. Two types are described. Type I is polymicrobial, with aerobes and anaerobes; it is more common in diabetics and immunocompromised individuals. Type II is caused by a single organism, and occurs in any age group and in patients who are not chronically ill. Group A streptococci are most common, and CA-MRSA is also a cause, although it appears to be less virulent. Initial symptoms may be vague (e.g., malaise, fever, body aches, nausea, diarrhea). There may initially be diffuse or fusiform swelling of an extremity, or it may appear to be a simple cellulitis or wound infection. Physical findings may not be obvious initially, and pain out of proportion to physical findings can be an early clinical indicator. Eventually, the skin turns violaceous or ecchymotic. Anesthesia may develop over the involved tissue because of infarction of superficial nerves. Subsequent inflammation may result in the classic sign of "woody" subcutaneous tissues.

Skin infections in the perineum warrant extra caution. *Fournier gangrene* is the term given to necrotizing polymicrobial infections of the perineum. Fournier gangrene progresses rapidly to extend to the entire perineum or abdominal wall. It can be recognized by severe pain, tenderness, and induration.

Myonecrosis, myositis, and pyomyositis refer to infections of muscle, which are rare. They may result from local spread of an adjacent infection, penetrating trauma, vascular insufficiency, or hematogenous spread. Clostridial myonecrosis, also known as gas gangrene, has two forms, a more common traumatic form and a rare spontaneous form. The traumatic form typically occurs from an injury that results in an interruption in the blood supply, and crush injuries are often implicated. The infection is most commonly due to *Clostridium perfringens,* a gram-positive spore-forming bacillus that is ubiquitous in nature, including the human body. Inoculation of the organism into tissue with low oxygen tension allows proliferation. Exotoxins destroy tissue, contribute to shock, and may cause intravascular hemolysis, with anemia and disseminated intravascular coagulation (DIC). Patients present with severe pain. The skin may initially be pale, then bronze, and eventually purplish red. Hemorrhagic bullae may develop. Soft tissue gas may not be present initially. Systemic toxicity and shock ensue when aggressive treatment is not initiated early and sometimes occur despite aggressive treatment. The spontaneous form of clostridial myonecrosis is very rare and occurs without any inciting wound. It is usually due to *Clostridium septicum* and occurs in patients with bowel disease, such as colon cancer. Synergistic nonclostridial myonecrosis is a related syndrome, usually seen in the immunocompromised.

Anaerobic streptococcal myositis usually results from trauma or is a postoperative complication. It resembles clostridial myonecrosis but has a more insidious course. It is caused by anaerobic streptococci, including *Peptostreptococcus,* but the infection may also include group A streptococci and *S. aureus*.

Spontaneous gangrenous myositis—also known as spontaneous streptococcal gangrenous myositis, group A streptococcal necrotizing myositis, or streptococcal myonecrosis—is rare but aggressive and fatal in most cases. It occurs spontaneously, without trauma, in immunocompetent hosts. Gangrenous necrosis of skeletal muscle then results in severe pain, with tense local swelling.

Pyomyositis is a deep abscess within striated muscle resulting from the hematogenous spread of bacteria in the setting of muscle injury. It is usually due to *S. aureus,* including CA-MRSA, and is more common in those who are immunocompromised. Mortality is less than 10%.

Differential Diagnosis and Diagnostic Testing

A necrotizing infection should be considered when a patient with a skin or soft tissue complaint presents with a rapidly progressing course or pain out of proportion to clinical findings. It should also be considered when the patient appears systemically ill (tachypnea, hypotension) or has tachycardia not explained by fever or dehydration. Crepitance or radiographic air is diagnostic of a necrotizing infection unless there is another explanation (e.g., recent surgery).

Phlegmasia cerulea dolens is iliofemoral vein thrombosis, which can be confused with necrotizing fasciitis. Arterial insufficiency causes gangrene, and it may be difficult to determine whether infection is present in severe or chronic cases. Similarly, compartment syndrome can be confused with necrotizing infection or coexist with it.

The diagnostic gold standard is the characteristic appearance of the tissue by direct visualization in the operating room. Some surgeons may elect to perform an exploration at the bedside.

The use of blood tests as part of scoring systems to help differentiate necrotizing infections from other skin infections has been proposed (e.g., Laboratory Risk Indicator for Necrotizing Fasciitis [LRINEC]). While laboratory values and scoring systems can assist in risk stratification, given the catastrophic consequences of delayed diagnosis and lack of validation, they should not be used alone to guide clinical decision making. The diagnosis of necrotizing infection remains clinical. Universal laboratory screening of well-appearing patients with uncomplicated skin and soft tissue infections is not recommended to evaluate for this rare condition.

Plain radiographs may show air in the soft tissues, but absence of this finding does not rule out necrotizing infection. Ultrasound examination can visualize the abscess of pyomyositis and evaluation for subcutaneous thickening, air, and fascial fluid (STAFF exam) has been proposed as a rapid modality for diagnosis, especially in unstable patients. CT and MRI may show compelling evidence of a necrotizing infection but can be time-consuming and delay definitive management. There is no established optimal use of imaging in these cases. The decision to pursue imaging depends on a patient's clinical status and the consistency of their presentation with a necrotizing soft tissue infection. If clinical suspicion is high, the diagnosis should not be ruled out solely based on any imaging modality.

Management and Disposition

Patients with suspected necrotizing infections should be treated for sepsis, with IV fluids as indicated by their hemodynamics and prompt administration of broad-spectrum antimicrobials. A good empiric regimen is clindamycin plus a broad-spectrum β-lactam such as piperacillin-tazobactam (gram negatives, anaerobes, *Streptococcus* spp., *Pseudomonas aeruginosa*) plus vancomycin (*S. aureus*, MRSA). Clindamycin, in addition to providing bacterial coverage, may reduce bacterial toxin (virulence proteins) synthesis and reduce disease severity.[23] Maximal doses of all antibiotics should be used.

When a necrotizing infection is suspected, a surgeon should be consulted in tandem with the diagnostic workup. The patient should be prepared for the operating room by being made NPO, ordering coagulation studies, and a type and screen. Repeated operative débridement is often needed. Fasciotomies are often necessary because these syndromes are associated with elevated compartment pressures, which contribute to myonecrosis. The efficacy of hyperbaric oxygen in the management of necrotizing infections is unproven, and treatment should not delay surgery.

TOXIC SHOCK SYNDROMES

Clinical Features

The main systemic, toxin-mediated, bacterial skin syndromes are streptococcal toxic shock syndrome, staphylococcal toxic shock syndrome, and staphylococcal scaled skin syndrome. These are caused by bacterial exotoxins known as superantigens because they cause a severe and pathologic host immune system response by stimulating T lymphocyte activation and functioning as mitogens in vitro. Systemic disease results from the immune system's response to the toxin, but may be accompanied by or simply resemble bacteremic septic shock (Table 126.3).

Streptococcal Toxic Shock Syndrome

Streptococcal toxic shock syndrome (TSS) is a severe, toxin-mediated syndrome that rapidly progresses to shock, with multiorgan failure and death. Identified in the mid-1980s, this syndrome is caused by group A streptococci, often in the setting of a severe soft tissue infection. Most victims were previously healthy. Rarely, TSS can occur as a complication of disseminated varicella (chickenpox).

Invasive group A streptococcal infections are often due to M-type isolates with potent exotoxins. Signs and symptoms are caused by pyrogenic exotoxins A and B. These act as superantigens and cause overactivation of T cells with a massive release of cytokines, including interleukins and tumor necrosis factor.

Patients may have an influenza-like prodrome with nausea, vomiting, diarrhea, myalgias, and chills. High fever, hypotension, and tachycardia are typical. Altered mental status with confusion is common. A diffuse rash is present in 10% of cases, which may make differentiation from staphylococcal TSS more difficult.

On presentation, the patient has a severe streptococcal infection; necrotizing fasciitis is present in 50% of cases. Pain is often out of proportion to physical findings. Most patients present with shock or develop it within 4 to 6 hours. Bacteremia is common, with positive blood cultures in about 60% of cases. Serious multisystem complications are common, including DIC, acute renal failure, and acute respiratory distress syndrome. In contrast to staphylococcal TSS, which is infrequently fatal, about 30% to 80% of patients diagnosed with streptococcal TSS die. Epidermolysis, typical of staphylococcal TSS, is not characteristic of the streptococcal variety.

TABLE 126.3 Comparison of Features of Streptococcal Toxic Shock Syndrome (TSS), Staphylococcal Toxic Shock Syndrome, and Staphylococcal Scalded Skin Syndrome (SSSS)

Parameter	Streptococcal TSS	Staphylococcal TSS	SSSS
Organism	*Streptococcus pyogenes*	*Staphylococcus aureus*	*Staphylococcus aureus*
Toxin	Pyrogenic exotoxins	TSS type 1; enterotoxins A, B, C	Epidermolytic toxin A or B
Patient	Previously healthy	Previously healthy	Infant
Source	Necrotizing infection	Nasal or wound packing, tampon; infection not obvious	Skin flora
Rash	Erythematous rash in only 10%; stigmata of necrotizing infection present; exfoliation weeks later	Initially diffuse erythroderma, with exfoliation after 1–2 wk; mucosal hyperemia	Tender erythematous rash, localized blisters, extensive exfoliation if no antibodies to toxin; mucosa spared
Systemic illness	Hypotension, shock, multiorgan failure likely	Hypotension, shock, sometimes multiorgan failure	Fever, irritability
Mortality	30%–80%	<5%	<5%
Treatment	Critical care resuscitation, operative débridement	Critical care resuscitation	Wound care, hydration

Staphylococcal Toxic Shock Syndrome

Although staphylococcal TSS is not as severe as the streptococcal variety, it remains a life-threatening systemic illness. The classic presentation is of fever, rash, and hypotension, often in previously healthy patients. It was first described in 1978 and, beginning in 1980, there was an epidemic of cases associated with the use of highly absorbent tampons. Menses-associated cases have since declined dramatically when these tampons were eliminated from the market, although tampon use remains a risk factor.

Nonmenstrual cases, which currently account for about 50% of cases, are associated with various conditions, including surgical procedures (e.g., rhinoplasty, abortion), nasal packing, burns, injection drug use, and the postpartum state. To the emergency clinician, menstrual and nonmenstrual staphylococcal TSS appear similar, and the source infection is often not readily apparent. Of note, prevention of TSS was a traditional indication for systemic antibiotic therapy after nasal packing for epistaxis, but recent evidence has suggested that this is not necessary, and topical antibiotics may be a preferred approach.

S. aureus exotoxins are superantigens that can activate large numbers of T lymphocytes, resulting in the massive release of inflammatory mediators, including interleukins, tumor necrosis factors, and interferon. Toxic shock syndrome toxin 1 (TSST-1) is associated with most menstrual cases. A lack of antibody against this toxin has been demonstrated in patients with menstrual staphylococcal TSS. Episodes of recurrent staphylococcal TSS have been reported in patients who do not mount a long-term antibody response, and it has been postulated that the toxin may interfere with antibody generation against itself.

Patients often have an acute onset of fever, chills, malaise, myalgia, muscle tenderness, and diffuse blanching macular rash that is not pruritic. There may be nausea, vomiting, or diarrhea. Patients may have fever and altered mental status.

Severe hypotension may ensue as a result of massive vasodilation and fluid shifts out of the intravascular space. Toxic cardiomyopathy may also contribute to low blood pressure. Hypotension or rhabdomyolysis may cause acute tubular necrosis. Anemia, thrombocytopenia, and leukocytosis are common, and DIC may develop. Desquamation of the skin, including the palms and soles, eventually occurs 7 to 14 days after onset. The overall mortality is below 5% with aggressive supportive care.

Staphylococcal Scalded Skin Syndrome

Staphylococcal scalded skin syndrome (SSSS) is a desquamating skin disorder caused by exfoliating toxins produced by *S. aureus*. A disease of infants, it is rare in older children and adults. It can cause outbreaks in nurseries and daycare centers. SSSS was historically known as fourth disease and as Ritter's disease in newborns.

SSSS is caused by certain strains of *S. aureus*, including CA-MRSA, that produce epidermolytic toxin A or epidermolytic toxin B. These toxins probably act as proteases that target the protein desmoglein 1 on the stratum granulosum layer of the epidermis. Whether they meet the T lymphocyte mitogenic criterion for a superantigen has been a subject of debate.

The severity of the disease ranges from a few blisters at the site of infection to exfoliation of most of the body. People with preexisting toxin antibodies develop the localized form, in which toxin is found in the wound periphery; those without preexisting toxin antibodies develop the generalized form, in which toxin spreads through the bloodstream. Cultures of the bullae are negative unless they are contaminated or secondarily infected.

Typically, a young child presents with fever, irritability, and tender red rash. The erythema progresses to bullae formation and subsequent exfoliation of the affected skin. The skin exhibits the Nikolsky sign, which is separation of the epidermal layer of skin on gentle stroking. Desquamation may be patchy or sheet-like, leaving the skin denuded, with a red moist base and predisposing it to secondary infection. Perioral, perianal, and flexural skin may be affected more severely. Mucous membranes are spared. SSSS is not associated with multisystem illness and typically does not lead to shock. Mortality is usually a result of complications from comorbid conditions or superimposed infection.

Differential Diagnosis and Diagnostic Testing

Streptococcal TSS should be suspected in any patient presenting with shock, especially if the patient was previously healthy. Diagnostic criteria for streptococcal TSS include the presence of group A streptococcal infection, hypotension, and two of the following: renal impairment, liver abnormalities, acute respiratory distress syndrome, coagulopathy, necrotic soft tissue infection, and rash. These criteria were developed for epidemiologic purposes; failure to meet all criteria should not exclude the clinical diagnosis in suspicious cases.

Staphylococcal TSS should be considered in any patient presenting with diffuse rash and hypotension. The diagnosis is made on the basis of the clinical presentation. The characteristic rash often raises suspicion and ultimately aids in establishment of the diagnosis. Isolation of *S. aureus* is not necessary for the diagnosis to be made; in fact, blood cultures are positive in a small minority of cases. In severe cases, laboratory abnormalities are those resulting from shock and organ damage.

Early SSSS may be difficult to differentiate from bullous impetigo. The lack of mucosal involvement helps differentiate SSSS from toxic epidermal necrolysis and Stevens-Johnson syndrome. Other differential considerations include Kawasaki syndrome, Rocky Mountain spotted fever, meningococcemia, leptospirosis, and heatstroke.

Management

Streptococcal and staphylococcal TSS require critical care resuscitation. In streptococcal TSS, immediate surgical consultation for operative débridement of necrotizing infections is critical. In staphylococcal TSS, any potential source of infection should be removed, such as tampons or wound packing, and all postoperative wounds should be explored for infection. Clindamycin and vancomycin should be administered. Gram-negative coverage should be added when the diagnosis of TSS is uncertain because the clinical picture overlaps with that of septic shock.

IV immune globulin has theoretical benefit, but its efficacy has not been shown in clinical trials. It is a reasonable option in cases of presumed staphylococcal TSS unresponsive to IV fluids and vasopressors, but is not commonly employed in the ED setting. There has been conflicting evidence on its efficacy for the treatment of streptococcal TSS. SSSS is treated with antibiotics active against *S. aureus*, including MRSA. Wound care and hydration are important.

Disposition

Patients with suspected TSS should be admitted, usually to the intensive care unit, for IV fluids, antibiotics, and close monitoring due to the potential for decompensation. Patients with necrotizing soft tissue infections associated with streptococcal TSS usually require surgical débridement.

Children with mild SSSS may be considered for outpatient management with oral antibiotics and close follow-up. Those with more severe skin involvement often need admission for pain control, temperature regulation, and fluid and electrolyte management. Severely affected patients may need intensive or burn center care. With proper supportive care and antibiotic treatment, the prognosis is excellent, with an overall mortality of less than 5%. Scarring is rarely severe.

OTHER INFECTIONS WITH SKIN MANIFESTATIONS

Borrelia burgdorferi is the spirochete that causes Lyme disease, endemic in the United States, especially in New England. It produces a characteristic targetoid rash known as erythema migrans, which emerges one week on average after the infecting tick bite. The targetoid appearance results from central clearing of the erythema. However, 20% of Lyme disease patients do not report a rash, and the rash does not always have the characteristic round and targetoid appearance.

Another spirochete, *Treponema pallidum* (syphilis), is an increasingly rare cause of rash. The primary lesion of syphilis is a painless ulcer at the inoculation site, known as a chancre, with raised borders and regional lymphadenopathy. The chancre appears days to months after infection and resolves in approximately 1 month. Secondary syphilis develops weeks to months later in about 25% of infected patients. It involves a rash that can take any form other than vesicular and includes the palms and soles; there is usually diffuse lymphadenopathy. Syphilis is uncommon in the United States, although about 10,000 cases still occur annually.

Rocky Mountain spotted fever, caused by *Rickettsia rickettsii,* is even more uncommon, diagnosed only about 2000 times each year in the United States. A few days after a bite by a dog tick or wood tick, the characteristic rash begins on the wrists and spreads everywhere, including the palms and soles. It starts macular and becomes petechial and then dusky. Of those infected, 10% never develop a rash. The untreated mortality for Rocky Mountain spotted fever approaches 25%, but treated patients do well.

Cutaneous anthrax is transmitted from animal products of infected animals, such as wool or pelts, to exposed areas of veterinarians and farmers. A spore of the gram-positive anaerobe *Bacillus anthracis* enters a break in the skin and, after an incubation period of about 1 week, a vesicle forms. This ruptures, leaving a shallow-based ulcer with a raised border. The lesion progresses to painless necrosis and the characteristic eschar. Severe surrounding edema is due to bacterial toxins. The lesions may be confused with recluse spider bites. Unlike the case with inhalational anthrax, treated cases do well, and even untreated cases have a mortality rate of less than 20%.

Tularemia is a rare disease resulting from exposure to animals such as rodents, rabbits, and hares and is endemic in much of the United States, especially the south central states. The ulceroglandular form is most common and involves an influenza-like illness with a single raised ulcer that has a mild central eschar formation. The lesion itself is raised, rather than the border, which might suggest anthrax.

The floor of the mouth is a dangerous location for soft tissue infections. Severe infections may progress to Ludwig angina, in which the floor of the mouth becomes severely indurated. Ludwig angina can be fatal due to airway obstruction. Broad-spectrum antibiotics are indicated. Steroids may reduce swelling. Intubation should be considered and a difficult airway anticipated.

Scabies is a skin infestation of the parasitic mite *Sarcoptes scabiei.* It is endemic worldwide and can cause institutional outbreaks. Lesions are most prominent on the dorsal aspect of the hand and in intertriginous areas. It is diagnosed by visualization of characteristic burrows and, in ambiguous cases, by microscopy of skin scrapings. It is treated with topical permethrin or a single dose of oral ivermectin (200 µg/kg). Norwegian scabies, also known as crusted scabies, is an aggressive infestation in the immunocompromised; it is treated with permethrin and ivermectin.

Cat-scratch disease results from *Bartonella henselae* infection after a cat bite or scratch. Its hallmark is regional lymphadenopathy that appears weeks after a primary lesion at the site of inoculation. Treatment is with a standard 5-day course of azithromycin, with a double dose on day 1.

Strongyloidiasis is caused by infection with the parasitic helminth *Strongyloides stercoralis.* Skin lesions can appear years after infection and are urticarial or serpiginous. A rapidly extending burrow that is pruritic and erythematous is diagnostic; this finding, due to rapid migration of larvae in the skin, is known as larva currens (running larva). Such findings or unexplained eosinophilia in people who have lived in Southeast Asia or tropical Africa should prompt consideration of strongyloidiasis. Diagnosis is by an enzyme-linked immunosorbent assay performed on serum. Detection is important because, unlike other nematodes, strongyloides can complete its life cycle in the human host, leading to lifelong infection. When the infected patient becomes immunosuppressed by medications or illness, the strongyloides hyperinfection syndrome can result and is often fatal.

Cutaneous larva migrans is another serpiginous skin lesion caused by migrating larvae. In this case, the organism is hookworm, and the site is typically the foot or buttock; it is often seen after a vacation on the beach in Mexico. Treatment is with a single dose of ivermectin 200 mg/kg.

Cutaneous leishmaniasis is common in many parts of the world and is found on every continent except Australia and Antarctica. It is caused by protozoans of the genus *Leishmania* and is transmitted by sandflies. Lesions are most common on the face and are painless, ulcerative, and disfiguring. Papules in returning travelers and immigrants should raise suspicion of myiasis (botfly) and, rarely, dracunculiasis (Guinea worm).

The references for this chapter can be found online at ExpertConsult. com.

127

Sepsis Syndrome

Nathan I. Shapiro and Alan E. Jones

KEY CONCEPTS

- Sepsis is a progressive disease due to a dysregulated inflammatory cascade, leading to organ dysfunction and circulatory compromise in severe cases.
- Older adults, immunocompromised and neutropenic patients, and patients with multiple comorbidities are at increased risk for the development of sepsis syndromes.
- A thorough history, physical examination, and laboratory testing should guide the diagnostic evaluation.
- Early treatment should focus on appropriate identification, improvement of tissue perfusion (through the administration of fluids and vasopressor medications), improvement of tissue oxygenation (through administration of oxygen and positive-pressure ventilation), administration of antibiotics, and early identification of infections requiring surgical management.
- Prompt administration of antibiotics is essential and should be based on the suspected source of infection.

FOUNDATIONS

Background

Sepsis syndrome represents the body's host response to an infection. The causative agent and host's activated inflammatory cascade overwhelm the body's defenses and regulatory systems, leading to disruption in homeostasis. Tachycardia, tachypnea, fever, and immune system activation are common manifestations. If the body is unable to overcome this insult, cellular injury, tissue damage, shock, multiorgan failure, or death may ensue.

In 1992, the American College of Chest Physicians and Society of Critical Care Medicine issued a consensus statement to establish uniform criteria defining the sepsis syndromes. The goal was to create a common nomenclature for disease classification and systematic comparisons across studies of septic patients. The term *systemic inflammatory response syndrome* (SIRS) is defined as two or more of the following: tachycardia, tachypnea, hyperthermia or hypothermia, high or low white blood cell count, or bandemia. Sepsis is the combination of infection plus SIRS, severe sepsis is sepsis plus organ dysfunction, and septic shock is sepsis plus hypotension, defined as a systolic blood pressure below 90 mm Hg, not responsive to a fluid challenge (Box 127.1). This nomenclature is intended to provide clinicians and researchers with a common classification. Efforts to validate this classification scheme in the emergency department (ED) population have demonstrated that the term *sepsis,* when characterized by fulfilling the SIRS criteria alone, is overly sensitive and nonspecific and does not convey an increased mortality risk. SIRS is not specific because it can be present in noninfectious inflammatory states and in localized infections that are not inclined to lead to sepsis, such as streptococcal pharyngitis or viral illnesses. However, organ dysfunction and shock have been shown to portend worse outcomes.

The Third International Consensus Definitions Task Force (SEP-3) is a group who revisited the sepsis definitions and published a set of revised definitions.[1] The quick SOFA (qSOFA) score emerged as a risk stratification tool for the Emergency Department (ED).[2] The qSOFA score uses three clinical criteria with each receiving one point if present: respiratory rate of 22 breaths or less per minute, altered mental status, and hypotension defined by a systolic blood pressure (SBP) 100 mm Hg or less. A qSOFA score of two or greater was associated with an increased risk of mortality. The definitions group proposed using a suspected infection plus a qSOFA of 2 or greater to help identify patients with potential sepsis in the non-ICU setting. Subsequent validation studies have called the accuracy into question; ultimately it appears that it is a reasonable tool that is less sensitive and more specific than the original sepsis criteria. However, consensus is lacking as to whether it should be used to define sepsis.[3]

Bacteremia may be present, but positive cultures are not obligatory in the diagnosis of sepsis. Culture-negative and culture-positive septic populations have similar outcomes in patients with similar illness severity. Pneumonia, abdominal abscess with viscus perforation, and pyelonephritis are common primary causes of sepsis. Gram-positive organisms account for 25% to 50% of infections, gram-negative organisms for 30% to 60%, and fungi for 2% to 10%. The distribution varies with the study and, more importantly, with host factors such as the status of the host immune system, age of the patient, recent hospitalizations, and presence of indwelling vascular catheters.

The health status of the host is an important risk factor in the development and progression of sepsis. Older adults and those with multiple comorbidities may be more susceptible to developing a systemic infection. Chemotherapy-induced neutropenia, acquired immunodeficiency syndrome, and steroid dependency increase susceptibility to sepsis. Increased use of indwelling devices such as intravascular catheters, prosthetic devices, and endotracheal tubes also contribute to the risk of systemic infection and sepsis.

Pathophysiology

Sepsis results from the complex interaction of detection molecules, signaling molecules, and numerous inflammatory and coagulation mediators in response to infection. Although our understanding of the pathophysiologic process of sepsis has evolved, it remains incomplete. The initial host response is to mobilize inflammatory cells, particularly neutrophils and macrophages, to the site of infection. These inflammatory cells then release circulating molecules, including cytokines, which trigger a cascade of other inflammatory mediators that result in a coordinated host response. Synthesis of the components of the cascade is increased at many steps along the pathway. If these mediators are not appropriately regulated, sepsis will occur. In the setting of

BOX 127.1 Definitions of Sepsis

- Bacteremia (fungemia)—presence of viable bacteria (fungi) in the blood, as evidenced by positive blood cultures
- Systemic inflammatory response syndrome (SIRS)—at least two of the following conditions: oral temperature > 38°C (100.4°F) or < 35°C (95°F); respiratory rate > 20 breaths/min or partial pressure of arterial carbon dioxide ($Paco_2$) < 32 mm Hg; heart rate > 90 beats/min; leukocyte count > 12,000/dL or < 4000/dL; or >10% bands
- Sepsis—systemic inflammatory response syndrome (SIRS) that has a proven or suspected microbial source
- Septic shock—sepsis with hypotension that is unresponsive to fluid resuscitation plus organ dysfunction or perfusion abnormalities, as listed for severe sepsis
- Multiple organ dysfunction syndrome (MODS)—dysfunction of more than one organ, requiring intervention homeostasis

Adapted from: Bone R, Balk RA, Cerra FB, et al. Definitions for sepsis and organ failure and guidelines for the use of innovative therapies in sepsis. The APP/SCCM Consensus Conference Committee. American College of Chest Physicians/Society of Critical Care Medicine. *Chest.* 1992;101:1644-1655.

ongoing toxin release, a persistent inflammatory response occurs, with ongoing mediator activation, cellular hypoxia, tissue injury, shock, multiorgan failure, and potentially death.

Mediators of Sepsis

Host response and pathogen characteristics are both important in the pathogenesis of sepsis. More than 100 discrete markers have been identified and attributed to the sepsis cascade, but the true culprits have not been clearly identified.[1] A pathogen is sensed by pattern recognition receptors, most notably Toll-like receptors, located on the surface of the white blood cell. The resulting host-pathogen interaction activates the inflammatory and coagulation cascades. The subsequent inflammatory signaling occurs through cytokines, chemokines, and other soluble mediators, including increased circulating levels of the interleukins IL-1, IL-6, and IL-8 and tumor necrosis factor alpha (TNF-α). Activation of the clotting cascade may result in increased D-dimer levels and decreased circulating levels of protein C.

In benign conditions, a self-limited response helps clear the pathogen. If the innate immune response is inadequate, mediators create a procoagulant state. Coagulation and fibrinolytic components are proinflammatory, precipitating a worsening cycle of procoagulant and proinflammatory mediators. Propagation of this cascade ultimately contributes to end-organ damage and often to disseminated intravascular coagulation (DIC). If it is not effectively reversed, the process leads to cellular hypoxia, organ dysfunction, shock, and death.

The primary mediators are cytokines that are primarily proinflammatory, antiinflammatory, or growth-promoting. The molecular mechanisms whereby they are regulated are not well understood. An initial cytokine, TNF-α, is found in serum approximately 90 minutes after the administration of endotoxin to healthy volunteers. IL-6 and IL-8 reach peak levels at approximately 120 minutes. The main proinflammatory cytokines include IL-1, TNF-α, and IL-8. The primary antiinflammatory cytokines are IL-10, IL-6, transforming growth factor-β, soluble receptors to TNF, and IL-1 receptor antagonist (IL-1RA). If the resultant inflammatory response is adequate, the infection is controlled and cleared. If the response is deficient or excessive, however, a persistent and worsening cascade is produced, ultimately leading to (once again) shock, organ failure, and potentially death.

Instability in vascular tone has become increasingly important in understanding the pathophysiologic mechanism of sepsis. Vasopressin, also known as antidiuretic hormone, is a naturally occurring hormone that is essential for cardiovascular stability. It is produced as a prohormone in the hypothalamus. The hormone is stored in the pituitary gland and released in response to stressors such as pain, hypoxia, hypovolemia, and hyperosmolality. In severe sepsis, there is a brief rise in circulating vasopressin levels followed by a prolonged and severe suppression. This pattern of secretion is different from other forms of shock, in which vasopressin levels remain elevated. Vasopressin has numerous physiologic effects, including vasoconstriction of the systemic vasculature, osmoregulation, and maintenance of normovolemia.

Nitric oxide (NO) is a gas that has an important role in septic shock, regulating vascular tone by an indirect effect on smooth muscle cells. NO also contributes to platelet adhesion, insulin secretion, neurotransmission, tissue injury, and inflammation and cytotoxicity. Its half-life is short (6–10 seconds), and it easily diffuses into cells. Although its mechanisms of action are not well understood, it seems to be a key mediator of sepsis. Animal data have shown that nitric oxide synthase, the enzyme that produces NO, is upregulated in cases of sepsis. Enhanced NO production is thought to contribute to the profound vasodilation found in patients in septic shock.

In the setting of ongoing inflammatory activation, the mediators of sepsis continue to be produced, and the cascade is perpetuated. Unless it is appropriately and rapidly controlled, the ultimate effect is a sequence of events starting with cellular dysfunction and ultimately leading to tissue damage, organ dysfunction, and death.

Organ System Dysfunction

The organ dysfunction that results from sepsis is central to the pathogenesis of the disease. The mortality of patients with sepsis increases as the number of failing organs increases (Fig. 127.1A). In one large study, the mortality rate was 1% for sepsis patients with no organ dysfunction, whereas the rates for patients with dysfunction of a single organ, two organs, three organs, and four or more organs were 6%, 13%, 26%, and 53%, respectively (see Fig. 127.1B).

Neurologic Impairment. Patients with sepsis may display neurologic impairment manifested by altered mental status and lethargy, commonly referred to as septic encephalopathy. The incidence has been reported as between 10% and 70%. The mortality rate in patients with septic encephalopathy is higher than that in septic patients without significant neurologic involvement. Although the pathophysiologic process has not been clearly defined, contributing factors may include direct bacterial invasion, endotoxemia, altered cerebral perfusion or metabolism, metabolic derangements, multiorgan system failure, and iatrogenic injury. In addition, impaired renal or hepatic function in the absence of overt organ failure has been shown to correlate with encephalopathy.

Cardiovascular Dysfunction. Cardiovascular dysfunction is common with sepsis. The cardiovascular dysfunction and failure arise from direct myocardial depression and distributive shock. Gram-negative, gram-positive, and killed organisms can cause myocardial depression. The direct insults of the toxic mediators as well as the mobilization of host mediators of sepsis produce a distributive shock. Early in sepsis, a hyperdynamic state develops, characterized by increased cardiac output and decreased systemic vascular resistance. Although the cardiac output is increased, it is at the expense of ventricular dilation and decreased ejection fraction (EF). Vigorous fluid resuscitation usually increases preload and, secondarily, EF, thereby improving the cardiac index. Much of the cardiovascular compromise from septic shock is reversible, and normal cardiovascular function usually returns within 10 days.

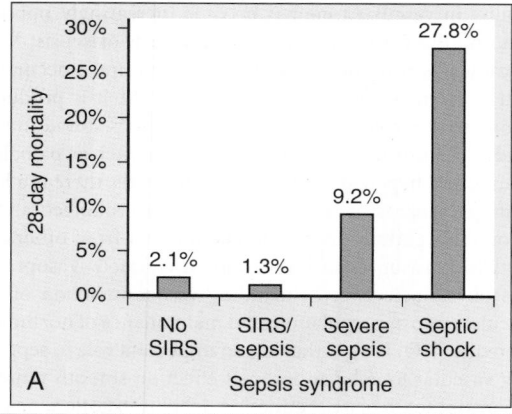

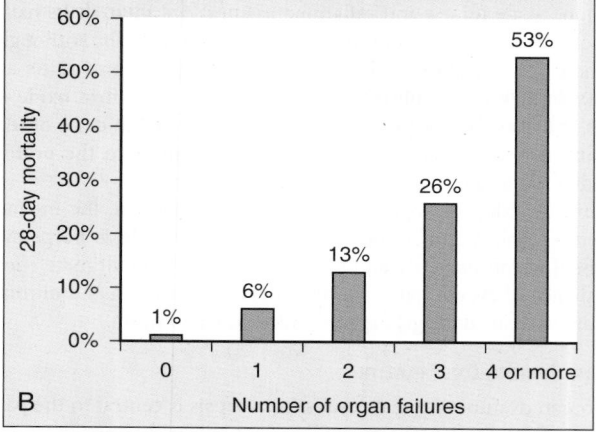

Fig. 127.1 Mortality rates by sepsis syndrome (A) and number of organ dysfunctions (B). *SIRS,* Systemic inflammatory response syndrome.

Pulmonary Involvement. Involvement of the lung is often seen in the inflammatory response to infection. These effects are apparent, irrespective of the primary infection that caused sepsis. Early infiltration with neutrophils, surfactant dysfunction, and edema gives way to monocyte infiltration and fibrosis. Significant right-to-left shunting, arterial hypoxemia, and intractable hypoxemia occur. The resulting morbidity is high and is a common endpoint to sepsis-related deaths.

Sepsis produces a highly catabolic state and places significant demands on the respiratory system to maintain the acid-base status. At the same time, airway resistance may be increased, and muscle function is impaired. Irrespective of whether pneumonia is the cause of sepsis, a common pulmonary endpoint is acute respiratory distress syndrome (ARDS). ARDS is defined clinically and correlates with the pathologic finding of diffuse alveolar damage (see Chapter 2). Because of alveolar-capillary membrane damage, fluid accumulates in the alveoli. Rather than being a diffuse disease, ARDS is a heterogeneous process that results in interspersed damaged and normal alveoli.

Gastrointestinal Effects. Splanchnic blood flow is dependent on mean arterial pressure because there is relatively little autoregulation. Therefore, hemodynamic dysfunction may have a profound effect on viscus metabolism. A shock state causes significant deleterious effects on a hollow viscus and its oxygen supply. A prolonged ileus may accompany hypoperfusion and persist beyond the perfusion deficit.

Solid organ involvement is also common. Even in the previously normal host, elevations in aminotransferases and bilirubin levels are common early in sepsis. The liver has also been implicated in the pathogenesis of sepsis; some of the mediators of sepsis are produced by the liver.

Endocrine Disorders. An absolute or relative adrenal insufficiency is common in sepsis. Depending on the balance of circulating cytokines, augmentation or suppression of the hypothalamic-pituitary axis is possible. IL-1 and IL-6 both activate the hypothalamic-pituitary-adrenal axis. TNF-α and cortistatin depress pituitary function. Other factors that may contribute to adrenal insufficiency in sepsis include decreased blood flow to the adrenal cortex, decreased pituitary function, and decreased pituitary secretion of adrenocorticotropic hormone due to severe stress. As a result of these interactions, the hypothalamic thermoregulatory mechanism may be reset, and temperature fluctuations may develop.

Hematologic Abnormalities. Sepsis causes abnormalities in many parts of the coagulation system. Endotoxin, TNF-α, and IL-1 are the key mediators. Pathologic activation of the extrinsic (tissue factor–dependent) pathway, protein C, protein S, and fibrinolysis lead to consumption of essential coagulation factors, causing DIC. The activation of the coagulation cascade produces fibrin deposition and microvascular thrombi. If these depositions are not corrected, they can compromise organ perfusion and contribute to organ failure. Tissue factor expression on monocytes is increased. This results in fibrin deposition and perhaps contributes to an increased incidence of multiorgan failure due to microvascular thrombi.

Protein C has been identified as an important modulator of inflammation and coagulation in patients with sepsis. Impairment of the protein C–dependent anticoagulation pathway is critical to the development of the thrombotic complications of sepsis. In healthy people, protein C is activated by a combination of thrombin and thrombomodulin. The activation of protein C results in the downregulation of many portions of the coagulation cascade, including release of tissue factor, inactivation of factors VIIIa and Va, and stimulation of fibrinolysis. It is possible that protein C activation in early sepsis is impaired because of an inflammatory cytokine–mediated downregulation of thrombomodulin. As a result, a consumptive coagulopathy ensues. This leads to increased fibrin deposition and a resulting upregulation of the fibrinolytic pathway, as identified by low plasma levels of the fibrinolytic proteins and increased fibrin split products. This sequence of events leads to consumption of coagulation factors and DIC. In late sepsis, the fibrinolytic system is suppressed.

Genetic Factors

There has been increasing evidence that genetics are a risk factor for the outcome of sepsis. An individual may contain a set of individual characteristics or polymorphisms that may affect the ways in which he or she responds to sepsis in general, or perhaps there may be differences in response to specific sepsis therapeutics. Identifying and understanding these differences in an individual's genetic makeup is likely to lead to tailored approaches to diagnosis and therapy. The impact of genetics on future treatment modalities for sepsis remains unclear, but the prospect of customized genetic therapy for sepsis is a promising early development.

CLINICAL FEATURES

Symptoms and Signs

The approach to a patient with sepsis relies on identification of the presence of a systemic infection and localization of the source of the initial infection. This allows appropriate treatment directed to the source of infection. Often, the source is not readily apparent, but early identification of the septic state allows implementation of broad-spectrum antibiotics.

The septic patient may manifest signs of systemic infection through tachycardia, tachypnea, hyperthermia or hypothermia and, if severe, hypotension. Very early in the patient's presentation, vital sign changes such as tachycardia and tachypnea may be first indicators of sepsis. If the patient is in shock, a rapid assessment that excludes other causes, such as hypovolemic or cardiogenic shock, is essential to the proper initial treatment. A septic patient will often have flushed skin with warm, well-perfused extremities secondary to the early vasodilation and hyperdynamic state. Alternatively, the severely hypoperfused patient with advanced shock may appear cyanotic. A complete detailed clinical examination will help the emergency clinician determine the cause of the shock state (see Chapter 3). These are classic signs; however, these findings may not be manifested in a septic patient, and signs and symptoms may be subtle or absent.

Both underlying comorbidities and the cause of sepsis should be considered. Risk factors such as immunocompromised states (e.g., acquired immunodeficiency syndrome, malignant disease, diabetes, splenectomy, concurrent chemotherapy), older age, debilitation, high-risk environments for iatrogenic infections (e.g., acute care hospitalizations, long-term care facilities), and multiple comorbidities should be considered.

The respiratory system is the most common source of infection in the septic patient (see Chapter 62). A history of a productive cough, fevers, chills, upper respiratory symptoms, sore throat, or ear pain should be sought. Physical examination should also include a detailed evaluation for focal infection, such as exudative tonsillitis, sinus tenderness, tympanic membrane injection, and crackles or dullness on lung auscultation. Also, pharyngeal thrush should be noted as a potential marker of an immunocompromised state.

The gastrointestinal system is the second or third (depending on the study) most common source of sepsis. A history of abdominal pain, including its description, location, timing, and modifying factors, should be sought. Further history, including the presence of nausea, vomiting, and diarrhea and time of the last bowel movement should be noted. A careful physical examination, looking for signs of peritoneal irritation, abdominal tenderness, and hyperactive or hypoactive bowel sounds, is critical in identifying the source of abdominal sepsis. Particular attention should be paid to physical findings suggestive of common sources of infection or disease—Murphy sign indicating cholecystitis, pain at McBurney point indicating appendicitis, left lower quadrant pain suggesting diverticulitis, or rectal examination revealing a rectal abscess or prostatitis.

The neurologic system should be evaluated for signs of meningitis, encephalitis, or epidural abscess, including nuchal rigidity, fevers, and change in consciousness (see Chapter 95). Lethargy or altered mentation may indicate primary neurologic disease or may be the result of decreased brain perfusion.

The genitourinary (GU) history includes queries about the presence of flank pain, dysuria, polyuria, discharge, Foley catheter placement, and genitourinary instrumentation. However, one must also remember that GU infection is a common source of infection in older patients and is a common offender in patients with nonspecific symptoms. Obstructed nephrolithiasis with associated urinary tract infection is a potentially lethal source of infection that can advance rapidly without decompression by nephrostomy.

Rarely, sexually transmitted infections may be the cause of sepsis. The genital examination could reveal ulcers, discharge, penile or vulvar lesions, or the woody induration of Fournier gangrene. Cervical motion tenderness indicates pelvic inflammatory disease, and adnexal tenderness in a toxic-appearing woman may represent a tubo-ovarian abscess. Tampons are rarely a cause of toxic shock syndrome, but when no other source of septic shock is found, a retained tampon should be considered.

The musculoskeletal history includes the presence of any localizing symptoms to a particular joint. Redness, swelling, and warmth over a joint, especially if there is a decreased range of motion in that joint, may be signs of septic arthritis and may mandate arthrocentesis. The skin should be examined for evidence of cellulitis, abscess, wound infection, or traumatic injury. Deep injuries, foreign bodies, and fasciitis may be difficult to identify clinically. The emergency clinician should look for crepitus, bullae, or skin edema extending beyond areas of erythema that may indicate the presence of an aggressive, gas-forming organism (see Chapter 126). Back pain and fever may be signs of an epidural abscess. Local lymphadenopathy, swelling, and streaking should also be noted as signs of an advancing infection. Petechiae and purpura may represent a *Neisseria meningitidis* infection or DIC. Generalized erythroderma and rash may represent an exotoxin from pathogens such as *Staphylococcus aureus* and *Streptococcus pyogenes*.

A history of fevers or chills in the setting of injection drug use, artificial heart valve, or mitral valve prolapse should increase the suspicion for endocarditis. The emergency clinician should suspect endocarditis in the presence of a murmur or other stigmata of endocarditis (e.g., splinter hemorrhages, Roth's spots, Janeway's lesions) (see Chapter 69).

Emergency clinicians must identify the severity of illness in patients with infection and initiate early resuscitation for those with the potential of becoming critically ill. Although a patient may meet SIRS criteria, this alone has little predictive value in determining the severity of illness and mortality. There are many scoring systems that have been developed to risk-stratify illness severity. Most scoring systems are not clinically relevant and not routinely used. The Mortality in Emergency Department Sepsis (MEDS) score is one proposed method to risk stratify ED patients with sepsis. The MEDS prediction rule assigns point values to specific clinical characteristics (Table 127.1). The total score can be used to assess risk of death. Thus, the greater the number of risk factors, the more likely a patient is to die during hospitalization. Although typically not calculated for all patients, the elements of the score may be identified and considered as a red flag when risk-stratifying a patient.

TABLE 127.1 Mortality in Emergency Department Sepsis (MEDS) Prediction Rule

Risk Factor	Odds Ratio for Death	Meds Score (Points)
Terminal illness (death within 30 days)	6.1	6
Tachypnea or hypoxia	2.7	3
Septic shock	2.7	3
Platelet count < 150,000/mm^3	2.5	3
Bands > 5%	2.3	3
Age > 65 yr	2.2	3
Pneumonia	1.9	2
Nursing home resident	1.9	2
Altered mental status	1.6	2

Risk of Death	Total Meds Score (% of Sepsis Deaths)
Very low	0–4 (1.1%)
Low	5–7 (4.4%)
Moderate	8–12 (9.3%)
High	13–15 (16.1%)
Very high	>15 (39%)

DIAGNOSTIC CONSIDERATIONS

Differential Diagnoses

The sepsis syndromes represent a spectrum of disease and clinical presentations. Often, noninfectious sources can cause a syndrome that mimics that of sepsis; thus, one must keep in mind a broad differential diagnosis when approaching these patients (Box 127.2). A detailed history and physical examination are the first steps in narrowing the differential diagnosis to identify the true source.

Diagnostic Testing

Diagnostic studies are used to identify the type and location of the infecting organisms and define the extent and severity of the infection to assist in focusing therapy. As a result, the diagnostic approach should be tailored to the particular patient.

BOX 127.2 Differential Diagnosis of Sepsis and Septic Shock

Sepsis
Dehydration
Acute respiratory distress syndrome
Anemia
Ischemia
Hypoxia
Congestive heart failure
Vasculitis
Toxicologic
    Poisonings
    Overdose
    Drug-induced
    Neuroleptic malignant syndrome
Pancreatitis
Hypothalamic injury
Disseminated intravascular coagulation
Anaphylaxis
Metabolic
Hyperthyroidism
Diabetic ketoacidosis
Adrenal dysfunction
    Environmental
    Burn
    Heat exhaustion or stroke
Trauma
Blood loss
Cardiac contusion

Septic Shock
Hypovolemic shock
Acute blood loss
Severe dehydration
Cardiogenic shock
Pulmonary embolus
Myocardial infarction
Pericardial tamponade
Tension pneumothorax
Vasogenic shock
Anaphylaxis
Paralysis

Laboratory Testing

Hematology. The white blood cell count can be an indicator of inflammation and activation of the inflammatory cascade. Leukocytosis is associated with infection and is incorporated in the consensus definition of sepsis; however, it is often insensitive and nonspecific, limiting its value in the ED. The febrile neutropenic patient has been shown to be at increased risk for severe infection. Thus, a neutrophil count of less than 500 cells/mm^3 should prompt consideration for admission, isolation, and empirical intravenous (IV) antibiotics in most chemotherapy patients. A bandemia (≥5%–10% bands on a peripheral smear) represents the release of immature cells from the bone marrow and may be a sign of infection and inflammation. Like the white blood cell count, it is an imperfect indicator of infection. The absence of leukocytosis or bandemia does not preclude the possibility of severe sepsis nor does their presence confirm it. The hemoglobin level should be determined to ensure adequate oxygen delivery in shock. Platelets are an acute-phase reactant and may be elevated in the presence of infection. Conversely, a low platelet count may be seen in patients with sepsis and septic shock. Thrombocytopenia, elevated prothrombin time, elevated activated partial thromboplastin time, decreased fibrinogen, and increased fibrin split products are associated with DIC and severe sepsis syndrome.

Blood Chemistry. Electrolyte abnormalities should be identified and corrected. A low bicarbonate level suggests acidosis and inadequate perfusion. An elevated anion gap acidosis in the setting of sepsis syndrome commonly represents lactic acidosis or diabetic ketoacidosis, but other causes need to be ruled out. An elevated serum creatinine concentration or decreased glomerular filtration rate signals renal dysfunction or failure, which, if due primarily to sepsis, indicates organ failure and a worse prognosis. Calcium, magnesium, and phosphorus levels should be checked.

An elevated lactate level is associated with inadequate perfusion, shock, and poorer prognosis. In one study, the mortality rate correlated with the venous lactate level—a lactate level of 0 to 2.5 mg/dL was associated with a 5% mortality rate, a lactate level of 2.5 to 4.0 mg/dL, 9% mortality, and a lactate level greater than 4 mg/dL, 28% mortality. A blood gas assessment is helpful in identifying and classifying acid-base disturbances, with metabolic acidosis suggesting inadequate tissue perfusion. Liver function tests can be used to identify liver failure or dysfunction. An elevated bilirubin level may suggest the gallbladder as a cause of sepsis. An elevated lipase level may represent pancreatitis as the cause of SIRS. Procalcitonin and C-reactive protein are biomarkers sometimes used in the diagnosis and prognosis of sepsis. The literature primarily supports procalcitonin in serial measurements and for antibiotic stewardship, but the role for procalcitonin in the ED has not been clearly delineated.

Urinalysis. Urinalysis is another essential laboratory test, especially in older patients with higher risk of urinary tract infection who may not manifest localizing symptoms of infection. Urinalysis is likewise important to rule out infection in patients with renal colic or ureteral obstruction.

Microbiology. Proper blood, urine, sputum, cerebrospinal fluid, and other tissue culture samples are important in guiding therapy. Although the results of culture are not helpful in the initial management, culture samples ideally should be obtained before the administration of antibiotics in the patient with sepsis. The initiation of antibiotic therapy should not be delayed significantly while waiting for culture samples to be obtained. Studies have suggested that the yield of initial blood cultures is low (5%–10%), but this is probably an artifact of the lack of reliable discriminatory guidelines for obtaining blood culture samples in the ED. Among patients with clinical sepsis, only 30% to 40% of patients will have positive cultures. The results of initial microbiologic tests, including Gram staining whenever possible, will help guide subsequent antibiotic treatment. Initial empirical therapy should be broad spectrum to allow early treatment of all likely organisms.

Special Procedures

Historically, a central venous pressure (CVP) line was thought helpful in guiding fluid resuscitation in sepsis patients. We do not recommend the routine use of CVP to determine fluid responsiveness. When available, arterial lines can be useful for close monitoring of hypotensive patients, especially when one or more vasopressors are being titrated to maintain an adequate blood pressure. However, they are not routinely placed in the ED. The technology of noninvasive or minimally invasive cardiac output monitoring is evolving and, where available, may help guide fluid administration by evaluating cardiac output alone or in conjunction with a fluid challenge or passive leg raise approach. Cardiac ultrasound, while unproven, is also commonly used to assess volume status and cardiac function.

Radiology

Imaging studies are generally used to identify the source of infection. A chest radiograph should be considered in patients with suspected sepsis syndrome, looking not only for a focal infiltrate representing pneumonia but also for the bilateral infiltrates indicative of ARDS. An upright chest radiograph should be considered for suspected bowel perforation to detect free air under the diaphragm. The presence of pneumomediastinum is suggestive of esophageal perforation and current or impending mediastinitis.

Soft tissue plain radiographs of infected areas can be obtained, looking for air in the soft tissues associated with necrotizing or gas-forming infection, although plain x-rays are not sensitive for tissue infection. Periosteal thickening or bone erosion may be seen on plain radiographs of patients with osteomyelitis; a bone scan may be diagnostic. Computed tomography (CT) of superficial infections may be more helpful to quantify the extent of infection further and identify abscesses that are not readily evident on physical examination. A CT scan of the abdomen and pelvis may identify abdominal or pelvic pathologic lesions, provided there is no clear clinical indication for immediate operative intervention. Suspected disease, such as diverticulitis, appendicitis, necrotizing pancreatitis, microperforation of the stomach or bowel, or formation of an intra-abdominal abscess, may be best diagnosed by a CT scan. A head CT scan can identify septic emboli from endocarditis or increased intracranial pressure from a mass and should be considered before a lumbar puncture is performed. An abdominal ultrasound examination may be indicated for suspected cholecystitis, and a pelvic ultrasound examination may be indicated for tubo-ovarian abscess or endometritis. If endocarditis is suspected, a transesophageal cardiac ultrasound study may be performed for the detection of any valvular vegetations. Magnetic resonance imaging (MRI) can be useful to identify soft tissue infection, such as necrotizing fasciitis or epidural abscess.

MANAGEMENT

Early detection and appropriate treatment can reduce the mortality from sepsis. The primary goal is timely administration of appropriate antimicrobial therapy—or interventional source control as required—and maintenance of adequate tissue oxygenation and perfusion through titrated resuscitation. With early detection and early resuscitation there is increasing evidence that the natural history of sepsis can be altered. Initial resuscitation, including appropriate airway management, IV access, oxygen, early and appropriate antibiotics, fluid resuscitation,

and vasopressor support, remains the foundation on which new efforts may be applied.

From a historical perspective, Rivers and associates[2a] provided compelling evidence supporting the importance of this concept when they published a protocol of standardized timely and titrated care being used to guide resuscitation in the ED. This randomized, double-blind, placebo-controlled study showed a 16% mortality reduction in patients with severe sepsis and septic shock. The protocol, termed *early goal-directed therapy* (EGDT), measures targeted goals and uses a resuscitation algorithm to guide the resuscitation. The theory behind the protocol was to normalize preload and blood pressure and prevent tissue hypoxia by matching oxygen delivery with consumption. Use of this protocol, which facilitated earlier and more aggressive fluid resuscitation through the use of increased fluids, increased blood products, increased use of dobutamine, and greater degree of normalization of tissue hypoxia, reduced mortality at their center. The interventions in combination were likely responsible for the better outcomes in the intervention group.

The principles of EGDT, as well as efforts such as the Surviving Sepsis Campaign, helped underscore the importance of early identification and timely resuscitation.[3] However, until 2014, the evidence in support of the formal EGDT protocol was only in the form of the original single-center trial and subsequent observational efforts. Subsequently, the ProCESS, ProMISE, and ARISE studies were large multicenter trials that sought to validate the value of EGDT.[4,5] Each of the trials showed no mortality benefit to EGDT as compared to usual resuscitation measures; thus, although EGDT is one strategy to consider, it is not a superior approach. It is important to underscore, however, that the usual care groups in these newer trials were all identified early, received antibiotics, and received generous amounts of fluids (on average, approximately 40–60 mL/kg in the first 6 hours across the trials), supporting the principle that early identification of sepsis, early antibiotics, and carefully titrated resuscitation should remain a core tenant.

Respiratory Support

Altered mental status is common in patients in septic shock, and patients may require rapid airway protection. Because patients with impending respiratory failure use a disproportionately large amount of energy for the muscles of respiration, improved oxygen delivery to other organs may be achieved by mechanical ventilation, sedation, and paralysis. Although there are no clear intubation guidelines, hypercapnia, persistent hypoxemia, airway compromise, and profound acidosis are valid indicators for intubation.

In addition to airway protection, intubation and mechanical ventilatory support provide positive-pressure ventilation. Pulmonary compliance is often low in ARDS, resulting in increased airway pressures to maintain oxygen delivery. The ARDSNet trial established the benefit of low tidal volumes (6 mL/kg) and plateau pressures of 30 cm H_2O or below in mechanically ventilated patients to prevent iatrogenic lung damage (see Chapter 2). Maintenance of a relatively low plateau pressure with higher positive end-expiratory pressure is an effective way to increase arterial oxygen delivery.

Cardiovascular Support

Fluid Resuscitation

Patients with sepsis are often administered IV fluid to maintain adequate perfusion. The primary reasons for this intravascular hypovolemia are venodilation and diffuse capillary leak. Initial therapy for adults with septic shock should generally be up to 30 mL/kg of isotonic crystalloid. Additional fluid replacement should be titrated to clinical parameters such as heart rate, blood pressure, change in mental status, capillary refill, cool skin, and adequate urine output (0.5–1 mL/kg/hr). Colloids are as effective as crystalloids, but they are more expensive and less readily available. Balanced salt solutions (e.g., lactated Ringers) have been shown to have beneficial effects over normal saline, due primarily to adverse renal effects associated with normal saline. Evidence suggests that balanced solutions are likely as good or better than normal saline; thus, we recommend the use of balanced solutions for sepsis resuscitation.

Although one should be increasingly vigilant in watching for fluid overload in patients who are predisposed, such as older adults, those with congestive heart failure (CHF), or those with renal impairment, these patients are not precluded from volume resuscitation as described previously. Efforts to identify ways to measure regional perfusion more directly, such as direct measurement of splanchnic blood flow, have been proposed, but are not commonly used in clinical practice. Even in the absence of global hypoxia and impaired tissue perfusion, there is evidence that regional hypoperfusion and ischemia exist.

Vasoactive Drug Therapy

Use of mean arterial pressure alone as an indicator of overall efficacy of therapeutic intervention is not always sufficient. A mean arterial pressure of 65 mm Hg has been recommended in otherwise healthy, normovolemic adult patients but must be correlated with other indicators of adequate perfusion, such as mental status and urine output. Patients with previously uncontrolled hypertension may require a mean arterial pressure of 75 mm Hg or even higher. If appropriate fluid resuscitation has failed to maintain end-organ perfusion, vasopressor support may be required (Table 127.2).

The 2016 Surviving Sepsis Campaign guidelines provided consensus recommendations for treatment of septic shock.[6] Norepinephrine should be used as the initial vasopressor, with the addition of epinephrine or vasopressin to norepinephrine as adjuncts. Vasopressin has not been shown to improve outcomes when added to norepinephrine in refractory septic shock, but there is no evidence of harm. As such, the optimum role for vasopressin is unclear. Once the mean arterial pressure is adequately supported, dobutamine should be used as the primary inotropic agent if myocardial dysfunction is evident. Patients requiring vasopressors and inotropes require frequent reassessment and medication titration, as needs can change greatly during the first few hours of resuscitation.

Norepinephrine. Norepinephrine is predominantly α-agonist with some β_1-agonism with minimal β_2 activity and primarily functions to increase systemic vascular resistance and cardiac output. In a large study examining patients with varied causes of shock, norepinephrine was associated with fewer adverse events (particularly arrhythmias) compared with dopamine. Dopamine was also associated with a higher mortality rate in patients with cardiogenic shock. In another meta-analysis, norepinephrine was shown to be superior to dopamine in both in-hospital and 28-day mortality. Compared with dopamine in septic patients, norepinephrine increases glomerular filtration and

urine output equally well. We recommend norepinephrine as the first-line vasopressor for septic shock, either as a sole vasopressor or in conjunction with other agents. Norepinephrine can be started at 3 to 5 µg/min and titrated to achieve the goal mean arterial pressure.

Dopamine. Dopamine is the immediate precursor of norepinephrine and epinephrine. It is primarily an α-, β_1-, and dopaminergic agonist. Dopamine was previously thought to improve renal outcomes, but it has not been shown to reduce mortality or decrease dialysis dependence, and should not be used for these indications. Persistent tachycardia, decreased partial pressure of arterial oxygen, and increased pulmonary artery occlusion pressure are common side effects of dopamine use. We do not recommend the routine use of dopamine if other vasopressors are available.

Vasopressin. Vasopressin is a naturally occurring peptide that is synthesized as a large prohormone in the hypothalamus. In states of septic shock, there is an early surge of vasopressin followed by a profound drop in circulating vasopressin levels. In a well-designed randomized trial, investigators demonstrated no change in mortality for patients with severe sepsis when vasopressin was added to catecholamine vasopressors. Vasopressin should not be used as the sole initial therapy for refractory septic shock. However, vasopressin does not increase pulmonary vascular resistance, making it a useful adjunct in patients with pulmonary hypertension, obstructive shock secondary to PE, or right ventricular dysfunction.

Epinephrine. Epinephrine is a potent mixed α- and β-agonist. Epinephrine infusion is also associated with increased oxygen consumption, increased systemic lactate concentrations, and decreased splanchnic blood flow. The rise in the lactate level is short term, and there is no evidence regarding its long-term effects. As a result of all the possible adverse effects of epinephrine, it is currently recommended only for those patients who are unresponsive to other vasopressors. Epinephrine can be a good adjunct for patients with combined septic and cardiogenic shock, given its vasopressor and inotropic activity.

Phenylephrine. Phenylephrine is a selective α_1-agonist, increasing systemic vascular resistance without significant changes in cardiac output. It can produce reflexive bradycardia or suppression in cardiac output. A single small study has shown that phenylephrine is effective in restoring perfusion in patients with septic shock refractory to dopamine or dobutamine. Another small study has demonstrated that phenylephrine is less effective than norepinephrine in the treatment of hypotension in septic patients; however, there was no difference in other measured hemodynamic parameters, including oxygen delivery. Phenylephrine does not impair cardiac and renal function and may be a good choice when significant tachyarrhythmia limits the use of other agents.

Dobutamine. Dobutamine is a mixed α- and β-agonist. In dosage ranges from 2 to 28 µg/kg/min, the cardiac index is increased at the expense of heart rate. In addition, decreased splanchnic blood flow is common. Dobutamine should be used in patients with depressed cardiac index and persistent hypoperfusion in spite of adequate volume expansion and the use of other vasopressor agents. Dobutamine decreases systemic vascular resistance, and therefore should not be used as the sole agent in a hypotensive patient. One study has suggested that survival in sepsis is associated with the patient's increase in stroke volume in response to dobutamine.

Bicarbonate

Bicarbonate supplementation was previously the standard treatment for patients with presumed lactic acidosis. Current consensus is that it should be reserved for severe acidemia (pH < 7.0–7.2) because there

TABLE 127.2	Dosing of Vasoactive Therapy
Drug	**Dosage**
Dobutamine	2–15 µg/kg/min
Epinephrine	5–20 µg/min
Norepinephrine	3–30 µg/min
Phenylephrine	2–300 µg/min
Vasopressin	0.01–0.04 units/min

TABLE 127.3   Suggested Initial Antibiotic Management[a]

Infection	Modifying Factors	Antibiotic
Sepsis, unknown source	Immunocompetent	Antipseudomonal cephalosporin *plus* aminoglycoside or fluoroquinolone, *or* antipseudomonal penicillin *plus* aminoglycoside or fluoroquinolone, *or* carbapenem *plus* aminoglycoside or fluoroquinolone
	Anaerobic infection	Add metronidazole or clindamycin to above regimen.
	Methicillin-resistant *Staphylococcus aureus* (MRSA)	Add vancomycin to above regimen.
	Neutropenia	Antipseudomonal penicillin *plus* aminoglycoside or fluoroquinolone, *or* carbapenem *plus* aminoglycoside or fluoroquinolone
	Splenectomy	Cefotaxime *or* ceftriaxone
Pneumonia	Immunocompetent	Second- or third-generation cephalosporin *plus* second-generation macrolide *or* fluoroquinolone
	Legionella suspected	Azithromycin, fluoroquinolone, or high-dose erythromycin
Abdominal infection	Immunocompetent	Ampicillin *plus* aminoglycoside *plus* metronidazole
	Multidrug-resistant organism suspected	Carbapenem, *or* piperacillin-tazobactam *plus* aminoglycoside
	Urinary tract source	Fluoroquinolone, *or* third-generation cephalosporin, *or* ampicillin *plus* aminoglycoside
Cellulitis	Nonnecrotizing fasciitis	Cefazolin *or* nafcillin
	MRSA possible	Vancomycin
	Necrotizing fasciitis (surgical drainage)	Ampicillin-sulbactam, piperacillin *plus* aminoglycoside *plus* clindamycin, *or* carbapenem
Intravenous catheter infection (remove catheter)	Outpatient-acquired	Third-generation cephalosporin
	MRSA suspected	Add vancomycin.
	Fungal infection	Amphotericin B
Cerebrospinal infection	Immunocompetent	Ceftriaxone *plus* vancomycin
	Older adult or immunocompromised patient	Add ampicillin.
Injection drug abuse	MRSA not suspected	Cefazolin *or* nafcillin *plus* aminoglycoside
	MRSA suspected	Vancomycin *plus* aminoglycoside

[a]Pending microbiologic identification of organism and sensitivity.

may be a paradoxical decrease in intracellular pH as a result of diffusion of soluble carbon dioxide across the cell membrane. Alternatively, hyperventilation has been suggested to help increase systemic pH.

Antibiotics

Early antibiotic therapy should target the nidus of infection if known. If the patient's condition permits, appropriate culture specimens should be obtained before the administration of broad-spectrum antibiotics (Table 127.3). Surgically correctable conditions, such as intra-abdominal abscesses, perforated viscus, retained products of conception, or retained foreign body (e.g., a tampon), should be treated concurrently. Antibiotics should be administered as soon as possible in patients with serious infections. Although some observational studies and national benchmarks have called for the administration of antibiotics within a predefined time period of 3 hours from ED presentation, a comprehensive meta-analysis failed to support an association between antibiotics administered after 3 hours and mortality.[7] Thus, early antibiotics are important, but their exact timing remains undefined.

In the absence of an obvious source of infection, the use of broad-spectrum antibiotics is recommended. The specific agent depends on many variables, including institutional preference and local resistance patterns. As results from cultures become available, therapy should be modified. There is no consensus about the need for double or triple antibiotic coverage for particular organisms, although it is common

practice to double-cover virulent organisms, such as *Pseudomonas aeruginosa*, as well as areas commonly infected with multiple organisms, such as the peritoneum. With increasing rates of methicillin-resistant organisms, combinations that include nonpenicillin choices may be warranted.

Steroid Therapy

It has been nearly 40 years since the first treatment attempts to block inflammation in sepsis. Because sepsis involves a systemic inflammatory response, corticosteroids are a logical treatment modality as anti-inflammatory agents. Physicians have been working for decades to prove or disprove their value. Steroids appear to be more effective in reducing the amount of time patients spend in a hypotensive state, and moderate-quality evidence suggests a mortality benefit, especially in the most critically ill patients.[8-10] However, the optimum timing, dose, drug, and method of administration (continuous or bolus dosing) remains unknown. At this time, we believe that the role of steroid therapy in sepsis remains controversial and recommend their use when there is refractory cardiovascular insufficiency, despite fluid and vasopressor therapy.

DISPOSITION

Once ED management is complete, patients who are deemed at increased risk should be admitted to the hospital into a setting that is deemed appropriate for the severity of the patient's condition. For example, in patients who remain hypotensive, are on vasopressors, or who are unstable and require more frequent monitoring, the intensive care unit may be appropriate. Other patients who are more stable but still require monitoring and perhaps IV therapy may be admitted to a hospital ward. Finally, in certain cases, patients initially meeting sepsis criteria but who are not severely ill (e.g., young patients with pharyngitis) may be appropriate for discharge.

The references for this chapter can be found online at ExpertConsult.com.

PART IV

Environment and Toxicology

128

Hypothermia, Frostbite, and Nonfreezing Cold Injuries

Ken Zafren and Daniel F. Danzl

ACCIDENTAL HYPOTHERMIA

KEY CONCEPTS

- Patients with hypothermia should be actively rewarmed whenever possible. Specific indications for active rather than passive rewarming include trauma, cardiovascular instability, temperature below 32°C (89.6°F), poor rate of passive rewarming, and endocrine insufficiency.
- Rewarming methods should be chosen to minimize core temperature afterdrop.
- If tachycardia is out of proportion to core temperature then hypoglycemia, hypovolemia, or an overdose should be considered.
- The effects of most medications are temperature dependent. Overmedication to achieve an effect when the patient is cold could cause toxicity during rewarming.
- Laboratory coagulation tests are performed at 37°C (98.6°F). Despite clinically obvious coagulopathy, measures of coagulation will be deceptively normal. Treatment for coagulopathy is to rewarm the patient.
- There are no safe predictors of serum electrolyte levels. Hypothermia enhances the cardiac toxicity of hyperkalemia and obscures premonitory electrocardiographic changes.
- Failure to rewarm despite good technique should suggest infection, endocrine insufficiency, or a futile resuscitation.

Foundations

Background and Importance

Reported reanimations of profoundly cold victims in prolonged cardiac arrest and the emergence of targeted temperature management (formerly called "therapeutic hypothermia") after cardiac arrest have made hypothermia a compelling topic. The lowest recorded core temperature in accidental hypothermia with successful resuscitation in an adult is 13.7°C (56.7°F) in a 29-year-old Norwegian physician. Cardiopulmonary resuscitation was initiated at the scene. The 9-hour resuscitation included 179 minutes of cardiopulmonary bypass. The lowest recorded core temperature with successful resuscitation in a child is 11.8°C in a 2-year-old boy who had an unwitnessed cardiac arrest. CPR was administered for 135 minutes. He was weaned off ECMO after 22 hours.[1] Profoundly cold patients have been resuscitated with full neurologic recovery after CPR for as long as 9 hours.[2] The lowest

possible temperature with neurologically intact survival in accidental hypothermia is not known. The lowest temperature in a survivor of induced hypothermia was long considered to be 9°C (48.2°F). Recently rediscovered journal articles from the early 1960s document survival after much lower induced core temperatures, as low as 4°C (39.2°F) measured using esophageal probes.

The treatment of accidental hypothermia has been controversial throughout history. The Bible recounts the truncal rewarming of King David by a damsel. Various remedies, including rubbing extremities with hot oil, were mentioned by Hippocrates, Aristotle, and Galen.

Cold weather has had a major impact on military history. Hannibal lost nearly half of his army of 46,000 while traversing the Alps in 218 BCE. The winter of 1777 took its toll on Washington's troops at Valley Forge. Napoleon's chief surgeon, Baron Larrey, reported that only 350 of the 12,000 men in the 12th division survived the cold during their retreat from Russia in 1812. Those soldiers who were rapidly rewarmed closest to the campfire died. Many lessons were relearned during World Wars I and II when pilots and U-boat crews perished in the cold waters of the North Atlantic.

Cold-related tragedies also affect civilians, including hunters, skiers, climbers, boaters, swimmers, and survivors of natural disasters. Hypothermia can occur in a wide range of climates and seasons. Large numbers of cases occur in urban settings. Indoor hypothermia in elderly patients is an increasing problem.[3] Primary hypothermia fatalities can be classified as accidental, homicidal, or suicidal. Death certificate data have underreported mortality from secondary hypothermia, in which cold complicates systemic diseases. As a result, the overall impact of cold on mortality from cardiovascular and neurologic disorders is greatly underestimated.

Anatomy, Physiology, and Pathophysiology

Hypothermia is defined as a core temperature below 35°C (95°F). Many variables contribute to the development of accidental hypothermia. Exposure, old age, poor health, inadequate nutrition, and various medications and intoxicants can decrease heat production, increase heat loss, or interfere with thermoregulation. Compensatory responses to heat loss through conduction, convection, radiation, and evaporation are often overwhelmed by exposure, even in healthy persons. Medications and central nervous system problems can also interfere with thermoregulation.

Temperature Regulation

Human basal heat production increases with ingestion of food or calorie containing fluids, muscle activity, fever, and acute cold exposure. Cold stress increases preshivering muscle tone, potentially doubling heat production. Maximal heat production, primarily due to shivering, lasts only a few hours because of fatigue and glycogen depletion.

Shivering thermogenesis increases the basal metabolic rate up to five times, markedly increasing oxygen consumption. Shivering begins at a normal core temperature when the skin is cooled. Shivering intensity is modulated by the posterior hypothalamus and the spinal cord. The preoptic anterior hypothalamus orchestrates nonshivering heat conservation and dissipation. Heat loss occurs by radiation, conduction, convection, respiration, and evaporation. The most common causes of accidental hypothermia are convective heat loss to cold air and conduction and convection in cold water. Heat loss increases up to five times in wet clothing. Conduction and convection in cold water can increase heat loss by a factor of 25.

Individuals with greater amounts of subcutaneous fat lose heat more slowly than thin people. Convective losses increase with shivering. Respiration and evaporation cause heat loss in the warming of inspired air and by insensible evaporation from the skin and lungs.

Cutaneous and respiratory heat losses are markedly influenced by the ambient temperature, air motion, and relative humidity. Greater losses occur in cool, dry, windy environments. When there is no sweating, most heat loss is through radiation and convection. Convective losses are significant in immersion-induced hypothermia. Children cool faster than adults because they have higher ratios of surface area to mass. Chronic cold exposure may result in thermal acclimatization (Fig. 128.1).

When the core temperature ranges from 37°C to 30°C (98.6°F to 86°F), vasoconstriction, shivering, and nonshivering basal and endocrine thermogenesis generate heat. From 30°C to 24°C (86°F to 75.2°F), the basal metabolic rate decreases, and shivering is absent. At temperatures below 24°C (75.2°F), autonomic and endocrine mechanisms for heat conservation become inactive. The pathophysiologic characteristics of hypothermia are described in Table 128.1.

Cardiovascular System

Initial tachycardia is followed by progressive bradycardia, although periods of tachycardia sometimes occur. The pulse decreases by 50% at 28°C (82.4°F). If the degree of tachycardia is inconsistent with the core temperature, consider associated conditions such as hypoglycemia, drug ingestion, and hypovolemia.

The bradycardia of hypothermia results from decreased spontaneous depolarization of cardiac pacemaker cells and is refractory to atropine. The electrocardiographic features of hypothermia include the

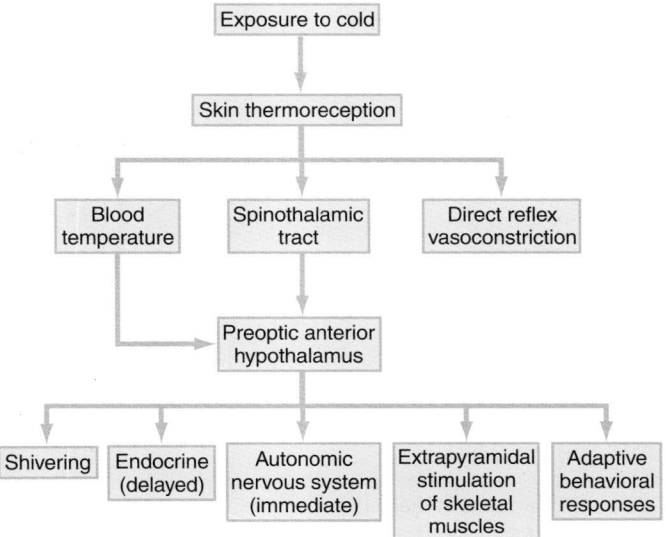

Fig. 128.1 Physiology of cold exposure.

TABLE 128.1	Physiologic Characteristics of the Four Zones of Hypothermia	
State	**Core Temperature °C (°F)**	**Characteristics**
Cold-stressed	37–35 (98.6–95)	Shivering and increased metabolism
Mild	35 (95)	Increased shivering thermogenesis; increase in metabolic rate
	34 (93.2)	Normal blood pressure; maximum respiratory stimulation; ataxia, and apathy
	33 (91.4)	Amnesia
Moderate	32 (89.6)	Stupor; 25% decrease in oxygen consumption
	31 (87.8)	Increased shivering thermogenesis
	30 (86)	Atrial fibrillation and other dysrhythmias; poikilothermia; pulse and cardiac output two-thirds normal; insulin ineffective; Progressive decrease in level of consciousness; loss of consciousness can be seen
	29 (85.2)	Progressive decrease in pulse, and respiration; pupils dilated
Severe	28 (82.4)	Ventricular fibrillation susceptibility; 50% decrease in oxygen consumption and pulse
	27 (80.6)	Loss of reflexes
	26 (78.8)	Major acid-base disturbances; no reflexes or response to pain
	25 (77)	Cerebral blood flow one-third normal; cardiac output 45% normal; pulmonary edema may develop
	23 (73.4)	No corneal or oculocephalic reflexes
	22 (71.6)	Maximum risk of ventricular fibrillation; 75% decrease in oxygen consumption
	20 (68)	Lowest resumption of cardiac electromechanical activity; pulse 20% of normal
	19 (66.2)	Flat electroencephalogram
	13.7 (56.7)	Lowest accidental hypothermia survival in an adult
	11.8 (53.2)	Lowest accidental hypothermia survival in a child
	4.2 (39.6)	Lowest therapeutic hypothermia survivor

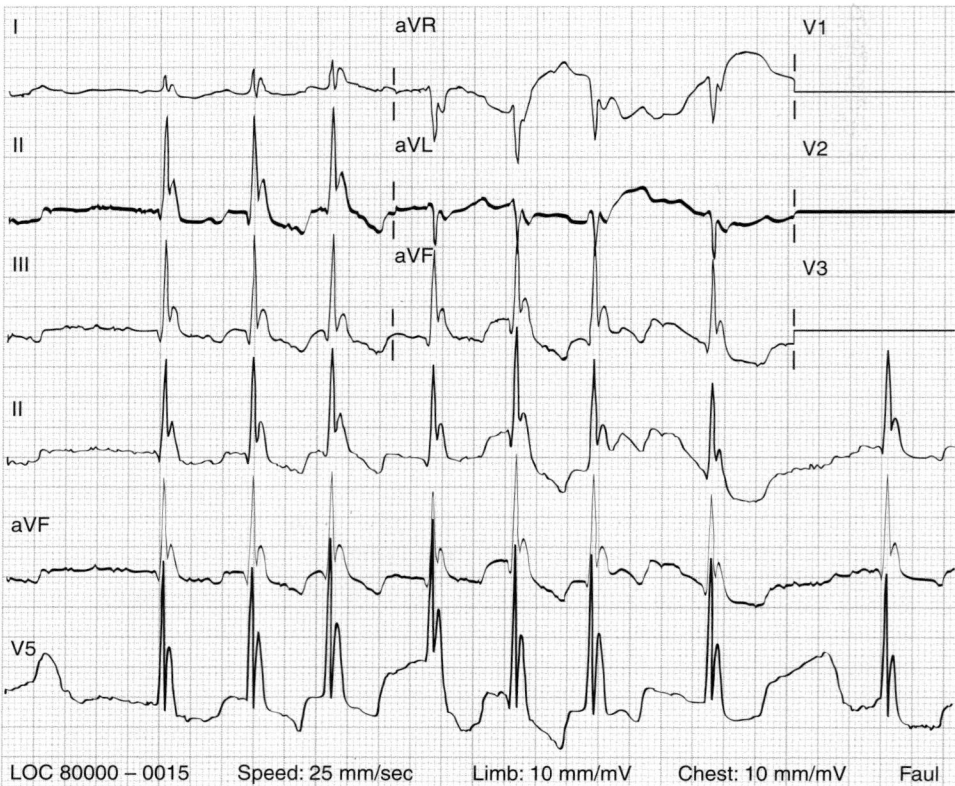

Fig. 128.2 Hypothermic J waves.

Osborn (J) wave seen at the junction of the QRS complex and ST segment with core temperatures below 32°C (89.6°F; Fig. 128.2). J waves are neither unique to hypothermia nor of any prognostic value. J waves are normally upright in aVL, aVF, and the left precordial leads. J waves can also be seen during local cardiac ischemia, with sepsis or CNS lesions, and hypercalcemia. J waves may resemble myocardial injury current and may not be recognized by ECG computer interpretations. This can result in misguided thrombolysis, which could exacerbate preexistent coagulopathies. Hypothermia can also cause electrocardiographic changes that mimic Brugada syndrome.

Atrial and ventricular dysrhythmias are common in moderate or severe hypothermia. Because the conduction system is more sensitive to the cold than the myocardium, cardiac cycle prolongation occurs. As hypothermia worsens, the PR interval, then the QRS interval, and finally the QTc interval become prolonged. Even in the absence of shivering, increased muscle tone may obscure P waves or produce artifacts. Atrial fibrillation is common when the core temperature is below 32°C (89.6°F). Sinus atrial or junctional rhythms also occur. Atrial fibrillation usually converts spontaneously during rewarming, but mesenteric embolization is a hazard. Ventricular fibrillation (VF) may be caused by tissue hypoxia, physical jostling, electrophysiologic or acid-base disturbances, or autonomic dysfunction. Asystole and VF can occur spontaneously when the core temperature falls below 25°C (77°F), but vital signs may persist well below 24°C (75.2°F).

The term *core temperature afterdrop* refers to a decrease in an individual's core temperature after removal from the cold. Temperature equilibration by conduction of heat from the core to the cooler peripheral tissue contributes to afterdrop, but countercurrent cooling of blood perfusing cold tissues in the periphery before returning to the warmer core results in a greater decrease in the core temperature. Active external rewarming of the extremities abolishes peripheral vasoconstriction

and reverses arteriovenous shunting. In one human experiment, cooling followed by immersion in a warm bath produced a 30% fall in mean arterial pressure, with a 50% decrease in peripheral vascular resistance.

Core temperature afterdrop is clinically relevant in the treatment of patients with large temperature gradients between the core and periphery. Large afterdrops can occur in severely hypothermic patients if frostbitten extremities are thawed before the core is rewarmed.

Central Nervous System

Hypothermia progressively depresses the CNS. Significant alteration of brain electrical activity begins below about 33.5°C (92.3°F). The electroencephalogram becomes silent at about 19°C to 20°C (66.2°F to 68°F). Cerebral autoregulation is maintained with an increase in vascular resistance until about 25°C (77°F). In severe hypothermia, there is a redistribution of blood flow to the brain. Like the heart, the brain has a critical period of tolerance to hypothermia.

Renal System

Exposure to cold induces diuresis, regardless of the state of hydration. The kidneys excrete a large amount of dilute urine that is essentially glomerular filtrate and does not clear nitrogenous waste products. Severe hypothermia causes relative central hypervolemia due to peripheral vasoconstriction. Cold diuresis may act as a volume regulator to diminish the capacitance vessel overload. Cold water immersion can further increase urinary output by 3.5 times.

Respiratory System

Hypothermia initially stimulates respiration, followed by a progressive decrease in the respiratory minute volume. Carbon dioxide production decreases 50% with an 8°C (14.4°F) decrease in temperature. Stimuli for respiratory control are altered in severe hypothermia and carbon dioxide

BOX 128.1 Factors Predisposing to Hypothermia

Decreased Heat Production
Endocrine failure
Hypopituitarism
Hypothyroidism
Diabetes
Insufficient fuel
Hypoglycemia
Malnutrition
Marasmus
Kwashiorkor
Extreme exertion
Neuromuscular inefficiency
Age extremes
Impaired shivering
Inactivity
Lack of adaptation

Increased Heat Loss
Environmental
Immersion
Nonimmersion
Induced vasodilation
Pharmacologic
Toxicologic
Erythrodermas
Burns
Psoriasis
Ichthyosis
Exfoliative dermatitis
Iatrogenic
Emergency deliveries
Cold infusions
Heatstroke treatment

Impaired Thermoregulation
Peripheral failure
Neuropathy
Acute spinal cord transection

Diabetes
Central neurologic failure
Central nervous system trauma
Cerebrovascular accident
Toxicologic
Metabolic
Subarachnoid hemorrhage
Pharmacologic
Hypothalamic dysfunction
Parkinson disease
Anorexia nervosa
Cerebellar lesion
Neoplasm
Congenital intracranial anomalies
Multiple sclerosis

Miscellaneous Associated Clinical States
Recurrent hypothermia
Episodic hypothermia
Sepsis
Pancreatitis
Carcinomatosis
Cardiopulmonary disease
Vascular insufficiency
Uremia
Paget's disease
Giant cell arteritis
Sarcoidosis
Shaken baby syndrome
Multisystem trauma
Shapiro's syndrome
Wernicke-Korsakoff syndrome
Hodgkin disease

retention with respiratory acidosis can occur. Hypercapnia increases core temperature cooling during snow burial. Other pathophysiologic factors that adversely affect the respiratory system include viscous bronchorrhea, decreased ciliary motility, and noncardiogenic pulmonary edema.

Predisposing Factors

Factors that predispose to hypothermia include decreased heat production, increased heat loss, and impaired thermoregulation (Box 128.1). Hypothermia can occur even in warm conditions.

Decreased Heat Production. Decreased thermogenesis may be due to endocrine dysfunction, such as hypopituitarism, hypoadrenalism, or myxedema. Myxedema coma is several times more common in women and up to 80% of women with myxedema coma are hypothermic. Hypothyroidism is often occult, with no history of lassitude, dry skin, arthralgias, or cold intolerance. Hypoglycemia can predispose to hypothermia. Another cause of decreased heat production is malnutrition, with a decrease in subcutaneous fat. Severe malnutrition with wasting contributes to heat loss. Kwashiorkor is less of a risk due to the insulating effect of hypoproteinemic edema.

Neonates are at particular risk of hypothermia due to large surface area–to–mass ratio, relatively little subcutaneous tissue, and inefficient shivering. Additionally, neonates do not have behavioral defense mechanisms. Acute neonatal hypothermia is common after emergency delivery or resuscitation and has also been reported after abandonment of infants. Hypothermic neonates are lethargic, fail to thrive, and have a weak cry. Many have paradoxically rosy cheeks. Hypothermia that occurs after 72 hours of life is often due to septicemia. Hypothermia can occur in shaken baby syndrome and may be a factor in some cases of sudden infant death syndrome.

Most older adults are capable of normal thermoregulation, but conditions such as immobility and systemic disease may interfere with heat production and conservation. Geriatric autonomic dysfunction may cause an inability to sense cold, abnormal adaptive behavioral responses, and decreased peripheral blood flow.

Increased Heat Loss. Patients with erythrodermas, such as psoriasis, exfoliative dermatitis, ichthyosis, eczema, and burns, can have increased peripheral blood flow. Iatrogenic causes of heat loss include exposure during resuscitation, cold or room temperature infusions, overcooling of patients with heatstroke, and overzealous burn treatment.

Ethanol is metabolized slowly in hypothermia and interacts with thermoregulatory neurotransmitters. Ethanol may directly suppress the activity of the posterior hypothalamus and mammillary bodies. Cutaneous heat loss increases through vasodilation and shivering thermogenesis is decreased. Ethanol is the most common cause of excessive heat loss in urban settings. Aging is associated with an increased sensitivity to the hypothermic actions of ethanol. Intoxicated persons may be incapable of adaptive behavior to avoid cold and can be impaired by hypothermic alcoholic ketoacidosis.

Impaired Thermoregulation. Thermoregulation can be impaired centrally, peripherally, or metabolically. Skull fractures, particularly basilar fractures, and chronic subdural hematomas are associated with central impairment. Other causes include strokes, neoplasms, anorexia nervosa, and Hodgkin and Parkinson diseases. The final common pathway in these disorders may be centrally mediated vasodilation. Cerebellar lesions can produce choreiform inefficient shivering.

In therapeutic or toxic doses, antidepressants, mood stabilizers, antipsychotics, anxiolytics, and general anesthetics interfere with thermoregulation by impairing centrally mediated vasoconstriction. Other overdoses, including by organophosphates, opioids, sedative hypnotics, barbiturates, and carbon monoxide, predispose to hypothermia.

Peripheral thermoregulatory failure occurs in neurogenic shock after acute spinal cord transection. In spinal cord injury, disruption of the autonomic nervous system eliminates vasoconstriction. The patient effectively becomes poikilothermic and can rapidly become hypothermic. Neuropathies and diabetes are also peripheral causes of heat loss. Abnormal plasma osmolality may cause hypothalamic dysfunction in uremia, lactic acidosis, diabetic ketoacidosis, and hypoglycemia.

Trauma

After trauma, hypotension, immobility in a cold environment, and hypovolemia predispose to hypothermia. In patients with major injuries, shivering is decreased or absent, causing skin and core temperatures to fall. Thermoregulation is impaired, and heat production decreases.

Hypothermia may exacerbate blood loss by inducing coagulopathy due to impaired activity of coagulation factors and enhanced plasma fibrinolytic activity, with decreased function and sequestration of platelets. Hypothermia in trauma is a risk factor for multiorgan dysfunction. Traumatic injuries may be missed if hypotension or neurologic findings such as areflexia or paralysis are misattributed to hypothermia. Major risk factors for hypothermia in trauma patients include extremes of age, severe injury, intoxication, large transfusion requirements, and prolonged field, emergency department (ED), and operating room times.

Hypothermia can protect the brain from ischemia only when induced before shock develops. This reduces adenosine triphosphate (ATP) use while ATP stores are nearly normal. In trauma patients, ATP stores are already depleted.

Clinical Features

Appreciation of subtle presentations facilitates the early diagnosis of mild to moderate hypothermia. Vague symptoms include hunger, nausea, confusion, dizziness, chills, pruritus, and dyspnea (Box 128.2). During outdoor activities, individuals may simply become uncooperative, uncoordinated, moody, or apathetic. Indoors, older patients may exhibit confusion or become less communicative and may display lassitude or a flat affect. Progression of mental deterioration or motor skill

impairment may mimic dementia. Symptoms such as slurred speech and ataxia may resemble symptoms of stroke or intoxication. Some older adults have a decreased ability to sense cold and fail to take adaptive action.

Paradoxical undressing has been widely reported in hypothermic patients. This final preterminal effort may be related to peripheral vasoconstrictive changes of hypothermia. Hypothermic patients who have paradoxically undressed have been mistaken for victims of sexual assault or thought to have a psychiatric disorder. In urban settings, hypothermia is most commonly associated with alcohol consumption or underlying illness. Other causes include stroke, drug overdose, psychiatric emergency, and major trauma.

Neurologic manifestations vary widely. A progressive decrease in the level of consciousness is usually proportional to the degree of hypothermia. Some patients, however, continue to be verbally responsive and display intact reflexes at 27°C to 25°C (80.6°F to 77°F).

Eye movement abnormalities and extensor plantar responses do not correlate directly with the degree of hypothermia. Cranial nerve signs may be seen with bulbar damage from central pontine myelinolysis. Above 22°C (71.6°F), it should be assumed that nonreactive dilated pupils reflect inadequate tissue perfusion rather than hypothermia.

Neuromuscular examination may reveal stiff posture, pseudo–rigor mortis, or opisthotonos. Reflexes are usually hyperactive to 32°C (89.6°F) and then become hypoactive, disappearing around 26°C (78.8°F). Cremasteric reflexes are absent because the testicles are already retracted. The plantar response usually remains flexor until 26°C (78.8°F). The knee jerk reflex is the last reflex to disappear and the first to reappear with rewarming. Diagnosis of CNS disorders, including spinal cord lesions, may be obscured by hypothermia. From 30°C to 26°C (86°F to 78.8°F), both contraction and relaxation phases of the reflexes are equally prolonged. If intact, the ankle jerk is helpful to diagnose hypothermic myxedema. Myxedema characteristically prolongs the relaxation phase more than the contraction phase.

Psychiatric disorders do not improve when the patient is cold. Mental status alterations can include anxiety, perseveration, neurosis, and psychosis. Individuals who are functional in warm conditions may decompensate in cold weather. Hypothermia-induced psychiatric presentations and suicide attempts are commonly misdiagnosed.

Differential Diagnoses

The differential diagnosis of hypothermia is broad and includes hypothyroidism, hypopituitarism, diabetes, hypoglycemia, malnutrition, intracranial and spinal cord injuries, and sedative-hypnotic and alcohol intoxication (see Box 128.1). Hypothermia is also common in patients with Wernicke encephalopathy. Hypothermia can mask the usual clinical triad of ophthalmoplegia, confusion, and truncal ataxia. Intravenous thiamine can be diagnostic and therapeutic.

Hypothermia occurs in conjunction with infections, most commonly overwhelming gram-negative sepsis, pneumonia, meningitis, and encephalitis. Other infections that can lead to hypothermia include bacterial endocarditis, brucellosis, malaria, syphilis, typhoid, miliary tuberculosis, and trypanosomiasis.

Medical conditions associated with hypothermia include carcinoma, pancreatitis, peritonitis, and cerebrovascular disease. Low cardiac output resulting from myocardial infarction can induce hypothermia. Fetal and maternal bradycardia and hypothermia may result from magnesium sulfate infusion during preterm labor. Hypothermia can cause delayed recovery from neuromuscular blockade. Although many conditions can cause or be associated with accidental hypothermia, there is no true differential diagnosis of accidental hypothermia once the diagnosis has been established by core temperature measurement.

BOX 128.2 Presenting Signs of Hypothermia

Head, Eye, Ear, Nose, Throat
Mydriasis
Decreased corneal reflexes
Extraocular muscle abnormalities
Erythropsia (altered color perception)
Flushing
Facial edema
Epistaxis
Rhinorrhea
Strabismus

Cardiovascular
Initial tachycardia
Subsequent bradycardia
Dysrhythmias
Decreased heart tones
Hepatojugular reflux
Jugular venous distention
Hypotension

Respiratory
Initial tachypnea
Adventitious sounds
Bronchorrhea
Progressive hypoventilation
Apnea

Gastrointestinal
Ileus
Constipation
Abdominal distention or rigidity
Poor rectal tone
Gastric dilation in neonates or in adults with myxedema

Genitourinary
Anuria
Oliguria
Polyuria
Testicular torsion

Neurologic
Depressed level of consciousness
Ataxia
Hypesthesia

Dysarthria
Antinociception
Amnesia
Initial hyperreflexia
Anesthesia
Hyporeflexia
Areflexia
Central pontine myelinolysis

Psychiatric
Impaired judgment
Perseveration
Mood changes
Flat affect
Altered mental status
Paradoxical undressing
Neuroses
Psychoses
Suicide
Organic brain syndrome

Musculoskeletal
Increased muscle tone
Shivering
Rigidity or pseudo–rigor mortis
Paravertebral spasm
Opisthotonos
Compartment syndrome

Dermatologic
Erythema
Pernio
Pallor
Frostnip
Cyanosis
Frostbite
Icterus
Popsicle panniculitis (inflammation of the cheeks; also called "cold panniculitis")
Sclerema (hardening of subcutaneous tissue)
Cold urticaria
Ecchymosis
Necrosis
Edema
Gangrene

Diagnostic Testing

Except in mild cases of hypothermia, initial laboratory evaluation should include glucose level, complete blood cell count, comprehensive metabolic panel, serum lipase level, and coagulation studies. Blood urea nitrogen and creatinine levels should be checked because renal failure may occur after rewarming in patients with chronic hypothermia. Arterial or venous blood gases, if obtained, should not be temperature-corrected. A serum ethanol level and urine toxicology screen may be helpful based on history or when a depressed level of consciousness is inconsistent with the degree of hypothermia. Thyroid function studies, cardiac markers, and serum cortisol levels may also be indicated.

Acid-Base Balance. Blood gas analyzers warm blood to 37°C (98.6°F), increasing the partial pressure of dissolved gases. This results in arterial blood gases with higher oxygen and carbon dioxide and lower pH than in vivo values. Attempting to maintain a corrected pH at 7.4 and arterial partial pressure of carbon dioxide ($Paco_2$) at 40 mm Hg during hypothermia depresses cerebral and coronary blood flow and cardiac output and increases the incidence of VF. The ideal acid-base goal is an uncorrected pH of 7.4 and $Paco_2$ of 40 mm Hg.

Cold blood buffers poorly. In normothermia, pH decreases by 0.08 unit for every 10-mm Hg increase in $Paco_2$. At 28°C (82.4°F), the decrease in pH doubles. Because the neutral point of water at 37°C (98.6°F) is a pH of 6.8, the normal 0.6-unit pH offset between blood and intracellular water should be maintained at all temperatures (Fig. 128.3). Intracellular electrochemical neutrality ensures optimal

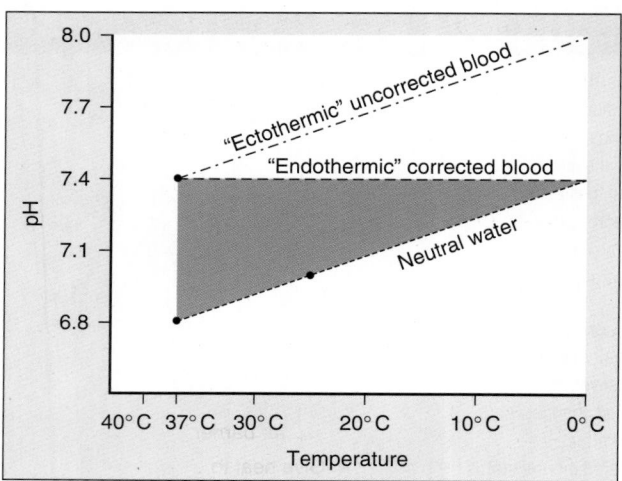

Fig. 128.3 Neutrality reflects the pH of water at any given temperature. The pH of water is 6.8 at 37°C (98.6°F) and 7.0 at 25°C (78.8°F). The physiologically ideal intracellular-to-extracellular, 0.6-unit pH offset will be maintained if the arterial pH is kept at 7.42, uncorrected for temperature.

enzymatic function at all temperatures. Relative alkalinity affords myocardial protection and improves the heart's electrical stability.

Hematologic Evaluation. The hematocrit can be deceptively high due to decreased plasma volume. The hematocrit increases 2% for every 1°C (1.8°F) fall in temperature. A low-normal hematocrit level in a moderately to severely hypothermic patient should suggest acute or chronic blood loss.

Splenic, hepatic, and splanchnic sequestration in hypothermia decreases leukocyte and platelet counts. As in normothermia, a normal white blood cell count does not exclude infection, especially if the patient is debilitated, alcoholic, myxedematous, or at either extreme of age.

Frequent evaluation of serum electrolyte levels during rewarming is essential. There are no safe predictors of values or trends. Changes occur in membrane permeability and in the sodium-potassium pump. The patient's preexisting physiologic status, severity and chronicity of hypothermia, and method of rewarming alter the serum electrolyte values.

The plasma potassium level is independent of hypothermia. Hyperkalemia can be associated with metabolic acidosis, rhabdomyolysis, or renal failure. Hypothermia enhances the cardiac toxicity of hyperkalemia and obscures premonitory electrocardiographic changes. Hypokalemia is most common with chronic hypothermia. It results from potassium entering muscle, rather than potassium diuresis. A decline in the serum potassium level despite a decreasing serum pH is caused by intracellular pH fluxes greater than extracellular pH fluxes.

Conditions associated with hypokalemia include preexisting diabetic ketoacidosis, hypopituitarism, inappropriate secretion of antidiuretic hormone, previous diuretic therapy, and alcoholism. If the serum potassium level is less than 3 mEq/L, provide supplementation during rewarming.

Blood urea nitrogen and creatinine levels are elevated with preexisting renal disease or decreased clearance. Because of hypothermic fluid shifts, hematocrit and blood urea nitrogen levels are poor indicators of actual fluid status.

The blood glucose level may provide a subtle clue to the chronicity of hypothermia. Acute hypothermia initially elevates the blood glucose level by catecholamine-induced glycogenolysis, diminished insulin release, and inhibition of cellular membrane glucose carrier systems.

Subacute and chronic hypothermia produce glycogen depletion, leading to hypoglycemia. Hypoglycemia can also develop during rewarming in acute hypothermia. Symptoms of hypoglycemia can be masked by hypothermia. A cold-induced renal glycosuria neither implies hyperglycemia nor guarantees normoglycemia.

When hyperglycemia persists during rewarming, suspect hemorrhagic pancreatitis or diabetic ketoacidosis. Actively rewarm patients with diabetic ketoacidosis past 30°C (86°F) because insulin is ineffective below 30°C (86°F). Correction of hypoglycemia corrects the level of consciousness only to the level consistent with the degree of hypothermia.

Severe hypothermia also causes serum enzyme level elevation because of the ultrastructural cellular damage. Rhabdomyolysis is commonly associated with cold exposure. Ischemic pancreatitis may result from the microcirculatory shock of hypothermia. Decreased pancreatic blood flow then activates proteolytic enzymes, increasing the serum lipase level.

Hypothermic Coagulation. A physiologic hypercoagulable state can occur with hypothermia and can be associated with a disseminated intravascular coagulation (DIC)–type syndrome. The cause may be catecholamine or steroid release, circulatory collapse, or release of tissue thromboplastin from cold, ischemic tissue.

Coagulopathies also occur because the enzymatic activity of the activated clotting factors is depressed by the cold. Clotting prolongation is proportional to the number of steps in the cascade. Because kinetic tests of coagulation are performed in the laboratory at 37°C (98.6°F), there is a disparity between clinically evident coagulopathy in vivo and deceptively normal prothrombin times, partial thromboplastin times, and international normalized ratios reported by the laboratory. The only effective treatment is rewarming, not administration of clotting factors.

Leukopenia and thrombocytopenia usually reverse with rewarming. Clinically significant coagulopathies can still occur, particularly in association with trauma and volume resuscitation. Cold-induced thrombocytopenia may be from direct bone marrow suppression or from splenic and hepatic sequestration. Platelet thromboxane B2 production is also temperature dependent, which can result in decreased platelet function and adhesion.

Elevated blood viscosity seen in hypothermia may be exacerbated in patients with cryoglobulinemia or cryofibrinogenemia, especially in older patients. Cryofibrinogen, a cold-precipitated fibrinogen, is associated with collagen vascular diseases, carcinomas, and coliform sepsis. Cold hemagglutination from cold agglutinins produces hemolysis or agglutination with thrombosis, which might explain the increase in coronary and cerebral thromboses in winter.

Imaging

If the patient is not alert and there is suspicion of trauma, standard trauma imaging is indicated, including an extended focused assessment with sonography in trauma (eFAST) and computed tomography (CT) scan of the head. CT scanning of the abdomen and pelvis may show pancreatic calcifications, unsuspected pneumoperitoneum, small bowel dilation from hypothermia-induced mesenteric vascular occlusion, or colonic dilation associated with myxedema coma.

Management

General Measures

Patients who are cold, stiff, and cyanotic, with fixed pupils, inaudible heart tones, and no visible thoracic excursions, can still be successfully resuscitated. Unexpectedly, a few patients have revived in the morgue while awaiting autopsy.

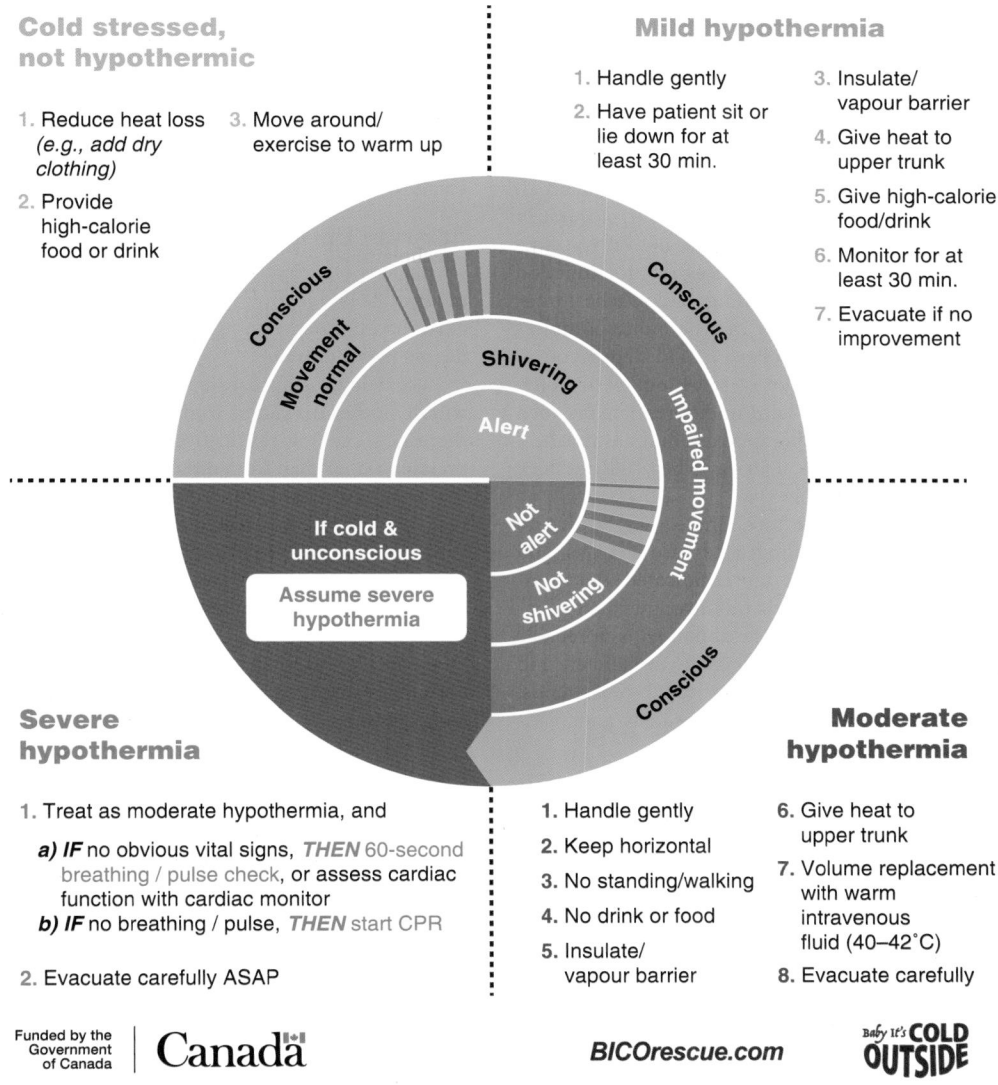

Assess cold patient

1. From outside ring to center: Assess consciousness, movement, shivering, alertness
2. Assess whether normal, impaired or no function
3. The colder the patient is, the slower you can go, once patient is secured
4. Treat all traumatized cold patients with active warming to upper trunk
5. Avoid burns: Following product guidelines for heat sources; check for excessive skin redness

Cold stressed, not hypothermic

1. Reduce heat loss (e.g., add dry clothing)
2. Provide high-calorie food or drink
3. Move around/ exercise to warm up

Mild hypothermia

1. Handle gently
2. Have patient sit or lie down for at least 30 min.
3. Insulate/ vapour barrier
4. Give heat to upper trunk
5. Give high-calorie food/drink
6. Monitor for at least 30 min.
7. Evacuate if no improvement

Conscious · Movement normal · Shivering · Alert · **Conscious** · Impaired movement

Not alert · Not shivering

If cold & unconscious

Assume severe hypothermia

Conscious

Severe hypothermia

1. Treat as moderate hypothermia, and
   a) IF no obvious vital signs, *THEN* 60-second breathing / pulse check, or assess cardiac function with cardiac monitor
   b) IF no breathing / pulse, *THEN* start CPR
2. Evacuate carefully ASAP

Moderate hypothermia

1. Handle gently
2. Keep horizontal
3. No standing/walking
4. No drink or food
5. Insulate/ vapour barrier
6. Give heat to upper trunk
7. Volume replacement with warm intravenous fluid (40–42°C)
8. Evacuate carefully

Funded by the Government of Canada | **Canada**

BICOrescue.com

Baby It's **COLD OUTSIDE**

Fig. 128.4 "Cold card" for treatment of cold patients.

Pertinent history includes information about preexisting cardiac, pulmonary, neurologic, or endocrine disease. The duration of exposure, outdoor conditions, circumstances of discovery, associated injuries, and predisposing conditions should be documented. Initial management should emphasize prevention of further heat loss. Specific goals of prehospital care include adequate insulation, avoidance of core afterdrop, gentle handling, and transport in a horizontal position.[4] Hypothermic patients should be actively rewarmed in the field, if possible.[4]

A graphic flowchart to assist with clinical staging of hypothermia and to guide treatment is available as a "cold card" (Figure 128.4).[5]

A patient who is unresponsive and not shivering should be treated for severe hypothermia. At core temperatures below 32°C (89.6°F), expect an irritable myocardium, a large temperature gradient between the core and periphery, and relative hypovolemia.

In the ED, hypothermia should be confirmed and monitored with continuous core temperature evaluation. Clinically, the rectal temperature is most widely used. However, it lags behind core temperature changes and is influenced by lower extremity temperatures and probe placement. The probe should be inserted to 15 cm and not placed into cold feces. Epitympanic temperature equilibrates rapidly with core temperature and is closest to the hypothalamic temperature. Most epitympanic probes are not suitable for field use.[4] Infrared thermography (tympanic temperature) is too unreliable be used, except to exclude hypothermia. So-called temporal artery thermometers are often random number generators and unreliable for clinical use. If the airway is protected, an esophageal probe placed in the lower third of the esophagus, an average of 24 cm below the larynx in adults, is the ideal method for continuous core temperature monitoring. If the probe is placed higher, the reading can be falsely elevated by inhalation of heated oxygen. An esophageal probe without markings can have tape placed on the proximal part to mark the correct depth of insertion.

Hand-held Doppler may be useful to establish the presence of a spontaneous pulse. Bedside echocardiography should precede chest compressions. Pulse oximetry is usually unreliable in hypothermia with peripheral vasoconstriction. It is often not possible to obtain an accurate reading. End-tidal carbon dioxide measurements accurately assess tissue perfusion and tracheal tube placement, but only at normal temperatures. Commercially available devices do not function when humidified air is used for airway rewarming. Endotracheal intubation or placement of a supraglottic airway may be indicated unless the patient has intact protective airway reflexes. Cold depression of ciliary activity allows for the accumulation of secretions with frothy sputum and chest congestion. It may be hard to differentiate between bronchorrhea and pulmonary edema. Fiberoptic or blind nasotracheal intubation can be useful to avoid a surgical airway when cold-induced trismus is present.

Dysrhythmias during intubation are rare. These may be due to failure to preoxygenate, mechanical jostling, acid-base changes, and electrolyte level fluctuations. A nasogastric tube is indicated after endotracheal intubation because decreased gastric motility and gastric dilation are common. Physical examination of the abdomen is unreliable because cold can induce rectus muscle rigidity. Many moderately and severely hypothermic patients have decreased or absent bowel sounds. It is important to evaluate the patient for an associated ileus, pancreatitis, or occult trauma.

In moderate and severe hypothermia, indwelling urinary catheters are useful to monitor urine output and help determine the severity of vascular fluid shifts.

Cardiac monitoring should be continuous. If central venous access is required, avoid insertion of the catheter tip into the heart, which can irritate the myocardium and precipitate dysrhythmias. Arterial catheters for continuous monitoring of intra-arterial blood pressure may be helpful in profoundly hypothermic patients. Placement of a pulmonary artery catheter risks perforation of a cold, stiff, pulmonary artery and is not recommended in the emergency department.

Volume Resuscitation

Patients with moderate or severe hypothermia are usually volume depleted. They are prone to thromboembolism resulting from increased viscosity. During rewarming, the total plasma volume is usually high, but the circulatory plasma volume is usually low due to increased peripheral vascular resistance. Rapid volume expansion can be lifesaving, especially in hypothermic neonates. Adult patients with moderate or severe hypothermia should initially receive a 500-mL fluid challenge of warmed normal saline. Avoid lactated Ringers solution because the cold liver metabolizes lactate poorly. Fluids administered via the intravenous (IV) route should be warmed to 40°C to 42°C (104°F to 107.6°F). If a commercial fluid or blood warmer is not

available, IV fluids can be heated in a standard microwave. Shake the fluid bag before administration to avoid hot spots. Avoid rapid central venous administration, which may produce myocardial thermal gradients. Another option in vasoconstricted patients is administration via the intraosseous route. Countercurrent heat exchangers effectively heat crystalloids and blood from 10°C to 35°C (50°F to 95°F). There can be significant conductive heat loss through IV tubing, especially with long lengths of tubing at slow flow rates. It is preferable to administer fluids as boluses to effect rather than as drips.

Normally, hypothermia increases natriuresis. Preexisting gastrointestinal losses or previous diuretic treatment can also contribute to sodium loss. Patients with a normal sodium level and osmolality may have preexisting sodium overload as a result of cirrhosis, nephrosis, or congestive heart failure. However, most patients will be free-water depleted, elevating the sodium level and osmolality. Hemoconcentration due to decreased plasma volume, fluid shifts, and increased vascular permeability usually is present. Hemodilution can occur from parenteral crystalloid administration, but a low hematocrit can also result from acute hemorrhage or preexisting anemia.

Advanced Life Support

During hypothermic cardiac arrest, cardiac output and cerebral and myocardial blood flows are much less than those during normothermic closed chest compressions. Metabolic demands, however, are also less during hypothermia.

Blood flow during cardiopulmonary resuscitation (CPR) in patients with hypothermia differs from flow during normothermia. In normothermia, some flow results from phasic alterations in the intrathoracic pressure rather than from direct cardiac compression. In hypothermia, the heart is a passive conduit, and phasic alterations in the intrathoracic pressure are exerted equally on all cardiac chambers. The mitral valve remains patent during systole, and blood continues to circulate through the left side of the heart. This explains an observation of a thoracotomy in a patient who ultimately survived severe hypothermia: "the heart was found to be hard as stone and it is hardly conceivable how effective external cardiac massage could have been." There have been many neurologically intact survivors after prolonged closed chest compressions.

Chest wall elasticity and pulmonary compliance are decreased with cold. More force is needed to depress the chest wall sufficiently to generate adequate intrathoracic pressure gradients. Powered thoracic compression devices are useful during prolonged resuscitations pending decisions about extracorporeal rewarming.

Apparent rigor mortis and fixed dilated pupils are not reliable criteria for withholding CPR in a hypothermic patient. Accurately diagnosed dependent lividity is a sign of death even in hypothermia, although previous guidelines have stated the contrary. Because intermittent flow may provide adequate support during evacuation, CPR should not be withheld just because continuous compressions cannot be ensured.[6]

Rescuers should initiate CPR in accidental hypothermia unless do-not-resuscitate status is known, obviously lethal injuries are present, chest wall depression is impossible, signs of life are present, or rescuers are endangered.[4] If possible, verify that there is no spontaneous mechanical cardiac activity with bedside ultrasonography before chest compressions are initiated.

Pharmacologic Treatment

The efficacy of most medications is temperature dependent. Protein binding increases during hypothermia. Liver metabolism is decreased. Large doses could be required to achieve a therapeutic response. Toxic levels could develop with rewarming. In severe hypothermia, withhold medications until the patient is warmed, and then leave longer intervals between doses. No medication should be given orally because of the patient's decreased gastrointestinal motility. Intramuscular medications are also contraindicated because of poor absorption from vasoconstricted sites.

Cardiovascular Medications. The effects of hypothermia on the autonomic nervous system are variable. In primates, sympathetic response increases rapidly to cooling from 37°C to 31°C (98.6°F to 87.8°F) and then switches off at about 29°C (84.2°F). This suggests that modest catecholamine support might be useful below 29°C (84.2°F).

Pharmacologic manipulation of the pulse and blood pressure should be avoided. Epinephrine and other vasoconstrictors may be dysrhythmogenic and have a minimal effect on the maximally constricted peripheral vasculature. There are no clear indications for vasopressors although, in animal models, the return of spontaneous circulation after induced VF below 30°C (86°F) is higher after the administration of vasopressors.

Inotropes are usually not necessary to support blood pressure. Inotropic support may be considered in disproportionately hypotensive patients who do not maintain a mean arterial pressure of 60 mm Hg in response to volume replacement and rewarming.

Atrial dysrhythmias are common below 32°C (89.6°F), associated with a slow ventricular response. Atrial fibrillation is common but self-limited and typically converts spontaneously during rewarming. Beta blockers and calcium channel blockers are contraindicated unless there is a rapid ventricular response.

Preexisting, chronic, premature ventricular contractions can be suppressed during hypothermia and recur during rewarming. Most hypothermia-induced dysrhythmias convert spontaneously during rewarming. Asystole that develops during rewarming is not as ominous as asystole in normothermic patients. For VF, defibrillation should be attempted at the usual energy level. Successful defibrillation has been reported at 20°C (68°F) but attempted defibrillation is often unsuccessful until the core temperature is above 30°C (86°F). If a defibrillation attempt is unsuccessful, active rewarming should be initiated while continuing CPR. Defibrillation can be attempted occasionally during rewarming. Once the core temperature is above 30°C (86°F), further attempts can be made.[7]

The ideal approach to ventricular dysrhythmias in the hypothermic patient has not been well studied. Lidocaine and propranolol have minimal hemodynamic effects during hypothermia. Their efficacy in the treatment of ventricular dysrhythmias appears limited. In a canine model of severe hypothermic VF, neither amiodarone nor bretylium was effective. Human chemical defibrillations with bretylium tosylate in cases of severe hypothermia have been reported. Recurrent VF was controlled by isoproterenol in one reported case.[8] Amiodarone can cause torsades de pointes by QT prolongation and its safety during accidental and induced hypothermia is not known.

In hypothermia, at least one Group 1 antidysrhythmic agent, procainamide, increases the incidence of VF. Another drug in the same group, quinidine, can prevent VF during induced profound hypothermia and during cardiac manipulation at 25°C to 30°C (77°F to 86°F). Transvenous cardiac pacing is hazardous for bradydysrhythmias in hypothermia. External pacing may be worth trying in the rare setting of profoundly disproportionate bradycardia. Transcutaneous pacing has been used to facilitate continuous arteriovenous rewarming in perfusing patients by raising the systolic blood pressure above 60 mm Hg. Other active rewarming techniques do not require specific pressure gradients.

Antibiotics. Hypothermia compromises host defenses and predisposes to infection. In hypothermia, the usual signs of infection, including fever, are absent. Shaking chills from sepsis may be mistaken for shivering. Suspect CNS injury or infection if a patient's mental status remains altered, despite rewarming.

In hypothermic children younger than 3 months, empirical antibiotics are indicated after cultures have been obtained. There are no reliable clinical or laboratory indicators of infection, but bradycardia, anemia, uremia, and high serum glucose levels, as well as leukocyte abnormalities, are common clues. The role of empirical antibiotics in adults is less clear. Although gram-negative septicemia may cause hypothermia, coexistent infections from gram-positive cocci, Enterobacteriaceae, and oral anaerobes are common.

Older adults with thermoregulatory failure have a high risk of mortality and should be considered septic until proven otherwise. Routine empiric antibiotics are warranted in hypothermia only in geriatric patients. Administer antibiotics if the clinical picture is consistent with septic shock or if there is failure to rewarm. Cellulitis, myositis, bacteriuria, or infiltrate on chest x-ray warrants immediate antimicrobial therapy. In an urban setting, infection is the leading cause of failure to rewarm and subsequent mortality.

Failure to Rewarm. Cold abolishes adrenal responsiveness to adrenocorticotropic hormone (ACTH). A false diagnosis of decreased adrenal reserve is possible. The increase in ACTH level seen in hypothermic individuals may be a neurogenic or emotional response to the cold.

Acute cold stress initially stimulates cortisol secretion. There may already be a very high level as a result of underlying stress. In clinical series, total serum cortisol levels are commonly elevated; however, the active free fraction is decreased due to increased protein binding. Failure to rewarm may be due to adrenocortical insufficiency or steroid dependence. If either condition is suspected, administer 100 mg IV of hydrocortisone.

Empirical treatment with thyroxine is reserved for patients thought to have myxedema. Thyroid hormone should be replaced if there is a history of hypothyroidism, suggestive neck scar, or failure to rewarm. After thyroid function study samples have been drawn, levothyroxine, 250 to 500 µg IV, can be slowly administered over several minutes. Daily injections of 50 to 100 µg are necessary for 5 to 7 days. Hydrocortisone (100–200 mg) should be added to the first several liters of crystalloid fluid. The absorption of oral or intramuscular levothyroxine is variable. IV administration has a smooth effect after the onset of action at 6 to 12 hours. This will be manifested by improvement in vital signs and rewarming rate. Half the dose is converted by the peripheral tissues into L-triiodothyronine (T_3). An underlying infection can also compromise thermogenesis.

Rewarming

There are no published controlled studies comparing rewarming methods in hypothermia. Rigid treatment protocols are not evidence-based. The emergency clinician should choose specific methods on a case-by-case basis, taking into account availability, institutional resources, and clinical experience.

Passive External Rewarming. Spontaneous passive external rewarming is noninvasive. It is the treatment of choice for patients with mild hypothermia when active rewarming is not available. The patient should be able to generate sufficient metabolic heat to maintain an acceptable rate of spontaneous rewarming. Older adults are commonly glycogen-depleted, have central hypovolemia, and are not capable of normal cardiovascular or metabolic homeostasis.

The normal processes of heat dissipation are minimized by passive external rewarming. Cessation of evaporation and convection is coupled with insulation against further radiation of heat. This technique simply involves covering the patient with an insulating material in a favorable atmospheric condition. The ambient temperature should exceed 21°C (69.8°F). When the air is stationary, less heat is lost to conduction, convection, and radiation.

BOX 128.3   Indications for Active Rewarming

Cardiovascular instability
Mild to severe hypothermia
Inadequate rate of rewarming or failure to rewarm
Endocrine insufficiency
Trauma
Traumatic or toxicological peripheral vasodilation
Secondary hypothermia impairing thermoregulation

Shivering is the most effective thermoregulatory neuromuscular response to cold in humans. Without shivering, endogenously generated metabolic heat is insufficient to raise the core temperature. When the core temperature exceeds 32°C (89.6°F), unless complete glycogen depletion occurs, the major source of heat production is shivering thermogenesis.

Recommended rewarming rates vary between 0.5°C and 2.0°C/hr (0.9°F and 3.6°F/hr). The rewarming rate should be rapid enough to avoid prolonged exposure to dysrhythmias. Below 32°C (89.6°F), humans are functionally poikilothermic. Shivering is ineffective below 32°C (89.6°F) and absent below 30°C (86°F).

Active Rewarming. Active rewarming is the direct transfer of exogenous heat to the patient. It can be accomplished by external or internal techniques. Active rewarming is useful in mild hypothermia to decrease metabolic requirements of rewarming and improve thermal comfort.

In moderate to severe hypothermia, cardiovascular instability and decompensation require prompt elevation of the core temperature while minimizing afterdrop (Box 128.3). Defibrillation is rarely successful at temperatures below 28°C (82.46°F). Active rewarming is indicated with strokes and other conditions that impair CNS control of thermoregulation. Active rewarming is also indicated for patients when endogenous thermogenesis is insufficient or when glycogen depletion is present, usually from endocrine causes that include hypopituitarism, adrenal insufficiency, hypothyroidism, and Wernicke encephalopathy. Active rewarming is recommended in diabetic ketoacidosis because the core temperature must be elevated above 30°C (86°F) before insulin becomes effective.

Pharmacologically induced peripheral vasodilation or acute spinal cord transection prevents sufficient thermogenesis and requires active rewarming. Patients with severe hypothermia do not necessarily require invasive extracorporeal rewarming techniques, especially if they have a sustained perfusing rhythm.

Aggressive treatment of hypothermia is indicated in infants. Rapid rewarming is advantageous because it minimizes energy expenditures. Hypothermic neonates have been successfully rewarmed using minimally invasive methods. A neonate with a core temperature of 14.8°C (58.6°F) receiving CPR made a full neurologic recovery after being rewarmed by active external rewarming (AER), warmed IV fluids, and heated, humidified ventilator gases.

Active External Rewarming. Early concern with AER was sparked after a 1961 study, in which 20 of 23 patients died. Retrospective analysis of clinical series has shown widely varying mortality rates with AER. Various methods conduct heat directly to the skin. Rewarming options include plumbed garments that circulate warm fluids, hot water bottles, heating pads, forced air warming systems, and radiant sources. Thermal injury to vasoconstricted hypoperfused skin is a potential hazard with local heat application.

Forced air warming systems efficiently transfer heat. They can be used in field conditions or in the ED. These devices circulate hot air through a blanket. The air flows through apertures on the patient's side, allowing convective transfer of heat. Hypotension and core temperature afterdrop are not seen in forced air warming for accidental hypothermia in the ED. Like all active methods, forced air warming decreases shivering and is able to transfer large amounts of heat while minimizing afterdrop. Other options include thermoregulatory systems that circulate warm water through energy transfer pads.

Arteriovenous anastomosis (AVA) rewarming is a unique, noninvasive, AER technique. Exogenous heat is provided by immersion of distal extremities (upper extremities to the elbows and lower extremities to the knees) in hot (44°C to 45°C [111.2°F to 113.6°F]) water. The heat opens the AVAs, which are 1 mm below the epidermal surface in the digits. As a result, there is an increased flow of warmed venous subcutaneous blood returning directly to the heart. The forearms and calves must be included for this technique to be effective. The AVA technique was designed for use on ships and is not practical in most situations. In addition, many patients cannot tolerate the very hot water. Burns of vasoconstricted skin are a potential hazard.

Previously healthy patients with acute hypothermia are optimal candidates for AER. They have minimal dehydration and pathophysiologic circulatory changes. If AER is used, and the extremities are vasoconstricted, the heat source should be applied preferentially to the thorax rather than to the extremities. Application of heat to the extremities increases the cardiovascular load by increasing the metabolic requirements of the peripheral musculature. The depressed cardiovascular system may not be able to meet the demands, resulting in cardiovascular collapse.

Combining truncal AER with core rewarming can also be successful. The provision of heated humidified oxygen and warmed IV fluids, in addition to AER, may help prevent hypoxia, metabolic acidosis, core temperature afterdrop, and hypotension. If AER is used to treat moderate or severe hypothermia, it can be combined with one or more active core rewarming techniques.

Active Core Rewarming. Many methods achieve active rewarming of the core. These techniques minimize the risk of rewarming collapse in patients with core temperatures below 32°C (89.6°F).

Airway Rewarming. Airway rewarming with heated humidified oxygen is a simple and inexpensive method that can be used as an adjunct to other forms of active rewarming in moderate or severe hypothermia, although it is ineffective on its own. Airway rewarming improves oxygenation, helps avoid afterdrop, stimulates pulmonary cilia, decreases viscosity of pulmonary secretions, and reduces cold-induced bronchorrhea. Pulmonary absorption of moisture does not adversely affect surfactant or increase pulmonary congestion.

The respiratory tract is a limited site for heat exchange, but heated humidified oxygen increases blood oxygen content and temperature in the pulmonary circulation. The myocardium is perfused by warmer oxygenated blood, decreasing intermittent temperature gradients.

Sufficient minute volume and complete humidification are necessary for maximal heat delivery. Because dry air has low thermal conductivity, ventilation with warm dry air provides negligible heat. Increases in rewarming rates from 1°C to 4.5°C/hr (1.8°F to 8.1°F/hr) have been reported with heated humidified oxygen. The larger increases are unlikely to be true. Increases in warming rates with endotracheal intubation are higher than those with a mask. Positive-pressure ventilation with a mask can be used but has not been studied.

Maintenance of sufficient oxygenation is important in moderate to severe hypothermia. In patients on cardiopulmonary bypass cooled to 28°C to 30°C (82.4°F to 86°F), the capacity of hemoglobin to unload oxygen to the tissue is less than half that found in normothermic patients. Despite lower metabolic requirements, this decreased functional hemoglobin, combined with a depressed respiratory minute volume, results in minimal oxygen reserves. Some patients maintain a level of spontaneous respiration appropriate to depressed carbon dioxide production. This may not be the case in patients with coexisting toxicologic, traumatic, or metabolic depression of the respiratory center.

Providing heated, humidified oxygen to a patient with spontaneous respiration requires a heated cascade nebulizer. An immersion heater can be connected to a hose with a warming wire. Because patients with a depressed level of consciousness do not complain of pain, it is essential to check the temperature of the inspired air frequently with an in-line temperature probe. The gas temperature should be maintained at 42°C to 45°C (107.6°F to 113°F). Most heater modules require modification to allow the temperature to reach 42°C to 45°C (107.6°F to 113°F). Modified heater modules should be labeled to avoid routine use. Most humidifiers will not exceed 41°C (105.8°F) close to the patient outlet with a 2-m tubing length. Strategies to circumvent the 41°C (105.8°F) ceiling include reduction of tubing length, addition of more heat sources, disabling of the humidifier safety system, and placement of the temperature probe outside the patient circuit. Because of the modest clinical benefit in stable patients, it is probably not worth the effort to circumvent the 41°C (105.8°F) ceiling. The only report of thermal airway injury was in a patient ventilated by endotracheal tube for 11 hours with 80°C (176°F) inhaled gas.

Peritoneal Dialysis. Peritoneal dialysis delivers dialysate at 40°C to 45°C (104°F to 113°F). Heat is conducted directly to intraperitoneal structures through the posterior parietal peritoneum and the solid viscera and through the hemidiaphragms to the heart and lungs. A double-catheter system with suction at the outflow can theoretically increase flow to about 6 L/hr. Two liters are infused, retained for 20 minutes, and then aspirated. In practice, it can be difficult to recover all of the infused fluid. This lowers the achievable flow rate. Rewarming rates average 1°C to 3°C/hr (1.8°F to 5.4°F/hr).

An additional benefit of peritoneal dialysis is hepatic rewarming, which reactivates detoxification and conversion enzymes. Serum electrolyte levels should be monitored because peritoneal dialysis can exacerbate preexisting hypokalemia. Peritoneal lavage is useful primarily in severe cases in combination with other rewarming techniques for patients without spontaneous perfusion but has also been used alone in patients undergoing CPR for whom extracorporeal circulation was thought to be contraindicated due to coagulopathy or was not available.

Heated Irrigation. Heat transfer from irrigation fluids is usually limited due to the minimal surface area available for heat exchange. Gastric or colonic irrigation can cause fluid and electrolyte level fluxes and are not recommended. An esophageal heat transfer device with closed circulation of heated water is practical and has been used successfully for rewarming in hypothermia.[9]

Closed thoracic lavage can be useful in severe hypothermia. Two large-bore thoracostomy tubes are inserted into one or both hemithoraces. One is inserted anteriorly in the second or third intercostal space at the midclavicular line, the historical classic site for needle thoracostomy. The other is inserted between the fifth and sixth intercostal spaces in the posterior axillary line, the usual site for tube thoracostomy. Normal saline heated to 40°C to 42°C (104°F to 107.6°F) is infused into the superior tube. The inferior tube is used for drainage. Left-sided tube insertion in perfusing patients risks causing VF. Efficiency of the heat transfer varies with flow rate and dwell times. Pleural adhesions can prevent adequate infusion and can result in a tension hydrothorax. Adequate drainage should be ensured to prevent intrathoracic hypertension.

Thoracic lavage is usually reserved for the severely hypothermic patient who does not respond to standard techniques or the patient with another indication for a chest tube. It should be combined with other rewarming modalities in potentially salvageable cardiac arrest patients. However, thoracic lavage has been used successfully in patients requiring CPR when extracorporeal circulation was not available. The rate of rewarming averages 3°C/hr (5.4°F/hr).

Mediastinal irrigation and direct myocardial lavage should be considered only in patients without spontaneous perfusion. The procedure requires a standard left lateral thoracotomy incision. The pericardium is not incised unless an effusion or tamponade is present. The heart is bathed in 1 to 2 L of an isotonic solution heated to 40°C (104°F) for several minutes. The fluid is removed and the lavage is repeated. Internal defibrillation is attempted at intervals of 2°C (3.6°F) after the myocardial temperature exceeds 26°C to 28°C (78.8°F to 82.4°F). When a perfusing rhythm is achieved, lavage is continued until the myocardial temperature exceeds 32°C (89.6°F). A median sternotomy approach allows ventricular decompression in addition to direct defibrillation. Open cardiac massage of a cold, rigid, and contracted heart may not generate flow.

Endovascular Rewarming. Another active core rewarming option uses endovascular warming devices that are intended for therapeutic cooling and subsequent rewarming of comatose, resuscitated, cardiac arrest patients.[10] These systems involve femoral vein catheterization with a closed-loop catheter that has a thermostat at the tip. If the core temperature is below 30°C (86°F), the fail-safe feature on the console must be circumvented to allow rewarming.

Diathermy. Truncal diathermy involves the conversion of energy waves into heat. Large amounts of heat can be delivered to deep tissues with ultrasonic and low-frequency microwave irradiation. Frostbite, burns, significant edema, and the presence of all types of metallic implants and pacemakers are contraindications. In spite of successes in piglets, infants, and a few adults, diathermy is still experimental.

Extracorporeal Blood Rewarming. The four common extracorporeal techniques to rewarm blood are venovenous rewarming, hemodialysis, continuous arteriovenous (AV) rewarming, and extracorporeal circulation–cardiopulmonary bypass (CPB and extracorporeal membrane oxygenation [ECMO]); Table 128.2).

In venovenous rewarming, blood is removed, ideally by a large peripheral venous catheter, heated to 40°C (104°F) and returned through a second venous catheter. Flow rates are 150 to 400 mL/min. The circuit is simple and efficient. There is no oxygenator, and the system does not provide circulatory support. Volume infusion is an option to augment inadequate cardiac output.

Standard hemodialysis is a widely available, practical rewarming technique. It is portable and efficient and can also be used to treat electrolyte abnormalities, renal failure, or intoxication with a dialyzable substance (e.g., ethylene glycol, methanol).

Continuous AV rewarming is an option if the blood pressure is at least 60 mm Hg, which may be maintained, if necessary, with CPR. AV rewarming involves the use of percutaneously inserted femoral arterial and contralateral femoral venous catheters. Heparin-bonded tubing circuits obviate the need for systemic anticoagulation. The blood pressure of a spontaneously perfusing, traumatized, hypothermic patient creates a functional arteriovenous fistula by diverting part of the cardiac output from the femoral artery through a commercially available countercurrent heat exchanger. The heated blood is then returned with admixed heated crystalloids through the femoral vein. Continuous AV rewarming avoids the need for specialized equipment and a perfusionist, which are necessary for cardiopulmonary bypass. The average rate of rewarming is 3°C to 4°C/hr (5.4°F to 7.2°F/hr). Because the catheters are 8.5 Fr, the patient should weigh at least 40 kg.

Extracorporeal circulation, also called *extracorporeal life support* or ECLS, refers to cardiopulmonary bypass or ECMO. In one review, the

TABLE 128.2 Extracorporeal Blood Rewarming Options

Options	Considerations
Venovenous circuit	Central venous catheter to central venous or peripheral catheter rewarming
	No oxygenator, circulatory support
	Flow rates, 150–400 mL/min
	Rate of rewarming 2°C–3°C/hr (3.6°F–4.5°F)
Hemodialysis circuit	Single- or dual-vessel cannulation; stabilizes electrolyte or toxicologic abnormalities
	Exchange cycle volumes 200–500 mL/min
	Rate of rewarming 2°C–3°C/hr (3.6°F–5.4°F/hr)
Continuous arteriovenous rewarming circuit	Percutaneous 8.5-Fr femoral catheters
	Requires blood pressure of 60 mm Hg systolic
	No perfusionist, pump, anticoagulation
	Flow rates, 225–375 mL/min
	Rate of rewarming, 3°C–4°C/hr (5.4°F–7.2°F/hr)
Cardiopulmonary bypass circuit	Full circulatory support with pump and oxygenator
	Perfusate-temperature gradient, 5°C–10°C/hr (9°F–18°F/hr)
	Flow rates, 2–7 L/min (average, 3–4 L/min)
	Rate of rewarming up to 9.5°C/hr (18.9°F/hr)

Adapted from: Danzl DF. Hypothermia and frostbite. In Kasper D, Fauci A, Hauser S, et al, eds. *Harrison's Principles of Internal Medicine*, ed 20. New York: McGraw-Hill; 2018.

mean temperature increase was 9.5°C/hr (17.1°F/hr) with CPB. ECMO appears to reduce the risk of intractable cardiorespiratory failure or severe pulmonary edema after rewarming.

The major advantage of extracorporeal circulation in perfusing patients is the preservation of flow if mechanical cardiac activity is lost during rewarming. Other candidates are patients who do not respond to less invasive rewarming techniques, those with completely frozen extremities, and those with rhabdomyolysis accompanied by major electrolyte disturbances. In some European centers, severely hypothermic patients without obvious trauma are admitted directly to the operating suite for extracorporeal circulation.

Very rapid rates of rewarming do not necessarily improve survival, but slow rewarming increases hospital mortality.[11] Complications of rapid rewarming include DIC, pulmonary edema, hemolysis, and acute tubular necrosis. Extracorporeal circulation can provide cardiovascular support in hemodynamically unstable patients.

Extracorporeal rewarming should be considered in hypothermic cardiac arrest patients if there are no contraindications to CPR.[12] A realistic assessment of the risk-benefit ratio for debilitated patients with secondary hypothermia should be made. Discontinue resuscitation if frozen or clotted intravascular contents are identified.

Disposition

Previously healthy patients who have mild primary accidental hypothermia (35°C to 32°C [95°F to 89.6°F]) usually rewarm easily. They can be safely discharged if a warm environment is available. Patients with mild hypothermia associated with trauma are more difficult to rewarm and require admission.

Patients with severe hypothermia (<32°C [89.6°F]) generally require admission to an intensive care setting. These patients should be evaluated for the presence of underlying medical disorders (see Box 128.1).

Cardiac monitoring should be considered for patients with persistent toxicologic or metabolic abnormalities and should be used for patients with cardiovascular instability or an inadequate rate of rewarming. Transfer of patients to tertiary care centers is generally not mandatory, but severely hypothermic patients may be most easily managed in facilities capable of extracorporeal circulation.

Because human physiologic responses are variable, it is difficult to predict outcomes. The type and severity of the underlying or precipitating disease process are major determinants.[13] The age of the patient is a weak predictor of mortality. Trauma, infection, and toxin ingestions unpredictably affect survival. Outcome prediction based on the Glasgow Coma Scale score is unreliable. Significant predictors of poor outcome include asphyxia, prehospital cardiac arrest, low or absent blood pressure, elevated blood urea nitrogen level, and need for endotracheal or nasogastric intubation in the ED. Patients with hypothermic cardiac arrest due to alcohol intoxication may have better neurologic outcomes than patients with hypothermic cardiac arrest from other causes.

In the past, the treatment dictum was that *"no one is dead until they are warm and dead."* Now we realize that some patients are cold and dead. It would be useful and humane if they could be safely identified. The search for a valid triage marker of death continues. Grave prognostic indicators include evidence of intravascular thrombosis (fibrinogen < 50 mg/dL), ammonia levels greater than 250 mmol/L, and cell lysis (hyperkalemia > 10–12 mEq/L). In hypothermia with asphyxia in avalanche victims, hyperkalemia greater than 7 mEq/L is a reliable indicator of death.[14]

FROSTBITE AND NONFREEZING COLD INJURIES

KEY CONCEPTS

Frostbite

- Premature termination of thawing in 37°C to 39°C (98.6°F to 102.2°F) water is a common error. Reperfusion of completely frozen tissue may be painful, requiring parenteral analgesia.
- The early formation of clear blebs is more favorable than delayed formation of hemorrhagic blebs, which reflect damage to the subdermal vascular plexi.
- Advise patients that accurate prediction of eventual tissue loss is not always possible at presentation, despite imaging.
- Thrombolysis may salvage severely frostbitten tissue if given within 24 hours of thawing.

Nonfreezing Cold Injuries

- Immersion injuries should be rewarmed slowly and not above 30°C (86°F).
- Gentle cooling of nonfreezing cold injuries may be helpful to relieve pain and edema.
- Pernio can be treated by drying and gentle massage. The skin should not be warmed above 30°C (86°F).

FROSTBITE

Foundations

Background and Importance

Unlike other mammals that live outside the tropics, humans are susceptible to local cold injuries. Local cold injuries may occur in conjunction with systemic hypothermia. Frostbite involves tissue freezing with formation of ice crystals in the tissues. Immersion injury (trench foot) is a nonfreezing injury that results from exposure to wet cold.

Pernio (chilblains) is a nonfreezing injury that occurs in susceptible individuals, usually after repetitive exposure to dry or damp cold.

Historically, frostbite has been a disease of wars. Frostbite caused over 1 million casualties in World Wars I and II and the Korean War. Trench foot was common in the world wars and during the conflict in the Falkland Islands. Frostbite and immersion injuries are risks for anyone who ventures outdoors in severely cold conditions for recreation or work. Homeless or displaced people are also at risk, especially during cold winter months and disasters.

Anatomy, Physiology, and Pathophysiology

The human body attempts to maintain a core temperature of about 37°C (98.6°F). Skin cooling activates the anterior hypothalamus, causing catecholamine release, thyroid stimulation, shivering thermogenesis, and peripheral vasoconstriction. People are physiologically adapted to tropical conditions. In cold conditions, humans have a limited ability to protect themselves against decreased core temperature. Behavioral responses are far more effective if adequate clothing or shelter is available.

Cutaneous circulation is one of the keys to maintenance of a constant core temperature. Baseline cutaneous circulation greatly exceeds nutritional requirements. In warm conditions, the skin acts as a radiator to shed excess heat. Cold-induced vasoconstriction can reduce flow to as low as 10% of baseline without damage to the skin.

During cold stress, peripheral vasoconstriction limits radiant heat loss. Acral skin structures (including fingers, toes, ears, and nose) contain a plethora of arteriovenous anastomoses. These anastomoses shut down in the cold, causing drastic reductions in blood flow. This so-called life-versus-limb mechanism is a means of preventing systemic hypothermia.

Cooling of digits to about 15°C (59°F) results in maximal peripheral vasoconstriction, with minimal blood flow. Continued cooling to about 10°C (50°F) produces cold-induced vasodilation (CIVD, also called "the hunting response"), a counterbalance to cold-induced vasoconstriction. Vasodilation follows 5- to 10-minute cycles, interrupting vasoconstriction and protecting the extremity. Inuits, Lapps, and other northern peoples have stronger CIVD than do individuals from tropical regions. There is evidence of adaptation, with more robust CIVD in response to cold, in addition to genetic control.

Frostbite occurs only when the tissue is supercooled to well below 0°C (32°F). The required temperature is at least −4°C (24.8°F) and may be as low as −10°C (14°F) under some conditions. Tissue injury occurs due to structural damage to cells from ice crystal formation and due to microvascular thrombosis and stasis. In the prefreeze phase, tissue temperatures drop below 10°C (50°F), and cutaneous sensation is lost. Before ice crystals form, microvascular vasoconstriction can occur, with endothelial leakage of plasma into the interstitium. In the freeze-thaw phase, the timing, location, and rate of ice crystal formation depend on conditions. Wind and moisture increase the freezing rate. The phases vary with the extent and rapidity of the cold response and may overlap (Box 128.4).

Except in extremely cold conditions, ice crystal formation initially occurs extracellularly. Water then exits the cells to maintain osmotic equilibrium. Cellular dehydration increases the intracellular osmolarity and electrolyte concentrations. After approximately one-third of the cellular volume is lost, the cell collapses and dies, even if there was no direct structural damage from ice crystals. Extracellular crystallization increases the tissue pressure on cell membranes and vascular structures. Sludging, stasis, and cessation of flow occur at the capillary level.

A third phase, progressive microvascular collapse, first affects venules, then arterioles. Red blood cells sludge and form microthrombi during the first few hours after the tissues are thawed. Factors that decrease flow include hypoxic vasospasm, hyperviscosity, and direct endothelial cell damage. Ischemic conditions extend the surrounding

---

BOX 128.4 Freezing Injury Cascade

Prefreeze Phase
Superficial tissue cooling
Increased viscosity of vascular contents
Microvascular constriction
Endothelial plasma leakage

Freeze-Thaw Phase
Extracellular fluid ice crystal formation
Water movement across cell membrane
Intracellular dehydration and hyperosmolality
Cell membrane denaturation or disruption
Cell shrinkage and collapse

Vascular Stasis and Progressive Ischemia
Vasospasticity and stasis coagulation
Arteriovenous shunting
Vascular endothelial cell damage and prostanoid release
Interstitial leakage and tissue hypertension
Necrosis, demarcation, mummification, or slough

aExtremely rapid cooling produces more initial intracellular than extracellular ice crystallization.

---

injury. Plasma leakage and arteriovenous shunting result in thrombosis, increased tissue pressure, ischemia, and necrosis.

Progressive dermal ischemia is partially mediated by thromboxane. Prostaglandins are found in clear vesicles. When subdermal vascular plexi are injured, hemorrhagic blisters develop, which also contain prostaglandins. Arachidonic acid breakdown products released from underlying damaged tissue into blister fluid include prostaglandins and thromboxane. These mediators produce platelet aggregation, vasoconstriction, and leukocyte immobilization.

Injury to the microvasculature is the ultimate determinant of progressive tissue damage. Endothelial cells are very susceptible to freezing injury. After thawing, the vasculature may be temporarily patent. Platelet and erythrocyte aggregates promptly clog and distort the vasculature. Intense vasoconstriction and arteriovenous shunting occur at the interface between normal and damaged tissue. Injured viable vasculature remains distorted. Local arteritis, medial degeneration, and intimal proliferative thickening occur. Nerve and muscle tissues are more susceptible than connective tissue to cold injury. Nonviable hands and feet can be moved after thawing if the tendons are intact.

Edema progresses for 48 to 72 hours after tissue is thawed. Necrosis becomes apparent as edema resolves. The dry gangrene carapace of frostbite is superficial in comparison to arteriosclerosis-induced, full-thickness gangrene. Although the historical surgical aphorism was "frostbite in January, amputate in July," advances in imaging modalities can accelerate the identification of the demarcation between viable and nonviable tissue.

The extent of peripheral cold injury is determined by the type and duration of cold contact with the skin (Box 128.5). Risk factors include physiologic, mechanical, psychological, environmental, and cardiovascular factors.

Any condition affecting judgment can jeopardize a physiologically tropical human. Cold injuries are often due to psychiatric impairment or intoxication, primarily ethanol intoxication. Ethanol also produces peripheral vasodilation, which increases heat loss. Blunting of self-protective instincts can cause people to put themselves at increased risk by not wearing appropriate clothing or finding shelter in cold conditions.

Although air is a poor thermal conductor, the combination of cold and wind (wind chill index) markedly increases heat loss. Direct skin contact with good thermal conductors such as metal, water, and volatile liquids

BOX 128.5   Predisposing Factors

Physiologic
Genetic
Core temperature
Previous cold injury
Lack of acclimatization to altitude
Dehydration
Overexertion
Trauma—multisystem, extremity
Dermatologic disease
Physical conditioning
Diaphoresis, hyperhidrosis
Hypoxia

Mechanical
Constricting or wet clothing
Tight boots
Vapor barrier, neoprene liners
Inadequate insulation
Immobility or cramped positioning

Psychological
Mental status
Fear, panic
Attitude
Peer pressure

Fatigue
Intense concentration on tasks
Hunger, malnutrition
Intoxicants

Environmental
Ambient temperature
Humidity
Duration of exposure
Wind chill factor
Altitude and associated conditions
Quantity of exposed surface area
Heat loss—conductive, evaporative
Aerosol propellants
Cardiovascular
Hypotension
Atherosclerosis
Arteritis
Raynaud syndrome
Anemia
Sickle cell disease
Diabetes
Vasoconstrictors, vasodilators

increases the rate and extent of tissue destruction. Commercial aerosol spray propellants, such as propane and butane, and carbon dioxide in fire extinguishers are potentially hazardous. Liquid oxygen and Freon can also cause frostbite. Overenthusiastic application of ice or frozen gel packs for soft tissue injuries can cause frostbite, with tissue loss. Contact with dry ice or vapor coolant sprays such as chloroethane can also cause frostbite.

Clinical Features

The term *frostnip* refers to a superficial freezing injury manifested by transient numbness and tingling that resolves after rewarming. No tissue destruction occurs. The most common, nearly universal, presenting symptom of frostbite is numbness. All patients have initial sensory deficits of light touch, pain, or temperature. Anesthesia is produced by intense vasoconstrictive ischemia and neurapraxia, usually in acral areas and distal extremities. Fingers, toes, nose, ears, and penis are the specific areas at the greatest risk. Patients often complain of clumsiness and report so-called "block of wood" sensations in the extremities. Complete anesthesia in a cold digit suggests a severe injury.

Initial presentation of frostbite is often deceptively benign. Most patients do not arrive in the emergency department (ED) with frozen insensate tissue. Frozen tissue feels hard and appears mottled or violaceous white, waxy, or pale yellow (Fig. 128.5). In severe cases, it is not possible to roll the dermis over bony prominences. Rapid thawing in warm water results in an initial hyperemia, even in severe cases (Fig. 128.6). After thawing, there is usually partial return of sensation until blebs form.

Favorable initial symptoms after rewarming include normal sensation, warmth, and color. Soft pliable subcutaneous tissue suggests a superficial injury. A residual violaceous hue after rewarming is ominous (Figs. 128.7 and 128.8). Early formation of large blebs with relatively clear fluid that extend to the tips of the digits (Fig. 128.9) is more favorable than a delayed appearance of smaller, more proximal hemorrhagic vesicles that are produced by damage to subdermal vascular plexi (Fig. 128.10). Bullae and vesicles usually form in 1 to 24 hours.

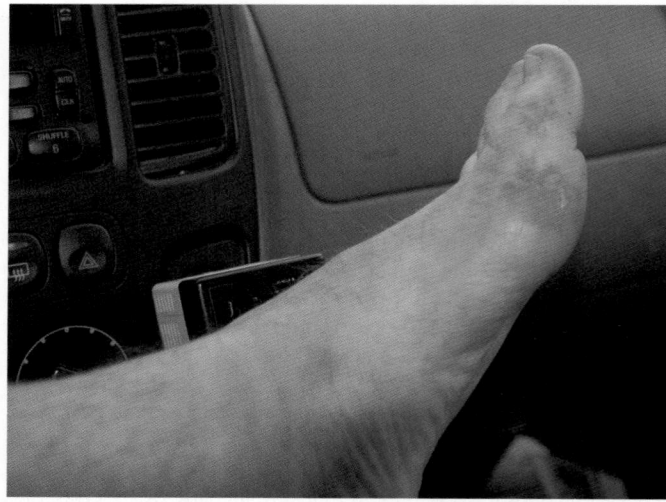

Fig. 128.5 Frostbite that is still frozen. The victim is thawing the foot using a car heater. This technique is not advisable due to a high likelihood of causing further damage. (Courtesy Dr. Nicholas Kanaan.)

Lack of edema formation suggests significant tissue damage. Postthaw edema usually develops within 3 hours. In severe cases, frostbitten skin forms a black dry eschar that mummifies, with demarcation between living and dead tissue (Figs. 128.11 and 128.12). The appearance may be misleading as live tissue often extends distally deep to the eschar.

Historically, frostbite, like burns, was classified into degrees of injury. Anesthesia and erythema were considered to be first-degree frostbite. Superficial vesiculation surrounded by edema and erythema indicated second-degree frostbite. Third-degree frostbite produced deeper hemorrhagic vesicles. Fourth-degree injuries extended into subcutaneous tissues, including bones and muscles.

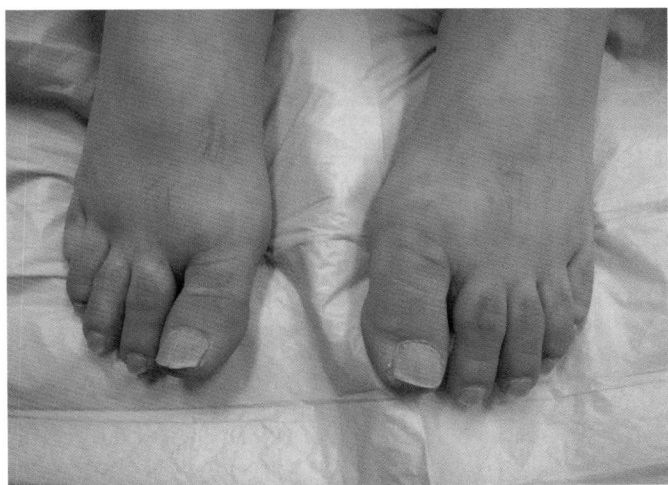

Fig. 128.6 Severe frostbite of the toes immediately after thawing. The injury appears deceptively benign. (Courtesy Dr. Ken Zafren.)

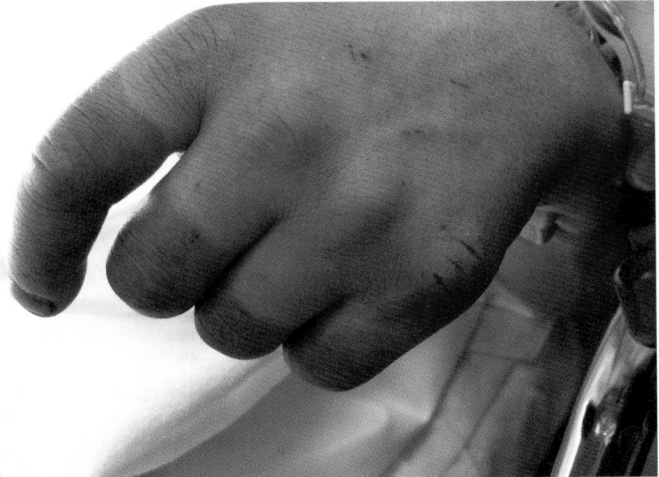

Fig. 128.7 Early appearance of severe frostbite of the hand after thawing. A purple color and absence of blisters are very unfavorable prognostic signs. (Courtesy Dr. Ken Zafren.)

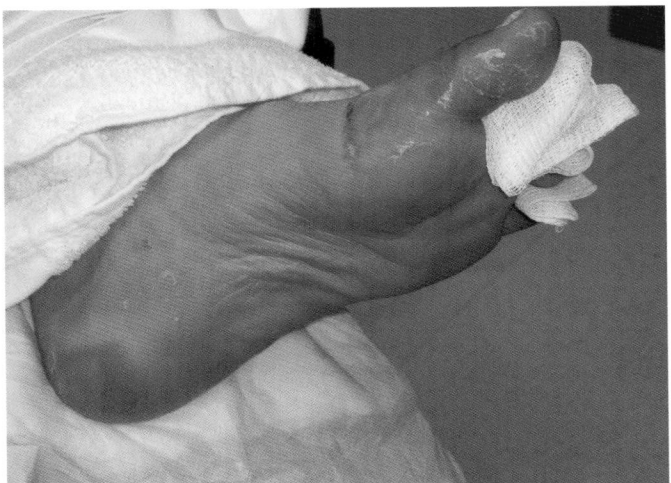

Fig. 128.8 Early appearance of severe frostbite of the foot. A purple color and absence of blisters are very unfavorable prognostic signs. (Courtesy Dr. Ken Zafren.)

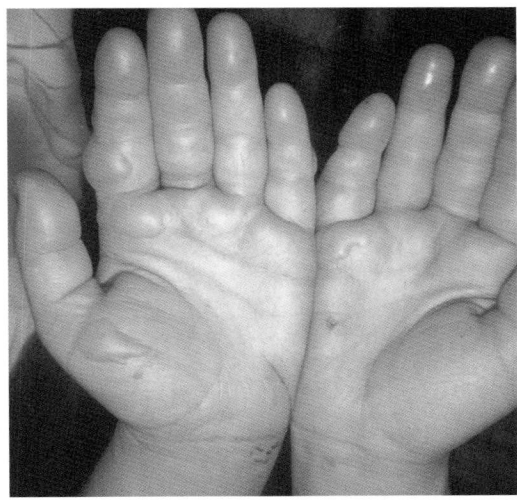

Fig. 128.9 Frostbite with clear vesiculations. (Courtesy Dr. William Mills, Jr.)

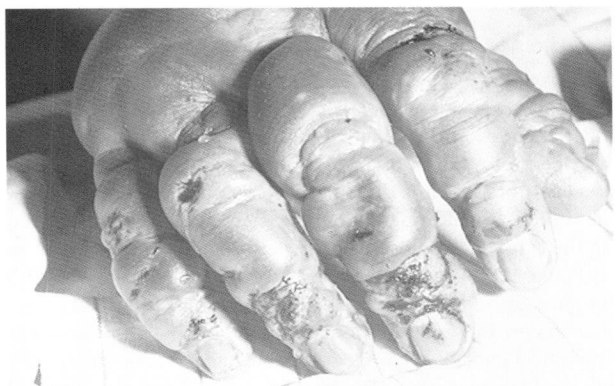

Fig. 128.10 Severe frostbite with early hemorrhagic vesicles. (Courtesy Dr. William Mills, Jr.)

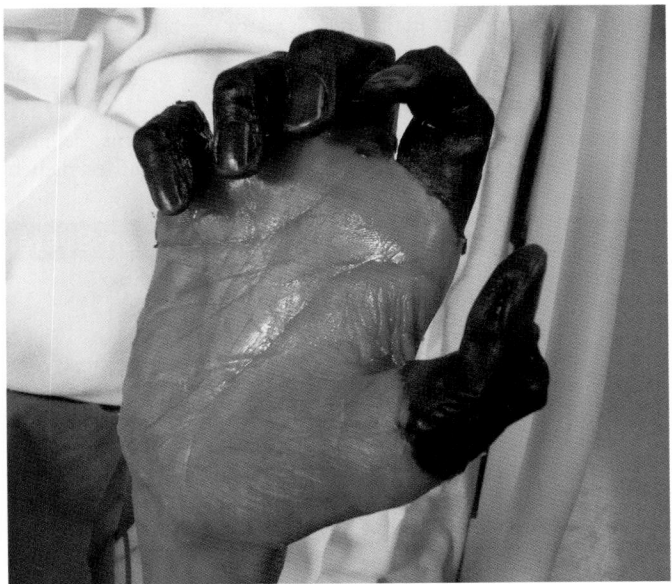

Fig. 128.11 Severe frostbite of the hand. Dry gangrene is clearly demarcated. There was significant tissue loss. (Courtesy Dr. Ken Zafren.)

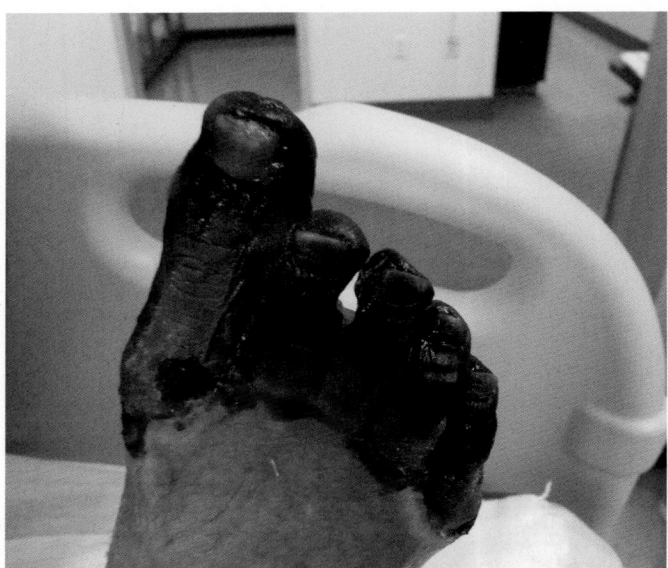

Fig. 128.12 Severe frostbite of the foot. Dry gangrene is clearly demarcated. There was significant tissue loss. (Courtesy Dr. Ken Zafren.)

Classification by degrees is a poor method of predicting the amount of tissue damage and is therapeutically misleading. A simpler, more useful classification divides frostbite into superficial (mild) frostbite, which does not result in tissue loss, and deep (severe) frostbite, which causes loss of tissue. It is difficult to predict the amount of tissue loss at the time of initial presentation. The best method is clinical staging using the extent of cyanosis immediately after rapid thawing in warm water (Table 128.3). In Grade 1 frostbite there is no cyanosis, predicting no amputation and no sequelae. In Grade 2, cyanosis limited to the distal phalanx predicts only soft tissue amputation and sequelae involving the nails. In Grade 3, cyanosis of the intermediate and proximal phalanges predicts bone amputation and functional sequelae. In Grade 4, cyanosis over the carpal or tarsal bones predicts limb amputation with severe functional sequelae.

Significant pain usually accompanies reestablishment of perfusion. A dull continuous ache evolves into a throbbing sensation in 48 to 72 hours. This may persist until tissue demarcation occurs weeks later. Short-term and long-term sequelae are common (Box 128.6).

Differential Diagnoses

The differential diagnosis of frostbite is limited. Burns, cellulitis, gangrene from causes other than freezing, vascular injuries, diabetic neuropathies, and pressure necrosis can resemble frostbite, but can usually be distinguished based on history. Severe, nonfreezing, cold injuries that have been complicated by pressure necrosis with or without infection, can also mimic frostbite. After spontaneous thawing, before edema develops, frostbitten areas may appear deceptively normal for a few hours.

Diagnostic Testing

Except in patients being considered for thrombolytic therapy, diagnostic imaging has a limited role in the emergency care of patients with frostbite. Ancillary diagnostic imaging techniques can be used to help grade the severity of injury, but no technique consistently predicts tissue loss at the time of initial examination.

Patients with frostbite should undergo laboratory testing and imaging, as indicated for coexisting conditions and injuries. Plain radiographs of frostbitten extremities can be used to diagnose fractures due to trauma. Follow-up radiographs may begin to demonstrate abnormalities due to frostbite 4 to 10 weeks after injury.

Patients being considered for thrombolytic therapy may undergo computed tomography angiography (CTA), magnetic resonance angiography (MRA) or Doppler ultrasound, for intra-arterial therapy or radionuclide scanning for intravenous (IV) therapy. Otherwise, angiography or scintigraphy should be delayed. In pediatric patients, magnetic resonance imaging (MRI) of developing hyaline cartilage can demonstrate physial injury, which has the largest impact on longitudinal growth.

Management

Prehospital

Napoleon's Surgeon General, Baron Larrey, first recorded the disastrous effects of the freeze-thaw-refreeze cycle. During the 1812 to 1813 Russian campaign, soldiers would thaw frozen extremities directly over open fires, only to burn them or have them refreeze, with resulting tissue destruction. Unfortunately, the formation of gangrene was misattributed to rapid thawing. Gradual thawing, often including friction massage with snow, became the standard treatment regimen until the 1950s. In 1961, William Mills, Jr., popularized rapid thawing in warm water after extensive research with severe Alaskan frostbite cases.

Field rewarming of frozen tissue is rarely practical. If possible, remove wet or constricting clothing and immobilize and insulate affected areas. Massage is not efficacious and increases tissue loss. Frozen parts should be kept away from dry heat sources, such as heated forced air during transport.

In general, the longer tissue has been frozen, the greater the extent of cellular damage. However, rewarming should not be initiated in the field if there is any possibility that thawing will be interrupted

TABLE 128.3	Frostbite Classification System			
Frostbite injuries of the extremities	Grade 1	Grade 2	Grade 3	Grade 4
Extent of initial lesion at day 0 after rapid rewarming	Absence of initial lesion	Initial lesion on distal phalanx	Initial lesion on intermediary and proximal phalanx	Initial lesion on carpal/tarsal
Bone scanning at day 2	Useless	Hypofixation of radiotracer uptake area	Absence of radiotracer uptake area on the digit	Absence of radiotracer uptake area on the carpal/tarsal
Blisters at day 2	Absence of blisters	Clear blisters	Hemorrhagic blisters on the digit	Hemorrhagic blisters over carpal/tarsal
Prognosis at day 2	No amputation	Tissue amputation	Bone amputation of digit	Bone amputation of the limb ± systemic involvement ± sepsis
	No sequelae	Fingernail sequelae	Functional sequelae	Functional sequelae

From: Cauchy E, Chetaille E, Marchand V, Marsigny B. Retrospective study of 70 cases of severe frostbite lesions: a proposed new classification scheme. *Wilderness Environ Med.* 2001;12:248.

BOX 128.6 Sequelae of Frostbite and Nonfreezing Cold Injuries

Neuropathic
Pain
    Phantom pain
    Complex regional pain syndrome
    Chronic pain
Sensation
    Hypesthesia
    Dysesthesia
    Paresthesia
    Anesthesia
Thermal sensitivity
    Heat
    Cold
Autonomic dysfunction
    Hyperhidrosis
    Raynaud syndrome

Musculoskeletal
Atrophy
Compartment syndrome
Rhabdomyolysis
Tenosynovitis

Stricture
Epiphyseal fusion
Osteoarthritis
Osteolytic lesions
Subchondral cysts
Necrosis
Amputation

Dermatologic
Edema
Lymphedema
Chronic or recurrent ulcers
Epidermoid or squamous cell carcinoma
Hair or nail deformities

Miscellaneous
Core temperature afterdrop
Acute tubular necrosis
Electrolyte fluxes
Psychological stress
Gangrene
Sepsis

---

or incomplete or that tissue will refreeze during evacuation. Tissue refreezing is disastrous. It is better to walk to safety on frozen feet if rescue will be delayed. When evacuation is not possible, rapid field rewarming, preferably in water at 37°C to 39°C (98.6°F to 102.2°F), may be the best option.

Emergency Department

Prethaw. Stabilize hypothermia and other life-threatening conditions before warming frostbitten extremities.[15] Do not delay treatment while waiting for the results of laboratory and radiographic studies. Most patients are volume-depleted, partly due to poor oral intake and hypothermia-induced cold diuresis, and volume replacement with crystalloid at 40°C (104°F) to decrease blood viscosity and sludging is indicated.

Thawing by Immersion in Warm Water

Rapidly rewarm completely frozen or partially thawed tissue by immersion in gently circulating water that is carefully maintained at a temperature of 37°C to 39°C (98.6°F to 102.2°F). A whirlpool is ideal, but any large container can be used for the hands or feet. Do not let frostbitten areas bump or rub against the side of the container. Water warmer than 39°C (102.2°F) does not thaw significantly faster but causes more pain. Tissue can suffer thermal injury when the water temperature exceeds 42°C (107.6°F). Rewarming should be continued until distal erythema is noted. The part should have return of color and feel pliable, which usually requires 15 to 30 minutes of submersion. Active gentle motion is encouraged during rewarming, but the tissue should not be massaged. Premature termination of rewarming results in a partial thaw, with increased tissue damage.

Parenteral analgesia is often indicated during rewarming. Reperfusion may be intensely painful, with throbbing, burning pain and tenderness. Sensation is usually diminished after thawing until it disappears with bleb formation.

Patients with completely frozen extremities are usually hypothermic and at risk for significant fluid and electrolyte fluxes during rewarming. The acute thawing of large amounts of distal musculature can extinguish peripheral vasoconstriction, resulting in a sudden return of cold, hyperkalemic, acidotic blood to the central circulation. This can produce core temperature afterdrop, with ventricular fibrillation. In the most severe cases, extracorporeal rewarming should be used (Box 128.7). Rewarm frostbitten extremities only after the hypothermic patient has been stabilized.

Postthaw. We elevate injured extremities to minimize edema formation, apply sterile dressings loosely, and handle frostbitten areas gently. Due to cold-induced anesthesia, soft tissue injuries are often not appreciated by the patient or emergency clinician. Persistent cyanosis in the extremities after a complete thaw may reflect increased compartment pressure. Tissue should be monitored carefully, although decompressive fasciotomies are usually not necessary during initial treatment.

Although there is no definitive supporting evidence, we recommend the use of topical aloe vera with oral aspirin or ibuprofen. Topical aloe vera every 6 hours inhibits thromboxane when applied directly to frostbitten areas. Aspirin and ibuprofen inhibit the arachidonic acid cascade, although there is no evidence of efficacy for either agent. Some experts prefer ibuprofen because it may also cause fibrinolysis. However, aspirin is also used widely. There is no convincing data showing improved tissue salvage with any of these agents.

Large clear blisters can be left intact, débrided or aspirated. We débride broken or intact nonhemorrhagic blisters. Hemorrhagic blisters are aspirated rather than débrided. When hemorrhagic blisters are débrided, secondary desiccation of deep dermal layers may extend the injury.

Although there is no demonstrated benefit of penicillin for streptococcal prophylaxis, it is used routinely in some centers. We recommend against prophylactic antibiotics for frostbite unless there is associated gross contamination or crush injury. Tetanus can occur after frostbite. Administer tetanus prophylaxis per usual wound care guidelines.

Thrombolytic therapy has been used to treat microvascular thrombosis in frostbite. In one retrospective study, IV tissue plasminogen activator (tPA) and heparin reduced predicted digit amputations in severe frostbite. In other studies, intra-arterial tPA decreased the incidence of amputations when administered within 24 hours of thawing.[16,17]

Thrombolysis should be reserved for patients with severe injuries (Grade 3 or 4) likely to produce significant tissue loss. Frostbite that has not undergone freeze-thaw-refreeze can be treated using tPA within 24 hours of thawing if there are no contraindications to thrombolysis. There is no standard dosing regimen. With intra-arterial tPA, angiography is performed with intra-arterial vasodilators, such as papaverine,[18] nitroglycerin,[17] and nicardipine.[19] If flow is not reestablished, intra-arterial, catheter-directed tPA can be infused with a bolus of 2 to 4 mg followed by an infusion of 0.5 to 1 mg/hr. Heparin is also given at 500 units/hour via the intra-arterial catheter. Angiograms are repeated every 8 to 12 hours. Treatment is stopped when perfusion is restored or up to 48 hours.

Intra-arterial thrombolysis should only be performed in centers that have intensive care capabilities and are familiar with the technique. An alternative approach that appears to have equal efficacy uses systemic IV thrombolytic therapy. After thawing, a technetium-99m triple phase bone scan can be performed. One regimen uses a loading dose of alteplase 0.15 mg/kg IV over 15 minutes followed by an infusion of 0.15 mg/kg/hour for 6 hours. If technetium scanning is available, a repeat technetium scan can be used to evaluate reperfusion. Treatment with alteplase is followed by enoxaparin 1 mg/kg subcutaneously twice daily for 14 days. Intravenous tPA for frostbite is an option at smaller hospitals where tPA is available for myocardial infarction or stroke.

Prostacyclin has vasodilatory properties that mimic a chemical sympathectomy. The risk of amputation was significantly lower in a controlled trial of patients with severe frostbite who received IV Iloprost (a prostacyclin analog not currently available in the United States) with aspirin after thawing. Selected patients with severe frostbite were also treated with recombinant tPA. We recommend treatment with Iloprost, if available for Grade 2 to 4 frostbite injury. It should be infused within 48 hours of thawing, combined with tPA in appropriate settings for Grade 3 to 4 frostbite injury in patients seen within 24 hours who meet the indications for tPA. Iloprost is safe enough that it can be used in prehospital settings if necessary.

There are many unproven therapies for frostbite, including low-molecular-weight dextran, vasodilator therapy, and phenoxybenzamine. Hyperbaric oxygen may accelerate demarcation but has not been shown to increase tissue salvage in severe frostbite.[20]

Chemical or surgical sympathectomies do not decrease tissue loss. Surgical sympathectomy produces a smoother initial clinical course but no long-term benefits, with the possible exception of decreased long-term pain. Forearm nerve blocks produce a chemical sympathectomy that increases finger skin temperature. Although prehospital wrist blocks may achieve rapid pain control with rewarming, there have been no systematic studies of outcomes.

Disposition

Patients with superficial frostbite can be safely discharged to a warm place unless there is another indication for admission. Consult social services if the patient is undomiciled. All other patients with significant frostbite are best admitted for further evaluation and treatment. Transfer or further consultation is indicated when the admitting service lacks experience in the care of frostbite. At hospitals not capable of giving intravenous tPA, patients who meet the criteria for thrombolysis should be transferred to a suitable facility if thrombolysis can be initiated after transfer within 24 hours of thawing.

NONFREEZING COLD INJURIES

Foundations

Background and Importance
Nonfreezing cold injury occurs when tissue fluids have not frozen. The most common nonfreezing cold injury is immersion injury, often referred to as *trench foot*, although the hands may also be affected. This is a significant threat during recreational activities and military expeditions in cold wet climates.

Anatomy, Physiology, and Pathophysiology
Trench foot is produced by prolonged exposure to wet cold at temperatures too high to cause frostbite. It usually develops slowly over several days and results in neurovascular damage. Immersion injury commonly develops while a person is wearing socks that are wet from immersion in water.

Immersion injury can also occur from sweat, especially with the use of neoprene socks, vapor barrier boots, or constrictive gaiters. People who soak their feet for hours in cool water for pain relief are also at risk. Bullae and tissue loss in immersion injury are due to pressure necrosis with or without infection rather than to cold injury. Most patients with severe immersion injury are military personnel who have worn boots continuously for days or weeks. Prevention of immersion injury may require frequent drying of feet and socks.

Pernio (chilblains) is a form of cold injury that often follows repetitive exposure to cold in susceptible individuals. Chilblains can also occur without exposure to cold in individuals who have underlying diseases, such as systemic lupus erythematosus (SLE).

Clinical Features

Immersion Injury
Immersion injury is classically described as progressing through four stages. In the first stage (during cold exposure), numbness is the most

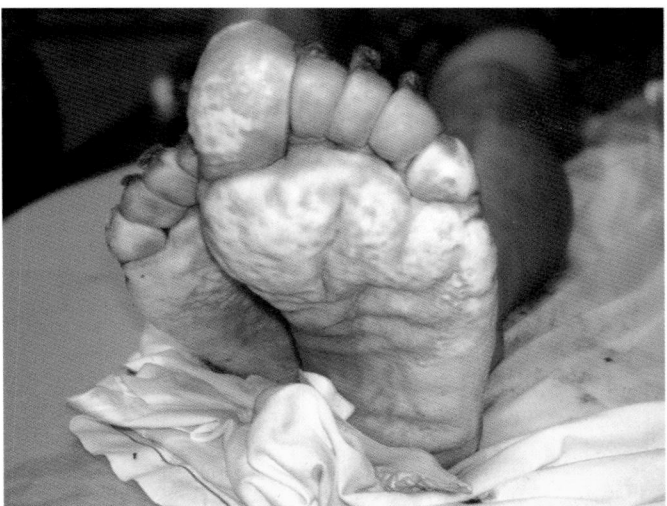

Fig. 128.13 Nonfreezing cold injury (trench foot, immersion foot) in a homeless man in the emergency department, shortly after removal of wet socks and shoes. (Courtesy Dr. Ken Zafren.)

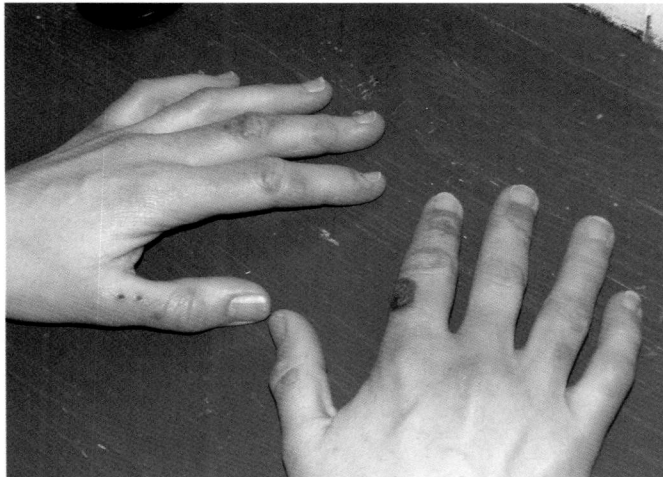

Fig. 128.14 Pernio in a woman who was working in an unheated high-altitude clinic. (Courtesy Dr. Alice Murray.)

common symptom. The extremities may appear bright red, but soon become pale or white due to extreme vasoconstriction (Fig. 128.13). There is no pain or swelling at this stage.

In the second stage (following cold exposure) after removal from a cold environment and during rewarming, peripheral blood flow slowly returns, and the extremities become a mottled pale blue. This change may be subtle in highly pigmented skin. The extremities remain cold and numb, although pain and edema can result from active rewarming. This stage usually lasts for a few hours, but occasionally persists for several days.

In the third stage (hyperemia), blood flow increases markedly. The extremity suddenly becomes hot and red, with bounding pulses, while the microcirculation is sluggish, as evidenced by prolonged capillary refill. Dependent redness (rubor) with pallor on elevation may occur due to vasomotor paralysis. At the same time, numbness gives way to severe pain with hyperalgesia, even to light touch. Edema often develops. In severe cases associated with pressure necrosis, bullae, like those seen in frostbite, can form. In cases associated with tissue loss, necrosis becomes evident. The third stage may last weeks to months.

In the fourth stage (following hyperemia), the limb generally appears normal except in cases with tissue loss, but pain may persist. Tissue that was necrotic in the third stage becomes gangrenous and is lost. This stage can last from weeks to years or be permanent. Most cases of immersion injury present to the ED during the first or second stage, but pain that is often resistant to usual pain medications may be a presenting complaint during later stages.

Short- and long-term sequelae of cold immersion injury are similar to those of frostbite, although only the most severe immersion injuries are associated with tissue loss (see Box 128.6).

Pernio

Chilblains, or cold sores, appear within 24 hours of exposure and most often affect the face, dorsa of the hands and feet, and pretibial areas (Fig. 128.14). Young women with Raynaud phenomenon, SLE, or antiphospholipid antibodies are at increased risk. Persistent vasospasm and vasculitis result in burning, pruritus, erythema, and mild edema. Plaques, blue nodules, and ulcerations can develop. These painful

lesions usually last 1 to 2 weeks but can persist much longer if there are repeated exposures to cold.

Differential Diagnoses

Frostbite can mimic nonfreezing cold injury but can usually be diagnosed by history. Frostbite and nonfreezing cold injuries can also occur together. Warm immersion injuries, including jungle foot (paddy foot) or tropical immersion foot, may appear similar to immersion injuries due to wet cold, but resolve with drying and elevation within a few days.

Pernio has a wide differential diagnosis. The diagnosis is usually clear when pernio is associated with recent cold exposure. Cases of suspected pernio with uncertain cause should prompt a search for underlying conditions, such as SLE.

Diagnostic Testing

Intraepidermal nerve fiber density measurement can be used to assess the severity and guide management of immersion injury in patients with neuropathic symptoms. Diagnostic testing in patients with pernio is directed toward finding an underlying condition.

Management

Immersion Injury

Treat hypothermia, if present, before treating nonfreezing cold injuries. Provide volume replacement with warm IV fluids if the patient is clinically volume depleted. Immersion injuries should be allowed to rewarm slowly to room temperature. Rapid rewarming or rubbing may worsen the injury. No medications are known to be helpful. Local cooling, often in a cool room with a fan, lowers metabolic requirements and improves pain and edema. Cooling should be continued until hyperemia resolves. Pain after rewarming is common and usually responds poorly to most pain medications. Amitriptyline (50–100 mg orally at bedtime) is the treatment of choice.

Pernio

There is no standard treatment for pernio. We recommend drying the skin if it is damp and gentle massage if the patient can tolerate it. Avoid warming the skin above 30°C (86°F). Pernio is very painful and may require opioid analgesia. Nifedipine (20–60 mg daily) is the only medication that has been shown to be potentially effective in the treatment of severe pernio.

Disposition

Many patients with significant immersion injury require admission for pain control, as well as social service assistance with activities of daily living. Patients with mild immersion injuries can be discharged if there are no other indications for admission and the patient can be released to a warm environment. Patients with pernio are usually managed as outpatients.

The references for this chapter can be found online at ExpertConsult. com.

129

Heat Illness

Melissa A. Platt and Timothy G. Price

FOUNDATIONS

Background and Importance

Humans have been plagued by heat illness throughout recorded history. Heat illness has the potential to affect all age groups and population types. Older adults and the poor (who often lack adequate air conditioning and nutrition) are susceptible to heat illness during environmental extremes and heat waves. Those with preexisting disease are also prone to heat illness. It is estimated that at least 10 times as many heat aggravated illnesses occur in patients with comorbid conditions such as coronary artery disease, cerebrovascular disease, and diabetes.[1] Children are also susceptible to heat stressors because of their higher surface area-to mass ratios. They also have lower sweat rates per gland. Military personnel, athletes, including American football players, and those who occupationally exert themselves in heat, are also at risk.

For an accurate heat illness diagnosis, information about living conditions, occupation, access to water, strenuous physical activity, acclimatization, and current environmental temperatures need to be ascertained. Heat illness is often associated with military exercises, athletic events, occupation, and recreational activities. A recognition of the microclimates conducive to heat illness including military tanks, tents in the sun, engine rooms, mines, hot tubs, saunas, and automobile interiors, is also important. In the United States, nearly 40 children die each year from hyperthermia after being left alone in a motor vehicle.[2]

Anatomy, Physiology, and Pathophysiology

Heat Production

Humans are essentially biochemical furnaces that burn food to fuel with a complex array of metabolic functions. These chemical reactions consume substrate, generate usable energy, and produce byproducts that must be eliminated for continued operation of the system. Water and carbon dioxide are produced and eliminated in large quantities, as well as urea, sulfates, phosphates, and other chemical byproducts. These reactions are exothermic and combine to produce a basal metabolic rate that amounts to approximately 100 kCal/h for a 70-kg person. In the absence of cooling mechanisms, this baseline metabolic activity would result in a 1.1°C (2°F) hourly rise in body temperature.

Heat production can be increased 20-fold by strenuous exertion. Rectal temperatures as high as 42°C (107.6°F) have been recorded in trained marathon runners, without ill effects. Metabolic factors (hyperthyroidism and sympathomimetic drug ingestion) can dramatically increase heat production. Environmental heat not only adds to the heat load but also interferes with its dissipation. The physics of heat transfer as it relates to human physiology involves four mechanisms—conduction, convection, radiation, and evaporation.[3]

Conduction. This is the transfer of heat energy from warmer to cooler objects by direct physical contact. Air is a good insulator; therefore, only approximately 2% of the body heat loss is by conduction. In contrast, the thermal conductivity of water is at least 25 times that of air.

Convection. This is heat loss to air and water vapor molecules circulating around the body. As the ambient temperature rises, the amount of heat dissipated by convection becomes minimal. Once the air temperature exceeds the mean skin temperature, heat is gained by the body. Convective heat loss varies directly with wind velocity. Loose-fitting clothing maximizes convective, and also evaporative, heat loss.

Radiation. This is heat transfer by electromagnetic waves. Although radiation accounts for approximately 65% of heat loss in cool environments, it is a major source of heat gain in hot climates. Up to 300 kCal/h can be gained from radiation when someone is directly exposed to the hot summer sun.

Evaporation. Evaporation is the conversion of a liquid to the gaseous phase. Evaporation of 1 mL of sweat from the skin cools the body by 0.58 kCal. In humans, heat loss through sweat evaporation is the principal means of heat loss during exercise and the dominant means of dissipating heat via the skin when ambient air temperatures exceed skin temperature. Panting mammals such as dogs have an oropharyngeal countercurrent flow mechanism *(carotid rete mirabile)* that results in selective cooling of the brain. In humans, respiratory and countercurrent mechanisms are minimal sources of heat loss.

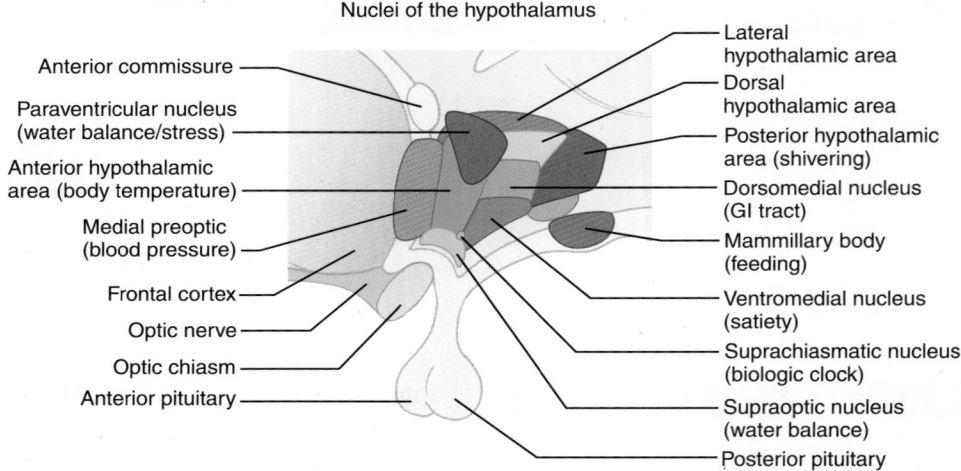

Fig. 129.1 Preoptic Anterior Hypothalamus. (Adapted from Nuclei of the hypothalamus. bhavanajagat.files. wordpress.com/2012/07/nuclei-of-hypothalamus.jpg.)

Heat Regulation

The regulation of body temperature involves three distinct functions—thermosensors, a central integrative area, and thermoregulatory effectors.

Thermosensors. Temperature-sensitive structures are located peripherally in the skin and centrally in the body. However, skin temperature changes correlate poorly with changes in the rate of heat loss. Thermosensitive neurons, located in the preoptic anterior hypothalamus, are activated when the temperature of the blood circulating through that area exceeds a set point (Fig. 129.1).

The skin temperature affects heat loss when a person resting in a warm environment initiates sweating, even though the core temperature remains constant. In contrast, changes in core temperature are more dominant than skin temperature changes in producing heat-dissipating responses.

Central integrative area. The central nervous system (CNS) interprets information received from the thermosensors to instruct thermoregulatory effectors properly. The concept of a central thermostat where an alteration shifts effector thresholds in the same direction fits a variety of clinical situations. For example, fever, the circadian rhythm of temperature variation, and the difference in rectal temperature after ovulation can be explained by variation of a thermal set point.

Thermoregulatory effectors. Sweating and peripheral vasodilation are the major mechanisms whereby heat loss can be accelerated. In a warm environment, evaporation of sweat from the skin is the most important mechanism of heat dissipation. Heat loss from the skin by convection and radiation is maximized by increased skin blood flow to facilitate sweating.

Humans possess apocrine and eccrine sweat glands. Apocrine glands are concentrated in the axillae and produce milky sweat, rich in carbohydrate and protein. They are adrenergically innervated and respond to emotional stress as well as to heat. Most glands producing so-called thermal sweat are eccrine glands. These are cholinergically innervated and distributed over the entire body, with the largest number on the palms and soles. Eccrine sweat is colorless, odorless, and devoid of protein. Individuals exercising in hot environments commonly lose 1 or 2 L/h of sweat. A loss of up to 4 L/h is possible with strenuous exercise.

Cooling is best achieved by evaporation from the body surface; sweat that drips from the skin does not cool the body. Each liter of completely evaporated sweat dissipates 580 kCal of heat. The ability of the environment to evaporate sweat is termed *atmospheric cooling power* and varies primarily with humidity, but also with wind velocity. As humidity approaches 100%, evaporative heat loss ceases.

The vascular response to heat stress is cutaneous vasodilation and compensatory vasoconstriction of the splanchnic and renal beds. These vascular changes are under neurogenic control and allow heat to be dissipated quickly and efficiently, but they place a tremendous burden on the cardiovascular system. To maintain blood pressure, cardiac output increases dramatically. For this reason, saunas and hot tubs may be dangerous for patients with cardiac disease. Cardiovascular and baroreceptor reflexes also affect skin blood flow. Reduced forearm sweating and vasodilation have been observed in severely dehydrated subjects exercising in a warm environment.

Acclimatization

Acclimatization is the constellation of physiologic adaptations that occur in a normal person as the result of repeated exposures to heat stress. Daily exposure to work and heat for 100 min/day results in near-maximal acclimatization within 7 to 14 days.[4] This is characterized by an earlier onset of sweating (at a lower core temperature), increased sweat volume, and lowered sweat sodium concentration. Acclimatization is hastened by modest salt deprivation and delayed by high dietary salt intake.

The cardiovascular system plays a major role in acclimatization and endurance training, largely resulting from an expansion of plasma volume. Heart rate is lower and associated with a higher stroke volume. Other physiologic changes include earlier release of aldosterone, although acclimatized individuals generate lower plasma levels of aldosterone during exercise heat stress. Total body potassium depletion of up to 20% (500 mEq) by the second week of acclimatization can occur as a result of sweat and urine losses, coupled with inadequate repletion.

Although many similarities exist among thermoregulatory responses to heat and exercise, the well-conditioned athlete is not necessarily heat-acclimatized. For heat and exercise-induced adaptive responses to be maintained, heat exposure needs to continue intermittently, at least on 4-day intervals. Plasma volume decreases considerably within 1 week in the absence of heat stress.

Predisposing Factors

Advanced age, psychiatric conditions, chronic disease, obesity, and certain medications increase the risk for classic heatstroke during periods of high heat and humidity. Adequate fluid intake is essential. Older adults often overdress during hot weather conditions. Heat loss is maximized by light, loose-fitting garments.

Exertional heatstroke is most likely to occur in young healthy people involved in strenuous physical activity, especially if they have not acclimatized to environmental factors that overwhelm heat-dissipating mechanisms. For example, wrestlers frequently fast, restrict food and fluid intake, and exercise vigorously wearing vapor-impermeable clothing in an effort to maintain or drop their current weight class. Pre-existing illness may not increase the risk of exertional heat stroke.[5] Fluid intake is the most critical variable. Dehydration can be minimized by education on work-rest cycles and fluid consumption, and through provision of cool flavored fluids.

The goal is to maximize voluntary fluid intake and gastric emptying so that fluid can rapidly enter the small intestine, where it is absorbed. Gastric emptying is accelerated to 25 mL/min by large fluid volumes (500 to 600 mL) and cool temperatures (10°C to 15.8°C [50°F to 60.4°F]). High osmolality inhibits gastric emptying; osmolality of less than 200 mOsm/L is optimal. Most commercially available electrolyte solutions contain excessive sugar. Hydration can be monitored by measurement of body weight before and after training or athletic competition. An athlete with a loss of 2% to 3% body weight (1.5 to 2 L in a 70-kg man) should drink extra fluid and be permitted to compete only when his or her body weight is within 0.5 to 1 kg (1 or 2 pounds) of the starting weight on the previous day. A weight loss of 5% or 6% represents a moderately severe deficit and usually is associated with intense thirst, scant dark-colored urine, tachycardia, and increase in rectal temperature of approximately 2°C (3.6°F). These athletes should be restricted to light workouts after hydration until they return to normal weight. A loss of 7% or more of body weight represents severe water depletion; participation in sports should not be permitted until the athlete is evaluated by a physician or sports trainer. The administration of salt tablets during strenuous exercise can cause delayed gastric emptying, osmotic fluid shifts into the gut, gastric mucosal damage, and hypernatremic dehydration. A 6-g sodium diet is sufficient for successful adaptation for work in the heat, with sweat losses averaging 7 L/day. Excessively high salt intake in relation to salt losses in sweat during initial heat exposure can impair acclimatization because of the inhibition of aldosterone secretion. Excessive salt ingestion can also exacerbate potassium depletion.

Evaporative cooling can be lost when clothing inhibits air convection and evaporation. Water evaporated from clothing is much less efficient for body cooling than water evaporated from the skin. Loose-fitting clothing or ventilated fishnet jerseys allow efficient evaporation. Light-colored clothing reflects rather than absorbs light.

The heat dissipation mechanisms of the body are analogous to the cooling system of an automobile (Fig. 129.2). Coolant (blood) is circulated by a pump (heart) from the hot inner core to a radiator (skin surface cooled by the evaporation of sweat). Temperature is sensed by a thermostat (CNS), which alters coolant flow by a system of pipes, valves, and reservoirs (vasculature). Failure of any of these components can result in overheating.

Effective circulation requires an intact pump and adequate coolant levels. β-adrenergic blocking agents or calcium channel blockers may prevent an increase in cardiac output sufficient to produce the necessary peripheral vasodilation to dissipate heat. Dehydration caused by gastroenteritis, diuretics, or inadequate fluid intake predisposes to heat illness. Individuals working in the heat seldom voluntarily drink as much fluid as they lose and replace only approximately two-thirds

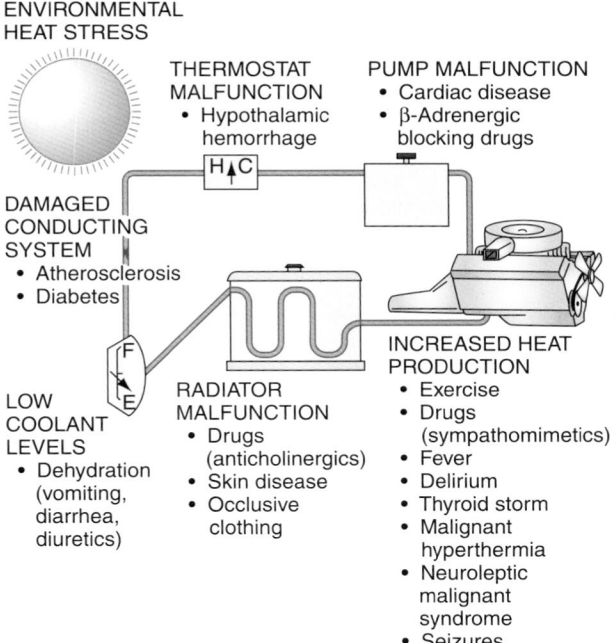

Fig. 129.2 Predisposing factors for heat illness, an automotive analogy.

of net water loss (so-called voluntary dehydration). Dehydration alone increases body temperature at rest by increasing the work of the sodium-potassium adenosine triphosphatase pump, which accounts for 25% to 45% of the basal metabolic rate. This is particularly true in cases of hypernatremic dehydration. The pipes and valves of the coolant system may be abnormal in diabetic or older patients with extensive atherosclerosis.

Radiator function depends on the skin and sweat glands. Occlusive, vapor-impermeable clothing hinders evaporative and convective cooling. Anticholinergic medications and stimulant drugs of abuse interfere with sweating and contribute to heat illness. Various skin diseases, including miliaria (prickly heat rash), extensive burns, scleroderma, ectodermal dysplasia, and cystic fibrosis, are risk factors. Anhidrosis can also be secondary to central or peripheral nervous system disorders.

Increased heat production causing heat illness most often accompanies exercise in a hot humid environment. When heat and humidity are extreme, exertion is not necessary to produce heat-related problems. Several indices help objectify heat strain. These indices can be divided into two categories, heat scales based on meteorologic parameters and those that combine environmental and physiologic parameters.

The wet bulb globe temperature heat index is an excellent meteorologic measure of environmental heat stress (Box 129.1). It measures the effects of temperature, humidity, and radiant thermal energy from the sun. When climatic conditions exceed 25°C (77°F) wet bulb, even healthy people are at high risk during exercise. Above 28°C (82.4°F), exercise and strenuous work should be avoided or limited to extremely short periods of time.

Fever Versus Hyperthermia

It is diagnostically and therapeutically important to identify patients suffering from a febrile response rather than heat illness. Fever does not cause primary pathologic or physiologic damage to humans and does not require primary emphasis in the therapeutic regimen, which is directed at the underlying disease state. If temperature-related physiologic changes such as febrile seizures and tachycardia compromise a patient with marginal cardiac reserve, the temperature should be artificially regulated with antipyretics. In contrast, antipyretics are not effective against heat illness and are **not** recommended to control environmental hyperthermia.

MINOR HEAT ILLNESSES

Miliaria Rubra

Miliaria rubra, also known as prickly heat, lichen tropicus, and heat rash, is an acute inflammatory disorder of the skin that occurs in hot and humid climates. It is the result of the blockage of sweat gland pores by macerated stratum corneum and secondary staphylococcal infection. The acute phase is characterized by vesicles in the malpighian layer of the skin, caused by dilation and rupture of the obstructed sweat gland ducts.

Clinical Features

Miliaria produces intensely pruritic vesicles on an erythematous base. The rash is confined to clothed areas, and the affected area is often completely anhidrotic. During the next week, a keratin plug develops and fills these vesicles, causing a deeper obstruction of the sweat gland duct. The obstructed duct then ruptures a second time, producing a deeper vesicle within the dermis. This is known as the profunda stage, and it can persist for weeks. Profunda vesicles are not pruritic and closely resemble the white papules of piloerection. Chronic dermatitis is a common complication (Fig. 129.3).

Differential Diagnoses

Alternative diagnoses include contact dermatitis, cellulitis, and allergic reactions. A heat exposure history and distribution of the rash will solidify the diagnosis.

Diagnostic Testing

Laboratory data is not indicated with miliaria.

Management and Disposition

Miliaria rubra can be prevented by wearing light, loose-fitting, clean clothing and avoiding situations that produce continuous sweating. Avoid routine use of talcum or baby powder. Gentle exfoliation may help to remove debris that occlude the eccrine sweat ducts. However, soap may cause additional skin irritation. Topical corticosteroids, such as hydrocortisone 2.5% or triamcinolone 0.1% twice a day for one to two weeks, may decrease pruritus and inflammation but is not required for the resolution of miliaria. Patients can be discharged with dermatologic or primary care follow-up.

Heat Cramps

Heat cramps are brief, intermittent, and often severe muscle cramps occurring typically in muscles that are fatigued by heavy work or

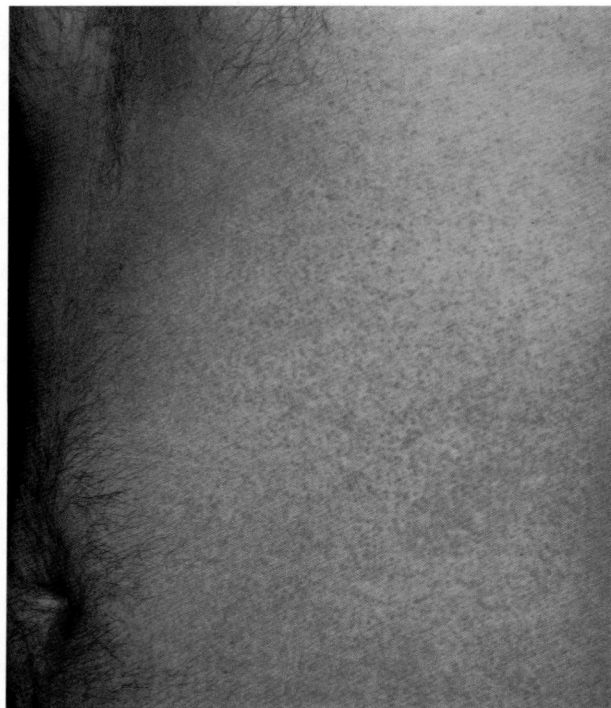

Fig. 129.3 Prickly Heat. (From Habif TP. *Clinical Dermatology: A Color Guide to Diagnosis and Therapy.* 3rd ed. St. Louis: Mosby; 1996.)

prolonged exercise. Heat cramps appear to be related to a salt deficiency. They usually occur during the first days of work in a hot environment and develop in persons who produce large amounts of thermal sweat and subsequently drink copious amounts of hypotonic fluid.

Clinical Features

Athletes, roofers, steelworkers, coal miners, field workers, and boiler operators are among the most common victims of heat cramps. Heat cramps tend to occur after exercise, when the victim stops working and is relaxing (Box 129.2). In this respect, they differ from the cramps experienced by athletes during exercise, which tend to last for several minutes, are relieved by massage, and resolve spontaneously.

Differential Diagnoses

Heat cramps are occasionally confused with hyperventilation tetany, which can occur during heat exhaustion. Hyperventilation tetany can be distinguished by the presence of carpopedal spasm and paresthesias in the distal extremities and perioral area.

Diagnostic Testing

Heat cramps accompanied by systemic symptoms may be part of salt depletion heat exhaustion. Check serum electrolyte levels as heat cramp victims often exhibit hyponatremia and hypochloremia.

Rhabdomyolysis or resultant renal damage is not present with isolated heat cramps.

Management and Disposition

Heat cramps are rapidly relieved by salt solutions. Many commercially available flavored electrolyte solutions are available. Mild cases without concurrent dehydration are treated orally with a 0.1% or 0.2% salt solution (two to four 10-grain salt tablets [56 to 112 mEq] or ¼ to ½ teaspoon of table salt dissolved in 1 quart of water), which is the general limit of palatability. Severe cases respond rapidly to an infusion of normal saline. Salt tablets are gastric irritants, delay gastric emptying, and are not recommended as treatment. Although most patients do not seek medical treatment, most patients with heat cramps may be safely discharged after the administration of balanced salt solutions and clinical improvement.

Heat Edema

It is presumed that hydrostatic pressure and vasodilation of cutaneous vessels, combined orthostatic pooling, lead to vascular leak and accumulation of interstitial fluid in the lower extremities. Simultaneously, the aldosterone level increases in response to the heat stress and perceived central volume deficit.

Clinical Features

Swollen feet and ankles are often reported by non-acclimatized individuals, especially older adults, who encounter climatic stresses of tropical and semitropical areas. They commonly have schedules that involve long periods of sitting or standing. The edema is usually minimal, is not accompanied by any significant impairment in function or ambulation, and often resolves after several days of acclimatization.

Differential Diagnoses

Differentiate heat edema from congestive heart failure, liver disease states, nephrosis, lower extremity infections, and deep venous thrombosis.

Diagnostic Testing

Awareness of this clinical presentation prevents overly vigorous diagnostic and therapeutic intervention. A brief diagnostic evaluation to rule out thrombophlebitis, lymphedema, or congestive heart failure may be appropriate, but invasive diagnostic techniques are not indicated.

Management and Disposition

Pharmacologic therapy is not indicated, and diuretic therapy is not effective. Simple leg elevation or thigh-high support hose should be used. In most individuals, the problem resolves through adequate acclimatization or with the individual's return to a temperate climate. Given its benign nature, patients with heat edema can be safely discharged with outpatient follow-up.

Heat Syncope

Individuals adapt to a hot, humid environment by dilation of cutaneous vessels to deliver heat to the body surface. Thus, an increased portion of the intravascular pool is located in the periphery at any given time. Increasing blood flow to compliant cutaneous veins raises skin vascular volume at the expense of thoracic blood volume. The combination of volume loss and peripheral vasodilation can result in inadequate central venous return, a concomitant drop in cardiac output, and cerebral perfusion inadequate to maintain consciousness.

Clinical Features

Heat syncope is a multifactorial disorder that results in a temporary loss of consciousness in the presence of heat exposure. Older adults have a special predilection for this disorder, due to reduced cardiovascular reserve and blunted baroreceptor reflexes.

Differential Diagnoses

The diagnosis of heat syncope requires the appropriate clinical setting and exclusion of other possible causes of syncope, given a patient's age and underlying medical disorders such as cardiovascular and neurological causes (see Chapter 11).

Diagnostic Testing

Heat syncope can be precipitated by an underlying metabolic or cardiac disorder, so cardiac monitoring, electrocardiography, and hemoglobin determination are warranted. Other tests are individualized based on clinical suspicion following a thorough history and physical examination (see Chapter 11).

Management and Disposition

This disorder is self-limited and placing the patient in a horizontal position is generally curative. Older patients with comorbidities may require admission to address cardiac or neurologic etiologies. These individuals are at risk for recurrent heat syncope and should be advised to move around often, flex leg muscles repeatedly when standing stationary, avoid protracted standing in hot environments, and assume a sitting or horizontal position when prodromal warning symptoms or signs occur.

MAJOR HEAT ILLNESSES

Heat Exhaustion
Foundations

Background and importance. Heat exhaustion (heat prostration) is a clinical syndrome characterized by volume depletion that occurs under conditions of heat stress. Two types of heat exhaustion are classically described, water depletion and salt depletion.

Anatomy, physiology and pathophysiology. Water depletion heat exhaustion results from inadequate fluid replacement by individuals working in a hot environment and incapacitated individuals without free access to water. Those working in the heat seldom drink as much as they lose, and this voluntary dehydration results in progressive hypovolemia. Left untreated, heat exhaustion caused water depletion will progress to heatstroke because they are a continuum of the same disease.

Salt depletion heat exhaustion takes longer to develop than the water depletion form. It occurs when large volumes of thermal sweat are replaced by water with too little salt. It differs from heat cramps in that systemic symptoms occur. Symptoms are similar to those seen in water depletion heat exhaustion; the body temperature usually remains normal or minimally elevated.

Clinical Features

The symptoms and signs associated with both types of heat exhaustion are variable and include weakness, fatigue, frontal headache, impaired judgment, vertigo, nausea and vomiting and, occasionally, muscle cramps (Box 129.3). Orthostatic dizziness and syncope can occur. Sweating persists and may be profuse. The core temperature is only moderately elevated, usually below 40°C (104°F). Signs of severe CNS dysfunction (e.g., altered mental status) are not present.

Differential Diagnoses

Mild heat exhaustion and full-blown heatstroke represent extremes of the spectrum of heat illness, and intermediate cases may prove difficult to differentiate. Heat exhaustion should not be diagnosed in the

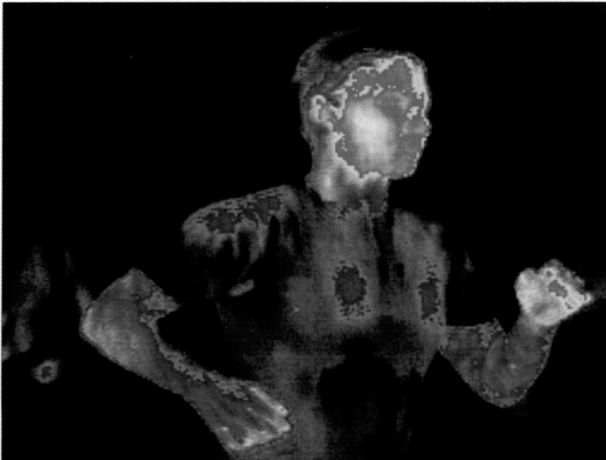

Fig. 129.4 Human Infrared Image. Note that the palms and face are substantially warmer than the rest of the body. (From Auerbach PS. *Wilderness Medicine*. 6th ed. Philadelphia: Mosby/Elsevier; 2012.)

presence of major CNS dysfunction (e.g., seizures, coma) or severe hyperthermia (40.5°C [105°F]).

Diagnostic Testing

This syndrome is characterized by hyponatremia, hypochloremia, and low urinary sodium and chloride concentrations. Determine a serum creatine kinase (CK) level and renal function. Measurement of hepatic transaminase levels may prove helpful. Elevations to several thousand units can be seen in patients with heat exhaustion or in healthy runners after a marathon.

Management

Pure forms of either type of heat exhaustion are rare, and most cases of heat exhaustion involve mixed salt and water depletion. Heat exhaustion is primarily a volume depletion problem, and rapid recovery follows fluid administration. Decisions regarding the type of fluid and electrolyte replacements should be based on serum electrolyte level measurements and the estimation of hydration status by clinical and laboratory parameters.

Patients with significant volume depletion or electrolyte abnormalities require IV fluids. If the patient is orthostatic, normal saline should be administered until vital signs normalize. Free water deficits should be replaced slowly over 48 hours to avoid a decrease of serum osmolality of more than 2 mOsm/h. Overly rapid correction of hyponatremia can result in cerebral edema and seizures.

Disposition

Young, otherwise healthy patients who do not have significant laboratory abnormalities and who respond rapidly to hydration do not require hospitalization. These patients should be instructed to drink plenty of fluids and avoid heat stress for 24 to 48 hours. Older patients, particularly those with cardiovascular disease or other chronic diseases, may benefit from more cautious inpatient fluid and electrolyte replacement and frequent reassessment (Box 129.4).

Heatstroke

Foundations

Background and importance. In the previously discussed forms of heat illness, although the body temperature rises, homeostatic thermoregulatory mechanisms remain intact. Heatstroke is the catastrophic life-threatening emergency that occurs when these mechanisms fail. This results in the elevation of body temperature to extreme levels, usually higher than 40.5°C (105°F), producing multisystem tissue damage and organ dysfunction.

Anatomy, physiology and pathophysiology. As heatstroke develops, energy will be insufficient to sustain thermoregulatory mechanisms, resulting in dramatic increases in core temperature and the clinical manifestations of heatstroke. Tissue damage is a function of a complex interaction of body temperature, exposure time, workload, tissue perfusion, and individual factors. The exact temperature at which cellular damage begins to occur in an individual patient varies. With rapid intervention, full recovery is possible, despite rectal temperatures up to 46.5°C (115.7°F).

Neurologic dysfunction is a hallmark of heatstroke, and cerebral edema is common. Other pathologic changes include petechiae in the walls of the third and fourth ventricles and marked cerebellar Purkinje cell damage.[6,7] Interestingly, the hypothalamus, the predominant site of central thermoregulatory control, is usually not damaged. Long term neurological impairment, such as motor, cerebellar or cognitive, is common.[6,7]

Heat stress creates tremendous demands on the cardiovascular system, and patients who succumb to heatstroke show signs of circulatory failure. Although such pathologic changes are common, cardiac damage alone is not lethal.

Prolonged heat stress produces impressive increases in skin blood flow (peripheral vasodilation) and a reduction of the thermal gradient between the core and the skin (Fig. 129.4). Functional hypovolemia is avoided by compensatory vasoconstriction of the splanchnic and renal vasculatures. The resulting splanchnic and renal ischemia may explain the nausea, vomiting, and diarrhea observed in runners after a marathon. Hepatic damage is a consistent feature of heatstroke, and its absence should cast doubt on the diagnosis.

If severe heat stress continues, compensatory splanchnic vasoconstriction will eventually fail, resulting in reduced mean arterial pressure and a continued cascade of exaggerated systemic inflammatory responses. Failure to perfuse the skin with heated blood from the core results in a dramatically increased rate of heat storage. This produces elevated intracranial pressure, which, in combination with the reduction in mean arterial pressure caused by failure of compensatory

BOX 129.5 Heatstroke: Diagnosis

- Exposure to heat stress, endogenous or exogenous
- Signs of severe central nervous system dysfunction (coma, seizures, delirium)
- Core temperature usually >40.5°C (105°F), but may be lower
- Hot skin common, and sweating may persist
- Marked elevation of hepatic transaminase levels

TABLE 129.1 Characteristics of Classic Versus Exertional Heatstroke

Exertional	Classic
Healthy	Predisposing factors or medications
Younger	Older
Exercise	Sedentary
Sporadic	Heat wave occurrence
Diaphoresis	Anhidrosis
Hypoglycemia	Normoglycemia
DIC	Mild coagulopathy
Rhabdomyolysis	Mild CK level elevation
Acute renal failure	Oliguria
Marked lactic acidosis	Mild acidosis
Hypocalcemia	Normocalcemia

CK, Creatine kinase; DIC, disseminated intravascular coagulation.

TABLE 129.2 Medications Associated With Heat Stroke

Drug Class	Examples
Anticholinergics	Atropine
	Benztropine
	Oxybutynin
	Scopolamine
Antidepressants	Tricyclics
Antiemetics	Metaclopramide
	Prochlorperazine
	Promethazine
Antiepileptics	Topiramate
	Zonisamide
Antihistamines	All
Antihypertensives	Beta blockers
	Calcium channel blockers
Antipsychotics	All
Diuretics	Hydrochlorothiazide
	Furosemide
	Spironolactone
Ergogenic Aids	Anabolic steroids
	Creatine
	Ephedra
Sympathomimetics	Amphetamines
	Cocaine
	Methylphenidate

splanchnic vasoconstriction, conspires to produce a decrease in cerebral blood flow. This results in the major CNS dysfunction characteristic of heatstroke.

Clinical Features

The onset of heatstroke is sudden, and the patient's level of consciousness is altered. Prodromal symptoms lasting minutes to hours occur in approximately 20% of cases. These are non-specific and may include weakness, dizziness, nausea, vomiting, anorexia, frontal headache, confusion, drowsiness, disorientation, muscle twitching, ataxia and signs of cerebellar dysfunction, along with possible psychiatric symptoms, ranging from anxiety and irritability to psychosis. These prodromal symptoms are reminiscent of the description of heat exhaustion. Heat exhaustion, particularly the water depletion variety, can progress to heatstroke if untreated.

The usual manifestations of heatstroke include hyperpyrexia above 40.5°C (105°F), profound CNS dysfunction, and hot skin (Box 129.5). Persistent sweating can be observed in patients with rectal temperatures of 41.5°C to 42.4°C (106.7°F to 108.3°F). Importantly, the cessation of sweating is not the cause of heatstroke, and continued sweating does not preclude the diagnosis.

Although in heatstroke the core temperature is elevated above 40.5°C (105°F), significant cooling may occur in the out-of-hospital setting, and the first temperature obtained in the emergency department (ED) may not represent the original maximum core temperature.

Classic heatstroke versus exertional heatstroke. The two forms of heatstroke, classic (epidemic) heatstroke (CHS) and exertional heatstroke (EHS), may have significantly different presentations and manifestations (Table 129.1).

CHS occurs during periods of sustained high ambient temperatures and humidity, such as during summer heat waves. Victims are often fixed income older adults who live in underventilated dwellings without air conditioning. Debilitated patients who have limited access to oral fluids may develop heat exhaustion due to water depletion, which progresses to heatstroke if untreated. Victims of CHS commonly suffer from chronic diseases, substance abuse, or psychiatric conditions which predispose to heat illness. Such patients are often prescribed medications (diuretics, antihypertensives, neuroleptics, anticholinergics) that impair the ability to tolerate heat stress (Table 129.2). Sweating ceases in most CHS patients. The central venous pressure (CVP) is usually elevated. The combination of elevated CVP with right-sided cardiac dilation suggests high output cardiac failure. These changes are expected because skin blood vessels dilate to dissipate heat; however, this low peripheral vascular resistance can persist in patients after reduction of body temperature to nearly normal. Pulmonary edema may also be present. Factors such as advanced age, hypotension, altered coagulation status, lactic acidosis, and the necessity for endotracheal intubation on arrival at the ED predict a poor outcome, despite successful cooling measures.

In contrast, patients with EHS are usually young and healthy individuals whose heat-dispelling mechanisms are overwhelmed by endogenous heat production. Athletes and military recruits are typical victims. Rhabdomyolysis and acute renal failure, rarely seen in patients with CHS, are common in patients with EHS. Sweating is present in 50% of cases of EHS. Hypoglycemia may occur as the result of increased glucose metabolism and hepatic damage, resulting in impaired gluconeogenesis. Coagulopathy is common. Hyponatremia with serum sodium levels of less than 130 mmol/L has been detected in summer hikers in the Grand Canyon; many were found to have neurologic symptoms or seizures.

Patients with heatstroke usually have hyperdynamic cardiovascular systems with low peripheral vascular resistance, tachycardia (up to 180 beats/min), and an elevated cardiac index. Elevation of cardiac troponin is not uncommon with CHS; however, it is rarer in EHS. Respiratory alkalosis is a physiologic response to active or passive heating and may be severe enough to produce tetany. Although most patients with CHS have respiratory alkalosis, those with EHS usually have a relatively pure lactic acidosis. Lactic acidosis is associated with a poor prognosis in cases of CHS but not necessarily with EHS.

Signs of profound CNS dysfunction dominate the early course of CHS and EHS. Delirium or coma is characteristic, but virtually any neurologic abnormality, including bizarre behavior, opisthotonos, hallucinations, decerebrate rigidity, oculogyric crisis, and cerebellar dysfunction, can be seen. Convulsions occur in up to 75% of patients and can be precipitated by therapeutic cooling maneuvers. Profound muscle rigidity with tonic contractions, coarse tremor, and dystonic movements can mimic seizures. Pupils may be fixed and dilated, and the electroencephalogram may be isoelectric. All of these changes are potentially reversible with rapid intervention, although permanent damage, including cerebellar deficits, hemiplegia, dementia, and personality changes, may still occur in severe cases.[6,7]

Both CHS and EHS cause the hemoglobin-oxygen dissociation curve to shift to the right. An increase in the temperature denatures the bond between oxygen and hemoglobin, decreasing the concentration of oxyhemoglobin. Aberrations in coagulation are common in patients with severe heatstroke, and their presence is a poor prognostic sign.[8] Abnormal hemostasis is manifested clinically by purpura, conjunctival hemorrhage, melena, bloody diarrhea, hemoptysis, hematuria, myocardial bleeding, or hemorrhage into the CNS. Pancreatitis is described, with elevated serum amylase and lipase levels. Diarrhea, probably caused by intense splanchnic vasoconstriction, is commonly seen. Cooling aggravates the diarrhea, creating an unpleasant treatment dilemma.

Differential Diagnoses

Heatstroke occurs when the thermoregulatory responses are overwhelmed and fail. If the patient is evaluated as this is occurring, differentiation between heat exhaustion and heatstroke is difficult. If heatstroke cannot be excluded, efforts to cool the patient should begin immediately. Only after the initial assessment and cooling are initiated is the differential diagnosis relevant. When a history of collapse under conditions of heat stress is present, rapid improvement in mental status and blood pressure with cooling essentially eliminates alternative diagnoses. Consider other causes of fever and coma such as infectious causes if the temperature does not respond, and the patient does not recover neurologically (Box 129.6).

Meningitis and encephalitis. These can masquerade as heatstroke. In patients with heatstroke, the spinal fluid should be clear, with occasional lymphocytic pleocytosis and elevated protein levels. Cerebral falciparum malaria, which has a clinical picture of high fever and encephalitis, is seen in tropical areas where heat illness can also occur.

Thyroid storm. In patients with thyroid storm, the clinical symptoms resemble those of heatstroke. It should be suspected if the thyroid gland is enlarged or nodular, but a normal thyroid gland does not exclude the diagnosis. Thyroid function test results are elevated, but these may not be available on an emergency basis. Fortunately, thyroid storm is rare,

---

BOX 129.6 Differential Diagnoses of Heatstroke

- Central nervous system hemorrhage
- Toxins, drugs
- Seizures
- Malignant hyperthermia
- Exercise-induced hyponatremia
- Neuroleptic malignant syndrome
- Serotonin syndrome
- Thyroid storm
- High fever, sepsis
- Encephalitis, meningitis

---

and some critical aspects of treatment, such as rapid cooling, coincide with those for heatstroke.

Drug-induced heat illness. This is an important consideration, particularly anticholinergic poisoning. Differentiation may be difficult because heatstroke and anticholinergic poisoning cause hyperpyrexia, hot and dry skin, tachycardia, and abnormal mental status. Constricted pupils are present in many heatstroke patients. Mydriasis should be present in patients with anticholinergic poisoning, and its absence argues strongly against this diagnosis. Typhoid fever, typhus, delirium tremens, and hypothalamic hemorrhage all produce a symptom complex similar to that of heatstroke.

Drug overdose of sympathomimetics or stimulants, such as amphetamines, cocaine, and phencyclidine, can cause fatal hyperpyrexia. A high ambient temperature is associated with a significant increase in mortality from cocaine overdose. Many younger patients who die of hyperthermia test positive for cocaine. Heatstroke can occur with delirium resulting from ethanol withdrawal. Aspirin and clopidogrel attenuate the skin vasodilatory response and shifts the onset of peripheral thermoeffector mechanisms toward a higher body temperature during exercise heat stress. Heatstroke occurs in well-trained military soldiers and athletes who ingest dietary supplements containing ephedra or the ergogenic aid creatine. Some antipsychotics also cause suppression of thirst recognition. Individuals with a history of heatstroke, with or without an inherent aberration that predisposed them to the initial episode, are at increased risk for a recurrence.

Exercised associated hyponatremia. Symptoms of hyponatremia, especially exercised associated hyponatremia, can be mistaken for heat exhaustion or heat stroke. Although not a true heat related illness, it may be difficult to differentiate from exertional heat illnesses due to overlapping symptoms of collapse, dizziness, weakness, and in severe cases, mental status changes. However, severe hyperthermia (40.5°C) should not be present.[9]

Neuroleptic malignant syndrome. This disorder is induced by antipsychotic medications and is characterized by muscle rigidity, severe dyskinesia or akinesia, hyperthermia, tachycardia, dyspnea, dysphagia, and urinary incontinence. Although the so-called "lead pipe rigidity" and hyperthermia are reminiscent of malignant hyperthermia, the putative mechanism is different. Dopamine receptor blockade in the corpus striatum caused by butyrophenones (e.g., haloperidol) and similar agents produces severe muscle spasticity and dystonia, leading to the overproduction of heat in patients with NMS (see Chapter 150).

Serotonin syndrome. This can also mimic heatstroke because of the elevated body temperature tremors, clonus, and CNS alterations that occur. Serotonin syndrome is classically a triad of mental status changes, autonomic hyperactivity, and neuromuscular abnormalities (e.g., clonus) secondary to increased CNS serotonergic activity. A history of recent exposure to an illicit drug or interaction with a therapeutic medication is an important clue.

Diagnostic Testing

Most standard measurements of body temperature vary significantly from the actual core temperature. Oral thermometry is affected by mouth breathing and is a poor approximation of the body's core. Rectal thermometry is less variable but responds to changes in core temperature slowly. Thermistors that are inserted 15 cm into the rectum, and not within stool, offer continuous monitoring of temperature and have less variability. Although rectal measurements are slower to respond to changes in core temperature than tympanic temperature readings, rectal measurements are not biased by head skin temperature. An esophageal thermistor positioned adjacent to the heart is another option. Do not use alternative methods such as oral, aural canal, tympanic, or skin to measure body temperature in patients with heatstroke.

The hematologic evaluation should include arterial blood gas determination, complete blood cell and platelet counts, liver transaminases, electrolyte values (including calcium), glucose, blood urea nitrogen, and serum creatinine levels. Hypoglycemia with a serum glucose level less than 65 mg/dL is often found in cases of EHS. With the risk of acute rhabdomyolysis, serum creatine kinase and myoglobin levels should be measured, and urinalysis performed. Severe heatstroke can induce disseminated intravascular coagulation (DIC). Measure prothrombin and partial thromboplastin times, international normalized ratio, and fibrin degradation products. Obtain serum cardiac troponin levels. Metabolic acidosis is common, especially in patients with EHS. Serum lactate levels are usually elevated and may persist or even worsen with improved extremity perfusion.

Acute renal damage is common. The initial urine specimen, usually obtained by catheterization, is a scant, brownish, turbid fluid resembling machine oil. Microscopic examination reveals proteinuria, with abundant granular casts and red blood cells. Acute oliguric renal failure complicates 25% to 30% of EHS cases and 5% of CHS cases. The glomerular filtration rate, renal plasma flow, urine flow, and sodium excretion diminish markedly during exercise. Heavy physical exertion in hot climates produces acidic and maximally concentrated urine, which can result in acute oliguric renal failure in combination with hypotension and myoglobinuria.

Because heatstroke patients are prone to liver failure, aspartate transaminase (AST), alanine transaminase (ALT), lactate dehydrogenase (LDH), and liver other enzyme levels should be monitored. Elevation typically occurs within 24 hours. Hepatic transaminase level elevations may be diagnostically helpful. In most febrile states that include altered mental status or coma, these enzyme levels will be normal or minimally elevated, although they are usually dramatically elevated early in the course of heatstroke. Hepatic damage is consistently featured in heatstroke. Hepatic injury is evidenced by markedly elevated levels of hepatic aminotransferases (serum AST and ALT). Elevation can be into the tens of thousands. Early experimental models have shown that high-mobility group box 1 (HMGB1) as a mediator of systemic inflammation is elevated in heatstroke, and its inhibition may be liver-protective. Jaundice typically appears 24 to 72 hours after the onset of severe heatstroke and gradually precedes if the victim survives. Survivors generally have no permanent impairment of liver function.

Management

Cooling. Immediate cooling is the cornerstone of treatment. If heatstroke cannot be excluded, begin cooling immediately. In EHS, it is usually best to follow the "cool first, transport second" guideline.[10,11]

BOX 129.7   Cooling Modalities to Lower Body Temperature in Heatstroke

Preferred
Evaporative cooling with large circulating fans and skin wetting
Ice water immersion

Adjuncts
Ice packs to axillae and groin
Cooling blanket
Peritoneal lavage (unproven efficacy in humans)
Rectal lavage
Gastric lavage
Cardiopulmonary bypass

Cooling should not be delayed in order to remove all clothing; this can be done simultaneously with cooling efforts.[12] Patients who present to the hospital with heatstroke have high mortality rates ranging from 20% to 65%, and mortality increases significantly when cooling is delayed. Insert a rectal thermistor probe as soon as possible and monitor the patient's temperature continuously.

Immersion in ice water results in a rapid reduction of core temperature to below 39°C within 10 to 40 minutes. Vigorous skin massage to maintain cutaneous circulation has been advocated, but there is no evidence that this is clinically efficacious. Ice water immersion presents many logistical challenges and may hamper resuscitative efforts especially in the ED. The lack of adequate space or drainage, the need for monitoring, rapid facilitation of patient entry and exit from the immersion tank create unique challenges. Environmental safety concerns surrounding management of spilled ice and water in proximity to electrical equipment is an additional concern. For EHS, it is most beneficial when it is preplanned and available for mass participation events during the warm season such as in medical tents in close proximity to the participants.[13] The military has recognized the difficulties with ice water immersion in remote military exercises and have adapted to ice water sheets draped over the patient. It can be initiated at the scene using skin lavage with ice water slurry and chilled intravenous saline.[14]

Evaporative cooling is also recommended because it is effective, easy to perform, noninvasive, and less likely to interfere with other patient care activities than other cooling techniques. The patient is stripped of all clothing, and tepid tap water is sprayed while fans blow air continuously over the body, causing evaporative cooling. One reported method of evaporative cooling uses a body cooling unit on which the patient lies suspended on a net surface while being sprayed with atomized 15°C (59°F) water from above and below. Air warmed to 45°C to 48°C (113°F to 118.4°F) is blown over the skin surface at a rate of 3 m/min. This approach maximizes evaporative and convective cooling by maintaining cutaneous vasodilation and avoiding heat generation caused by shivering. Vasoconstriction from ice water immersion may be beneficial to hypotensive patients and may be better than evaporative cooling for victims in shock who have poor peripheral circulation. Discontinue cooling measures when the patient's body temperature reaches 39°C (102.2°F) to avoid "hypothermic overshoot."[15] Continuous monitoring is necessary to maintain the core temperature at 37°C to 38°C (98.6°F to 100.4°F).

Cooling modalities other than evaporation and immersion are considered adjunctive treatments (Box 129.7).[16] Application of ice packs to high heat transfer areas (e.g., neck, groin, axillae) is commonly used. Cooling blankets may be a useful adjunct but will not produce rapid cooling if used exclusively. Cold irrigant gastric or rectal lavage will not provide significant heat exchange if used as the primary cooling modality. Antipyretics have no role in the treatment of heat-related illness. The clinical efficacy of dantrolene has not been established in the setting of heat stroke.

Resuscitation. Mortality correlates with the elevated temperature duration and number of dysfunctional organ systems, with an increased risk of death if patients present with anuria, coma, or cardiovascular failure. Aspiration and seizures are common in patients with heatstroke, and airway control is indicated. Hypoxemia may occur because of aspiration, pneumonitis and pulmonary infarction, hemorrhage, or edema. Metabolic demands are high, and normal pulmonary ventilation may be inadequate in this setting.

Crystalloid fluid resuscitation is essential. Circulatory fluid requirements are modest in some cases, averaging 1200 mL of isotonic crystalloid solution in the first 4 hours. Pulmonary edema occurs in patients with heatstroke and can be exacerbated by overzealous fluid administration. The use of a CVP catheter to monitor fluid resuscitation may be deceptive. Most patients have a hyperdynamic circulation with a high cardiac index, low peripheral vascular resistance, and elevated CVP as a result of high output cardiac failure. These patients may require only modest IV fluids because cooling produces vasoconstriction and increases blood pressure. Hypotension is common in patients with heatstroke and is usually caused by peripheral vasodilation resulting in high-output cardiac failure in addition to dehydration. Blood pressure usually rises with cooling. If this does not occur, or if the invasively monitored patient has a low CVP, a fluid challenge of 250 to 500 mL of isotonic intravenous fluid should be given rapidly while blood pressure, pulse, and urine output are monitored. Fluid replacement is continued until the blood pressure reaches 90/60 mm Hg or the CVP exceeds 12 mL H_2O. On occasion, patients exhibit hypodynamic responses with a low cardiac index, elevated CVP, and hypotension. These patients may be cyanotic, whereas patients with hyperdynamic circulation are initially pink. This clinical observation can be helpful in identifying patients who may respond to catecholamines.

A variety of tachyarrhythmias commonly occur during heatstroke. These usually resolve with cooling, and electrical cardioversion should be avoided until the myocardium is adequately cooled. The use of α-adrenergic agents such as norepinephrine is not recommended because they promote vasoconstriction without improving cardiac output or perfusion, decrease cutaneous heat exchange, and may exacerbate ischemic renal and hepatic damage. Atropine and other anticholinergic drugs that inhibit sweating should be avoided.

The pathophysiologic processes of heatstroke and fever differ, so antipyretics are not indicated and may be harmful. Salicylates, particularly in large doses, may worsen hyperthermia by uncoupling oxidative phosphorylation and aggravating coagulopathies. Large doses of acetaminophen can result in further hepatic damage.

If rhabdomyolysis is present, maintenance of urinary output of at least 2 mL/kg/h is recommended. Consider urinary alkalinization (higher than a pH of 6.5) early in patients with acidemia, dehydration, or underlying renal disease. After volume repletion, administration of mannitol may be considered to increase intravascular volume and increase the glomerular filtration rate. Mannitol, however, should not be used in an oliguric patient. Persistent anuria, uremia, or hyperkalemia is an indication for consideration of hemodialysis.

Cooling modalities that drastically lower skin temperature may induce violent shivering; this increases metabolic heat production and may impede cooling. Intravenous benzodiazepines are the treatment of choice for shivering. The administration of neuroleptics, like chlorpromazine, should be avoided. These agents have anticholinergic properties that can interfere with sweating and cause hypotension or precipitate seizures. Many patients are extremely agitated during the initial cooling period. Short-acting benzodiazepines can be used for sedation and to control seizures. Barbiturates are less desirable as their metabolism is altered by hepatic dysfunction and they may exacerbate hypotension.

Coagulopathies can occur during the first day of illness but are more common on the second and third days. Initial treatment after cooling should include replacement therapy with fresh-frozen plasma and platelets while monitoring for laboratory signs of DIC (hypofibrinogenemia, elevated fibrin split products, prolonged prothrombin time, and thrombocytopenia). The bleeding diathesis seen in patients with heatstroke may be the result of fibrinolysis. Although α-aminocaproic acid can impede fibrinolysis, administration of this compound is associated with rhabdomyolysis, and its use is not recommended.

Disposition

Admission to an intensive care setting may be necessary. Heat stroke victims can have long term sequela from heat stroke that may not be readily apparent in the initial stages. Follow-up after hospitalization is needed. Patients with more complex end-organ damage (e.g., renal failure requiring dialysis) will require transfer to a center with more comprehensive tertiary care capabilities.

The references for this chapter can be found online at ExpertConsult.com.

130

Electrical and Lightning Injuries

Paul Chen and Alice Kidder Bukhman

FOUNDATIONS

Background and Importance

Electrical injuries are uncommon but can cause significant morbidity and mortality. Toddlers and younger children experience low-voltage injuries in the household as the result of contact with electric sockets and cords. Adolescents and young adults more frequently experience high-voltage injury from contact with electric lines outside of houses. Another peak occurs in the third to fourth decade of life, almost exclusively in men with occupational injuries due to high-voltage encounters with power lines and, to a lesser extent, from electric tools. Worldwide, electrical injuries comprise less than 5% of admissions to burn units, but in developing countries this proportion is much higher at 25%.[1] Forensic reports of deaths caused by electrical injury show that the overwhelming majority of victims are men and most deaths are accidental, with a minority attributed to suicide or homicide.[2]

Anatomy, Physiology, and Pathophysiology

Electrical Injury

Current and Voltage. *Joule's law*, which describes the amount of thermal energy applied to tissues from electricity, is described by the formula

$$P = I^2RT$$

where P is thermal energy, I the current, R the resistance, and T is the duration (time) that the electricity is applied. Current is the flow of electrons down an electrical gradient and is measured in units of amperage. Current is the most important factor in determining the degree of energy transmitted, but it is rarely known in a given exposure. Instead, voltage is used as a proxy for current. According to *Ohm's law*, current (I) is directly proportional to the voltage (V) of the source and inversely proportional to the resistance (R) of the material through which it flows (I = V/R).

Injuries are conventionally classified as being caused by high- or low-voltage sources, with 1000 V as the dividing line. In North America, household sources are low voltage, typically 120 or 240 V. High-voltage injuries, such as those caused by electrical power lines or occupational accidents, are characterized by partial to full-thickness skin burns, deep tissue destruction, and potential cardiac or respiratory arrest. High-voltage injuries are associated with higher rates of death, and more associated traumatic injuries, such as extremity fractures, blunt head injuries, and spinal cord injuries.[1,2] Low-voltage exposure causes less surface damage, but may be equally lethal, particularly in cases in which skin resistance is low, such as when immersed or exposed to water.

Current Type. Electrical sources create current that flows in one direction (*direct current, DC*) or alternates direction cyclically at varying frequencies (*alternating current, AC*). The few systems in the United States that use DC include batteries, automobile electronics, and railroad tracks. Exposure to DC most frequently causes a single, strong, muscular contraction. This may throw the victim back from the source in a way that limits duration of exposure but can result in other traumatic injuries. AC is more commonly used (e.g., household currents) because it conveniently allows for an increase or decrease of power at transformers. It is more dangerous than DC of similar voltage because amperage above the so-called "let-go" current will cause muscular tetanic contractions. Because the flexor muscles of the upper extremities are stronger than extensor muscles, these contractions pull the victim closer to the source resulting in prolonged exposure. Box 130.1 shows the physical effects of different amperage levels at a common 60-Hz AC exposure.

Capacitors store electric charge in circuits, and discharge from these devices may result in sudden bursts of very large amounts of electrical

BOX 130.1 Physical Effects of Different Amperage Levels[a]

1 mA—barely perceptible
6–9 mA—usual range of let-go current
16 mA—maximum current that an average person can grasp and let go
20 mA—paralysis of respiratory muscles
100 mA—ventricular fibrillation threshold
2 A—cardiac standstill and internal organ damage

[a] At 60-Hz AC exposure.
From Centers for Disease Control. Worker deaths by electrocution: a summary of NIOSH surveillance and investigative findings. www.cdc.gov/niosh/docs/98-131/pdfs/98-131.pdf.

BOX 130.2 Resistance of Body Tissues[a]

Lowest
Nerve
Blood vessels
Muscle
Skin
Tendon
Fat
Bone
Highest

[a] Lowest to highest.

energy. Injury from a capacitor may occur even when the electrical device is not energized or plugged in into an electrical source.

Resistance of Tissue Affected. Resistance is the degree to which a substance resists the flow of current; when resistance goes down, current increases. Resistance varies among body tissues. Neurovascular tissues are good conductors of electricity, whereas skin, tendons, fat, and bone are relatively poor conductors (Box 130.2). Current that is initially unable to pass through skin will create thermal energy and cause significant burns. As the skin blisters and deteriorates, its resistance decreases. Once current is through the skin, it can pass easily along lower resistance structures, causing deep tissue injury which may not be immediately evident. As a result, the degree of burns seen on the surface of the skin typically underestimates the damage occurring below the surface. As current strength increases, the relative resistance of tissues ceases to determine the pathway of current, and the entire body functions as a conductor. Current may also jump across skin surfaces in a behavior termed *arcing*, resulting in prominent burns across flexor surfaces.

Within a given tissue, resistance differs based on the fluid and electrolyte content of cells. Dry skin offers the largest resistance, up to 100,000 ohm (Ω) in thick, calloused skin, but dermal resistance decreases to as little as 1000 Ω when wet. This explains why electrical injuries are generally worse in the setting of water.

Path Taken by Current Through the Body. The pathway followed by electrical current determines morbidity and mortality. The entrance and exit sites of the electrical current typically demonstrate greater evidence of skin damage, with full-thickness burns commonly encountered. These sites are properly referred to as the *source and ground contact points*. A patient may have one or multiple source and ground contact points. The most common points of source contact are the hands, wrists, and arms, but children also present with burns from oral contact with electric cords or sockets. The most common ground contact points are the heels of the feet.

Electrical current passing through a limb causes greater local tissue damage than current passing through the trunk because the smaller cross-sectional area limits the ability to dissipate heat. However, current passing through the trunk results in greater mortality due to the involvement of more vital cardiothoracic organs. Transthoracic pathways (arm to arm) are more likely to generate dysrhythmias and have higher mortality rates than vertical currents (leg to arm) or straddle pathways (leg to leg).

Duration of Contact. The degree of tissue damage is directly proportional to the duration of exposure for all voltage levels. Exposure times greater than the length of one cardiac cycle tend to generate dysrhythmias, likely in a manner analogous to the R-on-T phenomenon.

Lightning Injury

Although the same basic scientific principles of electricity apply to lightning, there are several major differences. Lightning strikes involve hundreds of millions of volts, significantly more than those from electrical sources. In contrast, the duration of contact is drastically shorter, averaging 30 microseconds. As a result, current flow is altered, with most of the energy passing over rather than through a victim (termed the "flashover effect"). This reduction in penetration explains why lightning strikes paradoxically result in less destruction to tissues compared with lower-voltage electrical injuries.

Lightning takes various forms, described as streaked, forked, ribbon, sheet, or beaded. The most unusual form is ball lightning, which appears as a globe, rolls along structures, and may even pass through open doors or windows. Strikes occur from cloud to cloud, cloud to ground, and less commonly, ground to cloud.

Lightning may strike a person directly or indirectly. A person's chances of being struck are increased by wearing or carrying metal objects (such as golf clubs or umbrellas) or other conductors. Current from lightning may reach the body indirectly by traveling through a tree or other object (contact voltage), through the ground or even through the air from a struck object (side flash, or splash injury). Side flashes may travel as far as 30 meters.

The risk of injury from a ground strike is increased when one contact point on the victim (e.g., the right foot) is closer to the strike than a second contact point (e.g., the left foot), thus creating a potential difference. This is referred to as the "stride voltage" and is likely responsible for cattle deaths in a pasture after a thunderstorm. Hence, when out in the open during a storm, risk of a lightning strike can be reduced by placing an insulating material, such as a raincoat, between the ground and the body and assuming the lightning position, a squatting configuration with the feet together, or by curling up in a ball on the ground to reduce the number of contact points. Box 130.3 lists safety tips for avoiding lightning strikes.

Injury occurs from the force of a strike, blunt trauma when the victim is thrown, the superheating of metallic objects in contact with the patient, barotrauma, or penetrating trauma from shrapnel.

Conducted Energy Weapons

Conducted energy weapons (CEW), commonly known as Tasers or stun guns, are now widely used in law enforcement. These weapons deliver brief bursts of high-voltage, low-amperage direct current. Although CEWs have been associated with several high-profile police-involved fatalities, a clear causal link between their use and a death has not been established.

The most commonly known CEWs are the Taser (Axon Enterprise, Inc.) (Fig. 130.1). These weapons consist of a hand-held unit with two barbs (Fig. 130.2) with connecting cables that are deployed by the user at distances of up to 25 feet. The units typically lodge in the skin or

BOX 130.3 Tips to Avoid Lightning Strike

- Seek shelter inside an enclosed building or metal-topped automobile.
- Avoid large flat, open areas or hilltops.
- Avoid contact with metal objects and remove metal objects, such as jewelry or hairpins.
- Avoid trees, boats, and open water.
- If caught on open ground, curl up on your side with hands and feet close together to reduce contact points, or squat with feet together. If possible, place a rubber raincoat under your body or feet to reduce ground current effects.
- If in a forest, seek shelter under a thick growth of shorter trees.
- If indoors, avoid the use of wired phones and contact with plumbing or electrical appliances.

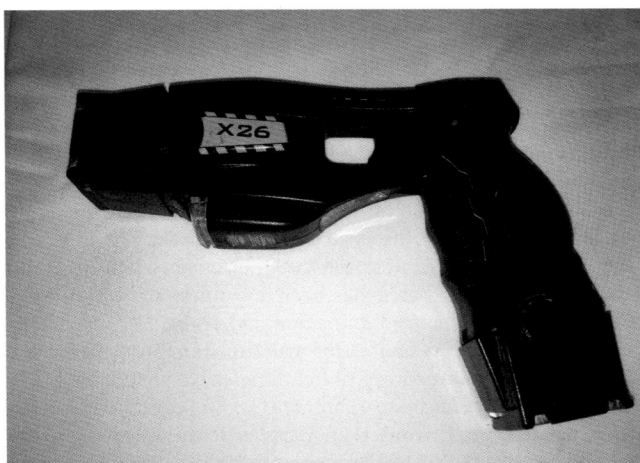

Fig. 130.1 Commonly used conducted energy weapon—Taser X26.

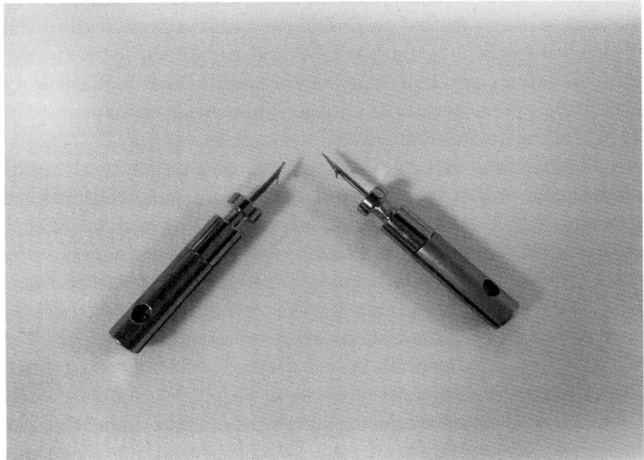

Fig. 130.2 Taser barbs that deliver electrical burst, causing neuromuscular incapacitation.

clothing and then automatically deliver a 5-second burst of energy. Further energy bursts can be delivered at the user's discretion. When these barbs lodge in the person at a distance from one another, they cause an energy arc that results in general muscle contraction and neuromuscular incapacitation (NMI). Newer devices have been developed to create a larger barb spread at close range to maximize the arc distance and more readily induce NMI.

BOX 130.4 Types of Burns Associated With Electrical Injury

Entrance and exit site burns
Arc burns, kissing burns
Thermal burns
Flash burns

CEWs may also include a touch-stun mode, in which direct contact of the weapon to the person is required to deliver an electrical energy pulse. In these cases, the barbs are not deployed, and the subject experiences localized pain but will not undergo NMI.

CLINICAL FEATURES

Electrical Injury

At the cellular level, current causes damage to cell membranes and alters membrane solubility, leading to electrolyte abnormalities and cellular edema. This process, termed *electroporation*, eventually leads to irreversible cell damage and death. At the tissue and organ levels, electrical current produces damage when electrical energy is converted to thermal energy. Electrical injury rarely causes immediate death, but when it does, it is often due to current-induced cardiac arrest (ventricular fibrillation or asystole), respiratory arrest due to respiratory muscle paralysis, or brainstem injury. Commonly reported delayed complications of electrical injuries include sepsis, acute renal failure, wound infections, and amputations.[3]

Lightning Injury

In contrast to electrical injury, lightning injuries involve very brief exposure to high-voltage energy. General effects are thus quite different than electrical injury, with deep muscle injury being much less common. Instead, lightning more commonly causes blunt traumatic injuries or cardiopulmonary arrest from transient stunning and disruption of the pacemaker cells and brainstem.

Skin

Electrical Injury. Most electrical injuries result in skin burns, which fall into one or more of four patterns (as described in Box 130.4). The relatively high resistance of skin in many cases leads to significant partial- or full-thickness burns at entrance and exit sites, most commonly seen over the upper extremities, particularly at the hand and wrist. The skull is another common source contact point. Visible burns may be insignificant in comparison to the damage that occurs beneath the surface and, as a result, are associated with significantly greater morbidity than simple thermal burns involving a similar surface area. Because of this, use of the Parkland formula or other fluid resuscitation equations tend to under-resuscitate these patients. Burns at entrance and exit sites will typically have a punctate appearance, with central depression and necrosis surrounded by a hyperemic border.

Arc burns, or so-called "kissing burns" (Fig. 130.3), occur when electricity jumps from skin surface to skin surface, typically across flexed areas of the body. Temperatures may reach 3500°C (6332°F) and cause severe damage. Arc burns are usually noted across the volar forearm and elbow and along the inner arm and axilla.

In cases in which clothing ignites and catches fire, patients also experience thermal burns. Flash burns are skin burns caused by brief, intense flashes of light, electrical current, or thermal radiation. Cutaneous burns across the chest and upper abdomen indicate a transthoracic current and portend a worse prognosis.

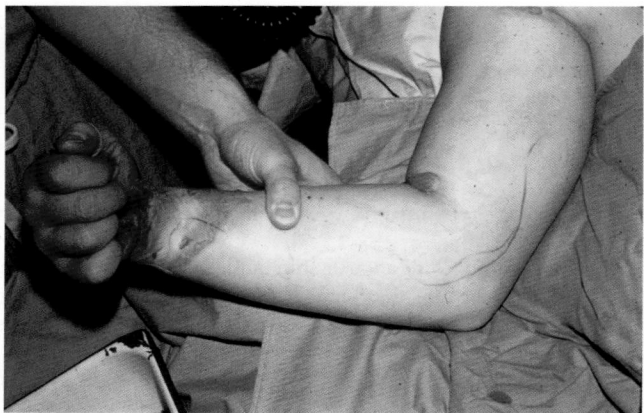

Fig. 130.3 Kissing burn. (Courtesy Dr. Mary Ann Cooper.)

Fig. 130.4 Lightning burn. (Courtesy Dr. Mary Ann Cooper.)

Lightning Injury. Roughly 90% of lightning strike victims suffer skin burns, but less than 5% are deep burns. Although the voltages involved in a strike are substantial, most of the voltage will pass over rather than through the body in what is called a flashover effect. Moreover, the duration of contact is so brief that significant damage does not usually occur. Skin resistance is typically lessened by rain or perspiration, contributing to the flashover effect, where current preferentially flows over the integument rather than through it (i.e., following the path of least resistance). The result is the arborescent or fernlike patterns of erythematous streaks (typically first-degree burns) that have been termed *Lichtenberg figures* (Fig. 130.4). Deeper burns may occur at the direct point of contact or wherever metal is involved (due to superheating), such as with a belt buckle or jewelry. Clothing may catch on fire, resulting in thermal burns. Unlike conventional high-voltage electrical exposures, exit wounds are generally not seen, and the overall effects are much less severe.

Cardiovascular

Electrical Injury. Cardiac or respiratory arrest is the most common cause of death immediately following electrical injury. High-voltage exposures are associated with higher rates of cardiac complications, although low-voltage exposures can also cause cardiac arrest.[2] Traditionally, it is believed that AC causes ventricular fibrillation and DC causes asystole. In reality, exposure to either type of circuit is associated with both dysrhythmias, especially at higher voltages. Respiratory arrest may occur as a result of tetanic paralysis of the thoracic respiratory muscles and diaphragm or as a result of damage to

the brainstem respiratory centers. Prolonged apnea in these situations can lead to hypoxic cardiac arrest.

Most dysrhythmias are seen immediately following electrocution. These include life-threatening dysrhythmias, but more frequently involve sinus tachycardia or bradycardia, atrial fibrillation, and ectopic beats. A variety of electrocardiographic abnormalities may be present, including transient ST elevation or depression that does not correlate with myocardial ischemia or infarction. Injury to coronary arteries or directly to the myocardium may result in infarction, but this is rare. Nonspecific cardiac biomarker levels (e.g., creatine kinase) are frequently elevated in the period following electrical injury, but this is usually due to skeletal muscle injury and is only rarely related to cardiac damage. Dysrhythmias may also appear in a delayed fashion, with case reports of fatal dysrhythmias, although the limited available studies suggest the risk is very low.[4,5,6]

Lightning Injury. The most severe effects of lightning strike are cardiac and respiratory arrest. The massive surge is analogous to defibrillation and can result in asystole or nonperfusing ventricular rhythms, with the latter likely more common than previously thought.[7] The actual pacemaker cells are typically not permanently damaged. Thus, with recovery, the intrinsic pacemaker activity of the heart brings about a resumption of cardiac activity. However, a lightning strike can result in stunning of the respiratory center of the medulla and brainstem, causing central apnea. This respiratory arrest is thought to often last longer than the cardiac standstill itself, which may lead to hypoxic cardiac arrest. Research into the actual effects of lightning on humans is limited but it has been hypothesized that the strike leads to a state of suspended animation and cessation of metabolism in all cells, including the brain. This may explain reports of successful resuscitation and full recovery of lightning strike victims after being apneic and pulseless for up to 15 minutes and following resuscitations lasting up to 8 hours. This observation has led to the practice of treating the "apparent dead" first at the scene of a multiple-victim lightning strike because early resuscitative efforts may prevent death.

Lightning has also been linked to a variety of less ominous dysrhythmias, such as atrial fibrillation, most of which resolve with time. Lightning strikes can also cause QT prolongation which can persist for weeks after the incident.[7] A lightning strike in close proximity to a patient with an automatic implantable cardioverter defibrillator can cause firing of the device. The longer-term effect of a strike on the integrity of the device is not clear.[7]

A number of electrocardiographic changes, usually with gradual resolution, have been reported (Box 130.5). ST segment elevation and depression and T wave inversions suggestive of myocardial ischemia have been widely reported, and may be the result of cardiac contusion, hypoxia-induced infarction, transient coronary vasospasm or actual coronary thrombosis. Given this wide differential diagnosis, the role of immediate coronary interventions is not yet established.[7]

Head and Neck

Electrical Injury. Ocular involvement is common following exposure to electrical current, with cataracts being the most frequent manifestation. Other forms of injury include vitreous and anterior chamber hemorrhages, retinal detachment, macular lacerations, ocular foreign bodies, and corneal or conjunctival burns. Injury to structures of the ear is less common, but sensorineural deafness can be seen as a result of nerve damage. Patients frequently develop vertigo, which may be transient or persistent. Toddlers and young children sustain orofacial injuries after chewing or sucking on electrical cords or from lingual contact with sockets. Full-thickness burns may be sustained on the mucous membranes and lips, with destruction to the tongue and teeth as well. Injuries to the oral commissure produce cosmetic difficulties and, more significantly, delayed labial artery bleeding which typically occurs 2 to 3 days after injury when the resultant eschar separates from the wound.

Lightning Injury. The most common ocular event after lightning strike is the development of cataracts, occurring immediately or in a delayed fashion. Damage to almost every part of the eye has been described. Fixed and dilated or asymmetrical pupils due to autonomic dysfunction may accompany a strike, a finding that by itself should not obviate the need for resuscitative efforts.

The tympanic membranes of patients involved in lightning events are commonly ruptured due to the shock wave and blast effect produced by the rapid expansion of the air as lightning passes through it. Bleeding and cerebrospinal fluid leaks may accompany this injury. Other effects include hearing loss, tinnitus, vertigo, and nystagmus. Specific injuries include avulsion of the mastoid process, ossicle damage, rupture of the Meissner membrane, and strial degeneration.

Extremities

Electrical Injury. Neurovascular bundles have low resistance and are particularly prone to damage from electrical current. Muscle necrosis occurs primarily or is secondary to compromise of the blood supply. Vascular injury is most prominent at the intimal and medial layers. Involvement of the intima results in immediate coagulative necrosis and thrombosis. Injury to the media causes aneurysmal dilation, and occasionally artery rupture and hemorrhage, and may occur months after the injury. Decreases in tissue perfusion lead to edema and tissue death. Areas of infarction may be distributed sporadically throughout the injured region, with areas of surviving tissue adjacent to necrotic tissue.

Muscle that initially appears viable may deteriorate over days and weeks, especially in the periosteal regions. Rhabdomyolysis may occur from muscle breakdown and patients should be aggressively hydrated to prevent acute kidney injury (see "Management" section). Endothelial and smooth muscle function are depressed for many weeks following the initial injury, contributing to a hypercoagulable state that increases the risk of delayed deep venous thrombosis. The combination of tissue edema and perfusion defects makes compartment syndrome likely, necessitating emergent fasciotomy or possible amputation. Compartment syndrome and rhabdomyolysis are risk factors for late arterial rupture.[8] Cyanosis or pulselessness may be transient or may indicate permanent damage; in a similar fashion, limbs that appear initially well perfused may later necrose. Bony injury is common because bone is highly resistant to electrical current flow. This generates large amounts of heat resulting in periosteal burns and osteonecrosis. Fractures and dislocations often occur as a result of the patient being thrown or propelled (particularly with DC current) or from the strength of muscular contractions (AC current).

Nervous System

Electrical Injury. Electrical injury damages the central and peripheral nervous systems. The most common immediate central symptoms are altered mentation, seizure, or coma. Seizures may occur

as an isolated event or as a chronic seizure disorder. Vascular injury may cause cerebral infarction, and secondary trauma may result in intracranial hemorrhage. Cerebral venous sinus thrombosis has been reported.

Patients may experience transient spastic paralysis with accompanying sensory deficits immediately following electrical injury. Delayed and chronic manifestations include ascending paralysis, transverse myelitis, and amyotrophic lateral sclerosis (ALS). Peripheral neuropathies are a common result, most often involving the median and ulnar nerves.

Unlike other complications, rates of neuropsychological sequelae are equal in low- and high-voltage injuries. Immediately after injury, sleep disturbances and anxiety are particularly common. Other short-term complications include depressed mood, flashbacks, dizziness, nightmares, and memory and concentration impairments. Longer-term neuropsychiatric sequelae include posttraumatic stress disorder and major depressive disorder.[9] A post–electrical and lighting injury syndrome has been described and features both prominent memory and executive function deficits as well as other miscellaneous features such as depression and social withdrawal.[10]

Lightning Injury. A wide variety of very serious neurologic effects follow lightning strike. Apnea, due to effects on the medullary respiratory center, may persist for several hours. Direct trauma may result in skull fractures, intracerebral and extracerebral hematomas and hemorrhages, cerebral edema, and elevated intracranial pressure. More common findings include transient loss of consciousness, amnesia of the event, and transient paresthesias and paralysis of the extremities. This later phenomenon, called *keraunoparalysis* is characterized as a flaccid paralysis, usually accompanied by marked vasomotor changes that result in extremities that appear cyanotic, mottled, and pulseless. The lower extremities are more commonly involved, and the typical prognosis is recovery within minutes to days.

Prolonged loss of consciousness may be related to trauma or hypoxia. "Miracle" recoveries have been documented, despite prolonged cardiac arrest and apnea. Conversely, death may occur rapidly from massive brain edema and herniation. Permanent peripheral nerve damage can occur. Other neurologic sequelae include seizures, cerebellar ataxia, Horner syndrome, cognitive dysfunction, facial nerve palsy, neuritis, and neuralgia.

Some psychiatric effects are predictable, usually anxiety and a logical fear of thunderstorms. Other negative effects are similar to those experienced with electrical injury, including memory loss and concentration deficits, prolonged depression, sleep disturbances, nightmares, nocturnal enuresis, and separation anxiety. Hysterical blindness, deafness, and muteness have been described.

Other Viscera

Electrical Injury. Extensive muscle damage may result in significant myoglobinuria, subsequent renal failure, and life-threatening hyperkalemia. These complications are more likely in patients who are hypotensive or volume-depleted. Stress ulcers are a common gastrointestinal complication. Uncommon but severe intra-abdominal injuries include a ruptured hollow viscus and necrosis of the pancreas or gallbladder. Pulmonary edema is rare. Although early fatalities are due to respiratory and cardiac arrest, delayed deaths occur from sepsis, pneumonia, and renal failure. For obstetric patients, the overall risk to the fetus is low, but a spontaneous abortion can occur. Secondary trauma may lead to placental abruption.

Lightning Injury. The lungs, gastrointestinal tract, and other internal organs may suffer injury from blunt trauma or a blast effect. Strikes to the face may produce damage to the tongue and oral structures, esophagus, and trachea. Various fractures, dislocations, and soft tissue injuries occur. Myoglobinuria is relatively unusual due to the brief duration of contact.

Vasomotor changes may occur at the time of the strike and can last for variable periods. Mottling or cyanosis appears, and pulses may be absent. Although dramatic in appearance, these typically resolve without intervention. Vascular changes mimic those seen in compartment syndromes, but fasciotomy is generally not indicated. When pregnant women are struck by lightning, the effects on the fetus are not predictable therefore, depending on the dates of gestation, maternal-fetal monitoring is generally recommended.

Conducted Electrical Weapon. Patients who present after receiving a CEW barb discharge may have local injury to the skin and nearby superficial structures, such as vessels, nerves, and bones. Most barbs penetrate the chest or back, but barbs may also lodge in the face, eyes, or genitals. These patients may also sustain injuries from muscle contraction or falls due to NMI. Traumatic brain injury and spinal compression fractures in osteopenic patients as a result of CEW discharge have been described. However, the overall occurrence of injuries due to this mechanism is rare, occurring in less than 0.5% of CEW deployment subjects.[11] Patients who have received CEW touch-stun exposure may develop skin irritation or minor contact burns.

Current literature indicates that there is no evidence of cardiac ischemia, dysrhythmias, or structural cardiac damage to patients who have received CEW exposure of less than 15 seconds, and who are otherwise asymptomatic, awake, and alert. Most CEW exposures from law enforcement are less than 15 seconds, suggesting that the risk of cardiac complications is very low.[11]

DIFFERENTIAL DIAGNOSES

Electrical Injury

Most electrical injuries are self-evident, except in unwitnessed water-related exposures where there may be no skin burns. In such cases, patients may present with cardiac arrest, dysrhythmias, or altered mentation. Victims of known electrical injury who present with altered mentation may be suffering from electrical injury of the central nervous system, associated traumatic brain injury, or underlying metabolic disease.

Lightning Injury

In cases in which lightning strikes are not witnessed, these injuries should be suspected in patients presenting from the outdoors with altered mentation or cardiac arrest in the setting of a recent thunderstorm. Other clues include the presence of typical skin burn patterns, clothing that has been blasted off, singed or has melting of metal pieces such as zippers or grommets. Other suggestive findings are listed in Box 130.6. Differential diagnoses of altered mentation in lightning strike victims are the same as with other high-voltage injuries.

BOX 130.6 Findings Suggestive of a Lightning Strike

Clothing wet from rain
Tears or disintegration of clothing
Multiple victims
Typical arborescent pattern of erythema or superficial linear or punctate burns
Tympanic membrane injury
Cataracts, especially in a younger patient
Magnetization of metallic objects on the body or clothing
Electrocardiographic changes

DIAGNOSTIC TESTING

Electrical Injury

No evidence-based guidelines direct the ancillary testing of electrical injury victims. Testing is not required for victims of low-voltage electrical injuries who are asymptomatic or have minimal localized symptoms. Evaluation for underlying injury should be undertaken in patients who have been exposed to high-voltage sources. In addition, those victims who have lost consciousness or present with altered mentation or neurologic deficits, have entrance and exit wounds or more than superficial partial-thickness burns, cardiac dysrhythmias or other significant symptoms should be fully evaluated, regardless of the source voltage. Because the location and extent of injury cannot be predicted clinically, we recommend electrocardiography, a complete blood count, basic serum electrolytes, serum myoglobin and troponin, blood urea nitrogen, serum creatinine levels, and urine analysis, testing for myoglobinuria. Patients with suspected intra-abdominal injury from electrical current or associated trauma should have hepatic transaminases and pancreatic enzyme levels (lipase) measured and coagulation studies performed. Radiographs of injured extremities are indicated if there is significant pain, deformity, swelling or bony tenderness following trauma. Computed tomography or magnetic resonance imaging should be used when intracranial, spinal, intra-abdominal or pelvic injuries are clinically suspected. There is little evidence to guide further workup of patients with significant troponin elevations, but we recommend 12 to 24 hours of telemetry monitoring and an echocardiogram for those with a troponin rise thought to signify myocardial damage.[5] The utility of prolonged cardiac monitoring in patients with an electrical exposure is unclear, as most studies show delayed cardiac dysrhythmias are rare.[4] However, we recommend a period of observation for 12 to 24 hours in any patient who sustained a high-voltage electrocution as well for those who suffered loss of consciousness, or have a dysrhythmia or abnormal ECG on arrival to the ED.

Lightning Injury

The Wilderness Medical Society has recommended that an electrocardiogram (ECG) be obtained on lightning strike victims with high-risk indicators, such as suspected direct strike, loss of consciousness, focal neurologic complaint, chest pain or dyspnea, associated traumatic injuries, pregnancy, or burns of the cranium or legs or on more than 10% of the total body surface area. Cardiac markers are often elevated in victims of lightning strikes, but they do not correlate with myocardial injury and are not prognostic. Patients will often have been thrown or propelled by the force of the lightning and a detailed examination looking for signs of secondary trauma is indicated. Compared to electrical injuries, lightning strikes are much less likely to result in compartment syndrome or rhabdomyolysis and when these occur, it is often a result of a traumatic injury rather than from the strike itself. A thorough eye and ear exam should be performed because lightning current can affect the lens as well as the tympanic membranes, which can often burst due to the acoustic blast wave.

Patients without any obvious sequalae should still receive follow-up care, as a large percentage of lightning survivors will experience some neurocognitive sequelae. Regional burn centers are often equipped to further evaluate and refer these patients.

Conducted Electrical Weapon

In patients who are awake and alert, asymptomatic, and have had CEW exposure of less than 15 seconds, no specific diagnostic testing is required to evaluate for cardiac injury, electrolyte imbalance, renal abnormalities, or acid-base disturbances. Similarly, evidence has not shown any clinically significant rise in lactate or CK levels, and we do not recommend testing in this patient population. Additionally, routine

EKG, cardiac monitoring, or echocardiography are not recommended in this patient population. However, patients may have underlying conditions that precipitated the use of the CEW, including but not limited to altered mental status, intoxication, or psychiatric conditions, and they should undergo diagnostic testing as guided by their presentation and past medical history. Additionally, patients should be evaluated for secondary traumatic injury and undergo appropriate trauma evaluation.

MANAGEMENT

Electrical Injury

Low-voltage electrical injuries associated with minimal signs and symptoms generally require only local wound treatment and patient reassurance. The treatment of other patients is directed at the organ systems involved.

Patients who present in cardiopulmonary arrest should be resuscitated, regardless of cardiac rhythm, because favorable outcomes have been documented even with patients presenting in asystole. Patients with electrocardiographic signs of cardiac injury or dysrhythmias and patients with more than minimal local signs and symptoms should be monitored in the emergency department (ED), observation unit, or inpatient setting, depending on the extent and severity of associated injuries. Dysrhythmias are treated according to advanced cardiovascular life support (ACLS) guidelines. Hypotensive patients should be evaluated for possible blood loss from associated traumatic injuries. Hypotension may also be caused by third spacing of intravascular volume secondary to electrical injury of deep tissues, so fluid management is similar to that of crush injuries, often requiring more fluid than typically recommended by thermal burn wound protocols. Intravenous crystalloid fluids are given to maintain adequate urine output (over 100 mL/hr in adults and 1.5 to 2 mL/kg/hr in young children). Serum potassium levels should be closely monitored in patients with acute renal injury or myoglobinuria.

Although AC causes thrombotic injury to blood vessels, DC can result in transient vasospasm that results in extremities that appear cyanotic, mottled, and pulseless. This should be kept in mind when deciding when vascular surgical intervention is indicated. Skin and vascular findings are likely to resolve with supportive care only but, if significant thrombosis (immediate or delayed) develops, amputation may be required. The presence of pulseless and mottled extremities may limit the ability to detect hypotension with standard devices, and central monitoring or arterial lines may be required to accurately assess volume status.

Patients with myoglobinuria should be monitored with determination of serial serum myoglobin levels and renal function studies. The management of rhabdomyolysis is discussed in Chapter 116. Injured extremities require burn wound management (see Chapter 54). These injuries should be monitored for the development of compartment syndromes (see Chapter 41).

Lightning Injury

Lightning strike victims who present without symptoms or signs of injury, including those with minor first-degree burns, do not require treatment in the ED unless their electrocardiograms show signs of ischemia or concerning dysrhythmias. Patients who present with altered mentation or significant symptoms are approached in a manner similar to that used for victims of high-voltage electrical injury. However, a few differences should be noted. Lightning strikes can result in a spectrum of peripheral and central neurologic injuries, including pupils that are fixed and dilated in the absence of irreversible brain injury. This factor should be kept in mind when deciding when to discontinue resuscitative efforts in patients who present in cardiac arrest. Lightning strikes can cause extensive catecholamine release or autonomic stimulation, resulting in transient hypertension and tachycardia that can be treated with β-adrenergic blockers and hydralazine or with alpha-2 adrenergic agonists such as clonidine, to reduce adrenergic excesses.

Conducted Electrical Weapon

Patients injured by CEWs rarely require intervention. Patients with barb injury should have evaluation of the barb penetration site, and most will not require additional treatment beyond removal and localized wound care. For those who sustain barbs to the face, eyes, or genitals, specialist consultation and operative removal may be required. In those patients with touch-stun exposure, local wound care is recommended.

DISPOSITION

Electrical Injury

Asymptomatic patients who present after low-voltage exposures may be safely discharged home. Other patients are monitored and treated in the ED, observation unit, or inpatient setting, depending on their clinical status and extent and severity of identified injuries. There is some debate around the need for prolonged cardiac monitoring of patients, with most studies showing that the risk of delayed dysrhythmia is very low. A reasonable approach is to observe patients with loss of consciousness, dysrhythmia, high-voltage exposure, ECG abnormality or significant troponin increase on telemetry for 12 to 24 hours. Patients with significant burns should be stabilized and transferred to a burn unit, if available.

Pediatric patients with oral electric injuries are usually hospitalized for hydration, wound and pain management, and plastic surgery consultation. Patients with minor burns confined to the oral commissure can be discharged with close follow-up but should be provided with information regarding the possibility of delayed labial artery bleeding, which can be managed by the parents with direct wound pressure and return visit instructions.

Pregnant patients should receive a period of fetal monitoring when gestational age–appropriate. Women who are subsequently discharged should be counselled regarding the remote risk of spontaneous abortion and referred for high-risk obstetric follow-up care.

Patients may experience delayed neuropsychiatric sequelae, so discharge instructions with a neurologic referral may be provided.

Lightning Injury

The Wilderness Medical Society has recommended that victims of direct lightning strikes and those with an abnormal ECG be monitored with telemetry for a minimum of 24 hours. Other patients can be discharged but should be counselled regarding the need to seek further care if they develop delayed-onset symptoms, which can be cardiopulmonary, neurologic, psychiatric, ophthalmologic, or otolaryngologic in nature.

Conducted Electrical Weapon

Unless there is a concomitant condition present that requires further care or admission, routine cardiac monitoring, ED observation, or hospitalization is not recommended for patients who are awake, alert, and asymptomatic who have had CEW exposure less than 15 seconds.

For patients who have had CEW exposure for greater than 15 seconds, there is limited experience and no clear guidelines exist, so an observation period of 6 to 8 hours is a reasonable approach.

ACKNOWLEGMENTS

The authors wish to acknowledge and thank Kelly P. O'Keefe and Rachel Semmons for their valuable contributions, expertise, and authorship of this chapter in previous editions.

The references for this chapter can be found online at ExpertConsult.com.

Scuba Diving and Dysbarism

David A. Peak

FOUNDATIONS

Background and Importance

Underwater free diving has been practiced for more than 5000 years both commercially and for recreation. Diving bells physically provided access to air and protection from pressure at depths to divers and have been described as far back as the 4th century BCE. The earliest artificial underwater breathing devices were restrictive to shallow water because of pressure constraints. In the 1940s, Cousteau and Gagnan introduced a self-contained underwater apparatus (SCUBA) and buoyancy control device (BCD), which revolutionized the ability of divers to safely dive to moderate depths. Diving has increased exponentially since that time among commercial, military, and especially recreational activities which now account for approximately 9 million participants per year in the United States alone, with several hundred thousand new divers trained per year. As a result of its recreational popularity, injuries related to diving have also increased.[1,2] According to the Divers Alert Network (DAN), which is the diving industry's largest association dedicated to diving safety, there are approximately three injuries of any kind per 100 dives and up to 10% of these are fatal. This represents a small but clinically relevant subpopulation of dives.

The symptoms and signs of diving-related illness, also known as *dysbarisms*, began to be recognized as diving became increasingly accessible. The ailment became known as *caisson disease,* named after the large diving bell commonly used for submersion. Construction workers on the Brooklyn Bridge (constructed between 1870–1880) termed the disorder "the bends," because the symptoms often caused the victim to bend forward in pain. The first clinical description by Bert in 1878 correctly attributed the disease to nitrogen gas coming out of solution in the tissues during decompression, which led to the recommendation of slow ascents for pressurized workers and the development of the first recompression chambers.

Most divers use compressed air, open-circuit scuba equipment at depths of less than 130 feet of seawater (fsw). Systems with artificial mixtures of various gases, however, are used to extend the depths to which divers can descend or the duration that a diver may safely remain submerged. Other variations of supplying air for divers include closed-circuit and semiclosed-circuit diving apparatus (called "rebreathers") that use calcium hydroxide to absorb expired carbon dioxide and add oxygen to the decarboxylated gas before rebreathing and allow more efficient and safe diving.

Physiology and Pathophysiology

The leading cause of death among divers is from drowning accidents. Scuba divers may also encounter emergencies common to environmental exposures (e.g., hypothermia, sun exposure, motion sickness, bites, envenomation, and physical trauma). They are also subject to the unique injuries related to pressure at depth.[3] The pathophysiologic mechanism of diving or dysbarisms can be separated into two broad categories: (1) Barotrauma which is related to pressure and; (2) Decompression illness which is related to gas bubbles. Barotrauma can be related to the speed of descent and ascent but is almost completely independent of time of depth. Bubble formation (primarily nitrogen) during and immediately after ascent as well as nitrogen narcosis are both dependent on being at depth for an extended period of time. Therefore, it is useful when treating a patient with an acute diving injury to know the recent dive history because it can assist the clinician in narrowing down the differential diagnoses. For instance, a recreational diver who was at a moderate depth for only a few minutes can still have a major barotrauma-related dive injury but would not have had time to accumulate enough gas or nitrogen in their tissues to cause symptoms.

Familiarity with several of the laws of physics that define the properties of liquids and gases (Table 131.1; Figs. 131.1 to 131.5) is useful when discussing diving pathophysiology. Boyle's law explains diver-related barotrauma and states that at constant temperature, the absolute pressure, and the volume of gas are inversely proportional ($PV = k$). In other words, as pressure increases (with descent), the gas volume is reduced; as the pressure is reduced (with ascent), the gas volume increases. A diver needs to descend only 33 feet in seawater to double the atmospheric pressure, an increase of 23 mm Hg per foot of depth. Abrupt changes in the volume of air-containing parts of the body (e.g., ears, sinuses, and lungs) are at risk of barotrauma with the extreme pressure changes of the environment. These include barotrauma associated with an inability to equalize, mask squeeze, or

TABLE 131.1 Laws of Physics

Gas Law	Formula	Significance
Pascal's law: A pressure applied to any part of a liquid is transmitted equally throughout.	$\Delta P = \varrho g\ (\Delta h)$ ΔP is the hydrostatic pressure. ϱ is the fluid density. g is acceleration due to gravity. Δh is the height of fluid.	Pressure increases in a contained space are transmitted throughout; significant for IEBT and MEBT (see Fig. 131.1)
Boyle's law: At a constant temperature, the absolute pressure and the volume of gas are inversely proportional. As pressure increases, the gas volume is reduced; as the pressure is reduced, the gas volume increases.	$P1 \cdot V1 = P2 \cdot V2$	Relates to change in the volume of a gas caused by the change in pressure due to depth, which defines the relationship of pressure and volume in breathing gas supplies (see Fig. 131.2)
Charles' law: At a constant pressure, the volume of a gas is directly proportional to the change in the absolute temperature.	$V1/T1 = V2/T2$	Increasing pressure (filling a scuba tank) causes heat; cooling a tank decreases the pressure (see Fig. 131.3)
The general gas law combines these concepts to predict the behavior of a gas when the factors change.	$P1 \cdot V1/T1 = P2 \cdot V2/T2$ P1 is the initial pressure. V1 is the initial volume. T1 is the initial temperature. P2 is the final pressure. V2 is the final volume. T2 is the final temperature.	A means of relating pressure, volume, and temperature together in one equation when variables are not constant
Dalton's law: The total pressure exerted by a mixture of gases is equal to the sum of the pressures (partial pressures) of each of the different gases making up the mixture, with each gas acting as if it alone is present and occupies the total volume.	$PTotal\ 3\ P1 + P2 + P3 + \ldots + Pn$	Nitrogen under pressure acts as if other gases are not present (see Fig. 131.4)
Henry's law: The amount of a gas that will dissolve in a liquid at a given temperature is directly proportional to the partial pressure of that gas.	$e^p = e^{kc}$ e is approximately 2.7182818 (the base of the natural logarithm). p is the partial pressure of the solute above the solution. c is the concentration of the solute in the solution. k is the Henry's law constant.	More nitrogen is taken into solution (e.g., serum) at high pressures than comes out of solution at lower pressures (see Fig. 131.5)

IEBT, Inner ear barotrauma; *MEBT,* middle ear barotrauma.

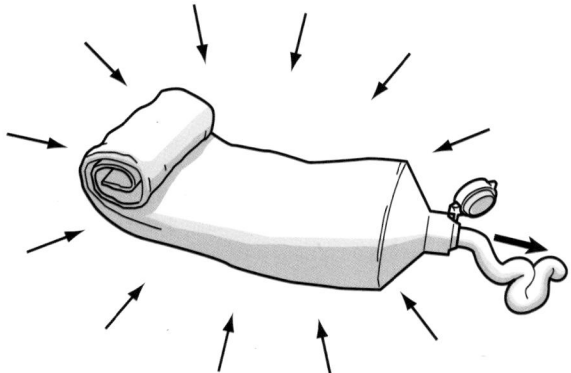

Fig. 131.1 Pascal's law. A pressure applied to any part of a liquid is transmitted equally throughout.

barotrauma to the ears and sinuses during descent, as well as barotrauma related to ascent (usually associated with breath-holding) including pneumomediastinum, pneumothorax, and arterial gas embolism. Fractional changes in volume are greater near where the proportional pressure changes are highest, which is generally in more shallow water.

Henry's law explains decompression illness and states that the amount of any gas that dissolves in a liquid at a given temperature is directly proportional to the partial pressure of that gas. At higher ambient pressures, an increasing concentration of each component gas of the inhaled air will dissolve in solution until a new steady-state concentration is achieved. Therefore, the length of time the diver is breathing the gas at the increased pressure and the inherent solubility of the gas also govern the quantity of a particular gas that dissolves. The dissolved gas remains in solution as long as the pressure is maintained. As the diver ascends, however, increasingly more of the dissolved gas comes out of solution. A rapid ascent may reduce the pressure at a rate higher than the body can accommodate, and the bubbles (particularly nitrogen) may accumulate and disrupt body tissues and systems, a phenomenon termed *decompression sickness* (DCS). This is similar to the rapid opening of a bottle of a carbonated beverage which allows bubbles of carbon dioxide to rapidly come out of solution.

Safe diving practice includes a controlled ascent rate (i.e., through the use of safe decompression tables or submersible dive computers), during which the gas is carried to the lung vascular bed and is exhaled before it accumulates to form significantly large or numerous bubbles in the tissues. This is similar to how opening of a soda bottle slowly reduces agitated bubbling of the contained carbonated liquid.

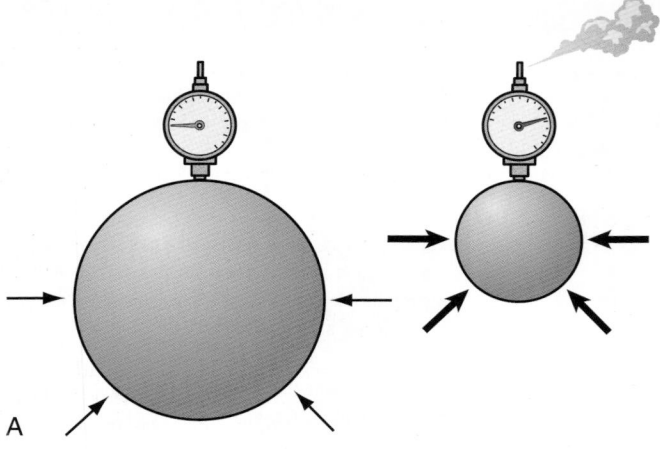

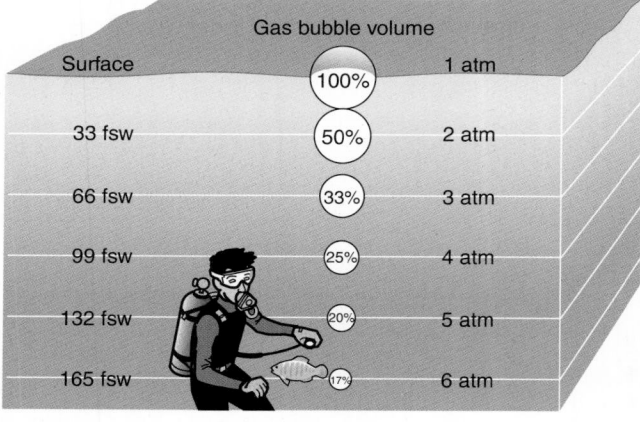

Fig. 131.2 Boyle's law. (A) At a constant temperature, the absolute pressure and the volume of gas are inversely proportional. (B) As pressure increases, the gas volume is reduced; as the pressure is reduced, the gas volume increases. *fsw,* Feet of seawater.

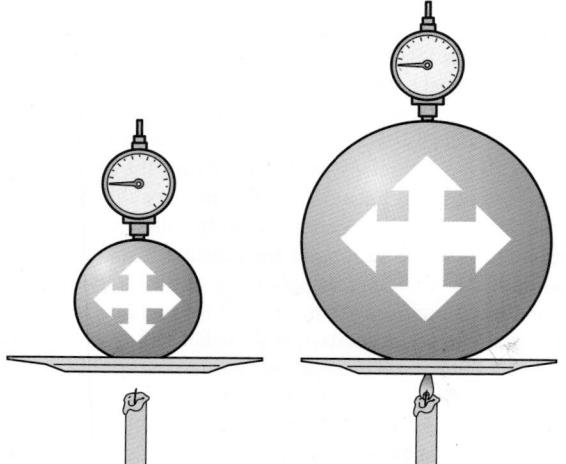

Fig. 131.3 Charles' law. At a constant pressure, the volume of a gas is directly proportional to the change in the absolute temperature.

CLINICAL FEATURES

The clinical features of the injuries and maladies related to diving will be presented in this section based on when the symptoms are likely to

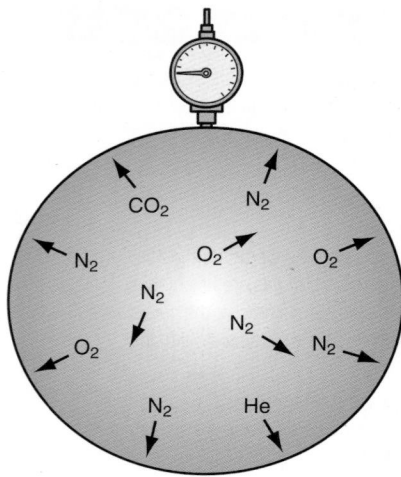

Fig. 131.4 Dalton's law. The total pressure exerted by a mixture of gases is equal to the sum of the pressures (partial pressures) of each of the different gases making up the mixture, with each gas acting as if it alone is present and occupies the total volume. *CO2,* Carbon dioxide; *He,* helium; *N2,* nitrogen; *O2,* oxygen.

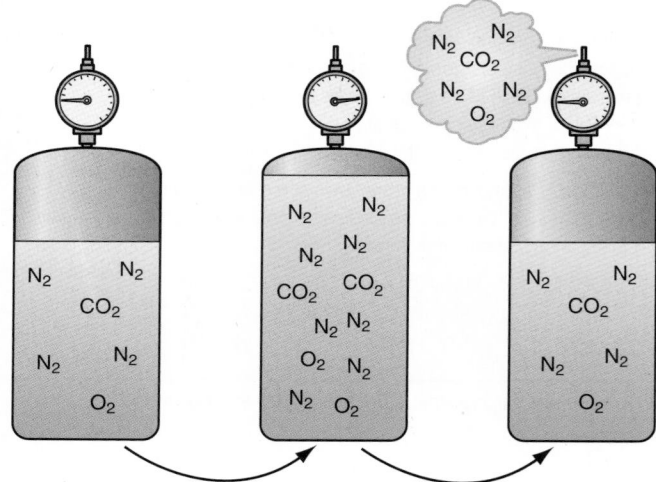

Fig. 131.5 Henry's law. The amount of a gas that will dissolve in a liquid at a given temperature is directly proportional to the partial pressure of that gas. *CO2,* Carbon dioxide; *N2,* nitrogen; *O2,* oxygen.

start during a dive, first those that occur on descent, then those that occur at depth, and finally those that occur upon surfacing. This organization is used to help the clinician stratify the likelihood of a specific disorder based on when the symptoms started during the dive. Box 131.1 lists the recommended components of a focused dive history.

Disorders Related to Descent/Barotrauma

Middle Ear Barotrauma

Middle ear barotrauma (MEBT), also known as *barotitis or ear squeeze,* is the most common complaint of scuba divers. In a survey of over 750 recreational divers, over half experienced pain related to mild ear barotrauma multiple times during their dives. Most of these were minor pains associated with descent that resolve with equalization maneuvers with no long-term effects.[4-6]

The middle ear is an air-filled space with solid bone walls except for the tympanic membrane (Fig. 131.6). In the auditory system, the eustachian tube is the only anatomic passage to the external environment. During descent, there is an increase in external pressure that

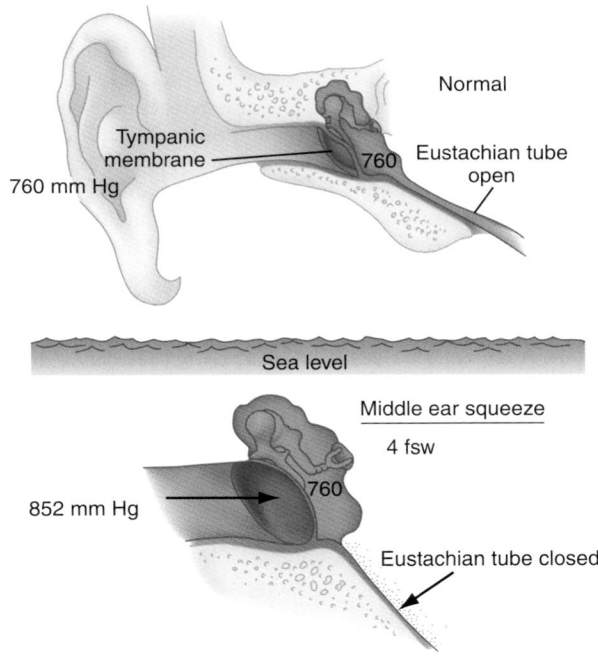

Fig. 131.6 Middle ear barotrauma symptoms include fullness and pain caused by stretching of the tympanic membrane. (From: Van Hoesen KB, Bird NH. Diving medicine. In Auerbach PS, ed. *Wilderness Medicine*, ed 6. Philadelphia: Elsevier; 2012: 1529.)

exerts inward pressure against the tympanic membrane (TM). This occurs when the eustachian tube (ET) does not effectively allow air to flow into the middle ear space to equalize pressure. The ET can become blocked and eventually locked in place by a combination of pressure differential and tissue inflammation or edema.

During a diving descent, there is increasing external and inward pressure against the tympanic membrane unless air enters the middle ear via the eustachian tube (ET) to maintain equal pressure across the tympanic membrane. Typically, a diver performs various equalization maneuvers to force air into the middle ear through the ET. The ET may become blocked or collapse related to the pressure differential or inflammation, making subsequent attempts at equalization virtually impossible. This is typically painful and may be associated with

tinnitus; some patients develop transient vertigo. Further descent without successful equalization can cause the TM to collapse inward and rupture. The pain may or may not resolve as the TM ruptures. Rupture of TM can cause asymmetric caloric stimulation by exposure of the middle ear to cold water, inducing a transient nystagmus and vertigo. This can become life-threatening if the diver panics or becomes disoriented. The pressure of the water in the middle ear may also lead to a facial palsy in certain individuals where the seventh cranial nerve passes through this space.

External Ear Barotrauma

External ear barotrauma is less common than MEBT and can be caused by an obstruction of the external auditory canal (e.g., cerumen, ear plugs) which can trap air in the canal instead of filling with water. This may lead to localized pain or hemorrhages within the wall of the external auditory canal on examination. These symptoms are generally self-limited.

Inner Ear Barotrauma

IEBT is trauma occurring as a result of a pressure differential between the middle and inner ear spaces. Inner ear barotrauma (IEBT) results in damage to the cochleovestibular apparatus. It is less common than MEBT (reported as 0.5% lifetime incidence in divers) but is associated with greater morbidity. If the diver is unable to equalize the middle ear during descent, pressure is transmitted across the labyrinthine windows (oval and round) leading to inner ear hemorrhage. Intralabyrinthine membrane tears which effect the Reissner, tectorial or basilar membranes can also occur or cause a tear of the labyrinthine windows, leading to perilymphatic fistula formation (PLF). Fifty percent of these injuries are mixed cochlear and vestibular, 40% are isolated cochlear, and 10% isolated vestibular.

Symptoms associated with IEBT include variable hearing loss, severe vertigo, nausea, tinnitus, and fullness in the affected ear. Signs include severe nystagmus, positional vertigo, ataxia, and vomiting. The degree of sensorineural hearing loss is variable. Distinguishing IEBT from inner ear DCS can be challenging but should not delay recompression in a patient in whom the diagnosis is unclear.

Reverse Middle Ear Squeeze

Reverse middle ear squeeze is the opposite of middle squeeze and occurs during ascent. As the pressure lessens, a pressure gradient can cause the TM to bulge outward and even rupture causing pain. This is much less common than middle ear squeeze during descent.

Barosinusitis

After ear barotrauma, the second most common diving-related physical disturbance is sinus barotrauma. In a survey of over 750 recreational divers, 35% experienced sinus pain related to barotrauma on more than one occasion while diving. Most of these were minor pains associated with descent that resolve with equalization maneuvers and have no long-term effects. The air-filled maxillary, frontal, and ethmoidal sinuses are susceptible to volume-pressure changes on ascent or descent; the most commonly affected is the maxillary sinus, followed by the frontal. The most common symptoms are facial pain and epistaxis. Obstruction of the sinus ostia for any reason (e.g., mucosal thickening, polyps, pus, or deviated septum) predisposes to the inability to equalize and sinus barotrauma.[5-6]

Alternobaric Vertigo

Alternobaric vertigo is a common but usually transient, self-limited vertigo secondary to asymmetric ear pressure transmitting from the middle ear to the inner ear. It is not thought to have long-term effects.

Facial Barotrauma or Mask Squeeze

During descent, a negative pressure develops within the diving mask that may increase to the point of damaging surrounding tissues if the diver does not exhale into the mask in order to equalize the pressures within and outside the mask. "Mask squeeze" is a type of facial barotrauma injury that occurs more commonly in novice divers or in masks that cannot be exhaled into (e.g., free diving masks) The difference in pressure inside and outside the mask can lead to barotrauma to the contents inside the mask leading to injury of blood vessels and tissue of the eyes and face. This can lead to facial and conjunctival edema, diffuse petechial hemorrhages on the face, and subconjunctival hemorrhages which are generally self-limited. Rarely, optic nerve damage can result from severe facial barotrauma. Recent eye surgery or preexisting glaucoma may increase the risk of injury.

Disorders Arising at Depth

Nitrogen Narcosis

Nitrogen narcosis (known as *rapture of the deep*) is a phenomenon that occurs when exposed to the intoxicating increases of partial pressures of nitrogen and is considered a significant contributing factor in diving-related accidents. Narcosis is characterized by an impairment of psychomotor coordination and alterations in mood (such as euphoria or increased anxiety) and behavior (lowering of inhibitions and impairment in reasoning). Symptoms require time at depth and may become apparent at a depth of 100 ft (30 m) and increase with further increases in depth. Use of mixed gases with lower concentration of nitrogen is recommended for technical, military, commercial or sport diving to deeper depths. The effects of nitrogen narcosis resolve with gradual and controlled ascent to shallower depths.

Oxygen Toxicity

At elevated partial pressures for extended periods, oxygen can be toxic to the central nervous system (CNS) or lungs. Oxygen becomes toxic to the CNS when its partial pressure exceeds 1.6 atmosphere absolute (ata). Oxygen partial pressures below 1.4 ata are unlikely to produce CNS toxicity. A diver breathing compressed air would attain a partial pressure of 1.6 ata of oxygen at a depth of 218 fsw. This far exceeds the depth to which most recreational divers would dive. Most professional divers prevent oxygen toxicity by breathing mixed gases with decreased oxygen and nitrogen content to decrease the possibility of oxygen toxicity (and nitrogen narcosis). This requires special equipment and advanced training.

Pulmonary oxygen toxicity (low-pressure oxygen poisoning) can occur after 24 hours of exposure to partial pressures of oxygen in excess of 0.6 ata. The symptoms of pulmonary oxygen toxicity include a burning sensation or pain on inspiration and coughing. Pulmonary function gradually becomes normal after the exposure is terminated, but pneumonitis and permanent fibrosis are possible. CNS oxygen toxicity symptoms include headache, dizziness, irritability, anxiety, visual changes, extremity tingling or twitching, tinnitus and hearing abnormalities, nausea, and seizures. It can cause drowning and death. It is extremely unlikely that a sport diver would ever be exposed for the duration that is required to produce toxicity; however, long exposures to higher levels of oxygen, such as those administered for certain recompression protocols, may lead to oxygen toxicity. In a 20-year single hyperbaric center study of over 18,000 patients, only 0.02% of patients experienced seizure activity.[5] Most hyperbaric centers use intermittent "air breaks" during hyperbaric treatment sessions in which the patients breath air with a normal Pao_2 to give their bodies a break from high oxygen levels and prevent toxicity.

Contaminated Air

Rarely, other gases, such as carbon monoxide and carbon dioxide, can contaminate the air that is compressed into a tank. This can happen if the compressor intake is placed too close to the compressor's engine exhaust. As in the case of oxygen and nitrogen, the partial pressure of these contaminants in the tissues increases dramatically with depth, potentiating their clinical effects. The symptoms of hypercarbia or carbon monoxide poisoning are thus more severe at elevated partial pressures. Hypercarbia will also increase a diver's susceptibility to CNS oxygen toxicity.

Rebreathers are used by recreational divers to recirculate the gas used by the diver after replacing oxygen and removing carbon dioxide. The major advantages are extended dive times and diminished accumulation of bubbles. Rebreathers use absorbent material to remove carbon dioxide from the circuit. A hose rupture allowing seawater contamination of the circuit may create a caustic alkaline-based liquid containing calcium or sodium hydroxide, which can cause burns to the mouth, throat, and airways.

Disorders Arising on Ascent

Alternobaric Vertigo

Alternobaric vertigo (ABV) results from an inability to equalize pressure within the middle ear during ascent and affects up to 25% of divers. ABV is based on asymmetrical pressure changes in the middle ear that are transmitted through the oval and round window to the vestibular system, resulting in a sensation of spinning and loss of orientation. This profound but transient sense of vertigo during ascent may be associated with nausea and vomiting but is not thought to lead to major morbidity or mortality. Unlike those of IEBT, the symptoms are self-limited.

Barodontalgia

On occasion, air that is trapped beneath a poorly filled dental cavity or within a dental abscess and expands on ascent, leading to dental pain. This condition affects up to 10% of divers but is relatively benign and self-limited.

Gastrointestinal Barotrauma

Serious gastrointestinal barotrauma is a rare condition in scuba divers. It results from the expansion of bowel gas in the small intestine and colon on ascent after diving. Predisposing factors include consumption of carbonated beverages, large meals, or gas-producing foods before diving, as well as performance of the Valsalva maneuver in the head-down position. Symptoms include eructation, flatulence, bloating, and crampy abdominal pain. In divers with inguinal or other abdominal hernias, the potential for expansion of trapped gas within the hernia exists, and expansion may result in incarceration or strangulation. Gastric rupture has been reported. Although gastrointestinal barotrauma is a rare entity, it should be suspected in the diver-patient with a provocative history and acute abdominal pain.

Pulmonary Barotrauma

Without continuously expiring on ascent, the lungs of a scuba diver who takes a full breath at 33 fsw would have to expand to double their volume by the time they reached the surface (based on Boyle's law). However, expansion of the alveoli is limited. Breath-holding during ascent with resultant expansion of lung volumes and pressure can force gas bubbles across the alveolar-capillary membrane and cause the wall of the alveoli to rupture. This can occur with as little a change in depth from 3 to 4 feet (or pressure difference of 80 mm Hg) and *does not* require being at depth for a prolonged time period.

In fact, the greatest risk for pulmonary barotrauma occurs in less than 10 feet of water. Therefore, it is important for the clinician to consider this disease entity in patients with symptoms even after exposure to shallow depths for a short period. Pulmonary barotrauma can result in the following four conditions: pneumothorax, pneumomediastinum, subcutaneous emphysema, and alveolar hemorrhage. Risk factors elicited from the dive and medical history may suggest the diagnosis of pulmonary barotrauma. In most cases, fast ascent, panic, problems in regulating proper buoyancy, or running out of air precipitates an uncontrolled ascent with breath-holding.

Patients with restrictive and obstructive lung diseases are at increased risk. Asthmatics have a twofold-increased risk for pulmonary barotrauma compared with the general diver population. Box 131.2 lists six mechanisms that contribute to the increased risk in asthmatics,[8] who should be instructed not to dive unless they are completely free of symptoms. Box 131.3 summarizes the recommendations from the multiple national scuba governing agencies, as well as expert consensus.[6]

Pneumomediastinum and subcutaneous emphysema result when air crosses the alveolar endothelium and dissects into the pulmonary interstitium. Most commonly, air travels into the neck, mediastinum, or pericardium. The manifestations of pneumomediastinum may include fullness or pain in the neck, palpable subcutaneous crepitance, and a change in voice quality. Unless evidence of either hemodynamic instability or airway compromise exists, interstitial air or subcutaneous emphysema is not a life-threatening condition.

Pulmonary barotrauma-induced pneumothorax occurs when air from alveoli crosses the visceral pleura. A tension pneumothorax is a rare complication. The symptoms and signs of a pneumothorax secondary to pulmonary barotrauma are similar to a pneumothorax of any other cause.

Pulmonary barotrauma can also cause alveolar hemorrhage. Patients may present with hemoptysis coincident with chest pain and dyspnea. Chest radiography may reveal an interstitial infiltrate. If alveolar gas invades the pulmonary veins and enters the systemic circulation it can cause arterial gas embolism (AGE) which is discussed later.

Decompression Sickness

The term *decompression sickness (DCS)* refers to a spectrum of clinical illnesses resulting from the formation of small bubbles of nitrogen gas in the blood and tissues on ascent. The clinical expression of DCS depends on the location, destination, and degree of nitrogen bubble formation in blood and tissues. Small, usually asymptomatic venous gas emboli are common in the ascending diver after ascent and for the first several hours after ascent and are usually filtered by the lungs without apparent permanent damage. Persistent intravascular bubbles, however, may elicit inflammatory cascades, cytokines, the complement system, platelet aggregation, and thrombosis. They can also induce mechanical obstruction leading to ischemia and hypoxia resulting in major pathology and even death. Nitrogen is highly fat soluble, and the heavily myelinated white matter of the CNS is at particular risk for DCS.

The incidence of DCS ranges from 1 per 1000 dives to 1 in 20,000 dives based on previous studies, but may be underreported because some divers may not present to a health care professional. The potential for development of DCS increases with the length and depth of diving. Other risk factors may include age, obesity, fatigue, heavy exertion, dehydration, fever, cold ambient temperatures after diving, diving at high altitude or flying soon after diving. The risk of DCS is 2.5 times greater for men than for women, possibly due to risk-taking behaviors. A patent foramen ovale (PFO) or other left-to-right shunt (e.g., atrial septal defect) is a risk factor for increased susceptibility to DCS and larger defects are likely to be more relevant.[7,8,9] Sixty-five percent of divers who present with serious DCS have a PFO. Most sport divers do not undergo screening for PFO with echocardiographic bubble studies.

The United States Navy dive tables estimate the amount of nitrogen that accumulates in the body during a dive to a particular depth and duration. The tables calculate a maximal dive time, called the *no-decompression limit.* If the no-decompression limits are exceeded, underwater decompression stops are recommended. Many sport scuba divers use submersible dive computers to calculate maximum dive times in lieu of the tables. These tables and computers are meant to reduce the likelihood of exceeding the solubility of nitrogen at sea level to produce DCS. The diver still must ascend in a slow, controlled manner to allow the gradual release of nitrogen. Off-gassing continues after the diver has surfaced. Repetitive dives within several hours result in accumulation of tissue nitrogen and shorter no-decompression limits. Because dive tables are based on several assumptions about nitrogen elimination, even strict adherence to these tables does not guarantee that DCS will not occur. It is important for emergency clinicians to realize that divers can develop DCS even when they are within these calculated no-decompression limits.

DCS typically is manifested within hours after surfacing. Approximately 40% of symptoms occur within 1 hour after diving, 60% within 3 hours, 80% within 8 hours, and 98% within 24 hours. Flying shortly after diving or ascending to altitude, however, may cause symptoms in patients later than expected, and some patients may present days after diving with DCS.

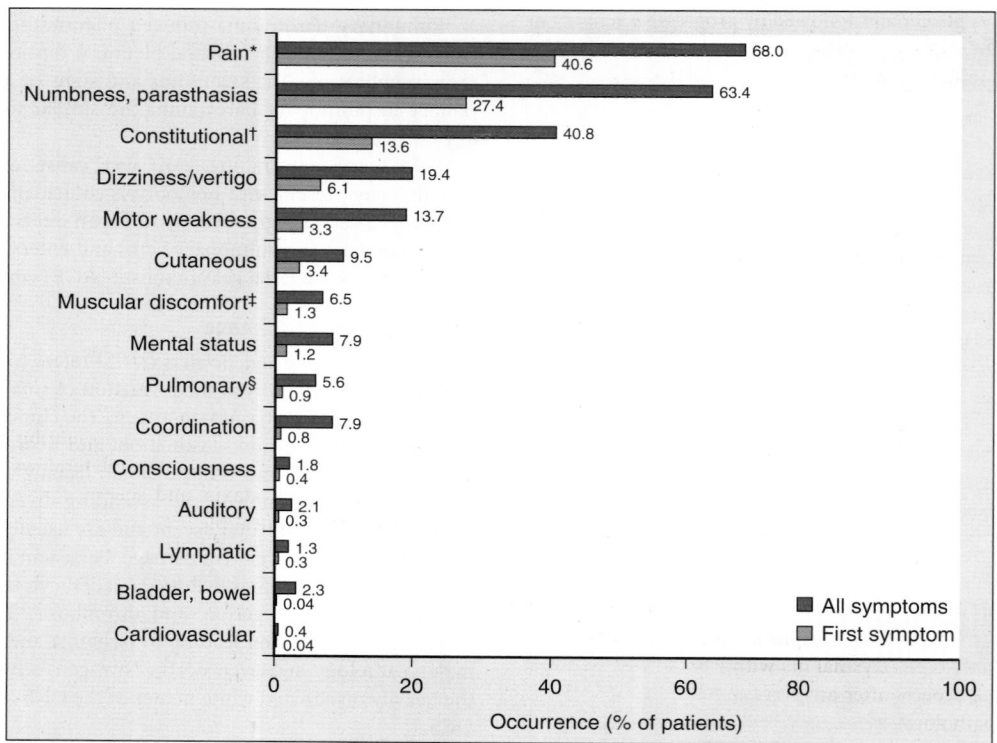

Fig. 131.7 Classification of initial and of all eventual manifestations of decompression illness in 2346 recreational diving accidents reported to the Divers Alert Network (DAN) from 1998 to 2004. *For all instances of pain, 58% consisted of joint pain, 35% muscle pain, and 7% girdle pain. Girdle pain often portends spinal cord involvement. †Constitutional symptoms included headache, lightheadedness, inappropriate fatigue, malaise, nausea or vomiting, and anorexia. ‡Muscular discomfort included stiffness, pressure, cramps, and spasm but excluded pain. §Pulmonary manifestations included dyspnea and cough. (From: Vann RD, Butler FK, Mitchell SJ, et al. Decompression illness. *Lancet.* 2011;377:153-164.)

Traditionally, DCS has been divided into two categories, type I and type II. Type I DCS is considered less severe and affects the musculoskeletal system, skin, and lymphatic vessels. Type II DCS involves any other organ system and typically involves neurologic, vestibular or pulmonary symptoms. The more inclusive decompression illness (DCI) or "decompression-related illness" is now also used to encompass DCS I, DCS II, and arterial gas embolism (AGE). This simplified DCI terminology can aid clinicians to more rapidly select the necessary intervention since all types of decompression illness require recompression. DCS I, DCS II, and AGE can also coexist. The symptoms of DCS may be subtle and resolve by the time of evaluation. A distribution of the initial most common symptoms is presented in Figure 131.7.

Divers experiencing more minor type I DCS generally experience joint pains. The elbow and shoulder joints are most commonly affected. Local tenderness and erythema are uncommon. The placement of a blood pressure cuff inflated to 150 to 200 mm Hg on an affected joint produces relief of pain and helps confirm the diagnosis; however, the sensitivity of this maneuver has been reported to be as low as 60%. Mild skin irritation or pruritus may also be consistent with more minor type I DCS. Lymphatic obstruction by air bubbles can also occur, causing extremity edema, but is still considered type I DCS. (Fig. 131.8).

Patchy cyanotic marbling of the skin, known as *cutis marmorata* was previously considered as part of type I DCS, but more recent literature suggests that this reticular rash may be related to CNS-related changes in vasomotor regulation and may be more closely related to type II DCS.[10] This update has been reflected in the Divers Alert Network website information as well. Cutis marmorata may begin as

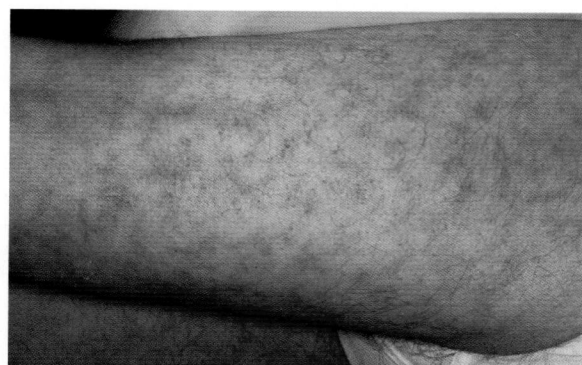

Fig. 131.8 Marbling of the thigh in cutaneous decompression sickness (DCS). (From: Maeyens E. Aquatic skin disorders. In: Auerbach PS, ed. *Wilderness Medicine.* ed 6. Philadelphia: Elsevier; 2012: 1665.)

severe pruritus and progress into an erythematous rash and then skin mottling which commonly involves the trunk and torso but does not follow a dermatomal distribution. Type II DCS includes symptoms that can involve the CNS, the inner ear, and the lungs. The CNS is particularly susceptible to decompression illness because of its high lipid content. The spinal cord, especially the upper lumbar area, is more often involved than cerebral tissue. Symptoms of spinal DCS include limb weakness or paralysis, paresthesias, numbness, with low back and abdominal pain. Limb symptoms often begin as a distal prickly sensation that advances proximally, followed by progressive sensory or motor loss. Urinary retention, bladder and fecal incontinence, and priapism may also occur. Unlike patients with spinal cord trauma, patients experiencing DCS may have patchy or unequally distributed sensory and motor findings.

Spinal DCS can occur alone or in combination with cerebral, inner ear, or pulmonary symptoms. Cerebral symptoms include mild to moderate headache, blurred vision, diplopia, dysarthria, unusual fatigue, inappropriate behavior, dizziness and a sense of detachment. Loss of consciousness in CNS DCS is rare (in marked contrast to AGE).

Inner ear DCS is commonly called *the staggers*. Approximately one-third of patients that present with DCS report cochlear vestibular symptoms. The symptoms of inner ear DCS are the same as those of IEBT and include nausea, dizziness, vertigo, nystagmus, and hearing loss. Vestibular symptoms predominate with only about a quarter of patients experience hearing loss or tinnitus. This can usually be distinguished from IEBT because the onset occurs during ascent or after surfacing.

Pulmonary DCS is commonly called *the chokes*. All divers are exposed to some degree of microbubble emboli to the lungs on ascent. The progression to symptoms depends on the number and volume of bubbles. The deposition of venous gas emboli in the pulmonary arterial circulation produces progressive dyspnea, cough, and chest pain. The cough may progress to paroxysmal fits with worsening pain. This is usually a progressive process after ascent as opposed to pulmonary barotrauma-related pathology which generally occurs immediately after ascent.

The physical examination of patients suffering from pulmonary DCS may reveal cyanosis and hypotension in association with increased central venous pressure and pulmonary arterial pressure. The condition may progress to respiratory arrest.

DCS may be particularly dangerous to a developing fetus of a scuba diving mother because the majority of the fetal circulation bypasses the pulmonary bed through the foramen ovale and the ductus arteriosus. This bypass prevents the fetal lungs from acting as a filter for microbubbles. In addition, venous gas emboli may appear in the fetal circulation before they are apparent in the maternal circulation. Data on the effects of diving on pregnant women suggest a higher incidence of low-birth-weight infants, prematurity, congenital malformations, stillbirths, and spontaneous abortions. There are no safe-diving tables that would protect a fetus from DCS; therefore, pregnant women should be advised to refrain from scuba diving.

Arterial Gas Embolism

AGE can be caused by barotrauma with air forced across the alveolar-capillary membrane through the pulmonary venous circulation into the arterial system. Alternatively, venous bubbles can cross into the arterial circulation from a left-to-right shunt. Barotrauma-related AGE from air bubbles forced across the alveolar-capillary membrane into the pulmonary venous circulation through the left atrium and ventricle and then into the arterial circulation can be immediately life-threatening. It is one of the most common causes of death in divers and is usually related to an uncontrolled ascent with breath-holding and does not require a significant time at depth. Even at a relatively shallow depth, a diver can elicit significant barotrauma with rapid surfacing, especially with breath-holding. Clinical symptoms and signs are the result of mechanical obstruction by gas bubbles. AGE can also result from a right-to-left shunt of venous bubbles, such as in a diver with a PFO, and often presents with symptoms consistent with type II DCS. AGE may occur alone or in conjunction with DCS.

Although air bubbles may embolize to any organ, the coronary and cerebral arteries are associated with the most serious consequences.

Emboli to the coronary arteries may cause cardiac ischemia, myocardial infarction, dysrhythmias, or cardiac arrest. Dysrhythmias may also be indirectly caused by centrally mediated autonomic dysfunction from cerebral emboli. Mechanical occlusion of the cerebral vasculature from emboli, most commonly to the anterior and middle cerebral arteries, causes a variety of symptoms and signs similar in appearance to an acute stroke. Large volumes of intracardiac bubbles can mechanically displace blood in the ventricles, leading to a precipitous fall in cardiac output with resultant hypotension and cardiac arrest.

The clinical manifestations of AGE may be sudden, dramatic, and life-threatening. Any diver breathing compressed air at any depth underwater and who surfaces unconscious or who loses consciousness within 10 minutes of reaching the surface should be assumed to be suffering from AGE. The most common presentation of AGE includes a global alteration of consciousness, headache, dizziness, convulsions, and visual changes. Other common presenting symptoms and signs include cranial nerve symptoms, unilateral weakness, unilateral or bilateral sensory loss, ataxia, and speech changes. Pulmonary symptoms, including dyspnea, pleuritic chest pain, and hemoptysis, occur in up to a quarter to half of cases.

Pulmonary Edema

Pulmonary edema while scuba diving was first reported in the 1980s. An increase in afterload (from vascular hyper-reactivity, possibly triggered by cold water) combined with an increase in preload (from the hyperbaric underwater environment) are likely causes.

DIFFERENTIAL DIAGNOSES

Most diving injuries have limited differential diagnoses that include medical disorders and trauma unrelated to dysbarism. The differential diagnoses of IEBT include inner ear DCS, ABV, and isolated MEBT with a rupture of the tympanic membrane. It is relatively easy to distinguish IEBT from MEBT and ABV because the vestibular symptoms associated with the last two entities are transient and self-limited (Table 131.2). When IEBT occurs simultaneously with MEBT, the presence of both may be documented by an audiogram, which demonstrates both a conductive and a sensorineural hearing loss.

The differentiation of IEBT from inner ear neurologic DCS is crucial because the treatments differ. IEBT is considered classic when symptoms begin during descent or the diver relates a history of difficulty equilibrating or performing a vigorous Valsalva maneuver. Inner ear DCS usually presents within 15 minutes to 2 hours after ascent, and usually includes a dive profile which approached no-decompression limits. A trial of recompression therapy is prudent if concerns for DCS exist.

Differential diagnoses of pulmonary DCS include AGE. Table 131.3 provides factors that differentiate the two conditions. Although the treatment of both requires recompression therapy, they can be differentiated by the timing of the onset of symptoms. Almost all cases of AGE present within the first 10 minutes of surfacing, whereas DCS presents more typically well after 10 minutes upon surfacing: 40% of pulmonary DCS symptoms begin within 1 hour of surfacing, 60% within 3 hours, 80% within 8 hours, and almost all within 24 hours.

Diagnostic Testing

Most diagnostic imaging and laboratory studies are not useful in diving- and dysbarism-related injuries and should not delay transfer for definitive recompression therapy. Focused history concerning the dive profile, including the depth and length of the dive and other details of the dive profile (including rapid ascent) and a careful assessment of when the symptoms first occurred, may provide

TABLE 131.2 Middle Ear Barotrauma, Inner Ear Barotrauma, and Alternobaric Vertigo

	Middle Ear Barotrauma	Inner Ear Barotrauma	Alternobaric Vertigo
Symptoms	Ear pain during descent	Ear pain during descent	Ear pain during ascent
	Hearing loss	Hearing loss	Transient hearing loss
	Possible transient vertigo	Severe vertigo and nausea	Nausea
Signs	Conductive hearing loss	Nystagmus	Nystagmus
	TM injury	Emesis	Emesis
	Unilateral face paralysis	Ataxia	TM injury
		Romberg sign	
		Neural hearing loss	

TM, Tympanic membrane.

TABLE 131.3 Decompression Sickness Versus Arterial Gas Embolism

Decompression Sickness	Arterial Gas Embolism
Dive History	
Depth and length dependent	Independent of dive profile
Decompression limits approached	Rapid ascent
Flying after diving	Inexperience
Diving at altitude	Out of air
Risk Factors	
Fatigue	Obstructive lung disease
Dehydration	Emphysema
Fever, hypothermia	Mucus plugging
Obesity	Patent foramen ovale (PFO)
Strenuous activity	
Symptoms and Signs	
Progressive onset	Rapid onset
Spinal symptoms predominate	Cerebral symptoms predominate
Headache	Headache
Unusual fatigue	Loss of consciousness
Limb weakness or paralysis	Confusion
Paresthesias	Convulsions
Abdominal pain	Motor or sensory loss
Urinary retention	Cardiac dysrhythmias or arrest
Fecal incontinence	
Periarticular joint pain	
Skin marbling	
Vertigo or nystagmus	
Treatment	
Recompression	Recompression

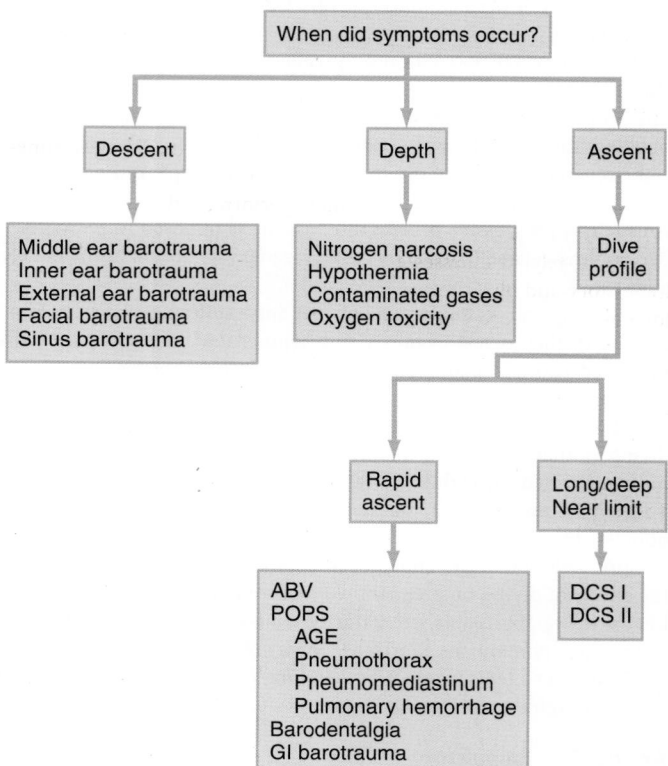

Fig. 131.9 The approach to the injured diver. *ABV,* Alternobaric vertigo; *AGE,* arterial gas embolism; *DCS,* decompression sickness; *GI,* gastro-intestinal; *POPS,* pulmonary overpressure syndrome.

important diagnostic clues (see Box 131.3). In making the diagnosis of a dive injury, it is helpful to think of the injuries in terms of occurring during descent, while at depth, or during ascent (Fig. 131.9). Because recompression therapy is time sensitive, it is more important to concentrate on treatment decisions rather than on securing a definitive diagnosis.

Pulmonary barotrauma can also cause alveolar hemorrhage. Patients may present with hemoptysis coincident with chest pain and dyspnea. Chest radiography may reveal an interstitial infiltrate or pneumothorax. An untreated pneumothorax is considered an absolute contraindication for recompression therapy and will need to be managed prior to treatment. Magnetic resonance imaging (MRI), computed tomography (CT), and single-photon emission CT with technetium (Tc-99m)–labeled hexamethyl propylene amine can identify the bubbles of CNS DCS. However, *no* imaging studies are sensitive enough to exclude DCS, and normal imaging results should not delay transfer for definitive therapy. DCS can cause right-sided strain on an electrocardiogram and decreased end-tidal carbon dioxide level. Even after ascent from very shallow saturation dives, microbubbles in the venous circulation can be routinely detected by M-mode ultrasonography; however, their presence does not necessarily correlate with symptoms.

TABLE 131.4 Important Contact Information

Divers Alert Network Head Quarters	Phone Number	Website
DAN America Emergency Hotline	1-919-684-9111	www.diversalertnetwork.org
DAN America nonemergency line (Monday to Friday 8:30 a.m. to 5:00 p.m. Eastern time)	1-919-684-2848 or 1-800-446-2671	
DAN Europe	+3906-4211-5685	www.daneurope.org
DAN South Africa	+27-10-209-8112	www.dansa.org
DAN Asia-Pacific	+61-39886-9166	www.danap.org
DAN Japan	+81-3-3812-4999	www.danjapan.gr.jp

DAN, Divers Alert Network.

MANAGEMENT

Patients with stable vital signs and suspected dive injuries should receive 100% oxygen until the clinician can exclude pulmonary barotrauma or decompression illness. Normobaric 100% oxygen can improve outcomes and should be provided until the patient can be treated definitively. Patients with unstable vital signs or in cardiac arrest should be treated according to advanced cardiac life support (ACLS) guidelines. The clinician should conduct a focused history, including elements summarized in Box 131.1, and then perform a thorough physical examination.

Diving-related illnesses are diagnosed and treated on the basis of the history and physical examination, with several resources available for emergent advice. The Divers Alert Network (DAN), located at Duke University in Durham, North Carolina, is a membership association that provides courses on diving-related emergencies and publishes data on diving accidents and fatalities. DAN provides a 24-hour medical emergency hotline at 1-919-684-9111 (collect calls are accepted) and a nonemergency advisory line Monday through Friday, 8:30 a.m. to 5 p.m. Eastern time, at 1-919-684-2948 or 1-800-446-2671 (Table 131.4). In addition, DAN international contacts are in Europe, Brazil, Japan, Asia Pacific, and southern Africa. DAN maintains a website with links to key information at www.diversalertnetwork.org. DAN uses a telephone intake form, the DAN On-Site Neurological Assessment for Diver's History (Fig. 131.10).

The United States Navy has its current diving manual (6th edition) available at its website, www.usu.edu/scuba/navy_manual6.pdf. This manual contains readily accessible information describing diving principles, equipment, operations, and recompression.

Diving Disorders Requiring Recompression Therapy

Diving disorders that require recompression therapy are listed in Box 131.4. Early consultation with a hyperbaric specialist is recommended. Treatment with 100% normobaric oxygen during recovery, assessment, and transfer is recommended. Treatment with 100% oxygen replaces inert gases in the lungs with oxygen by establishment of a large gradient from the tissues to the alveoli, removal of inert gases is enhanced, and bubble size is reduced. In addition, oxygen administration treats the tissue hypoxia created by the accumulation of gas bubbles.

Dehydration may increase the seriousness of DCS. Diving appears to be associated with dehydration and hemoconcentration in many studies. Intravenous fluids may be administered to divers suspected of having nonpulmonary ("chokes") DCS. Overly aggressive hydration in divers with pulmonary DCS may worsen pulmonary edema and is discouraged. Similarly, fluid overload should be avoided in patients with suspected cerebral or spinal cord edema or AGE. If given, fluids should be administered to ensure a urinary output of 0.5 mL/kg per hour.

The goals of recompression therapy are to reduce the mechanical obstruction of air bubbles, to facilitate the washout of nitrogen by increasing the tissue-blood nitrogen gradient, and to increase oxygen delivery to ischemic tissue. Recompression is the only definitive treatment of DCS and AGE and is most effective if administered early. Treatment of DCS or AGE should not be withheld even if a significant time delay in transferring a patient to a hyperbaric chamber is anticipated. Although delayed recompression is less effective than immediate recompression in serious cases, the time beyond which recompression offers no benefit is not well documented.

Hyperbaric therapy for AGE is also considered time sensitive. Patients with AGE who are recompressed within 5 hours of surfacing have a mortality rate of 5%, and there is an extremely low risk of morbidity among the survivors. If recompression is delayed by 5 hours or more, the mortality rate increases to 10%, with 50% morbidity. Although spontaneous resolution of symptoms may occur in patients with AGE, all patients should be recompressed. The rationale is that although microbubbles may clear from the cerebral circulation, secondary capillary edema and swelling may be further ameliorated by recompression.

Similarly, the prognosis for DCS when it is treated with recompression is generally good but depends on the severity of symptoms at onset, and the delay to recompression. A delay to definitive recompression treatment is associated with a worse outcome in cases of severe DCS. Patients can obtain some benefit from recompression, however, even if treatment is initiated more than 24 hours after the dive. Recompression therapy for DCS initiated as late as 10 to 14 days after exposure has been associated with improved outcomes.

Recompression for DCS and AGE may be performed in a multiplace chamber with one or more in-chamber attendants or within a monoplace chamber. Monoplace chambers are compact, lightweight, and more widely available than multiplace chambers, but most monoplace chambers cannot be pressurized beyond 3 ata (100 fsw) or deliver air-oxygen mixtures. The most common recompression schedule is the United States Navy treatment (or an equivalent procedure). With this protocol, the diver is compressed to 2.8 bar (60 fsw pressure) while breathing 100% oxygen. The time to complete treatment is 4 hours 45 minutes, not including descent and ascent time.

Ground transport to a hyperbaric facility is preferred to air transportation, if feasible, because an increase in altitude lowers the ambient pressure and allows microbubbles to expand. If air transportation must be used, it is recommended maintain cabin pressure at less than 1000 feet. Commercial aircraft are typically pressurized to a cabin altitude of 5000 to 8000 feet in cruise flight (30,000 feet). Many of these aircraft are capable of near–sea level cabin pressures if flying no higher than 15,000 to 20,000 feet. Because helicopters are not pressurized, it is recommended that they maintain an altitude of no more than 500 feet during transport of a diving accident victim.

DAN *DAN On-Site Neurological Assessment for Diver's History*

Last Name:_____ First Name:_____ MI: _____

Date: (mm/dd/yy):_____ Time: (hh:mm)_____

COMPLETED BY:_____

How do you feel? _____

Symptoms? _____

Did symptoms start during descent, on bottom, during ascent, or after surfacing? _____

_____

Dive profile, breathing gas, ascent and time of surfacing, recent dive history _____

_____

_____

_____

Unusual features of dive (eg, out of air, rapid ascent) _____

Decompression computer, table _____

Difficulty with middle ear equalization?_____

Numbness, tingling? Where?_____

Pain? Where? What makes it better or worse?_____

Rate the pain on a scale of 0 (no pain) to 10 (the worst pain imaginable)_____

Shortness of breath?_____

Ringing or buzzing in ear?_____ Decreased hearing?_____

Dizziness? Vertigo?_____
"Vertigo" implies a sensation of the world spinning around. Vague "dizziness" is not vertigo.

Weakness?_____

Difficulty walking? If so, is this due to difficulty with balance or leg weakness?_____

Nausea, vomiting?_____ Able to urinate?_____

From "observer" (eg, dive buddy, companion) _____

Confirm dive profile_____

His/her version of events _____

_____

_____

Did the diver breach safe procedures (eg, ascent rate, out of air, was he/she breathing during ascent)?

_____

Has the diver been acting inappropriately?_____

Was there loss of consciousness, seizure?_____

Fig. 131.10 The Divers Alert Network (DAN) On-Site Neurological Assessment for Diver's History.

BOX 131.4 Diving Disorders That Require Recompression Therapy

Decompression sickness type I
Decompression sickness type II
Arterial gas embolism (AGE)
Contaminated air (carbon monoxide poisoning)

In addition to recompression therapy, several adjunctive treatments are proposed in the treatment of DCS and AGE. The treatment or prevention of hypothermia may increase tissue perfusion and prevent off-gassing. Anticoagulants to prevent deep venous thromboembolism may be considered in patients with paralysis with long transport times. Intermittent pneumatic compression devices are alternative therapeutic measures. Seizures may be managed with standard doses of benzodiazepines; however, mannitol should be avoided. Spinal DCS patients often develop urinary retention requiring bladder catheterization.

Urinary catheter (and endotracheal tube) balloons should be inflated with saline (not air) before recompression therapy is initiated.

The head-down position (Trendelenburg) has traditionally been advocated to prevent migration of intra-arterial bubbles to the brain, however, it may actually result in worsening cerebral edema and intracranial pressure and is no longer recommended. Transport of the patient with AGE in a flat supine position is recommended to maximize arterial-venous flow.

Suspected carbon monoxide poisoning from contaminated air supplies in a diving environment should be treated immediately with high-flow normobaric 100% oxygen and may require hyperbaric oxygen therapy if neurologic symptoms are present. Consultation with a hyperbaric specialist or medical toxicologist is recommended.

Diving Disorders Not Requiring Recompression Therapy

Diving disorders that do not require recompression therapy are summarized in Box 131.5.

External Ear Barotrauma

Treatment of external ear barotrauma includes cleaning of the external canal and removal of foreign bodies. Earplugs should not be worn when diving.

Middle Ear Barotrauma

Prevention of MEBT requires that the diver equalize the pressure in both middle ears. Any diver who cannot clear both ears on the surface should not dive. The diver should not perform a forceful Valsalva maneuver during descent or ascent to clear the ears because of the risk of ABV, round or oval window rupture (descent), or pulmonary barotrauma (ascent). The prophylactic use of pseudoephedrine (60 mg taken orally 30 minutes before diving) or oxymetazoline nasal spray may reduce the incidence and severity of MEBT. The use of these medications to facilitate diving with symptoms of an upper respiratory infection, however, is not recommended. Antihistamines should be avoided before diving because these agents induce dry mouth when breathing compressed air and drowsiness. Sinusitis and upper respiratory infections increase the likelihood of suffering barotitis. Diving should be avoided during and for 2 weeks after the resolution of an upper respiratory infection. Persistent symptoms may require otolaryngology consultation.

Treatment of uncomplicated serous otitis from MEBT includes topical nasal vasoconstrictors, such as phenylephrine and oxymetazoline

hydrochloride, and repeated Frenzel maneuvers to displace the fluid through the eustachian tube. The *Frenzel maneuver* is performed by pinching the nose, placing the tongue on the roof of the mouth, as far forward as possible, and gently moving the back of the tongue upward, as when starting to swallow. This is repeated as many times as necessary until equalization occurs. If the physical examination reveals a ruptured tympanic membrane, prophylactic treatment should also include an oral antibiotic. Oral steroids (prednisone) may speed recovery when a seventh nerve palsy is diagnosed in conjunction with a perforated tympanic membrane, although this disorder is typically self-limited. Diving must also be suspended until the tympanic membrane heals to prevent calorically induced vertigo. Outpatient follow-up with an otolaryngologist is recommended.

Internal Ear Barotrauma

A conservative treatment approach to IEBT includes bed rest for 5 to 7 days with the head elevated, avoidance of straining or the Valsalva maneuver, and decongestants to facilitate drainage of the middle ear. Early surgical intervention may benefit patients with total or near-total hearing loss but is not effective in isolated high-frequency hearing loss.[11] All patients with suspected IEBT should be referred to an otolaryngologist, because IEBT suggests significant injury to the cochleovestibular system.

Barosinusitis

Treatment of barosinusitis is typically conservative, including the use of decongestants and occasionally, antibiotics. If symptoms persist, referral to an otolaryngologist should be considered. The patient should be advised not to dive until any underlying respiratory infection or acute inflammatory process has resolved.

Facial Barotrauma

The victim of facial barotrauma may have a dramatic appearance, but the condition is usually benign and requires no specific treatment. The patient should be advised not to resume diving until facial edema resolves.

Nitrogen Narcosis

Nitrogen narcosis symptoms should resolve on ascending as the partial pressure of nitrogen decreases. Persistent symptoms should prompt a search for other causes, such as DCS, cerebral AGE, contaminated air, and near drowning.

Pulmonary Barotrauma

With the exception of AGE, none of the pulmonary barotrauma disorders (pneumothorax, pneumomediastinum, subcutaneous emphysema, and alveolar hemorrhage) require recompression therapy. Treatment with 100% oxygen may aid in the resolution of these disorders. Tube thoracostomy may be required for divers undergoing recompression therapy to prevent a tension pneumothorax. Catheter aspiration of the pneumothorax may be an acceptable alternative to tube thoracostomy if the patient does not receive positive-pressure ventilation or recompression therapy.

The evaluation and management of pneumomediastinum includes observation, monitoring, and serial chest radiographs to ensure that no coexisting pneumothorax develops. One hundred percent oxygen therapy may hasten the resolution of symptoms.

Alternobaric Vertigo

Oral and intranasal decongestants may be indicated if symptoms persist. Myringotomy is occasionally required. Outpatient follow-up with otolaryngology is recommended for persistent symptoms.

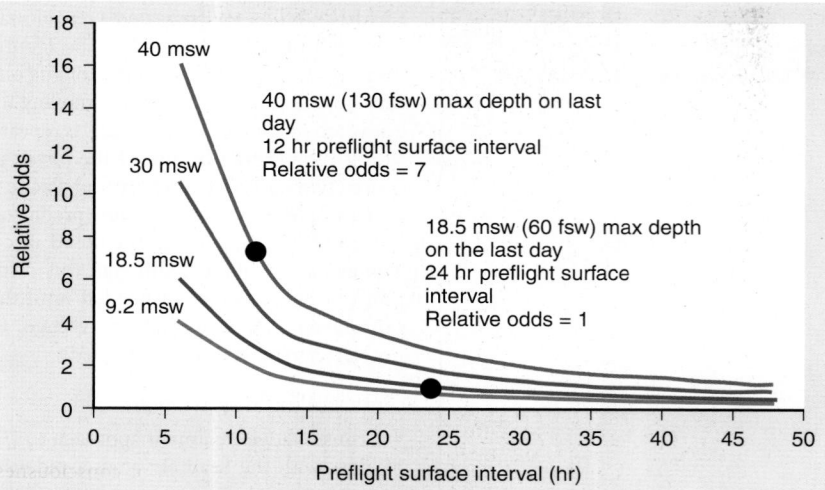

Fig. 131.11 The risk of decompression sickness (DCS) relative to flying. *fsw,* Feet of seawater; *msw,* meters of seawater. (From: Freiberger JJ, et al. The relative risk of decompression sickness during and after air travel following diving. *Aviat Space Environ Med.* 2002;73:983.)

DISPOSITION

Divers should be aware that commercial airliners may be pressurized to a cabin altitude of 5000 to 8000 feet in cruise flight. Many cases of DCS have a delay in the onset of symptoms in divers who fly after diving even if they are symptom-free before departure. Divers who experience DCS symptoms before departure and still elect to fly, are more likely to have type II DCS, less likely to achieve complete relief after recompression, and more likely to have residual symptoms for up to 3 months.

The relative risk for development of DCS increases with longer dive times at significant depth and shorter preflight surface intervals (Fig. 131.11). Flying should be delayed for at least 12 hours after diving if less than 2 hours of total dive time was accumulated in the preceding 48 hours. For multiple-day, unlimited diving, flying should be delayed for at least 24 hours. Patients recompressed after DCS or AGE should not fly for at least 72 hours.

United States Navy guidelines recommend that the patient not return to diving for 7 days after recompression for type I DCS and for 4 weeks after type II DCS. Divers who experiences DCS type II symptoms or AGE should be discouraged from future diving again and may referred to dive specialist for further recommendations.

After treatment for pulmonary barotrauma or DCS, divers should be referred to a dive specialist to consider if they require further evaluation to determine if there are any preexisting conditions (e.g., bullae, PFO or left-to-right shunts) prior to diving. A history of any major diving-related injury is a clear risk factor for future events.

The author wishes to thank Richard L. Byyny and Lee W. Shockley for their valuable contributions and expertise in previous chapter editions.

The references for this chapter can be found online at ExpertConsult. com.

High-Altitude Medicine

N. Stuart Harris

FOUNDATIONS

Background and Importance

Acute high-altitude illnesses result from exposure to low oxygen states caused by low atmospheric pressure (hypobaria). Syndromes of the brain and lung are the primary clinical manifestations of high-altitude illness. They result from ascent too rapid to allow for adequate acclimatization. Cerebral forms of altitude illness occur as a continuum, from common and benign acute mountain sickness (AMS), to rare, but potentially lethal high-altitude cerebral edema (HACE). High-altitude pulmonary edema (HAPE) is the primary lung syndrome. HAPE is the leading cause of death from altitude illness.

All forms of altitude illness have their origins in acute oxygen insufficiency due to hypobaria. All can be treated with oxygen and descent. Although the percentage of atmospheric oxygen is a constant 20.9%, as elevation increases, atmospheric pressure decreases and with it, oxygen availability. Human physiology is adaptable when given sufficient time to acclimatize by gradual ascent. Rapid ascent to elevations greater than 8,000 feet prevents adequate acclimatization and can lead to debilitating and deadly high-altitude illnesses. On the summit of Mt. Everest (8848 m), the partial pressure of inspired oxygen (Pio_2) is only 29% of the sea-level value. Although gradual ascents (over weeks) of Mt. Everest without oxygen are not uncommon, a rapid ascent to the same summit would result in loss of consciousness and death. Gradual ascent reduces symptoms and can save lives. Serious altitude illness typically follows from unheeded warning symptoms of mild altitude illness. The importance of patient and public education to reduce the morbidity and mortality of serious altitude illness cannot be overstated.[1]

Epidemiology

It is estimated that approximately 40 million individuals worldwide live above 8,000 feet. These individuals do not suffer acute altitude illness. Instead, it is the individual who rapidly travels to high altitude (whether for skiing, climbing, or travel) who is at the greatest risk. In the United States alone, approximately 35 million visitors travel to high-altitude recreation areas every year. Internationally, millions more travel to high mountain ranges in Europe, Asia, Africa, and South America, placing these transient sojourners at risk.[2]

The incidence and severity of altitude illness are directly related to elevation and rapidity of ascent. Other variables include prior acclimatization, individual genetic susceptibility, sleeping elevation, and duration of stay. Rapid ascent to 8000 feet is associated with an approximately 25% incidence of AMS, whereas a rapid ascent (1 or 2 days) to 14,410 feet on Mt. Rainier has rates as high as 67%. Rapidity and mode of ascent also matter; trekkers who fly into the Khumbu region to explore the Mt. Everest region are more likely to develop AMS (47%) than those who trek in from lower elevations (23%).

HACE is much less common than AMS, occurring in less than 1% of rapid ascents to more than 14,000 feet. Although rare, it carries a grave prognosis if not quickly recognized and treated. The incidence of HAPE varies from 0.01% to 2% but may be as high as 15.5% if flown directly to 14,500 feet without a chance to acclimatize at a lower altitude. Both HAPE and HACE are more common with a longer duration of visit (more than 2 days) and higher sleeping altitude.

Age may be a relative risk factor. Most studies of children suggest that they have the same incidence of AMS as adults. Younger individuals (younger than 20 years old) are more likely to have HAPE, although HAPE is extremely rare in children younger than 2 years old. Gender does not affect the incidence of AMS; however, women may have less risk for development of HAPE. No relationship appears to exist between AMS development and timing of the menstrual cycle.

The number of older travelers visiting mountain resorts is increasing. Many of these individuals have underlying health problems, including lung disease, heart disease, and hypertension. Despite these conditions, the risk for AMS in adults older than 50 years old may be less than in younger age groups. Nevertheless, there are indications that elders may not react well to acute high-altitude exposure. Pulmonary vital capacity decreases by one-third in elders ascending from sea level to 14,000 feet for 1 week, producing a large decrease in both oxygen saturation and maximal oxygen uptake during altitude-related exercise.

Definitions

Moderate altitude is between 5000 and 8000 feet of elevation. Rapid ascent to this altitude may result in mild, transient symptoms, but severe altitude illness is uncommon. *High altitude* is between 8000 and 14,000 feet. Although most people do not experience significant arterial oxygen desaturation until they reach higher altitudes, high-altitude illness is common with rapid ascent above 8000 feet, and individuals with underlying medical problems may be predisposed to develop altitude illness at lower levels. The pathophysiologic effects of high altitude begin when the oxygen saturation of the arterial blood begins to fall below the 90% level. The sigmoidal shape of the oxyhemoglobin dissociation curve prevents a significant fall of arterial oxygen saturation (SaO_2) in most individuals until an altitude of approximately 12,000 feet. At this altitude, the steep portion of the curve is encountered, and marked oxygen desaturation may occur with relatively small increases in altitude (Fig. 132.1). Some predisposed individuals may desaturate to less than 90% at altitudes as low as 8000 feet. *Very high altitude* is between 14,000 to 18,000 feet. At this elevation, the likelihood of altitude illness is high, and the risk of serious altitude illness (HAPE and HACE) increases. *Extreme altitude* is above 18,000 feet. Although climbers using careful acclimatization schedules can transiently tolerate this elevation, complete acclimatization generally is not possible and long durations above this level result in progressive deterioration. Given limitations in physiologic reserves, climbers who become incapacitated at this elevation typically are dependent on others to survive.

Environmental Considerations

Barometric pressure decreases logarithmically as the altitude rises. The pernicious effects of altitude are due to hypobaric hypoxia; as atmospheric pressure decreases the partial pressure of oxygen (PO_2) decreases. Due to centrifugal forces, the earth is slightly flatter at the poles and bulging at the equator. The atmospheric envelope that surrounds the earth has a similar shape; therefore, at any one elevation the barometric pressure tends to be lower at higher latitudes than at the equator. Although subtle, the physiologic reserves are so limited

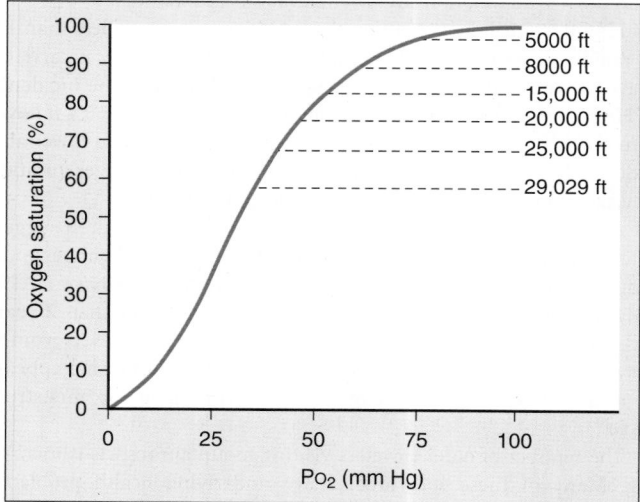

Fig. 132.1 Oxygen-hemoglobin dissociation curve. Approximate oxygen saturations are marked for several altitudes. *PO2,* Partial pressure of oxygen. (Data for 15,000 to 29,029 feet from: Sutton JR, et al. Operation Everest II: oxygen transport during exercise at extreme simulated altitude. *J Appl Physiol.* 1988;64:1309.)

at extreme elevations that it has been calculated that if Mt. Everest happened to be at a more northern latitude, it would be impossible to climb without supplemental oxygen.

The atmospheric envelope also undergoes seasonal variations in local thickness. In the winter, barometric pressures tend to be lower making "relative altitudes" physiologically higher. Local weather can also significantly affect the barometric pressure. A low-pressure front can reduce the barometric pressure 12 to 40 mm Hg and so increase the "relative altitude" by 500 to 2,500 feet. At extreme elevations these changes can be physiologically relevant. High-altitude illness can occur even where mountains appear distant. Although the South Pole is on a flat, barren plain, it rests at approximately 9300 ft and severe altitude illness caused by rapid transport from sea-level research facilities is not uncommon.[3]

Anatomy, Physiology, and Pathophysiology
Acclimatization

Exposure to acute hypobaric hypoxia results in myriad physiologic responses that act to improve oxygenation. *Acclimatization* is both immediate (within minutes the carotid bodies sense hypoxemia) and continuous over months (hemoglobin increases may continue over more than 6 weeks). It involves multiple systems from mitochondrial function, protein synthesis to respiratory, cardiovascular, renal, and hematologic responses. Acclimatization begins as the oxygen saturation of arterial blood falls below sea-level values. The altitude at which this occurs depends on the rate of ascent, the duration of exposure, and the individual's physiology. Individuals with preexisting conditions that limit cellular oxygen delivery and pulmonary reserves may have a decreased altitude tolerance. Most healthy, unacclimatized visitors to high altitude will not desaturate significantly (to less than 90%) until they reach elevations higher than 8000 feet.

The risk of high-altitude illness depends, in part, on an individual's inherent ability to acclimatize. Some people acclimatize easily without having any clinical symptoms. Others may transiently have AMS during acclimatization and a few develop severe altitude illness. This variability involves many genetic and epigenetic factors that influence acclimatization. Previous successful acclimatization may be predictive of future responses for adults in similar conditions, but this may not be the case for children.

One of the most fundamental physiologic changes that occurs during acclimatization is an increase in minute ventilation. Within minutes of exposure to high altitude, the peripheral chemoreceptors in the carotid bodies sense hypoxemia resulting from the decrease in the partial pressure of oxygen in alveoli (PAO_2) and signal the respiratory control center in the medulla to increase ventilation. Increased minute ventilation causes a decrease in the partial pressure of carbon dioxide in alveolus ($PACO_2$). As described by the alveolar gas equation, for any given inspired oxygen tension, the level of ventilation determines alveolar oxygen: as the $PACO_2$ decreases, PAO_2 correspondingly increases (Box 132.1). This increased ventilation in response to hypoxic challenge is known as the *hypoxic ventilatory response (HVR).* The magnitude of the HVR varies among individuals and may be genetically predetermined. HVR may also be inhibited or stimulated by numerous

BOX 132.1	**Alveolar Gas Equation**
$PAO_2 = PIO_2 (PACO_2/R)$	
PAO_2	Partial pressure of oxygen in alveolus
PIO_2	Partial pressure of oxygen in inspired air
$PACO_2$	Partial pressure of carbon dioxide in alveolus
R	Respiratory quotient

factors, including ethanol consumption, sleep medications, caffeine, cocoa, prochlorperazine, and progesterone.

As minute ventilation increases, carbon dioxide exhalation increases. Within minutes, a resulting respiratory alkalosis acts on the central respiratory center to limit further increases in ventilation. To compensate for this respiratory alkalosis, the kidneys begin to excrete bicarbonate. Acetazolamide enhances this excretion. Gradual, progressive renal excretion of bicarbonate allows ventilation to rise slowly, reaching a maximum after 6 to 8 days at a given altitude. An individual's HVR is related to their ability to acclimatize. A low HVR and relative hypoventilation are implicated in the pathogenesis of both AMS and HAPE. For the majority of people with intermediate HVRs, however, ventilatory drive appears to have no predictive value for AMS development.

The stress of acute hypoxia leads to rapid release of catecholamines. This results in increased cardiac output and elevations in heart rate, stroke volume, blood pressure, and venous tone. Except at extreme altitudes, acclimatization over weeks results in the gradual return of the resting heart rate to near sea-level values. Continued resting tachycardia is evidence of poor acclimatization. As the altitude increases, the maximal heart rate capacity decreases. At the limits of acclimatization, maximal and resting heart rates converge. Ultimately, for most individuals it is pulmonary, not cardiac reserves that limit high-altitude performance.

The hematopoietic response to high-altitude acclimatization includes an increase in both hemoglobin and the number of red blood cells. As a result of fluid shifts into the extravascular space, hemoglobin concentration increases up to 15% after rapid ascent to high altitude. Long-term acclimatization leads to an increase in plasma volume and total blood volume. Within hours of ascent, erythropoietin is secreted in response to hypoxemia which in turn stimulates the production of red blood cells, leading to new circulatory red blood cells in 4 or 5 days. During the next 2 months, red blood cell mass increases in proportion to the degree of hypoxemia.

Hypoxemia also results in an increase in 2,3-diphosphoglycerate, causing a rightward shift of the oxyhemoglobin dissociation curve, which favors a release of oxygen from the blood to the tissues. This is counteracted by the leftward shift of the oxyhemoglobin dissociation curve caused by the respiratory alkalosis from hyperventilation. The net result is a negligible change in the oxyhemoglobin curve. Some individuals with mutant hemoglobin and high oxygen-hemoglobin affinity are found to acclimatize more efficiently than their normal counterparts at moderate altitudes.

Physiologic Response to Hypobaric Hypoxia

Although acute hypoxia elicits a broad array of physiologic responses, the clinical syndromes of high-altitude illness predominantly affect the brain and lungs. Hypobaric hypoxia's effects on central nervous system homeostasis give rise to AMS and HACE. AMS is the common, benign form that unheeded, can develop into rare, but potentially lethal HACE. HAPE results from overly exuberant increases in pulmonary arterial pressures that lead to stress failures of the delicate pulmonary capillary beds.

Although discrete physiologic responses occur within minutes of exposure to acute hypoxia, the clinical syndromes of high altitude typically require hours to days to manifest themselves. AMS can develop within 4 to 8 hours of acute exposure to hypobaric hypoxia. HACE and HAPE typically occur 2 to 4 days after exposure to high altitude. Because hypobaric hypoxemia occurs within minutes of arrival, it cannot be the direct cause of high-altitude illness. Instead, it appears to be the initiating factor for a complex pathologic process that leads to the development of the various clinical syndromes. The proposed

mechanisms for the development of AMS, HAPE, and HACE are represented schematically in Figure 132.2.

HVR is the first response to insufficient oxygen, leading to increased minute ventilation. A robust HVR tends to be protective by encouraging compensatory ventilation. A limited HVR leads to relative hypoventilation and inadequate response to the hypoxemia of high altitude.

Centrally mediated periodic breathing associated with high-altitude exposure may result in periods of apnea during sleep, causing severe arterial oxygen desaturation, which further exacerbates hypoxemia. Significant hypoxemia initiates multiple systemic responses that involve the circulatory, pulmonary, endocrine, and central nervous systems.

Hypoxemia alters fluid homeostasis, resulting in generalized fluid retention followed by the shift of fluid into the intracellular spaces. This is manifested by peripheral edema, decreased urinary output, decreased central vascular volume, and increased body weight in patients with AMS. Several different mechanisms may account for these fluid shifts, including arginine vasopressin levels and centrally mediated sympathetic stimulation. Arginine vasopressin levels are elevated in some cases of AMS and HAPE and decreased in others. Aldosterone, plasma renin, and atrial natriuretic levels are higher in people with AMS.

HAPE results from hypoxia-induced acute pulmonary hypertension leading to stress failure of pulmonary capillaries with consequent alveolar and interstitial edema. Although exercise and cold stress at altitude may increase hypoxemia and exacerbate pulmonary hypertension, the hypoxic pulmonary vasoconstrictive response (HPVR) acts as the primary mediator. HPVR results in pulmonary arterial smooth muscle contraction within the typically low-pressure pulmonary arterial system, with consequent increases in pulmonary arterial pressures within minutes. The HPVR can vary widely between individuals and can even vary widely in different regions of the lungs of the same individual. This unevenness of pulmonary vasoconstriction within the lung is thought to contribute to the pathophysiology of HAPE. In patients with HAPE, exaggerated pulmonary arterial pressures (mean pressure 36 to 51 mm Hg) occur. Uneven vasoconstriction forces the pulmonary hypertension to be transmitted to delicate capillary vessels in an asymmetrical fashion, leading to the failure of capillary endothelium with resultant alveolar and interstitial edema. This uneven edema explains the patchy nature of the infiltrate seen on a chest radiograph with HAPE. Although elevated pulmonary arterial pressure is the sine qua non of HAPE, even marked acute pulmonary hypertension is not alone sufficient to cause HAPE.

The mechanism for the uneven vasoconstriction in HAPE may be due to decreased nitric oxide bioavailability at the pulmonary tissue level. That HAPE has its origins in acute pulmonary hypertension and resultant over-perfusion is supported by studies revealing that pharmacologic agents that limit excessive rises in pulmonary artery pressure prevent HAPE.

Once mechanical injury and pulmonary edema occur, other factors come into play. Acute inflammatory mediators appear and likely contribute to worsening lung function. As alveolar fluid accumulates, impairment in a patient's transepithelial sodium transport may decrease their ability to clear alveolar fluid worsening HAPE. Sodium channel–mediated alveolar fluid clearance is upregulated by inhaled beta-adrenergic agonists, which have been proven to decrease risk of HAPE.

Preexisting inflammation may also be a risk factor for HAPE. Particularly in children, preexisting respiratory infection during ascent to high altitude increases susceptibility to HAPE. Inflammation may "sensitize" the pulmonary endothelium to mechanical injury and increase susceptibility to alveolar fluid accumulation and HAPE during ascent.

The definitive etiology of the cerebral forms of altitude illness remains unclear. Evidence suggests that clinical manifestations of AMS

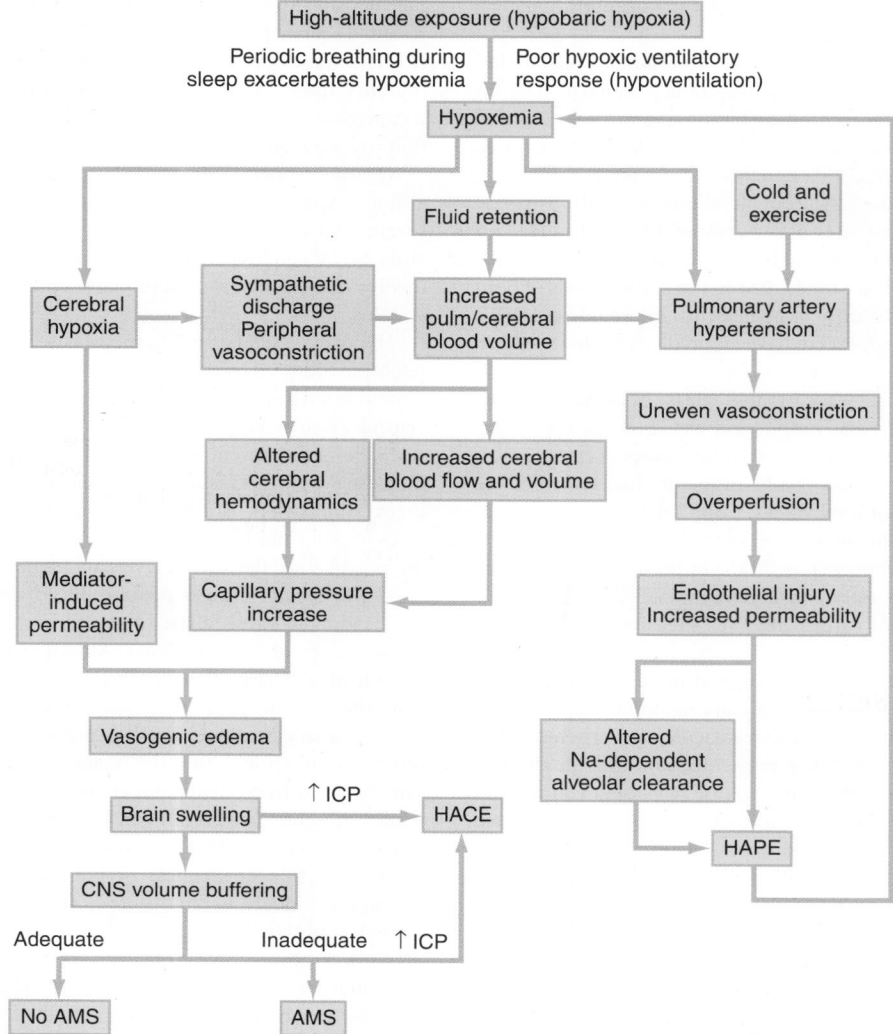

Fig. 132.2 Flowchart of proposed mechanisms for the development of acute mountain sickness *(AMS)*, high-altitude pulmonary edema *(HAPE)*, and high-altitude cerebral edema *(HACE)*. *CNS,* Central nervous system; *ICP,* intracranial pressure.

and HACE result from the combined effects of altered cerebral hemodynamics and inflammatory mediators. Within minutes of exposure to hypoxia, cerebral vasodilation occurs with increased arterial blood velocity and volume. Hypocapnia (secondary to increased ventilation) creates a countervailing cerebral vasoconstriction, however, the overall effect is one of increased cerebral blood flow. Given the rigid confines of the skull, increases in intracranial blood volume require compensatory changes in the brain and cerebral spinal fluid or intracranial pressures will increase. CNS hypoxemia leads to impaired vascular autoregulation, causing increased pressures within the brain's capillary beds. In addition, systemic hypertension from strenuous exercise at high altitude may overwhelm the brain vasculature, resulting in transcapillary leakage and vasogenic edema. In susceptible individuals, these hemodynamic changes are likely to contribute to clinical manifestations of AMS and HACE.

Additional circumstances, however, may be necessary for the development of vasogenic edema and clinical symptoms. Inflammatory mediators may contribute to edema formation. Vascular endothelial growth factor, the inducible form of nitric oxide synthase, reactive cytokines, mitochondrial dysfunction, and free radical formation may alter brain endothelial permeability. The roles that these play in the pathophysiologic process of altitude illness remain unclear.

The role of vasogenic edema in AMS is still under investigation. Magnetic resonance imaging (MRI) of subjects acutely exposed to hypoxia reveal similar signal changes in both subjects with and without clinical AMS. In patients with HACE, MRI studies reveal characteristic white matter changes consistent with vasogenic edema that correlate with symptoms. Although still an area of active research, AMS and HACE pathophysiology is likely due to disturbances in the blood-brain barrier through a combination of mechanical factors and biochemical mediation of permeability.

In severe AMS, MRI studies have revealed cytotoxic edema to present. Rather than being the primary mechanism of severe AMS or HACE, this cytotoxic edema is likely secondary to increased cell ischemia resulting from initial hemodynamic changes, vasogenic edema, biochemical mediators, and increased ratios of brain volume to intracranial space. Increasing data highlight the independent role of hypobaria in the development of AMS and on physiologic responses, including heart rate.[4] In experiments where subjects are exposed to identical levels of alveolar oxygen deprivation, subjects exposed to normobaric hypoxia (by decreasing fraction of inspired oxygen [Fio_2]) alone have much lower AMS incidence than subjects exposed to a hypobaric hypoxia.

The "tight fit" hypothesis was proposed more than three decades ago to explain AMS development and its inherent individual susceptibility. This theory suggests that individuals are more susceptible to AMS and HACE as their ability to accommodate increased hypoxia-related intracranial blood volume and cerebral edema decrease. As brain volume increases from increased cerebral blood volume, the volume-buffering capacity of the central nervous system may prevent an immediate rise of intracranial pressure. As brain volume increases, the intracranial cerebrospinal fluid (CSF) is displaced through the foramen magnum into the spinal canal. Increased absorption of CSF by the arachnoid villi and decreased CSF production also occur. Individuals with less intracranial and intraspinal CSF buffering capacity have less compliance, and so experience larger increases in intracranial pressure, and become more symptomatic (i.e., manifested as AMS) from mild brain swelling. The tight fit hypothesis is supported by lumbar puncture, MRI, and computed tomography (CT) studies. More recently, optic nerve sheath ultrasonography has emerged as an early, noninvasive diagnostic tool to assess intracranial pressure. Increasing intracranial pressure correlates directly with optic nerve sheath diameter (ONSD). Studies have demonstrated that elevated intracranial pressure is associated with AMS and HACE.

ACUTE MOUNTAIN SICKNESS

Clinical Features

AMS is a clinical diagnosis. As defined by the Lake Louise Criteria, the diagnosis of AMS requires a patient to have recently ascended to an elevation to 8000 feet, with report of a headache *plus* at least one of the following symptoms: gastrointestinal upset (anorexia, nausea, or vomiting), general weakness or fatigue, or dizziness or lightheadedness (Box 132.2).[5] The headache may vary from mild to severe, is generally bitemporal and throbbing in nature, and is worse during the night and on awakening or when suddenly becoming upright. Anorexia and nausea, with or without vomiting, are common, and the other symptoms described can range in severity from mild to incapacitating. The disturbance of sleep caused by periodic breathing is common in all visitors to high altitudes but may be exacerbated in the setting of AMS. The symptoms of AMS develop within a few hours after arrival at high altitude and generally reach maximum severity between 24 and 48 hours, followed by a gradual resolution. Most individuals become symptom-free by the third or fourth day. Patients with continued symptoms should not ascend until symptoms abate, and descent and alternative diagnoses should also be considered.

Given its subjective nature, AMS is difficult to definitively diagnose in infants and pre-verbal children. AMS may be manifested by increased fussiness, decreased playfulness, decreased appetite, and sleep disturbance. Although AMS, or a change in environment, sleeping accommodation, or eating habits may result in a fussy, unhappy child, the differential diagnosis for these nonspecific findings must remain broad. If occult bacteremia or another serious illness is suspected in a young child, descent to lower altitude for an appropriate diagnostic and treatment regimen is recommended.

Differential Diagnoses

AMS is a clinical diagnosis without objective diagnostic physical findings, therefore a broad differential diagnosis when treating these nonspecific symptoms is prudent (Box 132.3). Less common, but lethal etiologies of headache, nausea, and fatigue must be considered before the relatively benign diagnosis of AMS is made. Any evidence of ataxia or altered mentation suggests HACE or other malignant etiology and mandates immediate descent. Benign focal neurologic findings and transient global amnesia have been described at altitude but should be assumed to be malignant in etiology until proven otherwise. Acute carbon monoxide (CO) poisoning should also be considered in high-altitude settings and is most commonly detected in poorly ventilated shelters near campfires, stoves or gas-powered generators used for heat, cooking, and fuel. Physiologically, when coupled with hypobaric hypoxia, carbon monoxide exposure is more dangerous in cold high-altitude locations than in other environments. Although dyspnea on exertion is universal and expected at high altitudes, dyspnea at rest suggests HAPE and warrants a careful examination for pulmonary edema.

Diagnostic Testing

Serial measurement of ONSD using ultrasound has demonstrated that subjects with symptoms and signs of worsening AMS or HACE have enlarged ONSDs on serial measurements, which may prove a useful adjunct in the diagnosis and monitoring of AMS and HACE (Fig. 132.3). Given significant individual variability in ONSD, isolated ONSD ultrasonography at a single point in time has little utility in the diagnosis of AMS.

Management

Patients with AMS should not ascend to a higher sleeping altitude until symptoms resolve to allow acclimatization to occur. Continued ascent exacerbates the underlying pathologic processes and may lead to severe AMS or lethal HACE. If patients develop neurologic abnormalities

---

BOX 132.2 Acute Mountain Sickness

Incidence: 12% to 67%, varies widely with elevation, rate of ascent, and individual susceptibility; rare below 8000 feet, most common with rapid ascent to altitudes above 10,000 feet.

Symptoms and signs: Headache, anorexia, nausea, fatigue, dizziness.

Treatment: Mild cases are usually self-limited and do not require treatment; discontinue ascent, rest. For moderate cases, administer acetazolamide; ibuprofen, aspirin, or acetaminophen for headache; Zofran or prochlorperazine for nausea; supplemental oxygen if available; descend if persistent or severe; add dexamethasone in severe cases.

Prevention: Gradual ascent to allow acclimatization; high-carbohydrate diet, avoidance of ethanol or smoking; acetazolamide if ascent is rapid or known history of recurrent acute mountain sickness (AMS).

BOX 132.3 Acute Mountain Sickness Differential Diagnosis

- Tension headache
- Viral syndrome
- Alcohol intoxication/toxidrome
- Carbon monoxide (CO) poisoning
- Dehydration
- Caffeine withdrawal
- Migraine headache
- Infectious (meningitis, encephalitis/viral syndrome)
- Intracranial hemorrhage or mass
- Central nervous system aneurysm
- Venous sinus thrombosis
- Abdominal process (e.g., gastroenteritis)
- Acute angle closure glaucoma/ocular process

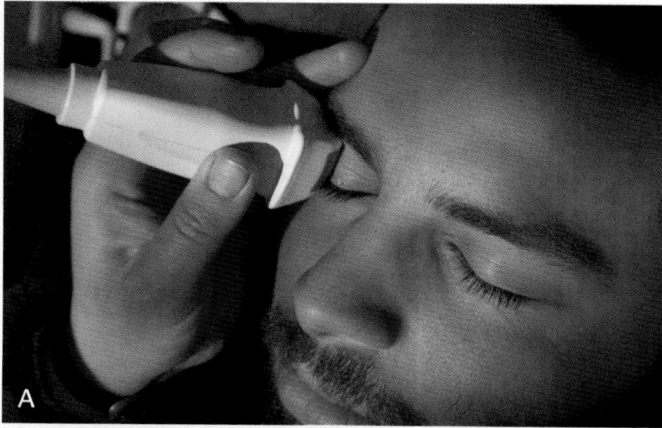

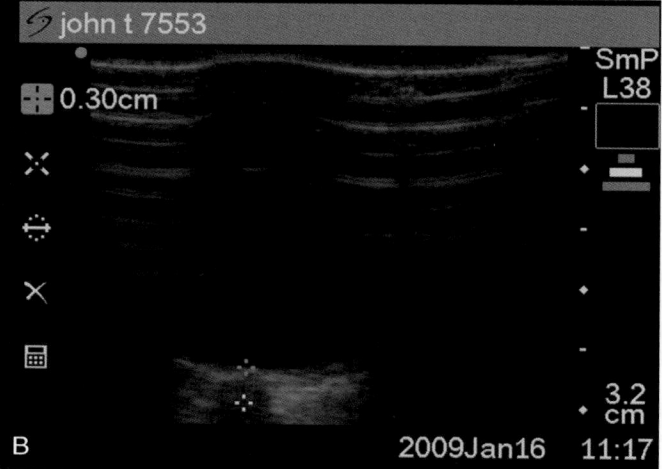

Fig. 132.3 Diagnostic image of optic nerve sheath ultrasonography. (A) Probe positioning: This study is typically performed with the subject supine and with eyes closed. The probe is placed on the closed lid, lateral of the center of the pupil, and adjusted until a longitudinal, cross-sectional image of the optic nerve (deep to the retina) is obtained. For clarity, this figure does not show the use of ultrasound gel, occlusive dressing, or a high-frequency (7- to 10-MHz) linear probe. (B) Optic nerve sheath ultrasonogram with measurements. (Courtesy N. Stuart Harris, MD.)

(e.g., ataxia or altered mentation) or evidence of severe pulmonary edema, immediate descent is indicated.[6]

Mild AMS may be treated by symptom management and cessation of ascent until acclimatization occurs. This may take 1 to 4 days. AMS that becomes worse or does not respond to maintenance of altitude, rest, and pharmacologic intervention necessitates descent. A descent of as little as 500 feet may be sufficient. Descent of 1500 to 3000 feet effectively reverses high-altitude illness in most cases. Descent should be continued until symptom improvement is seen, and efforts to minimize exertion should be instituted during the descent.[7]

Oxygen Therapy

All forms of altitude illness, including AMS, are effectively treated with supplemental oxygen. In mild AMS, supplemental oxygen may be helpful but is not essential. For severe forms of altitude illness, oxygen can be lifesaving. In resort settings, oxygen can often be rented directly from the hotel or condominium. For AMS, low flow oxygen (1 to 2 L/min), including small amounts during sleep, is often sufficient. In the wilderness, oxygen tanks are cumbersome, heavy, and are usually unavailable in adequate quantities. To overcome this, remote clinics often use solar-powered oxygen generators. In resource-limited settings, oxygen therapy is reserved for the more serious manifestations of high-altitude illness. Hyperbaric therapy with a portable fabric chamber that simulates descent is also effective.

Analgesics and Antiemetics

Symptomatic treatment of headache and nausea can be beneficial during the course of mild AMS. Aspirin, ibuprofen, and acetaminophen are useful for the treatment of high-altitude headache. Narcotic analgesics should be avoided because of depression of the hypoventilation response (HVR) and respiratory drive during sleep. For nausea and vomiting, prochlorperazine, unlike other antiemetics, stimulates the HVR and is preferred.

Acetazolamide

Periodic breathing causes insomnia, which is best treated with the respiratory stimulant acetazolamide.[8] Doses of acetazolamide as low as 62.5 mg to 125 mg bid may prevent intermittent breathing and eradicate insomnia.[9] Most benzodiazepines and other sedative-hypnotics should be avoided because of their tendency to decrease ventilation during sleep. Even individuals who have previously used diazepam at lower altitudes without difficulty describe unusual reactions, including agitation, hallucinations, and disorientation when this agent is used at high altitude. Studies suggest that low doses of benzodiazepines in combination with acetazolamide are safe at high altitude and can improve sleep quality and reduce episodes of nocturia without increasing oxygen desaturation. Nonbenzodiazepine sleep agents (such as zolpidem and zaleplon) do not depress ventilation and may prove useful in AMS-related insomnia.

Acetazolamide accelerates acclimatization and, if given early in the development of AMS, may rapidly resolve symptoms. Although the optimal dose has not yet been definitively established, a dose of 250 mg of acetazolamide at the onset of symptoms and repeated twice daily is effective therapy for AMS. The treatment of AMS in children is not formally studied, but anecdotal experience supports the use of acetazolamide in children. The dose for children is 2.5 mg/kg/dose every 6 to 8 hours or 125 mg given twice daily to a maximum of 250 mg.

Acetazolamide has myriad beneficial effects. By acting as a carbonic anhydrase inhibitor, it enhances renal bicarbonate diuresis and so improves renal correction of the ventilation-related respiratory alkalosis by causing continued increased ventilation and arterial oxygenation. It improves sleep by decreasing nocturnal period breathing. Acetazolamide also acts as a diuretic and so attenuates fluid retention common in patients with AMS. It lowers CSF volume and pressure, which may play an additional role in its therapeutic effect. In addition, it has positive effects beyond its role as a carbonic anhydrase inhibitor, with beneficial chemoreceptor effects on ventilatory drive, alterations of cerebral blood flow, relaxation of smooth muscles, and upregulation of fluid resorption in the lungs.

The most common adverse reactions to acetazolamide are paresthesias and polyuria. Less common reactions include nausea, diarrhea, drowsiness, tinnitus, and transient myopia. Carbonic anhydrase inhibition at the tongue causes dysgeusia, altering the flavor of carbonated beverages, including carbonated beers (of note, nitrogenated beers are unaffected). Acetazolamide is a sulfa compound and carries a low risk of cross-reactivity for individuals with an allergy to sulfa antibiotics. Patients with known sulfonamide allergy may consider administration of a trial dose of acetazolamide in a controlled environment before ascent. Acetazolamide is contraindicated in patients with a history of anaphylaxis or severe skin reactions to any sulfa-containing medication, and it should be avoided in breast-feeding mothers and pregnant women.

Dexamethasone

Dexamethasone is an effective alternative treatment of moderate to severe AMS. An initial dose of 8 mg followed by 4 mg every 6 hours is recommended. As a treatment option, concurrent use with acetazolamide is advocated by some to promote acclimatization. Dexamethasone is known to have antiinflammatory properties. Additionally, it may reduce cerebral blood flow and block the action of vascular endothelial growth factor. Reduction of AMS symptoms with the use of dexamethasone may be the result of these or its euphoric effects. Prophylactic use of dexamethasone should generally be reserved for use in individuals forced to rapidly ascend (e.g., professional mountain search and rescue operations). Although dexamethasone effectively relieves the symptoms of AMS, unlike acetazolamide, it does not enhance acclimatization. If used as a prophylactic agent to allow ascent beyond physiologic acclimatization, acute cessation can result in rapid onset of severe altitude illness. For treatment, use should be limited to patients with acetazolamide intolerance or more advanced cases of AMS, especially to help facilitate descent. Common side effects of dexamethasone include gastrointestinal irritation, gastritis, esophagitis, altered mood, and gastroesophageal reflux disease (GERD). Dexamethasone should not be used for more than 3 days for this indication because more serious side effects such as GI bleed and altered mental status with aberrant behavior have been described.

Disposition

Individuals with AMS may resume their ascent after symptoms resolve. Consider prophylactic acetazolamide if they are to further ascend. Further elevation gain should be halted if symptoms recur.

Prevention

The symptoms of mild AMS are generally benign and well-tolerated. For some, however, they are unpleasant and debilitating to the point that travel, business, or vacation plans are interrupted. Up to 50% of individuals with AMS report a decrease in activity.

The best method of prevention is a gradual or staged ascent that allows adequate time for acclimatization; however, the time constraints of many vacationers and inexperienced guides often make such an ascent profile unrealistic. The 19th-century climbing adage, "Climb high, sleep low," is born of experience: during acclimatization, hypoxic nadirs encountered during sleep are much greater than those during waking hours. Decreased respiratory drive during sleep can lead to increasing symptoms of poor acclimatization. Ideally, the first night should not be spent at an altitude higher than 9200 feet, with a subsequent increase (to a new sleeping altitude) of not more than 1600 feet each night. One extra night of acclimatization (at the same sleeping altitude) should be added for every 3000 to 5000 feet of altitude gain above 10,000 feet. Excursions to higher altitudes during the day with a return to a lower sleeping altitude aid in successful acclimatization.

Pre-exposure to artificially hypoxic environments to prompt acclimatization and to decrease symptoms of high-altitude illness have been studied. Pre-exposure regimens (typically in normobaric, hypoxic tents) lasting less than 8 to 12 hours appear to offer limited protection from subsequent altitude exposure.

Mild to moderate exercise likely aids acclimatization; however, overexertion can contribute to the development of AMS. Maintaining adequate hydration—targeting relatively clear (dilute) urine and normal urine output—is also recommended. No data support recommendations for hyperhydration that is sometimes promoted in the lay literature. In fact, consumption of excessive amounts of free water may lead to hyponatremia and possibly complicate altitude illness. Balanced electrolyte solutions are recommended (premixed or prepared with purified water).

The elevation goal, rate of ascent, and prior history of altitude illness should be considered in the assessment of the risk for development of altitude illness and the choice of prevention strategies (eTable 132.1). Individuals in low-risk situations should not need medications for prophylaxis. Ascent should be gradual to prevent illness. In some cases, such as arrival at a high-altitude airport (e.g., Lhasa, Tibet, 11,995 ft) or the immediate dispatch of rescue personnel to high altitude, a slow or staged ascent is not possible. Mountain climbers commonly ascend at rates that are higher than recommended, and some individuals continue to suffer AMS symptoms despite gradual ascent. Individuals who have a known susceptibility to the development of AMS and those for whom slow ascent is impractical fall into the moderate- and high-risk categories and should consider prophylactic medication in addition to gradual ascent.

Numerous studies demonstrate the effectiveness of acetazolamide in prevention of AMS in adults. Lower dosages provide prophylaxis similar to that of higher dosages with fewer adverse reactions. A dose of 125 mg twice daily starting 24 hours before ascent and continuing for the first 2 days at high altitude is effective. When compared with higher doses, this dose has a lower likelihood of noxious side effects. Although it is unstudied, the recommended dosage of acetazolamide for AMS prophylaxis for children is 2.5 mg/kg/dose up to 125 mg total given twice daily, and this weight-based approach may reduce side effects in smaller adults. Ibuprofen compared with acetazolamide is equally efficacious in preventing headache.

Dexamethasone also prevents AMS. The lowest effective prophylactic dosage is 2 mg every 6 hours or 4 mg every 12 hours. Some patients experience the rapid onset of AMS after dexamethasone is discontinued. Dexamethasone does not facilitate acclimatization but rather reduces nausea and enhances mood. In most cases, dexamethasone use should be reserved for treatment of AMS rather than for prophylaxis. Military or rescue personnel rapidly ascending to high altitude and individuals with acetazolamide intolerance are candidates for prophylaxis with dexamethasone. The combination of acetazolamide and dexamethasone may be more effective than either drug alone.

Oxygen is an effective prophylactic modality for rescue personnel. Adequate supplies should be available to ensure the safety of all team members for the entire duration of the rescue. Air drops of oxygen can be lifesaving when weather or terrain prevents the immediate arrival of rescue personnel.

HIGH-ALTITUDE PULMONARY EDEMA

Clinical Features

HAPE is the most common fatal manifestation of severe high-altitude illness (Box 132.4). Although HAPE is uncommon below 10,000 feet, it can occur and even be fatal at altitudes below 8000 feet. Episodes occurring between 8000 and 10,000 feet are usually related to heavy exercise or comorbidities; but at higher altitudes, pulmonary edema can also occur at rest or with light activity.

Some individuals are susceptible and experience HAPE with each ascent to altitude, but many patients have a single episode of HAPE and subsequently are able to return to high altitude without a recurrence. Less commonly, those with multiple previously uneventful high-altitude exposures may still develop HAPE. Individuals, especially children and young adults, who have been residents at high-altitude locations for extended periods may have pulmonary edema develop on re-ascent from a trip to low altitude. This phenomenon has been termed *reentry HAPE*.

The initial symptoms of HAPE typically begin insidiously 2 to 4 days after arrival at high altitude. Most cases occur during the second night, but HAPE may develop rapidly, with early symptoms apparent after just a few hours at high altitude. Marked dyspnea on exertion, fatigue with minimal-to-moderate effort, prolonged dyspneic recovery time, and dry cough are early manifestations of the disease. The symptoms of AMS usually occur concurrently with the development of HAPE.

As the HAPE patient deteriorates, usually through the night, the dyspnea intensifies with effort and is unrelieved by rest. Dyspnea at rest is a red flag warning. The cough may become productive of copious amounts of clear, watery sputum. Hemoptysis may be seen in severe cases. As the condition intensifies, cerebral edema or simply severe hypoxemia may cause central nervous system dysfunction, such as ataxia and altered mentation. Coma may follow and precede death in a few hours if immediate oxygen therapy and descent are not instituted.

The physical examination reveals a few rales in patients with mild HAPE, usually found in the region of the right middle lobe, progressing to unilateral or bilateral rales and then to diffuse bilateral rales, rhonchi, and gurgles audible without a stethoscope. Neck veins are not distended. Cyanosis of the nail beds alone may progress to severe central cyanosis. Tachypnea and tachycardia become more pronounced as severity increases. Elevated temperatures are common, and a concurrent respiratory tract infection is occasionally seen, especially in children.

Differential Diagnoses

It is prudent to maintain a wide differential diagnosis in assessing patients with acute dyspnea at high altitude (Box 132.5). Although HAPE occurs at high altitude, so does acute coronary syndrome, pulmonary embolism (PE), congestive heart failure (CHF), and pneumonia.

Pneumonia can be misdiagnosed in the setting of HAPE because the symptoms and signs of pneumonia are similar to those of HAPE. The incidence of pneumonia and the common organisms responsible for pneumonia at high altitude are understudied, but visitors to high altitudes may be predisposed to acquire bacterial infections because of impaired T-lymphocyte function. Treat patients for HAPE who present with symptoms compatible with pneumonia at high altitude. Initiate antibiotics if there is doubt about the diagnosis of HAPE versus pneumonia. Because of decreased respiratory reserves and mild immunosuppression coincident with high-altitude exposure, the treatment of any serious pulmonary infection at high altitude requires oxygen, descent, and antibiotics.

High-altitude bronchitis ("Khumbu cough") and pharyngitis are common problems among climbers. They may result from the increased ventilation of cold, dry air across the upper airway mucosa, causing mucosal inflammation. Copious sputum production is sometimes seen, and antibiotic therapy is rarely helpful. Coughing spasms may be severe and require treatment with antitussives. Other therapeutic measures include hydration, lozenges, and steam inhalation.

Death from PE at high altitude is described. Given frequent travel involving long plane flights prior to many vacations at high altitude, patients may often have increased risk of deep vein thrombus (DVT) and PE. Additional predisposing factors for DVT include acute hyperviscosity due to increased hematocrit, dehydration, and forced stasis due to sleeping and sheltering in confined spaces, particularly during inclement weather conditions. The symptoms and signs of PE can mimic those of HAPE; however, embolic disease tends to have a more rapid onset, and pleuritic chest pain is a more prominent feature.

Diagnostic Testing

Ultrasonography

Ultrasound machines are portable, require limited training for effective use in this setting, and use non-ionizing radiation. As a result, serial assessments can easily be performed to gauge response to treatment. Given their portability, limited power requirements, and instant access to diagnostic data, they are the preferred modality for many remote clinical settings.

Thoracic ultrasonography allows rapid, accurate assessment for acute pulmonary edema at the bedside (Fig. 132.4). The presence of "lung comet tails" (also called *B-lines*) on thoracic ultrasound indicates extravascular water, is reproducible, quantifiable, and has been inversely correlated with oxygen saturation and clinical status in HAPE patients. The use of ultrasonography to estimate pulmonary artery pressure is an established modality for early detection and diagnosis of HAPE. Demonstration of high pulmonary artery pressures with normal left ventricular function is associated with HAPE and HAPE susceptibility.

Chest Radiographs

In HAPE patients, chest films reveal patchy alveolar infiltrates with areas of clearing between the patches. Unilateral infiltrates may be present in mild cases; however, bilateral infiltrates are seen in more advanced cases, most commonly involving the right mid-lung fields (Fig. 132.5). Pleural effusion is rare but may be present in severe cases. The extent of the edema on the chest radiograph roughly parallels the clinical severity. Of note, the radiographic findings of cardiomegaly, bat-wing distribution of infiltrates, and Kerley B-lines, which are typical of cardiogenic pulmonary edema, are generally absent in cases of HAPE.

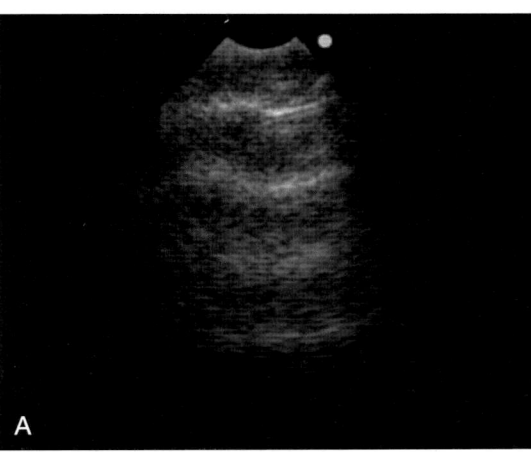
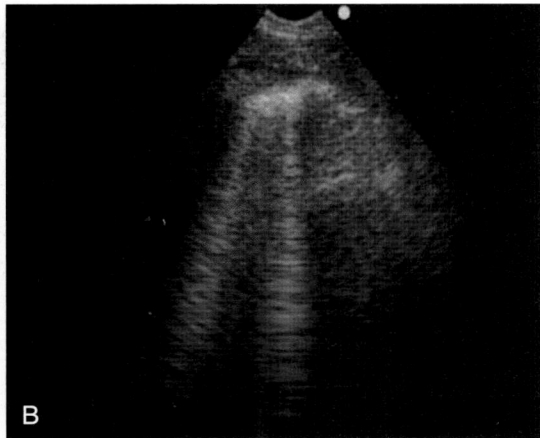

Fig. 132.4 Diagnostic image of thoracic ultrasound of lung with high-altitude pulmonary edema (HAPE). (A) Normal lung tissue is uniform "snowstorm." (B) B-lines, also known as "comet tails," are present in this patient with HAPE. They are defined as echogenic, coherent, wedge-shaped signals with a narrow origin in the near field of the image, arising from the pleural line and extending to the edge of the screen. B-lines indicate pulmonary interstitial fluid (edema). Views obtained using *low* frequency, curved probe and B-mode imaging. (Courtesy American College of Chest Physicians.)

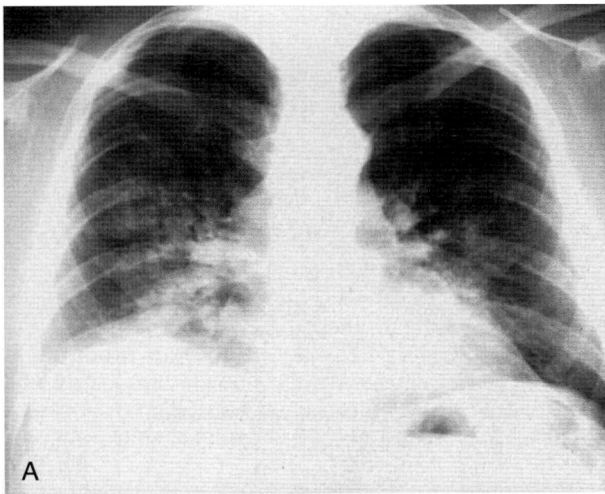
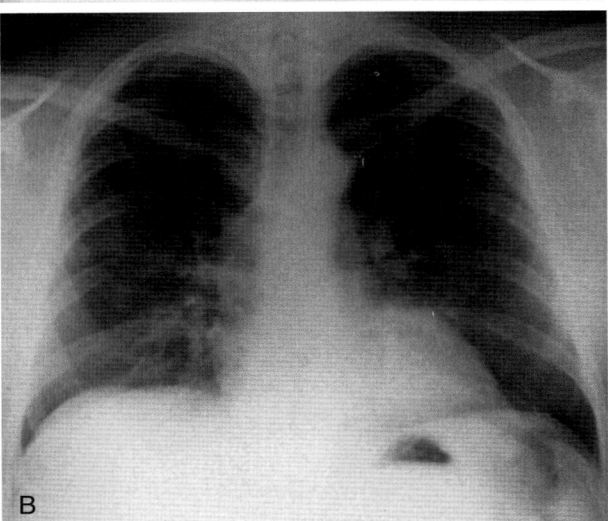

Fig. 132.5 Diagnostic image of chest radiograph of a patient with high-altitude pulmonary edema (HAPE). (A) Before treatment. (B) After treatment. (Courtesy Richard Nicholas, MD.)

Radiographic evidence of HAPE clears rapidly after initiation of treatment; some mild cases may clear in 4 to 6 hours, and most clear by 24 hours. Radiographs of patients with severe HAPE may reveal infiltrates that persist for as long as 2 weeks, even though the clinical symptoms have resolved.

Electrocardiogram and Echocardiogram

An electrocardiogram reveals tachycardia and evidence of right-sided heart strain, including right axis deviation, P wave abnormalities, tall R waves in the precordial leads, and S waves in the lateral leads. Hemodynamic studies reveal increased pulmonary vascular resistance, elevated pulmonary artery pressures, and normal pulmonary wedge pressures. Echocardiographic studies demonstrate high estimated pulmonary artery pressures, pulmonary vascular resistance, and normal left ventricular function.

Management
Descent

In remote settings, where oxygen and medical expertise may be unavailable, immediate descent to treat HAPE may be lifesaving. Delay of descent (e.g., waiting hours for rescue personnel to initiate evacuation) can lead to rapid HAPE progression and death. Descents of 3000 feet are generally adequate for a rapid recovery; however, descent should continue until symptoms resolve.

Oxygen Therapy

To minimize cold- or exercise-induced pulmonary hypertension, HAPE patients should be kept warm and should minimize exertion (Fig. 132.6). Patients with mild cases of HAPE under expert supervision have been successfully treated at altitude with oxygen, medications, and 1 or 2 days of bed rest. Oxygen administration increases the rate of improvement. Moderate cases can be treated without descent if bed rest, experienced providers, and adequate supplies of supplemental oxygen are available. Any treatment plan that does not include descent necessitates serial examinations by clinicians with experience in management of high-altitude illness.

If difficult terrain or weather conditions hamper efforts to descend, oxygen administration (or hyperbaric therapy) can be a lifesaving measure. If immediate evacuation to lower altitudes

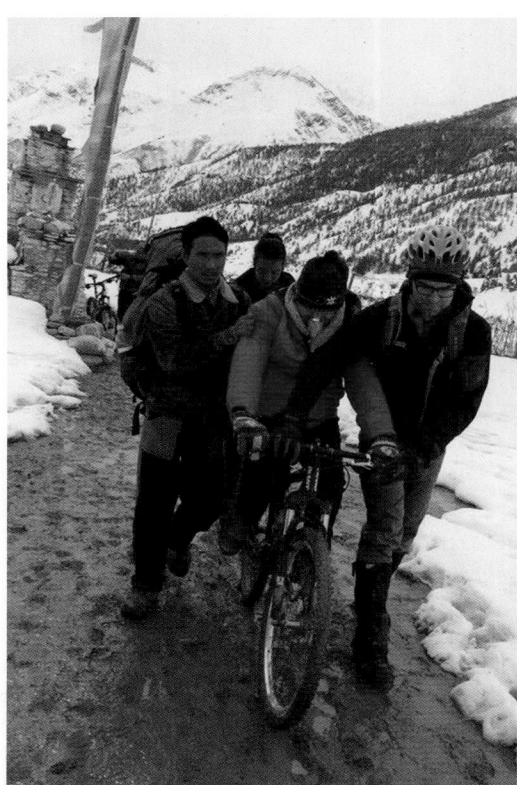

Fig. 132.6 Clinical photograph of high-altitude pulmonary edema (HAPE) patient being treated with immediate descent in rural Nepal. Patient is provided with oxygen and descending with minimal exertion. (Courtesy Lara Phillips, MD.)

will be delayed, rescue personnel should air drop oxygen supplies. Deliver oxygen at rates of 6 to 8 L/min by mask to victims with severe HAPE until clinical improvement is seen. As patients improve, flow rates can then be lowered until recovery or descent is completed with a goal peripheral oxygen saturation greater than 90% likely sufficient. Delivery of oxygen with a continuous positive airway pressure mask will decrease work of breathing and improve alveolar fluid clearance.

Hyperbaric therapy simulates descent by increasing the available oxygen at a given altitude, as the amount of oxygen available is a function of the percentage of inspired oxygen multiplied by the barometric pressure. Although preferred with oxygen, if supplies are low, hyperbaric therapy may be employed without administration of supplemental oxygen. Several portable, lightweight (approximately 15 pounds), fabric hyperbaric chambers are available. They are pressurized manually (Fig. 132.7) and generate approximately 103 mm Hg (2 psi) above the ambient pressure. This simulates a descent of 4000 to 5000 feet at moderate altitudes, and at the summit of Mt. Everest it would simulate a descent of approximately 9000 feet. These devices can be lifesaving in patients with HAPE and HACE. They should only be used as a temporizing treatment when descent is not immediately feasible. Some previously nonambulatory patients are able to descend under their own power after a few hours of treatment in these hyperbaric chambers.

Most of the pharmacotherapies used for HAPE treatment derive their presumed efficacy from studies examining their abilities to prevent HAPE in a "HAPE-susceptible" subject population. There are few robust studies directly examining pharmacologic treatments for HAPE. Oxygen and descent remain the mainstays in treatment.

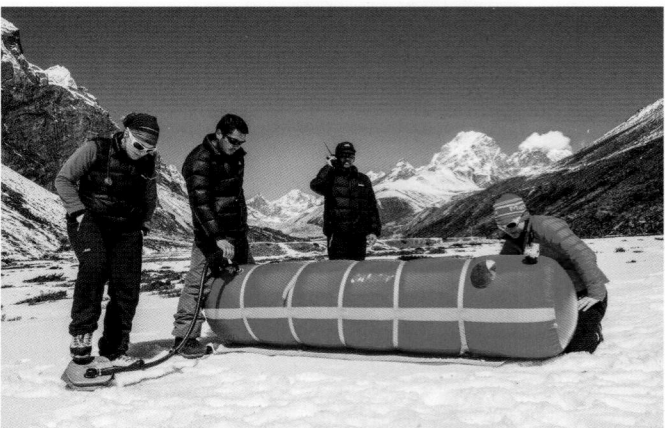

Fig. 132.7 Clinical photograph of Gamow bag, a lightweight, portable hyperbaric chamber used for rapid treatment of severe altitude illness. Note the attached foot-operated pressure pump. (Courtesy Reuben Tabner.)

Nifedipine

In addition to oxygen and descent to treat HAPE, medications that lower pulmonary artery pressure, pulmonary blood volume, and pulmonary vascular resistance or enhance alveolar fluid clearance may be useful adjuncts. Unlike pulmonary edema secondary to acute CHF, HAPE results from increased pulmonary vascular tone. It does not result from excessive intravascular volume or failed cardiac pump function. As such, diuretic therapy has no role in the treatment of HAPE and may further exacerbate volume loss in patients who are already intravascularly depleted.

One of the better studied agents for both prophylaxis and treatment of HAPE is the calcium channel blocker nifedipine. Acting as a pulmonary vasodilator, nifedipine is especially useful when oxygen is not readily available or descent is impossible. Nifedipine does not improve pulmonary hemodynamics as much as oxygen or descent do, and it does not have an additive effect when it is administered with oxygen. Treatment with 30 mg of a slow-release nifedipine preparation administered twice daily is recommended. Patients should be monitored for the development of hypotension during nifedipine administration.

Other Medications

Although phosphodiesterase type 5 inhibitors (including tadalafil and sildenafil) are known to be useful for HAPE prevention, are widely used, and are unlikely to cause acute harm in this indication, they remain unstudied for HAPE treatment. Alveolar fluid clearance is upregulated by beta-adrenergic agonists in animal models, and inhaled beta-agonists (salmeterol 125 µg inhaled twice daily) have been used anecdotally for therapy of HAPE.

The mainstay of HAPE treatment remains immediate oxygen administration (when available) and descent. Nifedipine treatment is recommended if these treatments are unavailable. No compelling evidence suggests the concurrent use of these medications with oxygen has additional benefit beyond the use of oxygen alone.

Disposition

Mild to moderate cases of HAPE can be treated with oxygen, rest, and careful monitoring. Experienced clinicians in recreational areas at moderate altitudes (e.g., Colorado ski resorts or dedicated high-altitude clinics in Nepal) administer oxygen and observe HAPE patients to ensure adequate oxygenation. These patients are then discharged to their local lodging with supplemental oxygen and monitored for improvement or deterioration. In severe HAPE, or milder cases that do not improve with therapy, descent is warranted. Rapid recovery is usually seen after descent to lower altitudes, and observation of the patient in the emergency department to ensure adequate room air oxygenation is generally adequate. On occasion, admission to the hospital is indicated to maintain the SaO_2 greater than 90%. In the hospital, continuous positive airway pressure may improve gas exchange and decrease work of breathing in HAPE patients. Hypocapnia, alkalosis, and radiographic evidence of HAPE may persist for several days. Thoracic ultrasound allows for frequent reassessments and has been shown to closely follow resolving edema and increasing oxygen saturations.

If oxygen saturation can be maintained at greater than 90% on room air and clinical improvement is apparent, the patient can be discharged. If the patient requires air travel to return home (cabin pressures equal approximately 8000 feet), additional recovery time before travel or arrangement for supplemental oxygen administration is advised. Assessment for structural cardiac abnormalities with echocardiography is indicated if a heart murmur is detected in a patient with HAPE. An evaluation for underlying congenital heart disease is warranted after an episode of HAPE in a young child.[10]

Patients may be able to re-ascend (generally in 2 to 3 days) when symptoms resolve and oxygen levels remain acceptable off supplemental oxygen at rest and with mild exercise. Re-ascent with pulmonary vasodilator medication may be considered.

Prevention

As with all forms of serious altitude illness, two key teaching points are the most effective means of prevention and must be understood by the patient: (1) a gradual or staged ascent to allow sufficient time to acclimatize is critical, and (2) immediate cessation of further ascent at the onset of symptoms can be lifesaving. Individuals with a prior history of HAPE should also avoid extreme exertion during the first 2 days at altitude. Consider prophylactic therapy with nifedipine (30 mg extended release twice daily for 3 days) in patients with a prior history of HAPE. Less evidence exists to support the routine use of other pulmonary vasodilators for HAPE prevention.

Phosphodiesterase type 5 inhibitors are selective pulmonary vasodilators that increase cyclic guanosine monophosphate availability. Sildenafil (40 mg every 8 hours) and tadalafil (10 mg every 12 hours) have been found to be effective in preventing HAPE in HAPE-susceptible subjects. The phosphodiesterase type 5 inhibitors have the added benefit that they are less likely than calcium channel blockers to induce systemic hypotension. However, as with other indicated uses, they should not be administered to individuals concurrently taking nitroglycerin.

Although high-quality data are lacking, a few additional medication options may be considered for prevention. Dexamethasone (8 mg every 12 hours) started 2 days before ascent may prevent HAPE. To enhance alveolar fluid clearance, salmeterol 125 μg inhaled twice daily may be used as an adjunct to nifedipine in patients with a history of HAPE, although side effects are common at this high inhaled dose. Finally, clinical experience suggests that acetazolamide aids in acclimatization and prevents HAPE, with additional benefits of reducing hypoxic pulmonary vasoconstriction.

HIGH-ALTITUDE CEREBRAL EDEMA

Clinical Features

HACE is the least common but most lethal form of high-altitude illness (Box 132.6). Death from HACE typically occurs above 12,000 feet. Mild AMS can progress to severe HACE with coma in as few as 12 hours. Although severe symptoms usually develop within 1 to 3 days, they may not occur until 5 to 9 days. HACE is characterized by

---

> ### BOX 132.6 High-Altitude Cerebral Edema
>
> Incidence: Lower than 1% or 2%, uncommon as a pure entity; usually associated with the presence of severe AMS and HAPE.
> Symptoms and signs: Ataxia, severe headache, nausea and vomiting, altered mentation, seizures, coma.
> Treatment: Immediate evacuation to a lower altitude; oxygen, bed rest, dexamethasone (8 mg PO or IV, then 4 mg q6h). Hyperbaric therapy if unable to immediately descend.

AMS, Acute mountain sickness; *HAPE*, high-altitude pulmonary edema.

> ### BOX 132.7 High-Altitude Cerebral Edema Differential Diagnoses
>
> - Acute cerebral vascular accident (CVA)/transient ischemic attack
> - Intracranial hemorrhage
> - Hypoglycemia
> - Carbon monoxide (CO) poisoning
> - Meningitis/encephalitis
> - Hypothermia
> - Intracranial mass
> - Vertebral/carotid dissection or stenosis
> - Acute toxidrome—alcohol, other
> - Acute alcohol withdrawal/delirium tremens
> - Seizure
> - Transient global amnesia

---

evidence of global cerebral dysfunction. The symptoms of severe AMS (headache, fatigue, and vomiting) as well as those of HAPE (cough and dyspnea) are often present. Patients with HACE invariably have had prior, unheeded symptoms of worsening AMS over hours to days. HACE-specific signs include ataxia, slurred speech, and altered mental status, which can range from mild emotional lability or confusion, to hallucinations and worsening obtundation that may advance to coma and death. Less commonly, generalized seizures and rarely, focal neurologic deficits may occur. HACE can also occur in children.[11]

Altered mental status and cerebellar ataxia are the most sensitive signs of early HACE. The early appearance of ataxia reflects the particular sensitivity of the cerebellum to hypoxia. Ataxia alone is an indication for immediate descent. Retinal hemorrhages are common and rarely of clinical significance. Papilledema and occasionally cranial nerve palsy also occur in the setting of increased intracranial pressure.

Differential Diagnoses

Paroxysmal onset of symptoms should prompt consideration of other etiologies, such as hypothermia, hypoglycemia, CO poisoning, and acute cerebral vascular accidents (CVAs) (Box 132.7). A cerebral vascular lesion is suggested by abrupt onset, presence of a dense hemilateral palsy, a lack of preceding symptoms of AMS, or the persistence of signs despite adequate treatment of high-altitude illness.

Diagnostic Testing

Without advanced imaging, differentiating between HACE and acute CVA may be difficult – regardless, both are acute neurologic emergencies. Although not common, the occurrence of cerebral thrombosis and transient ischemic attacks, in the absence of high-altitude illness, have been documented at high altitude. Subsequent MRI studies of patients with HACE reveals white matter changes consistent with vasogenic edema (Fig. 132.8).[12]

Management

Successful therapy for HACE requires early recognition and immediate descent. Administer high-flow oxygen, if available. Oxygen alone reduces intracranial blood flow at high altitude. Steroid therapy is recommended and may result in recovery from HACE without neurologic deficits. The initial dose of dexamethasone is 8 mg parenterally or orally in mild cases, followed by 4 mg every 6 hours.

Patients with severely altered levels of consciousness require tracheal intubation. Increase oxygenation, both by increasing Fio_2 and barometric pressure by descent or hyperbaric treatment. Hyperventilation, diuretics (e.g., furosemide), and hypertonic solutions (e.g., mannitol) have been used to manage severely elevated intracranial pressure, but extreme caution is warranted. Many patients with HACE are already volume depleted from poor fluid intake; diuretic use could compromise adequate intravascular volume and reduce cerebral perfusion pressure.

Hyperbaric treatment of HACE is also effective and may result in temporary improvement and allow self-rescue and descent. Conversely, coma may persist for several days even after descent to lower altitudes.

Disposition

When safe and feasible, immediate descent is essential. If immediate descent to definitive care is an option, placing HACE patients in a hyperbaric device may only delay the more comprehensive care available in the hospital setting.

Long-term neurologic deficits including ataxia and cognitive impairment have been reported after recovery from acute episodes of HACE. Both transient and long-lasting neurobehavioral impairments can occur in mountaineers after climbing to extreme altitude without experiencing clinical HACE. Because of the potential for long-lasting neurologic injury, the clinician must maintain awareness of the early manifestations of HACE. Early treatment of HACE generally results in good outcomes, but after coma is present, the mortality rate exceeds 60%. Patients who have suffered HACE should be referred to a neurologist for further evaluation.

SPECIAL CONSIDERATIONS

High-Altitude Retinal Hemorrhage

High-altitude retinal hemorrhage (HARH) is the most common type of retinopathy in visitors to high altitude. These hemorrhages are common at altitudes above 17,500 feet, although they can occur at lower levels.

The exact incidence of HARH is unknown because most patients are asymptomatic, with HARH noted only on retinoscopy. HARH is not generally related to the presence of mild AMS but does seem to be related to strenuous exercise at high altitude. At any altitude, in the setting of severe HAPE or HACE, retinal hemorrhages are commonly noted, but the mechanism remains unclear.

Hemorrhages usually spare the macula (Fig. 132.9) and most often resolve without treatment in 2 or 3 weeks. With macular involvement, central scotomas may be noticed and only gradually resolve. In some cases, these visual defects are permanent. HARH is more likely to occur among individuals with a previous history of such hemorrhages and those on anticoagulation therapy. The underlying risk remains unclear. They usually do not pose a contraindication to return to high altitude unless the macular region is involved. Altitude related changes in intraocular pressure are not associated with AMS.

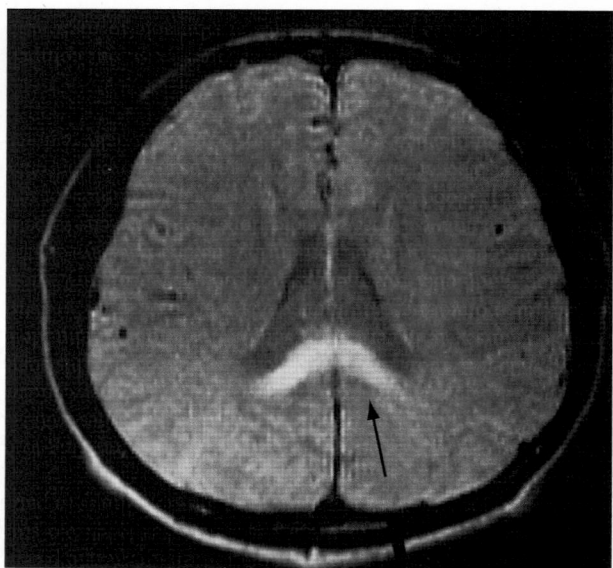

Fig. 132.8 Diagnostic image of axial proton-weighted magnetic resonance image of a mountain climber with high-altitude cerebral edema (HACE). The *arrow* demonstrates the markedly increased signal (edema) in the splenium of the corpus callosum. (Courtesy Peter Hackett, MD.)

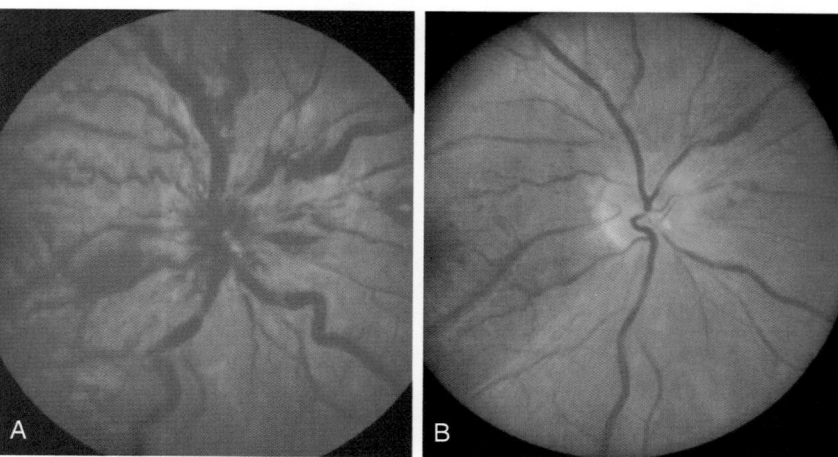

Fig. 132.9 Diagnostic image of high-altitude retinal hemorrhages (HARHs). (A) Acute. (B) After 1 week of resolution. (Courtesy Charles Houston, MD.)

Carbon Monoxide Poisoning

CO poisoning is not uncommon at altitude, typically from the use of fires and combustion stoves to keep warm or to prepare food in the high-altitude environment. CO poisoning at altitude can be more devastating because of preexisting hypobaria-induced hypoxia. As CO avidly binds to hemoglobin, it prevents oxygen transport and exacerbates tissue hypoxia. CO poisoning and AMS are clinically indistinguishable. If suspected, immediate removal of the patient from the potential CO source with assay of carboxyhemoglobin levels using co-oximetry or lab testing is indicated. Importantly, empirical treatment with oxygen hyperbaria will benefit both conditions. If CO poisoning is suspected, test the patient's affected indoor space and assess other victims who may have been exposed. If testing is not available, the patient should not return to the enclosed space and should descend or use supplemental oxygen, if available.

ALTITUDE AND UNDERLYING MEDICAL CONDITIONS

Individuals with preexisting diseases such as sickle-cell disease, moderate to severe chronic obstructive pulmonary disease (COPD) and coronary artery disease (CAD) may have a more difficult time acclimatizing, because these disease states can be aggravated by the hypoxic atmosphere at higher elevations. eBox 132.1 describes the risk associated with travel to altitude in individuals with a variety of underlying comorbidities.

Respiratory Illnesses

Travelers with COPD have underlying anatomic and physiologic changes that predispose them to development of hypoxemia, sleep apnea, pulmonary hypertension, and ventilation disorders at even moderate altitudes. COPD is a risk factor for the development of AMS. Although oxygen saturation remains more than 90% in a healthy, awake individual until an altitude of 8000 feet, patients with COPD may desaturate below 90% at lower altitudes. High altitude increases hypoxic pulmonary vasoconstriction and may potentiate the development of cor pulmonale, which is known to adversely affect survival at sea level. Individuals with chronic COPD should be advised of the potential need for oxygen supplementation when traveling to moderate altitude, especially if they are already using oxygen at sea level or if dyspnea or fatigue becomes worse. Use of a pulse oximeter can guide the need for increased oxygen supplementation.

Patients with asthma, on the other hand, may have fewer problems at altitude because of decreased ambient allergens and pollutants as well as decreased airflow turbulence. Even those with exercise-induced bronchospasm do not have worsening symptoms while exercising at 5000 feet. In addition, AMS incidence is not increased in asthmatics. People with asthma traveling to higher elevations should continue their usual medications and carry a rescue supply of bronchodilators and steroids.

Patients who ascend to high altitude with preexisting primary or secondary pulmonary hypertension are considered HAPE susceptible, and those with primary pulmonary hypertension are considered at increased risk for HAPE. Patients with known pulmonary hypertension should be advised against travel to higher elevations. If travel cannot be avoided, supplemental oxygen should be used. Prophylactic sustained release nifedipine, 30 mg twice daily for the duration of the stay at altitude, can decrease the risk of HAPE. Phosphodiesterase type-5 inhibitors and dexamethasone may also be used.

Cardiovascular

Individuals with a history of CHF, CAD, dysrhythmias, or coronary bypass surgery are infrequently studied in the high-altitude setting. In theory, people with diseased myocardium should avoid high altitude because of decreased environmental oxygen availability. No studies report increased mortality in visitors to these locations, however. To the contrary, long-term residents at high altitude may be protected from coronary artery disease (CAD) by increased collateral vessel formation or a decrease in the development of atherosclerosis.

All travelers have increased sympathetic activity on initial exposure to high altitude. In patients with heart disease, the resultant increase in heart rate and blood pressure increases cardiac work and myocardial oxygen consumption, which could increase angina symptoms and dysrhythmias. Although both cardiac rhythm abnormalities and ST segment and T wave electrocardiographic changes are reported, none of these changes are associated with clinical evidence of myocardial ischemia. Limited data suggest no increased risk for sudden cardiac death or myocardial infarction at altitudes up to 8000 feet in patients with asymptomatic CAD. When individuals with stable angina are exercised, there is conflicting evidence for the probability of inducing malignant dysrhythmias. Travelers with heart disease who ascend to moderate altitudes do not appear to have an increased incidence of AMS.

Travelers with mild stable CAD should be advised to ascend gradually, to limit activity especially in the first few days at elevation, and to continue anti-anginal and antihypertensive medications. Individuals who have more severe, symptomatic coronary disease or those in a high-risk group (low ejection fraction, abnormal stress test results, and high-grade ventricular ectopy) should avoid travel to high altitudes. Ascent to moderate elevations can be suggested on an individual basis with the previously mentioned precautions. Individuals with heart failure who travel to altitude may require increased use of diuretics to promote diuresis and acclimatization. Patients previously prescribed nitroglycerin should be instructed not to take phosphodiesterase type-5 inhibitors. Acetazolamide prophylaxis may be useful to speed acclimatization and to prevent AMS and its accompanying fluid retention.

Hypertension

High-altitude travel produces a rapid, mild increase in blood pressure and heart rate in healthy individuals because of increased sympathetic tone. This increase is maximal at 2 or 3 weeks, and returns to baseline values over time because of a downregulation of adrenergic receptors if one stays at high altitude or upon descent to sea level. No studies demonstrate an increased predisposition for altitude illness in patients with underlying hypertension.

The incidence of hypertension in sea-level dwellers traveling to high altitude is 10% to 25%. On travel from sea-level to low altitudes (3000 feet), no differences are noted in either normotensive or hypertensive individuals. Above 9800 feet, more significant increases may occur. This suggests that people with severe hypertension should travel to high altitude only under careful monitoring. For individuals who have mild preexisting hypertension, additional treatment is not routinely necessary. Monitor patients with moderate hypertension during the first few days at altitude and continue all antihypertensive medications. For hypertensive patients with a rapid rise in blood pressure who will be staying at altitude for several weeks, an alpha-blocker, nifedipine, or angiotensin-converting enzyme inhibitor are recommended agents to add to the patient's daily regimen.

Seizures

Numerous reports of altitude-provoked seizures exist, but compelling epidemiologic data are lacking. Seizures attributable to high altitude are typically generalized tonic-clonic in nature and a new-onset focal seizure at altitude should prompt a thorough evaluation for a structural brain lesion. Several pathophysiologic mechanisms are implicated. These include sleep deprivation from periodic breathing, hyperventilation, and the direct effect of hypobaric hypoxia. These mechanisms are postulated to induce a metabolic state that lowers the seizure threshold.

Seizures not responding to supportive care can be treated with benzo-diazepines. Should an epileptic who is already taking seizure medicine experience a breakthrough seizure at altitude, standard seizure evaluation is warranted, and acetazolamide at 125 to 250 mg twice daily may be added. Acetazolamide itself has antiepileptic properties and may ameliorate the altitude-related metabolic derangements. As discussed previously, any patient with seizure activity at high altitude should also be assessed for possible HACE.

Sickle Cell Disease

In patients with sickle cell disease, exposure to even low to moderate altitudes (4000 to 6500 feet) will provide additional hypoxic stress. Up to 20% of patients with hemoglobin sickle cell and sickle cell–thalassemia disease may experience a vaso-occlusive crisis, even under pressurized aircraft conditions. Oxygen is therefore advised for air travelers who have sickle cell disease.

Although most people with sickle cell trait remain asymptomatic, this subgroup can experience the development of left upper quadrant pain as a result of splenic ischemia or infarction.

Pregnancy

Studies of permanent high-altitude residents in Colorado and Peru show an increased incidence of complications in maternal, fetal, and neonatal life. Infants born at high altitude have a lower birth weight compared with infants born at sea level because of a combination of factors, including altitude-related effects on fetal growth, changes in uterine blood flow, and increased premature births. As supported by evolutionary genetic studies, patient ethnicity is relevant. At the same elevation, newborns of recently immigrated Han Chinese have lower birth weights than indigenous Tibetans.

Pregnancy-induced hypertension, proteinuria, and peripheral edema (manifestations of toxemia and preeclampsia) are more common at high altitudes and may also be related to maternal and uterine hypoxemia. Although hypertension in pregnancy is more common at high altitudes, no evidence exists for an increase in spontaneous abortions, abruptio placentae, or placenta previa.

Travel by pregnant women to moderate altitudes appears to be safe, but caution is advised for lowland women with normal pregnancies who wish to travel above 13,000 feet, for pregnant women who wish to remain at high altitude for a prolonged period, and for women with complicated or high-risk pregnancies.

Radial Keratotomy

Patients with a history of radial keratotomy may experience hyperopic (farsighted) visual changes with ascent above 9000 feet. This results from corneal swelling from ambient hypoxia because the cornea is markedly sensitive to both systemic and ambient oxygen tension. In normal corneas, this swelling is uniform. After radial keratotomy, the swelling is exacerbated and inconsistent secondary to the pattern of the incisions. Photorefractive keratotomy and LASIK, which use laser techniques that do not produce incisions but instead shave the cornea and corneal stroma, respectively, do not result in similar problems.

ACKNOWLEDGMENT

The author would like to acknowledge Drs. Benjamin Honigman, Michael Yaron, Ryan D. Paterson, and Christopher B. Davis for their contributions to previous editions of this chapter.

The references for this chapter can be found online at ExpertConsult.com.

Drowning

David B. Richards

FOUNDATIONS

Background and Importance

Traditionally, the terminology describing drowning injuries has been confusing and impractical. In the past, *drowning* referred to death within 24 hours of suffocation from submersion in a liquid, whereas *near-drowning* described victims who survived at least 24 hours past the initial event regardless of the outcome. The World Health Organization (WHO) published a new policy defining drowning to clarify documentation and to better track drowning injuries worldwide. *Drowning* was defined as "the process of experiencing respiratory impairment from submersion/immersion in liquid." Furthermore, the WHO policy states, "Drowning outcomes should be classified as: death, morbidity, and no morbidity; the terms wet, dry, active, passive, silent, and secondary drowning should no longer be used." Also, the term *near-drowning* should not be used, and the associated term *drowning with a fatal outcome* should be abandoned.

Immersion syndrome refers specifically to syncope resulting from cardiac dysrhythmias on sudden contact with water that is at least 5°C lower than body temperature. The risk is proportional to the difference between body temperature and water temperature. Wetting of the face and head before entrance into the water may prevent the inciting sequence of events. Putative mechanisms for the syndrome are vagal stimulation leading to asystole and ventricular fibrillation secondary to QT prolongation after a massive release of catecholamines on contact with cold water. The resultant loss of consciousness leads to secondary drowning.

Each year an estimated 360,000 people die of drowning worldwide, a rate of approximately 40 individuals an hour, most of whom are children. Low- and middle-income countries account for more than 90% of all drowning deaths and a disproportionate share of years of life lost. Drowning is among the top ten causes of mortality for children and young people worldwide.

In the United States, drowning is the tenth most common cause of unintentional death, accounting for 3709 deaths (1.1 per 100,000) in 2017. Among children 1 to 4 years old, drowning is the leading cause of injury mortality; for 5- to 9-year-olds, it is second only to motor vehicle crashes.[1]

The incidence of drowning with nonfatal outcomes is not well documented. The Centers for Disease Control and Prevention (CDC) estimates that for every child who dies by drowning in the United States, another five receive emergency department (ED) care for a drowning event, and half of these children require hospitalization.[2] Among all age groups, an estimated one to four hospitalizations secondary to nonfatal drownings occur for every drowning death. The economic implications of drowning injuries are profound. In Australia, drowning-related injuries have the highest average lifetime cost ($40,000 USD per patient) of any injury type.

Drownings occur in domestic settings such as swimming pools, hot tubs, bathtubs, large buckets, and rainwater tanks and in all forms of natural bodies of water. A review of all drowning deaths among individuals younger than 20 years old in the United States during a 1-year period revealed that 55% of infants younger than 1 year old drown in bathtubs, and nearly 16% drown in large household buckets. Most (56%) children 1 to 4 years old drown in artificial pools, whereas most (63%) deaths among older children occur in natural bodies of fresh water.

Because of natural disasters, the incidence of drowning injuries and fatalities is rising. In disasters such as floods and tsunamis, older populations are disproportionately affected. A study from hurricane Katrina found that 49% of fatalities were in people 75 years old or older.

Age, gender, and race affect incidence of drowning. Toddlers (1–3 years old) and those over 80 years old are at greatest risk of death by drowning, with annual incidences of 2.5 and 2.1 per 100,000, respectively. Males account for almost 75% of victims.[1] Indigenous American and Alaska Native children between 1 and 4 years old have the highest annual incidence of drowning mortality (3.8 per 100,000), and black teenagers between 11 and 12 years old drown in swimming pools at ten times the rate of white children of the same age. The risk of death by drowning for all ages of the American Indigenous and Alaska Native population is 80% higher than the United States population as a whole.[3,4]

Ethanol consumption in proximity with water is a major risk factor for drowning. Acute ethanol intoxication may be a contributing factor in up to 50% of drownings among adults and adolescents.[5] The risk of death from drowning while using watercraft is directly proportional to an operator's blood ethanol concentration (BEC). The odds ratios of fatality from drowning follow a trend from 2.8 for a BEC of 1 to 49 mg/dL to 37.4 for a BEC of 150 mg/dL or greater compared with sober case controls.

Drowning in the United States is seasonal, with most occurring during the summer months. Two-thirds of pediatric deaths occur between the months of May and August. Drowning injuries are 48% more likely to occur on weekends than weekdays and drowning victims older than 20 years old are most often participating in water sports or using watercraft.[6]

The relationship between swimming ability and the risk of drowning is unclear. No direct evidence exists to suggest that inexperienced swimmers are more likely to drown. On the contrary, skilled swimmers have greater exposure time in water and may be more prone to drowning incidents.

Numerous medical conditions confer an increased likelihood of drowning injury. Seizure disorders increase the chance of drowning among children and adolescents nearly 20-fold and longitudinal studies of patients with epilepsy found that 10% of deaths were due to drowning. Autism and other developmental and behavioral disorders increase risk in children as well. Immersion in cold water extends the QT interval, thus increasing the risk of dysrhythmias in individuals with baseline prolonged QT syndrome.

Anatomy, Physiology, and Pathophysiology

Unexpected submersion triggers breath-holding, panic, and a struggle to surface. Air hunger and hypoxia develop, and the victim begins to swallow water. As breath-holding is overcome, involuntary gasps result in aspiration. The quantity of fluid aspirated, rather than the composition, determines subsequent pulmonary system derangement.

The pathophysiologic differences between freshwater and saltwater aspiration with respect to resultant electrolyte imbalance, hemolysis, and fluid compartment shifting do not occur until the amount of aspirated water is significantly more than the typical drowning victim aspirates. In one review of the hospital treatment of drowning victims, no patient required emergent intervention for a significant electrolyte abnormality. Aspiration of 1 to 3 mL/kg of either fresh water or saltwater destroys the integrity of pulmonary surfactant, leading to alveolar collapse, atelectasis, noncardiogenic pulmonary edema, intrapulmonary shunting, and ventilation-perfusion mismatch. Profound hypoxia and metabolic and respiratory acidosis ensue, leading to cardiovascular collapse, neuronal injury, and ultimately death.

The classic hypothesis was that 10% to 15% of drowning victims die without aspiration of a significant amount of water. Death from such dry drowning purportedly results from severe laryngospasm causing hypoxia, convulsion, and death without entry of fluid into the lungs. An exhaustive review of the literature failed to corroborate this hypothesis. Dry drownings more appropriately reflect deaths from other causes (e.g., fatal cardiac dysrhythmias and severe hypothermia) than from simple submersion.

Many factors may influence the pathophysiologic sequence of events in drowning and affect the chance of survival, including age, water temperature, duration and degree of hypothermia, diving reflex, and effectiveness of resuscitative efforts. Children have a lower ratio of body mass to surface area and, therefore, develop hypothermia more quickly and to a greater degree after immersion in cold water than adults do. Hypothermia lowers cerebral metabolic rate and is neuroprotective to some extent for victims of submersion injury. Despite dramatic case reports of patients surviving prolonged submersion in cold water with full neurologic recovery, hypothermia is generally a poor prognostic finding. Cold-water immersion speeds the development of exhaustion, altered consciousness, and cardiac dysrhythmia. The *diving reflex*, an involuntary physiologic response to cold submersion that includes apnea, bradycardia, and increased peripheral vascular resistance, may play a protective role in infant and child submersions. The diving reflex works to shunt blood centrally to the heart and brain, thereby prolonging the duration of submersion tolerated without central nervous system (CNS) damage. The evidence to date, however, has not shown a clear correlation between outcome and water temperature.

CLINICAL FEATURES

History and Physical Examination

Many drowning episodes are witnessed. Toddler drownings are an important exception, however, often occurring because of a lapse in supervision. Signs of pulmonary injury may be obvious in a drowning victim who is hypoxic, cyanotic, and in respiratory distress or arrest. More subtle clues, such as increased respiratory rate and audible rhonchi, rales, or wheezes on pulmonary auscultation, should alert the clinician to evolving respiratory compromise. Drowning victims swallow a significantly greater volume of water than is aspirated, and gastric distention from positive-pressure ventilation during rescue is common. As a result, 60% of patients vomit soon after a drowning event. Aspiration of gastric contents greatly compounds the degree of pulmonary injury and increases the likelihood that acute respiratory distress syndrome (ARDS) will ensue. In addition, aspiration of particulate contaminants such as mud, algae, sewage, and bacteria may obstruct the smaller bronchi and bronchioles and greatly increase the risk of infection (both bacterial and fungal in nature).

Victims with CNS injury may present with symptoms ranging from mild lethargy to coma with fixed and dilated pupils. CNS injury results from the initial hypoxic or ischemic insult and from the cascade of reperfusion injury that follows reestablishment of cerebral blood flow after a cardiopulmonary arrest. The release of inflammatory mediators and the generation of oxygen free radicals in the post-resuscitative period contribute to cytotoxic cerebral edema, compromise of the blood-brain barrier, and increased intracranial pressure.

Cardiac dysrhythmias may incite drowning or develop as a consequence. Hypoxemia, acidosis, and, potentially, hypothermia are the primary factors responsible for dysrhythmias ranging from ventricular tachycardia and fibrillation to bradycardia-asystole. Electrolyte disturbances are rarely significant enough to be dysrhythmogenic.

Other clinical sequelae of drowning may include acute renal injury, which is present on admission in approximately 50% of patients as the result of lactic acidosis; prolonged hypoperfusion; and, in some instances, rhabdomyolysis. Hypothermia-related coagulopathy or disseminated intravascular coagulation (DIC) may occur.

Prognostic Factors

Many factors help predict patients who will survive a drowning injury neurologically intact. Hypoxia, which is usually dependent on submersion time, is the most important factor related to outcome and subsequent quality of life in drowning victims. Drowning victims who arrive in the ED alert with normal hemodynamics are unlikely to experience neurologic impairment. Victims younger than 3 years old, submersion for longer than 5 to 10 minutes, and initiation of cardiopulmonary resuscitation (CPR) more than 10 minutes after rescue portend a poor prognosis. Adverse neurologic findings on initial presentation do not preclude full neurologic recovery, although in general, patients whose duration of submersion or resuscitation exceeds 10 minutes have an unfavorable outcome.[7] With the exception of victim age, however, such measurements are often unknown or inaccurately estimated at the time of a patient's arrival in the ED. On arrival, objective findings associated with an unfavorable prognosis include hypothermia, severe acidosis, unreactive pupils, a Glasgow Coma Scale score of 3, and asystole or the need for ongoing CPR. Neurologically intact survival is reported for individual patients even with several of these factors present; however, none of the proposed scoring systems using combinations of these variables has 100% predictive power.

Children who present with an abnormal head computed tomography (CT) scan (e.g., intracranial bleed, cerebral edema) within the first 24 hours have a nearly 100% mortality rate. Furthermore, an abnormal head CT scan at any time is associated with poor outcome (persistent vegetative state (PVS), post-coma unresponsiveness (PCU) or death).

DIFFERENTIAL DIAGNOSES

The precipitants of a drowning, such as drug or ethanol intoxication, cardiac arrest, hypothermia, hypoglycemia, seizure, and attempted suicide or homicide, should be considered in patients found unresponsive in water. For pediatric victims, child abuse or neglect should also be considered a potential cause. Potential head or cervical spine injury is an important consideration in drowning associated with diving injuries or trauma.

DIAGNOSTIC TESTING

Initiate cardiac monitoring and obtain an electrocardiogram (ECG) to determine the presence of significant dysrhythmias, QT prolongation, or ischemia. Monitor pulse oximetry, capnography, and arterial or venous blood gases closely for signs of hypoxemia, hypercarbia, and acidosis. Blood glucose, serum creatinine, and electrolyte values should be obtained, although serum creatinine concentration and electrolyte levels are usually normal on initial presentation. Similarly, complete blood count is often normal with the exception of leukocytosis. Serum ethanol levels and urine toxicology screening may be appropriate for illicit drugs, depending on the circumstances of the drowning. Subsequently, evidence of renal failure, hepatic dysfunction, and DIC may be noted on laboratory testing.

The initial chest radiograph is often unremarkable and may underestimate the severity of pulmonary injury. Infiltrates or pulmonary edema may be evident within hours; therefore, repeat radiographs are indicted with persistent respiratory symptoms. Initial chest radiographs are often unremarkable even in the setting of serious and evolving pathologic processes.

Electroencephalography to assess for seizure activity should be performed, if available, in the obtunded drowning victim. Head CT scans are rarely initially contributory unless significant trauma or other pertinent injury is suspected. Magnetic resonance imaging (MRI) of the brain may predict neurologic outcome after drowning, but its prognostic value is not optimal until 3 or 4 days have elapsed and is therefore not indicated in the emergency setting.

MANAGEMENT

Salient details of the events surrounding the incident should be ascertained rapidly from family, friends, or EMS personnel. Resuscitation of pulseless and apneic patients should be attempted initially in most cases because bystander estimates of total submersion time are often inaccurate. The clinical presentation of severe hypothermia often mimics death, and functional recovery is possible for hypothermic individuals submerged for significant periods of time.

For a victim without measurable vital signs or signs of life, outcome depends on the interval preceding CPR.[8] Since most cases are hypoxia-driven cardiac arrests, CPR with assisted ventilations may be more effective than compression-only CPR, although this has not been well studied. Mouth-to-mouth ventilation while in the water should be attempted but not at the cost of prolonging the extrication.[9] Chest compressions are impractical before extrication but should be initiated as soon as the individual is placed on a solid surface, such as a boat deck, poolside, or beach.

Cervical spine injuries are rare in drowning victims. Patients more likely to have cervical spine injuries tend to have either clinical signs of serious trauma or a history of motor vehicle crash, fall from height, or diving into the water. Unless such factors are present, routine cervical spine immobilization for submersion victims is not warranted.

On arrival in the ED, cardiac monitoring and continuous pulse oximetry should be established. A core temperature obtained with a low-reading probe is indicated for any unstable or lethargic patient. Values obtained by use of infrared ear thermometry are unreliable in drowning victims. Rewarming of a hypothermic patient may suffice for hemodynamic stabilization and improvement in mental status. A spontaneously breathing patient should be monitored for signs of developing pulmonary injury.

As with any patient, expected clinical course, mental status and objective determination of the adequacy of oxygenation and ventilation should determine the decision for tracheal intubation. If an arterial blood gas is obtained, a partial pressure of carbon dioxide ($Paco_2$) greater than 50 mm Hg should warn the clinician that intubation and lung protective ventilation is likely needed. Patients unable to maintain oxygen saturation greater than 90% despite high-flow supplemental oxygen, require positive airway pressure to increase alveolar recruitment, decrease intrapulmonary shunting, and reduce ventilation-perfusion mismatch. In awake patients, this may be accomplished by face or nasal mask (continuous positive airway pressure), but the risk of potential gastric distention, vomiting, and aspiration should be considered. Otherwise, tracheal intubation and lung-protective ventilation are indicated. The hemodynamic consequences of positive end-expiratory pressure should be monitored carefully, because increased intrathoracic pressure may compromise venous return and cardiac output. Decreased cranial venous return may impede cerebral perfusion.

No consensus exists with regard to the appropriate length of resuscitative effort for hypothermic drowning victims in the ED. The safest parameter is to continue until the core temperature reaches at least 32°C to 35°C, because cerebral death cannot be diagnosed accurately in severely hypothermic patients with temperatures below this level. This parameter may not always be practical, however, because brain-dead patients are often poikilothermic.

The administration of corticosteroids in the setting of drowning and potential ARDS does not improve outcome. Barbiturate-induced coma, diuresis, neuromuscular blockade, and hyperventilation do not improve neurologic outcome and, particularly in the case of hyperventilation, may be harmful. Similarly, empirical antibiotics do not increase survival and should be administered only to the patient who was submerged in grossly contaminated water or who shows signs of infection or sepsis.

Interventions, such as induced or permissive hypothermia, aimed at attenuation of reperfusion injury after anoxic brain insult are the focus of intense investigative effort. Drowning victims in cardiac arrest are usually colder than 30°C and require warming. Comatose patients who have been resuscitated after reasonable submersion time regardless of rhythm should not be rewarmed above 34°C. Rewarming only up to 34°C followed by a 24-hour mild hypothermic treatment before normothermia is reached may be advantageous because of decreased pulmonary reperfusion injury and reduced secondary brain injury. Emerging resuscitation literature indicates an emerging role for therapeutic hypothermia in drowning victims.[10]

DISPOSITION

Symptomatic patients should be admitted for treatment. Patients with a history of apnea, unconsciousness, intoxication, or hypoxia and any patients who manifest cardiac dysrhythmias or an abnormal chest radiographs also require admission. Patients who are asymptomatic on presentation to the ED, maintain normal room air oxygen saturation, and have no chest radiograph abnormalities can be discharged safely after an observation period of 8 hours.[11,12] Careful instructions about symptoms or signs of delayed pulmonary complications are necessary, and the patient should be discharged in the care of a competent adult.

Preventive Efforts and Discharge Education

For survivors of a drowning episode, discharge instructions with a focus on parental education and future preventative measures are critical. Canadian research has shown that drowning was in the top three causes of death and costs per hospitalization for youths under the age of 19 years and identified prevention of drowning as a high-yield priority.[13] An Australian study highlighted this by demonstrating a $830 million annual economic burden in Australia alone.[14] In low-income countries, drowning deaths (particularly in children) are on the rise. In high-income countries, drowning morbidity and mortality are on the decline although the exact causes of this decline are unclear. An increased public awareness of preventive measures and an emphasis on public education with regard to bystander CPR and the dangers of ethanol use in conjunction with water-related activities are contributing significantly to the reduction in fatalities, in some locations by over 80%.

Parental education about the danger of pediatric drowning is an important focus of preventive efforts. Inadequate supervision of children playing in or near water is one of the most common causes of pediatric submersion death, underscoring the importance of increasing awareness of the need for constant oversight of children in this setting. Most pediatric submersion injuries in swimming pools occur at the victim's home. In most cases, the child is last seen in the house, is left unattended for a moment, and enters the pool on an unfenced side closest to the home with no audible splash or screaming. Fully circumferential fencing with functioning door locks or latching mechanisms of residential pools is a current recommendation of the American Academy of Pediatrics (AAP). Drowning or submersion is 3.7 times more likely in a nonfenced pool than in a properly fenced pool. In Australia, safety legislation is associated with a 30% reduction in drowning rates in young children. Unfortunately, legislation requiring appropriate fencing is poorly adhered to, and only 40% of households are compliant. Legislation requiring personal floatation device usage in recreational boaters in Australia has resulted in a significant decrease in drowning deaths.

Effective approaches to prevention efforts in low- and middle-income countries differ from those in high-income countries.[15] Data from almost 100,000 children in Bangladesh either entered into swim lessons or kept in a common supervision area in the community showed relative risks of drowning of 0.072 and 0.181, respectively. Both interventions were found to be extremely cost effective.[16]

Emergency care providers are a vital resource for enhancement of public awareness of the importance of these measures. The literature supports the concept that education in the ED highlighting drowning prevention can have a positive impact on patient and family awareness of steps to lessen the likelihood of catastrophic drowning injury.

The references for this chapter can be found online at ExpertConsult. com.

Radiation Injuries

Jillian L. Theobald and J. Marc Liu

FOUNDATIONS

Background and Importance

Radiation is energy that travels through space in the form of a particle or wave.[1] It is produced by radioactive decay of an unstable atom (radionuclide or radioisotope) or by the interaction of a particle with matter. *Particle radiation* consists of particles that have mass and energy and may carry an electric charge. Examples of particle radiation include alpha particles (helium nuclei), protons, beta particles (electrons ejected from the nucleus), and neutrons. *Electromagnetic radiation* consists of photons that have energy but no mass or charge. Radiation can be either ionizing or nonionizing depending on its energy and ability to penetrate matter. Electromagnetic radiation varies by frequency and wavelength as shown in Figure 134.1.

Radioactive decay (radioactivity) is the process by which a nucleus of an unstable atom loses energy by emitting ionizing radiation in the form of high-energy particles or rays. Radioactive decay can emit particles (e.g., alpha and beta) or rays such as gamma or x-rays. Gamma rays and x-rays are high-energy photons that differ in their place of origin: gamma rays are emitted from the nucleus, whereas x-rays are produced as the result of changes in the positions of electrons orbiting the nucleus.

The type and rate of radioactive decay varies by radionuclide. The rate of decay is measured by the radioactive half-life (the time for half the radioactive nuclei in any sample to undergo radioactive decay) and varies from a few microseconds to billions of years. Radiation exposure can be external (e.g., exposure to x-rays) or internal, resulting from the inhalation, ingestion, or injection of radioisotopes.

Radiation Measurements

The four different but interrelated units for measuring radiation (radioactivity, exposure, absorbed dose, and dose equivalent) are shown in Table 134.1. These units are also commonly expressed as fractions of whole units using the terms and abbreviations milli (m; 1/1000th) and micro (μ; 1/1,000,000th).[1]

Radiation Protection

The principles of radiation protection include time, distance, shielding, and quantity. Reducing the time of radiation exposure will reduce the absorbed dose. The intensity of radiation is a function of distance from the source and follows the inverse square law: the dose of radiation decreases inversely with the square of the distance. For instance, if you double the distance from the source you decrease the radiation exposure by a fourth. Shielding is the placement of an absorber (material that reduces radiation) between the person and the source. The effectiveness of shielding varies with the type of the radiation. For example, alpha particles can be stopped by a thin piece of paper or even the dermal cells in the outer layer of the skin, whereas thick, dense shielding like lead or concrete is necessary to protect against gamma rays. Limiting the quantity of radioactive material in the work area will also decrease exposure. National and international regulatory bodies set acceptable limits for occupational and population exposures to radiation.

Radiation Sources

Ionizing radiation and radioactive substances are natural and permanent features of the environment. The average annual radiation dose per person in the United States is 6.2 mSv (620 mrem). Fifty percent of this average dose comes from background radiation and 48% from medical procedures. The major sources of background radiation are radon and thoron (37%), cosmic radiation (5%), naturally occurring internal radioisotopes (e.g., potassium-40 [5%]), and terrestrial background radiation (3%). The major medical sources include computed tomography (CT; 24%), nuclear medicine (12%), interventional fluoroscopy (7%), and conventional radiography and fluoroscopy (5%). The remainder of the average annual radiation dose comes from occupational and consumer sources.[2]

Radon is a naturally occurring radioactive gas that is formed from the radioactive decay of uranium. Radon can accumulate in homes and is the second leading cause of lung cancer in the United States after tobacco exposure.[3] Radon exposure is estimated by measuring radon

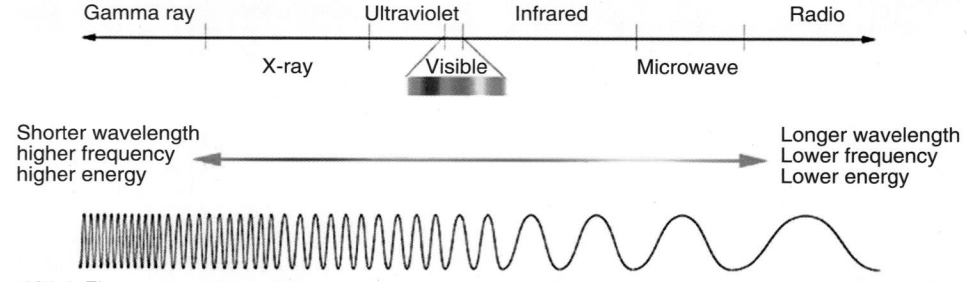

Fig. 134.1 Electromagnetic radiation varies by frequency and wavelength. (National Aeronautics and Space Administration: Imagine the universe: the electromagnetic spectrum. Available at: http://imagine.gsfc.nasa.gov/science/toolbox/emspectrum1.html.)

TABLE 134.1	Radiation Units Description and Conversion Factors			
Measure	**Description**	**United States Units**	**International Units**	**Conversion**
Radioactivity	Amount of ionizing radiation released by a material	Curie (Ci)	Becquerel (Bq)	1 Bq = 2.7 × 10⁻¹¹ C
Exposure	Amount of radiation traveling through air	Roentgen (R)	Coulomb (C)/kg	1 C/kg = 3875.9 R
Absorbed dose	Amount of radiation absorbed by a person	Radiation absorbed dose (Rad)	Gray (Gy)	1 Gy = 100 rad
Dose equivalent (effective dose)	Combines the amount of radiation absorbed with the tissue damaging potential of the type of radiation	Roentgen equivalent man (Rem)	Sievert (Sv)	1 Sv = 100 rem

levels in the air using inexpensive and readily available kits. If indoor levels of radon are 4 pCi/L or greater, then the US Environmental Protection Agency (EPA) recommends that the homeowner consult a certified radon mitigation specialist to reduce radon air levels in the home.

Although radiation-related incidents are rare, the consequences of exposure or significant internal contamination can be fatal. The Radiation Emergency Assistance Center at Oak Ridge National Laboratory maintains a worldwide registry of serious radiation incidents. Between 1944 and 2012, there have been 454 radiation incidents recorded worldwide. The greatest numbers of serious exposures have occurred with sealed sources, which include brachytherapy sources used in radiation oncology and industrial radiography devices (n = 214), followed by x-ray devices (n = 86). Radioisotopes used in medical diagnosis and therapy have caused approximately 10% of major radiation incidents.

Serious nuclear power incidents include the Fukushima Daiichi disaster (2011), the Chernobyl disaster (1986), Three Mile Island (1979), and the SL-1 accident (1961). The radioisotopes most commonly released from nuclear reactor accidents include iodine, cesium, and strontium. Chernobyl had the largest number of radiation-related injuries. About 150 individuals who received very high whole-body doses were treated for acute radiation sickness; 28 of these died within a relatively short time, and approximately 20 more have since died from radiation-related diseases.[4] Radiation to the thyroid from radioisotopes of iodine released during the Chernobyl event has caused several thousand cases of thyroid cancer, with children being the most susceptible population.

The detonation of nuclear bombs has the greatest potential to produce mass casualties. The acute and long-term effects following the bomb blasts in Hiroshima and Nagasaki in 1945 (18 and 22 kilotons) have been well documented. Today's nuclear weapons are orders of magnitude potentially more devastating. Another threat is the detonation of a low-yield nuclear bomb by terrorists. A 10-kiloton nuclear detonation within a city in the United States would result in a zone of destruction of more than 2 miles from ground zero and would expose hundreds of thousands of people to radiation.[5] A more likely terrorist scenario is the explosion of a *dirty bomb*. A dirty bomb is the combination of a conventional explosive with a radioisotope. The radioisotopes most likely to be used in a dirty bomb are cesium-137, cobalt-60, or strontium-90.[6] Although the acute radiation risks from a dirty bomb detonation are low, the localized residual radiation contamination would likely cause widespread panic.

Anatomy, Physiology, and Pathophysiology

The biologic effects of radiation exposure are determined by the type of radiation, the total dose, the dose rate, the volume of tissue or anatomic body part irradiated, and individual susceptibility factors. The amount of energy released in matter (linear energy transfer) varies by type of radiation. Different types of radiation are assigned a quality factor (QF) based on their ability to produce biologic damage in exposed tissue. The higher the QF, the more biologically damaging the radiation is. Gamma rays, x-rays, and beta particles have a QF of 1. Alpha particles (internal exposure only) have a QF of 20, whereas neutrons have a QF range of 3 to 20, depending on their energy.

Ionizing radiation includes particles and photons that have sufficient energy to detach electrons, thus causing ionization of the atoms that they encounter. Alpha particles, beta particles, and neutrons are examples of particle ionizing radiation. Only the high-frequency portion of the electromagnetic radiation spectrum (gamma rays, x-rays, and far-ultraviolet) has sufficient energy to produce ionization. Other frequencies and wavelengths (near-ultraviolet, infrared, microwaves, radio waves, and very or extremely low frequency radiation) are considered *nonionizing*. The health effects of exposure to nonionizing radiation depend on the frequency and wavelength. For example, ultraviolet light can produce sunburns, visible light (such as lasers), can produce corneal and retinal burns, and microwaves can produce heating of body tissues.

TABLE 134.2 Systemic Radiation Effects Based on Dose

Dose (gray)			
12 +	→ Bone Marrow Suppression	Neurovascular syndrome onset	Multiple organ failure
11			Probable death
10			Consider stem cell transplants
9			
8			
7			LD 50/60 with supportive care
6		Gastrointestinal syndrome onset	
5			LD 50/60 without treatment
4			
3			
2			≈100% survival without treatment
1		Hematopoietic syndrome onset	
0			

Adapted from: The Medical Aspects of Radiation Incidents; originally published by ORISE and REAC/TS under contract number DE-AC05-06OR23100 between the US Department of Energy and ORAU, 2013.

The effects of ionizing radiation on tissue can be *direct* or *indirect*. Direct effects include single- and double-strand DNA breaks. Indirect effects act through generation of free radicals that then attack other molecules in the cell. Cells vary in their sensitivity to radiation. In general, cells that are undifferentiated, divide quickly, and have high metabolic activity are most radiosensitive. Examples of these types of cells include bone marrow stem cells, lymphocytes, spermatogonia, ovarian cells, intestinal crypt cells, and epidermal basal cells. Less radiosensitive tissues and organs are made up of cells with little or no turnover such as connective tissue or the central nervous system. The effects of radiation can be *deterministic* or *stochastic*. Deterministic effects are those in which the severity of injury is a function of dose (e.g., bone marrow suppression). Stochastic or probabilistic effects are those in which the probability of an effect, rather than its severity, is a function of dose. An example of a stochastic effect is the development of radiation-induced cancer.

For external exposure, the site of the body that is irradiated (e.g., bone marrow vs. upper extremity) is an important determinant of the resulting effects. For internal exposure, the biodisposition of the radioisotope, its radiologic and biologic half-lives, as well as the types of radioisotopes produced during radioactive decay are important determinants of the effects. *Biodisposition* refers to the absorption, distribution, metabolism, and excretion of a radioisotope.

The *effective half-life* reflects both the radiologic and biologic half-life and can be calculated as 1/effective half-life = 1/biologic half-life + 1/physical half-life.[7] For example, iodine-131 has an approximate biologic half-life of 57 days and a radiologic half-life of 8 days. The resulting effective half-life is approximately 7 days.

Radioisotopes will have their greatest effects at the sites in the body where they are concentrated. For example, radioiodine concentrates in the thyroid gland and the resulting effects, such as thyroiditis or thyroid cancer, occur at the site of concentration.

Routes of Exposure

An individual can be exposed to radiation by one or a combination of three processes: irradiation, incorporation, and contamination.

Irradiation occurs when an object or person is exposed to a radioactive source. An object does not become radioactive unless neutron activation occurs. When a person is irradiated, such as a patient who has just received a CT scan or x-ray, no hazard exists to medical personnel who come into contact with the patient.

Contamination is the presence of radioactive matter on or in an object. Contamination usually occurs externally but may be internal if the radioactive material is ingested or inhaled with continued radiation emitted by the contaminating substance. However, in almost all cases, contamination is not an acute threat to the life of the patient or the health care provider, and its presence should not preclude institution of lifesaving measures. The radioactive particulate matter may emit radiation with an effect that is directly related to the time of exposure, distance from the source, and type of contamination.

Incorporation occurs when a radioactive material is taken up by a tissue, cell, or organ. This can occur through ingestion, inhalation, or absorption via an open wound.

CLINICAL FEATURES

Acute Radiation Syndrome

Acute radiation syndrome (ARS) occurs after a patient is exposed to whole body radiation. ARS from external or internal exposure to radiation varies in nature and severity by dose, dose rate, dose distribution, and individual susceptibility. There are three phases to ARS: prodromal, latent, and manifest illness. The progression and patterns of symptoms and signs of the phases of ARS can overlap. The timing of the progression through the phases can be accelerated with increasing radiation doses.[8]

In the *prodromal phase,* initial symptoms are typically nonspecific, and include anorexia, nausea, vomiting, and fatigue. This phase is useful to help predict the severity of the radiation injury. The presence, onset, and frequency of nausea and vomiting, although nonspecific, can serve as a prognostic factor. Early onset or persistent nausea and vomiting as well as the presence of diarrhea, indicate a more severe radiation injury.

The *latent phase* is a period of initial symptom improvement. Patients may even become symptom-free. Those victims with lethal radiation doses may not have a symptom-free period and progress from the prodromal phase directly to the manifest illness phase.

The *manifest illness phase* has three sub-syndromes that may occur and overlap depending on the radiation dose received (Table 134.2). All organs are affected by radiation. However, the relative sensitivities of the organ systems exposed to radiation determines the clinical symptoms. Tissues with greater rates of cellular division, particularly the hematopoietic and gastrointestinal systems, are most radiosensitive.

TABLE 134.3   Local Irradiation Symptoms by Dose

Threshold Dose (Gy)	Symptoms	Time To Onset (Days)
3	Epilation	14 to 18
6	Early erythema	14 to 21
10	Dry desquamation	25 to 30
15	Wet desquamation	20 to 28
>20	Ulceration and necrosis	>21

The hematopoietic sub-syndrome is the first sub-syndrome seen. This sub-syndrome can appear at doses greater than 1 Gy and typically results in bone marrow suppression. At doses less than 1 Gy (100 rem), most cells survive but may be susceptible to radiation-induced cancer.[9] Lymphocytes are the first cell line to decrease and with high doses of radiation this drop will occur sooner and with greater severity. The hematopoietic system in children has been estimated to be more than twice as radiosensitive as in adults.[10]

The gastrointestinal sub-syndrome begins to occur at doses nearing 6 Gy, about 1 week after exposure. Patients will display nausea, vomiting, gastrointestinal bleeding, malabsorption, and fluid losses, potentially leading to hypovolemia and cardiovascular collapse. These symptoms are due to death of the intestinal epithelial precursor cells and resultant denuding of the intestinal epithelial surface. Thrombocytopenia and immunosuppression from the accompanying hematopoietic sub-syndrome also predispose patients to infection and bleeding.[11]

The neurovascular sub-syndrome results from doses greater than 10 Gy and is typically lethal. Patients will develop irritability, altered mental status, seizures, prostration, ataxia, and hypotension. Coma and death usually occur within a few hours. Because of the high dose of radiation needed to produce these findings, patients often die without experiencing a latent phase.[11]

Local Radiation Injury

Cutaneous involvement can occur following a radiation exposure. It can be one component of ARS with other organ involvement or it can occur alone.[11] Radiation injury limited to the skin and the tissues located directly beneath the area of injury is termed a *local radiation injury (LRI)*. This injury typically happens after a patient handles or has close contact with an industrial radioactive source. LRI can also result from medical testing or therapy, such as fluoroscopy, nuclear medicine studies, and CT scans.[12] Inflammation, oxidative damage, and damage to the microvasculature are all involved in the pathophysiology of LRI. Hair loss occurs after exposure to 3 Gy, and erythema is seen after exposure to 6 Gy. Wet desquamation, a loss of epithelial thickness and integrity leading to fluid loss, occurs after 15 Gy, and necrosis occurs after 20 to 25 Gy of localized skin exposure (Table 134.3).[13,14]

DIFFERENTIAL DIAGNOSES

The initial signs and symptoms following radiation exposure are nonspecific and include anorexia, nausea, vomiting, and fatigue. In the absence of an exposure history, these symptoms in the prodromal phase of acute radiation sickness can be confused for gastroenteritis with its long list of differential diagnoses. Neutropenia seen after whole body radiation exposure also has many other etiologies, including viral infections, medication-induced, certain autoimmune or oncological disorders, and nutritional deficiency.

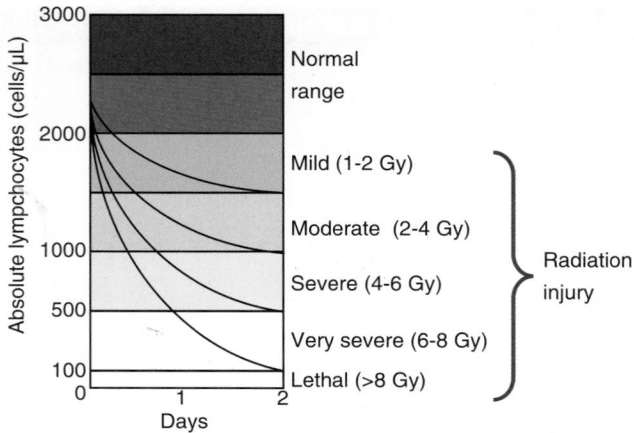

Fig. 134.2 Lymphocyte decrease over time following radiation injury. (Adapted from: Andrews GA, Auxier JA, Lushbaugh CC. The importance of dosimetry to the medical management of persons exposed to high levels of radiation. In: *Personal Dosimetry for Radiation Accidents.* Vienna: International Atomic Energy Agency; 1965.)

The severe symptoms following high-dose radiation injury resulting in the neurovascular sub-syndrome can occur with any catastrophic cardiovascular or neurologic event. Local radiation injuries can appear similar to thermal or sun exposure burns but differ in their progression over time.

DIAGNOSTIC TESTING

If contamination with radioactive material is a possibility, then the patient should be surveyed with a contamination survey instrument (e.g., Geiger Muller detector). These very sensitive detectors measure the presence of radioactive material in counts per minute. There are a variety of other radiation detection devices that are designed to measure field strength in units of mrem/hour or μSv/hour. These latter types of instruments are most often used to measure radiation fields at an incident scene or "hot zone." The hospital radiation safety officer should be consulted to assist in performing radiation surveys of potentially contaminated patients or objects.

Quantifying the absorbed dose of radiation can be challenging, especially in the emergency department (ED). Information on the radiation source, field strength, time of exposure, distance, shielding, and routes of exposure is often incomplete. Although radiation doses can be reconstructed at a later time by health physicists, emergency clinicians will most often rely on biodosimetric tools, such as time to vomiting and lymphocyte depletion kinetics. These online tools are available at www.remm.nlm.gov/ars_wbd.htm#vomit.

A baseline complete blood count (CBC) with differential and absolute lymphocyte count should be obtained and repeated every 6 hours for the first 24 hours and at least daily thereafter. The absolute lymphocyte count at 48 hours after exposure is a good predictor of radiation injury (Fig. 134.2). If the absolute lymphocyte count at 48 hours is greater than 1200 cells/μL, it is unlikely that the patient has received a clinically significant dose of radiation. If the absolute lymphocyte count falls between 100 and 500 cells/μL at 48 hours, a significant or even lethal dose of radiation should be suspected. A level in this range is an indication for neutropenic precautions.[11] Thrombocytopenia and anemia may develop weeks later because these cell lines are less radiosensitive. Serum lipase, liver function tests, and C-reactive protein (CRP) should also be obtained and repeated daily. If the patient has been internally exposed to radioisotopes, rather than just external radiation,

TABLE 134.4 Available Resources for Assistance and Consultation During a Radiation Incident and Informational Resources

Organization	Contact	Website
Consultative		
Radiation Emergency Assistance Center/Training Site (REAC/TS)	24-hour emergency number: (865) 576-1005	www.orau.gov/reacts
Armed Forces Radiobiology Research Institute	24-hour military emergency response resource: (301) 295-0530	http://afrri.usuhs.edu
Chemical/Biological Hotline of the National Response Center	24-hour federal point of contact: (800) 424-8802	http://nrc.uscg.mil/
Informational		
US Department of Human and Health Services: Radiation and Emergency Medical Management		http://remm.hhs.gov
Center for Disease Control and Prevention: Radiation Emergencies		http://emergency.cdc.gov/radiation/
World Health Organization: Radiation Emergencies		www.who.int/ionizing_radiation/a_e/en/

obtain nasal and mouth swabs and collect 24-hour urine and feces specimens for radiation bioassay.[7] Hospital nuclear medicine departments may have equipment that can be adapted and used for the diagnosis of internal contamination (e.g., thyroid scanners and gamma cameras).

MANAGEMENT

Prehospital Care

Gathered information regarding the exposure event includes: the numbers and types of patients potentially affected, the radionuclide involved, the route of exposure, and the estimated dose of radiation. Multiple triage guidelines exist to help guide transport and decontamination of individuals in the prehospital setting and are available to the public (Table 134.4).[15,16] Most communities will have a disaster plan for radiation incidents, which should be activated if a significant number of patients are involved.

Decontamination should be initiated at the scene. Patients with abnormal vital signs need partial decontamination, such as clothing removal, at the scene before expeditious transportation to an ED or medical facility. Unstable patients, however, should be rapidly transported in lieu of decontamination measures. Pre-arrival contact and up-to-date information should be provided to the receiving hospital as far in advance as possible to facilitate preparations and local safety measures. If the community disaster plan has a designated hospital for radiation-contaminated victims, patients should be transported directly to that facility, bypassing other hospitals less equipped to care for these complicated patients.

Emergency Department

Preparation

The chaos that occurs following radiation exposure incidents highlights the need for a community disaster plan with a predetermined incident command structure empowered to make decisions about evacuation and other issues concerning the at-risk population. On notification of the numbers and types of patients involved in a radiation exposure, incident commanders make a decision about implementation of a full disaster plan versus a limited response. The hospital radiation control officer should be contacted immediately. The radiation control officer monitors all patients and medical personnel with a radiation counter and supervises the "clean-up" and routing of patients to minimize "tracking," or spread, of contamination. Information dissemination to the public is critical. Timely and accurate information and instructions should be given to a public relations representative for dissemination to the news media to minimize the chaos and paranoia that inevitably result from such incidents.

External Contamination

Radiation contamination is *not* an acute threat to the life of the patient, first responder or health care provider, and its presence does not preclude institution of lifesaving measures. If standard precautions are taken, the risk to the health care providers is minimal. This was true for the providers caring for Alexander Litvinenko, a former agent of the Federal Security Service of the Russian Federation who was poisoned with a radioactive substance. It was 3 weeks before it was determined that he was internally contaminated with polonium 210.[17] Because the risk is minimal, care for life-threatening conditions and evaluation for severe traumatic injuries takes precedence over decontamination measures. A general approach to the patient exposed to radiation developed by the Radiation Emergency Assistance Center/Training Site of Oak Ridge Associates Universities is shown in Figure 134.3.

When a person is irradiated without any contamination, as in a patient who has just received a CT scan or x-ray, no hazard exists to medical personnel and the patient may be handled like any other emergency patient.

If a patient is determined to be contaminated with radioactive material by survey with a radiation counter (such as a Geiger counter), then they require decontamination. Universal precautions, including rubber gloves, eye protection, hair covers, shoe covers, and respirators (if airborne contamination is suspected), are effective in protecting personnel and the work area from contamination. The only variation from standard precautions is to wear two sets of gloves and to change the outer pair when appropriate to avoid cross-contamination.[15] Removing the patient's clothing and placing it in a plastic bag is paramount because exposed garments are responsible for 70% to 90% of the radiation from the patient.[15] If possible, soap and water cleansing of exposed skin should be performed. All materials, including wash water, should be placed in containers and labeled as radioactive waste. After decontamination, a repeat survey is performed. Decontamination is repeated until the patient's radiation reading is equal to or below two times the background radiation level. If decontamination methods are causing damage or injury to the skin, they should be discontinued regardless of the patient's radiation survey results.[7]

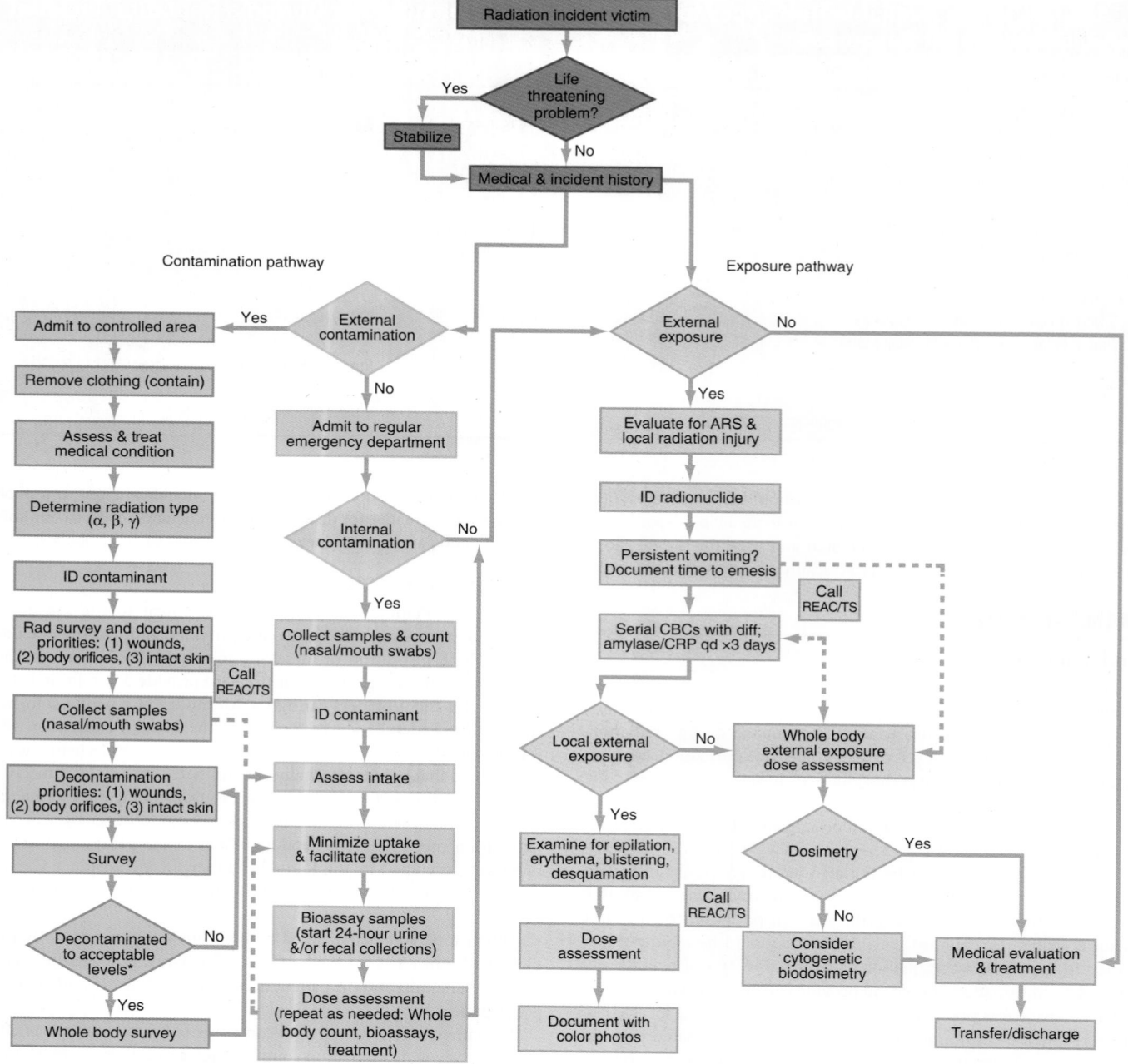

Fig. 134.3 Radiation patient treatment algorithm. *, <2–3× Natural background or no reduction in counts, medical priorities dictate stopping decontamination, health physics consultation warranted. *ARS,* Acute radiation syndrome; *CBC,* complete blood count; *CRP,* C-reactive protein; *diff,* differential; *ID,* identification; *qd,* on prescription; *REAC/TS,* Radiation Emergency Assistance Center/Training Site. (Used with permission and originally published by ORISE and REAC/TS under contract number DE-AC05-06OR23100 between the US Department of Energy and ORAU.)

Wounds can be decontaminated with saline or water. Using high pressure for irrigation is more important than the type of irrigation solution.[18] Remove foreign bodies and safely set these aside for further analysis. Repeat irrigation until the survey reveals decreased wound radiation. If further attempts at decontamination do not result in a decreased amount of radiation in the wound, then clinicians can proceed with standard medical treatment or surgical closure. Attempts to surgically decontaminate the wound should be avoided because this will potentially cause more localized damage.[19]

Internal Contamination

Assessing a patient for internal contamination can be difficult because most beta and alpha emitters will not be detectable with standard handheld survey devices. If a patient is externally contaminated, they have a higher risk of being internally contaminated. For internally contaminated patients, management focuses on decreasing absorption, enhancing elimination, and blocking distribution to target organs.[7] Treatment directed at internal contamination by particular radionuclides can include potassium iodide for radioactive iodine exposures,

TABLE 134.5 Radionuclides of Interest, Primary Decay Pattern, Half-Life, Major Routes of Exposure, and Recommended Treatment

	Name	Isotope	Decay	Half-Life	Route of Exposure	Treatment
University Five	Carbon 14	^{14}C	β	5700 years	Inhalation Ingestion	N/A
	Phosphorus 32	^{32}P	β	14 days	Inhalation Ingestion Skin	Phosphorus
	Iodine 125	^{125}I	γ	59 days	Inhalation Ingestion	KI
	Iodine 131	^{131}I	β, γ	8 days	Inhalation Ingestion	KI
	Californium 252	^{252}Cf	α, γ	2.6 years	Inhalation Ingestion	DTPA
Industrial Three	Iridium 192	^{192}Ir	β, γ	74 days	Inhalation Ingestion	DTPA
	Cesium 137	^{137}Cs	β, γ	30 years	Inhalation Ingestion	Prussian Blue
	Cobalt 60	^{60}Co	β, γ	5.3 years	Inhalation	DTPA
Military Five	Tritium	^{3}H	β	12 years	Inhalation Ingestion Skin	Water Diuresis
	Uranium 235	^{235}U	α	700 million years	Inhalation Ingestion	Bicarbonate
	Uranium 238	^{238}U	α	4.5 billion years	Inhalation Ingestion	Bicarbonate
	Plutonium 239	^{239}Pu	α	24,000 years	Inhalation	DTPA
	Americium 241	^{241}Am	α	430 years	Inhalation Skin	DTPA

DTPA, Diethylenetriaminepentaacetate; KI, potassium iodide.

bicarbonate for uranium, Prussian blue for cesium, and DTPA for plutonium and transuranics (Table 134.5).

Acute Radiation Syndrome

Hematopoietic Sub-Syndrome. Colony-stimulating factors (cytokines) that induce bone marrow hematopoietic cells to proliferate may have substantial benefit with little risk to victims who are predicted to have moderate or severe bone marrow failure. Cytokine therapy should be started for the following reasons: a greater than 2 Gy dose exposure, decrease in lymphocyte count, or if leukopenia is expected to last more than 7 days. Cytokines are started within 24 hours of exposure and continued until the absolute lymphocyte count is above 1000 cells/μL. Bone marrow transplant is considered for patients who continue to have prolonged leukopenia (2 to 3 weeks) in spite of cytokine treatment; however, the patients must not have other significant organ involvement.[11] Prophylactic antibiotics are given in accordance with the Infectious Disease Society of America recommendations for neutropenia.[19]

Gastrointestinal Sub-Syndrome. Treatment for the gastrointestinal sub-syndrome is largely supportive with antiemetics (preferably serotonin receptor antagonists such as ondansetron), antidiarrheals, fluid resuscitation, antibiotics, and monitoring for signs of gastrointestinal perforation.

Neurovascular Sub-Syndrome. Patients who develop signs and symptoms consistent with this sub-syndrome within the first 24 hours should be provided palliative comfort care, because they likely sustained a lethal dose of radiation.

Local Radiation Injury

Patients who sustained an LRI are managed in a manner similar to thermal burn patients.[14,20] Treatment at a burn center is preferred for débridement and wound care. Eventual extremity amputation may be necessary in patients who present with symptoms such as pain and erythema shortly after radiation exposure. Due to the chronic vascular injury and the potential for even minor trauma to the area to recapitulate the injury, the following are important in the treatment of LRI: topical corticosteroids, hyperbaric oxygen (HBO) therapy, pentoxifylline and vitamin E therapy, and appropriate wound care. New treatments currently under investigation include gene therapy, topical administration of growth factors, and laser therapy.[20]

Psychological Consequences

The general public harbors a profound fear of radiation and its effects on the body. Radiation is one of the most dreaded components of a terrorist attack or industrial disaster.[21] People are fearful of the long-term effects of radiation exposure, such as cancer, and especially with their children. This fear can lead to ostracizing people or things associated with the event. Furthermore, those who develop ARS or other illnesses related to radiation may have significant fear and depression requiring psychological posttraumatic support. Moreover, both health care providers and communities as a whole are also at risk for psychological effects from a radiation incident. As a result, proper information dissemination to the public and incorporation of behavioral health professionals early into the disaster response are extremely important.

DISPOSITION

The disposition will depend in part on the scale of the event and the availability of medical resources. A mass casualty event may place a strain on surge capacity, requiring disaster triage and resource rationing. Fortunately, large-scale radiation events are rare, and most radiation incidents have generated small numbers of patients requiring emergency or intensive care. The time of onset to vomiting can be useful in determining likelihood of survival. Patients who experience vomiting within 2 hours of exposure will require hospitalization and careful medical observation, because they are likely to have sustained life-threatening doses of radiation. Patients with severe burns and those requiring surgical management should be transferred to a burn unit, preferably within 72 hours from the time of radiation exposure.

ADDITIONAL RESOURCES

Many resources are available for both assistance in diagnosing and managing radiation injuries and for reporting of incidents. Table 134.4 lists resources that can help guide diagnosis and treatment of radiation emergencies and provide evidence-based information for those without formal radiation medicine expertise.

The authors wish to thank and acknowledge Daniel O. Hryhorczuk for his expertise and contributions to this chapter in previous editions.

The references for this chapter can be found online at ExpertConsult. com.

Care of the Poisoned Patient

Timothy J. Meehan

KEY CONCEPTS

- Toxidromes are constellations of signs and symptoms based primarily on vital signs and neuropsychiatric functions that are characteristic manifestations of certain toxic exposures. Recognition of the presence of a toxidrome can suggest a potential intoxicant and guide early interventions and management strategies. Examples of toxidromes include sympathomimetic, antimuscarinic, cholinergic, sedative-hypnotic, and opioid categories.
- Qualitative urine drug assays have limited roles in the clinical setting and are inferior to quantitative serum levels in terms of guiding specific therapy.
- Syrup of ipecac is not indicated in the emergency department (ED) care of a poisoned patient. Gastric lavage is not part of routine care. When given in a timely fashion (1-hour post ingestion), activated charcoal may be indicated for potentially lethal agents in alert, cooperative patients as noted in Figure 135.1. Whole-bowel irrigation is rarely useful for management of poisoned patients but is potentially helpful for specific poisonings, such as metals, illicit drug packets, or sustained-release medications.
- Serum alkalinization enhances urinary drug elimination for certain drugs and is indicated for significant poisoning caused by salicylates, phenobarbital, and methotrexate.
- Hemodialysis is best suited to remove poisons of low molecular weight, low protein binding, and high water solubility; examples include methanol, ethylene glycol, lithium, and salicylates.
- Regional Poison Control Centers (US: 1-800-222-1222) or a medical toxicologist can assist with antidotal therapy and may help facilitate patient disposition.
- If the motivation behind the toxic exposure was self-harm, a psychiatric consultation is warranted. Patients with substance use disorders should be referred to a detoxification center or designated program.

PRINCIPLES OF TOXICITY

Most poisoned patients seen in the emergency department (ED) are adults with intentional drug overdoses. The second most common scenario involves accidental poisoning in children, which actually represents the majority of calls to regional poison control centers.[1] Additionally, other frequent causes of toxicity include: illicit drugs of abuse, accidental poisoning from pharmaceutical agents (drug-drug interactions as well as chronic toxicity), environmental exposures, and envenomations. Occupational chemical exposures, both industrial and agricultural, represent other important sources of potential toxicity. In the ED, it is important to evaluate and recognize scenarios where there may be immediate or delayed toxicity, in order to guide strategies for decontamination, enhanced drug elimination, and administration of antidotes when indicated.

When evaluating a patient with a particular ingestion, essential historical points include: the agent itself, the route of exposure, the amount ingested, possible co-ingestants, and the timing of the exposure. Knowing these facts can help make a determination regarding the expected course of care in the ED and help to mobilize diagnostic and therapeutic resources.

CLINICAL FEATURES

Toxicologic History and Physical

Oftentimes, the poisoned patient may be altered, obtunded, or uncooperative with the examiner. This leaves the history limited to that which can be gleaned from witnesses, such as paramedics or family, and the information generated from physical examination findings over which the patient does not have conscious control.

Historical information should be pulled from all available sources. A family member or friend may offer insight into the circumstances behind the patient's exposure (e.g., intentional or accidental). Information regarding what medications or substances were available to the patient, and the timing of ingestion also is important. Paramedics should bring in all medication bottles present at the scene, not just the patient's prescribed medications or alleged ingestion; if they do not, someone should be sent to the patient's dwelling to retrieve them. Frequently, confusion as to what exactly was ingested can occur (e.g., ibuprofen mistaken for aspirin or acetaminophen) and this can lead a provider down the wrong path. A patient attempting suicide may intentionally mislead the ED staff, or medications may have been stored in mislabeled containers. Other sources of potentially useful information include state controlled-substance registries, pharmacy records, and previous medical records. Accessing the patient's text-messaging history also may be helpful, if the patient consents to this or if friends and family provide this collateral information of their own accord.

For chemical exposures in either the home or workplace, avoid exposure to other individuals in the ED. Proper identification of the substance is important to initiate care and obtain product safety information, such as a Material Safety Data Sheet. Consequently, one could consider taking a picture of the label including any precise chemical

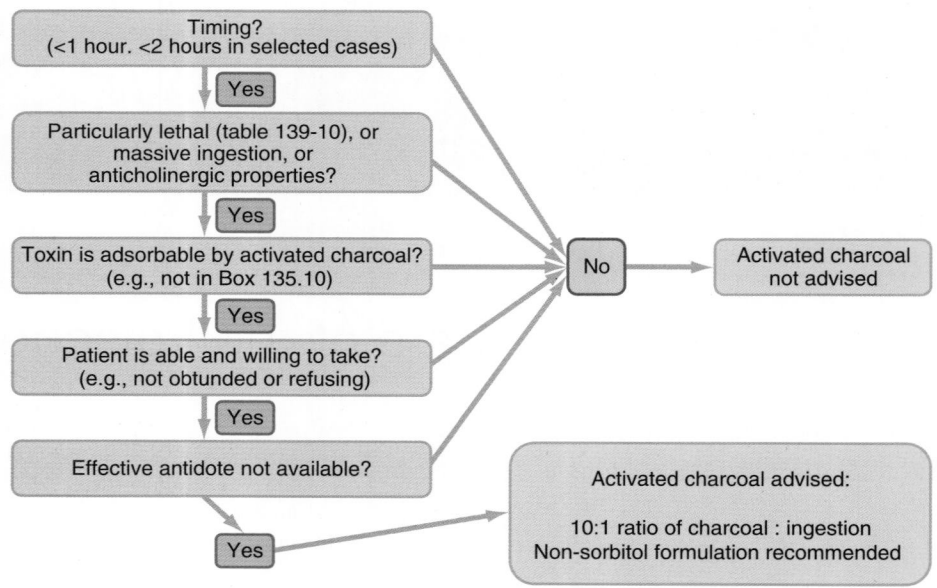

Fig. 135.1 Indications for early administration of activated charcoal 1 hr post-ingestion.

BOX 135.1 Agents Affecting Pupil Size

Miosis (COPS)
Cholinergics, clonidine, carbamates
Opioids, organophosphates
Phenothiazines (antipsychotics), pilocarpine, pontine hemorrhage
Sedative-hypnotics

Mydriasis (SAW)
Sympathomimetics
Anticholinergics
Withdrawal syndromes

Toxicology acronyms listed in Boxes (135.1–12) were created and previously published by Timothy B. Erickson (used and modified with permission.)

BOX 135.2 Agents Causing Coma or Seizures

Coma (LETHARGIC)
Lead, lithium
Ethanol, ethylene glycol, ethchlorvynol
Tricyclic antidepressants, thallium, toluene
Heroin, hemlock, hepatic encephalopathy, heavy metals, hydrogen sulfide, hypoglycemics
Arsenic, antidepressants, anticonvulsants, antipsychotics, antihistamines
Rohypnol (sedative hypnotics), risperidone
Gamma-hydroxybutyrate (GHB)
Isoniazid, insulin
Carbon monoxide, cyanide, clonidine

Seizures (OTIS CAMPBELL)
Organophosphates, oral hypoglycemics
Tricyclic antidepressants
Isoniazid, insulin
Sympathomimetics, strychnine, salicylates
Camphor, cocaine, carbon monoxide, cyanide, chlorinated hydrocarbons
Amphetamines, anticholinergics
Methylxanthines (theophylline, caffeine), methanol
Phencyclidine (PCP), propranolol
Benzodiazepine withdrawal, botanicals (water hemlock, nicotine), bupropion, GHB
Ethanol withdrawal, ethylene glycol
Lithium, lidocaine
Lead, lindane

---

numbers; if a substance is brought to the ED, take appropriate steps to avoid further exposure, such as sealing in an airtight container.

Poisoned patients are frequently unwilling or unable to participate in an interactive physical examination. The toxicologic physical examination, therefore, rests upon observing factors that do not require cooperation to elicit. Many ingested substances can cause derangement of the pulse, respiratory rate, as well as blood pressure. Rapid and accurate recording of the patient's vital signs, including pulse oximetry and a rectal core temperature, should be done and repeated at appropriate intervals depending on the suspected toxin. Patients with hemodynamic instability or obtundation should be considered for continuous monitoring, at least initially until stabilized. The overall level of consciousness, pupillary size, and presence or absence of seizure activity may suggest a particular agent (Boxes 135.1 and 135.2). Examination of the skin and mucous membranes with particular attention to discoloration and level of moisture may suggest poisoning by any of several agents (Box 135.3); it may also reveal evidence of injection drug abuse, such as "track marks" or ulcerations from "skin popping." A careful neurologic examination focusing on the level of muscle tone, clonus, or hyperreflexia can assist in the diagnosis of serotonin syndrome or neuroleptic malignant syndrome (NMS). Certain intoxicants may have particular odors associated with them; the presence of such an odor ought to alert the clinician to the possibility of poisoning by one of

these agents (Table 135.1); however, the absence of a characteristic smell does not exclude it.

Toxidromes

Toxidromes are constellations of signs and symptoms based on autonomic and neurochemical processes that can suggest a particular class of exposure and direct management and therapy. The five traditionally described entities include the sympathomimetic, anticholinergic (antimuscarinic), cholinergic, sedative/hypnotic, and opioid toxidromes.

BOX 135.3   Agents Causing Skin Findings

Diaphoretic Skin (SOAP)
Sympathomimetics
Organophosphates
Acetylsalicylic acid or other salicylates
Phencyclidine (PCP)

Dry Skin
Antihistamines, anticholinergics

Bullous Lesions or Blisters
Barbiturates and other sedative-hypnotics
Mustard gas
Snakes and spiders

Flushed or Red Appearance
Anticholinergics, niacin
Boric acid
Carbon monoxide (in morbid states)
Cyanide (rare)

Cyanosis
Ergotamine
Nitrates
Nitrites
Aniline dyes
Phenazopyridine
Dapsone
Agent causing hypoxemia, hypotension, or methemoglobinemia

Acneiform Rash
Bromides
Chlorinated aromatic hydrocarbons

TABLE 135.1   Agents With a Characteristic Odor

Odor	Possible Source
Bitter almonds	Cyanide
Carrots	Cicutoxin (water hemlock)
Fruity	Diabetic ketoacidosis, isopropanol
Garlic	Organophosphates, arsenic, dimethyl sulfoxide (DMSO), selenium
Gasoline	Petroleum distillates
Mothballs	Naphthalene, camphor
Pears	Chloral hydrate
Pungent aromatic	Ethchlorvynol
Oil of wintergreen	Methylsalicylate
Rotten eggs	Sulfur dioxide, hydrogen sulfide
Freshly mowed hay	Phosgene

In addition, withdrawal disorders, serotonin syndrome, and NMS have been well described.

Sympathomimetic

This toxidrome is defined by a state of sympathomimetic excess, typically causing those effects expected from the "fight or flight" reaction. Patients are often in an altered state and may be delusional—especially with ingestion of substituted amphetamines, such as *N*-methyl-3,4-methylenedioxyamphetamine (MDMA: "ecstasy" or "molly") or synthetic cannabinoids. Patients typically present with hypertension, tachycardia, and tachypnea. They may also be hyperthermic as a consequence of an increased metabolic rate. Mydriasis and diaphoresis may also be present. In severe overdoses, derangement of cardiac output can occur. Decreased diastolic filling time coupled with dysrhythmogenesis can result in circulatory collapse and shock, which may be refractory to fluid resuscitation and pressor agents.

Anticholinergic

The anticholinergic toxidrome is frequently encountered, because many pharmaceuticals have antimuscarinic properties. It manifests as a consequence of blocking normal cholinergic tone, causing an alteration in the normal homeostatic balance between the sympathetic and parasympathetic arms of the autonomic nervous system. This allows the sympathetic side to function unopposed and generates a state of relative sympathomimesis. Therefore, many of the symptoms attributable to the anticholinergic toxidrome—delirium, hyperthermia, mydriasis, and cutaneous flushing—share similarity with the sympathomimetic toxidrome. In contrast, because the secretory glands of the skin and mucous membranes contain muscarinic acetylcholine receptors, these patients are typically dry and not diaphoretic as found in the sympathomimetic toxidrome. The typical signs and symptoms can be recalled by the mnemonic "mad as a hatter, hot as a hare, blind as a bat, red as a beet, and dry as a bone." Patients with severe anticholinergic toxicity are often altered and may be delusional, often requiring sedation in the emergency department (see Management section).

Cholinergic

The cholinergic toxidrome results from overstimulation of the parasympathetic portion of the autonomic nervous system, which maintains the "rest and digest" functions. These patients typically have "fluids coming from every orifice" as a consequence of increased glandular secretion, and present with diaphoresis, urination, miosis, bronchorrhea, emesis, lacrimation, lethargy, and salivation (Box 135.4). Agents of concern are primarily anticholinesterase agents, such as organophosphates and carbamate insecticides. These substances are readily available as pesticides; but they have also been engineered as weapons of mass destruction, typically referred to as nerve gases (e.g., sarin gas) and more recently the novel or *Novichok* agents. It is important to rapidly recognize this toxidrome because patients frequently die from excessive bronchorrhea, effectively drowning in their own secretions, unless timely antidotal therapy and cholinesterase regenerators are given.

Nicotine poisoning from tobacco can occur in children who ingest detritus, such as used cigarettes or chewing tobacco, as well as liquids from electronic cigarettes.[2] Nicotine stimulates the nicotinic acetylcholine receptors in the autonomic nervous system. This is the first postsynaptic step in both the sympathetic and parasympathetic subsystems. Given the role of nicotine in both the central and peripheral autonomic nervous systems, the clinical picture in these poisonings may resemble both sympathomimetic and cholinergic toxidromes as noted in Box 135.4.

Sedative/Hypnotic

This toxidrome primarily presents with sedation and occurs on a spectrum depending on the particular substance, route, and potency. In severe ingestions, a state of general anesthesia may be reached with loss of muscle tone and airway protective reflexes. Additionally, overdose can be severe enough to cause hypothermia through suppression of muscular thermogenesis. The sedative/hypnotic toxic syndrome is well known in the ED, largely because ethanol intoxication is frequently seen. Other agents such as benzodiazepines and barbiturates will also cause a similar picture, as will illicit substances such as

BOX 135.4   Toxidrome Symptoms

Cholinergic
Muscarinic (DUMBELLS)
Diarrhea, diaphoresis
Urination
Miosis
Bradycardia
Bronchorrhea
Emesis
Lacrimation
Lethargic
Salivation

Nicotinic: Days of Week
Mydriasis
Tachycardia
Weakness
Tremors
Fasciculations
Seizures
Somnolence

Anticholinergic
Hyperthermia (HOT as a hare)
Flushed (RED as a beet)
Dry skin (DRY as a bone)
Dilated pupils (BLIND as a bat)
Delirium, hallucinations (MAD as a hatter)
Urinary retention (DRY as a bone)
Tachycardia

Opioid
Acute Intoxication/Overdose
Miosis
Hypoventilation
Depressed mental status/coma

Withdrawal
Withdrawal
Diarrhea
Mydriasis
Goose flesh
Tachycardia
Lacrimation
Hypertension
Yawning
Cramps
Hallucinations
Seizures (with ethyl alcohol [ETOH] and benzodiazepine withdrawal)

Sympathomimetic
Hyperthermic
Flushed
Diaphoretic
Mydriatic
Agitated
Tachycardic
Seizures

gamma-hydroxybutyrate (GHB). The incidence of concomitant traumatic injuries (from falls or syncope) may be high in these patients, and providers should exclude their presence.

Opioid

Similar to sedative/hypnotics, the opioid toxidrome also involves sedation and a diminished respiratory drive. With the notable exception of pentazocine and propoxyphene, this toxidrome causes pupillary miosis. The diagnosis is confirmed by noting a rapid response to naloxone, a direct opioid receptor antagonist. However, because certain opioids have higher potencies, a lack of response to this reversal agent does not exclude opioid intoxication. Furthermore, this is a clinical diagnosis because not all opioids will be detectable by the standard drug screen (discussed later).

Serotonin Syndrome

A state of serotonergic excess defines this toxidrome, and it is often precipitated by the addition of a new serotonergic agent or a substance that interferes with the metabolism of a previously tolerated agent. Typically described with selective serotonin reuptake inhibitors (SSRIs) and monoamine oxidase inhibitors (MAOIs), it has been reported with cyclic antidepressants, atypical antipsychotics; and nonpsychiatric medications such as tramadol and ondansetron. Serotonin syndrome typically occurs within hours to days of introduction of a new medication, although it has been described in a delayed fashion due to the prolonged half-lives of some antidepressants. The manifestations of serotonin syndrome include altered mental status, agitation, autonomic instability (hyperthermia, diaphoresis, hypertension), and most notably, neuromuscular abnormalities (hyperreflexia and clonus).

BOX 135.5   Altered Mental Status

AEIOU
Alcohol/acidosis
Encephalopathy/electrolytes
Infection
Opioids/overdose
Uremia

Tips
Trauma
Insulin (hypoglycemia/hyperglycemia)
Psychosis
Seizure/stroke

Neuroleptic Malignant Syndrome

Similar to serotonin syndrome, NMS also presents with altered mental status, agitation, autonomic instability, severe hyperthermia, and neuromuscular abnormalities. Unlike serotonin syndrome, however, peripheral muscular effects tend toward rigidity and hyporeflexia rather than clonus and hyperreflexia. It is due to dopaminergic depletion secondary to chronic use of dopamine antagonists, such as antipsychotics.

DIFFERENTIAL DIAGNOSES

Frequently, poisoned patients have some level of delirium as part of their presentation. As such, excluding other causes of altered mental status while initiating appropriate toxicologic therapy is appropriate (Box 135.5). Any "intoxicated" patient presenting to the ED should

BOX 135.6 Predicting Toxicity from Vital Signs

Bradycardia (PACED)
Propranolol (β-blockers), poppies (opioids), propoxyphene, physostigmine
Anticholinesterase drugs, antiarrhythmics
Clonidine, calcium channel blockers
Ethanol or other alcohols
Digoxin, digitalis

Tachycardia (FAST)
Free base or other forms of cocaine, Freon
Anticholinergics, antihistamines, antipsychotics amphetamines, alcohol withdrawal
Sympathomimetics (cocaine, caffeine, amphetamines, phencyclidine [PCP]), solvent abuse, strychnine
Theophylline, tricyclic antidepressants (TCAs), thyroid hormones

Hypothermia (COOLS)
Carbon monoxide
Opioids
Oral hypoglycemics, insulin
Liquor (alcohols)
Sedative-hypnotics

Hyperthermia (NASA)
Neuroleptic malignant syndrome (NMS), nicotine
Antihistamines, alcohol withdrawal
Salicylates, sympathomimetics, serotonin syndrome
Anticholinergics, antidepressants, antipsychotics

Hypotension (CRASH)
Clonidine, calcium channel blockers
Rodenticides (containing arsenic, cyanide)
Antidepressants, aminophylline, antihypertensives
Sedative-hypnotics
Heroin or other opioids

Hypertension (CT SCAN)
Cocaine
Thyroid supplements
Sympathomimetics
Caffeine
Anticholinergics, amphetamines
Nicotine

Rapid Respiration (PANT)
Phencyclidine (PCP), paraquat, pneumonitis, phosgene
Acetylsalicylic acid (ASA) and other salicylates
Noncardiogenic pulmonary edema, nerve agents
Toxin-induced metabolic acidosis

Slow Respiration (SLOW)
Sedative-hypnotics (barbiturates, benzodiazepines)
Liquor (alcohols)
Opioids
Weed (marijuana)

---

have the reversible causes of altered mental status excluded, such as hypoglycemia and nutritional deficiencies.[3] Trauma is frequently coincident with intoxication, so a careful unclothed examination looking for evidence of head trauma and other traumatic injuries should be part of the initial evaluation.

The physical examination may also reveal findings that could suggest specific intoxicants, as noted in Box 135.6. The most important diagnostic approach is maintaining a broad differential diagnosis of both toxicologic and non-toxicologic causes for the patient's presentation and avoid making a premature conclusion to the case. In these cases, differential diagnoses may be extremely broad such as when ingestion of a toxin is not known or felt unlikely.

DIAGNOSTIC TESTING

Diagnostic testing is guided by the clinical findings and suspected toxin(s) involved. When a patient presents with altered mental status and hyperthermia, testing may focus on differentiating a toxic cause from thyrotoxicosis or acute infectious diseases. Patients with intoxication and evidence of trauma may require evaluation for head trauma as a cause of their altered mental status. In many instances, it is known that the patient has a potentially toxic exposure but some or all of the involved toxins have not been implicated or identified. The approaches to individual toxins and syndromes are outlined in the relevant chapters. In the setting of an unknown overdose or exposure, a broad array of laboratory testing is often used to screen for abnormalities and potentially elucidate the clinical picture. The diagnostic studies routinely checked are: complete blood count, serum chemistry with renal function, liver function tests, urinalysis (with a pregnancy test if appropriate), urine toxicology screen, serum ethanol concentration, arterial blood gas, serum lactate, and a bedside glucose.

BOX 135.7 Commonly Available Serum Drug Levels

Acetaminophen
Acetylsalicylic acid (salicylate)
Carbamazepine
Carbon monoxide
Digoxin
Ethanol
Ethylene glycol
Iron
Isopropyl alcohol
Lead
Lithium
Methanol
Methotrexate
Phenobarbital
Phenytoin
Valproic acid

Based on these results, or when the ingestion is known, other tests such as specific serum concentrations may be obtained; Box 135.7 lists those drug levels commonly available in most hospitals. When assays for a particular agent are not available, or are not performed on site, empirical treatment generally begins before results are available. Reference laboratories are available to analyze specific and unique assays, but the turn-around time is often delayed and not clinically applicable in the emergency department.

If the blood gas shows the presence of a metabolic acidosis, calculating the anion gap can further refine the possible etiologies.

The calculation is: [Na] – ([HCO$_3$] + [Cl]). The normal range is 8 to 12 mEq/L.

Metabolic acidosis without an anion gap typically results from loss of bicarbonate (diarrhea, renal tubular acidosis) or gain of chloride-containing compounds (ammonia, calcium chloride). Metabolic acidosis associated with an anion gap results from an increase in unmeasured serum anions and suggests several specific toxins and disease states (Box 135.8).

When ingestion of a toxic alcohol (such as methanol, ethylene glycol, or isopropanol) is suspected, calculating the osmolal gap may be helpful because early in the poisoning course the patient may be minimally or non-acidemic. Furthermore, urine fluorescence is not sufficiently sensitive to be reliable and its absence cannot be used to "rule out" ethylene glycol ingestion. The osmolal gap is discussed in Chapter 136.

Toxicology "screens" may also be helpful in diagnosing an unknown ingestion, provided that the limitations of these panels are understood. Blood toxicology screens can be falsely negative if the ingested drug has a short half-life and the sample is not drawn soon enough after the exposure. Urine toxicology screens are more reliable, because they typically have a longer time period for positive detection, typically 24 to 72 hours. Urine toxicology screens typically include phencyclidine (PCP), cocaine, opioids, amphetamines, and cannabinoids; however, these can vary among institutions, so knowing what is available in one's facility is important in interpreting a positive or negative screen. The urine screen is also a qualitative, not a quantitative test; as such, a positive result does not necessarily imply acute toxicity. A urine toxicology screen can be falsely positive due to cross-reactivity between agents (such as a "positive" phencyclidine or PCP screen in the setting of dextromethorphan ingestion). Alternatively, urine screens can be falsely negative if the substance ingested does not cross-react with the tested analyte—such as methadone, which does not cross-react with the opiate component of the urine toxicology screen (Table 135.2). Ultimately, the diagnosis of intoxication is clinical; urine drug screening may be confirmatory but should

BOX 135.8 Substances Causing Wide Anion-Gap Acidosis

Metal Acid Gap

M Methanol, Metformin, Massive overdose
E Ethylene glycol
T Toluene
A Alcoholic ketoacidosis
L Lactic acidosis
A Acetaminophen (large overdose)
C CO, Cyanide, Colchicine
I Isoniazid (INH), Iron, Ibuprofen
D Diabetic ketoacidosis (DKA)
G Generalized seizure inducing drugs
A ASA (salicylates)
P Paraldehyde, Phenformin

TABLE 135.2 Urine Drug Screen Limitations

Assay	False Positive	True Positive (Therapeutic Use)	False Negative
Amphetamines	Many; some clinically relevant ones include: Amantadine, Bupropion, Labetalol, Promethazine, Ranitidine, Trazodone	ADHD medications: Dextroamphetamine, methamphetamine; Phenylephrine; Pseudoephedrine	"Designer amphetamines"; Molly; Ecstasy
Benzodiazepines	Sertraline, Oxaprozin		Alprazolam; Flurazepam; Midazolam; "Z" drugs (zolpidem, zaleplon, zopiclone, eszopiclone)
Cannabinoids	Dronabinol, Efavirenz, PPI	Medical marijuana; CBD oil (contaminant)	Synthetic marijuana: K2/Spice
Opiates	Dextromethorphan, Diphenhydramine, Quinolones		Synthetic opioids: Demerol, fentanyl, methadone, propoxyphene; Semisynthetic opioids (may have some cross-reactivity): Hydrocodone, hydromorphone, oxycodone
Phencyclidine (PCP)	Dextromethorphan, Diphenhydramine, Ibuprofen, Tramadol	Ketamine	
Cocaine	Coca leaf tea	Cocaine-containing anesthetics (topical TAC)	

ADHD, Attention deficit hyperactivity disorder; *PPI,* proton pump inhibition; *TAC,* tetracaine, adrenaline (epinephrine), and cocaine.

not supplant clinical evaluation and judgment nor should it delay therapy.

In addition to the blood work discussed earlier, one should obtain an electrocardiogram (ECG) if the patient is tachycardic or bradycardic or may have ingested a cardiotoxic agent that can prolong the QRS complex or QT intervals, such as cyclic antidepressants, antimalarials (e.g., chloroquine), and antipsychotic agents. Table 135.3 provides guidance regarding for which patients an ECG should be obtained.

MANAGEMENT

The general management of a poisoned patient involves providing appropriate supportive care, undertaking decontamination, enhancing elimination, and providing specific antidotal therapy when indicated. Specific strategies will be discussed at length in the following chapters regarding specific poisons. However, the basic framework remains the same.

Antidotes do not exist for every potential poisoning, and thus supportive care is the cornerstone of managing the poisoned patient. Providing resuscitation by ensuring airway protection and adequacy of ventilation while maintaining the circulatory status of the patient with crystalloids and vasopressor support is the prime focus. If the airway is compromised or in danger of becoming so, or if the respiratory effort is insufficient to maintain appropriate ventilation, intubation is usually the preferred course (with special care in the situation of a salicylate poisoning, which is discussed in Chapter 139).

Vascular access needs to be obtained, with peripheral or central venous catheters, intraosseous lines are also viable access points from the toxicologic perspective, because there are no known contraindications to antidotal therapy through this route. Once supportive care has been initiated and the patient stabilized, one should then progress to a systematic assessment of decontamination strategies, enhanced elimination, focused therapy (antidotes), and obtaining consultation.

Decontamination

Decontamination is the process of preventing systemic absorption. In the case of ocular or dermal exposure, this is achieved by copious irrigation with water, after removal of contaminated clothing to expose the area. Water irrigation is not used for metallic potassium, magnesium, or sodium (found in "tracer" ammunition, for example), because these can ignite on contact with water. Instead, in these very rare exposures, the area should be covered with petroleum jelly or mineral oil.

SYRUP OF IPECAC

Inducing emesis with syrup of ipecac is not indicated in the care of any poisoned patient in the ED. Syrup of ipecac use is associated with significant side effects (e.g., dehydration due to intractable vomiting) and complications (e.g., aspiration pneumonitis, Mallory-Weiss tears, and gastric rupture). There are also insufficient data and evidence showing improvement in clinical outcomes with poisonings.[4]

GASTRIC LAVAGE

Gastric lavage, the process of directly removing an ingested substance from the stomach using a 30 Fr or larger orogastric tube, also has little data or evidence showing its efficacy and should not be performed routinely for the treatment of poisoned patients. Given the risks of aspiration and esophageal trauma, the American Association of Poison Centers suggests it only be employed "within an hour of ingestion of a potentially life-threatening poison which does not adsorb to activated charcoal or for which no antidote exists" and, even then, in a center with "sufficient expertise" to perform the procedure safely.[5] Only a rare overdose (such as colchicine) will meet all these criteria; and hence, despite its once widespread use, gastric lavage is mostly of historical interest only.

SINGLE-DOSE ACTIVATED CHARCOAL

Historically, single-dose activated charcoal (SDAC) has been the mainstay of gastric decontamination in medical toxicology. Activated charcoal is a carbonaceous substance that has been exposed to high heat and steam—i.e., "activated"—which results in a large surface area to volume ratio. This provides ample surface space for intralumenal ingested substances to adsorb, and thus decreases absorption into the body. Current understanding of the role of activated charcoal in poison management is based on pharmaco-toxicologic data (lethality, availability of antidotes, or alternative detoxification therapies); pharmacokinetics (area under the concentration versus time curve in controlled volunteer studies); clinical trials in patients with overdose; and collective, empirical clinical experience.[6] Studies involving healthy volunteers ingesting small (safe) doses of various agents do not accurately replicate the overdose (large ingestion) situation, so are of limited value. In addition, there are very few appropriately designed clinical studies assessing the benefit from SDAC. Therefore, due to the lack of convincing evidence demonstrating benefit in clinical outcome in human overdose, we do not recommend

TABLE 135.3 Toxicologic Electrocardiogram Manifestations

Segment/Interval	Appearance	Agent(s)	Segment/Interval	Appearance	Agent(s)
P wave	Absent	Digoxin Cholinergics Hyperkalemia	QT/QTc	Prolonged	Antipsychotics (typical and atypical), citalopram, hydrofluoric acid, methadone, ethylene glycol (oxalate byproduct)
	Notched	Quinidine			
PR interval	Prolonged	Beta-antagonists, calcium-channel antagonists, magnesium, lacosamide	T wave	Peaked	Hydrofluoric acid (hyperkalemia)
				Flattened	Lithium
QRS interval	Prolonged	Type 1 antidysrhythmics, cocaine, diphenhydramine, tricyclic antidepressants	U wave		Barium, beta-agonists, lithium, methylxanthines (caffeine, theophylline), toluene
ST segment	Scooped	Digoxin ("Salvador Dali's moustache")			

the routine use of activated charcoal following ingestion.[7] We do, however, recommend its use in certain overdose scenarios.

Although few studies have shown a reduction of morbidity or mortality attributable to activated charcoal administration, and there have been reports of pulmonary aspiration of activated charcoal with serious patient harm, these aspiration events have occurred in a minority of patients receiving activated charcoal; therefore it is considered a relatively low-risk intervention. With certain toxic exposures, SDAC administration may be reasonable after a consideration of the risk versus benefit for the patient in the context of the quantity and toxicity of the ingested substance, the time elapsed between ingestion and treatment, and the availability of alternative antidotes or decontamination procedures (e.g., hemodialysis). Benefits include decreasing primary absorption or binding during enterohepatic recirculation of a potentially toxic xenobiotic. These benefits are more likely to occur if:

- The activated charcoal is administered within one hour after ingestion, *and*
- The patient is alert, able, and willing to cooperate with administration, and anticipated to remain alert and protective of airway reflexes, *and either*
  - The substance ingested has high toxicity or is a toxic sustained-release agent, *or*
  - There is evidence of a massive ingestion of a toxic agent (e.g., salicylates)

If the patient is sedated, has an unprotected airway, or is unwilling to drink the charcoal suspension, administration is contraindicated. This may be particularly true for young children with limited ability to drink the slurry. Furthermore, one should not place a nasogastric tube solely to administer activated charcoal, because of the risk of aspiration or direct instillation of activated charcoal into the lungs, thus changing the risk-benefit ratio.

Considering all of this information, how does one decide whether activated charcoal is indicated in a specific overdose? First, the ingested drug must have a high potential for toxicity and lethality. These drugs are listed by class in Box 135.9. If the drug ingested has low toxicity (e.g., ibuprofen, diazepam), or there is an effective antidote available (e.g., *N*-acetylcysteine for acetaminophen, digoxin immune fab for digoxin), activated charcoal administration is not advised.

Second, the ingestion must be recent. For most overdoses, this means that the activated charcoal needs to be administered within one hour of the ingestion. For certain overdoses (sustained-release products, anticholinergic agents, massive ingestions), either because of pharmacokinetics or the quantity ingested, activated charcoal may be given up to 2 hours after ingestion. Many patients arrive at the ED more than 2 hours after the ingestion or ingest the drugs over a period of several hours, often with alcohol, and do not meet this time requirement. Third, the ingestion must be amenable to adsorption by activated charcoal. This eliminates rapidly absorbed toxins (e.g., alcohols) and those agents listed in Box 135.10. Fourth, the patient must be alert and anticipated to remain alert and be willing to take the activated charcoal slurry voluntarily. An algorithm guiding the administration of activated charcoal is shown in Figure 135.1. We recommend consultation with a regional poison center or medical toxicologist if there is uncertainty regarding the indications for activated charcoal.

Activated charcoal historically has most often been given in a dose of 50 to 100 grams (or 1.0 g/kg in young children), but we advise customizing the dose to the dose of the ingested agent by administering activated charcoal in a weight ratio of 10:1 (ratio of activated charcoal to drug).

WHOLE BOWEL IRRIGATION

In certain ingestions such as extended-release preparations, illicit drug packets, or metals (e.g., iron and lead), continuous whole-bowel irrigation may be indicated. Whole bowel irrigation (WBI) is performed with a balanced polyethylene glycol solution that does not participate in fluid exchange nor become absorbed into the body. To be effective, it requires a rate of 2 liters per hour in an adult; consequently, this will require nasogastric tube placement.[8] However, if a patient is critically ill, has hypoperfusion of the gut, or has obstruction of the bowel, WBI is contraindicated because there have been reports of increased morbidity and mortality in these clinical settings.

Enhanced Elimination

Once a toxin has been absorbed into the body, it undergoes metabolism and elimination primarily via hepatic and renal pathways. Certain substances are amenable to enhancing these elimination pathways either ex vivo as is the case with hemodialysis and its related therapies, or in vivo as is the case with multiple-dose activated charcoal (MDAC) and urinary alkalinization.

Hemodialysis and its related therapies are best suited to remove poisons of low molecular weight, low protein binding, and high water solubility; examples include toxic alcohols, lithium, and salicylates, as listed in Box 135.11. All forms of extracorporeal removal have been studied and found to be efficacious; the selection of a specific type of

---

BOX 135.9 Potentially Lethal Toxins Where Early Activated Charcoal Administration May Be Indicated

The Killer Cs
Cyanide
Colchicine
Calcium channel blockers
Cyclic antidepressants
Cardio glycosides
Cyclopeptide mushrooms (*Amanita phalloides*)
Cocaine
Cicutoxin (water hemlock)
Salicylates

BOX 135.10 Substances That Do *Not* Bind to Activated Charcoal

Phails
Pesticides
Heavy metals
Acids/alkalis
Iron
Lithium
Solvents

BOX 135.11 Dialyzable Toxins

Stumbled
Salicylates
Theophylline
Uremia
Metformin/methanol
Barbiturates
Lithium
Ethylene glycol
Depakote (valproic acid—in massive overdose)

elimination modality ought to be made based on patient-specific factors and early consultation with a nephrologist in conjunction with a medical toxicologist or poison control center.[9]

MULTIPLE-DOSE ACTIVATED CHARCOAL

Unlike preventing absorption of a drug as is the case for SDAC, multiple dose activated charcoal (MDAC) is intended to facilitate removal of a toxin that has already been absorbed. MDAC decreases xenobiotic absorption and elimination half-life when large amounts of the toxin are ingested and dissolution is delayed (e.g., concretions, bezoars, or extended release formulations). It also is believed to create a hemoperfusion substrate for the gut wall microcirculation to permit "gastrointestinal dialysis," which generates a concentration gradient into the stool for certain poisons, which are then eliminated by defecation. In addition, certain drugs are excreted in the bile, then reabsorbed by the gut, only to be re-excreted in the bile, a process called *enterohepatic circulation*. MDAC also may interfere with reabsorption of these drugs by binding them during their transit of the gastrointestinal tract. Drugs with significant enterohepatic circulation are listed in Box 135.12. As with SDAC, MDAC administration may cause pulmonary aspiration and intestinal obstruction. Aspiration is best avoided by applying the same conditions for administration as for SDAC—patient is awake, alert, and cooperating and is anticipated to remain so. Obstruction is more difficult to predict and prevent, although avoidance in situations with delayed gut motility (e.g., critical illness, opioid or anticholinergic effects) is recommended to reduce this risk.

When MDAC is indicated, the initial loading dose of an activated charcoal–to–xenobiotic ratio of 10:1 is followed by subsequent doses of 50% of the initial dose every 4 to 6 hours for up to 24 hours. MDAC may be discontinued when the patient's measurable serum levels are no longer considered in the toxic range. Take care to only use non-sorbitol containing formulations when administering MDAC; sorbitol, a non-absorbable sugar added to charcoal slurries to enhance palatability, can induce significant fluid shifts and cause profound electrolyte abnormalities (particularly in children) such as hypernatremia when a large amount is ingested, as in the case of MDAC.

SERUM ALKALINIZATION

Certain water-soluble drugs such as salicylates, methotrexate, and phenobarbital will undergo ion-trapping and enhanced urinary elimination if the serum is sufficiently alkalinized. This is especially important with salicylate poisonings, because alkalinization not only promotes elimination but also prevents salicylate crossing the blood-brain barrier into the central nervous system (CNS). Monitor the serum pH and bicarbonate level, as well as the urinary pH, with the goal being a serum pH of approximately 7.5 and a urinary pH of approximately 8.0. Also ensure that the serum potassium level is normal, because alkalinization will cause an intracellular shift of potassium and consequently increase urine reabsorption of potassium by excreting hydrogen ions into the urine; this will eliminate the pH gradient and dissipate the

benefits of this process. To accomplish this, combine 150 mEq (3 amps) of 8.4% sodium bicarbonate into a liter of dextrose 5% in water (D5W) and add potassium (20 to 40 mEq total) to the intravenous fluid as well. This solution should be infused at a rate not to exceed 250 mL/hour. Barring concerns for fluid overload (particularly in elderly and renal failure patients) we recommend infusing at 250 mL an hour.

INTRAVENOUS FAT EMULSION (INTRALIPID)

Intravenous fat emulsion (IFE) is utilized for poison-induced cardiogenic shock or intractable seizures. This therapy was first described for treatment of toxicity from local anesthetics, such as bupivacaine. IFE is proposed to work primarily by two separate mechanisms: (1) the lipid sink and (2) enhanced cardiac metabolism.[10] The lipid sink theory posits that fat-soluble drugs are "soaked up" and removed from the site of toxicity, effectively increasing the volume of distribution for a fat-soluble drug. This is the predominant theory behind the use of IFE. A second theory involves optimization of cardiac metabolism. The heart under physiologic circumstances prefers free fatty acids; in times of stress, it switches to glucose metabolism for energy. A dose of IFE theoretically provides a large supply of free fatty acids to optimize energy use in the heart. In addition to providing supplemental energy for myocytes, IFE may also enhance activation of cardiac calcium channels.

Indications for IFE are not universally agreed upon. In addition to anesthetic agents, successful resuscitations have been described with refractory B-blocker overdose, calcium channel blockers, cyclic antidepressants, and bupropion and cocaine toxicity. Although originally described as a treatment for overdose patients in cardiac arrest, several reports now exist describing the successful use of IFE in critically ill patients prior to circulatory collapse and cardiac arrest. Dosing for IFE also varies in the literature. If indicated, we recommend an initial bolus of 1.5 mL/kg of 20% lipid solution given over 2 to 3 minutes followed by an infusion of 0.25 mL/kg/min over 30 to 60 minutes, based on the most commonly recommended and described protocols; this can be given via peripheral, central, or intraosseus access.

With the exception of local anesthetic systemic toxicity (LAST), where IFE is considered front-line therapy, intralipids should only be administered to overdoses when resuscitative efforts have been refractory to other more conventional therapies (e.g., vasopressor agents, sodium bicarbonate, calcium, high-dose insulin-dextrose therapy). When considering administration of IFE therapy to an unstable overdosed patient, consultation with a medical toxicologist or regional poison center is recommended.

Despite recent enthusiasm for IFE, its use has associated complications, including extreme lipemia resulting in lab interference with blood tests (complete blood counts, chemistries, and coagulations studies), as well as acute pancreatitis, and acute respiratory distress syndrome.[11]

Focused Therapy

Although the majority of poisonings require supportive care alone, in selected ingestions specific antidotal therapy may be available. Evidence and experience support the use of several antidotes, which should be available either immediately (e.g., hospital stocked) or rapidly accessed (e.g., transported within a few hours). These antidotes and their indications can be found in Table 135.4, and their use is discussed in the relevant chapters.[12]

Toxicology Consultation

Most poisoning cases are straightforward and appropriately handled by the emergency clinician. When the poisoning is severe, high risk,

---

BOX 135.12 Substances Amenable to Multiple-Dose Activated Charcoal

ABCDQ

Aminophylline/theophylline
Barbiturates
Carbamazepine/concretion forming drugs (e.g., salicylates)
Dapsone
Quinine

TABLE 135.4   Selected Antidotes and Their Indications

Antidote	Indication (Poison)
N-acetylcysteine	Acetaminophen
Fomepizole (4-MP)/ethanol	Methanol/ethylene glycol
Oxygen/hyperbarics	Carbon monoxide
Naloxone	Opioids, clonidine
Physostigmine	Anticholinergics
Atropine/pralidoxime (2-PAM)	Organophosphates
Methylene blue	Methemoglobinemia
Nitrites/hydroxycobalamin	Cyanide
Deferoxamine	Iron
Dimercaprol (BAL)	Arsenic, lead
Succimer (DMSA)	Lead, mercury
CaEDTA	Lead
Fab fragments	Digoxin, crotalids
Glucagon	β-blockers
Sodium bicarbonate	Salicylates, tricyclic antidepressants
Insulin/Glucose, calcium	Calcium channel antagonists, B-blockers
Dextrose, glucagon, octreotide	Oral hypoglycemic agents
Pyridoxine (vitamin B$_6$)	Isoniazid (INH)
Intravenous fat emulsion	Local anesthetic systemic toxicity
	Certain fat-soluble medications

2-PAM, 2-pralidoxime; *4-MP,* 4-methylpyrazone; *BAL,* British antilewisite; *CaEDTA,* calcium ethylenediamine tetracetate; *DMSA,* dimercaptosuccinic acid.

involves unfamiliar or multiple toxins, or occurs in a patient with significant comorbidity, we recommend consultation with a Poison Control Center or, if available, a medical toxicologist. Consultation can assist the bedside clinician in the determination of an unknown ingestion, critical management decisions, or whether an antidote or invasive procedure, such as hemodialysis, is advisable.

In the United States, a national toll-free phone number has been established that will route a practitioner to their nearest Poison Control Center. This number is 1-800-222-1222.[1]

DISPOSITION

Patients with severe toxicity (for example seizures, persistent cardiovascular instability, airway compromise, or significant metabolic derangements) should be admitted to an intensive care setting. Patients who are asymptomatic on arrival but have ingested a potentially dangerous substance or an extended-release preparation that could cause significant deterioration in their clinical status, ought be admitted to either an inpatient setting or an observation unit for 24 hours, or until peak toxicity has passed and the patient is physiologically stable. For patients who are asymptomatic after an ingestion of a minimally toxic substance and for whom other ingestions and psychiatric issues have been addressed, discharge after the ED visit, which typically takes at least 4 to 6 hours, is appropriate.

If the motivation behind the ingestion, was suicidality, or self-harm, a psychiatric consultation is warranted. If a suicidal patient is to be admitted medically for observation, it is important to ensure that a dedicated sitter or other type of secure environment is available to prevent any further patient inflicted self-injury.

The references for this chapter can be found online at ExpertConsult.com.

136

Toxic Alcohols

Michael E. Nelson

KEY CONCEPTS

- The classic finding of an elevated osmolar and anion gap should raise suspicion of methanol or ethylene glycol toxicity but may not be present depending on the timing of ingestion. Early ingestion has a high osmolar gap without acidosis, and late ingestion has acidosis without an osmolar gap.
- Serum osmolarity is calculated by the following equation:

  Calculated osmolarity $(mOsm/kg) = 2Na^+ + (BUN/2.8) + (glucose/18) + (ethanol/4.6)$

  The measured osmolar gap is the difference between the measured serum osmolality and calculated serum osmolarity, with a normal range of −15 to +10 mOsm.
- It is important to note that a normal osmolar gap does not exclude toxic alcohol ingestion.
- Initiate therapy based on strong clinical suspicion of exposure to methanol or ethylene glycol. Block alcohol dehydrogenase preferably with fomepizole, but ethanol can be used if fomepizole is unavailable.
- The main priorities in toxic alcohol exposure are correction of acidosis using bicarbonate solution and hemodialysis, inhibition of the production of toxic metabolites, and elimination of the parent alcohol and its toxic metabolites.
- The presence of acidosis indicates the accumulation of the toxic metabolites of methanol (formic acid) and ethylene glycol (glycolic and oxalic acid). Consult nephrology for emergent hemodialysis to correct acid-base disturbances and remove the parent compound as well as its toxic metabolites.
- Severe acidosis is a poor prognostic factor, with high mortality rates in methanol and ethylene glycol ingestions. A comatose state at the time of presentation also is associated with a higher mortality outcome.
- The findings of an elevated osmolar gap with ketonemia or ketonuria and no development of acidosis indicate isopropanol ingestion. Patients can have a prolonged period of inebriation and can be comatose. Alcohol dehydrogenase inhibition is not indicated in these cases.
- Hypotension and gastrointestinal bleeding are poor prognostic factors in isopropanol ingestion.
- Diethylene glycol can result in acidosis and renal failure and should be managed similarly to ethylene glycol poisoning with fomepizole and hemodialysis.

Ethyl alcohol (ethanol) is ubiquitously consumed worldwide on a daily basis and contributes to a multitude of acute and chronic disease processes and traumatic events. Although ethanol certainly can be viewed as a toxic alcohol, its use, abuse, and related conditions are discussed in Chapter 137. This chapter focuses on methanol, ethylene glycol (EG), and isopropyl alcohol (IPA; isopropanol).

METHANOL

Foundations

Methanol (methyl alcohol; CAS 67-56-1; H_3COH) is a clear, volatile, colorless, slightly sweet-tasting alcohol at room temperature. It is also known as wood alcohol due to methanol being produced from the destructive distillation of wood. Methanol is mainly used as a solvent or octane booster in gasoline. It is manufactured frequently as an intermediate in chemical reactions. As a solvent, it is present in many items found in the home, including cleaning solutions, adhesives, enamels, stains, dyes, and paint removers. Methanol is also commonly found in windshield washer fluid, antifreeze (particularly brake line antifreeze), embalming fluid, and fuel for camp stoves.

Many mass methanol poisonings have occurred throughout history, including outbreaks in Estonia (2001), Norway (2002–2004), the Czech Republic (2012), Libya (2013), Kenya (2014), Nigeria (2015), and Iran (2018).[1,2] Despite vast knowledge and experience with methanol, these outbreaks demonstrate the diagnostic challenge and difficulty in treating these patients. In 2018, 1828 single substance exposures to methanol were reported to US poison centers. The vast majority were unintentional exposures (89.4%), with few major complications (1.6%) and only 11 deaths.[3] These data, however, rely on voluntary reporting and likely underrepresent the true burden of methanol exposures and mortality outcomes from forensic data in the United States.

Principles of Toxicology

Methanol is rapidly absorbed from the gastrointestinal (GI) tract with an average absorptive half-life of 5 minutes and reaches peak concentration in 30 to 60 minutes. While the majority of exposures occur through oral ingestion, occupational and recreational inhalation of methanol from cleaning and cooling fluids has resulted in toxicity causing neurologic dysfunction and necessitating antidote therapy and hemodialysis (HD).[4–6] Transdermal exposure as well can lead to significant methanol toxicity. High-risk occupations for exposure to methanol include painting, varnishing, lithography, printing, and glazing.

Methanol itself has very low toxicity, but its metabolism results in toxic metabolites, in particular, formic acid, which dissociates into formate and hydrogen ions. Methanol is primarily metabolized in the liver by alcohol dehydrogenase (ADH) into formaldehyde. Formaldehyde is then metabolized by aldehyde dehydrogenase (ALDH) very rapidly, with a half-life of 1 to 2 minutes, into formic acid (Fig. 136.1). Formic acid can combine with tetrahydrofolate (THF) to form 10-formyl THF, which can be metabolized into carbon dioxide and water.

Elimination of methanol is mainly characterized via zero-order kinetics in the poisoned patient but does have first-order metabolism

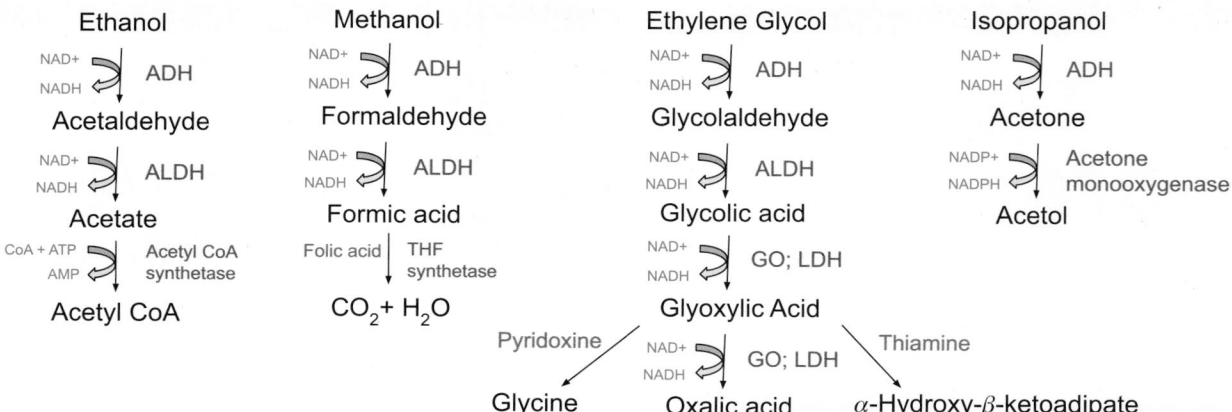

Fig. 136.1 Metabolism of alcohols. *ADH,* Alcohol dehydrogenase; *ALDH,* aldehyde dehydrogenase; *AMP,* adenosine monophosphate; *ATP,* adenosine triphosphate, *GO, Glycolate oxidase, LDH,* lactate dehydrogenase, *NAD+,* nicotinamide adenine dinucleotide; *NADH,* reduced form of nicotinamide adenine dinucleotide, *THF,* tetrahydrofolate.

at very low concentrations, with an elimination half-life of about 2 to 3 hours at low concentrations. Small amounts of methanol are eliminated by the renal and pulmonary systems.

At toxic concentrations, the elimination half-life of methanol is nearly 24 hours. The metabolite, formic acid, has a half-life of nearly 20 hours. With ADH inhibition by concurrent consumption of ethanol or administration of fomepizole, the half-life of methanol extends upward to more than 50 hours. With dialysis, the half-life of methanol is approximately 3 to 4 hours.

Formic acid will accumulate due to its slower metabolism as it exceeds the elimination rate. Formic acid binds iron efficiently, resulting in mitochondrial cytochrome oxidase inhibition, and interferes with oxidative metabolism in a manner similar to that of cyanide, carbon monoxide, and hydrogen sulfide. The dissociation of formic acid into formate and hydrogen ions leads to acidosis. The interference of oxidative metabolism, combined with acidosis, further promotes lactate production and worsens the acidotic state. Decreasing pH promotes formic acid diffusion across cell membranes, in particular to the central nervous system (CNS). Also, inhibition of cytochrome oxidase by formic acid is potentiated with decreasing pH. The net effect of this vicious cycle, coined the "*circulus hypoxicus,*" is tissue hypoxia and inhibition of intracellular respiration.[7] Further mechanisms of toxicity include free radical formation, lipid peroxidation, and impairment of antioxidant reactions.

Formic acid uniquely targets the optic disk of the retina and retrolaminar optic nerve, potentially due to the high amount of blood and cerebrospinal fluid (CSF) flow through the choriocapillaris. These cells are more susceptible to cellular hypoxia due to low levels of mitochondria and cytochrome oxidase, making formic acid oxidation slower in the eye compared to the brain.[8] Inhibition of mitochondrial cytochrome oxidase results in decreased adenosine triphosphate (ATP) production, leading to myelin sheath damage and loss of vision. Worsening acidosis potentiates these effects by enhancing the diffusion of formic acid across cell membranes into the neurons.

The basal ganglia and subcortical white matter are affected by formic acid in a similar manner to the ocular toxicity. Neuroimaging and autopsy findings classically demonstrate putamen hypodensity, with hemorrhages and necrosis. Bilateral putamen changes are not specific to methanol toxicity and can be found in Wilson disease, Leigh disease, Kearns-Sayre syndrome, toxic encephalopathy (e.g., carbon monoxide, cyanide, hydrogen sulfide), hemolytic-uremic syndrome, and

hypoxic-ischemic injury. The severity of findings and extent of necrosis on imaging do not necessarily correlate with clinical outcomes. The vulnerability of the basal ganglia to formic acid toxicity may be due to its high metabolic activity, with poor venous drainage and inadequate arterial flow.

Clinical Features

Clinical signs and symptoms of methanol intoxication typically involve the GI tract, CNS, and optic system. Shortly after exposure, patients appear similar to other alcohol ingestions, with GI irritation, inebriation, and CNS depression. Methanol has a less inebriating effect than ethanol but causes similar slurred speech, ataxia, confusion, and CNS depression. Abdominal discomfort and vomiting occur from mucosal irritation, and patients can develop acute pancreatitis. Severe mucosal irritation can also result in hemorrhagic gastritis. A latency period, ranging from 1 to 72 hours, depending on the amount ingested, can occur with the improvement of inebriation symptoms and development of visual symptoms as methanol metabolizes and formic acid accumulates.

As formic acid accumulates, the most characteristic feature is some degree of visual disturbance, including seeing spots with blurred vision (commonly referred to as "snowstorm vision"), altered visual fields, and blindness. Visual disturbances occur in 30% to 70% of patients.[9] Early ophthalmologic findings include reduced pupillary response to light and hyperemia of the optic disc. Peripapillary retinal edema and loss of optic disk cupping follow and often lead to decreased visual fields and central scotomata. Retinal dysfunction can be reversible. Blurred vision from formic acid induced retinal injury, is typically transient, and vision recovers. Optic atrophy and optic neuropathy suggest a poor prognosis for visual recovery. The incidence of ophthalmologic abnormalities correlates directly with the degree of acidosis. Long-term visual sequelae are associated with visual deficits at presentation, coma, and brain lesions on imaging.[10,11]

As acidosis progresses, compensatory tachypnea develops. Acidosis can be profound, with many patients presenting with an arterial pH less than 7.0 and serum bicarbonate level less than 10 mEq/L. Tachycardia is often noted, but patients rarely have significant cardiac dysrhythmias. Also, shock, seizures, myoglobinuria, and rhabdomyolysis have been reported. Death typically results from respiratory failure and sudden respiratory arrest, with cerebral edema and multiorgan failure.

TABLE 136.1	Causes of Elevated Osmolar and Anion Gaps		
Osmolar Gap	**Anion Gap (A Cat Piles Mud)**	**Double Gap**	**Distinguishing Features**
Methanol	**A**lcoholic ketoacidosis	Methanol	Vision loss—methanol
Ethylene glycol	**C**yanide, carbon monoxide, colchicine	Ethylene glycol	Hypocalcemia and calcium oxalate crystalluria—
Isopropanol	**A**cetaminophen (large ingestion)	Diabetic ketoacidosis	ethylene glycol
Ethanol	**T**oluene	Alcoholic ketoacidosis	Hyperglycemia, ketonuria—diabetic ketoacidosis
Mannitol	**P**araldehyde	Uremia	Normal or low glucose level, ketonuria—alcoholic
Acetone	Propylene glycol	Septic shock	ketoacidosis
Glycerol	Phenformin	Multiorgan failure	Positive blood cultures, lactic acidosis—septic
Propylene glycol	**I**soniazid, iron, ibuprofen		shock
Sorbitol	**L**actic acidosis (e.g., sepsis, ischemia)		
Fructose	**E**thylene glycol		
Diatrizoate (IV dye)	**S**alicylates		
Acetonitrile	**M**ethanol, metformin		
Ethyl ether	**U**remia		
Hyperlipidemia	**D**iabetic ketoacidosis		
Hyperproteinemia			
Diabetic ketoacidosis			
Alcoholic ketoacidosis			
Sick Cell Syndrome			
Uremia			
Multiorgan failure			
Septic shock			

Prognosis after methanol ingestion correlates with the degree of acidosis, time to presentation, and initiation of treatment. The strongest predictor of morbidity and mortality is the degree of acidosis, with high mortality rates observed at a pH less than 7.0. A comatose state at presentation also portends a worse outcome with high mortality rates and long-term neurologic sequelae.[12] Aggregated data from mass methanol poisoning events demonstrate that a comatose state with a pH less than 6.74 has an 83% mortality rate and 100% of survivors had neurologic sequelae, while non-comatose patients with a pH greater than 7.0 had a 5% mortality rate and only 16% of survivors had neurologic sequelae.[12] Patients that survive the acute toxicity of methanol can have permanent complications, including blindness and neurologic deficits. A Parkinson-like extrapyramidal syndrome, with bradykinesia, tremor, and dementia, can occur. These findings are generally associated with necrosis of the putamen and subcortical white matter on neuroimaging studies. Other neurologic sequelae include polyneuropathy, encephalopathy, ataxia, and cognitive deficits. Permanent vision deficits and evidence of brain hemorrhages on magnetic resonance imaging (MRI) are associated with decreased quality of life in survivors of methanol poisoning.[13]

Differential Diagnoses

The differential diagnoses for methanol intoxication are broad, making it difficult to detect, particularly at the initial presentation. The inebriated state of the patient can easily be confused with ethanol intoxication. Further causes of altered mental status (AMS) include hypoglycemia, hypoxia, carbon dioxide narcosis, infections, trauma, seizures, metabolic disturbances, endocrinopathies, and encephalopathy. Poisoning or intoxication by other substances, including opiates, carbon monoxide, sedative-hypnotics, and benzodiazepines, often presents with AMS. The GI irritation can occur with ethanol intoxication and with other intra-abdominal pathologies, such as gastritis and pancreatitis.

After ingestion of methanol, serum osmolality will be elevated and can lead to an elevated osmolar gap. Other substances that contribute to an elevated osmolar gap include EG, isopropanol, ethanol, mannitol, glycerol, propylene glycol (PG), sorbitol, fructose, diatrizoate (IV dye), acetonitrile, and ethyl ether (Table 136.1). Additionally, hyperlipidemia, hyperproteinemia, and sick cell syndrome cause an increase in the osmolar gap by decreasing the measured sodium concentration.[14]

As the parent compound methanol is metabolized, the production of formic acid results in an elevated anion gap (AG) acidosis. In addition to methanol, causes of AG acidosis include lactic acidosis of varying causes (e.g., sepsis, ischemia), diabetic ketoacidosis, alcoholic ketoacidosis, uremia, inborn errors of metabolism, and toxins (e.g., salicylates, isoniazid, iron, carbon monoxide, cyanide, metformin, toluene, paraldehyde, PG, and EG; see Table 136.1). Worsening acidosis, despite adequate fluid hydration and no evidence of underlying ischemia producing lactic acidosis, should raise the concern for toxic alcohol ingestion.

The presence of a so-called double gap (elevated osmolar and AGs) is classically described for toxic alcohol ingestion. Many other situations, however, can cause a similar picture, including diabetic ketoacidosis, alcoholic ketoacidosis, renal failure, multiple organ failure, and septic shock (see Table 136.1). This double gap picture is also dependent on the timing of presentation because early presenters will have only an osmotically active parent compound and late presenters will have acidosis without an elevated osmolar gap (Fig. 136.2).[15]

The development of ocular manifestations with worsening acidosis is a strong indicator of methanol poisoning. Other toxins, however, can cause ophthalmologic conditions and blindness such as cinchonism with quinine intoxication, but this lacks the elevated osmolar and AGs. Cortical blindness can occur with various causes of toxic leukoencephalopathy, including carbon monoxide, hydrocarbons, steroids, metals (organic mercury), and various chemotherapeutic agents (e.g., carboplatin, cisplatin).

Diagnostic Testing

The classically described presentation of toxic alcohol ingestion includes an AG metabolic acidosis and an elevated osmolar gap. Due

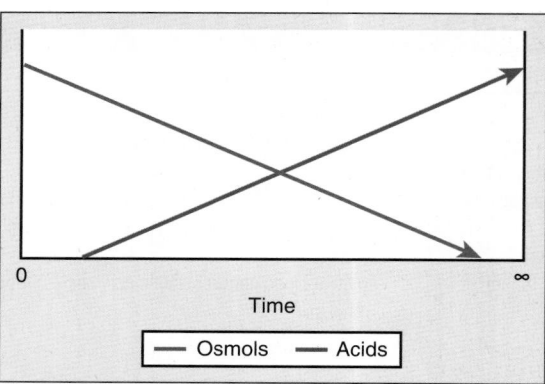

Fig. 136.2 Relationship of osmotically active parent alcohol to acid metabolite over time. (Adapted and modified with permission from Mycyk MB, Aks SE. A visual schematic for clarifying the temporal relationship between the anion gap and the osmol gaps in toxic alcohol poisoning. *Am J Emerg Med.* 2003;21:333–335.)

to the latency period of methanol metabolism, a normal AG does not exclude methanol ingestion. The AG is commonly calculated by the following equation:

$$AG = [Na^+] - ([HCO_3^-] + [Cl^-])$$

with a normal AG of 8 to 12 mEq/L. Decreased albumin can falsely elevate the AG; the AG can be corrected by using the Figge equation:

$$AG\ corrected = AG + (2.5 \times [44 - measured\ serum\ albumin]),$$
$$(albumin\ expressed\ as\ g/dL)$$

Mortality correlates highly with the degree of acidosis and formate concentration rather than with a specific methanol concentration. Visual dysfunction occurs with a formate concentration greater than 20 to 30 mg/dL. Indicators for a poor prognosis include a formate concentration of more than 50 mg/dL and a pH less than 7.0

Many formulas exist for calculating serum osmolarity, but the most commonly used is the following:

$$Calculated\ osmolarity\ (mOsm/L) = 2Na^+ + (BUN/2.8) +$$
$$(glucose/18) +$$
$$(ethanol/4.6)$$

where blood urea nitrogen (BUN), glucose, and the ethanol concentrations are measured in mg/dL. The difference between measured serum osmolality and calculated serum osmolarity is as follows:

$$Osmolar\ gap = measured\ osmolality\ (mOsm/kg) -$$
$$calculated\ osmolarity\ (mOsm/L)$$

If using the International System of Units (SI units), there are no corrections, and the various serum levels are simply added or subtracted. The normal osmolar gap has been arbitrarily defined as normal if it is less than 10 mOsm. However, a wide range of osmolar gaps is observed in the population, from −15 to +10 mOsm. As a result, individuals who begin with a negative osmolar gap can have significantly elevated concentrations of toxic alcohols but have a so-called normal osmolar gap. Many other substances can contribute to an osmolar gap and can be misleading. Also, if patients are acidotic, the parent compound (methanol, EG) has been metabolized into its respective acid and does not contribute to the osmotic load. Thus, a normal osmolar gap cannot exclude toxic alcohol ingestion. Methanol, however, is more likely than EG to have an elevated osmolar gap. An extremely elevated osmolar gap (>20–25 mOsm)

however is highly suspicious for toxic alcohol ingestion.[16–18] In methanol ingestions, the metabolite formic acid can be measured using enzymatic analysis but this test is not routinely available.[14,19]

Neuroimaging with MRI and computed tomography (CT) can be performed for patients with AMS. The most consistent finding for methanol poisoning is bilateral necrosis of the putamen. However, this finding is not specific for methanol poisoning, and neuroimaging is typically normal in the first 24 hours after methanol exposure because findings typically lag behind clinical symptoms. Patients with evidence of putaminal necrosis on imaging are at risk for an irreversible Parkinson-like extrapyramidal syndrome and chronic disability limiting daily functioning.[13] The measurement of visual evoked potentials (VEP) is sensitive to detect impairment in the optic system.[8]

Ultimately, the definitive diagnosis requires laboratory confirmation of the presence of methanol. Once toxic alcohol ingestion is suspected, directly measure methanol and EG concentrations and begin empirical therapy. Peak methanol concentrations less than 20 mg/dL are generally not associated with toxicity, but peak methanol concentrations greater than 50 mg/dL indicate significant and serious exposure. Peak methanol concentrations occur shortly after ingestion due to rapid GI absorption. Due to the variability of the timing of patient presentation, the methanol level interpretation must be based on clinical findings (e.g., AMS, vision complaints) as well as additional laboratory findings (e.g., metabolic acidosis, elevated osmolar gap). Depending on the location of the practice and laboratory capabilities, specific serum concentrations of methanol or EG may not be readily attainable in most hospitals, and blood specimens may need to be transported to regional reference laboratories for emergent analysis.

Management

Alcohols are rapidly absorbed from the GI tract, so GI decontamination has limited to no value. Gastric suctioning via a nasogastric or orogastric tube may be considered in a large volume exposure (such as an entire bottle of windshield washer fluid or antifreeze) in someone who presents immediately after ingestion, but there is no evidence to support routine use and gastric lavage is generally not recommended. Activated charcoal is not indicated for toxic alcohol ingestions. Aside from standard stabilization and resuscitation, the main priorities in toxic alcohol exposure are correction of acidosis, inhibition of the production of toxic metabolites, and elimination of the parent alcohol and its toxic metabolites. Therapy should be initiated based on strong clinical suspicion. Treatment should not be delayed while waiting for specific serum concentrations to be determined.

Because the degree of acidosis correlates with severity and outcome, treat a serum pH less than 7.3 with intravenous (IV) sodium bicarbonate to normalize the pH. Worsening acidosis from formic acid accumulation potentiates mitochondrial cytochrome oxidase inhibition and anaerobic metabolism, also generating lactic acidosis. Based on supporting patient data, correction of acidosis likely improves outcomes and ophthalmologic symptoms. Bicarbonate can be administered via intermittent boluses, combination of a bolus and infusion, or infusion alone based on the severity of symptoms. Administer bolus sodium bicarbonate at 1 to 2 mEq/kg and infuse 150 mEq/L of sodium bicarbonate in 5% dextrose at 1.5 to 2 times the maintenance fluid rate until normalization of the serum pH (7.35–7.45). Large amounts of bicarbonate may be necessary for even partial correction of acidosis due to metabolism of the parent alcohol into its toxic acid. With bicarbonate administration, monitor for the development of hypernatremia and hypokalemia. The use of bicarbonate should not deter definitive elimination of the parent alcohol and its toxic metabolites via HD.

Prevent the further production of formic acid by inhibiting ADH with fomepizole (methylpyrazole, 4-MP) or ethanol. Fomepizole is preferable due to its safety profile and ease of administration, with a

> ## BOX 136.1 Criteria for Initiation of Alcohol Dehydrogenase Blockade for Methanol or Ethylene Glycol Poisoning
>
> Documented plasma methanol or EG concentration ≥20 mg/dL
> *or*
> History of ingestion of methanol or EG and an osmolar gap >10 mOsm/L
> *or*
> Strong clinical suspicion of ingestion of methanol or EG and at least two of the following:
> 1. Arterial pH <7.3
> 2. Serum bicarbonate <20 mEq/L (mmol/L)
> 3. Osmolar gap >10 mOsm/L
> 4. Urinary oxalate crystals present (for EG ingestion)

EG, Ethylene glycol.

> ## BOX 136.2 Fomepizole Dosing
>
> - Loading dose—15 mg/kg IV
> - Maintenance dose—10 mg/kg IV every 12 h for up to 48 h
> - After 48 h—15 mg/kg every 12 h
> - If undergoing HD—same doses as above, but start maintenance schedule 6 h after loading dose and then administer every 4 h during HD

sevenfold reduction in adverse drug event rate versus ethanol.[9,18,20] No contraindication exists for fomepizole use except for a severe allergic reaction, but currently, there have been no reported cases.[18] Most adverse reactions to fomepizole are transient and do not require discontinuation of treatment.[21] Specific indications for initiating ADH blockade are a documented methanol or EG concentration more than 20 mg/dL, documented history of methanol or EG ingestion with an osmolar gap more than 10 mOsm/L, or suspected methanol or EG ingestion with an arterial pH less than 7.3, serum carbon dioxide (bicarbonate) level less than 20 mmol/L, or oxalate crystalluria (Box 136.1).

In clinical practice, however, initiate fomepizole therapy with a strong clinical suspicion for serious ingestion, and send for confirmatory levels, because a delay in ADH blockade can lead to the development of acidosis and deleterious consequences. Fomepizole dosing involves a loading dose of 15 mg/kg followed by 10-mg/kg doses every 12 hours, up to 48 hours. After 48 hours, give 15 mg/kg every 12 hours because repeated dosing of fomepizole induces its own cytochrome P-450 metabolism. Of note, the fomepizole dosing frequency does need to be adjusted with HD (Box 136.2). Side effects of fomepizole include headache, nausea, dizziness, phlebitis, and reversible liver transaminase level elevation. One case of hypotension and bradycardia due to the rapid infusion of fomepizole has been described.[15,20]

If fomepizole is not available, and ethanol therapy is used to inhibit ADH, maintain serum ethanol concentrations between 100 and 150 mg/dL. The affinity of ADH for ethanol is 10 times greater than for methanol. Ethanol dosing is complex, however, and can cause worsening CNS and respiratory depression, with hypotension, vomiting, phlebitis, and hypoglycemia, particularly in children or malnourished individuals.[18,20] Given the widespread availability of fomepizole and its safety profile versus that of ethanol, the dosing of IV ethanol is not discussed here because its routine use is not recommended with the exception of mass outbreaks or lack of fomepizole availability.[12,22] With ADH inhibition, the half-life of methanol is significantly extended

upward of 50 hours. Patients who present early after methanol ingestion without acidosis can potentially be treated with ADH inhibition alone but may have prolonged hospitalizations due to the extended half-life of the parent compound.

Elimination of the parent alcohol via HD is the mainstay of therapy in severe toxic alcohol ingestions, and consultation with a regional poison center or medical toxicologist will help determine whether the patient is a candidate. HD serves multiple purposes in that it removes the parent alcohol and its metabolites, corrects acidosis, and aids in fluid management and cardiovascular stabilization. Additionally, it can shorten the course and cost of hospitalization, particularly in methanol ingestions, due to methanol's long half-life.[11] Intermittent HD is preferred over continuous renal replacement therapy (CRRT) but CRRT is acceptable if HD is not available.[15,23]

HD is indicated for acidosis (pH < 7.3), renal failure, vision abnormalities with methanol exposure, electrolyte imbalances unresponsive to conventional therapy (i.e., hyperkalemia), hemodynamic instability, and methanol or EG concentration more than 50 mg/dL.[15] Traditional endpoints for discontinuing HD or ADH inhibition are a normal acid-base status and methanol-EG concentration less than 20 mg/dL.[15] Ophthalmologic disturbances are not an indication for continued dialysis after correction of the acid-base disturbance and removal of methanol. There is no specific treatment for methanol-induced persistent optic nerve injury. Formic acid is converted to carbon dioxide and water via THF synthetase; therefore, folinic acid (leucovorin) may aid in formic acid elimination, but there have been no human trials to support its efficacy. The recommended dose is 1 mg/kg (maximum dose: 50 mg) of folinic acid IV every 4 to 6 hours until methanol has been eliminated and the acidosis resolves. The use of folinic acid (leucovorin) should not deter emergent HD if indicated.

Disposition

Admission is generally necessary for patients being treated for methanol exposure. Consult with nephrology early for possible HD. If HD is not available, administer fomepizole and transfer the patient to an institution where emergent HD can be initiated. Consult the regional poison center (1-800-222-1222) or a medical toxicologist to guide management. Consult an ophthalmologist to evaluate visual fields and the retina for methanol-induced ocular injury within 24 hours. Patients with a methanol concentration less than 20 mg/dL and no clinical symptoms or laboratory abnormalities may be discharged. If the patient has psychiatric issues or intent of self-harm, a psychiatric consultation is indicated.

ETHYLENE GLYCOL

Foundations

EG (ethane-1,2-diol, CAS 107-21-1, $C_2H_6O_2$) is a colorless, odorless, sweet-tasting liquid. It is a common component of antifreeze and de-icing solutions because it lowers the freezing point of water. Additional sources of EG include hydraulic brake fluids, industrial solvents, foam stabilizer, paints, and cosmetics. Because EG has a sweet taste, it is often substituted for ethanol and has led to mass poisonings historically. In 2018, 6599 single substance exposures to EG were reported to US poison centers. Most of these were unintentional (82%) but resulted in roughly 10.5% of patients having moderate to severe effects and a total of 19 deaths.[3] Like methanol, the data rely on voluntary reporting and likely underestimate the true burden of EG exposures and mortality outcomes.

EG is rapidly absorbed from the GI tract with peak blood levels occurring within 1 to 4 hours after ingestion. EG is highly water-soluble and, unlike methanol or isopropanol, is not volatile at room temperature. Thus, transdermal and pulmonary absorption of EG are extremely limited, and toxicity from these routes of exposure is not expected or observed.

Metabolism of EG primarily occurs in the liver via the conversion of ADH into glycolaldehyde, which is rapidly converted by ALDH into glycolic acid. Glycolic acid is further metabolized into glyoxylic acid (glyoxylate) and oxalic acid (see Fig. 136.1). The conversion of glycolic acid into glyoxylic acid is slow, and the accumulation of glycolic acid generates a profound metabolic acidosis. Pyridoxine and thiamine are cofactors in the metabolism of glyoxylic acid; however, given the slow conversion of glycolic acid to glyoxylic acid, these cofactors likely do not contribute significantly to EG detoxification. A small amount of oxalate will precipitate with calcium to form calcium oxalate crystals. These metabolic oxidation steps result in the conversion of nicotinamide adenine dinucleotide (NAD^+) to nicotinamide adenine dinucleotide (NADH). The increase of NADH to NAD^+ converts pyruvate to lactate and generates lactic acidosis.

Calcium oxalate crystals precipitate in the proximal renal tubules and are the main contributing factor in the development of acute tubular necrosis and renal failure. Calcium oxalate deposits also occur in the brain, intestinal mucosa, lungs, heart, and spleen, although the contribution of these deposits to the clinical picture is less clear. Further findings of EG toxicity include diffuse petechial hemorrhages in the heart, lungs, and brain, as well as the development of cerebral edema. Myonecrosis and rhabdomyolysis can occur. The chelation of calcium by oxalate can lead to systemic hypocalcemia.

Elimination of EG occurs mainly in the liver, but roughly 20% to 25% of EG is excreted unchanged in the urine. The reported half-life of EG ranges from 3 to 9 hours, but when metabolism is inhibited by ethanol or fomepizole, the half-life increases up to 20 hours. With HD, the half-life of EG is about 2 to 3 hours, depending on flow rates.

Clinical Features

The clinical picture of EG toxicity is typically divided into three stages: (1) acute neurologic stage; (2) cardiopulmonary stage; and (3) renal stage. As with methanol, delayed neurologic sequelae are described. An extreme amount of clinical variability occurs, stages may overlap, and mortality may occur at any stage. Poor prognostic factors at admission include hyperkalemia, severe metabolic acidosis, renal failure, seizures, coma, and delays in treatment. Seizures are highly prognostic for death.[20] The co-ingestion of ethanol can delay the onset of symptoms.

EG is a gastric irritant and can produce nausea and vomiting shortly after ingestion. The acute neurologic stage occurs over 30 minutes to 12 hours after ingestion with EG, producing inebriation and euphoria similar to ethanol. In severe poisonings, CNS depression can progress to coma, hypotonia, and seizures. Additional findings include nystagmus, ataxia, and myoclonic jerks. Cerebral edema can develop from calcium oxalate crystal deposition and cytotoxic damage contributing to CNS depression.

The cardiopulmonary stage occurs 12 to 24 hours after ingestion, with patients developing tachycardia with severe metabolic acidosis and compensatory tachypnea. The acidosis occurs from the generation of glycolic acid. Hypoxia with pulmonary edema and acute respiratory distress syndrome (ARDS) can cause hypoxia. Multiorgan failure with circulatory collapse can occur, and most deaths ensue during this stage.

The renal stage occurs 24 to 72 hours postingestion with the development of acute renal failure (ARF) from calcium oxalate crystal deposition. Conscious patients may complain of flank pain and have costovertebral tenderness. Hematuria and proteinuria can occur. Renal failure can be anuric, oliguric, or nonoliguric. Renal dysfunction frequently necessitates HD and, in some cases, for months after exposure. Renal function usually returns to normal following EG intoxication,

but occasionally renal damage can be permanent. Long-term HD is rarely necessary.

Delayed neurologic sequelae commonly present as bulbar palsy from 5 to 20 days after ingestion, with cranial nerve VII being most commonly implicated. Other cranial nerve involvement has been documented; clinical findings include ophthalmoplegia, diplopia, nystagmus, facial droop, facial sensory loss, hearing loss, dysphagia, and vertigo.[24] The term *facial auditory nerve oxalosis* has been used to describe this delayed syndrome and its predilection to affect cranial nerves VII and VIII noted on autopsy. In addition to the cranial nerves, an autonomic nerve dysfunction has been described, with postural hypotension and gastroparesis. The exact pathogenesis for these neurologic findings is unclear, but postulated mechanisms include calcium oxalate deposition resulting in mechanical nerve injury, inflammatory response causing nerve dysfunction, and depletion of thiamine and pyridoxine cofactors. Neuroimaging studies can demonstrate the focal infiltration of calcium oxalate with inflammation and necrosis of the basal ganglia. Despite significant MRI pathology, individuals with neurologic complications can have a full recovery.[25]

Differential Diagnoses

The differential diagnoses for EG intoxication are broad and similar to methanol. See earlier, "Methanol: Differential Diagnoses," for a more in-depth explanation, especially regarding the initial presentation of inebriation and AMS, proceeding through elevated osmolar and AGs (see Table 136.1).

Unlike methanol, however, the hallmark of EG toxicity involves renal failure with calcium oxalate crystalluria. Many other substances cause ARF, including antimicrobials (e.g., aminoglycosides, vancomycin, sulfa-based drugs, ciprofloxacin, penicillins, polymixins), nonsteroidal antiinflammatory drugs, angiotensin-converting enzyme inhibitors, angiotensin II receptor blockers, HMG-CoA reductase inhibitors, antivirals (e.g., acyclovir, foscarnet, antiretrovirals), amphotericin B, chemotherapeutics (e.g., methotrexate, cisplatin, ifosfamide), diethylene glycol (DEG), bisphosphonates, radiocontrast media, heavy metals, proton pump inhibitors, lithium, and acetaminophen. Calcium oxalate crystalluria is not specific for EG and is only present in up to 50% of cases of EG ingestion. Healthy individuals with excess dietary intake of vitamin C or foods rich in oxalate (e.g., garlic, tomatoes, spinach, rhubarb, and tea) may have incidental calcium oxalate crystalluria.

Xenobiotic-induced hypocalcemia can occur from proton pump inhibitors, bisphosphonates, other phosphate-containing substances (e.g., laxatives and sodium phosphate), loop diuretics, glucocorticoids, calcitonin, cisplatin, pentamidine, interferon-alfa, fluorides (e.g., hydrofluoric acid), citrate, phenytoin, phenobarbital, carbamazepine, estrogens, and ethylenediaminetetraacetic acid. Hypocalcemia, metabolic acidosis, ARF, and calcium oxalate crystalluria, however, strongly suggest EG toxicity. Ultimately, the definitive diagnosis requires laboratory confirmation of EG concentrations in blood or serum.

Diagnostic Testing

Diagnostic testing for EG is similar to that for methanol; for a more detailed discussion of AG acidosis and elevated osmolar gap calculations, see earlier, "Methanol: Diagnostic Testing." The contribution of EG to the osmolar gap is relatively small compared to other alcohols, and an EG concentration of 50 mg/dL will only cause an 8- to 10-mOsm rise in the osmolar gap. Thus, an elevated osmolar gap can suggest EG ingestion, but a normal gap does not exclude it.

Glycolic acid is structurally similar to lactate and can cause a false positive lactate elevation in laboratory equipment using a lactate oxidase-based system measuring hydrogen peroxide generated from the metabolism of lactate to pyruvate. These machines tend to be

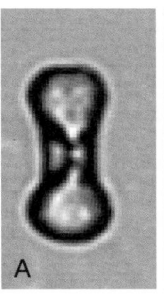 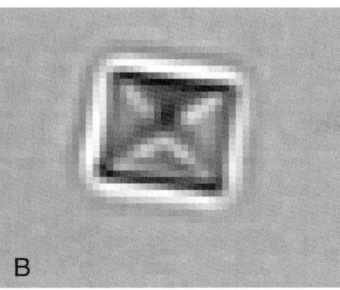

Fig. 136.3 Calcium oxalate crystals. Illustrated are calcium oxalate monohydrate (A) and dihydrate (B) crystals in the urine. The monohydrate whewellite crystals typically are needle-like or dumbbell-shaped and strongly birefringent, whereas the dihydrate weddellite crystals are octahedral, envelope-shaped, and weakly birefringent.

point-of-care tests such as whole blood arterial or venous blood gas analyzers. This can create a "lactate gap" in EG ingestion where a point-of-care lactate is extremely elevated but a formal laboratory analysis of lactate using a lactate dehydrogenase system is markedly less.[26,27]

Calcium oxalate crystalluria can be of two major forms, needle-shaped calcium oxalate monohydrate or polyhedron-shaped calcium oxalate dihydrate crystals. The calcium oxalate monohydrate crystals may be mistaken for hippuric acid crystals. Crystals can be found in the urine 4 to 8 hours after exposure. Additional urinary findings include hematuria and proteinuria (Fig. 136.3).

Fluorescein dye is often added to antifreeze agents to assist in the detection of automobile radiator leaks, so patients who ingest anti-freeze EG-containing agents may exhibit urinary fluorescence under a Woods lamp. Urinary fluorescence, however, is neither specific nor sensitive for diagnosing or excluding EG intoxication. The fluorescence of gastric contents soon after EG ingestion may be more definitive.

The EG concentration itself does not predict severity as much as it depends on the timing of presentation and initiation of intervention. Serum EG concentrations greater than 50 mg/dL, however, are associated with serious ingestion and toxicity. The degree of acidosis (particularly a pH <7.2–7.3) does predict an increase in the creatinine level and mortality outcome. A peak EG concentration less than 20 mg/dL is generally not associated with significant toxicity.

In EG intoxication, the serum glycolic acid concentration is the driving force for acidosis. Glycolic acid concentrations greater than 99 mg/dL are strongly associated with severe CNS toxicity and mortality. Levels greater than 76 mg/dL have nearly 100% sensitivity for predicting ARF.[28] Glycolic acid levels greater than 60 mg/dL could be an indication for HD, but this is not well validated.[28] Serum glycolic acid concentrations typically are not readily available in a timely fashion to aid in most clinical situations and only a small percentage of reference laboratories perform this test.[28]

Management

Many of the management principles of EG toxicity overlap with those of methanol. EG, like methanol, is rapidly absorbed from the GI tract; thus, gut decontamination has a limited to no role in EG ingestion. Correction of metabolic acidosis with sodium bicarbonate (pH < 7.3) may increase the urinary excretion of EG and delay calcium oxalate-induced ARF. Initiate ADH blockade, preferably with fomepizole, as soon as possible to prevent the development of toxic metabolites (see Boxes 136.1 and 136.2). Ethanol therapy can be used if fomepizole is unavailable, although its routine use is not recommended. Consider HD for the indications stated earlier, particularly for an acid-base imbalance and renal failure. EG, however, has a shorter half-life than

methanol, and patients without acidosis or renal compromise can be managed with fomepizole alone, thus preventing the need for HD in adult and pediatric patients. Continue treatment until serum EG concentrations are less than 20 mg/dL, and a normal acid-base status is present.

Pyridoxine and thiamine are cofactors in EG metabolism. Pyridoxine aids in the conversion of glyoxylic acid metabolism to glycine. Thiamine stimulates conversion of glyoxylic acid to α-hydroxy-β-ketoadipate (see Fig. 136.1). No clinical data, however, support the effectiveness of these cofactors in otherwise healthy patients with EG ingestion. These cofactors should be given to patients with vitamin deficiencies, such as alcoholics and malnourished individuals. The recommended adult doses are thiamine 100 mg IV daily, and pyridoxine 100 mg IV daily, for 2 days. If patients have symptomatic hypocalcemia (interval changes on the electrocardiogram and dysrhythmias), replete with calcium gluconate or calcium chloride as needed.

Disposition

Admission is generally necessary for patients being treated for EG exposure. Consult nephrology early for possible HD. If HD is not available, initiate ADH inhibition and transfer the patient to an institution where emergent dialysis is available. Consult the regional poison center (1-800-222-1222) or a medical toxicologist to guide management. Patients with an EG concentration less than 20 mg/dL and no laboratory abnormalities or clinical symptoms may be discharged. If the patient has psychiatric issues or intent for self-harm, a psychiatric consultation is indicated.

ISOPROPYL ALCOHOL

Foundations

IPA (isopropanol, 2-propanol, CAS 67-63-0, C_3H_7OH) is a clear, colorless liquid with a fruity odor and bitter taste. IPA is found in numerous household and commercial products, including rubbing alcohol, antifreeze, disinfectants, cleaning solutions, skin and hair products, and hand sanitizers. IPA is commonly used as a solvent for industrial applications. It is the second most commonly ingested alcohol after ethanol. Exposures to IPA, either as a single substance or combined with other substances, reported to US poison centers have ranged from about 15,000 to 21,000 cases/year.[3] In 2018, 12,730 single substance IPA exposures occurred, with 82% unintentional in nature, 1% having moderate to major effects, and zero deaths, reflecting a low case-fatality rate.[3]

Isopropyl alcohol is rapidly absorbed from the GI tract with peak plasma concentrations occurring within 30 minutes. Oral ingestion is the major route of exposure, but absorption can occur transdermally, rectally, or via inhalation. Children are especially susceptible to systemic symptoms from the dermal application of IPA used to reduce fever.

Metabolism occurs primarily in the liver by ADH into acetone. Acetone is metabolized to acetol (hydroxyacetone) by acetone mono-oxygenase (see Fig. 136.1). Further metabolic products include PG, methylglyoxal, lactate, formate, and acetate. Many of these minor metabolic products are then converted to glucose. Acetone reaches a peak plasma concentration from 7 to 30 hours postexposure and has a half-life of up to 24 hours. IPA follows first-order kinetics, with a half-life of 2.5 to 8 hours. ADH inhibition increases the half-life to 16 to 27 hours. Elimination primarily occurs via the kidneys, with up to 20% of IPA excreted unchanged in the urine.

Isopropyl alcohol directly acts as a CNS depressant and is considered to be twice as inebriating as ethanol. Acetone can also contribute to CNS depression. A concomitant respiratory depression can occur with profound CNS depression. With larger doses, peripheral vasodilation and decreased cardiac inotropy can cause hypotension. Topical exposure leads to corneal de-epithelialization, with dermal irritation.

Clinical Features

Isopropyl alcohol irritates mucosal surfaces, and GI effects typically occur early after ingestion. Nausea, vomiting, and abdominal pain typically ensue, but hemorrhagic gastritis, hematemesis, and significant blood loss can result with larger ingestions. As with other alcohols, pancreatitis is a potential complication. Aspiration of IPA can cause hemorrhagic tracheobronchitis and pulmonary edema.

CNS depression ranges from lethargy to stupor or coma. Headache, dizziness, ataxia, hypotonia, hyporeflexia, dysarthria, and seizures have been reported. Pupil size is variable, but miosis is commonly observed. Loss of consciousness is associated with respiratory depression, hypoxia, and aspiration pneumonitis. Hypotension and hypothermia can occur with very large ingestions. Hypotension signifies severe poisoning with increased mortality risk. Injuries from prolonged immobilization with CNS depression can lead to compartment syndrome and rhabdomyolysis. Myoglobinuria can cause ARF. Hypoglycemia has not been reported with IPA as it has for other alcohols. Dermal contact causes a defatting dermatitis with drying and cracking of the skin, and pediatric patients can sustain chemical burns. Ketosis without acidosis is a classic finding in IPA ingestion.

Differential Diagnoses

Patients with significant IPA ingestion appear intoxicated similar to ethanol. IPA will elevate the osmolar gap but, unlike methanol and EG, not the AG. See earlier, "Methanol: Differential Diagnoses" for causes for AMS and an elevated osmolar gap. As IPA is converted to acetone, ketosis will occur. Ketosis is present in conditions such as diabetic ketoacidosis, alcoholic ketoacidosis, starvation ketosis, salicylism, and cyanide and acetone ingestion. Those chronically dependent on ethanol may consume IPA to prevent alcohol withdrawal and can have a mixed picture of alcoholic ketoacidosis with IPA ingestion.[29] ARF can develop from rhabdomyolysis but the differential for ARF is extensive.

Diagnostic Testing

The most common laboratory abnormality is ketosis without acidosis and euglycemia. As IPA is metabolized, acetone accumulates. Acetone does not elevate the AG, but IPA and acetone do contribute to the osmolar gap. Acetone can be detected within 30 minutes in serum and within 3 hours in urine postexposure. Acetone can interfere with the assay for creatinine and cause a pseudo-renal failure measurement with an isolated elevated creatinine but normal BUN level. If patients are hypotensive from a large IPA ingestion, lactic acidosis can occur, which can then cause a confounding AG acidosis.

The measurement of the IPA concentration is the definitive method of diagnosis. Occasionally, IPA can be detected in patients with acetonemia not exposed to IPA because acetone is converted to IPA in vivo. Serum concentrations of IPA do not correlate well with clinical outcomes—deaths have been reported with concentrations as low as 20 mg/dL. The scant data available suggest that a concentration of more than 50 mg/dL is associated with toxicity, and some authors suggest HD for levels greater than 400 mg/dL, hypotension, or lactic acidosis, although there has been no clear evidence for these recommendations[9]

Management

Supportive care is the mainstay of therapy for IPA ingestion. There is no role for GI decontamination. Wash the skin with soap and water for dermal contamination. Provide proton pump inhibitors (e.g., pantoprazole, 80 mg IV push and a drip at 8 mg/h for 72 hours, or until the patient can tolerate oral foods and fluids) for hemorrhagic gastritis. Consult gastroenterology for endoscopy to exclude other causes of upper GI bleeding or to intervene for persistent bleeding causing hemodynamic instability, necessitating transfusion, or worsening clinical condition. For deeply comatose patients, airway protection is indicated. Hypotension generally responds to IV crystalloid solution. For significant hypotension, initiate 1 to 2 L of normal saline as a bolus infusion, followed by repeated 500-mL boluses at 30-minute intervals until a mean arterial pressure (MAP) of 65 mm Hg is achieved. If the target MAP cannot be achieved or maintained with 4 L of normal saline boluses, start a norepinephrine infusion and titrate to the target MAP. Additional vasopressor support can be added with fluids, as needed. If the patient is persistently hypotensive, despite standard resuscitative measures, HD is indicated. ADH blockade with fomepizole or ethanol is not indicated because this will only prolong the hypotensive and CNS depressant effects of IPA.

Disposition

Due to IPA's rapid absorption on its onset of action, patients who are stable and alert 6 hours after ingestion are unlikely to develop significant complications and can be monitored until no longer clinically intoxicated and discharged from the emergency department (ED). Patients with significant inebriation or AMS should be admitted as an inpatient or placed in an observation unit for 24 hours. Consult gastroenterology for patients with hemorrhagic gastritis for endoscopy. Consult nephrology for patients with a comatose state or refractory hypotension for HD. Consult the regional poison center (1-800-222-1222) or medical toxicologist to help guide management.

OTHER ALCOHOLS OF CLINICAL SIGNIFICANCE

DEG is an odorless, viscous, sweet-tasting liquid commonly used as a solvent. It is found in brake fluid, antifreeze, lubricants, wallpaper strippers, and artificial fog machine solutions. Most exposures to DEG occur in epidemics in which DEG is substituted in pharmaceutical preparations for more expensive glycols. The first epidemic occurred in the United States in 1937, with DEG being used as a solvent for sulfanilamide, and led to the passing of the 1938 Federal Food, Drug, and Cosmetic Act requiring drug manufactures to demonstrate product safety prior to marketing. Other epidemics include those in South Africa (1969), Spain (1985), Nigeria (1990), Bangladesh (1990–92), Haiti (1996), India (1998), Panama (2006), and Nigeria (2008). DEG toxicity resembles that of EG, with initial GI irritation and CNS depressant effects, followed by metabolic acidosis. ARF without urinary calcium oxalate crystals occurs. Patients who survive ARF, unlike EG, typically require lifelong HD. Neurologic symptoms develop 5 to 10 days postingestion and can include lethargy, cranial neuropathies, peripheral polyneuropathies, and quadriparesis. DEG is metabolized into 2-hydroxyethoxyacetic acid and does not metabolize into EG, as once believed. Management is similar to that of methanol and EG and includes ADH blockade and early consideration for HD.[9,18]

PG is commonly used as a solvent in various pharmaceutical products and in antifreeze and hydraulic fluids. Common medications that use PG as a diluent include IV phenytoin, lorazepam, diazepam, etomidate, nitroglycerin, phenobarbital, hydralazine, and trimethoprim-sulfamethoxazole.[30] PG is metabolized to lactic acid and can produce metabolic acidosis. Also, it can contribute to an elevated osmolar gap. Because PG has a short half-life, the osmolar gap rapidly returns to normal once the medication diluent or exposure is discontinued.

Underlying renal insufficiency and hepatic dysfunction increase the risk for toxicity. Case reports have noted acute kidney injury from proximal tubular necrosis with PG toxicity. Additionally, PG toxicity can mimic a systemic inflammatory response syndrome and cause a confounding picture, with an elevated osmolar and AG triggering exploration for methanol and EG exposure. Approximately 20% of intensive care unit patients on continuous lorazepam infusions can have some degree of PG toxicity. Treatment typically involves stopping the offending agent, but HD and ADH blockade can be considered for severe acidosis and metabolic abnormalities.[9]

The references for this chapter can be found online at ExpertConsult. com.

137

Alcohol-Related Disease

John T. Finnell

As eloquently stated by Paracelsus in the 16th century, "all substances are poisons; there is none which is not a poison. The right dose differentiates a poison from a remedy."

FOUNDATIONS

Excess alcohol consumption places a significant burden on individuals and society. Globally, alcohol consumption is the seventh leading risk factor for both death and the burden of disease and injury. 2016 data from the World Health Organization (WHO) state that 5.3% of all deaths globally were attributable to alcohol consumption.[1] The overall costs associated with alcohol use represent more than 1% of the gross national product in high- and middle-income countries, with the costs of social harm (e.g., violence and road accidents) being far greater than health costs alone. In short, except for tobacco, alcohol accounts for a higher burden of disease than any other drug.[2]

From 2002 to 2010,[3] the rate of emergency department (ED) visits for alcohol-related diagnoses increased by 38%. In addition to the number of visits, current National Hospital Ambulatory Care survey data indicates that the total time and the length of stay (LOS) for ethanol-related visits are increasing as well.[4]

Twenty-seven percent of the US population admits to alcohol misuse.[5] Alcohol misuse accounts for more than 100,000 deaths in the United States every year, making it the fourth leading preventable cause of death in the United States and the 12th leading cause of death overall and is associated with over 200 diseases.[5,6] Alcoholism permeates all levels of society. Studies reveal a complex association between alcohol consumption and socioeconomic status (SES),[7] where people of lower SES show greater susceptibility to the damaging effects of alcohol.

Alcohol use and misuse also have social and financial costs, with estimates of over $220 billion in societal costs in the United States annually.[8] The literature refers to harmful, hazardous, and risky drinking interchangeably as a pattern of drinking that increases the risk of harm for the person consuming alcohol or others. The International Classification of Disease 10th Revision (ICD-10), draft ICD-11, and the *Diagnostic and Statistical Manual of Mental Disorders 4th Edition* (DSM-4) use the term "alcohol dependence." Alcohol dependence is a result of repeated use leading to a person having impaired control over the use of alcohol despite physical, psychological, and social harms. The fifth edition of the Diagnostic and Statistical Manual (DSM-5) combines diagnostic criteria for alcohol abuse and dependence under the term "alcohol use disorder," with severity modifiers of "mild," "moderate," or "severe," based on the number of criteria met. DSM-5 AUD of moderate or greater severity is essentially equivalent to DSM-4 and ICD-10 criteria for alcohol dependence. DSM–5 integrates alcohol abuse and alcohol dependence into a single disorder called alcohol use disorder (AUD), with mild, moderate, and severe sub-classifications.

At least 24% to 31% of ED patients meet National Institute Alcohol Abuse and Alcoholism (NIAAA) criteria for "at-risk" or heavy drinking. At-risk drinking is defined as an average of 14 or more standard drinks/week or 5 or more per occasion for men and 7 or more drinks weekly or 3 or more per occasion for women and people older than 65 years. (Table 137.1: Terms and Definitions of Unhealthy Alcohol Use.[9])

Patients, their families, and society, in general, should be aware that AUDs are not a result of any individual weakness or moral failing but arise from a complex interaction of individual, social, cultural, and biological factors. Most people with AUD are difficult to identify because they are likely to have jobs and families and to present with general complaints, such as malaise, insomnia, anxiety, sadness, or a range of medical problems.

In 2013, the US Preventive Services Task Force (USPSTF) recommended that clinicians screen adults 18 years or older for alcohol misuse and provide brief behavioral counseling interventions to those engaged in risky or hazardous drinking behaviors.[10] Of the available screening tools, the USPSTF determined that 1-item to 3-item screening instruments have the best accuracy for assessing unhealthy alcohol use in adults 18 years or older. These instruments include the abbreviated Alcohol Use Disorders Identification Test–Consumption (AUDIT-C) and the NIAAA-recommended Single Alcohol Screening Questionnaire (SASQ).[9] This high

TABLE 137.1   Terms and Definitions of Unhealthy Alcohol Use

Term	Source	Definition
Low-risk use/lower-risk use	ASAM	Consumption of alcohol below the amount identified as hazardous and in situations not defined as hazardous
Risky/at-risk use	NIAAA	Consumption of alcohol above the recommended daily, weekly, or per-occasion amounts but not meeting criteria for alcohol use disorder
		For all women and men 65 years or older: No more than 3 drinks/day and no more than 7 drinks/week for men (21 to 64 years): No more than 4 drinks/day and no more than 14 drinks/week
		Should avoid alcohol completely: Adolescents, women who are pregnant or trying to get pregnant, and adults who plan to drive a vehicle or operate machinery, are taking medication that interacts with alcohol, or have a medical condition that can be aggravated by alcohol
		For adolescents: NIAAA defines moderate- and high-risk use based on days of alcohol use in the past year, by age group:
		Moderate risk:
		Ages 12–15 years: 1 day/year
		Ages 16–17 years: 6 days/year
		Age 18 years: 12 days/year
		Highest risk:
		Age 11 years: 1 day
		Ages 12–15 years: 6 days
		Age 16 years: 12 days
		Age 17 years: 24 days
		Age 18 years: 52 days
Unhealthy use	ASAM	Any alcohol use that increases the risk or likelihood of health consequences (hazardous use [see below]) or has already led to health consequences (harmful use [see below])
Hazardous use	WHO	A pattern of substance use that increases the risk of harmful consequences; in contrast to harmful use, hazardous use refers to patterns of use that are of public health significance, despite the absence of a current alcohol use disorder in the individual user
	ASAM	Alcohol use that increases the risk or likelihood of health consequences; does not include alcohol use that has already led to health consequences
Harmful use	WHO	A pattern of drinking that is already causing damage to health; the damage may be either physical (e.g., liver damage from chronic drinking) or mental (e.g., depressive episodes secondary to drinking)
		The description for *ICD-10* code F10.l, also labeled "Alcohol Abuse" in the 2018 *ICD-10-CM* codebook
	ASAM	Consumption of alcohol that results in health consequences in the absence of addiction
Alcohol use disorder	DSM-5	A maladaptive pattern of alcohol use leading to clinically significant impairment or distress, as manifested by 2 (or more) of the following, occurring within a 12-month period:
		1. Having times when the patient drank more, or longer, than intended
		2. More than once wanted to cut down or stop, tried It, but could not
		3. Spending a lot of time drinking or being sick/getting over the aftereffects of drinking
		4. Wanting to drink so badly that they could not think of anything else
		5. Found that drinking (or being sick from drinking) often interfered with taking care of home or family responsibilities, caused problems at work, or caused problems at school
		6. Continuing to drink even though it was causing trouble with family and friends
		7. Given up or cut back on activities that were important or interesting in order to drink
		8. More than once gotten into situations while or after drinking that increased the chances of getting hurt (e.g., driving, swimming, unsafe sexual behavior)
		9. Continued to drink even though it was causing depression or anxiety, other health problems, or causing memory blackouts
		10. Having to drink much more than previously in order to get the desired effect, or finding that the usual number of drinks had much less effect than previously
		11. Experiencing the symptoms of withdrawal after the effects of alcohol were wearing off, such as trouble sleeping, shakiness, restlessness, nausea, sweating, racing heart, or seizure
		Severity is determined based on the number of symptoms present:
		Mild: 2–3 symptoms
		Moderate: 4–5 symptoms
		Severe: ≥6 symptoms

(Continued)

TABLE 137.1   Terms and Definitions of Unhealthy Alcohol Use—cont'd.

Term	Source	Definition
Binge drinking/heavy drinking	NIAAA	A pattern of drinking that brings blood alcohol concentration levels to 0.08 g/dL, which typically occurs after 4 drinks for women and 5 drinks for men-in about 2 h
Episodes[a]	SAMHSA	Drinking ≥5 alcoholic drinks on the same occasion on at least 1 day in the past 30 days
Heavy drinking	SAMHSA	Drinking ≥5 drinks on the same occasion on each of ≥5 days in the past 30 days
Alcohol dependence	WHO/ICD-10-CM	≥3 of the following at some time during the previous year:
		A strong desire or sense of compulsion to take the substance
		Difficulties in controlling substance-taking behavior in terms of its onset, termination, or levels of use
		A physiological withdrawal state when substance use has ceased or been reduced, as evidenced by the characteristic withdrawal syndrome for the substance; or use of the same (or a closely related) substance with the intention of relieving or avoiding withdrawal symptoms
		Evidence of tolerance, such that increased doses of the psychoactive substance are required in order to achieve effects originally produced by lower doses (clear examples of this are found in alcohol- and opiate-dependent individuals who may take daily doses sufficient to incapacitate or kill nontolerant users)
		Progressive neglect of alternative pleasures or interests because of psychoactive substance use, increased amount of time necessary to obtain or take the substance, or to recover from its effects
		Persisting with substance use despite clear evidence of overtly harmful consequences, such as harm to the liver through excessive drinking, depressive mood states consequent to periods of heavy substance use, or drug-related impairment of cognitive functioning; efforts should be made to determine that the user was actually, or could be expected to be, aware of the nature and extent of the harm
Abbreviations: ASAM. American Society of Addiction Medicine; DSM-5. Diagnostic and Statistical Manual of Mental Disorders, Fifth Edition; ICD-10-CM. International Classification of Diseases. Tenth Revision Clinical Modification NIAAA. National Institute on Alcohol Abuse and		Alcoholism; SAMHSA. Substance Abuse and Mental Health Services Administration; WHO. World Health Organization.

[a] According to the American Society of Addiction Medicine, the preferred term; is "heavy drinking episode."
Data from US Preventive Services Task Force, Curry SJ, Krist AH, et al. Screening and Behavioral Counseling Interventions to Reduce Unhealthy Alcohol Use in Adolescents and Adults: US Preventive Services Task Force Recommendation Statement. *JAMA*. 2018;320(18):1899–1909.

burden of alcohol-related injury and disease indicates a need to increase awareness of AUD and its effective treatment options (see Box 137.3).[11]

Metabolism of Alcohol

While some alcohol is absorbed in the stomach, the vast majority is absorbed in the small intestine. It is distributed uniformly to all organ systems, including the placenta. Although 2% to 10% of alcohol is excreted through the lungs, urine, and sweat, most is metabolized to acetaldehyde, primarily by alcohol dehydrogenase (ADH). The oxidation of alcohol is a complex process involving three enzyme systems, all contained in the hepatocyte. Acetaldehyde is then quickly converted to carbon dioxide and water, primarily through aldehyde dehydrogenase (ALDH). The common forms of ADH decrease the alcohol concentration in blood by about 4.5 mmol/L ethanol/h (the equivalent of about one drink/h):

$$\text{Ethanol ADH} \xrightarrow[\text{NAD}\to\text{NADH}]{\text{Alcohol hydrogenase}}$$
$$\text{Acetaldehyde ADH} \xrightarrow[\text{NAD}\to\text{NADH}]{\text{Alcohol dehydrogenase}}$$
$$\text{Acetyl coenzyme A} \xrightarrow[\text{Cycle}]{\text{Critical acid}} CO_2 + H_2O$$

where NAD is nicotinamide adenine dinucleotide and NADH is reduced nicotinamide adenine dinucleotide.

At least two variations of ADH genes (*ADH1B*2* and *ADH1C*1*) produce a slightly more rapid breakdown of alcohol and therefore potentially faster production of acetaldehyde, which is rapidly metabolized by *ALDH2*. However, about 40% of Asian people (Japanese, Chinese, and Koreans) have an inactive *ALDH2* mutation that results in much higher acetaldehyde levels after drinking than normal. About 10% of people who are homozygous for this gene form cannot drink alcohol without becoming sick and have almost no risk of AUD, whereas those who are heterozygous have a relatively low rate of AUD.

An alternative pathway, the microsomal ethanol-oxidizing system (MEOS), is induced by chronic alcohol exposure. The primary component of the MEOS is the molecule cytochrome P_{450}, which exists in several variants. The variant most important for alcohol metabolism is cytochrome P_{450} 2E1 (CYP2E1). Many effects of alcoholism are produced by the toxic byproducts (hydrogen, acetaldehyde), acceleration of the metabolism of other drugs, and activation of hepatotoxic compounds by these metabolic pathways.

Although the liver is the major site of ethanol metabolism, other tissues contribute to its metabolism. ADH is found in the gastric mucosa, but the gastric metabolism of alcohol is decreased in women and those of Asian descent. This increased bioavailability of ethanol or decreased first-pass metabolism may explain the greater vulnerability of women to acute and chronic complications of alcohol.

Alcohol metabolism has two elimination rates. The alcohol elimination rate approximates zero-order kinetics (constant rate) for lower

TABLE 137.2 Physiologic Effects and Blood Ethanol Levels

Blood Ethanol Concentration (mg/dL)	Effects[a]
20–50	Diminished fine motor control
50–100	Impaired judgment, impaired coordination
100–150	Difficulty with gait and balance
150–250	Lethargy, difficulty sitting upright without assistance
300	Coma in the novice drinker
400	Respiratory depression

[a]These effects are for the occasional drinker. Chronic drinkers can function at much higher alcohol concentrations because of tolerance. On the other hand, patients may become comatose with low levels of alcohol in mixed alcohol-drug overdose.

ethanol levels and first-order kinetics (amount of drug removed over time is proportional to the concentration of the drug) for higher levels, especially in chronic alcoholics; most likely, through induction of the MEOS pathway, the elimination rate is increased at higher blood levels.

The absorption and elimination rates of alcohol vary by individual and depend on many factors. There is enormous variation among patients in the rate of elimination of ethanol from the blood, ranging from 9 to 36 mg/dL/h in published data. Although the clearance rate may be as high as 36 mg/dL/h in some chronic drinkers, 20 mg/dL/h is a reasonable rate to assume in a typical intoxicated ED patient.

Physiologic effects vary directly with the blood alcohol level (Table 137.2). Diminished fine motor control and impaired judgment appear with alcohol concentrations as low as 20 mg/dL (0.02 mg%), but wide individual variability exists. Chronic alcoholics can exhibit impressive tolerance. The blood alcohol concentration of a person cannot be accurately determined without quantitative testing. More than 50% of the adult population is obviously intoxicated with a level of 150 mg/dL (0.15 mg%). As the ethanol level rises, the patient's level of consciousness declines, eventually ending in a coma. Death is caused by aspiration or respiratory depression.

CLINICAL FEATURES

Alcohol Withdrawal Syndrome

Alcohol is a central nervous system (CNS) depressant. Chronic alcohol use results in a down-regulation of γ-aminobutyric acid (GABA) receptor activity and disinhibition of the dopaminergic reward pathway.[12] This down-regulation of GABA receptors is thought to lead to an increase in the desirable effects of alcohol and vulnerability for dependence due to the presence of increased synaptic GABA. The hallmark of alcohol withdrawal is CNS excitation, with increased cerebrospinal fluid, plasma, and urinary catecholamine levels. Alcohol withdrawal syndrome (AWS) is a continuum of syndromes that begins after a decrease in the amount of intake of ethanol. Therefore, only a reduction, not the abrupt cessation, of ethanol intake may result in withdrawal.

AWS is often divided into three sets of symptoms. The first set consists of autonomic hyperactivity, which appears within hours of the last drink and usually peaks within 24 hours.

Symptoms may occur as early as 6 hours after cessation of or a significant decrease in alcohol intake and usually peaks at 24 to 36 hours. It is characterized by mild autonomic hyperactivity—anorexia, nausea,

BOX 137.1 DSM-5 Criteria for Withdrawal Delirium (Delirium Tremens)

Criteria for Alcohol Withdrawal

Cessation of or reduction in heavy and prolonged use of alcohol
At least two of eight possible symptoms after reduced use of alcohol:
- Autonomic hyperactivity
- Hand tremor
- Insomnia
- Nausea or vomiting
- Transient hallucinations or illusions
- Psychomotor agitation
- Anxiety
- Generalized tonic-clonic seizures

Criteria for Delirium

Decreased attention and awareness
Disturbance in attention, awareness, memory, orientation, language, visuospatial ability, perception, or all these abilities change from the normal level and fluctuate in severity during the day
No evidence of coma or other evolving neurocognitive disorders

From the American Psychiatric Association. *Diagnostic and Statistical Manual of Mental Disorders.* 5th ed. Washington DC: American Psychiatric Publishing; 2013.

vomiting, anxiety, coarse tremor, tachycardia, hypertension, hyperreflexia, and sleep disturbances such as insomnia and vivid dreams.

The second symptom set includes additional neuronal excitation, with epileptiform seizures and global confusion, usually occurring within 24 to 48 hours of abstinence and usually peaks at 50 hours after cessation of or a significant decrease in alcohol intake but occasionally takes up to 5 days. The syndrome is characterized by pronounced anxiety, insomnia, irritability, tremor, anorexia, tachycardia, hyperreflexia, hypertension, fever, decreased seizure threshold, visual and auditory hallucinations, and finally delirium.

The third set of symptoms features delirium tremens or alcohol withdrawal delirium (AWD). While only 5% of patients hospitalized for alcohol withdrawal have delirium tremens, this syndrome is a life-threatening manifestation of alcohol withdrawal and consists of gross tremor, frightening visual hallucinations, profound confusion, agitation, and a hyperadrenergic state characterized by a temperature above 101°F (≈38.5°C), blood pressure higher than 140/90 mm Hg, and tachycardia. It seldom appears before the third post abstinence day.

The criteria for withdrawal delirium, as described in Box 137.1, are delirium and alcohol withdrawal. Alcohol withdrawal is the most common alcohol-related illness that may require inpatient admission and is associated with adverse events such as uncontrolled agitation with the potential for over-sedation, generalized seizures, and prolonged hospital stay.[3] Emergency clinicians should be familiar with the commonly used withdrawal rating instrument known as the Clinical Institute Withdrawal Assessment of Alcohol Scale, revised (CIWA-Ar). See Table 137.3.

Alcohol-Related Seizures

Patients presenting to the ED with seizures should be questioned about alcohol intake (Box 137.2). Of seizure patients presenting to an ED, 20% to 40% will have their seizures related to alcohol use or abuse. The primary consideration in the initial care of seizure patients who regularly consume alcohol is the recognition of treatable, life-threatening causes. Alcohol may act in one of several ways to produce seizures in

TABLE 137.3   **Clinical Institute Withdrawal Assessment of Alcohol Scale, Revised (CIWA-Ar)**

Components of Scale	Most Severe Manifestations
Nine items[a]	
• Nausea or vomiting	Constant nausea with vomiting
• Tremor	Severe tremor, even with arms extended
• Paroxysmal sweats	Drenching sweats
• Anxiety	Acute panic
• Tactile disturbances (e.g., itching, numbness, sensation of bugs crawling on or under the skin)	Continuous hallucinations
• Auditory disturbances (e.g., sensitivity to sound, hearing things that are not there)	Continuous hallucinations
• Visual disturbances (e.g., sensitivity to brightness and color, seeing things that are not there)	Continuous hallucinations
• Headache, sensation of a band around the head	Extremely severe headache
• Agitation	Pacing during most of an interview with clinician or thrashing about
One item—orientation and clouding of sensorium[b]	

[a]Scored on a scale ranging from 0 (no symptoms) to 7 (most severe symptoms).
[b]Scored on a scale ranging from 0 (no symptoms) to 4 (disoriented with respect to place or person).
Adapted from Sullivan JT, Sykora K, Schneiderman, J, et al. Assessment of alcohol withdrawal: The revised Clinical Institute Withdrawal Assessment for Alcohol scale (CIWA-Ar). *Br J Addict.* 1989;84:1353–1357.

BOX 137.2   **Differential Diagnosis of Alcohol-Related Seizures**

Withdrawal (alcohol or drugs)
Exacerbation of idiopathic or posttraumatic seizures
Acute intoxication (e.g., amphetamines, anticholinergics, cocaine, isoniazid, organophosphates, phenothiazines, tricyclic antidepressants, salicylates, lithium)
Metabolic (e.g., hypoglycemia, hyponatremia, hypernatremia, hypocalcemia, hepatic failure)
Infectious (e.g., meningitis, encephalitis, brain abscess)
Trauma (e.g., intracranial hemorrhage)
Cerebrovascular accident
Sleep deprivation
Noncompliance with anticonvulsants

---

patients by its partial or absolute withdrawal after a period of chronic intake by, an acute alcohol-related metabolic disorder (e.g., hypoglycemia, hyponatremia), an acute event leading to cerebral trauma, precipitation of seizures in patients with idiopathic or posttraumatic epilepsy, or lowering of the seizure threshold in patients with prior existing intracerebral disease states.

Alcohol Withdrawal Seizures

Withdrawal seizures may occur 6 to 48 hours after the cessation of drinking. Of patients with seizures, 90% have one to six generalized tonic-clonic seizures, and 60% experience multiple seizures within a 6-hour period. The incidence of partial seizures, common with posttraumatic epilepsy, is increased during alcohol withdrawal. The term *alcohol withdrawal seizure* is reserved for seizures with these characteristics. The term *alcohol-related seizure* is used to refer to all seizures in the aggregate associated with alcohol use, including this subset of alcohol withdrawal seizures.

Alcoholic Hallucinosis

Alcoholic hallucinosis is clinically distinct from delirium tremens and is characterized by hallucinations presenting within 12 to 24 hours of abstinence and resolve within 24 to 48 hours, in contrast to delirium

tremens that presents at least 48 to 72 hours after abstinence. Hallucinations are typically visual, although tactile hallucinations have been described. Alcoholic hallucinosis is also generally not associated with autonomic instability such as tachycardia, hypertension, or hyperthermia.

Cardiovascular Effects

Acute and chronic ethanol consumption can affect the mechanical function of the heart, produce dysrhythmias, and exacerbate coronary artery disease (CAD). It may alter myocardial function by direct toxic effects, by associated hypertension, or indirectly by altering specific electrolytes. Acute intoxication can decrease cardiac output in alcoholic and nonalcoholic patients with preexisting cardiac disease (see Table 137.4).[13]

Studies have linked moderate alcohol consumption (two drinks/day in men and one drink/day in women) with a reduced risk of cardiovascular disease.[14–16] There is a strong biological plausibility that moderate wine consumption may have a positive effect on organs and systems. Whether the positive effect of wine on health is attributed to ethanol, to wine micro-constituents, or to their synergistic effect, is still unanswered.[17] Low to moderate alcohol consumption decreases platelet aggregation, raises plasma levels of endogenous tissue plasminogen activator, and lowers insulin resistance and likely poses little cardiovascular risk.[14]

Heavy alcohol consumption has a detrimental effect on those with preexisting CAD. It reduces exercise tolerance, induces coronary vasoconstriction, and raises heart rate and blood pressure. These patients also have a significantly higher incidence of peripheral arterial disease.[18] The additive cardiovascular effects of ethanol and nicotine contribute to dysrhythmias and sudden death in patients with CAD.[19]

Alcohol abuse is a known risk factor for the development of alcoholic cardiomyopathy which presents as a dilated cardiomyopathy that can lead to heart failure.[14,20] Heavy drinkers have increased odds of having a prolonged QTc interval and supraventricular dysrhythmias.[21] Supraventricular (usually atrial fibrillation) and ventricular (usually transitory ventricular tachycardia) dysrhythmias, commonly referred to as "holiday heart," have been documented in alcoholic patients who have been drinking heavily. Tachydysrhythmias as a result of episodic

TABLE 137.4 Cardiovascular Effects of Alcohol

Condition	Probable Relationship With Alcohol		Potential Epidemiological Consequences
	Lighter drinking[a]	Heavier drinking[b]	
Dilated Cardiomyopathy	Unrelated	One (of several) causes; ? requires cofactors	↑ risk of HF, AF, cardioembolic stroke and HS if on ACs
Systemic HTN	Little or none	Probably causal in susceptible persons	↑ risk of HF, AF, IS, and HS
CAD	Protective	? less protective or ↑ risk	↑ risk of HF, cardioembolic stroke, and AF; ↑ risk of HS if on ACs
Supraventricular arrhythmia	Little or none	Probably a causal factor, especially with binges	↑ risk of cardioembolic stroke, and HS if on ACs
HS	? unrelated or slight ↑ risk	↑ risk	Disability and ↑ risk of VTE
IS	Protective	Probable ↑ risk; varies with subtype	Disability and ↑ risk of VTE
Heart failure	Indirectly protective	Varies with underlying CV condition	Disability and ↑ risk of VTE

AC, Anticoagulant; *AF*, atrial fibrillation; CAD, coronary artery disease; *HS*, hemorrhagic stroke; *HTN*, hypertension;; *IS*, Ischemic stroke; VTE, venous thromboembolism; cv, cardiovascular; ↑, increase; ↓, decrease; ?, possibly.
[a]Less than three standard-sized drinks per day; [b]Three or more standard-sized drinks per day.
Data from Klatsky AL. Alcohol and cardiovascular diseases: where do we stand today? *J Intern Med.* 2015;278(3):238–250.

drinking commonly revert to sinus rhythm with abstinence and do not require immediate intervention if the patient is hemodynamically stable.

Pulmonary Effects

There is a clear and statistically significant relationship between alcohol consumption and the risk of community-acquired pneumonia (CAP). Consuming drinks that contain 10 to 20 g of alcohol per day is linked to an 8% increased risk of acquiring CAP.[22] Pneumococcal pneumonia is the most common type of pneumonia in both healthy individuals and heavy alcohol users. In addition, *Klebsiella pneumoniae* also is increased in people with AUD and seems to cause disproportionate rates of lung infection and high mortality in this population.[23]

For centuries, it has been known that people with AUD are more likely to have pulmonary infections such as pneumonia and tuberculosis. Over the past two decades, it has become clear that other conditions such as RSV and ARDS also are linked to high-risk alcohol consumption.[23]

Gastrointestinal and Hepatic Effects

Esophagus and Stomach
Alcoholic patients have a higher incidence of esophagitis, gastric cancer, and esophageal carcinoma than in the general population. Acute alcohol ingestion also decreases lower esophageal sphincter pressure, delays gastric emptying, and disrupts the normal gastric mucosal barrier. Alcohol consumption, because of its inherent toxicity, has been shown to eliminate infection of the gastric mucosa by *Helicobacter pylori*. Forceful or persistent emesis can lead to a Mallory-Weiss tear or more severely, Boerhaave syndrome.

Gastrointestinal Bleeding
Alcohol is closely associated with gastrointestinal (GI) bleeding. Causes and contributing factors include Mallory-Weiss tears, esophagitis, esophageal varices, acute and chronic gastritis, thrombocytopenia, portal hypertensive gastropathy, qualitative and quantitative platelet disorders, and prolonged clotting times. Alcohol may exacerbate gastric mucosal damage when it is combined with nonsteroidal antiinflammatory drugs (NSAIDs), but ethanol itself is not a risk factor for peptic ulcer disease. Peptic ulcer disease is the most common cause of bleeding in alcoholic patients with upper GI hemorrhage, as well as in those who do not regularly consume alcohol.

Liver Damage
Hepatic damage has been recognized for centuries as the hallmark of chronic alcohol abuse. Above a certain quantity, alcoholic consumption can elicit a spectrum of liver lesions among which steatosis is present in nearly all drinkers who consume in excess of 40 g/day regularly.[24] The activation of the immune system with the production of cytokines such as tumor necrosis factor-alpha is one of the earliest events in many types of liver injury. This cascade stimulates Kupffer cells and the production of other cytokines that together enlist inflammatory cells, kill hepatocytes, and initiate healing through fibrogenesis.

Alcoholic liver disease is the most common liver disorder in the Western Hemisphere and, along with hepatitis C (HCV), is a leading cause of liver transplantation. Alcohol use is associated with more persistent HCV infection and more extensive liver damage than no alcohol use because of interactions between alcohol use and HCV that affect immune responses, cytotoxicity, and oxidative stress.[2] No safe level of alcohol consumption has been determined for patients with HCV.[2]

Alcoholic Hepatitis
Alcoholic hepatitis is a pro-inflammatory chronic liver disease that is associated with high short-term morbidity and mortality (25% to 35% in 1 month) in the setting of chronic alcohol use.[25] It is a clinical syndrome characterized by right upper quadrant pain, a tender enlarged liver, fever, jaundice, leukocytosis, and altered liver function test results. aspartate transaminase (AST) levels are usually less than 400 IU/L, and ALT levels are typically less than half the AST level. It is associated with profound immune dysfunction with a primed but ineffective immune response against pathogens.[26]

Alcoholic hepatitis has a range of clinical manifestations from mildly symptomatic hepatomegaly to fulminant hepatic failure. The severity of the disease can be estimated in the ED by a prolonged prothrombin time/international normalized ratio (INR) or with the use of the Maddrey discriminant factor. The ABIC (**a**ge, **b**ilirubin, **I**NR, **c**reatinine) score and model for end-stage liver disease (MELD) are also helpful in predicting mortality in these patients.

Cirrhosis

The causal association between alcohol intake and alcoholic liver disease has been well documented, yet liver cirrhosis develops in only 10% to 20% of heavy drinkers.[2] Cirrhosis is the disruption of the normal architecture of the liver by scarring and regenerating nodules of parenchyma. Alcoholism is the most common cause of cirrhosis in the United States and is responsible for approximately 48% of all cirrhotic-induced deaths.[27] Alcoholic cirrhosis usually requires 10 to 15 years of chronic drinking, often punctuated by one or more episodes of acute alcoholic hepatitis. The clinical outcome is determined by the development of complications of portal hypertension and hepatic dysfunction. Alteration of the normal hepatic architecture by fibrosis and nodule formation may eventually lead to portal hypertension. Portal hypertension may be complicated by ascites and esophageal varices. Although cirrhosis is irreversible, its progression may be halted with abstinence.

Pancreatitis and Malabsorption

The association of ethanol with acute and chronic pancreatitis is well established, but the exact pathogenesis is unclear. Hypotheses include reflux of duodenal contents and bile into the pancreatic duct, obstruction by a plug of pancreatic juice rich in proteins, and a direct toxic effect of ethanol.

The diagnosis of alcoholic pancreatitis can be difficult because asymptomatic alcoholics may have an elevated amylase level. Conversely, up to 30% of patients with acute alcoholic pancreatitis have an amylase value within normal limits. The serum lipase level rises after amylase, remains elevated longer, and is a more reliable indicator of alcoholic pancreatitis, especially when it is more than three times the normal range.

Neurologic Effects

Neuropathy. A symmetric sensorimotor polyneuropathy is common with chronic alcohol abuse, usually in the lower extremities. It is thought to be a combination of nutritional deficiency with thiamine or vitamin B_{12} deficit and a direct neurotoxic effect of alcohol. Burning pain and paresthesia are common complaints. Findings on physical examination include loss of light touch, decreased pinprick sensation, and reduced lower extremity deep tendon reflexes. Distal muscle weakness is a delayed finding. The neuropathy may lead to nonhealing ulcers on the feet. Treatment of alcoholic neuropathy is abstinence, adequate diet, and thiamine. Complete recovery is rare.

So-called "Saturday night palsy" or "honeymooner's syndrome" is a wrist drop caused by radial nerve compression. The patient usually has spent the night with his or her arm drooped over the back of a chair, bench, or companion; compressing the radial nerve against the humerus producing neurapraxia. Loss of function due to radial nerve neuropraxia usually returns after a few weeks to months.

Wernicke-Korsakoff Syndrome. There are high rates of dementia reported in patients with AUD, and up to 25% when all types of severe cognitive impairment are considered. Previously, two main disorders were described: Wernicke-Korsakoff syndrome (WKS) and alcohol-related dementia (ARD). Now, the DSM-5 introduces major neurocognitive disorder as an alternative term to dementia, with a subtype related to substance or medication use. WKS and ARD could be a direct result of alcohol neurotoxicity or the consequence of a concurrent underlying pathology (such as thiamine deficiency) or both (neurotoxicity associated with nutritional deficiencies).[28]

Although they are similar pathologically and are caused by thiamine deficiency, Wernicke and Korsakoff syndromes are clinically distinct. Wernicke encephalopathy, a medical emergency with a mortality rate of approximately 17%, remains a clinical diagnosis and is often unrecognized. Contemporary criteria require two of these signs—dietary deficiencies, oculomotor abnormalities (nystagmus being the most common), cerebellar dysfunction, and an altered mental state or mild memory impairment. Mental abnormalities include lethargy, inattentiveness, abulia, and impaired memory, progressing without treatment to coma.

Korsakoff psychosis or amnesic state also called an alcohol-induced persisting amnestic disorder, is a disorder with recent memory impairment, inability to learn new information or recall previously learned information, apathy, and confabulation. Although it is common, confabulation is not essential for the diagnosis. Whereas 80% of patients with acute Wernicke's encephalopathy have Korsakoff syndrome, age older than 40 years and many years of heavy alcohol use are additional risk factors.

Treatment of WKS consists of abstinence, adequate diet, and thiamine. The ophthalmoplegia and nystagmus usually have a good response to thiamine administration within hours to days. The ataxia and mental changes may take days to weeks to improve and usually have a poorer prognosis. Less than 25% of patients show any real recovery, 50% show some recovery, and the remainder show no response, despite adequate thiamine replacement. Because magnesium is a cofactor for this enzyme system, its serum levels should be corrected. Patients with WKS require admission with thiamine and magnesium repletion.

Alcoholic Cerebellar Degeneration

Characterized by ataxia of the extremities, cerebellar ataxia of alcoholism results in a wide-based stance and uncoordinated gait. Lower extremity involvement predominates, although the arms may rarely be involved. Pathologic changes consist of the degeneration of elements in the cerebellum, especially the Purkinje cells. The diagnosis is based on history, physical examination, and findings on magnetic resonance imaging or computed tomography (CT), which shows severe cerebellar atrophy. Treatment consists of abstinence, adequate nutrition, and thiamine.

Infectious Disease

Chronic alcohol exposure depresses the development and expression of cell-mediated immunity. This depression may contribute to the high incidence of head, neck, and upper GI cancers in alcoholics. The suppression of macrophage function by alcohol reduces the reticuloendothelial system's ability to clear particles. This may contribute to spontaneous bacteremia, spontaneous bacterial peritonitis, pneumonia, and tuberculosis.

The most common infection in alcoholism is pneumonia. Although alcoholic patients may contract a variety of bacterial pneumoniae, *Streptococcus pneumoniae* is still the most common organism. Periods of alcoholic stupor with incomplete glottic closure and subsequent aspiration can lead to aspiration pneumonia or lung abscess. *K. pneumoniae,* classically associated with alcoholism, is currently more common in patients with cytotoxic chemotherapy, hematologic malignant disease, and transplantation than in the chronic alcoholic. Chronic alcohol consumption increases the risk and severity of chronic infections with HIV; hepatitis C virus (HCV); and *Mycobacterium tuberculosis.*[29]

Endocrine Effects

Alcohol dependence adversely affects many endocrine systems. Peripheral thyroid hormone dysfunction and central hypothalamic-pituitary-thyroid axis deregulation are seen. Male hypogonadism and feminism are seen in chronic male alcoholics. Alcohol's effects on the testes and hypothalamus decrease testosterone production in men. Alcohol may cause impotence by CNS sedation, secondary depression, or decreased testosterone production. Decreased testosterone, increased estrogen (in patients with liver disease), and increased prolactin levels can lead to decreased libido, feminization, and gynecomastia in male alcoholics and to abnormalities in lactation and menstruation in women. In female alcoholics, increased levels of testosterone and estrogen are found. Estrogen replacement therapy may increase hormonal levels threefold and thus increase the risk of cholelithiasis and breast cancer.

Metabolic Effects

Carbohydrates

Alcohol-induced hypoglycemia occurs in up to 4% of chronic alcoholics. Coma, seizures, hemiparesis, and a variety of other neurologic signs have been described in patients presenting with alcohol-induced hypoglycemia. Starvation, depletion of liver glycogen stores, decreased plasma cortisol levels, the impaired release of growth hormone, and inhibition of gluconeogenesis contribute to this phenomenon.

Hyperglycemia and diabetes may be found in chronic alcoholism. Alcohol abuse can lead to chronic pancreatitis, resulting in the underproduction of insulin by the damaged pancreatic cells. Alcohol also impairs peripheral glucose utilization, causing relative insulin resistance (similar to type 2 diabetes).

Lipids

Ethanol increases the hepatic synthesis of triglycerides. Abstinence is necessary to reverse elevated triglyceride levels. Except for its relationship to fatty infiltration of the liver, the clinical significance of this hyperlipidemia is unknown.

Electrolytes

Ethanol has numerous effects on electrolytes and mineral metabolism, as summarized in Table 137.5. Hyponatremia and hypokalemia are common in active drinkers. Vomiting, diarrhea, magnesium depletion, malnutrition, and metabolic alkalosis contribute to these abnormalities.

Alcoholism is the most common cause of severe magnesium deficiency in adult outpatients. Magnesium deficiency is seen in 30% of alcoholics as a result of malabsorption, malnutrition, diarrhea, vomiting, and increased urinary losses. Oral magnesium supplementation in chronic alcoholics improves liver function test results, electrolyte balance, and muscle strength.

Hypocalcemia is common in alcoholic patients with magnesium depletion. The mechanism is related to diminished parathyroid hormone secretion, decreased tissue responsiveness to parathyroid hormone, decreased vitamin D metabolism, and decreased calcium release from bone, which is independent of parathyroid hormone. Correction of magnesium depletion is necessary to restore calcium to normal levels. Hypoalbuminemia, pancreatitis, or vitamin D deficiency also contribute to low serum calcium levels or low total-body stores of calcium in alcoholic patients.

Hypophosphatemia is found in up to 50% of hospitalized patients with alcoholism. Phosphorus depletion results from malnutrition, vomiting, respiratory alkalosis, diarrhea, enhanced release of calcitonin, phosphate-binding antacids, and urinary loss (related to vitamin D deficiency and secondary hyperparathyroidism). Hypophosphatemic patients often have low magnesium levels. Rehydration, carbohydrate repletion, and parenteral alimentation further exacerbate phosphorus depletion. Glucose bolus and infusions have been shown to produce a significant fall in serum inorganic phosphate levels. Severe hypophosphatemia (<1 mg/dL) has been associated with acute respiratory failure, myocardial depression, CNS irritability, dysfunction of erythrocytes, leukocytes, and platelets, and rhabdomyolysis.

Although chronic alcoholics who require admission often have potassium, magnesium, and phosphate depletion, empirical treatment with potassium and phosphate is discouraged. Serum levels and renal function should be determined first. Unintended hyperkalemia and hyperphosphatemia can produce significant morbidity, and phosphate infusion exacerbates hypocalcemia if present. Because most magnesium is intracellular, a normal serum magnesium level does not rule out decreased total-body magnesium stores. If the serum level is normal, total-body levels may still be low. As long as renal function is adequate, empiric magnesium treatment can be considered. Abstinence and a proper diet resolve electrolyte and nutritional deficiencies in the alcoholic patient who is healthy enough to be treated as an outpatient.

Alcoholic Ketoacidosis

Twenty-five percent of patients who are admitted to the hospital with an alcohol-related disorder develop alcoholic ketoacidosis.[30] Alcoholic ketoacidosis occurs most frequently in severe chronic alcoholics who have had a recent binge followed 1 to 3 days later by protracted vomiting, decreased food intake, dehydration, and abstinence. Nausea, vomiting, and abdominal pain are common presenting complaints. Serum glucose levels are usually less than 200 mg/dL. Normal blood pH may be found despite ketonemia because of coexisting respiratory alkalosis and metabolic alkalosis.

Treatment of alcoholic ketosis consists of the administration of normal saline, glucose, and thiamine with correction of hypokalemia. This can be accomplished with 5% dextrose in normal saline and 30 mEq of potassium chloride or 30 mEq of oral potassium. If no serious complicating illness is present, ketosis is often reversed within 12 to 24 hours of treatment.

Hematologic Effects

Chronic alcohol use is associated with significant alterations in the immune system that predispose people to viral and bacterial infections and cancer development. The alcoholic presents with myriad hematologic abnormalities. The direct toxic effect of ethanol and its metabolites, secondary nutritional deficiency, and hepatic disease, individually or in combination, affect red blood cells, white blood cells, platelets, hemostasis, and the immune system.

Anemia

Several mechanisms cause anemia, which is common in the alcoholic. Megaloblastic anemia resulting from folate deficiency is the most common anemia in alcoholics. The mean corpuscular volume (MCV) is typically increased but may be normal when iron deficiency coexists. Malnutrition, the inability of the cirrhotic liver to store folate, excessive urinary loss, and malabsorption decrease folate stores. Alcohol accelerates the development of megaloblastic anemia in individuals with depleted folate stores (MCV > 100 fL) by less clearly defined mechanisms.

Iron deficiency anemia is common and is usually a result of blood loss from the GI tract. With iron deficiency anemia, the serum iron level is decreased, total serum iron-binding capacity is elevated, and serum ferritin level is decreased. Alcoholics frequently have chronic inflammatory diseases that produce anemia of chronic disease.

Leukocyte Abnormalities

Leukopenia is common in alcoholic patients and has several possible causes. Sepsis, folate deficiency, and hypersplenism all lead to a decreased white blood cell count. Alcohol has a direct toxic effect on white blood cell production in the bone marrow. Granulocyte mobilization (chemotaxis) and adherence are also impaired, resulting in decreased inflammatory responses.

TABLE 137.5 Electrolyte Disturbances[30]

Disturbance	Mechanism or Cause	Comment	Treatment
Acid-Base			
Alcoholic ketoacidosis	Anion-gap metabolic acidosis due to decrease in insulin: glucagon ratio	Increased NADH:NAD ratio favors formation of/3-hydroxybutyric acid	Administer 5% dextrose in 0.9% (normal) saline and treat other disorders if present
Lactic acidosis	Increased NADH:NAD ratio due to ethanol metabolism	Average lactate level 3 mmol/L consider sepsis or thiamine deficiency with higher levels	Administer 5% dextrose in 0.9% (normal) saline and treat other disorders if present
Hyperchloremic normal-gap metabolic acidosis	Indirect loss of bicarbonate due to loss of ketoacid salts in urine	Regeneration of bicarbonate by kidneys repairs deficit	Provide conservative management
Metabolic alkalosis	Vomiting	Increase in anion gap greater than decrease in bicarbonate concentration when combined with alcoholic ketoacidosis	Restore volume of extracellular fluid with chloride-containing fluids, correct hypokalemia
Respiratory alkalosis	Alcohol withdrawal, chronic liver disease, pain, sepsis	Often the primary disorder in a mixed acid-base disturbance	Administer benzodiazepines for alcohol withdrawal; treat underlying disorders
Hypophosphatemia	Alcohol-induced urinary loss, magnesium deficiency, acidemia, increased parathyroid hormone level, nutritional deficiency, decrease in gastrointestinal absorption, cellular shift due to insulin release, respiratory alkalosis, β_2-adrenergic stimulation	Muscle weakness, rhabdomyolysis, tissue ischemia, hemolysis, cardiac dysfunction; urine phosphate excretion >100 mg/24 h r or fractional excretion ≥5% indicates renal wasting	Oral supplements preferred; for complications, administer 42–67 mmol phosphate over 6 to 9 hr, not to exceed 90 mmol/day to avoid decrease in calcium and magnesium levels
Hypomagnesemia	Alcohol-induced urinary loss, phosphate deficiency, nutritional deficiency, decreased gastrointestinal absorption, cellular shift due to insulin release, respiratory alkalosis, β_2-adrenergic stimulation	Persistent renal wasting can last several weeks, accounting for recurrence of hypomagnesemia after initial correction; urinary magnesium excretion >25 mg/ 24 h or fractional excretion >2% indicates renal wasting	Oral supplements preferred; intravenous magnesium indicated in patients with arrhythmias or neuromuscular irritability
Hypocalcemia[†]	Decrease in parathyroid hormone level and resistance due to magnesium deficiency, alcohol-induced urinary loss, vitamin D deficiency	Correct for a low albumin concentration as follows: corrected calcium=serum calcium in mg/dL + [0.8× (4.0-serum albumin in g/dL)]; bicarbonate therapy can decrease ionized fraction	Correct the magnesium deficit; correct the deficiency in vitamin D
Hypokalemia	Urinary loss due to coupling of increased distal sodium delivery and increased aldosterone level, magnesium deficiency, diarrhea, cellular shift due to insulin release, correction of acidosis, respiratory alkalosis, β_2 adrenergic stimulation	A low or normal potassium level in patients with rhabdomyolysis suggests a significant underlying total-body deficit of potassium; urinary potassium >30 mmol/24 h or urinary potassium: creatinine ratio >13 (in millimoles of potassium per gram of creatinine) indicates renal wasting	Oral supplements preferred; for complications, administer intravenous potassium chloride at 10–20 mmol/h; administer potassium before Bicarbonate in patients with acidemia
Hyponatremia	Increased release of vasopressin due to volume depletion; decreased solute excretion in beer potomanía	Increased risk of osmotic demyelination	Restore volume and increase protein intake; limit rate of correction to 6–8 mmol in first 24 hours, to slow rate with 5% dextrose in water, desmopressin, or both

Data from Palmer BF, Clegg DJ. Electrolyte Disturbances in Patients with Chronic Alcohol-Use Disorder. *N Engl J Med.* 2017;377(14):1368–1377.

Platelet Disorders

Thrombocytopenia can occur with folate deficiency, marrow suppression, sepsis, disseminated intravascular coagulation, or splenic sequestration. The direct toxic effects of alcohol decrease measured survival time and impair the production of platelets in the bone marrow, but marrow toxicity rarely reduces the platelet count below 30,000/mm³. Qualitative platelet function is also impaired. Binge drinking is associated with a reactive thrombocytosis potentially responsible for acute stroke and sudden death.

Hemostasis

Alcoholic patients have a bleeding diathesis for many reasons, including thrombocytopenia, qualitative platelet disorders, deficient production of hepatic clotting factors, GI variceal formation, and vitamin K deficiency. Bleeding associated with coagulation abnormalities may require fresh-frozen plasma for the immediate correction of coagulation factor depletion; vitamin K (10 mg IV) takes 6 to 10 hours to reverse the vitamin K–dependent factors II, VII, IX, and X. Because of poor diet and impaired hepatobiliary function, alcoholics may have insufficient vitamin K storage and benefit from vitamin K delivery. However, alcoholic patients with profound liver failure are unable to produce the precoagulation factors II, VII, IX, X, and IV, so vitamin K therapy is ineffective. Platelet transfusions should be started in the ED for adult patients with active bleeding when the platelet count is less than 50,000/mm³.

Oncologic Effects

While alcohol itself is not carcinogenic, its metabolite, acetaldehyde, has emerged as an important contributor; it can form stable DNA adducts, trigger mutations in tumor suppressors and oncogenes, and interfere with DNA repair. Over 5% of all new cancer occurrences and 6% of all cancer deaths worldwide were estimated to be attributable to alcohol.[31,32]. Alcohol consumption has been highly associated with specific oncological diseases such as oral, pharyngeal, laryngeal, esophageal, hepatic, colorectal, and breast cancers.[31,32]

Hypothermia

Acute alcohol ingestion is one of the most common precipitating factors for accidental hypothermia and occurs in 33% to 75% of patients presenting with a core temperature below 35°C (95°F). Alcohol exacerbates hypothermia of other causes, with depressed hypothalamic thermoregulation, peripheral vasodilation producing heat loss, CNS depression, sepsis, inability to shiver, hypoglycemia, and increased risk of environmental exposure. Hypothermia may be the presentation of Wernicke syndrome, possibly caused by lesions of the posterior hypothalamus, hypoglycemia, or sepsis.

Psychiatric Effects

Depression and antisocial personality are the two most common psychiatric disorders that correlate with alcoholism, with a prevalence of 30% to 60% in most studies. Of alcoholic men admitted to a psychiatric ward, approximately 40% have another psychiatric disorder unrelated to substance abuse—in particular, antisocial personality disorder, schizophrenia, mood disorders, and anxiety disorders.

Mental illness and substance use often co-occur and heavy alcohol use and AUDs are known risk factors for violence.[33] Secondary depression may be caused by alcoholism, or the primary affective disorder may be present with secondary alcoholism. Mild depressive symptoms are also common in alcohol withdrawal. Alcoholism, major depression, and antisocial personality all predispose to suicide, and interaction among the three is particularly dangerous, but the acute risk on any given day is difficult to assess.[34] Alcohol increases the lifetime risk of suicide, with over 15% of all alcoholics eventually dying by suicide.

Toxicologic Effects

Alcohol has long been known to have additive or even synergistic effects with several drugs including opioids and sedative hypnotic agents. Acute intoxication decreases the rate of drug metabolism, which is partially explained by competition for the same enzymatic process in the liver. Ethanol increases aspirin-induced prolongation of bleeding time and reduces the metabolism of warfarin, leading to increased anticoagulant effects. There is an increased risk of upper GI bleeding when alcohol is combined with NSAIDs.

Disulfiram and Similar Reactions

Most patients pretreated with disulfiram (Antabuse) who then consume even small amounts of alcohol experience an extremely unpleasant reaction. These patients have a hypersensitivity to ethanol and experience a direct response within 15 minutes, lasting 30 minutes to several hours. The reaction consists of skin flushing on the head that spreads to the trunk, along with nausea, vomiting, headache, chest and abdominal discomfort, diaphoresis, vertigo, palpitations, and confusion. A severe reaction may produce hypotension, seizures, and dysrhythmias. The disulfiram-ethanol reaction is thought to occur by the accumulation of acetaldehyde secondary to inhibition of the ALDH enzyme, which may be deficient in many Asians, or another unknown toxic factor. The common ink cap mushroom (*Coprinopsis atramentatia*), while nontoxic when ingested alone, causes a similar disulfiram reaction if consumed with alcohol. Treatment for disulfiram reaction is generally observation, cardiac monitoring, an antiemetic for symptoms, and intravenous (IV) fluids.

Other Considerations—Patient Groups Affected

Adolescents. Excessive high school and college drinking continues to be prevalent and problematic. Approximately 1.2 million youths aged 12 to 17 met the criteria for SUDs in 2015 (5% of this population).[35] Alcohol is by far the most commonly used substance among youth, with 37% of 18-year-olds endorsing alcohol use and 24 % reporting being drunk in the past month.[36] Alcohol is the most commonly used drug and is a common contributor to the leading cause of death, unintentional injury, homicide, and suicide among adolescents (10 to 20 years old) in the United States.

Adolescent onset of alcohol use has been associated with an increased risk for developing an AUD later in life.[37] Although underage youth may drink less often than adults, they typically drink in larger quantities than adults when they do drink, and often binge drink.[38] Binge drinking, as defined by the NIAAA, is a pattern of alcohol consumption that brings blood alcohol concentration to .08 g/dL, which typically occurs following the intake of five or more standard alcohol drinks by men and four or more by women over a period of approximately 2 hours. In 2011, the NIAAA produced a two-question Youth Alcohol Screening Tool which asks about the frequency of alcohol consumption and friends' alcohol use in the past year (Table 137.6).[39]

Older Patients. Alcohol use is a growing public health concern for elderly adults. Elderly patients, meaning patients ages 65 years and older, comprise the fastest-growing portion of the US population. By 2040, the elderly will comprise more than 20% of the total population. Compared with all other substances, alcohol is the most commonly used among the elderly, and thus, the risks of drinking by older individuals will undoubtedly become an increasing issue as this population rises over the coming decades.[40]

Common screening tests (e.g., the CAGE questionnaire) tend to be less sensitive in this age group. Alcohol may exacerbate underlying disease by masking anginal chest pain, worsening hypertension, and inducing dysrhythmias. Older adults who consume low to moderate levels of alcohol, however, may have a decreased risk for the development of dementia and heart failure.

Older patients are more likely to have neuropsychiatric complications of alcoholism, such as sleep problems, anxiety, depression, and dementia. Alcohol is involved in one-third of suicides in older adults. Older subjects also perform less well than younger subjects on tests of perception and attention when under the influence at all blood alcohol levels. This may result in an increased risk of fractures from falling and osteoporosis. However, evidence has suggested that compared with abstinence, consumption of up to one drink/day is associated with a decreased risk of osteoporotic hip fracture, and there is a beneficial effect of moderate alcohol consumption on bone density.

Pregnant Women. There is no known safe level of alcohol consumption during pregnancy. Alcohol is a known teratogen that can impact fetal growth and development during all stages of pregnancy. The current recommendation from the American College of Obstetricians and Gynecologists, Center for Disease Control (CDC),

TABLE 137.6　The NIAAA Youth Alcohol Screening Tool

Age:	First Question:	Second Question:
Elementary School (ages 9–11)	Friends: Any drinking? "Do you have any friends who drank beer, wine, or any drinking containing alcohol in the *past year?*"	Patient: Any drinking? "How about you —have you *ever* had more than a few sips of beer, wine, or any drink containing alcohol?
Middle School (ages 11–14)	Friends: Any drinking? "Do you have any friends who drank beer, wine, or any drinking containing alcohol in the *past year*	Patient: How many days? "How about you—in the *past year, on how many days* have you had more than a few sips of beer, wine, or any drink containing alcohol?"
High School (ages 14–18)	Patient: How many days? in the *past year, on how many days* have you had more than a few sips of beer, wine, or any drink containing alcohol?"	Friends: How much? "If your friends drink, *how many drinks* do they usually drink on an occasion?"

Surgeon General, and medical societies from other countries all recommend complete abstinence during pregnancy.[41]

Alcohol readily crosses the placenta with fetal blood alcohol levels approaching maternal levels within 2 hours of maternal intake. There are a wide variety of developmental defects that result from alcohol exposure, including brain abnormalities, CNS dysfunctions, and growth deficiencies of developing organs and body systems. These adverse effects on the developing fetus are known collectively as fetal alcohol spectrum disorders (FASDs).[42] FASDs cause dysfunctions in learning, emotion, cognition, motor performance, and can lead to behavioral as well as social problems.[42] FASDs are characterized by a triad of CNS defects, including mild to moderate mental retardation, dysmorphology, involving mostly facial structures, and growth deficiencies, usually consisting of short stature and microcephaly. FASDs are now considered the most common identifiable source of mental retardation. Children exposed to prenatal alcohol exhibit increased activity levels, cognitive and attention deficits, perseverative behavior, and language and motor problems, which persist into adulthood.

Alcohol has the ability to freely pass through a lactating mother's milk and thus lactating mothers who decide to continue to drink should avoid breastfeeding 3 to 4 hours after moderate to high consumption of alcohol.[41]

Trauma

Injury is a leading cause of death in those between the ages of 1 and 44 years, accounting for more than 50 million injuries/year and approximately 26,000 deaths/year. In the United States, alcohol is the major risk factor for virtually all categories of intentional and unintentional injury. In addition to increasing the frequency and severity of the injury, alcohol consumption significantly impacts the management of the trauma victim. Alcohol intoxication often complicates the initial assessment of injury severity, resulting in an increased need for invasive diagnostic and therapeutic procedures (e.g., intubation and ventilation, CT imaging, intracranial pressure monitoring).

Alcohol may diminish the patient's capacity to respond to hemorrhagic shock by altering hemodynamic effects and the acid-base balance. Volume depletion as a result of the diuretic effect of alcohol or vomiting can impair the reserve of the intoxicated trauma patient. Peripheral vasodilation caused by alcohol may contribute to hypotension and hypothermia. Although these effects may be transient, they underscore the need for early and adequate fluid resuscitation in these patients. Intoxicated patients with severe non-neurologic trauma may have lower blood pressures and carbon dioxide levels, indicative of compensatory hyperventilation, on hospital arrival compared with sober patients. More importantly, a poorly understood cardiac depressant effect also increases the depth of shock and volume requirements

for resuscitation. Alcohol-induced skin vasodilation may be accompanied by an increase in skeletal muscle, mesenteric, and renal bed constriction and left ventricular stroke work. Thus, the overall effect on systemic vascular resistance and blood pressure may be balanced.

Intoxication renders the signs and symptoms of intra-abdominal and retroperitoneal injury less reliable than usual. If the risk of an intra-abdominal injury exists, further evaluation (e.g., diagnostic ultrasonography, CT imaging) should be considered. Alcohol intoxication predisposes to abdominal wall laxity and therefore less protection from blunt trauma. These patients are also likely to have full stomachs, increasing the risk of gastric injury after trauma and predisposing to vomiting and aspiration, especially during acute airway management. The fatty liver changes in alcoholism can result in hepatomegaly. Portal hypertension in alcoholics may produce splenomegaly. These organs can become more vulnerable to the effects of trauma because of their enlarged size, protrusion beneath the protection of the ribs, and increased intracapsular pressure.

The American College of Surgeons Committee on Trauma requires screening for problem drinking for designation at a level I or II trauma center. In addition, level I trauma centers must provide intervention for identified problem drinkers. Although many institutions use blood alcohol levels to determine at-risk drinking in trauma patients, the Alcohol Use Disorders Identification Test (AUDIT) offers a practical alternative (Box 137.3).[43]

DIFFERENTIAL DIAGNOSIS

Acute alcohol intoxication is a diagnosis of exclusion. Before it is assumed that a patient's behavior is caused only by alcohol, other conditions should be considered, particularly co-ingestion of other substances and pharmaceutical agents, head trauma, and infection. Hypoglycemia, hypoxia, carbon dioxide narcosis, mixed alcohol-drug overdose, ethylene glycol poisoning, isopropanol or methanol poisoning, hepatic encephalopathy, psychosis, severe vertigo, postictal state, and psychomotor seizures can be manifested in a manner similar to that of ethanol intoxication.

AWS can initially be confused with acute schizophrenia, encephalitis, drug-induced psychosis, thyrotoxicosis, anticholinergic poisoning, and withdrawal from other sedative hypnotic agents. Alcohol withdrawal and alcohol-induced hypoglycemia also present with similar clinical presentations.

DIAGNOSTIC TESTING

Determination of a blood ethanol level is not routinely necessary in caring for the intoxicated patient when there is clear evidence of

BOX 137.3 AUDIT-C Questions

1. How often did you have a drink containing alcohol in the past year?
   a. Never (0 points)
   b. Monthly or less (1 point)
   c. Two to four times a month (2 points)
   d. Two to three times per week (3 points)
   e. Four or more times a week (4 points)
2. How many drinks containing alcohol did you have on a typical day when you were drinking in the past year?
   a. 0–2 (0 points)
   b. 3–4 (1 point)
   c. 5–6 (2 points)
   d. 7–9 (3 points)
   e. 10 or more (4 points)
3. How often did you have six or more drinks on one occasion in the past year?
   a. Never (0 points)
   b. Less than monthly (1 point)
   c. Monthly (2 points)
   d. Weekly (3 points)
   e. Daily or almost daily (4 points)

Adapted from Miller LB, Brennan-Cook J, Turner B, et al. Utilizing an Evidence-Based Alcohol Screening Tool for Identification of Alcohol Misuse. *J Addict Nurs.* 2018;29(2):90–95.

alcohol intake (e.g., confirmation by the patient). When the mental status is sufficiently altered that an adequate history cannot be obtained, there is evidence of head trauma, or the patient fails to improve (detoxify) as expected, a serum ethanol level or measurement by a breathalyzer should be determined. If the degree of obtundation is not commensurate with the measured (or breathalyzed) level, and other laboratory test results (e.g., toxicology screen, electrolyte levels, metabolic profile) do not explain the altered mental status, a head CT scan is indicated. Adequate history from paramedics, patient, and family members, serial physical examinations (especially mental status), and bedside testing, such as serum glucose level and oximetry, can help clarify the clinical situation and guide further testing.

Blood tests can be useful if the history is in doubt and can also help patients recognize that alcohol has adversely affected their health. The utilization of direct metabolites of ethanol is considered more accurate biomarkers of recent alcohol consumption. Three of these biomarkers, ethyl glucuronide (EtG), ethyl sulfate (EtS), and phosphatidylethanol (PEth), are gaining acceptance, although they are not currently available for routine testing.[5,44]

Tests of liver function that measure AST and ALT levels can identify heavy drinking and AUDs with sensitivities of 25% to 45% and specificities as high as 90%. A ratio of AST to alanine transaminase (ALT) higher than 2 suggests that alcohol is the cause of liver injury.

Laboratory Tests

In the apparently intoxicated patient with altered mental status, the serum glucose level, usually as a point of care test, should be measured to assess for hypoglycemia. In the alcoholic patient, electrolyte levels and acid/base status should be determined to look for hypomagnesemia, hypophosphatemia, hyponatremia, and metabolic acidosis. A complete blood count is obtained to evaluate for anemia, leukopenia, and thrombocytopenia and a serum lipase level to evaluate for pancreatitis if the patient has severe upper abdominal pain or tenderness, especially if accompanied by vomiting. A complete blood count, peripheral smear, platelet count, reticulocyte count,

thrombin time, prothrombin time and INR, and partial thromboplastin time help evaluate episodes of significant alcohol disease-induced bleeding.

Liver function tests are followed in a serial manner in cases of alcoholic hepatitis. An electrocardiogram (ECG) is indicated for tachydysrhythmias or chest pain (e.g., holiday heart, acute ischemia). A CT scan of the head or cervical spine imaging may be indicated if head trauma or seizures are suspected or confirmed or if the patient's mental status does not improve in step with the metabolism of alcohol. A chest radiograph is obtained to rule out cardiomyopathy, infectious pneumonia, or aspiration pneumonitis.

Alcohol Screening Questionnaires

Detection of risky drinking behaviors can be through clinical history or the administration of short alcohol screening tools in the ED setting. The screening tools with superior sensitivity and specificity are the SASQ, AUDIT, and AUDIT-Consumption (AUDIT-C), see Box 137.3.

As part of the initial assessment and in alignment with national recommendations, computerized screening programs could be used as an effective method for detecting at-risk alcohol use in ED patients. Identification of AUD and brief, sentinel event advice in the ED can be an effective and cost-effective method to reduce levels of alcohol consumption and alcohol-related harm.

The SASQ From the NIAAA can be used to streamline the screening process—it includes only 1 question: "How many times in the past year have you had x or more drinks in a day?" (where x is 5 for men and 4 for women).

MANAGEMENT

Comatose or stuporous patients may require assisted ventilation and intubation. If the bedside serum glucose level identifies hypoglycemia, IV glucose, as $D_{50}W$ or an infusion of D_5W, is indicated. Patients with evidence of poor nutrition should receive thiamine, 100 to 250 mg IM or IV once daily for 3 to 5 days. If an opioid overdose is suspected, naloxone may be diagnostic and therapeutic. Because magnesium is a necessary cofactor for thiamine metabolism, consider administering magnesium, 2 g IV. When possible, hypoglycemia should be documented before the empirical administration of glucose. With the airway maintained and respirations supported, the patient's liver eventually metabolizes the alcohol, and most patients recover.

Intoxicated patients who do not appear capable of appropriate decision making require evaluation and treatment in the ED, regardless of their willingness to cooperate. It is incumbent on the emergency clinician to establish that the patient understands the nature of the problem, whether intoxication alone or intoxication in the context of acute illness or injury and is capable of making reasoned and responsible decisions about care. Inappropriate discharge and failure to diagnose are two common areas of liability in the treatment of the alcohol-dependent patient. Discharge can be considered when a patient is clinically sober enough to be able to dress, walk, make reasonable decisions, and function independently, as judged and well documented by the treating emergency clinician. When possible, it is ideal to have another sober adult who is willing to take responsibility for and remain with the patient for the next 24 to 48 hours. Once clinically sober and cleared for discharge, patients should be reminded not to drink and drive.

Alcohol Withdrawal Syndrome

Family, friends, bystanders, or paramedics often give more reliable historical data than the patient does. Accurate vital signs are essential; this may require a rectal temperature. Hyperthermia, hypothermia, tachypnea, or tachycardia may suggest serious disorders that often accompany the alcohol-dependent patient. A rapid and thorough physical examination should be performed, with attention to the level of consciousness, signs of hepatic failure, or coagulopathy. Signs of trauma are sought, as well as a thorough neurologic examination.

The AWS should be promptly recognized and treated. The CIWA-Ar is a validated tool for symptom-based prescribing of benzodiazepines for alcohol withdrawal. Scores on the CIWA-Ar ranges from 0 to 67; scores lower than 8 indicate mild withdrawal symptoms that rarely require the use of medications, scores from 8 to 15 indicate moderate withdrawal symptoms that are likely to respond to moderate doses of benzodiazepines, and scores higher than 15 indicate severe syndromes that require close monitoring to avoid seizures and AWD (or delirium tremens).

Pharmacologic Treatment

Patients suffering from alcohol withdrawal should receive pharmacologic intervention along with supportive care. The ideal drug for alcohol withdrawal should have a rapid onset, a wide margin of safety, metabolism not dependent on liver function, and limited abuse potential. Although no one drug class meets all these requirements, benzodiazepines are clearly the mainstay of treatment.

Benzodiazepines. Benzodiazepines have anticonvulsant activity, dose-dependent respiratory and cardiovascular depressive effects, and and be given IV/IM if necessary. By interacting with receptors linked to the GABA-associated chloride ion channel, benzodiazepines substitute for the withdrawal of the GABA-potentiating effect of alcohol and abate withdrawal signs and symptoms. Numerous benzodiazepines have been studied, but there is no evidence of the clear superiority of any one benzodiazepine.

Lorazepam has good bioavailability with the oral, intramuscular, and IV routes. It may be given via an IM injection in agitated patients with no IV access. The half-life of lorazepam is ~12 hours and it does not have any active metabolites.. Excessive sedation, confusion, and ataxia are potential complications of all benzodiazepines with prolonged half-lives. Lorazepam is metabolized (conjugated) in the liver, yielding inactive products. Although the half-life of lorazepam increases in patients with cirrhosis or liver failure, it is much shorter than the increase with chlordiazepoxide. The elimination of lorazepam is only minimally altered in patients with renal failure and in older adults. Lorazepam may be given IV in a dose of 1 to 4 mg, depending on the severity of the withdrawal. Dosing can be repeated at 5 to 15-minute intervals for patients in severe withdrawal. Although it is not ideal, an intramuscular dose of 1 to 4 mg can be used every 30 to 60 minutes until the patient is calm and then every hour, as needed, for light somnolence.

Diazepam is another commonly used benzodiazepine to treat patients with alcohol withdrawal. When given IV, it has a rapid onset (1 to 3 mins) and a duration of 1 to 2 hours, though its half-life can be increased significantly in patients with liver dysfunction. Since diazepam has a more rapid onset than lorazepam, its dosing interval can be much shorter. One such dosing strategy involves giving diazepam 5 mg IV every 5 to 10 minutes for patients with major withdrawal symptoms. The dose can be repeated in 5 to 10 minutes. If the second dose of 5 mg is not working, consider 10 mg for the third and fourth doses every 5 to 10 minutes. If this is not effective, consider 20 mg for the fifth and subsequent dose until adequate sedation has been obtained.

Butyrophenones. Haloperidol, a dopamine antagonist, can be considered in patients with major alcohol withdrawal or delirium tremens and acute agitation or behavioral issues not responding to IV benzodiazepines. However, antipsychotics should never be used alone or as a first-line treatment for alcohol withdrawal as they do not treat the underlying pathophysiology. Haloperidol has little effect on myocardial function or respiratory drive, and its safety and efficacy by the IV, intramuscular, or oral route in the ED has been established.

The typical dose is 2 to 5 mg q4–8h prn; q1h may be required with acute agitation; but not to exceed 20 mg/day. Haloperidol has no anticonvulsant properties; however, extrapyramidal effects may be seen. Caution should be used in patients who may be susceptible to a prolonged QTc interval. Droperidol has effects and risks similar to those of haloperidol and remains a safe and effective treatment for acutely agitated patients in the ED. The recommended adult dose is 2.5 mg IV/IM; additional doses of 1.25 mg may be given to a desired effect if the clinical benefit outweighs the potential risk.

Other Agents. Patients being treated for major alcohol withdrawal may be given thiamine (100 mg IV) and magnesium (2 g IV). Although magnesium sulfate does not decrease the severity of withdrawal symptoms, the incidence of delirium, or seizures, it carries no significant risk with adequate renal function. For patients who require intubation for refractory withdrawal or for other reasons, an infusion of propofol or a benzodiazepine should be initiated to treat the patient's alcohol withdrawal.

Neurologic Examination

New-Onset Seizures

Patients with new-onset, alcohol-related seizures should be thoroughly evaluated. This includes alcoholics who claim to have had seizures but for whom no documentation or appropriate evaluation is available. Metabolic disorders, toxic ingestion, infection, and structural abnormalities should also be considered.

If the initial physical examination findings, imaging studies, and laboratory test results are within normal limits, patients who remain seizure-free and symptom-free, with no sign of withdrawal after 4 to 6 hours of observation, may be discharged. It may be unclear whether the patient has had a pure alcohol withdrawal seizure or a new-onset seizure disorder in the setting of alcohol ingestion. Long-term treatment with antiepileptic drugs is not useful in unprovoked new-onset seizures that have resolved or when a clear relation to alcohol consumption can be identified.

Optimal outpatient treatment includes follow-up and referral to a detoxification or rehabilitation program. Ideally, the assistance of a reliable family member or friend who is not a drinking partner and can remain with the patient for at least 1 or 2 days is helpful.

Prior History of Seizures During Withdrawal

The risk of seizure increases significantly in alcoholic patients with manifestations of alcohol withdrawal who relate a history of alcohol withdrawal seizure. Detoxification with benzodiazepines reduces alcohol withdrawal seizures and should be initiated early because most seizures occur within the first 24 hours after alcohol withdrawal. An initial dose of 2 mg of lorazepam or 5 mg of diazepam can be given IV. These doses frequently need to be repeated, as noted in the Benzodiazepine section.

Abnormal Neurologic Examination

New-Onset Partial Seizures. Partial seizures account for up to 50% of alcohol-related seizures. Conversely, approximately 20% of patients with partial alcohol-related seizures have structural lesions— hematomas, tumors, vascular abnormalities, or stroke. These primary causes of partial alcohol-related seizure, such as prior head trauma, may be easily missed in the history taking. As a result, an emergent CT scan of the head is indicated to evaluate new-onset partial seizures. The patient with a history of a focal alcohol-related seizure who has been previously evaluated does not require an emergency CT scan provided a return to baseline occurs promptly.

Patients Taking Anticonvulsants. A patient currently taking antiepileptic drugs for an antecedent seizure disorder who presents with a seizure while intoxicated falls into a different category. Such an episode could be an isolated event in a usually compliant patient without a history of chronic alcohol abuse. In this patient, a seizure in the setting of a subtherapeutic antiepileptic drug level may represent the consequences of noncompliance with antiepileptic medication, co-ingestants, or sleep deprivation versus alcohol withdrawal seizure.

DISPOSITION

Most patients with acute alcohol intoxication are managed in the ED or observation unit and then discharged home. Patients who achieve sufficient sobriety to be ready for discharge are offered detoxification or alcohol treatment programs. Most alcoholics suffer from a combination of medical, psychiatric, and social problems. Hospitalization may be necessary to diagnose and treat these multiple problems. Moreover, with alcoholics who are no longer able to care for themselves, hospitalization is often dictated for this reason alone. Unfortunately, many managed care and Medicaid plans limit or do not cover inpatient detoxification. In choosing medical versus psychiatric admission, a medical illness usually takes priority. Optimal outpatient therapy for chronic alcoholics includes the involvement of concerned family or friends to ensure that the patient takes his or her medications properly, keeps follow-up appointments, abstains from alcohol, and maintains an adequate diet. Alcoholic patients who undergo outpatient treatment need close supervision; therefore, a follow-up clinic appointment within 24 to 48 hours should be considered.

Acute Intoxication

Acute intoxication alone seldom requires admission. However, a combined alcohol-drug overdose or associated medical, psychiatric, or social problems may require hospitalization. Acute alcohol intoxication is a diagnosis of exclusion reached after adequate observation to ensure that the altered mental status resolves and that the patient is hemodynamically stable.

Alcohol levels that may be tolerated by an adult can be lethal in children. It is prudent to admit young pediatric patients with acute intoxication and ensure close psychosocial follow-up for adolescent patients. Children presenting with hypoglycemia or medical complications should be admitted. Child abuse or neglect should always be considered.

Alcohol Withdrawal

Outpatient treatment consists of lorazepam, 1 to 2 mg TID tapered over 3 to 6 days, chlordiazepoxide, 25 to 100 mg TID tapered over 3 to 6 days, or diazepam, 30 mg once daily tapered over 5 days, depending on the severity of symptoms. Adequate diet, abstinence, and participation in a rehabilitation program in the community are also desirable. Any patient requiring 300 mg of chlordiazepoxide or 60 mg of diazepam/day to control withdrawal should be considered for admission.

Patients with signs of major withdrawal (fever, hallucinations, confusion, extreme agitation) require admission for close monitoring, serial neurological checks, and repeated medication dosing. Risk factors for clinical deterioration in patients with moderate to severe withdrawal include older patients who may be at greater risk for delirium tremens and may not tolerate the systemic stress of major withdrawal. Patients with delirium tremens generally require ICU admission. Criteria for ICU admission may also include patients with hemodynamic instability, electrolyte or acid-base disturbance, persistent hyper or hypothermia, rhabdomyolysis, renal insufficiency, and co-morbid conditions such as severe infection or pancreatitis.

Patients with mild alcohol withdrawal can be observed in the ED. After 4 to 6 hours of observation and treatment, the alert-oriented patient whose vital signs, physical examination findings, and results of laboratory analysis are within normal limits may be released with appropriate medications and aftercare instructions. Nevertheless, the patient can benefit from treatment for the underlying disease of alcoholism and should be advised or referred accordingly.

Seizures

The alcoholic patient with a first-time, alcohol-related seizure may be discharged to a suitable social situation in these situations: (1) when the patient's alcohol withdrawal is mild and controlled by supportive care or low-dose benzodiazepines; (2) the diagnostic evaluation, including a head CT scan, is unremarkable; (3) the patient has had fewer than two seizures; and (4) the patient has been observed to be alert and oriented, with stable vital signs and physical examination findings, normalized laboratory study results since the last seizure, and appropriate outpatient follow-up can be ensured.

Patients with a documented history of alcohol-related seizures can be discharged if they have had no more than two alcohol-related seizures during a 6-hour period, with a lucid interval between seizures, and are observed to be seizure-free and at baseline mental and physical status for at least 6 hours after their last alcohol-related seizure. Three to five brief, self-limited seizures may occur with alcohol withdrawal seizures. We recommend prolonged observation in the ED or observation unit for patients with two or more seizures because of the potential for deterioration to status epilepticus. Such patients should be observed until at least 6 hours have passed since their last seizure and they have a normal mental status and neurologic examination.

Patients with partial seizures or focal neurologic findings on physical examination require admission unless these findings have been previously documented. Patients with seizures associated with head trauma or mixed alcohol-drug withdrawal are admitted. Status epilepticus or recurrent seizures during ED observation indicate a lack of seizure control and require further hospitalization, often in a critical care setting.

Psychiatric and Social Problems

Alcoholic patients requiring admission with acute intoxication, alcohol-related seizure, alcohol withdrawal, or medical or surgical disorders are usually best managed in acute care units rather than by a general psychiatric service. Some psychiatric and social conditions in the alcoholic can be better handled on a general psychiatric unit—psychosis, exacerbation of schizophrenia, depression with suicidal tendencies, any patient who is a danger to self or others, or alcoholic hallucinosis with an otherwise clear sensorium.

Patients who are no longer able to care for themselves may also require admission. Although these patients' ultimate destination is a rehabilitation center or a border care program, hospitalization may be necessary to rule out medical or psychiatric illness and treat impending withdrawal symptoms. Patients who wish to stop drinking are usually referred to a detoxification unit for treatment of impending withdrawal.

Psychosocial interventions are the basis of long-term treatment, but medications are also often used. However, the data surrounding the use of medications are weak.[45] The FDA has approved three medications for alcohol dependence in the United States: disulfiram, naltrexone, and acamprosate. A fourth drug, nalmefene (oral), is approved throughout the European Union and is taken on an "as needed" basis prior to anticipated drinking occasions.

Other medications for AUDs have shown limited efficacy, and there is a high degree of variability in treatment response. Baclofen for the long-term treatment of alcohol dependence shows no clear-cut evidence from randomized, double-blind studies.[1,45] Gabapentin is used as monotherapy or as an add-on pharmacotherapy in outpatient settings in the control of alcohol consumption and craving and in helping patients achieve abstinence.[46] Ondansetron may show benefit in early-onset but not in late-onset alcoholics. Risperidone for agitation has minimal effects on vital signs with or without a benzodiazepine, suggesting that risperidone is a safe option for patients presenting with acute agitation even in the setting of alcohol intoxication.[47]

Brief intervention and screening (SBIRT—*s*creening, *b*rief *i*ntervention, and *r*eferral to *t*reatment) can reduce alcohol consumption and is feasible and effective in the ED.[48] An ultra-BI (less than 10 minutes face-to-face time) or employing technology such as computers and mobile phones reduces previously identified barriers to ED clinician utilization.[49] Internet-based interventions show promise for reducing alcohol consumption, especially among those meeting criteria for hazardous or harmful drinking. Telephone contact after the ED visit may be another effective tool to screen injured patients for hazardous drinking and offer a brief intervention while avoiding interruptions to patient flow. Providing internet-based interventions is more effective than no intervention at all to reduce binge drinking among college-aged students. The Internet could be an economic and acceptable form of delivering brief interventions and is a preferred approach to reach binge drinkers in college.[50]

Most communities have an Alcoholics Anonymous (AA) chapter or treatment center for anyone who desires help with alcohol. Sobering centers can have a prominent role in the care for those with acute alcohol intoxication, particularly those individuals with chronic public intoxication who are likewise homeless. In smaller communities, clergy or social workers can usually arrange rehabilitation. Psychosocial treatments such as brief counseling, motivational enhancement therapy, the community reinforcement approach, guided self-change, behavior contracting, and social skills training were among the top ten most effective interventions for AUDs, together with various pharmacological interventions.

The references for this chapter can be found online at ExpertConsult. com.

138

Acetaminophen

Michael Ganetsky

KEY CONCEPTS

- Acetaminophen concentration should be measured in patients with intentional oral overdoses. Acetaminophen poisoning is relatively silent clinically until serious hepatotoxicity ensues.
- Repeated supratherapeutic dosing of acetaminophen can lead to life-threatening toxicity.
- Use the acetaminophen concentration on the nomogram at 4 hours or later post-ingestion to determine whether *N*-acetylcysteine (NAC) therapy is indicated for acute ingestions.
- IV NAC is preferable to PO NAC. When initiating NAC, continue it until the protocol is completed with adequate clearance of acetaminophen, and there is no evidence of liver injury. If there is evidence of liver injury or acetaminophen concentration remains >10 µg/mL, continue NAC until acetaminophen is undetectable, clinical signs of liver injury have resolved, and liver enzymes are declining (aspartate aminotransferase [AST] <1000 IU/L).
- For maximum benefit, NAC treatment should not be delayed beyond 8 hours after ingestion. If more than 8 hours have passed since ingestion, initiate treatment with ongoing assessment of the amount of ingestion (serial serum acetaminophen levels) and development of hepatotoxicity (elevated transaminases, coagulopathy, and encephalopathy).
- Late or prolonged administration of NAC is beneficial even with low or absent acetaminophen concentrations if hepatotoxicity is evident.
- NAC is safe in pregnancy and is used in the same protocol as for the non-pregnant patient.

FOUNDATIONS

Acetaminophen (known internationally as paracetamol) is one of the most important toxins encountered in emergency care because of its ready availability, high potential lethality, and absence of symptoms in the early period after acute ingestion, during which administration of the antidote is most effective. Acetaminophen is found as an isolated product or in combination medications for the treatment of pain and febrile illness. An intravenous (IV) formulation is also available. Given its widespread availability and occult clinical presentation, acetaminophen toxicity is a concern in the vast majority of intentional ingestions, as well as with repeated supratherapeutic dosing, prescription drug misuse, and use by patients with alcohol use disorder. Acetaminophen toxicity is one of the leading causes of hospital admission, antidote use, and fatalities from oral poisonings in the United States.[1]

Protocols have been established for the assessment and management of acute and chronic acetaminophen ingestion through decades of research and experience; however, controversy continues to exist, and management of acetaminophen exposures continues to evolve.

Acetaminophen is absorbed rapidly, with peak plasma concentrations generally occurring within 1 hour and complete absorption within 4 hours. Once absorbed, acetaminophen inhibits prostaglandin E_2 (PGE_2) synthesis, leading to antipyresis and analgesia. Inhibition of PGE_2 synthesis is either by direct cyclooxygenase-2 (COX-2) inhibition or inhibition of membrane-associated prostaglandin synthase.

In therapeutic doses, 85% to 90% of acetaminophen is conjugated or sulfated into nontoxic metabolites that are excreted in the urine (Fig. 138.1).[2] A small percentage (<5%) is oxidized by cytochrome P_{450} 2E1 (CYP2E1) (and to a lesser extent 1A4 and 3A4) to a highly cytotoxic metabolic intermediary, *N*-acetyl-*p*-benzoquinone imine (NAPQI).[2] In therapeutic doses, NAPQI is short-lived, combining rapidly with glutathione and other thiol-containing compounds to form nontoxic metabolites that are excreted in the urine. With typical therapeutic acetaminophen dosing, glutathione stores and the ability to regenerate glutathione easily detoxify any NAPQI that is produced.

After large acute ingestions or repeated supratherapeutic ingestions, the amount of NAPQI produced begins to overwhelm glutathione stores and the liver's ability to regenerate glutathione, leading to unbound NAPQI. The highly reactive electrophile NAPQI covalently binds to cell proteins in the liver, which initiates a cascade of events that leads to hepatic cell death. Renal injury may also occur with or without liver injury and may be mediated by renal cytochrome P_{450} (CYP) enzymes or activation of prostaglandin synthase.

Acetaminophen-induced liver damage initially occurs in hepatic zone III (centrilobular), because oxidative metabolism is concentrated in this area. With severe toxicity, necrosis of the entire liver parenchyma may occur. The clinical effects of acetaminophen toxicity are the result of fulminant liver failure rather than a direct acetaminophen effect. These effects include multiorgan failure, systemic inflammatory response syndrome, hypotension, cerebral edema, and death. In the setting of massive ingestions, patients can present with altered mental status and metabolic acidosis. They typically have serum acetaminophen concentrations greater than 300 to 500 mg/L, and are at increased risk of developing hepatotoxicity despite early NAC administration.[3,4]

The principal therapy for acetaminophen toxicity is *N*-acetylcysteine (NAC),[5] which is effective via two separate mechanisms. Soon after overdose, NAC serves as a glutathione precursor and a sulfur-containing glutathione substitute (see Fig. 138.1) binding to, and thereby detoxifying, NAPQI. NAC may also decrease NAPQI formation by enhancing acetaminophen conjugation with sulfate to nontoxic metabolites.

Even after acetaminophen hepatotoxicity is evident, NAC acts as a free-radical scavenger and an antioxidant and alters hepatic microcirculation and oxygen delivery. In patients with acetaminophen-induced hepatic failure, IV NAC decreases the rates of cerebral edema, hypotension, and death even when no detectable acetaminophen remains in the serum.[5,6]

CLINICAL FEATURES

Adolescent and adult patients typically present after an acute, intentional ingestion of acetaminophen, either alone, or in combination with other drugs. Patients with chronic toxicity fall into two main categories: persistent supratherapeutic dosing (>4 g/day over 48 to 72 hours) or therapeutic or regular use in the presence of comorbidities that predispose to acetaminophen-induced hepatic injury. This latter group includes chronic alcohol users, patients with dehydration, malnutrition, and those taking other potentially hepatotoxic agents (e.g., isoniazid, valproic acid). Patients with chronic toxicity typically present with abdominal pain, anorexia, nausea, vomiting or new onset of jaundice. Careful questioning about acetaminophen use in patients with unexpected transaminitis is important, particularly when the cause of the abnormalities is not clear. Early after acute acetaminophen ingestion, patients are asymptomatic or have mild nonspecific symptoms

(e.g., nausea, vomiting, anorexia, malaise, and diaphoresis) (Table 138.1). Liver injury becomes evident after a period of 8 to 36 hours as an elevation in aspartate transaminase (AST).[2] Once liver injury has ensued, patients may develop right upper quadrant (RUQ) pain or tenderness, vomiting, and jaundice. AST concentrations continue to rise rapidly and usually peak in 2 to 4 days, corresponding to maximal liver injury. Alanine transferase (ALT), prothrombin time (PT), and bilirubin typically begin to rise and peak several hours after AST values. With severe toxicity, AST, ALT, and PT may all be elevated within 24 hours (Fig. 138.2). With maximal liver injury, patients develop signs and symptoms consistent with fulminant liver failure, including metabolic acidosis, coagulopathy, and hepatic encephalopathy. Death may occur from hemorrhage, adult respiratory distress syndrome, sepsis, multiorgan failure, or cerebral edema. The risk of renal injury increases with the severity of hepatic injury (known as the hepatorenal syndrome), occurring in 1% to 2% of patients without hepatotoxicity and in 25% of patients with severe hepatotoxicity.

If hepatotoxic patients recover, aminotransferases return to baseline concentrations over a 5- to 7-day period (see Fig 138.2), although complete histologic resolution of liver injury may take months. Once histologic recovery is complete, there are no long-term sequelae to the liver and patients are not at risk for chronic hepatic dysfunction.

Differential Diagnoses

Until excluded, acetaminophen should be considered a co-ingestant in patients with intentional oral overdoses regardless of whether they state that they ingested acetaminophen. Other causes of injury in patients with elevations in aminotransferases, bilirubin, prothrombin time and international normalized ratio (PT/INR), or creatinine, include acute tubular necrosis, rhabdomyolysis, ischemic hepatitis, alcoholic hepatic disease, cyclopeptide-containing mushroom toxicity, viral hepatitis, and Wilson disease. Other hepatic toxins include valproic acid, isoniazid (INH), statins, herbal medications (such as chaparral and pennyroyal oil), vinyl chloride, and polychlorinated biphenyls.

DIAGNOSTIC TESTING

The goals of patient assessment after acetaminophen ingestion are (1) the determination of the patient's risk, (2) diagnostic testing, and (3) treatment with the antidote NAC when indicated.

We recommend serum acetaminophen testing for intentional ingestion patients, whether or not they report acetaminophen ingestion. Patients with a known acetaminophen exposure should have the following laboratory testing: serum acetaminophen concentration at four hours post-ingestion, serum salicylate concentration (since patients often confuse these over-the-counter analgesics), AST, ALT, bilirubin, PT/INR, bicarbonate (screening for metabolic acidosis), and creatinine (to assess renal function). If a patient has signs of liver injury (elevated

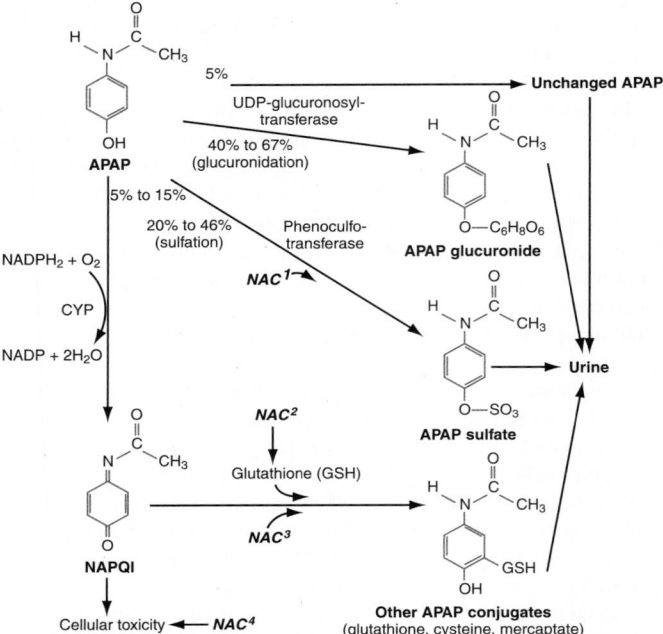

Fig. 138.1 Acetaminophen *(APAP)* metabolism and *N*-acetylcysteine *(NAC)* mechanisms of action. *NAC[1]* enhances sulfation; *NAC[2]* serves as a glutathione (GSH) precursor; *NAC[3]* is a GSH substitute; *NAC[4]* may reduce systemic toxicity. *CYP,* Cytochrome P_{450}; *NAPQI,* N-acetyl-*p*-benzoquinone imine; *UDP,* uridine 5'-diphospho. (Modified from Hendrickson RG: Acetaminophen. In Hoffman RS, et al, editors: *Goldfrank's Toxicologic Emergencies*, ed 10. New York: McGraw-Hill Education; 2015: 448.)

Stage	Time Course	Name	Symptoms	Signs
1	0 to 12 (up to 24 to 36) hours	Preinjury	Nausea, vomiting, anorexia, malaise	Elevated serum acetaminophen concentration
2	8 to 36 hours	Liver injury	Nausea, vomiting, RUQ abdominal tenderness	Aminotransferase elevation (AST begins to rise 8 to 36 hours after ingestion)
3	2 to 4 days	Maximum liver injury	Liver failure (encephalopathy, coagulopathy, hemorrhage, acidosis)	Hemorrhage, ARDS, sepsis/SIRS, multiorgan failure, cerebral edema
4	>4 days	Recovery	None	Complete hepatic histologic recovery

TABLE 138.1 Time Course and Clinical Stages of Acetaminophen Toxicity

ARDS, Acute respiratory distress syndrome; *AST,* aspartate transaminase; *RUQ,* right upper quadrant; *SIRS,* systemic inflammatory response syndrome.

AST or ALT), a venous blood gas and serum lactate should be measured. Acetaminophen exposures may be classified as acute or chronic, and each type requires different testing and risk assessment. An acute ingestion is defined as a single ingestion or a series of ingestions within an 8-hour period. All other ingestions, including accidental repeated supratherapeutic ingestions and intentional ingestions spread over longer than 8 hours, are considered to be chronic.

Risk Assessment With Acute Acetaminophen Ingestion

The initial diagnostic strategy of an acute ingestion is well-established. The first step is to determine the patient's risk of developing acute liver injury. Patients who report an acute intentional ingestion of acetaminophen should have laboratory risk stratification regardless of the reported amount ingested, because history alone is not reliable. In an otherwise healthy adult patient, ingestions of less than 10 grams in total or 150 mg/kg (approximately thirty 325 mg [regular strength] or twenty 500 mg [extra strength] tablets for an 70 kg adult) in an acute ingestion will not cause significant liver toxicity. A serum acetaminophen concentration should be checked in all intentional overdose patients, regardless of whether they report taking it, unless it is certain that the patient could not have had access to acetaminophen. Acetaminophen has been detected in the serum of up to 8% to 10% of patients with intentional ingestions who deny acetaminophen ingestion. Also, there is a high prevalence of unrecognized acetaminophen toxicity among subjects presenting with indeterminate acute liver failure.

Once an acute acetaminophen overdose is identified, establish the time of ingestion as accurately as possible using all available information. If no accurate time of ingestion can be determined, it is best to assume the earliest possible time of ingestion or to begin NAC therapy empirically if the time of ingestion is indeterminate.

A serum acetaminophen concentration 4 hours post-ingestion, or as soon as possible after 4 hours, determines the need for antidotal therapy by plotting the serum acetaminophen concentration against the time since ingestion on the treatment nomogram (Fig. 138.3). A serum acetaminophen concentration above the treatment line (that starts at 150 μg/mL at 4 hours and decreases to 4.7 μg/mL at 24 hours), indicates need for treatment with NAC. If the serum acetaminophen concentration is below the treatment line and the highest risk scenario has been assumed for the time of ingestion, then the patient requires no antidotal therapy. Use of the treatment line is indicated for otherwise healthy patients presenting after single acute ingestions. Alternative approaches in patients with alcohol use disorder, patients with

co-ingestions of antimuscarinic agents, patients with unknown ingestion times, and after IV formulations have been suggested, but these are not supported by trial data.[2] In a patient with an antimuscarinic (i.e., diphenhydramine) co-ingestion who has an elevated serum acetaminophen concentration at 4 hours that does not meet criteria for treatment, we recommend rechecking an acetaminophen concentration at 8 hours to ensure that appropriate clearance has occurred with no delayed absorption.

Measurement of serum acetaminophen concentration prior to 4 hours post-ingestion is not indicated. There is insufficient evidence to support claims that a serum acetaminophen concentration of less than 10 μg/mL between 1 and 4 hours excludes significant ingestion of acetaminophen. Absorption of acetaminophen may not be complete prior to 4 hours, and serum acetaminophen concentrations measured prior to 4 hours cannot be plotted on the treatment nomogram. There is no known benefit to administering NAC before the recommended 4 to 8-hour window after ingestion. Patients treated with NAC within 8 hours after ingestion, even after very large overdoses, have no increased risk of hepatotoxicity regardless of their serum acetaminophen concentration. For patients who have developed hepatotoxicity at presentation, those with preexisting liver disease, or those in whom a serum acetaminophen concentration cannot be obtained prior to 8 hours after ingestion, a loading dose of NAC is recommended along with consultation with a medical toxicologist or poison center. (See Box 138.1 listing indications for a medical toxicology consultation)

Risk Assessment With Chronic Ingestion

With repeated or chronic exposure, risk assessment is more complex, and the treatment nomogram cannot be used. Determination of the need for NAC is based on assessment of the risk for hepatotoxicity and measurement of serum concentrations of acetaminophen and AST.

The risk of hepatotoxicity from chronic ingestion of acetaminophen increases with total dose of acetaminophen and the duration over which it has been ingested in supratherapeutic quantities. Laboratory testing for serum acetaminophen concentration and AST should be initiated in any patient who fits the criteria outlined in Table 138.2.

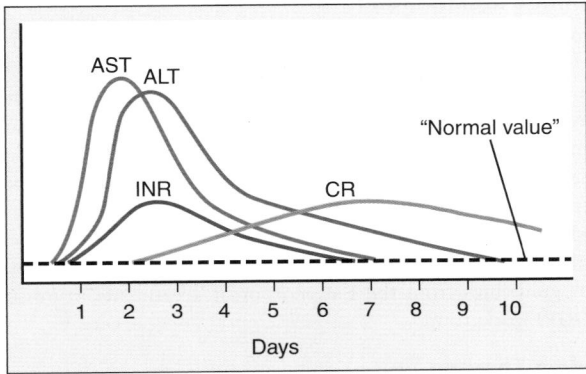

Fig. 138.2 A typical time course of rise, peak, and fall of laboratory values in patients with acetaminophen-induced hepatic dysfunction who survive. Peaks are not proportional. Not all laboratory abnormalities occur in all patients, and significant individual variation may occur. *ALT*, Alanine transaminase; *AST*, aspartate transaminase; *CR*, creatinine; *INR*, international normalized ratio. (Copyright Robert G. Hendrickson, MD.)

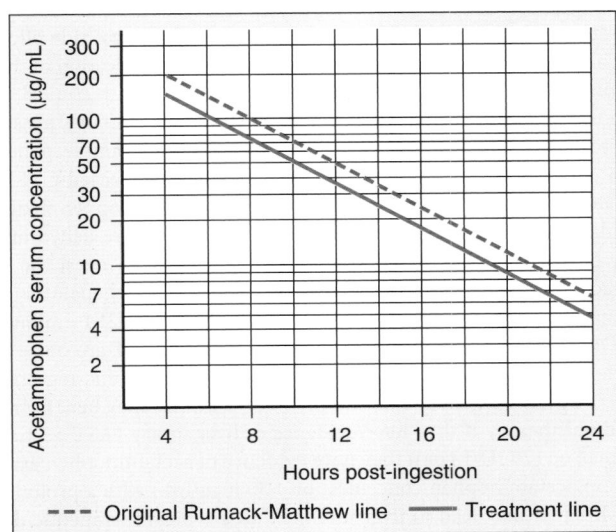

Fig. 138.3 Treatment nomogram for acute overdose. The lower treatment line should be used for treatment decisions. (Modified from Rumack BH, Matthew H: Acetaminophen poisoning and toxicity. *Pediatrics.* 1975;55:871.)

TABLE 138.2 **Indications for Initiating Testing for Serum Acetaminophen Concentration and Aspartate Transaminase in Chronic Acetaminophen Ingestions**

Age ≥6 years old;	Ingestion of >10 g/d (or >200 mg/kg/d) (whichever is smaller) over a 24-hour period
or	Ingestion of >6 g/d (or >150 mg/kg/d) (whichever is smaller) over a 48-hour period or longer
or	Symptomatic (e.g., RUQ pain/tenderness, jaundice, vomiting)
Children <6 years old;	Ingestion of >200 mg/kg/d over a 24-hour period
or	Ingestion of >150 mg/kg/d over a 48-hour period
or	Ingestion of >100 mg/kg/d over a 72-hour or longer period
or	Symptomatic (eg, RUQ pain/tenderness, jaundice, vomiting)

AST, Aspartate transaminase; *RUQ,* right upper quadrant.

Ingestion of therapeutic amounts of acetaminophen appears to be quite safe, although subclinical transaminitis can occur. Studies of patients presenting after taking 4 grams per day have shown ALT elevation of greater than 3 times the upper limit of normal in up to one-third of patients at one week, although no subject had clinical side effects, and all recovered without antidotal treatment. The implication of these findings is unclear but could be helpful to explain certain clinical scenarios. Some patients may be at increased risk for liver injury, possibly due to genetic variation or to specific risk factors. For example, patients who chronically ingest INH or ethanol may have increased CYP2E1 activity and may be at higher risk for chronic acetaminophen toxicity. Similarly, patients who are malnourished or have severe dehydration may be at higher risk for hepatotoxicity. Patients who ingest the liquid acetaminophen formulation may have lower risk of hepatotoxicity because the common diluent, propylene glycol, is a CYP2E1 inhibitor.[7]

Once serum acetaminophen concentration and AST are obtained, further risk assessment is necessary. Patients with chronic ingestions (e.g., >4 grams/day over a period of 48 to 72 hours) may benefit from antidotal therapy if they have evidence of liver injury (AST >2 times normal, or 120 IU/L) *or* if they have evidence of acetaminophen excess (serum acetaminophen concentration >30 mcg/mL) with a prolonged half-life that may lead to liver injury. After a typical therapeutic dose of acetaminophen, serum acetaminophen concentration peaks at less than 30 μg/mL and declines to less than 10 μg/mL at 4 hours. In patients who are asymptomatic, who have a minimal AST elevation, who do not report an intentional ingestion, we recommend a recheck

of serum aminotransferases after 4 hours. If there is not a sharp increase as would be expected to occur with acetaminophen acute liver injury, NAC therapy is not indicated.

Risk Assessment in Pregnant Women

The risk assessment and diagnostic approach to pregnant women is the same as for nonpregnant women. In acute overdoses, a serum acetaminophen concentration should be drawn and plotted on the treatment nomogram. NAC therapy should be initiated if the serum acetaminophen concentration plots above the treatment line. With chronic exposure, the same criteria strategy as outlined earlier should be instituted.

MANAGEMENT

Stabilization and Supportive Care

The mainstay of management is antidotal therapy with NAC, complemented by supportive measures. Supportive care includes management of co-ingestions, nausea and vomiting, hepatic injury, and renal dysfunction related to acetaminophen poisoning. Treatment of these problems is based on general treatment principles and is not acetaminophen-dependent (see Chapters 76 and 83). When questions exist regarding initiation of NAC or there are confounding clinical issues present (e.g., preexisting liver disease), clinicians may consult with a regional poison center (1-800-222-1222 in the United States) or a medical toxicologist for advice.

Decontamination

Activated charcoal (AC) effectively binds acetaminophen in vitro, and some studies have suggested that early administration of AC (within 1 to 2 hours post-ingestion) may decrease the number of patients that require antidotal therapy. In massive ingestions (≥40 grams), AC was shown to decrease acetaminophen concentrations and rate of hepatotoxicity up to 4 hours after ingestion.[3] However, many patients have co-ingestions that may depress mental status, and patients with severe acetaminophen poisoning often develop vomiting and are not able to tolerate AC. Given the lack of demonstrated efficacy in terms of improved outcomes from single-dose AC and the existence and availability of a very effective antidote, we do not recommend the routine use of AC for acetaminophen overdose, except in circumstances where the patient is asymptomatic and AC administration may prevent need for NAC, such as pediatric accidental ingestions.

Enhanced Elimination

Hemodialysis is not routinely used for acetaminophen overdose, because there is a highly effective antidote with good clinical outcomes when given within 8 hours of ingestion. However, acetaminophen is removed by hemodialysis, which may be helpful when the absorbed acetaminophen burden is sufficient to cause hepatotoxicity despite standard doses of NAC.[4] We recommend consultation with a poison center or medical toxicologist and nephrologist for initiation of hemodialysis for patients presenting following an acute massive ingestion with the characteristics outlined in Box 138.2. These are based on consensus guidelines from the Extracorporeal Treatments in Poisoning (EXTRIP) workgroup.[8]

Antidote Therapy

N-Acetylcysteine

NAC should be administered as early as possible when the acetaminophen concentration obtained at or after 4 hours post-ingestion is determined to be above the treatment line. NAC is also indicated when the liver function tests are noted to be elevated in a chronic

BOX 138.2 **Indications for Emergent Hemodialysis Following Acute Acetaminophen Ingestion**

- If the serum acetaminophen concentration >1000 mcg/mL and NAC is NOT administered
- If the patient presents with altered mental status, metabolic acidosis, an elevated lactate, and a serum acetaminophen concentration >700 mcg/mL and NAC is NOT administered
- If the patient presents with an altered mental status, metabolic acidosis, an elevated lactate, and a serum acetaminophen concentration >900 mcg/mL even if NAC is administered[a]

[a] NAC therapy should be continued during hemodialysis.

supratherapeutic ingestion. NAC is highly efficacious at preventing hepatotoxicity when administered at any time within 8 hours after an acute ingestion; delaying more than 8 hours after ingestion increases the risk of hepatotoxicity (Fig. 138.4).

NAC can be administered by mouth (PO) or IV. Both methods are efficacious in most situations, with advantages in favor of IV administration. All formulations of NAC (PO or IV) are effective when started within 8 hours of ingestion, with reductions in effectiveness when started between 8 and 24 hours post-ingestion. The risk of liver injury (i.e., AST >1000 IU/L) in patients treated with NAC within 8 hours is less than 1% and the mortality rate approaches zero (see Fig. 138.4).[9]

Once liver failure is evident (e.g., acidosis, coagulopathy, encephalopathy) NAC is given intravenously. IV NAC decreases the risk of hypotension, cerebral edema, and death in patients with acetaminophen-related hepatic failure. Oral NAC should only be used if IV NAC is not available. Even when there is no acetaminophen detectable in the serum, if a patient has AST greater than 1000 IU/L and there is a history or suspicion for acetaminophen ingestion or exposure, NAC should be started because there is evidence it decreases the need for liver transplantation and overall mortality.[6] There is an acetaminophen protein adducts assay in development that can discriminate liver injury due to acetaminophen and in the future may help to determine when NAC is indicated in the setting of liver failure with no detectable acetaminophen concentration in the serum.[10]

The main differences between IV and PO NAC are in their side effect profiles (Table 138.3). Approximately 5% of patients treated with IV NAC develop significant anaphylactoid reactions, although rates of up to 30% have been reported in prospective trials. The majority of these reactions are mild and self-limited consisting of sneezing, transient skin rashes, and flushing. More severe reactions have been reported in less than 1% of patients and include angioedema, bronchospasm, hypotension, and rarely death. Symptoms occur within 30 minutes of the start of the loading infusion. These anaphylactoid reactions are dose, rate, and peak NAC concentration dependent.[9]

Anaphylactoid reactions are less frequent with PO NAC. Skin rash, serious systemic reactions, and anaphylactic reactions are rarely reported with the PO formulation. However, approximately 15% of patients receiving PO NAC vomit (versus 7% with IV NAC), delaying timely antidote delivery. PO NAC is extremely unpalatable largely due to a sulfur or "rotten egg" odor and taste. Palatability may be improved by administering NAC diluted with either soda or juice and serving it in a covered container through a straw. Any dose that is vomited within 1 hour of administration should be repeated. If vomiting occurs, an antiemetic such as ondansetron can be trialed, but antiemetics administered prophylactically are not indicated.

Anaphylactoid reactions to IV NAC are typically mild (e.g., flushing) and occur during the initial loading infusion. Mild reactions can

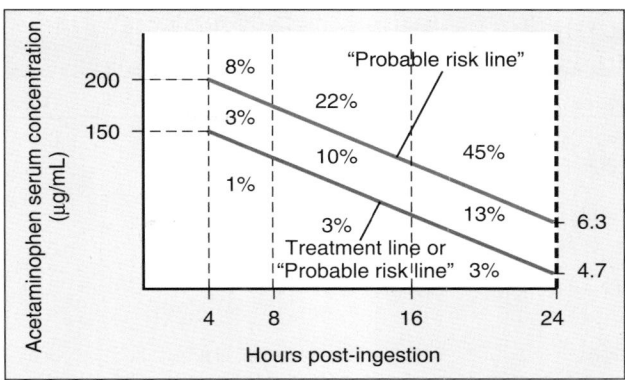

Fig. 138.4 Risk of liver injury (alanine transaminase >1000 IU) based on initial acetaminophen concentration and time to administration of oral *N*-acetylcysteine (NAC). (Adapted from Rumack BH: Acetaminophen hepatotoxicity: the first 35 years. *J Toxicol Clin Toxicol.* 2002;40:3.)

TABLE 138.3 **Side Effect Profile for *N*-Acetylcysteine Formulations**

N-Acetylcysteine Formulation	Common Side Effects	Severe Side Effects
PO NAC	Vomiting (13%), inability to tolerate due to smell	Very rare
IV NAC	Mild anaphylactoid reactions (e.g., rash, flushing, pruritus, vomiting), 2% to 18%	Severe anaphylactoid reactions (e.g., hypotension, bronchospasm), <1%

IV, Intravenous; *NAC, N*-acetylcysteine; *PO, per os* (by mouth).

be managed with parenteral diphenhydramine, 25 mg IV, without stopping the infusion. If hypotension develops, we recommend slowing or pausing the infusion, giving a 500 mL fluid crystalloid bolus, and administering diphenhydramine, 25 mg IV, and restarting the NAC infusion at a slower rate. For reactions persisting despite these steps, administer methylprednisolone 80 mg IV and treat as indicated for severe allergic reaction. Epinephrine is rarely required. These reactions require observation and treatment, but do not preclude subsequent doses, and treatment with diphenhydramine should be continued.[11]

Use in Pregnancy

Acetaminophen crosses the placenta, but the fetus in the first trimester of development is only at risk for injury if the mother suffers hepatotoxicity because fetal CYP enzymes have not fully developed. If the fetus is near-term (third trimester of development), there is a risk for direct fetal and neonatal hepatotoxicity, because the liver is more developed at this stage. Treating the mother with NAC is safe and effective, and NAC effectively crosses the placenta. NAC is used with the same protocols as for the nonpregnant patient. We recommend IV NAC when treating a pregnant patient. IV administration circumvents first-pass metabolism, therefore likely delivering higher doses to the fetus via higher maternal serum concentrations.

Duration of Therapy

There are two well-established protocols for NAC administration in cases of acute acetaminophen toxicity, depending on the route of administration: a 21-hour IV protocol and a 72-hour PO protocol. The standard IV NAC protocol in adults is a loading dose of 150 mg/kg up to a maximum of 15 gm in 200 mL of dextrose 5% in water (D5W)

TABLE 138.4 Inpatient Predictors of the Severity of Illness in Patients With Acetaminophen Toxicity

Score	Predictive Variables	Outcome Predicted	Notes
Kings College Criteria	pH <7.3 *or All three:* • Cr >3.3 *and* • INR >5 (or PTT >100s) *and* • Encephalopathy more than grade III (patient comatose)	Death or transplant	Arterial pH is measured *after* fluid resuscitation. The presence of any one of the Cr, INR, encephalopathy variables alone has a lower specificity for transplant than all 3 combined, but still has significant sensitivity to prompt consideration of transfer to transplantation center.
APACHE II	APACHE II score >20	Death or transplant	Confounders include co-ingested medications that may alter the APACHE II score.
Lactate	Lactate >3.5 mmol/L prior to resuscitation	Death or transplant	Lactate was drawn a mean of 55 hours after ingestion. The predictive ability of an early lactate draw is unknown.

APACHE II, Acute Physiology and Chronic Health Evaluation II; *Cr,* creatinine; *INR,* international normalized ratio; *PTT,* partial thromboplastin time.

infused over 60 minutes followed by a first maintenance dose of 50 mg/kg (up to a maximum of 5 gm) in 500 mL D5W infused over 4 hours. This is followed by a second maintenance dose of 100 mg/kg (up to a maximum of 10 gm) in 1000 mL D5W infused over 16 hours (6.25 mg/kg/hour).

Oral NAC is given as a 140 mg/kg loading dose, either by mouth or by enteral tube. Starting 4 hours after the loading dose, 70 mg/kg is given every 4 hours for an additional 17 doses (total treatment duration of 72 hours).

Several other regimens, including 48 hours IV, 36 hours IV, 36 hours PO, and 20 hours PO protocols are described; however, none of these are generally accepted as standard of care.[9] Recently, a "two-bag" protocol has been developed as an alternative to the 21-hour IV NAC protocol: 200 mg/kg NAC (in 500 ml D5W or 0.9% saline) over 4 hours followed by 100 mg/kg NAC (in 1 L D5W or 0.9% saline) over 16 hours. This protocol has demonstrated fewer adverse reactions and fewer medication errors with similar efficacy as the 21-hour protocol and is now being used in many centers.[12-14] Until further clinical trials are conducted to prove the clinical efficacy of these alternative dosing regimens, we recommend using the traditional 21-hour IV protocol.

Patients with very large acetaminophen ingestions may develop hepatotoxicity despite early and appropriate NAC dosing, and we recommend early consultation with a medical toxicologist in such cases (see Box 138.1.) We also advise consultation with a nephrologist or transfer to a capable center for possible hemodialysis for patients with the characteristics outlined in Box 138.2. Patients with hepatic failure and persistently elevated serum acetaminophen concentrations that do not decrease as expected are also at risk of failing NAC therapy. There have been various recommendations to increase NAC dosing based on very elevated 4-hour concentrations, but none are universally accepted. One recommendation is to increase the NAC rate to 12.5 mg/kg/hr (200 mg/kg NAC in 1 L over 16 hours) when the concentration is greater than the 300 μg/mL at 4 hour treatment line.[15] We do not recommend routinely using this dosing regimen until further

clinical trials are conducted proving its clinical efficacy or unless recommended in consultation with a medical toxicologist..

For delayed, chronic, or supratherapeutic dosing toxicity, NAC therapy should continue until acetaminophen is undetectable in the serum (<10 mcg/mL) and signs of liver injury have resolved (i.e., no encephalopathy, improvement of the coagulation profile with INR <2.0, resolution of metabolic acidosis, and AST less than 1000 IU/L with a downward trend).

DISPOSITION

Asymptomatic patients who meet criteria for treatment should be treated with NAC, which is started in the ED and continued in a medical inpatient unit or an ED observation unit. The motivation behind any ingestion needs to be evaluated, and psychiatric consultation obtained when appropriate.

Patients showing evidence of hepatotoxicity and those at risk for fulminant hepatic failure may require admission to a monitored bed or an ED or inpatient intensive care unit. These patients require frequent neurologic checks, monitoring of vital signs, and repeated laboratory studies.

Need for Transplantation

The King's College Criteria are the most commonly accepted decision rule for determining risk for needing liver transplantation.[16] Clinical rules for identifying patients at risk for developing fulminant hepatic failure are listed in Table 138.4, and patients meeting these criteria should be transferred to a tertiary care center that specializes in the management of patients with hepatic failure with potential need for liver transplant.

We would like to acknowledge the scholarly contributions of the previous edition authors, Robert G. Hendrickson and Nathanael J. McKeown

The references for this chapter can be found online at ExpertConsult. com.

139

Aspirin and Nonsteroidal Agents

Benjamin W. Hatten

KEY CONCEPTS

- In the overdose setting, salicylates are profoundly toxic and can be fatal. Salicylate overdose requires vigilant assessment and treatment. The other nonsteroidal antiinflammatory drugs (NSAIDs) generally have self-limited toxicity and respond to supportive measures. There is no specific antidote for any of these drugs.
- Salicylism should be considered in the differential diagnosis of altered mental status, particularly in the elderly.
- Acidemia signifies loss of respiratory compensation and acceleration of toxicity.
- The Done nomogram is no longer used and is not recommended in the evaluation and treatment of salicylate toxicity.
- Salicylate concentrations and blood gas draws should occur every 2 hours until the serum salicylate level is less than 30 mg/dL and is steadily declining at least 10% between assays in the absence of measures to enhance elimination.
- Potassium stores are rapidly depleted in patients with salicylate intoxication and should be repleted with a goal serum level of 4.5 to 5.0 mEq/L (4.5–5.0 mmol/L).
- When possible, mechanical ventilation should be avoided in cases of severe salicylate poisoning. Acidosis may rapidly worsen due to loss of adequate ventilation during the intubation procedure, and it is difficult to maintain ventilation at the level of physiologic hyperventilation.
- If intubation is necessary, a bolus of sodium bicarbonate (50 to 100 mEq) should be given before intubation and post-intubation; minute ventilation should be increased to match pre-intubation respiratory compensation.
- Enhanced elimination through urinary alkalinization with an intravenous sodium bicarbonate drip should be initiated in acute toxicity with a serum level >30 mg/dL.
- Consultation with nephrology and preparation for emergent hemodialysis should occur if the salicylate concentration is above 80 mg/dL or is rising rapidly.
- Hemodialysis is recommended for signs of pulmonary or cerebral edema, coma, seizures, hepatic failure, renal failure, circulatory collapse, or refractory metabolic acidosis along with acute serum levels greater than 100 mg/dL and chronic levels over 40 mg/dL.
- Altered mental status in the setting of salicylate toxicity warrants IV dextrose supplementation.
- Most NSAID overdoses are asymptomatic or cause only minor gastrointestinal symptoms.
- Ibuprofen, along with other propionic acid derivatives, has been associated with sporadic cases of aseptic meningitis.
- The management of NSAID overdose is supportive, and there is no specific antidote. Hemodialysis is reserved for patients with massive overdose (>400–500 mg/kg) and pH <7.1.
- Patients who have ingested a pyrazolone or fenamate require observation for possible seizures for 8 to 12 hours following ingestion.

ASPIRIN

Principles of Toxicity

Overview

Aspirin, or acetylsalicylic acid, is widely consumed for its analgesic, antiinflammatory, and antiplatelet effects. Although its therapeutic use is ubiquitous, salicylate toxicity is not a benign condition and causes a complex set of life-threatening metabolic derangements with significant morbidity and mortality.

Epidemiology

In 2017, twenty-three deaths were reported to United States Poison Control Centers due to aspirin alone.[1] This is consistent with reports to Poison Control Centers of twenty to thirty deaths per year for the past decades. One analysis identified salicylate toxicity as the most common preventable death due to poisoning that reached medical attention, suggesting an opportunity to impact mortality through proper management.[2] Elderly patients with chronic medical problems and young patients diagnosed with an acute illness are particularly at risk for delay in diagnosis with consequent severe adverse clinical effects.[3] In addition, increasing age has been identified as an independent predictor of severe outcomes and has been associated with lower peak levels in fatal cases.[4,5]

Salicylate-Containing Products

Aspirin is the most common salicylate-containing product. Other potential sources of salicylate toxicity include topical salicylates, analgesic balms, oil of wintergreen, willow bark, Alka Seltzer®, and bismuth subsalicylate. Ingestion of oil of wintergreen is of particular concern given that 1 mL of 98% solution contains the equivalent of 1.4 grams of aspirin.[6]

Pathophysiology

Salts of salicylic acid are rapidly absorbed intact from the gastrointestinal (GI) tract with appreciable serum concentrations typically occurring within 30 minutes after ingestion of a therapeutic dose with peak levels delayed from 2 to 4 hours. Large ingestions frequently slow gastric emptying. Aspirin, particularly enteric-coated preparations, tends to form concretions or bezoars in the stomach. These properties often result in prolonged absorption with rising serum levels for 12 hours or more.[3]

In the intestinal wall, liver, and red blood cells, aspirin is hydrolyzed to free salicylic acid, which reversibly binds to albumin. Free salicylate is eliminated by renal excretion. At therapeutic salicylate concentrations, elimination follows first-order kinetics. Once serum salicylate concentrations are greater than 30 mg/dL, elimination follows zero-order kinetics. The metabolic pathways become saturated, and the pH-sensitive urinary excretion of salicylic acid determines the half-life, prolonging significantly (up to 15 to 30 hours) with large overdoses.[3]

The initial physiologic effect of salicylates is direct stimulation of the medullary respiratory center. In addition, salicylic acid increases the sensitivity of the respiratory center to pH and partial pressure of carbon dioxide (PCO_2). Hyperventilation develops early, subsequently becoming a compensatory mechanism for metabolic acidosis. Prolonged high serum concentrations eventually depress the respiratory center. Respiratory alkalosis is compensated by the buffering capacity of the hemoglobin-oxyhemoglobin system, the exchange of intracellular hydrogen ions for extracellular cations, and the urinary excretion of bicarbonate. Loss of bicarbonate decreases buffering capacity and exacerbates the degree of metabolic acidosis (Box 139.1).[3]

Toxicity results primarily from salicylate interference with aerobic metabolism by uncoupling of mitochondrial oxidative phosphorylation. Inhibition of the Krebs cycle increases production of pyruvic acid and increases conversion to lactic acid. Increased lipid metabolism generates ketone bodies. Metabolic rate, temperature, tissue carbon dioxide, and oxygen consumption are increased. Tissue glycolysis predisposes to hypoglycemia, particularly in children. Inefficiency of anaerobic metabolism results in decreased production of adenosine triphosphate, with energy released as heat causing the hyperthermia frequently attributed to salicylate poisoning.

Only nonionized particles can cross the lipophilic cell membrane and accumulate in the brain and other tissues. Because salicylic acid has a pK_a of 3.5, the majority of salicylate is ionized and unable to enter tissue at the physiologic pH of 7.4. However, as serum pH decreases, more particles become un-ionized and cross the cell membrane and blood-brain barrier, markedly increasing the movement of salicylate into the tissues and central nervous system (CNS).

The rapid depletion of potassium stores in salicylate toxicity is caused by multiple factors. Immediate losses occur due to vomiting, which is secondary to stimulation of the medullary chemoreceptor trigger zone. In addition, increased renal excretion of sodium, bicarbonate, and potassium occurs as a compensatory response to the respiratory alkalosis, and salicylate-induced increased permeability of the renal tubules causes further loss of potassium. A final factor is inhibition of the active transport system, secondary to uncoupling of oxidative phosphorylation.[6]

Salicylate-related decreases in renal blood flow or direct nephrotoxicity may cause acute nonoliguric renal failure. Drug-induced, inappropriate secretion of antidiuretic hormone may also affect renal function. The exact mechanism by which salicylates increase alveolar capillary membrane permeability is not clearly defined. Theories include inhibition of prostacyclin, changes in platelet-vessel interaction, and neurogenic influences.

In adults, risk factors for salicylate-induced pulmonary edema include age greater than 30 years old, long-term cigarette smoking, chronic salicylate ingestion, metabolic acidosis, neurologic symptoms, and serum salicylate concentration greater than 40 mg/dL. Risk factors in children include high serum salicylate levels (>80 mg/dL), large anion gap acidosis, decreased serum potassium concentration, and low pCO_2.

Salicylates severely affect the CNS in two ways. First, there is a poorly elucidated aspect of toxicity that ultimately results in cerebral edema. This pathway is presumably related to increased energy requirements, acidemia, and direct cellular toxicity. Second, the consumption of glucose in the brain may outpace the supply. This occurs even in the face of normal serum glucose. One or both of these mechanisms can cause altered mental status, seizures, and coma.

At moderate to high tissue burden, salicylates induce a classic finding of toxicity—tinnitus, or the sensation of ringing in the ears. This phenomenon is due to a combination of central and peripheral effects. Cochlear toxicity is thought to be the result of alterations in N-methyl-D-aspartate (NMDA) activity, decreased blood flow, and increased membrane permeability. Cochlear toxicity combines with hyperactivity in the auditory cortex to cause tonotopic shifts where upper and lower frequency sounds are perceived in the 10 to 20 hertz tinnitus range, and sounds within this range become hyperacute. Salicylate-induced hearing disturbance may take days to resolve after the tissue burden normalizes.

At therapeutic dosing, salicylates increase bleeding risk via irreversible inhibition of platelet cyclooxygenase (COX). In overdose, vitamin K epoxide reductase is inhibited in a manner similar to warfarin. This acquired coagulopathy prolongs prothrombin time measurements and is associated with a substantial risk of clinically significant bleeding.[7]

Physiologic changes of aging predispose elderly patients to toxicity from chronic therapeutic ingestion. Decreased liver blood flow limits biotransformation of salicylate, and decreased renal function reduces salicylate clearance. Chronic ingestion decreases albumin binding, increasing the free salicylate that can enter the cell, and allows salicylates more time to pass through the blood-brain barrier. Therefore, a patient with chronic salicylate toxicity and a serum concentration of 40 mg/dL may be more ill than a patient with an acute ingestion and serum concentration of 80 mg/dL.

Clinical Features

Salicylate toxicity initially generates gastrointestinal (GI) distress followed by tachypnea with an accompanying respiratory alkalosis, tinnitus, and hearing disturbances due to concentration-dependent reversible ototoxicity, diaphoresis, and an evolving anion gap acidosis. As the toxicity progresses, hyperthermia, coagulopathy, cerebral and pulmonary edema, cardiovascular collapse, and, ultimately, death occur. Chronic poisoning may be more subtle, manifesting as a waxing and waning combination of the above manifestations of toxicity.[6]

Differential Diagnoses

Salicylism mimics sepsis, CNS infection, withdrawal syndromes, and alcoholic or diabetic ketoacidosis. This is especially true in chronic toxicity given that the serum salicylate concentration is relatively low. Thus, the severity of poisoning is often not recognized or not fully appreciated. In addition, co-ingestion is common, so evaluation for other toxic exposures is warranted. Other pain relievers and fever reducers such as acetaminophen and ibuprofen are often confused with aspirin by patients. Other toxins that cause a metabolic acidosis with an elevated anion gap include colchicine, iron, isoniazid, methanol, ethylene glycol, metformin, and cyanide. Other toxins that can cause tinnitus include aminoglycosides, loop diuretics, opioids, methotrexate, cisplatin, and antimalarial agents containing quinine.

Diagnostic Testing

The serum salicylate concentration, acid-base status, serum potassium, and glucose are key diagnostic studies. Be mindful of the laboratory units of measurement when interpreting salicylate levels. Serum salicylate concentrations are reported as mg/dL, mg/L, or mmol/L by various labs but are listed in mg/dL in this text. The Done nomogram, historically used for aspirin toxicity, should not be used to determine prognosis or treatment of the salicylate-poisoned patient.

Measure an initial salicylate concentration on arrival with a second sample obtained 2 hours later. A low initial salicylate level may be deceptive as early salicylate levels have not been shown to predict severity of outcome.[4] Obtain concentrations every 2 hours to monitor for continued absorption, which may be prolonged. Serum salicylate levels should be repeated every 2 hours until three consecutive levels are less than 30 mg/dL and are declining by at least 10% to 20% on each measurement while the patient is no longer undergoing therapy to enhance elimination. In one series, 3.5% of cases demonstrated peak serum levels greater than 30 mg/dl despite a nondetectable initial level with the longest interval from ingestion to detection of 225 minutes.[8] Thus, given sufficient clinical suspicion, continue to obtain salicylate levels up to 4 hours post-ingestion even if the initial level is undetectable.

Acid-base status can change quickly, and monitoring of pH every 2 hours is important to guide treatment. Use early and frequent arterial or venous blood gas determinations in symptomatic patients to rapidly assess acid-base and compensatory status. Developing acidemia portends severe disease. The pH begins to drop when the patient is unable to compensate for acidemia. Lactic acid accumulates, and serum bicarbonate is consumed. A serum lactate greater than 2.25 mmol/L is a predictor of severe outcome.[4] When serum pH is less than 7.4 and both PCO_2 and bicarbonate level are low, hemodynamic instability rapidly develops.[6]

A metabolic panel is necessary to guide electrolyte replacement (with a focus on serum potassium) and to assess renal function and glucose metabolism. However, anion gap determination on a metabolic panel is not a substitute for obtaining a salicylate level or measuring the pH. Measurement of protime/INR will assist in guiding vitamin K therapy in the setting of coagulopathy. A serum acetaminophen concentration should also be obtained to screen for ingestion of this common, clinically occult analgesic overdose.

Management

Stabilization and Supportive Care

Accurate ascertainment of vital signs is the initial step in assessment, including oxygen saturation, respiratory rate, and a reliable temperature. Chest auscultation can provide evidence of pulmonary edema, and altered mental status may suggest CNS toxicity. Dehydration occurs early in salicylate intoxication because of the hypermetabolic state, and initial fluid requirements may be as high as 4 to 6 L. Fluid administration should be guided by the patient's apparent deficit to maintain urine output of 2 to 3 mL/kg/hr. Correct potassium depletion to maintain a serum level between 4.5 and 5.0 mEq/L (4.5–5.0 mmol/L).[6]

Unless the patient is rapidly decompensating, early mechanical ventilation should be avoided in the aspirin poisoned patient. Similar to diabetic ketoacidosis, it is difficult to artificially achieve adequate minute ventilation that sufficiently matches the patient's own respiratory compensation. In addition, the loss of ventilation during the intubation procedure results in rapid loss of respiratory compensation and

BOX 139.2 Treatment of Acute Salicylate Poisoning

Treat dehydration; maintain urine output at 2 to 3 mL/kg/hr.
Correct potassium depletion with goal serum level of 4.5–5.0 mEq/L.
Consider oral activated charcoal (AC); 25 grams every 2 to 4 hours for two to four doses if tolerated.
Alkalinize urine with goal urine pH of 7.5 to 8.0.
  Infuse bicarbonate drip: 132 to 150 mEq (three 50-mL ampules of 7.5% or 8.4% sodium bicarbonate ($NaHCO_3$) in 1 L of dextrose 5% in water (D5W) + 40 mEq of potassium chloride (KCl) running at 2 to 3 mL/kg/hr.
  Allow serum pH up to 7.55.
  Do not attempt forced diuresis.
Initiate hemodialysis if any of the following occur:
  Altered mental status, coma, seizure
  Renal failure
  Hepatic failure
  Pulmonary edema or respiratory failure
  Severe acid-base imbalance (pH <7.1 to 7.2)
  Deterioration in condition
  Need for intubation
  Failure of urine alkalinization
  Rapidly rising salicylate level
  Serum salicylate concentration ≥100 mg/dL after acute ingestion
  Serum salicylate concentration ≥40 mg/dL after chronic ingestion
Administer intravenous (IV) dextrose 0.5 to 1 g/kg IV for any central nervous system (CNS) abnormalities (altered mental status, coma, agitation, seizure).

worsening acidemia. If the patient is critically ill and requires intubation, worsening of acidosis during apnea is potentially harmful. Thus, we recommend bolus administration of 50 to 100 mEq (1 to 2 amps) of sodium bicarbonate ($NaHCO_3$) immediately prior to the procedure irrespective of the serum pH to temporarily compensate for a respiratory acidosis in addition to the bicarbonate drip being administered for enhanced elimination. Attempt to adjust the tidal volume post-intubation to optimally match the pre-intubation PCO_2 level. In addition, establish an elevated minute volume and obtain frequent arterial blood gases to guide ventilator management to maintain respiratory compensation.[6]

Decontamination

Activated charcoal (AC) has been shown to reduce salicylate absorption in both animal studies and human volunteer trials. Evidence in the overdose setting is less clear. We recommend administering multiple-dose oral AC (25 to 50 gm via a nasogastric tube) every 2 to 4 hours for 2 to 4 doses if the patient's GI distress, mental status, and hemodynamic stability can tolerate, because large salicylate ingestions tend to form gastric concretions. AC is not used in chronic salicylate poisoning because the presentation occurs long after absorption from the GI tract.[6]

Enhanced Elimination

Specific treatment of salicylate toxicity has two objectives: (1) to correct fluid deficits and acid-base abnormalities and (2) to increase excretion (Box 139.2). Because salicylates have a low pK_a and are renally excreted, alkaline urine traps the salicylate ion and increases excretion. Urine alkalinization is advisable in patients with salicylate levels greater than 30 mg/dL, significant acid-base disturbance, or increasing salicylate levels. This is most often achieved via administration of a bicarbonate drip: 132 to 150 mEq (three 50 mL ampules) of 7.5% or 8.4% $NaHCO_3$ in 1 L of dextrose 5% in water (D5W) plus 40 mEq of potassium chloride (KCl) running at 2 to 3 mL/kg/hr. Salicylate clearance varies in direct proportion to renal flow rate but increases exponentially with pH. A urine pH of at least 7.5 to 8.0 is ideal to increase excretion. Urine alkalinization is difficult to achieve because the excretion of salicylic acid in the urine decreases urine pH. In addition, potassium depletion must be corrected to attain alkaline urine as the kidney exchanges hydrogen for potassium in the setting of hypokalemia, further acidifying the urine. In most patients, a serum pH of up to 7.55 is well tolerated. Forced diuresis should not be performed, because it does not significantly increase salicylate excretion and may potentiate fluid overload, as well as cerebral and pulmonary edema.[3,6]

Hemodialysis is highly effective in treating severe salicylate toxicity. It is indicated for patients with any of the following: serum salicylate levels greater than 100 mg/dL in acute and over 40 mg/dL in chronic salicylate poisoning; altered mental status, including coma; seizure; endotracheal intubation (other than for co-ingestions); renal or hepatic failure; pulmonary edema; severe acid-base imbalance (pH <7.1 to 7.2); rapidly rising serum salicylate level; and failure to respond to more standard treatments previously described. Of note, the levels recommended here are the maximum levels permissible for initiation of hemodialysis. Early consultation with nephrology to prepare for hemodialysis should occur prior to reaching a serum salicylate concentration of 100 mg/dL. In one series, over half of peak levels in fatal cases were less than 100 mg/dl. A concentration of 80 mg/dL, or even lower if concentrations are rising rapidly, should prompt nephrology consultation or transfer to a higher level of care with extracorporeal capabilities in anticipation of emergent hemodialysis.[3,5,6,9]

Greater salicylate concentration on the fetal side of the placenta and relative fetal acidemia contribute to fetal distress from maternal salicylate poisoning. Salicylate poisoning during pregnancy is associated with fetal demise, and therefore the mother should be treated expeditiously. Consultation with an obstetrician to facilitate delivery of the distressed fetus in the third trimester of pregnancy is indicated if the fetus is viable.[3]

Antidote Therapy

There is no specific antidote for salicylate toxicity. Central hypoglycemia may be responsible for altered mental status in the setting of salicylate toxicity. In all cases of altered mental status, even in the face of a normal serum glucose measurement, supplemental intravenous (IV) dextrose (0.5 to 1 gm/kg) should be administered. Additional glucose supplementation may be required and should be administered in response to recurrent altered mental status.[6]

In the setting of major bleeding with elevated protime/INR measurements, administer prothrombin complex concentrate along with vitamin K 5 to 10 mg IV. Platelet transfusion may also be helpful in the setting of bleeding to correct irreversible platelet inhibition.

Disposition

In patients with acute intoxication, hospital admission to an intensive care setting is recommended for pulmonary edema, CNS symptoms (other than tinnitus), seizures, pH less than 7.3, electrolyte disorders, dehydration, renal insufficiency, or increasing serum levels during serial testing. In patients with chronic intoxication, low serum salicylate concentrations (40 mg/dL) may accompany severe salicylism. These patients should be admitted to a monitored setting for observation, serial serum levels, and metabolic assessment. Consultation with a medical toxicologist may allow for emergency department (ED) observation management of the salicylate poisoned patient not requiring hemodialysis.

In patients with acute ingestion, repeated serum salicylate measurements are essential to determine that the serum concentration

is decreasing before the patient is discharged. Serum salicylate levels should be repeated every 2 hours until three consecutive levels are both less than 30 mg/dL and decreasing by at least 10% to 20% on each measurement when no longer undergoing therapy to enhance elimination. In addition, the patient should not be symptomatic (aside from residual tinnitus) at the time of discharge. With any case of intentional overdose, psychiatric evaluation is recommended.[3,6]

NONSTEROIDAL AGENTS

Principles of Toxicity

The nonsteroidal antiinflammatory drugs (NSAIDs) have analgesic, antiinflammatory, and antipyretic activities. Ibuprofen and naproxen, both propionic acid derivatives, are available over the counter in the United States and are the most commonly encountered NSAIDs. The therapeutic antiinflammatory effect of the NSAIDs is achieved by inhibition of cyclooxygenase (COX) and consequent blockade of prostaglandin production.[10]

NSAIDs are almost completely absorbed from the upper small intestine after oral administration. NSAIDs are highly bound to plasma proteins and therefore have small volumes of distribution (0.10 to 0.17 L/kg). They are eliminated by hepatic biotransformation. Metabolites are typically inactive with the notable exception of phenylbutazone. Plasma half-lives are relatively short (1 to 4 hours), except for naproxen (12 to 15 hours), oxaprozin (25 to 50 hours), piroxicam (45 hours), and phenylbutazone (50 to 100 hours). Elimination half-lives are not substantially prolonged in overdose.[11]

Clinical Features

Most NSAID overdoses are asymptomatic or cause only minor gastrointestinal symptoms. Ibuprofen is the most common NSAID ingested in overdose. Such exposures typically follow a benign, self-limited course. Symptomatic overdose occurs only after ingestion of at least 100 mg/kg, and symptoms develop within 4 hours of ingestion. Life-threatening toxicity is rare with most cases limited to mild GI disturbance that resolves in hours. Less common clinical effects include metabolic acidosis, muscle fasciculations, mydriasis, diaphoresis, hyperventilation, bradycardia, hypotension, dyspnea, tinnitus, and rash. Rare cases of coma, seizure, hypotension, and metabolic acidosis have been reported in acute massive overdoses (>400–500 mg/kg).[11]

Renal dysfunction is seen only after large acute overdose and in association with a period of relative hypovolemia with hypotension. It is usually reversible and generally responds to supportive measures. There are sporadic cases of acute liver injury with a predominantly hepatocellular pattern. This occurs both in therapeutic and supratherapeutic NSAID exposure. Diclofenac was the most common agent identified in a North American acute liver injury registry whereas nimesulide presented the highest risk. Both ibuprofen and ketoprofen were also identified as culprits in a European study.[12,13]

All propionic acid derivatives have been associated with sporadic cases of aseptic meningitis. This complication is most common with ibuprofen. It occurs in an idiosyncratic fashion—both in overdose and with therapeutic dosing.

Mefenamic acid, a fenamate, is associated with a high rate of CNS toxicity in overdose compared to other NSAIDS. In particular, there is a high incidence of seizures, which occur 2 to 8 hours after supratherapeutic ingestion. Rapid recovery is the rule with supportive care and IV doses of benzodiazepines administered in the case of seizure activity.[14]

Phenylbutazone, a pyrazolone, is now rarely prescribed because of its association with aplastic anemia and agranulocytosis. Although phenylbutazone overdose is rare, the course is much more severe than with other NSAIDs. Severely poisoned patients have early onset of GI distress, coma, seizure, hyperthermia, hyperventilation, alkalosis or acidosis, hypotension, electrocardiographic abnormalities, or cardiac arrest. Late sequelae of severe poisoning (2 to 7 days) include renal, hepatic, and hematologic dysfunction. The clinical course is prolonged compared with that of other NSAID poisonings, reflecting the long elimination half-lives of phenylbutazone and its principal metabolite, oxyphenbutazone.

Differential Diagnoses

Given that NSAID overdoses rarely cause substantial morbidity and are almost never fatal, the differential diagnosis should focus on toxicity due to possible co-ingestions. Patients often confuse NSAIDs with other pain relievers and fever reducers, including acetaminophen and salicylates. Other over-the-counter medications that can cause GI distress include iron preparations, vitamins, herbal supplements, as well as acetaminophen and salicylates.

Diagnostic Testing

Plasma NSAID concentrations are not clinically useful and are rarely available in the ED. With larger overdoses (>100 mg/kg), a complete blood count, metabolic profile, and assessment of renal function are recommended. Because patients often confuse and mix pain relievers, screening serum acetaminophen and salicylate levels are also recommended.

Management

Stabilization and Supportive Care

The management of NSAID overdose is largely supportive, and there is no specific antidote. Pyrazolone (e.g., phenylbutazone) and fenamate (e.g., mefenamic acid) toxicity is associated with significantly higher morbidity and may require more supportive care measures, including control of seizures with benzodiazepines, crystalloid fluid resuscitation, correction of electrolyte disturbances, and ventilatory support. Hypotension is managed with a 1 to 2 L bolus of normal saline or lactated Ringer solution, which may be repeated or supported by infusions at two to three times maintenance rate. If perfusion compromise persists, initiate a vasopressor, such as norepinephrine, and titrate to maintain an adequate mean arterial pressure for perfusion. Although it is rarely indicated and understudied, extracorporeal membrane oxygenation (ECMO) has been used to successfully manage refractory hypotension after massive ibuprofen overdose.

Decontamination

There is no evidence supporting the use of gastric emptying, AC or whole bowel irrigation in NSAID overdoses.

Enhanced Elimination

Because of high protein binding and rapid metabolism, enhanced elimination is not useful in most cases. In the rare case of a massive overdose (>400–500 mg/kg) with pH less than 7.1, hemodialysis should be considered to correct acidemia. Consultation with a nephrologist or transfer to a facility capable of emergently dialyzing the patient is indicated. In this situation, hemodialysis may also remove the free drug once protein binding is overwhelmed. Plasmapheresis has been attempted in severe phenylbutazone poisoning.

Antidote Therapy

There is no specific antidote for NSAID poisoning.

Disposition

Patients who are mildly symptomatic or asymptomatic for more than 4 hours after an NSAID overdose do not require further medical care. Patients who have ingested a pyrazolone or fenamate require observation for possible seizures for 8 to 12 hours after ingestion. Those with CNS symptoms, acidosis, or renal insufficiency and who require further supportive care should be admitted for ongoing treatment. Patients with mild to moderate symptoms may be observed in the ED until they are asymptomatic or improving. Patients for whom the ingestion represents a suicidal gesture should undergo psychiatric assessment.

The references for this chapter can be found online at ExpertConsult. com.

140

Anticholinergics

Jason A. Hoppe and Andrew A. Monte

PRINCIPLES OF TOXICOLOGY

Overview

Anticholinergic agents cause toxicity through inhibition of muscarinic, nicotinic, parasympathetic, or sympathetic acetylcholine receptors. Nicotinic receptor inhibition and ganglionic acetylcholine inhibition at parasympathetic and sympathetic locations are covered in Chapter 152. This chapter will focus on antimuscarinic effects and toxicity. The terms *anticholinergic* and *antimuscarinic* are used synonymously though the mechanism of toxicity is more accurately described by the term "antimuscarinic," and thus that term will be used in this chapter.

Antimuscarinic effects are due to competitive inhibition of acetylcholine at muscarinic receptors. Muscarinic receptors are found on peripheral postganglionic cholinergic nerves in smooth muscle (intestinal, bronchial, and cardiac), the secretory glands (salivary and sweat), the ciliary body of the eye, and the central nervous system (CNS).

Antimuscarinic agents have been used medicinally from antiquity to the present day. Mandrake plant remains were found in the coffin of Tutankhamen, the Old Testament of the Bible references its use as an aphrodisiac, and antimuscarinic plants were used as anesthetics in Greek and Roman settlements in the 1st century. Atropine, hyoscyamine, and scopolamine are naturally occurring tertiary amine antimuscarinic agents that remain in wide clinical use today. The tertiary amine structure allows the agent to cross the blood-brain barrier; therefore, these agents may precipitate CNS toxicity. Quaternary amine antimuscarinic agents, such as the anti-sialagogue glycopyrrolate, have been developed to mitigate CNS side effects due to their limited ability to cross the blood-brain barrier, though mild delirium may occur in the setting of a large overdose.

CLINICAL FEATURES

Over 600 compounds contain antimuscarinic activity, including prescription drugs, over-the-counter drugs, and plants. The effects of muscarinic receptor blockade are utilized for clinical purposes including pupillary dilation, antispasmodics, sleep aids, treatment of motion sickness, allergic reactions, drying of airway secretions, reactive airway disease, treatment of bradycardia, treatment of Parkinsonism, and the management of urinary incontinence and bladder spasm. The agents that most commonly precipitate antimuscarinic toxicity, such as H1 antihistamines and some antipsychotics, often affect several neurotransmitters and receptor systems in addition to antagonism at muscarinic receptors. This may complicate the clinical presentation and some clinical symptoms may be unique to the specific etiologic agent (Box 140.1).

Antimuscarinic toxicity has both central and peripheral manifestations (Fig. 140.1). Peripheral muscarinic antagonism causes tachycardia, hypertension, hyperthermia, mydriasis, dry mouth, lack of sweating, skin flushing, decreased bowel motility, and urinary retention. Central nervous system blockade of muscarinic receptors may produce delirium characterized by confusion, mumbling speech, agitation, hallucinations, hand picking gestures, myoclonus, tremor, and coma. Manifestations of the toxidrome are frequently incomplete and either peripheral or central components may predominate depending upon which antimuscarinic agent is involved, the dose, and the individual patient (Table 140.1). In one large series of antimuscarinic poisoning, only 28% of patients had all three classic manifestations of tachycardia, dry skin/axilla, and mydriasis. Therefore, most patients will not present with all of these features.[1] Duration of toxicity may be prolonged (18–72 hours) depending on the specific agent, dose, and the pharmacologic effect of delayed gastric emptying.[1]

DIFFERENTIAL DIAGNOSES

The differential diagnosis of altered mental status is broad. Consider antimuscarinic toxicity when there is a history of exposure or if there are physical exam findings consistent with the antimuscarinic toxidrome (Box 140.2).

DIAGNOSTIC TESTING

Laboratory

Patients with mild toxicity, a reliable history of exposure, and symptoms consistent with antimuscarinic toxicity do not require specific laboratory testing. Patients with an unclear history of exposure, other potential etiologies, moderate to severe toxicity or hyperthermia should be evaluated for causes of altered mental status and end-organ toxicity including: serum glucose, electrolytes, cardiac biomarkers, renal function, creatinine kinase to evaluate for rhabdomyolysis, and acid-base status. Patients with an overdose of unclear history should be evaluated for co-ingestion since antimuscarinic agents are often formulated with other potentially toxic agents. Serum acetaminophen and salicylate levels should be measured. Physostigmine may be used as a diagnostic test (see section on management).

Electrocardiogram

An electrocardiogram (ECG) should be obtained in cases of suspected tricyclic antidepressant or diphenhydramine toxicity to assess for possible sodium channel blockade (widened QRS interval > 120 ms or terminal R wave in lead aVR > 3 mm). Prior to the use of physostigmine, an ECG should be reviewed for bradycardia or atrioventricular (AV) block which would preclude the use of the antidote.

BOX 140.1 Signs and Symptoms of Antimuscarinic Toxicity

Mydriasis: "blind as a bat"
Altered mental status: "mad as a hatter"
Dry mucous membranes: "dry as a bone"
Dry, flushed skin: "red as a beet"
Hyperthermia: "hot as hades"
Urinary retention: "full as a flask"
Decreased bowel sounds/ileus
Tachycardia

MANAGEMENT

Stabilization

Initial management should focus on evaluation and stabilization of cardiovascular and neurologic toxicity. Sodium bicarbonate boluses of 50 mEq (1 amp) in adults and 1 to 2 mEq/kg in children should be given for evidence of sodium channel blockade with a QRS interval greater than 120 msec. Benzodiazepines should be considered for treatment of agitation and recurrent seizures. Patients with drug-induced hyperthermia should be treated with rapid cooling with progression to paralysis, ventilation and airway control, with sedation, when noninvasive cooling measures fail.

Decontamination

Most patients do well with symptomatic care alone. Gastric decontamination with activated charcoal may be considered though the risk of aspiration due to CNS depression or seizures generally outweigh the benefits. Activated charcoal may decrease ongoing absorption in patients that have ingested antimuscarinic plants or patients with decreased gastric motility. Theoretically this may decrease symptom duration. If considered, activated charcoal should only be administered early in the clinical course in awake, cooperative patients with a low risk of seizures or aspiration. There is little role for gastric lavage in antimuscarinic poisoned patients. There is no role for dialysis.

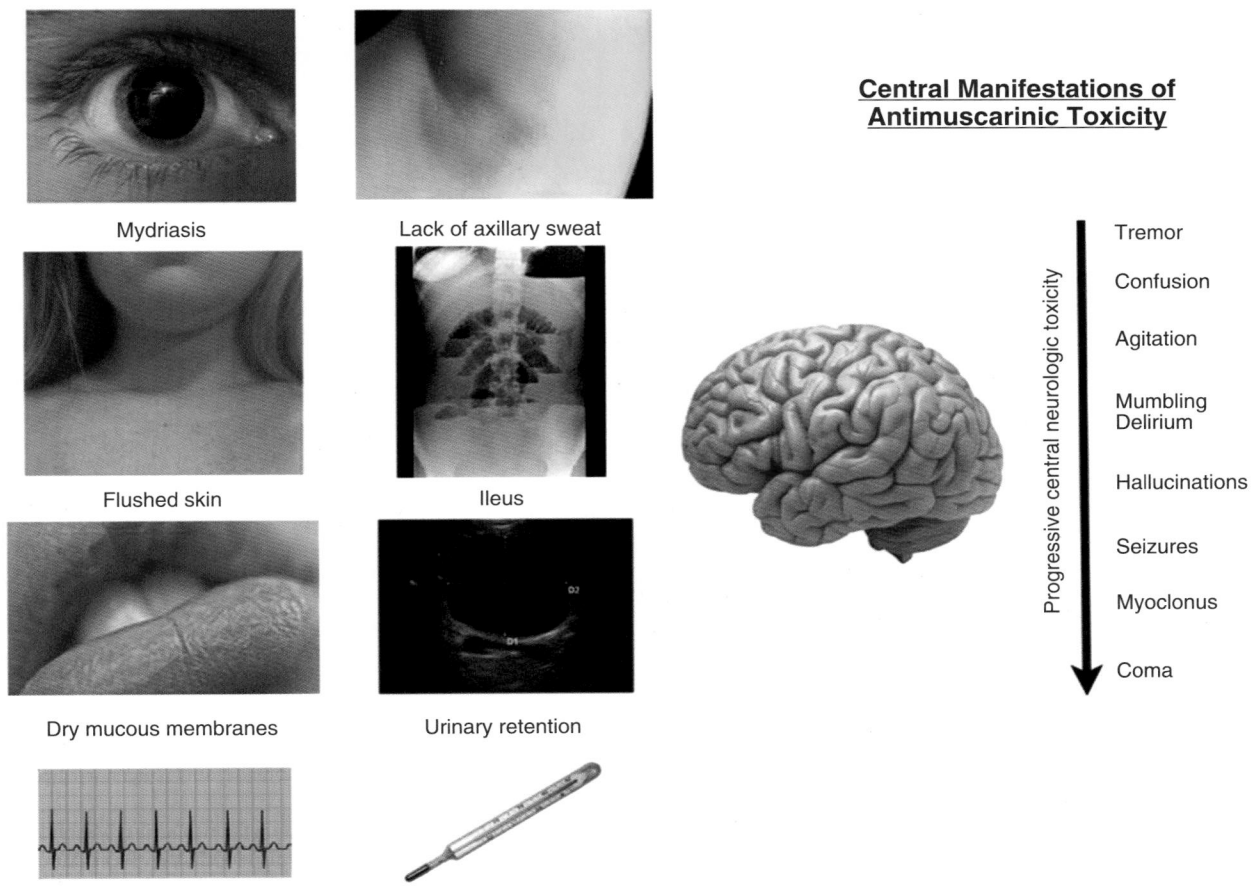

Peripheral Manifestations of Antimuscarinic Toxicity

Mydriasis

Lack of axillary sweat

Flushed skin

Ileus

Dry mucous membranes

Urinary retention

Tachycardia and hypertension

Hyperthermia

Central Manifestations of Antimuscarinic Toxicity

Progressive central neurologic toxicity

Tremor
Confusion
Agitation
Mumbling Delirium
Hallucinations
Seizures
Myoclonus
Coma

Fig. 140.1 Signs and symptoms of antimuscarinic toxicity.

TABLE 140.1   Specific Antimuscarinic Agents and Their Unique Clinical Manifestations

Antimuscarinic Agent	Toxic Dose	Unique Clinical Manifestations and Receptors Antagonized.
Datura spp.	Seeds contain high concentrations of hyoscyamine and scopolamine. The toxic dose depends upon the species and the mode of ingestion. In general 5 to 10 seeds may be toxic.	Classic peripheral and central antimuscarinic features M_1
Diphenhydramine	2.5 mg/kg, >10 mg/kg may result in cardiovascular and neurologic toxicity	CNS depression, QRS prolongation and ventricular dysrhythmias, seizures M_1, H_1, Na^+ channels
Doxylamine	>20 mg/kg associated with rhabdomyolysis	CNS depression, seizures, rhabdomyolysis M_1, H_1
Tricyclic antidepressants (TCA)	2.5 mg/kg, >10 mg/kg may result in cardiovascular and neurologic toxicity.	CNS depression, QRS prolongation, ventricular dysrhythmias, seizures, hypotension, antimuscarinic symptoms may manifest late in the course. M_1, H_1, α_1, Na^+ channels
Atypical antipsychotics	Varies depending upon agent.	CNS depression, hypotension, antimuscarinic symptoms may manifest late in the course. M_1, H_1, α_1, D_2, 5-HT_{2A}

M_1, Muscarinic; D_2, dopamine; 5-HT_{2A}, serotonin; H_1, histamine; α_1, alpha adrenergic.

BOX 140.2 Common Differential Considerations With Overlapping Signs and Symptoms of Antimuscarinic Toxicity

Differential Diagnosis Considerations
Toxicological
Sympathomimetic toxicity
Serotonin toxicity
Neuroleptic malignant syndrome
Lithium toxicity
Antidepressant toxicity
Antipsychotic toxicity

Central Nervous System
Intracranial hemorrhage
Seizure
Infectious
Sepsis
CNS infections

Metabolic
Hyperthyroid
Encephalopathy
Psychiatric
Delirium
Dementia
Bipolar disorder

BOX 140.3 Antimuscarinic Reversal Agent: Physostigmine

Physostigmine Salicylate
Indications: Diagnosis and treatment of antimuscarinic toxicity.
Contraindications: narrow angle glaucoma, AV blockade, bradycardia, and seizures due to current overdose.
Adverse effects: bradycardia, seizure, vomiting
Route: IV or IM.
Kinetics/dynamics: Time of onset: within 5 to 10 minutes following IV administration, 20 to 30 minutes following IM administration. Half-life: 16 ±3 minutes. Plasma cholinesterase inhibition 84 ±5 minutes.
Adult dosing: 1 to 2 mg bolus slowly (no faster than 1 mg/min). Start infusion at 1 mg/hour titrated every 30 minutes to clinical effect. Pediatric dose: 0.02 mg/kg (max 0.5 mg/dose) IV over 5 min, repeat every 5 min PRN (max total dose: 2 mg)

Pharmacologic Intervention and Antidote Treatment

Control of delirium is the most common reason for emergency intervention in antimuscarinic poisoned patients. Sedation or antidotal treatment should be considered in patients whose delirium places them at risk of physical harm; falling out of bed, becoming combative with staff, need for physical restraints, or pulling out intravenous (IV) access necessary for treatment. Sedation can be accomplished with IV benzodiazepines, such as lorazepam (0.05–0.1 mg/kg), midazolam (0.05–0.1 mg/kg), or diazepam (0.1–0.5 mg/kg), titrated every 15 minutes to sedation. However, benzodiazepines are inferior to physostigmine for control of delirium and agitation.[1]

Physostigmine salicylate is the antidote for antimuscarinic toxicity. It may be used for diagnostic and therapeutic purposes (see Box 140.3 for indications, contraindications, and dosing). Physostigmine is a tertiary amine carbamate that reversibly inhibits cholinesterases in both peripheral and central nervous systems.[1] This allows for acetylcholine accumulation and subsequent competition with the antimuscarinic blocking agent occupying the receptor. It has a short half-life, approximately 20 minutes,[1] though inhibition of the esterase, which yields the pharmacodynamic effects, lasts considerably longer with a half-life of 80 minutes.

When used diagnostically in an antimuscarinic poisoned patient, a response is expected rapidly, within 10 minutes. Near complete reversal of delirium is expected in a matter of minutes and may decrease the need for more invasive testing, such as lumbar punctures (to exclude meningitis) or neuroimaging. Therefore, if antimuscarinic poisoning is considered, appropriate doses of physostigmine may be considered early in the course.

Physostigmine may be used for treatment of delirium. Multiple observational studies have found that patients with antimuscarinic poisoning have delirium controlled with physostigmine in a large proportion of cases, 79% to 96%.[2-4] Further, benzodiazepines controlled agitation in only 24%, were ineffective for reversal of delirium in antimuscarinic poisoned patients, and were associated with a longer time to recovery.[1] A prospective observational study of 154 poisoned patients reported the odds of delirium control with physostigmine were six times greater than non-antidotal treatment.[3] Importantly, a retrospective study of 1815 patients with antimuscarinic toxicity within a clinical toxicology registry found a significantly decreased rate of intubation (1.9% versus 8.4%, OR 0.21) with physostigmine alone when compared to other treatments.[4]

Repeat dosing of physostigmine may be necessary in severely symptomatic patients. In case series of patients with antimuscarinic poisoning receiving the antidote, 30% to 39% needed re-dosing within 5.5 hours and the longest time between the first and last dose was 6.5 hours.[5] This suggests patients that remain asymptomatic beyond 6.5 hours are unlikely to have recurrence of symptoms. Severely poisoned patients requiring frequent re-dosing, such as *Datura stramonium* poisoned patients, may benefit from an infusion of the antidote. We recommend that the dose for the intravenous infusion be the same dose required for reversal of delirium, given per hour. The infusion should be stopped every 4 to 6 hours to reevaluate for ongoing need of the antidote.

Adverse drug events associated with physostigmine are manifestations of excess acetylcholine at neuromuscular junctions and thus can approximate cholinergic poisoning.[5] Symptoms may include salivation, nausea, vomiting, diarrhea, bradycardia, bronchospasm, muscular weakness, or seizures.[2,5] Physostigmine use in antimuscarinic patients is associated with very low rates of adverse events (5% to 9%), with serious events attributable to the underlying overdose, rather than the antidote.[2,5] However, it is advisable to avoid physostigmine in patients who have had a seizure temporally related to the overdose. Adverse drug events may be more common in antimuscarinic poisoned patients treated with benzodiazepines compared with physostigmine, largely due to airway complications secondary to respiratory depression associated with high-dose benzodiazepines.

Physostigmine has traditionally been contraindicated in patients with tricyclic antidepressant (TCA) overdose. This is based on a few well-publicized case reports that subsequently discouraged use of the antidote. The consistent ECG manifestations in these cases were AV blockade and bradycardia. The role of physostigmine as an etiology of the subsequent cardiac dysrhythmias has been questioned given that tricyclic antidepressants have inherent cardiac toxicity. Many patients in case series examining the safety and efficacy of physostigmine were found to have ingested TCAs.[2,3] This suggests that the antidote may be used safely when tricyclic antidepressant toxicity is manifested as antimuscarinic delirium, which occurs at low doses or late in the course. We, however, do not recommend use of physostigmine in the treatment of acutely TCA poisoned patients with cardiovascular toxicity.

Use of the antidote should be avoided in overdosed patients with bradycardia or AV block.

Overall, physostigmine should be considered as a safe diagnostic and therapeutic intervention in patients with antimuscarinic toxicity without overdose-induced seizure, AV blockade, or bradycardia, especially when the antimuscarinic-induced delirium places the patient or staff at risk.

DISPOSITION

Most patients do improve with supportive care alone (sedation, hydration, temperature control, and observation). Length of observation and need for admission depend on the agent, the dose, the intent, and the patient. Antimuscarinic agents slow gut motility, which increases the time to peak symptoms. As such, long-acting agents, plant seeds, or large ingestions should be considered for extended observation of up to 24 hours even if asymptomatic. Patients at extremes of age are at increased risk for toxicity and should be considered for observation over a similar period of time. Patients with an unreliable history or concern for self-harm should have extended observation and psychiatric consultation.

Observation at Home

Asymptomatic reliable patients with low-dose accidental exposures are safe to be observed at home by a trustworthy adult.

Emergency Department Observation

Patients with mild toxicity, normal mental status, normal vital signs, and small ingestions can potentially go directly home or may be observed in the ED for 4 to 6 hours for resolution of symptoms.

Hospital Admission

Patients with large ingestions or moderate toxicity (abnormal vital signs, altered mental status) should be observed for progression of toxicity or until symptoms improve. Ingestion of large amounts of pills or plant seeds should be expected to require prolonged observation (up to 24 hours) due to decreased gastrointestinal motility.

ICU Admission

Patients with agitated delirium, hyperthermia, dysrhythmia or seizures will benefit from intensive care unit admission for monitoring, redosing of reversal agents, and airway control if high doses of sedatives or additional physostigmine administration is necessary.

Consultations

Medical toxicology or poison center consultation should be considered when there are questions about exposure, diagnosis, or the appropriateness of antidotal therapy.

The references for this chapter can be found online at ExpertConsult. com.

141

Antidepressants

Michael D. Levine and Anne-Michelle Ruha

KEY CONCEPTS

- Although rarely used for depression, MAOIs are used in the treatment of Parkinson disease.
- Because serious symptoms can occur after a lengthy latent period, patients with reported MAOI overdose should be admitted for 24 hours, regardless of symptoms. Toxicity is characterized by tachycardia, hypertension, and CNS changes, and later cardiovascular collapse.
- The primary manifestations of TCA toxicity are seizures, tachycardia, hypotension, and intraventricular conduction delay. IV sodium bicarbonate should be administered for QRS prolongation.
- SSRIs are relatively benign in overdose and generally managed with supportive care alone.
- SNRI ingestions can result in seizures, tachycardia, and occasionally intraventricular conduction delay.
- The hallmark feature of serotonin syndrome is lower extremity rigidity with spontaneous or inducible clonus, especially at the ankles.
- Serotonin syndrome is primarily treated with supportive care, including discontinuation of the offending agent, and benzodiazepines.

PRINCIPLES OF TOXICITY

Depression is one of the most common medical conditions in the United States and is associated with significant morbidity. Worldwide, depression is the third leading cause of disability.[1] Whereas many treatment strategies are used in the management of depressed patients, pharmacotherapy remains a cornerstone of modern practice. Modern antidepressant therapy hinges on the monoamine hypothesis, which suggests that depressive symptoms are mediated through an imbalance of the dopaminergic, noradrenergic, and serotonergic systems.[1] Consequently, numerous antidepressant classes have emerged in an attempt to increase synaptic monoamine concentrations.

In the early 1950s, isoniazid and iproniazid were introduced for the treatment of tuberculosis. Shortly after, it was noted that these patients had improved mood, which was attributed to the ability of iproniazid to inhibit monoamine oxidase (MAO). Iproniazid subsequently became one of the first drugs used specifically as an antidepressant.[2] This led to the advent of other monoamine oxidase inhibitors (MAOIs). In 1956, the antidepressant effect of imipramine, a tricyclic agent, was recognized, and it was marketed the following year. The MAOIs and tricyclic antidepressants (TCAs) became the mainstay for treatment of depression for several decades until the advent of the safer selective serotonin reuptake inhibitors (SSRIs) and serotonin-norepinephrine reuptake inhibitors (SNRIs).

The morbidity of antidepressants in overdose varies greatly by specific class. Overall, however, there were more than 132,000 overdoses on antidepressants reported to United States poison control centers in 2017. Despite representing only 5.2% of calls, they accounted for 9.4% of fatalities.[3]

MONOAMINE OXIDASE INHIBITORS

MAO is located on the outer mitochondrial membrane and is responsible for breakdown of cytoplasmic catecholamines. Monoamine oxidase type A (MAO-A) primarily deaminates serotonin and norepinephrine; monoamine oxidase type B (MAO-B) primarily deaminates phenylethylamine.[2] Tyramine and dopamine are metabolized equally by both isoenzymes.[2] Whereas most tissues contain both isozymes, MAO-A is primarily found in the placenta, sympathetic nerve terminals, and intestinal mucosa; MAO-B is found primarily in platelets and the basal ganglia.

Drugs targeting the MAO system can act as specific or nonspecific inhibitors. The first-generation MAOIs are nonselective and irreversible. Drugs belonging to this class include phenelzine, isocarboxazid, and tranylcypromine. The second-generation MAOIs can preferentially inhibit either MAO-A or MAO-B.

MAOIs have fallen out of favor for treatment of depression due to side effects from adverse drug and food interactions. However, their use in treatment of Parkinson disease is increasing.

Drugs that selectively inhibit MAO-B disproportionately increase dopamine concentrations in the striatum.[2] Selegiline is an irreversible MAO-B inhibitor used in the treatment of Parkinson disease. Importantly, the selectivity for MAO-B is only present at low doses.[4]

Rasagiline is also an irreversible inhibitor of MAO-B and has similar clinical efficacy as selegiline.[5] Furthermore, unlike selegiline, which is metabolized to L-methamphetamine, rasagiline is not metabolized to an amphetamine derivative. Table 141.1 summarizes the MAO-inhibitors currently available for use in the United States. In addition to its antibiotic properties, linezolid, an oxazolidinone class antibiotic, is a reversible inhibitor of MAO, producing significant inhibition of MAO-A.

As a class, MAOIs are rapidly absorbed from the gastrointestinal tract and are bound extensively to plasma proteins. With overdose, the MAOIs initially stimulate release of neurotransmitters from the presynaptic neuron but later inhibit their release.

Clinical Features

Patients may develop toxicity from an MAOI either as a result of an interaction with a medication or food, or because of an overdose. Depending on the scenario that leads to toxicity, the clinical presentation may vary. Obtaining a thorough medication history is critical to establishing the diagnosis of MAOI toxicity. After acute overdose, a patient may remain asymptomatic for up to 24 hours before life-threatening toxicity develops. After this asymptomatic period, hyperadrenergic symptoms, including tachycardia, hypertension, and hyperthermia, can develop. Seizures, rhabdomyolysis, coma, and

TABLE 141.1	Summary of Monoamine Oxidase Inhibitor Agents Currently Available.		
Generic Name	**Route**	**Selectivity**	**FDA-Approved Uses**
Tranylcypromine	Oral	Nonselective	Depression
Phenelzine	Oral	Nonselective	Depression
Isocarboxazid	Oral	Nonselective	Depression
Selegiline	Oral or transdermal patch	MAO-B at lower doses; MAO-A at higher doses	Depression, Parkinson disease

FDA, U.S. Food and Drug Administration; MAO-A, monoamine oxidase type A; MAO-B, monoamine oxidase type B.

ultimately cardiovascular collapse can occur once presynaptic catecholamines are depleted.

Patients who take nonselective MAOIs in therapeutic doses are at risk for food-drug interactions. Tyramine is an indirectly acting sympathomimetic amine that is present in foods including aged cheeses, red wine, smoked or pickled and aged meats. Usually, tyramine is metabolized in the gut and liver by MAO, rarely causing systemic effects. When MAO-A is inhibited, tyramine is absorbed systemically and enters presynaptic vesicles, ultimately causing release of norepinephrine and serotonin into the synapse, leading to a hypertensive crisis. This tyramine syndrome, which can occur within minutes to hours of ingestion of foods with high tyramine content, is characterized by headache, hypertension, flushing, and diaphoresis. This syndrome can occur up to 3 weeks after discontinuation of a nonselective MAOI. Although it is theoretically possible, this syndrome is rare with therapeutic use of MAO-B inhibitors. A drug-drug interaction may result when MAOIs are combined with other agents that have serotonergic effects. A variety of prescription and over-the-counter medications may interact with MAOIs to produce a constellation of symptoms referred to as *serotonin syndrome* (see later section). This syndrome may be life-threatening, therefore the use of medications with serotonin-potentiating activity should be avoided in patients taking MAOIs.

Differential Diagnoses

The differential diagnosis for MAOI toxicity includes sympathomimetic drugs of abuse such as cocaine and amphetamine derivatives, anticholinergic (or antimuscarinic) toxicity (e.g., diphenhydramine, cyclic antidepressants, anti-Parkinson drugs, and jimson weed), and methylxanthine toxicity (e.g., theophylline and caffeine). Other toxicologic considerations include acute withdrawal states (e.g., ethanol and benzodiazepines), neuroleptic malignant syndrome (NMS), and the serotonin syndrome from other serotonergic drug combinations. Nontoxicologic causes to consider include environmental hyperthermia or heatstroke, febrile illness from infectious causes (e.g., meningitis and encephalitis), pheochromocytoma, carcinoid syndrome, thyroid storm, and hypertensive emergency.

Diagnostic Testing

Laboratory abnormalities are nonspecific but can include hyperglycemia and leukocytosis, secondary to a hyperadrenergic state, and elevated creatine kinase due to rhabdomyolysis. Immunoassay urine drug screens that are commonly used in the emergency department do not detect MAOIs, and even gas chromatography–mass spectroscopy of urine may fail to detect the presence of an MAOI. Patients taking selegiline will test positive for methamphetamine because methamphetamine is a metabolite. Spectral analysis is needed to differentiate illicit methamphetamine from selegiline.

Symptomatic patients presenting after an MAOI overdose should have an electrocardiogram (ECG) to assess the QT and QRS intervals and for evidence of cardiac ischemia. Patients with chest pain should be evaluated for myocardial infarction. Measurement of serum glucose

and electrolytes are indicated if the patient is obtunded. Because of the potential for intracranial hemorrhage in the setting of severe MAOI-induced hypertension, patients with a seizure or focal neurologic deficit should undergo a non–contrast-enhanced head computed tomography (CT) scan.

Management

As with most intoxications, supportive care is paramount. Central nervous system (CNS) excitation should be treated with intravenous (IV) administration of benzodiazepines such as lorazepam and diazepam in titrated doses. Lorazepam may be given IV in a dose of 1 to 4 mg, depending on the severity of symptoms. Dosing can be repeated at 5- to 15-minute intervals for patients with severe toxicity. Alternatively, diazepam, 5 mg IV every 5 to 10 minutes, can be given until the patient is stabilized. Hyperthermia should be treated with external cooling using evaporative techniques and strategic ice packing. Antipyretics such as acetaminophen or nonsteroidal antiinflammatory medications have no role in the management. Hyperthermia that persists, despite administration of benzodiazepines and external cooling measures, may need intubation, ventilation, and chemical paralysis with a nondepolarizing neuromuscular blocker, such as rocuronium (0.6 to 1.2 mg/kg IV). The use of succinylcholine is discouraged as this may cause hyperkalemia if rhabdomyolysis has occurred, and fasciculation from succinylcholine may further increase metabolic heat production. Furthermore, many of these patients are already acutely hyperkalemic, which is a relative contraindication to succinylcholine. Mild hypertension should not be treated, but sustained severe hypertension (e.g., systolic blood pressure exceeding 200 mm Hg or a diastolic exceeding 100 mm Hg) is best managed with a rapid onset, short-acting agent such as phentolamine (titrated slowly by repeated IV doses of 1 mg every 3 minutes) or nitroprusside (0.25 to 0.5 mcg/kg/min by IV infusion). Treatment should target a 25% reduction in the mean arterial pressure. Hypotension should first be managed by volume resuscitation with normal saline. Persistent or severe hypotension requires treatment with infusion of a direct-acting catecholamine such as norepinephrine or epinephrine. Because hypotension and cardiovascular collapse after MAOI overdose are due to catecholamine depletion, the use of indirect-acting agents such as dopamine are not likely to be beneficial. Extracorporeal elimination methods such as hemodialysis are also unlikely to be beneficial because of extensive protein binding and large volume of distribution of MAOIs.

Patients presenting with a tyramine reaction may have spontaneous resolution of symptoms within 6 hours. Severe hypertension higher than 200 mm Hg systolic with symptoms such as headache, flushing, or chest pain should be treated with phentolamine or nitroprusside. Patients with persistent severe headache and hypertension should have a head CT scan to assess for intracranial hemorrhage. Patients with chest pain should be evaluated for myocardial infarction (see Chapter 64).

Treatment of suspected serotonin syndrome is supportive (see later section) and consists primarily of benzodiazepine administration and active cooling measures.

Disposition

Patients presenting with an MAOI overdose should be admitted to a monitored setting for 24 hours due to the risk of delayed, rapid deterioration and development of hyperadrenergic symptoms. Asymptomatic patients chronically taking an MAOI who present out of concern for a possible drug-food interaction can be discharged after 6 hours if no signs of toxicity develop over that period. The care of any patient with suspected toxicity from an MAO inhibitor should be discussed with a medical toxicologist or poison control center (800-222-1222).

TRICYCLIC ANTIDEPRESSANTS

Principles of Toxicity

In the 1950s, imipramine became the first TCA used for the treatment of depression. Until the introduction of the SSRIs, TCAs remained the primary agents for treatment of depression. The therapeutic benefit of TCAs results from monoamine reuptake inhibition.[6] Whereas use of TCAs for treatment of depression has waned, use for other conditions, including treatment of migraines, various neuropathies, trigeminal neuralgia, and nocturnal enuresis has increased.

Clinical Features

Cyclic antidepressant toxicity can result from overdose of a TCA or drug interactions. Overdose is more commonly associated with life-threatening toxicity, but toxic effects can also occur when a TCA is combined with drugs that impair its metabolism through cytochrome P450. Tertiary amine TCAs such as amitriptyline, imipramine, and clomipramine are substrates of CYP2C19 and CYP1A2. Doxepin is also a substrate for CYP2D6. Drug-induced inhibition of these enzymes as well as genetic polymorphisms of these isoenzymes can decrease metabolism of these drugs, resulting in unexpectedly high serum concentrations and clinical toxicity. Conversely, inhibition of CYP2D6 and other P450 enzymes by these TCAs can also lead to increased serum concentrations of other drugs metabolized by the same enzymes. Because desipramine and nortriptyline are only weak CYP2D6 inhibitors, they cause fewer drug interactions. Another toxicity that can occur with TCAs is serotonin syndrome, which can result when a TCA is combined with another serotonergic drug such as an MAOI or SSRI.

Following a TCA overdose, clinical toxicity typically begins within 1 to 2 hours. When smaller quantities are ingested, symptoms may be minimal and resolve quickly; patients who take large amounts may deteriorate rapidly soon after ingestion. Severely poisoned patients typically have symptoms within 1 to 2 hours after ingestion, but nearly always by 6 hours after ingestion. Early cyclic antidepressant toxicity (within the first 2 hours) is primarily characterized by anticholinergic effects. These findings include dry mucosal membranes, urinary retention, and hot dry skin. Despite having potent antimuscarinic properties, the pupils are often small due to competing *alpha* effects. Patients may be alert and confused, severely agitated, hallucinating, or even deeply comatose. Speech is often rapid and mumbling in character. Seizures may occur and are likely to be multifactorial, resulting from increased synaptic monoamines, sodium channel inhibition, and gamma-aminobutyric acid (GABA) receptor antagonism. Early hypertension is common from the anticholinergic effects of the TCA and excess norepinephrine in the synapse from blockade of norepinephrine reuptake, but hypotension may also be due to alpha-receptor antagonism and also norepinephrine depletion.

Later (2 to 6 hours post ingestion), myocardial depression resulting from severe sodium channel antagonism may also lead to hypotension and bradycardia. Significant sodium channel blockade is associated with widening of the QRS interval. The degree of widening is prognostic for both arrhythmias and seizures.[7] Tricyclic antidepressants also

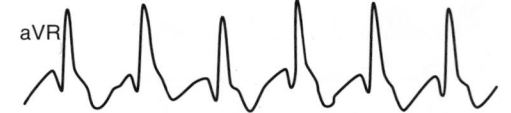

Fig. 141.1 Augmented vector right *(aVR)* demonstrating tall R wave.

block potassium efflux, which leads to a prolonged QT interval. Clomipramine and amitriptyline are especially associated with QT prolongation. Furthermore, clomipramine is associated with significant QT dispersion, which has been shown to be a risk for ventricular arrhythmias and mortality.[8] With severe poisoning, the combined effects of the TCA on various receptors and ion channels lead to depressed level of consciousness, seizures, hypotension, and wide-complex cardiac arrhythmias.

Chronic toxicity from drug interactions or decreased ability to metabolize the drug because of genetic polymorphism may be manifested in a less evident fashion. Confusion, urinary retention, and prolonged corrected QT (QTc) interval are common. Chronic toxicity presents more gradually and should be considered in any confused patient taking therapeutic doses of a cyclic antidepressant.

Differential Diagnoses

Many agents with anticholinergic properties produce similar clinical features as TCAs. Diphenhydramine and carbamazepine, in particular, can also produce seizure and sodium-channel blockade. Agents that produce sympathomimetic toxicity (e.g., cocaine, amphetamines) or serotonin syndrome (e.g., SSRIs, MAOIs) should be included in the differential diagnosis. Other drugs with sodium channel blockade, and hence a wide QRS complex, include the Vaughn-Williams class IA antidysrhythmics (e.g., procainamide, disopyramide, quinidine) and class IC antidysrhythmics (e.g., flecainide, encainide, and propafenone), along with amantadine, carbamazepine, cocaine, diphenhydramine, mesoridazine, and thioridazine. Propoxyphene and propranolol can also cause an intraventricular conduction delay by sodium channel blockade but typically cause a bradycardic rhythm rather than a tachycardic rhythm. The constellation of early anticholinergic symptoms, decreased level of consciousness followed by seizures, wide QRS and cardiovascular collapse, is highly suggestive of acute TCA overdose.

Diagnostic Testing

After overdose, the ECG can yield prognostic information. Early anticholinergic effects cause sinus tachycardia, which occurs uniformly before other effects. Whereas the serum tricyclic concentrations are not particularly beneficial in predicting adverse events, the ECG is prognostic. Historically, it is felt that QRS duration longer than 100 milliseconds is predictive of seizures, whereas QRS duration longer than 160 milliseconds is predictive of ventricular dysrhythmias, but hard evidence does not exist for either of these assertions. Additional findings on the ECG include a rightward shift of the terminal 40 milliseconds of the QRS complex seen as an R wave in augmented vector right (aVR) longer than 3 milliseconds. Figure 141.1 demonstrates lead aVR following a tricyclic ingestion. QT prolongation has less prognostic value than the QRS duration.

Urine drug of abuse screens commonly test for the presence of TCAs, but a positive test result suggests only use of a TCA or another xenobiotic that cross-reacts with the screen (e.g., antipsychotic medications, antimuscarinic agents, carbamazepine, or the muscle relaxant cyclobenzaprine). Quantitative serum tricyclic levels do not correlate well with severity of illness.

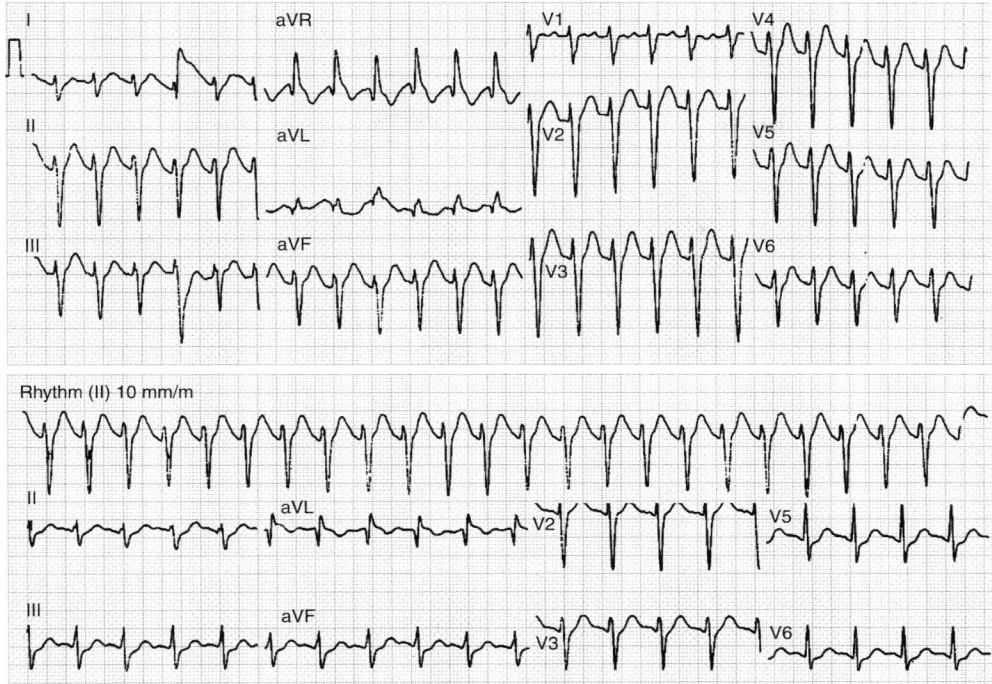

Fig. 141.2 *Top,* Initial 12-lead electrocardiogram (ECG) demonstrating substantial intraventricular conduction delay (QRS 141 milliseconds). *Bottom,* Repeated ECG after bicarbonate therapy. *aVF,* Augmented vector foot; *aVL,* augmented vector left; *aVR,* augmented vector right.

Management

Ensuring stability of the airway, with adequate ventilation, and volume repletion are of primary importance. There are no randomized controlled trials demonstrating improved patient-oriented outcomes and decreased mortality with activated charcoal administration in patients with cyclic antidepressant overdose. Nonetheless, because of the high lethality of the acute overdose, a patient who presents within 1 hour after an overdose and who is awake, alert, and cooperative and is not exhibiting any signs of toxicity (e.g., no tachycardia or intraventricular conduction delay) can be given oral activated charcoal. Patients who are not cooperative or who are not willing to drink charcoal should not have a nasogastric tube inserted for the sole purpose of administering charcoal. Due to risk of seizures with subsequent aspiration, activated charcoal is not routinely recommended in patients with an unprotected airway who are already exhibiting toxicity. There is no role for gastric lavage.

Patients with sinus tachycardia alone do not need specific treatment but should be monitored to detect QRS widening early in the clinical course. Early hypertension should not be treated. Hypotensive patients should first receive fluid resuscitation with an isotonic crystalloid. Patients who remain hypotensive should be treated with direct-acting vasopressors such as norepinephrine and epinephrine.

Hypertonic sodium bicarbonate is given only to treat specific evidence of sodium channel blockade such as a wide QRS and ventricular dysrhythmias.[7] Sodium bicarbonate should not be given strictly to treat tachycardia. Recommendations regarding the specific administration of sodium bicarbonate vary. We recommend a conservative approach by administering a bolus of 1 to 2 mEq/kg hypertonic sodium bicarbonate intravenous push (IVP) if the QRS interval exceeds 100 milliseconds. This dose may be repeated in 5 to 10 minutes if the QRS does not narrow. After IV bolus, a sodium bicarbonate infusion can be used to maintain a serum pH between 7.50 and 7.55.

Such an infusion can be created by the addition of 150 mEq sodium bicarbonate and 850 mL of dextrose 5% in water (D5W). The infusion should be created with a 5% dextrose solution, and not normal saline, due to the risk of hypernatremia with the latter. The infusion should be administered at twice the normal maintenance rate, titrating to QRS width and serum pH. Alternatively, infusions of 1 mEq sodium bicarbonate per milliliter of fluid may be used if volume overload is a concern. Additional IV boluses of sodium bicarbonate may be necessary if the QRS widens. The use of a bicarbonate-containing infusion should not be a substitute for IV sodium bicarbonate boluses for the initial treatment of intraventricular conduction delay. Figure 141.2 demonstrates a 12-lead ECG from a patient poisoned with a TCA before and after sodium bicarbonate therapy. If ventricular dysrhythmias persist despite maximal alkalinization (pH > 7.55), 3% hypertonic saline (in an adult) can be used. Class Ia or Ic antidysrhythmics should be avoided. Seizures are best treated with an IV benzodiazepine (lorazepam 1 to 4 mg IVP; diazepam 5 to 10 mg IVP) along with sodium bicarbonate. Refractory seizures can be treated with phenobarbital (15 to 20 mg/kg IV loading dose). Because seizure leads to acidosis and worsens the cardiac status, patients with intractable seizures who do not respond to benzodiazepines or phenobarbital should be rapidly paralyzed, intubated, and mechanically ventilated to prevent increasing metabolic acidosis.

Physostigmine, the antidote of choice for pure anticholinergic toxicity (see Chapter 140), is considered by many experts to be relatively contraindicated in the management of TCA overdose. Asystole has been reported after physostigmine use in TCA toxicity, particularly in patients with bradycardia and AV block. It is not advised to administer this agent to patients with QRS or QTc prolongation following TCA overdose. However, we recommend it be considered in patients with delirium of unclear etiology who are therapeutically taking anticholinergic agents and in whom toxicity is suspected, but only if there is no bradycardia, no history of seizures, and the PR, QRS, and QTc intervals are normal. Physostigmine (1 to 2 mg slow IV infusion over 5 minutes in adults) should be given with caution in a monitored setting, because it may exacerbate bradycardia, AV block, and seizures related to the overdose (see Chapter 140).

Intravenous lipid emulsion (ILE) therapy has gained interest recently for reversal of toxicity caused by lipophilic drugs, including TCAs.[9-10] Although the exact mechanism of ILE is not clearly defined, it likely involves redistribution of a lipophilic drug from the tissue receptors back into the vascular compartment in the context of a large bolus of concentrated lipid solution, the so-called *lipid sink phenomenon*.[10] Other mechanisms such as enhanced cardiac metabolism are also possible explanations. Because not all studies reveal beneficial effects from ILE in the treatment of TCA toxicity and due to the potential for iatrogenic harm, its use is currently reserved for life-threatening toxicity that remains refractory to sodium bicarbonate administration.[11] ILE should be administered only on advice of a medical toxicologist or regional poison center. If ILE is to be administered, there are several different dosing strategies. We recommend 1.5 mL/kg of a 20% lipid solution over 2 to 3 minutes. This bolus can be repeated once in 5 minutes if there is no clinical improvement. If clinical improvement does occur, the bolus may be followed by an infusion of 0.25 mL/kg/min.[12]

Complications of ILE include extreme lipemia resulting in interference with laboratory blood tests (complete blood counts, chemistries, and coagulation studies), as well as acute pancreatitis, and acute respiratory distress syndrome.[13]

Disposition

If the heart rate has not exceeded 100/minute for a sustained period of time (at least 10 to 15 minutes), ECG intervals are normal, level of consciousness is normal, and no seizures have developed within 6 hours of a TCA overdose, it is unlikely that toxicity will occur. The patient can be medically cleared from the ED for psychiatric evaluation and disposition if needed. Patients with signs of cyclic antidepressant cardiotoxicity, seizures, or coma should be admitted to an intensive care unit.

SELECTIVE SEROTONIN REUPTAKE INHIBITORS

Principles of Toxicity

In recent years, SSRIs have become the mainstay for treatment of depression. As implied by their name, these drugs prevent the presynaptic reuptake of serotonin without affecting the synaptic concentration of other monoamines. Some of the more commonly used SSRIs available today include escitalopram and its enantiomer citalopram, fluoxetine, fluvoxamine, paroxetine, and sertraline.

SSRIs have a wide therapeutic index. Most SSRIs undergo hepatic metabolism. There is considerable variability in their half-life; however, paroxetine has one of the shortest half-lives (17 hours) compared with fluoxetine, which has one of the longest half-lives (53 hours for parent drug, 240 hours for active metabolite).

Clinical Features

Overdoses of SSRI agents alone are usually well-tolerated and rarely fatal, with ingestions of up to 30 times the daily dose associated with few or no symptoms. Gastrointestinal upset and mild CNS depression can occur with large overdoses. Coma and seizures are rare, with incidences of approximately 2% for each. The incidence of serotonin syndrome after SSRI overdose is variable, but remains relatively uncommon in most series.

Citalopram overdose deserves special mention because of a reported higher rate of QTc prolongation and seizures compared with other SSRIs.[14] There has been some suggestion that the QT prolongation may be delayed with citalopram ingestion. However, there are not convincing data to support this delayed onset of toxicity. The risk of QT prolongation at therapeutic dosing may be over-stated.[15] In overdose, however, QT prolongation does appear to be dose-dependent. Despite a risk of QT prolongation, torsade de pointes associated with citalopram is relatively rare.[16] Escitalopram appears to be less toxic than citalopram, with a lower incidence of seizure and QT prolongation. Therapeutic administration of SSRIs may be associated with the syndrome of inappropriate antidiuretic hormone secretion (SIADH). Most cases of hyponatremia develop shortly after commencing use. The overall incidence is not well documented. Studies have documented that approximately 12% of elderly patients taking an SSRI may have SIADH.

Abrupt discontinuation of an SSRI may be associated with a mild withdrawal state, in which individuals feel anxious, jittery, and have some gastrointestinal upset. This withdrawal syndrome is not life-threatening.

Differential Diagnoses

The differential diagnosis for SSRI toxicity includes toxicity due to cyclic antidepressants, MAOIs, sedative hypnotics (e.g., benzodiazepines, barbiturates), SNRIs, neuroleptic agents, and atypical antipsychotics.

Diagnostic Testing

Diagnosis of SSRI toxicity is often dependent on obtaining a history of overdose. Clinical features of toxicity are similar to those seen after overdose of many other toxicants. An ECG can assess for conduction disturbances, especially QT prolongation. Specific SSRI levels are not performed by most hospital laboratories and do not influence management, although they may help confirm overdose retrospectively. A standard urine drug of abuse screen will not detect an SSRI.

Management

Treatment of an SSRI overdose is largely supportive. Activated charcoal has not been demonstrated to change outcomes following SSRI overdose but may be considered if the patient presents alert and cooperative within an hour of ingestion. Only rarely will patients require tracheal intubation because of loss of airway reflexes. For adult patients with a QTc interval greater than 500 msec, 2 grams of IV magnesium sulfate should be administered. IV administration of benzodiazepines (1 to 4 mg/kg of lorazepam via IV push; or 5 to 10 mg/kg diazepam via IV push) should be used to treat agitation and seizures.

Disposition

Patients who overdose with an SSRI who are asymptomatic after 6 hours of monitoring are unlikely to have toxicity. A patient who presents following an SSRI ingestion can be medically cleared after a six-hour observation period, assuming the patient has remained asymptomatic with a normal ECG. For citalopram or escitalopram, we recommend a repeat ECG be performed at the six-hour mark prior to providing medical clearance. Some advocate for extending this observation period to 12 hours following ingestions of more than 1000 mg of citalopram or escitalopram. Symptomatic patients should be admitted to a monitored care setting. Those patients with an intent of self-harm should be evaluated by a psychiatric service.

SEROTONIN-NOREPINEPHRINE REUPTAKE INHIBITORS AND NOREPINEPHRINE REUPTAKE INHIBITORS

Principles of Toxicity

Duloxetine, venlafaxine, desvenlafaxine, milnacipran, and levomilnacipran are collectively referred to as *serotonin-norepinephrine reuptake inhibitors (SNRIs).* All of these agents, except milnacipran, are approved for use in the United States for treatment of major depression. Milnacipran, despite being used as an antidepressant in Europe, is only approved for treatment of fibromyalgia in the United States. Some of these agents are also approved for other disorders. For example, venlafaxine can be used to treat panic disorder, generalized anxiety disorder, or social phobia, whereas duloxetine is also used to treat chronic musculoskeletal pain, diabetic neuropathy, fibromyalgia, and generalized anxiety disorder. Venlafaxine and its active metabolite desvenlafaxine are both available medicinally. The SNRIs may also produce dose-dependent inhibition of sodium channels. Reboxetine is an isolated norepinephrine reuptake inhibitor. It is also used for the treatment of depression.

Clinical Features

Unlike the SSRIs, which are relatively benign in overdose, ingestion of any of the SNRIs can be dangerous. Fatal ingestions have been described with virtually all of the SNRIs. The SNRIs may produce hyperadrenergic symptoms, including tachycardia and hypertension.[16] Rarely, hypotension can be observed after massive overdose.[17] Acute cardiac dysfunction, including impaired biventricular function, has been demonstrated following acute overdose.[17-18] Seizures can occur following ingestion of the SNRIs.[16] Unlike bupropion, however, which can have delayed onset of seizures, the onset of seizures following an SNRI ingestion is expected to occur within the first several hours post ingestion.

Rhabdomyolysis has been reported independent of seizure activity following ingestions of venlafaxine. Venlafaxine and desvenlafaxine overdoses can result in cardiovascular toxicity, manifesting as intraventricular conduction delay and ventricular dysrhythmias. Venlafaxine has also been associated with QT prolongation. In addition, based on their mechanism of action, serotonin syndrome may develop after ingestion of these agents.[16]

Differential Diagnoses

The differential diagnosis for SNRI toxicity includes toxicity due to cyclic antidepressants, MAOIs, sedative hypnotics, SSRIs, neuroleptic agents, bupropion, and atypical antipsychotic medications.

Diagnostic Testing

Specific drug levels are not rapidly available and do not aid management. An ECG can detect QRS or QT interval prolongation. SNRIs are not detected by urine drug of abuse screens, but venlafaxine and desvenlafaxine may be associated with a false-positive phencyclidine screen.[19] In cases of a venlafaxine ingestion, creatinine kinase and renal function tests should be obtained to assess for acute rhabdomyolysis. As with any multidrug ingestion, serum acetaminophen and salicylate levels should be measured.

Management

Care of the patient with an SNRI overdose is supportive, with focus on ensuring airway patency and adequate ventilation. While oral activated charcoal has not been clearly demonstrated to be beneficial in the setting of an SNRI overdose, if the patient presents within an hour and is awake and alert and cooperative, the use of charcoal can be considered. Hypotension (systolic blood pressure <90 mm Hg) should first be treated with a 20 cc/kg bolus of 0.9% normal saline. This bolus can be repeated if necessary. If hypotension still persists, a direct-acting vasopressor (such as epinephrine or norepinephrine) should be used. Intraventricular conduction delay with a widened QRS on ECG should be treated with sodium bicarbonate infusions (as previously described in the tricyclic antidepressants section). First-line treatment of seizures

is the IV administration of a benzodiazepine such as lorazepam, diazepam, or midazolam.

Disposition

Patients who are asymptomatic with a normal 12-lead ECG after an observation period of 6 hours can be cleared for discharge after appropriate psychiatric consultation. Patients with an intentional ingestion who develop manifestations of neurologic or cardiovascular toxicity (such as sedation, hypotension, or tachycardia) should be observed in a monitored setting. Those with profound CNS depression or hemodynamic instability warrant intensive care unit admission.

SEROTONIN MODULATORS AND STIMULATORS

Vilazodone and vortioxetine belong to a new class of antidepressants, referred to as serotonin modulators and simulators (SMS). While both of these drugs inhibit serotonin reuptake, they are also partial agonists at various serotonin receptors.[20-21] Clinical experience with these drugs in overdose is relatively limited. Unlike the SSRIs, in which serotonin syndrome is unlikely to occur with a single-agent ingestion, there are multiple case reports in which serotonin syndrome has been reported following isolated vilazodone ingestions.[21] In addition, gastrointestinal upset (e.g., vomiting), tachycardia, central nervous system depression, and seizures have been reported.[21-22]

The toxicologic differential diagnoses of these agents includes toxicity from the SNRIs, tricyclic antidepressants, bupropion, and trazodone. The primary aspects of management include ensuring the patient has adequate airway patency. Severe central nervous system depression may warrant intubation and mechanical ventilation. Seizures, should they occur, should be treated with benzodiazepines (e.g., lorazepam, diazepam, or midazolam). Hypotension should be first treated with rapid crystalloid fluid resuscitation. Refractory hypotension should be treated with a direct-acting vasopressor, such as norepinephrine or epinephrine. Patients who remain asymptomatic after a six-hour observation period can be medically cleared for psychiatric disposition.

MISCELLANEOUS ANTIDEPRESSANTS

Bupropion

Bupropion is an atypical antidepressant, belonging to a unique class (aminoketone).[23] It is widely used not only as an antidepressant, but also for smoking cessation. The primary mechanism of action is inhibition of dopamine and norepinephrine reuptake, but it also acts as a noncompetitive inhibitor of nicotinic acetylcholine receptors.[23]

Seizure activity is a dose-dependent phenomenon and can occur with therapeutic dosing or overdose of bupropion.[24] Seizures are relatively common after overdose and occur in approximately 30% of cases, the majority of which are initially tachycardic.[24-26] Sinus tachycardia, tonic-clonic seizures, and agitation are common after overdose.[24-26] Unlike many agents that produce seizures acutely following overdose, ingestion of extended-release bupropion can produce delayed onset seizures. The risk of seizures is not only dose dependent, but also preparation dependent; the immediate release is the least likely to cause seizures, whereas the XL preparation is the most likely.[27] Both QRS and QT prolongation can occur with toxicity.

Treatment is primarily supportive. Activated charcoal has not been clearly demonstrated to be beneficial in this setting, but its use can be considered if the patient is awake and alert and presents within one hour of ingestion. Patients with large overdoses may require endotracheal intubation and mechanical ventilation because of CNS and respiratory depression. Lorazepam, diazepam or midazolam are effective for terminating seizures. If seizures persist, phenobarbital or other GABA agonists may be used. Sodium bicarbonate (150 mEq IV or 3 mEq/ kg for pediatric patients) should be administered for any QRS prolongation, although because the mechanism of action of intraventricular conduction delay appears to be related to gap junction inhibition, rather than to sodium channel blockade, it tends to be less responsive to sodium bicarbonate therapy. Resuscitative ILE therapy, as well as extracorporeal membrane oxygenation (ECMO), has been described in anecdotal case reports of severely poisoned patients who are refractory to standard management measures.[28] Intravenous lipid emulsion should be undertaken only on the advice of a medical toxicologist or regional poison center (as described in the tricyclic antidepressant section).

Although pediatric patients may have seizures with accidental or exploratory ingestions, the risk of seizures is much less than in older children, where the exposure is typically the result of a suicidal attempt.[29] Nonetheless, because of the risk of delayed seizures, we recommend admission and monitoring for adult patients who ingest more than 450 mg of an ER or XL preparation or more than 8 mg/kg in pediatric patients.

Trazodone

Trazodone is an atypical antidepressant that is used for its hypnotic and anxiolytic properties. In addition to weakly inhibiting serotonin reuptake, it is a relatively strong blocker of the alpha$_1$ receptor.[30] Its use as an antidepressant has been historically somewhat limited by adverse effects, including orthostatic hypotension, priapism, and sedation. Priapism is probably a result of trazodone's alpha-antagonism, with an incidence of 1/100 to 1/10,000. Whereas many drugs are associated with priapism, particularly those with alpha-antagonism or inhibition of type 5 phosphodiesterase, trazodone is responsible for a disproportionate number of reported cases.

After overdose, sedation and hypotension due to vasodilation are expected. Priapism is not typically associated with overdose of trazodone. Prolongation of the QT interval may occur. Management is supportive, with airway protection, IV fluid resuscitation, and use of alpha-adrenergic agonists such as norepinephrine as needed for refractory hypotension. Activated charcoal has not been clearly demonstrated to be beneficial in this setting. If the patient is awake and alert, however, and presents within one hour of ingestion, its use can be considered.

Nefazodone

Nefazodone, a phenylpiperazine antidepressant, is structurally similar to trazodone. It acts as an antagonist at the 5-HT$_{2A}$ receptor, and chronic administration is associated with receptor downregulation. Nefazodone is associated with weak inhibition of norepinephrine and serotonin reuptake. It is metabolized to several active metabolites. After overdose, most patients remain asymptomatic. Antagonism of the alpha$_1$ receptor is responsible for the orthostatic hypotension that can occur. Treatment is primarily supportive.

SEROTONIN SYNDROME

Principles of Toxicity

Serotonin syndrome is a potentially lethal condition resulting from excess serotonin accumulation in the synaptic cleft.[31] This syndrome may occur after an isolated overdose of an SSRI, but it is more commonly a result of drug interactions, especially with drug combinations that raise synaptic serotonin concentrations by different mechanisms. Agonism of the 5-HT$_{2A}$ receptor appears to be largely responsible for this condition in humans.[31] Whereas numerous xenobiotics have been implicated in causing serotonin syndrome, some of the most

---

BOX 141.1   Xenobiotics Commonly Implicated in Serotonin Syndrome

Analgesics: Tramadol, meperidine, pentazocine
Drugs of abuse: Cocaine, amphetamine derivatives (e.g., methylenedioxymethamphetamine), lysergic acid diethylamide (LSD)
Monoamine oxidase inhibitors (MAOIs) (e.g., isocarboxazid, linezolid, phenelzine, moclobemide, selegiline)
Miscellaneous: Dextromethorphan, lithium, metoclopramide, St. John's wort
Selective serotonin reuptake inhibitors (SSRIs) (e.g., citalopram, escitalopram, fluoxetine, fluvoxamine, paroxetine, sertraline)
Serotonin-norepinephrine reuptake inhibitors (SNRIs) (e.g., milnacipran, venlafaxine)
Tricyclic antidepressants (TCAs) (e.g., amitriptyline, clomipramine, desipramine, doxepin, imipramine, nortriptyline)

---

common are the SSRIs, SNRIs, TCAs, MAOIs, dextromethorphan, amphetamines, and designer amphetamines, including methylenedioxymethamphetamine ("ecstasy"), cocaine, meperidine, lithium, tramadol, buspirone, lysergic acid diethylamide (LSD), and linezolid (Box 141.1). Serotonin syndrome is more likely to develop when drugs from different classes are combined, resulting in increased serotonin in the synaptic cleft from different mechanisms (e.g., increased release and impaired uptake).

Clinical Features

Serotonin syndrome is described as a triad of mental status changes, autonomic instability, and increased neuromuscular activity, but the condition exists along a spectrum; some patients have only mild tremor and diarrhea, whereas others exhibit life-threatening manifestations. Clinical features may include tremor, akathisia, gastrointestinal illness, clonus (inducible or spontaneous), rigidity, fever, seizures, and autonomic instability. The clonus is typically more pronounced in the lower extremities (most notably the ankles) than in the upper extremities. After an acute overdose of a serotonergic agent, symptom onset typically begins within several hours. With proper treatment, symptoms usually resolve within 24 hours but can persist for several days in severe cases.

Differential Diagnoses

The differential diagnosis of serotonin syndrome includes NMS, malignant hyperthermia, sympathomimetic toxicity, anticholinergic toxicity, strychnine toxicity, bupropion toxicity, and GABA withdrawal. Nontoxicologic considerations include thyroid storm, meningitis, idiopathic seizure, intracranial hemorrhage, and hypoglycemia.

Diagnostic Testing

There is no "gold standard" for the diagnosis of serotonin syndrome. Laboratory studies cannot be used to confirm or to exclude the diagnosis of serotonin syndrome. Rhabdomyolysis and hyperkalemia can occur as a result of increased neuromuscular activity, and these should be screened for as indicated on the basis of the clinical examination.

The Sternbach criteria were developed in the 1990s and became the first widely used diagnostic algorithm. Additional criteria, including the Hunter criteria and the Boyer and Shannon criteria, have been developed. The Hunter criteria (Box 141.2) appear to be more sensitive than the Sternbach criteria, with fewer false positives.

In general, a history of overdose or of recently starting an additional serotonergic agent along with clinical findings consistent with this diagnosis should raise the concern for serotonin syndrome.

BOX 141.2   The Hunter Criteria for Serotonin Syndrome

In the setting of exposure to a known serotonergic agent, serotonin syndrome can be diagnosed by the presence of any of the following:

- Spontaneous clonus
- Inducible clonus *and* agitation or diaphoresis
- Ocular clonus *and* agitation or diaphoresis
- Tremor and hyperreflexia
- Hypertonic with temperature >38°C *and* ocular clonus or inducible clonus

Management

Management is supportive, with removal of the offending agents being paramount. Mild cases may require only discontinuation of the agent and low-dose benzodiazepines (e.g., 5 to 10 mg of IV diazepam) for rigidity. More severe cases may require IV fluid resuscitation and large doses of benzodiazepines (e.g., 10 to 20 mg of IV diazepam, with titration in 10 mg aliquots) or other sedative-hypnotic agents to gain control of symptoms. Cyproheptadine, a 5-HT_{2A} antagonist, is an adjunctive therapy for more severe cases, but there are no randomized controlled trials demonstrating improved benefit with cyproheptadine over supportive care and benzodiazepines alone. If cyproheptadine is available, the syndrome is severe or refractory to treatment, and the clinician is confident with the diagnosis, we recommend a single oral dose of 12 mg of cyproheptadine for patients with serotonin syndrome. If anticholinergic toxicity remains on the differential diagnosis, cyproheptadine should not be given, because it can worsen anticholinergic toxicity. Patients with hyperthermia that does not respond promptly to sedation with benzodiazepines should receive a nondepolarizing neuromuscular blocking agent (e.g., rocuronium) during rapid sequence intubation. Typically, only a single dose of a long-acting neuromuscular blocking agent is required. If additional doses are required, we recommend a single IV dose of 10 mg of vecuronium.

Disposition

Patients with all but the mildest forms of serotonin syndrome should be admitted to a monitored care setting. Those with unresponsiveness, autonomic instability, hyperthermia, and rigidity should be admitted to an intensive care unit.

DISCONTINUATION SYNDROMES

After the abrupt discontinuation of certain antidepressants, patients can experience a withdrawal, or discontinuation, syndrome. Unlike potentially life-threatening GABA withdrawal from ethanol or benzodiazepines, the discontinuation syndrome from antidepressants is rarely life-threatening but can result in significant discomfort. One notable exception involves neonates born to mothers using TCAs, who can have serious, potentially life-threatening withdrawal. Antidepressant discontinuation syndrome does not always develop, but when it does, it typically starts within the first 3 days after therapy is stopped. This syndrome is difficult to distinguish from recurrence of the underlying depression, which has overlap of some symptoms.

Antidepressant discontinuation syndrome occurs with all major classes of antidepressants. Withdrawal from SSRIs involves both physical and psychological symptoms, most commonly nausea, lethargy, headache, and dizziness. The symptoms can be divided into six general categories: dysequilibrium (e.g., dizziness, ataxia), sleep disturbances, gastrointestinal symptoms, affective symptoms (e.g., irritability, anxiety), sensory symptoms (e.g., electric shock–like sensation, paresthesias), and general somatic symptoms (e.g., headache, tremor, anorexia, diaphoresis). The syndrome is more common after discontinuation of drugs with shorter half-lives (e.g., paroxetine) than of drugs with longer half-lives (e.g., fluoxetine). TCA withdrawal is similar to SSRI withdrawal, although sensory abnormalities and equilibrium disturbances are rare with TCA discontinuation. Non–life-threatening arrhythmias are rare after discontinuation of the TCAs.

Patients with mild withdrawal symptoms do not require any specific therapy. For those patients with more severe symptoms, treatment involves restarting of the antidepressant, followed by a gradual tapering dose.

The references for this chapter can be found online at ExpertConsult.com.

142

Cardiovascular Drugs

Jon B. Cole

CARDIOACTIVE STEROIDS (DIGOXIN)

KEY CONCEPTS

- Digoxin toxicity is often occult and should be considered in any patient who is on digoxin and presents with gastrointestinal or visual disturbance and a new dysrhythmia, conduction disturbance or hemodynamic instability, particularly in the setting of ingestion of a natural weight-loss supplement.
- Digitalis Fab is the specific antidote for digoxin toxicity and is dosed based on chronicity of poisoning; most patients require only 1 (chronic poisoning) or 2 (acute poisoning) vials. If full reversal is needed for patients in extremis, dosing is based on total body load of digoxin, not by patient weight.
- Indications for digitalis Fab include progressive and hemodynamically significant bradydysrhythmias and serum potassium >5.0 mEq/L, as summarized in Box 142.4. Of note, Fab therapy should be used before pacing or antidysrhythmic drugs.
- Hyperkalemia in acute digoxin toxicity is best treated with Fab fragments. Conventional treatment as for any other cause of hyperkalemia is also appropriate when Fab fragments are not immediately available. Hyperkalemia in chronic poisoning is likely multifactorial and should be treated with Fab fragments followed by usual hyperkalemia treatments as needed.

Foundations

Digoxin is derived from the Grecian foxglove plant, *Digitalis lanata* (Fig. 142.1); the trade name for digoxin (Lanoxin) is derived from the Latin name of this plant. Digitoxin, which is no longer in clinical use in the United States, comes from *Digitalis purpurea* (Fig 142.2).[2] Despite centuries of experience with digitalis preparations, chronic and acute poisonings still occur. Medication errors, including failure to account for drug-drug and disease-drug interactions (particularly kidney disease), account for a substantial number of poisonings.[3] Though the use of digoxin continues to be controversial, it is still commonly prescribed, particularly for patients with concomitant heart failure and atrial fibrillation.[4]

Digoxin is used therapeutically (1) to increase the force of myocardial contraction to increase cardiac output in patients with heart failure and (2) to decrease atrioventricular (AV) conduction to slow the ventricular rate in atrial fibrillation. The basis for its first effect is inhibition of membrane sodium-potassium–adenosine triphosphatase (Na^+, K^+-ATPase) pumps; this inhibition results in increased intracellular sodium and extracellular potassium concentrations.[5] This increase in intracellular sodium concentration results in dysfunction of the sodium-calcium ion exchanger, which normally extrudes intracellular calcium after systole. This subsequent increase in intracellular calcium concentration results in a larger amount of calcium pumped into the sarcoplasmic reticulum so that upon calcium release during subsequent action potentials, a larger amount of calcium is released into the cell, causing a more powerful contraction and thus increased stroke volume and subsequent cardiac output. Molecules containing an aglycone steroid moiety with this specific effect are classified as cardioactive steroids.[6] Cardiac glycosides (such as digoxin) are merely cardioactive steroids with additional sugar moieties attached to their steroid nucleus.[5] At therapeutic doses, the effects of digoxin on serum electrolytes are minimal. With toxic concentrations, digoxin paralyzes the Na^+, K^+-ATPase pump, potassium cannot be transported into cells, and serum potassium concentration can rise as high as 13.5 mmol/L.

Digoxin exerts direct and indirect effects on sinoatrial (SA) and AV nodal fibers. At therapeutic concentrations, digoxin indirectly increases vagal activity. At toxic concentrations, digoxin can directly block the generation of impulses in the SA node, depress conduction through the AV node, and increase the sensitivity of the SA and AV nodes to catecholamines. Catecholamines, whether endogenous or administered to treat bradydysrhythmias or hypotension, play an important role in digoxin toxicity. Because bradydysrhythmias and tachydysrhythmias can appear and alternate in the same patient, administration of antidysrhythmic agents to treat tachycardias may later contribute to more refractory bradycardias and AV block.

Digoxin also exerts three primary effects on Purkinje fibers: (1) decreased resting potential, resulting in slowed phase 0 depolarization and conduction velocity; (2) decreased action potential duration, which increases sensitivity of muscle fibers to electrical stimuli; and (3) enhanced automaticity resulting from increased rate of phase 4 repolarization and delayed after-depolarizations. These mechanisms account for an increase in premature ventricular contractions, which is the most common electrocardiographic manifestation of digoxin toxicity. At extremes of toxicity, these effects result in a hypersensitivity to mechanical and electrical stimulation. Interventions with pacemaker wires, catheters, and cardioversion can result in asystole, ventricular tachycardia, and ventricular fibrillation.

Unlike most cardiovascular drugs, digoxin can produce virtually any dysrhythmia or conduction block, and bradycardias are as common as tachycardias (Box 142.1). However, none is unique to digoxin, and because they can all occur in the setting of ischemic and other heart disease, digoxin toxicity remains a clinical rather than an electrocardiographic diagnosis.

The volume of distribution (V_d) of digoxin is 5 L/kg for adults but varies from 3.5 L/kg in premature infants to 16.3 L/kg in older infants. This indicates that only a small fraction of digoxin remains in the intravascular space, and the drug is highly concentrated in cardiac tissue. The myocardial-to-serum ratio at equilibrium ranges from 15 : 1 to 30 : 1.

The elimination half-life of digoxin, which is primarily excreted in the urine, is 36 hours.

Protein binding varies from 20% to 30% for digoxin. The significant protein binding and large volumes of distribution of digoxin suggest that hemodialysis, hemoperfusion, and exchange transfusion are ineffective. The long half-lives have therapeutic implications for temporizing measures such as pacemakers, atropine, and antidysrhythmic drugs compared to the more definitive treatment of Fab fragments.

Multiple drugs and disease states can alter absorption, V_d, protein binding, and elimination, rendering the heart more susceptible to digoxin toxicity. The factors listed in Box 142.2 are especially important risk factors in chronic intoxication.

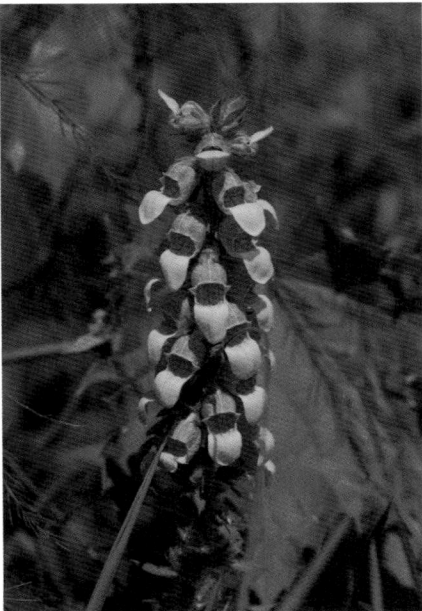

Fig. 142.1 The Grecian foxglove plant, *Digitalis lanata*, the source of digoxin. (Photos courtesy of Gary Bebeau and Friends of the Eloise Butler Wildflower Garden, Minneapolis, Minnesota.)

Clinical Features

The symptoms and signs of chronic digoxin toxicity are nonspecific. The most common symptoms are nausea, anorexia, and fatigue; but a variety of gastrointestinal, neurologic, and ophthalmic disturbances also occur (Box 142.3). Visual disturbances include decreased visual acuity, scotomata, photophobia, and chromatopsia (aberrations of color vision, classically yellow, but may occur in a variety of colors). Digoxin intoxication should be considered in any patient receiving maintenance therapy who has consistent symptoms, no matter how vague, particularly if presenting with new conduction disturbances or dysrhythmias.

There are significant differences between acute and chronic toxicity (Table 142.1). Chronic poisoning has an insidious onset and is accompanied by a higher mortality rate that is likely due in part to underlying heart disease and chronic accumulation of the toxin. In cases of chronic intoxication, the level with a 50% mortality (LL_{50}) is only 6 ng/mL. The LL_{50} for acute poisoning is much higher, especially in children. Although toxicity increases with greater body load, there is no clear correlation with amount ingested, especially in children, and many patients with large acute ingestions or high serum levels become only mildly symptomatic. The association of hyperkalemia with acute toxicity is more apparent given the mechanism of digoxin; either hypokalemia or hyperkalemia may occur with chronic toxicity.

Pediatric Considerations

Children with healthy hearts can tolerate massive acute oral ingestions and may not require Fab treatment. This excludes therapeutic errors, children who are taking digoxin therapeutically, and children with heart disease.

Medication errors account for the most common causes of preventable iatrogenic cardiac arrests. Therapeutic errors, especially accidental IV overdoses, often result in death within 1 to 4 hours.

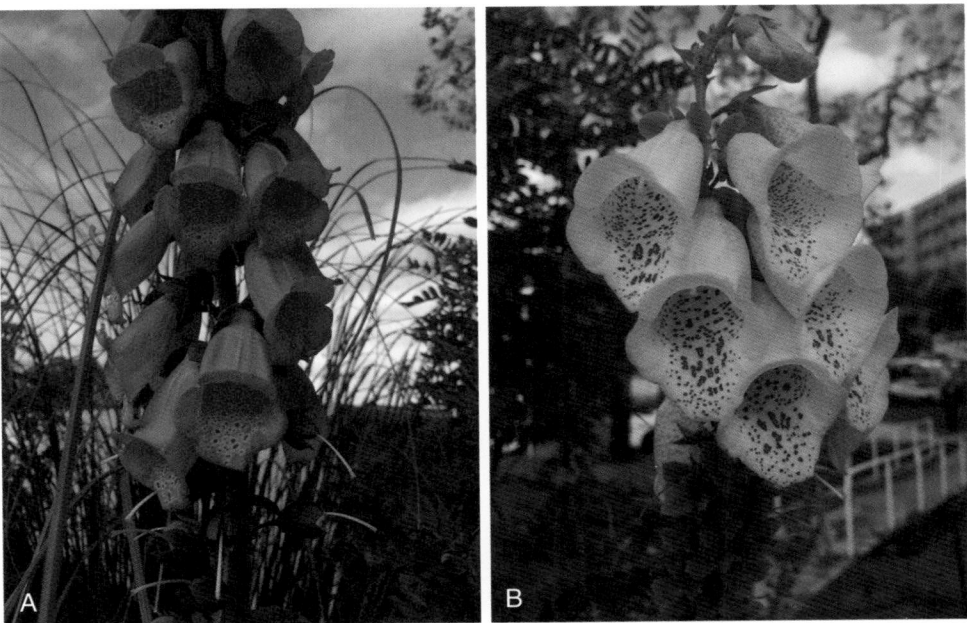

Fig. 142.2 The common foxglove plant *Digitalis purpurea*, the source of digitoxin. The flowers are typically purple but may also be white. White flowers may mature to purple or may remain white. (Photos courtesy of Ann Arens, MD.)

BOX 142.1   Dysrhythmias Associated With Digoxin Toxicity

Nonspecific Dysrhythmias
PVCs, especially bigeminal and multiform
AV heart blocks of all degrees
Sinus bradycardia
Sinus tachycardia
SA block or arrest
Atrial fibrillation with slow ventricular response
Atrial tachycardia
Junction (escape) rhythm
AV dissociation
Ventricular bigeminy and/or trigeminy
Ventricular tachycardia
Ventricular fibrillation

More Specific but Not Pathognomonic
Atrial fibrillation with slow, regular ventricular rate (AV dissociation)
Nonparoxysmal junctional tachycardia (rate usually 70–130 beats/min)
Atrial tachycardia with block (atrial rate usually 150–200 beats/min)
Bidirectional ventricular tachycardia

AV, Atrioventricular; *PVCs,* premature ventricular contractions; *SA,* sinoatrial.

BOX 142.2   Factors Associated With an Increased Risk of Digoxin Toxicity

Concomitant kidney injury or underlying kidney disease
Concomitant or underlying heart disease
    Congenital heart disease
    Ischemic heart disease
    Heart failure
    Myocarditis
Electrolyte disturbances
    Hyperkalemia
    Hypokalemia
    Hypomagnesemia
    Hypercalcemia
Alkalosis
Hypothyroidism
Sympathomimetic drugs (e.g., cocaine)
Cardiotoxic co-ingestions
    Beta-blockers
    Calcium channel blockers
    Class IA or IC antidysrhythmics (e.g., flecainide)
    Tricyclic antidepressants
Drug interactions (may increase serum digoxin concentration)
    Quinidine
    Amiodarone
    Erythromycin
    Nifedipine
Drug Interactions (may increase serum digoxin concentration and cause synergistic bradycardia)
    Verapamil
    Diltiazem

Signs and symptoms in children with digoxin poisoning are different than in adults (Table 142.2). Vomiting, somnolence, and obtundation are more common than in adults. Conduction disturbances and bradycardias are more common than ventricular dysrhythmias in children, especially following acute ingestion.

BOX 142.3   Noncardiac Symptoms of Cardioactive Steroid Intoxication

General
Weakness
Fatigue
Malaise

Gastrointestinal
Nausea and/or vomiting
Anorexia
Abdominal pain
Diarrhea

Ophthalmologic
Blurred or snowy vision
Photophobia
Chromatopsia (yellow, green, red, brown, blue vision changes)
Transient amblyopia, diplopia, scotomata, blindness

Neurologic
Dizziness
Headache
Confusion, disorientation, delirium
Visual and/or auditory hallucinations
Somnolence
Abnormal dreams
Paresthesias and/or neuralgia
Aphasia
Seizure

TABLE 142.1   Acute Versus Chronic Digoxin Poisoning

Acute	Chronic
Lower mortality	Higher mortality (LL_{50} = 6 ng/mL)
Bradycardia and AV block more common	Ventricular dysrhythmias more common
Typically, younger patients	Typically, elderly patients
Underlying heart disease generally less common, decreased morbidity and mortality	Underlying heart disease more common, increased morbidity and mortality

AV, Atrioventricular; LL_{50}, level with a 50% mortality.

Differential Diagnoses

No sign or symptom, including dysrhythmia, is unique to digoxin poisoning, so its differential diagnosis is broad. Intrinsic cardiac disease as well as other cardiotoxic drugs should be considered, particularly beta-blockers and calcium channel blockers. Cardioactive steroid poisoning from plants is rare in the United States but presents similarly to digoxin toxicity. Common examples include oleander (*Nerium oleander*) and lily-of-the-valley (*Convallaria majalis;* Fig. 142.3). Recently, there has been an increase in the use of natural products containing cardioactive steroids for the purpose of weight loss.[7] Several cardioactive-steroid containing plants have been purported to be "natural" agents for weight loss, including pong-pong seeds (*Cerebra odollam*) and yellow oleander (*Thevetia peruviana*), both of which have resulted in fatal poisonings.[8,9] Yellow oleander is particularly problematic in that its seeds bear a physical resemblance to the seeds of another minimally toxic plant (that does not contain cardioactive steroids but is also purported to aid in weight loss) commonly called candle nuts (*Aleurites moluccana*). The substitution of yellow oleander for candle nuts has resulted in at least one accidental fatality; it is likely other cases have gone unrecognized.[9] In some parts of the world, such as Southeast Asia and India, ingestion of plants containing cardioactive steroids (e.g., pong-pong or yellow oleander seeds) is a common method of suicide[10]; ingestion of 1 or 2 yellow oleander seeds has resulted in death.[6] Aconitine, a sodium-channel opening poison found in common Monkshood plants (*Aconitum napellus),* may also mimic digoxin poisoning.[11]

Central nervous system (CNS) depression or confusion may be due to various depressant drugs (e.g., opioids, sedative hypnotic agents, alcohol) and toxins, as well as infection, trauma, inflammation, and metabolic derangements. Visual disturbances caused by digoxin are binocular and are often not reported by the patient; they are not specific to digoxin poisoning. Methanol, metformin, ethambutol, ethyl chloride, quinine, and other antimalarial medications are all capable of producing visual disturbances. Gastrointestinal disturbances are common and nonspecific and may be misdiagnosed as gastritis, enteritis, or colitis.

Diagnostic Testing

Diagnosis and management rely on serum digoxin concentrations, but it is the steady state, rather than peak concentration, that correlates with tissue toxicity and is used to calculate antidote dosages. Peak concentrations after an oral dose of digoxin occur in 1.5 to 2 hours, with a range of 0.5 to 6 hours. Steady-state serum concentrations are not achieved until after alpha distribution, or 6 to 8 hours after a therapeutic or toxic dose and may be only 20% to 25% of the peak concentration. The ideal serum digoxin concentration for patients with heart failure is considered to be 0.7 to 1.1 ng/mL, although laboratory "normal ranges" are often reported up to 2.0 ng/mL. Serum steady-state digoxin concentrations of 1.1 to 3.0 ng/mL are difficult to interpret; that is, concentrations as low as 1.1 ng/mL have been associated with toxicity, and patients with levels up to 3.0 ng/mL can be asymptomatic. The incidence of digoxin-incited dysrhythmia reaches 10% at a concentration of 1.7 ng/mL and rises to 50% at a concentration of 2.5 ng/mL. Determination of a serum digoxin concentration measured too early after the last maintenance dose falsely suggests toxicity, especially in cases of chronic intoxication, in which significant morbidity and mortality can occur at levels of 2 to 6 ng/mL. After an acute massive overdose in a patient who is rapidly becoming symptomatic, however, it is impractical to wait 6 to 8 hours for the first measurement. It is unlikely that early concentrations exceeding 10 to 20 ng/mL will fade to clinical insignificance at 6 to 8 hours after ingestion.

Management

Fab Fragments (DigiFab)

The primary treatment of significant digoxin poisoning is the administration of digoxin-specific fragment antigen-binding (Fab) antibodies (DigiFab); all other interventions are considered complementary.

The mortality rate of digoxin poisoning before Fab fragment therapy was 23% despite all of the interventions described in this section.

TABLE 142.2	Age Difference in Digoxin Intoxication	
Adult	**Pediatric**
Toxic at lower concentrations	Asymptomatic at higher concentrations
Nausea, fatigue, and visual disturbances more common	Obtundation and vomiting more common
Tachydysrhythmias as common as blocks and bradydysrhythmias	Bradydysrhythmias and blocks more common
Allergic reactions to Fab fragments uncommon (<1%)	Allergic reactions extremely rare
V_d less variable (5–7.5 L/kg)	V_d more variable (3.5–6.0 L/kg in premature infants, 8.0–16.3 in infants 2–24 months old)

V_d, Volume of distribution.

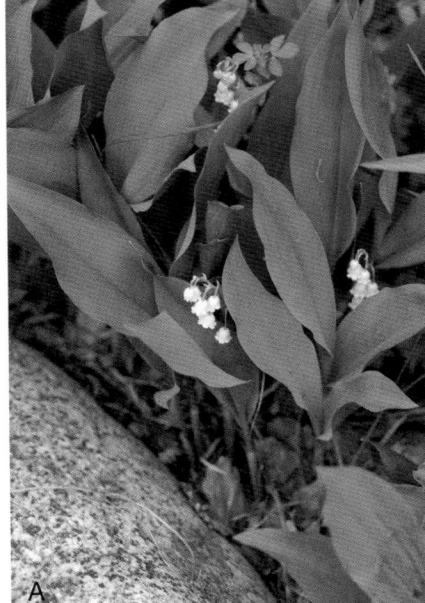
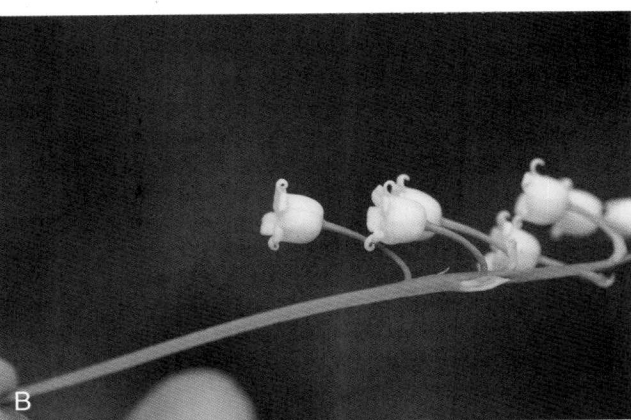

Fig. 142.3 Lily-of-the-valley (*Convallaria majalis*), which contains the cardiac glycoside convallatoxin. (Photos courtesy of Gary Bebeau and Friends of the Eloise Butler Wildflower Garden, Minneapolis, Minnesota.)

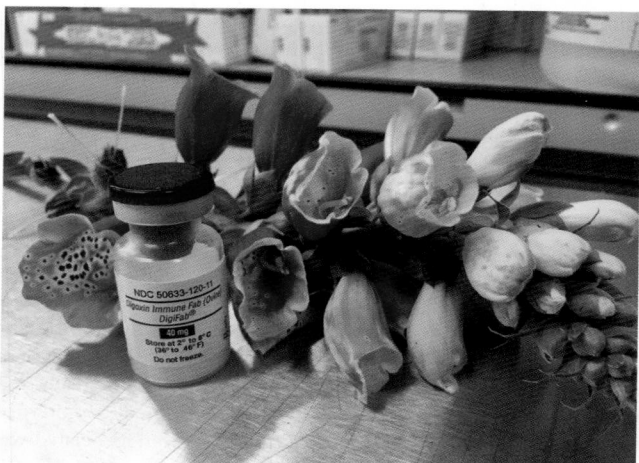

Fig. 142.4 A vial of digoxin antibody fragments (DigiFab) next to a cutting of *Digitalis purpurea*, demonstrating the darkening of the purple flowers as they age. (Photo courtesy of Laurie Wilhite, PharmD, CSPI.)

Fab fragment treatment is well established in both chronic and acute poisonings, with a successful response rate approaching 90%. Nonresponders usually receive Fab fragments too late, have concomitant poisoning, or are compromised by underlying comorbidities.

Digoxin antibodies are derived from sheep. Allergic reactions occur in less than 1% of cases but are slightly more common in patients with asthma. Reactions have included erythema, urticaria, and facial edema, all of which are responsive to the usual treatments for allergic reactions (e.g., diphenhydramine, corticosteroids, epinephrine). Other infrequent reactions when Fab fragments neutralize digitalis include hypokalemia, heart failure exacerbation, and increase in ventricular rate with atrial fibrillation. Two Fab fragment preparations were previously available; however, DigiFab is the only available product in the United States (Fig. 142.4). Previous products required a 0.22-μm membrane filter for proper use; such a filter is not required for DigiFab.

Fab fragment treatment is best reserved for cases of serious cardiovascular toxicity rather than for routine or prophylactic administration with higher than expected serum concentrations. Fab fragments should be used for a serum potassium level above 5.0 mEq/L or unstable dysrhythmias such as symptomatic bradycardia, ventricular dysrhythmias, or second- or third-degree heart block unresponsive to atropine. Fab fragment therapy should be used before transvenous pacing, because the latter is believed to carry a higher risk of ventricular dysrhythmia, although the evidence for this is mixed. Large acute overdoses (>0.1 mg/kg in a child or 10 mg in a healthy adult) are also likely to require Fab fragments.

The median time to initial response is 19 minutes after completion of the Fab infusion, but complete resolution of digitalis-induced toxic dysrhythmias may require hours. Late administration of Fab fragments has resuscitated up to 54% of patients who have suffered cardiac arrest secondary to digoxin toxicity. Fab fragments should be administered whenever hemodynamic compromise occurs in the setting of a digoxin-induced toxic dysrhythmia or heart block; a full list of indications is included in Box 142.4.

Dosing of Fab fragments is based both upon the patient's clinical status and acuity of poisoning. Patients in cardiac arrest, or in the midst of a life-threatening ventricular dysrhythmia, generally require full reversal. In chronic poisoning, however, the benefit of Fab fragments is less clear. Recently published prospective data on chronic digoxin-poisoned patients shows that small doses (median dose 1.5 vials) results in complete binding of free digoxin, with minimal improvement

---

BOX 142.4   Recommendation for Administration of Digoxin Antibody Fragments

1. Ventricular dysrhythmias more severe than PVCs
2. Progressive and hemodynamically significant bradydysrhythmias unresponsive to atropine
3. Serum potassium >5.0 mEq/L
4. Rapidly progressive rhythm disturbances or rising potassium
5. Co-ingestion of cardiotoxic drugs (for examples, see Box 142.2)
6. Ingestion of plant known to contain cardioactive steroids plus severe dysrhythmia or potassium >5.0 mEq/L
7. Acute ingestion of >10 mg or 0.1 mg/kg in a child *plus* any one of factors 1 through 6
8. Steady-state digoxin concentration > 6 ng/mL *plus* any one of factors 1 through 6

BOX 142.5   Sample Calculation of Digitalis Fab Fragments based on Ingested Dose

Case: A toxic-appearing 40-year-old woman has acutely ingested fifty 0.25-mg digoxin tablets.

$$\text{Body load} = \text{amount ingested}$$
$$\times\, 0.8 \text{ (bioavailability of digoxin tablets)} =$$
$$12.5 \text{ mg} \times 0.8 = 10 \text{ mg}$$
$$\text{Dose of digoxin Fab fragments (in vials)} = 10 \text{ mg} \div 0.5 \text{ mg bound per vial}$$
$$= 20 \text{ vials}$$

---

in clinically important parameters such as heart rate, blood pressure, or serum potassium.[12,13] These prospective data, which compared chronically digoxin-poisoned patients with similar physiologic parameters receiving Fab fragments with those who received supportive care only, showed no difference in vital signs, potassium, or mortality, despite complete binding of all available free digoxin. These data call into question the utility of Fab fragments in chronically poisoned patients. Nevertheless, in hemodynamically unstable patients, such as those with hypotension, treatment with Fab fragments is still considered the standard of care.

If the patient is in cardiac arrest, the maximum number of vials of Fab fragments available (up to 10) should be administered undiluted as an intravenous (IV) bolus. If, in acute or chronic toxicity, the patient is in a life-threatening ventricular dysrhythmia or heart block and the serum digoxin concentration *is unknown* but the amount of digoxin ingested is known, we recommend full reversal based upon the following concept: one vial of DigiFab contains 40 mg of Fab fragments, which bind 0.5 mg of digoxin (Box 142.5). In the same patient, if the steady-state serum digoxin concentration *is known*, we recommend full reversal with Fab fragments based upon the digoxin concentration utilizing the formula in Box 142.6. An exception to the above regimens is the case of yellow oleander poisoning, where a high case fatality rate and poor cross-reactivity of Fab fragments with the offending cardioactive steroids necessitates higher dosing. Therefore, with acute yellow oleander poisoning, 20 to 30 vials (if available) are recommended.

In hemodynamically stable patients, we recommend a more conservative dosing regimen of Fab fragments. The total body burden of digoxin is often overestimated. Furthermore, the incidence of life-threatening dysrhythmias, even in reported large ingestions, is low,

BOX 142.6 Sample Calculation of Digitalis Fab Fragments Based on Steady-State Digoxin Concentration

Case: A toxic-appearing 4-year-old child weighing 20 kg has a digoxin level of 16 ng/mL 8 hours after ingestion of an unknown number of digoxin tablets.

Dose (in number of vials) = (serum digoxin concentration
$$\times \text{ weight in kg}) \div 100$$
$$= (16 \times 20) \div 100$$
$$= \text{approximately 3 vials}$$

suggesting most patients do not require Fab fragments.[13] Pharmacokinetic modeling of digoxin toxicity suggests smaller doses of Fab fragments than previously recommended are adequate to reverse toxicity.[14] Therefore, in acute digoxin poisoning, if the patient has an indication for Fab fragments (see Box 142.4) but is not in an immediately life-threatening ventricular dysrhythmia or heart block, we recommend two vials, repeated as needed using clinical markers of toxicity such as evidence of shock or severe dysrhythmias. For similar patients with chronic poisoning, the recommended dose is one vial with a repeat dose at 60 minutes if the patient remains symptomatic. Earlier repeat dosing is reasonable if the patient becomes unstable.

Because most assays measure both bound and unbound drug, digoxin concentrations will be elevated for up to one week after Fab fragments administration, with values often greater than 100 ng/mL once Fab fragments have been administered. If laboratory measurement of free serum digoxin is available, these levels more accurately follow a patient's clinical status.

Electrolyte Correction

In cases of chronic toxicity, which may be exacerbated by hypokalemia, normalization of the serum potassium is an important early treatment. Potassium can be administered orally in the alert patient (which is safer) or intravenously at a rate of 20 mEq/hr or less.

In acute poisoning, serum potassium concentration may begin to rise rapidly within 1 to 2 hours of ingestion. Potassium should be withheld, even if mild hypokalemia is measured initially. The initial serum potassium concentration may in fact be a better predictor of mortality than the initial digoxin concentration. Before Fab fragments were available, up to 50% of the patients with serum potassium concentrations between 5.0 and 5.5 mEq/L died. In the setting of acute digoxin poisoning, we recommend initiating Fab fragment treatment based solely on a serum potassium concentration greater than 5 mEq/L.

The decision to administer calcium to patients with hyperkalemia and digoxin poisoning represents a clinical dilemma. Classic teaching is that in the setting of the increased intracellular calcium concentration from digoxin poisoning, administration of exogenous calcium will result in a "stone heart" (cardiac tetany) from excessive intracellular calcium. This concept has been in the literature since 1927, based primarily on animal studies. Documented cases of cardiac arrest after calcium administration are exceedingly rare, and the temporal relationship is dubious. More recent human data indicate that the IV administration of calcium for hyperkalemia in the setting of digoxin toxicity is safe. Unequivocally, however, the best treatment of hyperkalemia due to acute digoxin toxicity is Fab fragments. The treatment of hyperkalemia in a patient with chronic digoxin toxicity and renal failure is less clear. Patients with hyperkalemia and chronic digoxin poisoning often have multiple reasons for hyperkalemia in addition to digoxin toxicity (e.g., acute worsening of renal function, concomitant use of potassium-sparing diuretics). Furthermore in chronic digoxin-poisoned patients, even when full digoxin reversal is performed, potassium levels rarely

decline further than with supportive care alone.[13] Regardless, the evidence that calcium salts will be harmful in chronic digoxin poisoning is lacking. As such, treatment of hyperkalemia related to digoxin toxicity is similar in indication and approach to that for hyperkalemia from other causes after Fab fragments have been administered (see Chapter 114).

Hypomagnesemia enhances the effects of cardioactive steroids. Therefore, any patient with suspected poisoning should have serum magnesium concentrations measured. This is further supported by evidence of magnesium reversing digoxin-induced tachydysrhythmias. If significant magnesium depletion is present, 1 to 2 g of magnesium sulfate should be administered over 10 to 20 minutes (child: 25 mg/kg), followed by a constant infusion of 1 to 2 g/hr until magnesium concentrations are normal, accounting for concomitant kidney injury. We do not recommend administration of magnesium in digoxin-induced bradydysrhythmias and conduction blocks, because hypermagnesemia can impair impulse formation and AV conduction.

Atropine

Atropine is generally used for symptomatic bradycardia (pulse < 50 beats/min) and advanced AV block. We recommend using atropine as a temporizing measure for symptomatic patients while Fab fragments are being administered. We also recommend atropine for bradycardia refractory to Fab fragments. Standard dosing (0.02 mg/kg in children with a minimum of 0.1 mg; 1 mg IV in adults) should be used. Doses can be repeated every 3 to 5 minutes. In general, an external pacemaker should be readied once atropine has been administered.

Pacing and Cardioversion

Transvenous pacing is a mainstay of treatment for severe bradycardia. There is some evidence that the catheter may induce ventricular tachydysrhythmias in a myocardium made irritable by digoxin, although convincing studies on this question are lacking. Iatrogenic accidents of cardiac pacing are frequent (36%) in one study and can be fatal (up to 13%). Transvenous pacing should be used only if external pacing fails. Pacing usually is required only temporarily while waiting for Fab fragments to take clinical effect. Cardioversion in the setting of digoxin poisoning should be reserved for life-threatening dysrhythmias such as pulseless ventricular tachycardia or ventricular fibrillation.

Phenytoin and Lidocaine

Fab fragments are the preferred therapy for dysrhythmias, but a dysrhythmia may require intervention while Fab fragments are readied or until they begin to have effect after infusion.

Although both phenytoin and lidocaine are believed to be safe for control of tachydysrhythmias in the setting of digoxin toxicity, we prefer phenytoin. Indications for phenytoin include unstable tachydysrhythmias when Fab fragments are unavailable and unstable tachydysrhythmias that occur while waiting for Fab fragments to take effect. Phenytoin may enhance AV conduction. We recommend administering phenytoin in 100 mg boluses every 5 minutes until dysrhythmias improve or until the standard loading dose of 18 mg/kg is reached. No data exist to support or refute the substitution of fosphenytoin for phenytoin in this scenario. We recommend lidocaine only if the patient has a contraindication to phenytoin or if the maximum dose of phenytoin has been reached. When given, we recommend a loading dose of 1.5 mg/kg IV push, followed by an infusion of 1 to 4 mg/min (30 to 50 μg/kg/min), started at 1 mg/min and titrated up based on response to therapy. Most other cardiac drugs (isoproterenol, procainamide, amiodarone, beta-blockers, calcium antagonists) may worsen dysrhythmias or depress AV conduction in digoxin poisoned patients and should not be administered in this setting.

Extracorporeal Membrane Oxygenation

Extracorporeal membrane oxygenation (ECMO has been successfully used to treat cardioactive steroid poisoning, though cases are rare and data are limited.[15] Due to the relatively high survival rate in patients with cardiac arrest from digoxin poisoning treated with Fab fragments, we recommend ECMO in this instance only if Fab fragments are ineffective in establishing return of spontaneous circulation, or in the rare instance of cardiac arrest or refractory cardiogenic shock at an institution where ECMO is readily available, but high doses of Fab fragments are not.

Disposition

Patients who are symptomatic from digoxin toxicity with hyperkalemia, dysrhythmia, AV block, or significant comorbidity should be admitted to an intensive care unit after treatment with Fab fragments. Asymptomatic patients reporting an acute ingestion of digoxin should be observed for at least 12 hours of continuous cardiac monitoring. Chronically poisoned patients should be admitted to a monitored setting because they often have concomitant comorbidities and underlying heart disease.

BETA-BLOCKERS

KEY CONCEPTS

- Beta-blocker intoxication causes bradydysrhythmias and occasionally AV block.
- Noncardiac symptoms such as obtundation, seizures, and hypoglycemia may occur early in the course and are classically associated with propranolol toxicity.
- Volume expansion, atropine, calcium, and glucagon are early treatment measures, but absent a response, begin a high-dose insulin (HDI)/glucose infusion.
- When using HDI/glucose infusions, concentrated glucose solutions are recommended to avoid fluid overload.

Foundations

Principles of Toxicity

Beta-adrenergic blocking drugs (commonly referred to as beta-blockers) became widely used in Europe in the 1960s for treatment of dysrhythmias. Their antihypertensive effects were later appreciated. By the 1970s, they were one of the most widely prescribed classes of drugs in the United States. Current indications include supraventricular dysrhythmias, hypertension (although the drugs have fallen out of favor for this indication), angina, thyrotoxicosis, migraine, and glaucoma. Of the numerous beta-blockers available, overdose with propranolol has the highest fatality rate. In 2018, United States poison centers received more than 26,000 calls regarding beta-blocker exposures.[1] Over 1000 of these calls were regarding patients with life-threatening symptoms. While the vast majority of beta-blocker overdoses have favorable outcomes,[16] deaths from isolated ingestions still occur regularly.

Pathophysiology

Beta-blockers structurally resemble isoproterenol, a pure beta-agonist. They competitively inhibit endogenous catecholamines such as epinephrine at beta-adrenergic receptors, blocking the catecholamine effects of inotropy (increased myocardial contraction), dromotropy (enhanced cardiac conduction), and chronotropy (increased heart rate). These are all β_1 effects. Complex β_2 effects include vascular (smooth muscle relaxation and vasodilation), liver (glycogenolysis, gluconeogenesis), lung (bronchodilation), adipose tissue (release of free fatty acids), and uterus (smooth muscle relaxation) effects. Important additional properties, which vary from one beta-blocker to another, include cardioselectivity (β_1 selectivity), membrane-stabilizing activity (fast cardiac sodium channel blocking properties), lipophilicity, and intrinsic sympathomimetic activity (Table 142.3). Although cardioselectivity is masked in overdose, cardioselective beta-blockers such as atenolol, metoprolol, and esmolol still have lower mortality rates than that of propranolol.[1]

Beta-blockers are rapidly absorbed after oral ingestion, with peak effects varying among drugs (Table 142.3). Hepatic metabolism on first pass results in significantly less bioavailability after oral dosing than with IV injection (e.g., 1 : 40 for propranolol, 1 : 2.5 for metoprolol). Because volume of distribution for most beta-blockers generally exceeds 1 L/kg, hemodialysis is not efficacious for most beta-blocker overdoses.

Clinical Features

The most common initial clinical sign is bradycardia. Hypotension and unconsciousness are also common. While unconsciousness may be from a lack of brain perfusion due to cardiotoxic effects, beta-blockers (particularly propranolol) may also cause direct CNS depression and apnea. Hypoglycemia, due to blockade of the counter-regulatory effects of epinephrine, is often described, but rare. Though uncommon in all patients, hypoglycemia is more common in children than adults. In overdose, signs and symptoms are identical among beta-blockers, with the exception of propranolol which tends to cause seizures.[16] Much of propranolol's unique toxicity derives from its lipophilic nature combined with its membrane-stabilizing activity, which allows it to penetrate the CNS, causing obtundation, respiratory depression, and occasionally seizures. Of note, bronchospasm is rarely a problem in beta-blocker overdose, even with nonselective beta-blockers. The few cases of symptomatic bronchospasm respond to usual doses of nebulized bronchodilators.

Propranolol, nadolol, betaxolol, and acebutolol have membrane-stabilizing activity that impairs SA and AV node function and leads to bradycardia and AV block. Ventricular conduction is also depressed secondary to membrane-stabilizing activity (similar to tricyclic antidepressants or class IA/IC antidysrhythmics), which manifests as QRS widening on ECG, with ventricular dysrhythmias and cardiogenic shock. The intrinsic sympathomimetic activity of some beta-blockers (e.g., pindolol, oxprenolol, acebutolol, carteolol) can lead to some unusual manifestations such as ventricular dysrhythmias and tachycardia instead of bradycardia. Labetalol and carvedilol also block α_1-adrenergic receptors, giving an additional mechanism for hypotension and distributive shock, however clinically they present similarly to other beta blockers due to their respective $\beta : \alpha$ blockade ratios. Labetalol's beta-blockade is three times more potent via the oral route, and seven times more potent intravenously than its α-blockade. Carvedilol is even more beta-selective; its blockade of β_1 and β_2 receptors is 10 times more potent than α_1.

In contrast to digoxin, beta-blocker toxicity has a more rapid onset. Life-threatening CNS and cardiovascular effects can occur 30 minutes after oral overdose. With the exception of sotalol, which causes QT prolongation and torsades de pointes, toxicity from beta-blocker poisoning is usually apparent within 6 hours of ingestion. Patients ingesting delayed-release preparations, however, may remain asymptomatic for several hours, followed by a prolonged period of toxicity of up to 24 hours. For additional clinical features, see Table 142.5.

TABLE 142.3 Selected Pharmacologic Characteristics of Common Beta-Blockers

Drug	Time to Peak (hrs, oral form)	T1/2 (hrs)	V_d (L/kg)	Lipophilicity	Protein Binding (%)	MSA	ISA	Comments
Non-Selective Beta-Blockers								
Propranolol	1–4 (6–14 ERF)	4.0	4.0	+	93	Yes	No	Most fatalities
Nadolol	3–4	10–20	1.9	0	20	No	No	Dialyzable
Timolol	1–2	3–5	1.4–3.4	+	10	No	No	Dialyzable; available as ocular drops
Pindolol	1	3–4	3–6	+	51	Yes	Yes	
Labetalol	1–2	4–6	10	0	50	Yes	No	α_1-blockade
Oxprenolol	3	2	1.3	+	78	Yes	Yes	
Sotalol	2–4	7–18	1.6–2.4	+	0	No	No	Dialyzable, QT prolongation & risk of torsades de pointes
Carvedilol	5	6–10	1.5–2	+	95	No	No	α_1-blockade
Selective Beta-Blockers								
Metoprolol	1–2 (4–5 ERF)	3–4	5.5	+	12	No	No	
Atenolol	2–4	5–8	0.7	0	5	No	No	Dialyzable
Esmolol (IV only)	rapid	0.13	2	0	55	No	No	
Acebutolol	2–4	2–4	1.2	+	26	Yes	Yes	Dialyzable, QT prolongation & risk of torsades de pointes
Bisoprolol	2–4	10–12	2.9	0	30	No	No	
Betaxolol	1.5–6	12–22	5 - 13	0	55	No	No	

V_d, Volume of distribution; *T1/2*, elimination half-life; *MSA*, membrane stabilizing activity; *ISA*, intrinsic sympathomimetic activity; *ERF*, extended-release formulations.

Differential Diagnoses

The combination of bradycardia and hypotension suggests beta-blockade, calcium channel blockade, or digoxin poisoning. Centrally acting α_2-adrenergic agonists such as clonidine and tizanidine or imidazoline receptor agonists such as tetrahydrozoline and oxymetazoline may also cause this constellation of symptoms. Without a history of beta-blocker ingestion, the diagnosis can be challenging, especially when non-cardiac effects such as CNS depression and seizures predominate. Sodium channel poisoning with QRS widening can occur, suggesting other antidysrhythmic drugs or cyclic antidepressants. The differential diagnoses also include sedative-hypnotic drug overdose, hypoglycemic drug ingestion, opioid overdose, CNS injury or infection, various endocrine and metabolic disorders, sepsis, and acute myocardial infarction.

Diagnostic Testing

Diagnosis and management depend entirely on the clinical picture, and the only essential testing is a point-of-care glucose monitoring and a 12-lead electrocardiogram (ECG) with continuous ECG monitoring. Serum concentrations of beta-blockers correlate poorly with severity of intoxication and are not readily available. Most urine toxicology screens do not identify antidysrhythmic drugs and are not helpful. Known access of the patient to a beta-blocker and consistent clinical features such as bradycardia and hypotension should lead the clinician to consider beta-blocker intoxication and begin empirical treatment. Whereas some authors believe that a serum lactate concentration can help predict mortality in overdose patients,[17] this has not held true in pure beta-blocker ingestions.

Management

Immediate measures include IV fluids for hypotension, supplemental oxygen as needed for hypoxia, and monitoring of cardiac rhythm and respirations. Whole-bowel irrigation is cumbersome and because there is a lack of evidence for efficacy in clinical trials, we recommend against its use in beta-blocker poisoning.[18] The clinical efficacy of gastric lavage is also unproven, the procedure is cumbersome, and benefit is outweighed by procedural risks. Please see Chapter 135 for further information on gastrointestinal decontamination, including the use of activated charcoal.

Hypotension, Bradycardia, and Atrioventricular Block

The first step in the treatment of beta-blocker overdose is bolus administration of crystalloid fluids. In hypotensive patients, 20 to 40 mL/kg of normal saline or lactated Ringers solution can be infused. Further doses of isotonic fluids, however, can lead to pulmonary edema and should be avoided particularly in older patients with underlying

TABLE 142.4 Selected Pharmacologic Characteristics of Calcium Channel Blockers

Drug	Time to Peak (hrs, oral form)	T1/2 (hrs)	V_d (L/kg)	Protein Binding (%)	Comments
Non-dihydropyridines					
Verapamil	1–2 (5–11 ERF)	3–12	4	90	Most lethal in overdose; impairs contractility and AV conduction more than most other calcium channel blockers
Diltiazem	2–4 (10–18 ERF)	3–7.9	1.7–5.3	70–80	AV node suppression similar to verapamil, contractility inhibition generally less than verapamil
Dihydropyridines					
Amlodipine	6–12	30–50	21	98	Vasodilation; additional vasodilation from nitric oxide production
Nifedipine	1 (6–11 ERF)	1–5	1.4–2.2	92–98	Vasodilation
Nimodipine	1	1–2	0.94–2.3	95	Vasodilation
Nicardipine	0.5–2 (1–4 ERF)	8–9	0.64	95	Vasodilation
Clevidipine (IV only)	Rapid	0.25	0.17	>99.5	Formulated in lipid emulsion for infusion
Felodipine	2.5–5	10	10	99	Vasodilation
Isradipine	1–1.5	1.9–16	3	95	Vasodilation
Nisoldipine	4–14	7–12	4–5	99	Vasodilation
Amine Calcium Channel Blocker					
Bepridil	2–6	33–42	8	99	Blocks sodium channels as well; QT prolongation & risk of torsades de pointes; no longer sold in United States

V_d, Volume of distribution; *T1/2*, elimination half-life; *AV*, atrioventricular; *ERF*, extended-release formulations.

TABLE 142.5 Clinical Characteristic of Poisoning from Beta-Blockers and Calcium Channel Blockers

Organ System	Beta-Blockers	Calcium Channel Blockers
Cardiovascular	Bradycardia & hypotension	Bradycardia & hypotension in non-DHPs, tachycardia & hypotension with DHPs
Pulmonary	Apnea (likely central) Bronchospasm (rare)	Pulmonary edema
Neurologic[a]	Drowsiness/coma in lipophilic BBs, seizures possible, preserved consciousness in non-lipophilic BBs until shock ensues	Generally preserved mental status until shock ensues
Endocrine	Hypoglycemia (rare)	Hyperglycemia

[a]Regardless of lipophilicity, both classes may cause obtundation once shock ensues.
BB, Beta-blocker; *DHP*, dihydropyridine.

cardiac disease. Frequent monitoring of volume status, such as with point-of-care ultrasound (by measuring the diameter and collapsibility of various large vessels including the inferior vena cava and common carotid artery) is recommended to avoid volume overload. Atropine at standard doses noted earlier may be used for bradycardia but is rarely effective. We recommend atropine for a heart rate of less than 50 beats per minute with concomitant hypotension and symptoms of severe bradycardia such as weakness, drowsiness, or obtundation. Infusion of more potent drugs or cardiac pacing is often necessary, and we recommend that atropine is best used as a temporizing measure to the therapies noted later.

Calcium

The final common pathway for stimulation of beta-adrenergic receptors is an increase in intracellular calcium concentration, and deleterious effects on calcium transport may contribute to beta-blocker toxicity. Therefore, IV administration of calcium can be used for treatment of hypotension. One gram of calcium gluconate contains 4.65 mEq of elemental calcium, whereas 1 g of calcium chloride contains 13.4 mEq. Calcium chloride is an acidifying salt and can cause significant tissue damage and necrosis if extravasation at the IV site occurs. Thus, it should be administered through a central venous catheter (or a secure large-bore antecubital peripheral line if the patient is in extremis). Indications for calcium include hypotension unresponsive to crystalloid fluids or symptomatic bradycardia. Typically, the heart rate should be less than 60 beats per minute, while considering whether the patient may have relative bradycardia. We recommend an initial dose of 13 to 25 mEq of calcium in adults (1 to 2 g calcium chloride, 3 to 6 g calcium gluconate) infused over 10 minutes. Patients in extremis may receive the initial dose over one minute. If a response is observed, repeated doses may be given in 20 minutes, and a constant infusion may be started at 20 mg/kg/hr of calcium chloride (60 mg/kg/hr of calcium gluconate). If ionized calcium is measured instead of total calcium, we recommend not to exceed 1.5 times the upper limit of normal. The total serum calcium concentration can be as high as 18 mg/dL within 15 minutes after a bolus of just 5 mL of 10% calcium chloride, so calcium concentrations should be measured at least 30 minutes after bolus dosing has finished.

Glucagon

Glucagon has both inotropic and chronotropic effects and does not depend on beta-adrenergic receptors for its action; therefore, it has long been used for beta-blocker toxicity. It stimulates the production of intracellular cyclic adenosine monophosphate independently of the beta-adrenergic receptor. Furthermore, it helps counteract the hypoglycemia induced by beta-blocker overdose. Although not well studied, the initial recommended dose of glucagon is a 3- to 10-mg IV bolus (0.05 mg/kg for children). If a response occurs to glucagon, specifically if heart rate, blood pressure, or symptom improvement is observed, an infusion can be started at 3 to 5 mg/hr. Because glucagon is rarely used in large quantities, many hospitals may not stock enough glucagon to facilitate a long-term infusion. Additionally, glucagon is only available in 1 mg/1 mL vials that must be reconstituted, and preparation of it is labor-intensive and may be prolonged. Thus, clinicians administering glucagon should simultaneously ready themselves for additional therapies, such as high-dose insulin (HDI). We recommend glucagon for patients with bradycardia or hypotension not responsive to crystalloid fluids, atropine, and an initial bolus of calcium. In addition to stocking problems in most facilities, glucagon has a short (20-minute) half-life, and its effect is often transient. Vomiting is a common complication of glucagon, particularly if administered too rapidly, so the airway should be secured or monitored closely to prevent aspiration. With cumulative large doses, glucagon should be diluted in 5% glucose in water for constant infusion. Side effects also include hypokalemia. The response to glucagon alone is often inadequate, and glucagon is likely to be less effective than HDI for severe poisoning. From clinical experience, we find glucagon most useful as a transient therapy to bridge patients to HDI therapy, unless a glucagon bolus effectively resolves symptoms.

High-Dose Insulin

Despite glucagon's longer history for treatment of beta-blocker toxicity, HDI is a superior therapy. HDI is not a vasopressor; it is a potent inotrope with vasodilating properties.[19] The mechanism for HDI is not fully elucidated but probably involves both optimization of the use of carbohydrates for fuel by cardiac myocytes and modulation of intracellular calcium. HDI improves cardiac output significantly in beta-blocker toxicity from an increase in stroke volume more than heart rate.[20] Dosing of HDI is not universally agreed on; dosing in humans successfully treated with HDI has ranged from 0.5 to 22 U/kg/hr.[21] Human evidence for years was limited to case reports and small case series, however recommendations for HDI use with beta-blocker poisoning is increasing.[22] Multiple centers have reported favorable outcomes with HDI.[22,23] In the largest HDI study to date of 199 patients (103 of which were poisoned with beta-blockers), the overall survival was 84%. In this study, 21% of patients suffered cardiac arrest; however, of those experiencing arrest, 25% survived. Median peak HDI infusion in this study was 8 U/kg/hr. In beta-blocker poisoning, we recommend a bolus of 1 U/kg of regular insulin IV, followed by an infusion at 1 U/kg/hr titrated up by 2 U/kg/hr every 10 minutes (up to a maximum of 10 U/kg/hr) based on hemodynamic response to achieve adequate end-organ perfusion. Regardless of HDI dosing, we recommend that patients receive a bolus of 25 g glucose (1 traditional

"amp" of D50) prior to insulin administration unless the serum glucose is greater than 200 mg/dL. A dextrose infusion (preferably a concentrated solution such as D50)[22] is administered via a central line because patients receiving HDI therapy are at higher risk of fluid overload.[24] Glucose concentration should be monitored as frequently as every 15 minutes until a steady state of glucose use is achieved. Although glucose requirements in HDI are typically higher with beta-blockers than with calcium channel blockers,[22] in neither scenario do glucose requirements increase with increasing doses of insulin.[23] Potassium concentration should also be monitored closely and replaced as needed because patients may become hypokalemic. Clinicians should be aware that metabolic abnormalities are common in HDI; hypoglycemia occurs in 31% to 73% of patients and hypokalemia occurs in 29% to 82% of patients, though in both cases careful monitoring and replacement prevents adverse outcomes.[22,23] In addition, hypoglycemia is less common if concentrated glucose infusions are used.[22] We recommend HDI for patients experiencing hypotension despite crystalloid fluid, atropine, and a single bolus of calcium. We also recommend a central venous catheter and an arterial catheter be placed upon the decision to initiate HDI. Of note, the inotropic effects of HDI do not typically occur until 20 minutes after the insulin bolus. As such, patients may need the bridging therapies described above, while HDI takes effect.

Sodium Bicarbonate

Sodium channel blockade from beta-blockers with membrane-stabilizing activity such as propranolol occasionally causes QRS widening, which mechanistically should respond to sodium bicarbonate. Bicarbonate should be dosed at 1 to 2 mEq/kg IV as a bolus repeated every 3 to 5 minutes until the QRS narrows to less than 120 ms. It is our experience that this is typically a late or even moribund finding in propranolol overdose. We recommend sodium bicarbonate for patients poisoned with a membrane-stabilizing beta-blocker who have an acute change in QRS duration to greater than 120 ms and demonstrate clinical signs of shock.

Vasopressors and Other Inotropes

Catecholamines are indicated when mean arterial pressure (MAP) cannot be maintained at 60 mm Hg or above, despite use of crystalloid infusion, calcium, atropine, glucagon, and HDI. We recommend against the use of vasopressors before HDI, because animal data show worse outcomes with vasopressors than HDI,[25] or even placebo.[26] A clinical conundrum exists regarding the use of vasopressors for toxin-induced shock in that animal studies generally show no benefit or even harm, while human data (which is limited to case reports and case series) show generally favorable outcomes.[27] Recent data in pigs poisoned with propranolol demonstrate rapid death with a combination of norepinephrine and epinephrine, and that HDI was a superior therapy in terms of mortality.[25] HDI, however, did not confer universal survival, and in fact both survival and brain perfusion improved when norepinephrine was added to HDI.[25] Given the extensive body of evidence demonstrating the safety and effectiveness of norepinephrine in other forms of shock, we recommend it as our first-line vasopressor, titrated to a MAP of 60 mm Hg up to a dose of 0.5 mcg/kg/min. In the selection of cardioactive medications to supplement HDI, glucagon, and norepinephrine, we recommend early assessment of cardiac contractility with bedside echocardiography. If contractility and heart rate are adequate, therapeutic focus should shift to providing support with vasopressors. Our second-line vasopressor of choice is vasopressin, dosed at a constant infusion of 0.01 to 0.04 U/min. If the clinical picture is still uncertain, an assessment of systemic vascular resistance and cardiac output by either indirect or direct measurements is recommended to determine if either cardiogenic or distributive shock exists. We recommend third-line vasopressors or inotropes be chosen based upon these measurements used in conjunction with bedside echocardiography. Refractory cases of bradycardia may respond to an external or transvenous pacemaker. A pacemaker is particularly useful when cardiac contractility is vigorous, but bradycardia is persistent.

Intravenous Fat Emulsion (Intralipid)

Intravenous fat emulsion (IFE) is an adjunctive therapy for cardiotoxic shock. This therapy was first described for treatment of toxicity from local anesthetics such as bupivacaine.[28] The pharmacologic rationale for the use of IFE is discussed in Chapter 135. Enthusiasm for IFE for beta-blocker poisoning was high after the publication of positive animal studies and several case reports describing good outcomes,[29] but subsequent larger studies cast significant doubt on the effectiveness of IFE for oral overdoses, as in beta-blockers.[30,31] One study found that in 91% of published IFE cases, a concomitant resuscitative therapy was administered that could also explain the observed positive outcome.[30] A recent systematic review and collaborative expert panel found the evidence for non-local anesthetic poisoning to be of very low quality, and did not recommend in favor or against the use of IFE, even as a salvage therapy.[32] A national toxicology organization's position statement recently stated there is no standard of care to use or not use IFE for oral overdoses, and that in circumstances where there is significant hemodynamic instability secondary to a lipid-soluble drug, that IFE is a reasonable consideration for therapy. As such, we recommend IFE in patients with persistent bradycardia or hypotension not responding to IV fluids, calcium, HDI, and at least three vasopressors or inotropes at maximum recommended infusion rates and if extracorporeal membrane oxygenation (ECMO) is unavailable. Dosing for IFE is also not universally agreed upon.[33] We recommend an initial bolus of 1.5 mL/kg of 20% lipid solution given over 2 to 3 minutes, followed immediately by an infusion of 0.25 mL/kg/min. If a response occurs at this infusion rate, the infusion dose may be decreased to 0.025 mL/kg/min (1/10th the initial rate) to sustain lipemic serum for a longer period of time.[33,34] The 1.5 mL/kg bolus can be repeated up to two additional times for refractory shock or cardiac arrest, although clinicians should avoid exceeding 10 mL/kg unless hemodynamic compromise requires otherwise. Response, when it occurs, is typically within minutes of the bolus.

The use of IFE is associated with several complications, including extreme lipemia resulting in lab interference with blood tests (complete blood counts, chemistries, and coagulation studies), as well as acute pancreatitis, acute kidney injury, acute respiratory distress syndrome, fat overload syndrome, and cardiac arrest.[35]

Ventricular Dysrhythmias

Although it is uncharacteristic, ventricular tachydysrhythmias can occur following beta-blocker toxicity. Cardioversion and defibrillation are indicated for ventricular tachycardia and ventricular fibrillation, respectively, following American Heart Association guidelines. Pulsatile ventricular tachycardia can most safely be treated with lidocaine. For dosing recommendations, please see the Management of Cardioactive Steroids section of this chapter. Antidysrhythmic drugs, especially of classes IA and IC, should be avoided because they may potentiate AV block or be pro-dysrhythmic because of additive membrane-stabilizing activity. Sotalol, unlike other beta-blockers, has class III as well as class II effects causing prolongation of the QT interval and can induce torsades de pointes and other ventricular dysrhythmias. Overdrive

pacing with isoproterenol or a pacemaker and magnesium sulfate are specific therapies for torsades de pointes.

Extracorporeal Elimination and Circulatory Assistance

Hemodialysis or hemoperfusion may be beneficial for beta-blockers with lower V_d, lower protein binding, and greater hydrophilicity (see Table 142.3), though due to limited evidence[36] we recommend hemodialysis only if another indication for hemodialysis is present (e.g., severe metabolic acidosis, acute renal failure, fluid overload, hyperkalemia, or other electrolyte disturbances).

Unlike overdoses of other drugs, toxicity from cardiovascular drugs do not destroy tissue, and if circulation can be supported, complete recovery can be expected. Intra-aortic balloon pumps,[22] percutaneous left ventricular assist devices,[36-38] and cardiopulmonary bypass have all been successfully employed as salvage therapies. However, with the proliferation of extracorporeal cardiopulmonary resuscitation (eCPR) programs[39] the availability of ECMO for poisonings has increased substantially in the past decade.[15,40-43] As such, ECMO is our recommended mechanical support therapy in cases where patients have hypotension refractory to HDI, and at least three vasoactive agents or in cases with bradycardia or cardiogenic shock unresponsive to inotropes and a pacemaker.

Pediatric Considerations

Severe pediatric beta-blocker poisonings are rare. In the cases reported, CNS, cardiac, and metabolic toxicities are similar to those in adult overdoses. Symptomatic hypoglycemia, however, is more common in children and occurs even after therapeutic doses. Therefore, serum glucose concentration should be measured in children. Risk factors include young age, fasting state, and diabetes mellitus. Obtunded children should receive empirical glucose, 1 to 2 mL/kg of 25% glucose IV. In general, 5% glucose infusions have been sufficient to maintain euglycemia, especially with concomitant use of glucagon and catecholamines, which stimulate glucose release.

Seizures also occur in cases of pediatric beta-blocker overdose; hypoglycemia may be a contributing factor. They are more common with the lipid-soluble beta-blocker propranolol. Benzodiazepines in standard doses are generally effective. Children generally fare well after beta-blocker ingestion, with symptoms in only 2% of potential beta-blocker exposures.

Sequential Approach to Beta-Blocker Poisoning

The management of beta-blocker poisoning begins with a 20 mL/kg bolus of IV fluid, repeated once if needed (Table 142.6). Symptomatic bradycardia, typically a heart rate of 50 bpm or less in adults, should be treated with atropine, 1 mg every 3 minutes up to a total of 3 mg. If hypotension (systolic pressure <90 mm Hg) persists, 3 to 6 g of calcium gluconate should be infused over 10 minutes. If hypotension persists after calcium infusion, HDI should be initiated. Glucagon, given as a 5-mg bolus, can be used to bridge to HDI. One "amp" of D50 should be administered followed by 1 U/kg of regular insulin as a loading dose. An infusion of 25 g/hr of concentrated glucose should be initiated in addition to an infusion of insulin at 1 U/kg/hr. The insulin infusion should be increased by 2 U/kg/hr every 10 minutes until hypotension resolves or a maximum rate of 10 U/kg/hr is reached. Glucagon may be repeated during HDI titration if hypotension persists. If HDI does not resolve hypotension, norepinephrine should be administered starting at 0.1 mcg/kg/min and titrated up until hypotension resolves or until a maximum dose is reached. After maximal norepinephrine is reached, the clinician should reassess using bedside echocardiography and measurement of cardiac

TABLE 142.6 **Sequential Treatment Recommendations for Poisoning from Beta-Blockers and Calcium Channel Blockers**

Phase of Treatment	Beta-Blockers	Calcium Channel Blockers
Phase 1 (initial resuscitation; primarily bolus dose therapies)	Activated charcoal as indicated Isotonic fluid bolus 20–40 mL/kg Atropine Calcium Glucagon	Activated charcoal as indicated Isotonic fluid bolus 20–40 mL/kg Atropine Calcium
Phase 2 (stabilization; place central & arterial lines, consider cardiac output & SVR monitoring)	Place central & arterial lines HDI infusion Norepinephrine Vasopressin 3rd agent based on type of shock Pacemaker for bradycardia	Place central & arterial lines HDI infusion Norepinephrine Vasopressin 3rd agent based on type of shock Pacemaker for bradycardia
Phase 3 (salvage therapies)	IFE ECMO Other mechanical devices if ECMO not available	IFE Methylene blue ECMO Other mechanical devices if ECMO not available

HDI, High-dose insulin; *IFE*, intravenous fat emulsion; *SVR*, systemic vascular resistance; *ECMO*, extracorporeal membrane oxygenation.

output and systemic vascular resistance to determine if the patient needs additional inotropy, chronotropy, or vasotropy. If bradycardia is contributing to decreased cardiac output, we recommend a pacemaker; a transvenous approach will likely be necessary. Additional inotropes or vasopressors such as vasopressin, phenylephrine, epinephrine, dopamine, or dobutamine should be selected and titrated up based upon the patient's cardiac output and systemic vascular resistance. We recommend vasopressin as the second-line vasopressor at a steady-state infusion of 0.01 to 0.04 U/min. Once the patient has reached maximal doses on HDI and three vasopressors or catecholamines, depending on institutional availability we next recommend either IFE or ECMO; if ECMO is readily available, ECMO is preferred. If used, IFE may be dosed at 1.5 mL/kg IV of 20% lipid solution followed by an infusion as noted above. The bolus may be repeated; however, a maximal dose of 1000 mL of lipid solution should not be exceeded. A concern exists that if IFE and ECMO are used in tandem, clogging and malfunction of the membrane oxygenator from lipemia and fat agglutination is a concern.[44] Case reports[45] and in vitro data suggest this can occur, along with cracking of stopcocks and increased blood clotting in the circuits.[44] Nonetheless, the use of IFE is not a contraindication to ECMO. If IFE is used prior to ECMO, the infusion should be discontinued once the decision to cannulate has been made, and the perfusionist alerted that clogging of the oxygenator may occur so they may anticipate this complication.

Disposition

Patients who remain completely asymptomatic for 6 hours after an oral overdose of normal-release preparations can be safely discharged home if the overdose was accidental or referred for psychiatric evaluation if it was intentional. We recommend consultation with a poison control center or standard pharmacologic reference to confirm that peak effect of the beta-blocker in question has passed before psychiatric disposition (see Table 142.3). Patients ingesting sustained-release preparations should be admitted to a monitored bed; however, those who remain asymptomatic 8 to 12 hours after ingestion are unlikely to have toxicity. Patients with second or third-degree AV heart block, hypotension not responding to IV fluid administration, or who have hemodynamically significant dysrhythmias should be admitted to an intensive care unit.

CALCIUM CHANNEL BLOCKERS

KEY CONCEPTS

- Signs and symptoms of calcium channel blocker intoxication often occur early after overdose but may be significantly delayed with sustained-release products.
- AV block and bradydysrhythmias predominate with verapamil and diltiazem; dihydropyridine calcium channel blockers often present with tachycardia.
- Treatment is similar to beta-blockers, except glucagon is not recommended, and methylene blue is a reasonable option for vasoplegia unresponsive to maximum doses of norepinephrine and vasopressin.

Foundations

Principles of Toxicity

Verapamil and nifedipine, the earliest calcium channel antagonists, were introduced in Europe in the 1970s and in the United States in the early 1980s. Calcium antagonists have found many clinical applications: angina pectoris, hypertension, supraventricular dysrhythmias, hypertrophic cardiomyopathy, and migraine prophylaxis. Verapamil is the most lethal in overdose, but severe toxicity and death have been reported for most drugs of this class. In 2018, United States poison control centers received nearly 14,000 calls about calcium channel blockers.[1] Nearly 1200 of these calls were regarding patients with life-threatening symptoms.[1] In general, calcium channel blockers are more toxic than beta-blockers, likely because they cause both cardiogenic shock and vasoplegia.

Pathophysiology

Calcium channel antagonists block the slow L-type calcium channels in the myocardium and vascular smooth muscle, leading to coronary and peripheral vasodilation. They also reduce cardiac contractility, depress SA nodal activity, and slow AV conduction. In cases of overdose, verapamil has the deadliest profile, combining severe myocardial depression and peripheral vasodilation. Both verapamil and diltiazem act on the heart and blood vessels, whereas dihydropyridine calcium channel blockers (e.g., amlodipine) cause primarily vasodilation and subsequent reflex tachycardia due to subtle binding differences in the α1c subunit of L-type calcium channels. As with beta-blockers, selectivity is lost after overdose and toxicity is in four domains: negative effects on heart rate, contractility, conduction, and vascular tone, with the exception of dihydropyridine calcium channel blockers, which tend to result in tachycardia until severe toxicity occurs, when bradycardia ensues.

All calcium channel blockers are rapidly absorbed, although first-pass hepatic metabolism significantly reduces bioavailability (see Table 142.4). Onset of action and toxicity may occur as early as 30 minutes after ingestion. In contrast, the poisoning from sustained-release verapamil may not manifest for 12 hours or more. High protein binding and V_d greater than 1 to 2 L/kg make hemodialysis or hemoperfusion ineffective with calcium antagonists.

Clinical Features

Severe calcium antagonism eventually affects multiple organ systems, but cardiovascular toxicity is primarily responsible for morbidity and mortality. Hypotension and bradycardia occur early, and other rhythm disturbances include AV block of all degrees, sinus arrest, AV dissociation, junctional rhythm, and asystole. Dihydropyridine calcium channel blockers (e.g., amlodipine) often cause reflex sinus tachycardia from peripheral vasodilation. Calcium channel blockade has little effect on ventricular conduction; therefore, QRS widening is not seen early on. Ventricular dysrhythmias are also uncommon. A unique feature of calcium channel blocker poisoning is endocrine dysfunction. Like many drugs, calcium channel blockers lose specificity in overdose and thus interfere with other calcium channels within the body. As calcium influx triggers the release of insulin, patients poisoned with calcium channel blockers are often hyperglycemic. In addition, edema is a common side effect of calcium channel blockers at therapeutic doses. Edema occurs because of selective dilation of vessels on the afferent side of the capillary bed while suppressing normal regulatory responses that protect capillaries from hydrostatic pressure. At therapeutic doses, peripheral edema from calcium channel blockers is common; however, pulmonary edema may occur in overdose, which is likely due to a combination of drug effect and iatrogenic volume overload.[46,47] Nearly half of patients with severe amlodipine poisoning have non-cardiogenic pulmonary edema.[48] As with digoxin and beta-blocker overdose, nausea and vomiting are common but not specific. For additional clinical features, see Table 142.5. Like beta-blockers, calcium channel blockers cause early toxicity, and symptoms commonly occur within 6 hours of ingestion of normal-release preparations. Toxicity can be delayed 12 to 24 hours with sustained-release preparations.

Differential Diagnoses

Differential diagnoses are similar to that of digoxin and beta-blocker overdoses. Until characteristic rhythm disturbances supervene, many other toxic, metabolic, traumatic, and cardiovascular disorders can cause hypotension but less commonly bradycardia. The reflex tachycardia and distributive shock seen with dihydropyridine calcium channel blockers can mimic sepsis, volume depletion, or anaphylaxis.

Diagnostic Testing

Serum levels of calcium antagonists are not readily available nor do urine toxicology screens reliably detect this class of drugs. Glucose and electrolytes (including calcium and magnesium) should be measured. Hyperglycemia secondary to insulin inhibition occurs and correlates with severity of verapamil and diltiazem poisoning; it is unknown if the same is true in dihydropyridine overdose. If hyperglycemia is present with concomitant hypotension, we recommend HDI. Please see specific dosing recommendations later. A metabolic (lactic) acidosis can occur with prolonged hypotension and hypoperfusion.

An ECG should be promptly obtained, with special attention to atrial and ventricular rates and PR, QRS, and QT intervals. The ECG should be repeated when the patient's hemodynamic status changes.

Management

Initial management includes rapid establishment of vascular access, cardiac monitoring, and frequent blood pressure measurement. Please see Chapter 135 for further information on gastrointestinal decontamination, including the use of activated charcoal. For an algorithmic approach to management, see Table 142.6.

Hypotension and Bradycardia

Hypotension can be caused by myocardial depression, inadequate heart rate, or peripheral vasodilation. Atropine may be used for bradycardia but is rarely effective. We recommend atropine at the doses noted earlier for a heart rate of less than 50 beats per minute with concomitant hypotension and symptoms of severe bradycardia such as weakness, drowsiness, or obtundation. Atropine's effect has often been minimal and short-lived, and it is at best a temporizing intervention. A bolus of crystalloid (20 to 40 mL/kg or more) should also be infused early; however, care should be taken to avoid fluid overload given the additional risk of pulmonary edema with calcium channel blocker poisoning, particularly in elderly patients or those with underlying heart disease.

After the basic supportive therapies noted previously, expert consensus recommendations include calcium salts, HDI, and norepinephrine.[49] We recommend these three agents be administered in the sequential fashion noted for beta-blocker poisoning. We do not recommend glucagon in calcium channel blocker poisoning. It has no mechanistic advantage over epinephrine or other beta-agonists, and no good evidence exists to support its use in calcium channel blocker poisoning.

IFE (e.g., Intralipid) has been described in the use of calcium channel blockers. The proposed mechanisms are discussed in Chapter 135. Similar to beta-blockers, early animal studies and case reports were promising, while larger follow-up studies showed poor outcomes in human poisoning. The same collaborative expert panel on IFE noted earlier did not recommend in favor or against the use of IFE in calcium channel blocker poisoning, even as a salvage therapy.[32] As such, we recommend IFE in patients with persistent cardiogenic shock not responding to IV fluids, calcium, HDI, and at least three vasopressors or inotropes at maximum recommended infusion rates if extracorporeal membrane oxygenation (ECMO) is not immediately available.

Methylene blue is an emerging therapy for calcium channel blocker poisoning.[50] Although traditionally used as a reducing agent for the treatment of methemoglobinemia, methylene blue is also a vasoconstrictor. Specifically, it inhibits the enzyme guanylyl cyclase, resulting in decreased production of cyclic guanosine monophosphate (cGMP) and inhibition of endothelial smooth muscle relaxation, causing an increase in systemic vascular resistance.[51] Methylene blue is particularly intriguing for the treatment of amlodipine poisoning, because amlodipine specifically causes an increase in nitric oxide production, which leads to increased cGMP and vasodilation as noted earlier. Data are limited to a small number of animal studies and human case reports,[52,53] and thus far suggest improvement is limited to hemodynamic parameters and not overall mortality.[51] Methylene blue was inferior to IFE in a rat model of amlodipine poisoning,[54] nor did it improve outcomes when compared to norepinephrine in a pig model of amlodipine poisoning.[55] We recommend the use of methylene blue only as an alternative salvage therapy for vasoplegic shock refractory to infusions of HDI, maximal norepinephrine, and vasopressin. Dosing involves a 1- to 2-mg/kg bolus of a 1% methylene blue solution followed by an infusion of 1 mg/kg for up to 6 hours. Recently angiotensin II was FDA-approved for the treatment of vasodilatory shock;[56] its use in poisoning from calcium channel blockers (and poisoning in general) is limited to case reports requiring further study.[57] The use of angiotensin II would be a reasonable treatment for refractory vasodilatory shock in lieu of methylene blue, or as an additional therapy for profound vasoplegia refractory to maximal infusions of an α_1-adrenergic agonist (e.g., norepinephrine, phenylephrine) and vasopressin.

Pediatric Considerations

Nifedipine, verapamil, and probably other drugs in its class join the short list of medications that can kill a child with ingestion of a single tablet. Seizures may be more common in children than in adults and should be treated with benzodiazepines. Overall, death after calcium antagonist ingestion in children is rare. The IV route of administration, as with digoxin, is much more dangerous. Even therapeutic doses of IV verapamil are considered contraindicated in infants with supraventricular tachycardia because of cardiovascular collapse and cardiac arrest after injection which have been documented in case reports.[58]

Hyperglycemia occasionally occurs in children, but the elevation is usually short-lived. Although insulin has been administered in a small number of cases, it is generally not necessary unless HDI is required for hemodynamic compromise, because the hyperglycemia usually resolves spontaneously within 24 to 36 hours.

There are case reports of children in refractory shock secondary to drug toxicity who have been treated with intra-aortic balloon counterpulsation or cardiac bypass, though ECMO has gained favor as the mechanical support device of choice.[58] Aside from the differences previously noted, the presentation in children is similar to that in adults: rapid onset of toxicity with CNS depression, bradydysrhythmias (except for dihydropyridine calcium channel blockers), and hypotension.

Disposition

Because the peak effect of normal-release calcium channel blockers commonly occurs in 90 minutes to 6 hours, patients who are totally asymptomatic for 6 hours after an ingestion of immediate-release medication can be safely discharged if accidental, or according to psychiatric recommendations if intentional. Symptomatic patients or those who ingested delayed-release preparations should be admitted for at least 24 hours of continuous cardiac monitoring. Persistently hypotensive, bradycardic patients who do not respond to conventional therapy require intensive care monitoring.

CLONIDINE AND OTHER CENTRAL ALPHA-2 AGONISTS

KEY CONCEPTS

- Clonidine poisoning may mimic opioid poisoning and is best treated with crystalloid fluids followed by an infusion of norepinephrine.
- In patients at low risk for opioid dependence, naloxone, given as a 10 mg bolus from a single syringe, is recommended for obtundation.

Foundations

Clonidine is a central acting α_2-adrenergic and imidazoline agonist initially approved by the FDA as a treatment for hypertension in 1974. Since that time, its use has expanded to treat conditions such as attention deficit hyperactivity disorder (ADHD), pheochromocytoma, and withdrawal from opioids, ethanol, and nicotine. It is also used in spinal and epidural anesthesia. Based on its mechanism of action, it mimics clinical features of both opioid poisoning and poisoning from digoxin, beta-blockers, or calcium channel blockers. In 2018 United States poison centers received over 10,000 calls regarding clonidine exposures with over 2,000 suffering life-threatening effects.[1] Clonidine poisoning appears to be increasing in children.[59]

Clinical Features

Clonidine exerts its effects by binding to presynaptic α_2-adrenergic receptors in the brain, inhibiting neurons in the nucleus tractus solitarius, causing decreased norepinephrine release. This leads to bradycardia, hypotension, decreased mental status, miosis, and occasionally hypothermia. Clonidine is also an agonist at imidazole receptors; imidazoline receptors are located throughout the body, but their activation in the brain, specifically in the rostral ventrolateral medulla, causes unconsciousness, bradycardia, and hypotension, potentially exacerbating the α_2-adrenergic effects of clonidine.[60] Although clonidine overdose presents with bradycardia, hypotension, and coma, most cases have favorable clinical outcomes.[61]

Differential Diagnoses

There is a wide overlap between the clinical effects of central α_2-agonists such as clonidine and imidazole agonists. Individual drugs that are agonists at either or both receptors may belong to disparate classes. Therefore, antihypertensive medications (e.g., guanabenz, α-methyldopa), ADHD medications (e.g., guanfacine), muscle relaxers (e.g., tizanidine), and topical vasoconstrictors in dermatologic (e.g., brimonidine),[62] ocular, and nasal settings (e.g., tetrahydrozoline, oxymetazoline, and naphazoline)[63] all have similar systemic effects in overdose. The presentation of miosis and obtundation may be mistaken for opioid or sedative-hypnotic overdose, and the combination of bradycardia and hypotension may mimic digoxin, beta-blocker, or calcium channel blocker poisoning. Pontine hemorrhage should also be considered in the differential diagnoses.

Diagnostic Testing

Clonidine and other similar drugs are not routinely screened for in most blood or urine drug screens. Clonidine poisoning is a clinical diagnosis. An ECG should be obtained to evaluate for heart block and to evaluate the QRS and corrected QT (QTc) intervals, and the patient should be placed on continuous cardiac monitoring and pulse oximetry. Small doses of naloxone may help differentiate clonidine poisoning from opioid poisoning; however, if large doses are required, this may be less helpful diagnostically because large doses of naloxone have been reported to reverse clonidine toxicity.

Management

Supportive care is the mainstay of therapy for clonidine poisoning. Monitoring as described earlier is essential. Hypotension should be treated with boluses of 20 mL/kg of isotonic fluid. The concern for pulmonary edema is less than with beta-blocker or calcium channel blocker poisoning, thus the clinician can be more liberal with IV fluid administration in clonidine poisoning. We recommend treating hypotension with up to 60 mL/kg of isotonic fluid. If hypotension is worsening or persistent at a level of inadequate organ perfusion despite adequate fluid resuscitation, a catecholamine is indicated. There are no human randomized trials comparing various catecholamines in clonidine poisoning; however, because the underlying pathophysiology is a lack of systemic norepinephrine, we recommend norepinephrine initiated as 0.1 mcg/kg/min and titrated to a MAP of 60 mm Hg. When blood pressure stabilizes, downward titration of norepinephrine is initiated, with a goal of maintaining adequate organ perfusion with the least necessary dose, ultimately weaning the patient off the vasopressor entirely.

Several authors have suggested naloxone may be a useful therapy in clonidine poisoning. Clonidine causes the spontaneous release of β-endorphin, an endogenous opioid. It is likely naloxone's antagonism of β-endorphin's opioid effects that causes reversal of CNS depression in clonidine poisoning. Although case reports of naloxone successfully reversing clonidine poisoning exist, they are rare and inconsistent. Our clinical experience is that naloxone is rarely effective for clonidine poisoning in adults, however recent data suggest clonidine may be an effective treatment in children. In a study of 51 somnolent children poisoned with clonidine, 40 (78%) woke upon administration of naloxone.[64] The authors noted greater success when 10 mg of naloxone was administered as a bolus from a single syringe, rather than a titrated approach. Because the precipitation of opioid withdrawal can be dangerous, in patients at high risk for opioid dependence we recommend escalating doses of naloxone of 0.2 mg, 0.4 mg, 2 mg, and then 10 mg if the patient is obtunded. If there is no concern for opioid dependence, we recommend naloxone be given as a 10-mg rapid bolus from a single syringe, regardless of the patient's age or size.

Disposition

Clonidine's peak effects occur 2 to 4 hours post-ingestion. Its half-life is between 5 and 13 hours. Therefore, patients with normal vital signs and mental status 4 hours post-ingestion may be discharged home if the overdose was accidental or to an appropriate psychiatric facility if intentional. Patients with persistent vital sign abnormalities or altered mental status should be admitted to a unit capable of continuous cardiac and oximetry monitoring. Patients requiring vasopressor support or with severe obtundation should be admitted to a critical care unit.

NITRATES, NITRITES, AND METHEMOGLOBINEMIA

KEY CONCEPTS

- Nitrates are contraindicated in patients who have recently taken phosphodiesterase inhibitors for erectile dysfunction.
- Patients with a methemoglobin concentration of 25% and symptoms of anemia should be treated with methylene blue.

Foundations

Principles of Toxicity

Nitrates (nitroglycerin, isosorbide mononitrate and dinitrate) are widely used as vasodilators in the treatment of heart failure and ischemic heart disease. They augment coronary blood flow, as well as reduce myocardial oxygen consumption by reducing afterload. At lower doses nitrates primarily dilate veins, but at higher doses they also dilate arteries. In addition, many exposures occur in young adults, usually male, who inhale various alkyl nitrites (amyl, butyl, isobutyl, or ethyl nitrite) in the hope of enhancing or prolonging sexual pleasure. Because of the sound they make when broken open, these products are commonly known as "poppers."[65]

Nitrates are occasionally found in rural well water contaminated by livestock or fertilizer runoff. Oral nitrates may be converted to nitrites in the gastrointestinal tract, especially in infants up to 4 months old. Nitrites, and to a lesser extent, nitrates themselves, have substantial oxidizing power and may oxidize the ferrous (Fe^{2+}) ion in hemoglobin to its ferric (Fe^{3+}) state, causing methemoglobinemia. Methemoglobin is incapable of carrying oxygen, thus it alters the shape of the hemoglobin-dissociation curve shifting it to the left, causing functional anemia via impaired oxygen delivery.

Clinical Features

Hypotension is a common complication. Typically, it is accompanied by reflex tachycardia unless the patient also has taken another agent such as a beta-blocker that slows chronotropy. Even in therapeutic doses, rapid dilation of meningeal arterioles causes headache, often leading to patient noncompliance.

Patients suffering nitrate-induced methemoglobinemia have symptoms related to impaired oxygen delivery. The concentration of methemoglobinemia and the speed with which it is achieved are directly proportional to symptom severity. Cyanosis occurs commonly when the percentage of methemoglobin exceeds 10%. Inspection of the patient's blood upon venipuncture reveals "chocolate-colored" blood due to the spectrum of light absorbed by methemoglobin; this typically occurs at a methemoglobin concentration greater than 15%. Higher concentrations of methemoglobin may result in fatigue, dyspnea, weakness, dizziness, drowsiness, syncope, coma, seizures, and death.

Differential Diagnoses

The differential diagnosis of nitrate poisoning includes all other vasodilating drugs such as diuretics, angiotensin-converting enzyme (ACE) inhibitors, and dihydropyridine calcium channel blockers, as well as oxidative phosphorylation uncouplers such as cyanide and carbon monoxide. Non-toxicologic conditions capable of mimicking nitrate poisoning include sepsis and anaphylaxis. The differential diagnosis of methemoglobinemia includes hypoxia, as well as other hemoglobinopathies such as sulfhemoglobinemia.

Diagnostic Testing

No specific mandatory diagnostic testing is recommended for nitrate poisoning. For patients with suspected methemoglobinemia, an oxygen challenge should first be attempted. If the patient is cyanotic and high-flow oxygen at 15 L/min by non-rebreather mask does not improve cyanosis, blood co-oximetry should be performed to determine the percentage of methemoglobin in the blood. If methemoglobinemia is confirmed, a hemoglobin concentration should be obtained. If anemia is present, smaller concentrations of methemoglobin may be clinically significant because the functional anemia of methemoglobinemia is synergistic with absolute anemia. Most humans have, at baseline, a methemoglobin percentage of 1% to 3%. Symptoms do not typically occur until concentrations of 10% or more.

Clinicians should be wary of interpreting pulse oximetry in the setting of methemoglobinemia. Pulse oximeters function by reading the absorbance of light at wavelengths of 660 and 940 nm, which are selected to separate oxy and deoxyhemoglobin. Methemoglobin absorbs light at both these wavelengths more than either oxy or deoxyhemoglobin. This results in unreliable pulse oximetry that typically reads near 85%, regardless of the patient's oxygenation status.

Management

Nitrate poisoning usually responds to supine positioning, IV fluids, and reduction of dose or removal of the offending agent. Hypotension is usually transient. Low-dose vasopressors are occasionally needed, but it is best to avoid them in the setting of acute coronary syndrome.

Review of the therapeutic use of nitrates offers insight into poisoning. For example, IV nitroglycerin infusions are used commonly in patients with acute pulmonary edema for afterload reduction. Infusions are usually initiated at 5 to 10 μg/min, but rates of 300 mcg/min or greater may be used. These doses may be beneficial in patients with pulmonary edema accompanied by acute hypertension, but hypotension may develop suddenly. IV nitroglycerin has a rapid offset of action, so excessive fall in blood pressure usually responds to reduction or termination of the infusion.

Use of nitrates is contraindicated in patients who have recently taken certain drugs for erectile dysfunction, such as sildenafil (Viagra) or tadalafil (Cialis). These drugs inhibit type 5 phosphodiesterase, relaxing vascular smooth muscle, which can prolong and intensify the vasodilating effects of nitrates causing severe hypotension. If blood pressure does not normalize with IV fluids and cessation of the nitrate infusion, norepinephrine should be cautiously titrated to a MAP of 60 mm Hg, beginning at 0.1 mcg/kg/min.

Treatment of patients with methemoglobinemia involves supportive care such as supplemental oxygen and IV fluids as needed. More severely poisoned patients should be treated with IV methylene blue. Methylene blue is an oxidizing agent. However, in the presence of the red blood cell enzyme nicotinamide adenine dinucleotide phosphate (NADPH) methemoglobin reductase, it is reduced to leukomethylene blue, which then reduces methemoglobin back to hemoglobin. We recommend an intravenous dose of 1 to 2 mg/kg of 1% methylene blue solution for patients with a methemoglobin concentration greater than 25% and any symptoms of functional anemia. The infusion should be given over 5 minutes to reduce pain at the IV access site. A clinical response should occur within minutes of infusion. If cyanosis does not resolve in 1 hour, a second infusion of 1 mg/kg can be repeated. At doses exceeding 7 mg/kg, the oxidizing power of methylene blue becomes great enough that it may paradoxically worsen methemoglobinemia or cause hemolysis; thus, multiple or excessive doses are not recommended.

Disposition

Patients with refractory hypotension despite therapeutic measures discussed in the preceding section should be admitted to a monitored setting. We recommend all patients receiving methylene blue be admitted, as some poisons that cause methemoglobinemia have half-lives that exceed that of methylene blue. If the patient remains unstable and persistently cyanotic or hypoxic, or requires repeat doses of methylene blue, they should be admitted to a critical care setting.

The references for this chapter can be found online at ExpertConsult.com.

143

Caustics

Christopher Hoyte

KEY CONCEPTS

- Health care workers caring for patients with caustic exposures should adhere to universal precautions to prevent additional exposure.
- All symptomatic patients should undergo endoscopy and be should be observed for at least 24 hours.
- Asymptomatic patients can undergo endoscopy in the emergency department or be discharged with close follow-up monitoring.
- Gastric emptying or GI decontamination is not indicated for the majority of caustic ingestions.
- Concentration and pH are the most important characteristics of a substance to predict esophageal and gastric injury.
- Button batteries lodged in the airway or esophagus require endoscopic retrieval.

FOUNDATIONS

Caustic or corrosive agents have the potential to cause tissue injury on contact with mucosal surfaces. Both strong acids and alkalis are capable of causing corrosive chemical injury. Alkalis are proton acceptors and result in the formation of conjugate acids and free hydroxide ions. Lye is an example of an alkali and refers to both sodium hydroxide (NaOH) and potassium hydroxide (KOH). Ammonia (NH_3) is another common alkaline corrosive. Acids are proton donors; they dissociate into conjugate bases and free hydrogen ions in solution. Acidic caustics include hydrochloric acid (HCl) and sulfuric acid (H_2SO_4). The injury from caustic agents typically increases with a pH below 3 or above 11. Other chemicals that have caustic properties include phenol, formaldehyde, iodine, and concentrated hydrogen peroxide. This chapter discusses oral exposure. Dermal and inhalational exposures are discussed in Chapter 55 and Chapter 148, respectively.

More than 40,000 exposures involving caustic agents occur in the United States every year.[1] Nearly 75% of reported caustic ingestions are intentional for the purpose of self-harm.[1] Accidental ingestions occur typically among the pediatric and elderly populations. Transfer and storage of cleaners in alternative containers that may not be "child proof," such as jars, soda bottles, and sports drink containers, contribute to unintentional ingestion. Intentional ingestions may have a greater degree of oropharyngeal sparing because of rapid swallowing but have a higher likelihood of serious injury.

Principles of Toxicity

Some household products, such as liquid drain cleaners, continue to have high concentrations of alkali (30% KOH) or acid (93% H_2SO_4) (Table 143.1). These products often do not have concentration or content information available on the label, making it difficult for clinicians to determine the severity of exposure. Industrial, agricultural (dairy pipeline cleaners containing liquid NaOH and KOH in concentrations of 8% to 25%), and swimming pool chemicals also contain caustics in high concentrations.

Crystals and solid particles can have prolonged tissue adherence, causing more severe injury. Household detergents such as laundry powders and detergent pods (LDPs) and dishwasher detergents containing silicates, carbonates, and phosphates have the potential to induce caustic burns and strictures, even when ingested unintentionally. These ingestions are limited by immediate oral pain, usually causing them to be spit out sooner than a liquid agent. The ingestion of granular automatic dishwashing detergents or brightly colored laundry detergent capsules or "pods" can be associated with devastating injuries.[2] Compared to children with traditional non-LDP exposures, LDP exposures are associated with a higher incidence of toxicity including central nervous system depression and respiratory compromise with failure. Whether the toxicity observed with LDP exposures is due to other ingredients in the products, pH, concentration, tensile strength, or the delivery vehicle remains unclear.

Crystal drain cleaners have lye concentrations as high as 74% NaOH and may cause proximal esophageal injury. Liquid dishwashing detergents and laundry detergents have a pH higher than 12, but because the titratable alkaline reserve is low, tissue equilibration occurs quickly, and there is less risk of injury after ingestion.

Liquid household bleach typically contains dilute (3% to 5%) sodium hypochlorite (NaOCl), and ingestion rarely causes consequential injury. Industrial-strength bleach, however, contains significantly higher concentrations of NaOCl, which are more likely to cause esophageal necrosis. Toilet bowl cleaners contain HCl concentrations as high as 26%. General-purpose anticorrosive cleaners, such as 31% hydrochloride acid (HCl), are sold in gallon containers for home use and as swimming pool cleaners.

The alkali powder in air bags can cause ocular burns. Perfume unintentionally sprayed in the eyes can be caustic. Cement is alkaline and causes topical burns, typically on the knees and hands. Although hair relaxer creams contain NaOH and have a pH of 11.2 to 11.9, injuries after ingestion are usually mild.

Caustic ingestions may occur when methamphetamine is produced from over-the-counter medications and household chemicals. H_2SO_4, HCl, NaOH, ammonium hydroxide, anhydrous ammonia, and metallic lithium are all used in the clandestine production of methamphetamine. Severe caustic injuries occurring from ingestion of these agents can cause stricture formation, esophageal resection, and the need for colonic interposition.

Many medication pills can cause injury when they come in contact with the esophageal mucosa for prolonged periods. Patients who take medications in the supine position or who take pills without water are at higher risk of pill esophagitis. The pills most likely to adhere are doxycycline, tetracycline, potassium chloride, antimalarials, and aspirin.

TABLE 143.1 **Household Cleaning Products That Contain Caustic Chemicals**

Application	Product (Manufacturer), Chemical
Drain cleaner, liquid	Heavy Duty Liquid Drain Opener (Share), H₂SO₄ 93%
	Drain Out Extra (Iron Out), KOH 30%
	Liquid-Plumr (Clorox), NaOH 0.5% to 2%, NaOCl 5% to 10%
	Maximum Strength Drain Opener (Enforcer), KOH 1% to 10%, NaOCl <5%
	Drain Care Professional Strength Drain Opener, NaOH 5% to 15%
Drain cleaner, crystals	Heavy Duty Crystal Drain Opener (Roebic), NaOH 100%
	Crystal Drain Opener (Rohyme), NaOH 74%
	Crystal Drain Out (Iron Out), NaOH 30% to 60%
	Drano Pipe Cleaner (Johnson), NaOH 54%
Oven cleaner	Easy-Off Heavy Duty Oven Cleaner (Reckitt), NaOH 4% to 6%
Rust remover	Rust Remover/Carpet Care (Johnson Wax Professional), HCl 10%
	Rust Stain Remover (Whink), hydrofluoric acid 2.5% to 3%
	Rust Stripper (Certified), NaOH 50% to 75%
	Naval Jelly Rust Dissolver (Loctite), phosphoric acid 25% to 30%
Toilet bowl cleaner	Instant Power Toilet Bowl Cleaner (Scotch), HCl 26%
	Bowl and Porcelain Cleaner (Cleanline), HCl 0.10%
	Bowl/Tile/Porcelain Cleaner (Share), phosphoric acid 15% to 25%
	Husky 303 Toilet Bowl Cleaner, HCl 23%
	Misty Bolex Bowl Cleaner, HCl 26%
Swimming pool cleaner	Muriatic acid, Aqua Chem (Recreational Water), HCl 31%

H₂SO₄, Sulfuric acid; *HCl,* hydrochloric acid; *KOH,* potassium hydroxide; *NaOCl,* sodium hypochlorite; *NaOH,* sodium hydroxide.

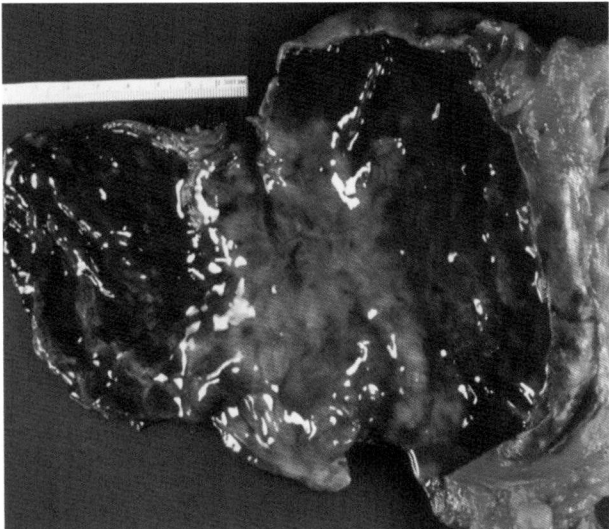

Fig. 143.1 Gastric mucosa after ingestion of 35% potassium hydroxide (KOH).

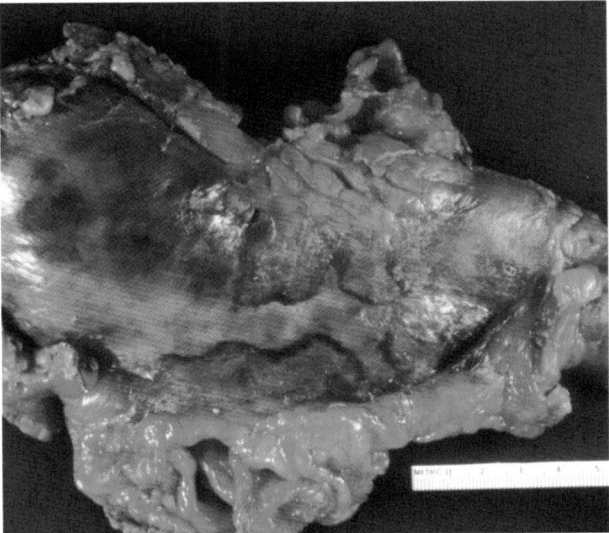

Fig. 143.2 Gastric serosa after ingestion of 35% potassium hydroxide (KOH).

Although uncommon, potassium chloride is particularly dangerous and can cause esophageal perforation with devastating communication with the aorta, left atrium, and bronchial artery.[3]

Pathophysiology

Factors that influence the extent of injury from a caustic exposure include type of agent, concentration of solution, volume, viscosity, duration of contact, pH, and presence or absence of food in the stomach. The titratable acid/alkaline reserve of an alkali or acid correlates with the ability to produce tissue damage. Concentrated forms of acids and bases generate heat, resulting in superimposed thermal injury.

Acidic compounds desiccate epithelial cells and cause coagulation necrosis. An eschar is formed that limits further penetration. Because acids tend to have a strong odor and cause immediate pain on contact, the quantity ingested is usually limited. Because of resistance of squamous epithelium to *coagulation necrosis*, acids are thought to be less likely to cause esophageal and pharyngeal injury, although severe esophageal and laryngeal injury still occur, particularly with intentional ingestions.[4] In many case series, acid ingestion results in equal esophageal and gastric mucosal injury.[4] Acids can also be absorbed

systemically, causing metabolic acidosis as well as damage to the spleen, liver, biliary tract, pancreas, and kidneys from perforation and direct local contact.

Alkaline contact, in contrast to acids, causes *liquefaction necrosis*, fat saponification, and protein disruption, allowing further penetration of the alkaline substance into the tissue. The depth of the necrosis depends on the concentration of the agent. A concentration of 30% NaOH in contact with tissue for one second results in a full-thickness burn. Alkalis are colorless and odorless, and unlike acids, they do not cause immediate pain on contact. Alkaline ingestions typically involve the squamous epithelial cells of the oropharynx, hypopharynx, and esophagus. The narrow portions of the esophagus, where pooling of secretions can occur, are also commonly involved. Alkalis may also cause gastric necrosis (Figs. 143.1 and 143.2), intestinal necrosis, and perforation. The esophagus can also be injured (Fig. 143.3). Burns below the pylorus carry a 50% mortality compared with 9% for burns above the pylorus.[5]

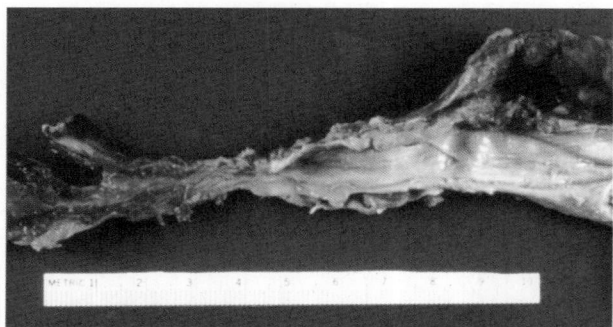

Fig. 143.3 Esophagus after ingestion of 35% potassium hydroxide (KOH).

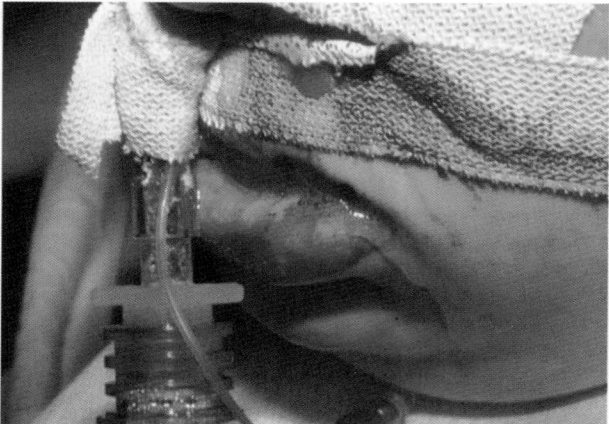

Fig. 143.4 Lip burn after exposure to 35% potassium hydroxide (KOH).

Caustic damage occurs in four phases. Initially, necrosis occurs, with invasion by bacteria and polymorphonuclear leukocytes. Vascular thrombosis follows, increasing the damage. During the next two to five days, superficial layers of injured tissue begin to slough. The tensile strength of the healing tissue may be low for up to three weeks after the caustic exposure, greatly increasing the chance of delayed perforation in some cases. Between one week and several months, granulation tissue forms, collagen is deposited, and reepithelialization occurs in the burn area. Esophageal strictures may form during a period of weeks to years from contraction of the scar.

Caustic injury is categorized as first, second, and third degree, similar to a thermal burn, by appearance on endoscopy. The initial depth of injury found on esophagoscopy correlates with the risk of stricture formation. Grade I injury consists of edema and hyperemia. Grade II injury can be further divided into grade IIa, which is non-circumferential, and grade IIb, which is nearly circumferential. Overall, grade II injuries are characterized by superficial ulcers, whitish membranes, exudates, friability, and hemorrhage. Grade III injury is associated with transmural involvement with deep injury, necrotic mucosa, or perforation of the stomach or esophagus. Although grade I injuries do not progress to stricture, 15% to 30% of all grade IIa injuries and up to 75% of circumferential grade IIb injuries of the esophagus develop strictures. With grade III injury, up to 90% result in stricture. Recently, the formation of strictures is decreasing for both grade II and grade III injury, possibly because of the type and caustic intensity of the substance ingested.[4]

CLINICAL FEATURES

Airway edema and esophageal or gastric perforations are the most emergent issues. Laryngeal edema begins in minutes and occurs over several hours. Systemic toxicity, hypovolemic shock, and hemodynamic instability with hypotension, tachycardia, fever, and metabolic acidosis are ominous signs. Small ingestions of potent substances can be as serious as larger ingestions. More than 40% of patients reporting to have "only taken a lick or sip" have esophageal burns. Patients with acid or alkali ingestions present with similar initial constellation of signs and symptoms. Oral pain, abdominal pain, vomiting, and drooling are common. Patients can have wheezing and coughing, respiratory distress, hoarseness, odynophagia, dysphagia, stridor, and dysphonia. Chest pain is common. Visible burns to the face, lips, and oral cavity may be seen (Fig. 143.4), although these signs are not always clinically reliable.[5,6] Skin burns can occur from spillage or secondary contamination after vomiting. Peritoneal signs suggest hollow viscus perforation or contiguous extension of the burn injury to adjoining visceral areas. Oropharyngeal burns alone are not predictive of more distal injury, but drooling, odynophagia, dysphagia, vomiting, and stridor, especially in combination, are highly predictive of significant lesions. Tracheal necrosis is one of the most frequent causes of death after caustic ingestion.

Dysphagia usually subsides in three to four days. Patients with significant esophageal burns, particularly those that are circumferential, may develop esophageal stricture; 80% of strictures become apparent in 2 to 8 weeks. Symptoms include dysphagia and food impactions. Strictures that become symptomatic early are generally more severe. In one study of 86 adults admitted to the hospital after caustic ingestion, 18 had complications with strictures and 6 died.

Patients with significant esophageal injury have a thousand-fold increase in esophageal carcinoma, which develops 40 to 50 years after the caustic ingestion. Long-term, 2% of patients who ingest caustics develop esophageal cancer and nearly 3% of esophageal cancer patients have a history of caustic ingestion.

Significant acid ingestions may be devastating and result in a higher mortality rate than alkali ingestions. The fulminant course of some acid ingestions may be due to systemic absorption of the acid, resulting in metabolic acidosis (which may also be the result of extensive tissue necrosis), hemolysis, and renal failure. Ingestion of glacial acetic acid (80% acetic acid) is common among certain ethnic populations as a suicidal gesture or accidental ingestion during food preparation, resulting in systemic complications, including renal and hepatic insufficiency, hemolysis, and disseminated intravascular coagulation. Ingestion of H_2SO_4 and HCl typically does not cause these systemic complications.

On clinical evaluation, the goal is to identify the extent and severity of the burn. In evaluation of a patient, the history should include the time, amount, type of product ingested, and presence of suicidal intent, if any. Patients who are suicidal may minimize their symptoms or understate the ingestion. Physical examination addresses all of the above described features and should focus on the oropharynx, supraglottic area, airway, and gastrointestinal (GI) tract.

DIFFERENTIAL DIAGNOSES

The ingestion of a caustic agent is most often reported upon presentation by patient or family member. When this is not known, the differential diagnosis is essentially that of abdominal discomfort, nausea, and vomiting, until typical mucosal injury becomes apparent. Mucosal injuries can be the result of various causes. The presence of early shock or altered mental status soon after ingestion of a caustic agent should prompt the search for other causes. Gastroenteritis from the ingestion of heavy metals (e.g., iron, arsenic, inorganic mercury) and hydrocarbons can result in similar clinical effects as seen in caustic ingestions. Other GI conditions such as gastric perforation, esophageal rupture, esophagitis, and gastroesophageal reflux disease should be considered.

Patients suffering from allergic reactions progressing to anaphylaxis and angioedema can present with irritation and inflammation of the throat and larynx mimicking a caustic ingestion. Infectious sources such as aspiration pneumonitis, croup (laryngotracheobronchitis), and epiglottitis can present in a similar manner as well.

DIAGNOSTIC TESTING

Product labels are important in confirming the concentration of chemicals. If the product with the label is brought by the patient or family, call the regional poison center for product information, look up the contents, or test the pH with litmus paper.

Evaluation of the severity of caustic ingestion and determination of the likelihood of deterioration or serious injury is based on examination of the upper airway, the esophagus, and the chest and abdomen. Examination of the oral pharynx is optimized by direct visualization. Nasopharyngoscopy, after appropriate application of a vasoconstrictor (e.g., phenylephrine) and local anesthesia (e.g., 4% lidocaine), determines the extent of injury and edema posterior to the tongue and in the supraglottic area and the glottis itself. Flexible endoscopy is used to evaluate the esophagus and stomach, after completion of the airway evaluation. Computed tomography (CT) scan is much more sensitive than plain radiography for identification of perforation of the GI tract, and both chest and abdomen are scanned when there is concern for serious injury (see earlier criteria). CT scan of the chest and the abdomen is able to detect evidence of perforation, such as mediastinal and extraluminal air, with high sensitivity.[7,8,9] Another benefit of CT is the ability to evaluate surrounding tissues that cannot be directly visualized during endoscopy due to technical challenges or safety.[7,8] Although chest and abdominal radiography are often used in the early stages to determine whether perforation has occurred, they are insensitive and these tests are not indicated if CT scanning is available.

Patients with significant injury (such as grades IIb or III) may have perforations difficult to detect during endoscopic evaluation. Thus, delayed (approximately 24 hours post ingestion) esophagram with water-soluble contrast medium may detect perforations by the presence of extravasation of contrast. If there is a high clinical suspicion, we recommend barium in the case of a nondiagnostic water-soluble contrast study that does not demonstrate a leak because barium is more radiopaque. Esophageal dilation, widening of the pleuroesophageal line, and pleural reflection displacement all portend impending perforation.

Laboratory studies should evaluate for metabolic acidosis, coagulation profile, hemoglobin, and electrolyte derangements. Some ingested acids are absorbed from the gastric mucosa and subsequently hydrogen ion disassociation occurs. The accumulation of the anionic species in the vascular space contributes to an elevation in ion gap. Ingestion of acids such as HCl result in a non-anion gap metabolic acidosis because both the dissociated hydrogen and chloride ions contribute in the measurement of the anion gap. Typically, alkalis are not absorbed from the gastric mucosa into the vascular space. A lactic acidosis can result, however, due to esophageal or gastric injury and necrosis. Therefore, in the setting of significant acid or alkali ingestion, serum pH and chemistry for serum bicarbonate analysis are indicated to determine the degree of acidosis. In cases of intentional overdose, co-ingestants should be considered and measured diagnostically if levels are available and clinically indicated.

Hydrofluoric acid exposures, whether by inhalation, ingestion, or dermal contact (hand size or larger), are notorious for the effect of absorbed fluoride, resulting in hypocalcemia, and require immediate cardiac monitoring to assess for corrected QT (QTc) prolongation, torsades de pointes, or other ventricular dysrhythmias. Rapid cardiac deterioration can occur in these cases. Serum calcium, potassium, and magnesium levels should also be determined in these cases.

The depth and extent of injury cannot be predicted based on signs and symptoms alone. Patients with signs and symptoms (vomiting, drooling, stridor, or dyspnea) of intentional ingestion should undergo endoscopy within 12 to 24 hours to define the extent of the disease. Endoscopy is contraindicated, however, in patients with likely or known perforation. Endoscopy performed too early may miss the extent or depth of tissue injury. Wound softening in the subacute phase when the likelihood of perforation is greatest makes late endoscopy (after 24 hours) more hazardous. Wound strength is weakest between day 5 to day 14 and the time of greatest risk for perforation. Early endoscopy has been studied and shown to be beneficial. Early endoscopy and GI tract evaluation permits more rapid administration of nutritional support. However, it is advised that the endoscopy be terminated at the level of the most proximal circumferential burn, particularly if the burn is severe, to avoid iatrogenic perforation. A soft feeding tube or silk string can be placed in the esophagus, when burns are present, for future dilation.

MANAGEMENT

Early and continuous hemodynamic monitoring is indicated. All contaminated clothing should be removed to prevent ongoing injury to the patient as well protection of health care personnel. Appropriate personal protective equipment (PPE) and hazardous waste disposal should be used.

After a caustic ingestion, little can be done to attenuate the severity of the tissue injury. Early endotracheal intubation or upper airway endoscopic examination is warranted when there are indications of upper airway injury on nasopharyngoscopy. If there are significant symptoms or signs, such as respiratory distress, stridor, or voice alteration (hoarseness, muffling), intubation is often necessary early in the course of evaluation, before edema and secretions both threaten the airway and make intubation difficult or impossible. For this reason, upper airway examination is often done with an intubating bronchoscope so that if significant injury and edema are identified, intubation can be accomplished during performance of the bronchoscopic examination. Blind nasotracheal intubation is contraindicated. When oral intubation is planned, a video laryngoscope should be used to provide optimal view with the least amount of tissue trauma. If significant symptoms and signs are present, intubation can be anticipated to be difficult, and awake flexible endoscopy is the method of choice.

After the airway is secured, persistent hypoxia and an increasing arterial-alveolar gradient warrant early bronchoscopy. Patients should have intravenous fluid resuscitation (20 to 40 mL/kg 0.9% normal saline bolus). Oropharyngeal and GI injury secondary to caustic ingestion can result hypotension because of fluid shift from the intravascular to the interstitial space. Intravenous access should be established and a bolus of 30 mL/kg of isotonic crystalloid, usually normal saline, should be administered. Standard measures of resuscitative progress such as heart rate and urine output should be monitored closely. In alert patients who are not vomiting and can tolerate liquids, small volumes (1 to 2 cups) of water or milk can be considered within the first 5 minutes after ingestion. Because injuries occur almost immediately, later dilution is not warranted. Forcing of fluids is never indicated. Attempts to neutralize the ingested corrosive with weak acids or alkalis can cause possible thermal reactions and worsen the injury.

GI decontamination after caustic ingestion is generally not indicated and can be hazardous. Inducing emesis is absolutely contraindicated given the risk of re-induction of the caustic agent into the esophagus, oropharynx, and airway. Activated charcoal is contraindicated as well, because it has little effect and will interfere with the endoscopist's view and assessment.

Careful nasogastric aspiration may decrease the amount of acid absorbed and may be useful in the setting of significant (massive) acid ingestions presenting within 30 to 45 minutes after the event, given the ominous natural history of many of these cases and the lower risk of esophageal perforation compared with alkali ingestion.

Exceptions to the general rules of gastrointestinal decontamination regarding caustics are noted in the management of zinc chloride ($ZnCl_2$) and mercuric chloride ($HgCl_2$). Both may result in severe systemic toxicity due to cationic metal injury. The local caustic effects, while of concern, are less consequential than the effects after systemic absorption. Thus, prevention of systemic absorption should be the primary action followed by direct assessment and management of the local effects. Initial management to prevent systemic absorption includes decontamination with gentle nasogastric tube aspiration and administration of activated charcoal.

Surgical consultation is indicated for free air, peritonitis, increasing and severe chest and abdominal pain, and hypotension. The decision to perform surgery in patients with caustic ingestions is generally clear. Endoscopic or diagnostic imaging evidence of perforation, severe abdominal rigidity, or persistent hypotension are all indications for surgical intervention. Hypotension is a grave clinical finding and often indicates perforation or significant blood loss. Additionally, elevations in prothrombin and partial thromboplastin times, as well as acidemia, are associated with severe caustic injury.

There remains controversy regarding the use of corticosteroid therapy in the management of grade IIb circumferential esophageal burns due to caustic injury. A dated prospective study of 83 children with grade IIb esophageal burns compared a short (3 day) course of high-dose methylprednisolone to placebo and found a statistically significant decrease in stricture formation in the high-dose steroids group. Prior to this study, the medical literature suggested no benefit of corticosteroids because there was no demonstrated significant decrease in stricture formations after grade IIa, IIb, or III esophageal burns, but there was increased risk for hemorrhage, infectious complications, severe esophagogastric necrosis, and prepyloric ulcer formation. Steroids can also mask early signs of inflammation and inhibit resistance to infection. Accordingly, they are not indicated to reduce the extent of esophageal injury. Controversy also surrounds the administration of steroids in patients with airway edema secondary to caustic ingestion. There are no controlled studies evaluating this practice, and the same downside risks exist as for steroid use for esophageal stricture. Airway edema can be fatal, however, and a single dose of a potent corticosteroid might mitigate some of the edema with minimal risk to the patient. We recommend dexamethasone 10 mg IV when there is indication of airway edema.

Prophylactic antibiotics are not indicated. Patients with proven perforation should have an emergent surgical consultation.

The risk of perforation from esophageal dilation is decreased if the initial procedure is delayed beyond 4 weeks post-ingestion. At this time, healing, remodeling, and potential stricture formation in the esophagus have already taken place. Following perforation, patients develop clinical symptoms such as dyspnea or chest pain in the setting of associated subcutaneous emphysema or pneumomediastinum. Diagnostic imaging is recommended to identify the perforation and provide information for emergent surgical repair. Patients with stricture formation require long-term endoscopic follow-up for the presence of neoplastic changes of the esophagus that may occur with a delay of several years to decades.

DISPOSITION

Asymptomatic patients can undergo endoscopy in the emergency department. Those patients with grades 0 or I injury may be discharged home after 4 to 6 hours of observation with close follow-up monitoring with appropriate gastroenterology or otolaryngology consultants.[9] They can have a liquid diet for 24 hours and then gradually transition to soft food over the next 3 days and to a full diet thereafter if progressing well.

Surgical intervention is required in cases of hollow viscus perforation; early exploration may also be warranted in cases of suggested full-thickness burns.[9] Symptomatic patients, particularly those with potential for airway compromise, or high-grade esophageal or gastric injuries, require admission to an intensive care unit. If endoscopy is unavailable, the patient should be transferred to a tertiary care facility where it can be performed. Psychiatric evaluation is indicated in patients with intentional ingestion.

SPECIAL CASES

Ocular alkali exposures are true ophthalmologic emergencies. Immediate irrigation with at least 2 L of normal saline per eye is indicated in almost all cases except frank perforation. Management is described in Chapter 57. Dermal caustic exposures can also result in significant burn injuries (see Chapter 55). Clothing removal, copious irrigation, and local wound débridement are the most important initial treatment measures.

Povidone-Iodine

Povidone-iodine (Betadine) is used as a surgical scrub and is not a caustic agent, but ingestion of tincture of iodine can cause severe GI injury and is potentially life-threatening. Gastric irrigation with starch or milk in these cases may convert iodine to the much less toxic iodide. Either of these agents is most likely to be effective if administered within the first 30 to 45 minutes post ingestion. The goal is to convert the gastric effluent to a dark blue or purple hue.

Phenol and Formaldehyde

Ingestion of phenol or formaldehyde can also cause severe caustic injury to the GI tract. Both phenol and formaldehyde are general protoplasmic poisons and can cause protein denaturation and coagulation necrosis. Systemic symptoms, including dysrhythmias, hypotension, seizures, and coma, may also result from phenol ingestion. Acidosis may be prominent after formaldehyde ingestion because of its metabolism to formic acid. Phenol is well absorbed through the skin, and dermal exposure may result in burns and systemic toxicity. Although dermal decontamination of phenol exposures with low–molecular-weight polyethylene glycol has been suggested, there is no evidence that it is superior to irrigation with water, which is more readily accessible.

Hydrogen Peroxide

Ingestion of concentrated (>30%) hydrogen peroxide (H_2O_2) may cause GI burn injuries and the formation of gas emboli. Radiographic evaluation for the presence of gas in the chest or abdominal cavities, including the portal system, should be performed in symptomatic patients or those who ingest concentrated H_2O_2. Hyperbaric oxygen has been used successfully to treat gas emboli from H_2O_2 ingestion.

Button Batteries

Button (disk) batteries and conventional alkaline cylindrical batteries pose potential obstructive and chemical hazards if they are ingested. Ingestion of large (25-mm) wafer-sized button batteries was a common problem in the past, but the smaller button batteries of today are less likely to cause esophageal obstruction. Button batteries are usually made of a metallic salt (lithium, mercury, nickel, zinc, cadmium, or silver) bathed in NaOH or KOH. Obstruction can cause pressure necrosis, caustic injury due to leakage of alkaline medium, or electrical injury. Caustic injury is much less common. Ulceration, perforation, and possible fistula formation occur but are uncommon. Heavy-metal toxicity in this setting has not been reported with newer-generation of disk batteries.

Evaluation of button battery ingestions includes radiography to assess the position of the foreign body. Batteries lodged in the airway or esophagus require expeditious removal. Single gastric or intestinal batteries can be treated with watchful waiting, generally in the patient's home. Checking the stool for passage of the batteries is recommended. Follow-up radiographs should be obtained one week after ingestion if the battery has not passed. If the patient becomes symptomatic with acute abdominal pain or exhibits GI bleeding, expedited reassessment is indicated.

The references for this chapter can be found online at ExpertConsult. com.

144

Cocaine and Other Sympathomimetics

Michael A. Chary and Timothy B. Erickson

KEY CONCEPTS

- Excessive use of stimulants can lead to *sympathomimetic toxicity*, manifesting as tachycardia, hypertension, mydriasis, diaphoresis, hyperthermia, hyperreflexia, and agitation. If untreated, sympathomimetic toxicity can lead to seizures, coma, and death.
- Administration of benzodiazepines is the key therapeutic intervention for sympathomimetic toxicity. Ketamine, olanzapine, and butyrophenones are alternative adjuncts if the cause of severe agitation is not clearly sympathomimetic toxicity.
- Worsening hyperthermia portends imminent death. Reduce body temperature rapidly by external cooling, sedation, and, if needed, paralysis.
- Anti-hypertensives are adjuncts to benzodiazepines. Antihypertensives do not treat as many aspects of sympathomimetic toxicity as do benzodiazepines, however, and short-acting antihypertensive agents (e.g., phentolamine, nitroglycerin, nicardipine, clevidipine) are preferred.
- Wide-complex rhythms secondary to stimulants (cocaine, bupropion) may respond to intravenous sodium bicarbonate administration.
- Cocaine body packers who develop toxicity need emergent surgical intervention to limit bowel necrosis and life-threatening sequelae caused by leaking packets.
- Novel psychoactive substances (e.g., MDMA, bath salts) combine stimulant, hallucinogenic, and psychedelic effects. They generally produce longer-lasting and more intense effects than cocaine or amphetamine.
- Screen for hyponatremia in patients with sympathomimetic or serotonin toxicity.
- If the clinical presentation does not fit the history (e.g., ingested cocaine but hypoxic and somnolent), consider a contaminant or alternate cause. Contaminants change rapidly and vary by geographic region. Consult a medical toxicologist or regional poison control center.

FOUNDATIONS

Sympathomimetics are substances that activate the sympathetic nervous system (Box 144.1). These substances stimulate release (amphetamine, phenethylamines) or decrease reuptake (cocaine, amphetamine, phenethylamines) of neurotransmitters (serotonin, norepinephrine, dopamine, epinephrine). As a result, these neurotransmitters remain in synapses longer and activate neuronal pathways more strongly and persistently.[1] Stimulants cause an acute upper effect—euphoria and increased energy. Excessive use can lead to sympathomimetic toxicity—tachycardia, hypertension, mydriasis, diaphoresis, hyperthermia, hyperreflexia, and agitation. If untreated, sympathomimetic toxicity can lead to seizures, coma, and death.

This chapter reviews the epidemiology, pathophysiology, and treatment of stimulant toxicity. Over the past two decades, many designer chemicals have emerged with properties that combine traditional drug classes. Some are stimulants and hallucinogens. Others are stimulants and sedatives. Toxicity from a stimulant, whatever its pedigree, manifests as overactivation of the nervous and cardiovascular systems. The primary goals of clinical intervention are to decrease activation of the sympathetic nervous system by sedating the patient, identify end-organ toxicity, and involve a medical toxicologist to guide further management for more complicated cases.

Cocaine

Cocaine is the canonical ubiquitous stimulant drug of abuse. The indigenous people of South America chew the cocoa leaf (*Erythroxylon coca*) for energy. Spanish colonists initially banned chewing cocoa leaves, but soon acknowledged their ergogenic properties, legalizing and taxing cocoa leaf production in the 16th century. In 1855, Friedrich Gaedcke isolated pure cocaine. This three-century delay partly reflects the difficulty in keeping cocaine warm and dry while shipping it across the Atlantic Ocean. Soon after, cocaine became a popular ingredient in beverages, pharmaceuticals, and tonics. In the 19th century, physicians such as Carl Koller and William S. Halsted explored the use of cocaine as an anesthetic, exploiting its unique ability to block sodium channels and constrict blood vessels. Victorian literature mentions cocaine's ability to "stave off the ennui of existence," and it was notably used by the character Sherlock Holmes to keep him stimulated between cases. In 1914, the U.S. Congress passed the Harrison Narcotics Tax Act, which required a physician's order to dispense cocaine and narcotics.

Epidemiology

General statistics on drug use may not distinguish between people who have ever used cocaine, those who have used in the last year, or those who have used in the last week. As a result, these studies combine different populations: the regular user, the sporadic user, the heavy user, the sampler, adults, and adolescents. Any of these groups may experience an overdose of cocaine, although anecdotal experience suggests that inexperienced drug users with psychiatric comorbidities are the population most at risk for cocaine toxicity. Regular use of cocaine accelerates vascular pathology, including coronary artery arteriosclerosis. It is more useful for the clinician to consider incidence or prevalence in terms of the at-risk population. Most information on novel psychoactive substances comes from observational studies on social media, which rarely can identify the exposure or fully define the population.

The prevalence of people in the world who reportedly used cocaine was 13 million in 2012 (0.18%), increasing to 18 million (0.24%) in 2016.[2] The fraction of 8th graders in the United States who reportedly used cocaine was 0.9%, nearly four times the global average. The fraction of 12th graders who used cocaine was 3.8%, again, nearly four times the global average.[3]

In the emergency department (ED), cocaine use is associated with up to 20% of drug misuse-related deaths in the United States[4,5] and between 20% and 50% in the European Union. These data may underestimate the incidence of morbidity and mortality attributable to cocaine, especially in trauma patients.[6] In 2017, drug overdose deaths involving cocaine increased by more than 33%, with almost 14,000 Americans dying from an overdose involving cocaine. From 2016 to 2017, the largest relative and absolute rate changes for cocaine-involved overdoses among racial/ethnic groups were highest among non-Hispanic Blacks. The highest death rate for overdoses involving cocaine in 2017 also occurred among Non-Hispanic Blacks.[7]

Formulation

Unpurified cocaine paste is converted to more usable forms of cocaine. The crystallized freebase of the cocaine alkaloid is known as crack cocaine. It is inhaled with a "crack pipe" designed to tolerate the high temperature required to volatilize pure cocaine. The high lipid solubility and rapid transport from the lungs into the brain contribute to crack's rapid onset of action (Table 144.1). The water-soluble salts of cocaine (i.e., cocaine hydrochloride and cocaine sulfate) are available as a white crystalline powder that is inhaled intranasally or dissolved and injected intravenously. Oral administration is rare except for among those patients who are smuggling or concealing drugs.

Pathophysiology

Cocaine decreases the clearance of dopamine, epinephrine, norepinephrine, and serotonin from synapses between nerve cells or between nerve cells and muscle cells (Fig. 144.1). Decreased clearance allows these neurotransmitters to stay bound to post-synaptic receptors longer, leading to autonomic stimulation (all four neurotransmitters), euphoria (dopamine and serotonin), and a sensation that things are more salient, or important, than they might be otherwise (dopamine) (see Box 144.1). Norepinephrine causes vasoconstriction by stimulation of alpha-adrenergic receptors on vascular smooth muscle. Epinephrine increases myocardial contractility and heart rate through stimulation of beta$_1$-adrenergic receptors. In addition to catecholamine release, the reuptake of these stimulatory neurotransmitters from synaptic clefts is inhibited, altering the normal balance between excitatory and inhibitory tones in the central nervous system (CNS). Subsequent stimulation propagates peripheral catecholamine release. Reuptake of serotonin is similarly inhibited and can cause serotonergic excess, as well.

Cocaine is also a local anesthetic. It blocks sodium channels, slowing nerve impulses from neuronal pain fibers by prolonging the upstroke of the action potential. Along with adrenergic stimulation, this can precipitate tachydysrhythmias such as supraventricular or, with severe sodium channel blockade, ventricular tachycardia. A clinical marker for heart sodium channel blockade is the duration of the QRS on a 12-lead electrocardiogram (ECG). QRS durations longer than 100 ms in a patient with a previously unremarkable ECG suggests sodium channel blockade. The prognostic value of the QRS in patients with preexisting bundle branch blocks or who are actively paced is less known.

The half-life of cocaine is approximately 90 minutes. Cholinesterases in the plasma and liver metabolize cocaine to the inactive metabolites—ecgonine methyl ester and benzoyl ecgonine. In the presence of ethanol, cocaine is metabolized to cocaethylene, which has the same effects as cocaine,[8] giving rise to the observation that ethanol prolongs rather than counteracts cocaine's effects. Genetic differences in the phenotypic expression of plasma cholinesterases may explain the variation across individuals in susceptibility to cocaine toxicity. Most standard urine drug screens in the ED test for benzoylecgonine, which is a metabolite only of cocaine. It can be detected in the urine within 4 hours after using cocaine and remains detectable, depending on the laboratory threshold, for up to 7 days after use.

Amphetamine and Its Derivatives

Amphetamines are structurally distinct from cocaine even though they have similar effects. They are in fact structurally more similar to dopamine than cocaine. The word "amphetamine" is an abbreviation of **a**lpha-**m**ethyl**ph**en**et**hyl**amine**. Phenethylamine is the parent compound from which amphetamines, catecholamines, cathinones (bath salts), and novel psychoactive substances such as methylenedioxymethamphetamine (MDMA) can be derived.

Amphetamines were discovered while chemists John K. Smith and Mahlon Kline were trying to develop a cheaper alternative nasal decongestant to ephedrine. Beginning in 1929, dextroamphetamine was sold as Dexedrine. It was made a prescription drug in 1959, however, owing to concerns over its addictive potential. The racemic mixture is sold as Adderall. Amphetamine-based psychostimulants with abuse potential include illicit drugs, such as methamphetamine and ecstasy, and prescription stimulants, as well. Prescription stimulants, used to treat conditions such as attention-deficit/hyperactivity disorder (ADHD), are commonly misused.

Epidemiology

Rates of overdose deaths from all psychostimulants have been increasing since 2010. More than 10,000 Americans died from an overdose involving psychostimulants with abuse potential in 2017, which was a

---

BOX 144.1	Clinical Effects of Sympathomimetics

Central nervous system (CNS) excitation
Diaphoresis
Hypertension
Hyperthermia
Increased motor tone
Mydriasis
Tachycardia

TABLE 144.1 Cocaine Pharmacology by Route of Administration

Route	Formula	Onset of Action	Peak Effect	Duration
Inhalation	"Crack"	8–12 s	2–5 min	10–20 min
Intranasal	Cocaine HCl	2–5 min	5–10 min	30 min
Intravenous	Cocaine HCl	Seconds	10–20 min	60–90 min
Oral	Cocaine HCl	30–60 min	60–90 min	Unknown
"Skin popping"	Cocaine HCl	Unknown	Unknown	Unknown

HCl, Hydrogen chloride.

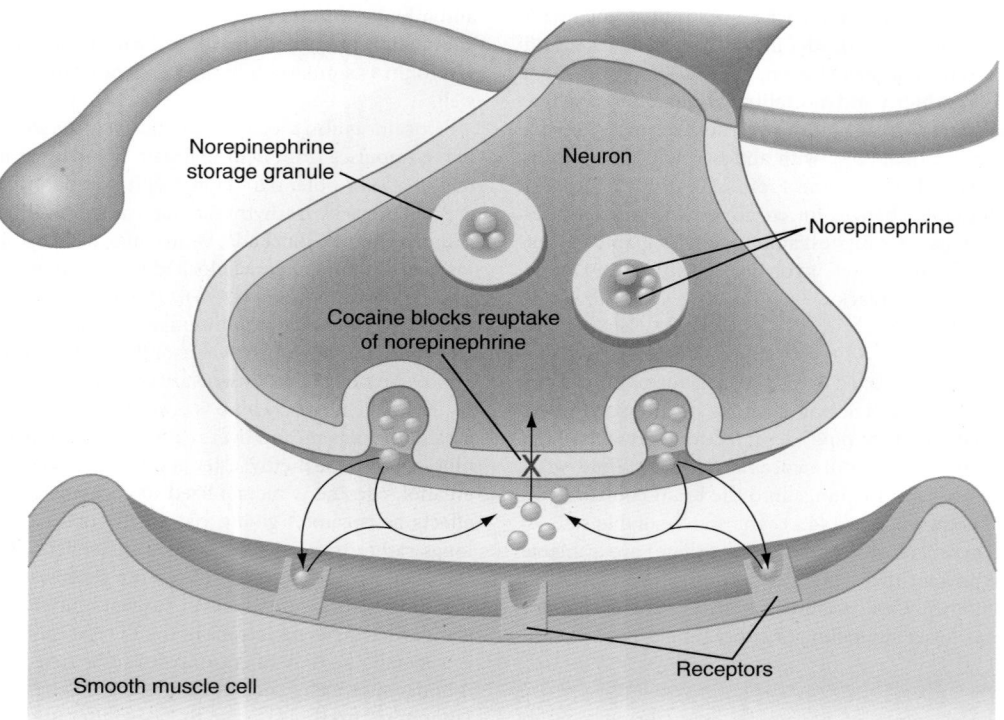

Fig. 144.1 How cocaine increases sympathetic tone by increasing neurotransmitters in the synapse.

nearly 40% increase over the previous year. From 2016 to 2017, non-Hispanic whites had the greatest percent increase in the death rate for overdoses involving psychostimulants, while the largest absolute rate change in psychostimulant-involved overdoses was in American Indian/Alaska Native (AI/AN) populations. AI/AN also experienced the highest death rate for overdoses involving psychostimulants in 2017.

The highest rate increases of psychostimulant-related overdose deaths were in the Midwest region in 2017, while the overall rate was highest in the West. However, the highest overdose death rates were in West Virginia and Alaska.[7]

Methamphetamine

Methamphetamine (methyl amphetamine) was discovered shortly after amphetamine, also as an alternative to ephedrine. Like amphetamine, it was extensively used during the Second World War, to the point that German soldiers called it "Stuka-Tabletten," referring to the pilots of the Stuka dive bombers. The effects of methamphetamine, also known as "crank" and "crystal meth," last longer. Some paranoid delusions persist for 24 hours. The production of methamphetamines requires metal salts. Lead toxicity from the drug being inappropriately produced has been reported. Injuries during illicit methamphetamine production or police raids include exposure to anhydrous ammonia, hydrochloric acid, sodium hydroxide, ether, and ephedrine, as well as burns and explosions in "meth labs." Amphetamines are usually ingested orally as pills, but can be crushed and injected, as well.

Pathophysiology

Amphetamines act by multiple mechanisms to increase norepinephrine, epinephrine, dopamine, and serotonin levels in the brain. They increase the amount of neurotransmitter released per action potential, decrease the rate of clearance from the synaptic cleft, and decrease the rate of enzymatic inactivation. The subsequent CNS

stimulation results in sympathomimetic effects nearly identical to those from cocaine, but the effects generally last longer and are less intense. Patients are at risk for hyperthermia, hypertensive emergencies, dysrhythmias, myocardial ischemia, and hyperkalemia associated with rhabdomyolysis.[9] In contrast to cocaine, amphetamines do not block sodium channels. Although urine drug screens can identify amphetamines, they are of little utility in the treatment of an intoxicated patient.

Phenylethylamines, which are closely related in molecular structure to amphetamines, include the "2C" and "NBOMe" drugs, named for the location of specific structural elements along the amphetamine backbone.[10] These have powerful serotonergic, hallucinogenic effects, and patients can present with adrenergic toxicity and behavioral agitation. The brominated form (street-named "Bromo-DragonFLY" due to its structural similarity to a dragonfly) is associated with a necrotizing angiitis that can compromise blood flow to the limbs.[11] Limb or digit pain in such patients warrants comprehensive monitoring and evaluation for vasospasm and tissue ischemia.

Ephedrine and Ephedra

Ephedra is a plant-based medicinal preparation from the herb Ephedra sinica. It is an evergreen shrub-like plant native to Asia and also grows in southwestern United States. Ephedra, also known as the Chinese herbal product Ma Huang, has been associated with strokes and deaths in adolescent users. People have used ephedra for centuries in China for colds, fever, flu, headaches, asthma, nasal congestion, and wheezing. Ephedrine is the main active ingredient in ephedra. In 1997, in response to mounting concern over cardiovascular side effects, the U.S. Food and Drug Administration (FDA) banned products containing 8 mg or more of ephedrine alkaloids and required all ephedra-containing products to disclose the health risks of heart attack, stroke, and death.

Ephedra is widely used by athletes as a performance-enhancing drug, despite a lack of evidence that it improves athletic performance.

Its use has been completely banned from all sports competitions since 2003. Bitter orange is marketed as a "safer" herbal alternative to ephedrine. It contains p-synephrine, which is demethylated ephedrine. At the dose amounts generally available, bitter orange appears to have neither stimulant nor cardiotoxic effects.[12] Ephedrine (and its diastereomer pseudoephedrine) can also be used as a precursor in the manufacture of methamphetamine by dehydrating it. Ephedrine and its stereoisomer, norpseudoephedrine, cross the blood-brain barrier and lead to the release of noradrenaline and dopamine in the substantia nigra.

Caffeine

Caffeine (1,3,7-trimethylxanthine) is a widely consumed psychoactive substance noted for its ergogenic and prokinetic effects. It is a common component of energy drinks and weight loss supplements. It is also a reported adulterant in cocaine, MDMA, and many novel psychoactive substances. In one analysis of 512 street samples of cocaine from Brazil, caffeine concentration ranged between 40% and 60% by weight.[13] Caffeine potentiates the euphoric effects of cocaine in mice.[14] Caffeine is an adenosine antagonist, binding to post-synaptic adenosine receptors throughout the body. Toxic doses of caffeine (greater than 100 mg/kg, or roughly one cup of coffee per kilogram) may induce status epilepticus and tachydysrhythmias refractory to standard treatment regimens requiring hemodialysis.[15]

Novel Psychoactive Substances

Novel psychoactive stimulants are structural variants of amphetamine that combine hallucinogenic, euphoric, and stimulant properties to strike balances between auditory hallucinations, visual hallucinations, paranoia, euphoria, dysphoria, and dissociation.[16] A general rule of thumb used by informal chemists is that aromatic substitutions increase the hallucinogen/entactogen effects and aliphatic substitutions increase the stimulant effects.

Novel psychoactive stimulants are often combined with ethanol or sedatives to mitigate anxiety or dysphoria, or to prolong the perceptual alteration.[17] Novel psychoactive substances are a broader category including synthetic cannabinoid receptor agonists (K2, synthetic marijuana). This chapter does not discuss those substances as they are conceptually closer to cannabis than stimulants.

Data on the usage of most novel psychoactive substances are lacking. Epidemiologists have used wastewater analysis to quantify exposure,[18] but it is difficult to estimate usage from this method. From questionnaires, the use of mephedrone, a bath salt (cathinone), seems more prominent in the United Kingdom than the United States, where 0.5% of people aged 16 to 59 reported using mephedrone at least once in 2015 to 2016.[19]

There is a similar trajectory between derivatives of amphetamine overtaking amphetamine and derivatives of fentanyl overtaking the parent compound fentanyl. In both cases, the derivatives are often more potent than the unmodified compounds, have narrower therapeutic indices, and are generally not detected on standard drug screens. In addition, novel combinations such as methamphetamine contaminated with fentanyl (street named "goofballing") are emerging.

Ecstasy

MDMA (ecstasy, Molly) is a derivative of amphetamine. It is the canonical entactogen. An entactogen produces experiences of emotional communion, oneness, relatedness, emotional openness—that is, empathy or sympathy. The molecular structure of MDMA is in between amphetamine and serotonin, explaining its combination of sympathomimetic and serotonergic features. The term "Molly" (short for molecular) is used to describe a product with a higher concentration of MDMA, although these products may contain merely caffeine or placebos. User reports are, therefore, often unreliable in determining true exposure.

MDMA can precipitate hyponatremia via drug-induced syndrome of inappropriate antidiuretic hormone secretion (SIADH). MDMA and its metabolite increase the release of vasopressin (anti-diuretic hormone), which in the setting of high free water intake, results in free water retention.[20] Patients with MDMA-induced hyponatremia demonstrate urine with high osmolality and sodium. Chronic use of MDMA and its variants (MDA) may cause irreversible neurologic damage to serotonergic neurons in mice.[21]

Bath Salts

Bath salts are derivatives of cathinone, an active ingredient in the leaves of khat or qat (*Catha edulis*). Cathinone is, itself, a phenethylamine derivative. Khat leaves also contain methcathinone, a similarly potent sympathomimetic.

Bath salts were first encountered in Japan in the early 2000s. The ease of synthesis and modification of specific functional groups of the parent cathinone make these drugs particularly difficult to regulate.[22,23] This led to a cat-and-mouse dynamic between internet vendors and regulatory agencies. Most initial bath salts contained mephedrone (4-methyl methcathinone). Once regulatory agencies developed tests for mephedrone, the composition of bath salts rapidly changed to include methylone, ethylone, butylone, pyrovalerone, methylenedioxypyrovalerone (MDPV), methcathinone, and ethcathinone. One cathinone, bupropion (Wellbutrin), is approved for medical use in the United States.

Bath salts may be ingested, inhaled, or injected and can result in severe agitation, sympathomimetic effects, hyperthermia, and rhabdomyolysis. One in vitro study suggests that cathinones and MDMA may have direct myotoxic effects by increasing the permeability of the outer mitochondrial membrane.[24] Smoking khat typically results in little toxicity because cathinone is heat labile. Numerous fatalities have been reported, causing the U.S. Drug Enforcement Administration (DEA) to categorize these agents as illegal Schedule I substances.[25] Synthetic cathinones are usually not detectable on routine urine drug screens. Treatment is similar to that of cocaine and amphetamine toxicity and includes adequate dosing of benzodiazepines for agitation with diazepam, lorazepam, or butyrophenone antipsychotic agents, such as haloperidol and droperidol (see Management, Pharmacologic Sedation for Agitation section).

Some users of synthetic methcathinone demonstrate an extrapyramidal syndrome similar to Parkinson disease with elevated manganese concentrations, presumably resulting from contamination during production. Chelation therapy is, in general, not useful in treating the parkinsonism associated with manganese toxicity.

Kratom

Kratom is a tropical tree (*Mitragyna speciosa*) native to Southeast Asia. Its leaves contain psychotropic compounds, the most studied of which are mitragynine and 7-hydroxymitragynine. Kratom is not currently an illegal substance and can be readily acquired over the internet. It is sometimes sold as an extract, gum, or green powder in packets labeled "not for human consumption." Kratom was traditionally chewed or brewed in a tea in a fashion similar to coca leaves. Mitragynine and 7-hydroxymitragynine exert opioid effects at low doses and stimulant effects at higher doses. This has led to the usage of kratom as a means to treat opioid withdrawal or to address problematic opioid use. There is one report of possible kratom use presenting as opioid intoxication requiring sedation after naloxone, similar to cocaine "speedballing," or cocaine contaminated with heroin.[26]

Clinical Features

The treatment of sympathomimetic toxicity begins with recognition of high-risk symptoms. The imminent life-threatening nature may necessitate treatment before the most likely cause is established. Risk-stratification begins with recognition of high-risk features of sympathomimetic toxicity, which are described in this section.

The sympathomimetic toxidrome refers to the constellation of tachycardia, hypertension, hyperthermia, tachypnea, mydriasis, diaphoresis, tremor, hyperactive bowel sounds, agitation, psychosis, and seizures. These clinical signs reflect overactivation of the sympathetic nervous system by sympathomimetic substances.

Sympathomimetic toxicity is an acute phenomenon with abnormal vital signs. Ingestions that do not develop abnormal vital signs after an appropriate period of monitoring may be medically cleared. Toxicity can range from mild tachycardia or agitation, depending on the amount ingested and the potency of the medication.

A patient with mild toxicity is alert and awake but may be diaphoretic, tachycardic, mydriatic, or hypertensive without organ damage. A patient with severe toxicity may be agitated, combative, or hyperthermic. Patients may present with focal acute pain syndromes, circulatory abnormalities, acute hypertension, coronary vasospasm, or seizures.

Additives, contaminants, or other drugs may create a mixed picture. Patients may combine intravenous (IV) heroin and cocaine ("speedballing"), presenting with signs of opioid toxicity but manifesting signs of cocaine toxicity after they receive naloxone. Patients may combine cocaine or crack cocaine with ethanol to elongate cocaine's euphoric effects.

The clinical presentation of sympathomimetic toxicity depends on the dose, route of administration, coingestants, and time elapsed between ingestion and presentation. Initial assessment should focus on rapidly fatal complications including hyperthermia, hypertensive emergencies, cardiac dysrhythmias, and hyponatremia.

Hyperthermia

Cocaine-toxic patients have increased motor tone and generate excessive heat. Vasoconstriction and salt and water depletion can compromise cooling, resulting in life-threatening hyperthermia with core temperatures exceeding 106°F (41°C). Delay in recognition and management increases the likelihood of death. Even with a normal temperature, increased motor tone can release intramuscular (IM) creatine kinase (CK), with rhabdomyolysis and its attendant renal and electrolyte complications. Acute psychomotor agitation with delirium increases the risk of hyperthermia.

Hypertensive Emergencies

Acute cocaine-induced hypertension can injure the cardiovascular and CNS systems. Reported sequelae include aortic dissection, pulmonary edema, myocardial ischemia and infarction, intracranial hemorrhage, stroke, and infarction in the distribution of the anterior spinal artery.[27] Vasospasm can also compromise perfusion. Intestinal infarctions and mesenteric ischemia can occur, particularly in body packers with large oral ingestions. Other local ischemic events include retinal vasospasm, renal infarctions, and placental insufficiency and infarction in the gravid uterus.

Cardiac Dysrhythmias

Sinus tachycardia is the most common rhythm. Atrial fibrillation and other supraventricular tachycardias can occur as a result of the surge in catecholamines. Life-threatening dysrhythmia may occur suddenly, heralded by abrupt diminution of cardiac output and loss of consciousness. Torsades de pointes from hypokalemia due to potassium shifting into the cells or wide-complex tachycardias from blockade of fast sodium channels on the myocardium may deteriorate into poorly perfusing or fatal ventricular rhythms. Transient conduction abnormalities consistent with a Brugada-type pattern are associated with cocaine, although some cases may be unmasking previously undiagnosed pathology. Hyperkalemia from rhabdomyolysis and myocardial ischemia can also cause dysrhythmias.

Cocaine Use Disorder, Stimulant Use Disorder

Cocaine's effects on the CNS can lead to craving behavior and cocaine use disorders that lead to secondary harm (cellulitis from injection, trauma, and sexually transmitted infections due to accessing drugs by risky means). Paranoia, either drug-induced or from underlying psychiatric illness, may occur even after the acute effects of the drug subside. Similar to phencyclidine (PCP), the neuropsychiatric effects of cocaine can alter behavior and judgment, increasing the risk of violent injuries.

Cardiomyopathy

Cocaine may precipitate heart failure by increasing the risk of myocardial ischemia and by direct injury to the myocardium.[28] The incidence of cardiomyopathy attributable to cocaine use is not well known, but case studies suggest that one should treat cardiomyopathy due to cocaine use just as cardiomyopathy from any other cause and encourage cessation of sympathomimetics.[29]

Washout

Those who binge on sympathomimetics have a prolonged activation of the sympathetic nervous system and reward pathways. This prolonged activation depletes catecholamine stores, disrupts salt/water balance, and may lead to malnutrition as eating falls to the wayside in the face of desire for cocaine. After a cocaine binge, users may experience cocaine washout, an obtunded state where the user is profoundly sedated but arousable and oriented when aroused, with normal vital signs or a mild sinus bradycardia. Users of MDMA report "suicide Sundays," where those who reported using MDMA on Friday night felt profoundly depressed on Sunday.

Nontoxicologic sequelae

Complications also arise from the route of administration. Inhalation may cause oropharyngeal burns. Inhaling and suppressing the cough reflex may precipitate spontaneous pneumothorax, pneumopericardium, or pneumomediastinum. Intranasal cocaine use is associated with sinusitis and nasopalatine necrosis or perforation. IV users have a high risk of infection with blood-borne viruses, local abscesses, and systemic bacterial infections, including *Clostridium botulinum* and endocarditis. Transdermal injection of cocaine, or "skin popping," has similar types of complications, especially skin abscesses. For chronic users, addiction or psychological dependence is mediated through specific dopaminergic neurotransmitter pathways. Although there are no well-defined syndromes constituting cocaine withdrawal, patients have strong cravings for the drug or a general feeling of dysphoria that is not physiologically life-threatening.

Some of the toxicity associated with cocaine is due to the unintentional ingestion of adulterants, rather than the formulation of cocaine or route of administration. Of a case series of 97 patients with serum cocaine levels, 31 had one of the following: atropine, phenacetin, hydroxyzine, ketamine, lidocaine, or tetramisole.[30] An analysis of 615 samples from two drug seizures in the United States identified the following contaminants: caffeine (31%), quinine/quinidine (25%), levamisole (12%), acetaminophen (8%), and procaine (8%).[31]

Levamisole is an older adulterant, related to tetramisole, used to dilute cocaine. Neither levamisole nor tetramisole is psychoactive;

rather, they have a similar consistency to cocaine. Levamisole was used to treat pediatric nephritic syndrome and rheumatoid arthritis until it was withdrawn from the market due to hematological complications and vasculopathy. Agranulocytosis, vasculopathy with thrombosis, dermal ulcers, and purpura, often affecting the earlobes, occurred from unintentional exposure to levamisole. A case series of 50 patients reports the development of long-lasting anti-levamisole antibodies that contribute to a serum sickness-like illness.[32] Clenbuterol is a beta-agonist with a similar appearance to cocaine that is used to dilute the amount of cocaine to sell more units. Clenbuterol inhalation or injection may precipitate tachydysrhythmias and hypokalemia.

DIFFERENTIAL DIAGNOSES

The differential diagnoses of the sympathomimetic toxidrome can be split into toxicologic and non-toxicologic causes. One useful rule of thumb is that all vital signs are "revved-up" in frank sympathomimetic toxicity. The heart rate, blood pressure, core temperature, and respiratory rate are all elevated.

Other causes of tachycardia are usually normotensive or hypotensive, for example tachydysrhythmias or hemorrhage. Thyroid storm presents similarly to the sympathomimetic toxidrome because thyroxine also activates the sympathetic nervous system.

A current medication list can help identify possible coingestants. Thought disorders and auditory hallucinations are not typically present, unlike acute psychotic or manic episodes (Box 144.2). It can be difficult to distinguish cocaine toxicity from withdrawal from sedative-hypnotics (benzodiazepines, ethanol, baclofen, gamma-hydroxybutyrate). A history of abstinence from sedative-hypnotics after heavy use may suggest sedative-hypnotic withdrawal if there is documented prior use and no other compelling explanation.

Toxicity from other sympathomimetic agents such as amphetamines, amphetamine derivatives, and PCP can present similarly to cocaine toxicity. Cocaine toxicity generally causes more frequent cardiotoxic effects (acute myocardial infarction, cardiac dysrhythmia, aortic dissection) than amphetamines or PCP.[33] One should also include myocardial ischemia, hyperkalemia, and drug-induced sodium channel blockade (e.g., cyclic antidepressants) in the differential for cocaine-induced wide-complex tachycardia.

Designer amphetamines such as MDMA are more likely than cocaine to cause hyponatremia, either from SIADH or excessive intake of free water. Patients abusing methamphetamine also tend to have more muscle wasting, malnutrition, and poor dental hygiene than chronic cocaine users. PCP toxicity may be distinguished by the presence of multidirectional nystagmus and highly combative behavior.

Like cocaine, patients with antimuscarinic poisoning (such as diphenhydramine, atropine, and jimsonweed; see Chapter 140) may present with agitation, tachycardia, hypertension, and mydriasis. Findings of acute urinary retention and dry mucous membranes distinguish the anticholinergic from the sympathomimetic toxidromes.

The hyperthermic state induced by cocaine toxicity should be further differentiated from classic and exertional heat stroke. Heat stroke tends to have more ambient environmental factors, dehydration, and more profound changes in mental status than cocaine toxicity. Serotonin toxicity (previously called serotonin syndrome) is often precipitated by the addition of a new serotonergic agent or a substance that interferes with the metabolism of a previously tolerated agent. Serotonin toxicity is most commonly reported with selective serotonin reuptake inhibitors (SSRIs) and monoamine oxidase inhibitors (MAOIs), but it has also been reported with cyclic antidepressants and atypical antipsychotics. The cardinal signs of serotonin toxicity include altered mental status and autonomic instability (hyperthermia,

BOX 144.2 Differential Diagnosis of Agitated Delirium

Endocrine disease
   Thyrotoxicosis
Heatstroke
Infections
   Bacterial or viral meningitis or encephalitis
Psychiatric
   Acute mania
   Acute schizophrenia
Metabolic causes
   Electrolyte abnormalities
   Hyperammonemia
   Hypoglycemia
   Hypoxia
   Uremia
Postictal state
Structural lesions of the CNS
   Hemorrhage
   Mass
   Stroke
   Trauma
Toxicologic causes
   Amphetamines and derivatives
   Anticholinergics
   Caffeine
   Cocaine
Lithium
Neuroleptic malignant syndrome (NMS)
   PCP, ketamine
   Sedative-hypnotic withdrawal
   Serotonin toxicity
   Sympathomimetics, stimulants
   Synthetic cannabinoid receptor agonists

CNS, Central nervous system; PCP, phencyclidine.

diaphoresis, labile blood pressure) with hyperreflexia and clonus. The neuromuscular findings in serotonin toxicity are more prominent in the lower extremities, in contrast to many motor disorders, which prefer the upper extremities or spread diffusely. The agitation described with serotonin syndrome is less organized and the patient is unlikely to be ambulatory or severely combative. The onset is typically abrupt in the setting of serotonergic drug interactions or overdose. The finding of clonus is an important differentiating feature, because this is present in serotonin syndrome but absent in cocaine toxicity. Similar to serotonin toxicity, neuroleptic malignant syndrome (NMS) also presents with altered mental status, hyperthermia, and agitation. However, unlike serotonin toxicity, peripheral muscular effects tend toward rigidity and decreased reflexes rather than clonus and hyperreflexia. This is due to dopaminergic depletion from the use of dopamine antagonists, such as the older or classic antipsychotic agents. Patients presenting with NMS generally have a gradual course of hypokinesis and increasing resting muscle tone in the setting of escalating antipsychotic use. The alteration in mental status is more commonly a catatonic state.

DIAGNOSTIC TESTING

Urine drug screening (UDS) for cocaine is accurate but unlikely to change treatment in the ED, except to provide diagnostic clarity when cocaine toxicity is suspected (e.g., young, otherwise healthy adult with chest pain) to substantiate exposure in cases of abuse or neglect, to confirm cocaine as the unknown substance in body packers, or to exclude acute cocaine toxicity in an acutely paranoid patient. Most urine drug screens in the ED for cocaine are an immunoassay for benzoyl ecgonine, a chemical produced only by the metabolism of cocaine. Benzoyl ecgonine persists in the urine for 3 to 7 days after last use, depending on the detection limits. Despite popular belief, the local anesthetic lidocaine does not produce a false-positive cocaine screen.[34]

Urine Drug Screening for Amphetamines and Amphetamine Derivatives

The urine drug screen for amphetamine is less useful for providing diagnostic clarity in the ED than the urine drug screen for cocaine. In contrast to cocaine's unique structure, amphetamine, as described above, serves as a starting point for many FDA-approved medications (Adderall [amphetamine salts], Vyvanse [lisdexamfetamine], Wellbutrin [bupropion]) and novel psychoactive substances (cathinones [bath salts], NBOMes, and methamphetamine). The common starting point of these medications and novel psychoactive substances may lead to a false positive result, more accurately termed a cross-reaction. As an example, some beta blockers such as metoprolol are reported to cause a false-positive amphetamine screen.[35]

Electrocardiogram

An ECG screens for dysrhythmias, conduction abnormalities, and ischemia, and can provide insights into hyperkalemia or hypokalemia, as well as sodium channel blockade. Sodium channel blockade, which manifests as a QRS duration longer than 100 milliseconds, can precipitate wide-complex tachycardia by slowing myocardial depolarization. Cyclic antidepressants and cocaine share class IA antidysrhythmic effects with QRS widening and resultant QT prolongation. The prognostic value of QRS widening in the context of a bundle branch block is not known.

The evaluation of chest pain in cocaine ingestion is challenging because cocaine toxicity can precipitate myocardial ischemia via coronary vasospasm. Chronic cocaine use also accelerates arteriosclerosis, which itself can precipitate myocardial ischemia. Young patients may also demonstrate early repolarization, further complicating interpretation. Serial ECGs may be helpful to identify dynamic processes.

A chest radiograph may identify aspirated foreign bodies, pneumothorax, or pneumomediastinum from inhalational barotrauma when these are suspected, but is not required in most cases.

CK, a nonspecific marker for muscle injury, is often elevated with cocaine use. In users with myalgias, a serum CK and urine for myoglobin is checked to screen for rhabdomyolysis. Original data on cocaine-related coronary syndromes used CK-MB as a cardiac marker. This is now supplanted by troponin I, T, or the newer generation high sensitivity troponin assays, as for all patients evaluated for possible ischemic chest pain. Most patients presenting with troponin elevation and chest pain after cocaine use had angiographically proven obstructive coronary disease, often of a single vessel, but almost 20% have normal angiography.[36]

Even though the sensitivity and specificity of troponin cardiac markers for cocaine-related chest pain is unknown, we recommend that patients with cocaine use be evaluated for chest pain in a similar fashion as chest pain patients without cocaine use. Decisions regarding further investigation are based on the characteristics and course of the chest pain and results of serial troponin measurements and ECGs. We do not recommend routine use of diagnostic coronary computed tomographic angiography (CTA) in the evaluation of patients with chest pain in the context of acute cocaine use.

> **BOX 144.3 Initial Evaluation of Patients With Sympathetic Stimulation**
>
> Rapid assessment of vital signs, especially core temperature
> Exclude hypoxia, hypoglycemia, and hyponatremia
> Pharmacologic sedation with benzodiazepines
> Electrocardiogram (ECG)
> Urinalysis
> Serum creatine kinase (CK)

Severe persistent headache despite normalization of blood pressure may be caused by a subarachnoid hemorrhage (SAH) and warrants evaluation (see Chapters 16 and 33).

In the rare event that a cocaine user presents with agranulocytosis or digital discoloration suggestive of levamisole, a "send-out" or reference laboratory evaluation for urine levamisole by gas chromatography–mass spectrometry can be performed. The sample is ideally obtained within 48 hours after last use.

MANAGEMENT

The altered mental status associated with the sympathomimetic toxidrome ranges from agitated to belligerent behavior. A severely poisoned patient may be combative and unable to cooperate in assessment of vital signs. Agitated delirium is associated with up to a 10% mortality rate. Actions taken during these first stages of the encounter are crucial (Box 144.3) even though the patient remains undifferentiated. Sedation with benzodiazepines serves multiple purposes. It treats agitation and reduces heat production by muscle, heart rate, blood pressure, and the overall adrenergic surge of cocaine or sympathomimetic toxicity.

In the severely agitated patient, immediate administration of IM benzodiazepines while the patient is transiently restrained may be necessary. Once more under control, staff can obtain a complete set of vital signs (including temperature), a bedside glucose measurement, and IV access. If a chest restraint is used, a mesh vest is preferred over a jacket to help limit hyperthermia. Immediate pharmacologic sedation with IM or IV administration of benzodiazepines may be necessary (see next section), which, in adequate doses, restores inhibitory tone to the CNS and decreases excessive sympathetic outflow to peripheral tissues. Sedation also facilitates measurement of vital signs (particularly core temperature), continuous electrocardiographic monitoring, and completion of the physical examination.

Pharmacologic Sedation for Agitation

Benzodiazepines are the mainstay of treatment of cocaine-induced agitation. Diazepam has a rapid onset of action, is easily titratable, and has active metabolites for a sustained effect. Diazepam can be administered intravenously in increments of 5 to 10 mg every 5 minutes in adults until sedation is achieved. Lorazepam, administered 1 to 2 mg intravenously every 5 minutes, is also an acceptable option. Midazolam in 1 to 2 mg doses IV is more rapid in onset with a shorter duration of effect. The endpoint of benzodiazepine administration in sympathomimetic toxicity is normalization of vital signs and motor tone. Persistently increased motor tone reflects an inadequate benzodiazepine dose, even if the patient appears somnolent. In that case, additional doses of diazepam, lorazepam, or midazolam can be given, with close monitoring of the patient's respiratory status.

If IV access is not possible because of agitation, IM midazolam 5 to 10 mg is the preferred approach and may be repeated every 10 to 20 minutes until the patient can be controlled. Lorazepam is a less-preferred alternative because it takes longer to reach peak concentration (5 vs. 15 minutes) and clears less rapidly than midaz-olam, increasing the risk of respiratory depression. Ethanol is a common coingestant. The combination of ethanol and benzodiazepines depresses respiration more than either alone. A prudent course is to give the medication and observe for an objective response, redosing after an appropriate interval. In all patients, titration of the benzo-diazepine is important, allowing the clinician to observe the effects of one dose (usually 5 minutes) before an additional dose is given. After sedation is achieved, the patient is closely observed to ensure that the patient's respiratory status is stable when peak sedation effect is achieved.

Benzodiazepines provide the cleanest pharmacologic approach to treating the agitated patient as they bind to one receptor system. However, benzodiazepines may precipitate paradoxical reactions in the pediatric and geriatric populations and may be suboptimal treatments if the ultimate diagnosis of the agitated patient is a psychotic disorder that might benefit from an antipsychotic agent.

Ketamine has been used to treat the acutely agitated patient in the ED[37] and in the prehospital setting.[38-40] Ketamine, like midazolam and haloperidol, can be administered intramuscularly with reliable onset and duration of action. Ketamine is an NMDA-antagonist that induces a dissociative state. It also produces modest increases in heart rate (on the order of 10 beats/min) and blood pressure (10 to 20 mm Hg systolic) when used in 0.3 to 0.5 mg/kg doses. Aripiprazole and ketamine reduced the time to seizure in a mouse model of cocaine toxicity.[41] A systematic review identified 330 subjects with amphetamine toxicity treated with an antipsychotic and documented a low incidence of adverse effects, including two episodes of coma and QT prolongation, with one episode of each: hypotension, NMS, cardiac arrest, and death.[42]

If the cause of delirium is unclear, careful attention to the patient's respiratory status avoids the respiratory depression caused by excessive benzodiazepine administration in the presence of other sedating agents, such as ethanol or opioids.

Most cocaine-induced agitation responds to adequate doses of benzodiazepines. The dose of benzodiazepine required to treat excessive sympathetic tone may exceed 10 times the typical dose used for anxiolysis or relaxation of musculature. Butyrophenone antipsychotic agents (e.g., haloperidol and droperidol) are rapidly effective and generally safe for drug-induced psychosis or agitation states from sympathomimetic agents, including cocaine, amphetamines, and PCP when used in patients with stable vital signs (also discussed in Chapters 13 and 90). They may, however, worsen hyperthermia and tachydysrhythmias, because of their anticholinergic properties. Haloperidol, given 2 to 5 mg IM, may be repeated every 20 to 30 minutes with consideration of other agents after a total of 10 mg. Although not approved for IV use, this route is widely used but should only be considered in the psychotic patient with stable vital signs with close cardiac monitoring in 5-mg doses to a maximum dose of 15 mg. The sedative dose for droperidol is 2.5 to 5 mg IM. Droperidol has a box warning from the FDA for QT prolongation and potentially torsades de pointes. However, most reported cases of butyrophenone-induced dysrhythmias have been in individuals receiving large doses for prolonged periods, such as hours to days, or in elderly populations (older than 60 years). These medications lack the respiratory depression potentially caused by other agents and may be beneficial in some cases when rapid sedation is required. For these reasons, the butyrophenones remain effective agents for treatment of drug and sympathomimetic-induced agitation in carefully selected patients.

Hyperthermia

Cocaine-induced hyperthermia must be treated with rapid cooling (Box 144.4). Patients who sustain elevated core temperatures above

---

BOX 144.4 Management of Stimulant-Induced Hyperthermia

Cooling
Early identification of elevated core temperature
Large-bore IV access with rapid infusion of crystalloid
Sedation and muscle relaxation with benzodiazepines
Rapid cooling within 20–30 minutes
Paralysis and intubation if necessary

Monitoring and Diagnostics
Urine output via Foley catheterization
Laboratory analysis for organ function
  Serum chemistries, creatinine, CK
  Liver function
  PT, PTT, fibrin split products
  Bacterial cultures
  Urinalysis for myoglobinuria
Neuroimaging if etiology unclear

aIdeally with ice water immersion.
bConsider lumbar puncture or antibiotic therapy, especially in injection drug users.
CK, Creatine kinase; *IV,* intravenous; *PT,* prothrombin time; *PTT,* partial thromboplastin time.

106°F (41°C) for more than 20 minutes will likely develop disseminated intravascular coagulation (DIC) followed by fatal multisystem organ failure. It is crucial to reduce core temperature to 102°F (38.8°C) as soon as clinically possible, ideally within 20 minutes or less. Cooling blankets are insufficient. Ice water submersion in a portable tub is preferred when available, although some favor wet sheets with large circulating fans.[43] These patients require continuous temperature monitoring and fluid resuscitation as judged by standard measures. Invasive cooling techniques are often delayed and inadequate against the vasoconstrictive effects of cocaine and other adrenergic agents. Patients should have continuous monitoring of their core temperature with a rectal probe. Heat generated by agitation and increased muscle tone can be terminated by adequate use of benzodiazepines, as described earlier, with neuromuscular paralysis and intubation as required. If paralysis is needed, we recommend rocuronium, 1 mg/kg, over succinylcholine. Succinylcholine and cocaine are metabolized by the same plasma enzyme—plasma cholinesterase. Concomitant use may prolong the effects of each drug. Succinylcholine may also worsen hyperkalemia due to rhabdomyolysis.

Acute Hypertensive Emergencies

The goal in cocaine-induced hypertensive emergencies is to lower blood pressure by counteracting alpha-adrenergic vasoconstriction. Benzodiazepines are the first line treatment. These agents restore the CNS inhibitory tone throughout the body, including the heart. We also recommend phentolamine, a direct alpha-adrenergic antagonist, given as repeated IV doses of 1 mg every 3 minutes with continuous blood pressure monitoring. If two doses fail to reduce the mean arterial pressure by at least one-third, increase each following dose by 1 mg up to 5 mg/dose until the mean arterial pressure is reduced by at least one-third. Phentolamine lasts roughly 45 minutes. Alternative agents include hydralazine, nitroglycerin, and short-acting IV calcium channel antagonists like nicardipine or clevidipine (see Chapter 70). We prefer shorter-acting antihypertensives because they can be discontinued as toxicity subsides without risk of overshoot, which may be deleterious if the patient also has a SAH or aortic dissection attributable to cocaine.

It had been previously recommended to avoid beta-adrenergic antagonists (beta blockers) in treating cocaine-induced hypertension because unopposed α-receptor activity would precipitate coronary artery spasm and hypertension. This concern was based on data that patients undergoing cardiac catheterization demonstrated decreased coronary artery diameter in the presence of injected (mainlined) cocaine and beta-adrenergic antagonists. In two retrospective studies, beta-blocker use was not associated with clinically significant hypertension, troponin elevation, or adverse events in patients presenting with acute cocaine toxicity.[44,45] A meta-analysis of five studies found no differences between patients treated with or without beta-blockers for either myocardial infarction or overall-cause mortality. Another meta-analysis found no significant difference in the odds of myocardial infarction or overall-cause mortality in patients who received a beta-blocker versus not. This second meta-analysis did not explicitly control for whether the patients were currently prescribed a beta-blocker and shared one study with the first meta-analysis.

One way to reconcile previous concerns with the evidence is to recognize that most beta blockers are also alpha-adrenergic antagonists. Beta-blockers may be a useful adjunct in treating cocaine-associated hypertension, but the clinician should be aware that beta-blockers do not treat the other toxic effects of cocaine, which are generally responsive to adequate doses of benzodiazepines. As a result, while not contraindicated, we do not postulate that beta-blockers provide a clinical benefit in this setting and do not recommend their routine use in patients presenting with cocaine-induced hypertension.

Dysrhythmias

Dysrhythmias from cocaine may be atrial or ventricular. Atrial fibrillation and supraventricular tachycardias attributable to cocaine will respond to benzodiazepines. Calcium channel blockers or beta blockers can be used if rapid atrial rhythms fail to respond to sedation, cooling, and volume resuscitation, but negative ionotropic agents (e.g., beta-1 preferential antagonists, verapamil, diltiazem) should be used with caution as cocaine is directly cardiotoxic.

Important considerations in the differential diagnosis of a wide-complex tachycardia include hyperkalemia, sodium channel blockade (cyclic antidepressants and cocaine), and myocardial ischemia. In cocaine body packers or patients presenting with cocaine-induced adrenergic toxidrome, abrupt development of a wide-complex tachycardia with a pulse should be treated with empirical sodium bicarbonate, 1 to 2 mEq/kg IV bolus, with closely recorded cardiac monitoring to observe for QRS narrowing.[46] If hypotension and QRS prolongation do not improve with sodium bicarbonate, consult a medical toxicologist to discuss possible intravenous lipid emulsion therapy. Intravenous lipid emulsion therapy was reported as "life-saving" in case reports of cocaine toxicity. However, the absence of rigorous trials prevents the American Association of Clinical Toxicologists (AACT) from recommending routine use in these cases.[47] Fluid and electrolytes should be corrected as indicated. Close monitoring is required for patients with a preexisting or unmasked Brugada-type conduction pattern.

Hyponatremia

Treatment for sympathomimetic-induced hyponatremia (e.g., MDMA) is the same as that for SIADH from other causes and includes fluid restriction and hypertonic saline (if seizing). Normal saline may worsen hyponatremia by inadvertently increasing free water retention. To our knowledge, treatment with V2-receptor antagonists has not been described for these patients.

Cocaine-Related Chest Pain

The causes of cocaine-related chest pain are diverse (Box 144.5), including aspirated foreign bodies or pneumothorax or pneumomediastinum from inhalational barotrauma. Fever and shortness of breath

> **BOX 144.5   Causes of Stimulant-Induced Chest Pain**
>
> **Cardiac Chest Pain**
> Coronary stent thrombosis
> Endocarditis
> Ischemia, infarction
>   During acute intoxication
>   After acute intoxication
> Left ventricular apical ballooning
> Pericarditis
>
> **Noncardiac**
> Aortic dissection
> Foreign body aspiration
> Infection
> Pneumomediastinum
> Pneumopericardium
> Pneumothorax
> Pulmonary infarction
> Intestinal ischemia or infarct

should prompt consideration of pneumonia, pulmonary infarction, or endocarditis with septic pulmonary emboli in IV drug abuse.

Cocaine acutely induces coronary vasoconstriction while increasing myocardial oxygen demand. Platelet aggregation is enhanced through thrombogenic and antifibrinolytic pathways. These cumulative effects can result in coronary insufficiency. Cigarette smoking acutely exacerbates these conditions. Chronic cocaine use may accelerate atherogenesis and induce left ventricular hypertrophy.[48] All of these factors contribute to myocardial ischemia or infarction. Of nonfatal myocardial infarctions in patients aged 18 to 45 years, 25% are attributed to cocaine, even after adjustment of other known cardiac risk factors.[49]

Identification of a patient with a cocaine-related coronary syndrome is difficult. Patients may present hours to days after use, possibly because of vasoactive metabolites. The patient may deny drug use and have atypical chest pain. Almost one-third of cocaine-using patients with elevated serum enzymes have pleuritic chest pain. There are no clear predictors for patients at risk for cocaine-related coronary syndrome, including the patient's age, route of drug use, time to presentation, and preexisting risk factors for coronary artery disease. In the setting of cocaine-related chest pain, risk stratification by thrombolysis in the myocardial infarction (TIMI) score may not adequately identify patients at risk for 30-day adverse outcomes. Cocaine history alone, however, in low-risk asymptomatic patients assessed by coronary CTA is generally not associated with increased risk of coronary artery disease. Patients with positive serum biomarkers for myocardial infarction often have significant angiographic stenosis. Of patients without positive serum markers, up to 20% may still have significant disease by angiography. Other predictors of significant disease in this group included elevated cholesterol concentration and prior diagnosis of coronary disease or myocardial infarction. Patients with previous coronary stent placement are at higher risk of thrombosis with cocaine use.

As for most complications of cocaine use, benzodiazepines decrease myocardial oxygen demand by limiting peripheral stimulation and should be given early to patients presenting with cocaine-induced chest pain, especially when signs of adrenergic excess are present. Aspirin and nitrates should be administered as for any case of suspected ischemic chest pain. In patients meeting electrocardiographic criteria for myocardial infarction with persistent chest pain and hypertension and a clear history of acute cocaine intoxication, coronary vasodilation with IV phentolamine (1 mg) can be given slowly over 3 minutes if available. This dose can be repeated, if needed, as long as the patient's blood pressure remains stable. Morphine sulfate can be used to treat chest pain. Patients with persistent chest pain and ST segment changes strongly suggestive of myocardial infarction can be considered for percutaneous intervention or thrombolytic therapy, assuming there are no contraindications, such as uncontrolled severe hypertension.[48]

In contrast to non-cocaine-induced myocardial ischemia or infarction, beta-adrenergic antagonists, including labetalol, are generally not recommended with acute cocaine toxicity because coronary vasoconstriction may be exacerbated. In patients with cocaine-related coronary syndromes who are not acutely toxic, alpha-adrenergic vasoactive metabolites may be responsible. Outcomes of uncomplicated chest pain due to cocaine are generally good. Current guidelines for care of the patient with an acute coronary syndrome that is unrelated to cocaine do not recommend immediate administration of beta-adrenergic antagonists, but rather within the first 24 hours. As such, in patients with known or suspected cocaine-related myocardial infarction with or without ST segment elevation, there is little role for beta-adrenergic antagonists in the ED and we do not recommend their routine use. Such patients warrant further evaluations of coexisting atherosclerotic heart disease and clinical reevaluation prior to consideration of this therapy. Administration of beta-adrenergic antagonists on discharge is controversial, especially if cocaine use is likely to continue, and we advise against this routine practice.[44]

Heparin can be given, but fibrinolytic therapy is not well studied. Some mechanisms of cocaine-induced myocardial infarction would be expected to respond to fibrinolytic agents. Patients failing to respond to treatment with nitrates and phentolamine who have a known coronary artery disease or a previous ECG confirming new ST segment elevations are candidates for cardiac catheterization or fibrinolysis, if necessary. The same contraindications apply as those for non-cocaine-induced myocardial infarction. Nuclear imaging studies also may provide more diagnostic information, but their use is best considered in consultation with cardiology. Patients presenting with chest pain after cocaine use and an ECG with definitive or new ST elevations should have prompt evaluation by a cardiologist for potential cardiac catheterization intervention when such services are available.

Antiplatelet and glycoprotein IIb/IIIa inhibitors and calcium channel antagonists seem to be of benefit to some patients with myocardial infarction or ischemia of atherosclerotic origin. Theoretically, these agents may counter some of the platelet aggregation enhanced by cocaine, but data investigating their use are lacking.

Patients with cocaine-related chest pain without other cardiac risk factors who have normal ECGs and cardiac biomarkers are at low risk for myocardial infarction. The role of provocative testing in these patients is not well established.

In summary, cocaine-induced coronary ischemia is managed with benzodiazepines, nitrates, and vasodilators, preferably phentolamine. As with non-cocaine-using patients presenting with acute ischemic chest pain, we recommend use of aspirin, heparin, and antiplatelet agents in conjunction with interventional therapy as indicated.

Interventions to cease cocaine use are warranted. For patients with documented coronary artery disease, cessation of cocaine use is imperative. In studies, cocaine users presenting with chest pain who subsequently continued cocaine use after ED discharge were more likely to have recurrent ED visits than were those who stopped subsequent use.

SPECIAL TOPICS

Body Packers

A body packer is an individual who intentionally ingests a large amount of an illicit substance in multiple carefully wrapped packages to transport that substance from an area of production to an area of distribution or consumption. The substances are often wrapped tightly into condoms or other latex products and sometimes coated in wax.

Body packing is most extensively described with cocaine. Each packet can contain nearly 10 g of cocaine. Packers may swallow as many as 150 packets. To quiet peristalsis, the packer may be forced to take antimotility drugs (loperamide, diphenoxylate-atropine). On arrival at the patient's destination, a cathartic is often taken to stimulate gastrointestinal passage of the product for subsequent delivery and distribution. Body packers are likely to know the exact number of packets they ingested but may be reluctant to share that information. Treatment should be specific for each group of drugs, whether it is opioids, cocaine, or amphetamine. Surgical interventions are indicated for obstruction of the intestines or package rupture. Legal consultation should be obtained because of the legal complexity of body packing cases.

A body packer may present without symptoms to the ED. Diagnosis is made by history. The patient may not be forthcoming, owing to the presence of law enforcement or fear of retribution by the packer's handlers. The patient should be placed on continuous cardiac monitoring, with large-bore IV access. An abdominal radiograph may qualitatively confirm foreign bodies, but cannot be used to count packets. Plain radiographs do not reliably detect small or loosely packed packets; computed tomography may be warranted if suspicion is high.

The main step in body packer management is to ensure that the patient passes all of the swallowed packages.[49] We recommend whole-bowel irrigation with polyethylene glycol to facilitate passage. Endoscopic retrieval is generally discouraged because the packets may rupture during the procedure, but it has been done on occasion.[50] Patients stating that they swallowed a larger number of packets than are passed or who refuse to reveal the number ingested should have continued bowel irrigation, observation, and repeated studies. Subsequent computed tomography (CT) scans or contrast studies may be required to evaluate for remaining packets.[50] However, these radiographic studies may fail to detect isolated packets that contain potentially fatal quantities of cocaine.

Rupture of a single cocaine packet can be fatal. Each packet contains almost 10 times the lethal dose. Cocaine body packers with retained packets should be admitted to a monitored setting with a plan to facilitate removal of the packets via whole bowel irrigation. There is no indication for surgical intervention to remove drug packets from the gastrointestinal tract of an asymptomatic patient.[2] If the patient develops sympathomimetic toxicity and abdominal pain or signs of a bowel obstruction, surgery should be consulted for evaluation of urgent removal.[51,52] When evidence of cocaine toxicity is manifested, rapid surgical intervention may be the only way to rescue these patients. Benzodiazepines, neuromuscular blockade, or sodium bicarbonate administration (for wide-complex tachycardia) do not address the imminently ischemic gut.

All packets passed in the stool, through endoscopic procedures, or in the operating room should be counted carefully and promptly given to law enforcement officials. If law enforcement is not yet involved, hospital legal counsel or risk management and the hospital ethics committee may be helpful in determining the handling of the packets. If the patient fails to improve after passage of all packets intact, one should consider alternative diagnoses. As an example, one case identified a body packer with HIV who presented with tachypnea, tachycardia, mydriasis, and a temperature of 102° F. He was found to have pulmonary infiltrates on computed tomography and was eventually diagnosed with pneumococcal pneumonia.[53]

Body Stuffers

A "body stuffer" attempts to conceal evidence of possession of illicit substances by internally concealing the drug while being pursued by law enforcement officials. Stuffing usually is by ingestion. It may also involve vaginal or anal concealment. In contrast to packing, stuffing is usually an unplanned event that involves a spontaneous insertion of small amounts of poorly packaged material. The substances are often swallowed in poorly sealed vials or glassine packets that may not be evident on radiographs. In general, patients ingest nonlethal doses and are asymptomatic. For cooperative asymptomatic oral body stuffers, the role of gastric decontamination is not well studied. We recommend activated charcoal if presenting within 3 hours after ingestion to bind and sequester any contents leaking into the GI tract. Monitoring, as described earlier with body packers, should be performed if the quantity ingested is of concern or if signs of toxicity develop. Due to lower doses and less potential lethality, the vast majority of body stuffers will not require whole bowel irrigation therapy as do body packers. Body stuffers rarely have fatal events, and these patients usually have symptoms in the first 8 hours. Asymptomatic patients who are unwilling to disclose events or cooperate with care should have monitoring in the ED regardless of status of police custody. However, if the patient is not under arrest, they are free to decline therapy and leave the ED against medical advice if they can demonstrate clear understanding of the risks, including sudden death, of leaving with retained packets. Although the ideal period of observation is uncertain, 8 to 12 hours is reasonable with admission if the patient develops signs or symptoms of toxicity. Patients with suspected vaginal or anal concealment who are asymptomatic and without signs of toxicity who refuse a physical examination should be assessed for capacity and observed in the ED as outlined earlier. Any judicial warrants for an invasive examination against the patient's will should carefully involve risk management and hospital legal counsel, because these are forensic requests and not medically emergent in the asymptomatic patient.

DISPOSITION

Most patients with sympathomimetic toxicity are young adults with a clear history of single substance ingestion. If there are no signs of end-organ damage, they may be discharged once vital signs and mental status return to baseline after a period of observation of 4 to 6 hours.

Patients who respond quickly to one to two doses of sedation, have no concerning elements in their history or presentation, and exhibit no evidence of end-organ toxicity may be safely discharged once their vital signs and mental status return to baseline. Concerning elements in the history include the presence of coingestants, concern for drug packing, human trafficking, or prior episodes of endocarditis. Some patients may be extremely lethargic from catecholamine depletion, even if not in frank washout. It is prudent to discharge them with a responsible adult. Patients may be open to drug counseling and referral while in the ED.

Patients with chest pain (Box 144.6) and who show dynamic changes on the ECG, troponin elevation, dysrhythmias, or pulmonary edema and patients requiring vasodilators or reperfusion should be admitted to a coronary care unit or a telemetry unit. These patients require further evaluation of the extent of preexisting reversible ischemia and intervention to encourage cessation of drug use. Patients in whom the chest pain is felt to be less likely attributable to cocaine (e.g., frequent user with no change in pattern of use with chest pain) may be treated and risk-stratified according to standard screening for risk factors as with non-cocaine chest pain (see Chapter 64).

> **BOX 144.6   Admission Criteria for Cocaine-Related Chest Pain**
>
> Cardiogenic shock
> CHF
> Dysrhythmias or conduction abnormalities
> Electrocardiographic changes
> Elevated myocardial enzymes
> Multiple risk factors for CAD
> Persistent chest pain, dyspnea, or abnormal vital signs
> Preexisting CAD or stent placement
> Requiring vasodilating pharmacotherapy
> Persistent symptoms

CAD, Coronary artery disease; *CHF*, congestive heart failure.

In patients with no other risk factors for cardiovascular disease, cocaine use is not associated with an increased likelihood of coronary disease after adjustment for age, race, sex, and other risk factors for coronary disease.[48] Complications such as congestive heart failure and ventricular dysrhythmias typically manifest within the first 4 to 6 hours. Young patients who present after resolution of chest pain with normal and unchanging ECGs, no dysrhythmias and few or no risks of coronary artery disease are likely to have a good outcome. Prior studies have demonstrated that these low- to intermediate-risk patients with cocaine-associated chest pain can be safely discharged after 8 to 12 hours of observation. The goal of a more recent study was to determine the safety of an 8-hour protocol for ruling out myocardial infarction in patients who presented with cocaine-associated chest pain. Application of an abbreviated cardiac enzyme protocol (at 0, 2, 4, and 8 hours) after presentation with continuous cardiac monitoring, resulted in the safe and rapid discharge of patients presenting to the ED with cocaine-associated chest pain.

Body packers need to be observed until all packets have passed. Ideally, these patients have had several packet-free stools, a reliable packet count consistent with the ingestion, and a normal CT scan or contrast radiographic study. Body stuffers who receive activated charcoal, have normal ECGs, and remain asymptomatic with normal vital signs after 6 to 12 hours of observation may be discharged.

There are special considerations for the pediatric patient. There should be a low threshold to admit the pediatric patient in whom the intent of the ingestion is unclear, even if the patient demonstrates no current sympathomimetic toxicity. An unintentional ingestion by an adolescent of one to two short-acting sympathomimetics (e.g., Adderall) may be treated as above. An intentional ingestion not for suicidal purposes of a similar amount may be similarly discharged if evaluation by social work uncovers no other concerns and the clinician of records feels that it is a safe discharge. Any toddler presenting with sympathomimetic toxicity should be evaluated by social work and may require admission until a safe discharge can be assured. Involve a medical toxicologist early to guide clinical care and to provide insight with critically ill patients or when expanded testing is needed for forensic or medicolegal concerns.

We would like to acknowledge the scholarly efforts and expertise of the previous edition authors Drs. Rama B. Rao and Robert S. Hoffman.

The references for this chapter can be found online at ExpertConsult.com

145

THC and Hallucinogens

Whitney Barrett and Janetta L. Iwanicki

Hallucinogens include many types of drugs and chemicals with different associated effects, including action at serotonin receptors, dopamine receptors, and glutamate N-methyl-D-aspartate receptors. Diagnosis and management are based primarily on the history and physical examination, with hallmarks of therapy including supportive care, a calm quiet environment, and sedation with benzodiazepines. Severely agitated patients may benefit from butyrophenone antipsychotic agents such as haloperidol and droperidol.

Screening tests for hallucinogenic drugs of abuse are of limited value in the acute management of intoxicated patients. Novel synthetic hallucinogens continue to emerge. These drugs are rarely detected by screening tests, and cases of toxicity may occur in regional outbreaks. Patients with phencyclidine (PCP) toxicity can have unpredictable, violent behavior, and may sustain traumatic injuries. They may require rapid sedation to decrease danger to the patient and health care providers. For hyperthermic patients, sufficient sedation to decrease neuromuscular hyperactivity may require intubation, paralytics, and active external cooling. Extreme agitation is less common with abuse of ketamine and methoxetamine. The care of patients intoxicated from cannabis and synthetic cannabinoids consists of prevention of injury and reassurance for those who have panic reactions. High doses of antiemetics may be necessary to treat the nausea and vomiting associated with synthetic cannabinoids and heavy daily cannabis use, referred to as the "cannabinoid hyperemesis syndrome." The central nervous system and physiologic effects of mescaline use are similar to those of lysergic acid diethylamide (LSD) derivatives, but more vivid hallucinations can occur. Nausea and vomiting are pronounced and almost always precede the hallucinogenic effects.

The term *hallucinogen* is used to describe a variety of xenobiotics causing altered perception. A hallucination is defined as perception of an object or sensation that does not exist in reality. However, most drugs do not produce actual hallucinations. Drugs that are classified as hallucinogens are more likely to cause illusions, or misperceptions of real objects. Some hallucinogens are called psychedelics, a subset that alters cognition and perception. Hallucinogens work by several mechanisms, including stimulating the serotonergic 5-HT$_{2A}$ receptor, hyperactivation of the dopamine D2 receptor, and blockade of the glutamate N-methyl-D-aspartate (NMDA) receptors. This chapter describes serotonergic agents, dissociative agents, and selected plants and fungi. Sympathomimetic agents are discussed in Chapter 144.

SEROTONERGIC AGENTS

Principles of Toxicity

Serotoninergic agents are a broad category of compounds that share structural similarities with serotonin (5-hydroxytryptamine [5-HT]) or enhance serotonergic tone within the body, predominantly by their action at the 5-HT$_{2A}$ serotonin receptor subtype. These agents include various lysergic acid derivatives (lysergamides) and tryptamines (indolealkylamines). Serotonin-like agents produce changes in thought, mood, perception, and consciousness. Orientation to person, place, and time is usually preserved, but severe intoxication may cause delirium, disorientation, and altered levels of consciousness. Patients may present to the emergency department (ED) because of an acute panic reaction, excessive ingestion, or accidental exposure (e.g., children or adults who have ingested the drug unknowingly). Unlike opioids, there is no addictive component in psychedelics and no euphoria-dysphoria cycle, as occurs with sympathomimetic drugs such as cocaine. The rapid development of tolerance also limits the effect of repeated doses.

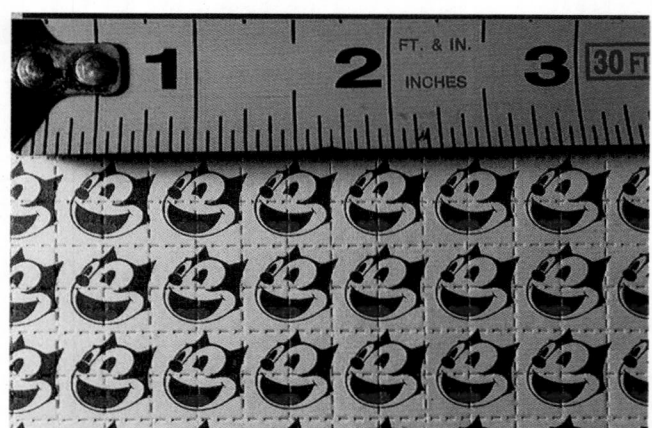

Fig. 145.1 LSD blotters (Felix the Cat). (Photo by Jon, copyright 2001, Blotterart.com. Accessed at www.erowid.org.)

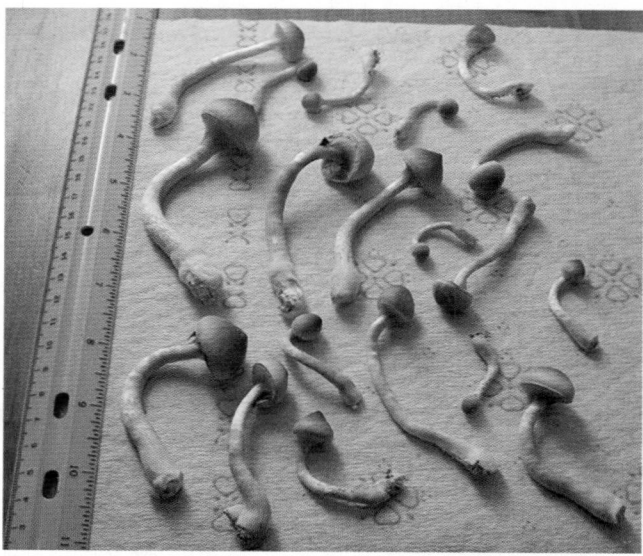

Fig. 145.2 *Psilocybe cubensis* mushroom. (Photo by Gweedo, copyright 2003. Accessed at www.erowid.org.)

Lysergamides

Lysergic acid diethylamide (LSD), or acid, is a potent psychedelic drug. Doses of 1 to 1.5 µg/kg produce psychedelic effects. The typical dose taken for an "acid trip" is approximately 25 to 100 µg. LSD is sold as a tablet (microdot), liquid, powder, gelatin square (or "windowpane"), and blotter acid. Sheets of blotting paper are sprayed with LSD, dried, and perforated into small squares. Graphics are incorporated onto the blotting paper in designs that include cartoon characters (e.g., Felix the Cat, Bart Simpson) and geometric designs (Fig. 145.1). Each sheet is composed of hundreds of squares that are placed sublingually or eaten whole. Massive ingestions are rare. Drug paraphernalia recently sold and touted as "LSD" does not actually contain lysergic acid diethylamide but synthetic cannabinoids.

In addition to synthetic LSD, several plants contain lysergic acid amide (LSA) similar in structure and action to LSD. These plants include the Hawaiian baby wood rose (*Argyreia nervosa*), Hawaiian wood rose (*Merremia tuberosa*), morning glory (*Ipomoea violacea*), and ololiuqui (*Rivea corymbosa*). Intoxication may result after ingestion of the seeds, extract, or tea.

Tryptamines

Tryptamines may be synthetic or natural compounds. For centuries, Native Central and South Americans have used tryptamine-containing beverages such as ayahuasca in their religious ceremonies. This beverage is brewed from a combination of plants containing dimethyltryptamine (DMT) and 5-methoxy-*N,N*-dimethyltryptamine (5-MeO-DMT), as well as harmine alkaloids with monoamine oxidase inhibitor effects that increase the bioavailability of orally ingested DMT. Ayahuasca has gained recent popularity in Europe and North America.

Psilocybin and psilocin are naturally occurring tryptamines found in some species of *Psilocybe* (Fig. 145.2), *Panaeolus,* and *Conocybe* mushrooms. Psilocybin remains active when the mushrooms are dried or cooked. Street psilocybin sold as pills or capsules is frequently substituted with phencyclidine (PCP) or LSD. Naturally occurring tryptamines are also found in the parotid glands of the *Bufo* toad species. The venom of the Sonoran Desert or Colorado River toad (*Bufo alvarius*) contains 5-MeO-DMT. Smoking of the dried venom results in psychoactive effects.

Designer tryptamines such as α-methyltryptamine, diisopropyltryptamine, and diisopropyl-5-methoxytryptamine (street named foxy or foxy methoxy) have been synthesized and are orally active. The effects of these synthetic derivatives are similar to those of naturally occurring tryptamines.

Clinical Features

In Western society, psychoactive agents are taken for internal mental exploration or, more commonly, for recreation. Effects include loss of boundaries between the user and environment, the sensation that colors and sounds are distorted and intensified, the sensation that perceptions are occurring via unusual pathways such as synesthesia, and the perception that usual objects appear novel, fascinating, or awe-inspiring. Users are usually aware that they are under the influence of the drug. A sense of euphoria is common, but it may alternate with an intense dysphoric experience that is accompanied by paranoia (e.g., illusions of dying or being born).

Acute panic reaction is a common adverse reaction to psychedelics. Paranoid delusions and fear of impending death can also occur. Behavior may be agitated or withdrawn. Sympathomimetic effects include mydriasis, tachycardia, hypertension, and in severe cases, hyperthermia. Mydriasis seems to parallel the intensity of the trip. The individual's altered perceptions may result in lack of awareness of dangers in the environment, resulting in injury. Psychosis after LSD trips has been reported, and schizophrenia (overt or borderline) may worsen. Transient depression sometimes occurs after LSD use. Flashbacks, or posthallucinogen perceptual disorder, are transient episodes of altered consciousness that occur months or years after LSD ingestion. Hyperactivity may also be seen, with marked auditory and visual hallucinations. Massive ingestions may result in coma and decreased responsiveness to painful stimuli. Fixed and dilated pupils, diaphoresis, vomiting, hyperthermia, rhabdomyolysis, coagulopathy, and seizures may result.

Euphoria and a distortion of reality usually occur after ingestion of one to five *Psilocybe cubensis* mushroom caps. In contrast to peyote (discussed later), vomiting is unusual. Larger doses (5–20 *P. cubensis* mushrooms) produce colorful visual hallucinations. Few adverse reactions occur, and the incidence of bad trips or panic reactions is lower than with LSD. Rarely, seizures, coma, and hyperthermia have been reported after psilocybin use.

Differential Diagnoses

Alcohol, other drugs and mixed ingestion are a possible source of the patient's symptoms, especially with coma or marked physiologic changes. Cocaine, PCP, amphetamines, and anticholinergic agents should be considered. Acute psychosis and schizophrenic breaks may also appear similar to a psychedelic reaction. Finally, nontoxicologic diagnoses are crucial to rule out, including central nervous system infection, intracranial mass or bleed, and partial complex seizures.

Diagnostic Testing

Often, patients are in a panic or are brought in by a worried companion who may be aware of the use of hallucinogenic substances. A focus on history, especially from collateral information sources, and physical exam are important to make the diagnosis. Most patients require no laboratory testing, but a basic metabolic profile, serum ethanol, and serum glucose levels may be helpful in patients with unclear ingestions, co-ingestants, or underlying psychiatric disorders. Toxicology screening and specific testing for psychedelics is not available in a timely fashion in most clinical settings, and rarely changes management.

Management

Reassurance and supportive care are the cornerstones of management. If patients are a danger to themselves or others, they may need to be sedated with benzodiazepines (see below) or physically restrained temporarily to permit sedation. There is no specific antagonist to the effects of serotonergic agents. Empathetic reassurance in a calm, quiet environment with decreased external stimuli is an effective therapeutic modality. The drug effects typically last for hours, but most patients return to baseline after the acute effects.

Benzodiazepines are the mainstay of treatment for hallucinogenic drug-induced agitation. Diazepam, lorazepam, and midazolam have all been successfully used in this setting. Diazepam can be administered via the intravenous (IV) route in increments of 5 to 10 mg every 5 minutes in adults until sedation is achieved. Diazepam has a rapid onset of action, is easily titratable, and has active metabolites for a sustained effect. Lorazepam, 1 to 2 mg IV every 5 minutes is also an acceptable option. Additional doses of lorazepam or diazepam should be titrated to effect, until the patient is calm and relaxed. There is no true maximum dose of these medications. For an adult patient in whom IV access is not possible because of agitation, intramuscular (IM) midazolam, 5 to 10 mg, can be administered to facilitate subsequent interventions. In all patients, titration of the benzodiazepine is important. The emergency clinician should observe the effects of one dose (usually 5 minutes) before an additional dose is given. After sedation is achieved, the patient should be closely observed to ensure that respiratory status is stable when the peak sedation effect is achieved.

The vast majority of patients with hallucinogen-induced agitation respond clinically to adequate doses of benzodiazepines. Butyrophenone antipsychotic agents, such as haloperidol and droperidol, are rapidly effective and generally safe for drug-induced psychosis or agitation states from other drugs, including cocaine, amphetamines, and phencyclidine (also discussed in Chapters 144 and 150). Haloperidol, given 2 to 5 mg IM, may be repeated every 20 to 30 minutes with consideration of other agents after a total of 10 mg. Although not approved for IV use, this route is widely used but may be considered in the psychotic or severely agitated patient with stable vital signs with cardiac monitoring in 5-mg doses to a maximum dose of 15 mg. The recommended sedative dose for droperidol is 2.5 to 5 mg IM. Of note, droperidol has a black box warning from the U.S. Food and Drug Administration (FDA) for QT prolongation and potentially torsade de pointes. However, most reported cases of butyrophenone-induced dysrhythmias have been in individuals receiving large doses for prolonged periods, such as hours to days, or in elderly populations (older than 60 years). These medications lack the respiratory depression potentially caused by other agents and may be beneficial in some cases when rapid sedation is required. For these reasons, the butyrophenones remain effective agents for

treatment of more severe hallucinogenic-induced agitation in carefully selected patients.

Disposition

The majority of patients with anxiety or panic reactions can be verbally deescalated, with little clinical intervention. Acutely toxic patients who respond to sedation and do not have complications can be discharged after the acute toxicity stage resolves. We recommend discharging them accompanied by a non-intoxicated, responsible family member or friend. Patients who persist with confused or paranoid behavior should be observed until their mental status returns to baseline. Patients with altered mental status that does not normalize after 8 to 12 hours of observation in the ED, or who present after a massive ingestion with medical complications, require admission to a monitored setting for serial reassessments. Patients with self-destructive behavior or in need of addiction counselling may benefit from psychiatric intervention.

DISSOCIATIVE AGENTS

Principles of Toxicity

Dissociative hallucinogens describe a cohort of agents that result in symptoms that include dissociation from the environment that frequently have analgesic and amnestic properties. The agents in the category of dissociative hallucinogens have effects on multiple receptors that result in their unique properties, but the common thread among this group is their activity at the N-methyl-D-aspartate (NMDA) receptor. The NMDA receptor is found on neurons and normally functions as an ion channel that is activated by glutamate or glycine but modulated by various other substances that bind to the receptor. When open, it allows cations to flow into the nerve cell and propagate an impulse. The NMDA receptor in the brain is thought to play an important role in neuronal plasticity and memory. Phencyclidine (PCP) and ketamine are the two main agents included in the class of dissociative hallucinogens, although dextromethorphan and methoxetamine have emerged as drugs of abuse and have some similar symptoms of toxicity. All of these are similar in chemical structure and pharmacologic effects and at least part of their activity is on the NMDA receptor and more specifically as channel blocking agents. Despite being simple molecules, PCP, ketamine, dextromethorphan, and methoxetamine have complex pharmacology that includes activity on the NMDA receptor, dopamine-norepinephrine-serotonin reuptake pump, sigma opioid receptor, and cholinergic receptors. The combination of these pharmacologic effects, duration of the effects, and amount of agent used all contribute to the ultimate presentation and management of these patients.

Phencyclidine

PCP was initially marketed for use as a general anesthetic; however, severe emergence reactions rapidly led to its recall. In 1978, PCP was classified as a Schedule I drug. Despite well-described negative sensory effects and psychiatric effects, PCP became a common drug of abuse in the 1960s. PCP was sold as the PeaCePill, which was consumed orally and also as Angel Dust. In the mid-1970s, PCP was the most common cause of recreational drug–related emergencies, and in some regions it resulted in more hospitalizations than alcohol and schizophrenia combined.[1] Its popularity eventually decreased because of unpredictable effects, long clinical course, dysphoria, and association with violence; however, over the past decade, there has been a resurgence of PCP use.

PCP causes variable effects depending on dose. At low doses, users can experience sight and sound distortion as well as feelings of invulnerability. At high doses, users can experience hallucinations and catatonia. Violent behavior and profound psychiatric effects can be seen initially or as part of an emergence phenomenon. PCP is well absorbed from any oral, nasal, or rectal mucous membrane and can be insufflated or smoked. It can be injected IM, subcutaneously, or IV. Ingested PCP is well absorbed, with an onset of action between 15 and 60 minutes. When smoked, PCP produces symptoms within 5 minutes, with peak activity in 15 minutes. Intoxication with PCP usually lasts 8 to 16 hours but can be prolonged in chronic users. Although enterohepatic recirculation has been proposed, a more likely cause of these prolonged effects in chronic users is gastrointestinal concretion or delayed release from lipid stores.

Ketamine

Ketamine was developed shortly after PCP in an effort to find a sedative with similar hemodynamic stability and properties as PCP that was shorter acting and without the severe emergence phenomenon commonly seen with PCP. It was first trialed in humans in 1964 and since then has become a relatively common medication with multiple indications, including as a sedative for procedural sedation, an induction agent for rapid sequence intubation (RSI), treatment of acute agitation, and treatment of depression. As a drug of abuse, ketamine is known as Vitamin K, Special K, kit kat, and cat valium; however, preparations available on the street are often adulterated with various stimulants. The most common route of use of street ketamine is by insufflation, but subcutaneous and IM injection and even rectal infusions are performed to achieve a level of intoxication or high, known as the K-hole. Similar to PCP, effects of ketamine are dose dependent and can range from mild disorientation and illusions to catatonia or complete dissociation. Ketamine is approximately an order of magnitude less potent than PCP. With ketamine, the intensity of intoxication is less pronounced, although in larger doses the effects may parallel those of PCP. Duration of action of ketamine is typically shorter, with symptoms lasting approximately 1 hour after insufflation but up to 4 to 8 hours after an oral dose. It is important to point out that chronic ketamine users, even at low doses, can experience persistent psychiatric symptoms similar to schizophrenia.[2] In addition, chronic users of ketamine both as a substance of abuse and under medical direction, have a high incidence of urologic complications such as urinary frequency and nocturia. PCP and ketamine are both highly lipid-soluble agents that undergo extensive metabolism in the liver and are eventually excreted in the urine.

Methoxetamine

Methoxetamine is a derivative of ketamine known as Special M, MXE, Mexxy, and ROFLcopter, and has been sold as a legal high and an alternative to ketamine, with reports of a lower risk of the urologic complications seen with chronic ketamine use which may make it preferable to a minority of users.[3] It is readily available on the internet as an agent often labeled as "research chemicals" and with the warning "not for human consumption." Symptoms of intoxication are similar to those seen with ketamine but may also have an increased risk of neuronal toxicity.[4] Methoxetamine appears to have a slower onset and longer duration of action than ketamine.

Dextromethorphan

Dextromethorphan is not truly a dissociative agent, but at higher doses than medically indicated dextromethorphan and its major metabolite, dextrorphan, act as an NMDA receptor antagonist that produces dissociative hallucinogenic effects similar to ketamine and PCP. With the availability of concentrated pill formulations, abusers of dextromethorphan can ingest large doses without having to drink large volumes of the less palatable cough syrup formulation. Particularly popular in the adolescent community, dextromethorphan is known as DXM, robo, skittles, triple C, and red hots. Although dextromethorphan is typically classified as an opioid, it also has a complex pharmacology. Structurally,

DMX is similar to the opioids and is the methylated dextroisomer of the opioid analgesic levorphanol. Dextromethorphan not only antagonizes the NMDA receptor, resulting in its dissociative effects, but it also inhibits the uptake of serotonin, and drug interactions with selective serotonin reuptake inhibitors and monoamine oxidase inhibitors have been reported. At high dosages, dextromethorphan is an agonist at the sigma opiate receptor, and naloxone has been reported to reverse intoxication.

Clinical Features

The desired effects of dissociative agents include changes in and pleasant intensification of sensory perceptions such as a euphoric "out of body experience." In this setting, patients seldom come to the attention of emergency care providers. However, more distressing symptoms are very common, especially with PCP, and frequently result in patients or friends seeking emergency treatment. Patients with PCP intoxication presenting to EDs can have a wide spectrum of findings, including sympathomimetic signs and symptoms. Behavior may be bizarre, lethargic, agitated, confused, or violent. A blank or catatonic stare is relatively common. Vital signs frequently demonstrate moderate tachycardia and hypertension, with some patients also having hyperthermia. Physical exam can demonstrate pupils that are midsized and reactive, although there may be miosis or mydriasis. Vertical and horizontal nystagmus are often present and considered a hallmark sign of PCP intoxication. Less commonly, rotary nystagmus may be noted with PCP toxicity but should prompt a consideration for another etiology such as head injury or intracranial lesion. Additionally, bizarre posturing, grimacing, and writhing may be seen.

In more severe intoxications, other findings include ataxia, muscle rigidity, increased deep tendon reflexes, increased secretions, bronchospasm, hyperthermia, and seizures. Up to 40% of PCP patients may be violent and combative, and control of these patients may be one of the most challenging encounters in the ED. Superhuman strength is possible because of the dissociative and analgesic action of PCP. Rarely, severe hypertension with PCP overdose has caused intracerebral hemorrhage.

Hyperthermia from PCP can range from mild to life-threatening and high-output congestive heart failure has been reported. Acute rhabdomyolysis and acute myoglobinuric renal failure are also seen due to muscle damage from seizures, extreme muscle activity such as struggling against restraints, or prolonged immobility. Respiratory depression, apnea, and cardiac arrest have also been described.

Although dextromethorphan has activity at opioid receptors, the typical triad of opioid intoxication—miosis, respiratory depression, and mental status depression—is not generally encountered. Similar to meperidine, dextromethorphan may result in mydriasis through paralysis of the ciliary body with intoxication. Typical clinical findings include lethargy, agitation, slurred speech, ataxia, diaphoresis, hypertension, nystagmus, nausea, vomiting, and hallucinations.

Differential Diagnoses

PCP, ketamine, methoxetamine, and dextromethorphan intoxication can mimic other drugs of abuse and intoxicants or can mimic organic causes of the behavior. Sympathetically mediated vital sign changes can be found with numerous other agents, including cocaine, amphetamine, and LSD. Antimuscarinic compounds, such as diphenhydramine, benztropine, and tricyclic antidepressants, can also produce the tachycardia and altered mental status found with PCP or ketamine.

There are many organic causes of symptoms such as altered mental status, tachycardia, and agitation commonly found with dissociative hallucinogens. Trauma and specifically head injuries and intracranial hemorrhage should be considered. Medical etiologies include meningitis (viral or bacterial), heatstroke, salicylate poisoning, thyrotoxicosis, and sepsis. Underlying psychiatric disease, especially if it exists in combination with substance abuse, can be very difficult to distinguish. The provider should be cautious about ascribing symptoms to substance use or abuse without considering other etiologies.

Diagnostic Testing

Many hospital laboratories use radioimmunoassays that can detect urinary PCP with a detection limit of 5 ng/mL. Urine may be positive for PCP for 2 to 4 days after use and can be positive for more than 1 week. Serum screening for PCP is of little clinical benefit because levels correlate poorly with symptoms. Several substances, including dextromethorphan, may cross-react with urine screens for PCP because of their structural similarities. Chlorpromazine, methadone, mesoridazine, ketamine, diphenhydramine, venlafaxine, meperidine, and tramadol may also cross-react with some assays, causing false-positive results. If the ingestion is known or suspected to be dextromethorphan because of the prevalence of combination medications, a serum acetaminophen level should be obtained.

If patients have not been hyperthermic and have no signs of trauma, laboratory or other diagnostic tests are generally not needed. With acutely symptomatic patients, a complete metabolic profile, renal function, and creatine phosphokinase (CPK), serum glucose, and ethanol levels should be measured. Workup for any other disease processes should also be pursued as directed by presentation. For patients with acute mental status changes that persist beyond the expected natural course, computed tomography of the head is indicated.

Of particular note, because dextromethorphan is typically formulated as a hydrobromide salt, chronic use may result in spurious hyperchloremia with a low or negative anion gap due to interference of chloride analysis by the bromide ion in the laboratory autoanalyzer.

Management

Prehospital treatment should follow usual protocols for management of agitated patients. The threat of violence to prehospital care providers from patients with PCP intoxication is important to recognize and prehospital systems should have both chemical and physical restraint protocols in place that maximize the safety of providers, patients, and bystanders. Sometimes, awaiting more help or awaiting providers who can use chemical sedation is better than engaging with these patients without adequate support. Extreme agitation, although possible, is less common with ketamine and methoxetamine. Especially when these patients have been sedated prior to hospital arrival, prehospital providers can often provide critical information regarding the patient and notify ED providers of potential trauma or other issues associated with patient care and presentation at the scene.

Sedation of patients under the influence of dissociative hallucinogens is often the first challenge. Chemical sedation is preferred to physical restraint with PCP or ketamine intoxication to reduce the incidence of rhabdomyolysis. Temporary physical restraint may be necessary to ensure patient and medical staff safety until chemical restraint has been achieved. A well-coordinated team with security personnel involvement should apply restraints simultaneously to all four extremities and the body. Assessment of mental status may not be as reliable after chemical sedation, but the benefits of protecting the patient, staff, and other patients in adjacent rooms far outweigh the disadvantages.

As discussed earlier with hallucinogenic agents, butyrophenones such as haloperidol and droperidol can be given IM with a rapid response, avoiding the danger of IV establishment. Haloperidol, 5 to 10 mg IM or IV, is usually effective but can be titrated at 10- to 15-minute intervals until the patient is calm. The sedative dose for droperidol is 2.5 to 5 mg IM. These agents may antagonize the CNS receptor sites that

are responsible for much of the violent behavior in these individuals. These medications lack the respiratory depression potentially caused by other agents and may be beneficial in some cases when sedation is required. Droperidol and haloperidol are sometimes withheld because of the FDA black block warning about QT prolongation. It is important to note that most cases of this have been seen in patients receiving higher doses than those recommended here, given repeatedly over a longer period of time, and in patients greater than 60 years old. For these reasons, butyrophenones are still considered safe and effective agents in controlling agitated patients. Benzodiazepines such as lorazepam, 2 to 4 mg IV or IM, or diazepam, 5 to 10 mg IV, or midazolam 5 to 10 mg IM may also be used to treat agitation (see Chapters 144, 150, and 185).

Any effects of dissociative hallucinogens should be managed with symptomatic and supportive care. Hyperthermia and seizure are two of the more common severe complications. Hyperthermia is common in severe cases of PCP poisoning. All patients with significant symptoms, psychosis, or history of violent behavior should have their core temperature measured. Individuals with hyperthermia should be treated with rapid sedation to decrease neuromuscular hyperactivity and heat production. Rapid sequence intubation may be required to allow for adequate sedation and active, evaporative cooling measures (see Chapter 129). Renal status and creatine kinase level should also be monitored to detect rhabdomyolysis and myoglobinuric renal failure.

Dextromethorphan poisoning may cause agitation, or it can present with somnolence due to the opiate effects of the agent. Respiratory depression may respond to IV administration of naloxone; however, the dissociative effects of the drug do not typically respond to naloxone. Similar to mild cases of other dissociative hallucinogens, patients generally improve within 4 to 6 hours post ingestion.

Disposition

For nonviolent patients with dissociative agent intoxication, a quiet holding room is ideal for 4 to 6 hours of observation. Patients with violent behavior or obtundation sometimes require admission to the hospital, especially if they have developed significant renal insufficiency, rhabdomyolysis, require respiratory monitoring, or if their temperature does not normalize. Many of these patients, even when presenting with significant symptoms, can be medically cleared within 12 to 24 hours.

CANNABIS AND SYNTHETIC CANNABINOIDS

Principles of Toxicity

Cannabis (marijuana) is the most common federally illegal drug in the United States. It was used medicinally in ancient times for conditions such as colic and asthma and has been federally illegal since 1937. However, as of 2020, fifteen states (Alaska, Arizona, California, Colorado, Illinois, Maine, Massachusetts, Michigan, Montana, Nevada, New Jersey, Oregon, South Dakota, and Washington) and the District of Columbia have passed legislation to legalize recreational cannabis, and 29 additional states have legalized medical cannabis.

Cannabis sativa and *Cannabis indica* plants are some of the earliest plants grown by humans. Bioactive substances derived from these plants are collectively called cannabinoids. The seedless flowering tops of the female plant are referred to as sinsemilla and are the commonly grown form of cannabis in the United States. The resin from the flowers is made into hashish. Cannabis is smoked, vaporized, or eaten blended into foods. Δ^9-Tetrahydrocannabinol (THC) is the main psychoactive agent of the more than 61 cannabinoid compounds and approximately 300 other substances present in the cannabis plant, and cannabidiol (CBD) is the major nonpsychoactive component. THC has been associated with some of the adverse effects of cannabis use, including

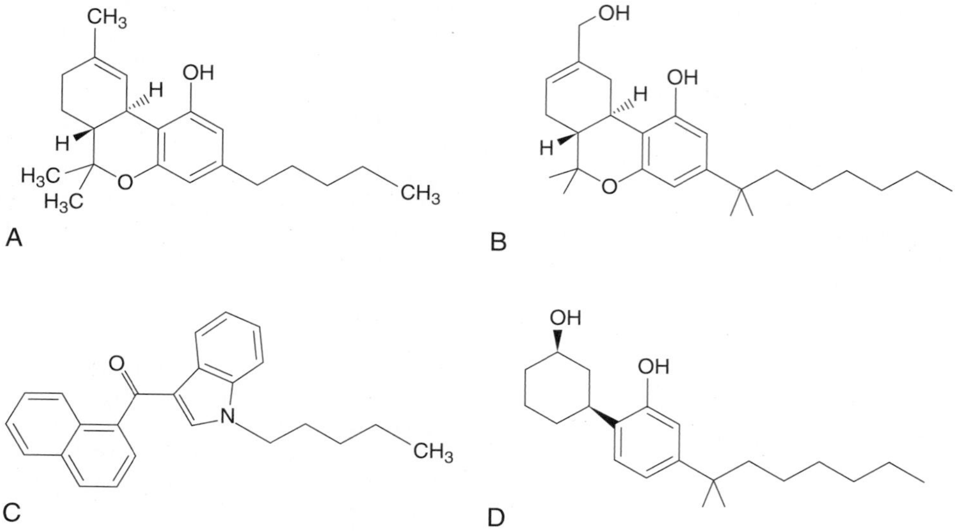

Fig. 145.3 Cannabinoid structures. (A) Δ⁹-Tetrahydrocannabinol. (B) HU-210. (C) JWH-018. (D) CP-47,497.

increased agitation, anxiety, and potential for psychosis. Neuroimaging studies have shown that co-ingestion with CBD may modulate and decrease some of these effects, leading to concerns that newer, high-potency, THC-predominant strains of cannabis may lead to a higher-risk chemical profile of these plants.[5]

Synthetic cannabinoids have also become readily available. These products are often marketed as novelty herbal incense and labeled "not for human consumption." They typically come in resealable foil packages and contain various plant leaves sprayed with a solvent mixture of one or several synthetic cannabinoid compounds. Products have names such as Spice, K2 Summit, Banana Cream Nuke, Yucatan Fire, Genie, Black Mamba, Crazy Clown, and many others depending on the region of the country. The Drug Enforcement Administration (DEA) issued an order in 2011 to list five synthetic cannabinoids—JWH-018, JWH-073, JWH-200, CP-47,497, and cannabicyclohexanol—into Schedule I of the Controlled Substances Act (CSA) to avoid an imminent hazard to public safety. Previously, only one synthetic cannabinoid (HU-210), a structural analogue of THC, was listed as such. In 2014, another four compounds—PB-22, 5F-PB-22, AB-FUBINACA, and ADB-PINACA—were also listed as Schedule I after outbreaks of severe illness in several states. Because numerous synthetic cannabinoids are available, producers of spice products can simply replace a scheduled cannabinoid with others that are not on the Schedule I list, which minimizes the impact of scheduling by the DEA on long-term availability because the demand for the cannabinoid products remains high.

Cannabinoids act primarily at cannabinoid receptors CB1R, found mostly in the CNS, and CB2R, found primarily on peripheral immune cells. Discovery of these cannabinoid receptors and experiences in states with medical cannabis availability have led to interest in further exploration of the therapeutic potential of cannabinoids (Fig. 145.3).

Clinical Features

Smoking cannabis, either in the dried plant form or by smoking or vaporizing resins, extracts, or oils, leads to rapid and predictable signs and symptoms. Ingestion can cause delayed and sometimes unpredictable effects. The most common effects from smoking of cannabis include alteration of mood and usually relaxation and euphoria. The only reliable physiologic effects are a mild increase in heart rate and conjunctival injection. Other acute peripheral changes include urinary

retention, decreased testosterone levels, and decreased intraocular pressure. Short-term memory is impaired, and the ability to perform complex tasks may be adversely affected. Many users report excessive appetite after cannabis use. Peak blood levels occur within 8 minutes of inhalation, with rapid distribution into tissues, especially tissues with a high lipid content. The duration of perceived effects is usually 2 to 4 hours when the drug is smoked.

Oral ingestion of cannabis edibles may be associated with longer duration of effect (≥6–12 hours), and patients with a massive oral cannabis ingestion may develop profound ataxia, vomiting, agitation, anxiety, and CNS depression requiring medical care. Edible products often carry high concentrations of THC in relatively small portion sizes and, due to a delayed onset of effect up to 4 hours after ingestion, patients may ingest escalating amounts of product while awaiting the onset of psychoactive effects.[6]

Pediatric exposures to cannabis may lead to hypothermia, ataxia, nystagmus, tremor, tachycardia, injected conjunctiva, and labile affect. Oral ingestion of potent cannabis in children can produce rapid onset of drowsiness, hypotonia, lethargy, and less commonly seizures. Large ingestions can lead to coma and airway obstruction and respiratory compromise requiring intubation and ventilatory assistance.[7] Pediatric exposures have been rising with the legalization of cannabis in several states.[8]

Whereas intoxications with cannabis and synthetic cannabinoids may have some similarities, significant differences have been described. First-generation synthetic cannabinoids such as JWH-018, JWH-073, HU-210, and CP-47 were commonly associated with tachycardia, agitation, nausea and vomiting, altered mentation, and hallucinations. Seizures were also noted with this group of cannabinoids. Second-generation synthetic cannabinoids such as ADB-PINACA and AB-FUBINACA have been associated with more profound agitation and aggression followed by CNS depression, seizures, tachycardia followed by bradycardia, hypertension followed by hypotension, and, less commonly, ischemic stroke and cardiac toxicity.

Additionally, synthetic cannabinoid use has been associated with an outbreak of anticoagulant toxicity.[9,10] In these cases, patients were exposed to brodifacoum and similar long-acting vitamin K antagonist anticoagulants that contaminated synthetic cannabinoids and presented with bleeding from multiple sites and bruising. Over 160 cases presented to hospitals in Illinois alone, with 4 reported deaths. Many other patients required long-term management with vitamin K supplementation and close follow-up.[9]

Differential Diagnoses

The presentation that most closely resembles that of cannabis and synthetic cannabinoid intoxication is acute psychosis. Some individuals with underlying and preexisting psychiatric disorders may progress to overt psychosis after heavy or first-time cannabis use. Because cannabis is so readily available, it is commonly a co-intoxicant used with ethanol and other psychotropic agents. Pediatric patients with unknown unintentional exposures may appear similar to patients with opioid or sedative hypnotic agent overdose, sepsis, meningitis, or metabolic disorders. Rarely, cannabis can be adulterated with other substances, such as PCP and other illicit drugs used concomitantly.

Diagnostic Testing

Cannabis screening is rarely helpful in the ED. Urinary metabolites of THC are detectable within 1 hour after smoking cannabis, but a positive result on a routine urine toxicology screen does not correlate with acute intoxication. Smoking a single "joint" can be detected for 72 hours when a cutoff level of 100 ng/mL is used, and positive urine levels may persist for 3 months after chronic cannabis use. Inadvertent or passive exposure to large amounts of second-hand cannabis smoke in enclosed areas may produce positive urine test results, depending on the laboratory cutoff levels used. False-positive urine screen results may be produced by efavirenz, ibuprofen, and naproxen. An exception to the utility of a urine drug screen for cannabis exposure in pediatric patients may be an unclear cause of altered mental status.

Of the synthetic cannabinoids, only HU-210 should trigger a positive THC immunoassay screen as a result of structural homology. The majority of other synthetic cannabinoids are structurally distinct from THC and do not result in positive THC immunoassay screens.

Management and Disposition

Care of patients intoxicated from cannabis and synthetic cannabinoids consists of prevention of injury and reassurance for those who have panic reactions. An extremely agitated patient can be sedated with oral or parenteral administration of benzodiazepines or antipsychotics. Antiemetics (e.g., ondansetron 4–8 mg IV, or metoclopramide, 10–20 mg IV) or butyrphenones (e.g., haloperidol or droperidol 0.625–2.5 mg IV) may be used to treat nausea and vomiting induced by the cannabinoid hyperemesis syndrome associated with the synthetic cannabinoids and heavy, daily cannabis use. Hot showers are often recommended for patients suffering these symptoms. The precise mechanism whereby hot bathing produces a rapid reduction in the symptoms of CHS is not clear, but thought to be related to a peripheral tissue receptor called TRPV1, a G-protein coupled receptor that has been shown to interact with the endocannabinoid system.[11] Capsaicin cream may also have some benefit in these cases through a similar mechanism and activation of TRPV1 receptors, although discomfort with its use may limit its utility. Children who are significantly symptomatic may require admission for a 24-hour observation period.

Other Agents

Mescaline

Mescaline is a naturally occurring phenylethylamine usually consumed in the form of peyote buttons, which are derived from the small, blue-green cacti *Lophophora williamsii* and *Lophophora diffusa* (Fig. 145.4). They grow in the deserts of the southwestern United States and Mexico.

Peyote has been used in religious ceremonies for 8000 years. Mescaline is also contained in the San Pedro cactus (*Trichocereus pachanoi*) of South America and is used ritualistically by Andean Native Americans.

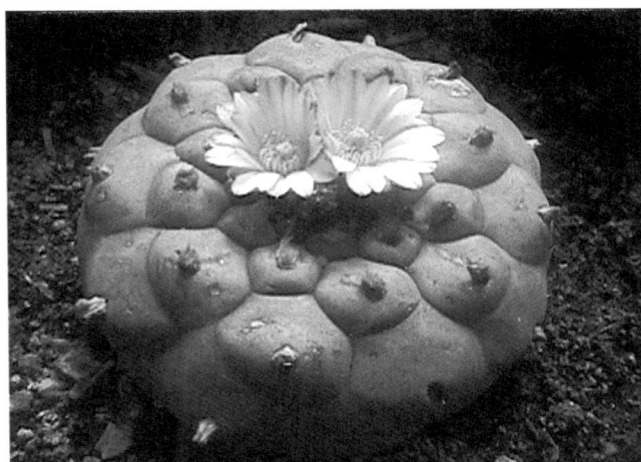

Fig. 145.4 *Lophophora williamsii* (peyote cactus). (Photo by Christopher B., copyright 2000. Accessed at www.erowid.org.)

These cacti contain many other alkaloids, some of which are also psychoactive. The use of peyote is legal for members of the Native American Church in some states. Adverse reactions (e.g., panic attacks) to peyote are rare in structured religious use. Mescaline has an onset of action of 45 to 60 minutes, with a duration of effect lasting 4 to 8 hours. The CNS and physiologic effects of mescaline use are similar to those of LSD, but more vivid hallucinations can occur. Nausea and vomiting are pronounced and almost always precede the hallucinogenic effects, which is an important aspect of the cleansing spiritual ritual.

Nutmeg

Nutmeg is a spice derived from the seed of the nutmeg tree, *Myristica fragrans*. Use of nutmeg as a natural and legal psychotropic agent was popularized in the 1960s. Despite lack of any in vivo human studies, myristicin and elemicin have been suggested as the agents responsible for intoxication because their chemical structure resembles that of mescaline. Reports of intoxication are uncommon. Ingestion of 5 to 30 g (1–4 tablespoons) of the spice is said to induce euphoria and hallucinations but is more likely to cause gastroenteritis.[12]

Salvia

Salvia divinorum, a perennial herb cultivated outdoors in mild climates, is a member of the mint (Lamiaceae) family. Common names for *S. divinorum* are diviner's sage, mystic sage, magic mint, sage of the seers, Sally-D, ska, and Maria Pastora. Although the plant has been used for divination and shamanism by the Mazatec Indians of Oaxaca, Mexico, *S. divinorum* has become popular in the past 20 years for recreational purposes because of its recognized hallucinogenic properties and hallmark "uncontrollable laughter" side effect. In 2004, the DEA listed *S. divinorum* as a drug of concern but, to date, *S. divinorum* and salvinorin A are not currently controlled under the CSA in the United States. Several states, however, have instituted or are considering legislation making possession, cultivation, and use of *S. divinorum* or its extracts illegal.

The active ingredient in *S. divinorum* is salvinorin A, a neoclerodane diterpene with selective agonist activity for kappa opioid receptors. Salvinorin A appears to have no activity at delta or mu opioid receptors. The threshold dose of salvinorin A to produce hallucinations is comparable to that of LSD. However, salvinorin A is distinct from more traditional hallucinogens because it does not bind to the 5-HT$_{2A}$ serotonin receptors, as is the case with LSD.

Salvia is usually chewed and spit out or swallowed, and it seems to be absorbed more readily from the oral mucosa than from the rest of the gastrointestinal tract. Effects produced as a result of oral mucosal absorption may persist for 1 hour. Dried leaves can also be smoked. Inhalation of smoke can produce symptoms within 1 minute that subside after 20 to 30 minutes. Sensations experienced are variable but include distortions of color and vision, laughter, and synesthesias, which are confusions of the senses, such as "seeing sounds or smelling colors." Salvinorin A is not detected by typical drug screening tests and is not known to cause interference with routine drug screens used in the clinical setting. Management of intoxication from *S. divinorum* is mainly supportive, with emphasis on injury prevention.[13] Use of naloxone, a nonspecific opioid receptor antagonist, may theoretically be helpful for the reversal of psychotropic manifestations.

Kratom

Mitragyna speciosa, or kratom, is a tree found in tropical and subtropical regions of Asia and Africa. The popularity of kratom has grown because of reports of its successful use to attenuate symptoms of opioid withdrawal. Because kratom remains easily obtainable, individuals are able to self-administer the perceived remedy, obviating the need for physician supervision. The safety of such a practice is unknown.

Although kratom extract contains more than 25 alkaloids, mitragynine is the most abundantly found in the plant. Mitragynine is an indole alkaloid with structural analogy similar to that of yohimbine and has agonist activity at mu and delta opioid receptors, producing euphoric, analgesic, and respiratory depressant effects. The respiratory depressant effects are more likely to occur when combined with opioids or other respiratory depressants. Despite its structural similarity to yohimbine, a selective antagonist of presynaptic α_2-adrenergic receptors, animal studies have suggested that mitragynine is also an agonist at postsynaptic α_2-adrenergic receptors and blocks 5-HT$_{2A}$ receptors.

Often, kratom is ingested in powder or capsule form. The leaves may also be chewed, smoked, or brewed into a tea. Psychotomimetic effects occur within 5 to 10 minutes of use and may persist for 1 hour, with stimulatory effects at lower doses and opioid effects at higher doses. Opioid properties include analgesic, antitussive, antidiarrheal, and emetogenic effects.[14]

Currently, there are no clinical diagnostic tests available to detect the presence of kratom alkaloids. Treatment of intoxication is supportive. Although coma and opioid activity have been demonstrated with kratom, the effectiveness of opioid antagonists in reversing its effects is inconsistent. A withdrawal syndrome characterized by anxiety, restlessness, and nausea treated with an opioid agonist and lofexidine (an α_2-agonist related to clonidine) has also been reported.

The issues regarding the safety and efficacy of kratom and its mitragynine constituent require additional research. The DEA classification of the Mitragyna alkaloids as Schedule I controlled substances is likely to impede further studies on kratom.[15]

Ibogaine

Ibogaine is a naturally occurring indole alkaloid found in the roots of the African rain forest shrub *Tabernanthe iboga*. For many centuries, iboga has been ingested by the indigenous peoples of western Africa as a remedy for fatigue, hunger, and thirst and as a sacrament in religious ceremonies. As with many plant-derived agents, ibogaine's physiologic effects are highly complex and may involve opioid, dopaminergic, serotonergic, glutaminergic, γ-aminobutyric acid (GABA)–ergic, glutamatergic, adrenergic, and cellular ion channel signaling systems.

Although ibogaine is classified as a Schedule I drug, it is still sought after as a treatment to ease opioid withdrawal and diminish craving of other abused drugs. The intensity of visual hallucinations from ingestion of iboga, in contrast to other hallucinogens, is described to be more pronounced with eyes closed. Since the first report in 1990,

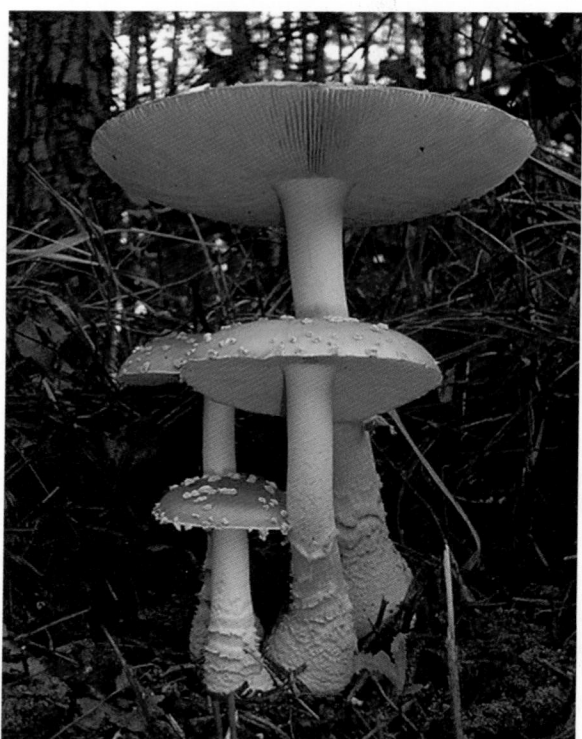

Fig. 145.5 *Amanita muscaria* mushroom. (Photo by Mark Shubert, copyright 2004. Accessed at www.erowid.org.)

there have been reported fatalities due to sudden cardiac death within 72 hours of ibogaine use. The mechanism appears to be blockage of the hERG/IKr channel, leading to marked QT prolongation and tachyarrhythmias. There are no specific detection tests for ibogaine, and diagnosis is dependent on a history of exposure because clinical findings are largely nonspecific. Management is predominantly supportive, although patients with markedly prolonged QT intervals and evidence of risk for torsades de pointes may require admission to a monitored setting, treatment with IV magnesium supplementation (magnesium sulfate, 2–4 g IV), electrolyte repletion, and overdrive pacing (either chemical with isoproterenol, or electric via transdermal or transvenous pacing) in severe cases.

Isoxazole Mushrooms

Isoxazole-containing mushrooms include *Amanita muscaria*, *Amanita pantherina*, *Amanita gemmata*, and *Amanita cothurnata*. *A. muscaria* has a red or yellow cap, with white warty structures on its surface, and grows in forests of aspen, birch, fir, or pine trees (Fig. 145.5). It has been used in Siberia for centuries and is often described in folklore and fairy tales (also see Chapter 153).

The active ingredients are the isoxazole derivatives ibotenic acid and its decarboxylation product, muscimol, which are structural analogues of the endogenous neurotransmitters glutamic acid (excitatory) and GABA (inhibitory) and are thought to act at these respective receptor sites. The excitatory effects characterized by elation, giddiness, hyperactivity, muscle tremors, and distortion of space and time begin approximately 30 minutes to 2 hours after ingestion and are likely to be mediated by ibotenic acid. Following is a phase of tiredness and deep sleep, in which it may be difficult to arouse the patient. During this phase, vivid hallucinations and manic excitement may oscillate with periods of deep sleep. The duration of effect is up to 12 hours. Management of the excitatory phase is similar to that of other hallucinogens previously described in this chapter, consisting of supportive care, a low stimulus environment, and benzodiazepine administration. Prolonged sleep with *A. muscaria* ingestion requires only observation and supportive care. Tonic-clonic seizures are reported, but occurrences are rare. In general, adult patients more often experience GABA-dominant symptoms, and pediatric patients more often experience glutamic acid-dominant symptoms.

Paradoxically, there has been a high incidence of mistreatment of *A. muscaria* ingestion with atropine because the name implies that it contains muscarine, a cholinergic toxin. However, the amount of muscarine is miniscule. Atropine may exacerbate the anticholinergic effects associated with isoxazole mushrooms. It is important to differentiate isoxazole-containing *Amanita* mushrooms from the potentially deadly hepatotoxic cyclopeptide-containing *Amanita* mushrooms, of which *Amanita phalloides* is a member.

The references for this chapter can be found online at ExpertConsult.com.

146

Iron and Heavy Metals

Jillian L. Theobald and Mark B. Mycyk

IRON

Foundations

Iron poisoning used to be the leading cause of poisoning death in children. In 1997 the U.S. Food and Drug Administration (FDA) required warning labels and implemented changes in the packaging of iron supplements after which there was an abrupt decrease in the number of poisonings and deaths. Although the FDA rescinded its strict packaging restrictions on iron supplements in 2003, iron poisoning currently remains relatively uncommon. In 2017, there were 6033 calls to poison centers concerning iron exposures and there were two deaths. Calls regarding multivitamins containing iron were much more common, resulting in 11,157 calls but no deaths.[1]

Iron is an important metal that is essential to the function of hemoglobin, myoglobin, and many cytochromes and enzymes. Certain disease states result from too much or too little iron, such as hemochromatosis and anemia, respectively. Iron is absorbed mostly in the small intestine. Depending on total body stores, as little as 10% or as much as 95% of the ingested iron is taken into cells. In the cell, iron has three pathway options: storage bound to ferritin, transfer to the serum where it is bound to transferrin, or loss when the intestinal cell is sloughed off. Under normal conditions only 15% to 35% of the iron-binding capacity of transferrin is used. The total iron-binding capacity (TIBC), a crude measure of the ability of serum proteins (including transferrin) to bind iron, ranges from 300 to 400 µg/dL. Normal serum iron concentrations range from 50 to 150 µg/dL. When iron concentrations rise after a significant overdose, transferrin becomes saturated. Excess iron circulates free and unbound in the serum. Unbound iron is directly toxic to target organs.

Iron has two distinct toxic effects: (1) direct caustic injury to the gastrointestinal mucosa, and (2) impaired cellular metabolism, primarily of the heart, liver, and central nervous system (CNS). The caustic effects of iron on the gut cause the initial symptoms of vomiting, diarrhea, and abdominal pain. Hemorrhagic necrosis of gastric or intestinal mucosa can lead to bleeding, perforation, and peritonitis. Metabolic acidosis occurs when unbound iron moves into cells and localizes near the mitochondrial cristae, resulting in uncoupling of oxidative phosphorylation and impairment of adenosine triphosphate synthesis. Hydration of the iron molecule creates an excess of unbuffered protons, worsening metabolic acidosis. Cell membranes are injured by free radical–mediated lipid peroxidation. Hypotension occurs as iron increases capillary permeability and leads to both arteriolar and venodilation. Direct myocardial toxicity decreases cardiac output. These effects, combined with severe gastrointestinal fluid losses, can lead to shock, cardiovascular collapse, and death.

In an iron overdose, determining the amount of elemental iron ingested is most important, because cellular toxicity depends on the effects of elemental iron. Different formulations of iron salts contain different percentages of elemental iron (Table 146.1). The total amount of elemental iron ingested can be approximated by multiplying the estimated number of tablets by the fraction of elemental iron contained in the tablet. Ingestions of less than 20 mg/kg of elemental iron usually causes no symptoms. Ingestion of 20 to 60 mg/kg results in mild to moderate symptoms, and ingestion of more than 60 mg/kg may lead to severe morbidity and mortality. Newer forms of iron are carbonyl iron and iron polysaccharide: both are non-ionic and associated with lower toxicity. Neither form is directly corrosive. The conversion to the iron ion, which is responsible for toxicity, is very slow in these newer preparations. There are no reported cases of serious toxicity or death from the ingestion of the non-ionic compounds.

Clinical Features

The clinical effects of acute iron poisoning have traditionally been divided into five stages (Table 146.2). The timing of each stage varies for individual patients. The severity of phase 4 is primarily dose-related, and it is usually during this phase that fatality occurs.

Differential Diagnoses

Many toxins are irritating to the gastrointestinal tract and can cause nausea, vomiting, and diarrhea. Hemorrhagic gastroenteritis in the setting of an ingestion history should raise suspicion for caustic ingestions, ethanol, toxic alcohols, salicylates, ibuprofen, colchicine, and other heavy metals, such as arsenic, inorganic mercury, and iron.

Diagnostic Testing

The presence of early gastrointestinal symptoms suggests a potentially serious ingestion, whereas absence of gastrointestinal symptoms is usually reassuring. A serum iron concentration measured at 3 to 5 hours after ingestion is the most useful laboratory test to evaluate the potential severity of an iron overdose. Sustained-release or enteric-coated preparations may have erratic absorption, so the serum concentration should be repeated at 6 to 8 hours after ingestion. Peak serum iron below 350 µg/dL is generally associated with minimal toxicity; 350 to 500 µg/dL with moderate toxicity; and above 500 µg/dL with severe toxicity. Because iron is rapidly cleared from the serum and deposited in the liver, the concentration of iron after a substantial ingestion may be deceptively low if it is measured several hours after its peak absorption. TIBC is an inaccurate test and is not useful to gauge the severity of iron poisoning.

A screening abdominal radiograph may also be helpful to confirm a recent large ingestion and should be interpreted in the context of serum levels, as described later. Most tablets that contain a significant amount of elemental iron are radiopaque (Fig. 146.1). False-negative radiographs may occur with chewable, liquid, and completely dissolved iron compounds, so negative radiography should not be used to exclude iron ingestion in cases of suspected or witnessed ingestion. Repeated radiographs can also demonstrate the efficacy of gastrointestinal decontamination efforts.

Management

Stabilization and Supportive Care

Early hypotension is often due to GI losses and should be treated with intravenous fluids. Later, direct toxic effects on the cardiovascular system occur and are best treated with vasopressors. Patients with mental status depression and concern for airway protection should be intubated and mechanically ventilated.

Decontamination

Oral activated charcoal does not bind iron. Gastric lavage and ipecac are ineffective and not recommended. Iron tablets clump together as their outer coatings dissolve, often forming large pharmacobezoars. Whole bowel irrigation (WBI) is the preferred method of decontamination for significant iron tablet ingestions, especially when confirmed by radiograph, but WBI is not useful in cases of liquid or chewable iron.[2] Early, rapid decontamination of the gastrointestinal system may obviate the need for or shorten antidotal therapy duration.

For significant ingestions, especially when the number of tablets identified by abdominal radiography indicates a likely toxic dose, WBI with a polyethylene glycol–electrolyte solution (PEG-ELS) should be initiated.[2] The solution should be administered through a nasogastric tube. The recommended rate of administration of PEG-ELS is 500 mL/hr in children 9 months to 6 years old, 1000 mL/hr in children 6 to 12

TABLE 146.1	Common Iron Preparations
Compound	**Percentage of Elemental Iron**
Ionic Compounds	
Ferrous sulfate	20
Ferrous fumarate	33
Ferrous gluconate	12
Non-Ionic Compounds	
Carbonyl iron	100
Iron polysaccharide	46

TABLE 146.2 Clinical Manifestations of Iron Toxicity Following an Acute Overdose[a]

	Phase	Clinical Features	Mechanism of Toxicity
1	Gastrointestinal (6 hours)	Vomiting Diarrhea Hematemesis Hematochezia	Corrosive effect of iron on the gastrointestinal mucosa
2	Latent (6 to 24 hours)	Resolution of gastrointestinal symptoms Tachycardia Acidosis Depressed mental status	Ongoing cellular toxicity and organ damage
3	Systemic (12 to 24 hours)	Return of gastrointestinal symptoms Acidosis Leukocytosis Coagulopathy Renal failure Lethargy or coma Cardiovascular collapse	Iron distributes to the tissues with worsening cellular toxicity and organ damage
4	Hepatic (2 to 5 days)	Fulminant liver failure Coagulopathy	Rapid absorption from portal system with resultant oxidative damage
5	Obstructive (3 to 6 weeks)	Pyloric or bowel scarring Obstruction	Healing of the injured gastrointestinal mucosa

[a]Typical duration of symptoms post-ingestion is also given.

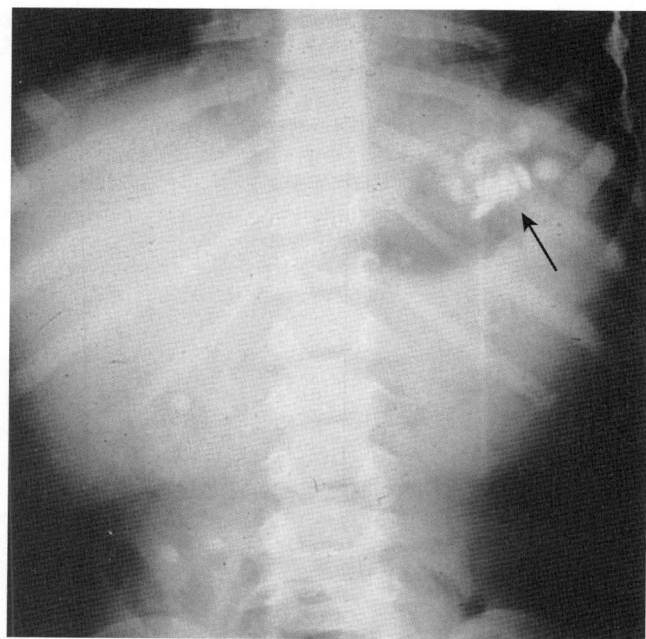

Fig. 146.1 Radiopaque iron tablets *(arrow)* seen on abdominal radiograph. (From: Craig SA. Radiology. In: Ford MD, Delaney KA, Ling LJ, et al, editors. Clinical Toxicology. Philadelphia: WB Saunders: 2001; p 62.)

years old, and 1.5 to 2 L/hr in adolescents and adults. WBI is continued until the rectal effluent is clear and there is no radiographic evidence of pill fragments.[2] This technique has been used in children, adolescents, and pregnant women without serious complications or electrolyte disturbances. Common side effects include nausea, vomiting, abdominal cramping, and bloating. WBI is contraindicated in the presence of bowel obstruction, perforation, ileus, or hemodynamic instability.[2]

Enhanced Elimination

Hemodialysis and hemoperfusion are not effective in the removal of iron because of its large volume of distribution. Early exchange transfusions have been used with some success for severely symptomatic patients. However, this should only be considered in patients who are not responding to standard chelation therapy.

Antidotal Therapy

Deferoxamine is the antidote for iron toxicity. Deferoxamine chelates iron to form the water-soluble compound ferrioxamine, which is renally excreted. Deferoxamine binds to free iron and will not chelate iron from hemoglobin, transferrin, or ferritin. Patients with an iron concentration above 500 μg/dL and those who, regardless of level, are exhibiting severe signs and symptoms of iron toxicity (metabolic acidosis, lethargy, hypotension, or signs of shock) require chelation. Pregnancy is not a contraindication to deferoxamine therapy. However, the prepregnancy weight should be used to calculate the ingested dose. Because of its short half-life, deferoxamine is administered as a continuous intravenous infusion starting at 5 mg/kg/hr and titrated to the typical goal rate of 15 mg/kg/hr, as tolerated, for 24 hours. Infusion rates of up to 35 mg/kg/hr have been reported, but this should only be considered following consultation with a toxicologist. More rapid administration of deferoxamine can lead to hypotension, which is managed by reducing the initial rate of the infusion and then slowly increasing it to the desired rate. Prolonged deferoxamine infusion has been associated with acute respiratory distress syndrome (ARDS) and also with *Yersinia* sepsis. The pulmonary complications are usually related to high dose deferoxamine for durations longer than 24 hours.

Category	Source
Pediatric	Lead dust
	Paint in old homes
	Parent's occupation
	Imported toys or candies
	Foreign body ingestion (fishing weights, toys)
Occupational	Construction, particularly old home remodeling
	Lead smelters
	Battery recycling, repair, and manufacturing
	Firing range instructors
	Automobile mechanics
	Plastics manufacturing
Recreational	Moonshine
	Ceramics
	Home and car remodeling
	Painting
Other	Herbal remedies
	Retained lead bullets

TABLE 146.3 Sources of Lead Exposure

Disposition

The asymptomatic patient who is reliably known to have ingested less than 40 mg/kg of elemental iron does not need additional therapy and can be discharged home after appropriate poison prevention counseling with reliable care takers. In patients who ingest more than 40 mg/kg, an iron concentration should be obtained at 3 to 5 hours post-ingestion and also 6 to 8 hours post-ingestion. If peak iron remains less than 300 μg/dL, is not rising, and the patient is asymptomatic during 6 hours of observation, the patient can be discharged home. If the patient is exhibiting signs of severe toxicity, even if the ingested dose is unknown, or meets criteria for deferoxamine chelation therapy, admission to an intensive care unit with poison center or toxicologist consultation is advised. If indicated, a psychiatric consultation should be requested.

LEAD

Foundations

Lead poisoning remains one of the most common and preventable environmentally mediated problems in the United States. The elimination of leaded gasoline and the ban on leaded paint in households in the 1970s exponentially reduced the number of lead poisonings in the United States. However, the Center for Disease Control and Prevention (CDC) estimates that approximately 535,000 children, aged 1 to 5 years old, still have elevated blood lead levels (BLLs) from various environmental exposures.[3] Immigrant and refugee children are at much greater risk for lead poisoning than children born in the United States because of exposures prior to arrival in the United States.[4,5] Adult lead poisoning has been decreasing over time and the CDC reported that in 2013, 20.4 per 100,000 adult workers had BLLs of 10 mcg/dL or greater, down from 26.6 in 2010.[6] Given the continued wide use of lead in industry, there are many potential sources of exposure. Retained bullet fragments are another important source to investigate[7] (Table 146.3).

Most lead exposures occur by ingestion in children and workplace inhalation in adults. Dermal absorption may also occur but is much less significant. Children and pregnant women absorb almost four times the amount of ingested lead than other adults. Once absorbed, lead is bound to red bloods cells and slowly distributes to the soft tissues where it is eventually stored, primarily in bone. The half-life of lead in the red blood cell is approximately 30 days, but once in the bone, the half-life can last decades. Lead easily crosses the placenta,

TABLE 146.4   Typical Blood Lead Levels and Correlative Signs and Symptoms in Children and Adults

Level (µg/dl)	SYMPTOMS	
	Adults	Children
10	None	Decreased IQ
		Decreased hearing
		Decreased growth
20	Increased protoporphyrin	Decreased nerve conduction velocity
	No symptoms	Increased protoporphyrin
30	Increased blood pressure	Decreased vitamin D metabolism
	Decreased hearing	
40	Peripheral neuropathies	Decreased hemoglobin synthesis
	Nephropathy	
	Infertility (men)	
50	Decreased hemoglobin synthesis	Lead colic
70	Anemia	Anemia
		Encephalopathy
		Nephropathy
100	Encephalopathy	Death

IQ, Intelligence quotient.

and maternal blood levels correlate with umbilical cord blood levels.[8] Neonatal lead exposure also occurs through breast milk. Most lead is ultimately excreted in the urine and bile.

There is no biologic role for lead in the human body. Lead complexes with sulfhydryl groups of proteins, which can alter enzyme and receptor function and distort structural proteins. Lead is also structurally similar to calcium and interferes with calcium-dependent cellular processes. Its toxic effects are most prominent in the hematopoietic and neurologic systems.

Clinical Features

The clinical features of lead poisoning are broad and often nonspecific (Table 146.4). Symptoms depend on the BLL, whether the patient is an adult or child, and whether the exposure is acute or chronic. Although all organ systems are affected, the most sensitive are the hematologic, vascular, and nervous systems. Lead inhibits heme biosynthesis, and the classic manifestation of hematopoietic lead toxicity is anemia. Anemia may be either normochromic or hypochromic. Chronic kidney disease and hyperuricemic gout ("saturnine gout") can also result from elevated BLLs. Chronic kidney disease consequently may worsen underlying anemia. Lead poisoning is associated with chronic hypertension. In the peripheral nervous system, segmental demyelination and degeneration of motor axons result in peripheral neuropathies. Wrist-drop and foot-drop are characteristic of adult lead poisoning but rarely seen today.[9] Importantly, lead toxicity can cause neuropsychiatric disorders. Many are difficult to distinguish during an emergency department (ED) evaluation, so collaboration with a primary care physician is essential to identify new cognitive deficits. In children, elevated BLL is associated with decreased intelligence quotient (IQ) scores, hyperactivity, decreased attention span, overaggressive behavior, learning disabilities, and criminal behavior. Severely high BLLs may present with lead encephalopathy associated with increased capillary permeability and cerebral edema.

Differential Diagnoses

The differential diagnoses of lead poisoning are broad, and because the symptoms of early poisoning are nonspecific, lead poisoning today is often initially not considered or misdiagnosed. Lead poisoning could be confused for neuropathies (such as carpal tunnel or Landry-Guillain-Barré syndrome) or abdominal or urologic pathologies (such as gastroenteritis, nephrolithiasis, or appendicitis).[9,10] The subtle neuropsychiatric signs in children can also be misdiagnosed as attention deficit hyperactivity disorder or other behavioral disturbances. Therefore, it is necessary to consider lead poisoning in the appropriate circumstance, particularly where another diagnosis is not established as the primary cause of the presentation.

Diagnostic Testing

Lead toxicity rarely presents primarily to the ED. Most patients encountered in the ED have been referred for management of an elevated screening BLL measured in a clinic or workplace surveillance program. Some patients may seek ED care following an ingestion of a leaded foreign body or with worrisome symptoms following a possible environmental exposure. Diagnostic testing should consist of a venous BLL, including those cases referred in for an abnormal screening test. Capillary screens (such as finger or heel sticks) may be falsely elevated. If the patient is symptomatic, other tests include a complete blood cell count, basic metabolic panel, liver and renal function tests, and urinalysis. A peripheral smear classically shows basophilic stippling, but this finding is relatively rare. Because lead-containing objects and paint chips are radiopaque, abdominal radiographs can confirm acute ingestion and determine the need for bowel decontamination. In cases of altered mental status, seizures, or coma, a computed tomography (CT) scan of the head may show cerebral edema associated with acute lead encephalopathy and can assist in ruling out other causes of these neurologic signs. In children, plain radiographs of the wrist and knees classically demonstrate increased metaphyseal activity termed *lead lines* that are characteristic of chronic exposures. However, such x-rays are not routinely obtained in the ED.

Management

Stabilization and Supportive Care

The most important treatment step in lead poisoning is removing the patient from the source. This is the only treatment needed in most cases of lead poisoning. Determining the exact source often requires the collaborative assistance of a primary care physician, social worker, and the department of public health. Recent data suggest urban patients at risk for lead poisoning are also at risk for asthma; the environmental evaluation for lead and asthma risks is similar, so ensuring follow-up with a primary care provider to assess the risk for both problems is essential.

Decontamination

Oral activated charcoal does not bind lead. If an abdominal radiograph demonstrates lead within the gastrointestinal tract—particularly the stomach and small intestine—then bowel decontamination should be performed. This can be done with WBI or repeated doses of polyethylene glycol (see the Iron section for dosing regimen).

Antidotal Therapy

Children. Treatment for lead toxicity rarely is commenced in the ED, but the decision to admit for chelation or source control may be indicated after consultation with the poison control, a medical toxicologist, or the primary care provider. Regardless of the BLL, eliminating the source of exposure remains the most important priority. Evidence indicates no significant benefit from chelation for children with a BLL lower than 45 µg/dL as long as the source of exposure is controlled. A BLL less than 44 µg/dL in a patient who is asymptomatic or minimally symptomatic requires a medical and environmental evaluation to identify the source, stop further exposure, and have scheduled repeat BLLs done as per current Centers for Disease Control (CDC) and public health guidelines. Caregiver education about concerning symptoms and sources of lead exposure should be coupled with close follow-up with a primary caregiver for all patients with a detectable BLL. An environmental evaluation can often be arranged with the local public health department.

Blood lead levels of 45 to 69 µg/dL in patients without vomiting or CNS symptoms can be managed in the outpatient setting with oral succimer (2,3-dimercaptosuccinic acid [DMSA]; Chemet). The initial dose of succimer is 10 mg/kg every 8 hours for 5 days, then 10 mg/kg every 12 hours for 14 days (maximum 500 mg per dose for children). The most common adverse reactions include nausea, vomiting, diarrhea, and transient elevations in liver transaminase levels. Although succimer has been FDA-approved only for children, it is effective and can be used in adults with lead poisoning. Table 146.5 summarizes available chelating agents with indications and doses. Any patient treated on an outpatient basis should be discharged to a lead-free environment.

Patients with a BLL of 69 µg/dL or higher require hospitalization and parenteral chelation therapy, even if asymptomatic. Evidence of encephalopathy, regardless of BLL, requires admission for parenteral chelation therapy. Consultation with a medical toxicologist, regional poison center, and pediatrician is indicated. Dimercaprol (or British antilewisite [BAL]) is given via a deep intramuscular injection as 4 mg/kg every 4 hours for children and adults. Adverse reactions to BAL include nausea, vomiting, urticaria, pyrexia, hypertension, and hemolysis in patients with glucose-6-phosphate dehydrogenase deficiency. Because BAL is diluted in peanut oil, it is contraindicated in patients with peanut allergies. In cases of encephalopathy, intravenous calcium disodium ethylenediaminetetraacetic acid (CaNa$_2$EDTA) should be initiated with the second dose of BAL. Starting treatment with CaNa$_2$EDTA may paradoxically increase lead transport across the blood-brain barrier. The dosage of CaNa$_2$EDTA for adult and pediatric patients with acute lead encephalopathy is 1500 mg/m²/day (approximately 50 to 75 mg/kg/day) given by continuous intravenous infusion for 5 days (maximum of 1000 mg per day for children and 3000 mg per day for adults). Adverse reactions include renal tubular injury and chelation of other metals, especially iron and zinc. CaNa$_2$EDTA should be given only with adequate urine flow or with hemodialysis in the patient with renal failure. For patients with a BLL more than 69 µg/dL but no signs of encephalopathy, the dosage of

CaNa$_2$EDTA is 50 mg/kg/day or 1000 mg/m²/day, given in two to four divided doses for up to 5 days without the need for concurrent BAL therapy.

Adults. The treatment of adults with chronic poisoning is based primarily on symptoms and threshold BLLs established by workplace regulatory agencies. In the asymptomatic adult or the patient with only mild clinical symptoms, the only intervention needed is cessation of exposure. According to the Occupational Safety and Health Administration (OSHA) lead standard, workers with serum lead levels above 40 µg/dL should be removed from work. If encephalopathy or severe symptoms are present, then hospitalization and chelation therapy with combined BAL and CaNa$_2$EDTA, as with children described previously, are indicated. Pregnant women should be treated in accordance with adult treatment guidelines. Lead does cross the placenta and can accumulate in the fetus. Newborn infants of exposure mothers may require chelation as well.

Disposition

Families of asymptomatic children with BLLs less than 45 µg/dL and asymptomatic adults should be counseled on how to avoid further exposure and given close follow-up with their primary care provider for a repeat BLL and exposure risk evaluation.

Patients who require oral chelation can be discharged home if they can tolerate succimer and if it can be ensured they do not return to a lead-contaminated environment. The health department should conduct an environmental assessment and testing of other family members so that the primary source of lead exposure can be identified, and further exposure prevented. Follow-up should be arranged with a pediatrician, medical toxicologist, or occupational medicine physician.

Patients who are significantly symptomatic, have worrisome CNS symptoms, and any children with a BLL of 69 µg/dL or higher require hospitalization for environmental exposure evaluation and parenteral chelation therapy.

ARSENIC

Foundations

Arsenic has an infamous history as an agent of homicide and been implicated in mass environmental poisonings.[11] Currently, arsenic exposure is primarily environmental and occupational. Arsenic is found in smelters and electric power plants that burn arsenic-rich coal; in the production of glass and microcircuits; and in rodenticides, fungicides, insecticides, paint, tanning agents, defoliants in the cotton industry, and wood preservatives. Arsenic is also still used for medicinal purposes in the treatment of trypanosomiasis, amebiasis, and leukemia. Importantly, significant concentrations of heavy metals including arsenic, lead, and mercury have been found as contaminants in ayurvedic medications.[12] Arsenic has also been reported in resource challenged countries with large environmental poisonings via well water.

Arsenic exists in different forms: elemental, organic, inorganic, and gaseous. Elemental arsenic (As) is a metal that is poorly water soluble and considered nontoxic. Organic arsenic, found in shellfish, is also generally nontoxic to humans. Of the two inorganic forms, trivalent arsenite (As^{3+}) is more toxic than the pentavalent arsenate (As^{5+}) form.[13] Absorbed arsenic is bound by hemoglobin, leukocytes, and plasma proteins. It is cleared from the intravascular compartment within 24 hours and concentrates in the liver, kidneys, spleen, lungs, and gastrointestinal tract. Arsenic crosses the placenta and can also accumulate in the fetus. Inorganic arsenic interferes with normal cellular metabolic function, energy generation, and induces apoptosis. Arsenic also generates reactive oxygen species and induces oxidative damage in the cell.[13] Gaseous arsenic in the form of arsine (AsH$_3$) is colorless, almost odorless, and extremely toxic. It is lethal at 250 ppm

TABLE 146.5 Chelators

Chelator	Dosage	Indications	Contraindications	Adverse Effects
Deferoxamine	15 mg/kg/hr up to 24 hours (titrate up slowly because of hypotension)	*Iron* level >500 g/dL or systemic symptoms	Severe renal disease Anuria	Rate-related hypotension Pulmonary complications if given for >24hrs Increased incidence of *Yersinia* and *Mucormycosis* infections
Dimercaprol (BAL)	*Lead encephalopathy:* 4 mg/kg deep IM injection every 4 hours for 5 days in children and adults *Arsenic (severe):* No established regimen; consider 3 mg/kg IM every 4 hours for 48 hours, then twice daily for 7 to 10 days *Mercury:* 5 mg/kg IM first, then 2.5 mg/kg every 12 to 24 hours for 10 days	*Lead* level >70 µg/dL or encephalopathy *Arsenic:* Symptomatic patient with known exposure *Mercury:* Inorganic	Peanut allergy Organic mercury poisoning Hepatic insufficiency	Pain at injection site Hypertension and tachycardia Nausea, vomiting Headache Fever (especially in children) Nephrotoxicity in the setting of an acidic urine
CaNa$_2$EDTA	1500 mg/m^2/day continuous intravenous infusion 50 mg/kg/day or 1000 mg/m^2/day in two to four divided doses for up to 5 days if less severe symptoms	*Lead* level of 70 µg/dL or encephalopathy (given after first dose of BAL)	Severe renal disease Anuria Hepatitis	Nephrotoxicity Transient increase in AST/ALT
Succimer (DMSA)	10 mg/kg every 8 hours for 5 days, then every 12 hours for 14 days (maximum 500 mg per dose for children)	*Lead* level of 45 to 69 µg/dL *Arsenic:* If tolerated orally for subacute and chronic toxicity *Mercury:* Acute and chronic	None	Nausea, vomiting Diarrhea Metallic taste Transient increase in AST/ALT
D-Penicillamine	*Lead:* 1–1.5 g/d (children: 20–30 mg/kg/d), in 3 or 4 divided doses for 1–6 months. To minimize adverse reactions, start at 250 mg/d (children: 10 mg/kg/d) and increase to 50% during week 2 and to a full dose by week 3. The maximum adult daily dose is 2 g. *Elemental or Inorganic Mercury (not effective for Organic):* 250 mg (5 mg/kg) every 6 hours for 1–2 weeks *Arsenic:* 25 mg/kg every 6 hours for 5 days	*Lead* level of 45 to 69 µg/dL, succimer not tolerated *Arsenic:* Only if BAL and DMSA are unavailable *Mercury:* If BAL and DMSA are unavailable or not tolerated	Penicillin allergy	Leukopenia Thrombocytopenia Enuresis Abdominal pain
DMPS (investigational)	*Oral:* 100–200 mg (50–100 mg in children) every 6–8 hours, tapered over days to weeks *Parenteral (preferred for acute ingestions):* 5 mg/kg/dose IM or slow IV push every 6–8 hours; day 1, every 8–12 hours; day 2, every 12–24 hours; day 3, until 24-hour urine is <50 mcg/L	*Lead* (chronic) *Arsenic* *Mercury*		Nausea, vomiting Headache Fatigue Rash, pruritis

Note: Indications for chelation and dosing regimens may change. Consult with a medical toxicologist or regional poison center for the most up-to-date recommendations.

BAL, British antilewisite; *CaNa$_2$EDTA,* calcium disodium ethylenediaminetetraacetic acid; *DMPS,* dimercapto-1-propanesulfonic acid, *DMSA,* 2,3-dimercaptosuccinic acid; *IM,* intramuscular; *AST,* alanine transaminase; *ALT,* aspartate transaminase.

and causes massive hemolysis. The excretion of arsenic and its metabolites occurs primarily through the kidneys.

Clinical Features

Acute Arsenic Toxicity

Gastrointestinal effects including nausea, vomiting, abdominal pain, and diarrhea predominate as the initial manifestations of acute exposure to inorganic arsenic. The diarrhea has often been described as "rice water–like" and difficult to differentiate from diarrhea induced by *Vibrio cholerae* infection. These symptoms can be so severe that

they progress to hematemesis and hematochezia. The patient can also develop multisystem organ failure and cardiac conduction disturbances (Box 146.1). In cases of severe poisoning, cardiovascular collapse and death ensue. Early arsenic poisoning may be misdiagnosed as gastroenteritis or sepsis. For those who survive the initial gastrointestinal illness, chronic effects of arsenic poisoning appear weeks to months later. These include characteristic white lines that transverse the nailbeds running parallel to the lunula (also known as Aldrich-Mees lines; Fig. 146.2), painful sensorimotor neuropathy, and hyperkeratosis of the palms and soles.

BOX 146.1   Acute Effects of Arsenic Poisoning

Gastrointestinal
Severe gastroenteritis; hematemesis or hematochezia
Jaundice
Pancreatitis
Dysphagia
Hepatomegaly

Cardiovascular
Third spacing with shock
Sinus or ventricular tachycardia
Prolonged QT interval, ST depression, T wave inversion
Torsades de pointes
Pericarditis

Respiratory
Pneumonia
Pulmonary edema
Acute respiratory distress syndrome
Respiratory failure

Renal
Proteinuria
Hematuria
Oliguria
Renal failure

Neurologic
Headache
Drowsiness
Delirium
Coma
Encephalopathy
Seizures

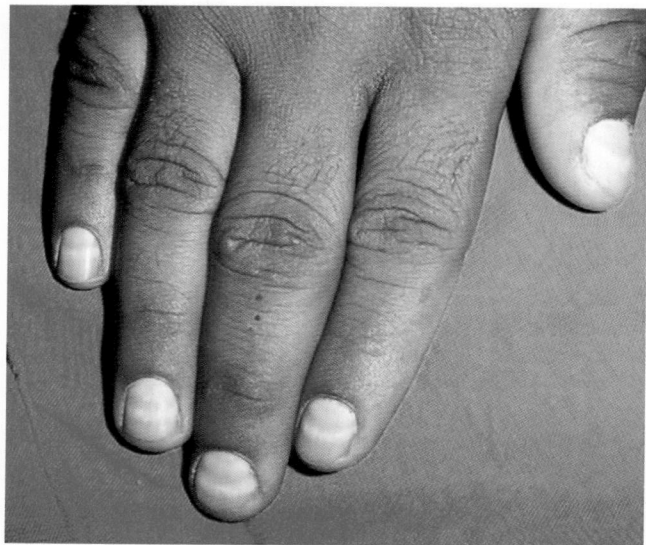

Fig. 146.2 Aldrich-Mees lines seen on the fingernails of a patient. (From: Chauhan S, D'Cruz S, Singh R, et al. Mees' lines. Lancet. 2008;372[9647]:1410.)

100 µg/day or 50 µg/L necessitates treatment. Seafood contains organic arsenic (arsenobetaine), which can significantly increase total urine arsenic concentrations, but arsenobetaine does not result in human toxicity. For this reason, patients should refrain from eating seafood, specifically shellfish, before testing, and the laboratory should be asked to specify the type of arsenic measured. Most patients referred to the ED for management of abnormal urine arsenic tests are not arsenic toxic; their urine tests are falsely abnormal because laboratories do not routinely differentiate between organic and inorganic arsenic. In cases of chronic arsenic poisoning or remote exposure, the serum and urine arsenic levels may no longer detect abnormal concentrations of arsenic.

Other laboratory results may suggest arsenic poisoning. Anemia, leukocytosis or leukopenia, and erythrocyte basophilic stippling may be seen. The results of renal function tests may be abnormal, demonstrating proteinuria, hematuria, and pyuria. Serum alanine transaminase, aspartate transaminase, and bilirubin levels may be elevated.

Arsenic in the gastrointestinal tract is radiopaque and can appear on a radiograph, although sensitivity is limited by its rapid absorption and the ensuing gastroenteritis.

Chronic Arsenic Toxicity

Chronic exposure to arsenic, typically through contaminated drinking water or occupational exposure, is associated with cardiovascular disease, diabetes mellitus, and both benign and malignant dermatologic disease.[14,15] Patients chronically exposed to arsenic have an increased risk of bladder, kidney, liver, and lung cancer.[16]

Arsine Gas

Acute exposure to arsine gas is characterized by severe hemolysis that is also associated with renal tubular injury. Signs of toxicity are usually evident within minutes to hours after exposure. Gastrointestinal symptoms are common, and CNS and liver dysfunction can occur.

Differential Diagnoses

Acute arsenic poisoning is often misdiagnosed as viral or bacterial gastroenteritis or gastrointestinal bleeding. Hemorrhagic gastroenteritis in the setting of an ingestion history should raise suspicions for caustic ingestions, ethanol, toxic alcohols, colchicine, heavy metals, and iron. Obtaining an environmental and occupational exposure history is important to help discern the etiology of the patient's symptoms.

Diagnostic Testing

To diagnose arsenic poisoning accurately, a 24-hour urine collection should be done. Spot urine samples are inaccurate and should not guide therapy. Normal arsenic concentrations are 5 µg/L or less in blood or less than 50 µg/day in a 24-hour urine collection. Any urine level above

Management

Stabilization and Supportive Care

Initial management of arsenic poisoning should address life-threatening conditions with supportive care of shock, dysrhythmias, and seizures. Fluid resuscitation helps maintain kidney perfusion early after arsine gas exposures.

Decontamination and Enhanced Elimination

As is the case with other metals, oral activated charcoal does not adsorb arsenic and is not recommended. Hemodialysis may remove some arsenic in the setting of acute renal failure. Exchange transfusions or plasma exchange can be done early after a severe arsine exposure. These treatments should be initiated in the intensive care setting for critically ill patients and in consultation with a medical toxicologist and nephrologist.

Antidotal Therapy

Acute Arsenic Poisoning. With a confirmed history of exposure in a symptomatic patient, chelation should start as early as possible without waiting for laboratory confirmation. Intramuscular BAL is the preferred chelator in patients who are critically ill as described for lead poisoning. Succimer can be given orally, but its use is often limited by the severe gastroenteritis resulting from arsenic poisoning. D-Penicillamine has a high side effect profile and is much less effective than BAL or succimer, so should be used only when BAL or succimer are unavailable. Table 146.5 summarizes available chelating agents with indications and doses. Chelation is not useful for arsine gas exposures. With arsine gas poisoning, exchange transfusion, continuous veno-venous hemodialysis, and plasma exchange have been used to remove arsine, which is tightly bound to erythrocytes.[17]

Chronic Arsenic Poisoning. Treatment of chronic arsenic toxicity should begin in a symptomatic patient after confirmation of elevated urinary arsenic levels. Oral chelation with succimer (DMSA) is the treatment of choice. Workers should modify their habits to avoid further exposure, and repeated monthly 24-hour urine collections can follow arsenic excretion dynamics. Prolonged chelation treatment in patients with chronic exposure but no detectable arsenic in blood or urine has not been proven to be effective.

Disposition

Patients who are severely ill and those receiving parenteral chelation for acute arsenic toxicity should be admitted to an intensive care setting. Patients with chronic arsenic exposure who are mildly symptomatic can be discharged home after removal from the source of exposure. Close follow-up with occupational medicine or a medical toxicologist should be arranged. Patients who are asymptomatic with a normal physical examination and vital signs can be discharged home.

MERCURY

Foundations

Mercury is a shimmering silver metal, familiar to most as one of the few metals that is liquid at room temperature in its elemental form. It has a long history of medicinal uses as an antiparasitic, a diuretic, a cathartic, an antiseptic, and a preservative in many older vaccines.[18]

Significant poisoning can occur in the home and in the workplace.[18] Mercury has many industrial uses that include the manufacture of fluorescent lights, batteries, polyvinyl chloride, and in paints as a biocide. Recently, artisanal small-scale gold mining has become a significant source of global mercury pollution and toxicity.[19] For these reasons, mercury is a common environmental pollutant of air and water.[20] This has led to restrictions in the consumption of fish caught in many local waters, especially by pregnant women and children.

Like other metals, mercury exists in different forms: elemental, organic, and inorganic. Toxicity depends on the form of mercury. The most familiar form of mercury is elemental or metallic mercury, also known as *quicksilver*. A common route of exposure to elemental mercury is the inhalation of volatilized vapor during the goldmining extraction process or after vacuuming up a spill. After inhalation, metallic mercury is retained in the lungs and can result in pneumonitis and acute respiratory distress syndrome. Later systemic absorption may also occur leading to CNS and renal toxicities.[21] Subcutaneous and intravenous injections also cause poisoning from systemic absorption.[22] Elemental mercury is not well absorbed by the gastrointestinal tract and toxicity is unlikely by this route.[23]

Inorganic mercury salts have two different valences: Hg^{1+} (mercurous) and Hg^{2+} (mercuric). Ingestion of either salt leads to significant gastrointestinal and renal toxicity. Inorganic salts have a direct corrosive effect on the gastrointestinal tract resulting in third spacing and hemorrhage.

The organic mercury compounds are categorized as either short chain (alkyl) or long chain (aryl). The major route of exposure to organic mercury is through ingestion, but these compounds are also

TABLE 146.6   Mercury Poisoning and Clinical Manifestations Based on Route of Exposure and Form of Mercury

Type of Mercury and Route of Exposure	Signs and Symptoms
Inhalation of elemental mercury	Hypoxemia, dyspnea, chest tightness Fever, chills Burning in mouth and throat Nausea, vomiting, bloody diarrhea Renal tubular necrosis
Subacute or chronic inhalation of metallic mercury	Metal fume fever Neuropsychiatric symptoms Renal dysfunction Skin changes
Ingestion of inorganic mercury salts	Severe hemorrhagic gastroenteritis, shock, hypovolemia, third spacing Acute tubular necrosis
Subacute or chronic inhalation of mercury	Neurasthenia, erethism, acrodynia
Organic mercury exposure (methyl-, diethyl-)	Delayed neurologic problems (ataxia, tremor, dysarthria) Visual field constriction Hearing loss Spasticity Hyperreflexia

ARDS, Acute respiratory distress syndrome.

readily absorbed through the skin. Organic forms classically result in delayed neurotoxicity, and most documentation describing this form of toxicity comes from large population exposures.[24] Concerns about mercury poisoning from excessive fish consumption are extrapolations from those exposures.

Like lead, mercury has no known physiologic role in the human body. Mercury binds covalently to sulfhydryl groups, disturbing multiple cellular enzyme functions. Nephrotoxicity results from oxidative damage, cytoskeletal alterations, and increased autophagy in the kidney.[25] Mercury exposure affects both the cardiovascular system and the CNS. Mercury may lead to hypertension and other cardiovascular problems.[26] Mercury also increases reactive oxygen species in the nervous system, leading to cellular damage.[24] Although mercury was previously used as a preservative in various vaccines, it is important to note the dose in those vaccines was relatively low, and mercury has not been proven to be a cause of autistic spectrum disease.

Clinical Features

The clinical manifestations of mercury poisoning depend on the acuity of the exposure, the route of exposure, and the chemical form of mercury (Table 146.6).

Differential Diagnoses

Hemorrhagic gastroenteritis in the setting of an ingestion history should raise suspicions for caustic ingestion, heavy metals, and iron. Respiratory distress from elemental mercury inhalation can also be mistaken for pneumonia, asthma, or influenza. The vague neurotoxic symptoms of mercury may also be confused with lead-induced neurocognitive deficits and encephalopathy. Obtaining an environmental and occupational exposure history is important to help discern the etiology of the patient's symptoms.

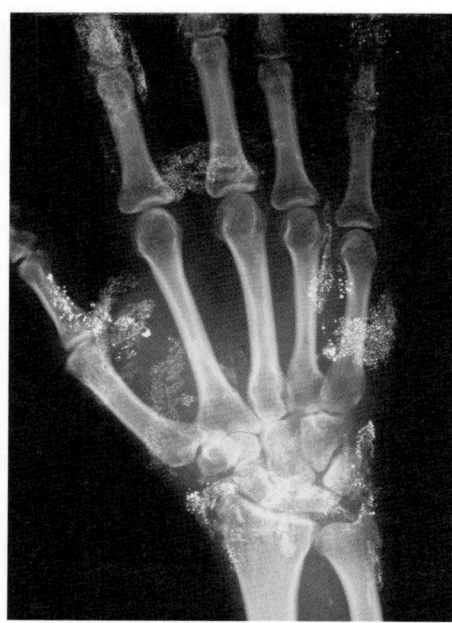

Fig. 146.3 Radiograph of the hand showing elemental mercury deposits in the subcutaneous tissue of a patient who was injecting chronically subcutaneously. (Courtesy Dr. Steven Aks.)

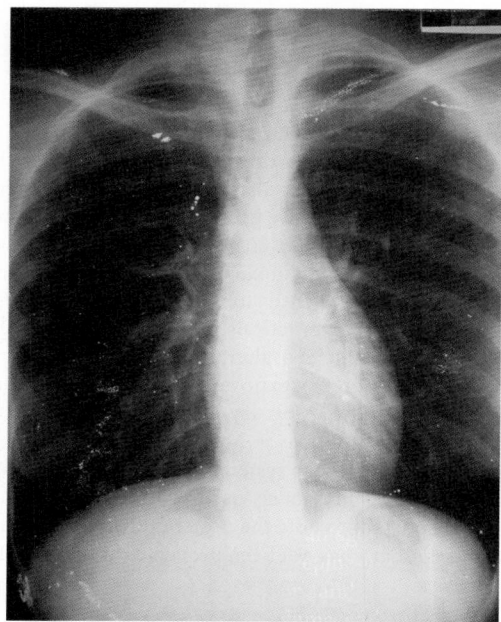

Fig. 146.4 Radiograph of the chest showing elemental mercury deposits in a patient who was chronically injecting the metal subcutaneously. (Courtesy Dr. Steven Aks.)

Diagnostic Testing

Measurement of a 24-hour urine mercury concentration is the most helpful test in confirming exposure and monitoring the effectiveness of chelation therapy. For organic mercury compounds, which undergo little urinary excretion, serum concentration should be used to confirm the diagnosis. A "normal" mercury concentration is considered to be less than 10 μg/L in the blood or less than 20 μg/L in the urine. Blood concentrations above 35 μg/L and urine concentrations above 150 μg/L require intervention. Fish can be contaminated with mercury, especially larger predatory fish and those from certain bodies of water known by local health departments to be most polluted. Individuals eating these locally caught fish may have elevated mercury levels. Elemental (metallic) mercury is radiopaque on plain radiographs, which can be ordered in cases of ingestion or dermal injection of elemental mercury (Figs. 146.3 and 146.4).

Management

Stabilization and Supportive Care

Initial management in the acutely poisoned patient is removal from the source and supportive care regardless of the type of mercury or route of exposure. There is no role for prophylactic antibiotics or steroids.

Decontamination

Oral activated charcoal and other gastrointestinal decontamination strategies are not recommended.

Enhanced Elimination

For acute inhalational exposures, the patient should be removed from the source of exposure and supportive management provided. Suction and postural drainage are indicated in cases of acute aspiration of metallic mercury. Self-injection of metallic mercury may require surgical débridement of infiltrated tissue.[22]

Antidotal Therapy

BAL is used for clinically significant acute inorganic mercury intoxication. BAL is contraindicated for patients poisoned with organic methylmercury compounds because it may increase transport of mercury across the blood-brain barrier.[27] Succimer (DMSA) has been used for both acute and chronic mercury poisoning and may be the best available chelator for methylmercury. D-Penicillamine may also be used but should only be administered if no additional mercury is present in the gastrointestinal tract, because mercury absorption from the intestinal lumen may be enhanced by the penicillamines. Table 146.5 summarizes available chelating agents for mercury poisoning with indications and doses.

Disposition

Ingestion of inorganic mercury in patients with any symptoms warrants admission for further evaluation and supportive treatment. Patients who self-inject metallic mercury may need surgical consultation for surgical débridement; this may be done as an outpatient if no symptoms or signs are evident. Patients with signs of neurotoxicity from organic mercury require admission. Asymptomatic patients with exposure to any form of mercury warrant environmental counseling, and those with exposure from excessive fish consumption need primary care or medical toxicology follow-up as outpatients for dietary counseling and further testing as indicated.

The references for this chapter can be found online at ExpertConsult. com.

147

Hydrocarbons

George Sam Wang and Jennie Alison Buchanan

KEY CONCEPTS

- Aspiration is the major toxic risk of hydrocarbon poisoning.
- Hydrocarbons may cause systemic toxicity, burns, cardiac dysrhythmias, altered mentation, and seizures depending upon the specific agent, dose, and duration of exposure.
- Gastrointestinal decontamination is potentially harmful in cases of hydrocarbon ingestion and is contraindicated.
- Hydrocarbon inhalant abuse can cause central nervous system (CNS) and cardiotoxic effects.
- In most cases of hydrocarbon ingestion or inhalation, symptomatic care with observation and monitoring are the cornerstones of management. There are no specific antidotes for hydrocarbons. Patients with pulmonary symptoms should have a chest radiograph.
- Symptoms of toxicity, especially aspiration, can be delayed, so asymptomatic patients should be observed for 6 hours and given instructions to return if symptoms develop after discharge.

FOUNDATIONS

Overview

Hydrocarbons are a diverse group of organic compounds that contain hydrogen and carbon (Table 147.1). Most hydrocarbons (such as gasoline) are byproducts of crude oil and are therefore called *petroleum distillates*. Essential oils such as turpentine or wormwood are derived from plants. Hydrocarbons are used as solvents and diluents in many products, including household cosmetics and chemicals, pesticides and fuels. The two main categories of hydrocarbons are aliphatic (straight chain structures, such as propane) and aromatic (cyclic structures, such as toluene). Hydrocarbons can also have multiple nonorganic side chains. For example, halogenated hydrocarbons will have at least one bromide, chloride, fluoride, or iodide moiety (e.g., carbon tetrachloride). Finally, hydrocarbons are used as a solvent base for many toxic chemicals, such as insecticides, carburetor cleaner (methanol), and heavy metals, which in turn can cause separate distinct syndromes of poisoning. Although there is a wide variety of toxic hydrocarbons, the majority of human exposures are confined to petroleum distillates.

Human exposure, both intentional and unintentional, to hydrocarbons is a common problem. In 2018, U.S. poison centers reported over 28,500 exposures to hydrocarbons accounting for over 1% of all calls with 121 major outcomes and 20 deaths.[1] Over the prior decade, there were approximately 4000 pediatric exposures to hydrocarbons per year, and almost 10% were hospitalized.[2] It is estimated that nearly 10% of the United States population aged 12 years and older have used an inhalant for its psychoactive properties.[3] Toxic exposure to hydrocarbons is dermal, inhalational, or via ingestion (with potential for aspiration). Inhalational exposures are typically due to either intentional abuse of volatile hydrocarbons (huffing, sniffing, dusting or bagging) or household and workplace exposures. Ingestions are mostly accidental pediatric exposures, which can lead to aspiration pneumonitis. Dermal exposures are from household or workplace use of hydrocarbon-based agents and are rarely intentional.

Pathophysiology

Hydrocarbons are local gastrointestinal irritants, but acute toxicity usually manifests through effects on three main target organs: lungs, heart, and central nervous system (CNS). Most ingestions of hydrocarbons do not lead to serious systemic toxicity but localized gastrointestinal symptoms such as abdominal pain, vomiting, and diarrhea may occur. Exceptions include halogenated or aromatic hydrocarbons, and hydrocarbons containing metals or pesticides, which are capable of causing significant CNS, hepatic, or renal toxicity. Despite the fact that there are thousands of different types of hydrocarbons, their potential for acute toxicity depends on a few physical properties:

- Viscosity is the capacity to resist flow or change. Low-viscosity hydrocarbons, such as gasoline, lamp oil, and furniture polish, spread rapidly into the airway, with high risk of aspiration toxicity. Lubricants and mineral oil, conversely, have high viscosity and low aspiration potential.
- Volatility is a measure of a liquid's ability to evaporate to a gas or vapor. Hydrocarbons with high volatility can displace alveolar oxygen and cause hypoxia. Butane and propane are examples of hydrocarbons with high volatility.
- Surface tension is the capacity for a liquid to adhere to a surface. Low surface tension, like low viscosity, enables a substance (e.g., turpentine) to disperse easily and may lead to pulmonary toxicity.
- Chemical side chains or substitutions often increase potential toxicity. These include metals (e.g., lead), halogens (e.g., the chloride ions in carbon tetrachloride), and those found on aromatic structures (e.g., the CH_3 groups in toluene and xylene). Halogenated hydrocarbons may cause cardiotoxicity.
- Lipophilicity enhances blood brain barrier penetration resulting in CNS effects.

Pulmonary Pathophysiology

The primary target organ for direct toxicity is the lung. Fatalities after ingestion usually occur because of accompanying aspiration. As noted above, hydrocarbons with high volatility, low viscosity, and low surface tension are especially dangerous (Box 147.1).[2-4]

Hydrocarbons penetrate into the lower airways, producing bronchospasm and direct injury to pulmonary alveoli and capillaries leading to an inflammatory response and pneumonitis.[2,4] Hydrocarbons

TABLE 147.1   Spectrum of Hydrocarbon Toxicity

Type	Example	Use	Pathophysiology	Comments
Aliphatic petroleum distillates	Methane, propane, butane, gasoline, kerosene, mineral spirits, mineral oil, naphtha, mineral seal oil, diesel oil, n-hexane	Fuels, liquid fuels, solvents, furniture polish, degreasers, multiple uses in chemical industry	Asphyxiants causing hypoxia and CNS depression Abused inhalants Pneumonitis when aspirated CNS depression n-Hexane causes peripheral neuropathy	Sudden death from inhalation abuse Viscosity and volatility determine spectrum of toxicity Mineral seal oil has high aspiration potential Poor gastrointestinal absorption
Aromatic petroleum distillates	Toluene, xylene, benzene	Used in plastics, pharmaceutical, rubber, chemical, and solvent industries, degreasers	Highly volatile, lung aspiration Absorbed from gastrointestinal tract Abused inhalants	Inhaled toluene causes renal tubular acidosis Benzene causes aplastic anemia, leukemia
Essential oils	Turpentine, pine oil, oil of wintergreen, pennyroyal	Solvents, household disinfectants, incense	Well absorbed from gastrointestinal tract	Gastrointestinal and CNS toxicity Wintergreen with methylsalycylates Pennyroyal can lead to hepatotoxicity
Halogenated hydrocarbons	Methylene chloride, chloroform, carbon tetrachloride, trichloroethylene, Freon, methylbromide, lindane, DDT	Solvents cleaning fluids, degreasers, fire extinguishers, paint strippers, fumigants	Multisystem toxicity (CNS, renal, hepatic, cardiac) Inhalant abuse Highly lipid soluble	Methylene chloride metabolized to carbon monoxide after ingestion, absorbed through the skin resulting in burns Carbon tetrachloride is radiopaque and can lead to hepatotoxicity Insecticides absorbed through skin
Related chemicals	Phenol, creosols	Disinfectants	Very corrosive	Phenol causes severe skin burns, and systemic toxicity including metabolic acidosis

CNS, Central nervous system; DDT, dichlorodiphenyltrichloroethane.

BOX 147.1   Qualities of Hydrocarbon That May Lead to Aspiration and Pneumonitis

- High volatility
- Low viscosity
- Low surface tension

also impair surfactant lipid production and function, leading to alveolar instability and collapse, decreased compliance, and impaired gas exchange. These mechanisms lead to alveolar dysfunction, ventilation-perfusion mismatch, and hypoxemia, which can progress to respiratory failure. Lipoid pneumonia can also develop after hydrocarbons coalesce in alveoli and become encapsulated by fibrous tissue. This has been reported in adults siphoning gasoline and from fire-eating performances and is known as "fire-eater's lung."[5-7]

Central Nervous System Pathophysiology

Most inhalant forms of hydrocarbons cause CNS depression. Products used for recreational mood alteration include glues and adhesives, aerosols, anesthetics, cleaning agents, solvents, and gases. After respiratory exposure, hydrocarbons passively diffuse through the pulmonary alveolus, are absorbed in blood and tissues, and cross the blood-brain barrier. Experimental data suggest that effects occur through binding of hydrocarbons with various neurotransmitter receptors, including glutamate/N-methyl-D-aspartate (NMDA), gamma-aminobutyric acid (GABA), dopamine, and opioids.[3] The inhalation route avoids hepatic first-pass metabolism and generates high CNS concentrations. With an isolated single exposure, these effects usually have a rapid onset of intoxication and short duration of effect. Chronic use of inhaled hydrocarbons can cause severe abnormalities in nervous system function,

which include deficits in memory, attention, and judgment, peripheral neuropathy, cerebellar degeneration, neuropsychiatric disorders, chronic encephalopathy, and dementia. More than 50% of patients who abuse toluene for greater than 10 years will have cerebral cortical atrophy (Fig. 147.1) with histologic changes that include loss of neurons, diffuse gliosis, and axonal degeneration.[3] CNS depression can also occur through ingestion of some hydrocarbons, such as tea tree oil.

Cardiac Pathophysiology

Hydrocarbons can precipitate sudden death, usually in the setting of intentional inhalation. These compounds are thought to produce myocardial sensitization to endogenous and exogenous catecholamines by inhibition of calcium signaling, which precipitates ventricular dysrhythmias and myocardial dysfunction. Hypoxemia is also thought to be a contributing factor. Cardiac dysrhythmia occurs disproportionately among those using halogenated and aromatic hydrocarbons (e.g., difluoroethane). Halogenated hydrocarbons can be found in refrigerant propellants and air spray cleaners commonly used for computer keyboard cleaning. Prolonged use can lead to cardiac structural damage and may impede normal cardiac electrical function

Other Organ Systems

Toxicity related to hydrocarbons also has been reported for other organ systems. Recognized syndromes include toluene-induced renal tubular acidosis, benzene-induced bone marrow toxicity and leukemia, delayed methylene chloride–induced carbon monoxide poisoning, and chlorinated hydrocarbon–induced centrilobular hepatic necrosis.[1] Direct skin exposure to certain hydrocarbons can cause defatting dermatitis, contact dermatitis, or chemical burns. Intentional intravenous injection of hydrocarbons such as kerosene has led to both localized caustic and necrotic effects, and systemic effects including renal or

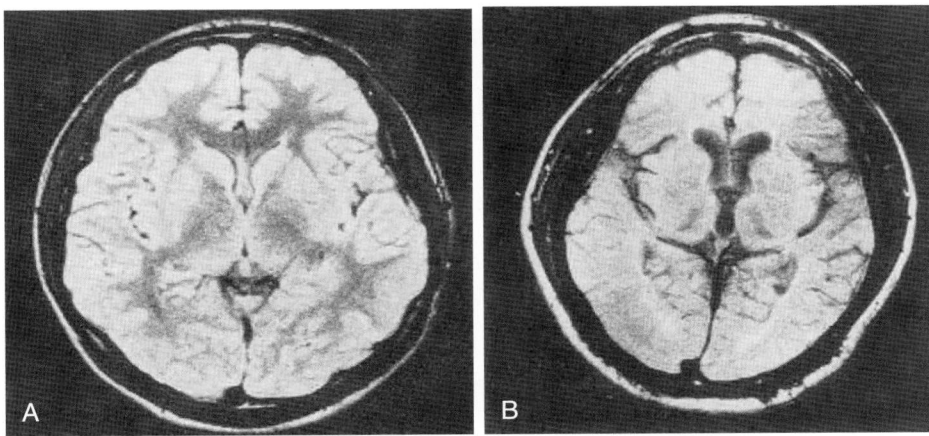

Fig. 147.1 Brain magnetic resonance imaging (MRI) of an individual with no history of inhalant abuse (A) and a patient with a history of chronic toluene abuse (B). (From NIDA Research Report [NIH 05-3818].)

hepatic toxicity, systemic inflammatory response syndrome (SIRS), hemolysis, seizures, pulmonary injury, cardiovascular toxicity, and death.[8] Huffing can lead to localized increased vascular permeability, which can lead to angioedema, or localized frostbite when refrigerants or freon are abused (Fig. 147.2).[9]

CLINICAL FEATURES

After oral ingestion of hydrocarbons, severe poisoning is most often related to aspiration. This manifests with progressive respiratory symptoms, including cyanosis, coughing, grunting, noisy respirations, and increased work of breathing. A patient may initially have mild symptoms and then develop tachypnea, dyspnea, bronchospasm, wheezing, rales, and fever after several hours.[2,4] A change in mental status can be a manifestation of hypoxia or hypercapnia, but it is also a direct effect of the hydrocarbon itself. In extreme cases, respiratory failure can require intubation. Various additives or solutes can produce symptoms independently (e.g., seizures from camphorated hydrocarbons, cyanosis from nitrite-induced methemoglobinemia, or delayed carbon monoxide poisoning from methylene chloride exposure[10]). Pesticides are often dissolved in a hydrocarbon base. With pesticide exposures, it can be difficult to distinguish acute respiratory distress syndrome induced by hydrocarbon aspiration from bronchorrhea induced by organophosphate toxicity (see Chapter 152).

Hydrocarbon solvent abuse is common and associated with various paraphernalia, such as plastic bags used for "bagging" (a method of pouring or spraying hydrocarbons in a bag or container and then inhaling deeply) and hydrocarbon soaked cloth used for "huffing" (a method in which abusers inhale through a saturated cloth).[9] Patients often have the distinctive odor associated with organic hydrocarbons. A characteristic coloration from spray paint (usually silver or gold because these paint colors contain higher concentrations of toluene) may be present over the mouth and nose or localized angioedema may occur, resulting in a "glue-sniffer's rash" (Fig. 147.3). These patients generally present to the emergency department (ED) with CNS intoxication and exhibit euphoria, agitation, hallucinations, confusion, or bizarre behavior. This may progress to CNS depression and seizures. In extreme cases, an individual who has inhaled solvents and then engaged in physical exertion, such as an altercation, may suddenly collapse in cardiac arrest, likely due to cardiac sensitization of endogenous catecholamines by hydrocarbons with ensuing dysrhythmias.[3] Chronic hydrocarbon inhalers may be brought to medical attention for behavioral problems or nonspecific medical symptoms caused by long-term

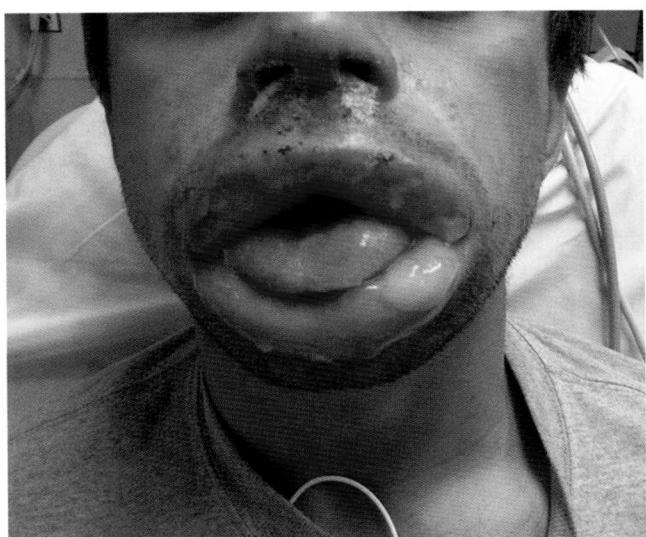

Fig. 147.2 Angioedema resulting from huffing computer cleaner. (From: Kurniali PC, Henry L. Inhalant abuse of computer cleaner manifested as angioedema. *Am J Emerg Med.* 2012;30:265.e3-5.)

exposure. These patients may share traits with the chronic ethanol user, with peripheral neuropathy (caused by, for example, *n*-hexane), cerebellar degeneration, and encephalopathy.[11]

Accidental dermal or inhaled (non-aspiration) respiratory exposure to hydrocarbons may occur in the workplace or home. Such exposures are rarely life-threatening. Most cases do not present for medical care.[1] The few patients who present to the ED typically will be asymptomatic or have transient nonspecific symptoms, such as headache, dizziness, or nausea. Those with significant respiratory exposure may have persistent pulmonary complaints and physical findings, such as coughing, wheezing, and cyanosis. Patients with significant acute dermal exposures may have localized pain and evidence of chemical burns consisting of erythema, swelling, angioedema, blistering, and dermal destruction (e.g., exposure to phenol).[3,9]

In the absence of aspiration, large-volume ingestion, or co-ingestion of another toxic substance, oral ingestion of most commonly available hydrocarbons is not associated with significant morbidity or mortality. Cough or tachypnea may be an early sign of pneumonitis or aspiration.

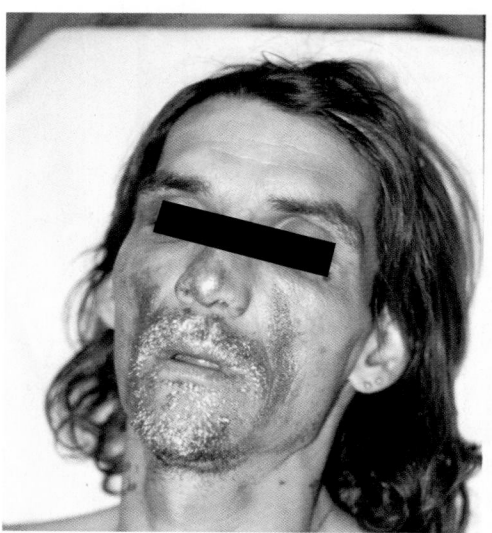

Fig. 147.3 Presentation of paint sniffer ("huffer") with paint around the face and sedation. (Courtesy Chris Tomaszewski, MD.)

DIFFERENTIAL DIAGNOSES

The history of exposure to a hydrocarbon, and the route or method of that exposure is usually straightforward. Additional history and examination should focus on other ingredients and possible aspiration, especially if the agent is ingested. Symptoms of aspiration include cough, dyspnea, and shortness of breath. Signs of significant pulmonary exposure include tachypnea, tachycardia, wheezing, and hypoxemia. Differential diagnosis depends upon the route of exposure, which primarily includes inhalation and ingestion, and the likelihood of co-intoxicants. CNS depressants such as ethanol and sedative-hypnotics can mimic the altered mental status of hydrocarbon ingestion. For hydrocarbon pneumonitis, pulmonary irritants; organophosphates, salicylates, and paraquat poisonings; and viral or bacterial pneumonia, may all produce a similar clinical presentation, but a focused history usually will lead to the correct diagnosis. In the scenario of the recreational abuser inhaling a particular agent, multiple drugs of abuse are often present, which can confound the clinical evaluation. Furthermore, hydrocarbon products may contain other constituents leading to specific toxicities. Behavioral disorders and confusion can be caused by hypoxia and respiratory compromise, as well as by the drugs themselves. Hypoglycemia, electrolyte abnormalities, and trauma should be considered as an etiology of altered mentation in these patients.

DIAGNOSTIC TESTING

The diagnosis is usually self-evident, and the exposure is often reported by the patient, supported by history of exposure and chemical odor. Ideally, the offending agent and container are brought to the ED. The local poison control center, medical toxicologist or material safety data sheet (MSDS) may identify and verify substances containing hydrocarbons. Hydrocarbons often are vehicles for other chemicals, and other exposures should be investigated.

CHAMP is a long-standing mnemonic used to help identify hydrocarbons and their additives with systemic toxicity (Box 147.2).

We do not recommend laboratory identification of specific hydrocarbons, which is difficult, time-consuming, and does not alter ED management. Other laboratory tests including electrolytes, complete blood count, and liver function tests can be performed to assess for renal tubular acidosis, electrolyte abnormalities (e.g., hypokalemia), bone marrow suppression, or liver injury caused by various hydrocarbons.[3] If essential oils such as oil of wintergreen (salicylates) or pennyroyal (liver toxicity) are ingested, specific relevant testing is performed. We recommend an electrocardiogram (ECG) in patients with a history of halogenated hydrocarbon use, dysrhythmias, syncope, or hemodynamic instability. Abnormal ECG findings may include premature ventricular contractions, QTc interval prolongation, or, in extreme cases, ventricular tachycardia or fibrillation.

Patients with pulmonary symptoms should have a chest radiograph and be observed for at least 6 hours with a repeat chest radiograph if there is worsening of their pulmonary status.[2,3]

MANAGEMENT

Dermal exposures to hydrocarbons can cause extensive burns, and exposed patients require early decontamination. Contaminated clothing should be removed, and the skin should be washed with soap and copious lukewarm water. Thermal injuries and chemical injuries are treated as described in Chapters 54 and 55.

In most cases of hydrocarbon ingestion or inhalation, symptomatic care along with observation and monitoring are the cornerstones of management. Gastrointestinal decontamination with gastric lavage or activated charcoal is not indicated. Most hydrocarbons are much more toxic to the lungs than to the gastrointestinal tract, and emesis or attempts at gastric emptying or decontamination may lead to aspiration and pulmonary toxicity.

Cardiac abnormalities are treated according to standard advanced cardiac life support (ACLS)/pediatric advanced life support (PALS) resuscitation with the exception of epinephrine administration. It is postulated that catecholamines worsen or precipitate cardiac dysrhythmias. This had led to recommendations for using short-acting beta blockers, such as esmolol, for hydrocarbon-induced refractory tachydysrhythmias. We recommend an initial bolus of 1 mg/kg IV over 30 seconds followed by an infusion starting at 50 mcg/kg/min (maximum of 300 mcg/kg/min) until resolution of the tachydysrhythmia. Epinephrine should be avoided in the acutely intoxicated patient for concern of precipitating an arrhythmia.[3] Patients with any history or ECG abnormalities concerning for cardiac involvement should be monitored on cardiac telemetry until symptoms resolve.

Significant hydrocarbon toxicity may lead to early and rapid decompensation of a patient's pulmonary, cardiac, and CNS functions. Monitoring in an intensive care or appropriate ED observation setting is indicated for patients with respiratory distress, significant oxygen requirements, those needing positive-pressure assistance or mechanical ventilation, tachydysrhythmias, cardiac conduction disturbance, or CNS depression. Patients with mild pulmonary symptoms (cough, minimal work of breathing, or low oxygen requirement) may be admitted to an inpatient unit for further observation. All other asymptomatic or minimally symptomatic patients should be observed with cardiac monitoring and pulse oximetry for a minimum of 6 hours and until asymptomatic. Indications for positive-pressure ventilation or mechanical ventilation include hypercarbia, severe respiratory distress, hypoxia unresponsive to noninvasive measures, or CNS depression. There are case reports and animal models using high-frequency jet ventilation, and extracorporeal membrane oxygenation in severe

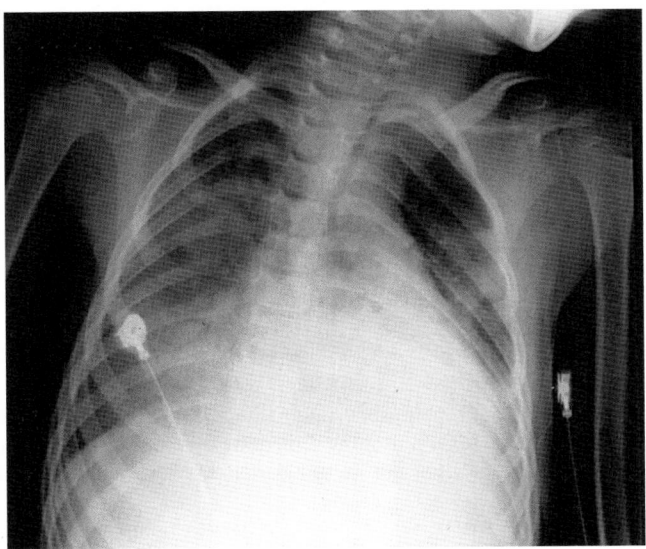

Fig. 147.4 Chest radiograph of a patient with hydrocarbon ingestion 6 hours after exposure.

cases of pneumonitis, with unproven clinical efficacy. Clinical decisions regarding these novel therapies should be made as in any other case of severe lung disease.[2-4] We recommend consideration of intrapulmonary administration of surfactant for severe hydrocarbon pneumonitis, using elevated oxygenation index, PaO_2/FiO_2 ratios, or poor lung compliance as indicators for use.[12] Consultation with a pulmonologist is advised for surfactant administration. Corticosteroids and antibiotics have not been shown to improve outcomes and are not indicated.[3]

DISPOSITION

Exposures to known, relatively benign hydrocarbons with minimal symptoms should have a 6-hour period of observation. Asymptomatic patients can be discharged home after appropriate psychiatric clearance, if indicated. If signs of pulmonary or systemic toxicity develop during the observation period (such as tachypnea and hypoxia), and a chest radiograph shows evidence of pneumonitis (Fig. 147.4), patients will require observation or hospital admission for at least 24 hours until symptoms have improved. Patients with CNS depression, history of dysrhythmia, significant respiratory distress including cyanosis, coughing, grunting, noisy respirations, and increased work of breathing should be monitored in the intensive care unit (Box 147.3).

Recreational inhalational users of hydrocarbons should be observed until clinical symptoms are improving or resolved. In most cases, if asymptomatic without complaints, the patient may be discharged after medical clearance for drug abuse counseling. Patients exposed to hydrocarbons with chemical side chains or substitutions have an increased incidence of systemic toxicity. These include metals (e.g., lead), halogens (e.g., the chloride ions in carbon tetrachloride), those found on aromatic structures (e.g., the CH_3 groups in toluene and xylene) and halogenated hydrocarbons, which can cause cardiotoxicity. These types of hydrocarbon exposures should be managed in conjunction with a poison control center or a medical toxicologist.

The references for this chapter can be found online at ExpertConsult.com.

148

Inhaled Toxins

Christopher W. Meaden and Lewis S. Nelson

KEY CONCEPTS

- An asphyxiant is any gas that displaces sufficient oxygen from the breathable air. Treatment consists of removal from exposure, supplemental oxygen, and supportive care.
- Highly water-soluble gases produce rapid irritation and predominantly upper respiratory tract effects, such as airway irritation. Poorly water-soluble gases, like phosgene, often produce delayed lower respiratory tract findings, such as bronchospasm or acute respiratory distress syndrome (ARDS).
- Carbon monoxide (CO) poisoning is confirmed by co-oximetry measurement. Cyanide poisoning is treated empirically when cardiovascular instability (e.g., hypotension), altered mental status, or a serum lactate greater than 10 mmol/L are present in a patient with a concerning history, such as a fire victim.
- Hydroxocobalamin is the preferred antidote for most cyanide-poisoned patients due to its efficacy, ease of use, and safety in patient with concomitant CO poisoning. Sodium thiosulfate may be administered concomitantly and may provide additional benefits.
- Patients with hydrogen sulfide poisoning generally respond to removal from exposure and ventilatory support.
- Normobaric oxygen therapy is sufficient to many patients with CO poisoning, but we recommend consultation with a hyperbaric (HBO) facility, poison control center, or medical toxicologist for consideration of HBO therapy under specific conditions. Indications for consultation and HBO treatment include patients with a carboxyhemoglobin (COHb) greater than 25% in the absence of clinical findings, a COHb greater than 15% or signs of fetal distress in pregnancy, or an elevated COHb level with one or more of the following: syncope, coma, altered mental status, abnormal cerebellar function, or a prolonged CO exposure with minor clinical findings.

Inhalational exposure to systemic toxins can be covert and indolent (as in occupational exposure to irritant photochemical smog) or overt and fulminant. The circumstances of the exposure, the presence of combustion or odors, and the number and condition of victims assist in the management. Despite the array of possible toxic inhalants, identification of a specific inhalant is generally unnecessary because therapy is based primarily on the clinical manifestations (Table 148.1).

SIMPLE ASPHYXIANTS

Foundations

Simple asphyxiants are inert and produce toxicity only by displacement of oxygen and lowering the fraction of inspired oxygen (FiO_2). Exposed patients remain asymptomatic if the FiO_2 is normal. Carbon dioxide and nitrogen are exceptions in that both can produce narcosis at elevated partial pressures, even though their predominant toxicological effect is simple asphyxiation. Since the introduction of catalytic converters, most deaths from the intentional inhalation of automotive exhaust result from simple asphyxiation, due to hypoxia, and not from carbon monoxide (CO) poisoning. Emerging methods of suicide secondary to gas inhalation are the inhalation of helium and charcoal burning.[1]

Clinical Features

Acute effects occur within minutes of the onset of hypoxia and are manifestations of ischemia. A fall in the FiO_2 from normal, 0.21 (i.e., 21%), to 0.15 results in autonomic stimulation (e.g., tachycardia, tachypnea, and dyspnea) and cerebral hypoxia (e.g., ataxia, dizziness, incoordination, and confusion). Dyspnea is not an early finding because hypoxemia is not nearly as potent a stimulus to the medullary respiratory center as are hypercarbia and acidemia. Lethargy from cerebral edema occurs as the FiO_2 falls below 0.1 (10%), and life is difficult to sustain at an FiO_2 below 0.06 (6%). Because removal from exposure terminates the simple asphyxiation and allows restoration of oxygenation and clinical improvement, most patients present with resolving symptoms. Failure to improve suggests complications of ischemia (e.g., seizures, coma, and cardiac arrest) and is associated with a poor prognosis.

Differential Diagnoses

Because the presenting complaints offered by most exposed patients are nonspecific (e.g., dizziness, syncope, and dyspnea), the differential diagnosis is extensive. A consistent history, particularly of a setting in which asphyxia is expected to occur such as in an enclosed space, an appropriate spectrum of complaints and a rapid resolution on removal from exposure are generally sufficient to establish the diagnosis.

Diagnostic Testing

Minimally, symptomatic patients do not require chest radiography or arterial blood gas (ABG) analysis. There is no need for toxicology testing unless the asphyxiation was an act of deliberate self-harm, in which in this case, we recommend selected screening for acetaminophen and any other relevant toxin implicated by history, physical examination, or observation. A definitive diagnosis ultimately requires scene investigation by a trained and suitably outfitted team with personal protective equipment (PPE). Determination of the exact nature of the gas is of limited clinical value but may have important public health implications.

Management

Management rarely requires specific therapy other than removal from exposure, administration of supplemental oxygen, and supportive care. Neurologic injury or cardiorespiratory arrest should be managed with standard advanced cardiac life support (ACLS) resuscitation protocols. Psychiatric consultation is indicated when the exposure was an act of deliberate self-harm.

TABLE 148.1 Common Inhaled Toxins

Inhalant	Source or Use	Predominant Class
Acrolein	Combustion	Irritant, highly soluble
Ammonia	Fertilizer, combustion	Irritant, highly soluble
Carbon dioxide	Fermentation, complete combustion, fire extinguisher	Simple asphyxiant; systemic effects
Carbon monoxide (CO)	Incomplete combustion, methylene chloride	Chemical asphyxiant
Chloramine	Mixed cleaning products (e.g., hypochlorite bleach and ammonia)	Irritant, highly soluble
Chlorine (Cl_2)	Swimming pool disinfectant, cleaning products	Irritant, intermediate solubility
Chlorobenzylidene malononitrile (CS), chloroacetophenone (CN)	Tear gas (Mace)	Pharmacologic irritant
Hydrogen chloride	Tanning and electroplating industry	Irritant, highly soluble
Hydrogen cyanide	Combustion of plastics, acidification of cyanide salts	Chemical asphyxiant
Hydrogen fluoride	Hydrofluoric acid	Irritant, highly soluble; systemic effects
Hydrogen sulfide	Decaying organic matter, oil industry, mines, asphalt	Chemical asphyxiant; irritant, highly soluble
Methane	Natural gas, swamp gas	Simple asphyxiant
Methylbromide	Fumigant	Chemical asphyxiant
Nitrogen	Mines, scuba diving (nitrogen narcosis, decompression sickness)	Simple asphyxiant; systemic effects
Nitrous oxide	Inhalant of abuse, whipping cream, racing fuel booster	Simple asphyxiant
Noble gases (e.g., helium)	Industry, laboratories	Simple asphyxiant
Oxides of nitrogen	Silos, anesthetics, combustion	Irritant, intermediate solubility
Oxygen	Medical use, hyperbaric conditions	Irritant, free radical; systemic effects
Ozone	Electrostatic energy	Irritant, free radical
Phosgene	Combustion of chlorinated hydrocarbons	Irritant, poorly soluble
Phosphine	Hydration of aluminum or zinc phosphide (fumigants)	Chemical asphyxiant
Smoke (varying composition)	Combustion	Variable, but may include all classes
Sulfur dioxide	Photochemical smog (fossil fuels)	Irritant, highly soluble

Disposition

Patients with manifestations of mild asphyxia, who recover after removal from the exposure can be discharged after 6 hours of observation if they are asymptomatic or minimally symptomatic with improvements. Patients at risk for complications of hypoxia, such as those presenting with significant signs or symptoms (e.g., altered mental status, coma, chest pain, electrocardiogram [ECG] changes) or with exacerbating medical conditions (e.g., cardiac disease, asthma), should be observed for 24 to 48 hours for the development or progression of post-hypoxic complications.

PULMONARY IRRITANTS

Foundations

The pulmonary irritant gases are a large and diverse group of agents that produce a common toxicological syndrome when they are inhaled in moderate concentrations. Although many of these gases can be found in the home, significant poisoning from consumer products is uncommon because of restrictions designed to reduce their toxicity. However, catastrophes such as the 1984 release of methyl isocyanate in Bhopal, India, which resulted in more than 2000 fatalities and 250,000 injuries, remain as an environmental risk. On a different scale, industrialization has increased ambient concentrations of sulfur dioxide, ozone, and oxides of nitrogen. These irritant gases frequently exacerbate chronic pulmonary disease.

Irritant gases dissolve in the respiratory tract mucus and alter the air-lung interface by invoking an irritant, or inflammatory response.[2]

When these gases are dissolved, most of them produce an acid or alkaline product, but several generate oxygen-derived free radicals that produce direct cellular toxicity (Fig. 148.1). The clinical effects of pulmonary irritants can be predicted by their water solubility (see Table 148.1).

Clinical Features

Highly, water-soluble gases rapidly impact the mucous membranes of the eyes and upper airway causing lacrimation, cough and nasal burning. Although their pungent odor and rapid onset of symptoms tend to limit significant exposure, massive or prolonged exposure can result in life-threatening laryngeal edema, laryngospasm, bronchospasm, or acute respiratory distress syndrome (ARDS). In contrast, because poorly water-soluble gases do not readily irritate the mucous membranes at low concentrations and some have a pleasant odor (e.g., phosgene's odor is similar to that of newly mown hay or freshly cut grass), prolonged breathing in the toxic environment allows time for the gas to reach deep into the alveoli. Even moderate exposure causes delayed irritation of the lower airway, alveoli, and parenchyma 2- to 24-hour after exposure. Initial effects may be mild, only to progress to overt respiratory failure and delayed ARDS during the ensuing 24 to 36 hours.[3] Gases with intermediate water solubility tend to produce syndromes that are a composite of the clinical features manifested with the other gases, depending on the extent of exposure. Massive exposure is most often associated with rapid onset of upper airway irritation and more moderate exposure with delayed onset of lower airway symptoms.

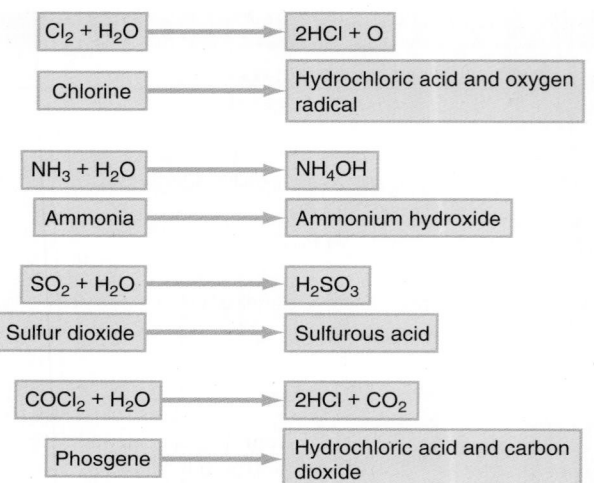

Fig. 148.1 Sample Reactions of Pulmonary Irritants Reacting With Water in the Lung. *Cl$_2$*, Chlorine; *CO$_2$*, carbon dioxide; *CoCl$_2$*, cobalt (II) chloride; *H$_2$O*, water; *H$_2$SO$_3$*, sulfurous acid; *HCl*, hydrochloric acid; *NH$_3$*, ammonia; *NH$_4$OH*, ammonium hydroxide; *O*, oxygen; *SO$_2$*, sulfur dioxide.

Differential Diagnoses

The typical symptoms of pulmonary exposure to an irritant gas are bronchospasm, cough, chest tightness, and acute conjunctival irritation. Presentation may mimic non-toxicological causes of pulmonary disease, but the history generally confirms the exposure to the irritant (Box 148.1). History may be particularly important if the patient presents with severe or advanced findings, such as ARDS, which can occur after many physiologic insults, including trauma and sepsis.

Diagnostic Testing

Inhalation of respiratory irritants may affect the upper airway, the lower airways and lungs, or both. Upper airway evaluation proceeds as described in the following Management section. Radiographic and laboratory studies are not useful in the evaluation of upper airway symptoms.

Oxygenation and ventilation are assessed by serial chest auscultation, pulse oximetry, and continuous capnography. Chest radiography is indicated for patients presenting with cough, dyspnea, hypoxia, or abnormal findings, such as rales or wheezes, on pulmonary examination. ABGs are reserved for patients who are more severely symptomatic, have hypoxia, or do not improve readily with oxygen therapy.

In general, it is neither possible nor necessary to test for the specific agent. There are no clinical tests that will differentiate the irritant to which a patient was exposed, although testing at the site by public health authorities may be performed for epidemiologic purposes. Knowing that an agent is highly water soluble will shorten the observation period for symptom development, whereas patients exposed to poorly water-soluble agents will require a more prolonged period of observation.

Management

Patients with no upper airway symptoms, normal voice, and no evidence of irritation (erythema) or burns on examination of the oral pharynx require no further upper airway evaluation but should be reexamined if symptoms or signs develop after the initial evaluation. Those with evidence of tissue irritation, such as oral or tongue edema, altered voice (raspy or muffled), stridor, or significant odynophagia or dysphagia require early examination by laryngoscopy and if severe,

should undergo early intubation because rapid progression of these injuries is expected. Laryngoscopy may be performed using a flexible laryngoscope, rigid video, or conventional laryngoscope with appropriate topical anesthesia and sedation as indicated (see Chapter 1). Patients with evidence of mild irritation of the larynx or supralaryngeal area (erythema, no edema, normal glottis) may be observed. Those with more severe findings are considered not to require early intubation, such as erythema with mild edema, should undergo repeat examination from 30 to 90 minutes after the initial examination or earlier, if symptoms or signs are worsening.

Bronchospasm generally respond to inhaled beta-adrenergic agonists. Data regarding the use of corticosteroids are limited and do not support clinical benefits in humans. Therefore, corticosteroids are not recommended unless the patient has underlying reactive airways disease.[3–5]

Patients exposed to chlorine or hydrogen chloride gas receive symptomatic relief from nebulized 2% sodium bicarbonate solution.[6] This solution is prepared by diluting a given volume of standard 8.4% sodium bicarbonate solution with three equivalent volumes of sterile water and administering it in 3 to 5 mL aliquots with standard nebulizer equipment. There are no studies on the recommended dosing regimen, but if successful after its first use, providing it every 30 minutes as needed for symptom relief, for up to 6 hours, is a reasonable approach. Nebulized bicarbonate will not alter the inflammatory cascade so it will not have significant effect on the progression of pulmonary injury. ARDS, if identified, is managed as described in Chapter 2.

Disposition

Patients exposed to highly water-soluble gases (see Table 148.1) can be discharged if they are asymptomatic or symptoms are minimal and improving. After exposure to intermediate or poorly water-soluble gases, asymptomatic patients should be observed for increasing dyspnea for 6 hours before final disposition. Regardless of the solubility, patients with prolonged gas exposure, exposure to highly concentrated gases, exposure in a closed space or those with high-risk medical conditions (e.g., underlying pulmonary disease, extremes of age, and poor follow-up) should be observed in an inpatient setting or observation unit for 24 hours. Patients with upper airway findings on examination should be observed in the emergency department (ED) or an intensive care unit (ICU) until there is clear evidence that the process is subsiding. All discharged patients should receive instructions for signs and symptoms of pulmonary deterioration.

SMOKE INHALATION

Foundations

According to a 2019 report by the National Fire Protection Association, an average of 2,620 deaths and 11,220 injuries occur per year in residential fires in the United States.[6] Many of these casualties do not suffer serious cutaneous burns but rather die of smoke inhalation. This is a variant of irritant injury in which heated particulate matter and adsorbed toxins injure normal mucosa. In addition, CO and cyanide are systemic toxins often considered in conjunction with the smoke inhalation syndrome because of their common origin.

Even at temperatures between 350°C and 500°C, air has such a low heat capacity that it rarely produces lower airway damage. The greater heat capacity of steam (approximately 4000 times than that of air), or heated soot suspended in air (i.e., smoke) can transfer heat and cause injury deep within the respiratory tract.

The nature of the fuel determines the composition of its smoke, and because fires involve variable fuels and burning conditions, the character of fire smoke is often undefined to the emergency clinician. Irritant toxins produced by the fire are adsorbed onto carbonaceous particles that are deposited in the airways and damage the mucosa through mechanisms similar to those of the irritant gases.

Clinical Features

Thermal and irritant-induced laryngeal injury may produce cough, voice alteration, or stridor, but these findings are often delayed. Soot and irritant toxins in the airways can produce early cough, dyspnea, and bronchospasm. Subsequently, a cascade of airway inflammation results in ARDS with failure of pulmonary gas exchange. The time between smoke exposure and the onset of clinical symptoms is highly variable and dependent on the nature of the exposure. Deaths that occur rapidly after exposure are caused by asphyxia, airway compromise, or metabolic poisoning (e.g., CO and cyanide). Singed nasal hairs and soot in the sputum suggest substantial exposure, but significant exposure and injury can occur with neither of these being present.

Differential Diagnoses

With the obvious exposure history to smoke inhalation, the differential diagnosis is limited, however, cyanide and carbon monoxide should always be considered as discussed below. Although it is often unclear whether smoke inhalational injuries are thermal or irritant, the differentiation is clinically irrelevant, as the management approach remains the same. Concomitant physical injuries such as "burns" or trauma may complicate the metabolic picture.

Diagnostic Testing

Airway patency should be evaluated early. Airway management is as described earlier for inhaled pulmonary irritants. If evidence of significant airway exposure is present, such as carbonaceous sputum or a hoarse voice, the airway should be examined by laryngoscopy and secured if signs of injury or compromise are noted. Pulmonary injury is assessed through auscultation and chest radiography for signs of alveolar filling or hyperinflation. Oxygenation should be assessed by co-oximetry, because blood gas analysis and pulse oximetry may be inaccurate in CO-poisoned patients (see discussion in the Carbon Monoxide section later). Co-oximetry will provide a blood carboxyhemoglobin (COHb) level, and we recommend testing for every patient, unless the smoke exposure was brief and in an open space. Metabolic acidosis, particularly when serum lactate concentration is greater than 8 mmol/L and the COHb is not significantly elevated, suggests concomitant cyanide poisoning.[7]

Management

The acute management of a patient with smoke inhalation, is identical to that with other irritant inhalational injuries. Early assessment of the airway and early intubation, as indicated, are critical because deterioration may be occult and rapid. Patients with no upper airway symptoms, normal oropharyngeal, nasopharyngeal examination, no voice alteration, and normal swallowing, may be observed and reevaluated if symptoms develop. Patients with symptoms or findings should be evaluated early stage by laryngoscopy. Simply observing these patients for deterioration can result in airway compromise requiring rapid and potentially difficult airway intervention. Despite a lack of evidence supporting their effectiveness, inhaled beta-adrenergics are widely used for patients with dyspnea or wheezing. Because these agents may provide benefit with little likelihood of harm, we recommend at least one dose of a beta-adrenergic agonist for patients with symptoms of bronchospasm. Both subjective (patient-reported) and objective (respirometry) assessment may be used to determine whether these agents appear to benefit a particular patient, and guide the use of additional doses. Optimal supportive care and maintenance of adequate oxygenation (e.g., suctioning and pulmonary toilet) are the most important aspects of care. Bronchoscopy with bronchoalveolar lavage is frequently recommended to clear debris and toxins from the distal airways. We do not recommend the use of corticosteroids, by inhalation or systemically, because there is no evidence of clinical benefit and they are potentially harmful in patients with cutaneous burns. Ibuprofen, antioxidants, exogenous surfactant, and high-frequency ventilation yield, variably improved survival in experimental and clinical trials but none are considered as standard care.[8] Antibiotics should be used only in patients with suspected bacterial infection.

Disposition

Patients who are intubated should be admitted to the ICU or burn unit, depending on the extent of the cutaneous burns or respiratory tract injury. Patients with upper airway symptoms or signs, but without concerns for airway loss, should undergo repeat airway examination for 6 hours, preferably in an ICU. Patients with prolonged closed-space exposure or lower airway findings, such as rales or carbonaceous sputum, should be admitted to an ICU, and observed for at least 24 hours while assessing for the development of signs of lower respiratory tract injury. Transfer considerations to a higher level of care at another institution or to a burn center should be based on local resources, consultation with the specialty center, an assessment of the risks of transfer, and existing protocols. Patients that should be considered for transfer include those with burns greater than 10 percent body surface area, burns that involve the face, hands, genitalia, perineum, or major joints, and those with third degree burns. See Chapter 54 for further discussion.

CYANIDE AND HYDROGEN SULFIDE

Foundations

Instead of directly affecting the airway and lungs, these poisons cause effects at the cellular level. Hydrogen cyanide is a gas with many commercial uses, particularly in synthetic fiber manufacture and fumigation. Gaseous hydrogen cyanide is occasionally noted to have the odor of bitter almonds. Cyanide in its salt form (e.g., sodium or potassium) is important in metallurgy (e.g., jewelry) and photography and is much safer to work with because of its low volatility. When cyanide salts are dissolved in water, hydrogen cyanide, a gas, can be produced, particularly under acidic conditions. Cyanide is metabolically released *in vivo* from precursors (cyanogens) such as amygdalin, found in apricot and other *Prunus* species pits, and from nitriles, a group of chemicals with many commercial uses.

H_2S poisoning most often occurs in petroleum refinery and sewage storage tank workers. A more recent means of suicide involves generation of H_2S from sulfur-containing products, such as detergent, mixed with acids in an enclosed space, such as an automobile.[9] On occasion, well-intentioned but ill-prepared pre-hospital rescuers become victims emphasizing the need for proper training and equipment. H_2S has a noxious odor similar to that of a rotten egg, which becomes unnoticeable with extremely high concentrations or prolonged exposure (a process called "olfactory fatigue").

Gaseous cyanide is rapidly absorbed after inhalation and is immediately distributed to the body tissues. Inhibition of oxidative metabolism by binding to cytochrome c oxidase (or Complex IV) of the electron transport chain within the mitochondria which occurs within some seconds. The poisoned tissue rapidly depletes its adenosine triphosphate (ATP) reserves and ceases to function (Fig. 148.2). Cyanide has no evident effect on other oxygen-binding enzyme systems, most notably hemoglobin. This is probably explained by the oxidation state of its iron moiety; cyanide binds only to oxidized iron (Fe^{3+}), whereas deoxyhemoglobin contains reduced iron (Fe^{2+}).

H_2S exerts its toxic effects both as a pulmonary irritant, and as a cellular poison. Its deadly metabolic effects are produced by a mechanism identical to that of cyanide.[10] However, H_2S's spontaneous dissociation from the mitochondria is rapid, allowing most patients to survive after brief exposure.

Clinical Features

Tissue hypoxia occurs within minutes, with the exact onset dependent on the route, dose or concentration, and nature of the exposure. Dysfunction of the heart and the central nervous system that is the organ systems most sensitive to hypoxia and it is a characteristic of cyanide poisoning, manifested as coma, seizures, dysrhythmias, and cardiovascular collapse. Metabolic acidosis develops as a result of diffuse cellular dysfunction and this is associated with an elevated serum lactate concentration. Despite popular belief, cyanosis is not a characteristic clinical finding. Given the extreme toxicity of cyanide, mild acute poisoning is uncommon. Patients with acute H_2S poisoning have similar clinical manifestations, although generally recover by the time of arrival to the ED due to its spontaneous mitochondrial dissociation.

Because cyanide and H_2S prevent tissue extraction of oxygen from the blood, the oxygen content of venous blood remains high, approaching that of arterial blood. Clinically, this may appear as the "arterialization" or brightening of venous blood to resemble arterial blood. A comparison of the measured (by co-oximetry) venous and arterial oxygen contents may assist in the diagnosis of cyanide poisoning. A

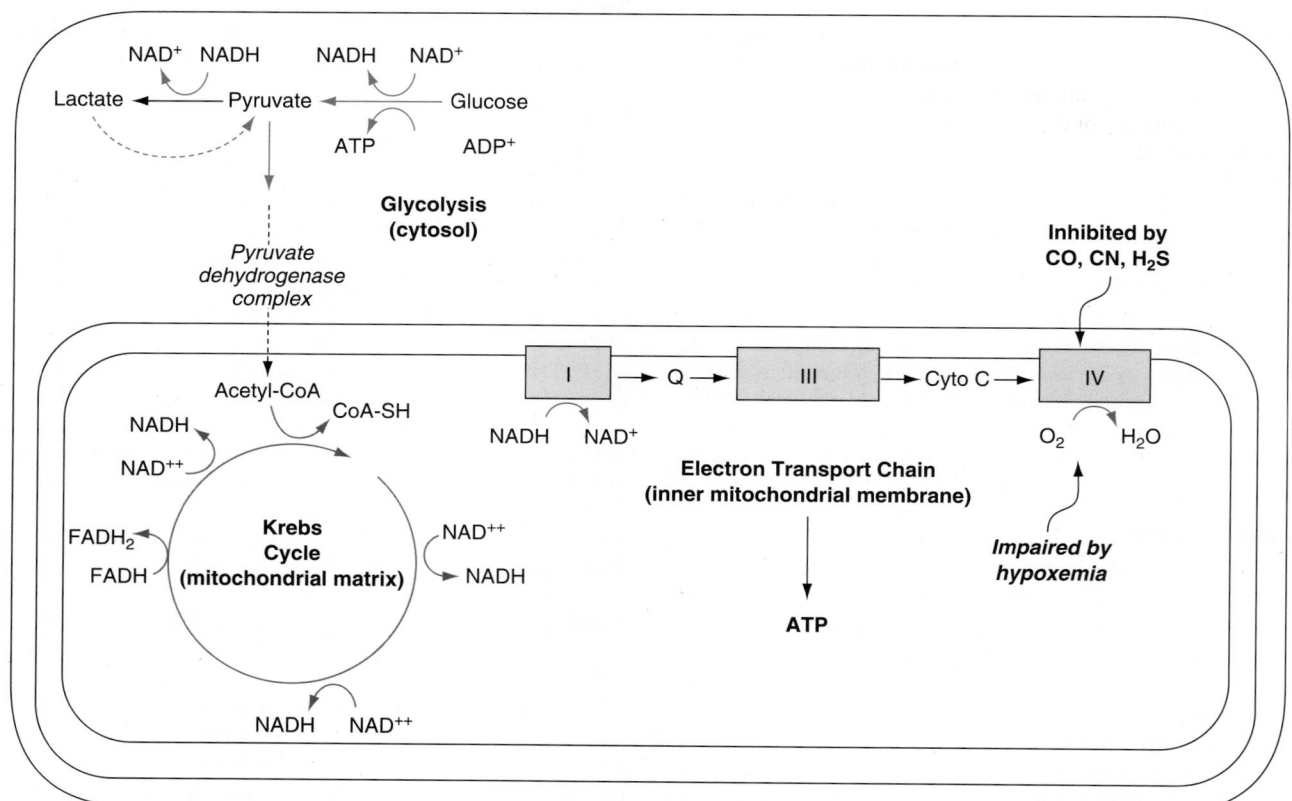

Fig. 148.2 The Complete Metabolism of a Molecule of Glucose to Energy Is Complex but Occurs in Two Broad Steps. The first step, anaerobic glycolysis, which occurs in the absence of oxygen, generates pyruvate, nicotinamide adenine dinucleotide (NADH), and adenosine triphosphate (ATP). Pyruvate then enters the Krebs cycle to create potential energy in the second step, through the reduction of NAD^+ to NADH and flavin adenine dinucleotide (FADH) to $FADH_2$. Fatty acid metabolism and protein metabolism produce $FADH_2$ and NADH, which also requires conversion to ATP. These conversions occur in the mitochondrial membrane, where oxidative phosphorylation is linked to the electron transport chain, the last phase of which involves the transfer of electrons to molecular oxygen to form water. Cyanide (CN), hydrogen sulfide (H_2S), and carbon monoxide (CO) bind to and inhibit the last step, the Fe^{3+}-containing cytochrome-aa_3 oxidase in Complex IV, preventing further oxidation of NADH. This in turn hinders the Krebs cycle because the required regeneration of NAD^+ does not occur, and glucose metabolism is forced to end at pyruvate. For energy production to continue, NADH donates its electrons to pyruvate, creating lactate, and sufficient NAD^+ is regenerated for glycolysis to progress. Ultimately, energy failure and end-organ damage occur. *CoA,* Coenzyme A; *H_2O,* water; *IV,* intravenous; *O_2,* oxygen.

low arterial-venous oxygen difference is suggestive, but not pathognomonic of cyanide poisoning and its absence does not exclude the diagnosis.

Patients surviving cyanide or H_2S poisoning may have persistent or delayed-onset neurologic syndromes identical to those noted in patients with CO poisoning or post-cardiac arrest.

Differential Diagnoses

Rapid cardiovascular collapse, hypotension, bradycardia, ventricular dysrhythmias, and seizures in a fire victim should suggest profound hypoxia, cyanide poisoning, severe CO poisoning, or a combination.[11] In patients without an exposure history, the differential diagnosis is vast and includes CO poisoning, asphyxiants, and other toxicologic and non-toxicologic causes.

Diagnostic Testing

Unlike with CO poisoning, pulse oximetry and ABG analysis are accurate in cases of isolated cyanide or H_2S poisoning. An increased anion gap metabolic acidosis and hyperlactatemia are usually present. A lactate concentration greater than 8 mmol/L is highly predictive of cyanide poisoning in the appropriate clinical context.[6,12] CO and cyanide are fellow travelers, so an elevated COHb level in a fire victim warrants consideration of concomitant cyanide poisoning. The presence of severe clinical findings and metabolic acidosis with a low COHb level is particularly concerning for cyanide poisoning. The result of a blood cyanide determination is usually delayed, to be of use in the ED, but it can be useful for confirmation and documentation purposes. Technology exists for immediate cyanide determination but is not widely available. Testing for H_2S is not clinically available, and support for the diagnosis of H_2S exposure would come primarily from on-scene testing.

Management

The diagnosis of cyanide poisoning usually cannot be confirmed rapidly, and therapy is almost always empirical. Treatment should not be delayed pending the COHb level or other laboratory tests in patients with suspected acute cyanide poisoning. Patients removed from a fire environment who have cardiovascular instability, altered mental status, or a serum lactate greater than 8 mmol/L should receive cyanide treatment regardless of the COHb concentration.

Hydrogen Cyanide

The accepted goal of therapy is to reactivate the cytochrome oxidase system by providing an alternative binding site for the cyanide ion. There are two types of antidotal therapy for cyanide. The preferred antidote is hydroxocobalamin, which takes advantage of the high affinity of cobalt for cyanide. On binding of cyanide, cyanocobalamin, or vitamin B_{12}, is formed. The initial dose is 5 g intravenously (IV) over 15 minutes for adults and 70 mg/kg IV for children, up to an adult dose, and can be repeated once if an incomplete response is noted. Thiosulfate, 12.5 g in adults (250 mg/kg in children), can be considered in combination with hydroxocobalamin (via a separate IV line) in severe cases of cyanide toxicity, but the benefit of this is not well established. The known adverse effects of hydroxocobalamin are mild and include hypertension in those not cyanide poisoned and a bright red discoloration of the patient's skin and urine. Inexperienced clinicians often mistake this side effect as an "allergic" reaction to the drug. The drug's red color can interfere with certain spectrophotometric laboratory tests, including COHb and possibly serum lactate. Therefore, blood samples should be obtained before the administration of the first dose of hydroxocobalamin.

The cyanide antidote kit, an alternative therapy for toxicity, contains three components (amyl nitrite, sodium nitrite, and sodium thiosulfate). The cyanide antidote kit produces a high-affinity source of ferric ions (Fe^{3+}) for cyanide to bind. Its administration can be impractical or dangerous, particularly for nonhospital providers due to the means by which it is administered (i.e., amyl nitrite capsules are crushed between the fingers and placed under the victim's nose and may be inadvertently inhaled by rescuers). Because animal models and clinical evidence in humans demonstrate that sodium thiosulfate alone in combination with oxygen offers substantial protection, this should be the initial therapy administered by paramedics and during mass poisoning events if ample supplies of hydroxocobalamin are not available. Antidotes should not completely replace other resuscitation measures, including high-flow oxygen and removal of the patient from the source of exposure.

Methemoglobin (MetHb) formation results from the nitrites found in the kit. Inhaled amyl nitrite and IV sodium nitrite are both effective, but amyl nitrite should only be administered to patients in the absence of IV access. Caution should be taken to minimize the provider's exposure to the volatile amyl nitrite because dizziness, hypotension, or syncope may occur. The dose of sodium nitrite for a previously healthy adult is 300 mg (10 mL of a 3% solution) given over 2 to 4 minutes. Dosing instructions for anemic patients and children are supplied with the kit. Cyanide has a high affinity for MetHb and readily leaves cytochrome oxidase to form cyanmethemoglobin, which is metabolically inactive. Additionally, the nitrites are vasodilators, and this may be mechanistically important in their therapeutic effect by enhancing blood flow to the liver for clearance. However, hypotension may complicate a rapid infusion.

Both free serum cyanide and cyanmethemoglobin are converted by sulfur transferase (rhodanese) to thiocyanate, which is renally eliminated. Because the rate of rhodanese function increases with the availability of a sulfur donor, the third component of the antidote kit is the sulfur-containing compound sodium thiosulfate. The adult dose is 12.5 g IV, which is provided as 50 mL of a 25% solution (250 mg/kg sodium thiosulfate up to an adult dose in children). In general, few if any adverse effects are associated with proper doses. The nitrite components of the cyanide antidote kit should be avoided in fire victims with known or suspected simultaneous CO and cyanide poisoning because both CO and MetHb reduce oxygen delivery to the tissues. The use of the thiosulfate component alone in this subset of patients is recommended if hydroxocobalamin is not available (Box 148.2).

There are insufficient clinical data to fully support the use of one cyanide antidote over the other. We recommend hydroxocobalamin because of its ease of use and presumed superior safety in CO-poisoned fire victims.[12] Direct comparison to thiosulfate alone in this population has not been and likely never will be performed, but animal models and case reports suggest that hydroxocobalamin is superior.[13] When possible, we recommend administering both hydroxocobalamin and thiosulfate, with the priority given to hydroxocobalamin, and not administering them through the same IV due to incompatibility.[14]

Hydrogen Sulfide

Because the bond between H_2S and cytochrome oxidase is rapidly reversible, removal from exposure and standard resuscitative techniques are usually sufficient to reverse H_2S toxicity. Use of the nitrite portion of the cyanide antidote kit is suggested to create MetHb for patients with severe or prolonged toxicity. Sodium thiosulfate is unnecessary because H_2S is not detoxified by rhodanese. Hydroxocobalamin also binds sulfide, and has been shown to decrease sulfide concentrations, but has not been shown to be clinically effective for H_2S poisoning. There is no defined role for hyperbaric oxygen (HBO) therapy in cases of H_2S toxicity.

BOX 148.2 Cyanide Antidotes

Hydroxocobalamin[a]
Adults: 5 g IV over 15 min[b]
Children: 70 mg/kg up to 5 g[b]

Cyanide Antidote Kit (Two Parts)
1. MetHb inducers[c]
   Amyl nitrite (inhalational, prehospital) *or*
   Sodium nitrite ($NaNO_2$) 3% solution IV over 2–4 min IV
       Adults: 10 mL (300 mg)
       Children: See labeling information with kit
2. Cyanide detoxification
   Sodium thiosulfate (NaS_2O_3) 25% solution IV
       Adults: 50 mL (12.5 g)
       Children: 250 mg/kg up to 12.5 g

[a]Thiosulfate (see text) can be concomitantly administered for patients with severe clinical effects.
[b]A second dose may be administered in patients with an incomplete response.
[c]Withhold nitrites if an elevated blood carboxyhemoglobin (COHb) is suspected to be present (e.g., fire victims).
IV, Intravenous; *MetHb,* methemoglobin.

Disposition

Patients with symptomatic cyanide or H_2S poisoning should be admitted to a critical care unit and observed for complications of tissue hypoxia. These patients should also be evaluated for delayed neuropsychiatric findings.

CARBON MONOXIDE

Foundations

CO remains a common cause of morbidity and mortality worldwide with an estimated incidence of 137 cases per million annually.[15] CO is generated through incomplete combustion of virtually all carbon-containing products. Structure fires (e.g., wood), clogged vents for home heating units (e.g., methane), and use of gasoline-powered generators indoors are examples of the myriad means through which patients are poisoned by CO. Appropriate public health authorities (e.g., fire department and Department of Health officials) should be informed immediately about any potential public health risks that are identified during the care of a CO-exposed patient.

CO interacts with deoxyhemoglobin to form COHb, which cannot carry oxygen. Hemoglobin binds CO tightly and forms a complex that is only slowly reversible. This allows the exposed individual to accumulate CO, even with exposure to low ambient concentrations. Although binding of hemoglobin is historically described as the mechanism of CO poisoning, it is relevant only in profoundly CO-poisoned patients because a simple reduction in oxygen-carrying capacity due, for example, to anemia would not cause similar symptoms. However, for pregnant patients, the fetus is at increased risk because it is relatively hypoxic compared with the mother. CO shifts the oxyhemoglobin dissociation curve to the left in such a way that even if oxygen is bound to hemoglobin, its unloading to tissues is impaired. In muscle, CO binds myoglobin, preventing its normal function. This likely contributes to the development of atraumatic rhabdomyolysis.

CO affects cellular oxygen use at the tissue level. Similar to cyanide, it inhibits the final cytochrome complex involved in mitochondrial oxidative phosphorylation. This results in a switch to anaerobic metabolism and ultimately in cellular death.

Delayed-onset neurologic complications may be a manifestation of the hypoxic insult, and reperfusion injury and lipid peroxidation related to platelet-induced nitric oxide release may play a significant role.[16] By alteration of the platelet-associated nitric oxide cycle, the microvascular endothelium of the central nervous system undergoes free radical–mediated injury, resulting in localized inflammation and dysfunction. Animal models and human reports suggest that loss of consciousness during CO exposure is a risk factor for the development of delayed neurologic sequelae.

Clinical Features

Severe CO toxicity and cyanide poisoning have identical clinical presentations of chemical asphyxia: altered mental status, including coma and seizures; unstable vital signs, including hypotension and cardiac arrest; and metabolic acidosis. Unlike cyanide poisoning, however, mild CO poisoning occurs frequently, with headache, nausea, vomiting, dizziness, myalgia, and confusion as common presenting complaints. The neurological assessment in these patients may yield normal findings or may demonstrate focal findings or subtle perceptual abnormalities. The often-touted "cherry-red" skin color in patients with cyanide or CO poisoning is a postmortem finding and is not noted in living patients.

Delayed neurologic sequelae is a well-documented phenomenon after CO exposure; the frequency varies from 10% to 30%, depending on the definition and the sensitivity of the test used for their detection. Patients have a variety of neurologic abnormalities after an asymptomatic period, ranging from 3 to 240 days.[17] The delayed neurologic effects can be divided into those with readily identifiable neurologic syndromes (e.g., focal deficits and seizures) and those with primarily psychiatric or cognitive findings (e.g., apathy and memory deficits). Although the delayed neuropsychiatric sequelae require formal neuropsychiatric testing to be detected, the impact of these abnormalities on the patient's daily function may be significant. Risk factors that predict the development of delayed neurologic sequelae include extremes of age and loss of consciousness. Because most CO-poisoned patients reaching the ED survive with minimal intervention, prevention of delayed neurologic and neuropsychiatric sequelae is a major goal of therapy.

Differential Diagnoses

Mild-to-moderate CO poisoning is a difficult diagnosis to establish clinically, and patients are easily misdiagnosed as having a benign headache syndrome or viral illness. CO poisoning should be suspected in patients with persistent or recurrent headache, especially if a group of people have similar symptoms or if the headache improves soon after the person leaves an exposure site.

Patients with severe CO poisoning may present with coma or cardiovascular collapse, both of which have a broad toxicologic, metabolic, infectious, medical, and traumatic differential diagnosis. The medical history, physical examination, and standard laboratory testing are easily able to exclude many of these diagnoses. Given the relatively protean manifestations of CO poisoning and the potentially serious consequences of misdiagnosis, particularly if the patient returns to the contaminated environment, we recommend specific measurement of CO by co-oximetry of an arterial or venous blood sample when the clinician considers CO poisoning as a possible cause for the patient's presentation.

Diagnostic Testing

Suspicion of CO poisoning relies on the history and physical examination findings. Co-oximetry, an inexpensive and readily available spectrophotometric laboratory method that can distinguish between normal hemoglobin, COHb, and MetHb, confirms exposure to CO.

Other laboratory tests only exclude other diagnoses. Severity of poisoning may not correlate with COHb levels because prolonged exposure to low levels can be fatal with a low measured COHb, but a brief, high-concentration exposure can produce a high COHb level with minimal symptoms.

The standard blood gas (ABG or venous blood gas [VBG]) analysis is a poor screening test for CO poisoning other than to identify the presence of a metabolic acidosis and a normal partial pressure of oxygen (P_{O_2}). CO impairs binding of oxygen to hemoglobin but does not affect the amount of oxygen dissolved in blood. Because the P_{O_2} is a measure of dissolved oxygen, it is normal in patients with CO poisoning. The calculated oxygen saturation will be normal even in the presence of significant CO poisoning. Most pulse oximeters are unable to identify CO poisoning because COHb is misinterpreted as oxyhemoglobin. Newer pulse co-oximeters are capable of noninvasively detecting COHb as well as methemoglobinemia.[18]

Management

Treatment begins with oxygen therapy, which serves two purposes. First, the half-life of COHb is inversely related to the P_{O_2}; it can be reduced from approximately 5 hours at room air to 1 hour by providing supplemental 100% oxygen. HBO therapy (at 3 atmospheres) further reduces the half-life to approximately 30 minutes. Alteration of the kinetics of COHb is relevant only to patients with extremely elevated COHb levels (e.g., over 50%). Even then, only a minority of patients can be treated sufficiently and rapidly enough for HBO to be lifesaving. A sufficient P_{O_2} can be achieved with HBO to sustain life in the absence of adequately functioning hemoglobin, but this is helpful only when the COHb is extremely elevated. Thus, the primary indication for HBO is not to prevent mortality but rather to prevent delayed neurologic sequelae.

There is controversy regarding the benefit of HBO because the effect is not immediate (as with life and death) and outcome assessment requires close follow-up and sophisticated testing. Several evidence-based reviews have asserted the limited role for HBO, although this conclusion is disputed.[17] Evidence suggests that HBO helps prevent the development of delayed neuropsychiatric and neurologic sequelae after CO poisoning, with a decrease of delayed neurologic sequelae from approximately 12% to less than 1% with its use. When HBO administration is delayed for more than 6 hours after exposure, its efficacy appears to decrease, suggesting the need for rapid implementation. A meta-analysis performed on randomized controlled trials showed a lower risk of impaired memory in patients who received HBO versus those who did not. The meta-analysis also revealed that HBO treated patients had an improvement in their neuropsychlic scores of block design and trail making when compared to patients treated with normobaric oxygen.[19]

Given the implications of poor tissue oxygenation with COHb and the relative safety of HBO, a patient with a neurologic abnormality or cardiovascular instability (e.g., syncope, altered mental status, seizures, myocardial ischemia, and dysrhythmias) is a candidate for HBO (Box 148.3). This should be tempered by the need for transport, often over long distances, for HBO therapy to be obtained. The decision about HBO therapy should not be strictly based on the COHb level, which correlates only weakly with poisoning. Patients with prolonged low-level exposure have a "soaking" phenomenon, in which extremely high tissue concentrations of CO occur with relatively low COHb levels. Thus, patients with consequential clinical findings that are considered to be related to CO poisoning should receive HBO despite relatively low COHb levels.

In addition to the use of HBO in patients with obvious signs of tissue hypoxia or syncope, we recommend referral for HBO for asymptomatic patients with a COHb level of 25% or greater. The decision

BOX 148.3 Recommendations for Hyperbaric Oxygen

Carboxyhemoglobin (COHb) (varies by local standards) independent of clinical findings
>25% with normal clinical findings
>15% in pregnancy or fetal distress
or an elevated COHb with one or more of the following findings:
Syncope
Coma
Seizure
Altered mental status (GCS < 15) or confusion
Abnormal cerebellar function
Prolonged CO exposure with minor clinical findings ("soaking")

CO, Carbon monoxide; *GCS*, Glasgow Coma Score.

to perform HBO therapy should be made in the context of transport and other medical requirements, including need for transfer to a burn center which may delay or prevent HBO therapy unless implemented at the burn center. If doubt remains, consultation with a medical toxicologist, poison center, or the HBO treatment specialist will guide decision-making. Because fetal CO poisoning is associated with dysfunction and death and HBO therapy appears to be safe in pregnancy, we recommend HBO therapy in a pregnant woman with a COHb level of 15% or greater regardless of symptoms. Further study is still needed to define the optimal duration, pressure, and frequency, as well as the cost-benefit and risk-benefit relationships of HBO therapy. At this time, discussion with a regional HBO center or poison control center is advisable. Patients with elevated COHb levels who do not require HBO should be treated with normobaric oxygen delivered by a tight-fitting non-rebreather face mask at a flow rate of 15L/min until the symptoms resolve and the COHb levels fall to normal.

Simultaneous Carbon Monoxide and Cyanide Poisoning (Fire Victims)

Concurrent toxicity from CO and cyanide is widely reported and a major factor in the mortality associated with smoke inhalation.[20] Victims who present with coma and metabolic acidosis can have severe CO poisoning, cyanide poisoning, or both. Nitrite-induced methemoglobinemia, which further reduces the tissue oxygen delivery, may be detrimental to patients with elevated COHb levels or otherwise impaired oxygen delivery.

Sodium thiosulfate, administered without nitrites, or hydroxocobalamin should be given to all smoke inhalation victims with coma, hypotension, severe acidosis, or cardiovascular collapse in whom cyanide poisoning cannot be rapidly excluded.

Disposition

The decision to transfer a patient to an HBO facility should consider the time delay to therapy, patient issues (e.g., hemodynamic instability, burns, and age), and potential transport-related complications. Patients with minor clinical effects that resolve can be discharged with dedicated follow-up. Those with signs of end organ effects, such as chest pain or altered mental status, if not transferred for HBO, should be admitted for observation. All patients exposed to CO require close follow-up for delayed neurologic sequelae.

The references for this chapter can be found online at ExpertConsult. com.

Lithium

Jillian L. Theobald and Steven E. Aks

FOUNDATIONS

Lithium has been used therapeutically since the mid-1800s, when it was initially prescribed to treat gout. Lithium compounds were also historically used therapeutically: lithium bromide as a hypnotic, lithium iodide to treat syphilis, and lithium chloride introduced as a table salt alternative for heart failure patients in the 20th century. Ultimately, multiple deaths led to removal of lithium chloride from the US market. In 1970, lithium was approved for the treatment of bipolar disorder, and it remains one of the most effective agents for both depressive and manic symptoms. Lithium is the only drug treatment for bipolar disorder that is associated with a reduced risk of suicide.[1]

Lithium is a monovalent cation with a narrow therapeutic range, and significant toxicity can result when outside of this range. Lithium largely has no effect when given in therapeutic doses to patients without mood disorders. Despite its long history of therapeutic use, the complex and multimodal mechanism of action of lithium is still not fully understood. Its efficacy in the treatment of psychiatric illnesses is thought to be due to the modulation of neurotransmitters, which has downstream effects through cell signaling and molecular mechanisms.[2]

Lithium is rapidly absorbed from the gastrointestinal tract and peaks in the serum 1 to 2 hours after ingestion of immediate-release preparation and 4 to 5 hours with sustained-release preparations. Absorption and peak concentrations can be delayed in overdose situations, with ingestion of sustained-release formulations, or when concretions form in the gut. Once absorbed, lithium enters the serum followed by a delayed distribution to the tissues. In therapeutic dosing, lithium reaches a steady state within 6 hours after the last dose. Therefore lithium levels must be interpreted in the context of the patient's last dose. Lithium is not metabolized and is excreted unchanged in the urine. Any decreases in renal excretion because of conditions such as dehydration, hyponatremia, or renal dysfunction will lead to increases in serum lithium levels.

CLINICAL FEATURES

Lithium toxicity is categorized into acute, acute on chronic, or chronic toxicity. Evaluation of the potentially lithium toxic patient requires knowledge of whether the patient was previously taking lithium, the timing of the last dose, and the amount of drug ingested. The clinical features of lithium toxicity depend on whether it is acute or chronic in nature (Table 149.1). Acute toxicity usually follows a recent ingestion in a patient who is not therapeutically taking lithium and manifests early with gastrointestinal symptoms such as vomiting and diarrhea. Neurologic consequences of an acute lithium overdose include seizures, altered mental status, tremors, hyperreflexia, clonus, or fasciculations. They occur several hours later, after lithium redistributes to the central nervous system. In some cases with delayed-release lithium, neurologic symptoms may occur 12 or more hours after ingestion. These neurologic consequences are similar to chronic lithium toxicity. Chronic toxicity is caused by a relatively gradual increase in serum lithium level in a patient who is regularly taking lithium. This can either be from reduced excretion, renal insufficiency, or a dose adjustment. Chronic lithium toxicity causes predominantly neurologic symptoms with minimal to no gastrointestinal symptoms. Acute-on-chronic toxicity occurs when a patient with a stable steady-state lithium level takes a substantial additional amount of lithium, intentionally or accidentally. These patients present with signs and symptoms of both acute and chronic toxicity. Either acute or chronic toxicity can result in cardiac conduction abnormalities with T-wave inversions being the most common electrocardiogram (ECG) finding.[3]

Long-term chronic use of lithium can lead to nephrogenic diabetes insipidus and hypothyroidism. Both conditions are reversible with discontinuation of the medication and respond well to conventional management.[4] Hypercalcemia and hyperparathyroidism also can occur and reverse upon discontinuation of lithium.[5] Patients chronically taking lithium can develop the syndrome of irreversible lithium-effectuated neurotoxicity (SILENT). Patients with SILENT will often have persistent cerebellar and brain stem dysfunction, dementia, and extrapyramidal signs even after lithium use has been discontinued for days to weeks.[6] Use of lithium during early pregnancy may increase the risk for cardiovascular abnormalities in the fetus.[7]

DIFFERENTIAL DIAGNOSES

Lithium toxicity is nonspecific and may present in a manner similar to many systemic and neurologic disorders, so obtaining a history of lithium use or ingestion is critical to making the diagnosis. Nausea and vomiting are common with viral or bacterial gastrointestinal

TABLE 149.1   Clinical Features of Lithium Toxicity

Clinical Features	TYPE OF TOXICITY	
	Acute	**Chronic**
Gastrointestinal[4]	Nausea Vomiting Diarrhea	Mild or nonexistent
Neurologic[8]	Similar to chronic toxicity, occurs several hours after lithium distribution to the brain	Tremors Clonus Hyperreflexia Extrapyramidal symptoms Altered mental status Somnolence Coma Seizures
Cardiac[2]	Sinus node dysfunction AV blockade Brugada pattern on ECG Ischemic changes on ECG QTc prolongation	

AV, Atrioventricular; *ECG,* electrocardiogram.
Modified from Won E, Kim YK. An oldie but goodie: lithium in the treatment of bipolar disorder through neuroprotective and neurotrophic mechanisms. *Int J Mol Sci.* 2017;18(12):2679. https://doi.org/10.3390/ijms18122679; Davis J, Desmond M, Berk M. Lithium and nephrotoxicity: a literature review of approaches to clinical management and risk stratification. *BMC Nephrol.* 2018;19(1):305; Thanacoody R, Caravati EM, Troutman B, et al. Position paper update: whole bowel irrigation for gastrointestinal decontamination of overdose patients. *Clin Toxicol.* 2015;53(1):5–12.

BOX 149.1   Diagnostic Testing for Lithium

Serum lithium level
Serum electrolytes
Creatinine concentration or a glomerular filtration rate (GFR)
Electrocardiogram (ECG)
If the clinical picture dictates:
   Acetaminophen/salicylate levels
   Thyroid function tests

---

syndromes, early pregnancy, various abdominal pathologies, acute neurologic events, and other toxic ingestions. The neurologic manifestations of lithium toxicity (tremors, hyperreflexia, altered mental status, and seizures) may prompt consideration of withdrawal syndromes (alcohol or benzodiazepines), sympathomimetic toxicities (cocaine and amphetamines), and serotonin syndrome.

DIAGNOSTIC TESTING

Serum lithium levels should be obtained in all patients who are taking lithium, or have access to lithium, and present with potential toxicity. Because of the insidious and nonspecific nature of chronic lithium toxicity, a serum lithium level is also advisable in any patients who is on lithium maintenance therapy, regardless of their reason for presentation (Box 149.1). Therapeutic serum concentrations of lithium are between 0.6 and 1.2 mEq/L. Serum lithium levels are in a steady state approximately 6 hours after ingestion of a therapeutic dose and should be interpreted in the context of when the last dose was taken. In overdose situations, peak concentrations can occur beyond 6 hours. We recommend obtaining serum lithium concentrations every 2 to 4 hours until two consecutive declining measurements are observed. Serum electrolytes should be obtained because lithium can cause alterations in calcium and sodium, most commonly hypercalcemia and hypernatremia. An assessment of the patient's renal function either by a serum creatinine concentration or a glomerular filtration rate should also be performed. If there is clinical concern for thyroid dysfunction, then thyroid studies should be obtained. In patients presenting with an acute intentional ingestion, both acetaminophen and aspirin levels should be sent to evaluate for possible coingestants. Finally, an ECG

should be obtained and cardiac monitoring initiated in patients presenting with an acute or chronic overdose. An ECG also should be obtained for patients on chronic lithium therapy, given the propensity of lithium to cause conduction abnormalities.

MANAGEMENT

Stabilization and Supportive Care

No specific antidote exists for lithium toxicity therefore supportive care and enhanced elimination are the mainstays of treatment. Most patients who are lithium-toxic are dehydrated because of gastrointestinal losses in acute toxicity or from underlying dehydration and lithium-induced diabetes insipidus, leading to chronic toxicity. Crystalloid solution (lactated Ringers solution) should be infused as a 1 L bolus followed by a continuous infusion at 150% of the calculated maintenance rate if there are no contraindications, such as congestive heart failure. Volume expansion also enhances renal elimination of lithium. Electrolyte abnormalities, such as hypernatremia and hypercalcemia, if significant, should be corrected (see Chapter 114).

Decontamination

Activated charcoal does not bind lithium. Furthermore, we do not recommend the use of whole bowel irrigation (WBI) in routine lithium ingestions. Although a position paper suggests that WBI can be considered after massive overdose, there is only scant evidence that WBI can decrease the amount of lithium absorbed in nontoxic doses, and there is no clinical evidence of benefit in overdose.[8] Similarly sodium polystyrene resins (e.g., Kayexalate) have been proposed to assist in the elimination of lithium by sodium-lithium exchange; however, due to limited binding capacity, large volumes are needed to have any significant reduction in lithium levels. There are no studies demonstrating an actual impact on clinical outcome, the risks outweigh the benefit, and we do not recommend the use of ion-exchange resins in lithium poisoning.[9]

Enhanced Elimination

Because lithium is primarily excreted unchanged by the kidney, early initiation of intravenous crystalloid solution, as described earlier, enhances elimination. Diuretics are contraindicated, because they can cause worsening dehydration, with further impairment of renal function, and also can enhance renal reabsorption of lithium.

Lithium is highly dialyzable, and hemodialysis is indicated for patients exhibiting signs of severe lithium toxicity (Box 149.2). Patients with severe neurologic toxicity (e.g., altered mental status, clonus, hyperreflexia, and seizures) should undergo hemodialysis to reduce serum lithium levels to less than 1.0 mEq/L.[10] In addition, hemodialysis is indicated for patients with impaired renal function or those who cannot tolerate intravenous fluids. There is little high-quality evidence in favor of dialysis based solely on serum lithium concentration. A Cochrane review concluded that there is insufficient evidence to determine which lithium-intoxicated patients might benefit from hemodialysis.[11] Based on our experience and available evidence, we recommend

---

BOX 149.2   Indications for H Somnolence

Hemodialysis in Lithium Poisoned Patients

Severely symptomatic patients
Unable to tolerate crystalloid fluid resuscitation
Renal impairment
Acute or chronic toxicity: Levels >5 mEq/L
Neurotoxicity including tremors, clonus, altered mental status, somnolence, seizures

---

dialysis for serum levels greater than 5 mEq/L[12] or for patients with signs of severe neurologic lithium toxicity, particularly tremor, clonus, altered mental status, and seizure, regardless of the serum concentration. Serum lithium concentrations can rise or rebound after dialysis sessions; therefore a steady state concentration should be determined at 6 hours post procedure.

DISPOSITION

Disposition depends largely on the extent of clinical toxicity and the psychiatric status of the patient. Patients manifesting clinical signs of neurotoxicity such as tremors, altered mental status, and seizures should be admitted. Patients with an acute overdose complicated by significant cardiologic or neurologic symptoms and high (>5 mEq/L) or increasing supratherapeutic serum lithium levels should undergo hemodialysis. Patients with significant altered mental status or seizures, and those requiring dialysis should be monitored in an intensive care which may require early transfer to a hospital with this capability. In these cases, we recommend consultation with a regional poison center or medical toxicologist. Patients with overdoses of sustained-release lithium should also be placed in an observation unit or hospitalized for serial monitoring of lithium concentrations until at least two consecutive declining serum levels are documented. Patients who remain asymptomatic with normal physical examination findings and serum lithium levels in the therapeutic range 6 hours after ingestion of immediate-release lithium preparations or 12 hours after a sustained-release preparation can be discharged or cleared for psychiatric evaluation. Women taking lithium who present to the emergency department with newly diagnosed pregnancy should be referred to an obstetrician for fetal evaluation and monitoring and to discuss the risk benefit profile of lithium use during pregnancy.

The references for this chapter can be found online at ExpertConsult. com.

150

Antipsychotics

Jessica Monas and Aaron B. Skolnik

KEY CONCEPTS

- Antipsychotics are commonly categorized into typical, or first-generation antipsychotics (FGAs) with primary antagonism to dopamine receptors, and atypical, or second-generation antipsychotics (SGAs) which include serotonin receptors as a target. Aripiprazole is an example of a third type of antipsychotic that acts as a partial agonist at dopamine sites.
- Extrapyramidal symptoms are common side effects of antipsychotics. First line treatment is benztropine or diphenhydramine. Lorazepam may be used in refractory cases.
- The most common presentation of an antipsychotic overdose is central nervous system (CNS) depression. Treatment focuses on supportive care, airway management, and cardiac monitoring.
- QT prolongation and *torsades de pointes* are potential complications of antipsychotic overdose but may also occur with therapeutic use.
- Clozapine is associated with potentially life-threatening agranulocytosis. Treatment includes cessation of the medication, treating potential infections, and supportive care.
- Neuroleptic malignant syndrome (NMS) is characterized by altered mental status, hyperthermia, muscle rigidity, and autonomic instability. Treatment includes supportive care with airway management, benzodiazepines, muscular rigidity management, and evaporative cooling methods for hyperthermia.

FOUNDATIONS

Background

In 1950, promethazine was synthesized in an effort to develop antihistamines, but it was also found to potentiate the effects of anesthetics and was widely used. An attempt to derive similar drugs led to the synthesis of chlorpromazine. It was discovered that patients treated with this became sedate and apathetic and it was termed a *neuroleptic*. Chlorpromazine was first used to successfully treat a patient with psychosis in 1952 and helped to pave the way for the modern treatment of mental illness. Prior to the development of antipsychotics, pharmacotherapy for psychosis had focused on tranquilization rather than modification of disease.

In 1956, clozapine was synthesized. It demonstrated that a drug could treat psychosis without significant extrapyramidal effects and became the precursor of the *atypical* antipsychotics. Clozapine was initially removed from market in 1974 due to agranulocytosis but was reintroduced in 1990 with mandatory monitoring because of its clinical efficacy in treatment-resistant schizophrenia.[1]

The term *neuroleptic* has since been replaced with *antipsychotic*, because newer agents are less sedating. Antipsychotic use has expanded beyond schizophrenia and schizoaffective disorders to include supplemental treatment for major depressive disorder, bipolar disorder, anxiety disorders, behavioral changes associated with dementia, and psychoses related to substance use disorders and withdrawal. In the past decade, antipsychotic prescribing has dramatically increased, including off-label and nonpsychosis use.[2-5] In 2018, nearly 50,000 exposures attributable to antipsychotics were reported to poison control centers in the United States. In conjunction with sedatives and hypnotics, antipsychotics comprised the group of drugs with the greatest increase per year in serious adverse outcomes and human ingestions.[6]

Pathophysiology

Antipsychotics have been categorized according to their mechanism of action as well as their clinical effect. All antipsychotics have dopamine receptor antagonism. Typical, or first-generation antipsychotics (FGAs) focused on dopamine blockade as a primary target with subsequent adverse extrapyramidal effects. FGAs are sometimes classified as low-potency or high-potency based on their affinity for the dopamine D_2 receptor subtype (Box 150.1). Atypical, or second-generation antipsychotics (SGAs) were developed to combine with serotonin receptor antagonism (5-hydroxytryptamine type 2A) to decrease neurologic side effects and also treat negative symptoms of thought disorders. More recent development of partial dopamine agonism, such as aripiprazole and brexpiprazole, led to the phrase "third-generation" antipsychotic, but this term has not been readily accepted.[7,8] In 2019, the US Food and Drug Administration (FDA) approved a novel first-in-class antipsychotic, lumateperone, that acts synergistically though serotonergic, dopaminergic, and glutaminergic modulation.[9] Lumateperone has been shown to improve depressive as well as psychotic symptoms.[10] In general, low-potency FGAs are the most sedating. Movement disorders are a significant adverse effect of this class of medication, with SGAs having lower frequency. Although neuroleptic malignant syndrome (NMS) can occur with all antipsychotics, it occurs less often with SGAs.[11]

Antipsychotic medications are widely used for both psychiatric and nonpsychiatric purposes. The antiemetic effects of prochlorperazine, promethazine, and droperidol result from blockade of dopamine receptors of the chemoreceptor trigger zone of the medulla. Prochlorperazine and droperidol are thought to improve migraine headaches by inhibiting dopamine-mediated trigeminovascular activation. Olanzapine has been used for fibromyalgia and the treatment of other chronic pain.[12,13] Chlorpromazine is the historical drug of choice for singultus or intractable hiccups, although other antipsychotics are also used.[14] Although haloperidol, pimozide, and aripiprazole are the only FDA-approved treatments for Tourette syndrome, other SGAs have been recommended.

Toxicity

Toxicity of antipsychotic drugs can be divided into three categories: exaggerated pharmacologic effects seen in acute overdose, undesired clinical effects seen in therapeutic use such as extrapyramidal syndromes, and idiosyncratic effects such as NMS.

In addition to D_2 receptor antagonism, most antipsychotics take effect at other receptors and ion channels. These include alpha-1 adrenergic, muscarinic, and histamine H_1 receptor antagonism, as well as fast voltage-gated sodium, and delayed potassium rectifier channel blockade.

Alpha antagonism may result in orthostatic hypotension. Muscarinic antagonism can produce minor side effects in therapeutic use or anticholinergic toxicity in acute overdose including cognitive impairment. Histaminergic blockade can produce sedating effects in both therapeutic use and overdose.

Phenothiazine antipsychotics such as chlorpromazine are structurally related to tricyclic antidepressants (TCAs), exhibiting sodium channel blockade that may lead to wide complex dysrhythmias. Many agents inhibit potassium rectifying currents resulting in QT prolongation and, potentially, torsades de pointes. The degree of prolongation varies between antipsychotics and can increase in a dose-dependent manner, with ziprasidone and iloperidone having the highest risk, and aripiprazole and brexpiprazole the lowest.[15] QT prolonging effects may be worsened in chronically ill patients and with concomitant use of other QT-prolonging drugs.[15,16] Although a direct correlation between degree of QT prolongation and risk of torsades de pointes has not been well

established, antipsychotics are associated with increased risk of sudden death that is worsened with comorbid cardiac disease and in elderly patients.[17] In addition, psychotic disorders alone increase the risk of sudden death.[18] Therapeutic use of clozapine has been linked to myocarditis and cardiomyopathy that may be accompanied by eosinophilia.[19]

Antipsychotic drugs block dopamine receptors at multiple regions within the brain. Mesolimbic D_2 blockade produces the desirable effect of reducing positive symptoms of schizophrenia. However, similar degrees of D_2 receptor blockade in the nigrostriatal pathway also produce the undesirable extrapyramidal symptoms (EPSs). This includes dystonia, akathisia, and drug-induced parkinsonism, which may be immediate or delayed in onset. SGAs have lower affinity for the dopamine receptors and add-in serotonin receptor antagonism, both of which are thought to reduce EPSs. The propensity of antipsychotics to produce EPSs is also inversely proportional to the agent's muscarinic receptor antagonism.[20] Rapid dissociation from the D_2 receptor has been hypothesized to reduce the risk of EPS; however, data suggest that association rates may also play a factor.[21,22]

Tardive syndromes (TSs) encompass the hyperkinetic and hypokinetic movements that result after delay from exposure to dopamine-blocking drugs. Tardive dyskinesia (TD) may develop after prolonged use of these medications and has been reported with all antipsychotics. One proposed pathophysiological mechanism is chronic dopamine receptor blockade in the nigrostriatal pathway leading to D_2 receptor upregulation and hypersensitivity to dopamine. Genetic factors are also thought to play a significant role in the development of TD.

NMS is a rare, idiosyncratic reaction to antipsychotic medications, the pathophysiology of which is less understood. It can be severe and, if unrecognized or undertreated, can lead to permanent neurologic sequalae and death. NMS is thought to result from D_2 receptor blockade in the nigrostriatum and hypothalamus, which can lead to rigidity and hyperthermia, with downstream dysregulation of the autonomic nervous system. It has more recently been suggested that NMS may be due to a direct toxic effect of the drug on the musculoskeletal fibers.

Clozapine-associated agranulocytosis is rare, with an incidence of approximately 1%, which drops to 0.38% with routine white blood cell count monitoring.[23] A more recent meta-analysis found that this does not occur more frequently with clozapine than with other antipsychotics.[24] The classic proposed mechanism is a direct cytotoxic effect on bone marrow mesenchymal stromal cells. An alternate suggested etiology is that it may be related to an autoimmune process.

Antipsychotic use has also been associated with weight gain, dyslipidemia, glucose intolerance, metabolic syndrome, and new-onset diabetes mellitus.[23] Numerous observational and case-control studies indicate an increased risk of venous thromboembolism (VTE) with antipsychotic use. Multiple hypotheses regarding the mechanism include drug-induced sedation, weight gain, enhanced platelet aggregation, antiphospholipid antibody level increase, and the possibility that thought disorders may cause a predisposition. The risk of VTE may also be highest within the first 3 months of antipsychotic therapy initiation.

CLINICAL FEATURES

Acute Overdose

In overdose, antipsychotics produce signs and symptoms that are exaggerations of their pharmacologic profile. Most patients develop symptoms within a few hours post ingestion. Paliperidone has a unique delayed-delivery system, and late onset of symptoms has been reported.[25] Central nervous system (CNS) depression is common, ranging from mild sedation to coma. Anticholinergic delirium and agitation may result from drugs with antimuscarinic effects (Box 150.2). Airway reflexes can be impaired and respiratory depression can occur after overdose. Pupils may be of variable size; anticholinergic effects promote mydriasis, whereas miosis, resulting from alpha-antagonism, may mimic opioid toxicity. Orthostatic hypotension is also a common finding resulting from alpha-adrenergic blockade. Variable evidence suggests that antipsychotics lower seizure threshold; however, with the exception of clozapine, seizures rarely occur in overdose. Acute EPSs have also been reported in overdose.

Acute Extrapyramidal Syndromes

Acute dystonia presents with involuntary spasms of antagonistic muscle groups most often involving facial, neck, back, or limb muscles. This results in trismus, facial grimacing, dysarthria, tongue and lip distortion, torticollis, or oculogyric crisis. Half of patients who develop acute dystonia do so within 48 hours of receiving the implicated drug. Symptoms may develop rapidly or may be delayed hours to days, although most acute dystonia develops within 5 days of drug administration. Recurrent dystonic reactions may occur, even following a single dose of an antipsychotic. *Laryngeal dystonia*, a rare but life-threatening form of dystonia, manifests as dyspnea, stridor, choking sensation, or respiratory distress and has been reported with both FGAs and SGAs.[26] Increased risk of death due to choking has been reported in patients treated for schizophrenia; both FGAs and SGAs have been associated with dysphagia.

Akathisia (from Greek, *"unable to sit"*) is characterized by subjective feelings of internal restlessness associated with objective motor findings, including repetitive foot shuffling, truncal shifting, or pacing. Akathisia usually develops within hours to days of initiating or increasing the dose of an antipsychotic. Studies of emergency department (ED) patients have demonstrated a lower incidence of akathisia and other EPSs with SGAs. *Rabbit syndrome* is a perioral, tongue-sparing dyskinesia in which rhythmic lip and nose movements resemble the chewing movements of a rabbit. Rabbit syndrome is primarily associated with FGA drugs but has also been case reported with SGAs.

Drug-induced parkinsonism, manifest by bradykinesia, masklike facies, shuffling gait, rigidity, and tremor, may occur in up to 60% of patients treated with antipsychotics and frequently develops 2 to 4 weeks after initiating treatment. Ninety percent of cases develop within 3 months.

Tardive Syndromes

TSs refer to delayed-onset motor and nonmotor syndromes induced by prolonged use of dopamine antagonists, including antipsychotic medications. TSs include dystonia, akathisia, motor, sensory syndromes, and classic TD. TD refers to the repetitive, rapid, involuntary orofacial, limb, trunk, or pelvic movements first described in 1964. The risk of TD with sustained antipsychotic treatment is estimated to be approximately 5% per year and may be higher in the elderly. Prevalence is estimated at approximately 20% of psychiatric patients undergoing long-term treatment. Reduction of the antipsychotic dose or a change to an alternative agent should be considered, in consultation with the patient's psychiatrist. Two drugs, valbenazine and deutetrabenazine, were FDA approved for the treatment of TD in 2017.

Neuroleptic Malignant Syndrome

NMS is a serious idiosyncratic drug reaction that is potentially life threatening. NMS typically develops during the first 2 weeks of therapy but has occurred during long-term drug regimens. The incidence of NMS has been reported to range from less than 1% to 3% among patients exposed to antipsychotics. The unadjusted mortality rate of NMS has been estimated at approximately 5%. Males are approximately 50% more likely to develop NMS, with peak overall incidence between the ages of 20 and 25 years old. Other risk factors include recent dose changes, cumulative drug dosage, high-potency antipsychotics, parenteral formulations, polypharmacy, prolonged physical restraint, dehydration, hyperthermia, prior brain injury, family history of catatonia, muscle channelopathies, and previous episodes of NMS. Cotreatment with two antipsychotics is associated with increased risk for NMS.[27] Although highly potent FGAs are most frequently the culprit in NMS, all antipsychotics have been implicated, including SGAs. NMS caused by SGAs is associated with a lower incidence, decreased severity, and lower mortality than that caused by FGAs.[11] Abrupt withdrawal from dopaminergic agents used to treat Parkinson disease (i.e., levodopa/carbidopa) may cause a potentially fatal syndrome that is clinically indistinguishable from NMS, termed the parkinsonism-hyperpyrexia syndrome.

NMS is characterized by the tetrad of altered mental status, muscular rigidity, hyperthermia, and autonomic instability (Table 150.1). Other features of NMS may include sialorrhea, dysarthria, dysphagia, metabolic acidosis, generalized slowing on electroencephalogram (EEG), coagulopathy, rhabdomyolysis, deep venous thrombosis, pulmonary embolism, and acute kidney injury. Laboratory studies are typically notable for markedly elevated creatinine kinase (>1000 IU/mL), leukocytosis, and nonspecific elevation of inflammatory markers such as C-reactive protein (CRP) and erythrocyte sedimentation rate (ESR).

Most patients have the cardinal features of NMS within 1 to 2 weeks after starting an antipsychotic or abruptly increasing the dose. Of note, the signs of NMS may develop gradually and in any order. Clinicians should discontinue all antipsychotics, other dopamine antagonists, and other psychotropic drugs in patients with suspected NMS. Acute care in the ED includes airway management as required, intravenous (IV) fluid resuscitation, correction of metabolic disturbances, and supportive care with rapid cooling methods for hyperthermia. Administration of benzodiazepines is also indicated depending on the patient's clinical severity and response to treatment (see dosing recommendations in Management section). Most episodes of NMS resolve with appropriate care within 2 weeks after cessation of the offending medication; however, symptoms may wax and wane for months.

Cardiovascular Toxicity

The most common cardiac effect of these medications is sinus tachycardia with a normal QRS duration. A few FGAs can cause QRS prolongation; however, coingestions should be considered. QT prolongation was once considered a "class effect" of all antipsychotic medications. More recent literature has identified significant differences among the antipsychotics with respect to potential for QTc prolongation and torsades de pointes during therapeutic dosing or in overdose. At therapeutic doses, the highest risk of QT prolongation occurs with pimozide and sertindole. The only antipsychotics without any effect on QT in therapeutic use are brexpiprazole, cariprazine, and lurasidone.[28]

TABLE 150.1   Prevalence of Suggested Diagnostic Criteria for Neuroleptic Malignant Syndrome

Criterion	Prevalence
Exposure to a dopamine antagonist or withdrawal of a dopamine agonist within 72 h:	
Hyperthermia (>38°C) on at least two occasions, measured orally	98%
Rigidity	97%
Mental status alteration	97%
Creatinine kinase elevation (at least 4 times the upper level of normal)	95%
Sympathetic nervous system lability, defined as at least two of the following:	
Blood pressure elevation (SBP or DBP ≥25% above baseline)	61%[a]
Blood pressure fluctuation (≥20% DBP change or ≥25% SBP change in 24 h)	
Diaphoresis	98%
Urinary incontinence	
Hypermetabolic state (heart rate ≥25% and respiratory rate ≥50% above baseline)	88%[b]
Negative evaluation for other toxic, metabolic, infectious, or neurologic causes	

[a]Elevated or labile blood pressure.
[b]Tachycardia.
DBP, Diastolic blood pressure; SBP, systolic blood pressure.
Modified from Gurrera RJ, Caroff SN, Cohen A, et al. An international consensus study of neuroleptic malignant syndrome diagnostic criteria using the Delphi method. *J Clin Psychiatry.* 2001;72:1222–1228.

Antipsychotic use has also been associated with an overall increased risk of cardiopulmonary arrest and death.[17]

Myocarditis has been reported in less than 1% of patients taking clozapine. The majority of cases develop in the first 2 months of treatment, with the incidence decreasing 10-fold over 12 months of treatment. A nonspecific, flulike prodrome frequently precedes the onset of myocarditis by days to weeks. The spectrum of disease ranges widely, from subclinical, asymptomatic disease to decompensated heart failure with case-fatality reported between 10% and 30%.

Agranulocytosis

Clozapine can produce life-threatening agranulocytosis in approximately 1% of exposed patients; the highest risk occurs between 1 and 5 months after starting the drug and decreases with subsequent duration of treatment. By 1 year, the risk of agranulocytosis approaches that of chlorpromazine (0.1%). With monitoring and treatment, attributable mortality is approximately 1 in 10,000. Agranulocytosis has not been reported after acute clozapine overdose. Agranulocytosis and neutropenia have been reported with many FGAs and SGAs. A recent meta-analysis of controlled trials suggests that the risk of neutropenia associated with clozapine is not greater than that associated with other antipsychotics.[24] With early recognition, antipsychotic-induced neutropenia typically resolves within 3 to 4 weeks of discontinuing the drug.

Seizures

The risk of new-onset seizures among patients treated with antipsychotics is up to 2.5-fold higher than the background rate in the untreated population, suggesting antipsychotic medications lower the seizure threshold.[29] The prevalence of psychosis in persons with epilepsy may be threefold greater than that of nonepilepsy controls, with a pooled prevalence estimate of 6%. The prescription of antipsychotic drugs to persons with epilepsy is therefore necessary and safe when indicated, even though most antipsychotics may reduce the seizure threshold.

DIFFERENTIAL DIAGNOSES

Antipsychotic toxicity may present similarly to clinical conditions and agents that produce altered mental status, seizures, anticholinergic toxidrome, orthostatic hypotension, QT prolongation, or torsades de pointes, such as TCAs. The differential diagnosis of NMS includes malignant catatonia, serotonin syndrome, heatstroke, sympathomimetic toxicity, acute salicylate poisoning, and other medical conditions (Table 150.2). Consider malignant hyperthermia in patients receiving inhalational anesthetics or succinylcholine.

DIAGNOSTIC TESTING

Quantitative blood levels of antipsychotics are neither readily available nor helpful in the ED setting. As with any patient who presents with suspected drug toxicity, blood glucose concentration, serum acetaminophen level, and directed toxicologic screening are recommended. Aspiration is common among patients with depressed mentation; chest radiography should be performed in hypoxic patients.

An electrocardiogram (ECG) should be obtained in all patients with suspected overdose and in those taking antipsychotics therapeutically with symptoms concerning for cardiotoxicity, because the ECG may predict adverse cardiovascular events.[30] If QT prolongation is present, serum sodium, potassium, calcium, and magnesium levels should be measured.

Patients who have NMS, EPSs with marked muscle rigidity, or prolonged seizures are at risk for rhabdomyolysis. In such patients we recommend serum creatinine kinase, assessment of renal function, and urine myoglobin measurements.

Patients who are severely hyperthermic (>40°C) are at risk for multi-system organ failure and disseminated intravascular coagulation. Because severe salicylate poisoning can cause CNS toxicity and hyperthermia due to uncoupling of oxidative phosphorylation, we recommend a serum salicylate level, in addition to serum transaminases and coagulation studies.

Patients taking antipsychotic medications who present with unusual infections or fever without a source should be evaluated for neutropenia, as the (low) risk appears to be similar for clozapine and other antipsychotics.[24]

Second-generation antipsychotics are associated with new-onset diabetes mellitus (including adult diagnosis of previously latent autoimmune diabetes) and diabetic ketoacidosis (DKA). This typically occurs within 1 year from the onset of treatment and may occur in the absence of weight gain. Most of these patients will subsequently require insulin for long-term blood glucose management.[31] Patients in whom DKA is clinically suspected should have blood glucose and pH, serum electrolytes, and serum or urine ketone testing. Salicylism can also produce a clinical picture that mimics DKA.

Other tests, such as brain computed tomography, lumbar puncture, and drug screens may be helpful in some cases to exclude other diagnoses or establish a comorbid condition but are not indicated when

TABLE 150.2	Differential Diagnoses of Neuroleptic Malignant Syndrome[a]			
Disease	**Proposed Mechanism**	**Differentiating Factor**	**Time Course**	**Treatment**
Neuroleptic malignant syndrome (NMS)	Impaired thermoregulation in hypothalamus and basal ganglia due to due to dopamine blockade Downstream autonomic nervous system dysfunction	Antipsychotic use Muscle rigidity	Gradual over several days Waxing and waning course	Stop offending medication Hydration Active cooling IV benzodiazepines Nondepolarizing neuromuscular blockade Limited evidence: Dantrolene Dopamine agonists (e.g., bromocriptine) Consider ECT for refractory cases
Serotonin syndrome	Excess serotonin levels in CNS	Medications (usually a combination) that increase serotonin levels (e.g., SSRIs, MAOIs, lithium, dextromethorphan, meperidine, tramadol) Muscle rigidity (lower > upper extremities) Muscular or ocular clonus	Usually rapid after introduction of new medication or increase in dose	Stop offending medication Hydration Active cooling IV benzodiazepines Cyproheptadine
Malignant or lethal catatonia	Severe manifestation of schizophrenia, mood disorders, other psychiatric disorders, or neurological conditions Multiple mechanisms proposed	Occurs in absence of antipsychotic administration May be clinically indistinguishable from NMS	Gradual, typically over several days	Hydration Active cooling IV benzodiazepines ECT
Sympathomimetic toxicity	Hyperadrenergic state Extreme psychomotor agitation	Occurs in absence of antipsychotic administration Cardiovascular toxicity may be prominent Muscular hyperactivity in lieu of rigidity	Subacute, typically over hours	Hydration Active cooling IV benzodiazepines Alpha-antagonists Vasodilators
Malignant hyperthermia	Mutations in ryanodine receptors or dihydropyridine receptors allow uncontrolled calcium release from sarcoplasmic reticulum	Occurs after administration of inhalational anesthetic or succinylcholine Muscle rigidity	Sudden Provoked by administration of anesthetic	Stop anesthetic Hyperventilation with 100% oxygen Active cooling Dantrolene
Heatstroke	Impaired physiologic mechanisms for heat dissipation (classical) Environment or exercise elevates body temperature beyond range of cooling mechanisms (exertional)	Environmental exposure History Muscle rigidity rare	Subacute, typically over hours	Hydration Active cooling Prevent shivering

[a]Other clinical entities to consider in the differential diagnosis of NMS include CNS infection, status epilepticus (including nonconvulsive status), alcohol or sedative hypnotic withdrawal, hypocalcemia, hypoglycemia, hyponatremia, intracranial hemorrhage, other poisoning (e.g., anticholinergics, nicotine, salicylates, strychnine, theophylline), sepsis, tetanus, thalamic infarct, thyroid storm, and psychotic agitation.
CNS, Central nervous system; *ECT*, electroconvulsive therapy; *IV*, intravenous; *MAOI*, monoamine oxidase inhibitor; *SSRI*, selective serotonin reuptake inhibitor.

the historical context and presentation support uncomplicated antipsychotic toxicity as the cause.

MANAGEMENT

General

Treatment of antipsychotic overdose is supportive. Endotracheal intubation and mechanical ventilation may be required in patients with severe CNS depression or respiratory distress. Dextrose should be given to patients with hypoglycemia. Neither gastric emptying nor activated charcoal is indicated for antipsychotic toxicity. See Chapter 135 for a discussion of the roles of activated charcoal and other methods of gastric decontamination.[32]

If sedation and miosis suggest possible opioid intoxication, a trial of intranasal or IV naloxone is warranted. We recommend administering naloxone 0.04 to 0.4 mg intravenous push (IVP) every 2 to 3 minutes in escalating doses and, if effective, titrating to return of normal oxygenation and ventilation. If a naloxone infusion is required, it may be started at two-thirds of the total dose required to restore respiration per hour and titrated to clinical effect.

Anticholinergic Toxidrome

Physostigmine has been used to treat anticholinergic (antimuscarinic) delirium from antipsychotic overdoses. Contraindications to physostigmine include reactive airway disease and cardiovascular disease (including any intraventricular conduction delay, QRS widening, bradycardia, or heart block). Physostigmine will usually cause a decrease in heart rate through enhanced vagal tone. We recommend avoiding its use in patients who present with seizures, because physostigmine may precipitate additional seizures. In adult patients who have obvious central anticholinergic delirium with agitation, we use physostigmine 1 to 2 mg IV, infused over 5 minutes in the absence of contraindications. In patients in whom agitated delirium is present but the toxidrome is unclear, we recommend lorazepam 1 to 2 mg IV every 10 to 15 minutes titrated to mild sedation. The delirium reversal effect of physostigmine is usually short lived (45 to 60 minutes), with delirium recurring in 30% to 90% of complete responders. The use of physostigmine for reversal of anticholinergic delirium does not preclude the use of benzodiazepines for agitation and vice versa.

Seizures

Antipsychotic-induced seizures may be short and self-limited and may not require pharmacologic treatment. For multiple seizures or status epilepticus, first line treatment is lorazepam 0.1 mg/kg (maximum 4 mg) given intravenously. This dose may be repeated in 5 minutes if seizures have not terminated. Refractory seizures unresponsive to lorazepam can be treated with phenobarbital (10 to 20 mg/kg IV loading dose) or propofol infusion may be administered (80 to 200 mcg/kg/min in healthy adults <55 years old). Use of phenobarbital or propofol in these dosages will likely require endotracheal intubation and initiation of continuous EEG monitoring, if available.

Acute Extrapyramidal Syndromes

Dystonia will often respond within 30 minutes to diphenhydramine (25 to 50 mg) or benztropine (1 to 2 mg) intravenously, intramuscularly, or orally. Lorazepam (1 to 2 mg IV) may also be effective in patients who do not respond within 1 hour to diphenhydramine or benztropine. IV lorazepam may be repeated in 15 to 20 minutes if dystonia is not improved. The first line treatment for akathisia is modification of the antipsychotic regimen. In the acute setting, clinicians may start by giving benztropine (1.5 to 8 mg total daily dose, divided) until symptoms improve. If sufficient improvement in symptoms is not achieved, propranolol (40 to 80 mg total daily dose, divided) or mirtazapine (15 mg/day) can be added.[33] Treatment of drug-induced parkinsonism includes minimizing the effective antipsychotic dose. Acute therapy begins with an anticholinergic agent, dosed as for dystonia and akathisia.

Cardiotoxicity

Cardiac monitoring is recommended in patients who are symptomatic or those with ECG abnormalities until the symptoms are resolving or ECG intervals have normalized. Sinus tachycardia with normal ECG intervals is expected in overdose and does not need to be treated unless secondary cardiac injury is present. Widening of the QRS due to sodium channel blockade is uncommon and is managed similarly to cyclic antidepressant toxicity. We recommend sodium bicarbonate 1 to 2 mEq/kg IVP, which may be repeated every 3 to 5 minutes until QRS narrowing occurs. Boluses may be repeated or an infusion of 150 mEq/L of sodium bicarbonate in 5% dextrose in water may be infused at 1.5 times the calculated maintenance rate and titrated to a goal blood pH of 7.45 to 7.55.

Hypotension is generally mild and typically responds to IV sodium chloride bolus and infusion. We prefer sodium chloride as the crystalloid in these cases because the sodium ion may be beneficial in the context of sodium channel blockade. If hypotension is severe, or persists after 2 L of isotonic crystalloid, a direct-acting vasopressor with alpha-adrenergic agonism should be initiated. We recommend a norepinephrine IV infusion, started at 0.1 mcg/kg/min and titrated to maintain mean arterial pressure greater than 65 mm Hg.

Correction of hypokalemia, hypomagnesemia, and hypocalcemia shortens the QT interval. Adults with a QTc greater than 500 msec or transient torsade de pointes should be given 1 to 2 g of magnesium sulfate IV. Treatment of sustained torsades de pointes includes IV magnesium sulfate up to 4 g total, defibrillation, overdrive pacing, or isoproterenol (see Chapter 65).[34] Any drugs that prolong the QT interval should be avoided.

ED treatment of clozapine-induced myocarditis is supportive. Clozapine treatment should be discontinued when the diagnosis is suspected.

Neuroleptic Malignant Syndrome

Treatment of NMS consists of supportive care and discontinuation of all dopamine-blocking medications. Agitation, psychomotor hyperactivity, and muscle rigidity should be treated with liberal doses of IV benzodiazepines. Lorazepam is administered at a dose of 1 to 2 mg IV every 5 to 10 minutes, until muscle rigidity improves. Refractory cases or patients at risk for aspiration can be managed with intubation and neuromuscular blockade with a nondepolarizing agent (e.g., rocuronium). Hyperthermia should be managed with IV fluids and evaporative cooling. To facilitate evaporative cooling, the patient's bare skin is continually misted with water while a cooling fan blows air continuously across the skin surface. The goal of cooling is a reduction in core temperature to less than 39°C within 30 minutes. If rhabdomyolysis is present, it is treated as described in Chapter 116 with IV fluids, urinary alkalinization, and mannitol depending on the clinical severity.

The dopamine agonists bromocriptine and amantadine (both available only in enteral formulations) have been successfully used in the treatment of NMS, although the quality of evidence is low. Dopamine agonists also carry a theoretical risk of worsening psychosis and are not recommended as a first line treatment. Dantrolene has also been used for the treatment of muscle rigidity. However, as rigidity in NMS is believed to originate in the CNS rather than in myocytes, dantrolene offers no mechanistic advantage over benzodiazepines and nondepolarizing neuromuscular blockade. We do not recommend dantrolene as part of routine treatment of NMS, although it may be administered for refractory, severe rigidity.

Electroconvulsive therapy (ECT) may be used in cases of NMS refractory to pharmacologic treatment. Evidence for efficacy is limited, although it is proposed as a treatment of choice in malignant catatonia, which may be indistinguishable from NMS. One of the primary advantages of ECT is that it may continue to be used when use of antipsychotic drugs is precluded by possible NMS.

Venous thromboembolism (VTE) disease is a prominent cause of morbidity and mortality in NMS. Patients with NMS should receive pharmacologic VTE prophylaxis.

DISPOSITION

Patients with NMS and overdose patients with hemodynamic instability, coma, torsades de pointes, or airway compromise should be admitted to an intensive care unit. Patients with a prolonged QT interval of any magnitude should have at least 12 hours of cardiac monitoring to ensure that the interval prolongation is resolving and QTc is less than 500 ms. Patients with minimal signs of toxicity should be observed for at least 6 hours from the time of ingestion, with hospitalization for persistent or worsening signs and symptoms. Criteria for hospital discharge include return of baseline mental status and normalization of vital signs with resolution of metabolic and electrocardiographic abnormalities. Psychiatric consultation may be necessary to assess the risk of harm to self or others. Patients with acute dystonia resolved by diphenhydramine or benztropine should continue the drug for 48 hours to prevent recurrence. Patients with drug-induced parkinsonism who must continue antipsychotic medications may need to use anticholinergic agents long term. Such patients should be discharged with benztropine 1 to 2 mg by mouth twice daily for at least 48 hours and should be referred to their treating physician, who may reduce the antipsychotic dose or change treatment regimens as necessary. Patients should be informed that benztropine, diphenhydramine, and other antipsychotic medications have anticholinergic effects, so combination therapy may increase symptoms of dry mouth, blurred vision, and urinary retention.

The references for this chapter can be found online at ExpertConsult.com.

151

Opioids

Jenna Karagianis Nikolaides and Trevonne M. Thompson

KEY CONCEPTS

- The opioid toxidrome includes three prominent findings—central nervous system depression, miosis, and, most importantly, respiratory depression—but presentations may be variable.
- A negative urine screen is often unreliable, and absence of detection should not deter a diagnosis of opioid intoxication when clinical findings support it.
- Airway protection, oxygenation, ventilation, and early administration of the reversal agent naloxone are the cornerstones for management of patients with opioid toxicity.
- The duration of action of many opioids, especially after overdose, is significantly longer than that of naloxone. Patients responsive to naloxone should be observed for recurrence of respiratory depression because they may require additional doses of naloxone.
- Naloxone distribution, prescription drug monitoring programs, and initiation of buprenorphine with a referral to addiction treatment programs are ways in which the medical profession is trying to combat the epidemic of opioid-related deaths.
- Opioid withdrawal syndrome does not include altered cognition. Patients with known or suspected opioid withdrawal who also have altered mental status should be evaluated for an alternative cause of altered cognition.

PRINCIPLES OF TOXICITY

Opiate is the term for natural agents derived from the poppy plant that have morphine-like pharmacological effects. Examples of opiates include morphine and codeine. Opioid is the more inclusive term, which refers to any synthetic, semisynthetic, or natural agent that has morphine-like properties. Some common semisynthetic opioids are heroin, hydrocodone, oxycodone, hydromorphone, oxymorphone, and buprenorphine. Some common synthetic opioids are fentanyl, methadone, and meperidine. Both "opiate" and "opioid" are terms derived from "opium," which was the Greek word for the juice of the poppy plant (Papaver somniferum).

Opioids are among the world's oldest known drugs. The therapeutic use of opioids has been a practice since ancient times, with the primary goals being sedation and analgesia. Opioids act on receptors in the central nervous, cardiovascular, pulmonary, and gastrointestinal systems and can also be used therapeutically for their antitussive and antidiarrheal effects.

Pain is a common reason why patients present to the emergency department (ED). Since the Joint Commission placed increased attention on pain management and hospitals increased their emphasis on patient satisfaction, there has been a proliferation in the number of opioid prescriptions written by physicians, including emergency providers. This trend did not lead to an actual improvement in overall patient satisfaction, but rather led to a flood of available opioids into the wider population.[1] According to the Centers for Disease Control and Prevention (CDC),

there was a 300% increase in the sale of opioid analgesics from 1999 to 2011. As the medical profession recognized the severity of the subsequent epidemic of deaths due to opioids, the CDC issued new opioid prescribing guidelines[2] in 2016 and prescription rates began to decline.[3]

Opioid-related fatalities continued, however, because of a concomitant rise in illicit heroin use, and a heroin supply that has been mixed with a family of synthetic opioids such as fentanyl. According to the CDC, the death rate from heroin overdose increased five-fold from 2010 to 2017.[4] There has also been a change in demographics of heroin use. Formerly involving primarily inner-city minority populations, in recent years, the use of heroin has spread geographically beyond urban areas[5] and has increased among men and women, in most age groups and at all income levels. Some of the greatest increases have occurred in women, the privately insured, and people with higher incomes.[6] It is now believed that prescription analgesics can be a gateway to heroin use. During 2000 to 2013, approximately three out of four new heroin users reported having misused prescription opioids prior to using heroin.[5]

The wider availability of opioids has affected each population group. This has been especially concerning for pediatric patients, because analgesic prescriptions written for adults can end up in the hands of children and adolescents. From 1999 to 2016, there was an approximate threefold rise in the mortality rate of pediatric opioid poisonings, resulting in the deaths of nearly 9000 children and adolescents.[7] Unintentional opioid overdose is also a growing concern among chronic pain patients, geriatric patients, and obese patients because risk is increased by polypharmacy, medical comorbidities, and sleep apnea.

Opioids come in three forms: synthetic, semisynthetic, and natural opiates. There are prescription versions of all three forms, which are available in many different preparations, including tablets, liquids, patches, and even lollipops. Prescription opioids are commonly packaged as combination preparations with acetaminophen, ibuprofen, and aspirin, and have historically existed in combination with atropine and camphor. Other prescription oral preparations are formulated with opioid-receptor antagonists, such as naloxone, which has little oral bioavailability to prevent illicit use and intentional alteration for intravenous (IV) misuse. There are also prescription drugs that are not chemically classified as opioids, but which have opioid receptor agonist properties, such as tramadol and tapentadol.

Illicit opioids also exist in all three forms. Table 151.1 details some of the known street names for opioids sold illicitly.[8,9] Street names are often unreliable, however, because they tend to be regional and are subject to dealers who attempt to market or rebrand their product to cater to their target population. Heroin (diacetylmorphine), a semisynthetic opioid, is the most widespread street preparation, but recent years have seen a rise in synthetics, such as fentanyl, fentanyl analogues, and other novel substances such as U-47700, often mixed with or mislabeled as heroin. Synthetic opioids have also proliferated in the form of counterfeit pills due to increased demand for prescription opioids on the illicit

TABLE 151.1 Street Names for Illicitly Obtained Opioids

Opioid	Street Names
Heroin	Dope, Smack, H, Horse, Junk, Skag, Skunk, Brown Sugar, White Horse, China White
Heroin + acetaminophen and diphenhydramine	Cheese
Codeine ± acetaminophen	Captain Cody, Cody, Lean, Schoolboy, T-threes, cough syrup
Codeine + promethazine + soft drinks and hard candy	Purple Drank, Sizzurp
Codeine + glutethimide	Doors & Fours, Loads, Pancakes and Syrup
Fentanyl	China White, China Girl, Apache, Dance Fever, Friend, Goodfella, Jackpot, Murder 8, Tango and Cash, TNT
Hydrocodone ± acetaminophen	Vike, Watson-387
Hydromorphone	D, Dillies, Footballs, Juice, Smack
Meperidine	Demmies, Pain Killer
Methadone	Dollies, Amidone, Fizzies
Methadone + MDMA	Chocolate Chip Cookies
Morphine	M, Morph, Miss Emma, Monkey, White Stuff
Oxycodone ± acetaminophen	O.C., Oxycet, Oxycotton, Oxy, Hillbilly Heroin, Percs
Oxymorphone	Biscuits, Blue Heaven, Blues, Mrs. O, O Bomb, Octagons, Stop Signs
Pentazocine	Yellow Footballs

MDMA, N-methyl-3,4-methylenedioxyamphetamine.

drug market.[10] Consequently, the U.S. Drug Enforcement Administration (DEA) added "Fentanyl-Related Substances" to the list of Schedule I drugs in 2018, making it illegal to manufacture, distribute, or possess fentanyl analogs.[11]

Illicit opioid preparations can be contaminated by the byproducts from the manufacturing process, adulterated with additives to change the preparation's pharmacological effects, and diluted with inert substances to increase bulk. The most commonly found additional substances are sugars and starches, talcum powder, caffeine, over-the-counter medications (such as diphenhydramine), prescription medications (including other opioids, quinine, benzodiazepines, and other psychoactive medications such as antipsychotics),[12,13] other illicit drugs (such as cocaine), heavy metals, and spore-forming infectious agents.[14,15] Toxicity can occur as a consequence of intentional overdose, recreational misuse, or as an adverse effect of therapeutic use. Although different opioids have receptor preferences in therapeutic doses, this specificity is lost at higher doses.

Opioids are well absorbed via gastrointestinal, IV, intramuscular (IM), mucocutaneous, and subcutaneous routes of administration. Depending on the lipid solubility of the specific opioid, they can also be absorbed through nasal, buccal, pulmonary, or a specifically formulated transdermal delivery system.[16] In general, toxicity is less pronounced but more prolonged when ingested than with parenteral administration. In therapeutic doses, an ingested opioid is absorbed in the small intestine within 1 to 2 hours. In toxic doses, delayed gastric emptying prolongs the absorption and clinical effects of the opioid.

Most opioids have a large volume of distribution. Different opioids and their metabolites cross into the blood-brain barrier due to variations in lipid solubility. All opioids undergo hepatic metabolism and renal elimination. Thus, changes in hepatic or renal function will alter drug clearance, which could prolong clinical and toxic effects of the specific opioid.

CLINICAL FEATURES

The hallmarks of the opioid toxidrome are central nervous system (CNS) depression, respiratory depression, and miosis. Miosis is caused by stimulation of μ receptors in the Edinger-Westphal nuclei of the third cranial nerve. This effect may be unreliable or masked by coingestants and, thus, respiratory depression is the essential feature of opioid intoxication. Respiratory depression is caused by opioids' effect on the medullary respiratory center via suppressing its sensitivity to hypercapnia and overriding the hypoxic drive. When combined with CNS depression, prolonged hypopnea can lead to hypoxia, causing further neurologic complications and death. Long-term opioid use is known to cause dependence and appears to contribute to central sleep apnea, as well as structural and functional changes in the brain.

Acute lung injury can be seen in opioid overdose, and pulmonary edema can cause further hypoxia. This manifests as desaturations on pulse oximetry, despite an adequate respiratory rate, with rales auscultated on lung examination. The cause of acute lung injury in opioid overdose is not clearly elucidated but may be related to a capillary leak phenomenon.

Other signs and symptoms commonly associated with opioids include relative bradycardia, mild hypotension, pruritus, skin flushing, nausea, vomiting, and bowel dysfunction. Hypotension, pruritus, and flushing are caused by nonallergic histamine release—an effect more pronounced with morphine. Nausea and vomiting are frequently seen, even in therapeutic doses of opioids, and are responsive to antiemetics and more potent opioids. Decreased gastrointestinal motility, delayed gastric emptying, constipation, and ileus are all commonly described with the spectrum of opioid-induced bowel dysfunction.

The skin should be examined in a patient exhibiting the opioid toxidrome because it may give diagnostic clues as to which opioids have been used. Look for the presence of fentanyl patches over the entire body, including in the oropharynx and other bodily orifices. If IV puncture sites or scars from "skin popping" (a process where opioids are injected subcutaneously) are detected, these findings could be signs of illicit opioid use.

Certain opioids have unique clinical findings due to their chemical structure or to their route of exposure (Table 151.2). Propoxyphene is associated with sodium channel blockade properties, causing QRS widening, in addition to PR and QT interval prolongation, which led to its withdrawal from the market. Methadone is known to block the human ether-a-go-go-related gene (hERG) as well as potassium channels, causing QTc prolongation. Propoxyphene, meperidine, and tramadol have been associated with hypertonicity, myoclonus, and seizures. Meperidine, methadone, tramadol, and fentanyl inhibit serotonin reuptake and are associated with serotonin syndrome. Sensorineural hearing loss has been reported with both acute and chronic use of heroin, methadone, and hydrocodone, thought to be due to direct ototoxicity. Heroin has also been found to be associated with Parkinsonian-like symptoms. A practice known as "chasing the dragon," where heroin is heated in aluminum foil and the vapor inhaled, has been found to be associated with spongiform leukoencephalopathy, with symptoms including psychomotor retardation, dysarthria, ataxia, and tremor.

Patients who hastily ingest loosely packaged bags of illicit drugs are known as "body stuffers." Patients who internally conceal dense and meticulously packaged packets of illicit drugs for the purpose of trafficking across international borders are known as "body packers." Heroin is a common drug seen in both stuffers and packers. Both populations are at risk for severe and prolonged opioid toxicity if the

TABLE 151.2   Special Clinical Properties of Certain Opioids

Effect	Opioid
QRS widening, sodium channel blockade	Propoxyphene
QT widening, potassium channel blockade	Methadone
Seizures	Propoxyphene, meperidine
Serotonin syndrome	Meperidine, methadone, tramadol, fentanyl
Hearing loss, ototoxicity	Methadone, hydrocodone, heroin
Spongiform leukoencephalopathy Parkinsonism	Heroin via "chasing the dragon" or inhalation of heroin vapor

packets leak or rupture. Heroin "stuffers" however, generally do not ingest enough to cause serious effects when compared to "packers," who may have several-fold lethal amounts of concentrated product in their gastrointestinal tract.

DIFFERENTIAL DIAGNOSES

The diagnosis of opioid intoxication is usually based on history, vital signs, and physical examination, with recognition of its characteristic toxidrome: hypopnea, stupor, and miosis. All of these findings are not consistently present, and the clinical picture may be complicated by cointoxicants. The essential finding in opioid intoxication is respiratory depression. Other intoxications may present similarly, such as clonidine, guanfacine, tetrahydrozoline, valproic acid, gamma-hydroxybutyrate, ethanol, sedative hypnotics, and atypical antipsychotics. Nontoxicologic considerations include pontine stroke or hemorrhage.

DIAGNOSTIC TESTING

No laboratory test or drug screen should be relied upon by the emergency clinician to make the diagnosis of opioid toxicity. The presence of the toxidrome and rapid response to naloxone are the two most important diagnostic clues. End-tidal carbon dioxide and oxygen saturation monitoring may be helpful for recognition of respiratory depression and hypoxia but are not as necessary as observation of the patient's respiratory rate.

A 12-lead electrocardiogram is a useful diagnostic for identifying QRS widening, as seen in propoxyphene use, or for QTc prolongation, as seen in methadone use. If the patient exhibits audible pulmonary rales on examination, then a chest radiograph is useful to evaluate for the presence of acute lung injury. If the opioid preparation is unknown, then acetaminophen and salicylate levels should be measured, because many prescription opioids are sold as combination preparations with these pain relievers. Hypoglycemia is the only consistent laboratory abnormality found in opioid toxicity. It is generally mild but can contribute to the decreased level of consciousness seen in opioid overdose. In addition, a serum ethanol level should be measured.

If needed for confirmation, a urine drug screen can be obtained once the patient has been stabilized. Nonetheless, a negative urine screen can be unreliable, and absence of detection should not deter a diagnosis of opioid intoxication when clinical findings support it. Opiates or opioids that metabolize to opiates, such as morphine, codeine, and heroin, are reliably detected on most qualitative antibody-based enzymatic immunoassay urine toxicology screens. Some semisynthetic and synthetic opioids, such as oxycodone, methadone, and fentanyl,

however, are often missed on typical urine drug screens unless they are specifically measured. A urine test result can remain positive for up to 72 hours after last use, depending on the half-life of the drug used. A large poppy seed ingestion can lead to a positive opiate screen, although federal workplace testing guidelines have raised the confirmatory morphine concentration threshold to 2000 ng/mL to avoid positive screens for commonplace poppy seed ingestions in food sources. Advanced screening methods detecting for 6-monoacetylmorphine, a specific metabolite of heroin, can be used to confirm heroin use, although this test is generally not available in the ED setting.

MANAGEMENT

Stabilization and Supportive Care

The ED clinician should direct efforts at stabilizing the patient's airway, oxygenation, and ventilation. This can be accomplished with a combination of basic supportive measures and titrated use of naloxone. Patients with acute lung injury may require oxygen and positive-pressure modalities, such as bi-level positive airway pressure (BiPAP), continuous positive airway pressure (CPAP), or mechanical ventilation with positive end-expiratory pressure (PEEP).

Decontamination

Because many opioids are extended-release preparations and can also delay gastric motility, activated charcoal has been used in the past but there are no data to support or refute the effectiveness of this practice. Additionally, naloxone is a highly effective antidote for opioid overdose, and sedation from opioid intoxication could conceivably lead to charcoal aspiration. Hence, activated charcoal administration should be considered on a patient-specific basis, but we generally discourage its use in patients with opioid intoxication. Gastric lavage similarly is not recommended because the risks outweigh the benefits. Whole bowel irrigation is not generally useful, but it can be considered for body packers (see Chapter 135).

Enhanced Elimination

As mentioned previously, most opioids have a large volume of distribution. There are no clinically effective techniques for enhanced or extracorporeal elimination of opioids.

Antidote Therapy

Naloxone is a competitive opioid antagonist that rapidly reverses the effects of opioid intoxication. Because of the rapid clinical response, it can also aid in the diagnosis of opioid overdose. Naloxone is ineffective orally because its bioavailability is minimal due to first-pass hepatic metabolism. It is effective via IV, subcutaneous, intramuscular (IM), intranasal (IN), inhalational, and endotracheal routes. It is indicated when an opioid-intoxicated patient has significant CNS or respiratory depression.

In the ED, naloxone is usually administered intravenously with empirical dosing. The dose widely ranges from 0.04 to 15 mg, depending on the amount and formulation of the opioid taken, the patient's weight, and whether the patient is opioid dependent. In general, it is best to start with low doses and to increase each subsequent dose as needed to alleviate respiratory depression. The exception to this rule is the arrest or near-arrest situation where opioids are the suspected cause. In this scenario, recommended starting doses are 0.4 to 4.0 mg IV. In chronic opioid users, the minimal effective naloxone dose should be used so as not to precipitate acute withdrawal. In this population, when respiratory status is adequate, we recommend starting with doses of 0.04 mg of naloxone, followed by titration of subsequent doses. Acute opioid withdrawal can be unpleasant for the habituated patient, but it is not considered life-threatening. Furthermore, naloxone has an excellent safety profile. The clinician should not be reluctant to dose naloxone as needed, even if opioid withdrawal symptoms develop, in order to ensure adequate patient oxygenation and ventilation.

Naloxone's onset of action, when administered intravenously, is less than 2 minutes, and the duration of action is anywhere between 20 minutes and 2 hours, which is shorter than the duration of action of most opioids. Reversal of respiratory depression usually occurs at low doses, but dosing may be repeated until the desired effect is achieved. If respiratory depression is not reversed after the administration of high doses of naloxone (10 to 15 mg), then it is unlikely that opioid intoxication is the cause of the symptoms. If naloxone does reverse the symptoms but the patient later develops recurrent respiratory depression, then repeated naloxone doses, a continuous naloxone infusion, or endotracheal intubation should be considered. When starting a naloxone infusion, one-half to two-thirds of the bolus dose that effectively reversed intoxication is given hourly, although individual patient responses may vary depending on dose, tolerance, and dependency. This is usually enough to maintain an adequate respiratory effort without producing withdrawal.

In situations where IV access is not easily obtained, naloxone can also be given via IM, IN, IO, or nebulized routes. IN naloxone has proved a viable alternative to IV administration, especially for prehospital providers and nonmedical bystanders. It is available as 0.4 mg/mL and 1 mg/mL solutions, in vials or prefilled syringes, delivered into each nostril using an atomizer device, or as a 4 mg/0.1 mL prepackaged nasal spray.[17] Nebulized naloxone—2 mg of naloxone is mixed with 3 mL of saline—has also been shown to be a safe, effective, and gradual way to reverse opioid intoxication in both the ED and prehospital settings. Care must be taken in selecting the optimal patient for nebulized naloxone. A patient with profound respiratory depression, such as a respiratory rate of less than six breaths per minute or cyanosis, will not receive enough naloxone via a nebulizer to obtain the desired clinical effect.

Nalmefene and naltrexone are opioid antagonists with longer half-lives and duration than naloxone. Nalmefene's duration of action is 4 to 10 hours. Naltrexone is available in an oral preparation, with a duration of action between 24 to 72 hours, and as an extended-release injectable solution, with a duration of action of up to 30 days. We do not recommend their use in the ED because of concern for inducing a prolonged withdrawal state. Naloxone bolus and titration remains the treatment of choice for opioid reversal in the acutely intoxicated patient.

DISPOSITION

Patients who present with heroin toxicity can be successfully treated in the ED. Opioid intoxicated patients who use longer-acting opioids may require an admission to an observation unit. Body stuffers who remain asymptomatic after 6 hours of observation may be discharged. Asymptomatic body packers, however, require admission until all packets have been successfully passed or retrieved. If an overdose is severe, involves multiple drugs, or requires multiple doses of naloxone, naloxone infusion, or endotracheal intubation, then intensive care unit (ICU) admission is appropriate.

The observation period following the administration of naloxone is dependent on the opioid implicated in the poisoning. Overdoses of long-acting opioids or sustained-released opioid preparations will require longer observation periods. In cases of heroin-only overdose, an observation period of up to 4 hours is generally sufficient. After an appropriate observation period, if there are no signs of recurrent toxicity and no concerns for longer-acting coingestants, the patient may be discharged. When indicated, the patient may require a psychiatric evaluation or be referred for substance misuse counseling and an appropriate treatment program.

In recent years, as the opioid overdose epidemic has grown, there have been increased efforts to expand access to naloxone as a public health measure intended to save lives. Most states have passed laws to widen the availability of naloxone to family, friends, and other potential bystanders of an overdose.[18] Community and hospital-based initiatives have worked to educate opioid users and bystanders on signs of overdose, train them for out-of-hospital naloxone use, and then distribute or prescribe naloxone directly to patients or bystanders.[19,20] Both IN and IM auto-injector delivery methods have been used.[21] The number of naloxone prescriptions dispensed from retail pharmacies increased substantially from 2012 to 2018.[22] These programs are showing that providing overdose education and naloxone distribution has decreased opioid overdose mortality.[19,23] Prescribing take-home naloxone is one intervention that the emergency provider can provide to reduce the harm caused by opioids.

Another evolving public health effort is the use of prescription drug monitoring programs (PDMPs), which are currently available in 49 U.S. states, the District of Columbia, and Guam.[24] To decrease the opioid burden in the community, the emergency provider can use these programs to access a patient's prescription opioid history prior to prescribing a new opioid upon discharge. However, while there is some evidence to suggest that states with more robust PDMPs have less overdose deaths,[25] inconsistent implementation has resulted in mixed results regarding the impact PDMPs have on prescribing[26] and on overdose deaths.[27] There have been several proposed solutions, such as improving the technology and its integration into electronic medical records, which may make PDMPs a more useful public health tool in the ED setting.[28]

WITHDRAWAL

Withdrawal occurs in tolerant patients when opioids are abruptly withheld or an antagonist is administered. In withdrawal, the patient goes into a hyperadrenergic state. The symptoms include yawning, piloerection, CNS excitation, tachypnea, mydriasis, tachycardia, hypertension, nausea, vomiting, diarrhea, abdominal cramps, and myalgias. CNS excitation takes the form of restlessness, agitation, dysphoria, and insomnia. Cognition and mental status are usually unaffected. In general, opioid withdrawal is uncomfortable but not life-threatening. As with opioid toxicity, no diagnostic test exists for acute opioid withdrawal. It is diagnosed based on the patient's symptoms, signs, and a history of prior opioid use.

Treatment for the withdrawing patient in the ED has historically been supportive and symptom-based: IV fluids, electrolyte replacement, and antiemetics. Clonidine, an alpha$_2$-agonist, can be used to suppress sympathetic hyperactivity and shorten the duration of withdrawal. However, there are now increased efforts by EDs to use buprenorphine, a long-acting partial opioid agonist approved by the U.S. Food and Drug Administration (FDA) for opioid use disorder, to not only control withdrawal, but to also initiate as a maintenance therapy in the ED as a bridge to long-term addiction treatment.[29] For an emergency provider to be able to prescribe buprenorphine at discharge, additional training to get an X-waiver applied to his or her DEA license is required. Methadone, a full opioid agonist, can also palliate withdrawal and has federal prescribing restrictions, as well. Even without a waiver, emergency providers are permitted to initiate the administration of either buprenorphine or methadone for 72 hours to patients under their care for the purposes of transitioning patients to outpatient treatment through an opioid treatment program or addiction medicine specialist.[30] Opioid withdrawal alone typically does not require inpatient treatment, but some patients with severe symptoms and other comorbidities may require admission. It has been documented that patients who ultimately die from an opioid overdose sharply increase their ED utilization prior to their death.[31] Therefore, treating withdrawal in the ED setting gives emergency providers a sentinel opportunity to engage patients in treatment and long-term recovery.[32]

The references for this chapter can be found online at ExpertConsult.com.

152

Pesticides

Katherine Louise Welker and Trevonne M. Thompson

Pesticide is a general term that refers to all pest-killing agents. It includes insecticides, herbicides, rodenticides, and fungicides. In this chapter, several classes of pesticides will be discussed, as well as their importance in the emergency department (ED) setting (Table 152.1).

ORGANOPHOSPHATE INSECTICIDES

Foundations

Organophosphates are a class of insecticide that work by inhibiting cholinesterases, including acetylcholinesterase and pseudocholinesterase. This is both the mechanism of their efficacy as insecticides, as well as their toxicity in humans. Inhibition of cholinesterases results in accumulation of acetylcholine at multiple receptors within the autonomic nervous system, such as the sympathetic and parasympathetic ganglionic nicotinic sites, postganglionic cholinergic sympathetic and parasympathetic muscarinic sites, skeletal muscle nicotinic sites, and central nervous system sites (Fig. 152.1).[1]

Organophosphates are lipid soluble and are absorbed through dermal, gastrointestinal, and respiratory routes. This can lead to deposition in fat tissues, allowing for possible toxicity from acute and chronic, low-level exposures. Some organophosphates have active metabolites that can result in delayed toxicity.

For a discussion of chemical warfare nerve agents (e.g., sarin gas and novel "*Novichok*" agents), see Chapter 55.

Clinical Features

Organophosphate toxicity is represented by the "SLUDGE" or "DUMBELS" syndrome (these are acronyms, which are explained in Box 152.1) manifested by accumulation of acetylcholine at receptor sites. The clinical features in any given case are attributable to the location of the receptors affected, the properties of the specific organophosphate product (predominance of nicotinic versus muscarinic effects), and the dose of the exposure. Muscarinic acetylcholine accumulation leads to salivation, lacrimation, urinary incontinence, defecation, emesis, bronchospasm, bronchorrhea, and bradycardia. Nicotinic acetylcholine accumulation leads to tachycardia, tachydysrhythmias, and skeletal muscle fasciculations.

At the neuromuscular junction, excess acetylcholine causes hyperstimulation of the muscles with secondary paralysis, and when the diaphragm is affected, cholinesterase poisoning leads to respiratory arrest. Sympathetic stimulation can lead to diaphoresis. A combination of sympathetic stimulation, involvement of the *N*-methyl-D-aspartate (NMDA) receptor, and enhanced acetylcholine concentrations can induce seizures.[2,3]

Pulmonary edema can occur in organophosphate poisoning and should not be confused with bronchorrhea or bronchospasm. Pulmonary edema results from many factors, including the release of inflammatory mediators and increased vascular permeability. Bronchospasm and bronchorrhea are mediated by both central and local mechanisms involving acetylcholine. Pulmonary edema, bronchospasm, bronchorrhea, and the aforementioned respiratory muscle paralysis all contribute to respiratory failure.

Although the classic clinical picture of acute organophosphate poisoning is more apparent, toxicity from gradual, cumulative exposure may be subtle. These patients commonly exhibit vague confusion or other central nervous system complaints; mild visual disturbances; or chronic abdominal cramping, nausea, and diarrhea.

A unique feature of organophosphate insecticides is the process called *aging*, the irreversible conformational change that occurs when the organophosphate is bound to the cholinesterase enzyme for a prolonged time. This causes the clinical effects to persist for periods of days to weeks. The time to aging varies by the specific product involved. Once an enzyme has aged, an oxime antidote (as discussed under Antidote Therapy) cannot regenerate the cholinesterase.

Differential Diagnoses

Differential diagnoses for acetylcholinesterase inhibitor poisoning are limited. Carbamate pesticides, carbamate medications (e.g., rivastigmine), nicotine and other nicotine alkaloids, and cholinomimetics (e.g., pilocarpine) are xenobiotics that can cause a similar constellation of symptoms. There are few medical conditions included in the differential diagnosis: viral and bacterial gastroenteritis, as well as conditions causing exaggerated vagal response (e.g., inferior wall myocardial infarction with pulmonary edema) and conditions that cause exaggerated sympathetic responses (e.g., thyroid storm or pheochromocytoma).

Diagnostic Testing

Patients who present with the classic cholinergic toxidrome should be treated empirically without waiting for laboratory confirmation of decreased cholinesterase activity. Known or suspected exposures to organophosphates can be evaluated by assessing plasma and erythrocyte (red blood cell [RBC]) cholinesterase concentrations. These concentrations are not generally available in real-time clinical settings and are usually sent out to regional reference laboratories for analysis.

In acute toxicity, plasma cholinesterase levels decrease first. In chronic, low-level exposure, however, plasma enzyme levels may be normal, but RBC cholinesterase may still be decreased. This is because plasma cholinesterases can recover in 4 to 6 weeks, whereas RBC cholinesterases can take as long as 12 weeks to recover. Other laboratory studies should focus on the evaluation of pulmonary, cardiovascular, and renal function, as well as fluid and electrolyte balance. A measurement of acid-base status should be performed, because patients with metabolic acidosis have higher mortality rates.[1] Both initial hyperglycemia and hypoglycemia in organophosphate-poisoned patients have been shown to be associated with increased mortality and severity of toxicity.[3] Other prognostic tools such as the Glasgow Coma Scale or the Poison Severity Score vary by type of organophosphate and are generally of little clinical utility.[2]

Management

Treatment of organophosphate poisoning is directed toward four goals: (1) decontamination, (2) supportive care with an emphasis on respiratory stabilization, (3) reversal of acetylcholine excess, and (4) reversal

TABLE 152.1 Pesticide Classes and Examples	
Pesticide Class	**Example(s)**
Organophosphates	Parathion, malathion
Carbamates	Aldicarb, carbaryl
Chlorinated hydrocarbons	Dichlorodiphenyltrichloroethane (DDT), gamma-hexachlorocyclohexane (lindane)
Substituted phenols	2,4-dinitrophenol (DNP)
Chlorophenoxy pesticides	2,4,5-trichlorophenoxyacetic acid (2,4,5-T), 2,4-dichlorophenoxyacetic acid (2,4-D)
Bipyridyl pesticides	N, N′-dimethyl-4,4′-bipyridinum dichloride (paraquat), 1,1′-ethylene-2,2′-bipyridyldiylium dibromide (diquat)
Pyrethrins/pyrethroids	Permethrin
Glyphosate	N-(phosphonomethyl)glycine
Insect repellent	N, N-Diethyl-meta-toluamide (DEET)

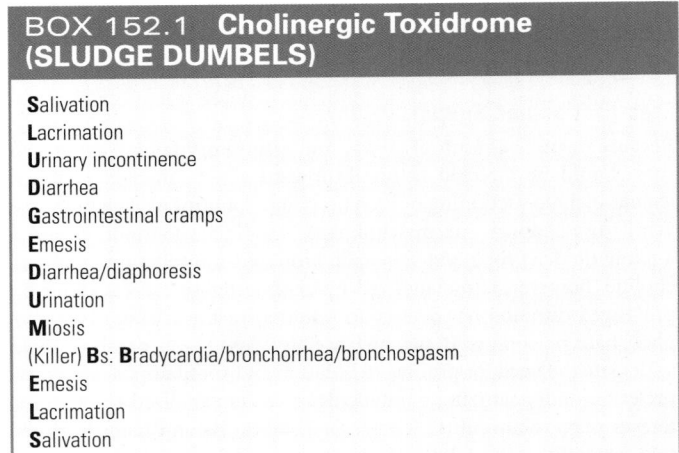

BOX 152.1 Cholinergic Toxidrome (SLUDGE DUMBELS)

Salivation
Lacrimation
Urinary incontinence
Diarrhea
Gastrointestinal cramps
Emesis
Diarrhea/diaphoresis
Urination
Miosis
(Killer) **B**s: **B**radycardia/bronchorrhea/bronchospasm
Emesis
Lacrimation
Salivation

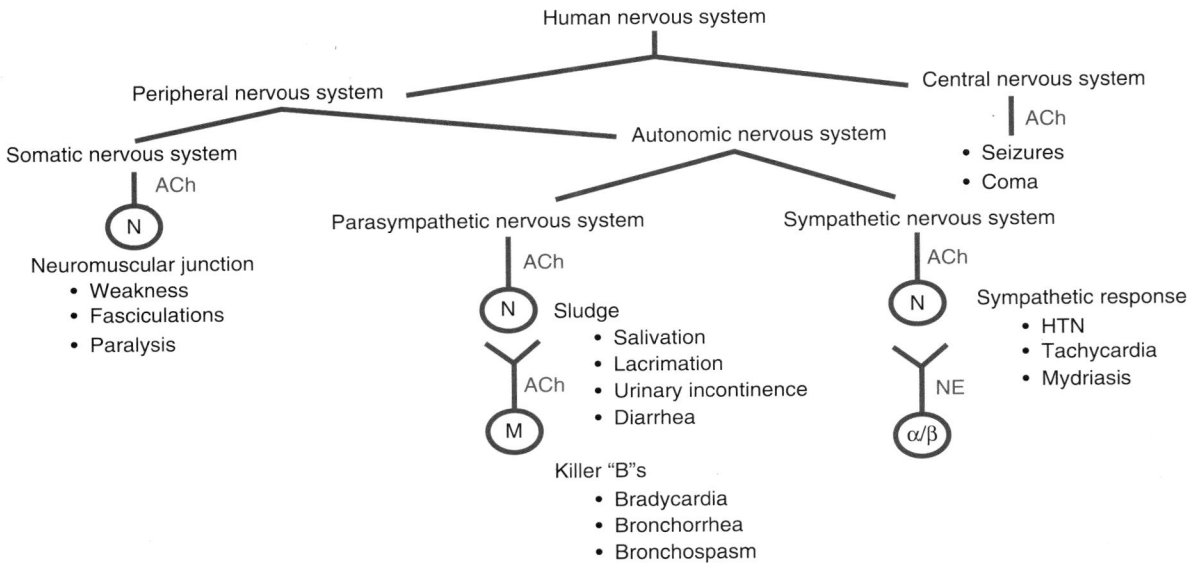

Fig. 152.1 Cholinergic Effects on Nervous System. *ACh*, Acetylcholine; *HTN*, hypertension; *M*, Muscarinic; *N*, nicotinic; *NE*, norepinephrine.

of toxin binding at receptor sites on the cholinesterase molecule. The severity of the patient's signs and symptoms, as well as antidote availability, will guide management.

Decontamination

Decontamination begins in the out-of-hospital setting to prevent further absorption and to protect care providers. Because dermal absorption is likely, removal and destruction of clothing and thorough flushing of exposed skin limits absorption and toxicity. Alternatively, dermal decontamination can be done with dry agents, such as military resins, flour, sand, or bentonite. Due to availability and ease of flushing with water, we recommend this as the primary method of decontamination. Caregivers are at risk for contamination from splashes or handling of contaminated clothing. Personnel may be rotated to limit their exposure to either multiple contaminated patients or patients extensively contaminated (or contaminated with a high concentration product). Caregivers should use universal precautions (level C PPE), which includes a full-face air purifier cartridge mask, eye shield, and protective clothing including a chemical-resistant suit, boots, and nitrile or butyl rubber gloves. In the case of ingestion, neither gastrointestinal decontamination procedures (such as gastric lavage) nor activated charcoal are of benefit. Cholinergic agents are rapidly absorbed and profuse vomiting and diarrhea are seen early in ingestion, negating any beneficial effect of additional gastrointestinal decontamination. Equipment, but not skin, may be washed with a 5% hypochlorite solution.

Stabilization and Supportive Care

Because death is a result of airway and respiratory failure, supportive care should be directed primarily toward airway management and should include suctioning of secretions and vomitus, oxygenation, and ventilatory support. Succinylcholine, 1.5 mg/kg, is commonly used as a paralytic drug for rapid-sequence orotracheal intubation. Succinylcholine, however, is metabolized by cholinesterases and may have a prolonged duration of effect (4 to 6 hours) in the setting of organophosphate poisoning. If succinylcholine is used as a paralytic drug, anticipate the need for prolonged sedation and ventilatory support. We prefer a nondepolarizing paralytic drug not metabolized by cholinesterases (e.g., rocuronium, 1 mg/kg). Tachycardia and tachydysrhythmia generally resolve by treating the underlying cholinergic excess and should not be treated symptomatically (e.g., with beta blockers). Patients with agitation, seizures, and coma should be treated with adequate doses of a benzodiazepine after the airway has been secured and ventilatory support established.

Enhanced Elimination

There is no role for enhanced elimination or extracorporeal techniques of removal, such as hemodialysis, in organophosphate poisoning.

Antidote Therapy

Definitive treatment for organophosphate poisoning is focused on decreasing the amount and effect of acetylcholine at its various receptor sites. This begins with atropine, which is a competitive inhibitor of acetylcholine at muscarinic receptors. The atropine dose for the treatment of organophosphate poisoning is 1 to 3 mg (0.05 mg/kg in children) intravenously with doubling of each subsequent dose every 5 minutes until there is control of the muscarinic effects, particularly reduction in airway secretions. Atropine may initially be administered intramuscularly until intravenous or intraosseous access is obtained. Depending on the specific organophosphate product involved and the degree of poisoning, patients may require as much as 200 to 500 mg of atropine during the first hour. Once the patient has been stabilized with appropriate "atropinization," an infusion is initiated to provide

10% to 20% of the total cumulative dose needed to obtain symptom control per hour. Tachycardia and mydriasis may occur at these atropine doses but are not an indication to discontinue therapy. However, excessive administration of atropine may cause the typical symptoms of the anticholinergic toxidrome. The endpoint of atropinization is drying of respiratory secretions, easing of respiratory effort, and normalization of respiratory rate. Early and rapid atropinization is associated with better control of seizures and reduced mortality in animal models. The recommended atropine dosing regimen can easily exhaust available hospital supplies, and arrangements for alternative sources should be discussed with the appropriate hospital personnel early in the case of an organophosphate poisoning. Other anticholinergic medications, such as diphenhydramine and anticholinergic ophthalmic drugs, have been studied in rodents and may be considered a "last resort" alternative in humans if intravenous atropine is scarce or exhausted. Atropine is not active at nicotinic receptor sites and will not reverse skeletal muscle effects, such as respiratory muscle paralysis.

The second part of the treatment of organophosphate poisoning is the use of an oxime to regenerate acetylcholinesterase function. Oximes bind to the organophosphate-cholinesterase complex, causing a conformational change that allows for the cholinesterase to resume normal function. There are currently five oximes in common use worldwide: pralidoxime (2-PAM), trimedoxime (TMB-4), obidoxime chloride (Toxogonin), methoxime, and asoxime chloride (HI-6). Pralidoxime is the product commonly available in the United States. There are controversies regarding the use of oximes related to dosing, duration of treatment, time to therapy initiation, and effectiveness in treating neurologic symptoms. Despite these controversies, we recommend oximes for the treatment of moderate or severely poisoned patients, defined as those who require multiple, large doses of atropine. Indications for oxime treatment include respiratory depression or failure, muscle fasciculations, seizures, dysrhythmias, hemodynamic instability, or the use of large amounts or repeated doses of atropine to completely control signs and symptoms of organophosphate intoxication. We recommend administering pralidoxime as a 1 to 2 g bolus (25 to 50 mg/kg in pediatric patients) over 30 minutes, which can be repeated as needed (up to hourly) based on response (improved mental status and respiratory and heart rate, as well as decreased secretion). Even higher doses may be required. Alternative dosing options are 2 g bolus over 20 minutes followed by an infusion of 500 mg/h for up to 7 days; 1 g/h every 4 hours; or 30 mg/kg followed by infusion of 8 mg/kg/h (Table 152.2). Oximes can be given intravenously or intramuscularly (as with standard military autoinjectors).

Novel treatments for organophosphate and nerve agent poisoning are under investigation. At present, pyridostigmine is the most commonly used prophylactic drug. Other prophylactics include tablets containing pyridostigmine, trihexyphenidyl and benactyzine, as well as a transdermal patch containing H-series oximes (HI-6).

Disposition

Most patients who present to the ED after significant organophosphate exposure should be admitted to a monitored setting. The effects of organophosphate intoxication can be prolonged. If plasma cholinesterase levels are available, they may be useful for treatment and disposition decisions. Asymptomatic or minimally symptomatic patients with normal or minimally depressed cholinesterase levels may be discharged after 6 hours with close outpatient follow-up to ensure that progressive toxicity does not occur. Patients who present with significant symptoms (e.g., seizures, acute respiratory compromise associated with depressed cholinesterase levels) require admission and continuous monitoring, usually to an intensive care unit (ICU). Patients may have rebound toxicity several days after apparently

TABLE 152.2 Specific Treatment Dosing

Agent	Indication	Adult Dose	Pediatric Dose	Route	Comments
Atropine	Organophosphate toxicity	1–3 mg	0.05 mg/kg	IV, IM	Double dose every 5 min until effect
Pralidoxime	Organophosphate toxicity	1–2 g bolus	25–50 mg/kg	IV, IM	Given over 30 min Dose can be repeated based on response

IM, Intramuscular; *IV,* intravenous.

satisfactory response to initial treatment. This may occur for many reasons, including persistent release of organophosphates from lipid stores. Poisoning with fenthion is of particular concern because initial symptoms could be mild and progress to life-threatening intoxication over time.

The intermediate syndrome (IMS) can occur after the acute intoxication from organophosphates has resolved. IMS manifests with delayed muscle paralysis, including in respiratory muscles, which can occur 24 to 96 hours after the resolution of the cholinergic crisis. The precise cause of IMS is not well documented. Delayed peripheral neuropathy may occur 7 to 21 days after acute organophosphate intoxication.[4] Therefore, close patient follow-up, including a neurological evaluation, is important after stabilization. Finally, those patients with acts of self-harm or suicidal intent require psychiatric consultation once medically stabilized.

Carbamate Insecticides

Carbamates are acetylcholinesterase inhibitors whose toxicological picture is similar to organophosphates. There are two important differences: (1) short duration of effect (minutes to 48 hours) and (2) the process of aging does not occur. Decontamination, supportive care, airway management, and atropinization are usually adequate for treating patients poisoned with these compounds. Severe toxicity, including respiratory depression and seizures, can occur. Because carbamates do not cross the blood-brain barrier as readily as organophosphates, neurotoxicity is less likely. Dosing of atropine is the same as for organophosphates, but the duration of treatment is usually less. There is controversy regarding the use of oximes in carbamate poisoning. We recommend the use of oximes only when the poisoning is severe (as defined for organophosphates) or if the provider cannot differentiate carbamate from organophosphate poisoning.

Chlorinated Hydrocarbons Insecticides

Foundations

Dichlorodiphenyltrichloroethane (DDT) is the best-known example of chlorinated hydrocarbon insecticides. This class is also known as *organochlorine insecticides.* DDT was developed in the late 1800s and first used widely in World War II to reduce mosquito populations in an attempt to prevent transmission of typhus and malaria. It was found to be effective and stable and led to the development of other similar insecticides that were used in agricultural, industrial, and residential settings. Their widespread and indiscriminate use, long half-life, and persistence in the environment resulted in adverse ecologic effects that lead to a ban on most chlorinated hydrocarbons. In the United States, gamma-hexachlorocyclohexane (also known as *lindane*) is a chlorinated hydrocarbon insecticide available as a pharmaceutical drug for the second-line treatment of head lice and scabies. Many U.S. states have banned lindane and restricted its use to physician prescription only.

Principles of Toxicity

Chlorinated hydrocarbon insecticides are highly lipid soluble. They are readily absorbed via dermal, respiratory, and gastrointestinal routes and are stored in fatty tissues. This storage allows for toxicity from repeated, low-level exposure. Lindane toxicity often occurs from excessive dermal exposure or accidental oral exposure.

Chlorinated hydrocarbon insecticides affect neuronal voltage-gated sodium channels. They are also gamma-aminobutyric acid (GABA) antagonists. This results in hyperexcitability and irritability of both central and peripheral neurons. Chlorinated hydrocarbons increase susceptibility to ventricular tachydysrhythmias, as well, because of increased myocardial sensitivity to circulating catecholamines.

Clinical Features

The primary clinical feature of chlorinated hydrocarbon insecticide toxicity is neurologic excitation. This includes muscle fasciculations, ataxia, tremors, delirium, weakness, paresthesias, and, in severe toxicity, paralysis, seizures, and death. Mild premonitory symptoms are not always present prior to serious neurological manifestations; patients can present initially with seizure activity. Hyperthermia can result from muscle fasciculations and seizures. Metabolic acidosis, respiratory failure, and acute renal failure can also occur. Chronic exposure can cause liver toxicity, arrhythmias, menstrual changes, and neuropsychological effects. The most important clue to diagnosing exposure to chlorinated hydrocarbons is a detailed history because there is no specific clinical toxidrome.

Differential Diagnoses

The defining features of chlorinated hydrocarbon insecticide toxicity are neuro-excitation and seizure. Differential diagnoses are broad, including any disorder or toxic exposure that can lead to seizures (e.g., organophosphates, isoniazid, theophylline, sympathomimetic agents, lead, ethanol, and benzodiazepine or alcohol withdrawal).

Diagnostic Testing

The diagnosis of chlorinated hydrocarbon insecticide poisoning is determined by history and clinical features. Some reference laboratories can measure chlorinated hydrocarbons from fat or plasma samples, but this will not be readily available during emergency treatment. An electrolyte panel, creatinine kinase, and blood gas should be measured on patients with known or suspected acute poisoning.

Management

Decontamination

The first step in chlorinated hydrocarbon insecticide toxicity is decontamination. Remove all clothing and wash the skin and hair with soap and water. Ingested chlorinated hydrocarbons are rapidly absorbed by the gastrointestinal tract; therefore, decontamination with activated charcoal has no clinical effectiveness.

Stabilization and Supportive Care

The main objective in treating chlorinated hydrocarbon toxicity is cessation of seizures. Benzodiazepines and barbiturates are the mainstays of therapy to treat seizures. Chlorinated hydrocarbons can cause myocardial sensitization that can lead to ventricular tachydysrhythmias, which are most commonly seen around the time of seizure activity due to a catecholamine surge. Beta-adrenergic antagonists (e.g., intravenous metoprolol, 5 mg boluses every 5 minutes) are recommended for treating any life-threatening tachydysrhythmias (e.g., ventricular tachycardia and fibrillation). Prolonged seizures can lead to hyperthermia. Seizure control with benzodiazepines and external cooling with evaporative cooling methods should be implemented if severe hyperthermia is present. Other complications such as metabolic acidosis, rhabdomyolysis, and acute kidney injury are treated with intravenous crystalloid hydration and, in the case of rhabdomyolysis, alkalinization, as described in Chapter 116.

Enhanced Elimination

There is no role for enhanced elimination of chlorinated hydrocarbon insecticides in the ED.

Antidote Therapy

There is no known antidotal therapy for chlorinated hydrocarbon insecticides.

Disposition

Patients who present symptomatic with chlorinated hydrocarbon insecticide poisoning require admission for evaluation, monitoring, and treatment of neurologic and metabolic derangements.

SUBSTITUTED PHENOLS

Foundations

Dinitrophenol (DNP), pentachlorophenol, and dinitrocresol belong to a class of compounds called *substituted phenols* and have been used as dyes, wood preservatives, photograph developers, and insecticides. DNP was previously used as a weight loss medication but has not been available by prescription since the 1930s because of fatalities associated with its use. DNP is currently used as a weight loss supplement and is readily available over the internet. It can be easily obtained from online nutritional supplement retailers and is available in powder, capsule, and crystalline form. The most common route of exposure is oral, but substituted phenols can also be absorbed dermally or inhaled.

Principles of Toxicity

Substituted phenols uncouple oxidative phosphorylation. This results in decreased adenosine triphosphate (ATP) formation and increased heat generation, which is the mechanism of action for DNP in weight loss because calories are burned excessively. DNP also stimulates glycolysis, which, along with the uncoupling of oxidative phosphorylation, increases lactic acid production.

Clinical Features

Patients with acute toxicity from substituted phenols present with hyperthermia, tachycardia, diaphoresis, and tachypnea. Neurologic signs and symptoms include confusion, agitation, seizures, and coma. Rhabdomyolysis, myocardial injury, acute kidney injury, and hepatic damage can occur in acute toxicity. These patients can progress to cardiovascular collapse and death. Dermal exposure can cause a yellow discoloration of the skin and corrosive injury.

Differential Diagnoses

Patients suffering from the toxic effects of substituted phenols will appear to have sympathomimetic excess. This leads to a broad differential diagnosis that includes toxicologic, infectious, and environmental considerations, such as cocaine and amphetamine toxicity,

TABLE 152.3 Differential Diagnoses for Substituted Phenol Poisoning

Toxicological	Infectious	Environmental
Cocaine	Meningitis	Hyperthermia
Salicylates	Encephalitis	Heat stroke
Amphetamines/MDMA	Sepsis	
Caffeine		
Other sympathomimetics		

MDMA, N-methyl-3,4-methylenedioxyamphetamine.

encephalitis, and heat stroke (Table 152.3). Since substituted phenols act by uncoupling oxidative phosphorylation, salicylate toxicity should also be considered in the differential diagnosis. An accurate history is important to the diagnosis of substituted phenol intoxication.

Diagnostic Testing

Diagnostic testing focuses on the metabolic disturbances and potential organ damage associated with acute substituted phenol toxicity. Serum electrolytes and renal function are to be assessed. Liver studies should be performed, and creatinine kinase is measured to assess for rhabdomyolysis. An electrocardiogram (ECG) and laboratory assessment for myocardial injury with serial cardiac markers (troponin) is advised for any patient with symptoms consistent with myocardial ischemia.

Management

Decontamination

Patients who present with dermal exposure should have their clothing removed and skin washed with soap and water. Because of the potential lethality of phenol-containing compounds with no effective antidote, a patient presenting within 1 hour of an acute oral ingestion who is alert and cooperative should be given oral activated charcoal (at least 100 g in adults).

Stabilization and Supportive Care

Supportive care is the mainstay of treatment for substituted phenol toxicity. Patients with hyperthermia (temperature >102.5°F) should be cooled with evaporative cooling, a cooling blanket, cold intravenous fluids, and strategically placed ice packs. Patients should be given adequate crystalloid fluid resuscitation and electrolyte derangements should be corrected. This is especially important in hyperthermic patients. Agitation and seizures should be treated with benzodiazepines, such as lorazepam (1 to 2 mg intravenous push [IVP]) or diazepam (5 to 10 mg IVP).

Enhanced Elimination

There is no known role for enhanced elimination in substituted phenol toxicity.

Antidote Therapy

There is no known antidote for acute phenol poisoning.

Disposition

Patients who manifest symptoms after substituted phenol exposure should be admitted for intensive cardiac and neurologic monitoring and treatment. A patient who presents asymptomatically after an exposure should be observed for 8 to 12 hours and may be safely discharged if they remain asymptomatic over that period of time.

CHLOROPHENOXY HERBICIDES

Foundations and Principles of Toxicity

Chlorophenoxy compounds are effective herbicides for broad-leaved weeds. This class of herbicides includes 2-methyl-4-chlorophenoxyacetic acid (MCPA), methylchlorophenoxypropionic acid (MCPP), and 2,4-dichlorophenoxyacetic acid (2,4-D). Chlorophenoxy herbicides are widely used in both commercial and residential settings.

Chlorophenoxy herbicides are absorbed through the gastrointestinal tract, skin, and respiratory tract. Most cases of toxicity, however, result from ingestion. Skeletal muscle is the primary organ of toxicity, although the exact mechanism of action is not well defined. Proposed mechanisms of action include direct cell membrane damage, forming analogues of acetyl-CoA and acting as false cholinergic messengers, and at high doses, uncoupling of oxidative phosphorylation.[5]

Clinical Features

Ingestion of chlorophenoxy herbicides can result in gastrointestinal symptoms that include vomiting, abdominal pain, diarrhea, oropharyngeal burning, and gastrointestinal hemorrhage. Other symptoms include muscle fasciculations, weakness, myotonia, and decreased tendon reflexes. Myotonia and fasciculations may lead to rhabdomyolysis and metabolic acidosis.[5]

Differential Diagnoses

Severe toxicity from chlorophenoxy herbicides is rare. When symptoms are present, other possible diagnoses include other causes of acute myopathy. When gastrointestinal symptoms are present, viral and bacterial gastroenteritis, ingestion of caustic substances, organophosphate, and carbamate exposure are other considerations.

Diagnostic Testing

Testing for chlorophenoxy herbicides is not available in the emergency setting. Diagnostic testing should focus on assessing skeletal muscle damage and its consequences. Measurement of creatinine kinase, electrolyte profile, renal function, liver function, and acid base status are indicated.

Management

Decontamination

In the case of a dermal exposure, remove the clothing and wash the skin with soapy water. Because chlorophenoxy herbicides are rapidly absorbed via the gastrointestinal tract and vomiting may occur early, activated charcoal is not indicated.

Stabilization and Supportive Care

Supportive care with fluid resuscitation is the mainstay of treatment for patients symptomatic after chlorophenoxy herbicides.

Enhanced Elimination

In the rare event of a critically ill patient (patients requiring ventilator, hemodynamic support, and those with seizures, hyperthermia, or significant metabolic derangements) who presents after chlorophenoxy herbicide poisoning, urinary alkalinization or hemodialysis can be used to enhance elimination.

Antidote Therapy

There is no known antidote for chlorophenoxy herbicide toxicity.

Disposition

A patient who presents with muscular symptoms after chlorophenoxy herbicide toxicity should be admitted and carefully monitored for progression of symptoms. A patient who is asymptomatic at presentation should be monitored for 6 hours. If no symptoms develop, the patient can be safely discharged home.

BIPYRIDYL HERBICIDES

The bipyridyl (also called *dipyridyl*) herbicides paraquat and diquat are extremely effective contact herbicides that are widely used throughout the world. Paraquat is particularly toxic to humans and is under strict regulation in the United States. Diquat is less toxic and is subject to less regulation.

Foundations and Principles of Toxicity

Paraquat causes the production of superoxides created during cyclic oxidation-reduction reactions in tissues. This causes oxygen radical damage that results in cell death.[6] Paraquat selectively concentrates in the lungs, regardless of the route of exposure, because of an uptake mechanism in alveolar cells. High concentration of oxygen in the pulmonary system increases the extent of paraquat-induced oxygen radical injury; therefore, the lungs are the major target in paraquat poisoning. Paraquat exposure can lead to adult respiratory distress syndrome, progressive pulmonary fibrosis, and respiratory failure. Paraquat damages other organ systems by the same oxygen radical injury effect, including the liver, kidneys, heart, and central nervous system. Diquat has a similar mechanism of action but does not accumulate in the lungs as does paraquat. Diquat concentrates in the kidneys and often results in renal failure. Paraquat is absorbed through the skin, gastrointestinal tract, and respiratory tract. Diquat is poorly absorbed through intact dermis.

Clinical Features

Paraquat and diquat are corrosive and can cause vomiting and caustic injury to the oropharynx, esophagus, and gastrointestinal tract. Dermal exposure can cause corrosive injury to the skin. Systemic toxicity from both paraquat and diquat poisoning will often progress to multiorgan failure and death. This is especially true for paraquat, which can be fatal in small amounts. Patients who survive systemic toxicity from paraquat often develop a progressive pulmonary fibrosis 1 to 3 weeks after the exposure. The clinical course, however, is dependent on the dose of the exposure.

Differential Diagnoses

Bipyridyl herbicides are corrosive and the differential diagnosis encompasses other caustic agents (e.g., acids and alkalis), insecticides (organophosphates and carbamates), and pulmonary toxic chemotherapy agents (e.g., bleomycin). The subsequent systemic toxicity and multiorgan failure with bipyridyl herbicide poisoning could be attributable to other sources of similar symptoms, such as sepsis and acute respiratory distress syndrome (ARDS).

Diagnostic Testing

The cornerstone of diagnosing bipyridyl herbicide poisoning lies in the history of exposure. There is a colorimetric test to detect diquat and paraquat in urine that can be useful but is not readily available in the United States. Serum concentrations of bipyridyl herbicides can be measured but are generally not available in a time frame useful in the ED; however, the concentration paired with the time of ingestion can be used for mortality prognostication.

Multiorgan failure is possible after bipyridyl herbicide poisoning. Laboratory evaluation for respiratory, renal, hepatic, metabolic, and cardiovascular toxicity is indicated. Serial chest radiographs and arterial blood gases are recommended for symptomatic patients.

Management
Decontamination
Dermal exposure should be treated by removing soiled clothing and washing the skin with water. In general, gastrointestinal decontamination is not indicated in the case of caustic ingestions. Because bipyridyl herbicides, particularly paraquat, can cause systemic toxicity in small amounts, gastrointestinal decontamination may be warranted in these cases of ingestion. We recommend at least 100 g activated charcoal or Fuller's earth (in certain international settings) if an alert patient presents early, within 1 hour of the ingestion, because this toxicity has high morbidity and mortality without any antidotal therapy.

Stabilization and Supportive Care
Upper airway corrosive injury can lead to an obstructed airway. Orotracheal intubation is necessary when there is any concern for pending obstruction. Because of the oxygen radical damage, supplemental oxygenation should be targeted to an oxyhemoglobin saturation of 90% to 95%, and excessive supplemental oxygen should be avoided. Supportive care for multiorgan failure is indicated based on the clinical circumstances.

Enhanced Elimination
The use of hemodialysis to increase the elimination of paraquat or diquat is controversial. If renal failure, metabolic acidosis, or electrolyte imbalance develops as a result of the poisoning, hemodialysis is indicated.

Antidote Therapy
There is currently no specific antidotal therapy for bipyridyl herbicide poisoning. Antioxidants, immune modulators, and corticosteroids have been incompletely evaluated as options for therapy to prevent the delayed pulmonary fibrosis. There is currently insufficient data to recommend specific antidotal treatment in the ED.

Disposition
Due to potential high lethality, patients presenting with bipyridyl poisoning require admission to an ICU setting. As with any pesticide or herbicide exposure, those patients with acts of self-harm or suicidal intent require psychiatric consultation once medically stabilized.

PYRETHRIN AND PYRETHROID INSECTICIDES

Pyrethrins are naturally occurring insecticides derived from the chrysanthemum plant. Pyrethroids are synthetic derivatives of pyrethrins that are more stable in the environment.

Foundations and Principles of Toxicity
In humans, pyrethrins block voltage-gated sodium channels, voltage-gated calcium channels, and the chloride channels on GABA receptors. Toxicity in humans, however, is not common. Pyrethrins and pyrethroids are used both as commercial insecticides and pharmaceutically to treat human infestations of scabies and lice (e.g., permethrin). Pyrethrins and pyrethroids are poorly absorbed dermally but are well absorbed via gastrointestinal and respiratory routes.

Clinical Features
Toxicity from pyrethrins and pyrethroids is rare. Allergic and sensitivity reactions can be seen with exposure. Skin exposure can result in erythema. Inhalation can result in rhinitis, sneezing, oral mucosa irritation, cough, dyspnea, wheezing, and chest pain. Nausea, vomiting, abdominal pain, and diarrhea can occur after ingestion; in severe cases, this can contribute to metabolic acidosis.[7] With massive ingestions, the patient is at risk for neurological symptoms, such as numbness, tremors, ataxia, paralysis, seizures, and cerebral infarction.[8]

Differential Diagnoses
Sensitivity reactions seen with exposure to pyrethrins and pyrethroids can mimic allergic reactions or contact dermatitis from other etiologies.

Diagnostic Testing
There are no laboratory or diagnostic tests specific to poisoning from pyrethrins and pyrethroids in the ED setting.

Management
Decontamination
In the case of dermal exposure, clothing should be removed and skin washed with water.

Stabilization and Supportive Care
Skin reactions should be treated symptomatically with histamine blockers, such as diphenhydramine. Wheezing should be treated with beta agonists. Neurologic symptoms can be treated with benzodiazepines as needed (lorazepam, 1 to 2 mg IVP; diazepam, 5 to 10 mg IVP).

Enhanced Elimination
There is no role for enhanced elimination in pyrethrin and pyrethroid poisoning.

Antidote Therapy
There is no known antidotal therapy for pyrethrin and pyrethroid poisoning.

Disposition
Most cases of pyrethrin and pyrethroid exposure will not demonstrate signs of toxicity and can be safely discharged from the ED. Patients with massive ingestions should be observed for 24 hours for the development of neurologic symptoms. Any patient with neurologic symptoms should be admitted to a monitored setting.

GLYPHOSATE

Glyphosate is one of the most commonly used pesticides in the United States. It is a nonselective, contact herbicide that interferes with amino acid synthesis in plants. Recent in vitro studies have shown that glyphosate causes DNA damage and mitochondrial-driven apoptosis, resulting in potential human toxicity.[9] There is much controversy regarding whether glyphosate is associated with cancer in humans; however, this issue is less pertinent to the ED management in an acute exposure.[10,11]

Foundations and Principles of Toxicity
Glyphosate is poorly absorbed dermally. It is absorbed through the gastrointestinal tract. Concentrated solutions (40%) can cause mucosal injury. The residential concentration is 1%. Human acute toxicity is thought to be due to the surfactant included in the glyphosate preparation. Unintentional ingestion of glyphosate generally results in mild

gastrointestinal symptoms. Hypotension, renal failure, respiratory distress, and death can occur from intentional, massive ingestions.

Clinical Features

Patients who present with dermal exposure to glyphosate will likely have no signs of toxicity. However, one case of a large exposure (unclear if inhalational or dermal) resulted in vasculitic peripheral neuropathy.[12] Most ingestions of dilute preparations cause only mild gastrointestinal symptoms. Patients ingesting large volumes of dilute solutions or moderate volumes of concentrated solutions may develop sore throat, nausea, vomiting, abdominal pain, hyperthermia, respiratory distress, acute lung injury, renal failure, and coma. Metabolic acidosis may develop as a result of cardiovascular compromise. Poor prognostic features include altered mental status, hyperkalemia, and renal failure.

Differential Diagnoses

The differential diagnosis of glyphosate poisoning includes caustic ingestions and other causes of respiratory distress or cardiovascular compromise from other pesticides (e.g., organophosphates and carbamates) and herbicides (e.g., paraquat and diquat).

Diagnostic Testing

The key to the diagnosis of glyphosate poisoning is to obtain an accurate history of exposure. An electrolyte profile is recommended to assess for hyperkalemia. A creatinine concentration assesses for renal injury. If respiratory distress is present, a chest radiograph should be performed. We recommend measuring acid-base status with a venous or arterial blood gas to assess extent of respiratory compromise and for comparison with serial measurements to ascertain whether the patient is clinically improving or deteriorating.

Management

Decontamination

With dermal exposure, remove the clothing and wash the skin with water. Gastrointestinal symptoms are generally present with significant ingestions, and activated charcoal is not indicated.

Stabilization and Supportive Care

The mainstay of management of acute glyphosate exposure is supportive care. Provide airway management and cardiovascular support as indicated by the symptom profile. Hyperkalemia can be managed by standard measures.

Enhanced Elimination

There is no role for enhanced elimination in the management of glyphosate poisoning.

Antidote Therapy

There is no known antidote for glyphosate poisoning.

Disposition

Patients who demonstrate symptoms after glyphosate ingestion should be admitted for further management. Patients who present after unintentional exposures of small amounts or low concentrations of glyphosate can be discharged from the ED after a 6-hour observation period.

DEET

N, N-diethyl-m-toluamide, or DEET, is not technically a pesticide. It is the most widely used insect repellant used throughout the world. DEET is available in concentrations ranging from 5% to 100%, and it primarily repels mosquitoes and ticks. The American Academy of Pediatrics recommends 30% as the maximum concentration for use in children and does not recommend use of DEET in infants younger than 2 months old. It is available as lotions, aerosols, pump sprays, roll-on applicators, and impregnated towelettes. Concentrated DEET solutions (up to 100%) can cause plastic products, such as sunglasses and water bottles, to melt with contact.

Foundations and Principles of Toxicology

DEET is lipid soluble and is well absorbed when applied to the skin or ingested. Repeated exposure, skin wounds or abrasions, sweating, and elevated skin temperature increase absorption. DEET affects the central nervous system at the GABA receptors in humans.

Clinical Features

Most exposures to DEET result in minimal or no symptoms. Prolonged skin contact may lead to contact dermatitis, and prolonged contact with higher concentrations can lead to skin blisters. Ingestion of DEET can result in nausea, vomiting, and oral mucosal irritation. Ingestion or excessive skin exposure can lead to headache, liver injury, lethargy, respiratory depression, seizures, and coma.

Differential Diagnoses

The differential diagnosis for DEET poisoning includes any infectious (malaria, encephalitis) toxicological (pesticides, organophosphates, carbamates), metabolic, or neurologic abnormality that could cause seizures and depressed mental status.

Diagnostic Testing

There is no specific test for DEET poisoning that is useful in the ED.

Management

Decontamination

In patients with excessive or prolonged skin exposure to DEET, wash the skin with water. Gastrointestinal decontamination has no role in DEET ingestions because of rapid absorption and the potential for seizure activity.

Stabilization and Supportive Care

Supportive care is the mainstay of treatment for a DEET-poisoned patient. Seizures should be treated with benzodiazepines (lorazepam, 1 to 2 mg IVP; diazepam, 5 to 10 mg IVP) and are generally self-limited.

Enhanced Elimination

There is no role for enhanced elimination with DEET exposure.

Antidote Therapy

There is no known antidote for DEET poisoning.

Disposition

Any patient with acute neurologic symptoms after DEET exposure should be admitted. An asymptomatic patient after an oral ingestion or a patient with localized skin reaction can be discharged after a 6-hour observation period.

RODENTICIDES

Foundations

There are hundreds of rodenticides available throughout the world with variable toxicity (Table 152.4). Rodenticides are implicated in self-harm attempts, malicious poisonings, and accidental ingestions. In the United States, anticoagulants, or superwarfarin-type, are the most common rodenticides, accounting for over 90% of exposures. They are

TABLE 152.4 Rodenticides (Acronym: RATS PANIC)

	R SUPER WARFARINS	AT FLUORACETAMIDE	S STRYCHNINE	P PHOSPHORUS	A ALUMINUM[1]	NIC NICOTINAMIDE
Rodenticide		SMFA, fluoroacetamide 1080–1972; banned in 1972 Today: Sheep collars	Moles, gophers, pigeons Adulterant in heroin and cocaine	Yellow (white) phosphorus	Aluminum and zinc phosphide ("rice tablet")	Vacor: 2% PNU banned in 1979
Mechanism		Irreversible TCA cycle inhibitor (fluorocitrate is "suicide inhibitor")	Competitive inhibitor of glycine binding (increased neuronal excitability)	Corrosive, cellular poison Combusts at room temp	Unknown (inhibit electron transport chain, release phosphine gas with moisture and gastric acid)	Unknown (antagonizes nicotinamide axons and injures pancreatic cells)
Effects		GI: Nausea/vomiting/ diarrhea/pain Respiratory distress Seizures Cardiotoxicity Hypotension	"Awake seizure" Risus sardonicus Opisthotonus Hyperthermia, rhabdomyolysis	Respiratory "Phossy jaw" GI ("smoking" stool), liver failure Neuro, cardio Eye Skin (burns)	Delayed pulmonary edema, ARDS, GI, neurologic, cardio, hepatic, adrenal Refractory hypotension Metabolic acidosis	Nausea/vomiting Orthostatic hypotension Diabetes mellitus Neuropathy, coma
Diagnosis		Electrolytes, BUN/Cr, calcium, LFTs ECG, MRI Levels not helpful acutely	Cramps, awake seizure, electrolytes, BUN/Cr, CPK, ABG, serum levels do not correlate with toxicity	Garlic odor Burns (skin fluoresces) BUN/Cr, calcium, LFTs UA ABG, chest x-ray, ECG	Fishy/garlic odor BUN/Cr, electrolytes, LFTs ABG, chest x-ray	History Sudden orthostatic hypotension or DM Electrolytes, glucose, BUN/Cr
Treatment		Decontaminate Activated charcoal Supportive care	Stabilization and supportive care Limit stimulation Benzodiazepines for seizures, analgesia	PPE Decontaminate Sand or water over solid phosphorus	Benzodiazepines for seizures, steroids for adrenal dysfunction, magnesium for refractory arrhythmia	IVFs, activated charcoal Nicotinamide Insulin Steroids
Disposition		ICU for CNS, CV symptoms—more than rapid death	ICU if symptomatic Symptoms several hours (supportive care)	Likely ICU admission if significant exposure Isolation (patient and secretions)	Observe at least 72 hours for delayed effects	Admit for delayed neurologic symptoms Neuropathy/DM after several days

Modified from the original acronym created by Jack Snyder, MD.
ABG, Arterial blood gas; *ARDS,* acute respiratory distress syndrome; *BUN/Cr,* blood urea nitrogen/creatinine; *CNS,* central nervous system; *CPK,* creatine phosphokinase; *CV,* cardiovascular; *DM,* diabetes mellitus; *ECG,* electrocardiogram; *GI,* gastrointestinal; *ICU,* intensive care unit; *IVF,* intravenous fluids; *LFT,* liver function test; *MRI,* magnetic resonance imaging; *PNU,* N-3-pyridylmethyl-N'-p-nitrophenyl urea; *PPE,* personal protective equipment; *SMFA,* sodium monofluoroacetate; *TCA,* tricarboxylic acid; *UA,* urine analysis.
Hassan NAM, Madboly AG. Correlation between serum creatine phosphokinase and severity of acute organophosphorus poisoning: a prospective clinical study (2012–2013). *IOSR J Environ Sci Toxicol Food Tech.* 4(5):18–29, 2013.

long-acting, anti-vitamin K anticoagulants. Examples are brodifacoum, diphacinone, bromadiolone, chlorophacinone, and difenacoum.

Principles of Toxicology

Superwarfarins competitively inhibit vitamin K and the hepatic synthesis of vitamin K-dependent coagulation factors II, VII, IX, and X. These anticoagulants can also damage capillary walls, increasing permeability and fragility and exacerbating bleeding. Effects are prolonged in these long-acting anticoagulants—half-life of 150 hours versus 15 hours in first generation warfarins, leading to toxic effects that can last for months. All significant toxicological exposures are via ingestion, and all warfarins are well absorbed orally.

Clinical Features

Initially, patients can by asymptomatic and remain so for as long as 72 hours after ingestion, even with large ingestions. Alternatively, signs of gastrointestinal irritation can predominate early in the course of poisoning, and symptoms appear as early as 8 hours after exposure. They can then present with bleeding anywhere in the body, as evidenced by ecchymosis, epistaxis, hemarthrosis, gingival bleeding, menorrhagia, and hematuria. Life-threatening effects are massive gastrointestinal bleeding and intracranial hemorrhage.

Differential Diagnoses

The differential diagnosis includes supratherapeutic doses of warfarin, advanced stages of hepatic failure, disseminated intravascular coagulation, hemophilia, oncological diseases, and other hematological disorders that can present with similar bleeding symptoms.

Diagnostic Testing

Measure hemoglobin/hematocrit, platelets, prothrombin time (PT)/ international normalized ratio (INR), and partial thromboplastin time (PTT). Additionally, obtain blood type and screen as well as crossmatch (if actively bleeding). PT/INR might not be abnormal until 48 hours after ingestion; a normal INR at 48 hours essentially excludes a significant ingestion. Although most rodenticides are not commonly measurable, brodifacoum level is available at many reference labs (<4 to 10 ng/mL is normal and generally does not cause coagulopathy).

Management

Decontamination

If a patient presents within 1 hour after reported massive ingestion of superwarfarin, we recommend oral activated charcoal in a 10:1 activated charcoal to poison ratio. If the dose ingested is unknown, 100 g is an appropriate dose. Do not perform gastric lavage, because, in addition to a lack of clinical efficacy, it adds the additional risk of inducing gastrointestinal bleeding with insertion of a large orogastric tube.

Stabilization and Supportive Care

With massive blood loss, fluid resuscitation and transfusion are necessary. Packed RBCs to replace blood loss, fresh frozen plasma to improve coagulation profile, and four-factor prothrombin complex concentrate (PCC) are proven to be beneficial and are considered first-line treatments. Another option shown to be beneficial is recombinant activated factor VII.

Enhanced Elimination

There is no role for enhanced elimination in superwarfarin toxicity.

Antidote Therapy

Vitamin K_1, (as opposed to K_3 or K_4), is the preferred antidote, or reversal agent, because other forms are not effective and have potential for toxicity. Although vitamin K_1 will reliably reverse anticoagulation, it should not be given prophylactically; toxicity is determined by derangement in INR. This therapy requires 6 hours to take effect and, therefore, is not used for immediate reversal. This pharmacokinetic principle explains the usual vitamin K dosing regimen of every 6 hours. Prolonged treatment with doses as high as 800 mg daily has been required in massive overdoses.

Disposition

The majority of patients with small warfarin-based rodenticide ingestions (e.g., children tasting two to three pellets) can be discharged home with outpatient follow-up in 48 to 72 hours. Patients presenting with reported large intentional ingestion of superwarfarins (i.e., an entire box or bait tray) should be admitted for at least 48 hours, at which time an INR should be checked (minimum time after ingestion to check INR is 48 hours). In patients with coagulopathy, admission is required until all bleeding has subsided, and the patient is maintained on a vitamin K regimen for desired INR. On an outpatient basis, these patients may require monitoring of their coagulation profile for 4 to 6 weeks with the longer-acting superwarfarin products. Patients with acts of self-harm or suicidal intent require psychiatric consultation once medically stabilized.

The references for this chapter can be found online at ExpertConsult. com.

153

Plants, Herbal Medications, and Mushrooms

Christopher S. Lim and Steven E. Aks

PLANTS

FOUNDATIONS

The nutritional, therapeutic, psychoactive and toxic properties of botanicals have made their usage pervasive since antiquity. The earliest documented use of plants for medicinal purposes can be found in Sumerian clay tablets that describe the use of over 200 different plants in the treatment of various maladies. Ancient Greeks recognized the lethal effects of botanicals, sentencing Socrates to death by ingestion of a poison hemlock-based liquid. The recreational abuse and medicinal use of opium poppies highlight the wide-ranging role plants have played throughout history.

Exposures to plants comprise over 42,000 calls nationally to US poison centers, with over half of cases involving pediatric patients less than 6 years of age. Over 85% of plant exposures are accidental ingestions. The overwhelming majority of plant exposures result in minimal toxicity and death is exceedingly rare.[1] Plant exposures reported to US poison centers have been decreasing over the past three decades, ranking 3rd and comprising 9% of all exposures in 1983, but ranking 22nd and making up only 2% of all exposures in 2018. The most common plant exposures resulting in severe and occasionally fatal poisonings involve those with anticholinergic, antimitotic, cardiotoxic or convulsive properties.[1]

CLINICAL FEATURES

The vast majority of plants are considered non-toxic (Table 153.1). However, serious toxicity can result from certain plant exposure (Table 153.2). Toxicity does not correlate well with taxonomy, and plants within the same genera may have varying toxic profiles. Further complicating matters, the severity of exposure may depend on the method of exposure (chewed, swallowed, smoked or injected) and which part of the plant was ingested (berries, leaves, or stems). For example, although all parts of the water hemlock plant are considered toxic, cicutoxin is most concentrated in the root of the plant. The majority of serious or fatal outcomes occur when adults intentionally consume botanicals for suicidal or recreational intent. A focused history and physical exam should be aimed at identifying the etiology of the present illness and to identify any toxidrome common to botanical exposures.

DIFFERENTIAL DIAGNOSES

Patients with plant ingestions present with vomiting and diarrhea and should be differentiated from food poisoning, viral or bacterial gastroenteritis, and pesticide poisoning (often sprayed on plants). Those patients presenting with altered mental status should be differentiated from patients co-ingesting hallucinogenic, stimulant, or opioid drugs of abuse.

DIAGNOSTIC TESTING

Although specific concentrations of botanical toxins are not routinely available at most institutions, evaluation of electrolytes, renal and liver functions, transaminases, and complete blood count should be performed in patients with potentially toxic exposures. An electrocardiogram (ECG) and cardiac monitoring should be performed to identify any dysrhythmias. Efforts at botanical identification should be made to determine the potential toxicity of any exposure. Patients should not be routinely relied upon for botanical identification. Mistaken identification by patients and family members is a frequent cause of accidental ingestion of toxic botanicals and can lead to toxicity and inappropriate disposition from the emergency department (ED).[2-4] Most emergency medical staff struggle to correctly identify even common house plants. Instead, family members or friends should be asked to bring in or send digital photographs of the involved plant, which can then be compared to reliable reference photographs or sent to local botanical experts or regional poison centers for proper identification.

MANAGEMENT

Ipecac for forced emesis and gastric lavage in botanical poisoning is not indicated. There is little evidence of clinical benefit of activated charcoal, and we do not recommend its routine use in botanical poisoning. A few exceptions can be made in patients who present within 1 hour of ingestion of a potentially life-threatening exposure (see Table 139.12).

TABLE 153.1 Non-toxic Plants

Common Name	Botanical Name	Common Name	Botanical Name
Abelia	Abelia spp.	Creeping Charlie (houseplant)	Pilea nummulariifolia, Plectranthus australis
African daisy	Gerbera jamesonii	Creeping Jennie	Lysimachia nummularia
African violet	Saintpaulia ionantha	Crocus (Spring ONLY)	Crocus spp.
Aglaonema	Aglaonema spp.	Dahlia	Dahlia spp.
Aluminum plant	Pilea cadierei	Dandelion	Taraxacum officinale
Alyssum	Slyssum spp.	Day lily	Hermocallis spp.
Aralia	Dizygotheca elegantissima	Donkey's tail	Sedum morganianum
Areca palm	Chrysalidocarpus lutescens	Dracaena	Dracaena spp., Cordyline spp.
Artillery plant	Pilea spp.	Dragon tree	Dracaena draco
Asparagus fern	Asparagus setaceus	Easter lily	Lilium longiflorum
Aspidistra	Aspidistra spp.	Echeveria	Echeveria spp.
Aster	Callistephus chinensis, Townsendia sericea	Emerald feather	Asparagus densiflorus sprengeri
Astilbe	Astilbe japonica	Eugenia	Eugenia cyanocarpa, Syzygium cuminii
Baby's breath	Gysophila paniculate	False aralia	Dizygotheca elegantissima
Baby's tears	Hypoestes phyllostachya, Soleirolia soleirolii	Fatsia	Fatsia japonica
Baby's toes	Centaurea cyanus	Ferns	Davallia canariensis, Davallia fejeensis, Rumohra adiantiformis, Asplenium spp.
Bachelor's buttons	Centaurea cyanus		
Balsam	Impatients spp.	Ficus	Ficus benjamina
Bamboo	Phyllostachys aurea	Fig	Ficus carica
Basket vine	Aeschynanthus spp.	Fingernail plant	Aregelia spp.
Beauty bush	Kolkwitzia amabilis	Firecracker flower	Crossandra spp.
Begonia	Begonia goegoensis, Cissus spp.	Firecracker vine	Menettia bicolor
Bird's nest fern	Asplenium nidus	Fittonia	Fittonia spp.
Bleeding heart vine	Clerodendrum spp.	Florida beauty	Dracaena spp.
Blood leaf plant	Iresine spp.	Flowering quince	Chaenomeles spp.
Boston fern	Nephrolepis spp.	Forsythia	Forsythia spp.
Bromeliad	Vriesea hieroglyphica	Friendship plant	Billbergia spp., Pilea involucrate
Brunch berry	Cornus canadensis	Fuchsia	Fuchsia spp.
Butterfly bush	Buddleia davidii	Gardenia	Gardenia jasminoides
Button fern	Pellaea rotundifolia	Gazania	Gazania spp.
Calathea	Calathea spp.	Geranium	Pelargonium spp.
Camellia	Camellia japonica, Thea japonica	Glory tree	Clerodendrum thomsoniae
Candle plant	Plectranthus oetendahlii	Gloxinia	Gloxinia perennis, Sinningia speciosa
Cape primrose	Streptocarpus spp.	Golddust plant	Alyssum spp., Aucuba japonica
Cast iron plant	Aspidistra elatior	Goldfish plant	Hypocyrta spp.
Cattail	Typha latifolia	Hawthorn	Crataegus spp.
China doll	Leea spp.	Hemlock tree	Tsuga spp. (not to be confused with Conium or Cicuta spp.)
Chinese evergreen	Aglaonema modestum		
Christmas cactus	Cactaceae	Hens and chicks	Echeveria spp., Sempervivum tectorum
Coleus	Coleus spp.	Hibiscus	Hibiscus spp.
Columbine	Aquilegia spp.	Honey locust	Gleditsia triacanthos
Coral bells	Kalanchoe uniflora	Honeysuckle	Lonicera fragrantissima
Cordyline	Cordyline spp.	Hosta	Hosta spp.
Corn plant or cornstalk plant	Dracaena fragrans	Hoya	Hoya spp.

Continued

TABLE 153.1   Non-toxic Plants—cont'd

Common Name	Botanical Name
Ice plant	Aptenia cordifolia, Lampranthus spp., Mesembryanthemum cordifolium
Impatients	Impatients spp.
Iron plant	Aspidistra spp.
Jade plant	Portulacaria afra
Janet Craig plant	Dracaena deremensis
Japanese aralia	Fatsia japonica
Japanese lantern	Hibiscus schizopetalus
Japanese snowbell	Styrax japonica
Kalanchoe	Kalanchoe spp.
King and queen fern	Asplenium spp.
Lavendar	Lavandula officinalis
Lilac	Syringa spp.
Linden tree	Tilia americana
Lipstick plant	Aeschynanthus spp.
Magnolia	Magnolia spp.
Maidenhair fern	Adiantum decorum
Maple tree	Acer spp.
Maranta	Calathea spp., Maranta spp.
Marigolds (except Marsh Marigolds)	Calendula spp.
Maternity plant	Kalanchoe spp.
Mexican snowball	Echeveria spp.
Mimosa	Albizia julibrissin
Mock orange	Philadelphus spp., Pittosporum tobira
Monkey plant	Ruellia makoyana
Mosaic plant	Fittonia argyroneura
Mother fern	Asplenium spp.
Mother of thousands	Kalanchoe pinnata
Mountain grape	Mahonia spp.
Mulberry tree or bush	Morus spp.
Nasturtium	Tropaeolum spp.
Neanthebella	Chamaedorea elegans
Nerve plant	Fittonia spp.
Norfolk Island pine	Araucaria heterophylla
October plant	Sedum sieboldii
Old man of the mountains	Hymenoxys grandiflora
Orchid	Cattleya spp., Cymbidium spp., Epidendrum spp., Oncidium spp.
Painted lady	Echeveria spp.
Panda plant	Kalanchoe tomentosa
Parlor palm	Chamaedorea elegans
Passion vine, purple	Gynura aurantiaca
Patient Lucy	Impatients spp.

Common Name	Botanical Name
Peacock plant	Calathea makoyana, Kaempferia spp.
Peperomia	Peperomia spp.
Petunia	Petunia spp.
Phlox	Phlox spp.
Piggyback plant	Tolmiea menziesii
Pilea	Pilea spp.
Pine trees	Pinus spp.
Pitcher plant	Darlingtonia californica
Pittosporum	Pittosporum spp.
Plantago	Plantago major
Plush plant	Echeveria spp., Kalanchoe spp.
Pocketbook plant	Calceolaria spp.
Poinsettia	Euphorbia pulcherrima
Polka Dot plant	Hypoestes phyllostachya
Pony Tail plant	Beaucarnea recurvata
Potentilla	Potentilla spp.
Prayer plant	Maranta leuconeura
Pregnant plant	Kalanchoe pinnata
Propeller plant	Crassula cultrate
Purple passion	Gynura aurantiaca
Pyracantha	Pyranchantha spp.
Queen's tears	Billbergia spp.
Rabbit's foot	Maranta leuconeura
Rainbow plant	Billbergia spp.
Red bud	Cercis canadensis
Red hot poker	Kniphofia spp.
Resurrection plant	Selaginella lepidophylla
Rex-begonia vine	Cissus discolor
Ribbon plant	Dracaena sanderiana
Rosary vine	Ceropegia woodii, Crassula rupestris
Rose, rosehips	Rosa spp. (except Rosa rugose)
Rose of Sharon	Hibiscus syriacus
Rubber plant	Ficus elastica
Salvia	Salvia spp.
Sedum	Sedum spp.
Sensitive plant	Mimosa pudica
Sentry palm	Howea forsterana
Silk tree	Albizia julibrissin
Silver bell	Halesia spp.
Silver berry	Elaeagnus spp.
Silver dollar plant	Astrophytum asterias, Crassula arborscens
Silver evergreen	Aglaonema spp.
Silver king	Aglaonema spp.

TABLE 153.1 Non-toxic Plants—cont'd

Common Name	Botanical Name	Common Name	Botanical Name
Silver vine	Actinidia polygama	Tiger lily	Lilium spp.
Snapdragon	Antirrhinum majus	Tulip tree	Liriodendron tulipifera, Spathodea campanulata
Snowball bush	Viburnum spp.	Umbrella plant	Eriogonum umbellatum
Spider aralia	Dizygotheca elegantissima	Umbrella tree	Magnolia tripetala
Spider flower	Cleome spp., Hermocallis spp., Tibouchina spp.	Velvet plant	Gynura aurantiaca
Spiraea	Astilbe japonica	Viburnum	Viburnum spp.
Spirea	Spirea spp.	Wandering Jew	Zebrina pendula
Spruce tree	Picea spp.	Wax flower	Stephanotis floribunda
Staghorn fern	Platycerium spp.	Wax plant	Hoya spp.
Starfish flower	Stapelia spp.	Wild strawberry	Fragaria spp.
Stone face	Lithops spp.	Willow	Salix spp.
String of buttons	Crassula rupestris	Yellow wood	Cladrastis lutea, Rhodosphaera rhodanthema
Striped inch plant	Callisia spp.	Yucca plant	Yucca spp.
Swedish ivy	Plectranthus australis	Zebra plant	Aphelandra squarrosa, Calanthea zebrina, Cryptanthus zonatus
Sword fern	Polystichum munitum	Zinnia	Zinnia spp.
Teddy bear plant or vine	Cyanotis kewensis		

TABLE 153.2 Toxic Plants

Common Name	Botanical Name	Toxic Effects
Ackee tree	Blighia sapida	Hypoglycemia, gastrointestinal, neurologic
Almond, apricot, cherry, plum, peach	Prunus spp.	Cyanogenic
American mistletoe	Phoradendron spp.	Gastrointestinal
Angel trumpet	Brugmansia suaveolens	Anticholinergic
Autumn crocus, meadow or wild saffron	Colchicum autumnale	Gastrointestinal, multi-organ
Azalea	Azalea spp.	Cardiovascular
Betel nut	Areca catechu	Cholinergic
Bird-lime, blue thistle	Atractylis gummifera	Hepatic
Bitter orange	Citrus aurantium	Cardiovascular, neurologic
Black locust	Robinia pseudoacacia	Gastrointestinal
Buckeye	Aesculus glabra	Gastrointestinal, neurologic
Calabar bean	Physostigma venenosum	Cholinergic
Cassava	Manihot exculentus	Cyanogenic
Castor bean	Ricinus communus	Gastrointestinal, multi-organ
Cayenne pepper	Capsicum spp.	Dermatologic, mucosal irritant
Chysanthemum, dandelion	Chrysanthemum spp.	Dermatologic
Cinchona	Cinchona spp.	Cardiovascular, cinchonism
Common, white or pink oleander	Nerium oleander	Cardiovascular[a]
Deadly nightshade	Atropa belladonna	Anticholinergic
Dumbcane, mother-in-law plant	Dieffenbachia spp.	Dermatologic, mucosal irritant
Elderberry	Sambucus nigra	Gastrointestinal, metabolic
Elephant ear, angel wings, heart of Jesus	Caladium spp.	Dermatologic, mucosal irritant
Ergot	Claviceps purpurea	Cardiovascular, neurologic, oxytocic

TABLE 153.2   Toxic Plants—cont'd

Common Name	Botanical Name	Toxic Effects
Eucalyptus	Eucalyptus spp.	Dermatologic, gastrointestinal
European or true mandrake	Mandragora officinarum	Anticholinergic
Fava bean	Vicia fava	Hematologic
Foxglove	Digitalis spp.	Cardiovascular[a]
Glory lily	Gloriosa superba	Gastrointestinal, multi-organ
Golden chain or rain	Laburnum anagyroides	Gastrointestinal, neurologic
Grass pea	Lathyrus sativus	Neurologic, skeletal
Green tomato	Lycopersicon spp.	Gastrointestinal, neurologic, anticholinergic
Guarana	Paullinia cupana	Neurologic, cardiac
Henbane, hyoscyamus	Hyoscyamus niger	Anticholinergic
Holly	Ilex spp.	Gastrointestinal
Ipecac	Cephaelis ipecacuanha, Cephaelis acuminata	Gastrointestinal
Jequirity pea, rosary or prayer bead	Abrus precatorius	Gastrointestinal, neurologic
Jimsonweek, angel's trumpet	Datura Stramonium	Anticholinergic
Khat	Catha edulis	Cardiovascular, neurologic
Larkspur	Delphinium spp.	Cardiovascular, neurologic
Lily of the valley	Convallaria majalis	Cardiovascular[a]
Mad honey	Rhododendron spp.	Gastrointestinal, cardiac
Madagascar periwinkle, vinca	Catharanthus roseus	Gastrointestinal
Marijuana, hashish, pot	Cannabis	Neurologic
Mayapple	Podophyllum emodi, Podophyllum peltatum	Multi-organ
Milkweed	Asclepias spp.	Cardiovascular[a]
Monkshood, Wolfsbane	Aconitum napellus	Cardiovascular, neurologic
Nightshade (various), potato	Solanum spp.	Anticholinergic
Opium poppy	Papaver somniferum	Neurologic, respiratory
Peace lily	Spathiphyllum spp.	Dermatologic, mucosal irritant
Peyote, mescal	Lophophora williamsii	Neurologic
Philodendron	Philodendron spp.	Dermatologic, mucosal irritant
Pilocarpus	Pilocarpus jaborandi, Pilocarpus pinnatifolius	Cholinergic
Pink-eyed cerbera, sea mango, suicide tree, pong pong tree	Cerbera spp.	Cardiovascular[a]
Poison hemlock	Conium maculatum	Neurologic, pulmonary
Poison ivy, poison oak, poison sumac	Toxicodendron spp.	Dermatologic
Pokeweed	Phytolacca americana	Gastrointestinal
Poplar	Populus spp.	Salicylism
Pothos	Epipremnum aureum	Dermatologic, mucosal irritant
Queen sago, indu	Cycas circinalis	Neurologic
Rattlebox	Crotalaria spp.	Hepatotoxic
Red squill	Urginea maritima, Urginea indica	Cardiovascular[a]
Spider plant	Chlorophytum comosum	Dermatologic, mucosal irritant
Tansy	Tanacetum vulgare	Neurologic
Tobacco	Nicotiana spp.	Gastrointestinal, neurologic
Tonka beans	Dipteryx odorata, Dipteryx oppositifolia	Hematologic

TABLE 153.2	Toxic Plants—cont'd	
Common Name	**Botanical Name**	**Toxic Effects**
Tubocurare, curare	*Chondrodendron spp., Curarea spp., Strychnos spp.*	Neurologic
Tullidora, buckthorn	*Karwinskia humboldtiana*	Neurologic, respiratory
Umbrella tree	*Schefflera spp., Brassaia spp.*	Dermatologic, mucosal irritant
Water hemlock	*Cicuta maculata*	Neurologic
Water hemlock	*Oenanthe crocata*	Neurologic
White cedar	*Thuja occidentalis*	Neurologic
Wormwood, absinthe	*Artemisia absinthium*	Neurologic
Yellow oleander	*Thevetia peruviana*	Cardiovascular[a]
Yew	*Taxus spp.*	Cardiovascular

[a]Cardioactive steroid.

of the plant is not immediately known and treatment should be focused on symptom-based, supportive care. This includes maintenance of a patent airway, intravenous fluids and vasopressors for hypotension, active cooling for hyperthermia, and benzodiazepines for agitation and seizures. Management of specific categories of botanicals is outlined in the following sections.

DISPOSITION

Any patient with signs of severe toxicity, especially those involving the cardiovascular and neurologic systems, should be managed in the ED until symptoms and signs are resolving, or they are admitted to an intensive care setting. Patients with exposure to unknown plants can be discharged after 6 hours of cardiac monitoring if they are hemodynamically stable and otherwise asymptomatic. This period of observation should be extended to 24 hours if pre-existing cardiovascular or other concerning medical problems exist or an exposure to a plant of serious toxicity is suspected.

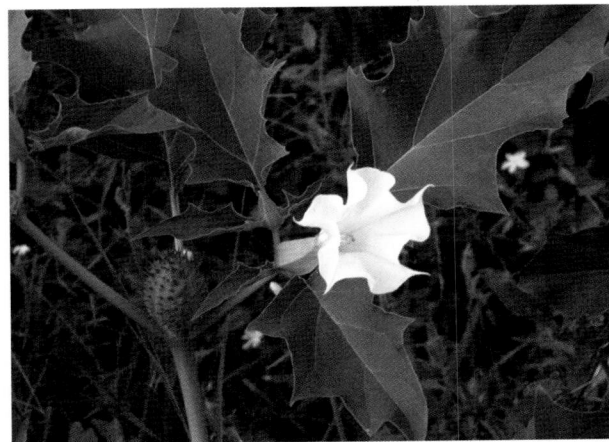

Fig. 153.1 *Datura stramonium* (jimson weed). (Courtesy Steven Setzer.)

PLANT CATEGORIES

Anticholinergics
Foundations

Principles of toxicity. Datura stramonium (Jimson weed, angel's trumpet) (Fig. 153.1) and *Atropa belladonna* (deadly nightshade) are the most frequently encountered plants with anticholinergic toxins. They contain scopolamine, hyocyamine and atropine. All parts of the plant contain toxic alkaloids, but they are most concentrated in the seeds of *D. stramonium* and the fruit and leaves of *A. belladonna.*

Clinical features. Ingestion can cause the antimuscarinic syndrome of agitation, diminished gastrointestinal (GI) motility, dry skin, flushing, hallucinations, hyperthermia, mydriasis, tachycardia, and urinary retention.[5,6] *D. stramonium* is commonly abused for its hallucinogenic properties, whereas berries from *A. belladonna* have been mistaken for the common blueberry (*Vaccinium arctostaphylos*) resulting in poisonings.

Differential diagnoses. The differential diagnosis of antimuscarinic toxicity includes toxicity from pharmaceutical agents such as diphenhydramine, benztropine, cyclic antidepressants, antipsychotics, and antiparkinson medications. Sympathomimetic drugs such as cocaine and amphetamines will also cause similar toxic symptoms but typically present with diaphoresis instead of dry skin, which is typical of the antimuscarinic toxidrome.

Diagnostic testing. Symptomatic patients with altered mental status or abnormal vital signs should have a screening ECG to assess corrected QT (QTc) and QRS intervals, serum electrolytes, glucose, creatinine phosphokinase (CPK) and renal function.

Management. Management should be focused on supportive care, including active cooling for hyperthermia and benzodiazepines for agitation. Recommended agents include diazepam, 5 to 10 mg IV, or lorazepam, 1 to 2 mg IV. Additional doses can be administered every 10 minutes until the patient is calm and able to cooperate with care. The use of a cholinesterase inhibitor, such as physostigmine (0.5 to 2 mg in adults; 0.02 mg/kg in children), is recommended for severe anticholinergic toxicity (see Chapter 140).[6]

Disposition. Mildly symptomatic patients can be observed in the ED for 6 to 8 hours and discharged from the ED. Severely poisoned patients with refractory antimuscarinic symptoms should be admitted to a monitored setting for 24 hours.

Antimitotic Toxins
Foundations

Principles of toxicity. Colchicum autumnale is also known as autumn crocus, meadow saffron, or wild saffron, and contains the toxic alkaloid colchicine. Colchicine inhibits microtubule formation, leading to disruption of mitosis, intracellular transport mechanisms and cell structure. *C. autumnale* is often mistaken for *Allium ursinum* (wild garlic), leading to fatal, unintentional ingestions. Pharmaceutical colchicine is most commonly used to treat acute gouty arthritis. Serious toxicity from pharmaceutical colchicine is seen at doses greater than 0.5 mg/kg, and it is invariably lethal at doses of 0.8 mg/kg.

Clinical features. The clinical course of colchicine poisoning is typically divided into three phases of illness.[7] The first phase is marked by GI symptoms, such as severe vomiting, diarrhea, abdominal pain, hypovolemia, and electrolyte disturbances. Multi-organ failure ensues in the second phase, with manifestations of cardiac dysrhythmia, adult respiratory distress syndrome (ARDS), pancytopenia, liver failure, rhabdomyolysis, and sepsis. Death usually occurs during this second phase. The third phase is recovery from the poisoning.

Differential diagnoses. Patients presenting in the first phase of illness may be misdiagnosed as having gastroenteritis or food poisoning. In the second phase, colchicine poisoning mimics many serious disorders and is treated similarly with supportive interventions based on the type and severity of the patient's presentation. Obtaining a history of ingestion is critical to making the correct diagnosis but will not significantly alter the treatment plan. Patients with pancytopenia should be differentiated from patients with sepsis, leukemia, or oncological disorders—obtaining the history of ingestion may avoid invasive testing, such as a bone marrow biopsy.

Diagnostic testing. Laboratory data should include a complete blood count to assess for pancytopenia. Additional labs include serum electrolytes, renal and liver function tests as well as a screening ECG. Serum colchicine levels can be sent out to reference laboratories for analysis, but the results are time consuming and should not alter or delay emergency care.

Management. There is no specific therapy for colchicine poisoning, and management consists primarily of supportive care. There is no commercially available antidote for colchicine poisoning in the United States, and supportive care is ineffective in those who ingest a lethal dose. Thus, efforts to prevent gastric absorption by administration of activated charcoal should be made for those who ingest a potentially lethal dose of colchicine and present within 1 hour of ingestion.

Disposition. Patients presenting with GI symptoms but normal laboratory testing may be discharged home after 6 to 8 hours of hydration and observation in the ED. Patients with cardiac dysrhythmias, pancytopenia, liver dysfunction or renal failure require admission to a monitored setting. Patients with pancytopenia require admission and isolation precautions to avoid sepsis and secondary nosocomial infections.

Cardiac Glycosides
Foundations

Principles of toxicity. Cardiac glycosides bind to cell transmembrane Na^+-K^+-ATPases, which, in turn leads to a rise in intracellular Ca^{2+} concentrations, causing decreased automaticity and increased contractility. Common plants that contain cardiac glycosides include *Convallaria maalis* (lily of the valley), *Digitalis* spp. (foxglove) (Fig. 153.2), *Nerium oleander* (common, pink or white oleander) (Fig. 153.3), and *Thevetia peruviana* (yellow oleander).

Clinical features. Similar to digoxin poisoning, patients with exposure to cardiac glycosides can present with GI symptoms, generalized weakness, altered mental status, bradydysrhythmias, tachydysrhythmias, and hypotension. Toxicity and treatment of cardiac glycosides are also discussed in Chapter 142.

Differential diagnoses. The differential diagnoses of cardiac glycoside plant poisoning is broad and includes pharmaceutical toxicity with digoxin, calcium channel blockers, beta blockers, and clonidine. Additionally, other cardiogenic bradydysrhythmias (atrioventricular [AV] blocks and sick sinus syndromes) should be considered.

No sign or symptom, including dysrhythmia, is unique to digoxin poisoning, so the differential diagnosis is broad. Intrinsic cardiac

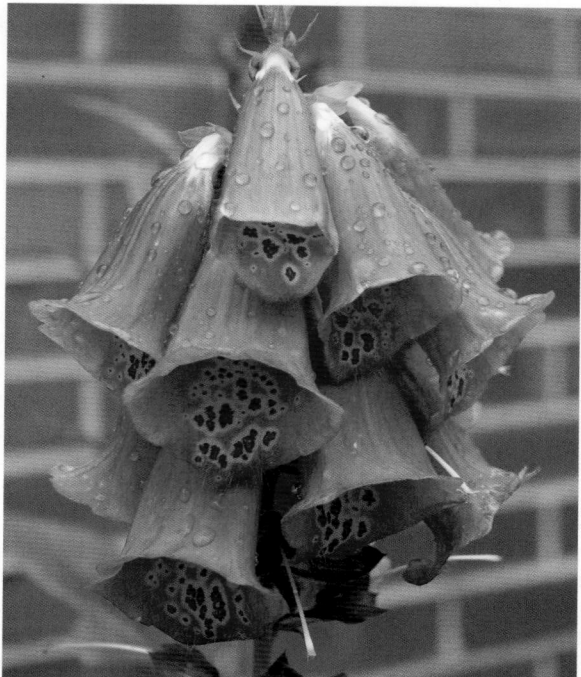

Fig. 153.2 *Digitalis purpurea* (foxglove). (Courtesy Christopher Lim.)

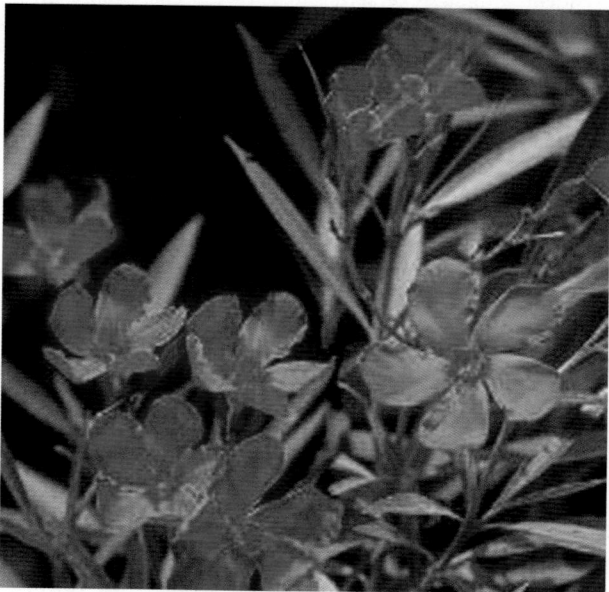

Fig. 153.3 Nerium oleander. (Courtesy Steven Setzer.)

disease, as well as other cardiotoxic drugs, should be considered. Cardioactive steroid poisoning from plants is rare but presents similarly to digoxin toxicity. Common examples include oleander (*N. oleander*, see Fig. 147.2) and lily of the valley (*Convallaria majalis*, see Fig. 147.3). Aconitine, a sodium-channel opening xenobiotic found in common monkshood (*Aconitum napellus*), may also mimic digoxin poisoning. Central nervous system (CNS) depression or confusion may be due to various depressant drugs (opioids, major tranquilizers, sedative hypnotic agents) and toxins, as well as infection, trauma, inflammation, and metabolic derangements. Visual disturbances caused by digoxin are binocular and are often not reported by the patient; unfortunately, they are not specific to digoxin poisoning. Methanol, metformin, ethambutol, ethyl chloride, quinine, and other anti-malarial medications are all capable of producing visual disturbances. GI disturbances are common and nonspecific and may be misdiagnosed as gastritis, enteritis, or colitis.

Diagnostic testing. Patients should have an ECG performed, and serum electrolytes should be evaluated with attention to potassium because cardiac glycoside-poisoned patients are susceptible to hyperkalemia. A serum digoxin concentration can be measured, but correlates poorly with the degree of toxicity and should be used only to confirm exposure.

Management. The cornerstone of therapy is digoxin-specific antibody fragments (Fab) and should be administered in any patient displaying serious toxicity (heart rate <40 beats/min, sinus arrest or exit block, atrial tachydysrhythmia, ventricular dysrhythmia, second- or third-degree AV block, hypotension, and/or serum potassium level >5.0 mEq/L).[8] The optimal dose is not established and may be dependent on several variables (e.g., plant species, amount, route of exposure, and part of plant ingested).[8,9] Studies from yellow oleander poisoning suggest higher dose requirements of digoxin immune Fab with plant cardiac glycoside poisoning than with pharmaceutical digoxin poisoning. A reasonable approach considers the patient's clinical status. If the patient is in cardiac arrest or unstable, we suggest an initial 20 vials IV of Fab fragment. For stable patients, we recommend an initial 10 vials IV. Patients should be re-evaluated every hour for the need of additional doses. Cardiac pacing, atropine, beta-adrenergic agents are without demonstrated benefit and should only be considered adjunctive therapies.

Disposition. Symptomatic patients with bradycardia, hypotension, altered mental status, or hyperkalemia are admitted to a monitored setting. Those requiring digoxin-specific Fab should be admitted to an intensive care setting with cardiology and medical toxicology consultation.

OTHER CARDIOTOXIC PLANTS

Rhododendron species contain grayanotoxin, which can be found in concentrated levels in the honey that is produced from the nectar. Often referred to as "mad honey," poisonings can result in GI symptoms, hypersalivation, diaphoresis, and cardiac effects. Grayanotoxin binds to cell membrane sodium channels, preventing voltage-dependent inactivation, thereby holding cells in a depolarized state. This is thought to increase the vagal tone. The cardiac manifestations mainly consist of bradydysrhythmias (including sinus bradycardia, AV blocks, and atrial fibrillation with slow ventricular response) and hypotension, leading to symptoms of dizziness and syncope.[10,11] It has even been implicated as a cause of myocardial infarction.[12] In addition to IV fluids for hypotension, atropine and cardiac pacing have been used successfully in the treatment of mad honey toxicity.[10,11]

Taxus species (Fig. 153.4), commonly known as yew, are coniferous trees and shrubs that are often cultivated for ornamental landscaping. They contain several toxic components, including taxine pseudoalkaloids that cause sodium and calcium channel blockade. The most serious effects are on the cardiovascular system, and manifestations include hypotension, dysrhythmias, and cardiac arrest.[13,14] Management of toxicity is largely supportive. The successful use of extracorporeal membrane oxygenation (ECMO) for severe and refractory cardiotoxicity and hypotension has been reported.[13,15]

Aconitium spp. (monkshood, wolfsbane) contain aconitine and other related alkaloids. Similar to grayanotoxins, aconitine binds and prevents inactivation of voltage-gated sodium channels of myocardial and neural cells. Thus, the main features of poisoning are neurological (paresthesias, weakness) and cardiovascular (hypotension,

dysrhythmias).[16] Management includes supportive care and standard therapy for dysrhythmias.[17]

Cicutoxin
Principles of Toxicity

Both *Cicuta* spp. (Fig. 153.5) and *Oenanthe crocata* are commonly known as water hemlock and contain toxins responsible for the hallmark presentation of intractable and life-threatening seizure activity. Seizures are thought to occur from non-competitive gamma-aminobutyric acid (GABA) antagonism.

Clinical Features

Initial features of poisoning may include vomiting, abdominal pain, confusion, weakness, and dizziness. Prolonged seizures can further complicate the clinical course, leading to rhabdomyolysis, hyperthermia, acidosis, hypoxia, cerebral edema, and eventual cardiopulmonary arrest.

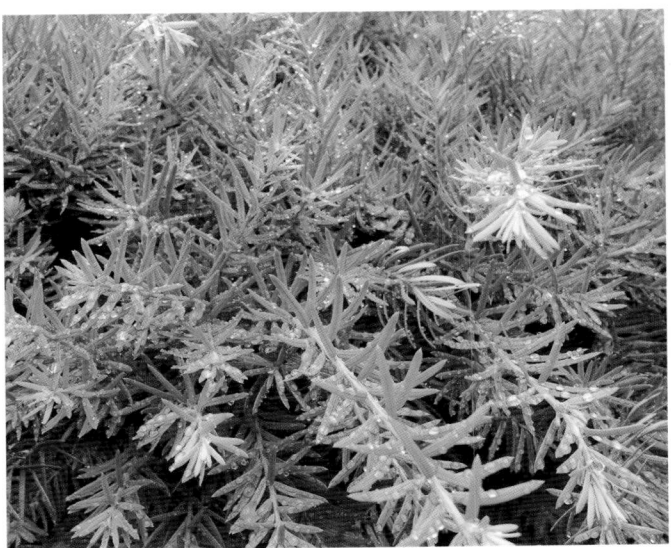

Fig. 153.4 *Taxus media* (yew). (Courtesy Christopher Lim.)

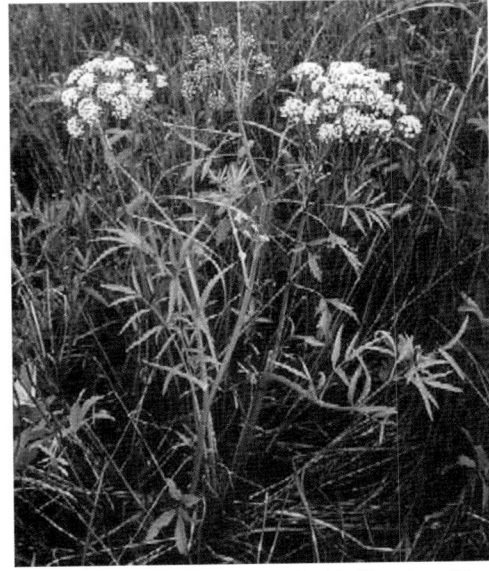

Fig. 153.5 *Cicuta maculata* (water hemlock). (Courtesy Steven Setzer.)

Differential Diagnoses

Water hemlock is often confused for edible plants (e.g., carrots, parsnips, turnips), leading to unintentional poisonings. Other neurotoxic agents should be considered including organophosphates, isoniazid (INH), cyclic antidepressants, methyl xanthines, tramadol, sympathomimetic toxicity, and ethanol and benzodiazepine withdrawal. Seizure disorders, hypoglycemia, head trauma, and brain lesions are also diagnostic considerations.

Diagnostic Testing

History is essential to identify the toxin as the cause of the new onset seizure, thus obviating the need for further diagnostic testing. Serum electrolytes exclude hypernatremia, hyponatremia, hypocalcemia, or hypoglycemia as a cause of the confusion or seizures and hypokalemia as a cause of the weakness. Serum CPK and creatinine evaluate for rhabdomyolysis and renal impairment. A toxicology screen, especially a serum ethanol level, help identify or exclude alternate causes of the confusion. An ECG should be performed to assess intervals if an electrolyte disturbance or overdose is suspected.

Management

The mainstay of management is seizure control with benzodiazepines (lorazepam, 1 to 2 mg IV, or diazepam, 5 to 10 mg IV, repeated every few minutes until seizure activity ceases). If seizure activity is not controlled with benzodiazepines, treatment is similar to that of other toxicologic causes of status epilepticus (see Chapter 88).

Disposition

Patient with altered mental status and seizures should be admitted to an intensive care setting. Those who are asymptomatic after 6 to 8 hours of observation in the ED may be discharged home.

OTHER TOXIC PLANTS

Nicotinic toxin

Conium maculatum (poison hemlock) (Fig. 153.6), *Nicotian tabacum* (Fig. 153.7), and *Nicotiana glauca* (wild or tree tobacco) contain alkaloids capable of producing nicotinic-cholinergic poisoning. They contain the toxins coniine and coniceine (*C. maculatum*), and anabasine (*N. glauca*) that stimulate nicotinic acetylcholine receptors on the autonomic nervous system and neuromuscular junction. Clinical effects can include hypersalivation, vomiting, diarrhea, muscle fasciculation, and agitation; toxicity can progress to profound weakness, paralysis, respiratory failure, hypotension, rhabdomyolysis, and renal failure.

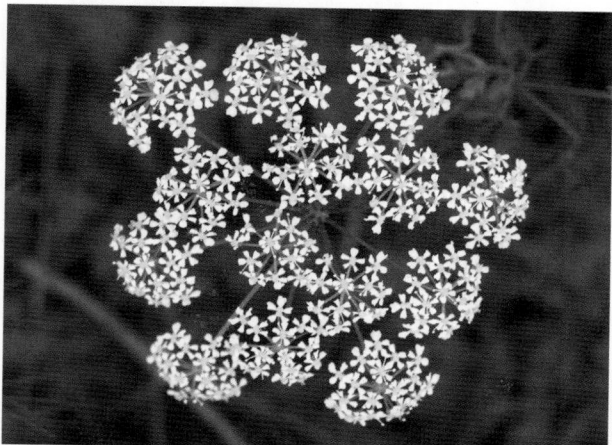

Fig. 153.6 *Conium maculatum* (poison hemlock). (Courtesy Steven Setzer.)

There is no specific antidote, and treatment should be aimed at ventilatory support for those with respiratory distress or muscle fatigue and those who cannot adequately oxygenate. Treatment should be continued until resolution of respiratory muscle fatigue and airway stabilization.[18,19]

Raphides

Raphides are needle-shaped, calcium oxalate crystals and have been observed in over 200 plants. Common plants that contain calcium oxalate crystals include the species from the genera *Dieffenbachia* (dumb cane, mother-in-law plant) (Fig. 153.8), *Philodendron*, *Spathiphyllum*, and *Brassaia* spp. Dieffenbachia plants are commonly found in homes and offices due to their attractive appearance, low cost and resistance to neglect. Ingestions can result in vomiting, and mucosal irritation,

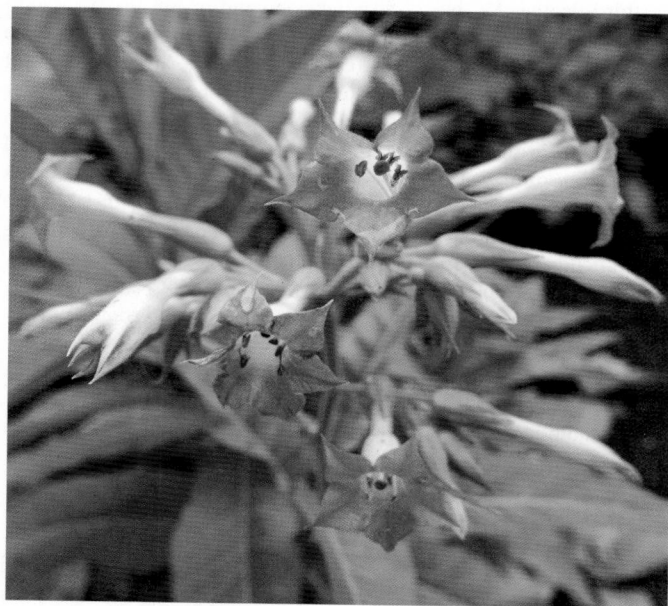

Fig. 153.7 *Nicotiana tabacum* (tobacco). (Courtesy Christopher Lim.)

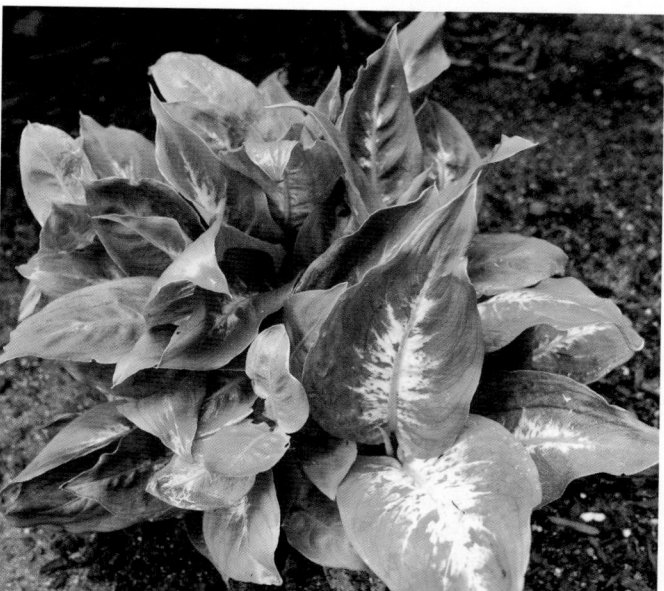

Fig. 153.8 *Dieffenbachia amoena* (dumb cane). (Courtesy Christopher Lim.)

ulceration and edema that can lead to compromise of the airway in severe ingestions. Dermal exposures may lead to contact dermatitis.[20]

Treatment is supportive including maintenance of a patent airway. The use of corticosteroids and antihistamines are considered adjunctive therapies, but they have not been shown to improve outcomes in mild cases of exposure. However, we recommend the administration of diphenhydramine (25 to 50 mg intravenous push [IVP]) and dexamethasone (4 to 8 mg IVP) for the rare cases of respiratory distress with significant airway edema following ingestion of specific raphide plants.

Toxalbumins

Abrus precatorius (jequirity pea, rosary, or prayer bead) (Fig. 153.9) and *Ricinus communis* (castor oil plant) contain the toxins abrin and ricin, respectively, that inhibit ribosomal protein synthesis, leading to cell death. Seeds of *A. precatorius* are distinctive, bright red or orange seeds with black caps that are often used in jewelry or rosaries. Castor beans are light brown and mottled, with dark brown spots. Seeds or beans swallowed whole with the hard outer shell intact typically prevent absorption of significant toxin. Chewed or crushed seeds or beans may release the toxin and cause local toxicity in the GI tract, leading to gastroenteritis, abdominal pain, dehydration, and electrolyte disturbances.[21,22]

Rarely, abrin or ricin is absorbed systemically, and symptoms may progress to severe neurologic toxicity (seizure, coma, cerebral edema, demyelinating encephalitis), multi-organ failure, and death. Purified ricin derived from the castor bean is highly toxic and lethal in small doses. It has been used historically as a biologic weapon, implicated in the assassination of Bulgarian journalist Georgi Markov in the 1970s, and discovered at a Washington DC postal service facility in 2001. There is no effective antidote, vaccine, or other therapy for the treatment of prevention of abrin or ricin poisoning. Treatment consists of fluid resuscitation, vasopressor agents for hypotension, and correction of electrolyte imbalances with neurotoxic symptom precautions.

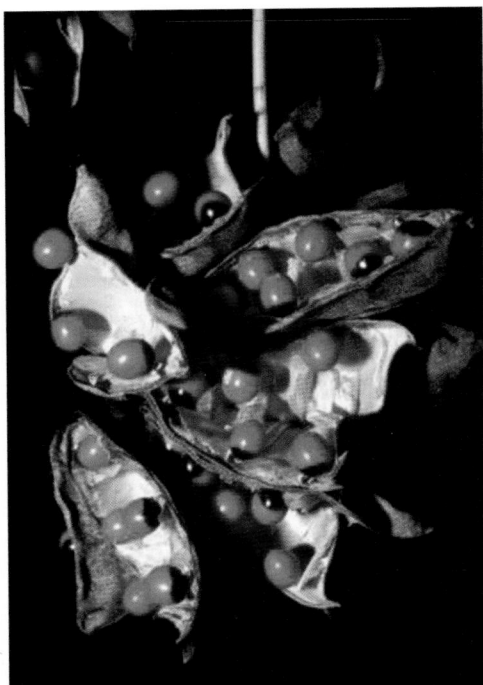

Fig. 153.9 *Abrus precatorius* (jequirity pea or rosary pea). (Courtesy Steven Setzer.)

MUSHROOMS

FOUNDATIONS

Mushrooms represent a wide range of species with regional variation. In this section, we will consider the mushrooms of toxicologic significance. The categories of poisonous mushrooms are grouped according to the types of illness or organ-specific toxicity. Another important perspective is that the most common species of toxic mushrooms belong to the GI irritant group and generally do not cause life-threatening illness. Distinguishing the GI irritant group from the more serious groups is the challenge for the treating emergency clinician.

According to data from 2018 as reported by the American Association of Poison control centers, there were a total of 6318 mushrooms exposures. The majority of the ingested mushrooms were never identified (5138). Four mushrooms from the cyclopeptide group, nine from the hallucinogenic group, one from the muscimol-containing group, and one from the orellarine group resulted in major effects. There were five fatalities from mushroom exposures in this database.[1]

CLINICAL FEATURES

An important clinical consideration is the onset of symptoms after a mushroom ingestion. In general, the GI irritants will develop symptoms in the first 2 to 3 hours after ingestion. Some of the most lethal mushrooms will cause symptoms on a delayed basis, such as *Amanita phalloides*, or *Gyromitria esculenta*, at 6 to 8 hours after ingestion.[23] There are some exceptions that are highlighted later in the chapter.

DIFFERENTIAL DIAGNOSES

Many mushrooms are edible and considered delicacies, such as puffballs or morels. However, there are many look-alikes, and foragers must be certain that they identify correct species to avoid morbidity and mortality. The differential diagnosis with mushroom poisoning includes gastroenteritis, pancreatitis, hepatitis, acute renal failure, hallucinogenic poisonings, anticholinergic and cholinergic poisonings, disulfiram toxicity, and food poisoning.

DIAGNOSTIC TESTING

Identifying the mushroom ingested is extremely helpful to the treating team. It is beyond a realistic scope for emergency clinicians to be able to identify mushrooms, and it is wise to coordinate with poison control centers and local mycologists to identify mushrooms in real time. Smart phone digital identification by sending images to mycologists via a poison control center model has been shown to be accurate in identifying mushrooms. Attempts at mushroom identification should be made, particularly if a patient presents with a delayed onset of symptoms.

Routine testing includes complete blood count, urinalysis, and basic metabolic profile with specific attention to renal function and measures of dehydration. Liver enzyme and tests of liver function should be obtained if cyclopeptide or gyromitrin poisoning is suspected.

MANAGEMENT

The general management of mushroom poisoning focuses on symptom-based supportive care. There is no proven outcome benefit from administration of activated charcoal for patients with mushroom ingestion. We recommend activated charcoal only if it can be administered within 1 hour of the ingestion and the clinician suspects ingestion of a potentially life-threatening mushroom (e.g., cyclopeptide- or gyromitrin-containing species). We do not recommend gastric emptying by any method. Because many toxic mushrooms can cause vomiting or diarrhea, it is important that these patients are fluid resuscitated and rehydrated until they can tolerate oral liquids.

DISPOSITION

Patients should be admitted for 24 hours when the ingestion of a potentially life-threatening mushroom has occurred. For hepatotoxic mushrooms, transferring the patient to a tertiary care center with liver transplantation capabilities should be considered. For suspected or confirmed GI irritant mushroom ingestion the patient can be safely discharged after the GI symptoms are controlled and oral fluids are tolerated.

MUSHROOM CATEGORIES

Hepatotoxic Mushrooms
Principles of Toxicity

The two major categories of mushrooms that can cause life-threatening hepatotoxicity include cyclopeptide-containing mushrooms such as *A. phalloides*, or certain *Lepiota* species of mushrooms. The *Gyromitra* species also cause hepatotoxicity but have other symptoms distinct from the cyclopeptide-containing mushrooms.

Clinical Features

The cyclopeptide-containing mushrooms will cause an onset of GI symptoms 6 to 8 hours after ingestion. This includes nausea, vomiting, diarrhea, and abdominal pain. Over the next 1 to 2 days, the patient will develop increasingly severe hepatic injury and encephalopathy.

Differential Diagnoses

In patients with cyclopeptide-containing mushroom toxicity with elevations in liver aminotransferases, bilirubin, partial thromboplastin time (PTT)/international normalized ratio (INR), or creatinine, other sources of injury should be considered, including acute tubular necrosis, rhabdomyolysis, ischemic hepatitis, alcoholic hepatic disease, viral hepatitis, and Wilson's disease. Other hepatotoxic considerations include poisoning with acetaminophen, valproic acid, INH, statins, herbal medications (e.g., pennyroyal oil, pyrrolizidine alkaloids), vinyl chloride, and polychlorinated biphenyls.

Diagnostic Testing

Poisoning is evidenced by rising liver enzymes and worsening measures of liver function (rising bilirubin and increased INR). Hyperammonemia can also be seen in severe toxicity. These markers should be followed serially during the hospital course. Also, because patients may develop a hepatorenal syndrome, creatinine and blood urea nitrogen should be measured.

Management

Many therapies have been tried for cyclopeptide-containing mushrooms. Initial decontamination measures with oral activated charcoal are recommended if the patient presents within 1 hour of ingestion and has not already vomited. Suggested therapies in the literature that may be immediately available include *N*-acetylcysteine (NAC), high dose IV penicillin, and early hemodialysis or hemoperfusion.[23] NAC is thought to work via hepatoprotective effects, and animal studies indicate that amatoxins deplete glutathione stores. IV NAC dosing regimens are similar to those administered to acetaminophen poisoned patients (see Chapter 138). High dose penicillin is thought to work by displacing

amatoxin uptake by the hepatocytes. Experimental antidotes such as thioctic acid, silibinin, and *polymyxin* B, have been more commonly used in Europe. Silibinin, the main isomer of silymarin, found in milk thistle, is currently available as an investigational agent. It works as an antioxidant, free radical scavenger, and can restore glutathione stores.[24] If a cyclopeptide-containing mushroom has been ingested, we suggest mobilizing silibinin by calling the regional poison control center to coordinate management and prioritization of agents. The use of oral milk thistle extract, a common health supplement product, has been reported in areas where the IV formulation is not available. However, its use has not been adequately studied to be routinely recommended as a therapeutic option. Patients who progress to fulminant hepatic failure despite appropriate supportive care may ultimately require liver transplantation.[25] Consultation with a transplant center should be initiated early in the course of management.

Disposition

Patients showing evidence of severe hepatotoxicity and those at risk for fulminant hepatic failure should be admitted to an intensive care unit. These patients require frequent neurological checks, continuous vital sign monitoring, and serial laboratory studies. If a patient presents with established hepatotoxicity, transferring to a tertiary-care center that specializes in the management of patients with hepatic failure with liver transplant capabilities is recommended.

Gyromitrin-containing Mushrooms
Principles of Toxicity

Gyromitrin-containing species are also known as the *false morel*. Like the cyclopeptide-containing mushrooms, these can also cause significant hepatotoxicity[26] but may also cause neurotoxicity, particularly seizures and altered mental status. The mechanism for seizures is similar to INH by causing deficiency of pyridoxine and inhibiting the action of glutamic acid decarboxylase. This prevents the formation of GABA, an inhibitory neurotransmitter.[27] These mushrooms can also induce some degree of oxidant stress, which can clinically manifest as methemoglobinemia.

Clinical Features

Similar to the cyclopeptide-containing group, gyromitrin mushrooms can cause delayed nausea, vomiting, diarrhea, and hepatotoxicity, but most notably manifest with generalized seizure activity.

Differential Diagnoses

The highly sought-after *true morel* is an edible delicacy and is considered nontoxic. The *false morel* has a close resemblance and can be found in similar regions. Other causes of seizures and neurotoxicity should be considered, including INH poisoning, sympathomimetic toxicity, intracranial bleeds, brain mass lesions, and underlying seizure disorders. Other causes of methemoglobinemia include ingestion of nitrate and nitrate-containing compounds, local anesthetic agents, dapsone, and inborn errors in metabolism.

Diagnostic Testing

In patients presenting with seizure activity, obtaining a history of toxic ingestion obviates the need for most diagnostic testing. Because there is potential for hepatoxicity, serial liver transaminases should be monitored. Serum electrolytes should be monitored for protracted vomiting or diarrhea. A screening methemoglobin level is also recommended.

Management

Management of gyromitrin-induced seizures should include IV pyridoxine, as recommended for INH poisoning, with 5 g as an empirical dose (see

Chapter 124). Clinically significant methemoglobinemia can be managed with methylene blue, although this is a rare occurrence. Methylene blue dosing is typically 2 mg/kg IV, which can be repeated within 30 to 60 minutes as needed. (See Chapters 55 and 148 for dosing of methylene blue.)

Disposition

Patients with altered mental status and seizures requiring pyridoxine therapy should be admitted to an intensive care setting. Those who are asymptomatic after 6 to 8 hours observation the ED may be discharged home.

OTHER MUSHROOM CLASSES

Cholinergic Agonists

True cholinergic agonists are rarely encountered in the clinical setting. *Clitocybe dealbata*, also known as "the sweater," is one of these mushrooms. If ingested, clinical symptoms of cholinergic excess may be seen. Muscarinic effects recalled by the mnemonic SLUGBAM, can be useful. **SLUGBAM** stands for **S**alivation, **L**acrimation, **U**rination (excessive), **G**astrointestinal effects (nausea, vomiting, and diarrhea), **B**radycardia/bronchorrhea/**b**ronchospam, **A**bdominal cramps, and **M**iosis. Treatment is supportive, but atropine can be used for excessive cholinergic symptoms, as described in Chapter 152. Unlike organophosphates, there is no role for oxime therapy.

Disulfiram Reaction-Inducing Mushrooms

Coprinus atramentarius and other *Coprinus* species contain the toxin coprine that can inhibit aldehyde dehydrogenase similar to disulfiram. If ingested along with ethanol, it can lead to a disulfiram-like reaction including nausea, vomiting, diarrhea and flushing. Treatment is generally supportive, including IV hydration and antiemetics, such as prochlorperazine, or ondansetron (Fig. 153.10).

Hallucinogenic Mushrooms

There are a wide variety of mushrooms that can lead to hallucinations. Some common examples include the *Psilocybe* and *Conocybe* species. These are direct hallucinogens and contain psilocybin and related compounds. Psilocybin is found in a wide range of mushrooms. These are well known to be available for purchase online and in "grow at home" kits.[28] Possession of these types of mushrooms has recently been decriminalized in the State of Colorado.

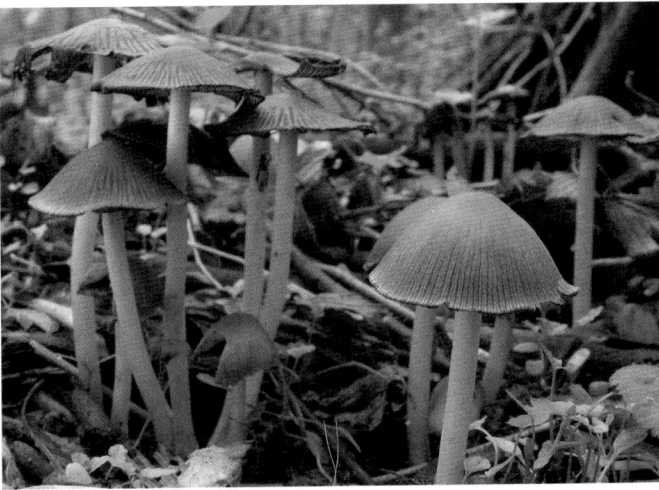

Fig. 153.10 Coprinus atramentarius (Courtesy Joe McFarland.)

The ibotenic acid and muscimol containing mushrooms can also lead to hallucinations. *Amanita muscaria* is an important example of this class. Others include *Amanita pantherina* and *Gemmata* species. Ibotenic acid acts similarly to glutamate and can have excitatory effects. Muscimol has inhibitory effects and works as a GABA agonist. These mushrooms are used for their hallucinogenic effect and both CNS excitation and depression can be seen.

Overdose of these mushrooms can lead to nausea, vomiting, diarrhea, abdominal pain, dry mouth, dilated pupils, tachycardia, agitation, delirium, coma and seizures.[29] The mainstay of treatment of hallucinogenic mushrooms is providing a low-stimulus environment where the effects can dissipate. Benzodiazepines are generally effective in treating the agitation and tachycardia (lorazepam, 1 to 2 mg IVP; diazepam, 5 to 10 mg IVP). Antipsychotic agents can be used for prolonged hallucinations not improved with benzodiazepines (e.g., haloperidol, 2 to 5 mg IM or droperidol, 1.25 to 2.5 mg IM).

Gastrointestinal Irritants

There are hundreds of species of mushrooms that are GI irritants. These mushrooms will cause irritation to the GI tract within 2 to 3 hours of ingestion. Some commonly encountered species of GI irritants include *Boletus* sp., *Chlorophyllum molybdites*, *Lactarius* sp, and *Omphalotus* sp. Nausea, vomiting, diarrhea, and crampy abdominal pain will be the typical presenting symptoms. The course is generally self-limited, but care should be taken to monitor patients with prolonged symptoms or with significant fluid losses.

Another consideration with mushrooms ingested that cause GI symptoms is that the mushroom will be contaminated with pesticides or metals. Therefore, the symptoms may not be from the mushroom itself but from the chemical contaminant.

Renal Insufficiency

Two species of mushrooms can potentially lead to direct renal toxicity. In Europe, the *Cortinarius* species of mushrooms have been associated with renal failure.[30] Similar to the deadly cyclopeptide and gyromitirin-containing mushrooms, symptoms commonly occur on a delayed basis and as long as 2 weeks after ingestion. This mushroom is not generally found in the US.

A more problematic mushroom that is found in the Pacific Northwest is the *Amanita smithiana* mushroom. The toxin contained in this mushroom is allenic norleucine, which can have serious nephrotoxic effects. This mushroom leads to GI symptoms early after ingestion, and thus violates the general rule that serious poisoning follows delayed onset of GI symptoms. GI symptoms can begin between 2 and 12 hours after ingestion. Treatment is generally supportive, including fluid bolus followed by maintenance. However, with acute renal failure, metabolic acidosis, and electrolyte imbalances, hemodialysis may be required.

Rhabdomyolysis-Inducing Mushrooms

Another mushroom that can cause toxicity on a delayed basis is *Tricholoma equestre* (commonly referred to as the "man on horseback" or "yellow knight" mushroom). It can cause weakness, fatigue, and muscle pain 24 to 72 hours after ingestion. This mushroom can cause clinically significant rhabdomyolysis. Serial serum CPK levels should be followed to monitor for rhabdomyolysis and development of renal failure. Treatment is supportive with IV hydration and alkalinization therapy.

HERBAL MEDICATIONS

Although much of the world's population has used herbal products as medicine for centuries, its growing popularity in the United States has been a relatively recent trend. Since the passage of the Dietary Supplement Health and Education Act (DSHEA) in 1994, the number of herbal products on the market has sharply increased from 4000 to 90,000 in 2014.[31] It is estimated that nearly 40 million US adults use herbal products with sales exceeding $5 billion annually.

PRINCIPLES OF TOXICITY

The DSHEA established herbal products as food, and unlike pharmaceuticals, they are not subject to rigorous regulations and do not need to demonstrate efficacy or safety for commercial sale. As a result, ingredients and their concentrations are often unknown, and controlled clinical trials and toxicologic testing are not routinely performed. The consumer may believe that herbal medications undergo strict regulation and testing, and are safer and more efficacious than pharmaceuticals. This misperception, combined with a lack of proper dosing and scheduling regimen, may lead to misuse and over-use of herbal medications. Factors that further contribute to adverse events include inherent toxicity, contamination and adulteration of products, and herb-drug interaction.[32] Studies show that most people who use herbal medications in addition to prescribed medications will do so without consulting or notifying their health care providers.

Clinical research in the area of herb-drug interaction is lacking.[33] Most pharmaceutical drugs undergo hepatic biotransformation and inactivation via the cytochrome P_{450} enzymes. Herb-drug interactions typically stem from alteration of this system, leading to increased or decreased drug concentration. Herbal medications may also affect drug transporters, such a p-glycoprotein, and further modify pharmacodynamics. Herb-drug interactions are best documented in the use of St. John's Wort (Hypericum perforatum) (Fig. 153.11).[34] It induces cytochrome P_{450}, family 3, subfamily A (CYP3A), which metabolizes approximately 50% of available US pharmaceuticals, leading to decreased drug concentrations.

CLINICAL FEATURES

Many herbal medications possess toxicity inherent to the botanical from which they are derived (Table 153.3). Adverse effects can range from allergic reactions to cardiovascular and hepatic toxicity.[35–39] The Food and Drug Administration (FDA) banned the sale of Ma Huang (Ephedra sinica) in 2004 after reports of serious cardiovascular events and death related to its sympathomimetic effects. Many herbal medications, including Germander (Teucrium chamaedrys), Pennyroyal oil (Mentha pulegium

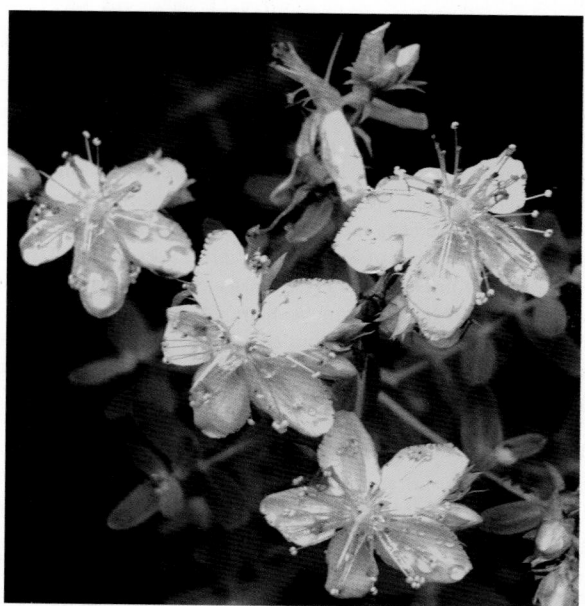

Fig. 153.11 Hypericum perforatum (St. John's wort). (Courtesy Christopher Lim.)

TABLE 153.3 Mushrooms

Early Onset Symptoms (First 2–3 h)

Clinical Category	Symptoms	Treatment
Gastrointestinal irritants (Boletus sp., Chlorophyllum sp., Lactarius sp.)	Nausea, vomiting, diarrhea	Supportive care
Hallucinogens (Psilocybe and Conocybe sp., Amanita muscaria, Amanita pantherina)	Agitation, hallucinations	Benzodiazepines Low stimulus environment
Disulfiram (Coprinus sp.)	Nausea, vomiting, diarrhea, abdominal cramping, flushing	Supportive
Cholinergic (Clitocybe sp.)	SLUGBAM (Salivation, lacrimation, Urination, GI Distress, Bronchorrhea, Bradycardia, Bronchospasm, Abdominal cramps, Miosis)	Atropine
Renal (Amanita smithiana)	Renal insufficiency (GI symptoms early)	Supportive Hemodialysis

Late Onset Symptoms (>4–5 h)

Mushroom Group Hepatotoxic	Symptoms	Treatment
Cyclopeptide-containing (Amanita phalloides, Amanita bisporigera, Lepiota sp., Galerina sp.)	Hepatic failure, symptoms begin 6–8 h post-ingestion	Supportive, NAC, Dialysis, Penicillin, Thioctic acid Silibinin, Liver transplant
Gyromitrin (Gyromitra esculenta)	Hepatic failure, Seizures, Supportive, Vitamin B6, Methylene blue	Methemoglobinemia
Renal (Cortinarius sp.)	Delayed onset renal failure	Supportive, Dialysis
Rhabodomyolysis (Tricholoma equestre, Russula subnigricans)	Muscle pain, weakness, fatigue	Supportive, hydration, Hemodialysis

and *Hedeoma pulegoides*), and those containing pyrrolizidine alkaloids are associated with hepatotoxicity.[39] Most herbal medications that possess inherent toxicity can have adverse maternal-fetal effects, and we advise against the routine use of herbal medications during pregnancy.

Some herbal medications increase bleeding risk by altering the pharmacokinetics of anticoagulants, such as warfarin, or having a synergistic effect with antiplatelet agents and anticoagulants.[40] The concurrent use of several herbal medications, such as St. John's wort, with other serotonergic drugs can potentially contribute to the development of serotonin syndrome. Kava Kava *(Piper methisticum)* and Valerian *(Valerian officinalis)* have been shown to potentiate the GABA-mediated CNS depression from alcohol consumption.

DIFFERENTIAL DIAGNOSES

Due to the unregulated nature of herbal medications, contaminants and adulterants are often present and sometimes result in toxicity. In addition to fillers and substituents, contamination with heavy metals, pesticides and other harmful materials has been found in herbal medications. Certain metals are believed to have therapeutic properties. Lead is the most commonly reported heavy metal contaminant, but arsenic, cadmium, and mercury poisoning after herbal medication use have been described as well.[32] Additionally, there are many examples reported in the literature of toxicity from herbal medications adulterated with pharmaceuticals.

DIAGNOSTIC TESTING

Diagnostic studies in patients presenting with herbal medication toxicity include a complete blood count, coagulation profile, serum electrolytes, glucose, hepatic, and renal function tests. In addition, acetaminophen and salicylate levels should be measured along with urinary heavy metal screens, targeting lead, arsenic, and mercury.

MANAGEMENT

Treatment is largely supportive, with hydration, bleeding control if coagulopathic, cardiac dysrhythmia treatment, and targeted antidote therapy (e.g., NAC, heavy metal chelation therapy; see Chapter 146).

DISPOSITION

The majority of patients with herbal medication toxicity will be mildly symptomatic with GI symptoms and normal diagnostic testing. These patients can be observed and hydrated in the ED and safely discharged home. Patients with systemic toxicity including hepatic, renal, cardiac or multi-organ failure require admission for monitoring and consultation from appropriate services.

The references for this chapter can be found online at ExpertConsult. com.

154

Sedative-Hypnotics

Daniel L. Overbeek and Timothy B. Erickson

KEY CONCEPTS

- Supportive care, with a focus on respiratory depression, is the foundation of management of all sedative-hypnotic ingestions.
- Benzodiazepines are commonly used medications both medically and recreationally. Coingestions with other sedative-hypnotic agents can potentiate their neurologic and respiratory effects.
- Barbiturate medications are less commonly prescribed, and intoxications are infrequent. Most patients recover with supportive care alone.
- A positive urine toxicology screen for benzodiazepines or barbiturates does not prove a causal linkage between the drug and the current clinical condition.
- We do not recommend routine use of flumazenil for benzodiazepine toxicity, particularly in chronic benzodiazepine users in whom flumazenil can precipitate seizures. Due to the short duration of action of flumazenil, when administered, patients should be monitored closely for recurrence of respiratory depression.
- Chloral hydrate toxicity may result in sedation and cardiotoxicity, principally in the form of supraventricular tachycardias, which are best treated with a short-acting beta blocker.
- Withdrawal from sedative-hypnotic use, including benzodiazepines, barbiturates and gamma hydroxybutyrate (GHB), can be life threatening. Management often requires high doses of benzodiazepines or barbiturates.

FOUNDATIONS

The sedative-hypnotic toxidrome encompasses depressed mental status, decreased respiratory rate, and suppressed response to stimuli. Within this chapter, we will discuss a variety of medications and agents that can induce a sedative-hypnotic toxidrome at therapeutic or toxic doses. Also, the general treatment recommendations and specific considerations for individual agents will be presented.

Most sedative-hypnotics have effects mediated through the gamma-aminobutyric acid (GABA) neurotransmitter system. GABA is the primary inhibitory neurotransmitter, and the GABA-A receptor is a protein complex found on postsynaptic membranes in the CNS. Structurally, it consists of several distinct receptor sites surrounding a chloride ion (Cl^-) channel (Fig. 154.1), which is opened by GABA binding. The resulting flow of Cl^- into the cell increases the negative resting potential, hyperpolarizing and stabilizing of the membrane. The net effect is a diminished ability of the nerve cell to initiate an action potential, inhibiting neural transmission. There are separate receptor sites for barbiturates and for benzodiazepines and a third site that binds GABA, ethanol, and meprobamate. Increasing either the frequency or duration of GABA stimulation in the nervous system causes most of the effects seen in the sedative-hypnotic toxidrome, including blunted responses to stimuli and sedation.

Sedative-hypnotic drugs, especially benzodiazepines, are among the most widely prescribed classes of drugs[1] (Table 154.1) and are the most commonly prescribed drugs used in suicide attempts. Pediatric patients comprise 10% of benzodiazepine overdose cases. With the significant proliferation of opioid usage, prevalence of combined benzodiazepine and opioid toxicity with significant risk of respiratory compromise has increased significantly.[2]

BENZODIAZEPINES

Clinical Features

Benzodiazepines are widely used medically for their antiepileptic, sedative, and anxiolytic properties. Prior to benzodiazepines, barbiturates were the primary sedative-hypnotics used, but they have been overwhelmingly supplanted by benzodiazepines and other, newer agents.

Benzodiazepines produce sedative, hypnotic, anxiolytic, and anticonvulsant effects by potentiating the GABA-A receptor in the presence of GABA.[3-5] In contrast, barbiturates can directly increase Cl^- conductance. This may account for the relative safety of benzodiazepines in comparison with barbiturates.

At therapeutic dosage, the GABA effects of benzodiazepines cause euphoria, anxiolysis, and drowsiness. Mild toxicity includes CNS depression, ataxia, slurred speech, nystagmus, and impaired cognition. Most benzodiazepine overdoses follow a relatively benign clinical course. Larger overdoses may cause respiratory depression, which may require intervention. The respiratory depression is less severe than with barbiturates, especially if benzodiazepines are the only substance ingested. Coingestants with sedative properties, particularly ethanol or opioids, can markedly potentiate the respiratory depression caused by benzodiazepines.[6] Loss of muscle tone leads to upper airway obstruction and increased airway resistance. Hypoventilation is often the first sign of severe respiratory depression, and may be masked by oxygen supplementation, which can maintain adequate oxyhemoglobin saturation. Capnography can be useful in detecting early signs of hypoventilation.

Cardiac toxicity or hypotension from pure benzodiazepine overdose is rare. Other potential complications include aspiration pneumonia and pressure necrosis of skin and muscles. Intravenous solutions of diazepam and lorazepam contain the diluent propylene glycol, which is metabolized to lactate, and prolonged or high-dose infusions of these preparations can cause lactic acidosis. Patients with renal or hepatic insufficiency are at increased risk for this complication.

Most pediatric patients have symptoms within four hours of benzodiazepine ingestion. Ataxia is the most common sign of toxicity, occurring in 90% of pediatric patients. Respiratory depression occurs in fewer than 10% of pediatric cases, and hypotension is rarely reported in children.

Benzodiazepines were previously identified as pregnancy category D, noting some risk, but that they should be used when indicated based on a risk-benefit analysis (see Chapter 175 regarding drug therapy for the pregnant patient). There are some studies showing risks, but these are difficult to analyze as most patients involved were also exposed to other psychiatric medications.[7] In the acute setting, when needed for management of emergent conditions including seizures, the benefits of short term acute use likely outweigh the complications to the mother and fetus.[8,9] Management of seizures during pregnancy is discussed in Chapter 173. The management of benzodiazepine toxicity during pregnancy follows the standard approach, including supportive care and respiratory support, with the recognition of an increased risk of respiratory and mental status depression in the fetus if delivery is required.

Novel synthetic benzodiazepines are procured from a variety of internet sites or other illicit sources, and the true content of the product received is unknown to the user. Limited information is available about many of these agents. Management should be similar to the known pharmaceutical benzodiazepines, recognizing the increased likelihood of coingestants, as discussed in the following.[10,11]

Pharmacokinetics

Benzodiazepines are rapidly absorbed orally. Intramuscular use of chlordiazepoxide and diazepam is limited by erratic absorption, but lorazepam and midazolam are predictably absorbed after intramuscular injection. Parenteral and rectal administration of benzodiazepines provide faster time to onset than oral ingestion and can be used for antiepileptic and sedative indications. After absorption, benzodiazepines distribute readily, and rapidly penetrate the blood-brain barrier. In plasma, benzodiazepines are highly protein bound.[12,13]

Benzodiazepines are metabolized in the liver. Lorazepam, oxazepam, and temazepam are directly conjugated to an inactive, water-soluble glucuronide metabolite that is excreted by the kidney. Other benzodiazepines must first be converted by the hepatic cytochrome P450 system. Many benzodiazepines, including chlordiazepoxide and diazepam, are metabolized to active compounds that are then conjugated and excreted. The long elimination half-lives of up to 120 hours of these intermediates can cause accumulation in the body with repeated dosing and prolong the sedative effects of these benzodiazepines.[13] Alprazolam and midazolam are converted to hydroxylated intermediates that are rapidly conjugated and excreted, but do not contribute significantly to the overall effect of the drug.[12]

Cytochrome P450 metabolism may be significantly impaired in elderly patients or those with liver disease, leading to prolonged elimination of benzodiazepines. Coingestion of drugs that inhibit P450 metabolism (e.g., cimetidine, ethanol) also prolongs the half-lives of benzodiazepines.[12]

Differential Diagnoses

Benzodiazepine overdose is usually suspected or diagnosed by clinical presentation. Many patients are able to interact appropriately with providers and can provide supporting information. Atypical or focal neurological findings suggest the presence of other conditions, such as intracranial events (e.g., intracerebral hemorrhage, cerebral ischemia). Profound coma or cardiopulmonary instability is rare with pure benzodiazepine overdose and should prompt the search for coingestants, such as opioids, ethanol, phenobarbital, choral hydrate, or a cyclic antidepressant. Non-toxicologic metabolic causes of CNS depression,

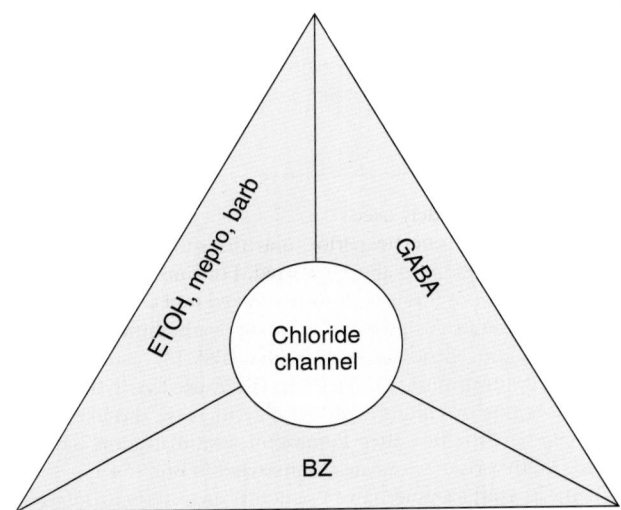

Fig. 154.1 The gamma-aminobutyric acid (GABA) receptor complex. *BZ*, Benzodiazepine binding site; *GABA*, GABA binding site; *ETOH, mepro, barb*, binding sites for ethanol, meprobamate, and barbiturates, respectively.

TABLE 154.1 Benzodiazepines

Name	Usual Dose	Oral Peak (Hours)	Half-Life (Hours)	Parent Metabolite Activity
Alprazolam (Xanax)	0.25–0.5 mg	1–2	6–27	Inactive
Chlordiazepoxide(Librium)	5–25 mg	0.5–4	5–30	Active
Clonazepam (Klonopin)	0.25–0.5 mg	1–2	18–50	Inactive
Clorazepate (Tranxene)	7.5–15 mg	1–2	1–3	Active
Diazepam (Valium)	2–10 mg	0.5–1	20–50	Active
Estazolam (Prosom)	1–2 mg	2	8–28	Inactive
Flurazepam (Dalmane)	15–30 mg	0.5–1	2–3	Active
Halazepam (Paxipam)	20–40 mg	1–3	14	Active
Lorazepam (Ativan)	0.5–2 mg	2–4	10–20	Inactive
Midazolam (Versed)	10–20 mg	1–2	1.5–3	Active
Oxazepam (Serax)	10–30 mg	2–4	5–20	Inactive
Quazepam (Doral)	7.5–15 mg	2	39–41	Active
Temazepam (Restoril)	7.5–30 mg	1–2	3–19	Inactive
Triazolam (Halcion)	0.125–0.25 mg	1–2	1.5–5.5	Inactive

such as hypoglycemia or hyponatremia should also be considered. The broader differential of CNS depression includes conditions described in Chapters 12 and 13.

Diagnostic Testing

Sedative-hypnotic toxidromes are clinical diagnoses, and most laboratory testing will not be helpful in determining the appropriate care for the patient. Any patient with altered mental status should have a blood glucose level rapidly determined. Qualitative immunoassays for benzodiazepines in urine are available, but do not aid management decisions and cannot provide definitive information regarding the cause of the altered mental status. Because most screening tests detect a specific benzodiazepine metabolite, including nordiazepam or oxazepam glucuronide, some benzodiazepines (including clonazepam, lorazepam, midazolam, and alprazolam) will not be detected on many standard urine drug tests. A positive urine drug screen for benzodiazepines indicates exposure or use but does not identify intoxication or indicate a specific agent and does not confirm benzodiazepine exposure as the cause of the clinical presentation. The positive screen also does not provide information regarding the timing of the benzodiazepine exposure. Serum drug concentrations are not routinely available and do not correlate with clinical severity.[14]

Adjunct testing should be used as clinically indicated, including computerized topography (CT) imaging when concerned for head trauma or intracranial hemorrhage. The benzodiazepine antagonist flumazenil should not be routinely administered to patients with suspected benzodiazepine overdose or coma of unknown origin solely for diagnostic purposes.[15]

MANAGEMENT

Stabilization and Supportive Care

Initial stabilization, including endotracheal intubation when necessary, should not be delayed by the administration of an antidote. Most benzodiazepine overdoses can be managed expectantly with observation and supportive care alone. Neither gastrointestinal (GI) decontamination or administration of activated charcoal is indicated in benzodiazepine ingestion. Close respiratory monitoring is indicated to guide respiratory interventions and end tidal carbon dioxide (CO_2) monitoring can be a useful adjunct. Naloxone should be administered in cases of suspected opioid coingestion (see further discussion of opioid overdoses in Chapter 151).

Antidote Therapy

Flumazenil, a nonspecific competitive antagonist at the benzodiazepine receptor, can reverse benzodiazepine-induced sedation after general anesthesia, procedural sedation, and confirmed benzodiazepine overdose. However, the risks of flumazenil usually outweigh the benefits in patients with benzodiazepine toxicity. Therefore, flumazenil is not recommended for the routine reversal of sedative overdose in the ED.[15] Theoretic benefits of flumazenil use include cost savings and avoidance of procedures and tests (such as endotracheal intubation and CT scans). However, several clinical studies have failed to demonstrate these benefits in practice.[15] Benzodiazepine toxicity has a low mortality rate with supportive care, shifting the risk benefit analysis away from the use of flumazenil in routine cases.

There are also risks associated with flumazenil; it can precipitate acute withdrawal in patients who are chronically dependent on benzodiazepines, leading to significant complications including status epilepticus. Similarly, this antidote is hazardous when it is given to patients who have coingested seizure-inducing drugs (such as cocaine or a tricyclic antidepressant) because of loss of the benzodiazepine's

BOX 154.1 Use of Flumazenil

Indications
Isolated benzodiazepine overdose in non-habituated user (e.g., accidental pediatric exposure)
Reversal of conscious sedation

Absolute Contraindications
Suspected coingestant that lowers seizure threshold (e.g., tricyclic antidepressants, cocaine, lithium, methylxanthines, isoniazid, propoxyphene, monoamine oxidase inhibitors, bupropion, diphenhydramine, carbamazepine, cyclosporine, chloral hydrate)
Patient taking benzodiazepine for control of a potentially life-threatening condition (e.g., seizures)
Concurrent sedative-hypnotic withdrawal
Seizure activity or myoclonus
Hypersensitivity to flumazenil or benzodiazepines
Patient with neuromuscular blockade

Relative Contraindications
Chronic benzodiazepine use, not taken for control of life-threatening condition
Known seizure disorder not treated with benzodiazepines
Head injury
Chronic alcoholism

protective anticonvulsant properties and the subsequent ineffectiveness of benzodiazepines to abort a seizure if one occurs. Seizures after the administration of flumazenil should be treated with the administration of barbiturates or propofol. Cardiac dysrhythmias (principally paroxysmal supraventricular tachycardia [PSVT]) can occur after flumazenil administration. Coingestants that cause dysrhythmias, such as carbamazepine or chloral hydrate, may increase the likelihood of cardiac effects. Fatalities after flumazenil administration have been reported.[15] Other risk factors are summarized in Box 154.1.

When benzodiazepine-naive patients ingest benzodiazepines alone in overdose (as occurs in young children), the risks associated with flumazenil are lower.[15] In cases of benzodiazepine overdose by a non-benzodiazepine habituated patient, flumazenil use combined with close monitoring and repeated or infusion-based dosing, may obviate the need for intubation and mechanical ventilation. We recommend basing this decision on a balance of risks/benefits for the particular patient and the reliability that the patient is a novice benzodiazepine user. This approach extends to the setting of unintended over-sedation by benzodiazepines for procedural sedation. In these cases, as patients are often nonbenzodiazepine-dependent, flumazenil would likely have a lower risk of complications.

The initial adult dose of flumazenil is 0.2 mg given intravenously over 30 seconds. A second dose of 0.2 mg may be given, followed by 0.2 mg dose at 1-minute intervals to a total of 1 mg. In children, the initial dose is 0.01 mg/kg (up to 0.2 mg). Because the duration of action of flumazenil is short (45 to 75 minutes), re-sedation occurs in up to 65% of patients and requires either re-dosing or continuous infusion (0.25 to 1.0 mg/h). It is important to note that flumazenil reverses the CNS depressant effects of benzodiazepines more than it reverses the respiratory depression.

In summary, benzodiazepine overdose requires primarily supportive care, assisted ventilation, and if severe, intubation. Flumazenil may precipitate seizures or acute withdrawal and should be used only in highly selected cases (such as to reverse procedural sedation, or to treat young children with a clear history of inadvertent benzodiazepine ingestion). When flumazenil is used, close monitoring of oxy-hemoglobin saturation and overall ventilatory status (ideally including end-tidal CO_2) is necessary because of the risk for recurrent respiratory depression or resedation.[15]

Disposition

Patients remaining asymptomatic after 4 to 6 hours of ED observation following benzodiazepine ingestion may be medically cleared. For cases of deliberate overdose, appropriate psychiatric consultation should be obtained. Patients presenting with respiratory depression and coma should be given oxygen, ventilatory support, and admission to a monitored setting, such as an ED Observation Unit, or monitored inpatient unit.

Benzodiazepine Withdrawal Syndrome

Abrupt discontinuation of a benzodiazepine in a chronic user results in a characteristic constellation of symptoms similar to ethanol withdrawal (Box 154.2). Risk for withdrawal is a function of both the dose of benzodiazepine and the duration of its use. Continuous treatment for more than 3 to 4 months is generally required before a patient is at risk for withdrawal. With abrupt discontinuation of a benzodiazepine, the most severe withdrawal symptoms occur within several days to a week. Treatment of withdrawal consists of restarting benzodiazepines in the acute setting and, if refractory, phenobarbital or propofol administration to treat withdrawal symptoms. Patients who have experienced withdrawal symptoms after cessation of benzodiazepine use may require benzodiazepine tapers to avoid symptomatic withdrawal.

BARBITURATES

Clinical Features

Barbiturates, once commonly prescribed as sedative-hypnotic agents, are generally used now only for management of some seizure disorders and withdrawal states. Mortality from barbiturate poisoning declined from approximately 1500 deaths per year in the 1950s to fewer than five fatalities in 2017.[16]

Barbiturates are addictive, producing physical dependence and a potentially life-threatening withdrawal syndrome similar to that of benzodiazepines. Whereas tolerance to the mood-altering effects of barbiturates develops rapidly with repeated use, tolerance to the lethal effects including respiratory depression develops more slowly, and the risk of severe toxicity increases with the dose escalation that often accompanies continued use.

Barbiturates depress the activity of excitable cells, especially those in the central nervous system (CNS), by enhancing the activity of GABA. In acute overdose, barbiturates decrease neural transmission in autonomic ganglia, the myocardium, and the GI tract, also inhibiting the response to acetylcholine at the neuromuscular junction.

Barbiturates produce dose-related depressive effects ranging from mild sedation to coma and respiratory arrest. Mild barbiturate toxicity manifests with drowsiness, slurred speech, ataxia, unsteady gait, nystagmus, emotional lability, and impaired cognition. In severe acute intoxication, CNS depression progresses from stupor to deep coma and respiratory arrest. The life threat in severe barbiturate toxicity is

respiratory depression, from direct barbiturate action on the respiratory centers in the medulla. Because respirations can be rapid but shallow, the degree of hypoventilation may not be apparent on clinical examination, and pulse oximetry or capnography may be needed to detect the ventilation compromise. Barbiturate-induced respiratory depression can be significantly potentiated by the addition of other respiratory depressants, particularly opioids. High barbiturate levels depress GI motility, delaying drug absorption. As the drug is metabolized and blood levels drop, peristalsis and drug absorption may increase, causing drug levels to rise again.

Therapeutic doses cause anxiolysis and euphoria, and mild decreases in pulse rate and blood pressure, similar to sleep. With toxic doses, more significant hypotension occurs from direct depression of the myocardium along with pooling of blood in a dilated venous system. Peripheral vascular resistance is usually normal or increased, but barbiturates interfere with autonomic reflexes, which then do not adequately compensate for the myocardial depression and decreased venous return. Barbiturates can precipitate severe hypotension in patients whose compensatory reflexes are already maximally stimulated, such as those with heart failure or hypovolemic shock. Barbiturates also decrease cerebral blood flow and intracerebral pressure. Although hypnotic doses of barbiturates do not affect gastric emptying, higher doses can decrease GI smooth muscle tone and peristaltic contractions, delaying gastric emptying.

Hypotension is common in patients with severe intoxication, along with a normal or increased heart rate. Barbiturate overdose is also associated with noncardiogenic pulmonary edema or acute lung injury. Altered pulmonary capillary permeability can be caused by hypoperfusion, hypoxia, or a direct effect of the drug.

Barbiturates are classified according to their onset and duration of action (Box 154.3). Only long-acting preparations have anticonvulsant effects in doses that do not cause sedation. Short- and intermediate-acting preparations are almost completely metabolized to inactive metabolites in the liver, whereas 25% of a phenobarbital (long-acting) dose is excreted unchanged through the kidney.

Barbiturates cross the placenta with fetal levels approaching those of the mother. They are also excreted in low concentration in breast milk. Use during pregnancy is associated with birth defects (category D).

Barbiturate withdrawal syndrome includes tremors, hallucinations, seizures, and delirium, which is similar to the delirium tremens of ethanol withdrawal or benzodiazepine withdrawal discussed previously. However, severe withdrawal occurs only after dependence on short- or intermediate-acting barbiturates (e.g., pentobarbital, secobarbital, amobarbital, or butalbital). Because these drugs are less commonly used, this syndrome is now rare.

Differential Diagnoses

Mild barbiturate toxicity mimics ethanol intoxication and that of other sedative-hypnotic agents such as benzodiazepines. Barbiturate intoxication causes relatively more respiratory depression and hypotension than ethanol compared to benzodiazepine toxicities. Chloral hydrate overdose is marked by greater cardiotoxicity (discussed later in this chapter). Gamma-hydroxybutyrate (GHB) produces coma just like barbiturates, but resolution of the coma occurs much more rapidly. Opioids cause similar sedation with a greater degree of respiratory depression, which reverses rapidly with the administration of naloxone. Other common antiepileptic agents (such as, carbamazepine, phenytoin, and valproic acid) will cause sedation similar to barbiturates with acute overdose. As with any patient exhibiting depressed mental status, metabolic causes (such as, hypoglycemia or hyponatremia) and intracranial events (such as, cerebral ischemia or hemorrhage) should be excluded.

BOX 154.2 Benzodiazepine Withdrawal Symptoms

Nonspecific
Anxiety, depression, insomnia, tremor, tachycardia, sweating

Severe (Rare)
Visual hallucinations, delirium, seizures

BOX 154.3   Barbiturates

Ultrashort Acting
Methohexital (Brevital)
Thiopental (Pentothal)

Short and Intermediate Acting
Pentobarbital (Nembutal)
Secobarbital (Seconal)
Amobarbital (Amytal)
Aprobarbital (Alurate)
Butabarbital (Butisol)
Butalbital (Fiorinal)

Long Acting
Phenobarbital (Solfoton, Luminal)
Mephobarbital (Mebaral)

Diagnostic Testing

Generally, laboratory testing is not helpful in the acute management of barbiturate toxicity, except to exclude metabolic or electrolyte disorder. A positive urine screen establishes only qualitative exposure to a barbiturate but does not prove that the drug is present in toxic amounts and should not be relied on to explain decreased mental status. A quantitative serum phenobarbital level can be obtained to document toxicity (therapeutic levels range 10 to 40 mcg/mL) but rarely guide management. Other than phenobarbital, barbiturates have high volumes of distribution, so serum levels do not accurately reflect CNS concentrations or correlate with clinical severity and these levels are not rapidly available.

A chest radiograph can detect noncardiogenic pulmonary edema, acute lung injury or aspiration pneumonia. Computed tomography (CT) of the head may be helpful in comatose patients with evidence of trauma, focal neurologic signs, papilledema, or no otherwise identifiable cause of stupor and coma.

Because the electroencephalogram may be silent as a result of barbiturate overdose, in patients with coma, brain death should not be determined if phenobarbital is present in the serum at therapeutic levels or higher.[17]

MANAGEMENT

Supportive Care and Stabilization

Barbiturates have no specific antidote, and management is supportive care, particularly with respect to the cardiovascular and respiratory systems. Severely intoxicated patients are unable to protect their airway and have a decreased ventilatory drive. Supplemental oxygen may suffice for patients with mild to moderate overdose, but intubation and mechanical ventilation is often required. Fluid replacement should be limited to maintain a systolic blood pressure above 90 mm Hg and adequate urine output as patients may be at risk of pulmonary edema.

Gastrointestinal Decontamination

Gastric emptying by lavage is not indicated. High barbiturate levels depress GI motility, delaying drug absorption. As the drug is metabolized and blood levels drop, peristalsis and drug absorption may increase, causing drug levels to again rise. Although multidose activated charcoal increases clearance of phenobarbital via hepato-enteric circulation and may shorten the duration of clinical toxicity, there is no convincing evidence it results in improved outcome over supportive care alone and we do not recommend its routine use.

Enhanced Elimination

Because phenobarbital is a weak acid (pKa 7.2), alkalinization of the urine will increase the amount of drug present in ionized form, minimizing tubular reabsorption and increasing drug clearance. Short- and intermediate-acting barbiturates are not significantly affected by pH changes in this range. Alkalinization may interfere with the ability of the drug to diffuse across intestinal mucosa from the gut into the blood. There is limited evidence, regarding the clinical benefits of alkalinization in the setting of barbiturate toxicity,[18] and we do not recommend its routine use.

Despite a lack of compelling data demonstrating, its benefit in acute phenobarbital overdose, hemodialysis is a legitimate option for severe phenobarbital toxicity.[19,20] Phenobarbital is 40% to 60% protein bound, and newer, high-efficiency dialyzers using high blood flow rates provide drug clearance greater than that achieved by hemoperfusion. Cases with pharmacokinetic data have documented significant elimination of barbiturates with hemodialysis. Although rarely indicated, we recommend hemodialysis for acute phenobarbital toxicity (persistent serum levels over 100 mcg/mL) in the presence of prolonged coma, refractory hypotension, renal or cardiac failure, metabolic acidosis, or inadequate response to less invasive measures (such as supportive care and mechanical ventilation).[19] Although potentially efficacious with severe toxicity, we are not aware of studies assessing the role of extracorporeal membrane oxygenation (ECMO) in cases of refractory barbiturate poisoning, and until further studied, would not recommend its use over hemodialysis.

Disposition

Asymptomatic patients presenting after barbiturate ingestion should be observed for 6 hours for mental status changes, slurred speech, ataxia, hypotension, and respiratory depression. Symptoms generally occur within 1 hour of ingestion. Patients who remain asymptomatic and have no significant complicating coingestants can be discharged or referred for psychiatric evaluation. Patients who are symptomatic after 6 hours should be admitted to a monitored setting in hospital or an ED observation unit for respiratory monitoring and supportive care. Those with persistent hypotension, severe depression of mental status, or respiratory depression requiring intubation and ventilator support will need intensive care monitoring. Psychiatry or social services consultation is undertaken when the patient with intentional ingestion is medically cleared.

INDIVIDUAL MEDICATIONS

Zolpidem, Zaleplon, and Zopiclone

Zolpidem (Ambien), zaleplon (Sonata), and zopiclone (Imovane) differ in structure from the benzodiazepines and act selectively at the benzodiazepine receptor, producing sedation without many of the side effects seen with benzodiazepines. They have modest anxiolytic, muscle relaxant, and anticonvulsant properties. Significant drug interactions are rare.[21] Transient visual disturbances, transient global amnesia, hallucinations, and somnambulism can occur in patients with normal levels of consciousness with both zolpidem and zaleplon. Over ingestion of zolpidem is limited by vomiting, which may occur after a supratherapeutic dose. Both zolpidem and zaleplon are rapidly eliminated and lack active metabolites. A controlled-release formulation of zolpidem (Ambien CR) is also available. The dual-layered tablet releases an immediate dose of zolpidem, followed by a slow, extended release from the inner layer to maintain plasma zolpidem concentrations. Overdoses with the controlled-release formulation mirror those of the immediate-release preparation, with only small differences in the likelihood of drowsiness, hallucinations, and ataxia. Of the three "Z-drugs," zopiclone has the longest duration of action, and may have longer duration of symptoms in toxic ingestions.

Zolpidem overdose is managed by supportive care. Fatalities from isolated zolpidem overdose are rare[21] and are associated with coingestants, particularly other sedative-hypnotics or antipsychotics. Drowsiness is the most common symptom; coma and respiratory failure are rare, despite overdoses of up to 40 times the normal dose. Intubation may be required for airway protection or ventilatory support, particularly if there are coingestants that exacerbate respiratory depression. Zolpidem overdose in children which generally follows a similarly benign course. Drowsiness, ataxia, and hallucinations generally resolve within eight hours. Patients who remain asymptomatic after six hours can be discharged.

Adverse effects with therapeutic zaleplon use include headache, anterograde amnesia, and transient visual hallucinations. Overdose information is limited, but patients generally experience CNS depression and mild hypotension. Flumazenil administration is not advised.[21] The blue-green discoloration of gastric contents, oral cavity, and urine after zaleplon overdose is attributed to the indigo carmine dye present in zaleplon's capsule shell.

Minimal data are available on the toxicity of zopiclone, which is not currently available as a commercial product in the United States. There have been multiple reported deaths with zopiclone ingestion;[23] however most of these have associated coingestants. Zopiclone has a notably high prevalence of toxicity in areas where its prescription is uncontrolled. General principles should follow the sedative-hypnotics discussed previously, including supportive care with respiratory intervention when indicated.

Eszopiclone

Eszopiclone (Lunesta) has been marketed in the United States for treatment of insomnia. It is the S-isomer of racemic zopiclone, which has been used for decades outside the United States. Eszopiclone has a structure unrelated to that of benzodiazepines or barbiturates.

The mechanism of eszopiclone's action involves a specific GABA-A receptor close to or coupled with the benzodiazepine receptor. Eszopiclone is rapidly absorbed, with a peak serum level at 1 hour and a half-life of 6 hours. It is metabolized in the liver to minimally active metabolites. The maximum hypnotic dose is 3 mg. It is recommended that elderly patients and those with hepatic insufficiency be treated with a lower (1 mg) dose.

Adverse effects with therapeutic use of eszopiclone include drowsiness, dizziness, dry mouth, unpleasant taste, nausea, and vomiting. Auditory and visual hallucinations have been reported. Experience with eszopiclone overdose is limited. Treatment is supportive. CNS depression may be prolonged and pronounced in elderly patients. Most reported eszopiclone ingestions had mild to moderate symptoms.

Buspirone

Buspirone (BuSpar) is often prescribed for generalized anxiety disorder because of its lack of sedative effect. Even when combined with ethanol, CNS depression is minimal. Buspirone acts on the serotonin (5HT-1A) receptor and antagonizes dopamine (D2) receptors, unlike the mechanism of action of benzodiazepines discussed above. There are rare case reports of toxicity in overdose, including a death reported in single-drug buspirone overdose.[16] A withdrawal state after discontinuation has not been reported. Due to the low toxicity in most situations, supportive care is sufficient for buspirone overdose.

Flunitrazepam

Flunitrazepam (Rohypnol) has been used in Europe, Asia, and Latin America for insomnia and preoperative sedation. Although it has never been manufactured or sold commercially in the United States, flunitrazepam has been documented in many sexual assaults or "date

rape" incidents. Flunitrazepam has been an active agent in the illicit drug market, where it is used to alter the effects of other drugs, including ethanol, heroin, and cocaine.

Flunitrazepam has 10 times more affinity than diazepam for benzodiazepine receptors. CNS depression occurs within 30 minutes. The drug is most frequently ingested with alcohol, producing additional disinhibition and amnesia. Despite marked CNS depression, patients can usually be aroused with noxious stimuli. The half-life of the drug is 16 to 36 hours, but coma can be prolonged for up to 48 hours. Management should include monitoring for hypoxia, hypoventilation, and aspiration; airway protection and ventilatory support can be provided when indicated. Flunitrazepam is easily obtained outside the United States and on the Internet. The drug is not detected on routine urine drug screens, but if needed as evidence, a urine sample should be obtained and the local or state police crime laboratory contacted to arrange specific testing. Metabolites of flunitrazepam can be detected in the urine up to 72 hours after exposure.

Chloral Hydrate

Clinical Features

Chloral hydrate has a low therapeutic ratio and can produce significant, potentially fatal toxicity. It is used in rare cases, but chloral hydrate is occasionally prescribed as a sedative in the elderly and for children undergoing hospital and outpatient procedures.[24,25] The use has decreased significantly with the availability of other procedural sedation medications with wider therapeutic indices. The oral hypnotic in adult is of dose 0.5 to 1.0 g. The pediatric sedation dose is 25 to 50 mg/kg orally 30 minutes prior to the procedure, with a maximum dose of 1000 mg.

The toxic oral dose is approximately 10 g in adults and may be as little as 1.5 g in children. The toxic effects of chloral hydrate include CNS and respiratory depression, GI irritation, cardiovascular instability, hepatitis, and proteinuria.[24] The combination of deep coma and cardiac dysrhythmia without hypoxia is characteristic of severe cases. Chloral hydrate decreases myocardial contractility, shortens the cardiac refractory period, and increases the sensitivity of myocardium to catecholamines. Dysrhythmias can be fatal, and include atrial fibrillation, supraventricular tachycardia, ventricular tachycardia, multifocal premature ventricular contractions, torsades de pointes, ventricular fibrillation, and asystole.

A citrus or pear-like odor to the patient's breath or gastric contents may suggest the diagnosis. Findings consistent with chloral hydrate toxicity include miosis, muscle flaccidity, diminished deep tendon reflexes, hypoventilation, hypotension, and hypothermia. Chloral hydrate is a GI irritant and causes nausea, vomiting, esophagitis, hemorrhagic gastritis, and, rarely, GI perforation or necrosis. Transient hepatic or renal dysfunction can also occur.

Chloral hydrate is rapidly absorbed from the GI tract. The primary active metabolite of chloral hydrate, trichloroethanol, has a barbiturate-like effect on GABA-A receptors and is responsible for most of the CNS depression seen with significant overdose. Metabolism to trichloroethanol occurs via the enzyme alcohol dehydrogenase with an onset of action of 20 to 30 minutes. Trichloroethanol is long acting, and its half-life can be significantly prolonged after overdose as the metabolic pathways become saturated.

Chloral hydrate and ethanol in combination (historically referred to as a "Mickey Finn") potentiate each other's effects to produce rapid loss of consciousness. Chloral hydrate increases the half-life of ethanol by competitively inhibiting the enzyme alcohol dehydrogenase, and the metabolism of ethanol generates nicotinamide adenine dinucleotide (NADH), a cofactor for the conversion of chloral hydrate to trichloroethanol.

Differential Diagnoses

Mild chloral hydrate toxicity can mimic many other sedative-hypnotics, including ethanol, benzodiazepines or barbiturates, with drowsiness, ataxia, and lethargy. More severe toxicity can mimic other cardiotoxic agents, including tricyclic antidepressants and cocaine. Hypomagnesemia can also induce torsades de pointes, as can QTc prolonging agents such as antipsychotics or methadone.

Management

The key to management is support of cardiorespiratory functions. Intubation may be required for airway protection, or to support ventilation, and oxygenation if there is significant depression of respiratory function. Avoid naloxone or flumazenil, which may precipitate ventricular dysrhythmias and will not have reversal effects. Because chloral hydrate, like other chlorinated hydrocarbons, sensitizes myocardium to catecholamines, epinephrine and norepinephrine should also be avoided. Standard type I antidysrhythmic agents, such as quinidine (1a) and lidocaine (1b), do not appear effective against chloral hydrate–induced cardiac ectopy. The treatment of choice for chloral hydrate-induced tachydysrhythmias is a beta-blocker. A short-acting agent, such as esmolol, can be used with an initial bolus of 1 mg/kg IV over 30 seconds followed by an infusion starting at 50 mcg/kg/min (maximum of 300 mcg/kg/min) as an intravenous infusion until resolution of the tachydysrhythmia. Torsades de pointes should be treated with intravenous magnesium or overdrive pacing, as described in Chapter 65. Patients with refractory hypotension or persistent unstable dysrhythmia despite supportive therapy can be treated with hemodialysis.

Disposition

Patients with acute chloral hydrate overdose should be observed in the ED until clinically stable, alert, oriented, and ambulatory. In cases of prolonged altered mental status, respiratory depression, hypoxia, or evidence of cardiotoxicity (e.g., PSVT, QRS widening, QTc prolongation, torsades de pointes), the patient should be admitted to a monitored setting. If the intent of the overdose was self-harm, psychiatric consultation is indicated once the patient is medically stabilized.

OVER-THE-COUNTER SLEEP AIDS

Over-the-counter (OTC) sleep aids, currently available in the United States, contain either diphenhydramine or doxylamine. Many preparations also contain acetaminophen or aspirin, added to achieve nighttime pain relief. The availability and frequent use of these agents may explain why overdose is so common. Diphenhydramine and doxylamine are first generation H-1 antihistamines that also have hypnotic, antimuscarinic, and weak local anesthetic properties. They act as competitive antagonists of H-1 histamine receptors and cause sedation by inhibiting the actions of acetylcholine on muscarinic receptors in the CNS. They also have sodium channel blocking effects which can cause QRS prolongation. Patients generally experience anticholinergic toxidromes, including tachycardia, dilated pupils, red and dry skin, and delirium. Further discussion of antimuscarinic toxicity is found in Chapter 140.

GAMMA-HYDROXYBUTYRATE

Clinical Features

Originally synthesized in the 1960s as an anesthetic, GHB was later discovered to be a naturally occurring metabolite of GABA. GHB had been used clinically to treat narcolepsy, alcohol addiction, opioid withdrawal, and depression.[26] GHB quickly distributes across the blood-brain barrier where it exerts its main toxic effects.[27]

The FDA approved GHB for the treatment of narcolepsy under the trade name Xyrem (sodium oxybate, 0.5 mg/mL) as a schedule III drug. The sale and manufacture of GHB is otherwise banned in the United States yet illicit use of GHB has increased, along with its precursors gamma-butyrolactone (GBL) and 1,4-butanediol (1,4-BD). There is a wide variety of "street names" that have been associated with GHB (Box 154.4).

GHB remains a popular drug of abuse. Some individuals take GHB for its purported muscle-building and fat-burning actions, others for its psychoactive effects. The drug's euphoria-producing properties make it popular at "raves" (large, crowded parties with energetic dancing to rhythmic music). Self-treatment of insomnia with GHB has been reported and can cause dependence. CNS depression, amnesia, and disinhibition caused by mixing of GHB with ethanol make this combination a potential agent in "date rape" situations. After overdose, a call for medical assistance is often delayed because of the false belief that victims need only to "sleep off" their intoxications. Death occurs most often in the prehospital setting, both from direct effects of the drug and increased the risk for fatal traumatic accidents. Combined intoxication with ethanol occurs in most fatal cases.

GHB binds to specific GHB receptors and at high concentrations to GABA-B receptors. The complex interaction between these two receptors may explain the paradoxical manifestations of GHB toxicity with somnolence alternating with agitation.

GHB is lipophilic and rapidly absorbed. Onset of symptoms occurs within 15 to 30 minutes, and peak plasma levels are reached within 20 to 60 minutes. Unlike GABA, GHB readily crosses the blood-brain barrier. The half-life of GHB is 30 minutes but may increase at high doses.

As underground clandestine laboratories often synthesize liquid GHB by mixing and heating butyrolactone and sodium hydroxide, careless preparation can result in residual unreacted alkali, causing significant caustic injury when the liquid is ingested.

Chemical precursors to GHB are also commonly abused with similar toxic effects. GBL is an industrial solvent that is rapidly absorbed after ingestion and it is metabolized within minutes to GHB by peripheral and hepatic lactonases. Before conversion to GHB, GBL itself is inactive and has no sedating effects. It produces a clinical syndrome similar to that of GHB ingestion, but its effects are more pronounced and prolonged.

1,4-BD is converted after ingestion to GHB by the enzyme alcohol dehydrogenase. Like GBL, it is used as an industrial solvent. Clinical findings are similar to those of GHB. When 1,4-BD and ethanol are ingested together, ethanol acts as a competitive inhibitor of alcohol dehydrogenase, so the toxic effects of 1,4-BD are delayed and prolonged, and the risk of death is increased.

BOX 154.4 Gamma-Hydroxybutyrate Street Names

Grievous bodily harm (GHB)	Liquid G
Georgia home boy (GBH)	Somatomax
Gib	Soap
Natural sleep-500	Salty water
Gamma-OH	Scoop
Gamma hydrate	Sodium oxybate
Liquid X	Easy lay
Organic Quaalude	Cherry menth
Liquid E	Fantasy
Liquid ecstasy	G-Riffick

Differential Diagnoses

The differential diagnoses of GHB intoxication is broad including other sedative-hypnotics (such as barbiturates or benzodiazepines), OTC sleep aids, antimuscarinic agents, opioids, ethanol, ketamine, chloral hydrate, and designer amphetamines.

Poisoning with other sedative-hypnotics can produce a similar clinical picture. Unique to GHB, however, is the relatively rapid resolution of symptoms. In the absence of a coingestant such as ethanol, most patients will be functionally awake within 3 to 4 hours. Nearly all patients recover fully within 8 hours. Prolonged coma should prompt a search for another toxicological or non-toxicological cause. Cardiac effects and refractory seizures are rare and suggest the presence of other agents or etiologies.

Diagnosis of GHB intoxication is based on the history and clinical course, as clinical laboratory testing is not readily available. Rapid recovery from coma or periods of agitation alternating with periods of decreased level of consciousness is its characteristic. Hypothermia may occur with prolonged coma. In the presence of coma, bradycardia with or without hypotension can occur and may respond to auditory or tactile stimulation alone. Miosis with or without nystagmus may be seen. Because emesis occurs in about 50% of cases, obtunded patients are at risk for aspiration pneumonitis. Apparent seizure activity may actually represent random myoclonic movements of the face and extremities. Severity is dependent on the dose and the concurrent use of alcohol or other psychoactive drugs.

Diagnostic Testing

GHB is not detected on routine urine toxicology screens. If laboratory confirmation is required, specimens must be collected early in the clinical course, and sent for gas chromatography–mass spectroscopy. The drug may be detected in urine up to 12 hours after ingestion. In most cases, the toxicology laboratory test is not available for patient management. Pulse oximetry and end-tidal capnometry can be used to monitor respiratory status, and adjunct testing can be used to rule out alternative diagnoses.

Management

The management strategy for GHB toxicity follows the same principles as the other sedative-hypnotics discussed previously. Supportive care including respiratory and ventilatory support is critical. Because of rapid absorption and the high incidence of emesis with GHB overdose, there is no indication for gastric decontamination. Intubation for airway protection may be required by patients with significant CNS depression or hypoxia. There is a high prevalence of coingestants with recreational use of GHB. Physostigmine should not be used for GHB intoxication, based on reported adverse events, particularly in the setting of polydrug use.

Disposition

Because of GHB's short half-life, symptoms of intoxication generally resolve while the patient is still in the ED. The patient generally regains consciousness spontaneously within 3 to 4 hours. No delayed toxicity is expected unless there are coingestants. Patients should be counseled about the seriousness of GHB intoxication, withdrawal potential with chronic use, and discharged home with reliable caretakers.

Additional monitoring and observation for up to 12 to 24 hours should be provided in the setting of ingestions of either GBL or 1,4-BD as toxicity can be prolonged and more severe, as well as less predictable.

Withdrawal

Patients who abruptly stop GHB or its precursors after chronic frequent use can experience a severe and potentially life-threatening withdrawal syndrome. Because of the short half-life of GHB, symptoms of withdrawal begin within several hours of the last dose. The typical patient will have been using these products for weeks or months, in frequent repetitive doses, to avoid withdrawal symptoms.[28]

Withdrawal symptoms are similar to withdrawal from other sedative-hypnotics, including benzodiazepines. Mild withdrawal is manifested with anxiety, tremor, and insomnia. This can progress to confusion, delirium, overt psychosis, paranoid ideation, hallucinations (visual, aural, or tactile), and autonomic instability. Diagnosis relies on a history of symptoms beginning after abrupt cessation of use of these products. The differential diagnosis includes withdrawal from other sedative-hypnotic agents, delirium tremens, sympathomimetic toxicity, serotonin syndrome, neuroleptic malignant syndrome, CNS infection, and thyroid storm.

Initial treatment begins with high-dose benzodiazepines with doses escalated as required for agitation. However, GHB withdrawal may involve depleted levels of GABA. Because the effect of benzodiazepines requires the presence of GABA, they may be less effective in control of GHB withdrawal. Barbiturates, such as pentobarbital or phenobarbital, which do not need GABA to be effective, are often required in cases of severe withdrawal. These patients often require admission to an intensive care unit for titrated sedation, as well as to observe for development of seizures, rhabdomyolysis or hyperthermia.

ACKNOWLEDGMENTS

We would like to acknowledge the valuable contributions of the previous edition authors Drs. Andrea Carlson and Leon Gussow.

The references for this chapter can be found online at ExpertConsult.com.

Special Populations

155

Care of the Pediatric Patient

Stephen John Cico and Derya Caglar

FOUNDATIONS

Emergency clinicians assess and manage pediatric patients from newborns to adolescents. Of the 146 million annual US emergency department (ED) visits, 27.4 million (19%) are for children younger than 15 years.[1] Twenty-two percent of children have at least one ED visit per year. Infants have higher per capita ED utilization than other age groups, with 98.7 visits/100 infants.[1] More than 80% of pediatric patients are seen in general EDs, requiring all emergency clinicians to be skilled in the assessment, treatment, and stabilization of pediatric illnesses and injuries.[2]

Children can present diagnostic and management challenges due to their anatomic, physiologic, and developmental differences from adult patients. Understanding these differences is crucial to the recognition and appropriate treatment of many pediatric emergencies. In addition, caring for the pediatric patient also involves active participation from caregivers.

Pathophysiology

Children exhibit different patterns of illness and injury because of their unique physiologic and anatomic characteristics. Illness and injury patterns not only differ between pediatric and adult patients, but also vary in children by age. In addition to changes in cognitive and behavioral development, temperature regulation, airway anatomy, cardiovascular physiology, immune function, and the musculoskeletal system all change as children grow. Furthermore, pediatric patients may present to the ED with previously undiagnosed congenital disorders. Drug dosing and choice of medications also depend on patient size and physiology.

Assessment should begin with a review of vital signs, evaluating for early signs of physiologic decompensation. Normal heart rate and respiratory rate vary by age (Table 155.1). Normal blood pressure also varies by age, height, and gender (Box 155.1; Table 155.2). Abnormal vital signs should be repeated and persistently abnormal vital signs quickly addressed.

Temperature Regulation

Infants and young children have a larger surface area–to–mass ratio, resulting in more heat loss to the environment than in adolescents and adults. Maintenance of a stable body temperature can be a significant metabolic demand for young infants, especially those stressed by injury or illness. Maintain a neutral thermal environment for children during the physical examination and while performing procedures. Patients exposed briefly for examinations and interventions should be covered as soon as possible to avoid excessive heat loss. Critically ill young infants should be placed under radiant warmers. Overhead warming lights are useful for older infants and children who require prolonged exposure for resuscitation and procedures.

Airway

The pediatric airway differs in a number of ways from an adult airway.[3,4] Compared to the adult airway, the pediatric larynx is more

TABLE 155.1 Normal Pediatric Vital Signs

Age (Years)	Respiratory Rate (Breaths/Min)	Heart Rate (Beats/Min)
<1	30–60	100–160
1–2	24–40	90–150
2–5	22–34	80–140
6–12	18–30	70–120
>12	12–16	60–100

From Dieckmann R, Brownstein D, Gausche-Hill M, eds. *Pediatric Education for Prehospital Professionals.* Sudbury, MA: Jones & Bartlett; 2013.

BOX 155.1 Hypotension in the Pediatric Population by Age

0–28 days: 60 mm Hg
1–12 months: 70 mm Hg
1–10 years: 70 mm Hg + (2× age in years)

From American Heart Association: American Heart Association emergency cardiovascular care (ECC) guidelines, 2010. https://www.ahajournals.org/doi/10.1161/circ.102.suppl_1.I-291.

TABLE 155.2 Pediatric Blood Pressure by Age

Age (Years)	50TH PERCENTILE (MM HG) Girls	Boys	HYPERTENSION–95TH PERCENTILE (MM HG) Girls	Boys
1	86/40	85/37	104/58	103/56
5	93/54	95/53	110/72	112/72
10	102/60	102/61	119/78	119/80
15	110/65	113/64	127/83	131/83

aFor children at the 50th percentile for height.
Modified from The National High Blood Pressure Education Program Working Group on Children and Adolescents: The fourth report on the diagnosis, evaluation, and treatment of high blood pressure in children and adolescents. https://www.ncbi.nlm.nih.gov/pmc/articles/PMC4074640/ and https://www.nhlbi.nih.gov/files/docs/resources/heart/hbp_ped.pdf

anterior and cephalad, and the epiglottis is composed of more flexible cartilage, making it floppy. The relatively larger occiput in infants and young children can cause neck flexion in the supine position, leading to potential airway obstruction. To open the airway, particularly during intubation attempts, a towel roll placed under the shoulders may be needed to align the laryngeal, pharyngeal, and oral airway axes (Fig. 155.1). Infants and young children also have relatively large tongues, which may lead to airway obstruction during periods of changes in muscle tone, such as during a seizure. Use of a nasopharyngeal airway can alleviate the obstruction by allowing a clear passage of inhaled gases. In addition, airways in children are much smaller in diameter and much more easily obstructed with secretions. Because young infants preferentially breathe through their noses, respiratory distress can develop from copious nasal secretions. Thus, suctioning the nose and upper airway can dramatically diminish an infant's work of breathing.

Cardiovascular System

Healthy children have compensatory mechanisms to maintain blood pressure, even when cardiac output is decreasing. Children have the ability to increase their heart rate and vasoconstrict peripherally to shunt blood centrally, while very young children have limited ability to increase their cardiac contractility. Hypotension is a late finding of shock in previously healthy children, and interventions should ideally occur before the onset of hypotension.[5] The earliest sign of cardiovascular compromise in most patients is tachycardia. Unfortunately, tachycardia is nonspecific and may be due to fever, pain, or anxiety. Repeated assessment of the heart rate can be helpful. In a crying child, a true resting heart rate can be obtained by leaving the pulse oximeter on until the child is calm. Unexplained tachycardia in a calm or sleeping child should be investigated for the cause of the tachycardia. The quality of the pulse is also helpful. A thready peripheral pulse associated with tachycardia should be considered a sign of shock. Bradycardia in ill children is especially ominous and may signal impending cardiopulmonary failure.

Musculoskeletal System

Growing children have musculoskeletal injury patterns different from those of adults. Ligaments are stronger relative to the immature bone, so children are more likely to fracture bones than sprain ligaments. The weakest part of a growing child's bone is the physis, or growth plate. If tenderness is present on examination, physeal injuries should be considered in children with normal radiographs. Treatment of fractures in children should consider future growth potential. For example, certain physeal injuries can lead to long-term growth disturbances, whereas greater degrees of angulation are acceptable in many fractures due to the increased potential for bone remodeling.

Immunologic System

Due to their immature immune system, young infants are at increased risk of serious bacterial infections. Febrile infants younger than 1 month are a particularly high-risk group and have a 10% or higher rate of serious bacterial infection.[5] For this reason, the evaluation of infants with fever differs from the evaluation of older children and adults; the evaluation varies by age and vaccination status (see Chapter 161).

Pharmacologic Considerations

Medications for children are calculated using weight-based dosing, with attention to the maximum medication dose. Suggested safeguards to prevent calculation-based dosing errors in children include pharmacy review of medication orders, computerized order entry, use of templated order forms, and length-based resuscitation tapes to reduce calculation errors.[6] One easily remedied potential error is the inadvertent calculation of a drug dose on the basis of weight in pounds, not kilograms, leading to a more than twofold overdose. Therefore, ED scales and electronic charts should be programmed to report weight only in kilograms.[7]

In addition to potential dosing errors, certain frequently used medications in older children and adolescents should not be given to young infants. For example, ceftriaxone is not recommended for infants younger than 28 days because it can displace bilirubin from albumin, leading to kernicterus or bilirubin-induced neurologic dysfunction (BIND). Although not well studied, the use of ibuprofen in infants younger than 6 months has not been approved by the US Food

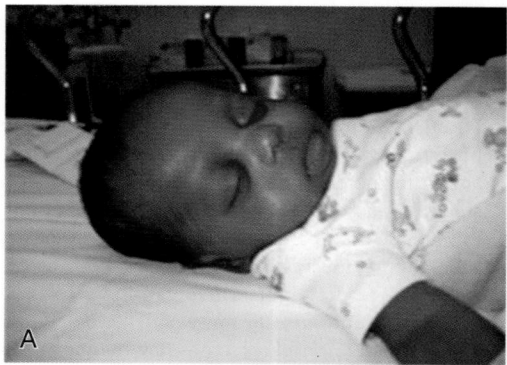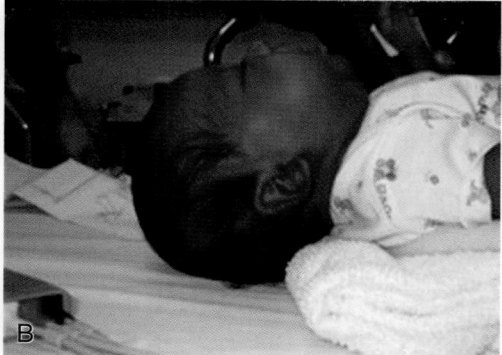

Fig. 155.1 Infant With Neck in Flexed Position (A) and After Placement of a Shoulder Roll (B). (From Santillanes G, Gausche-Hill M. Pediatric airway management. *Emerg Med Clin North Am.* 2008;26:961–975.)

and Drug Administration because of the theoretical risk of kidney and liver injury.

Developmental Considerations

Assessment of pediatric patients requires an understanding of normal developmental milestones. Table 155.3 lists basic developmental milestones in the first 2 years of life. Variation in the rate at which children develop can be normal or may signal neurodevelopmental delays. Therefore, the parent's report of the child's developmental history and normal behavior is extremely important. Injuries identified should also fit the developmental milestones of a child. Injuries that fall outside of the normal developmental patterns should raise the consideration of non-accidental trauma/child abuse.[8]

Young Infants

Infants younger than 2 months are especially challenging to assess because they have a limited behavioral repertoire. They may not make eye contact nor have a social smile. Normal behavior includes sleeping, crying, quiet alert time, feeding, and stooling. A change in any of these activities may indicate serious disease. Increased sleeping or crying or decreased interest in feeding may herald a serious illness, such as sepsis or an underlying cardiac or metabolic disorder.

Infants (<12 Months)

Infants typically develop a social smile and track close objects by 2 to 3 months of age. After 6 months, infants may develop significant stranger anxiety, making the physical examination challenging. Whenever possible, examining the infant in the parent's lap, with the infant initially facing away from the examiner, can mitigate anxiety and facilitate physical examination. Bubbles or interactive toys can distract infants and may help keep them calm.

Toddlers (1- to 2-Year-Olds)

Toddlers have variable reactions to a physical examination. A toddler may provide a limited history due to their narrow expressive language skills (e.g., only pointing to the location of pain). Some are fearful and will not cooperate, whereas others are curious and cooperate more easily with the examination. In a stable patient, begin the encounter standing or sitting at a distance from the child while taking the history. Speaking in a soothing voice and distracting the child with toys or other interesting objects can facilitate the examination. Emergency clinicians should interact with the parents, because this will be perceived by the child as a sign of endorsement and indicate that the parents are involved with the emergency care. Conversely, toddlers will often negatively react to parental anxiety.

TABLE 155.3	**Developmental Milestones in Typically Developing Children Up To 2 Years of Age**	
Age (Months)	Gross Motor	Visual-Motor, Social, and Language
1	Raises head from prone position	Visually follows to midline, alerts to sound, regards face
2	Lifts chest off table	Smiles socially, recognizes parent, follows object past midline
4	Rolls over	Laughs, orients to voice
6	Sits unsupported	Babbles
9	Pulls to stand, cruises	Says "mama" and "dada" indiscriminately, plays games such as pat-a-cake
12	Walks alone	Two words other than "mama" and "dada"
15	Creeps upstairs, walks backward	Uses 4–6 words
18	Runs	Uses 7–10 words, knows five body parts
24	Walks up and down stairs independently	50-word vocabulary, two-word sentences

Adapted from Engorn B, Flerlage J. *The Harriet Lane Handbook.* 20th ed. Philadelphia: Elsevier Saunders; 2015.

Preschoolers (3- to 5-Year-Olds)

Preschool-age children have increasing language skills. Like toddlers, their receptive language skills exceed their expressive language skills, and they often understand more than is realized. Preschoolers should be included in the conversation when possible. Emergency clinicians should be cautious about talking to the parents about procedures or diagnoses in front of the preschool child, even if the child seems not to be paying attention or not to understand. Like toddlers, preschool children vary greatly in their cooperation with the physical examination. Providing limited options, such as sitting with the parent or on the gurney, or choosing which ear should be examined first, may give the child a sense of control and improve cooperation. Distraction with stories, videos, or games on a smartphone or other devices can also facilitate the physical examination. The young child will build up anxiety awaiting a procedure. For this reason, clinicians should provide children with simple concrete explanations of procedures only immediately before and during the procedure. Preschool children may perceive illness or painful procedures as punishment for their actions, making simple explanations of what and why it is occurring even more important.

School-Age Children

Some questions during the history should be directed at the school-age child, because many can provide much of the history themselves. At this age, children are often cooperative with the examination, but may regress when they are frightened or in pain. Additionally, children at this age become increasingly modest, and conscious attempts should be made to provide privacy.

School-age children may develop anxiety and attempt to negotiate or stall when a painful or unpleasant examination or procedure is planned, particularly if there is a long delay between the explanation and procedure. Firm but reassuring explanations of what will happen are important. Appropriate concrete explanations include the sequence of events and what physical sensations the patient will experience. It is also crucial to involve parents in the process to provide not only a candid explanation of the procedure itself, but also anticipated reactions from their child. When available, child life specialists are particularly helpful with this age population, using play and education to prepare children for anxiety-provoking procedures.

Adolescents

Adolescents will be able to provide much, if not all, of the history. However, despite desired independence from their parents, adolescents may regress in times of stress. It is therefore important to elicit the concerns of the adolescent and parent, and to ensure that both understand the diagnosis and plan. The adolescent should be given a chance to speak to the emergency clinician without the parent in the room. Any sensitive questions, such as those about drug use, alcohol consumption, tobacco and vaping, and sexual activity should be asked privately. State laws vary on confidentiality and ages of consent, so it is important for emergency clinicians to know those specifics which may be applicable to their patients.

Adolescents can generally be examined in a manner similar to that for adults. They may or may not prefer to have a parent present during the physical examination, and providers should clarify the patient's preference. Adolescents are often extremely modest, and attempts should be made to preserve privacy with the examination in a private room, when possible, with exposure of only the body part being examined.

EVALUATION

Triage

Pediatric-specific triage systems are important to avoid overtriage and undertriage of children. The application of adult-specific vital signs to children will lead to an inappropriate triage level classification or inadvertently trigger inappropriate sepsis alerts. In addition, signs and symptoms of serious illness may be subtle in infants and very young children, requiring those providing the initial triage assessment to be familiar with normal pediatric physiology and development.

Triage systems with pediatric modifications include the Emergency Severity Index, Paediatric Canadian Triage and Acuity Scale, Manchester Triage System, and Australasian Triage Scale. No triage system has been clearly demonstrated to be superior, and data on reliability and validity are limited for all triage systems. The Emergency Severity Index, Manchester Triage System, and Paediatric Canadian Triage and Acuity Scale have been demonstrated to be valid for pediatric patients.

The Emergency Severity Index has been updated by the Emergency Nurses Association and has pediatric specific resources.[9]

History

In critically ill or injured patients, the SAMPLE history can be used to obtain a focused history quickly (Box 155.2). The SAMPLE history reminds providers to ask for **S**igns and symptoms, **A**llergies, **M**edications, **P**ast medical history, **L**ast meal, and **E**vents surrounding the illness or injury.

A more detailed history will be guided by the patient's presenting complaint. In preverbal children, symptoms will often be inferred by the caregiver based on the child's behavior. Parents are often very perceptive and may notice subtle changes in behavior that are not immediately evident to a healthcare provider.

Additional age-specific questions may be indicated. In neonates, pregnancy and birth history will help identify risk factors for conditions such as hyperbilirubinemia (e.g., prematurity, ABO incompatibility), infection (e.g., maternal fever during labor, early or prolonged rupture of membranes, maternal group B streptococcus [GBS] status), and respiratory illnesses (e.g., prematurity, meconium aspiration, need for supplemental oxygen or mechanical ventilation). The emergency clinician should also inquire about results of the newborn screen if available. Each state screens for a different panel of disorders determined by their public health board. Most of the conditions included in newborn screening can lead to serious health problems if not recognized and treated shortly after birth. Prompt identification and management of these conditions may be able to prevent life-threatening complications.

In infants and toddlers, urine output, quantified by the number of wet diapers, helps determine hydration status. This can be especially helpful in breast-feeding newborns, whose intake is difficult to quantify. Vaccination status is important in infants and children presenting with symptoms such as fever (e.g., risk of bacteremia) and rash (e.g., risk of varicella, measles). Drug, alcohol, and e-cigarette use, as well as the sexual history, become important in adolescents who have increased risk-taking behaviors and should be questioned in a private setting, not in front of the caregiver.

Pediatric Assessment Triangle

Rapid recognition of the critically ill child is a crucial skill. The pediatric assessment triangle (PAT) assists emergency clinicians in assessing children quickly and is an orderly approach for formulating an initial impression of the child's overall status from the door of the examination room (Fig. 155.2). The three components of the PAT are (1) appearance, (2) work of breathing, and (3) circulation to the skin. On the basis of the initial PAT, the emergency clinician can distinguish the "sick" from the "well" child rapidly. Table 155.4 summarizes the findings that may be noted on each of the three sides of the triangle, and Table 155.5 summarizes interpretation of the PAT.

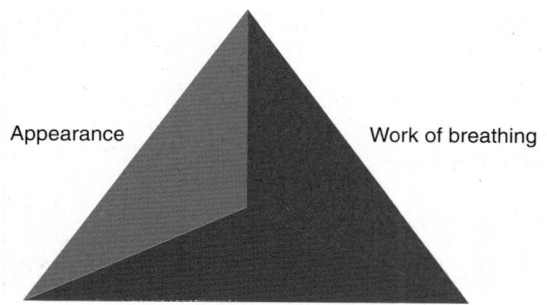

Fig. 155.2 Pediatric Assessment Triangle.

TABLE 155.4 Pediatric Assessment Triangle Abnormal Findings

Appearance	Work of Breathing	Circulation to the Skin
Tone—poor tone, floppy infant	Abnormal sounds—stridor, grunting, snoring, wheezing	Pallor
Interactiveness—irritability, poor responsiveness to surroundings	Abnormal positioning—sniffing, tripoding, refusal to lie down	Delayed capillary refill time (>2 s) Mottling
Consolable—inability to be consoled by parent	Retractions	Cyanosis
Look, gaze—poor attention, lack of normal tracking	Head bobbing	Petechiae
Speech, cry—weak cry, or no cry with environmental stimuli	Nasal flaring	

Adapted from Dieckmann R, Brownstein D, Gausche-Hill M, eds. *Pediatric Education for Prehospital Professionals.* Sudbury, MA: Jones & Bartlett; 2013.

TABLE 155.5 Interpretation of the Pediatric Assessment Triangle General Impression of Condition

Physiologic State	Appearance	Work of Breathing	Circulation to the Skin
Respiratory distress	Normal	Abnormal	Normal
Respiratory failure	Abnormal	Abnormal	Normal-abnormal
Compensated shock	Normal	Normal	Abnormal
Decompensated shock	Abnormal	Normal-abnormal	Abnormal
Brain injury or dysfunction	Abnormal	Normal	Normal
Cardiopulmonary failure	Abnormal	Abnormal	Abnormal

Adapted from Dieckmann R, Brownstein D, Gausche-Hill M, eds. *Pediatric Education for Prehospital Professionals.* Sudbury, MA: Jones & Bartlett; 2013.

Work of Breathing

The work of breathing should be observed ideally when the child is calm. Children may have increased work of breathing with retractions without facial signs of respiratory distress, therefore, the emergency clinician should ask the parent to remove the clothing so the chest wall can be observed for retractions. Infants and children with respiratory distress may assume the sniffing position in an attempt to decrease their work of breathing. The tripod position is an ominous sign of severe respiratory distress.

The quality of the voice or cry may be a clue to airway and respiratory disease or compromise. For example, children with croup have a hoarse voice, and children with peritonsillar abscesses may have a have muffled or so-called "hot potato" voice. Abnormal breath sounds may be audible without a stethoscope.

Signs of respiratory compromise include stridor, audible wheezing, retractions, grunting, and snoring respirations. Retractions may be seen in the suprasternal, supraclavicular, intercostal, and subcostal areas (Fig. 155.3). Nasal flaring is an attempt to decrease airway resistance (Fig. 155.4). Head bobbing (the use of neck muscles to assist respiration) and seesaw breathing (ineffective breathing pattern, in which the abdomen moves outward while the chest moves inward during inspiration) are signs of impending respiratory failure. As the child tires and nears complete respiratory failure, the respiratory rate falls and the work of breathing may diminish.

Normal pediatric respiratory rates are inversely related to age due to younger children's increased metabolic rates and lower tidal volume reserves. Because children normally function near their maximum tidal volume capacity, relatively small increases in metabolic demands (e.g., fever) can result in an elevated respiratory rate. As a result, abnormal respiratory patterns may provide clues about a nonrespiratory illness. Effortless tachypnea may be a sign of shock from any cause, whereas deep rapid breathing without other auscultative findings may be compensation for a metabolic acidosis. Children who are tachypneic despite normothermia should be evaluated for respiratory and nonrespiratory causes. Neurologic disorders may also lead to abnormal respiratory patterns (e.g., bradypnea and irregular respiration in the setting of increased intracranial pressure).

Appearance

Observation of the child from a distance allows the provider to assess the patient's overall status without upsetting the child. The mnemonic TICLS (*t*one, *i*nteractiveness, *c*onsolability, *l*ook and gaze, *s*peech and cry) summarizes the components of the assessment of overall appearance. Observation of the infant or child interacting with his or her parents provides many clues about the child's overall status. An ill infant with a vacant or glazed look can be distinguished from an alert infant who responds to environmental stimuli. An infant who is awake but lying motionless on a gurney is much more concerning than an active infant who moves all the extremities. Irritability is an early sign of inadequate brain perfusion. This may be followed by lethargy and then coma as perfusion is further compromised.

The quality of the cry is another helpful clue. A persistently high-pitched or irritable cry is concerning for central nervous system disease, such as meningitis. A normal overall appearance suggests that oxygenation, ventilation, and perfusion are adequate.

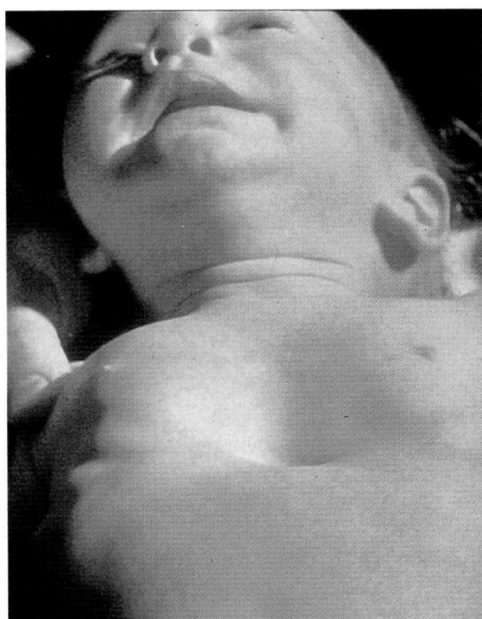

Fig. 155.3 Intercostal Retractions in a Child With Respiratory Distress.

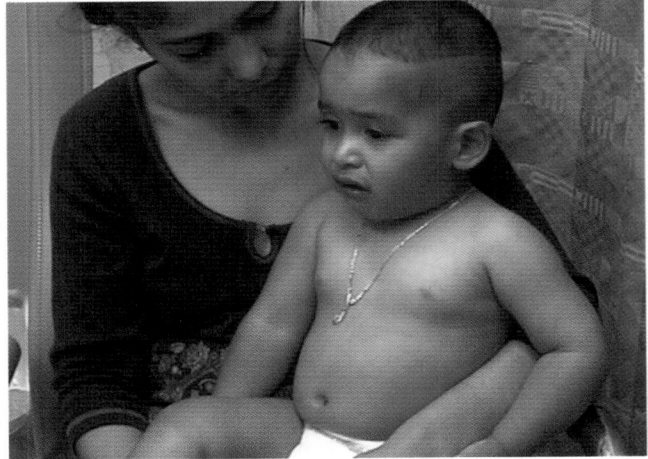

Fig. 155.4 Nasal Flaring in a Child With Respiratory Distress From Lower Airway Obstruction.

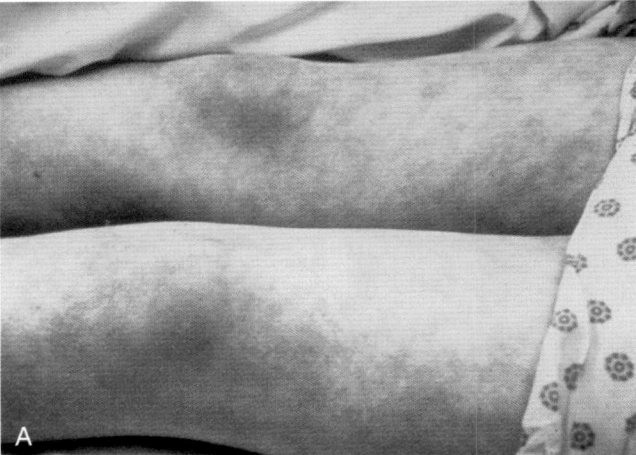

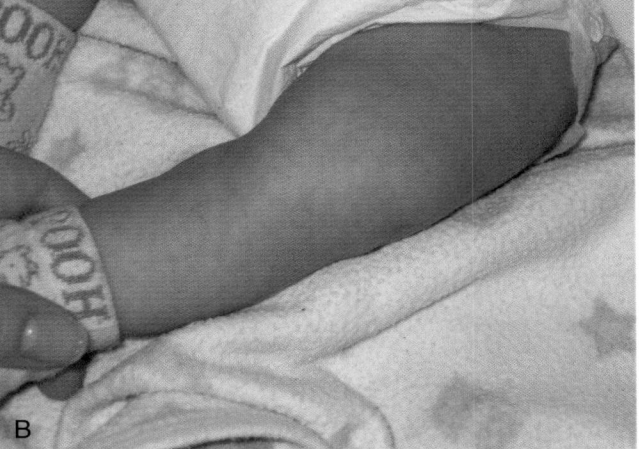

Fig. 155.5 Infant with skin mottling (A) and cutis marmorata (B).

Circulation to the Skin

Visual inspection of the skin can provide clues to overall cardiovascular status. Early compensated shock is characterized by peripheral vasoconstriction and shunting of blood to the brain and other vital organs. At this stage, skin appears pale but remains warm to the touch with delayed capillary refill time (>2 seconds). If the shock state is not corrected, the patient may become mottled, with cold extremities (Fig. 155.5A). Mottling is a random pattern of vasoconstriction in adjacent capillary beds in the skin. This is not to be confused with cutis marmorata, a regular lacy pattern on the skin caused by vascular instability (see Fig. 155.5B). Cutis marmorata is a normal finding in young infants in a cool environment. In contrast to infants with mottling, infants with cutis marmorata will be otherwise well-appearing, and the skin findings will diminish or disappear if the infant is placed in a warm environment. Cyanosis may be present normally in children with congenital heart disease but, if cyanosis is a new finding for the patient, it is almost always indicative of respiratory failure or decompensated shock.

Length-Based Resuscitation Tape

Ideally an actual body weight in kilograms should be used for determination of medication dosing in children. An accurate weight may not be available for critically ill children especially for those that require immediate resuscitation. Use of a color-coded, length-based resuscitation tape gives an estimate of the child's weight. Each color on the tape corresponds to a weight range that corresponds to an ideal body weight for length. Medication doses and appropriate equipment are listed on the tape for each weight range. Use of the length-based resuscitation tape avoids error-prone calculations of medication dosages and equipment sizes in the high-stress setting of a pediatric resuscitation. In addition, pediatric resuscitation equipment organized by weight ranges minimizes the need to search for appropriately sized equipment.

Physical Examination

As in adults, the physical examination in critically ill or injured children will focus initially on airway, breathing, and circulation, with abnormalities in these systems corrected before a complete physical examination is performed. In any infant or toddler with respiratory complaints, observing the child breathing with the shirt removed will allow the most reliable assessment of the work of breathing. The respiratory rate should be manually counted for a minimum of 30 seconds, due to periodic breathing, and also because the rate on the monitor

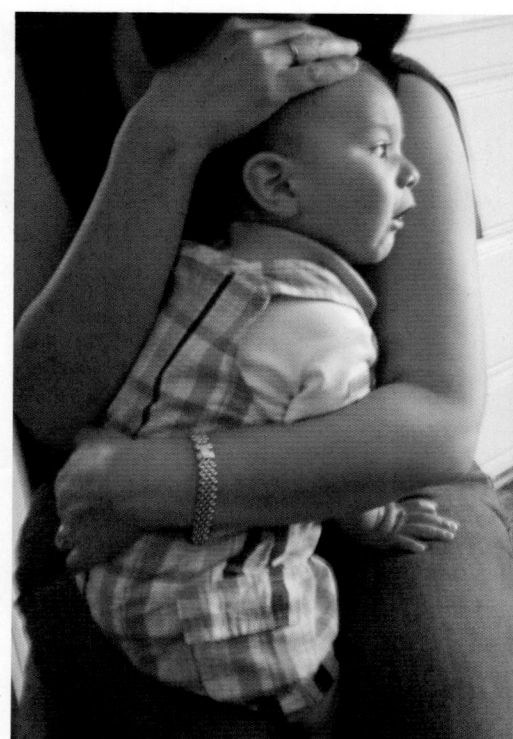

Fig. 155.6 Toddler Being Held for Otoscopic Examination of the Ears.

can be unreliable. In infants and young children with some degree of respiratory distress, observation of respiratory status and pulse oximetry during feeding or sleeping can be helpful when deciding on further observation and admission.

In infants and young children, the physical examination should not be performed in a head-to-toe fashion. Auscultation of the heart and lungs and palpation of the abdomen should be performed before other more frightening or uncomfortable parts of the examination. Although, ideally, the emergency clinician should palpate the child's abdomen, occasionally a fearful child will cry so much it is impossible to determine if the child has abdominal tenderness or guarding. In these cases, observing the parent palpate the abdomen may be helpful. Although parents cannot be relied on to examine for masses or organomegaly, they can elicit pain with palpation and feel for guarding.

Examination of the ears, oropharynx, or area of injury should occur toward the end of the physical examination. Providers can try to ease a child's fear by first demonstrating the examination on a parent, older sibling, or stuffed animal. For the ear examination, the parent can hold the young child in his or her lap, with one arm around the head and one arm around the child's body and arms (Fig. 155.6). Young children can often be coaxed into opening the mouth wide enough for examination of the oropharynx without use of a tongue depressor. The examination can be turned into a game by asking the child to open his mouth and pant "like a puppy" or see if she or he can touch the tongue to the chin. The exam of the groin in young girls or boys can be facilitated by having them sit in a frog leg position in the parent's lap. Children should be reassured of the safe environment with the provider and caregiver but also should be counseled to understand the difference between the examination and inappropriate touching by others.

SPECIFIC DISORDERS

The most common reasons for infants and children to present to EDs are respiratory illness, fever, and injury. Causes of serious illness and injury vary by age. Respiratory illnesses are the most common reason for infant hospitalization after the immediate neonatal period. Asthma and appendicitis are the most common reasons for hospitalization of school-age children, and affective disorders are the most common cause of adolescent hospitalizations.

This section focuses on complaints specific to the pediatric population and complaints in which the differential and approach vary significantly from those in adult populations.

Common Neonatal Complaints

Neonates may present with a variety of previously undiagnosed genetic, anatomic, and metabolic conditions. In addition to the very limited behavioral cues displayed by newborns, parents of newborns are frequently anxious and may not know what behaviors or patterns are normal.

Concerns about feeding are common. Neonates typically feed every 2 to 3 hours. Bottle-fed neonates take about 2 to 3 ounces per feed, whereas breast-feeding neonates typically spend 10 to 15 minutes on each breast each feed. Newborns, especially those who are exclusively breast-fed, can lose up to 10% of their birth weight during the first 7 days of life. Birth weight should be regained by day 10, with a subsequent weight gain of 20 to 30 g/day for the first 3 months of life. Providers should clarify feeding routines with caregivers. Infants with excessive weight loss or failure to gain weight may have underlying metabolic, cardiac, or infectious causes or be victims of abuse or neglect.

Small amounts of regurgitation of breast milk or formula are normal in infants and generally are not concerning if the amount is stable, the infant is gaining weight, and emesis is not bilious. Larger volume emesis should be evaluated. Common benign causes include overfeeding and inadequate burping, but providers should consider other serious causes, such as pyloric stenosis, malrotation with volvulus, intussusception, and nonaccidental trauma (head or abdominal). Bilious emesis in a neonate should always prompt further investigation with imaging.

Another common concern is the frequency and consistency of bowel movements. Although infants typically have soft stools multiple times a day, it can be normal for exclusively breast-fed infants to stool as infrequently as once every 5 to 7 days. Straining during a bowel movement is also commonly seen and may occur after transition from breast milk to formula. In infants presenting with constipation, a history of failure to stool in the first 24 hours of life is concerning for Hirschsprung's disease—aganglionic segments of the colon that fail to relax.

Urate crystals may also form in the first week of life. Families often come to the ED with concerns for neonatal hematuria upon seeing these reddish "brick stained" deposits in the diaper. Though benign, these are most commonly seen in babies who have some degree of dehydration, especially in mothers who are breastfeeding and have not quite established a good milk supply.

Neonatal Intensive Care Unit Graduate

Gestational rather than chronologic age is typically used for premature infants in whom development is often delayed. Due to their immature immune function relative to infants of the same chronologic age, premature infants are at increased risk for recurrent respiratory infections. Chronic lung disease is a common complication in extremely premature infants (gestational age <28 weeks). Such infants frequently have a baseline tachypnea and increased work of breathing and may require supplemental home oxygen. Parental report of changes in work of breathing, activity, feeding pattern, and level of alertness can be clues to serious illness, such as sepsis or underlying metabolic abnormalities.

Respiratory syncytial virus (RSV) immunoglobulin (palivizumab) prophylaxis is recommended for certain high-risk infants during peak season.[10] During RSV season, the timing of the last RSV immunoglobulin injection given should be ascertained when a premature infant presents with fever, cough, or rhinorrhea. Palivizumab is administered monthly and, if a dose has been missed, the physician should have a higher level of suspicion for RSV infection.

Children With Special Health Care Needs

The assessment of children with chronic illnesses and other special health care needs is especially challenging. Although specialty care is often provided at pediatric EDs affiliated with tertiary children's hospitals, a greater absolute number of the most complex pediatric patients are cared for within general EDs, likely due to regional proximity and easier access to care. This emphasizes the need for general EDs to be prepared to care for this vulnerable population[3,11]. Parents or other daily caregivers can provide helpful information on baseline behavior and mental status, and the caregiver's input should be sought.

However, a parent's knowledge and recollection of detailed medical information may be limited, especially during times of high stress. Parents may forget medication names or concentrations, details of previous hospital admissions, and current treatment plans. An Emergency Information Form (EIF) that summarizes chronic medical conditions, medications, medical devices, and other critical information can be used for children with special health care needs.[12] These forms can quickly provide critical information to the ED provider, assisting in the early management and stabilization of the child until more detailed records are obtained. ED staff can request that specialists affiliated with their hospitals provide EIFs for complex patients to facilitate rapid and appropriate emergency treatment.

Children with autism or sensory processing disorders may have a particularly difficult time in the loud and unpredictable environment of the ED. Day-to-day life for a child with an autism spectrum disorder can become extremely regimented, and knowing what is going to happen may help the encounter go more smoothly and decrease patient and family stress. Asking what sensory sensitivities the child experiences with touch, noise, and lighting will help guide the best approach to evaluating and treating the patient.[13]

Child Abuse

Nonaccidental trauma should be in all patients presenting with injuries and complaints, such as altered mental status and apparent life-threatening events. Unfortunately, abusive injuries are frequently not recognized at the initial health care encounter, leaving children at high risk for future and more serious injuries and death. Historical clues to nonaccidental trauma include mechanisms inconsistent with the injury pattern or a history inconsistent with the developmental level of the child (Box 155.3). Physical examination clues for abuse include presence of bruises in young precruising or nonambulatory infants and unusual locations of bruises, such as the trunk, ear(s), and neck (the so-called TEN regions) (Box 155.4). The TEN-4 Rule for bruising states that bruising in children under the age of four in any of the TEN regions, or any bruising under 4 months of age, should raise suspicion for non-accidental trauma. Fractures in children younger than 12 months without a significant witnessed trauma mechanism are especially concerning (see Chapter 172).

BOX 155.3 Historical Features Causing Concern for Child Abuse

History lacking in details
Inconsistency—details change with repeated questioning
History inconsistent with child's developmental status
Reported mechanism inconsistent with injury

BOX 155.4 Physical Examination and Radiologic Findings Concerning for Abuse

Any bruises in young precruising infants
Patterned ecchymosis, burns, or skin marks (abrasions, lacerations)
Bruises on the ears, trunk, inner thighs, neck, or groin
Posterior oropharynx bruising or lacerations
Posterior rib fractures
Classic metaphyseal fractures
Any fracture in a nonambulatory child
Fractures in different stages of healing

OTHER CONSIDERATIONS

Consent for Emergency Care

In general, parent or guardian consent is required for the evaluation and treatment of minors, and emergency clinicians should attempt to notify parents or guardians and obtain consent. However, in emergency situations, evaluation and stabilization cannot be delayed while awaiting consent. The Emergency Medical Treatment and Active Labor Act has mandated that patients presenting for emergency care receive a medical screening examination and, if an emergency medical condition is identified, patients should receive the care required to stabilize the condition (see Chapter e7). Thus, all minors presenting to the ED require an examination to determine if an emergency medical condition exists. If a condition that is threatening to life or health exists, treatment should be provided under the doctrine of implied consent. If an emergency medical condition is not suspected after a screening examination, nonemergent care should be delayed until guardian consent is obtained, unless the minor is legally able to consent for care. Patients in foster care or who are in child protective services custody should have a medical screening examination, but consent for treatment beyond emergency medical conditions may need to be obtained from a state representative.

The circumstances under which minors can consent for their own care vary from state to state, but minors can generally consent if they are emancipated or if they are seeking treatment for mental health issues, drug or alcohol abuse, contraception, pregnancy, or testing for or treatment of sexually transmitted infections. Minors are generally considered emancipated if married, on active duty in the military, or living independently and economically independent from their parents. Some states recognize minors as emancipated if they are pregnant or a parent. Many states recognize that a mature minor, generally 14 years or older, can consent for care if sufficient intelligence and maturity is displayed to make a reasonable and voluntary choice. The process for determining mature minor status varies from state to state.

Pediatric-Ready Emergency Department

Preparation to care for infants and children of all ages involves not only ED staff training but also stocking pediatric medication formulations, equipment, and supplies in appropriate sizes for the premature neonate to the adult-sized adolescent. The American College of Emergency Physicians, American Academy of Pediatrics, and Emergency Nurses Association have developed joint guidelines for the care of children in the ED.[14-16] The guidelines include recommendations for necessary personnel, protocols, medications, equipment, and supplies. Surveys have found that EDs frequently lack the items recommended in the guidelines.[3] One strong recommendation in the guidelines is the appointment of physician and nurse coordinators for pediatric emergency care.[14-16]

Pediatric emergency readiness also requires a plan for continuing care of critically ill and injured children. Small community hospitals often do not have pediatric intensive care units or access to pediatric subspecialists. Therefore, a plan for transfer of patients whose needs exceed available resources is necessary. Receiving hospitals and a mechanism for transporting critically ill pediatric patients should be identified in advance. Overall mortality for critically ill children is reduced in pediatric ready facilities.[17]

Pediatric-Friendly Emergency Department

One topic that has received increasing attention is pain and anxiety management in pediatric patients. Procedural pain is frequently undertreated in infants. Appropriate use of sedation, anesthesia, analgesia, and nonpharmacologic methods of pain management can increase the patient's cooperation and increase visit satisfaction for the child and parent. Children have significant anxiety and fear surrounding medical procedures, leading to additional challenges in performing procedures successfully. In addition to reducing pain and anxiety during the acute visit, adequate pain control is likely to have long-term benefits. Multiple studies have demonstrated that inadequate procedural pain control can lead to increased pain perception with future painful procedures.

A variety of options are available to minimize pain associated with blood draws and intravenous line starts, including vapocoolants, topical anesthetics, and needle-free jet injection of anesthetics.[18] Topical anesthetics can also decrease the pain of an anesthetic injection before a lumbar puncture and other procedures. Topical application of a lidocaine, epinephrine, and tetracaine mixture has been shown to have comparable efficacy to injected anesthesia for facial and scalp lacerations. The combination of sucrose and radiant warmth can provide effective analgesia to newborns.[19] Child life specialists are particularly helpful and, when available, should be used to provide play therapy and education to frightened children, allowing the provider to focus on the procedure. Child life providers are trained in the developmentally appropriate use of nonpharmacologic distraction techniques such as bubbles, songs, books, videos, and video games to decrease anxiety, tools that can also be adopted by department staff.[18] In young children, the use of anxiolytic medications or procedural sedation may be appropriate for procedures that could be accomplished with local anesthesia in older patients.

Providers should encourage and support the family's presence during pediatric procedures and resuscitations.[20] Children are stressed when separated from their parents and their presence can reassure and calm the child. Studies have shown that a family's presence also decreases anxiety levels in family members.[20] Their presence during unsuccessful cardiopulmonary resuscitation is perceived by families as beneficial in the grieving process. Studies have shown that with well-implemented policies, a family's presence does not interfere with resuscitation.[20]

Families present during resuscitations should have a family support person assigned who can explain procedures and answer questions. Ideally, families are briefed on what to expect before entering the resuscitation room. Social workers and Child Life specialists can provide expertise and support, helping families understand what is happening to their child, guide them through procedures, and support them through critical illness and death. Guidelines have been developed to assist emergency clinicians in implementing family presence protocols at their institutions.[21]

The references for this chapter can be found online at ExpertConsult. com.

156

Pediatric Airway Management

Joshua Nagler and Nathan W. Mick

KEY CONCEPTS

- Pediatric advanced airway management is a relatively rare skill to perform in most emergency departments (EDs), and skill maintenance is difficult based solely on clinical practice.
- There are several anatomic differences that impact pediatric airway management, and these occur mostly in the very young child (<2 years of age). Infants have a large occiput and a high, anterior airway, which impacts positioning during intubation. The narrowest portion of the pediatric airway is at the level of the cricothyroid membrane which means a foreign body could be lodged below the cords. They are also more dependent on diaphragmatic excursion for ventilation, thus gastric insufflation can result in difficulty with rescue ventilation.
- Children are prone to desaturation due to their high metabolic rate and their lungs' small functional residual capacity, making preoxygenation and maintenance of oxygenation during intubation attempts crucial.
- The cognitive burden inherent in dealing with the large age/size spectrum in pediatrics can be overcome with reference aids that organize equipment selection and drug dosing based on length/age/size. Formulas have been developed to aid in selection of the correct endotracheal tube (ETT) size and determine appropriate depth of ETT insertion. For estimation of uncuffed tube sizes in children older than 1 year old: ETT size = 4 + (age in years/4). Subtract 0.5 in size for cuffed tubes. To estimate the depth of ETT insertion (the so-called "lip to tip" distance), multiply the ETT size × 3 (e.g., a 5.0 ETT would be inserted to 15 cm at the lip).
- Rapid sequence intubation (RSI) is the preferred method of airway management in the vast majority of pediatric cases in the ED.
- Compared to adults, children are more prone to desaturation over the time it takes for a neuromuscular blocking agent (NMBA) to take effect. Use of high-flow nasal cannula during the apneic period of RSI has not been well studied in children in the emergency setting, but we recommend its use at 1 to 2 L/min/year of age to a maximum of 15 Lpm. Because children desaturate more rapidly than adults, we recommend that assisted ventilation (coordinated with the child's respiratory efforts if not yet fully paralyzed) be initiated if oxygen saturation drops below 95%.
- Video laryngoscopy is an evolving technology for use in pediatrics and assists in visualization of the airway but may prolong time to intubation.
- Surgical airway techniques differ in infants and young children, necessitating a needle technique that is different from the older child or adult. This technique provides a mechanism to oxygenate the "can't intubate, can't ventilate" child, but should not be relied on as a definitive airway.

FOUNDATIONS

Background and Importance

Pediatric airway management is an uncommon, but critical resuscitation skill. Acquisition and retention of necessary skills is difficult when relying solely on clinical practice. Although the skills required to perform advanced airway management between adults and children are similar, there are anatomic and physiologic nuances of pediatric patients. These differences are most prevalent in the first 2 years of life and necessitate modifications to the "typical" intubation approach in older adolescents and adults. Additionally, because of the size and weight spectrum inherent in the pediatric patient population, there is a large spectrum of equipment and medication dosages.

Even in large children's hospitals, there are few opportunities to perform endotracheal intubation as part of clinical practice. Of 1000 pediatric emergency department (ED) patients, 1 to 3 will require intubation, compared to 1 out of 100 adults. Many providers will leave residency training with fewer than 10 pediatric intubations and will not routinely intubate children as part of their clinical practice after training. At the same time, pediatric intubation success and skill mastery improves with increasing experience. Operating room studies demonstrate first-pass intubation success rates are less than 50% after 10 airways but rise to more than 90% after 50 intubation attempts. Fortunately, through experience with older patients, most emergency clinicians can recognize critical illness and have the skills necessary to manage the pediatric airway. These translational skills can be augmented using a simulated environment or with dedicated training in the operating room. Developing a systematic approach to pediatric airway management, while recognizing the anatomic and physiologic differences in the young child, is critical to success and will help to eliminate much of the anxiety associated with performing a time-dependent, infrequent critical procedure.

ANATOMY

There are several anatomic differences in pediatric patients that directly impact airway management (Table 156.1). These differences are most notable in the first 2 years of life; children 2 to 8 years old represent a transitional stage where the anatomy becomes more adult-like, yet there remains variability with medication dosing and equipment size selection.

By correctly positioning the patient, the oral, pharyngeal, and laryngeal axes can be aligned to visualize the glottis during direct laryngoscopy. The small infant has a relatively large head and occiput in relation to their body size. This can cause slight flexion at the neck when the patient is lying supine, impeding the ability to visualize the glottis. The patient should be positioned so that a line drawn through the external auditory canal and the anterior shoulder is horizontal and parallel to the bed (Fig. 156.1). In the infant (younger than 6 months old), this is accomplished by placing a towel roll under the patient's shoulders, elevating the body, and overcoming the neck flexion associated with their large occiput. In the small child (6 months to 5 years old), correct positioning can likely be achieved without the need for support. In the older child/adolescent, the head is smaller in relation to the size of the body, and the head may need to be elevated. As long as cervical spine

TABLE 156.1   Anatomic Differences in Pediatric Airway Management

Anatomic Difference	Implications for Airway Management	Solution
Large occiput and head	Neck position flexed when lying supine and flat on stretcher	Shoulder roll required for optimal positioning of young infant
Large tongue	May occlude airway in the unconscious or obtunded patient	Jaw thrust and oral or nasopharyngeal airway useful adjuncts during airway management
High, anterior airway	Visualization of the vocal cords may be difficult	Correct positioning prior to laryngoscopy critical
Upper airway anatomy and narrow subglottic region	Upper airway prone to dynamic collapse and inflammation (e.g., croup)	Cuffed tubes safe, and sometimes preferred, as long as cuff pressure monitored
Large tonsils and adenoids	Prone to bleeding with manipulation	Blind nasotracheal intubation relatively contraindicated younger than 10 years old
Small cricothyroid membrane	Surgical cricothyrotomy difficult	Needle cricothyrotomy recommended in infants and young children
Large stomach, dependence on diaphragmatic excursion for ventilation	Insufflation of the stomach during BMV can compromise ventilation	Use orogastric or nasogastric tube for decompression

BMV, Bag-mask ventilation.

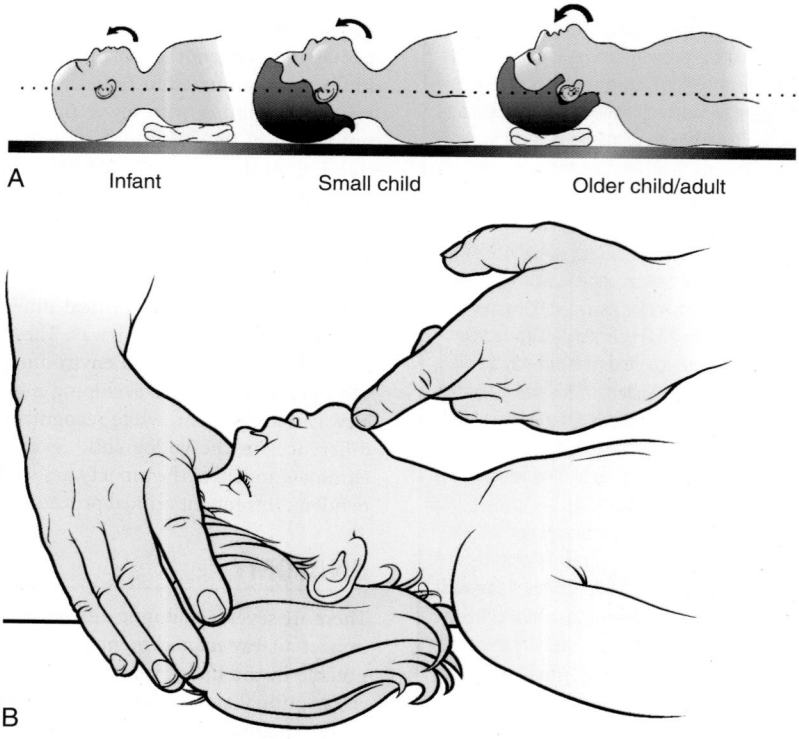

Fig. 156.1 Correct positioning of a pediatric patient to ensure optimal airway alignment utilizing a line passing through the external auditory canal and the anterior shoulder. (A) The small infant requires a shoulder roll to achieve optimal positioning, the small child typically requires neither a shoulder roll nor head support, and the older child/adolescent may require head support. (B) In this small child, a line drawn through the external auditory canal and the anterior shoulder reveals the child to be in good position without support. Slight extension of the head results in the achievement of the sniffing position. (Used with permission: Walls R, Murphy M. *Manual of Emergency Airway Management*, ed 4. Philadelphia: Lippincott Williams & Wilkins; 2012.)

injury is not suspected, correct positioning combined with slight head extension will optimize conditions for direct laryngoscopy.

Infants and children have large tongues relative to the size of their mouths and tend to have a large, floppy epiglottis. Because of these differences in anatomy, they are prone to obstruction when sedated or obtunded, and manipulation of the epiglottis during direct laryngoscopy is frequently required to achieve intubation. Practically, these differences may necessitate the use of an oral or nasopharyngeal airway during bag-mask ventilation (BMV) to bypass the large tongue. Furthermore, a straight (Miller) laryngoscope blade may better manipulate the floppy epiglottis.

The vocal cords and glottic opening are situated at the level of the first cervical vertebrae in infants, gradually dropping to the C3 to C4 level by age 7, and further descending to the C6 level by late

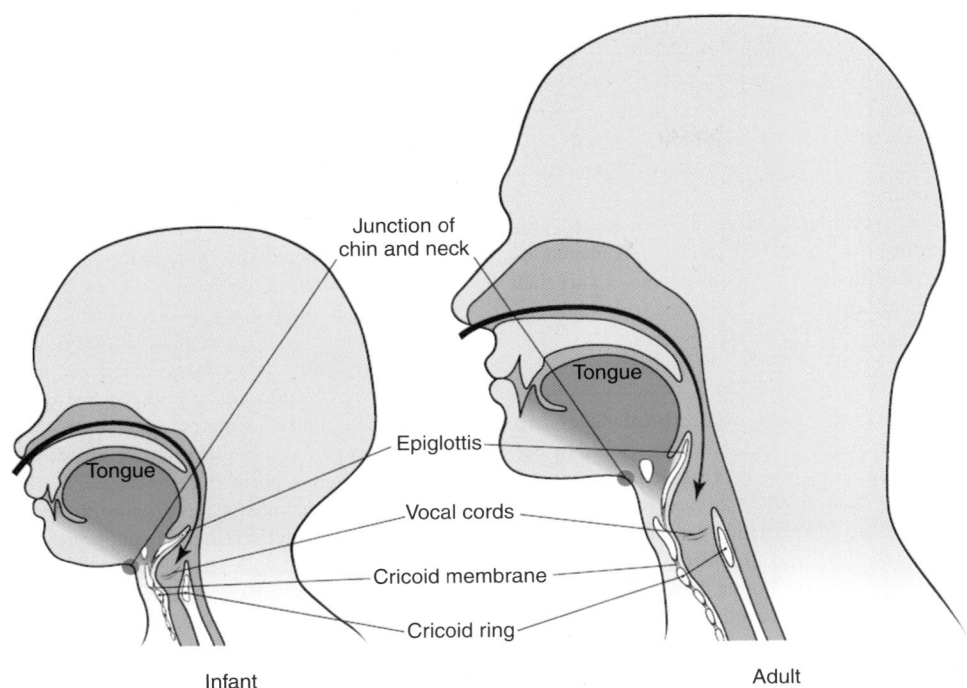

Fig. 156.2 High, anterior airway of the small child. Anatomic difference in the relation of the glottis in the small child compared with the adult.

adolescence. Therefore, the airway is higher and more anterior in small infants than what is encountered in adults, making correct positioning prior to direct laryngoscopy critical to ensure success of intubation (Fig. 156.2).

Historically the narrowest portion of the pediatric trachea was felt to be subglottic at the cricoid ring. However, recent studies using airway CT in anesthetized pediatric patients have confirmed prior MRI and bronchoscopy findings demonstrating anatomic narrowing at the level of the vocal cords and an elliptical-shaped subglottic region.[1,2] Because of the non-distensible nature of the cricoid cartilage, the subglottic region functionally remains the narrowest in the spontaneously breathing child.

The unique anatomy of the pediatric upper airway has traditionally led to the use of uncuffed endotracheal tubes (ETTs) in the small child. Support for uncuffed tubes came at a time when the cuffs were relatively stiff and there was not a reliable, easy way to identify high cuff pressures that can lead to subglottic tracheal injury. Current cuff technology can accurately measure cuff inflation pressures, and we recommend using cuffed tubes for intubation of children, particularly in instances of high airway pressures or poor compliance (e.g., asthma, pneumonia, and acute respiratory distress syndrome [ARDS]).[3-5] Utilizing a cuffed ETT may obviate the need to replace and upsize a tube when there is significant air leak that impacts ventilation, avoiding the risk of losing an already secured airway.

The pediatric trachea is more flexible and prone to dynamic collapse. In addition to implications with positioning during assisted BMV and intubation, the trachea can narrow due to upper airway pathology (e.g., croup, bacterial tracheitis). In cases of upper airway pathology, keeping the patient in a calm and quiet environment is important. Children with "complete" upper airway obstruction often respond well to positive pressure via BMV, which can act to stent open the upper airway. Heliox, typically a 70% to 30% mixture of helium to oxygen, can help decrease a child's work of breathing by increasing laminar flow in partially obstructed airways. Where available, a trial of heliox may be considered in cases of partial upper airway obstruction (e.g., croup), although it has been found no more effective than racemic epinephrine or humidified oxygen in reducing the level of distress in these patients.[6]

The anatomic variations in children impact recommendations in pediatric airway management. Children have relatively prominent tonsillar and adenoidal tissue that is prone to bleeding with even minor trauma. Thus, blind nasotracheal intubation is relatively contraindicated and not routinely recommended in pediatric patients younger than 10 years old. Anatomic landmarks in the neck may be difficult to identify in young infants and children with short necks, and the cricothyroid membrane is small. Thus, needle cricothyrotomy is the recommended invasive airway of choice rather than surgical cricothyrotomy in emergency department settings when the airway cannot otherwise be managed with BMV, intubation or supraglottic device.

Finally, small children are dependent on diaphragmatic excursion for ventilation and have relatively large stomachs and low gastroesophageal sphincter tone. They are predisposed to gastric insufflation during BMV, which can impede diaphragmatic motion and compromise ventilation. Use of cricoid pressure in infants and young children is controversial and not well supported in the literature. If gentle cricoid pressure is used during BMV to reduce gastric insufflation and chest rise is poor, we recommend release of cricoid pressure to see if effective ventilation can then be maintained. We recommend placement of a nasogastric or orogastric tube and aspiration of air immediately following endotracheal intubation, or before intubation attempts if the abdomen is becoming distended and impeding ventilation during BMV.

PHYSIOLOGY

Owing to a high metabolic rate and low functional residual lung capacity, young children are prone to quick desaturation once apneic, even with adequate preoxygenation. Whereas a fully preoxygenated adult with healthy lungs may not desaturate below 90% for a full 6 minutes, a normal healthy 10-kg child may fall below 90% in half that time and a sick infant may desaturate in less than 1 minute. Thus, careful attention to preoxygenation is crucial. Additionally, use of nasal cannula (1–2 L/min/year of age to a maximum of 15 L/min) during the apneic period may help support oxygenation until intubation can be achieved. BMV should be provided between intubation attempts when oxygen saturation levels start to decline below 95%.

Children have a large extracellular fluid volume compared with adults. Many of the drugs used to facilitate endotracheal intubation (sedatives and paralytics) need higher per kilogram doses and their duration of action may also be shorter when compared with adults.

EQUIPMENT

The cognitive burden that occurs when caring for a critically ill child is significant. Equipment selection and medication dosing should be calculated based on weight and size, which can vary tremendously across the spectrum of pediatric patients, from the 3 kg newborn to the 100 kg adolescent. Every ED that cares for pediatric patients should have airway equipment stocked, accessible, and organized by age and size to facilitate easy use. There are numerous mobile device and computer applications, as well as color-coded length-based systems, which can be utilized to simplify medication and equipment selection (Fig. 156.3). Regardless of method, elimination of the reliance on rote memorization lessens the cognitive burden of caring for pediatric patients across the age/size spectrum, particularly during periods of high stress.

There are several "formulas" that are useful in selecting the appropriate equipment for pediatric patients. To determine ETT size, a number of methods are used. Measure the length of the child with a length-based resuscitation tape that has tube sizes based on length and weight recorded on the tape, or use of age-based formulas for a child older than 1 year old:

$$4 + (\text{age in years}/4)$$

Example: 4-year-old patient

$$4 + (4 \text{ years}/4) = 5.0 \text{ uncuffed ETT}$$

or

4.5 *cuffed* ETT (subtract 0.5 from above formula for cuffed tube sizing)

ETT depth of insertion (lip to tip distance) can be visualized during intubation by watching the vocal cord marker go past the vocal cords, or estimated by use of the Broselow-Luten tape or by the following formula:

$$3 \times \text{uncuffed tube size} = \text{lip to tip distance (midtrachea)}$$

Example: 5.0 ETT

$$3 \times 5.0 = 15 \text{ cm depth of insertion}$$

MANAGEMENT

Decision Making

For a child who is effectively stabilized using noninvasive means (such as BMV), the additional benefit of a secure airway needs to be weighed against the risk of potential difficulty or complications. Failure to successfully oxygenate or ventilate a child by other means forces immediate action, whereas other conditions allow medical interventions and recurrent assessments over time to determine if advanced airway management is required.

Overall, an equal number of pediatric intubations in the ED are performed on trauma and nontrauma patients.[7] Indications for pediatric intubation can be placed into four categories: (1) inability to oxygenate and ventilate; (2) inability to maintain or protect the airway; (3) potential for clinical deterioration; and (4) facilitation of necessary diagnostic studies, procedures, or for safe patient transport (e.g., high risk of decompensation on route).

Respiratory compromise is a leading contributor to morbidity and mortality in the pediatric population, and more likely than a primary cardiac disease to be the cause of arrest. Respiratory failure can result from intrinsic pulmonary disease or from conditions with infectious, neuromuscular, traumatic, toxicologic, or environmental etiologies. Respiratory failure is a clinical diagnosis, identified by characteristic examination findings and supported by noninvasive measurement of oxygenation (pulse oximetry) and ventilation (capnography). Blood gas analysis can also be informative but should not be relied upon to determine need to perform necessary advanced airway management.

Signs of partial obstruction (sonorous or stridulous airway noises) or complete obstruction (inability to phonate or produce audible breath sounds in a patient with adequate respiratory effort) suggest an inability to maintain the airway and should prompt immediate basic airway maneuvers, including airway repositioning or insertion of oral and nasal airways to help stent open the upper airways. Suctioning and removal of any foreign material might also be required. When these efforts are ineffective, patients may require an advanced airway. For patients with severely depressed mental status, the loss of protective airway reflexes may necessitate airway control, regardless of the ability to maintain the airway. For example, the use of a Glasgow Coma Score (GCS) of 8 or less is often cited as an indication for intubation in head-injured patients. Systemic illness, toxicologic exposure, and other etiologies of central nervous system (CNS) depression may also increase risk of aspiration; the presence of a gag reflex correlates poorly with GCS and the risk of aspiration. Thus, testing for a gag is not recommended, because it may increase the risk of vomiting and subsequent aspiration.

When airway compromise is progressive (e.g., from acute thermal injury), airway management should be initiated early to avoid increased difficulty later in securing the airway. Similarly, patients with systemic illnesses (e.g., sepsis) may require intubation to maximize oxygen delivery and decrease the metabolic demands of increased work of breathing.

Children often require sedation to perform diagnostic testing, such as computed tomography (CT), magnetic resonance imaging (MRI), or invasive procedures. The risk of airway compromise during procedural sedation is greater in patients with significant illness or medical instability. Therefore, securing the child's airway may be necessary to ensure safety during the procedure, particularly in circumstances where accessibility for assessment and intervention may be compromised (e.g., a patient under surgical drapes or tunneled into a CT or MRI scanner). Because many acutely ill and injured children will require transfer to a pediatric tertiary care center, the stability of the patient's overall condition and risk of airway compromise should be carefully considered. Securing the airway prior to transfer can obviate the need for emergent advanced airway management in a less controlled setting.

Rapid Sequence Intubation

Rapid sequence intubation (RSI) is the preferred method to perform endotracheal intubation in children, provided no contraindications exist. We do not recommend attempting emergency pediatric endotracheal intubation with sedation only as studies have demonstrated higher success and lower complications rates with RSI. A small number of medications are used for pretreatment, sedation/induction, and neuromuscular blockade during ED pediatric RSI (Table 156.2).

GENERIC PEDIATRIC RSI

zero – 10+ min.	**Preparation**	
	Preoxygenation	100% O₂
	Apneic preoxygenation (1-2 lpm per year of age to a max of 15 lpm)	
	Pre-Intubation Optimization	Atropine*
	Paralysis with Induction	Etomidate, SCh or Rocuronium
zero	**Positioning**	Consider shoulder roll for infants < 6 months
zero + 15 sec.	**Placement with Proof**	Intubate
	Confirm placement clinically and with ETCO₂ detection	
zero + 45 sec.	**Post-Intubation Management**	Sedation and analgesia
zero + 1 min.	Paralysis only if necessary	

* optional, used principally for infants less than one year of age

the.**difficult airway**course™

theairwaysite.com

The Broselow Luten zones for PEDIATRIC DRUGS AND EQUIPMENT

ZONE	3kg	4kg	5kg	PINK	RED	PURPLE	YELLOW	WHITE	BLUE	ORANGE	GREEN
Length (cm)	46–52	52–57	57–61	61–67	67–75	75–85	85–97	97–109	109–121	121–133	133–146
Weight (kg)	3	4	5	6–7	8–9	10–11	12–14	15–18	19–23	24–29	30–36
PRETREATMENT											
Atropine	0.06 mg	0.08 mg	0.1 mg	0.13 mg	0.17 mg	0.2 mg	N/A	N/A	N/A	N/A	N/A
INDUCTION											
Etomidate	0.9 mg	1.2 mg	1.5 mg	2 mg	2.5 mg	3.2 mg	4 mg	5 mg	6.3 mg	8 mg	10 mg
Ketamine	6 mg	8 mg	10 mg	13 mg	17 mg	20 mg	26 mg	33 mg	42 mg	53 mg	66 mg
Propofol	9 mg	12 mg	15 mg	20 mg	25 mg	32 mg	40 mg	50 mg	63 mg	80 mg	100 mg
PARALYSIS											
Succinylcholine	6 mg	8 mg	10 mg	13 mg	17 mg	20 mg	26 mg	33 mg	40 mg	53 mg	66 mg
Rocuronium	3 mg	4 mg	5 mg	7 mg	9 mg	10 mg	13 mg	17 mg	21 mg	27 mg	33 mg
MAINTENANCE*											
Vecuronium	0.3 mg	0.4 mg	0.5 mg	0.7 mg	0.9 mg	1 mg	1.3 mg	1.7 mg	2.1 mg	2.7 mg	3.3 mg
Lorazepam	0.15 mg	0.2 mg	0.25 mg	0.3 mg	0.4 mg	0.5 mg	0.6 mg	0.8 mg	1 mg	1.3 mg	1.6 mg
EQUIPMENT											
ET Tube (mm)	3.5 unc/3.0 cuff	3.5 unc/3.0 cuff	3.5 unc/3.0 cuff	3.5 unc/3.0 cuff	3.5 unc/3.0 cuff	4.0 unc/3.5 cuff	4.5 unc/4.0 cuff	5.0 unc/4.5 cuff	5.5 unc/5.0 cuff	5.5 cuff	6.0 cuff
Lip-Tip (cm)	9–9.5	9.5–10	10–10.5	10–10.5	10.5–11	11–12	12.5–13.5	14–15	15.5–16.5	17–18	18.5–19.5
Suction	8 F	8 F	8 F	8 F	8 F	8–10 F	10 F	10 F	10 F	10 F	12 F
L-Scope blade	1 St.	1 St.	1 St.	1 St.	1 St.	1 St.	2 St./Cvd.	2 St./Cvd.	2 St./Cvd.	2–3 St./Cvd.	2–3 St./Cvd.
Stylet	6 F	6 F	6 F	6 F	6 F	6 F	10 F	10 F	10 F	14 F	14 F
Oral Airway	50 mm	50 mm	50 mm	50 mm	50 mm	60 mm	60 mm	60 mm	70 mm	80 mm	80 mm
NP Airway	14 F	14 F	14 F	14 F	14 F	18 F	20 F	22 F	24 F	26 F	26 F
ETCO₂ Detector	PED	PED	PED	PED	PED	PED	PED	ADULT	ADULT	ADULT	ADULT
BVM (min vol mLs)	450	450	450	450	450	450	450	450–750	750–1000	750–1000	1000
LMA	1	1	1	1.5	1.5	2	2	2.5	2.5	2.5	3
VENTILATION											
Tidal Volume mL	20–30	24–40	30–50	40–65	50–85	65–105	80–130	100–165	125–210	160–265	200–330
Frequency (BPM)	20–25	20–25	20–25	20–25	20–25	15–25	15–25	15–25	12–20	12–20	12–20
Insp. time (sec)	0.6	0.6	0.6	0.6	0.6	0.7	0.7	0.7	0.8	0.8	0.8

* optional, used principally for infants less than one year of age

* Midazolam and propofol can be used for post-intubation sedation. Dosing is on the other side of the card.

INTUBATION CONSIDERATIONS IN CHILDREN

Insertion Depth — see color chart
Ventilator Settings
 FiO₂: 100%
 PEEP: 5 cm H₂O initial
 PIP: 20–30 cm H₂O
 Inspiratory Time: see color chart
 Tidal Volume* and RR: see color chart
Post Intubation — Secure tube at lip and stabilize neck

*Tidal volume of 6–10 mL/kg frequently used, but assess patient to determine there is chest rise and distal air entry on exam. Adequate tidal volume typically requires PIP of at least 15 cm H₂O if lung compliance is normal.

Fig. 156.3 The Broselow-Luten zones for pediatric drugs and equipment. *BVM,* bag-valve mask; *ETco₂,* end-tidal carbon dioxide; *ETT,* endotracheal tube; *Fio₂,* fraction of inspired oxygen; *LMA,* laryngeal mask airway; *NP,* nasopharyngeal; *PED,* pediatric; *PEEP,* positive end-expiratory pressure; *PIP,* peak inspiratory pressure; *RR,* respiratory rate; *RSI,* rapid sequence intubation; *SCh,* succinylcholine. (Reproduced with permission from the Airway Management Education Center, The Difficult Airway Course: Emergency 2020.)

TABLE 156.2   Common Rapid-Sequence Intubation Medications in Children[a]

Medication	Dosage	Comments
Premedications		
Atropine	0.02 mg/kg	Not routinely used in RSI. Consider use in young infants (<1 year of age) Should be given for preexisting or periprocedure bradycardia not responsive to oxygenation and ventilation
Lidocaine	1.5 mg/kg	Not routinely used in RSI. Very limited pediatric-specific data to support use in increased ICP Needs to be given 3 minutes prior to laryngoscopy No data for bronchodilatory effect in children
Induction Agents		
Etomidate	0.3 mg/kg	Rapid and reliable sedation Preserves hemodynamics Known to cause adrenal suppression even with single dose, although limited data on impact on clinical outcome Consider stress dose hydrocortisone with use No analgesic properties
Ketamine	1 to 2 mg/kg	Causes release of endogenous catecholamines May support hemodynamics in hypotensive patients Beta-agonist effect may help with bronchodilatation, favoring its use in asthma Preserves airway reflexes and respiratory drive Can be used without NMBA for "awake sedated look" in suspected difficult airways
Propofol	3 mg/kg	Rapid onset, short acting May cause hypotension Apnea possible Higher dose recommended in infants No analgesic properties
Midazolam	0.3 mg/kg	Higher dosing required than used for antiepileptic dosing or anxiolysis At induction dosing, may cause hypotension Often used concomitantly with opioids No analgesic properties
Fentanyl	1 to 5 mcg/kg	Often used with midazolam Lower dosing (1–2 mcg/kg) recommended for shock or hemodynamic concerns
Paralytics		
Rocuronium	1 to 1.2 mg/kg	Nondepolarizing agent Equivalent onset as succinylcholine but longer duration of action No specific contraindications in patients suitable for RSI
Vecuronium	0.1 mg/kg	Nondepolarizing agent Slower onset of action than rocuronium Suitable alternative for rocuronium if more readily available
Succinylcholine	0–11 years: 2 mg/kg >11 years: 1.5 mg/kg Double the dose when given IM	Fasciculations without clinical relevance in children Shorter duration than rocuronium Very low risk of bradycardia with IV induction agents used in ED (see earlier) Risk of hyperkalemia and arrest in patients with known and undiagnosed myopathies and neuromuscular disease
Sugammadex	16 mg/kg (full reversal dose)	Rapid reversal agent for rocuronium or vecuronium Neuromuscular blockade generally reversed within 3 minutes

[a]RSI medications can be given intraosseous (IO) when IV access cannot be obtained.
ED, Emergency department; *ICP,* intracranial pressure; *IM,* intramuscular; *IV,* intravenous; *NMBA,* neuromuscular blocking agent; *RSI,* rapid sequence intubation.

Pretreatment

The goal of pretreatment medications is to attenuate the physiologic responses to laryngoscopy and intubation, or to mitigate the adverse effect of pharmacologic agents used for sedation or neuromuscular blockade; however, data are limited with regard to the benefit of pretreatment medications in children. Use of these agents needs to be weighed against the potential for procedural delays and drug errors that can occur with the administration of medications requiring weight-based dosing. This is particularly relevant during high stress situations, such as the management of critically ill children. Two drugs have been used for pretreatment in pediatrics: (1) atropine to prevent bradycardia related to vagal tone, and (2) lidocaine to attenuate the reflex sympathetic response in patients with concern for increased intracranial pressure (ICP); however, their use today is not routinely recommended.

Infants, particularly younger than 1 year old, have higher intrinsic vagal tone than older children or adults. Atropine serves as a vagolytic and can reduce the risk of bradycardia resulting from laryngoscopy in this age group. There is an association between the use of succinylcholine and bradycardia. Data suggest that this risk may be tied to use with select inhaled anesthetics (e.g., halothane) and with newer induction agents the incidence of succinylcholine-related bradycardia is very low.[8] Given the limited available evidence, routine use of atropine for patients receiving succinylcholine during RSI is not necessary.[9] Atropine may be helpful for bradycardia that exists prior to intubation, but it should only be considered once hypoxia-induced bradycardia is excluded and maximal oxygenation achieved.

Data on the effectiveness of lidocaine in blunting the sympathetic response to laryngoscopy in patients with suspected elevated ICP are limited to case series and extrapolated from adult experience. Literature reviews have failed to identify a benefit in adult head injured patients, and no supporting data exist in pediatric populations. Therefore, we do not recommend the routine use of lidocaine.

Sedatives

Sedatives rapidly induce unconsciousness and facilitate intubation. Providers should choose sedatives based on their efficacy, adverse effect profile, and clinical situation. In particular, providers should pay careful attention to the hemodynamic profile of these agents, to minimize the risk of clinical deterioration during RSI.

Etomidate is a common sedative used for pediatric RSI. It has reliable efficacy and pharmacokinetics and a stable hemodynamic profile. Etomidate may suppress adrenal corticosteroid synthesis transiently. However, no convincing data exist to suggest that administration of a single dose during intubation influences clinical outcome. Pediatric advanced life support (PALS) guidelines have included precautions against "routine use" in septic shock, and suggest consideration of stress dose hydrocortisone when etomidate is used.

Ketamine is a dissociative anesthetic with reliable and rapid onset. Its use is well established for procedural sedation and analgesia in pediatrics. It causes an endogenous release of catecholamines, making it appealing for patients with hypotension or shock. Adverse reactions to ketamine include vomiting, laryngospasm, myoclonus, and emergence phenomenon. Although ketamine is a known sialagogue, the coadministration of atropine is unlikely to be of help during RSI given that the onset of action for the drying effects of atropine may take up to 20 minutes. Ketamine has been shown to increase ICP, although the significance of this on clinical outcome is unclear, as it can also support cerebral perfusion pressure.[10,11] The catecholamine release with ketamine may lead to the beta-agonist effect of bronchodilation, making it an ideal drug for patients with bronchoconstriction. This same benefit may not apply to conditions such as bronchiolitis, in which airway edema and debris are the primary etiology of airway obstruction. Ketamine is the preferred sedative for children in septic shock requiring RSI because of its ability to maintain mean arterial pressure.[12]

Propofol has rapid and profound sedative properties, that when combined with its short duration of action, make it an ideal induction agent. However, as a vasodilator and myocardial depressant, propofol is not recommended in patients with tenuous hemodynamics, including hypovolemia or shock. Propofol may also compromise cerebral perfusion if mean arterial pressure is rapidly reduced.

Benzodiazepine dosing is higher for RSI induction than when used as an anticonvulsant or during procedural sedation. For example, 0.3 to 0.4 mg/kg of midazolam may be required to achieve sufficient sedation. Alternatively, benzodiazepines may be used in conjunction with opioids, such a fentanyl, but the combination can compromise hemodynamics.

Neuromuscular Blocking Agents

Neuromuscular blocking agents (NMBAs) are used to relax airway musculature and block airway protective reflexes during laryngoscopy to facilitate the passage of an ETT. The aim is rapid onset of action to limit the time without spontaneous or assisted ventilation. Succinylcholine and rocuronium are the most commonly used NMBAs for emergent pediatric RSI.[13] Understanding the specific benefits and risks of each is helpful in creating an airway management plan.

Succinylcholine has a rapid onset of action of 30 to 60 seconds and duration of action of 3 to 8 minutes. It is the oldest, and often the most familiar, NMBA for emergency clinicians, and has a long track record of safe and effective use. Higher doses (2 mg/kg) are recommended in neonates and infants compared to 1.5 mg/kg for adolescents. Providers should be aware of several side effects and potential risks of succinylcholine. Muscle fasciculations result from the depolarizing effect of this agent, although young children may not have large enough muscle mass to result in clinically observable effects. Succinylcholine can cause hyperkalemia, which can be fatal in a number of clinical conditions (see Table 156.2). In many patients, high-risk diagnoses are known or suspected; however, published case series have described succinylcholine use in infants with undiagnosed myopathies leading to hyperkalemia arrest. As a result, a US Food and Drug Administration (FDA) black box warning exists for the use of succinylcholine in children, although given the rarity of these conditions, exception has been allowed for emergency use. Given this waiver, succinylcholine is still the most commonly used NMBA in pediatric emergency airway management.[7] Other serious but rare adverse effects of succinylcholine use in children include masseter spasm and malignant hyperthermia, which are most commonly associated with concurrent halothane use. Masseter spasm is a rare side effect of succinylcholine administration in children and can be terminated by the administration of a competitive neuromuscular blocking agent (NMBA).

Rocuronium is the most common nondepolarizing NMBA used in emergency pediatric airway management. Pediatric data suggest that rocuronium at a dose of 1.2 mg/kg has equivalent efficacy in time to intubation conditions as succinylcholine. The duration of action, however, is much longer with a time to return of spontaneous respirations of anywhere from 20 to 90 minutes. The primary advantage of nondepolarizing agents is the absence of the risks (e.g., hyperkalemia) associated with depolarizing agents. The longer duration of action can be of concern if the airway cannot be secured or in patients in whom rapid return of examination findings (e.g., neurologic examination) is important. However, it may also have advantages if subsequent management may include imaging, additional vascular access, initial ventilator management, or other procedures. A reversal agent (sugammadex) for rocuronium exists that can limit its duration of action to less than that of succinylcholine.

DEVICES AND TECHNIQUES

Basic Airway Management

The priority in pediatric airway management is establishing effective oxygenation and ventilation. For children with hypoxemia but effective ventilation and without concern for increased work of breathing, passive supplemental oxygen delivery may be sufficient. For mild hypoxemia in children who will not tolerate a nasal cannula or face mask, "blow-by" oxygen using a mask, shovel, or plastic funnel attached to oxygen tubing aimed toward the face are options. Nasal cannula can provide more consistent oxygen delivery, particularly in infants who are preferential nasal breathers. High-flow nasal cannula is increasingly being used to deliver supplementary oxygen to pediatric patients. The heated and humidified delivery allows higher flow rates without discomfort, and the absence of a need for a tight seal makes application easier than other forms of noninvasive ventilation.[14] Simple face masks can be used, whereas non-rebreather masks provide maximal passive oxygen delivery in spontaneously breathing patients.

When ventilation is of concern or a child's work of breathing is excessive, assisted ventilation may be required with a bag and mask. Effective assisted ventilation requires: (1) a patent airway and (2) an effective mask seal. Opening the airway is accomplished with positioning of the child, avoiding flexion of the neck from a large occiput or from downward pressure on the face when applying the mask. Application of basic airway maneuvers including a head tilt–chin lift maneuver or a jaw thrust can be of further help. Placement of nasopharyngeal and oral airways can be of value when the airway is being partially or completely obstructed, often by the tongue or soft palate. Oral airways are only tolerated in patients with depressed mental status, either pharmacologically induced or related to underlying pathophysiology. To create an effective mask seal, the provider first needs to select the appropriate size mask. An ideal fitting mask is large enough to cover the nose and open mouth but should not allow air leak across the bridge of the nose or off the base of the chin. Emergency clinicians should deliver appropriate volume and pressure breaths. There may be a tendency in an acute situation to deliver a much larger tidal volume than is appropriate for the size of the child, which may result in barotrauma. Gentle rise of the chest accompanied by clinical improvement are key clinical features of effective BMV. The bag-mask device should be squeezed just until chest rise is initiated and then released. The emergency clinician may time ventilation by stating "squeeze, release, release" which slows ventilation rate and may reduce complications from hyperventilation and gastric insufflation during rescue ventilation. Cricoid pressure has limited utility, primarily in reducing gastric insufflation, and should be used with caution in children. Too much cricoid pressure can compress the pliable pediatric trachea, leading to iatrogenic upper airway obstruction. Cricoid pressure should be lightened or released if felt to impede BMV.

Advanced Airway Management

Chapter 1 covers a detailed approach to RSI. The general approach to the procedure is identical to that of an adult, although there are several pediatric considerations worthy of mention.

Preparation

Passive oxygen delivery devices, self-inflating bags and masks, oral and nasal airways, laryngoscope blades, ETTs, stylets, and rescue devices all come in varying sizes to match the anatomy of the child. Generally having at least two sizes of ETTs (estimated size as well as a half size smaller) available during the procedure is prudent. Having a systematic approach to identifying the correct equipment prior to initiating the procedure can eliminate errors and failed attempts in critical situations. Potential resources include a length-based resuscitation system, pediatric resuscitation cards (Fig. 156.3), print or online textbooks, and mobile device applications.

Preoxygenation

As described earlier, young children desaturate much more quickly than adolescents or adults. In a patient with sufficient respiratory effort,

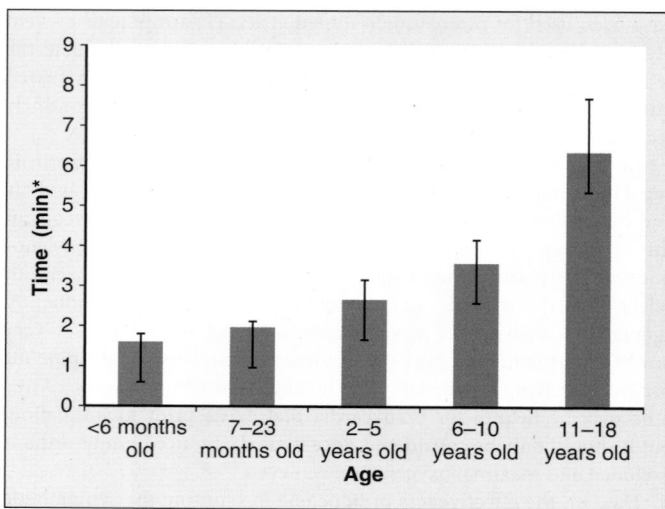

Fig. 156.4 Time to desaturation in preoxygenated healthy children. (American Society of Anesthesiologists Classification 1 [ASA 1] patients undergoing elective surgery.) *Time from administration of neuromuscular blocking agent (NMBA) to desaturation to 90%, with no ongoing supplemental oxygen or respiratory support. (Adapted from: Patel R, Lenczyk M, Hannallah RS, et al. Age and the onset of desaturation in apnoeic children. *Can J Anaesth.* 1994;41:771-774.)

preoxygenation with maximal passive oxygen delivery (i.e., a non-rebreather mask) for 2 to 3 minutes may be sufficient in healthy children. However, patients requiring emergency intubation often have compromised pulmonary function or respiratory effort and may benefit from a more prolonged preoxygenation time. A technique of using vital capacity breaths for more rapid preoxygenation will be difficult to accomplish in children who may not be cooperative with this technique. Even with appropriate preoxygenation, a significant percentage of young children will desaturate during intubation attempts, particularly those with underlying respiratory illness or when intubation attempts are prolonged (Fig. 156.4).[15] Due to children's propensity to quickly drop oxygen saturations during intubation attempts, we recommend utilizing apneic oxygenation using nasal cannula during RSI. A number of nasal cannula flow rates for apneic oxygenation in children have been proposed.[8] As a simplified approach in infants and children, we recommend 1 to 2 L/min/year of age to a maximum of 15 L/min for children to help prevent the drop in oxygen saturation during the apneic period of RSI. Positive-pressure ventilation with bag-mask device should be considered at the first sign of desaturation, and we recommend it be initiated when oxygen saturation drops below 95%. Once oxygen saturation has improved, additional attempts can begin.

Positioning

As described previously, age-appropriate positioning is required during laryngoscopy and endotracheal intubation. Alignment of the oral, pharyngeal, and tracheal axes greatly facilitates visualization. In neonates and infants, a shoulder roll is often required; toddlers and school-age children are usually best aligned in the neutral recumbent position; and adolescents will often require elevation of the head similar to adults.

Placement of Tube

When performing direct laryngoscopy, straight blades placed beneath the epiglottis are preferred in infants and younger children to lift the larger pediatric epiglottis and bring the vocal cords into line of sight. Alternatively, an appropriately sized laryngoscope blade placed into the

TABLE 156.3	Common Post-Intubation Sedation/Analgesia in Children		
Medication	**Bolus Dosing**	**Drip**	**Comments**
Lorazepam	0.05 to 0.1 mg/kg		Long-acting sedative/amnesic Often used in combination with analgesic
Midazolam	0.5 to 2 mg/kg	0.05 to 0.1 mg/kg/h	Short-acting sedative/amnestic Often used in combination with analgesic
Fentanyl	1 to 2 mcg/kg	1 to 3 mcg/kg/h	Short-acting analgesia Preserves hemodynamic stability
Morphine	0.05 to 0.1 mg/kg	0.05 to 0.1 mg/kg/h	Longer-acting analgesic May cause histamine release
Ketamine		0.1 to 1 mg/kg/h	Bolus dosing not recommended for prolonged ongoing sedation May be helpful in status asthmaticus
Propofol	0.5 to 1 mg/kg	25 to 250 mcg/kg/min	No analgesic properties Prolonged infusion in children can lead to profound acidosis and rhabdomyolysis
Dexmedetomidine		0.2 to 0.7 mcg/kg/h	Associated with significant cardiovascular effects (including bradycardia, hypotension, AND hypertension) Limited data on safety in infants (<5 kg)

vallecula can engage the hyoepiglottic ligament to elevate the epiglottis in most pediatric patients.[7] In younger children, emergency clinicians may tend to insert the laryngoscope blade too deeply, resulting in retroglottic or esophageal placement and unnecessary airway trauma. With this in mind, emergency clinicians should start the intubation procedure by placing the laryngoscope blade just to the base of the tongue and lift up to view the airway anatomy. Identify structures progressively, first directly identifying the base of the tongue and the epiglottis prior to insertion of the straight blade underneath the epiglottis or the curved blade into the vallecula to visualize the vocal cords. If no laryngeal structures are identified due to inadvertent deep insertion, the blade should be slowly withdrawn under visualization, and the cords or the epiglottis will often fall into view.

Given the superior position of the larynx in children, use of a stylet is often helpful in guiding the ETT into the glottic opening. This is particularly true during videolaryngoscopy, where the delivery of the endotracheal tube to the glottic opening is often performed under *indirect* visualization. Given the relatively small size of the oropharyngeal cavity, the tube should be placed from the 3 o'clock position, often with an assistant applying lateral traction to the child's lip to provide more room for tube insertion.

There is a tendency to insert the ETT too far in the young child in whom the distance from the vocal cords to the tracheal carina may just be a few centimeters.[16] Right mainstem intubation is difficult to appreciate on auscultation, particularly in the infant whose breath sounds are easily transmitted throughout the chest. Using a pediatric resuscitation resource as described earlier, or the formula (tube size × 3 = depth [cm] at the lip) can approximate insertion depth. Under direct visualization, the vocal cord markers on the tube should rest just below the glottic opening, or the cuff observed to pass just beyond the vocal cords.

Post-Intubation Management

Optimally, the ETT should be visualized to pass into the glottic opening. If vocal cords are not seen, passage of the tube below the epiglottis and above the posterior cartilages indicates ETT placement into the glottic aperture, but should be subsequently assessed clinically in conjunction with other confirmatory tests. Visible chest wall rise, auscultation of breaths sounds in both axillae, absence of gurgling noise in the epigastrium (i.e., exclusion of esophageal placement), and improving

oxygenation are all used to confirm tube position. However, end-tidal carbon dioxide ($ETco_2$) detection, either with a colorimetric device or capnography, is the most reliable and accurate measure of correct tube placement. Waveform capnography is preferred for monitoring pediatric ventilation and for determination of correct airway placement.

If waveform capnography is not available, then pediatric colorimetric $ETco_2$ detectors are available for children weighing less than 15 kg in whom smaller tidal volumes may result in less apparent detection using adult-sized devices. Detection of $ETco_2$ confirms the ETT is in the tracheobronchial tree; however, it does not discriminate between intubation of the trachea and the right mainstem bronchus. In patients in cardiac arrest, CO_2 delivery to the lungs is markedly reduced and gas exchange is compromised, therefore CO_2 may not be detectable. Here, an esophageal detector device or bulb may be used to confirm tracheal placement in children who weigh more than 20 kg. Point-of-care ultrasound has been introduced as a real-time modality for detecting bilateral lung sliding, diaphragm excursion, and cuff position in the trachea.[16] However, a chest radiograph is still considered standard of care to confirm appropriate position.

Even small movements of the child's head can result in accidental displacement of the tube: flexion of the neck can advance the tube into a mainstem bronchus, whereas neck extension can lead to unintended extubation. After intubation, the ETT should be secured and, as much as is possible, the child's head and neck kept still. Most sedatives used for induction will wear off before rocuronium; therefore post-intubation sedatives should be administered after the airway has been secured. Table 156.3 lists common drugs used for post-intubation sedation in the pediatric population. Decisions regarding continued neuromuscular blockade can be made based on clinical context, including desire for return of clinical examination, ventilation management strategies, need for additional procedures or diagnostics studies, and need for interfacility transfer.

Video Laryngoscopy

Video laryngoscopy is an emerging approach to pediatric airway management. Much as in adults, data support improved laryngeal views with video laryngoscopes, with particular benefit in cases where there is difficulty visualizing the vocal cords, or Cormack-Lehane airways classified as grade 3 (only epiglottis seen) or grade 4 (neither epiglottis nor glottis seen). In addition, video laryngoscopy allows for shared

TABLE 156.4	Video Laryngoscopy Devices for Use in Pediatrics				
Device	**Description**	**Monitor**	**Disposable**	**Recording**	**Sizes**
C-MAC	Traditional Miller and Macintosh shaped blades Allows for direct or indirect (video projection) laryngoscopy	7" LCD monitor or 2.4" pocket monitor	Reusable blades or disposable blades	SD card in 7" monitor Pocket monitor also allows recording	Miller (size 0, 1, 2) Macintosh (size 0, and 2 to 4) D-Blade (pediatric and adult sizes)
GlideScope	Blades with 60-degree angulation Different models GVL, AVL (advanced video technology) GlideScope Go (handheld)	7" LCD monitor or 3.5" portable screen	Reusable blades Video batons with single use blades	DVR or USB depending on model	Newly available Miller 0 and 1 blades GVL Blades (size 0, 1, 2, 2.5, 3, and 4) Macintosh blades (size 3 and 4)
Airtraq	Different models Disposable blade with reusable optics Fully disposable optical laryngoscope, no electronics Channeled device (provides guide for ETT to pass around curvature of airway)	Direct view eyepiece or 2.6" camera hood with wi-fi capabilities	Disposable single-use devices Reusable optics with disposable blades available in adult sizes only	Phone adapter or wi-fi camera	Size 0 (infant) Size 1 (pediatric) Size 2 (small) Size 3 (regular)
King Vision	Handheld videolaryngoscope, disposable channeled and unchanneled blades	2.4" LCD display	Reusable display and video adapter, disposable blades	Video output capability, no internal recording	Size 1 (unchanneled) Size 2 and 3 (channelled and unchanneled)

AVL, Advanced video laryngoscopy; *DVR*, digital video recording; *ETT*, endotracheal tube; *GVL*, GlideScope video laryngoscope; *LCD*, liquid crystal display; *SD*, secure digital; *USB*, universal serial bus.

viewing by multiple providers, which permits real-time guidance and supervision during tracheal intubation. Currently, data on the use of video laryngoscopy in pediatric patients are largely limited to the anesthesia literature or performance in simulated scenarios, although emergency medicine studies focused on use in children are emerging. Data consistently show that video laryngoscopy improves visualization, and newer data suggest it may also improve first-pass success.[18,19] Importantly, video laryngoscopy has been shown to have a faster learning curve than direct laryngoscopy. This may be particularly important for airway management in children, given the infrequency with which pediatric airway management is performed in the ED.

Video laryngoscopes for use in pediatrics are becoming increasingly available. Many are smaller adult models, which permit use in older children. Currently, there are a limited number of devices available with a complete range of sizes that allow for use across all pediatric ages, from neonates to adolescents. There are unique advantages, potential drawbacks, and subtleties in technique for using each (Table 156.4). The decision regarding which device to use is ultimately based on availability, operator preference, operator experience, and patient-specific attributes that may favor a given approach.

Airway Rescue Devices for Children

The overall success rate for advanced airway management in children is more than 99%, so the need for rescue device use is fortunately rare. Nonetheless, it is imperative to have a contingency plan for circumstances in which a provider cannot secure the airway. Bag-mask ventilation is a critical, and often underestimated, skill for establishing adequate oxygenation and ventilation in pediatric patients. A recent retrospective study on nontraumatic out-of-hospital pediatric cardiac arrest found improved survival to hospital discharge among children who received BMV by emergency medical services (EMS) compared to children who received either endotracheal intubation or supraglottic device (SGD).[20] Additionally, a study of children with in-hospital

cardiac arrest found no difference in survival to hospital discharge among children receiving either ETI or BVM.[21] Alternative strategies to manage the airway when intubation cannot be accomplished using traditional techniques include SGDs or optical approaches to improve glottic visualization.[22,23] SGDs have been demonstrated to be a reliable way to establish oxygenation and gas exchange in the normal and difficult pediatric airway, as well as during resuscitation. First-generation devices have been used in anesthesia for decades. Newer, second-generation devices often include a channel that allows gastric decompression. In addition to the gastric channel, some current SGDs have alternative construction that may be advantageous in pediatrics.[24] For example, the Air-Q does not have aperture bars and uses a shorter wider tube to allow passage of an ETT through the lumen. The I-gel uses a thermoplastic elastomer that molds to the airway as it warms from body temperature. This allows a tighter seal and avoids complications related to cuff hyperinflation.

In most cases, SGDs are easily and rapidly placed, with more than 90% success rate on first attempts; devices sized for neonates and young infants are the most difficult to place. Placement technique is similar to adults with two potential differences: (1) some studies have demonstrated improved placement success and fewer complications when using a rotational approach with traditional laryngeal mask airways (LMAs); and (2) insertion of the SGD with the cuff partially inflated may facilitate placement and help it mold to the shape of the pharynx. SGDs are available in all sizes from neonatal to adolescent ages but data are limited on their use in emergency settings. The Combitube is not recommended for those under 4 feet tall.[25,26]

Pharyngeal sealers, also called *esophageal blockers,* are double-balloon devices in which the tip is placed into the upper esophagus, and ventilation occurs between one balloon occluding the proximal esophagus and another occluding the airway above the glottis. In small children, laryngeal tubes (and laryngeal mask airways) may cause folding of the epiglottis, leading to iatrogenic airway obstruction and significant air leaks, requiring repositioning or another modality to secure the airway.

A number of pediatric devices beyond video laryngoscopes are available to facilitate visualization and intubation in cases of difficult airways. Flexible fiberoptic scopes can be effective, although extensive experience is required, and young children may not be cooperative with awake approaches. This approach is most commonly used by anesthesia or otorhinolaryngology, often in the operating room. Similarly, fiberoptic stylets are available in pediatric sizes to facilitate visualization with intubation. As with video laryngoscopes, gaining experience with the technique for a given device prior to use in the stressful scenario of a difficult or failed airway is critical.

Pediatric Surgical Airway Techniques

In the rare case of the "can't intubate, can't ventilate" child, a surgical airway represents the final airway option. This can occur if direct/video laryngoscopy has failed and the emergency clinician is unable to maintain oxygenation and ventilation via BMV or a rescue device, such as an SGD. In this case, direct access to the airway through the neck is the only option. Surgical techniques are challenged by limited optimal visualization or palpation of anatomic landmarks in infants and young children; therefore, we recommend needle cricothyrotomy in these children.

Experience in surgical airway techniques is limited in small children, with most of the published literature representing case reports, operating room experience, or animal studies. Needle-based rescue procedures should be considered an "oxygenation" strategy rather than a "ventilation" strategy, because progressive hypercarbia will inevitably ensue, limiting the utility of this technique for long-term use. Animal models suggest that a needle cricothyroidotomy will provide approximately 30 to 45 minutes of adequate oxygenation.

To perform a needle cricothyroidotomy, the provider places a large needle catheter (e.g., 14-gauge) through the anterior neck into the airway, ideally entering through the cricothyroid membrane. However, difficulty identifying landmarks by palpation or even ultrasound in young children with short, adipose-rich necks may make determination of the exact level of airway entry difficult. The needle is then removed, and the catheter can be connected to the adaptor from a 3.0-mm ETT, which is then connected to a standard bag device. If a 3.0-mm ETT is not available, an adaptor from a 7.0-mm ETT can be placed into a 3-mL syringe with the plunger removed; this can then be attached directly to the catheter. The bag is then squeezed to provide oxygen delivery, allowing prolonged time between breaths for the passive exhalation phase. Alternatively, commercially available oxygen tubing set-up (e.g., ENK modulator, Cook Inc.) can be used with oxygen flow set at 1 L/min for every year of age. These techniques are preferred to true "jet" ventilation, which uses a much higher-pressure oxygen source and has a greater potential for iatrogenic injury. Open surgical cricothyrotomy or percutaneous Seldinger-based cricothyrotomy, performed in the same way as in an adult, is reserved for children *in whom anatomic landmarks can be found* and in whom the cricothyroid membrane is larger. The literature does not support a specific age cutoff for needle cricothyrotomy versus surgical cricothyrotomy, but needle cricothyrotomy should be performed when indicated in infants and small children (<6 years of age or older depending on anatomic landmarks).

OUTCOMES

The majority of pediatric intubations performed in the ED are successful. Despite the relative rarity of the procedure, there is significant overlap in the techniques and strategies used in adult airway management. There are a limited number of anatomic and physiologic differences that can be learned and mastered. The cognitive burden associated with the procedure can be overcome by length/size-based systems or readily available electronic applications to allow the clinician to focus on the critical actions necessary to successfully manage the airway.

The references for this chapter can be found online at ExpertConsult.com.

157

Pediatric Sedation and Analgesia

Huma Shaikh and Corrie E. Chumpitazi

KEY CONCEPTS

- Patients of all ages experience pain, including infants, neonates, and premature babies.
- Oligoanalgesia, the inadequate treatment of pain, has many short-term and long-term consequences: worse patient outcomes, increase in patient's pain threshold, and development of chronic pain.
- Pain management may include a combination of techniques: analgesics, topical anesthetics, local anesthetic injections, oral sucrose in infants, and nonpharmacologic interventions.
- Nonpharmacologic interventions to decrease pain or anxiety include parental presence; physical measures, such as heat or cold therapy and splinting for musculoskeletal injuries; and behavioral or cognitive measures, such as distraction and play therapy.
- Topical anesthetics are recommended to decrease the pain of minor procedures, such as venipuncture or IV cannulation.
- Techniques for decreasing the pain of intradermal injections include topical agent prior to the intradermal injection; slowly injecting warmed, buffered local anesthetic solution from within the wound with the smallest gauge needle possible; and limiting the number of needle punctures.
- When using large amounts of local anesthetics in small children or infants, calculate the drug dose to avoid toxicity; a 1% solution = 1 g/100 mL or 10 mg/mL.
- Procedural sedation and analgesia (PSA) requires pre-sedation evaluation; sufficient monitoring (during and after the procedure) by qualified individuals capable of dealing with any adverse events that may occur; age-appropriate equipment (including airway equipment) and medications (including reversal agents and advance life support drugs); and discharge criteria for when the patient is fully awake, returns to baseline with normal vital signs, and is able to be discharged in the care of a responsible adult.
- Overall, preprocedural fasting is not necessary for most emergency patients, because large studies show no clinically significant differences with airway complications, emesis, or other adverse effects between groups of patients stratified by their preprocedural fasting status.
- Choice of sedative and analgesic for PSA depends on many variables including patient factors and the procedure to be done. Slow titration of medications can achieve the desired level of sedation and analgesia while minimizing risk of adverse events.

SEDATION

Foundations

Sedation is a controlled reduction of environmental awareness. Sedation is a continuum that begins with minimal, moving to moderate, then deep sedation, and may proceed to general anesthesia.

Definitions[1,2]

- *Anxiolysis* is a state of decreased apprehension concerning a particular situation in which the patient's level of awareness does not change.
- *Analgesia* refers to the relief of pain without the intentional alteration of mental status, such as occurs in sedation. An altered mental state may be a secondary effect of the medications administered for this purpose.
- *Minimal sedation* (e.g., anxiolysis) is a drug-induced state during which patients respond normally to verbal commands. Although cognitive functions and coordination may be impaired, ventilatory and cardiovascular functions are unaffected.
- *Moderate sedation/analgesia* (formerly called "conscious sedation") refers to a drug-induced depression of consciousness during which patients respond purposefully to verbal commands, either alone or accompanied by light tactile stimulation. Reflex withdrawal from the painful stimulus is NOT considered a purposeful response. No interventions are required to maintain a patent airway, and spontaneous ventilation is adequate. Cardiovascular function is usually maintained.
- *Dissociative sedation* is a trancelike cataleptic state induced by the dissociative agent ketamine and characterized by profound analgesia and amnesia, while protective airway reflexes, spontaneous respirations, and cardiopulmonary stability are maintained.
- *Deep sedation/analgesia* describes a drug-induced depression of consciousness during which patients cannot be easily aroused but respond purposefully after repeated or painful stimulation. The ability to independently maintain ventilatory function may be impaired. Patients may require assistance in maintaining a patent airway, and spontaneous ventilation may be inadequate. Cardiovascular function is usually maintained.
- *General anesthesia* is a drug-induced loss of consciousness during which patients are not arousable, even with painful stimulation. The ability to independently maintain ventilatory function is usually impaired. Patients require assistance in maintaining a patent airway, and positive-pressure ventilation may be required because of depressed spontaneous ventilation or drug-induced depression of neuromuscular function. Cardiovascular function may be impaired.
- *Procedural sedation and analgesia (PSA)* are techniques of administering a sedative or dissociative agent, usually along with an analgesic, to induce a state that allows the patient to tolerate painful or unpleasant procedures while maintaining adequate spontaneous cardiorespiratory function. It is intended to result in a depressed level of consciousness that allows the patient to maintain oxygenation and airway control independently and continuously.

The goal of PSA is to alleviate the anxiety, pain, and suffering associated with medical procedures. PSA is an essential part of emergency medicine practice and part of the core curriculum for emergency medicine training programs. Providers should be prepared to appropriately manage the airway and in rare instances intubate if sedation becomes deeper than expected.

Specific Issues

Preparation

The patient's American Society of Anesthesiology (ASA) physical status classification should be calculated prior to procedure (Table 157.1) and airway assessed, for example, using the Mallampati score (see Chapter 1) to identify potential difficulties. Children with special needs, anatomic airway abnormalities, moderate to severe tonsillar hypertrophy, and current or recent upper respiratory illness present increased risk and require additional consideration.[1,3] ASA classes I and II are considered appropriate candidates for minimal, moderate, or deep sedation.[1-3] Staff are encouraged to consult with appropriate subspecialists (e.g., pediatric anesthesiologist) if there is a question of sedation adverse events because of an underlying medical/surgical condition (e.g. Pierre Robin syndrome). Those aged less than 3 months or with weight less than 5 kg are at increased risk for sedation adverse events.

There should be at least one provider, in addition to the provider performing the procedure, who is responsible to monitor appropriate physiologic parameters and assist in any needed supportive or resuscitation measures.[1-3] Pulse oximetry and capnography readings should be continuously monitored; depth of sedation, heart rate, blood pressure, and respiratory rate should be recorded at regular intervals. Although there are scales for assessing the depth of sedation in pediatric patients, continuous monitoring is more important than any specific measurement on a sedation scale. Although there is no evidence of benefit in young healthy individuals, cardiac monitoring has been shown useful in those with a cardiac history and older patients. Thus, we recommend continuous cardiac rhythm monitoring, especially for high-risk patients (e.g., preexisting cardiovascular disease or a history of dysrhythmias) or high-risk procedures (e.g., cardioversion).

Providers administering pediatric procedural sedation should have training and skills in airway management and be ready to rescue the patient from a deeper level than intended for the procedure, since it is common for children to pass easily into a deeper level of sedation. In addition to monitoring equipment and oxygen, age-appropriate suction, bag-valve-mask, and intubating equipment should be available and readied prior to administering medications. The SOAP-ME mnemonic provides an equipment checklist for sedation[3]:

Size-appropriate suction catheters (connected, checked, and with suction turned on)

Oxygen supply (connected to bag and turned on)

Airway: Size-appropriate airway equipment (appropriate size mask and intubation supplies)

Pharmacy: Advanced life support medications and antagonists

Monitors: Size-appropriate oximeter, end-tidal carbon dioxide monitor, and blood pressure cuff

Equipment or drugs for a particular case

Children over age 4 can benefit from simple information about what to expect for their procedure. Explaining the steps, as well as what they might see or feel, being shown the medical supplies (e.g., irrigation solution), and offering realistic options for their procedure help them feel in control. Similarly, parents should be prepared for where to sit and how they can assist with positioning or distraction. A child's ability to control behavior and cooperate for a procedure depends on chronologic age and cognitive/emotional development.

TABLE 157.1 American Society of Anesthesiologists Physical Status Classification

Class	Description	Examples	Sedation Risk
I	Normal and healthy patient	No past medical history	Minimal
II	Mild systemic disease without functional limitations	Mild asthma, controlled diabetes	Low
III	Severe systemic disease with functional limitations	Pneumonia, poorly controlled diabetes mellitus, hypertension or seizure disorder	Intermediate
IV	Severe systemic disease that is a constant threat to life	Advanced cardiac disease, renal failure, sepsis	High
V	Moribund patient who may not survive without procedure	Septic shock, severe trauma	Extremely high
VI	A declared brain-dead patient whose organs are being removed for donor purposes		

Preprocedural Fasting

The ASA has guidelines for preoperative fasting in healthy patients of all ages undergoing elective procedures. In patients undergoing PSA in the emergency department (ED), the evidence indicates that preprocedural fasting does not decrease the risk of emesis or aspiration, as noted in the American College of Emergency Physicians (ACEP) clinical policy.[1,2] Recent studies in pediatric patients do not find any evidence of association between vomiting and shortened fasting time, and no patients were found to have aspiration.[4] Therefore, adherence to the ASA preoperative fasting guidelines for procedures is not necessary in ED patients undergoing PSA.

Supplemental Oxygen and Capnography During Procedural Sedation and Analgesia

Use of supplemental oxygenation has been shown to decrease the incidence of desaturation in pediatric patients from 17% to 10%, although it may delay the recognition of hypoventilation or apnea. Oxygen desaturation and delay in assisted ventilation events can be significantly reduced with the use capnography.[5] Close capnography monitoring can detect hypoventilation early, prior to a drop in pulse oximetry, irrespective of use of supplemental oxygen.[3] ACEP and AAP clinical policy recommend capnography be routinely used to monitor ventilation in children undergoing PSA.[1-3]

Specific Medications

Table 157.2 details specific PSA sedative agents commonly used in infants and children. Patient age, preexisting conditions, and anticipated level of pain or anxiety should guide choice of sedative. Providers should administer drugs by slow intravenous (IV) titration to decrease the risk of adverse events, including hypotension and respiratory depression. For intranasal medications or nitrous oxide use, employing a Child Life specialist or the parents to assist with

PART V Special Populations

TABLE 157.2 Commonly Used Sedatives for Procedural Sedation in Children and Infants

Sedative[a]	Route	Dose[b]	Usual Dose[c]	Maximum Dose	Onset	Duration	Side Effects	Advantages/Comments[a]
Dexmedetomidine	IN	2–4 mcg/kg/dose	3 mcg/kg/dose	200 mcg (100 mcg/nare)	30 min	60–90 min	Decreased HR and BP	Contraindication with heart block, severe renal or hepatic impairment or use of beta blockers
Etomidate	IV	0.1–0.3 mg/kg	0.2 mg/kg PSA	0.4 mg/kg	<1 min	3–10 min	Pain on injection, myoclonic movements, adrenal insufficiency (prolonged use)	Minimal CV/respiratory depression
Ketamine[d]	IV	1–2 mg/kg initial (repeat 0.5–1 mg/kg for longer procedures)	1.5 mg/kg initial PSA		1 min	15 min	Sympathomimetic effects (↑HR, ↑BP) Nausea, vomiting Emergence reaction Laryngospasm (rare)	Warn parents of nystagmus as an expected effect. Has analgesic effect CV/respiratory stability bronchodilator (use in asthmatics) Battlefield use/disasters
Ketamine	IM	4 mg/kg	4 mg/kg 2 mg/kg if <2 years old		5 min	30 min	(Same as above) Higher risk of nausea	(Same as above)
Ketamine	IN	3–9 mg/kg			10 min	60 min	(Same as above)	(Same as above)
Midazolam[e]	IV	0.05–0.1 mg/kg (6 months to 5 years old or adult) 0.025–0.05 mg/kg ≥6 years old) Give slowly 1–2 mg over ≥2 min and titrate to effect	If giving with fentanyl, may dose at 0.02 mg/kg	0.6 mg or 6 mg if ≤5 years old and 10 mg if >6 years old	5 min	30 min	Paradoxical agitation, vomiting, coughing, hiccups, dizziness, respiratory depression, apnea so use lower dose if given with opioids or respiratory depressants	Protective in seizure patients ↓ICP, CBF, ↓LV filling pressure may benefit cardiac patients Mild CV effects unless hypovolemic Reversed by antagonist flumazenil
Midazolam	IN	0.2–0.5 mg/kg	0.2 mg/kg	10 mg	<10 min		(Same as above)	(Same as above)
Pentobarbital[f]	IV	1–6 mg/kg	1–2 mg/kg initial, repeat 3–5 min to desired effect or max dose	100 mg/dose	1–2 min	15–60 min	CV/respiratory depression, paradoxical agitation, extravasation can cause tissue necrosis Contraindication: Porphyria	↓IOP, ↓ICP, used to treat status epilepticus Use in head injury/neurology patients Can use if malignant hyperthermia

Drug	Route	Dose			Onset	Duration	Cautions/Contraindications	Comments
Propofol	IV	0.5–1.5 mg/kg (repeat 0.5 mg/kg every 3–5 min for longer procedures)	Variable, may be 1 mg/kg	None	<1 min	5–15 min (mean 8 min)	CV/respiratory depression; Use with caution if shock/low BP/impaired cardiac function; Caution if allergy to eggs, soybean oil, EDTA[g]	Rapid onset/recovery; No dose change if renal or liver disease; Can use if malignant hyperthermia
Nitrous oxide	Inhalation	Dose is 30%–70% mixture	Commercially available in 50%:50% mixture	70%	1–2 min	15–20 min	Contraindications: Trapped air (bowel obstruction, pneumothorax, emphysema, air emboli)	Need a scavenger system and proper ventilation, potential for abuse, chronic exposure may have adverse effects

[a]Other agents used for sedation, e.g., DPT (meperidine [Demerol], promethazine [Phenergan], and chlorpromazine [Thorazine]) IM should be avoided because there are better, newer agents for sedation with fewer side effects. Chloral hydrate has been used in the past but is used infrequently at present because there are other better options.

[b]Doses will vary with the individual patient; these are some generally recommended starting doses. Some patients will need greater than the typical maximum dose, whereas others may be sedated with less than the usual dose. It is best to titrate the dose in all patients.

[c]Be especially cautious in at-risk patients. At-risk patients include those patients with significant heart disease, including heart failure or pulmonary hypertension, liver disease, renal failure, and patients at the extremes of age (infants, particularly neonates and the geriatric patient). It may be prudent in these patients, to "start low and go slow."

[d]Ketamine's effect on ICP is discussed in the text. Previously ketamine was thought to be contraindicated if there was an increase in ICP. However, recently, this concept has been challenged. If ketamine is given PO or PR, higher doses are needed with less predictable effect and increased side effects so PO and PR routes are not recommended.

[e]Midazolam may be given by several routes including IV, IM, IN, PO, and PR. The PO and especially PR routes of administration have more variable absorption and effects, so they are not commonly used.

[f]Pentobarbital can be given PO or PR or IM, but onset and duration are longer with more variable effect, so IV is preferred.

[g]Although the manufacturer's labeling lists egg allergy as a contraindication, available studies (mostly retrospective) and an American Academy of Allergy, Asthma, and Immunology statement have suggested that propofol may be used safely in soy- or egg-allergic patients (AAAAI [Lieberman 2015]; AAAAI 2019; Asserhoj 2016; Dziedzic 2016; Murphy 2011). In patients with more severe soy or egg allergy, some experts recommend the use of an alternative anesthetic or a small trial dose of propofol prior to full dose administration (Sicherer 2020).

BP, Blood pressure; CBF, cerebral blood flow; CV, cardiovascular; EDTA, ethylenediaminetetraacetic acid; HR, heart rate; ICP, intracerebral pressure; IM, intramuscular; IN, intranasal; IOP, intraocular pressure; IV, intravenous; LV, left ventricular; PO, per oz. (by mouth); PR, per rectum; PSA, procedural sedation and analgesia; RSI, rapid sequence intubation.

distraction, music, or other cognitive behavioral modalities may be advantageous.

Propofol. Propofol has several advantages for PSA; it has a rapid onset in 30-60 seconds, is short acting, and has antiemetic properties. Its side effects include hypotension and respiratory depression. However, studies have shown safe administration in the ED for sedation by physicians who are skilled in airway management and resuscitation of patients that may enter deeper sedation or respiratory distress.[6] Although the dosing of propofol varies from 0.5 to 2 mg/kg, an initial dose of 0.5 to 1.0 mg/kg should be administered and titrated to effect with additional doses, usually in increments of 0.5 mg/kg.

Ketamine. Ketamine, a dissociative anesthetic, has sedative, amnestic, and analgesic properties. Ketamine maintains cardiovascular and respiratory stability, has minimal respiratory depression, and maintains protective airway reflexes in patients with spontaneous respirations. Ketamine's sympathomimetic effects include increased blood pressure, heart rate, cardiac output, and bronchodilation, making it the preferred sedative in patients with asthma.

Apnea is rare with ketamine (0.8% incidence), but has been associated with very high doses, rapid administration, and co-administration with narcotics or other respiratory depressants. Ketamine increases salivary secretions, which may increase the incidence of laryngospasm, especially in oral procedures; however laryngospasm can typically be resolved with simple airway maneuvers.[7] Laryngospasm is usually transient and responds to repositioning of the head, supplemental oxygen administration, gentle suctioning if secretions are the irritant, and positive pressure ventilation with a bag-valve mask. Although rarely needed, the use of a paralytic at lower doses than required for intubation (e.g., succinylcholine given at 10% of a paralytic dose) has been shown to break laryngospasm when the above measures fail. Rapid sequence intubation is rarely needed, but a last resort option to treat laryngospasm.

Ketamine may be given intravenously, intramuscularly, per os (by mouth; PO), or intranasal (IN). For IV administration in pediatric patients, initial doses range from 1.0 to 2.0 mg/kg, with further bolus doses of 0.5 to 1 mg/kg titrated to desired effect. Intramuscular (IM) dosing is an option when IV access is unobtainable; dosing ranges from 4 to 5 mg/kg. The disadvantages of IM ketamine include a higher rate of vomiting, longer recovery time, and lack of IV access in the event of complications requiring IV medication administration (e.g., paralytics). IN ketamine can be used in dosing ranges from 3-9 mg/kg/dose with onset of action between 5 and 10 minutes. As with all intranasal medications, the optimal intranasal dose per nare is 0.5 to 1 mL.[8]

Use of Ketamine in Patients With Head Injury. Multiple studies have dispelled the myth that ketamine increases intracranial pressure (ICP). Ketamine may even have beneficial effects on the brain, including protection against seizures, cerebral ischemia, and secondary brain injury related to hypotension.[9]

Ketamine Recovery Agitation: Use of Benzodiazepines. Emergence reaction or recovery agitation refers to agitation (which may include floating sensation, vivid pleasant dreams, nightmares, hallucinations or delirium) that can occur after waking up or emerging from ketamine. Pediatric studies have not demonstrated benefit in routine use of benzodiazepines to prevent recovery agitation, likely due to their own adverse effects; although rare, they can cause paradoxical agitation. A large pediatric study showed no significant difference in the report of agitation in patients receiving ketamine and benzodiazepine versus ketamine alone.[10] As no pediatric studies to date have shown benefit, we do not recommend that midazolam be routinely given as an adjunct to ketamine in children. However, when recovery agitation occurs, children can be treated with midazolam (0.03 mg/kg; up to a maximum of 5 mg for ages 6 months to 5 years old, or a maximum cumulative dose of 10 mg for children greater than 5 years old).

Emergence reactions occur more frequently in patients greater than 16 years of age, females, shorter operative procedures, large doses, and individuals with psychiatric disorders. Providers should consider an alternate agent or ketamine plus midazolam for older teens and children with psychiatric illness; schizophrenia is an absolute contraindication. Children typically emerge from the sedated state in the format that they achieve sedation; all children, but teenagers especially, may benefit from the use of positive visualization, music, massage, or other distraction techniques in preparation for sedation.

Use of Anticholinergics With Ketamine. Ketamine stimulates tracheobronchial and salivary secretions. However, studies have shown that the co-administration of anticholinergic medications is associated with an increase in the odds of adverse events.[9] Providers may consider anticholinergics for children undergoing an airway examination (e.g., fiberoptic laryngoscopy) to improve visibility, or in patients with clinically significant hypersalivation or an impaired ability to mobilize secretions, but it should not routinely be used.

Glycopyrrolate is the preferred anticholinergic over atropine; it is a more potent anti-sialagogue and has fewer tachy-dysrhythmias. Unlike atropine, glycopyrrolate does not cross the blood brain barrier, so has no central nervous system (CNS) side effects. CNS side effects of atropine range from drowsiness to coma and include headache, nervousness, insomnia, excitement, dizziness, disorientation, hallucinations, and ataxia. Headache is the only CNS side effect listed for glycopyrrolate.

Use of Antiemetics with Ketamine. Vomiting with ketamine sedation in children is common.[10] Vomiting usually develops during recovery, when patients are alert and can clear their airways. Slow IV administration over several minutes may mitigate this response. Risk is higher among adolescents and patients receiving high doses or IM administration. Although ondansetron is associated with a small decrease in the incidence of vomiting associated with ketamine sedation in children, ondansetron is also associated with other adverse effects, including QT prolongation and serotonin syndrome. We recommend reserving treatment with ondansetron for patients who develop nausea or vomiting during recovery from ketamine.

Ketofol: Ketamine Plus Propofol. The combination of ketamine with propofol has the potential to provide benefits of both sedatives. The combination allows for lower doses of each medication, which may theoretically minimize adverse effects of either sedative alone. The incidence of hypotension from propofol alone has been shown to be lessened when combined with ketamine.[10,11] However, studies have not shown significant differences in rates of respiratory depression between co-administration versus either sedative alone.[10–12]

Ketamine and propofol (ketofol) can be dosed at 0.5 mg/kg to 0.75 mg/kg for each drug via separate syringes. For short procedures, re-dosing is usually not needed. For longer procedures, if the sedation is wearing off, propofol is usually re-dosed (due to its shorter half-life) at 0.1 to 0.5 mg/kg IV.

Dexmedetomidine. Dexmedetomidine is an effective sedative, anxiolytic and analgesic that does not cause respiratory depression.[13] A loading dose poses the risk of bradycardia and hypotension due to α_2-agonist effects on the sympathetic ganglia.[13] Lack of amnesia can be a concern in certain situations, however, this can be managed with the addition of low dose benzodiazepines. Use of dexmedetomidine in addition to propofol has been shown to decrease cardiovascular, respiratory, and agitation-related adverse effects.[14] Dexmedetomidine can be used intranasally at 2 to 3 mcg/kg/dose (max 100 mcg/nare). An additional 1 mcg/kg/dose may be administered in 30 minutes (max cumulative dose 4 mcg/kg). Contraindications include heart block, severe renal or hepatic impairment, or use of a beta blocker.

Nitrous Oxide

The use of inhaled nitrous oxide in the pediatric emergency setting has been well established for mildly painful or distressing procedures. Although the exact mechanism of action is not known, sedation is likely achieved due to a noncompetitive inhibition of the NMDA-receptor and analgesia via central opioid and opioid-like receptors. Concentrations between 50% and 70% are commonly used, with best effect to side effect ratios seen with inhalation times less than 30 minutes. The combination of inhaled nitrous oxide and IN fentanyl obviates painful and time-consuming IV access insertions and delivers a short recovery time.[15] Another study in a pediatric emergency department found fewer adverse reactions and lower length of stay in patients treated with inhaled nitrous oxide and IN fentanyl, as compared to ketamine and midazolam, with no difference in efficacy between groups.[16]

Post-Sedation Monitoring

Once the procedure is complete and the painful stimuli are removed, patients are at risk of hypoventilation or hypoxia. Monitoring should continue until the patient has met predetermined discharge criteria, which should include normal vital signs and baseline mental and physical status. Once fully awake, patients should be discharged to the care of a responsible adult. Patients should receive predeveloped age-appropriate PSA discharge instructions.

Outcomes

Adequately treating anxiety and pain results in greater procedural success rates; improved patient and caregiver satisfaction; decreased likelihood of the patient developing chronic pain; and improved patient outcomes. Patients at increased risk of adverse events during PSA include the following: the very young or very old; those with comorbidities (e.g., cardiopulmonary diseases) or craniofacial abnormalities (e.g., Down syndrome and Pierre Robin syndrome); the morbidly obese; and those with a higher ASA physical status classification (see Table 157.1).

PAIN MANAGEMENT

Foundations

Pain is defined as an unpleasant visceral or somatic experience or sensation associated with actual, potential, or perceived tissue damage. Pain receptors, termed *nociceptors,* are the free nerve endings of a sensory neuron that convert mechanical, thermal, or chemical stimuli into electrical activity, and initiates an impulse that travels along the neuron and then on to the dorsal horn of the spinal cord (Fig. 157.1). Input from various peripheral nerves and additional sensory stimuli are processed, undergoing integration and modulation in the dorsal horn of the spinal cord, and then transmitted up the spinal cord to the CNS (Fig. 157.2).

There are two types of pain: nociceptive or neuropathic. Nociceptive pain occurs when tissue injury or inflammation stimulates intact pain receptors. Nociceptive pain can be further divided into visceral pain (i.e., of internal organs) and somatic pain (i.e., of the skin, soft tissue, and musculoskeletal structures). Neuropathic pain occurs when there is abnormal functioning or stimulation of damaged sensory nerves. Children with severe developmental impairment may have central neuropathic pain or pain secondary to visceral hyperalgesia.

Neuropathic pain is typically burning, searing, tingling, shooting, or electric in quality. Nociceptive somatic pain is generally described as sharp and well localized. However, pain in deeper structures (e.g., bones, joints, or tendons) can cause achy, diffuse, or radiating pain. Nociceptive visceral pain is typically poorly localized, deep, and aching. Chronic pain is a maladaptive response in which the pain persists after the original injury or illness has resolved.

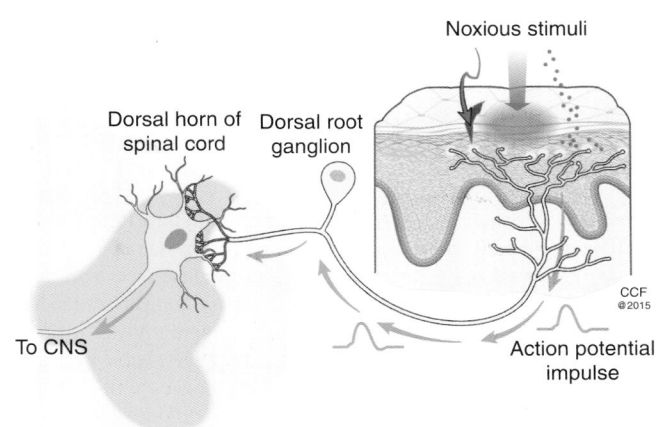

Fig. 157.1 Nociceptors. *CNS,* Central nervous system. (Figure illustration by Department of Medical Art and Photography—Cleveland Clinic and Mr. Dave Schumick with permission.)

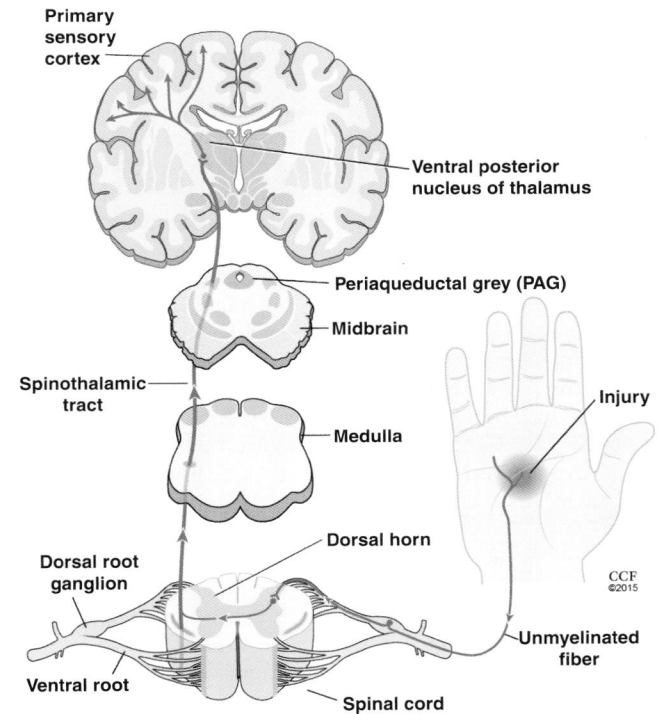

Fig. 157.2 Pain Pathway. (Figure illustration by Department of Medical Art and Photography—Cleveland Clinic and Mr. Dave Schumick with permission.)

Specific Issues

Pain Assessment

Patient self-report is the most accurate measure of pain severity. Pain assessments can be used to guide pain management. Pain scales should be age-specific; subjective or self-reporting scales can start being used at 3 years of age, depending on developmental level. Children younger than 3 years old do not have the cognitive or verbal skills needed to communicate levels of pain and, thus, require behavioral or psychological pain scales. Behavioral pain scales rely on the observation of specific child or infant behaviors. Some of the parameters used in behavioral pain scales include facial expressions, consolability, interaction level, limb responses, trunk motor responses, and verbal responses. Behavioral and physiologic pain scales combine behavioral observations and physiologic parameters (e.g., vital signs) to obtain a score.

The numeric rating scale (NRS) and the visual analogue scale (VAS) are commonly used self-report scales that have been found to have reliability and validity. With the VAS, patients are asked to place a mark on a 10-cm line with descriptors along the line. With the NRS, patients are asked to rate their pain severity on a scale from 0 to 10 or 0 to 100, with 0 being no pain and 10 or 100 the worst pain possible. Horizontal lines are preferred rather than vertical lines because scores are more normally distributed. Patients with poor hand-eye coordination, visual acuity or hand dexterity have difficulty completing the VAS.

As noted, the use of pain scales is based on age. Adolescents and adults can rate their pain using an NRS or VAS. Older children (8 to 11 years old) can also use an NRS or VAS. Younger children (3 to 8 years old) can quantify their pain using a faces pain scale, most commonly, the Faces Pain Scale–Revised (FPS-R)[17]. The Premature Infant Pain Scale (PIPP) is used to assess pain in premature infants. The Crying, Requires oxygen, Increased vital signs, Expressions, and Sleeplessness (CRIES) scale is for infants. The Faces, Legs, Activity, Cry, Consolability (FLACC) pain scale can be used for infants and toddlers. The Children's Hospital of Eastern Ontario Pain Scale (CHEOPS) and the Observational Scale of Behavioral Distress (OSBD) may be used for toddlers and young children.

Nonverbal children with neurological impairment, irrespective of age, cannot self-report their pain. The child's caregiver generally knows his or her typical behavior patterns, both at baseline and in response to stimuli or needs. Behaviors that may indicate pain include facial expressions (e.g., grimacing), vocalizations (crying or moaning), inconsolability, increased movement, increased tone or posture (e.g., stiffening or arching), and uncharacteristic or atypical behaviors (e.g., withdrawal, lack of expression, or even laughing). The revised FLACC (r-FLACC) scale is one pain scale designed for use in children with cognitive impairment.

We recommend that all patients have a pain assessment and that the FLACC scale be used in infants to age 3 years of age and those with developmental delay and nonverbal of any age, the FPS-R scale be used in children 3 to 8 years of age, and the NRS used in children 8 years of age or older.

Nonpharmacologic Techniques

Nonpharmacologic interventions should be routinely used with pharmacologic therapy for pain management; this includes physical comfort measures and distraction techniques. Patients should be given basic first measures, including the application of splints or immobilization to stabilize fractures and dislocations; cold packs can help reduce swelling and provide topical analgesia. Hypnosis is accepted by the American Medical Association as a medical therapy and has been used to treat anxiety, as well as acute and chronic pain. Children may be more easily hypnotized compared to adults. Studies indicate that hypnosis is efficacious in pediatric patients for painful medical procedures, headaches, sickle cell disease, chronic pain, and even in cancer treatment.[18] In non-ED settings, acupuncture and acupressure has also been used as a nonpharmacologic method for pain management.

Techniques that distract from pain should be tailored to patients based on their age and developmental stage.[19] Younger children may not yet comprehend verbal reassurance, and thus benefit more from distraction techniques. Distractions include playing games, blowing bubbles or looking at books. Older children can use music, video games, cartoon videos, and books to distract from pain and reduce anxiety. Preliminary research suggests that the high-tech virtual reality that uses multiple sensory inputs may be effective in decreasing pain.

Educated in human growth, development, and psychology, Child Life specialists are invaluable team members of any pediatric ED. Child Life specialists help children effectively cope with illness or injury and the emotional stressors of healthcare and hospitalization through play, preparation, education, and distraction. A study of children undergoing suturing in the ED found that having a Child Life specialist involved lessened the emotional distress for children.[20] Child Life services have resulted in lower self-reported pain in children receiving peripheral IV placement and greater family satisfaction with the ED visit.[21]

Perhaps one of the most important and common nonpharmacologic methods for limiting the anxiety and pain of the child or infant is parental presence during the procedure. Techniques used in infants include nonnutritive sucking, breastfeeding, skin-to-skin contact (kangaroo care), and oral sucrose. Skin-to-skin care is a safe, effective measure to reduce distress in term and preterm neonates based on composite pain scores. Sucrose water (2mL of 25% glucose solution) administered by pacifier or oral syringe has been shown to effectively decrease pain in infants 3 months old and younger undergoing painful procedures. To optimize pain reduction and recovery in infants, a combination of interventions should be used before, during, and after painful procedures.

Pharmacologic Techniques

Topical Anesthetics. Used in conjunction with other methods for decreasing pain, topical anesthetics may decrease the need for systemic analgesics or local anesthesia. Topical anesthetics can be used for venipuncture, IV cannulation, minor surgical procedures, wound care, suturing, and lumbar puncture. Topical anesthetics are painless to apply and do not distort tissue (e.g., for cosmetically important facial lacerations). Needleless, they also avoid the risk of needle sticks.

Different topical anesthetics can be used on intact skin or broken skin (Table 157.3), as well as mucosal surfaces. Vasoconstrictors, such as epinephrine, increase anesthetic efficacy and duration of effect. While traditionally not used at an end-arteriolar blood supply (e.g., fingertip), the risk of irreversible ischemia is very low. Common formulations used for intact skin (e.g., prior to venipuncture) are eutectic mixture of local anesthetics (EMLA), liposome encapsulated lidocaine (LMX), and vapo-coolants. Lidocaine, epinephrine (adrenaline), tetracaine (LET), and cocaine (TAC) can be used for open wounds. Due to the potential for cocaine toxicity, we recommend using other topical anesthetics instead of TAC. EMLA has been associated with methemoglobinemia, seizures, and respiratory depression with excessive skin application. Methemoglobinemia is associated with the prilocaine component of EMLA and is more likely to occur in patients with glucose-6-phosphate dehydrogenase (G6PD) and those on methemoglobinemia-inducing medications.

The use of topical anesthetic agents (e.g., lidocaine and benzocaine) on mucosal surfaces for teething pain or stomatitis has been associated with overdose toxicity, including seizures, respiratory depression, cardiovascular events, and death. These adverse events have led to a recent black box warning for viscous lidocaine, and the U.S. Food and Drug Administration (FDA) recommendation against using over-the-counter (OTC) topical anesthetics for teething pain. We recommend not using topical anesthetics on mucosal surfaces in infants and young children. For teething pain, use a chilled (not frozen) teething ring or have the caregiver gently massage the gums with a finger. Children with stomatitis can be treated with acetaminophen or nonsteroidal anti-inflammatory drugs (NSAIDs).

The topical vapo-coolants or refrigerant anesthetic sprays have similar uses to topical anesthetics (Table 157.4). Two commonly used vapo-coolants are ethyl chloride, which is flammable, and 1,1,1,3,3 pentafluoropropane/1,1,1,2 tetrafluoroethane, which is nonflammable

TABLE 157.3 Topical Anesthetic Agents for Application to Intact Skin or Open Wounds

Topical Agent[a,b,c]	Composition	Sites	Time to Efficacy	Administration	Comments	Contraindications
Eutectic mixture of local anesthetic agents (EMLA)	Lidocaine 2.5% Prilocaine 2.5% 1:1 mixture	Intact skin	Onset: 60 min Peak: 120 min Max ≤ 4 h Max 1 h in children ≤ 3 months	Apply 5–10 g in thick layer Cover with semiocclusive dressing	Dose[d]: 0–3 months old or <5 kg: maximum 1 g per 10 cm^3 3–12 months and >5 kg: maximum 2 g per 20 cm^3 1–6 years and >10 kg: maximum 10 g per 100 cm^3 7–12 years and >20 kg: maximum 20 g per 200 cm^3	Infants EGA <37 weeks, <1 year if susceptible to methemoglobinemia or on methemoglobin-inducing agents (sulfonamides, nitrates, primaquine, others) Use with caution if age <3 months old, heart block, or severe hepatic disorder
Liposome encapsulated lidocaine (LMX)	Lidocaine 4% (LMX4) or 5% (LMX5) (previous name: ELA Max)	Intact skin	Onset: 30–60 min	Apply 2.5 grams in thick layer Cover with semiocclusive dressing	Max dose: 4.5 mg/kg/dose, not to exceed 300 mg/dose	Same as for lidocaine
Lidocaine, epinephrine, and tetracaine (LET)	Lidocaine 4% Epinephrine 0.1% Tetracaine 0.5%	Open dermis	20–30 min	Apply 5 mL to cotton ball, place in wound, cover with semiocclusive dressing, apply gentle pressure to infiltrate tissue		Area of compromised blood supply, or end-arteriolar blood supply
Vapo-coolant (PainEase) (other common vapo-coolant is ethyl chloride)	1,1,1,3,3 pentafluoropropane, 1,1,1,2-tetrafluoroethane (nonflammable and ozone friendly so is preferred over ethyl chloride)	Intact dermis Open dermis	Almost instantaneously, 4–10 s	Hold the spray can 3–7 inches from site, spray for 4–10 s or until blanching occurs	Inexpensive Can use on intact or open dermis (such as, laceration) Should perform procedure quickly since effect wears off rapidly (within 1 min) Can be reapplied	Area of compromised blood supply, insensitive skin cold intolerance or hypersensitivity

[a]Tetracaine, adrenaline (epinephrine), and cocaine (TAC) is a topical anesthetic used on open dermis, but because of the potential toxicity due to the cocaine component as well as for legal and regulatory issues, it has been replaced by other topical anesthetics.
[b]Tetracaine topical (Ametop) has been used in adults and reported in the literature in pediatric patients, but according to Pediatric and Neonatal Lexi-drugs for tetracaine topical under dosing, "Children: safety and efficacy has not been established" so it is not included in this list.
[c]Use of topical anesthetic agents on mucosal surfaces in infants and young children, as for teething pain or stomatitis, has been associated with serious adverse events, including seizures, respiratory depression, and death, so they are not included on this list. The American Academy of Pediatrics (AAP) recommends using a chilled (not frozen) teething ring or gently rubbing/massaging with the caregiver's fingers for teething pain. The U.S. Food and Drug Administration (FDA) recommends against using topical over-the-counter (OTC) medicines for teething pain. Such OTC products may contain up to 20% local anesthetic, such as 20% benzocaine, which is 200 mg/mL. This can be compared with the usual concentration of local anesthetics for subdermal injection for suturing, such as 2% lidocaine, which is 20 mg/mL for a tenfold increase to 200 mg/mL for 20% concentration.
[d]The dose of EMLA® varies by age and weight, with the maximum amount of intact skin in cm^3 over which the cream can be applied and the length of time allowed for skin contact specified.
EGA, Estimated gestational age.

and ozone friendly. A meta-analysis study showed that vapo-coolant spray significantly reduced pain during IV cannulation in comparison to placebo spray or no treatment.[22] To be effective, application should include correct distance 3 to 7 inches from the skin site, a steady spray covering the specific area (about as large as a quarter for a venipuncture or IV cannulation), and adequate spray time for 4 to 10 seconds or until the skin begins to turn white, whichever comes first. Vapo-coolants have also been used to alleviate myofascial pain, muscle pain, and musculoskeletal injury pain. Vapo-coolants have immediate onset.

Although the anesthetic effect subsides within a minute, it can be reapplied.

The J tip is a needleless jet injector that uses pressurized gas for the delivery of local anesthetic. J tip lidocaine delivery has been found effective in decreasing the pain of peripheral IV catheter insertion. In one study of neonatal patients in the ED requiring lumbar punctures, jet delivered lidocaine was not found to be more effective in reducing pain than topical anesthetic cream, however, advantages included quick onset of action and increased success rate.[23] Devices used for

TABLE 157.4 Common Local Anesthetics

Local Anesthetics[a]	Maximum Dose[b] (mg/kg)	Onset (min)	Duration[c] (Average) (min)
Amides[d]			
Long Duration			
Bupivacaine (Marcaine)	2	10	200
Etidocaine (Duranest)	3	3	200
Moderate Duration			
Lidocaine (Xylocaine)	4–4.5	5	100
Mepivicaine (Carbocaine)	4–4.5	3	100
Prilocaine (Citanest)	5	5	100
Amides With Epinephrine			
Lidocaine with epinephrine	7	5	120
Mepivicaine with epinephrine	7	5	120
Esters[d]			
Short Duration			
Chloroprocaine (Nesacaine)	8	5	45
Procaine (Novocain)	7	18	40
Long Duration			
Tetracaine (Pontocaine)	1.5	15	200

[a]Use of commercially available brand names does not imply endorsement of any medication or product. They are included because individuals may be more familiar with commercial or brand names than the specific drug or category of drugs.

[b]Maximum dose is based on ideal body weight.

[c]Duration is affected by binding (e.g., ↑ protein binding produces ↑ duration) and concentration (↑ concentration ↑ duration). 2% lidocaine has greater duration than 1% lidocaine.

[d]In case of a true immunoglobulin E (IgE) anaphylaxis, which is very rare, to one class of local anesthetics the other class may be used (e.g., if allergy to esters, then one can use amides and vice versa). If there is an allergy to all "caines" (both amides and esters), then one can use benzoyl alcohol or diphenhydramine. Benzoyl alcohol is preferred over diphenhydramine.

Derived from multiple sources including Berde CB, Strichartz GR. Local anesthetics. In: Miller RD, Cohen NH, Eriksson LI, et al., eds. *Miller's Anesthesia*. 8th ed. Philadelphia: Elsevier; 2015:1028–1054.

injection of local anesthetics are often associated with minor local skin side effects (such as, erythema or bruising) and may produce an audible "pop" when used, which could frighten a young child. One study in pediatric patients found that a vibrating cold device showed equal effectiveness in reducing pain and distress during IV cannulation as 4% topical lidocaine cream and is an acceptable alternative due to speedy time to onset.[24]

Local Anesthetics

Local anesthetics reversibly block sodium channels, which inhibits the propagation of nerve impulses (Fig. 157.3). Local anesthetics fall into one of two classes: amides and esters. Amides can be remembered as the prefix before the ending "caine" will have the letter "I" (e.g., lidocaine and bupivacaine). Local anesthetics are also classified by duration

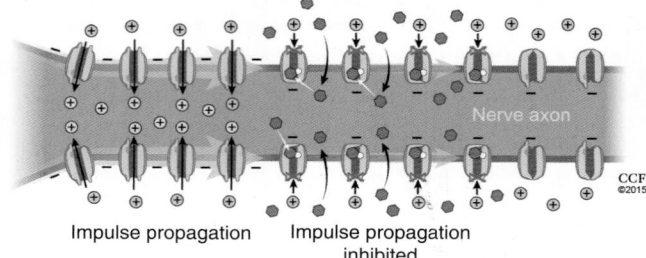

Fig. 157.3 Local Anesthetics Mechanism of Action. Local anesthetics reversibly block sodium channels. (Figure illustration by Department of Medical Art and Photography—Cleveland Clinic and Mr. Dave Schumick with permission.)

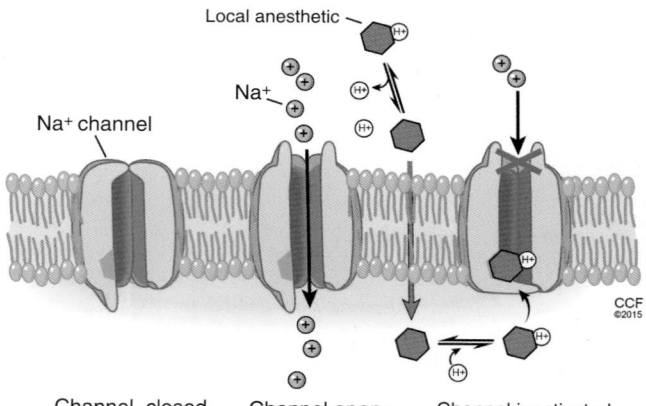

Fig. 157.4 Local Anesthetics Mechanism of Action. Local anesthetics blocks transmission of nerve impulse by binding to the receptor within the sodium channel and inactivating it. H^+, Hydrogen ion; Na^+, sodium ion. (Figure illustration by Department of Medical Art and Photography—Cleveland Clinic and Mr. Dave Schumick with permission.)

of action. Local anesthetics that are tightly protein bound to a receptor in the sodium channel (e.g., bupivacaine and tetracaine) have a longer duration of action than less tightly bound anesthetics (e.g., procaine and prilocaine). Greater concentrations of the local anesthetic will also increase the duration of action.

Potency refers to the degree to which the individual local anesthetic blocks transmission in the neural tissue (Fig. 157.4).

When added to a local anesthetic, epinephrine lengthens the duration of the anesthesia, slows systemic absorption, and aids in controlling local bleeding Although the risk is currently being questioned for epinephrine-containing local anesthetics, we recommend generally avoiding in end-arterial fields (e.g., digits) and in patients with vascular pathology (e.g., Buerger's disease or digital vascular injury) who are at high risk for ischemia. Techniques for decreasing injection pain are described in Box 157.1.

The vasoconstrictor reaction is the most common adverse reaction to a local anesthetic. It occurs when an epinephrine-containing local anesthetic is injected into a highly vascular space. The patient suddenly feels a rapid heartbeat and becomes anxious and panicky from rapid absorption of epinephrine. This reaction ends quickly and is not a true allergy.

True immunoglobulin E (IgE)-mediated anaphylaxis to local anesthetics is very rare, especially to the amide class. Reported allergies to amides are more likely to be a reaction to epinephrine or an allergy to one of the preservatives (e.g., methylparaben). There is no cross-reactivity between amides and esters, and they contain

Use a topical agent prior to the injection

Use smallest gauge needle possible (generally, a 27- to 30-gauge needle)

Use warmed solution: Warmed to 98.6°F–102°F (37°C–39°C)

Inject slowly

Inject into the subcutaneous space, not the dermis

Minimize the number of punctures

Inject from within open wounds, do not inject through the adjacent intact skin

Buffer the local anesthetic: Mix 1% lidocaine with 8.4% sodium bicarbonate solution in a ratio of 9 parts lidocaine to 1 part sodium bicarbonate (Mixing bupivacaine with bicarbonate can cause precipitation of the anesthetic and is not recommended.)

different preservatives. For patients with a known true allergy to lidocaine, a benzyl alcohol solution (made by adding 0.2 mL of 1:1000 epinephrine to a 20 mL vial of normal saline containing 0.9% benzoyl alcohol) can be used. Diphenhydramine is no longer recommended because it is a tissue irritant and can cause local necrosis.

Serious toxicity from local anesthetics is due to their effects on the CNS and to the cardiovascular system (CVS). Early signs of toxicity include numbness or tingling of the lips, metallic taste, muffled hearing, and tinnitus. These symptoms often portend the onset of drowsiness, seizures, status epilepticus, and coma. Direct myocardial depression and pump failure can occur, especially if the patient is on beta blockers or calcium channel blockers; heart block and asystole can also occur. If cardiac arrest is known or presumed to be from local anesthetic toxicity, length of resuscitation should take into consideration time for the negative cardiac effects to wear off. Any of the local anesthetics can have these adverse effects, especially when exceeding recommended doses.

Compared to the amides, the esters have a higher incidence of allergic reactions. Procaine and benzocaine are metabolized to para-aminobenzoic acid (PABA), which has been associated with rare anaphylactic reactions. The metabolites of prilocaine and benzocaine have been associated with methemoglobinemia. Bupivacaine has a higher cardiac toxicity profile than other local anesthetics, but bupivacaine is still widely used and generally safe and effective when used as recommended. In general, the choice of local anesthetic depends more on duration and personal preference than a marked advantage of one specific drug or anesthetic class.

Nerve Blocks. A nerve block is regional anesthesia attained by the injection of a local anesthetic agent near a nerve, nerves, or nerve plexus supplying a particular area. There may be a fairly well circumscribed region of anesthesia (e.g., a wrist or ankle block) or an entire limb, termed *major regional anesthesia.* Nerve blocks are often used to provide anesthesia prior to procedures (e.g., reduction of fractures or dislocations and suturing large lacerations). This approach has the advantage of limiting the amount of lidocaine or other anesthetic needed, decreasing the possibility of reaching toxic levels of the local anesthetic. The use of ultrasound-guided nerve blocks in the ED has been increasing due to the increased safety and efficacy found with sonographic visualization of structures. Although there has been much literature on the use of nerve blocks for adults in the ED, there are relatively few studies dealing with the use of nerve blocks for pediatric patients in the ED.

Complications that can occur with any nerve block include needle breakage (more likely with very small and long needles or if needles are bent to perform the block; e.g., posterior superior alveolar block),

needle damage to anatomic structures (e.g., nerves, vessels, viscera, pleura, other structures), neurotoxicity, vascular complications (e.g., hematoma formation, intra-arterial injection), infection, and bleeding. With any nerve block, providers should review the appropriate anatomy (particularly if performed infrequently), be careful not to exceed maximum doses of anesthetics, and calculate the maximum dose based on actual, not ideal, body weight. Mixing lidocaine and bupivacaine will give both a rapid onset and longer duration nerve block.

Nonopioid Systemic Analgesics. Nonopioid systemic analgesics (Table 157.5) include acetaminophen (paracetamol), which has analgesic and antipyretic effects but does not have any anti-inflammatory effects. There is no need for any dosage change for mild renal or hepatic impairment. If therapeutic doses are used and there is no alcohol abuse or preexisting liver disease, then hepatic toxicity is rare. Acetaminophen is an excellent choice for the treatment of mild pain, in combination with opioids for moderate to severe pain, and has several methods of administration, including the IV route. Indications for the IV use of acetaminophen include patients with pain or fever who are unable to take oral medications and those who have impaired gastrointestinal (GI) absorption.

The NSAIDs have analgesic and antiinflammatory properties. NSAIDs inhibit cyclooxygenase (COX)-1 and COX-2, which decreases the synthesis of prostaglandins, thereby elevating the threshold for nociceptor activation. Nonselective NSAIDs inhibit both COX-1 and COX-2. Side effects of COX-1 inhibition include GI bleeding, renal failure, and platelet dysfunction. In pediatric patients, ibuprofen is the NSAID of choice, because it has fewer side effects than other NSAIDs. NSAIDs may be more effective than acetaminophen at reducing pain from inflammation associated with tissue injury.

Aspirin has analgesic, antipyretic, and anti-inflammatory effects. However, aspirin is not recommended in children and infants due to risk of Reye syndrome, a rapid-onset encephalopathy associated with hepatic dysfunction and seizures; for this reason, aspirin should not be used in any individual with chicken pox or flu symptoms.

Opioid Analgesics. Opioids, previously termed *narcotics,* produce analgesia by binding to opioid receptors in the brain, brainstem, spinal cord, and peripheral nervous system. The main adverse effect of opioids is a dose-dependent respiratory depression with blunting of the responses to hypoxia and hypercarbia; this effect is potentiated when co-administered with other sedative medications. Other side effects are primarily GI (e.g., constipation, nausea, vomiting), urinary retention, and pruritus.

There are many routes of administration of opioids. IM is not recommended secondary to injection pain and variable IM absorption. IN administration is useful for quick pain relief in children who have moderate-to-severe pain without established IV access. IN fentanyl has been shown to be effective in treatment of acute pain in children as young as 6 months.[25] IV is used for patients with severe pain and titrated to effect to avoid adverse events.

Morphine and fentanyl are the commonly used opioids used to treat acute and breakthrough pain in pediatric patients. Hydromorphone, though less commonly used, is useful to treat children with chronic pain or opioid tolerance, such as in sickle cell disease. Codeine is a weak opioid that has an increased incidence of side effects compared to other opioids. It is no longer recommended in children because of genetic variability in the metabolism and risk of respiratory depression in fast metabolizers. Meperidine is not recommended due its possible CNS toxicity (e.g., seizures, hallucinations, and psychosis) at therapeutic doses and its risk of serotonin syndrome.

Opioid Prescribing and Use. In 2017, the Department of Health and Human Services declared a public health emergency due to the opioid crisis. Although there is no evidence-based literature documenting

TABLE 157.5   Systemic Analgesics

Systemic Analgesic[d,e]	Route[c,f]	Dose (Pediatric)[a]	Dose (Adult)[b]	Maximum Dose[c]	Formulations and Notes	Comments
Nonopioid[b]						
Acetaminophen (Paracetamol) (Tylenol)	PO	Child/infant 10–15 mg/kg dose every 4–6 h. Child 6–11 years old: 325 mg dose every 4–6 h	≥12 years old/ adults 650 mg every 4–6 h 1000 mg every 6 h (maximum 4000 mg daily)	Child single dose 15 mg/kg. Total daily dose: Lesser of 75 mg/kg or 4000 mg. Not more than 5 doses daily	PO solution or suspension: 160 mg/5 mL, 500 mg/15 mL. Tablets/gelcaps: 325 mg, 500 mg. Chewable or ODT: 80 mg, 160 mg, 325 mg	Analgesic. Antipyretic. No anti-inflammatory effect has been associated with liver failure. Hepatotoxicity is usually associated with excessive dose. Do not exceed maximum daily dose
	PR	10–20 mg/kg dose every 4–6 h	325–650 mg every 4–6 h	Child total daily dose: Lesser of 75 mg/kg/day or 1625 mg/day	80, 120, 325, 650 mg	(Same as above)
Acetaminophen (Ofirmev)	IV	Adolescents >50 kg: 650 mg every 4 hours or 1000 mg every 6 hours	≥50 kg: 650 mg every 6 h or 1000 mg every 6 h	If <50 kg: Single dose 15 mg/kg, total daily dose <75 mg/kg/day. ≥50 kg: Single dose 1000 mg daily. Total daily dose: 4000 mg	10 mg/mL (100 mL vial)	(Same as above). More expensive, can be used in NPO patients
Ibuprofen (Advil, Motrin)	PO	6 months old to 5 years old: 5–10 mg/kg dose every 6–8 h	≥12 years old/ adults 400–600 mg every 4–6 h or 800 mg every 8 h	<12 years old Single dose: 400 mg. Total daily dose: 40 mg/kg up to 1600 mg. Adults: Total daily dose 3200 mg	Suspension: 50 mg/1.25mL, 100 mg/5 mL. Tablets: 100, 200, 400, 600, 800 mg. Chewable tab: 100 mg	Analgesic. Antipyretic. Anti-inflammatory. Side effects: GI bleeding, renal failure, and platelet dysfunction; most side effects occur with the chronic use of nonselective NSAIDs
Ketorolac (Toradol)	IV or IM	0.5 mg/kg dose every 6–8 h	Child >50 kg and adult 15 mg	15 mg/dose. Total daily dose: 120 mg	Doses up to 60 mg can be given but are not recommended because doses higher than 15 mg have no greater efficacy but have more incidence side effects	(Same as for ibuprofen). Therapy should not be more than 5 days
Opioids: Oral With or Without Acetaminophen[b]						
Hydrocodone	PO	0.1–0.2 mg/kg dose every 4–6 h. Usual dose: 0.15 mg/kg	Child ≥50 kg and adult: 5–15 mg every 4–6 h, usual dose 10 mg	No more than 6 doses/day. 60 mg total daily dose	24-h extended-release tablets: 20, 30, 40, 60, 80, 100, 120 mg capsules. 12-h extended-release tablets: 10, 15, 20, 30, 40, 50 mg	Weak opioid. Preferred over codeine. Generally hydrocodone is given in combination with acetaminophen

TABLE 157.5   Systemic Analgesic—cont'd.

Systemic Analgesic[d,e]	Route[c,f]	Dose (Pediatric)[a]	Dose (Adult)[b]	Maximum Dose[c]	Formulations and Notes	Comments
Hydrocodone and acetaminophen[j] (Lorcet, Vicodin)	PO	0.1–0.2 mg/kg dose every 4–6 h (based on hydrocodone component) Usual dose: 0.15 mg/kg	Child ≥50 kg and adult: 10 mg hydrocodone every 4–6 h	No more than 6 doses/day or recommended acetaminophen daily dose, 60 mg hydrocodone total daily dose	Elixir: hydrocodone 10 mg/acetaminophen 300 mg/15 mL Solution: Hydrocodone 7.5 mg/acetaminophen 325 mg/15 mL Tablets: Hydrocodone 2.5 mg/acetaminophen 325 mg Hydrocodone 7.5 mg/ acetaminophen 325 mg Hydrocodone 10 mg/ acetaminophen 325 mg Hydorcodone 5 mg/ acetaminophen 300 mg Hydrocodone 7.5 mg/ acetaminophen 300 mg Hydrocodone 10 mg/ acetaminophen 300 mg	Weak opioid Preferred over codeine Generally hydrocodone is given in combination with acetaminophen
Oxycodone	PO	Age >6 mo: 0.1–0.2 mg/kg dose every 4–6 h Usual dose: 0.15 mg/kg	Child ≥50 kg and adult: Immediate release: 5–10 mg every 4–6 h	Initial: 5 mg/dose oxycodone	Solution: 5 mg/5 mL Concentrate: 100 mg/5 mL Capsule: 5 mg Tablets: 5, 7.5, 10, 15, 20, 30 mg 12-h extended-release tablets: 9, 10, 13.5, 15, 18, 20, 27, 30, 36, 40, 60, 80 mg	Strong opioid Preferred over hydrocodone Generally oxycodone is given in combination with acetaminophen Sustained release form is available but is usually not given for acute pain in the ED setting
Oxycodone and acetaminophen[j] (Endocet, Percocet, Roxicet)	PO	Age >6 mo: 0.1–0.2 mg/kg dose every 4–6 h Usual dose: 0.15 mg/kg (based on oxycodone component)	Child ≥50 kg and adult: Immediate release: 5–10 mg every 4–6 h	Initial: 5 mg/dose oxycodone Total daily dose: Based on acetaminophen component	Solution: Oxycodone 5 mg/ acetaminophen 325 mg/5 mL (Roxicet), oxycodone 10 mg/acetominophen 300 mg/5 mL Tablets: Oxycodone 5 mg/ acetaminophen 325 mg (Roxicet5), oxycodone 2.5 mg/acetaminophen 325 mg, oxycodone 7.5 mg/acetaminophen 325 mg, oxycodone 10 mg/ acetaminophen 325 mg, oxycodone 2.5 mg/ acetaminophen 300 mg, oxycodone 5 mg/ acetaminophen 300 mg, oxycodone 7.5 mg/ acetaminophen 300 mg, oxycodone 10 mg/ acetaminophen 300 mg	Strong opioid Preferred over hydrocodone Generally oxycodone is given in combination with acetaminophen
Opioids: Oral[b] Hydromorphone (Dilaudid, Exalgo)	PO	Child <50 kg: 0.03–0.08 mg/kg dose every 3–4 h	Child ≥50 kg and adults; opioid naive: 1–2 mg every 3–4 h	Varies: Depends on whether opioid naive or opioid tolerant	Oral liquid: 1 mg/mL Tablets: 2, 4, 6, 8 mg 12-h Extended release tablets: 8, 12, 16, 32 mg	More potent (×5) than morphine No histamine release and fewer side effects than morphine Sustained release form is available but is usually not given for acute pain in the ED setting

Continued

PART V Special Populations

TABLE 157.5 Systemic Analgesic—cont'd.

Systemic Analgesic[d,e]	Route[c,f]	Dose (Pediatric)[a]	Dose (Adult)[b]	Maximum Dose[c]	Formulations and Notes	Comments
Morphine (Duramorph, Kadian, MS Contin)	PO	Child <50 kg: 0.2–0.5 mg/kg/dose every 3–4 h (immediate release)	Child ≥50 kg and adults: 15–20 mg every 3–4 h		Solution: 10 mg/5 mL, 20 mg/5 mL, 20 mg/mL Tablets: 15 mg, 30 mg 12-h Extended-release tablets: 15, 30, 60, 100, 200 mg 24-h Extended release tablets: 10, 20, 30, 45, 50, 60, 80, 100, 120 mg	Potent opioid Side effect: May cause histamine release (some prefer other opioids for this reason) May be the most commonly use opioid in pediatric patients Sustained release forms available but generally not given for acute pain in the ED
Tramadol (Synapryn, Ultram)	PO	Child ≥ 4 years old: 1–2 mg/kg dose every 4–6 h	Adolescents and adults: 50–100 mg every 4–6 h	Maximum of 100 mg/dose Total daily dose: lesser of 8 mg/kg/day or 400 mg/day	Solution: 5 mg/mL Tablets: 50, 100 mg 24-h extended-release tablets or capsules: 100, 200, 300 mg	Weak opioid; related to codeine; preferred over codeine Less respiratory depression than other opioids Mechanism of action: Central inhibition of norepinephrine and serotonin reuptake, weak affinity for mu receptors
Opioids: Parenteral[b]						
Fentanyl (Abstral, Actiq, Duragesic, Fentora, Lazanda, Onsolis, Subsys)	IV	<50 kg: 1–2 mcg/kg every 1–2 h	Child ≥50 kg and adults: 25–100 mcg/dose every 1–2 h	1–2 µg/kg/dose	Note: Fentanyl is µg or micrograms/kg dose (unlike other opioids which are milligrams or mg/kg per dose), also shorter half-life so given more frequently	More potent (70–100×) than morphine Side effect: Chest wall rigidity with high doses given rapidly More rapid onset and shorter duration than morphine and other opioids
Hydromorphone (Dilaudid, Exalgo)	IV	<50 kg: 0.015 mg/kg every 3–6 h	Child ≥50 kg: 0.2–0.6 mg every 2-4 h	May need higher doses in opioid tolerant patients		More potent (×5) than morphine No histamine release and fewer side effects than morphine
Morphine (Duramorph, Kadian, MS Contin)	IV	<50 kg: 0.05 mg/kg every 2–4 h	Child ≥50 kg and adults: 2–5 mg every 2–4 h	Infants: 2 mg/dose Children 1–6 years: 4 mg/dose Children 7–12 years: 8 mg/dose Adolescents: 10 mg/dose		IM is not recommended because of painful administration, variable absorption, and lag time to peak effect Repeated subcutaneous causes local pain, irritation and induration (see also PO)

[a]Typical doses and maximums are listed. This may not apply to all individuals. Patients differ greatly in their responses to medications, especially opioids. Response may vary due to many factors including age (very young and elderly), previous or chronic exposure to opioids (opioid naive or opioid tolerant), and initial pain severity, so opioids should be titrated to effect.

[b]Use of commercially available brand names does not imply endorsement of any medication or product. They are used because health care providers may be more familiar with brand names than the specific drug name or category or drugs.

[c]There are many routes of administration of opioids, but IM is not recommended, because the injection is painful and has variable absorption and, thus, variable efficacy and unpredictable side effects.

[d]Codeine and meperidine are not included in this table, because they are not preferred and other options are available with fewer side effects.

[e]Oral transmucosal fentanyl is not included in the table, because the fentanyl lollipop was associated with a high incidence of side effects, including nausea, vomiting, and respiratory depression, so it was removed from the market.

[f]Rectal suppositories are available for hydromorphone but are not recommended due to variable absorption.

[g]Other analgesics, such as remifentanil, have been administered for analgesia as part of procedural sedation and analgesia (PSA) but has not yet gained widespread popularity so is not included in the table.

[h]Transdermal patches are available for various medications including lidocaine (Lidoderm), opioids, fentanyl (Duragesic), and buprenorphine (Butrans), but these are generally for chronic pain. They may be encountered in patients with chronic pain, such as cancer patients, but are not generally used for the treatment of acute pain in the ED.

[i]If hydrocodone, oxycodone, or morphine are in the extended release or sustained form, which is for chronic pain, the tablets should be swallowed whole and should not be moistened, dissolved, cut, crushed, broken, or chewed, because this changes the formulation from sustained release to immediate-acting, which can lead to an acute overdose.

[j]Note: Both hydrocodone (Hysingla ER, Zohydro) and oxycodone (Oxecta, OxyContin, Roxicodone) are available in formulations without the acetaminophen component, with the same dosage of hydrocodone or oxycodone, respectively, as for the combinations with acetaminophen. However, they are not frequently prescribed in these formulations without the acetaminophen.

ED, Emergency department; *GI*, gastrointestinal; *IM*, intramuscular; *IV*, intravenous; *NPO, nil per oz.* (nothing by mouth); *NSAID*, nonsteroidal anti-inflammatory drug; *ODT*, orally disintegrating tablets; *PCA*, patient-controlled analgesia; *PO, per oz.* (by mouth); *PR*, per rectal.

a clear superiority of opioid versus nonopioid analgesics, there are multiple adverse effects and consequences for both the individual and the community associated with opioid use, misuse, and abuse. Thus, we recommend that opioids be reserved for more severe pain or pain refractory to other analgesics rather than for routine prescription. If opioids are indicated, they should be given at the lowest effective dose for a limited duration (e.g., 3 days), and the prescriber should consider the patient's risk for opioid use, abuse, or diversion.[26]

Low Dose Ketamine for Treatment of Pain. Low dose ketamine has been successfully used in adults and pediatric patients for the treatment of acute pain.[27] Doses for the treatment of acute pain are lower than those used for sedation and vary. A commonly used dose is 0.15 mg/kg (range 0.1 to 0.2 mg/kg). Higher doses (e.g., 0.3 mg/kg) have been associated with a higher incidence of side effects. Continuous infusions have also been used, in the range of 0.1 to 0.2 mg/kg/h. A randomized control study in children with vaso-occlusive pain crises showed that low dose ketamine had a rapid decrease in pain when compared to morphine.[28] Low dose ketamine was more likely to develop side effects (37.5% vs 3.3% with morphine), with nystagmus and dysphoria being the most common; all side effects were transient and non-life threatening.

Reversal Agents. Naloxone is used for the reversal of opioids effects on the mu receptors (e.g., sedation and respiratory depression). Although the half-life is about 1 hour, the clinically effective duration of action may be much less (e.g., 20 to 60 minutes). Due to longer half-lives of many opioids, re-dosing or an infusion of naloxone is often needed with opioid overdoses. The usual dose for full reversal of opioid intoxication is 0.1 mg/kg/dose with an initial maximum dose of 2 mg. The dose may be repeated every 2 to 3 minutes if there is no response. The IV route is preferred, but intraosseous (IO) can be used if there is no IV line. It may also be given intramuscularly or subcutaneously, but the onset of action may be delayed, especially if there is poor perfusion. Naloxone may be administered intranasally at a dose of 2 mg (1 mg per nare) for adolescents (13 years old and older) and is often given by emergency medical service (EMS) in the field or at home for acute opioid overdoses. Naloxone can also be administered endotracheally at 2 to 3 times the initial IV dose. For reversal of respiratory depression with therapeutic opioid doses, lower doses may be used with an initial dose of 0.001 to 0.005 mg/kg/dose with some recommending 0.001 to 0.015 mg/kg/dose intravenously, intramuscularly, or subcutaneously; the dose is titrated to effect or repeated every 2 to 3 minutes as needed until the desired response is obtained.

Flumazenil antagonizes the action of the benzodiazepines at the gamma-aminobutyric acid (GABA) receptor. It has a half-life of about 1 hour, but the clinically effective duration of action may be much less (20 to 60 minutes). Flumazenil can only be given intravenously. Flumazenil may be given when there is an acute overdose of benzodiazepines which were administered for clinical reasons, and only in a patient who is not benzodiazepine habituated. In individuals who overdose on benzodiazepines, it is likely that they are habituated and on benzodiazepines chronically. In these cases, flumazenil can precipitate benzodiazepine withdrawal with status epilepticus and even death. Thus, except in the acute iatrogenic overdose setting, the use of flumazenil is not recommended. Patients who co-ingest benzodiazepines and tricyclic antidepressants may develop intractable seizures after flumazenil administration. Thus, use of flumazenil should be reserved for patients with an uncomplicated benzodiazepine overdose, no evidence of tricyclic antidepressant use (e.g., no electrocardiogram [ECG] findings and no anticholinergic signs and symptoms), no history of seizure disorder, and no history of benzodiazepine habituation. For benzodiazepine reversal with procedural sedation or anesthesia, the initial dose of flumazenil for infants, children, and adolescents is 0.01 mg/kg (maximum 0.2 mg), which may be repeated after 45 seconds and then every minute up to 4 additional doses. The maximum total cumulative dose is 1 mg or 0.05 mg/kg, whichever is lower. Flumazenil is used infrequently and has a black box warning; we recommend its use only for patients requiring benzodiazepine reversal with procedural sedation or anesthesia (e.g., airway compromise due to oversedation).

Outcomes

There are moral, ethical, legal, and regulatory reasons to adequately treat pain. Oligoanalgesia, the failure to adequately treat pain, continues despite increasing literature demonstrating that pain is too often undertreated. Children and infants, the elderly, individuals with limited cognitive ability, and ethnic and social minorities have a greater risk of oligoanalgesia. The negative consequences of undertreating pain include decreasing the patient's pain threshold and predisposing patients to developing chronic pain syndromes. Inadequate analgesia may lead to harmful physiologic consequences, including an increase in stress hormones and increased sympathetic outflow. This results in an increase in catabolism, myocardial oxygen consumption, production of carbon dioxide, and peripheral vascular resistance, as well as an impaired immune response.

The Joint Commission (TJC) mandates that hospitals adapt a pain management quality improvement program, which includes the measurement, documentation, and therapy for pain. Patient satisfaction and the patient experience are gaining greater importance, and the Centers for Medicare and Medicaid Services (CMS) and the National Committee on Quality Assurance require public reporting of patient satisfaction data for participating health plans. In the future, hospital and physician payment will be based on patient outcomes, as well as patient satisfaction. The positive relationship between adequate treatment of pain and patient satisfaction has been documented for all ages of patients, including children and infants. Eliminating or minimizing the pain of medical procedures can also lead to greater procedural success rates.

The references for this chapter can be found online at ExpertConsult. com.

158

Pediatric Resuscitation

Joshua S. Easter

KEY CONCEPTS

- Unlike adults, most cardiac arrests in children arise from respiratory etiologies. Therefore, emphasis is first on oxygenation and ventilation.
- Detection of a child's pulse may be difficult; if a brachial pulse is not definitively present after 10 seconds of palpation, initiate cardiopulmonary resuscitation (CPR).
- Hypotension is a late finding in pediatric shock and requires immediate intervention to prevent cardiac arrest. Progression from tachycardia to bradycardia in a child is often a harbinger of imminent arrest.
- Although few studies support recommendations for exact rate, depths, and ratios of compressions to ventilations in pediatric CPR, emergency clinicians should perform rapid compressions over the lower sternum with minimal interruptions. The hand encircling technique is recommended for infants requiring chest compressions and the two-hand approach in mid sternum for older children. In the emergency department (ED), we recommend 15 compressions to 2 ventilations for children less than 8 years and 30 compressions to 2 ventilations for older children.
- Verbal and quantitative feedback improves compressions and ventilations.
- Advanced airway management (i.e., endotracheal intubation) may be harmful for children in arrest in the ED. If attempted, physicians should strive for minimal interruptions in compressions and to ventilate at 8 to 10 breaths/min. High quality bag-mask ventilation is a reasonable alternative to advanced airway maneuvers.
- If ventricular fibrillation or pulseless ventricular tachycardia arise, defibrillate at 2 J/kg as soon as possible. While preparing the equipment and charging, continue to perform high quality compressions. Administer subsequent defibrillations at escalating energy doses of 4 J/kg and then 10 J/kg.
- Early administration of epinephrine for non-perfusing rhythms may improve survival.
- Empiric administration of medications to children in arrest worsens outcomes. Reserve medications for specific indications, for example, bicarbonate administration for hyperkalemia.

- Knowledge of the child's approximate weight is necessary to administer the appropriate medication doses and to utilize the appropriate equipment. Determine actual weight in kilogram and estimate weight based on parental report or the child's length.
- Prompt vascular access is critical in a resuscitation. Intraosseous access tends to be the easiest and fastest, but care should be taken that the needle is not residing in the subcutaneous tissue. Central venous access is resource intensive and not necessary in the first few hours of a resuscitation.
- Except in specific circumstances, resuscitations greater than 30 minutes are unlikely to yield favorable outcomes for pediatric arrest.
- After return of circulation, maintain normothermia and avoid hypotension.
- Current definitions of sepsis are based on consensus and primarily for research purposes.
- Systemic inflammatory response syndrome (SIRS) criteria are sensitive but not specific for identifying sepsis in children.
- Hypotension should prompt administration of 20 to 60 mL/kg fluids and likely vasopressors.
- Most children with septic shock have cold shock and therefore epinephrine (0.05 mcg/kg/min) is the first line vasopressor.
- Protocols bundling intravenous fluids, antibiotics, and blood culture acquisition in septic children improve outcomes.
- Brief resolved unexplained events (BRUEs) involve alterations in breathing, tone, or behavior that last less than 1 minute before resolving spontaneously. Children appear well on presentation to the ED, and there are no elements of the history that suggest a particular etiology for the event.
- Low-risk BRUEs occur in children that were born greater than 32 weeks, are greater than 60 days of age, have had no prior BRUEs, and CPR was not required during the event. These children require an assessment and brief observation in the ED, little or no diagnostic testing, and may be discharged with close follow-up.

CARDIAC ARREST

Foundations

Background

Pediatric cardiac arrest is rare, but the consequences are dire when considering lost years of life and productivity. The incidence and survival of pediatric cardiac arrest varies with the location of the arrest, the patient's age, and the mechanism (Table 158.1). Most cardiac arrests encountered in the emergency department (ED) occur outside the hospital, from medical causes in infants and traumatic causes in older children. In children, cardiac arrest is most prevalent in infants,

occurring primarily in children less than 3 months of age. The incidence of atraumatic cardiac arrest in older children is 30 to 50 times less common than infants and adults. Overall, survival following cardiac arrest in children is low; however, it is improving, and certain groups have higher likelihoods of survival. Infants survive infrequently (6%) but older children survive (14%) comparably to adults (11%).[1] The frequency of survival with good neurologic outcome has been estimated at 6% to 12%.

Pediatric resuscitations are relatively rare, limiting clinicians' proficiency. In a review of resuscitations at a busy pediatric ED, less than half of emergency physicians had completed any critical care procedures

TABLE 158.1 Differences in Cardiac Arrest Pathophysiology, Presentation, and Management by Age

	Infant	Child	Adult
Incidence (per 100,000)	75	5	141
Survival (%)	6	14	11
Etiology	Respiratory	Respiratory > Trauma	Cardiac
Rhythm	Asystole, bradycardia	Asystole	Ventricular fibrillation or tachycardia
Early Focus	Compressions, Ventilations		Defibrillation
Location for pulse check	Brachial	Carotid	Carotid
Compression technique	Hands encircling chest	2 hands	2 hands
Compression depth	1.5 inches	2 inches	2 inches
Defibrillation dose (monophasic)	2J/kg, then 4J/kg, and then 10 J/kg		200 J
Epinephrine dose	0.1 mg/mL		0.1 mg/mL

(e.g., cardioversion, intubation, intraosseous line placement) in the preceding year. No physicians had performed cardiac pacing, needle cricothyrotomy, diagnostic peritoneal lavage, thoracentesis, arterial line placement, and venous cutdown line placement. In the absence of actual clinical experience, emergency clinicians often rely on didactic resuscitation courses. However, knowledge retention after these courses is poor. As a result, many emergency clinicians remain uncomfortable managing critically ill children.[2–4] This discomfort can lead to insufficient interventions for fear of harming a child, or alternatively, excessive interventions that stress resources, families, and clinicians.

Pathophysiology

Most atraumatic cardiac arrests in children arise from respiratory etiologies, particularly respiratory failure, drowning, and asphyxia. Children commonly progress from respiratory failure to shock, and finally to bradycardia and loss of circulation. Pediatric advanced life support (PALS) guidelines have largely focused on the treatment of these respiratory emergencies. However, population-based studies suggest cardiac causes account for approximately a third of pediatric medical arrests. Another 21% of pediatric arrests follow trauma. These frequencies are in stark contrast to adults, where two-thirds of arrests are attributed to cardiac etiologies. The differences in the etiology of arrests between adults and children have significant implications for management; arrests from respiratory causes require an emphasis on ventilatory support, oxygen delivery, and maintenance of perfusion, whereas arrests from cardiac causes require a more directed emphasis on restoring perfusion and treatment of underlying dysrhythmias (see Table 158.1).

The most common presenting pediatric arrest rhythm is asystole, occurring in two-thirds of children. Pulseless electrical activity and bradycardia are the next most common presenting rhythms. Unlike adults, ventricular fibrillation and tachycardia are rare, occurring in 9% of children in cardiac arrest. These dysrhythmias can arise with prolonged resuscitation and are more common in adolescents and children with congenital heart disease.

With return of circulation after cardiac arrest, reperfusion induces a cascade of physiologic changes that increase morbidity. During the initial minutes after return of circulation, there is not adequate substrate for aerobic metabolism leading to accumulation of free radicals and cellular necrosis. Children may also develop a sepsis like syndrome, with increased cytokines and endotoxin producing capillary leak and coagulopathy. This may lead to hypotension and multiple organ dysfunction. In the hours following return of circulation, nearly half of children may also develop reversible myocardial dysfunction, producing pulmonary edema, hypotension, or arrhythmias.[5]

Clinical Features

The absence of a pulse, respiratory effort, and responsiveness constitute cardiac arrest. While identifying respiratory effort and responsiveness are relatively straightforward, detecting a pulse in a pediatric patient can be difficult. Physicians identified the presence of a pulse when one was not present in one quarter of children undergoing extracorporeal membrane oxygenation (ECMO). Moreover, emergency clinicians require extended time to determine if a pulse is present in a child, with an average of 9 (±6) seconds to detect a brachial pulse and 29 (±14) seconds to determine that a pulse was not present. Current guidelines suggest lay people should initiate cardiopulmonary resuscitation (CPR) in children without performing a pulse check; any child that is unresponsive and apneic should receive CPR. For emergency clinicians, if no pulse is detected in 10 seconds, CPR should be initiated without delay; the adverse effects of delayed CPR outweigh the effects of CPR for an apneic, unresponsive child with a weak pulse.

The ideal location for palpation of a child's pulse is unclear. There are few studies comparing sites, and they are conducted in the operating room with conflicting results. In infants, the carotid pulse can be difficult to detect compared to the brachial or femoral pulse. In adolescents, the carotid is the easiest location to identify a pulse. In children in cardiac arrest, auscultation of the heart or palpation of the apical impulse can be misleading; patients with pulseless electrical activity can have an apical impulse or auscultated heartbeat without central pulses or adequate perfusion.

Recognizing Imminent Arrest

Anticipating impending cardiac arrest allows for early interventions that may prevent progression. Abnormal vital signs, based on age-specific norms, are often the best indicator of imminent arrest in an ill child. These values can be difficult to remember, but physicians can recognize several key features (Box 158.1). While tachycardia and tachypnea are commonly present in children with relatively benign febrile illnesses, hypotension or ill appearance should prompt immediate intervention.

Management

The paucity of pediatric out-of-hospital cardiac arrests limits available evidence on its management. Most pediatric guidelines are consensus-based and much is extrapolated from adult data.[6–8] The American Heart Association (AHA) guidelines for management are illustrated in

BOX 158.1   Worrisome Vital Sign Findings in Children

Blood Pressure

Systolic blood pressure <70 mm Hg + (2 × age in years) is hypotension (less than fifth percentile for age)

Respiratory Rate

Respiratory rate >60 breaths/min is tachypnea

Declining respiratory rate in previously tachypneic patient can represent improvement *or* fatigue and imminent respiratory failure

Fever

Each 1°C (1.8°F) of fever increases heart rate by only 10 beats/min and respiratory rate by 2–5 breaths/min

End-Tidal Carbon Dioxide

Progressive increase or decrease precede desaturation and respiratory failure

Fig. 158.1. Neonatal resuscitation guidelines (see Chapter 159) should be used for newborns and for neonates within the first weeks of life, after which these pediatric guidelines are applicable for children until puberty (i.e., axillary hair in males and breasts in females).

Compressions-Airway-Breathing

During the initial no-flow state of cardiac arrest, the priority is initiation of flow. This priority has prompted a change in the sequence of "airway-breathing-compressions (A-B-C)" to "compressions-airway-breathing (C-A-B)." This avoids delays in the initiation of blood flow and may render bystanders to an arrest more likely to provide CPR. This is particularly helpful in children; bystander CPR improves pediatric survival but is infrequently administered.[9] Although the A-B-C approach is still considered preferred in children, it is feasible to begin with the C-A-B approach and still provide timely ventilations; a simulated pediatric respiratory arrest model found no delays in the initiation of ventilations with the C-A-B approach compared to the A-B-C approach. Moreover, the C-A-B approach led to prompter recognition of cardiac arrest. If untrained bystanders are reluctant to provide ventilations, children with out-of-hospital cardiac arrest should still receive chest compressions without delay. In the ED, with multiple professionals available, compressions should be administered concurrently with ventilations.

Compressions. High quality compressions improve outcomes but are rarely performed. When administered appropriately, compressions generate one-third of a child's normal cardiac output and a coronary artery perfusion pressure of 10 mm Hg. In a prospective, observational study of in-hospital pediatric arrest, one half of children received the recommended rate of chest compressions and one fifth received the recommended depth per AHA guidelines. In an academic pediatric ED study, 87% of compressions exceeded 100 per minute. However, only 40% complied with recommended compression to ventilation ratios, and there were frequent pauses in compressions.[10]

The location of compressions influences cardiac output. Infants' hearts reside inferior to the lower third of their sternums. In these younger children, encircling the chest with both hands and compressing the lower part of the sternum with the thumbs while squeezing the thorax with the remaining fingers yields greater cardiac output than compression with two fingers. In video review of infant CPR, this approach yielded more accurate compression rates compared to a one handed technique.[11] The AHA suggests utilizing the one hand approach to administer compressions to children 1 to 8 years old, but

a study of simulated compressions suggested a two-handed technique, identical to that performed on adults, is easier and generates higher pressures. When feasible, a resuscitation board placed under children receiving chest compressions improves compressions; at a minimum, the child should be supine on a firm surface.

The ideal compression depth and rate is unknown, but the AHA recommends pushing "hard and fast." Compressions should be deep enough to achieve optimal cardiac output without being so deep as to cause injuries to other vital organs. Attempts to increase depth excessively can result in leaning, which reduces coronary artery perfusion pressure and cardiac output. Guidelines suggest compressing the chest an estimated one-third of the anteroposterior diameter of the child. However, this estimating method has led to relatively deeper compressions than recommended in adults, and it can be extremely difficult to assess proportional anteroposterior compression depth during CPR. As a result, it is more practical to focus on absolute depths; we recommend 1½ inches in infants and 2 inches in older children.

Similarly, the exact rate of compressions to generate ideal cardiac output is unclear. Rates more than 100 compressions per minute improve cardiac output, coronary artery perfusion pressure, and survival compared with rates less than 90 compressions per minute in children. However, attempts to exceed 120 compressions per minute diminish perfusing pressures.[12] High quality compressions diminish after 2 minutes. At this point, emergency clinicians may deny fatigue and be able to maintain the rate of compressions, but depth of compressions decreases substantially. This reduction in quality worsens with time. In adults, pauses in compressions yield substantial drops in coronary artery perfusion pressure, and pauses more than 20 seconds increase the odds of mortality by 50%. A recent study of in-hospital pediatric arrest found that brief pauses (median of 2.4 seconds) did not lead to significant reductions in intra-arterial pressures.[13] Nevertheless, pauses in compressions should be minimized. When pauses are necessary to switch compressors, check rhythms, or provide defibrillation, they should be kept as brief as feasible.

Finally, the appropriate ratio of compression to ventilations is unknown. Animal models indicate the amount of ventilation required during CPR is much lower than with a normal perfusing rhythm, likely due to the lower cardiac output in CPR. The AHA recommends 30:2 compressions to ventilations for single rescuers and 15:2 for two rescuers. However, 15:2 ratios may yield insufficient compressions per minute in older children, and we recommend 30:2 ratios for children greater than 8 years. If an advanced airway is in place, ventilations should be delivered at 8 to 10 breaths per minute and should not interrupt compressions. Overventilation can be dangerous, but is common; in an observational study at a busy pediatric ED, 70% of CPR involved ventilations in excess of recommendations.[10]

Notably, although resuscitation guidelines provide exact rates, depths, and ratios of compressions to ventilations, these recommendations are largely based on consensus. There are no randomized control studies comparing the impact of exact ratios, frequencies, or depths of compressions on survival. Rather than focusing on strict adherence to exact guidelines, we recommend focusing on promptly recognizing the need for compressions and then administering rapid compressions over the lower sternum with minimal interruptions. Practice is critical to maintaining quality, as most individual clinicians have limited real patient experience; in a busy pediatric ED, clinicians averaged 3 minutes of compressions per year.[14,15]

The AHA recommends feedback, as it improves the quality of compressions. Quantitative feedback is most helpful because qualitative assessments can be difficult. During simulated arrests, emergency clinicians significantly overestimated compression depth and rate while underestimating pauses. Accelerometers and force

Pediatric cardiac arrest algorithm – 2020 update

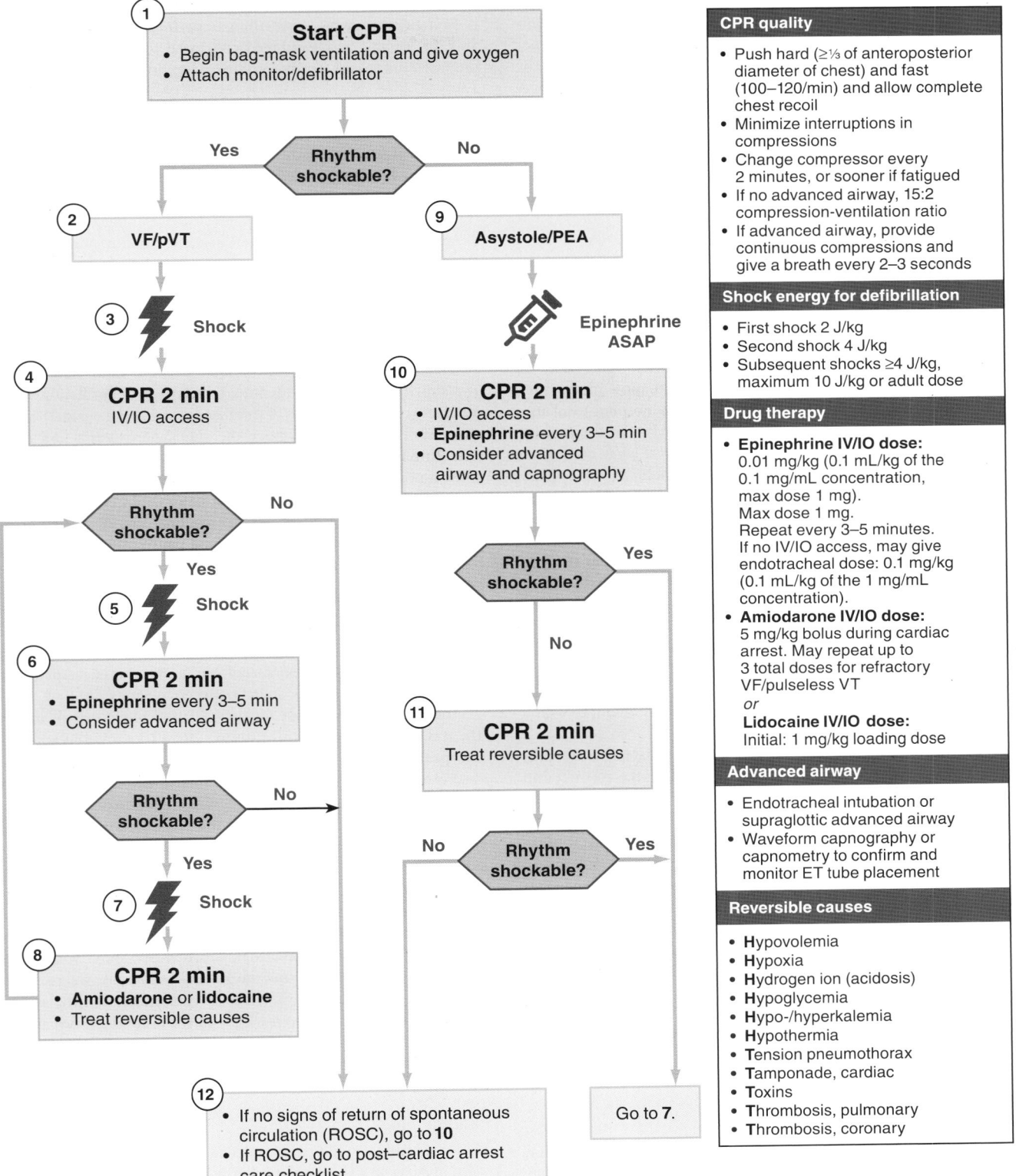

Fig. 158.1 The American Heart Association (AHA) Guidelines Algorithm for Management of Infants and Children in Cardiopulmonary Arrest. *CPR,* Cardiopulmonary resuscitation; *ETT,* endotracheal tube; *IO/IV,* intraosseous/intravenous; *PEA,* pulseless electrical activity; *ROSC,* return of spontaneous circulation; *VF/VT,* ventricular fibrillation/pulseless ventricular tachycardia.

sensors provide real-time data on compression rate and force. These feedback devices improve adherence with compression guidelines amongst children in simulated cardiac arrest.[16] The presence of a coach providing verbal feedback augments feedback devices in simulated arrests.[17-19] End-tidal carbon dioxide (ETCO$_2$) also serves as an adjunct measure of the adequacy of compressions.[20,21] In the low-flow state of CPR, the flow of venous blood to the lungs serves as the rate-limiting step for the elimination of CO$_2$ as opposed to ventilation. As a result, exhaled CO$_2$ increases with cardiac output, and the AHA recommends titration to greater than 20 mm Hg, although an observational study of in-hospital pediatric arrest found levels greater than 20 mm Hg were not associated with survival.[22] Despite proven benefits, less than 5% of hospitals employ feedback devices regularly during resuscitation.

Ventilation. Although life-threatening airway emergencies in children are rare, most critical illness in children stems from respiratory etiologies; therefore, focus is largely on effective ventilation and oxygenation. The appropriate method to ventilate children in arrest is unclear, as advanced airway management with endotracheal intubation may not improve outcomes compared to bag-mask ventilation. A randomized trial of intubation versus mask ventilation in the pre-hospital setting found no difference in survival to hospital discharge (OR = 0.82; 95% CI, 0.61 to 1.1) for tracheal intubation versus bag-mask ventilation alone. A large observational study in Japan confirmed these results.[23] In contrast, a retrospective review of an airway registry suggested endotracheal intubation was associated with reduced survival (OR = 0.39; 95% CI, 0.26 to 0.59). While this may stem from complications associated with pre-hospital pediatric intubation, results are similar for in-hospital pediatric arrest. An observational study of 2294 children found intubation was associated with reduced survival (RR = 0.89; 95% CI, 0.81 to 0.99).[24] The lack of benefit of pre-hospital advanced airway management may extend to supraglottic devices, with a retrospective study showing reduced survival (OR = 0.32; 95% CI, 0.12 to 0.84).[25] Advanced airway management may reduce survival by leading to interruptions in compressions; a review of pediatric ED intubation attempts found pauses in over half of attempts with a median duration of 25 seconds.[26]

As a result of this evidence, the 2019 PALS update recommends bag-mask ventilation for pre-hospital arrest.[6] While the AHA found insufficient evidence to create a guideline for the ED, we extrapolate from the pre-hospital and in-hospital evidence and recommend emergency physicians focus on delivering high quality bag-mask ventilation. This requires the appropriate equipment (mask size and airway adjuncts) as well as deliberate practice.[7] If advanced airway management is attempted during resuscitation, care should be taken to avoid prolonged interruptions in compressions. In addition, patients should receive only 8 to 10 breaths/min via the advanced airway without interruptions in compressions. A more in-depth discussion of pediatric airway management can be found in Chapter 156.

Compression-Only Cardiopulmonary Resuscitation

Compression only CPR is utilized in adults, but the benefits in children are less apparent. For arrests secondary to ventricular fibrillation, as are common in adults, patients often have a reservoir of oxygen in their lungs and can maintain adequate arterial partial pressure of oxygen (PaO$_2$) for 5 minutes with compressions alone. In contrast, animal studies of arrests from respiratory causes show that compression-only CPR leads to rapid depletion of oxygen reservoirs and increased CO$_2$ and lactate. In a large observational study of children, conventional CPR was associated with improved survival compared to compression-only CPR.[27] For children with cardiac etiologies to their arrest, survival was similar with both approaches. As children commonly suffer

respiratory etiologies for their arrest, and there are multiple providers available in the ED, conventional CPR should be the norm.

Bystander CPR improves outcomes, but only half of children receive it. Bystanders may be more willing to perform compression-only CPR, and this should be encouraged compared to no CPR. Compression-only CPR improved survival compared to no CPR (OR = 3.3, 95% CI, 1.9 to 5.7).[9,28]

Defibrillation. Although ventricular fibrillation and pulseless ventricular tachycardia are rarely the presenting rhythm in children, they arise at some point during one quarter of pediatric resuscitations. Children with these rhythms are more likely to survive. Defibrillation applies asynchronous current to the heart to restore a perfusing rhythm. While out-of-hospital arrest studies demonstrated that shorter durations between onset of a shockable rhythm and defibrillation improved survival, a recent observational study of in-hospital pediatric arrest found time to defibrillation was not associated with survival (RR = 0.99; 95% CI, 0.94 to 1.1).[29] This may reflect the abrupt recognition of arrest and initiation of CPR in-hospital, which may mitigate the survival benefit of rapid defibrillation. In the setting of conflicting evidence, in the ED we recommend prompt defibrillation as soon as a shockable rhythm is identified. Delays in defibrillation of over 3 minutes arise in nearly half of simulated shockable arrests. These delays stem from failure to recognize the shockable rhythm and difficulty operating the defibrillator.[30] While awaiting defibrillation, emergency clinicians should focus on administering high quality compressions without interruptions until the defibrillator is placed and charged.

Pediatric specific equipment is available for defibrillation. Both paddles and pads provide adequate energy, assuming gel is placed on the paddles and pads are firmly attached to the chest wall. Optimal pad size has not been well defined in the pediatric population; pads can be used according to the manufacturer's size recommendations and should fit on the child's chest without touching. Anteroposterior and anterolateral positioning of pads provide equivalent energy to the heart. If pediatric pads are not available, apply adult-sized pads anteroposteriorly and minimize contact between the pads.

The optimal energy dose for defibrillation in children is uncertain. The AHA recommends administering 2 to 4 J/kg initially, whereas the European Resuscitation Council recommends 4 J/kg. Dosing based strictly on weight often leads to lower than anticipated energy delivery. Theoretically, a higher dose per kilogram may overcome this variability and ensure adequate energy reaches the heart. However, multiple small studies have not identified any association between energy dose and survival.[31] The primary disadvantage of higher energy doses is damage to the myocardium, but animal studies suggest long-term myocardial necrosis only occurs with doses more than 10 J/kg. The only circumstance where a child would receive such high doses is if adult pads are utilized with an infant. Nevertheless, when presented with an infant in ventricular fibrillation and no other equipment, we recommend employing the adult pads.[32] We also recommend starting defibrillation at 2 J/kg, increasing to 4 J/kg with the second defibrillation, and increasing to 10 J/kg for third and subsequent shocks. There is no difference in survival between monophasic and biphasic defibrillation in children.

Pharmacology

There are no high-quality randomized control studies showing improvement in survival to hospital discharge or neurologic outcome with any medications administered during pediatric cardiac arrest. Observational studies suggest that prompt administration of epinephrine may improve return of circulation and mortality for non-traumatic out-of-hospital cardiac arrest in children; each minute from emergency medical service (EMS) arrival until administration of epinephrine reduced

TABLE 158.2 Medications for Pediatric Cardiac Arrest

Medication	Indications	Dose (mg/kg)	Comments
Epinephrine	Asystole, PEA, bradycardia, VF, pulseless VT	0.01	0.1mg/mL formulation Higher doses of epinephrine may decrease survival May increase harm with bradycardia
Atropine	Bradycardia	0.02	Not for routine use in PEA, asystole 0.02 mg/kg
Amiodarone	VF, VT, SVT	5	Unclear if superior to lidocaine for VF, VT
Lidocaine	VF, VT	1	Avoid in WPW
Procainamide	SVT refractory to adenosine, stable VT	10–15	First line for SVT in WPW May be more effective than amiodarone for SVT Do not give in patients receiving amiodarone, torsades de pointes, or prolonged QT Can cause hypotension
Adenosine	SVT	0.1	First line therapy for stable SVT Avoid in WPW, wide complex tachycardia, long QT Potentially unreliable through IO route
Dextrose	Hypoglycemia	0.5–1 g/kg, maximum 25 g	D10W: 5mL/kg, D25W: 2mL/kg, D50W: 1mL/kg Do not administer empirically
Calcium chloride	Hyperkalemia, hypocalcemia, calcium channel blocker overdose	20	Not for routine use Calcium chloride provides more bioavailable calcium but requires central line
Sodium bicarbonate	Hyperkalemia, TCA overdose	1 mEq/kg	Not for routine use
Magnesium sulfate	Torsades de pointes, hypomagnesemia	Maximum single dose: 2g	Not for routine use

D10W, Dextrose 10% in water; *D25W*, dextrose 25% in water; *D50W*, dextrose 50% in water; *PEA*, pulseless electrical activity; *SVT*, supraventricular tachycardia; *TCA*, tricyclic antidepressant; *VF*, ventricular fibrillation; *VT*, ventricular tachycardia; *WPW*, Wolff-Parkinson-White.

survival 9%.[33–36] Doses of epinephrine greater than 0.01 mg/kg do not improve survival. Pre-filled code cart epinephrine syringes may lead to substantial overdoses in infants.[37] The benefits of epinephrine may not extend to *non*-pulseless events, with a recent observational study showing decreased survival (RR = 0.79; 95% CI, 0.74 to 0.85) with epinephrine administration within the first 10 minutes of resuscitation for children with bradycardia and poor perfusion.[38]

There is mounting evidence to suggest that certain commonly administered medications are associated with decreased survival and poorer neurologic outcome. Bicarbonate continues to be used in two thirds of pediatric in-hospital arrests despite evidence suggesting empiric administration is associated with decreased survival (OR = 0.80; 95% CI, 0.65 to 0.97).[39] Similarly, calcium is administered in nearly half of pediatric in-hospital cardiac arrests, despite an association with decreased survival and poorer neurologic outcome. Atropine is also often administered inappropriately, including in 1 of every 5 out-of-hospital pediatric arrests.[40] These drugs should be reserved for specific indications (Table 158.2).

The ideal drug for ventricular tachycardia and pulseless ventricular tachycardia remains unclear, with recommendations extrapolated from adult data. A prospective study of in-hospital pediatric arrest with shockable rhythms found that there were no differences in return of circulation or mortality (RR = 1.0; 95% CI 0.63 to 1.6) between lidocaine and amiodarone.[41] The implications of this study for out-of-hospital cardiac arrest are uncertain. Without further evidence or consensus, either agent seems appropriate.

Dosing of medications during pediatric cardiac arrest can be difficult; accurate administration requires correct estimation of weight, determination of weight-based dose, and conversion of weight to volume. Time spent on these tasks increases clinicians' cognitive load and errors. Estimations based on length (Broselow-Luten) or upper

extremity circumference (Mercy TAPE) are better than estimates based on appearance or age, but may underestimate weight in obese children or overestimate in underweight children.[42] Parents tend to be more accurate than these estimation methods.[43] Regardless, these estimates do not eliminate all dosing errors because clinicians still have to calculate volumes of medications. Utilization of color coded, prefilled syringes corresponding to the weight, or precalculated medication charts or applications based on a standardized formulary may mitigate these dosing errors.[44]

Confirmation of weight estimates reduces errors. Often in the rush of resuscitation, inaccurately estimated weights result in inappropriate equipment and medications. The finger counting method can confirm an estimated weight. The clinician counts age on the left hand, starting with 1 on the thumb and counting by odd numbers to 9 on the small finger (i.e., 1–3–5–7–9 years of age). Weight in kilograms is counted on the right hand, starting with 10 kg and counting by 5 to 30 kg on the small finger (i.e., 10 kg–15 kg–20 kg–25 kg–30 kg). Fingers are matched between hands to estimate weight based on age. To prepare appropriate equipment and medications, emergency clinicians should ask EMS providers for the child's approximate weight.

Vascular Access. The particular site of vascular access is less important than its timely acquisition. Peripheral venous and intraosseous drug administration produce similar onset of drug action and peak levels for the commonly administered resuscitation drugs.[45] Prolonged delays are common in the ED; nearly half of children in the resuscitation area of an ED required greater than 90 minutes to obtain vascular access.[46]

For children in arrest or imminent arrest, an immediate attempt to obtain intraosseous access saves time. Intraosseous access is more successful and faster with minimal complications compared to peripheral or central access in critically ill patients.[47] Directing the needle away

TABLE 158.3 Monitoring After Return of Circulation

Parameter	Assessment	Goal	Action
Oxygen	Arterial blood gas; continuous pulse oximetry	SpO_2 94%–99% PaO_2 80–200 mm Hg	Titrate FiO_2
Carbon dioxide	Continuous capnography	$PaCO_2$ 35–45 mm Hg	Adjust respiratory rate
Perfusion	Arterial line; lactate; urine output	Avoid SBP <70 + 2 × age	20 mL/kg of isotonic fluid; norepinpehrine 0.1–2 mcg/kg/min
Heart rhythm	Continuous cardiac monitor	Avoid arrhythmias	Treat if arise; no prophylaxis
Glucose	Blood glucose	Avoid glucose <60	Dextrose
Temperature	Continuous core temperature	<38	Antipyretics; cooling blanket
Sedation		Avoid shivering	Fentanyl; midazolam
Seizure	EEG	Termination of seizure	Midazolam; phenytoin or levetiracetam

EEG, Electroencephalogram; *SBP,* systolic blood pressure.

from the growth plate during insertion reduces the risk of injury to the growth plate; long-term follow up has shown minimal adverse impact on bone growth from intraosseous placement alone. Monitoring of the insertion site allows detection of compartment syndrome, which can arise from excessive insertion of fluids into a needle misplaced in the subcutaneous tissue. Powered intraosseous insertion devices, such as the EZ-IO (Vidacare), may decrease insertion times and improve the frequency of successful insertion; although, other powered devices that require calibration, such as the Bone Injection Gun (WaisMed) may delay insertion and reduce the frequency of success. Manual placement may avoid insertion through the posterior cortex in children less than 8 kg.[48] In young children, the tibia and femur are preferred, because their marrow cavity is well developed. When administering fluid through an intraosseous line, manual pressure is helpful to overcome the resistance of the marrow cavity. Multiple injections of smaller (10 mL) syringes of fluid (i.e., "flushes") can resuscitate infants and small children through an intraosseous needle. Surveys suggest physicians often unnecessarily delay attempts at intraosseous access while attempting peripheral or central access. Central line access should typically be reserved for children requiring prolonged vasopressors. The femoral vein is the easiest site of cannulation in young children.

Termination of Resuscitation. There are no universal criteria to guide the termination of a pediatric resuscitation. Emergency clinicians are less comfortable terminating efforts in children than adults, often resulting in prolonged, futile resuscitations that increase stress on families and staff. There are anecdotal reports of children surviving with good neurologic outcome after prolonged resuscitations, but these often involve in-hospital arrests or arrests with prompt access to extracorporeal membrane oxygenation (ECMO). Several variables, including length of resuscitation, unwitnessed arrest, initial cardiac rhythm, administration of multiple doses of epinephrine, administration of atropine, and $ETCO_2$ less than 10 mm Hg have been associated with low survival and poor neurologic outcome.[49,50] However, none of these variables possess sufficient discriminative ability to provide absolute cutoffs for termination of resuscitation. Perhaps the most predictive variable is duration of resuscitation; a multicenter retrospective analysis indicated that for every additional minute of pediatric CPR, the frequency of survival decreased by 2.1%. For traumatic arrest, guidelines suggest prehospital termination after 30 minutes of unsuccessful resuscitation.[51] A recent large retrospective study of pediatric arrest following traffic accidents found that when CPR was necessary for greater than 15 minutes, less than 1% of children survived and all had poor neurologic outcome.[52] Such guidelines do not exist for atraumatic arrest. Guidelines designed for adults, such as the Termination of Resuscitation rule, fail to predict survival in children adequately and should not be employed.[53] Outside of family wishes and specific clinical situations where prolonged resuscitation may be beneficial (e.g., hypothermia with drowning or electrocution, in-hospital arrest, or prompt access to ECMO), we recommend considering termination of resuscitation after 30 minutes for atraumatic causes and 15 minutes for traumatic causes. This approach can minimize suffering for the patient, family, and staff.

E-CPR

When readily available, physicians should also consider ECMO early in an arrest course. Although initial studies suggested ECMO provided greater benefits for patients with underlying cardiac disease, a retrospective analysis also identified benefits for children with non-cardiac etiologies of their arrest. Pediatric critical care centers performing high volumes of ECMO and with rapid response teams to initiate timely cannulation have better outcomes. ECMO also should be considered for children with return of circulation but refractory shock, particularly cardiogenic shock.

Post-Arrest Care

For children with return of circulation, several actions may improve survival and neurologic outcome. Focus should shift to treating the underlying etiology of the arrest, minimizing brain injury, and improving end-organ perfusion. This requires monitoring oxygen, carbon dioxide, blood pressure, temperature, glucose, and urine output (Table 158.3).

Blood Pressure

Hypotension develops in over half of children following in-hospital cardiac arrest and predicts increased mortality. A single episode of hypotension (<5th percentile for age) within the first 6 hours after arrest is associated with decreased survival (OR = 0.39; 95% CI, 0.20 to 0.74).[54] More frequent episodes of hypotension further reduce survival. Arterial pressure monitoring facilitates early detection of hypotension; we recommend it for children with hypotension or protracted courses in the ED. While avoidance of hypotension (<5th percentile for age, estimated as systolic blood pressure <70 + age × 2) reduces mortality, the ideal blood pressure target is unknown.

It is also not clear if augmentation of blood pressure with intravenous fluids or vasopressors mitigates the mortality risk. Although vasopressors can help maintain end-organ perfusion in the setting of post-arrest myocardial dysfunction, in observational studies their use has not improved survival. There are no randomized studies of comparing the performance of particular vasopressors for pediatric post-arrest care. In the absence of strong evidence, we administer intravenous fluid boluses and norepinephrine or push dose epinephrine to maintain systolic blood pressure greater than 5th percentile. Norepinephrine causes fewer arrhythmias than dopamine in adults and is the preferred first-line vasopressor in the post-arrest period. Push dose epinephrine can augment blood pressure while a norepinephrine drip is prepared. Concurrent administration of dobutamine may be necessary to achieve hemodynamic stability in patients with refractory cardiogenic shock.

Ventilation and Oxygenation

Significant alterations in oxygenation and ventilation may also increase mortality. These are quite common; less than one fifth of children have normal oxygen and carbon dioxide levels when measured during the first 6 hours after return of circulation. Confirming the results of a prior smaller study focused on pediatric cardiac arrest, a recent large study of 6250 critically ill children found that severe hyperoxemia ($PaO_2 \geq 300$ mg Hg) increased mortality (OR = 1.5, 95% CI, 1.1 to 2.1) and recurrent hyperoxemia further increased mortality (OR = 2.5, 95% CI, 1.6 to 3.9).[55] Ventilator settings should be adjusted to maintain oxygen saturations above 94%, while avoiding PaO_2 levels greater than 300 mm Hg. Hypocapnia induces cerebral vasoconstriction, exacerbating ischemia. Meanwhile, hypercapnia leads to vasodilation and cerebral edema. While end tidal CO_2 measurement may allow assessment of trends in carbon dioxide levels, alteration in alveolar dead space in the post arrest period may lead to end tidal CO_2 not accurately representing $PaCO_2$. Therefore, we measure CO_2 directly with a blood gas. Notably, studies of post-arrest oxygenation and ventilation are limited by the timing of oxygen and carbon dioxide measurement, and therefore the true impact of abnormalities on survival is not clear. Nevertheless, in the absence of strong evidence, we recommend adjusting ventilator settings in the post-arrest period to normalize carbon dioxide and oxygen levels.

Targeted Temperature Management

Maintaining normothermia is most important. Theoretically, hypothermia reduces many of the complications seen with reperfusion after cardiac arrest by reducing metabolic demand and free radical production. However, two large randomized control trials of targeted temperature management in children failed to show benefit for children who received induced hypothermia. In a randomized trial of 260 children with out-of-hospital cardiac arrest, targeted temperature management to 33°C (range of 32°C to 34°C) with automated cooling blankets for 120 hours demonstrated no difference from therapeutic normothermia (target temperature of 36.8°C, range of 36°C to 37.5°C) in survival or favorable neurologic outcome (RR = 1.59; 95% CI, 0.89 to 2.85).[56] A subsequent randomized controlled study of 329 children with in-hospital cardiac arrest was terminated early because targeted temperature management to 33°C with the same protocol did not improve survival (RR = 0.92; 95% CI, 0.67 to 1.3).[57] When the in-hospital and out-of-hospital studies were combined to increase the power of the study, targeted temperature management to 33°C continued to show no benefit on survival or favorable neurologic outcome, including in subgroup analyses.[58] These studies were multicenter without standardization regarding other elements of post-arrest care, potentially limiting the conclusions. The 2019 PALS update endorses targeted temperature management or avoidance of hyperthermia as "reasonable" options.[6] In the absence of strong evidence, we recommend monitoring core temperature and focusing on the avoidance of hyperthermia (target temperature of 36°C to 37.5°C) with external cooling and antipyretic medications. If cooling is employed, children should not be allowed to reach temperatures less than 32°C, which increases mortality.[59]

Glucose

In response to the stress of cardiac arrest, alterations in glucose levels are also common. In theory, significant hyperglycemia produces an osmotic diuresis, which impairs perfusion. In critically ill children not suffering from cardiac arrest, hyperglycemia worsens outcomes. However, in pursuit of euglycemia with insulin administration, children often become hypoglycemic. Critically ill children randomized to a lower target glucose (80 to 110 mg/dL) had more frequent episodes of profound hypoglycemia but similar mortality and duration of intensive care unit (ICU) stay compared to higher glucose levels (150 to 180 mg/dL).[56] In the absence of strong evidence in post-arrest care, we recommend targeting modest glucose control (80 to 180 mg/dL) and vigilant avoidance of hypoglycemia.

Arrhythmia and Seizures

Children may develop arrhythmias or seizures following reperfusion. Premature atrial or ventricular contractions are most frequent, particularly with vasopressor administration, and do not require therapy. In contrast, ventricular arrhythmias may arise and require prompt administration of antiarrhythmics (see Table 158.3). Seizures arise in 10% of children, with over two thirds of cases evolving into status epilepticus.[60] As seizures are associated with poor neurologic outcome, consensus guidelines recommend continuous electroencephalogram (EEG) monitoring as soon as possible to detect non-convulsive status, which is common.[61-63] While there are no randomized trials in children seizing after arrest, we recommend benzodiazepines, followed by fosphenytoin or levetiracetam, for seizures.

Family Presence

We endorse the recommendation from the American College of Emergency Physicians (ACEP) and American Academy of Pediatrics (AAP) that physicians offer family the opportunity to be present during their child's resuscitation. The limited evidence to support this recommendation is primarily descriptive or survey-based. Most families want to be present for the resuscitation of their child, and when asked after being present, they report that they would repeat the experience, even if their child died. Families report their presence helps them appreciate the efforts of clinicians, facilitates their understanding of the gravity of the situation, and facilitates the grieving process. In contrast, surveyed physicians frequently are reluctant to have families present, often mistakenly assuming families will impede care. In the only randomized study of family presence during trauma resuscitations in a pediatric ED, 93% of physicians reported increased stress from family presence. However, the adverse effects of family presence seemed limited to stress on the physician. No differences were detected in clinical care, and other studies have confirmed that family presence rarely hinders care. In most situations, the benefits to the family of being present outweigh the increased stress on clinicians.

Structured programs for family presence during resuscitations are helpful. Families should be counseled on anticipated events prior to entering the resuscitation. They should be informed that their presence in the resuscitation is their decision; although, they can be asked to leave if they impede medical care. Designated nurses or social workers with training in grief counseling and free of clinical responsibilities should focus on the family, explaining steps in the resuscitation and answering questions.

SEPTIC SHOCK IN THE PEDIATRIC PATIENT

Foundations

Background

Sepsis is the leading cause of death in children worldwide. Globally, 8% of children in the ICU have severe sepsis with mortality approaching 25%.[64] Young age (<1 month), immunosuppression, chronic debilitating disease, presence of invasive devices, and genitourinary anomalies increase the risk of sepsis and severe disease.[65,66] Rates of sepsis have increased over time, likely due to increased recognition. Mortality has decreased, likely a result of immunizations and the implementation of consensus recommendations. While these guidelines are not grounded in strong evidence, EDs in the United States implementing these guidelines have reduced mortality and length of stay. Nevertheless, variation and uncertainty persist for multiple elements of ED sepsis management, particularly the optimal approaches to screening, diagnosis, fluid administration, and vasoactive therapy.

Pathophysiology

Sepsis arises when immune dysregulation following an infection promotes pro and anti-inflammatory cascades that may manifest in vasodilation, myocardial depression, activation of the complement system, disseminated intravascular coagulation, and increased production of nitric oxide. Infection tends to arise from common bacterial and viral pathogens in the lungs, blood, urine, or the skin, with the most likely organism depending on the location of the infection and patient risk factors. Immunosuppressed children may develop less common bacterial or fungal infections. Unchecked, infections progress to shock with end-organ hypoperfusion and then multisystem organ failure.

Clinical Features

The diagnosis of sepsis is difficult, with numerous definitions in the literature. Definitions were derived from consensus only and were primarily established for research purposes. For example, the presence of SIRS criteria (abnormal temperature or white blood cell count and tachycardia or tachypnea) plus infection constitutes sepsis per guidelines, but many children with non-life threatening infections display SIRS criteria.[67] Differentiating these patients from patients with early sepsis is crucial, as delays in treatment of sepsis adversely impact outcomes. While definitions of sepsis were revised in adults to improve clinical application during the latest consensus conference (Sepsis-3), pediatric definitions have not been significantly revised in the last fifteen years. We extrapolate from the adult evidence and recommend strong consideration of sepsis in children with concern for infection, SIRS criteria, and any physical examination or laboratory findings of decreased perfusion or organ dysfunction.[68] Systematic screening allows for early detection of sepsis, but clinician assessment is necessary to confirm concern for sepsis and the need for treatment.

Most individual physical examination findings demonstrate poor diagnostic accuracy for sepsis. Hypotension is the most reliable indicator of septic shock and impending organ dysfunction, but it tends to develop late in the disease course, as children are able to maintain their blood pressure through tachycardia and vasoconstriction. In contrast to adults, hypotension is not universally present with pediatric septic shock. Other potential signs of organ dysfunction may be present, including toxic appearance, altered mental status, loss of consciousness, seizures, or respiratory failure. The combination of hypotension and delayed capillary refill together portended the highest mortality in a large study of patients transported to a pediatric ICU. Other findings, such as dry mucus membranes, sunken eyes, decreased urine output, height of fever, or rigors, have poor diagnostic accuracy for sepsis or shock.

Multiple scoring systems exist to identify early sepsis and predict outcomes. Similar to adults, the Quick Sequential Organ Failure Assessment (qSOFA) score may help identify patients with organ dysfunction. qSOFA includes altered mental status, hypotension, and tachypnea. In two large retrospective studies, an age adjusted qSOFA had lower sensitivity but much better specificity compared to SIRS for predicting mortality from pediatric sepsis.[69,70] Other scoring systems, such as the quick Pediatric Logistic Organ Dysfunction-2 Score (qPELOD2) have poorer diagnostic accuracy.[71]

Consensus guidelines define septic shock as hypotension refractory to administration of ≥40 mL/kg of intravenous fluids in one hour. From a practical perspective, we recommend considering any child with hypotension (blood pressure <5th percentile for age) to be in shock. While children may develop cold or warm shock, it is difficult to differentiate these processes without invasive monitoring. Laboratory testing may augment the diagnosis, but treatment should not be delayed if there is high clinical suspicion for sepsis. Venous blood gas can identify a metabolic acidosis and elevated lactate. In an observational study of children with SIRS, lactate greater than 4 mmol/L in the ED was associated with increased 30 day mortality (OR = 3.3; 95% CI, 1.2 to 9.2).[72] Efforts should be made to identify the source of the infection in order to target therapy. Bacteremia and urinary tract infections are common, so blood and urine cultures should be obtained from all patients. Risk-stratification strategies in a research setting include RNA expression profiling and novel serum biomarkers. These techniques hold promise in the future for more objective and systematic assessment to enable clinicians to distinguish children with more benign viral illness from those with early septic shock.

Management

The pillars of emergency treatment of pediatric sepsis are: (1) timely establishment of intravascular access; (2) rapid fluid resuscitation titrated to patient condition; (3) appropriate, broad-spectrum antibiotics; and (4) individualized vasoactive agents directed to reverse shock (Table 158.4).

The 2020 pediatric Surviving Sepsis Campaign guidelines strongly recommend antibiotic administration as soon as possible and within 1 hour of recognition of septic shock.[73] Delays in appropriate antimicrobial therapy increase mortality and prolong organ dysfunction in pediatric patients with severe sepsis or septic shock.[74] For children with sepsis-associated organ dysfunction but not shock, guidelines recommend antibiotic administration as soon as possible and within 3 hours of recognition. This allows time to acquire laboratory studies to help differentiate sepsis from other infections. Acquisition of blood cultures should not delay administration of antibiotics. While host factors, suspected source, and local susceptibility patterns should guide antibiotic selection, children with septic shock or organ dysfunction typically require broad spectrum antibiotic therapy in the ED. For otherwise healthy children with community acquired sepsis, a third-generation cephalosporin, such as ceftriaxone, is often appropriate. For chronically ill children or hospital acquired sepsis, an antipseudomonal cephalosporin, such as cefepime; a carbapenem, such as meropenem; or extended spectrum penicillin, such as piperacillin/tazobactam is appropriate. Additional antibiotics may be required in children at risk for drug resistance. Antibiotics can later be tailored to culture results. There is not strong evidence to suggest that children with sepsis require multiple antibiotics targeting the same organism, although multiple antibiotics may be appropriate in certain high-risk scenarios, such as septic shock in immunocompromised children. If available, an infectious disease physician can help guide antibiotic therapy for complex patients.

Septic shock in children is most frequently marked by relative or absolute hypovolemia; outcomes from shock in children are improved when the shock state is reversed as early as possible. Cohort studies have demonstrated improved mortality and hospital length of stay in septic children with hypotension or organ dysfunction treated with 40 to 60 mL/kg of intravenous (IV) fluid in the first hour. A highly publicized randomized controlled trial in African children with severe infection, but not hypotension, demonstrated increased mortality in patients receiving 20 to 40 mL/kg in the first hour compared to no fluid. This outcome likely is specific to the setting, as there were limited resources and a high frequency of malaria and anemia. In another single, small study, rapid administration of fluid bolus in less than 10 minutes increased the risk of needing mechanical ventilation. We follow the 2020 Surviving Sepsis guidelines and administer up to 40 to 60 mL/kg in the first hour.[75,76] Fluid resuscitation should be goal-directed and continue until vital signs and signs of perfusion improve, which may necessitate administration of multiple 10 to 20 mL/kg boluses.

TABLE 158.4 Bundled Management of the First Hour of Septic Shock

	Key Features	Sample Regimen
Antibiotics	Broad spectrum; MRSA coverage if indwelling catheter; Pseudomonas coverage if nosocomial infection	Cefepime 50 mg/kg +/– Vancomycin 20 mg/kg
Fluids	Large bore intravenous access; Bolus isotonic fluid; Monitor fluid responsiveness	20 mL/kg lactated Ringers over 10 min
Vasopressors	Hypotension refractory to fluids	Epinephrine 0.05 mcg/kg/min
Cultures	Blood, urine cultures; Viral testing based on clinical suspicion; Should not delay antibiotics	2nd blood culture if indwelling line
Monitoring	Frequent bedside assessments for signs of fluid overload	Cardiorespiratory monitoring; arterial line for hypotension; not routinely need central venous pressure, mixed venous saturation

MRSA, Methicillin-resistant Staphylococcus aureus.

Concomitant with fluid administration, clinicians should monitor children for signs of fluid overload and reduce or stop fluids for any signs of pulmonary edema (e.g., tachypnea) or new hepatomegaly. Notably, hypoperfusion may persist despite correction of hypotension. Similarly, tachycardia may persist despite restoration of perfusion. In resource limited settings, clinicians should be cautious about reflexively administering excessive amounts of fluid, and guidelines recommend a maximum of 40 mL/kg over the first hour.[73] Most children will not require invasive monitoring in the ED to assess fluid responsiveness.

We recommend prompt acquisition of large bore intravenous access via an intravenous or intraosseous line and fluid bolus administration early in presentation. Fluid can be administered using a "push-pull" inline syringe, rapid infuser, or pressure bag to achieve a goal of administering each 20 mL/kg crystalloid fluid bolus over 10 to 20 minutes, followed by reassessment and potentially additional boluses (Fig. 158.2). There is conflicting evidence from two large retrospective studies about the benefits of balanced fluids, such as lactated Ringers, versus normal saline.[77,78] When data from these studies was combined it showed decreased mortality with balanced fluids. Based on this result and other studies in adults, the 2020 pediatric guidelines recommend administration of balanced fluids.[73] There is *insufficient* evidence to support routine administration of albumin or starches in the resuscitation of children in septic shock in the ED.

If shock does not improve with administration of 60 mL/kg of isotonic fluid, or if signs of fluid overload develop in the setting of ongoing hypoperfusion, children should receive **vasoactive agents**. Epinephrine or norepinephrine may serve as the first-line agent in pediatric septic shock. In two small studies, epinephrine was associated with more rapid resolution of shock and decreased mortality compared to dopamine.[79,80] Therefore, epinephrine (0.05 mcg/kg/min) is our standard first-line agent. If the child's status does not improve with the initial agent, then a second vasopressor should be administered. There is no evidence to guide the choice of the second agent. We initiate vasoactive agents in any pediatric patient with septic shock and hypotension lasting more than 1 hour, regardless of the amount of fluid delivered.

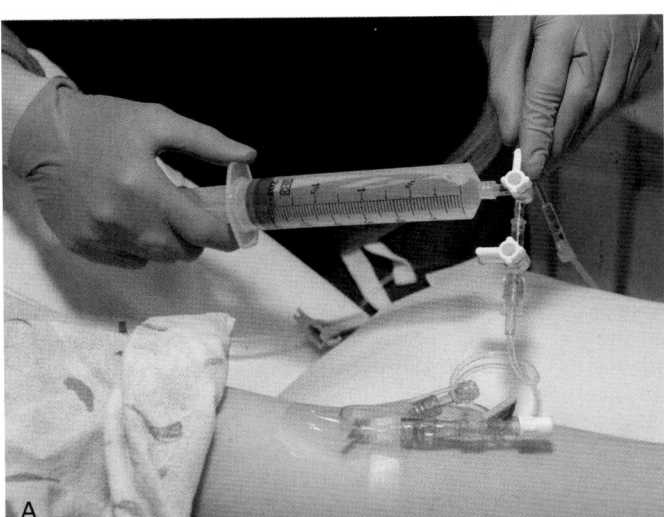
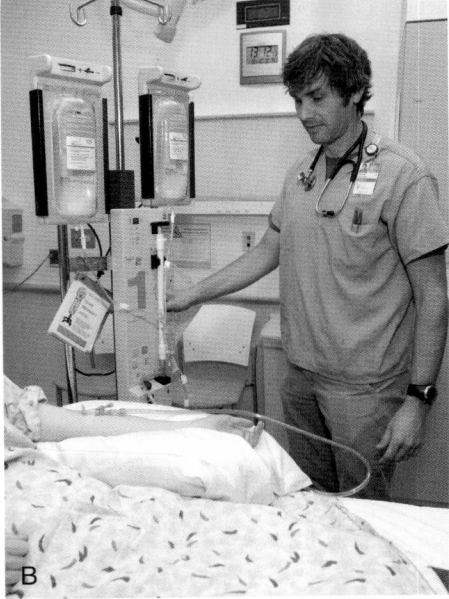

Fig. 158.2 (A) Using a 60-mL syringe with an inline three-way stopcock is an effective way to deliver rapid fluid boluses, particularly in patients less than 25 kg where a bolus is not easily dosed by a standard fluid bag. (B) Rapid infusers and pressure bags rapidly deliver fluid boluses when a full bag is an appropriate dose. (Courtesy Tia Brayman, Children's Hospital Colorado.)

Obtaining central venous access in an ill child is an uncommon procedure in most EDs, and it is a frequent source of delayed care in pediatric septic shock. Instead, we recommend rapid vascular access in critically ill children with large bore peripheral IV catheters or an intraosseous device. Vasoactive infusions can be administered through a peripheral IV catheter to correct shock until a central venous catheter can be placed safely.

Critical illness-related corticosteroid insufficiency is moderately prevalent in pediatric sepsis, and nearly half of septic children receive exogenous **corticosteroids**.[64] However, there is insufficient evidence to support or refute this practice. A small retrospective study found increased mortality with hydrocortisone administration to children with catecholamine resistant shock.[81] Nevertheless, based on larger studies in adults, we administer hydrocortisone (50 to 100 mg/m² or 1 to 2 mg/kg, maximum 100 mg/dose) for children in shock refractory to fluids and vasoactive agents. The 2020 pediatric sepsis guidelines state hydrocortisone may be considered under these circumstances.[73]

Although, like adults, children with sepsis may be prone to stress hyperglycemia, they are also prone to hypoglycemia due to their limited glycogen stores. Tight and conventional **glycemic control** has shown equivalence in critically ill children; a large trial is currently underway to determine optimal glucose control strategies. We recommend correction of hypoglycemia and cautious use of insulin with frequent glucose monitoring for blood glucose levels more than 180 mg/day (10.0 mmol/L).

Combining the aforementioned therapies into a **bundle** appears to improve outcomes. A large prospective, multicenter, observational study found that administration of a bundle of antibiotics and fluids coupled with acquisition of blood cultures within one hour reduced mortality (OR = 0.59; 95% CI, 0.38 to 0.93).[82] Notably, administration of each individual element within one hour was not associated with decreased mortality. The 2020 pediatric Surviving Sepsis guidelines recommend a bundled approach for children with signs of organ dysfunction.[73] EDs should establish protocols to ensure acquisition of a blood culture and administration of a fluid bolus and antibiotics within one hour. Despite a mandate at participating hospitals in the aforementioned study to complete the bundle within one hour, less than one in four children met this mandate. Therefore, EDs should have continuing quality improvement measures which facilitate and encourage use of a bundled protocol.

Monitoring Response to Therapy

There are limited options to assess response to therapy beyond the physical examination. Clearance of lactate may reflect reversal of tissue hypoxia. In a small prospective observation study, children whose lactate decreased to less than 2 mmol/L within 3 to 4 hours had less organ dysfunction (RR = 0.46; 95% CI, 0.29 to 0.73).[83] Passive leg raise may predict fluid responsiveness, but there are no large studies in pediatric sepsis. Transthoracic echocardiography may establish a role in refractory septic shock in the future; small studies suggest between 41% and 71% of children have myocardial dysfunction.[84,85] Currently there is insufficient evidence to support routine ED utilization of other modalities for treatment response, including mixed venous oxygen saturation monitoring, central venous pressure, biomarkers, or non-invasive cardiac output monitors.[86]

Brief Resolved Unexplained Events
Background

In 2016, the American Academy of Pediatrics published consensus guidelines creating a new term, BRUE, to describe infants less than 1 year of age presenting with transient alterations in their breathing, appearance, or behavior that cannot be explained based on their

TABLE 158.5 Brief Resolved Unexplained Event Compared to Apparent Life-Threatening Event

	BRUE	ALTE
Defining characteristics	Change in breathing, tone, color	
Other elements	Possible alteration in consciousness	Apnea; possible choking, gagging
Perception	Concerning to clinician	Concerning to lay observer
Etiology	Unexplained	Unexplained or GERD, seizure, infection, etc.
Age	<1 year	<1 year
Duration	<1 min	Any
History	Unrevealing	May identify etiology
Vital signs	Normal	May be abnormal
Physical examination	Normal	May identify etiology

ALTE, Apparent life-threatening event; *BRUE*, brief resolved unexplained event.

history or physical examination.[87] BRUE has supplanted apparent life-threatening event (ALTE), a term that was too broad in scope to be clinically useful. BRUE is more precise and allows for the establishment a low-risk group of infants that do not require further evaluation. The hallmark of a BRUE is that the cause for the event is unclear. As a result, children with potential explanations for their presentation are not classified as having BRUEs, e.g., a child with a transient episode of cyanosis in the setting of congestion is not a BRUE.

Clinical Features

With a BRUE, a child may have changes in breathing, tone, or responsiveness. Breathing may be absent, decreased, or irregular, potentially leading to central cyanosis or pallor. This does not include acrocyanosis, perioral cyanosis, rubor, or periodic breathing, which are commonly encountered in healthy infants. Infants may have increased or decreased tone, although this does not include hypertonia with crying or straining, which is normal.

There are multiple differences between BRUEs and ALTEs (Table 158.5), but the primary distinction is that the emergency clinician cannot determine any potential etiology for a BRUE. On presentation to the ED, the infant appears well without any examination abnormalities. Therefore, to determine if an event constitutes a BRUE, clinicians should focus on historical circumstances before, during, and after the event. Certain features may suggest a common or dangerous etiology and indicate the event does not represent a BRUE (Table 158.6).

If no etiology for the event is apparent, BRUEs can be classified further into high or low risk events. Low-risk infants are those born ≥32 weeks and greater than 60 days of age with no prior BRUEs, and CPR (by a health care provider) was not performed during the event. If these features are present, infants are potentially at higher risk of recurrent events or adverse outcomes. Several retrospective studies have confirmed the diagnostic accuracy of these criteria.[88,89]

Management

As the concept of BRUE is relatively new, there is not strong evidence to guide management. However, evidence extrapolated from children with ALTEs suggests that testing low-risk BRUEs is low yield, and we recommend limiting routine testing to an electrocardiogram, which

TABLE 158.6 Presenting Features of Common Conditions Leading to Transient Alterations in Breathing, Responsiveness, or Color in Infants

Condition	Potential Features
GERD	Choking, gagging, vomiting, after feed; Often turn red; Brief apnea
Respiratory infection (RSV, pertussis)	Congestion, cough; Tachypnea; Adventitial lung findings
Seizure	Convulsions; Altered consciousness; Eye deviation
NAT (brain hemorrhage)	Delayed presentation; Inconsistent history; Signs of trauma; Head circumference >95th percentile
Bacterial infection (UTI, bacteremia, meningitis)	Fever; Lethargy; Irritability

GERD, gastroesophageal reflux disease; NAT, nonaccidental trauma; RSV, respiratory syncytial virus; UTI, urinary tract infection.

displayed high sensitivity for arrhythmias and structural heart disease in children with ALTE. While cardiac abnormalities are rare causes of BRUEs, an electrocardiogram is safe, inexpensive, and easy to obtain. For children with signs of central apnea during their event, we consider pertussis testing, as infants may develop apnea before they manifest other respiratory symptoms.

Guidelines explicitly discourage routine acquisition of other tests, including blood, CSF, radiography, EEG, echocardiogram, or testing for gastroesophageal reflux disease (GERD). Moreover, typically viral respiratory testing, urinalysis, or neuroimaging are not necessary for low-risk infants. These guidelines appear to have reduced testing over time.[90,91] There is no definitive evidence about the benefit of ED observation or pulse oximetry measurement, but we observe low-risk infants for 2 to 4 hours in the ED with intermittent pulse oximetry assessments.

There is little evidence for the management of high-risk BRUEs. We agree with a recently proposed tiered approach.[92] To determine occult etiologies for a high-risk BRUEs, we recommend obtaining a respiratory viral panel, hematocrit, glucose, bicarbonate, and lactic acid, as well as a feeding evaluation and screen for non-accidental trauma, to be completed by a social worker. If the evaluation is unrevealing, we recommend the patient be admitted for further evaluation and continued monitoring. Where ED resources are limited or in high demand, some children may require admission to complete this evaluation. This approach is derived from consensus and has not been studied.

Disposition

Low-risk BRUEs are unlikely to benefit from hospitalization and therefore guidelines recommend discharge from the ED with outpatient follow-up within 24 hours. Parents may be reluctant to return home, but a recent meta-analysis may provide reassurance.[93,94] Pooling of data from 3,005 infants found no increased risk of death following a BRUE.[95] There is no evidence to support outpatient cardio-respiratory monitoring.

The references for this chapter can be found online at ExpertConsult. com.

Neonatal Resuscitation

Ryan D. Kearney

- Resuscitation should be anticipated for all deliveries; 10% of newborns will require some resuscitation, and 1% will require advanced life support interventions after birth.
- Predictable indications for resuscitation include hypoxia, hypothermia, hypoglycemia, hypovolemia, prematurity, maternal infection, and adverse effects of maternal medication.
- Drying, warming, positioning, and stimulating the infant are sufficient resuscitative measures for most deliveries.
- Adequate ventilation will reverse most bradycardia, while oxygenation with more than 21% fraction of inspired oxygen (FiO_2) is not indicated for most neonatal resuscitations.
- The Neonatal Resuscitation Program (NRP) resuscitation algorithm provides a proven guide for management and its implementation has shown to improve short- and long-term outcomes, including neurodevelopment.
- Routine tracheal suctioning of vigorous and nonvigorous infants born through meconium-stained amniotic fluid is no longer recommended.
- Weight-based epinephrine and volume expanders are rarely required.
- Significant hypovolemia is rare in neonates. Hemorrhage is one of the few predictable situations in which volume expansion improves newborn outcome.
- Preterm infants and those born to mothers with suspected infection, including chorioamnionitis, should receive empirical antibiotic therapy. An acceptable regimen includes dual therapy with ampicillin and gentamicin.
- Any neonate with persistent cyanosis or signs of respiratory distress (e.g., grunting, nasal flaring, and tachypnea) should be assisted by continuous positive airway pressure (CPAP) or positive pressure ventilation (PPV). Endotracheal intubation should be performed in several situations, such as when bag-mask ventilation is ineffective or prolonged, chest compressions are performed, an extremely low birth weight infant is born, and tracheal suctioning for meconium in infants results in failure to improve, despite effective PPV.
- Chest compressions are rarely required, because bradycardia generally responds to effective ventilation. However, compressions should be started for a heart rate (HR) less than 60 beats/min despite oxygen and adequate ventilation for 30 seconds.
- The umbilical vein is the preferred route of immediate vascular access, followed by peripheral veins, peripherally inserted central catheter lines, and the femoral vein. Intraosseous (IO) line placement can be problematic in neonates.
- No reliable and widely adopted set of parameters has been identified for newborns who should not receive resuscitative efforts. Unless there is clear family, parent, and health care provider agreement, resuscitation efforts should ensue.
- Infants receiving appropriate resuscitation efforts nonetheless showing no signs of life after 10 minutes may have further efforts withheld, particularly when this decision is in accord with parental preference.
- All newborns requiring intravenous (IV) line placement, medication administration, chest compressions, or endotracheal intubation should be transferred to an appropriate neonatal intensive care unit.

FOUNDATIONS

Approximately 10% of newborns require some assistance at birth, with 1% requiring extensive resuscitative measures.[1] Knowledge of neonatal physiology, appropriate equipment, and procedural skills is essential to successful resuscitation. Preparation for neonatal resuscitation requires an understanding of how it differs from pediatric and adult resuscitation:

1. Newborns have rapidly changing, dynamic cardiopulmonary physiology, with a unique range of normal vital signs.[2,3]
2. Neonatal resuscitation is almost entirely respiratory (not cardiac) management.[2]
3. Neonates require special and dedicated equipment.

TRANSITION FROM FETAL TO EXTRAUTERINE LIFE

The successful transition from fetal to extrauterine life requires three major cardiorespiratory changes: (1) removal of fluid from unexpanded alveoli to allow ventilation; (2) lung expansion and establishment of functional residual capacity (FRC); and (3) redistribution of cardiac output to provide lung perfusion. Failed development of adequate ventilation or perfusion leads to persistent shunting, hypoxia and, ultimately, a deleterious reversion to fetal physiology.[2]

In utero, fetal nutrient and gas exchange is dependent on the placenta, a temporary organ with remarkably low vascular resistance, as well as the maternal circulation. As a result of its low resistance, the placenta receives approximately 30% of total fetal cardiac output between 18 and 41 weeks of gestation. In contrast, fluid-filled fetal alveoli have increased vascular resistance, leading to poor perfusion of the developing lung. The pulmonary arterial bed is so vasoconstricted that the fetal lung receives only 40% of right ventricular output and approximately 10% of total cardiac output; most of the right ventricular output is shunted from the pulmonary artery through the ductus arteriosus to the descending aorta.[4,5] An additional right-to-left shunting occurs at the level of the foramen ovale, with relatively oxygen-rich blood shunted from the right to left atrium. Fig. 159.1 illustrates normal intracardiac fetal circulation. Reversal of these two shunts is essential to the successful transition into extrauterine life and is facilitated by the significant drop in pulmonary vascular resistance that occurs at birth. The first step in this process is alveolar fluid clearance.

Removal of this fluid is partially accomplished by vaginal delivery, which provides some compression of the fluid out of the alveoli into the bronchi, trachea, and pulmonary capillary bed. The remaining fluid is largely evacuated by the first few breaths, with the quality of the first few breaths crucial to establishing adequate ventilation. Alveolar expansion requires the generation of high intrathoracic pressures and the presence of surfactant to maintain alveolar patency. Because the lung is one of the last organs to reach structural and functional maturity,

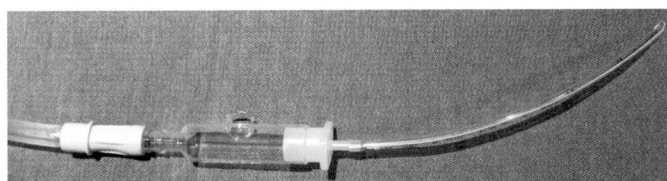

Fig. 159.1 Meconium Aspirator With Suction and 3.0 Uncuffed Endotracheal Tube (ETT) Attached. (Courtesy Seattle Children's Hospital, Seattle, WA.)

interruptions in this coordinated physiologic process, although rare, should be nonetheless anticipated in all deliveries, particularly those outside of the delivery room.[6]

After the first few breaths, pulmonary vascular resistance decreases as a result of alveolar oxygen exposure. Simultaneously, clamping of the umbilical cord removes the placenta from circulation, predictably increasing systemic vascular resistance. Shunting through the ductus arteriosus reverses as systemic vascular resistance increases; this usually ceases altogether by 15 hours of age as the ductus arteriosus also constricts. This reversal of flow redirects all right ventricular output to the lungs. However, hypoxia or acidosis can cause the pulmonary vascular bed to constrict again, and, when severe or prolonged, recurrent pulmonary vascular constriction can cause the ductus arteriosus to reopen. The reinstitution of fetal circulation, with its attendant shunting, leads to ongoing hypoxia and is termed *persistent fetal circulation*.[2] When indicated, resuscitation facilitates the first few breaths, prevents and reverses ongoing hypoxia and acidosis, and assists the newborn in the transition to extrauterine life.

SPECIFIC ISSUES

Indications for Resuscitation

At least one person, whose exclusive role is to ensure safe transition of the newborn, should be present for all deliveries, including those that occur outside the delivery room. Any infant born outside of a delivery room should be anticipated to need resuscitation.[1–3] Although minimal intervention may be required, a standardized approach should still be followed. Some specific conditions increase the likelihood that additional resuscitative efforts will be required.

Hypoxia

Even in the uncompromised newborn, it can take 10 minutes for blood oxygen saturation to reach normal extrauterine levels.[1] Pulse oximetry may assist in determining hypoxemia, but it may take several minutes for a reliable waveform to be achieved.[7,8] In utero or intrapartum asphyxia (pathologic lack of oxygen to the fetus before or during delivery) can precipitate a sequence of events that results in primary or secondary apnea. With initial hypoxia, rapid gasps are followed by cessation of respirations (primary apnea) and, if prolonged, decreased heart rate (HR). Ostensibly normal respiratory effort does not ensure adequate ventilation. However, bradycardia in the newborn (HR < 100 beats/min) almost always reflects inadequate ventilation and oxygenation. As such, bradycardia is a major indicator of hypoxia.[1,2] Simple stimulation is required at the onset of primary apnea to stimulate ventilation and reverse bradycardia. If asphyxia persists, the newborn takes several final deep, gasping breaths, followed by cessation of respirations (secondary apnea); this is accompanied by worsening bradycardia, refractory to simple stimulation, and eventually hypotension. For newborns with secondary apnea, more vigorous and prolonged resuscitation is needed to restore ventilation and adequate circulation.[2]

Hypothermia

Drying and warming the newborn are vital to initial resuscitation because the newborn's inability to maintain normothermia (>36.5°C [97.7°F]) has potentially dire consequences. Newborns cannot generate heat by shivering, cannot retain heat due to low fat stores, and have excess heat loss due to their large surface-to-volume ratio. Exacerbating these challenges in the immediate postpartum period, newborns have an acutely elevated metabolic rate, are covered with amniotic fluid, and are suddenly exposed to a relatively cool environment. Body temperature rapidly decreases, with hypothermia accelerating metabolic acidosis, oxygen consumption, hypoglycemia, and apnea.[1–3] Prematurity and very low birth weight status exacerbate these consequences and require extra efforts to mitigate.[1]

Hypoglycemia

Poor glycogen stores, coupled with immature hepatic enzymes, place the normal newborn at increased risk for hypoglycemia. Hypoglycemia is particularly common in premature and small-for-gestational-age newborns, as well as those born to diabetic mothers. Hypoglycemia may also be a response to other factors, including respiratory illness, hypothermia, polycythemia, asphyxia, and sepsis. Hypoglycemia can be asymptomatic or may cause an array of symptoms, including apnea, color changes, respiratory distress, lethargy, jitteriness, seizures, acidosis, and poor myocardial contractility.[9,10] A low blood glucose level, particularly when prolonged, recurrent, or associated with hyperinsulinism, has been associated with adverse neurologic outcomes[9]; correction of hypoglycemia, if detected expeditiously, improves outcomes.[11] Neonatal hypoglycemia is generally defined as a blood glucose level less than 40 mg/dL, although this number serves as more of a guideline than a strict cutoff. All newborns exhibiting signs of hypoglycemia, with glucose levels less than 40 mg/dL, should receive intravenous (IV) glucose. *Of note, bedside glucometers tend to underestimate plasma glucose levels by approximately 10 mg/dL.*[10]

Hypovolemia

Clinically significant hypovolemia is rare and usually secondary to blood loss. Risk factors include known maternal hemorrhage during delivery, prematurity, newborns with overt shock, and initiation of cardiopulmonary resuscitation (CPR).[1–3,12] Hemorrhage can lead to respiratory depression and overt shock in the newborn, whether secondary to abruptio placentae, placenta previa, umbilical cord accident, or trauma. In the newborn, hemorrhage is one of the few situations in which fluid resuscitation and volume expansion improves outcomes. At the time of birth, mean arterial pressure should be equivalent to known or estimated gestational age. Examination findings consistent with hypovolemia or hemodynamically significant hemorrhage include pallor, despite oxygenation, weak pulses with a rapid HR, and poor response to resuscitation.[1–3]

Prematurity

Premature infants, especially those born before 34 weeks of gestational age, are uniquely at risk due to their pulmonary immaturity and susceptibility to hypothermia. Those requiring delivery room CPR have increased risk of mortality, intraventricular hemorrhage, periventricular leukomalacia, early sepsis, and retinopathy of prematurity.[13] For these reasons, in utero transfer of high-risk pregnant women to tertiary centers possessing expertise and experience with premature infant resuscitation has been associated with improved neonatal outcomes.[14] Intubation should be performed for the premature newborn in respiratory distress, which is clinically suggested by retractions, desaturation, or tachypnea.[15] In certain cases, surfactant may be delivered via an endotracheal tube (ETT) shortly after birth.

MECONIUM-STAINED AMNIOTIC FLUID

Meconium-stained amniotic fluid (MSAF) indicates potentially significant newborn stress prior to delivery. Aspiration of meconium and its consequences can be avoided, or at least significantly limited, by rapid intervention. Previous recommendations stipulated suctioning meconium from the newborn's airway after delivery of the head but before delivery of the shoulders (intrapartum suctioning). However, there appears to be no benefit from intrapartum suctioning.[16,17] Therefore current recommendations no longer advise routine intrapartum suctioning of newborns with MSAF. To prevent aspiration of meconium, previous recommendations also stipulated tracheal suctioning of all nonvigorous newborns with MSAF immediately on delivery and before any other resuscitative efforts (including drying and stimulation). However, routine endotracheal intubation in nonvigorous and vigorous term, meconium-stained newborns has shown no benefit, including the incidence of meconium aspiration syndrome (MAS), pneumothorax, oxygen need, stridor, seizure, or hypoxic ischemic encephalopathy.[18] Standard measures to support adequate ventilation and oxygenation should be initiated for all infants born through MSAF, with a small subset eventually needing endotracheal intubation, as warranted.[1]

The most recent recommendations from the American Heart Association for the practice of tracheal suctioning after delivery for meconium aspiration is that it should be performed only if indicated for signs of airway obstruction secondary to meconium that do not improve despite standard resuscitative measures, including warming and drying and initiation of effective positive pressure ventilation (PPV). When performing tracheal suctioning, a meconium aspirator (see Fig. 159.1) should be attached to the appropriate-sized ETT and connected to wall suction at 100 mm Hg or less. On intubation by direct laryngoscopy, the ETT is then withdrawn while suction is applied. Serial reintubation with suctioning should be repeated to remove obstructing meconium or until the infant becomes vigorous, which is usually accomplished after two rounds. If bradycardia or apnea persists beyond two passes, ongoing resuscitation should include bag-mask ventilation (BMV) and consideration of endotracheal intubation to secure the airway. In tertiary centers with skilled providers, eventual lung lavage with surfactant for babies born through MSAF is likely to reduce duration of hospital stay, mechanical ventilation, and need for extracorporeal membrane oxygenation.[19]

Maternal Factors

Infection

Maternal infection (chorioamnionitis) is a particularly common trigger for premature delivery; premature infants are themselves more susceptible to infection. Therefore IV antibiotics should be administered after obtaining blood cultures, and a complete blood count should be carried out in all infants born before 37 weeks of gestation.

Medications

Medications provided to the mother during labor or illicit drugs taken before delivery, usually opioids, can promote newborn respiratory depression. Maternal opioid administration or antenatal drug abuse should be considered in any newborn with isolated respiratory depression that persists, despite a seemingly successful initial resuscitation. As in adults, opioid-induced respiratory depression could be reversed with naloxone.[1,20] However, naloxone may precipitate acute withdrawal and seizures in the newborn of an opioid-dependent mother; thus naloxone is not recommended in the initial resuscitation of the newborn.[3,21] Suspected opiate toxicity in the newborn should be treated with support of oxygenation and ventilation rather than pharmacologic reversal. This should include use of a bag-mask device and, if necessary, intubation.

Withholding and Discontinuing Resuscitation

No reliable and widely adopted set of parameters has been identified for newborns who should not receive resuscitative efforts.[22] A recent systematic review attempted to identify international consensus surrounding this medically and ethically complex scenario—worldwide, resuscitation is not typically recommended for neonates with a confirmed gestational age less than 23 weeks.[23] In high-income countries, there is increasing resuscitative efforts and postnatal intervention for babies with confirmed trisomies 18 and 13, highlighting the importance of timely counseling to ascertain parental values and expectations.[24] Parental request has been shown to be the most important factor determining resuscitative efforts for newborns at 22 to 25 weeks of gestation; most neonatologists consider a gestational age more than 25 weeks of gestation as the cutoff for obligatory resuscitation, even with parental refusal.[23] In the setting of uncertain gestational age and unclear or conflicting parental wishes, the recommendation is to initiate resuscitation. Similarly, if prognosis is uncertain at the time of delivery, resuscitation should be attempted until additional data can be obtained and parental wishes have been considered. Outside the delivery room, every attempt should be made to stabilize the neonate until further resuscitation would clearly not improve the likelihood of survival with acceptable morbidity. Neonates with no signs of life (asystole, apnea) after 10 minutes of resuscitation have high mortality or severe lifelong developmental delay, and resuscitation can be terminated.[25] This is a rare and inherently challenging decision to make and should account for availability of local resources and personnel skill, transportation needs and options, and parental preference. However, enhanced resuscitation techniques and postresuscitation therapeutic hypothermia have recently shown promise, even for neonates with a 10-minute APGAR score of zero.[26,27] In one notable cohort of term neonates receiving CPR and subsequent hypothermia, more than 50% were found to have normal developmental trajectory by 18 months of age,[26] highlighting the importance of dialogue with the parent(s) and acknowledgment of their feelings regarding the risks of morbidity. Parents should actively participate in the decision to continue or withdraw resuscitative efforts in cases in which there is prognostic uncertainty. For infants with a low 10-minute APGAR score but showing some signs of life, especially when aligned with parental preference, resuscitation efforts should continue until futility is determined. Although not absolute, we recommend considering terminating resuscitative efforts for infants with no signs of life after 10 minutes of resuscitation.

SPECIAL ANATOMIC ANOMALIES

Diaphragmatic Hernia

In addition to pulmonary hypoplasia, neonates with diaphragmatic hernias have exquisitely reactive pulmonary vascular beds, predisposing them to potentially fatal pulmonary vasospasm in the immediate and late postnatal period.[28] Examination findings concerning for congenital diaphragmatic hernia include barrel chest, ipsilateral absence of breath sounds, tracheal or point of maximum cardiac impulse displacement, and scaphoid abdomen. BMV will distend the stomach, which is usually intrathoracic, further worsening respiratory distress. The neonate should be immediately intubated if a prenatal diagnosis of diaphragmatic hernia is known or if a diaphragmatic hernia is diagnosed on the chest radiograph (Fig. 159.2).

Myelomeningocele and Omphalocele

Infants with myelomeningocele should never be placed supine but instead be placed prone or on the side to avoid pressure on the defect

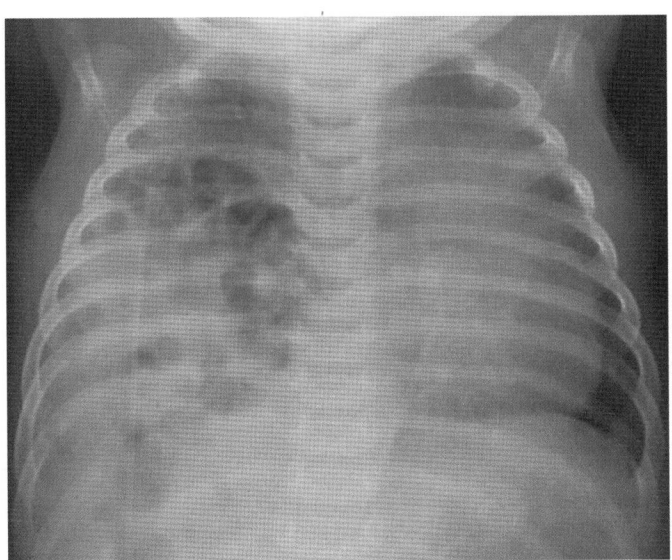

Fig. 159.2 Chest Radiograph Reveals Right-Sided Congenital Diaphragmatic Hernia. (Courtesy Seattle Children's Hospital, Seattle, WA.)

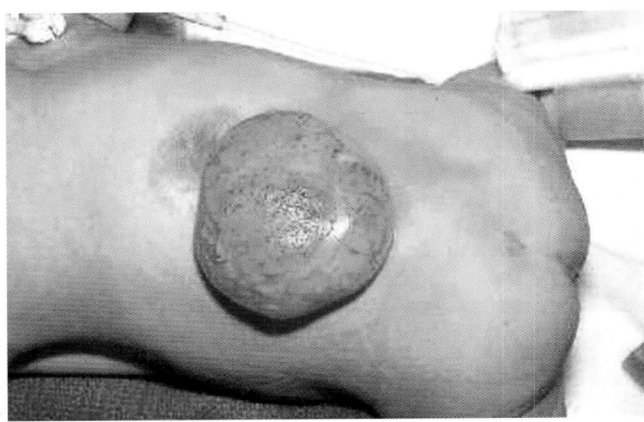

Fig. 159.3 Preoperative myelomeningocele, highlighting the obvious anatomic challenges and sensitivities required in resuscitation of neonates with this condition. (From Elbabaa SK, Luciano MG. Myelomeningocele and associated anomalies. In: Benzel E, editor. *Spine Surgery: Techniques, Complication Avoidance and Management*, 3rd edition. Philadelphia: Saunders; 2012. Figure 117-1.)

(Fig. 159.3). Resuscitation should proceed from this modified position. For unclear reasons, myelomeningocele seems to be associated with an elevated risk for latex allergy, usually necessitating efforts to avoid latex sensitization in these neonates.[29] The spinal defect should be gently wrapped with sterile gauze pads soaked in warm sterile saline and enclosed with plastic wrap.[30] Infants with gastroschisis or omphalocele should be resuscitated as needed, and these defects should also be covered with an occlusive plastic wrapping to decrease water and heat loss.[31] These newborns often require parenteral maintenance fluid infusion, orogastric tube for gastric decompression, and antimicrobial prophylaxis with IV antibiotics.[31]

Choanal Atresia

Because newborns are obligate nose breathers, bilateral choanal atresia causes upper airway obstruction and often severe respiratory distress. Choanal atresia can be rapidly diagnosed by the inability to pass a catheter through either naris into the posterior oropharynx. An oral airway device can bypass the obstruction. Special attention should be paid to a thorough physical examination of these infants because they often have multiple congenital anomaly syndrome.

Pierre Robin Sequence

The hallmark of this abnormality is profound micrognathia, resulting in glossoptosis (retraction or downward displacement of the tongue) and cleft palate. Therefore Pierre Robin sequence confers a high risk for significant upper airway obstruction. A nasal or oral airway should be able to bypass the obstruction; if not, intubation may be necessary. Given the technical challenges of performing endotracheal intubation on a patient with Pierre Robin sequence, fiberoptic intubation is often needed, although prone positioning and a laryngeal mask airway (LMA) or other supraglottic airway device can be attempted to support ventilation.[32] Consultation with anesthesiology or otolaryngology may be required.

Congenital Cardiac Disease

Echocardiographic evidence of congenital heart disease (CHD) is as high as 5% for term newborns.[33] However, critical CHD, defined as requiring surgery, catheter-based intervention, or death in the first 28 days of life, is present in only 1 to 2 per 1000 term births.[33] Stereotypic

examination findings seen in critical CHD include a blood pressure gradient between the upper and lower extremities, weak femoral pulses, central cyanosis, pathologic murmur, and hepatomegaly. These signs of cardiogenic shock in a newborn may be fairly indistinguishable from those of severe sepsis and respiratory failure. Resuscitation of a newborn with known or suspected critical CHD should therefore include standard ventilatory management, as well as empiric antimicrobial therapy.[34] Cardiomegaly on a chest radiograph is more likely consistent with cardiogenic shock. Some common laboratory findings include polycythemia and unexplained acidosis. Many newborns with critical CHD have a ductal-dependent lesion and are likely to experience profound physiologic decompensation—defined by severe metabolic acidosis, seizure, cardiac arrest, or renal or hepatic injury—on closure of the ductus arteriosus.[35] Prostaglandin E_1 (PGE_1) should be used in lesions with ductal-dependent systemic or pulmonary blood flow (Box 159.1).[36] In case of an uncertain diagnosis or in preparation for transport to a specialized facility, prostaglandin should be started via continuous IV infusion. A second peripheral IV is recommended to treat the possible adverse effects of prostaglandin: hypotension, tachycardia, and apnea. Continuous alprostadil should begin soon after birth,[36] with gradual dose titration to a maximum of 0.1 μg/kg/min. For a more in-depth discussion on CHD, see Chapter 165.

Newborn Resuscitation Algorithm

Preparation

To maximize the effectiveness of resuscitation, all emergency departments should have an age- and weight-appropriate prestocked drug pack, standardized equipment (Box 159.2), and staff trained on newborn resuscitation.[1,3] There are several pediatric length-based resuscitation tape (e.g., Broselow, PAWPER) that can be used to determine equipment size and drug dosages for newborn resuscitation of infants weighing 3 kg or more.[37,38] A dedicated neonatal resuscitation cart, organized according to the Neonatal Resuscitation Program (NRP) algorithm, increases the speed of equipment retrieval and is preferred by providers to other organizing schemes.[39] When available, additional maternal information (Box 159.3) can help to anticipate resuscitation needs so that appropriate staff, equipment, and disposition plans can be expeditiously managed.

Universal precautions, including gown, gloves, and eye protection, should be followed during neonatal resuscitations. An external heat source should be turned on early and the table warmed prior to the

BOX 159.1 Ductal-Dependent Congenital Cardiac Lesions

Ductal-Dependent Pulmonary Blood Flow
Critical pulmonary stenosis, atresia
Severe tricuspid stenosis, atresia
Severe tetralogy of Fallot

Ductal-Dependent Systemic Blood Flow
Hypoplastic left heart syndrome
Critical aortic stenosis
Interrupted aortic arch

BOX 159.2 Equipment Checklist for Neonatal Resuscitation

1. Gown, gloves, and eye protection (universal precautions)
2. Timing device
3. Blankets (to warm and dry infant)
4. Plastic wrap (for omphalocele, gastroschisis, possibly premature infant)
5. Radiant warmer
6. Bulb syringe
7. Suction and suction catheters (sizes 5, 8, and 10 Fr)
8. Self-inflating (450 and 750 mL) and flow-inflating (250 and 450 mL) bags
9. Masks (premature, newborn, and infant sizes)
10. Laryngoscope with straight blades (nos. 00, 0, and 1)
11. Endotracheal tubes with stylets (2.5, 3.0, 3.5, and 4 mm), uncuffed
12. Scissors and tape to stabilize endotracheal tube
13. Pediatric CO$_2$ detector
14. Meconium aspirator
15. Umbilical catheters (3.5 and 5 Fr)
16. Hemostats, sterile drapes and gloves, povidone-iodine solution, scalpel, umbilical tape, suture, and three-way stopcock for umbilical vessel catheterization

BOX 159.3 Maternal History Questions

1. What is the estimated gestational age?
2. Is this a multiple gestation?
3. Is meconium present?
4. Is there a history of vaginal bleeding?
5. Were medications given or drugs taken?
6. Was there documented maternal fever?
7. Did mother have routine prenatal care? If so, were any abnormalities seen on prenatal ultrasonography?

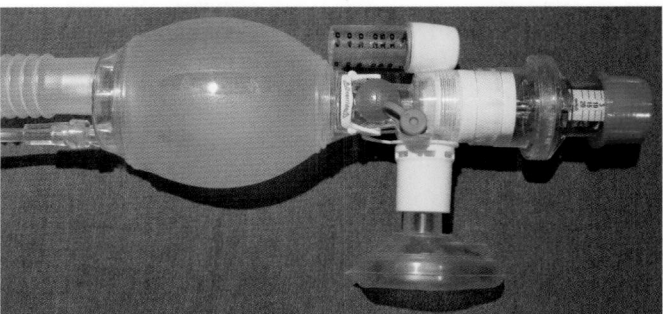

Fig. 159.4 Appropriate Self-Inflating Resuscitator With Appropriate Neonatal-Sized Mask Attached. This device has additional functionality with manometer and single-use positive end-expiratory pressure (PEEP) valve attachments. (Courtesy Seattle Children's Hospital, Seattle, WA.)

TABLE 159.1 Endotracheal Tube Size by Birth Weight and Gestational Age

Birth Weight (kg)	Gestational Age (Weeks)	ETT Tube Size (mm, Uncuffed)	Depth of Insertion (cm)
<1	<28	2.5	7
1–2	28–34	3	8
2–3	34–38	3.5	9
3+	38+	3.5–4	10

ETT, Endotracheal tube.
Adapted from American Academy of Pediatrics; American Heart Association. *Neonatal Resuscitation Textbook.* 6th ed. Elk Grove Village, IL: American Academy of Pediatrics; 2016.

As part of their shared NRP curriculum, the American Heart Association and American Academy of Pediatrics, with the International Liaison Committee on Resuscitation, have developed a newborn resuscitation algorithm (Fig. 159.5). This stepwise approach is detailed later.[1-3] However, if a term neonate is crying and appears to have good tone, she or he can be warmed, dried, and returned to the mother for ongoing care and evaluation, without any additional resuscitation efforts.[1]

Dry, Warm, Stimulate, Position, Suction, and Assess Need for Further Intervention

Hypothermia increases metabolic demand and oxygen consumption, which can render seemingly effective resuscitation efforts futile. To prevent hypothermia and its more subtle sequelae, all newborns should be dried immediately on delivery and placed under a radiant heat source. In the case of crying term infants with normal tone, this may be accomplished by simple drying and skin to skin contact with the mother.[1] Wet blankets should be replaced with dry blankets and preferably warm linens, but the baby should be left uncovered to facilitate radiant warming and team access. All resuscitation techniques are designed to be performed with these temperature-controlling efforts in place.[1] The supine neonate should be further positioned to maximize air entry and avoid obstruction of airflow. Due to a relatively large occiput and anterior glottic opening, airway patency is best achieved with the neck in slight extension. A slightly extended position that aligns the posterior pharynx, larynx, and trachea is best accomplished by placing a rolled diaper or small towel under the infant's shoulders. Placement under the neck is not useful. However, a towel that is too large and under the shoulders can also lead to airway occlusion due to hyperextension of the neck.

start of resuscitation. Hypothermia is an independent risk factor for neonatal mortality worldwide.[40-42] Similarly, hyperthermia is a risk factor for neonatal encephalopathy and correlates with respiratory depression, cerebral palsy, and mortality. Correct equipment size is essential; in particular, respiratory supplies are most likely to be used and key to most resuscitative efforts. Appropriately sized self-inflating devices (Fig. 159.4) decrease complications from overventilation, prevent injury, and limit the inability to ventilate due to improper mask fit. When available, and in the hands of experienced providers, flow-inflating devices have the added ability to deliver continuous positive airway pressure (CPAP), control ventilation pressure with greater precision, and ensure a proper fit. Table 159.1 lists the recommended ETT sizes by birth weight and gestational age.

Neonatal Resuscitation Algorithm

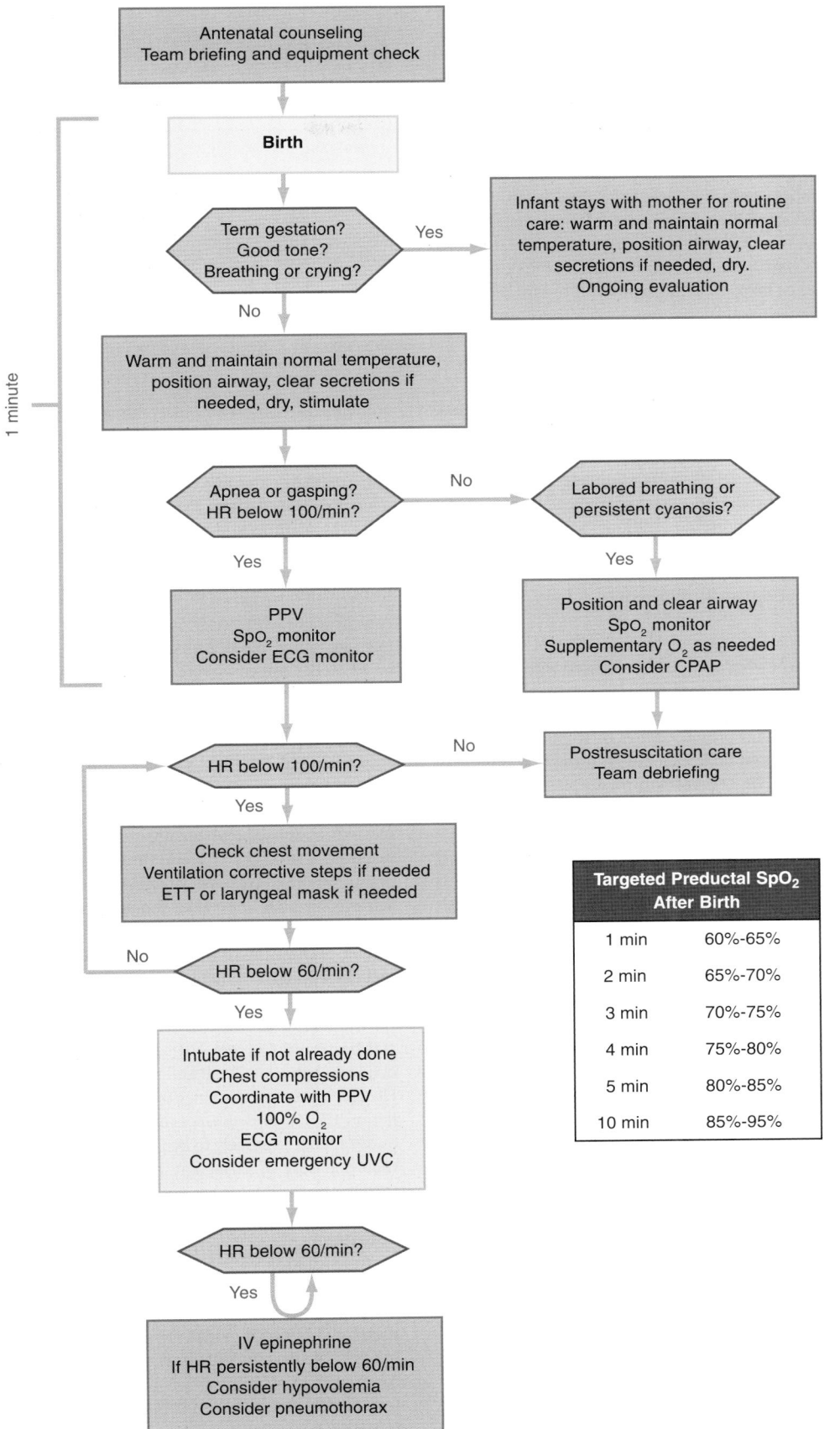

Fig. 159.5 Algorithm for Neonatal Resuscitation. *ECG,* Electrocardiogram; *ETT,* endotracheal tube; *HR,* heart rate; *PPV,* positive pressure ventilation; *UVC,* umbilical vein cannula. (Adapted from Wyckoff MH, Aziz K, Escobedo MB, et al: Part 13: neonatal resuscitation: 2015 American Heart Association Guidelines Update for Cardiopulmonary Resuscitation and Emergency Cardiovascular Care. *Circulation.* 2015;132:S543–S560.)

Only if meconium is present and the newborn has poor tone, poor respiratory effort, or bradycardia (HR < 100 beats/min) after 1 minute of appropriate PPV should the trachea be suctioned with an ETT and meconium aspirator attachment. Poor respiratory effort and obvious obstruction from secretions should otherwise be treated with bulb or mechanical suction (~100 mm Hg wall suction). Upper airway suctioning, including that performed with a bulb syringe, should be reserved only for newborns with these signs because suctioning has been associated with decreased lung compliance, bradycardia, and lowered cerebral blood flow velocity.[1] When suction is indicated, the NRP protocol should be followed, with the mouth suctioned first, followed by the nose. This sequence helps to avoid aspiration of oral secretions if the neonate inspires after nasal suctioning. Overly vigorous or deep suctioning should be avoided because it can cause significant vagal stimulation, and subsequent bradycardia or apnea.[2,43] Because NRP recommendations stipulate suctioning with less than 100 mm Hg, emergency clinicians should be judicious with syringe use because even standard delivery bulb syringes produce a negative pressure that can easily exceed this threshold.[43]

For most term neonates, these measures stimulate breathing sufficiently and may be all that is required to resuscitate a newborn. If adequate respirations are still not present, additional stimulation should be given. This is best done by flicking the soles of the feet and rubbing the back; more forceful efforts could prove harmful. If stimulation and warming efforts prove inadequate, PPV is required, followed by intubation, if necessary.

Time is an important component of NRP guidelines. Within the first 60 seconds of life, the newborn should be assessed with simultaneous warming, drying, and stimulation; if necessary, upper airway clearance should be performed (see Fig. 159.5). If the HR is less than 100 beats/min or if the newborn has primary apnea or respiratory distress, PPV and pulse oximetry should be initiated within the first minute of life. If bradycardia worsens (HR < 60 beats/min), despite adequate ventilation, chest compressions should be initiated. HR calculation can be manual—by palpation of the pulse at the base of the umbilicus or auscultation of cardiac sounds—with pulse oximetry, or most accurately with a standard electrocardiography (ECG) lead.[44] Three-lead ECG is more acute in identifying true bradycardia, as pulse oximetry and palpation of the umbilical pulse have been found to underestimate a newborn's HR.[1] Persistent bradycardia is usually secondary to inadequate ventilation. Thus intubation is recommended in the event that chest compressions are indicated.

Routinely counted at 1, 5, and 10 minutes of life, the APGAR score (Table 159.2) is a composite that reflects HR, respiratory effort, muscle tone, reflex irritability, and color. The score is primarily for assessing the need for (1 minute) and efficacy of (5 minute) ongoing resuscitative measures. In the setting of modern algorithm-based resuscitation, low 5- and 10-minute APGAR scores are associated with increased mortality because they identify infants who are failing medical management.[44] Muscle tone and reflex irritability do not significantly aid in the assessment of the newborn during resuscitation.[44,45]

Instead, HR and respiratory effort are the important indicators and should be continuously monitored. Skin color is a poor indicator of oxyhemoglobin saturation during the first several minutes of life while the transition from fetal to infant circulation ensues.[46–48] In this brief period, pulse oximetry may be a useful tool to assess the oxygenation status of the newborn.[8] However, level of oxygen saturation should take into account normal postductal saturations after birth. An oxygen saturation of 60% would be the targeted normal preductal saturation for 1 minute of life and may not reach 90% or more until 10 minutes of life (see Fig. 159.5). Pulse oximeter should be placed on the baby's right wrist or hand to measure preductal saturations after birth. NRP

TABLE 159.2 APGAR Score[a]

Sign	POINTS		
	0	1	2
Heart rate (beats/min)	Absent	Slow (<100)	≥100
Respirations	Absent	Slow, irregular	Good, crying
Muscle tone	Limp	Some flexion	Active, good flexion
Reflex irritability	No response	Grimace	Cough, sneeze
Color	Blue, pale	Pink body, blue hands and feet	Pink

[a]Calculate at 1, 5, and 10 minutes of life.

guidelines recommend pulse oximeter use in only a few select situations—anticipated resuscitation, prolonged PPV use, persistent central cyanosis, and use of supplemental oxygen.[1] We recommend preparing pulse oximetry and ECG monitoring as a standard approach for all ED neonatal resuscitations. Precipitous deliveries are infrequent, yet high-risk presentations and newborns are likely to require accurate HR and pulse oximeter measurements to guide resuscitation.

Ventilation, Oxygen, Intubation

Any neonate with persistent cyanosis or signs of respiratory distress (e.g., grunting, nasal flaring, tachypnea) should be assisted by CPAP or PPV. For apnea, severe respiratory distress, or HR less than 100 beats/min, BMV (with a manometer, if available) should be initiated. The first breaths often require higher pressures (30 to 40 mm Hg) to remove lung fluid, with the adequacy of ventilation assessed by chest rise. An initial sustained breath of 2 to 5 seconds may further increase FRC and promote clearance of lung fluid, but several clinical trials and meta-analyses have yet to prove the efficacy and safety of this technique.[49–52] Subsequent breaths generally require 20 mm Hg of peak inspiratory pressure.[1,2] To minimize barotrauma and the incidence of pneumothorax, excessive pressures (defined as more than needed to achieve adequate chest rise) should be avoided. An appropriately sized mask with a tight seal (covering the mouth and nose, but not the eyes), proper positioning of the newborn, and use of pressure to attain correct chest wall movement are essential for effective ventilation. Unless otherwise dictated by blood gas levels, recommended ventilation rates are 40 to 60 breaths/min, aimed at achieving a HR greater than 100 beat/min. Current NRP guidelines recommend PPV but do not delineate between CPAP and positive end-expiratory pressure (PEEP). However, preterm neonates (<33 weeks' gestation) receiving single-inflation CPAP (pressure-controlled inflation at 20 cm H_2O for 10 seconds) appear less likely to be intubated at 72 hours of age, receive more than one dose of surfactant, or develop bronchopulmonary dysplasia (BPD). When BMV is required for more than 2 minutes, an orogastric tube should be placed to prevent respiratory compromise from gastric distention.[2]

Resuscitation with 100% oxygen is no longer recommended.[3,53–56] There is reduced mortality in infants resuscitated on room air, with no obvious evidence of harm.[54] Resuscitation-induced hyperoxia results in increased oxidative stress, including direct cardiac and renal injury.[57] Neurologic outcomes appear improved by resuscitation with room air versus 100% oxygen, likely due to a reduction in cerebral free radical generation.[1,3,56,58] Current NRP guidelines recommend initiating resuscitation with room air and then blending to increasing oxygen concentrations, as needed. An updated guideline suggests it is reasonable to initiate resuscitation in preterm newborns (less than 35

BOX 159.4 Intubation Corrective Action and Deterioration Mnemonics

MR SOPA

M: Mask adjustment
R: Reposition airway
S: Suction mouth and nose
O: Open mouth
P: Pressure increase
A: Airway alternative

DOPE

D: Displacement of ETT
O: Obstruction of ETT
P: Pneumothorax
E: Equipment failure

ETT, Endotracheal tube.

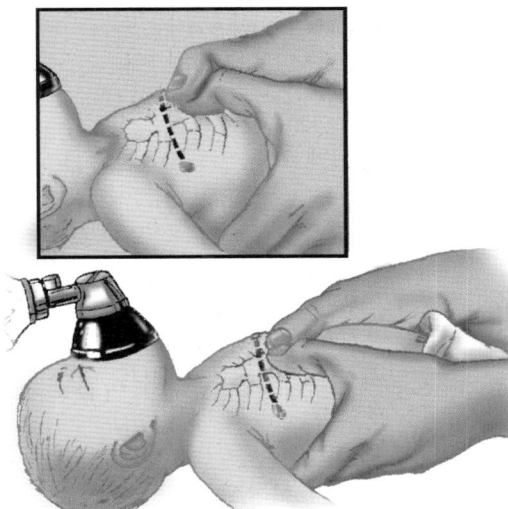

Fig. 159.6 The preferred way to provide chest compressions on a newly born neonate is called two thumbs-encircling hands. This method is best when one rescuer can provide chest compressions and another can ventilate the patient. The two thumbs are placed over the sternum and below an imaginary line between the nipples. If the newborn is very small, the two thumbs can overlap. (From From Gregory GA: In: *The Anesthesiology, The Mother and Newborn.* Edited by Shinder SM, Moya F. Baltimore, Williams and Wilkins, 1974.)

weeks' gestation) with 21% to 30% fraction of inspired oxygen (FiO_2) and titrate to goal saturations.[3] Unless needed to achieve target oxygen saturations, 100% oxygen should be used only for newborns with bradycardia of less than 60 beats/min after 90 seconds (see Fig. 159.5). Attempts to restore adequate ventilation are often more beneficial than increasing the oxygen concentration.

Endotracheal intubation is indicated at several points during neonatal resuscitation—tracheal suctioning for meconium in infants with failure to improve, despite effective PPV; if BMV is ineffective or prolonged; when chest compressions are performed; and for extremely low birth weight infants or infants with anatomic anomalies (e.g., diaphragmatic hernia). Traditional direct laryngoscopy and video laryngoscopy are both reasonable options, with video-assisted techniques consistently having improved views but slightly longer total intubation times.[59–61] Confirmation of proper ETT placement should include detection of expired carbon dioxide using capnography. Although ultrasonography can show appropriate ETT positioning in the term infant, the gold standard remains plain radiography.[62–66]

If acute deterioration occurs shortly after intubation, equipment should be immediately checked. Consider the DOPE and MR SOPA mnemonics when trying to determine the cause of the deterioration (Box 159.4). In the absence of an obvious explanation, it is safest to extubate the newborn and promptly ventilate with a BMV device by an experienced provider. Needle aspiration of the chest may be considered for treatment of a possible pneumothorax, particularly if unequal breath sounds are appreciated upon extubation, ventilatory pressures are inexplicably high, or a neonate's condition fails to improve with effective ventilation.

If ETT intubation is indicated but is technically challenging, the LMA has been shown to be effective for ventilating full-term newborns.[67–69] However, there are limited data on LMA use in preterm infants (<2000 g or <34 weeks' gestation) in the setting of MAS or during CPR.

Chest Compressions

Bradycardia (HR < 100 beats/min) is a reliable indicator of clinically significant hypoxia. Fortunately, most neonates with bradycardia respond promptly to effective ventilation. If a neonate has an HR less than 60 beats/min, despite oxygen and adequate ventilation (good air movement and chest rise) for at least 30 seconds, chest compression should be started.[1,2,70] Compressions should be performed at a rate of 90/min, coordinated with 30 breaths/min for a total of 120 events/min. The preferred neonatal resuscitation compression-to-ventilation ratio is 3:1. If the provider is certain that the cardiac arrest has a primary cardiac cause, a compression-to-ventilation ratio of 15:2 may be considered.[1,3] The preferred method for performing chest compressions, the two thumb-encircling hands technique, is as follows: the fingers of both hands encircle the chest and support the back, with the thumbs of both hands placed side by side or one over the other on the sternum, just below the nipple line (Fig. 159.6).[71,72]

The depth of compression is one-third the anteroposterior diameter of the chest.[2] Spontaneous respirations and HR should be assessed every 30 seconds, attempting to minimize interruptions, when possible, with coordinated chest compressions and ventilation continuing until the HR is at least 60 beats/min.[1,2] A yellow color change on a colorimetric CO_2 monitor or increase in end-tidal CO_2 values during PPV administration often precedes a significant rise in HR and should be used, when available.

Vascular Access

The umbilical vein is the preferred route of immediate vascular access because it can be easily identified and cannulated. Umbilical vein access can have serious complications (e.g., infection, portal vein thrombosis), so the umbilical vein cannula (UVC) should be removed by the accepting neonatologist after the infant has been stabilized and additional venous access has been obtained.[73] Other vascular access routes include peripheral veins, peripherally inserted central catheters, and the femoral vein.[74] Intraosseous (IO) access can be problematic in neonates (especially premature infants) because of bone fragility and the small size of the IO space. However, in simulated resuscitation, placement of an IO line has been shown to be almost 1 minute faster than a UVC, even for skilled providers. Preferred IO access sites in newborns include the distal femur (midline; ≈1 cm above the superior border of the patella, with the leg in extension) and the proximal tibia (≈2 cm below the tuberosity and 1 cm medially on the tibial plateau). If vascular access cannot be achieved, certain drugs including epinephrine, can be given through the ETT, although this is not the optimal route.

TABLE 159.3   Resuscitation Medications

Medication	Concentration	Dose	Route	Comments
Epinephrine	0.1 mg/mL	0.01–0.03 mg/kg (0.1–0.3 mL/kg)	IV (preferred) or ETT	
Dopamine	Varies	Continuous infusion at 5 μg/kg/min; increase to 20 μg/kg/min as needed.	IV	
Glucose	$D_{10}W$	2–4 mL/kg	IV	Avoid higher concentrations
Volume expanders	O-negative packed RBCs	10 mL/kg	IV	Give over 5–10 min for acute bleeding; repeat as needed
	Normal saline	10 mL/kg	IV	Give over 5–10 min; repeat as needed
	Lactated Ringers	10 mL/kg	IV	Give over 5–10 min; repeat as needed
Ampicillin	Varies	100 mg/kg	IV, IM	
Gentamicin	Varies	4 mg/kg	IV, IM	If neonate less than 35 weeks gestational age: 5 mg/kg
Cefotaxime	Varies	50 mg/kg	IV, IM	

$D_{10}W$, 10% dextrose in water; *ETT*, endotracheal tube; *IM*, intramuscular; *IO*, intraosseous; *IV*, intravenous.

Medications

Few neonates require pharmacotherapy during resuscitation. Medications (Table 159.3) are primarily indicated for bradycardia or asystole unresponsive to effective ventilation and chest compressions, as well as hemorrhage (maternal, fetal, or placental) that necessitates fluid resuscitation.[1–3]

Epinephrine. Epinephrine is indicated for asystole and persistent bradycardia (<60 beats/min) despite effective ventilation with 100% oxygen and ongoing coordinated chest compressions. Although it may be given by ETT, IV is the preferred epinephrine administration route. The recommended IV dose is 0.01 to 0.03 mg/kg, or 0.1 to 0.3 mL/kg, of a 0.1 mg/mL solution. Unlike epinephrine use in adult patients, weight-based dosing with no known minimum is required for neonates. Repeat doses may be given every 3 to 5 minutes.[1,2] If administered via an ETT, higher doses (0.05 to 0.1 mg/kg) with a 0.1 mg/mL solution are indicated, but the safety and efficacy of this practice have not been rigorously evaluated.[1,2,74–76] Unlike many adult resuscitations, sodium bicarbonate is not routinely used,[77,78] although it may be beneficial in the neonatal intensive care unit (NICU) setting when ventilation is known to be adequate.[1,79]

Volume Expanders. When indicated, volume expansion is accomplished with packed red blood cells (Rh-negative type O blood), normal saline, or Lactated Ringers solution given in IV boluses of 10 mL/kg over 5 to 10 minutes. During resuscitation of premature infants, rapid administration of volume expanders should be avoided because this practice has been associated with increased incidence of intraventricular hemorrhage.[2] Higher-volume (e.g., 20 mL/kg) fluid boluses are recommended for full-term infants. Boluses may be repeated several times, as indicated by the ongoing response to resuscitative efforts.

Antibiotics. Antibiotics are not indicated in the initial resuscitation phase but may be required once the neonate has been stabilized. When suspected, sepsis should be treated with broad-spectrum antimicrobial therapy directed against the most likely pathogens. The most common bacterial pathogens implicated in early-onset neonatal sepsis are a heterogeneous group that includes group B *Streptococcus* (GBS), *Escherichia coli*, *Klebsiella* spp., *Enterobacter* spp., and *Listeria*. In the United States, where GBS and *E. coli* represent the most common newborn pathogens, a recommended empirical antibiotic regimen is ampicillin (100 mg/kg IV) plus an aminoglycoside (usually gentamicin, 4 mg/kg).[80] Reasonable alternative regimens include ampicillin with a third-generation cephalosporin, but there is evidence that several members of the latter group predispose a neonate to invasive candidiasis. Because ceftriaxone can increase the risk of kernicterus, cefotaxime (50 mg/kg IV) is preferred.

Glucose. Concomitant hypoglycemia should be considered and promptly treated in a neonate requiring ongoing resuscitation. Hypoglycemia is most easily diagnosed by rapid bedside glucose testing or serum glucose level measurement. Neonates with a glucose level less than 40 mg/dL and with symptoms of hypoglycemia—irritability, tremors, jitteriness, apnea, tachypnea, seizures, cyanosis, lethargy, poor feeding—require treatment with IV glucose. Standard therapy is 2 to 4 mL/kg of 10% dextrose in water $(D_{10}W)$/kg as well as starting a continuous infusion of $D_{10}W$ at 80 to 100 mL/kg/day.[10] Higher concentrations of glucose (e.g., 25% dextrose in water, $D_{25}W$) are hyperosmolar and should be avoided. If the newborn can safely tolerate feeds, oral glucose solution, maternal breast milk, or formula should be given by mouth (PO) on demand. Repeat glucose measurement should be obtained 10 to 20 minutes after glucose administration. Asymptomatic neonates with hypoglycemia should be encouraged to feed more often and are treated with IV glucose only if glucose levels fall precipitously (<25 mg/dL at birth to 4 hours of age or <35 mg/dL at 4 to 24 hours of age).[10]

Dopamine. Dopamine is indicated only when signs of shock (e.g., poor peripheral perfusion, weak pulses) are still present, despite adequate volume replacement. Given as a continuous infusion beginning at 5 μg/kg/min, dopamine may be increased to 20 μg/kg/min as necessary, before additional inotrope support is indicated.

Therapeutic Hypothermia

When moderate to severe hypoxic-ischemic encephalopathy is suspected, selective cerebral hypothermia in asphyxiated infants may protect against brain injury.[1,81–89] Therapeutic hypothermia of 33.5°C to 34.5°C (92.3°F to 94.1°F) in this population can lower mortality and improve the likelihood of normal neurologic outcome at 18 months. Current NRP guidelines recommend therapeutic hypothermia for patients with suspected early neonatal asphyxia. Symptoms of possible evolving brain injury include abnormal levels of consciousness, seizures, hypotonia, and hyporeflexia. Established protocols generally recommend the initiation of cooling within 6 hours of birth, for a total of 72 hours, followed by gradual rewarming over at least 4 hours. Neonates meeting eligibility criteria should be transferred to facilities capable of providing this specialized care. Emergency clinicians and families should be aware that the risks associated with therapeutic hypothermia include thrombocytopenia and hypotension.

DISPOSITION

Early consultation with a neonatologist can assist in the resuscitation and postresuscitation phases of care. Once a neonate is stabilized, the monitoring of oxygenation, ventilation, perfusion, temperature, and glucose level continues. Neonates who require extensive resuscitation (i.e., obtaining venous access, medication requirement, or endotracheal intubation) should be transported to a NICU by personnel skilled in neonatal resuscitation. If feasible and safe, parents should be allowed to see, touch, and hold the newborn before transport.

OUTCOMES

Safety

Advanced life support skills are critical for successful neonatal resuscitation yet are far from routine for most emergency clinicians. For example, in a cohort of almost 5000 births in Norway, only 19 infants required intubation and 10 were given chest compressions.[90] An important step toward improving outcomes is team adherence to NRP guidelines. Highlighting the importance of safety, an essential component of the new NRP curriculum is the inclusion of simulation.[91] Simulation in neonatal resuscitation allows for a multidisciplinary team to practice behavioral and teamwork skills, not only individual technical skills, in a safe environment.[92] Implementation of an integrated Team Strategies and Tools to Enhance Performance and Patient Safety (TeamSTEPPS) and NRP curriculum improves communication and helps to prevent incorrect medication dosing and inadequate chest compression depth. Furthermore, routine (and unannounced) simulation-based neonatal resuscitation training has been shown to improve provider self-confidence, knowledge, and both technical and nontechnical skills.[93,94]

Effectiveness

In the hands of trained emergency clinicians, neonates requiring advanced resuscitative efforts receive improved PPV, decreased time to vascular access, and shortened time to first IV medication. Deliberate training has been shown to improve ability to perform the key first steps of resuscitation—stimulation, positioning and neck-extension, PPV effectiveness, and HR assessment.[95] Provider level improvements are seen worldwide with the implementation of guideline-based care.[96] Analyses of the NRP program, which has now trained more than 5 million providers in the United States alone, suggests fewer high-risk infants experience a drop in APGAR score from 1 to 5 minutes, with many actually showing an improvement since implementation. However, resuscitation is not without potential pitfalls.

Complications

Relatively common complications post neonatal resuscitation include hypoglycemia, transient tachypnea of the newborn, MAS, pneumothorax, electrolyte disturbances, significant hyperbilirubinemia, and sepsis. These conditions are associated with increased NICU admission rates, as well as morbidity and mortality.[97,98] Additional perinatal risk factors relevant to resuscitation that are associated with length of NICU stay include: placental abruption, assisted delivery, small for dates, gestational age less than 37 weeks, low 5-minute APGAR score, and need for intubation at birth.

The need for chest compressions and CPR is a known prognostic marker for increased rates of morbidity and mortality in neonates.[99] Undergoing CPR at delivery increases the likelihood of pneumothorax, sepsis, severe intraventricular hemorrhage, and death.[100] Unfortunately, these complications have also been associated with poor long-term neurodevelopment outcomes.[100] However, the implementation of neonatal resuscitation protocols appears to improve neurodevelopment outcomes, but data from randomized trials are lacking.[101]

The references for this chapter can be found online at ExpertConsult. com.

Pediatric Trauma

Sonia Singh and James F. Holmes

FOUNDATIONS

Injury is the leading cause of death among children 1 to 18 years of age in the United States, accounting for over 10,000 deaths and 9 million annual emergency department (ED) visits.[1] Motor vehicle collisions (MVCs) account for more than half of all pediatric trauma deaths, whereas nonfatal injuries are primarily due to unintentional falls.[1] Mechanisms of injury vary by patient age, and certain mechanisms result in specific injury patterns (e.g., sports and concussions). Blunt mechanisms account for over 95% of childhood injuries. The trauma history, as well as the initial response, determine injury risk and response required. Criteria for trauma center transport (primary triage) and trauma team activation (secondary triage) are primarily based on expert consensus and an area ripe for further research. Although the examination of the injured patient is standardized, diagnostic testing should be tailored to avoid unnecessary testing while assessing for important injuries.

Anatomy and Physiology

Children have distinct anatomy and unique physiology that impact their evaluation and management (Box 160.1). Force is more widely distributed throughout the child's body, making multi-system injuries more likely in children. The younger a patient is, the higher their surface area to weight ratio, resulting in a greater potential for heat loss. As injured patients are at increased risk of hypothermia, this is especially true in children.

Normal ranges for pediatric vital signs vary greatly and should be readily available in the ED (Chapter 155). A child's physiologic response to injury is different from the adult's, depending on the age and maturation of the child and severity of the injury. Children have a high capacity to maintain blood pressure despite significant hemorrhage; hypotension is a late finding with blood loss exceeding 30% of total blood volume. The younger the child is, the less their ability to increase cardiac contractility. Thus, a young child's cardiac output is primarily determined by heart rate and systematic vascular resistance. Compensated shock should be considered and promptly addressed when a child is tachycardic, especially if capillary refill is delayed. Changes in heart rate, blood pressure and extremity perfusion commonly precede cardiorespiratory failure and should prompt resuscitation.

CLINICAL FEATURES

Initial Assessment and Primary Survey

Most children evaluated in the ED are minimally injured and require limited diagnostic evaluation after the standard history and physical evaluation. In those with *major* trauma, cardiac and pulse oximetry monitoring, supplemental oxygen, frequent vital sign measurements, intravenous (IV) access, and laboratory testing are often needed. Immediately after prehospital notification, preparation should include assigning team member functions, preparing necessary equipment, and donning protective clothing. Color-coded length-based tape measures are often used to provide initial estimates of patient weight, equipment size and medication dosages, but important equipment sizes are in Box 160.2.

The initial trauma assessment is designed to rapidly identify and treat life- or limb-threatening injuries. Treatment of these injuries

BOX 160.1 Important Anatomic Differences in Adults and Children: Implications for Pediatric Trauma Management

- The child's head-to-body ratio is greater, the brain is less myelinated, and cranial bones are thinner, resulting in more serious head injuries.
- The child's internal organs are more susceptible to injury based on more anterior placement of the liver and spleen, and less protective musculature and subcutaneous tissue mass.
- The child's kidney is less well protected and more mobile, making it susceptible to deceleration injury.
- The elasticity of the child's chest wall allows for pulmonary injury without rib fracture.
- Children have a more tenuous spinal cord blood supply and a greater elasticity of the vertebral column, predisposing them to unique spinal cord injuries including SCIWORA.

SCIWORA, Spinal cord injury without obvious radiographic abnormality.

BOX 160.2 Specific Equipment Size Estimates for Pediatric Trauma

Endotracheal Tube (ETT) Size Estimates (Sizing in Millimeters Internal Diameter) and Depth
- Endotracheal (cuffed) tube size (mm) = (Age in years/4) + 3.5
- An ETT 0.5 mm larger and 0.5 mm smaller than the calculated size should also be ready at the bedside
- ETT tube depth = tube size × 3

Chest Tube Size (Diameter) = 4 × the ETT Size

Orogastric, Nasogastric, or Foley Size (Diameter) = 2 × ETT Size

precedes the continuation of the evaluation. The initial assessment and resuscitation occur simultaneously over the initial 5 to 10 minutes of care. Similar to adults, the elements of the primary survey for children are remembered as *A, B, C, D, E,* and *F.*[2] Patient deterioration warrants repeat of the primary survey to identify the cause and institute treatment.

A—Airway and Cervical Spine Stabilization

Children have important anatomic considerations that impact the management of the pediatric airway (Chapter 156). The patient is initially evaluated for possible airway obstruction or inability to maintain their airway. Gurgling or stridor may indicate upper airway obstruction. Maxillofacial trauma, blood, swelling, or vomitus may also obstruct the airway, and efforts are made toward clearing the oropharynx of debris. Initial attempts to open the airway include a jaw-thrust maneuver. If an open airway cannot be established and maintained by noninvasive means, endotracheal intubation (ETI) should be performed. Unless the neck has been cleared of injury, cervical spine immobilization should be maintained with in-line immobilization when airway maneuvers are performed.

Indications for ETI in a pediatric trauma patient include (1) inability to ventilate with bag-mask ventilation (BMV) or the need for prolonged airway control, (2) Glasgow Coma Scale (GCS) score ≤8, (3) respiratory failure from hypoxemia or hypoventilation, and (4) worsening decompensated shock resistant to initial fluid resuscitation. Rapid sequence intubation is the preferred method for ETI in severely injured children, and includes both sedative medications (e.g., ketamine or etomidate) and paralytic medications (e.g., succinylcholine or rocuronium), see Chapter 156. Although unlikely to do harm, premedication with fentanyl or lidocaine to blunt the rise of intracranial

pressure (ICP) is not evidence-based, and we do not recommend its use for this purpose.

B—Breathing and Ventilation

Breath sounds and adequacy of chest rise should be assessed. Adequate ventilation is dependent upon airway patency and sufficient air exchange. Pulse oximetry measures the adequacy of oxygenation, but not ventilation. Continuous end-tidal carbon dioxide capnography better informs ventilatory status but should be interpreted in conjunction with the respiratory wave form. For example, a child with a low capnography reading could either be taking slow shallow breaths (e.g., hypoventilation), or may be breathing deeply and rapidly (e.g., hyperventilation). Many factors may compromise ventilatory function in an injured child, including depressed sensorium, airway obstruction, painful respirations, diaphragmatic fatigue, and direct pulmonary injury.

In a young child, chest rise occurs in the lower chest and upper abdomen, and both should move concordantly. Discordant motion or *paradoxical breathing* is a sign of impending respiratory failure. Respiratory rates that are very fast or very slow may indicate impending respiratory failure; tachypnea may also be due to shock or inadequate pain control. If assisted ventilation is necessary, BMV should be initiated with only the volume necessary to cause the chest to rise. In addition to a potential increased risk of vomiting and aspiration, excessive bagging volumes (i.e., hyperventilation) can lead to gastric distension (Fig. 160.1). As the stomach distends, the diaphragm can push into the thoracic cavity, causing increased intrathoracic pressures, decreased venous return, and hypotension. Gastric decompression may be performed with either an orogastric tube or nasogastric tube (if no evidence of facial trauma).

C—Circulation and Hemorrhage Control

Shock occurs when the body is unable to maintain adequate tissue perfusion. Normal systolic blood pressure does not exclude shock. The pediatric vasculature maintains normal blood pressure by constricting peripheral arteries and progressively increasing systemic vascular resistance. Signs of poor perfusion (cool distal extremities, decreased peripheral pulse quality, and delayed capillary refill) are signs of pediatric shock, even when blood pressure is normal (Box 160.3). External hemorrhage should be sought and controlled with direct pressure. IV access should be established and blood collected for laboratory testing (see following).

Vascular access is best obtained by placing two large-bore IV lines, ideally in the upper extremities (lower extremity sites may be used if needed). If obtaining vascular access is unsuccessful or delayed in the critically injured patient, intraosseous (IO) access is a safe, quick, and reliable procedure to access the vascular space and is recommended prior to attempting a central line. The preferred site for IO placement is the proximal medial tibia, just below (and directed slightly away from) the growth plate; other potential locations include the proximal humerus, the flat area of the anterior distal femur, or the distal tibia. Once IO access is obtained, it should be stabilized and secured. More than one IO needle may need to be placed (in separate bones); IV access may be easier after initial fluid resuscitation and vascular volume expansion. IO placement in a fractured extremity is contraindicated. Medications and blood products can be administered through an IO line similar to an IV. Central line placement in young children is difficult, with frequent complications, and should be avoided if possible. If absolutely necessary, ultrasound-guided femoral line placement is our preferred initial option. Much less commonly used vascular access techniques include a venous cut-down, or a central line into the intrajugular, supraclavicular, or subclavian vein. Venous cutdown is a

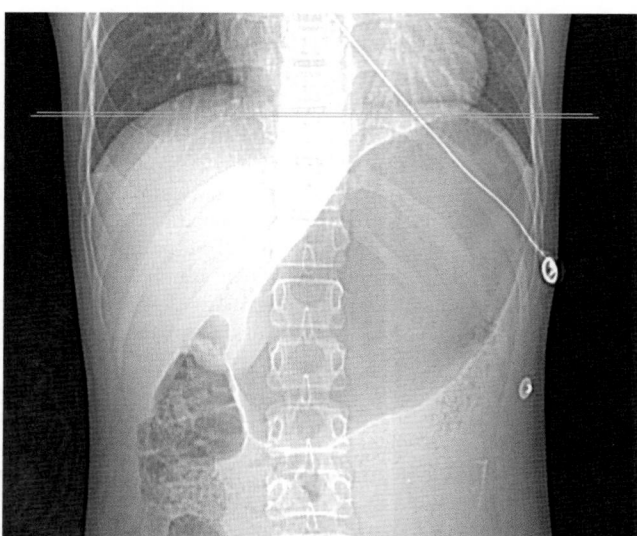

Fig. 160.1 CT (Scout) Demonstrating Gastric Distention in a Child Having Swallowed Large Amounts of Air from Crying. Severe Gastric Distention Can Harm Diaphragmatic Excursion and Impact Ventilation.

BOX 160.3   Circulation Assessment and Treatment in Critical Pediatric Trauma Patients

Assessment
- Tachycardia, delayed capillary refill, decreased peripheral pulses, tachypnea or bradypnea, and altered sensorium may indicate volume loss prior to hypotension.
- Vital signs, monitored every 5 min during the initial assessment.
- Continuous oximeter and cardiac monitor.

Treatment and Interventions for Hypovolemic Shock from Trauma
- Place two large-bore IV lines (above and below diaphragm if indicated).
- Intraosseous line placement if peripheral venous access is difficult.
- Bolus with 20 mL/kg of warm normal saline/lactated Ringers and repeat if necessary.
- Consider intubation and ventilation to decrease work of breathing.
- Transfuse 10 mL/kg pRBC for hemorrhagic shock secondary refractory to crystalloid.

IV, Intravenous; *pRBC,* packed red blood cells.

---

skill not often performed and is rarely needed to obtain vascular access in the pediatric trauma patient. If performed, the greater saphenous vein at the ankle is the preferred site. In the rare occasion that a neonate presents after trauma, an umbilical vein cannulation can be attempted in infants up to 10 days old if there is enough of an umbilical stump to perform the procedure.

Fluid resuscitation in pediatric trauma patients begins with a 20 mL/kg bolus of warm isotonic crystalloid solution over 10 minutes. A second bolus of 20 mL/kg of warm isotonic crystalloid is given for those who do not initially improve or stabilize. If the patient continues to require fluid resuscitation after two boluses, warmed, packed red blood cells (pRBCs) at 10 mL/kg should be transfused, while identifying and treating any sources of hemorrhage. In cases of massive transfusion (blood products >40 mL/kg in an adolescent or >50 mL/kg in a child/infant), it is important to add plasma and platelets to correct coagulopathy. Adult patients undergoing massive transfusion are

BOX 160.4   Disability: Neurologic Assessment and Treatment

Assessment
- Level of consciousness: Use AVPU scale and age-appropriate GCS
- Pupil size and reactivity
- Movement in all extremities and tone
- Posturing and reflexes

Treatment and Interventions
- Stabilize spinal column with spinal immobilization techniques.
- Rapid Sequence intubation for GCS scores ≤8
- Cranial CT scan all with GCS scores less than 15 and neurosurgical consultation as needed.
- With signs of herniation, elevate head of the bed and 3% hypertonic saline 2–5 mL/kg IV (or mannitol 0.5–1.0 g/kg IV).
- Maintain CPP of at least 40 mm Hg in children.

AVPU, Alert, verbal, painful, unresponsive; *CPP,* cerebral perfusion pressure; *CT,* computed tomography; *ETI,* endotracheal intubation; *GCS,* Glasgow Coma Scale; *IV,* intravenous; *Pco$_2$,* partial pressure of carbon dioxide, *RSI,* rapid sequence induction.

---

resuscitated with plasma, platelets, and pRBCs in a 1:1:1 ratio.[3] Less data exists for this strategy in the pediatric trauma population as data is conflicting,[4,5] although many centers now resuscitate children with a 1:1 plasma: pRBC ratio. In adult patients with significant traumatic hemorrhage, tranexamic acid is now routinely used to stabilize clot and limit blood loss. Although frequently used in non-traumatic pediatric surgery, use of tranexamic acid in injured children is rare.[6] The dosage in injured children (15 mg/kg over 20 minutes, then 2 mg/kg/h for 8 hours or 30 mg/kg over 20 minutes, then 4 mg/kg/h for 8 hours) is currently under study.[7]

D—Disability Assessment

A rapid neurologic and mental status evaluation is performed to assess neurologic status. The assessment of disability in pediatric trauma patients is described in Box 160.4. The alert, verbal, painful, unresponsive (AVPU) system and the GCS (Table 160.1) are utilized to assess neurologic status. The modified pediatrics GCS (used in pre-verbal children) performs similarly to the standard GCS in older children (see Table 160.1). Children's higher metabolic demands result in higher oxygen consumption and glucose utilization; a rapid bedside glucose level should be checked in any child with altered mental status after trauma.

E—Exposure and Environment

Trauma patients should have each body area fully exposed for evaluation; preverbal children are particularly high risk for missed injuries. However, children are often embarrassed or shy about physical exposure. In the stable patient, body areas can be examined in sections, keeping other parts covered from view. Compared to adults, children are also more susceptible to insensible heat and fluid loss due to their greater surface to mass ratios and should be kept normothermic, as hypothermia increases morbidity and mortality. Hypothermia contributes to metabolic acidemia and has direct adverse effects on cardiac inotropy, chronotropy, catecholamine responsiveness, platelet function, and both renal and hepatic drug clearance.

Interventions to maintain normothermia include increasing ambient temperature, administering warmed humidified oxygen, and warming all infused fluids, especially all blood products. Head wraps and convective warmers or radiant heat sources are adjuncts in

TABLE 160.1 Glasgow Coma Scale Score and Modified Pediatric Glasgow Coma Scale (For Those <2 Years)

BEST EYE OPENING RESPONSE

Score	>2 Years Old	<2 Years Old
4	Spontaneous	Spontaneous
3	To verbal command	To voice
2	To pain	To pain
1	None	None

BEST MOTOR RESPONSE

Score	>2 Years Old	<2 Years Old
6	Follows commands	Spontaneous movement
5	Localizes pain	Withdraws to touch
4	Withdraws to pain	Withdraws to pain
3	Abnormal flexion to pain (decorticate)	Abnormal flexion to pain (decorticate)
2	Abnormal extension to pain (decerebrate)	Abnormal extension to pain (decerebrate)
1	None	None

BEST VERBAL RESPONSE

Score	>2 Years Old	<2 Years Old
5	Oriented and converses	Coos/babbles
4	Confused conversation	Irritable/cries
3	Inappropriate words	Cries to pain
2	Incomprehensible sounds	Moans
1	None	None

aTotal score key for traumatic brain injury: severe, ≤8; moderate, 9 to 12; mild, 13 to 15.

newborns and infants, as well as older children with mild hypothermia (temperature <36°C). The exposure phase of the survey is often the appropriate time to concurrently begin initial imaging and further diagnostic testing (see following).

F—Family

We recommend the option of family members present during the initial resuscitations, a practice often preferred by families in both traumatic and non-traumatic pediatric resuscitations. A social worker or other qualified staff member dedicated to the family should be available to help explain treatments, answer questions, and provide emotional support.

Secondary Survey

A systematic secondary survey should follow the primary survey and necessary interventions, and should consist of an organized, complete head to toe assessment to detect additional injuries. Significant historical findings are collected at this time and can be remembered by the mnemonic AMPLE (Box 160.5). Key points of the ongoing assessment of the patient, after the secondary assessment, are summarized in Box 160.6.[2]

BOX 160.5 Ample History

A—Allergies
M—Medications
P—Past medical history
L—Last meal
E—Events and Environment

BOX 160.6 Tasks to Be Completed After the Secondary Survey

- Continuous monitoring of vital signs
- Provision of analgesia, and continuous reassessment of pain
- Antibiotics and tetanus as appropriate
- Ensure urine output of 1 mL/kg/h
- Begin transport process if the patient will obviously need transport

If patient instability prohibits completion of the secondary survey, this should be communicated to the next caregivers. Tertiary surveys are now completed on all trauma patients within 24 hours of admission.

Physical Examination

During the secondary survey, a head-to-toe examination should be carefully performed. Specifics of the head examination include inspection and palpation of the skull (fontanelle) and facial bones, assessing pupillary size and reactivity, and evaluation of extraocular movements. In possible nonaccidental trauma, funduscopic examination may reveal retinal hemorrhages. A fluorescein examination may reveal occult eye injury in the crying child.

Cervical spine immobilization should be maintained until the patient's neck is cleared of injury. Patients in spinal immobilization should be removed from the backboard with spinal motion restriction maintained. When the patient is log-rolled for backboard removal, the thoracic and lumbar spinous processes are individually palpated, evaluating for tenderness or step-offs. To protect them from further injury, obtunded patients and those with signs or symptoms of thoracic or lumbar spine injuries should be carefully moved and positioned until imaging or clinical assessment provides a more definitive assessment.

Chest assessment involves visual inspection for wounds and flail segments, palpation for tenderness or crepitus, and auscultation for breath sounds. The abdominal examination consists of inspection for evidence of abdominal wall trauma and palpation for the presence of tenderness. A "seat belt sign," consists of erythema, abrasions, or ecchymosis extending across the chest or abdomen from the seat belt (see below). Abdominal tenderness is present in approximately 75% of alert children with an intra-abdominal injury; however, the reliability of the abdominal examination decreases drastically in patients with GCS scores less than 14. Digital rectal examination should only be performed to evaluate rectal tone in suspected spinal cord injury, or if the integrity of the rectum is in question. Testing the injured child's stool for occult blood is not useful and we do not recommend this. All pelvic bones should be assessed for stability and tenderness. Although rare in children, urethral injuries may result in perineal, scrotal, penile, or lower abdominal hematomas, or blood at the urethral meatus. If there is a concern for urethral injury, a retrograde urethrogram should be completed prior to insertion of a urinary catheter to avoid further injury.

Extremity examination evaluates for deformities, skin disruptions, neurologic deficits, and abnormal perfusion. Fractures may be stabilized with splinting before definitive management. Careful and recurrent vascular and neurologic examinations should be performed and documented, especially after interventions such as splinting or reduction.

Trauma patients should be reexamined throughout their time in the ED to ensure their condition is stable, their pain is controlled, and no injuries are missed. When possible, ambulation can expose additional injuries not identified with previous examinations. Up to 70% of injuries with delayed diagnosis in pediatric trauma are orthopedic.[8]

Pain Assessment

Pain assessment and control is an essential part of any trauma patient's management. Analgesic medications, immobilization of injured extremities, and non-pharmacologic techniques should all be considered. Please refer to Chapter 157 for further discussion of pain control in children.

DIAGNOSTIC TESTING

Laboratory Testing

Laboratory testing is used to guide resuscitation, monitor blood loss, and screen for particular injuries, but should be tailored to avoid unnecessary testing. Patients at risk for hemorrhage should have a type and screen in addition to hemoglobin measurements. In acute hemorrhage, hemoglobin requires time to equilibrate and does not initially correlate with severity of blood loss. Serial hemoglobin measurements are not useful to screen for occult injuries; however, serial measurements may identify ongoing blood loss in patients with undifferentiated hypotension. In children with solid organ injuries, serial hemoglobin measurements are routinely performed, but the exact timing and utility is unclear.[9,10] Liver transaminases are useful to screen for hepatic injury, as they immediately elevate following liver injury. Children with GCS scores ≤13, hypotension, open or multiple bony fractures, or major tissue wounds are at risk for coagulopathy and should be screened with coagulation studies (INR and aPTT). Urinalysis is used to assess for blood (see below). Older pediatric trauma patients should be assessed for substance abuse and depression as contributing factors to the traumatic event. Post-pubertal females or those Tanner stage greater than 3 should be tested for pregnancy. Other than glucose testing in patients with altered mental status, serum electrolytes are routinely measured, but of limited initial use.

Radiologic Imaging

In the severely injured patient, we recommend performing an anteroposterior chest radiograph and a focused assessment with sonography for trauma (FAST), particularly if hypotensive. Plain films should be performed following the primary survey (routinely after the patient is rolled to their side, backboard removal and radiograph plates placed under the patient). An initial chest radiograph screens for immediate life-threatening thoracic injuries, but misses more subtle thoracic injuries. The FAST can be performed after the primary survey (or in conjunction if multiple providers), and evaluates for the presence of intraperitoneal and pericardial fluid. In hemodynamically unstable children, the FAST has good test characteristics for detecting intraabdominal hemorrhage and can guide further management. The extended FAST (eFAST) examination incorporates the addition of lung views to evaluate for pneumothorax or hemothorax, but has yet to be proven useful in children. A plain pelvis radiograph may identify major pelvic disruptions, but should only be performed in patients who are hypotensive or have unstable pelvic bone examinations. In these patients, the pelvic radiograph may guide the use of a pelvic binder to limit further hemorrhage.

Further imaging should be obtained based on findings from the history and physical examination. Computed tomography (CT) has substantially changed the trauma patient evaluation, as it provides rapid injury identification and details to guide treatment. However, CT carries the risk of radiation-induced malignancy, which is greater in children than adults due to their higher organ sensitivity and longer life expectancy. Data suggests the risk of radiation-induced malignancy is 1 per 5000 to 10,000 cranial CT scans and 1 per 300 to 600 abdominal CT scans. Girls are more sensitive to CT radiation than boys. CT use has rapidly increased in injured children and is highly variable, and CT scans are more commonly obtained in children treated at adult or mixed trauma centers than pediatric trauma centers.[11] In an effort to improve and provide evidence-based care, investigators have developed clinical decision instruments that align CT use in injured children with need (see following).

DISPOSITION

The primary role of the emergency physician is to evaluate and stabilize the severely injured patient before admission or transfer to a facility able to provide the necessary care. Moderately to severely injured pediatric patients of all ages have improved outcomes in pediatric trauma centers.[12,13] For patients requiring transport to a pediatric trauma center, the emergency clinician should not delay transfer for extensive radiologic testing. There should be direct communication between the emergency physician and the accepting doctor, and all radiologic imaging, notes and laboratory results should accompany the patient. Technology now allows images to be transported via the cloud for immediate review by a trauma specialist, which has the potential to decrease unnecessary trauma transfers. Parents should be informed of the reason for the transfer and the exact location to which the child is being taken.

SPECIFIC INJURIES

Head Injury

Traumatic brain injury is the leading cause of death and disability in children older than 1 year of age in the United States.[14] Infants and toddlers are more prone to falls from standing height; school-age children are involved in sports injuries and MVCs; and children of all ages are subject to the sequelae of assault or abuse.

Important anatomic variations lead to differences in pediatric and adult head trauma. The cranial vault of a child is larger and heavier in proportion to the total body mass, predisposing young children to high degrees of torque that are generated by forces along the cervical spine axis. Sutures within the pediatric skull are both protective and detrimental to the outcome of head injury; although the cranium may be more pliable relative to traumatic insult, forces transmitted internally can result in parenchymal injury in the absence of skull fractures. The pediatric brain is less myelinated, with higher water content, predisposing it to shearing forces and higher risks for diffuse axonal injury and post-traumatic seizures.

Clinical Features

The height of the fall and the quality of the surface at the point of impact are important risk factors associated with severity of injury. Most children fall from standing height, but impact with an object can increase the localized force despite the short distance. In MVCs, the type of restraint used should be evaluated because unrestrained and improperly restrained children are at increased risk of serious injury. Several methods are available for evaluating mental status of head-injured patients, including the AVPU system and the GCS score.[15] The

GCS score should be modified for preverbal children (see Table 160.1). The "pediatric" GCS performs similarly to the adult GCS in verbal children.[16] In addition to assessing the child's mental status and examining the head for signs of trauma (including hematomas, lacerations and signs of skull fracture), the child and parents should be questioned on risk factors for intracranial hemorrhage, including loss of consciousness, mechanism of injury, behavior since the event, vomiting, and headache.

A brief seizure that occurs immediately after an insult (with a rapid return to a normal level of consciousness) is commonly called an *impact seizure*. Most children with post-traumatic seizures should undergo cranial CT scanning, but if the CT and the child's mental status are both normal, the child may be safely discharged home.[17]

The examination of a moderate to severely head-injured child includes strict attention to the ABCs (airway, breathing, and circulation). As the pediatric brain is highly sensitive to hypoxia and hypoperfusion, maintenance of oxygenation and blood pressure reduces further insult and optimizes the chance of functional recovery. Cerebral perfusion pressure (CPP) is adequate only in the face of a normal mean arterial pressure (MAP). Conceptually, CPP is equal to MAP minus ICP: CPP = MAP – ICP. As MAP is reduced, so is CPP. Therapy should target a CPP greater than 40 mm Hg and ICP less than 20 mm Hg.[18] Localized CPP at the site of injury and surrounding areas may vary greatly and be difficult to detect. Common symptoms and signs of raised ICP in infants and children are listed in Box 160.7. Herniation syndromes in children are similar to those in adults and described in Chapter 33.

Concussion. A *concussion* is a functional brain injury seen after a blow to the head or body, a fall, or another injury that "shakes" the brain within the skull. Radiographic studies should be obtained if there are findings suggestive of intracranial hemorrhage, but imaging solely for concussion is not recommended, as standard structural radiographic studies are normal, and current imaging for concussion is primarily experimental.[19]

Patients who sustain concussive insults may have somatic, cognitive, affective, or sleep symptoms. All children with concussive symptoms should be monitored for progression of symptoms by their primary care physician or a concussion recovery specialist. Treatment recommendations for concussion are a source of current research, as prior recommendations of bed rest are not beneficial.[20] Currently, we recommend a period of 24 to 48 hours of rest followed by increasing physical activity.

Scalp injuries. Bleeding from scalp wounds is often profuse and can lead to hemodynamic compromise in infants and small children if not quickly controlled. Early hemostasis prevents ongoing blood loss and should be addressed during the initial examination of the trauma patient. Scalp injuries in infants and children may also involve the development of three injury complexes. For these injury complexes to be better understood, the layers of the *skin*, *connective tissue*, *aponeurosis*, *loose areolar tissue*, and *periosteum* (SCALP) should be considered (Fig. 160.2). *Caput succedaneum* refers to a hematoma in the connective tissue layer. This is freely mobile and crosses suture lines. A *subgaleal hematoma* refers to a hematoma that is within the loose areolar tissue above the periosteum. Lastly, *cephalohematoma* refers to a collection of blood under the periosteum. Because the periosteum adheres tightly to the various suture lines, cephalohematomas do not cross them.

Skull fractures. In children, skull fractures occur in many different configurations. Simple linear non-depressed fractures rarely require therapy, are associated with good outcomes, and do not routinely require hospitalization in isolation. Factors associated with poor outcomes include the presence of a fracture overlying a vascular channel (especially the middle meningeal artery), a depressed fracture,

BOX 160.7 **Symptoms and Signs of Increased Intracranial Pressure in Infants and Children**

- Headache
- Stiff neck
- Photophobia
- Altered state of consciousness
- Persistent emesis
- Cranial nerve abnormalities
- Papilledema
- Hypertension, bradycardia, and hypoventilation
- Infants: paradoxical irritability, split sutures, full fontanelle, and "setting sun sign"
- Decorticate or decerebrate posturing

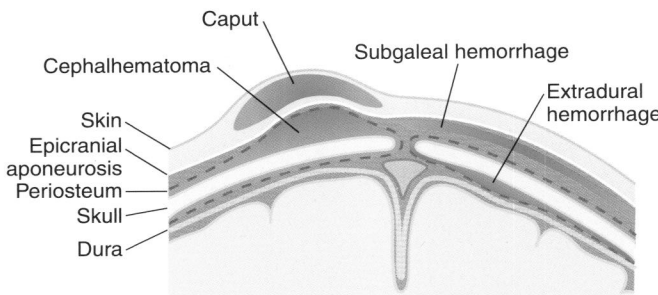

Fig. 160.2 Sites of Extracranial Hemorrhages in the Infant. (From Volpe JJ. *Neurology of the Newborn.* 4th ed. Philadelphia: WB Saunders; 2001.)

or a diastatic fracture. Diastatic fractures are defects which extend through suture lines and can lead to leptomeningeal cysts and "growing fractures." Leptomeningeal cysts are more common in children younger than 3 years old and may form after a skull fracture with a dural tear. "Growing fractures" develop when leptomeninges herniate through a dural tear, causing bony erosion around the fracture site.

Signs of basilar skull fractures in children are similar to adults and include the presence of periorbital subcutaneous hematoma (raccoon eyes), posterior auricular ecchymosis (Battle's sign), and CSF rhinorrhea or otorrhea. Both raccoon eyes and Battle signs take hours to days to develop, and therefore an absence of these signs does not rule out basilar skull fracture.

Cerebral contusions. Cerebral contusions are often the result of coup and countercoup forces and manifest as multiple microhemorrhages. Patients often have associated symptoms, which include an altered level of consciousness, severe headache, vomiting, or focal deficits on neurologic assessment.

Epidural hematoma. Epidural hematomas are typically caused by bleeding from the meningeal vessels and are often associated with overlying skull fractures. The classic presentation of an epidural hematoma is the triad of head injury, followed by a lucid interval, and rapid deterioration as the hematoma expands and compresses the brain.

Subdural hematoma. Subdural hematomas are often secondary to the rupture of bridging veins. Subdural hematomas most commonly occur in patients younger than 2 years of age, and less than half have associated skull fractures. Chronic subdural hematomas are associated with nonaccidental injury or "shaken baby syndrome," the result of accelerating and decelerating forces within the cranial vault from the violent shaking of a child. Subdural hematomas at multiple sites, over areas other than the convexities, in the posterior fossa, or the posterior interhemispheric fissure should raise suspicion for nonaccidental trauma. See Chapter 172 for a more in-depth discussion on nonaccidental trauma.

Diagnostic Testing

Skull radiographs. Clinicians have historically used skull radiographs as a screen for skull fractures in young patients with scalp hematomas. Due to the limited sensitivity of skull radiographs and the increased use of CT scanning in head trauma, skull radiographs are now rarely obtained. Skull radiographs may be considered for part of a skeletal survey in the evaluation of child abuse; to evaluate functioning of a ventricular peritoneal shunt; or to identify suspected foreign bodies underlying scalp lacerations.

Cranial computed tomography. Cranial CT provides substantial information but should be balanced with the risk of radiation. Substantial research has now identified various risk factors for

intracranial hemorrhage. The Pediatric Emergency Care Applied Research Network (PECARN) head injury decision instrument was derived in over 42,000 children and validated in a separate population of over 15,000 children.[21] The decision instrument provides evidence based guidelines for children with blunt head trauma (Fig. 160.3). Patients with no risk variables are at very low risk for intracranial injury and should not undergo cranial CT imaging. Furthermore, most patients with only a single risk variable can be observed in the ED and safely discharged after improvement, decreasing CT utilization. However, as the number of PECARN variables increase, risk increases and CT scanning becomes warranted.

Management and Disposition

Alert patients with normal cranial CT scans and normal neurologic examinations may be discharged home. Those with no PECARN risk variables, and those with a single risk factor who clinically improve after a period of observation, can also be discharged home. Reliable caretakers should be given specific return precautions for any focal

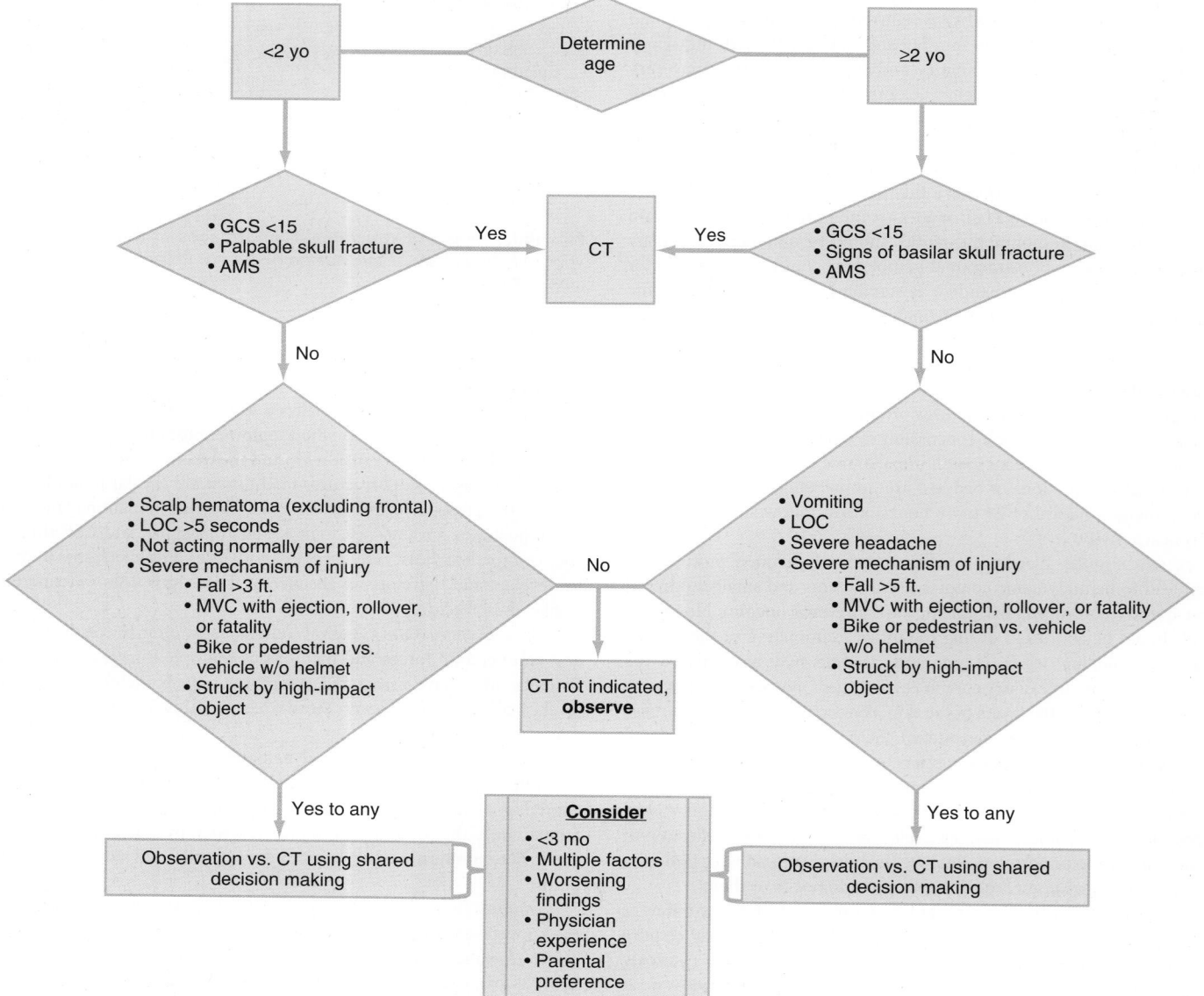

Fig. 160.3 PECARN Head Injury Chart. *AMS,* Altered mental status; *CT,* computed tomography; *GCS,* Glasgow Coma Scale; *LOC,* loss of consciousness; *MVC,* motor vehicle collision.

deficit, lethargy, worsening of symptoms, or alteration of consciousness. Children with intracranial hemorrhage or skull fractures should be evaluated by a neurosurgeon.

Skull fractures. Historically, children with skull fractures are routinely admitted to the hospital. However, alert children with linear, non-depressed skull fracture are unlikely to benefit from hospitalization. In selected cases after neurosurgical consultation, discharge with close outpatient follow-up and return precautions may be acceptable.[22] Skull fractures depressed more than the width of the skull are often repaired surgically. Basilar skull fractures require observation, but no specific therapy unless a persistent CSF leak is identified.

Severe traumatic brain injury. Prehospital BVM is recommended over ETI for support of ventilation and oxygenation. In the ED, ETI is performed in those with rapid deterioration, inability to protect their airway, or GCS scores ≤8. Recommendations for the treatment of children with moderate to severe head injuries are provided and regularly updated by the Brain Trauma Foundation (Box 160.8).[18] Standardization of care with early identification of impending herniation, emergency management of raised ICP, neuroimaging and neurosurgical involvement for appropriate use of ICP monitors improves outcomes.[18] In patients with suspected intracranial hypertension, treatment measures should include elevation of the head of the bed to 30 degrees, appropriate analgesia and sedation, controlled mechanical ventilation with $PaCO_2$ 35 to 40 mm Hg, hemoglobin maintained greater than 7 g/dL, normothermia (35 to 38°C), correcting any coagulopathy, and adequate intravascular volume with normal saline boluses.[18] Management of suspected acute herniation includes administering 3% hypertonic saline between 2 and 5 mL/kg over 15 minutes.[18] Mannitol (0.5–1 g/kg IV) is also used in this setting, but data is insufficient in the pediatric population to support its use. Serial neurologic examinations are the most reliable indicators of clinical deterioration and impending herniation. Repeat cranial CT scanning should be based on clinical assessments and not routinely performed.[18] We recommend a 7-day course of anticonvulsants (phenytoin or levetiracetam) for children with moderate to severe head injury to prevent early post-traumatic seizures. Prophylaxis beyond 7 days is not warranted. If a seizure does occur, rapid treatment with benzodiazepines is indicated.

Vertebral and Spinal Cord Injury

Foundations

Due to anatomic differences in the cervical spine, vertebral and spinal cord injury patterns vary with the age of the patient (Box 160.9) and are most commonly from falls, followed by MVCs. Thoracic and lumbar spine fractures are more common and characterized by compression fractures, whereas burst fractures are rare in children.[23] Cervical spine fractures are rare, especially in children less than 8 years. In this age group, cervical spine injuries are usually C3 or above.[24] As anatomic features of the cervical spine approach adult patterns between ages 8 and 10 years, injuries are more common in the lower cervical spine, and by age 15 years, the injury spectrum is similar to adult patients.

The anatomic differences between children and adults (see Box 160.9) lead to higher cervical cord injuries and an increased incidence of cord injury without bone involvement.[25] Thus, spinal cord injury without obvious radiographic abnormality (SCIWORA) is more common in children.[26] SCIWORA is a misnomer in this era of magnetic resonance imaging (MRI), because most injuries traditionally described as SCIWORA are identified on MRI but not plain radiographs. Treatment and prognosis of cervical spine injury depend on the neurologic presentation and extent of MRI findings. Whenever a cervical spinal injury is identified, careful attention should be paid to the entire spine as multilevel injuries occur frequently.[23]

BOX 160.8 Emergent Management of Severe Traumatic Brain Injury Pertinent to the Emergency Department

- ICP monitoring is suggested for severe TBI with a threshold for treatment of less than 20 mm Hg.
- Excluding increased ICP based on a normal cranial CT in comatose children is not recommended.
- Target CPP is 40–50 mm Hg.
- Bolus 3% hypertonic saline for increased ICP at 2–5 mL/kg IV over 15 min.
- Avoid fentanyl and midazolam boluses during ICP crises.
- Seizure prophylaxis to prevent early post-traumatic seizures with (phenytoin or levetiracetam).
- Avoid prophylactic hyperventilation (PaCO2 <30 mm Hg).
- Prophylactic hypothermia and corticosteroids are not recommended.

CPP, cerebral perfusion pressure; *ED*, emergency department; *ICP*, intracranial pressure; *IV*, intravenously; *Paco₂*, arterial carbon dioxide partial pressure; *TBI*, traumatic brain injury.
Kochanek PM, Tasker RC, Carney N, et al. Guidelines for the Management of Pediatric Severe Traumatic Brain Injury, Third Edition: Update of the Brain Trauma Foundation Guidelines, Executive Summary. *Pediatr Crit Care Med.* 2019;20:280-289.

BOX 160.9 Anatomic Differences in the Pediatric Cervical Spine

- Cervical spine fulcrum changes from C2 to C3 in toddlers to C5 to C6 by 8–12 years old.
- Relatively larger head size, resulting in greater flexion and extension injuries.
- Relatively large occiput in children younger than 2 years old leads to flexion of cervical spine if they are laid flat on standard backboard without support under their scapula and pelvis.
- Smaller neck muscle mass with ligamentous injuries more common than fractures.
- Anterior wedge appearance of cervical vertebral bodies is common.
- Increased flexibility of interspinous ligaments.
- Flatter facet joints with a more horizontal orientation.
- Incomplete ossification, making interpretation of bony alignment difficult (synchondrosis).
- Uncinate processes do not calcify until approximately 7 years old.
- Basilar odontoid synchondrosis fuses at 3–7 years old.
- Apical odontoid epiphyses radiographically apparent at 7 years old but may not fuse until approximately 12 years old.
- Posterior arch of C1 fuses at 4 years old.
- Anterior C1 arch may not be visible until 1 year old and fuses at 7–10 years old.
- Neural arches fuse to body by approximately 7 years old.
- Posterior arches fuse by 3–5 years old.
- Epiphyses of spinous process tips may mimic fractures.
- Predental space less than 5 mm in those less than 8 years and less than 3 mm in those ≥8 years.
- Pseudosubluxation of C2 on C3 seen in 40% of children up to 10 years and can be identified by an intact Line of Swischuk (Fig. 160.4).
- Prevertebral space size varies with phase of respiration.

Clinical Features

Although all trauma patients should be examined for vertebral injuries, significant head, neck, or back trauma, high-speed MVCs, or falls from a height onto the head should heighten suspicions. After the initial evaluation and stabilization, the cervical region can be definitively examined. Gentle palpation of the spine for tenderness or bony deformity can be performed to clinically assess the spine in alert children with otherwise normal neurologic exams. The facial response of a younger child to pain is often more indicative of injury than their verbal response. The neurologic examination in a pediatric patient can be difficult, but several factors should be evaluated in a patient with suspected spinal cord injury. Paralysis, paresthesia, and priapism are highly correlated with spinal cord injuries. Symptoms of paralysis or paresthesia, even if completely resolved at the time of examination, should be considered an indication of spinal cord injury. Spontaneously resolved deficits from an initial stretching of the cord with a rapid deceleration mechanism may return several days later from subsequent cord edema (as commonly described in patients with SCIWORA).[26]

Pediatric presentations of spinal cord injury syndromes are similar to adults and are detailed in Chapter 35. Spinal cord injuries are described as complete or incomplete, depending on the presence or absence of sensory and motor function. Incomplete lesions have preservation of some sensory or motor function below the injury level. Incomplete cord injury has a better prognosis.

Diagnostic Testing

Radiographic recommendations for potential cervical spine injuries are a source of current research and substantial variability. The National Emergency X-Radiography Utilization Study (NEXUS) criteria are often used to clear the cervical spine in adults (see Chapter 35). However, of the 34,069 patients enrolled in NEXUS, only 3065 (9.0%) were less than 18 years of age, and only 30 (0.98%) of these children had cervical spine injuries. Although the NEXUS decision rule identified all patients less than 18 years of age with cervical spine injury, only four children with injuries were younger than 9 years of age, and none were younger than 2 years of age. In a retrospective case-control study, the PECARN reviewed 540 records of children less than 16 years of age with cervical spine injury to identify 8 factors associated with cervical spine injury: altered mental status (including intoxication), focal neurologic findings, any neck pain, torticollis, substantial torso injury, conditions predisposing to cervical spine injury, diving mechanism, and high-risk motor vehicle crash. Children with none of these factors were at very low risk of cervical spine injury.

With limited research to direct pediatric cervical spine clearance, emergency physicians have developed reasonable practice variations in the use of specialist consultation and choice of imaging modalities. We recommend institutions develop multidisciplinary agreements on pediatric cervical spine clearance; establishing protocols has been shown to decrease time to clinical clearance and reduce unnecessary radiation exposure in children. We believe it is reasonable to follow a recent consensus statement and diagnostic algorithms published by the Pediatric Cervical Spine Clearance Working Group, consisting of 15 pediatric orthopedic surgeons, 3 pediatric emergency medicine physicians, 3 pediatric neurosurgeons, 2 pediatric trauma surgeons, and 2 pediatric radiologists.[27] Based on literature and expert opinion, the authors recommend clinical clearance in children with GCS scores 14 to 15, with minor mechanisms of injury (see following), no midline spine tenderness with full range of motion, normal head position, no associated neurological deficits, no painful distracting injuries, hypotension, or intoxication.[27] Patient not meeting all of these criteria should receive cervical spine imaging, starting with plain radiographs that should include a lateral view at minimum. We also agree with this group that a child who is able to maintain focus during an examination can have their cervical spine clinically cleared, despite other significant injuries. However, any child with a visible or known "substantial" injury to the chest, abdomen, or pelvis should have imaging.[27] High risk mechanisms of injury that should prompt imaging include an axial load, clotheslining injury, high-speed MVCs, suspected nonaccidental trauma, or a fall from a height of more than 10 feet. Thus, any alteration of mental status, focal sensory or motor abnormalities, neck pain, the presence of midline neck

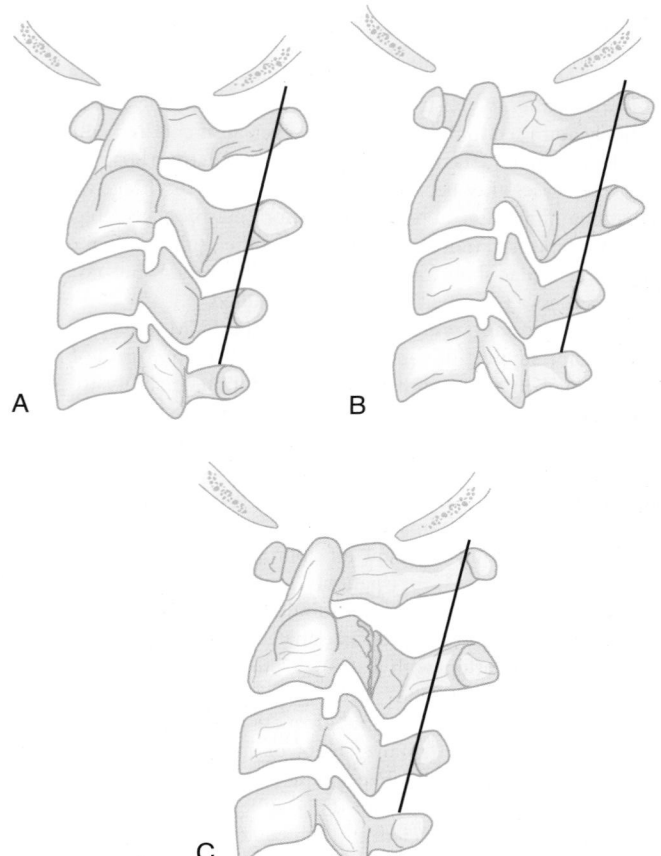

Fig. 160.4 Spinolaminar Line. Use only to access anterior displacement of C2 on C3. A line is drawn from the cortex of the spinous process of C1 to the cortex of the spinous process of C3, and the relationship of the spinous process of C2 is noted. (A) Normal line passing through the cortex of C2. (B) Normal line passing within 1.5 mm of the cortex of C2. (C) Abnormal line passing more than 1.5 mm anterior to the cortex of C2, suggesting underlying fracture of posterior elements of C2. (From American Academy of Pediatrics and American College of Emergency Physicians. *APLS: The Pediatric Emergency Medicine Resource.* 4th ed. Sudbury, MA: Jones and Bartlett Publishers; 2004.)

tenderness or torticollis, limited cervical range of motion or substantial distracting injuries on physical examination, warrant further imaging.[27] To reduce radiation exposure from CT, plain cervical spine radiographs are initially recommended in children with GCS scores 14 to 15 whose cervical spines cannot be clinically cleared.[27] Plain radiographic evaluation consists of lateral and anteroposterior views. In children older than 8 years, an open-mouth odontoid view should be added. The sensitivity of cervical spine plain radiographs is variable, as interpretation in children may be challenging due to the anatomic changes occurring with growth (see Box 160.9).

An essential criterion for radiographic clearance of the cervical spine is complete visualization of all seven cervical vertebrae to the C7 to T1 interface. The pre-dental space should be less than 5 mm in children younger than 6 years old, and the prevertebral soft tissue space should not be greater than one-half the vertebral body width above C4, and not greater than the width of the vertebral body at C6. The four cervical radiographic lines should be evaluated and the atlanto-occipital alignment assessed for dislocation (Fig. 160.4). Pseudo-subluxation of C2 on C3 in children up to age 10 years, occurs in approximately 40% of patients. Subluxation can be differentiated from pseudo-subluxation by the posterior cervical line and the relationship of the spinolaminar line

(line of Swischuk) to the anterior cortical margin of the spinous process at C2 (see Fig. 160.4). This line should maintain its integrity with no more than 1.5 mm of deviation. Although exceptions to this occur, an abnormal line of Swischuk is usually a pathologic finding and should prompt further investigation, typically with specialist consultation.

In children with GCS scores less than 14, we recommend cervical spine CT be obtained at the time of cranial CT imaging.[27] Alternatively, in children less than 3 years of age with GCS scores less than 14, cervical spine CT of C1–C2/C3 can be obtained with plain radiographs of the remaining cervical vertebral. Spine consultation should be obtained in children with injuries found on initial imaging. MRI may be obtained for ongoing concerns or to further delineate spinal cord injury.

Young children are at risk for occipital cervical junction injuries (atlanto-occipital disassociation). Although many of these injuries are immediately fatal, early detection and immobilization are important to prevent further morbidity and mortality. A Power's ratio greater than 1 on imaging indicates atlanto-occipital dislocation (Fig. 160.5). Traumatic atlantoaxial rotatory subluxation should be suspected in an injured child with torticollis. Classically, it is differentiated from muscular, non-traumatic torticollis by history, time course, and the absence of palpable spasm of the sternocleidomastoid muscle on the side contralateral to the direction in which the chin is pointing. When an atlantoaxial rotatory subluxation is suspected, plain radiographs or CT of the cervical spine are indicated. In children with upper cervical spine tenderness, it is prudent to consider a fracture of the synchondrosis between the odontoid and C2. This can be difficult to diagnose on plain radiographs, but it is often recognized as a subtle anterior tilt to the odontoid on C2. A CT scan with sagittal reconstructions can confirm the diagnosis. Children with peripheral neurologic abnormalities should be initially screened with CT or plain radiographs, but undergo MRI if findings persist. If a cervical spine ligamentous or cord injury is suspected with a negative CT scan, we recommend obtaining an MRI. Depending on the scenario and resources, patients with continued neck pain or tenderness despite negative plain radiographs or CT may require spine consultation, MRI, or treatment with a cervical collar and 1 to 2 week outpatient follow-up. The use of cervical spine flexion and extension radiographs to evaluate for ligamentous injury in the acute setting is often limited by the child's pain with neck ranging.

Management

Direct spinal cord injury results in a potentially irreversible injury. Indirect injury results from preventable or reversible injury secondary to ischemia, hypoxemia, and cord edema. Resuscitation of a patient with spinal cord injury should focus on prevention or minimization of the indirect causes of injury to the cervical spine. Spinal injury management begins prehospital, and most injured children arrive with adequate spine immobilization. In transport, the child who requires spinal immobilization should be placed in a stiff cervical collar, a rigid backboard, and external fixation using head blocks, cloth tape, or straps to provide adequate precautions. Appropriate padding should be placed under the shoulder blades of the patient to approximate neutral alignment of the cervical spine and help prevent pressure-related injury. Smaller children can be immobilized in their car seats.

In the ED, spinal immobilization should be maintained throughout the initial trauma evaluation. However, even when thoracic or lumbar fractures exist, patients should be expeditiously removed from the backboard to prevent discomfort and morbidity. Sliding boards (smooth movers) can be used to move patients onto scanner tables and back to their trauma beds.

Breathing should be assessed to determine the presence of hypoventilation, as patients with spinal cord injury may have diminished diaphragmatic activity or intercostal muscle paralysis. Supplemental

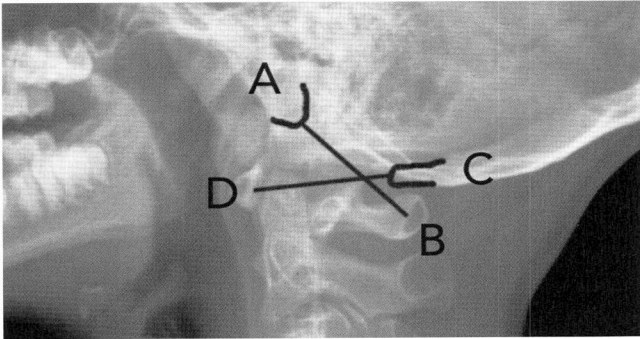

Fig. 160.5 Power's Ratio is Calculated as the Ratio of the Distance From the Basion (Midpoint of the Anterior Margin of the Foramen Magnum) *(A)* to the Anterior Cortex of the Posterior Arch of the Atlas *(B)* Divided by the Distance From the Opisthion (Midline Point of the Posterior Margin of the Foramen Magnum) *(C)* to the Posterior Cortex of the Anterior Arch of the Atlas *(D)*. A Ratio of Ab:cd Greater than 1 Indicates an Atlanto-Occipital Dislocation. The Figure Shows a Normal Power's Ratio.

oxygen should be provided, and ventilatory assistance considered in patients with hypoventilation or altered mental status.

Spinal shock is the loss of spinal reflexes below the site of injury, and generally resolves in 1 to 24 hours as spinal reflexes return below the site of injury. Neurogenic shock typically occurs with spinal cord injuries above the mid-thoracic level, and should only be considered once hemorrhagic shock has been excluded. Patients with neurogenic shock lose their sympathetic tone, manifested as hypotension and bradycardia. Treatment includes fluid administration, parasympathetic receptor blocking agents (e.g., atropine), and vasopressors with chronotropic, vasoactive, and inotropic characteristics (e.g., norepinephrine). Corticosteroids are no longer recommended in spinal cord injury. Early spine consultation is critical in children with potential spine injury to determine the need for further imaging and treatment, including possible need for transfer with continued spinal immobilization.

Cardiothoracic Injury

Foundations

Thoracic injuries are the second leading cause of death in injured children.[1] Most serious pediatric thoracic injuries are caused by blunt trauma (MVCs or pedestrian accidents). Considering the typical forces associated with blunt trauma, isolated chest injury is relatively infrequent in children. Those with penetrating chest trauma often die from primary vascular injuries which are rare following blunt mechanisms.

Pediatric ribs are less calcified than adults, resulting in more rib flexibility. This results in fewer rib fractures and more energy from the trauma transmitted internally. The presence of actual rib fractures in children suggests high energy and substantially increases the risk of morbidity and mortality. Pediatric rib fractures are generally treated with supportive care, but additional injuries should be sought. Rib fracture in infants should raise suspicion for abuse.[28]

Because of their unique anatomy and respiratory physiology (see Chapter 155), children have an increased risk for early decompensation after chest injury. A child's chest wall circumference does not change substantially during respiration, impairing their ability to increase forced vital capacity. Due to this and their increased metabolic demands, children normally function near maximum tidal volume capacity. As a result, children primarily increase ventilation by increasing their respiratory rate. Thus, anything that impedes a child's ability to increase ventilatory rate can significantly compromise ventilation, as with diaphragmatic impairment from gastric over-inflation (see Fig. 160.1). Finally, infant diaphragmatic muscle fibers predispose them to muscle fatigue and sudden apnea.

Diagnostic Testing

Plain chest radiography is the initial screening test for thoracic injury and is indicated in children with hypotension, tachypnea, or abnormal thoracic examinations, including any auscultatory abnormalities. This diagnostic test, however, fails to identify 50% of thoracic injuries. Chest CT has greater sensitivity, but exposes the child to substantial radiation, results in increased costs, and has demonstrated limited impact on outcomes.[29] Indications for contrast enhanced chest CT include the need to evaluate for trachea-bronchial or aortic/great vessel injury.[29] Unfortunately, further indications for thoracic CT are not well identified.

Pneumothorax. Traumatic pneumothoraces are less common in children and often associated with a hemothorax. Patients present with symptoms of chest pain, shortness of breath with evidence of chest wall abrasions or ecchymosis. Decreased breath sounds may not be appreciated in children with a pneumothorax because of the extensive transmission of breath sounds in the chest and upper abdomen. Initial anteroposterior supine chest radiography fails to identify half of pneumothoraces. Thoracic ultrasound has higher sensitivity, and chest CT is the gold standard.

Pneumothorax treatment includes the placement of an appropriately sized tube thoracostomy (see Box 160.2) in the mid-axillary line. Chest radiographs should confirm the eyelets of the chest tube are within the chest wall cavity. The chest tube is then attached to an under-water sealed suction device to drain the pneumothorax. A small, simple pneumothorax (<20% volume) in a spontaneously breathing alert, hemodynamically stable child may be observed. Occult pneumothoraces (visualized only on CT or ultrasound and not on plain radiography) are also routinely observed. All pneumothoraces undergoing observation should be treated with high flow oxygen to speed resolution. Children with occult pneumothoraces under positive pressure ventilation may also be observed, but rapid treatment should be available for any decompensation.

Pulmonary air leaks occurring through a one-way valve can cause a tension pneumothorax (Fig. 160.6). Increasing amounts of trapped air within the pleural cavity force the mediastinal structures toward the opposite side, compromising cardiac output. The mediastinal shift forces the trachea to the opposite side, with distention of the neck veins from the decreased venous return to the heart. This results in hypoxia, hypotension, and fluid-refractory shock. Most patients with tension pneumothorax have severe respiratory distress, decreased breath sounds (often bilaterally), and a shift in the point of maximal cardiac impulse. Immediate treatment includes angiocatheter (14 gauge) decompression in the second intercostal space in the midclavicular line or a tube thoracostomy in the fourth intercostal space anterior to the mid-axillary line.

An open pneumothorax occurs when the injured chest wall allows the bi-directional flow of air through the wound. The equalization of pressures between the atmosphere and the chest cavity prevents adequate lung expansion. As a result, ventilation and oxygenation can be severely impaired. In the prehospital setting, a bandage applied over an open pneumothorax wound and taped on three sides, as a temporizing measure, allows air to escape during expiration but not to enter during inspiration.

Management of an open pneumothorax is determined by the size of the chest wall defect and the amount of respiratory compromise. A simple, small, open pneumothorax in a breathing patient may be treated by covering the chest wall defect with an occlusive dressing, such as sterile petroleum gauze, and performing a separate incision for

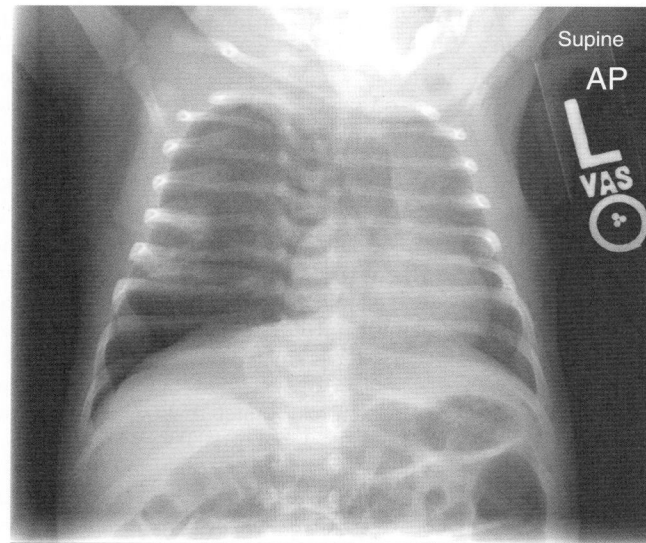

Fig. 160.6 Plain radiograph demonstrating a right sided tension pneumothorax with shift of the mediastinal structures to the left. The mediastinum is more mobile in children resulting in rapid ventilatory and circulatory collapse when under tension.

the chest tube. Defects that are too large to seal adequately and patients with ventilatory failure are candidates for intubation with mechanical ventilation in addition to the chest thoracostomy.

Hemothorax. Significant bleeding may occur as a result of injury to intercostal vessels, the internal mammary vessels, or lung parenchyma. Clinically, patients have decreased breath sounds and dullness to percussion on the affected side. Approximately 50% of pneumothoraces have concomitant hemothoraces. As hemothoraces collect in the most dependent portion of lung, they are better visualized on upright films as opposed to the standard anteroposterior radiograph. The only sign of hemothorax on a supine radiograph may be a slightly less radiolucent appearance on the affected side of the chest. Although small hemothoraces are observed, significant hemothoraces are treated with tube thoracostomy. In the supine patient with a simple pneumothorax, chest tubes are directed superiorly; in hemopneumothorax, however, they are directed posteromedially. Repeat chest radiographs should be obtained to confirm tube position and document lung expansion.

Massive hemothorax is rare in children and is associated with severe mechanisms of injury (high-velocity MVCs, falls from extreme heights, or gunshot wounds). Indications for open thoracotomy include evacuated blood volumes greater than 15 mL/kg of blood immediately on placement of the chest tube, persistent blood loss (exceeding 2 to 4 mL/kg/h over 3 hours), persistent hemodynamic instability or continued air leak.

Pulmonary contusion. Both penetrating and blunt thoracic trauma may cause pulmonary contusions, the most common thoracic injury in children. The compliance of the rib cage in children makes them susceptible to the development of pulmonary contusion, even in the absence of external signs of chest trauma. Injury to capillary membranes allows blood to collect within the interstitial spaces, resulting in hypoxia and respiratory distress. If bleeding is severe, both oxygenation and ventilation can be impaired. Initial chest radiographs underestimate the degree of injury and chest CT better delineates the insult. Treatment includes close monitoring, as these injuries evolve and patients can progress to respiratory distress over hours. The majority can be treated, however, with observation and supplemental oxygen as needed. Most resolve without sequelae, but those that progress can require positive pressure ventilation or even extracorporeal membrane oxygenation. Prophylactic steroids and antibiotics are of no known benefit.

Traumatic diaphragmatic hernia. Traumatic diaphragmatic hernias are exceedingly rare. Mechanisms causing these injuries usually involve a sudden increase in intra-abdominal pressure. The degree of symptoms is dependent on the extent of abdominal herniation into the pulmonary space. Most commonly, the herniation occurs on the left side, as the liver hinders the herniation of bowel on the right (Fig. 160.7). Initial management involves placement of a nasogastric tube to decompress the stomach. In cases of severe respiratory distress, intubation with mechanical ventilation is indicated. BMV should be avoided whenever possible, as this can cause distension of the herniated contents in the chest. Surgery is required for definitive repair.

Cardiac and vascular injuries. Although cardiac injuries following trauma are rare, cardiac contusion is the most common injury of the heart but is frequently without symptoms and not diagnosed. Patients often have chest wall tenderness or may report generalized chest pain; tachycardia is the most common finding. No consensus exists on the need and type of evaluation, but most providers screen those at risk with an electrocardiogram. In symptomatic patients (unexplained hypotension) an echocardiogram is indicated and may be diagnostic. Screening with cardiac enzymes is generally not warranted, but normal high sensitivity troponin measurements make the diagnosis unlikely. Patients with significant myocardial contusions should be monitored closely for the development of dysrhythmias and impaired myocardial function; however, in most cases no sequelae occur.

Cardiac tamponade is an immediately life-threatening condition, as extravasated blood fills the pericardial space and impairs cardiac filling during diastole. It presents with tachycardia, distant heart sounds, narrow pulse pressure, jugular venous distention, and pulsus paradoxus. In the scenario of profound hypovolemia, venous distention may be absent. The final common pathway involves the development of cardiopulmonary failure and pulseless electrical activity. The FAST examination (or dedicated echocardiogram) can rapidly identify tamponade (Fig. 160.8), provide an estimate of the pericardial effusion and diastolic dysfunction, and guide therapy. In critical patients with tamponade, emergency pericardiocentesis should be performed to drain the fluid from the pericardial sac. However, this is often inadequate, depending on the volume of blood and the presence of a subpericardial clot. Therefore, a definitive thoracotomy or pericardial window is often required to evacuate the pericardium adequately and repair the primary injury. Penetrating cardiac wounds and tamponade are survivable if recognized early.

Commotio Cordis results from blunt trauma to the anterior chest wall, which causes cessation of normal cardiac function. The patient may have an immediate dysrhythmia or ventricular fibrillation that is refractory to resuscitation efforts. Significant morbidity and mortality are associated with this disorder. Although most patients recover completely, some require extended treatment with antiarrhythmic agents, cardiac pacemaker placement, inotropic agents, or an intra-aortic balloon pump. In patients with prolonged cardiac instability, cardiogenic shock and death may occur despite maximal therapeutic intervention. Aortic and large vessel injuries are fortunately quite rare in young children but begin to increase in adolescents as mediastinal and vascular anatomy more closely resembles adults.

ED thoracotomy is more effective for penetrating trauma; it may be considered for patients with thoracic trauma who deteriorate to cardiopulmonary arrest despite maximal resuscitation. Because their injuries are more likely to be from penetrating mechanisms, adolescents have the best response to intervention.[30] In patients with penetrating chest trauma with cardiopulmonary resuscitation (CPR) for less than 15

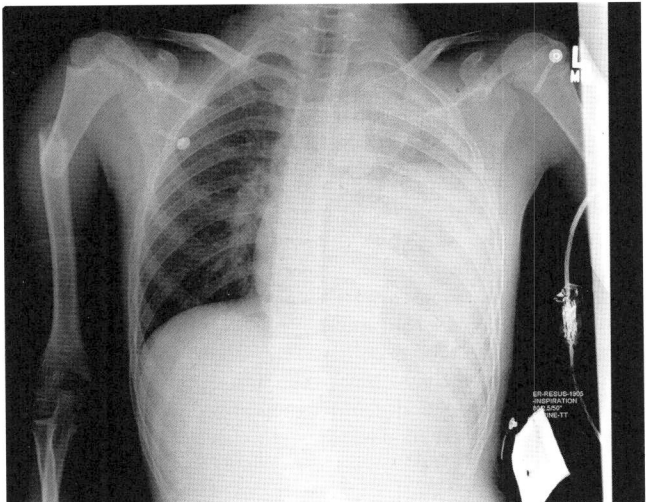

Fig. 160.7 Chest Radiograph with Herniation of the Stomach into the Left Thoracic Cavity. Care should be taken in these patients as the absence of breath sounds on the left may be mistaken for a pneumothorax. Chest tube placement could be complicated if the stomach was punctured during the procedure.

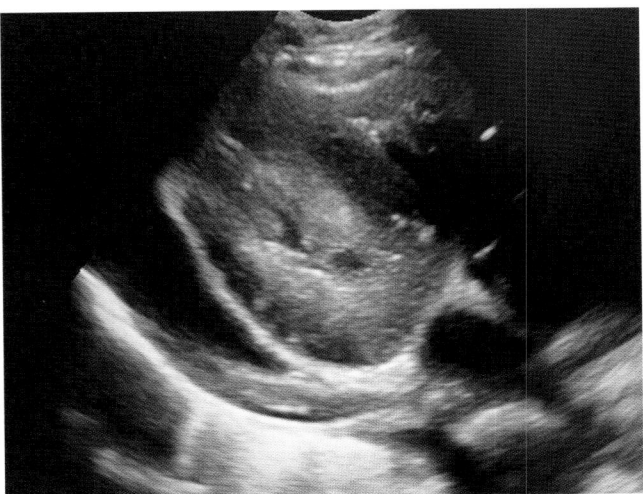

Fig. 160.8 FAST Examination Demonstrating Pericardial Tamponade in a Young Child with unexplained hypotension following a motor vehicle collision. This image resulted in immediate transport to the operating suite for life saving repair of a right atrial perforation in an otherwise uninjured child.

minutes, a left anterior thoracotomy may be warranted. Suggested contraindications to ED resuscitative thoracotomy after out-of-hospital CPR include (1) blunt trauma with CPR for longer than 10 minutes with asystole and no signs of life on presentation without ultrasound evidence of cardiac tamponade and (2) penetrating trauma with CPR for greater than 15 minutes and asystole with no signs of life on arrival without ultrasound evidence of cardiac tamponade.

Abdominal and Pelvic Injury

Foundations

After head and thoracic injuries, abdominal injury is the third leading cause of traumatic death in children.[1] Blunt trauma in MVCs is most lethal, causing more than half of abdominal injuries. Certain injury patterns are more common in children due to their unique activities or anatomy. These range from handlebar-inflicted abdominal injuries (Fig. 160.9) to crush injuries from television toppling. "Lap belt" injuries are most common in children and adolescents, and are characterized by intestinal injuries and "Chance" (horizontal) spinal fractures. Sports-related abdominal injuries often involve an isolated organ, as a result of a direct blow. Finally, abdominal injury is second only to head injury as a cause of death in child abuse cases.

A child's anatomy lends protection from some abdominal injury patterns, while predisposing children to other types of injuries. Children have proportionally larger solid organs, less subcutaneous fat, and less protective abdominal musculature than adults. Children have relatively larger kidneys with fetal lobulations, predisposing to renal injury. Children also have a flexible cartilaginous rib cage that allows for significant excursion of the lower chest wall, permitting compression of the abdominal organs. The combination of these factors provides the basis for the differences in abdominal injury patterns seen between children and adults.

Clinical Features

The rate of abdominal tenderness in alert children with intra-abdominal injuries is similar to that in adults, suggesting that the reliability of the abdominal examination is no different. However, the abdominal examination does become increasingly unreliable in children with significant head injuries (GCS scores <13).

Signs and symptoms of abdominal injury in children include tachypnea (from impaired diaphragmatic excursion and increased metabolic demands), abdominal tenderness, and signs of shock. Patients with abdominal wall injury (e.g., erythema, ecchymosis, abrasions) are much more likely to have intra-abdominal injuries. Abdominal distention is a common nonspecific finding that is often the result of swallowing air (e.g., from crying) after a painful event and not usually from massive hemorrhage (see Fig. 160:1).

Pelvic injuries are uncommon in young children due to their pliable pelvis and relatively larger shielding intraabdominal organs. To exclude injury, pelvic bone stability should be assessed in cases of abdominal trauma, including a genital examination searching for signs of injury. Rectal examination should only be performed in patients with a concern for specific injuries: spinal injury to assess rectal tone; or lower abdominal/pelvic trauma to evaluate rectal integrity.

Diagnostic Testing and Management

In patients with suspected abdominal injuries, management and resuscitation should be carefully planned to balance identification of all clinically important injuries and avoiding unnecessary testing. A careful history and physical examination can risk stratify patients for further evaluation. The PECARN abdominal injury rule risk stratifies children with abdominal trauma for intraabdominal injuries (Fig. 160.10). Children without any PECARN risk variables should not undergo abdominal CT, whereas CT is indicated for most with high risk variables. We recommend that children at intermediate to low risk undergo a period of observation, laboratory screening and FAST examination. Screening laboratory tests considered useful in children include elevated liver enzyme levels (serum aspartate aminotransferase [AST] >200 U/L or serum alanine aminotransferase [ALT] >125 U/L, hematuria, or an initial hematocrit <30%).

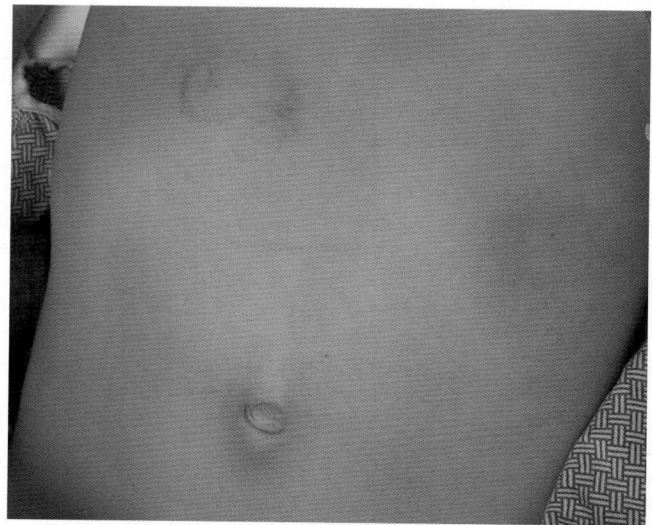

Fig. 160.9 Handlebar Injury in a Child Who Fell Off a Bike. Due to the location, the child sustained a liver laceration, but this mechanism often results in pancreatic or duodenal injuries when striking the epigastrium.

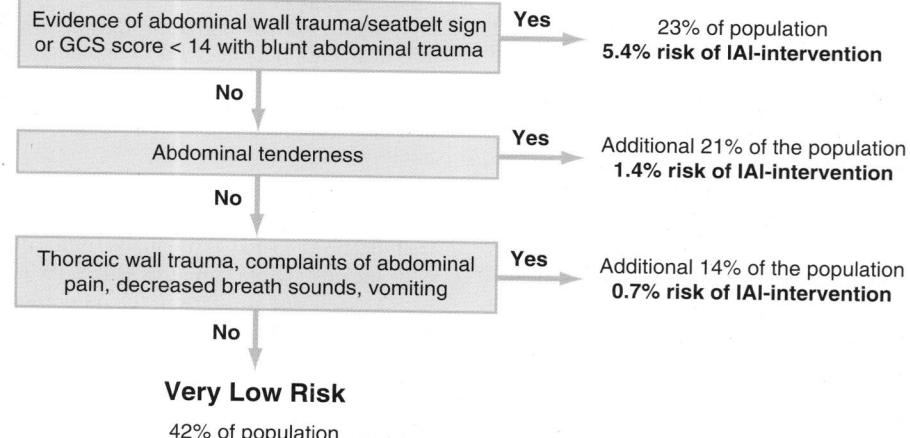

Fig. 160.10 PECARN abdominal injury rule provides evidence-based guidance for abdominal CT use in children. Children at 5.4% risk of injury undergoing intervention are considered at high risk, whereas those at 1.4% or 0.7% are considered at intermediate and low risk, respectively. Children without any risk factors are unlikely to benefit from CT. (Holmes JF, Lillis K, Monroe D, et al. Identifying children at very low risk of clinically important blunt abdominal injuries. *Ann Emerg Med.* 2013;62:107–16.e2)

The FAST examination evaluates the right upper quadrant (Morison's pouch), left upper quadrant and pelvis for intraperitoneal fluid. Although Morison's pouch is the most sensitive location for intraperitoneal fluid in adults, fluid is equally identified in the pelvis and Morison's pouch in children. Unfortunately, FAST has a lower sensitivity for intraperitoneal fluid in children than in adults, leading to uncertainty in its appropriate use.[31] Observational data suggests FAST safely decreases CT in children, however, the single randomized controlled trial in children did not demonstrate any clinical benefit with FAST.[32] Use of the FAST, however, did appropriately decrease the clinical suspicion of intra-abdominal injury, suggesting further study is warranted.[32] The finding of intraperitoneal hemorrhage on FAST does not mandate laparotomy, but if positive, ED abdominal CT is warranted. In hemodynamically unstable children, FAST quickly identifies an abdominal source of hemorrhage and can expedite care.[31]

The diagnostic test of choice to assess for intra-abdominal injury in stable patients at significant risk of intra-abdominal injury is abdominal CT. Abdominal CT scans should be performed with IV contrast; oral contrast is not necessary.[33]

Non-operative management of patients with solid organ injuries was pioneered in children. Now, patients with known sources of bleeding are routinely treated with observation, transfusion, and even arterial embolization instead of surgery.[34,35] Indications for laparotomy include intra-abdominal injuries with hemodynamic instability unresponsive to fluid resuscitation, transfusion greater than 50% of total blood volume, treatment of gastrointestinal injuries, penetrating abdominal trauma, and peritonitis.

Pelvic bone imaging is indicated in children with hemodynamic instability, decreased levels of consciousness, pelvic bone tenderness or instability, hematuria or significant distracting injuries (e.g. femur fracture).[36] If abdominal CT scan is already planned, plain pelvic radiographs are unnecessary, as the sensitivity of plain pelvic radiographs is less than 80%[37] with no additional information to CT. A CT should be considered for children with a strong suspicion for pelvic fracture (severe pain, inability to walk) but normal plain pelvic radiographs.

Splenic injury. The spleen is the most commonly injured abdominal organ. Findings include left upper quadrant abdominal pain that may radiate to the left shoulder. The presence of costal margin tenderness increases the risk of splenic injury, although isolated costal margin tenderness is very low and further evaluation is usually unnecessary.[38] Splenic injuries are best identified and characterized by abdominal CT scans.

Most splenic injuries are managed with simple observation, but surgical consultation should be obtained.[34,35] Almost all patients with splenic injury are admitted, but those with minor (Grade I or II injuries) managed on the ward.[39] Patients with more severe injuries are typically observed in the intensive care unit.[39] Delayed splenic hemorrhage occurs in a small subset of patients, and includes rupture of subcapsular hematomas. To maintain immunocompetency, every effort is made to avoid splenectomy and salvage the spleen.

Hepatic injury. The liver is the second most commonly injured abdominal organ. Abdominal tenderness especially in the right upper quadrant suggests injury. Similar to the left costal margin, tenderness to the right costal margin is associated with hepatic injury, but when present in isolation does not warrant CT imaging.[38] Patients with low-grade injuries are managed on the ward, while high grade injuries are typically admitted to the intensive care unit.[39] Following hepatic injuries, AST levels are usually greater than ALT levels. However, since AST degrades faster than ALT, AST will often be lower than ALT in hepatic injuries greater than 12 hours old.

Renal injury. Due to unique anatomic differences, the pediatric kidney is more susceptible to injury: potential remnant fetal lobules;

increased organ mobility with rapid deceleration mechanisms; and lack of protective abdominal musculature. Because of its retroperitoneal location, signs and symptoms of kidney injury are often less obvious and more diffuse than those of other abdominal organ injuries. Flank pain and posterior costal margin tenderness increase risk of injury. Fortunately, patients are readily screened for renal injury by urinalysis. Those without hematuria are unlikely to have significant urinary system injury. Gross hematuria requires abdominal CT scanning as the risk of intra-abdominal injury is approximately 50%. The degree of microscopic hematuria warranting imaging, however, is controversial, as investigators have suggested cutoffs ranging from 5 to 100 RBC/hpf. We recommend ED providers consider hematuria in context with other findings, as isolated asymptomatic microscopic hematuria is unlikely to yield an important injury on CT. For most patients, initial CT scan of the abdomen to assess for genitourinary injury is indicated when there is gross hematuria, microscopic hematuria with additional risk variables (e.g., abdominal pain or evident pelvic trauma), and penetrating injury to the abdomen (with or without hematuria).

Gastrointestinal injury. Approximately 15% of children with intra-abdominal injuries will have gastrointestinal injuries. These injuries range from simple serosal tears or intestinal wall hematomas that often do not require specific intervention, to intestinal perforation and bowel devascularization which require prompt surgical therapy. Fortunately, alert children with severe gastrointestinal injuries have significant abdominal examination findings. Historically, CT had insufficient sensitivity to identify children with gastrointestinal injuries. With improvement in CT technology, abdominal CT now demonstrates abnormalities in approximately 95% of children with gastrointestinal injuries. Abdominal CT findings suggestive of gastrointestinal injuries include intraperitoneal air, bowel wall thickening, bowel wall enhancement, mesenteric infiltration, and vascular contrast extravasation. With improved CT technology, isolated intraperitoneal fluid, once thought to be an ominous sign, is now known to be a common finding in children without diagnosed intra-abdominal injury. Asymptomatic children with normal abdominal examinations and small amounts of isolated intraperitoneal fluid may be observed and ultimately discharged from the ED with appropriate return precautions.

Pancreatic injury. Fortunately, pancreatic injury is rare, occurring in 5% of children with intra-abdominal injuries, but less than 1% of children undergoing abdominal CT scanning. Despite improvements in CT technology, this injury remains difficult to diagnose, as CT has a sensitivity of only 50% for pancreatic injury and fails to correctly grade the injury. Lipase and amylase are poor initial screening labs but increase 24 to 48 hours after pancreatic injury. Most injuries are managed non-operatively, but significant morbidity can occur in those with severe pancreatic trauma.

Penetrating injury. Penetrating wounds to the abdomen usually require rapid evaluation by a surgeon and consideration for operative intervention. Gunshot wounds generally result in more damage and higher mortality than stab wounds. With hemodynamic instability or peritonitis, urgent laparotomy is indicated. Depending on clinical findings, management options for the hemodynamically stable patient include further evaluation with abdominal CT scan; local wound exploration to determine violation of the peritoneum; diagnostic laparoscopy; and observation. In modern practice, diagnostic peritoneal lavage has been supplanted by other diagnostic modalities, including CT and diagnostic laparoscopy.

Straddle injuries. Straddle injuries occur when the child falls, striking their genitals and perineum on a hard object, most commonly bicycles and playground equipment. Injuries are typically localized to the genitalia and perineum, and physical examination is usually sufficient to identify the extent of injury. Pain and anxiety, however, may limit the ability to adequately examine the area, often requiring sedation. Child abuse should be ruled out, especially if the injury is unlikely from blunt trauma (e.g., rectal or posterior fourchette tears). We recommend observing children with straddle injuries to confirm the ability to void and assess for hematuria. Scrotal ultrasound is recommended for significant scrotal edema or tenderness. Children who should receive referral for definitive care include those with extensive lacerations, vaginal bleeding, large hymenal tears, scrotal laceration through the dartos layer, or evidence of urethral injury.

Pelvic fractures. While pelvic fractures are less common in children than adults, pelvic avulsion fractures are significantly more common in children, especially as related to sports. More severe pelvic fractures are the result of high energy mechanisms, and frequently associated with other injuries. Genitourinary injuries are found in 10% of children with pelvic fractures. Orthopedic consultation is recommended to determine further treatment.

MUSCULOSKELETAL INJURIES

Musculoskeletal injuries are a common ED complaint for children. Pediatric injury patterns differ substantially from those of adults, as children have strong ligaments and growing, less dense bones covered in a thicker periosteum. The Salter-Harris fracture classification characterizes fracture patterns unique in children. In cases where the skin is disrupted at the site of the fracture, the fracture is considered open; the wound should be irrigated and IV antibiotics covering gram-positive skin flora administered. Antibiotics with gram-negative coverage are added in those with more complicated fractures. Fractures with vascular deficits require emergent reduction and splinting, but those with normal neurovascular examinations should be splinted until definitive care. A detailed discussion of these types of injuries is found in Chapter 170.

The references for this chapter can be found online at ExpertConsult.com.

Pediatric Fever

Nathan W. Mick

FOUNDATIONS

Background

Fever is the most common chief complaint of pediatric patients presenting to the emergency department (ED). Most cases of fever are viral in origin, benign in course, and resolve spontaneously. Management of children with fever varies by the age of the child, with the following common divisions: 0 to 28 days old, 1 to 2 months old, 2 to 3 months old, 3 to 6 months old, 6 to 36 months old, and 3 years old to adulthood. Understanding that risk is a continuum, these divisions reflect differing immunologic and vaccination milestones, as well as a spectrum of age-specific pathogens.

Anatomy, Physiology, and Pathophysiology

Fever is defined as any elevation in body temperature of 100.4°F (38.0°C) or above. The most reliable method to measure temperature is with a rectal thermometer and is the preferred method of measurement in high-risk groups, such as infants 0 to 3 months old. However, the rectal route should not be used in patients who are potentially immunocompromised (e.g., children receiving cytotoxic chemotherapy) because of the risk of mucosal damage leading to bacteremia. The cutoff for a clinically significant fever (i.e., one that may trigger a laboratory evaluation) varies with the age and immunologic status of the child. A rectal temperature of 100.4°F (38.0°C) is considered a clinically significant fever in an infant younger than 3 months, often warranting laboratory evaluation; however, a toddler with a temperature of 103.1°F (39.5°C) and an upper respiratory infection may not need any evaluation beyond a thorough history and physical examination.

Causes of fever vary with the age of the child (Table 161.1). The majority of pediatric fever is due to infections, and most infections are attributable to a viral source. (See Chapter 120 for a discussion of COVID-19 in children) Upper respiratory infections, viral gastroenteritis, croup, bronchiolitis, stomatitis, roseola, infectious mononucleosis, and varicella are all known causes of fever. Most viral illnesses are benign and self-limited, but infection with measles, herpes simplex virus (HSV), or respiratory syncytial virus (RSV) can lead to significant morbidity and mortality, particularly in the first month of life.

Bacterial disease is also an important cause of fever in children. Serious bacterial infection (SBI) is defined as the presence of pathogenic bacteria in a previously sterile site and includes urinary tract infection (UTI), bacteremia, meningitis, osteomyelitis, bacterial gastroenteritis, bacterial pneumonia, cellulitis, and septic arthritis. The risk of SBI in febrile infants younger than 3 months old with a temperature of at least 100.4°F (38.0°C) is between 6% and 10%; children younger than 28 days old have the highest incidence.[1] Hyperpyrexia (rectal temperature ≥40.0°C) is associated with a higher risk of SBI.[2] Pathogens change during early infancy, with vertical transmission of organisms such as group B streptococcus, *Listeria monocytogenes,* and HSV more common in neonates. By 1 to 2 months of age, organisms such as *Streptococcus pneumoniae, Neisseria meningitidis,* and urinary pathogens *(Escherichia coli* or *Enterococcus)* become more common. In all children younger than 3 months old, the urinary tract is the most common site of infection, followed by bacteremia and meningitis.

Children younger than 3 months old may present with an apparent viral syndrome and still harbor SBI. Levine and colleagues studied 1248 infants younger than 60 days old who had temperatures above 100.4°F (38.0°C). Of these children, 22% were positive for RSV. Overall, children with documented RSV had a lower incidence of concomitant SBI than those without RSV (12.5% vs. 7%), but there was no significant difference in rates of SBI in those younger than 28 days old (14.2% in RSV-negative vs. 10.1% in RSV-positive). Most of the bacterial infections were UTIs. Older children 3 to 36 months old with recognizable viral syndromes (e.g., croup, bronchiolitis, varicella, stomatitis) have a very low incidence of bacteremia; in over 1300 patients with a temperature above 102.2°F (39.0°C) who had a recognizable viral syndrome, the risk of bacteremia was 0.2%.

Occult bacteremia describes the presence of pathogenic bacteria in the bloodstream of a well-appearing febrile child in the absence of a focus of infection; it was first described as a clinical entity in the 1970s. The term typically refers to children 3 to 36 months old who are highly febrile (>102.2°F [39.0°C]) but appear well. Before the adoption of the conjugate vaccines against *Haemophilus influenzae* type b and *S. pneumoniae,* the incidence of bacteremia in this population was approximately 5%. Vaccination has proved remarkably effective, nearly eradicating *H. influenzae* type b as a significant pathogen and greatly

TABLE 161.1   Etiology of Fever in Children

Age	Bacterial Causes	Viral Causes	Other
0–8 days old	Group B streptococcus	HSV	Bundling (skin temperature only)[a]
	Listeria monocytogenes	Varicella	Environmental
	Escherichia coli	Enteroviruses	
	Chlamydia trachomatis	RSV	
	Neisseria gonorrhoeae	Influenza	
1–3 months old	*Haemophilus influenzae*	Varicella	
	Streptococcus pneumoniae	Enteroviruses	Environmental
	Neisseria meningitidis	RSV	
	E. coli	Influenza	
3–36 months old	*S. pneumoniae*	Varicella	Leukemia
	N. meningitidis	Enteroviruses	Lymphoma
	E. coli	RSV	Neuroblastoma
		Influenza	Wilms' tumor
		Mononucleosis	
		Roseola	
		Adenovirus	
		Norwalk virus	
		Coxsackievirus	
3 years old to adulthood	*S. pneumoniae*	Varicella	Leukemia
	N. meningitidis	Enteroviruses	Lymphoma
	E. coli	RSV	Neuroblastoma
	Group A streptococcus	Influenza	Wilms' tumor
		Mononucleosis	Juvenile rheumatoid arthritis
		Roseola	
		Adenovirus	
		Norwalk virus	

[a]Bundling may raise skin temperature but does not change rectal temperature. Irrespective of how measured, a fever in this high-risk population should not be attributed to bundling alone.
HSV, Herpes simplex virus; *RSV,* respiratory syncytial virus.

reducing the burden of pneumococcal disease (Fig. 161.1).[3,4] Currently, the rate of occult bacteremia is less than 1%, with pathogens such as *N. meningitidis* becoming proportionally more prevalent. Urinary pathogens, occurring in 5% of febrile children younger than 2 years old, continue to be a common source of bacterial illness in infants and children. Risk factors include female sex, absence of another apparent source of infection, fever higher than 102.2°F (39.0°C), white race, and for boys, uncircumcised status.

Bacterial illness in school-age children and adolescents includes focal infections, such as streptococcal pharyngitis, cellulitis, and pneumonia, as well as bacteremia and meningitis. *N. meningitidis* has a bimodal distribution, with the highest incidence in children younger than 12 months old (9.2/100,000 population). A second peak occurs

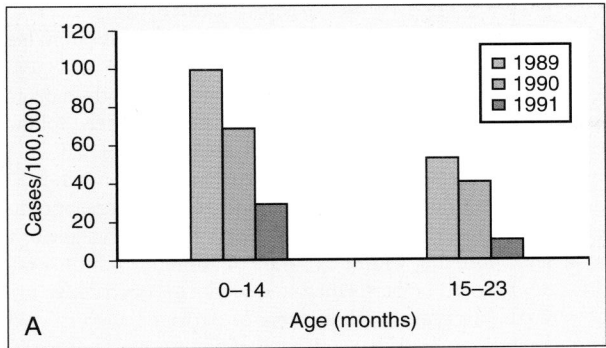

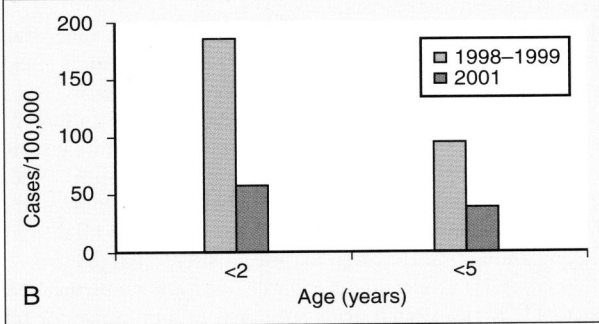

Fig. 161.1 Decline in incidence of occult bacteremia after the introduction of the conjugate vaccine against *Haemophilus influenzae* (A) and *Streptococcus pneumoniae* (B).

during adolescence, when the rate of illness is 1.2/100,000 population, with a significant proportion of cases occurring in college students who reside in a dormitory setting (3.2/100,000 population).

Although it is much less common than in viral or bacterial infection, fever can also be a presenting sign of autoimmune diseases, such as juvenile rheumatoid arthritis or Kawasaki disease. Central nervous system (CNS) lesions such as brain tumors also can infrequently manifest with fever.

The body's ability to fight infection varies with age. Maternal antibodies confer some protection after birth, but the infant's immune system is initially inadequate, particularly T-cell function and the ability to mount an immunoglobulin G response to infection. Their immature immune system and exposure to certain pathogens during the birthing process (e.g., group B streptococcus, *Chlamydia trachomatis*, *Neisseria gonorrhoeae*) places the newborn at particularly high risk for SBI. Young infants are also at risk for disseminated infection because they are unable to mount the immune response needed to prevent bacterial spread. Thus, a simple cellulitis, mastitis, omphalitis, or, rarely, gonococcal eye disease, can lead to sepsis or seeding of the CNS. Immune function improves during the first 2 to 3 months of life, as does the ability to assess a child clinically. Infants begin the primary series of vaccinations against acquired infections, such as *S. pneumoniae* and *H. influenzae*, at 2 months of age, providing further protection against common bacterial pathogens. As a result, empirical testing and treatment give way to more selective evaluations above 2 to 3 months old.

Clinical Features

History taking should focus on the length of illness, localizing symptoms (e.g., headache and neck pain [meningitis or encephalitis] or ear pain [otitis media]), exposure to ill contacts, travel history, and pertinent past medical history. For infants younger than 28 days old, document birth history, including gestational age and the presence of potentially transmittable maternal infections (HSV or group B streptococcus). Document immunization status, sick contacts, use of antipyretics before evaluation, and prior use of antibiotics. Defervescence after acetaminophen administration has not been shown to reliably exclude bacteremia in children of any age. Prior antibiotic use may mask the classic findings in diseases, such as meningitis. Cough and congestion may suggest pneumonia or viral upper respiratory infection, whereas a harsh, barking, or seal-like cough is often a predominant complaint in viral laryngotracheitis (croup). Parents may report vomiting and diarrhea as a component of gastroenteritis, or the presence of sore throat and lymphadenopathy with viral or streptococcal pharyngitis. Decreased oral intake or decreased urine output is a frequent complaint in gastroenteritis but may also be seen in patients with stomatitis because painful oral aphthous ulcerations prevent fluid intake. A history of lethargy, irritability, or altered mental status can occur with severe dehydration but should raise concern for meningitis or encephalitis. A rash occurs in many viral illnesses (e.g., roseola) but may be seen in life-threatening conditions, such as meningococcemia, Rocky Mountain spotted fever, and toxic shock syndrome (TSS).

The physical examination of the febrile child should begin with a complete set of vital signs, including pulse oximetry. Hypoxia or significant respiratory distress (e.g., tachypnea, grunting respirations, nasal flaring, or retractions) may accompany sepsis or pulmonary infection. Stridor can be seen with croup but also can occur with retropharyngeal abscess, epiglottitis, or bacterial tracheitis. Signs of shock, such as hypotension and poor peripheral perfusion, should be noted. Children typically mount a tachycardic response to fever, and hypotension is often a late and dire finding. Tachycardia is often due to the fever itself, but tachycardia out of proportion to the degree of fever can be seen with early shock, myopericarditis, and dehydration. Estimations of heart rate increase based on fever in infants younger than 12 months old (i.e., heart rate increases linearly by 9.6 beats/min with each 1°C increase in body temperature) should be used with caution and clinical signs of sepsis evaluated before attributing tachycardia to fever alone. Once oxygenation, ventilation, and perfusion have been assessed and deemed adequate, the physical examination should focus on a thorough search for focal infection. In young infants, particularly those younger than 3 months old, and in children who lack immunocompetence, fever may be the only presenting sign of SBI, including meningitis. The physical examination in this age group is insufficiently sensitive to exclude SBI, and emergency clinicians should not be falsely reassured by a normal physical examination in young children. Those who do appear toxic may have decreased tone, poor skin turgor, poor tracking, increased or decreased respiratory effort, a weak cry or suck, or delayed capillary refill times. The neonate who refuses to feed should have a full SBI evaluation, irrespective of temperature. See Chapter 155.

Diagnostic Testing

Numerous laboratory and radiographic studies can be used to evaluate the febrile child. In general, testing should be directed at the identification of the source and complications of infection. Several guidelines exist for the evaluation of febrile children, although there is marked variation in adherence to these guidelines. Office-based practitioners have been found to follow published guidelines only 42% of the time in the evaluation of febrile children. Clinicians with less experience and those based in the hospital tend to order more tests compared with more experienced clinicians and those practicing in an office setting, respectively. The use of institutional clinical decision rules and guidelines can help streamline appropriate testing.[5,6]

White Blood Cell Count

An elevated white blood cell (WBC) count (>15,000/mm^3) can be an indicator of bacteremia but is also present in many viral illnesses. Leukopenia (<5000/mm^3) can also be a sign of SBI or early sepsis. Pneumococcal infection is classically associated with leukocytosis, whereas infection with *N. meningitidis* and *H. influenzae* may be present even with normal WBC counts. In children with fever greater than 102.2°F (39.0°C), Lee and colleagues found that the rate of pneumococcal bacteremia increased from 0.5% with a WBC count between 10,000 and 15,000/mm^3 to 3.5% if the WBC count was 15,000 to 20,000/mm^3 and up to 18% with a WBC count above 30,000/mm^3. More extreme leukocytosis is associated with an increased risk of bacterial infection, particularly lobar pneumonia, and a WBC count of above 25,000/mm^3 should prompt consideration of a chest radiograph unless another definitive source is apparent.[7]

The WBC differential diagnosis has also been used to risk-stratify febrile children in various models; an increase in polymorphonuclear leukocytes increases the risk of bacterial disease. A rise in polymorphonuclear leukocytes is also seen early in some viral infections. An absolute neutrophil count (ANC) above 10,000/mm^3 suggests an increased risk of pneumococcal bacteremia in febrile children (0.8% for children with an ANC below 10,000/mm^3 vs. 8% for children with an ANC above 10,000/mm^3). Routine screening of all febrile children greater than 3 months of age with bloodwork has not been shown to be cost-effective in the post-vaccination era. The vast majority of acute febrile illness is due to self-limited viral infection. If the decision is made on clinical grounds to obtain a WBC and if it is abnormal (<5000/mm^3 or >15,000/mm^3) or the ANC is greater than 10,000/mm^3, then we recommend screening for occult bacteremia with a blood culture, understanding that leukocytosis is neither perfectly sensitive nor specific for bacterial illness. We also recommend treatment with ceftriaxone for incompletely immunized children who have a WBC of more than 15,000/mm^3.

Inflammatory Markers

Both C-reactive protein (CRP) and procalcitonin have been studied as markers of bacterial infection. The utility of the measurement of inflammatory markers is dependent on the cutoff level assigned for clinical significance with lower values having higher sensitivity but lower specificities. Procalcitonin greater than 0.5 ng/mL is highly specific for SBI, though some clinicians use a lower cutoff (>0.2 ng/mL) to increase sensitivity. Both CRP and procalcitonin appear to be more sensitive and specific than the WBC alone, although the lack of widespread availability limits the usefulness of procalcitonin clinically at this time.[8,9]

Blood Culture

Many centers obtain blood for culture during intravenous (IV) catheter placement after sterile preparation of the skin has been performed. Although this eliminates a second venipuncture solely to obtain blood for culture, in children, the rates of contamination with this technique are higher than a sterile straight stick (9.1% vs. 2.8%). The risks of contamination should be weighed against the ability to obtain blood through a separate venipuncture. The yield of a single blood culture in infants and small children is actually good. The routine sending of more than one sample is generally not needed, and bacteremia is often accurately detected even if only 0.5 to 1 mL of blood is obtained. The advent of automated blood culture systems has led to the identification of true pathogens more quickly than by traditional methods, often within 24 hours. Pathogens isolated in the first 24 hours are more likely to be true pathogens than are bacteria isolated after 24 hours.[10]

Urinalysis and Urine Culture

UTIs are common causes of bacterial illness in febrile children, occurring in 5% of infants 2 to 24 months old with fever 100.4°F (38.0°C) or higher. Accurate documentation of UTI is imperative both to diagnose the cause of a fever and to identify those infants who need follow-up radiographic imaging to exclude anatomic abnormalities that will predispose them to further infection. It is currently recommended that febrile infants with documented UTIs undergo renal ultrasonography to evaluate for urinary tract anomalies. For infants with signs of urosepsis or not improving within 24 hours of antibiotic administration, an ultrasound should be performed to evaluate for obstructive uropathy or rare complications, such as renal or perirenal abscesses. Voiding cystourethrography is not indicated after the first febrile UTI in children unless renal ultrasonography reveals evidence of high-grade vesicoureteral reflux or scarring.

The only reliable method to obtain urine in a non-toilet-trained child is bladder catheterization or suprapubic aspiration. Bladder catheterization is the preferred method in *almost all* cases. Bag collection of urine is notoriously unreliable; up to 85% of cultures from bag specimens will be falsely positive (defined as a culture growing a single organism with >10^5 colony-forming units [CFUs]/mL or a mix of two or more organisms), which then places these children at risk for unneeded, potentially painful, and expensive follow-up diagnostic testing and antibiotics. However, for select patients, bagged urine may be obtained, and if results do not indicate infection, no further studies are needed.[11] A clean catch urine specimen is appropriate for toilet-trained children.

UTI is defined as the combination of bacteriuria and pyuria. Bacteriuria in the absence of WBCs on microscopic examination represents asymptomatic bacteriuria. Urine is typically analyzed with a dipstick, followed by microscopic analysis of a centrifuged specimen of urine. An "enhanced" urinalysis, which is an examination with a hemocytometer of an unspun specimen of urine for pyuria (defined as >10 WBCs per high-power field) or the presence of any bacteria per high-power field in Gram stain of unspun urine has a negative predictive value of 99.8%, perhaps making urine culture unneeded if pyuria and bacteriuria are absent by use of the enhanced urinalysis method. However, many centers are not using this enhanced method. Because dipstick and microscopic analysis have lower sensitivities, most experts recommend sending urine for culture in high-risk groups (febrile girls <24 months old, uncircumcised boys <12 months old, and circumcised boys <6 months old).

A positive urine culture is defined as the growth of more than 50,000 CFU/mL of a single uropathogen in urine obtained via catheterization or suprapubic aspirate.

Lumbar Puncture

A sample of cerebrospinal fluid (CSF) should be obtained from any child with signs and symptoms of meningitis. Fluid should be obtained with the smallest spinal needle possible (typically a 22-gauge) and sent for cell counts, manual differential diagnosis, Gram staining, culture, and measurement of CSF protein and glucose concentrations. Meningoencephalitis due to HSV is a potential cause of fever, particularly in neonates; if suspected, CSF should be sent for HSV polymerase chain reaction (PCR) testing. Panel-based nucleic amplification tests that detect a wide array of viral and bacterial pathogens can also be useful but should be coupled with traditional CSF cultures as they do not identify every possible pathogen and do not give information on antibiotic susceptibility.[12,13] The CSF in bacterial meningitis typically contains more than 1000 WBCs/mL, although there is considerable overlap in the CSF profile of bacterial and viral meningitis, making a determination of viral or aseptic meningitis difficult on the basis of

CSF parameters, such as cell count, protein, and glucose; thus, CSF culture of a pathogenic bacterium is the "gold standard." A prediction rule has been developed and validated to differentiate bacterial from aseptic meningitis in children 29 days to 19 years old who have CSF pleocytosis. Children *without* any of the following criteria have a low risk (0.1%) of bacterial meningitis: positive CSF Gram stain, CSF ANC of 1000 cells/mL or more, CSF protein concentration of at least 80 mg/dL, peripheral blood ANC of 10,000 cells/mL or more, and history of seizure before or at the time of presentation. This may obviate the need for empirical antibiotic therapy and hospital admission in some children who are at low risk for bacterial meningitis.[14]

Contraindications to lumbar puncture include cellulitis over the proposed site of puncture, cardiopulmonary instability, bleeding diathesis, or platelet count below 50,000/µL, focal neurologic deficits, and signs of increased intracranial pressure, including papilledema. In these patients, lumbar puncture should be deferred until the child is stable, and blood should be obtained for culture while the child is treated empirically, recognizing that up to 50% of children with meningitis will not have bacteremia.

CSF contaminated by blood (i.e., a traumatic lumbar puncture) can make interpretation of cell counts and differential diagnoses difficult. In these cases, fluid should be obtained for Gram stain and culture and the child hospitalized and treated presumptively for meningitis until culture data are available.

Stool Studies

Stool studies are indicated in patients in whom bacterial gastroenteritis may be a cause of fever. A stool guaiac test for blood, as well as Gram stain for WBCs, should be performed. The presence of more than five WBCs per high-power field in the stool of a febrile child should trigger a culture of stool for *Salmonella, Shigella, Campylobacter,* enterotoxigenic *E. coli,* and *Yersinia* species. Patients with sickle cell disease are at particular risk for focal complications, such as osteomyelitis from *Salmonella* infection (see Chapter 167).

Chest Radiography

Chest radiographs may be useful in the evaluation of the febrile child and are indicated when hypoxemia, respiratory distress, tachypnea, or focal findings on lung examination are present. Children younger than 6 months old may present with tachypnea as the sole finding of bacterial pneumonia. Occult pneumonia can also occur in a small percentage of children, particularly in the highly febrile child (>102.2°F [39.0°C]) without an apparent source of fever and an elevated ANC. Studies done prior to universal vaccination against pneumococcus demonstrated a relatively high rate of pneumonia in highly febrile children who had leukocytosis more than 20,000/mm³ (26%). Since the advent of universal vaccination, the number of occult pneumonias has declined (15% to 9%) but is not yet low enough to recommend not obtaining radiographs on highly febrile children with leukocytosis or elevated ANC and no other apparent source of infection. Point of care lung ultrasound has been shown to compare favorably to chest radiographs in multiple studies when used for the diagnosis of pneumonia.[15]

Rapid Viral Antigen Testing

Many clinical laboratories have the ability to perform rapid viral antigen testing, either individually or as part of a panel for such common pediatric viral illnesses as influenza A and B, parainfluenza, rhinovirus, and RSV. The presence of a viral "source" for the fever in an ill child may obviate the need for expensive, painful, and lengthy diagnostic evaluations for bacterial processes. Of patients aged 2 months to 21 years old who present with classic signs and symptoms of influenza, more than half have been shown to have positive rapid assays for

influenza, leading to fewer antibiotics prescribed. A large multicenter trial of febrile infants 60 days old or younger revealed a decreased risk for SBI (2.5% vs. 11.7%) if the infant was influenza positive.

RSV is also a frequent cause of fever in children. As previously noted, RSV decreases but does not completely eliminate the risk of SBI in children. This is especially true of UTI in infants younger than 28 days old. Routine testing for RSV has not been shown to affect outcomes at the individual patient level.[16] Given the exceedingly low rates of bacteremia and meningitis, it is reasonable to consider a selective, de-escalated evaluation (i.e., urine and urine culture only) of well-appearing infants who have positive viral testing in the ED. Ill-appearing infants or neonates (28 days old and younger) should still undergo a full evaluation for SBI.

Management

Approach to the Febrile Infant and Child

The initial approach to any child with a febrile illness is a rapid assessment for evidence of cardiopulmonary compromise or shock. Significant respiratory distress, hypoxemia unresponsive to supplemental oxygen, or altered mental status may necessitate intubation by rapid sequence induction and mechanical ventilation. Evidence of shock (poor perfusion, hypotension, altered mentation) should be quickly treated with fluid resuscitation. An IV or intraosseous line should be placed, and the initial resuscitative fluid should be 20 mL/kg of isotonic crystalloid. This should be repeated to a total of 60 mL/kg over 60 minutes if signs of hypovolemia persist, followed by vasopressor therapy (dopamine 1 to 20 µg/kg/min or norepinephrine 0.05 to 2 µg/kg/min titrated to blood pressure) to maintain blood pressures.

Every effort should be made to obtain appropriate specimens for culture (blood and urine) before antibiotic administration, even in the critically ill child. Lumbar puncture may be deferred in the critically ill child until stabilization occurs. Empirical antibiotic therapy should be directed at the most likely causative organisms based on age. Sterilization of the CSF starts to occur once antibiotic administration has been initiated—within 15 minutes to 2 hours in patients with meningococcal meningitis and within 4 to 10 hours in patients with pneumococcal meningitis. However, antibiotics should not be delayed awaiting successful lumbar puncture. Antibiotics will not affect PCR or bacterial antigen test results.

Infants 0 to 28 Days Old

Children presenting with a temperature of 100.4°F (38.0°C) or higher who are younger than 28 days old are at particularly high risk for bacterial illness, with rates as high as 12%.[17] Often, fever is the only manifestation of potentially life-threatening disease, with other signs and symptoms that may be exceedingly subtle. This has led to a conservative approach to diagnostic testing, empirical antibiotic therapy, and hospitalization in this age group, even if the child appears well.

Children in this age group often present with nonspecific complaints, such as irritability, lethargy, poor feeding, and grunting. Besides fever, other signs of serious illness include a bulging fontanel, mottled extremities, petechiae, and tachypnea. Bacterial pathogens in this age group include *E. coli,* group B streptococcus, *L. monocytogenes, and less commonly, N. meningitidis, S. pneumoniae.* Viral pathogens, including RSV and HSV, are also important considerations. Neonatal HSV infection carries a high degree of morbidity and mortality and should be considered in any febrile neonate who appears ill, presents with fever and seizure, has cutaneous vesicles on physical examination, has evidence of transaminitis or coagulopathy, or has a maternal history of genital herpes. HSV meningoencephalitis should also be considered in patients with fever and CSF pleocytosis but a negative CSF Gram stain. The highest risk period for HSV disease is between 2 and 12 days old

(Fig. 161.2). Other noninfectious causes of a septic-appearing neonate include inborn errors of metabolism, the acute salt-wasting crisis associated with congenital adrenal hyperplasia, and undiagnosed ductal-dependent congenital heart disease.

Because of the high risk of bacterial pathogens and the difficulty in the clinical assessment of children younger than 28 days old (neonate), febrile neonates require a thorough diagnostic evaluation, including a complete septic evaluation. This consists of a complete blood count (CBC) with differential, blood culture, urinalysis and urine culture, and lumbar puncture. Lumbar puncture is indicated in this age group even in the presence of a UTI because of the risk of concomitant meningitis. All neonates should be admitted to the hospital with empirical antibiotics while awaiting culture results. Appropriate parenteral antibiotic regimens include ampicillin (50 to 100 mg/kg every 6 to 12 hours) plus either gentamicin (4 to 5 mg/kg every 24 to 48 hours) or cefepime (50 mg/kg every 8 to 12 hours). Ceftriaxone should be avoided in infants younger than 28 days old because ceftriaxone causes bilirubin to be displaced from its protein binding sites and has a theoretical risk of inducing acute bilirubin

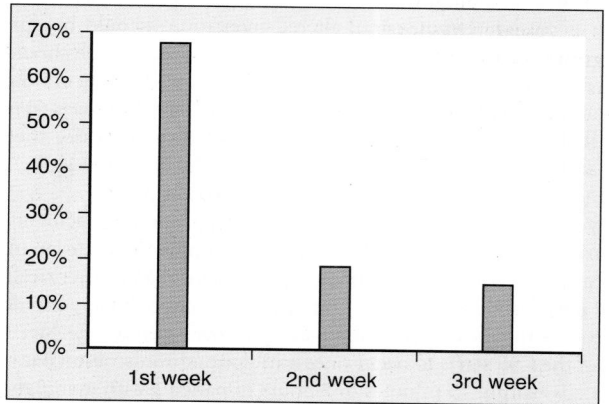

Fig. 161.2 Age at Presentation for Neonatal Herpes Simplex Virus (HSV) Infection.

encephalopathy. Empirical acyclovir should be added if risk factors for HSV disease exist or a pleocytosis is found in the CSF (20 mg/kg every 8 hours if adequate renal function).

Infants 29 to 90 Days Old

Although there is a relative consensus as to the evaluation and management of febrile infants younger than 28 days old, there is debate about the appropriate evaluation for slightly older febrile infants. Ill-appearing children of any age should have a complete sepsis evaluation performed and be admitted to the hospital with empirical antibiotic therapy. Appropriate antibiotic therapy for high-risk children includes coverage of neonatal pathogens, such as *L. monocytogenes* and group B streptococci, as well as coverage against *H. influenzae*, *N. meningitidis*, and *S. pneumoniae*. Ampicillin (50 to 100 mg/kg every 6 to 12 hours based on gestational age and renal function) plus ceftriaxone (50 mg/kg every 12 hours) are two reasonable options. Vancomycin, 10 to 20 mg/kg IV every 6 to 8 hours, should be considered if *S. pneumoniae* resistant to penicillins and cephalosporins is suspected.

Historically, various strategies (herein referred to as the *Rochester, Philadelphia, and Boston criteria*) for the evaluation of well-appearing children have been reported, compared, and retested in the literature. Each strategy has unique features, including the definition of fever (100.4°F [38.0°C] vs. 100.8°F [38.2°C]), the study population (0 to 3 months old, 1 to 2 months old, and 1 to 3 months old), the clinical and laboratory variables studied, and the disposition (hospitalization with or without antibiotics or outpatient treatment with or without antibiotics). Each strategy seeks to identify a set of low-risk criteria that, if met, identify patients that may forgo further testing or empirical antibiotic therapy. The three main strategies are highlighted in Table 161.2. Baraff synthesized the recommendations of the Rochester, Philadelphia, and Boston criteria into an algorithm for the management of the previously healthy febrile infant 29 to 90 days old (Fig. 161.3). To be low risk, the child had to have been previously healthy with an uncomplicated nursery stay, to be nontoxic clinically, and to have no focal source of bacterial infection. Low-risk laboratory criteria in this schema included a normal WBC count (between 5000 and 15,000 WBCs/mm^3), fewer than 1500 bands/mm^3, normal urinalysis (negative Gram stain and

TABLE 161.2	Summary of Major Strategies for the Management of Febrile Infants Younger Than 3 Months Old		
	Philadelphia	**Rochester**	**Boston**
Age	29–60 days old	<60 days old	28–89 days old
Temperature	>100.8°F (38.2°C)	>100.4°F (38.0°C)	>100.4°F (38.0°C)
Examination	Well, no focus	Well, no focus	Well, no focus
Laboratory values (define low risk)	WBCs >15,000/mm^3	WBCs 5000–15,000/mm^3	WBCs <20,000/mm^3
	Band/neutrophil ratio <0.2	Absolute band count <1500	UA <10 WBCs/hpf
	UA <10 WBCs/hpf (negative Gram stain)	UA <10 WBCs/hpf	CSF <10 WBCs/hpf
	CSF <8 WBCs/hpf (negative Gram stain)	Stool <5 WBCs/hpf (if obtained)	Chest radiograph normal (if obtained)
	Chest radiograph normal, stool negative (if obtained)		
High risk	Admission + IV antibiotics	Admission + IV antibiotics	Admission + IV antibiotics
Low risk	Home, no antibiotics	Home, no antibiotics	Home, empirical antibiotics
Performance	Sensitivity 98% (92%–100%)	Sensitivity 92% (83%–97%)	Sensitivity not available
	Specificity 42% (38%–46%)	Specificity 50% (47%–53%)	Specificity not available
	PPV 14% (11%–17%)	PPV 12% (10%–16%)	PPV not available
	NPV 99.7% (98%–100%)	NPV 98.9% (97%–100%)	NPV 94.6%

CSF, Cerebrospinal fluid; *IV*, intravenous; *NPV*, negative predictive value; *PPV*, positive predictive value; *UA*, urinalysis; *WBC*, white blood cell; *WBCs/hpf*, white blood cells per high-power field.

<5 WBCs per high-power field), and negative CSF Gram stain and cell counts (<8 WBCs/mm³), if obtained. When diarrhea was present, fewer than 5 WBCs per high-power field was the threshold for low risk. Since this publication, numerous variations of these historical criteria have been developed, modified, and tested.[18–21] All seek to identify criteria that categorize febrile young infants into "high risk" and "low risk" groups based on historical features (e.g., prematurity, prior antibiotic exposure, past medical history), physical examination findings (e.g., hyperpyrexia, focal infection) and laboratory parameters (e.g., elevated or depressed WBC, elevated procalcitonin, elevated CRP). Studies evaluating the various permutations of the evaluation of a febrile infant all perform similarly, emphasizing consistent use of a set of criteria is more critical than which set of criteria are used. The use of an evidence-based guideline to standardize the evaluation and disposition of young infants has been shown to reduce costs.

An infant who meets "low risk" criteria can be appropriately managed in several ways. For instance, one management strategy may call for a CBC, blood culture, urinalysis, and urine culture. If the results reveal the patient to be at low risk, the child may be discharged without antibiotics with close outpatient follow-up. If results are abnormal, the patient should receive a lumbar puncture and antibiotics. Another option, based on the Boston criteria, calls for a complete sepsis evaluation, including lumbar puncture, followed by empirical treatment with or without ceftriaxone (50 mg/kg IV or intramuscularly [IM]) and reevaluation within 24 hours. Generally, antibiotics should not be administered unless a complete sepsis evaluation is performed (including a lumbar puncture); children treated with antibiotics will not have reliable culture results if performed much later.

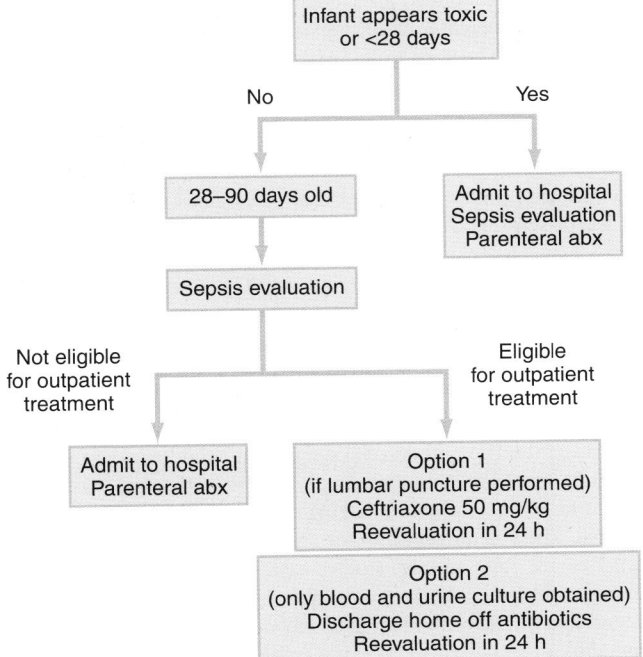

Fig. 161.3 Sample Algorithm for the Management of Febrile Infants Younger than 3 Months Old. To be eligible for outpatient treatment, the following should be met: white blood cell (WBC) count 5000 to 15,000 cells/mm³, urinalysis is negative, lumbar puncture without pleocytosis or bacteria on Gram stain, able to return for care if necessary, reliable outpatient follow-up, no focal infection present (i.e., cellulitis, omphalitis), and chest radiograph and stool studies negative if obtained. *abx,* Antibiotics.

Infants 3 to 36 Months Old

Most cases of fever in children 3 to 36 months old represent self-limited viral illnesses. Common causes of fever in this age group include viral upper respiratory infections, croup, bronchiolitis, stomatitis (typically caused by HSV or coxsackievirus), gastroenteritis, roseola, and fifth disease (parvovirus B19 infection). Focal infections, such as pyelonephritis, periorbital cellulitis, bacterial pharyngitis (group A streptococcus), septic arthritis, retropharyngeal abscess, meningitis, and bacterial pneumonia, also become more common in this age group. Typically, these focal infections are apparent on the basis of history and physical examination findings, and diagnostic testing and treatment should be directed accordingly.

The history in this age group should focus on the duration of illness, associated symptoms that may focus the evaluation, immunization history (particularly vaccination for *H. influenzae* type B and pneumococcus), and sick contacts. A thorough physical examination is essential to rule out serious focal infection, such as meningitis. Young children may demonstrate inconsolable irritability or lethargy as the sole manifestation of meningitis; furthermore, classic meningeal signs, such as nuchal rigidity, are seen in less than 27% of infants (0 to 6 months old) with bacterial meningitis.

Prior research has focused on the assessment of children in this age group for the presence of occult bacteremia. It was found that a small percentage of highly febrile children (>102.2°F [39.0°C]) 3 to 36 months old were bacteremic. These children were noted to be highly febrile but lacked any localizing signs of infection. No historical or physical examination findings were sufficiently sensitive or specific to identify cases of occult bacteremia, making universal diagnostic testing necessary. A typical evaluation included a CBC and blood culture, and empirical antibiotic therapy was prescribed for children with WBC counts above 15,000/mm³. Empirical antibiotics were justified on the basis of studies that revealed treatment with antibiotics prevented focal sequelae of bacteremia, such as meningitis, and shortened the duration of fever. Before almost universal immunization against *S. pneumoniae*, the rate of occult bacteremia was approximately 3%, and although pneumococcal bacteremia resolved without therapy up to 75% of the time, a small proportion of children had sepsis or focal infections, such as meningitis. Pneumococcal meningitis has a high degree of morbidity and mortality, including permanent neurologic disability, hearing loss, and death.

Since the advent of PCV7 (conjugate pneumococcal vaccine) and most recently PCV13, the number of invasive pneumococcal infections caused by vaccine-serogroup isolates among eight children's hospitals in the United States has decreased more than 75% among children younger than 24 months old. Because of the decline in invasive pneumococcal disease, young children with fever of unknown source no longer require blood culture; instead, clinical judgment should select high-risk populations that might benefit from testing and treatment. Although the incidence of pneumococcal bacteremia has declined in infants 3 to 36 months old because of the deliberate campaign to vaccinate, infants 3 to 6 months old have not yet completed the primary series of immunizations against *S. pneumoniae* and to a lesser extent against *H. influenzae*. Despite being "incompletely vaccinated" at this age, the rate of bacteremia is exceedingly low, and we do not recommend routine screening in this age group. The 13-valent conjugate pneumococcal vaccine (PCV-13) for routine childhood vaccinations provides expanded coverage. The additional six serotypes included in PCV13 were responsible for more than 60% of the cases of invasive pneumococcal disease in the years preceding the release of the updated vaccine schedule.[22] Despite these vaccine advances, there are approximately 90 serotypes that are capable of infecting humans, and

Fever algorithm (3–36 months old)

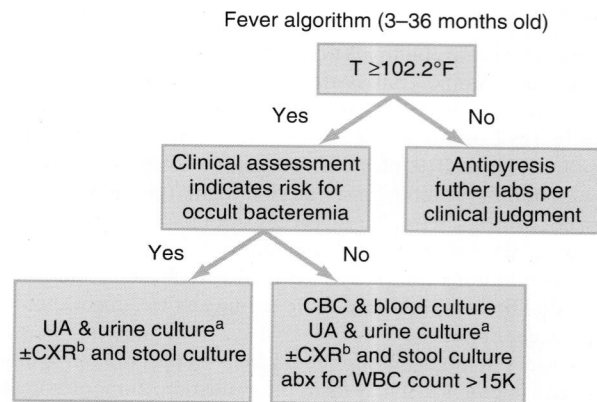

Fig. 161.4 Sample algorithm for the management of febrile infants 3 to 36 months old. ᵃFemales <24 months old; circumcised males <6 months old, uncircumcised males <12 months old. ᵇCXR for symptoms or WBC >20,000/mm³. *abx*, Antibiotics; *CBC*, complete blood count; *CXR*, chest x-ray; *T*, temperature; *UA*, urinalysis; *WBC*, white blood cell.

continued bacterial surveillance is necessary to ensure that other serotypes do not rise in incidence to fill the void left by vaccination.

No clinical prediction algorithm correctly identifies all patients with meningococcal disease. Additional signs and symptoms that may suggest meningococcemia are purpuric rash, bandemia, limb pain, and exposure to a person with the disease. A flow diagram for the evaluation of febrile infants 3 to 36 months old is presented in Fig. 161.4.

Children 3 Years Old to Adulthood

The incidence of occult bacteremia decreases after 3 years of age. Focal infections such as streptococcal pharyngitis, septic arthritis, pneumonia, peritonsillar abscess (most often in adolescents), and cellulitis become more common. Viral pathogens are also common, such as infectious mononucleosis. Infection with atypical pathogens, such as *Mycoplasma pneumoniae*, should also be considered in children presenting with pneumonia. Skin infections secondary to community-acquired methicillin-resistant *Staphylococcus aureus* (MRSA) are also becoming more common and should be considered in children who present with pyogenic skin infection and skin abscesses. Community-acquired MRSA occurs in all age groups but has clustered among such children as wrestlers (associated with contaminated wrestling mats) and football players (infected equipment). Appropriate therapy includes incision and drainage of the abscess cavity. Based on recent studies that demonstrate improved primary resolution, decreased recurrences, and decreased spread, we recommend antibiotic therapy in addition to incision and drainage, especially for patients with large abscesses (>5 cm), cellulitis, or fever.[23] Antibiotic selections should be based on local resistance patterns but could include trimethoprim-sulfamethoxazole or clindamycin for younger children and doxycycline for children 8 years old or older.

There is a second peak in incidence of meningococcal disease in adolescent children with an attack rate of 1.2 infections per 100,000 population. As opposed to infants, adolescents with meningococcal infection are more likely to present with meningococcemia (40% vs. 20%) and shock (69% vs. 27%) and to have a fatal outcome (22.5% vs. 4.6%). Meningococcal infections often manifest with one of three clinical syndromes: meningitis, bacteremia, or a combination of the two. College students residing in dormitories are at particular risk for infection, with attack rates of 3.2/100,000 population.

Meningococcal infection is often rapidly progressive, presenting with fever, headache, and a stiff neck. Shock, altered mental status or frank coma, petechiae or purpura, seizures, and myalgias are also common. Some of the first signs of meningococcal infection include leg pain, cold hands and feet, and abnormal skin mottling. Children

exposed to a patient with meningococcemia, particularly those with close contact with nasopharyngeal secretions, and who have any of the presenting signs, should receive a full septic evaluation, admission to the hospital, and empirical treatment with antibiotics until results of blood and CSF cultures. Appropriate initial therapy for children suspected of having meningococcal infection is ceftriaxone 100 mg/kg IV.

In January 2005, the U.S. Food and Drug Administration (FDA) approved the quadrivalent meningococcal conjugate vaccine (Menactra) for use in adolescents. This vaccine is a polysaccharide-protein conjugate directed against the four serotypes that cause most cases of invasive meningococcal disease in humans. The Advisory Committee on Immunization Practices recommends vaccination of adolescents at their 11- or 12-year-old well-child checkup, and the American Academy of Pediatrics (AAP) has also advised that all college freshmen living in dormitories be vaccinated. The use of the vaccine is associated with a 67% decrease in invasive disease and a 66% decrease in carriage rates. Younger children with anatomic or functional asplenia, those with complement component deficiencies, and children who travel reside in other countries where the disease is hyperendemic should be vaccinated. Based on age, a number of vaccines for the prevention of meningococcal disease are available (www.cdc.gov/vaccines/schedules/hcp/imz/child-adolescent.html).

SPECIFIC DISORDERS

Febrile Seizures

Febrile seizures are a common cause of convulsions in children younger than 5 years old.[24] They are defined as a seizure accompanied by a fever without the presence of CNS infection. They typically occur in infants and children 6 months to 5 years old. It is thought that the at-risk period is the rapid rise or defervescence of a fever rather than the absolute height of the fever. The subsequent risk of epilepsy after a febrile seizure is a common parental worry, although studies have shown that the risk is only slightly increased. The risk of epilepsy in the general population is thought to be 0.5% to 1%, whereas the risk in a patient who has had a febrile seizure is 1% to 2%. Although they are generally benign in course, febrile seizures can rarely be the presenting complaint of infants and children with CNS infection, such as meningitis. Febrile seizures are classified as either simple or complex. Simple febrile seizures are brief (<15 minutes), single, and nonfocal or generalized tonic-clonic. Complex febrile seizures are prolonged, recurrent (more than one within 24 hours), focal, prolonged, or occur outside the typical age range.

Differentiation of a benign febrile seizure from one that heralds CNS infection can be difficult. The AAP has published consensus guidelines for the evaluation and management of febrile seizures. Laboratory and radiographic evaluation should be directed at finding the source of the fever, not driven by the seizure itself. The AAP suggests that a lumbar puncture be performed in any child with signs of meningeal irritation after the first febrile seizure and be considered in symptomatic children who are incompletely immunized or have received prior antibiotic therapy.

Routine referral for neuroimaging or electroencephalography is not indicated. There is also no role for antiepileptic therapy after a single febrile seizure. Retrospective studies have shown that the incidence of meningitis after the simple or complex febrile seizures is exceedingly low and that infants with meningitis will demonstrate signs of sepsis or meningitis after the seizure, making empirical lumbar puncture based solely on a febrile seizure unnecessary.[25,26] Febrile status epilepticus, in contrast to a simple or even complex febrile seizure, carries a higher risk of meningitis and lumbar puncture should be performed in these cases. See Chapter 169 for a more in-depth discussion on pediatric seizures.

Fever and Petechiae

The presence of a petechial rash in the setting of a febrile illness is concerning for the possibility of meningococcal infection, although the vast majority are due to a viral cause. The incidence of meningococcal infection has been found to be 7% to 11% in patients hospitalized with fever and petechiae. The rate of bacteremia of any cause was found to be much lower (1.9%) in an ED population. The differential diagnosis of fever and petechiae also includes disseminated intravascular coagulation, Rocky Mountain spotted fever, pneumococcal bacteremia, *Streptococcus pyogenes* infection, various viral infections, idiopathic thrombocytopenic purpura, Henoch-Schönlein purpura, and leukemia. Petechiae can also be caused mechanically by a tourniquet, retching, or violent coughing. Petechiae due to vomiting or coughing are typically confined to the skin above the nipple line, but petechiae caused by SBI can have any distribution.

Because of the risk of serious illness in children with fever and petechiae, blood should be obtained for CBC, CRP, and culture. Patients with associated pharyngitis should undergo testing for group A streptococcus infection. Among patients presenting to a pediatric ED with a temperature higher than 100.4°F (38.0°C) and petechiae, an abnormal WBC count (<5000 WBCs/mm³ and >15,000 WBCs/mm³) or abnormal coagulation studies have been shown to be predictive but not diagnostic of invasive bacteremia. We recommend that children with fever and petechiae and an abnormal WBC, high band count, or elevated CRP be admitted and treated for presumptive bacterial infection until blood cultures result. Well-appearing children with normal WBC, CRP, and coagulation studies are unlikely to have invasive bacteremia and can be discharged without antibiotic therapy with close outpatient follow-up.

Kawasaki Disease (Mucocutaneous Lymph Node Syndrome)

Kawasaki disease is one of the most common vasculitides in childhood and should be considered in any infant or child with prolonged fever (greater than 4 days).[27] Accurate diagnosis is important because the main complication of Kawasaki disease is the development of coronary artery aneurysms. Some patients will present with "incomplete Kawasaki disease," which occurs when not all diagnostic criteria are met. Despite the lack of classic findings, these children are still at risk for coronary complications. Laboratory abnormalities found in cases of Kawasaki disease include leukocytosis, thrombocytosis (platelet counts as high as 1,000,000/mm³), and evidence of systemic inflammation with elevation in the erythrocyte sedimentation rate and CRP level.

Children with suspected Kawasaki disease should be hospitalized and receive therapy with intravenous immune globulin (IVIG; 2 g/kg infused during 10 to 12 hours) and aspirin (initial dose 80 to 100 mg/kg daily divided every 6 hours). Pediatric cardiology consultation for echocardiography is also indicated (see Chapter 165 for a more complete discussion of Kawasaki's Disease and Chapter 120 for a discussion on multi-inflammatory syndrome in children [MIS-C]).

Toxic Shock Syndrome

TSS refers to the toxin-mediated clinical syndrome that occurs from *S. aureus*, although a similar illness is caused by group A streptococcus. The toxin implicated in TSS is an exotoxin termed *TSS toxin 1*. The syndrome is classically associated with tampon use by menstruating women, although cases also occur in males and prepubertal girls from other sources of infection with *S. aureus*.

Clinical manifestations of TSS include fever (>102°F [38.9°C]), hypotension, diffuse erythroderma, and multisystem involvement. Patients may present with vomiting or diarrhea, severe myalgias, oropharyngeal hyperemia, or altered mental status. Laboratory abnormalities are common and include elevated creatine kinase, elevated blood urea nitrogen or creatinine, transaminitis, and thrombocytopenia. The Centers for Disease Control and Prevention (CDC) has developed a set of findings for case definition (Box 161.1).

Treatment of TSS involves fluid resuscitation because these patients typically have immense requirements and antistaphylococcal antibiotic

---

BOX 161.1 Centers for Disease Control and Prevention Case Definition for Toxic Shock Syndrome

Fever: Temperature >102°F (38.9°C)

Hypotension: Systolic blood pressure 90 mm Hg for adults or less than fifth percentile by age for children <16 years old; orthostatic drop in diastolic blood pressure by 15 mm Hg

Orthostatic syncope or dizziness

Diffuse erythroderma

Desquamation: 1–2 weeks after onset of illness, particularly involving palms and soles

Multisystem involvement (three or more of the following organ systems):
- Gastrointestinal: Vomiting or diarrhea at onset of illness
- Muscular: Severe myalgia or creatine kinase elevation more than two times the normal upper limit
- Mucous membranes: Vaginal, oropharyngeal, or conjunctival hyperemia
- Renal: Blood urea nitrogen or serum creatinine more than two times the normal upper limit, or pyuria (>5 WBCs/high-power field)
- Hepatic: Bilirubin or transaminases more than two times the normal upper limit
- Hematologic: Platelets <100,000/L
- CNS: Disorientation or alterations in consciousness without focal neurologic signs in the absence of fever and hypotension

Negative results on the following tests, if obtained:
- Blood, throat, or CSF cultures for another pathogen (blood cultures may be positive for *Staphylococcus aureus*)
- Serologic tests for Rocky Mountain spotted fever, leptospirosis, or measles

Criteria for a probable case include a patient with temperature >102°F (38.9°C), hypotension, diffuse erythroderma, desquamation (unless the patient dies before desquamation can occur), and involvement of at least three organ systems. A probable case is a patient who is missing one of the characteristics of the confirmed case definition.

CNS, Central nervous system; *CSF*, cerebrospinal fluid; *WBC*, white blood cell.

---

therapy with clindamycin (20 to 40 mg/kg/day in three divided doses) and vancomycin (10 to 20 mg/kg IV every 6 to 8 hours).

Fever in Children With an Underlying Chronic Medical Illness

Oncology Patients

Children with cancer, particularly those undergoing treatment with cytotoxic chemotherapy, are at particular risk for sepsis and bacterial infection. These life-threatening infections are most common during periods of profound neutropenia. Neutropenia is defined as an ANC of less than 500/mL or an ANC of less than 1000/mL that is falling. Children with cancer also frequently have central venous catheters, predisposing them to central line-associated bloodstream infections.

Causative organisms include both gram-positive and gram-negative bacteria. Staphylococci and streptococci as well as *Pseudomonas* are frequent pathogens. Often, patients with focal infection may not present with classic signs because of their leukopenia. Focal infections specific to cancer patients include stomatitis and typhlitis, which is a necrotizing enterocolitis of the terminal ileum and cecum.

Children presenting with fever and possible neutropenia should receive a prompt evaluation with a goal of arrival to antibiotic therapy of fewer than 60 minutes.[28] Blood should be obtained for a CBC and manual differential diagnosis as well as culture. Once appropriate laboratory studies are obtained, empirical antibiotic therapy should be initiated without waiting for the laboratory results. Appropriate monotherapy antibiotic regimens include cefepime, 50 mg/kg IV every 8 to 12 hours based on gestational age and renal function, or ceftazidime, 50 mg/kg IV every 8 hours. Vancomycin, 10 to 20 mg/kg every 6 to 8 hours, should be added for staphylococcal coverage in children with suspected central line infections or skin and soft tissue infections. Children with fever and neutropenia are rarely treated as outpatients; in very select cases and in consultation with an oncologist, ceftriaxone 50 mg/kg IV may be given every 24 hours with close follow-up.

Patients With the Acquired Immunodeficiency Syndrome

Children with the acquired immunodeficiency syndrome (AIDS) are at risk for bacterial infection due to a whole host of different organisms—some common, some uncommon. Infections specific to AIDS include cryptococcosis and infection with *Mycobacterium tuberculosis, Mycobacterium avium-intracellulare,* and *Pneumocystis jiroveci (carinii).* Viral infections, such as cytomegalovirus and Epstein–Barr virus infections, are also common.

Laboratory evaluation should be directed by the history and physical examination. Early initiation of broad-spectrum antibiotic therapy is warranted.

Sickle Cell Disease

Febrile children with sickle cell disease are at particular risk for overwhelming infection. In fact, infection is the most common cause of sickle cell-related death, occurring in up to 40% of patients with sickle cell disease who die. Recurrent episodes of splenic infarction lead to functional asplenia early in life. Thus, these patients are at particular risk for infection with encapsulated organisms, including *S. pneumoniae* and *H. influenzae.* Because of this risk of bacterial disease, it is recommended that all children with sickle cell disease be completely immunized. Prophylaxis with penicillin is recommended in children younger than 5 years old, after which it can be safely discontinued in children who have not had a prior severe pneumococcal infection or surgical splenectomy. The dose of penicillin is 125 mg orally twice daily until 3 years old (at about 14 kg) and 250 mg orally twice daily after 3 years old.

High-risk criteria for bacterial infection include toxic appearance, temperature higher than 104°F (40°C), abnormal WBC count (<5000 or >30,000 WBCs/mm³), and noncompliance with penicillin prophylaxis. Sickle cell patients are at particular risk for *Salmonella* osteomyelitis. All patients presenting with a temperature higher than 100.4°F (38.0°C) and sickle cell disease should have a blood specimen drawn for CBC, reticulocyte count, and culture. A reticulocyte count is important because many infections (e.g., parvovirus B19) can induce a life-threatening aplastic crisis. Infection also predisposes children with sickle cell disease to acute chest syndrome. Common causes of infection include *C. pneumoniae, M. pneumoniae,* RSV, *S. aureus,* and *S. pneumoniae.* Further laboratory and radiographic evaluation should be directed by the presenting history and physical examination findings.

As defined earlier, high-risk patients should be admitted for further evaluation and antibiotic therapy. Low-risk patients may be treated with a single dose of IV or IM antibiotics, typically ceftriaxone 50 mg/kg, and discharged to close outpatient follow-up. All patients should be reevaluated within 24 hours or sooner if the clinical condition deteriorates.

Osteomyelitis typically manifests as fever and bone pain. As patients with sickle cell disease may have frequent bone pain due to vaso-occlusive crisis, the diagnosis can be difficult. All patients should have a blood specimen drawn for CBC with differential diagnosis, erythrocyte sedimentation rate, and culture; a radionuclide bone scan or magnetic resonance imaging (MRI) may help localize the infection. If *Salmonella* infection is suspected, a stool sample should be sent for culture.

Congenital Heart Disease

Children with congenital heart disease are at high risk for cardiovascular complications in the setting of febrile illness. Often, relatively minor viral illness can produce significant changes in cardiac function or make it difficult for children to be compliant with their oral medications. Children with congenital heart disease are also at risk for infective endocarditis. Infective endocarditis is heralded by fever and possibly a changing or worsening cardiac murmur. The modified Duke criteria for the diagnosis of endocarditis are presented in Box 161.2.

BOX 161.2   Modified Duke Criteria for the Diagnosis of Infective Endocarditis

Major Criteria

Blood cultures positive for IE
  Typical microorganism for IE from two separate blood cultures
  Viridians streptococci
  Streptococcus bovis, including nutritional variant strains
  HACEK group: *Haemophilus* species, *Actinobacillus actinomycetemcomitans, Cardiobacterium hominis, Eikenella* species, and *Kingella kingae*
  Staphylococcus aureus
  Community-acquired enterococci, in the absence of a primary focus; *or*
  Persistently positive blood culture, defined as recovery of a microorganism consistent with IE from blood samples drawn more than 12 hours apart; *or*
  All of three or a majority of four or more separate blood cultures, with first and last samples drawn at least 1 hour apart
  Single blood culture positive for *Coxiella burnetii* or antiphase I immunoglobulin G antibody titer >1:800
Evidence of endocardial involvement
Echocardiogram positive for IE
  TEE recommended in patients with prosthetic valves, rated at least "possible IE" by clinical criteria, or complicated IE (paravalvular abscess); TTE as the first test in other patients[a]

Definition of positive echocardiogram
Oscillating intracardiac mass on valve or supporting structures, in the path of regurgitant jets, or on implanted material in the absence of an alternative anatomic explanation; *or*
Abscess; *or*
New partial dehiscence of prosthetic valve
New valvular regurgitation (increase in or change in preexisting murmur not sufficient)

Minor Criteria

Predisposition: Predisposing heart condition or injection drug use
Fever: 100.4°F (38.0°C)
Vascular phenomena: Major arterial emboli, septic pulmonary infarcts, mycotic aneurysm, intracranial hemorrhage, conjunctival hemorrhages, Janeway lesions
Immunologic phenomena: Glomerulonephritis, Osler nodes, Roth spots, rheumatoid factor
Microbiologic evidence: Positive blood culture but not meeting major criterion (excluding single positive cultures for coagulase-negative staphylococci and organisms that do not cause endocarditis) or serologic evidence of active infection with organism consistent with IE

IE, Infective endocarditis; *TEE,* transesophageal echocardiography; *TTE,* transthoracic echocardiography.
[a] Echocardiographic minor criteria eliminated.

Endocarditis is typically caused by *S. aureus,* viridans streptococci, *Streptococcus bovis,* enterococci, or infection with organisms from the HACEK group (*Haemophilus* species, *Actinobacillus actinomycetemcomitans, Cardiobacterium hominis, Eikenella* species, and *Kingella kingae*). Children with suspected endocarditis should have blood culture specimens drawn and be admitted to the hospital for treatment and echocardiography. The American Heart Association recommends that initial antibiotic therapy be with ceftriaxone, 100 mg/kg IV or IM every 24 hours, or vancomycin, 10 to 20 mg/kg IV Q6-8H. Therapy is typically continued for at least 4 weeks. Ceftriaxone can be combined with gentamicin, 3 to 6 mg/kg IV divided every 8 hours (if renal function is normal), if shorter treatment duration (2 weeks) is desired. See Chapter 165 for a more complete discussion.

Ventriculoperitoneal Shunts

Children presenting with fever in the setting of ventriculoperitoneal shunts are at risk for shunt infection. If shunt infection is suspected, based on the presence of altered mental status or signs of meningismus, neurosurgical consultation should be obtained and a sample of CSF obtained. This is typically accomplished by sterile aspiration of fluid from the shunt reservoir. *S. aureus* and *Staphylococcus epidermidis* are the usual causative organisms. If an altered mental status is present, a computed tomography (CT) scan should be obtained to assess ventricular size. Children with suspected shunt infection are typically managed as inpatients, and antibiotics should begin as soon as possible.

The references for this chapter can be found online at ExpertConsult.com.

162

Pediatric Upper Airway Obstruction and Infections

Emily Rose

KEY CONCEPTS

Respiratory arrest precedes most pediatric cardiac arrests. Quick recognition of an airway problem and intervention in potentially life-threatening upper airway obstruction in children are critical.

Retropharyngeal Abscess

- This is a potentially life-threatening emergency in young children with signs of upper airway obstruction or meningismus; a retropharyngeal abscess is often related to oral trauma.
- Retropharyngeal abscess is most frequently caused by *Staphylococcus aureus,* group A streptococci, and anaerobes. Treatment is admission, IV antibiotics, and for more severe cases, surgical drainage.

Epiglottitis

- Epiglottitis may be caused by many bacteria or local injury. In the post–*Haemophilus influenzae* type b vaccine era, the incidence of pediatric epiglottitis has decreased, and epiglottitis is now more likely in older patients.
- Clinical features of epiglottitis are often subtle, such as in the older adolescent, (e.g., sore throat out of proportion to physical findings, anterior neck tenderness), but may also be dramatic, as in infants and young children (i.e., drooling, stridor, toxicity, severe respiratory distress).

Croup

- Viral croup is the most common infection of the upper airway in young children.
- Glucocorticoids (usually given as a single oral dose of dexamethasone) reduce symptoms, hospitalizations, and length of stay in the emergency department (ED).

- Treatment of moderate to severe croup includes vaporized epinephrine in addition to glucocorticoids. Patients can be discharged from the ED after a posttreatment observation period. We recommend discharge after a period of observation, if the child is free of resting stridor and distress and has access to follow-up care.

Bacterial Tracheitis

- Suspect bacterial tracheitis when an upper respiratory infection (URI) progresses to acute toxicity and marked respiratory distress and stridor. Standard treatment for croup may be tried, but usually does not significantly improve the patient's symptoms. Antibiotic therapy should include a cephalosporin plus coverage for *S. aureus*, which is the most common cause of this infection.
- Bronchoscopy is diagnostic and therapeutic and should be emergently performed.

Airway Foreign Body

- Complete obstruction due to an airway foreign body requires emergent life support procedures for removal of the foreign body.
- Plain films may be negative in aspirated foreign bodies. Bronchoscopy should be performed with a clinical suspicion of aspiration.
- Emergency cricothyroidotomy may be required for obstructed patients who cannot be intubated or ventilated as a lifesaving temporizing measure; needle cricothyroidotomy is preferred for infants and young children because of the challenges in identifying landmarks and associated complications of surgical cricothyrotomy.

FOUNDATIONS

Respiratory distress from upper airway obstruction is a rare but potentially a catastrophic emergency in young children. Causes include acute infectious processes, congenital anomalies, or a foreign body in the airway or esophagus. Children are predisposed to respiratory failure due to increased airway resistance (small, compressible airway), low functional residual capacity, high oxygen metabolism, which leads to quicker fatigue, and shorter safe apnea time, with precipitous hypoxia.

Clinical presentations of children with upper airway disease vary with cause, predisposing factors, and age at presentation:

- Acute infections of the upper airway range from relatively mild distress and self-limited signs and symptoms, to the abrupt onset of a rapidly progressive airway obstruction.
- Undiagnosed congenital anomalies of the airway and surrounding structures may be manifested as chronic or progressive stridor, or simply difficulty with feeding.

- An infant with a congenital airway anomaly in whom an acute airway infection develops is at higher risk for decompensation and respiratory failure.
- Upper airway obstruction from a foreign body in the airway or esophagus can cause partial or complete airway obstruction and may require urgent, advanced, airway management skills.

CLINICAL FEATURES

Recent history and observation of the child typically provide clues to the cause of the airway obstruction. Important items to elucidate in the history include the following:

- Onset and duration (acute vs. chronic)
- Associated symptoms (e.g., respiratory distress, fever, toxicity, drooling, cyanosis, neck stiffness, or torticollis)
- Progression with age (number of bouts and severity of "croup" with increasing age)

- Exacerbating factors (supine vs. prone position, upper respiratory infection [URI], crying)
- Feeding abnormality or dysphagia
- Prior airway procedures, such as intubation in the neonatal period
- Choking episode indicating possible foreign body aspiration
- Baseline noises, quality of cry and voice to assist the emergency clinician in pinpointing the location of obstructive lesion

Initial observation can be quickly assessed utilizing the Pediatric Assessment Triangle (see Chapter 155). Observation and physical examination should include vital signs (respiratory rate, heart rate, oxygen saturation) and indicators of increased work of breathing (retractions, flaring, grunting, stridor, wheezing) to gauge the severity of distress. Observe the character and timing of stridor, as well as the symmetry and quality of breath sounds. Respiratory failure is identified by the presence of extreme distress: hypoventilation or hyperventilation; altered mental status; pale, mottled, or cyanotic skin color; or hypotonia. Stridor may not be present in respiratory failure due to the lack of airflow.

Stridor (from the Latin, *stridulus,* indicating creaking, whistling, or grating) is the classic sound associated with upper airway obstruction. Stridor is a harsh vibratory sound of variable pitch caused by partial airway obstruction or collapse and the resultant turbulent airflow through some portion of the airway, from the nose to the trachea. Stridor is described by timing in the respiratory cycle (inspiratory, expiratory, biphasic) and quality (coarse or high-pitched; Table 162.1). Inspiratory stridor is usually associated with obstruction above the glottis, expiratory stridor with intrathoracic obstruction, and biphasic stridor typically with a critical or fixed obstruction at any level. Stridor character differs by cause and anatomic location (Fig. 162.1).

Snoring or stertor is low-pitched inspiratory noise caused by nasal or nasopharyngeal obstruction. Stertor and stridor can coexist. Stridor from the pharynx, such as from a peritonsillar abscess (PTA), tends to have a sonorous, gurgling, and coarse quality. The voice may be altered and have a muffled or "hot potato" quality to it. High-pitched inspiratory stridor occurs in the supraglottic and immediate subglottic trachea, as in croup and laryngomalacia. The voice may sound hoarse or weak, but a normal voice may be heard, even with a laryngeal cause of stridor.

Biphasic stridor is heard with inspiration and expiration and usually suggests a fixed lesion. Examples include laryngeal webs and vocal cord paralysis. Stridor from the lower part of the trachea is usually expiratory, such as in bacterial tracheitis or aspirated foreign bodies (Fig. 162.2).

Diagnostic Testing and Management

Definitive airway management takes precedence in an acute airway emergency. An individualized diagnostic evaluation can be undertaken in a less critical, stable patient with an uncertain diagnosis. Lateral and anteroposterior radiographs of the soft tissues of the neck may be helpful to assess the adenoid and tonsillar size, contour of the epiglottis, thickness of the retropharyngeal soft tissue space, vallecula, aryepiglottic folds, and tracheal air column (Fig. 162.3). The child's head should be positioned in extension and film taken during inspiration. However, plain radiographs are commonly misleading and may be normal, even with significant underlying pathology. Chest views assess the heart size, trachea and bronchi, location of the aortic arch, and presence of other pulmonary pathologic processes.

Additional studies may be indicated in specific settings. Bedside fiberoptic nasopharyngoscopy allows for the visualization and assessment of the supraglottic structures and vocal cords and can assist with intubation when indicated. Esophagography can define lesions compressing the airway and trachea; computed tomography (CT),

TABLE 162.1 Causes of Stridor: Anatomic Location, Sound, and Quality

Features (Structures)	Supraglottic (Nose, Pharynx, Epiglottitis)	Glottic (Larynx, Vocal Cords)	Subglottic Trachea (Lower Trachea)
Sound	Sonorous (stertor)	Biphasic stridor	High-pitched stridor
	Gurgling		Inspiratory stridor
	Coarse		Expiratory stridor (if intrathoracic)
	Expiratory stridor		
Congenital	Micrognathia	Laryngomalacia	Subglottic stenosis
	Pierre Robin syndrome	Vocal cord paralysis	Tracheomalacia
	Treacher-Collins syndrome	Laryngeal web	Tracheal stenosis
	Macroglossia	Laryngocele	Vascular ring
	Down syndrome		Hemangioma cyst
	Storage diseases		
	Choanal atresia		
	Lingual thyroid		
	Thyroglossal cyst		
Acquired	Adenopathy	Papillomas	Croup
	Tonsillar hypertrophy	Foreign body	Bacterial tracheitis
	Foreign body		Subglottic stenosis
	Pharyngeal abscess		Foreign body
	Epiglottitis		
Positional stridor	Micrognathia, macroglossia		Laryngomalacia

magnetic resonance imaging (MRI), or bronchoscopy may be needed to evaluate the upper airway.

Specific Disorders

Supraglottic Airway Diseases

The supraglottic portion of the airway includes the nose, pharynx, epiglottis, and surrounding structures. Diseases of the nose and pharynx are commonly associated with noisy congested breathing and respiratory distress. Congenital lesions involving these structures may cause mild symptoms at baseline, but dramatic distress when there is a superimposed infectious process. Congenital lesions include choanal atresia, macroglossia, micrognathia, thyroglossal duct cyst, and lingular thyroid. Acquired causes of supraglottic disease include a nasal foreign body, nasal polyps, hypertrophic tonsils and adenoids, epiglottitis, retropharyngeal abscess (RPA), PTA, pharyngitis, mononucleosis, and upper airway foreign body. The most common conditions are discussed in the following sections.

Congenital Lesions

Choanal atresia. All infants are obligate nose breathers; they breathe nasally when the mouth is closed to allow breathing while feeding. In choanal atresia, the most common congenital anomaly of

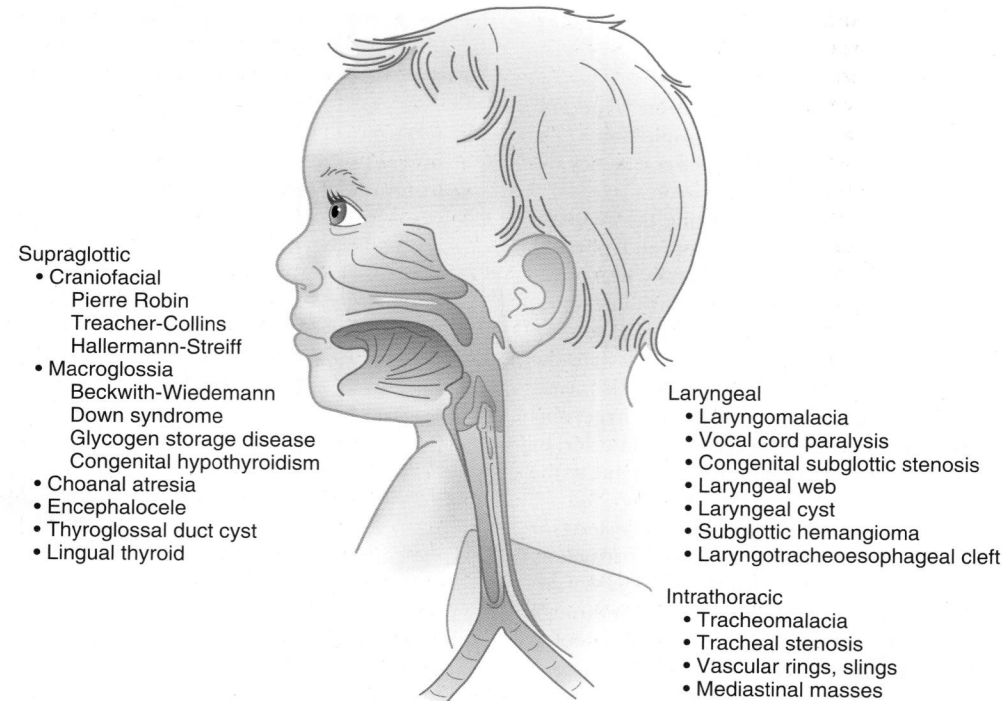

Fig. 162.1 Regions and Associated Diseases of the Pediatric Upper Airway. (From Simon NP, Simon N. Evaluation and management of stridor in the newborn. *Clin Pediatr [Phila]*. 1991;30:211.)

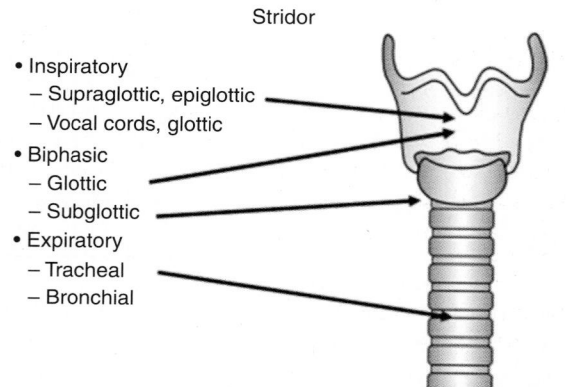

Fig. 162.2 Level of Obstruction Correlates with Phase of Stridor. (From Ida JB, Thompson DM. Pediatric stridor. *Otolaryngol Clin North Am*. 2014;47:795–819.)

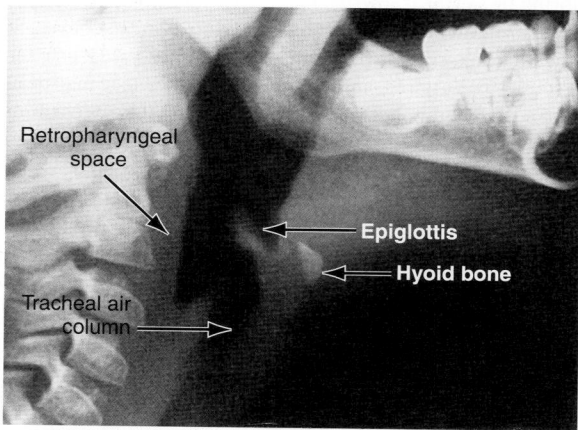

Fig. 162.3 Normal Appearance of Upper Airway Structures on a Lateral Neck Radiographic Study. Note the hyoid bone, epiglottis, retropharyngeal space, and tracheal air column.

the nose, there is persistence of the bucconasal membrane or a bony septum in the posterior naris. The posterior aspect of the infant's soft palate extends downward and contacts the tip of the epiglottis. Bilateral choanal atresia is a life-threatening emergency that is almost always identified early, as neonates become acutely distressed and cyanotic at birth. Immediate airway management is with oral airway and definitive surgical correction of the obstructing membrane. Unilateral choanal atresia is often initially undetected. Infants may present in respiratory distress with a URI when the normal patent naris is obstructed by swelling or secretions. Immediate nasal suction should be performed along with urgent referral for surgical repair.

Macroglossia. Macroglossia, an abnormally large tongue that protrudes posteriorly into the hypopharynx, is associated with conditions such as Down syndrome, glycogen storage disease, and congenital hypothyroidism. The increased secretions with a URI exacerbate underlying obstruction and may induce stridor or labored breathing. Good head positioning with nasal suctioning should be performed to relieve the obstruction.

Micrognathia. With micrognathia, an abnormally small mandible posteriorly displaces the normal-sized tongue (e.g., Pierre Robin and Treacher-Collins syndromes). Obstructive symptoms typically worsen when supine.

Pharyngitis

Infection is the most common cause of sore throat in children. Viruses cause the majority of infections. Certain viruses have characteristic features such as coxsackie A viruses that manifest as herpangina or hand, foot, and mouth disease. Herpes simplex more commonly causes stomatitis and less commonly may cause pharyngitis. *Streptococcus pyogenes* (Group A streptococcus) is the most common bacterial infectious etiology (see Chapter 19). Diphtheria can cause a thick exudative tonsillar membrane. Acetaminophen (15 mg/kg/dose q4h) or ibuprofen (10 mg/kg/dose q6h) is sufficient supportive treatment for most causes of pharyngitis.

Peritonsillar Abscess

PTA is the most common deep neck infection and usually occurs in older children and teenagers. Drooling and a muffled, hot potato voice is common, but severe respiratory distress is unusual. PTA is associated with trismus (in two out of three patients), bulging or asymmetry of the tonsils, and deviation of the uvula away from the abscess side (in 50% of patients). Throat pain may radiate to the ear. Treatment involves antibiotics and incision and drainage or needle aspiration. Antibiotics alone are insufficient management for an abscess but may resolve a phlegmon or cellulitis.[1] Surgical intervention typically removes the majority of purulence, but additional antibiotics are recommended to clear the remaining infection.

PTAs are typically polymicrobial. Predominant bacterial species are *S. pyogenes* (group A streptococcus), *Staphylococcus aureus* (including Methicillin-resistant *S. aureus* [MRSA]), and respiratory anaerobes. Posterior pharynx ultrasonography can confirm the diagnosis and guide treatment.[2,3] A CT scan may be indicated if extension of infection is suspected. Any drainage effort should take great care to avoid puncture of the carotid artery (the carotid artery lies 25 mm posterolateral to the tonsillar pillar in children >12 years). Approximately 10% to 20% of patients have recurrent PTAs.

Mononucleosis

Infectious mononucleosis, caused by the Epstein-Barr virus (EBV), can lead to mucosal edema and an exudative pharyngitis. Uncommonly, massive tonsillar enlargement can occur and create upper airway distress. EBV IgM antibody is the preferred test for infective mononucleosis (>90% sensitive), particularly in children younger than 4 years who are less likely to generate heterophile antibodies with primary EBV infection. In older children and adults, the heterophile antibody can be detected in 50% of patients within the first week of illness and in 60% to 90% in weeks 2 and 3.

In addition to airway management and general supportive care, there may be additional benefits of steroids in reducing tonsillar edema and pain.[4] Although steroids decrease pharyngitis symptoms, it is important to consider an underlying lymphoid malignancy. Children often present with sore throat prior to malignancy diagnosis. Treatment with glucocorticoids prior to the diagnosis of leukemia may delay leukemia diagnosis, increase the risk of tumor lysis syndrome, complicate risk stratification, and ultimately result in fatal complications. Therefore, great caution should be exercised in using glucocorticoids in children and adolescents and should be avoided in children younger than 14 years or in a child who has any signs of possible lymphoid malignancy such as lymphadenopathy, hepatosplenomegaly, rash, or abnormal complete blood count.

Retropharyngeal Abscess

A RPA is a potentially life-threatening airway emergency resulting from infection of the retropharyngeal soft tissue space. The retropharyngeal space is a potential space between the posterior pharyngeal wall and prevertebral fascia that extends from the base of the skull to the level of T2. It is rich in lymph tissue that drains the nose, pharynx, sinuses, and ears. An abscess may result from direct trauma from a fall with a hard object in the mouth that penetrates the soft tissue, suppuration of

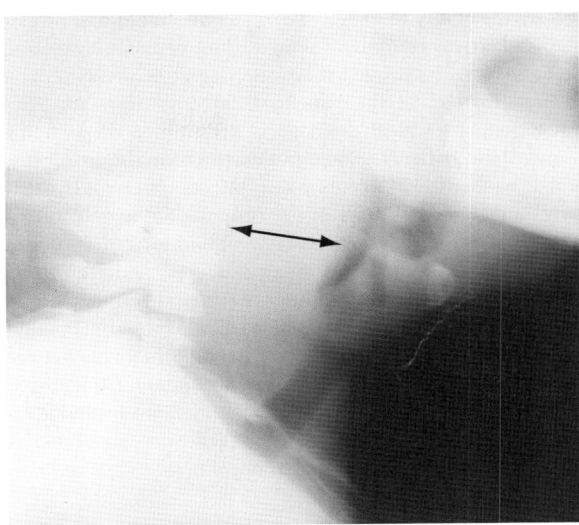

Fig. 162.4 Retropharyngeal Abscess. Note the widened retropharyngeal soft tissue space *(double arrow)*.

lymph nodes, contiguous spread of infection, or hematogenous seeding. RPA is usually a disease of young children because the lymphatic chains are prominent in the young and atrophy before puberty; RPA in older children often occurs after inciting trauma. These infections are commonly polymicrobial, with *Streptococcus* and anaerobes being the most commonly isolated organisms. MRSA is increasing in incidence and is commonly associated with severe infections such as jugular venous thrombosis or mediastinal extension.

Clinical features. Retropharyngeal infections typically progress from cellulitis to organized phlegmon to mature abscess. Presenting symptoms may vary. Common signs and symptoms include fever, sore throat, neck stiffness or nuchal rigidity, torticollis, trismus, neck swelling, drooling, stridor, and muffled voice. Stridor and respiratory distress may occur if a large abscess compresses the trachea; the clinical appearance can resemble that of epiglottitis. Reluctance to extend the neck and an unwillingness to look side to side is often seen with RPA and may help differentiate it from other supraglottic infections. With less obvious signs of airway obstruction, patients can exhibit a mixture of symptoms, including fever, neck stiffness, and generalized toxicity, which may suggest meningitis or sepsis. Other serious complications of a RPA include aspiration pneumonia, mediastinitis, and empyema.

Diagnostic testing. Careful evaluation of airway patency takes precedence in the management of a child with a presumed RPA. Examination of the pharynx may reveal bulging of the posterior pharyngeal wall. A soft tissue lateral view of the neck may be helpful to establish the diagnosis; in the normal patient, the width of the retropharyngeal space should not exceed the diameter of the adjacent vertebral body (Fig. 162.4). The soft tissue width should not be larger than 7 mm at C2, regardless of the patient's age. At C6, this distance should not exceed 14 mm in children younger than 15 years and 22 mm in adults. Most patients will demonstrate retropharyngeal thickening on the lateral neck radiograph. An air-fluid level may be present with perforation or anaerobic infections. Redundant soft tissue of the retropharyngeal space complicates the interpretation of lateral neck films in young infants with an RPA. Artefactual widening of a normal retropharyngeal space is commonly seen when the radiograph is taken with the head and neck in flexion or during exhalation. CT scanning of the neck (thin cuts to T2) may be beneficial in delineating the size and extent of an abscess and determining possible impingement on airway structures. The ability to tolerate lying supine should first be assessed, and staff and airway equipment should be immediately available.

Management. The size of the abscess, degree of airway obstruction, and overall toxicity of the patient dictate management. The need for intubation or surgical drainage is determined on an individual basis, and these patients generally benefit from the involvement of an otolaryngologist. Intubation can be complicated by distorted anatomy and can lead to abscess rupture. Some retropharyngeal infections respond to intravenous (IV) antibiotics and do not require surgical drainage.[5] Features that suggest abscess and require surgical intervention include imaging findings of scalloping of the abscess wall, rim enhancement, and lesions larger than 2 cm. The decision to admit and provide a trial of antibiotic therapy should be made between the emergency clinician and otolaryngology consultant. Clindamycin and a third-generation cephalosporin are recommended antibiotic therapy. Vancomycin or linezolid should be added with suspected MRSA infection, resistant cases, or with systemic illness.

Ludwig's Angina

Ludwig's angina is a rapidly spreading, woody induration or brawny cellulitis of the sublingual, submandibular, and submaxillary spaces, with the potential for airway obstruction. Most patients have dental sources of infection, which are usually polymicrobial. The spread of infection is direct and not via the lymphatics, so involvement is typically bilateral and without associated lymphadenopathy. Hallmark signs include enlargement and elevation of the tongue above the lower teeth, a tender woody induration in the sublingual space, trismus, and odynophagia. Ludwig's angina can create a functional upper airway obstruction or respiratory distress through significant swelling and direct airway compression. Subsequent abscess formation may occur. CT evaluates the extent of infection but MRI may better delineate soft tissue involvement. Treatment involves broad-spectrum IV antibiotics with anaerobic coverage, airway support, and admission for close monitoring. Otolaryngology and anesthesia consultants may facilitate planning and support if an emergent airway is required.

Epiglottitis

Although still a feared pediatric emergency, acute epiglottitis has declined markedly in incidence since the widespread administration of the *Haemophilus influenzae* type b vaccine in the 1980s.

Foundations. Epiglottitis is an invasive bacterial disease that causes inflammation and edema of the epiglottis, aryepiglottic folds, arytenoids, and surrounding supraglottic tissues. As these structures become inflamed and distended, they protrude downward and over the glottic opening. Supraglottic swelling reduces the upper airway caliber and causes turbulent airflow during inspiration (stridor). The epiglottis may also act as a ball valve, obstructing airflow during inspiration but permitting exhalation. This traditional profile of *H. influenzae* type b (Hib) in young children has changed; the overall incidence has decreased, and now epiglottitis is relatively more common in older children and adults. However, Hib is still the most common infectious cause of epiglottitis in children and can occur in fully immunized children. Additional causes include other *H. influenzae* types (A, F, nontypeable), streptococci, *S. aureus* (including methicillin-resistant strains), and *Neisseria meningitidis*.[6,7] Immunocompromised children may have other infections such as *Pseudomonas aeruginosa* and *Candida* spp. Noninfectious causes are rare and include thermal injury from swallowing hot liquids, steam inhalation, caustic ingestions, allergic reactions, foreign body and irritant injuries, and lymphoproliferative disorders.

Clinical features. Epiglottitis is classically acute in onset. It is marked by high fever, intense sore throat, toxicity, and rapid

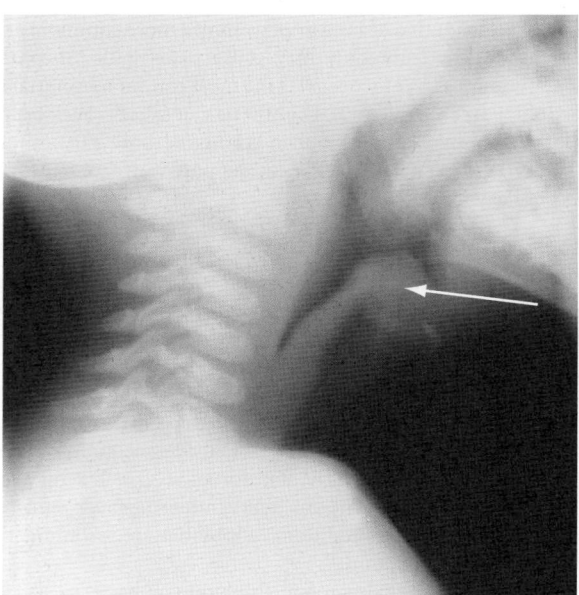

Fig. 162.5 Epiglottitis. Note the thumbprint sign of the epiglottis *(arrow)* and thickened aryepiglottic folds.

progression. Children with epiglottitis appear anxious and maintain a sniffing or tripod position, with the jaw jutting forward and the neck extended to maximize airway patency. As symptoms worsen, cough and phonation are usually absent. Drooling is prominent because of an inability to swallow. Toxicity, altered mental status, dyspnea, stridor, retractions, and fever are common initial symptoms; the diagnosis is often delayed and is associated with a significantly increased mortality rate. Croup is a common misdiagnosis made in young children and those without prominent drooling and difficulty swallowing. The older patient is less likely to show dramatic signs of upper airway obstruction compared with the younger child because the diameter of the airway is larger and thus takes a greater degree of swelling to produce symptoms. These patients often complain of a sore throat that is out of proportion to physical findings and may also exhibit tenderness on palpation of the anterior neck. Epiglottitis caused by bacteria other than *H. influenzae* tends to have a slower onset and is less likely to cause airway compromise. Epiglottic abscess may occur, particularly in adolescents. Patients with immunodeficiency may develop necrotizing epiglottitis.

Diagnostic testing. When epiglottitis is strongly suspected, a lateral neck radiograph can be helpful to confirm the diagnosis and should be evaluated for an enlarged epiglottis (thumbprint sign; Fig. 162.5), thickened aryepiglottic folds, lack of air in the vallecula, and dilated hypopharynx. However, up to 70% of all patients with epiglottitis have normal radiographic findings. Careful observation of a child in consultation with an otolaryngologist is essential, and clinicians skilled in airway management should accompany the patient at all times; the risk of obstruction is particularly high in younger children with smaller airways.

Management. For the younger child, the importance of securing the airway takes precedence over diagnostic evaluation. A stable patient who is maintaining a patent airway and adequate oxygenation should not be moved or repositioned for examination, laboratory tests, or radiography. Such patients should be carefully transported to a setting where definitive airway management can be achieved in a controlled fashion, generally the operating room. Adolescents with epiglottitis generally have signs and symptoms of adults and do not often require airway stabilization. These patients can be managed as inpatients in a pediatric intensive care unit (PICU) setting with IV antibiotics but do

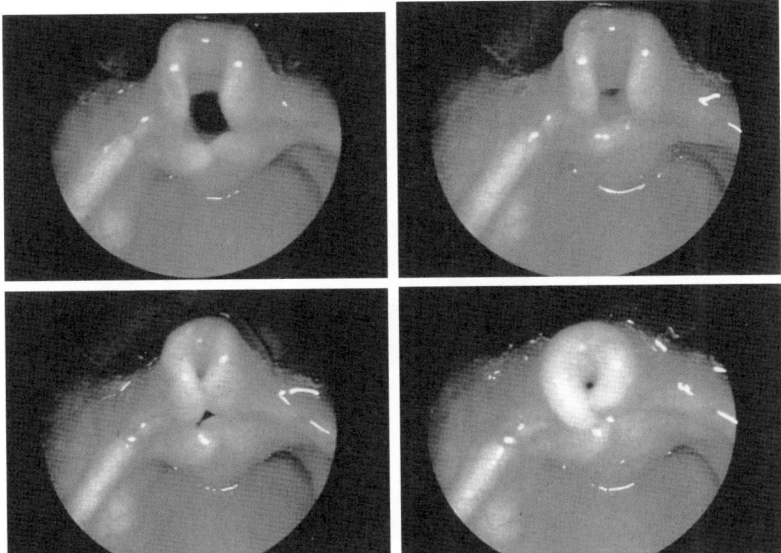

Fig. 162.6 Laryngomalacia. Note the progressive obstruction with inspiration as the epiglottis and surrounding structures collapse into the glottic opening.

not require immediate airway management unless signs and symptoms dictate that this is the case.

Unstable patients with respiratory failure require assisted ventilation. Bag-mask ventilation should be attempted first and, if successful, continued until intubation can be performed. If neither bag-mask ventilation nor intubation is successful, needle cricothyroidotomy or tracheostomy may be indicated. Regardless of the approach to securing the airway, it is prudent for the emergency clinician to consult other experts in airway management rapidly, such as an anesthesiologist (fiberoptic intubation), otolaryngologist, or general surgeon (surgical approaches), so that a plan of approach can be made and morbidity minimized. Patients often remain intubated for 3 to 5 days in order for antibiotic therapy to reduce inflammation and surrounding tissue edema. A second- or third-generation cephalosporin is recommended.

Trauma and Burns

Thermal injury from facial burns and inhaled smoke or steam and trauma to the face and neck can create physical findings similar to those of infectious epiglottitis. Rapidly progressive stridor, drooling, an unwillingness to lie flat, and a swollen inflamed epiglottis may occur. Aspiration of hot liquids is the most common cause of airway burns in infants and young children. Toddlers are particularly prone to inhalation of hot liquids because they can eat and drink independently without initially being attentive to temperature. The initial physical examination of the oropharynx may be relatively normal. The airway should be secured early in suspected laryngeal edema, as progression and obstruction can occur rapidly. Bronchodilators may help with bronchospasm; steroids are not recommended.

Allergic Reactions

Acute allergic reactions may cause rapid supraglottic edema with respiratory distress and stridor. Food is the most common precipitant in infants and children. Children with peanut allergies and those with atopy and asthma have higher mortality rates. The treatment of anaphylaxis is epinephrine. Intramuscular epinephrine (1 mg/mL solution) at 0.01 mg/kg up to 0.5 mg per dose is initial management and may be repeated twice. IV epinephrine (0.1 mg/mL solution) at a 0.001 mg/kg bolus followed by 0.1 to 1 mcg/kg/min up to 10 mcg/min

may be necessary for patients in shock with anaphylaxis. IV fluids and oxygen should be administered. Racemic epinephrine may be given to reduce airway edema and other bronchodilators may be given for epinephrine-resistant bronchospasm. H1 and H2 antihistamines and steroids are commonly given for symptomatic relief but do not act rapidly enough to effectively treat anaphylaxis. Intubation may be required and should be considered early for acute airway obstruction unresponsive to epinephrine. On discharge from the hospital, all patients with anaphylaxis should be given a prescription for an epinephrine auto-injector (0.15 mg for children <30 kg; 0.3 mg for older children) and instructed in its use. Follow-up with the primary care physician for allergist referral and a medical alert bracelet is also recommended.

Diseases of the Larynx

The larynx and vocal cords are commonly involved with obstructing airway disease. Many obstructing conditions are congenital lesions, including laryngomalacia, laryngeal web, and vocal cord paralysis. Acquired lesions include laryngeal papillomas.

Congenital lesions. Laryngomalacia is the most common cause of chronic stridor in infants and accounts for 60% to 75% of congenital laryngeal anomalies. It is a result of incomplete development of the supporting cartilage of the larynx. With inspiration, the long floppy epiglottis, arytenoids, and aryepiglottic folds are drawn into the larynx and create a partial obstruction (Fig. 162.6). Baseline inspiratory stridor begins several weeks after birth and worsens with supine positioning, neck flexion, and increased respiratory effort (crying, URI). Laryngomalacia is rarely associated with significant respiratory distress, feeding difficulties, or failure to thrive. Most patients experience complete resolution of symptoms by 2 years of age and are treated conservatively. Fiberoptic bronchoscopy is used to confirm the diagnosis and identify the existence of coexisting or synchronous anomalies (e.g., subglottic stenosis, tracheomalacia). Surgical intervention is warranted in severe cases in which the child suffers from apneic events, respiratory compromise, pulmonary hypertension, or failure to thrive.[8]

Vocal cord paralysis is the second most common cause of chronic stridor in infants. Bilateral vocal cord paralysis results in severe respiratory distress and stridor and typically requires intervention for airway

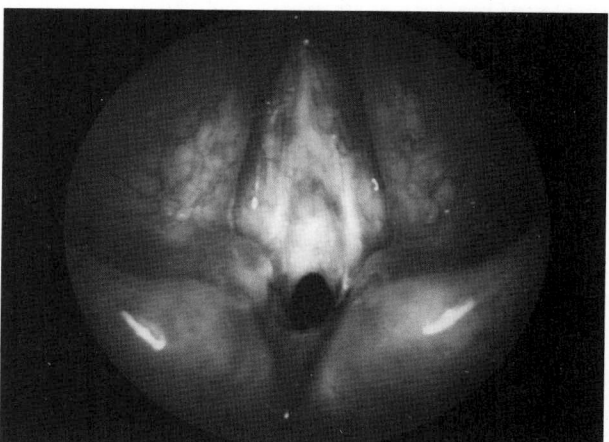

Fig. 162.7 Large Laryngeal Web.

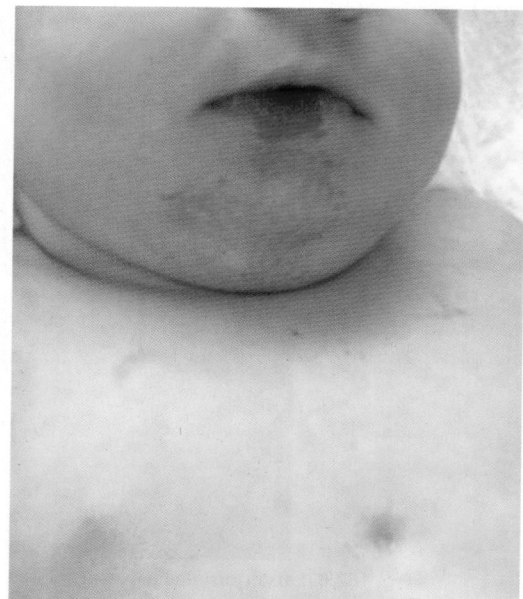

Fig. 162.8 2-month-old infant with a facial hemangioma in the beard distribution. This patient was also found to have a subglottic hemangioma. (From O-Lee TJ, Messner A. Subglottic hemangioma. *Otolaryngol Clin North Am.* 2008;41:903–911, viii–ix.)

protection; it is often associated with serious central nervous system abnormalities, such as Arnold-Chiari malformations. Unilateral vocal cord paralysis is usually left-sided and related to traction on the left recurrent laryngeal nerve at birth or compression from mediastinal structures. Infants with unilateral vocal cord paralysis have a hoarse weak cry, feeding difficulties, and aspiration. Stridor often worsens with distress and improves with positioning the affected side down. Most children improve with voice and speech therapy and do not require invasive treatment.

A laryngeal web results from failure of complete canalization of the airway. Most webs lie between the cords and appear as a partial anterior fusion (Fig. 162.7). The spectrum of symptoms reflects the size of the web. Small webs may cause a hoarse weak cry and mild stridor. Larger, more complete webs are associated with aphonia and severe respiratory distress.

Congenital laryngotracheal (subglottic) stenosis is a result of a congenital defect in canalization of the subglottic trachea. Deformity of the cricoid ring is usually seen. Infants with severe stenosis have stridor at birth. Milder lesions may be asymptomatic until additional obstruction from infection or inflammation occurs. Subglottic stenosis is also an acquired condition that occurs after prolonged intubation or blunt trauma to the neck.

A subglottic hemangioma is a less common cause of stridor and subglottic airway obstruction in infants. The infant is usually asymptomatic at birth, but stridor (which may be biphasic) and cough develop within the first few weeks to months of life. Symptoms generally peak at 6 months as a result of rapid growth of the infant and hemangioma during the first months of life. Respiratory symptoms worsen with crying and agitation. Cutaneous hemangiomas are seen in approximately 50% of cases (often in a beard distribution; Fig. 162.8). Hemangiomas of the airway may be seen on plain film as an asymmetric lesion along the tracheal air column. Endoscopy is diagnostic (Fig. 162.9).

Acquired lesions

Laryngeal papillomas. Laryngeal papillomas are the most common benign laryngeal neoplasm in children and the second most common cause of hoarseness. They are typically acquired after exposure to human papillomavirus via vertical transmission from an infected mother. Multiple lesions are generally present and usually occur in the vocal cords but may involve any part of the larynx. Hoarseness, abnormal cry, and inspiratory stridor commonly occur by 3 to 4 years of age. Symptoms can progress to severe respiratory distress as the lesions enlarge and obstruct the larynx. Multiple ablation procedures are often required and malignant transformation may rarely occur.

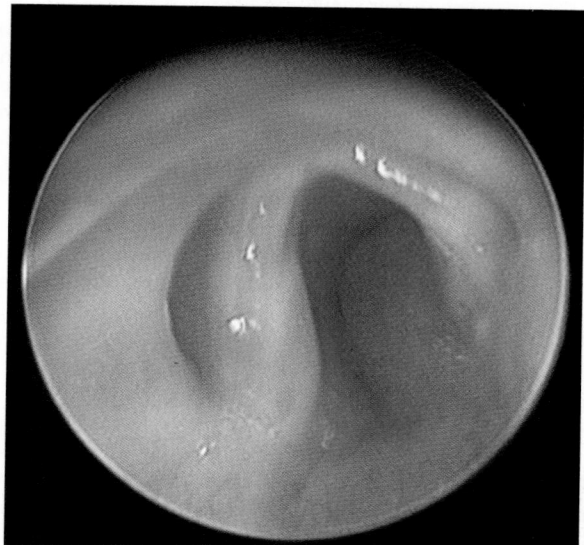

Fig. 162.9 Subglottic Hemangioma Seen on Endoscopy. (From Ida JB, Thompson DM. Pediatric stridor. *Otolaryngol Clin North Am* 2014;47:795–819.)

Subglottic tracheal disease. The subglottic trachea is the origin of the high-pitched inspiratory sound commonly associated with upper airway obstruction. The subglottic space is elliptical-shaped and completely surrounded by the cricoid ring. This anatomy predisposes this part of the airway to obstruction. Subglottic narrowing or stenosis can result from a congenital anomaly, inflammation from infection, and trauma associated with prolonged intubation.

Viral Croup

Foundations. Croup (laryngotracheobronchitis) is the most common infectious cause of upper airway distress and obstruction

TABLE 162.2 Simplified Differential Diagnosis of Upper Airway Symptoms

Condition	Distinguishing Features
Anaphylaxis	Abrupt onset, associated trigger, other organ system involvement
Croup	URI symptoms, acute onset of barky cough, stridor, no distinct positional preference
Bacterial tracheitis	Fever, toxicity, prolongation of symptoms, lack of response to croup treatment
Epiglottitis	Drooling a predominant symptom, patient desire to remain sitting. Muffled voice (but hoarseness typically absent), cough absent, anxiety
Retropharyngeal abscess	Fever, toxicity, torticollis, neck pain/stiffness, +/– drooling, +/– muffled voice
Foreign body aspiration	History of choking episode, absence of URI symptoms or hoarseness, +/– drooling
Peritonsillar abscess	Sore throat, trismus, muffled voice, pharyngeal erythema and edema, uvular deviation

URI, Upper respiratory tract infection.

in childhood. It accounts for more than 90% of all cases of stridor in children. It usually occurs between 6 and 36 months of age but can be seen from early infancy through school age. Croup is rare in children greater than 6 years of age. Parainfluenza virus accounts for 50% to 75% of cases; respiratory syncytial virus, influenza A and B viruses, and rhinovirus cause the remainder. Measles can also cause croup and should be considered in unvaccinated children. The clinical picture of croup associated with influenza is more severe than with parainfluenza. Croup is caused by inflammation, exudates, and edema of the loosely adherent mucosal and submucosal tissues of the subglottic space. The inflamed mucosa expands into the airway lumen because the cricoid cartilage forms a complete cartilaginous (nonexpanding) ring in this part of the trachea. In severe disease, the airway may be narrowed to as little as 1 to 2 mm.

Clinical features. Croup is diagnosed clinically. A 1- to 3-day prodrome of mild fever and URI symptoms is followed by a fairly abrupt onset of barky cough, hoarse voice, and high-pitched inspiratory stridor. The barky cough is the predominant presentation in infants and young children, whereas older children tend to present primarily with hoarseness. The cough lasts an average of 3 days and all symptoms typically resolve in 4 to 7 days. A simplified differential diagnosis for croup is shown in Table 162.2. Scoring systems have been developed for the assessment of croup; these include an evaluation of worsening stridor, retractions, cyanosis, heart rate, and respiratory rate. Although a formal croup score is often not assigned in many clinical settings, the determination of mild, moderate, or severe croup should be based on careful evaluation of these five signs as well as on mental status and air movement. See Fig. 162.10 for a clinical treatment algorithm based on croup severity.

Mild croup is characterized by an intermittent barky cough, stridor with agitation but not at rest, mild tachypnea, and tachycardia. A child with mild croup is minimally distressed and well hydrated and has normal mental status. Moderate croup is characterized by audible stridor at rest, worsening stridor with agitation, barky cough, and increased work of breathing (retractions, tachypnea, and tachycardia). A patient with moderate croup may be fussy but is alert, interactive, and comforted by parents. Hypoxia is rare in mild or moderate croup. When hypoxia is seen, it may signify concomitant lower respiratory disease, another disease process, or severe croup. Mild croup occurs in 85% of

children; fewer than 1% of children have severe croup. Laboratory tests are nondiagnostic, and radiographic studies of the neck do not change management nor are they sensitive or specific. The classic x-ray finding is a steeple sign—a tapered narrowing of the normal shouldered appearance of the subglottic trachea—which can be seen in those with croup and also in patients without the disease.

Management. Glucocorticoids reduce symptoms, decrease the need for aerosolized epinephrine, and result in fewer readmissions to the ED and shorter ED and hospital stays. Oral dexamethasone (0.15 mg/kg to 0.6 mg/kg, max 10 to 16 mg) is the preferred agent and can improve symptoms within two hours. The IV form of dexamethasone is more concentrated than the oral formulation and can be given orally. Severe cases or patients with oral intolerance may be given the same dose IM/IV. Lower dosing (0.15 mg/kg) has been shown to be as effective as a higher dose (0.6 mg/kg) in most cases. However, there is some evidence that patients with more severe obstruction benefit from the higher dose.[15,16] Inhaled budesonide (2 mg/dose) is also effective but more expensive, so it is not routinely used. Prednisolone may be as effective as dexamethasone in milder cases but should not be used in patients with significant symptoms due to the shorter duration of action.[9]

Aerosolized epinephrine, which reverses edema and relieves acute symptoms through vasoconstriction in the subglottic mucosa, should be given to children with stridor at rest or with significant respiratory distress. It is a temporizing measure with a quick onset of action (<10 minutes) and a duration of up to 2 hours. The L form of epinephrine is the active isomer and has the same degree of safety and efficacy as racemic epinephrine; either form may be used. Nebulized L-epinephrine (1:1000 solution) dosing is 0.5 mL/kg (max, 5 mL) *or* racemic epinephrine (2.25% solution) is 1.125 mg/kg (max, 11.25 mg/dose or 0.5 mL/dose); either should be diluted in 2 to 3 mL of NS and given via nebulizer over 15 minutes. Patients with stridor at rest who receive inhaled epinephrine should be observed in the ED to ensure no recurrence of severe symptoms. The amount of time needed to observe these patients is controversial, but patients are unlikely to deteriorate beyond 3 hours. We recommend that patients be observed in the ED for 2 to 3 hours after epinephrine administration to ensure that stridor and respiratory distress do not recur.

Heliox (i.e., concentrations of helium: oxygen at 80:20, 70:30, or 60:40) may improve resistance to gas flow and thus decrease work of breathing in young children with moderate to severe croup. Heliox has been shown to improve symptoms temporarily (in the first hour), but the benefits are not sustained (after two hours). Heliox (with nebulized epinephrine) may be considered to avoid intubation in young children with moderate to severe increased work of breathing, although studies to date have not been powered to assess its effect on this rare outcome.[10] Cool mist has not been demonstrated to improve outcomes and there is insufficient evidence to support its routine use.

Most children with croup can be safely discharged, provided respiratory distress and resting stridor have resolved.[11] A small percentage of patients with croup require admission. Several factors may impact the decision to admit a child with moderate croup, such as the severity of symptoms at initial evaluation, persistence of respiratory distress, stridor at rest, hypoxia, poor response to treatment, dehydration, history suggesting airway disease or recurrent croup, young age (<6 months), difficulty with feeds, and poor social support (Box 162.1).

Severe croup is rare (<1%) and associated with signs of impending airway obstruction and respiratory failure—fatigue, hypoxia, hypercapnia, abnormal mental status, and extreme respiratory distress. In the rare case in which intubation is required, an endotracheal tube (ETT) at least a half-size smaller than expected for the child's size is often necessary. If the ETT that can be passed is too small to allow adequate ventilation, tracheostomy may be required.

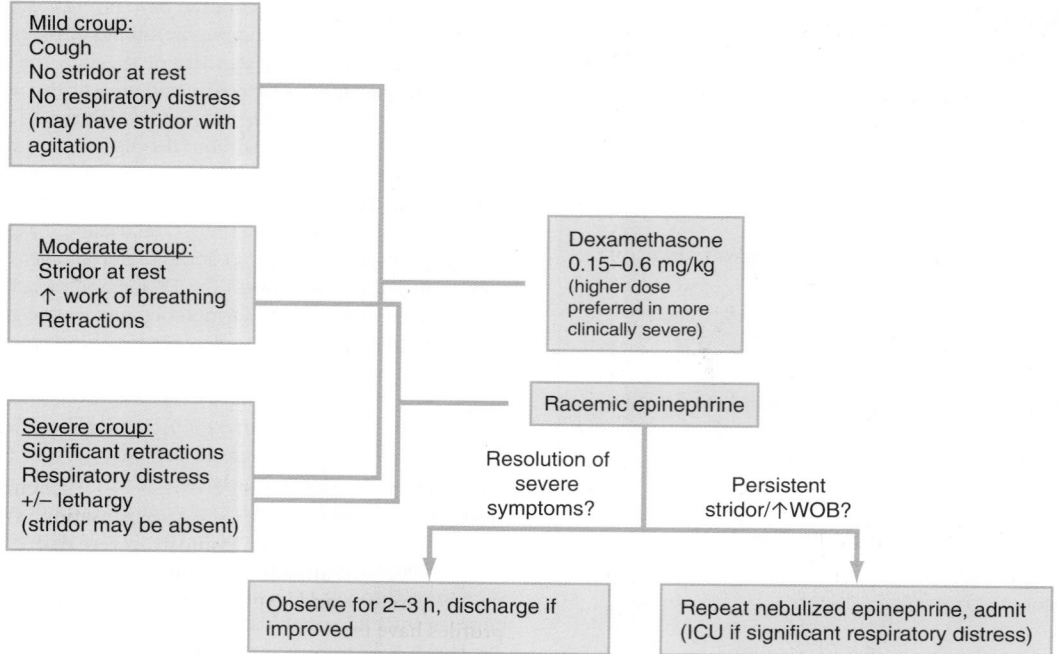

Fig. 162.10 Simplified Croup Treatment Algorithm Based on Presenting Signs, Symptoms, and Severity. (Rose E, ed. *Pediatric Emergencies: A Practical, Clinical Guide.* New York, NY: Oxford University Press; 2021)

BOX 162.1   Croup: Indications for Admission

Severe respiratory distress or failure
Unusual symptoms (hypoxia, hyperpyrexia)
Dehydration
Persistence of stridor at rest after aerosolized epinephrine and steroids
Persistence of tachycardia, tachypnea
Complex past medical history (prematurity, pulmonary, cardiac disease)

Spasmodic or Atypical Croup

Spasmodic or atypical croup is a somewhat indistinct clinical entity with many features that overlap those of viral croup. There is no consensus on the definition, but the term *atypical croup* is often used to describe numerous recurrent episodes or croup in children outside the expected age group. An association with allergy, atopy, airway hyperreactivity, asthma, and gastroesophageal reflux has been described. Airway lesions (most commonly subglottic stenosis) may be present and contribute to the pathophysiology.[12]

Diseases of the Trachea

Obstruction of the trachea distal to the subglottic space can be a result of congenital and acquired lesions.

Congenital lesions

Tracheomalacia. Tracheomalacia results from abnormally soft, undeveloped supporting cartilage of the tracheal rings. Primary or congenital tracheomalacia is seen in otherwise healthy term newborns, as well as in infants with conditions such as Down syndrome and DiGeorge syndrome. Healthy infants with isolated disease have a good prognosis because symptoms improve as the cartilage strengthens with growth. Secondary disease is associated with extrinsic compression of the trachea (e.g., vascular rings, tumor, nodes, and cysts). Tracheomalacia should be suspected in patients with a history of stridor that increases during the first few weeks of life and worsens with agitation, supine positioning, and infection. Plain radiographs

are nondiagnostic but dynamic studies, such as fluoroscopy, may be helpful. Patients should follow up with primary care for outpatient monitoring of symptoms.

Tracheal stenosis. Tracheal stenosis is a congenital anomaly that results from complete tracheal rings. Infants have persistent stridor and respiratory distress. Because the tracheal diameter is fixed, symptoms worsen with agitation and age.

Tracheal compression. Tracheal compression may also occur externally from vascular anomalies or mediastinal lesions (Fig. 162.11). A vascular ring is an anomaly of the aortic arch and related vessels in which a ring of vessels encircles the trachea, esophagus, or both. Examples of vascular rings include a double aortic arch, right aortic arch with a persistent left ligamentum arteriosum, anomalous innominate artery and anomalous left common carotid artery, left pulmonary artery, or aberrant right subclavian artery. Stridor, wheezing, dyspnea, and cough are common initial symptoms and are frequently mistaken as a URI. Many patients with vascular rings have additional cardiovascular anomalies and further work up is often indicated. Other associated mediastinal lesions that can compress the trachea include esophageal duplication cysts, bronchogenic cysts, mediastinal cyst, teratomas, lymphomas, and lymphadenopathy.

Vascular rings. Infants with vascular rings typically present with persistent, unexplained respiratory and feeding problems. A chest radiograph revealing an abnormal (right-sided) aortic arch may suggest the diagnosis in the ED; barium esophagography has traditionally been considered to be the single most important diagnostic procedure in patients with complete vascular rings (Fig. 162.12). Additional studies, such as CT, MRI, angiography, or bronchoscopy, may be indicated based on symptoms and associated risk factors for co-morbidities.

Bacterial tracheitis

Foundations. Bacterial tracheitis, also referred to as bacterial laryngotracheobronchitis, pseudomembranous croup, is a serious cause of stridor and airway obstruction in children. The epidemiology of upper airway infections has changed since widespread immunization for *H. influenzae* and the use of steroids for croup. This has increased the relative frequency of bacterial tracheitis as a cause of respiratory

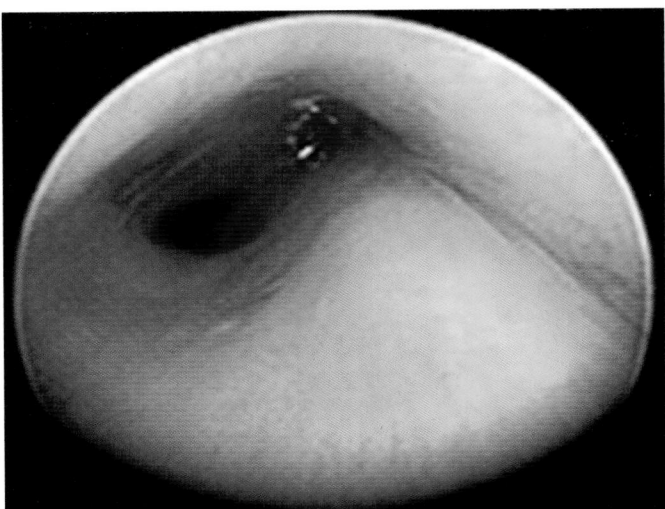

Fig. 162.11 External Vascular Compression of the Trachea Seen on Endoscopy. (From Ida JB, Thompson DM. Pediatric stridor. *Otolaryngol Clin North Am.* 2014;47:795–819.)

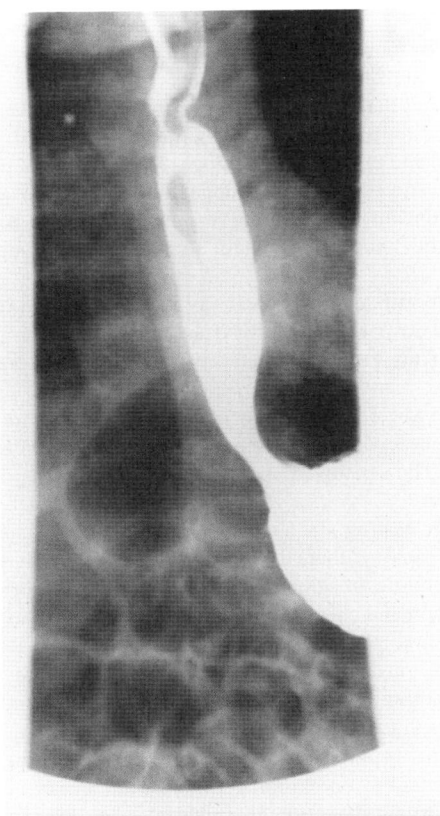

Fig. 162.12 Barium Esophagogram. Note the indentation of the esophagus caused by an encircling vascular ring.

failure from upper airway infection. Bacterial tracheitis is three times more likely to cause respiratory failure than epiglottis and viral croup combined. Bacterial tracheitis usually affects younger children but may occur at any age.

The pathogenesis of bacterial tracheitis is severe inflammation of the tracheal epithelium and the production of thick mucopurulent secretions. The lining of the trachea forms a loosely adherent membrane that may become necrotic and slough, occluding the lumen. Microabscesses may be present in the tracheal mucosa. Perforation and pneumomediastinum have been described. Traditionally, *S. aureus* (including MRSA) has been the organism primarily responsible for bacterial tracheitis, but many causative bacteria have been reported. Fungal tracheitis in immunocompromised individuals portends a grave prognosis.

Clinical features. The classic presentation of bacterial tracheitis is a toxic child with high fevers and rapidly worsening stridor that fails to improve with racemic epinephrine. Symptoms may overlap with those of croup and epiglottitis (Table 162.3). Most patients experience a viral prodrome of fever, barky cough, and stridor. These symptoms typically intensify as the bacterial superinfection grows on damaged tracheal epithelium. The child appears toxic, and signs of airway obstruction and respiratory failure may develop acutely. Less commonly, primary bacterial tracheitis may occur with a fulminant onset and rapid progression to acute respiratory distress. Features that suggest bacterial tracheitis include a viral prodrome followed by acute decompensation, symptoms atypical for croup (e.g., high fever, cyanosis, severe distress), poor response to the usual treatment of croup (e.g., nebulized epinephrine), and inspiratory and expiratory stridor. Changes in bacteriologic profiles have produced less virulent but more prolonged infections, increasing the diagnostic challenge.[13]

Diagnostic testing. The evaluation of a toxic-appearing child with bacterial tracheitis should be conducted expeditiously. Laboratory tests are nondiagnostic. The white blood cell count is often normal or slightly elevated, and blood cultures are rarely positive in bacterial tracheitis. Lateral and anteroposterior views of the neck and chest may be helpful. Findings on plain radiographs include subglottic narrowing, a ragged edge of the usually smooth tracheal air column, and a hazy density within the tracheal lumen, mimicking the appearance of airway foreign bodies. The epiglottis and supraglottic structures appear normal. In addition, the chest radiograph may reveal coexisting pneumonia. Bronchoscopy is both diagnostic and therapeutic and should be performed emergently (Fig. 162.13); this procedure allows visualization of the supraglottic structures and larynx, exclusion of other diseases, suctioning of tracheal secretions and debris, and establishment of an artificial airway.

Management. Severe distress may rarely require immediate intubation and suctioning in the ED, although airway management in the operating room is preferred. Endoscopic tracheal débridement may result in significant clinical improvement and allow the child to be managed without intubation. Serial endoscopy may be needed to manage secretions. Endotracheal intubation is required in children with respiratory distress and hypoxia. Patients should be admitted and receive supplemental oxygen, fluid resuscitation, and broad-spectrum antibiotics.

Broad antibiotic coverage is recommended with an antistaphylococcal agent (e.g., vancomycin, clindamycin) plus a third-generation cephalosporin (e.g., ceftriaxone). Alternatively, an antistaphylococcal agent plus ampicillin-sulbactam may be used. In penicillin-allergic patients, vancomycin or clindamycin plus a quinolone should be administered (ciprofloxacin if *Pseudomonas* is a concern or levofloxacin if *Streptococcus pneumoniae* is suspected). Although 7 to 10 days is usually sufficient, longer courses of antibiotics may be necessary for children with extra-tracheal infection or persistent tracheal inflammation. Complications of bacterial tracheitis include toxic shock syndrome, septic shock, renal failure, postintubation pulmonary edema, acute respiratory distress syndrome, and the need for reintubation. Residual subglottic stenosis has been described.

TABLE 162.3   Comparison of Croup, Epiglottitis, and Bacterial Tracheitis

Parameter	Croup	Epiglottitis	Bacterial Tracheitis
Peak age	6 months–3 years	5–7 years, but can be seen throughout childhood	3–5 years, but seen throughout childhood
Pathologic features	Subglottic inflammation, edema	Inflammation and edema of the epiglottis, aryepiglottic folds	Bacterial superinfection with inflammation of the tracheal mucosa, copious mucopurulent secretions obstructing the trachea
Organisms	Parainfluenza virus, RSV, adenovirus, influenza	*Haemophilus influenzae*, group A beta-hemolytic streptococcus, *Staphylococcus aureus*, *Streptococcus pneumoniae*	*S. aureus* or mixed flora
Clinical features	Onset follows URI prodrome consisting of croupy cough, hoarse voice, low-grade fever, inspiratory stridor	Rapid progression of high fever, toxicity, drooling, stridor	Several-day prodrome of croup-like illness progressing to toxicity, inspiratory and expiratory stridor, marked distress
Laboratory and radiographic findings	Steeple sign on PA view of the neck or normal	Thumbprint sign on the lateral aspect of the neck, thickened aryepiglottic folds, loss of air in the vallecula	Normal upper airway structures, shaggy tracheal air column
Management	Steroids uncommon, aerosolized epinephrine	Intubation, antibiotics	Intubation common, antibiotics rare, intubation

PA, Posteroanterior; *RSV,* respiratory syncytial virus; *URI,* upper respiratory infection.

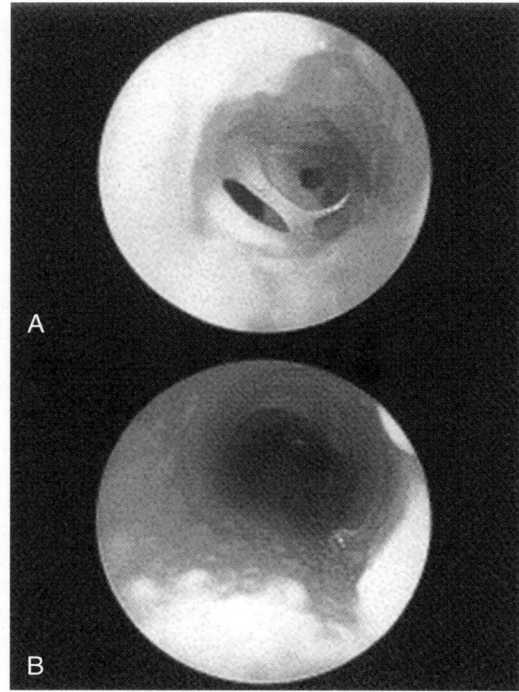

Fig. 162.13 Thick Tracheal Membranes Seen on Rigid Bronchoscopy in Bacterial Tracheitis. (A) Thick adherent membranous secretions. (B), The distal tracheobronchial tree is unremarkable. (From Salamone FN, Bobbitt DB, Myer CM, et al. Bacterial tracheitis reexamined: is there a less severe manifestation? *Otolaryngol Head Neck Surg.* 2004;131:871–876.)

Foreign Bodies

Airway foreign body

Foundations. Asphyxia from airway obstruction by an airway or esophageal foreign body is a common cause of death in children. Round foods (e.g., peanuts, grapes, raisins, and hot dogs) are especially common. Conformable objects are the most difficult to manage and remove, and balloons, including those made from hospital gloves, are the objects most likely to result in death.

Large objects that lodge in the upper airway and trachea cause dramatic signs of upper airway obstruction (e.g., dyspnea, drooling, stridor, cyanosis) and carry the worst prognosis. Objects that pass through the subglottic space typically will lodge in a bronchus, usually the right mainstem bronchus, or in a more terminal part of the airway. These objects may be "coughed up" again and cause sudden upper airway obstruction.

Clinical features. An upper airway foreign body can cause partial or complete obstruction. Clinical signs of complete obstruction include poor air exchange, inability to speak, ineffective cough, severe distress, and cyanosis. Foreign body aspiration that has settled in the lower airways may have subacute symptoms, such as unilateral wheeze, or may present later (days to years) as recurrent pneumonia. The sensitivity of a witnessed choking episode varies in the literature.

Diagnostic testing. In a child with an aspirated foreign body in the upper airway, there is often no time, nor is it prudent, to perform diagnostic imaging. In a stable patient, a portable lateral neck radiograph and chest radiograph may be obtained as long as the patient is allowed to maintain a position of comfort. Radiographic findings suspicious for foreign body aspiration include radiopaque materials, mediastinal shift, emphysema, and atelectasis. A normal chest radiograph cannot rule out a nonradiopaque foreign body. CT scan and virtual bronchoscopy (a reformatted three-dimensional CT image that generates intraluminal views of the airway and bronchi) may be used to aid diagnosis in equivocal cases. Diagnostic flexible bronchoscopy is indicated with significant clinical suspicion of foreign body aspiration, despite normal imaging.

Management. An acute obstructing upper airway foreign body requires emergent intervention with basic life support maneuvers. Choking infants younger than 1 year should be given five back blows delivered between the shoulder blades, followed by five chest thrusts with the head held below the trunk. Abdominal thrusts should not be performed in infants and may injure abdominal organs. Blind finger sweeps may push the object further into the airway and are no longer recommended.

The Heimlich maneuver is used in conscious children older than 1 year; chest compressions should be delivered to unconscious children. If there is no chest rise with assisted ventilation with a bag-mask device, advanced airway techniques are indicated. Laryngoscopy should be performed to attempt visualization and foreign body removal with pediatric Magill forceps. If the obstructing foreign body cannot be visualized, it may be pushed distally into the right mainstem bronchus with an ETT to ventilate the non-obstructed portion of the lung. Recruiting additional expertise from an otolaryngologist, anesthesiologist, or general surgeon may be needed.

A patient who is adequately oxygenated and is moving air should be initially allowed to maintain a preferred position, continue coughing to clear the obstruction, and breathe spontaneously until operative management can be arranged. Paralysis with rapid sequence induction should be avoided if the patient is maintaining a patent airway; with paralysis, the airway tone may be lost, and a partial obstruction can become complete.

Can't Intubate, Can't Ventilate Scenari. Surgical cricothyrotomy is not generally recommended for infants and young children younger than 8 to 10 years. The anatomy changes with growth (i.e., the larynx is high and cricothyroid membrane small), and it may be difficult to locate pertinent anatomy until a child is of school age.[14] Trachea compressibility also increases complication risk. Needle cricothyrotomy may be performed in children, but significant CO_2 retention limits its effectiveness; it is a temporizing measure used as a bridge to a more definitive, secure airway.

Commercial percutaneous transtracheal ventilation kits are available, but homemade kits can be constructed using tools readily accessible in the ED. A 14- to 18-gauge angiocatheter (the size of the catheter does not affect the rate of turbulent gas flow) is inserted in the cricothyroid membrane and connected to a 3-mL syringe (without the plunger) to a 7.5-mm ETT adaptor (or a 3.0-mm ETT connector directly to the angiocatheter). These homemade kits are rigid and may easily become dislodged. Alternative setups include using IV tubing—attaching IV tubing to the angiocatheter, cutting the tubing, and attaching a 2.5-mm ETT connector—or directly connecting oxygen tubing to the catheter with a Y connector or three-way stopcock. Bag-mask ventilation (recommended in children <5 years) can be performed through the ETT adaptor at 10 to 12 breaths/min to minimize barotrauma by allowing for passive exhalation. Percutaneous transtracheal ventilation (in children ≥5 years) is given at an oxygen flow rate of 1 L/min/year of age with a 1:4 inspiration-to-expiration ratio (I:E). Adults should receive oxygen from the wall source at 15 L/min (50 to 58 psi) and children at a rate of 10 to 12 L/min (25 to 35 psi). Complete airway obstruction does not allow for passive exhalation and necessitates a reduction of bag-mask ventilation rate to five or six breaths/min or an I:E ratio of 1:8 to 10 as a temporizing measure. Complications of needle cricothyrotomy include barotrauma and damage to adjacent structures. See Chapter 156 for further discussion.

The references for this chapter can be found online at ExpertConsult.com.

163

Pediatric Lower Airway Obstruction

Richard J. Scarfone and Jeffrey A. Seiden

ASTHMA

KEY CONCEPTS

- No single asthma score has been universally adopted to assess the degree of illness or treatment responses. However, most scores include some combination of respiratory rate, degree of wheezing, inspiratory-to-expiratory ratio, use of accessory muscles, and oxygen saturation.
- Chest x-ray (CXR) is not required for wheezing children, even for those who are febrile, are wheezing for the first time, or require hospitalization. CXR is indicated for those with a history of choking, focal chest findings, extreme distress, subcutaneous emphysema, diagnostic uncertainty relative to respiratory illness, or with clinical findings suggestive of a cardiac etiology.
- Albuterol delivered by metered-dose inhalers with spacers (MDI-S) is as effective as that delivered by nebulizers for children with acute asthma. The mode of delivery is largely chosen on the basis of cost and ability to achieve the goal of three treatments within the first hour of care. Per the 2007 National Heart Lung and Blood Institute guidelines, a high dose (4–12 puffs) of a short-acting beta-agonists (SABAs) metered-dose inhaler (MDI) with a spacer has "equivalent bronchodilation" to nebulized treatment.
- Levalbuterol does not lead to better emergency department (ED) outcomes compared with racemic albuterol. Racemic albuterol, at a substantially lower cost, should remain the drug of choice for children with acute asthma exacerbations.
- Dexamethasone is as effective as prednisone in the ED treatment of acute asthma. Dexamethasone is associated with fewer doses, less vomiting, and greater compliance.
- Continuously nebulized albuterol, corticosteroids, magnesium sulfate, and parenteral SABA are cornerstones of therapy for moderately to severely ill children with asthma.

Foundations

Background and Importance

A recent national survey found that one in 12 children had asthma; however, the prevalence among non-Hispanic black children was 16%.[1] Asthma is associated with significant morbidity, with approximately 17% of children with asthma requiring emergency department (ED) or Urgent Care management and 5% needing to be hospitalized annually[1]

Anatomy, Physiology, and Pathophysiology

Asthma is a lower airway disease marked by bronchoconstriction, mucosal edema, and pulmonary secretions. Upper respiratory infections (URIs) associated with copious rhinorrhea, a common trigger of an asthma exacerbation, may significantly increase airway resistance in young children. Because children have compliant chest walls and horizontally located ribs, their ability to use the thorax to increase tidal volume is limited; thus, ventilation is highly dependent on diaphragmatic movement. Also, as functional residual lung capacity increases with age, minute ventilation is largely rate-dependent in young children and may quickly lead to fatigue. An infant younger than 12 months has an oxygen consumption index that is double that of an adult. Increased airway resistance and a compliant chest wall predispose infants to tachypnea, increased work of breathing, and increased oxygen consumption. As a result, the infant with respiratory distress may rapidly develop hypoxemia, precipitating bradycardia and cardiopulmonary arrest.

Clinical Features

All acutely wheezing children arriving for ED care should be attached to a cardiorespiratory monitor and have oxygen saturation determined by pulse oximetry. For children with hypoxia, supplemental oxygen should be provided while the emergency clinician begins the clinical assessment.

History

To initiate appropriate therapy quickly, based on the degree of illness, a concise history should be obtained upon patient arrival, followed by a physical examination that focuses on the cardiopulmonary system. An abbreviated history should include questions about the child's age, duration and severity of symptoms, recent medication use, and hospitalizations, including the need for intensive care unit (ICU) care or intubation. The parents should be able to relate how the severity of this attack compares with that of previous exacerbations. A history of difficulty sleeping, eating, or speaking suggests a moderate to severe exacerbation. Names, doses, and frequency of asthma medications, as well as preexisting conditions, should be documented.

After starting therapy, a more comprehensive history should include questions about asthma triggers, such as URIs, cigarette smoke, allergies, and exercise. Frequent ED visits or hospitalizations due to asthma may indicate poorly controlled asthma. The impact of asthma on the child's life may be gauged by the monthly frequency of daytime or nighttime symptoms, including cough, as well as missed days of school or restricted activity. A child with persistent asthma marked by frequent symptoms should be receiving daily anti-inflammatory therapy. Family and social histories should focus on asthma, cystic fibrosis, or atopic disease, and on the adequacy of support systems at home.

Physical Examination

The targeted examination includes assessing vital signs, mental status, and cardiopulmonary systems. A child who is anxious, restless, or lethargic may be hypoxic. The oxygen saturation, sometimes referred to as the "fifth vital sign," should be determined soon after ED arrival for any child with respiratory distress, and supplemental oxygen should be provided for values 92% or less. No single asthma score has

TABLE 163.1　Differential Diagnosis of Asthma

Condition	Distinguishing Characteristics
Infectious	
Bronchiolitis	Infant, preceding upper respiratory infection, seasonal, no history of atopy, no family history of asthma
Laryngotracheobronchitis (croup)	Inspiratory stridor, barky cough, fever, response to humidified air or racemic epinephrine
Pneumonia	Focal wheezing, rhonchi, rales, grunting, fever
Tuberculosis	Diffuse adenopathy, weight loss, prolonged fever
Bronchiolitis obliterans	Prolonged cough or chest pain, inhalational exposure to toxin
Anatomic or Congenital	
Gastroesophageal reflux	Frequent emesis, weight loss, aspiration
Cystic fibrosis	Diarrhea, weight loss, chronic cough, salty sweat
Congestive heart failure	Rales, murmur, gallop, hepatosplenomegaly, cardiomegaly, or pulmonary vascular congestion on chest radiograph
Tracheoesophageal fistula	Choking, coughing, cyanosis with feeds
Mediastinal mass	Chest pain, mediastinal density on chest radiograph
Vascular ring	Stridor, cyanosis, apnea, high-pitched brassy cough, dysphagia
Acquired	
Foreign body aspiration	History of choking, toddler, asymmetric pulmonary examination, unilateral hyperinflation on chest radiograph
Anaphylaxis	Abrupt onset, urticarial rash, angioedema, sensation of throat "tightening," history of allergies

been universally adopted to assess the degree of illness or treatment responses. However, most scores include some combination of respiratory rate, degree of wheezing, inspiratory-to-expiratory ratio, use of accessory muscles, and oxygen saturation. These scores can assist in assessing the pretreatment degree of illness and tracking the response to therapy.

Assessing the work of breathing should include a careful inspection of the chest and neck; rarely, an associated pneumomediastinum or pneumothorax will produce subcutaneous air. Severely ill children may have wheezing that is audible without a stethoscope or have no wheezing ("silent chest") due to critically limited aeration. Asymmetric wheezing suggests pneumonia, pneumothorax, or a foreign body. More anxiety-provoking parts of the examination, such as otoscopy, should be delayed until treatment is well underway.

Differential Diagnoses

The differential diagnosis for childhood asthma includes bronchiolitis, laryngotracheobronchitis (croup), pneumonia, cardiac disorders (e.g., myocarditis), and gastroesophageal reflux (Table 163.1).

Bronchiolitis is the disease that is most commonly confused with asthma, and the two are not easily distinguished by examination findings alone. Children with bronchiolitis are typically younger and have

symptoms associated with viral illness. Children believed to have bronchiolitis but who have some combination of food allergies, atopic dermatitis, or a strong family history of asthma should receive bronchodilator therapy to determine if their wheezing is reversible. Croup may have a viral or allergic cause and affects children from infancy through early school age. Clinical presentation is marked by an abrupt onset of a harsh barky cough and inspiratory stridor. Symptoms are typically worse at night. Asthma will not be manifested with stridor alone, but a subset of children with croup may present with stridor and wheezing. Children with pneumonia may sometimes present with a component of wheezing, although rales and rhonchi are the usual auscultative findings. Infants and young children with pneumonia may also have a high fever, cough, grunting, nasal flaring, retractions, and an asymmetric lung examination. Children with pulmonary edema secondary to congenital cardiac disease or myocarditis may present with wheezing and rales, often associated with a cardiac murmur and hepatomegaly. A history of weight loss and sweating with feeds may also indicate a cardiac etiology (see Chapter 165).

Diagnostic Testing

Most children with wheezing have asthma or bronchiolitis and do not need imaging or laboratory studies. Performing an arterial blood gas (ABG) analysis is rarely indicated for most children with acute asthma but may be useful among those with severe bronchospasm and signs of respiratory failure despite initial therapy. A high or apparently normal partial pressure of carbon dioxide ($Paco_2 \geq 40$ mm Hg) in a child with hypoxia and retractions indicates impaired ventilation and impending respiratory failure. Alternatively, a young child who suddenly appears 'calm' with decreased respiratory effort may be developing hypercarbia and altered mental status from respiratory fatigue; an elevated $Paco_2$ helps differentiate this child from those finally able to rest from improved aeration. Measurement of the peak expiratory flow rate (PEFR) is a means of obtaining an objective assessment of exacerbation severity. However, up to two-thirds of children greater than 5 years are unable to complete PEFR testing during an asthma exacerbation. When feasible, the PEFR should be measured with the child standing and the best of three attempts recorded.

URIs marked by low-grade fever and coughing are common triggers of asthma exacerbations. These signs overlap with those found among children with pneumonia, making it difficult to determine the necessity of obtaining a CXR. No set of predictors has been found that can accurately identify children likely to have radiographic abnormalities. Emergency clinicians frequently obtain a CXR for children in the ED with asthma but rarely are pneumonia or other unsuspected diagnoses discovered, even if the child has never wheezed before.

It should not be routine practice to obtain a CXR for wheezing children, even for those who are febrile, wheezing for the first time, or requiring hospitalization. Performing chest radiography is indicated for those with a history of choking, focal chest findings, extreme distress, subcutaneous emphysema, or diagnostic uncertainty of respiratory versus or suspected cardiac etiology. Reassessment after SABA treatment to evaluate for resolution of focal findings may further decrease the need to obtain a CXR.

Management

Children can be stratified by degree of illness based on the physical examination (Fig. 163.1).

Mild Exacerbation

A mild exacerbation is characterized by alertness, slight tachypnea, expiratory wheezing only, a mildly prolonged expiratory phase, minimal accessory muscle use, and oxygen saturation of greater than 95%. Some children may have 1 or 2 of these features that are more

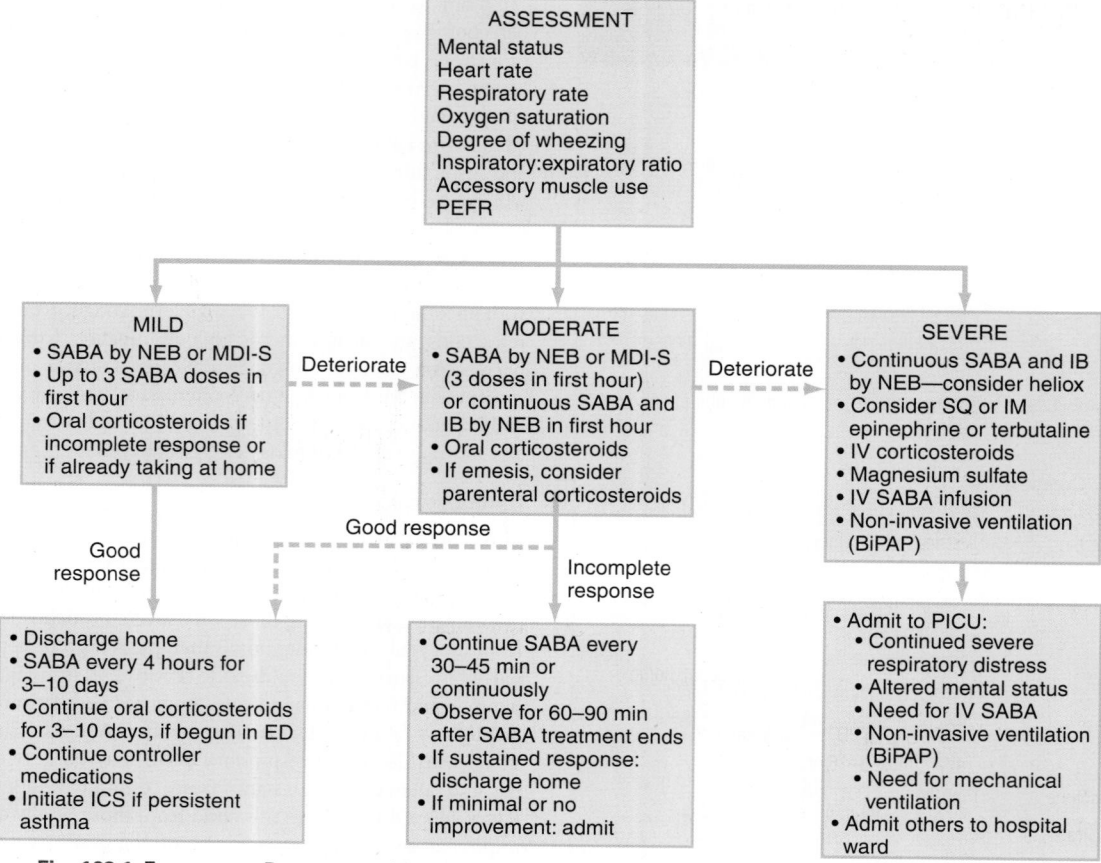

Fig. 163.1 Emergency Department Management of Acute Asthma. *ED,* Emergency department; *IB,* ipratropium bromide; *ICS,* inhaled corticosteroids; *IM,* intramuscular; *MDI-S,* metered-dose inhaler with spacer; *NEB,* nebulizer; *PEFR,* peak expiratory flow rate; *PICU,* pediatric intensive care unit; *SABA,* short-acting β₂-agonist: *SQ,* subcutaneous.

characteristic of a moderate exacerbation, yet still be judged as mildly ill overall. Usually, patients with a mild exacerbation will only require SABA therapy, and the Expert Panel of the National Heart, Lung, and Blood Institute (NHLBI) recommends that it be given every 20 minutes in the first hour of care. Children with mild exacerbations often improve promptly with just one or two SABA treatments and many are managed without corticosteroids (CS). However, CS may be given to mildly ill children who have received home SABA doses prior to presentation or to those who do not respond promptly to SABA therapy (see later, "Moderate Exacerbation").

Racemic albuterol has become the SABA of choice for the treatment of children with acute asthma. Options for the mode of delivery include a small-volume nebulizer (NEB) and metered-dose inhaler (MDI)-S. Most emergency clinicians use NEBs to administer SABA, regardless of illness severity. NEBs provide a passive means of receiving aerosolized medication because precise coordination between respiration and aerosol delivery is not needed; additionally, anticholinergic medication and humidified oxygen may be delivered concurrently. However, medication delivery via NEBs is inefficient, with only about 10% of the drug delivered to the small airways. Also, the administration takes about 10 minutes, increasing respiratory therapy time and costs.

On the other hand, spacers used with an MDI provide a reservoir of medication that is available to be inhaled. Therefore, precise coordination between actuation and inhalation is not needed, and there is no need for breath-holding. After each actuation, children should take five to eight breaths. Drug deposition in the oropharynx and systemic

absorption are reduced with the use of a spacer and decreased administration time may result in reduced costs. Face mask–equipped spacers are available for children too young to use the spacer's mouthpiece, although mouthpieces are preferable for older children to decrease nasal filtering of the drug.

Numerous clinical trials and meta-analyses over the past three decades have consistently demonstrated that albuterol delivery by MDI-S is as effective as NEBs among children of all ages and degrees of illness[2]. In some studies, MDI-S use was associated with a greater reduction in wheezing and lower hospitalization rates. The American College of Chest Physicians and American College of Asthma, Allergy, and Immunology have concluded that either NEBs or MDI-S are appropriate for the delivery of SABA in the ED.

Nebulized racemic albuterol should be administered at a dose of 0.15 mg/kg with a maximum dose of 5 mg, while optimal dosing for albuterol administered by MDI-S is not as well defined. Multiple puffs of SABA delivered by MDI-S seem to be well tolerated, even by young children. Children 1 to 4 years of age treated with six puffs of albuterol by MDI-S have been shown to have less tachycardia than those treated with 2.5 mg of albuterol by NEB. Per the 2007 NHLBI guidelines, a high dose (4 to 12 puffs) of a SABA MDI with a spacer has "equivalent bronchodilation" to NEB treatment. We recommend two to eight puffs, depending on weight (Table 163.2).

Another consideration in the use of SABA is the potential role of levalbuterol. Racemic albuterol is an equal mix of the active *R*-albuterol and inactive *S*-albuterol. *R*-Albuterol produces bronchodilation as well

TABLE 163.2 Recommended Doses of Medications for Acute Asthma

Medication	Dosage
Albuterol	0.15 mg/kg/dose (0.03 mL/kg/dose, max, 5 mg)
Continuous albuterol	0.5–1.0 mg/kg/h by nebulization (max, 15 mg/h)
Albuterol by metered-dose inhaler	Dose not well established
• ≤10 kg	2–4 puffs
• 11–19 kg	4–6 puffs
• ≥20 kg	6–8 puffs
Levalbuterol	Half the recommended albuterol doses
Ipratropium bromide	
• ≤20 kg	250 µg/dose
• >20 kg	500 µg/dose
L-Epinephrine (1:1000) or terbutaline (1.0 mg/mL)	0.01 mg/kg (max, 0.5 mg) 0.01 mg/kg (max, 0.25 mg)
IV terbutaline	10 mcg/kg IV over 10 minutes Every 30 minutes, may increase infusion by 0.3 µg/kg/min to max of 5 µg/kg/min
Prednisone	2 mg/kg (max, 60 mg), in ED 1 mg/kg/dose bid (max, 30 mg/dose), home therapy
Dexamethasone	0.3–0.6 mg/kg PO, two or three doses 24 hours apart (max, 8–16 mg/dose)
IV methylprednisolone	1 mg/kg (max, 125 mg)
IV magnesium sulfate	50–75 mg/kg over 20 min (max, 2g)

IM, Intramuscular; *IV*, intravenous; *PO*, by mouth; *SC*, subcutaneous.

as tachycardia and tremors, and *S*-albuterol had been long thought to be inert. However, there is some evidence that *S*-albuterol may increase reactivity to histamine, have proinflammatory effects, and exhibit characteristics of a typical contractile agent. There is also preferential retention of *S*-albuterol in the lungs of healthy volunteers; this may account for diminished effectiveness with frequent dosing. On the other hand, levalbuterol is pure *R*-albuterol without the *S* component. In theory, levalbuterol should be more effective than racemic albuterol at 50% of the dose (same amount of *R*-albuterol) because there are no competing harmful effects from the *S* isomer. However, studies assessing the use of levalbuterol for the treatment of children with acute asthma have not consistently demonstrated this theoretic advantage.

In an early study, the ED use of levalbuterol was associated with a decreased need for hospitalization. Subsequently, other randomized trials comparing the ED use of the two drugs failed to find a levalbuterol benefit and at least one clinical trial failed to demonstrate benefit with continuously nebulized levalbuterol. The cost of levalbuterol is more than 10 times that of racemic albuterol. Until there are more compelling data to demonstrate conclusively that the additional costs of levalbuterol are offset by clinical benefits, racemic albuterol is the drug of choice for children with acute asthma exacerbations.

Children sustaining clinical improvement 60 minutes after the most recent SABA treatment may be discharged; SABA should be weaned over the next 3 to 7 days. If prednisone was administered in the ED, it may be continued as 3 to 5 days of prednisone (1 mg/kg once or twice per day; maximum, 60 mg); however, compliance is not as good as with dexamethasone. Children treated with dexamethasone in the

ED should be provided either one or two additional doses to be taken 24 and 48 hours after the ED dose. The recommended dose is 0.3 to 0.6 mg/kg once per day with a maximum of 8 to 16 mg. Children should continue all other asthma controller medications, including inhaled corticosteroids (ICSs).

For those who are not already receiving ICSs, it is unclear if prescribing them at ED discharge leads to improved short-term outcomes, such as fewer ED relapses within 72 hours. Some have found "insufficient evidence that ICS therapy provides additional benefit" when added to systemic corticosteroids at ED discharge. Rather than prescribing ICS to prevent ED relapse, prescribing may be considered to help achieve longer-term symptom relief for patients with persistent disease marked by frequent coughing or wheezing, frequent exacerbations requiring the use of SABA, or recurrent visits to the ED. ICS are safe and well tolerated at recommended doses and may be given concurrently with systemic corticosteroids. In addition to prescribing medications, emergency clinicians should also provide asthma education at discharge. Some EDs provide standardized information to families with a video or DVD while they undergo ED therapy. Descriptions of how to identify and avoid asthma triggers, a written asthma action plan explaining proper steps to take in response to an asthma flare, a review of discharge medications, and instruction on proper MDI-S use should be included. Follow-up asthma care is recommended within 1 to 4 weeks.

Moderate Exacerbation

In general, a moderate exacerbation is characterized by alert tachypneic children who have wheezing throughout expiration, an inspiratory-to-expiratory ratio of 1:2, and significant use of accessory muscles. Typically, the oxygen saturation will be 92% to 95% and the PEFR will be 41% to 70% of personal best. As with children experiencing milder attacks, the cornerstone of therapy is SABA therapy. Other medications include ipratropium bromide and corticosteroids.

Ipratropium bromide, an anticholinergic agent, blocks reflex bronchoconstriction caused by stimulation of airway cholinergic receptors. It is available as an MDI and as an NEB solution for nebulization that may be mixed directly with albuterol. The combination therapy of a SABA with ipratropium bromide has been demonstrated to be more effective than a SABA alone (i.e., lower hospitalization rates and improvements in asthma scores and pulmonary function test results).

The clinical benefits of ipratropium bromide may be delayed for up to 60 minutes. However, it is inexpensive and free of adverse effects because less than 1% is systemically absorbed. Ipratropium bromide should be given to children with moderate to severe exacerbations. Two to three doses may be mixed with three doses of albuterol and delivered continuously by NEB for 1 hour (Table 163.3). This means of administration, although not superior in efficacy to delivery of albuterol and ipratropium bromide by MDI-S, more consistently achieves the goal of three treatments in the first hour of care, as opposed to giving intermittent treatments every 20 minutes. Alternatively, intermittent therapy may be provided for moderately ill children by giving 4 to 8 puffs of ipratropium bromide every 20 minutes in the first hour, along with albuterol via MDI-S.

Moderately ill children who continue with dyspnea or significant work of breathing or poor aeration after the first hour of albuterol and IB therapy need continued albuterol therapy. Children treated with continuously nebulized SABAs have lower rates of hospitalization, greater improvements in PEFR, and similar rates of adverse events compared with those treated intermittently. Additionally, continuous NEB therapy will result in less respiratory therapy, nursing time, and costs, has been shown to be safe, and may benefit the sickest patients the most.

The prompt use of corticosteroids can decrease the need for hospitalization and should be administered early for patients with moderate disease. Although oral prednisone has historically been the corticosteroids of

TABLE 163.3 Short-Acting β₂-Agonists in Acute Asthma.

	Mild	Moderate	Severe
Delivery method	Intermittent NEB or MDI-S	Intermittent by NEB or MDI-S (3 doses in first hour) or continuous by NEB for 1 hour	Consider subcutaneous or intramuscular therapy; continuous by NEB
Comments	Most patients will need one or two treatments; allows MDI-S teaching; no IB needed	Continuous is not superior to MDI-S; easier to adhere to NHLBI guidelines for the first hour of therapy: concurrent IB therapy more easily delivered	Better outcomes in severe asthma

IB, Ipratropium bromide; *MDI-S,* metered-dose inhaler with spacer; *NEB,* nebulizer; *NHLBI,* National Heart, Lung, and Blood Institute.

choice in the ED treatment of acute asthma, recent studies demonstrate that oral dexamethasone has equivalent efficacy.[3] Dexamethasone has the advantage of having a substantially longer half-life (36 to 72 hours) than prednisone (18 to 36 hours), permitting a shorter treatment course with less vomiting and greater compliance. At this point, the optimal dose and duration of dexamethasone therapy are being established. Dose ranges from 0.3 to 0.6 mg/kg/dose are commonly used, with maximum doses of 8 to 16 mg[4]. Following the initial ED dose, patients typically receive either one or two additional doses, each spaced apart by 24 hours.

Most children with moderate asthma exacerbation can be managed without the insertion of an IV line. Intramuscular therapy is a reasonable option for children who vomit orally administered corticosteroids. The use of ICS, in addition to systemic corticosteroids, for the ED treatment of acute asthma is an area of ongoing research; at this point, we do not recommend its routine use.

A suggested approach to the management of children with moderately acute asthma is summarized in Fig. 163.1. After 1 hour of therapy, a clinical reassessment should be made; evaluation at this time is more accurate than the assessment at ED arrival in predicting the need for hospitalization. Those who worsen despite the first hour of therapy are likely to need continuously nebulized albuterol and hospitalization. In contrast, children with markedly decreased wheezing and work of breathing with improved aeration may be monitored without SABAs to assess for clinical deterioration. The disposition decision can then be made after the child has been observed for 90 to 120 minutes from their last SABA dose. The disposition decision should take into consideration the frequency of prior hospitalizations and ED visits and issues regarding compliance and support systems. ED discharge medications and education are the same as outlined for those with mild exacerbations.

There is a third group of children who are improved after the first hour of therapy but are not well enough to be discharged home. In a study of children treated with prednisone and 2 hours of SABA therapy who met criteria for admission at the 2-hour point, less than 50% were hospitalized when SABA therapy was continued for an additional 2 hours, and none returned to the ED within 48 hours of discharge. To avoid unnecessary hospitalizations, we recommend observing patients who do not otherwise decline for a total of 3 to 4 hours from ED arrival prior to making the disposition decision.

Severe Exacerbation

A severe exacerbation is characterized by restlessness or lethargy, extreme tachypnea and tachycardia, audible wheezing, inspiratory-to-expiratory ratio exceeding 1:2, significant use of accessory muscles, and oxygen saturation less than 92%. Some older children with a severe exacerbation may have bradypnea due to a prolonged expiratory phase, and auscultated wheezing may be absent with markedly decreased aeration. The PEFR will typically be less than 40% predicted, although most children will be too ill to use a peak flow meter.

Fig. 163.1 outlines the approach to the management of severely ill children. They should be attached to a cardiorespiratory monitor and blood pressure cuff, with continuous monitoring of oxygen saturation by a pulse oximeter. As with moderately ill children, supplemental oxygen and continuously nebulized albuterol and ipratropium bromide should be provided soon after arrival. Nearly all severely ill children will require more prolonged therapy with continuously nebulized albuterol, as outlined above. To achieve an oxygen saturation of 92% or greater, it may be necessary to use a non-rebreathing facemask. Severely ill children may be too sick to tolerate oral medications and may need IV medications. A dose of methylprednisolone or dexamethasone should be given as soon as an IV line is established.

For children with very poor inspiratory flow, nebulized SABAs may not be effectively delivered to the smallest airways; short inspiratory time, low inspiratory pressures, and a prolonged exhalation phase will impair the delivery of inhaled medications. In these cases, subcutaneous or intramuscular terbutaline or epinephrine may be considered. Terbutaline has the advantage of being a more selective agent with fewer side effects, such as tremors, vomiting, or palpitations. This treatment can be of particular benefit for very ill and anxious young children who are uncooperative with the inhalation treatments. There are no data to suggest that one mode of administration is superior to the other, although intramuscular epinephrine therapy is recommended for children with bronchospasm due to anaphylaxis. If it is more readily available, an epinephrine autoinjector is effective for this subset of patients. Subcutaneous or intramuscular therapy may be repeated every 10 to 15 minutes, as needed, in extreme cases. If IV access is already established, instead of the subcutaneous or intramuscular therapy outlined above, the patient may be treated with a bolus of 10 µg/kg of IV terbutaline.

Meta-analyses have determined that the use of magnesium sulfate results in improved outcomes for adults and children. In particular, children with a suboptimal response to initial SABA therapy who are subsequently treated with magnesium have significantly greater improvements in pulmonary function compared with those treated with placebo. In contrast, magnesium has not been found to be efficacious as a component of initial therapy for children with moderate to severe exacerbation when given prior to judging the response to early albuterol therapy.

Magnesium is inexpensive and has minimal adverse effects. Hypotension may be minimized by slowly infusing the dose over 20 minutes. Magnesium (50 to 75 mg/kg over 20 minutes; maximum, 2 g) should be given to moderately ill patients who have a suboptimal response to SABAs, IB, and CS, as well as for all severely ill children.

There are insufficient data to make recommendations for the use of continuously infused IV SABAs. Potential adverse effects from use of continuously infused IV SABAs are substantial and include dysrhythmias, hypertension, and hypokalemia. Continuously infused IV SABAs should not be used except for impending respiratory failure, a situation in which the risk-benefit ratio shifts toward favoring their use.

Heliox is a low-density mixture of helium and oxygen that results in less turbulent flow through narrowed airways. Theoretically, heliox may decrease the work of breathing, resulting in less respiratory muscle fatigue and a lower likelihood of ventilatory failure. Heliox has not been found beneficial in all asthma exacerbations, but it may be considered for severely ill children who are not responding to more conventional therapy.

Although there is little in the literature to support the use of non-invasive ventilation (NIV), such as bilevel positive airway pressure (BiPAP), in the management of severe asthma in children, clinicians have employed it with good success to avoid the need for mechanical ventilation. Theoretically, the positive pressure of NIV can ease inhalation and decrease the alveolar collapse associated with exhalation. For a child who remains severely ill despite the previously outlined treatment, the risk-benefit ratio favors the use of BiPAP. The need for mechanical ventilation of the severely ill patient should take into account the entire clinical picture, including illness severity, response to therapy, and ABG results. However, the ABG results should not be used solely to make this decision. The child with an initial pH of 7.10 and a $PaCO_2$ of 55 mm Hg who shows marked improvement with IV SABA therapy may not require ventilatory assistance, whereas the child with a pH of 7.18 and $PaCO_2$ of 50 mm Hg who appears fatigued and is not responding to therapy will likely need mechanical support. Ketamine is a bronchodilator and is the drug of choice for sedation and analgesia of the asthmatic child who requires intubation.

Since mechanical ventilation can result in air trapping and baro-trauma, enough expiratory time should be allowed for air exit from the lungs. Permissive hypercapnia describes one strategy to prevent baro-trauma; it minimizes tidal volumes and respiratory rates to decrease peak inspiratory pressures.

BRONCHIOLITIS

KEY CONCEPTS

- An infant younger than 12 months has an oxygen consumption index double that of an adult and with bronchospasm, may rapidly develop hypoxemia, bradycardia, and cardiopulmonary arrest.
- Bronchiolitis is a clinical diagnosis based on a history of prodromal upper respiratory infection symptoms in an infant or young child, followed by findings on physical examination of wheezing (often with shifting crackles) and increased work of breathing. The value of diagnostic imaging and laboratory evaluation is limited, and these measures should not be used routinely.
- All febrile infants in the first month of life should undergo testing and evaluation for serious bacterial infection and be empirically treated with antibiotics, regardless of respiratory syncytial virus (RSV) status or presence of clinical bronchiolitis.
- A urinalysis and culture should be performed for febrile infants between 1 and 3 months of age who are known to be RSV-positive or have clinical bronchiolitis. The decision to obtain blood or cerebrospinal fluid cultures and give empirical antibiotics should be made on an individual basis (see Chapter 161).
- The management of infants with bronchiolitis focuses largely on supportive measures, and most patients able to tolerate oral hydration can be managed as outpatients. There are currently no consistently effective pharmacologic therapies for bronchiolitis (including SABA, corticosteroids, or antibiotics).
- Despite reports that more than 50% of infants may be prescribed corticosteroids when diagnosed with bronchiolitis, well-designed controlled trials have demonstrated no benefit for their use in rates of admission, clinical scores, or any other clinical outcomes.
- High-flow nasal cannula (HFNC) and continuous positive airway pressure (CPAP) may have some utility in preventing the need for endotracheal intubation, but the evidence is limited and so the use of these modalities should be reserved only for patients with moderate to severe bronchiolitis.
- Disposition from the ED for bronchiolitis depends on the assessment of multiple risk factors, including young age, prematurity, significant hypoxemia, and severe tachypnea, which may predict a more severe clinical course.

Foundations

Bronchiolitis is an acute infectious disease that results in inflammation of the small airways in children younger than 2 years of age. This process is manifested clinically as wheezing and crackles and increased work of breathing, along with the typical signs and symptoms of a URI. Nearly all children are affected by the viruses that cause bronchiolitis at least once during their first 2 years of life, but it is more common for infants younger than 12 months to manifest clinical signs of bronchiolitis.

Bronchiolitis is a seasonal disease, with most cases occurring between November and April in temperate climates. Bronchiolitis is rarely fatal, and severe cases are associated with a number of risk factors, including low birth weight, prematurity, chronic lung disease, and congenital heart disease. Many viruses are implicated as the underlying cause of bronchiolitis, but respiratory syncytial virus (RSV) is estimated to cause up to 70% of cases in previously healthy children. Other viruses commonly isolated are parainfluenza, human metapneumovirus, influenza, adenovirus, bocavirus, and rhinovirus.

Most respiratory viruses that cause bronchiolitis in children are transmitted from one host to another by fomites spread from hand to nose or by droplets produced by sneezing or coughing of respiratory secretions. Shedding of the virus often begins before the onset of significant clinical symptoms and can continue for 2 to 3 weeks in an immunocompetent infant. The typical incubation period is 2 to 8 days from the time of initial contact.

Anatomy, Physiology, and Pathophysiology

In an infected patient, viral replication often begins in the epithelial cells of the upper airway before spreading to the mucosal surfaces of the lower respiratory tract. The infected epithelial cells are generally destroyed by lysis or apoptosis, which results in the desquamation of these cells and the release of host inflammatory mediators. Affected lungs demonstrate epithelial cell necrosis, monocytic inflammation and edema of the peribronchial tissues, and mucus and fibrin plugging of the distal airways on histologic examination. These findings translate into the clinical findings of wheezing and lower airway obstruction in an infant with bronchiolitis. Younger infants, whose distal airways are of smaller caliber and who lack active immunity to most respiratory viruses, are prone to more severe clinical symptoms. Severe lower airway obstruction leads to air trapping and atelectasis, resulting in mismatched ventilation and perfusion and hypoxemia. In addition, younger infants are at increased risk for fatigue, leading to hypercarbia and respiratory failure.

Clinical Features

Infants with bronchiolitis are typically younger than 12 months and present during the winter months. The first symptoms are generally those of a URI, such as nasal congestion and copious rhinorrhea. This is followed within a few days by a tight cough, often associated with difficulty in feeding. Some parents will report audible wheezing as well. Approximately one-third of patients admitted with bronchiolitis will have a fever. Very young infants may present with a history of apnea, which may precede the onset of typical symptoms of respiratory infection. The emergency clinician should ascertain information about the infant's hydration status, including the amount and frequency of oral intake, urine output, vomiting, and diarrhea.

Comorbidities, such as congenital heart disease, chronic lung disease, and prematurity, can have a significant impact on the clinical course of bronchiolitis. A past history or family history of wheezing or atopy may make the diagnosis of asthma more likely, particularly in the older infant; daycare attendance and household contacts with respiratory symptoms favor a diagnosis of bronchiolitis.

TABLE 163.4   Suggested Bronchiolitis Assessment Tool

Parameter	DEGREE OF BRONCHIOLITIS		
	Mild	**Moderate**	**Severe**
Feeding	Normal	Less	Poor
Sao$_2$ in room air	≥95%	92%–94%	<92%
Respiratory rate (breaths/min)	<60	60%–70%	>70
Retractions	None or minimal	Intercostal	Substernal
Accessory muscle use	None	None	Neck or abdominal
Wheeze	None or minimal	Moderate expiratory	Severe inspiratory-expiratory; audible without a stethoscope
Air exchange	Good, equal breath sounds	Localized, decreased breath sounds	Multiple areas of decreased breath sounds

Common vital sign abnormalities include fever, tachycardia, tachypnea, and hypoxia. The oxygen saturation (Sao$_2$) of any moderately or severely ill infant should be obtained soon after ED arrival as an adjunct to the physical examination. With the use of pulse oximetry, an ABG analysis is generally unnecessary to assess a patient's oxygenation. Thus, carrying out ABG analysis should be reserved for those with severe disease and impending respiratory failure to measure the extent of hypercarbia and respiratory acidosis.

Nasal flaring and retractions are visible signs of respiratory distress. Lung auscultation often reveals decreased air movement, rales, rhonchi, wheezing, and a prolonged expiratory phase. Irritability or lethargy, particularly in young infants, indicates a more severe disease. Children can be stratified into mild, moderate, and severe categories based on the physical examination findings (Table 163.4). The combination of poor feeding and increased insensible fluid losses often has an impact on an infant's hydration status. A careful assessment of the anterior fontanel, mucous membranes, capillary refill time, and skin turgor can help identify dehydration.

The worst phase of the illness generally occurs in the first few days and children admitted for bronchiolitis have a median length of hospital stay of 2 to 3 days. However, the entire course of illness can last much longer, with a median duration of 12 days. Coughing and noisy breathing, in particular, can last for more than 4 weeks.

Acute bacterial otitis media is the most common associated illness, with a prevalence of up to 60%. The bacterial pathogens are similar to those recovered in other children with acute otitis media and should be treated accordingly. Other concurrent bacterial infections are rare.

Young infants with fever and bronchiolitis present a unique dilemma for the emergency clinician. The rate of serious bacterial infections (SBIs), defined as UTI, bacteremia, bacterial meningitis, or bacterial enteritis, among all febrile infants younger than 8 weeks is as high as 12%. However, in infants with documented RSV infection or clinical bronchiolitis at the time of ED presentation, the incidence of an SBI is substantially lower. Due to their particularly high level of SBI risk, all febrile infants in the first month of life should undergo a complete laboratory evaluation for SBI and be empirically treated with antibiotics, regardless of RSV status or presence of clinical bronchiolitis. For infants between 1 and 3 months of age who are known to

be RSV-positive or have clinical bronchiolitis, we recommend catheterized urinalysis and culture for rectal temperatures above 38°C (100.4°F), since nearly all concomitant SBIs in this age group are UTIs. Urine testing should also be considered for febrile infants with bronchiolitis who are older than 3 months of age, particularly for those with high-risk features for a UTI: temperatures over 39°C (102.2°F), fever for greater than 24 hours, females, and nonblack race.[5] Additional testing to obtain culture specimens of cerebrospinal fluid and blood may be done selectively. Assuming a normal urinalysis and no concern for bacteremia or meningitis, these infants will not typically require empiric antibiotic therapy for presumed SBIs; decisions to treat with antibiotics should be made on an individual basis, considering the degree of ill appearance and comorbidities.

Apnea is commonly reported in young infants with bronchiolitis, especially among those who are hospitalized. Of admitted patients, nearly 5% will have apnea during the hospital stay. Risk factors for the development of in-hospital apnea include post-menstrual age ≤43 weeks, low birth weight, and a history of apnea reported by the caregiver.[6] The absence of all these risk factors has a high negative predictive value for the development of in-hospital apnea.

Differential Diagnoses

Asthma is the condition that has the most clinical overlap with bronchiolitis. Physical examination findings alone cannot often distinguish the two. Younger age, presentation during the winter months, antecedent URI symptoms, and absence of a prior or family history of atopic disease and wheezing suggest bronchiolitis as the cause of wheezing in an individual patient. Some infants will have clinical features consistent with both conditions. For example, a 12-month-old may present in July with a URI and wheezing for the first time. For this child, a clinician may choose to initiate SABA therapy in the ED but continue it only if the child has a favorable response. Conditions that should be differentiated from bronchiolitis are summarized in Table 163.1.

Diagnostic Testing

Bronchiolitis should be diagnosed primarily on the basis of history and physical examination findings. In general, expensive viral diagnostic testing is not warranted for the majority of patients, although confirmation of a viral cause of the illness may eliminate the need for further laboratory evaluation in young infants with fever. (See Chapter 161 for a comprehensive overview of recommendations for pediatric fever.)

There is tremendous variability in the use of diagnostic imaging, with some centers reporting that chest radiographs are obtained for more than 70% of infants hospitalized with bronchiolitis. In children with clinical findings typical for bronchiolitis, however, radiographic imaging is rarely helpful. Hyperinflation, atelectasis, and peribronchial cuffing are the radiography findings most commonly associated with bronchiolitis. In ambulatory patients with acute lower respiratory infections, obtaining a chest radiograph does not affect the clinical outcome but has been associated with increased use of unnecessary antibiotics. Furthermore, the chance of identifying an alternative diagnosis from a chest x-ray is less than 1%. Diagnostic imaging may be helpful in patients with severe distress, significant hypoxia, or an atypical presentation. We agree with the clinical practice guideline published by the American Academy of Pediatrics in 2014 that "when clinicians diagnose bronchiolitis on the basis of history and physical examination, radiographic or laboratory studies should not be obtained routinely."[7]

Management

Whereas the diagnosis of bronchiolitis is fairly straightforward, the management of children with the disease often presents emergency clinicians with confusing and controversial dilemmas. The literature

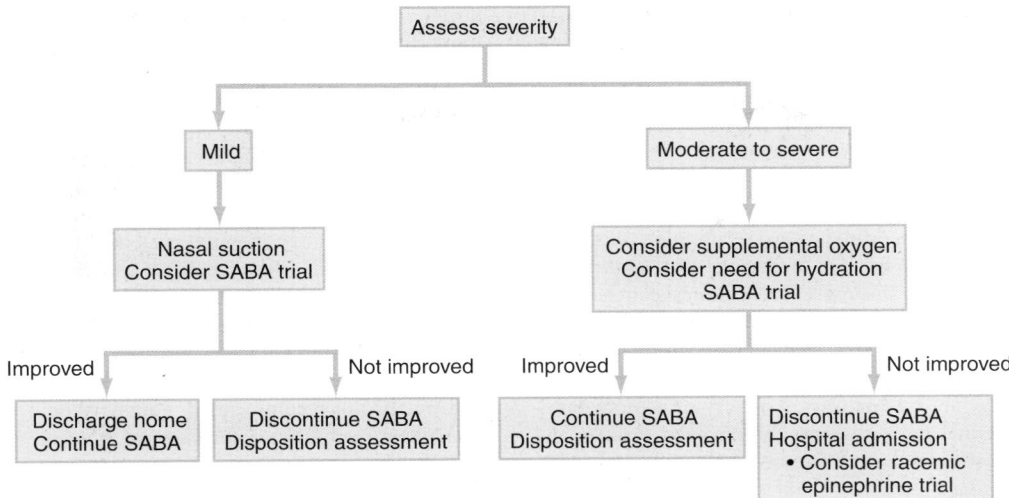

Fig. 163.2 Emergency Department Management of Bronchiolitis. *SABA*, Short-acting β₂-agonist.

is often contradictory, making it difficult to reach a consensus. As a result, there is wide practice variation in the management of bronchiolitis. However, it is clear that a consistent, evidence-based approach to this disease can lead to more efficient and effective care. Supportive care, such as nasal suctioning, providing hydration and supplemental oxygen, is the cornerstone of therapy for affected children A management strategy, stratified by the patient's initial degree of illness, is outlined in Fig. 163.2.

SABAs are the treatment of choice for children with wheezing due to asthma. However, the evidence supporting their use in wheezing caused by bronchiolitis is considerably less favorable. Treatment with SABAs has no significant effect on rates or duration of hospitalization. Conversely, adverse effects such as tachycardia, decreased oxygen saturation, flushing, and hyperactivity occur more frequently in children treated with SABAs. Thus, we do not recommend the routine use of SABAs for bronchiolitis; instead, we recommend a trial of such medications to determine if a patient has a beneficial clinical response *only* if it is unclear whether the patient has asthma or bronchiolitis.

Similar controversy exists with respect to the use of racemic epinephrine in the treatment of bronchiolitis. We recommend that a trial of nebulized epinephrine be considered for a select group of infants with moderate to severe distress who might otherwise require more invasive interventions (e.g., endotracheal intubation) secondary to disease severity. As with SABAs, nebulized epinephrine should be continued only for those patients who demonstrate a clinical benefit. There is currently no sufficient evidence to recommend the use of other bronchodilators, such as anticholinergic agents, for young children with wheezing and suspected bronchiolitis.

Many of the symptoms of bronchiolitis are a result of increased and thickened respiratory secretions. A great deal of literature supports the use of nebulized hypertonic saline in the treatment of cystic fibrosis, in which clearance of thickened secretions is vital. Although there is not yet enough evidence to recommend the routine use of nebulized hypertonic saline in the ED for bronchiolitis, several studies have suggested that it is a safe medication that may reduce the length of stay for some hospitalized children.

Systemic corticosteroids are a well-established and effective treatment of wheezing due to acute asthma. Despite reports that more than 50% of infants may be prescribed corticosteroids when they are diagnosed with bronchiolitis, well-designed controlled trials have demonstrated no benefit for their use in terms of rate of admission,

clinical score, or any other outcome. Thus, our recommendation is that emergency clinicians not use corticosteroids for the treatment of bronchiolitis.

Whereas infants with severe bronchiolitis, who require intensive care and mechanical ventilation, frequently have concurrent or secondary bacterial infections, this is an uncommon complication for most children. There is no evidence for the routine use of antibiotics for bronchiolitis, and they should be reserved for patients with identified bacterial infections.

High-flow nasal cannula (HFNC) is a treatment modality that utilizes heated and humidified air flow with FiO_2 ranging from 21% to 100% to deliver variable degrees of positive airway pressure. By increasing the intraluminal diameter of airways, HFNC can stabilize unsupported airways and relieve air trapping and hyperexpansion. In addition, HFNC can improve alveolar gas exchange by increasing the transpulmonary pressure gradient. Finally, the delivery of heated and humidified air decreases the metabolic demand on the patient. While a few small studies suggest that non-invasive positive pressure ventilation (e.g., CPAP) may be helpful in avoiding endotracheal intubation in severe disease, a Cochrane meta-analysis failed to find sufficient evidence for its use in children with bronchiolitis.[8] A randomized trial of HFNC vs. standard oxygen therapy demonstrated that patients treated with HFNC had fewer escalations of care due to treatment failure.[9] However, the definition of treatment failure in this study is controversial and not widely accepted. A meta-analysis of the available literature regarding HFNC in bronchiolitis concluded that there is not sufficient evidence to show significant benefit from HFNC when compared with standard oxygen therapy or nasal CPAP.[10] While awaiting results from larger, well-designed clinical trials, we believe the risk/benefit ratio favors utilizing HFNC and other forms of non-invasive positive pressure ventilation for patients with moderate to severe disease and judging the response by assessing rate and work of breathing.

Prophylaxis

Although emergency clinicians generally do not have a role in the administration of preventive medications, they should be aware that selected infants will be receiving prophylactic management. Palivizumab (Synagis) consists of monoclonal antibodies against RSV. Whereas RSV-specific immune globulin is not effective for treating the acute disease process, palivizumab is effective in reducing hospitalization rates for RSV in certain high-risk populations; it is recommended for most children younger than 24 months with chronic lung disease, congenital heart disease, or prematurity and is administered as a monthly intramuscular injection during the high-prevalence months. The emergency clinician should be aware that although preventive treatment has been initiated, treated infants with signs of bronchiolitis may still have RSV infections.

Disposition

Because bronchiolitis is a dynamic disease, evaluations at a single point in time may not be sufficient to estimate its severity fully; thus, serial examinations are necessary. A number of demographic and clinical features have been associated with a more severe clinical course. These factors include age younger than 12 weeks, history of prematurity, ill appearance, hypoxemia (SaO_2 <95%), tachypnea (>70 breaths/min), and significant atelectasis on the chest radiograph (when obtained). In addition to younger age and prematurity, a history of hemodynamically significant congenital heart disease, chronic lung disease, and immunocompromised state has been associated with higher morbidity and mortality among inpatients.

Ultimately, the emergency clinician should assess more than just the child's degree of respiratory distress. Patients should be admitted if they are unable to maintain oral hydration due to respiratory symptoms, difficulty with feeds due to increased work of breathing, or copious nasal secretions requiring frequent deep suctioning. The family or caregiver should be able to continue supportive measures at home and have access to medical care. Discharge instructions should include 24-hour follow-up with a primary care provider or emergency clinician for reevaluation. For the small subset of children who are treated with and had a sustained clinical improvement to SABA therapy, this treatment should be continued at home every 4 hours, as needed. Although home oxygen therapy for selected patients with mild to moderate disease has demonstrated success in reducing inpatient hospitalization, primarily in high-altitude conditions, this practice requires careful coordination of care and resources, which may not be feasible in all practice settings. Furthermore, its application to children at sea level is still unclear and thus is not recommended. Parents should be instructed to seek immediate medical care for signs of worsening respiratory distress, including poor feeding, retractions, increased tachypnea, lethargy, and irritability.

The references for this chapter can be found online at ExpertConsult. com.

164

Pediatric Lung Disease

Eric R. Schmitt

KEY CONCEPTS

- Determining the causative agent of pneumonia by clinical presentation and radiographic findings is not reliable; empirical treatment is based on guideline recommendations and likely pathogens.
- Causative agents vary by age; viral agents predominate, especially in younger children, and *Streptococcus pneumoniae* is the leading bacterial cause outside of the neonatal period.
- Infants and younger children with pneumonia may have subtle or nonspecific symptoms and signs on presentation, and fever may be the only sign of disease.
- First line therapy for the treatment of bacterial pneumonia in children is amoxicillin for an outpatient and ceftriaxone or ampicillin for an inpatient.
- Pertussis should be considered in a young infant with a staccato cough or episodes of cyanosis.
- In patients with cystic fibrosis, defects in chloride transport across the airway epithelium result in reduced ciliary clearance of thickened mucus, which leads to an increased likelihood for pneumonia, especially that caused by *Pseudomonas aeruginosa*.
- Cystic fibrosis may respond favorably to bronchodilator therapy and mucolytics, such as inhaled *N*-acetylcysteine.
- Patients with bronchopulmonary dysplasia have increased airway resistance, decreased lung compliance, and obstructive lung disease; reactive airway disease and pneumonia are common in these patients.

SPECIFIC DISORDERS

Pneumonia

Foundations

Although upper respiratory tract infections are more common, children frequently develop lower respiratory tract infections, most notably pneumonia and bronchiolitis. Bronchiolitis (see Chapter 163– Pediatric Lower Airway Obstruction) is primarily seen in children younger than 2 years old and manifests as wheezing and congestion due to a viral infection. Pneumonia is an inflammation of the lung tissue that is most often due to an infection but occasionally may follow a noninfectious insult. The diagnosis of pneumonia is made by clinical signs and symptoms and is often aided by an abnormal chest radiograph demonstrating pulmonary infiltrates (Fig. 164.1).[1] The clinical presentation of pneumonia is variable, ranging from a mild illness to life-threatening disease. A specific organism may be suggested by clinical and radiographic findings, but determination of a precise causative agent is not always possible given the limitations of diagnostic testing, nor is it critical in an emergency setting, as initial treatment is empiric. Infection rates for pneumonia in children vary inversely with age, averaging 40/1000 in preschool-age children and decreasing gradually to 7/1000 in 12- to 15-year-olds.[2] Most deaths from pneumonia result from bacterial infections.

The causative organisms vary with the age of the child. Overall, viral agents cause up to 90% of all pneumonias and are more common in younger children.[3] Bacteria predominate in neonates but become less frequent in toddlers and older children. Outside the neonatal period, the incidence of bacterial agents is stable throughout different age groups. *Chlamydia trachomatis* is a unique cause of pneumonia in infants 3 to 19 weeks of age. *Bordetella pertussis* classically occurs in infants younger than 1 year but may occur in older children and adolescents. *Mycoplasma pneumoniae* is one of the most common causes of pneumonia among children older than 5 years but may also be seen in younger children.[3] *Chlamydophila* (formerly *Chlamydia*) *pneumoniae* is also seen more often in children older than 5 years but may cause infection in younger children.

Among bacteria, group B streptococci and gram-negative bacilli predominate in neonates. Although rare, *Ureaplasma urealyticum* and *Listeria monocytogenes* may cause illness in infants younger than 2 months. *Streptococcus pneumoniae* is the leading bacterial cause of pneumonia in all age groups beyond the newborn period, whereas *Staphylococcus aureus* and *Haemophilus influenzae* are less common causative agents. A vaccine against *H. influenzae* type b first became available in 1985, and incidence of disease has decreased markedly with widespread immunization of infants and young children. In 2010, the 13-valent pneumococcal vaccine (Prevnar 13, Wyeth Pharmaceuticals, NY) replaced the heptavalent pneumococcal conjugate vaccine Prevnar (Wyeth). Prevnar 13 is recommended for the primary series at 2, 4, and 6 months of age, with a fourth booster dose given at 12 to 15 months of age. Vaccination is highly efficacious, with 85% protection against serotype-specific cases of pneumococcal pneumonia, decrease in carriage rates of the included serotypes in daycare settings, and even some protection against viral pneumonia (possibly due to frequent concomitant infection of viral pneumonia with pneumococcal infection).[2,4,5]

Less common bacterial agents include group A streptococci, *Neisseria meningitidis,* and anaerobic bacteria (usually in the setting of aspiration pneumonia). Unusual causes of pneumonia include *Pseudomonas aeruginosa, Legionella pneumophila, Pneumocystis jiroveci,* and rickettsial infections. The incidence of *Mycobacterium tuberculosis* has been increasing in the United States, particularly in urban and low-income areas and among non-White racial or ethnic groups. Infants and adolescents are at highest risk in the United States.[6] Respiratory syncytial virus (RSV) and parainfluenza are the most frequent viral agents in infants younger than 1 year.[3] Viruses that may be responsible for neonatal pneumonia include rubella, cytomegalovirus (CMV), and herpes simplex virus. Other viral agents include influenza, adenovirus, rhinovirus, enterovirus, measles, varicella, and Epstein-Barr virus. In addition, immunocompromised hosts are susceptible to mixed and opportunistic infections, including bacterial, viral (CMV, varicella), protozoan (*P. jiroveci*), and fungal disease (*Coccidioidomycosis*, etc.).

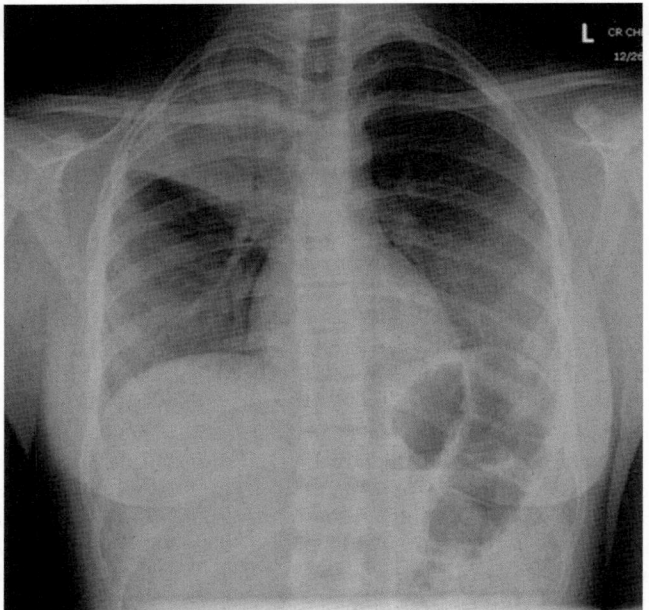

Fig. 164.1 Radiograph showing a right upper lobe consolidation with air bronchograms in a 13-year-old. (Courtesy Dr. Eric R. Schmitt.)

TABLE 164.1	Tachypnea as Defined by the World Health Organization for the Clinical Diagnosis of Pneumonia	
Patient Age	**Respiratory Rate**
Younger than 1 year	Greater than 50 breaths/min
1–5 years old	Greater than 40 breaths/min
Older than 5 years	Greater than 30 breaths/min

The lung is protected from infection by a variety of local and systemic immune mechanisms. Passively acquired maternal antibodies are important in protection against *S. pneumoniae* and *H. influenzae* infections during the first few months of life. Children with altered protective mechanisms are at increased risk for development of pneumonia; this includes children with congenital anatomic abnormalities (e.g., cleft palate, tracheoesophageal fistulas, pulmonary sequestration, congenital cystic adenomatoid malformation), immune deficiencies (e.g., congenital, acquired, medication induced), neurologic alterations that predispose to aspiration (e.g. coma, seizures, cerebral palsy, general anesthesia), and alterations in quality of secreted mucus (cystic fibrosis [CF]).

Bacterial pneumonia and mycoplasma infections are usually transmitted person to person by droplet aspiration. Asymptomatic upper airway colonization often occurs in children and may spread infection to other children. Much less commonly, bacterial pneumonia may result from hematogenous spread from a distant focus or during primary bacteremia. Viral agents that cause pneumonia proliferate in the upper respiratory tract and spread contiguously to involve the lower respiratory tract. Viruses such as varicella, CMV, herpes simplex, Epstein-Barr, measles, and rubella also may infect the lungs through hematogenous spread.

Clinical Features

Clinical symptoms and signs of pneumonia in pediatric patients vary with patient age, specific pathogen, and disease severity.[2] Infants younger than 3 months of age generally have respiratory symptoms, such as tachypnea, cough, retractions, and grunting, but may show only nonlocalizing symptoms, such as isolated fever or hypothermia, vomiting, poor feeding, irritability, and lethargy. Toddlers with *S. pneumoniae* infection may have nonspecific symptoms, such as high fever and lethargy, without significant respiratory symptoms. In general, signs and symptoms in children become more specific with increasing age, although pneumonia may have only subtle manifestations in any child.[1] Systemic symptoms include fever and chills, headache, rigors, and malaise. Symptoms of lower respiratory tract disease may include cough and wheezing. Pleural irritation often causes chest pain, but the

child may also complain of pain in the abdomen or neck. Vomiting (often posttussive) and poor oral intake are common.

Key historical factors include birth and immunization history (particularly pneumococcal and *H. influenzae* type b vaccination), sickle cell status, history of previous pneumonia or frequent infections, and presence of underlying chronic disease. Children with known respiratory (e.g., bronchopulmonary dysplasia [BPD], CF) or cardiac disease tend to have more severe courses of illness; children with a primary or acquired immunodeficiency are also prone to more severe and fulminant disease from common, uncommon, and opportunistic pathogens.

The physical examination should begin with the general appearance and breathing pattern. A full set of vital signs, including oxygen saturation, should be obtained on arrival. Fever is often present but may be low grade or absent. Important findings include hydration status, perfusion, and level of alertness and interaction. Abnormal cardiovascular parameters may indicate dehydration or, rarely, shock. Tachypnea, although not universal, is the most sensitive indicator of pneumonia and may be the only manifestation in younger children. The World Health Organization (WHO) has published guidelines for the clinical diagnosis of pneumonia in developing countries and cites tachypnea and retractions as indicators of lower respiratory disease (Table 164.1).

Other manifestations of lower airway disease include cough, wheezing, or signs of increased work of breathing: nasal flaring, retractions, grunting, and accessory muscle use. The characteristics of the cough may aid in the diagnosis; a staccato cough in an infant may indicate pneumonia caused by *C. trachomatis* or *B. pertussis*. The patient's lungs should be auscultated, and findings may include rales, wheezing, or diminished breath sounds. Although these may be present in younger children, the findings are much less consistent and may be masked by poor inspiratory effort or noisy upper airway sounds. Pleural irritation can cause abdominal tenderness or meningismus, and pulmonary hyperinflation may cause downward displacement of the liver and spleen. Extrapulmonary exam findings may include rhinorrhea, pharyngitis, or exanthem with viral infections. Conjunctivitis can be seen with chlamydial pneumonia, whereas pharyngitis and exanthems are associated with *M. pneumoniae*.

Several complications of pneumonia may result from local and systemic effects of the infection, with the most common systemic complication being dehydration. Pleural effusion or empyema is usually associated with bacterial pathogens (notably *S. pneumoniae, H. influenzae,* and *S. aureus*) but are occasionally seen with mycoplasma, viral, and tuberculosis pneumonia. Similarly, lung abscess, pneumatocele, and pneumothorax are local complications primarily seen with bacterial disease, particularly with *S. aureus*. Extensive pulmonary involvement, regardless of the causative agent, may lead to hypoxia, progressive respiratory deterioration, and multiple organ failure (Fig. 164.2). Apnea in isolation without other symptoms can occur in infants younger than 3 months and is usually associated with viral (especially RSV), chlamydial, and pertussis infections. Additional infectious foci may develop from concomitant bacteremia (e.g., meningitis, epiglottitis, pericarditis, septic arthritis, soft tissue infections). Viral or bacterial

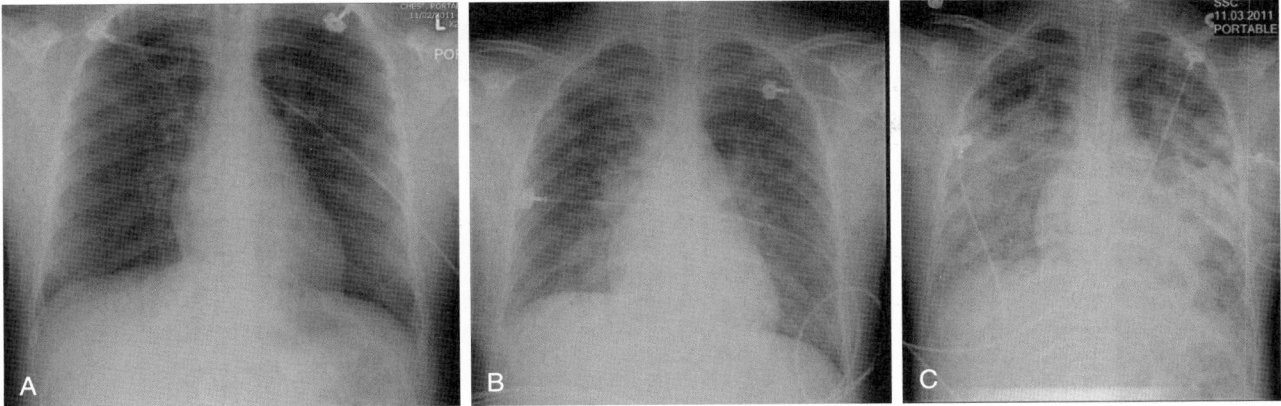

Fig. 164.2 An 11-year-old presented in respiratory distress; radiographs at presentation (A), 4 hours later following resuscitation (B) showing the development of diffuse bilateral infiltrates, and after intubation (C) as the patient rapidly progressed to respiratory failure. (Courtesy Dr. Eric R. Schmitt.)

pneumonia is rarely associated with meningitis, encephalitis, arthritis, rhabdomyolysis, and hemolytic uremic syndrome.

Differential Diagnoses

Unfortunately, no single finding can reliably differentiate pneumonia from other causes of respiratory distress in children.[7] The major conditions to be differentiated in children with pneumonia include bacterial pneumonias, viral disease, other unusual infectious causes (mycobacterial, protozoal, fungal), and noninfectious pathologic conditions (Box 164.1). Common infectious causes classically present with certain historical, clinical, and laboratory findings (Table 164.2). However, the broad spectrum of illness for each condition makes a definitive diagnosis difficult for any individual patient, and no specific feature can reliably differentiate bacterial from nonbacterial pneumonia. Providers should consider a bacterial cause in a child with a temperature higher than 39°C (102.2°F), clinical toxicity, lobar infiltrate, or pleural effusions (Fig. 164.3). Host factors, epidemiology, clinical presentation, and judicious use of diagnostic tests can establish a likely diagnosis and appropriate empiric management.

Bacterial Pneumonia

S. pneumoniae is one of the most frequently seen bacterial causes of pneumonia in children. Children with immunodeficiency, chronic renal disease, and functional or anatomic asplenia and Native Americans are at increased risk for *S. pneumoniae* infections. *S. aureus* pneumonia, although less common, tends to cause a more severe pneumonia and should be considered in any patient who is unusually ill appearing or presenting with respiratory failure or shock.[8] Children with foreign body aspiration, immunosuppression, or concomitant skin infections are at increased risk for *S. aureus* pneumonia. Progression of the disease is rapid, and empyema (90%), pneumatocele (50%), and pneumothorax (25%) are common complications (Fig. 164.4).

Before widespread immunization, *H. influenzae* type b was the second most common bacterial cause of pneumonia. However, its incidence has decreased by 90% since the advent of effective immunization. *H. influenzae* was previously considered a disease of younger children, but most cases now occur in older children.[9] Although clinically indistinguishable from *S. pneumoniae* pneumonia, *H. influenzae* pneumonia historically had a higher incidence of associated pleural effusions (25% to 75%) and bacteremia (75% to 95%).

Although still uncommon, the incidence of group A streptococcal pneumonia has increased since the 1980s. Group A streptococcal pneumonia may occur sporadically and may be a complication

---

BOX 164.1   Noninfectious Diagnoses for Patients Presenting With Lung Disease

Radiologic technique
- Inadequate inspiration
- Breast shadow
- Thymus
- Underpenetration

Primary pulmonary
- Asthma
- Bronchiectasis
- Atelectasis
- Bronchopulmonary dysplasia
- Cystic fibrosis
- Pulmonary sequestration
- Congenital cystic adenomatoid malformation
- α_1-Antitrypsin deficiency

Aspiration
- Foreign body
- Chemical
- Recurrent, caused by anatomic or physiologic disorders

Primary cardiac
- Congenital heart disease
- Congestive heart failure

Pulmonary infarction
- Sickle cell vaso-occlusive crisis
- Pulmonary embolism

Collagen vascular disorders

Acute respiratory distress syndrome

Pleural effusion

Neoplasm

---

of varicella infection. It is typically a severe illness with abrupt onset, rapid progression to toxicity, and high fatality rate (30% to 60% fatality rate reported in a study of all ages).

In bacterial pneumonia beyond the neonatal period, fever is almost universal (often >39°C [102.2°F]). Patients usually have a cough and tachypnea disproportionate to fever and may also appear relatively toxic (e.g., pallor, poor tone, lethargy, delayed capillary refill). Focal lung findings (rales, wheezes, and decreased or bronchial breath sounds) are easier to appreciate in older children, whereas the physical examination in a younger child may be completely unrevealing.

TABLE 164.2 Pneumonia Syndromes

Typical Feature	INFECTIOUS CAUSE			
	Bacterial	Viral	Chlamydial	Mycoplasmal
Historical				
Age	Any	Any	4–16 weeks	5–18 years
Fever	High (>39°C [102.2°F])	Low grade	Usually none	Low
Onset	Abrupt, often after upper respiratory infection	Gradual	Gradual	Gradual
Cough	Productive	Nonproductive	Staccato	Hacking
Associated symptoms	Chest pain; focal infarct	Myalgias, rash, sore throat, coryza	Conjunctivitis	Headache, sore throat, rash
Physical	Toxic appearance			
Lungs	Confined rales	Diffuse rales, wheeze, stridor	Diffuse rales, rare wheeze	Unilateral rales
Chest radiograph				
Infiltrate	Lobar or segmental	Interstitial	Diffuse, interstitial	Lobar or diffuse
Pleural effusion	Occasional	Rare	None	Rare
Other	Pneumatocele; abscess	Hyperinflation, atelectasis	Hyperinflation	
Laboratory test results	Increased WBC granulocytosis	Normal or increased WBC count, lymphocytosis	Normal WBC count, eosinophilia	Normal WBC count
Pathogens (common)	*Streptococcus pneumoniae* *Haemophilus influenzae* *Staphylococcus aureus* <2 months—group B streptococcus; gram-negative enterics; *Listeria monocytogenes*	RSV, parainfluenza, influenza, adenovirus, enterovirus	*Chlamydia trachomatis*	*Mycoplasma pneumoniae*

RSV, Respiratory syncytial virus; *WBC,* white blood cell.

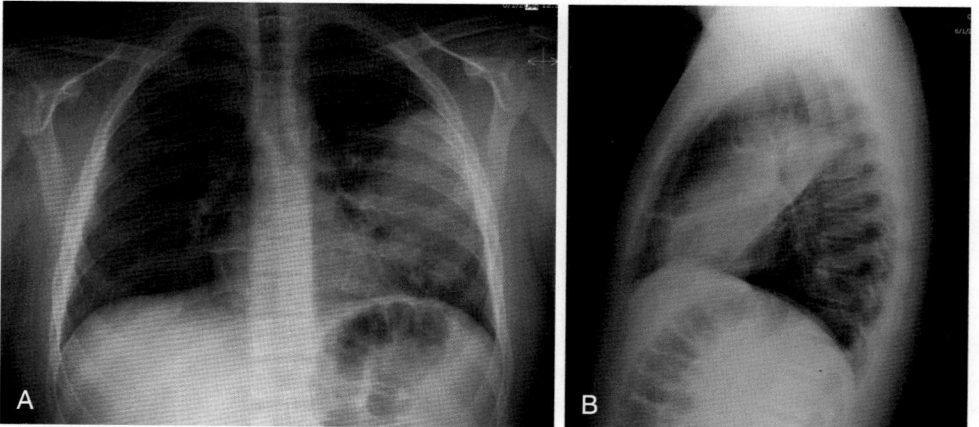

Fig. 164.3 Posteroanterior (A) and lateral (B) radiographs of a left upper lobe consolidation in a 15-year-old with pneumococcal pneumonia. (Courtesy Dr. Eric R. Schmitt.)

Viral Pneumonia

Viral pneumonia is more common in the winter season and generally has a gradual onset, often with associated cough, congestion, and low-grade fever. Tachypnea may be the only physical finding; however, retractions, rales, and wheezing are common. Grunting, cyanosis, lethargy, dehydration, and apnea are seen in more severely affected children.

Radiographic findings typically include hyperinflation and peribronchial thickening, with a diffuse increase in interstitial findings (Fig. 164.5). Patchy areas of consolidation may be present, representing lobular atelectasis or alveolar pneumonia (Fig. 164.6). Although lobar consolidation and small pleural effusions may occur in viral pneumonia, these findings are more consistent with a bacterial cause.

Children do not require chest radiography or viral testing to make the diagnosis of viral pneumonia, particularly in a child who presents during the winter months with fever, cough, congestion, and wheezing. Most viral pneumonias resolve without therapy; however, because of the possibility of secondary bacterial infection and the difficulty in differentiating between bacterial and viral pneumonia, antibiotics should be considered for a more severely ill child.[10] Complications seen with viral pneumonia include dehydration, local progression of the disease, bronchiolitis obliterans, and apnea (usually in the first 3 months of life).

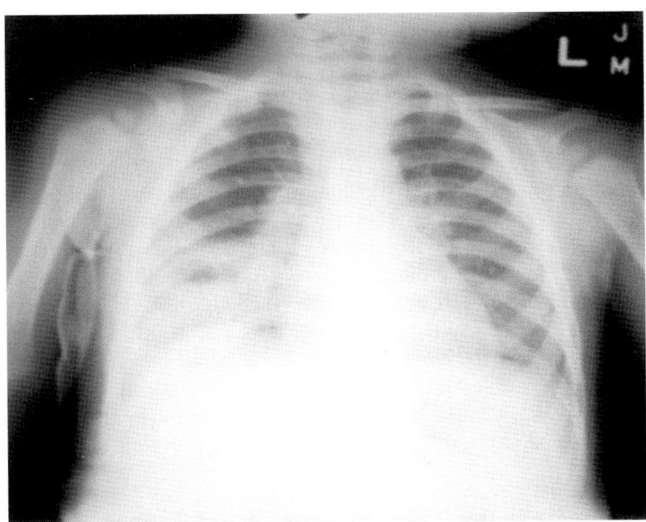

Fig. 164.4 Radiograph showing staphylococcal pneumonia, with empyema and abscess on the right. (Courtesy Dr. Brianna Enriquez and Dr. Marianne Gausche-Hill.)

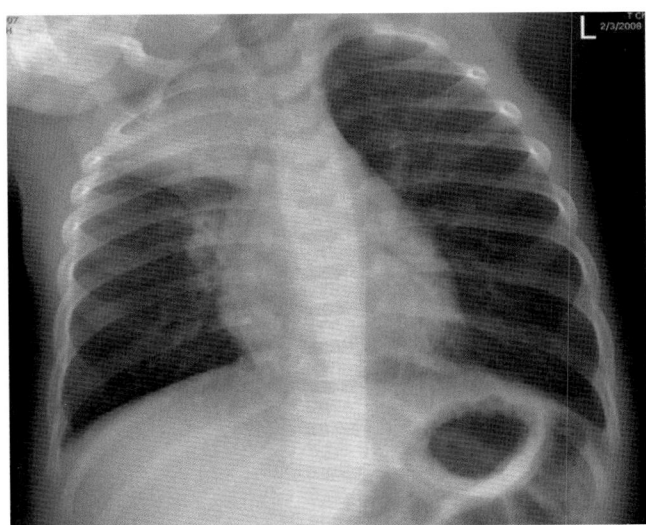

Fig. 164.6 Radiograph showing right upper lobe atelectasis and bilateral interstitial infiltrates in a 9-month-old. (Courtesy Dr. Eric R. Schmitt.)

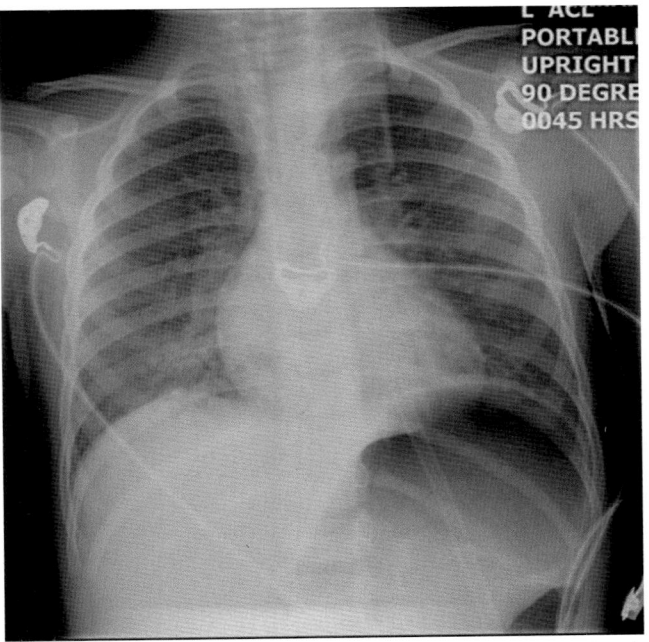

Fig. 164.5 Radiograph of a 3-year-old with viral pneumonia showing hyperinflation, peribronchial thickening, and diffuse interstitial infiltrates. (Courtesy Dr. Eric R. Schmitt.)

Mycoplasma Pneumonia

Mycoplasma pneumonia accounts for 10% to 20% of all pediatric pneumonias. It occurs more commonly in 5- to 18-year-olds, but can be seen in younger children (although rare in infants younger than 1 year).[3] Onset is classically gradual and insidious, but some patients may have an abrupt onset of symptoms. Prodromal symptoms include fever, headache, and malaise, followed several days later by a nonproductive, hacking cough. Associated symptoms of infection may include hoarseness, sore throat, and chest pain; coryza is unusual.

Children with mycoplasma pneumonia generally appear nontoxic and may have rales or, less often, wheezing. Patient may have associated pharyngitis, cervical lymphadenopathy, conjunctivitis, or otitis media.

A rash is present in 10% of patients but can take various forms: urticaria, erythema multiforme, maculopapules, or vesicles. *Mycoplasma* infection is typically benign and self-limited but can play a significant role in the exacerbation of asthma and may cause chronic pulmonary structural abnormalities (e.g., pneumatocele, pleural effusion, pneumothorax, or bronchiectasis). Physical findings are generally less impressive than the radiographic picture. Radiographic findings typically show lower lobar consolidation, but scattered segmental infiltrates and interstitial disease can also be seen (Fig. 164.7). Pleural effusions are uncommon. The white blood cell (WBC) count is usually normal.

Because specific testing and treatment is not applicable to the emergency department (ED) setting, infection is diagnosed clinically and treated empirically. Cold agglutination is rarely used nowadays and is not accurate, particularly in patients younger than 12 years old. Diagnosis may be confirmed with acute and convalescent antibody titers; however, patients may take 4 to 6 weeks to seroconvert, and some patients may fail to mount an immune response altogether. Multiplex polymerase chain reaction (PCR) panels can demonstrate the vital etiology and also bacterial causes including *M. pneumoniae*. Complications of mycoplasma pneumonia are varied, but unusual, and include hemolytic anemia, hemolytic uremic syndrome, myopericarditis, neurologic disease (e.g., meningoencephalitis, Guillain-Barré syndrome, transverse myelitis, and cranial neuropathy), rhabdomyolysis, arthritis, and Stevens-Johnson syndrome.[11,12]

Chlamydia Pneumonia

C. trachomatis is a common sexually transmitted organism that causes cervical infection in 2% to 30% of pregnant women. It is transmitted from the genital tract of infected mothers to their newborn infants, resulting in conjunctivitis in 22% to 44% and pneumonia in 5% to 20%.[13] An infant with pneumonia caused by *C. trachomatis* presents at 3 to 19 weeks of age after colonization at birth. The illness usually begins with nasal congestion followed by cough. In 50% of cases, conjunctivitis precedes the onset of respiratory symptoms. The infant is often afebrile and alert but tachypneic, with a repetitive staccato cough that may interfere with feeding or sleeping. It can resemble the paroxysms of pertussis and occasionally precipitates episodes of alarming respiratory distress. Mild retractions and diffuse inspiratory rales may be noted on chest examination; expiratory wheezing is usually absent or minimal. Middle ear abnormalities are present in 50% of cases.

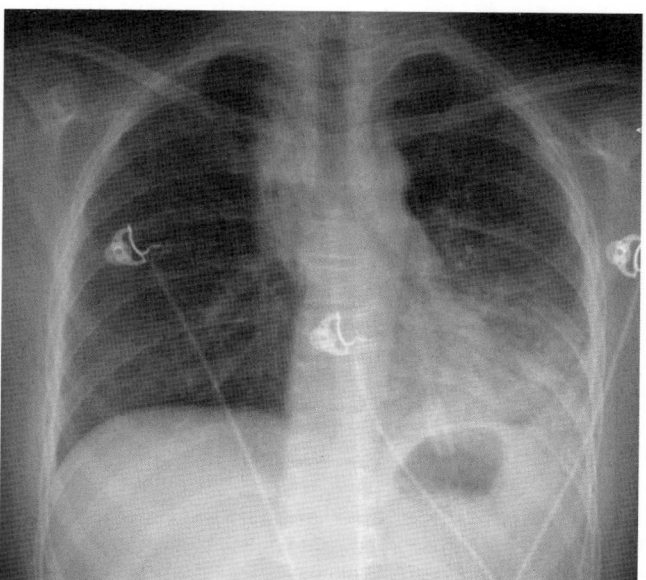

Fig. 164.7 Radiograph of a 12-year-old showing a left lower lobe infiltrate consistent with mycoplasma pneumonia. (Courtesy Dr. Eric R. Schmitt.)

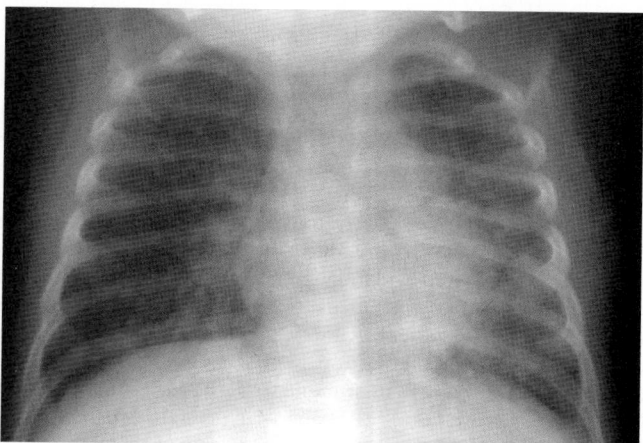

Fig. 164.8 Radiograph showing chlamydial pneumonia in an infant. Note the symmetric interstitial infiltrates. (Courtesy Dr. Michael Diament.)

Chest radiograph usually shows hyperinflation with bilateral and symmetric, diffuse, interstitial infiltrates (Fig. 164.8). Nucleic acid amplification tests have replaced other detection methods (e.g., culture, direct fluorescent antibody tests) because of their higher sensitivity and specificity. Chlamydial pneumonia is often a mild illness but may rarely be complicated by apnea and hypoxemia. Treatment with erythromycin may shorten the course; however, the disease tends to be protracted, and cough and tachypnea can persist for weeks despite antibiotic treatment.

C. pneumoniae is a species of *Chlamydia* that is antigenically, genetically, and morphologically distinct from other *Chlamydia* species. *C. pneumoniae* infection is transmitted from person to person, may play a role in respiratory tract infections in infants and young children, and may cause mild illness or asymptomatic infection in children and adults. Like *Mycoplasma, C. pneumoniae* may play a greater role in pediatric pneumonia than was previously thought. It has been reported to cause sore throat, fever, headache, pertussis-like cough, pneumonia,

and influenza-like illness.[14] Outbreaks have been reported in schools, daycare centers, military camps, adolescents, and families. Infection with *C. pneumoniae* can trigger acute episodes of wheezing in children with asthma. Infection can be confirmed with PCR testing.

Aspiration Pneumonia

Aspiration pneumonia may be due to mechanical, chemical, or bacterial causes. Bacterial aspiration occurs in children with anatomic abnormalities and central nervous system disturbances that impair normal swallowing or protective airway reflexes.[15] Pulmonary damage results from chemical (e.g., stomach acid) and bacterial (e.g., gastrointestinal and upper respiratory organisms) insults. Within several hours of the aspiration, the child may have the onset of cough, tachypnea, and fever. Physical examination commonly reveals rales and wheezing, with cyanosis as the disease progresses. Radiographic findings include both localized (right middle lobe or lower lobe) and diffuse/bilateral infiltrates.

Pneumonia in the Immunocompromised Patient

Children with chronic disease and congenital, acquired, and iatrogenic immunodeficiencies are susceptible to the aforementioned respiratory pathogens and to a multitude of opportunistic organisms, including *P. jiroveci*, CMV, and fungi. Presenting symptoms may be similar to those in normal hosts; however, the course tends to be more rapid, severe, and fulminant. While awaiting organism identification and the results of culture, patients should be hospitalized for monitoring, supportive therapy, and treatment with intravenous antibiotics active against a broad spectrum of organisms. Invasive sampling for diagnosis of potentially treatable organisms may need to be considered if the patient fails to improve after initial therapy.

Diagnostic Testing

Radiography. A chest radiograph is unnecessary in children without comorbid conditions who have no fever, tachypnea, or focal findings on auscultation, because they are unlikely to have pneumonia. Chest radiography can also be deferred in a well-appearing child who has pneumonia based on clinical presentation (fever, tachypnea, abnormal lung auscultation). We recommend that any child who appears ill or in whom the diagnosis is unclear receives radiographic evaluation, with chest radiography. A clear chest radiograph (without infiltrate) is sufficient to exclude pneumonia in the majority of children.[16,17] However, an infiltrate may not be initially apparent in a dehydrated child with suspected pneumonia, only becoming visible on subsequent imaging after rehydration (see Fig 162.2).

Although great variability exists, bacterial pathogens classically produce alveolar infiltrates in a lobar distribution (Fig. 164.9) but may produce diffuse interstitial infiltrates. Viral and chlamydial infections tend to appear as diffuse interstitial infiltrates, commonly with hyperinflation and atelectasis (see Fig. 164.5). Chest radiographs can identify multilobar disease, pleural effusions, pneumatoceles, and pneumothorax (see Fig. 164.4). Hilar adenopathy may indicate tuberculosis or malignant neoplasm.

Lateral decubitus radiographs in patients with pleural effusions can help assess effusion size and loculation. Computed tomography (CT) may be useful to provide greater detail of effusions and lung abnormalities in critically ill children with complicated pneumonia, or when alternative pathology is suspected based on the plain radiograph (Fig. 164.10). Routine CT of the chest to establish the diagnosis is not recommended.

Ultrasound. Recent studies have examined the utility of lung ultrasound for the diagnosis of pneumonia in children.[18] Most studies use highly skilled sonographers with specific training in pediatric thoracic ultrasound, and this level of expertise is not widely available.[19] When performed by a skilled sonographer, ultrasound has sensitivity similar to chest radiography, although it may not be as specific.[20] Ultrasound predicts the presence of consolidation on chest radiography; the best correlation occurs when the consolidation measures greater than 1 cm on ultrasound.[21,22] When available, a positive ultrasound study may safely allow for the reduction of chest radiography.[23]

Laboratory Studies. Children with pneumonia are at risk for hypoxemia and should undergo pulse oximetry to determine oxygen saturation; arterial or venous blood gas analysis should be reserved for patients in significant distress or respiratory failure to monitor respiratory status or response to therapy. A complete blood count (CBC) is not useful in differentiating between viral and bacterial pneumonia and should not be obtained unless the results will change management. We do not recommend blood cultures in otherwise well-appearing children with uncomplicated pneumonia, because they are unlikely to be helpful.[24] Blood cultures may be considered in ill-appearing hospitalized patients.[8,25] Sputum cultures are technically difficult in younger children and should not be routinely obtained.[18]

Patients with pleural effusions that are enlarging or compromising respiratory function should undergo thoracentesis for diagnostic and therapeutic purposes. Although parapneumonic effusions are most suggestive of bacterial infection, they also occur with mycoplasmal and

occasionally with viral infections. The fluid should be sent for Gram staining and culture (anaerobic and aerobic bacterial), cell count and differential, total protein level, pH, and glucose concentration. Interpretation of pleural fluid in children follows adult guidelines (see Chapters 62 and 63). Cultures for rare pathogens may be considered if the initial assessment is not diagnostic or specific risk factors are identified. Bronchoscopy with bronchoalveolar lavage may be useful in a child who is severely ill or refractory to treatment.

Rapid antigen testing for RSV is not indicated unless the result would change management (e.g., risk stratification in a young infant with fever, or to cohort for inpatient treatment).[26] A real-time influenza PCR assay may be helpful for atypical cases when the use of antivirals is being considered.[18] However, influenza may be diagnosed clinically during times of high prevalence (i.e., a higher likelihood of a false negative influenza assay). Children at higher risk (e.g., children <2 years or those with significant comorbid disease) should be empirically treated with antivirals without confirmatory testing. Although most pediatric patients with tuberculosis do not have pulmonary symptoms, testing for tuberculosis should be considered for patients with lobar pneumonia, pulmonary effusions, or hilar adenopathy, especially in immunocompromised children or children who have recently immigrated from less developed countries.

Management

Treatment of pneumonia in a pediatric patient consists of appropriate antimicrobial use and supportive therapy (Table 164.3). Because of the difficulty in identifying a specific pathogen, antibiotic choice is generally empirical. The three most important factors in directing management are the patient's age, likely pathogen, and degree of illness.

Infants Younger Than 2 Months. An infant younger than 2 months with pneumonia should usually be admitted to the hospital and monitored with continuous pulse oximetry for signs of needed respiratory support; apnea and respiratory failure may be precipitous. This age group is immunologically immature, and signs of sepsis may be subtle. We recommend blood, urine, and cerebrospinal fluid cultures before the initiation of antibiotics when possible (see Chapter 161). In infants younger than 1 month, ampicillin, plus ceftazidime, or gentamicin (recommended in premature infants) are appropriate choices; ampicillin and ceftriaxone should be used for infants 1 to 2 months of age. If *C. trachomatis* or *B. pertussis* is suspected, the infant should also be treated with azithromycin or erythromycin (given the association of erythromycin with infantile hypertrophic pyloric stenosis, we recommend azithromycin when available).

Infants 2 to 3 Months of Age. Blood and urine cultures should be obtained for infants 2 to 3 months of age. The decision to perform a

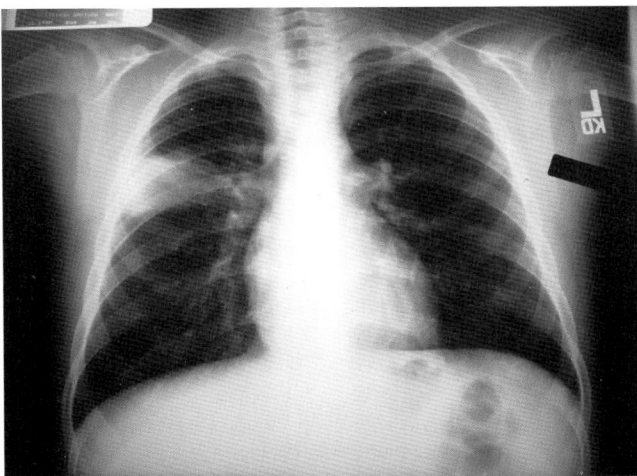

Fig. 164.9 Radiograph showing pneumococcal pneumonia, with infiltrate in the right upper lobe. (Courtesy Dr. Marianne Gausche-Hill.)

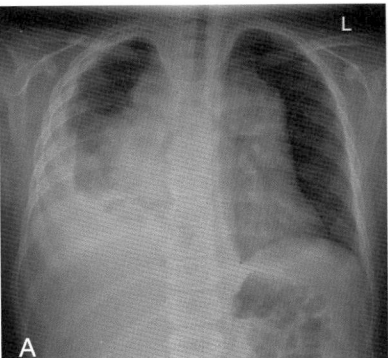
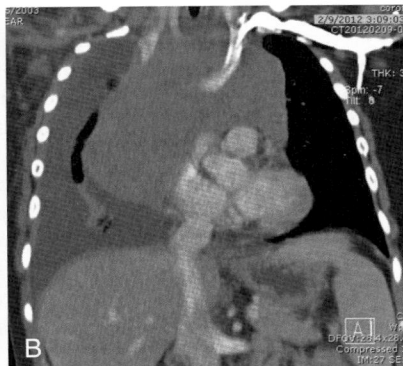
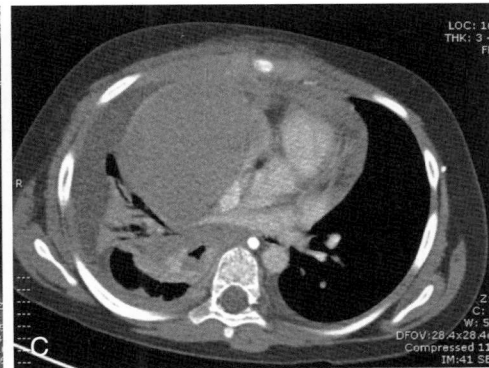

Fig. 164.10 Radiograph (A) of an 8-year-old that was initially interpreted as a right-sided pneumonia with effusion; coronal (B) and axial (C) computed tomography images demonstrate a large mediastinal mass later determined to be a T-cell lymphoma. (Courtesy Dr. Eric R. Schmitt)

TABLE 164.3   Empiric Antibiotic Treatment of Bacterial Pneumonia

Age Group	Most Frequent Pathogens	Outpatient Treatment	Inpatient Treatment
Neonate (<4 weeks)	Group B streptococcus, *Escherichia coli*, other gram-negative bacilli		Ampicillin (150–200 mg/kg/day every 6 hours) + ceftazidime (100 mg/kg/day every 12 hours) *or* Gentamicin (2.5 mg/kg daily) Avoid ceftriaxone.[a]
4 weeks–3 months	*Streptococcus pneumoniae, Haemophilus influenzae, Chlamydia trachomatis* (if afebrile)	Azithromycin (10 mg/kg on day 1, 5 mg/kg daily on days 2–5) *or* Erythromycin (50 mg/kg/day every 6 hours)	Ampicillin (150–200 mg/kg/day every 6 hours) + ceftriaxone (50 mg/kg daily)
	Bordetella pertussis (if afebrile and prolonged cough)	Azithromycin (10 mg/kg on day 1, 5 mg/kg daily on days 2–5)	Azithromycin (10 mg/kg on day 1, 5 mg/kg daily on days 2–5)
3 months–4 years	*S. pneumoniae, H. influenzae*, group A streptococcus	Amoxicillin (75–90 mg/kg/day every 12 hours) *or* Amoxicillin–clavulanic acid (90 mg/kg/day of the amoxicillin component every 8 hours) *or* Cefuroxime (20-30 mg/kg/day every 12 hours)	Ceftriaxone (50 mg/kg daily) *or* Ampicillin (150–200 mg/kg/day every 6 hours) In critically ill patients add: clindamycin (40 mg/kg/day every 6 hours) *or* vancomycin (10–20 mg/kg IV every 6–8 hours) for coverage of MRSA[b]
	Mycoplasma pneumoniae	Azithromycin (10 mg/kg on day 1, 5 mg/kg daily on days 2–5) *or* Clarithromycin (15 mg/kg/day every 12 hours)	Azithromycin (10 mg/kg on day 1, 5 mg/kg daily on days 2–5) *or* Erythromycin (20 mg/kg/day every 6 hours)
	B. pertussis (if afebrile and prolonged cough)	Azithromycin (10 mg/kg on day 1, 5 mg/kg daily on days 2–5)	Azithromycin (10 mg/kg on day 1, 5 mg/kg daily on days 2–5)
≥5 years	*M. pneumoniae, Chlamydophila pneumoniae*	Azithromycin (10 mg/kg on day 1, 5 mg/kg daily on days 2–5) *or* Clarithromycin (15 mg/kg/day every 12 hours)	Azithromycin (10 mg/kg on day 1, 5 mg/kg daily on days 2–5) *or* Erythromycin (20 mg/kg/day every 6 hours)
	S. pneumoniae, H. influenzae	Amoxicillin (75–90 mg/kg/day every 12 hours) *or* Amoxicillin–clavulanic acid (90 mg/kg/day of the amoxicillin component every 8 hours) *or* Cefuroxime (20–30 mg/kg/day every 12 hours)	Ceftriaxone (50 mg/kg daily) *or* Ampicillin (150–200 mg/kg/day every 6 hours) In critically ill patients add: clindamycin (40 mg/kg/day every 6 hours) *or* vancomycin (10–20 mg/kg IV every 6–8 hours) for coverage of MRSA[b]
	B. pertussis (if afebrile and prolonged cough)	Azithromycin (10 mg/kg on day 1, 5 mg/kg daily on days 2–5)	Azithromycin (10 mg/kg on day 1, 5 mg/kg daily on days 2–5)

[a]Ceftriaxone is not preferred in neonates due to risk of hyperbilirubinemia, particularly in premature infants.
[b]*MRSA*, Methicillin-resistant *Staphylococcus aureus*.

lumbar puncture depends on clinical suspicion of central nervous system infection. Ampicillin and ceftriaxone should be given for an infant 2 to 3 months old. If *C. trachomatis* or *B. pertussis* is suspected, the infant also should be treated with azithromycin or erythromycin. Supportive therapy in this age group consists of fever control and hydration. As with infants under 2 months of age, we recommend admission for infants 2-3 months of age, as they are only partially protected against *S. pneumoniae* and *H. influenzae* with one dose of vaccinations.

Infants and Children Older Than 3 Months. In an older child, pneumonia should be categorized into likely bacterial, viral, or mycoplasmal. The emergency clinician should base the presumptive causative diagnosis on clinical and radiographic findings (if obtained). A toxic child with high fever and lobar consolidation is likely to have a bacterial process, whereas a child with a disease of gradual onset, low-grade fever, and interstitial infiltrate with air trapping is more likely to have a viral process.

A well-appearing infant or preschool-age child with isolated pneumonia may be treated with outpatient oral antibiotics. In an infant beyond the neonatal period or a preschool-age child, high-dose amoxicillin is the first line agent and will treat susceptible *S. pneumonia.*[27] Amoxicillin–clavulanic acid is a second line agent and includes some gram-negative and methicillin-sensitive *S. aureus* coverage. Oral cephalosporins are relatively poorly absorbed and highly protein-bound, resulting in inferior pharmacokinetics as compared with amoxicillin; we recommend their use be reserved for penicillin-allergic patients. Azithromycin should not be used to treat *S. pneumoniae*, because there is significant resistance, but it is appropriate therapy for presumed atypical pneumonias in this age group. Azithromycin is the antibiotic of choice in a school-age child or adolescent, in whom *M. pneumoniae* and *C. pneumoniae* are more common. Uncomplicated bacterial pneumonia often has a rapid response to antibiotics; a stagnant or worsening clinical picture should prompt further investigation (e.g., postobstructive pneumonia from an unrecognized foreign body).

Children with neurologic or anatomic abnormalities who aspirate oral or gastric contents are susceptible to pneumonia, predominantly from anaerobes. Penicillin (100,000 to 250,000 units/kg/day every 4 to 6 hours) and clindamycin are appropriate first line antibiotic choices. In seriously ill patients or patients not responding, agents such as metronidazole (40 mg/kg/day every 6 hours) and cefoxitin (80 to 160 mg/kg/day every 4 to 6 hours) may be administered. Nosocomial infections should be treated with antibiotics also active against aerobes and gram-negative bacilli. Children with significant aspiration should be admitted to the hospital, and supportive therapy should include hydration, supplemental oxygen, and oropharyngeal suctioning.

Disposition. Well-appearing children who can maintain hydration and are not in respiratory distress should be considered for outpatient management. Oral antibiotic therapy is appropriate if there is concern for bacterial etiology. Children treated as outpatients should be reevaluated within 24 to 48 hours.[2] Inpatient hospitalization for parenteral antibiotic therapy should be considered for patients who are dehydrated or clinically worsening; a repeat chest radiograph may reveal progression of disease or development of a pleural effusion.

Indications for hospitalization at the time of diagnosis include a toxic appearance, vomiting or dehydration, respiratory compromise (e.g., distress, hypoxia, or inadequate ventilation), multilobar disease, pleural effusions, impaired immune function, and unreliable social environments. Strong consideration should be given to hospitalization of children younger than 6 months, because they are more prone to complications of bacterial pneumonia than older children. Supportive therapy for the inpatient should include maintenance of hydration, fever control, supplemental oxygen, ventilatory assistance, and pleural fluid drainage, as indicated. Parenteral antibiotic therapy should be administered until clinical improvement.

Long-term management of a child with pneumonia should include a clinical reevaluation 2 to 3 weeks after diagnosis. If the child had a prompt response to therapy and is well at the follow-up evaluation, a repeat radiograph is unnecessary at this time. If the child had a complicated course (e.g., pleural effusion) or residual symptoms or if the illness is not the child's first episode of pneumonia, a chest radiograph can ensure resolution.

Pertussis

Pertussis, or whooping cough, is a respiratory tract infection, classically seen in infants younger than 6 months. The incidence of pertussis increased in the 1980s and 1990s, especially in adolescents and adults, likely due to waning immunity.[28] More recently, inconsistent immunization has led to epidemics in vulnerable populations.[29]

Pertussis disease is characterized by three clinical stages—catarrhal stage, paroxysmal stage, and convalescent stage. Pertussis begins with mild upper respiratory tract symptoms and cough; this *catarrhal stage* usually lasts 1 to 2 weeks. The disease progresses to severe paroxysms of a staccato cough (*paroxysmal stage*), followed by posttussive emesis, and may be accompanied by periods of cyanosis and apnea in infants younger than 6 months. The classic whoop is rare, occurring in only 6% of patients and generally seen in children older than 2 to 3 years. Fever is often absent, and the examination findings are remarkably normal between paroxysms. The paroxysmal stage lasts 2 to 4 weeks and is followed by a *convalescent stage*, during which symptoms gradually wane. The duration of the illness in more complicated cases may be 6 to 10 weeks. Immunization is only 80% effective in providing immunity after three doses, making pertussis possible in immunized infants.[30]

The WBC count (if obtained) is usually elevated, often with a marked lymphocytosis. The chest radiograph may show a shaggy, right-sided heart border or have clear lung fields. *B. pertussis* is a fastidious organism, making culture difficult. The organism is most easily recovered in the catarrhal or early paroxysmal stages. Cultures may be negative during the first week or after the fourth week of illness in immunized patients or in patients treated with antibiotics. The PCR assay has been increasingly used for the detection of *B. pertussis*, because of its high sensitivity and more rapid turnaround time than culture.

Pertussis is a particularly severe disease in the first year of life and is often complicated by apneic episodes; less common complications include seizures, secondary bacterial pneumonia, encephalopathy, and death.[31] Pertussis has been increasing in incidence among immunized children and young adults who have waning immunity. The illness in these older patients does not follow the classic stages as described earlier; patients have a mild but prolonged course (often lasting 3 weeks or more), with a dry cough as the predominant symptom.

Because of the risk of apnea, we recommend that all children younger than 3 to 6 months with presumed pertussis be observed in the hospital for monitoring and supportive care, and treated with azithromycin or erythromycin. Antimicrobials have no effect on disease progression after the beginning of the paroxysmal stage but limit the spread of organisms. Vaccination of all health care workers and the general adult population with tetanus, diphtheria, and pertussis (Tdap) is recommended and has been shown to decrease rates of pertussis in infants.

Cystic Fibrosis

CF is an autosomal recessive disease caused by a mutation in the CF transmembrane conductance regulator (*CTFR*) gene. In Whites, approximately 1 in 25 is a carrier, and the disease has an incidence of 1 in 2500 births. The disease also is present (in decreasing incidence) in Hispanics, Native Americans, African Americans, and Asians. Progressive lung disease and infection account for most of the morbidity and nearly all the mortality in those with CF.[32] Defects in chloride transport across the airway epithelium result in reduced ciliary clearance of thickened mucus, decreased antimicrobial effect of the airway surface, increased bacterial adherence, and innate secretion of inflammatory cytokines. All these factors result in a unique sensitivity to bacterial infection of the airway.

Chest radiographic findings of CF include emphysema, peribronchial thickening, bronchiectasis, and focal infiltration, which may be linear or nodular (Fig. 164.11). Identification of the pathogens involved is crucial to the effective treatment of pulmonary infections in CF patients (usually through sputum culture), although early childhood pneumonias in patients with CF are predominantly caused by *S. aureus* and *H. influenzae*. With the emergence of methicillin-resistant *S. aureus* (MRSA), careful attention should be paid to antibiotic coverage. Patients receiving antistaphylococcal prophylaxis may be at increased risk for pseudomonal infections. By 18 years of age, 80% of patients are permanently colonized with *P. aeruginosa*. Acute infective exacerbations generally are managed by oral and intravenous antimicrobial drugs, typically a penicillin (e.g., ticarcillin or piperacillin) or ceftazidime, combined with an aminoglycoside for synergistic effects. If a patient's previous sputum culture results are available, antibiotic coverage for the last known bacterial pathogen should be used. Resistant strains may benefit from imipenem or meropenem, and patients should often be hospitalized for the course of therapy.[33] *Burkholderia cepacia* is a significant pathogen in CF patients and has been associated with an accelerated decline in clinical status and increased mortality. Antimicrobial coverage is similar to that for *Pseudomonas*, although resistance is common and the existence of differing colonization and resistance patterns of patients with CF necessitates respiratory isolation from other susceptible individuals.

Clearance of the thick mucoid secretions is important for treatment. Patients may respond favorably to bronchodilator therapy and to mucolytics, such as inhaled *N*-acetylcysteine, in the acute setting. Chest physiotherapy provided by a high-frequency oscillator device is often used. A flutter valve or positive expiratory pressure mask may be of assistance for improved mucoid clearance. Short-term control of

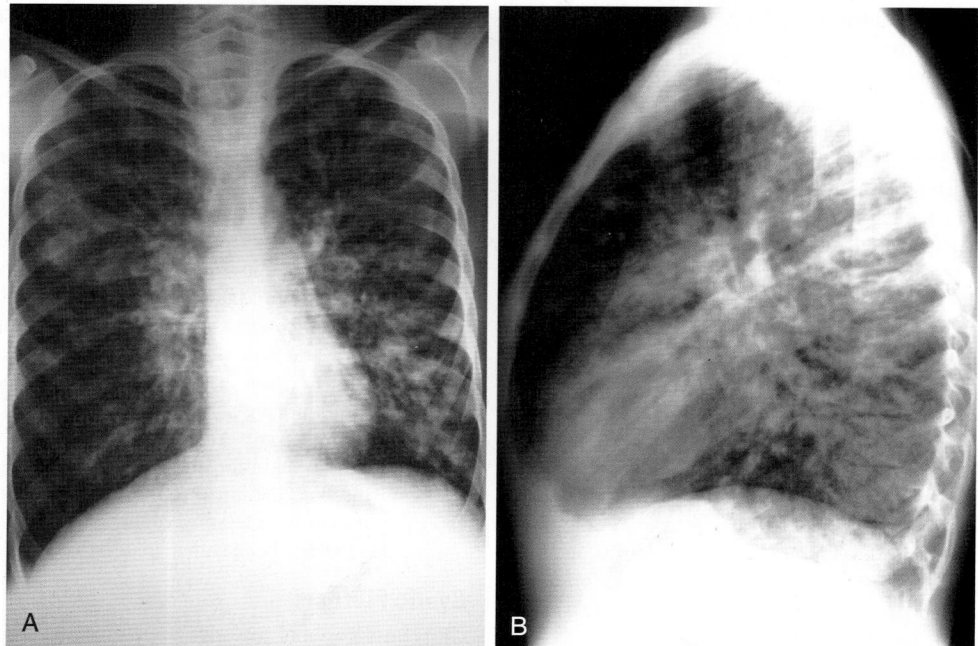

Fig. 164.11 Posteroanterior (A) and lateral (B) radiographs of a teenager with cystic fibrosis. Note emphysema and nodular infiltrates. (Courtesy Dr. Michael Diament.)

inflammation may be obtained by inhaled corticosteroids. Given the complicated nature of these patients and the need for individualized treatment plans, we recommend early consultation with a pediatric pulmonologist.

Bronchopulmonary Dysplasia

BPD is defined as the need for supplemental oxygen 28 days postnatally.[34] BPD is a common cause of diffuse lung disease in infants. Approximately 40% of children with a birth weight less than 1000 g will develop BPD. The severity of disease is related to several factors, including degree of prematurity, use of peripartum steroids, damage incurred by ventilation in the neonatal period, and nutritional status.[35] Infants with BPD have greatly increased rates of hospitalization because of respiratory illness in the first year of life, approaching 65% in infants born weighing less than 1000 g.

Immunizations are used to help prevent pneumonia in patients with BPD. All infants 6 to 23 months old should receive the influenza vaccine during the appropriate season. The 13-valent pneumococcal vaccine and *H. influenzae* type b vaccine are especially important for the prevention of bacterial pneumonia. Monthly prophylaxis against RSV with the monoclonal immunoglobulin palivizumab should be administered to carefully selected patients because it reduces the incidence of RSV disease and risk of subsequent hospitalization.

Patients with BPD have increased airway resistance, decreased lung compliance, and obstructive lung disease. Pneumonia in patients with BPD may be complicated by a reactive airway component. If complicated by pneumonia, radiographs show marked hyperinflation and infiltrates (Fig. 164.12). Inhaled bronchodilators may be efficacious, although these medications may worsen air exchange in patients with

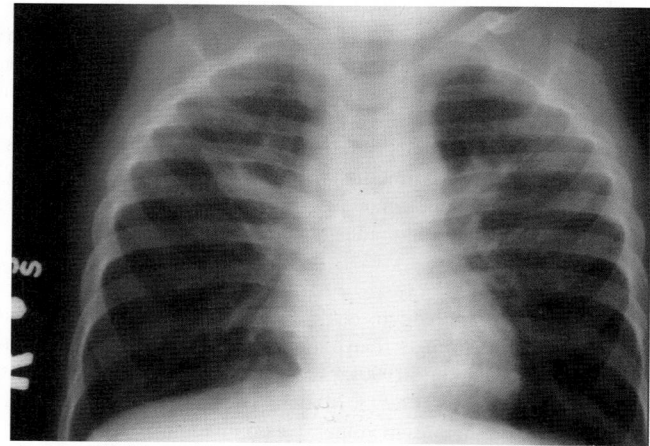

Fig. 164.12 Radiograph of a child with bronchopulmonary dysplasia showing findings of chronic lung disease and hyperinflation. (Courtesy Dr. Michael Diament.)

concomitant airway malacia. Hypoxia and hypercarbia are common, despite an increased respiratory effort. Patients with severe BPD may be receiving long-term diuretic therapy to improve lung mechanics; care should be taken not to confuse pneumonia with cor pulmonale, which can occur in younger infants with chronic supplemental oxygen requirements.

The references for this chapter can be found online at ExpertConsult. com.

165

Pediatric Cardiac Disorders

Timothy Horeczko

FOUNDATIONS

Children with cardiac disorders present to the emergency department (ED) in one of two scenarios. In the first scenario, the child presents with an exacerbation or complication of an already known underlying cardiac disorder. Early consultation with the child's cardiologist along with comparisons of the child's previous and most recent diagnostic studies are very useful in the evaluation and management phases.

The second scenario represents more of a challenge to the emergency clinician: the child with an undiagnosed congenital or acquired cardiac disorder who presents with concerning signs and symptoms (Box 165.1).

Fetal and Neonatal Circulation

During fetal development, blood oxygenated by the placenta flows to the fetus through the umbilical vein, bypasses the fetal liver through the ductus venosus, and returns to the fetal heart through the inferior vena cava. From the inferior vena cava, blood enters the right atrium and is preferentially shunted to the left atrium through the patent foramen ovale (Fig. 165.1). Fetal pulmonary vascular resistance (PVR) is higher than fetal systemic vascular resistance (SVR); this forces deoxygenated blood to mostly bypass the fetal lungs (see Fig. 165.1). From the left atrium, blood flows to the left ventricle and the aorta. The oxygenated blood ejected through the ascending aorta is preferentially directed to the fetal coronary and cerebral circulations.

The proportion of returning deoxygenated blood from the superior vena cava that empties into the right atrium and then right ventricle is pumped into the pulmonary artery. This poorly oxygenated blood enters the aorta through the patent ductus arteriosus and mixes with the well-oxygenated blood in the descending aorta. The mixed blood in the descending aorta then returns to the placenta for oxygenation through the two umbilical arteries.

Once the infant is delivered and the umbilical cord is cut, expansion and aeration of the lungs cause a decrease in PVR, which enhances pulmonary blood flow. Increased global oxygenation causes a physiologic closure of the umbilical arteries, umbilical vein, ductus venosus, and ductus arteriosus. Increasing pulmonary blood flow to the infant's left atrium promotes closure of the foramen ovale. Complete anatomic closure of the foramen ovale does not occur until about 3 months of age. Although the ductus arteriosus functionally closes at about 10 to 15 hours of life, complete anatomic closure does not occur until 2 to 3 weeks of life.

In the absence of any congenital cardiac defects, these transitional circulatory changes pose no physiologic problems to the infant. However, closure of the ductus arteriosus can be life-threatening in neonates with cardiac defects that depend on the patency of the ductus arteriosus for survival.

Pathophysiology of Cardiovascular Compensatory Responses

The young myocardium is inefficient and unable to increase contractility in response to demand.[1] When more cardiac output is needed, infants and children respond with an increase in heart rate; therefore, bradycardia is an ominous sign that connotes a severely compromised cardiac output. Children develop the adult capacity to increase contractility by 8 to 10 years of age.

A decrease in stroke volume can be caused by a weak "pump," decreased volume in the circulation, or both. As stroke volume decreases, a compensatory increase in the heart rate is needed to preserve normal cardiac output. The most common cause of decreased stroke volume in children is hypovolemia from dehydration. Other causes of decreased stroke volume in children are listed in Box 165.2.

CLINICAL FEATURES

Tachycardia is the first compensatory cardiovascular response to decreases in stroke volume. If tachycardia alone is not enough to maintain a normal cardiac output, the next compensatory physiologic mechanism to preserve perfusion is an increase in the SVR. This change in SVR is exhibited as an increase in the diastolic blood pressure, which in turn creates a narrowed pulse pressure. The clinical examination findings of the extremities of a child with an increased SVR include pallor, mottling, cool skin, delayed capillary refill time (>2 seconds), and weak or thready distal pulses.

Pathophysiology of Cyanosis

Cyanosis is a clinical sign caused by the preponderance of deoxygenated blood in the capillary beds, most readily observed in the mucous membranes, conjunctiva, nail beds, and skin. For cyanosis to be evident clinically, there must be at least 4 to 5 g/dL of deoxyhemoglobin admixed in the blood; this usually correlates with an oxygen saturation of approximately 80% to 85%. However, children with anemia—even if hypoxic—may not show overt signs of cyanosis (i.e., the critical mass of deoxygenated hemoglobin is not met to manifest cyanosis clinically). Central cyanosis results from a decrease in pulmonary ventilation and oxygenation, a decrease in pulmonary perfusion, the shunting of deoxygenated blood directly into the systemic circulation, or the presence of abnormal hemoglobin. Cyanosis in the neonate may be due to a variety of cardiac, pulmonary, hematologic, or toxic causes. Cardiac causes of cyanosis include congenital lesions with right-to-left shunts and cardiac lesions with decreased or increased pulmonary blood flow. Common pulmonary causes of cyanosis include bronchiolitis, pneumonia, and pulmonary edema. Methemoglobinemia is a hematologic cause of cyanosis.

Clinical Features of Cyanosis

Central cyanosis involves the lips, tongue, and mucous membranes; peripheral cyanosis (acrocyanosis) involves the hands and feet. Acrocyanosis is a common mostly benign finding in neonates caused by cold stress and peripheral vasoconstriction. Infants with cyanosis due to a congenital heart defect may not exhibit as much respiratory distress compared with the infant with cyanosis due to a pulmonary cause. Thus, a cardiac cause of central cyanosis should be suspected in a child who appears "comfortably blue." Another important clinical clue to the cause of central cyanosis is that cyanosis of cardiac origin usually worsens with crying, whereas cyanosis due to a pulmonary cause may

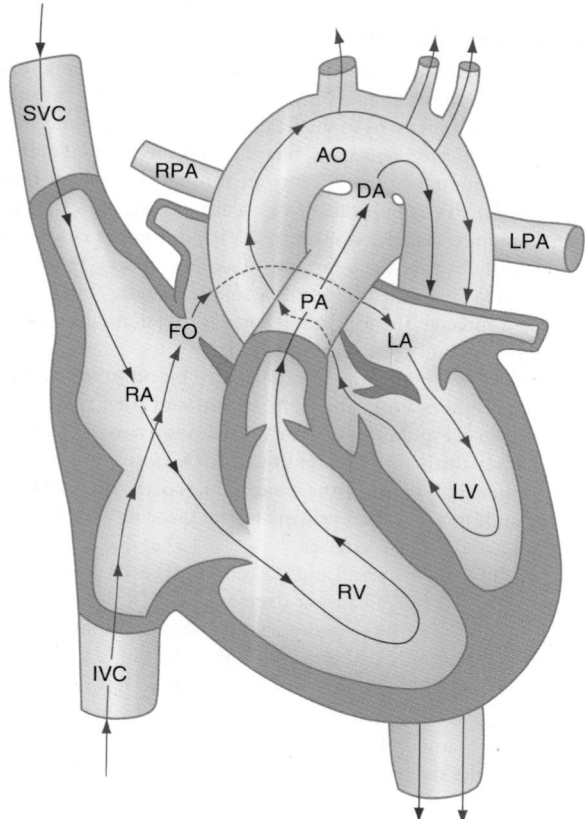

Fig. 165.1 Normal intracardiac fetal circulation: Physiologic shunting through the patent foramen ovale *(FO)* and the patent ductus arteriosus *(DA)*. Oxygenated blood from the placenta *(red arrows)* reaches the right atrium *(RA)* through the inferior vena cava *(IVC)*. This well-oxygenated blood is preferentially shunted from the RA across to the left atrium *(LA)* through the FO and is then ejected out the left ventricle *(LV)* to the ascending aorta *(AO)*. Deoxygenated blood *(blue arrows)* returning from the superior vena cava *(SVC)* preferentially travels from the RA into the right ventricle *(RV)* and then out through the main pulmonary artery *(PA)*. Because of the high pulmonary vascular resistance (PVR) in the fetal lungs, this deoxygenated blood bypasses lungs and enters the descending aorta through the DA. Thus the areas of the fetal body that are perfused by arteries proximal to the DA receive well-oxygenated blood, whereas those areas of the body that are perfused by arteries distal to the DA receive blood with a mixed oxygenation. *LPA,* Left pulmonary artery; *RPA,* right pulmonary artery.

improve. Cyanotic congenital heart defects with right-to-left shunting will demonstrate a minimal improvement with supplemental oxygen, whereas cyanosis of a purely pulmonary origin typically exhibits a significant improvement with supplemental oxygen (Table 165.1).

History

Infants with an underlying congenital heart disorder may be detected with a thorough history targeting key question (Box 165.3). Additional

TABLE 165.1 Clinical Clues to Help Distinguish Between Cardiac and Pulmonary Causes of Central Cyanosis[a]

	Cardiac Etiology	Pulmonary Etiology
Respiratory status	May be "comfortably blue"	Respiratory distress
Response to crying	Worsening cyanosis	Improved cyanosis
Response to oxygen	Minimal or no improvement	Improvement with oxygen

[a]Cyanosis due to severe pulmonary disease (e.g., severe pneumonia, tension pneumothorax, acute chest syndrome of sickle cell disease) may not show significant improvement with supplemental oxygen, but these children will also typically exhibit severe respiratory distress along with clinical cyanosis.

BOX 165.3 Key Elements to Elicit in the History of a Child With a Known Cardiac Disorder

Cardiac Diagnosis
Congenital or acquired disorder?
Any episodes of previous decompensation? (If so, are the current signs and symptoms similar to or different from those previous episodes?)

Oxygen Issues
Currently receiving home oxygen supplementation (continuous or only during feedings and sleep)?
Baseline oxygen saturation (room air or while receiving home oxygen)?
Any recent need for increasing the amount of supplemental oxygen?

Medications
Names and dosages of all current medications (cardiac and noncardiac medications)?
Were any of these cardiac medications stopped recently (by the cardiologist or parental noncompliance)?
Any recent increases in the cardiac medications (reasons for the increase, previous dosage versus the current dosage, and the date this dosage was increased)?
Any new cardiac medications added recently and the reason for these additions?
Recent digoxin level if the patient is receiving daily digoxin therapy?

Results of Most Recent Studies (Chest Radiograph, Electrocardiogram, Echocardiogram, and Cardiac Catheterization)
When were the last studies performed, and what were the results?
Why were those studies performed (routine follow-up studies or obtained because of decompensation from baseline, or a planned evaluation for an upcoming surgical procedure)?

Surgical Procedures
Previous procedures and complications?
Any future planned procedures?

history including diaphoresis during feeds and poor weight gain may signal early congestive heart failure (CHF). The cause of the infant's hypoxia—cardiac or pulmonary—may be ascertained by the age at onset and the events surrounding a change in color. For example, an infant who sweats during feeding may exhibit a splanchnic steal from anomalous coronary arteries, causing transient ischemia, pain, color change, and diaphoresis that resolve after eating. A child with an undiagnosed congenital heart defect resulting in CHF and pulmonary edema may take longer to feed, frequently pausing to catch his or her breath, with subsequent poor weight gain and gradually increasing work of breathing. Respiratory tract infections are common during childhood and may cause an acute deterioration in a child with an underlying cardiac disorder. In turn, children with congenital heart disease (CHD) with large left-to-right shunts and increased pulmonary blood flow tend to have a higher incidence of lower respiratory tract infections. Acute respiratory distress in these patients may be from a combination of pulmonary and cardiac factors (e.g., CHF).

Chest Pain

Common causes of pediatric chest pain are musculoskeletal chest wall pain, asthma exacerbation, pneumonia, pleurisy, gastritis, and gastroesophageal reflux. Precordial catch syndrome (also known as *Texidor's twinge*) presents as a sharp, focal pain, usually located in the left periapical area of the chest wall. It occurs suddenly, is often worsened by inspiration, and is not associated with dyspnea. The child may report that the pain "took my breath away" or that "I was afraid to move"; the pain typically resolves within a few minutes and is not associated with dysrhythmias or other sequelae.

Chest pain or syncope on exertion should be investigated for an underlying cardiac condition, especially if there is a positive family history of sudden unexplained death in young adulthood. Myocardial injury may also be secondary to drug abuse (e.g., cocaine, methamphetamines, synthetic or over-the-counter drugs of abuse). Pulmonary embolism is a possible cause of chest pain, especially in pregnant adolescent girls, patients taking oral contraceptive agents, or those with blood dyscrasias. The rare, though life-threatening, condition of aortic dissection should be considered as a cause of chest pain in a patient with physical examination findings suggestive of a collagen vascular disorder, such as Marfan syndrome.

Physical Examination
General Appearance and Pulses

Clinicians can use the Pediatric Assessment Triangle (PAT) to evaluate the child's overall appearance: alertness and interaction with the environment (mental status); presence of retractions, nasal flaring, or posturing (breathing); and skin color including perfusion (circulation) (see Chapter 155). All four extremities should be palpated for the presence and quality of pulses. In infants, feel for the brachial and femoral pulses. Bounding pulses are typically present in infants with a patent ductus arteriosus. Coarctation of the aorta should be suspected in any child with strong or unequal pulses in the upper extremities and weak pulses in the lower extremities. A child presenting with CHF and shock will have weak and thready pulses in all extremities.

Vital Signs and Blood Pressures

A mild resting tachypnea or tachycardia may be the only clinical clue to an underlying cardiovascular disorder. A simplified table of normal pediatric vital signs may be used at the bedside (Table 165.2).

To measure blood pressure accurately, use a cuff that covers two-thirds of the upper arm or thigh. A cuff that is too narrow will overestimate the patient's true blood pressure; conversely, a cuff that is too large will underestimate the true blood pressure. Measure blood pressures in both arms in children with a suspected cardiac disorder. Coarctation of the aorta

TABLE 165.2   Pediatric Vital Signs and Pertinent Formulas for Estimation of Blood Pressure

SIMPLIFIED PEDIATRIC VITAL SIGNS

Age Group	Average Normal Heart Rate (beats/min)	Respiratory Rate (breaths/min)
Newborn to 1 year	140	40
1–4 years	120	30
4–12 years	100	20
>12 years	80	15

FORMULAS TO CALCULATE THE ESTIMATED NORMAL BLOOD PRESSURES IN CHILDREN 1 YEAR OLD AND OLDER

Estimated average systolic blood pressure (SBP): [age in years × 2] + 90 mm Hg
Estimated average diastolic blood pressure: ⅔ × [estimated SBP]

MINIMUM ACCEPTABLE SYSTOLIC BLOOD PRESSURE FOR AGE (LOWER FIFTH PERCENTILE)

Newborn to 1 month	60 mm Hg
1 month to 1 year	70 mm Hg
1–10 years	[Age in years × 2] + 70 mm Hg
>10 years	90 mm Hg

BOX 165.4   A Pathologic Etiology of a Heart Murmur Should Be Suspected With Any of the Following Criteria

Diastolic murmurs
Systolic murmurs that are louder than a grade 3/6, continuous, or associated with a thrill
Murmurs that are associated with abnormal heart sounds (clicks, rubs, or gallop rhythms)
Presence of cyanosis or respiratory distress
Bounding pulses or weak pulses
Abnormalities on the electrocardiogram (ECG)
An abnormal cardiac silhouette, abnormal pulmonary vascularity, or cardiomegaly on the chest radiograph

BOX 165.5   Auscultation Locations of Common Systolic Murmurs in Children

Left Upper Sternal Border (Pulmonic Area)
Pulmonic valvular stenosis
Atrial septal defects (ASDs; due to an increased pulmonic flow)
Innocent pulmonic ejection murmur
Neonate pulmonic flow murmur
Patent ductus arteriosus (a continuous, "machinery" sounding murmur)

Left Lower Sternal Border
Innocent vibratory Still murmur
Ventricular septal defects (VSDs)
Endocardial cushion defects
Tetralogy of Fallot
Hypertrophic cardiomyopathy

Apex
Innocent vibratory Still murmur
Mitral regurgitation
Aortic stenosis
Hypertrophic cardiomyopathy

Right Upper Sternal Border (Aortic Area)
Aortic stenosis
Coarctation of the aorta

(proximal to the origin of the left subclavian artery) may present with a left arm blood pressure significantly lower than the right arm. Measure blood pressures in the thighs in any child with a suspected aortic coarctation or with documented hypertensive blood pressures in the upper extremities. The presence of femoral pulses does not rule out the possibility of a coarctation of the aorta. Because of the lack of well-designed blood pressure cuffs for the legs, blood pressures in the thighs can be 10 to 20 mm Hg higher than the blood pressures in the upper extremities. Therefore, blood pressures in the lower extremities that are lower than blood pressures in the upper extremities suggest coarctation of the aorta. Pulse oximetry readings lower in the legs than in the upper extremities suggests either a coarctation of the aorta or a right-to-left-shunt across a patent ductus arteriosus.

Cardiac Auscultation

Listen for the intensity and degree of splitting of the S_2 heart sound (closure of the pulmonic and aortic valves). In normal children, both aortic closure and pulmonic closure of S_2 should be heard along the left upper sternal border. A widely split and fixed S_2 suggests a physiologic problem from either a constant volume overload to the right side of the heart (e.g., atrial septal defect [ASD]) or a pressure overload to the right side of the heart (e.g., pulmonic stenosis). An ASD classically presents as a widely split and fixed S_2. The intensity of the S_2 component may be louder than normal in the child with pulmonary hypertension.

The third heart sound (S_3) is best heard along the lower left sternal border or the apex and may be a normal finding in children and young adults. An S_3 is produced by a rapid filling of the ventricles and is heard during early diastole, just after the S_2 sound. A loud S_3, however, is pathologic and due to dilated ventricles from volume overload (e.g., CHF and large ventricular septal defects [VSDs]). The fourth heart sound (S_4) occurs late in diastole, just before the S_1 sound. The finding of an S_4 is due to a decrease in compliance of a stiff, hypertrophic ventricle, best heard at the apex with the patient in the left lateral decubitus position (Box 165.4).

Cardiac murmurs are produced by turbulent blood flow through the heart and may not be associated with an underlying cardiac defect. The location, intensity, quality, timing, and radiation of the murmur determine whether the murmur is suggestive of an underlying cardiac pathologic condition. Although systolic murmurs can be present without any underlying anatomic abnormalities, diastolic murmurs are always considered pathologic in nature. Murmurs may be difficult to appreciate in the noisy ED setting, especially in tachycardic children. However, the location of the murmur may be a valuable clinical tool in determining the underlying anatomic origin of the murmur (Box 165.5).

Murmurs without any underlying anatomic abnormalities or hemodynamic significance are termed *innocent* or *functional murmurs*. All innocent murmurs are associated with normal ECGs and normal chest radiographs. Two of the most common innocent murmurs encountered in the pediatric population are the neonatal pulmonic flow murmur (peripheral pulmonic stenosis murmur) and Still's murmur. The pulmonic flow murmur of the neonate is due to the relatively thin walls and angulation of the right and left pulmonary arteries at birth. This systolic murmur is best heard at the left upper sternal border with radiation throughout the entire chest, axilla, and back. It usually disappears by 3 to 6 months of age. Persistence of a systolic murmur in the pulmonic area beyond this period raises the possibility of pathologic pulmonary arterial stenosis.

Still's murmur is a common innocent murmur found in children between 2 and 6 years of age. Best heard along the left midsternal border, this murmur has a vibratory, musical, or twanging quality from turbulent flow. The distinct quality of Still's murmur distinguishes it from the harsher quality of a VSD murmur. The intensity of Still's murmur increases in the supine position, or with fever, excitement, exercise, or anemia; like most murmurs, it is best heard with the bell of the stethoscope.

DIAGNOSTIC TESTING

Hyperoxia Test

The hyperoxia test may help differentiate between cardiac and pulmonary causes of central cyanosis. This test consists of assessment of the rise in arterial oxygenation with the administration of 100% oxygen. An arterial blood gas is measured after several minutes on high-flow oxygen (100% oxygen). When the child is breathing high-flow oxygen, an arterial oxygen partial pressure (Pao_2) of more than 250 mm Hg virtually excludes hypoxia due to CHD—a "passed" hyperoxia test. An arterial oxygen reading of less than 100 mm Hg (in a child without obvious pulmonary disease) is consistent with a right-to-left shunt and is highly predictive of CHD—a "failed" hyperoxia test. Values of 100 to 250 mm Hg may indicate lesions with intracardiac mixing. Pulse oximetry is not an appropriate substitute for an arterial blood gas analysis; it is not sensitive enough to determine "pass" or "fail" of the test, because a child breathing high-flow oxygen and registering 100% on pulse oximetry may actually have a Pao_2 anywhere between 80 and 680 mm Hg. Prolonged administration of 100% oxygen may cause some theoretic problems, such as, closure of the ductus arteriosus in infants with critical left-sided heart obstructions or pulmonary vasodilation (which could potentially worsen pulmonary vascular congestion). However, oxygen should not be initially withheld in critically ill infants based on this concern alone; rather, clinicians should closely monitor the response to oxygen in infants with suspected CHD.

Laboratory Analysis

Patients with CHF exacerbation may exhibit respiratory acidosis (low pH and high $Paco_2$), in addition to a low Pao_2 due to respiratory fatigue; this may initially be clinically subtle. In contrast, children with compensated cyanotic congenital heart defects may have a normal pH despite a (chronically) low Pao_2. Chronic mild hypoxemia causes a chronic mild acid load on the respiratory, renal, and blood buffer systems; acute illness, such as a respiratory infection, can rapidly cause a decompensation in this fragile balance, resulting in a worsening acidosis. Patients with congenital heart defects who are not experiencing respiratory compromise are unlikely to exhibit elevation in $Paco_2$.

Children with cyanotic CHD often partially compensate with an acquired polycythemia. Hemoglobin and hematocrit levels can also help determine if a child with CHF has pallor due to CHD or high-output failure from anemia. Serum electrolyte values may be helpful in the evaluation of children with acute dysrhythmias, suspected metabolic acidosis, or chronic diuretic therapy. We recommend that patients with a known congenital heart defect or an acquired cardiac disorder (e.g., Kawasaki disease, acute rheumatic heart disease, myocarditis, pericarditis, and cardiomyopathy) who present with dysrhythmias, syncope, chest pain, or unexplained shortness of breath be assessed with cardiac biomarkers and an ECG.

Chest Radiography

Three important features of the chest radiograph (Fig. 165.2) are the cardiac size (cardiothoracic ratio), the cardiac shape (silhouette), and the degree of pulmonary vascular markings. The easiest method to gauge heart size in children is to determine the cardiothoracic ratio: compare the largest transverse diameter of the cardiac shadow on the posteroanterior view of the chest radiograph with the widest internal diameter (measured from the inside rib margin at the widest point above the costophrenic angles) of the chest. The films should be obtained during maximal inspiration whenever feasible. Of note, the cardiothoracic ratio is not very accurate in preverbal children, in whom a good inspiratory view is rarely obtained.

The normal cardiothoracic ratio in children is 50% to 55%. A cardiac silhouette that is larger than normal may be due to a shunt lesion,

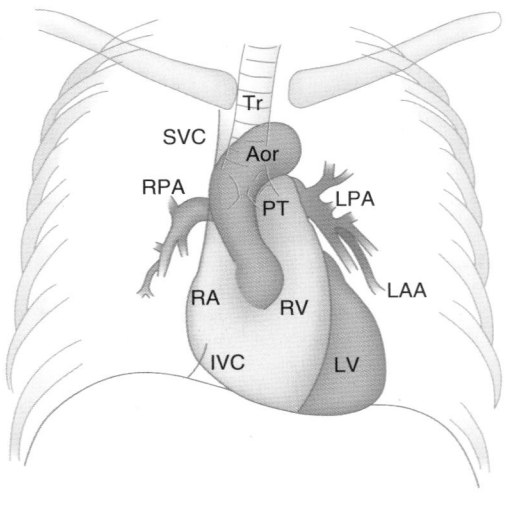
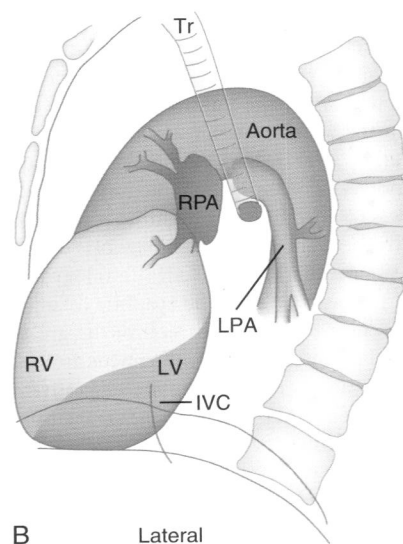

A Posteroanterior   **B** Lateral

Fig. 165.2 Diagrammatic representations of the anatomy of the chest radiograph. (A) Normal heart in a young man, posteroanterior projection. (B) Right lateral projection of a normal heart in a young man. *Aor*, Aorta; *IVC*, inferior vena cava; *LAA*, left atrial appendage; *LPA*, left pulmonary artery; *LV*, left ventricle; *PT*, pulmonary trunk; *RA*, right atrium; *RPA*, right pulmonary artery; *RV*, right ventricle; *SVC*, superior vena cava; *Tr*, trachea.

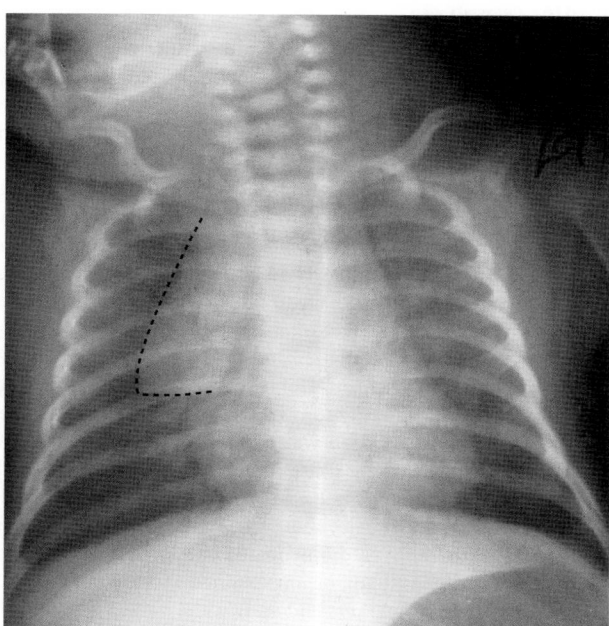

Fig. 165.3 Thymic shadow demonstrating the "sail sign" along the right cardiac border *(dotted line)*.

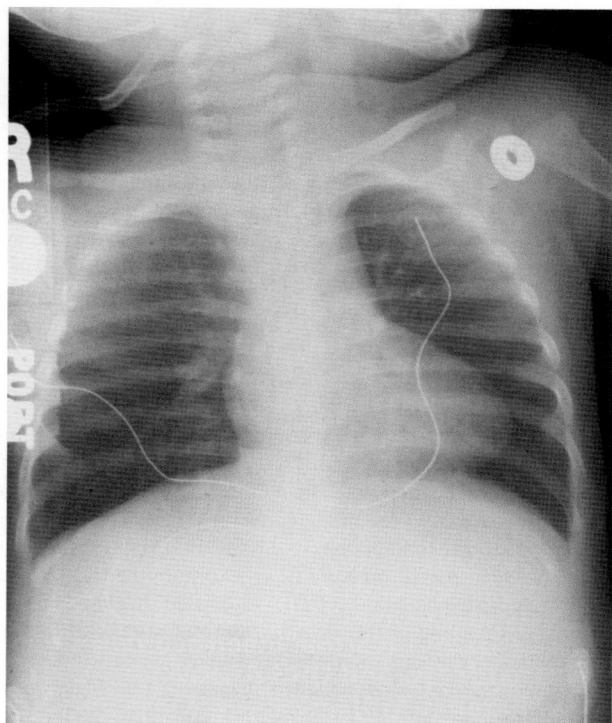

Fig. 165.4 The classic boot-shaped heart of tetralogy of Fallot.

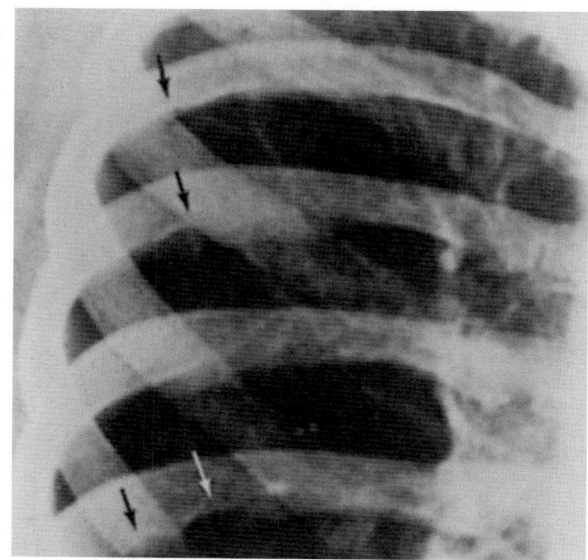

Fig. 165.5 Rib notching *(arrows)* in an 11-year-old girl with coarctation of the aorta. (From: Park MK. *Park's Pediatric Cardiology for Practitioners*, ed 6. Philadelphia: Elsevier/Saunders; 2014: 67-74. Figure 4-9 from: Caffey J. *Pediatric X-ray Diagnosis*, ed 7. Chicago: Mosby; 1978.)

cardiomegaly, or pericardial effusion. An enlarged heart shadow on a chest radiograph more reliably reflects a volume overload rather than pressure overload. The cardiac size can be falsely increased in infants by the presence of the thymus, seen in the mediastinum on the chest radiograph from birth until about 5 years of age. The thymic borders are typically wavy in appearance and sometimes can be seen as the classic "sail sign" along the superior right border of the heart (Fig. 165.3). The thymic shadow may not be visible radiographically in infants during times of physiologic stress, but should reappear when the infant recovers.

The three classic cardiac silhouettes seen in patients with congenital heart defects are the "boot-shaped heart" of tetralogy of Fallot (Fig. 165.4), the "egg-on-a-string" silhouette of transposition of the great arteries, and the "snowman-shaped" or "figure-of-eight" heart of total anomalous pulmonary venous return.

The degree of pulmonary vascular markings is a key factor in the differential diagnosis of congenital heart defects. Increased pulmonary vascularity is present when the pulmonary arteries appear enlarged and are visible in the lateral third of the lung fields or the lung apices. Another marker of increased pulmonary vascularity is seen on the posteroanterior view of the chest radiograph: the diameter of the right pulmonary artery in the right hilum is wider than the internal diameter of the trachea. The differential diagnosis of a cyanotic infant with decreased vascular markings includes Tetralogy of Fallot, pulmonary atresia, and tricuspid atresia. The cyanotic infant with increased vascular markings may have transposition of the great arteries, total anomalous pulmonary venous return, or truncus arteriosus. Increased vascular markings in an acyanotic infant are suggestive of an endocardial cushion defect, VSD, ASD, or patent ductus arteriosus.

In a normal left-sided aortic arch, the aorta descends to the left of the midline and slightly displaces the tracheal air shadow toward the right of midline above the level of the carina. With a right-sided aortic arch, the tracheal air shadow may be midline or deviated toward the left. A right-sided aortic arch is found in up to 25% of the children with tetralogy of Fallot. Rib notching secondary to increased collateral blood flow along the intercostal vessels can sometimes be appreciated between the fourth and eighth ribs in older children with undiagnosed coarctation of the aorta (Fig. 165.5) but is rarely visualized in children with coarctation of the aorta who are younger than 5 years old.

Electrocardiography

Electrocardiographic findings in infants and children change with the child's age (Table 165.3). At birth, muscle mass of the right ventricle is greater than that of the left ventricle; this is demonstrated by right axis deviation on the neonatal ECG. By the end of the first month of life, the left ventricle assumes dominance. By 6 months old, the left ventricular to right ventricular mass ratio is 2 : 1, which then reaches the adult ratio of 2.5 : 1 by adolescence. The durations of the PR interval, QRS complex, and QT intervals increase with age.

Left axis deviation is present when the QRS axis is less than the lower limit of normal for the child's age; it occurs with left ventricular hypertrophy and left bundle branch block. Right axis deviation is present when the QRS axis is greater than the upper limit of normal for the child's age; this is seen with right ventricular hypertrophy and right bundle branch block. A "superior" QRS axis (0 to −180 degrees with an S wave in aV_F greater than the R wave) may be suggestive of an endocardial cushion defect or tricuspid atresia.

Some common indications for ECG in a pediatric patient include chest pain, dyspnea, syncope, palpitations, suspected dysrhythmias, or an underlying cardiac disorder. A rare but potentially fatal congenital cardiac abnormality detected by ECG, anomalous origin of the left coronary artery from the pulmonary artery (ALCAPA), will show ischemic changes. Infants may have a history of poor feeding, irritability, and failure to thrive. Older children and adolescents may have acute-on-chronic ischemic symptoms. Anyone of any age with ALCAPA may suddenly present with cardiogenic shock secondary to myocardial ischemia. Evidence of volume overload seen on ECG includes: right atrial enlargement (also seen with ASD, atrioventricular [AV] canal defects, tricuspid atresia, Ebstein anomaly, and severe pulmonary stenosis); and right ventricular hypertrophy (also seen with pulmonary stenosis, Tetralogy of Fallot, transposition of the great arteries, VSD with pulmonary stenosis or pulmonary hypertension, coarctation of aorta [CoA] in the newborn, pulmonary valve atresia, and hypoplastic left heart syndrome).

Biochemical Markers

As in adults, cardiac troponin T (cTnT) and cardiac troponin I (cTnI) are highly sensitive and specific in children for myocardial damage. Reference values are slightly higher for neonates younger than 3 months of age; normal and indeterminate values will depend on the bioassay used. The indications for troponin testing in children include suspected cardiac ischemia (of any etiology), myocarditis, and myocardial dysfunction in sepsis syndrome. Several studies have supported the use of plasma B-type natriuretic peptide (BNP) levels in the assessment and management of CHF in adults. Elevated BNP levels have demonstrated a similar correlation in children with CHF. BNP levels also correlate with the clinical symptoms of heart failure and ejection fraction.

SPECIFIC DISORDERS

Congenital Heart Disease
Foundations
Although a large percentage of CHD is now detected with prenatal ultrasound, pulse oximetry before discharge from the nursery is currently a standard screening for CHD, and its false-negative rate is very low.[2]

Clinical Features
Age, severity of symptoms, and time of presentation of a child with CHD vary by the specific defect, complexity, severity, and timing of the normal physiologic changes that occur as the fetal circulation transitions to that of a neonate (Table 165.4). The more severe or complex

TABLE 165.3 Normal Electrocardiographic Values (PR, QTc, and QRS Axes) in Infants and Children

Age	PR INTERVAL Average (Upper Limit)	QRS DURATION Average (Upper Limit)
0–1 month	0.10 (0.12)	0.05 (0.07)
1 month to 1 year	0.10 (0.14)	0.05 (0.07)
1–3 years	0.11 (0.15)	0.06 (0.07)
3–8 years	0.13 (0.17)	0.07 (0.08)
8–12 years	0.15 (0.18)	0.07 (0.09)
12–16 years	0.15 (0.19)	0.07 (0.10)
Adult	0.16 (0.21)	0.08 (0.10)

The corrected QT (QTc) interval should not exceed:
0.45 second in infants <6 months old
0.44 second in children and adolescents

NORMAL QRS AXES IN INFANTS AND CHILDREN

Age	Mean Degrees (range)
1 week to 1 month	+110 (+30 to +180)
1–3 months	+70 (+10 to +125)
3 months to 3 years	+60 (+10 to +110)
>3 years	+60 (+20 to +120)
Adults	+50 (−30 to +105)

NORMAL T WAVE AXIS IN INFANTS AND CHILDREN

Age	Leads V_1 and V_2	Lead Av_f	Leads I, V_5, and V_6
Birth to 1 day	+/−	+	+/−
1–4 days	+−−	+	+
4 days to adolescent	−	−	+
Adolescent to adult	+	+	+

+, Upright T wave; −, inverted T wave.

TABLE 165.4 Symptomatic Presentation of Congenital Heart Defects and Time of Presentation

Defect	Time of Presentation
CONGENITAL HEART DEFECTS THAT PRESENT WITH CYANOSIS	
Transposition of the great arteries	Birth to 2 weeks
Total anomalous pulmonary venous return	Birth to 2 weeks
Tricuspid atresia	Birth to 2 weeks
Ebstein anomaly of the tricuspid valve	Birth to 2 weeks
Truncus arteriosus	Birth to 2 weeks
Pulmonary atresia	Birth to 2 weeks
Hypoplastic right heart syndrome	Birth to 2 weeks
Hypoplastic left heart syndrome	Birth to 2 weeks
Tetralogy of Fallot	Birth to 12 weeks
CONGENITAL HEART DEFECTS THAT PRESENT WITH SHOCK	
Coarctation of the aorta	From first week on
Aortic stenosis	From first week on
CONGENITAL HEART DEFECTS THAT PRESENT WITH CONGESTIVE HEART FAILURE	
Ventricular septal defects (VSDs)	From 4 weeks on
Patent ductus arteriosus	From 4 weeks on

CHD lesions may not be clinically apparent immediately after birth. As the ductus arteriosus begins to close in the first several weeks of life, cardiac defects with obstructive lesions of the pulmonary or systemic circulations will be unmasked, and these infants will present with acute cyanosis, shock, or both. In general, the more severe the anatomic defect is (i.e., lack of pulmonary blood flow or lack of systemic blood flow), the earlier in life these conditions will be manifested with cyanosis and shock.

Differential Diagnosis

Many children with CHD do not fit neatly into a single pattern; some have mixed defects. The exact anatomic diagnosis of a CHD is dependent on echocardiography, cardiac catheterization, or advanced imaging; establishment of the exact anatomic diagnosis is seldom possible in the ED setting.

Diagnostic Testing

The emergency clinician should rely on several key elements of the clinical evaluation in addition to findings on the chest radiograph and ECG to narrow the diagnostic possibilities. Pattern recognition may be helpful (Box 165.6). For example, the presence of cyanosis, a grade 3/6 systolic ejection murmur best heard at the mid left sternal border, a boot-shaped heart, and a decreased pulmonary blood flow on the chest radiograph with evidence of right ventricular hypertrophy on the ECG suggest Tetralogy of Fallot.

Management

The majority of children who present to the ED in shock have volume depletion or sepsis. These patients should receive rapid repeated fluid boluses of 20 mL/kg. Children with poor perfusion and suspected CHD, however, should receive smaller aliquots of 10 mL/kg to avoid precipitation or exacerbation of CHF. This is especially important in the neonate with undifferentiated shock. In these cases, give the initial 10 mL/kg bolus and assess for effect. If the child is improved or no worse, give more fluids. Be judicious in suspected CHD and ready to provide inotropic support or positive pressure ventilation, either by noninvasive or endotracheal means.

CHD that is manifested within the first 2 to 3 weeks of life with a sudden onset of cyanosis or cardiovascular collapse is typically due to ductal-dependent cardiac lesions (Box 165.7). Closure of the ductus arteriosus in these patients interrupts blood flow either to the lungs, producing cyanosis (e.g., tricuspid atresia) *or* to the systemic circulation, producing shock (e.g., hypoplastic left heart syndrome). To maintain an open ductus arteriosus and promote mixture of oxygenated and deoxygenated blood, prostaglandin E_1 (alprostadil) is typically started at 0.05 to 0.1 µg/kg/min. A known adverse reaction to a PGE_1 infusion is apnea (30%). Assiduous monitoring of the child's respiratory drive is essential with PGE_1 administration. Although some small studies endorse the omission of endotracheal intubation of neonates on a PGE_1 infusion, endotracheal intubation should be considered for these infants, especially before inter-facility transport.

Children with cardiac conditions are at risk of post-intubation cardiovascular collapse due to positive pressure ventilation, increased intrathoracic pressures, and decreased venous return (e.g., cyanotic heart disease is often preload dependent). To support cardiac output and SVR (which mitigates a right-to-left shunt), ketamine is the preferred induction agent along with a non-depolarizing metabolically neutral neuromuscular blocker, such as rocuronium. Not only will intubation provide a secure airway, but controlled ventilation will also help decrease the infant's work of breathing, shunting much needed cardiac output and metabolic demands from the overtaxed respiratory apparatus. Other adverse reactions to a PGE_1 infusion include fever,

seizures, bradycardia, hypotension, flushing, and decreased platelet aggregation.

Acyanotic Congenital Heart Defect

Foundations

Acyanotic CHD can be further subdivided (Fig. 165.6) into obstructive lesions (e.g., pulmonic stenosis, aortic stenosis, coarctation of the aorta) and lesions characterized by left-to-right shunting with an associated increase in pulmonary blood flow (e.g., VSDs, ASDs, patent ductus arteriosus, endocardial cushion defects). These acyanotic lesions

---

BOX 165.6 **Clinical Clues to Aid in the Diagnosis of Congenital Heart Disease**

Presence or Absence of Central or Peripheral Cyanosis?
Central cyanosis with minimal respiratory distress ("comfortably blue") is suggestive of CHD more than of a purely pulmonary etiology.

Abnormalities in Cardiac Auscultation?
Murmurs: Systolic versus diastolic, location, and radiation
Quality of S_1, S_2, and the presence of any clicks or gallops

Change in the Degree of Central Cyanosis With Crying?
Worsening of cyanosis with crying suggests a cardiac rather than a purely pulmonary etiology.

Response of Pao_2 to the Hyperoxia Challenge (Administering 100% Oxygen)?
Purely pulmonary causes of cyanosis: Pao_2 should rise to levels above 250 mm Hg
Cyanotic CHD associated with an increased pulmonary blood flow: Pao_2 may occasionally reach as high as 150 mm Hg
Cyanotic CHD associated with a decreased pulmonary blood flow: Pao_2 will not rise above 100 mm Hg

Chest Radiograph Abnormalities?
Cardiac size and shape (one of the three classic cardiac silhouettes)?
  Boot-shaped heart: Tetralogy of Fallot
  Egg-on-a-string silhouette: Transposition of the great vessels
  Snowman-shaped or figure-of-eight heart: Total anomalous pulmonary venous return

Degree of Pulmonary Blood Flow?
Increased (acyanotic): ASD, Eisenmenger syndrome, VSD, patent ductus arteriosus, endocardial cushion defects
Increased (cyanotic): Transposition of the great arteries, total anomalous pulmonary venous return, hypoplastic left heart syndrome, truncus arteriosus
Decreased or normal (acyanotic): Pulmonic stenosis, aortic stenosis, coarctation of the aorta
Decreased (cyanotic): Tetralogy of Fallot, severe pulmonic stenosis, Ebstein anomaly, tricuspid atresia, pulmonary atresia, hypoplastic right heart syndrome

Electrocardiographic Abnormalities?
Evidence of chamber enlargement: right ventricular hypertrophy, left ventricular hypertrophy, biventricular hypertrophy, right atrial hypertrophy, or left atrial hypertrophy
An abnormal superior QRS axis is suggestive of endocardial cushion defect or tricuspid atresia.

ASD, Atrial septal defect, *CHD,* congenital heart disease; *Pao2,* arterial oxygen partial pressure; *VSD,* ventricular septal defect.

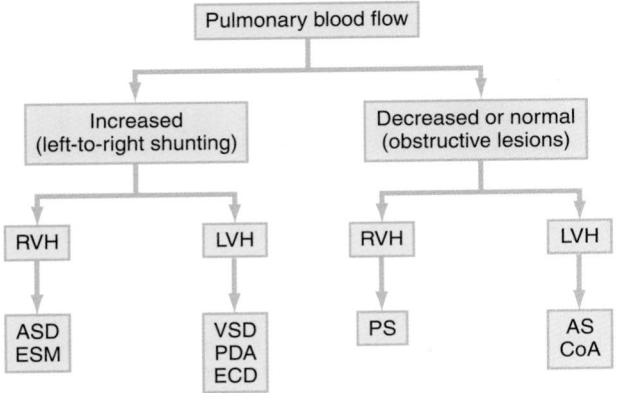

Fig. 165.6 Clinical clues to diagnosis of acyanotic congenital heart defects. *AS,* Aortic stenosis; *ASD,* atrial septal defect; *CoA,* coarctation of the aorta; *ECD,* endocardial cushion defect; *ESM,* Eisenmenger syndrome; *LVH,* left ventricular hypertrophy; *PDA,* patent ductus arteriosus; *PS,* pulmonic stenosis; *RVH,* right ventricular hypertrophy; *VSD,* ventricular septal defect.

usually present within the first 6 months of life with symptoms of CHF; however, ASDs can remain asymptomatic until adulthood.

Specific Disorders

Ventricular Septal Defect. VSD is the most common congenital cardiac defect and accounts for 20% to 25% of all cases of CHD. Spontaneous closure occurs in 30% to 40% of all VSDs overall and in 50% to 70% of smaller VSDs.

Clinical Features. Symptoms from a VSD are dependent on its size, and the degree of pulmonary vascular resistance present. Most VSDs are clinically asymptomatic (minimal or no left-to-right shunting) immediately after birth because of normal, relatively higher pulmonary vascular resistance. By 6 to 8 weeks of age, pulmonary vascular resistance naturally decreases. If a VSD is present, then left-to-right shunting can occur, and its typical systolic murmur may be appreciated.

Small VSDs may remain completely asymptomatic throughout childhood. In contrast, by 2 to 3 months of age some infants with large VSDs may experience an abnormally high pulmonary blood flow, and signs and symptoms of CHF (e.g., poor feeding and poor growth). Older children with VSDs may present with decreased exercise tolerance or recurrent pulmonary infections. If moderate to large VSDs are not corrected surgically, by 6 to 12 months of age irreversible changes occur in the pulmonary vasculature; high pulmonary vascular resistance is established, possibly resulting in pulmonary hypertension. Subsequently, high pulmonary vascular resistance increases right atrial and right ventricular pressures. If a large VSD is also present, the direction of the shunt is reversed, now right-to-left. The previous left-to-right shunt would have been tolerated relatively well. Once the reversal is established—a right-to-left shunt—poorly oxygenated blood flows into the systemic circulation with resulting degrees of cyanosis, called Eisenmenger syndrome.

Diagnostic Testing. The chest radiograph in children with small VSDs may be entirely normal. Cardiomegaly with increased pulmonary vascular markings is usually present with untreated moderate-to-large VSDs. The ECG of moderate-sized VSDs typically reveals left ventricular hypertrophy, but biventricular hypertrophy may be present in VSDs with large left-to-right shunting.

Management. All VSDs, regardless of the size of the defect, are at risk for bacterial endocarditis because of the high velocity of turbulent blood flow through them, and thus, should be repaired.

Traditional closure of VSDs required open heart surgery. Today, however, a transcatheter closure technique that avoids the inherent risks and complications of open heart surgery and cardiopulmonary bypass has supplanted traditional methods.

Atrial Septal Defect. ASDs account for 5% to 10% of all cases of CHD. The majority of infants and children with ASDs remain clinically asymptomatic until adulthood. Spontaneous closure has been reported in up to 40% of the cases within the first 5 years of life.

Clinical Features. Large ASDs or those associated with comorbid conditions, such as bronchopulmonary dysplasia, can be manifested with symptoms of CHF and pulmonary overcirculation (e.g., dyspnea with feedings, poor weight gain, and frequent lower respiratory tract infections). The majority of ASDs are discovered when a suspicious murmur is detected on a routine physical examination: a widely split and fixed S$_2$ is a characteristic finding of ASDs.

Diagnostic Testing. The chest radiographs of children with ASDs will reveal varying degrees of cardiomegaly, right atrial and right ventricular enlargement, and a prominent main pulmonary artery segment and increased pulmonary vascular markings. The ECG will show right axis deviation and right ventricular hypertrophy. All patients with unrepaired ASDs will have symptoms if pulmonary hypertension develops. Patients with large ASDs that are not detected and repaired are at risk for development of Eisenmenger syndrome. Unlike VSDs, uncomplicated ASDs are not associated with high risk of bacterial endocarditis because of the lower turbulence and velocity of blood flow through the atrial defect.

Management. Traditionally, ASDs required open heart surgery to place a patch over the septal defect. Newer therapies include septal occlusion devices placed by the transcatheter approach.[3] Antiplatelet therapy during the 6-month period after placement of the device is typically given and is safe and effective in preventing thrombus formation on the surface of the septal occluder.

Eisenmenger Syndrome

Clinical Features. Eisenmenger syndrome can occur in any large left-to-right shunt defect. Left uncorrected, irreversible changes in the pulmonary arterioles lead to pulmonary vascular obstruction and pulmonary hypertension. As the degree of pulmonary hypertension increases, PVR may then begin to exceed SVR. This causes right-sided pressures to exceed those on the left, causing right-to-left shunting. The reversal in the direction of shunt flow produces cyanosis. Other clinical features of patients who have Eisenmenger syndrome include chest pain, dyspnea on exertion, and hemoptysis.[4]

Coarctation of the Aorta

Foundations. Nearly 50% of patients with coarctation of the aorta also have an associated bicuspid aortic valve. The area of coarctation can occur proximal to the insertion of the ductus arteriosus (preductal type) or distal to the insertion of the ductus arteriosus (most common, postductal type).

Clinical Features. The severity of symptoms and age at time of presentation are dependent on the location of the coarctation, the degree of narrowing, and the presence of any other associated cardiac defects. Infants with the rarer, preductal type of coarctation of the aorta may also exhibit differential cyanosis if the ductus arteriosus remains open. With differential cyanosis, the upper half of the body is perfused with well-oxygenated blood supplied by the left ventricle and the ascending aorta. However, the lower half of the body will appear cyanotic, being largely perfused by right-to-left shunting of deoxygenated blood from the patent ductus arteriosus into the descending aorta. Infants with the preductal type of coarctation of the aorta will present with signs of circulatory failure and shock when the ductus arteriosus begins to close. The clinician should search for a "brachial-femoral delay" by palpating both pulses simultaneously.

Most of the asymptomatic cases of the more common postductal coarctation of the aorta are diagnosed as a result of a cardiology referral for a systolic murmur or a hypertension evaluation, but infants with severe postductal coarctation of the aorta can also present during the first few weeks of life with signs of circulatory failure and shock. If a child is discovered to have hypertension on a routine physical examination, obtain blood pressure measurements in the lower extremities to assess the possibility of coarctation of the aorta. Coarctation of the aorta should be suspected if the systolic blood pressure in the right arm is 15 to 20 mm Hg higher than that in the legs. If the systolic pressure in the right arm is higher than that in the left arm, the area of coarctation is probably preductal and located proximal to the origin of the left subclavian artery. In general, diastolic blood pressures are similar in the upper and lower extremities, although lower extremity pressures often have higher measured values due to use of smaller blood pressure cuffs meant for arms.

Diagnostic Testing. The chest radiograph will most often reveal a normal cardiac silhouette and normal pulmonary vascular markings, but notching along the lower borders of the posterior fourth to eighth ribs due to the pressure of the dilated collateral vessels may be exhibited in children older than 5 years of age. The ECG typically reveals a left axis and left ventricular hypertrophy. Suspected cases of coarctation of the aorta should be imaged with transthoracic echocardiography or cardiac magnetic resonance imaging to confirm and define the coarctation. In stable patients, this can be done on an outpatient basis.

Management. Definitive surgical repair of coarctation of the aorta involves angiography or stenting of the narrow aortic lumen; resection of the narrowed section of the aorta with an end-to-end anastomosis may be necessary. Complications of undiagnosed cases are related to resultant hypertension, and can include heart failure, hypertensive encephalopathy, and intracranial hemorrhages.

Cyanotic Congenital Heart Diseases

Foundations. Cyanotic CHDs are a result of either decreased pulmonary blood flow to the lungs or right-to-left shunting of desaturated blood directly into the systemic circulation (Fig. 165.7). The classic cyanotic CHDs can be remembered by the five Ts: truncus arteriosus, transposition of the great arteries, tricuspid atresia, Tetralogy of Fallot, and total anomalous pulmonary venous return. Other forms of cyanotic CHD include Ebstein anomaly, pulmonary atresia, severe pulmonary stenosis, hypoplastic left heart syndrome, and hypoplastic right heart syndrome. Many of these cyanotic heart

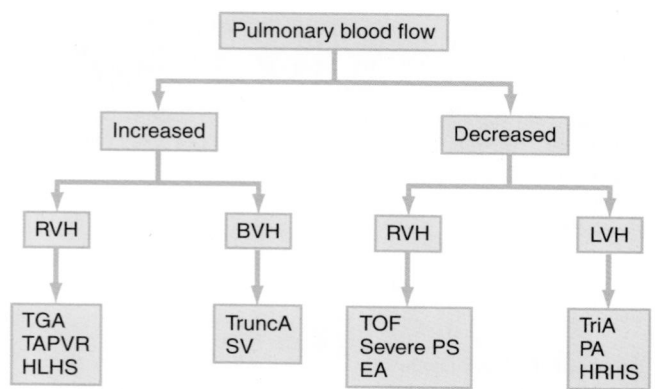

Fig. 165.7 Clinical clues to diagnosis of cyanotic congenital heart defects. *BVH,* Biventricular hypertrophy; *EA,* Ebstein anomaly; *HLHS,* hypoplastic left heart syndrome; *HRHS,* hypoplastic right heart syndrome; *LVH,* left ventricular hypertrophy; *PA,* pulmonary atresia; *PS,* pulmonary stenosis; *RVH,* right ventricular hypertrophy; *SV,* single ventricle; *TAPVR,* total anomalous pulmonary venous return; *TGA,* transposition of the great arteries; *TOF,* Tetralogy of Fallot; *TriA,* tricuspid atresia; *TruncA,* truncus arteriosus.

lesions are routinely detected either on prenatal ultrasound or in the nursery; only Tetralogy of Fallot is covered in this section.

Tetralogy of Fallot

Foundations. Tetralogy of Fallot is the most common cause of cyanotic CHD beyond infancy. It arises from a single embryologic defect in which the subpulmonic conus fails to expand, resulting in four abnormalities (Fig. 165.8): (1) right ventricular outflow tract obstruction; (2) large, unrestrictive, misaligned VSD; (3) overriding aorta that receives blood flow from both ventricles; and (4) right ventricular hypertrophy secondary to the high pressure load placed on the right ventricle by the right ventricular outflow tract obstruction. These anatomic defects collectively result in decreased pulmonary blood flow and varying degrees of right-to-left shunting of deoxygenated blood across the VSD. Tetralogy of Fallot is often associated with other cardiac defects, such as right-sided aortic arch, ASD, and anomalous origin of the left coronary artery.

Clinical Features. The degree of cyanosis and the age at presentation are directly dependent on the degree of right ventricular outflow tract obstruction. Infants with Tetralogy of Fallot typically have worsening of their cyanosis during crying and feeding. Older children with tetralogy of Fallot may have cyanotic exacerbations during periods of physical exertion. Infants with milder forms of right ventricular outflow tract obstruction may be acyanotic, and sometimes referred to as having a "pink" Tetralogy of Fallot. Infants with severe right ventricular outflow tract obstruction exhibit profound cyanosis within the first few days of life; they may even require PGE$_1$ infusion to preserve pulmonary blood flow by left-to-right shunting from the aorta into the main pulmonary artery through the patent ductus arteriosus.

The physical examination can reveal varying degrees of cyanosis, and a systolic ejection murmur along the left sternal border. Chronic hypoxemia results in a compensatory polycythemia and varying degrees of clubbing of the fingers and toes.

Diagnostic Testing. The chest radiograph of a patient with cyanotic Tetralogy of Fallot (see Fig. 165.4) shows decreased pulmonary vascular markings and a boot-shaped heart (secondary to a concave main pulmonary artery segment along the superior aspect of the left border of the heart). The heart size in Tetralogy of Fallot is normal; a right-sided aortic arch may be seen in 25% of the cases. The ECG of cyanotic Tetralogy of Fallot reveals right ventricular hypertrophy and a right axis deviation. Children with pink Tetralogy of Fallot may not

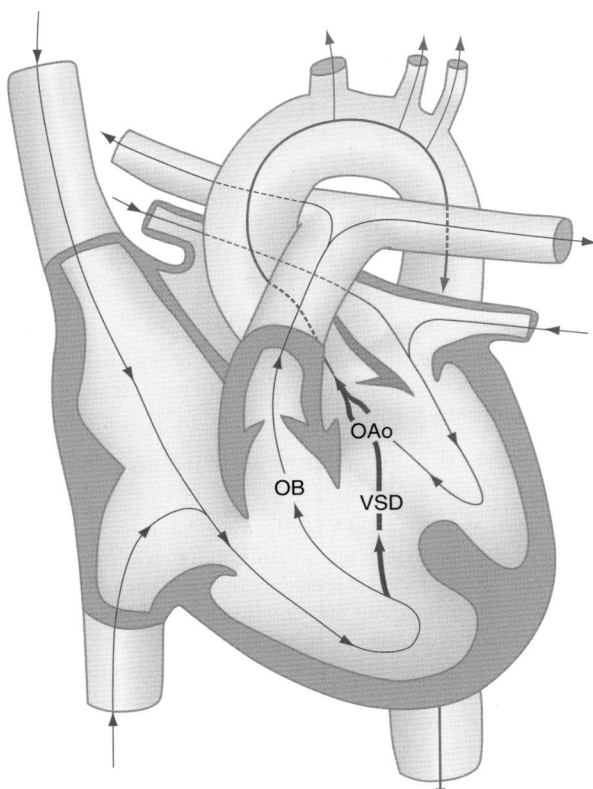

Fig. 165.8 Diagrammatic representation of the right-to-left shunting that occurs in Tetralogy of Fallot. Some of the deoxygenated blood *(thick blue arrow)* in the right ventricle is shunted across the ventricular septal defect *(VSD)* into the left ventricle. This deoxygenated blood mixes with the well-oxygenated blood from the lungs *(red arrow)*. The blood that is ejected out through the overriding aorta *(OAo)*, therefore, contains blood of mixed oxygenation *(purple arrows)*. The amount of deoxygenated blood that is shunted through the VSD *(thick blue arrow)* is dependent on a combination of factors, including the severity of right ventricular outflow tract obstruction *(OB)*, the size of the VSD, and the degree of systemic vascular resistance (SVR). When the SVR falls (as occurs during a tet spell), more deoxygenated blood from the right ventricle will be shunted across the VSD into the systemic circulation, which results in hypoxia, metabolic acidosis, and worsening cyanosis.

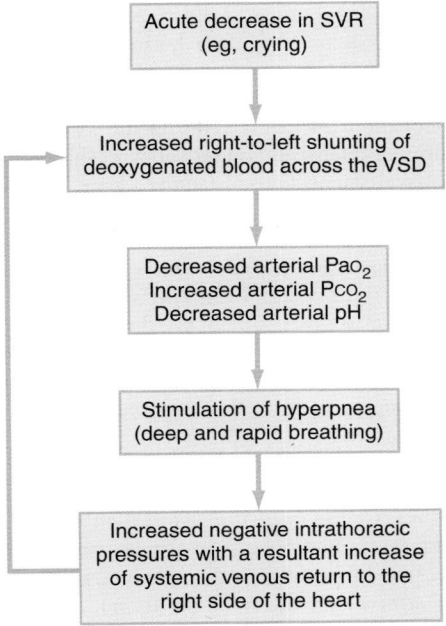

Fig. 165.9 Pathophysiologic mechanisms of a hypoxic (tet) spell. *PaO$_2$*, Arterial oxygen partial pressure; *PCO$_2$*, partial pressure of carbon dioxide in the arterial blood; *SVR*, systemic vascular resistance; *VSD*, ventricular septal defect.

BOX 165.8 Management of Tetralogy of Fallot Hypoxic Spells

Place the child in the knee-to-chest position to increase the systemic vascular resistance (SVR), which decreases the right-to-left shunt across the ventricular septal defect (VSD).

Provide supplemental oxygen (limited value by itself).

Morphine: 0.1 to 0.2 mg/kg IV or IM

Fentanyl: 1 μg/kg/dose IV or IM as an alternative to morphine

Fentanyl: 1.5–2 mcg/kg/dose intranasally (anatomic limit of 1 mL solution per naris)

Midazolam: 0.2 to 0.3 mg/kg/dose intranasally (anatomic limit of 1 mL solution per naris)

Sodium bicarbonate: 1 mEq/kg IV if suspected or documented acidosis

Consider ketamine: 1 to 2 mg/kg IV or 3 to 5 mg/kg IM

Consider propranolol: 0.1 to 0.2 mg/kg IV

Consider phenylephrine: 0.01 to 0.02 mg/kg IV

IM, Intramuscular; *IV*, intravenous.

---

initially exhibit any degree of right ventricular hypertrophy, but these acyanotic variations of Tetralogy of Fallot gradually develop into the cyanotic form by 1 to 3 years old.

A potentially life-threatening complication of Tetralogy of Fallot is the so-called *tet spell*, also known as a hypercyanotic or hypoxic spell. These episodes occur most commonly in infants, with a peak incidence between 2 and 4 months old.

Any event that suddenly lowers the SVR (such as crying or defecation), hypovolemia, or tachycardia will promote a large right-to-left shunt across the VSD, beginning the vicious circle of a hypoxic spell. The large right-to-left shunt through the VSD bypasses the lungs, which then causes a decrease in the Pao$_2$, an increase in the Pco$_2$, and a fall in the arterial pH. These metabolic changes then stimulate the respiratory centers in the brain to produce hyperpnea (deep and rapid respirations), which increases the negative intrathoracic pressure during inspiration, causing an increase in the systemic venous blood return to the right side of the heart. This increased volume of blood in the right ventricle is then shunted through the VSD by the combination of the existing right ventricular tract outflow obstruction and the acute

decrease in the SVR. This in turn further decreases the arterial oxygen saturation, perpetuating the hypoxic spell (Fig. 165.9).

These hypoxic spells are characterized clinically by periods of hyperpnea, prolonged crying, and worsening cyanosis. Limpness, seizures, cerebrovascular accidents, and even death have been reported with more severe tet spells. During a tet spell, the intensity of the murmur decreases because of less blood flow through the right ventricular tract obstruction and more blood being shunted from the right ventricle to the left ventricle through the VSD.

Management. The overall treatment goals for tet spells are to increase the SVR, to abolish the hyperpnea, and to correct the metabolic acidosis (Box 165.8). Give supplemental oxygen and increase the child's SVR by placing him or her in a knee-to-chest position; older children may be placed in the squatting position, if tolerated. Both maneuvers are believed to increase SVR and to decrease the pathologic right-to-left shunting of blood. Analgesics should be given to calm the child, decrease the catecholamine surge, and decrease the respiratory rate. Morphine (0.1 to 0.2 mg/kg) intramuscularly has been a traditional option but has the possible untoward effect of systemic vasodilation (further decreasing the SVR) by endogenous histamine release. Fentanyl and midazolam are newer options without the potential risk of endogenous histamine release. Both may be given via the intranasal route and may be less distressful than intramuscular morphine. Ketamine (1 to 2 mg/kg IV or 3 to 5 mg/kg IM) is a good choice for its analgesic and sedative effects; it is an excellent choice to improve SVR. In the event of clinically suspected or documented (pH <7.4) metabolic acidosis, sodium bicarbonate (1 mEq/kg IV) may be given to break the cycle of hypoxemia, acidosis, and worsening hypotension and perfusion. Most infants respond to these measures and exhibit an improvement in their oxygenation and a decrease in their degree of cyanosis.

An infant whose condition does not improve with these measures may require a vasopressor (such as phenylephrine) to increase the SVR and thereby decrease the degree of right-to-left shunting across the VSD. An intravenous fluid bolus may also be considered to increase the volume of blood flow through the pulmonary artery. If the aforementioned pharmacologic interventions are not successful, consider propranolol 0.1 to 0.2 mg/kg IV (0.01 to 0.2 mg/kg IV) administered slowly and repeated if needed every 10 to 15 minutes (possibly reduces infundibular spasm at the right ventricular outflow tract) or phenylephrine (5 to 20 mcg/kg IV) administered slowly and repeated if needed every 10 to 15 minutes (alpha-antagonist to increase SVR).

Palliative surgical procedures to increase the amount of blood flow temporarily to the pulmonary arteries are performed in infants with severe cyanotic Tetralogy of Fallot. The most commonly performed procedure is the modified Blalock-Taussig shunt, in which an anastomosis is created between the subclavian artery and the ipsilateral pulmonary artery. Definitive surgical repair consists of closing the VSD and opening the right ventricular outflow tract obstruction by resection of the infundibular tissue. The mortality rate is 5% to 10% within the first 2 years after definitive surgical repair in uncomplicated Tetralogy of Fallot cases. Complications that can occur after definitive surgical repair include complete heart block, ventricular dysrhythmias, and right bundle branch block (secondary to the right ventriculotomy).

Postoperative Complications of Congenital Heart Defects

A variety of postoperative complications can be seen in patients who present to the ED weeks to months after cardiac surgery: thrombosis of a shunt conduit with decreased flow; increased shunt conduit flow with resultant CHF; atrial and ventricular dysrhythmias; heart block; myocardial ischemia; and endocarditis. The size of the cardiac silhouette and the degree of pulmonary blood flow on the chest radiograph may provide valuable clues as to whether there is an increased or decreased blood flow through a surgical conduit that was created to provide an improvement in blood flow to the pulmonary system. Comparison of the child's other postoperative chest radiographs can help determine whether there has been a change in the heart size and pulmonary vascularity.

The post-pericardiotomy syndrome is an inflammatory pericarditis that can occur 1 to 6 weeks after any surgical procedure that involved a pericardiotomy. An immunologic inflammatory response is characterized by fever, chest pain, and pericardial effusion. A pericardial friction rub may be heard, depending on the amount of fluid that accumulates in the pericardial sac. The chest radiograph may reveal an enlarged cardiac silhouette, and the echocardiogram will confirm the diagnosis. Pericardiocentesis is rarely required but may be necessary if the amount of pericardial effusion is significant enough to cause

> **BOX 165.9   Conditions Associated With an Increased Risk of Severe or Fatal Respiratory Syncytial Virus Infections**
>
> Cyanotic or complex congenital heart defects
> Pulmonary hypertension
> Prematurity (especially those infants with bronchopulmonary dysplasia or chronic lung disease)
> Immunodeficiency states

pericardial tamponade. The majority of cases of post-pericardiotomy syndrome will resolve within 2 to 3 weeks with bed rest and nonsteroidal anti-inflammatory medication.

Respiratory Syncytial Virus Infections in Infants and Children With Congenital Heart Defects

Respiratory syncytial virus (RSV) is the most common cause of lower respiratory tract infections in infants and children worldwide, with the majority of children infected at least once by 2 years of age. Reinfection occurs commonly throughout life. Children with CHD who have RSV infections tend to have a higher rate of intensive care unit (ICU) admissions and require mechanical ventilation more frequently than those children who do not have CHD. RSV infection in a child with CHD carries a 40% mortality rate (Box 165.9).

Congestive Heart Failure
Foundations

CHF occurs when cardiac output is unable to meet the hemodynamic and metabolic demands of the body. Although there is a wide array of causes of CHF, the primary cause in infants and children is CHD. Other causes of CHF include the anomalous left coronary artery in infants, myocarditis, endocarditis, rheumatic heart disease, pericardial effusions, anemia, cardiomyopathies, systemic hypertension, hypothyroidism, hyperthyroidism, electrolyte imbalances, endocrine disorders, cardiac toxins, and dysrhythmias that compromise cardiac output.

CHF can result from a derangement in any of the four primary determinants of normal cardiac function: (1) excessive preload (e.g., large left-to-right shunts and severe chronic anemia); (2) decreased cardiac contractility (e.g., myocarditis); (3) excessive afterload (e.g., left-sided obstructive lesions); and (4) rhythm abnormalities that compromise cardiac output or stroke volume (e.g., paroxysmal supraventricular tachycardia and severe forms of heart block). The treatment of CHF depends on which of these four primary determinants of normal cardiac function are compromised. For example, inotropic agents and diuretics may be required in a child with volume overload and decreased cardiac contractility, whereas vasodilatory agents may be required in a child with CHF due to an increased afterload.

Clinical Features

Clinical manifestations of CHF depend on the exact pathophysiologic cause of the CHF; common presenting signs and symptoms include tachycardia, gallops (especially an S_3), tachypnea with rales, hepatomegaly, peripheral edema, and decreased peripheral perfusion of the extremities. Wheezing and a chronic cough may also be the presenting symptoms of CHF.

Diagnostic Testing

The chest radiograph typically reveals an enlargement of the cardiac silhouette and varying degrees of pulmonary congestion. An echocardiogram will be able to assess the ejection fraction, as well as to identify underlying anatomic defects. BNP may be helpful in differentiating cardiac from pulmonary causes of dyspnea in children.[5]

Management

Acute stabilization of any child who presents with CHF includes administration of supplemental oxygen and agents to augment cardiac contractility and to improve cardiac output. Children with respiratory distress due to pulmonary congestion may benefit from elevation of the head and upper torso—if available, place the infant in a car seat. Continuous positive airway pressure (CPAP) or biphasic positive airway pressure (BiPAP) ventilation via mask or nasal cannula (nasal CPAP) may be useful initially to decrease work of breathing and avert the need for endotracheal intubation. Children who present in severe respiratory distress secondary to pulmonary edema may require intubation to support oxygenation and ventilation. Plasma BNP levels have been used also to monitor the response to treatment regimens in patients with CHF.

Diuretics and inotropic agents may be considered. Furosemide (0.5 to 1 mg/kg) is the most common loop diuretic used to increase renal perfusion and to improve urine output. In contrast to adults, nitroglycerin is not first-line therapy for CHF in children. Children are much more sensitive to the drug's potent vasodilatory effects than adults, and they can experience profound and rapid hypotension with administration of nitroglycerin.

In the past, dopamine was administered for undifferentiated shock in children; however, other agents with less arrhythmogenic side effects are available. Increasingly, guidelines advocate for an approach based on etiology and pathophysiology. Norepinephrine is a good choice as a first-line vasopressor for pediatric decompensated cardiogenic shock due to its effectiveness in supporting SVR. Dobutamine may be added for its selective cardiac inotropic effects. Epinephrine is also potent inotrope and chronotrope that increases the SVR.

Amrinone and milrinone, most commonly used in the ICU setting, may be added to an inotrope to promote forward blood flow via peripheral vasodilatory effects. These agents have been used to improve cardiac index in septic shock and to prevent low cardiac output states for children with CHD. Side effects of these medications include profound hypotension, dysrhythmias, hypersensitivity reactions, fever, hepatotoxicity, and thrombocytopenia.

Pediatric Dysrhythmias

Foundations

The most common cause of cardiopulmonary arrest in infants and children is the untreated progression of respiratory failure or shock, rather than a primary cardiac dysrhythmia. Accordingly, the most common arrest rhythm is asystole or bradycardia rather than ventricular fibrillation or ventricular tachycardia.

The most common dysrhythmia in children is supraventricular tachycardia, which occurs most commonly in infants and young children. Although supraventricular tachycardia can spontaneously occur in infants without any underlying structural cardiac defects, ventricular tachycardias, in contrast, are typically due to an underlying myocardial abnormality.

Clinical Features

Rhythm disturbances in infants can be manifested with symptoms, such as fussiness, lethargy, poor feeding, pallor, respiratory distress, or cardiogenic shock. Older children present with chest pain, palpitations, difficulty in breathing, or syncope. The type and degree of severity of the presenting signs and symptoms should be taken into account in the evaluation and management of the specific dysrhythmia in each case (Box 165.10).

BOX 165.10 Conditions Associated With a High Risk for Development of Dysrhythmias

Congenital heart defects (uncorrected defects and postoperative complications)
Congenital complete heart blocks (e.g., maternal systemic lupus erythematosus)
Myocarditis
Rheumatic heart disease
Kawasaki disease with involvement of the coronary arteries
Cardiomyopathy
Prolonged QT syndrome
Aberrant atrioventricular conduction pathways (e.g., Wolff-Parkinson-White syndrome)
Electrolyte abnormalities (e.g., potassium, calcium, and magnesium disturbances)
Commotio cordis
Profound hypothermia
Hypoxia

Management

Children who exhibit electrocardiographic evidence of conduction abnormalities (e.g., Mobitz type II second-degree heart block, complete heart block, prolonged QT intervals, or aberrant conduction, such as the Wolff-Parkinson-White syndrome) may require emergent management, depending on symptoms and hemodynamic status.

Although some medications can be used to treat only atrial tachycardia (e.g., adenosine for supraventricular tachycardia) or ventricular tachycardia (e.g., lidocaine for ventricular tachycardia), amiodarone and procainamide can be used for an array of both atrial and ventricular dysrhythmias, including supraventricular and ventricular tachycardia.

Bradydysrhythmias

Sinus Bradycardia. Bradycardia is defined as a heart rate that is slower than the lower limit of normal for a child's age. Clinically significant bradycardia in children is a heart rate slower than 60 beats/minute and associated with poor systemic perfusion. An athletic adolescent may have a resting baseline heart rate lower than 60 beats/minute, requiring no treatment if asymptomatic with good perfusion.

Bradycardia is poorly tolerated in infants and children because they are not physiologically capable of increasing their stroke volume to maintain an adequate cardiac output in the face of significant bradycardia. **The most common cause of symptomatic bradycardia in infants and children is hypoxia.** First, ensure adequate oxygenation and ventilation. Epinephrine is the first-line medication for treatment of symptomatic bradycardia in children that is not responsive to appropriate oxygenation and ventilation. If additional doses of intravenous or intraosseous epinephrine are required to treat symptomatic bradycardia, the dose should remain at standard dosing (0.01 mg/kg). Atropine is indicated for vagally induced bradycardia or treatment of primary atrioventricular block. Atropine will have no effect on the denervated heart (e.g., after cardiac transplantation). If vascular access is not available, both epinephrine and atropine can be administered through the tracheal tube, although the intravenous route is preferred.

Other causes of bradycardia include hypothermia, increased intracranial pressure, heart blocks (congenital and acquired), denervated heart status after cardiac surgery, hypothyroidism, sick sinus syndrome, and various medications and toxins (e.g., digoxin, beta-blockers, calcium channel blockers, and cholinergic agents). Children with presyncopal or syncopal symptoms or poor perfusion with Mobitz type II second-degree atrioventricular block, complete third-degree heart block, or sick sinus syndrome should be paced.

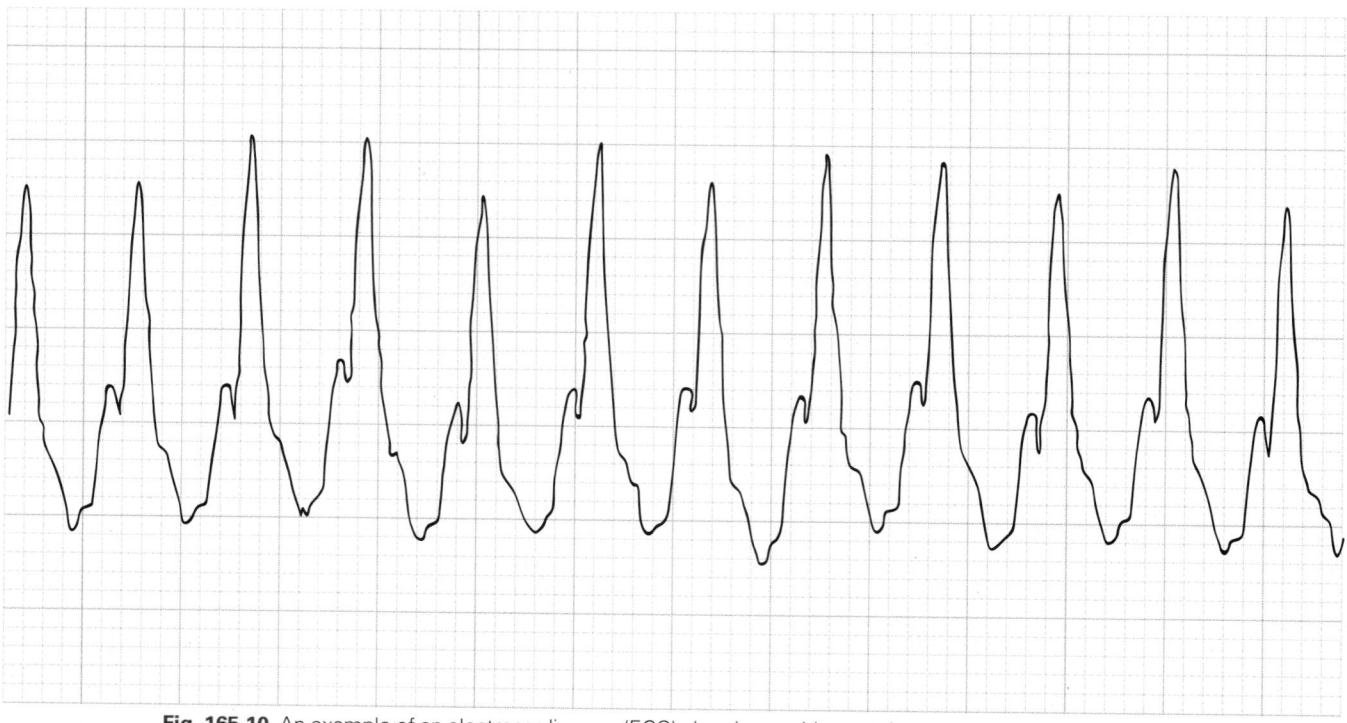

Fig. 165.10 An example of an electrocardiogram (ECG) showing a wide-complex supraventricular tachycardia at a rate of approximately 270 beats/minute in an infant with Ebstein anomaly of the tricuspid valve. This infant was in supraventricular tachycardia for approximately 2 days and presented with an acute exacerbation of her congestive heart failure (CHF), as evidenced by the cardiomegaly on the chest radiograph (see Fig. 165.11). Note that the cardiothoracic ratio in this infant is approximately 70%.

Tachydysrhythmias

Supraventricular Tachycardia. Supraventricular tachycardia is the most common symptomatic dysrhythmia in infants and children. No cardiac abnormalities are found in approximately half of cases; the Wolff-Parkinson-White syndrome is present in only 10% to 20%. The type of supraventricular tachycardia that occurs most commonly in infants and children involves a reentrant mechanism that uses an accessory pathway and the atrioventricular node (i.e., atrioventricular reentrant tachycardia [AVRT]). The *orthodromic* reentry phenomenon involves the normal antegrade conduction from the atria to the ventricles down the atrioventricular node, with retrograde conduction back from the ventricles to the atria by the accessory pathway. Orthodromic conduction will produce a narrow–QRS complex supraventricular tachycardia. The less common reentry mechanism is the *antidromic* form in which conduction from the atria to the ventricles first goes antegrade down the accessory pathway then retrograde back to the atria by the atrioventricular node. Antidromic conduction will produce a wide–QRS complex supraventricular tachycardia. Supraventricular tachycardia in a child with a preexisting bundle branch block can also result in a wide-complex supraventricular tachycardia. The ECG in Figure 165.10 reveals a case of a wide-complex supraventricular tachycardia in a child with Ebstein anomaly of the tricuspid valve who also presented with CHF (Fig. 165.11).

Clinical Features and Diagnostic Testing. Supraventricular tachycardia is most likely with heart rates above 180 in young children and 220 in infants, without beat-to-beat variability (Fig. 165.12 and Table 165.5). Although healthy infants can generally tolerate supraventricular tachycardia with heart rates approaching 300 beats/minute, supraventricular tachycardia may begin to produce signs of CHF and shock if left untreated. Older children with supraventricular tachycardia commonly present with palpitations, difficulty in breathing, and chest discomfort.

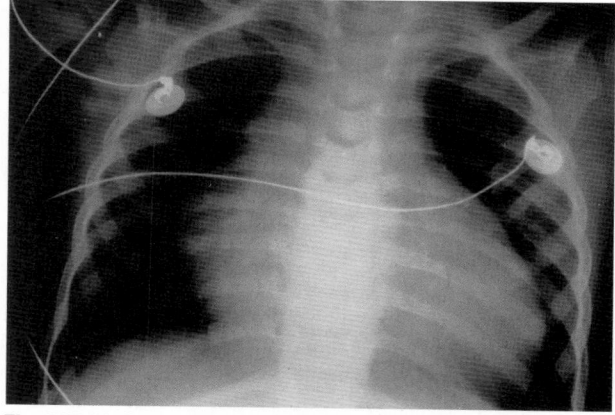

Fig. 165.11 Chest radiograph of same infant as in Figure 165.10.

Management. The emergency clinician should quickly initiate synchronized cardioversion (0.5 to 1 J/kg) for children in supraventricular tachycardia (SVT) with signs of poor perfusion, such as altered mental status, delayed capillary refill, pallor, cyanosis, or hypotension (i.e., decompensated shock). If the child does not convert with this initial cardioversion attempt, the energy dose can be doubled up to 2 J/kg on subsequent attempts. If the child is hemodynamically stable, vagal maneuvers, then adenosine, may be attempted initially before cardioversion; a continuous rhythm strip should be run to document the response to each conversion attempt. Vagal maneuvers (e.g., blowing into a syringe) can be attempted before adenosine administration in the child with hemodynamically stable supraventricular tachycardia. Application of ice to the face has been demonstrated to be a fairly effective method of converting supraventricular tachycardia in infants and children.

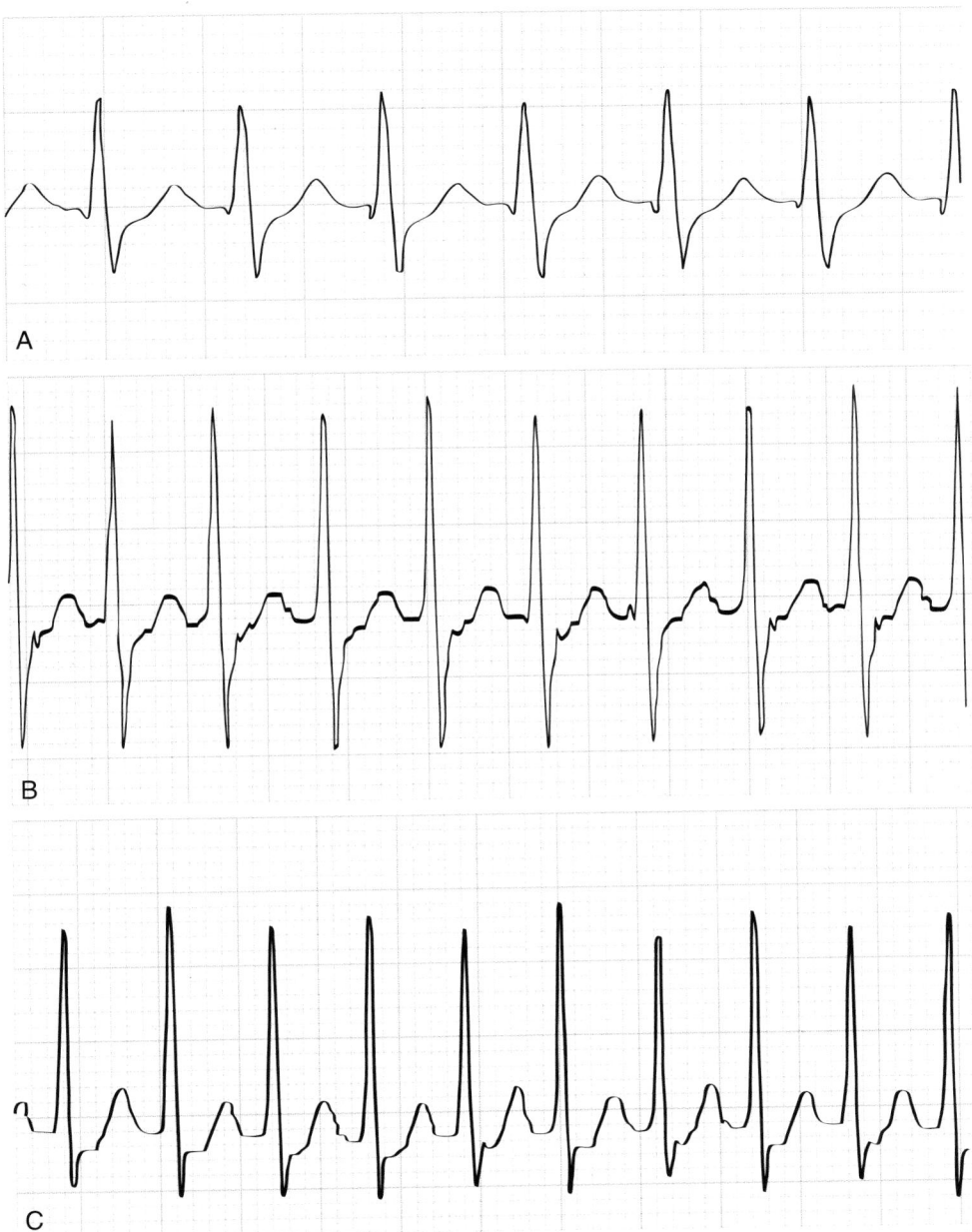

Fig. 165.12 Three electrocardiographic examples of classic narrow-complex supraventricular tachycardia in children. The heart rate is approximately 240 beats/minute in the first two examples (A and B) and approximately 270 beats/minute in the third example (C).

TABLE 165.5 Clinical and Electrocardiographic Features to Differentiate Sinus Tachycardia From Supraventricular Tachycardia in Children		
	Sinus Tachycardia	**Supraventricular Tachycardia**
Precipitating events	Dehydration, fever, pain	No precipitating event
P waves on electrocardiogram (ECG)	Present	Absent
Heart rate varies with activity	Yes	No
Beat-to-beat variability	Yes	Constant R-R intervals
Heart rate in infants (beats/minute)	Usually <220	Usually >220
Heart rate in children (beats/minute)	Usually <180	Usually >180

One method to perform this maneuver is to fill a plastic bag or surgical glove with a slurry of crushed ice and water, which is then placed over the infant's forehead, eyes, and bridge of the nose for 10 to 15 seconds. Placement of the ice bag should not occlude the nose or mouth. External ocular pressure should be avoided. Carotid massage is less effective and is not recommended as a vagal maneuver in infants or children.

The initial dose of adenosine in children is 0.1 mg/kg with a maximum initial dose of 6 mg. If this initial dose of adenosine fails to convert the supraventricular tachycardia, the dose is then doubled to 0.2 mg/kg with a maximum of 12 mg/dose. This 0.2 mg/kg dose of adenosine may be repeated once. Elective cardioversion with procedural sedation may be required in children who fail to convert with adenosine. Adenosine-induced wide-complex tachycardia (secondary to an occult accessory conduction pathway) is an uncommon complication (Fig. 165.13). Amiodarone may be given at a loading dose of 5 mg/kg

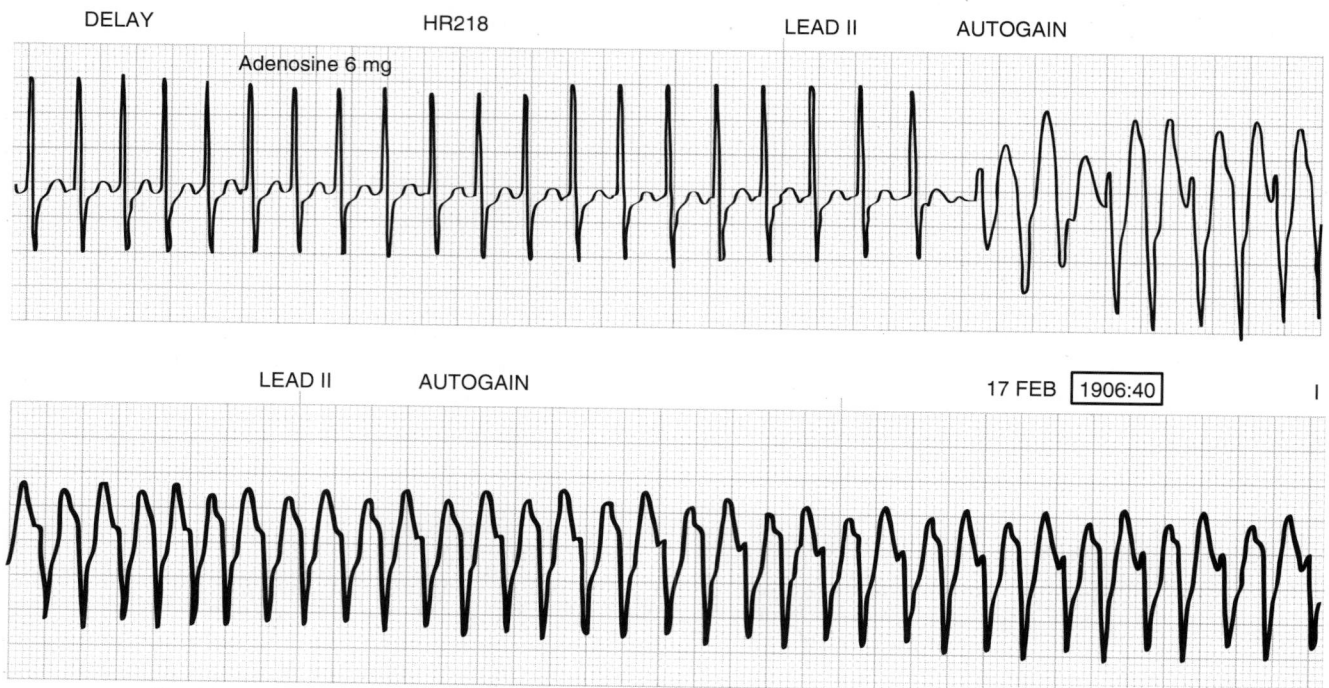

Fig. 165.13 An example of adenosine-induced wide-complex tachycardia. A dose of 6 mg of adenosine was administered to this previously healthy 15-year-old girl who presented with a 6-hour history of palpitations. She had no previous cardiac problems except for intermittent palpitations in the past that always resolved spontaneously without any medical interventions. Once adenosine blocked the conduction through the atrio-ventricular node, a wide-complex tachycardia appeared on the electrocardiogram (ECG), which was probably due to antegrade conduction through an accessory pathway. During the 30 seconds of this wide-complex tachycardia, the patient remained alert with excellent perfusion parameters. This wide-complex tachycardia then spontaneously converted to normal sinus rhythm. Although the patient's postconversion ECG did not reveal an accessory pathway, Holter monitoring 1 month later detected the classic electrocardiographic findings of Wolff-Parkinson-White syndrome.

over 20 to 60 minutes, then continued at 5 mcg/kg/min. Verapamil should be avoided altogether in infants and children, and not given to those younger than 2 years old because of the risk of profound hypotension and cardiovascular collapse in this age group. Once the patient has converted to sinus rhythm, a 12-lead ECG should be obtained to assess for the possibility of Wolff-Parkinson-White syndrome or any other underlying conduction abnormalities that may have predisposed the child to development of the supraventricular tachycardia.

Atrial Flutter and Atrial Fibrillation. Both atrial flutter and atrial fibrillation are rare in children and are usually associated with underlying heart conditions (e.g., CHD, status post–open heart surgical procedures that involved the atria, myocarditis, and digoxin toxicity). Hemodynamic stability depends on the ventricular response. As in adults, children with hemodynamically unstable atrial flutter or atrial fibrillation should be electrocardioverted. The initial treatment priority in patients with hemodynamically stable atrial flutter and atrial fibrillation is first to slow the rate of the ventricular response with medications such as diltiazem, beta-blockers, or digoxin. IV calcium channel blockers and IV beta-blockers often cause complete heart block and should not be given concurrently.

If the patient who presents with atrial flutter or atrial fibrillation is known to have an underlying Wolff-Parkinson-White syndrome, the four medications that should be avoided are the A-B-C-D medications (adenosine, amiodarone, beta-blockers, calcium channel blockers, and digoxin); all of these medications preferentially block conduction down the atrioventricular node, leaving the accessory pathway open to conduct the atrial tachycardia to the ventricles at a potentially lethal rate.

Safer alternatives are amiodarone, procainamide, or cardioversion. Procainamide is preferred to amiodarone as there have been reports of VF following amiodarone administration in WPW. Consultation with the cardiologist and initiation of anticoagulation should also be considered.

Ventricular Tachycardia. The majority of children with ventricular tachycardia have an underlying condition, such as post–cardiac surgery status, myocarditis, prolonged QT syndrome, drug or toxin exposures (e.g., cyclic antidepressants), or electrolyte abnormalities. The treatment of ventricular tachycardia will depend on hemodynamic status of the patient. Torsades de pointes is a unique type of polymorphic ventricular tachycardia characterized by QRS complexes that change in polarity and amplitude. Prolonged QT syndrome, underlying congenital cardiac defects, hypomagnesemia, and various medications (e.g., cyclic antidepressants) have been identified as known causes of torsades de pointes. The treatment of choice is intravenous magnesium at an initial dose of 25 to 50 mg/kg, up to the adult dose of 2 g over 2 minutes. Class IA (i.e., procainamide) and class III (i.e., amiodarone) antidysrhythmic agents are contraindicated in the treatment of torsades de pointes because these agents are capable of prolonging the QT interval, which can precipitate the degeneration of the torsades de pointes into a lethal rhythm.

Special Resuscitation Situations in Children

Children with single-ventricle physiology (e.g., hypoplastic left heart syndrome and double-outlet right ventricle physiology) after a palliative shunting procedure should be given standard resuscitation care. Heparin may be used in the pre-arrest or arrest of infants with a systemic-to–pulmonary artery shunt or right ventricle–to–pulmonary artery shunt to halt thrombus propagation in this low circulatory flow state. A target oxyhemoglobin saturation (SpO_2) of approximately 80% is preferred in these children. End-tidal carbon dioxide readings after resuscitation may lag behind, because varying pulmonary blood flow changes do not necessarily reflect cardiac output. The goal is to provide adequate preload with judicious fluids to balance systemic and pulmonary blood flow. If available, extracorporeal membrane oxygenation should be considered.

Children with a history of pulmonary hypertension should also receive standard resuscitation management. Preload should be optimized with isotonic saline boluses. Inhaled nitric oxide in the ICU may be given to reduce PVR. Early contact with the child's cardiologist and cardiothoracic surgeon is instrumental in the post-resuscitative care of children with CHD.

Bacterial Endocarditis

Foundations

Although bacterial endocarditis most commonly occurs in children with an underlying CHD or an acquired cardiac lesion (e.g., acute rheumatic valvular heart disease), it can also occur in patients with no underlying anatomic defects of the valves or endocardium.

Cardiac lesions that carry this higher risk include VSD, aortic valvular stenosis, tetralogy of Fallot, single-ventricle states, bicuspid aortic valves, prosthetic valves, and postoperative systemic-to-pulmonary shunts. Isolated secundum ASD carry a much lower risk for bacterial endocarditis because the shunt flow through the ASD is typically of a much lower velocity (Box 165.11).

Clinical Features

The early clinical manifestations of bacterial endocarditis are nonspecific. The child may simply present with only fever and tachycardia (see Box 165.11). A new heart murmur is present in less than 50% of the bacterial endocarditis cases. Common presenting signs are fever (99%), petechiae (21%), changing murmur (21%), dental caries (14%), and hepatosplenomegaly (14%). Less common signs are CHF (9%), splinter hemorrhages (5%), Roth spots (5%), and Osler nodes (4%).

Diagnostic Studies

Diagnostic studies for a child with suspected bacterial endocarditis include a complete blood cell count, C-reactive protein (CRP) assessment, measurement of erythrocyte sedimentation rate (ESR), three blood cultures, chest radiography, and electrocardiography. *Streptococcus viridans* and *Staphylococcus aureus* are the two most common offending organisms recovered from the blood cultures of children with bacterial endocarditis. Studies have shown that in children with CHD, 60% of the cases caused by staphylococcal species are methicillin resistant and associated with increased risk of mortality. Formal echocardiography is typically done as an inpatient.

Management

In some patients, antibiotic prophylaxis to prevent endocarditis is recommended. Box 165.12 lists the cardiac conditions for which endocarditis prophylaxis is recommended and Box 165.13 lists the procedures for which these patients should receive antibiotic prophylaxis. In children with suspected acute bacterial endocarditis, antibiotics should be started immediately after blood culture samples have been obtained. Although the choice of intravenous antibiotics depends on the suspected source of seeding and the child's immune status, a commonly recommended regimen includes an aminoglycoside plus a penicillinase-resistant penicillin, such as oxacillin. If methicillin-resistant *Staphylococcus* is suspected, vancomycin should also be included in the initial empirical antibiotic regimen. Surgical intervention may be required to remove septic vegetations, or valve replacement is sometimes necessary. Further reading on endocarditis may be found in Chapter 69.

Pericarditis

Foundations

Pericarditis is an inflammatory process within the pericardial sac that may not be associated with a pericardial effusion. In the majority of cases, pericarditis in children is self-limited and follows a benign clinical course. A sudden increase or a large amount of fluid within this

---

BOX 165.12 Cardiac Conditions for Which Endocarditis Prophylaxis Is Recommended

Prosthetic cardiac valve or prosthetic material used for cardiac valve repair
Previous infective endocarditis
Congenital heart disease (CHD)[a]
Unrepaired cyanotic CHD, including palliative shunts and conduits
Completely repaired congenital heart defect with prosthetic material or device during the first 6 months after the procedure[b]
Repaired CHD with residual defects at the site or adjacent to the site of a prosthetic patch or device (which inhibit endothelialization)
Cardiac transplantation recipients who have cardiac valvulopathy

[a] Except for those conditions above, antibiotic prophylaxis is no longer recommended for any other form of CHD.
[b] Prophylaxis is reasonable because endothelialization of prosthetic material occurs within 6 months after the procedure.
From: American Heart Association. Prevention of infective endocarditis: guidelines from the American Heart Association. *Circulation.* 2007;116:1736.

BOX 165.11 Clinical Conditions in Which Bacterial Endocarditis Should Be Suspected in a Child With an Underlying Anatomic Cardiac Defect

Fever of unknown etiology
A change in the quality of the preexisting heart murmur or the presence of a new heart murmur
Development of a neurologic deficit (secondary to central nervous system emboli)
New-onset microscopic hematuria
Splenomegaly
Petechiae
Splinter hemorrhages involving the conjunctiva, nail beds, palms, or soles
Myalgias

BOX 165.13 Procedures for Which Endocarditis Prophylaxis Is Recommended

All dental procedures that involve manipulation of gingival tissue or the periapical region of teeth or perforation of the oral mucosa[a]
Consider prophylaxis for incisional procedures on the respiratory tract, infected skin, or musculoskeletal tissue only for high-risk patients

[a] The following procedures do not need prophylaxis: routine anesthetic injections through noninfected tissue, dental radiographs, placement of removable prosthodontic or orthodontic appliances, adjustment of orthodontic appliances, placement of orthodontic brackets, shedding of deciduous teeth, and bleeding from trauma to the lips or oral mucosa.

pericardial sac can cause a tamponade-induced decrease in stroke volume, resulting in diminished cardiac output and hypotension.

The most common causes of pericarditis include bacterial and viral infections; other causes are ARF, systemic lupus erythematosus, uremia, post-pericardiotomy syndrome, leukemia, lymphoma, and tuberculosis. Approximately 30% of pericarditis cases are due to bacteria, such as pneumococcus, *S. aureus,* meningococcus, and *Haemophilus influenzae.* Viral causes are most common, but a specific viral pathogen is recovered in only 20% to 30% of cases. Viral causes include coxsackieviruses, echoviruses, adenovirus, Epstein-Barr virus, and influenza viruses.

Clinical Features

The presenting signs and symptoms of pericarditis depend on the cause of the pericarditis, as well as on the amount of fluid that has accumulated within the pericardial sac. Chest pain that varies with position is a common complaint with pericarditis; pain is exacerbated with inspiration and the supine position but relieved when the patient sits up or leans forward. Tachycardia is also a common finding in patients with pericarditis and may be the only clue to the diagnosis. Other findings

include fatigue, tachypnea, neck vein distention, pulsus paradoxus, hepatomegaly, lower extremity edema, and thready distal pulses if heart failure is present. Cardiac auscultatory findings can include a harsh-sounding friction rub or diminished or muffled heart tones if there is a significant amount of fluid within the pericardial sac. A pericardial friction rub, if present, is best heard when the patient sits up or leans forward. The friction rub of pericarditis can be distinguished from a pleural friction rub by having the patient hold his or her breath during auscultation. The friction rub of pericarditis will remain present during breath-holding, while the pleural friction rub will no longer be heard.

The chest radiograph in a child with pericarditis may not reveal an enlarged cardiac silhouette. If there is a large collection of fluid within the pericardial sac, the heart shadow on the chest radiograph will resemble a "water bottle" silhouette. Approximately 50% of pericarditis cases have some associated pleural effusion.

The classic electrocardiographic findings of viral pericarditis include diffuse ST segment elevation and diffuse T wave inversions. The classic electrocardiographic changes associated with pericarditis evolve through four phases (Fig. 165.14). During the initial phase,

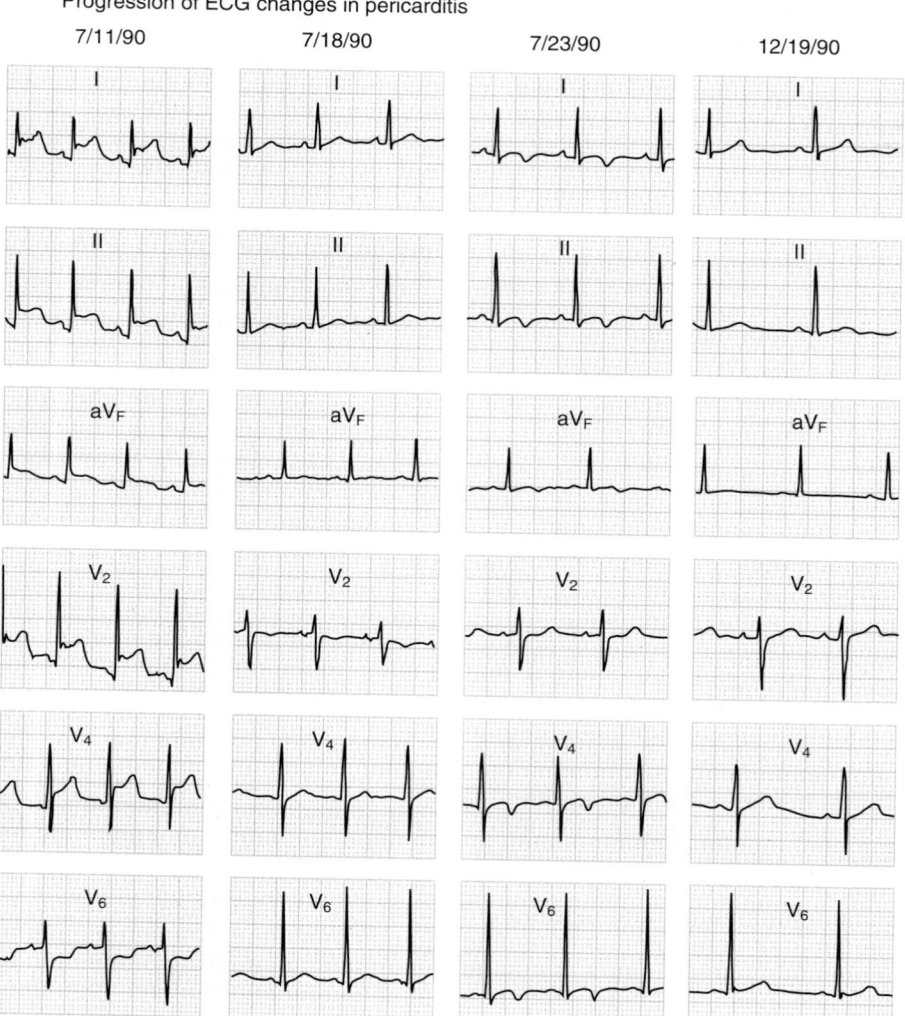

Fig. 165.14 The classic electrocardiographic progression of a patient with pericarditis. First phase: Diffuse ST segment elevation. Second phase: ST segments back to isoelectric but decreased T wave amplitude. Third phase: T wave inversion. Fourth phase: Complete resolution. Notice that the first three phases of the electrocardiographic abnormalities of pericarditis in this patient are evident during the first 2 weeks of his illness. A follow-up electrocardiogram (ECG) obtained 5 months later reveals a complete resolution of all the previous electrocardiographic abnormalities.

there is diffuse ST segment elevation secondary to subepicardial inflammation; PR segment depression may also be seen. During the second phase, the previously elevated ST segments begin to return to isoelectric baseline, and the T wave amplitudes begin to decrease with flattening of the T waves. During the third phase, although the ST segments are now back to isoelectric baseline, the T waves are inverted. The fourth and final phase demonstrates complete resolution of the ST segment and T wave abnormalities. Diminished electrocardiographic voltages in all leads can also occur if there is a significant amount of fluid accumulated within the pericardial sac.

Diagnostic Studies

Ultrasound will confirm both the presence and the amount of accumulated fluid within the pericardial sac. Although echocardiography cannot accurately quantify the exact amount of fluid that has accumulated within the pericardial space, the presence of an anterior and posterior fluid collection is suggestive of a large collection.

Management

The management of a child with pericarditis depends on both the suspected cause, severity of symptoms, and amount of fluid that has accumulated within the pericardial space. Patients with fever, respiratory distress, or signs of CHF should be admitted and an echocardiogram emergently performed. An emergency pericardiocentesis is required in those patients with signs of acute cardiac tamponade. Fluid that is aspirated from the pericardial space should be sent for routine cell counts, Grams stain, and cultures. Antiinflammatory agents and appropriate antibiotics should be initiated on the basis of the suspected cause. Steroids are reserved for refractory cases that are not responsive to these agents and should be considered only after an infectious etiology is ruled out. See also Chapter 68 for more on pericarditis.

Myocarditis
Foundations

In the United States, the most common cause of myocarditis is viral; adenovirus and enteroviruses account for the majority of cases.[7] Other viral causes include echoviruses, influenza, coxsackie, adenovirus, varicella-zoster, Epstein-Barr, cytomegalovirus, and hepatitis B virus. Bacterial causes include *Corynebacterium diphtheriae, Streptococcus pyogenes, S. aureus, Mycoplasma pneumoniae, Borrelia burgdorferi,* and meningococcus. Noninfectious causes include Kawasaki disease, acute rheumatic fever (ARF), collagen vascular disorders (e.g., systemic lupus erythematosus), toxins (e.g., cocaine and doxorubicin), endocrine disorders (e.g., hyperthyroidism), and drug-induced hypersensitivity (e.g., penicillins, sulfonamides, phenytoin, carbamazepine).

Clinical Features

Viral myocarditis usually has a gradual onset with preceding upper respiratory tract infection. Clinicians should consider myocarditis in infants and children with symptoms out of proportion to the typical course of a benign cause, such as a viral syndrome. Early in its course, the only sign of myocarditis may be tachycardia. Tachycardia that is disproportionate to the degree of fever should alert the emergency clinician to the possibility of myocarditis. Other presenting signs and symptoms include fever, myalgias, fatigue, tachypnea, wheezing, abdominal pain, and chest pain. More severe cases of myocarditis can even have signs and symptoms of acute CHF and various dysrhythmias. The physical examination may reveal a new murmur, a gallop rhythm, or a pericardial friction rub with muffled heart tones (if the myocarditis is also accompanied by pericarditis and subsequent pericardial effusion). In general, these are sick children with vague symptoms.

Diagnostic Testing

The evaluation and management of the child with myocarditis depend on the suspected cause and presenting signs and symptoms. Blood cultures and viral titers should be considered in infectious and postinfectious cases. Appropriate antibiotics should be initiated immediately in cases with suspected bacterial origin. The chest radiograph may be normal in very mild cases, but cardiomegaly will be evident in more advanced cases. The electrocardiographic findings are usually nonspecific and can include low-voltage, nonspecific ST segment abnormalities, T wave inversions, atrioventricular block, and various other dysrhythmias. Creatine kinase-MB, cTnT, cTnI, CRP, and ESR may be elevated.

Bedside echocardiography can evaluate for effusion, tamponade, and global function. The goal of treatment is to maintain adequate cardiac output and to control any associated dysrhythmias.

Management

Children who present in CHF with poor perfusion (e.g., lethargy, delayed capillary refill, poor urine output, or hypotension) will likely require inotropic support, positive-pressure ventilation, or diuretics. The role of intravenous immunoglobulin (IVIG) in pediatric myocarditis is unclear.[8] The use of beta-blockers is contraindicated, and the routine use of immunosuppressive agents remains controversial.[9,10] Although the majority of children with acute viral myocarditis make a full recovery, a few patients will progress to dilated cardiomyopathy, which is characterized by dilated ventricles and impaired systolic contractility. See Chapter 68 for more on myocarditis.

Kawasaki Disease
Foundations

Kawasaki disease, originally described as mucocutaneous lymph node, has emerged as a significant cause of acquired cardiac disease in children in the United States. This febrile, exanthematous, multisystem vasculitis is seen most commonly in children younger than 5 years old. Up to 20% of untreated children have some degree of coronary artery abnormalities.[11] Although the exact cause of this vasculitis of small- and medium-sized vessels remains unknown, early clinical recognition and initiation of high-dose aspirin and IVIG improve the morbidity and mortality rates of Kawasaki disease in children.

Clinical Features

In addition to fever, the physical examination of a child with Kawasaki disease may reveal the typical findings as listed in Box 165.14 and illustrated in Figure 165.15. The classic features of Kawasaki disease may be manifested simultaneously or in series of days; a careful history and physical examination may elucidate the need for further testing. In addition, very young children may not have a classic presentation and require further investigation. All children with suspected Kawasaki disease, with either classic or incomplete features, should undergo echocardiography for detection of the presence and degree of coronary aneurysm.[11]

Incomplete Kawasaki Disease. The classic presentation of Kawasaki disease is a clinical diagnosis of four or more of the five criteria in a child who is febrile 5 days or more. However, these strict criteria may miss a substantial number of children who present with incomplete Kawasaki disease. Any child may have an incomplete presentation, but this is mostly seen in infants younger than 6 months old.

Current criteria recommend that in a child who is febrile 5 days or more, the presence of two or three criteria should prompt further testing. We recommend that a CRP of 3 mg/dL or more or an ESR of 40 mm/hr or more prompt further laboratory investigations; children with elevated inflammatory markers should be empirically treated

BOX 165.14   Diagnostic Criteria for Kawasaki Disease

- Fever for 5 days or more
- At least four of the five following physical examination findings:
  1. Bilateral, nonexudative bulbar conjunctival injection (bilateral scleral injection with perilimbic sparing)
  2. Oropharyngeal mucous membrane changes (pharyngeal erythema, red and cracked lips, and a strawberry tongue)
  3. Cervical lymphadenopathy (with at least one node >1.5 cm in diameter)
  4. Peripheral extremity changes (diffuse erythema and swelling of the hands and feet during the acute phase or periungual desquamation during the convalescent phase of the illness); this diffuse palmar erythema seen in Kawasaki disease is in contrast to the discrete macular lesions of various viral illnesses (e.g., measles) that can sometimes be seen on the palms and soles
  5. A polymorphous generalized rash (nonvesicular and nonbullous); there is no specific rash that is pathognomonic for Kawasaki disease
- In a child with four or more criteria, the diagnosis may be made on day 4 of the fever.

(Box 165.15). During their hospital stay, children should receive an echocardiogram to assess for coronary aneurysms.

Children with a CRP of less than 3 mg/dL and an ESR of less than 40 mm/hr may be observed daily and reassessed without treatment; serial ESR and CRP should be obtained daily on an outpatient basis. Infants 6 months of age or younger are more likely to present with incomplete Kawasaki disease and are more susceptible to giant coronary artery aneurysm formation. For this reason, irrespective of general well appearance or lack of clinical findings, infants 6 months of age or younger with fever lasting for 7 days or more should undergo supplemental laboratory testing and undergo echocardiogram when inflammatory markers are abnormal.

Kawasaki disease is postulated to be caused by an infectious agent that enters the respiratory tract and initiates an oligoclonal immunoglobulin A response, which activates lymphocytes, cytokines, and proteinases that weaken vessel walls and predispose the entire circulation to aneurysms. Approximately 25% of patients have mild diffuse myocardial inflammation. This occurs during the acute febrile period and is characterized by tachycardia, a gallop, and nonspecific ST-T wave changes. Up to 5% of the children also exhibit some degree of CHF during this acute phase of their illness; this carditis usually resolves when the fever resolves. Pericardial effusions also occur in up to 20% to 40% of cases. Mild mitral and aortic regurgitation is seen in 1% to 2% of untreated cases on echocardiographic examinations. This phase of the disease is mild and self-resolving.

Differential Diagnoses

Measles can mimic Kawasaki disease (i.e., a febrile illness with red eyes, a rash, and erythema of the oropharynx). The measles rash classically begins on the head and face and progresses caudally. The rash of Kawasaki disease typically begins on the trunk and then spreads to the face and extremities; it may be polymorphous, but not bullous or vesicular.

The palmar lesions of measles are discrete macular lesions (see Fig. 165.15F), whereas the palmar finding in children with Kawasaki disease is diffuse erythema, which may later desquamate (see Fig. 165.15C).

There are many imitators of Kawasaki disease. For example, Kawasaki disease can present with nausea, vomiting, and abdominal pain in a febrile child, which may be mistaken for a surgical abdomen. A febrile irritable child with Kawasaki disease may have a cerebrospinal fluid pleocytosis and be misdiagnosed with viral meningitis.

Streptococcal disease, including pharyngitis and scarlet fever, can be confused with Kawasaki disease, but conjunctivitis and swelling of the hands and feet are unusual for streptococcal disease. Other infectious or autoimmune causes that mimic Kawasaki disease include Rocky Mountain spotted fever, leptospirosis, Stevens-Johnson syndrome, and juvenile rheumatoid arthritis.

Management

The main goal of treatment during the acute febrile phase of Kawasaki disease is to provide supportive care and to decrease the inflammation of the myocardium and coronary arteries. IVIG and high-dose aspirin have an additive effect and, when initiated within 10 days from the onset of the illness, can substantially decrease the progression to coronary artery dilation and aneurysm formation compared with aspirin therapy alone.[12] The combination results in a more rapid resolution of fever and the other indicators of acute inflammation.[12] However, despite prompt treatment with IVIG and high-dose aspirin, 2% to 4% of children still have coronary artery abnormalities.[11]

The current IVIG regimen involves an infusion of 2 g/kg over 10 to 12 hours. Side effects include hypotension, nausea, vomiting, headache, and seizures. Close cardiac monitoring during the IVIG infusion is recommended. The 5% to 10% of children who receive IVIG and experience a persistent or recurrent fever after the initial dose of IVIG may be given a second infusion at the same dose. Approximately two-thirds of children who fail to respond to the initial dose of IVIG will improve with the second infusion.

Aspirin is initiated at 80 to 100 mg/kg/day orally divided into an every-6-hour dosing regimen until the child is afebrile for 48 to 72 hours. Prompt diagnosis and treatment leads to rapid symptomatic improvement in 90% of cases and prevents coronary aneurysm formation in 95%.

The follow-up of children with Kawasaki disease depends on the degree and presence of carditis and coronary artery abnormalities detected on the initial echocardiogram. Other imaging modalities used to follow aneurysmal parameters include electron-beam computed tomography, coronary magnetic resonance angiography, and computed tomography. Those children with more severe cardiac abnormalities should have close follow-up by a cardiologist experienced in Kawasaki disease.

Acute Rheumatic Fever
Foundations

ARF, one of the most common causes of acquired heart disease in children, is the result of a delayed immune reaction to a group A streptococcal infection. In the United States, ARF most commonly occurs in children 5 to 15 years old, with an attack rate of 0.3% in children with an untreated streptococcal infection. Although this disease affects multiple organ systems, carditis is the most serious complication.

Clinical Features

The diagnosis of ARF is based on the Jones criteria (Box 165.16). In addition, there must also be evidence of an antecedent streptococcal infection, which can be documented by a positive throat culture, a positive rapid streptococcal antigen test finding, or an elevated antistreptolysin O (ASO) titer. The ASO titer begins to rise 1 to 3 weeks after streptococcal infection, peaks at 3 to 5 weeks, and reliably falls to baseline after 6 months. The diagnosis of ARF is made in a patient with a documented antecedent streptococcal infection who exhibits either two major criteria or one major plus two minor criteria.[13]

The most common presenting major criterion is migratory polyarthritis, which commonly involves the larger joints of the extremities, as well as the

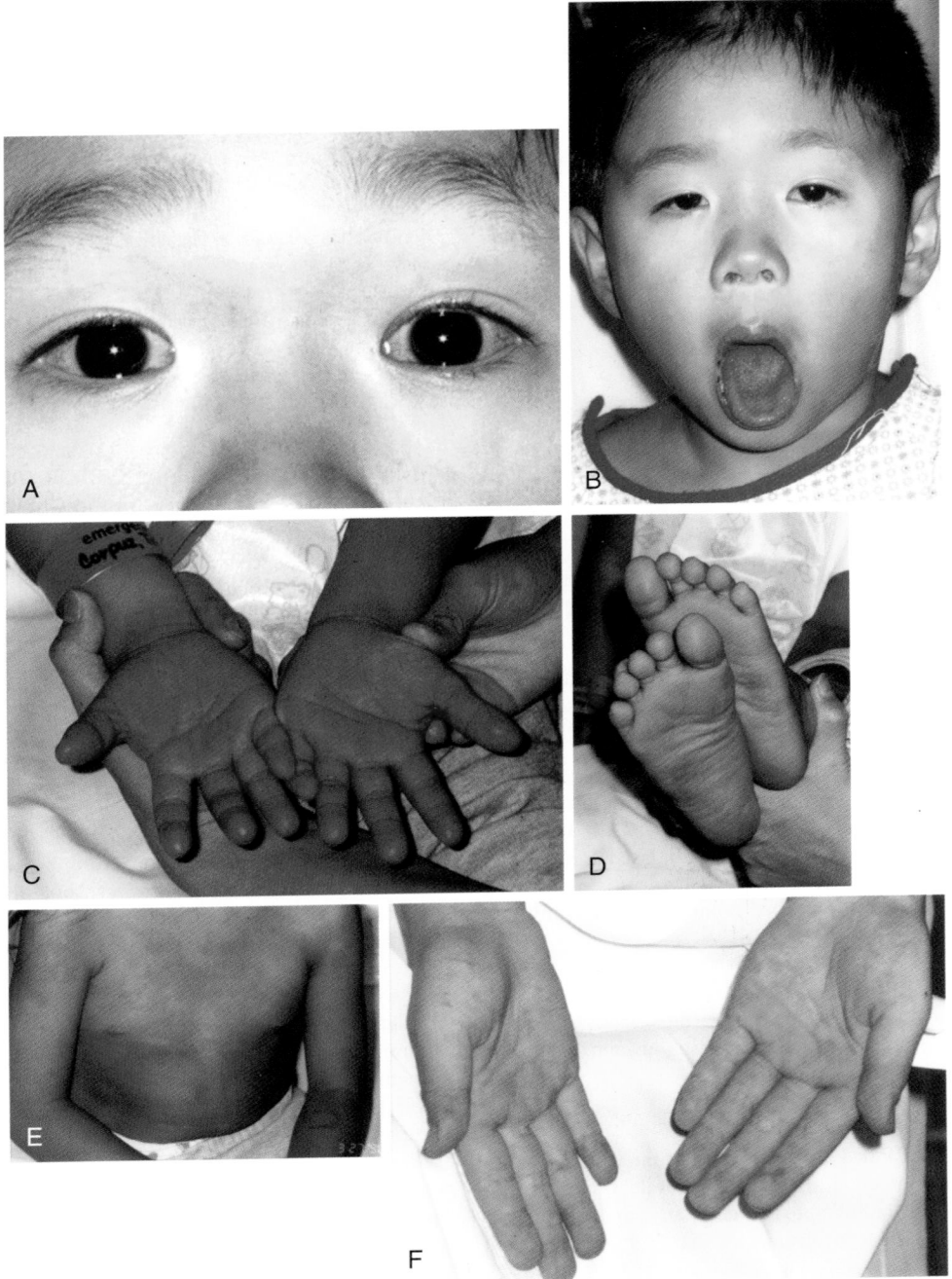

Fig. 165.15 Classic physical examination findings of Kawasaki disease. Note the bilateral nonexudative scleral injections (A) with perilimbic sparing (the thin margin of white sclera around the cornea), red and cracked lips with a strawberry tongue (B), diffuse palmar erythema (C), red soles (D), and polymorphous exanthem (E). The diffuse palmar erythema of Kawasaki disease (C) is distinct from the palmar findings seen in other viral illnesses, such as the discrete macular lesions on the palms in this child with measles (F).

BOX 165.15 Supplemental Laboratory Criteria for Kawasaki Disease

Albumin ≤3 g/dL
Anemia for age
Platelet count of ≥450,000/mm³
White blood cell (WBC) count ≥15,000 mm³
Elevation of alanine aminotransferase
Sterile pyuria of ≥10 WBCs per high-power field

smaller tarsal joints in the foot and the smaller carpal joints in the hand. The carditis of ARF most commonly involves valvulitis of the mitral and aortic valves, which clinically is manifested as occult mitral or aortic insufficiency. The murmur of mitral insufficiency is characterized as a holosystolic murmur best heard over the apex with radiation to the axilla. The murmur of aortic insufficiency is characterized as a diastolic murmur that is best heard over the base of the heart. Innocent murmurs that are normally exacerbated with fever can be mistaken for the murmurs of mitral or aortic insufficiency.

Other cardiac manifestations of ARF include CHF, pericarditis, and various degrees of heart block. The two dermatologic major criteria (erythema marginatum and subcutaneous nodules) and chorea occur less commonly than the migratory polyarthritis and carditis. Chorea may occur as the only manifestation of ARF. If arthritis is used as a major component, arthralgia cannot be used as a minor component to make the diagnosis. Likewise, if carditis is used as a major component, a prolonged PR interval cannot be used as a minor component.[13]

Differential Diagnoses

The differential diagnosis of ARF includes myocarditis, bacterial endocarditis, Lyme disease, systemic lupus erythematosus, juvenile rheumatoid arthritis, serum sickness, and septic arthritis.

Diagnostic Testing

In addition to the ECG, CRP or ESR levels, and documentation of an antecedent streptococcal infection, the diagnostic evaluation of ARF should also include a chest radiograph, as well as an echocardiogram to evaluate the degree of cardiac involvement.

Management

The acute management of ARF should focus on stabilization and treatment of any of the symptomatic cardiac manifestations of the illness, such as CHF or tamponade due to a pericardial effusion. Treatment should also include appropriate antibiotic therapy to eradicate the streptococcal infection, bed rest, and antiinflammatory agents for arthritis. Steroids should be used in the treatment of carditis only under direction of a cardiologist. Monthly injections of benzathine penicillin G provide prophylaxis against recurrent attacks; alternative regimens include oral penicillin administered twice daily and, for penicillin-allergic patients, twice daily oral erythromycin. Prophylaxis is required until 18 years of age but can be continued for life, depending on the degree of cardiac involvement and risk of recurrence.[13]

Cardiac Causes of Sudden Death in Young Athletes

The most common cardiovascular cause of sudden death in the athlete is hypertrophic cardiomyopathy, accounting for up to 36% of the cardiovascular-related cases (Box 165.17). Brugada syndrome is uncommonly diagnosed in childhood.[13]

Specific Disorders

Congenital Coronary Artery Anomalies. Although there are a variety of congenital coronary artery anomalies, the most common potentially lethal lesion is the anomalous left coronary artery, in which the left main and right coronary arteries both arise from the right sinus of Valsalva. Individuals with this particular anomaly have a 46% incidence of sudden death, with more than 85% of the known cases of sudden death occurring during exercise. Congenital coronary artery hypoplasia is another uncommon cause of exercise-induced sudden death. Any athlete with exertional syncope or chest pain should be evaluated by a cardiologist for the possibility of a congenital coronary artery anomaly. If an anomaly is detected and surgically corrected, the athlete may resume full activity and participation in competitive sports.

Marfan Syndrome. Clinical manifestations of the disease include tall and slender habitus, striae atrophicae, disproportionately long extremities compared with the trunk, scoliosis, pectus excavatum or carinatum, and lens dislocation. Approximately 50% of patients with Marfan syndrome have cardiac manifestations, such as mitral valve prolapse or aortic dilation. The most serious cardiac complication of Marfan syndrome is the progressive dilation of the aorta with the potential risk of aortic rupture, which most commonly involves the descending portion of the aorta. Therefore, patients with Marfan syndrome should be prohibited from participation in contact sports. Those individuals who are known to have aortic dilation should also be prohibited from participation in any competitive sports regardless of the degree of contact involved. All patients with Marfan syndrome with or without cardiac involvement on their initial evaluation should be observed by a cardiologist with serial imaging studies of the aorta by echocardiography, magnetic resonance imaging, or computed tomography.

Hypertrophic Cardiomyopathy. Obstructive hypertrophic cardiomyopathy involves a thickened muscular intraventricular septum that bulges into the left ventricle and impedes forward flow, causing chest pain, shortness of breath, pre-syncope, or syncope. The nonobstructive form, which occurs when the thickened septum does not block forward flow, occurs in only 0.2% of the general population, yet it is the single most common cardiac cause of sudden death in the young athlete. Sudden death in previously asymptomatic individuals with hypertrophic cardiomyopathy occurs during moderate or severe physical exertion. The proposed pathophysiologic mechanism of sudden death during exertion in these individuals is thought to be a transient decrease of blood flow out through the aorta or dysrhythmia originating from the hypertrophied ventricular myocardium.

Clinical Features. Some individuals with hypertrophic cardio-myopathy have experienced previous "warning" episodes of chest pain, dyspnea, syncope, or palpitations during vigorous activities. A family history of sudden unexplained death in young adults should also alert the clinician to the possibility of hypertrophic cardiomyopathy. The majority of young athletes who die of this condition have the nonobstructive form of hypertrophic cardiomyopathy. The classic loud systolic ejection murmur that is present with the obstructive form may not be heard during the routine pre-sports physical examination.

If a systolic murmur along the lower left sternal border is heard on the routine screening physical examination of a young athlete, a Valsalva maneuver may help differentiate the murmur of aortic ste-nosis from the systolic murmur associated with the obstructive form of hypertrophic cardiomyopathy. During the Valsalva maneuver, the venous blood return to the heart is decreased, which in turn tran-siently reduces the left ventricular size. The transient reduction in the size of the left ventricle will increase the degree of obstruction and thus an increase in the intensity of the systolic murmur heard with the obstructive form of hypertrophic cardiomyopathy. In contrast to this, the systolic murmur of aortic stenosis will decrease in intensity during a Valsalva maneuver because of the transient reduction of blood flow through the stenotic aortic valve.

Current recommendations for pre-sports screening include a detailed family and personal history of known or suspected heart dis-ease, physical examination, and 12-lead ECG. If any suspicion remains, further evaluation (e.g., echocardiography, Holter monitoring, other imaging studies) and referral to a cardiologist are indicated.

Diagnostic Testing. The electrocardiographic findings in hyper-trophic cardiomyopathy show left ventricular hypertrophy and left atrial enlargement. Other findings include prominent Q waves in the inferolateral leads and diffuse T wave inversions. The most accurate study for the diagnosis of hypertrophic cardiomyopathy is the echocardiogram, which will demonstrate various degrees of left ventricular hypertrophy and involving the ventricular septum in up to 90% of the cases. Patients with echocardiographic evidence of hypertrophic cardiomyopathy should receive serial echocardiographic examinations to monitor progression.

Management. No pharmacologic therapy has been proven to prevent sudden death. Beta-blockers exert negative inotropic effects, attenuate adrenergic-induced tachycardia, improve myocardial oxygen supply-and-demand, and improve diastolic filling. The use of digoxin is contraindicated in patients with hypertrophic cardiomyopathy because its positive inotropic effect may worsen the left ventricular outflow obstruction. Sudden death in patients with hypertrophic cardiomyopathy is thought to be due to exertion-induced ventricular fibrillation or pulseless ventricular tachycardia. Therefore, all individuals diagnosed with hypertrophic cardiomyopathy, as well as those with an equivocal diagnosis of hypertrophic cardiomyopathy, should not participate in vigorous activities and competitive sports.

A transaortic septal myomectomy may be considered for patients with severe symptoms unresponsive to medical therapy. For subopti-mal surgical candidates, implantation of a dual-chamber pacemaker may improve symptoms by decreasing the left ventricular outflow tract gradient.

Long QT Syndrome. Both the Jervell–Lange-Nielsen (congenital deafness) and the Romano-Ward syndromes are inherited disorders characterized by a prolonged QT interval and associated with sudden death. The corrected QT (QTc) interval in normal individuals should not exceed 0.44 second in children or 0.42 second in adolescents. Individuals with QTc intervals longer than 0.55 second have a higher risk of sudden death. Prolongation of the QT interval predisposes the individual to ventricular tachycardia, torsades de pointes, and ventricular fibrillation, which is often initiated by a premature ventricular contraction occurring during the prolonged repolarization phase. In addition to the inherited syndromes of prolonged QT intervals, other causes of prolonged QT intervals include hypocalcemia, hypokalemia, hypomagnesemia, myocarditis, and medications (e.g., procainamide, erythromycin, cyclic antidepressants, phenothiazines, quinidine, and organophosphates).

Clinical Features. Symptoms in the young athlete that are suggestive of QT prolongation include exercise-induced palpitations, chest pain, syncope, dizziness, and atypical seizures. The young athlete who has any of these symptoms should be evaluated by a cardiologist, especially if the family history is positive for sudden unexplained death, cardiac problems, syncope, or deafness. Any young athlete who has been diagnosed with a prolonged QT syndrome should be prohibited from participation in competitive sports and vigorous activities. The growing popularity and presence of AEDs in public places and at sporting events can potentially save the lives of those athletes who suddenly collapse because of an underlying prolonged QT syndrome–induced nonperfusing ventricular dysrhythmia.

Management. Treatment of a prolonged QT interval depends on the cause. Underlying metabolic disorders should be corrected, and medications that induce prolongation of the QT interval should be discontinued. Magnesium sulfate is the drug of choice in the treatment of torsades de pointes. Lidocaine is the safest medication for patients with prolonged QT interval–induced ventricular tachycardia or fibrillation. Anti-dysrhythmic agents that can prolong the QT interval, such as procainamide and amiodarone, should be avoided. Beta-blockers have been used to prevent sudden ventricular dysrhythmias in those patients with the familial forms of QT prolongation. Adjunctive treatment in these selected patients also includes the insertion of pacemakers or internal defibrillators.

Commotio Cordis. Commotio cordis occurs after a high-impact trauma to the chest, as in a high-speed motor vehicle collision or a baseball to the sternum. The impact occurs during the vulnerable repolarization period of the cardiac cycle, mechanically inducing ventricular fibrillation. This phenomenon most commonly occurs in children between 5 and 15 years old with no known predisposing cardiac conditions. Although commotio cordis most commonly occurs in baseball, it has also been reported to occur in ice hockey, lacrosse, softball, and fist fights. The majority of patients who sustain commotio cordis do not survive unless rapidly treated with defibrillation. If an AED is not immediately available and the patient is completely unresponsive with no pulse after sustaining a direct blow to the chest, a chest thump during CPR should be attempted.

The author would like to thank Alson Inaba, M.D. for his work on previous editions of this chapter.

The references for this chapter can be found online at ExpertConsult.com.

166

Pediatric Gastrointestinal Disorders

Patrick J. Maloney

FOUNDATIONS

Gastrointestinal (GI) symptoms are common among pediatric patients presenting to the emergency department (ED). Because young children lack the knowledge, social skills, and vocabulary to describe and localize their symptoms, the signs and symptoms commonly attributed to the GI tract, such as abdominal pain, nausea, anorexia, and vomiting, are often nonspecific and ill-defined. As a result, their evaluation and management may be challenging.

Pediatric gastrointestinal disorders may be divided into different groups on the basis of their unique pathophysiologic mechanisms (Table 166.1). Several disorders occur as normal variants of early neonatal and infant development (e.g., neonatal jaundice, gastroesophageal reflux, hypertrophic pyloric stenosis). Others result from congenital malformations (e.g., malrotation, Meckel diverticulum) or genetic abnormalities (e.g., Hirschsprung disease). Idiopathic or poorly explained disorders include necrotizing enterocolitis (NEC), intussusception, Henoch-Schönlein purpura (HSP), and inflammatory bowel disease (IBD). The child's age can also help identify common causes of abdominal pain. Infants, for example, may have disorders such as NEC, hypertrophic pyloric stenosis, or intussusception, whereas older children are more likely to present with appendicitis, pancreatitis, or biliary tract disease.

SPECIFIC DISORDERS

Neonatal Jaundice

Foundations

Bilirubin is formed by the breakdown of heme-containing proteins, primarily hemoglobin. Unconjugated bilirubin binds to albumin and

TABLE 166.1 Differential Considerations for Abdominal Pain by Age

Classification By Cause	Infancy	Childhood	Adolescence
Mechanical	Malrotation with midgut volvulus Intussusception Incarcerated hernia Meckel diverticulum Hirschsprung disease	Constipation Incarcerated hernia Meckel diverticulum Bowel obstruction	Constipation Incarcerated hernia Meckel diverticulum Bowel obstruction
Inflammatory or infectious	Necrotizing enterocolitis	Gastroenteritis Appendicitis Henoch-Schönlein purpura Pancreatitis Gastritis Biliary tract disease	Gastroenteritis Appendicitis Henoch-Schönlein purpura Pancreatitis Gastritis Biliary tract disease
Genitourinary	Urinary tract infection	Urinary tract infection	Urinary tract infection Nephroureterolithiasis Pregnancy, ectopic Pelvic inflammatory disease Testicular or ovarian torsion
Other or atypical	Colic Occult trauma (abuse) Toxic ingestions Munchausen syndrome by proxy	Pneumonia Diabetic ketoacidosis Sickle cell Toxic ingestions Occult trauma (abuse) Munchausen syndrome by proxy	Pneumonia Diabetic ketoacidosis Sickle cell Toxic ingestions Occult trauma (abuse) Munchausen syndrome or Munchausen syndrome by proxy

TABLE 166.2 Differential Considerations for Hyperbilirubinemia in Infants

Classification by Cause	Unconjugated (Indirect)	Conjugated (Direct)
Benign, physiologic	Physiologic jaundice of the newborn Breast milk jaundice	
Hemolysis	ABO incompatibility Physiologic breakdown of birth trauma hematoma (cephalhematoma) Intracranial/intraventricular hemorrhage Spherocytosis, elliptocytosis Sickle cell anemia Thalassemia Glucose-6-phosphate dehydrogenase deficiency Pyruvate kinase deficiency	
Infectious	TORCHS infections Urinary tract infection Sepsis	TORCHS infections Urinary tract infection Gram-negative sepsis Listeriosis Tuberculosis Hepatitis B Varicella Coxsackievirus infection Echovirus infection HIV infection
Obstructive	Meconium ileus Hirschsprung disease Duodenal atresia Pyloric stenosis	Biliary atresia Choledochal cyst Bile duct strictures Inspissated bile syndrome Neonatal hepatitis Alagille syndrome Byler disease Congenital hepatic fibrosis
Metabolic or genetic	Galactosemia Congenital hypothyroidism Crigler-Najjar syndrome Gilbert syndrome	Galactosemia Tyrosinemia Glycogen storage disease type IV Niemann-Pick disease Wolman disease Gaucher disease Cholesterol ester storage disease α_1-Antitrypsin deficiency Cystic fibrosis Dubin-Johnson syndrome Neonatal hypopituitarism Zellweger syndrome Donohue syndrome (leprechaunism) Rotor syndrome
Miscellaneous		Drugs and toxins Parenteral nutrition

CMV, Cytomegalovirus; *HIV*, human immunodeficiency virus; *TORCHS*, toxoplasmosis, other infections, rubella, CMV, herpes, syphilis.

is carried to the liver, where it is conjugated by glucuronyl transferase and excreted into bile. While jaundice in adults is usually a conjugated hyperbilirubinemia, resulting from primary hepatobiliary disease, neonatal jaundice is usually the result of extrahepatic causes and results in an unconjugated hyperbilirubinemia (Table 166.2). There are typically three physiologic factors that contribute to neonatal jaundice: (1) increased bilirubin production, (2) decreased clearance and excretion, and (3) increased enterohepatic resorption. Conjugated hyperbilirubinemia in neonates, on the other hand, is less common and always pathologic.

Nearly every newborn develops an unconjugated serum bilirubin level greater than 1 mg/dL— the normal upper limit in adults—during the first week of life. Jaundice, the yellow discoloration of the skin and sclera, becomes clinically noticeable when the total bilirubin level rises above about 5 mg/dL. Risk factors for the development of severe hyperbilirubinemia in the neonate include prematurity, isoimmune-mediated hemolysis (ABO incompatibility), sepsis, cephalohematomas, dehydration, and inherited abnormalities, such as hereditary spherocytosis and glucose-6-phosphate dehydrogenase (G6PD) deficiency.

Unconjugated bilirubin crosses the blood-brain barrier, where it causes cell death. At levels greater than approximately 20 to 25 mg/dL, there is an increased risk of bilirubin-induced neurologic dysfunction (BIND). Kernicterus refers to the chronic, irreversible, long-term neurologic sequelae of BIND.

Jaundice during the newborn period is usually the result of an immature metabolism of bilirubin. This benign self-limited jaundice is termed *physiologic jaundice of the newborn*, occurring in approximately 50% of normal newborns. Although it varies based on ethnicity, total bilirubin levels typically peak between two and five days of life, and the yellow discoloration of the skin usually resolves by the first two weeks of life.

Breast milk jaundice is the second most common cause of neonatal jaundice. The exact pathophysiology is uncertain, but it may be hormonally mediated or related to increased enterohepatic resorption of bilirubin. Breast milk jaundice is typically characterized by a mild unconjugated hyperbilirubinemia that peaks a bit later than physiologic jaundice and may persist for several weeks to months. Other causes of jaundice vary significantly (see Table 166.2)

Clinical Features

Healthy infants are born with normal bilirubin levels that gradually increase to a peak level of 6 mg/dL on approximately the third day of life and then decline to normal levels within 2 weeks. Infants with hyperbilirubinemia usually begin life with similarly low bilirubin levels but exhibit a faster rise in bilirubin levels over the first few days of life. Physiologic jaundice is rarely present on the first day of life, meaning that a total bilirubin level greater than 5 mg/dL within the first 24 hours of life is almost always pathologic. Children with breast milk jaundice typically demonstrate the same gradual increase seen with physiologic jaundice, but levels continue to increase and peak at around 10 to 21 days of life. Elevated levels may persist for 3 to 10 weeks before gradually declining.

Toxic levels of bilirubin (dependent on age, but in general >20 mg/dL) may be associated with neurotoxicity and encephalopathy, termed *bilirubin-induced neurologic dysfunction* (BIND), and the development of kernicterus. Symptoms of BIND include poor feeding and lethargy, sometimes progressing to muscle rigidity, opisthotonos, seizures, and death. Other potential clinical manifestations are cerebral palsy, sensorineural hearing loss, and gaze abnormalities (usually upward gaze limitations).

Acute bilirubin encephalopathy (ABE) refers to the early and potentially reversible signs and symptoms of the hyperbilirubinemia, including somnolence, poor feeding, hypertonia or hypotonia, and a high-pitched cry. If untreated, symptoms can progress to lethargy, hypertonia, backward arching of the neck and trunk (retrocollis and opisthotonos, respectively), fever, irritability, and apnea. Ultimately, this can lead to seizures and death. Survivors may have chronic, permanent coordination problems, cerebral palsy, hearing loss, and learning disabilities. If treated, some or all of these symptoms may be reversible. Ultimately, the management of neonatal jaundice aims to prevent the development of BIND and kernicterus.

Differential Diagnoses

Once the diagnosis of neonatal jaundice is established based on physical exam and laboratory confirmation of an elevated unconjugated bilirubin level, focus should be directed to identifying and managing the

---

BOX 166.1   Indications for Evaluation of Jaundiced Infants

Jaundice appearing within 24 hr of birth
Elevated direct (conjugated) bilirubin level
Rapidly rising total serum bilirubin unexplained by history or physical examination
Total serum bilirubin approaching exchange level or not responding to phototherapy
Jaundice persisting beyond 3 weeks of age
Sick-appearing infant

---

physiologic factors contributing to the derangement. The birth history may reveal prematurity or a history of birth trauma–related cephalohematomas. Review of the maternal and infant perinatal records may identify maternal-child blood type (ABO) incompatibility or other risk factors for isoimmune-mediated hemolysis. A detailed history of feeding patterns, urine output, and stool appearance may identify poor nutritional intake, poor weight gain, and dehydration. The presence of hyper- or hypothermia may suggest the presence of infection/sepsis. The family history may identify siblings or other relatives with a history of jaundice or genetic or metabolic disorders. Table 166.2 presents additional differential considerations for jaundiced infants.

Diagnostic Testing

Physiologic and breast milk jaundice are the most common causes of neonatal jaundice; pathologic causes and indications for evaluation of hyperbilirubinemia are listed in Box 166.1. Transcutaneous bilirubin meters can be used to quickly measure bilirubin levels through the skin in otherwise well-appearing neonates who are beyond 24 hours, but within 7 days, of life. Infants who have previously undergone phototherapy, those with known risk factors for hemolysis, and those with high transcutaneous levels (based on the meter manufacturer's recommended product range) should also have serum levels sent.[1] Initial serum testing can also determine fractionated levels of total versus direct (conjugated) bilirubin.

We recommend that further laboratory evaluation include a complete blood count (CBC) with a peripheral smear and Coombs test to determine immune-mediated major blood group incompatibility, if not previously known. Diagnostic testing in ill-appearing infants includes finger stick blood glucose measurement, electrolyte panel, urine assay for reducing substances, serum ammonia levels, ketones, lactate and evaluation for infection. Conjugated hyperbilirubinemia is always pathologic, resulting from biliary atresia, other biliary obstructive pathology, severe infections, toxins, or inborn errors of metabolism.

Management

The treatment of infants with unconjugated hyperbilirubinemia centers on the prevention of kernicterus. Because oral intake stimulates enterohepatic circulation and decreases bilirubin levels, feeding (including breast-feeding) should be encouraged. Phototherapy is the initial intervention used to reduce the total bilirubin level in affected infants. Guidelines for the use of phototherapy, based on age, risk factors for developing BIND, and bilirubin level, have been established and recommended by the American Academy of Pediatrics (AAP) (Fig. 166.1). BiliTool (www.bilitool.org) is an additional online resource that utilizes the same AAP guidelines to help clinicians assess the risk of developing hyperbilirubinemia in late preterm and full term infants.

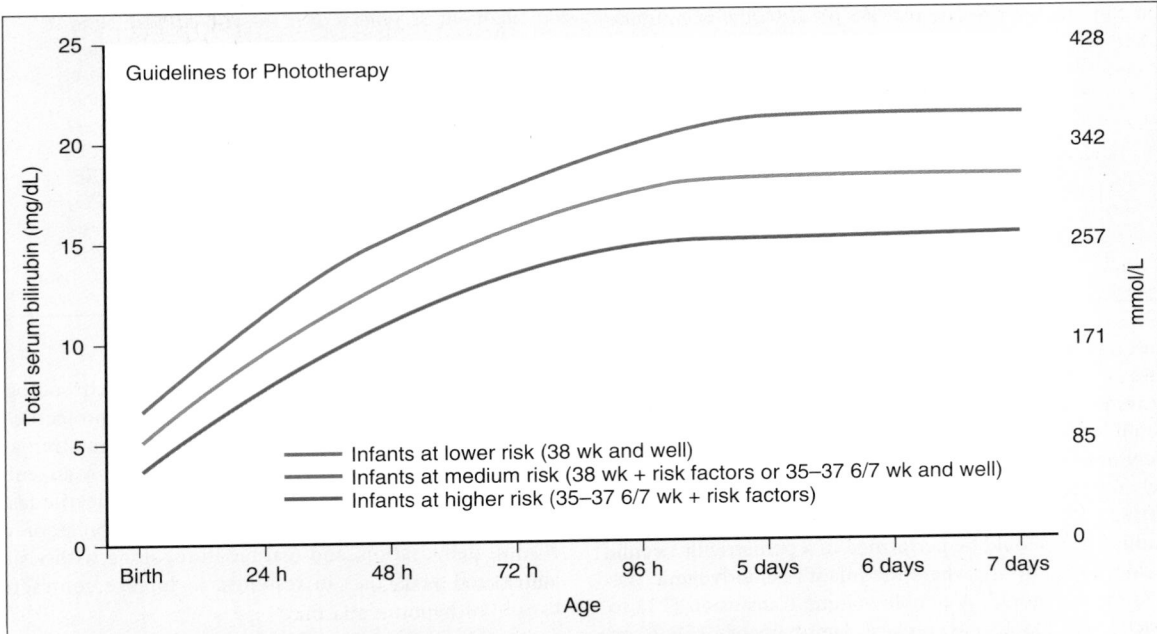

- Use total bilirubin. Do not subtract direct reacting or conjugated bilirubin.
- Risk factors = isoimmune hemolytic disease, G6PD deficiency, asphyxia, significant lethargy, temperature instability, sepsis, acidosis, or albumin <3.0 g/dL (if measured).
- For well infants 35–37 6/7 wk, can adjust TSB levels for intervention around the medium risk line. It is an option to intervene at lower TSB levels for infants closer to 35 wk and at higher TSB levels for those closer to 37 6/7 wk.
- It is an option to provide conventional phototherapy in hospital or at home at TSB levels 2–3 mg/dL (35–50 mmol/L) below those shown, but home phototherapy should not be used in any infant with risk factors.

A

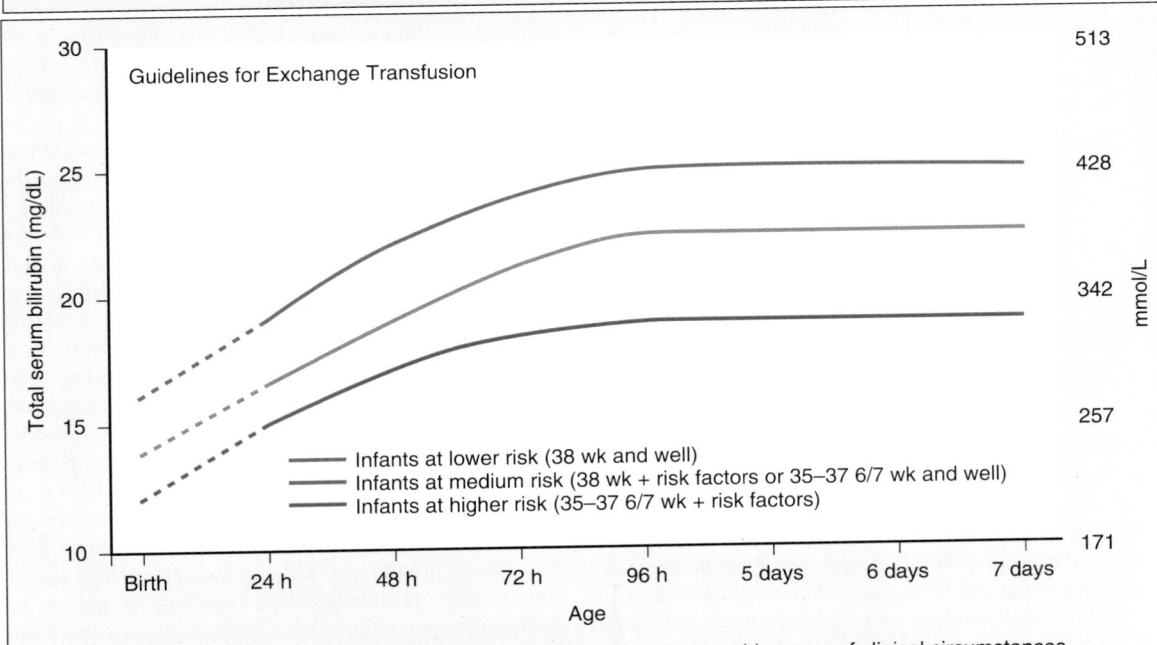

- The dashed lines for the first 24 hours indicate uncertainty due to a wide range of clinical circumstances and a range of responses to phototherapy.
- Immediate exchange transfusion is recommended if infant shows signs of acute bilirubin encephalopathy (hypertonia, arching, retrocollis, opisthotonos, fever, high-pitched cry) or if TSB is 5 mg/dL (85 mmol/L) above these lines.
- Risk factors = isoimmune hemolytic disease, G6PD deficiency, asphyxia, significant lethargy, temperature instability, sepsis, acidosis.
- Measure serum albumin and calculate B/A ratio (see legend).
- Use total bilirubin. Do not subtract direct reacting or conjugated bilirubin.
- If infant is well and 35–37 6/7 wk (median risk), can individualize TSB levels for exchange based on actual gestational age.

B

Fig. 166.1 (A) Guidelines for phototherapy in hospitalized infants at 35 weeks or more of gestation. Note that these guidelines are based on limited evidence. The guidelines refer to intensive phototherapy, which should be used when the total serum bilirubin (TSB) exceeds the line indicated for each category. Infants are designated higher risk because of the potential negative effects of the conditions listed on albumin binding of bilirubin, the blood-brain barrier, and the susceptibility of the brain cells to damage by bilirubin. (B) Guidelines for exchange transfusion in infants at 35 weeks or more of gestation. Note that these suggested levels represent a consensus but are based on limited evidence. Exchange transfusion is recommended if the TSB continues to rise or remains above these levels, despite intensive phototherapy. *B/A*, Bilirubin/albumin; *G6PD*, glucose-6-phosphate dehydrogenase. (From: American Academy of Pediatrics Subcommittee on Hyperbilirubinemia. Management of hyperbilirubinemia in the newborn infant 35 or more weeks of gestation. *Pediatrics.* 2004;114:297-316.)

Infants with severely elevated bilirubin levels are at greatest risk for developing BIND. Exchange transfusions are the most effective and rapid way to remove bilirubin. Indications for exchange transfusion include bilirubin level above age-specific threshold recommended by the AAP guidelines (see Fig. 166.1), failure of phototherapy (i.e., the bilirubin level continues to rise despite intensive phototherapy), and jaundiced infants with signs and symptoms of BIND. The procedure is time-consuming and should be performed in a pediatric or neonatal intensive care unit (NICU), where the infant's hemodynamic status may be closely monitored. A double-volume transfusion (180 to 190 mL/kg packed red blood cells) replaces approximately 85% of an infant's blood volume and reduces the total bilirubin level by at least 50%. It is performed by serially removing small aliquots of the infant's blood, typically no more than 5 to 10 mL/kg and replacing it with a similar volume of packed red blood cells until the total transfusion volume is achieved.

Disposition

Infants with bilirubin levels greater than established age- and risk factor-specific levels should receive phototherapy (Fig 166.1A). Infants who appear ill, are below their expected weight for day of life, cannot maintain oral intake, or require exchange transfusion (Fig 166.1B) should undergo hospital admission for phototherapy, IV hydration, and on-going evaluation. Home phototherapy is an option for infants who are otherwise well-appearing, have reliable caregivers with access to emergency care, and can receive follow-up within 24 hours.[2] All infants with direct hyperbilirubinemia should be admitted to the hospital for evaluation of the cause, treatment of sepsis or other treatable cause, and consultation with subspecialist (e.g., pediatric gastroenterology) as indicated.

Hypertrophic Pyloric Stenosis

Foundations

Hypertrophic pyloric stenosis is the most common cause of infantile GI obstruction beyond the first month of life. This condition occurs in 1 of every 250 live births, although rates and trends vary significantly by region. Boys are affected at four times the rate of girls. Approximately one-third of cases occur in first-born children. Prematurity and infant exposure to macrolide antibiotics are additional risk factors.[3] Hypertrophic pyloric stenosis tends to have familial patterns, but the exact pattern of inheritance is unclear.

Affected infants are born with a normal sized pylorus that enlarges as time progresses. The exact cause is unknown, although hypertrophy seems to be stimulated by feeding. As the pylorus enlarges, a progressive gastric outlet obstruction develops, and vomiting ensues. Vomiting causes loss of fluid and gastric acid (hydrogen and chloride ions). As dehydration and electrolyte derangements worsen, the kidney attempts to retain hydrogen ions in exchange for potassium, resulting in the classic hypochloremic-hypokalemic metabolic alkalosis.

Clinical Features

Infants classically present at 2 to 6 weeks of chronologic age, with gradually progressive vomiting that becomes projectile but remains nonbilious. Early in the disease process, infants remain vigorous, with a ravenous appetite. They rapidly finish an entire feeding, only to regurgitate the entire volume in a projectile fashion. In the later stages of the disease, infants may exhibit poor weight gain, clinical dehydration, and malnutrition, along with visible waves of abdominal peristalsis in response to intense contractions against the obstruction.

Diagnostic Testing

Infants may have a palpable pylorus in the right epigastrium on abdominal examination, commonly referred to as an "olive." Because access to ultrasound is now readily available in the developed world, pyloric stenosis is generally diagnosed earlier compared to decades ago, and the "olive" is now palpated in only a minority of infants who present later in the disease course. Laboratory derangements reflect a state of dehydration and electrolyte loss through vomiting—a hypochloremic metabolic alkalosis (serum bicarbonate [HCO_3] levels $\geq$29 mmol/dL and chloride levels $\leq$98 mmol/dL), although these abnormalities may be absent early in the disease course.

Hypertrophic pyloric stenosis may be confirmed by ultrasonography or fluoroscopic upper GI series (UGI). Ultrasonography is often the first diagnostic modality of choice because it is simple, readily available, and without serious complications such as aspiration. Upper GI series may be preferred when there is bilious vomiting and concern for more distal bowel obstruction. With both modalities, reported accuracy is greater than 95%. On ultrasound, the pylorus appears thickened (pyloric muscle thickness > 4 mm; pyloric diameter > 14 mm) and elongated (>19 mm), which is diagnostic (Fig. 166.2). On UGI series, a characteristic string sign, reflecting passage of contrast material through the narrowed pyloric sphincter, may also be evident. In advanced stages with complete obstruction at the pylorus, plain films may reveal a distended, air-filled stomach.

Differential Diagnoses. Vomiting in infants is common, and the differential diagnosis is broad. Usually, infants present early in the disease progression and are well-appearing, and the common consideration is differentiating hypertrophic pyloric stenosis from gastroesophageal reflux. Reflux classically begins shortly after birth and remains relatively constant. Infants with pyloric stenosis typically have progressively worsening emesis beginning around 2 or 3 weeks of life. In advanced stages, it occurs with every feed and is often described as projectile.

Infants who present with sudden onset of severe vomiting and bilious emesis, or who are ill-appearing, should be evaluated for other surgical emergencies, including malrotation with midgut volvulus, duodenal atresia, and necrotizing enterocolitis. With reflux and pyloric stenosis, emesis is rarely bilious.

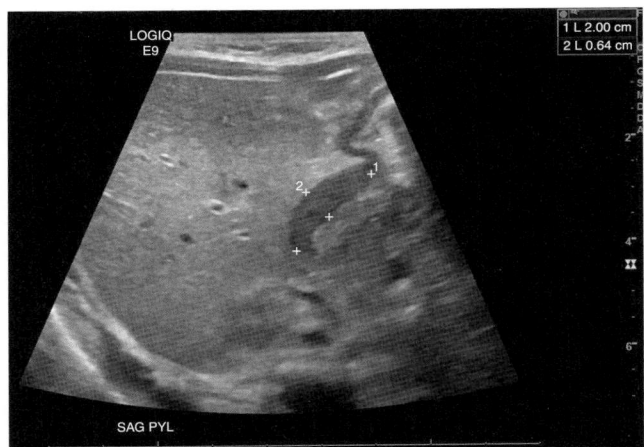

Fig. 166.2 Ultrasound of the abdomen revealing an elongated (20 mm) and thickened (6 mm) pylorus muscle consistent with hypertrophic pyloric stenosis. Normal pylorus muscle measurements are: pyloric muscle thickness < 4 mm; pyloric diameter <14 mm; pylorus length <19 mm. (Courtesy Dr. Patrick J. Maloney)

Many causes of vomiting do not have a true GI origin, including sepsis, metabolic disturbances (e.g., diabetic ketoacidosis), increased intracranial pressure, urinary tract infections, inborn errors of metabolism, adverse medication reactions or side effects, and drug intoxications. Differential considerations for vomiting in children vary by age (Table 166.3).

Management

Treatment consists of fluid and electrolyte replacement and surgical consultation. Hypertrophic pyloric stenosis is not a true surgical emergency but may be a fluid and electrolyte emergency. Fluid resuscitation should begin with repeated boluses of 20 mL/kg of normal saline as necessary to treat dehydration and hypovolemic shock.[4] Potassium supplementation (KCl, 0.5 to 1 mEq/kg IV over 1 to 2 hours) is often necessary. Definitive management is surgery. The corrective procedure, called a pyloromyotomy, may be performed open, referred to as the Ramstedt pyloromyotomy, or laparoscopically. Associated mortality is rare.

Disposition

Most children are best managed with hospital admission for rehydration and correction of electrolyte abnormalities in conjunction with urgent imaging and surgical consultation.

TABLE 166.3 Differential Considerations for Vomiting by Age

Classification by Cause	Infancy	Childhood	Adolescence
Mechanical	Gastroesophageal reflux Malrotation with midgut volvulus Pyloric stenosis Meckel diverticulum Intussusception Bowel obstruction Incarcerated hernia Tracheoesophageal fistula	Constipation Incarcerated hernia Meckel diverticulum Bowel obstruction	Constipation Incarcerated hernia
Inflammatory or infectious	Necrotizing enterocolitis Gastroenteritis Sepsis Henoch-Schönlein purpura Meningitis Pneumonia Otitis media	Gastritis or gastroenteritis Otitis media Appendicitis Pancreatitis Henoch-Schönlein purpura Biliary tract disease	Gastroenteritis Appendicitis Pancreatitis Gastritis Biliary tract disease
Genitourinary	Urinary tract infection	Urinary tract infection	Urinary tract infection Pregnancy Testicular or ovarian torsion
Central nervous system	Hydrocephalus Intracranial hemorrhage Intracranial tumor	Migraine headache Hydrocephalus Intracranial hemorrhage Intracranial tumor Reye syndrome	Migraine headache Hydrocephalus Intracranial hemorrhage Intracranial tumor Glaucoma
Metabolic	Diabetic ketoacidosis Congenital adrenal hyperplasia Urea cycle defects Organic acidurias Amino acidopathies Fatty acid oxidation disorders	Diabetic ketoacidosis Urea cycle defects Fatty acid oxidation disorders	Diabetic ketoacidosis
Other or atypical	Occult trauma (abuse) Toxic ingestions Munchausen syndrome by proxy	Sickle cell Toxic ingestions Occult trauma (abuse) Munchausen syndrome by proxy	Sickle cell Toxic ingestions Occult trauma (abuse) Munchausen syndrome or Munchausen syndrome by proxy

Malrotation with Midgut Volvulus

Foundations

Malrotation of the intestines occurs in 1 in 500 live births and has a male predominance of at least 2 : 1. Among infants with malrotation, symptomatic volvulus of the midgut occurs in the first month of life in approximately one-third, in the first year of life in approximately one-half, and before the age of 5 years in 75% of children. Rarely, patients born with intestinal malrotation develop midgut volvulus later in life as adults. Some remain asymptomatic. When midgut volvulus does occur, the mortality rate may be as high as 10% with surgical intervention.

During embryologic development, the GI tract rotates around the superior mesenteric artery. As it completes the rotation, the duodenum forms a C-loop and is fixed to the retroperitoneum in the left upper quadrant at the ligament of Treitz. The cecum becomes similarly fixed in the right lower quadrant. Thus, the duodenum and cecum normally come to lie widely separated and are firmly fixed in position by peritoneal attachments called Ladd bands. They are only loosely connected by a broad-based mesentery. In cases of malrotation, the duodenum and cecum do not rotate completely, remain closely positioned, and are suspended in the midgut region by the mesenteric vascular stalk. This unusually close proximity results in a short stalk of mesentery that easily twists on itself, resulting in obstruction of the distal duodenum and bowel ischemia and necrosis secondary to compression of the superior mesenteric artery.

Clinical Features

The hallmark presentation of acute midgut volvulus associated with intestinal malrotation is sudden-onset bilious emesis and abdominal distention in an infant. Affected infants usually appear quite ill and may present in shock. Any yellow or green pigmented staining of the vomitus suggests the presence of bile. When bile is initially produced, it is bright yellow and turns green only with time and oxidative exposure. Therefore, differential coloring of bile-stained emesis, yellow versus green, is not predictive of a surgical condition.

Diagnostic Testing

Plain radiographs may demonstrate nonspecific signs of a small bowel obstruction, including dilated loops of proximal small bowel with air-fluid levels and a paucity of bowel gas distally (Fig. 166.3). The diagnostic procedure of choice to identify midgut volvulus is a limited upper GI contrast series, revealing an abnormal position of the duodenal

C-loop, which fails to normally cross the midline from right to left (Fig. 166.4), and a characteristic corkscrew appearance of the more distal small bowel (Fig. 166.5).

Ultrasonography, usually performed to evaluate for hypertrophic pyloric stenosis, may reveal an abnormal orientation of the superior mesenteric artery and vein (the vein is abnormally positioned anteriorly or to the left of the artery (Fig. 166.6) or a whirlpool sign caused by the vessels twisting around the mesenteric stalk, causing an echogenic twisting pattern.[5] CT is usually not recommended because it carries the risk of additional radiation without benefit of improved diagnostic ability over upper GI series.

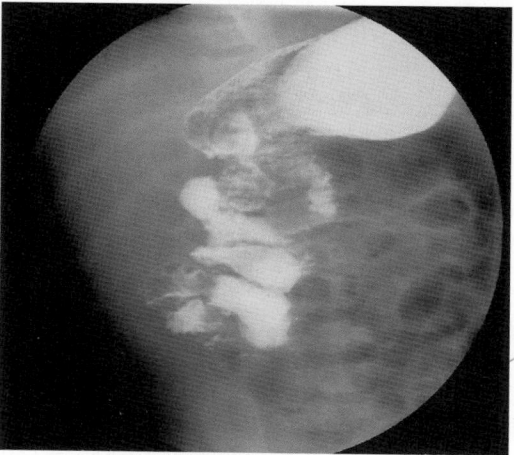

Fig. 166.4 Upper gastrointestinal film, obtained in the same infant as in Fig. 166.3, reveals abnormal positioning of the duodenal C-loop to the right of the spinal column, consistent with malrotation. (Courtesy Dr. Mark A. Hostetler.)

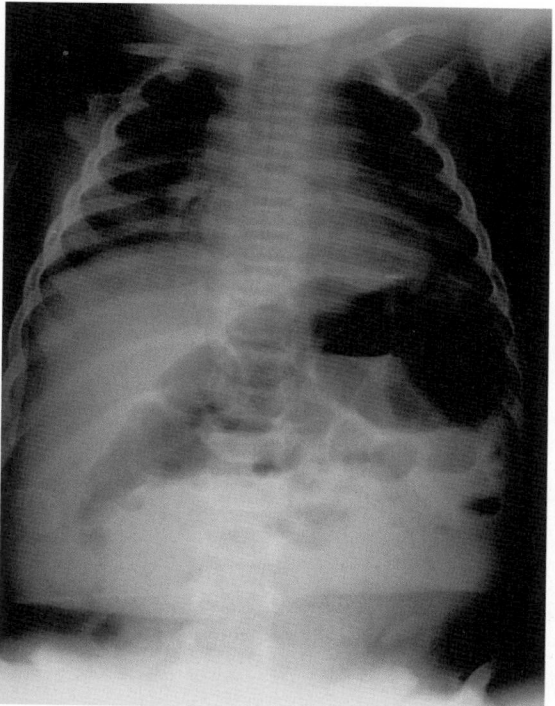

Fig. 166.5 Spot film from the upper gastrointestinal series obtained in the infant in Fig. 166.3. This radiograph shows the characteristic corkscrew appearance seen on small bowel follow-through in patients with malrotation. (Courtesy Dr. Mark A. Hostetler)

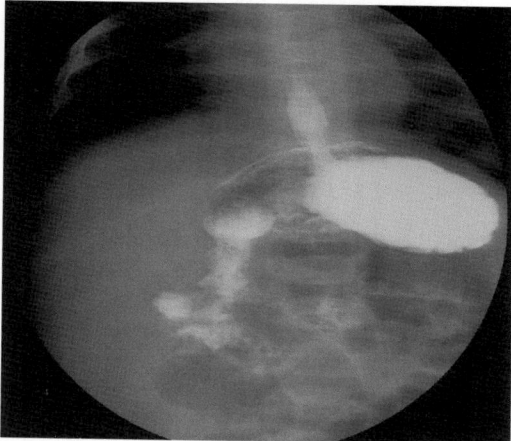

Fig. 166.3 Upright abdominal radiograph obtained in an infant with bilious vomiting illustrates dilated loops of small bowel and a paucity of bowel gas distally, consistent with proximal obstruction secondary to malrotation with midgut volvulus. (Courtesy Dr. Mark A. Hostetler.)

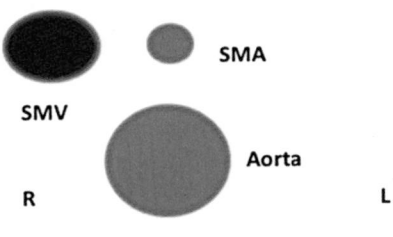

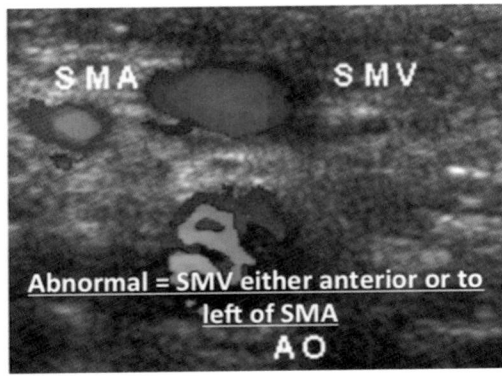

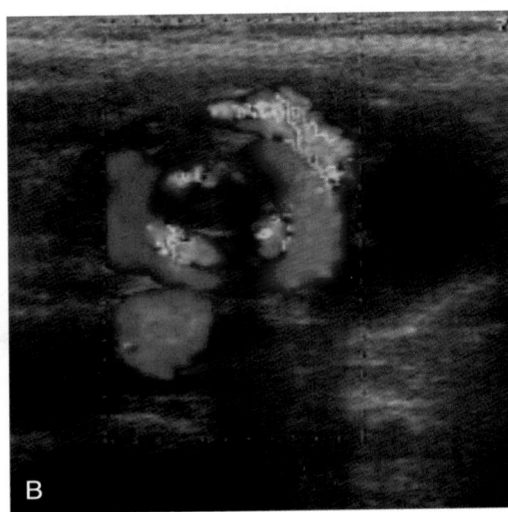

Fig. 166.6 Ultrasonographic findings in malrotation with midgut volvulus. (A) Abnormal orientation of mesenteric vessels associated with malrotation with midgut volvulus. Normally, the superior mesenteric vein (SMV) is positioned to the right of the superior mesenteric artery (SMA). In malrotation, the vein is abnormally positioned anteriorly or to the left of the artery. (B) Whirlpool sign caused by the vessels twisting around the mesenteric stalk, resulting in an echogenic twisting pattern. *AO,* Aorta. (Courtesy Dr. Patrick J. Maloney.)

Differential Diagnoses

Vomiting in childhood, especially infants, is common and occurs across a wide spectrum of illnesses (see Table 166.3). Causes vary by age, progression of symptoms, and vomitus appearance. In children less than one year old, sudden onset of bilious vomiting is an ominous sign and should prompt emergent evaluation for acute bowel obstruction, including malrotation with midgut volvulus. Gastroesophageal reflux disease (GERD) and hypertrophic pyloric stenosis typically cause nonbilious emesis in relatively well-appearing infants. NEC may also present with obstructive signs and symptoms, including bilious emesis and abdominal distention. However, unlike malrotation with volvulus, NEC is characterized radiographically by diffusely dilated loops of small bowel and the presence of air within the bowel walls, termed *pneumatosis intestinalis.*

Management

Emergent pediatric surgical consultation should be obtained for any neonate or infant with bilious vomiting, even before diagnostic studies have been completed. In acute midgut volvulus, operative intervention should be rapid to save the bowel from necrosis.

Intravenous (IV) access should be obtained, and laboratory studies should include blood glucose level, a CBC with differential, electrolyte values, and renal and liver function tests. If there are clinical signs of shock, repeated fluid boluses of 20 mL/kg of normal saline or lactated Ringers solution should be given until adequate circulation has been established.

BOX 166.2 Empirical Antibiotic Regimens for Enteric Bacterial Pathogens

Regimen
- Piperacillin-tazobactam + gentamicin
- Piperacillin-tazobactam + gentamicin + vancomycin
- Ampicillin + gentamicin + metronidazole
- Ampicillin + ceftriaxone + metronidazole
- Meropenem

Dosing
- Piperacillin-tazobactam: 200–300 mg/kg/day of piperacillin component q6–8 hours
- Gentamicin: 3–7.5 mg/kg/day in divided doses based on age/renal function
- Ampicillin: 200 mg/kg/day q6h
- Vancomycin: 10–20 mg/kg IV q6–8h
- Metronidazole: 30–40 mg/kg/day q8h
- Ceftriaxone: 50 mg/kg/day once daily
- Meropenem: 60 mg/kg/day q8h

Ill-appearing infants should receive empirical broad-spectrum antibiotic coverage for enteric bacterial pathogens (Box 166.2). A nasogastric or orogastric tube should be placed to decompress the proximal bowel and stomach. A limited upper GI series should also be emergently obtained but should not delay resuscitation and surgical consultation.

Disposition

Patients with a confirmed or equivocal diagnosis should be admitted with emergent surgical consultation.

Necrotizing Enterocolitis
Foundations

Necrotizing enterocolitis (NEC) is the most common gastrointestinal emergency in neonates. However, because most affected infants are premature and acquire the condition in the NICU, NEC usually is not usually encountered in the ED setting. NEC does occur in a small subset of late preterm and full-term infants, although most of them have other underlying illnesses and rarely are discharged from the NICU prior to the onset of disease. Complications in children who survive NEC, which are often encountered in the ED, include strictures, fistulas, and short gut syndrome.

The exact pathophysiologic mechanism of NEC is unclear but is likely multifactorial. The primary pathophysiologic event is inflammation or injury to the intestinal wall. Prematurity is the most common and universally accepted risk factor, as 90% of all affected infants are born prematurely.

Clinical Features

Infants with NEC usually first develop feeding intolerance and bilious or nonbilious emesis. In the more advanced stages of the disease, infants may appear extremely ill with hematemesis, hematochezia, fever, and shock. Abdominal radiographs may show intestinal dilation, pneumatosis intestinalis, or intestinal perforation.

Differential Diagnoses

Feeding intolerance and vomiting are common and nonspecific findings in neonates. However, unlike most infants with GERD, pyloric stenosis, and other relatively benign or self-limited causes of vomiting, infants with NEC are usually quite ill-appearing. GERD classically begins shortly after birth and remains relatively constant in character. Pyloric stenosis–related vomiting does not begin until 2 to 3 weeks of age and then gradually increases in severity and forcefulness, but these infants rarely appear acutely toxic. Bilious vomiting, while common in NEC, requires careful consideration to rule out other obstructive pathology, including malrotation with midgut volvulus, especially in children born at or near full term. The appearance of the plain radiographs may help differentiate NEC and volvulus. Volvulus is associated with dilated, air-fluid loops of small bowel proximally and a paucity of bowel gas distally, whereas the hallmark of NEC is diffusely dilated loops of small bowel and pneumatosis intestinalis.

Diagnostic Testing

Plain abdominal radiographs are the imaging study of choice in NEC. Radiographs may show nonspecific signs reflecting the presence of small bowel obstruction (dilated, air-fluid filled loops of bowel), bowel ischemia (intramural bowel wall gas, called pneumatosis intestinalis, or air within the portal system and biliary tract), or bowel perforation (pneumoperitoneum). Pneumatosis intestinalis (Fig. 166.7) is pathognomonic for NEC and is present in 75% of patients. No individual laboratory test is diagnostic or specific for NEC, but may reflect dehydration, electrolyte derangements, and sepsis.

Management

Patients suspicious of having NEC should receive nothing by mouth (NPO), with placement of an orogastric or nasogastric tube for

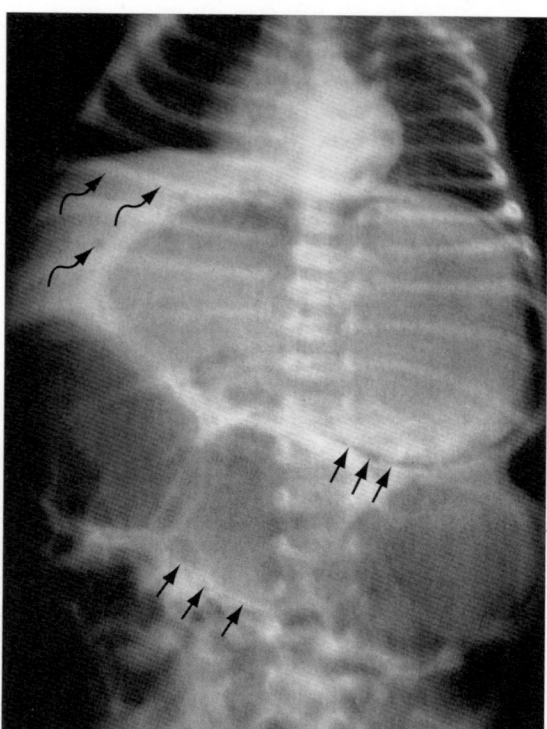

Fig. 166.7 Plain radiograph obtained in an infant with necrotizing enterocolitis. *Straight arrows* indicate air within the wall of the small bowel and gastric mucosa (pneumatosis intestinalis and gastralis). *Curved arrows* indicate air in the biliary tree (portal venous gas). (Courtesy Dr. Mark A. Hostetler.)

decompression of the stomach and small bowel. Because these patients are frequently hemodynamically unstable and may have periods of apnea or significant respiratory distress, intubation may be needed. IV or intraosseous access should be established; laboratory studies should include a CBC with differential, electrolyte panel, glucose, renal and liver function tests, and type and screen. Blood and urine cultures should be obtained. Fluid resuscitation with 20 mL/kg boluses of normal saline or lactated Ringers solution should be repeated until adequate circulatory volume has been reestablished. Vasoactive agents such as epinephrine, or norepinephrine are indicated for patients in refractory shock. Broad-spectrum antibiotic coverage is indicated (see Box 166.2). Emergent pediatric surgery consultation should be obtained in all cases because perforation and bowel necrosis may not be immediately evident on plain radiographs. Mortality is very high (30% to 50%) despite appropriate management.

Disposition

Children thought to have NEC require admission to an ICU and should have emergent pediatric surgical consultation.

Gastroesophageal Reflux
Foundations

Gastroesophageal reflux (GERD) refers to the symptomatic regurgitation of stomach contents into the esophagus, with or without vomiting. Reflux occurs as a result of an incompetent lower esophageal sphincter. Reflux is a normal physiologic event in infants, and essentially all infants experience intermittent reflux during at least the first six months of life. When reflux causes troublesome symptoms or complications, it is referred to as GERD. Chronic reflux of gastric contents into the esophagus may result in esophagitis, chronic cough, aspiration, and failure to thrive if severe.

Clinical Features

Reflux and GERD generally begin shortly after birth and resolve with time, usually by the age of one year. Clinical manifestations occur along a wide spectrum of disease, ranging from asymptomatic to occasional episodes of spitting up to severe persistent vomiting and failure to thrive. Sandifer syndrome, although rare, refers to the stereotypical opisthotonic movements highly suggestive of severe GERD. Chronic GERD may cause chronic cough, recurrent stridor, and persistent wheezing. GERD may even be implicated in infants who experience "brief resolved unexplained events" that include symptoms of respiratory distress or apnea, transient color change (i.e., pallor, cyanosis), and possibly a change in muscle tone (flaccidity or rigidity), although evidence of this direct causation is lacking.[6]

Differential Diagnoses

Children with GERD exhibit nonbilious emesis that begins shortly after birth and is relatively constant over time. Unlike pyloric stenosis, vomiting is usually neither progressive nor projectile. Most children with GERD of milder severity continue to gain weight. Unlike midgut volvulus and other causes of small bowel obstruction, the emesis associated with GERD should never have a yellowish-green or darker pigmented appearance. In addition, the presence of hematemesis or hematochezia or significant abdominal tenderness or distension should prompt considerations other conditions than GERD.

Diagnostic Testing

In the ED, the diagnosis of GERD is typically made on the basis of the history and physical examination. Well-appearing infants with nonbilious vomiting, a normal physical exam, and an adequate weight gain trajectory may cautiously be diagnosed with GERD presumptively. However, ill-appearing infants in whom the diagnosis is uncertain may benefit from additional diagnostic studies; these tests, such as esophageal pH probes, barium swallow studies, and direct visualization by endoscopy, are not routinely available in the ED and should be conducted in consultation with a pediatric gastroenterologist.

Management

Most infants respond to conservative lifestyle modifications, such as smaller feedings, frequent burping, formula thickened with cereal, and a semiupright position after feeding. Parents should avoid using a car seat to maintain a semiupright position during and after feeding because these devices have actually been shown to exacerbate reflux rather than alleviate it.

Pharmacologic regimens are not recommended for infants with uncomplicated reflux (so-called "happy spitters"). Although lacking supportive evidence, acid suppression can be used, but should be reserved for those with more severe symptoms, such as esophagitis, weight loss, or significant irritability, in whom more conservative lifestyle modifications have failed.[7] Severe and refractory cases occasionally require pediatric surgical consultation for Nissen fundoplication.

Disposition

Most children may be discharged home safely with conservative measures. Children with more severe symptoms or poor weight gain should be referred to a pediatrician or pediatric gastroenterologist for testing and additional pharmacologic management. Those with severe dehydration, weight loss, or failure to thrive should be admitted.

Intussusception

Foundations

Intussusception refers to the invagination of part of the intestine into itself. It is the most common cause of intestinal obstruction in children younger than 2 years, occurring most frequently in infants 5 to 12 months of age. Most cases of intussusception in children are idiopathic and occur in otherwise healthy children.

The exact cause of intussusception is unclear, but the most prevalent theory relates to a lead point that causes telescoping of one segment of the intestine into another. Bowel wall edema develops, resulting in mechanical obstruction, vascular compromise, and, ultimately, bowel wall ischemia and necrosis.

Intussusception may occur at any point along the GI tract, but ileocolic intussusceptions are most common in children. In younger children, lead points are usually the result of enlarged Peyer patches secondary to a recent viral infection. In children older than 5 years, pathologic lead points, including HSP vasculitis, Meckel diverticulum, lymphoma, polyps, postsurgical scars, celiac disease, and cystic fibrosis, are more common. Ileoileal intussusception occurs more frequently in children with HSP.

Clinical Features

The classic triad of clinical findings in intussusception consists of abdominal pain, a palpable sausage-shaped abdominal mass, and bloody stools, described as "currant jelly" in appearance. All three features are present in a minority of patients, however. Abdominal pain is the most common symptom. Affected children experience cyclic episodes of severe abdominal pain as waves of peristalsis cause bowel dilation adjacent to and proximal to the involved bowel. These episodes typically last 10 to 15 minutes and occur in intervals of 15 to 30 minutes. During the painful episode, children may be irritable and inconsolable, often drawing the legs up to the abdomen and screaming in pain. Vomiting is usually present. Blood, gross or occult, may or may not be present in the stool.[8] Diarrhea containing mucus and blood constitutes the classic "currant jelly stool," a relatively infrequent and late finding. Occasionally, children present with atypical symptoms, including altered level of consciousness and profound lethargy, rather than the more typical abdominal pain syndrome.

Differential Diagnoses

Differential considerations for abdominal pain in children by age are listed in Table 166.1. A slow progressive onset of pain is more likely to be associated with appendicitis, constipation, or pancreatitis. A sudden onset of severe pain is usually associated with acute bowel obstruction, such as intussusception or volvulus, or acute vascular compromise, as seen with torsion of a testicle or ovary. Infants and children with intussusception classically have severe intermittent colicky pain.

Diagnostic Testing

Initial screening radiographs of the abdomen may be obtained, but findings are usually nonspecific. Images should be examined for signs of small bowel obstruction, including dilated small bowel loops followed by a paucity of gas in a decompressed colon. Perforation may demonstrate free air within the peritoneum. More specific, although less commonly seen, signs on radiograph include evidence of a soft tissue mass or mass effect in the right abdomen, a "target sign" (representing air in the intussusceptum as it telescopes into adjacent bowel), and a "meniscus sign" (representing air compressed like a meniscus from invaginating bowel, Fig. 166.8). Plain radiographs may be obtained to rule out perforation which would preclude nonoperative reduction but cannot be used to exclude intussusception. The common clinical scenario is that radiographs reveal indeterminate or nonspecific findings, which do not exclude the diagnosis.

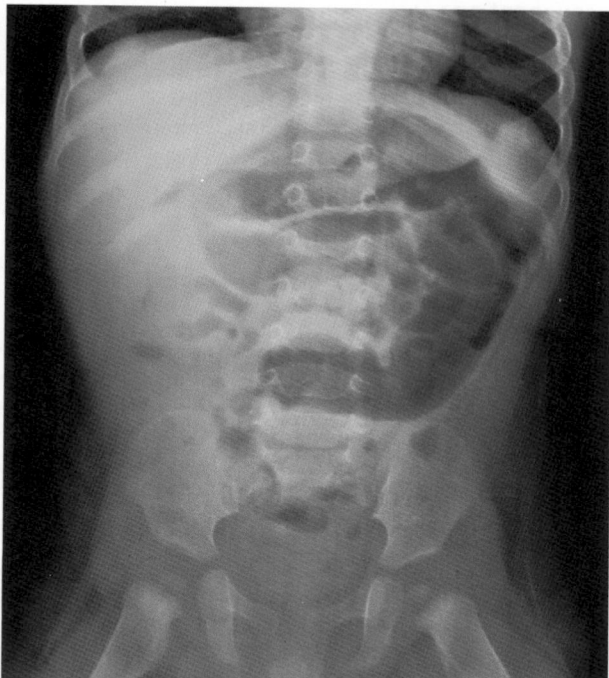

Fig. 166.8 Plain radiograph obtained in a child with crampy abdominal pain and vomiting, later confirmed to have intussusception. Findings include a poorly defined soft tissue density in the right upper quadrant, obscuration of the liver edge, and focally dilated loops of small bowel, consistent with an acute obstructive process (intussusception). (Courtesy Dr. Mark A. Hostetler.)

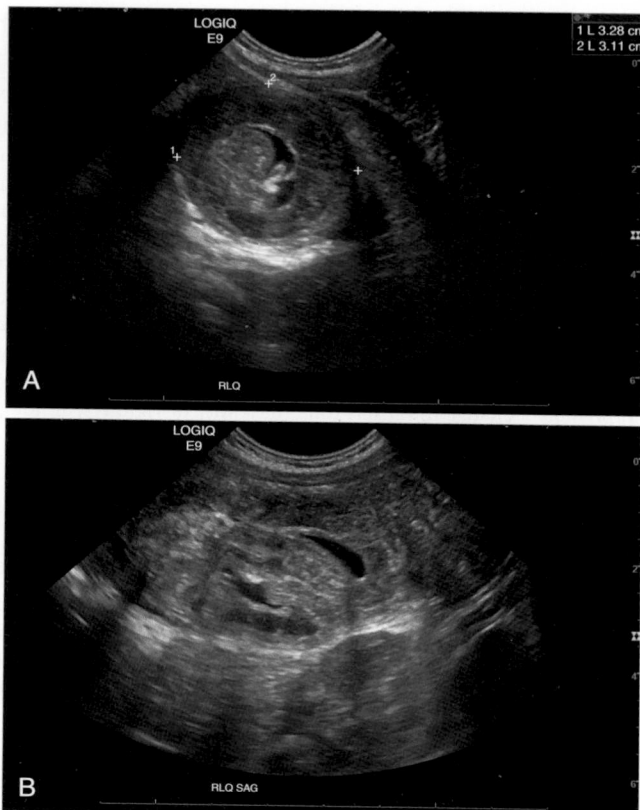

Fig. 166.9 Abdominal ultrasound examination in a child with colicky abdominal pain and vomiting, later confirmed to have intussusception. (A) On the transverse view, findings include a complex mass with a multilayered or rolled appearance (i.e., "target sign"). (B) In the long view, the ileum can be seen protruding up into the cecum, forming the intussuscipiens-intussusceptum complex. (Courtesy Dr. Patrick J. Maloney.)

When performed by skilled hands, ultrasound is highly sensitive and specific and the initial imaging modality of choice. The classic finding is a "target sign" (also referred to as a "bull's eye" or "doughnut sign"), which refers to visualization of the telescoping intestinal wall in the transverse or cross-sectional view. When visualized in the longitudinal plane, it is referred to as the "pseudo–kidney sign" (Fig. 166.9). Alternatively, contrast enemas have the advantage of being diagnostic and therapeutic. Occasionally, in children with the triad of paroxysms of pain, vomiting, and blood in the stool, contrast enemas may be safely done as first-line therapy (Fig. 166.10). Air-contrast enemas are equally efficacious and may be favored over contrast enemas due to speed of performing and efficacy.[9] Either type of enema requires readily available consultation by a pediatric surgeon in the event that reduction is unsuccessful or iatrogenic perforation occurs.

Management

IV fluids should be given in repeated boluses of 20 mL/kg of normal saline until adequate intravascular volume has been achieved. Children should be maintained on NPO status. Prompt surgical consultation is recommended. Diagnostic and therapeutic interventions depend on the location and resources available. Patients may undergo an initial ultrasound examination or, if history and plain film findings are highly suggestive of intussusception, may go directly to therapeutic enema.

The overall success rate for an air-contrast or barium enema approaches 90%. Surgical intervention is indicated in cases of prolonged intussusception with signs of perforation or shock or if enema reduction is unsuccessful. A severe, acutely life-threatening complication of air-contrast enema reduction is intestinal perforation with tension pneumoperitoneum.

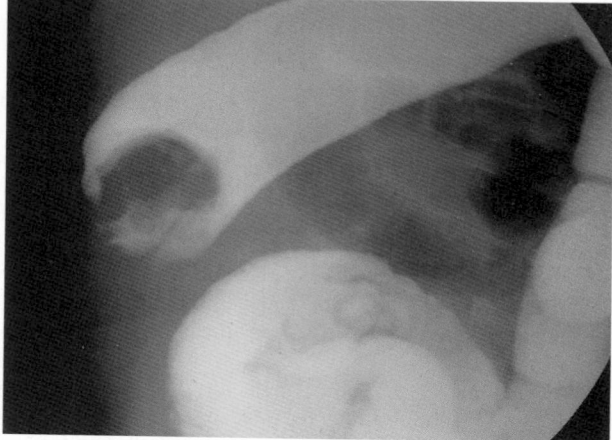

Fig. 166.10 Contrast enema image obtained in a child with intussusception shows a sharp cutoff where the contrast material meets the intussusceptum and acute obstruction. (Courtesy Dr. Mark A. Hostetler.)

Intussusception recurs within the first 48 hours after successful reduction in a very small minority of patients. Therefore, a short observation period (6 hours) is safe, and children who are able to tolerate oral fluids may be discharged home.[10]

Disposition

Children with suspected intussusception should receive definitive imaging with ultrasonography or enema. Confirmed intussusception requires reduction with enema or surgery.

Hirschsprung Disease
Foundations

Hirschsprung disease accounts for approximately 20% of cases of partial intestinal obstruction in early infancy. It occurs at a rate of 1 in 5000 live births and is four to five times more common in boys. Cases are usually sporadic in occurrence but may be associated with Down syndrome or other congenital anomalies.

Hirschsprung disease refers to congenital aganglionosis of the colon—that is, an absence of ganglion cells in the myenteric plexus of the distal colon. The anus is invariably involved, with aganglionic bowel usually extending proximally 4 to 25 cm. The absence of colonic ganglion cells interferes with that segment's ability to relax, creating a functional obstruction. Stool accumulates proximal to the level of obstruction and produces dilation of the colon, referred to as megacolon.

Clinical Features

Neonates with Hirschsprung disease often present in the newborn nursery with failure to pass meconium; however, a spectrum of disease is recognized, and presentation may be later in life. Affected infants brought to the ED usually have a history of chronic constipation. Digital rectal exam may cause an explosive passage of stool, sometimes referred to as the "squirt sign." Vomiting, irritability, poor weight gain, failure to thrive, and abdominal distention may be present. Children who appear ill with fever should be evaluated for other serious pathology, including enterocolitis, inflammatory bowel disease, and toxic megacolon.

Differential Diagnoses

Constipation is one of the most common causes of abdominal pain and vomiting in children. During the first few months of life, normal infants may have stool frequencies that range from one per feeding to one every few days, with breast-fed infants having more frequent stools than formula-fed infants. Truly pathologic causes of constipation are uncommon. In addition to Hirschsprung's disease, alternative etiologies for constipation include cystic fibrosis, infantile botulism, and hypothyroidism.

Diagnostic Testing

Plain films of the abdomen are usually nonspecific and may reveal evidence of fecal impaction with proximal obstruction, air-fluid levels, and a dilated colon. Barium enema studies revealing a narrowed aganglionic segment of distal colon with proximal dilation is highly suggestive of Hirschsprung disease. The diagnosis is confirmed by biopsy or manometry.

Management

Initial management should focus on ensuring adequate fluid and electrolyte status. Abdominal films should be obtained. With evidence of acute obstruction, such as marked bowel dilation, decompression with a rectal tube may acutely relieve symptoms. Definitive therapy of Hirschsprung disease is surgical, with resection of the aganglionic segments.

Disposition

Unless a child appears ill, most constipated children may be managed safely on an outpatient basis often with pediatric gastroenterology consultation.

Meckel Diverticulum
Foundations

Meckel diverticula are remnants of the omphalomesenteric duct and contain bowel wall, with 60% containing heterotopic tissue, usually gastric mucosa. Bleeding occurs when acid secretion from the ectopic gastric mucosa causes ulceration and erosion of the surrounding small bowel mucosa. Meckel diverticulum is the most common congenital malformation of the small intestine.

Meckel diverticula traditionally follow the "Rule of 2's": the diverticulum is approximately 2 cm wide, 2 cm long, and located within 2 feet of the ileocecal valve; moreover, the condition occurs in 2% of the population, and only 2% of affected patients ever become symptomatic; of symptomatic patients, 50% manifest symptoms by the age of 2 years, and most present by the age of 20 years.

Clinical Features

The classic presentation of a Meckel diverticulum is massive, painless rectal bleeding. Some children may have complaints of abdominal cramping. The abdominal examination is usually benign. The blood is often described as brick red but may range from melena to bright red. Complications may include intussusception, obstruction, perforation, and peritonitis.

Differential Diagnoses

Massive GI bleeding is uncommon in childhood. Children commonly eat or drink substances containing red dyes that lead to changes in the stool's color that may be mistaken for hematochezia. In addition, bismuth subsalicylate (e.g., Pepto-Bismol), iron, and spinach may cause black stools falsely appearing melanotic. A Hemoccult test of stool or Gastroccult test of emesis can confirm the presence or absence of blood, although false positives and negatives do occur.

Similar to adults, the location of bleeding may be theorized on the basis of the appearance of the blood. Hematemesis suggests bleeding proximal to the ligament of Treitz. Melena results from bleeding beyond the ligament of Treitz but proximal to the ileocecal valve. Hematochezia implies bleeding from the colon. Occasionally, in young children, GI transit time may be rapid enough for an upper GI source to cause hematochezia.

In neonates, the cause of GI bleeding is usually never identified. In young breast-fed neonates, an Apt test may be performed to differentiate fetal from swallowed maternal blood. Nursing mothers should be asked about cracked bleeding nipples. Milk protein allergy is another common cause of GI bleeding in infancy. Affected children are typically younger than 6 months, with a history of sudden-onset, mucoid, blood-streaked stools. Table 166.4 lists the differential considerations for GI bleeding in children by age.

Diagnostic Testing

A technetium-99m (^{99m}Tc) scan, also called a Meckel scan, is the diagnostic modality of choice and has an accuracy of 90% when ectopic gastric mucosa is present, since technetium has an affinity for gastric mucosa. A computed tomography (CT) scan of the abdomen may be performed to look for signs of inflammation or obstruction. Definitive diagnosis is confirmed by laparoscopy or laparotomy.

Management

Management of GI bleeding begins by assessing the child's circulatory status administering volume resuscitation as indicated. In cases of minimal or mild bleeding in otherwise healthy and well-appearing children, laboratory studies are unlikely to be useful. The child may be referred to urgently see a pediatric gastroenterologist as an outpatient. When there is concern for more serious disease, screening laboratory

TABLE 166.4   **Differential Considerations in Gastrointestinal Bleeding by Pediatric Age Group**

Classification by Cause	Infancy	Childhood	Adolescence
Factitious	Swallowed maternal blood Dyes in foods and beverages Vaginal origin Urinary origin	Dyes in foods and beverages Swallowed nasopharyngeal blood Vaginal origin Urinary origin	Dyes in foods and beverages Swallowed nasopharyngeal blood Vaginal origin Urinary origin
Upper gastrointestinal tract	Necrotizing enterocolitis Intussusception Gastroenteritis Gastritis	Esophagitis Gastroenteritis Gastritis Peptic ulcer disease	Esophagitis Gastroenteritis Gastritis Peptic ulcer disease
Lower gastrointestinal tract	Necrotizing enterocolitis Intussusception Gastroenteritis Milk allergy Vascular malformation	Gastroenteritis Intussusception Meckel diverticulum Inflammatory bowel disease Vascular malformation Henoch-Schönlein purpura Hemolytic-uremic syndrome Colitis	Gastroenteritis Intussusception Meckel diverticulum Inflammatory bowel disease Vascular malformation Henoch-Schönlein purpura Hemolytic-uremic syndrome Polyps Colitis
Rectal	Rectal fissure	Rectal fissure	Rectal fissure Hemorrhoids Trauma
Other or atypical	Bleeding dyscrasia Occult trauma (abuse) Toxic ingestions Munchausen syndrome by proxy	Bleeding dyscrasia Toxic ingestions Occult trauma (abuse) Munchausen syndrome by proxy	Bleeding dyscrasia Toxic ingestions Occult trauma (abuse) Munchausen syndrome or Munchausen syndrome by proxy

studies should include a CBC, coagulation studies (e.g., prothrombin time, partial thromboplastin time), and type and screen. A pediatric surgeon should be consulted.

Disposition

Children with massive GI bleeding suspicious for Meckel diverticulum should undergo a Meckel scan, usually after admission to a pediatric intensive care setting. Children with minor bleeding may be discharged home after consultation with a surgeon and with close follow-up. Children with ongoing active bleeding should be hospitalized.

Henoch-Schönlein Purpura

Foundations

HSP, also known as anaphylactoid purpura, is a hypersensitivity vasculitis with immune complex deposition with immunoglobulin A. Although most well-known for its characteristic petechial to purpuric rash, HSP is a systemic vasculitis affecting any vessels.

HSP is commonly associated with abdominal pain, palpable purpuric rash, arthralgias, and renal disease. Its incidence is highest among children 4 to 11 years of age. It more commonly occurs during the spring season following viral upper respiratory infections.

Clinical Features

Patients are usually diagnosed clinically on the basis of the classic palpable purpuric rash located on the buttocks and lower extremities (Fig. 166.11). Up to 70% of patients have GI complaints, including abdominal pain, nausea and vomiting, diarrhea, intestinal bleeding, and ileoileal intussusception. Laboratory findings are significant for a lack of thrombocytopenia. Microscopic hematuria occurs in half of patients. The syndrome is often relapsing and remitting for several weeks and may be associated with arthralgias. Neurologic involvement is uncommon.

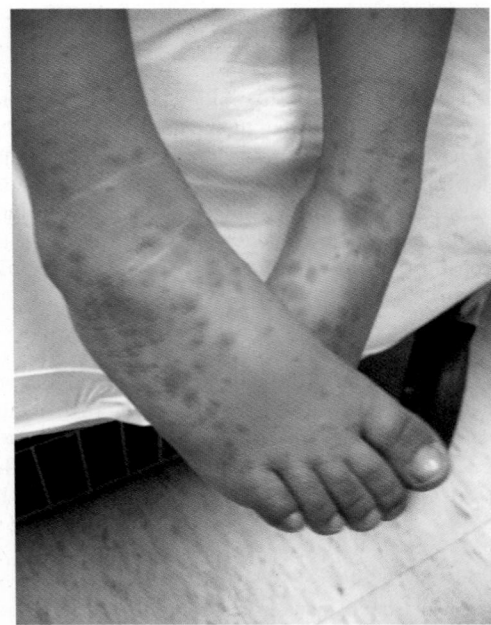

Fig. 166.11 Henoch-Schönlein purpura in a 7-year-old child. Note the typical red-purple rash on the lower extremities. (Courtesy Dr. Marianne Gausche-Hill.)

Differential Diagnoses

Patients with HSP do not have thrombocytopenia. This differentiates HSP from most other clinical diseases associated with petechiae or purpura, including meningococcemia. In addition to a thrombocytopenia, patients with meningococcemia are typically febrile and ill-appearing. The classic triad of palpable purpura, abdominal pain, and hematuria in an otherwise well-appearing and afebrile child with a normal platelet count is most likely to be HSP.

Diagnostic Testing

Patients are usually diagnosed clinically on the basis of the classic rash. All children diagnosed with HSP should have a urinalysis for evaluation of renal involvement, which manifests as white cells, red cells, casts, and protein in the urine. Those with apparent renal involvement should have serum electrolyte and creatinine levels measured. Patients with an uncertain diagnosis should have a CBC with differential, coagulation studies, blood culture, and sedimentation rate. Children diagnosed with HSP who have worrisome abdominal pain should be evaluated for intussusception.

Management

Most children with HSP require only supportive management. Mild and moderate pain is usually well controlled with nonsteroidal anti-inflammatory drugs (NSAIDs) or acetaminophen. Glucocorticoids reduce the pain associated with HSP but have not been shown to affect the other disease complications, including nephropathy. Prednisone, at a dose of 1 mg/kg/day (maximum, 60 mg), is reserved for patients with severe symptoms, including severe abdominal pain, GI bleeding, hematuria, or severe arthralgias.

Disposition

Most patients can be managed symptomatically with close outpatient observation and follow-up. Indications for hospital admission include uncertain diagnosis to exclude the possibility of meningococcemia, severe abdominal pain, and intractable vomiting. Those with compromised renal function should have a nephrology consultation and be considered for admission, particularly if presenting with hypertension.

Inflammatory Bowel Disease

Foundations

Inflammatory bowel disease (IBD) comprises two disorders: ulcerative colitis and Crohn disease. Ulcerative colitis is an inflammatory disease primarily involving the mucosa and submucosa of the rectum and distal colon. Crohn disease is a transmural inflammatory disease that may involve any portion of the intestinal tract. Chronic inflammation may result in the formation of an abscess, fistula, or stricture. Crohn disease is commonly associated with extraintestinal manifestations, especially in children.

Most patients with IBD do not experience symptoms until adolescence or adulthood. However, a small subset do develop symptoms before the age of 20 years. IBD is rare in children younger than 1 year of age.

Clinical Features

Although patients experiencing complications of IBD frequently present to the ED, the diagnosis is rarely made in this setting. Usually, children with known disease present in the midst of an acute flare, commonly associated with increased frequency of diarrheal stools, bloody diarrhea, abdominal pain, and occasionally fevers. Patients with toxic megacolon or intestinal perforations demonstrate significant abdominal tenderness with peritonitis and are usually febrile, volume-depleted, and ill-appearing.

Diagnostic Testing

Acute IBD flares are usually diagnosed clinically based on the history of present illness and physical exam. There are no laboratory or radiologic tests that are specific for acute IBD flares, and basic laboratory studies, including CBC with differential and electrolyte panel, usually reflect dehydration, inflammation, and possible anemia. The erythrocyte sedimentation rate (ESR) and C-reactive protein (CRP) levels may be beneficial in the diagnosis and management because most patients have elevated levels at the time of diagnosis as well as with acute flares. Plain radiographs are helpful when evaluating for intestinal perforation and toxic megacolon.

Differential Diagnoses

There are a large number of differential considerations for abdominal pain, vomiting, and GI bleeding (see Tables 166.1, 166.3, and 166.4). Gastroenteritis is the most common consideration in this clinical scenario. Children experiencing their first episode of IBD and children outside the usual age at presentation are much more likely to be misdiagnosed with acute gastroenteritis.

Management

Management in the ED begins with attention to volume status and resuscitation with repeated boluses of 20 mL/kg of normal saline or lactated Ringers solution until the volume status is adequate. Acute exacerbations should be treated in conjunction with a gastroenterologist. Corticosteroids (e.g., prednisone, 1 mg/kg/day; maximum dose, 60 mg/day) are usually recommended for mild to moderate exacerbations. Other agents commonly used include sulfasalazine and azathioprine, among other immunosuppressive agents. Patients with suspected toxic megacolon require IV broad-spectrum antibiotic therapy (see Box 166.2) and surgical consultation.

Disposition

Children not diagnosed with IBD but who have recurrent GI symptoms or a family history of IBD should be referred to a pediatric gastroenterologist for further evaluation. With acute flares, indications for admission include dehydration, toxic or ill appearance, and inability to tolerate oral fluids. Children with evidence of toxic megacolon should have a surgical consultation.

Gastrointestinal Foreign Bodies

Foundations

GI foreign bodies usually are seen in children younger than 5 years of age and in those with developmental delays. Coins, small toys, magnets, batteries, and jewelry are the most common esophageal foreign bodies in children, compared to food boluses in adults. Most ingestions in children are accidental.

The vast majority of swallowed foreign bodies pass through the entire GI tract without complications. However, foreign bodies commonly become lodged in one of three areas of normal physiologic narrowing within the esophagus: (1) the upper esophageal sphincter (cricopharyngeus muscle)/thoracic inlet (C6-T1); (2) the aortic arch/tracheal bifurcation (T4-6); and (3) the lower esophageal sphincter/diaphragmatic hiatus (T10-11). Of objects that successfully pass into the stomach, 80% to 90% also pass through the entire GI tract without complications.

Clinical Features

Many accidental ingestions are unwitnessed. Children may gag as they attempt to swallow the object. Objects aspirated into the respiratory tract generally produce persistent coughing, wheezing, increased work of breathing, and respiratory distress. Children who swallow objects which then become lodged within the esophagus may remain asymptomatic or develop a wide spectrum of symptoms, including food refusal, persistent gagging, drooling, or continuous dry heaves. Some esophageal foreign bodies may cause local airway compression, resulting in stridor, wheezing, and respiratory distress. Complications such as esophageal or intestinal perforation are more likely to occur when foreign bodies have been impacted for an extended period of time; symptoms include progressive dysphagia, pain, respiratory distress, and fever.

Swallowed lithium button batteries warrant special mention. Button batteries lodged in the esophagus cause severe mucosal erosions, burns, and mediastinitis in as little as 2 hours, most likely as a result of the electrical current discharged from these batteries. Gastrointestinal or pediatric surgical consultation for emergent foreign body removal is warranted. Button batteries in the stomach usually pass without complications and do not require removal unless they fail to pass the pylorus within 48 hours of ingestion. The National Capital Poison Center operates a 24/7 website (www.poison.org/battery) and hotline (800-498-8666) for battery ingestion cases.

On occasion, objects successfully pass into the stomach, but are too large to pass through the pylorus. As a general rule, objects longer than 5 cm and wider than 2 cm are less likely to pass the pylorus spontaneously. Persistent vomiting may herald obstruction. If not removed, foreign bodies may, over time, result in erosion, perforation, infection, stricture, or fistula formation.

Diagnostic Testing

Plain radiography is the most common method of diagnosing and locating foreign bodies. Classically, coins and button batteries in the esophagus project en face (round) in the frontal (coronal/AP or PA) view (Fig. 166.12). When coins or button batteries are lodged

in the upper airway, they will project on end in the frontal view. Occasionally, it may be difficult to differentiate the appearance of a coin from a button battery radiographically. A button battery will typically have a distinctive double-rim contour on radiographs (Fig. 166.13).

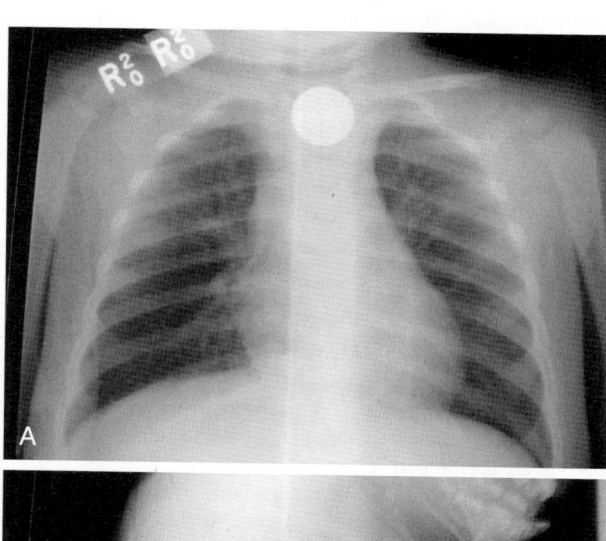
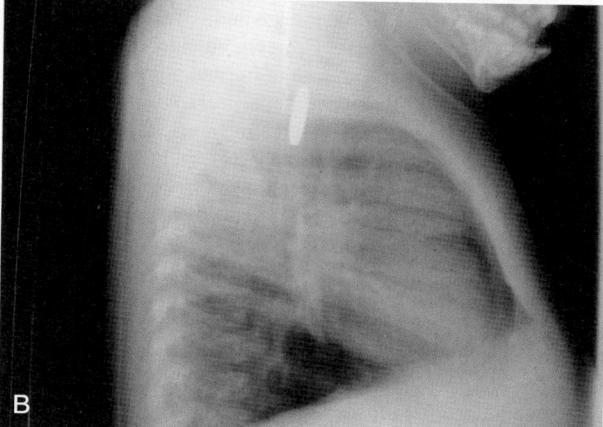

Fig. 166.12 Plain radiographs obtained in a child with an esophageal coin foreign body. Posteroanterior (A) and lateral (B) views show the expected orientation for a coin lodged in the esophagus. (Courtesy Dr. Mark A. Hostetler.)

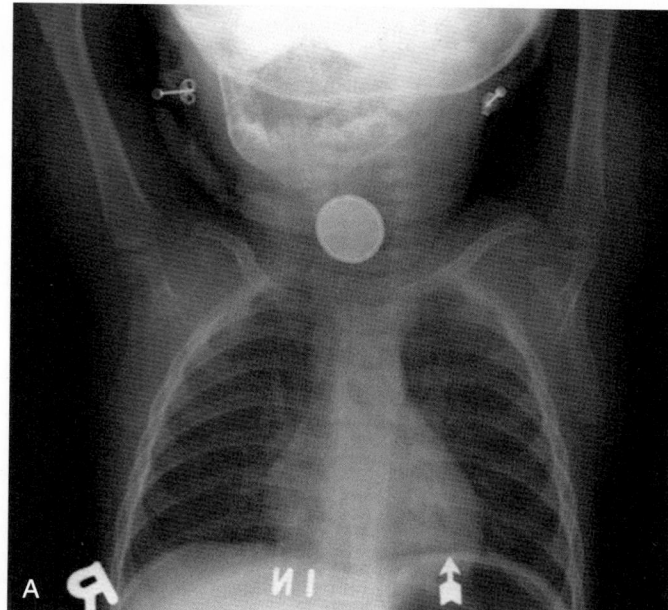
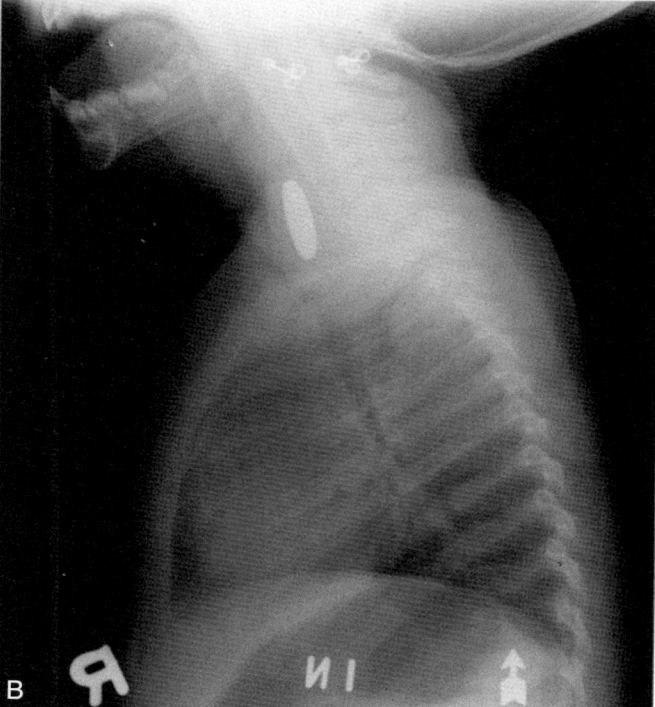

Fig. 166.13 Esophageal button battery. It may be difficult to differentiate the appearance of a coin from a button battery radiographically. However, a button battery will typically have a distinctive double-rim contour on radiographs, as seen in this posteroanterior radiograph. (From: Lin VYW, Daniel SJ, Papsin BC. Button batteries in the ear, nose and upper aerodigestive tract. *Int J Pediatr Otorhinolaryngol.* 2004;68:473-479.)

Differential Diagnoses

Not all foreign bodies are radiopaque and visible with standard radiography. Patients who remain symptomatic require further contrast-enhanced imaging or direct visualization.

Management

Most GI foreign bodies will spontaneously pass without complications. In general, small objects that successfully pass into the stomach do not require further treatment or routine serial imaging. Button batteries and multiple magnetic objects represent two exceptions. Patients with button batteries located in the stomach should have serial films to ensure successful passage beyond the pylorus. Ingestion of multiple magnets or a single magnet plus a second metallic object may result in the objects attaching to each other across bowel wall, resulting in bowel necrosis and perforation. Therefore, multiple magnets or a single magnet plus another metallic object located within the stomach are typically removed urgently by endoscopy because they are more likely to require more complicated surgical removal if allowed to pass beyond the pylorus. However, if they have already passed into the small bowel in a well-appearing, asymptomatic patient without any signs of bowel obstruction or peritonitis observation and serial radiographs are recommended. Surgical consultation for removal should be obtained if there are signs of bowel necrosis, obstruction, perforation, or peritonitis.

Asking parents to check the child's stool for a passed foreign body is rarely productive. The timing of intervention for foreign body removal is based largely on the type of object, location, duration, and symptoms. With the exception of button batteries, which should be removed emergently within 2 hours, esophageal foreign bodies may be removed urgently within 24 hours. Blunt objects, such as coins, in the esophagus of asymptomatic children may be observed for 12 to 24 hours because many of them will pass spontaneously into the stomach. Indications for more emergent removal are listed in Box 166.3.

The preferred method to remove esophageal foreign bodies varies by institution; flexible endoscopy is most common and has a high success rate. Other options include fluoroscopic Foley catheter removal, bougie advancement into the stomach, and removal by rigid bronchoscopy under general anesthesia in the operating room.

Disposition

Esophageal foreign bodies require removal, as described previously. Once foreign bodies have passed into the stomach, most pass without complications, and no specific follow-up is usually necessary. Abdominal pain, food aversion, and intractable vomiting may suggest a retained gastric foreign body warranting repeat radiography. Button batteries in the stomach and multiple magnets constitute exceptions. Button batteries in the stomach necessitate follow-up films in 24 hours to document passage beyond the pylorus, even in asymptomatic

---

BOX 166.3 Indications for Emergency Removal of Gastrointestinal Foreign Bodies

- Signs of respiratory distress
- Evidence of esophageal obstruction (inability to swallow secretions)
- Lithium button batteries in the esophagus
- Sharp or long (>5 cm) objects in the esophagus or stomach
- Multiple magnets or single magnet plus another metallic object within esophagus or stomach
- Signs or symptoms of intestinal inflammation, obstruction or perforation
- Esophageal foreign bodies impacted for >24 hr or for an unknown amount of time

---

children. When multiple magnets are suspected of being within the stomach, urgent endoscopy and removal is warranted. When they have passed the pylorus but there is no evidence that they have attached to each other across bowel wall causing tissue necrosis and/or perforation, close observation and serial radiographs is recommended. If there are clinical concerns for bowel necrosis, obstruction, or perforation, surgical consultation is emergently necessary.

Appendicitis

Foundations

Appendicitis is the most common surgical condition involving the abdomen and the most common nontraumatic surgical emergency in children. It develops in approximately 1 of every 15 people during their lifetime. The peak age of incidence is between 9 and 12 years, and it is uncommon in children younger than 5 years of age.

The appendix is a blind pouch that may become obstructed, resulting in edema, vasocongestion, inflammation, ischemia, infarction, necrosis, and perforation. In adults, a thicker appendiceal wall resists perforation, and a well-developed omentum aids in walling off the infection to prevent its diffuse spread. Children have neither, so rupture tends to occur earlier, and diffuse peritonitis develops more readily.

Morbidity and mortality related to acute appendicitis increase significantly if the appendix ruptures prior to operative management. Therefore, the goal of management is diagnosis and operative management prior to appendiceal perforation. Perforation seems to be directly related to the duration of symptoms. In children, the rate of appendiceal perforation varies inversely with age. Perforation is highest among children younger than 5 years, among whom more than 50% are ruptured at the time of surgery. This likely reflects, at least in part, the fact that preschool children have a limited ability to describe their symptoms and often present for evaluation later in the disease course.

Clinical Features

Patients classically present with a constellation of symptoms that includes abdominal pain, nausea, vomiting, and anorexia. Symptoms are gradually progressive over the first 24 hours. Abdominal pain is usually first described as vague, crampy, and periumbilical. Pain becomes more severe, constant, and localized to the right lower quadrant as the disease progresses. Fever usually develops later or not at all. A subset of patients may have a multiphasic course to their illness, with symptom resolution followed several days later by the development of fever, chills, and abdominal pain. This likely represents spontaneous appendiceal rupture and formation of an abscess.

The physical examination may reveal several typical findings. In patients with inflammation surrounding the appendix, peritoneal findings that localize to the right lower quadrant are classic. Pain occurs with movement; patients may be unwilling to jump up and down, and tapping their heels may cause abdominal pain. Bowel sounds are usually decreased or absent. Rebound tenderness may be elicited in the right lower quadrant. The Rovsing, psoas, and obturator signs are difficult to assess in young children and should not be relied on due to their poor sensitivities and specificities. The absence of the classic signs and symptoms of appendicitis unfortunately does not exclude the diagnosis, especially in younger children.

Diagnostic Testing

Appendicitis may be diagnosed clinically on the basis of the history and physical findings alone in children with a classic constellation of findings. Patients with an equivocal presentation should undergo a diagnostic evaluation. There are no sufficiently sensitive or specific laboratory tests that alone can confirm or exclude the diagnosis of acute appendicitis. Screening studies may include a CBC with differential,

CRP, urinalysis, electrolyte levels, and renal and liver function testing. Pregnancy testing, vaginal wet mount, and gonorrheal and chlamydial testing should be considered in postpubertal females. Most children with acute appendicitis have an elevated white blood cell count (>10,000 × 10⁶/L), absolute neutrophil count, or an elevated CRP level (>0.6 mg/dL). Because none of these tests are sufficiently sensitive or specific, they should not be exclusively used to diagnose or exclude appendicitis. Acute appendicitis occasionally causes a mild sterile pyuria (<5 to 10 white blood cells/high-power field in the absence of bacteria) related to local inflammation of the right ureter.

Several clinical scoring systems have been developed to assist in the evaluation of appendicitis. The most widely studied prospectively include the Alvarado score, Pediatric Appendicitis Score, and Refined Low-Risk Appendicitis Rule. Each system relies on a combination of clinical factors and laboratory values to risk-stratify children into low-, moderate-, and high-risk categories for appendicitis. Unfortunately, none of these have been shown to be sensitive and specific enough to be recommended alone for widespread clinical use.

Diagnostic imaging options include plain films of the abdomen, ultrasonography, and CT. Plain films have limited value in appendicitis and are not recommended in the routine evaluation. Occasionally, an appendiceal fecalith will be evident (Fig. 166.14). Although the presence of an appendicolith in a child with acute abdominal pain is essentially pathognomonic for acute appendicitis, it is present in less than 10% of cases.

Ultrasonography is routinely recommended as the first-line imaging modality in suspected appendicitis. It has the advantages of lacking ionizing radiation and the ability to evaluate ovarian anatomy. Ultrasonographic findings consistent with appendicitis include an enlarged, noncompressible appendix (wall thickness > 2 mm; total appendix diameter > 6 mm) that is painful during scanning (Fig. 166.15A, B). Appendiceal ultrasound has a sensitivity and specificity of more than 90% when the appendix is successfully visualized. Unfortunately, the ability to visualize the appendix adequately with ultrasound is limited in obese children and highly user-dependent.

In the child in whom the appendix is not visualized or findings are equivocal with ultrasonography, clinical observation with serial examinations or CT imaging may be undertaken. CT in general has high sensitivity and specificity for unruptured and ruptured appendicitis, and the use of IV contrast improves sensitivity slightly. Limited appendiceal

CT protocols decrease the ionizing radiation exposure without sacrificing sensitivity or specificity. The increased use of CT has been shown to reduce the negative laparotomy rate without increasing the risk of perforation.

Differential Diagnoses

Differential considerations for abdominal pain by age are listed in Table 166.4. Mesenteric adenitis is the most common imitation of appendicitis. Similar to appendicitis, it often is associated with significant diffuse tenderness that may localize in the right lower quadrant. Children with mesenteric adenitis lack true peritoneal signs, however.

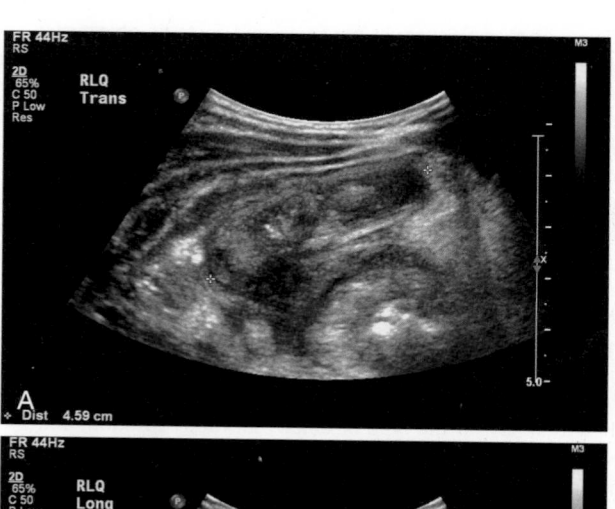

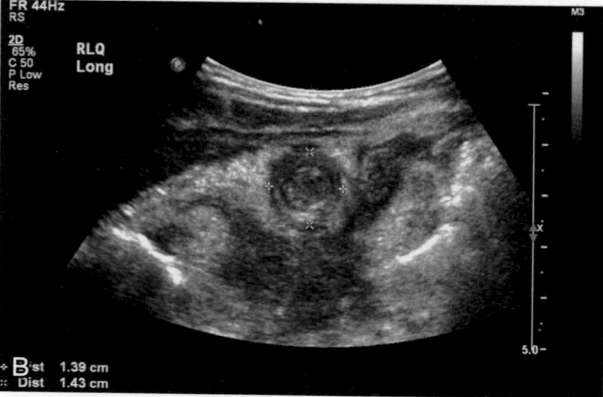

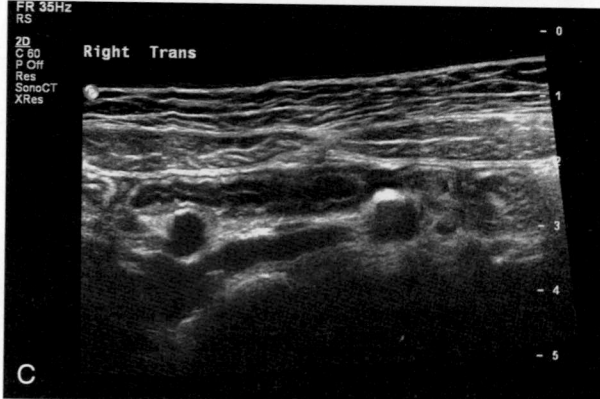

Fig. 166.15 Ultrasound images obtained in children with appendicitis. Findings include an enlarged, noncompressible, tubelike structure in the longitudinal view with an appendicolith (A), an enlarged noncompressible structure seen in cross section (B) and, in another patient, an enlarged, poorly compressible structure with a moderate amount of free fluid consistent with acute perforation (C). (Courtesy Dr. Mark A. Hostetler.)

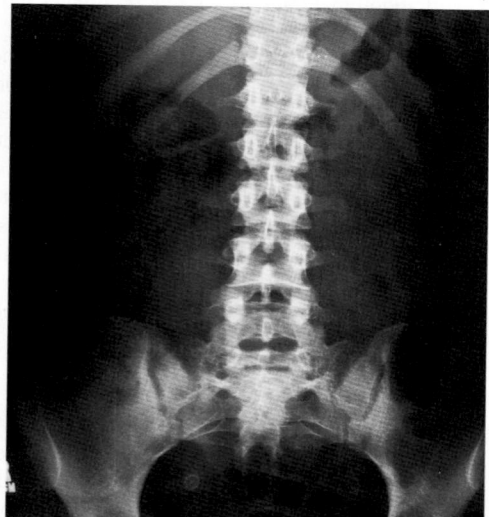

Fig. 166.14 Fecalith in a child with appendicitis. (Courtesy Dr. Marianne Gausche-Hill.)

Mesenteric adenitis usually follows a viral illness and results from non-specific inflammation of the mesenteric lymph nodes.

Girls of reproductive age merit consideration of gynecologic pathology, including ectopic pregnancy, ovarian torsion, ovarian cyst, pelvic inflammatory disease, and tubo-ovarian abscess. Testicular torsion may manifest with nausea, vomiting, and abdominal pain, but the testicular examination is usually grossly abnormal in these boys. Boys with abdominal pain on the side of an undescended testis should be evaluated for torsion of an intra-abdominal testicle. Group A streptococcal pharyngitis may also present with abdominal pain and mimic appendicitis.

Management

Definitive management of acute appendicitis is open or laparoscopic appendectomy. The exact timing of surgery is controversial but should optimally be performed within 12 to 24 hours of diagnosis. Most patients benefit from IV fluids and parenteral administration of opioid pain medications and antiemetics. Opioids are safe and effective and do not alter the diagnostic accuracy of the physical examination. Patients with a nonperforated appendicitis should receive a single dose of parenteral antibiotics (Box 166.4) 30 to 60 minutes prior to surgery to decrease the risk of wound infection and intra-abdominal abscess formation. Patients with suspected perforation, signs or symptoms of sepsis, or unusual delay in surgical management should receive empirical broad-spectrum IV antibiotics (see Box 166.2) in the ED and continued postoperatively.

While appendectomy remains the standard of care in most cases of acute appendicitis, nonoperative management with parenteral antibiotics and observation alone is an emerging option in a subset of older children with uncomplicated disease. Nonoperative management typically results in fewer days of disability and overall decrease health care costs.[11]

Disposition

Children with appendicitis should be hospitalized for appendectomy. Patients with nonspecific signs and symptoms in whom imaging studies are nondiagnostic should be observed for a period of 12 to 24 hours with serial examinations or, with adequate family and social support, discharged home with careful instructions to return for reexamination.

Pancreatitis
Foundations

Pancreatitis is uncommon in childhood, especially in children younger than 10 years. In adults, pancreatitis is most commonly associated with

---

BOX 166.4   Empirical Antibiotic Regimens for Acute Appendicitis

Regimen
- Cefoxitin
- Ceftriaxone + metronidazole
- Cefotetan
- Gentamicin + clindamycin or metronidazole (penicillin-allergic patients)
- Piperacillin-tazobactam

Dosing
- Cefoxitin: 40 mg/kg IV; maximum dose, 2000 mg
- Ceftriaxone: 50 mg/kg IV; maximum dose, 2000 mg
- Metronidazole: 10 mg/kg IV; maximum dose, 500 mg
- Cefotetan: 40 mg/kg IV; maximum dose, 2000 mg
- Gentamicin: 2–7.5 mg/kg/day
- Clindamycin: 10 mg/kg IV; maximum dose, 900 mg
- Piperacillin-tazobactam: 80–100 mg/kg of the piperacillin component, max 4.5 g

---

alcohol abuse and biliary tract disease. In children, pancreatitis is usually caused by trauma, infection, structural anomalies, systemic disease, and drugs or toxins. Idiopathic causes account for 30% of cases. Biliary disease should be considered in adolescents and teenagers.

The common pathophysiologic pathway of acute pancreatitis is inflammation, edema, and autodigestion of pancreatic tissue by pancreatic enzymes. In severe cases, the inflammatory cascade may progress to necrotizing or hemorrhagic pancreatitis. Other complications include the formation of abscesses, pseudocysts, and fistulas.

Clinical Features

Abdominal pain is the hallmark of pancreatitis in adults and children. Patients typically present with complaints of severe, constant epigastric pain that worsens gradually and radiates to the back. Nausea, vomiting, diarrhea, fevers, irritability, and lethargy are also described. Patients have significant abdominal tenderness in the epigastric area.

Diagnostic Testing

Screening laboratory studies reveal an elevation in the serum lipase level. The degree of elevation and serial changes are not always directly related to disease severity. Evidence of liver inflammation (i.e., elevated aspartate transaminase and alanine transaminase levels) and elevated bilirubin and alkaline phosphatase levels may be seen in patients with associated hepatobiliary disease. Plain films of the abdomen commonly show an ileus pattern, often with a sentinel loop of dilated small bowel in the left upper quadrant. An ultrasound study or CT may be helpful to evaluate anatomy for congenital malformations, biliary tract disease, pseudocyst, or abscess formation. In patients with respiratory distress, a chest radiograph may identify a secondary pleural effusion.

Differential Diagnoses

Slow progressive onset of pain is more likely to be associated with appendicitis, constipation, and pancreatitis. Sudden onset of severe pain is usually associated with acute intestinal obstruction, such as intussusception or midgut volvulus, or vascular occlusion, as seen with testicular or ovarian torsion. Differential considerations for abdominal pain in children by age are listed in Table 166.4.

Management

Patients should receive volume replacement and electrolyte correction and be maintained on an NPO status. IV fluids are given in repeated boluses of 20 mL/kg of normal saline until adequate vascular volume has been established. Patients should receive adequate symptomatic relief with parenteral narcotics and antiemetics. Steroids and antibiotics are not indicated.

Disposition

Children with acute pancreatitis should undergo hospitalization. Children with known or recurrent disease, who are able to self-hydrate and have adequate analgesia, may be managed as outpatients in select cases.

Biliary Tract Disease
Foundations

Biliary tract disease is uncommon in childhood and has causes that differ from those in older individuals. Cholestasis in the neonatal period is usually associated with biliary atresia, biliary cysts, infections, and other metabolic and genetic disorders. Gallstones in children are usually associated with hemolytic disease (e.g., sickle cell disease), cystic fibrosis, total parenteral nutrition, sepsis, and dehydration. Acute acalculous cholecystitis has been associated with Rocky Mountain spotted fever and a variety of bacterial infections, including those due to *Salmonella* and *Shigella* organisms. Hydrops of the gallbladder (i.e., fluid distention of the gallbladder from chronic cystic duct inflammation or obstruction without inflammation or infection) is associated with viral upper respiratory or GI infections, Kawasaki disease, streptococcal pharyngitis, mesenteric adenitis, nephrotic syndrome, and leptospirosis.

Pigment gallstones stones are more common in childhood; cholesterol stones are uncommon prior to adolescence. Pigment stones result from the excess breakdown of red blood cells and are usually seen in those with hemolytic anemia, such as sickle cell disease and spherocytosis. Adolescents may form cholesterol gallstones in association with oral contraceptives, pregnancy, or obesity.

Clinical Features

Similar to adult patients, pediatric patients usually present with postprandial right upper quadrant pain associated with fever, nausea, and vomiting. Jaundice occurs in one-third of patients.

Diagnostic Testing

Biliary tract disease is usually associated with elevations in alkaline phosphatase, liver transaminases, and bilirubin levels; however, absence of elevations does not exclude the diagnosis. An elevated white blood cell count is nonspecific. Although only 15% of gallstones in adults are calcified and visible on plain radiographs, 50% of stones in children are radiopaque. Ultrasonography is the imaging modality of choice. It not only can determine the presence of gallstones, dilation of the gallbladder and common bile duct, gallbladder wall thickness, and pericholecystic fluid, but can also reproduce pain on compression of the gallbladder (sonographic Murphy sign). When ultrasound findings are equivocal or normal and clinical suspicion is high, cholescintigraphy biliary tract imaging (HIDA [hepatobiliary iminodiacetic acid] scan) can further assess the functional status of the gallbladder. Magnetic resonance cholangiopancreatography (MRCP) can assess the intrahepatic and extrahepatic ducts.

Differential Diagnoses

Pediatric biliary tract disease is uncommon in children and requires consideration of an underlying or coexistent disease. Differential considerations are listed in Table 166.4.

Management

Asymptomatic patients with incidental findings of gallstones require no further therapy in the ED and may be referred to a surgeon for outpatient care. Febrile patients and those with intractable pain or nausea and vomiting require hospital admission, fluid resuscitation, IV antibiotics, and surgical consultation. Laparoscopic cholecystectomy is considered safe and effective in children.

Disposition

Indications for hospital admission for biliary disease include pain control, need for IV hydration, fever, and need for operative management.

The references for this chapter can be found online at ExpertConsult.com.

167

Pediatric Infectious Diarrheal Disease and Dehydration

Patricia Padlipsky and William White

KEY CONCEPTS

Identification of Pathogen

- Stool studies are not indicated in most uncomplicated cases of acute gastroenteritis (AGE). Exceptions are those cases in which specific treatment, specific prophylaxis, or health precautions are required, or in which the patient has systemic involvement, underlying medical complications, or dysenteric features.
- Antibiotics are not required for most cases of uncomplicated acute bacterial enteritis. Antibiotics are recommended routinely for *C. difficile*, *Giardia intestinalis,* and *E. histolytica*. Antibiotics can be considered for *Campylobacter, Cryptosporidium,* traveler's diarrhea, and *Shigella* (because antibiotics have been shown to decrease diarrhea and eradicate organisms in the stool).
- Patients with Shiga toxin–producing *E. coli* (STEC) should not empirically receive antibiotics, because they may increase the risk of hemolytic-uremic syndrome (HUS).
- Testing for fecal leukocytes is a useful initial test because it may support a diagnosis of invasive disease. This test should be considered in children with diarrhea who are febrile or have mucus or blood in the stool. If the test result is positive, stool culture is indicated to further guide management.

Oral Rehydration

- Most patients with mild to moderate dehydration can be treated with oral rehydration therapy (ORT). Resumption of feeding with age-appropriate diets should begin as soon as vomiting subsides. Routine fasting with infectious diarrhea is not recommended.

Dehydration Assessment

- The degree of volume depletion is estimated from the history and physical examination findings. The desired volume of oral rehydration solution is calculated as 30 to 50 mL/kg for mild dehydration and 60 to 80 mL/kg for moderate dehydration; 25% of the volume of oral rehydration solution is to be replaced every hour (100% over 4 hours). Continue to replace ongoing losses with 10 mL/kg for each diarrheal stool and 2 mL/kg for each vomiting episode. Patients who fail an oral rehydration trial of 4 to 8 hours in the emergency department (ED) should be admitted for intravenous hydration.

Severe Dehydration

- In severe dehydration, 20 mL/kg of 0.9% saline (or other appropriate isotonic crystalloid solution) given intravenously or intraosseously should reverse signs of shock within 5 to 15 minutes. Repeated boluses of 20 mL/kg are indicated until clinical improvement occurs, but volume requirements greater than 60 mL/kg without signs of improvement suggest other conditions, such as septic shock, hemorrhage, capillary leak with third-space fluid sequestration, and adrenal insufficiency. Rapid correction of sodium derangements in dehydration can lead to central nervous system complications.

DIARRHEA

Foundations

Background and Importance

Acute infectious diarrhea is a common illness seen around the world. Acute diarrhea is generally self-limiting in industrialized nations but can have significant morbidity and mortality for the elderly, very young, and immunocompromised patients. In underdeveloped countries, diarrheal diseases are a significant cause of death. According to the Global Burden of Disease Study 2016, diarrhea was found to be the eighth leading cause of death among all ages, responsible for more than 1.6 million deaths worldwide. Approximately half a million of the deaths from diarrhea worldwide occurred among children younger than 5 years of age, making it the third leading cause of death in children less than 5 years of age globally.[1,2] The rotavirus vaccine in the United States and internationally has markedly reduced pediatric diarrhea-associated emergency department (ED) visits, hospitalizations, and deaths.

Acute diarrhea is defined as the abrupt onset of abnormally high fluid content in the stool, with increased volume or frequency. As supported by the World Health Organization (WHO), "acute" diarrhea has a sudden onset and lasts no longer than 14 days; "chronic" or "persistent" diarrhea lasts longer than 14 days. This classification is important for epidemiologic studies and to identify the most likely offending organism. Protracted diarrhea has different causes, poses unique problems in management, and has a prognosis different from that of acute diarrhea. Acute infectious diarrhea can occur with or without vomiting. When it occurs with vomiting, it is often referred to as *acute gastroenteritis (AGE).*

Anatomy, Physiology, and Pathophysiology

Up to 9 L of exogenous fluid and endogenous secretions enter the adult proximal bowel each day, and proportionally even more in children. Ninety percent of fluid is absorbed in the small bowel and the remainder in the large bowel. Water follows osmotic gradients created by active and passive transport of electrolytes, sugars, and amino acids into the bloodstream by the following mechanisms:

- Sodium chloride absorption in the small bowel, with an exchange of cations (Na^+/H^+) and anions (Cl^-/HCO_3^-).
- Electrogenic sodium absorption in the colon, but also in the small intestine, wherein Na^+ enters the cell through an electrochemical gradient; this mechanism is often damaged in acute diarrhea.
- Sodium co-transport mechanism in the small bowel. Na^+ absorption is coupled with the absorption of glucose, amino acids, and peptides. This mechanism often remains intact during acute diarrhea illness, making oral rehydration possible.

Pathophysiology

Infectious agents cause diarrhea by adherence, mucosal invasion, enterotoxin production, and cytotoxin production. Under normal circumstances, the absorptive processes for water and electrolytes predominate over secretion, resulting in net water absorption. Diarrhea occurs when this balance is disrupted, either as a result of increased secretion from the gastrointestinal tract, decreased absorption of fluids, or from inflammation.

Secretory diarrhea is the result of increased intestinal secretion of water into the gut lumen or an inhibition of absorption. For example, *Vibrio cholera* produces an enterotoxin, resulting in increased chloride and bicarbonate secretion. Secretory diarrhea is characterized by the absence of expected reduction in stool volume with fasting, a stool pH above 6, and the absence of reducing substances in the stool. Other bacteria that produce enterotoxins include *Salmonella, Shigella, Escherichia coli,* and *Clostridioides difficile.*

Osmotic diarrhea is caused by the presence of poorly absorbed solutes from altered bacterial gut flora, damage to the mucosal absorptive surface, or ingestion of substances. These substances create an osmotic gradient across the bowel lumen, resulting in intraluminal movement of water and electrolytes. Typical acute viral gastroenteritis produces injury to the small bowel epithelium with consequent disruption of microvilli, decreasing the absorptive area, and preventing normal fluid, electrolyte, and nutrient absorption. The illness is compounded if the colon is unable to compensate for the large fluid volume. Osmotic diarrhea is often characterized by diarrhea that decreases or stops with fasting, a stool pH below 6, and the presence of reducing substances in the stool.

Inflammatory processes can cause destruction of villous cells or dysfunction of cellular transporters, leading to loss of fluids and electrolytes, as well as mucus, proteins, and blood in the intestinal lumen. *Dysentery,* diarrhea associated with blood and mucus in the stool, implies a compromised bowel wall. Acute inflammation, caused by enteroinvasive organisms such as *Salmonella, Shigella,* and *Campylobacter,* leads to infiltration of the gastrointestinal tract by neutrophils, which release a host of enzymes and factors causing both increased secretion and decreased absorption by the intestinal tract. Although blood loss may be clinically appreciable, it is usually less significant than fluid and electrolyte losses. Infectious diarrhea can present with significant signs of dehydration and electrolyte abnormalities.

Pediatric patients have several physiologic factors that predispose them to more severe complications from vomiting and diarrhea. As a result of their relatively larger extracellular fluid compartments, children can lose proportionately more fluids through the gastrointestinal tract. Furthermore, the turnover of fluids and solute in infants and young children can be three times that of adults. This rapid turnover of fluids is the result of higher metabolic rates, increased body surface area to mass index, and higher body water content. Children also have limited stores of metabolic substrates such as fat and glycogen, limited ability or desire to access fluids when ill, and a more limited ability to conserve water through their kidneys compared to adults. These factors make children more susceptible to large fluctuations in

fluid, electrolytes, and nutrients, resulting in hypoglycemia, electrolyte abnormalities, dehydration, and shock.

Some groups are at higher risk for developing serious complications of infectious diarrhea (e.g., invasive disease, bacteremia, and sepsis). These include premature infants, very-low-birth-weight infants (up to a year), young infants (younger than 3 months old), immunosuppressed or malnourished children, and those with chronic underlying conditions. Recent hospitalization, treatment with broad-spectrum antibiotics, and travel to developing countries are additional risk factors.

Clinical Features

Infectious diarrhea can present with diarrhea alone or accompanied by vomiting (i.e., acute gastroenteritis [AGE]). Signs and symptoms usually begin 12 to 72 hours after contracting the infectious agent. If due to a viral agent, the condition usually resolves within 1 week. See Box 167.1 for a list of common signs and symptoms. The history and physical examination should help differentiate acute infectious diarrhea from other causes of vomiting and diarrhea and help estimate the degree of dehydration. History and physical examination can sometimes aid in determining the type of pathogen responsible, although this will rarely affect management. Box 167.2 summarizes important information to gather from the history.

Vital signs should be assessed relative to age norms. The evaluation of the child should begin with looking at the child from across the room in a position of comfort, noting the patient's overall appearance, responsiveness, activity, and work of breathing (see Chapter 160). A head-to-toe physical examination of the patient should focus on signs of dehydration that may indicate another cause for the diarrhea (e.g., otitis media, pyelonephritis, appendicitis, diabetic ketoacidosis), or signs that indicate the disease may have become extraintestinal or systemic—bone pain (osteomyelitis), altered mental status (meningitis), petechiae (hemolytic-uremic syndrome [HUS]).

Acute infectious diarrhea in developed countries is often self-limited. The clinical presentation, course of illness, and treatment depends on the etiology of the diarrhea and the host. In the United States, viruses are responsible for most cases of acute infectious diarrhea, with bacteria causing only 7% to 10% of cases in children. Parasites are uncommon in the immunocompetent patient, unless they have traveled to endemic areas. Table 167.1 lists the most common viruses, bacteria, and protozoa that can cause acute infectious diarrhea in children in the United States.[3-6]

Specific Etiologies

Viruses. In the United States and Europe, the majority of cases of diarrhea are caused by viral pathogens, with incidence peaking in the winter. The most common of these are rotavirus and norovirus. See Table 167.2 for presentation and associated characteristics.

BOX 167.1   Common Signs and Symptoms in Patients With Acute Infectious Diarrhea

Diarrhea—frequent, loose, watery, mucousy, bloody, or foul smelling
Nausea
Decreased appetite
Weight loss
Vomiting
Headache
Abdominal pain or cramps
Fever
Malaise
Signs of dehydration (see Dehydration section)

TABLE 167.1 Common Causes of Childhood Infectious Diarrhea in Developed Countries

Viruses (70% to 80%)	Bacteria (10% to 20%)	Protozoa (<10%)
Rotavirus	*Salmonella* species	*Cryptosporidium*
Norovirus and	*Shigella* species	*Giardia intestinalis*
Sapovirus	*Campylobacter jejuni*	*Entamoeba histolytica*
Astrovirus	*Yersinia enterocolitica*	
Adenovirus	*Escherichia coli,* ETEC,	
	Clostridium perfringens	
	Clostridium difficile	
	Staphylococcus aureus	
	Vibrio cholera	
	Vibrio parahaemolyticus	

ETEC, Enterotoxigenic *E. coli.*

Rotavirus (RV) continues to be the leading cause of diarrhea and significant morbidity worldwide among children younger than 5 years old. Neurologic symptoms, most commonly seizures, occur in 2% to 3% of children with rotavirus infection.[7] The chronically ill or malnourished child often fails to repair damaged intestinal epithelium post rotavirus infection, leading to a vicious cycle of malnutrition and progressive epithelial injury.

With the introduction of the rotavirus vaccine, there has been a significant decrease in the incidence of RV in the United States.[8-10] According to the CDC, norovirus is now the most common cause of diarrheal illness in children. Two live rotavirus oral vaccines, RotaTeq (RV5) (Merck & Co., Inc.) licensed in 2006 and Rotarix (RV1) (GlaxoSmithKline Biologicals) licensed in 2008, are now approved and are given widely for prevention of rotavirus gastroenteritis. Since the introduction of the RV vaccine in the U.S., a biennial pattern has emerged, with small, short seasons in late winter/early spring,[11] and annual hospitalizations have declined among U.S. children younger than 5 years of age by 80% to 90%.[11,12] It is estimated that since the introduction of the RV vaccine, an estimated 177,000 hospitalizations, 242,000 ED visits, and 1.1 million outpatient visits for diarrhea have been averted among

children younger than 5 years of age.[13] The decrease in hospitalization and ED visits is also decreasing in many other countries as the use of the RV vaccine spreads globally.[14,15]

The current rotavirus vaccines were not associated with intussusception in large pre-licensure trials. There continues to be controversy over whether an increase in intussusception does occur. Some postlicensure studies done in the United States, Canada, Korea, Africa, Brazil, and Taiwan agree with the prelicensure trials showing no increase in intussusception with the RV vaccines.[16-21] However, recent postlicensure surveillance data in the United States[22-24] and internationally[25-27] indicate there is an increased risk of intussusception from the currently licensed RV vaccines. These studies found that most of the increased risk occurs within the first week after the first dose but may occur up to 21 days after the first dose. Although there may be a slight increased risk of intussusception following the oral vaccines, the Centers for Disease Control and Prevention (CDC) and the World Health Organization still recommend the rotavirus vaccine as the benefits of the RV vaccine in preventing severe RV disease far outweigh the risk of intussusception. Parents should be made aware of the risk, the early signs and symptoms of intussusception, and the need for prompt care if they develop.[13]

Human Caliciviruses (Norovirus and Sapovirus). According to the CDC Burden of Norovirus Illness in the United States,[28] each year, norovirus causes approximately 20 million cases of acute gastroenteritis, leading to 1.7 to 1.9 million outpatient visits and 400,000 ED visits, primarily in young children. It also contributes to about 56,000 to 71,000 hospitalizations and 570 to 800 deaths, mostly among young children and the elderly. Norovirus is now the leading cause of acute gastroenteritis among U.S. children less than 5 years of age.[29] Norovirus AGE is associated with more frequent and prolonged vomiting, but less fever, than AGE caused by rotavirus. Seizures are the most common central nervous system (CNS) complication, whereas encephalopathy is possible but rare.[30] Clinical manifestations for sapovirus are similar to those of norovirus.[31]

Astrovirus has a worldwide distribution and has been found in up to 17% of sporadic cases of nonbacterial AGE in children. It accounts for only 2.5% to 9% of severe childhood AGE requiring hospitalization. In healthy children, it is an illness of short duration, although asymptomatic shedding continues up to several weeks after symptom resolution. In the immunocompromised patient, astrovirus infections have been associated with extraintestinal disease, encephalitis, and meningitis.[32,33]

Adenovirus is well known for causing infections of the respiratory tract along with pharyngitis, otitis media, and pharyngoconjunctival fever. Enteric adenovirus serotypes (31, 40 and 41) cause gastroenteritis, accounting for 2% to 4% of cases of acute infectious diarrhea in children. In healthy people, infection with one adenovirus type may confer type-specific immunity or at least lessen symptoms associated with reinfections. Asymptomatic shedding of the virus for months is common.[34]

The mainstay for treatment of viral enteritis is supportive care with rehydration and electrolyte correction.

Bacteria. The common bacterial organisms causing acute diarrhea in U.S. children along with their presentations and associated characteristics are listed in Table 167.3, and their treatment is listed in Table 167.4.

Nontyphoidal *Salmonella* (NTS) is the most common cause of laboratory confirmed cases of enteric disease. The CDC estimates that approximately 1.35 million illnesses and 420 deaths occur annually in the United States due to NTS. In a recent study, the most commonly reported human isolates were *Salmonella* Enteritidis, Typhimurium, Newport, Heidelberg, and Javiana; these 5 serotypes accounted for 62% of U.S. *Salmonella* infections.[35] The incidence of NTS is highest in children less than 4 years of age. Infection can result in an asymptomatic carrier state, AGE, bacteremia, invasive disease, or a disseminated abscess syndrome.

TABLE 167.2   Viruses Causing Diarrheal Illness: Characteristics and Associated Symptoms

	Age	Season	Lasts	Incubation Period	How Spread	Length of Excretion	Abdominal Pain	N/V	Fever	Diarrhea Characteristics	Diagnostics
Rotavirus	<5 years old	Winter and spring	4 to 8 days	Less than 48 hours (1 to 3 days)	Mainly Fecal-oral (can stay on surfaces for weeks to months) or respiratory secretions	Up to 21 days	±	++	±; ⅓ have high fever	Watery; large volume	ELISA and latex agglutination most commonly used; PCR most sensitive
Norovirus	<5 years old	Anytime; colder months	2 to 3 days (up to 5 days)	12 to 48 hours	Fecal-oral; contaminated food and water	5 to 7 days after onset of symptoms; up to 3 weeks	++	++ (some may not vomit)	±	Abrupt onset; watery	RT-PCR testing available; CIDT
Astrovirus	<4 years old	Late winter; early spring	2 to 5 days	1 to 4 days	Fecal-oral	Few days after symptoms resolve	±	+	++	Watery; large volume	CIDT now available
Adenovirus	<4 years old	All year	5 to 12 days	3 to 10 days	Fecal-oral	Most contagious first few days; asym excretion for months	±	+	Low grade	Watery	Commercial test available

Key: ++, common; +, occurs; ±, variable.

N/V, Nausea/vomiting; *ELISA,* enzyme-linked immunosorbent assay; *PCR,* polymerase chain reaction; *RT-PCR,* reverse transcription polymerase chain reaction; *CIDT,* culture-independent diagnostic test.

Data from: World Gastroenterology Organization. *World Gastroenterology Organization global guidelines: acute diarrhea in adults and children: a global perspective.* Available at: www.worldgastroenterology.org/guidelines/global-guidelines/acute-diarrhea/acute-diarrhea-english; and Kimberlin DW, Brady MIT, Jackson MA, Long SS, editors. *Red Book: 2018-2021 Report of the Committee on Infectious Disease,* 31st ed. Itasca, IL; American Academy of Pediatrics; 2018.

TABLE 167.3 Bacteria Causing Diarrheal Illness: Characteristics and Associated Symptoms

	Who Affected	Incubation (range)	Duration of Illness	How Spread	Length of Excretion	Abdominal Pain	N/V	Fever	Diarrhea Characteristics	Other Characteristics	Diagnostic Tests
Salmonella species	<4 years old	12 to 36 hours (6 to 72 hours)	2 to 7 days	Foods from animals; contaminated water; infected reptiles, amphibians, rodents, and mammals	Up to 12 weeks in children <5 years old	++	+	++	Mild to severe; can have blood or mucus	Bacteremia can occur, focal infections in 10%	Stool culture; CIDT starting to be used
Salmonella typhi	Travelers	7 to 14 days (3 to 60 days)	Requires antibiotics	Contaminated food or water	Chronic carriers	++	+	++	Not main problem; mild diarrhea	Gradual onset; HA, malaise, anorexia; HSM, rose spots, dactylitis, ams	Blood, bone marrow, or bile culture
Shigella species	≤5 years old	1–3 (1 to 7 days)	48 to 72 hours	Fecal-oral, contaminated food/water, objects	1 to 4 weeks, antibiotics may shorten excretion	++	++	++	Mild to severe: watery to mucoid with or without blood	Can have systemic symptoms; neurological symptoms; tenesmus; Fecal PMNs often positive	Stool culture; improved with fresh stool, CIDT have high sensitivity; high false-positive rate
Campylobacter	<4 years old	2 to 5 days	5 to 7 days; 15% can relapse or have prolong or severe disease	Ingestion of contaminated foods; fecal-oral in the very young; greatest in acute phase	2 to 3 weeks without treatment; 2 to 3 days with treatment	++ Can mimic appendicitis or intussusception	+	++ Infants may not have fever	Watery to mucoid/bloody	Malaise; can have febrile symptoms before GI symptoms; Infants may have bloody diarrhea and no fever; Can mimic acute inflammatory bowel disease	*C. jejuni* and *C. coli* from stool culture; CIDT, don't differentiate species
Yersinia enterocolitica	<5 years most common	4 to 6 days (1 to 14 days)	Variable; usually few days but diarrhea up to 2 weeks	Contaminated food or water; contact with animals, person to person is rare	Average 2–3 weeks (up to 2–3 mos if untreated)	+	±	++	Often with blood and mucus	Pseudoappendicitis syndrome; Fecal PMNs often positive; Bacteremia: <1 year old, excessive iron storage, immunosuppressed	Stool culture; need to specify
Clostridium difficile	>24 months	Not really known. Colitis usually starts 5 to 10 days after starting antibiotics (up to 10 weeks)	Variable	Fecal-oral or environment	Unknown	+	−	+ Low grade	Mild: watery diarrhea to pseudomembranous colitis; mucus in stool		EIA detection of toxins NAAT good sensitivity and specificity
Clostridium perfringens	Any age	8 to 12 hours (6 to 24 hours)	24 hours	Catered foods	As long as illness persists	++ Crampy, epigastric	−	−	Sudden onset; watery diarrhea	Common in healthy people's stool; Treatment not necessary; short course	High spore count in stool; Commercially available kits

Continued

TABLE 167.3 Bacteria Causing Diarrheal Illness: Characteristics and Associated Symptoms—cont'd.

	Who Affected	Incubation (range)	Duration of Illness	How Spread	Length of Excretion	Abdominal Pain	N/V	Fever	Diarrhea Characteristics	Other Characteristics	Diagnostic Tests
Staphylococcus aureus	Any age	2 to 4 hours (30 minutes to 8 hours)	1 to 2 days	Contaminated food that remains at room temperature for hours	Short time	+	++	± Low grade	Watery	Violent onset of nausea/vomiting; can have mild hypothermia	Culture stool or vomitus EIA or PCR detect enterotoxin
Vibrio cholera	Traveled to endemic area	1 to 3 days (hours to 5 days)	3 to 7 days	Contaminated food and water (shellfish; raw vegetables)	Short time	±	±	±	Large amounts watery diarrhea; stool colorless with flecks of mucus; rice water appearing	Dehydration, hypokalemia, metabolic acidosis and shock within 4 to 12 hours; coma, seizures, hypoglycemia	Stool culture; need to request
Vibrio parahaemolyticus	All ages	23 hours (5 to 92 hours)	2 to 5 days	Seawater; undercooked seafood	Not excreted	++	±	± Low grade	Acute onset Watery stools	Liver disease, low gastric acidity, immunosuppressed increased risk	Lab needs to be notified when test; can test stool, blood, or wounds
E. coli (STEC)	All ages	3 to 4 days (1 to 8 days)	Usually 7 days	Contaminated food or water with human or animal feces; person to person occurs		++	+	– Sometimes low grade	Bloody or nonbloody	Stool becomes bloody after 3 to 4 days; can cause HUS Shiga toxin produced	Stool culture; must request test for *E. coli* O157 EIA for Shiga toxin if available
E. coli (EPEC)	<2 years old; RLAs and travelers	10 hours to 6 days	Usually few days but variable	Contaminated food or water with human or animal feces		–	–		Watery, usually mild	Can become chronic and cause growth retardation No toxin produced	Not widely available
E. coli (ETEC)	Infants in RLAs and travelers of all ages	10 hours to 6 days	1 to 5 days	Contaminated food or water with human or animal feces; person to person occurs		+	–	±	Watery	Uncommon in the U.S. Enterotoxin produced	Not widely available
E. coli (EIEC)	All ages	10 hours to 6 days	Variable	Contaminated food or water with human or animal feces		±	–	+	Usually watery without blood or mucus; dysentery can occur	Related to *Shigella* can cause similar dysenteric illness	Not widely available
E. coli (EAEC)	All ages	10 hours to 6 days	Variable	Contaminated food or water with human or animal feces		±	–	±	Watery, occasionally bloody	Enterotoxin and cytotoxin Associated with prolonged diarrhea; becoming more common in U.S.	Not widely available

Key: ++, common; +, occurs; ±, variable; –, not common.
CIDT, Culture-independent diagnostic test; *EAEC*, enteroaggregative *Escherichia coli*; *EIA*, enzyme immunoassay; *EIEC*, enteroinvasive *E. coli*; *EPEC*, enteropathogenic *E. coli*; *ETEC*, enterotoxigenic *E. coli*; *HA*, headache; *HUS*, hemolytic-uremic syndrome; *GI*, gastrointestinal; *NAAT*, nucleic acid amplification test; *NV*, nausea/vomiting; *PCR*, polymerase chain reaction; *PMN*, polymorphonucleocyte; *RLA*, resource limited area; *STEC*, Shiga toxin-producing *E. coli*
Data from: World Gastroenterology Organization. *World Gastroenterology Organisation global guidelines: acute diarrhea in adults and children: a global perspective.* Available at: www.worldgastroenterology.org/guidelines/global-guidelines/acute-diarrhea/acute-diarrhea-english; and Kimberlin DW, Brady MIT, Jackson MA, Long SS, editors. *Red Book: 2018-2021 Report of the Committee on Infectious Disease,* 31st ed. Itasca, IL; American Academy of Pediatrics; 2018.

TABLE 167.4   Treatment Recommendations for Common Bacteria Causing Acute Infectious Diarrhea in Children

	Routine Treatment	Treatment Indicated—High-Risk Groups	Antibiotic	Comments
Salmonella non-typhi	No; treatment prolongs excretion; does not shorten disease	Infants <3 months old, prolonged illness, chronic GI disease, neoplasms, hemoglobinopathies, HIV, immunosuppression, localized invasive disease (osteomyelitis, abscess, meningitis) or bacteremia	Susceptibility is known Oral: Amoxicillin 25–50 mg/kg divided every 8 hours IV: Ampicillin 200 mg/kg divided every 6 hours (max 8 g/d) Oral: TMP-SMX 10 mg/kg divided every 12 hours (max 160 mg/dose) Susceptibility not known or areas of high resistance or invasive disease or bacteremia IV or IM: Ceftriaxone 50–75 mg/kg q24h (max 2 g) or Oral or IV: Azithromycin 10–20 mg/kg (max 500 mg/dose) or Oral: Adult—[a]Ciprofloxacin 500 mg/dose every 12 hours, Children—[a]Ciprofloxacin 20–40 mg/kg divided every 12 hours (max 1 g/day)	Blood cx before initiating antibiotics. Bacteremia: Treat for 10 to 14 days Localized invasive disease: Treat for 4 weeks (6 weeks if meningitis) and begin with IV medications Aminoglycosides not recommended for invasive disease Drug of choice, route of administration, and duration of therapy based on susceptibility of organisms, site of infection, host and clinical response
Salmonella typhi	Yes	All patients with enteric fever Delirium, stupor, coma, or shock	Start with IV medications; change to oral when susceptibility is known Ceftriaxone 50–75 mg/kg q24h (max 2 g) or [a]Ciprofloxacin 20–40 mg/kg divided every 12 hours (max 1g/day)	Multidrug resistance is common 10- to 14-day treatment Check susceptibilities Azithromycin for uncomplicated disease Consider: Dexamethasone IV 3 mg/kg, followed by 1 mg/kg every 6 hours for 48 hours; relapse is common
Shigella species	No; usually self-limited but treatment decreases diarrhea and eradicates organism from stool	Severe disease, bacteremia, dysentery, immunosuppression Less ill and able to tolerate PO (See Oral dosing)	IV: Ceftriaxone 50 mg/kg (max 2 g) for 5 days (≥ 17 years old) or [a]Ciprofloxacin 20–30 mg/kg/day divided bid or Azithromycin 20 mg/kg/day (max 500 mg) Oral: Azithromycin 12 mg/kg for first day, then 6 mg/kg for days 2 to 5 or [a]Ciprofloxacin 20 mg/kg divided every 12 hours for 5 days	Oral route preferred when possible and disease is not serious TMP-SMX and ampicillin only if isolated strain is susceptible because of high resistance Amoxicillin less effective because of rapid absorption from GI tract; avoid fluoroquinolones if MIC >0.12 even if says susceptible.
Campylobacter jejuni	Variable	Variable recommendations. Most children will resolve on own.	Oral: Azithromycin 10 mg/kg for 3 days (max 500 mg/dose) or Erythromycin 40 mg/kg/day divided every 6 hours (max 2g/day) for 5 days	Shorten duration of illness and excretion of organisms and prevent relapse if given early Resistance to fluoroquinolones is frequent
Yersinia enterocolitica	No; although can be considered as it decreases shedding of the organism;	Neonates, septicemia or extraintestinal sites of infection; immunocompromised host	Oral: TMX-SMX 10 mg/kg divided every 12 hours or Oral or IV fluoroquinolone[a], 10 mg/kg/day of TMP component: Ciprofloxacin 20 mg/kg divided every 12 hours or IV: Ceftriaxone 50 mg/kg qd	Usually resistant to penicillin and first generation cephalosporins Antibiotics do decrease the duration of fecal excretion but do not decrease length of diarrhea Extraintestinal disease treat for 4 weeks. Usually susceptible to tetracycline and doxycycline
C. difficile	Yes	Symptomatic patients Severe disease, underlying intestinal tract disease, and those who don't respond to oral metronidazole use vancomycin	Stop antimicrobial therapy Oral or IV: Metronidazole 30–40 mg/kg/day for at least 10 days (maximum dose 500 mg/dose) if failure to respond in 5 days then: Oral: Vancomycin 40 mg/kg /day divided every 6 hours for at least 10 days (maximum 125mg/dose	25% relapse after treatment, usually responds to second course; IV vancomycin is not effective Do not give antimotility agents; if no abdominal distention and severe disease use Vanco PO and metronidazole IV. If ileus or toxic colitis add vancomycin (1–3 years old: 250 mg/50 mL q6h; 4–9 years old: 375 mg/75 mL q6h; ≥10 years old: 500 mg/100 mL q6h) NS enema until improved

Continued

TABLE 167.4   Treatment Recommendations for Common Bacteria Causing Acute Infectious Diarrhea in Children—cont'd.

	Routine Treatment	Treatment Indicated—High-Risk Groups	Antibiotic	Comments
Vibrio cholera	No	Patients with moderate to severe disease	Oral: Doxycycline[a] 4.4 mg/kg/day divided bid or Azithromycin 20 mg/kg single dose or Tetracycline[a] 50 mg/kg/day divided every 6 hours (maximum 3 g/day) for 3 days	Susceptibility testing recommended Treatment decreases duration of diarrhea and eradicates bacteria from stool; Cipro not recommended in children high treatment failures
V parahae-molytica	No	Severe diarrhea, septicemia Consider in patients <8 years old	Third-generation cephalosporin and doxycycline[a] TMX-SMX and aminoglycoside	
E. coli	No for STEC infection or concern for STEC	Severe watery diarrhea in a traveler to RLA	Azithromycin 10 mg/kg qd ×3 days, ciprofloxacin 30 mg/kg/day divided BID ×3 days[a]	Treating patients with STEC may increase risk for HUS

[a]Fluorquinolone: ciprofloxin recommended for greater or equal to 17 years unless benefits outweigh the risks. Tetracyclines/doxycyclines are not recommended in children younger than 8 years because of teeth staining, but the benefit of using the drug may outweigh the risk of teeth staining. Each case is considered separately. Ciprofloxacin recommended for greater or equal to 17 years unless benefits outweigh the risks.

GI, Gastrointestinal; *HIV,* human immunodeficiency virus; *HUS,* hemolytic-uremic syndrome; *IM,* intramuscular; *IV,* intravenous; *PO, per os* (by mouth); *RLA,* resource limited area; *STEC,* Shiga toxin–producing *E. coli, TMP-SMX,* trimethoprim-sulfamethoxazole.

Data from: Kimberlin DW, Brady MIT, Jackson MA, Long SS, editors. *Red Book: 2018-2021 Report of the Committee on Infectious Disease,* ed 31. Itasca, IL: American Academy of Pediatrics; 2018; and Hughes HK, Kahl LK, editors. *The Harriet Lane Handbook: A Manual for Pediatric House Officers,* ed 21. Philadelphia: Saunders; 2018.

Salmonellae invade the mucosa of the distal small intestine and the colon; they produce a cholera-like enterotoxin and a cytotoxin, which can cause significant diarrhea and fluid and electrolyte abnormalities similar to patients with documented cholera. Fever in NTS patients usually lasts about 48 hours, and patients with prolonged fever may have intermittent bacteremia. Patients with *Salmonella* bacteremia are at increased risk for developing extraintestinal infections, seen in up to 10% of patients with *Salmonella* bacteremia. Infants, the elderly, patients with hemoglobinopathies, and the immunosuppressed are at highest risk for invasive disease. Extraintestinal sites of infection can result in endocarditis, vascular infections, cholecystitis, hepatic and splenic abscesses, urinary tract infections, pneumonia, meningitis, septic arthritis, and osteomyelitis.[36]

Although uncommon, *Salmonella* serotype *typhi* is only found in humans and can cause a bacteremic illness often referred to as *enteric* or *typhoid fever.* Although uncommon in the United States, *S. typhi* is endemic in many resource-limited countries. Typhoid fever may be acquired during international travel and appear as a nonspecific febrile illness in young children in whom sustained or intermittent bacteremia may occur. Constipation can be the presenting symptom and is often seen early in the course of the disease, but diarrhea can also occur. If *S. typhi* is suspected, blood, bone marrow or bile should be cultured, because stool cultures are often negative.[35]

Treatment of noninvasive NTS infection is usually supportive. Antimicrobial treatment is only recommended for infants younger than 3 months and people with chronic gastrointestinal disease, malignant neoplasms, hemoglobinopathies, HIV infections, or other immunosuppressive illnesses or therapies. If treatment is started for presumed disease, stool and blood cultures should be obtained prior to initiating antibiotics. On the other hand, for children with *S. typhi* infection, antibiotics *are* recommended. Relapse of enteric fever occurs in up to 17% of patients and requires retreatment. Treatment failures have occurred in people treated with cephalosporins, aminoglycosides, and furazolidone, despite in vitro testing indicating susceptibility.[36]

Among *Shigella* isolates reported in industrialized nations, most are *Shigella sonnei* (84%). *Shigella flexneri, Shigella boydii,* and *Shigella dysenteriae* account for the remainder.[37] *S. sonnei* is the most common cause of dysentery in the United States. Extraintestinal symptoms and signs are relatively common in children with *Shigella* infection, including hallucinations, confusion, and seizures. Reactive arthritis (Reiter syndrome) can occur weeks after the infection. Rare complications of *Shigella* infection include bacteremia, HUS, toxic megacolon, pseudomembranous colitis, and encephalopathy (Ekiri syndrome). The risk of septicemia increases in neonates, malnourished children, and with *S. dysenteriae.* There is some evidence that antibiotic treatment is effective in shortening duration of diarrhea and hastening eradication of organisms from feces.[37] Drug-resistant *Shigella* has been rapidly increasing; resistance to first-line drugs, ampicillin and trimethoprim-sulfamethoxazole, has become so high that emergency clinicians must rely on alternative drugs like ciprofloxacin and azithromycin. However, over the last 5 years, resistance to these medications has also increased drastically. According to the CDC, both ciprofloxacin and azithromycin resistance has increased from approximately 2% to over 20%. Of particular concern are frequently reported outbreaks of multidrug-resistant *Shigella* among men who have sex with men.[38,39]

Campylobacter species cause a significant proportion of diarrheal disease worldwide, with 1.5 million annual U.S. cases and children younger than 5 years most commonly infected. Of the five types, *C. jejuni* and *C. coli* are the most common.[40,41] In neonates and young infants, bloody diarrhea without fever can be the only manifestation of infection. Febrile seizures can occur in young children before any gastrointestinal symptoms are present. The clinical presentation may be similar to acute appendicitis or intussusception. Severe or prolonged disease can mimic inflammatory bowel disease. Bacteremia is uncommon but can occur in children, including neonates. Immunocompromised hosts can have prolonged, relapsing, or extraintestinal infections. Immunoreactive complications include Guillain-Barré syndrome, reactive arthritis, myocarditis, pericarditis, and erythema nodosum.[41] Antibiotic treatment is recommended for those with severe invasive disease, those at increased risk for severe disease, and for those with prolonged excretion of the bacteria. According to the CDC and the World Health Organization, most healthy children will recover without antibiotic treatment. Azithromycin and erythromycin do shorten the duration of the illness and excretion of the organisms if susceptible. Resistance to antibiotics is increasing. Over 10% of isolates are resistant to azithromycin and erythromycin and over 35% are resistant to ciprofloxacin in the United States. Therefore, if using culture-independent diagnostic tests (CIDT) tests to diagnosis *Campylobacter*, cultures are recommended to confirm diagnosis and for susceptibility information.[38]

Yersinia enterocolitica is a relatively uncommon cause of simple self-limited diarrhea and vomiting in the United States. According to the CDC, there has been a recent increase in the incidence, most likely from CIDT results. *Y. enterocolitica* most often affects children younger than 5 years of age. As many as 6% of older children and adults may present with an appendicitis-like illness, with right lower quadrant tenderness, usually as a result of reactive mesenteric adenitis. Antibiotics are indicated for the immunocompromised patient with enterocolitis and in cases of septicemia or extraintestinal infections. Isolates are often resistant to first-generation cephalosporins and most penicillins. Bacteremia is the major complication of *Y. enterocolitica*, occurring mostly in children less than 1 year of age and in older children with predisposing conditions, including excessive iron storage (e.g., deferoxamine use, sickle cell disease, and beta-thalassemia) and immunosuppressive states. Extraintestinal manifestations of *Y. enterocolitica* are rare. Postinfectious sequelae include erythema nodosum, reactive arthritis, and proliferative glomerulonephritis, most often associated with older children and adults with HLA-B27.[42]

Humans acquire *C. difficile* from their environment or via the oral-fecal route, which can lead to infection. The disruption of the body's normal flora, often as a result of antimicrobial treatment, leads to overgrowth of *C. difficile*, toxin production, and disease development. Exposure to antibiotics is the most important risk factor for *C. difficile*.[43] Penicillins, cephalosporins, clindamycin, and fluoroquinolones are associated more commonly with *C. difficile* infection, whereas sulfonamides, tetracyclines, vancomycin, metronidazole, and aminoglycosides are less commonly linked in children. Pediatric patients who are exposed to multiple antibiotics from different classes in the previous 30 days have been shown in recent studies to be associated with severe and recurrent *C. difficile* infection.[44] Other risk factors include acid-suppressing medications, such as proton pump inhibitors, and use of gastrointestinal feeding tubes.[45]

C. difficile infections cause a spectrum of illnesses ranging from asymptomatic to watery diarrhea to pseudomembranous colitis.[46] Clinical illness is rare before 12 to 24 months of age. Asymptomatic infants can be colonized with *C. difficile*; carriage rates vary by age and range from 37% in neonates to less than 3% by age 2 years.[46,47] *C. difficile* should be considered in children 1 to 3 years old, but only after other causes of diarrhea (particularly viral) are excluded.[47] Endoscopic findings of pseudomembrane and friable rectal mucosa are sufficient to diagnose *C. difficile* at any age. This is helpful when trying to determine if a child younger than 3 years old is colonized or has disease. The endoscopic findings are diagnostic of disease. Complications include toxic megacolon and intestinal perforation. Severe or fatal disease is more common in neutropenic patients with leukemia, infants with Hirschsprung disease, and patients with inflammatory bowel disease.[46,47,48]

See Tables 167.3 and 167.4 for presentation and associated characteristics and treatment recommendations for *Clostridium perfringens*, *Staphylococcus aureus*, *V. cholera*, and *Vibrio parahaemolyticus*.[48-51]

Each year, the WHO Global Burden of Foodborne Diseases reports over 300 million illnesses and nearly 200,000 deaths caused by *E. coli* diarrheagenic infections. *E. coli*, part of the normal flora in the lower gastrointestinal tract, includes five species types recognized to cause acute diarrheal disease. The enterohemorrhagic *E. coli* (EHEC) strain is also known as Shiga toxin–producing *E. coli* (STEC). While there are 50 other serotypes that can cause illness, *E. coli* O157:H7 is the prototype and most virulent of the EHEC and is the one more commonly reported in industrialized countries. Outbreaks have been linked to ground beef, petting zoos, contaminated apple cider, raw fruits and vegetables, and ingestion of water in recreational areas. The infectious dose is low, and person-to-person transmission does occur.[51] In 2016, 52 state and regional public health laboratories reported 5441 cases of culture-confirmed STEC infections. Compared with 2015, the incidence of both STEC O157 and non-O157 infections in 2016 was higher (9% and 15% increase respectively).[52]

HUS, a triad of microangiopathic hemolytic anemia, thrombocytopenia, and renal insufficiency, is a serious complication of EHEC infection and occurs in up to 15% of children with *E. coli* O157:H7.[51] The overall incidence of HUS caused by a diarrheal pathogen (usually STEC) is estimated to be 2.1 cases per 100,000 persons per year, with a peak incidence in children younger than 5 years old (6.1 cases per 100,000 per year). HUS typically develops as diarrhea is resolving, usually at 7 days but may be up to 3 weeks after the onset of the illness.[51] Patients often present with pallor, weakness, irritability, and oliguria or anuria. Patients with HUS can develop neurologic complications, such as seizures, coma, and cerebral vessel thrombosis. Approximately 50% of patients who have HUS will require dialysis, and 3% to 5% die. Indicators that may predict poor outcome for patients with HUS include white blood cell counts greater than 20,000, oliguria or anuria, normal or high hematocrits ($\geq$10.8 g/dl), low sodium less than 128 mEq/L, or presence of a respiratory tract infection within 3 weeks of the diagnosis.[52-54]

A serious risk posed by hemorrhagic colitis is the rapid loss of fluids, which can cause electrolyte abnormalities and result in poor perfusion and end-organ damage. Patients should receive adequate amounts of intravenous (IV) fluids (or by mouth if able to take in enough) to restore intravascular volume (monitor urine output, capillary refill time, blood pressure, pulse, and mental status), and electrolyte abnormalities should be corrected. Fluids should be continued and ongoing losses replaced, with possible admission for ongoing treatment and monitoring of electrolytes, complete blood cell count, blood urea nitrogen (BUN), and creatinine. Evidence from a recent study suggests that patients with HUS who received early volume expansion (increase of body weight by 12.5%) had lower rates of central nervous system involvement, less need for dialysis or intensive care support, and fewer days of hospitalization. These patients also had significantly better long-term outcomes in renal and extrarenal sequale.[55]

Controversy continues to exist about the indications for antibiotic treatment of STEC infections due to a possible association with an increased risk of HUS. To date, there are no controlled trials to support or disprove this association with HUS and the most recently published observation studies found that at least some classes of antimicrobial agents were associated with HUS. Experts continue to advise not prescribing antibiotics for children with *E. coli* 0157 enteritis or a clinical picture strongly suggestive of STEC infection, because no benefit has been found from the use of antibiotics. See Tables 167.3 and 167.4 for presentation and associated characteristics and treatment recommendations for other *E. coli* infections.

Protozoa. Protozoa can also cause diarrhea in children but are responsible for less than 1% of all cases of acute infectious diarrhea in the United States (Tables 167.5 and 167.6). The most common protozoa causing diarrhea are *Cryptosporidium*, *Giardia intestinalis*, and *Entamoeba histolytica*.

Cryptosporidium hominis is the most common of the *Cryptosporidium* species to infect humans. The parasite is protected by an outer shell that allows it to survive outside the body for long periods of time and makes it very tolerant to chlorine disinfection. While this parasite

TABLE 167.5 Protozoa: Presentation and Associated Characteristics

	Who Affected	Incubation	How Spread	Length of Excretion	Abdominal Pain	Nausea/ Vomiting	Fever	Diarrhea Characteristics	Other Chara- cteristics	Diagnostic Tests
Cryptosporidium hominis	All ages	3 to 14 days	Contaminated water; fecal-oral	Immunocompetent: up to 2 weeks Immunosuppressed: Months	±	+	±	Frequent, nonbloody, diarrhea	Fatigue, anorexia and weight loss	DFA for detection of oocysts in stool
Giardia intestinalis	1 to 9 years old	1 to 3 weeks	Fecal-oral, contaminated water or food	Weeks to months	++	+	−	Acute watery diarrhea; foul smelling, flatulence	Can be protracted, abdominal distention, anorexia; FTT, anemia	EIA and DFA tests available; EIA with high sensitivity and specificity
Entamoeba histolytica	Immigrants or visitors to endemic areas	2 to 4 weeks (few days to months)	Fecal-oral; contaminated food or water; sexual transmission	Can excrete for years if untreated	+	±	<½	Colitis to dysentery	Gradual onset of symptoms over 1 to 3 weeks; tenesmus; weigh loss is common	Trophozoites or cysts in stool; serial specimens often necessary; EIA commercially available

Key: ++, common; +, occurs; ±, variable; −, not common.

DFA, Direct fluorescent antibody; EIA, enzyme immunoassay; FTT, failure to thrive.

Data from: World Gastroenterology Organization. *World Gastroenterology Organization Global Guidelines: acute Diarrhea in Adults And Children: A Global Perspective.* Available at: www. worldgastroenterology.org/guidelines/global-guidelines/acute-diarrhea/acute-diarrhea-english; and Kimberlin DW, Brady MIT, Jackson MA, Long SS, editors. *Red Book: 2018-2021 Report of the Committee on Infectious Disease,* ed 31. Itasca, IL: American Academy of Pediatrics; 2018.

TABLE 167.6	Treatment Recommendations for Common Protozoa Causing Infectious Diarrhea in Children			
	Treatment Routinely Recommended	**When Treatment Indicated—High-Risk Groups**	**Antibiotic Indicated**	**Comments**
Cryptosporidium	Not for immunocompetent	If treat: Children >1 year old HIV-positive, organ transplant	Nitazoxanide for children 1 to 3 years old: 100 mg/dose every 12 hours for 3 days 4 to 11 years old: 200 mg q12h x3 days >12yo: 500mg Q12H x3 days	
Giardia intestinalis	Yes	Most require treatment Children >1 year old Children ≥3 years old	Oral: Metronidazole 15–30 mg/kg/day divided every 8 hours for 5 to 10 days (maximum 250 mg /dose) Nitazoxanide: oral use same doses as for Cryptosporidium Tinidazole 50 mg/kg single dose (maximum 2 g/dose)	FDA has not approved of metronidazole for *Giardia* but is least expensive, poor palatability; not as effective as other 2. Symptom recurrence attributed to reinfection, lactose intolerance, immunosuppression, insufficient treatment or drug resistance Second course with same drug should be effective
Entamoeba histolytica	Yes	Asymptomatic excreters Mild to severe intestinal or extraintestinal disease	Oral: Drug of choice: Iodoquinol 30 to 40 mg/kg/day divided every 8 hours for 7 days (maximum 2 g) or Paromomycin 25 to 35 mg/kg/day divided every 8 hours for 7 days Drug of choice: Metronidazole 35 to 50 mg/kg/day divided every 8 hours for 7 to 10 days (max dose 750 mg/dose) or Tinidazole (>3 years old) 50 mg/kg/day for 3 days or 5 days for severe disease followed by Iodoquinol 30 to 40 mg/kg/day divided every 8 hours for 20 days (maximum 2 g) or Paromomycin (if no intestinal obstruction)(same dose as above)	Metronidazole is not effective against cysts. Do not give antimotility agents or corticosteroids Iodoquinol and paromomycin should be taken with meals

Data from: Kimberlin DW, Brady MIT, Jackson MA, Long SS, editors. *Red Book: 2018-2021 Report of the Committee on Infectious Disease*, ed 31. Itasca, IL: American Academy of Pediatrics; 2018; and Hughes HK, Kahl LK, editors. *The Harriet Lane Handbook: A Manual for Pediatric House Officers*, ed 21. Philadelphia: Saunders; 2018.

can be spread in several different ways, water (drinking water and recreational) is the most common way to spread the parasite. In the United States, *Cryptosporidium* is a leading cause of waterborne disease among humans. In the immunocompromised patient, chronic, severe diarrhea can develop and result in malnutrition, dehydration, and death. Cryptosporidiosis should be considered in any patient with solid organ transplant or HIV with diarrhea. Cryptosporidiosis can lead to an increase in tacrolimus levels in transplant patients, leading to acute renal injury. Because shedding can be intermittent, at least three stool specimens collected on separate days should be examined before considering test results to be negative. Treatment is usually supportive. However, the U.S. Food and Drug Administration (FDA) has approved a 3-day course of nitazoxanide oral suspension for the treatment of immunocompetent children older than 1 year of age.[56]

Infection with *Giardia intestinalis* is limited to the small intestine and biliary tract. It is the most common intestinal parasitic infection of humans in the United States and globally. Asymptomatic infection is common. Humans are the main reservoir, although it has been found in the stool of dogs, cats, cattle, rodents, and other animals. These animals can contaminate water with stool containing cysts that are infectious for humans. Epidemics from person-to-person transmission occur in childcare centers and in institutions for people with developmental delay. Treatment includes correction of dehydration and electrolyte abnormalities and antibiotics. If therapy fails, a course can be repeated with the same drug. Relapse is common in the immunocompromised

host, who often requires prolonged treatment. Patients with hypogammaglobinemia or lymphoproliferative disease are at higher risk of giardiasis and more difficult to treat. Patients with acquired immunodeficiency syndrome (AIDS) often respond to standard therapy. Treatment of asymptomatic carriers is not recommended except in households of patients with hypogammaglobinemia or cystic fibrosis.[57]

E. histolytica can be found worldwide but is more prevalent in the lower socioeconomic population and in developing countries, where the prevalence of amebic infection may be as high as 50% in some communities. In the United States, amebiasis is most common in people who have traveled to or immigrants from tropical places with poor sanitation, people who live in institutions with poor sanitary conditions, and men who have sex with men.[58] Symptoms can become chronic and may mimic inflammatory bowel disease. Complications include fulminant colitis, toxic megacolon, and ulceration of the colon and perianal area, rarely with perforation. Complications are more common in patients treated inappropriately with corticosteroids or antimotility drugs. Ultrasonography, computed tomography, and magnetic resonance imaging can identify liver abscesses and other extraintestinal sites of infection. Because complete eradication of intestinal infection is difficult, follow-up stool examination is recommended after completion of therapy. Asymptomatic household members with stools positive for *E. histolytica* should also be treated.[59]

See Tables 167.2, 167.3 and 167.5 for common signs and symptoms of the different viruses, bacteria, and protozoa.

Complications

The complications of acute diarrheal illness are reflected primarily in abnormalities of fluid, electrolytes, acid-base status, and systemic complications (bacteremia, osteomyelitis, polyarthritis, and HUS). Hypoglycemia and metabolic acidosis are common in younger children, yet manifested with nonspecific signs and symptoms, such as tachypnea and decreased activity. With severe illness or illness superimposed on underlying chronic conditions, children may present with weakness, lethargy, respiratory distress, shock, anuria, cardiac dysrhythmia, seizure, or coma. Children with early signs of shock (e.g., persistent tachycardia, hyperpnea, irritability, and lethargy) should have their intravascular volume restored before decompensation occurs.

Diagnostic Strategies

Acute diarrhea in children is usually a self-limited mild disease; it can, however, cause significant fluid and electrolyte abnormalities with serious consequences. Indications for medical evaluation of children with diarrhea have been proposed (Box 167.3). The principal goals of the ED evaluation are to identify and to correct fluid, electrolyte, acid-base, and nutrient deficits that may result from vomiting, diarrhea, or decreased oral intake, and to determine which children would benefit from admission.

Children who present with mild to moderate disease can often rehydrate orally and require no diagnostic testing. In children with moderate to severe dehydration from acute diarrhea (with or without vomiting) who require IV fluids, we recommend assessing serum electrolyte, bicarbonate, urea/creatinine, and glucose levels. Laboratory tests to estimate hydration status have been found helpful only when markedly abnormal, with no single test definitive for dehydration. Children who are critically ill or hemodynamically unstable should have intravenous/intraosseous hydration started immediately along with a finger-stick blood glucose and serum electrolytes.

Testing for fecal leukocytes may be useful to support a diagnosis of invasive disease and should be considered in children with diarrhea who are febrile or have mucus or blood in their stool. Many children with acute diarrhea caused by *Salmonella* or *Shigella* organisms will have fecal leukocytes in the stool. Fecal leukocytes are also found in patients with *Campylobacter*, *Y. enterocolitica*, invasive *E. coli*, and *V. parahaemolyticus*. Although a negative test does not rule out invasive disease, a positive test (more than five fecal leukocytes per high-power field) increases the likelihood of an invasive pathogen and should be followed with a stool culture.

Stool culture is not indicated in most cases of uncomplicated AGE. Stool cultures should be obtained when needed to guide specific therapy, hospitalization, or infection control measures. We recommend stool cultures in patients with systemic involvement, underlying chronic medical conditions, dysenteric features, or a prolonged course (longer than 2 weeks). Many hospital laboratories do not include testing for *E. coli* O157:H7 or *Y. enterocolitica* in their routine stool culture, thus the emergency clinician should order these tests separately. According to the CDC, all stools submitted for testing for *Salmonella*, *Shigella*, and *Campylobacter* (routine stool culture) should be cultured for *E. coli* O157:H7. These stools should also be simultaneously assayed for non-O157 STEC with tests that detect the Shiga toxins or the genes encoding these toxins. In immunosuppressed patients, patients with chronic disease, infants younger than 3 months, or children with possible bacteremia or localized invasive disease, a complete blood count, stool studies, blood and urine cultures, chest x-ray, and lumbar puncture should be considered. For patients with more than 2 weeks of watery diarrhea, consider sending stool for enzyme-linked immunoassay for rotavirus; consider ova and parasites in those with a history of travel to an endemic area.

There is an increase use of culture-independent diagnostic tests for diagnosing intestinal infections: bacterial, viral, and protozoan. CIDTs work by detecting the presence of a specific antigen or genetic sequence of an organism. CIDTs do not require isolation or identification of living organisms. Consequently, these tests can be conducted more rapidly and yield results within a few hours. However, they do not produce bacterial isolates that are needed to distinguish between strains and subtypes of bacteria, information needed to detect and prevent outbreaks, track antibiotic resistance, monitor disease trends, and assess prevention measures. The CDC is encouraging clinical laboratories to do cultures when CIDTs are positive and considering ways to make follow-up cultures easier and cheaper for clinical laboratories. The CDC is encouraging companies to design their CIDTs in a way that keeps the bacteria alive so they can be cultured if the test is positive. The CDC is also adapting their surveillance systems, such as the Foodborne Disease Active Surveillance Network or FoodNet, to include infections diagnosed only by CIDTs.[60]

Differential Diagnoses

Most children with diarrhea or vomiting have a relatively benign cause of their illness, but more serious diagnoses should be considered and ruled out. A few disorders causing diarrhea may be life-threatening in children: intussusception, HUS, pseudomembranous colitis, appendicitis, toxic megacolon, and in very young infants, the congenital secretory diarrheas. See Tables 167.7 and 167.8 for other conditions that may cause vomiting and diarrhea.

Management

The American Academy of Pediatrics (AAP), The European Society of Pediatric Gastroenterology and Nutrition, and the WHO all recommend oral rehydration solution as the treatment of choice for children with mild to moderate dehydration (see the Dehydration section). In addition to fluid resuscitation, the priorities in ED management of children with diarrhea are to consider and rule out potential causes of diarrhea, assess for and treat underlying fluid and electrolyte deficits and potential complications, determine which patients require prolonged treatment or hospitalization, and arrive at a microbiologic diagnosis when indicated. Tables 167.4 and 167.6 list the common infectious agents of diarrhea and their recommended treatment.

Antibiotics are not needed in viral gastroenteritis or in most cases of uncomplicated bacterial gastroenteritis in healthy patients. Antibiotics are routinely recommended for *C. difficile*, *Giardia intestinalis*, and *E. histolytica* and can be considered in *Shigella*, *Campylobacter*, and

---

BOX 167.3   Indications for Medical Evaluation of Children With Acute Diarrhea

Young age (e.g., <6 months old or weight <8 kg)

History of premature birth, chronic medical conditions, or concurrent illness

Fever to ≥38°C for infants <3 months or ≥39°C for children 3 to 36 months old

Visible blood or mucus in stool

High output, including frequent and substantial volumes of diarrhea

Persistent vomiting

Caregiver's report of signs consistent with dehydration (e.g., sunken eyes or decreased tears, dry mucous membranes, or decreased urine output)

Change in mental status (e.g., irritability, apathy, or lethargy)

Suboptimal response to oral rehydration therapy (ORT) already administered or inability of the caregiver to administer ORT

Modified from: King CK, et al. Managing acute gastroenteritis among children: oral rehydration, maintenance, and nutritional therapy. *MMWR Recomm Rep.* 2003;52:1.

TABLE 167.7 Common Causes of Vomiting in Children

Etiologic Category	Clinical Syndromes
Central nervous system (CNS)	Infections, space-occupying lesion
Gastrointestinal	Obstruction, peritonitis, hepatitis, liver failure, appendicitis, pyloric stenosis, midgut volvulus, intussusception, inborn errors of metabolism
Drug	Ingestion, overdose, drug effect
Endocrine	Addisonian crisis, diabetic ketoacidosis, congenital adrenal hyperplasia
Renal	Urinary tract infection, pyelonephritis, renal failure, renal tubular acidosis
Cardiac	Congestive heart failure of any cause
Infection	Pneumonia, acute otitis media, sinusitis, sepsis
Other	Psychogenic, respiratory insufficiency

TABLE 167.8 Common Causes of Diarrhea in Children

Etiologic Category	Clinical Syndromes
Gastrointestinal	Malabsorption (e.g., milk intolerance, excessive fruit juice), inflammatory bowel disease, irritable bowel syndrome, short gut syndrome
Drug	Ingestion, overdose, drug effect
Endocrine	Thyrotoxicosis, addisonian crisis, diabetic enteropathy, congenital adrenal hyperplasia
Renal	Urinary tract infection, pyelonephritis
Infection	Pneumonia, acute otitis media, sinusitis, sepsis
Other emergencies	Intussusception, appendicitis, hemolytic uremic syndrome (HUS), pseudomembranous colitis, toxic megacolon, and in very young infants, the congenital secretory diarrheas
Other	Parental anxiety, chronic nonspecific diarrhea

Cryptosporidium. Premature babies (younger than 1 year old), neonates, young infants, and patients with immunosuppression, chronic diseases, and articular or valve prostheses are at increased risk for developing complications from pathogens causing acute diarrhea (e.g., bacteremia, sepsis, invasive disease, extraintestinal disease). Antibiotics should be considered in these populations based on severity of presentation and in consultation with appropriate specialists (e.g., pediatric infectious disease specialist, pediatric oncologist, or pediatric cardiologist). Children with bloody diarrhea are at higher risk for complications, including sepsis and other systemic diseases, and should be considered for admission. In the majority of cases, empirical antimicrobial agents should not be administered while awaiting culture results. Antimicrobial therapy may not be indicated, even when culture results are positive, and antibiotics may increase the risk for developing HUS if the offending agent is STEC.[61] For severe watery diarrhea in a traveler to a developing country, azithromycin or a fluoroquinolone may be considered.[51]

Antidiarrheal compounds that impair gastrointestinal motility, such as loperamide (Imodium), diphenoxylate, and atropine (Lomotil), can prolong and exacerbate disease and have no role in the treatment of acute infectious diarrhea in young children. These agents may also cause lethargy, paralytic ileus, toxic megacolon, CNS depression, coma, and even death.[61]

Probiotics have been studied extensively over the past several years for the treatment of acute infectious diarrhea. Studies done in the past showed that probiotics, especially *Lactobacillus rhamnosus* (LGG), decrease the duration of diarrhea by approximately one day. Recent studies evaluating specific probiotics (i.e., *Lactobacillus reuteri*,[62] *Lactobacillus casei* variety rhamnosus,[63] and *Bifidobacterium lactis*[64]) found a modest decrease in duration, frequency of diarrhea, and length of hospital stay in patients with acute infectious diarrhea. The European Society of Gastroenterology, Hepatology, and Nutrition recommend that only LGG and *S. boulardii* be considered in the treatment of AGE in children as an adjunct to oral rehydrating solution.[65] Recommendations for children in the Asia–Pacific region have also strongly supported the use of LGG and *S. boulardii* as adjunct treatments to oral rehydration therapy for gastroenteritis.[66] However, the PECARN Probiotic Study Group recently published a large prospective, randomized, double-blind trial involving over 900 children 3 months to 4 years of age with acute gastroenteritis. They found that the children receiving LGG did not benefit with respect to the duration or frequency of vomiting or diarrhea, the rate of household transmission, or the duration of day-care or work absenteeism.[67] No studies have found any significant side effects in probiotics used in otherwise healthy children. However, it is recommended that caution be used for premature infants, immunocompromised and critically ill patients, and those with central venous catheters, cardiac valvular disease, and short–gut syndrome.[66] Further research is needed to establish efficacy, safety, and dosing of probiotics for children with acute infectious diarrhea.

Zinc deficiency is common in developing countries and occurs in most parts of Latin America, Africa, the Middle East, and south Asia. During the past 10 to 15 years, studies have shown that zinc supplementation given to children living in developing countries has decreased the duration and severity of diarrhea illness. A recent Cochrane review of 33 published studies including over 10,000 children found zinc supplementation may be effective in reducing the duration of diarrhea in children older than 6 months in areas where zinc deficiency and moderate malnutrition are prevalent.[68] The WHO recommends zinc supplementation (10 to 20 mg/day for 10 to 14 days) for all children younger than 5 years old with AGE, although few data exist to support this recommendation for children in developed countries.

Disposition

Most cases of childhood diarrhea can be managed on an outpatient basis by continuing breastfeeding, routine formula, or diet specific for age. Supplemental maintenance electrolyte solutions may be given or recommended to purchase over the counter. Before discharge from the ED, careful and specific instruction about the signs and symptoms of expected improvement or complications should be given to the parents or caregiver. Instructions should address proper hygiene and hand-washing techniques to prevent others from contracting the illness. Follow-up by the patient's primary care physician should be timely and address concerns of worsening of the condition and potential complications. Hospitalization should be considered in children at high risk for complications: infants, especially those younger than 3 months old; very-low-birth-weight infants; children with chronic medical problems; children with electrolyte abnormalities who require IV repletion; children with severe dehydration; and children with dysentery. Hospitalization may also be warranted in cases of protracted vomiting, diarrhea with losses in excess of fluid administration, worsening clinical status despite therapy, presence of an underlying condition that would complicate therapy, or suspected systemic involvement. Very-low-birth-weight infants, because of low physiologic reserve and immature immune system, are at the highest risk for complications of AGE in the first year of life.

TABLE 167.9   Isonatremic, Hyponatremic, and Hypernatremic Volume Depletion

Volume Depletion Type	Sodium and Water Balance	Pathologic Causes	Fluid Shifts	Osmotic CNS Complications
Isonatremic (Na 130–150 mEq/L)	Balanced loss of sodium and free water	GI fluid loss with or without replacement	None	None
Hyponatremic (Na <130 mEq/L)	Greater sodium loss	GI fluid loss with excess free water replacement, cerebral salt wasting, syndrome of inappropriate antidiuretic hormone (SIADH)	Shift to intracellular space; Depleted intravascular volume (appears more ill than history suggests)	Cerebral edema, seizures
Hypernatremic (Na >150 mEq/L)	Greater free water loss, associated with severe dehydration	GI losses with hypertonic fluid replacement or poor breastfeeding, excess insensible losses, diabetes insipidus	Shift to extracellular space; preserved intravascular volume (appears less ill than history suggests)	Cerebral dehydration (risk for bridging vein injury and thrombus)

CNS Complications From Rapid Correction	Skin Turgor on Exam	Management
None	Normal or tenting	Mild-moderate: oral rehydration therapy; severe: Rapid infusion of 20 ml/kg isotonic saline to restore perfusion, then oral rehydration therapy or maintenance IV fluid to resolve fluid loss
Osmotic demyelination syndrome (central pontine myelinolysis)	Tenting	Rapid infusion of 20 mL/kg isotonic saline to restore perfusion, then correction of sodium over 24–48 hours, avoid correction >10 mEq/L/day
Cerebral edema	Doughy	Rapid infusion of 20 mL/kg isotonic saline to restore perfusion, then correction of sodium over 24–48 hours, avoid correction >10 mEq/L/day

DEHYDRATION

Foundations

Anatomy and Physiology

The average adult male and female bodies are comprised of approximately 60% and 50% water, respectively. Total body water is divided between the extracellular (one-third) and intracellular compartments (two-thirds). The extracellular compartment is further divided into interstitial fluid (three-quarters) and plasma (one-quarter). Interstitial fluid serves as a reservoir to replenish intravascular plasma volume in hypovolemia. Water makes up over 70% of an infant's total body weight; the majority of this "extra" fluid resides in the extracellular compartment. Because infants excrete far more water than adults per body weight (100 mL/kg versus 40 mL/kg daily), they require far more water per body weight to maintain homeostasis. As a result, infants and children are more vulnerable to rapid volume depletion from decreased water intake or increased output.

Pathophysiology

Volume depletion management and complications depends on serum sodium concentration (Table 167.9). The most common clinical presentation is isonatremic volume depletion with hypernatremic volume depletion being less common than isonatremic or hyponatremic volume depletion.

Metabolic acidosis often accompanies pediatric dehydration due to AGE through several mechanisms: bicarbonate loss in the stool, starvation causing ketone production, decreased tissue perfusion leading to anaerobic metabolism and lactic acid production, and decreased hydrogen ion excretion from poor renal perfusion. For the majority of patients, the acidosis is easily reversed by oral or parenteral volume replacement.

Clinical Features

The severity of dehydration is usually measured as the acute weight loss (presumably fluid loss) as a percentage of pre-illness total body weight.

TABLE 167.10   Clinical Assessment of Degree of Dehydration

Signs and Symptoms	Mild (3% To 5%) (30 to 50 mL/kg)	Moderate (5% To 10%) (60 to 100 mL/kg)	Severe (>10%) (90 to 150 mL/kg)
Dry mucous membrane	±	+	+
Reduced skin turgor (pinch retraction)	–	±	+
Depressed anterior fontanel	–	+	+
Mental status	Alert	Irritable	Lethargic
Sunken eyeballs	–	+	+
Hyperpnea	–	±	+
Hypotension (orthostatic)	–	±	+
Increased pulse	–	+	+
Capillary refill	<2 seconds	>2 seconds	>2 seconds

+, Present; –, absent; ±, variable.
Adapted from: Barkin RM, Rosen P. *Emergency Pediatrics*, ed 5. St Louis: Mosby; 1999.

Dehydration of 3% to 5% or more is considered significant and can often be identified by history and physical examination (Table 167.10). Because pre-illness weights are neither generally available nor reliably reported, the clinician should rely on historical information and physical examination findings to assess the severity of dehydration. Parental reports of decreased oral intake, urine output, and tear production are of significant value, with good sensitivity in detecting dehydration. In a child who is dehydrated, initial physical examination may reveal an

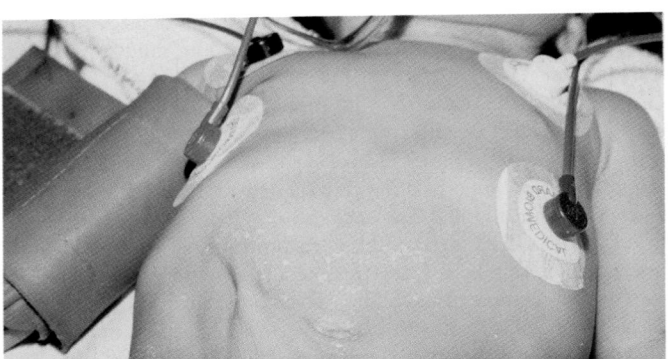

Fig. 167.1 Skin tenting. (Image courtesy of Dr. Stanley Inkelis.)

TABLE 167.11 Clinical Dehydration Scale

	0	1	2
	0: No Dehydration (<3%)	**1–4: Some Dehydration (≥3% to 6%)**	**5–8: Moderate Dehydration (≥6%)**
General appearance	Normal	Thirsty, restless, or lethargic but irritable when touched	Drowsy, limp, old, sweaty, or comatose
Eyes	Normal	Slightly sunken	Very sunken
Mucous membranes	Moist	"Sticky"	Dry
Tears	Present	Decreased	Absent

GORELICK SCALE

	No or Minimal Dehydration	**Moderate to Severe Dehydration**
General appearance	Alert	Restless, lethargic, unconscious
Capillary refill	Normal	Prolonged or minimal
Tears	Present	Absent
Mucous membranes	Moist	Dry, very dry
Eyes	Normal	Sunken, deeply sunken
Breathing	Normal	Deep, rapid
Quality of pulses	Normal	Thready, weak or impalpable
Skin elasticity	Instant recoil	Slow recoil, recoil >2 seconds
Heart rate	Normal	Tachycardia
Urine output	Normal	Reduced

Four-point scale (italics): Two signs or more ≥5%; three signs or more ≥10%.

Ten-point scale (including all): Three signs or more ≥5%; seven signs or more ≥10%.

Adapted from: Jauregui J, Nelson D, Choo E, et al. External validation and comparison of three pediatric clinical dehydration scales. *PLoS One.* 2014;9(5):e95739.

activity level lower than expected for age. The child may also appear weak or lethargic. If the fontanel is still open, it may be sunken. The eyes may appear sunken and the mucous membranes dry. However, if the child has recently had something to drink, the mucous membranes may falsely appear moist. Tachycardia and hyperpnea may be present. The skin over the trunk should be examined for tenting (Fig. 167.1; suggesting hyponatremia) or a doughy texture (suggesting hypernatremia). The three most useful signs to determine dehydration of more than 5% are prolonged capillary refill time, abnormal skin turgor, and abnormal respiratory pattern. However, clinical signs and symptoms of dehydration are variable and often subtle and determining the severity of dehydration is an ongoing challenge for emergency clinicians. Because individual signs are often inadequate for accurately diagnosing dehydration and estimating severity, most recent research has focused on noninvasive methods of dehydration assessment, including clinical scoring systems, bedside ultrasound, and laboratory testing.[69]

Clinical scoring systems have been developed by combining historical features and examination findings in an effort to better predict the presence and severity of pediatric dehydration. The Clinical Dehydration Score (CDS) and the Gorelick scale (Table 167.11) are the most widely used and well-studied. In 2015, a meta-analysis found both the CDS and Gorelick scale improve diagnostic accuracy over unstructured clinician assessment. However, with only approximately 80% accuracy, neither can definitively rule in or out dehydration in infants and children.[69] Falszewska and colleagues analyzed a cohort of 118 patients hospitalized for dehydration with the CDS, Gorelick, and WHO scales in 2017 and found only the CDS to be useful only in ruling in (LR 3.9) moderate dehydration (>6 %).[70] This suggests that additional clinical tools are needed to aid in the diagnosis of dehydration.

Diagnostic Strategies

The role of point-of-care ultrasound (POCUS) in the assessment of volume depletion in children is uncertain. Inferior vena cava (IVC) collapsibility has not been shown to correlate with dehydration in pediatric patients. IVC to aorta diameter ratio was analyzed in a population of 771 children with diarrhea and dehydration in a resource-limited environment in Bangladesh by Modi and colleagues; they found it has an unacceptably low sensitivity (67%) and specificity (49%) for evaluation for severe dehydration.[71] Current research suggests that the POCUS measurement of the ratio of the areas of the aorta to the IVC correlate with clinical dehydration scores and that this ratio changes in response to rapid IV fluid administration.[72,73] Further research is required before this application can be recommended for routine evaluation of dehydration in pediatric patients.

Laboratory tests are of little diagnostic value in the mildly dehydrated child, but they may be helpful in the severely dehydrated or

ill-appearing child to assess etiology, severity, and complications of dehydration. A serum electrolyte panel, BUN, serum creatinine, and blood glucose level are most likely to be clinically useful. Sodium concentration is important in identifying isonatremic, hyponatremic, and hypernatremic states for appropriate choice of therapy, but resuscitation and treatment should not be delayed for laboratory results. A low serum bicarbonate level may indicate bicarbonate loss in the stool or may reflect poor tissue perfusion. Children with dysentery, characterized by fever, bloody stools, and abdominal cramping, should have BUN and serum creatinine concentrations measured and stool culture specimens sent and examined for *E. coli* O157:H7 to identify potential cases of HUS. Serum glucose level is important because hypoglycemia is not uncommon in young children with AGE, and this test may help identify children with previously undiagnosed fatty acid oxidation disorders or other inborn errors of metabolism (e.g., galactosemia). Urine specific gravity and ketones are neither sensitive nor specific and should not be used in the assessment of pediatric dehydration.

TABLE 167.12 Differential Diagnosis of Volume Depletion

Fluid Loss Category	Potential Etiologic Disorders or Conditions
Renal	Diuretics, renal tubular acidosis, renal failure, urinary tract obstruction, diabetes insipidus, diabetes mellitus, hypothyroidism, adrenal insufficiency, renal trauma, salt-wasting nephritis
Extrarenal	Third spacing (pancreatitis, peritonitis, sepsis), skin loss (burns, cystic fibrosis), lung loss, congestive heart failure, liver failure, hemorrhage

BOX 167.4 Principles of Appropriate Treatment of Children With Diarrhea and Dehydration

Oral rehydration solutions should be used for rehydration.
Oral rehydration should be performed as rapidly as possible.
Unrestricted diet is recommended as soon as dehydration is corrected.
For breast-fed infants, nursing should be continued.
For formula-fed infants, diluted formula is not recommended. Special formula is not necessary.
Additional oral rehydration solution should be administered for ongoing diarrheal losses.

Modified from: King CK, et al. Managing acute gastroenteritis among children: oral rehydration, maintenance, and nutritional therapy. *MMWR Recomm Rep.* 2003;52:1.

Differential Diagnoses

Most commonly, dehydration in children results from diarrhea and vomiting caused by infectious gastroenteritis. Table 167.12 lists some other causes of dehydration that should be considered when the gastrointestinal tract is not primarily involved.

Management

Oral Rehydration Therapy

Oral rehydration therapy (ORT) is a safe and effective treatment of infants and children with mild to moderate dehydration. ORT may be instituted even if the patient continues to vomit or has diarrhea. However, children with severe dehydration, shock, lethargy, acute abdomen, suspected intestinal obstruction, sodium derangement, or significant underlying illness should receive IV fluids. Some of these principles are illustrated in Box 167.4.

The ORT period in the ED may span 4 to 8 hours and provides an opportunity to educate the family in skills of evaluating and treating childhood diarrhea. A number of oral rehydration solutions have been shown to be effective. The main ingredients are water, glucose, sodium chloride, citrate, and bicarbonate in various concentrations. In most situations, rehydration can be accomplished without the risk of causing hyponatremia or hypernatremia. Polymer-based carbohydrate solutions (derived from wheat or rice) continue to be investigated as an alternative to glucose-based solutions. A Cochrane review in 2016 showed that patients treated with polymer-based solutions compared with high osmolarity solutions (>310 mOsm/L) had cessation of diarrhea sooner.[74] Their comparison of polymer-based solutions to low osmolarity solutions (<270 mOsm/L, which describes most current oral rehydration solutions) trended towards faster resolution of diarrhea, but the study was not powered sufficiently to demonstrate

the effect. These data suggest that polymer-based and low osmolarity glucose solutions are both effective at treating mild to moderate dehydration.

In infants and children with minimal dehydration, treatment should be directed at maintaining hydration and nutrition with an age-appropriate diet. Freedman and colleagues showed that children age 6 months old to 60 months old with mild dehydration (CDS of 4 or less and with capillary refill < 2 seconds) from AGE given dilute apple juice in the ED and discharged with instructions for patient preference of hydration had significantly less treatment failure and less frequent need for IV fluids compared to children given oral rehydration solution in the ED and discharged with oral rehydration solution information.[75] This suggests that age-appropriate diet and fluids of patient preference is an effective alternative to oral rehydration solutions in patients with mild dehydration from AGE. Fluid intake should be increased, or oral rehydration can be administered to cover maintenance and to replace losses. Losses can be replaced at 10 mL/kg for each stool and 2 mL/kg for each emesis. Diet should not be restricted.

Children with mild to moderate dehydration should have their estimated fluid deficit replaced, often started in the ED and continued at home. The volume of ORT is calculated in the following manner:

1. Estimate the degree of volume depletion as mild or moderate with information from the history, clinical signs, and physical examination findings (see Tables 167.10 and 167.11).
2. Calculate the desired volume of oral rehydration solution as 30 to 50 mL/kg for mild (3% to 5%) and 60 to 80 mL/kg for moderate (6% to 9%) volume depletion.
3. Administer 25% of the volume of oral rehydration solution to be replaced each hour for the first 4 hours.
4. Replace ongoing losses at 10 mL/kg for each stool and 2 mL/kg for each emesis.
5. Monitor progress hourly and reevaluate frequently.

This technique requires that the ED have the facilities and personnel to observe and to monitor the patient for an extended time to determine the success or failure of ORT. The parent or other caregiver should be taught to administer ORT. Nursing personnel should instruct the parent in observation skills, methods of administration of the fluid, and types of fluid that are considered appropriate for children with vomiting and diarrhea. During the monitoring period, a child who is unable to tolerate intake of the prescribed volume of fluid at the expected rate should receive IV fluids. It is important to determine whether the failure is the result of the child's inability to ingest the fluid, excessive fluid loss through vomiting or diarrhea, or poor technique or motivation on the parent's part. It usually is possible to maintain the fluid administration rate in children who continue to vomit by administering small volumes frequently. This may require, for instance, use of a spoon or syringe to slowly drip the fluid by hand. Some success has been obtained with the use of nasogastric tubes; this method is often useful for prolonged fluid replacement in an inpatient setting, though its invasiveness limits its use.

The patient is reassessed at the end of the first few hours of ORT. If the clinical examination indicates adequate volume repletion, the child may be discharged home with further specific instructions for parents about maintenance fluid requirements with oral rehydration solution. If the child still exhibits mild or moderate volume depletion on clinical examination but no deterioration in status has occurred, another 2- to 4-hour trial may be warranted. If the child is unable to ingest the appropriate volume to keep up with ongoing losses, or if volume repletion is not adequate at the end of 8 hours, IV therapy and admission are recommended.

Ondansetron has become a useful adjunct in the treatment of AGE in the ED. Ondansetron, a selective 5-hydroxytryptamine type 3 receptor antagonist, acts at chemoreceptors in the peripheral and CNS to alleviate nausea. Ondansetron has been shown in a meta-analysis of numerous well-designed studies in children to reduce episodes of vomiting in the ED, improve oral intake in the ED, reduce the need for IV fluid rehydration, and reduce admissions.[76] Prescribing oral ondansetron for home use with good return precautions is safe in AGE, but multiple studies have shown it does not significantly change frequency of ED return visits.[77,78] Further research on patient-centered outcomes in this area is needed to evaluate the effectiveness of ondansetron prescriptions in outpatient management of dehydration.

Intravenous Therapy

Some dehydrated children brought to the ED may not qualify for ORT, and others may fail to improve with ORT. These patients include those with shock, severe dehydration, increasing deficit or clinical deterioration during ORT, intractable vomiting, hypoglycemia, or electrolyte derangements.

Patients are evaluated in accordance with their immediate (emergency phase), short-term (repletion phase), and long-term (early refeeding phase) needs.[79] During the *emergency* phase, the aim of fluid resuscitation is to restore circulatory volume. Fluid needs to be administered rapidly to prevent tissue hypoperfusion, end-organ damage, and death. During the *repletion* phase, fluid and electrolyte derangements are reversed, and ongoing losses are replaced. This phase lasts 24 hours. In the *early refeeding* phase, long-term needs are addressed in the next few days, during which the body recovers fluid, electrolyte, and nutritional homeostasis. Immediate and short-term therapies are initiated in the ED, with subsequent phases carried out in the inpatient setting or at home through the primary care physician. In clinical practice, this algorithm represents a continuum of care and not three separate phases.

Emergency Resuscitation Phase. Rapid reexpansion of the intravascular space is the goal of immediate resuscitation and can be achieved with an isotonic crystalloid solution. Administration of 20 mL/kg of 0.9% saline (or other appropriate isotonic crystalloid solution) intravenously at a rapid rate should result in reversal of signs of shock within 5 to 15 minutes. Avoid low sodium solutions such as lactated Ringers solution (Na 130 mEq/L) in isonatremic and hyponatremic volume depletion.[80] In critical situations, intraosseous routes should be used if venous access is not immediately available. Patients should be reevaluated periodically, and those with excessive deficits should receive repeated boluses of 20 mL/kg until clinical improvement occurs. Signs of recovery include normalization of blood pressure measurements, improvement of mental status, improvement of tachycardia and capillary refill time, and production of urine. Intravenous volume replacement greater than 60 mL/kg, without signs of improvement, warrants investigation for other conditions, such as cardiogenic shock, septic shock, hemorrhage, capillary leak with third-space fluid sequestration, adrenal insufficiency, and toxic shock.

A rapid determination of serum glucose is important. Children require glucose as an energy substrate and often have marginal stores available in illnesses. If the serum glucose concentration is low (<50 mg/dL), dextrose 0.25 to 0.5 g/kg should be rapidly administered intravenously or intraosseously. Glucose can be administered per the "rule of 50," whereby the percent dextrose multiplied by the number of mL per kilogram equals 50. For neonates, a 10% dextrose solution should be given at approximately 5 mL/kg. Children 1 month old to approximately 8 years old or 25 kg should be given 2 mL/kg of 25% dextrose. In children older than 2 years old, 1 mL/kg of 50% dextrose can be used. The higher tonicity 50% and 25% dextrose solutions have a risk of causing tissue necrosis if they extravasate during peripheral IV infusion. Ten percent dextrose is a safe and effective treatment for hypoglycemia

in all ages, and it has a lower tonicity if there is concern for extravasation in a peripheral IV. Glucose levels should be monitored (every 30 to 60 minutes until stable) to ensure improvement and to identify ongoing needs. Repeated episodes of hypoglycemia should raise concern for sepsis, adrenal insufficiency, fatty acid oxidation defects, or other inborn errors of metabolism.

Dehydration due to AGE in children often leads to metabolic acidosis and ketosis, in part due to reduced carbohydrate intake leading to free fatty acid breakdown. It has been hypothesized that the addition of dextrose to initial IV rehydration fluids in moderately to severely dehydrated children will stimulate insulin release, reduce free fatty acid breakdown and ketone production, and reduce ketone-induced nausea and vomiting. A meta-analysis of two studies that had 333 pooled, randomized patients to IV solutions with and without glucose, found no difference in hospitalization rates or ED return visits.[81] Further research focusing on patient-oriented outcomes is needed to determine whether dextrose should be included in the optimal rehydration regimen for moderately to severely dehydrated children requiring IV hydration.

Repletion Phase. Appropriate fluid therapy for the patient should be determined after initial resuscitation. Some patients may tolerate ORT; others may require ongoing parenteral hydration with 5% dextrose in half-normal normal at a weight-appropriate maintenance volume (Table 167.13), compensating for ongoing losses (10 mL/kg and 2 mL/kg for each diarrhea and vomiting episode, respectively). Potassium may be added to maintenance fluids once urine output is established and serum potassium levels are within a normal range. Overly rapid correction of serum sodium levels can lead to osmotic demyelination syndrome (central pontine myelinolysis) in hyponatremia and cerebral edema in hypernatremia.[80] Neurologic status and serum sodium concentration should be closely monitored and the amount of sodium content of repletion fluid adjusted to maintain a slow correction. Ongoing sodium losses should also be replaced. In addition to oral, IV, intraosseous, and nasogastric routes of fluid delivery, hyaluronidase-facilitated subcutaneous hydration (hypodermoclysis) offers yet another alternative for treatment of dehydration. A small-gauge catheter is inserted in subcutaneous tissue in an area without local neurovascular structures (e.g., between scapulae, anterior chest, deltoid, anterior/lateral thigh) and 20 ml/kg isotonic crystalloid can be infused. Hyaluronidase (150 units subcutaneously, independent of age or weight) breaks down hyaluronic acid, a chief component of the extracellular matrix that holds body tissues together and expedites the subcutaneous infusion. Subcutaneous hydration can be performed without hyaluronidase at a significantly reduced rate, limiting its utility in the ED. Certain medications, such as ondansetron and other antiemetics, can be administered by this route.[82] Subcutaneous hydration should be considered in mildly to moderately dehydrated children who are unable to tolerate oral fluids and who have difficult IV access; patients with severe dehydration should be evaluated for intraosseous or IV access.

TABLE 167.13 Holliday-Segar Method for Maintenance IV Fluids

Body Weight	MAINTENANCE RATE	
	mL/kg/day	mL/kg/hr
First 10 kg	100	4
Second 10 kg	50	2
Each additional kg	20	1

Modified from: Nalley CM. Fluids and electrolytes. In: Hughes HK, Kahl LK, editors. *The Harriet Lane Handbook: A Manual for Pediatric House Officers*, ed 21. Philadelphia: Saunders; 2018: 290-315.

Hospital-Acquired Hyponatremia. IV rehydration can lead to hyponatremia in children. This rare complication can lead to significant neurologic morbidity, including seizures, coma, and brain herniation or even death; children receiving IV fluids should have their neurologic status closely monitored. AAP clinical practice guidelines recommend use of isotonic saline for maintenance IV fluids, except in patients with voluminous watery diarrhea; in these patients, providers should consider hypotonic maintenance fluids to treat persistent free water loss with higher than normal maintenance rates.[83]

Disposition

Children with severe dehydration, intractable vomiting, inability to maintain oral hydration, severe metabolic acidosis or sodium derangement, or whose caregivers are unable to provide adequate care at home should be hospitalized. Observation status is often suitable for severely dehydrated children showing signs of improvement during their ED course.

The references for this chapter can be found online at ExpertConsult. com.

168

Pediatric Genitourinary and Renal Tract Disorders

Brittany Boswell and Anita A. Thomas

FOUNDATIONS

Genitourinary (GU) and renal tract emergencies in children are common. These issues span age and gender and have varying clinical presentations. Underlying pathology is due to both congenital and acquired disease. Careful history of present illness and family history can help guide a focused differential diagnosis. A complete physical is especially important in children who present with abdominal pain; in particular, a GU examination must be performed for any male that presents with abdominal pain because children may not be as forthright with GU complaints. The history and complete physical are key in guiding workup and management of renal and GU emergencies. This chapter outlines the most prevalent GU and renal disorders presenting to emergency clinicians.

SPECIFIC DISORDERS

Priapism

> **KEY CONCEPTS**
> - Ischemic priapism is a urologic emergency due to compartment syndrome of the penis and is managed with local analgesia with or without sedation, cavernosal aspiration, irrigation, and possibly injection with phenylephrine.

Foundations

Priapism is a pathologic painful penile erection, unrelated to sexual stimulation, lasting more than 4 hours. There are three types of priapism: low flow (ischemic), high flow (nonischemic), and stuttering (recurrent). Ischemic priapism is due to venous occlusion, leading to compartment syndrome of the penis, and is a *urologic emergency*. Nonischemic, or high flow priapism, is due to unregulated cavernosal blood flow, often due to trauma or arteriocavernous fistula, and is usually painless. In this subtype, oxygenation is preserved and can be managed conservatively. Lastly, stuttering priapism is due to recurrent episodes of ischemic priapism, lasting less than 4 hours. It is often self-limited, and primarily occurs in patients with sickle cell disease.

Clinical Features

Priapism is rare in pediatrics, although it may be underreported. It can occur at any age, even rarely, in the neonatal population.[1] Sickle cell disease accounts for 65% of all episodes of priapism occurring in children. Up to 89% of men with sickle cell disease have reported at least one episode of priapism before the age of twenty.[2] Patients present with painful rigidity of the corpus cavernosa and a soft glans (Fig. 168.1). Depending on the duration of the episode, one may see sequelae of ischemia such as erythema, other color change, or gangrenous appearance.

Differential Diagnoses

Priapism is a clinical diagnosis. The differential diagnosis of the underlying etiology is outlined in Table 168.1.[3] Laboratory testing can help determine an underlying etiology but is often not helpful in acute management. Complete blood count (CBC), reticulocyte count, and hemoglobin electrophoresis are useful in identifying undiagnosed sickle cell anemia. A cavernosal blood gas and color duplex ultrasonography can help differentiate the subtype of priapism.

Management

Determination of subtype and underlying etiology guide management of priapism. Ischemic priapism requires time-sensitive intervention. Conservative measures may be trialed in patients presenting before 4 hours: physical exercise, urination, and cold packs (except in sickle cell patients in which this may worsen priapism). In patients presenting after 4 hours, or in whom conservative measures have failed, additional treatment includes hydration, pain control, and local anesthesia. This should be followed with intracavernous irrigation of saline and injection of sympathomimetics to achieve detumescence. Various case reports have shown detumescence using procedural sedation alone with either ketamine or nitrous oxide.[4,5] A dorsal penile block with or without a ring block should be performed prior to intracavernous injection, using no more than 4 mg/kg of lidocaine without epinephrine (Fig. 168.2). After local anesthesia, corporal aspiration can be performed by using a 23- to 21-gauge butterfly needle in prepubescent males and a 19-gauge needle in adolescents; the needle should be inserted laterally, into the corpus cavernosum at 3 or 9 o'clock, avoiding the neurovascular bundle superiorly and the urethra inferiorly. Blood should be aspirated in 5 mL aliquots until it appears bright red followed by flush with 0.9% normal saline. A cavernosal blood gas can be sent using this sample. If detumescence is not achieved, the next step is intracavernosal injection of an alpha-adrenergic sympathomimetic agent, phenylephrine (100 mcg every 5 minutes, up to 1 hour.[6] If these measures fail, the patient should be considered for emergent urologic intervention with surgical shunt placement.

Contrary to ischemic priapism, management of stuttering and nonischemic priapism is not urgent, as many cases resolve spontaneously. Ultrasound may identify a fistula that may require arterial embolization or surgical ligation.[7]

Disposition

With successful detumescence, patients may be discharged home with close follow-up. Those who require ongoing injections of phenylephrine will likely need admission, especially if they have cardiac history. Patients who fail injection and require surgery should receive emergent urologic consultation and admission.

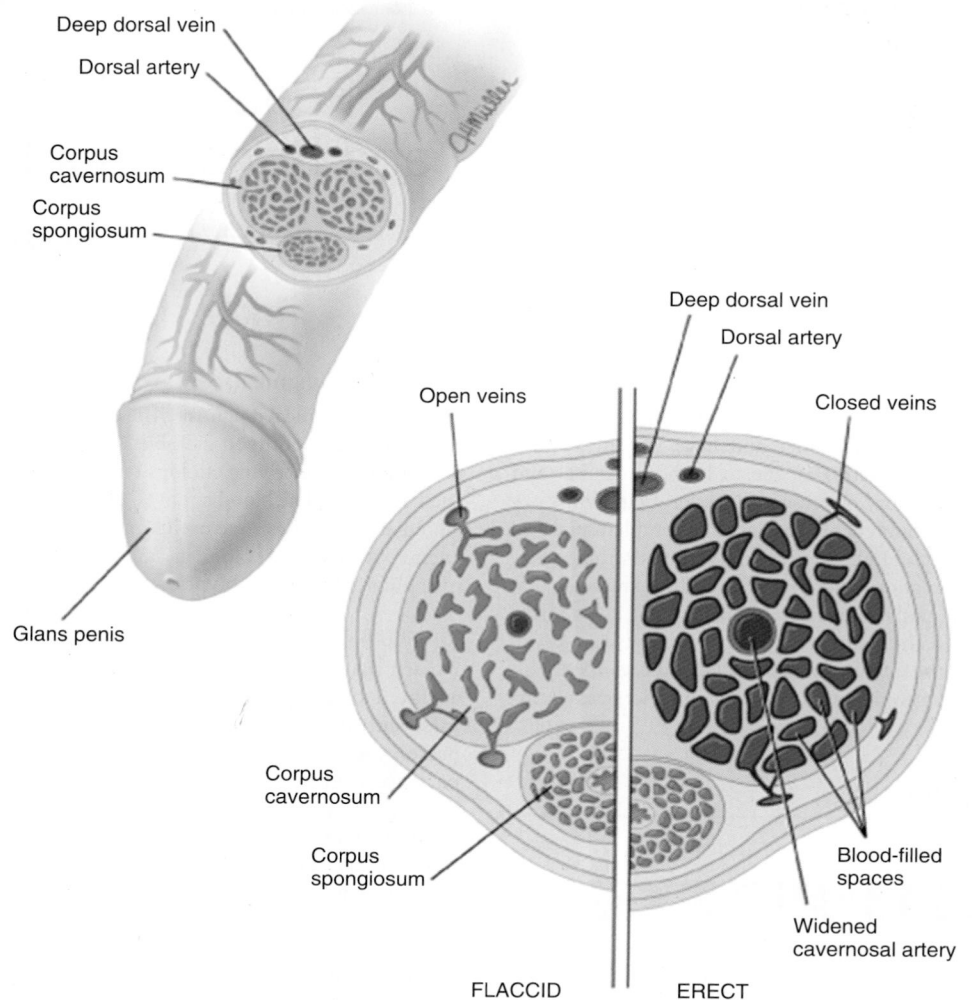

Fig. 168.1 Anatomy of the penis. (Reproduced with permission from: Field JJ, Vemulakonda VM, DeBaun MR. *Diagnosis and management of priapism in sickle cell disease.* www.uptodate.com/contents/diagnosis-and-management-of-priapism-in-sickle-cell-disease.)

TABLE 168.1	Differential Diagnosis of the Underlying Etiology of Priapism		
Ischemic	**Nonischemic**	**Medication Induced**	**Neonatal**
Hemoglobinopathy (SCD, thalassemia)	Trauma	PDE 5 inhibitor	Polycythemia
Leukemia	Hematologic (SCD, leukemia)	Hormone (testosterone)	Infection
Infection	Fabry disease	Antipsychotic	Forceps assisted delivery
Neurogenic	Iatrogenic (surgery)	Antidepressant	Respiratory distress syndrome
Toxin (scorpion, spider)		Antihypertensives	UAC manipulation
Henoch-Schönlein purpura		Alcohol, cocaine, marijuana	

Phimosis

KEY CONCEPTS

- Phimosis is usually physiologic, but is pathologic when associated with urinary retention, urinary tract infections, or balanoposthitis.

Foundations

Phimosis is a clinical diagnosis and defined as the inability to fully retract the prepuce beyond the glans penis. Parents or patients may describe a "balloon appearance" of the foreskin with urination. The majority of phimosis cases are physiologic. The ability to retract the prepuce increases with age, with 50% resolving by age one and 89% by age three.[8] Phimosis is pathologic when it leads to balanoposthitis, urinary tract infections (UTI), or urinary retention.

Diagnostic Testing

Asymptomatic patients do not require further workup, but those with pain on urination should have a urinalysis (UA) and culture to evaluate for urinary tract infection.

REGIONAL ANESTHESIA OF THE PENIS

A. Dorsal Nerve Block

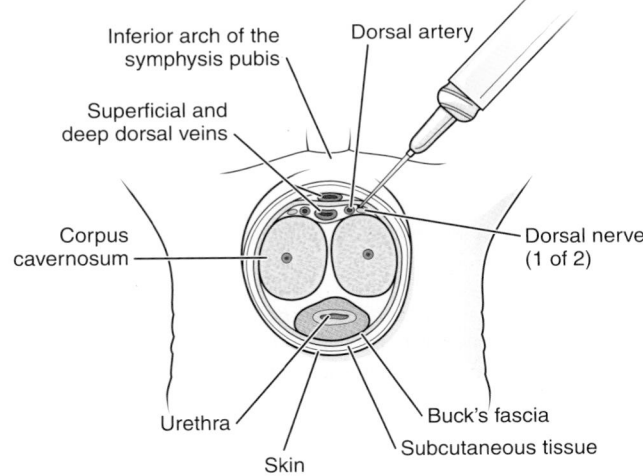

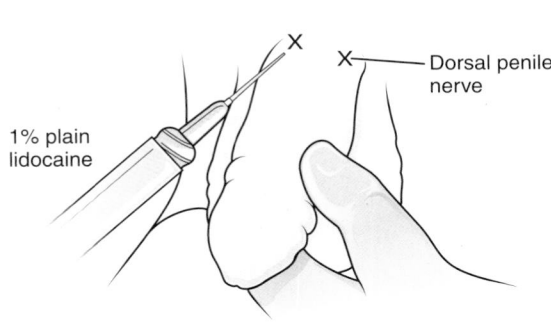

1. The penis has two dorsal penile arteries and two nerves running together and one dorsal penile vein in the midline. A *dorsal nerve block at the base of the penis will provide anesthesia of only the dorsum of the penis.*

2. To perform the dorsal block, inject at the base of the penis lateral to the midline at approximately the 10- and 2-o'clock positions.

B. Ring Block

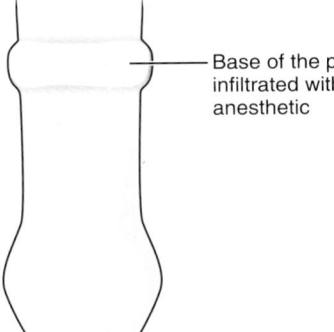

Alternatively, infiltrate subcutaneous lidocaine (without epinephrine) in a circumferential fashion for a ring field block at the base of the penis. This technique provides anesthesia to the entire distal end of the penis.

Fig. 168.2 Penile analgesia. (From: Davis JE, Silverman MA. Urologic procedures. In: Roberts JR, Custalow CB, editors. *Roberts and Hedges' Clinical Procedures in Emergency Medicine.* Philadelphia: Elsevier Saunders; 2014: 1113-1154.)

Management

Management of phimosis is conservative in most cases, but ongoing issues may require circumcision for definitive treatment. There is no general consensus among urologists on the care of phimosis.[9] Parents should be instructed on general hygiene measures of the uncircumcised penis and may practice gentle retraction beginning at 2 years of age. If there are minor recurrent issues with hygiene, infection, or urination, a course of 1% topical hydrocortisone or 0.1% topical triamcinolone applied BID for up to 12 weeks have similar rates of phimosis resolution.[8]

Disposition

Those with chronic UTIs, balanoposthitis, or issues with urination should be referred to urology for circumcision consideration. Patients who are able to urinate and have a reassuring physical examination can be managed as outpatients with primary care or urologic follow-up.

Paraphimosis

KEY CONCEPTS

- Paraphimosis is a urologic emergency wherein the foreskin of the penis is trapped at the corona, resulting in venous congestion and vascular compromise.

Foundations

Paraphimosis is a urologic emergency, wherein the foreskin of the penis is trapped behind the glans at the corona, resulting in engorgement,

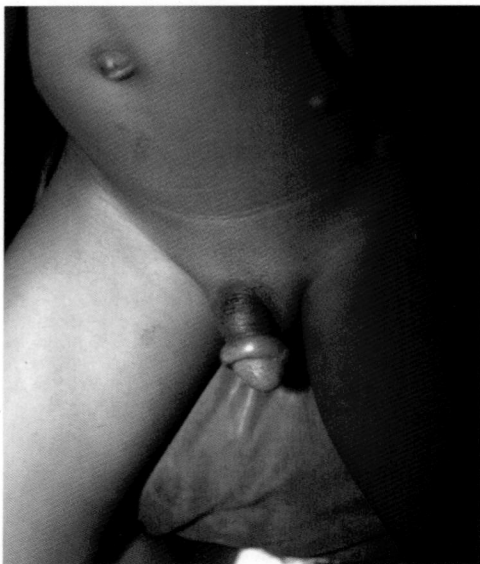

Fig. 168.3 Paraphimosis in a 4-year-old uncircumcised boy. (Courtesy Dr. Marianne Gausche-Hill.)

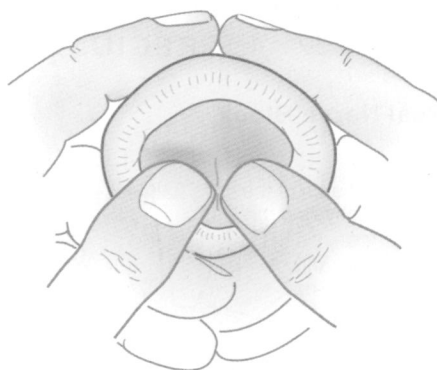

Fig. 168.4 Paraphimosis reduction. (Courtesy P.P. Kelalis.)

venous congestion, and vascular compromise. If left untreated, venous congestion and arterial compromise can lead to distal ischemia and even necrosis of the penis.

Clinical Features

History may reveal a recent penile examination, Foley catheter placement, parental attempts at hygiene, trauma, or recent sexual intercourse. This occurs more commonly in the uncircumcised male, but circumcised individuals who have excessive foreskin can develop paraphimosis. On examination, patients present with painful swelling of the penis with foreskin visibly retracted behind the glans. Any discoloration may indicate ischemia and compromised blood supply (Fig. 168.3).

Diagnostic Testing

The diagnosis is clinical, based on history and physical examination, and there is no role for blood work or imaging. The penis should be inspected for hair tourniquet, which can mimic symptoms of paraphimosis.

Management

Management is directed at replacing the foreskin back over the glans penis. In uncomplicated cases, the foreskin can be manually reduced. Ice packs are useful in decreasing edema but could worsen already compromised penile arterial flow. With manual reduction, gentle pressure is applied for 5 to 10 minutes, either by hand or with compression bandages. After applying pressure to reduce the edema, the provider should use two thumbs to gently press the glans, while pulling the foreskin into place (Fig. 168.4). Osmotic methods with sugar or 20% mannitol-soaked gauze can reduce edema prior to manual reduction.

If manual reduction is not successful, analgesia with dorsal penile block and procedural sedation may be required to facilitate the procedure. If unsuccessful, a dorsal slit may be required, using two clamps at the foreskin at 12 o'clock followed by an incision to release the constriction.[10] Ultimately, surgical circumcision by a urologist may be required.

Disposition

Patients with uncomplicated cases that are manually reduced can be discharged home with outpatient follow-up. The foreskin should be inspected for any abrasions, which should be treated with topical

bacitracin if found. Patients should not retract the foreskin for a week to avoid recurrence. Patients should be evaluated for need for definitive treatment with circumcision by urology. Patients with ischemia or necrosis should be admitted for pain control, antibiotics, and further care by urology.

Balanoposthitis

KEY CONCEPTS

- Inflammation of both the glans (balanitis) and foreskin (posthitis) is usually due to poor hygiene.

Foundations

Balanoposthitis is the inflammation of both the glans (balanitis) and foreskin (posthitis) of the penis, and is most common in young uncircumcised males. In pediatrics, the majority of cases are due to poor hygiene, with accumulated sebaceous material leading to bacterial or fungal overgrowth; however, there are also other infectious (fungal, bacterial, HPV, STIs) and noninfectious (contact dermatitis, chemical irritant, trauma) etiologies to consider.[11]

Patients present with localized pain, erythema, and sometimes dysuria due to local irritation. Penile discharge, rash, or lymphadenopathy raises suspicion for a sexually transmitted infection, such as *Neisseria gonorrhea* or *Chlamydia*, whereas oral ulcerations or arthralgias may point to a rheumatologic etiology, such as psoriasis or lichen sclerosis. The foreskin should be assessed for concomitant phimosis or paraphimosis.

Clinical Features and Diagnostic Testing

The diagnosis of balanoposthitis is clinical, based on history and physical examination. Additional evaluation for patients with dysuria, discharge, extragenital findings, or recurrent balanitis may include UA, STI testing, or glucose (to assess for diabetes in recurrent candidal balanitis).

Management

Management of balanoposthitis is mainly supportive and directed at adequate hygiene measures. Parents and teenagers should be educated on hygiene and care of the uncircumcised penis. Teenagers should also be provided with education on safe sex practices. Treatment should include coverage for both bacterial and fungal overgrowth, with topical bacitracin and topical nystatin (or clotrimazole), respectively. Inflammation can be managed with 0.5% hydrocortisone cream twice daily. In the event of overlying mild cellulitis, patients should be prescribed cephalexin, 25 to 50 mg/kg/day in divided doses for seven days.

Disposition

We recommend that children who are unable to urinate, have signs of systemic illness (e.g., fever), or evidence of more than a mild cellulitis be admitted for IV antibiotics and receive consultation from a urologist.

Complications of Circumcisions

KEY CONCEPTS

- Complications of circumcisions are rare, and most commonly involve minor bleeding.

Foundations

At times a controversial topic, circumcision rates are approximately 38% worldwide.[12] The most recent American Academy of Pediatrics Task Force Recommendations in 2012 concluded that there are lifelong benefits to circumcision that outweigh the risks of the procedure itself.[13] The rate of adverse events from circumcision is low at 1% to 4%.[12]

Management

The major postoperative circumcision complication is bleeding, which may reveal an underlying coagulopathy. Coagulants such as topical thrombin and local pressure should be applied to the circumcised area;[14] patients with a bleeding diathesis may warrant a hemoglobin check and coagulopathy studies, as well as fresh frozen plasma (FFP) or factor replacement. Urgent urologic consultation may be required.

Other immediate postoperative complaints include pain, concern for infection, or extremely rarely, a more severe injury to the penis. Pain usually self-resolves and should not require intervention; if a child is older than 6 months, nonsteroidal antiinflammatory drugs (NSAIDs) or acetaminophen may be trialed. As the circumcision dressing can contribute to urinary retention, patients are predisposed to a urinary tract infection. Those with symptoms should have a UA sent. Systemic infection is uncommon, but in the neonatal period may require a full septic workup with blood work, urine, and cerebrospinal fluid (CSF) studies. Delayed presentation may indicate postoperative adhesions or meatal stenosis. Adhesions or meatal stenosis require outpatient urology follow-up and potential repeat circumcision at a later date.

Penile Entrapment and Tourniquet Injuries

KEY CONCEPTS

- Foreskin injuries occur in pediatrics, and the goal is removal of the offending object to prevent further tissue damage.

Foundations

Penile injuries due to entrapment or hair tourniquet may present from childhood to adolescence and can result in neurovascular damage. Metallic rings used to improve sexual activity are placed by the patient, whereas zippers or hair are the result of accidental entrapment. These objects create damage by reducing vascular supply to the penis and can become a urologic emergency.[15]

Clinical Features and Diagnostic Testing

The patient will present with pain and swelling of penis. In the event of a hair tourniquet, the hair itself may be difficult to visualize. This does not require any lab testing or imaging, unless there is concern for underlying urethral injury, in which case a retrograde urethrogram may be required along with urology consult.

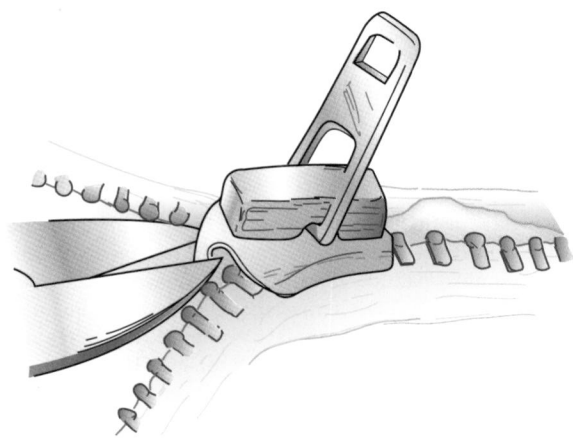

Fig. 168.5 Release of zipper entrapment by cutting of the median bar. (From: Snyder HM III, et al. Genitourinary trauma. In: Fleisher GR, Ludwig S, editors. *Textbook of Pediatric Emergency Medicine*, ed 4. Philadelphia: Lippincott Williams & Wilkins; 2000.)

Management

Management depends on the offending agent. Nonmetallic objects can be cut off with ring cutters or a saw, while using cooling agents to avoid burns to the skin.[15] Hair can be removed using a hair removal cream or by direct visualization and cutting the hair. Depending on the amount of edema, one may need to apply ice or compression before attempting removal. Pain control using a penile block will facilitate manipulation and removal of an object.

In the event of zipper entrapment, the zipper should be removed to free the foreskin from entrapment. There are 5 common methods to remove a zipper from the genitals: cutting the median bar with bone or wire cutters (Fig. 168.5); using a screwdriver to separate the teeth; application of mineral oil as lubricant; lateral compression of the fastener with pliers; and removal of the teeth with trauma sheers.[16] The cloth of the zipper should be cut close to the zipper teeth, which should release the underlying skin. Upon release, the underlying tissue may be damaged. If these techniques are unsuccessful, urology should be consulted for surgical intervention with circumcision as the last option.

Disposition

Most of these cases do not require surgical intervention and can be discharged home after the removal of the offending agent.

Epididymitis and Orchitis

KEY CONCEPTS

- Epididymitis is acute pain and swelling of the epididymis, lasting less than 6 weeks.
- Treatment of epididymitis is based on age and probability of underlying infection.
- Orchitis is pain and swelling of the testicle and is usually viral.

Foundations

Acute epididymitis is pain and swelling of the epididymis lasting less than 6 weeks, whereas orchitis is pain and swelling of the entire testicle. The etiology of the inflammation in epididymitis is due to infectious and noninfectious causes. Infectious causes vary by age of presentation. The most common cause in prepubescent males is viral infections. Adolescents may get epididymitis from *N. gonorrhoeae* or *C.*

trachomatis; other bacterial causes in this age group may be related to structural anomalies of the urinary tract.[17] Noninfectious causes may be due to a vasculitis (e.g., in Henoch-Schönlein purpura, see later), chemical irritation, or trauma. Orchitis is usually the result of bacterial or viral infection and is classically associated with mumps.

Clinical Features

Patients present with scrotal pain and swelling, with tenderness on physical examination. Patients may complain of nausea, vomiting, or referred abdominal pain. Urethral discharge may indicate a sexually transmitted infection (STI). Cremasteric reflexes should be intact, and one may see relief of pain with scrotal elevation (Prehn sign), although these elements *do not* rule out testicular torsion. Those with mumps may also present with viral symptoms, as well as lymphadenopathy and parotid gland swelling. Differential diagnosis should include epididymitis, orchitis, testicular torsion and torsion of the appendix testis, inguinal hernia, hydrocele, and varicocele.

Diagnostic Testing

Though the diagnoses of epididymitis and orchitis are clinical, UA and culture should be obtained to evaluate for pyuria. STI testing should be considered for all adolescents and those who are sexually active. Ultrasound (US) should be obtained in cases where testicular torsion is considered possible. US may show increased vascular flow to the epididymis. Patients with bacterial orchitis may rarely get a scrotal abscess, which would also be detected on ultrasound.

Management

Management of epididymitis and orchitis includes supportive care with analgesia, ice packs, and scrotal elevation. If there is concern for gonococcal STI, patients should be empirically treated with 500 mg IM ceftriaxone for patients <150 kg. If there is concern for chlamydial STI, treatment is with either doxycycline 100 mg PO BID for 7 days or azithromycin 1 g PO once.[18] Those with UA evidence of UTI should be treated for a complicated UTI according to local sensitivity patterns for *E. coli*. Scrotal abscess should receive antibiotics and consultation with urology.

Disposition

Most patients with uncomplicated epididymitis or orchitis can be discharged home with outpatient follow-up.

Testicular Torsion

KEY CONCEPTS

- Testicular torsion is a urologic emergency treated by detorsing the testis.
- Patients with classic symptoms and signs of testicular torsion should have an emergent urologic consultation for operative management.

Foundations

Testicular torsion is a urologic emergency associated with acute onset of scrotal pain. Testicular torsion should always be considered in acute scrotal pain, as delayed diagnosis can lead to loss of viability of testicular tissue and potentially loss of spermatogenesis. Testicular torsion can occur at any age, but in particular, has peaks in the neonatal and adolescent periods. Testicular salvage rates depend on time to presentation, as well as time to surgical intervention, with increased orchiectomy rates when blood flow is not restored within 6 hours of symptom onset.[19]

Testicular torsion can occur within the tunica vaginalis (i.e., intravaginally), constricting arterial blood flow, or within the scrotum (i.e.,

extravaginally). If there is inadequate fixation of the testicle, in which the tunica vaginalis completely covers the testis superior to the spermatic cord, this "bell clapper" deformity predisposes to torsion (Fig. 168.6). Other risk factors include cryptorchidism, trauma, familial history, or prior episodes.

Clinical Features

Patients with testicular torsion usually present with acute onset unilateral scrotal pain and edema, often associated with nausea and vomiting. Pain may radiate to the abdomen, and children may be embarrassed to note genital complaints; thus, even without a testicular complaint, a complete GU examination should be performed. Patients may have a high-riding, transverse, swollen testicle, with possible discoloration, and lack of cremasteric reflex on the affected side, though a normal cremasteric reflex *does not* rule out torsion.

Differential Diagnoses

Differential diagnosis includes torsion of the testicular appendage, which presents similarly, but usually occurs in prepubescent males with a more indolent course and less intense pain at the superior pole of the testis. Other considerations include orchitis, epididymitis, trauma, hydrocele, varicocele, inguinal hernias, or testicular tumors.

Diagnostic Testing

Testicular torsion is a clinical diagnosis, but scrotal ultrasound with Doppler can confirm the diagnosis when the testis is torsed. A UA may show hematuria or leukocytosis, which would be more indicative of epididymitis or orchitis. Doppler ultrasound may show decreased perfusion to the testicle or twisting of the spermatic cord.

Management

Urology should be consulted emergently for definitive surgical management. Once testicular torsion is confirmed, management requires surgical detorsion on the affected side, with either orchiopexy or orchiectomy if the testicle is not viable. Time to the operating room is directly related to testicular salvage, with less than 6 hours as most optimal.[19]

In the event of surgical delay, a bedside manual detorsion under analgesia can be attempted after discussion with urology. Because most torsion occurs medially, the testicle is rotated in an "open book" fashion, laterally until detorsion has occurred.[20] However, a small percentage of cases do torse laterally, so this maneuver could worsen symptoms in those cases. If manual detorsion fails, surgical management is warranted. For suspected testicular torsion that has detorsed and has normal findings or high flow (i.e., from reperfusion) on ultrasound, we recommend urology be consulted and surgery be considered to prevent recurrence.

Varicocele and Hydrocele

KEY CONCEPTS

- Consider reactive hydroceles in the setting of epididymitis, orchitis, testicular torsion, or testicular tumors.
- Consider abdominal mass or renal vein thrombosis in the event of right-sided varicocele.

Foundations

Painless scrotal swelling in children may occur secondary to a hydrocele or varicocele. A hydrocele occurs when peritoneal fluid accumulates within the tunica vaginalis; hydroceles are either communicating or noncommunicating with the peritoneal cavity. Hydroceles commonly

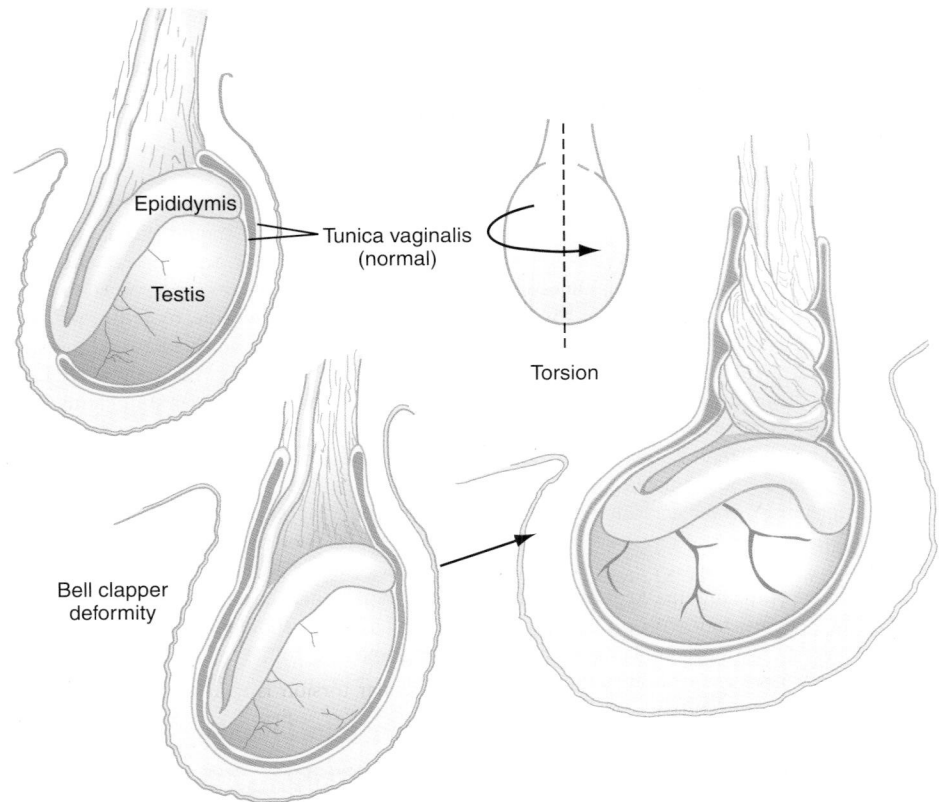

Fig. 168.6 Anatomy of testicular torsion. (From: Snyder HM III, et al. Pain—scrotal. In: Fleisher GR, Ludwig S, editors. *Textbook of Pediatric Emergency Medicine,* ed 4. Philadelphia: Lippincott Williams & Wilkins; 2000.)

occur in newborns and will spontaneously resorb by age one.[21] However, in older children, hydroceles may occur secondary to epididymitis, orchitis, torsion, or tumor. A varicocele is a collection of dilated veins in the pampiniform plexus, which surrounds the spermatic cord, and occurs in about 15% of adolescent males.[22] Primary varicoceles occur spontaneously, while secondary varicoceles occur due to some obstruction of venous outflow of the plexus. Most varicoceles are left-sided due to the 90-degree angle of drainage that occurs from the left spermatic vein to the left renal drain. A right-sided varicocele raises concern for intra-abdominal mass.

Clinical Features

If a hydrocele is communicating, painless scrotal swelling may increase when the patient performs a Valsalva maneuver. Transillumination will reveal clear fluid surrounding the testicle. Although varicoceles will also cause painless scrotal swelling, examination will reveal a "bag of worms" consistency on palpation, and a varicocele does not transilluminate. The differential for painless scrotal swelling includes hydrocele, varicocele, spermatocele, cyst, inguinal hernia, or testicular tumor. If there is pain, the differential includes reactive hydrocele secondary to epididymitis, orchitis, torsion, or a tumor.

Diagnostic Testing

If there is concern for testicular tumor, a CBC, lactate dehydrogenase (LDH), and uric acid would be reasonable. An ultrasound of the testes will be helpful to evaluate for torsion or mass. For right-sided varicoceles or those of sudden onset, we recommend patients undergo imaging with ultrasound with Doppler, CT, or MRI to evaluate for inferior vena cava thrombus, renal vein thrombosis, or abdominal mass.

Management and Disposition

Hydroceles in newborns can be managed expectantly as most will resorb on their own.[21] Outside the newborn period, there is moderate evidence that surgical correction of varicocele leads to improved sperm concentration and testicular volume.[23] Patients may be referred to urology for conservative management versus surgical repair with ligation or embolization; in the absence of an abdominal or testicular mass, these cases may be managed as outpatients.

Acute Idiopathic Scrotal Edema

KEY CONCEPTS

- Acute idiopathic scrotal edema (AISE) is rare and is a diagnosis of exclusion.

Foundations

Acute idiopathic scrotal edema (AISE) is a rare diagnosis characterized by acute scrotal erythema, swelling, and tenderness. It is a benign, self-limiting condition with an unclear etiology and is a diagnosis of exclusion. AISE generally affects prepubertal boys, though can affect males into adulthood.[24]

Clinical Features and Diagnostic Testing

Physical examination shows swelling, induration, and erythema of a unilateral testicle, which may or may not be tender. Diagnosis is via ultrasound and demonstrates edematous thickening and increased vascularity of the scrotal wall, but normal-appearing testes.

Management

Once more insidious causes have been ruled out, AISE generally resolves within a few days with NSAIDs and scrotal support.

Inguinal Hernia

KEY CONCEPTS

- Inguinal hernias can occur in males (intestines) and females (ovary more often than intestines).
- Manual reduction of inguinal hernia should be attempted, but definitive management is surgical repair.

Foundations

An inguinal hernia is a common cause of scrotal swelling in males and labial swelling in females, with indirect hernias accounting for just under 5% of full-term infants.[25] Risk increases with prematurity, low birth weight, and male gender. In males, an indirect hernia results from failed closure of the processus vaginalis, and usually contains intestines. In females, a hernia results from the failed closure of the canal of Nuck, and more often contains ovary rather than bowel. The greatest risk is with incarceration (inability to reduce the herniated contents), as well as strangulation (vascular compromise), of the herniated contents.

Clinical Features

Patients present with intermittent bulge of the inguinal region into the scrotum or labia, or a persistent bulge consistent with incarceration. Patients with a reducible bulge usually have no complaints of pain, whereas those with incarceration may have a significant amount of pain. The patient may also experience vomiting and diffuse abdominal pain from intestinal obstruction.

Differential Diagnoses

Differential diagnosis should include hydrocele, varicocele, testicular/ovarian torsion, or malignancy. The diagnosis is often clinical, but ultrasound with Doppler can assist in identifying herniated contents as well as ovarian flow in females.

Management and Disposition

Ultimately, surgery is needed for definitive repair. As long as the patient is clinically stable, manual reduction should be attempted with appropriate analgesia, by applying traction to the proximal inguinal canal with one hand and gentle pressure to the distal canal towards the abdomen with the other hand for up to 5 minutes. Incarcerated hernias with strangulation, as well as canal of Nuck hernias containing ovary, have high risk for bowel ischemia or ovarian torsion without prompt surgical intervention.[25] In the event of painless, reducible hernias without incarceration or strangulation, patients can be referred for surgery and outpatient evaluation.

Testicular Carcinoma/Tumors

KEY CONCEPTS

- Testicular tumors are the most common solid organ tumor in adolescents.
- Patients who have a hydrocele that does not transilluminate should have an ultrasound to investigate for an underlying mass.

Foundations

Although a small percentage of overall pediatric malignancies, testicular tumors are the most common solid organ tumor in adolescents, comprising 14% of all adolescent cancer.[26] Patients with cryptorchidism, prior testicular cancer on the contralateral side, or family history of cancer are all at increased risk. Most testicular cancers are teratomas, carcinomas, yolk sac tumors, Leydig cell tumors, or Sertoli cell tumors; however, lymphoma and leukemia can also metastasize to the testicle.

Clinical Features

Patients present with painless unilateral testicular swelling or mass. Some may describe an aching or pulling sensation, or abdominal pain. There may be a reactive hydrocele present, but the testis does not transilluminate with an underlying mass. Examination may demonstrate lymphadenopathy, hepatosplenomegaly, or gynecomastia.

Diagnostic Testing and Management

Diagnostic evaluation should include a CBC with differential, chemistry panel, LDH, uric acid, human chorionic gonadotropin (HCG), UA, and ultrasound. Labs are obtained to evaluate for cell line suppression, tumor lysis syndrome, or end-organ damage. Chest x-ray should be performed to rule out mediastinal mass with testicular metastasis. Tumor markers such as HCG, alpha fetal protein (AFP), luteinizing hormone (LH), and follicular stimulating hormone (FSH) can be sent and are helpful to the oncologist for further delineation of the underlying subtype. An ultrasound is necessary to identify solid tumor versus a cystic structure.

Once the workup is complete, pediatric oncology should be consulted for further management, including CT chest, abdomen, and pelvis for staging purposes, orchiectomy for histologic evaluation, and possibly retroperitoneal lymph node dissection or chemotherapy.[27] A testicular biopsy should not be performed due to concern for possible tumor seeding. Initial management may be inpatient, with long term outpatient follow-up.

Urinary Tract Infections

KEY CONCEPTS

- *E. coli* is the most common uropathogen isolated from urine cultures in patients with urinary tract infections (UTI).
- First time febrile UTI from 2 months to 2 years should have a renal bladder ultrasound.

Foundations

Urinary tract infection (UTI) is a common diagnosis in pediatrics and risk increases with age younger than 12 months, uncircumcised status, and anatomic obstruction or vesicoureteral reflux. The most common bacterial cause of UTI is *E. coli*, accounting for 80% of cases.[28]

Clinical Features

Patients present with dysuria, urgency, frequency, abdominal pain, fever, incontinence, or vomiting. In younger children, fever may be the only presenting symptom (see Chapter 161). Physical examination may reveal suprapubic tenderness; an upper tract infection may cause costovertebral angle or flank tenderness. GU examination should be performed to look for retained foreign bodies or signs of obstruction from phimosis or labial adhesions.

Differential Diagnoses

Differential diagnosis includes other sources of fever or abdominal pain, although those would not eliminate a concurrent UTI. Asymptomatic bacteriuria is a possibility in the event of colonization or gastroenteritis. In patients with pyuria but negative culture, consider balanitis, vulvovaginitis, or sexually transmitted disease. Also consider Kawasaki disease in the event of sterile pyuria.

Diagnostic Testing and Management

A urinalysis and urine culture should be obtained. A catheterized specimen is preferable in those who are not toilet trained to preserve a sterile sample. Blood work is not usually needed for otherwise well-appearing immunized children over 3 months of age. A UTI is diagnosed when there is pyuria or bacteriuria on UA, and at least 50,000 cfu/mL of a uropathogen cultured by catheterization.[29] Febrile infants with a UTI should receive renal bladder ultrasound, which may be performed as an outpatient, to assess for hydronephrosis or renal scarring. Once back to their usual state of health, infants with an abnormal ultrasound should undergo a voiding cysto-urethrogram to assess for reflux or obstruction.[29] See Chapter 161 for a comprehensive discussion on treatment of pediatric UTI.

Hematuria

KEY CONCEPTS

- Hematuria refers to >5 RBCs per high power field on UA.
- Gross hematuria is usually due to bladder or urethral bleeding, whereas microscopic hematuria is due to glomerular or tubular bleeding.

Foundations

Hematuria refers to red blood cells (RBCs) in the urine and can be either macroscopic or microscopic. While macroscopic hematuria is visible to the patient, microscopic hematuria refers to greater than 5 RBCs per high-power field. The prevalence of microscopic hematuria detected on two or more urinalysis samples in school age children is estimated at 1% to 2%, but in cases of isolated hematuria, 57% do not have underlying pathology.[30]

Irrespective of grossly visible or microscopic hematuria, patients should be assessed for trauma, queried for flank or abdominal pain, and inspected for bleeding from other sites. Patients with infection as the cause of hematuria may report fevers, dysuria, urgency, frequency, abdominal pain, or recent illness. Medical history should include documenting any sickle cell disease, bleeding disorders, medications, or family history of kidney disease. Physical examination should document other areas of bleeding/bruising (skin or mucosal), signs of renal impairment (hypertension, periorbital or lower extremity edema, pulmonary crackles), abdominal pain or masses, and GU examination to assess for external causes of bleeding (i.e., meatal, vaginal, or rectal sources). Causes of hematuria are categorized as extrarenal or intrarenal etiologies (Table 168.2).[30,31] Macroscopic hematuria is typically due to bladder/urethral damage, whereas microscopic hematuria is more commonly from glomerular or tubular damage.

Patients with hematuria have a UA with greater than 5 RBCs per high-power field. Proteinuria and RBC casts suggest glomerular damage. Patients with concern for hematuria, and dipstick positive for blood, but no RBCs on UA may have myoglobinuria from rhabdomyolysis. In patients with discolored urine but normal UA, consider certain foods (e.g., beets, rhubarb, berries) and medications (e.g., rifampin, nitrofurantoin, metronidazole).[31] Findings of leukocyte esterase, nitrite, or white blood cells (WBC) indicate urinary tract infection. WBC casts may be found in patients with pyelonephritis. In the context of recent throat or skin infection, a throat culture, anti-streptolysin O (ASO) titer, and complement levels may help diagnosis poststreptococcal glomerulonephritis. If there is greater than 3+ protein on UA, nephrotic syndrome should be considered and a basic metabolic panel (BMP) sent for electrolytes, creatinine, and albumin. If BMP reveals hypercalcemia, urine calcium levels should also be obtained, because hypercalciuria is a common cause of hematuria. If there is concern for lupus, erythrocyte sedimentation rate (ESR) and antinuclear antibodies (ANA) can be obtained. If the patient complains of flank or abdominal pain with hematuria, ultrasound or CT scan can help diagnose nephrolithiasis, renal vein thrombosis, nutcracker syndrome, or mass.

TABLE 168.2 Causes of Hematuria in Children

Extrarenal	Trauma
	Meatal stenosis or posterior urethral valves
	Menstrual or rectal bleeding
	Foreign body
	Cystitis, urethritis, epididymitis
Intrarenal	Pyelonephritis
	Nephrolithiasis or urolithiasis
	Poststreptococcal glomerulonephritis
	Acute interstitial nephritis
	Acute tubular necrosis
	Basement membrane glomerular disease
	Renal vein or artery thrombosis
	Recurrent familial hematuria
	Polycystic kidney disease
Systemic	Alport syndrome
	Henoch-Schönlein purpura
	Lupus
	Hemolytic uremic syndrome
	Mononucleosis
	Sickle cell disease/hemoglobinopathy
	Endocarditis
	Bleeding diathesis
	Medications (amitriptyline, chlorpromazine, radiocontrast dye)

If the patient has a history of trauma, we recommend a CT scan of the abdomen and pelvis be performed to evaluate for sources of injury and bleeding (see Chapter 160).

The management of hematuria depends on the etiology and may warrant subspecialty referral to nephrology, urology, or oncology. Well-appearing children with normal blood work, imaging, and no identifiable cause should be discharged to follow-up with their PCP for serial UAs to assess for persistent hematuria and need for further outpatient workup.

Nephrolithiasis

KEY CONCEPTS

- Clinical presentation in pediatrics may be more nonspecific than adults.
- Ultrasound is first-line imaging in diagnosis.
- Stones <6 mm will likely pass spontaneously.

Foundations

Nephrolithiasis, or kidney stones, is increasing in incidence across all ages. Calcium oxalate stones are the most common, followed by calcium phosphate, and less likely struvite, uric acid, and cysteine. Increased risk is associated with family history, low fluid intake, increased dietary sodium, urinary tract infections, metabolic abnormalities (hypercalciuria, hypocitraturia, renal tubular acidosis), anatomic abnormalities (ureteropelvic junction obstruction, posterior urethral valves), systemic disease (inflammatory bowel disease, nephrocalcinosis), genetic disease (cystinuria, cystic fibrosis), and medications (topiramate, acetazolamide, vitamin C).[32]

Clinical Features

Adolescents often present with colicky flank pain and hematuria, while younger children present with nonspecific abdominal pain or isolated hematuria which may lead to a delayed diagnosis. Patients may also complain of nausea, vomiting, or malaise. Children with concomitant UTI may complain of dysuria, urgency, and frequency. Some younger patients may be asymptomatic with stones detected incidentally. History should include any prior history of stones, UTIs (*Proteus* species are associated with struvite stones), congenital malformations, family history of nephrolithiasis, specific dietary constraints (ketogenic diet), and current medications.

Differential Diagnoses

In patients with intermittent abdominal pain, constipation, gastroenteritis, appendicitis, intussusception, testicular torsion, ovarian torsion, and cholelithiasis should be considered in the differential. In children with hematuria, consider urinary tract infection, trauma, and other causes of hematuria listed in Table 168.2.

Diagnostic Testing

Workup for suspected nephrolithiasis includes a UA with microscopy to evaluate for hematuria, crystals, and evidence of infection, as well as a BMP to evaluate for electrolyte abnormalities and acute kidney injury. Although hematuria is a common presenting symptom, up to 20% of patients with nephrolithiasis will not have hematuria on their UA. CBC with differential may be obtained if there is concern for infection or significant blood loss. Stones may be visualized using plain films, ultrasound, or non-contrast helical CT scans. Plain films will only detect radio-opaque stones; ultrasound will detect both radio-opaque and radiolucent stones but may miss smaller stones. CT scans will detect both types of stones, as well as small stones and ureteral stones. Renal bladder ultrasound is first-line imaging in children to avoid radiation, but with negative ultrasound and high suspicion, a non-contrast CT is diagnostic.

Management

Management of stones in pediatric patients focuses on pain control, as well as expectant management of stone passage versus surgical removal. In children with normal renal function, NSAIDS are preferred for pain relief, followed by opioids. Uncomplicated cases with adequate pain control, normal renal function, and stones of less than 6 mm can be discharged home, as they will likely pass the stone spontaneously.[33] For distal ureteral stones of less than 10 mm, the addition of medical expulsive therapy with tamsulosin (alpha antagonist) may increase successful expulsion.[33] Once passed, stones can be collected by families and sent for stone composition analysis. A 24-hour urine collection is recommended after the stone has passed, to evaluate for underlying metabolic abnormalities that may predispose to recurrence. Stone causing hydroureter or hydronephrosis and infected urine is a urologic emergency, requiring intravenous antibiotics and decompression, usually with ureteral stent or percutaneous nephrostomy tube.[33] Additional interventions may include extracorporeal shock wave lithotripsy, percutaneous nephrolithotomy, or ureteroscopy. Admission criteria for children with nephrolithiasis are any of the following: significant obstruction (unlikely to pass spontaneously), UTI with obstruction, persistent pain despite adequate therapy, persistent vomiting or inability to self-hydrate, struvite stones, failed conservative management, and patients with a solitary kidney.[34]

Renal Tumors

> ### KEY CONCEPTS
> - Wilms tumor is the most common renal tumor in children.
> - Patients often present with hematuria or an abdominal mass detected by caregivers.

Foundations

Renal tumors make up 7% of all pediatric cancers, of which Wilms tumor is the most common, followed by congenital mesoblastic nephroma (in children <12 months) and renal cell carcinoma (in children >5 years).[35,36] Certain syndromes such as Beckwith-Wiedemann, Denys-Drash, and WAGR, carry increased risk of developing Wilms tumor.

Clinical Features

Children with renal tumors often present with a palpable abdominal mass, but can also present with abdominal pain/distension, hematuria, or emesis. Vital signs may be normal or may reveal hypertension. In addition to renal tumors, the differential diagnosis includes other causes of abdominal mass such as hepatosplenomegaly, hydronephrosis, polycystic kidneys, cysts, abscesses, a full bladder, and constipation.

Diagnostic Testing

A suspected renal mass warrants laboratory workup, including CBC with differential and smear, complete metabolic panel (CMP), uric acid and LDH to assess for tumor lysis, urinalysis, and urine catecholamines (to help differentiate Wilms tumor from neuroblastoma). Renal ultrasound is preferred for diagnosis, followed by additional imaging with a CT, MRI, or PET scan for staging and surgical planning.

Management and Disposition

Once a renal tumor has been identified, pediatric hematology-oncology should be consulted for ongoing management. Children who are well-appearing with normal renal function may be discharged for outpatient follow-up after discussion with oncology, but often children will be admitted for expedited diagnostic workup and treatment planning.

Proteinuria

> ### KEY CONCEPTS
> - Trace or mild proteinuria may be seen in hypovolemia, fever, stress, or exercise.
> - Patients with moderate or severe proteinuria require workup with blood work, imaging, and nephrology consultation.

Foundations

Proteinuria is associated with renal pathology; however, trace or mild proteinuria is benign and generally asymptomatic. It is often seen with hypovolemia, fever or hypothermia, stress, seizures, or exercise. However, more insidious causes, such as nephrotic syndrome, can present with high levels of proteinuria (>1000 mg/m^2 per day, Table 168.3) and edema secondary to hypoalbuminemia less than 3 g/dL.[37] Glomerular filtration issues lead to the abnormal passage of albumin, a macromolecule, which is detected on urine dipstick. Tubular and overflow proteinuria are caused by extrusion of low-molecular-weight molecules, which are not typically detected on urine dipstick. Tubular proteinuria is associated with proximal tubular dysfunction, whereas overflow proteinuria, which is uncommon in children, occurs when tubular resorptive capacity is overwhelmed.

Clinical Features

The cause of proteinuria determines presentation. Edema commonly presents around the eyes (i.e., periorbital), in the lower extremities, and in the GU area. Eliciting a history of preceding illness (e.g., a recent streptococcal infection), weight changes, changes in urine output, and family history of kidney issues/autoimmune disease may assist in diagnosing the etiology of the proteinuria. If the patient has systemic

TABLE 168.3 Urine Dipstick Proteinuria

	Mild Proteinuria			Moderate Proteinuria	High Proteinuria
Negative	Trace	1+	2+	3+	4+
<15 mg/dL	15–30 mg/dL	30–100 mg/dL	100–300 mg/dL	300–1000 mg/dL	>1000 mg/dL

TABLE 168.4 Causes of Proteinuria

Glomerular	Tubular
Nephrotic syndrome	Heavy metal poisoning
Minimal change disease	Urinary tract infection
Glomerulonephritis	Diabetes-related glycosuria
Post-transplantation rejection	Proximal tubular acidosis
Transient	Phosphaturia
• Hypovolemia	Asymptomatic tubular proteinuria
• Hyperthermia	Genetic disorders
• Hypothermia	• Fanconi syndrome
• Seizures	
• Stress	
• Exercise	
• Postural/Orthostatic	
• Proteinuria only when upright	

TABLE 168.5 Normal Urine Protein-to-Creatinine Ratio

Age	Urine Pr/Cr
>2 years old	<0.2
6 months–2 years old	<0.5

Data from Gipson DS, et al. Complete remission in the Nephrotic Syndrome Study Network. *Clin J Am Society Nephrol.* 2016;11:81-89.

we recommend this decision be made in consultation with a pediatric nephrologist.

Poststreptococcal Glomerulonephritis (PSGN)

KEY CONCEPTS

- Patients with PSGN have a history of a preceding pharyngeal or skin infection in the past 2 to 6 weeks, respectively.
- Treatment of PSGN is supportive, with fluid restriction and diuretics for more significant disease.

Foundations

Poststreptococcal glomerulonephritis (PSGN) is the most common cause of pediatric glomerulonephritis globally and is caused by recent infection with group A beta-hemolytic streptococcus (GAS).[39] The exact mechanism is unclear, but it is believed to be caused by deposition of glomerular immune complexes, which leads to a decreased glomerular filtration rate from complement activation, and subsequent proteinuria.

Clinical Features

Generally, patients will present with a history of pharyngitis and fever about 2 weeks prior, or skin infection with fever up to 6 weeks prior.[39] PSGN symptoms can range from asymptomatic gross hematuria to acute nephritic syndrome with acute kidney injury including proteinuria, edema, hypertension, lethargy, cardiac arrhythmias, and renal failure. It occurs more frequently in males, patients ages 4 years to 12 years old, and is uncommon in children less than two years old.[39]

Diagnostic Testing

In children with PSGN, a urinalysis should be obtained and demonstrates hematuria (±RBC casts) and proteinuria, and sometimes pyuria. Generally, most children with PSGN do not have nephrotic range proteinuria. Lab values typically show an elevated BUN, low sodium, high potassium, elevated ASO, elevated IgG levels, and decreased C3 and decreased CH50 during the first 2 weeks of illness.[39] Complement levels generally return to normal within 4 to 8 weeks after initial presentation.[40]

If hematuria and nephritic symptoms persist beyond 2 weeks, clinical clues can point to diagnoses other than PSGN. Antecedent upper respiratory or gastrointestinal infection is often present in patients with IgA nephropathy or membranoproliferative glomerulonephritis

symptoms, such as joint pain or rash, this may point to an autoimmune process as the culprit.

In children, proteinuria is either glomerular or tubular; common causes are listed in Table 168.4.[37] False-positive proteinuria on urine dipstick is often related to alkaline or dilute urine, mucous, blood, vaginal or seminal secretions, or the presence of inflammatory cells (i.e., a urinary tract infection).[38]

Diagnostic Testing and Management

If a patient has mild proteinuria (≤2+ or ≤100 mg/dL), no further emergent testing is necessary. Patients with moderate proteinuria (≥3+ or ≥300 mg/dL), should have their blood pressure monitored, and a laboratory workup, including serum protein, serum albumin, electrolytes, BUN, creatinine, complement levels (C3 and C4), urine culture, antistreptolysin O (ASO), and urine protein-to-creatinine ratio (Pr/Cr). Random urine Pr/Cr correlates with a 24-hour urine collection and is easier to obtain, particularly in a pediatric patient. First morning void urine Pr/Cr is most accurate. Urine Pr/Cr greater than 3.0 is associated with nephrotic syndrome. We recommend pediatric nephrology consultation and follow-up for any child with moderate proteinuria or an elevated urine Pr/Cr value (Table 168.5).[37] Imaging such as a renal ultrasound may demonstrate anatomic abnormalities such as polycystic kidney disease, but can be completed on an outpatient basis.

Disposition

All children with proteinuria require follow-up with their primary care doctor for a reevaluation, including blood pressure monitoring and repeat UA. A pediatric nephrologist should determine the need for renal biopsy in children with moderate proteinuria.

We recommend hospital admission and pediatric nephrology consultation for children with significant proteinuria (3+), along with edema/ascites, hypertension greater than the 99th percentile, or renal dysfunction with elevation of greater than 50% of BUN or creatinine. Some children with new-onset mild nephrotic syndrome may be managed outpatient, particularly if well-appearing; however,

(MPGN). In IgA nephropathy, hematuria typically presents sooner (i.e., less than 5 days) after the preceding illness. Patients with MPGN have persistent hematuria and lab abnormalities of low complement and elevation in creatinine. Lupus nephritis and Henoch-Schönlein purpura (HSP) can present similarly, but can be differentiated by complement levels, with both C3 and C4 depressed in lupus nephritis, and normal complement levels in HSP. PSGN has a decreased C3 and generally has a normal C4 level, though a depressed C4 level can portend a poorer prognosis.[40] Hemolytic uremic syndrome (HUS) can also result in symptoms similar to PSGN, but has characteristic bloody diarrhea and is often associated with *E. coli* O157.

Management

PSGN is primarily managed supportively via fluid and salt restriction, often in consultation with a pediatric nephrologist. It is generally self-limited, with most creatinine levels returning to baseline about 3 to 4 weeks after initial manifestation. PSGN does not necessarily warrant antibiotic treatment, as the streptococcal infection has typically cleared by the time of presentation, although a streptococcal infection should be treated if still present. If hypertension or fluid overload develops, patients should be treated with calcium channel blockers or diuretics.

Diagnosis can be delayed if there is no history of antecedent infection or the patient does not have gross hematuria. In PSGN, the nephritis typically resolves within 1 to 2 weeks. Patients with persistent disease beyond 2 weeks should receive a pediatric nephrology consultation to determine additional diagnostic testing.

Most children with mild PSGN can be managed on an outpatient basis. Indications for pediatric nephrology referral and dialysis are outlined in Box 168.1.[41]

Nephrotic Syndrome

KEY CONCEPTS

- Nephrotic syndrome is defined by proteinuria, decreased albumin, hypertriglyceridemia, and edema.
- Patients have an increased risk for thrombosis and bacterial infections, especially *Streptococcus* and *E.coli*.

Foundations

Nephrotic syndrome occurs when impaired glomerular filtration leads to proteinuria (3+ or 4+ or >300 to 1000 mg/dL protein on urine dipstick) and hypoalbuminemia (<30 g/L or <3g/dL). As a result of this increased permeability, patients can present with significant edema. It can affect any age, although is most common in school-aged children and teenagers. The incidence in children is 2 to 7 per 100,000 children and it affects males more frequently (2 : 1).[42] Primary nephrotic syndrome is idiopathic and occurs without an inciting systemic illness while secondary nephrotic syndrome occurs due to systemic causes, such as infections, immune disorders, cancer, or medications. The

various types of nephrotic syndrome are listed in Box 168.2.[43] Most children have primary nephrotic syndrome, generally minimal change disease or focal segmental glomerulonephritis.

Clinical Features

Nephrotic syndrome is characterized by edema, although the presentation can vary from mild periorbital edema to anasarca. Some children can present without edema, but still have nephrotic range proteinuria. Nephrotic syndrome can be triggered by a recent upper respiratory illness or can present without incitement.[42] Some children can present with weight gain not recognized to be edema, and insidiously present with pulmonary edema or severe ascites. Children with nephrotic syndrome may have hypertension, hematuria, or oliguria, with resultant acute kidney injury, although acute renal failure is rare.

Children with nephrotic syndrome are at high risk for thrombosis with thromboemboli. Venous thrombosis can occur in the renal vein, sagittal sinus, or pulmonary artery.[42] Patients with nephrotic syndrome are also at higher risk for developing bacterial infections secondary to loss of immunoglobulins, and because they are often on corticosteroid treatment. Infections are the leading cause of morbidity and mortality in nephrotic syndrome, from spontaneous bacterial peritonitis, sepsis, and pneumonia resulting from *E. coli* and encapsulated organisms such as *Streptococcus pneumoniae*, *Haemophilus influenzae*, and Group B *Streptococcus*.

Diagnostic Testing

In suspected nephrotic syndrome, a urinalysis, protein : creatinine ratio, and serum labs including electrolyte, albumin, BUN, creatinine, CBC, and cholesterol should be checked. Nephrotic range labs are listed Box 168.3.[42] Labs generally reveal normal BUN and creatinine levels, but will have hypoalbuminemia, hyponatremia, hyperlipidemia, and can have hemoconcentration with elevated hemoglobin and hematocrit. Patients generally have normal complement levels, but if abnormal, other diagnoses should be considered.

Imaging such as chest x-rays and abdominal x-rays can demonstrate fluid overload with pulmonary edema and ascites. Abdominal ultrasound for nephrotic syndrome is otherwise nonspecific, but may demonstrate ascites or structural changes of the kidneys from chronic illness. Renal biopsy can characterize a specific nephrotic syndrome diagnosis, and is recommended for patients with hematuria, elevated BUN, persistent hypertension or renal dysfunction refractory to steroid treatment.

Differential Diagnoses

Primary renal disease such as glomerulonephritis and renal failure can also result in edema similar to nephrotic syndrome. These can be differentiated by gross hematuria, RBC casts in urine, elevated creatinine, or hypertension. Other causes of edema to consider include heart failure, drug-induced, liver failure/cirrhosis, cystic fibrosis, and other protein losing enteropathies such as malnutrition.

Management

Primary nephrotic syndrome can be treated with steroids (e.g., prednisone 2 mg/kg/day orally divided TID), with the duration determined by a pediatric nephrologist.[44] Some forms of nephrotic syndrome may be refractory to steroids, in which case subsequent steroid courses and renal biopsy may be warranted. Children with nephrotic syndrome require fluid and salt restriction. In ill-appearing patients with severe ascites or respiratory distress, furosemide 0.5 to 1 mg/kg and titrated based on response can be used as a diuretic. However, in spite of edema, children with nephrotic syndrome who appear hypovolemic or septic should receive fluid resuscitation with crystalloid. If patients develop chest pain, shortness of breath, abdominal pain, or extremity swelling/pain, thromboembolic complications should be considered. Children with significant ascites and pain should undergo paracentesis to assess for spontaneous bacterial peritonitis. Due to immunoglobulin loss and T-cell dysfunction, children with nephrotic syndrome are considered immunocompromised and if they present with a fever, can not only relapse but should also be hospitalized with blood cultures, respiratory viral studies if available, and initiation of antibiotic therapy effective against *S. pneumoniae* and *E. coli*.[44]

Disposition

As with many new-onset pediatric chronic illnesses, pediatric patients with new-onset nephrotic syndrome are generally hospitalized under the care of a pediatric nephrologist to expedite workup, treatment, and education. In mild cases, patients can be discharged home in consultation with a pediatric nephrologist. Patients who are ill-appearing with concern for thrombus, sepsis, shock, respiratory distress, worsening renal function, steroid-refractory disease, or infection should be hospitalized.

Acute Kidney Injury

KEY CONCEPTS

- Evaluation of fluid status in AKI is important in management strategies.
- Management is directed at correcting fluid and electrolyte derangements.

Foundations

Acute kidney injury (AKI) occurs when injury of renal tissue leads to alteration in fluid status, electrolyte imbalance, and poor elimination of waste, which can lead to chronic kidney disease and failure.[45] AKI is often multifactorial, but may be due to an underlying disease process, dehydration, medications, or toxins. AKI is often classified as prerenal, renal or postrenal (Table 168.6). Prerenal AKI is usually due to poor renal perfusion, renal AKI is due to intrinsic kidney parenchymal damage, and postrenal AKI is due to anatomic abnormality that prevents adequate drainage of the collecting system.

Clinical Features and Differential Diagnoses

Clinical presentation and differential diagnosis depend on the underlying etiology of AKI. Patients may have vital sign and physical

TABLE 168.6 Causes of AKI

Prerenal	Decreased renal perfusion: dehydration, hemorrhage, diuretics, burn, heart failure, sepsis, anaphylaxis
Renal	NSAIDs, ACE inhibitors, acute tubular necrosis, HUS, vasculitis (lupus, HSP), interstitial nephritis, malignancy, glomerulonephritis
Postrenal	Nephrolithiasis or urolithiasis, thrombosis, neurogenic bladder, medication-induced urinary retention, anatomic obstruction

examination findings consistent with dehydration (e.g., sunken fontanelle, dry skin, delayed capillary refill, dry mucous membranes). History may reveal poor oral intake, vomiting, diarrhea, or little to no urine output. History of sore throat or bloody diarrhea may point to poststreptococcal glomerulonephritis or hemolytic uremic syndrome (HUS), respectively. Medication history is important because many medications may be nephrotoxic. Patients may be edematous from fluid shifts and may have hematuria from renal injury.

Diagnostic Testing

Patients with suspected AKI should have a BMP drawn to assess for alterations in electrolytes, BUN, and creatinine. UA with microscopy may show hematuria or proteinuria depending on underlying etiology, and may have elevated specific gravity or ketones if the patient is dehydrated. RBC casts, WBC casts, or hyaline casts may also help identify glomerulonephritis, pyelonephritis, or acute tubular necrosis, respectively. Electrolyte abnormalities may be apparent such as hyponatremia, hyperkalemia, hyperphosphatemia and hypocalcemia. Elevated BUN and creatinine are hallmarks of AKI. If there are concerns for infection or HUS, CBC may identify leukocytosis, thrombocytopenia, or microangiopathic changes. Renal bladder ultrasound may be necessary to evaluate renal parenchyma, obstruction, and vessel thrombosis.

Management

Management of AKI is supportive and directed at correcting the underlying cause, as well as fluid and electrolyte abnormalities. Patients with prerenal or renal AKI may be fluid challenged with a 20 mL/kg normal saline (NS) bolus to assess for urine output response. Patients with nephrotoxic medication exposure would also benefit from fluid therapy, along with cessation of the exposure.[46] In patients with fluid overload or heart failure, fluids would worsen the clinical picture and pediatric nephrology should be consulted for diuretic management because furosemide is also nephrotoxic and could lead to hypotension in certain situations.[47] Severe electrolyte disturbances can lead to hyponatremic seizures or hyperkalemic cardiac arrhythmias. Hyponatremic seizures should be treated with 3% hypertonic saline at 3 to 5 mL/kg.

An electrocardiogram (EKG) also should be obtained in children with AKI. Hyperkalemia with QRS widening should be treated with calcium gluconate 30 to 60 mg/kg to stabilize the myocardium; additional hyperkalemia treatment includes dextrose (0.5 g/kg) and insulin (0.1 units/kg), albuterol, sodium bicarbonate (1 mEq/kg), kayexalate (1 g/kg) and Lasix (0.5–1 mg/kg). Dialysis may be necessary in cases of severe acidosis, electrolyte disturbances, toxic ingestions, fluid overload, or uremia.

Disposition

Pediatric patients with AKI warrant admission for fluid and electrolyte management; consultation with pediatric nephrology should be obtained for possible dialysis.

Hypertension

> **KEY CONCEPTS**
>
> - In children, blood pressure percentile is interpreted using sex, age, and height.
> - Blood pressure measurements are defined as normal, elevated, stage 1 hypertension, or stage 2 hypertension

Foundations

The prevalence of clinical hypertension in pediatrics is about 3.5%, and pediatric blood pressures (BP) are interpreted using sex, age, and height.[48] The definition of hypertension in children and adolescents differs from that of adults, and the most updated clinical guidelines for hypertension are outlined in Table 168.7.[48] If left untreated, children with hypertension are at increased risk of adult hypertension, cardiovascular disease, and metabolic syndrome.

Clinical Features

On presentation, children may be symptomatic or completely asymptomatic. If the initial BP is elevated, two separate BP measurements should be taken, and the three measurements averaged. If the patient still falls into one of the categories of hypertension, a thorough history should be completed including maternal complications at birth, gestational age, any umbilical vein catheter manipulation (risk of renal vein thrombosis), dietary salt intake, and family history. A physical examination, including 4-extremity blood pressure, is recommended to look for secondary signs of hypertension, such as coarctation of the aorta.

Differential Diagnoses

Children with confirmed hypertension greater than the ninety-fifth percentile should have follow-up with their primary care provider for ambulatory blood pressure monitoring. Patients with strong family history, elevated BMI, and poor dietary habits may have primary or essential hypertension. If this is not clear by history and physical examination, secondary causes of hypertension can be considered. Renovascular disease is the most common secondary cause of hypertension in children. Cardiac causes such as coarctation of the aorta also lead to hypertension in children and can go undiagnosed depending on the degree of narrowing. Other causes of secondary hypertension include sleep apnea, hormonal excess (e.g., catecholamines release of pheochromocytoma), genetic disease (neurofibromatosis 1), anatomic causes (renal artery stenosis), and medications/supplements (OCPs, stimulants, steroids).[48]

Diagnostic Testing

Laboratory evaluation for secondary causes of hypertension should include a BMP, lipid panel, and UA; other optional tests include renin, aldosterone, and urine catecholamines. Patients with a history of snoring and pauses in sleep can be referred for an outpatient sleep study. A urine toxicology screen can be helpful in patients suspected of drug abuse causing hypertension, but should not preclude urgent or emergency treatment. An ECG and echocardiography can assess for left ventricular hypertrophy or other structural causes of hypertension. Renal Doppler ultrasound is used to assess for renovascular disease, as well as renal artery stenosis or renal vein thrombosis.

Management and Disposition

Long-term goals in the treatment of hypertension in children include achieving a BP lower than the ninetieth percentile or less than 130/80 in adolescents to reduce end-organ damage and decrease the risk for cardiovascular disease in adulthood.[48] Lifestyle modifications that

TABLE 168.7	Definitions of Hypertension	
	Children Age 1–13 years	**Children Age >13 years**
Normal BP	<90th percentile	<120/80 mm Hg
Elevated BP	>90th percentile but <95th percentile	120/80 to 129/80
Stage I Hypertension	> 95th percentile to <95th percentile +12 mm Hg or 130/80 to 139/80 (whichever is lower)	130/80 to 139/80
Stage 2 Hypertension	>95th percentile + 12 mm Hg or >140/90 (whichever is lower)	>140/90

address diet, sleep, stress reduction, and physical activity are the initial management of choice for patients with elevated BP and asymptomatic stage I hypertension. If ongoing elevation persists despite lifestyle modifications, symptomatic stage I hypertension, or stage 2 hypertension, patients should undergo a diagnostic evaluation and pharmacologic treatment (with an ACE inhibitor, ARB, calcium channel blocker, or thiazide diuretic) with pediatric nephrology guidance and close follow-up.[48] Patients with stage 2 hypertension and end-organ damage such as encephalopathy, AKI, and heart failure are considered to have hypertensive emergency and should receive immediate reduction of BP by 25%. If the patient has stage 2 hypertension and remains symptomatic, or if the BP is greater than 30 mm Hg above the ninety-fifth percentile (>180/120 in adolescents), inpatient management is recommended.[48]

Henoch-Schönlein Purpura

> **KEY CONCEPTS**
>
> - HSP is a vasculitis that causes abdominal pain, GI bleeding, renal involvement, scrotal swelling, and arthralgias, and leads to an increased risk of intussusception
> - Consider inpatient admission for patients with HSP who cannot bear weight, cannot tolerate oral pain medications, or have GI bleeding or renal involvement.

Foundations

Henoch-Schönlein purpura (HSP) is the most common vasculitis in children and has an annual incidence of 10 to 20 per 100,000 children, peaking at age 4 to 6 years.[49] HSP is a small vessel IgA vasculitis which has the proclivity to affect any organ, but in particular causes issues with the gastrointestinal (GI) tract, skin, and kidneys. Its etiology is uncertain, but there may be an association with preceding upper respiratory tract illnesses since it is most commonly seen in the fall, winter, and spring and rarely in the summer months.

Clinical Features

Clinical manifestations are variable, and many sets of diagnostic criteria exist, but in general, the diagnosis is based on the tetrad of abdominal pain, nonthrombocytic palpable purpura, arthralgia, and renal involvement. Patients may present on a spectrum of mild to severe symptoms. The rash occurs in dependent areas of the buttocks and posterior legs and is typically palpable and purpuric. Gastrointestinal (GI) symptoms range from mild nausea and abdominal pain to severe GI bleeding and risk of intussusception. (See Chapter 166 for GI evaluation in patients with HSP.) Renal disease ranges from mild hematuria to more severe nephritis. Less common clinical manifestations also include scrotal edema, seizures, and interstitial lung disease.

Differential Diagnoses

Differential diagnosis may be broad depending on the patient presentation as some symptoms such as abdominal pain may be nonspecific. Given the purpuric nature of the rash, other causes of thrombocytopenia should be considered: sepsis, idiopathic thrombocytopenic purpura (ITP) or thrombotic thrombocytopenic purpura (TTP). Infection in the setting of rash and arthralgias can point to a strep infection, Lyme disease, or septic joint, as well as other rheumatic diseases. In patients with hematuria, a broad differential is necessary, as discussed in prior sections.

Diagnostic Testing

In patients with classic features of HSP, the diagnosis can be made clinically, as there is no diagnostic lab test. A UA is recommended to evaluate for renal involvement with hematuria. Patients with elevated blood pressure and hematuria should have a BMP to assess BUN and creatinine levels. CBC will be nonspecific and coagulopathy panels are generally normal. In patients with abdominal pain and/or GI bleeding, an ultrasound is recommended to assess for intussusception because these patients are at increased risk.

Management

Management of HSP is supportive and directed at symptomatic treatment. Pain can be treated with acetaminophen and NSAIDs (in the absence of severe renal involvement and ongoing GI bleeding). In general, patients who cannot bear weight due to arthralgias, pain not controlled with oral medications, ongoing GI bleeding, or renal involvement and signs of fluid overload should be admitted for pain control and fluid management. Use of glucocorticoids is controversial, as some evidence suggests improvement in GI sequelae but little benefit in preventing renal complications.[50]

Disposition

HSP nephritis may cause fluid overload, electrolyte derangements, and elevated blood pressure, requiring treatment with albumin, diuretics, and nephrology consultation. Milder cases of HSP may be managed outpatient with weekly PCP follow-up for BP and UA monitoring. Most cases resolve uneventfully, but some will have renal complications and recurrence.

Hemolytic Uremic Syndrome

KEY CONCEPTS

- Hemolytic uremic syndrome consists of a triad of acute kidney injury, thrombocytopenia, and microangiopathic hemolytic anemia, and is most frequently associated with E. coli 0157 Shiga toxin–producing bloody diarrhea.
- Care is mostly supportive with red blood cell transfusion, fluid and electrolyte management, and possibly renal replacement therapy.

Foundations

Hemolytic uremic syndrome (HUS) consists of acute kidney injury, thrombocytopenia, and microangiopathic hemolytic anemia, occurring secondary to an inciting etiology. Classification of HUS can be divided into either diarrhea positive, or typical HUS, versus diarrhea negative, or atypical HUS; 90% of cases are due to typical HUS secondary to Shiga toxin–producing E. Coli 0157, Shigella, or Streptococcus pneumoniae. The other 10% of cases are due to atypical HUS secondary to hereditary complement-mediated disease, pregnancy, malignancy, or medications.[51]

Clinical Features

Children often present with prodromal fever, abdominal pain, vomiting and diarrhea. After the first few days, the diarrhea progresses to bloody diarrhea and urine output may drop. Though rare, patients with HUS secondary to pneumococcal disease will present with fever, cough, and respiratory distress consistent with pneumonia. Patients with atypical HUS present with low urine output, signs of thrombocytopenia and anemia, and may also have neurologic complaints. Physical examination may reveal a petechial rash, pallor, and a tender abdomen.

Differential Diagnoses

Differential diagnosis includes other causes of thrombocytopenia and AKI, such as disseminated intravascular coagulation (DIC), TTP, or other vasculitides.

Diagnostic Testing

Laboratory studies recommended include a CBC with differential and smear to assess for microangiopathic anemia and thrombocytopenia, BMP to evaluate BUN and creatinine, as well as stool PCR to evaluate for E.coli O157 Shiga toxin. Coagulation studies can assess for DIC, and patients with fever and neurologic changes can have ADAMTS autoantibodies measured to diagnose TTP. Patients who are ill-appearing can have blood and urine cultures drawn, and those with altered mental status with severe thrombocytopenia may need a CT head scan to assess for intracranial hemorrhage.

Management

Management of HUS is largely supportive, with red blood cell transfusion for anemia, fluid and electrolyte management, and close monitoring for progression of AKI to renal failure, as dialysis may be required. Antibiotics should be avoided in E. coli O157 Shiga toxin–induced HUS, because it leads to lysis of more bacteria and can precipitate renal failure and need for dialysis. However, HUS cases due to pneumococcal disease should be treated with ceftriaxone and vancomycin.[52] Drugs that slow down GI transit, such as loperamide and opioids, should be avoided. Severe cases may have significant neurologic involvement due to intracranial hemorrhage, seizures, or altered mental status from uremia. Platelet transfusion may be required in clinically significant bleeding, but otherwise should be avoided due to ongoing consumption. Seizures can be treated with benzodiazepines. Atypical HUS has a higher risk of progression to end-stage renal disease, and may require dialysis, biologics such as eculizumab, plasmapheresis, and eventually require renal transplantation.[53]

Disposition

Overall, most patients will warrant inpatient admission for supportive care. Patients who fully recover should have yearly follow-up for close monitoring of hypertension and renal function.

The references for this chapter can be found online at Expert Consult.com.

169

Pediatric Neurologic Disorders

Marc Auerbach and Niyati Mehta

KEY CONCEPTS

- Altered mental status in children has a varied spectrum of clinical presentations, and may include any of the following: altered level of consciousness, excessive sleepiness, irritability, lethargy, and abnormal behavior.
- A careful and detailed history is instrumental in determining whether an event was a seizure.
- Status epilepticus constitutes a neurologic emergency that carries high morbidity and mortality rates. Initial treatment is typically with IV benzodiazepines, followed by fosphenytoin or levetiracetam. If the seizure continues to be refractory after a second-line agent, the patient may require airway management.
- A simple febrile seizure is generalized, lasts less than 15 minutes, and occurs in a neurologically and developmentally normal child between 6 months and 60 months of age.
- Breath-holding spells occur in children 6 months to 6 years of age, and are triggered by pain or emotional upset. After a trigger, the child becomes pale or cyanotic and may lose consciousness, sometimes with a brief period of clonic movements or opisthotonos that may mimic a seizure.
- Warning signs of secondary headaches include sudden onset, occurrence with straining or exertion, association with neurologic symptoms, change in headache pattern, nocturnal awakening, worsening in a recumbent position, and bilateral occipital headaches.
- If there are red flags on the history or physical exam, radiologic evaluation by computed tomography (CT), magnetic resonance imaging (MRI), or both may be necessary to rule out secondary causes of headache, such as intracranial hemorrhage, subarachnoid hemorrhage, brain tumor, or brain abscess.
- A toxicology screen is the test with the highest diagnostic yield for acute-onset ataxia in children.
- In children, 40% of ataxia cases are caused by acute cerebellar ataxia.

- Approximately 45% to 60% of all childhood brain tumors arise in the brainstem or cerebellum and can manifest with slowly progressive ataxia.
- When assessing an infant or child with motor weakness, it is important to distinguish presentations consistent with upper motor neuron pathology from lower motor neuron processes.
- Strokes represent a pediatric neurologic emergency and may be hemorrhagic or ischemic in nature. Imaging with CT or MRI can help confirm the diagnosis of stroke. Children with stroke may present with less specific signs such as headache, seizure, or alteration level of consciousness.
- Children presenting with suspected or confirmed strokes should be emergently transferred to a pediatric stroke center for timely consideration of therapies.
- Spinal cord compression is a medical emergency and requires prompt diagnosis and treatment. It may arise from trauma, infection and inflammation, or malignancy.
- The diagnosis of Guillain-Barré syndrome (GBS) is largely clinical, although lumbar puncture (LP) may be helpful in confirming the diagnosis. Patients with GBS are at risk for respiratory compromise and should be admitted to the hospital for observation and supportive care.
- The diagnosis of infant botulism is largely clinical. If there is high clinical suspicion, treatment should be initiated promptly, without awaiting laboratory confirmation. Given the risk of respiratory compromise, infants with botulism should be admitted to the hospital for observation and supportive care.
- Diagnosis of myasthenia gravis is often not confirmed in the ED. The disorder can often be treated on an outpatient basis, but patients with truncal involvement and concern for respiratory compromise should be admitted to the hospital for observation and supportive care.

SEIZURES

Foundations

Seizures are a common pediatric neurologic disorder presenting to the emergency department (ED); up to 10% of children suffer at least one seizure in the first 16 years of life, most of which are febrile seizures. A seizure is defined as a paroxysmal event characterized by temporary involuntary changes in the patient caused by excessive synchronous electrical neuronal discharges of a group of cortical neurons. The clinical manifestations of the seizures depend on the location of the neurons involved, and may include alterations in motor activity, behavior, level of consciousness, or autonomic function. Infants and children younger than 5 years are thought to be more susceptible to seizures due to an immature nervous system, in which excitatory neuronal activity predominates and inhibitory systems are undeveloped. A paucity of synaptic connections and alterations in the synthesis of neurotransmitters may also play a role. Epilepsy is commonly defined as the occurrence

of two or more unprovoked seizures. Provoked seizures are caused by an identifiable trigger and stem from a broad array of disturbances, including fever, metabolic derangements, and trauma (Table 169.1). Reflex seizures may be precipitated by a specific, identifiable stimulus, such as flashing lights on television or video games. Unprovoked seizures have no clear immediate precedent.

Clinical Features

The initial approach to the diagnosis and treatment of a pediatric patient with ongoing seizures involves resuscitation measures to ensure a patent and protected airway, adequate oxygenation and ventilation, stable circulation, and seizure control. The initial history should include duration of the seizures, preceding signs and *s*ymptoms, *a*llergies, current *m*edications, risk of ingestion, *p*ast medical history, *l*ast meal, and *e*vents preceding the seizure (SAMPLE). For patients who are no longer seizing on presentation, witnesses should be asked to provide a description of the event: type of body movements, accompanying

TABLE 169.1 Common Pediatric Presentations and Associated Differential Diagnoses

Pediatric Presentation	Underlying Diagnoses to Consider
Seizure	Infection (meningitis, sepsis, encephalitis)
	Metabolic derangement
	Ingestion
	Trauma
	Intracranial mass
	Antiepileptic dose or medication effect (in patient with known seizure disorder)
Altered mental status	Vascular event (stroke, arteriovenous malformation, intracranial bleed)
	Infection (meningitis, sepsis, encephalitis)
	Trauma
	Ingestion (toxin, medication)
	Seizures (clinical or subclinical)
	Structural/anatomic (intracranial mass/tumor, hydrocephalus)
	Metabolic derangements (e.g., diabetic ketoacidosis, hypoglycemia, urea cycle defect)
	Intussusception
Headache	Nonpathologic: due to stress, inadequate sleep, dehydration, fever, viral infection
	Migraine
	Trauma, concussion
	Intracranial pathology: mass, bleeding, hydrocephalus
	Infection (e.g., meningitis, sepsis, encephalitis)
Ataxia/disorders of balance	Postviral, postinfectious syndrome
	Intracranial mass
	Ingestion
	Metabolic disorders
Motor dysfunction, weakness	Vascular event (stroke)
	Spinal cord dysfunction (e.g., secondary to trauma, infection, autoimmune disorder)
	Infection-related (e.g., Guillain-Barré syndrome, Lyme disease, botulism)
	Idiopathic (Bell palsy)

Fig. 169.1 Café-au-lait spots as seen with neurofibromatosis. (From: Boyd KP, Korf BR, Theos A. Neurofibromatosis type I. *J Am Acad Dermatol.* 2009;61:1-16.)

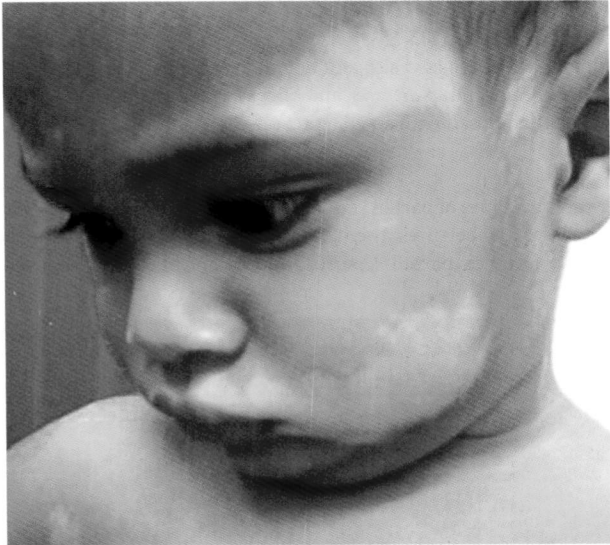

Fig. 169.2 Ash leaf spots as seen in tuberosclerosis. (From: Jindal R, Jain A, Gupta A, Shirazi N. Ash-leaf spots or naevus depigmentosus: a diagnostic challenge. *BMJ Case Rep.* 2013:2013.)

trauma, associated symptoms (e.g., urinary incontinence), duration, and postictal signs (e.g., period of sleepiness, lethargy or confusion). Patients with known seizure disorders should be asked about recent medication changes (i.e., new medications, missed doses, or dose adjustments) or any factors that may impact metabolism of medications (e.g., growth, diet change, illness, activity change).

The initial physical examination should focus on signs of systemic disease that can cause seizure, including evidence of meningitis or trauma and a review of the vital signs for hypertension or clinical toxidromes. After the seizure has resolved, a thorough examination should be completed, including a complete neurologic examination and funduscopic examination to assess for papilledema and retinal hemorrhages. Skin lesions may indicate a neurocutaneous disorder such as tuberous sclerosis or neurofibromatosis (Fig. 169.1 and 169.2) and café-au-lait spots or hypopigmented nevi. There is a high incidence of subclinical electrographic seizures in infants. Neonatal or infantile seizures may be subtle; apnea, sustained eye deviation, chewing, or limb bicycling movements may be the only apparent signs. Focal clonic movements are often associated with an underlying structural lesion in the brain.

If the presenting signs and symptoms are consistent with seizure activity, the seizure can then be classified by type based on the following three elements[1]: (1) location of onset (focal versus generalized); (2) level of consciousness/awareness (aware, impaired awareness, altered level of consciousness); and (3) motor versus nonmotor (i.e., staring, nonconvulsive status epilepticus, versus convulsive) (Table 169.2).

Generalized Seizures

Generalized seizures may be convulsive or nonconvulsive. A convulsive seizure may start focally and generalize secondarily. Convulsive status epilepticus is a true neurologic emergency defined as 5 minutes or more of continuous seizure activity (clinical or electroencephalographic) or recurrent seizure activity without return to baseline between seizures.[2] Refractory status epilepticus is defined as status epilepticus that does not respond to first- and second-line antiepileptics. Super-refractory status epilepticus is defined as status epilepticus that persists 24 hours or more. Super-refractory status epilepticus is associated with a risk of mortality (3%) and long-term morbidity, including recurrent seizures and cognitive-behavioral impairment.[3] The diagnosis of convulsive status epilepticus is usually obvious; however, the duration of the seizures is often underestimated because the intensity of the jerking tends to diminish with time. Status epilepticus occurs more frequently in children than in adults, particularly in those younger than 1 year. Medication changes, toxic ingestion, idiopathic epilepsy, metabolic derangements, and congenital abnormalities are common etiologies of pediatric seizures.

Nonconvulsive status epilepticus is marked by an altered mental status. Patients may demonstrate confusion, unresponsiveness, abnormal motor movements, twitches, lip smacking, automatisms, and sympathomimetic changes such as tachycardia, hypertension, and dilated pupils. An electroencephalogram (EEG) can confirm the diagnosis and should be obtained if nonconvulsive status is suspected. The most common type of generalized nonconvulsive seizure is absence seizures. Absence seizures are marked by a brief arrest of consciousness and movement, typically lasting 5 to 30 seconds; no postictal drowsiness occurs. It may be difficult to differentiate a brief complex partial seizure, in which a child may stare and not respond, from an absence seizure. Psychogenic nonepileptic seizures (PNES), caused by psychological factors, are events that look like generalized seizures but are not epileptic in nature. PNES are more common in patients with epilepsy, and patients with PNES are often later diagnosed with an epileptic seizure disorder.

Focal Onset

There are two types of partial (i.e., focal) seizures—complex and simple. In simple partial seizures, the patient experiences no change in mentation. In complex partial seizures, the patient experiences a change in level of awareness, and may exhibit bizarre behaviors, including staring, lip smacking, wandering, or picking at clothing. An important subcategory of focal seizures is composed of benign focal epilepsies of childhood, which are idiopathic in nature (i.e., they do not result from abnormalities in brain structure or injury to the brain). Benign focal epilepsies spontaneously resolve over time; benign childhood epilepsy with centrotemporal spikes (i.e., benign rolandic epilepsy) is most common and represents 10% to 20% of all childhood epilepsies.

The etiology of seizures can be divided into three categories—acute symptomatic, remote symptomatic, and idiopathic. Acute symptomatic seizures are provoked by an acute event such as fever. Remote symptomatic seizures are due to a preexisting or remote central nervous system (CNS) lesion such as cerebral palsy, neurocutaneous disorders, neurodegenerative disease, or a congenital brain malformation. Idiopathic seizures have no identifiable cause (Table 169.3).

Fever is the most common cause of acute symptomatic seizures. A febrile seizure is defined as a seizure occurring in the presence of fever without CNS infection or other cause and occurs in up to 5% of children. A simple febrile seizure is generalized, lasts less than 15 minutes, and occurs in a neurologically and developmentally normal child between 6 months and 60 months of age. Complex febrile seizures are diagnosed when multiple seizures occur during the same illness, the seizures are longer than 15 minutes, or the seizures have a focal component. Febrile seizures typically occur early in the course of illness; higher temperature or reduction of fever with antipyretics does not reduce the risk of seizure. Meningitis should be considered

TABLE 169.2	**Classification of Seizures**			
Onset	**Focal Onset**	**Generalized Onset**	**Unknown Onset**
Awareness	Aware Impaired awareness	Impaired awareness	Unsure of awareness
Other Features	Motor Nonmotor	Motor Nonmotor (Absence)	Nonmotor (Absence)
	May progress from focal to bilateral tonic-clonic (generalized)		*Unclassified seizures do not fit in any other category*

(Adapted from: Fisher RS, Cross JH, French JA, et al. Operational classification of seizure types by the International League Against Epilepsy: Position Paper of the ILAE Commission for Classification and Terminology. *Epilepsia.* 2017;58:522-530; and Trinka E, Cock H, Hesdorffer D, et al. A definition and classification of status epilepticus—Report of the ILAE Task Force on Classification of Status Epilepticus. *Epilepsia.* 2015;56:1515-1523.)

TABLE 169.3	**Causes of Seizures**	
CAUSE	**EXAMPLES**
Fever (febrile seizure)	
• Infectious process	Meningitis, encephalitis, brain abscess, other infectious process (viral or bacterial infections including viral URI, pneumonia, otitis media, AGE, UTI)
• Traumatic lesions	Cerebral contusion, hemorrhage (subdural, epidural, subarachnoid, intraparenchymal), impact seizure
Toxic conditions	Drug intoxication, drug withdrawal
Metabolic disturbances	Hypoglycemia, hyponatremia, hypernatremia, hypomagnesemia, hypocalcemia, hypophosphatemia, hepatic or renal disorder, inborn errors of metabolism (e.g., aminoacidurias, organic acidurias, mitochondrial disease)
Neoplastic disease	Brain tumors
• Vascular disorders	Arteriovenous malformation, subarachnoid hemorrhage, intraparenchymal hemorrhage, cerebral venous thrombosis, ischemic infarct, hypertensive encephalopathy
• Neurocutaneous disorders	Neurofibromatosis, tuberous sclerosis, Sturge-Weber syndrome
Neurodegenerative disorders—miscellaneous	Hypoxia, ventriculoperitoneal shunt malfunction, cerebral palsy, cerebral dysgenesis, primary epilepsy

in any patient with seizures and fever. However, a child whose mental status is normal before and after the seizure is very unlikely to have meningitis.[4] We recommend considering a lumbar puncture in infants younger than 6 months presenting with febrile seizures, especially those with complex features or who have other risk factors for bacterial meningitis (e.g., underimmunized, comorbid disease, immunocompromised).

Electrolyte derangements including hypoglycemia, hyponatremia, and hypernatremia are other common causes of acute symptomatic seizures in children. Hypoglycemia resulting in seizure may be the first presentation of an infant with an underlying metabolic disease. Dehydration is the most common cause of *hyper*natremia, whereas *hypo*natremia may be secondary to overdilution of infant formula—a feeding history should be obtained in infants with abnormal serum sodium levels. Hypocalcemia and hypomagnesemia may lead to muscle spasms, paresthesias, hyperactive reflexes, weakness, tetany, or seizures. Hypocalcemic seizures are a common cause of neonatal seizures.

Posttraumatic seizures occur in as many as 15% of children after head injury. Impact seizures, occurring within 1 hour of a head trauma, are often not associated with significant injury or with the development of epilepsy and therefore trigger diagnostic imaging with CT. It may be difficult to distinguish impact seizures from those associated with intracranial injury; existing clinical decision rules and electronic decision support systems should determine need for intracranial imaging.[5] Early posttraumatic seizures, occurring within the first week of injury, may arise from cerebral edema or intracranial hemorrhage or contusion.

Brain tumors and intracranial masses can present with seizures, depending on their location. However, infratentorial tumors, the most common location in the pediatric population, do not typically cause seizures. A seizure may be the presenting sign of stroke or vascular anomaly (discussed in more detail later in this chapter). Numerous drugs are known to cause seizures in children, especially in overdose. Cyclic antidepressants, cocaine and other stimulants, antihistamines, and isoniazid are the most common agents of drug-induced seizures. Seizures may occur during drug withdrawal from benzodiazepines or ethanol, usually within 48 hours of cessation.

Differential Diagnoses

Paroxysmal alterations in level of consciousness or motor activity may be confused with seizure activity in children (Table 169.4). Syncope can be mistaken for a seizure, as it is characterized by a sudden loss of consciousness and motor tone caused by a transient, global cerebral hypoperfusion. The patient may complain of lightheadedness and blurry vision or appear pale and sweaty prior to the event. Brief jerking movements with trembling or stiffening are common with syncopal events, but should not be prolonged, and postictal confusion or lethargy does not occur. Vasovagal syncope is common in otherwise healthy children and does not warrant further evaluation unless recurrent. Syncope or seizure-like events occurring during activities or associated with palpitations may be a presentation of potentially fatal cardiogenic syncope, such as prolonged QTc syndrome; patients should have an ECG obtained in their evaluation. Breath-holding spells occur in up to 5% of children and are triggered by pain or emotional upset. The first episode usually occurs between the ages of 6 and 18 months, with episodes recurring up to 6 years of age. After a trigger, the child becomes pale or cyanotic and may lose consciousness, sometimes with a brief period of clonic movements or opisthotonos. The average attack lasts approximately 40 seconds. A history of recurrent episodes associated with crying may be helpful in distinguishing these from seizures or brief resolved unexplained events. Migraines may mimic seizures or stroke, particularly when

TABLE 169.4 Disorders That Mimic Seizures

Age Group	Features
Neonates	Jitteriness
	Benign neonatal sleep myoclonus
	Nonepileptic apnea
	Opisthotonos
	Normal movement
Nonneonates	Breath-holding spells
	Rigors or chills
	Gastroesophageal reflux (Sandifer syndrome)
	Migraine
	Benign paroxysmal vertigo of childhood
	Syncope
	Neurovascular event
	Sleep disorders
	Sleep myoclonus
	Narcolepsy
	Nightmares, night terrors, somnambulism
	Movement disorders
	Tics or stereotypies
	Infantile shuddering attacks
	Paroxysmal choreoathetosis or dystonia
	Behavioral or psychiatric disturbances
	Psychogenic seizures
	Panic attack

they are accompanied by an aura, motor dysfunction, clouding of consciousness, or vomiting.

Disorders of sleep are distinguished by excessive daytime sleepiness or by disordered nighttime sleep. Patients with narcolepsy have daytime sleep attacks, sleep paralysis, hypnagogic hallucinations (i.e., vivid hallucinations while falling asleep), and cataplexy (i.e., sudden loss of motor tone). Cataplexy may be mistaken for atonic or absence seizures. Nocturnal enuresis may be a symptom of unwitnessed nighttime seizure associated with incontinence. In night terrors (pavor nocturnus), the child suddenly wakens, crying inconsolably, and is relatively unresponsive. The child returns to sleep and does not typically recall the event. Sleep walking (somnambulism) and sleep talking (somniloquy) are common among school-age children.

Movement disorders may mimic seizures. Tics are rapid, repetitive, brief involuntary movements that occur intermittently and in flurries. Those most commonly seen are eye blinking and head shaking. Patients do not lose consciousness. Sydenham chorea is an autoimmune-mediated systemic inflammatory response that occurs in association with a group A streptococcal pharyngitis infection. It typically manifests with irregular, nonrhythmic, involuntary jerking of the extremities and face, and may present during the acute phase of the streptococcal infection or as a latent manifestation months after the initial illness. Shudder attacks, with movements like the chill experienced when cold water runs down the back, are uncommon but easily mistaken for seizures. Paroxysmal choreoathetosis is an abnormal motor movement that may be spontaneous or triggered by the child's movement.

Behavioral or psychiatric disturbances can produce behaviors that may appear epileptic. Panic attacks may be mistaken for complex partial seizures, with a sudden sensation of intense fear accompanied by shortness of breath, dizziness, palpitations, sweating, choking, chest discomfort, and fear of dying. Psychogenic seizures or pseudoseizures are involuntary events that mimic seizures. Many children with psychogenic seizures also have epileptic seizures. Prolonged electroen-cephalographic with video monitoring may be necessary to differenti-ate an epileptic seizure from a psychogenic seizure.

Infants with gastrointestinal reflux may have Sandifer syndrome and appear to have seizure-like movements with episodes of abnormal posturing, arching of the back, and torticollis.

Management

The initial management of any actively seizing child involves ensuring patency of the airway, adequate oxygenation and ventilation, and sup-port of circulation. Oxygen should be applied via cannula or face mask, and intravenous (IV) or intraosseous (IO) access quickly obtained. Monitoring end-tidal carbon dioxide may be helpful to assess ventila-tory status. Patients with ongoing convulsions are at risk for hypoventi-lation and apnea, and preparations should be made to assist ventilation. The goal is to rapidly stop the seizure with antiepileptic medication while assessing for the underlying cause.

Hypoglycemia causing seizures in infants and children is treated with an IV bolus of 10% dextrose, 5 mL/kg, with repeat boluses as needed to normalize the serum glucose level. Severe symptomatic hyponatremia presenting with seizures is treated with the administration of 3% saline (3 mL/kg IV infused over 30 minutes) to raise the serum sodium chlo-ride level by 3 to 7 mEq/L. Hypernatremia should be corrected slowly over 48 hours. Hypocalcemia is treated with 10% calcium gluconate, 100 mg/kg IV over 5 to 10 minutes; the patient should be on a cardiac moni-tor during the infusion. Toxic ingestions are treated based on the specific toxin involved. Seizures caused by isoniazid (INH) poisoning are partic-ularly resistant to standard seizure treatment, yet respond to pyridoxine. The dose of pyridoxine is 1 g IV for every gram of INH ingested. When the quantity of INH ingested is unknown, 5 g IV may be administered to an adult and 70 mg/kg (maximum, 5 g) to a child at rate of 1 g/minute until seizure stops or maximum dose.

Status Epilepticus

Status epilepticus is a true medical emergency. The patient should be positioned to maximize ventilation and prevent aspiration; attempts should be made to immobilize the cervical spine if trauma is suspected. Oxygen should be administered by nasal cannula or face mask with a bag valve mask for positive pressure if ventilation is inadequate. A large suction catheter should be available to suction oropharyngeal secretions. In younger patients, the tongue may obstruct the airway; a nasopharyngeal airway should be used to improve ventilation unless there is significant facial trauma. Oral pharyngeal airways may lead to vomiting when the seizure resolves and are often not utilized in treat-ment of seizures. If there is evidence of increased ICP, the head of the bed should be elevated. In a prolonged seizure, treatment with multiple medications or increased metabolic demand may lead to respiratory failure, necessitating intubation. We suggest that noninvasive measures are used to support ventilation in the initial phases of treatment before moving to intubation. If the decision is made to intubate, a sedative agent with antiepileptic activity should be selected (e.g., propofol, ket-amine). In addition, a short-acting neuromuscular blocker (e.g., succi-nylcholine) is preferred to allow for monitoring of continued seizure activity as long as other contraindications to its use are not present.

Heart rate, blood pressure, respiratory rate, and pulse oximetry should be monitored and hyperthermia treated with antipyretics and cooling blankets. An IV line or, if an IV cannot be established, an IO line should be placed and blood samples sent for electrolyte values, glu-cose concentration (including rapid blood glucose test), calcium and magnesium levels, renal function tests, liver function tests, antiepilep-tic levels (when indicated), and CBC. Urine should be sent for toxicol-ogy. Metabolic abnormalities should be corrected.

Anticonvulsant treatment should begin as quickly as possible (Fig. 169.3).[6] Delays in the initiation of benzodiazepines of greater than 10 minutes is associated with higher frequency of death, longer seizure duration, and more complications.[7] Benzodiazepines, particularly lorazepam and diazepam, are the initial drugs of choice in the treat-ment of status epilepticus; they diffuse quickly into the CNS, rapidly terminating seizure activity 70% of the time. Hypotension, respiratory depression, and impaired consciousness may occur after administra-tion. Intranasal, buccal, or intramuscular routes may be used if IV or IO access cannot be obtained within the first 1 to 2 minutes of resusci-tation and are preferable to rectal administration. Recommended doses for these non-IV preparations are shown in Fig. 169.3.

A second dose of benzodiazepine should be administered only after 5 minutes of continued seizure activity following the first dose. If the seizure persists an additional 5 minutes after giving the second ben-zodiazepine dose, consider administering a third benzodiazepine dose and load with a second-line agent. The choices of second-line agents include levetiracetam, fosphenytoin, or valproic acid (Fig. 169.3).[6] There is limited evidence that one of these agents is preferred to the others. Recent controlled trials comparing phenytoin or phosphenytion to levetiracetam did not note a difference in the cessation of seizures.[8,9] One trial in Pakistan noted fewer adverse events and an improved efficacy for levetiracetam compared to phenytoin.[10] Valproic acid is contraindicated in the presence of liver disease, thrombocytopenia, or possible metabolic disease. There is limited evidence consisting of case reports that ketamine may be effective in treating refractory status epi-lepticus compared to conventional anesthetics and other agents.[11]

Fosphenytoin is a water-soluble phosphate ester of phenytoin that is rapidly converted in plasma to phenytoin. Unlike phenytoin, fos-phenytoin can be administered intramuscularly and with common IV solutions and is substantially less cardio-toxic and less sclerosing to the vasculature. In addition, it can be given three times more rapidly than phenytoin. Fosphenytoin achieves plasma concentrations similar to those achieved for phenytoin. If seizures continue after loading with a second-line agent, another second-line agent can be administered. We recommend a propofol or a midazolam infusion as third-line agent to induce a coma. Other options include phenobarbital, pentobarbi-tal, thiopental, or inhalant anesthetics. All have significant associated side effects and cause apnea, depressed consciousness, and hypoten-sion; these side effects are more pronounced in the presence of benzo-diazepines. Patients receiving these agents should receive continuous cardiorespiratory monitoring; staff and equipment should be readily available to support ventilation and advanced airway management.

Pediatric refractory status epilepticus is a high stakes and low frequency event and we recommend consultation with a neurologist when possible. Nonconvulsive status epilepticus is more difficult to recognize and often requires electroencephalography for diagnosis. Once the seizure has been effectively terminated, neuroimaging and lumbar puncture (LP) are often indicated to elucidate the cause of the seizure further.

Febrile Seizures

Children with simple febrile seizures do not require blood and urine testing other than as needed for the evaluation of fever source. An LP is not necessary in children older than 6 months with no signs of men-ingitis and no severe ill appearance before or after the seizure. If a child is less than 6 months or not fully immunized, an LP should be consid-ered. Electroencephalography, neuroimaging, admission, or specialty consultation is not required after a first simple febrile seizure. Children who fully recover after a simple febrile seizure can almost always be sent home. Guidance for families should include high likelihood of recurrence (>33%), the small increased risk for the development of

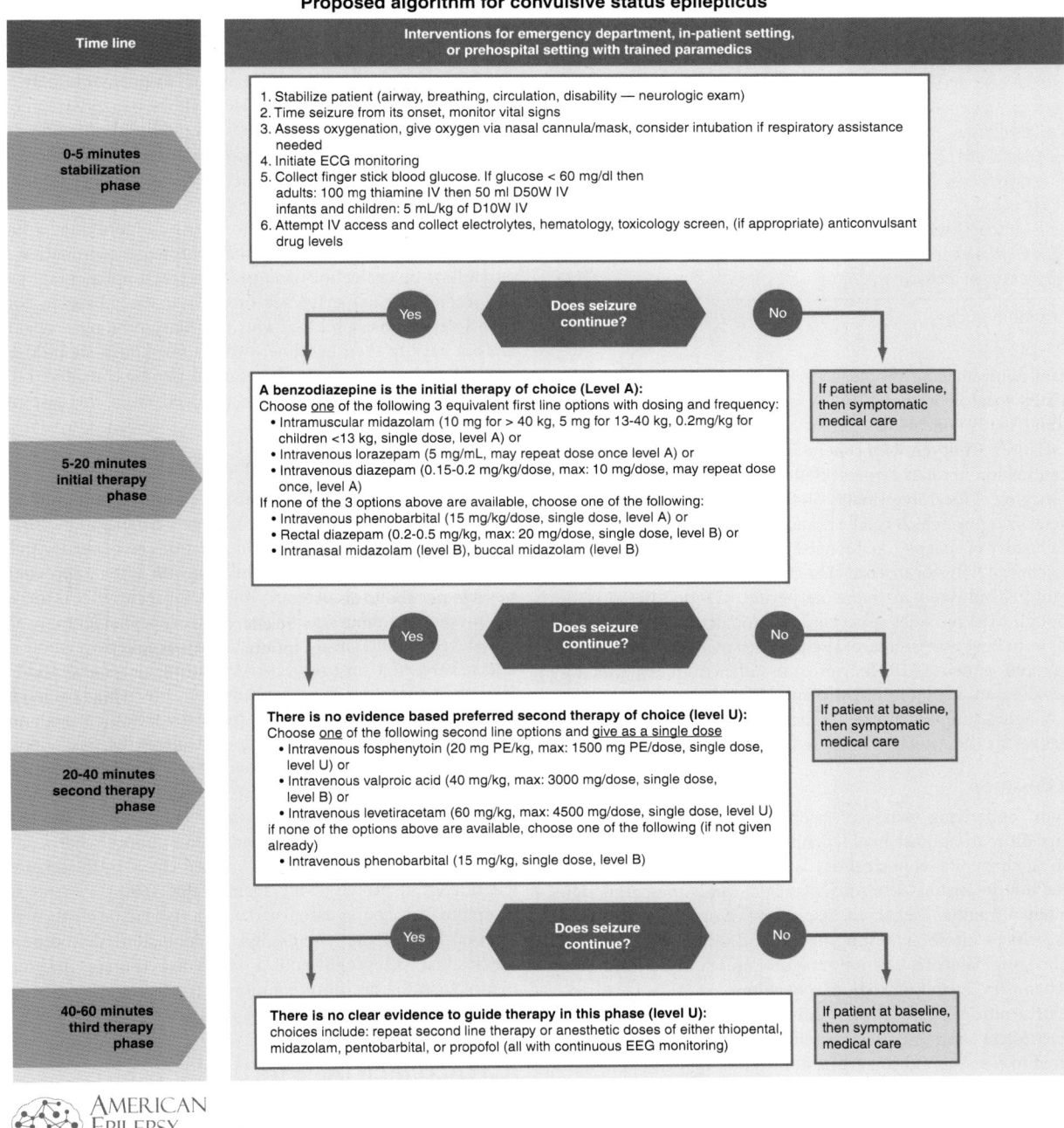

Fig. 169.3 Management of status epilepticus in infants >1 month of age and children. *IO,* Intraosseous; *IV,* intravenous. (Modified from: Glauser T, Shinnar S, Gloss D, et al. Evidence-based guideline: treatment of convulsive status epilepticus in children and adults: Report of the Guideline Committee of the American Epilepsy Society. *Epilepsy Curr.* 2016;16(1):48-61.)

afebrile seizures (2% to 5% or double the baseline risk), fever control, and emergency measures for seizure. Extensive anticipatory guidance and reassurance should be provided to the family with close follow-up with their pediatrician.

Afebrile Seizures

For infants and children older than 6 months who have had a first-time afebrile seizure and have returned to baseline, laboratory testing should be pursued in a targeted manner, based on clinical and historical findings. A seizure in the setting of recent vomiting, diarrhea or starvation may warrant examination of serum chemistries for possible electrolyte abnormalities. A toxicology screening history should be performed to explore any medications in the home and laboratory testing considered. A lumbar puncture should be considered for patients who present with unprovoked seizures and persistent abnormal mental status, do not return to baseline, or show signs of meningitis. An outpatient EEG may be appropriate in well-appearing children who have returned to baseline.

Emergent neuroimaging should be performed in infants and children with new focal neurologic deficits, persistent altered mental status (including status epilepticus), recent trauma, persistent headache, or partial seizures. Children with generalized unprovoked seizures and normal examination findings on presentation do not necessarily require emergent imaging. A focal abnormality on follow-up EEG may indicate a need for neuroimaging, which can be done on an outpatient basis. Children with a history of epilepsy do not need neuroimaging unless there is a change in clinical status or marked change in seizure pattern.

If imaging is indicated in the acute period, CT or MRI may be used. Although MRI provides superior anatomic detail, sedation may be needed, impeding assessment of the patient's mental status. When available, a rapid sequence MRI may provide sufficient information for the acute evaluation, with a full MRI planned for a later date.[12] Often the initial imaging study of choice, CT provides rapid imaging and is highly sensitive for the detection of acute blood and fractures.

Neonatal Seizures

The common underlying causes of neonatal seizures in infants <1 month of age differ from those in older children and adults (Box 169.1). In addition to congenital abnormalities, metabolic derangements, and birth-related injuries, neonatal seizures may be the only presenting sign of nonaccidental trauma. Diagnostic assessment of neonatal seizures is broad and includes metabolic testing (blood and urine), CSF analysis, and neuroimaging. Glucose, calcium, magnesium, and electrolyte levels (basic chemistry, including sodium, potassium, chloride, bicarbonate, blood urea nitrogen [BUN] and creatinine), and CBC should be obtained; lactic acid, ammonia, ketones, and pH determinations should be considered to assess for inborn errors of metabolism. Clinical assessment for meningitis is not reliable in young infants; thus, a LP should be performed and fluid sent for cell, protein, and glucose determinations, culture, and herpes simplex PCR assay. Head CT or MRI should also be performed when the neonate is stabilized. In the unstable neonate, a head ultrasound may be performed at the bedside to evaluate for a neurosurgical emergency until more definitive imaging can be obtained.

Empirical antibiotic coverage should be initiated if an LP is suggestive of bacterial meningitis. Antiviral therapy should be administered if there are clinical concerns for herpes encephalitis, including skin or mucosal findings, continued seizures with no other clear cause, or concerning maternal history; CSF red cells are a late and ominous finding. Electrolyte abnormalities, including hypoglycemia, hypomagnesemia, and hyponatremia, should be promptly corrected as described previously. If seizures are refractory to medical treatment, empirical treatment with pyridoxine, 15–30 mg/kg/day (not to exceed 500 mg/day), should be considered for the potential for a deficiency, and this dose can be repeated over the course of 30 minutes. This should be done with EEG monitoring, as clinical seizure detection in neonates is not reliable..

Phenobarbital is the usual drug of choice for neonatal seizures. However, there is increasing evidence of phenobarbital-induced neuronal apoptosis, even with a single dose, and evidence of memory and learning difficulties in rat models.[13] Due to its potential harm, other potential first-line agents for the treatment of neonatal seizures are currently being investigated. If seizures continue, fosphenytoin may be loaded. Refractory seizures may be treated with a benzodiazepine infusion. Neonates with a first-time seizures should be admitted for continuous cardiorespiratory monitoring and evaluation by a neurologist.

Disposition

Hospitalization is unnecessary for most children after a first unprovoked brief seizure, as long as the neurologic examination is normal and follow-up evaluation arranged. Electroencephalography and imaging studies can be performed on an outpatient basis in consultation with a neurologist. Children who have had a prolonged seizure, or who are not back to their baseline within a few hours, should be admitted to the hospital. Hospitalization should also be considered if adequate follow-up evaluation cannot be arranged or in the case of extreme parental anxiety.

Anticonvulsant Therapy at Discharge

The decision to start anticonvulsant prophylaxis should be done in consultation with a pediatric neurologist, balancing the risk of recurrent seizures against potential complications associated with long-term medication use. Two-thirds of children with a first unprovoked seizure never experience a recurrence. The risk for recurrence is increased with the presence of neuroimaging or electroencephalographic abnormalities, developmental delay, family history of epilepsy, remote symptomatic seizure, first seizure occurring during sleep, and Todd paralysis. If none of these risk factors are present, the 5-year recurrence risk is only 21%. There is no evidence that early treatment with anticonvulsant medications after a single seizure alters the risk of epilepsy, nor is there evidence to show that a single self-limited seizure causes neurologic sequelae. In light of these considerations, anticonvulsants are generally started after a second unprovoked seizure. The ED provider should only initiate a seizure medication upon discharge in consultation with a pediatric neurologist and is dictated by the seizure type and the side effect profile of the agent (Table 169.5). Patients with acute symptomatic seizures associated with a risk factor for recurrence (e.g., cerebral hemorrhage, meningitis, or contusion) should be treated in the hospital with prophylactic anticonvulsants under the guidance of a neurologist; the decision to continue treatment should be made once the patient is stable.

ALTERED MENTAL STATUS

Foundations

Altered mental status is a common and challenging pediatric presentation. Groupings of possible causes include vascular events (e.g., stroke, arteriovenous malformation with bleed), infection (e.g., meningitis, sepsis, encephalitis), trauma, toxic ingestion, anatomic or structural abnormality (e.g., intracranial mass or tumor), headache syndromes (e.g., acute confusional migraines, postconcussive syndrome), metabolic derangements, (e.g., DKA, hypoglycemia), intussusception, or subclinical seizures (see Table 169.1). Individual diagnoses associated with altered mental status will not be explored in full detail in this chapter. However, a guideline for approaching and managing pediatric patients in the ED with altered mental status will be presented.

Clinical Features

Altered mental status in children has a varied spectrum of clinical presentations and may include abnormalities in cognition, behavior, or memory. In children, these are manifested as an altered level of

TABLE 169.5 Commonly Used Anticonvulsants in Children

Drug	Seizure Type	Typical Daily Dose (mg/kg)	Therapeutic Level (µg/mL)
Carbamazepine (Tegretol)	Partial, GTC	10–20 (max 1000 mg/day)	4–12
Ethosuximide (Zarontin)	Absence	15–30 (max 1500 mg/day)	1.5–10
Phenobarbital	Partial, GTC	3–6	15–40
Phenytoin (Dilantin)	Partial, GTC	4–10	10–20
Valproic acid (Depakene, Depakote)	Atonic, GTC	15–40	40–120
Lamotrigine (Lamictal)	Partial, GTC, absence, Lennox-Gastaut syndrome	5–15 (1–5 if taking valproic acid)	Not routinely measured
Levetiracetam (Keppra)	Partial, GTC, myoclonic	20–60	Not routinely measured
Topiramate (Topamax)	Partial, GTC, myoclonic, Lennox-Gastaut syndrome	5–9	Not routinely measured
Clonazepam (Klonopin)	GTC, atonic, myoclonic	0.05–0.2	Not routinely measured

Starting doses for each drug may be lower than typical daily dose, and typical daily doses may fall outside the ranges noted in accordance with the child's underlying medical conditions and other medications.

GTC, Generalized tonic-clonic.

consciousness, excessive sleepiness, irritability, lethargy, or abnormal behavior. The nature of the altered mental status (e.g., lethargy versus coma), as well as the time course and concurrent findings (e.g., fever or focal neurologic signs), should guide evaluation. Information obtained in the history may be critical to diagnoses of trauma, toxic ingestion, atypical migraine, or infection.

During the initial assessment of an altered infant or child, vital signs can be essential to understanding the underlying diagnosis. Heart rate, blood pressure, and respiratory rate, for example, may provide information about conditions such as toxic ingestion (e.g., hyperpnea with salicylate ingestions), elevated intracranial pressure (e.g., Cushing triad), or metabolic derangements, such as diabetic ketoacidosis (often presenting with tachycardia and hyperpnea). Level of consciousness may be readily assessed using the AVPU scale: *a*lert (alert and spontaneously interactive), *v*erbal (responds to verbal cues), *p*ainful (responds only to painful stimuli), *u*nresponsive (unresponsive to all external stimuli). Additionally, identifying focal neurologic deficits and the presence or absence of fever will aid in the diagnostic evaluation.

Special consideration should be given to conditions that need emergent treatment or can lead to substantial morbidity or mortality. Examples include meningitis, intracranial bleed, toxic ingestion, and stroke. In infants less than one month old, the absence of fever does not eliminate the possibility of a serious bacterial infection and these infants often demonstrate vague findings: decreased tone, poor feeding, weak suck, increased sleepiness, or fussiness, with or without abnormal vital signs. In the ill-appearing or altered infant, clinical signs are often nonlocalizing and, therefore, can present a diagnostic challenge. In this age group, there are few distinguishing features to differentiate sepsis from meningitis, metabolic derangements, or an acute abdomen.

Differential Diagnoses

The breadth of differential diagnoses associated with altered mental status in children involves a broad spectrum of potential management interventions in the ED. The mnemonic AEIOUTIPS, as outlined in Box 169.2, can assist the emergency clinician in the differential diagnosis and determining priorities for management. With the recent legalization of marijuana in many states, there has been an increase in the presentation of altered mental status due to cannabinoid ingestion in infants and children.[14] With the current opioid epidemic, ingestion or cutaneous exposure to opioids should be considered in all pediatric cases of altered mental status.

BOX 169.2 AEIOU TIPS Mnemonic for Altered Mental Status in Children

A–ammonia, alcohol, atypical migraine, abuse
E–electrolytes, epilepsy, encephalitis
I–insulin (hypoglycemia), intussusception, inborn errors of metabolism
O–oxygen (hypoxia), opiates, overdose
U–uremia
T–trauma, tumor
I–infection
P–poisoning, psychiatric
S–seizure, sepsis, subarachnoid hemorrhage

Diagnostic Testing

After evaluation and stabilization of the airway, breathing, and circulation, priorities include obtaining a bedside glucose test, rapid IV access, and laboratory testing. A point-of-care electrolyte test or blood gas can quickly assess pH, sodium, and lactate levels. Toxicology screens are warranted when a toxidrome or a risk of exposure are identified, but should not delay empiric treatment. Emergent imaging by CT or MRI should be obtained when focal neurologic deficits are present in conjunction with a history suggestive of an acute intracranial process (headaches, trauma). When inflicted head injury is suspected as an etiology of altered mental status in an infant, a head CT should be obtained. The need for a LP should be considered based on vaccination history, exposures, immunologic state, and physical exam. Antibiotic and antiviral therapy for the patient with suspected bacterial meningitis should not be delayed by a LP. If the history or physical examination raises any concern for an acute abdominal process, abdominal ultrasound should be performed to evaluate for intussusception, as its presentation is often nonspecific and can present as altered mental status alone.

Management

After the initial resuscitation, including stabilization of the airway, breathing, and circulation, data obtained by the history, physical examination, and point of care labs often dictate the first steps in management. If lab values indicate hyperglycemia, hypoglycemia, or other electrolyte imbalances, early measures should be aimed at correcting these. If the abdominal examination reveals significant tenderness, a radiograph or ultrasound should be obtained to evaluate for surgical etiologies, including intussusception, perforation or obstruction. In ill-appearing children for which a surgical cause is suspected, we recommend emergent surgical consultation. Head imaging may also help guide early management. If there is a concern for toxic ingestion, efforts will quickly be directed at the correction of perturbations associated with the offending agent (e.g., naloxone for opioids).

When bacterial meningitis is in the differential diagnosis of altered mental status, but not highly suspected, it is reasonable to consider risk stratification of the patient to determine if antibiotics can be withheld until obtaining further information (e.g., CSF, white cell count). Finally, acyclovir should be administered to an ill or febrile infant with a history of maternal herpes simplex virus (HSV) infection, presence of vesicles on the skin, seizures, or focal neurologic signs. If a child lives or has visited an area that is endemic with infections associated with altered mental status, further evaluation and treatment should be considered (e.g., malaria, Lyme disease).

Disposition

All patients with persistent altered mental status should be admitted to the hospital for additional evaluation and monitoring for improvement or worsening. In selected cases, when the altered mental status is self-limited, the patient may be observed and discharged home with close follow-up with a primary care provider.

HEADACHES

Foundations

Headache is a common problem in children and adolescents, with 40% of children experiencing a headache by 7 years, and 75% by 15 years of age. Migraine, one of the most common causes of headache in childhood, has a prevalence of up to 20% by 15 years of age. Although most pediatric patients have benign causes of headaches, a thorough history and physical examination should be conducted to evaluate for serious and time-sensitive underlying pathologies. The history and physical should guide decisions related to the need for emergent neuroimaging.

Clinical Features

Headaches can be classified into five temporal patterns—acute, acute recurrent, chronic progressive, chronic nonprogressive, and mixed. An acute headache is new in onset and different from previous headaches; it can herald a broad range of conditions, ranging from a viral illness to subarachnoid hemorrhage. An acute headache with weakness, seizures, speech difficulty, ataxia, or neurologic deficits should prompt evaluation of time-sensitive conditions, such as a stroke.[15] Acute recurrent headaches are periodic events separated by pain-free intervals. Chronic progressive headaches continue over weeks to months. They can signify serious medical disorders, such as brain tumors or arteriovenous malformations. Chronic nonprogressive headaches usually occur for years and are classified as primary headaches (as opposed to secondary symptomatic headaches, which are caused by an underlying medical problem). Mixed headaches are acute recurrent headaches (e.g., migraines) superimposed on a pattern of daily chronic nonprogressive headaches.

The primary goal of the ED evaluation is to differentiate life-threatening causes of headaches, such as strokes or brain tumors, from primary headaches, such as migraines or tension headaches. The child's history is the most important component to an accurate diagnosis. The patient and family members should be asked about specific factors related to the headache, such as time of onset, duration, location, laterality, quality (e.g., sharp, dull, throbbing, or aching), relieving and exacerbating factors, precipitating factors (e.g., poor sleep, hunger, or specific foods), and associated symptoms (e.g., nausea, vomiting, or photophobia).

The emergency clinician should focus on a detailed history of the neurologic system to identify any related symptoms (e.g., vomiting, lethargy, ataxia, seizures, weakness, or visual disturbances) and a general review of other organ systems. Warning signs of secondary headaches include sudden onset, occurrence with straining or exertion, association with neurologic symptoms, worsening in a recumbent position, headache pattern change, nocturnal awakening, and bilateral occipital headaches. Additional information related to the past medical history (e.g., history of recent head trauma, neurologic or psychiatric disorders, hospital admissions, medications) should also be obtained, as well as any family history of headache syndromes. For those patients with a history of loss of developmental milestones, serious causes including central nervous system tumors should be considered.

The physical examination should be thorough to evaluate for infectious, toxic, and structural causes for the headache (e.g., strep pharyngitis, cannabinoid ingestion, tumor). Height, weight, and head circumference should be compared with standard percentiles and the child's previous growth history; a change in the rate or direction of head growth may indicate an intracerebral mass or hydrocephalus. The blood pressure should be carefully measured, with the use of age-appropriate cuff size and percentiles for age; hypertension may be a sign of increased ICP. An infant's fontanelle should be palpated for size and fullness, as well as auscultated for bruits associated with arteriovenous malformations. A skin examination should be performed to look for stigmata of neurocutaneous disorders, such as neurofibromatosis (café-au-lait spots; see Fig. 169.1) or tuberous sclerosis (ash leaf spots; see Fig. 169.2). The neurologic examination should begin with assessment of the child's mental status and overall development. For infants, observing their level of alertness, age-appropriate social interaction, overall tone, and general vigor is an essential component of the initial neurologic evaluation. Nonspecific findings such as irritability, fussiness, or poor feeding may be the only presenting signs in infants with headache. The neurologic examination should include a complete assessment: cranial nerves; gait analysis (when possible); cerebellar, sensory, and motor function testing; and evaluation of deep tendon reflexes. The ophthalmologic examination should include pupillary reactivity, visual acuity, extraocular movements, and funduscopic evaluation for papilledema or retinal hemorrhages. Observation of interactions between the patient and family may provide clues to potential family problems, depression, anxiety, or child abuse.

Differential Diagnoses

Headaches may be primary (e.g., migraines and cluster headaches) or secondary to an underlying disease process. The list of differential considerations for secondary headaches is extensive and should be considered in the context of the child's history and physical examination (Table 169.6).

Acute Headache

The acute headache is a common problem in children and adolescents and accompanies many infectious processes. In the absence of other signs of CNS involvement (e.g., nuchal rigidity, alteration in level of consciousness, or focal neurologic findings), headaches in febrile children usually do not constitute evidence of CNS infection; nonspecific viral illnesses or dehydration represent the most common diagnoses in children presenting to the ED with an acute headache.

Although far less common, arteriovenous malformations can be a trigger for a new severe headache. Intracranial arteriovenous malformations are structurally unstable and thus susceptible to spontaneous rupture. In children, the abrupt onset of a severe headache in the absence of trauma (especially when accompanied by focal neurologic findings) suggests an acute intracranial bleed, and a head CT should be

TABLE 169.6 Differential Diagnosis for Secondary Headache

Cause	Features
Trauma	Intracranial bleed
	Concussion
	Skull fracture
Structural	Neoplasm
	Arteriovenous malformation
	Congenital malformation
	Hydrocephalus
Systemic	Hypertension
	Metabolic (e.g., diabetes and ketoacidosis)
Infection	Meningitis
	Abscess
	Encephalitis
	Sinusitis
	Influenza
	Pyelonephritis
	Group A streptococcal pharyngitis
Toxic	Medication
	Ingestion

performed. Localized acute headaches without focal neurologic findings may be due to sinusitis, otitis media, dental disorders, or traumatic head injury. Headache associated with trauma should be carefully investigated for the possibility of subdural or epidural hematomas, fractures, and leptomeningeal cysts (a "growing" skull fracture, usually in a child <3 years of age, with a history of recent trauma). Ophthalmologic problems, such as astigmatism, refractory errors, eye strain, and squint, are occasionally responsible for headaches in children.

Chronic Progressive Headache

Chronic progressive headaches in children often signify underlying pathology. The development of increased ICP can be caused by brain tumors, hydrocephalus, impaired venous drainage, brain abscess, or intracranial bleeding. Headache that awakens the child from sleep (related to increased CSF production in the later hours of sleep), is present on first awakening, or is associated with early morning emesis is a classic symptom of increased ICP and suggests an intracranial mass or hydrocephalus. In the setting of an abnormal intracranial entity, such as a mass or CSF obstruction, impaired venous outflow in the supine position leads to excess volume inside the skull, generating elevated pressure. The physical examination may show signs of increased ICP—vital sign changes, including hypertension, bradycardia, and irregular respirations (i.e., Cushing triad); papilledema; brisk reflexes; cranial nerve deficits; positive Babinski sign; or decreased level of consciousness—as well as focal symptoms related to the location of the lesion (e.g., hemiparesis, ataxia, visual field deficits).

Headaches are more likely to be the first symptom of a brain tumor in older children, but may be a later finding in younger children. Frequently, there are associated symptoms: nausea, vomiting; visual effects, problems with walking, weakness, loss of developmental milestones, changes in personality or school performance, or speech changes. As symptoms progress and evolve, the diagnosis of a brain tumor is often made after one or more clinical visits for headache. Loss of developmental milestones can be a potential sign of a brain tumor in infancy and childhood. Neurologic findings in children newly diagnosed with brain tumors may include papilledema, abnormal eye movements, ataxia, abnormal tendon reflexes, abnormalities on the visual examination, or less specific signs of increased ICP.

Clinical findings of pseudotumor cerebri (i.e., idiopathic intracranial hypertension or benign intracranial hypertension) are secondary to the increased ICP and include papilledema (with or without sixth cranial nerve palsy) and visual field deficits. Idiopathic intracranial hypertension (i.e., pseudotumor cerebri) is more common in females and obese individuals, and in younger children can be associated with medications (e.g., vitamin A, steroids, birth control pills, tetracycline). Neuroimaging is normal in idiopathic intracranial hypertension and the LP usually demonstrates elevated pressure, greater than 25 cm H_2O, and normal CSF protein and glucose levels. Neuroimaging should precede LP when increased ICP is suspected. We suggest any neuroimaging performed in the evaluation of idiopathic intracranial hypertension to include imaging of the venous sinuses, as cerebral sinovenous thrombosis (CSVT) can present similarly. Treatment is usually with diuretics, with or without an initial LP for therapeutic removal of CSF.

Brain abscess can result from meningitis, head trauma, chronic otitis media, sinusitis, or septic embolization in children with congenital heart disease. Focal neurologic signs, as well as fever and headache, may be present, but the patient may look surprisingly well. CT of the head without contrast enhancement is not sufficiently sensitive when an abscess is considered in the differential, but may be obtained; CT with and without contrast enhancement or MRI should be performed. CSF findings usually include a mild leukocytosis (10–200 leukocytes/mm^3), slightly elevated protein level, and normal glucose level. The CSF smear and culture do not usually reveal any organisms.

A subdural hematoma, epidural hematoma or intraparenchymal bleed are associated with head trauma. Headaches in these patients may evolve and progress over a relatively short time period. Symptoms include those associated with increased ICP, seizures, and focal neurologic deficits. The diagnosis is confirmed by neuroimaging.

Chronic progressive headache also can be a symptom of systemic diseases, such as hypertension, collagen vascular disease, hypothyroidism, Lyme disease, mononucleosis, or inborn errors of metabolism.

Migraine Headache

The diagnosis of migraine is based on symptoms of recurrent headaches separated by pain-free intervals. Migraine headaches are multifactorial in cause, with environmental and genetic contributions. The principal mechanism of migraine headaches is thought to involve a primary dysfunction of the brain in which a wave of spreading cortical neuronal depression is accompanied by vascular changes. Derangement of the trigemino-vascular reflex results in alterations of regional blood flow, and this neurovascular interaction is thought to contribute to neurogenic inflammation and the development of migraine headaches. Serotonin (5-hydroxytryptamine [5-HT]) may be a key mediator in this cascade of events, and serotonin agonists have been shown to relieve migraine pain.

Pediatric migraines may last from 2 to more than 72 hours and are more often bilateral than unilateral, which is more common in adults. Photophobia and phonophobia may be more difficult to assess in the young child or infant. Occipital headaches are rare and should raise clinical suspicion for a diagnosis other than migraine. Migraine headaches are classified primarily into migraine with and without an aura. Migraine without an aura, also known as common migraine, is the most frequent type of pediatric and adolescent migraine and includes the following criteria: more than 5 attacks that last 2 to 72 hours (untreated or unsuccessfully treated), accompanied by nausea, vomiting, photophobia or phonophobia, and including a minimum of 2 of the following criteria: unilateral or bilateral location, pulsing quality, moderate to severe intensity, and aggravated by routine physical activities.

Migraine with an aura, previously known as classic migraine, is diagnosed when at least two attacks fulfilling the diagnosis of migraine occur accompanied by a variety of sensory warning symptoms, such as flickering lights (scintillations), obscuration or loss of vision (scotoma), and tingling or numbness (paresthesias). The aura typically develops over 5 or more minutes and completely resolves within 60 minutes.

Migraine variants or atypical migraines are more common in children. Hemiplegic migraine is characterized by the sudden onset of hemiparesis or hemiplegia, along with headache in the contralateral hemisphere. Even though symptoms usually last for hours or even days, patients are rarely left with permanent deficits. These patients often receive imaging on initial presentation to exclude other diagnoses. Ophthalmoplegic migraine is characterized by severe unilateral eye pain and headache, followed by ipsilateral third nerve palsy of variable degree. Rarely, the fourth or sixth cranial nerve, rather than the third nerve, may be affected. Basilar artery migraine, also common in children, is manifested with a combination of visual symptoms (e.g., transient bilateral blindness, blurred vision) and visual hallucinations, vertigo, ataxia, loss of consciousness, and drop attacks. An acute confusional state can be associated with migraines and is characterized by changes in personality, orientation, or behavior. The so-called Alice in Wonderland syndrome includes perceptions of distortion in body images and shapes; objects appear much larger (macropsia) or smaller (micropsia) before, during, or after the headache.

Migraine variants are not uncommon and can be misdiagnosed. Abdominal migraine is characterized by recurrent abdominal pain, nausea, vomiting, and recurrent headaches. Benign paroxysmal vertigo of childhood (distinct from benign paroxysmal positional vertigo) is manifested as headache accompanied by the sudden onset of vertigo, pallor, and nystagmus. Paroxysmal torticollis is defined as recurrent episodes of head tilt associated with headache, nausea, and vomiting. Of note, this is a diagnosis of exclusion; children with a head tilt, vomiting, and headache should first be evaluated for a posterior fossa lesion. Ocular migraine is characterized by transient monocular visual blurring to blindness with bright flashes of light.

The incidence of seizures is higher in patients with migraine than in the general population. Although epilepsy and migraine headache are distinct clinical syndromes, they share several characteristics, such as aura, vertigo, nausea, pallor, loss of consciousness, drowsy postictal state, confusion, and transient focal neurologic deficits. Headache as the sole manifestation of a seizure is uncommon; however, headaches frequently follow tonic, tonic-clonic, and brief complex partial seizures. Bilateral frontal throbbing headaches may follow episodes of status epilepticus. Further neurologic evaluation, including electroencephalography, may occasionally be necessary to distinguish between these two syndromes.

Chronic Nonprogressive Headache

Chronic nonprogressive headache is commonly seen in the adolescent population. Included in this category are muscle contraction and conversion headaches. The International Headache Society classification of headaches refers to these types of headaches as tension headaches. This type of headache includes the following symptoms: bilateral or unilateral, nonthrobbing, pressing, or bandlike tightness of mild to moderate intensity, and the absence of nausea, vomiting, and aura. Tension headaches are further classified as episodic (10–15 episodes/month lasting 30 minutes to 7 days) or chronic (>15 episodes/month for more than 6 months).

Cluster Headache

Cluster headache is a distinctive headache syndrome that is more common in males and rare in those younger than 10 years. Cluster headache is characterized by one to several attacks recurring each 24 hours, during several weeks to months. Headache-free periods between

> ### BOX 169.3 Indications for Radiologic Imaging in Patients With Headache
>
> **Strongly Indicated If:**
> Abnormal neurologic examination findings
> Signs and symptoms of elevated intracranial pressure
> Meningeal signs plus focal neurologic findings or altered mental status
> Progressive or new focal neurologic signs
> Significant head trauma
> Severe nocturnal headaches that awaken the patient from sleep or are present on awakening
> Severe (characterized by patient as "worst headache of my life") headaches; new or of increasing frequency and duration
> Presence of ventriculoperitoneal shunt
> Chronic progressive headache
>
> **Consider If:**
> Headache or vomiting on awakening
> Unvarying location of headache, especially occipital
> Persistent headache plus no family history of migraine
> Neurocutaneous syndrome
> Age < 3 years (limited verbal skills)

clusters may last months to years. The pain is throbbing, severe, and unilateral; occurs over the same orbito-temporal region, and is associated with ipsilateral scleral injection, lacrimation, nasal stuffiness, and sometimes a partial Horner's syndrome (enophthalmos, ptosis, miosis, and anhidrosis, unilateral, affecting sympathetic innervation of the eye). The pain lasts 30 minutes to several hours and can occur at any time of day or night.

Diagnostic Testing

Although many patients presenting to the ED with headache do not require neuroimaging or laboratory evaluation, if neuroimaging is obtained, MRI provides superior anatomic detail compared with CT, and is particularly useful in the detection of abnormalities in the sella turcica, posterior fossa, and cervicomedullary junction. MRI/A is also better for detecting arteriovenous malformations and low-grade tumors. CT scanning, however, is superior to MRI for the detection of acute blood and skull fractures, and therefore is often the modality of choice in the ED. Indications for the use of neuroimaging are presented in Box 169.3.

An LP is indicated for the diagnosis of an infectious process, subarachnoid hemorrhage not detected by CT, or idiopathic intracranial hypertension. In general, radiologic imaging should precede an LP on any patient with a headache or other red flags (e.g., early morning headaches and vomiting, progressively worsening headaches, or focal neurologic findings).

Chronic progressive headaches may be a symptom of a systemic disease. Guided by the history and physical examination, laboratory tests may include CBC, urinalysis, erythrocyte sedimentation rate, antinuclear antibody testing, liver function studies, thyroid function studies, serum lipid assay, serum magnesium concentration, lactate concentration, pyruvate concentration, and Lyme disease titers.

Management

Treatment of primary childhood headaches includes attention to initial pharmacologic management, as well as reassurance, removal of potential triggers, and initiation of a behavioral management program. The most important aspect of management is a thorough history and physical examination, past medical history of migraines or systemic disease, and targeted diagnostic evaluation for potentially life-threatening causes.

In addition to the use of standard oral analgesics, abortive treatment for children presenting to the ED with migraine headaches generally involves IV fluid hydration with a normal saline bolus, nonopioid analgesics (e.g., ibuprofen or IV ketorolac), and antiemetic (e.g., metoclopramide or prochlorperazine).[16] When migraines are refractory to traditional treatments or last over 72 hours, a neurologic consultation and admission should be considered.

Disposition

Children with primary headaches do not usually need hospitalization unless the diagnosis is uncertain and a serious cause of secondary headache is being considered. On discharge from the ED, patients may be given a variety of treatment recommendations while stressing the importance of close follow-up with a primary care provider for ongoing management of migraines.

Nonmedical interventions may have some impact and should be strongly considered. These include avoidance of triggers, placement of the child in a darkened room (with minimal or no extraneous noise), avoidance of hypoglycemia by feeding during a migraine, avoidance of caffeinated beverages (except for possible use as a migraine medication during an episode), application of a cool compress on the forehead, use of a gentle fan, breathing exercises, and relaxation techniques. Patients should be encouraged to keep a headache diary after discharge to track the duration, triggers, medication effects, and other characteristics of their headaches. Common triggers include insufficient or irregular sleep patterns, dehydration, missed meals, various psychosocial stressors, and certain foods (e.g., chocolate, processed meats, alcohol, hard cheeses, red wine, monosodium glutamate, yeast extracts, nuts, figs, aspartame, and sauerkraut).

In general, there are several outpatient treatment options available for acute migraine or other headache syndromes in children. For most patients, symptom relief can be achieved by oral analgesics such as acetaminophen or ibuprofen, along with rest, hydration, and avoidance of triggers. In other cases, additional abortive or prophylactic agents are needed, and the decision to initiate these agents should be deferred to a follow-up visit with the primary provider or neurologist. Treatment may include vasoconstrictors, sedatives, triptans, caffeine, dopamine antagonists, antiemetics or combination therapies. The placebo effect of many medications is high in children with migraines.

PEDIATRIC ATAXIA

Foundations

Ataxia comes from the Greek word *ataktos,* meaning "lacking order," and describes a pathologic abnormality of organization or modulation of movement. Congenital ataxia is associated with CNS macro or micro structural abnormalities. Acquired ataxia can be acute, episodic, or chronic. The chronic ataxias are usually caused by inherited metabolic or genetic disorders. Usually, ataxia is caused by cerebellar dysfunction, but lesions in the corticospinal tract or dorsal columns of the spinal cord may also be causative.

Clinical Features

Most children with ataxia are seen in the first few days after onset, usually because of a refusal to walk, unsteadiness of arm movements, or sudden development of a wide-based so-called drunken gait. The history should identify any recent infection, injury, inadvertent drug ingestion, or other family members with similar symptoms. Mental status is usually normal in cases of postinfectious ataxia; if abnormal, the possibility of ingestion, acute disseminated encephalomyelitis, or stroke should be considered. Nystagmus is common if the cerebellum is affected. Papilledema or cranial nerve palsies suggest hydrocephalus or a CNS lesion.

BOX 169.4 Causes of Childhood Ataxia

Acute cerebellar ataxia
Acute postinfectious demyelinating encephalomyelitis
Brainstem encephalitis
Drug ingestion
Guillain-Barré syndrome
Metabolic disorders
Aminoacidopathies
Mitochondrial disorders
Organic acidopathies
Urea cycle disorders
Migraine headaches
Multiple sclerosis
Neoplasm
Opsoclonus-myoclonus syndrome
Recurrent and chronic genetic ataxias
Seizures
Stroke
Vertebral artery dissection

Differential Diagnoses

Box 169.4 delineates common causes of pediatric ataxia. Approximately 40% of ataxia cases in children are caused by acute cerebellar ataxia. Boys are more commonly affected, with the highest incidence at the ages of 2 to 4 years. A history of recent illness with multiple causative agents is seen in 70% of patients, but varicella virus is the most common, associated with up to 26% of cases. The disease is thought to be due to an autoimmune phenomenon leading to cerebellar demyelination. Symptoms and signs are maximal at the onset, with the extremities more seriously affected than the trunk, and range from unsteadiness and wide-based gait to complete inability to walk. Mental status is normal, and nystagmus is common. Fever and seizures are uncommon outcomes.

Acute postinfectious demyelinating encephalomyelitis can also cause ataxia and occurs in the recovery phase of a viral illness or vaccination. It is distinguished from acute cerebellar ataxia by alteration in consciousness and multifocal neurologic deficits, as well as by fever and frequent occurrence of seizures. Brainstem encephalitis can involve the cerebellum, causing ataxia in association with focal neurologic abnormalities and respiratory irregularities. Potential causative agents include Epstein-Barr virus, *Listeria monocytogenes,* and enteroviruses.

Acute childhood ataxia can also be due to pharmacologic drug toxicity (e.g., anticonvulsants, benzodiazepines, alcohol, or antihistamines), or less commonly, from exposure to organic chemicals or heavy metals. The ataxia is usually accompanied by lethargy, confusion, and inappropriate speech or behavior, and nystagmus may be present.

Over half of all childhood brain tumors arise in the brainstem or cerebellum and can be manifested with slowly progressive ataxia. Acute decompensation can occur, with the development of hydrocephalus or hemorrhage into the lesion.

Head injuries with cerebellar contusion or hemorrhage can cause ataxia. Posterior circulation strokes are rare in children but should be considered after neck trauma, with possible vertebral artery dissection as a cause of the ataxia. Spontaneous vertebral artery dissections have also been reported in children.

The opsoclonus-myoclonus syndrome—ataxia; rapid, chaotic, multidirectional eye movements; and myoclonic jerks of the extremities, head, trunk, and face—is usually a presenting manifestation of neuroblastoma or ganglioneuroblastoma. Ataxia is thought to be due to a paraneoplastic autoimmune phenomenon involving cross-reactivity of tumor and cerebellar antigens.

Ataxia can be seen in patients with basilar migraine and can be associated with vertigo, hemiparesis, cranial nerve dysfunction, nausea, vomiting, or headache. Loss of sensory input to the cerebellum can cause a sensory ataxia. Clinical manifestations include a Romberg sign, decreased deep tendon reflexes, and impaired proprioception and vibration sense. Of patients with Guillain-Barré syndrome (GBS), 15% have sensory ataxia. In the Miller-Fisher variant of GBS, the triad of ataxia, areflexia, and ophthalmoplegia of vertical gaze is characteristic.

Transient ataxia can be present in the ictal or postictal phase of seizures. Repeated attacks of ataxia can be the presenting manifestation of multiple sclerosis. Inborn errors of metabolism can also manifest with ataxia, acutely or intermittently, depending on dietary intake or the presence of other illness. Inborn errors of metabolism should be considered when ataxia is accompanied by lethargy, encephalopathy, vomiting, diarrhea, loss of muscle tone, or unusual body odor, as in urea acid cycle defects (e.g., aminoacidurias) or defects in pyruvate and lactate metabolism. Ataxia is associated with other inherited diseases such as Niemann-Pick, Tay-Sachs, and Wilson diseases.

The two most common genetic disorders associated with ataxia are Friedreich ataxia and ataxia-telangiectasia. Friedreich ataxia is a disorder of autosomal recessive inheritance characterized by progressive gait and limb disturbance. Affected patients demonstrate dysarthria, lower limb areflexia, proprioceptive sensory loss, and high-arched feet (pes cavus). Ataxia-telangiectasia is a disorder of recessive inheritance manifested as a truncal ataxia in infancy that leaves most patients wheelchair-bound by the age of 12 years. Oculocutaneous telangiectasias usually appear by the age of 3 to 5 years. These patients also demonstrate dysarthria, nystagmus, dystonic posturing, myoclonic jerks, and accelerated aging.

Diagnostic Testing

An accurate diagnosis for pediatric ataxia is dependent on a complete history and thorough physical examination, including testing of gait and cerebellar function. Urine and serum toxicology studies are the highest yield laboratory studies and should be performed on all patients.[17] CT and MRI findings are usually normal in patients with postinfectious ataxia, but demyelination, tumor, hydrocephalus, or traumatic injuries may be identified. Neuroimaging should be ordered if a patient has focal neurologic deficits in the setting of ataxia, but may be deferred in other patients if they have close follow-up.[18,19] CSF analysis may show mild pleocytosis or lymphocytosis in acute postinfectious ataxia; findings are normal in most other cases.

Admission for electroencephalography should be considered in patients with altered consciousness and fluctuating clinical signs of ataxia. Urinary catecholamine levels can be assayed for diagnosis of neuroblastoma. Additional testing may include a CBC, liver function tests, glucose, ammonia, lactate, pyruvate, and ketone levels, and determination of acid-base status. The four most high-yield tests are for levels of glucose, lactate, ketones, and ammonia. If all four of these are normal, it is unlikely that there is an inborn error. Any other laboratory tests should be ordered in consultation with a specialist and may include plasma and urinary amino acids, urine organic acids, CSF lactate, or serum biotinidase levels.

Management

Children with ataxia can be managed, depending on the cause, as outpatients with consultation with the primary care physician and/or pediatric neurology. Management of these patients often requires consultation in the ED by infectious disease or neurology specialists. Most children with acute postinfectious cerebellar ataxia recover completely,

and treatment is supportive. Improvement is typically seen within 1 week, and the vast majority recover completely within 2 to 4 weeks. Some children exhibit persistent gait disturbances, ataxia, and delayed speech development.

Disposition

Children with persistent ataxia usually need hospital admission and consultation with a pediatric neurologist to identify causes of the ataxia not evident on the ED evaluation.

PEDIATRIC VERTIGO

Foundations

Vertigo, also discussed in Chapter 15, is defined as an illusion of movement, a sensation that the external world is revolving around an individual (objective vertigo) or that the affected person is revolving in space (subjective vertigo). Vertigo is well recognized to occur in the pediatric age group and has many potential causes. Disease processes that affect the balance of the vestibular, visual, and proprioceptive systems can cause vertigo by impairing the neural activity of the vestibular nucleus. Diseases of the ear, eighth cranial nerve, neck, brainstem, or eye can lead to vertiginous symptoms. Vertigo is characterized as central or peripheral, depending on whether the cause is in the CNS.

Clinical Features

Vertigo is often described as dizziness. There may be a history of sudden falls, grasping for support, or unwillingness to move. A review of systems should include those related to the ear, such as otalgia, hearing loss, and tinnitus. Other important historical features that should be determined include headache, loss of consciousness, head trauma or barotrauma, and family history of migraine or seizure disorders.

Diagnostic Testing

Patients can be divided into those who have hearing loss and those who have normal hearing. In the group with hearing loss, further characterization of the loss as conductive or sensorineural (using the Weber and Rinne tests) can help localize the peripheral lesion to the middle ear, labyrinth, or eighth cranial nerve.

Differential Diagnoses

Although vertigo is not as common in the pediatric age group as in adults, it has many potential causes (Box 169.5). It usually is helpful to separate conditions that cause vertigo into those with and without associated hearing loss.

Benign paroxysmal vertigo of childhood is defined by the repeated occurrence of vertiginous episodes lasting seconds to minutes, with occasional vomiting. In addition to being pale and diaphoretic, preverbal children may appear fearful, grasping onto a caregiver's leg for stability. This entity usually remits spontaneously within months to years. The most frequent cause of benign paroxysmal vertigo of childhood is a migraine headache, with vertigo occurring as the aura of an episode.

Patients with basilar artery migraines may also present with vertigo, hemiparesis, ataxia, palsies of the third, sixth, or seventh cranial nerve, drop attacks, and blindness in various combinations, followed by migraine headache. Children with benign paroxysmal vertigo of childhood or basilar migraines usually have a family history of migraine headaches.

Benign paroxysmal positional vertigo is rare in children, but can occur spontaneously as well as after trauma. It may present as early as in the second decade of life. It is believed to be due to otoliths that have moved out of their normal positions in the utricle and is corrected by canalith repositioning maneuvers (e.g., the Epley maneuver).

BOX 169.5 Causes of Pediatric Vertigo

Central Vertigo
Atrioventricular malformations
Brain abscess
Chiari malformations
Demyelinating disorders
Encephalitis
Meningitis
Migraine headaches
Neoplasm
Seizures
Trauma

Peripheral Vertigo
Alport syndrome
Benign paroxysmal torticollis
Benign paroxysmal vertigo of childhood
Benign positional vertigo
Cholesteatoma
Diabetes mellitus
Labyrinthine dysplasia or aplasia
Labyrinthine concussion
Labyrinthitis
Lyme disease
Otitis media, suppurative and serous
Ototoxins
Ocular disorders
Pendred syndrome
Perilymphatic fistula
Stenosis of the internal auditory canal
Syphilitic inner ear disease
Thyroid disease
Trauma
Usher syndrome
Vestibular neuronitis
Waardenburg syndrome (genetic disorder associated with deafness, widespaced eyes)

Ménière disease, caused by hydrops of the semimembranous labyrinth, is a syndrome of vertigo, fluctuating hearing loss, and tinnitus, and is responsible for up to 4% of cases of pediatric vertigo. Vestibular neuronitis, thought to be caused by viral infections, is manifested as vertigo without hearing loss. A preceding cold is found in 60% of patients. It is manifested with severe vertigo that resolves in a few days, after which the child will have vertigo only with rapid head movements, which persists for weeks or months until central compensation occurs.

Labyrinthitis is an inflammatory process involving the inner ear membranous labyrinth; it manifests with vertigo, hearing loss, and tinnitus. Cytomegalovirus, rubella virus, and rubeola viruses are common causative agents. Bacterial labyrinthitis usually occurs in association with meningitis and should be suspected in any ill child with vertigo and high fevers, especially in combination with a perforated tympanic membrane. Neurofibromatosis can be manifested with vertigo if it involves the superior vestibular nerve. Other genetic syndromes such as Alport syndrome are also associated with vertigo (see Box 169.5).

Ototoxic drugs, such as aminoglycosides and chemotherapeutic agents, can cause vertigo, usually in association with hearing loss. Cerebellar and brainstem lesions can also cause vertigo. Cranial nerve deficits associated with vertigo may indicate a brainstem lesion or tumor. Vertigo is the presenting symptom in up to 10% of cases of multiple sclerosis.

For most patients, the cause of vertigo cannot be established during their ED visit. A complete physical examination, including an otologic and neurologic evaluation, should be performed, including evaluation for nystagmus and cerebellar testing. Having the child hop and stand from a seated position on the floor, with eyes open and closed, can reveal vestibular dysfunction. Signs of other disease processes, such as café-au-lait spots in neurofibromatosis, may aid in the diagnosis.

Laboratory tests in the vertiginous patient should be dictated by the history and physical examination, and may include glucose and electrolyte levels, thyroid function tests, and viral titers or serologic studies (e.g., for Lyme disease or syphilis). CT or MRI is indicated for patients with a suspected underlying CNS abnormality (i.e., central vertigo).

Management

Management of the vertiginous patient depends on the underlying cause, which may not be evident in the ED. For acute symptomatic relief, vestibular suppressants such as meclizine and diazepam may be helpful. Patients with a positive Dix-Hallpike test should receive canalith repositioning maneuvers.

Disposition

Patients with suspected CNS infection, focal neurologic deficits, abnormal mental status, or inability to ambulate or tolerate oral fluids or medications should be admitted. Patients should follow up with their primary care provider and a neurologist or otolaryngologist for follow-up testing if vertigo persists.

MOTOR DYSFUNCTION

Acute weakness or motor abnormalities in the pediatric patient can result from pathology at a variety of levels in the neural axis. A complete neurologic assessment can indicate the location of pathology—upper motor neuron (i.e., motor neurons originating in the cerebral cortex or brainstem) or lower motor neuron (i.e., spinal cord anterior horn cells, peripheral nerves, neuromuscular junction, and the muscle itself). Generally, upper motor neuron pathology creates spasticity, increased tone, hyperreflexia, and no fasciculations. Lower motor neuron abnormalities result in decreased tone, poor reflexes, and muscle fasciculations.

STROKE

Foundations

Stroke is characterized by the acute and persistent onset of focal neurologic deficits. Less common in children than adults, pediatric strokes often go unrecognized, leading to delays in diagnosis and treatments. Often the cause of focal neurologic symptoms in children are stroke mimics (e.g., atypical migraine); however, the emergency clinician must always consider stroke in this differential, especially in those children with risk factors for stroke. Underlying conditions that predispose children to stroke include sickle cell disease, structural cardiac anomalies, homocystinuria, and moyamoya disease (Box 169.6). Vascular malformations, such as arteriovenous malformations, may cause hemorrhagic stroke or subarachnoid hemorrhage.

Strokes are classified as ischemic or hemorrhagic. In ischemic stroke, there is an interruption of blood supply to a particular area of the brain, resulting in hypoxic injury. In hemorrhagic stroke, the rupture of a blood vessel or an abnormal vascular structure causes focal damage. Hemorrhagic strokes are more common in children than adults, and often stem from unstable arteriovenous malformations.

BOX 169.6   Risk Factors for Pediatric Stroke

Cardiac
Congenital heart defects
Valvular heart disease
Right-to-left shunts
Cardiomyopathy
Endocarditis, myocarditis
Arrhythmia
Cardiac tumors
Cardiac surgery

Hematologic Disorders and Coagulopathies
Anemia
Sickle cell disease
Dehydration
Idiopathic thrombocytopenia purpura (ITP)
Thrombotic thrombocytopenic purpura (TTP)
Hemolytic uremic syndrome (HUS)
Thrombocytosis
Polycythemia
Disseminated intravascular coagulation
Leukemia or other neoplasm
Congenital and acquired coagulation disorders
Pregnancy and the postpartum period
Vasculitis, vasculopathies
Systemic lupus erythematosus
Polyarteritis nodosa
Takayasu arteritis
Kawasaki disease
Moyamoya syndrome, disease

Infection
Meningitis, encephalitis
Mastoiditis, otitis media
HIV

Varicella
Syphilis
Tuberculosis
Systemic infection

Metabolic, Miscellaneous
Homocystinuria
Fabry disease
Organic acidemia
Hyperlipidemia
Mitochondrial encephalopathy with lactic acidosis and strokelike episodes syndrome
Menkes disease

Other Vascular
Vasospasm (subarachnoid hemorrhage)
Migraine
Carotid ligation (e.g., extracorporeal membrane oxygenation)
Fibromuscular dysplasia
Cervicocephalic arterial dissection
Arteriovenous malformation
Arteriography
Hereditary hemorrhagic telangiectasia
Sturge-Weber syndrome
Intracranial aneurysm

Trauma (Including Nonaccidental)
Blunt and penetrating cervical trauma

Brain Tumor
Drugs
Cocaine
Amphetamines
Oral contraceptives
L-asparaginase

Clinical Features

Manifestations of stroke in infants and children are widely variable due to the potential affected areas of the brain, as well as the child's age and developmental level. Unlike adults who typically present with hemiparesis or localizable focal neurologic deficits, children often present with less specific symptoms such as headache, seizures, or altered level of consciousness. Seizures at stroke onset occur in 20% of pediatric cases, especially in those younger than 6 years of age.[20] The middle cerebral and anterior cerebral arteries are usually affected in children with stroke, generating upper extremity hemiplegia and lower extremity weakness, respectively. The posterior circulation, although less commonly involved, may produce ataxia, nystagmus, or vertigo, along with hemiparesis and hemianopsia.

Diagnostic Testing

Imaging of the brain can confirm the diagnosis of stroke in infants and children. A non-contrast head CT scan can reveal the presence of a bleed, but may not show evidence of ischemia if the stroke took place in the preceding 24 hours. Early consultation with a pediatric neurologist is prudent in children with a suspected stroke. Urgent MRI and MR angiography (MRA) are indicated if there is no evidence of hemorrhage on head CT and clinical suspicion for stroke remains high. If the child does not have a predisposing condition for stroke, additional

laboratory evaluation may be helpful, including a CBC and coagulation studies, inflammatory markers, chemistry and lipid panels, and toxicology screen. Electrocardiography and echocardiography can reveal structural abnormalities associated with intracardiac shunts and clots.

Management

Initial pediatric stroke management is directed at stabilization of the airway, breathing, and circulation and controlling any seizure activity. To prevent secondary brain injury, hypoxemia and hypotension should be avoided. When present, hypertension should be managed with consideration of possible increased ICP, particularly in the setting of a hemorrhagic stroke. Blood pressure should be slowly reduced while maintaining cerebral perfusion pressure. The metabolic demands of the brain should be minimized by controlling seizures, fevers, pain, and agitation. Any hyperglycemia or hypoglycemia should be corrected, particularly in the setting of an ischemic stroke.

Additional therapy and definitive treatment of stroke in children are ultimately dictated by the type and extent of the stroke. Although data are limited for the use of thrombolytics and thrombectomy in pediatric stroke, effective utilization has increased in the last decade. When the clinical suspicion for acute ischemic stroke is high and the patient is presenting within the window for consideration of thrombolysis (currently 4.5 hours) or thrombectomy (currently 24 hours),[21] the patient should be transferred emergently to a stroke center that has the capacity to effectively manage pediatric stroke. In the case of hemorrhagic stroke, neurosurgical intervention is often needed for intracranial decompression, blood evacuation, or control of active bleeding. For children with sickle cell disease, blood transfusion or exchange transfusion should be considered, in consultation with a hematologist and neurologist, to decrease the circulating level of hemoglobin S.

DISORDERS OF THE SPINAL CORD

Foundations

Disorders of the spinal cord may arise from within the spinal cord itself or from extrinsic causes, such as trauma or malignancy. Acute compression of the spinal cord is a medical emergency; rapid accurate assessment of children with acute spinal cord abnormalities can directly affect patient outcomes. Trauma, spinal masses, and infection or inflammation can all cause acute spinal cord compression. The mechanism of compression may be due to direct mass effect (e.g., from a tumor) or related to edema or hemorrhage from infection or trauma. Epidural abscesses are a common infectious cause of acute spinal cord compression and are typically caused by hematogenous spread of bacteria.

Infection or inflammation may also affect the spinal cord intrinsically. Transverse myelitis is an inflammation of the full width of the spinal cord (involving variable lengths of the cord) that manifests with demyelinating lesions at any level of the cord. It is thought to be autoimmune-mediated, often following a recent infection. Transverse myelitis typically evolves over hours to days, but may develop over a few weeks. Specific infections associated with transverse myelitis include Epstein-Barr virus, cytomegalovirus, measles, *Campylobacter jejuni,* and *Mycoplasma pneumoniae.*

Clinical Features

Regardless of the cause of acute spinal cord dysfunction, patients will present with certain characteristic findings, including paraplegia, hyporeflexia, and sensory deficits (complete sensory loss or paresthesias) below the level of the spinal cord lesion. Also, if the distal portion of the cord is affected, patients will have bowel and bladder incontinence. In the case of transverse myelitis, the thoracic region is usually affected. Children may demonstrate lower extremity paresthesias or pain with progressive weakness, which may be asymmetric, over a period of hours to days, and possibly urinary retention. There is often a history of a recent viral-like illness. An acute onset of local back pain with neurologic deficits suggests spinal cord compression due to a bleed, trauma, or infection. With infectious causes, pain may be the first sign, before fever, neurologic deficits, or other systemic signs. With oncologic processes such as spinal tumors, children may have a more insidious onset of symptoms and have evidence of spinal cord compression in the absence of pain.

Diagnostic Testing

A thorough history and physical examination can help diagnose children with acute spinal cord compression. A careful neurologic examination should include strength, deep tendon reflexes, sensation, and evaluation of anal sphincter tone. In suspected spinal cord compression, priority should be on emergent neuroimaging with MRI of the spine while immobilizing the patient. The use of gadolinium assists in identifying acute infectious and inflammatory lesions. CT is less helpful, and plain spine radiographs are of little value. An LP should not be performed when spinal cord compression is suspected. LP can be helpful in evaluating transverse myelitis, but should be performed only after confirmed by MRI.

Management and Disposition

Initial management steps for the patient with spinal cord trauma include immobilization of the spine and immediate neurosurgical consultation. Children with an epidural abscess identified on MRI should receive IV antibiotics and neurosurgical consultation for decompression or drainage. Corticosteroids should be administered only in select cases and in conjunction with neurosurgical consultation.

S. aureus is the most common pathogen in epidural abscesses; thus, initial IV antibiotic therapy in the ED should include vancomycin to cover methicillin-resistant *S. aureus* (in addition to methicillin-sensitive *S. aureus* [MSSA]) and coverage of gram-negative bacilli with a third- or fourth-generation cephalosporin, such as ceftazidime, ceftriaxone, or cefepime. Consideration of additional anaerobic coverage is warranted for higher risk individuals (e.g., associated sinus disease). Patient-specific conditions such as recent surgery or hospitalization may warrant additional coverage.

Surgical drainage in conjunction with IV antibiotic therapy is the mainstay of treatment of epidural abscesses. For spinal masses, neurosurgical intervention is needed to decompress the cord and further elucidate the diagnosis. Supportive care is the underpinning of treatment for transverse myelitis; these children should be hospitalized for observation, IV corticosteroid therapy, and consideration of additional immunotherapy. Initiation of IV corticosteroid therapy in the ED and its specific dosing and timing for children with transverse myelitis should be discussed with a neurologist. Although there are no randomized controlled trials to demonstrate the efficacy of IV corticosteroids in transverse myelitis, consensus favors their use.

GUILLAIN-BARRÉ SYNDROME

Foundations

Guillain-Barré syndrome (GBS) is an acute, demyelinating polyneuropathy that typically presents as transient, symmetric, ascending paralysis. GBS is thought to be autoimmune-mediated—a recent infection triggers an immune response, which, in turn, provokes acute peripheral nerve demyelination. Classically, patients with GBS have both motor and sensory nerve demyelination.

Children of all ages may be affected; however, it is uncommon in young toddlers and infants. Often, there is a history of a preceding minor viral or gastrointestinal illness in the weeks prior to presentation. *Campylobacter jejuni* is the most common infectious agent associated with GBS. The differential diagnosis for GBS is broad; a careful history and detailed neurologic examination will help localize the pathology to the peripheral nerves rather than to the brainstem, brain, spinal cord, neuromuscular junction, or muscle itself. The relatively acute and typically symmetrical nature of GBS paralysis helps distinguish this diagnosis.

Clinical Features

Lower extremity pain, paresthesias, and weakness in any combination may be the initial presenting symptoms of GBS, followed by progressive ascending weakness of the lower extremities. The weakness may progress rapidly over hours to involve the trunk and the muscles of respiration. Deep tendon reflexes are typically diminished or absent at the time of presentation. Cranial nerve abnormalities may also be present; in the Miller-Fisher variant of GBS, they represent the main findings, with oculomotor palsies, ataxia, and areflexia in the absence of extremity weakness.

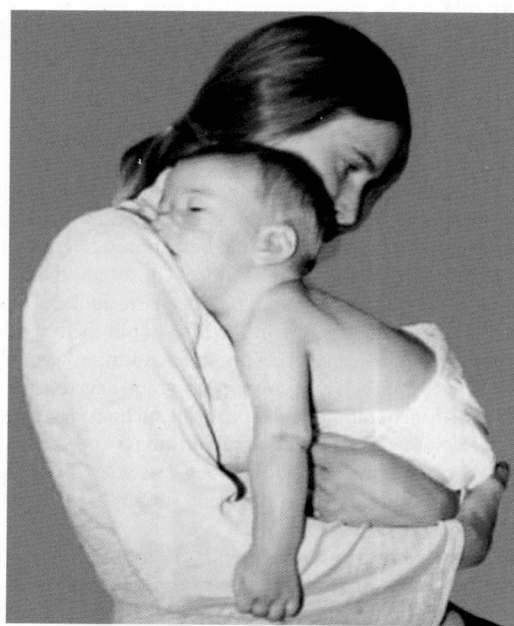

Fig. 169.4 Infant with hypotonia, as seen with botulism. (From: Arnon SS, Schechter R, Maslanka SE, et al. Human botulism immune globulin for the treatment of infant botulism. *N Engl J Med.* 2006;354:462-471.)

Diagnostic Testing

The diagnosis of GBS is largely clinical; however, a lumbar puncture can be helpful. CSF typically reveals an elevated protein level, with normal glucose, and white blood cell count, known as albumin cytologic dissociation.

Management and Disposition

Given the potential risk of respiratory compromise associated with progressive demyelination and weakness, patients with GBS should be admitted to the hospital for monitoring and supportive care. Bedside respiratory evaluations, such as forced vital capacity and negative inspiratory force trends, may be useful in predicting respiratory compromise. Treatment with plasma exchange and IV immunoglobulin may be used in severe cases.

INFANT BOTULISM

Foundations

Infant botulism typically affects infants younger than 6 to 8 months. It results from intestinal colonization with *Clostridium botulinum*. A neurotoxin produced by *C. botulinum* impairs acetylcholine release from the presynaptic membrane, thereby affecting skeletal muscle, smooth muscle, and autonomic function. Infants develop constipation and poor feeding, with subsequent hypotonia and weakness (Fig. 169.4), which may require respiratory support. Most United States cases of infant botulism are thought to arise from ingestion of environmental dust particles containing *C. botulinum* spores and may be associated with active construction areas in which there is disruption of the ground. Canned foods and honey are also potential reservoirs for *C. botulinum* spores.

Clinical Features

Infant botulism typically has an insidious onset of symptoms, commonly starting with constipation. Over time, infants develop poor feeding, lethargy, hypotonia, and weakness. On examination, infants may have decreased deep tendon reflexes, cranial nerve findings such as poor suck and gag, weak pupillary reflexes, or ptosis.

Diagnostic Testing

The diagnosis of botulism may be confirmed through isolation of botulinum toxin in the stool; however, this process may be delayed because infants are often constipated and laboratory processing times may be hours to days. As such, treatment should be initiated while awaiting confirmation of the toxin in a stool sample. Characteristic electromyography (EMG) findings of low-amplitude motor potentials of reduced duration can rapidly suggest the diagnosis.

Management and Disposition

Infants with botulism should be admitted to the hospital for supportive care, mechanical ventilation for depressed respiratory reflexes, and possibly nasogastric feeding. Botulism immune globulin is safe and effective and should be given IV as early as possible when the diagnosis is highly suspected, without awaiting confirmatory stool sample results. Initial dosing for botulism immunoglobulin in infants less than 1 year of age is 50 mg/kg of body weight in a single IV infusion.

MYASTHENIA GRAVIS

Foundations

Myasthenia gravis is an autoimmune disorder characterized by autoantibodies directed against the acetylcholine receptor of the neuromuscular junction. This action produces intermittent and fatigable weakness. Myasthenia gravis is usually seen in adults; however, there are three types that affect children—neonatal (transient), congenital, and juvenile. The juvenile form of myasthenia gravis presents similarly to the adult form and will be discussed here. Children with juvenile myasthenia gravis are more commonly female and of early school age.

Clinical Features

Patients typically have waxing and waning weakness of the skeletal and facial muscles, exacerbated by repetitive use of these muscles. Facial weakness with bilateral ptosis that fatigues throughout the day is a common initial presenting sign. Oculomotor, truncal, and extremity weakness may also be seen.

Diagnostic Testing

A history of fatigable weakness with predominantly facial muscle findings is suggestive of myasthenia gravis. Bedside testing using edrophonium is no longer available. Serologic testing for autoantibodies can aid in the diagnosis but will not be available in the ED. Electrophysiologic studies can be obtained upon admission or as an outpatient.

Management and Disposition

Myasthenia gravis may be life-threatening. Ventilatory support should be provided in the event of marked truncal weakness and respiratory failure, particularly in the setting of a concurrent illness which can exacerbate symptoms. In patients without risk of respiratory failure and in consultation with a neurologist, treatment may occur on an outpatient basis, with close symptom monitoring and oral cholinesterase inhibitor therapy.

The references for this chapter can be found online at ExpertConsult. com.

170

Pediatric Musculoskeletal Disorders

William B. Prince

KEY CONCEPTS

- The pediatric physis is the weakest part of the bone and more likely to separate before adjacent tendon or ligament tears, occurring more frequently during periods of rapid growth.
- Displaced supracondylar fractures are at greater risk for neurovascular injury and compartment syndrome. A lateral elbow radiograph with an elevated fat pad is suspicious for occult fracture.
- Transient synovitis has a peak presentation between 3 and 6 years of age. History, physical examination, radiographs, and laboratory values can help distinguish from septic arthritis and Lyme arthritis.
- Slipped capital femoral epiphysis (SCFE) is the posterior and inferior slippage of the proximal femoral epiphysis on the metaphysis, occurring through the epiphyseal plate. This condition affects boys at twice the rate of girls, occurring more commonly between 8 and 15 years of age. This prevalence is changing due to the increasing obesity rate.
- Lyme arthritis typically presents as mono-arthritis in two-thirds of cases, involving the knees 90% of the time. The knee tends to be swollen with limited range of motion, but pain varies and patients can usually still ambulate with a limp. Approximately 50% to 60% of patients not treated for early stages of Lyme will go on to develop Lyme arthritis, which can be their presenting symptom of the disease.
- Little League elbow describes a group of elbow injuries, including apophysitis, medical epicondylitis, and osteochondritis dissecans of the radial head and capitellum. The pediatric elbow is vulnerable to overuse injury, because it has multiple muscle and ligamentous attachments as well as six ossification centers that close at different ages of skeletal maturity.
- Apophyseal injuries of the hip occur at the multiple sites of muscle origination or insertion including on the pelvis. Athletes most at risk are dancers, distance runners, and those participating in kicking sports.
- Gymnast wrist is a chronic wrist pain affecting almost 80% of pediatric gymnasts at some point. Compressive loading and shearing forces cause physeal microfractures at the hypertrophic zone, causing physeal widening and metaphyseal irregularity in almost three-fourths of patients.

FOUNDATIONS

Anatomy and Physiology

Due to the dynamic developmental state occurring in growing children, the pediatric skeleton is unique compared to adults. The most unique feature of pediatric bones is the presence of the physis. This growth plate is composed of proliferating cartilage cells between the epiphysis and metaphysis. The physis is the weakest part of the bone and allows for distinctly different fracture patterns and injury mechanisms compared to adults. The physis can separate or fracture before the adjacent ligaments and tendons tear; similar injury mechanisms in adults which result in sprained ligaments can cause physeal injuries in children. These injuries are most common during periods of rapid growth and represent up to 18% of pediatric fractures.

The pediatric periosteum is thicker and stronger than mature periosteum, which can result in a reduction of fracture displacement. It is also physiologically active which allows for rapid healing and increased stability, making nonunion unlikely. Children have tremendous remodeling potential which allows for greater degrees of angulation or misalignment. If the child has at least 2 years of growth potential remaining, a fracture adjacent to a joint will remodel acceptably if the angulation is less than 30 degrees in the plane of motion.

Fracture Patterns

Immature bones are more porous and pliable, resulting in fracture patterns seen uniquely in pediatric injuries:

- Plastic deformity results in bowing of the bone without cortical disruption.
- Torus (buckle) fractures tend to occur from linear compression and result in buckling of bone without cortical disruption. These injuries are common at the metaphyseal-diaphyseal junction (Fig. 170.1).
- Greenstick fractures disrupt the cortex unilaterally, with periosteum on the compression side remaining intact (Fig. 170.2). The degree of acceptable angulation without reduction is age dependent. Children under 5 years of age can have up to 35 degrees of angulation on lateral radiograph and less than 10 degrees of angulation on AP views, whereas children 5 to 10 years old can tolerate up to 25 degrees on lateral and less than 10 degrees on AP view without need for reduction. Children older than 10 years of age can tolerate 5 to 20 degrees of angulation on lateral x-ray, presuming no angulation on AP view. Treatment for greenstick fractures generally involves casting for 4 to 6 weeks.
- Complete fractures transect both cortices of the bone; these include transverse (Fig. 170.3), spiral (Fig. 170.4), oblique, and comminuted (Fig. 170.5).
- Physeal fractures are not specific to pediatrics but are more likely during periods of rapid bone growth. The Salter-Harris classification is commonly used to delineate fracture patterns as they relate to the physis (Table 170.1). Concern for physeal injury stems from the potential for growth arrest and limb-length abnormalities. Nondisplaced Salter-Harris type I and II fractures (Fig. 170.6 and Fig 170.7) are generally low risk for these complications because the germinal layer of the physis is not commonly involved. These fractures can be splinted or casted with orthopedic follow-up within 1 week. Salter-Harris type III, IV, and V fractures (Fig. 170.8 through 170.10) are at greater risk for damage to the growth plate and are commonly unstable, requiring prompt orthopedic consultation. Types III and IV involve the joint surface and commonly require open reduction to maintain joint stability. Type V fractures are

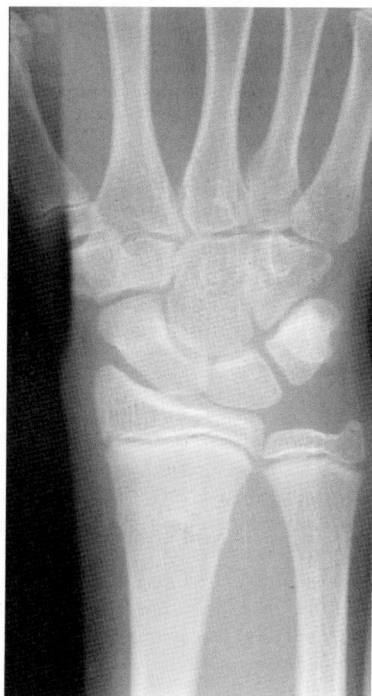

Fig. 170.1 Buckle fracture of the distal end of the radius.

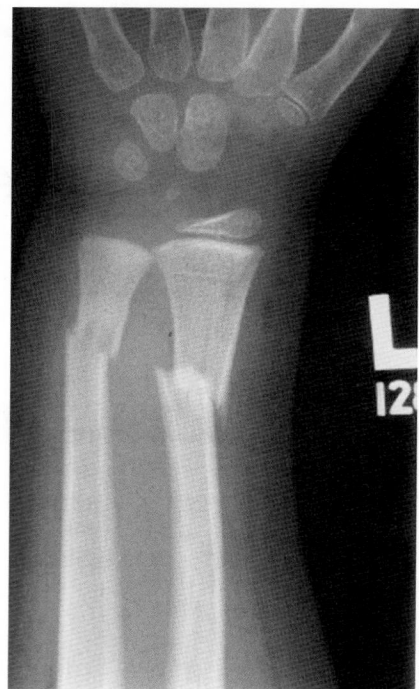

Fig. 170.3 Transverse fractures of the radius and ulna.

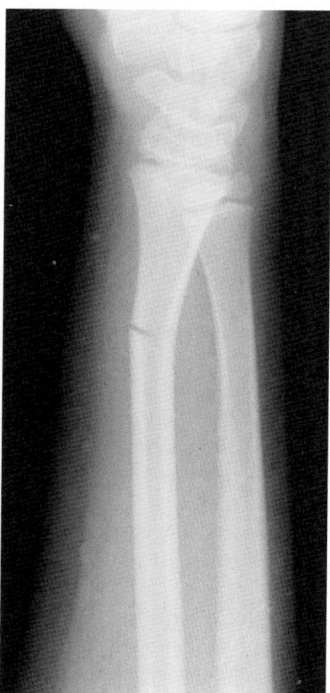

Fig. 170.2 Greenstick fracture of the radius.

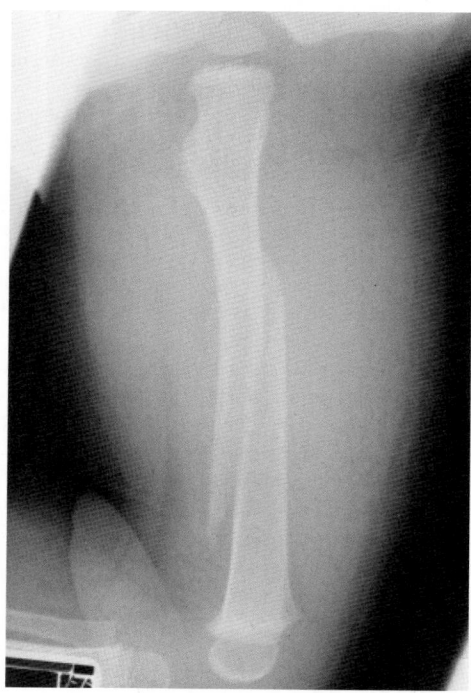

Fig. 170.4 Spiral fracture of the femur.

followed closely, as the risk for premature growth plate closure is high and surgical intervention is often needed.

SPECIFIC DISORDERS

Clavicle Fracture

Clavicle fractures are common in childhood but generally heal without complication. Most fractures occur between the middle and distal third of the bone. Mechanisms include birth trauma, direct trauma to the bone itself, and falls onto the shoulder. The bone's superficial lie allows for easy palpation when evaluating for pain or deformity. A clavicle fracture may be detected later in a neonate when a visible callus has formed around day 10 or per parent history of crying when being picked up.

The patient with a clavicle fracture commonly complains of pain at the clavicle and shoulder, often with neck and arm movement. An anteroposterior radiograph of the clavicle is sufficient for diagnosis

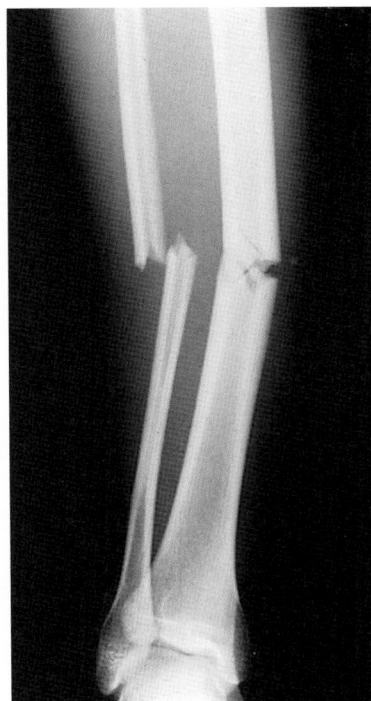

Fig. 170.5 Comminuted fractures of the tibia and fibula.

TABLE 170.1	**Salter-Harris Fracture Classification**	
Type	**Description**	
I	Fracture extends through the physis	
II	Fracture extends from the physis into the metaphysis (away from the joint space)	
III	Fracture extends from the physis into the epiphysis (toward the joint space)	
IV	Fracture extends from the physis into the metaphysis and epiphysis	
V	Crush injury of the physis	

(Fig. 170.11). Displacement of the affected shoulder along with crepitus and edema may be present upon inspection. The proximity of the clavicle to the subclavian vessels as well as the brachial plexus warrants a thorough neurovascular examination, especially in the setting of a displaced fracture. Complications can be seen in the setting of proximal fractures or posterior sternoclavicular displacement which can injure the trachea, esophagus, or cause pneumothorax.

Most children and adolescents with clavicle fractures only require supportive care and immobilization involving sling and swath for 4 to 6 weeks. However, recent studies suggest adolescents after 12 years of age have limited clavicular growth potential remaining and some surgeons have begun to use operative indications for adult patients in their pediatric population. Figure-of-eight splinting is not recommended due to risk of brachial plexus palsy with prolonged use. Newborns generally require no treatment following clavicle fractures from birth. Orthopedic consult should be obtained for clavicular fractures that are open, associated with neurovascular compromise, evidence of a floating shoulder (when associated with a scapular fracture), or with significant skin tenting.[1] An orthopedic referral should be considered in fractures that are comminuted, have a substantial degree of displacement, or in high-level athletes as surgery may facilitate a faster return to activity.

Supracondylar Fractures of the Humerus

Supracondylar humerus fractures are the most common fractures involving the elbow in pediatric patients. During childhood, the tensile strength of the ligaments surrounding the joint exceed that of the weaker bones themselves, which increases the likelihood for fractures rather than ligamentous injury. Typically the patient history involves a fall onto an extended arm, forcing the distal bone superiorly and posteriorly.

Radiographic evaluation of elbow injuries include an AP view of extended elbow (if possible), oblique view, and lateral flexed view. The elbow joint contains 6 cartilaginous ossification centers which can be easily mistake for fracture lines (Fig. 170.12). An acronym for remembering the order of appearance of the ossification centers is CRITOE (Table 170.2).

Injury mechanisms involving impact on flexed elbow result in anterior displacement of the distal fragment. Supracondylar fractures are classified as either flexion or extension injuries, of which the latter is more common. An AP and lateral radiograph are required to evaluate the degree of displacement and continuity of the cortex as defined by the Gartland classification (Table 170.3). Because subtle fractures can be difficult to visualize, the anterior humeral line can be used as indirect evidence of fracture (Fig. 170.13). A true lateral view should demonstrate a figure-of-eight appearance of the distal humerus, with intersection of the anterior humeral line with the posterior two-thirds of the capitellum. If this line intersects the anterior one-third of the anterior capitellum or is anterior to this structure, then a supracondylar fracture with posterior displacement of the distal fragment is suggestive. The Baumann angle, normally 70 to 75 degrees, can be helpful in detecting subtle fractures and is formed by a line drawn to follow the growth plate of the capitellum intersected with a line drawn down the center of the humerus (Fig. 170.14).

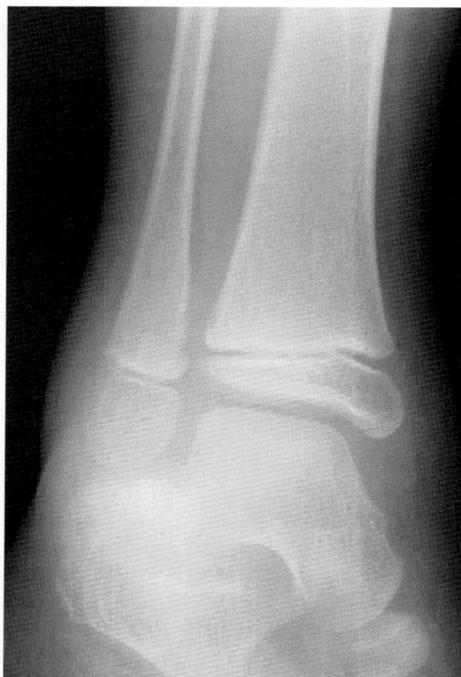

Fig. 170.6 Salter-Harris type I fracture of the fibula. Radiographic findings include soft tissue swelling over the growth plate and minimal physeal widening.

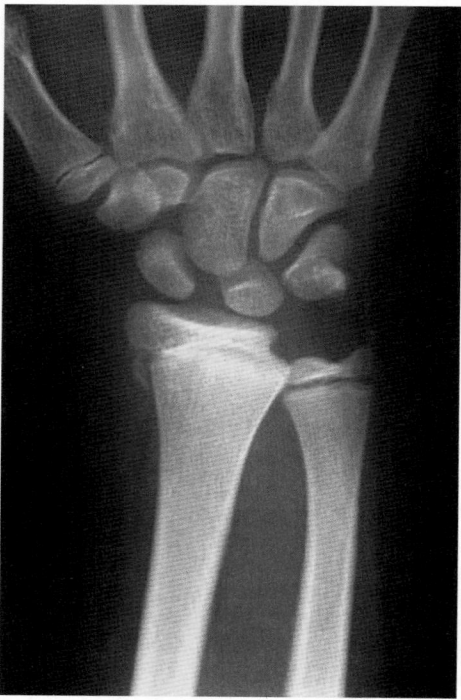

Fig. 170.7 Salter-Harris type II fracture of the radius.

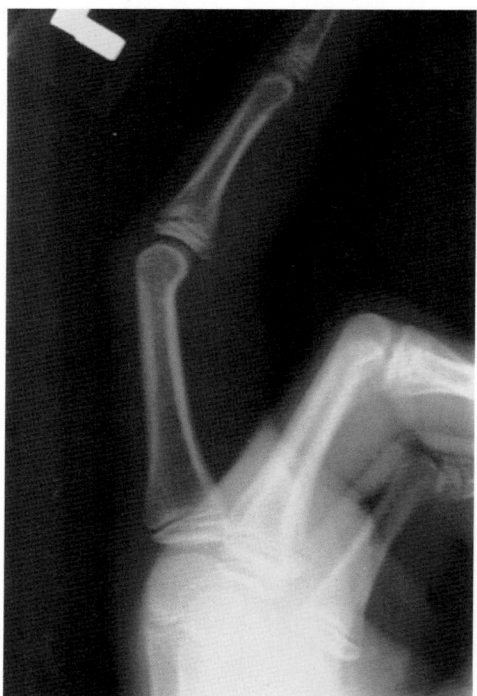

Fig. 170.8 Salter-Harris type III fracture of the middle phalanx.

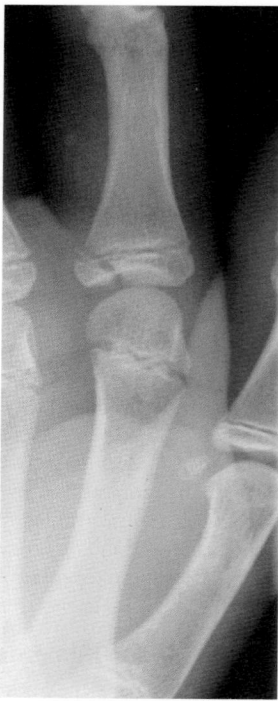

Fig. 170.9 Salter-Harris type IV fracture of the proximal phalanx.

Fat pads are markers for joint effusions or hemorrhage and raise suspicion for occult fracture. On a lateral radiograph with the elbow flexed at 90 degrees, the anterior fat pad demonstrates radiolucency anterior to the coronoid fossa. When thin, this can be a normal finding in children, but is considered a "sail" sign of occult fracture when bulging. The posterior fat pad is posterior to the distal humerus and always represents a pathologic effusion (Fig. 170.15).

The injured patient presents with a painful swollen elbow and typically holds the extremity in extension and slight pronation. Puckering, dimpling, or anterior bruising are indications that reduction may be difficult, as the anteriorly displaced fragment may have penetrated the brachialis muscle. Immediate assessment should include evaluating for neurovascular compromise by assessing capillary refill and palpating both radial and ulnar pulses. Signs of arterial compromise include the 5 "Ps": pain, pallor, pulselessness, paralysis, and paresthesias. Worsening

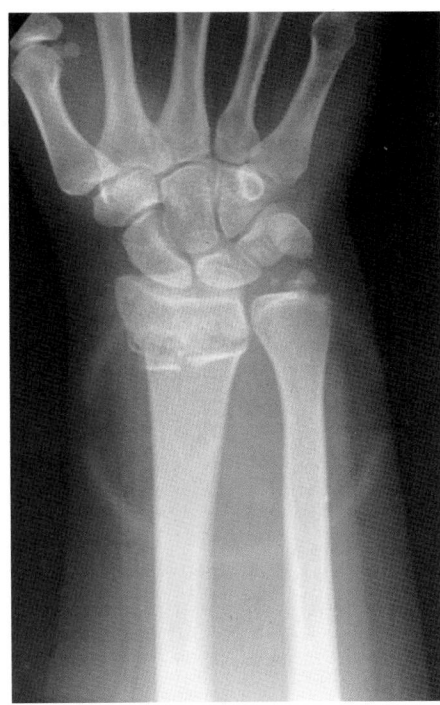

Fig. 170.10 Salter-Harris type V fracture of the distal end of the radius.

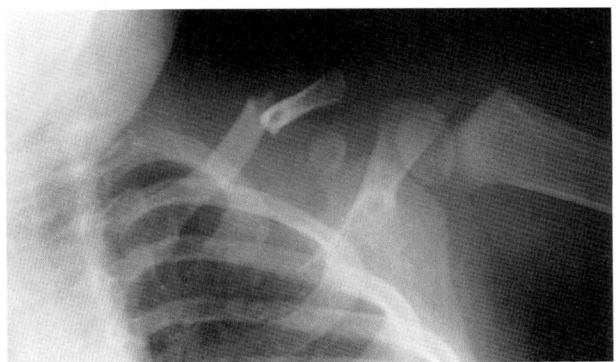

Fig. 170.11 Fracture of the middle third of the clavicle.

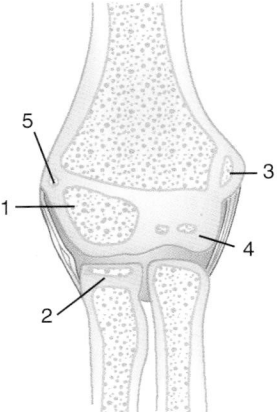

Fig. 170.12 Ossification centers of the elbow. *1,* Capitellum; *2,* radial head; *3,* medial epicondyle; *4,* trochlea; *5,* lateral epicondyle. (From: Connolly JF. *Depalma's Management of Fractures and Dislocations.* Philadelphia: WB Saunders; 1981.)

TABLE 170.2 Sequence of Ossification Around the Elbow: CRITOE

Ossification Center	Age at Appearance	Age at Closure (yr)
*C*apitellum	6–12 mo	14
*R*adial head	4–5 yr	16
Medial (*I*nternal) epicondyle	5–7 yr	15
*T*rochlea	8–10 yr	14
*O*lecranon	8–9 yr	14
Lateral (*E*xternal) epicondyle	9–13 yr	16

TABLE 170.3 Gartland Classification of Extension-Type Supracondylar Fractures

Type	Description
I	Nondisplaced fracture
II	Displaced fracture with intact posterior cortex
III	Displaced fracture with no cortical contact
IIIA	Posteromedial rotation of the distal fragment
IIIB	Posterolateral rotation of the distal fragment

Adapted from: Gartland JJ. Management of supracondylar fractures of the humerus in children. *Surg Gynecol Obstet.* 1959;109:145.

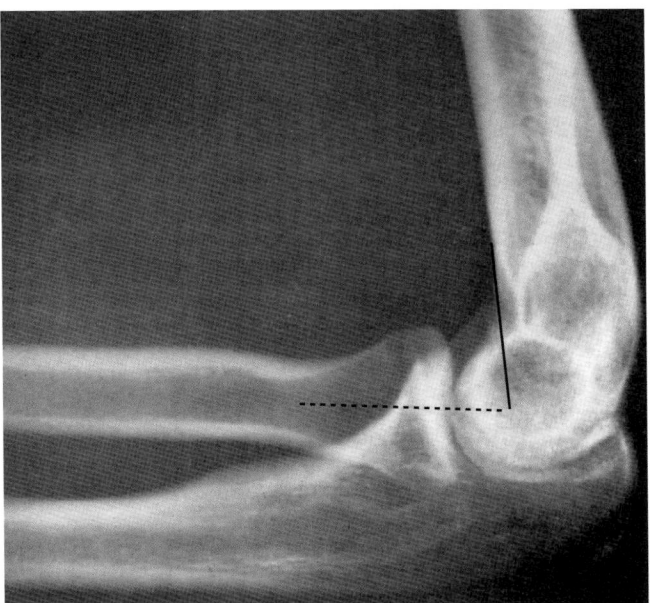

Fig. 170.13 Lateral radiograph demonstrating the bone relationships in a normal elbow. The anterior humeral line (*solid line*) and proximal radial line (*dashed line*) bisect the capitellum. (From: Weissman BN, Sledge CB. *Orthopedic Radiology.* Philadelphia: WB Saunders; 1986.)

pain or pain with passive extension of the fingers is a concerning sign of limb ischemia and can lead to Volkmann ischemic contractures. Emergent consultation with an orthopedic surgeon should be initiated and fracture reduced expeditiously in an attempt to restore blood flow (Fig. 170.16). Perfusion should be confirmed via radial artery signal by Doppler following closed reduction attempts; if reperfusion is unsuccessful, emergent vascular exploration is warranted to assess for and repair brachial artery injuries.

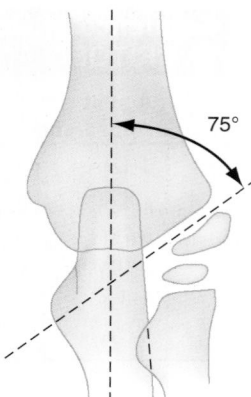

Fig. 170.14 Baumann angle in a normal elbow (anteroposterior radiograph). (From: Worlock P. Supracondylar fractures of the humerus: assessment of cubitus varus by the Baumann angle. *J Bone Joint Surg Br,* 1986;68:755.)

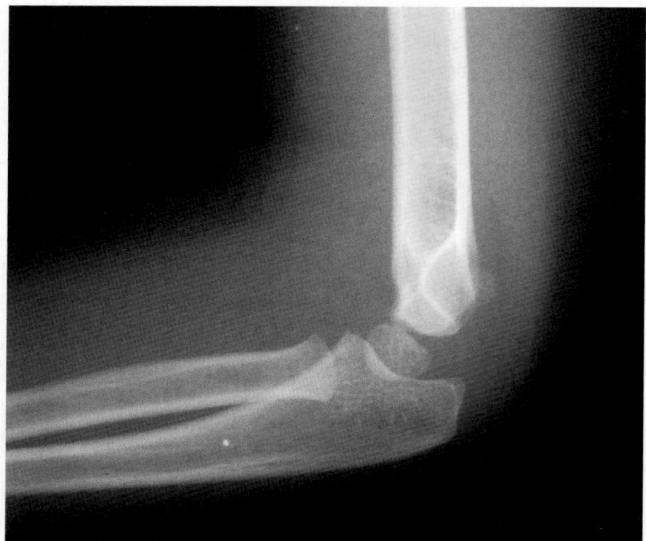

Fig. 170.15 Lateral radiograph of a supracondylar fracture with an anterior fat pad sail sign and posterior fat pad.

Because major nerves and arteries lie in proximity to the supracondylar region, a full motor and sensory function should evaluate for possible associated injury or entrapment. Major structures include radial, ulnar, and median nerves (Table 170.4). The median and radial nerves are commonly injured in extension injuries when the distal fragments are displaced posterior-laterally and posterior-medially, whereas the ulnar nerve is commonly affected with flexion injuries.

Supracondylar humerus fractures are the most common fractures treated surgically by pediatric orthopedic surgeons.[2] Management of Gartland type I fractures can be placed in a posterior long arm splint with the elbow flexed at 90 degrees and either neutral or pronated position. These patients should follow up with an orthopedist with 24 hours for evaluation and casting. Gartland type II and III fractures require emergent evaluation by an orthopedic surgeon. Type II fractures require closed reduction, but if greater than 90 degrees of flexion is required to maintain reduction, then stabilization with percutaneous pinning is advised. Treatment of type III supracondylar fractures includes admission and should include operative reduction and pinning, because they are prone to neurovascular compromise.

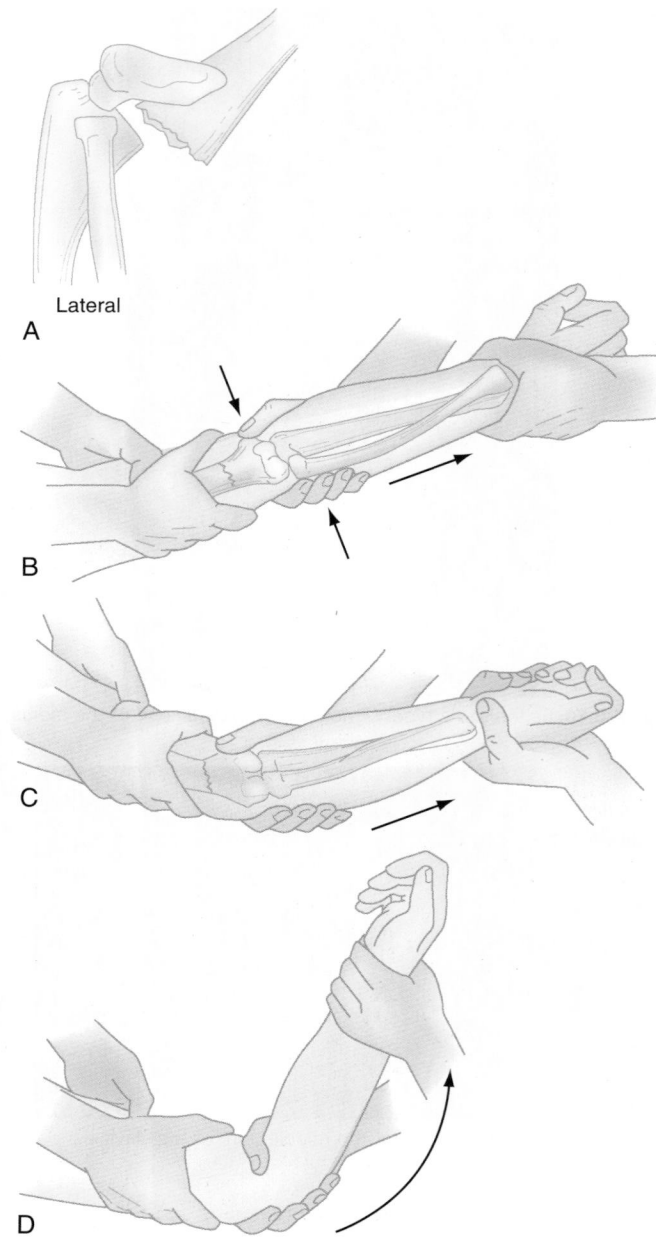

Fig. 170.16 Steps in reduction of a displaced supracondylar fracture. (A & B) The assistant fixes the arm of the patient while the emergency clinician grasps the patient's wrist and applies steady traction in line with the long axis of the arm while keeping the forearm in the neutral, thumb-up position. (C) If the distal fragment is displaced laterally, it is pushed inward with the emergency clinician's other hand. If it is displaced medially, it is pushed outward. Throughout manipulation, traction is maintained. (D) After length is restored and the medial and lateral displacement is corrected, the emergency clinician's thumb is placed over the anterior surface of the proximal fragment, with the fingers behind the olecranon, and the elbow is gently flexed. The arm is then immobilized with the forearm pronated; laterally displaced fractures are immobilized with the forearm supinated. (From: Geiderman JM, Magnusson AR. Humerus and elbow. In Rosen P, Barkin R, eds. *Emergency Medicine: Concepts and Clinical Practice,* ed 4. St. Louis: CV Mosby; 1998.)

Monteggia and Galeazzi Fracture-Dislocations

Monteggia fracture-dislocation represents a fracture of the proximal third of the ulna plus dislocation of the radial head (Fig. 170.17). Isolated ulna fractures are uncommon in children and can present as a plastic deformity of the ulna without obvious fracture. The radiocapitellar line, drawn down the radial shaft, should pass through the center of the capitellar ossification center on lateral elbow radiograph; radial head dislocations will disrupt this line (Fig. 170.18). In contrast, the Galeazzi fracture is characterized as a fracture of the distal radius and disruption of the distal radioulnar joint.

For both fracture types, orthopedic consultation is needed for closed reduction and casting. Management of the Monteggia fracture is predicated on recognizing the radial head dislocation, and reduction and stabilization of the ulnar fracture generally results in radial head reduction.[2] Failure to reduce the radial head over time can result in valgus instability of the elbow, arthritis of the elbow, and restricted forearm pronation.[2]

Nursemaid's Elbow

Nursemaid's elbow (i.e., radial head subluxation) occurs when the head of the radius is displaced from the annular ligament; it represents approximately 20% of pediatric upper extremity injuries, with a peak incidence between two and three years of age.[3] The typical mechanism occurs when axial traction is placed on the forearm, causing extension of the elbow and pronation. This movement permits subluxation of the radial head via partial tearing or entrapping of the annular ligament between the radial head and capitellum (Fig. 170.19).[3]

Patients generally present with unwillingness to use the affected arm, which is typically held against the body, slightly flexed at the elbow with the arm pronated. Edema, ecchymosis, or deformity are typically absent. Gentle palpation usually does not illicit pain of the long bones or elbow joint, although ranging the extremity can cause distress. The diagnosis of nursemaid's elbow is made clinically; AP and lateral radiographs of the elbow should be obtained if there is focal bony tenderness, ecchymosis, joint swelling, or a traumatic mechanism.

Two common techniques for reduction are supination/flexion and hyperpronation maneuvers. Both methods involve the examiner supporting the child's arm at the elbow by placing pressure with a finger on the radial head. In the supination/flexion maneuver, the examiner holds the forearm with their other hand and provides gentle traction while fully supinating and flexing the elbow in one motion. With hyperpronation, the examiner holds the affected arm's hand in a handshake grip and grips the elbow with the other hand. Hyperpronation of the forearm usually results in a palpable click over the radial head if reduction is successful.

TABLE 170.4 Neurologic Examination of the Distal Upper Extremity		
	EXAMINATION COMPONENT	
Nerve	**Motor**	**Sensory**
Radial	Wrist extension	Thumb and first finger web space
Ulnar	Wrist flexion and adduction	Little finger
Median	Wrist flexion and abduction	Thumb, index, and middle fingers
Thumb opposition	Radial aspect of palm of hand	
Anterior interosseous	Distal phalanx flexion (thumb and first finger)	None

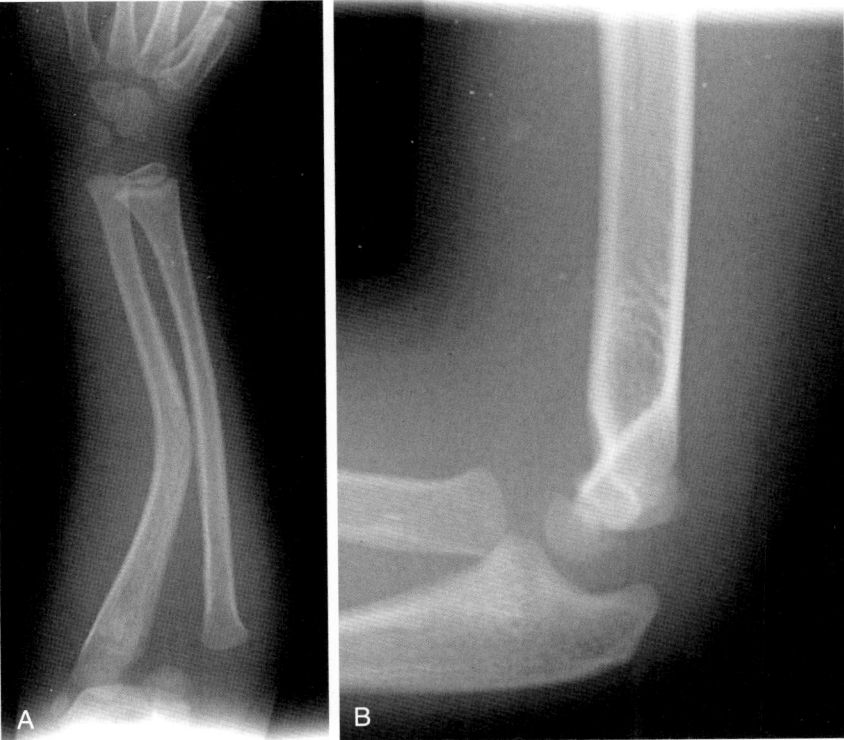

Fig. 170.17 (A) Anteroposterior view of the elbow revealing a distal ulna fracture with radial head dislocation. The radial head should align with the capitellum in all views. (B) Lateral view of the elbow demonstrating poor alignment of the radial head, with the capitellum consistent with Monteggia fracture-dislocation. (Courtesy Dr. Micheal Diament, Pediatric Radiology, Harbor-UCLA Medical Center, Torrance, CA.)

Both methods are effective, however, meta-analysis of randomized control trials have shown that hyperpronation is more effective, with a lower first attempt failure rate.[3] Recurrence is common and parents should be cautioned to avoid lifting the child by the arm or wrist, but may be taught to perform the maneuver themselves if it recurs.

Children typically begin using the arm normally within 15 minutes. If the child fails to move the extremity, repeat maneuvers may be attempted. However, if unsuccessful, radiographs should be obtained and the extremity placed in a long arm splint at 90 degrees. Pediatrician follow-up should be arranged within next 24 hours.

Toddler's Fracture

The toddler's fracture is a nondisplaced oblique fracture of the distal tibia that is the result of a minor fall or twisting mechanism, with a peak incidence between 1 and 4 years of age. Clinical diagnosis may be difficult, as the history may be vague and the physical examination

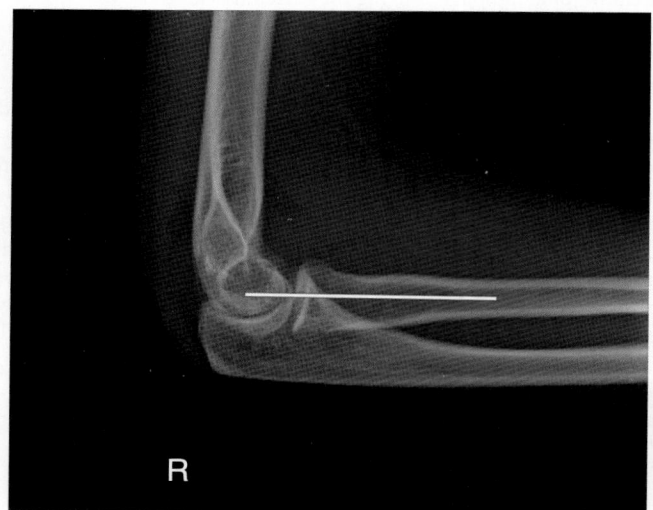

Fig. 170.18 Lateral elbow with a radiocapitellar line, which bisects the capitellum. (Courtesy D. Hanlon, MD, Pittsburg, PA)

is commonly nonspecific to a local injury. Typically, guardians report the child is limping or unwilling to bear weight; there may be a report of a minor fall. Tenderness may be elicited with palpation, but obvious swelling or deformity is uncommon. Gentle twisting of the lower leg may provoke pain.

Lower leg AP and lateral radiographs may reveal a subtle oblique lucency through the distal tibia terminating medially (Fig. 170.20). Because children have robust periosteum, any displacement can be minimal, making identification on radiograph difficult, and the fracture is often not initially visible. If suspicion for a toddler fracture is high, immobilization and reevaluation 2 weeks later will show callus formation on repeat radiographs from new periosteal growth. If available, ultrasound can be considered as an imaging modality to evaluate for fracture. Traditionally, immobilization involved a posterior long leg cast for 3 to 4 weeks, but recent studies have shown no differences in the clinical outcomes between various immobilization methods: casting, splinting, or a cast boot.[4] Casts should not extend above the knee on young toddlers, who are at risk for cast migration. Children are allowed to bear weight as tolerated after immobilization.

Nonaccidental Trauma

The National Child Abuse and Neglect Data System reported more than 680,000 children were victims of maltreatment and 1670 children died of abuse and neglect in 2015.[5] Of all these childhood fatalities 43.9% were victims of physical abuse exclusively or in combination with another maltreatment type and 74.8% of these children were less than 3 years of age.[5] Diagnosis of physical abuse can be elusive and missed identification can lead to additional injuries. An estimated 25% of children diagnosed with nonaccidental trauma (NAT) have a sentinel injury before their abuse diagnosis.[5] These data underscore the necessity for a thorough evaluation when there is a concerning history or physical findings for NAT. See Chapter 172 for a complete discussion on the evaluation of NAT.

Developmental Dysplasia of the Hip
Foundations

Developmental dysplasia of the hip (DDH) denotes a wide spectrum of clinical severity: neonatal instability, acetabular dysplasia, hip subluxation, and true dislocation of the hip. Laxity within the acetabulum refers

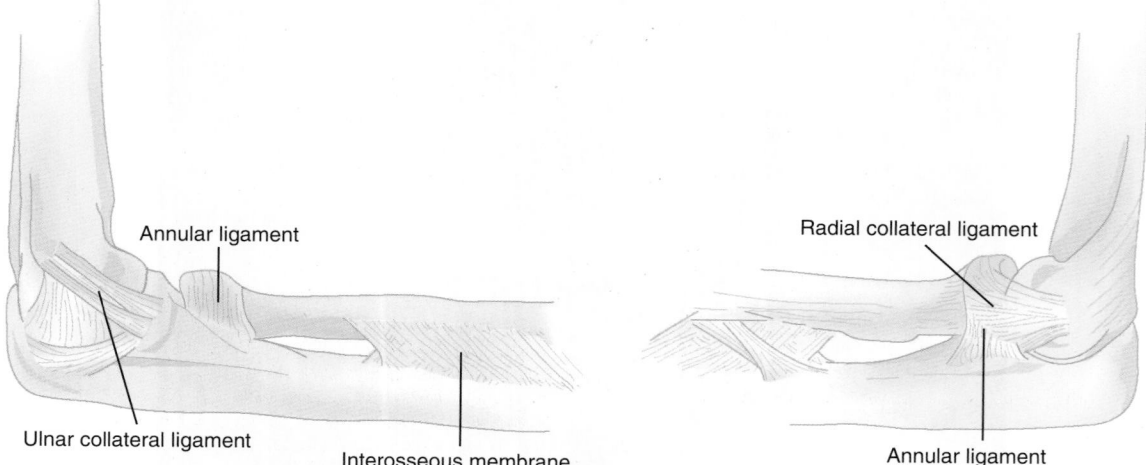

Annular ligament

Ulnar collateral ligament

Interosseous membrane

Radial collateral ligament

Annular ligament

Fig. 170.19 Nursemaid's elbow. In a nursemaid's elbow injury, the annular ligament around the radial head is dislodged as an axial force is applied. The ligament is then partially dislocated into the radiocapitellar joint when the arm is released. (From Simon R, Koenigsknecht S: *Emergency orthopedics, the extremities*, ed 2, Norwalk, CT, 1987, Appleton & Lange.)

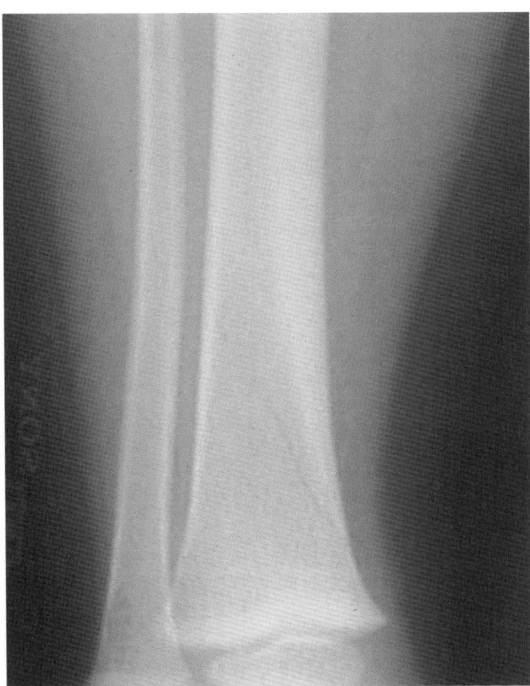

Fig. 170.20 Toddler's fracture.

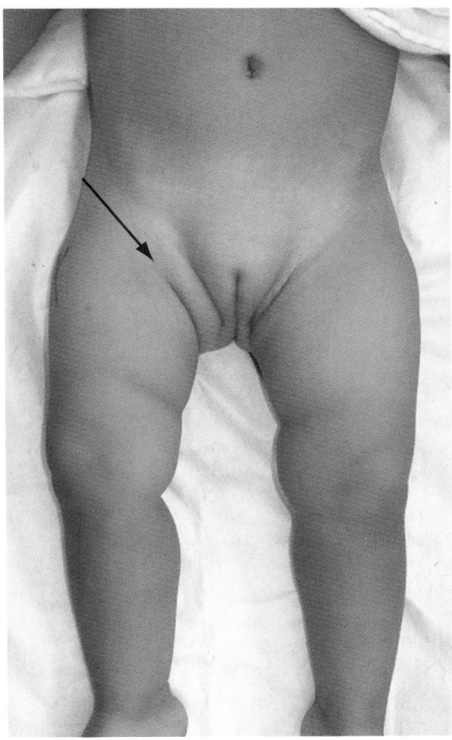

Fig. 170.21 A 21-month-old child with right hip dislocation. Note the asymmetrical skinfolds in the upper thigh (*arrow*). (From: Storer SK, Skaggs DL. Developmental dysplasia of the hip. *Am Fam Physician.* 2006;74:1310-1316.)

to instability, whereas dysplasia indicates some morphologic change in the acetabulum or proximal. With a subluxed hip, articular surfaces are in contact, but not concentrically aligned. With a hip dislocation, articular surfaces of the acetabulum and proximal femur are not in any contact.

Clinical hip instability occurs in 1% to 2% of term infants; up to 15% have findings on imaging studies.[6] Risk factors include breech presentation, female gender, family history, and incorrect lower extremity swaddling; risk factors are additive, with frank breech presentation and family history the two most important risk factors.[6]

Clinical Features

Signs of DDH may be present at birth or develop as the baby grows. Diagnosis is usually made during regular screening and surveillance by physical exams up to 6 months of age. Instability is the primary sign of DDH in the neonatal period; however, this quickly diminishes as muscle strength increases, leaving abduction asymmetry as the main clinical sign.

At less than 3 months of age, screening of newborns involves Ortolani and Barlow maneuvers. The Barlow test is done with the hip in 90 degrees of flexion and adduction; lateral pressure is put on the hip. In hip instability, a clunk can be felt as the femoral head falls out the back of the acetabulum, effectively dislocating. The Barlow test has no proven predictive value for future hip dislocation, and if performed frequently or forcefully, can create instability.[6] The AAP, in its 2016 clinical report on DDH, recommends that no posterior-directed force be applied during this procedure.[6] From a similar starting position, the Ortolani maneuver should transition smoothly from hip adduction into gentle anterior pressure on the trochanter while the hip is abducted; a clunk is felt if the hip locates into the socket.

Benign "hip clicks" without instability are clinically insignificant. This finding, which is secondary to soft tissue snapping over bony prominences, should be distinguished from "hip clunks," as detected in a positive Ortolani maneuver. A dislocated hip becomes fixed by 3 months of age, after which the usefulness and sensitivity of the Barlow and Ortolani tests are limited.[6]

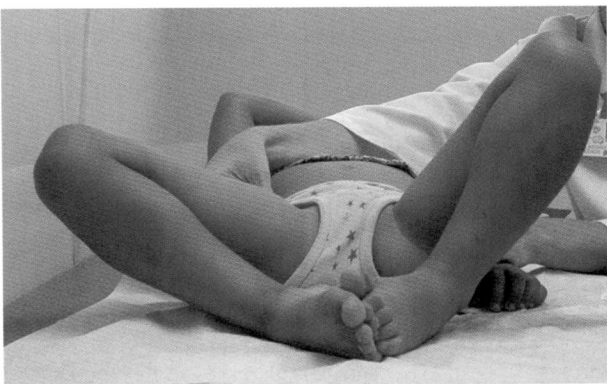

Fig. 170.22 A 3-year-old child with a left hip dislocation. Note the limited abduction. (From: Storer SK, Skaggs DL. Developmental dysplasia of the hip. *Am Fam Physician.* 2006;74:1310-1316.)

Restricted asymmetrical hip abduction may be found on physical examination. Limb length discrepancy (Galeazzi test), asymmetrical thigh or gluteal folds (Fig. 170.21), and limited or asymmetrical abduction (Fig. 170.22) raises suspicion for DDH. A positive Galeazzi test can be detected with the hips and knees flexed to 90 degrees, observing the vertical level of the knees (Fig. 170.23). Asymmetrical groin, thigh, and gluteal folds can be seen in up to 25% of normal infants and alone are not pathognomonic.[7] Once a child is walking, a dislocated hip may manifest as an abnormal gait.

Diagnostic Testing

Infants older than 4 weeks of age suspected of having DDH should undergo ultrasound, also recommended to diagnose clinically silent

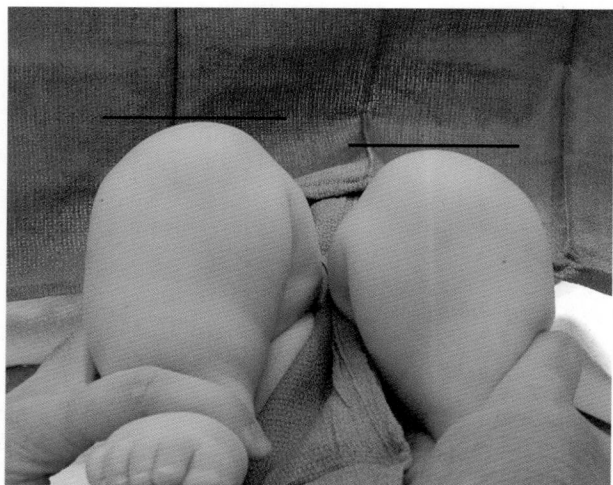

Fig. 170.23 Galeazzi sign in a 7-month-old girl with left hip dislocation. Apparent inequality of femur length is manifested as asymmetry in the level of the patient's knees. (From: Storer SK, Skaggs DL. Developmental dysplasia of the hip. *Am Fam Physician.* 2006;74:1310-1316.)

DDH in the high-risk infant from 6 weeks to 6 months of age.[6] Once the ossifying nucleus of the femoral head appears around 4 to 6 months of age, radiographs are more diagnostic than ultrasound. An AP radiograph of the pelvis with both legs extended in neutral position is sufficient to make the diagnosis (Fig. 170.24).

Management

Early detection of infants with suspected DDH and referral for bracing or casting can prevent the need for reconstructive surgery. Infants with suspected DDH should be referred after 4 weeks of age. An isolated positive Barlow result up to 2 weeks of age will generally stabilize on its own and can be followed with surveillance for an additional 4 to 6 weeks. Because 96% of pathologic changes found on ultrasound resolve spontaneously within the first 6 weeks of life, treatment can be safely delayed until that time if the hip is stable and not dislocated.

The treatment goal of DDH is concentric reduction and stabilization of the hip joint. If not treated, long-term consequences can include arthritis, back pain, and aseptic necrosis of the femoral head. If the hip is dislocated, the Pavlik harness (PH) is first-line treatment for reduction (Fig. 170.25). The PH is a safe and effective option during infancy for hips that are dislocated, located but unstable, or dysplastic.[8] The harness holds the hips in a flexed and abducted position, allowing for the femoral head to be reduced within the acetabulum. The P4 has a success rate of approximately 85% if treatment is initiated before 6 months of age.[8] If reduction with PH is not successful or in children older than 6 to 8 months, children should receive reduction in the OR followed by spica cast immobilization. Most children beyond 18 months of age require surgical reconstruction.

Pediatric Hip Pain

Children are susceptible to a number of hip disorders of varying degrees of severity (Box 170.1). Some of the conditions discussed can affect other joints in the body as well.

Transient Synovitis

Transient synovitis is a self-limited inflammatory process with a peak incidence between the ages of 3 and 6 years old, and more common in boys than girls. Caused by a benign nonpyogenic inflammatory response, it affects up to 3% of children, and is the most common hip disorder causing atraumatic limp in children.[9] The symptoms

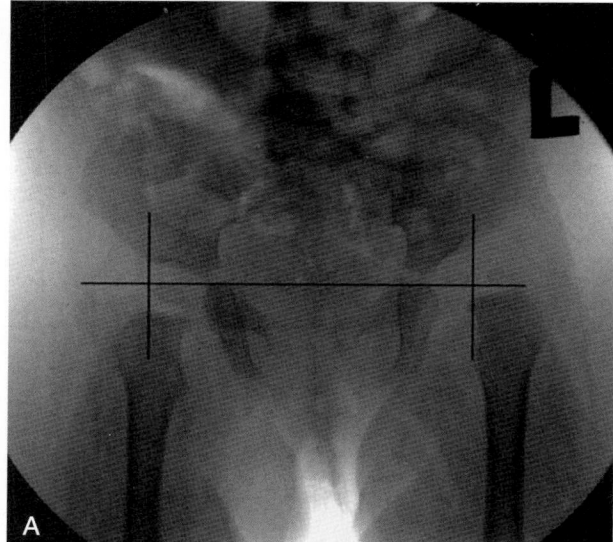

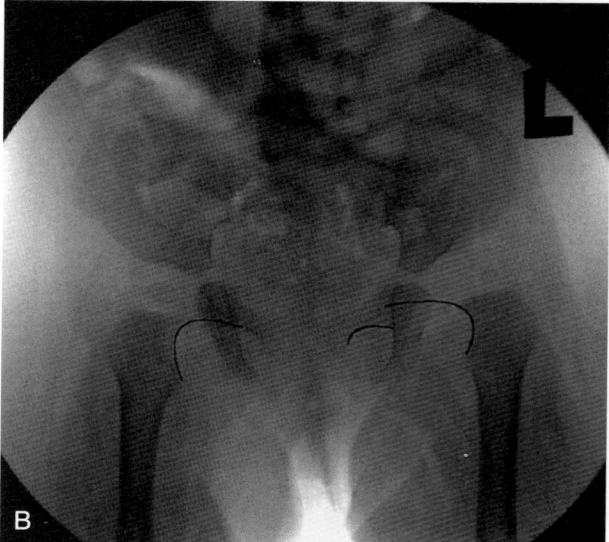

Fig. 170.24 Anteroposterior radiographs obtained in a 7-month-old girl with developmental dysplasia of the left hip. (A) The horizontal line is the Hilgenreiner line; the vertical lines are Perkin lines. Note that the femoral head on the right (normal) side lies in the inferomedial quadrant formed by those lines. The left hip is dislocated; its femoral head lies in the superolateral quadrant. (B) Shenton line is disrupted on the left (dislocated) hip. (From: Storer SK, Skaggs DL. Developmental dysplasia of the hip. *Am Fam Physician.* 2006;74:1310-1316.)

of transient synovitis often follow a viral respiratory illness, minor trauma, or allergic hypersensitivity. This condition may affect the hips or knees.

In a child presenting with a limp, transient synovitis should be distinguished from septic arthritis, because the latter can cause joint destruction if diagnosis is delayed. Generally, patients with septic joints have fevers and are unwilling to bear weight, whereas children with transient synovitis are rarely febrile and may limp but bear some weight. The leg of either condition is generally held in some flexion, slightly abducted and externally rotated due to the presence of an effusion. Transient synovitis often presents after a viral illness and the child may have no other symptoms; children with septic joints can appear ill.

Transient synovitis is a diagnosis of exclusion, involving history, physical examination, screening labs, and imaging to rule out a septic

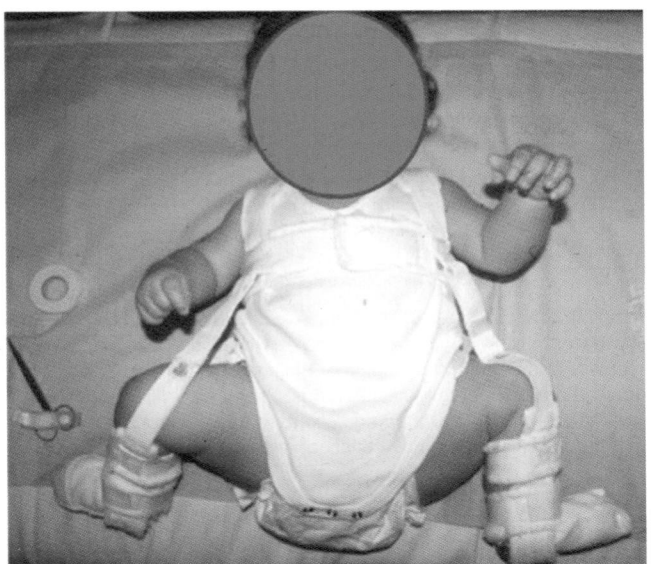

Fig. 170.25 Pavlik harness. (From: Clarke N, Taylor C. Diagnosis and management of developmental hip dysplasia. *Paediatr Child Health.* 2012;22(6):235-238.)

BOX 170.1   Causes of Hip Pain in Children

Trauma
Hip or pelvis fractures
Overuse injuries

Infection
Septic arthritis
Osteomyelitis
Myositis
Lyme disease

Inflammation
Transient synovitis
Juvenile rheumatoid arthritis
Rheumatic fever

Neoplasm
Leukemia
Osteogenic or Ewing sarcoma
Metastatic disease

Hematologic Disorders
Hemophilia
Sickle cell anemia

Miscellaneous
Legg-Calvé-Perthes disease
Slipped capital femoral epiphysis

joint. Because clinical features for these two entities can overlap, a set of four independent predictors of septic arthritis (Kocher criteria) can help evaluate the likelihood for septic joint: fever of 38.5°C or greater, inability to bear weight; erythrocyte sedimentation rate (ESR) of 40 mm/hr or greater; and peripheral white blood cell (CBC) count of 12,000 cells/μL or greater. The Kocher study found that the probability of septic arthritis in patients with one predictor was 3%; two predictors,

40%; three predictors, 93%; and all four, nearly 100%. Validation studies found a 2% chance of septic arthritis in patients with zero out of four predictors. Although not part of the original Kocher criteria, C-reactive protein (CRP), commonly used for additional risk stratification, has shown to be a better negative than a positive predictor of the disease. A CRP less than 1.0 mg/dL carries an 87% probability of *not* having septic arthritis. Inflammatory markers tend to be normal to mildly elevated in transient synovitis.

If septic arthritis cannot be reliably excluded in the differential, then we recommend ultrasound for initial hip imaging, because it is noninvasive and highly sensitive for detecting hip effusions. A hip ultrasound that is negative for joint effusion generally rules out septic arthritis; however, the presence of a hip effusion is nonspecific. Radiographs of the hip have limited utility in ruling in or out transient synovitis but can identify other pediatric hip disorders causing symptoms.

If transient synovitis is suspected, treatment includes symptomatic relief with nonsteroidal antiinflammatory drugs (NSAIDs) and joint rest. Return to activity is allowed as tolerated with improvement of pain. Close follow-up with primary care within 24 hours is recommended for continued monitoring for signs of septic arthritis. Symptoms of transient synovitis last 1 week or less in 67% of patients, and less than 1 month in an additional 21% of patients.

Acute Septic Arthritis

Septic arthritis is a bacterial joint space infection that can result in acute and chronic disability. Boys are affected twice as often as girls, and the lower extremities are most commonly involved; hips, knees, and ankles account for 80% of cases. Predisposing factors include trauma, preceding viral infection, immunodeficiency, hemoglobinopathy, hemophilia-induced hemarthroses, diabetes, intraarticular injections, surgery, and IV drug use.

The pediatric joint is most commonly infected through hematogenous inoculation via transphyseal vessels, as the blood flow is sluggish in metaphyseal capillaries. Contiguous spread of infection from osteomyelitis into the joint space is more common in infants and young children. The infection's inflammatory response leads to a high local cytokine concentration, which induces the host to release matrix metalloproteinases, which are collagen degrading enzymes. Bacterial toxins and lysosomal enzymes further damage the articular surface as soon as 8 hours after inoculation. Pressure ischemia and avascular necrosis cause additional joint destruction from increased capsular pressure.

Common bacterial etiologies for septic arthritis tend to be age specific (Table 170.5). The organisms most likely to cause bacteremia in a child are the most common organisms isolated from pediatric joint infections, including both methicillin-sensitive and methicillin-resistant *Staphylococcus aureus*. Community-acquired methicillin-resistant *S. aureus* (CA-MRSA) is isolated in up to 63% of cases. Some strains of CA-MRSA have been found to contain a gene encoding for the cytotoxin Panton-Valentine leucocidin (PVL), which is associated with complex infections, higher rates of septic shock, prolonged hospital stays, increased surgical interventions, and longer durations of antibiotic therapy.

In neonates, group B *Streptococcus* and gram-negative enteric organisms are common causes of infections. Neonates and adolescents share a risk for *Neisseria gonorrhoeae*, whereas children with sickle cell are at a greater risk for *Salmonella* infections. Other frequently isolated species include group A hemolytic *Streptococcus* and *Streptococcus pneumoniae*.

Septic arthritis can present similarly to transient synovitis, with a combination of fever, malaise, and immobility from pain when ranging the affected joint. Local erythema, warmth, and swelling may be noted in joints other than the hip. Hip infections commonly present with the

TABLE 170.5 Septic Arthritis Pathogens and Treatment

Age	Organism	Treatment
Birth–3 mo	Group B streptococcus (*Streptococcus agalactiae*) *Staphylococcus aureus* Gram-negative organisms *Neisseria gonorrhoeae*	Nafcillin 75–150 mg/kg/day q6h or oxacillin 75–100 mg/kg/day q6-8h, and cefotaxime 100–150 mg/kg/day q8h or cefepime 100 mg/kg/day q12h
3 mo–5 yr	*S. aureus* *Streptococcus pneumoniae* *Streptococcus pyogenes* *Kingella kingae* *Haemophilus influenzae*	Nafcillin, 150–200 mg/kg/day q6h or oxacillin 100–200 mg/kg/day q4–6h, and ceftriaxone, 50–100 mg/kg/day q12h[a]
5 yr–12 yr	*S. aureus* *S. pyogenes*	Nafcillin 150–200 mg/kg/day q6h or oxacillin 100–200 mg/kg/day q4–6h, and ceftriaxone 50–100 mg/kg/day q12h[a]
>12 yr	*S. aureus* *N. gonorrhoeae*	Nafcillin 150–200 mg/kg/day q6h or oxacillin 100–200 mg/kg/day q4–6h, and ceftriaxone 50–100 mg/kg/day q12h[a]

[a]Consider vancomycin, 45–60 mg/kg/day q6–8h, if methicillin-resistant *S. aureus* (MRSA) accounts for >10% local *S. aureus* isolates. Clindamycin 40 mg/kg/day q6–8h can be substituted for vancomycin if local *S. aureus* resistance to clindamycin is <10%.
Adapted from Liu C, Bayer A, Cosgrove SE, et al: Clinical practice guidelines by the Infectious Diseases Society of America for the treatment of methicillin-resistant *Staphylococcus aureus* infections in adults and children: executive summary. *Clin Infect Dis.* 2011;52:285; Gill P, Sanders JE. Emergency department management of pediatric Septic arthritis and osteomyelitis. *Pediatr Emerg Med Practice.* 2019;16:1-24; Kleinman K, McDaniel L, Molly M. *The Harriet Lane Handbook*, 22 edition, Elsevier, 2021, Philadelphia, PA.

TABLE 170.6 Proposed Guidelines for Synovial Fluid Interpretation

Positive	WBC >50,000 cells per microliter or Gram stain positive	%PMN >90	Pyogenic arthritis
Equivocal	WBC 20,000–80,000	%PMN >70	Lyme disease Tuberculosis
Negative	WBC < 5,000	%PMN <25	Transient synovitis Traumatic arthritis Reactive arthritis

Adapted from: Arson P, Posner J, Dooley RN, Cofin S, Jacobstein C, Lavelle J. This Children's Hospital of Philadelphia, Clinical Practice Guideline on Suspected Septic Arthritis. Last updated February 2017. Available at: http://www.chop.edu/clinical-pathway/septic-arthritis-suspected-clinical-pathway. Accessed February 2017.

K. kingae patients are commonly colonized and oropharynx PCR assay for the RTX toxin should be obtained if suspected.

In septic arthritis, plain radiographs of the affected joint are less likely to be helpful. In the acute setting, only soft tissue swelling may be noted. Radiographic changes including destruction of the articular cartilage and joint space narrowing can be seen in a chronic process, but not readily until 7 to 10 days after the infection has commenced. Ultrasound is a rapid and noninvasive method for detecting the presence of a joint effusion. This is particularly helpful when evaluating the hip or shoulders, which are not easily palpated for effusion. A negative ultrasound of the hip with absence of fluid generally rules out septic arthritis. MRI with and without gadolinium contrast is the optimal imaging modality for bone infections, which can help identify nearby osteomyelitis or pyogenic myositis. Between 15% and 50% of osteoarticular infections involve the joint *and* bone.

Definitive diagnosis of septic arthritis hinges on the evaluation of aspirated synovial fluid sent for Gram stain, cell count with differential, and aerobic and anaerobic cultures. Synovial fluid samples with WBC greater than 50,000/μL of which greater than 75% are polymorphonuclear cells (Table 170.6) is considered positive for septic arthritis. The synovial glucose concentration may be low (synovial fluid glucose/blood glucose ratio < 0.5). Culturing synovial fluid in aerobic blood culture bottles can improve detection of *K. kingae*.

Joint aspiration should be performed and treatment not delayed when septic arthritis is suspected. Empirical antibiotic therapy for septic arthritis is directed against the most likely organisms, as dictated by the patient's age and comorbid conditions (see Table 170.5). To improve bacterial identification, synovial and blood cultures should precede antibiotics; however, antibiotics should not be delayed in patients exhibiting signs of sepsis. Antibiotics have good penetrance into the joint, and synovial fluid concentrations are equivalent to serum concentrations within one hour. When treating gram-positive cocci, initial therapy is a penicillinase-resistant penicillin; however, in areas with high rates of CA-MRSA, therapy should include vancomycin or clindamycin (depending on local resistance patterns). Ceftriaxone should be added for gram-negative bacterial coverage, as well as *K. kingae*, Gonococcus, *Salmonella*, and *Borrelia burgdorferi* (Lyme disease). Optimal length for intravenous antibiotic treatment is generally 2 to 4 days, followed by transition to oral therapy if clinical symptoms are improving and CRP levels declining.

Timely decompression of the joint via open arthrotomy, irrigation, and débridement is the recommended treatment for septic arthritis. Due to risk of avascular necrosis, urgent intervention is particularly

joint in flexion, abduction, and external rotation. Patients may limp or refuse to bear weight. Infants may be irritable, lethargic, have pain when being handled, and refuse to feed. Neonatal hip infections commonly present with the joint in flexion and abduction with internal rotation.

Diagnosis of septic arthritis is made by history and physical examination, supported by laboratory studies and imaging, and confirmed by arthrocentesis. Initial blood work should include complete blood count with differential, CRP, ESR, and blood cultures. As discussed previously, some of these studies are included in the Kocher criteria, which helps differentiate between transient synovitis and septic arthritis. In septic arthritis, the ESR generally rises greater than 24 hours after the onset of infection symptoms, whereas the CRP rises quickly and is a better independent predictor of infection.

Kingella kingae arthritis deserves special mention, because the presentation is atypical for septic arthritis. *Kingella kingae* is an oral gram-negative bacterium, most commonly linked to septic arthritis in children less than 4 years of age. *K kingae* infections are often preceded by upper respiratory infections and tend to have a milder presentation than the typical septic arthritis, including lower to absent fever. *K. kingae* septic arthritis can present with a normal white blood cell count and normal acute-phase reactants, similar to transient synovitis.

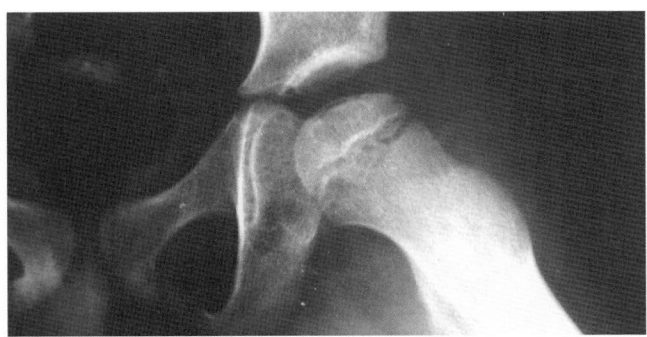

Fig. 170.26 Crescent sign (subchondral lucent zone) in early Legg-Calvé-Perthes disease. (Courtesy Dr. Marianne Gausche-Hill.)

indicated for septic arthritis of the hip. Less invasive cannula irrigation techniques are performed in some centers, but an open procedure is still recommended if concurrent bone infection or subperiosteal abscess is present.

Legg-Calvé-Perthes Disease

Legg-Calvé-Perthes Disease (LCPD) is an idiopathic necrosis of the capital femoral epiphysis and a form of osteochondrosis. The disorder is more common in boys, has a peak incidence in children aged 3 to 11 years, and presents with bilateral disease in 10% to 15% of patients.[7] The later the onset of the disease, the less favorable the outcome; patients older than 8 years old have poor outcomes.[7] The disease process involves a predominance of femoral head resorption compared to reformation, resulting in femoral head deformity and mechanical weakening.

Most children with LCPD present with a limp and may have the Trendelenburg sign, limited internal rotation and abduction of the hip. Early in the disease, hip motion is generally good. Pain is typically insidious in onset, experienced in the hip, or referred to the groin, thigh, or knee. Pain is worse with activity and relieved by rest. Disease progression can be variable but may include muscular atrophy of the buttocks, thigh, and calf, as well as limb length discrepancy up to 2.5 cm.[7]

Imaging of the hip should include AP pelvis and frog leg lateral radiographs. Early in the illness, the radiographs may be normal, but subtle changes may vary depending on the disease progression. If initial radiographs are normal, but symptoms concerning for LCPD persist for more than 6 weeks, then an MRI is recommended.[7] There are four phases of the disease: initial, fragmentation, reossification, and healed. In the initial phase, the femoral head loses blood supply. As bone dies, the medial joint space widens as the femoral head becomes less round due to subchondral collapse (Crescent sign) (Fig. 170.26). The hip joint becomes painful, stiff, and inflamed. In the fragmentation phase the epiphysis begins to fragment as new bone begins to form, reshaping the femoral head. The reossification phase includes continued bone density repair as the femoral head continues to reshape. In the healed stage, radiographs of the proximal third of the femur and femoral head may demonstrate residual deformities.

Children with concern for LCPD should be evaluated by an orthopedic surgeon. The goal of management is to keep the femoral head within the acetabulum. Treatment includes restriction of activity, physiotherapy, bracing, or surgery. The choice varies with the stage and onset of the disease.

Slipped Capital Femoral Epiphysis

Slipped capital femoral epiphysis (SCFE) is defined as the posterior and inferior slippage of the proximal femoral epiphysis on the metaphysis,

occurring through the epiphyseal plate (growth plate). This condition affects boys at twice the rate of girls, occurring more commonly between 8 and 15 years of age. The average age at diagnosis is 13.5 years for boys and 12 years for girls, presenting bilaterally in 18% to 50% of patients, although in most patients the second slip occurs within 18 months after the initial presentation.[7] SCFE is the most common hip disorder of adolescents, with a prevalence of 10.8 cases per 100,000 children. This prevalence is changing due to the increasing obesity rate, which data suggest is a contributing factor—63% of affected patients have weight in the 90th percentile or higher.[7]

The etiology of SCFE is felt to be multifactorial: obesity, periods of rapid growth, and endocrine disorders. Adolescent growth spurts and obesity contribute to the mechanical factors predisposing to epiphyseal sliding. Although increased mechanical load tends to increase bone strength, endocrine-related changes with obesity lead to a decreased overall bone mass. The most commonly observed endocrine abnormalities in SCFE patients are hypothyroidism, growth hormone deficiency, and chronic renal failure. Skeletal maturation is delayed in many SCFE patients.

Patients with SCFE generally present with limping and poorly localized pain to the hip, groin, thigh, or knee. Patients may have an antalgic gait or be unable to bear full weight on the affected leg. Limited internal rotation of the hip is common. Patients may have Drehmann sign, obligatory external rotation when the affected hip is flexed. Although the differential diagnosis for pediatric hip pain is broad, SCFE should be considered because a delayed diagnosis may result in a poorer prognosis.

Traditionally, SCFE is classified as preslip, acute slip, chronic slip, and acute on chronic slip. This classification is based on history, duration of symptoms, physical examination, and radiographs. Currently, however, a more clinically relevant method of classification is preferred based on stability of the physis and risk of avascular necrosis (AVN).[8] A SCFE is considered stable (90% of all slips) if the patient is able to ambulate with or without crutches; however, if the patient is unable to ambulate even with crutches, it is considered unstable.

If a stable SCFE is suspected on examination, then diagnostic radiographs should include anteroposterior and frog leg lateral views of both hips; for an unstable SCFE, anteroposterior and cross-table lateral views are recommended. Early in the course of the SCFE, the initial slippage is posterior and the AP view is generally normal in appearance or shows widening of the physis, whereas the lateral view is more diagnostic (Fig. 170.27). Signs of slippage on AP radiographs include evaluating the Klein line, a line drawn along the superior margin of the femoral neck. In a normal hip, the lines intersect with the epiphysis symmetrically; in a SCFE, the line does not intersect with the epiphysis (Fig. 170.28). MRI may be useful in diagnosing low-displacement forms of SCFE.

Slip severity can be graded using the Wilson method, which measures the relative displacement of the epiphysis on the metaphysis in a frog leg lateral radiograph. A mild slip involves epiphysis displacement less than one-third of the width of the metaphysis; a moderate slip shows displacement of one-third to one-half of the width; and a severe slip involves displacement greater than one-half of the width. Additional measurement of slippage can be made on a frog leg lateral radiograph with the epiphyseal shaft angle of Southwick (Fig. 170.29). This measurement involves drawing a line between the anterior and posterior tips of the epiphysis at the physeal plate level. A second line is drawn perpendicular to the epiphyseal line. A third line is then drawn along the midshaft of the femur. The epiphyseal shaft angle is formed by the intersection of the perpendicular and femoral shaft lines. The

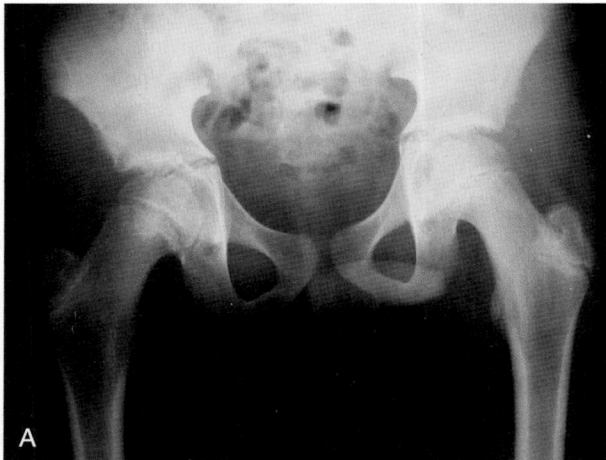

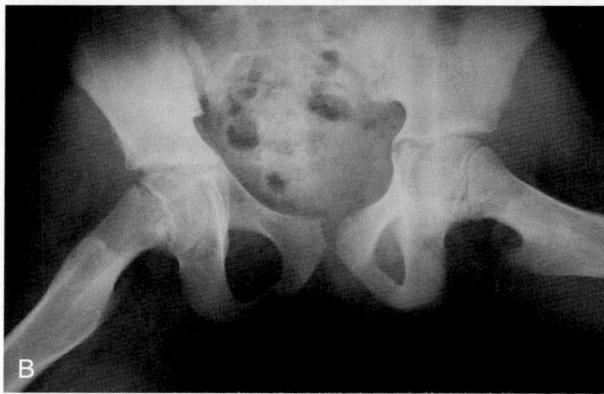

Fig. 170.27 (A) Anteroposterior radiograph of the pelvis with a unilateral slipped capital femoral epiphysis. Note widening of the physis on the right compared with the left. (B) Early inferior and posterior slippage is evident on the lateral view. (Courtesy Dr. Marianne Gausche-Hill.)

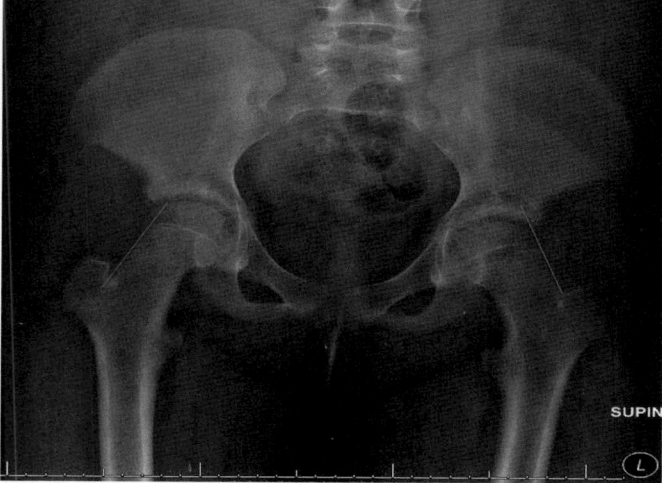

Fig. 170.28 Anteroposterior radiograph of the pelvis with a slipped capital femoral epiphysis. Note widening of the physis on the left and a greater distance from the lateral edge of the femoral epiphysis to the Klein line on the right than is seen on the left. A difference of more than 2 mm is diagnostic.

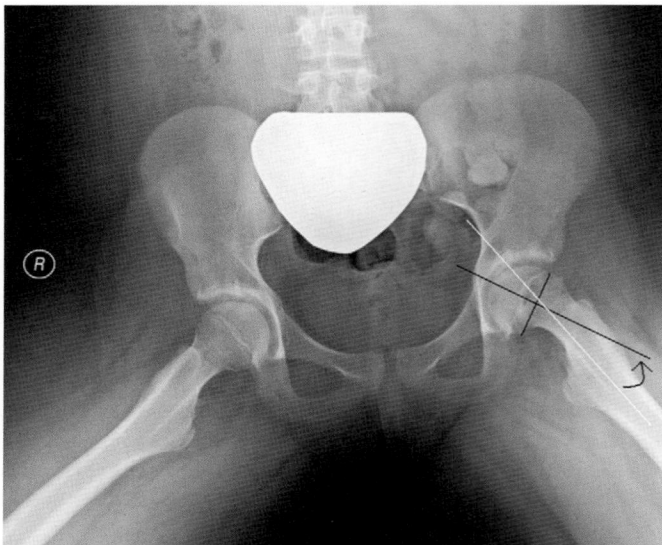

Fig. 170.29 Epiphyseal shaft angle of Southwick. On a lateral radiograph, a line is drawn from the anterior to the posterior epiphyseal edges and a second line is then drawn perpendicular to this line. A third line is drawn down the femoral diaphysis. The intersection between the perpendicular line and femoral shaft line is the epiphyseal shaft angle. The magnitude of slip displacement is the angle of the involved hip minus the angle of the normal hip. (From: Pinkowsky GJ, Hennrikus WL. Klein line on the anteroposterior radiograph is not a sensitive diagnostic radiologic test for slipped capital femoral epiphysis. *J Pediatr.* 2013;162f:804-807.)

degree of slip displacement is the angle of the involved hip minus the angle of the normal hip. A mild SCFE involves displacement of less than 30 degrees, a moderate slip is between 30 degrees and 50 degrees, and severe displacement is great than 50 degrees.[10]

Children diagnosed with SCFE should be made non-weightbearing and admitted or transferred for orthopedic intervention to prevent further slippage. The standard treatment for SCFE is in situ fixation with a single screw performing an epiphysiodesis. Fixation treatment goals are similar in stable and unstable SCFE; however, there is controversy regarding timing of surgery and value of reduction in the unstable type.

Secondary to blood supply disruption or hematoma formation, a vascular necrosis of the femoral epiphysis occurs in 20 to 50% of patients with unstable SCFE and is more common in severe displacement. Chondrolysis, the acute loss of articular cartilage, can be a complication of SCFE surgery, most often from pin penetration of the femoral head, causing joint stiffness and pain. The incidence of chondrolysis has decreased from 7 to 1% as SCFE surgical techniques have improved. Premature closures of the epiphyseal plate, as well as early onset degenerative changes, are common complications from SCFE.

Lyme Arthritis

Lyme disease is caused by the spirochete *Borrelia burgdorferi* and is now considered the most common vector-borne illness in North America and Europe, with a threefold increase in annual cases since 1992.[11] The primary vector is the *Ixodes* tick while in its nymph stage. The nymph stores the spirochetes in its midgut, which migrate to the salivary glands after the gut is engorged. An infected nymph must feed for at least 72 hours in order to transmit the disease.

The geographic distribution of Lyme disease has increased primarily into locations adjacent to recognized endemic areas, including New England, the Mid-Atlantic States, and Wisconsin (Fig. 170.30).[12] Two-thirds of cases

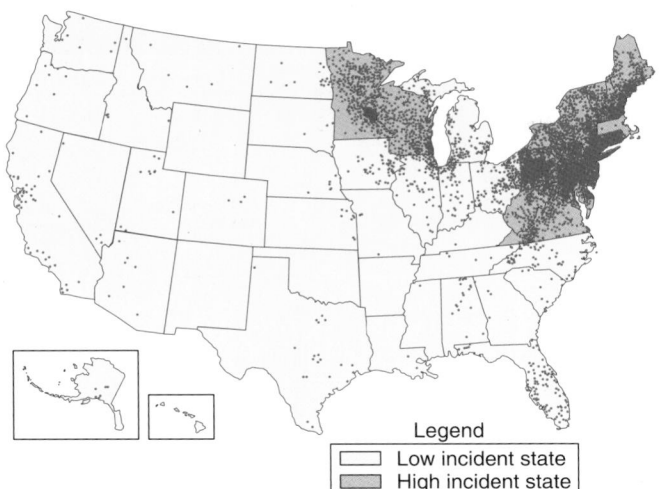

Fig. 170.30 Reported cases of Lyme disease in the United States, 2018. Each dot represents one case of Lyme disease and is placed randomly in the patient's county of residence. (From: Centers for Disease Control and Prevention. Reported Cases of Lyme Disease-United States, 2018. Retrieved from https://www.cdc.gov/lyme/datasurveillance/maps-recent.html.)

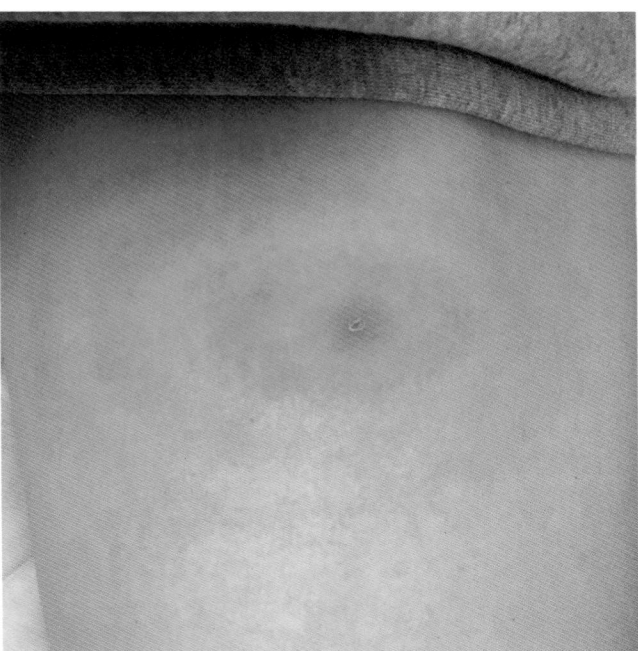

Fig. 170.31 Erythema migrans (EM) rash of the left inner thigh. EM is the most common early localized symptom of Lyme disease. (Courtesy Dr. William Prince, MD.)

of early Lyme disease occur in June, July, or August; however, because Lyme arthritis is a late manifestation (occurring weeks to months after initial infection), presentation is greatest in fall and winter months.[11]

Patients with Lyme disease have signs or symptoms correlating with disease progression: early localized, early disseminated, or late Lyme disease. Early localized disease is characterized by the erythema migrans (EM) lesion, the most common manifestation of Lyme disease in children.[13] This lesion begins as a red macule that expands over days to weeks to form an erythematous annular lesion with partial central clearing. The classic "bull's-eye" rash is seen less commonly (Fig. 170.31). Early disseminated disease may include multiple EM lesions, cranial nerve palsies (most commonly cranial nerve VII), lymphocytic meningitis, radiculitis, and carditis (AV block). Early disseminated disease may also include systemic symptoms such as low-grade fever, arthralgia, myalgia, headache, and fatigue. Approximately 50% to 60% of patients not treated for early stages of Lyme will go on to develop Lyme arthritis, which can be their presenting symptom of the disease. Late Lyme disease in children most commonly presents as arthritis.[13]

Lyme arthritis presents as monoarthritis in two-thirds of cases. If presenting as oligoarthritis, the knee is often involved; joint involvement is generally asymmetrical, involving a knee and another joint, such as the hip, shoulder, ankle, elbow, temporomandibular joint, or wrist. Patients can have acute joint swelling or intermittent and migratory arthralgias. The knee tends to be swollen, with limited range of motion, and the joint may be erythematous and warm to the touch. Pain varies, but patients can usually still ambulate with a limp.

Diagnosis of early Lyme disease can be difficult, because the immune system takes several weeks to develop antibodies after exposure to *B. burgdorferi*. Because the skin lesion is generally clinically identifiable, serology is not recommended for diagnosis in Lyme endemic areas. In fact, patients can still be seronegative, even after an erythema migrans rash develops.[12] However, by the time the late-stage symptoms of Lyme arthritis develop, immunoglobulin G serology for *B. burgdorferi* should be positive and is considered diagnostic in a patient from an endemic area with monoarthritis or oligoarthritis. Immunoglobulin M may wane and be negative at 30 days. Initial testing is performed using an ELISA screening followed by confirmatory Western blot test. A positive immunoblot result is defined as the presence of at least two 2 IgM bands or 5 IgG bands.[13]

In contrast to septic arthritis or rheumatic fever, the joint swelling, effusion, and stiffness in Lyme arthritis are disproportionate to the relatively mild degree of pain. Because of its insidious onset and subtle infectious symptoms, Lyme arthritis is commonly overlooked and mistaken for traumatic injury. Differentiating between Lyme arthritis, septic arthritis, and transient synovitis in the acute setting can be difficult, because many clinical symptoms overlap. Similar to delineating between septic arthritis and transient synovitis, a complete blood count with differential, ESR, and CRP can be helpful when determining risk for Lyme arthritis in an endemic area. Compared to Lyme arthritis, septic arthritis is more likely to have a history of fever, increased serum WBC count, and elevated CRP.[11] ESR levels are similar between Lyme arthritis and septic arthritis, and both are significantly elevated compared to transient synovitis.[14] Ultimately, serum markers for leukocytosis and inflammation alone are not reliable markers for distinguishing Lyme arthritis from transient synovitis or septic arthritis.[14]

To determine need for antibiotics or surgical intervention, children should undergo synovial fluid testing to rule out septic arthritis. Standard synovial fluid analysis includes cell count, Gram stain, culture, and, if indicated and available, *B. burgdorferi* PCR. Lyme arthritis elicits a synovial WBC count ranging between 10,000 to 50,000 cells per microliter, whereas septic arthritis is typically greater than 50,000 cells per microliter (see Table 170.6). PCR synovial fluid testing is often positive (40% to 96%) prior to antibiotic therapy but given the high specificity and sensitivity of serologic testing in late Lyme disease, it may not add any additional clinical value.

Antibiotic treatment for Lyme arthritis hastens resolution of symptoms and prevents long-term joint damage. Antibiotic recommendations for Lyme disease were updated in 2018 by the Infectious Disease Society of America, primarily pertaining to prophylaxis and treatment with doxycycline in children with early localized disease.[13] Doxycycline was previously not recommended in children less than 8 years of age due to

TABLE 170.7   Recommended Treatment of Lyme Disease in Children

Manifestation	First-Line Drugs	Alternative Drugs	Second-Line Drugs
Erythema migrans (single or multiple)	Amoxicillin 50 mg/kg/day TID PO × 14 days Doxycycline 2–4 mg/kg/day BID PO × 10 days	Cefuroxime 30 mg/kg/day BID × 14 days	Azithromycin 10 mg/kg daily × 10–14 days
Facial palsy	Amoxicillin 50 mg/kg/day TID PO × 14 days Doxycycline 2–4 mg/kg/day BID PO × 14 days		Azithromycin 10 mg/kg daily × 10–14 days
Meningitis	Ceftriaxone 100 mg/kg/day daily IV × 14 days Cefotaxime 180 mg/kg/day q8h IV × 14 days		
Carditis	Amoxicillin 50 mg/kg/day TID PO × 14–21 days Doxycycline 2–4 mg/kg/day BID PO × 14–21 days Ceftriaxone 100 mg/kg/day daily IV × 14-21 days Cefotaxime 180 mg/kg/day q8h IV × 14–21 days		
Arthritis	Amoxicillin 50 mg/kg/day TID PO × 28 days Doxycycline 2–4 mg/kg/day BID PO × 28 days		
Persistent arthritis after course of therapy	Retreat with one of above oral regimens	Ceftriaxone 100 mg/kg/day daily IV × 14–28 days Cefotaxime 180 mg/kg/day q8h IV × 14–28 days	

Adapted from: Sood S, Krause P. (2019). Lyme Disease. *Feigin and Cherry's textbook of pediatric infectious diseases*, 140;1246-1252.e2

the risk of dental staining. Evidence now suggests that doxycycline for 10 days, in the setting of early localized disease, is safe. However, the recommended oral antimicrobial treatment of Lyme arthritis calls for 28 days of doxycycline, and there are limited safety data on its use for greater than 21 days in children younger than 8 years old.[13] Treatment options for Lyme arthritis in children are listed in (Table 170.7). Patients with incomplete resolution of arthritis symptoms or relapse soon after treatment may be given a second 28-day course of oral therapy, or ceftriaxone parentally for 14 to 28 days if arthritis worsens.[13] The Infectious Disease Society of America recommends several months of observation after treatment due to anticipated slow resolution of inflammation.

Approximately 10% to 15% of patients treated for Lyme arthritis will have persistent synovitis for months to years, despite multiple courses of antibiotics.[13] This chronic arthritis is considered a postinfectious inflammatory process, with negative Lyme PCR from their synovial fluid; these patients may benefit from referral to a rheumatologist. Nonsteroidal antiinflammatory medications are reasonable for pain control; systemic steroids are not recommended.

Apophyseal Injuries

The apophysis is a cartilaginous structure on growing bones that serves as a site for tendon insertion. This site has a growth plate, with a slower rate of growth than the nearby epiphyseal plate. The apophysis is two to five times weaker than the surrounding structures, including the muscle tendon complex, ligaments, and bones. Rapid bone growth before adequate muscle lengthening contributes to increased tension at the apophysis. Although the age of onset varies, this injury is seen most commonly in the immature skeleton. Apophysitis results from a traction injury to the cartilage and bony attachment of tendons, most often as an overuse injury in children. Specific sports and activities have a predilection for specific apophyseal locations and may be secondary to a single trauma versus repetitive microtrauma.

Because many children are consistently playing year-round sports and nearly 44 million participate in more than one sport, overuse injuries in youth sports are increasing in prevalence.[15] Many children and adolescents will not recognize overuse injuries, due to insidious onset or misinterpretation of symptoms as simple fatigue or performance decline.

Osgood-Schlatter Syndrome

Osgood-Schlatter disease (OSD) is a condition in which the patellar tendon insertion on the tibial tubercle ossification center becomes inflamed due to repetitive tensile stress. It is more commonly seen in boys around 10 to 15 years of age and between 8 and 12 years in girls. Bilateral knees are affected in 20% to 30% of cases, but intensity of symptoms can vary in each knee.

Patients typically complain of a bony prominence and pain over the tibial tuberosity that is exacerbated by physical activity like running, jumping, and climbing stairs. Symptoms generally resolve without any treatment after natural closure of the physis, but some symptoms may persist if bone fragments do not fuse. Nonunion can occur in almost 10% of patients and generally results in anterior knee pain after minor activity, especially kneeling.

Diagnosis is based on history and clinical findings. Radiographs are not necessary but may aid in ruling out other causes of knee pain. A lateral knee radiograph may show blurred margins of the patellar tendon in the acute stage. After three to four months, bone fragmentation at the tibial tuberosity may be visible, and may later fuse during the chronic stage. Ultrasound may show pretibial swelling, fragmentation of the ossification center, insertional thickening of the patellar tendon, and excessive fluid collection in the infrapatellar bursa. Infrapatellar bursitis may be difficult to distinguish from OSD clinically, because the location of pain is similar; however, OSD should have tenderness with palpation of the tibial tuberosity.

Management of OSD focuses on reduction of pain and swelling over the tibial tuberosity. Activities that exacerbate pain should be limited for several months until symptoms resolve. Conservative management includes NSAIDs, ice, and exercises for the improvement of the quadriceps, hamstrings, and gastrocnemius muscles. In some cases, immobilization in a cast for 3 to 6 weeks may be necessary.

Sever Disease

The most common cause of heel pain in pediatric patients is calcaneal apophysitis, commonly called Sever disease. Similar to other overuse injuries, it is a result of repetitive microtrauma and inflammation at the site of the Achilles tendon insertion. Pain is felt at the posterior aspect of the calcaneus. This condition is primarily seen in pediatric athletes between 8 and 15 years of age, when the calcaneal physis is still an open growth plate. Bilateral involvement is seen in about 60% of cases. Sever disease can be associated with running and jumping sports.

Patients generally have no history of specific injury. Patients often report limping or walking on their toes to avoid putting weight on their heels. Physical examination includes tenderness at the lateral and medial aspects of the calcaneus. Compression of these sites can be diagnostic and is called the "squeeze test." X-rays of the heel may appear normal in the disease but radiographic findings can show increased density and fragmentation of the calcaneal apophysis.

Treatment for calcaneal apophysitis is universally conservative, including ice, NSAIDs, activity restriction, stretching, and heel cups. Stretching of the calf muscle is recommended, as it provides traction to the Achilles tendon, which may benefit from stretching during times of rapid bone growth. Arch taping has also been shown to decrease associated pain during ambulation. Recovery time varies according to the causative factors and treatment compliance. Activity restriction is recommended until the patient is pain free; full recovery is expected once skeletal maturity is reached.

Little League Elbow

Little League elbow is a term commonly used to describe a group of elbow injuries, including apophysitis, medial epicondylitis, and osteochondritis dissecans of the radial head and capitellum. The pediatric elbow is vulnerable to overuse injury because it has six ossification centers, closing at different ages of skeletal maturity, as well as multiple muscle and ligamentous attachments.[15]

Twenty-eight percent of youth pitchers report a history of elbow pain. Examination reveals localized tenderness and swelling over the medial epicondyle, and pain with resisted wrist flexion and forearm pronation. This condition is described as a valgus overload syndrome stemming from repetitive throwing imparting tensile force on the medial epicondyle and a compressive force at the lateral epicondyle. Medial injuries are most common, as the medial epicondyle is usually the last apophysis in the elbow to fuse.[15] Lateral epicondylitis of the elbow is felt to be tendinosis, worsened by wrist and finger extensor and supinator muscle contraction against resistance.

Radiographs may be normal in appearance, but commonly show focal lucency or sclerosis at the subchondral bone in the anterior aspect of the capitellum. Images may demonstrate fragmentation at the condyle, apophyseal avulsion, or widening at the medial epicondyle ossification center. MRI is the study of choice to fully delineate the extent of the injury.

The most important key to treatment is preventative, through adhering to proper pitch count guidelines by age and teaching proper mechanics.[16] Conservative treatment consists of ice, NSAIDs, and activity modification. Throwing can resume after symptoms have resolved, usually after 4 to 6 weeks. Operative intervention is indicated for displaced fractures > 5 mm, incarcerated fragments, or when associated with elbow dislocation.

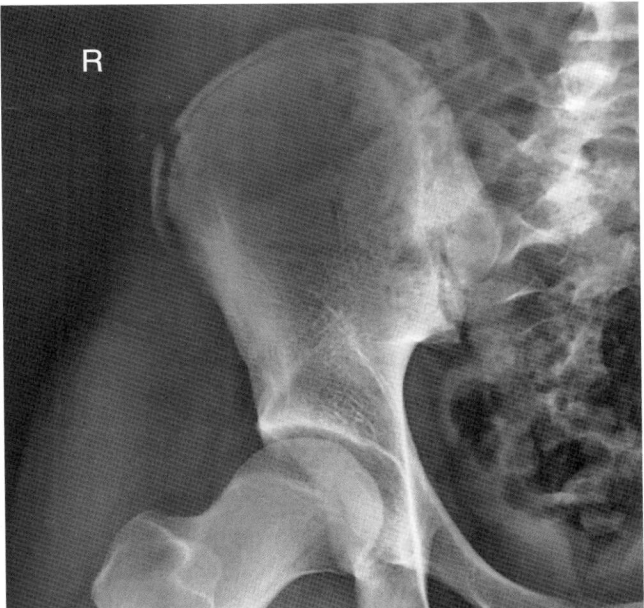

Fig. 170.32 Avulsion of the right anterior superior iliac spine in a child with hip pain after kicking a soccer ball. (Courtesy Dr. William Prince, MD.)

Apophysitis and Avulsion Fractures of the Hip

Apophyseal injuries of the hip occur at sites of muscle origination or insertion: iliac crest, anterior superior iliac spine, anterior inferior iliac spine, greater trochanter, lesser trochanter, ischial tuberosity, and pubic symphysis. Athletes most at risk include dancers, distance runners, and those in kicking sports. Patients most commonly present with pain at the tendinous insertion, which is commonly tender to palpation.

Radiographs may appear normal but can show mildly displaced avulsion fractures of the apophysis (Fig 170.32). Treatment for apophysitis includes activity restriction and stretching of associated muscles because this is a self-limited disorder that resolves by improving flexibility or when the apophyseal centers fuse when skeletal growth is complete. Avulsion fractures are generally treated conservatively with immobilization and slow resumption of activities. Surgery may be recommended for fragment displacement greater than 2 cm or for rapid rehabilitation of an athlete. Gradual return to pain-free activity may take several weeks to months.

Gymnast Wrist

Distal radial epiphysitis, also known as "gymnast wrist," is a chronic wrist pain affecting almost 80% of pediatric gymnasts at some point.[17] This injury is common to gymnasts who frequently bear weight through their upper extremities during events, such as the pommel horse and back handsprings. The overall weight load to the wrist ranges from 2 to 16 times the athlete's body weight, leading to distal radial growth plate injury in skeletally immature gymnasts.[17]

Compressive loading and shearing forces cause physeal microfractures at the hypertrophic zone. This leads to temporary ischemia which inhibits normal physeal calcification, causing physeal widening and metaphyseal irregularity. These radiographic abnormalities are seen in almost three-fourths of patients with the clinical diagnosis of gymnast wrist.[17]

Physical examination of the wrist is notable for tenderness over the distal radial physis, although range of motion of the wrist is generally normal.[15] Initial radiographs of the wrist may demonstrate widening of the distal radial physis, but a lack of bony edema, as this injury is due to chronic repetitive microinsults to the region (Fig 170.33).[15]

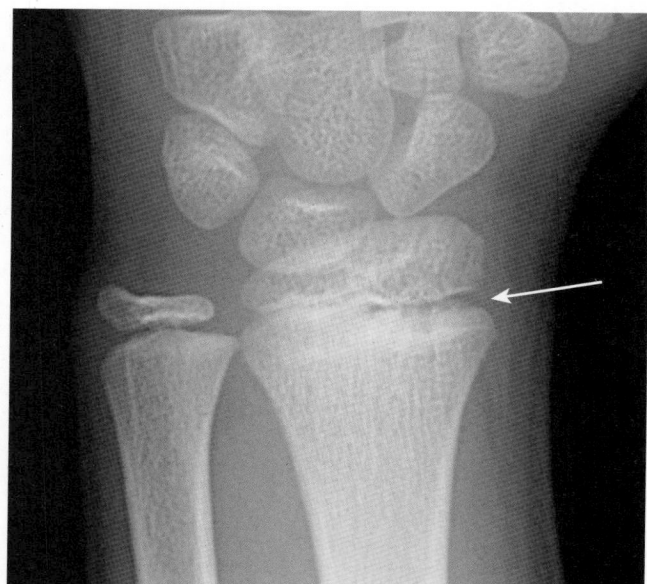

Fig. 170.33 Radiograph of 12-year-old female gymnast demonstrating mild physeal widening (*arrow*) of the distal radius with metaphyseal irregularity. (From: Paz DA, Chang GH, Yetto JM Jr, Dwek JR, Chung CB: Upper extremity overuse injuries in pediatric athletes: clinical presentation, imaging findings, and treatment. *Clin Imag.* 2015;39(6):954-964.)

Conservative treatment includes cessation from weightbearing activities until pain resolves, bracing of the wrist, and physical therapy. Premature closure of the distal radius physis can progress to bony deterioration, instability, and chronic arthritis if left untreated.[15]

The references for this chapter can be found online at ExpertConsult.com.

171

Pediatric Drug Therapy

Laurie Seidel Halmo and George Sam Wang

KEY CONCEPTS

- Awareness of differences in pediatric pharmacokinetics and specific drug toxicities is of critical significance for the safe and effective use of medications in children.
- Avoid prescription and over-the-counter (OTC) cough and cold medications in children because these agents have limited efficacy data and may cause harm.
- Counsel parents about the management of fever and appropriate indications and proper use of antipyretics.

- Perform a risk assessment (for prescription drug abuse and diversion) prior to prescribing opioid analgesics and, when indicated, limit prescribing to the lowest duration and amount possible.
- A multifaceted approach using clinical support systems and readily available reference tools is essential for the delivery of optimal emergent pediatric care.

FOUNDATIONS

Emergency clinicians are tasked with treating not only a wide age range of pediatric patients but also a wide spectrum of disease.[1,2] Nearly 75% of visits are associated with some form of pharmacotherapy during the visit or in the form of a prescription at discharge. Children may present to the emergency department (ED) with an acute life-threatening illness or injury. Although many children presenting for emergency care are otherwise healthy, children with complex medical needs and chronic illness account for an increasing number of ED encounters, many requiring some form of pharmacotherapy. At one tertiary care pediatric facility, 20% of their ED visits in a 2-year time frame were for children with chronic conditions. Pediatric patients are at high risk for medication errors and adverse drug events in the ED for a variety of reasons, including unique pharmacokinetic characteristics, lack of standard pediatric drug dosing and formulations, and weight-based dosing.[2]

PHARMACOKINETIC CONSIDERATIONS IN CHILDREN

Absorption

Absorption is the process in which a drug is transported from the site of administration (i.e., the GI tract for oral administration) to the systemic circulation. Children have unique differences that may lead to changes in drug absorption.[3] Figure 171.1 illustrates many of the key factors that account for pharmacokinetic differences between children and adults. For example, young children have higher gastric pH levels, which affects the bioavailability of acid-labile drugs (such as penicillins) to be absorbed in the stomach. They have decreased gastric emptying times, which prolongs exposure to medications before they pass the pylorus and may impact time to achieve peak concentrations. Variations in the intestinal tract also result in pharmacokinetic differences. The activity of drug-metabolizing enzymes on the intestinal border

vary as development occurs, and differences in gut flora can impact drug absorption in young infants. One commonality between children and adults is that drug absorption is often impaired in the setting of critical illness.

Absorption of drugs via a non-oral route can also vary significantly in children compared to adults. The topical route can result in increased absorption in children due to their relatively larger body surface area and increased skin vascularity. Additionally, children's skin contains more water and has a thinner stratum corneum. These factors make children more prone to increased absorption and risk for systemic toxicity from dermally applied drugs. Children have less muscle mass with associated weaker muscle contraction and reduced muscle blood flow. This can result in erratic absorption of intramuscular medications in young children.[3] Absorption of rectally administered medications also varies widely, depending on the age of the child and chemistry of the drug involved. However, this route can be used for medications when children are unable to tolerate or are refusing oral administration, such as for acetaminophen and diazepam. The ability to administer medications via the pulmonary route is particularly desirable in pediatric populations, given the high prevalence of respiratory conditions, such as asthma. At the same time, younger children may be less able to coordinate the use of a metered-dose inhaler to deliver these medications properly; parental assistance and adjunct devices such as spacers maximize efficacy by minimizing drug deposition in the oropharynx. There has been increasing experience in the use of intranasal preparation of analgesic, sedative, and anxiolytic medications in children. Medications that can be used intranasally include fentanyl, ketamine, dexmedetomidine, and midazolam.[4-9] This relatively noninvasive route of administration provides rapid absorption and clinical effect for circumstances requiring immediate pain control or sedation.

Distribution

Drug distribution is the movement of the drug after entering systemic circulation to the tissues of the body. Drug distribution can be impacted by circulation, proteins, extracellular fluid, and body composition. The

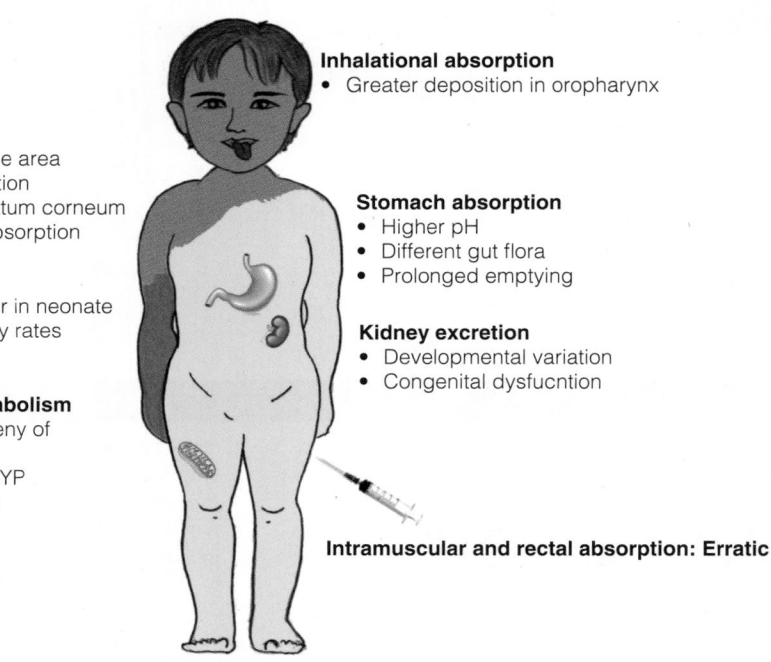

Inhalational absorption
• Greater deposition in oropharynx

Skin absorption
• Increased surface area
• Increased hydration
• Thickness of stratum corneum
• Net increased absorption

Stomach absorption
• Higher pH
• Different gut flora
• Prolonged emptying

Distribution
• Higher total body water in neonate
• Rising pediatric obesity rates

Kidney excretion
• Developmental variation
• Congenital dysfucntion

Mitochondrial metabolism
• Differential ontogeny of CYP enzymes
• Variation in non-CYP phase II enzymes

Intramuscular and rectal absorption: Erratic

Fig. 171.1 Major pharmacokinetic considerations in the pediatric patient. (Courtesy Voyo Wu.)

specific drug composition can also impact drug distribution greatly. Distribution can differ significantly in children, which has important clinical implications. Neonates and infants have higher total body water and larger volumes of distribution and extracellular fluid; therefore, dosing of medications such as aminoglycosides will differ in this age group, and drug concentrations should be closely monitored. The larger volume of distribution (Vd) may impact hydrophilic drugs and result in larger weight-based doses to achieve sufficient systemic concentrations. Free drug concentrations are also affected by relatively lower concentrations of plasma proteins (albumin, glycoprotein, globulins, etc.) in infants and young children. A consideration specific to neonates is the displacement of bilirubin from protein-binding sites by drugs such as ceftriaxone, which can lead to kernicterus. Consequently, these medications should be avoided until the blood-brain barrier matures. Table 171.1 presents examples of other commonly used medications in the practice of emergency medicine that carry pediatric-specific toxicities as a result of pharmacokinetic and other idiopathic differences.

Body composition can impact drug pharmacokinetics. Childhood obesity has reached epidemic proportions in the United States and worldwide, and significant knowledge gaps have led to a lack of guidance on how medications should be dosed in an obese pediatric patient.[10] Drugs should be cautiously administered in this patient population, especially for high-risk medications such as opioid analgesics and sedatives. Additionally, childhood obesity has resulted in more children being placed on medications, more commonly used in adults, for chronic conditions, such as anti-hypertensives and diabetes medications. Because these medications have been traditionally prescribed for adults, there are few guidelines and a significant paucity of safety and efficacy data in children, which can predispose them to adverse drug events.

Metabolism

Drugs are metabolized through various organs—most commonly the liver, but also in the kidneys and gastrointestinal mucosa. Phase 1 metabolism often involves oxidation or hydrolysis (often by

cytochrome P450 enzymes [CYP]), whereas phase 2 metabolism includes conjugation reactions such as glucuronidation and sulfation. Drug metabolism in neonates and infants can be diminished because of immature drug-metabolizing enzymes (Box 171.1). An example of toxicity due to differences in drug-metabolizing enzymes is the neonatal gasping syndrome. Benzyl alcohol, a common preservative for parenteral medications, is metabolized to benzoic acid, which is detoxified by glycine conjugation. Glycine conjugation is decreased in neonates and therefore benzoic acid accumulates when they are given drugs containing benzyl alcohol, leading to metabolic acidosis, respiratory distress, and cardiovascular collapse. As children approach adolescence, drug metabolism is generally the same as in adults.

Elimination

The two primary sites of drug excretion and elimination are the kidneys and liver. They rely on active and passive transport processes to clear drugs. However, the impact of age on many of these transporters remains unclear. Any underlying congenital or acquired hepatic or nephrotic disease will certainly impair drug clearance and drug interactions. In the neonate and infant, there is decreased renal blood flow and glomerular filtration for the first 6 months of life; tubular secretion is decreased for the first year. This pathophysiologic difference may impact renally eliminated drugs. An important example is gentamicin, where it has been demonstrated that using dosing regimens designed for older children and adults has resulted in significant toxicity.

OTHER CONSIDERATIONS

Drug Therapy in the Neonate

As previously mentioned, neonates are the subgroup of pediatric patients that differ the most with regard to physiology and drug pharmacokinetics; however, there is also the greatest paucity of pharmacologic data on this population. Emergency clinicians caring for neonates should consult drug references for specific prescribing information because dosing recommendations, administration, and

TABLE 171.1 Common Emergency Department Medications With Pediatric-Specific Toxicities

Medication	Pediatric-Specific Toxicity
Codeine	Ultrarapid CYP2D6 metabolism implicated in deaths in post-tonsillectomy patients and from breast milk excretion in infants. Not recommended for use in pediatrics
Antipyretics	Dosing errors led to 2011 US Food and Drug Administration (FDA) guidelines to reduce confusing labeling and package directions, elimination of infant formulation of acetaminophen
Aspirin	Reye syndrome associated with use during viral illness
Cough and cold medicines	FDA and Joint Advisory Panel warning for children <2 yr; expanded to 2–4 yr
Phenothiazines	Apnea risk (severe respiratory depression at wide range of doses)
Ceftriaxone	Calcium precipitation in patients <28 days, kernicterus
Doxycycline	Tooth discoloration
Trimethoprim-sulfamethoxazole	Bilirubin displacement may result in kernicterus in patients <2 mo

BOX 171.1 Maturation of Functioning Enzymes in the Pediatric Patient in Phase 1 and 2 Drug Metabolism

Phase 1 Drug Metabolism
- Birth: Cytochrome P450 (CYP)2D6 and CYP2C9
- 1 year: CYP3A4
- 10 years: CYP1A2

Phase 2 Drug Metabolism
- Birth: Glutathione S-transferase alpha 1 (GSTA1)
- 3–6 months: UDP glucuronosyltransferase family 1 member A1 (UGT1A1)
- 18 months: Glutathione s-transferases (GST)

contraindications differ in this age group. Early consultation with a neonatologist may be warranted, depending on the clinical scenario.

Neonates can also be exposed to and experience subsequent toxicity from pharmaceuticals via lactation. For example, the postpartum use of codeine in lactating mothers has been associated with toxicity in the newborn. This phenomenon has been linked to maternal CYP2D6 polymorphisms, which result in ultrarapid metabolism of codeine to morphine. High concentrations of morphine are excreted in the breast milk, which can cause toxicity in the infant. Although many medications are safely administered during breast-feeding, this underscores the importance of obtaining a complete maternal medication history when evaluating a breast-fed infant, as well as consulting a lactation reference when prescribing medications to nursing mothers. This can be difficult because there are limited human data regarding medication use in pregnancy, and multiple factors need to be considered, including maternal comorbidities, therapeutic alternatives, and preferences for continued breast-feeding. The National Library of Medicine maintains a Drugs and Lactation Database (LactMed) summarizing available evidence on medications and illicit drugs and their impact on the breast-feeding infant.[11]

Use of Antipyretics in Children

Fever is one of the most common presenting complaints for pediatric ED and urgent care visits.[12] An important distinction exists between fever, a controlled physiologic increase in body temperature that occurs when the hypothalamic temperature set point is increased in response to pyrogens, and hyperthermia, a pathophysiologic increase in body temperature that occurs when physiologic thermoregulatory mechanisms fail. Unlike fever, hyperthermia has the potential to cause serious harm and can be fatal; thus, hyperthermic children should be rapidly cooled and the underlying cause of their hyperthermia addressed. Antipyretics are not generally useful in managing hyperthermia, because antipyretics do not mechanistically address the underlying thermoregulatory dysfunction.

In contrast to hyperthermia, there is no evidence that fever is dangerous or detrimental to children. Fever as a response to infection has been conserved across vertebrates for hundreds of millions of years, and a growing body of evidence suggests that fever confers a survival benefit to hosts fighting an infection.[13] Even so, a recent survey study of parents found that most felt fever conferred no benefit to their child and that there were risks associated with being febrile.[14] This so-called "fever phobia" often leads to unnecessary administration of antipyretics which, unlike the fever itself, does confer some risk. Aside from the known adverse effects associated with antipyretics and with nonsteroidal antiinflammatory drugs in particular, therapeutic errors and accidental exploratory ingestions of antipyretics in children are relatively common.[15] Even when administered in a health care setting, antipyretic use in children can have unintended consequences; one study found that children with a temperature between 38°C and 39°C with otherwise normal vital signs who were given an antipyretic in the emergency department had a significantly longer length of stay compared to those who did not receive an antipyretic.[16]

Given the risks associated with antipyretic use and the lack of risk associated with fever, current recommendations focus on maintaining patient comfort and not on normalizing temperature. Even in patients who are critically ill with sepsis—to whom an antipyretic is often given because of a concern for the increased metabolic demands associated with being febrile—antipyretic administration was not associated with a decreased ICU length of stay in a randomized, placebo-controlled trial in adults; the same was true in a small pilot randomized, placebo-controlled trial in children.[17,18] As such, the primary goal of antipyretic administration should be to improve the patient's comfort. When emergency clinicians do prescribe an antipyretic in the ED, they should counsel parents regarding the safe and appropriate use of these medications on discharge. Ibuprofen should be avoided in infants younger than 6 months because of pharmacokinetic differences and ongoing renal development in this age group. Combined regimens or alternating therapy with acetaminophen and ibuprofen may be slightly more effective in alleviating discomfort and lowering body temperature; however, this approach is also more complicated and may predispose to medication errors, with small clinical benefit.[19] Table 171.2 presents manufacturer-recommended dosing for commonly used antipyretics and analgesics; Box 171.2 provides counseling points for parents regarding fever and antipyretic use.

Over-the-Counter Cough and Cold Medications

Cough and cold symptoms are complaints commonly encountered in pediatric ED patients, and over-the-counter (OTC) cough and cold medications containing various combinations of antitussives, antihistamines, decongestants, expectorants, and antipyretics have been widely used in children for decades. In 2007, a series of initiatives was launched to curb the use of these medications in young children due to a lack of efficacy data and mounting safety concerns.

TABLE 171.2   Common Antipyretics and Analgesics

Agent	Indication	Dose	Maximum
Acetaminophen	Analgesic, antipyretic	10–15 mg/kg PO, PR, q4–6h	75 mg/kg/day, never to exceed 3 g
Ibuprofen	Analgesic, antiinflammatory, antipyretic	10 mg/kg PO, q6–8h	40 mg/kg/day, never to exceed 3200 mg; not recommended for children <6 mo
Fentanyl	Analgesic	1 to 3 µg/kg IV, IO, IM, IN, SC	N/A
Morphine	Analgesic	0.1 mg/kg IV, IO, IM, SC	N/A

IM, Intramuscular; *IO*, intraosseous; *IV*, intravenous; *PO*, orally; *PR*, per rectum; *SC*, subcutaneous; *IN*, intranasal.

BOX 171.2   Counseling Tips for Parents and Caregivers for Safe Antipyretic Use

- Fever is a clinical sign that the body may be fighting infection and children should be monitored for signs of serious illness.
- Be sure the child maintains adequate hydration during febrile illness.
- Antipyretics should be given to minimize discomfort; if the child appears comfortable, he or she does not need an antipyretic.
- The use of combination products and alternating use of antipyretics can lead to dosing errors and therapeutic duplication.
- Do not use ibuprofen in children younger than 6 months.
- Do not use aspirin in children younger than 15 years due to the risk of Reye syndrome.
- Counsel caregivers and parents regarding appropriate weight-based dosing for the child.
- Recommend use of a calibrated measuring device to avoid dosing errors, showing milliliters ONLY.
- Store all medications, both OTC and prescription, out of the reach of children.

In October of that year, a joint panel meeting of the US Food and Drug Administration's (FDA) Nonprescription Drugs and Pediatric Advisory Committees voted to advise against the use of OTC cough and cold medications in children younger than 6 years. Later that month, the Consumer Healthcare Products Association (CHPA) issued a position statement and voluntarily withdrew OTC cough and cold products marketed for use in children younger than 2 years. In January 2008, the FDA formally recommended against the use of OTC cough and cold medicines in children younger than 2 years. The CHPA subsequently issued additional warnings against the use of these medications by children younger than 4 years. Currently, the American Academy of Pediatrics (AAP) advises against the use of OTC cough and cold medications in children younger than 6 years, and the FDA continues to review available data in consideration of changing the labeling for OTC cough and cold medications for all children aged 2 to 6 years.

Since these initial labeling changes were instituted, some studies have suggested that the use of OTC cough and cold medication in children under 6 years of age is declining. For example, one study found a significant decrease in the proportion of children under 2 years of age with bronchiolitis who had been given an OTC cough or cold medication in the week prior to their ED visit in 2007 to 2010 compared to 2004 to 2006.[20] Another study found that the national estimated number of ED visits for unsupervised exposures to cough and cold medications in children under 6 years of age decreased from 2010 to 2013 after having increased from 2004 to 2010.[21] There has also been a decrease in clinician recommendations for cough and cold medication use in children, though recommendations for use of antihistamines for cough and cold symptoms have increased.[22]

Despite this progress, numerous recent reports have documented that children under 4 years of age now consistently make up the largest proportion of children who suffer adverse events related to OTC cough and cold medication exposures in the years since the aforementioned labeling changes were introduced, despite the fact that the new labels state "do not use" in children under 4 years of age.[23-26] Emergency clinicians should be cognizant of current recommendations to avoid these medications in young children and educate parents regarding the dangers of OTC cough and cold medications; prescription cough and cold alternatives have similar safety and efficacy concerns. The most recent CHEST guidelines on this topic specifically recommend against the use of OTC cough and cold products for both children and adults with cough associated with the common cold.[27] Parents should also be counseled regarding alternative therapies, such as nasal suctioning and honey in children older than 1 year. Table 171.3 presents manufacturer-recommended dosing for commonly used medications in pediatric respiratory emergencies.

Opioid Analgesics

Opioid analgesics can be used safely and effectively in children for the management of moderate to severe pain in the ED and should not be withheld when indicated. However, the evolution of the opioid epidemic of the last 30 years has thrown into sharp relief the risks that opioid use—including therapeutic opioid use—can carry. Numerous studies have documented the large number of ED visits and hospital admissions for opioid-related adverse events in children over the past two decades, particularly in adolescents and in young children under 5 years of age.[28-31] In one study, there was no apparent deviation from the prescribed regimen in 71% of children presenting with an opioid-related adverse event.[30] Only in the last few years has the incidence of pediatric opioid exposures begun to fall; this decrease has mirrored the decrease in opioid prescriptions written for pediatric patients and likely reflects more conscientious opioid prescribing.[30-35] Among adolescents, risk factors that have been identified for development of adverse events related to opioid exposure include having a prescription for more than 30 days, concurrent benzodiazepine use, having a prescription for an extended-release or long-acting opioid, and having a preexisting mental health condition.[36,37] Several studies have also demonstrated that medical use of opioids during adolescence is associated with increased rates of opioid misuse later in life.[38,39] Opioid misuse during adolescence itself is not rare; one study found the prevalence of opioid misuse among high school seniors to consistently be between 10% and 15% from 2002 to 2013, and only recently has it begun to fall.[32] Another prospective study has further demonstrated that adolescents who nonmedically use opioids have higher odds of developing a formal substance use disorder at age 35.[39]

Certain opioids have additionally been described as having specific risks beyond the risks associated with opioid use in general. Codeine toxicity in those who are CYP2D6 ultrarapid metabolizers is a classic example. Codeine's analgesic effects are primarily due to its conversion

TABLE 171.3 Common Pediatric Emergent Respiratory Medications

AGENT	INDICATION	DOSE	MAXIMUM
Albuterol	Asthma	0.15 mg/kg (minimum dose 2.5 mg) INH 20 minutes for 3 doses, then 0.15–0.3 mg/kg up to 10 mg INH q1–4h PRN	Continuous dosing: • ≤10 kg: 7.5 mg/hr • 10–20 kg: 11.25 mg/hr • ≥20 kg: 15 mg/hr
Dexamethasone	Croup, Asthma	0.15–0.6 mg/kg PO, IV, IM	16 mg/dose
Diphenhydramine	Allergy, Urticaria	1–2 mg/kg PO, IV, IM	50 mg/dose
IM Epinephrine (1 mg/ml concentration)	Anaphylaxis	0.01 mg/kg IM	0.5 mg
Ipratropium	Asthma	250 µg INH if <20kg 500 µg INH if >20 kg	N/A
Magnesium	Severe asthma	50 mg/kg IV over 20 min	2 grams
Methylprednisolone	Asthma	1 to 2 mg/kg IV	80 mg/day
Prednisolone	Asthma	2 mg/kg PO	60 mg/dose
Racemic epinephrine	Croup	0.25–0.5 mL of 2.25% solution; as needed up to q30 min	N/A
Terbutaline	Severe asthma	0.01 mg/kg SC	0.4 mg/dose

IM, Intramuscular; *INH*, isoniazid; *IV*, intravenous; *PO*, orally; *SC*, subcutaneous.

to morphine by CYP2D6; ultrarapid metabolizers can therefore produce relatively large quantities of morphine in a short period of time and thus are at risk for toxicity. Toxicity, including death, has been documented in children who received codeine after a tonsillectomy or adenoidectomy for postoperative pain management; a black box warning was issued in 2013 for the use of codeine for postoperative pain in children who have undergone tonsillectomy or adenoidectomy.[40] In 2017, in response to these and other adverse events related to codeine exposure, the FDA formally stated that codeine was contraindicated for treatment of any pain or cough in children under 12 years of age, and added a new warning to codeine labels recommending against its use in children 12 to 18 years of age who are obese, have obstructive sleep apnea or have severe lung disease.[41] In 2018, the FDA went on to require that labels on prescription cough and cold medications containing codeine state that these products are contraindicated in children under 18 years of age. The FDA's mandate contraindicating the use of codeine-containing prescription cough and cold medications in children under 18 years of age was also extended to hydrocodone-containing products.[42] Hydrocodone, one of codeine's minor metabolites, was found in a recent study of pediatric adverse events related to exposures to hydrocodone- and codeine-containing cough and cold medications to be associated with a higher frequency of both fatal and nonfatal adverse events than codeine alone.[43]

Tramadol also deserves a special mention, because it has become increasingly implicated as one of the opioids associated with the highest risk of opioid toxicity among adolescents.[36,44] Tramadol is a prodrug like codeine and is similarly contraindicated for the treatment of pain in children under 12 years of age and for the treatment of postoperative pain in children under 18 years of age who have undergone tonsillectomy or adenoidectomy. It also carries the same warning as codeine recommending against its use in children 12 to 18 years of age who are obese, have obstructive sleep apnea or have severe lung disease. Both tramadol and codeine should be avoided in mothers who are breast-feeding because of the risk of serious adverse events, including death, in their breastfed infants.[41] Tramadol is additionally noteworthy for its well-described association with seizures in overdose.[45]

Unlike in adults, there is a paucity of guidelines for opioid use in the pediatric population. It is important for emergency clinicians to balance adequate analgesia with the risks associated with the use of prescription opioids. Use of nonpharmaceutical modalities and nonopioid alternatives (e.g., acetaminophen and nonsteroidal antiinflammatory drugs) should be used as primary therapy or as an adjunct to minimize the dose of opioids, including for conditions that historically were treated with opioids, such as fractures or acute pancreatitis. For example, a recent randomized, double blind, placebo-controlled trial of children 6 to 17 years old presenting to an ED with a musculoskeletal injury and a pain score of greater than 29 mm on a visual analog scale (VAS) found no difference in the proportion of children meeting the primary outcome of a VAS less than 30 mm, when comparing those who received morphine, morphine and ibuprofen, or ibuprofen alone. The only statistically significant difference found was in the mean reduction of VAS from baseline to 120 minutes after medication administration, which was significantly greater (a more reduced pain score) in children receiving ibuprofen alone compared to morphine alone.[46] There was also no significant difference in pain control among children treated with either morphine or ibuprofen for uncomplicated extremity fractures in an earlier randomized trial.

When an opioid is clearly indicated, clinicians should follow institution-based protocols, if available, for dosage and administration. Additional safeguards to mitigate risk of diversion and misuse include limiting prescriptions to the lowest effective dose for the shortest possible duration, and using the state prescription drug monitoring profile. Similarly, extended-release preparations should generally be avoided, as they are very rarely indicated for acutely painful conditions for which children present to emergency departments. While there are no national opioid prescribing guidelines for children, in 2016 the Centers for Disease Control and Prevention (CDC) published guidelines for opioid prescribing in adults, which state that clinicians "should prescribe no greater quantity than needed for the expected duration of pain severe enough to require opioids.... Three days or less will often be sufficient; more than seven days will rarely be needed."[47] Emergency physicians who supervise trainees should be aware that both the odds of receiving an opioid prescription at discharge and the odds of receiving an opioid prescription for a prolonged duration of time are greater if that prescription was written by an emergency medicine resident.[48-50] Similarly, the odds of receiving an outpatient opioid prescription were higher if the child was seen in a general emergency department compared to a pediatric emergency department.[51] In adolescent patients, it can be beneficial to use screening tools such as the CRAFFT to identify high-risk adolescents who may need closer follow-up[52] (Box 171.3).

BOX 171.3   CRAFFT for Substance Use Disorder[a]

C: Have you ever ridden in a **CAR** driven by someone (including yourself) who was high or had been using alcohol or drugs?

R: Do you ever use alcohol or drugs to **RELAX**, feel better about yourself, or fit in?

A: Do you ever use alcohol/drugs while you are by yourself, **ALONE**?

F: Do you ever **FORGET** things you did while using alcohol or drugs?

F: Do your family or **FRIENDS** ever tell you that you should cut down on your drinking or drug use?

T: Have you gotten into **TROUBLE** while you were using alcohol or drugs?

[a]http://crafft.org.

BOX 171.4   Best Practices for Prescribing Opioid Analgesics in the Emergency Department

- Assess if there is an indication for an opioid analgesic; nonopioid therapies and pharmaceuticals should be optimized and used as adjuncts, whenever possible.
- Perform a risk assessment for nonmedical use, particularly in adolescent patients.
- Consult state prescription drug monitoring programs and prior medical and pharmacy records whenever available.
- Short-acting opioids are preferred versus extended-release formulations.
- Use caution when combining opioid analgesics with other central nervous system depressants, such as benzodiazepines.
- Prescribe the lowest effective dose and limit duration of therapy to the shortest possible time.
- Provide instructions for the safe disposal of any unused medication.
- Arrange for close outpatient follow-up.
- Counsel parents and caregivers regarding signs of prescription drug abuse.

General recommendations for safe prescribing practices for opioid analgesics are presented in Box 171.4.

Medication Safety and Adverse Drug Events

Medication errors and adverse drug events are common among children cared for in an ED, with error rates in several studies reaching upwards of 30%.[2] This is in part due to characteristics inherent to emergency care, such as a lack of familiarity with individual patients who may be medically complex, and a chaotic environment where verbal orders may be used. Other factors also contribute to pediatric medication errors in all care settings. Because of legislative restrictions in pediatric drug research, many medications are used off label, with dosing based on experience and estimations rather than formal clinical trials. In one study, over 10% of ED visits included at least one off-label use of a medication for a child.[53] Even when a medication has pediatric data shown on the drug label, this information is often not clearly presented and may offer little guidance. For example, the age range for which a medication is formally approved is often not listed in the indications section of the labeling. Approved pediatric-specific dosing information, when available, is listed in another section of the label. To further complicate matters, labels very rarely have dosing listed for obese children; in one study, only 8% of acute care drugs had dosing information for obese children on the label, despite the fact that nearly 1 in 5 children in the United States is obese.[54,55]

The lack of pediatric-specific formulations is also a contributor to adverse drug events and poor patient adherence. Because pediatric formulations are not available for many medications, parents and clinicians may have to split fixed-dose adult tablets, or liquid formulations may need to be extemporaneously compounded, which introduces the potential for compounding and concentration errors. In addition, the poor palatability of adult formulations can lead to noncompliance; oral solutions, suspensions, and rapidly disintegrating and chewable tablets are often preferred. Parents should be counseled regarding proper measurement and administration of prescribed medications, and a dosing syringe using milliliter units should be provided. Payer formulary alerts can direct prescribers to choose an inappropriate alternative if the intended prescription is not covered by the patient's insurance. In one study at a single institution, 27% of payer formulary alerts were found to be inappropriate, and there were 24 specific instances of prescribing errors that were ultimately attributed to these alerts.[56]

Several other factors also contribute to adverse drug events in children. Weight-based dosing and calculations required for children introduce additional error-prone steps, particularly with emergent medications. In a randomized simulation study of residents in an emergency department, the use of a reference book that provided precalculated medication doses (as opposed to a card listing milligram per kilogram dosing) was found to significantly decrease the rates of ten-fold dosing errors, as well as dosing errors for medications administered via continuous infusions.[57] Another common error is calculating weight-based dosing using a patient's weight in pounds instead of kilograms. Despite the fact that numerous professional societies—including the American College of Emergency Physicians and the American Academy of Pediatrics—recommend obtaining scales that exclusively display weights in kilograms, multiple studies have demonstrated inconsistent adoption of this recommendation.[58,59] Medication reconciliation in pediatric patients is also often inaccurate, which can contribute to suboptimal therapy and adverse drug events. Parents and caregivers should be specifically asked about all prescription medications, OTC medications, homeopathic preparations, and dietary supplements. Details regarding dosage and schedule should also be obtained.

Ongoing attempts to mitigate these risks include the use of clinical pharmacists in the ED, separation of pediatric and adult care locations, and increased use of human factors and information technology solutions. In one study, after instituting 24-hour pharmacist coverage of an emergency department, 17% of pharmacist-reviewed orders were found to lead to a clinical intervention that otherwise may not have occurred.[60] The advent of hand-held wireless technology and gradual adoption of inpatient electronic health record (EHR) systems have generated many new reference options for pediatric pharmacology. Decision support tools in the EHR system, such as computerized physician order entry, have repeatedly been shown to decrease adverse events, in part because many are related to simple weight-based calculation errors.[2] At the same time, EHRs can also precipitate errors when clinicians "copy and paste" without critically evaluating data. The ultimate responsibility for medication dosing rests with the ordering clinician, dispensing pharmacist, and administering nurse. Simulation training for nurses has also been shown to decrease medication administration errors; a single 2-hour training in one study decreased the rate of serious medication administration errors from 2.5 events per month to 0.86 events per month.[61] Table 171.4 presents a selection of different types of decision support tools that can serve as a reference to emergency clinicians.

In recent years, prescription drug shortages have emerged as a threat to public health. According to the American Society of Health Systems Pharmacists, there were over 200 current drug shortages in the United States as of the end of 2019.[62] Drug shortages can lead to delayed treatment or no treatment even when treatment is indicated.

TABLE 171.4 Selected Pediatric Drug References[a]

Reference	Description	Examples
App store	Apps with calculators for common pediatric dosing; dosing recommendations provided for reference only	PediStat, palmPEDi, EMRA Pediatric Airway, PediCalc
Web-based	Web-based clinical information suites with medication dosing and company-provided evidence-based recommendations	Micromedex, Epocrates
EHR-based	Decision support tools and institutional guidelines incorporated into CPOE	Cerner, Epic, Allscripts
Reference text	Classic bedside reference texts for decision support and dosing information	Redbook, Harriet Lane, Tarascon, Broselow Tape

[a]This list is not all inclusive, nor does it carry a formal endorsement.

Sometimes, alternative medications are substituted that may be more toxic or less effective, and medication errors can occur when clinicians are forced to use less familiar therapeutic alternatives.[63] The reasons for the rising rates of prescription drug shortages are multifactorial, and it is anticipated that shortages will continue as a problem in the foreseeable future, despite mitigation efforts. Emergency clinicians should be cognizant of current drug shortages that may affect their practice and work to design protocols for the ethical distribution of available supplies of medications in short supply, as well as for safer use of therapeutic alternatives.

The references for this chapter can be found online at ExpertConsult. com.

172

Child Abuse

Daniel Lindberg

PHYSICAL ABUSE

KEY CONCEPTS

- The ultimate determination of whether abuse has occurred can take days or weeks. Emergency clinicians should focus on recognizing possible abuse, treating medical injuries, and establishing a safe disposition for the child.
- Completely undress infants and preverbal children for the physical examination; pay particular attention to the skin, ears, mouth and oral cavity, scalp, fontanel, and genitalia.
- Consider abuse routinely for sentinel injuries in young children without an independently witnessed traumatic mechanism. Sentinel injuries include the following: bruising in children younger than 6 months old; bruising on the torso, ears, neck, jaw, cheek, or eyelid; oral injuries; patterned cutaneous injuries; subdural hematoma; long-bone fractures in infants; intra-abdominal injuries; and rib fractures.
- Consider abuse for children when family violence (child abuse, intimate partner violence, elder abuse, or animal abuse) is recognized in the child's home.
- The goal of diagnostic testing is to identify additional clinically or forensically significant injuries or medical entities that may present similarly to abuse.
- Use objective, nonaccusatory, matter-of-fact statements to communicate concern for abuse.
- Emergency clinicians in the United States, Canada, and many other countries are legally mandated to report reasonable concerns for abuse to public child protective services (CPS) agencies.

FOUNDATIONS

Child physical abuse is a leading cause of death and disability for young children. In the United States (US), more than 120,000 children are victims of physical abuse leading to more than 550 preventable deaths each year.[1] This means that large pediatric centers will see several cases of physical abuse each month, while smaller, general emergency departments (EDs) may go several months without a single case.[2] Physical abuse is also commonly missed—approximately 30% of abusive head trauma and 20% of abusive fractures are missed on initial presentation.[3] Physical abuse is especially difficult to identify, because it predominantly affects preverbal children, particularly those younger than 6 months old.[1,4] Caregivers frequently omit or obscure the true history, and key portions of the physical examination (e.g., neurologic and musculoskeletal examinations) are limited. Early recognition of abuse therefore often depends on identifying subtle, minor, or self-limited injuries.[5-7] With these challenges, current practices are highly variable, and children are frequently returned to abusive environments.[2,8]

Overcoming these challenges is essential for abused children and their families. Because violence is a disease that affects entire households, recognition of abuse is important not only for the children themselves, but also for their siblings, parents, elders, and even pets.[9-13] For abuse survivors and those who share a violent household, the long-term health effects of toxic stress are severe, diverse, and widespread.

Role of the Emergency Clinician

It is rarely possible and almost never necessary to definitively diagnose abuse in the ED. Care of abused children involves the cooperation of medical, social, and law-enforcement agencies over weeks and months. Emergency clinicians are responsible for raising the initial concern for abuse and working with other professionals (e.g., general and child abuse pediatricians, CPS) to stratify risk, ensure safety, and arrange for ongoing care.

Most injuries in childhood are not the result of abuse, and unusual events may produce unusual or unusually severe injuries.[14] Inevitably, some children who are evaluated for abuse will ultimately be determined to have an innocent explanation for their injuries. To facilitate the evaluation and preserve the doctor-patient relationship, emergency clinicians should use nonaccusatory statements to explain the need for testing (Box 172.1). A routine, standardized approach to testing and reporting can improve abuse recognition and decrease racial and social disparities.[15-17]

CLINICAL FEATURES

The clinical features of physical abuse are listed in Box 172.2.

Social and Demographic Risk Factors

Understanding psychosocial and demographic risks is most important for primary prevention efforts.[18,19] Despite increased data, these factors are relatively insensitive and nonspecific and should not be used to confirm or exclude abuse. Serious physical abuse has been reported in every socioeconomic setting, and even in households with several risk factors, the vast majority of caregivers do not physically abuse their children. Nevertheless, poor or African American families remain disproportionately likely to be evaluated and reported for abuse, while abuse is more likely to be missed in White or affluent families.[20]

Physical abuse is more likely to occur with male caregivers, especially with new caregiving arrangements, or when the caregiver is an unrelated boyfriend.[21] Prior involvement with CPS, intimate partner violence, substance use, mental illness, poverty, and criminal history have been associated with increased risk for abuse, as has the use of negative descriptors of children.[22-25]

History

Abuse is challenging to recognize when a child presents with nonspecific symptoms and without a recognized traumatic injury. Fractures,

BOX 172.1 Communication Strategies

When Interviewing a Child About Abuse
- Open-ended, non-leading questions: "Tell me more about that.", "How did your body feel?", "Then what happened?"
- "What happens at your house when kids (or pets) get in trouble?"
- Frequently explain and ask permission: "I am going to ask you some questions about your health to make sure I provide the safest treatment. Is that ok? I'm going to examine your body to make sure you are healthy. Is that ok?"

To Introduce the Genital Examination for Young Children
- "I'm also going to examine your whole body to make sure that you are healthy. I'm going to look at your nose, your ears, your belly-button, and even under your undies."
- "This examination is ok because I'm a doctor, because your mother is here, and because your mother says it's ok."

After the Examination
- "Your body looks completely healthy and normal. This does not make me doubt what you told me. It does mean that no one, not your spouse, your friends, or even a doctor like me will know what happened by looking at you." Or, "Your body has some signs of injury, but these will heal very quickly, and in a few days, you will be completely back to normal. No one, not even..."
- "Despite what many people believe, doctors usually can't tell whether someone has had sex by looking at their body. In fact, in one study of teens that were pregnant, almost 90% had completely normal examinations."
- "In my opinion, someone stops being a virgin when they *choose* to have sex."

Nonaccusatory Statements of Abuse Concern
- "The injuries we've identified are more than we would expect from the event you've described."
- "Whenever we see injuries like this, we test for other injuries and medical conditions to be sure we're not missing something that could affect your child's health."
- "I want to make sure that your child is safe/that no one is hurting your child."
- "Have you ever been concerned that someone might have been rough with or might have injured your child?"

BOX 172.2 Red Flags for Physical Abuse

Psychosocial Factors (Nonspecific, Do Not Use to Exclude Abuse)
- Unrelated caregiver (especially boyfriend) or new caregiver relationship
- Family violence
- Mental health disorders
- Substance use disorders
- Describing the child negatively

Historical Factors
- Significant injuries with no or minor trauma
- Significant inconsistencies in history
- Unexplained delay in seeking care
- Significant injury attributed to pets or young children

Physical Examination Factors
- Bruising, frenulum or conjunctival injury in children <6 months old, or who are not "cruising"
- Bruising on the torso, ear, neck, angle of the jaw, cheek, or eyelid
- Patterned bruising or burns
- Immersion or cigarette burns

TABLE 172.1 The Pittsburgh Infant Brain Injury Score (PIBIS)

Applies to	• Age 30–364 days • Well-appearing • Afebrile (T <38.3°C) • No history of trauma
Who present with	• ALTE/BRUE/apnea • Vomiting without diarrhea • Seizures or seizure-like activity • Bruises/scalp swelling • Nonspecific neurologic symptoms/lethargy/fussiness/poor feeding
Score	• Abnormal skin exam (2 points) • Age >3 months (1 point) • Head circumference >85th percentile (1 point) • Hemoglobin <11.2 g (1 point)

Total points: 5; neuroimaging is recommended for children with scores of 2 or more.

abdominal injuries, and mild brain injuries can have a smoldering course of mild symptoms, such as irritability, vomiting, or decreased appetite or activity.[6,26] In these cases, identifying abuse is difficult and usually involves prolonged symptoms, additional clues on physical examination, known social risk factors, or prior concern for abuse. The Pittsburgh Infant Brain Injury Score (PIBIS) can be used in these cases to determine the need for neuroimaging (Table 172.1).[6]

Although still nonspecific, certain complaints should prompt consideration of abuse. A small percentage of children presenting with a brief, resolved, unexplained event (BRUE; formerly known as apparent life-threatening event (ALTE)) will have retinal hemorrhages or other abusive injuries. Occult fracture should be considered in young or preverbal children who present with decreased use of an extremity, fussiness, and localized tenderness or refusal to bear weight.

Regardless of the injury, unreasonable delay in seeking care should prompt concern for abuse. No precise time period defines an "unreasonable" delay, and physicians should consider the child's symptoms and progression of disease. A delay of several hours is not uncommon for children with nonabusive fractures or abdominal injury. Conversely, even a brief delay can be concerning in children with obvious signs and symptoms such as seizures, coma, or substantial burns.

Serious injury without a history of trauma, or with a history of only mild trauma (e.g., caused by the child themselves, a young sibling, or a pet) should raise a high level of concern for abuse. Nontrivial intracranial hemorrhage is extremely uncommon from short falls (e.g., from a bed or a couch) and does not result from choking on formula or saliva.[27-29] Abdominal and thoracic injuries rarely result from household falls, even with increased height or falls down stairs.

Physical Examination

To identify subtle signs of abuse, infants (i.e., children <12 months old) should be completely undressed during physical examination. The fontanel, scalp, ears, oropharynx, skin, and genitalia should be specifically examined. A growth chart can identify sudden increase in head circumference (a sign of intracranial injury) or failure to thrive.

Although bruises are very common in ambulatory children, *any* bruising in a child less than 6 months old, or that is not yet able to ambulate with assistance or "cruise," is highly concerning for abuse.[7,30]

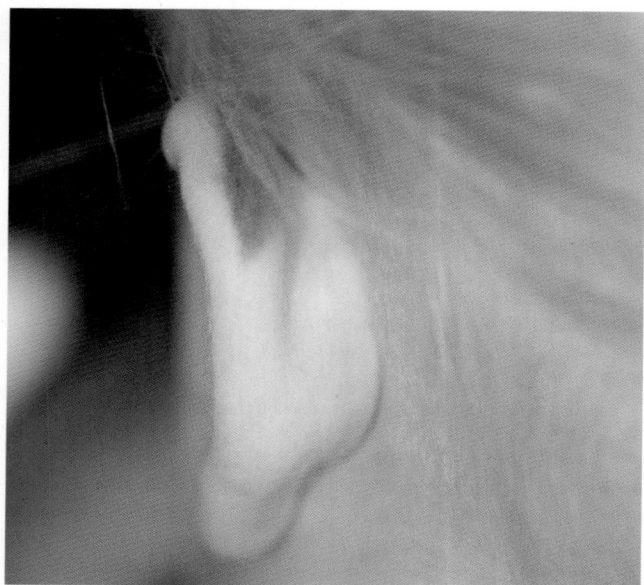

Fig. 172.1 Bruising to the helix of the ear is very concerning for abuse. (Courtesy John Melville, MD.)

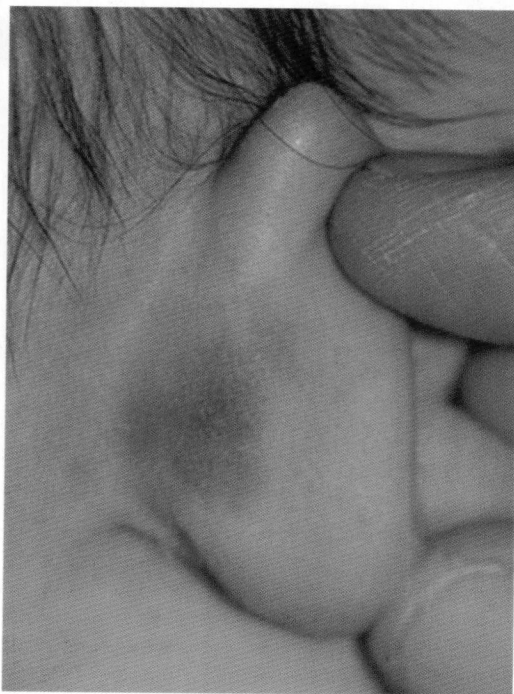

Fig. 172.2 Subtle bruising behind the child's ear can represent direct trauma or traction injury and should raise the level of concern for abuse. (Courtesy Daniel Lindberg, MD.)

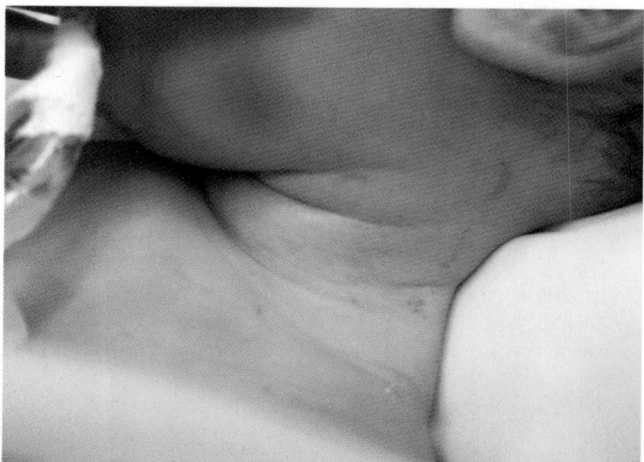

Fig. 172.3 Bruising to the neck and under the chin of an abused child. (Courtesy Carol Berkowitz, MD.)

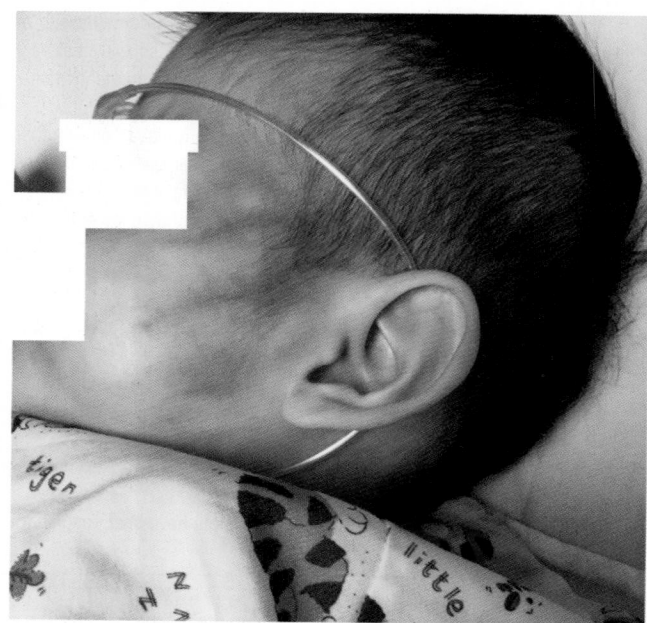

Fig. 172.4 Slap mark. The parallel, linear bruising results when capillaries rupture outward between fingers. (Courtesy John Melville, MD.)

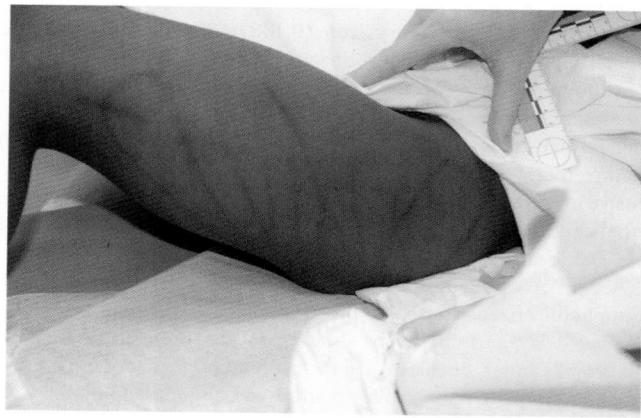

Fig. 172.5 Loop marks demonstrate contact injury from a looped cord. (Courtesy John Melville, MD.)

Of children younger than 6 months old referred for an abuse evaluation with apparently isolated bruises, 50% had additional injury (fracture, brain injury, abdominal injury) identified.

Even in children old enough to cruise, bruises to the TEN-4-FACESp regions (*T*orso, *E*ar, *N*eck, *A*ngle of the jaw, *C*heek, or *E*yelid, or *F*renulum or *S*cleral injury, or injury that is *p*atterned in children younger than 4 years old) should raise concern for abuse (Figs. 172.1 to 172.3).[31] Common patterns include bruises in the shape of a cord, belt, or hand (Figs. 172.4 to 172.6). Human bite marks are patterned bruises

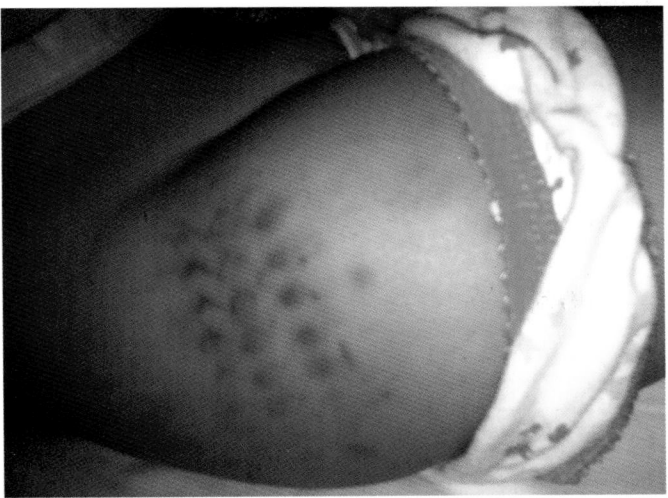

Fig. 172.6 Patterned bruising from a woven belt. (Courtesy Daniel Lindberg, MD.)

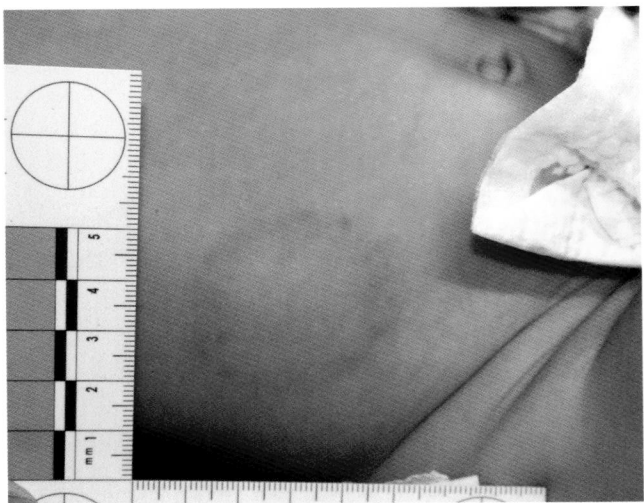

Fig. 172.7 Bite marks should be swabbed for DNA. (Courtesy John Melville, MD.)

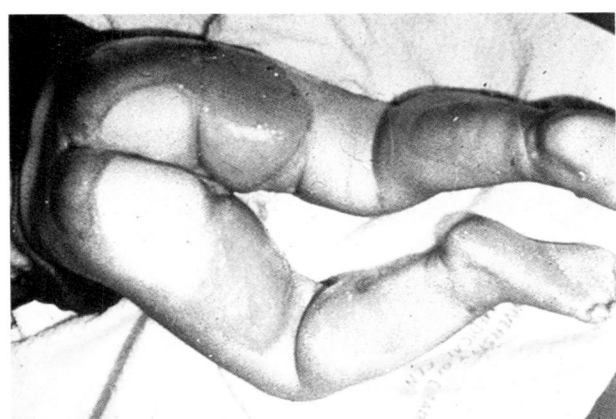

Fig. 172.8 Immersion burn. (Courtesy EMSC Slide Set, National EMSC Resource Alliance.)

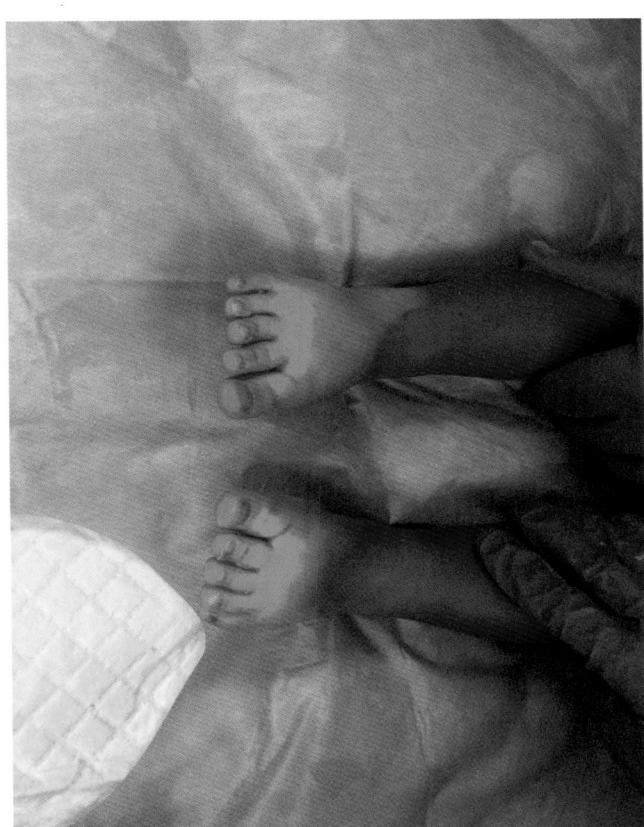

Fig. 172.9 Immersion burn of the feet after débridement. (Courtesy John Melville, MD)

in circular or paired semilunar rows (Fig. 172.7) and can be caused by adults or children. The ability of bite mark analysis to identify a biter is limited, so human bite marks should be swabbed to identify assailant DNA. Forensic evidence collection kits ("rape kits") used for sexual assault can be used to obtain, document, store, and transmit samples.

Abusive burns generally fall into three categories: immersion burns, contact burns, and cigarette burns. Immersion burns should be distinguished from pull-down scalds, which are very common in toddlers. Although pull-down scalds principally involve the upper body, immersion burns tend to involve the perineum or have a symmetric, stocking/glove distribution (Figs. 172.8 and 172.9). Abuse should also be considered when scalds affect a large body surface area, when sparing patterns suggest that the child was held in place, or when the incident is reported in the context of a toileting accident. For scald burns, CPS or law enforcement can measure the home's peak water temperature and the delay until peak temperature occurs. Although it takes several minutes to sustain a partial thickness burn from water at 120°F, the same burn can occur in seconds at 150°F.

As with bruises, emergency clinicians should consider abuse for young children with burns that take on the shape of an implement

(e.g., hair curler, grate, or lighter). Cigarettes can cause accidental or inflicted burns. Because the burning end of a cigarette can be more than 1000°F, inflicted burns are rarely superficial, and commonly result in crusted or ulcerated lesions between 8 to 10 mm (Figs. 172.10 and 172.11). Glancing or accidental contact with a cigarette can also cause superficial, linear burns.

Oropharyngeal injuries are also concerning in young children without a history of accidental trauma to the mouth or throat (Fig. 172.12). Tears of the lingual or labial frenula, or injuries to the lips, teeth, or soft palate should prompt an evaluation for abuse in children who are not yet walking and should increase concern, particularly when identified in evaluating children with other concerns of abuse.

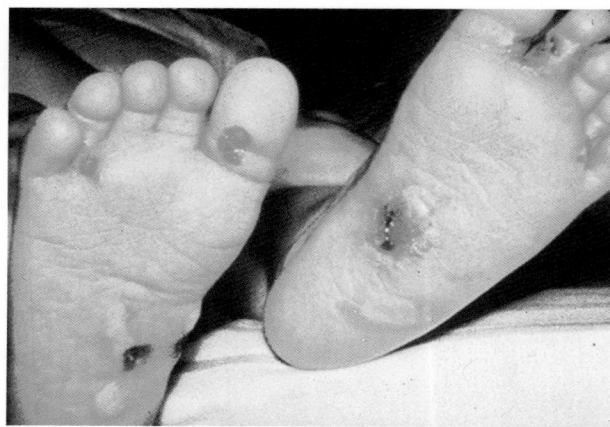

Fig. 172.10 Cigarette burns. (Courtesy EMSC Slide Set, National EMSC Resource Alliance.)

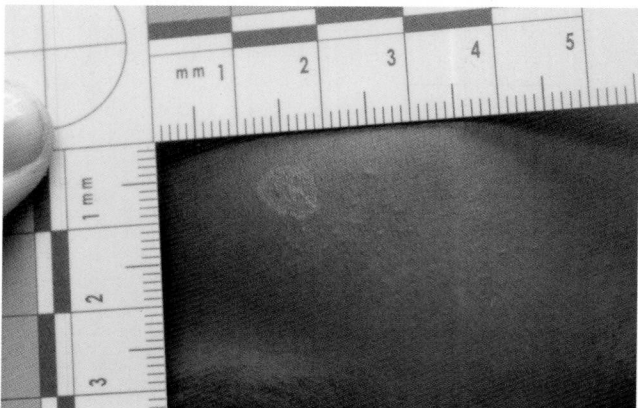

Fig. 172.11 Healing cigarette burn. (Courtesy of John Melville, MD)

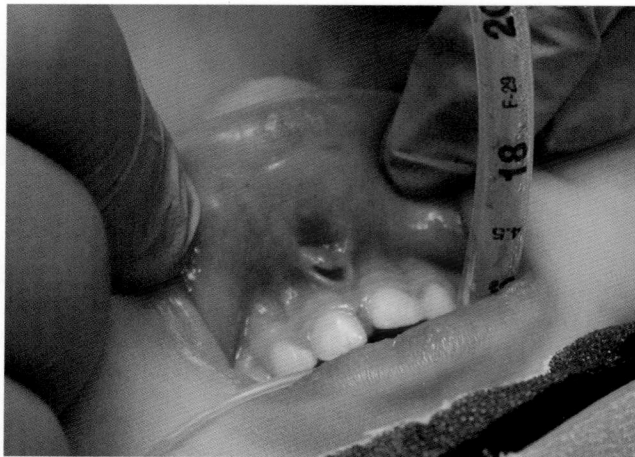

Fig. 172.12 Torn upper labial frenulum. (Courtesy John Melville, MD.)

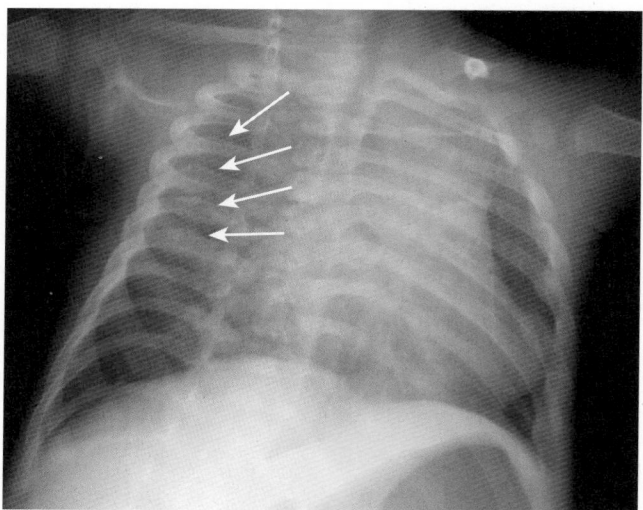

Fig. 172.13 Healing, posterior rib fractures. Right-sided, posterior rib fractures are indicated by the white arrows. Left-sided, lateral and posterior fractures are also present, and are better demonstrated by other views. (Courtesy Daniel Lindberg, MD.)

Sentinel Injuries

For many children, the concern for abuse is first raised by the unexpected or incidental identification of a traumatic injury. Abuse should routinely be considered when young children present with these injuries unless there is an independently verifiable history of major trauma (e.g., a motor vehicle collision).

Serious traumatic brain injury should prompt a concern for abuse in children younger than 3 years old, where abuse is the source of approximately one-third to one-half of all injuries excluding traffic collisions.[32,33] Subdural hematomas, parenchymal injuries, and multifocal injuries are especially concerning for abuse, whereas epidural hematomas and isolated intraventricular hemorrhages are more likely to be nonabusive.[32,34,35]

Long-bone fractures are concerning in infants; abuse is diagnosed in 30% to 60% of infants with radius, ulna, tibia, fibula, femur, or humerus fractures. Rib fractures (Fig. 172.13) are even more concerning, with abuse identified in more than 25% of children up to 36 months old, and more than 67% of infants.[36,37] Less common, fractures to the hands, feet, spine, pelvis, sternum, or scapula should be considered highly concerning for abuse in young children without a specific, independent history of significant trauma.

Classic metaphyseal lesions (CMLs) are subtle metaphyseal fractures that occur in the severely abused infants (Fig. 172.14). CMLs appear radiographically as chips or bucket handle lesions around the growth plate and are most commonly seen in the femur, humerus, and tibia.[38] No fracture is more specific for abuse than the CML, and identification should prompt a thorough evaluation for other injuries.[39-41]

Skull fractures in infants commonly raise the concern for abuse but, relative to the injuries listed earlier, are much less specific. Even in infants, linear, parietal skull fractures can result from very minor falls. Because skull fractures do not show signs of healing, birth-associated skull fractures can be clinically subtle and difficult to differentiate from acute injury. In series of infants with apparently isolated skull fractures, occult fractures were identified by skeletal survey in up to 5% of cases. Complex skull fractures–multiple fracture lines, fractures that cross suture lines, and those with substantial depression or widening—require more force or multiple impacts and are therefore more concerning. It is possible, however, for bilateral parietal fractures to result from a single impact to the cranial vertex.

Although spiral fractures were once thought to have high specificity for abuse, available data do not support this.[42] Indeed, spiral fractures of the tibia *in children learning to walk* (toddler's fractures) are among the few fractures in young children that do not require routine skeletal survey, even without a clear mechanism of trauma (see Chapter 170).

Intra-abdominal injuries in young children are concerning for abuse if not sustained as a result of a motor vehicle collision, accidental direct blow, or significant fall. Although hepatic injuries are the most

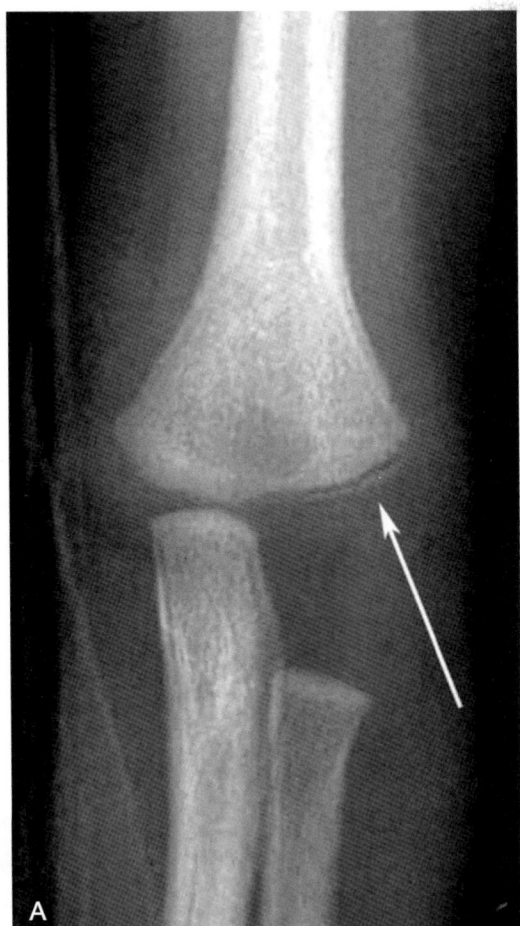

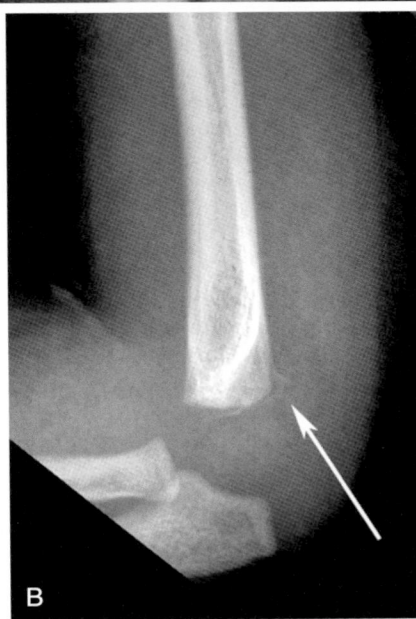

Fig. 172.14 (A) Classic metaphyseal fracture. In this anteroposterior view, the fracture assumes the "bucket handle" conformation. (B) In the lateral projection, the classic metaphyseal fracture appears as a chip. (Courtesy Daniel Lindberg, MD.)

common abusive injury identified, small bowel perforation and pancreatic injury are especially specific for abuse.[43]

TABLE 172.2 Differential Diagnoses (Not Exhaustive)

Presenting Injury	Diagnoses	Signs
Any	Accidental trauma	Minor injuries, walking children, history
	Birth trauma	Young infants
Fractures/bony injury	Osteomalacia of prematurity	Former significantly premature infants
	Osteogenesis imperfecta	Blue-gray sclera, family history
	Osteomyelitis	Fever (even minor)
	Congenital syphilis	Rash
Bruising/ hemorrhage	Congenital coagulopathy	Abnormal PT/PTT/platelets, family history
	Other cutaneous lesions	Failure to resolve with time
Burns	Phytophotodermatitis	Typical history
	Irritant burn	Exposure to senna, laxatives, irritants

Universal Screening

In an effort to reduce rates of missed physical abuse, some centers have implemented processes of "universal screening," in which the primary nurse documents whether there is concern for abuse in every child at the time they present for care. Nurses are prompted to consider historical and physical findings and to completely undress young children. In several large, population-based samples, universal screening has been shown to be feasible, to identify children with higher risk for abuse, and to increase reporting, but it has not yet been shown to decrease rates of missed abuse.[44-46]

DIFFERENTIAL DIAGNOSES

Because the diagnosis of abuse has a profound impact on a child, their family, and the alleged abuser, a variety of traumatic and medical conditions have been suggested to explain signs and symptoms of physical abuse (Table 172.2). These range from sincere attempts to distinguish abuse from rare but well-described medical entities, to the invention of new medical entities invoked only in legal settings or the lay press.[27,28,47-50] It is usually beyond the scope of an emergency clinician to test for such rare diseases or hypothetical entities unless there are specific signs or symptoms (e.g., the blue sclera of osteogenesis imperfecta) or a specific family history.

The most common entity to be differentiated from abuse is accidental injury. With few exceptions (e.g., the CML), most traumatic injuries that have been reported in the setting of abuse can also be seen with other severe forms of trauma. Isolated injuries reported in the context of an accidental trauma mechanism should be evaluated on a case-by-case basis to determine whether the identified injury matches the reported mechanism. Young children who have started to cruise or walk frequently may have unobserved short falls from standing height or furniture. Although the vast majority of these falls are benign, they can produce injury: isolated bruising to shins, elbows, or other hard body surfaces; linear skull fractures; toddler's fractures, buckle fractures of the distal femur; and clavicle fractures.

In the youngest infants, injuries from birth should be considered, because symptoms may only be recognized weeks after the child is discharged from the hospital. Skull fractures, cephalohematomas, and clavicle fractures are the most commonly identified, whereas asymptomatic subdural hematomas, rib fractures, and other extremity fractures are rarer. Retinal hemorrhages occur in approximately one-third of normal births and persist for 1 to 3 months.[51,52]

Bone fragility disorders should be considered in children with exclusively bony injuries. *Osteomalacia of prematurity* occurs in roughly 30% of extremely low-birth-weight infants and is commonly associated with fractures in the absence of significant trauma. Risk factors include exposure to prolonged parenteral nutrition, steroids or furosemide, and those with cholestasis or chronic lung disease. Minor forms of *osteogenesis imperfecta* can present with multiple unexplained fractures. Although the diagnosis can be made early in children with a family history or severe disease, some cases are only diagnosed in the course of an evaluation for abuse. Be alert for blue-gray sclera, especially if they persist beyond infancy, or family history of unexplained fractures, fragile teeth, congenital hearing problems, or short stature. Osteomyelitis and congenital syphilis can cause metaphyseal abnormalities and should be considered in children with even mild fever or rash.

In children whose injuries are confined to problems of bruising or bleeding, emergency clinicians should consider an undiagnosed coagulopathy. The American Academy of Pediatrics (AAP) has published guidelines for coagulopathy testing that will identify the vast majority of bleeding disorders.[53] Briefly, these children should have prothrombin time and international normalized ratio (PT/INR), partial thromboplastin time (PTT), Factors VIII and IX, and complete blood count (CBC).[53,54] Those with intracranial hemorrhage should have testing for D-dimer and fibrinogen. Because coagulopathy testing can take weeks or months, and because abuse is the more common etiology in children with isolated bruising and concern for abuse, the coagulation evaluation should not delay the evaluation for abuse, reporting to CPS, or safety planning.

Atraumatic cutaneous findings may be confused for isolated bruising, including congenital dermal melanosis (formerly "Mongolian spots"), other birthmarks, or even blue dye from clothing (diagnose and "cure" this with an alcohol wipe). Because bruising resolves over a few days, follow-up examinations with photo documentation can reliably distinguish most findings. In cases where an immediate decision is needed, preliminary data suggest that transcutaneous bilirubin testing might be useful.[55]

When children present with lesions concerning for abusive burns, emergency clinicians should consider phytophotodermatitis and irritant burns. Phytophotodermatitis is a skin reaction caused by sun exposure in the setting of photo-sensitizing substances such as citrus, parsnip, or celery juices. It can cause well-demarcated, patterned, burn-like, blistering lesions and the typical history can usually be elicited. Irritant burns can be caused by prolonged exposure to mild skin irritants, such as household bleach, which may not be uncomfortable to the child. Prolonged contact with stool in diapered children, especially after the use of Senna or other laxatives, can cause contact burns that look identical to immersion burns.[56]

DIAGNOSTIC TESTING

Protecting a child from an abusive caregiver may require proving that the child's injuries are the result of abuse. Identification of additional traumatic injuries suggests abuse, particularly when not explained by the initial history. Concomitant injuries may have important *forensic* significance, even when they do not require specific treatment. The clinical examination is insensitive, especially in very young children, for forensically significant injuries, such as healing fractures, CMLs, abdominal injuries, and even milder abusive head trauma.[57] To decrease testing disparities and improve abuse recognition, we recommend a routine testing strategy based on the level of concern for abuse and the child's presenting injuries (Table 172.3).[14,31,58,59]

Skeletal Survey

The radiographic skeletal survey is the oldest and most commonly used diagnostic test to identify occult traumatic injuries when there is concern for physical abuse. Depending on the population, skeletal surveys

TABLE 172.3   Recommendations for Occult Injury Testing

Diagnostic Test	Indications (With Concern for Abuse)
Skeletal survey	All patients <24 months old Consider in 24-60-month-olds
Neuroimaging (CT or MRI)	Signs/symptoms of traumatic brain injury History of assault to head or violent shaking <6 months old PIBIS score >1 (see Table 172.1)
Retinal examination	Patients with traumatic brain injury
AST/ALT	Patients <60 months old with significant injury (e.g., brain injury, torso injury, long-bone fracture)
Abdominal CT	History of assault to abdomen Signs/symptoms of abdominal injury AST or ALT >80 IU/L
Siblings and contacts	Skeletal survey for <24-month-old contacts of injured, abused children. Interview verbal children capable of participating
Toxicology testing (evidence is limited)	Altered mental status Evidence of substance use in the environment Abusive burns

ALT, Alanine transaminase; *AST,* aspartate transaminase; *CT,* computed tomography; *MRI,* magnetic resonance imaging.

identify additional fractures in approximately 10% to 25% of cases, with very low radiation exposure.[38,60] Guidelines recommend skeletal survey for all children younger than 24 months old with suspicion for abuse.[8,14,59,61,62] Skeletal surveys may be reasonable in children 24 to 60 months old, especially for those with limited mobility, decreased ability to communicate, and those 24 to 36 months old. Skeletal surveys require specialized technique, including at least 21 separate films and interpretation by an experienced radiologist.[63] A child should be transferred to an experienced center for skeletal survey rather than have an incomplete or inadequate series. There is no role for a single exposure "baby-gram" to identify occult fractures. A follow-up skeletal survey, repeated after at least 14 days, frequently identifies additional missed fractures and may clarify indeterminate findings (Box 172.3).

Neuroimaging (Computed Tomography or Magnetic Resonance Imaging)

Abusive head trauma is both the leading cause of death and disability in abused children, and the abusive injury most frequently missed by clinicians.[3] Head computed tomography (CT) or magnetic resonance imaging (MRI) should be undertaken in children with signs of brain injury—decreased mental status, external signs of impact to the head, bulging fontanel, seizure, coma, or focal neurologic findings.[57] We recommend neuroimaging also be performed in children younger than 6 months old when there is concern for abuse, even when the child is neurologically asymptomatic. In infants with nonspecific signs and symptoms, such as lethargy, seizure-like activity, or vomiting without fever or diarrhea, the PIBIS score should guide neuroimaging decisions (see Table 172.1). Because of the need to identify forensically significant injuries, the Pediatric Emergency Care Applied Research Network (PECARN) decision rule should not be used to identify children at low risk of injury when there is concern for abuse.[57,64] See Chapter 160 for a discussion on nonabusive pediatric head injury evaluation.

Because it is widely available, fast, and accurate, CT is currently the most widely used modality to diagnose abusive head trauma. Head CT should routinely include three-dimensional reformatting to identify

BOX 172.3   The Complete Skeletal Survey[63]

Appendicular Skeleton
Humeri (AP)
Forearms (AP)
Hands (PA)
Femurs (AP)
Lower legs (AP)
Feet (AP)

Axial Skeleton
Thorax (AP, lateral, L and R obliques)
Abdomen and pelvis (AP)
Lumbosacral spine (lateral)
Cervical spine (lateral)
Skull (frontal and lateral)

AP, Anteroposterior; *L,* left; *PA,* posteroanterior; *R,* right. American College of Radiology and the Society for Pediatric Radiology. ACR–SPR Practice Parameter for the Performance and Interpretation of Skeletal Surveys in Children. 2016; https://www.acr.org/-/media/ACR/Files/Practice-Parameters/Skeletal-Survey.pdf. Accessed January 16, 2020.

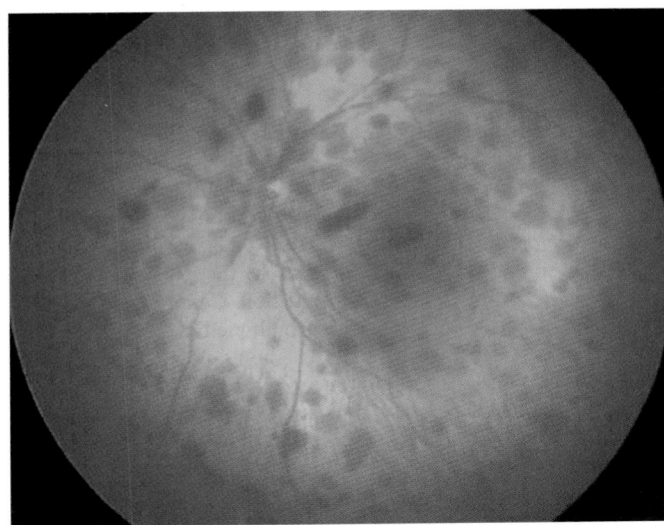

Fig. 172.15 Too numerous to count retinal hemorrhages in all layers that extend to the periphery—characteristic of abusive head trauma. (Courtesy of Daniel Lindberg, MD.)

subtle skull fractures that may be missed in the plane of the scan. These reformats do not require additional radiation exposure but do require reformatting before data are expunged.

Recently, MRI using faster, more motion-tolerant MRI sequences (fast MRI) has come to replace CT as the initial test for abusive head trauma in several centers.[65-69] In order to decrease radiation exposure, we recommend, as resources allow, rapid MRI in favor of CT for clinically stable children who do not require other CT imaging. Because rapid MRI is marginally less sensitive for skull fractures than CT, we recommend that a complete skeletal survey with skull radiographs be performed in children who undergo rapid MRI for concerns of abuse. Cranial ultrasound is not sufficiently sensitive to identify occult abusive injuries and is not recommended as an initial study for children with concern for abuse. In children with identified abusive head trauma, MRI of the brain and cervical spine is frequently performed several days after the initial CT scan to further delineate and assess progression of injury.[70]

Retinal Examination

Retinal hemorrhages identified in a child with head injury can significantly increase the recognition of abuse.[51] Although a wide range of diseases can cause mild retinal hemorrhages, numerous (>20), multilayered and extensive hemorrhages, or those associated with macular retinoschisis, are strongly associated with abusive head trauma (Fig. 172.15). Dedicated retinal examination by an experienced ophthalmologist is recommended for children with concern for abusive head trauma to characterize the hemorrhages and improve sensitivity.[51] Conversely, without radiographic evidence of brain injury, significant retinal hemorrhages are rare, and transfer or referral for specialty retinal examination should be considered optional in this group. Even in severe cases of abusive head trauma, retinal hemorrhages are absent in approximately 15% of cases; retinal examination should therefore not be used as an initial screening test to determine the need for neuroimaging.

Abdominal Injury Testing

Intra-abdominal injuries, ranging from obviously life-threatening to completely asymptomatic, are present in approximately 3% of children evaluated for physical abuse. Abdominal bruising, tenderness, or distention of the abdomen are present in approximately 50% of children with abusive abdominal injuries. In children with concern for abuse and aspartate transaminase (AST) or alanine transaminase (ALT)

greater than 80 IU/L, at least 20% had an intra-abdominal injury identified by CT scan or other definitive testing. Amylase and lipase have been recommended by some authors to increase sensitivity for abdominal injuries, but have not been shown to significantly improve yield beyond clinical examination plus AST and ALT. Although ultrasound can identify abdominal injuries, it is relatively insensitive; CT should be used to characterize injuries identified by ultrasound.

To assess for intra-abdominal injury, we recommend AST and ALT testing for children with concern for abuse unless there is obvious abdominal injury or history of direct abdominal trauma, in which case a CT scan should be performed. We also recommend CT scan with intravenous (IV) contrast be performed for those with AST or ALT greater than 80 IU/L. Because AST and ALT rapidly normalize, even in children with hepatic lacerations, trending of transaminases over time should not be used to determine the need for imaging. For this reason, it is also important that testing be completed during the initial evaluation.

Toxicology Testing

Children can ingest illicit drugs via malicious poisoning or neglectful exposure.[71-73] Centers with routine testing strategies identify illicit substances in approximately 5% to 10% of children with high levels of concern for abuse.[71] Because data are limited and the epidemiology of drug use is highly variable, there are currently no widely accepted guidelines for drug testing when there is concern for abuse. Currently, we recommend drug testing when children with high concern for abuse present with burns, altered mental status, or when substance use disorders are identified in the child's environment. Because rapid drug screens based on ELISA methodology are subject to high rates of false negatives, we recommend use of comprehensive testing based on mass spectroscopy.[71]

MANAGEMENT

Compared to children with nonabusive traumatic brain injury, as a group, children with abusive head trauma tend to have more severe injury, longer ICU stays, and higher mortality. Nonconvulsive seizures are identified in more than 30% of children with abusive head trauma, prompting some to recommend routine electroencephalogram (EEG) monitoring.[4,74] Otherwise, medical management of children with abusive traumatic injuries is generally the same as for nonabused children.

Beyond the management of the acute injuries themselves, management of abuse largely consists of protecting the child from further abuse.

Household Contacts

Violence is a disease that affects an entire household.[10,13,75,76] We recommend that emergency clinicians identify any other children who share a home where child abuse (or other forms of family violence) is identified.[9,12,59,75] Conversely, when child abuse is recognized, emergency clinicians should consider whether other family members or companion animals may be at risk and use the expertise of CPS to assist in bringing those at risk for evaluation. Contacts younger than 24 months, especially twins and other multiple births, should have a skeletal survey.[14] Older, verbal children should be interviewed about any reported trauma history, and to identify abusive disciplinary practices. In cases where there is significant concern for genetic diseases that mimic abuse, evaluation of biological siblings can help to establish the correct diagnosis.

Timing

Determining the age of an injury can affect the plausibility of an offered history and can assist law enforcement in identifying the perpetrator. In young children, multiple injuries of different ages are highly concerning for abuse. In many cases, the best way to determine the timing of an injury is based on when the child developed symptoms, independent witness reports, or images of visible injuries.

The best evidence for injury dating comes from fractures of endochondral bones (most bones except the skull). Signs of healing (e.g., periosteal reaction and callus formation) are rarely evident before 7 days and commonly seen within 10 to 14 days. Experienced radiologists can sometimes offer more nuanced estimates of fracture age. Multiple fractures of different ages are highly concerning for abuse.

Recent data suggest that the finding of too-numerous-to-count intraretinal hemorrhages reliably resolves within a few days. Thus, we recommend dedicated retinal examination occur within 24 to 48 hours in cases with concern for abusive head trauma; the patterns of retinal hemorrhages may be useful in estimating the time of injury.[77]

Conversely, emergency clinicians should be cautious not to estimate the age of bruises based on their appearance. Previously used dating systems were based on scant data and have poor accuracy when prospectively used to estimate bruise ages in children with known times of injury. Similarly, the CT appearance of subdural hematomas or other intracranial hemorrhages is of limited utility in estimating the age of injury. Although hyperdense "bright" blood is often thought to signify acute hemorrhage (and vice-versa), hyperacute bleeding, re-bleeding and mixing of blood and cerebrospinal fluid (CSF) probably account for their poor accuracy. Mixed density subdural hematomas have been described in several cases with a single traumatic episode, and therefore are not strong evidence for multiple episodes of trauma. In cases of severe traumatic brain injury, the onset of a child's symptoms is probably the most useful determination of timing of injury, especially when a child who had been acting normally suddenly becomes comatose.

Mandated Reporting

In the United States, Canada, and several other jurisdictions, emergency clinicians are mandated to report a reasonable concern of child maltreatment to public CPS agencies or law enforcement. These reports can mobilize social resources for family, expand the investigation of abuse beyond the hospital, and facilitate testing or protection for other children in the abusive environment. A final diagnosis of abuse is not required to trigger the mandate, and reporters generally have legal protection for reports made in good faith, even if a child is ultimately determined not to have been abused. In cases where there is reasonable concern for abuse, but where the final diagnosis is pending, emergency clinicians should be reassured that a mandated report need not automatically trigger the removal of a child from their home or the instigation of criminal proceedings. In many jurisdictions, the mandate to report can be satisfied by reporting to a designated child protection team who will complete the evaluation and determine the need for reporting.

Hospital social workers can assist with the reporting process. The exact procedure for reporting varies by jurisdiction, but instructions are usually accessible via an internet search for "report child abuse [location]." In preparing to report, gather the child and family's contact information, the identity and ages of any other children in the home, and the location where the abuse may have occurred (to determine reporting jurisdiction).

DISPOSITION

Many children with physical abuse will require hospital admission for treatment and stabilization of their injuries or identification of a safe environment. Children with concern for physical abuse may be discharged if: (1) injuries have been medically stabilized; (2) reasonable concerns for abuse have been reported as required by statute; and (3) a safe environment has been identified. In children who are otherwise stable for discharge, CPS should establish a temporary safety plan until testing can be completed.

Should caregivers attempt to leave the ED prior to the completion of an evaluation for abuse, emergency clinicians should follow their typical practice for parents seeking to leave against medical advice. If a caregiver demonstrates the capacity to make medical decisions, and has received the clinician's best advice, emergency clinicians and hospital staff should not seek to forcibly prevent them from leaving. Reasonable concerns for abuse should be reported in these circumstances as required by local statutes to CPS or law enforcement, which have the ability to implement secondary prevention.

SEXUAL ABUSE

KEY CONCEPTS

- ED evaluation of pediatric sexual assault should focus on time-dependent medical treatment and evidence collection. The ultimate determination of abuse likelihood can be deferred pending the forensic interview and additional investigation.
- A normal examination neither confirms nor excludes the possibility of abuse, and patients should be reassured that their body is normal and healthy.
- A genital examination should not be forced on a child. Most children can be referred for an examination when they are rested and prepared.
- Likelihood of obtaining forensic evidence decreases with time from assault. Evidence collection may be performed up to 7 days after sexual assault, depending on jurisdiction.
- Emergency contraception should be offered to pubertal females up to 120 hours after sexual assault.
- Prophylactic or empirical treatment for gonorrhea, chlamydia, and trichomonas should be offered to pubertal children, but treatment should be deferred in pre-pubertal children until infection is confirmed.
- When an investigation for sexual abuse is ongoing, caregivers and emergency clinicians should provide a believing, supportive environment if a child reports abuse or has questions but should not attempt to elicit a detailed narrative outside the context of the forensic interview.

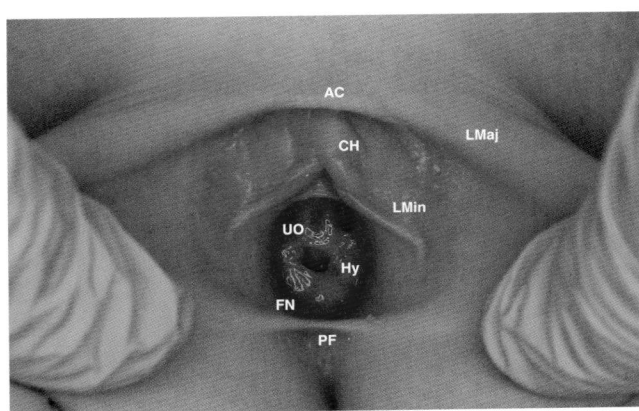

Fig. 172.16 Normal pre-pubertal hymen. This view is obtained by gentle outward (toward the examiner) traction on the labia. *AC*, Anterior commissure; *CH*, clitoral hood; *FN*, fossa navicularis; *Hy*, hymenal membrane (Note the thin, smooth membrane in this pre-pubertal child. Note also that the presence of the hymenal opening is entirely normal.); *LMaj*, labia majora; *LMin*, labia minora; *PF*, posterior fourchette. (Courtesy of Kathi L. Makoroff, MD.)

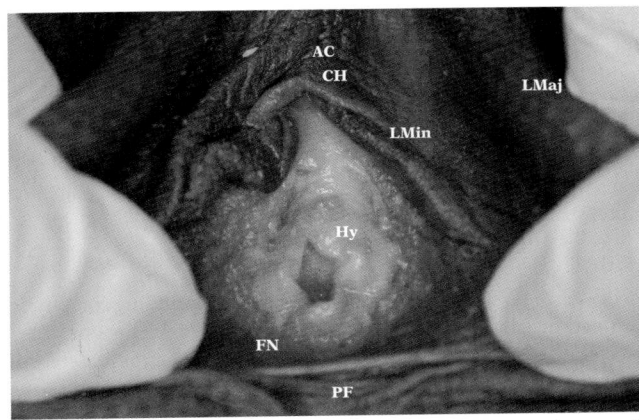

Fig. 172.17 Normal pubertal hymen. *AC*, Anterior commissure; *CH*, clitoral hood; *FN*, fossa navicularis; *Hy*, hymenal membrane (Note the thickened, redundant appearance in this pubertal adolescent); *LMaj*, labia majora; *LMin*, labia minora; *PF*, posterior fourchette. (Courtesy of Kathi L. Makoroff, MD)

FOUNDATIONS

Sexual abuse of children is common and under-recognized.[78] When surveyed as young adults, roughly 25% of women and 5% of men report some form of sexual abuse, with adolescents being at highest risk. These are likely under-estimates given the limitations of self-reporting. Perpetrators of sexual abuse are overwhelmingly male and can include family members, acquaintances, or strangers.

Especially in adolescents, the loss of control inherent in sexual abuse can be profoundly damaging. A trauma-informed approach can decrease anxiety and facilitate the evaluation. In school-aged or adolescent children (and adults) who have experienced sexual assault, emergency clinicians should seek to re-establish a sense of control whenever possible. For example, we recommend frequently explaining the purpose of each step of the process and asking for permission (examples, see Box 172.1). Respect a child's right to decline any part of the evaluation.

As with physical abuse, the bulk of the investigation in cases with concern for sexual abuse can occur outside of the ED. Urgent interventions include stabilization of medical injuries, evidence collection, post-exposure prophylaxis (PEP), arrangement of a safe environment, and CPS reporting. Evaluation of children more than 72 hours after possible abuse (or another period if mandated by law) can be deferred from the ED to an outpatient setting.[79] Completion of a full evidence collection kit can require more than an hour of undivided attention, and emergency clinicians responsible for multiple potentially unstable patients may benefit in partnering with a sexual assault/forensic nurse examiner (SANE/FNE) program or a subspecialty child abuse pediatrician.

Misconceptions about normal pediatric female genital anatomy (Figs. 172.16 and 172.17) are widespread among both patients and clinicians. The pre-pubertal hymen is thin, with a smooth edge. Normal configurations include annular or ring-shaped, crescent-shaped, and tulip-shaped, among many others. Although imperforate hymens exist and can cause symptoms in pubertal children, this is a rare abnormality. During puberty, the hymen becomes thickened and redundant (see Fig. 172.17).

Trafficking

Trafficking, or commercial sexual exploitation of children, occurs when someone engages a minor in any sex act that involves the exchange of something of perceived value, and can include the prostitution of children by others, "survival sex," or pornography.[80] Although reliable statistics on the prevalence and epidemiology of trafficking are limited, available evidence suggests that the large majority of trafficked children and adolescents in the United States are female and are US citizens.[81] Early data suggest that trafficking is more likely among adolescents who have history of substance use, run away from home, have been involved with law enforcement, had a traumatic injury (i.e., broken bone, loss of consciousness, significant wound), had an STI, or had more than 5 sexual partners.[80,82,83] When two or more of these risk factors are identified, clinicians should ask if anyone has asked or forced the patient to do something sexual with someone else, to do some sexual act in public (like dance in a strip club), to pose sexually for a photo or video, or if the patient has traded sex for something they needed.[84] Clinicians should take steps to ask these questions privately, because traffickers may pose as relatives, friends, or employers. The National Human Trafficking Resource Center maintains a hotline (1-888-3737-888) that can provide region-specific resources to clinicians or patients when there is concern for trafficking.

CLINICAL FEATURES

In contrast to physical abuse, most sexual abuse evaluations will be prompted by a patient or caregiver report. Genital bleeding or discharge should prompt consideration of sexual abuse even when no concern is raised in the history, and in pre-verbal children. Pregnancy or sexually transmitted infections (STIs) (gonorrhea, chlamydia, syphilis, trichomonas, or human immunodeficiency virus [HIV]) demonstrate evidence of sexual contact.[79,85-87] A diagnosis of pregnancy or STI in a young adolescent should prompt nonjudgmental questions about the child's sexual partners; some victims perceive abuse as consensual sexual activity with a boyfriend or girlfriend.

Caregivers sometimes bring children for evaluation based on concern for abnormal appearance of a child's genitalia (redness, size, or shape of vaginal or rectal orifices). Without other indications of abuse, these findings are extremely nonspecific and do not increase the likelihood of abuse.[88] In young children (2 to 6 years old), some sexual behaviors that are concerning to caregivers (e.g., touching genitals in public) are part of normal development, whereas others (e.g., inserting objects into the genitals) should prompt concern for sexual abuse. The AAP has published guidelines for the evaluation of several such sexual behaviors. In general, behaviors are less concerning if they are transient, few, and distractible. They are more concerning if they are persistent and resistant to parental distraction. When children engage in sexual actions or activity with each other, sexual abuse should be distinguished from sexual play by the presence of a significant difference in age or development, or the presence of coercion. Laws defining the age of consent for sexual activity and the age difference that constitutes statutory rape differ by jurisdiction.

History

Most cases of sexual abuse do not have diagnostic findings on physical examination, laboratory testing, or forensic evidence collection. Therefore, a child's history is usually the most important factor to determine social or legal interventions in cases of alleged sexual abuse. Forensic interviews, conducted by CPS, law enforcement, child advocacy centers, or child protection teams, are conducted to avoid suggestive or coercive questions. In most cases, these forensic interviews can take place after the initial ED evaluation, allowing emergency clinicians to limit their history to the information needed to identify medically significant injury or illness.

Forensic interviewing requires substantial training and ongoing peer review, and repeated interviews could "contaminate" evidence. For these reasons, we recommend that emergency clinicians, parents, and caregivers not attempt to obtain detailed narrative needed for prosecution outside the formal forensic interview.[79] However, adults should provide a safe, supportive, listening environment if the child approaches them with information or questions. Outcomes for sexually abused children are improved when they are believed and supported by their caregivers. Clinicians should transparently communicate that their ability to keep information confidential is limited in some cases by the legal mandate to report reasonable concerns for child abuse.[89]

In cases where a caregiver reports the initial concern for abuse, emergency clinicians should obtain the caregiver's history separated from the child. Document whether the child reported abuse; and if so, whether the report was spontaneous, or in response to questioning by the caregiver. Identify any additional children ("contact children") who share the environment where abuse may have occurred. If interviewing a child, avoid leading questions, and document both the question asked and the child's response.

Interviews should be conducted at an appropriate developmental level; most children younger than 4 years old will have limited ability to participate in the interview. Younger school-aged children may have difficulty with "when" questions, limiting the ability to determine the time elapsed from the last episode of abuse (needed to determine the need for an acute examination, evidence collection, or HIV PEP). Consider asking "where," "what," or "who" questions to understand the timeline. For example, a child who does not know what time or day something occurred may know whether it was day or night, a school day or a weekend, or during a specific holiday, event, or visit to a different home. It may be helpful to elicit the terms used by the child to describe different body parts.

Physical Examination

Most children who present to the ED with concern for sexual abuse should be offered a dedicated physical examination of the genitalia and rectum. With proper preparation, this examination need not be painful or distressing to the child (see Box 172.1). Conducting the examination on the lap of a trusted caregiver and in the context of other painless examination maneuvers (inspecting the nose, heart, and belly-button) can reassure the child. Limit exposure of the child's body to the area being examined.[89]

The pre-pubertal (non-estrogenized) hymen is exquisitely sensitive; touching it will almost certainly end the useful portion of your examination. For this reason, collection of internal vaginal and cervical swabs is not indicated in a pre-pubertal child and a speculum examination should not be conducted.[89]

To avoid additional trauma, a genital examination should not be forced on a reluctant child. In most cases, a child can return for an outpatient examination after food, rest, and preparation.[89] In the rare cases of substantial bleeding or concern for a medically unstable injury, a gynecologist should perform an examination under anesthesia.

To best expose the hymen and other relevant anatomy, pull the labia majora out (off the table or toward the examiner—not laterally) with the same force you would use to retract the cheek to examine the teeth. The posterior hymen, if not sufficiently visualized in this position, can sometimes be better seen in the "knee-chest" position, where the child is placed in a prone position on the examination table with her hips flexed so that the knees and chest are resting on the table. The posterior hymen is then visualized by laterally retracting the buttocks.[79]

If manipulation of the hymen is absolutely necessary, consider using the mucosal surface of the contralateral labia. Alternatively, a few drops of sterile saline can be used to "float" the posterior rim of the hymen and expose an area of interest. A colposcope can be useful to magnify, illuminate, and document examination findings. Data do not support the use of toluidine blue to identify mucosal injuries not apparent to the naked eye.[79] If photo-documentation is conducted, images should be maintained in a confidential format separate from the normal electronic medical record.

Even when concern for sexual abuse is high, most children will not have physical signs of genital or anal injury.[85] A wide array of nonspecific findings (e.g., erythema, periurethral bands, and bumps and notches of the hymen) should not be confused with evidence of sexual contact. (Table 172.4). Injuries that are indicative of trauma include bruising, petechiae, or abrasions on the hymen; acute lacerations of the hymen; vaginal lacerations; or complete transection of the hymen between 4 o'clock and 8 o'clock (Figs. 172.18 and 172.19). In adolescents capable of consensual sexual activity, no examination finding can distinguish consensual sexual activity from assault or rape.

Although the vast majority of physical examinations will be normal, even when performed soon after acute sexual assault, a normal examination does not exclude abuse. Children and families can be reassured that they are healthy and normal and that no one in the future (e.g., doctors, spouses) will know from looking at them that abuse has occurred. Some families have concern for an anatomic definition of virginity, although they are reluctant to broach the issue. Providers should emphasize that the child is anatomically normal and that the definition of virginity should depend on when someone *chooses* to have intercourse.

DIFFERENTIAL DIAGNOSES

Strep infection of the perineal skin and genitalia can produce redness, inflammation, and fissures. Vaginitis from infection or poor hygiene can result in vaginal discharge or dysuria. Isolated vaginal bleeding can be the result of urethral prolapse (beefy red protrusion inferior to clitoral hood) or lichen sclerosis (pale, irritated, thin, hypopigmented skin surrounding the genitalia; Figs. 172.20 and 172.21). Straddle injuries can produce bruising of the external genitalia (labia, perineum, and peri-urethral tissues) and are usually accompanied by a history of injury. In boys who are toilet training, a falling toilet seat can produce dorsal and ventral penile bruising similar to a bite mark.

TABLE 172.4   Significance of Genital Findings for Abuse

Normal Findings	Conditions Mistaken for Abuse	Findings Caused by Trauma and/or Sexual Contact
• Normal hymen variants (annular, crescentic, imperforate, micro-perforate, septate, redundant, with tissue tags, with bumps or mounds) • Hymenal notches or clefts between 3 and 9 o'clock • Superficial notches below 3 and 9 o'clock • Periurethral bands • Intravaginal ridges or columns • External hymenal ridge • Linea vestibularis • Diastasis ani • Perianal skin tags • Hyperpigmentation of the skin of the labia minora or perianal tissues in children of color • Dilated urethral orifice Findings commonly caused by other medical conditions: • Erythema • Increased vascularity • Labial adhesions • Friability of posterior fourchette • Vaginal discharge • Molluscum contagiosum • Anal fissures • Venous pooling • Anal dilatation from constipation, anesthesia, impaired muscular tone or post mortem	• Urethral prolapse • Lichen sclerosus • Vulvar ulcers • Erythema, inflammation or fissures from bacterial, viral, fungal, parasitic infection • Perineal groove • Rectal prolapse • Post mortem lividity	• Acute laceration(s) or bruising of labia, penis, scrotum, perianal tissues, or perineum • Acute laceration of the posterior fourchette or vestibule • Perianal or posterior fourchette scars (difficult to diagnose without documentation of the acute laceration) • Bruising, petechiae, or abrasions on the hymen • Acute laceration of the hymen • Vaginal laceration • Perianal laceration with exposure of tissues below the dermis • Healed hymenal transection/complete hymen cleft—a defect in the hymen between 4 and 8 o'clock that extends to the base of the hymen with no hymenal tissue discernible at that location • Evidence of female genital mutilation or cutting • Gonorrhea (genital, rectal or pharyngeal) • Syphilis • Chlamydia (genital or rectal) • Trichomonas • HIV (excludes transmission from blood transfusion) • Pregnancy • Semen found by forensic specimens

HIV, Human immunodeficiency virus.
Adapted from: Adams JA, Farst KJ, Kellogg ND. Interpretation of medical findings in suspected child sexual abuse: an update for 2018. *J Pediatr Adolesc Gynecol.* 2018;31(3):225-231.

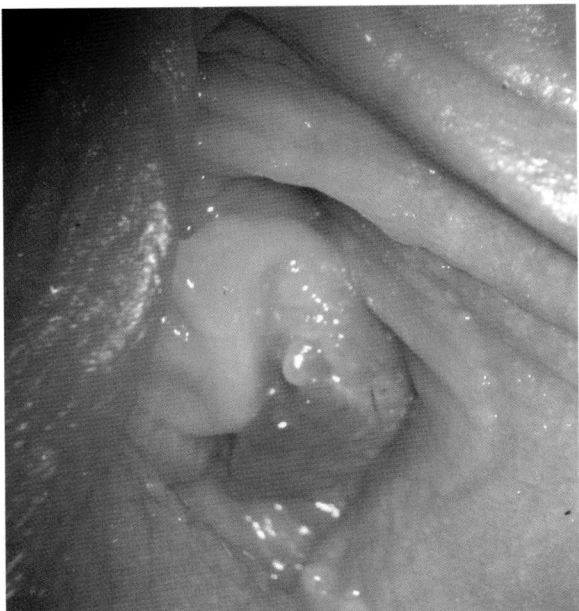

Fig. 172.18 Bruising to an estrogenized, pubertal hymen. Indicative of acute sexual contact. (Courtesy of Daniel Lindberg, MD.)

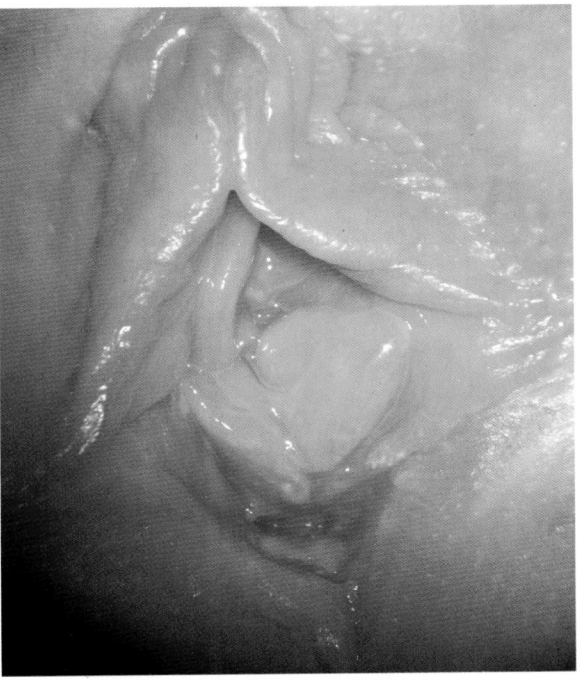

Fig. 172.19 Acute injury to the fossa navicularis in a pre-pubertal girl. The hymen is not well visualized. (Courtesy of Daniel Lindberg, MD.)

DIAGNOSTIC TESTING

The goal of diagnostic testing in the ED is to identify transient evidence of sexual assault or sexually transmitted diseases (Table 172.5). Beyond the history and physical examination, a forensic evidence collection kit ("rape kit") can provide evidence of sexual contact and identify the assailant if DNA is isolated. Evidence is more likely to be obtained soon after the assault with the majority of positive kits obtained within 24 hours, especially in pre-pubertal children. Forensic evidence collection is recommended for cases of assault with possibility of DNA transmission (semen, blood, or saliva) up to 72 hours from the assault, although some practitioners or jurisdictions are moving to a threshold of up to 7 days based on newer polymerase chain reaction (PCR)-based techniques.[89] Beyond 24 hours, specimens from the child's clothing are the most likely to retain evidence. Obtaining the child's underwear (even if not worn at the time of the assault) can recover DNA evidence beyond 24 hours and is relatively noninvasive. Although many kits require documentation of whether a child has eaten, defecated, urinated, or wiped prior to evidence collection, children should not be asked to defer these activities in service of evidence collection, and these considerations should not impact the decision to collect evidence.

Pregnancy testing is routinely obtained in pubertal females because emergency contraception (levonorgestrel or ulipristal; Plan B) is ineffective for established pregnancies. STI testing is undertaken for symptomatic patients or in cases with potential for subacute or chronic abuse. Determining which tests to obtain depends on the details of the child's potential exposure and their physical examination, as well as local disease prevalence, patient and parent preferences, and the availability of timely follow-up. In cases with concern for drug-facilitated sexual assault, blood (within 24 hours) or urine (within 120 hours), samples should be obtained and included in the evidence collection kit.[90] Emergency clinicians may benefit from case-by-case consultation with child abuse pediatrics or infectious disease colleagues.

In adolescents and adults, the prevalence of STIs is high enough to warrant routine screening for gonorrhea, chlamydia, and trichomoniasis using nucleic acid amplification testing (NAAT) methods, if acceptable to the patient. NAAT has improved sensitivity, lower cost, and can be collected more easily, relative to traditional cultures.[85,86,91] NAAT testing for gonorrhea and chlamydia has been endorsed by the Centers for Disease Control and Prevention (CDC) for urine or vaginal specimens in girls.[79,86] STI prevalence in pre-pubertal assault victims is lower (5% to 8%). The AAP recommends NAAT testing for gonorrhea, chlamydia, and trichomoniasis in pre-pubertal children when there is:[85-87,92]

- Penetration of the vagina or anus
- Abuse by a stranger
- Known STI or high-risk behavior (IV drug use, men who have sex with men, multiple sexual partners) in the perpetrator
- Contact of a child with a known STI
- Signs or symptoms of STI
- Prior diagnosis of another STI
- Reasonable need by the patient or family for reassurance

Currently, there are no guidelines to direct testing for syphilis, hepatitis B or C, or HIV in children following sexual assault. We recommend testing in children with any of the above risk factors, or with high community prevalence or incomplete hepatitis B vaccination. Initial screening for syphilis should be by rapid plasma reagin (RPR); hepatitis B screening should include hepatitis B surface antigen and hepatitis B virus (HBV) immunoglobulin M (IgM) core antibody. Testing for HIV and hepatitis B and C should be repeated 6, 12, and 24 weeks after sexual contact.[86]

MANAGEMENT

ED management should focus on the most time-dependent interventions: mandated reporting and PEP for pregnancy and HIV. When there is a reasonable concern for sexual abuse, reporting to CPS is mandatory for emergency clinicians in the United States, Canada, and many other countries. Some caregivers may strongly desire a report, even when the

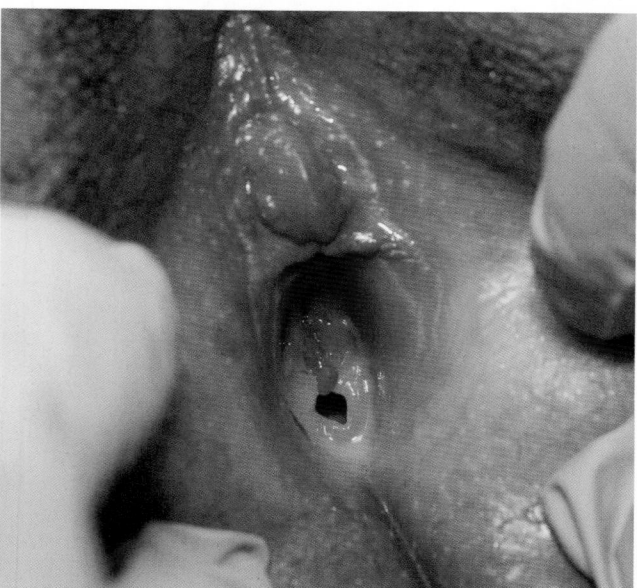

Fig. 172.20 Urethral prolapse. (Courtesy John Melville, MD.)

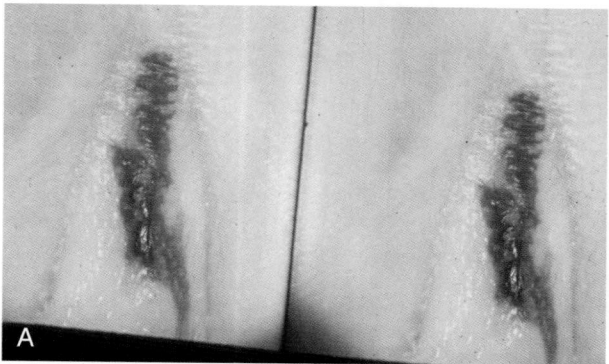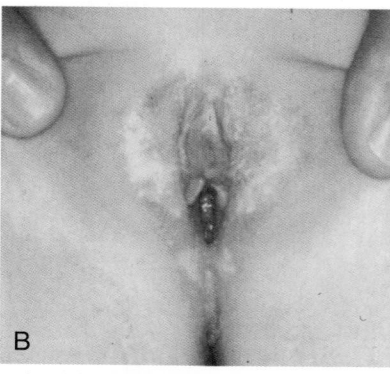

Fig. 172.21 (A and B) Lichen sclerosis. (Courtesy Carol Berkowitz, MD.)

TABLE 172.5 Indications to Offer Testing and Treatment in Cases With Concern for Sexual Abuse

Test/Intervention	Indication
Pregnancy testing	Pubertal females
Gonorrhea/chlamydia/trichomonas testing (NAAT)	All pubertal children
	Report of vaginal or anal penetration
	Physical examination findings of sexual contact or ejaculation
	Abuse by a stranger
	Symptoms of STI, or diagnosed STI in the patient or a contact child
	Known STI or risk in suspected assailant
	Patient or parent request
HBV, HCV, HIV, syphilis testing	As for gonorrhea (above) or:
	Absent or incomplete vaccination for hepatitis B
	High community prevalence
Forensic evidence collection ("rape kit")	Potential for DNA transmission (blood, semen, saliva)
	Abuse within 72 hours (or longer depending on local statutes)
Levonorgestrel (Plan B)	Non-pregnant, pubertal females <72 hours from assault
Ulipristal (Ella)	Non-pregnant, pubertal females <120 hours from assault
Empirical treatment for gonorrhea/chlamydia/trichomonas	Pubertal children
	Avoid treatment in pre-pubertal children without confirmation of infection
HIV PEP	Depends on local prevalence and case-specific details
	Consider consultation with infectious diseases or CDC hotline (800-933-3413)
Report to children's services	Reasonable concern for abuse

HBV, Hepatitis B virus; *HCV,* hepatitis C virus; *HIV,* human immunodeficiency virus; *PEP,* post-exposure prophylaxis; *STI,* sexually transmitted infection.

findings do not meet the threshold of a reasonable concern for abuse (as when the child presents for isolated nonspecific redness of the genitalia without a disclosure of abuse). Should the emergency clinician opt not to report these cases, caregivers can be advised that they have the option to report their concerns to CPS directly, independent of the health care provider.

Levonorgestrel (Plan B) should be offered to pubertal females within 72 hours (3 days) or ulipristal within <120 hours (5 days) of sexual assault. When taken within 72 hours, it can prevent up to 50% of pregnancies, although there is some potential to prevent pregnancy up to 120 hours after sexual assault. Because it works by suppressing ovulation, patients can be reassured that it will not terminate an established pregnancy.

The decision to offer PEP for HIV is complex and depends on the nature, timing, and likelihood of the sexual assault; local prevalence of HIV; and likelihood that the perpetrator is HIV positive. Although rates of HIV transmission in the course of sexual abuse are probably low, cases of HIV in children whose only risk factor is abuse have been reported.[86] Post-exposure prophylaxis is not effective if administered more than 72 hours after the assault. Consultation with infectious diseases specialists may be useful, and the CDC maintains a national telephone consultation service (1-800-933-3413) to provide real-time expert consultation to emergency clinicians with questions about HIV PEP.

Prophylaxis or empiric treatment for gonorrhea, chlamydia, and trichomonas should be offered to pubertal children but should be deferred for pre-pubertal children.[16] In pre-pubertal children, consensual sexual activity is impossible by definition, rates of STD are low, ascending infection is very uncommon, and follow-up is usually obtainable. For these reasons, the medical consequences of delayed treatment are low, but the forensic significance can be profound. Because infection with gonorrhea, chlamydia, or trichomonas is usually strong evidence of sexual abuse in pre-pubertal children, proof of infection can be essential to ensure the child's protection from ongoing abuse. Treatment prior to obtaining proof of infection can limit confirmatory testing and thwart protection efforts.

DISPOSITION

The vast majority of children evaluated for sexual abuse in the ED can be discharged to follow-up as outpatients. Follow-up is needed to arrange subsequent STI testing, ensure completion of HPV or hepatitis B vaccination, assess tolerance of HIV PEP, and arrange for mental health care. Medically stable patients can be discharged to a safe environment after obtaining appropriate testing and evidence collection. When the alleged assailant is a member of the child's household, CPS can arrange safety planning to ensure that a child has a safe place for discharge or that the alleged assailant is removed from the child's home.

The references for this chapter can be found online at ExpertConsult.com.

173

Complications of Pregnancy

Megan C. Henn and Michelle D. Lall

Acute complications of pregnancy can appear in all trimesters and pose challenges in diagnosis and management for the emergency clinician. Life-threatening disorders, such as ectopic pregnancy in early pregnancy, pregnancy-induced hypertension in mid to late pregnancy, and abruptio placentae in late pregnancy, are relatively common. Emergency clinicians must consider the signs and symptoms, stage of pregnancy, and hemodynamic stability of the patient in developing diagnostic and treatment strategies.

PROBLEMS IN EARLY PREGNANCY

Miscarriage Foundations

Miscarriage, the most common serious complication of pregnancy, is defined as the spontaneous termination of pregnancy before 20 weeks of gestation. Fetal demise after 20 weeks of gestation or when the fetus is more than 500 g is considered premature birth. Early pregnancy loss is defined as a nonviable, intrauterine pregnancy with either an empty gestational sac or gestational sac containing an embryo or fetus without fetal cardiac activity within the first 12 weeks and 6 days of gestation.

Early pregnancy loss is common, with 80% occurring in the first trimester, and it is seen in 10% of recognized pregnancies.[1] This estimation is likely low because it is difficult to measure those pregnancies lost before clinically confirmed but still recognized by the patient. Embryonic and fetal loss after implantation occur in up to one-third of detectable pregnancies. The risk of miscarriage rises with increasing maternal age (a fivefold increase in those >40 years compared with those 25 to 29 years), increasing paternal age, alcohol use, increased parity, history of prior miscarriage, poorly controlled diabetes mellitus and thyroid disease, obesity, low pre-pregnancy body mass index, maternal stress, smoking, alcohol, and caffeine consumption, and history of vaginal bleeding.

Approximately 25% of pregnant patients experience some bleeding. It is estimated that up to 50% of all women who have bleeding during early pregnancy miscarry before 20 weeks' gestation, although the risk is probably higher in the emergency department (ED) population.[2] Patients who have an intrauterine pregnancy with fetal cardiac activity visualized on ultrasound examination have a much lower risk of miscarriage (3% to 6%), although vaginal bleeding is a high-risk indicator, even when a viable fetus is present.[3] Those with a history of bleeding in singleton pregnancies who do not miscarry may have otherwise normal pregnancies, although they have an increased risk for preterm premature rupture of membranes, abruption, previa, stillbirth, and congenital abnormalities.[2]

Pathophysiology

Most miscarriages are due to uterine malformations or chromosomal abnormalities, which account for the majority that occur within 10 weeks of gestation. In some cases, the ovum never develops (anembryonic gestation). In most early miscarriages, fetal death precedes clinical miscarriage, often by several weeks. Although clinical symptoms of miscarriages are most common between 8 and 12 weeks of gestation, sonographic evidence in most cases demonstrates death before 8 weeks; if fetal viability can be demonstrated by cardiac activity and a normal sonogram, the subsequent risk of fetal loss decreases significantly.

Maternal factors that increase the risk of miscarriage include age greater than 30 years, congenital anatomic defects, uterine scarring, leiomyomas, and cervical incompetence. Other conditions associated with increased miscarriage rates include toxins (e.g., alcohol, tobacco, and cocaine), autoimmune factors, endocrine disorders, a prior history of miscarriage, and maternal infections.

Terminology

Miscarriage is broadly divided into four categories. The first is a *threatened miscarriage*, in which the patient presents with vaginal bleeding but is found to have a closed internal cervical os. The risk of miscarriage in this population is estimated at 35% to 50%, depending on the patient's risk factors and severity of symptoms. The second category is an *inevitable miscarriage* when the internal os is open. The third is an *incomplete miscarriage*, where the products of conception are present at the cervical os or in the vaginal canal. The last category is a *completed miscarriage*, which occurs when the uterus has expelled all fetal and placental material, the cervix is closed, and the uterus is contracted. A gestational sac should be visualized for diagnosis because the cervix may close after an episode of heavy bleeding and clot passage without or after only partial expulsion of the products of conception. Unless an intact gestational sac is passed and recognized, a completed miscarriage is diagnosed only after dilation and curettage (D&C) with pathologic confirmation of gestational products, demonstration by sonography of an empty uterus with a prior known intrauterine pregnancy (IUP), or reversion to a negative pregnancy test result. This may take up to several weeks after the initial presentation.

Missed abortion is a relatively obsolete term referring to the clinical failure of uterine growth over time. Instead, the terms *anembryonic gestation* (when no fetus is visualized on ultrasound), *first-* or *second-trimester fetal death* (failure to see fetal cardiac activity with at least a 5-mm crown-rump length), and *delayed miscarriage* are more appropriate.

Clinical Features

Patient history should include the estimated length of the gestation, time since the last menstrual period, symptoms of pregnancy, including evolution or loss of pregnancy symptoms, degree and duration of bleeding, presence of cramps, pain, or fever, and attempts by the patient to induce miscarriage. Although the history is important, it is not helpful in the classification of the type of miscarriage. In addition, the severity of symptoms does not correlate well with the risk of miscarriage, although cramping and passage of clots are thought more likely to occur as the miscarriage becomes inevitable.

The assessment of the patient who experiences first-trimester vaginal bleeding includes a careful abdominal examination to evaluate for tenderness or peritoneal irritation from a potential ectopic pregnancy and to determine the size of the uterus, which should not be palpable abdominally. A pelvic examination is performed to evaluate whether the cervix is closed or open, look for clots or the products of conception, determine the degree of vaginal bleeding, and assess uterine size and tenderness.

In the patient with second- and third-trimester bleeding, cervical probing should not be done because the uterus is more vascular, and the organized placenta may overlie the cervical os. Parous women normally have an open or lax external os, which is a finding of no significance. The adnexa may be enlarged, often unilaterally, because the corpus luteum is cystic or because the pregnancy is ectopic. Adnexal or uterine tenderness should always raise the possibility of an ectopic pregnancy. Much less commonly, pelvic inflammatory disease can cause uterine and adnexal tenderness during early pregnancy.

Differential Diagnoses

Ectopic pregnancy can masquerade as a miscarriage in the early stages of pregnancy and should always be considered in the differential diagnosis. Even in the patient with painless vaginal bleeding, the diagnosis of ectopic pregnancy must be considered. Early ultrasonography is indicated to locate the pregnancy in the patient who has bleeding or pain.

A small amount of bleeding occurs at the time of implantation of the blastocyst into the endometrium and, occasionally, at the time of the first missed menses. Molar pregnancy is also characterized by vaginal bleeding, usually during the late first trimester or second trimester. This condition can be identified by ultrasonography. Cervical and vaginal lesions can also cause local bleeding and can usually be seen on vaginal inspection.

TABLE 173.1 Landmarks for Gestational Age and β-hCG Level by Transvaginal Ultrasonography

Finding	Weeks From LMP	β-hCG (mIU/mL)
Gestational sac (25 mm)	5	1000
Discriminatory zone	5–6	1000–2000
Yolk sac	6	2000
Upper discriminatory zone	6–7	3000
Fetal pole	7	5700
Fetal heart motion	6–7	7000

β-hCG, Beta subunit of human chorionic gonadotropin; *LMP*, last menstrual period.
Adapted from: Ramsey E, Shilitto J. How early can fetal heart pulsations be detected reliably using modern ultrasound equipment? *Ultrasound.* 2008;16:193-195; and Sohoni A, Bosley J, Miss JC. Bedside ultrasonography for obstetric and gynecologic emergencies. *Crit Care Clin.* 2014 Apr;30(2):207-226.

BOX 173.1 Sonographic Criteria for Abnormal Pregnancy With Transvaginal Ultrasonography

No gestational sac at β-hCG level of 3000 mIU/mL
No yolk sac with gestational sac of 13 mm (or at 32 days since last menstrual period)
5-mm crown-rump length, with no fetal heart tones
No fetus, with gestational sac of 25 mm mean diameter
No fetal heart tones after gestational age of 10–12 wk
β-hCG, Beta subunit of human chorionic gonadotropin.

Adapted from: Dart RG. Role of pelvic ultrasonography in evaluation of symptomatic first-trimester pregnancy. *Ann Emerg Med.* 1999;33:310-320.

Diagnostic Testing

A hemoglobin level is useful to provide a baseline measurement and evaluate the degree of blood loss in women whose bleeding persists. In addition, the Rh type should be determined. Ultrasonography is the primary means of evaluating the health of the fetus as well as its location (Table 173.1). Because historical and clinical estimations of gestational age are often inaccurate, ultrasonography is useful to provide an accurate measure of fetal age and viability (Box 173.1).

Serial quantitative hCG levels are used to assess the health of the fetus if sonographic findings are indeterminate or if the gestational age is less than 6 to 7 weeks. The sonographic discriminatory zone is defined as the quantitative hCG level at which a normally developing IUP should reliably be seen. Discriminatory levels are operator- and equipment-dependent and vary by individual patient characteristics, but are usually considered to be 6500 mIU/mL for transabdominal ultrasonography and 1000 to 2000 mIU/mL for transvaginal ultrasonography. Ultrasonography can be performed or repeated when hCG levels rise to 1500 to 3000 mIU/mL. If hCG levels are level or decline, or if sonographic criteria for fetal demise are demonstrated (Box 173.1), the patient should be referred to an obstetrician for follow-up to ensure miscarriage completion and to assess for subsequent complications. Expectant management may be sufficient in the stable patient with threatened miscarriage, as long as ectopic pregnancy has been excluded.

Management and Disposition

Threatened Miscarriage. After assessment of hemodynamic status and management of blood loss, a patient with a threatened miscarriage requires very little specific medical treatment. Though expert opinions vary as to whether anti-D immune globulin should be administered to Rh-negative patients after a threatened or spontaneous miscarriage, we recommend administering anti-D immune globulin in the ED to all pregnant patients with bleeding. If anti-D immune globulin is administered, a 50-µg to 120-µg dose is used during the first trimester and a full 300-µg dose after the first trimester. Once evaluated for ectopic pregnancy, the need for a follow-up routine ultrasonogram should be discussed with the patient; the patient should be made aware that the potential for ectopic pregnancy exists until it is excluded by identification of an IUP. In the patient who is planning pregnancy termination, prompt referral should be encouraged and chorionic villi confirmed at the time of uterine evacuation.

Unless an IUP is diagnosed, the patient with threatened miscarriage should be given careful instructions on discharge to return if she has signs of hemodynamic instability, pain, or other symptoms that might indicate ectopic pregnancy. In conjunction with gynecologic colleagues, an ED protocol is useful to determine when follow-up sonographic evaluation and serial hCG measurements should be obtained since ultrasonography can be an inaccurate diagnostic tool if the hCG level is below 1500 mIU/mL, vaginal bleeding is significant, or sonographic findings do not include a fetal pole or yolk sac. The patient must be given explicit return precautions and close obstetrical follow-up is essential. Typically, serial hCG measurements are obtained between 48 to 72 hours after the initial ED visit and follow-up sonographic evaluation is obtained within 3 to 7 days of ED presentation.

Fifty percent or more of women with threatened miscarriage who are seen in the ED ultimately miscarry, and there is no proven treatment to prevent miscarriage. In most cases, spontaneous miscarriage is the body's natural method of expelling an abnormal or undeveloped (blighted) pregnancy. Thus, a major goal of early management should be patient education and support. Patients should be advised that moderate daily activities do not affect the pregnancy. Tampons, intercourse, and other activities that might induce uterine infection should be avoided as long as the patient is bleeding, and she should return immediately for fever, abdominal pain, or an increase in bleeding. Cramping from a known IUP can be safely treated with acetaminophen or oral synthetic narcotics, if needed. If the patient passes tissue, it should be brought to a provider to be examined for products of conception because differentiation of fetal parts or villi from decidual slough or casts is difficult.

Patient counseling is paramount with threatened miscarriage and education of the ED staff on this topic is critical. Determination of fetal viability can be helpful in reassuring the mother or preparing her for probable fetal loss. Miscarriages are associated with a grieving process, which is frequently more difficult because early pregnancy is unannounced, and early fetal death is not publicly recognized. Because many women consider that minor falls, injuries, or stress during the first trimester can precipitate miscarriage, patients should be reassured that they have done nothing to cause miscarriage. Patients should be made aware that miscarriage is common, grieving is normal, and counseling may be beneficial. A follow-up appointment should be scheduled after miscarriage to support the patient in resolving such issues.

Incomplete Miscarriage. Treatment of the patient with incomplete miscarriage includes expectant management, medical management, or surgical evacuation. When the miscarriage is incomplete, the uterus may be unable to contract adequately to limit bleeding from the implantation site. Bleeding may be brisk, and gentle removal of fetal tissue from the cervical os with ring forceps during the pelvic examination often slows bleeding considerably. Manual uterine aspiration performed in the ED may also be appropriate in cases of brisk uterine hemorrhage as a result of early pregnancy loss or retained products of conception up to 12 weeks gestational age.[4]

Completed Miscarriage. Management of patients with presumed completed miscarriage is more complicated. If the patient brings passed tissue with her, this should be sent to the pathology department for evaluation. Unless an intact gestational sac or fetus is visualized, it is rarely clear clinically whether miscarriage is complete. In women with a history consistent with miscarriage who have minimal remaining intrauterine tissue as determined by ultrasonography, expectant management is safe, but only if ectopic pregnancy can be excluded. If endometrial tissue is not seen with ultrasonography, bleeding is mild, and gestational age is less than 8 weeks, curettage is frequently unnecessary, and the patient can be safely observed by a gynecologist for serial hormonal assays. It is estimated that 65% of women with first-trimester miscarriage complete the miscarriage without intervention.[5] However, the need for later visits and procedures may be decreased by uterine curettage, particularly if the fetal pole or a gestational sac is visible on the sonogram at the time of evaluation. Medical management with misoprostol (800 µg intravaginal for one dose) instead of dilation and curettage is also an option and has a success rate of 80% to 91%.[5] The patient should be instructed to return if uncontrolled bleeding, severe pain or cramping, fever, or tissue passage occurs. Follow-up is recommended in 1 or 2 weeks to ensure that the miscarriage is complete.

After miscarriage, the patient should be advised that fetal loss can cause psychological stress. Follow-up in 1 or 2 weeks with a gynecologist should be provided. There is no conclusive evidence to support the use of antibiotics after D&C or miscarriage, and some evidence has suggested that the side effects of treatment may outweigh any potential benefit. For that reason, we do not recommend the routine use of antibiotics after a miscarriage. Ergonovine or methylergonovine (0.2 mg orally bid) can be used to stimulate uterine involution. The patient should be advised to return if signs of infection (e.g., fever, uterine tenderness) occur, bleeding resumes, or further tissue is passed.

Ectopic Pregnancy

KEY CONCEPTS

- An ectopic pregnancy can masquerade as a threatened miscarriage in the early stages of pregnancy and should always be considered in the differential diagnosis.
- Because the history and physical examination of the patient with ectopic pregnancy are insensitive and nonspecific, pelvic ultrasonography and determination of serum hCG levels are essential to locate the pregnancy in any patient who has abdominal pain or vaginal bleeding and a positive pregnancy test result.
- Ultrasonographic detection of an IUP is likely at hCG levels higher than 1500 to 2000 IU/L.

Foundations

Ectopic pregnancy is a pregnancy implanted outside the uterus, most commonly in the fallopian tube. It is increasing in frequency and the third leading cause of maternal death, responsible for 4% to 10% of cases.[6] Ectopic pregnancy is estimated to account for approximately 1% to 2% of all pregnancies, although national estimates of incidence are difficult to determine. Although the incidence of ectopic pregnancy is

Adapted from: Bouyer J, Coste J, Shojaei T, et al. Risk factors for ectopic pregnancy: A comprehensive analysis based on a large case-control, population-based study in France. *Am J Epidemiol.* 2003;157:185-194.

BOX 173.2 Risk Factors for Ectopic Pregnancy

Tubal surgery (for tubal sterilization or ectopic pregnancy)
Pelvic inflammatory disease
Smoking
Advanced age
Prior spontaneous abortion
Medically induced abortion
History of infertility
Intrauterine device

highest in women aged 25 to 34 years, the rate is highest among older women and women belonging to minority groups. Simultaneous intra-uterine and extrauterine gestations (heterotopic pregnancy) have historically been rare, occurring in approximately 1 in 4000 pregnancies; women who have undergone assisted reproduction techniques with embryo transfer are at high risk of one of the pregnancies being ectopic. The incidence of ectopic pregnancy among women presenting to the ED with vaginal bleeding or pain in the first trimester is approximately 10%, but may be as high as 16%.[7]

Pathophysiology

Implantation of the fertilized ovum occurs approximately 8 or 9 days after ovulation. Risk factors for an abnormal site of implantation include prior tubal infection (50% of cases), anatomic abnormalities of the fallopian tubes, assisted reproduction (especially multiple embryo transfers), and abnormal endometrium (host factors). This results in failure of the embryo to implant in the endometrium. The risk of ectopic pregnancy increases approximately threefold after a patient has had pelvic inflammatory disease (PID). If the patient is currently using an intrauterine device (IUD), increased risk can occur from complicating PID or from failure of the IUD to prevent pregnancy while preventing endometrial implantation. All forms of contraception, except the IUD and tubal sterilization, decrease the incidence of ectopic pregnancy. After an ectopic pregnancy, the risk of a subsequent ectopic pregnancy can be as high as 22%, depending on the characteristics and treatment of the ectopic pregnancy (e.g., location of implantation, surgical vs. medical management; Box 173.2).[8]

When abnormal implantation occurs in the fallopian tubes, on the ovaries, or in the cervix, the pregnancy usually grows at a less than normal rate, which can result in abnormally low or declining hCG production. Even if exceedingly low, a single hCG measurement cannot exclude the diagnosis of ectopic pregnancy. Blood leaks intermittently through the tubal wall or out the fimbrial ends, with spillage into the peritoneal cavity. Bleeding and other symptoms are usually intermittent. Three outcomes are possible: spontaneous involution of the pregnancy, tubal abortion into the peritoneal cavity or vagina, or rupture of the pregnancy with internal or vaginal bleeding. Implantation in the uterine horn (cornual pregnancy) is particularly dangerous because the growing embryo can use the myometrial blood supply to grow larger (10–14 weeks of gestation) before rupture occurs. Cornual pregnancy accounts for 2% to 4% of all ectopic pregnancies and can be difficult to identify by ultrasonography.[9]

Clinical Features

The classic clinical picture of ectopic pregnancy is a history of delayed menses, followed by abdominal pain and vaginal bleeding in a patient with known risk factors. Unfortunately, this history is neither sensitive nor specific. Risk factors for ectopic pregnancy are absent in almost half of patients. Of patients with symptomatic ectopic pregnancy, 15% to 20% have not missed a menstrual period, and occasionally the patient has no history of vaginal bleeding. Abdominal pain varies and can be described as crampy, intermittent, severe, or even absent.

The physical findings in ectopic pregnancy are likewise variable. Vaginal bleeding, uterine or adnexal tenderness, or both in the patient with a positive pregnancy test result should trigger consideration of ectopic pregnancy. Tachycardia is not always present, even with significant hemoperitoneum; the hemoglobin level is usually normal, and hypotension may be seen. The presence of peritoneal signs, cervical motion tenderness, or lateral or bilateral abdominal or pelvic tenderness indicates an increased likelihood of ectopic pregnancy. If peritoneal irritation is present, pain can preclude an accurate bimanual examination. Adnexal masses are palpated in only 10% to 20% of patients with ectopic pregnancy.

Vaginal bleeding is often mild. Heavy bleeding with clots or tissue usually suggests a threatened or incomplete miscarriage, although the patient with an ectopic pregnancy who has decreasing hormonal levels may experience endometrial sloughing, which can be mistaken for passage of fetal tissue. Passed tissue should be examined, as with cases of miscarriage, in tap water or saline (or under low-power microscopy). Unless fetal parts or chorionic villi are seen, ectopic pregnancy should not be excluded in the patient with bleeding or passage of tissue.

Differential Diagnoses

The spectrum of clinical presentations in ectopic pregnancy is wide, so the differential diagnosis includes essentially all first-trimester complications. Threatened miscarriage, the most common alternative diagnosis, can be recognized by sonographic evidence of an IUP, healthy or failed. Hypovolemia may be seen, particularly in incomplete miscarriage, but hypotension without significant vaginal hemorrhage is highly suggestive of ectopic pregnancy. Identification of fetal parts or chorionic villi in tissue expelled or obtained during D&C is useful to confirm a complication of IUP, although this is not sufficient to exclude ectopic pregnancy in a patient with an increased risk of heterotopic gestation, such as the patient undergoing assisted reproduction treatment.

A ruptured corpus luteum cyst should also be considered in the first trimester when bleeding is associated with peritoneal pain or irritation. The corpus luteum normally supports the pregnancy during the first 7 or 8 weeks. Rupture causes pelvic pain and peritoneal irritation. Ultrasonography is helpful if it reveals an IUP (except in patients with in vitro fertilization). During early gestation, when ultrasonography is nondiagnostic, free fluid is usually visible by ultrasonography, and serial observation may be required. If the patient is unstable, especially if an IUP cannot be identified by ultrasonography, laparoscopy or in rare cases laparotomy, may be required to differentiate between the two conditions.

Diagnostic Testing

Because the history and physical examination of the patient with ectopic pregnancy are insensitive and nonspecific, ancillary studies are essential to locate the pregnancy in any patient who has abdominal pain or vaginal bleeding and a positive pregnancy test result. Ultrasonography and hormonal assays are the most commonly used ancillary tests and advances in these technologies have allowed for more accurate detection and exclusion of ectopic pregnancy in patients with first trimester bleeding or pelvic pain. Laparoscopy may be the most efficient diagnostic tool in the hemodynamically unstable patient.

Ultrasonography. Ultrasonography is the primary method used to locate early gestation, establish gestational age, and assess fetal viability.

Transabdominal ultrasonography is most useful for identification of IUPs with fetal cardiac activity and exclusion of ectopic pregnancy, except in patients at high risk for heterotopic pregnancy because of infertility procedures. Transvaginal ultrasonography is more sensitive, recognizes IUP earlier than transabdominal ultrasonography, and is diagnostic in up to 80% of stable patients presenting in the first trimester. Transvaginal ultrasound requires operator training and can be limited by device availability and quality.

As home pregnancy tests and access to early ultrasound becomes more prominent, the risk of having a "pregnancy of unknown location" by ultrasound rises. Indeterminate sonograms, which demonstrate neither an IUP nor extrauterine findings suggestive of ectopic pregnancy, occur in approximately 20% of ED evaluations of women with first-trimester bleeding or pain. Ectopic pregnancy is more likely among this subgroup with indeterminate sonograms if the hCG level is less than 1000 mIU/mL and the uterus is empty. Endometrial debris and fluid in the uterus do not exclude ectopic pregnancy.

An indeterminate ultrasound study usually does not result in a diagnosis of normal pregnancy. In one series of more than 1000 pelvic ultrasound examinations, 53% of indeterminate ultrasound studies resulted in a diagnosis of embryonic demise, 15% were ectopic pregnancies, and only 29% had an IUP. However, correlation of sonographic results with quantitative hCG measurements can add to the predictive value. With no intrauterine pregnancy on transvaginal ultrasound and hCG greater than 1500 mIU/mL, ectopic pregnancy should be suspected keeping in mind that ectopic pregnancies can be discovered at any level of hCG. Normal pregnancy is unlikely if no gestational sac is seen by transvaginal ultrasonography with an hCG level higher than 1000 to 2000 mIU/mL, depending on the institution's discriminatory zone. Additional ultrasound findings that may predict early spontaneous abortion include crown rump length or fetal heart rate below the fifth percentile and fetal heart rate below 130 beats per minute.[10] The differential diagnosis includes miscarriage and ectopic pregnancy in these patients. Unfortunately, levels of approximately 1500 mIU/mL develop in only approximately 50% of patients with ectopic pregnancies (see Table 173.1). Sonographic findings in a patient with suspected ectopic pregnancy are listed in Box 173.3 and illustrated in Figures 173.1 to 173.5.

Hormonal Assays. Quantitative hCG levels serve two primary functions—serial levels can be used in the stable patient who can be observed as an outpatient, and a single level can be correlated with sonographic results for improved interpretation. Beginning 8 or 9 days after ovulation, serum hCG levels normally double every 1.8 to 3 days for the first 6 or 7 weeks of pregnancy. An initial quantitative level can be measured at the time of the ED visit, particularly if the sonogram is indeterminate or gestational age is estimated as less than 6 weeks. A repeated level should be measured 48 to 72 hours later. A doubling or rise of hCG by 66% generally indicates a viable intrauterine pregnancy, however approximately 15% of normal IUPs have a minimal rise in hCG, requiring a third serial test. A rapid decline in hCG tends to indicate miscarriage whereas a slow decline can indicate an ectopic pregnancy.

Single quantitative hCG levels can also be useful in conjunction with ultrasonography; normal IUPs should be visible transvaginally at 1000 to 2000 mIU/mL hCG or higher (see Table 173.1). A benign course for ectopic pregnancy cannot be assumed with low hCG levels. Ruptured ectopic pregnancies requiring surgery have been reported with very low or absent levels of hCG.

Serum progesterone levels have been studied as an additional or alternative marker to determine which patients need further evaluation and follow-up for possible ectopic pregnancy though it is not a standard tool in the ED. The progesterone level rises earlier than the

---

BOX 173.3 Sonographic Findings in the Patient With Suspected Ectopic Pregnancy

Diagnostic of Intrauterine Pregnancy
"Double" gestational sac
Intrauterine fetal pole or yolk sac
Intrauterine fetal heart activity

Diagnostic of Ectopic Gestation
Pregnancy in fallopian tube (see Fig. 173.1)
Ectopic fetal heart activity (see Fig. 173.2)
Ectopic fetal pole

Suggestive of Ectopic Gestation
Moderate or large cul-de-sac fluid without intrauterine pregnancy
Adnexal mass without intrauterine pregnancy[a]

Indeterminate
Empty uterus (see Fig. 173.3)
Nonspecific fluid collections (see Fig. 173.4)
Echogenic material
Abnormal sac (see Fig. 173.5)
Single gestational sac

[a] A complex mass is the most suggestive of ectopic pregnancy, but a cyst can also be seen with ectopic pregnancy.
Adapted from: Dart RG. Role of pelvic ultrasonography in evaluation of symptomatic first-trimester pregnancy. *Ann Emerg Med.* 1999;33:310-320.

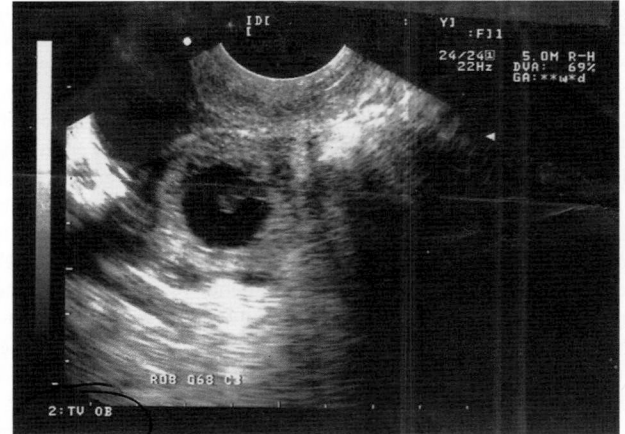

Fig. 173.1 Pregnancy in the fallopian tube, diagnostic of an ectopic pregnancy. (Courtesy Dr. Mary Ann Edens.)

hCG level in normal pregnancy and plateaus with levels higher than 20 ng/mL, so measurement of serial levels over time is not necessary. Levels below 5 ng/mL exclude a viable IUP with rare exceptions and can be used in combination with serum hCG ratios at presentation and 48 hours. Patients determined to have low risk of ectopic pregnancy by this algorithm can avoid additional testing and be managed conservatively.[11] A progesterone level should be sent when the hCG levels are low, ultrasonography is indeterminate, and the emergency clinician is considering consultation for D&C or laparoscopy.

Other Studies. Dilation and evacuation can be used in patients without a viable IUP or ectopic pregnancy on ultrasonography to differentiate intrauterine miscarriage from ectopic pregnancy. Identification of chorionic villi in endometrial samples is seen in approximately 70% of patients and excludes ectopic pregnancy, except in patients undergoing assisted reproduction. Identification of chorionic villi can be made, even in 50% of women with an empty uterus on ultrasonography, and limits the need for laparoscopy to exclude ectopic pregnancy in this population.

Although it is invasive, laparoscopy is extremely accurate as a diagnostic (and therapeutic) procedure for possible ectopic pregnancy. It is the diagnostic treatment of choice in unstable first-trimester patients with peritoneal signs and is also indicated in patients with peritoneal fluid or an ectopic gestation in the pelvic cavity. Medical alternatives for the management of ectopic pregnancy have resulted in decreased indications for laparoscopy in stable patients.

Management and Disposition

Unstable Patients. Approximately 20% of women with ectopic pregnancies manifest signs and symptoms warranting immediate intervention. This includes patients with hypovolemia, large amounts of peritoneal fluid, or an open cervical os. For patients with signs of hypovolemia, rapid volume resuscitation should be instituted with intravenous (IV) fluids and blood products as necessary, and a baseline hemoglobin level and type and crossmatch should be obtained. If the patient remains unstable, immediate surgery is warranted. Laparoscopy may be indicated for patients who stabilize with treatment or those who are hemodynamically stable but exhibit peritoneal signs on abdominal

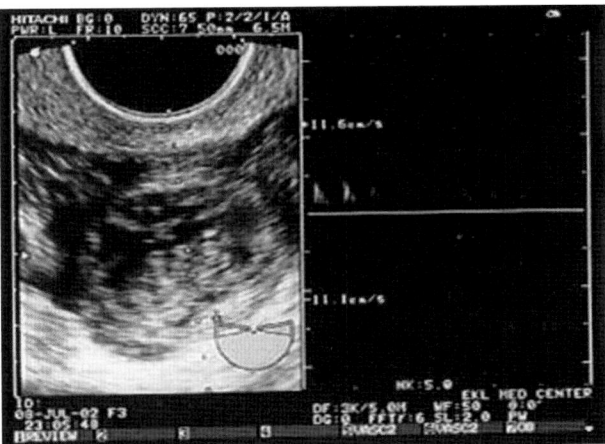

Fig. 173.2 Fetal heart movements detected by ultrasonography in the fallopian tube, diagnostic of an ectopic pregnancy. (Courtesy Dr. Mary Ann Edens.)

examination. One study has reported that identification of free fluid in the Morison pouch on bedside ultrasonography predicts the need for operative intervention in most cases in patients with suspected ectopic pregnancies. A D&C or evacuation procedure with examination of the endometrial contents for products of conception can be performed urgently in the unstable patient with an open cervical os. All patients with ectopic pregnancy who are Rh-negative should be given Rh immune globulin, 50 µg intramuscularly.

Stable Patients. In stable patients with first-trimester bleeding, the goal is to exclude ectopic pregnancy in a timely manner. In the patient with pain by history or examination or risk factors for ectopic pregnancy, ultrasonography should be performed before discharge.

In low-risk patients with minor symptoms or bleeding, ectopic pregnancy is still a possibility. In most cases, ultrasonography is the initial screening tool because it provides the most accurate and rapid information (Fig. 173.6). If an IUP is not seen, quantitative hCG levels help risk stratify these patients. In all cases, if the patient is discharged, careful instructions are given for symptoms that would require her earlier return. An alternative strategy uses hCG levels first. However, waiting times for the serum assay can increase ED length of stay. In addition, ultrasonography is usually diagnostic of IUP or ectopic pregnancy, even if the hCG level is less than 1000 mIU/mL.

A minority of patients have indeterminate sonographic results and hCG levels below 1000 mIU/mL. When the hCG levels never rise to the discriminatory zone, the differential diagnosis includes intrauterine fetal demise and ectopic pregnancy. Early D&C with identification of the products of conception can be useful in the patient with nonrising hCG levels to detect chorionic villi and confirm a failed IUP or strongly suggest ectopic pregnancy. Alternatively, hCG levels can be followed until they reach zero, particularly if initial levels are low.

Although laparotomy may be required for patients who have an ectopic pregnancy, an increasing number of surgeries are being performed through the laparoscope. Salpingostomy is preferred to salpingectomy if the patient is stable and the procedure is technically feasible. Overall, the advent of transvaginal ultrasonography has resulted in earlier diagnosis and a trend toward nonoperative management.

Medical management is a safe and cost-effective treatment for the stable patient with minimal symptoms, especially when future fertility is desired. Methotrexate (50 mg/m2 IM or 1 mg/kg IM, alternating with folinic acid) is the drug most commonly used to treat early ectopic pregnancy. It interferes with fetal DNA synthesis and causes destruction of rapidly dividing fetal cells and involution of the pregnancy. Medical treatment is used most often for patients who are hemodynamically stable, with a

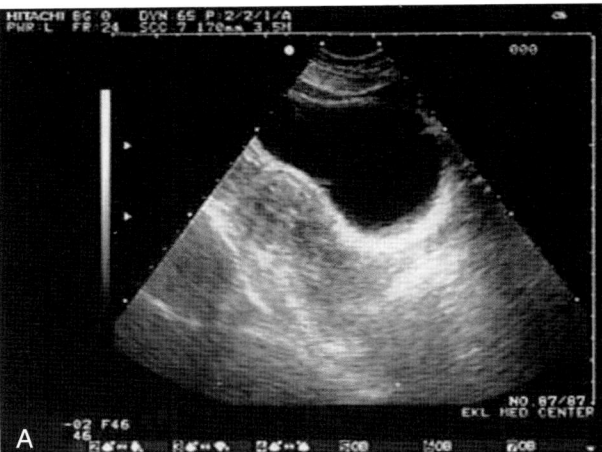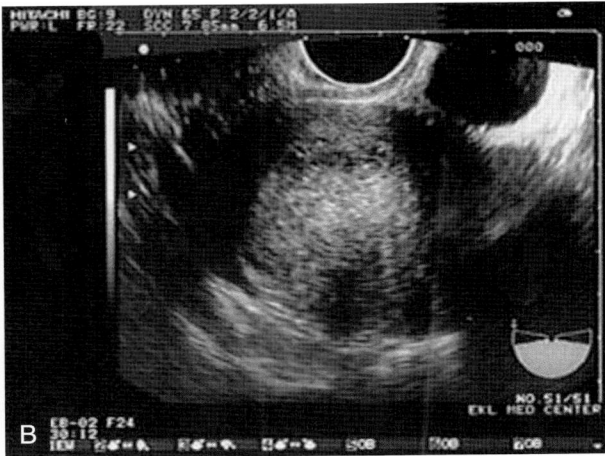

Fig. 173.3 Ultrasonogram showing an empty uterus, indeterminate for diagnosis of an ectopic pregnancy. (Courtesy Dr. Mary Ann Edens.)

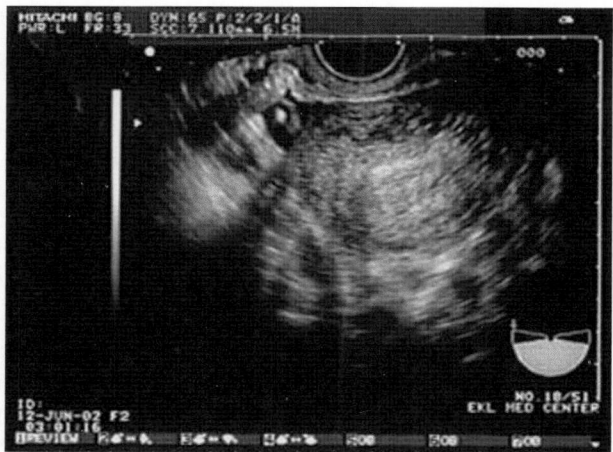

Fig. 173.4 Ultrasonogram showing fluid around the fallopian tube. (Courtesy Dr. Mary Ann Edens.)

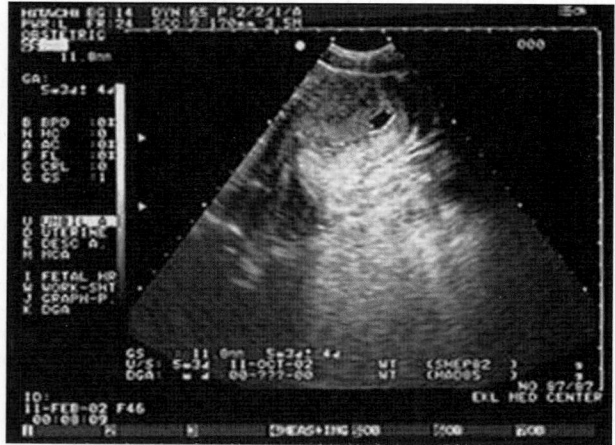

Fig. 173.5 Ultrasonogram showing a gestational pseudosac. (Courtesy Dr. Mary Ann Edens.)

tubal mass smaller than 3.5 cm in diameter, no fetal cardiac activity, and no sonographic evidence of rupture. Although there is no agreed on hCG cutoff for single-dose methotrexate, studies have suggested that increasing hCG levels are significantly correlated with methotrexate failure. Medical therapies are associated with an 85% to 93% success rate, with no significant difference between single- and multiple-dose protocols. Pelvic pain is common in patients receiving methotrexate (60%), even when it is used successfully. Indications of methotrexate failure and need for rescue surgery include decreasing hemoglobin levels, significant pelvic fluid, and unstable vital signs. All patients receiving methotrexate require close follow-up until the hCG level reaches 0, which may take 2 or 3 months.

Molar Pregnancy

Foundations

Molar pregnancy, also known as a hydatidiform mole, comprises a spectrum of diseases characterized by disordered proliferation of chorionic villi. In the absence of fetal tissue, the pregnancy is termed a *complete hydatidiform mole*. Complete moles are caused by the fertilization of an ovum without maternal DNA and the subsequent duplication of the haploid genome. The term *incomplete mole* refers to a mole that is caused by the fertilization of a normal ovum by two sperm. The duplication of the triploid karyotype causes some fetal tissue to be present, along with focal trophoblastic hyperplasia. In approximately

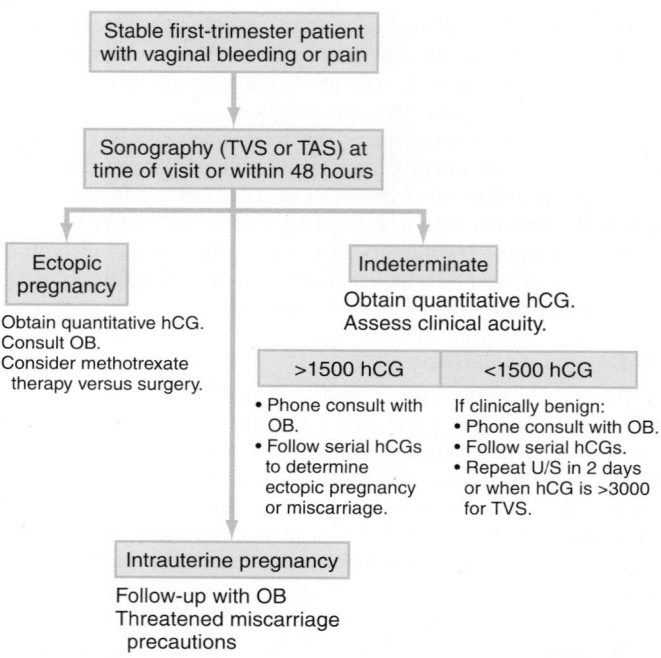

Fig. 173.6 Management of vaginal bleeding or pain in the stable first-trimester pregnant patient. *hCG*, Human chorionic gonadotropin; *OB*, obstetrics specialist; *TAS*, transabdominal sonography; *TVS*, transvaginal sonography; *U/S*, ultrasonography.

19% of molar pregnancies, neoplastic gestational disease develops, with persistence of molar tissue after the pregnancy has been evacuated.[12] Metastatic diseases can develop, requiring chemotherapy and intensive oncologic management.

Clinical Findings

Early molar pregnancy is usually not clinically apparent. The most well-described risk factor for the development of a molar pregnancy is extreme maternal age. Many patients present with abdominal pain, nausea and vomiting, or vaginal bleeding, and it may be difficult to differentiate these patients from those with threatened miscarriage or ectopic pregnancy by historical features alone. Patients sometimes seek treatment for apparent persistent hyperemesis gravidarum from high circulating levels of hCG, bleeding or intermittent bloody discharge, or respiratory distress; failure to hear fetal heart tones during the second trimester is the usual initial clue to diagnosis. If molar pregnancy spontaneously aborts, it is usually in the second trimester (before 20 weeks), and the patient or physician may note the passage of grapelike hydatid vesicles. Uterine size is larger than expected by date (by >4 weeks) in approximately 30% to 40% of patients. Theca lutein cysts may be present on the ovaries as a result of excessive hormonal stimulation, and torsion of affected ovaries can be seen.

Diagnostic Tests

The characteristic sonographic appearance of hydropic vesicles within the uterus, described as a snowstorm appearance, is highly suggestive of a diagnosis of molar pregnancy (Fig. 173.7). Alternatively, cystic changes are seen in partial molar pregnancies. In some cases, a partial molar pregnancy is detected only on pathologic examination of abortion specimens. Complications of molar pregnancy include preeclampsia or eclampsia, which can develop before 24 weeks of gestation, respiratory failure or distress from pulmonary embolization of trophoblastic cells, hyperemesis gravidarum, and uterine bleeding. Ultrasonography usually provides the diagnosis of a complete molar

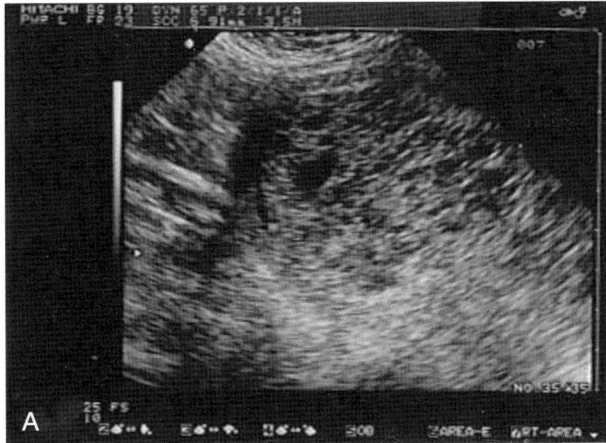

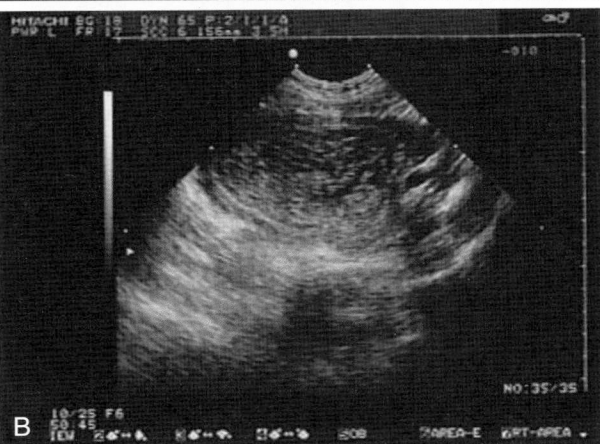

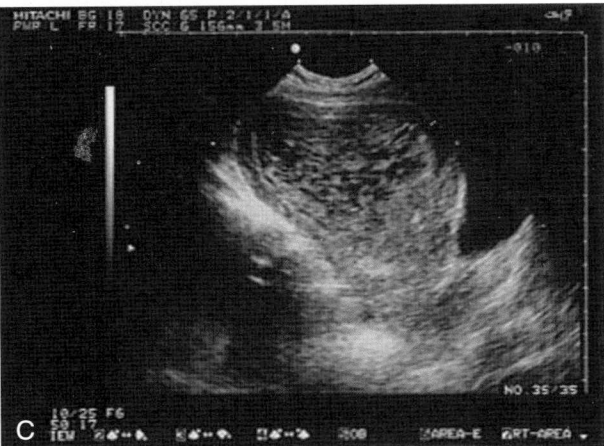

Fig. 173.7 Ultrasonogram showing molar pregnancy. (Courtesy Dr. Mary Ann Edens.)

pregnancy in the second-trimester patient who has "threatened miscarriage" or during sonographic assessment for fetal well-being and size. However, ultrasonography is only 58% sensitive, and diagnosis of a partial mole is made in only 17% of cases.[13] Up to two-thirds of molar pregnancies are diagnosed by pathologic specimens after miscarriage.

Management

Molar pregnancies are managed with uterine dilation and curettage (D&C). Following evacuation of a molar pregnancy, patients must be monitored in the outpatient setting for trophoblastic sequelae. Patients are at increased risk of an invasive mole, a benign tumor that invades

the uterine wall and metastasizes to the lungs or vagina, or choriocarcinoma, a malignant tumor that invades the uterine wall and metastasizes to the lungs, brain, and liver via the patient's vasculature. Patients who present to the ED with complications of bleeding metastases are managed with a combination of chemotherapy, radiation, and surgery.

COMPLICATIONS OF LATE PREGNANCY

Vaginal Bleeding in Later Pregnancy

KEY CONCEPTS

- Bleeding during the second trimester (14 to 24 weeks) is not benign and is associated with a 33% risk of fetal loss. Management is supportive and expectant because fetal rescue is impossible at this level of fetal immaturity.
- The major conditions associated with vaginal bleeding in the second half of pregnancy include abruptio placentae and placenta previa. Patient history, physical examination, and results of ultrasonography can be used to distinguish them.
- All patients with painless, second-trimester vaginal bleeding should be assumed to have placenta previa until proven otherwise. Digital or instrumental probing of the cervix should be avoided until the diagnosis has been excluded via ultrasound.
- Abruptio placentae consists of a wide spectrum of severity of symptoms and risk. Up to 20% of women will have no pain or vaginal bleeding. Assessment is generally based on clinical features, coagulation parameters, and signs of fetal distress.

Foundations

Bleeding during the second half of pregnancy occurs in approximately 4% of pregnancies. Only 20% of miscarriages occur after the first trimester, and the most important differential diagnoses after 12 to 14 weeks of gestation are abruptio placentae and placenta previa. The cause is often not determined, although occult marginal placental separations, which can be recognized only by placental inspection at delivery, are believed to come from a common source of bleeding above the cervix. Other causes of late vaginal bleeding include early labor, various cervical and vaginal lesions, lower genital tract infections, and hemorrhoids.

Bleeding during the second trimester before the fetus is potentially viable (14 to 24 weeks) is not benign. One-third of fetuses are ultimately lost when maternal bleeding occurs. Management is supportive and expectant because fetal rescue is not possible at this level of fetal immaturity. In the third trimester, vaginal bleeding is still associated with significant morbidity in approximately one-third of women; treatment includes consideration of urgent delivery.

Abruptio Placentae

Pathophysiology. Abruptio placentae is a separation of the placenta from the uterine wall and complicates roughly 1% of pregnancies. Small subclinical or marginal separations may go undetected until the placenta is examined at delivery and probably account for many of the other self-limited episodes of bleeding for which no diagnosis is made. In cases of nontraumatic abruptio placentae, spontaneous hemorrhage into the decidua basalis occurs, causing separation and compression of the adjacent placenta. Small amounts of bleeding may be asymptomatic and remain undetected until delivery. In other cases, the hematoma expands and extends the dissection. Bleeding may be concealed or may be clinically apparent if dissection occurs along the uterine wall and through the cervix. Placental separation may be acute or may be an indolent problem throughout late pregnancy.

Abruptio placentae is most clearly associated with maternal hypertension and preeclampsia. It is also more common with maternal age younger than 20 or older than 35 years of age, parity of three or more, unexplained infertility, history of smoking, thrombophilia, prior miscarriage, prior abruptio placentae, and cocaine use. Placental separation can also be associated with blunt trauma to the abdomen. In such cases, the cause appears to be shearing of a nonelastic placenta from the easily distorted elastic uterine wall at the time of traumatic impact. Intimate partner violence affects 4% to 8% of pregnancy and torso injuries are reported in 21.5% of cases placing the patient at risk for premature labor, abruption, uterine rupture, or fetal death. A significant etiology of trauma in pregnancy is motor vehicle accidents in which placental abruption may complication up to 40% of patients severely injured in a motor vehicle accident.[7]

Clinical Features. Vaginal bleeding occurs in 70% of patients with abruptio placentae. Blood is characteristically dark and the amount is often insignificant, although the mother may have hemodynamic evidence of blood loss. Uterine tenderness or pain is seen in approximately two-thirds of women; uterine irritability or contractions are seen in one-third. With significant placental separation, fetal distress occurs and the maternal coagulation cascade may be triggered, causing disseminated intravascular coagulation (DIC).

There is a wide spectrum of severity of symptoms and risk in placental separation. About 10% of women will present only with occult bleeding. Assessment is generally based on clinical features, coagulation parameters, and signs of fetal distress. Mild abruption is characterized by slight vaginal bleeding, little or no uterine irritability, absence of signs of fetal distress, and normal coagulation. As the separation becomes more extensive, it is associated with increased vaginal bleeding (or hidden maternal blood loss), increased uterine irritability with or without tetanic contractions, declining fibrinogen levels, evidence of fetal distress, and maternal tachycardia. In severe abruptio placentae (15% of cases), the uterus is tetanically contracted and very painful, maternal hypotension results from visible or concealed uterine blood loss, fibrinogen levels are less than 150 mg/dL, and fetal death can occur. Ultrasonography is insensitive in the diagnosis of abruptio placentae, often because the echogenicity of fresh blood is similar to that of the placenta. Symptomatic or even fetus-threatening abruption can occur in the presence of a normal sonogram.

Fetal distress and death occur in approximately 15% of patients with abruptio placentae by interruption of placental blood and oxygen flow. Risk of fetal death increases in proportion to the percentage of the placental surface involved and rapidity of separation. Fetal distress may result from the loss of placental blood flow, associated maternal hemorrhage (into the uterine cavity or externally), increased uterine tone, or resultant DIC. Maternal death can result, usually from coagulopathy or exsanguination. Fetomaternal transfusion can occur. Placental separation also predisposes the mother to amniotic fluid embolism.

Differential Diagnoses. The main alternative diagnosis in the woman with late-pregnancy bleeding is placenta previa, which is usually associated with painless, bright red bleeding and is excluded with ultrasonography. Lower genital tract or rectal lesions and blood-tinged cervical mucous plug are also considerations.

In the patient with abdominal pain but no vaginal bleeding, abruptio placentae with concealed hemorrhage must be distinguished from other causes of abdominal pain in later pregnancy—complications of preeclampsia, pyelonephritis, various liver diseases, gallbladder disease, appendicitis, and ovarian torsion. Uterine irritability caused by abruptio placentae can also be confused with early labor. If the patient has acute catastrophic hypotension, amniotic fluid embolus, with or without abruptio placentae, and uterine rupture must be considered.

Placenta Previa

Pathophysiology. Placenta previa, or implantation of the placenta over the cervical os, is the other major cause of bleeding episodes during the second half of pregnancy. The risk of placenta previa is increased with maternal age, smoking, multiparity, cesarean section, prior miscarriage or induced abortions, and preterm labor. Bleeding occurs when marginal placental vessels implanted in the lower uterine segment are torn, either as the lower uterine wall elongates or with cervical dilation near the time of delivery. Early bleeding episodes tend to be self-limited unless separation of the placental margin is aggravated by iatrogenic cervical probing or the onset of labor.

Clinical Features. Painless, fresh vaginal bleeding is the most common symptom of placenta previa. In approximately 20% of cases, some degree of uterine irritability is present, but this is generally minor. Vaginal examination usually reveals bright red blood from the cervical os. All patients with painless, second-trimester vaginal bleeding should be assumed to have placenta previa until proven otherwise. Digital or instrumental probing of the cervix should be avoided until the diagnosis is excluded via ultrasound because this can precipitate severe hemorrhage in a patient with asymptomatic or minimally symptomatic placenta previa. Speculum examination of the vagina and cervix should be limited to an atraumatic partial speculum insertion to identify whether the bleeding is coming from the cervical os (and a presumed placenta previa), hemorrhoids, or a vaginal lesion that might not require urgent management.

Most cases of placenta previa identified during the mid-trimester resolve by the time of delivery as the lower uterine segment elongates and the placenta no longer overlaps the cervical os. Central or total previa, which occurs in approximately 20% of cases, can, however, cause severe hemorrhage, with the risk of exsanguination for the fetus and mother.

Diagnostic Testing. Ultrasonography is the diagnostic procedure of choice for localization of the placenta and diagnosis of placenta previa. Accuracy is excellent, but visualization of the placenta and of the internal cervical os is required. The bladder should be emptied before examination for suspected placenta previa to avoid overdiagnosis of placenta previa. Transvaginal ultrasonography is safe and even more accurate for visualization of the relationships between the placenta and internal os.

Management. Patients who experience vaginal bleeding during late pregnancy require immediate obstetric consultation and arrangements for safe transfer to an appropriate obstetric facility. Initial management consists of maternal stabilization, with establishment of two large-bore intravenous (IV) lines and fluid resuscitation, as well as continuous fetal monitoring, if available. A baseline hemoglobin level should be determined, and blood should be sent for type and crossmatch. Baseline coagulation studies, including platelet count, prothrombin time, and partial thromboplastin time, should be performed, and the fibrinogen level and presence of fibrin split products should be determined. The normal fibrinogen level in pregnancy is 400 to 450 mg/dL; values below 300 mg/dL indicate significant consumption of coagulation factors.

Blood loss requiring transfusion can occur in patients with placenta previa or abruptio placentae. Fresh-frozen plasma or fresh whole blood may be needed because of the potential for a coagulopathy. Fetomaternal hemorrhage can occur with abruption. If the Rh-negative patient has not yet received her routine Rh immune globulin prophylaxis at 28 weeks, 300 µg of Rh immune globulin should be administered within 72 hours. Transfer to the obstetric unit should be expedited if the patient is stable, or it should be done after initiation of resuscitation if she is unstable. If transfer to another hospital is required, a high-risk transfer team should be used if bleeding is significant or the fetus is in distress. Assessment is best accomplished by obstetricians who are accustomed to the evaluation of late-pregnancy complications and who can perform an emergent cesarean section, if needed.

In the obstetrics unit, fetal monitoring is continued. Ultrasonography is used primarily to locate the placenta and diagnose placenta previa, but it may not be reliable in confirming the diagnosis of abruptio placentae. On occasion, subplacental hemorrhages of abruptio placentae can be seen, and changes in size of the collection can be monitored. If evidence of placenta previa is absent or equivocal, a vaginal examination is performed in the delivery suite, where an emergency cesarean section can be performed if uncontrolled bleeding is encountered.

Patients who have significant abruptio placentae may require early delivery—vaginal or surgical, depending on fetal status. If placenta previa is diagnosed or if abruptio placentae is considered mild, the patient is admitted for close monitoring. The goal is to support the patient, ideally until fetal maturity is demonstrated and a successful delivery can be accomplished.

Pregnancy-Induced Hypertension (Preeclampsia and Eclampsia)

KEY CONCEPTS

- Gestational hypertension occurs during pregnancy, resolves during the postpartum period, and is recognized by a new blood pressure reading of 140/90 mm Hg or higher.
- Preeclampsia is gestational hypertension after 20 weeks gestational age with proteinuria (>300 mg/24 hr) or signs of end-organ damage; eclampsia is the occurrence of seizures in a patient with signs of preeclampsia.
- The HELLP syndrome is a particularly severe form of preeclampsia characterized by *h*emolysis, *e*levated *l*iver enzyme levels (ALT and AST > 70 U/L), and *l*ow *p*latelet count (<100,000/mL).
- Because progression of preeclampsia to eclampsia is unpredictable and can occur rapidly, blood pressure control in the pregnant patient is of utmost importance.
- Magnesium sulfate has little antihypertensive effect but is the most effective anticonvulsant in the setting of eclampsia, preventing recurrent seizures while maintaining uterine and fetal blood flow.

Foundations

Hypertension is observed in up to 8% of pregnancies and is generally divided into several categories[14]:

- Gestational hypertension occurs during pregnancy, resolves during the postpartum period, and is recognized by a new blood pressure reading of 140/90 mm Hg or higher.
- Preeclampsia is gestational hypertension with proteinuria (>300 mg/24 hr).
- Eclampsia is the occurrence of seizures in a patient with signs of preeclampsia. Progression of preeclampsia to eclampsia is unpredictable and can occur rapidly.
- Pregnancy-aggravated hypertension is chronic hypertension with superimposed preeclampsia or eclampsia.
- Chronic or coincidental hypertension is present before pregnancy or persists for more than 6 weeks postpartum.

Approximately 2% to 7% of pregnancies are complicated by pregnancy-induced hypertension. The incidence of actual eclampsia has progressively declined but is still one of the major causes of maternal mortality. The risk of pregnancy-induced hypertension is greatest in women younger than 20 years, primigravidas and those with twin or molar pregnancies, those with hypercholesterolemia, pregestational diabetes, or obesity, or those with a family history of pregnancy-induced hypertension.

Pathophysiology

Gestational hypertension or preeclampsia is a vasospastic disease of unknown cause unique to pregnant women. Vasospasm, ischemia, and thrombosis associated with preeclamptic changes cause injury to maternal organs, placental infarction and abruption, and fetal death from hypoxia and prematurity. The cause of eclampsia is unknown, but recent studies have centered on vascular responsiveness to endogenous vasopressors in the preeclamptic woman. Vascular responsiveness is normally depressed during pregnancy, which is a high-output, low-resistance state. Gestational hypertension is characterized by an even greater elevation in cardiac output, followed by an abnormally high peripheral resistance as clinical manifestations of the disease develop. In patients with preeclampsia, the cardiac output eventually drops as peripheral resistance rises. The cause of these changes is not known, but endothelial dysfunction is purported to release vasoactive mediators and result in vasoconstriction. Antiplatelet agents during pregnancy have been reported to reduce the risk of development of preeclampsia, supporting the premise of an imbalance between levels of thromboxane and prostacyclin in preeclampsia.[14]

The vasospastic effects of gestational hypertension and preeclampsia are protean. The intravascular volume is lower than in normal pregnancy, central venous pressures are normal, and capillary wedge pressures are variable. Liver effects are believed to be due to hepatocellular necrosis and edema resulting from vasospasm. Renal injury causes proteinuria and may result in decreased glomerular filtration. Microangiopathic hemolysis may result from vasospasm, causing thrombocytopenia. Central nervous system (CNS) effects include microvascular thrombosis and hemorrhage, as well as focal edema and hyperemia.

Clinical Features

Signs and Symptoms. The patient with gestational hypertension has mild systolic or diastolic blood pressure elevation, no proteinuria, and no evidence of organ damage. Mental status assessment, testing of reflexes, abdominal examination, liver function studies, and coagulation studies yield normal results. Preeclampsia is associated with kidney changes and, in severe cases, other end-organ symptoms. Edema is often difficult to assess because pregnancy is normally associated with excess extracellular fluid and dependent edema, and it is no longer used as a criterion for preeclampsia. Proteinuria (300 mg/24 hr) is variable at any given time and may not be detectable in a random urine specimen.

In cases of severe preeclampsia, the diastolic blood pressure can exceed 110 mm Hg, proteinuria is more severe, and there is evidence of vasospastic effects in various end organs. CNS effects commonly include headache or visual disturbances. In preeclampsia, the patient will become hyperreflexive before seizures develop. Thrombocytopenia may be present, liver function test findings may be elevated, and the liver is often tender. Renal dysfunction may be indicated by oliguria and elevated creatinine levels in addition to proteinuria.

Complications

The HELLP syndrome, a particularly severe form of preeclampsia that develops in 5% to 10% of women who have preeclamptic symptoms, is characterized by *h*emolysis, *e*levated *l*iver enzyme levels (alanine transaminase [ALT] and aspartate transaminase [AST] > 70 U/L), and *l*ow *p*latelet count (<100,000/mL). Prothrombin time, partial thromboplastin time, and fibrinogen are normal, and blood studies reveal microangiopathic hemolytic anemia. Other complications of preeclampsia include spontaneous hepatic and splenic hemorrhage and abruptio placentae.

The most dangerous complication is eclampsia, which is the occurrence of seizures or coma in the setting of signs and symptoms of preeclampsia. Warning signs for the development of eclampsia include headache, nausea and vomiting, and visual disturbances. Elevated total leukocyte count, creatinine, and AST levels are also predictive of increased morbidity for the patient with severe preeclampsia. Particularly in early eclampsia before 32 weeks of gestation, seizures may develop abruptly, and hypertension may not be associated with edema or proteinuria. In postpartum women who have eclampsia, more than half (55%) have not been previously diagnosed with preeclampsia, and patients may present with headache, vision changes, elevated blood pressure, and seizures, often within 48 hours of delivery, but in up to 6 weeks after delivery and in rare cases up to 12 weeks postpartum.[15] After 48 hours postpartum and without predelivery signs of preeclampsia, other diagnoses, such as intracranial hemorrhage, should be considered. Maternal complications of eclampsia include permanent CNS damage from recurrent seizures or intracranial bleeding, renal insufficiency, and death.

The maternal mortality rate from eclampsia has been reduced to less than 1% with modern management. Perinatal mortality has also decreased, although it remains at 4% to 8%.[14] Causes of neonatal death include placental infarcts, intrauterine growth retardation, and abruptio placentae. In addition, fetal hypoxia from maternal seizures and the complications of premature delivery contribute significantly to fetal morbidity and mortality.

Differential Diagnoses

Peripheral edema is common in normal pregnancy, and it may be difficult to differentiate normal edema from that of early preeclampsia. Differentiation of gestational hypertension from preexistent hypertension is often impossible if no record of normal blood pressure is available. Seizures during pregnancy may be due to epilepsy as well as other intracranial catastrophes, such as thrombosis or hemorrhage.

Diagnostic Testing

The patient who has severe preeclampsia should have an IV line and fetal monitoring initiated. Blood testing includes a complete blood cell count, renal function studies, liver function tests, platelet count, coagulation profile, and a baseline magnesium level. The serum glucose concentration is determined in patients with seizures.

If a history of preeclampsia is not obtained or the symptoms are refractory to magnesium sulfate therapy, a computed tomography (CT) scan of the head is performed to exclude cerebral venous thrombosis or an intracranial hemorrhage, either of which can occur in pregnancy—with or without pregnancy-induced hypertension—and may require specific treatment. CT scan abnormalities can be seen in 50% of patients with eclampsia. Patchy hemorrhage and microinfarcts of the cortex are characteristic and may be due to loss of cerebral autoregulation in patients with severe pregnancy-related hypertension. Diffuse cerebral edema can also be seen.

Management

Mild Preeclampsia. The management of patients with mild preeclampsia includes documentation of blood pressure, reflexes, weight, and blood testing to ensure normal end-organ function. Accurate determination of gestational age by ultrasonography is needed to allow optimal management if symptoms progress. Limitation of physical activities, including bed rest, is the only demonstrated means of reducing blood pressure and allowing the pregnancy to be sustained longer. Definitive treatment is delivery of the fetus, although expectant management is standard in women at less than 34 weeks of gestation. Arrangement for close follow-up is important for patients who are not hospitalized.

Severe Preeclampsia. Hospitalization is recommended for patients with sustained hypertension above 140/90 mm Hg and signs of severe

BOX 173.4   Management of Eclampsia and Severe Preeclampsia

Control seizures with magnesium sulfate, 4–6 g given over 15–20 minutes, followed by 2 g/hr IV.
Control hypertension after seizure control if diastolic blood pressure >105 mm Hg; hydralazine (5–10 mg IV push, repeat q 2-4h) or labetalol (20 mg IV bolus, repeat q10 min PRN up to 300 mg/total dose)
Obtain initial laboratory studies to assess organ injury:
  Complete blood count and platelet count
  Liver function tests
  Blood urea nitrogen, creatinine
Monitor urine output; maintain at >25 mL/hr.
Limit intravenous fluid administration unless significant losses occur.
Avoid diuretics and hyperosmotic agents.
Perform a computed tomography scan of the head if consciousness is decreased or seizures persist, lateralizing signs are present, or there are other concerns.
Initiate steps to delivery.

Adapted from: Pritchard JA, Cunningham FG, Pritchard SA. The Parkland Memorial Hospital protocol for treatment of eclampsia: evaluation of 245 cases. *Am J Obstet Gynecol.* 1984;148:951-963.

preeclampsia. Baseline laboratory studies are recommended to identify end-organ effects in the liver, kidney, and hematologic systems. Both diuresis and antihypertensive therapy have been remarkably unsuccessful in improving fetal outcome or prolonging pregnancy. However, admission does allow the obstetrician to assess fetal age and well-being accurately, maternal organ function, and effect of bed rest on blood pressure before the optimal timing of delivery is decided.

Fulminant or severe preeclampsia, with marked blood pressure elevation (≥160/110 mm Hg) associated with epigastric or liver tenderness, visual disturbance, or severe headache, is managed in the same way as eclampsia (Box 173.4). The goal is prevention of seizures and permanent damage to maternal organs. Magnesium sulfate is given for seizure prophylaxis.

Seizures and coma are the hallmarks of eclampsia, the ultimate consequence of preeclampsia. As in all seizure patients, hypoglycemia, drug overdose, and other causes of seizures should be excluded with appropriate tests. Eclamptic seizures are controlled in almost all patients by administering magnesium sulfate, although the mechanism of action remains elusive. Magnesium has little antihypertensive effect but is the most effective anticonvulsant, preventing recurrent seizures while maintaining uterine and fetal blood flow. The goals of magnesium sulfate therapy are to terminate ongoing seizures and prevent recurrence. An IV loading dose of 4 to 6 g magnesium given over 15 to 20 minutes, followed by 2 g/hr IV, is recommended. Magnesium administration should be accompanied by clinical observation for loss of reflexes (which occurs at ≈10 mg/dL) or respiratory depression (which occurs at levels of 12 mg/dL, although actual serum magnesium levels are rarely monitored). The infusion should be stopped if signs of hypermagnesemia (loss of reflexes or respiratory depression as manifest by a decrease in the respiratory rate or an increase in end tidal CO_2 are seen. IV calcium gluconate, 1 g given slowly, will reverse the adverse effects of hypermagnesemia.

Despite ongoing controversy, the familiarity with magnesium sulfate and its physiologic advantages to the fetus, wide margin of safety, and high success rate in controlling seizures make it the first-line drug in patients with eclampsia. If seizures persist after the recommended doses of magnesium sulfate have been administered, the following agents may be used in the treatment of eclampsia in conjunction with obstetric consultation: lorazepam (2–4 mg IV for one dose, may repeat ×1 after 10–15 min), phenytoin or fosphenytoin (15–20 mg/kg IV ×1, may repeat at 10 mg/kg after 20 min), or levetiracetam (20–60 mg/kg IV, may repeat in 12 hours). In addition, a careful search for other causes of seizures (e.g., hypoglycemia and intracranial hemorrhage) should be instituted based on history and examination of the patient.[16]

Although magnesium sulfate is not a direct antihypertensive, the hypertension associated with eclampsia is often controlled adequately by stoppage of the seizures. Rapid lowering of blood pressure can result in uterine hypoperfusion, so specific antihypertensive treatment is initiated only if the diastolic blood pressure remains above 105 mm Hg or the systolic blood pressure remains above 160 mm Hg after control of seizures.[17] The goal is to lower maternal blood pressure by 15% to 20% with a systolic goal of 140 to 150 mm Hg and a diastolic goal of 90 to 100 mm Hg. Many patients do not require specific antihypertensive treatment after treatment with magnesium sulfate. The antihypertensives used most often by obstetricians are hydralazine (5–10 mg IV push, repeat q 2-4h) or labetalol (20 mg IV bolus, may repeat q10 min PRN up to 300 mg/total dose). Rapid-release nifedipine (10 mg PO) can be used if IV access is not immediately available. Other antihypertensive agents have not been well studied in this population because there are specific risks to uncontrolled lowering of blood pressure and loss of uteroplacental blood flow.

Although total body water in the eclamptic patient is excessive, intravascular volume is contracted, and the eclamptic patient is sensitive to further volume changes. Hypovolemia results in decreased uterine perfusion. Thus, diuretics and hyperosmotic agents should be avoided in these patients. Invasive monitoring has demonstrated that vasospasm is not reversed with IV fluid administration. Rather, excessive IV fluids increase extravascular fluid stores that are difficult to mobilize postpartum, resulting in a higher incidence of pulmonary edema in patients treated aggressively with fluid therapy. Invasive pulmonary artery pressure monitoring may be required for accurate fluid management in the eclamptic patient.

Amniotic Fluid Embolus

KEY CONCEPTS

- Amniotic fluid embolus should be suspected during the second or third trimester of pregnancy, particularly in the setting of uterine manipulation or contraction, when a patient experiences sudden onset of hypotension, hypoxia, and coagulopathy.
- Treatment of amniotic fluid embolus consists of supplemental oxygenation and ventilation, aggressive fluid resuscitation, inotropic cardiovascular support, and anticipation and management of consumptive coagulopathy.

Foundations

Amniotic fluid embolus is the release of amniotic fluid into the maternal circulation. This occurs during intense uterine contractions or uterine manipulation at areas of placental separation from the uterine decidua basalis (abruptio placentae) and triggers a rapidly fatal, anaphylactoid-type maternal response. Although amniotic fluid embolus usually occurs during labor, with the maternal mortality rate at 25% or higher, it can also occur after induced abortions, miscarriages, and spontaneously during the second and third trimesters. Amniotic fluid embolus can also occur after amniocentesis or in association with abruptio placentae after abdominal trauma. Although it is a rare syndrome, amniotic fluid embolus is the leading cause of cardiovascular collapse during labor.

Clinical Features

Amniotic fluid embolus should be suspected during the second or third trimester of pregnancy, particularly in the setting of uterine manipulation or contraction, when a patient experiences sudden hypotension, hypoxia, and coagulopathy. The embolization of amniotic fluid and the particulate matter suspended in it triggers a profound immunologic response when it enters the maternal circulation. The list of proposed mediators is extensive and includes histamine, endothelin, and leukotrienes. In survivors, DIC, acute respiratory distress syndrome, and left ventricular dysfunction develop. An initial seizure is seen in approximately 20% of patients. Bleeding diathesis may be the initial sign in some women, and DIC occurs in approximately 50% of cases.

Differential Diagnoses

Catastrophic pulmonary embolus, drug-induced anaphylaxis, and septic shock must be considered in the differential diagnosis. Seizures occur in patients with eclampsia, but hypertension rather than cardiovascular collapse is usually observed in that condition. Coagulopathy may be seen in patients with preeclampsia (HELLP syndrome), abruptio placentae, or other chronic coagulopathies seen in the nonpregnant patient.

Diagnostic Testing

When amniotic fluid embolus is suspected, a complete blood cell count, coagulation studies, arterial blood gas analysis, and chest radiograph are obtained. Urine output is monitored after urinary catheter placement. The diagnosis is usually made with certainty only at autopsy, with the finding of fetal hairs, squamous cells, and debris in the maternal circulation. Because squamous epithelial cells can be seen normally in the maternal pulmonary circulation, the typical clinical syndrome is also required for diagnosis.

Management

Amniotic fluid embolus is uncommon, so treatment recommendations are anecdotal and based on animal studies. The most helpful modalities appear to be high-flow oxygen, support of ventilation and oxygenation with intubation, aggressive fluid resuscitation, inotropic cardiovascular support, and anticipation and management of consumptive coagulopathy. Treatment usually requires invasive hemodynamic monitoring in an intensive care unit.

Rh (Anti-D) Immunization in Pregnancy

KEY CONCEPTS

- Rh immunization occurs when an Rh-negative woman is exposed to Rh-positive fetal blood. To prevent this, a dose of 50 µg of Rh immune globulin can be used if the patient less than 12 weeks of gestation. After 12 weeks, a 300-µg dose is recommended.

Rh immunization occurs when an Rh-negative woman is exposed to Rh-positive fetal blood. Sensitization occurs in up to 15% of Rh-negative women carrying Rh-positive fetuses. Small numbers of fetal cells enter the maternal circulation spontaneously throughout pregnancy, and the maternal immune system is triggered by as little as 0.1 mL of fetal-maternal hemorrhage. Fetal-maternal hemorrhage occurs in 3% to 11% of women with threatened abortions in the first trimester and approximately 45% during birth in the third trimester. To prevent this, anti-D immune globulin (RhoGAM) is routinely administered to Rh-negative mothers—if the father is Rh positive or his status is unknown—at approximately the 28th week of gestation to protect the mother from spontaneous sensitization, which occurs during the third trimester, and at the time of delivery. Transplacental hemorrhage can also occur during uterine manipulation, threatened miscarriage (even without fetal loss), spontaneous miscarriage, surgery for ectopic pregnancy, and amniocentesis, although the risk is not clear. Anti-D immune globulin should be administered when these events occur. A dose of 50 μg can be used if the patient is at less than 12 weeks of gestation, although many pharmacies carry only the 300-μg dose, which can also be given. After 12 weeks, a 300-μg dose should be given. The half-life of immune globulin is 24 days, and it needs to be administered within 72 hours of a sensitization event to prevent antibody development.

The Kleihauer-Betke test of maternal blood has been used to detect fetal cells in the maternal circulation. Unfortunately, the test is difficult to perform, not immediately available in most emergency laboratories, and only sensitive enough to detect 5 mL of fetal cells in the maternal circulation. Because only 0.1 mL of fetal cells is required to sensitize the mother, routine immune globulin administration has been recommended in situations likely to result in sensitization. Patients with third-trimester bleeding are not at increased risk of sensitization compared with patients with normal pregnancy. Thus, RhoGAM should be administered only if the patient did not receive her prophylactic dose at 28 weeks. In cases of blunt trauma to the uterus, the Kleihauer-Betke test should be ordered to detect the rare, large fetal transfusions that may require specific fetal blood therapy or administration of additional immune globulin to the mother. The standard dose (300 μg) is sufficient to prevent maternal immunization for fetal transfusions of up to 15 mL of red blood cells or 30 mL of whole blood.

MEDICAL AND SURGICAL PROBLEMS IN THE PREGNANT PATIENT

Clinicians should be aware of a variety of illnesses, related and unrelated to pregnancy, that may have altered symptoms, risk, and treatment in the pregnant patient (Tables 173.2 and 173.3). See also Chapter 174.

Abdominal Pain

KEY CONCEPTS

- Appendicitis is the most common surgical emergency in pregnancy. Clinical presentations may be atypical, leading to a misdiagnosis rate of 30% to 35% in pregnant patients. Right lower quadrant pain is the most common finding, especially early in pregnancy. Ultrasound, CT, and MRI are useful for the diagnosis.
- Cholelithiasis presents with similar symptoms to those in nonpregnant women and is similarly diagnosed through ultrasound. Surgery, if required, is optimally performed during the second trimester.
- During pregnancy, albumin levels decrease while alkaline phosphatase levels may increase up to double; amylase levels may also be slightly elevated.
- Hepatitis is the most common cause of liver disease in pregnancy; hepatitis E has increased maternal mortality and rate of fetal loss.
- Acute fatty liver of pregnancy is a rare disorder of the third trimester that can result in hepatic failure, complicated labor, and fetal mortality. Coagulopathy, jaundice, seizures, DIC, and hepatic encephalopathy may also result.
- Intrahepatic cholestasis of pregnancy typically presents with generalized pruritus and mild jaundice. Resolution occurs with delivery. Women are at increased risk for preterm delivery, meconium passage, and intrauterine fetal demise.

TABLE 173.2	**Differential Diagnosis of Abdominal Pain in Pregnancy**	
Diagnosis	**Gestational Age**	**Signs/Symptoms/ Diagnostic Testing**
Gynecologic		
Miscarriage	<20 wk; 80% <12 wk	Vaginal bleeding, pelvic pain, ultrasonography to confirm location, no fetal activity at 8 weeks, decreasing hCG level
Septic abortion	<20 wk	Fever, uterine tenderness
Ectopic pregnancy	<14 wk	Pelvic pain, hypotension
Corpus luteum cyst	<12 wk	Sudden focal peritoneal pain; no fever
Ovarian torsion	Especially <24 wk	Ischemic pain, episodic
Pelvic inflammatory disease	<12 wk	Very rare, pelvic pain, vaginal discharge
Chorioamnionitis	>16 wk	Tender uterus, fever, amniocentesis reveals white blood cells
Abruptio placentae	>16 wk	Focal uterine tenderness, fetal distress, variable bleeding
Preeclampsia	>20 wk	Hypertension, proteinuria, edema, right upper quadrant pain
Nongynecologic		
Appendicitis	Throughout	Guarding may be less prominent; location changes
Cholecystitis	Throughout	Confirm with ultrasonography
Hepatitis	Throughout	Confirm with liver function tests
Pyelonephritis	Throughout	Flank pain, fever, positive catheterized urinalysis

Appendicitis

Foundations. Appendicitis is the most common surgical emergency in pregnant patients. The incidence of appendicitis in pregnant patients is the same as that in nonpregnant patients, but delays in diagnosis contribute to an increased rate of perforation, which may result in fetal mortality and maternal morbidity. There is also an increased rate of other complications of appendicitis in pregnancy. A large, population-based study found an almost twofold increase in sepsis and septic shock, transfusion, pneumonia, bowel obstruction, postoperative infection, and length of stay longer than 3 days.[18] During the first half of pregnancy, diagnostic findings are usually similar to those in the nonpregnant woman, but the clinical picture becomes more atypical during the second half of pregnancy.

Traditionally, the appendix was thought to be displaced counterclockwise out of the right lower quadrant after the third month of gestation, with its ultimate location deep in the right upper quadrant, superior to the iliac crest (Fig. 173.8). However, even in the third trimester, the location changes from the right lower quadrant in less than 25% of pregnant patients. Displacement of the abdominal wall away from the abdominal viscera can result in difficulty in palpation of organs and loss of signs of parietal peritoneal irritation. The physiologic increase in white blood cell count and erythrocyte sedimentation rate in pregnancy should also be considered in the evaluation of the patient with possible appendicitis because these may confuse the overall clinical picture.

TABLE 173.3 Differential Diagnosis of Common Symptoms in Pregnancy

Diagnosis	Gestational Age	Signs, Symptoms, Diagnostic Testing
Vaginal Bleeding		
Miscarriage	<20 wk	Vaginal bleeding, pelvic pain, ultrasonography to confirm location, no fetal activity at 8 weeks, decreasing hCG level
Ectopic pregnancy	<14 wk	Pelvic pain, hypotension, evaluate with ultrasonography
Molar pregnancy	12-24 wk	No fetal heart tones, characteristic sonogram showing snow storm appearance
Cervical lesions	Throughout	Perineal and vaginal inspection
Vaginitis, cervicitis	Throughout	White blood cells on wet mount, with culture
Placenta previa	>16 wk	Ultrasonography to localize placenta
Abruptio placentae	>16 wk	Focal uterine tenderness, fetal distress, variable bleeding
Seizure		
Eclampsia	>24 wk	Blood pressure > 140/90 mm Hg; usually history of PIH, edema, proteinuria
Amniotic fluid embolus	>12 wk	Hypotension, respiratory distress, DIC
Epilepsy	Throughout	History; lack of PIH findings
Dyspnea		
Pulmonary embolus	Especially 6 wk prepartum and postpartum	Usual diagnostic studies including use of CT, Ventilation/perfusion studies, and extremity doppler ultrasound
Dyspnea of pregnancy	>24 wk	Exclude other causes
Pulmonary infection	Throughout	Examination; radiography
Amniotic fluid embolus	>12 wk	Uterine manipulation, bleeding diathesis, hypotension
Jaundice		
Cholestasis of pregnancy	>24 wk	Well patient; itching and jaundice
Hepatitis	Throughout	Abnormal liver function test results
Acute fatty liver	>24 wk	Rapid liver failure; coma, seizures, hypoglycemia
Bleeding Diathesis		
Eclampsia	>24 wk	Blood pressure > 140/90 mm Hg; proteinuria, edema, HELLP syndrome
Amniotic fluid embolus	>12 wk	Respiratory distress, cardiovascular collapse
Abruptio placentae	>20 wk	Uterine tenderness; vaginal bleeding; fetal distress

DIC, Disseminated intravascular coagulation; *hCG,* human chorionic gonadotropin; *HELLP,* hemolysis, elevated liver enzyme levels, low platelets; *PIH,* pregnancy-induced hypertension.

Clinical Features. The gastrointestinal symptoms of appendicitis, such as anorexia, nausea, and vomiting, mimic those of pregnancy, particularly during the first trimester, making such symptoms relatively nonspecific. Right-sided abdominal pain is the most constant finding, although this is less reliable later in pregnancy. Peritoneal signs are also most common during the first trimester. The absence of fever, leukocytosis, or tachycardia has been reported. The lack of these clinical findings in pregnant patients with appendicitis may be the result of a blunted inflammatory response caused by elevated maternal levels of pregnancy-related steroids. Pyuria without bacteriuria may be seen

These confounding factors contribute to the misdiagnosis rate for appendicitis of 30% to 35% overall in pregnancy, with a 40% to 50% rate of removal of normal appendix during the third trimester. In contrast to the relative safety of performing an exploratory laparotomy or laparoscopy during pregnancy, the risk of fetal loss and maternal morbidity from failure to diagnose appendicitis and perforation is considerable, so clinical vigilance is required, even in the absence of classic signs. In one study, in the setting of acute appendicitis, the relative risk of pregnancy loss at less than 20 weeks was 5.3, and was 6.0 at less than 24 weeks.[19] In later pregnancy, when peritoneal signs are often absent and the uterus obscures normal physical findings, diagnosis is frequently delayed, and the perforation rate may approach 25%.

Differential Diagnoses. Pyelonephritis, cholecystitis, nephrolithiasis, and pregnancy-related diseases such as ectopic pregnancy, round ligament pain, broad ligament pain, corpus luteum cyst leakage, and ovarian torsion should be considered in the patient who has right-sided abdominal pain. Pyelonephritis is the most common condition that is confused with appendicitis. During its migration, the appendix is located very near the kidney, resulting in a high incidence of sterile pyuria and flank pain (see Fig. 173.8). In cases of appendicitis, unless there is coincident urinary tract infection, the urine is free of bacteria, a feature distinguishing it from pyelonephritis. Salpingitis, another common misdiagnosis, is very rare in pregnancy, although it can occur before 12 weeks of gestation.

Diagnostic Testing. Leukocytosis is common in pregnant patients with appendicitis, although it is rarely high enough to distinguish it from the physiologic leukocytosis of pregnancy. A leukocytosis greater than 18,000 makes the diagnosis of appendicitis 10 times more likely.[19] Pyuria in a catheterized urine specimen suggests pyelonephritis, but may be seen in 20% of patients with appendicitis,[20] whereas bacteriuria is uncommon in appendicitis.

Ultrasonography with a graded compression technique may reveal a non-compressible tubular structure in the right lower quadrant consistent with appendicitis. Studies of the diagnostic value of

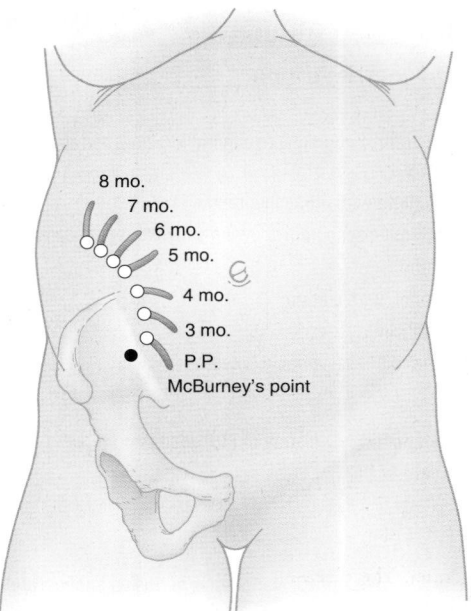

Fig. 173.8 Locations of the appendix during succeeding months of pregnancy. In planning an operation, it is better to make the abdominal incision over the point of maximal tenderness unless there is great disparity between that point and the theoretic location of the appendix. *P.P.,* postpartum. (From: Gabbe SG, Niebyl JR, Simpson JL, Galan HL. *Obstetrics: Normal and Problem Pregnancies.* New York: Churchill Livingstone; 2007.)

ultrasonography in the diagnosis of appendicitis are limited but have suggested that it has a high positive predictive value but a low negative predictive value.[21] Abdominal ultrasonography is recommended as the first imaging modality, followed by CT when ultrasound findings are inconclusive. Surgical, obstetric, and radiologic society guidelines agree that magnetic resonance imaging (MRI) is also useful in the evaluation of pregnant patients with suspected appendicitis (see Chapter 79).[21] Otherwise, laparoscopy or laparotomy is the diagnostic procedure of choice in the pregnant patient thought to have appendicitis. Early exploration is highly encouraged in pregnant patients because of the variability of clinical signs and increased fetal risk if diagnosis is delayed.

Management. The pregnant patient with suspected appendicitis should be hospitalized after consultation with a surgeon and obstetrician. Ultrasonography, MRI, or CT scan are diagnostic options. The patient should be kept on nothing by mouth (NPO) status, with IV fluid hydration to maintain intravascular volume. Although prompt surgery is required if the diagnosis is clear, in unclear cases the patient should undergo observation to allow for clarification of signs and symptoms. Patients undergoing observation are treated empirically with IV antibiotics, commonly piperacillin/tazobactam (3.375–4.5 g IV q6–8h) or ceftriaxone (2 g IV q24h) plus metronidazole (500 mg q8h).

Gallbladder Disease
Foundations
Cholelithiasis is present in approximately 5% of pregnant women and is the second most common non-obstetric surgical condition in pregnant patients. The natural history of asymptomatic cholelithiasis is believed to be similar to that in nonpregnant women, with less than 50% of patients with gallstones developing symptoms.

Changes in gallbladder kinetics are believed to be due to high pregnancy-related steroid levels. Progesterone decreases smooth muscle tone and induces gallbladder hypomotility and cholestasis, causing an increased risk of stone formation. In addition, pregnancy induces changes in bile composition and increased cholesterol secretion, thus increasing the incidence of cholesterol stone formation.

Clinical Features
The signs and symptoms of acute cholecystitis during pregnancy are the same as those in nonpregnant women. Epigastric or right upper quadrant pain and tenderness and nausea predominate. Leukocytosis must be interpreted carefully because of the normally increased white blood cell count seen in pregnancy. Likewise, a slightly elevated amylase level can be normal during pregnancy, and alkaline phosphatase, which is produced by the placenta, may be twice the nonpregnant level. A history of previous self-limited pain episodes associated with food intake suggests the diagnosis.

Differential Diagnoses
Pyelonephritis should be considered in the patient with right upper quadrant pain, with or without fever. During the third trimester, appendicitis can also be associated with right upper quadrant pain. Hepatitis and fatty liver infiltration occur in pregnancy; liver distention and inflammation associated with pregnancy-induced hypertension can also cause right upper quadrant pain. In addition, spontaneous intrahepatic bleeding can occur during late pregnancy, mimicking cholecystitis. Because of the potential for other serious diseases, diagnostic studies should be performed to verify a clinical diagnosis of symptomatic cholelithiasis and cholecystitis in pregnancy.

Diagnostic Testing
Ultrasonography is a reliable means of recognizing stones in the gallbladder, although it may not differentiate symptomatic from asymptomatic stones. In the patient with right upper quadrant pain, simultaneous sonographic evaluation of the liver is useful but technically difficult, particularly during the third trimester, when subcapsular liver hematomas and other intrinsic hepatocellular disease can occur but the liver may be obscured under the ribs.

Management and Disposition
The patient who has fever, leukocytosis, prolonged pain, or evidence of cholecystitis should be made NPO and given IV fluid hydration, adequate pain control, and broad-spectrum antibiotics. Some patients with uncomplicated cholecystitis can be managed medically. Patients with obstructive jaundice, gallstone pancreatitis, sepsis or failure to respond to conservative management are candidates for surgery (optimally, during the second trimester, if possible).[22] Approximately 40% of patients presenting with symptomatic cholelithiasis intrapartum require cholecystectomy during pregnancy, and recent evidence suggests that operative management compared to nonoperative management from uncomplicated disease has a reduced overall morbidity including reduced maternal and fetal complications.[22]

Discharge should be considered only for patients with uncomplicated and sonographically proven cholelithiasis who are not otherwise candidates for admission after consultation with an obstetrician. Pregnant patients with symptomatic cholelithiasis have a high rate of symptomatic relapse and increased severity of disease with each relapse. Early follow-up should be arranged, and the patient should be given careful instructions to return if she experiences fever, vomiting, or persistent pain.

Liver Disorders
Foundations
Pregnancy is associated with several unique liver abnormalities in addition to more usual hepatic diseases. Liver metabolism increases during

TABLE 173.4 Lab Abnormalities in Select Complications of Pregnancy

	WBC	Plt	BUN/Cr	AST/ALT	Alk Phos	PT/PTT	Fibrinogen	Bili	Other
Normal pregnancy	Mild ↑	nl	nl	nl	↑ (up to double)	nl	Nl	nl	nl LDH ↓albumin ↑amylase
Hepatitis				↑↑↑	Mild ↑	↑ (severe)		↑	Obtain: Acute hep panel APAP level
Acute fatty liver	↑	↓	↑	↑		↑	↓	↑	↑ Ammonia ↓glu +FSP
Preeclampsia HELLP		↓	↑ (severe preeclampsia)	↑		nl	nl		↓Hgb
Cholecystitis	↑			May be ↑	May be ↑				
Intrahepatic cholestasis				nl	↑↑ (7–10× nl)			↑	

pregnancy, but hepatic blood flow is unchanged, and little change occurs in liver function. Bilirubin, transaminase, and lactate dehydrogenase levels and prothrombin times are unchanged from those in the nonpregnant state. Albumin levels decrease secondary to an increase in maternal circulating plasma volume. Alkaline phosphatase levels may be up to double the nonpregnant values, and amylase levels may also be slightly elevated.

Hepatitis

Hepatitis is the most common cause of liver disease in pregnancy, accounting for 40% of cases of jaundice during pregnancy. Management and treatment are supportive and unchanged from those for nonpregnant patients. Hepatitis E is reported to have a more aggressive course in pregnancy, with an increased maternal mortality rate and rate of fetal loss. Maintenance of adequate nutrition is a priority. Vertical transmission of hepatitis B can occur if the disease is not recognized. Pregnant women should be vaccinated for hepatitis B. Prophylaxis should be administered to the newborn born to chronically infected mothers with both the hepatitis B vaccine (10 or 20 micrograms) as well as hepatitis B immune globulin (HBIG) given in 0.5 mL dose at birth. If no hepatitis vaccine is given, additional doses of HBIG are required at 3 months and 6 months.

Acute Fatty Liver

Pathophysiology. Acute fatty liver of pregnancy is a disorder of the third trimester that can result in hepatic failure, complicated labor, and fetal mortality. The disease is rare, occurring most often in primiparous patients and patients with twin gestations.

The cause of acute fatty liver of pregnancy is unknown, although studies have suggested that a deficiency in the fetus's fatty acid metabolism leads to an accumulation of hepatotoxic metabolites in the maternal circulation. On microscopic examination, fatty infiltration of the hepatocytes with edema and vacuolization can be seen, but there is no necrosis or inflammation. Liver function returns to normal after delivery if the patient can be supported through the acute phase. Although up to 50% of patients have signs of preeclampsia, the two are not clearly related. The diagnosis must be differentiated from viral hepatitis and HELLP syndrome, which have similar disease presentations and laboratory findings but, again, are not clearly related.

Clinical Features. Nausea and vomiting associated with malaise or jaundice during the third trimester should trigger consideration of a diagnosis of acute fatty liver. The right upper quadrant or epigastrium

is usually tender. The disease may progress to coagulopathy, jaundice, seizures, DIC, and hepatic encephalopathy. Hemorrhage from coagulopathy is the most common complication at delivery. The diagnosis is often delayed secondary to the multiple differential considerations.

Differential Diagnoses. Liver tenderness and coagulopathy usually suggest preeclampsia during the third trimester. Jaundice and increases in the ALT level are distinguishing features because they are unusual in cases of liver disease associated with pregnancy-induced hypertension. Similarly, rapid progression of hepatic failure, hypoglycemia, and coagulopathy are unlikely in cases of preeclampsia. Elevations in the creatinine level are more common in acute fatty liver of pregnancy. The patient with viral hepatitis is likely to have more marked elevations in transaminase levels. Drug-induced hepatic failure should be excluded by history and toxicologic screening for acetaminophen and other toxins, if appropriate. Cholecystitis may be distinguished by ultrasound examination but may also be characterized by right upper quadrant pain; it is not associated with coagulopathy or progressive liver failure (Table 173.4).

Diagnostic Testing. Typically, leukocytosis is present, the platelet count and fibrinogen level are low, prothrombin and partial thromboplastin times are elevated, and fibrin split products are present. Elevated bilirubin levels (a late finding), AST and ALT levels, and uric acid levels may be seen. Hypoglycemia and dehydration are frequently present. Additionally, elevated BUN and serum creatinine levels with associated oliguria may be seen. In contrast to Reye syndrome, the serum ammonia level is only mildly elevated. CT scan and liver ultrasonography may be normal, so liver biopsy is used to make the definitive diagnosis.

Management. The patient with acute fatty liver of pregnancy may require acute stabilization for seizures or coma. Hypoglycemia may occur, which is rapidly corrected with dextrose. Coagulation parameters should be assessed. Fluid resuscitation and replacement of clotting factors may be required, and the patient should be admitted to an obstetric service capable of managing this serious disease. The diagnosis is usually made with liver biopsy if the disease has not progressed to severe coagulopathy. Rapid delivery is usually advisable when the diagnosis has been established. Fresh-frozen plasma, platelet transfusions, and glucose may be needed to sustain the patient until delivery can be accomplished.

Intrahepatic Cholestasis

Pathophysiology. Intrahepatic cholestasis of pregnancy, also termed *idiopathic jaundice of pregnancy, icterus gravidarum,* or *pruritus gravidarum*, is a rare syndrome that occurs during the third trimester of pregnancy. It is the second most common cause of jaundice in pregnancy, after hepatitis. On histologic examination, the disease is characterized by cholestasis and dilated canaliculi in the biliary tree. The liver is normal. It is more common with increasing maternal age, multiple gestations, and in the winter months.

Clinical Features. Generalized pruritus and mild jaundice are the hallmarks of intrahepatic cholestasis of pregnancy. However, only 20% of patients present with this combination, and 80% present with pruritus alone. The pruritus usually begins in the palms and soles and ascends to the trunk. Although insomnia and fatigue occasionally accompany the pruritus, the patient appears nontoxic, without fever, vomiting, diarrhea, or significant malaise. The bilirubin level is rarely above 5 mg/dL, the alkaline phosphatase level can be elevated sevenfold to tenfold, and transaminase levels are in the normal range. Resolution occurs after delivery. Although maternal outcome is favorable, women with intrahepatic cholestasis of pregnancy are at increased risk for preterm delivery, meconium passage, and intrauterine fetal demise.

Differential Diagnoses and Management. Exclusion of more serious entities, such as viral hepatitis, acute fatty liver, drug-induced cholestasis, and complicated cholecystitis, is required. Outpatient management is appropriate, provided the diagnosis is clear and the patient has close obstetric follow-up. Some have advocated aggressive fetal surveillance and delivery after fetal lung maturity to improve the fetal outcome. Symptomatic treatment with antihistamines (chlorpheniramine 4 mg PO q4–6h) and ursodeoxycholic acid (300 mg PO BID) are considered first line; additional treatments including bile salts, guar gum, and benzodiazepines have been tried, with variable success.[23]

Nausea and Vomiting in Pregnancy

KEY CONCEPTS

- Nausea and vomiting in pregnancy are common and may be treated conservatively with diet modification and avoidance of environmental triggers. If conservative measures fail, Diclegis, a delayed-release combination of doxylamine, 10 mg, and pyridoxine (vitamin B_6), 10 mg, is the first-line pharmacologic agent for the treatment of nausea and vomiting in pregnancy.
- Hyperemesis gravidarum is defined as nausea and vomiting that cause starvation metabolism, weight loss, dehydration, and prolonged ketonemia and ketonuria. Initial management involves rehydration with IV fluids, antiemetics, and demonstration of ability to take oral hydration.

Normal Pregnancy

Nausea and vomiting are common in pregnancy, particularly from 6 to 20 weeks of gestation. Prevalence rates of nausea and vomiting are as high as 50% to 80%. Symptoms are usually self-limited and often resolve with lifestyle changes, such as diet modification and avoidance of environmental triggers. Although evidence supporting nonpharmacologic agents is mixed, in several randomized trials, ginger has been found to be effective. Treatment is recommended at a dose of 250 mg QID, in capsule or syrup form.

In women who fail conservative management, pharmacologic therapy may be initiated. The American College of Obstetricians and Gynecologists recommends doxylamine-pyridoxine (1–2 tab QD–BID), a delayed-release combination of doxylamine, 10 mg, and pyridoxine (vitamin B_6), 10 mg, as the first-line pharmacologic agent for the treatment of nausea and vomiting in pregnancy.[24] Multiple studies and the

Centers for Disease Control and Prevention (CDC) Birth Defect Monitoring Program data have demonstrated its safety and it is US Food and Drug Administration (FDA) approved for use in pregnancy.

If there are circumstances preventing the prescription of Diclegis, or in case of treatment failure, other antiemetics may be considered. Although the FDA has not explicitly approved metoclopramide (5–10 mg PO/IV/IM q 6h) or promethazine (12.5–25 mg PO/IV/IM/rectal q 4–6h, max 100 mg/day) for the treatment of nausea and vomiting in pregnancy, both drugs have been widely used and are generally considered safe. Ondansetron (4 mg PO/IV q8h) has also been widely used, though recent studies have suggested that ondansetron may be associated with an increased risk of fetal anomalies. However, the evidence is mixed and the prevalence of fetal anomalies associated with ondansetron use may not be significantly higher than the background 3% to 5% risk of fetal anomalies in the first trimester.[25] We recommend that ondansetron be used only when alternative antiemetics have failed and preferably after 10 weeks' gestation.[25]

Hyperemesis Gravidarum

Pathophysiology. Hyperemesis gravidarum occurs in approximately 1% of pregnant patients and is defined by nausea and vomiting that cause starvation metabolism, weight loss greater than 5% of total body weight, dehydration, and prolonged ketonemia and ketonuria. Without treatment, there is an increased risk of micronutrient deficiency and their respective sequelae to the patient (e.g., vitamin B_1 deficiency, Wernicke encephalopathy) and fetus (e.g., vitamin K deficiency, bleeding diatheses).[24]

The cause of hyperemesis gravidarum is not clear; associations have been made with increasing estradiol and hCG levels, as well as with maternal cytokines. Several studies have suggested an increased infection rate with *Helicobacter pylori* in patients with hyperemesis gravidarum; a nonteratogenic regimen for *H. pylori* treatment has been shown to decrease vomiting in hyperemesis patients.[26] Studies have also suggested that early treatment of nausea and vomiting of pregnancy may prevent progression to hyperemesis gravidarum.

Diagnostic Testing. Laboratory studies should assess volume status and reversible electrolyte abnormalities. A urinalysis screens for the presence of ketosis, elevated specific gravity, and infection. Serum chemistry assess the presence of hypokalemia, contraction alkalosis, elevated anion gap, or other metabolic abnormalities. Bilirubin and alkaline phosphatase levels can be mildly elevated but should return to normal after delivery. Hyperemesis may be complicated by liver disease and abnormal liver function test results, which are expected to resolve with supportive treatment.

Management. Initial management of hyperemesis involves rehydration with IV fluids (2 L of Ringer lactate [LR] at a rate of 500 ml/h), antiemetics (Diclegis is first line), and demonstration of ability to take oral hydration. Following the 2 liters of LR, expert consensus favors dextrose-containing IV fluids (D5/.45NS). Thiamine is administered before dextrose to prevent progression to Wernicke encephalopathy.[24] Dextrose-containing IV fluids are continued until ketones have cleared from the urine or the patient is able to tolerate oral intake. Patients who cannot tolerate oral intake should be admitted. Potassium and magnesium are repleted as needed. Antiemetics are used as previously described for nausea and vomiting in pregnancy. A short course of methylprednisolone (16 mg PO or IV q8h for 3 days) has been reported to be therapeutic for intractable hyperemesis; however, it is considered a last-line agent and its risk profile should be weighed carefully before administration.[24]

In women who cannot maintain their weight despite medical therapy, enteral nutrition via a nasogastric (NG) tube should be considered.

Thromboembolic Disease

KEY CONCEPTS

- Thromboembolic disease is a cause of maternal mortality in developed countries.
- CT angiography and lung scintigraphy (V/Q scan) are used for the diagnosis of pulmonary embolism (PE).
- Low-molecular-weight heparin is preferred for anticoagulation.

Foundations

Thromboembolic disease is associated with increased mortality in pregnancy and is among the most common causes of maternal death in developed countries. Pregnancy is a hypercoagulable state, with increased coagulation factors and stasis as pregnancy progresses and significant vascular trauma at the time of delivery. The risk of venous thrombosis increases during pregnancy to five or six times that of nonpregnant women. Although the risk is increased throughout pregnancy, it is highest during the first six weeks after delivery. Risk factors include smoking, obesity, age older than 35 years, hypercoagulable state, varicose veins, and prior superficial venous thrombosis. Women who deliver prematurely or have postpartum hemorrhage are also at increased risk.

Clinical Features

As in nonpregnant patients, clinical signs of pain, tenderness, and swelling are poor predictors of deep venous thrombosis (DVT) in pregnancy. The clinical diagnosis of pulmonary embolism (PE) is also difficult. Although tachypnea, tachycardia, dyspnea, and pleuritic pain are commonly associated with PE, the symptoms are nonspecific and may be associated with diverse diseases such as hepatic inflammation, pyelonephritis, and diaphragmatic impingement from a normal gravid uterus.

Diagnostic Testing

Deep Venous Thrombosis. Because of its widespread availability and avoidance of radiation, Doppler ultrasonography is the first-line test for the diagnosis of DVT. An abnormal study result is usually sufficient reason to treat the pregnant patient. However, normal leg study results can be seen with isolated iliac vein disease, which is common in pregnancy, and requires imaging with magnetic resonance venogram (MRV) or CT venogram (CTV) of the lower extremities for diagnosis. The risk of anticoagulation usually outweighs the risk of definitive studies when the diagnosis is equivocal.

Pulmonary Embolism. Currently, studies do not support the use of D-dimer tests in pregnancy to exclude the diagnosis of PE because this test may lack sufficient sensitivity in pregnant patients.[27] Chest radiography (shielding the pelvis and uterus) should be performed to exclude other disease processes that may mimic a PE. The diaphragm is normally symmetrically elevated during late pregnancy.

Magnetic resonance angiography (MRA) is considered a diagnostic modality of choice in pregnant patients because there is no risk of radiation exposure to the fetus.[27] MRA for PE is not often readily available for diagnosis of PE in the ED, therefore imaging with lung scintigraphy (V/Q scan) or CT angiography is recommended. The American Thoracic Society and The Society of Thoracic Radiology clinical practice guidelines for the evaluation of suspected PE in pregnancy suggest that chest x-ray be used as an initial evaluation and if chest x-ray is normal proceed to V/Q scan and if chest x-ray is abnormal, proceed to CTA.[27] Both have comparable performances for PE diagnosis during pregnancy. CTA delivers a lower fetal radiation dose but a higher maternal radiation dose when compared to V/Q scan.[27] However, the selection of the most appropriate test relies on local availability and expertise. In most EDs, the rapid availability of CTA makes it the diagnostic modality of choice for the evaluation of PE in pregnancy patients. Pulmonary angiography may be required if the diagnosis of PE is unclear after less invasive studies have been performed.

Management and Disposition

Warfarin (Coumadin) is contraindicated during pregnancy because of its teratogenic effects, high risk of abortions, and fetal hemorrhage. Heparinoids are used to treat thromboembolic disease during pregnancy. Unfractionated heparin carries a poorly understood risk of fetal osteoporosis, thrombocytopenia, prematurity, or miscarriage. In general, acute anticoagulation with IV heparin (80 units/kg bolus followed by 18 units/kg/hr) is followed by subcutaneous heparin (minimum 10,000 units subcutaneous q 12h), usually continued for 3 to 6 months postpartum in patients who have DVT or PE during pregnancy.

Patients receiving this treatment require laboratory testing every 1 or 2 weeks, and the efficacy of anticoagulation may be variable during pregnancy. We recommend low-molecular-weight heparin (enoxaparin 1 mg/kg subcutaneous q 12h) because it is considered safe in pregnancy and offers several advantages over unfractionated heparin. This includes decreased bleeding risk, reliable pharmacokinetics, decreased risk of heparin-induced thrombocytopenia, fixed dosages, less frequent dosing, and decreased risk of osteoporosis and thrombocytopenia. In patients with a history of DVT or PE, prophylaxis for subsequent gestations is usually recommended. Oral direct thrombin inhibitors (dabigatran) and anti-Xa inhibitors (rivaroxaban) should be avoided in pregnancy and lactation because there is insufficient data to evaluate the safety of these drugs to mother, fetus, and the breast-feeding neonate.[27]

Genitourinary Infections

KEY CONCEPTS

- Asymptomatic bacteriuria in pregnancy predisposes the patient to the development of symptomatic lower and upper tract genitourinary infections. Because up to 30% of women who have asymptomatic bacteriuria will have pyelonephritis if they are untreated, treatment of bacteriuria is cost-effective and important.
- Treatment of bacterial vaginosis is directed toward symptomatic relief for the patient and does not necessarily improve fetal outcomes. Management includes a 7-day course of either metronidazole or clindamycin.
- For the treatment of vulvovaginal candidiasis, oral azoles are contraindicated in pregnancy because of an association with adverse fetal outcomes. Treatment with vaginal azoles for 7 days during pregnancy is considered safe, with an estimated 80% cure rate.
- Of patients who have trichomoniasis, 50% are asymptomatic. Diagnosis is made by direct visualization of protozoans on a wet mount. The recommended treatment is metronidazole, a one-time dose of 2 g, for symptomatic patients only.
- Regarding the treatment of sexually transmitted diseases, in general, tetracyclines and quinolones are contraindicated in pregnant patients. Treatment of genital tract infections may be important for preventing preterm labor and decreasing transmission to the infant.
- *Chlamydia trachomatis* infection is the most common sexually transmitted disease in the United States and worldwide. Treatment during pregnancy or breast-feeding is azithromycin (single 1-g dose); a 7-day course of amoxicillin is an acceptable alternative.
- Women who have genital herpes during the third trimester have a 30% to 50% increased risk of fetal transmission compared to women with herpes simplex virus (HSV) infection in the first trimester (1%).
- Suppressive therapy can reduce the need for cesarean section in women whose first clinical episode of genital HSV occurred during pregnancy.

- Gonococcal arthritis is the most common manifestation of gonococcal dissemination. Diagnosis and treatment of gonococcal infections are unchanged by pregnancy; treatment includes cephalosporins or azithromycin.
- PID is rarely encountered in pregnancy and does not occur after the first trimester. Given the risk of endometrial infection in pregnancy and the need to consider other diagnoses, pregnant patients who have suspected PID require hospitalization and IV antibiotics.
- Chorioamnionitis is diagnosed by the findings of fever, maternal and fetal tachycardia, and uterine tenderness in a patient past 16 weeks of pregnancy. Patients are usually treated with IV ampicillin and gentamicin.

Urinary Tract Infection

Foundations. Asymptomatic bacteriuria in pregnancy predisposes the patient to the development of symptomatic lower and upper tract genitourinary infections. This has led to the US Preventive Services Task Force recommendation to screen for asymptomatic bacteriuria with urine culture for pregnant women at 12 to 16 weeks' gestation or at the first prenatal visit, if later (grade A recommendation). Uterine pressure exerted on the bladder and ureters, poor emptying of the bladder with voiding, and progesterone-induced smooth muscle relaxation that inhibits ureteral peristalsis appear to contribute to an increased risk of infection during pregnancy.

Prenatal screening of patients with asymptomatic bacteriuria in early pregnancy identifies approximately 95% of those at risk for subsequent bacteriuria during the pregnancy. Because up to 30% of women who have asymptomatic bacteriuria will have pyelonephritis if they are untreated, the treatment of bacteriuria is cost-effective and important. Antibiotic treatment may also reduce the risk of preterm delivery and low birth weight.

Clinical Features and Diagnostic Testing. The pregnant patient who presents with lower urinary tract symptoms (e.g., dysuria, frequency, urgency) or upper tract symptoms (e.g., fever, malaise, back pain) should have a pelvic examination and evaluation of an uncontaminated urine specimen. There is a predominance of right-sided symptoms during pregnancy, probably the result of increased mechanical forces on the right ureter, but left-sided flank pain or bilateral symptoms may be caused by pyelonephritis. Rarely, urinalysis may yield normal results or cultures may produce negative findings because of failure to report lower colony counts or because of complete obstruction of the involved ureter.

The major risk of asymptomatic and lower urinary tract infection is spread to the renal parenchyma. Acute pyelonephritis carries considerable morbidity in pregnancy, including maternal sepsis, permanent renal injury, and premature labor. The risk of prematurity can be minimized by effective treatment and continued monitoring for recurrence. The development of premature labor in the pregnant patient who has pyelonephritis is ominous; it can be prevented only by aggressive recognition and treatment earlier in pregnancy.

Differential Diagnosis. Vaginitis, herpes genitalis, chlamydial infection of the urethra, and ovarian torsion can masquerade as urinary tract symptoms. A history of external dysuria (burning at the perineum with urination) suggests herpes or vaginitis. A pelvic examination should be performed to obtain cervical culture specimens and identify perineal or vaginal causes of dysuria. Appendicitis, cholecystitis, pancreatitis, and liver diseases in pregnancy must be considered in the differential diagnosis of an upper urinary tract infection. Back pain may also be a sign of premature labor. Careful evaluation of an uncontaminated catheterized urine specimen is essential to the correct diagnosis.

Management. Patients with asymptomatic bacteriuria or lower urinary tract signs and symptoms should be treated with 7 to 10 days of an antibiotic that is active against common urinary pathogens and safe in pregnancy. The most common choices are a cephalosporin, such as cephalexin, 500 mg orally BID for 3 to 7 days; nitrofurantoin, 100 mg orally bid for 3 to 7 days; amoxicillin 500 mg TID for 7 days; or a sulfonamide, such as trimethoprim-sulfamethoxazole, 800/160 mg BID for 3 days (except during the third trimester). Clinicians should choose their antibiotic based on local antibiograms and consider factors such as cost, local availability, and side effects when selecting the best treatment option.

Patients with fever, back pain, and evidence of acute pyelonephritis in pregnancy are usually admitted for IV antibiotic administration. In such cases, IV hydration, obstetric consultation, and testing of urine cultures should be initiated. At least one parenteral dose of antibiotics should be given, with antibiotic coverage guided by known organism susceptibilities in a given hospital. Because the resistance of *Escherichia coli* to ampicillin is considerable in most regions, a cephalosporin, such as ceftriaxone, 1 g IV daily, is usually administered. Culture testing must be performed to ensure that the original choice of antibiotic was correct, and the patient must have a repeated culture and be observed closely after treatment.

Vaginitis

Bacterial Vaginosis. Bacterial vaginosis (formerly known as *Gardnerella* vaginitis or *Haemophilus vaginalis* vaginitis) is an overgrowth of multiple endogenous vaginal bacteria, in some cases producing excessive discharge and vaginal malodor. Prevalence rates for bacterial vaginosis in pregnancy are estimated at 15% to 20%. Bacterial vaginosis is associated with an increased risk of chorioamnionitis, subclinical PID, premature rupture of membranes, fetal prematurity, and postpartum endometritis after vaginal delivery. However, treatment of bacterial vaginosis is directed toward symptomatic relief for the patient and does not necessarily improve fetal outcomes. Management includes a 7-day oral course of metronidazole (500 mg BID) or 7-day oral course of clindamycin (300 mg BID). Intravaginal treatment is not recommended in pregnant patients.

Candida Albicans Vaginitis. The incidence of vulvovaginal candidiasis is increased during pregnancy by high levels of estrogen and other steroids. There is no association of *Candida* colonization with adverse pregnancy outcomes, so treatment is for relief of symptoms only. Oral azoles are contraindicated in pregnancy because of an association with adverse fetal outcomes. Treatment with vaginal azoles (intravaginal topical clotrimazole or miconazole) for 7 days during pregnancy is considered safe, with an estimated 80% cure rate.[28] Recurrent disease may require a vaginal culture to confirm the diagnosis and identify unusual *Candida* species (e.g., *Candida glabrata*) that may be resistant to conventional treatment. Longer treatment or treatment of a potential *Candida* reservoir in the patient's sexual partner(s) may also be required.

Trichomonas Vaginitis. Trichomoniasis is a sexually transmitted vaginitis caused by a protozoan parasite, *Trichomonas vaginalis*. Of patients who have trichomoniasis, 50% are asymptomatic. Symptoms include vaginal itching, malodorous discharge, and vaginal irritation. Diagnosis is made by direct visualization of protozoans on wet mount. Symptomatic pregnant women, regardless of pregnancy stage, should be tested and considered for treatment. The recommended treatment is metronidazole, 500 mg BID for 7 days.[28] Intravaginal treatment is not recommended in pregnant patients.

Sexually Transmitted Disease

Sexually transmitted diseases are treated in pregnant patients according to CDC guidelines.[29] In general, tetracyclines and quinolones are contraindicated in pregnant patients. Treatment of genital tract infections may be important in preventing preterm labor and decreasing transmission to the infant.

Chlamydia Trachomatis. Chlamydia trachomatis infection is the most common sexually transmitted disease in the United States and worldwide. Its prevalence is currently three to five times that of *Neisseria gonorrhoeae* infection. Clinical diagnosis is difficult during pregnancy because cervical mucus is usually cloudy and contains white blood cells, but urine sampling can be done and is equivalent to endocervical sampling in pregnancy infections. Routine chlamydia screening during pregnancy is important to prevent complications of preterm labor and postpartum endometritis, both of which are more common in patients who have chlamydial cervical infections. Additionally, repeat chlamydia screening should be considered in adolescent and young adult women and those who tested positive earlier in pregnancy.[29] Chlamydial infections of infants born to infected mothers include conjunctivitis and pneumonitis. Treatment during pregnancy or breastfeeding is azithromycin (single 1-g dose), which improves compliance and decreases gastrointestinal side effects; a 7-day course of amoxicillin (500 mg PO TID) is an acceptable alternative.

Neisseria Gonorrhoeae. Gonococcal infection of the cervix occurs in 1% of pregnant women.[30] Symptoms are similar to those in nonpregnant women. Salpingitis is rare but may develop during the first trimester from upper genital extension of cervical infection. Some practitioners believe that the incidence of the disseminated infection is increased in pregnant patients because of elevated progesterone levels and increased vascularity in the area of the cervix.

Gonococcal arthritis is the most common manifestation of gonococcal dissemination. Diagnosis and treatment of gonococcal infections are unchanged by pregnancy; treatment includes cephalosporins (ceftriaxone 250 mg IM) or azithromycin (single 2-g dose PO). Treatment of possible coexistent chlamydial infection is recommended for pregnant and nonpregnant women. The major complications of third-trimester gonococcal infection are neonatal gonococcal ophthalmia and sepsis.

Herpes Simplex. Herpes simplex virus (HSV) infections pose a risk in pregnancy to the mother and newborn. Women who have genital herpes during the third trimester have a 30% to 50% increased risk of transmission compared to those in the first trimester (1%). The virus can be transmitted prenatally through transplacental infection or ascending vaginal infection and by vaginal delivery, particularly when herpetic lesions are present. Infections in the neonate often are disseminated or involve the CNS, causing significant morbidity and mortality. In the ED, culture of new suspected herpetic lesions of the cervix, vagina, or perineum identifies patients at risk for perinatal complications. Although the risk of oral acyclovir (400 mg TID for 7–10 days) and valacyclovir (1 g BID for 7–10 days) use in pregnancy is not well known, it is recommended for first-episode genital herpes. Suppressive therapy can reduce the need for cesarean section in women whose first clinical episode of genital herpes simplex occurred during pregnancy but may not eliminate the need for cesarean section in women with recurrent herpes simplex. Treatment should be undertaken with obstetric consultation and careful patient monitoring.

Upper Genital Tract Infection

Pelvic Inflammatory Disease. PID is very rare in pregnancy and does not occur after the first trimester. The differential diagnosis includes ectopic pregnancy, septic abortion, and appendicitis, all of which are more common. In the patient with suspected infection, smears or cultures for *Chlamydia* and *N. gonorrhea* should be performed. Given the risk of endometrial infection in pregnancy and the need to consider other diagnoses, pregnant patients who have suspected PID require hospitalization and IV antibiotics.

Chorioamnionitis. Chorioamnionitis is the infection or inflammation of the placenta and fetal membranes. After 16 weeks of pregnancy, the chorioamniotic membranes adhere to the cervical os and may become infected. The risk is increased in women with preterm labor. Chorioamnionitis is diagnosed by the findings of fever, maternal and fetal tachycardia, and uterine tenderness in a patient past 16 weeks of pregnancy. Leukocytosis can be suggestive of chorioamnionitis but is not diagnostic. Patients should have blood specimens drawn for culture. Vaginal and cervical culture specimens for group B streptococci, *E. coli,* chlamydia, and gonorrhea should also be obtained. Urgent obstetric consultation should be obtained, and hospitalization for IV administration of antibiotics is required. Patients are usually treated with IV ampicillin (2 g q6 hr) and gentamicin (5 mg/kg q day).[31]

Endocrine Disorders

Thyroid Disorders

KEY CONCEPTS

- During pregnancy, the thyroid gland increases in size, requires more iodine, and produces more thyroid hormone than in the nonpregnant state.
- Hyperthyroidism, characterized by a suppressed TSH level and elevated T_4 and/or T_3 levels occurs in 0.1% to 0.4% of all pregnancies. Graves disease and hCG-mediated hyperthyroidism are the most common causes.
- When US women are diagnosed with hypothyroidism, the most common cause is Hashimoto (autoimmune) thyroiditis.
- Postpartum thyroiditis is characterized by transient hyperthyroidism or hypothyroidism, or both, in the postpartum period. Approximately 25% of these women develop permanent hypothyroidism in the subsequent 10 years.
- Hyperthyroidism may be associated with hydatidiform mole and usually resolves with evacuation of the mole.
- The diagnosis of hyperthyroidism is confirmed by a low (<0.1 mU/L) or undetectable (<0.01 mU/L) serum TSH level and levels of free T_3 and T_4 that exceed the normal range for pregnancy.
- Confirmation of hypothyroidism is based on an elevated serum TSH level, relying on trimester-specific TSH reference ranges.
- Propylthiouracil (PTU) is the preferred treatment of hyperthyroidism in the United States. For thyroid storm, dexamethasone and beta blockers are added, with the patient admitted to the intensive care unit.
- Hypothyroidism in pregnancy is managed with levothyroxine supplementation (1.6 μg/kg/day).

Foundations. Thyroid disorders are common in women of childbearing age. During pregnancy, however, this is associated with a range of adverse maternal and fetal outcomes, including spontaneous miscarriage, preeclampsia, heart failure, preterm delivery, intrauterine growth restriction, and stillbirth.[32] The evaluation and management of pregnant women with thyroid dysfunction parallel those of nonpregnant women but require attention to the physiologic changes to the thyroid gland that occur during pregnancy.

Normal pregnancy exerts stress on the thyroid gland. During pregnancy, the thyroid gland increases in size, requires more iodine, and produces more thyroid hormone than in the nonpregnant state. Moreover, maternal and fetal thyroid function are strongly linked, with maternal thyroxine accounting for a substantial portion of fetal thyroid function at birth.[32] Thyroid dysfunction in pregnancy can occur during pregnancy or the postpartum state.

Hyperthyroidism, characterized by suppressed thyroid stimulating hormone (TSH) levels, elevated triiodothyronine (T3) and/or thyroxine (T4), occurs in only 0.1% to 0.4% of all pregnancies.[33] Hyperthyroidism in pregnancy can be a result of any cause, but

Graves disease and hCG-mediated hyperthyroidism are the most common causes. Graves disease is an autoimmune process associated with thyroid-stimulating antibodies and usually becomes less severe during the later stages of pregnancy. hCG, which is homologous to TSH, has some thyroid-stimulating activity and may transiently cause hyperthyroidism in the first half of gestation. hCG-mediated hyperthyroidism is typically less severe than Graves disease–associated hyperthyroidism.

Hypothyroidism complicates 2% to 3% of pregnancies.[33] Although nutritional iodine deficiency is a common cause of hypothyroidism globally, it is rare in the United States. When women in the United States are diagnosed with hypothyroidism, the most common cause is Hashimoto (autoimmune) thyroiditis, in which autoantibodies cause destruction of the thyroid gland. Hypothyroidism is associated with adverse pregnancy effects, including preeclampsia, placental abruption, low birth weight, and an increased risk of stillbirth.

Postpartum thyroiditis is characterized by transient hyperthyroidism or hypothyroidism, or both, in the postpartum period. It is estimated that 5% to 10% of women have postpartum thyroiditis. Most women return to a euthyroid state within 1 year postpartum, but approximately 20% to 40% of these women develop permanent hypothyroidism in the subsequent 10 years.[33] The diagnostic triad consists of a lack of previous history of thyroid disorders, an abnormal TSH concentration during the first postpartum year, and the absence of TSH receptor antibodies (Graves disease) or a toxic nodule.

Clinical Features. The diagnosis of thyroid dysfunction during pregnancy is difficult because pregnancy itself can mimic the findings in mild to moderate hypothyroidism and hyperthyroidism.

Hyperthyroidism in pregnancy should be suspected when the patient exhibits disproportionate tachycardia, thyromegaly, exophthalmos, weight loss, or inadequate weight gain during pregnancy. Hyperthyroidism may be associated with hydatidiform mole and usually resolves with evacuation of the mole. Patients may present with signs of thyroid storm, including altered mental status, severe tachycardia, and signs of high-output heart failure (e.g., edema, dyspnea, orthopnea).

Like hyperthyroidism, *hypothyroidism* in pregnancy is difficult to diagnose. Signs such as edema, fatigue, and weight gain may be attributed to the pregnancy rather than thyroid dysfunction. Enlargement of the thyroid gland may be absent depending on the cause of the hypothyroidism. The diagnosis of hypothyroidism during pregnancy should be suspected when the patient exhibits edema, dry skin, hair loss, and a prolonged relaxation phase of deep tendon reflexes.

Patients with *postpartum thyroiditis* classically present with thyrotoxicosis 6 weeks to 6 months postpartum, followed by a hypothyroid state lasting up to 6 months. A euthyroid state returns by the end of the first postpartum year. However, most patients present with hyperthyroidism alone or lone hypothyroidism. The recurrence rate in subsequent pregnancy is estimated at 69%, and 25% of women eventually develop permanent hypothyroidism.

Differential Diagnoses. Thyroid dysfunction should be considered in the patient with nonspecific symptoms, including fatigue, anxiety, depression, and unexplained weight loss or weight gain. When a diagnosis of hypothyroidism or hyperthyroidism is recognized, their respective causes and differential diagnoses should be considered (see Chapter 117 for more detailed information).

Diagnostic Testing. Normal values of thyroid hormones vary based on stage of pregnancy. The diagnosis of hyperthyroidism is confirmed by a low (<0.1 mU/L) or undetectable (<0.01 mU/L) serum TSH level and levels of free T_3 and T_4 that exceed the normal range for pregnancy. Confirmation of hypothyroidism is based on an elevated serum TSH

level, relying on trimester-specific TSH reference ranges.[33] Overt hypothyroidism is defined as an elevated trimester-specific TSH, along with a decreased, trimester-specific free T_4 concentration. Subclinical hypothyroidism is defined as an elevated trimester-specific serum TSH concentration and a normal free T_4 concentration.

Management. Generally, no treatment is required for hCG-mediated hyperthyroidism. Treatment of pregnant women with overt hyperthyroidism due to Graves disease is of utmost importance because good fetal and maternal outcomes depend on controlling the mother's hyperthyroidism. Although thyroid ablation with radioactive iodine is contraindicated in pregnancy, medical treatments are available. Propylthiouracil (PTU) is the preferred treatment of hyperthyroidism in the United States. Methimazole is equally effective at treating hyperthyroidism in pregnancy but may be associated with fetal anomalies such as aplasia cutis, esophageal atresia, and choanal atresia. It is therefore not recommended as first-line treatment for hyperthyroidism in pregnancy.

Patients with symptoms of thyroid storm should be managed in an intensive care setting. Treatment with PTU (100 mg q8hr) should be initiated early.[33] Beta blockers such as propranolol (20–40 mg q6h) should be considered to control tachycardia; labetalol, esmolol, and propranolol have been used intrapartum.[33] A subtotal thyroidectomy may be considered once the symptoms of thyrotoxicosis are managed medically.

Hypothyroidism in pregnancy is managed with levothyroxine supplementation (1.6 μg/kg/day). Patients in the hypothyroid phase of postpartum thyroiditis require levothyroxine when they have a TSH level higher than 10 mU/L or between 4 and 10 mU/L with symptoms or active attempt at becoming pregnant. The hyperthyroid phase of postpartum thyroiditis is usually managed with a limited course of beta blockers.

Disorders of the Hypothalamic-Pituitary Axis

Foundations. The pituitary gland is normally enlarged in pregnancy due to estrogen stimulation. Disorders of the hypothalamic-pituitary axis may increase the incidence of maternal and fetal morbidity and mortality.

Pregnancy profoundly affects the hypothalamic-pituitary axis, resulting in increased circulating levels of cortisol and adrenocorticotropic hormone due to increased estrogen production. In contrast, levels of growth hormone decrease in pregnancy. Disorders of the hypothalamic-pituitary axis in pregnancy can result in adrenal insufficiency, Cushing syndrome, acromegaly, diabetes insipidus, and prolactinomas. Although these disorders are rare, they are associated with maternal morbidity (e.g., hypertension, hyperglycemia, eclampsia) and up to 20% fetal mortality.

Clinical Features. Disorders of the hypothalamic-pituitary axis usually present as an insidious set of chronic symptoms, many of which can mimic normal pregnancy, making diagnosis difficult. Symptoms vary depending on the specific disease but include fatigue, malaise, vomiting, weight gain or loss, amenorrhea, galactorrhea, and hyperprolactinemia. Normal pregnancy can be associated with slight decreases in the serum sodium level; more severe decreases in the serum sodium level may be signs of diabetes insipidus or adrenal insufficiency.

Diabetes insipidus may also be caused by pituitary infarction in the setting of severe obstetric hemorrhage (Sheehan syndrome). Advancements in the management and resuscitation of obstetric hemorrhage have made Sheehan syndrome increasingly rare, but it remains an important clinical consideration. The symptoms of Sheehan syndrome are dependent on the degree of the patient's hypopituitarism. Patients present with signs and symptoms that vary according to the deficient hormones. The failure of postpartum lactation and resumption of normal menstruation are strongly suggestive of Sheehan syndrome. Following postpartum hemorrhage, patients may have persistent tachycardia, hypotension, and latency between hemorrhage, and the onset of symptoms can vary, from months to years after pregnancy.

Diagnostic Testing. Diagnostic considerations vary according to the patient's presentation. Growth hormone levels are elevated in patients with acromegaly. Patients with adrenal insufficiency may present with hyponatremia and hyperkalemia, although these may be absent in many patients. MRI is helpful in the detection of prolactinoma or Sheehan syndrome.

Management. Stabilization consists of treatment of serious manifestations, such as hyperkalemia, tachycardia, and hypotension. Outpatient management is appropriate in the stable patient, provided there is urgent endocrinology follow-up.

Acknowledgment

We thank Dr. Sidhant Nagrani and Dr. Bisan Salhi for their contributions to previous editions of this chapter.

The references for this chapter can be found online at ExpertConsult. com.

174

Medical Emergencies During Pregnancy

Diane L. Gorgas and Robert Cooper

KEY CONCEPTS

Asthma

- The treatment goal for a pregnant woman with an acute asthma exacerbation is to prevent fetal hypoxia by keeping maternal oxygen saturation above 95%. Inhaled beta-agonists and corticosteroids are first-line emergency department treatment and are considered safe for use in pregnancy.

Cardiac Disease

- Hypertensive emergency in pregnancy is defined as acute-onset persistent hypertension with systolic blood pressure greater than 160 mm Hg or diastolic blood pressure greater than 110 mm Hg that is persistent for greater than 15 minutes. In these cases, antihypertensive therapy should be administered as soon as reasonably possible, and no later than 30 to 60 minutes after diagnosis with a target blood pressure of 140 to 150 mm Hg systolic and 90 to 100 mm Hg diastolic. The drugs of choice are oral nifedipine, IV hydralazine, and IV labetalol.
- The risk for acute coronary syndrome and acute myocardial infarction is increased in pregnant women compared to age-matched controls. The most common cause of AMI in the pregnant women is spontaneous coronary artery dissection. Treatment is similar to the nonpregnant agent, although P2Y12 receptor inhibitors should be avoided and fibrinolytic agent use should be carefully considered in women close to term.

Anemia

- Anemia in pregnancy is defined as a hemoglobin less than 11. Serum ferritin is the most accurate lab value for diagnosing iron deficiency anemia in pregnancy. Women with mild iron deficiency anemia can be started on daily iron supplementation while those with severe iron deficiency in the second and third trimester can be referred for IV iron infusion.
- Sickle cell disease causes maternal complications including more frequent pain crises, and increased risk of venous thromboembolism and preeclampsia. Treatment of pain crises is the same as in nonpregnant patients with the exception that hydroxyurea is contraindicated due to known teratogenicity.

Epilepsy

- Gravid patients with epilepsy have a tenfold risk of death compared to pregnant women without epilepsy. Many antiepileptic drugs (AEDs) have known teratogenicity and levetiracetam and lamotrigine are considered the safest agents during pregnancy. Treatment of status epilepticus is with benzodiazepines followed by a phenytoin as first-line AED and levetiracetam as second-line AED.

Endocrine

- Pregnant patients with type 1 diabetes mellitus (T1DM) are recommended to transition to insulin during gestation to achieve HgbA1C values <6%.

- Hypoglycemia is most common in the first trimester, and up to 40% of pregnancies are marked with at least 1 episode of severe hypoglycemia.
- Comorbid obesity increases the risk of cesarean section and venous thromboembolism.
- Graves disease commonly rebounds in the immediate postpartum period with thyrotoxicosis.
- Radioiodine is strongly contraindicated for the treatment of hyperthyroidism in pregnancy.
- All gravid patients with new-onset nephrolithiasis should be screened for hypercalcemia. Treatment of hypercalcemia with bisphosphonates is contraindicated in pregnancy.

Psychiatric Disorders

- Prenatal discontinuation of methamphetamines and other stimulants, although desirable, can cause depression and psychosis.
- Maternal and neonatal outcomes in women on opioid agnostic therapy show decreased rates of neonatal abstinence syndrome (neonatal opioid withdrawal syndrome).

Inflammatory Disorders

- Antiphospholipid syndrome (APS) in lupus patients is characterized by deep vessel clotting, pregnancy-related morbidity, and positive anticoagulant serum markers. Catastrophic APS has rapid-onset small vessel thrombosis, multiorgan dysfunction, and a high maternal mortality rate.

Renal Disease

- Management of chronic kidney disease (CKD) in pregnancy can be treated with intensified hemodialysis (increased length of treatment time or increased frequency) to improve fetal outcome.
- Patients post renal transplantation have fertility rates that return to normal within 6 months.

Infectious Disorders

- Moderate to severe anemia in pregnancy in an HIV-infected mother should prompt a workup for tuberculosis.
- During pregnancy, penicillin is the only known effective treatment for congenital syphilis, and pregnant patients with penicillin allergy should be desensitized and treated with penicillin.
- Lamivudine given in late pregnancy to women with high viral loads of HBV DNA reduces viral transmission when given in conjunction with HBV vaccine and immune globulin.
- Obstetric hemorrhagic complications, including DIC and shock and subsequent need for transfusion, are more common with HCV infection.

FOUNDATIONS

The physiologic changes that occur in pregnancy may exceed the patient's underlying compensatory mechanisms, resulting in initial symptom onset or rapid decompensation of medical illness during pregnancy. Certain chronic medical conditions also pose a serious threat to the mother's health or result in a poor fetal outcome. Finally, some medical illnesses result in a difficult delivery or the need for special resuscitation measures in the neonate.

The incidence of pregnancy in chronically ill patients has been increasing because of improved survival of patients with diseases such as diabetes, epilepsy, renal failure, obesity, and various cancers. Also, the demographics of pregnancy are changing in that maternal age at the time of first pregnancy is increasing. Advances in assisted reproduction, including in vitro fertilization and oocyte donation, have made it possible for older women—including those who are postmenopausal—to become pregnant. Older pregnant women experience an increased rate of antepartum and intrapartum complications and are more likely to have comorbid conditions such as cardiovascular disease.

The recognition of an unexpected or even expected pregnancy may occur in the setting of the emergency department (ED), and many interventions are time-sensitive, requiring treatment in the ED. All emergency clinicians should have an understanding of critical diagnostic and treatment possibilities when encountering a pregnant patient with a preexisting illness.

ASTHMA

Asthma exacerbations occur in up to 45% of pregnant asthmatics with almost half of those exacerbations requiring rescue oral corticosteroids or hospitalization.[1] Poorly controlled asthma is associated with an increased risk of preeclampsia or eclampsia, premature contractions, cesarean section, low birth weight, and small-for-gestational-age status. The risk of such complications varies with the severity of the disease and degree of control during pregnancy. Adverse perinatal outcomes increase with the severity of asthma during pregnancy. Controlling asthma during pregnancy leads to less intrauterine growth retardation and fewer adverse perinatal outcomes. It has been well documented that asthma may worsen, improve, or remain the same during pregnancy, but no studies have examined whether this is caused by changes in asthma triggers, treatment, or severity.

Maternal respiratory function changes can make it more difficult to recognize the decompensating pregnant asthmatic patient. Tidal volume and minute ventilation increase by 45% over the course of pregnancy resulting in an average PCO_2 of 32 mm Hg. The kidneys compensate and maintain an average bicarbonate level of 19 mEq/mL, which results in a compensated respiratory alkalosis with a serum pH between 7.40 and 7.45.

Many adverse perinatal outcomes associated with maternal asthma are thought to be due to fetal hypoxia. Thus, the overall goal of treatment is maintaining maternal oxygen saturations above 95%. Both the American College of Obstetrics and Gynecology (ACOG) and National Asthma Education and Prevention Program have clearly stated that it is safer to use asthma medications to treat pregnant women than to allow severe asthma symptoms and exacerbations to occur during pregnancy. Despite the support for aggressive asthma treatment from consensus guidelines, studies show variation in the amount of dispensed asthma medications before and during pregnancy.

The standard treatment for a pregnant asthmatic patient is the same as that for a nonpregnant patient with an asthma exacerbation. After history and the performance of a physical examination, the peak expiratory flow (PEF) or forced expiratory volume in 1 second (FEV_1)

should be measured. There is no significant change in the FEV_1/ FVC ratio throughout pregnancy and a decline in these values is of concern. Patients with an FEV_1 or PEF less than 50% of their predicted maximum are classified as having a severe exacerbation. An initial fetal assessment should be performed, including fetal heart tones and continuous electronic fetal monitoring with a biophysical profile if the pregnancy has reached viability. Supplemental oxygen should be given to all mothers with oxygen saturation below 95%.

Inhaled short acting β_2-agonists are the first-line treatment for an asthma exacerbation and can be given continuously, if needed, for a severe exacerbation. Adjunctive anticholinergic medications are considered and albuterol and can used as in nonpregnant patients. Long-acting selective β_2-agonists and inhaled corticosteroids can be added as controller medications on discharge from the ED.[2] Multiple studies have shown no increased risk of adverse perinatal outcomes from inhaled corticosteroids. Budesonide is the preferred agent in pregnancy.[3] Nonselective β-agonists such as epinephrine are generally avoided because of concern for uterine vasoconstriction. β-agonists are tocolytics and will often halt labor.

Oral corticosteroids are indicated for use in moderate to severe asthma exacerbations and should be prescribed for the same indications as in nonpregnant asthmatics. Despite these recommendations, in one study only 63% of pregnant women treated in the ED received systemic corticosteroids at discharge despite 100% of these women receiving inhaled β-agonists during their visit.[4] There is weak evidence that oral corticosteroid use increases the risk of preterm delivery and low-birth-weight infants; there is also conflicting evidence of an increased risk of orofacial clefts. The benefits of oral corticosteroid use for avoiding fetal hypoxia greatly outweighs the risk of adverse perinatal outcomes and all expert guidelines recommend oral corticosteroid use.

Second-line agents for asthma control (e.g., cromolyn sodium) are considered safe in pregnancy. In limited studies, magnesium has been shown to improve respiratory function in pregnant females with severe asthma exacerbations without adverse fetal outcomes.

CARDIOVASCULAR DISORDERS

Foundations

Heart disease in pregnant women is the leading cause of nonobstetric maternal deaths.[5,6] The proportion of maternal deaths due to cardiovascular disease has increased as pulmonary hypertension, cardiomyopathies, aortic dissection, and myocardial infarction have become more prevalent in pregnant women. The increase in blood volume due to pregnancy, along with the increases in preload, cardiac output, and oxygen consumption, can worsen or reveal cardiac disease in pregnant women. Because the signs and symptoms of acute coronary syndromes and heart failure (e.g., shortness of breath, mild chest pain, edema) can be seen in normal pregnancies, these entities are especially difficult to diagnose.

Hypertension

Chronic Hypertension

The definitions of hypertension and hypertensive crisis differ for pregnant and nonpregnant patients, as do the blood pressure values at which to start treatment. As opposed to the American College of Cardiology (ACC)/American Heart Association definition, chronic hypertension in pregnancy is defined as hypertension (>140 mm Hg systolic or > 90 mm Hg diastolic) diagnosed prior to pregnancy or before 20 weeks' gestation (Table 174.1).[7] Chronic hypertension in pregnancy increases the risk of superimposed preeclampsia, preterm delivery, intrauterine growth restriction, and cesarean section.

TABLE 174.1 Hypertensive Disorders of Pregnancy

	Chronic Hypertension	Gestational Hypertension	Preeclampsia	Chronic Hypertension With Superimposed Preeclampsia
Definition	Hypertension that antedates pregnancy[a]	Hypertension diagnosed after 20 wk of gestation in the absence of proteinuria or other evidence of preeclampsia	Hypertension that begins after 20 wk of gestation in association with new-onset proteinuria (>300 mg/24 hr) or symptoms below in the absence of proteinuria	Hypertension that antedates pregnancy in association with new-onset proteinuria
	Hypertension diagnosed before 20 wk of gestation		Decreased platelets, elevated liver transaminase levels, renal insufficiency, pulmonary edema	Sudden increase in proteinuria in woman with chronic hypertension[a] and proteinuria before 20 wk of gestation
				Hypertension that antedates pregnancy in association with sudden increase in blood pressure
	Comment—rarely, preeclampsia presents before 20 wk of gestation	Comment—may progress to preeclampsia; may also represent previously undiagnosed hypertension		Hypertension that antedates pregnancy in association with decreased platelets, elevated liver transaminase levels, renal insufficiency, pulmonary edema, or cerebral or visual symptoms

[a]Defined as blood pressure > 140 mm Hg systolic or > 90 mm Hg diastolic.
Adapted from: Nishimura RA, Otto CM, Bonow RO, et al, ACC/AHA Task Force Members. 2014 AHA/ACC guideline for the management of patients with valvular heart disease: a report of the American College of Cardiology/American Heart Association Task Force on Practice Guidelines. *Circulation.* 2010;129:e521e643.

Chronic hypertension of pregnancy is categorized as mild hypertension (systolic blood pressure of 140–159 mm Hg or diastolic blood pressure of 90–109 mm Hg) or severe hypertension (systolic blood pressure greater than 160 mm Hg or diastolic blood pressure greater than 110 mm Hg). Previously there was agreement that mild hypertension of pregnancy did not require treatment. However, tight control of blood pressure (goal diastolic blood pressure less than 85 mm Hg) has been shown to lower the frequency of severe maternal hypertension. There is no difference in the risk of pregnancy loss, high-level neonatal care, or overall maternal complication between "tight" and "less-tight" blood pressure control groups.[8] ACOG recommends that antihypertensive treatment be started when blood pressures are consistently higher than 160 mm Hg systolic and/or higher than 110 mm Hg diastolic. The European Society of Cardiology endorses treating chronic hypertension of pregnancy at 150/95 mm HG, though it sites a lack of evidence. Finally, the International Society for the study of Hypertension in Pregnancy endorses treating hypertension if blood pressures are consistently above 140/90 mm Hg.

The major risk posed by severe chronic hypertension is a progression to preeclampsia, which occurs in 25% of these pregnancies. Severe hypertension is associated with low birth weight, preterm delivery, elevated liver enzymes, and prolonged hospital stays as compared to women with chronic hypertension without severe hypertension.[9] Antihypertensive drugs are effective in preventing this progression. The first-line oral agents for the treatment of chronic hypertension are labetalol 200 to 1200 mg/day in 2 to 3 divided doses, nifedipine XL 30 to 120 mg/day, and methyldopa 500 to 3000 mg/day in 2 divided doses.

Hypertensive Emergencies

All major society guidelines define a hypertensive emergency as acute-onset persistent hypertension with systolic blood pressure greater than 160 mm Hg or diastolic blood pressure greater than 110 mm Hg that is persistent for greater than 15 minutes. In these cases, antihypertensive therapy should be administered as soon as reasonably possible, and no later than 30 to 60 minutes after diagnosis. Goal blood pressure is within the range of 140 to 150 mm Hg systolic and 90 to 100 mm Hg diastolic in order to prevent loss of cerebral autoregulation. IV labetalol, IV hydralazine, and oral nifedipine are all considered first-line treatment, with oral nifedipine indicated when IV access has not yet been established (Fig. 174.1).[10]

In 2013, ACOG changed its diagnostic criteria for preeclampsia to no longer require proteinuria. In the absence of proteinuria, preeclampsia is diagnosed as hypertension in the presence of thrombocytopenia, impaired liver function, pulmonary edema, visual disturbances, or the development of renal insufficiency.

Cardiac Disorders

Acute Coronary Syndromes

In a United Kingdom Registry, cardiac disease was the largest indirect cause of maternal death with ischemic heart disease accounting for more than one-fifth of cardiac mortality.[11] The mortality rate in pregnant women who have had an acute myocardial infarction (AMI) is from 5% to 7%. Pregnant women are two to four times more likely to have an AMI as compared to age-matched nonpregnant individuals. The number of older women becoming pregnant is increasing; pregnant women aged 40 years or older have a 30-fold greater risk for acute coronary syndrome (ACS) than pregnant women 20 years of age or younger. The incidence of AMI is highest during the last trimester and peripartum period with 21% of pregnancy related MIs occurring in the antepartum period.[12]

Multiple factors are hypothesized to increase the risk of AMI in pregnancy, including a prothrombotic state, increased myocardial oxygen demand secondary to increased cardiac output and heart rate, and decreased oxygen-carrying capacity secondary to physiologic anemia, which may precipitate angina. Hypertension, thrombophilia, anemia, diabetes, advanced maternal age, multiparous state, and smoking increase the risk of pregnancy-associated AMI.

Most cases of ACS in pregnancy are related to causes other than atherosclerosis. The most common cause of ACS is spontaneous coronary artery dissection (SCAD) accounting for anywhere from 23% to 43%

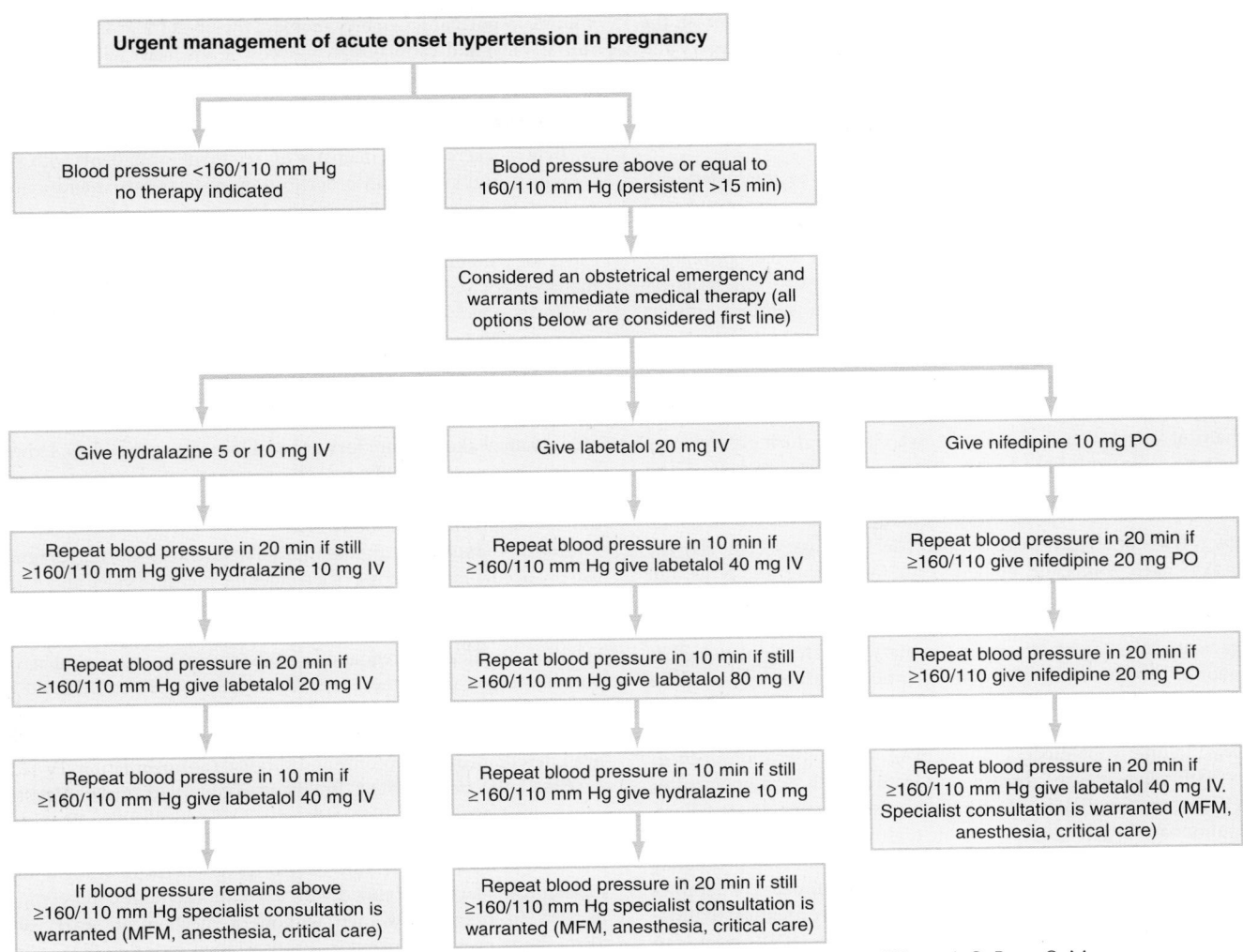

Fig. 174.1 Urgent management of acute-onset hypertension in pregnancy. (From: ElFarra J, C. Bean C, Martin, JN. Management of hypertensive crisis for the obstetrician/gynecologist. *Obstet Gynecol Clin North Am.* 2016;43, 623-637.)

of pregnancy-related MIs. In one study, 90% of patients presenting with a SCAD related AMI were postpartum while in another study 72% of SCAD related AMIs were postpartum.[13,14] Pulmonary embolus, reflux esophagitis, biliary colic, and aortic dissection are all more common than myocardial ischemia during pregnancy and should be considered in the differential diagnosis of the pregnant patient who presents with chest pain. Initial signs and symptoms of AMI, such as chest pain and shortness of breath, are often attributed to the normal physiologic changes of pregnancy.

The diagnosis of ACS is similar to that in nonpregnant patients, with certain exceptions. Electrocardiographic changes sometimes occur in normal pregnancies and delivery. These include T wave flattening, T wave inversion (mainly in lead III), and nonspecific ST changes during pregnancy, as well as ST depression during labor induction for cesarean section. As a result, an additional evaluation may be necessary. Echocardiography is useful in the correlation of suspicious electrocardiographic findings with wall motion abnormalities. The enzymatic diagnosis of myocardial infarction is unchanged, and a serial troponin rise suggests myocardial ischemia, even in preeclampsia.

Treatment of AMI during pregnancy is similar in most respects to treatment of the nonpregnant patient, with survival of the mother as the goal. Standard treatments including antiplatelet agents,

nitroglycerin, and beta blockers: antithrombotic agents are considered safe during pregnancy but the decision to use them should be made jointly by emergent consultation with a cardiologist and the patient's obstetrician. Angiotensin-converting enzyme (ACE) inhibitors, angiotensin receptor blockers, aldosterone antagonists, and statins are not advised until the postpartum period. Aspirin is the first-line antiplatelet agent. Clopidogrel has been studied in case reports with no adverse fetal outcomes and ACOG recommends that it can be used with caution, primarily after stenting. Ticagrelor, prasugrel, and bivalirudin are not recommended due to teratogenicity in animal studies. Heparin has long been the antithrombotic of choice for pregnant patients, although low-molecular-weight agents such as enoxaparin also do not cross the placenta and are considered efficacious and safe in pregnancy.

Cardiac catheterization with stenting is the treatment of choice for AMI in the pregnant patient and, with shielding, exposes the fetus to less than 1 radiation-absorbed dose (rad). However, both ACOG and the European Society of Cardiology recommend a conservative approach when considering cardiac catheterization in patients who may potentially have a coronary artery dissection. When a catheterization laboratory is unavailable, lifesaving thrombolytic therapy should not be withheld. Although thrombolytics do not cross the placenta, there is an increased risk of maternal hemorrhage and, in the setting of

AMI caused by coronary dissection, thrombolytic use can worsen the dissection. Because thrombolytic therapy precludes major surgery and epidural anesthesia in the hours to days immediately after administration, one must carefully consider whether to use these agents in pregnant women who are close to term, especially if the need for cesarean delivery is anticipated.

In the setting of peripartum AMI, labor should be conducted with continuous monitoring of the mother's hemodynamic status and fetal well-being. Assisted vaginal delivery is preferred unless there is an indication for cesarean section. Cesarean section avoids prolonged exertion by the mother but can subject the patient to general anesthesia if the use of antithrombotic agents precludes epidural catheter placement.

Valvular Heart Disease and Pulmonary Hypertension

Foundations. Valvular heart disease, including both native and mechanical valves, can lead to acute heart failure during pregnancy and is associated with both higher maternal and fetal mortality. The ability of patients to tolerate pregnancy without significant adverse effects depends on the type and severity of the lesion. Mild to moderate lesions (New York Heart Association [NYHA] classes I and II) are often associated with good outcomes for the mother and fetus. On the other hand, mitral stenosis (beyond class I), advanced aortic stenosis, and aortic and mitral lesions associated with moderate to severe ventricular dysfunction or pulmonary hypertension, as well as mechanical prosthetic valves requiring anticoagulation, can result in maternal mortality and require directed therapy and expert cardiology consultation.

Heart failure is the most common maternal complication in pregnancy with valvular heart disease, and women with cardiomyopathy, an NYHA functional class III or higher, pre-pregnancy heart failure, and pulmonary hypertension are at the highest risk. Diagnosing heart failure is challenging because women in the last months of pregnancy experience symptoms such as dyspnea on exertion, paroxysmal nocturnal dyspnea, orthopnea, and pedal edema that are identical to those of heart failure. Normal B-type natriuretic peptide (BNP) levels can be used to rule out heart failure in pregnant females but, because BNP levels increase twofold in pregnant females, a mildly elevated BNP level can be difficult to interpret.

Pulmonary Hypertension. Pregnancy is poorly tolerated by patients with pulmonary hypertension because the pulmonary circulation cannot cope with the increased stroke volume and cardiac output of pregnancy, causing pulmonary pressures to rise. This causes dyspnea, heart failure, and syncope. Mortality in pregnant women with pulmonary hypertension can approach 30%. Pregnancy is contraindicated, and patients early in pregnancy should be counseled about elective pregnancy termination.

The treatment of the pregnant patient with pulmonary hypertension focuses on diuresis and pulmonary vasodilation. Diuretics are indicated for the management of volume overload, and common diuretics—with the exception of spironolactone—are considered safe, although limited data exist regarding their effect on the fetus. Specific agents for treating pulmonary hypertension include endothelin receptor agonists (ERAs), phosphodiesterase inhibitors, and prostanoids. Phosphodiesterase inhibitors such as sildenafil and tadalafil, as well as the prostacyclin derivatives epoprostenol and treprostinil, are fetotoxic in animals; however, the benefits outweighs the risks, so they are regularly used in pregnancy. ERAs such as bosentan and ambrisentan are teratogenic.

Mitral Stenosis. Mitral stenosis is the most commonly encountered valvular lesion in pregnancy but is typically well tolerated except in moderate to severe disease. The increased resting heart rate and stroke volume in normal pregnancy increase the pressure gradient across the mitral valve and can cause symptoms of left heart failure, as well as atrial arrhythmias such as atrial fibrillation. The likelihood of maternal symptoms and worsening of cardiovascular status is directly related to the severity of disease.

Beta blockers are the mainstay of treatment for patients with symptomatic mitral stenosis in order to prevent tachycardia and maintain preload to overcome obstruction. Diuretics may also be used for patients with symptoms of heart failure. Surgical intervention is indicated for patients with refractory symptoms despite optimal medical management and in patients with pulmonary hypertension.

Aortic and Mitral Regurgitation. Mitral valve prolapse is the most common cause of mitral regurgitation in developed countries, whereas rheumatic heart disease is the most common cause worldwide. In most cases, chronic regurgitation lesions are well tolerated during pregnancy and may even improve because the reduced systemic vascular resistance of pregnancy allows more forward and less regurgitant flow. However, heart failure occurs in 20% to 25% of women with moderate or severe mitral regurgitation. When necessary, medical therapy consists of diuresis, digoxin, and vasodilators.

Aortic Stenosis. Symptomatic aortic stenosis during pregnancy usually occurs in the setting of a congenital bicuspid valve and patients with severe aortic stenosis may first become symptomatic during pregnancy. Patients with mild to moderate aortic stenosis tend to have uncomplicated pregnancies; conservative management is often possible, especially if the aortic valve area is greater than 1.0 cm^2. Patients with symptomatic aortic stenosis may respond to bed rest or preload reduction with diuretics. Severely symptomatic patients may need percutaneous valvotomy and surgical replacement.

Prosthetic Heart Valves. Pregnant women with mechanical heart valves are classified as high risk with a World Health Organization (WHO) risk classification III. The Registry of Pregnancy and Cardiac Disease (ROPAC) found that 82% of pregnancies in women with a mechanical heart valve ended with a live mother and child compared to 98% in pregnant women without a mechanical heart valve.[15] Thrombotic events occurred in 5% of women in the ROPAC registry with a mortality of 20%. Warfarin is the most effective anticoagulant in preventing maternal thromboembolic events. However, warfarin is considered teratogenic in the first trimester and is associated with a higher risk of fetal loss and fetal hemorrhage. Neither unfractionated heparin (UFH) nor low-molecular-weight heparin (LMWH) crosses the placenta and are not teratogenic. However, their use throughout pregnancy is not recommended due to the increased risk of thromboembolic events as compared to using UFH or LMWH in the first trimester, followed by warfarin for the remainder of pregnancy.[16]

Current anticoagulation recommendations in pregnant patients with prosthetic heart valves are to continue using warfarin until pregnancy has been achieved. If an international normalized ratio of 2.5 to 3.5 can be achieved with a warfarin dose less than or equal to 5 mg, the AHA/ACC and European Society of Cardiology Guidelines slightly prefer the use of warfarin throughout pregnancy after a full discussion with the patient about the benefits and risks of the therapy. If a dose more than 5 mg is required, UFH or LWMH is recommended in the first trimester, with warfarin being resumed for the second and third trimesters. Warfarin should again be replaced by UFH or LWMH several weeks before delivery.

HEMATOLOGIC DISORDERS

Anemia

Anemia is the most common medical complication of pregnancy and is associated with maternal mortality, perinatal mortality, preterm birth, low birth weight, and small-for-gestational-age infants. The classic clinical presentations of anemia include pallor, fatigue, and shortness of breath. Most anemia, however, is asymptomatic. The WHO defines anemia of pregnancy as a hemoglobin of less than 11 g/dL. The hemoglobin threshold for severe anemia requiring blood transfusions is typically considered to be less than 7 g/dL for gravid patients and less than 8 g/dL for postpartum patients. There are several types of anemia, but four types predominate: dilutional anemia, iron deficiency, folate deficiency, and sickle cell hemoglobinopathy.

Dilutional Anemia

Dilutional anemia is normally seen with pregnancy. In preparation for blood loss at delivery, blood volume increases by nearly 50% between weeks 6 and 34. This rapid blood volume increase, accompanied by a lag in red blood cell (RBC) production, results in a dilution of hemoglobin. The result is that the threshold for diagnosing anemia in gravid patients is slightly lower (11 g/dL) than in nongravid patients (12 g/dL). Hemoglobin concentrations typically reach their nadir between weeks 26 to 28 of pregnancy. Clinicians should consider that gravid patients with hemoglobin values of 13 to 15 g/dL have inadequate expansion of their plasma volume, which can result in outcomes like low birthweight and premature birth.

Iron Deficiency Anemia

Iron deficiency occurs in 18% of pregnancies in the United States (US) with iron deficiency anemia occurring in approximately 5%.[17] The risks of adverse pregnancy outcomes are correlated to the severity of the anemia. Studies show a higher risk of preterm birth and low birth weight in women with mild to moderate anemia. Severe anemia (<6 to 7 g/dL or 60–70 g/L) is associated with increased fetal mortality, abnormal fetal oxygenation, premature rupture of membranes, gestational hypertension, and reduced volume of amniotic fluid. The diagnosis of iron deficiency is difficult to make because many of the serum biomarkers typically used are affected by the changes in maternal physiology. Ferritin is the most sensitive test for iron deficiency in pregnancy, with a cutoff of 30 ng/mL showing a 92% sensitivity and a 98% specificity, but it is affected by the increased plasma volume in later pregnancy. Mean corpuscular volume, total iron-binding capacity, and transferrin are less sensitive and specific than ferritin for iron deficiency

The ACOG has developed guidelines for the management of iron deficiency anemia. Patients with an uncomplicated physiologic anemia who are not iron deficient can be expected to have good obstetric outcomes without therapy and do not require treatment. Patients presenting with mild iron deficiency anemia (i.e., a hemoglobin of 9–10.5 g/dL) should be treated with non–enteric-coated supplemental iron. A single daily dose of iron appears to be as effective as multiple-dosing regimens and decreases the risk for GERD, which is already heightened in pregnancy. Intravenous iron is not used in the first trimester, but is the treatment of choice for all iron deficiency anemia in the third trimester and severe iron deficiency anemia (hemoglobin < 9 g/dL) in the second trimester.

The evidence for the use of prophylactic supplementation in women with normal hemoglobin levels (>11 g/dL [110 g/L]) and normal iron stores (ferritin > 30 mg/dL [20 μg/L]) to prevent anemia in late pregnancy is mixed. However, recent studies demonstrate that prenatal iron supplementation reduces the risk of iron deficiency anemia at term. ACOG, the WHO, and other major health authorities recommend at least 30 mg of ferrous iron daily during pregnancy. Intermittent dosing at two to three times a week provides the same maternal and offspring benefits while reducing the risk of side effects like heartburn, constipation, and nausea.[18]

Folate Deficiency

Folate is critical to several intracellular processes associated with cell growth. However, due to the 5- to 10-fold increase in folate requirements during pregnancy, gravid patients are at risk for folate deficiency. Folate deficiency is one of a number of causes of megaloblastic anemia, which is the second most common anemia. The incidence of folate deficiency in pregnancy is low in high income countries but remains higher in other populations. The risk for development of folate deficiency is increased in patients with multiple gestations, short interpregnancy intervals, preexisting malnutrition, hyperemesis gravidarum, malabsorption syndromes, alcoholism, use of certain antiepileptic drugs, and diets lacking green leafy vegetables and animal protein. Low maternal folate stores have, most importantly, been linked to increased risk of neural tube defects, as well as increased risk of placental abruption, preterm birth and low birth weight, preeclampsia, and spontaneous abortion. As is the case for iron deficiency, effects on the fetus depend on the degree of anemia.

Iron deficiency and folate deficiency anemias often coexist, making the peripheral blood smear difficult to interpret. In cases of suspected folate deficiency, the measurement of serum and RBC folate levels is indicated. However, the serum folate level is noted to exhibit a rapid response to folate intake, and low levels may normalize within days after a folate-rich meal. Oral folate supplementation with 0.4 mg daily is routinely recommended for all women before conception, and 0.4 to 0.8 mg is recommended during pregnancy as the requirement for this micronutrient increases during gestation. ACOG recommends 1.0 mg for those women who have a known pregnancy-related folate deficiency. Women at higher risk for neural tube defects (e.g., neural tube defects in prior pregnancy) are advised to take much higher doses of folate, 4 mg daily for 1 month pre-conception and at least until 12 weeks gestational age under close supervision of their obstetrician. ACOG advises continuing oral folate supplementation throughout the second and third trimesters.

Sickle Cell Anemia

Sickle cell disease (SCD) is one of the major sources of maternal and fetal complications in the United States. Patients with SCD are subject to many chronic medical problems due to a variety of pathophysiologic mechanisms, including sickling of RBCs, anemia, immunosuppression caused by auto-splenectomy, and repeated transfusion. Median life expectancy is in the fifth decade for both genders affected by SCD, and female fertility is generally unaffected, so it is likely that the emergency clinician will encounter pregnant patients with the disease. Maternal complications are common in patients with SCD; these include preterm labor, premature rupture of membranes, maternal infections, more frequent pain crises, thrombosis, preeclampsia, and increased need for cesarean delivery. Due to these complications, pregnant women with SCD have a sixfold increased risk of maternal death compared with controls.

SCD also results in adverse effects on the fetus. Placental infarction and insufficiency are common, and the incidence of premature labor, small-for-gestational-age infants, and low-birth-weight infants is significantly increased in SCD pregnancies compared with normal controls. Perinatal mortality rates vary but are low in the setting of appropriate maternal and neonatal care.

Vasoocclusive crises and anemia occur more often in pregnancy and are the most common complications of SCD in pregnancy. Studies have also demonstrated that venous thromboembolisms occur 1.7 to 10 times more frequently in pregnant women with SCD. Recommended treatment is similar to that for the nonpregnant patient with a few exceptions. Hydroxyurea is not recommended for use in pregnancy because of potential teratogenicity, and nonsteroidal antiinflammatory drugs (NSAIDs) are avoided after 30 weeks of gestation.

General anesthesia can result in an increase in postpartum sickling complications, so regional anesthesia is preferred in the case of cesarean delivery. The use of supplemental iron and transfusion is controversial because of the potential for iron overload, alloimmunization, volume overload, and hyperviscosity syndrome.

Therapeutic transfusions should be given to patients with severe disease manifestations such as symptomatic anemia, cardiopulmonary instability, acute chest syndrome, intrapartum hemorrhage, and preeclampsia. In general, the goal with transfusion or exchange transfusion is to lower the percentage of hemoglobin S to 40% and achieve hemoglobin values of approximately 10 g/dL (110 g/L). Prophylactic red blood cell transfusions are often used in pregnant women with SCD without the indications for a therapeutic transfusion in order to decrease the frequency and severity of vaso-occlusive pain episodes during pregnancy.[19] Only low quality studies are available, but they show a reduction in maternal mortality, vasoocclusive pain episodes, pulmonary complications, and neonatal death. There is no consensus at this time whether the benefits of prophylactic transfusions outweigh the risks.

NEUROLOGIC DISORDERS

Epilepsy

Epilepsy is the most common neurologic complication of pregnancy but remains relatively rare, affecting less than 1% of all gestations. The treatment of epilepsy during pregnancy entails balancing the risk of increased frequency and duration of seizures to the mother and fetus against the teratogenic risks of antiepileptic drugs (AEDs).

Gravid patients with epilepsy have more than a tenfold increased risk of death compared to pregnant women without epilepsy. Pregnant women with epilepsy are also at increased risk for cesarean section, postpartum hemorrhage, hypertensive disorders and other adverse outcomes. Approximately 15% of patients experience an increase in seizure frequency during pregnancy. Delivery and the first 24 hours postpartum are the most likely times for a seizure to occur, with a nine-fold greater incidence of seizure than during pregnancy in general.

A decrease in plasma drug concentrations is expected due to pharmacokinetic alterations including decreased absorption, increased volume of distribution, elevated renal excretion, and induction of hepatic metabolism; many experts recommend that maternal plasma drug levels be monitored and compared to prepregnancy levels.[20] Antiepileptic medications also increase the clearance of medications, including oral contraceptives, making unintentional pregnancy a possibility. Patients who have nonconvulsive seizure disorders or who are seizure-free for a sufficient period of time before conception are candidates for nonpharmacologic observation because the risk of treatment with AEDs can outweigh the benefit. This decision should be deferred to the patient's primary physician or neurologist. However, there are obstetric complications related to prolonged seizure activity, and long-term treatment with an AED for most patients with seizures is warranted.

The primary complication of AED use in pregnancy is congenital malformations. Of primary concern is the risk for neural tube defects, facial clefts, cardiac anomalies, and cognitive defects with the older generation agents (e.g., valproate, carbamazepine, phenytoin) and several of the newer generation agents (e.g., gabapentin, topiramate). There is a two- to three-fold increase in the incidence of serious congenital malformations in offspring of epileptic mothers taking these agents. The risk is greatest with valproate and is also increased with AED polypharmacy and increased dose of individual agents. Recent studies have found that monotherapy with lamotrigine and levetiracetam does not have a higher risk of major congenital malformations than control.[21]

When compared to the older AEDs, levetiracetam performed as well at controlling seizures when used in monotherapy, while lamotrigine and topiramate, when used in monotherapy, showed worse seizure control. In the case of lamotrigine, this was due to increased renal clearance leading to variable levels. Because phenytoin, carbamazepine, valproate, and possibly other AEDs interfere with folate metabolism, oral supplementation with at least 0.4 to 1.0 mg/day is recommended for all women of childbearing age taking these drugs to help prevent congenital malformations such as neural tube defects. Enzyme-inducing AEDs such as carbamazepine, phenytoin, and phenobarbital have been reported to cause neonatal vitamin K deficiency and neonatal hemorrhage, but the American Academy of Neurology and American Epilepsy Society have noted that there is inadequate evidence to determine a definitive relationship.

Status epilepticus in pregnancy is relatively rare and can occur at any time during gestation, with a higher likelihood in the postpartum period. Any potential cause of seizure may result in status epilepticus, and recent studies have shown that eclampsia, posterior reversible encephalopathy syndrome, and cerebral venous thrombosis are all common causes. It may also occur in patients who have been seizure-free throughout pregnancy, and no specific risk factors for its occurrence have been identified. The risk of untreated status epilepticus to the mother and fetus clearly outweighs the potential for adverse teratogenic effects, and standard resuscitative measures, as well as drug therapy, are indicated. Benzodiazepines followed by levetiracetam are recommended.[22] Continuous fetal monitoring should be instituted as soon as possible to observe for signs of fetal hypoxia, and the mother should be positioned in the left lateral decubitus position to avoid the supine hypotensive syndrome.

Multiple Sclerosis

Multiple sclerosis (MS) affects approximately 400,000 Americans and is twice as common in women as in men. The peak age at onset is 20 to 35 years, which overlaps peak childbearing years. The disease is characterized by intermittent episodes of central nervous system (CNS) demyelination, with consequent neurologic impairment that follows a relapsing-remitting course. Progressive neurologic deficits and permanent disability develop in certain patients.

The frequency and severity of exacerbations of MS often improve during pregnancy, particularly during the third trimester. During the 3 months after delivery, the rate of relapse increases and then returns to the patients' pre-pregnancy baseline. Relapses are more likely in MS patients with higher disability at the time of pregnancy onset, as well as women treated with natalizumab and fingolimod.[23] However, it does not seem that postpartum relapses are related to the duration of disease or total number of relapses before conception.

MS patients with disease exacerbation are often treated with immunomodulators such as intravenous immune globulin (IVIG), corticosteroids, glatiramer acetate, and interferon beta. Small studies in gravid patients have shown that the use of IVIG during pregnancy and in the postpartum period is safe and may decrease the relapse rate. Likewise, the use of intermittent steroids in the postpartum period may decrease the likelihood of disease relapse. Glatiramer acetate may also be used in pregnancy as needed as studies have not shown any fetal toxicity.[24]

Spinal Cord Injury

Because spinal cord injury (SCI) occurs mainly in young people and usually does not impair fertility, there is a relatively large population of paraplegic and quadriplegic patients who become pregnant. The most common complication in pregnant women with SCI is urinary tract infection (UTI). One study showed that pregnant women with SCI were 26 times more likely to get a UTI than controls, while another found that 30% of gravid women with SCI developed pyelonephritis.[25] A high suspicion must be kept for UTIs in this population, as untreated infections carry an increased risk of fetal loss, prematurity, and maternal sepsis.

The hypercoagulable state of pregnancy, combined with chronic immobilization, results in an increased incidence of thromboembolic disease, with a nine times greater risk of venous thromboembolism versus control.

Autonomic dysreflexia is the most serious complication of SCI and occurs in up to 56% of women with high lesions (above T5-T6); it occurs with increased frequency during pregnancy. Autonomic dysreflexia is manifested as severe paroxysmal hypertension, headache, tachycardia, diaphoresis, piloerection, mydriasis, and nasal congestion. It is often precipitated by afferent stimuli from the hollow viscus such as the bladder, bowel, or uterus. Symptoms of autonomic dysreflexia often occur with uterine contractions during labor. However, labor may be difficult to detect because patients with spinal cord lesions below T10 to T12 have an intact uterine nerve supply and experience labor pains; however, with lesions above T10, labor may be imperceptible or experienced as only mild abdominal discomfort. Pregnant patients with SCI with symptoms of autonomic dysreflexia should be assessed for cervical dilation and have uterine contractions monitored. ED treatment is directed at the restoration of normal blood pressure with standard agents. Definitive therapy is with regional anesthesia. Spinal anesthesia and epidural anesthesia obliterate and prevent this response and should be used as soon as possible during labor for all women with SCI. Finally, it can be difficult to differentiate between the symptoms of autonomic dysreflexia and preeclampsia. In autonomic dysreflexia, symptoms such as hypertension will resolve once the stimuli to the skin or hollow viscus have been relieved; in preeclampsia, the symptoms and laboratory abnormalities are more likely to persist.

Myasthenia Gravis

Myasthenia gravis is a rare disorder in which autoimmune destruction of the postsynaptic cholinergic receptor results in profound muscle fatigability. The effect of pregnancy and the postpartum state on myasthenia gravis is unpredictable in the individual patient, but overall, approximately 25% to 50% of patients experience exacerbation of disease, with the remainder having improvement or no change in disease severity.[26] Disease exacerbations can occur anytime during pregnancy and the postpartum period and are not more likely in one trimester than in another. Additionally up to 15% of women will experience their first myasthenia symptoms in the pregnancy or postpartum period. Because of weight gain, anemia, and other physiologic adjustments of pregnancy that may result in fatigue, the distinction between normal pregnancy symptoms and myasthenia may be difficult.

Most deliveries are accomplished vaginally without complication in adequately treated patients; assisted and surgical delivery in these women is indicated mainly for obstetric reasons rather than for specific myasthenia-related care.[27] Between 10% and 20% of neonates born to mothers with myasthenia gravis have a transient neonatal myasthenia syndrome through the placental transport of acetylcholine receptor antibodies. There is no correlation between the severity of maternal disease and occurrence of neonatal myasthenia. The onset of neonatal myasthenia is typically within the first hours of life but may be delayed by a period of days. Manifestations include poor feeding and suck, diminished reflexes, hypotonia, and bulbar and respiratory muscle weakness. As in adults, the symptoms respond to cholinesterase

inhibitors, but treatment should be carried out in an intensive care unit setting.

Myasthenia crises during pregnancy present with typical symptoms of painless fluctuating weakness of skeletal muscles. Diplopia and ptosis are the most common early symptoms. When exacerbations do occur, treatment is no different from the treatment of nonpregnant patients. Acetylcholine esterase inhibitors, corticosteroids, IVIG, and plasmapheresis are all considered safe for the mother and fetus. Azathioprine and cyclosporine are considered second-line options for patients who are not controlled or who cannot tolerate corticosteroids. Assessment of pulse oximetry, forced vital capacity, and arterial blood gas parameters will guide respiratory therapy.

Magnesium sulfate is contraindicated for treatment of eclampsia in myasthenia gravis because of its neuromuscular blocking effects; barbiturates or phenytoin should be used instead.[27] Epidural anesthesia is also recommended to reduce pain and fatigue.

RENAL DISORDERS

Chronic kidney disease (CKD) can be silent well into its disease course and is more difficult to diagnose in pregnancy because of expected decreased blood urea nitrogen (BUN) and creatinine levels during pregnancy. For women with known renal disease, including end-stage renal disease (ERSD), on hemodialysis, conception rates have shown some improvement, but seem plateaued at roughly 10%.

CKD in and of itself is an independent risk factor for maternal and fetal complications. The degree of underlying renal dysfunction is a strong determinant of morbidity associated with pregnancy. Patients with moderate to severe renal dysfunction have a much higher risk of further decline in renal function, as well as adverse obstetric outcomes, including preeclampsia, placental abruption, fetal loss, preterm delivery, low birth weight, polyhydramnios, and increased need for cesarean section and neonatal intensive care. Worsening of underlying renal function is more likely in patients with a decreased glomerular filtration rate who also have associated proteinuria or hypertension. Because worsening renal function is manifested by hypertension and proteinuria, differentiation from preeclampsia can be difficult. In this setting, it is best to treat the patient for presumed preeclampsia, with the caveat that magnesium administration should be performed judiciously and carefully guided by serum magnesium levels.

Pregnant women with chronic renal failure require aggressive and timely management to optimize their chances for a successful gestation without causing further deterioration in renal function. One of the most successful tenets of CKD management in pregnancy is close control of blood pressure and monitoring for proteinuria. Thresholds for initiation of hemodialysis (HD) in pregnant patients are considered lower than those in nongravid patients. Intensified HD, through longer and/or more frequent dialysis sessions, offers improved maternal and neonatal outcomes.

Adverse pregnancy outcomes in HD patients include miscarriage, placental detachment, anemia, infections, premature rupture of membranes, polyhydramnios, preterm birth, uncontrolled arterial hypertension, preeclampsia/eclampsia, hemorrhage, need for a caesarean section and maternal death

For patients who are post–renal transplantation, fertility rates return to prerenal failure levels within 1 to 6 months post-transplantation, so pregnancy is not an uncommon finding in post-transplantation women of childbearing age. Obstetric outcomes for this patient population show live birth rates exceeding 70%, and adverse outcomes mostly associated with preterm births and with infants small for gestational age (SGA).

METABOLIC AND ENDOCRINE DISORDERS

Diabetes

General Management

Three types of diabetes affect pregnant patients—type 1, or insulin-dependent diabetes mellitus (T1DM); type 2, or non–insulin-dependent diabetes mellitus (T2DM); and gestational diabetes mellitus (GDM). The considerations for glycemic control in GDM are the same as those for T1DM and T2DM.

Both T1DM and T2DM are growing in prevalence, representing a challenge to the management of these high-risk obstetric patients. Technical advances in glycemic control have improved the potential for successful pregnancy outcomes, but euglycemic control is not the norm for these patient populations, especially given the tight control advised by ACOG.

Although T2DM is sometimes considered a more benign form of disease, the risk of pregnancy complications and fetal malformations is still significant and rates of elective cesarean section are increased compared to nondiabetic norms due to the development of neonatal macrosomia. Ideally, hemoglobin A_{1c} (HbA_{1c}) values should not be higher than 6%. T2DM patients are generally recommended to transition to insulin therapy to achieve tighter glycemic regulation during pregnancy.

T1DM does connote a much higher rate of preeclampsia, maternal mortality, premature delivery, neonatal hypoglycemia, congenital abnormalities and stillbirths. Preconception planning in this patient population is paramount, and tight glycemic control for at least 4 months prior to conception is recommended. Maternal and fetal complications are largely related to inadequate glycemic control and to the presence of vascular complications or severe renal insufficiency more than to the type of diabetes.

The effects of pregnancy on underlying diabetes vary by organ system. The data are limited, but pregnancy is not advised for diabetic patients with coronary artery disease because of the cardiovascular demands of pregnancy and high mortality rates of AMI during pregnancy. Given the likelihood of silent ischemic events in the diabetic population, atypical or vague presentations of angina or MI, including new-onset congestive heart failure should be carefully evaluated in those with preexisting known coronary artery disease, but also in any diabetic mother.

Patients with diabetic nephropathy are at increased risk for preeclampsia and the subsequent requirement for preterm delivery. Following progression of nephropathy closely in conjunction with aggressive blood pressure control and optimizing protein intake are strongly recommended.

Angioproliferation is a natural physiologic response in pregnancy, and because of this, diabetic retinopathy worsens acutely in 30% of DM1 and 12% of DM2 patients during pregnancy. Those at greatest risk for this are patients with high HbA_{1c} levels, hypertension, nephropathy, and active nonproliferative or proliferative retinopathy. New onset diabetic retinopathy during pregnancy occurs 10% of the time with DM1. Laser therapy of preexisting retinopathy is recommended before conception, as well as for pregnant patients with severe disease. Patients with known proliferative retinopathy should be counseled to avoid excessive, aggressive Valsalva maneuvers during labor to minimize the risk of retinal hemorrhages.

Autonomic neuropathy does not accelerate during pregnancy, with the exception of a possible increase in symptomatic severity of gastroparesis.

Hyperglycemic

Physiologically, insulin sensitivity increases in the first trimester, allowing for decreased insulin usage. This reverses in the second and third trimesters, ultimately increasing to 70% to 100% of baseline nonpregnant insulin requirements. The increased risk of diabetic ketoacidosis (DKA) results from intercurrent illness including hyperemesis, inadequate insulin administration, or iatrogenically from use of betamimetic medications for tocolysis, and use of corticosteroids to hasten fetal lung maturity, or from withholding insulin therapy for planned procedures. During pregnancy there is a continuous need for a basal rate of insulin, whether by insulin pump or long-acting (Lantus) insulin. Relying on a basic metabolic profile as screening for DKA in pregnancy (e.g., insulin glargine) can be dangerous. The serum pH may be deceptively normal in a pregnant patient with DKA because the initial pH tends to be higher in pregnancy as a result of physiologic hyperventilation. In addition, the serum glucose concentration may be normal or only moderately elevated. Screening with serum acetone or betahydroxybutarate is recommended for any pregnant DM patient with vague symptoms of headache, nausea, vomiting, or fatigue.

The treatment of DKA does not differ in pregnancy versus nonpregnant patients, except that fluid resuscitation and insulin therapy should be maintained in the presence of normoglycemia until bicarbonate levels return to normal, indicating that any lagging acidemia has cleared. Fetal viability and well-being should be assessed in all cases of maternal DKA. Fetal mortality associated with DKA can be as high as 35%.

Hypoglycemia

The risk for hypoglycemia is bimodal, mostly in the first trimester but also in the peripartum period. In the first trimester, insulin needs decrease and physiologic hormonal counter-regulation to hypoglycemia including glucagon, cortisol, and epinephrine surge is blunted. A contributing factor for some patients is the comorbid condition of gastroparesis, which can worsen hyperemesis gravidarum (HG); 18% to 40% of patients have at least 1 severe episode of hypoglycemia in the first trimester, almost always at night. Even subclinical hypoglycemia (sustained levels <85 mg/dl) can lead to low-birth-weight neonates, so ideal ranges for glycemic control are extremely tight between 90 to 120 mg/dl.

Fetal Effects

Diabetes has many deleterious effects on the fetus. The risk of congenital anomalies in infants of diabetic mothers (IDMs) is as high as 10%. The rate of congenital malformations in patients with prepregnancy diabetes is increased threefold or fourfold compared with the nondiabetic population, with anomalies being more likely in pregnant women with poor glycemic control. Macrosomia is the most likely factor leading to the need for cesarean section and has been associated with shoulder dystocia. Conversely, preeclampsia and placental infarction secondary to vascular disease may result in impaired fetal development and stillbirth. Diabetic patients are also at increased risk of spontaneous preterm delivery and labor-induced preterm deliveries. Neonatal complications seen at increased rates in infants of diabetic mothers (IDMs) include transient tachypnea of the newborn, neonatal hypoglycemia, hypocalcemia in the peripartum period, hyperbilirubinemia, polycythemia, cardiomyopathy, and respiratory distress as a result of fetal hyperinsulinemia. Elective delivery is indicated in the setting of poor metabolic control, significant diabetic complications, and fetal macrosomia with suspected birth weight more than 4500 g.

OBESITY

The incidence of obesity is increasing, and it has become the most common medical condition in women of childbearing age. It is an independent risk factor of poor outcomes, even without the comorbid conditions of diabetes, vascular disease, or hypertension. In early gestation, obesity is associated with spontaneous pregnancy loss and congenital anomalies. Increased insulin resistance in obese gravid patients can manifest clinically in late gestation as glucose intolerance and fetal overgrowth. At term, the risk of cesarean section is increased, threefold of that seen in the nonobese population because of inadequate contraction patterns in labor, leading to failure to progress, caused by an independent influence of obesity on myometrial activity, compounded by macrosomia.

Peripartum and postpartum, obese women have a more marked increased risk of venous thromboembolism and depression compared to nonobese counterparts. Meta-analysis has shown obesity to be an independent risk factor for infant death and neonatal asthma; this risk is proportional to increased body mass index (BMI). The BMI does not appear to be correlated with postpartum hemorrhage requiring intervention, severe maternal morbidity or maternal mortality, or spontaneous preterm delivery before 32 weeks of gestation.

THYROID DISORDERS

Hyperthyroidism

Hyperthyroidism affects less than 0.5% of all pregnancies, of which 85% are Graves disease. Because the symptoms of worsening hyperthyroidism resemble the physiologic changes expected during pregnancy in many respects, the diagnosis may not be immediately evident. In the first trimester, most gravid patients with Graves disease will experience a transient exacerbation, but improvement in later pregnancy. A postpartum rebound exacerbation is common.

Thyroid storm is the most serious manifestation of the disease and may be precipitated by stressors such as infection and delivery; it is manifested by fever, dysrhythmias, myocardial dysfunction, and circulatory collapse. Many of these symptoms appear similar to those of eclampsia, so obtaining TSH and free T4 levels on eclamptic patients is recommended. The symptom most helpful in differentiating thyrotoxicosis from thyroid storm is markedly altered mental status seen with thyroid storm. Untreated, mortality approaches 100%, but prompt recognition and aggressive therapy have lowered mortality to 20% to 30%. In addition to more general complications stemming from thyroid hormone excess, early (spontaneous abortion) and late (stillbirth) fetal loss, commonly as a result of placental abruption, are more common in hyperthyroid patients than in the general population.

The mainstay of treating hyperthyroidism consists of thyreostatic drugs. Propylthiouracil is recommended in the first trimester; there is an increased potential for adverse congenital drug effects from methimazole. Post organogenesis, in the second and third trimesters, methimazole is used to limit maternal hepatotoxicity. Most patients respond to pharmacologic manipulation, although thyroidectomy may be considered in severe cases in which patients cannot tolerate antithyroid medication or in the setting of medication failure. Radioiodine is strongly contraindicated during all stages of pregnancy because it will also destroy the fetal thyroid gland.

Additional therapy with beta blockade to mitigate the hemodynamic effects of sympathetic stimulation may be required in certain cases pending disease control with antithyroid medications. Iodide is considered class D in pregnancy because of fetal thyroid sensitivity to the medication; its use should be reserved for severe cases, with duration of therapy limited to days.

Graves disease places the fetus at risk for autoimmune-mediated thyroid dysfunction through placental transfer of maternal thyroid-stimulating immunoglobulins. Up to 20% of neonates of mothers with Graves disease and positive thyroid-stimulating immunoglobulin values have transient hyperthyroidism lasting 3 to 12 weeks. The condition gradually clears as maternal antibodies are metabolized.

Manifestations are potentially severe and include irritability, tachycardia, goiter, cardiomegaly, congestive heart failure, premature craniosynostosis, low birth weight, and failure to thrive.

Hypothyroidism

Overt hypothyroidism is often associated with infertility, so most cases seen during pregnancy are less severe. Subclinical disease forms can also be seen or may occur in patients already undergoing levothyroxine therapy for known disease. Undiagnosed subclinical hypothyroidism may become clinically apparent as the metabolic demands of pregnancy unmask deficient thyroid hormone levels. When signs and symptoms do occur, they are generally the same as those in the nonpregnant state. Myxedema coma is extremely rare but should be considered along with other causes of coma in a pregnant patient.

Patients who are already undergoing treatment for hypothyroidism should have therapy optimized pre-conception, but will also require an increased dosage of levothyroxine during pregnancy, especially during the first trimester, in which increases from 20% to 30% are usually required. Compared with euthyroid status, subclinical hypothyroidism in pregnancy is associated with higher rates of gestational hypertension, premature rupture of membranes, intrauterine growth restriction, and low-birth-weight infants; long-term, there is a decreased IQ of the child at age 6 years.

Adrenal Insufficiency

The most common reason for adrenal insufficiency in pregnancy is Addison disease. Early in pregnancy, Addisonian crisis can be mistaken for hyperemesis gravidarum because the clinical features and some electrolyte abnormalities are similar. Overall complications of Addison are greatest in the third trimester, when there is the biggest need for increased cortisol replacement. Careful monitoring of replacement steroids is important to avoid neonatal adrenal insufficiency. Addisonian crisis is precipitated in the gravid patient population by infection, trauma, surgery, delivery or any other significant metabolic stress.

Electrolyte Abnormalities

Gravid patients with primary hyperparathyroidism may develop hypercalcemia, which most commonly presents as nephrolithiasis. Indeed, all pregnant patients with new onset nephrolithiasis should be screened for hypercalcemia. The presence of untreated maternal primary hyperparathyroidism can lead to neonatal hypocalcemia which presents with intrauterine growth restriction, low birth weight, and or neonatal tetany secondary to suppressed development of parathyroid glands. Treatment of the condition is like that in the nongravid state, except that bisphosphonates are contraindicated in pregnancy.

SYSTEMIC INFECTIONS

Human Immunodeficiency Virus Infection

Seroprevalence of HIV infection in pregnant women is decreasing, with more than 8500 annually in 2006 to an estimated less than 5000 in 2018. Treatment of the seropositive HIV pregnant patient with opportunistic infections generally follows similar regimens to nonpregnant patients. There are limited data on specific therapy for opportunistic infections during pregnancy, but clinicians should consider that medication clearance may be affected by various pregnancy-related changes, including increased renal clearance, dilutional anemia, and fetal metabolism of medications. Maternal mortality is increased in HIV-positive mothers, including perinatal sepsis and sepsis related to abortion. Nonpregnancy-related infections, particularly tuberculosis, malaria, and pneumonia, are important causes of maternal death in HIV-infected pregnant or postpartum women.

In patients who are already taking antiretroviral therapy (ART) with good disease control (viral load <1000 copies/mL) at the time of pregnancy diagnosis, the current medication regimen should be continued. For those with a recent diagnosis of HIV, timing of initiation of ART is being reexamined, with a recent meta-analysis suggesting increased risk of preterm or very preterm infants, and low-birthweight neonates, compared to initiating treatment after conception.[28] In the absence of ART treatment, progression of maternal disease does not appear to accelerate during pregnancy, but disease progression is more rapid postpartum. Elective cesarean section is recommended in mothers with a viral load greater than 1000 copies/mL.

HIV does not appear to be an independent risk factor for pregnancy loss and pregnancies generally have good outcomes in patients who receive appropriate HIV treatment during pregnancy. Maternal HIV infection in women who have not received antiretroviral therapy is associated with preterm birth, low birthweight, small for gestational age, and stillbirth.

Vertical transmission of HIV infection (maternal to neonate) remains a monumental challenge in low resource countries with high HIV prevalence (notably sub-Saharan Africa), but is less prevalent in the US due to wide-ranging maternal HIV screening practices. In 2017, only 73 children under the age of 13 received a diagnosis of perinatally acquired HIV in the U.S. Patients presenting to the ED without prenatal care should be screened for HIV as a first point of contact, even if this is shortly after a precipitous delivery. Screening should consist of a rapid combination or fourth generation (antibody/antigen) test, followed by Nucleic Acid Tests (NATs) in high-risk individuals.

Tuberculosis

Comorbid infection or activation of latent tuberculosis (TB) during pregnancy can be challenging to diagnose because pregnancy may mimic and thus mask the symptoms of early tuberculosis (e.g., tachypnea and fatigue). Presenting symptoms in pregnancy are similar to those in the nonpregnant population, including cough, weight loss, fever, malaise, and fatigue. Moderate to severe anemia in an HIV-infected mother during pregnancy should prompt a workup for TB.

Tuberculosis does not appear to accelerate during pregnancy, nor does the pregnant state affect the site of infections. TB activation much more common in the postpartum period than in the prenatal period.

Infants born to TB-infected mothers have a twofold to threefold increased risk of prematurity and low birth weight and increased perinatal death. There is a well-defined constellation of neonatal clinical manifestations marked by cutaneous and mucosal lesions within the first week of life and a primary hepatic complex including caseating hepatic granulomas. These increased risks are highly associated with late diagnosis, inadequate treatment, and advanced disease. Pregnant women with active tuberculosis should begin therapy as soon as the diagnosis is established. The risk of transmission of the organism to the infant outweighs the risks of the drugs to the mother's own health.

The preferred initial treatment for pregnant women is the combination of INH, rifampin, and ethambutol, which has not been shown to be teratogenic. Rifampin and INH freely cross the placenta. Second-line drugs have higher risks of teratogenicity and require more judicious use.

Syphilis

The incidence of primary and secondary syphilis among US reproductive age women has steadily increased since the late 1990s and the incidence of congenital syphilis has shown a similar increase.

Syphilis causes numerous gestational complications, but its most significant sequela is congenital syphilis. This syndrome is characterized by hepatosplenomegaly, osteochondritis, jaundice, rash,

lymphadenopathy, rhinitis, Hutchinson teeth, and anemia. Infant mortality related to congenital syphilis is high. Fetal ultrasonography before the 20th week of gestation is indicated to assess for abnormalities consistent with congenital syphilis. Sonographic signs of fetal syphilis confer a higher risk of congenital syphilis at delivery, and few of these completely regress after sufficient treatment.

Treatment is identical to that given to nonpregnant patients, with the use of benzathine penicillin G appropriate for the disease stage. During pregnancy, penicillin is the only known effective treatment for congenital syphilis, and pregnant patients with penicillin allergy should be desensitized and treated with penicillin. Treatment failures leading to congenital syphilis are more likely in mothers with secondary syphilis, high Venereal Disease Research Laboratory or rapid plasma reagin test levels, and an interval from treatment to delivery of less than 30 days.

Viral Hepatitis
Hepatitis B

There are 14,000 new cases of hepatitis B reported annually in the United States, but this is likely an underestimation of disease burden, given the absence of symptoms in early infection. From 800,000 to 1.4 million people in the United States have chronic hepatitis B. Perinatal transmission is approximately 10% to 20% in women seropositive for HBV surface antigen (HBsAg) alone but approaches 90% in mothers who are seropositive for HBsAg and HBV envelope antigen (HBeAg); it is also more likely if the mother has acute infection during the third trimester. Of infants who have HBV infection, up to 90% become chronic carriers as adults and are at risk for complications such as cirrhosis and hepatocellular carcinoma.

Studies have suggested that lamivudine given in late pregnancy to women with high viral loads of HBV DNA reduces viral transmission when used in conjunction with HBV vaccine and immune globulin. Infants of HBsAg-positive mothers should receive hepatitis B immune globulin and the first dose of vaccine within 12 hours of birth. Two additional doses of vaccine are administered at a later date.

Hepatitis C

Between 2009 and 2019, there were 94,824 reported cases of maternal HCV infection among 31 million (0.30%) live births in the United States. The rate of maternal HCV infection increased from 1.8 to 4.7 cases per 1000 live births.[29]

Vertical transmission is rare in mothers with anti-HCV antibodies and no circulating HCV RNA. However, perinatal transmission is increased by the presence of HCV viremia, occurring in approximately 5% of cases. The transmission rate is even higher in the setting of co-infection with HIV; the rates of HCV co-infectivity with HIV are about 10-fold higher than that seen in non–HIV-infected mothers. Perinatal transmission is now the leading cause of HCV transmission to children in middle and high income countries. Cesarean delivery has not been shown to prevent HCV transmission. There is no available vaccine or immune globulin to prevent hepatitis C, and routine prenatal screening is not indicated.

Obstetrical hemorrhagic complications, including DIC and shock and subsequent need for transfusion are more common among HCV infection, with particularly high rates seen peripartum. HCV mothers have higher risk for stillbirth, Cesarean section, preterm birth, SGA. Co-infection with hepatitis B further increases each of these risks.

INFLAMMATORY DISORDERS

Inflammatory autoimmune diseases (IAIDs) have a strong female predilection with onset generally during the childbearing years.

Pregnancy can affect the course of IAIDs with variability: some conditions ameliorate (rheumatoid arthritis), some remain unchanged (Sjögren), and some worsen (SLE). Although all IAIDs are chronic diseases, acute manifestations of IAIDs can be severe, difficult to diagnose and challenging to address in a management plan. Active maternal disease during pregnancy is associated with adverse pregnancy outcomes. These adverse outcomes can be minimized through optimizing disease suppression regimens prior to conception, aggressively managing IAIDs during pregnancy, and aggressively treating emergent complications during pregnancy.

Systemic Lupus Erythematosus

SLE is most common encountered IAID in emergencies related to pregnancy. Maternal complications include lupus flares, hypertension (exacerbation of preexisting disease), nephritis, preeclampsia, and eclampsia. Elevated levels of lupus anticoagulant and antiphospholipid antibodies have emerged as markers of disease activity and are good predictors for adverse pregnancy outcomes. SLE-associated preeclampsia and eclampsia rates, recently as high as 15% to 20%, have been decreasing due to optimal prepregnancy management of active disease and adoption of low-dose aspirin therapy prior to 16 weeks' gestation.[30] Hypertension in SLE-associated pregnancy should lead to careful consideration of lupus glomerulonephritis versus preeclampsia, as both conditions are marked by increasing proteinuria. The presence of abnormal urine sediment, increasing titers of anti-DNA antibody, and decreasing levels of C3 and C4 suggest lupus nephritis.

The most common neurologic complication of SLE in pregnancy is cerebral venous sinus thrombosis. Common presenting symptoms include acute or subacute headache (80%), impaired consciousness (25%), ear complaints (21%), paresis (20%) and epileptic seizures (15%). Neurologic presentations may be associated with a subset of SLE patients who will test positive for antiphospholipid antibodies, and approximately half of these patients will develop thrombosis-related disorders of pregnancy, an antibody-mediated acquired thrombophilia. The most common arterial presentation is stroke; positive antiphospholipid antibody (aPL) test results are found in up to 20% of ischemic stroke patients younger than 50 years of age.

Antiphospholipid syndrome (APS) is characterized by (1) clinical manifestations of deep vessel clotting during pregnancy (2) pregnancy related morbidity, usually fetal or neonatal loss, and (3) confirmatory laboratory tests for lupus anticoagulant, anticardiolipin antibody of IgG and/or IgM isotype, and anti-β2–glycoprotein I antibody of IgG and/or IgM isotype.

The most common thrombotic presentation of APS is deep venous thrombosis (DVT) of the lower extremity. The most serious but rare thrombotic presentation of APS is catastrophic APS (CAPS). This condition is characterized by rapid-onset, small vessel thrombosis, multiorgan dysfunction or failure (renal, hepatic) and a high maternal mortality rate.

Adverse pregnancy outcomes related to IAIDs include fetal death (4%), neonatal death (1%), preterm delivery (9%), and SGA neonate (10%).[31] Baseline predictors of adverse outcomes included presence of lupus anticoagulant, antihypertensive use, an elevated Pregnancy Disease Activity Index score, and low platelet count. Pregnant women with these preexisting measures of active disease had an adverse outcome rate of 58% and neonatal mortality of 22%. Neonates born to patients with lupus are at increased risk of neonatal lupus as well as heart block if born to patients with positive SSA/SSB.

Corticosteroids are the mainstay of therapy for most rheumatologic complications or exacerbations. Aspirin has been advocated for all lupus-related pregnancies of more than 16 weeks' gestational age, and other NSAID regimens remain useful treatments for inflammatory

flares. Cytotoxic agents are considered second-line therapy for rheumatic diseases. Cyclophosphamide and methotrexate are both potent teratogens and abortifacients and should be avoided, especially in the first trimester. Azathioprine is a cytotoxic agent that appears to be much better tolerated in pregnancy.

PSYCHIATRIC DISORDERS

Schizophrenia, Bipolar Disorder, and Depression

Similar risks and management principles apply to both schizophrenia and bipolar disorders in pregnancy. In both disorders, abrupt discontinuation of medication leads to high relapse rates in pregnancy. Untreated bipolar disorder and schizophrenia are considered independent risk factors for congenital malformations.

Polypharmacy should be avoided in this patient population during pregnancy in that it contributes to both fetal and maternal risk of adverse outcomes. Sole treatment with second-generation antipsychotics is the recommended management, including intention to control disease with the lowest acceptable dose of any given agent.[32]

Up to 17% of pregnant women experience major depressive disorder, and 25% of pregnant women with bipolar disorder experience mood exacerbation. Anxiety and depression are associated with adverse pregnancy outcomes including preeclampsia, instrument-assisted delivery, and emergency C section.

Adverse neonatal outcomes include low birth weight and preterm delivery. The ill effects of depression in pregnancy can carry into the later newborn period and even into later childhood. Infants of mothers with significant depression show increased cortisol and norepinephrine levels, and decreased dopamine levels. Neonatal outcomes are manifest as altered EEG patterns. reduced vagal tone, and stress/depressive-like behaviors. Adverse pregnancy outcomes include an increased rate of premature deaths and neonatal intensive care unit admissions, and central adiposity in later childhood.[33] Major depressive disorder during pregnancy has had good responses to cognitive behavioral therapy, in addition to pharmacotherapy.

Eating Disorders

The peak incidence of eating disorders occurs during the childbearing years, so the likelihood of anorexia nervosa (AN) or bulimia nervosa (BN) complicating a pregnancy is high. The prevalence of an eating disorder during pregnancy is 7%. The overall prevalence of AN is approximately 1% of young adult women, with a mean age of onset of 17 years, and an overall prevalence of BN of 1% to 3% in the same population. Of all eating disorders, 90% begin before the age 25 years. The high incidence of amenorrhea in AN makes pregnancy less likely than in BN. Medical complications of AN include bradycardia, hypotension, orthostatic changes, hypothermia, mitral valve prolapse, and symptoms associated with electrolyte imbalance. Anemia and transaminitis are also seen.

Pregnancy can frequently precipitate a subclinical eating disorder or exacerbate a condition in remission. The loss of control of body image and weight gain are frequent inciting features for recurrence. Adverse pregnancy outcomes include increased rates of miscarriage, low birth weight, preterm birth, congenital malformations, and increased likelihood of cesarean section births. Inappropriate dieting, with subsequent folate deficiency, increases the rate of congenital neural tube defects. In the postpartum period, depression risk is increased threefold in mothers with a history of eating disorders.

Treatment of eating disorders during pregnancy focuses on the restoration of normal physiologic parameters, electrolyte replacement, and correction of ketosis. There are no recommended pharmacologic interventions for AN by the US Food and Drug Administration, but antidepressant therapy may be beneficial in those with exacerbations of BN.

Substance Dependence/Use Disorder

The prevalence of substance use disorder in pregnancy has been increasing, with major societal and personal costs. Substance dependence is frequently not identified during pregnancy unless self-reported, or an unplanned pregnancy is discovered during the evaluation of the mother for a substance-related disorder. This is particularly common in the ED, where women of childbearing age are seen frequently for associated complications and pregnancy is coincidentally identified during the visit.

The overall rate of substance use in pregnancy has been steadily increasing in the last 3 decades. According to a national survey conducted in the United States in 2012, 6% of pregnant women use illicit drugs, 9% drink alcohol, and 16% smoke cigarettes, resulting in over 380,000 offspring exposed to illicit substances, over 550,000 exposed to alcohol, and over one million exposed to tobacco in utero. These numbers do not begin to take into account the rapidly rising opioid epidemic un the United States.

The impact of substance use on pregnancy is determined by the following: (1) specific exposure (mono- vs. polysubstance use); (2) gestational timing; (3) duration of exposure; (4) dosing of exposure; and (5) other maternal comorbid conditions (e.g., smoking, general nutritional status). There is a strong association of substance use disorder with psychiatric conditions, particularly depression and psychosis.

Within this context, the terms *use disorder* and *dependence* will be used synonymously, although they are different clinical entities. Both conditions have the same impact on maternal and neonatal health and pregnancy-related complications.

Alcohol

Approximately 50% of women of childbearing age self-identify as alcohol users and 15% are binge drinkers. Nearly 2 million women annually are at risk for alcohol-exposed pregnancies, defined as women who are not using birth control, currently drinking, and are sexually active with a man. Once pregnancy has been identified, the rate of active alcohol consumption in gravid women drops to 7%, and binge drinking to lower than 2%. The true incidence of this disease may be severely underappreciated though. Unfortunately, pregnant women presenting to the ED are 75% less likely to be tested for drug or alcohol use than nonpregnant women.[34] Even when pregnant women present with psychiatric or substance abuse concerns, they are less likely to be screened for alcohol or drug use. Screening for alcohol use in pregnancy is recommended to identify at-risk pregnancies. Screening tools that assume the presence of alcohol intake yield more honest reporting from patients.

There is no safe threshold for alcohol intake during pregnancy, with intake as little as one drink per day being associated with increased rates of IUGR and low birth weight. Heavier consumption of alcohol at more than three drinks/day increases the rate of miscarriage, and more than five drinks/day increases the risk of intrauterine fetal demise two to three times that of nondrinking mothers. Alcohol consumption in pregnancy is the most preventable cause of developmental delay, with alcohol-exposed children having a 1.7-fold greater relative risk of mental retardation and a 2.5 times greater risk of delinquent behaviors.[35]

Congenital abnormalities associated with in utero alcohol exposure can be characterized within the fetal alcohol spectrum disorders. Fetal alcohol syndrome, the most severe of these, has a prevalence of up to 1/1000 births. It is characterized by at least one of a series of morphologic abnormalities in association with a history of heavy alcohol use (>three drinks/day), including midfacial hypoplasia, flat philtrum, low nasal bridge, epicanthal folds, shortened palpebral fissure, low-set ears, and microcephaly. It can also have ocular, cardiac, and skeletal manifestations.

Treatment of an alcohol-dependent mother is difficult. As with nonpregnant patients, withdrawal symptoms are likely to manifest 6 to 24 hours after last alcohol consumption. Any signs of withdrawal should prompt admission and continued management in an inpatient setting. There is a paucity of data on the risk of delirium tremens and major withdrawal in pregnant versus the nonpregnant population. There are also little data on the safety profiles of medications used to ameliorate withdrawal symptoms. The use of naltrexone, acamprosate, or disulfiram or the long-term use of benzodiazepines has not been studied in pregnancy.

Smoking

The long-term deleterious effects of smoking on fetal growth and development have been well documented, up to and including the risk of sudden infant death syndrome (SIDS). Chronic placental insufficiency and vasoconstriction lead to an increased risk of miscarriage, IUFD, preterm birth, IUGR, and clubfoot. Prenatal maternal smoking also has an association with severe bronchiolitis during infancy. Conversely, smoking decreases the risk of preeclampsia.

Treatment for tobacco addiction in pregnancy is largely behavioral and cognitive. Nicotine patches have not been associated with adverse maternal or newborn consequences when used in the second and third trimesters.

Cannabis

Cannabis is the most commonly used recreational drug in pregnancy. There is a maternal association with cannabis use and maternal anemia. Although marijuana use in pregnancy is not associated with any major congenital malformations or increased risk of IUFD, there is an association with low birth weight and need for placement into a neonatal ICU. Infants born to cannabis-using mothers show increased tremulousness, exaggerated startle responses, and high-pitched cries. These are some of the same features associated with neonatal abstinence syndrome (NAS) or Neonatal Opioid Withdrawal Syndrome (NOWS) discussed later in more detail (see "Opioids"). Cannabis is excreted in breast milk and has been associated with neurologic impairment during continued exposure.

Cocaine and Methamphetamines

The prevalence of stimulant use in pregnancy is likely being underrecognized. Maternal cocaine, methamphetamine, and stimulant use is independently linked to IUGR from impaired placental circulation and preterm birth less than 36 weeks' gestation, preeclampsia, IUFD, and increased incidence of cesarean section, gestational hypertension, and gestational diabetes mellitus. Cocaine use also increases the risk of placental abruption and infarction.

Infants of methamphetamine-addicted mothers have lower Apgar scores and increased rates of neonatal mortality and jaundice, but also morphologic difference in brain anatomy, with reduced subcortical volumes. The potential for adverse outcomes is increased in the presence of polysubstance use disorder or other confounding maternal risks, such as poor nutrition. Neonatal congenital abnormalities do not seem to be significantly increased with cocaine use, although there is a slight increased risk of cleft palate with cocaine exposure.

Discontinuation and abstinence are generally the main goals of treatment for pregnant persons addicted to methamphetamines, but immediate discontinuation can cause depression, fatigue, and psychosis. Treatment of a gravid patient who is acutely intoxicated with cocaine or methamphetamine may involve the judicious use of benzodiazepines and antipsychotics, weighing the risk-benefit ratio for treatment against the medical and psychiatric instability of the patient, but this is not always necessary. Methamphetamine is excreted in breast milk, so infant exposure continues after pregnancy.

Opioids

Roughly 7% of all pregnant patients use opioids, a significant increase over the last decade.[36] This has created a downstream effect of large numbers of addicted infants requiring neonatal intensive care. There is a significant risk of unintended pregnancy among opioid-addicted women, close to 90%, compared to the unintended pregnancy rate in the general population of 40%.[37] The ED is a likely site of entrance of the opioid-addicted gravid patient to the health care system.

There are no well-identified syndromes, congenital abnormalities, or teratogenic effects in infants of opioid-dependent mothers, although there is some association with cleft lip deformities and ventricular septal defects. Neonatal risks include IUGR, specifically symmetric smallness and small head circumference, and an increased risk of SIDS. Maternal risks of postpartum hemorrhage, preterm birth, and increased rates of cesarean section have been documented. The major complication in infants of opioid-addicted mothers is neonatal opioid withdrawal syndrome (NOWS), also known as neonatal abstinence syndrome (NAS), a constellation of physiologic and neurobehavioral changes noted in newborns of addicted mothers secondary to a sudden discontinuation of fetal exposure to substances. The syndrome is characterized by the following: (1) CNS disturbances, including excessive or continuous high-pitched crying, shortened postprandial sleep pattern, hyperactive newborn reflexes, tremulousness, and increased muscle tone, myoclonic jerks, or frank convulsions; (2) metabolic and respiratory abnormalities (e.g., sweating, hyperthermia, yawning, mottling, sneezing, nasal flaring, tachypnea); and (3) gastrointestinal disturbances (e.g., increased sucking, poor feeding, regurgitation or projectile vomiting, loose or watery stools). The Finnegan scale, developed in the 1970s, is still the mainstay of neonatal assessment for NOWS. Treatment of NOWS is supportive. The incidence of NOWS has grown rapidly in the past decade. These infants have a 97% admission rate to neonatal intensive care units.

A new generation of mothers and infants who sustained exposure to methadone, buprenorphine or naltrexone is upon us. Compared to mothers using opioids, those on agonist therapy had improved pregnancy outcomes and decreased risk of NOWS.

The references for this chapter can be found online at ExpertConsult. com.

175

Drug Therapy in Pregnancy

Valerie A. Dobiesz and Daniel W. Robinson

KEY CONCEPTS

- Chemically induced birth defects are responsible for approximately 1% to 3% of anomalous births.
- Gestational age is crucial in determination of the impact of any given exposure, especially during organogenesis (days 21–56 of fetal life), when major body organs are formed.
- Human data on teratogenicity and fetal toxicity of medications are often limited, and causal associations are difficult to determine, especially with newer medications.

- In general, the health of the fetus is directly related to the health of the mother, and drugs should be given when the maternal benefits outweigh the risks to the fetus.
- Certain medications should be avoided during pregnancy because they are known teratogens or cause potential toxic effects in the newborn; these include anticonvulsants, warfarin derivatives, NSAIDs, sulfonamides, fluoroquinolones, and ACE inhibitors. If there are no alternatives to these agents, it is recommended to use the lowest dose for the shortest duration possible.

FOUNDATIONS

More than 90% of women take at least one prescription or over-the-counter medication during pregnancy, and overall medication use during pregnancy has increased in the last 3 decades. One study revealed that only 22% of reproductive-aged women have pregnancy testing done when administered or prescribed potentially harmful or teratogenic medications in the emergency department (ED).[1] Unfortunately, the majority of research on the use of medications during pregnancy is insufficient to determine reliable and accurate risks to the mother and fetus, especially for newer agents. Only a few medications have been tested specifically for safety and efficacy during pregnancy. Prescribing medications during pregnancy must account for the physiologic changes associated with pregnancy as well as the benefits and risks to the mother and developing fetus.

The fetal age at exposure to a medication is crucial in determining its impact on the pregnancy. The fetus is most vulnerable to toxic insults during the time of organogenesis (days 21–56 of fetal life). Exposure during this period may result in major anatomic defects. Exposure after the period of organogenesis may affect the growth and development of the fetus. Functional development of the central nervous system (CNS) is affected when it is exposed to a CNS teratogen during the 10th to 17th weeks of pregnancy.

Major birth defects affect 3% to 5% of all live births. Most are of unknown cause, but 1% to 3% of these are thought to be due to pharmaceutical or environmental agents. A teratogen is any chemical, pharmacologic, environmental, or mechanical agent that can cause disruptive development of the conceptus. Included in this definition are functional impairment, growth restriction, and congenital malformations.

The process of establishing teratogenicity is tedious and often flawed. Animal research, although valuable in determining risk initially, is not always applicable to humans, and controlled prospective human studies are generally not performed for ethical reasons. As a result, much of our current knowledge on teratogenicity has been derived from less rigorous studies, which are inherently weak in establishing a causal relationship between a specific exposure and malformations. The genetic background of the fetus, timing and duration of the exposure, environmental factors, multiple exposures, nutritional deficits, maternal illness, and illicit drug use all contribute to the outcome of pregnancy. Large population studies are needed to understand the connection between the outcome of a pregnancy and in utero exposures. Finally, as in the case of diethylstilbestrol, teratogenicity may not be apparent for years after birth.

Classification of Teratogenic Risk

The FDA issued a final rule for drug labeling called the Pregnancy and Lactation Labeling Rule (PLLR) in June 2015. The PLLR changed the content and format of prescription drug labeling to help health care providers better assess the benefits and risks in counseling pregnant and nursing women who are taking medications. The rule requires the removal of letter categories (A, B, C, D, and X) and mandates labeling that includes a summary of data on the risks of a drug used during pregnancy, lactation, and the impacts on male and female reproduction. It requires the provision of current data supporting that summary, and any relevant information to help health care providers make informed decisions and counsel patients. The PLLR also mandates the label be updated when new information becomes available. Drugs already approved before this rule are being phased in. Currently, a number of clinical teratology resources that assign risk are available online, such as Clinical Pharmacology, TERIS, and Micromedex Reprotox (Shepard's *Catalog of Teratogenic Agents*).

Drug Transfer Across the Placenta

Drug transfer across the placenta usually occurs by simple passive diffusion or protein transport. A thin layer of trophoblastic cells is all that separates maternal from fetal circulation. The degree to which a drug gains access to fetal circulation depends on molecular size, ionic state, lipid solubility, and extent of protein binding. Drugs with a molecular mass of less than 5 kilodaltons (kDa) readily diffuse. Anionic substances diffuse through the lipid layer more readily than ionized forms.

A free drug diffuses more readily than a protein-bound drug. Because fetal pH is slightly more alkalotic than maternal pH, weak organic acids may become ion-trapped in the fetal circulation, increasing fetal exposure.

Drug Transfer During Lactation

Generally, drugs that are ingested or injected by the mother diffuse passively into milk and then back into the maternal circulation for excretion. The amount of drug diffusing into milk depends on many factors. Lipid-soluble and nonionic substances diffuse more readily, and highly protein-bound substances diffuse less readily. Whether a substance is concentrated in maternal milk or not, the neonate generally is able to detoxify it with no adverse effects, and only a few drugs pose a serious danger to a breast-feeding infant. The interruption of breast-feeding should not be advocated except in rare situations of known drug toxicity to the infant and in all cases of maternal critical illness.

Drug Therapy During Pregnancy

In general, the health of the fetus is directly related to the health of the mother. Physicians should not withhold lifesaving medications from pregnant patients because of a reported risk to the fetus and should resuscitate pregnant patients according to advanced life support guidelines. Physicians may also prescribe any agent when the maternal benefits outweigh the risks to the fetus. Included in this category are therapeutic medications for asthma, arrhythmias, status epilepticus, life-threatening overdoses, and human immunodeficiency virus (HIV) infection. When prescribing drugs to pregnant and lactating women, the benefits of treatment must be weighed against the inherent risks of treatment or disease. The drug with the lowest known toxicity should be chosen, and used at the lowest effective dose.

PHARMACOLOGIC THERAPY

Analgesic Agents

Over-the-counter analgesics are used commonly during pregnancy, with acetaminophen being used by at least two-thirds of pregnant women. Studies are emerging that call for a reassessment of the safety of these medications. Several studies report increasing use and adverse pregnancy outcomes with opioids, such as neonatal abstinence syndrome and birth defects (Table 175.1).

Acetaminophen

Acetaminophen (paracetamol) is the most widely used analgesic during pregnancy. It has not been associated with congenital malformations

TABLE 175.1 Analgesic Medications

Drug	Breast-Feeding	Clinical Risk Summary
Acetaminophen	Compatible, excreted in breast milk	CP, NHT; studies suggest increased risk of neurodevelopmental problems such as attention-deficit/hyperactivity-hyperkinetic disorder, cryptorchidism, childhood asthma/wheezing
Ibuprofen	Compatible, excreted in breast milk	CP, increased risk of spontaneous abortion at time of conception, association with structural cardiac defects and gastroschisis; risk in third trimester of premature closure of ductus arteriosus and subsequent primary pulmonary hypertension; potential increased risk of asthma with use in pregnancy
Aspirin	Potential toxicity, excreted in breast milk	CP; increased risk of spontaneous abortion at time of conception, avoid chronic or high doses in pregnancy; high doses may increase perinatal mortality, teratogenic effects; increased risk of gastroschisis in first trimester; increased risk of IUGR and fetal and maternal hemorrhage in third trimester; risk in third trimester of premature closure of ductus arteriosus and subsequent primary pulmonary hypertension; near-term use may prolong gestation, labor
Codeine	Potential toxicity Use with caution Excreted in breast milk, metabolized to morphine	LHS; congenital malformation data in humans are inconsistent; avoid prolonged use or high doses near term; may develop respiratory depression and/or withdrawal symptoms, neonatal abstinence syndrome
Oxycodone	Potential toxicity Use with caution Potential for SAR	LHS; use during organogenesis associated with low absolute risk of congenital birth defects; may result in preterm birth, poor fetal outcomes, NOWS
Morphine	Potential toxicity Usually compatible for short-term use Use with caution	CP; use during organogenesis associated with low risk of CBD; may result in preterm birth and poor fetal outcomes; prolonged maternal use during pregnancy may result in NOWS

CBD, Congenital birth defects; CP, crosses placenta; IUGR, intrauterine growth restriction; LHS, limited human studies; NHT, no human teratogenicity; NOWS, neonatal opioid withdrawal syndrome; SAR, serious adverse reactions.
Adapted data from: Lopes LM, Carrilho MC, Francisco RPV, Lopes MAB, Krebs VLJ, Zugaib M. Fetal ductus arteriosus constriction and closure: analysis of the causes and perinatal outcome related to 45 consecutive cases. *J Matern Fetal Neonatal Med*. 2016;29(4):638–645; ACOG Practice Bulletin No. 196: Thromboembolism in pregnancy. *Obstet Gynecol*. 2018;132(1):e1-e17; Shenai N, Shulman J, Gopalan P, Cheng E, Cerimele JM. Fetal outcomes in intentional over-the-counter medication overdoses in pregnancy. *Psychosomatics*. 2018;59(4):400-404; Mullins N, Galvin SL, Ramage M, et al. Buprenorphine and naloxone versus buprenorphine for opioid use disorder in pregnancy: a cohort study. *J Addict Med*. 2019;14(3):185-192; Acar S, Keskin-Arslan E, Erol-Coskun H, Kaya-Temiz T, Kaplan YC. Pregnancy outcomes following quinolone and fluoroquinolone exposure during pregnancy: A systematic review and meta-analysis. *Reprod Toxicol*. 2019;85:65-74; Mallah N, Tohidinik HR, Etminan M, Figueiras A, Takkouche B. Prenatal exposure to macrolides and risk of congenital malformations: a meta-analysis. *Drug Saf*. 2019;43(3):1-11; Sheehy O, Santos F, Ferreira E, Berard A. The use of metronidazole during pregnancy: a review of evidence. *Curr Drug Saf*. 2015;10(2):170-179; Committee Opinion No. 717: Sulfonamides, nitrofurantoin, and risk of birth defects. *Obstet Gynecol*. 2017;130(3):e150-e152; Alsaad AM, Kaplan YC, Koren G. Exposure to fluconazole and risk of congenital malformations in the offspring: a systematic review and meta-analysis. *Reprod Toxicol*. 2015;52:78-82; Floridia M, Dalzero S, Giacomet V, et al. Pregnancy and neonatal outcomes in women with HIV-1 exposed to integrase inhibitors, protease inhibitors and non-nucleoside reverse transcriptase inhibitors: an observational study. *Infection*. 2020;48(2):249-258.

and does not appear to increase the risk of adverse outcomes. There is weak evidence suggesting a link between maternal acetaminophen use in pregnancy with a higher risk of multiple neurodevelopmental problems including hyperkinetic disorders and attention-deficit hyperactivity disorder–like behaviors in children.[1a] Still, it is considered by most clinicians to be the safest analgesic and antipyretic medication currently available during pregnancy and lactation.

Nonsteroidal Antiinflammatory Drugs

Prostaglandin synthesis inhibitors, such as nonsteroidal antiinflammatory drugs (NSAIDs), taken in the first trimester may lead to increased risk of spontaneous abortions, although most of the studies showing this association are limited by not controlling for the conditions for which the medication was taken. The mechanism for this association is inhibition of prostaglandin production by NSAIDs, which is essential for embryonic implantation. Some epidemiologic and animal studies show an increase in ventricular septal defects and gastroschisis with NSAID use during pregnancy. When used in the third trimester, NSAIDs inhibit labor and may be used as tocolytic agents for premature labor. NSAID use in the latter part of pregnancy has been linked to a number of negative effects on the neonate, most notably premature closure of the ductus arteriosus, leading to neonatal pulmonary hypertension, and death.[2] Use in the latter part of pregnancy is therefore discouraged. NSAIDs in general appear to be safe during lactation.

Aspirin

Studies show a proposed increased risk of spontaneous abortion with aspirin use around the time of conception. Chronic or high doses of aspirin during pregnancy should be avoided and may affect maternal and newborn hemostasis and bleeding abnormalities, leading to increased perinatal morbidity and mortality. Aspirin use has been associated with premature closure of the ductus arteriosus causing primary pulmonary hypertension in the newborn, and neonatal death.[2] Low doses of aspirin (60 to 100 mg/day) may be beneficial in pregnancies complicated by systemic lupus erythematosus with antiphospholipid antibodies and those at risk for gestational hypertension and preeclampsia, as well as fetuses with intrauterine growth restriction (IUGR).[3] Aspirin is excreted into breast milk and its use is discouraged during breast-feeding due to risk of Reye syndrome.

Opiate Analgesics

In general, short-term, episodic use of opiates such as oxycodone, hydrocodone, morphine, and fentanyl appear to be safe in pregnancy. Their use near term, however, may result in respiratory depression of the neonate. Prescribing of narcotics for long periods may be associated with preterm birth, low birth weight, reduced infant head circumference, congenital malformations, sudden infant death, and neonatal abstinence syndrome.[4] Neonatal abstinence syndrome is characterized by CNS hyperirritability, autonomic nervous system dysfunction, and higher infant mortality. The short-term use of opiates during lactation appears to be safe, but nursing infants should be closely monitored for respiratory depression.

Rapid Sequence Intubation Agents

Data regarding the use of these agents during pregnancy are limited and have primarily been obtained from animal studies and retrospective human data. None of the agents has been consistently associated with congenital malformations or had adverse effects on the fetus (Table 175.2).

TABLE 175.2   Rapid Sequence Intubation Medications

Drug	Breast-Feeding	Clinical Risk Summary
Fentanyl	Compatible; may cause sedation or respiratory depression	CP; associated congenital birth defects; may cause neonatal respiratory depression, transient neonatal muscular rigidity, NOWS
Etomidate	Probably compatible	CP; animal studies show no teratogenicity; transient decrease in newborn cortisol levels of unknown clinical significance; LHS not harmful when used as induction agent
Propofol	Probably compatible, but not recommended	CP; animal studies show no malformations, LHS with no data on use in first and second trimesters; use at term appears to be safe, but high doses may be associated with neonatal CNS, respiratory depression
Thiopental	Probably compatible; use with caution	CP; LHS; animal studies show no congenital defects, even with high doses; may cause respiratory depression
Ketamine	Probably compatible; plasma levels undetectable after 12 hr	CP; used frequently in obstetrics, not associated with fetal developmental malformations; dose-dependent oxytocic effect; in high doses (>2 mg/kg), associated with uterine tetany; may increase maternal blood pressure and heart rate; may increase neonatal muscle tone or cause apnea and depression of the newborn, SAR usually dose-related
Midazolam	Use with caution Avoid with other CNS depressants	CP; animal studies show no congenital effects, even with high doses; LHS, human observational studies show no malformations, no data on use in first and second trimesters; use near term has resulted in adverse neonatal neurobehavior and neonatal respiratory depression
Succinylcholine	Probably compatible because of rapid hydrolysis	Not embryotoxic or teratogenic in animals; may result in neonatal apnea and partial or complete newborn paralysis in neonates with pseudocholinesterase deficiency
Rocuronium	Probably compatible; LHS	CP; LHS; animal data suggest low risk; newborn neuromuscular blockade is potential complication but probably rare, may have prolonged blockade when used with magnesium
Vecuronium	Probably compatible	CP; LHS; use late in gestation appear to carry little if any risk to the newborn; use lower doses if administering magnesium sulfate

CNS, Central nervous system; *CP,* crosses placenta; *LHS,* limited human studies; *NHT,* no human teratogenicity; *NOWS,* neonatal opioid withdrawal syndrome; *SAR,* serious adverse reactions.

Anticoagulants

Low-molecular-weight-heparin (LMWH) is preferred over unfractionated heparin and warfarin when indicated in pregnancy for therapeutic and prophylactic anticoagulation. Warfarin has the highest teratogenicity of the anticoagulants. The heparins, as a class, do not cross the placenta. All three anticoagulants are considered compatible with breast-feeding (Table 175.3).[5] Oral DTI (dabigatran) and anti-Xa inhibiitors (apixaban, rivaroxaban, edoxaban) have been extensively studied in pregnancy and therefore should be avoided.

Thrombolytic Agents

Alteplase, reteplase, urokinase, and streptokinase have been used successfully in pregnant women in cases of life-threatening pulmonary embolus, myocardial infarction, ischemic stroke, thrombosis of cardiac valve prosthesis, and deep venous thrombosis. Complication rates when used for these indications were similar compared to nonpregnant patients, and none of the live-born children had permanent defects. Recombinant tissue plasminogen activator does not cross the placenta. Poor fetal outcomes have been associated with poor maternal prognosis.

To date, no teratogenic effects have been reported in humans, but intrapartum maternal hemorrhage, fetal hemorrhage, spontaneous abortion, preterm delivery, and fetal death have been reported. Most thrombolytics are thought to be compatible with breast-feeding (Table 175.4).

Antidotes

There are limited human data on the risks of antidote use during pregnancy. Generally, antidotes should be used when there is a clear maternal indication and the potential benefits outweigh the possible risk (Table 175.5). In general, overdoses of medication with higher rates of placental transfer have increased potential for fetal toxicity.

N-Acetylcysteine

N-Acetylcysteine has been used successfully and without untoward effects in pregnant women who have overdosed on acetaminophen. No teratogenic effects have been reported, and pregnant patients who overdose on acetaminophen should be treated the same as nonpregnant patients.[6] It is most likely safe during lactation because it has been used in neonates without untoward effects.

Deferoxamine

Deferoxamine has been associated with developmental effects on ossification in some animal species. Experience in humans is limited, but

TABLE 175.3 Anticoagulant Medications

Drug	Breast-Feeding	Clinical Risk Summary
Warfarin	Compatible; however, caution advised when breast-feeding premature infants due to increased risk for intraventricular hemorrhage	CP; known dose-dependent teratogen affecting 4%–5% of exposed fetuses; greatest risk at gestational wk 6–9; fetal warfarin syndrome associated with corpus callosum agenesis, hypoplasia of nasal bones, midline dysplasia, optic atrophy and blindness; also associated with fetal osteogenesis, CNS malformations, fetal intraventricular hemorrhage, stillbirths, spontaneous abortions, abnormal development of bones, stippled epiphyses; school-age children exposed in utero had increased incidence of mild neurologic dysfunction
Heparin (UFH)	Compatible	DNCP; associated with maternal osteopenia, immune-mediated thrombocytopenia, maternal hemorrhage at delivery, requiring careful monitoring; has reduced bioavailability, shorter half-life, lower peak plasma concentrations during pregnancy; risk of antepartum bleeding ≈1%
Low-molecular-weight heparin	Compatible	DNCP; lower risk of osteoporosis than UFH has reduced bioavailability, shorter half-life, lower peak plasma concentrations during pregnancy; lower rate of bleeding, HIT, lower allergic response versus heparin; recommended over UFH for VTE

CP, Crosses placenta; DNCP, does not cross placenta; HIT, heparin-induced thrombocytopenia; UFH, unfractionated heparin; VTE, venous thromboembolism.
Additional data adapted from: ACOG Practice Bulletin No. 203. Chronic hypertension in pregnancy. *Obstet Gynecol.* 2019;133(1):e26-e50; ACOG Committee Opinion No. 767. Emergent therapy for acute-onset, severe hypertension during pregnancy and the postpartum period. *Obstet Gynecol.* 2019;133(2):e174-e180.

TABLE 175.4 Thrombolytic Medications

Drug	Breast-Feeding	Clinical Risk Summary
Alteplase	Compatible Unknown if excreted in breast milk	Embryocidal, not teratogenic, in animal studies; LHS; use if benefits to mother outweigh risks; has been used in human pregnancy with normal fetal outcomes, risk of hemorrhage at any time in gestation
Streptokinase	Use with caution; unknown safety	Use with caution; CP in minimal amounts; no fetal abnormalities reported; antistreptokinase antibodies cross the placenta
Reteplase	Probably compatible Use with caution Unknown if crosses into breast milk	Unknown if CP; risk for bleeding during labor and delivery; abortifacient, but no teratogenicity in animals; LHS; several cases of use with normal infants
Tenecteplase	Hold breast-feeding Unknown safety	Unknown if CP; use with caution, safety unknown; risk of bleeding during labor and delivery; toxicity to mother in animal studies; LHS
Urokinase	Probably compatible Unknown if excreted in breast milk	Probably acceptable in pregnancy; not fetotoxic or teratogenic in animal studies; unknown if CP; placental hemorrhage and separation may occur; increased risk of bleeding during pregnancy; LHS

CP, Crosses placenta; LHS, limited human studies.
Additional data adapted from: ACOG Committee Opinion No. 767: Emergent therapy for acute-onset, severe hypertension during pregnancy and the postpartum period. *Obstet Gynecol.* 2019;133(2):e174-e180; ACOG Practice Bulletin No. 212. Pregnancy and heart disease. *Obstet Gynecol.* 2019;133(5):e320-e356. doi:doi: 10.1097/AOG.0000000000003243; ACOG Practice Bulletin No. 190. Gestational diabetes mellitus. *Obstet Gynecol.* 2018;131(2):e49-e64.

TABLE 175.5   Antidotes

Drug	Breast-Feeding	Clinical Risk Summary
N-Acetylcysteine	Probably compatible unknown if excreted in milk so consider waiting 30 hr for elimination	CP; not teratogenic or embryotoxic in animal studies; LHS; no adverse fetal outcome when administered IV as antidote in acetaminophen overdose
Deferoxamine	Probably compatible Unknown if excreted in breast milk	LHS; no adverse toxic or teratogenic effects seen; animal studies show toxicity and teratogenicity (delayed ossification, skeletal anomalies)
Digoxin immune fragment	Probably compatible Unknown if excreted in breast milk	Unknown if CP; LHS; no adverse outcomes in fetus or newborn
Dimercaprol	Contraindicated Unknown if excreted in breast milk	Animal studies show teratogenicity; safety in pregnancy unknown; chelates essential elements including zinc, copper, and iron that may alter fetal development but LHS
Flumazenil	Probably compatible Unknown if excreted in breast milk	Unknown if CP, but may occur; animal studies show no teratogenicity or impaired fertility; LHS
Fomepizole	Hold breast-feeding	No animal or human studies; safety unknown
Hydroxocobalamin	Probably compatible, but monitoring of infant recommended	Animal studies showed no teratogenicity; LHS, safety unknown
Methylene blue	Probably compatible Unknown if excreted in breast milk	Epidemiologic evidence of teratogenicity; diagnostic intraamniotic injection resulted in hemolytic anemia, hyperbilirubinemia, methemoglobinemia, jejunal-ileal atresias
Naloxone	Probably compatible Unknown if excreted in breast milk LHS	CP; animal studies show no teratogenicity, no adverse fetal outcomes in human studies
Physostigmine	Probably compatible but safety unknown	Rarely used in pregnancy; no reports linking it with teratogenicity; safety unknown
Pralidoxime	Hold breast-feeding for 6 to 7 hr after dose	Rarely used in pregnancy; safety unknown; limited human case reports, with no adverse outcomes
Pyridoxine	Compatible	High doses appear to pose little risk to the fetus; no increased risk of malformations in first trimester in human trials
Succimer	Contraindicated Heavy metals may be excreted in breast milk, cause harm to newborn	Teratogenic and fetotoxic in animals; avoidance in first trimester recommended for pregnant women unless severe symptoms; LHS

CP, Crosses placenta; *LHS,* limited human studies.
Additional data adapted from: Lai T, Wu M, Liu J, et al. Acid-suppressive drug use during pregnancy and the risk of childhood asthma: A meta-analysis. *Pediatrics.* 2018;141(2):e20170889; McParlin C, O'Donnell A, Robson SC, et al. Treatments for hyperemesis gravidarum and nausea and vomiting in pregnancy: a systematic review. *JAMA.* 2016;316(13):1392-1401; Bonham CA, Patterson KC, Strek ME. Asthma outcomes and management during pregnancy. *Chest.* 2018;153(2):515-527; Chambers C. Over-the-counter medications: Risk and safety in pregnancy. *Semin Perinatol.* 2015;39(7):541-544.

has been used in pregnancy without adverse effect on the fetus. The effects of deferoxamine on the nursing infant are not known, but are probably compatible.

Digoxin Immune Fragment

There are very few case reports of the use of digoxin immune fragment (Fab) during pregnancy, so effects on the fetus are inconclusive. In cases of life-threatening digitalis overdose with arrhythmias, the benefits of treatment of the mother outweigh the risk to the fetus. Digoxin fab is probably safe for use during lactation.

Dimercaprol

Dimercaprol, or British antilewisite, is teratogenic in mice and has been associated with increased mortality, growth restriction, cleft facial features, cerebral herniation, and abnormal digits, but experience in humans is limited. In general, with heavy metal poisonings, the maternal benefits of treatment will outweigh the potential risks to the fetus. Breast-feeding is contraindicated in patients poisoned by heavy metals.

Flumazenil

No teratogenic effects have been reported with flumazenil in animals, and there are limited human data. Its use in pregnancy and lactation depends on the potential maternal benefit compared with possible

risks to the fetus and nursing infant. Because it has a short half-life, breast-feeding may resume after a few hours.

Fomepizole

Fomepizole use during pregnancy has not been studied in animals or humans. Its safety during pregnancy is not known. In cases of toxic alcohol poisoning, the benefits of treatment of the mother outweigh the possible risks to the fetus or nursing infant. Use of ethyl alcohol in these situations may be considered. Breast-feeding is not recommended during treatment.

Hydroxycobalamin

The effects of hydroxycobalamin on human pregnancy have not been studied, but benefits of its use in cyanide poisoning outweigh any risk to the fetus. Use is considered compatible with breast-feeding.

Methylene Blue

Historically, methylene blue was injected into the amniotic sac to identify twins and detect rupture of the membranes, but these practices were associated with hemolytic disease in the newborn, hyperbilirubinemia, and deep blue staining of the newborn. Methylene blue in pregnancy has also been associated with an increased incidence of intestinal obstruction and atresia in the newborn, primarily with intra-amniotic or intrauterine administration. Methylene blue has been used successfully in pregnant women with methemoglobinemia; however, the benefits of treatment should outweigh the risks of the therapy and must be considered. The effects of methylene blue on the nursing infant are expected to be minimal.

Naloxone

Naloxone readily crosses the placenta. Although it has not been associated with reproductive abnormalities, its use during pregnancy results in increased fetal wakefulness, increased fetal movement, and increased heart rate, effects attributable to the antagonism of fetal endorphins. In addition, its use in opiate-addicted mothers may precipitate withdrawal in mother and term fetus. The use of buprenorphine with naloxone in pregnant women with opioid use disorder has been found to be safe.[7] It is compatible with breast-feeding.

Physostigmine

Experience during pregnancy is limited, and its effects on the developing fetus are unknown. Use of physostigmine at term has been associated with only mild decreases in Apgar scores at 1 and 5 minutes. Physostigmine is thought to be safe with breast-feeding.

Pralidoxime

Experience with pralidoxime in pregnancy is limited, and its effects on fetal development are not known. In cases of organophosphate poisoning, the benefits to the mother generally outweigh the possible risk to the fetus. Breast-feeding can be resumed after 6 to 7 hours after the last dose.

Pyridoxine

Pyridoxine, vitamin B_6, has not been associated with any adverse developmental effects when given in high doses, and it is safe in lactation.

Dimercaptosuccinic Acid (Succimer)

Succimer has been linked to congenital defects in animal models, possibly because of its negative effects on zinc and copper metabolism. Experience with the use of succimer in human pregnancy is limited to case reports, and adverse effects are unknown. Breast-feeding is contraindicated in heavy metal poisoning.

Antiinfective Agents

Infections during pregnancy potentially affect outcomes as well as fetal development. In the first trimester, infections are a common cause of spontaneous abortion and, in the second or third trimester, they are the most common cause of low birth weight and preterm labor. Antimicrobial agents may also adversely affect the pregnancy. Aminoglycosides, for example, may be nephrotoxic and ototoxic to the mother and newborn, tetracyclines may result in dental staining of the developing fetus, and lincosamides may be skeletotoxic.

The penicillins, cephalosporins, and macrolide antibiotics are the drugs of choice for infections during pregnancy. Alternative classes of antibiotics are prescribed only if these have failed to control the infection or in cases of severe maternal intolerance to these drugs. The choice of antimicrobial therapy will depend on the gestational age of the pregnancy, severity of infection, and maternal tolerance for the drug used. Many drugs are secreted into breast milk. Potential problems for the neonate include direct effects on the neonate, changes in bowel flora, diarrhea, and potential interference with culture results (Table 175.6).

Antibiotics

Aminoglycosides

Aminoglycosides do not appear to have any structural teratogenic effects in humans. Kanamycin and streptomycin have been reported to cause ototoxicity in the mother and her offspring. There are no reports definitively linking in utero exposure to gentamicin, streptomycin,

TABLE 175.6	Antiinfective Medications	
Drug	**Breast-Feeding**	**Clinical Risk Summary**
Aminoglycosides	Probably compatible Excreted in breast milk Oral absorption poor	No definable structural risk of any aminoglycoside when exposed in utero; streptomycin—low incidence of ototoxicity with careful dosing
• First generation	Compatible	CP; NHT (most studies); conflicting studies on risk of congenital defects in first trimester
• Second generation	Compatible	CP; immune hemolytic reactions observed, especially with cefotetan
• Third generation	Compatible	CP; immune hemolytic reactions observed
• Fourth generation	Compatible	CP; LHS
Chloramphenicol	Potential toxicity (LHS) Excreted in breast milk	CP; may cause grey baby syndrome; idiosyncratic bone marrow suppression
Clindamycin	Compatible Excreted in breast milk	CP; no reports of fetal toxicity or malformations
Fluoroquinolones	Compatible Excreted in breast milk	Ciprofloxacin, ofloxacin, and levofloxacin CP; few reports of arthrotoxicity; risk of major malformations low; caution use during first trimester, risk of cardiac defects
Linezolid	Potential toxicity (LHS) Excreted in breast milk	No studies in pregnancy Use with caution
Macrolides	Compatible Excreted in low concentrations in breast milk	Estolate salt—may induce hepatotoxicity in pregnant patients; no risk of congenital heart malformations or pyloric stenosis, but use of erythromycin in infancy associated with pyloric stenosis
Metronidazole	Compatible Excreted in breast milk—but AAP recommends cessation of breast-feeding during use	CP; in vitro mutagen; NHT
Nitrofurantoin	Compatible	Caution advised with G6PD deficiency—may cause hemolytic anemia; limit use in later pregnancy

Continued

TABLE 175.6   Antiinfective Medications—cont'd

Drug	Breast-Feeding	Clinical Risk Summary
Penicillins	Compatible Small amount excreted in breast milk	CP; long-standing safety data
Sulfonamides	Compatible Excreted in breast milk Caution in newborns, infants with known G6PD deficiency	CP; adverse effects rare; most reports fail to demonstrate congenital malformations; concern for jaundice, hemolytic anemia, kernicterus; trimethoprim is folate antagonist—use with caution
Tetracyclines	Compatible Excreted in breast milk	CP; doxycycline poses little teratogenic risk; adverse effects on fetal bone development; discoloration of adult teeth; oxytetracycline shows neural tube defects, cleft palate, cardiac defects
Vancomycin	Compatible IV form found in breast milk, but, no oral absorption	No toxicity or teratogenicity found
Clotrimazole	Compatible	Systemic absorption from skin minimal; vaginal and topical formulations preferred over oral lozenge; NHT; avoid vaginal use during first trimester; some reports suggest increased risk of spontaneous abortions
Fluconazole	Compatible	High dose in first trimester associated with malformations; If necessary vaginal formulation preferred.
Ketoconazole	Compatible Excreted in breast milk	NHT, but teratogenicity seen in animal studies
Nystatin	Compatible Not excreted in breast milk	Poor systemic absorption from vaginal formulation (preferred route); often first-line therapy in pregnancy
Terbinafine	Potential toxicity Excreted in breast milk	LHS; Likely compatible
Isoniazid	Compatible Excreted in breast milk	CP; benefits of treatment outweigh risks; NHT
Ethambutol	Compatible Excreted in breast milk	CP; benefits of treatment outweigh risks; no adverse effects seen
Rifampin	Compatible Excreted in breast milk	CP; benefits of treatment outweigh risk; hemorrhagic disease of newborn
Acyclovir	Compatible Excreted in breast milk	CP—found in higher concentrations than in maternal blood; systemic use should be avoided unless benefits outweigh the risks; NHT
Valacyclovir	Compatible Excreted in breast milk	CP; LHS
Famciclovir	Potential toxicity	Unknown if crosses placenta or enters breast milk; LHS
Amantadine	Potential toxicity (LHS) Excreted in breast milk	CP; teratogenicity in animals; associated with cardiac malformations.
Oseltamivir	Compatible Excreted in breast milk but in low concentration	Benefits of treatment during gestation likely greatly outweigh risks; no congenital malformations identified

AAP, American Academy of Pediatrics; *CP,* crosses placenta; *G6PD,* Glucose-6-phosphate dehydrogenase; *LHS,* limited human studies; *LS,* limited studies; *NHT,* no human teratogenicity.
Additional data adapted from refs.[24-37]

tobramycin, and neomycin with ototoxicity or nephrotoxicity. Aminoglycosides are probably compatible with breast-feeding.

Cephalosporins

The first- to fourth-generation cephalosporins appear to be safe during pregnancy, although there have been no controlled studies examining their safety. Some cephalosporins are excreted into breast milk and may interfere with culture results in the evaluation of neonatal sepsis.

Chloramphenicol

Chloramphenicol is associated with bone marrow suppression and aplastic anemia. Apart from these complications, its use during pregnancy appears to have no effects on the developing fetus. Exposure to topical chloramphenicol during pregnancy appears to have no adverse effects. However, it is contraindicated at birth because chloramphenicol has

been associated with cardiovascular collapse in the neonate, the so-called gray baby syndrome. Chloramphenicol is secreted into the breast milk, and therefore not recommended for use during lactation.

Clindamycin

Clindamycin has not been associated with birth defects in humans or in animal studies. The American Academy of Pediatrics (AAP) considers clindamycin to be compatible with breast-feeding, although there is a rare association with bloody diarrhea in nursing infants.

Fluoroquinolones

Fluoroquinolones are linked to numerous toxic effects on bone and cartilage growth in animal models and are discouraged from use during pregnancy, particularly during the first trimester. Observational studies, however, have failed to demonstrate such a toxic effect on the human fetus. Meta-analyses have not found an association between fluoroquinolones and fetal malformations, preterm delivery, stillbirth, or spontaneous abortions.[8] Regardless, at this time, they are not recommended in the first trimester until further studies are done. Ciprofloxacin is compatible with breast-feeding, but data are inconsistent for other quinolones, and they are best avoided in lactation.

Linezolid

Linezolid is linked to embryonic death, decreased weight, and abnormalities in cartilage and ossification in animal studies, but human data are lacking. Its use in pregnant women should be limited to cases in which the maternal benefits outweigh possible risks to the fetus. Linezolid is likely compatible with breast-feeding.

Macrolides

Erythromycin is considered safe for use in pregnancy and compatible with breast-feeding. Some reports have linked erythromycin to pyloric stenosis and congenital heart defects. The estolate salt of erythromycin is associated with the development of hepatotoxicity in pregnant women and should be avoided. Clarithromycin is associated with an increased risk of fetal and embryonic death, as well as with congenital malformations in animal studies; this has not been shown in humans. Meta-analyses demonstrate a weak association between macrolides and congenital malformation but data are conflicting.[9] Azithromycin is poorly concentrated in breast milk and may be the preferred agent in lactating mothers.

Metronidazole

Metronidazole is mutagenic and carcinogenic in mice and rats. In humans, a number of studies have failed to demonstrate a clear association between metronidazole and congenital malformations when used in the first trimester of pregnancy. Metronidazole has been used during the second and third trimesters to treat bacterial vaginosis, with no untoward effects.[10] The use of metronidazole during lactation is discouraged because of its potential mutagenic and carcinogenic effects reported in rats, and its slow elimination from infants.

Nitrofurantoin

Though historically considered safe throughout pregnancy, except near term, there is some literature that associates nitrofurantoin use in the first trimester to a number of congenital abnormalities.[11] We recommend to avoid use in the first trimester, but can be used in the second and third trimesters. It is contraindicated in patients with glucose-6-phosphate dehydrogenase deficiency.

Penicillins

The first- to fourth-generation penicillins and their derivatives (including procaine, benzathine, clavulanate, sulbactam, and tazobactam) are considered safe for use in pregnancy, as is oral probenecid. Penicillins are considered safe during breast-feeding, but their use may interfere with culture results if evaluation is required for a neonatal fever.

Sulfonamides

Sulfamethoxazole, commonly combined with trimethoprim, is contraindicated in pregnancy because of an increased risk of neural tube defects and other congenital abnormalities, such as cleft palate. There is also an increased risk of cardiovascular and urinary tract malformations in the offspring of women treated with trimethoprim-sulfamethoxazole in the first trimester. Sulfonamides are contraindicated near term because of their association with kernicterus; they are excreted in breast milk and generally tolerated by a healthy neonate. They should be avoided, however, in ill or premature infants and in infants with hyperbilirubinemia or glucose-6-phosphate dehydrogenase deficiency.

Tetracyclines

Tetracycline and doxycycline readily cross the placenta. Tetracycline is associated with the development of fatal fatty liver in pregnant women. It chelates calcium, causing abnormalities in bone growth and staining of decidual teeth. It is associated with fetal genitourinary anomalies, inguinal hernias, and limb abnormalities. Tetracycline should therefore be avoided during pregnancy.

Doxycycline does not bind to calcium and is associated less with stained teeth than tetracycline. It does not appear to cause an increase in any type of congenital malformation. Despite these findings, doxycycline is not recommended in pregnancy.

Because tetracycline binds to breast milk calcium, only a small amount reaches the nursing infant, and it may be used for short periods (<10 days) during breast-feeding. Doxycycline does not bind to breast milk calcium and is present in greater quantities in breast milk. This could theoretically increase its side effects in the newborn. Its use in nursing infants is best avoided.

Vancomycin

Vancomycin has not been linked to birth defects in animals or in humans. Reports of auditory abnormalities and renal insufficiency in neonates of mothers treated with vancomycin are believed to be false positives because these abnormalities were resolved on retesting. Vancomycin is excreted into milk but not well absorbed by the GI tract. Its effects on the nursing infant have not been studied.

Antifungals

Nystatin has a long safety profile during pregnancy and lactation. It is poorly absorbed from skin, mucous membranes, and the GI tract and is considered the antifungal of choice for the treatment of mucocutaneous fungal infections. Clotrimazole, miconazole, and ketoconazole are considered second-line treatment of fungal infections. Fluconazole is teratogenic in high doses (>400 mg/day) and has been associated with spontaneous abortions and stillbirth as well as an increased incidence of craniofacial and cardiovascular defects in offspring and multiple abnormalities of the skeleton and cartilage. There are conflicting reports about the teratogenic effects, but expert recommendations suggest that a single dose of 150 mg one time during pregnancy after the first trimester is unlikely to be associated with teratogenesis.[12]

Ketoconazole, fluconazole, and itraconazole are excreted into breast milk. Because of the safe use of ketoconazole in neonates and the lack of negative reports, it is considered compatible with breast-feeding (see Table 175.6).

Antituberculous Agents

The incidence of tuberculosis is higher during pregnancy and postpartum than in the general population. Untreated tuberculosis places the mother, fetus, and family at greater risk than the use of antituberculous medications. Isoniazid, ethambutol, and rifampin cross the placenta and no association has been reported between these medications and major congenital malformations. Rifampin is associated with hemorrhagic disease of the newborn. Despite this adverse effect, it is considered first-line therapy for the treatment of tuberculosis. All three antituberculous medications are considered compatible with breast-feeding (see Table 175.6).

Antiviral Agents
Antiherpetic Drugs

Acyclovir readily crosses the placenta and reaches higher concentrations in fetal circulation than in maternal circulation. Neither acyclovir nor valacyclovir has been associated with congenital malformations or adverse effects on the offspring. Intravenous (IV) acyclovir is the drug of choice for life-threatening maternal herpes simplex virus infections, such as disseminated disease, herpes encephalitis, and varicella pneumonia, which carries a maternal mortality of 44% if untreated. For non–life-threatening genital herpes infection in pregnant women, acyclovir or valacyclovir may be used. Experience with famciclovir is limited and therefore it is not recommended for use in pregnancy. Because there are no reported adverse outcomes in infants of mothers taking acyclovir or in infants treated with acyclovir for disseminated herpes, it is considered safe during breast-feeding (see Table 175.6).

Antiinfluenza Drugs

Influenza in pregnancy carries a high risk of morbidity and mortality. Neuraminidase inhibitors, such as oseltamivir and zanamivir, are active against influenza A and B and are associated with improved outcomes. Oseltamivir is considered the treatment of choice for influenza in pregnancy and available safety data report no significant risk to the fetus. Antiviral therapy with M2 ion channel inhibitors, such as amantadine and rimantadine, is also effective against certain subtypes of influenza A but not influenza B. However, amantadine has been linked to various malformations, including cardiac defects in humans, and is considered teratogenic and embryotoxic in rats.

Oseltamivir appears to be safe in lactation. In addition to antiviral therapy, the Centers for Disease Control and Prevention (CDC) recommends that pregnant women receive the inactivated influenza vaccine at any point during pregnancy (see Table 175.6).

Anti-HIV Drugs

Mothers infected with human immunodeficiency virus (HIV) are treated with antiretroviral therapy (ART) in order to decrease mother-to-child HIV transmission as the viral load of the mother directly correlates with the risk of perinatal transmission. No specific pattern of birth defects has been described with the use of anti-HIV drugs,[13] but the drugs' mutagenesis and carcinogenesis and their long-term effects on the liver, heart, and reproductive system are yet to be determined.

Animal and human data suggest that didanosine, lamivudine, stavudine, zidovudine, and zalcitabine present a small risk of structural malformations and mitochondrial dysfunction in the developing fetus, but no specific pattern of birth defects has been described with protease inhibitors, such as ritonavir and nelfinavir. Despite potential risks, it is thought that the benefit from HIV treatment far outweighs the risk of these drugs and should not be withheld. In addition, zidovudine has been shown to reduce vertical and perinatal transmission of HIV from the mother to the fetus. Because of the risk of postnatal HIV transmission through milk, the CDC advises against breast-feeding by HIV-positive mothers.

Cardiovascular Agents

Antidysrhythmics

Atrial and ventricular arrhythmias are common during pregnancy. Most are benign; however, malignant degeneration occasionally occurs. All unstable tachycardias should be treated with electrical cardioversion and Advanced Cardiovascular Life Support (ACLS) guidelines. Stable patients may be treated medically, but the choice of drugs needs to be modified to protect the patient as well as the fetus from the drug's potentially harmful effects (Table 175.7).

Adenosine. Adenosine has been used safely throughout pregnancy and is the drug of choice for termination of maternal supraventricular tachycardia. Adenosine has also been used safely for termination of incessant tachycardia in the fetus. Adenosine is safe in lactation.

Amiodarone. Amiodarone contains large amounts of iodine and is associated with congenital goiter and transient neonatal hyperthyroidism and hypothyroidism. Amiodarone has been linked to many congenital abnormalities, including growth restriction, structural cardiac abnormalities, corneal deposits, and developmental

TABLE 175.7	Antidysrhythmic Medications	
Drug	**Breast-Feeding**	**Clinical Risk Summary**
Adenosine	Compatible	Many reports show compatibility during pregnancy; LHS; effects on fetus unknown, but teratogenicity or malformations not expected
Amiodarone	Contraindicated excreted in breast milk Concern for hypothyroidism	CP; linked to many congenital abnormalities; thyroid abnormalities, congenital goiter have been observed; contains high concentration of iodine; use only in refractory tachydysrhythmias
Digoxin	Compatible excreted in breast milk	CP; NHT; one of the safest antiarrhythmics during pregnancy
Quinidine	Probably compatible (LHS) Excreted in breast milk	CP; no teratogenic effects in humans reported; LHS
Lidocaine	Compatible excreted in breast milk	CP; animal studies—no harm; high doses near term associated with neonatal CNS depression, hypotonia, seizures, bradycardia
Procainamide	Probably compatible (LHS) Excreted in breast milk	LHS
Flecainide	Compatible Concentrated in breast milk	LHS; animal data suggest possible teratogenicity
Ibutilide	Probably compatible (LHS)	Unknown if CP; animal studies show teratogenicity, embryocidal events
Sotalol	Potential toxicity (LHS) Concentrated in breast milk. Conflicting reports	CP; may cause fetal bradycardia and/or IUGR

CP, Crosses placenta; *IUGR*, intrauterine growth restriction; *LHS*, limited human studies; *NHT*, no human teratogenicity.
Data adapted from refs.[38,39]

delay. It should be used only in refractory cases of supraventricular or ventricular tachycardias in the mother and incessant tachycardias in the fetus. Because of its high iodine content, excretion into milk, and long elimination half-life, amiodarone should not be used in nursing mothers.

Digoxin and Quinidine. Digoxin and quinidine are considered safe for use during pregnancy and lactation. Neither has been linked to congenital defects in humans or animals, and they are first-line agents for the treatment of significant maternal dysrhythmias. They have also been successfully used in fetal tachycardia. During lactation, digoxin and quinidine appear compatible with breast-feeding.

Lidocaine. Lidocaine rapidly crosses the placenta and becomes ion-trapped in the fetus. There is no evidence of a link between the use of lidocaine in the first trimester and any fetal developmental malformations. However, high doses used near term are associated with neonatal CNS depression, apnea, hypotonia, seizures, and bradycardia. Lidocaine is considered compatible with breast-feeding.

Procainamide. Procainamide has been safely used in the treatment of stable, wide-complex tachydysrhythmias during pregnancy. It is not associated with fetal developmental abnormalities and appears well tolerated when used for a short duration. It is associated with a high incidence of maternal antinuclear antibodies and the occurrence of a lupus-like reaction in humans. During lactation, procainamide and its metabolite, *N*-acetylprocainamide, are found in breast milk. The AAP considers its short-term use compatible with breast-feeding.

Flecainide. Flecainide has been used safely to terminate maternal and fetal tachycardia, but it is associated with fetal hyperbilirubinemia, hepatotoxicity, and loss of fetal heart rate variability. Flecainide has also been found to be teratogenic in some animal species, resulting in cardiac and musculoskeletal abnormalities. It is present in breast milk and the AAP considers it compatible with breast-feeding, despite limited experience.

Ibutilide. There are only a few case reports of the successful and safe use of ibutilide during the latter part of pregnancy in humans. In animals, however, ibutilide was found to be teratogenic and caused

TABLE 175.8 Antihypertensive Medications

Drug(s)	Breast-Feeding	Clinical Risk Summary
Angiotensin-converting enzyme inhibitors, angiotensin II receptor antagonists	Probably compatible, but variable safety	Use in second and third trimesters may cause teratogenicity, severe fetal/neonatal toxicity; reduce fetal renal function; associated with anuria, PDA, IUGR, prematurity, abnormal bone, lung development, renal failure, death
Esmolol	Safety unknown Appears to be low risk	LHS; not thought to cause structural anomalies; may result in persistent beta blockade of fetus or newborn[a]
Labetalol	Probably compatible Low excretion in breast milk	LHS; little risk to fetus except possibly in first trimester; most studies found no effect on fetal growth; IUGR and RPW may occur if used near delivery; newborn should be monitored for 24–48 hr for symptoms of beta blockade[a]
Metoprolol	Conflicting reports Concern for toxicity Excreted in breast milk	CP; LHS; no animal teratogenicity; may cause IUGR, RPW, and persistent beta blockade in newborns[a]
Propranolol	Conflicting reports Concern for toxicity	CP; NHT; fetal and neonatal toxicity may occur; may cause IUGR and RPW if used near delivery; newborn should be monitored for 24–48 hr for symptoms of beta blockade[a]
Amlodipine	Probably compatible, but safety unknown Neonatal myocardium sensitive to changes in calcium status Caution during breast-feeding	LHS; animal studies demonstrated fetotoxicity; safety unknown; case reports of IUGR, fetal death, neonatal rash
Diltiazem	Probably compatible, but safety unknown Neonatal myocardium sensitive to changes in calcium status Caution during breast-feeding	LHS; animal studies demonstrate fetotoxicity, teratogenicity; safety unknown
Nicardipine	Probably compatible but safety unknown LHS	Dose-related embryonic toxicity but not teratogenicity in animals; LHS; neonatal hypotension and acidosis reported, but safety unknown; causes hypotension, reflex tachycardia, PPH, tocolysis, headache, nausea, dizziness, flushing in pregnancy
Nifedipine	Probably compatible but safety unknown Advised to delay breast-feeding for 3–4 hr	LHS; safety unknown; NHT; has been used as a tocolytic agent; may potentiate neuromuscular blocking action of magnesium
Verapamil	Probably compatible	CP; animal studies show adverse effects on fetal growth and fetotoxicity, LHS; appears to be low risk during any stage of pregnancy
Furosemide	Probably compatible Caution advised May suppress lactation	CP; LHS; fetotoxic and teratogenic in animals; no significant alteration of amniotic fluid volume; monitor fetal growth because may cause higher birth weight
Hydrochlorothiazide	Compatible Excreted in breast milk May suppress lactation	CP; NHT; risks to fetus and newborn include hypoglycemia, thrombocytopenia, hyponatremia, hypokalemia, death; may inhibit labor by direct effect on smooth muscle
Nitroglycerin	Probably compatible Monitoring infants recommended	LHS; no adverse effects in animal studies; safety unknown, but appears safe; tocolytic
Nitroprusside	Potential toxicity	CP; LHS; adverse effects in animal studies, caution advised; transient fetal bradycardia noted; accumulation of cyanide in fetus may occur
Clonidine	Probably compatible May alter prolactin and oxytocin levels, affecting lactation	CP; LHS; safety unknown; no observed adverse fetal effects in humans; may develop sleep disorders later in life with prolonged use during pregnancy
Hydralazine	Probably compatible LHS Excreted in breast milk	CP; use with caution, no known congenital defects, but fetal toxicity associated with third-trimester use; meta-analysis on use in preeclampsia demonstrated more hypotension, placental abruption, cesarean section, maternal oliguria, adverse fetal heart rates, lower Apgar scores compared with labetalol or nifedipine
Methyldopa	Probably compatible	Long history of safety and efficacy in pregnancy

[a]Beta blockade = bradycardia, respiratory depression, and hypoglycemia.
CP, Crosses placenta; *IUGR*, intrauterine growth restriction; *LHS*, limited human studies; *NHT*, no human teratogenicity; *PDA*, patent ductus arteriosus; *PPH*, postpartum hemorrhage; *RPW*, reduced placental weight
Data adapted from refs.[40-45]

cardiac septal defects as well as skeletal dysgenesis in rats, especially when high doses were given. Ibutilide should be reserved for refractory cases in which the benefits of therapy outweigh any fetal risk. There are very few data about the risk during breastfeeding, though there is low bioavailability and likely low risk to the infant.

Sotalol. Sotalol has been used in pregnant women to treat atrial arrhythmias successfully and safely, as well as hypertension. It has also been successfully used to terminate fetal atrial tachycardias. It does not appear to have teratogenic effects in animals. Some of the negative effects of sotalol include bradycardia in the newborn, persisting for 24 hours. Sotalol is concentrated in milk but does not appear to result in bradycardia or hypotension in the nursing infant and, according to the AAP, it is compatible with breast-feeding.

Antihypertensives

Labetalol is the agent of choice for hypertensive emergencies in pregnancy (Table 175.8).[14]

Angiotensin-Converting Enzyme Inhibitors. Angiotensin-converting enzyme (ACE) inhibitors are contraindicated for use during pregnancy. Furthermore, ACE inhibitors are embryocidal in animals and increase the rate of stillbirths in some animal species. In humans, the most significant adverse fetal effects occur when used in the second and third trimesters. ACE inhibitor use in the first trimester is controversial; some studies suggest no increased risk whereas ACOG recommends against its use. Captopril and enalapril are considered compatible with breast-feeding.

Angiotensin II Receptor Antagonists. Angiotensin II receptor antagonists should be avoided during pregnancy because their use has been reported to result in fetal abnormalities similar to the abnormalities seen with ACE inhibitors, including renal agenesis, neonatal anuria, oligohydramnios, intrauterine growth restriction, persistent patent ductus arteriosus, abnormal ossification, and death. Their safety in lactation is unknown.

Beta Blockers. Beta blockers are a first-line treatment of hypertension in pregnancy.[15] They have not been associated with fetal malformations and appear to be safe when used for short periods. Adverse fetal effects include intrauterine growth restriction and a low placental weight. Beta blockers lacking intrinsic sympathomimetic activity, such as acebutolol, atenolol, nadolol, and propranolol, are more likely to be associated with these adverse effects. When beta blockers are given near term, they have been associated with persistent beta blockade in the newborn. Nonselective beta blockers, such as propranolol, also have resulted in neonatal hypoglycemia, respiratory depression, and hyperbilirubinemia in the newborn. These adverse effects are less common when a cardioselective beta blocker, such as atenolol or metoprolol, is used. Esmolol has been associated with fetal bradycardia, neonatal bradycardia and hypotonia, and fetal distress requiring emergent cesarean section. Beta blockers have variable effects on the nursing infant, and close monitoring of the infant for adverse effects is recommended.

Calcium Channel Blockers. Calcium channel blockers are effective treatments for hypertension and the termination of supraventricular rhythm disturbances during pregnancy. IV verapamil is useful to terminate fetal tachycardia, and IV nicardipine has been used for severe preeclampsia. In addition, some calcium channel blockers, such as nifedipine and diltiazem, are used as tocolytic agents. In laboratory animals, calcium channel blockers in the first trimester have been associated with a dose-dependent increase in embryonic mortality and skeletal abnormalities. To date, however, these abnormalities have not been seen in humans. Complications of calcium channel blocker use during pregnancy include maternal hypotension, tachycardia, and fetal distress, especially pronounced when sublingual nifedipine or IV nicardipine is used. The AAP considers these drugs compatible with breast-feeding.

Diuretics

Loop diuretics such as furosemide are indicated in the treatment of pulmonary edema due to congestive heart failure. In laboratory animals, furosemide has been linked to renal and skeletal abnormalities when used in pregnancy. These effects have not been seen in humans, but a slightly increased risk of hypospadias has been reported. Furosemide is secreted into breast milk but is considered compatible with breast-feeding.

Thiazide diuretics have been associated with hypoglycemia and electrolyte abnormalities in neonates when given near term and with an increase in meconium staining and perinatal mortality. Moreover, thiazide diuretics may have a direct effect on smooth muscle and inhibit labor. In general, these agents are considered safe during breast-feeding.

Nitrates. Nitroglycerin has not been shown to cause fetal harm in animal studies. Limited reports in humans have not shown any major effects on the fetus or neonate. Nitroglycerin is rarely used during pregnancy, but it appears to be a safe, effective, rapidly acting, and short-acting agent. Nitroprusside for the treatment of hypertensive emergencies in pregnancy has the same advantages and disadvantages as in nonpregnant patients. During prolonged administration of high doses, nitroprusside may result in cyanide toxicity and severe acidosis. It readily crosses the placenta, and fetal levels of cyanide can increase as high as twice maternal levels. Standard doses do not seem to subject the fetus to a major risk of toxicity but, with the availability of safer alternatives, notably labetalol, nitroprusside is considered a last resort agent. No data are available on its use during lactation

Clonidine. Clonidine has been safely used throughout pregnancy, but experience during the first trimester remains limited. It does not appear to be teratogenic in laboratory animals and does not increase fetal mortality. Transient neonatal hypertension has been reported with the use of clonidine in the treatment of neonatal abstinence syndrome. Its effects on breast-feeding neonates are unknown, but it is considered compatible with breast-feeding.

Hydralazine. Hydralazine use is associated with higher rates of maternal hypotension, placental abruption, and neonatal distress compared with labetalol. It is therefore no longer recommended as a first-line agent in the treatment of severe acute hypertension in pregnancy.[15] It may still be used as a second-line agent. Hydralazine is considered compatible with breast-feeding.

Methyldopa. Methyldopa has been safely used throughout pregnancy, and most reviews have not linked it to any teratogenic effects on the offspring or adverse effects on the pregnancy. The use of methyldopa has been associated with depression, which may limit its use in the peripartum phase. Methyldopa is compatible with breast-feeding.

Vasopressors

Vasopressors all have the potential to increase uterine vascular resistance, resulting in a proportional decrease in placental blood flow. ACOG currently recommends epinephrine as the vasopressor of choice in the treatment of vascular collapse during pregnancy (Table 175.9).[16]

Endocrine Agents
Diabetes Medications

Diabetes mellitus is associated with a number of congenital malformations involving multiple organ systems, as well as with a significant increase in perinatal morbidity. Glycemic control in pregnancy is therefore important and should be accomplished in a controlled manner, because hypoglycemia is also associated with adverse pregnancy outcomes. Insulin is the drug of choice for diabetes mellitus types 1 and 2 in pregnancy and gestational diabetes, if treatment is needed. Metformin is generally well tolerated but has rare serious adverse effects in non-pregnant and pregnant adults, including life-threatening metabolic acidosis and hepatitis. It has not been associated with fetal malformations in animals and humans (Table 175.10).[17]

TABLE 175.9 Vasopressors

Drug	Breast-Feeding	Clinical Risk Summary
Dobutamine	Probably compatible (LHS)	CP; LHS; animal data suggest low risk; no adverse effects on human fetuses found
Dopamine	Probably compatible (LHS)	LHS; used in maternal shock, including spinal shock due to spinal anesthesia; low-dose dopamine can be used to improve cardiac and urine output in patients with preeclampsia and oliguria, but has not been shown to improve mortality or renal function; animal studies suggest maternal toxicity, but no fetal teratogenicity found; decreases uterine blood flow
Epinephrine	Potential toxicity (LHS)	CP; NHT; preferred treatment agent for anaphylaxis, used for status asthmaticus and shock during pregnancy; associated with fetal anoxic injury, intracranial hemorrhage, and increased incidence of inguinal hernias; decreases uterine blood flow, which may lead to fetal anoxia
Norepinephrine	Potential toxicity (LHS)	CP; animal studies demonstrate malformation—situs inversus, cataracts, hemorrhages, bone abnormalities; increased incidence of cerebral hemorrhage; decreased placental flow and fetal anoxia, but overall effects unknown
Ephedrine	Potential toxicity	CP; NHT; effective in treatment of shock in pregnancy; compared to phenylephrine, ephedrine associated with higher heart rates, gastric upset, increased incidence of fetal acidosis; no major or minor malformations shown
Phenylephrine	Probably compatible (LHS)	Preferred agent to treat shock during pregnancy; severe hypertension during delivery when reacting to oxytocics or ergots; malformations when used in first trimester; use during late pregnancy, labor, or cesarean section may cause fetal anoxia, bradycardia due to uterine contractions, decreased uterine blood flow

CP, Crosses placenta; *LHS*, limited human studies; *NHT*, no human teratogenicity.
Data adapted from ref.[44]

TABLE 175.10 Diabetic Medications

Drug	Breast-Feeding	Clinical Risk Summary
Insulin	Compatible Degraded by infant's GI tract	Maternal hypoglycemia; DNCP; no observable effects found
Sulfonylureas	Compatible	Minimal amounts found in fetal circulation; no greater risk of adverse effects compared with insulin therapy; infant 200 g heavier with use of sulfonylureas; stop ≈2 wk before birth to prevent neonatal hypoglycemia
Metformin	Compatible Excreted in breast milk Monitoring advised	CP; NHT Less likely to experience maternal and neonatal hypoglycemia

CP, Crosses placenta; *DNCP*, does not cross placenta; *GI*, gastrointestinal; *NHT*, no human teratogenicity.
Data adapted from refs. [46,47,64]

TABLE 175.11 Thyroid Medications

Drug	Breast-Feeding	Clinical Risk Summary
Levothyroxine	Compatible Excreted in breast milk	Minimal transfer across placenta; treatment of choice for hypothyroidism in pregnancy; minimal side effects; maternal benefits outweigh risks to fetus
Potassium iodide	Compatible Excreted in breast milk	CP; reserved for thyrotoxic patients; easily taken up by fetal thyroid, resulting in prolonged fetal hypothyroidism and goiter
Propylthiouracil (PTU)	Compatible Excreted in breast milk	CP; causes fetal goiter, hypothyroidism, hepatic injury, death; preferred drug in the first trimester for hyperthyroidism in pregnancy; maternal benefits outweigh risk to fetus
Methimazole	Compatible Excreted in breast milk	CP; may cause a methimazole embryopathy—congenital skin defects, umbilical defects, preferred drug in the second and third trimesters

CP, Crosses placenta.

Thyroid Medications

Maternal hyperthyroidism is associated with an increased risk of spontaneous abortion, preterm labor, placental abruption, and maternal congestive heart failure. Effects of the disease on the offspring include intrauterine growth restriction, intrauterine fetal death, and neonatal goiter. Propylthiouracil (PTU) is the drug of choice in the first trimester and should be replaced with methimazole in the second and third trimester. Methimazole is associated with higher rates of congenital malformations such as choanal and esophageal atresia and therefore not recommended in the first trimester. PTU is associated with maternal hepatotoxicity. When used close to term the newborn may display hypothyroidism and a goiter. Methimazole and carbimazole have been associated with abnormal development of the skin, albeit inconsistently. Hypothyroidism in pregnancy may result in an increased risk for spontaneous abortion, intrauterine growth restriction, placental abruption, and fetal demise and has been associated with severe neurologic impairment of the offspring. Levothyroxine is the treatment of choice for hypothyroidism in pregnant women (Table 175.11).

Gastrointestinal Agents

Gastroesophageal reflux disease (GERD) occurs in up to 80% of pregnancies and peaks in the third trimester (Table 175.12). Another common condition during pregnancy is nausea and vomiting of pregnancy (NVP), which can affect up to 80% of women during pregnancy. NVP typically presents after 4 to 5 weeks' gestation and resolves before the beginning of the second trimester (see Antiemetic Medication section).

Antacids

H2 Receptor Antagonists. None of the H2 receptor antagonists has been linked to congenital malformation, and they all appear to be safe for the nursing infant. There are multiple reports in the literature, however,

TABLE 175.12 Gastrointestinal Medications

Drug	Breast-Feeding	Clinical Risk Summary
Famotidine	Probably compatible Secreted less than other H2 blockers Considered low risk	CP; no fetal toxicity or teratogenicity in animal studies[a]
Ranitidine	Probably compatible Considered low risk	CP; no toxicity or teratogenicity in animal studies; considered H2 blocker of choice due to efficacy and safety data; ranitidine-induced anaphylactoid shock has been reported[a]
Cimetidine	Compatible Has antiandrogenic activity, so use with caution	CP; no toxicity in animal studies, has some weak anti-androgenic activity that could result in feminism of male fetuses but no documented cases in humans[a]
Omeprazole	Potential toxicity LHS	CP; animal data show dose related embryonic and fetal mortality; low risk of fetal harm or teratogenicity; overall slightly higher rates of congenital malformations and stillborns after exposure in first trimester of pregnancy, but studies limited/unconfirmed[a]
Esomeprazole	Potential toxicity LHS Wait 5–7.5 hr after dose for breast-feeding to limit exposure Strontium formulations—should not be used	CP; LHS; some changes in bone morphology observed in animal studies; should be used with caution[a]; esomeprazole magnesium preferred over esomeprazole strontium
Lansoprazole	Potential toxicity Should be avoided	Unknown whether CP but likely; carcinogenic in animals; LHS; should be avoided in first trimester[a]
Pantoprazole	Probably compatible Potential for tumorigenicity and carcinogenicity in animals Caution advised	Animal and human data suggest low risk in pregnancy[a]

[a]Several studies have shown a possible link between in utero exposure to gastric acid suppressors and childhood allergy and asthma.
CP, Crosses placenta; *LHS*, limited human studies.
Data adapted from ref.[48-50]

TABLE 175.13 Antiemetic Medications

Drug	Breast-Feeding	Clinical Risk Summary
Pyridoxine	Compatible Excreted in breast milk	High doses pose little risk to fetus; vitamin B_6 deficiency common during pregnancy—pyridoxine required for good maternal and fetal health
Doxylamine, pyridoxine	Probably compatible, but sedative and antihistamine actions are potential concern	Safe in pregnancy, including first trimester; several meta-analyses demonstrated no increased risk of malformations, fetal abnormalities
Metoclopramide	Potential toxicity Concern for CNS effects but data lacking	CP; no association with adverse fetal and neonatal outcomes while with used during all stages of pregnancy
Prochlorperazine	Potential toxicity Use caution—may cause sedation, lethargy in infant	CP; LHS; fetal toxicity, teratogenicity in animals; adverse effects of extrapyramidal effects, agitation, hypertonia, hypotonia, tremor, somnolence, respiratory distress, feeding disorder reported in infants exposed during third trimester; considered low risk for mother and fetus if used occasionally in low doses
Promethazine	Probably compatible May cause sedation in infant	CP; LHS; reports of embryonic and fetal harm may be considered low risk for embryo, fetus; theoretical increased risk of respiratory depression in the newborn if given close to delivery, of unknown clinical significance
Ondansetron	Probably compatible Unknown safety	CP; animal, human data suggest low risk of birth defects; studies show inconsistent data on increased risk of cardiac anomalies and cleft palates

CP, Crosses placenta; *LHS*, limited human studies.
Additional data adapted from refs.[52,53]

linking in utero gastric suppression to an increased incidence of asthma and allergies during childhood, which require confirmation.[18]

Proton Pump Inhibitors. Studies on proton pump inhibitor (PPI) use in pregnancy are limited but several studies and a meta-analysis have found no association with an increased risk for major congenital birth defects, spontaneous abortions, or preterm delivery. Esomeprazole, lansoprazole, pantoprazole, and rabeprazole may be used during pregnancy. There are reports, however, of an increased incidence of GI, hepatic, and thyroid cancers in rats and mice. Several studies have demonstrated a possible link between in utero exposure to gastric acid suppressors and childhood allergic disorders and asthma. There are limited data in humans on the effects of PPIs on nursing infants. Breast-feeding should be avoided while taking PPIs.

Antiemetic Medications

Nausea and vomiting occur in up to 85% of all pregnant women between 6 and 12 weeks of gestation, but these symptoms are usually self-limiting. One-third of women with nausea and vomiting of pregnancy have clinically significant symptoms, and 3% will progress to hyperemesis gravidarum, which poses health risks to the mother and fetus. Despite these symptoms being common in pregnancy, there is a lack of high-quality evidence to support any particular intervention (Table 175.13).

Pyridoxine (Vitamin B_6), Doxylamine-Pyridoxine Combination. Pyridoxine is used alone, or in combination with doxylamine, an antihistamine, for the treatment of nausea and vomiting of pregnancy. Combination therapy of doxylamine and pyridoxine is FDA approved and fetal safety has been demonstrated in multiple epidemiologic studies.[19]

Phenothiazines. Phenothiazines, such as metoclopramide, prochlorperazine, and promethazine, are dopamine antagonists commonly used in the treatment of nausea and vomiting during pregnancy. Although there have been reports of increased risk of cardiac defects, these reports did not consider other factors, such as the mother's health, when the drug was reviewed. The bulk of evidence does not support a link to congenital abnormalities. The AAP cautions against their use in nursing mothers because they may cause sedation and other untoward effects.

Serotonin 5-HT₃ Receptor Antagonists. Dolasetron, granisetron, and ondansetron have not been consistently linked to any fetal malformations, although experience with the newer agents remains limited. Recent studies of ondansetron have suggested a low teratogenic risk; however, an increased risk for a cardiac septum defect and cleft palate is possible, but data are inconsistent, and has not been confirmed in other studies. The AAP considers these agents compatible with breast-feeding.

Neurologic Agents
Anticonvulsants
Maternal mortality is ten times higher in women with a seizure disorder. Pregnant women with a seizure disorder are at increased risk of spontaneous miscarriage, antepartum and postpartum hemorrhage, hypertensive disorders, induction of labor, cesarean sections, preterm birth, and fetal growth restriction. Pregnant women exposed to antiepileptic drugs (AEDs) have an increased risk of postpartum hemorrhage, induction of labor, fetal growth restriction, and admission to the NICU.

Newer-generation AEDs, lamotrigine and levetiracetam, have not been associated with increased risk of congenital malformations compared to controls but data are limited. Several anticonvulsants are known teratogens, and 30% of neonates exposed to commonly used anticonvulsants exhibit congenital anomalies. Monotherapies shown to have increased risk of congenital malformations are carbamazepine, ethosuximide, phenobarbital, phenytoin, topiramate, and valproate.

The risks for birth defects increase with the duration of exposure and with the number of agents used. Valproate is associated with the most frequent serious adverse effects on the pregnancy and fetus (20% incidence of serious adverse outcomes) compared with phenytoin, carbamazepine, and lamotrigine (11%, 8%, and 1%, respectively). Despite the risks, most practitioners believe that it is important to control seizures during pregnancy. Generalized seizures during pregnancy are associated with an increased risk of spontaneous abortion, hypoxic injury to the fetus, and impaired neuropsychological functioning. Monotherapy is the most appropriate option and is recommended at the lowest effective anticonvulsant dose. Dividing the daily dose to decrease peak plasma levels may be considered. Adjustment of the dosage upward may be required to maintain adequate seizure control.

Antipsychotics
These agents sometimes cause extrapyramidal side effects of the infants when exposed in utero. These effects are seen with use of the first- and second-generation antipsychotics. Haloperidol may cause limb defects when the mother is exposed during the first trimester, but data are inconsistent. This effect is not seen with other first-generation antipsychotics. Most second-generation antipsychotics do not show teratogenicity. The most commonly prescribed antipsychotics are olanzapine, risperidone, and quetiapine, which do not appear to cause consistent congenital defects (Table 175.14).

Migraine Medications
Ergot Alkaloids
Neither ergotamine nor dihydroergotamine are associated with teratogenic effects but are contraindicated in pregnancy because of their oxytocic effects and effects on uterine blood flow. In a number of animal studies, these alkaloids have been associated with intrauterine growth restriction, probably because of reductions in uteroplacental blood flow. They are also contraindicated during breast-feeding because of possible ergot poisoning of the nursing infant manifested by convulsions and gastrointestinal symptoms.

Triptans
Triptans have been found to be teratogenic in a number of animal species, but recent human studies appear to favor their safety during pregnancy. The AAP considers sumatriptan to be compatible with breast-feeding, especially if the breast milk is not used for 8 hours after the last dose.

Respiratory Agents
Antihistamines
Approximately 10% to 15% of women reportedly take an antihistamine during pregnancy. Chlorpheniramine, diphenhydramine, doxylamine, hydroxyzine, and meclizine are safe for the treatment of allergic reactions and as antiemetics in the treatment of nausea and vomiting during pregnancy. First-generation antihistamines are not recommended during breast-feeding because they are thought to inhibit lactation. In addition, serious adverse CNS effects, including seizures, have been reported to develop in neonates receiving antihistamines, especially when they are premature.

The newer-generation antihistamines, such as cetirizine and loratadine, also appear safe during pregnancy. These may be acceptable alternatives if the first-generation antihistamines are not tolerated or if the patient has severe allergies. The AAP has classified these drugs as compatible with breast-feeding (Table 175.15).

TABLE 175.14　Antipsychotic Medications

Drug	Breast-Feeding	Clinical Risk Summary
First Generation		
Haloperidol	Potential toxicity (LHS) Excreted in breast milk	CP; extrapyramidal symptoms can be seen in infants exposed in utero in the third trimester; limb defects seen with first-trimester exposure but data inconsistent
Droperidol	Potential toxicity (LHS)	CP; no effect on respiratory drive when given perinatally; no observed fetal or maternal SAR, risk of extrapyramidal signs with exposure in the third trimester
Second Generation		
Olanzapine	Potential toxicity (LHS) Concentrated in breast milk	CP; no teratogenicity or mutagenicity in animal studies; extrapyramidal effects noted in infants exposed in third trimester
Risperidone	Potential toxicity (LHS)	CP; extrapyramidal effects noted in infants exposed in third trimester

CP, Crosses placenta; *LHS*, limited human studies; *SAR*, serious adverse reactions.
Additional data adapted from refs.[58,59]

Asthma Medications

Asthma is the most common respiratory disorder in pregnancy. The prevalence of asthma in pregnancy is 8%, and one-third of pregnant asthmatics experience a worsening of their asthma that may progress to a critical asthma syndrome, including status asthmaticus and near-fatal asthma. Pregnant women with asthma are at risk for neonatal death, preterm birth, low-birth-weight infants, preeclampsia, and small-for-gestational-age infants. Asthmatic mothers may also have higher rates of antepartum/postpartum hemorrhage, placenta previa, placental abruption, chorioamnionitis, gestational diabetes, hypertensive disorders of pregnancy, cesarean section, and prolonged hospital stay compared with control mothers. Active asthma management during pregnancy is associated with improved maternal and fetal outcomes.[20]

Albuterol has the most safety data and is the treatment of choice for asthma in pregnancy. None of the β-adrenergic medications has been linked to fetal or congenital malformations, but some have been associated with significant cardiovascular and metabolic effects, which are transient and generally well tolerated by the fetus. Transient hyperglycemia followed by insulin secretion may also occur, resulting in neonatal hypoglycemia, especially in diabetic patients. Terbutaline, when used IV or orally in pregnant women, may result in maternal and fetal arrhythmias, maternal pulmonary edema, and death. The FDA has recommended a label change to add a warning against its use in preterm labor because safer β2-agonists and tocolytic agents are available. Long-acting β-agonists also appear to be safe during pregnancy. Albuterol is compatible with breast-feeding.

Ipratropium has not been found to be teratogenic in numerous animal models, but there are few data regarding its safety in human pregnancy. It is considered compatible with breast-feeding. Data on the use of leukotriene antagonists in pregnancy are limited (Table 175.16).

Corticosteroids

Inhaled corticosteroids are the main therapy for the prevention of asthma exacerbations during pregnancy. Budesonide has the greatest

---

TABLE 175.15 Antihistamine Medications

Drug	Breast-Feeding	Clinical Risk Summary
Chlorpheniramine	Probably compatible; use with caution: may cause sedation, irritability, disturbed sleep, hyperexcitability, excessive crying	LHS; no known congenital defects, low risk in pregnancy; recommended antihistamine in pregnancy, especially in first trimester[a]
Diphenhydramine	Probably compatible; use with caution, can be sedating; parenteral use contraindicated	LHS; animal and human studies demonstrate safety in pregnancy; association with cleft palate in one study; drug of choice if parenteral antihistamine is indicated[a]
Hydroxyzine	Probably compatible, LHS; not recommended with breast-feeding: may interfere with establishment of lactation	Contraindicated in 1st trimester; lower risk in 2nd and 3rd trimesters, if necessary to use; CP; teratogenic in animals, with high doses associated with developmental toxicity; low potential risk for fetus in humans; withdrawal or seizures noted in newborn exposed near term; possible increased risk of oral clefts, but limited data[a]
Meclizine	Probably compatible Safety unknown Occasional dose should not pose risk	Teratogenic in animals but not in humans; frequently used as antiemetic; considered low risk in pregnancy[a]
Cetirizine	Probably compatible Excreted in breast milk Not recommended—safety unknown	Animal studies—no teratogenicity; LHS; no evidence of increased risk of adverse fetal outcomes; may be used as alternative to oral first-generation antihistamine
Fexofenadine	Probably compatible excreted in breast milk	Animal studies—embryonic and fetal toxicity; no human studies available
Loratadine	Probably compatible considered antihistamine of choice in breast-feeding	Unknown if CP, but expected; no evidence of teratogenicity in animals or humans

[a]H1 blockers are not recommended for use in last 2 wk of pregnancy due to association with retrolental fibroplasia in premature neonates.
CP, Crosses placenta; *LHS*, limited human studies.
Data adapted from refs.[51]

TABLE 175.16 Asthma Medications

Drug	Breast-Feeding	Clinical Risk Summary
Ipratropium	Probably compatible, LHS May appear in breast milk	LHS; NHT; no teratogenicity in animals; recommended for use in severe asthma as additional therapy
Albuterol	Probably compatible, LHS Unknown if excreted in breast milk	May act as tocolytic; drug of choice for treatment of asthma; association with functional and neurobehavioral toxicity with prolonged use; may cause maternal and fetal tachycardia, hyperglycemia
Epinephrine	Potential toxicity, LHS Not known if excreted in breast milk	CP; teratogenic in animals; avoid during active labor and delivery—can delay labor progression; may lead to decrease in uterine blood flow with placental, uterine vasoconstriction
Terbutaline	Probably compatible Excreted in breast milk in small amounts	CP; NHT; may act as tocolytic; association with autism spectrum disorders (if used >2 wk); cardiac defects in first trimester; fetal tachycardia and hypoglycemia after parenteral use; avoid in early gestation, continuous use in second and third trimesters; may cause serious maternal cardiovascular events (e.g., increased heart rate, hyperglycemia, hypokalemia, cardiac arrhythmias, pulmonary edema and MI), death; black boxed warnings against use for prevention or prolonged use (beyond 2–3 days) of preterm labor

CP, Crosses placenta; *LHS*, limited human studies; *MI*, myocardial ischemia; *NHT*, no human teratogenicity.
Additional data adapted from refs.[60,61]

amount of safety data but others are also considered safe. Oral corticosteroids are the mainstay of therapy for acute exacerbations of asthma. Although they are not considered human teratogens, there may be a slightly increased incidence (0.1% to 0.3%) of orofacial clefts when systemic steroids are used during the first trimester. Furthermore, their use in the third trimester has been linked to an increased incidence of preterm delivery, low birth weight, preeclampsia, and cataracts in the newborn. Prednisone is considered safe during breast-feeding.

Decongestants

Decongestants with strong vasoconstrictive properties, such as phenylpropanolamine, phenylephrine, and pseudoephedrine, cause placental vasoconstriction and are not recommended during pregnancy.

Pseudoephedrine is one of the most commonly used over-the-counter medications in pregnancy, with 8% to 12% of pregnant women using it in the first trimester. They are often used as a combination product and therefore difficult to study. There are limited data suggesting that their use in the first trimester may result in an increased incidence of abnormalities typically associated with placental vascular disruption, such as gastroschisis and intestinal atresia. Recent evidence has supported the association of phenylephrine and endocardial cushion defect, phenylpropanolamine and ear defects, and phenylpropanolamine and pyloric stenosis with oral and intranasal decongestant use in the first trimester.[21] The risk, however, appears to be low. The AAP classifies pseudoephedrine as compatible with breast-feeding.

The references for this chapter can be found online by accessing the accompanying Expert Consult.website.

176

Labor and Delivery

Jeremy Rose and Erick Eiting

KEY CONCEPT

- Most ED deliveries require only basic equipment to cut and clamp the umbilical cord and dry and suction the infant. However, the ED should have additional equipment and trained staff should be available to care for a newborn requiring further resuscitation.
- Women in labor who present to the ED are generally best cared for in the obstetric suite. Women with the urge to push or with the head of the infant crowning are at imminent risk of delivery, which should take place in the ED.
- The Braxton Hicks contractions of false labor do not escalate in frequency or duration like the contractions of true labor. When in doubt, external electrical monitoring of uterine activity can rule out true labor.
- Preterm labor is defined as uterine contractions with cervical changes before 37 weeks of gestation. Treatment includes tocolytics and fetal maturation therapy combined with bed rest and hydration.
- Premature rupture of membranes (PROM) occurs after 37 weeks' gestation. Its management depends on several factors, including gestational age and fetal maturity, presence of active labor, presence of infection or placental abruption, and degree of fetal well-being or distress.
- Preterm PROM should be treated with antibiotics to prevent infection (chorioamnionitis).
- The first stage of labor averages 8 hours in nulliparous women and 5 hours in multiparous women. Throughout labor, ongoing assessment of fetal well-being is important, and continuous external electrical monitoring helps identify fetal distress.
- Ultrasonography provides crucial information regarding pending delivery, including fetal viability, lie, and presentation.
- The fourth stage of labor refers to the first hour after delivery of the placenta and is a critical period during which postpartum hemorrhage is most likely to occur.
- Deliveries complicated by dystocia, malpresentation, or multiple gestations are life-threatening emergencies. The emergency clinician should develop strategies to treat each of these potential complications of delivery. Please see the following link for a video demonstration of maneuvers used to treat shoulder dystocia: https://www.hopkinsmedicine.org/gynecology_obstetrics/education/training/shoulder-dystocia.
- When a prolapsed cord occurs with a viable infant, cesarean section is the delivery method of choice. If surgical delivery is available, maneuvers to preserve umbilical circulation should be instituted immediately. The mother is placed in the knee-chest position, with the bed in the Trendelenburg position, and instructed to refrain from pushing to avoid further compression of the cord. The presenting part is then manually elevated off the cord. Elevation is maintained until the baby can be delivered surgically.
- Uterine atony accounts for 75% to 90% of cases of postpartum hemorrhage. Administration of a uterotonic, such as oxytocin in conjunction with massage usually provide enough stimuli to control bleeding.
- Approximately 10% of postpartum hemorrhage cases are due to retained placental tissue. Treatment requires manual removal of the remnant placental tissue.
- Pelvic bleeding postpartum can be difficult to control without hysterectomy. When available, embolization of bleeding vessels by an interventional radiologist has reported success rates of 95% to 100%.
- Maternal complications of labor and delivery include obstetric trauma, uterine inversion and rupture, amniotic fluid embolism, coagulation disorders, and infections. Many of these problems can initially be managed in the ED while awaiting obstetric consultation.

FOUNDATIONS

Births in the emergency department (ED) remain a rare event. However, hospital closures and health system consolidation of services has left more hospitals without obstetric coverage, especially in rural areas. These practices have stressed the need for emergency clinicians to be familiar with labor, delivery, and their complications.

Limitations of the Emergency Department

The ED is a suboptimal location for the management of a complicated delivery. Unlike the obstetric suite, the ED may be lacking in appropriate resources, certain specialized equipment, and information about the patient's prenatal care. Cesarean section may be indicated to ensure a successful delivery in dire perimortem circumstances.

Epidemiology of Emergency Delivery

From 2014 to 2016, the perinatal mortality rate in the United States (US) was 6.00/1000 live births.[1] This is remarkably high, almost three times the rate of other similar countries in the developed world. Delivery complications and mortality occur with greater frequency in the ED, where the perinatal mortality rate is approximately 8% to 10%. There are multiple features of the high-risk ED delivery profile. The ED as a care environment is often selected by an obstetric population that subsequently may have unexpected complications. Psychosocial factors, such as drug or alcohol abuse, domestic violence, and lack of access to medical care, contribute to precipitous deliveries in pregnant women with little or no prenatal care. Antepartum hemorrhage, premature rupture of membranes (PROM), eclampsia, premature labor, abruptio placentae, malpresentation, and umbilical cord emergencies are overrepresented in the ED population.

Patient Transfer Considerations

Because of the high risk associated with ED delivery, patients should be transported to a facility that has obstetric and neonatal resources whenever possible. The transfer of a woman with an impending high-risk delivery to such a facility should be based on careful consideration of the risks and benefits. Transferring a pregnant patient with impending delivery can be disastrous for the mother and fetus and may actually violate federal law. Further consideration should be given to the level of care that the neonate will require after delivery, particularly in preterm (<36 weeks of gestation) deliveries, in which interval transfer for a higher level of care may be necessary.

NORMAL DELIVERY

Initial Presentation

Although the epidemiology and high complication rate associated with ED births demand caution, most are normal deliveries. Knowledge of normal labor and delivery mechanics aids safe vaginal delivery and facilitates the identification of complications.

Whenever a woman in the third trimester of pregnancy seeks treatment in the ED, the possibility that she is in labor must be considered. A wide array of nonspecific symptoms may herald the onset of labor. Abdominal pain, back pain, cramping, nausea, vomiting, urinary urgency, stress incontinence, and anxiety can be symptoms of labor. After 24 weeks' gestation, fetal viability is established and thus a medical screening exam should include assessment of both the mother and fetus. Risk factors for preterm labor include older maternal age and presence of systemic disease. This should be considered when treating pregnant patients, even with non–pregnancy-related complaints such as asthma.

Distinguishing False From True Labor

Braxton Hicks contractions, or false labor, must be differentiated from true labor. After 30 weeks of gestation, the previously small and uncoordinated contractions of the uterus become more synchronous and may be perceived by the mother. Braxton Hicks contractions do not escalate in frequency or duration, in contrast to the contractions of true labor. By definition, these contractions are associated with minimal or no cervical dilation or effacement. Examination should also reveal intact membranes. Care not to rupture the membranes is important to avoid inducing labor prematurely. Examination should be done in a sterile fashion to avoid introducing infection if the membranes have ruptured. If the diagnosis remains in doubt, external electrical monitoring of uterine activity can rule out true labor. Any discomfort associated with false labor is usually relieved with mild analgesia, ambulation, or change in activity.

Unlike false labor, true labor is characterized by cyclic uterine contractions of increasing frequency, duration, and strength, culminating in delivery of the fetus and placenta. In contrast to Braxton Hicks contractions, true labor causes cervical dilation to begin, marking the first stage of labor.

Bloody Show

At the onset of labor, the cervical mucous plug may be expelled, resulting in what is termed a *bloody show*. The bleeding associated with this process is slight (usually only a few dark red spots admixed with mucus) and is due to the increase in cervical vascularity that occurs in pregnancy. Bloody show is not a contraindication to vaginal examination for the determination of cervical effacement and dilation. If bleeding continues or is of a larger volume, more serious causes should be suspected, such as placenta previa and placental abruption, which are contraindications for a vaginal examination.

Stages of Labor
First Stage of Labor

The first stage of labor is the cervical stage, ending with a completely dilated, fully effaced cervix. It is divided into a latent phase, with slow cervical dilation, and an active phase, with more rapid dilation. The active phase begins once the cervix is dilated to 3 cm. Most women who deliver in the ED arrive while in the active phase of stage 1 or early stage 2 labor (Fig. 176.1). The duration of the first stage of labor averages 8 hours in nulliparous women and 5 hours in multiparous women. During this time, frequent assessment of fetal well-being is important, and continuous external electrical monitoring may help identify fetal distress, allowing for appropriate intervention.

The maternal examination provides a rough guide to gestational age. At 20 weeks' gestation, the uterine fundus reaches the umbilicus. Approximately 1 cm of fundal height is added per week of gestation until 36 weeks. At that time, the fundal height decreases as the fetus drops into the pelvis (Fig. 176.2). These estimates help establish gestational age rapidly.

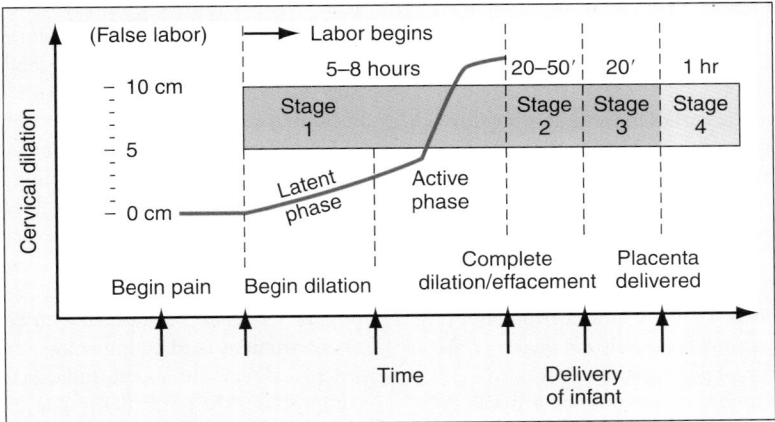

Fig. 176.1 Stages of labor and delivery. Stage 1, cervical stage; stage 2, fetal expulsion; stage 3, placental expulsion (20 minutes); stage 4, uterine contraction (1 hour postpartum).

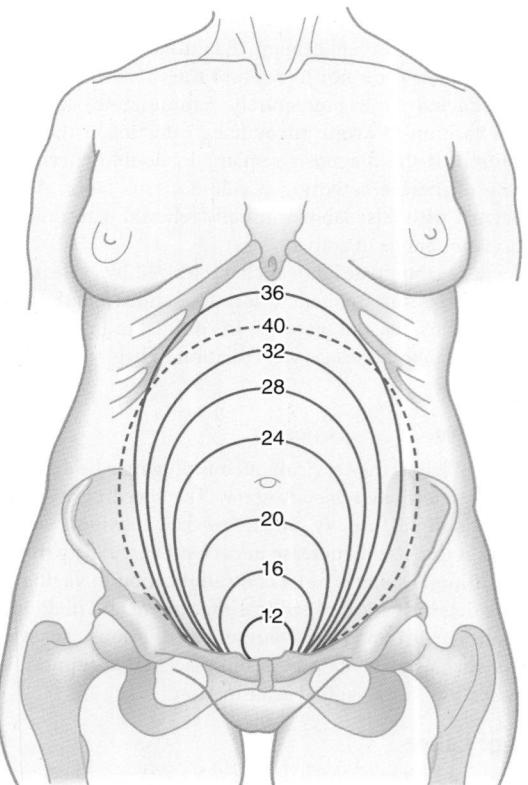

Fig. 176.2 Height of fundus by weeks of normal gestation with a single fetus. The dotted line indicates height after lightening. (Adapted from: Barkaukas V, et al. *Health and Physical Assessment.* St. Louis: Mosby; 1992.)

The abdominal examination with Leopold maneuvers may confirm the lie of the fetus (Fig. 176.3). Bedside ultrasound can be especially useful in determining fetal position. The determination of the stage of labor depends on examination of the cervix. A sterile approach using sterile gloves, sterile speculum, and povidone-iodine solution is indicated to prevent ascending infection. On pelvic examination, the clinician should determine the following:

- *Effacement* refers to the thickness of the cervix. A paper thin cervix is 100% effaced.
- *Dilation* indicates the diameter of the cervical opening in centimeters. Complete, or maximum, dilation is 10 cm.
- *Position* describes the relationship of the fetal presenting part to the birth canal. The most common position of the head is occiput anterior.
- *Station* indicates the relationship of the presenting fetal part to the maternal ischial spines (Fig. 176.4).
- *Presentation* specifies the anatomic part of the fetus leading through the birth canal.

In 95% of all labors, the presenting part is the occiput, or vertex. On digital examination, a smooth surface with 360 degrees of firm bony contours and palpable suture lines is noted. Palpation of the suture lines and the fontanels where they join allows the examiner to determine the direction the fetus is facing. Three sutures radiate from the posterior fontanel, and four radiate from the anterior fontanel (Fig. 176.5). The lateral margins are examined carefully for fingers or facial parts that indicate compound or brow presentations.

When the clinician suspects rupture of membranes, a sterile speculum examination is performed. This may reveal pooling of amniotic fluid, a fernlike pattern when the fluid is allowed to dry on a microscope slide, and the use of Nitrazine paper, which should turn blue, indicating an alkaline amniotic fluid (pH > 6). Although vaginal blood, cervical mucus, semen, and infection can interfere with results, sensitivities of Nitrazine paper and ferning for the detection of amniotic fluid are nearly 90%. If vaginal bleeding is evident, digital and speculum examination of the pelvis should be deferred until an ultrasound study can be obtained to rule out placenta previa.

Second Stage of Labor

The second stage of labor is characterized by a fully dilated cervix and accompanied by the urge to bear down and push with each uterine contraction. The median duration of this stage is 50 minutes in nulliparous women and 20 minutes in multiparous women, with the anticipation of a more rapid progression for low-birth-weight premature infants. A prolonged second stage of labor is associated with an increase in maternal complications, including postpartum hemorrhage, infection, and severe vaginal lacerations.

Antenatal Fetal Assessment. During labor and delivery, the identification of fetal distress and appropriate intervention can reduce fetal morbidity and mortality. There are currently three methods of assessing a fetus in utero: (1) clinical monitoring; (2) electrical monitoring; and (3) ultrasonography. External electrical monitoring and ultrasonography merit consideration for use in the care of women laboring in the ED. Both modalities provide real-time information that is helpful for the diagnosis of fetal distress and assistance with intrapartum decision making.

Electronic Fetal Monitoring. Electronic fetal monitoring uses tracings of the fetal heart rate and uterine activity. Documentation of organized cyclic uterine contractions helps confirm true labor and may help diagnose fetal distress. In combination with clinical data, this can portend fetal distress due to hypoxia and provide a window for intervention.

Uterine activity is measured transabdominally by a pressure transducer, creating a recording of the contraction frequency. Because the measurements are indirect, the strength of the contractions correlates poorly with the tracing. The tracings are position and placement sensitive.

Fetal heart rate tracings have several components that can be assessed—baseline heart rate, variability, accelerations, decelerations, and diagnostic patterns.

Baseline Heart Rate. This is the average fetal heart rate during a 10-minute period (in the absence of a uterine contraction) and is the most important aspect of fetal heart rate monitoring. Fetal bradycardia is defined as a baseline rate of less than 110 beats/min; fetal tachycardia is defined as a baseline rate of more than 160 beats/min.

Variability. This can be instantaneous (beat to beat) or long term (intervals ≥ 1 minute). Both types of variability are indicators of fetal well-being. Accelerations occur during fetal movement and reflect an alert mobile fetus. Decreased variability may indicate fetal hypoxemia and acidemia, or it may be a side effect of a wide array of drugs, including analgesics, sedative-hypnotics, phenothiazines, and alcohol.

Decelerations. Decelerations in fetal heart rate are more complicated and should be interpreted according to the clinical scenario. There are three types of deceleration—variable, early, and late (Fig. 176.6). These terms refer to the timing of the deceleration relative to the uterine contraction.

Variable and early decelerations are common and normally represent physiologic reflexes associated with head compression in the birth canal or intermittent cord compression. Variable decelerations that are persistent and repetitive usually indicate repeated episodes of umbilical cord compression. The resultant hypoxia and acidosis may cause fetal distress. Attempts to shift maternal and fetal weight off the umbilical cord by changing position are indicated. If variable decelerations continue, the

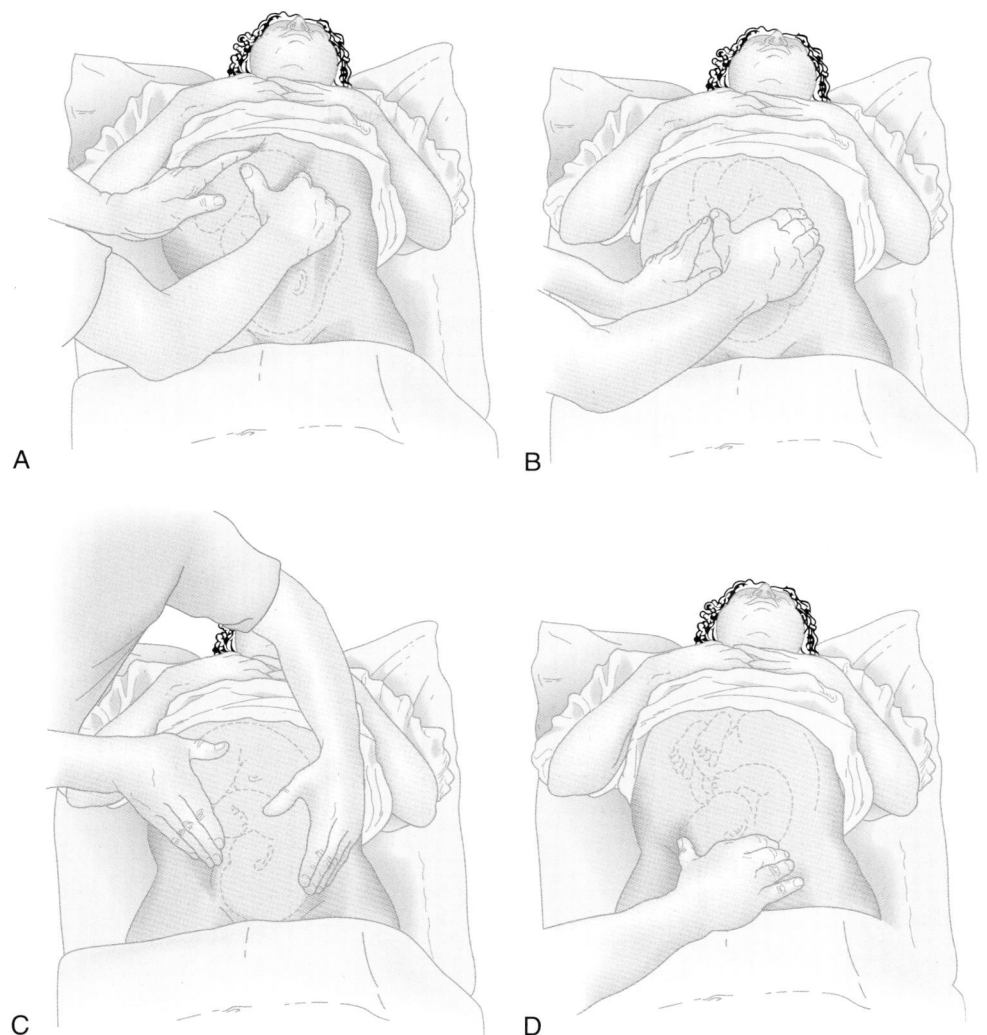

Fig. 176.3 Leopold maneuvers. (A) The first Leopold maneuver reveals which fetal part occupies the fundus. (B) The second Leopold maneuver reveals the position of the fetal back. (C) The third Leopold maneuver reveals which fetal part lies over the pelvic inlet. (D) The fourth Leopold maneuver reveals the position of the cephalic prominence. (Adapted from: Willson JR, et al. *Obstetrics and Gynecology*, ed 9. St. Louis: Mosby; 1991.)

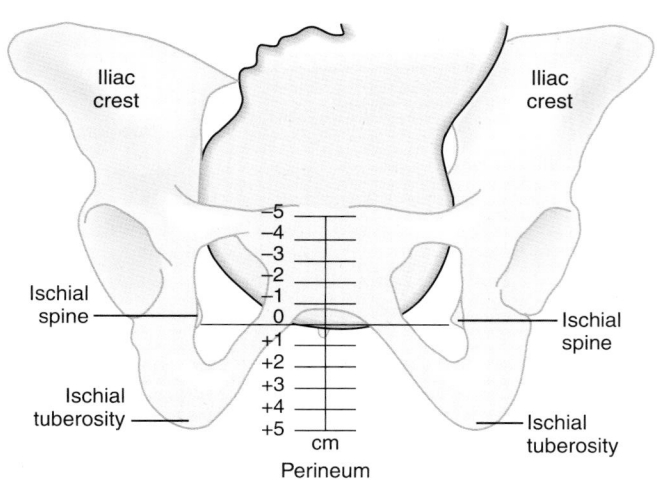

Fig. 176.4 Fetal stations. The level of the ischial spines is considered 0 station. The silhouette of the infant's head is shown approaching station +1. (Courtesy Ross Laboratories, Columbus, OH.)

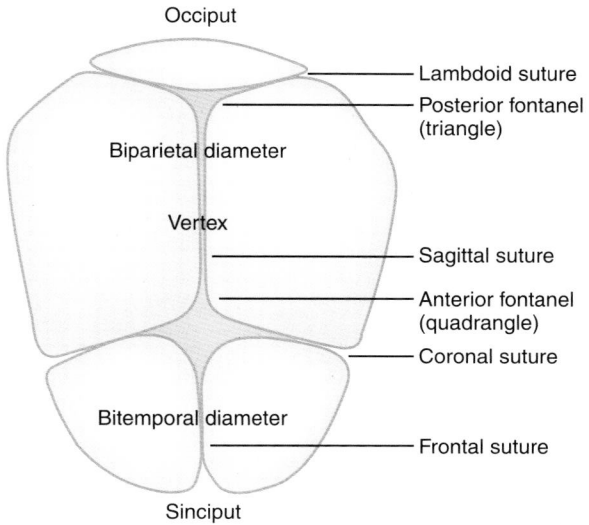

Fig. 176.5 Bony landmarks of the fetal skull. (Adapted from: Willson JR, et al. *Obstetrics and Gynecology*, ed 9. St. Louis: Mosby; 1991.)

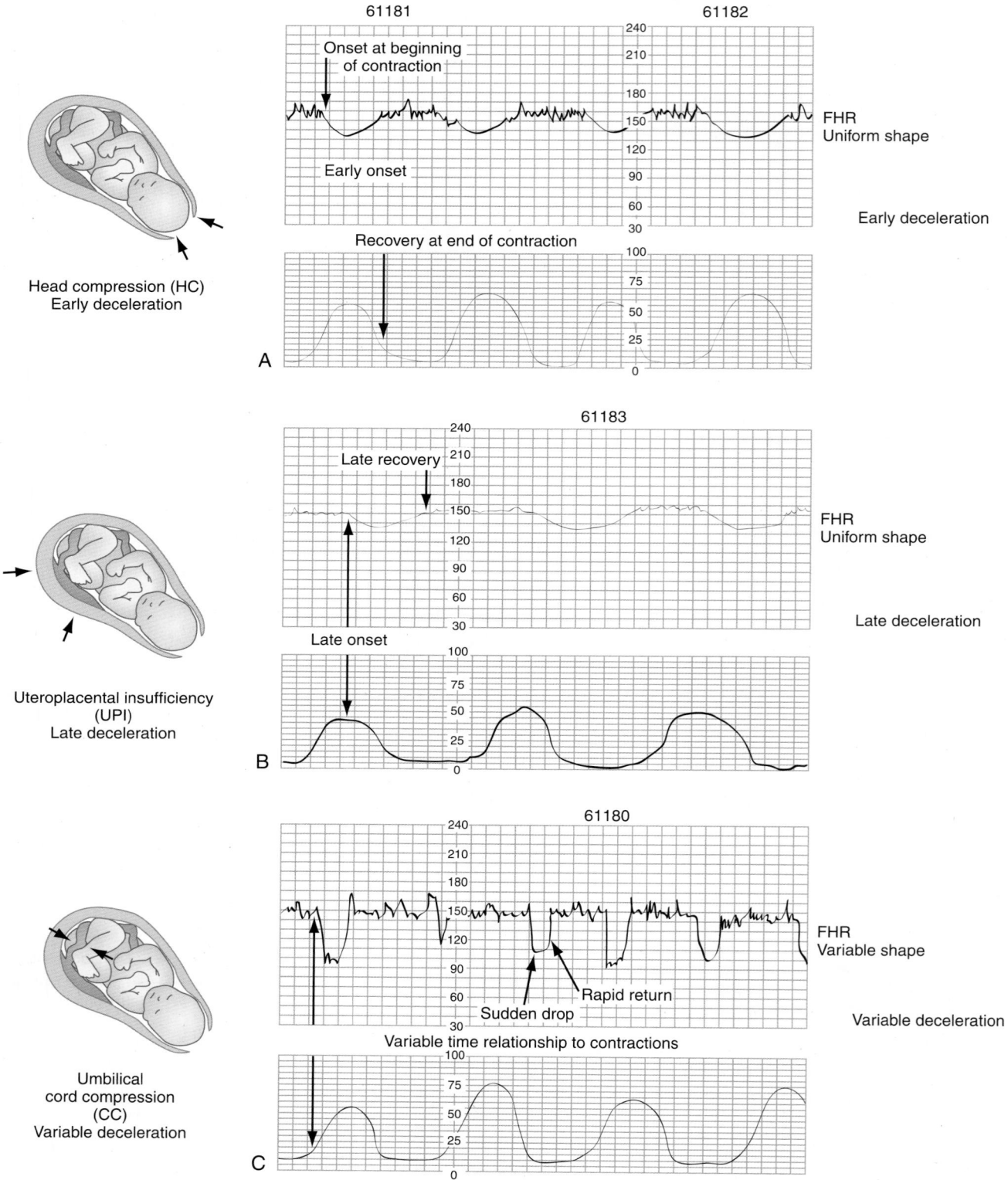

Fig. 176.6 Deceleration patterns of the fetal heart rate (FHR). (A) Early deceleration caused by head compression. (B) Late deceleration caused by uteroplacental insufficiency. (C) Variable deceleration caused by cord compression. (Modified from: Lowdermilk DL, et al. *Maternity and Women's Health Care*, ed 6. St. Louis: Mosby; 1997.)

situation warrants efforts to hasten the delivery or, if obstetric backup becomes available, to perform an emergency cesarean section.

Late decelerations are more serious and most often indicate uteroplacental insufficiency. The tracing contours are generally smooth, with the heart rate nadir occurring well after a maximal uterine contraction (typically, ≥30 seconds afterward). The lag, slope, and magnitude of late decelerations correlate with increasing fetal hypoxia. Late decelerations are particularly ominous in association with poor variability, nonreactivity, and baseline bradycardia. When these findings are present, immediate obstetric consultation for delivery is indicated to prevent further hypoxia.

Diagnostic Patterns. Finally, the emergency clinician should be aware of the significance of sinusoidal tracings. Tracings of this type have low baseline heart rates and little beat to beat variability. The sinusoidal tracing is an ominous finding that is often premorbid. The differential diagnosis includes erythroblastosis fetalis, placental abruption, fetal hemorrhage (trauma), and amnionitis.

Ultrasonography. In the third trimester or during labor, ultrasonography can provide crucial information pertaining to impending delivery, such as the number and position of fetus(es) and fetal heart rate. When a technician and radiologist are available, and if time permits, the gestational age, biophysical profile, amniotic fluid index, and a survey of fetal and placental anatomy may be obtained. The American College of Obstetricians and Gynecologists (ACOG) has published recommendations regarding the indications for ultrasonography in the third trimester (Box 176.1). The parameters of immediate interest in the ED are fetal viability (specifically in utero gestation and fetal heart rate), lie, and presentation. Transvaginal ultrasonography is relatively contraindicated in the peripartum period, particularly in the cases of premature rupture of membranes (PROM) and placenta previa.

Delivery. As stage 2 of labor progresses, preparation for delivery should be under way. A radiant warmer should be available and heated. Neonatal resuscitation adjuncts should be available, including a towel, scissors, umbilical clamps, bulb suction, airway equipment (oxygen, bag-mask device with appropriate-sized masks, and tools for endotracheal intubation), and equipment to achieve vascular access. Most deliveries require only basic equipment to cut and clamp the umbilical cord, suction the mouth and nose, and dry and stimulate the infant. A nurse should be at the bedside to coach and provide reassurance to the mother.

The mother is placed in the dorsal lithotomy position and prepared for delivery. The Sims position, or left lateral position with knees drawn toward the mother's chest and back to the physician, is also an acceptable position. The vulva and perineum are cleared and gently scrubbed with sterile water or saline. A repeated sterile examination to assess labor progression and confirm presentation may be performed. Firm digital stretching of the perineum, particularly posteriorly, may prevent tears and lacerations later in delivery.

BOX 176.1 Third-Trimester Ultrasonography: Possible Indications

Determine number of fetuses.
Establish fetal presentation.
Identify fetal heart motion.
Locate placenta.
Measure amniotic fluid.
Determine gestational age.
Survey fetal anatomy.
Diagnose cord prolapse.
Diagnose cause of third-trimester bleeding.
Rule out placental abruption.

Controlled coordinated expulsion with coaching to sustain each push aids with crowning and delivery of the head. The most vulnerable moment is when the fetal head begins to stretch and distend the perineum. Instructing the mother to pant and not push slows the passage of the head and shoulders. The modified Ritgen maneuver may be used to support the perineum and prevent maternal injury: In this technique, a towel-draped, gloved hand is used to stretch the perineum and gently exert pressure on the chin of the fetus. The second hand places pressure on the occiput superiorly, guiding the head into slight extension and positioning it so that its smallest diameter passes through the pelvic outlet. Calm communication between the physician and mother is the best way to maintain control of the delivery.

After the head is delivered, the physician allows the head to rotate toward the maternal thigh and clears the fetal face and airway. Next, the shoulders, usually anterior shoulder first, clear the perineum. The shoulders often deliver spontaneously, with little effort by the physician. Gentle downward traction on the head promotes delivery of the anterior shoulder. A subsequent upward motion pulls the posterior shoulder through the pelvic outlet. If delay occurs in delivery of the shoulders, the potential for shoulder dystocia should be considered.

As the infant clears the perineum, attention focuses on the umbilical cord. The infant should be kept low or at the level of the perineum to promote blood flow into the infant from the placenta. The cord is clamped and cut. Clamps should be placed 4 or 5 cm apart, with the proximal clamp 10 cm from the infant's abdomen. The cord should be cut at least 1 cm from the skin to ensure venous access if the neonate requires resuscitation. Suctioning of the nose and mouth at this time may reduce secretions that can cause increased airway resistance.

The infant is now clear of the mother and can be wrapped in towels and moved to the warmer. Gentle drying with a towel and suctioning usually provide sufficient respiratory stimulation. If not, flicking the soles of the feet and rubbing the back are other modalities. Apgar scores at 1, 5, and 10 minutes after birth should be documented.

Episiotomy. With a controlled delivery, routine performance of an episiotomy is not recommended. It should be performed only for specific indications, such as shoulder dystocia or breech delivery. An episiotomy should be done before excessive stretching of the perineal muscles occurs but near the time of delivery to avoid excessive bleeding. Common practice is to cut the episiotomy when the head is visible during a contraction and the introitus opens to a diameter of 3 or 4 cm. The literature currently recommends a mediolateral incision to avoid perineal tears and rectal involvement (Fig. 176.7).

Third Stage of Labor

The third stage of labor involves the delivery of the placenta and frequent checks of the tone and height of the uterine fundus. Signs of placental separation include the following: the uterus becomes firmer and rises; the umbilical cord lengthens 5 to 10 cm; or there is a sudden gush of blood.

These signs usually occur within 5 to 10 minutes of the delivery of the infant but may extend to 30 minutes. Beyond 18 minutes, the risk of postpartum hemorrhage increases and is up to six times more likely after 30 minutes. Although the placenta may be delivered expectantly, active management reduces the length of the third stage of labor and thereby decreases the risk of postpartum hemorrhage. Active management includes the administration of uterotonic gentle traction of the clamped umbilical cord with mild pressure applied above the symphysis pubis and uterine massage after delivery. Any attempt to deliver the placenta before it separates is contraindicated.

Examination of the umbilical cord and placenta is an essential part of the delivery process and any abnormalities should be noted at this

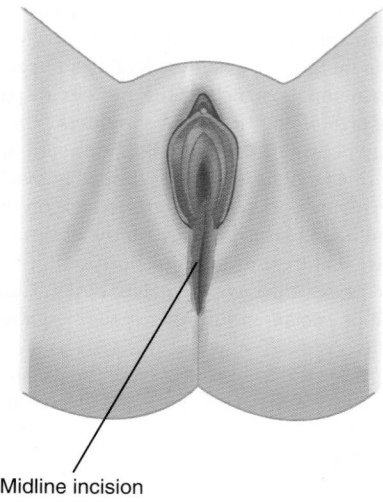

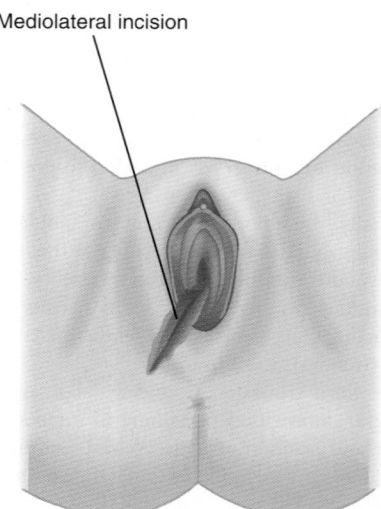

Mediolateral incision

Midline incision

Fig. 176.7 A mediolateral episiotomy incision is preferred to a strictly midline incision. (Adapted from www. aurorahealthcare.org/healthgate/images/exh44028a_ma.jpg.)

time. The umbilical cord is normally a three-vessel structure, with two umbilical arteries on either side of the single umbilical vein. A two-vessel cord (one umbilical artery) occurs in 1 of 500 deliveries. Common abnormalities of the placenta include accessory lobes and abnormal cord insertion. Visible clots adherent to the uterine aspect may indicate placental abruption and the discovery of an incomplete placenta or membranes should alert the clinician to the possibility of postpartum complications.

Fourth Stage of Labor

The fourth stage of labor refers to the first hour after delivery of the placenta and is a critical period during which postpartum hemorrhage is most likely to occur. The cervix and vaginal fornices should be inspected for deep lacerations as a result of delivery, and repair of any vaginal lacerations should be performed at this time.

Finally, oxytocin is infused to promote contraction of the uterus and control hemorrhage. The uterus is evaluated frequently for tone and massaged transabdominally if any sign of relaxation exists. Oxytocin should not be given before delivery of the placenta because this could result in the trapping of placental fragments or may hinder the delivery of an undetected twin.

THIRD-TRIMESTER COMPLICATIONS ASSOCIATED WITH DELIVERY

Obstetric problems in the third trimester often result in the initiation of labor. Premature labor, PROM, and third-trimester bleeding are relatively common complications. The fundamental question to be addressed in these settings is whether the fetus would fare better in utero or delivered.

Premature Labor

Premature or preterm labor and fetal immaturity are the leading causes of neonatal mortality. Preterm labor is defined as uterine contractions with cervical changes before 37 weeks of gestation. Many underlying conditions result in preterm labor, which is associated with 5% to 18% of all pregnancies and is the leading cause of neonatal death. Factors

---

BOX 176.2   Factors Linked to Preterm Labor

Demographic and Psychosocial
Extremes of age (>40 yr, teenagers)
Lower socioeconomic status
Tobacco use
Cocaine abuse
Prolonged standing (occupation)
Psychosocial stressors

Reproductive and Gynecologic
Prior preterm delivery
Diethylstilbestrol exposure
Multiple gestations
Anatomic endometrial cavity anomalies
Cervical incompetence
Low pregnancy weight gain
First-trimester vaginal bleeding
Placental abruption or previa

Surgical
Prior reproductive organ surgery
Prior paraendometrial surgery other than genitourinary (appendectomy)

Infectious
Urinary tract infections
Nonuterine infections
Genital tract infections (bacterial vaginosis)

---

linked to this problem include substance abuse, history of preterm delivery, multiple gestations, placental anomalies, infections, and lifestyle or psychosocial stressors (Box 176.2). The unexpected nature of premature labor often results in an ED visit. When delivery is not imminent, the patient can be moved to the obstetrics unit for further care.

Clinical Features

The diagnosis of preterm labor requires the identification of uterine activity and cervical changes before 37 weeks of gestation. Early maternal signs and symptoms include an increase or change in vaginal discharge, pain resulting from uterine contractions (sometimes perceived as back pain), pelvic pressure, vaginal bleeding, and fluid leak.

Diagnostic Testing

If uterine contractions and cervical changes are present, and the estimated fetal weight on ultrasonography is less than 2500 g, the diagnosis of premature labor is likely. The differentiation of false labor from true labor is best done by electrical monitoring. The initial evaluation of a woman with possible preterm labor includes urinalysis, complete blood count, and pelvic ultrasonography. If delivery is not imminent, these studies can be performed under monitoring in the ED or obstetrics area. Whenever possible, these patients should be transferred to a perinatal center with an associated intensive care unit.

Management

A viable fetus and healthy mother are indications for medical management directed toward the prolongation of gestation. Preterm labor should not be postponed with medical management in the cases of fetal compromise, major congenital anomalies, intrauterine infection, placental abruption, eclampsia, significant cervical dilation, or PROM.

The treatment of preterm labor involves multiple modalities and is usually performed outside the ED. Tocolytics and fetal maturation therapy combined with bed rest and hydration are used with the hope of prolonging pregnancy (Box 176.3). When tocolytics are indicated, they should be used in coordination with an obstetric consultant. These patients optimally should be transferred to an appropriate center before delivery, whenever possible, because medical management fails in more than 25% of preterm patients for whom it is attempted. The contraindications to tocolytics should be reviewed before initiation of these therapies (Box 176.4). Any patient receiving tocolytics needs to be monitored for signs of fetal distress. Terbutaline has been associated with serious maternal side effects and deleterious behavioral effects in the offspring after in utero exposure. Terbutaline should be limited to short-term inpatient use.

Premature Rupture of Membranes
Clinical Features

PROM is defined as rupture of the amniotic and chorionic membranes before the onset of labor. It affects 3% of all gestations. During pregnancy, the chorionic and amniotic membranes protect the fetus from infection and provide an environment that allows fetal growth and movement. The amniotic fluid is constantly exchanged by fetal swallowing and urination and umbilical cord transfer.

The word *premature* in PROM refers to rupture before labor, not to fetal prematurity. In 8% of PROM cases, the fetus is at or near term, and PROM may result in normal labor. When PROM occurs before 37 weeks, it is called preterm PROM and is associated with significant fetal morbidity and mortality. PROM is the inciting event in one-third of all preterm deliveries.

After the membranes rupture, the period from latency to the onset of labor varies. Longer latent periods are common earlier in pregnancy, and the latency shortens as gestational age increases. At term, labor is a desirable result of PROM, but with fetal immaturity, delivery would result in fetal complications.

Diagnostic Testing

The diagnosis of PROM can be established by the history and physical examination. In most cases, the patient suggests the diagnosis and usually is correct. The patient typically describes a spontaneous gush of watery fluid, followed by a mild persistent seepage. Urinary incontinence or excess vaginal or cervical secretions are occasionally confused with PROM.

Examination of women with potential PROM is performed under sterile conditions to prevent ascending infection. Direct digital examination of the cervix is avoided. The identification of amniotic fluid was previously discussed. Table 176.1 summarizes the bedside testing modalities available to confirm the diagnosis of PROM. Visualization of the cervix for a prolapsed cord or small fetal part is performed during the evaluation for effacement and dilation. Culture specimens for group B streptococci, *Chlamydia trachomatis,* and *Neisseria gonorrhoeae* should be obtained.

BOX 176.3 Commonly Used Tocolytic Agents

Magnesium sulfate
    4–6 g IV bolus over 20 min
    1–2 g/hr IV infusion
Terbutaline
    5–10 mg PO q4–6h
    0.25 mg SC q20min
    2.5–5 mcg/min increased every 20 min to max 25 mcg/min
Ritodrine[a]
    10 mg PO q2–4h
    10 mg IM q3–8h
    0.05–0.35 mg/min IV infusion
Isoxsuprine
    20 mg PO q6h
    0.2–0.5 mg/min IV infusion
Nifedipine
    10–30 mg PO q15–20 min for the first hour then 10–20 mg PO q4–8h

[a]Ritodrine and Isoxsuprine have been discontinued in the United States.

BOX 176.4 Contraindications to Tocolysis

Absolute
Acute vaginal bleeding
Fetal distress (not tachycardia alone)
Lethal fetal anomaly
Chorioamnionitis
Preeclampsia or eclampsia
Sepsis
Disseminated intravascular coagulopathy

Relative
Chronic hypertension
Cardiopulmonary disease
Stable placenta previa
Cervical dilation > 5 cm
Placental abruption

TABLE 176.1 Bedside Testing for Premature Rupture of Membranes

Method	Result
Nitrazine	Amniotic fluid (pH > 6.5) will turn Nitrazine paper blue; normal vaginal secretions (pH < 5.5) leave Nitrazine paper yellow
Ferning	Amniotic fluid crystallizes
Smear combustion	Amniotic fluid, when flamed, turns white and crystallizes; vaginal secretions caramelize, turn brown

Management

The management of PROM depends on several factors, including gestational age and fetal maturity, presence of active labor, presence or absence of infection, presence of placental abruption, and degree of fetal well-being or distress. In all cases, fetal heart rate monitoring, obstetric consultation, and admission are indicated. In the immature fetus (24–31 weeks of gestation), the initiation of specific treatment decisions aimed at accelerating fetal maturity should be made in coordination with the receiving obstetrician. This includes the possible administration of corticosteroids to promote pulmonary maturation. Patients with PROM between 31 and 33 weeks' gestation are usually managed expectantly and those at or beyond 34 weeks of gestation are generally delivered.

All patients with PROM should be assessed for intraamniotic infection. Infectious complications should be diagnosed and treated before the mother demonstrates overt clinical signs. We recommend treating preterm PROM with an initial dose of ampicillin (2 g IV) plus azithromycin (1 g PO) followed by ampicillin (2 g IV Q6h × 48h) plus amoxicillin 875 mg PO BID for 5 days.

Chorioamnionitis

Chorioamnionitis occurs when vaginal or cervical bacteria ascend into the uterus, instigating an inflammation of the chorion and amnion layers of the amniotic sac. It occurs in 1% to 10% of all pregnancies; risk factors include prolonged labor, PROM, excessive vaginal examinations, and recent amniocentesis. Box 176.5 summarizes the findings and evaluation of chorioamnionitis. Chorioamnionitis may result in

---

BOX 176.5 Chorioamnionitis Evaluation

Fluid in Vaginal Vault
Phosphatidylglycerol

Cervical Cultures
Escherichia coli and other gram-negative bacteria
Neisseria gonorrhoeae

Vaginal Cultures
Chlamydia spp.
Mycoplasma hominis
Group B streptococci
Ureaplasma urealyticum

Amniocentesis Studies
Gram stain (group B streptococci)
Culture
Glucose
Lecithin to sphingomyelin ratio

Maternal Signs and Symptoms
Premature rupture of membranes
Uterine tenderness
Fever
Tachycardia (maternal or fetal)
Malodorous vaginal discharge
Leukocytosis

Fetal Signs and Symptoms
Decreased activity
Abnormal biophysical profile (ultrasonographic examination)
Fetal tachycardia
Decreased variability of fetal heart rate

---

prolonged first- and second-stage labor and decreased responsiveness to oxytocin. Early aggressive treatment, even before evidence of infection occurs, decreases neonatal morbidity and delays delivery, allowing more time for fetal maturation.

Vertical Transmission of Human Immunodeficiency Virus

The antiretroviral drug zidovudine (AZT) has long been used to prevent vertical transmission of HIV during labor. With appropriate therapy, the risk of vertical transmission is well under 1%. Current guidelines do not recommend perinatal intravenous AZT for patients with well-controlled disease that are already taking oral antiretroviral medications.[2] If doubt exits as to a patient's HIV progression or medication compliance, AZT (2 mg/kg infused over 1 hour followed by a continuous infusion of 1 mg/kg/hour for 2 additional hours) should be started. Patients with unclear HIV status should be tested on presentation to the ED. Transmission may occur in the antepartum, intrapartum, or postpartum (breast-feeding) period. Because intrapartum transmission accounts for up to 75% of vertically transmitted HIV infections, antiretroviral therapy on presentation, even while labor progresses, can decrease vertical HIV transmission. Risk factors for transmission include high viral loads, prolonged rupture of membranes, maternal drug use, vaginal delivery, and breast-feeding.

Advances in point-of-care testing for HIV have resulted in the ability to make a preliminary diagnosis in a patient with HIV in the ED. Serologic confirmation is recommended, but emergent interventions can proceed on the basis of the bedside result. A positive HIV test result may, in some cases, allow a change in the method of delivery; cesarean section decreases the rate of HIV transmission compared with vaginal delivery methods.

COMPLICATED DELIVERY

Foundations

Deliveries involving dystocia, malpresentation, and multiple gestations are potentially life-threatening emergencies. The emergency clinician cannot solve these obstetric problems with cesarean section and will therefore face the prospect of an extremely high-risk vaginal delivery. As expected, these abnormal deliveries increase the risk of fetal and maternal complications. Aggressive attempts to obtain obstetric, neonatal, and anesthesia support are warranted. If the delivery proceeds in the ED, preparations for maternal and neonatal resuscitation need to be made proactively and rapidly.

Dystocia and Malpresentation

Dystocia, or abnormal labor progression, accounts for one-third of all cesarean sections and half of primary cesarean sections. Because rapid surgical resolution is unavailable to the emergency clinician, intrapartum management skills are required.

Dystocia can be divided into three categories of causative factors. Labor fails to progress when there are problems related to the pelvic architecture (the passage), fetal size or presentation problems (the passenger), and inadequate uterine expulsive forces. Although it is useful to consider these causes independently, dystocia is usually caused by a combination of factors. Presentation problems are particularly important because they become apparent during stage 2 of labor and require immediate action.

In order of increasing incidence, brow, face, shoulder, and breech presentations are the most common malpresentations (Table 176.2). True fetopelvic disproportion is much less common. Cesarean section is indicated when labor arrest or cord prolapse coexists with these presentations.

TABLE 176.2 Relative Incidence of Malpresentations

Malpresentation	Incidence
Breech presentation	1/25 live births
Shoulder dystocia	1/300 live births
Face presentation	1/550 live births
Brow presentation	1/1400 live births

Breech Delivery

Breech is the most common malpresentation, occurring in just less than 4% of all deliveries. Three types of breech presentation exist—frank, incomplete, and complete (Fig. 176.8; Box 176.6).

By convention, the presentation (frank, incomplete, and complete) is followed by the relationship of the fetus to the birth canal, with the fetal sacrum as a reference point. Correlated with this abnormal presentation are several factors, such as prematurity, multiparity, fetal abnormalities, prior breech presentation, polyhydramnios, and uterine abnormalities.

Overall, one-third of breech fetal deaths are believed to be preventable. Asphyxia is often due to umbilical cord prolapse or entrapment of the head. Other complications include labor arrest or brachial plexus injuries, and fetal head and neck trauma can occur if inappropriate delivery techniques are used. Scheduled cesarean section for these patients reduces the potential for an ED presentation. However, emergency clinicians should be prepared for vaginal delivery of breech presentations in the event of premature or unforeseen labor in the absence of immediate surgical services.

The mechanical problem with breech presentations is that the buttocks and legs do not provide a sufficient wedge, hindering cervical accommodation of the relatively larger head. In addition, because the presenting part does not occlude the cervical opening completely, umbilical cord prolapse may occur.

In the successful vaginal delivery of a breech presentation, the legs or buttocks are given time to dilate the cervix. This creates a tenuous appearing scenario where the baby's hips are delivered, but the shoulders and head are still inside the cervical OS. It appears as though the baby can simply be pulled free, but pulling on the hips will bring the shoulders through the OS, trapping the head and obstructing the labor. In fact, the clinician should take care to support, but not pull, the presenting part.

Diagnostic Testing

Before labor, *Leopold maneuvers* (see Fig. 176.3) facilitate the diagnosis of breech presentation. Active labor restricts the use of Leopold maneuvers, and a vaginal examination is required. Bedside ultrasound can help establish position if it is unclear. The differentiation of a vertex presentation from a breech presentation by tactile vaginal exam may be difficult. Whenever a fontanel is not identified on examination, a breech presentation should be suspected. It is helpful to remember that the face and skull have a complete circle of bone, whereas the anus is flanked by bone on only two sides.

If time permits, an ultrasound examination is indicated to distinguish the type of breech presentation, gestational age, fetal weight, and position of the fetal arms and neck. If the fetus has a hyperextended neck, vaginal delivery is associated with a high incidence of spinal cord injuries. If possible, labor should be delayed to allow cesarean section. Similarly, if the arms are over the head, they increase the dystocia when the head enters the birth canal.

Management

Premature infants in the breech position often deliver spontaneously without difficulty. As the infant comes to term, dystocia becomes increasingly common. With commitment to a vaginal delivery,

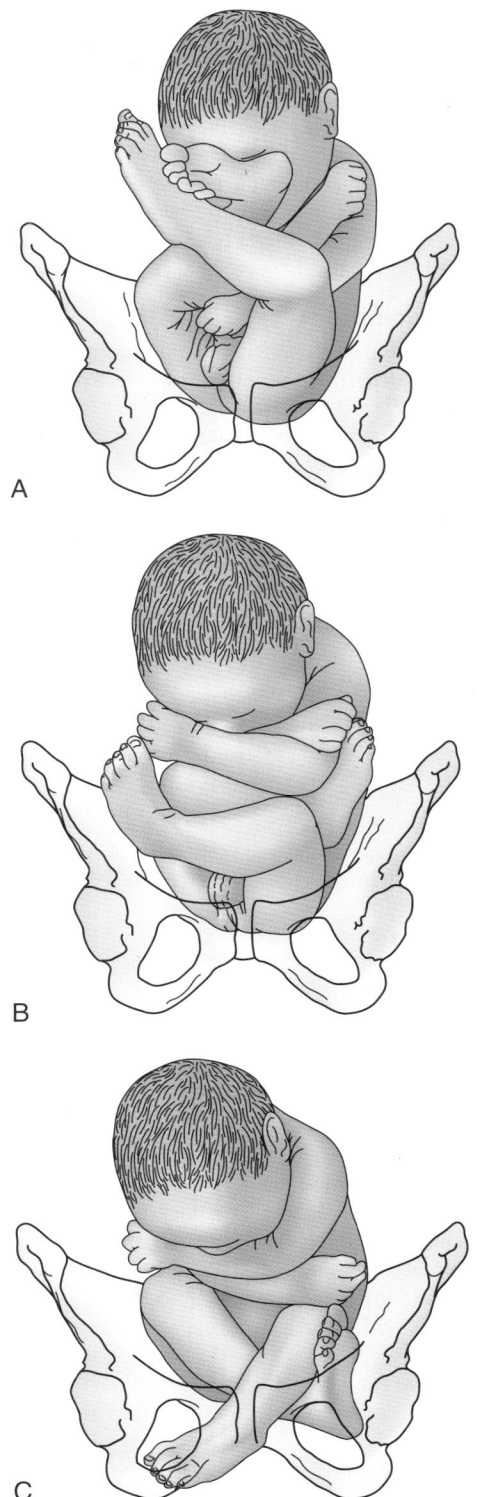

Fig. 176.8 Breech presentations. (A) Frank breech presentation. (B) Complete breech presentation. (C) Incomplete breech presentation. (Adapted from: Cunningham FG, et al. *Williams Obstetrics,* ed 19. Norwalk, CT: Appleton & Lange; 1993.)

knowledge of breech dystocia mechanics may allow atraumatic delivery. The key goals are to maximize the size of the passage and to minimize the dystocia of the after-coming head. Box 176.7 summarizes the actions associated with successful vaginal breech delivery.

The *Mauriceau maneuver* is the use of the fetal mouth to flex the fetal neck and draw in the chin. Because fetal neck extension is associated with cord injuries and worsening dystocia, this maneuver is useful to ensure a successful vaginal delivery. This maneuver should only be attempted once the fetal elbows and chin have entered the pelvic inlet to avoid inducing the Moro reflex, in which fetal head flexion results in the arms being suddenly extended. During this maneuver, the fetal pelvis should be supported to avoid abdominal injuries. A generous episiotomy may be necessary to facilitate the maneuver in a full-term infant. If the after-coming head cannot be delivered quickly, the chances of good fetal outcome are poor.

Shoulder Dystocia

Shoulder dystocia is the second most common malpresentation, occurring in 1.4% of all deliveries. In contrast to a breech presentation, which may be diagnosed in the antepartum period, shoulder dystocia develops in the intrapartum period. Maternal and fetal factors are associated with shoulder dystocia. Maternal factors include diabetes, obesity, and precipitous or protracted labor; fetal factors include macrosomia, postmaturity, and erythroblastosis fetalis. Shoulder dystocia responds well to a variety of intrapartum maneuvers; therefore, the skill involved during delivery is an important determinant of fetal outcome.

The consequences of shoulder dystocia can be devastating. As with a breech presentation, infant complications are more common and severe than maternal complications. Traumatic brachial plexus injuries, clavicular fractures, and hypoxic brain injury are all well-documented complications. Maternal complications are related to traumatic delivery and include vaginal, perineal, and anal sphincter tears, as well as urinary incontinence.

Diagnostic Testing

Shoulder dystocia is diagnosed clinically by the inability to deliver either shoulder. The fetal head may appear to retract toward the maternal perineum, otherwise known as the turtle sign. Traction on the head extends and abducts the shoulders, increasing the bisacromial diameter and worsening the dystocia. Fig. 176.9 shows the normal and abnormal

---

BOX 176.6 Breech Presentations

Frank Breech
60%–65% of all breech presentations
Hips flexed, knees extended
Buttocks act as good dilating wedge
Incidence of cord prolapse ≈0.5%

Complete Breech
Least common; occurs in ≈5% of all breech presentations
Hips and knees flexed
Buttocks act as good dilating wedge
Incidence of cord prolapse is 5%–6%

Incomplete Breech
25%–35% of all breech presentations
Incomplete hip flexion, single or double footling
Poor wedge
Increased incidence of prolapsed cord (15%–18%)

BOX 176.7 Vaginal Breech Delivery

Actions to Do as Able
Monitor fetal heart rate.
Obtain a focused history.
Diagnose a breech lie.
Determine cervical dilation and station.
Obtain an ultrasound or plain radiographic study.
Evaluate for prolapsed cord if there is spontaneous rupture of membranes.
Perform an episiotomy.
Flex knees and sweep out legs.
Pull out a 10- to 15-cm loop of cord (room to work) after the umbilicus clears the perineum.
Use the bony pelvis as a means of holding the infant.
Keep face and abdomen away from the symphysis and use rotation to deliver the more accessible arm.
Perform the Mauriceau maneuver.

Actions to Avoid
Inappropriate transfer with delivery en route
Misdiagnosis of cervical dilation
Iatrogenic rupture of membranes (cord prolapse)
Moving of patients or leaving them unmonitored
Traction on the fetus during delivery
Grasping of the fetus by the waist, causing abdominal organ injury
Arm entrapment over head
Neck hyperextension

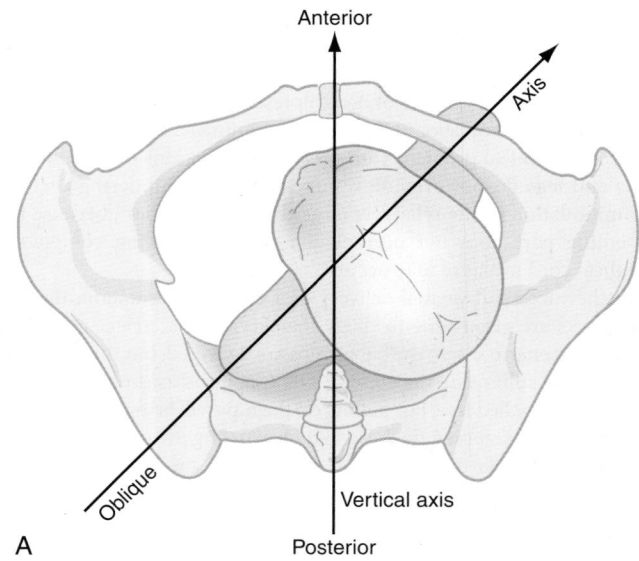

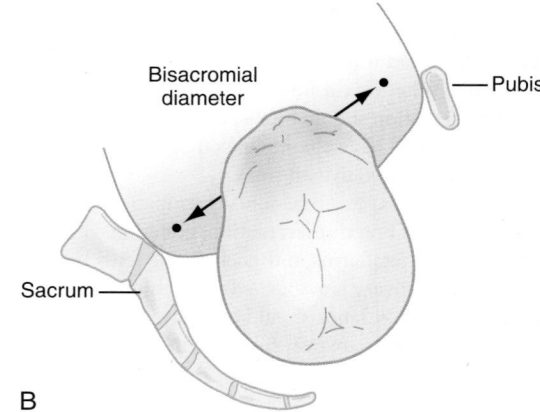

Fig. 176.9 (A) Normal delivery. As the fetal head rotates, the shoulders assume an oblique position and enter the pelvis one at a time. (B) Shoulder dystocia. Both shoulders attempt to clear the pelvis simultaneously, forcing the bisacromial diameter into the opening.

relationship of the shoulders to the birth canal and illustrates why the bisacromial diameter is an important element of fetal biometry.

Normally, the shoulders negotiate the maternal pelvis in sequential fashion, anterior shoulder first. With shoulder dystocia, both shoulders attempt to clear the maternal pelvis simultaneously. In addition to the turtle sign, examination often reveals that the fetal shoulders are on a vertical axis, rather than oblique. These findings, in combination with an arrested delivery, confirm the diagnosis of shoulder dystocia.

Management

When shoulder dystocia becomes evident, knowledge of intrapartum delivery maneuvers can be lifesaving. Successful vaginal delivery is most likely when a directed sequential approach to each maneuver is used. A rapid resolution of shoulder dystocia is important to avoid fetal asphyxia and resultant central nervous system injury. Obstetric and neonatology assistance may improve the outcome, and aggressive attempts to obtain assistance are warranted.

Initial attempts to resolve shoulder dystocia involve increasing the anteroposterior diameter of the passage. An episiotomy may be used for fetal maneuvering by allowing access to the posterior shoulder. Anteriorly, draining the bladder with a Foley catheter can generate room.

The most important first step is to use the *McRoberts maneuver* (Fig. 176.10). Maternal leg flexion to a knee-chest position may disengage the anterior shoulder, allowing rapid vaginal delivery to follow. This maneuver "walks" the pubic symphysis over the anterior shoulder and flattens the sacrum, helping the fetus pass through the birth canal, one shoulder at a time. This method, although requiring very little effort, is often successful in alleviating shoulder dystocia.

If the McRoberts maneuver fails to free the anterior shoulder, the application of suprapubic pressure may accomplish this by forcing the anterior shoulder to slip beneath the pubis or posterior shoulder to retreat into the hollow of the sacrum. Digital pressure on the posterior shoulder (through the episiotomy) may help facilitate posterior shoulder retreat. The use of the McRoberts maneuver and suprapubic pressure resolve most cases of shoulder dystocia.

If delivery is still impossible, the next step is to attempt the *Rubin maneuver* (Fig. 176.11). The goal of this maneuver is to decrease the bisacromial diameter by pushing the most accessible shoulder toward the fetal chest. Often, both shoulders assume the same attitude, decreasing the bisacromial diameter and allowing delivery. Attempts to manipulate the shoulders for the Rubin maneuver may be transabdominal, through the introitus (anterior shoulder), or through the episiotomy (posterior shoulder).

If the shoulders remain undeliverable, the next step is to use *Wood corkscrew maneuver*. In this process, the impacted shoulders are released through rotation of the fetus 180 degrees. Fetal rotation is achieved by pushing the most accessible shoulder in toward the chest. The fetal axilla can be snared with a digit, or a hand can be slid in along the fetal spine to sweep the hips and generate rotation. Wood corkscrew maneuver is difficult to perform but should be attempted before reaching for an arm.

If the fetus remains trapped and several attempts have failed to yield delivery, consideration of delivery of an arm is appropriate. A hand is introduced along the posterior aspect of the posterior shoulder. The posterior arm is swept across the chest, bringing the fetal hand up to the chin. Attempts to splint the humerus may prevent fractures and brachial plexus injuries. The fetal hand is grasped and pulled out of the birth canal across the face, delivering the posterior shoulder.

The mnemonic HELPER (Box 176.8) is useful to keep these steps organized and facilitate a sequential approach which will successfully deliver almost all cases of shoulder dystocia.

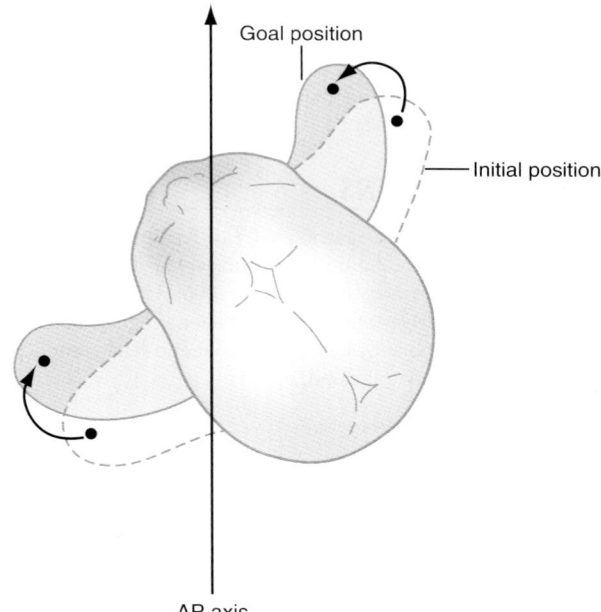

Fig. 176.11 Rubin maneuver decreases the bisacromial diameter. *AP,* Anteroposterior.

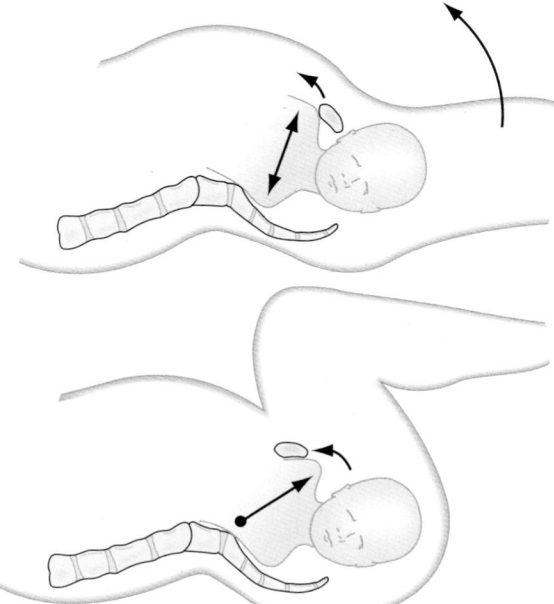

Fig. 176.10 McRoberts maneuver. *Top,* Bisacromial diameter pinned behind pubic symphysis. *Bottom,* Removing the maternal legs from the stirrups and putting the knees up to the chest act as a fulcrum to the pubic symphysis over the impacted anterior shoulder.

BOX 176.8 **HELPER Mnemonic for Shoulder Dystocia**
Help—obstetrics, neonatology, anesthesia
Episiotomy—generous, possibly even episioproctotomy
Legs flexed—McRobert maneuver
Pressure—suprapubic pressure, shoulder pressure
Enter vagina—Rubin maneuver or Wood maneuver
Remove posterior arm—Splint, sweep, grasp, and pull to extension.

Face, Brow, and Compound Presentations

Face and brow presentations yield a larger engaging aspect of the fetal head and predispose to labor arrest. Although these abnormal presentations can be diagnosed with ultrasonography or Leopold maneuvers, most are discovered during labor by vaginal examination. Approximately 50% are discovered during the second stage of labor.

The engaging diameter of the head in vertex position is approximately 0.8 cm less than a face presentation and 1.5 cm less than a brow presentation. Face presentations are described with the chin as a reference point (e.g., mentum anterior). Face presentation is managed expectantly. The obstetric adage—"if a face presentation is progressing, leave it alone"—is based on the fact that mentum anterior presentations usually deliver vaginally, and mentum transverse presentations frequently rotate to become mentum anterior. Brow presentations, occurring when the fetal head is partially flexed, also spontaneously convert to a vertex or face presentation in more than 50% of cases.

A persistent mentum posterior face and brow presentation cannot be delivered vaginally if the fetus is full term. The resultant labor arrest requires symphysiotomy or cesarean section. Prolongation of the second stage is the most common outcome of both these malpresentations at term. For the emergency clinician, this prolonged second stage may provide a window during which obstetric help may arrive.

Compound presentations are those in which an extremity enters the birth canal with the head or breech. Small and premature fetuses generally proceed to vaginal delivery without incident.

Labor arrest and umbilical cord prolapse are accepted indications for cesarean section in the setting of face, brow, and compound presentations. Manipulation of a compound presentation, including attempts to reduce the hand or arm, increases the rate of cord prolapse. Therefore, manipulation attempts are contraindicated. Cord prolapse rates are 10% to 20%, even without manipulation. Close monitoring and careful examination are indicated.

MULTIPLE GESTATIONS

Due to the increasing use and availability of fertility treatments, the incidence of multiple gestation pregnancies has been increasing. In 2013, twin deliveries accounted for 34/1000 births in the United States. Because multiple gestation deliveries have a higher incidence of preterm labor and low birth weights, maternal and fetal complication rates are correspondingly increased.

Diagnostic Testing

Most women with multiple gestations have the situation identified well before the third trimester. In patients who have had little or no prenatal care, bedside ultrasonography allows for a rapid diagnosis. The stages of labor for twins and other multiple gestations are similar to the stages for a singleton. Of importance to the emergency clinician is a relatively short latent phase of labor, with rapid progression to the active phase. The active phase is usually longer, however, and may allow time for obstetric assistance to arrive.

Vertex twin A and vertex twin B occur in approximately 42% of deliveries. One of the twins presents in a nonvertex position in approximately 35% to 40% of cases.[3]

Management

The presentation of twins is a key determinant for the safety of vaginal delivery. Twins who are vertex-vertex can be delivered vaginally, barring any other obstetric complication. If twin B is nonvertex, many obstetricians recommend cesarean section to prevent delivery-related complications for twin B. External cephalic version and breech extraction are possible maneuvers to facilitate precipitous vaginal delivery. Generally, if twin A is nonvertex, cesarean section is preferred. In such cases, efforts should be made to delay delivery until an operative approach can be used. Proceeding vaginally can result in the interlocking of twins, associated with a high mortality.

The interval between the delivery of twin A and twin B is variable. In most cases, twin B delivers in minutes. When twin B does not follow rapidly, in utero assessment is important to document fetal well-being. If fetal heart tracings are reassuring, the delivery of twin B (especially nonvertex) should not be hastened. Repeated ultrasonographic evaluation may also be used to confirm twin B's presentation and well-being.

After every ED delivery, particularly deliveries that are precipitous or that occur in the out-of-hospital setting, the mother should be examined for the possibility of twins. Ongoing labor may be confused with postpartum cramping, only to have twin B and all the potential complications surprise the emergency clinician. This is particularly relevant for women with inadequate prenatal care and low-birth-weight infants.

UMBILICAL CORD-RELATED EMERGENCIES

Umbilical cord–related complications can occur in normal and abnormal deliveries. Immediate intervention is required to prevent fetal morbidity and mortality. The spectrum of cord-related emergencies includes prolapsed cord, nuchal loops of the umbilical cord, body coils, cord knots, and entangled cords in monoamniotic twins. The cord length is believed to be proportional to fetal activity in utero during the first and second trimesters. Excess cord length increases the potential for umbilical cord complications of all types. Because the umbilical cord supplies the fetus with all its oxygen, interruption of cord circulation before establishment of fetal respiration is a life-threatening emergency. Fetal asphyxia caused by cord circulation compromise is potentially preventable with early recognition and intervention.

Umbilical Cord Prolapse

Clinical Features

Umbilical cord prolapse occurs when the umbilical cord precedes the fetal presenting part or when the presenting part does not fill the birth canal completely. Most cases of cord prolapse are unexpected and develop during the second stage of labor.

Cord prolapse has a variable rate of association with different fetal presentations. Compound, shoulder, and breech presentations yield gaps and a relatively poor dilating wedge. Table 176.3 summarizes the rates of umbilical cord prolapse with various fetal presentations. Malpresentations account for 50% of all cord prolapse cases and the prolapsed cord itself may be the first indication of a malpresentation. The reported incidence of cord prolapse ranges from 1.4 to 6.2/1000 deliveries, and associated perinatal mortality is estimated to be just below 10%.[4]

TABLE 176.3 Conditions Associated With Umbilical Cord Prolapse	
Presentation	**Incidence (%)**
Vertex	0.14
Breech	2.5–3.0
Frank breech	0.4
Complete breech	5
Incomplete breech	10
Shoulder	5–10
Compound	10–20
Face or brow	Rare

Diagnostic Testing

Umbilical cord prolapse may be overt or occult, requiring a pelvic examination to reveal the umbilical cord lying beside the presenting part. The diagnosis may also be made with Doppler ultrasonography. In most cases, the diagnosis is obvious, and the cord is encountered at the perineum or introitus.

Management

When a prolapsed cord occurs with a viable infant, cesarean section is the delivery method of choice. If surgical delivery is available, maneuvers to preserve umbilical circulation should be instituted immediately. The mother is placed in the knee-chest position, with the bed in the Trendelenburg position, and instructed to refrain from pushing to avoid further compression of the cord. The presenting part is then manually elevated off the cord. Elevation is maintained until the baby can be delivered surgically. The time from prolapse to surgical intervention is an important factor in fetal outcome. Perinatal mortality rates are higher for out-of-hospital cases versus those within a monitored setting, and outcomes correlate with time from diagnosis to delivery.

If timely surgical delivery cannot be performed, funic reduction—manual replacement of the cord into the uterus—and rapid vaginal delivery may be necessary. The same maneuvers to decrease cord compression should be used, pushing gently on the cord in a retrograde fashion, above the presenting part. Manipulation and cord trauma should be kept to a minimum because resultant vasospasm can cause fetal hypoxia. After funic reduction, the development of umbilical cord body coils or nuchal loops is common and should be anticipated.

Cord Entanglement

The umbilical cord can also become entangled with itself, spontaneously knotting. Umbilical cord knots are related to intrauterine movements early in pregnancy. Approximately 5% of stillbirths are found to have knots that are believed to have caused fetal demise. Despite this association, cord knots can persist without problems as long as perfusion is maintained.

Loose umbilical cord knots pulled tight at delivery may cause fetal distress. As with cord prolapse, this situation must be resolved quickly to prevent fetal asphyxia. Rapid delivery with avoidance of further cord traction optimizes fetal outcome. No specific interventions have been identified to deal with this problem.

Long umbilical cords are associated with true knots, as well as with entanglements and prolapse. Umbilical cord loops can be single or multiple and can occur around the neck or body. Because the fetal limbs are short and flexed in most presentations, they are rarely involved. Although generally benign, umbilical cord loops may result in fetal complications, such as nonreassuring fetal status and respiratory distress.

During delivery, loose nuchal cords should be reduced at the perineum. Loose body coils usually disentangle spontaneously. The reduction process may be aided by slipping them over the extremities or forward over the head. On occasion, loops are tight enough to impede delivery and cannot be reduced. The solution is to cut the clamped cord and deliver the infant rapidly. The high frequency of nuchal loops (one in five births) means that the emergency clinician should expect to encounter this problem.

MATERNAL COMPLICATIONS OF LABOR AND DELIVERY

Maternal complications of labor and delivery include postpartum hemorrhage, uterine inversion and rupture, amniotic fluid embolism, and infections. Although some are managed medically, severe complications threaten the reproductive future and life of the mother, thereby requiring emergent surgical intervention.

Postpartum Hemorrhage
Clinical Features

Postpartum hemorrhage is the most common complication of labor and delivery. Defined as hemorrhage of more than 500 mL after vaginal delivery, it accounts for up to 11% of obstetric deaths.[5] Postpartum hemorrhage is divided into two categories; the primary category includes blood loss that occurs within the first 24 hours, and the secondary category is hemorrhage 24 hours to 6 weeks after delivery. Because of maternal adaptations during pregnancy, the patient may not show signs of shock until more than 1500 mL of volume has been lost.

Differential Diagnosis and Management

The differential diagnosis of primary postpartum hemorrhage includes uterine atony, genital tract trauma, retained placental tissue, and coagulopathies, or the "four Ts"—*t*one, *t*rauma, *t*issue, and *t*hrombin.

Uterine Atony. Accounting for 75% to 90% of cases, the most common cause of serious immediate postpartum hemorrhage is laxity of the uterus after delivery. Normally, postpartum bleeding from the placental implantation site is limited by contraction of the myometrium, constricting the spiral arteries. If the uterus does not contract, ongoing hemorrhage will occur. Predisposing factors include overdistention of the uterus (e.g., multiple gestations, fetal macrosomia, polyhydramnios), prolonged labor, chorioamnionitis, use of tocolytics, and general anesthesia with halogenated compounds. As a diagnosis of exclusion, a physical examination to rule out obstetric trauma and retained products of conception should be performed before the diagnosis is reached. On examination, the uterus is palpable as a soft boggy mass.

After other causes have been excluded, therapy to augment myometrial contractions is instituted to prevent further hemorrhage. A two-handed uterine massage may stimulate uterine contractions. One hand exerts pressure transabdominally while the other supports the uterus through the introitus. Administration of a uterotonic, such as oxytocin in conjunction with massage usually provides enough stimuli to control bleeding. We recommend 10 units IM following the delivery of the placenta. Intravenous options include oxytocin 5 to 10 units initially followed by an infusion of 10 units/hr to a maximum of 40 units total. Blood is ideally typed, cross-matched, and available for resuscitation should these measures fail, with unmatched O negative blood used in true emergencies

Maternal Birth Trauma. Maternal birth trauma is the second most common cause of postpartum hemorrhage, accounting for up to 20% of cases. Associated factors include uncontrolled delivery, macrosomia, episiotomy, nulliparity, maternal coagulopathy, operative delivery, prolonged second stage of labor, preeclampsia, and malpresentation. Tears and lacerations may involve the perineum, rectum, cervix, vagina, vulva, and urethra. Blood vessels beneath the vulvar or vaginal epithelium can also be injured without frank hemorrhage, resulting in the formation of large contained hematomas. These hematomas may go unrecognized for hours, gradually enlarging and possibly resulting in hemorrhagic shock. Delayed postpartum hemorrhage at these sites can also occur and is often a diagnostic challenge. The physical examination may reveal uterine displacement (lateral or cephalad), and confirmation with ultrasound is helpful in stable patients. Management, decided in conjunction with specialists, may be expectant, involve bedside repair with absorbable suture, or require vascular embolization or surgical intervention, depending on the severity of clinical presentation.

Tears are classified by depth. First-degree tears involve the perineal skin and vaginal mucous membranes only. Second-degree tears extend through the skin into the fascia and muscles of the perineal body. Third-degree tears extend into the anal sphincter, whereas fourth-degree tears extend through all layers, including the rectal mucosa. Third- and fourth-degree tears should be repaired by an obstetrician in the operating room.

Retained Products of Conception. Approximately 10% of postpartum hemorrhage cases are due to retained placental tissue. Normally, the plane of cleavage between the zona basalis and zona spongiosa results in a clean separation of the placenta from the uterus. When this occurs, the placental tissue delivers as a single unit, without evidence of fragmentation. Any placental defect or evidence of accessory placental tissue may signify a retained cotyledon (part of the embryo). Retained fragments prevent myometrial constriction and result in hemorrhage. Aggressive traction on the placenta during stage 3 of labor can result in retained products of conception, which may cause immediate or delayed postpartum hemorrhage. Ultrasound may reveal an expanded endometrium or solid echogenic mass within the uterus, providing evidence of retention.

Treatment requires removal of the remnant placental tissue. Digital uterine exploration with blunt dissection of the fragments from the myometrium will also facilitate myometrial contractions. Abnormally adherent tissue will not be freed by this maneuver.

The terms *placenta accreta*, *placenta increta*, and *placenta percreta* describe various degrees of abnormal placental attachment to the uterus. In placenta accreta, the placenta adheres to the myometrium without invading the decidua basalis. In placenta increta, the villi extend into the myometrium, and in placenta percreta the placenta penetrates the full thickness of the myometrium.

The current incidence of placenta accreta is approximately 3/1000 deliveries, a relative increase from past decades. Associated risk factors include multiparity, prior cesarean sections, placenta previa, previous curettage, and uterine anomalies.

Coagulopathies. All women with postpartum hemorrhage should receive tranexamic acid (1 g IV) and should also be evaluated for disseminated intravascular coagulation (DIC). DIC can occur as a consequence of placental abruption, eclampsia, amniotic fluid embolism, postpartum infections, and dilution of clotting factors caused by aggressive volume resuscitation. Also, retained products of conception and dead fetal tissue contain excess thromboplastin, which can precipitate DIC. As with DIC from nonobstetric causes, bleeding is associated with hypofibrinogenemia, thrombocytopenia, and elevated levels of fibrin split products and D-dimer.

Appropriate management entails hemodynamic support and correction of coagulopathies. Recent investigations have reported the successful use of recombinant factor VIIa for severe cases of postpartum hemorrhage.

Uterine Exploration and Removal of the Placenta. In the presence of ongoing hemorrhage and retained products of conception, attempts to remove the placenta manually are indicated. The procedure entails risk of infection, perforation, and increased hemorrhage but may be the most expeditious way to control bleeding. Before beginning, the patient is placed on a monitor, vascular access is established, and blood products are secured. Also, a Foley catheter may be placed to reduce bladder distention and monitor urinary output. The umbilical cord is traced through the cervical os to the placenta, allowing the identification of a placental margin. The placental membranes are digitally perforated, and the placenta is gradually divided from the myometrium. After removal of the placenta, the uterus is explored for retained cotyledons. Removal of fragments that are still present may require curettage of the uterine cavity by an obstetrician. Placenta accreta, percreta, and increta may be diagnosed in this way because they are not digitally dissectible.

Once it is emptied, the uterus should be stimulated to contract with uterine massage, oxytocin, and prostaglandins. Prophylactic antibiotic administration at the time of manual placenta extraction has been debated, but is not supported by current evidence.[6]

Pelvic Vessel Embolization. Pelvic bleeding postpartum can be difficult to control. Hysterectomy as a solution results in infertility and brings with it all the complications of general anesthesia and major surgery. Embolization of bleeding vessels by an interventional radiologist is another option with reported success rates of 95% to 100%. The procedure does not require an anesthesiologist, operating room, or obstetrician and may be readily available on an emergent basis. Common sites of bleeding include the uterine artery, pudendal artery, and hypogastric artery. Because only the smallest involved branches are embolized, and recanalization usually occurs, future reproductive capability is generally preserved.

Uterine Packing. When uterine bleeding is severe and uncontrolled, and embolization or hysterectomy are not available, uterine packing may be used to tamponade the bleeding vessels. The procedure has limited morbidity and can be accomplished by inserting sterile gauze or a foley catheter into the uterine cavity.[7]

Opponents of packing point out that an atonic uterus may accommodate a large volume of packing without effective tamponade. Packing may also increase the risk of postpartum infection, even when prophylactic antibiotics are given. As with all uterine manipulation and instrumentation, some risk of perforation also exists. Nevertheless, when pelvic embolization and hysterectomy are not immediately available, uterine packing may be a lifesaving temporizing measure.

Uterotonic Agents. Although they are commonly applied on delivery of the placenta, uterotonic agents also have special application in the case of a postpartum hemorrhage. Uterotonics such as oxytocin and prostaglandins control bleeding by inducing myometrial contractions. Oxytocin, 10 units IM or IV, is recommended.

Hysterectomy. Rarely, hemorrhage continues, despite the interventions outlined. In the case of life-threatening obstetric bleeding, an emergency hysterectomy should be performed.

Uterine Inversion

Foundations

Uterine inversion, a serious complication of delivery that occurs during stage 4 of labor, complicates 1 in 2000 deliveries. The resultant postpartum hemorrhage can be severe and life-threatening, accounting for a maternal mortality rate of up to 15%. Uterine inversion complicates 1 in 2000 deliveries. Risk factors include excessive fundal pressure during delivery, forceful traction on the umbilical cord (especially in conjunction with a fundal placenta), placenta accreta, maternal congenital abnormalities of the uterus, use of magnesium sulfate in the antepartum period, and primiparity.

Clinical Features

The patient will complain of sudden, severe abdominal pain. The abdominal examination reveals tenderness and an absence of the uterine corpus, which is potentially visualized at the cervical os or bulging from the introitus. Profuse bleeding with hemodynamic instability can also occur. Ultrasound may assist in the diagnosis.

Management

Once uterine inversion is identified, the appropriate mobilization of resources should begin simultaneously with efforts to reestablish the correct anatomic position of the uterus. Initial management involves aggressive fluid resuscitation.

The highest likelihood for successful repositioning of the inverted uterus is immediately after inversion occurs. If the placenta is still adherent, it should not be removed until after repositioning. Removal of the placenta while the uterus is inverted is associated with excessive blood loss. The initial attempt to reposition the uterus should be to push the fundus upward through the introitus. Contraction of the cervical uterine segments can create a muscular ring, preventing repositioning. Therefore, all uterotonic agents should be withheld immediately on diagnosis of uterine inversion.

If initial attempts fail and a cervical ring develops, pharmacologic attempts to relax the uterus with sedation and tocolytics are indicated. Terbutaline (0.25 mg IV or SC) and magnesium sulfate (4–6 g IV over 15–20 min) have been used successfully to relax cervical rings. When the uterus has been repositioned, the muscle relaxants should be halted, and oxytocin and prostaglandin therapy restarted. Firm manual pressure through the introitus should be maintained until the cervical ring contracts. If all these measures fail, and surgical backup becomes available, halogenated anesthetics may be used to induce relaxation of the cervical rings, with or without an attempt at surgical repair. Once uterine inversion has resolved, an assessment must be made to screen for uterine perforation, adherent placenta, and vaginal lacerations.

Uterine Rupture

Foundations

Criticism of the high rate of cesarean delivery in the United States has led to advocacy of vaginal birth after cesarean (VBAC). The high success rate and relative safety of VBAC are countered partly by the risk of uterine rupture, which occurs in approximately 1% of VBAC deliveries following a single cesarean section.[8] The rate of rupture increases in women who have had multiple cesarean sections.

Clinical Features

Uterine rupture occurs late in pregnancy or as stage 1 of labor transitions to the active phase. Defined as a full-thickness uterine wall perforation, the severity of rupture ranges from simple scar dehiscence to complete fetal extrusion. It may be spontaneous but is most often linked to previous uterine surgery. Other risk factors for uterine rupture include multiple gestation, trauma, and prostaglandin administration. Minimal fetal extrusion results in a perinatal mortality rate of less than 1%, whereas complete extrusion results in a 10% to 20% mortality rate. Maternal death is rare, but significant hemorrhage complicates one-third of cases.

Diagnostic Testing

The diagnosis of uterine rupture may be difficult because pain is not always present. In fact, clinical presentation of uterine rupture ranges from abnormal fetal heart rate patterns to frank maternal hemorrhagic shock. Prolonged fetal heart rate deceleration, indicating fetal distress, is the most reliable sign of fetal extrusion. Ultrasound may reveal a protruding amniotic sac, hemoperitoneum, or the myometrial defect; however, good sensitivity data are lacking.

Management

If uterine rupture is suspected, delivery should be hastened to limit fetal hypoxia. Emergency cesarean section is the best method to speed delivery and repair the injury. ACOG guidelines for uterine rupture identify a 30-minute window of opportunity that maximizes fetal outcome. Note that uterotonic agents may exacerbate the rupture and are contraindicated.

Amniotic Fluid Embolism

Amniotic fluid embolism is a rare and catastrophic complication of labor and delivery. The incidence rate is estimated to be between 1 and 12/100,000 maternities. Although the mechanism is not well understood, it is thought to involve the spread of amniotic fluid through the maternal vasculature, activating a complement or anaphylactic cascade. Cesarean delivery, forceps- or vacuum-assisted delivery, uterine rupture, eclampsia, placenta previa, and placental abruption have been found to be associated with amniotic fluid embolism. The diagnosis is clinically evident during labor, during delivery, or within 48 hours of delivery. It is characterized by the sudden onset of hypoxia, coagulopathy or hemorrhage, seizure, fetal compromise, or cardiovascular collapse. DIC occurs in approximately 50% of cases, and maternal and fetal mortality rates are high. Treatment is generally supportive and may include assisted ventilation, central hemodynamic monitoring, vasopressors, and the administration of blood products.[9.]

Postpartum Venous Thromboembolism

Pregnancy increases the risk of venous thromboembolism five- to tenfold. The risk increase through pregnancy, but may actually be highest 3 to 6 weeks postpartum.[10] The diagnosis of pulmonary embolism in pregnancy has always been complicated, but recent clinical trials have suggested that an adjusted D-dimer can be used for otherwise low-risk patients.[11] The gold standard remains CT pulmonary angiogram; VQ scans are being performed increasingly less frequently, even in pregnancy. An in-depth discussion of thromboembolism can be found in Chapter 74.

Postpartum Endometritis

Puerperal infections affect 5% of all vaginal deliveries and 10% of all cesarean sections. Predisposing factors include operative delivery, prolonged rupture of membranes, lack of prenatal care, prolonged stage 2 labor, use of intrauterine monitoring, and frequent vaginal examinations. It is estimated that sepsis results in up to 15% of maternal deaths worldwide. Causative organisms for these infections include gram-positive cocci and gram-negative coliforms and, less commonly *Chlamydia* and *Mycoplasma* spp.

Endometritis is the most common puerperal infection, usually developing on the second or third day postpartum. Typically, the lochia has a foul odor, and the white blood cell count is elevated. Fever and abdominal pain indicate greater severity of infection, often warranting inpatient care and intravenous antibiotics. A coexistent surgical wound infection is often present. A search for retained products of conception is indicated, particularly if bleeding is present.

Treatment is empirical and is directed at gram-positive, gram-negative, and anaerobic organisms. We recommend a combination of clindamycin (900 mg IV Q8H) and an aminoglycoside (gentamicin 5 mg/kg Q24H). Most patients with postpartum endometritis require admission.

POSTPARTUM PROBLEMS

Peripartum Cardiomyopathy

For unclear reasons, the peripartum period is associated with the relatively sudden onset of cardiomyopathy in healthy women without evidence of prior cardiac disease. Estimates indicate that peripartum cardiomyopathy (PPCM) occurs in 1 of 2229 pregnancies; reported risk factors include advanced maternal age, preeclampsia, gestational hypertension, multiparity, and being African American. The cause is unknown.

Onset usually occurs days to weeks after delivery; symptoms range from mild fatigue to florid pulmonary edema. PPCM is often unrecognized in its milder form, leading to the consensus that the condition may be more prevalent than reported. Dyspnea on exertion, orthopnea, and fatigue may be easily misinterpreted as normal in the postpartum period, so vigilance in evaluating these symptoms is warranted.

Treatment includes the use of diuretics, vasodilators, and oxygen. Angiotensin-converting enzyme inhibitors are contraindicated if

PPCM occurs during the last month of pregnancy owing to teratogenicity but should be considered a mainstay of treatment postpartum. Hydralazine may be used before delivery to reduce afterload. Bromocriptine and pentoxifylline may also have roles in the treatment of PPCM. Cardiac function returns to normal in up to 30% of patients with PPCM during the following 6 months. Complications result in a mortality rate of approximately 15% worldwide. An in-depth discussion of cardiopathy can be found in Chapter 68.

Postpartum Depression

Considered underdiagnosed, postpartum depression is estimated to affect 10% to 15% of new mothers. Although often self-limited, the condition has important consequences for the mother, infant, and family. Risk factors include previously diagnosed depression, inadequate spousal support, adverse socioeconomic factors, life stressors, and emergency delivery.

Clinical Features

Postpartum depression patients present similarly to those with other major depressive disorders. Symptoms include depressed mood, anhedonia, loss of appetite, insomnia, fatigue, decreased concentration, feelings of guilt and worthlessness, and suicidal ideation. Most women with postpartum depression do not have vegetative signs or symptoms. Symptoms peak at 10 to 12 weeks postpartum, although some cases are diagnosed up to 1 year after delivery. When postpartum depression is unrecognized, these women are at high risk for suicide and may come to the ED with overdoses or other manifestations of a suicidal attempt.

Management

Early identification and referral are the key components of therapy. Dismissal of postpartum fatigue as normal, without consideration of the diagnosis of postpartum depression, can be disastrous. Not only does this condition contribute to marital discord, maternal risk for suicide, and even infanticide, but studies have shown that children of depressed mothers have an increased incidence of delayed cognitive, psychological, neurologic, and motor development. An in-depth discussion of depression can be found in Chapter 97.

The references for this chapter can be found online at ExpertConsult. com.

177

Trauma in Pregnancy

Valerie A. Dobiesz and Daniel W. Robinson

FOUNDATIONS

Trauma, both intentional and unintentional, occurs in up to 8% of all pregnancies and is the leading nonobstetric cause of maternal death.[1-3] The most common causes of injury in pregnancy are motor vehicle collisions (MVCs), interpersonal violence, and falls. Trauma in pregnancy increases the risk of spontaneous abortion, preterm rupture of membranes, preterm birth, uterine rupture, cesarean delivery, placental abruption, and stillbirth. Because some woman are not aware they are pregnant when they present to a trauma center, all women of reproductive potential should be screened for pregnancy.

Commonly used thresholds of fetal viability are an estimated gestational age between 22 and 24 weeks or an estimated fetal weight of 500 gr. Only viable fetuses are monitored, because no obstetric intervention will alter the outcome with a previable fetus. Counseling on proper seatbelt and alcohol/drug use as well as screening for interpersonal violence may help to reduce the morbidity and mortality rates for pregnant patients.[4] Although the essential principles of trauma management remain unchanged in the pregnant patient, there are special considerations in the management of these patients due to the gravid uterus altering the pattern of injury, and changes in physiology and anatomy that affect multiple organ systems. Although there are two lives involved, maternal life takes priority and fetal outcomes are directly correlated with early and rapid maternal resuscitation.[5]

Anatomic Changes in Pregnancy

The uterus remains an intrapelvic organ until approximately the 12th week of gestation. It reaches the umbilicus by 20 weeks and the costal margins by 34 to 36 weeks. At term, the uterus has often enlarged by 30 cm and has increased fifteen-fold in weight, which alters the normal anatomic location and function of multiple structures. The diaphragm progressively rises in pregnancy with compensatory flaring of the ribs, which may predispose to pneumothorax and a faster progression to tension pneumothorax. A thoracostomy done in the third trimester requires that the chest tube be placed one or two interspaces higher than the usual fifth interspace site to allow for diaphragm elevation.[6]

Abdominal viscera are pushed upward by the enlarging uterus and can alter the location of perceived pain. The gravid uterus itself tends to protect abdominal organs from trauma but substantially increases the likelihood of bowel injury from penetrating trauma to the upper abdomen. Conversely, the upward displacement of the bowel makes it less susceptible to blunt trauma. The stretching of the abdominal wall as pregnancy nears term modifies the normal response to peritoneal irritation (blunting of muscle guarding and rebound), potentially underestimating the extent and severity of maternal trauma despite intra-abdominal bleeding and organ injury.

In the first trimester, the bony pelvis shields the uterus and bladder. After the third month, these structures rise out of the pelvis and become vulnerable to direct injury. Both organs become hyperemic during pregnancy, and injury may lead to a marked increase in blood loss compared with similar injury in a nonpregnant patient. Ureteral dilation secondary to smooth muscle relaxation or from compression by the gravid uterus is often found on imaging studies but is not necessarily pathologic. The ligaments of the symphysis pubis and sacroiliac joints are loosened during pregnancy. As a result, a baseline diastasis of the pubic symphysis may exist that can be mistaken for pelvic disruption on radiographic studies.

Physiologic Changes

Cardiovascular

The normal cardiovascular changes of pregnancy can alter the clinical presentation and may either mimic or mask the recognition of shock or exacerbate the effects of traumatic hemorrhage (Table 177.1). Blood pressure declines in the first trimester, levels out in the second trimester, and then returns to nonpregnant levels during the third trimester. The decline in systole is small, 2 to 4 mm Hg, whereas diastole falls 5 to 15 mm Hg. Heart rate increases in pregnancy but does not rise by more than 10 to 15 beats per minute above baseline (mean of approximately 90 beats/min).

TABLE 177.1   Hemodynamic Changes of Pregnancy (Mean Values)

Parameter	Nonpregnant	Trimester 1	Trimester 2	Trimester 3
Heart rate (beats/min)	70	78	82	85
Systolic blood pressure (mm Hg)	115	112	112	114
Diastolic blood pressure (mm Hg)	70	60	63	70
Cardiac output (L/min)	4.5	4.5	6	6
Central venous pressure (mm Hg)	9.0	7.5	4.0	3.8
Blood volume (mL)	4000	4200	5000	5600
Hematocrit without iron (%)	40	36	33	34
Hematocrit with iron (%)	40	36	34	36
White blood cells (cells/mm³)	7200	9100	9700	9800

Data from: de Swiet M. The cardiovascular system. In: Hytten F, Chamberlain G, eds. *Clinical Physiology in Obstetrics*. Oxford: Blackwell Scientific Publications; 1980: 3-42; Colditz RB, Josey WE. Central venous pressure in supine position during normal pregnancy. Comparative determinations during first, second and third trimesters. *Obstet Gynecol*. 1970;36:769; Letsky E. The haematological system. In: Hytten RF, Chamberlin G, eds. *Clinical Physiology in Obstetrics*. Oxford: Blackwell Scientific Publications; 1980: 43-78; and Cruikshank DP. Anatomic and physiologic alterations of pregnancy that modify the response to trauma. In: Buchsbaum HJ, ed. *Trauma in Pregnancy*. Philadelphia: WB Saunders; 1979: 21-39.

A major contributor to maternal hypotension is the supine hypotensive syndrome. After 20 weeks' gestation, the enlarging uterus has risen to the level of the inferior vena cava, resulting in compression when the mother is supine. Aortocaval obstruction diminishes cardiac preload, which can decrease cardiac output and systolic blood pressure. In late pregnancy, it is common for the inferior vena cava to become completely occluded when the pregnant patient is supine. Hemodynamic improvement occurs when compression is relieved. In determining whether observed hypotension is related to positioning, the pregnant woman can be tilted 15 to 30 degrees onto her left side, or if unable due to injuries, the uterus can be manually displaced to the left by using two hands in order to relieve compression on the inferior vena cava. Elevating the patient's legs will improve venous return. Inferior vena caval compression can also lower central venous pressure (CVP) in the last two trimesters.

Blood volume gradually increases during pregnancy, starting at 6 to 8 weeks' gestation, to as much as 45% above normal, peaking at 32 to 34 weeks' gestation. Blood volumes become increasingly larger for multigravidas and for twin, triplet, and quadruplet gestations. With this increased circulatory reserve, clinical signs of maternal hypotension from acute traumatic bleeding may be delayed. Up to 35% of circulating blood volume may be lost before an injured pregnant patient exhibits signs or symptoms of shock.[5] By the beginning of the second trimester and throughout the remainder of pregnancy, cardiac output is increased 40% to 6 L/min. Blood flow to the uterus increases from 60 mL/min before pregnancy to 600 mL/min at term. This hyperdynamic state is needed to maintain adequate oxygen delivery to the fetus. Because the mother's total circulating blood volume flows through the uterus every 8 to 11 minutes at term, this can be a major source of blood loss in injury.

By the third trimester, there is also marked venous congestion in the pelvis and lower extremities, increasing the potential for hemorrhage from both bony and soft tissue pelvic injuries. Compression of the lower abdominal venous system by the gravid uterus increases peripheral venous pressure and blood volume in the legs, creating the potential for brisk blood loss from leg wounds and can exacerbate bleeding from attempts at central venous catheter placement.

Pulmonary

The pregnant woman at term has a reduced oxygen reserve due to a reduction in functional residual capacity caused by diaphragm elevation and an increase in oxygen consumption related to the growing fetus, uterus, and placenta. Mean arterial oxygen tension drops by 29% in pregnant women at term during 60 seconds of apnea compared with 11% in nonpregnant women. Labor further accelerates this decline. In addition, minute ventilation and tidal volume increase, leading to hypocapnia. Therefore, a partial pressure of carbon dioxide in the arterial blood ($PaCO_2$) of 35 to 40 mm Hg may indicate inadequate ventilation and impending respiratory decompensation in the pregnant patient. Maternal hypoxia rapidly leads to fetal hypoxia, distress, and possibly demise. There are no contraindications to rapid sequence intubation during pregnancy. Bag-valve-mask ventilation is more difficult in the pregnant patient due to weight gain and obesity. The incidence of difficult or failed intubations in obstetric anesthesia is four times higher than in surgical nonobstetric patients. Pregnant patients are considered difficult airways with potential for rapid desaturation due to decreased oxygen reserves, increased oxygen demands, upper airway edema, mucosal friability, increased Mallampati scores with increasing gestational age, and increased risk of aspiration. It is recommended that the emergency clinician use a difficult airway algorithm, prepare equipment in advance including rescue devices, call for help early if available, and optimize a ramped, head up, or reverse Trendelenburg position to optimize preoxygenation and apneic oxygenation in all pregnant patients.

Gastrointestinal

Gastroesophageal sphincter tone and gastrointestinal motility are decreased in pregnancy, thus increasing the possibility of aspiration in patients with altered level of consciousness, such as during intubation. Early gastric decompression should be performed in these circumstances.

SPECIFIC DISORDERS

Blunt Trauma

Physical examination is unreliable in predicting adverse outcomes in the pregnant woman with blunt trauma.[7] Risk factors predictive of the onset of contractions or preterm labor include gestational age greater than 35 weeks, assaults, and pedestrian collisions. Fetal mortality can be as high as 40% after maternal trauma, with most likely causes of fetal death occurring from placental abruption, maternal shock, and maternal death, in order of decreasing incidence. Risk factors significantly predictive of fetal death include ejection, motorcycle and pedestrian collisions, maternal death, maternal tachycardia, abnormal fetal heart rate, lack of restraints, and an injury severity score greater than 9 (see Chapter 32).

Unbelted or improperly restrained pregnant women are twice as likely to experience excessive maternal bleeding and increased maternal death with fetal death being three times more likely to occur. For low- to moderate-severity collisions (constituting 95% of all MVCs), proper restraint use, with or without air bag deployment, generally leads to acceptable fetal outcomes. For high-severity collisions, even proper restraint does not improve fetal outcome.

Pregnant crash-test-dummy trials show that improper placement of the lap belt over the pregnant abdomen causes a threefold to fourfold increase in force transmission through the uterus. The lowest force transmission readings through the uterus occur when a three-point seat belt is used properly. For correct position, the lap belt should be placed under the gravid abdomen, snugly over the thighs, with the shoulder harness off to the side of the uterus, between the breasts and over the midline of the clavicle. Women who receive information on seat belt use during pregnancy from a health care provider are statistically more likely to use seat belts and to use them properly than uninformed controls.

Interpersonal Violence

Women experiencing abuse in the year before or during a pregnancy are 40% to 60% more likely than nonabused women to report high blood pressure, vaginal bleeding, severe nausea, kidney or urinary tract infections, and hospitalization during that pregnancy.[4] Abused pregnant women are more likely to deliver preterm, and children of abused pregnant women are more likely to be born underweight. Children born to abused mothers are more likely than other children to require intensive care at birth. Physicians detect only a minority of interpersonal violence cases in pregnant women, which supports the need for routine screening for interpersonal violence in this population.[4]

Falls

Falls become more prevalent after the 20th week of pregnancy and roughly 25% of pregnant women will fall at least once while pregnant. Protuberance of the abdomen, loosening of pelvic ligaments, strain on the lower back, and fatigability are contributory factors. In a given pregnancy, about 2% of pregnant women sustain repeated direct blows to the abdomen from repetitive falls. Although repeated falls often trigger premature contractions, they seldom result in immediate labor and delivery.

Penetrating Trauma

The gravid uterus affects the injury pattern seen with penetrating trauma to the upper abdomen with the probability of harm to the bowel, liver, or spleen at almost 100%. When the entry site is anterior and below the uterine fundus, visceral injuries are less likely. Although the enlarging uterus can act as a shield against intra-abdominal injuries in the mother, it makes the fetus more susceptible to injury. A high fetal death rate from penetrating trauma to the uterus has been reported and is lower for maternal injuries above the uterus.

Fetal Injury

There is a high risk of fetal loss in the pregnant trauma patient. Poor fetal outcome is predicted by maternal hypotension and acidosis, and a fetal heart rate less than 110 beats/min. When the mother sustains life-threatening injuries, there is a 40% chance of fetal demise, compared with a less than 2% chance in cases of non–life-threatening maternal injuries. Disseminated intravascular coagulation (DIC), which may be caused by placental products entering the maternal circulation, is a significant predictor of fetal mortality. The American College of Obstetrics and Gynecology recommends a minimum of 4 hours of cardiotocographic fetal monitoring after maternal trauma because monitoring is useful in predicting fetal outcome.

Fatal fetal injuries from blunt trauma are usually the result of intracranial hemorrhage and skull fractures secondary to fractured maternal pelvic bones striking the fetal skull as a result of vertex lie.[8] Pelvic and acetabular fractures during pregnancy are associated with a high maternal (9%) and a higher fetal (38%) mortality rate. Both gunshot wounds and stab wounds to the uterus produce substantial morbidity and mortality to the fetus.

Placental Injury

The leading cause of fetal death after blunt trauma is placental abruption.[1] Placental separation results when the inelastic placenta shears away from the elastic uterus during sudden deformation of the uterus. Because deceleration forces can be as damaging to the placenta as direct uterine trauma, abruption can occur with little or no external sign of injury to the abdominal wall. Placental abruption inhibits the flow of oxygen to the fetus and causes in utero carbon dioxide (CO_2) accumulation, resulting in hypoxia and acidosis that leads to fetal distress. Sustained uterine contractions induced by intrauterine hemorrhage also inhibit uterine blood flow, further contributing to fetal hypoxia.

The diagnosis of abruption is made clinically. Classic clinical findings of abruption are vaginal bleeding, abdominal cramps, uterine tenderness, maternal hypovolemia (up to 2 L of blood can accumulate in the gravid uterus), or a change in the fetal heart rate; but many cases of placental abruption after trauma present without vaginal bleeding.

The most sensitive indicator of placental abruption is fetal distress, which can be detected with prompt fetal monitoring. In clinical settings without continuous fetal monitoring capabilities intermittent monitoring of FHR (e.g., every 15 minutes) is recommended, but early transfer should be arranged to a facility with obstetric and neonatal services as the definitive treatment may be surgical. Increased frequency of contractions is associated with abruption. Transabdominal ultrasonography has poor sensitivity for detection of placental abruption (24% sensitivity; 96% specificity).[9] Placental abruption hematomas have a variable appearance on ultrasound including homogenous and heterogenous consistency, and can be either hypo-, hyper-, or isoechoic compared to the placenta depending on the extent and chronicity of bleeding. If the abruption bleeds externally, there may be an insufficient quantity to be detected sonographically. Even with significant intrauterine blood accumulation, accurate ultrasonographic diagnosis may be difficult because of placental position (i.e., posterior) and confounding uterine or placental structural conditions. An ultrasound is useful in clinical practice despite the poor sensitivity because it can help identify other causes of abdominal pain or vaginal bleeding in the setting of trauma.

Placental abruption is associated with an increased risk of stillbirth (after 20 weeks) and preterm delivery (before 37 weeks) even with minor abruption. The extent of placental separation is correlated with the rate of stillbirth. A trial of expectant management with ongoing maternal and fetal monitoring is appropriate when mother and fetus are stable and with partial placental abruptions of less than 25%. This usually applies to fetuses of less than 32 weeks' gestation in which the likelihood of morbidity and mortality associated with prematurity makes delivery management risky. Expectant care in stable patients may allow further fetal maturation and improved outcome. An immediate cesarean section is recommended in cases of fetal distress from further placental separation. After 32 weeks' gestation, the risk of further placental separation outweighs the benefits of further fetal maturation, so intervention is indicated.

Women with placental abruption are more likely to have coagulopathies than those without abruption. The injured placenta can release thromboplastin into the maternal circulation, resulting in DIC, whereas the damaged uterus can disperse plasminogen activator and trigger fibrinolysis. The precipitation of DIC is directly related to the degree of placental separation. Severe clotting disorders rarely occur unless separation of the placenta is significant enough to result in fetal demise.

Uterine Injury

The most common obstetric complication caused by maternal trauma is uterine contractions. Myometrial and decidual cells, irritated by contusion or placental separation, release prostaglandins that stimulate uterine contractions. Progression to labor depends on the extent of uterine damage, the amount of prostaglandins released, and the gestational age of the pregnancy. The routine use of tocolytics for preterm labor is not recommended because most contractions stop spontaneously. Contractions that are not self-limited are often induced by some pathologic condition, such as underlying placental abruption, which is a contraindication to tocolytic therapy. Some studies describe this risk as relative and have used tocolysis successfully with careful evaluation and intensive monitoring to continue the pregnancy and enhance fetal maturity. The option to use tocolytics ends when cervical dilation reaches 4 cm or greater.

Traumatic uterine rupture is a rare event. It is most often caused by severe vehicular collisions in which pelvic fractures strike directly against the uterus. Uterine rupture may occur from stab wounds and gunshot injuries, but this is rare. Maternal shock, abdominal pain, easily palpable fetal anatomy caused by extrusion into the abdomen, and fetal demise are typical findings on examination. Diagnosing uterine rupture can be difficult. A fractured liver or spleen can produce similar signs and symptoms of peritoneal irritation, hemoperitoneum, and unstable vital signs. Optimal treatment, between suturing the tear or performing a hysterectomy, depends on the extent of uterus and uterine vessel tears and the importance of future childbearing.

DIAGNOSTIC TESTING

All women of childbearing potential presenting with trauma should be assessed for possible pregnancy.

Changes in Laboratory Values with Pregnancy

Increases in plasma volume greater than red blood cells cause a physiologic anemia of pregnancy (hematocrit 32% to 34% by the 32nd to 34th week). Despite the lower hematocrit, there is an overall increase in oxygen-carrying capacity because of an increased total red blood cell mass. Placental progesterone directly stimulates the medullary respiratory center, producing a lower $Paco_2$ (30 mm Hg) from the second trimester until term. The subsequent compensatory lowering of serum bicarbonate slightly reduces blood-buffering capacity during conditions of physiologic stress. A $Paco_2$ of 40 mm Hg in the latter half of pregnancy reflects inadequate ventilation and potential respiratory acidosis that could precipitate fetal distress.

Electrocardiographic changes include a left-axis shift averaging 15 degrees, caused by diaphragm elevation. Consequently, flattened T waves or Q waves in leads III and augmented voltage unipolar left limb lead may be seen (Fig. 177.1)

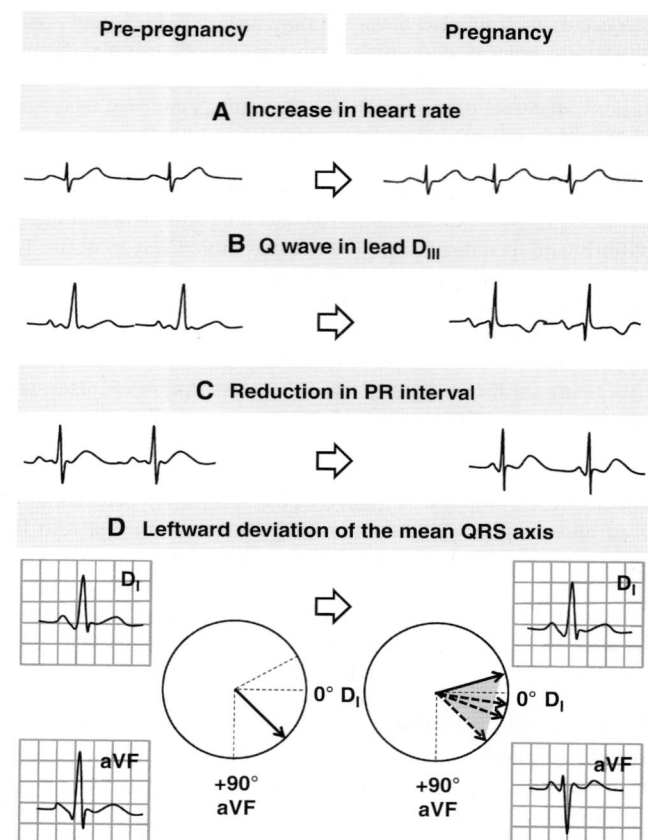

Fig. 177.1 EKG changes in pregnancy. (From: Angeli F, Angeli E, Verdecchia P. *Int J Mol Sci.* 2015;16(8):18454-18473; https://doi.org/10.3390/ijms160818454.)

Laboratory

Laboratory tests for a pregnant patient with trauma should include a complete blood count, basic electrolyte panel, urinalysis, blood type with Rh status, and coagulation studies including fibrinogen.[6] Patients who appear to be stable but have a low serum bicarbonate level may have occult maternal shock. Interpretation of bicarbonate results requires consideration of the physiologic changes that occur in the later stages of pregnancy as a result of respiratory alkalosis (see Chapter 173). Coagulation studies are important in directing management of patients with multisystem trauma or when the diagnosis of placental abruption is considered.

Kleihauer-Betke Test and Fetomaternal Hemorrhage

Fetomaternal hemorrhage (FMH), the transplacental bleeding of fetal blood into the normally separate maternal circulation, is a unique complication of pregnancy. MVCs, anterior placental location, and uterine tenderness are associated with an increased risk of FMH. Massive fetomaternal transplacental hemorrhage causes alloimmunization in Rh incompatibility but also endangers the fetus by causing severe fetal anemia, fetal distress, and possible exsanguination. ABO incompatibility causes less severe disease.

FMH most commonly occurs after 12 weeks' gestation, when the uterus rises above the pelvis and becomes susceptible to direct trauma.

The Kleihauer-Betke test quantifies the amount of FMH. Most laboratories screen for FMH of 5 mL or more, even though the amount of FMH sufficient to sensitize most Rh-negative women is much less than 5 mL. Therefore, it is advisable that all Rh-negative mothers who have a history of abdominal trauma receive one prophylactic dose of Rhesus immune globulin

(RhIG) within 72 hours of injury. Trauma patients at risk for massive FMH will have major injuries or abnormal obstetric findings, such as uterine tenderness, contractions, or vaginal bleeding. Rarely, the amount of FMH will exceed that covered by the maximum RhIG dose (300 μg). Because RhIG can effectively prevent Rh isoimmunization when administered as late as 72 hours after antigenic exposure, the results of the Kleihauer-Betke test are not immediately needed in the emergency department (ED).

Radiography

Adverse effects to the fetus are unlikely if radiation exposure is less than 50 mGy. Less than 1% of trauma patients are exposed to more than 30 mGy. Sensitivity to radiation is greatest during intrauterine development when the embryo undergoes organogenesis in weeks 2 to 15. However, the risk to the fetus of a 10-mGy exposure is thousands of times smaller than the spontaneous risks of malformations, abortions, or genetic disease. Intrauterine exposure to 50 mGy does not appear to cause a significant increase in congenital malformations, intrauterine growth retardation, or miscarriage but is associated with a 0.3% increased risk of childhood cancer and 2% risk of lifetime cancer. Pathologic conditions more readily appear with intrauterine radiation doses of 150 mGy or greater.

Providing information on radiation exposure from diagnostic radiographs is difficult. Fetal dose from computed tomography (CT) scans depends on the type of equipment used, the abdominal girth of the mother, and the fetal distance from the maternal skin. Diagnostic radiographic studies should be performed with regard for fetal protection, but necessary diagnostic studies of the traumatized pregnant patient should not be withheld out of concern for fetal radiation exposure.[10] Fetal irradiation should be minimized by limiting the scope of the examination and using technical means, such as shielding and collimation. Table 177.2 provides estimated radiation doses from various types of examinations.

Ultrasonography

Ultrasonography is the best modality for simultaneous assessment of the mother and fetus. It is useful in detecting major abdominal injury and establishing fetal well-being or demise, gestational age, and placental location. It obviates radiation risks, minimizes diagnostic delays, and provides high sensitivity for injury. The sensitivity of the focused assessment with sonography for trauma (FAST) examination in identifying intra-abdominal bleeding or pericardial bleeding is 61% to 83%, lower than the general population, but it has a specificity and negative predictive value of 99.7%.[11] Ultrasonography has low sensitivity (24%) but high specificity (96%) for placental abruption.[9] Limitations in accuracy include operator experience, patient obesity, the presence of subcutaneous air, and a history of multiple abdominal surgeries.[11]

Computed Tomography and Magnetic Resonance Imaging Scans

CT and, increasingly, magnetic resonance imaging (MRI) studies are used in evaluating abdominal trauma in pregnancy.[6] If ultrasonography is indeterminate and the patient's condition is stable, CT and MRI can identify specific organ damage. They are particularly useful in assessing penetrating wounds of the flank and back. CT can miss diaphragm and bowel injuries. Both of these studies carry the risk of moving the patient from the closely monitored environment of the ED to the radiography suite.

Radiation from CT is a concern in the pregnant trauma patient. However, with shielding, fetal exposure from head and chest CT scans can be kept below an acceptable 1-rad limit. CT of the abdomen can be performed with 4 mGy of exposure to the fetus. Abdomen and pelvic CT produces about 25 mGy of radiation to the fetus, which is well below the 50 mGy level, where a 2% increase in risk of cancer is seen without evidence of malformation to the fetus. Radiation exposure

TABLE 177.2 Estimated Fetal Radiation Dose From Conventional Radiographic and Computed Tomography Examination[21,22]

Imaging Study	Estimated Fetal Dose (mGy)[a]
Radiography	
Cervical spine (AP, lateral)	<0.001
Extremities	<0.001
Chest (PA, lateral)	0.0005–0.01
Thoracic spine	0.003
Abdomen (AP)	0.1–3.0
Lumbar spine (AP, lateral)	1–10
Computed Tomography	
Head or neck	0.001–0.01
Chest (routine)	0.01–0.66
Chest (pulmonary embolism protocol)	0.01–0.66
Abdomen	1.3–35
Pelvis	10–50
Abdomen and pelvis	13–25
CT angiography of the aorta	6.7–56
CT angiography of the coronary arteries	0.1–3
Nuclear Medicine	
Low-dose perfusion scintigraphy	0.1–0.5
V/Q scintigraphy	0.1–0.8
Myocardial perfusion with 99mTc-sestamibi	17
Myocardial perfusion with 99mTc-tetrofosmin	8.45

[a]The naturally occurring background radiation dose during pregnancy is 0.5 to 0.1 mGy.
AP, Anteroposterior; CT, computed tomography; PA, posteroanterior.
Data adapted from: Trada N, Dreizin D, et al. Imaging pregnant and lactating patients. Radiographics. 2015;35(6):1751-1765; Copel J, et al. Guidelines for diagnostic imaging during pregnancy and lactation. ACOG committee opinion number 723. Obstet Gynecol. 2017;130:e210-216.

ultimately depends on the patient, scanner, and technique used in performing the study (see Table 177.2).

When available, MRI is preferable to CT because it uses no radiation and has not been associated with significant fetal disease or disability, and it is more sensitive in diagnosing diaphragm and bowel injury.

SPECIAL PROCEDURES

Diagnostic Peritoneal Lavage

In unstable trauma patients with equivocal or negative findings on ultrasonography, diagnostic peritoneal lavage (DPL) may be considered in any trimester. It should be performed in conjunction with a trauma surgeon using an open technique above the uterus following placement of a nasogastric tube and Foley catheter. The gravid uterus, in the later trimesters, makes the procedure riskier and technically challenging.

MANAGEMENT

Management of the patient with multiple trauma is covered in Chapter 32. The following discussion focuses on the aspects of management unique to the pregnant patient.

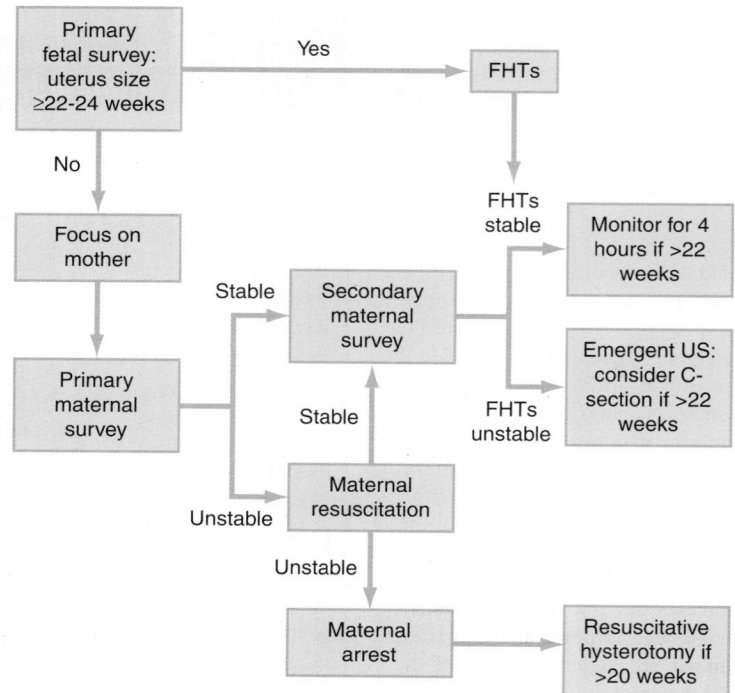

Fig. 177.2 Decision-making algorithm in emergency obstetric care. *C-section,* Cesarean section; *FHT,* fetal heart tone; *US,* ultrasonography.

Depending on the mechanism of trauma, maternal condition, and gestational age, the clinician should consider early notification or consultation with a trauma surgeon, obstetrician, neonatologist, or pediatrician (or all four) for a multidisciplinary approach. A fetal monitor, portable ultrasound, and neonatal resuscitation equipment should be immediately available. Tetanus toxoid and immune globulin have no detrimental effect on the fetus. The World Health Organization (WHO) specifically recommends vaccination during pregnancy. To prevent alloimmunization of a Rh-negative mother, administer one 50-µg dose of RhIG in the first trimester. It is sufficient because total fetal blood volume is only 4.2 mL by 12 weeks' gestation, and a 50 µg-dose covers 5 mL of bleeding. During the second and third trimesters, a 300-µg dose of RhIG is given, which protects against up to 30 mL of FMH. Beyond 16 weeks' gestation, the total fetal blood volume reaches 30 mL or more. Massive FMH likely exceeds the efficacy of one 300-µg dose of RhIG, so the Kleihauer-Betke test can be used to guide effective dosing.

Maternal Resuscitation

Primary Survey

The primary survey focuses on the mother. However, because two patients are present, it is reasonable to gather preliminary information about the age of the fetus at this time (Fig. 177.2).

Airway and Breathing. The general principles of airway management are discussed in Chapter 1. Oxygen therapy should be instituted early in the traumatized pregnant patient because she can quickly become hypoxic due to her reduced oxygen reserve and increased oxygen consumption. The fetus is vulnerable to any reduction in oxygen delivery. Supplemental oxygen is recommended throughout maternal resuscitation and evaluation with oxygenation saturation levels maintained above 95%.[6]

A secure airway enables proper oxygenation and negates the higher risk of aspiration in pregnancy. Rapid sequence intubation after preoxygenation of the pregnant patient is recommended. Data are limited on use of RSI agents during pregnancy but none have been consistently

associated with congenital malformations or adverse effects on the fetus. Mechanical ventilation settings need to be adjusted for increased tidal volumes and respiratory alkalosis, which is consistent with the physiologic $PaCO_2$ of 30 mm Hg in the last stage of pregnancy. No specific initial ventilation settings are recommended, but settings can be adjusted as clinically indicated and if the patient has ARDS clinicians can use the ARDS network guidelines.[12]

Circulation. Intravenous access with two large-bore catheters above the diaphragm is preferred. Maternal blood pressure and heart rate are not consistently reliable predictors of fetal and maternal hemodynamic stability. Due to an expanded circulating volume, the mother can hemorrhage without showing early signs of hypotension. Uterine blood flow is markedly reduced when maternal circulation is compromised. As a result, after an acute blood loss, uterine blood flow can be substantially decreased while maternal blood pressure remains normal. Consequently, the pregnant woman with borderline hemodynamic stability probably already has a jeopardized fetus. When traditional signs of shock appear, fetal compromise may be far advanced.

Fluid resuscitation with isotonic fluids should occur in all patients with suspected or observed significant blood loss. Type O-negative packed red blood cells are recommended for hemodynamically unstable trauma patients until type-specific blood products are available. Vasopressors are recommended only with refractory hypotension unresponsive to fluid resuscitation because of the adverse effect on uteroplacental perfusion.[6] A massive transfusion protocol should be initiated on all hemodynamically unstable patients in a 1 : 1 : 1 ratio of red blood cells, platelets, and plasma. Tranexamic acid is an antifibrinolytic agent used in trauma to reduce bleeding and mortality and should be administered within 3 hours of injury. Limited data are available on the safety of tranexamic acid in pregnancy but no adverse fetal events have been described. It is unknown if there is a mortality benefit with the use of tranexamic acid in pregnant trauma patients.[1,13]

Beyond 20 weeks' gestation, a left lateral tilt of 15 to 30 degrees or leftward manual displacement of the uterus using two hands is recommended to reduce compression on the inferior vena cava caused by the gravid uterus. A Foley catheter for measuring urine output provides further information on circulatory volume status.

With trauma in pregnancy, the primary survey is modified to assess uterine size and the presence of fetal heart tones if the patient is severely injured. Otherwise, this assessment belongs in the secondary survey. Uterine size, measured from the symphysis pubis to the fundus, is the quickest means of estimating gestational age. This distance in centimeters equals the gestational age in weeks (e.g., 24 cm = 24 weeks), which allows some early indication of fetal viability if delivery is necessary (Fig. 177.3). Usually, between 22 to 24 weeks is used as the cutoff point for fetal viability (Table 177.3). As a rough guide, the fetus is potentially viable when the dome of the uterus extends beyond the umbilicus. Fetal heart tones can be detected by auscultation at 20 weeks' gestation or by Doppler probe at 10 to 14 weeks. If either the uterus is less than 22 cm in size or fetal heart tones are absent, the pregnancy is probably too early to be viable, and treatment is directed solely at the mother.

Secondary Survey

The secondary survey involves a detailed examination of the patient but is also modified to gather additional information about the maternal abdomen and the fetus. Physical examination of the abdomen, frequently unreliable in the nonpregnant patient, is even more inaccurate

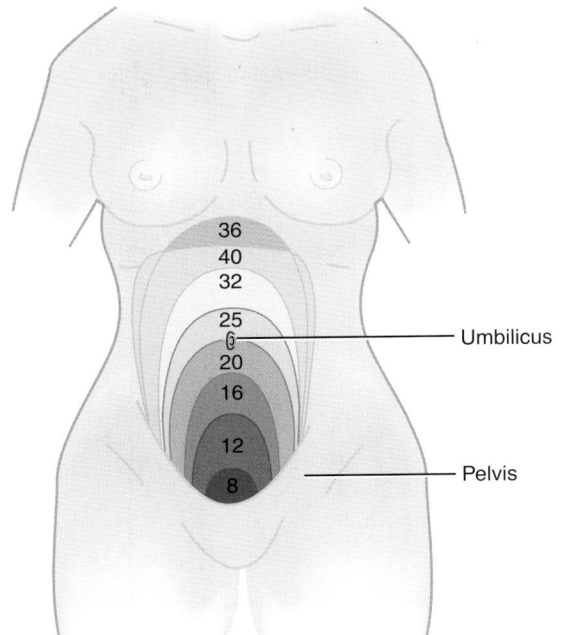

Fig. 177.3 Uterine size at different weeks of gestation. (From: Kravis TC, Warner CG, eds. *Emergency Medicine: A Comprehensive Review.* Rockville, MD: Aspen Publishers; 1979.)

with changing organ position, abdominal wall stretching in advancing pregnancy, and uterine contraction pains. Still, valuable information can be gathered about uterine tenderness, contraction frequency, and vaginal bleeding.

An external perineal examination should be performed. A sterile speculum examination is done in consultation with or by an obstetrician after placental previa has been ruled out by ultrasonography. A bimanual examination is avoided due to the risk of causing prelabor rupture of membranes or bleeding in cases of unidentified placenta previa. Vaginal bleeding suggests placental abruption, and a watery discharge suggests rupture of the membranes. Significant vaginal bleeding from intravaginal injuries can be temporized by packing with sterile moistened gauze. If the mechanism of injury is significant enough and the fetus is judged to be viable, early involvement of an obstetrician may enhance the fetal outcome.

Fetal Evaluation. Fetal evaluation in the secondary survey focuses on the fetal heart rate and detection of fetal movement. When the presence of fetal heart tones has been confirmed, intermittent monitoring of fetal heart rate is sufficient for the previable fetus. If the fetus is viable (i.e., 22 to 24 weeks or more), continuous external monitoring initiated quickly and maintained throughout all diagnostic and therapeutic procedures may be useful in directing management. Such monitoring can also benefit the mother, because fetal hemodynamics are more sensitive to decreases in maternal blood flow and oxygenation than are most measures of the mother. Fetal distress can be a sign of occult maternal distress. However, fetal distress and even demise can occur with seemingly minor maternal trauma. Signs of fetal distress include an abnormal baseline heart rate, decreased variability of heart rate, and fetal decelerations after contractions.

The normal fetal heart rate ranges from 120 to 160 beats/min; rates outside or trending toward these limits are ominous. Heart rate variability has two components. Beat-to-beat variability measures autonomic nervous function, whereas long-term variability indicates fetal activity. Heart rate variability increases with gestational age. The loss of beat-to-beat and long-term variability warns of fetal central nervous system depression and reduced fetal movement caused by fetal distress (Fig. 177.4).

Late decelerations are an indication of fetal hypoxia. These decelerations are relatively small in amplitude and occur after the peak or conclusion of a uterine contraction. By comparison, early decelerations are larger, occur with the contraction, and recover to baseline immediately after the contraction. Early decelerations may be vagally mediated when uterine contractions squeeze the fetal head, stretch the neck, or compress the umbilical cord. Variable decelerations are large, occur at any time, and are possibly caused by umbilical cord compression (Fig. 177.5).

Mother Stable, Fetus Stable

Minor trauma does not exempt the fetus from significant injury. It is estimated that up to 3% of all minor trauma results in fetal loss,

TABLE 177.3	**Fetal Viability in Trauma**	
Weeks of Gestation	**6-Month Survival (%)**	**Survival With No Severe Abnormalities (%)**
22	0	0
23	15	2
24	56	21
25	79	69

Data from: Morris JA Jr, et al. Infant survival after cesarean section for trauma. *Ann Surg.* 1996;223:481.

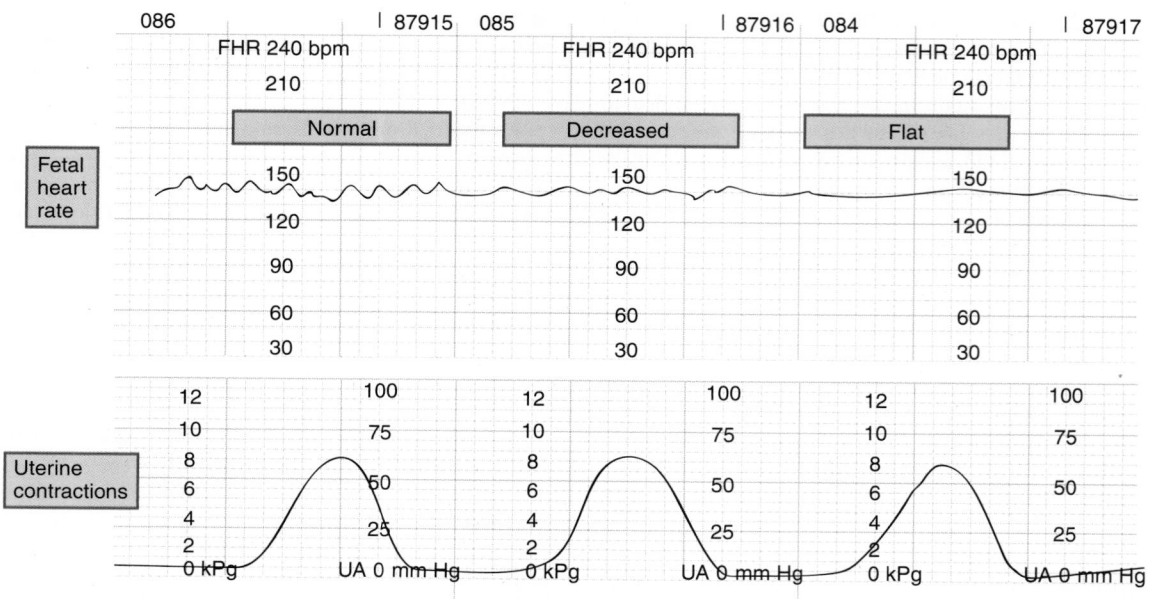

Fig. 177.4 Types of fetal heart rate variability. *bpm,* Beats per minute; *FHR,* fetal heart rate; *UA,* uterine activity.

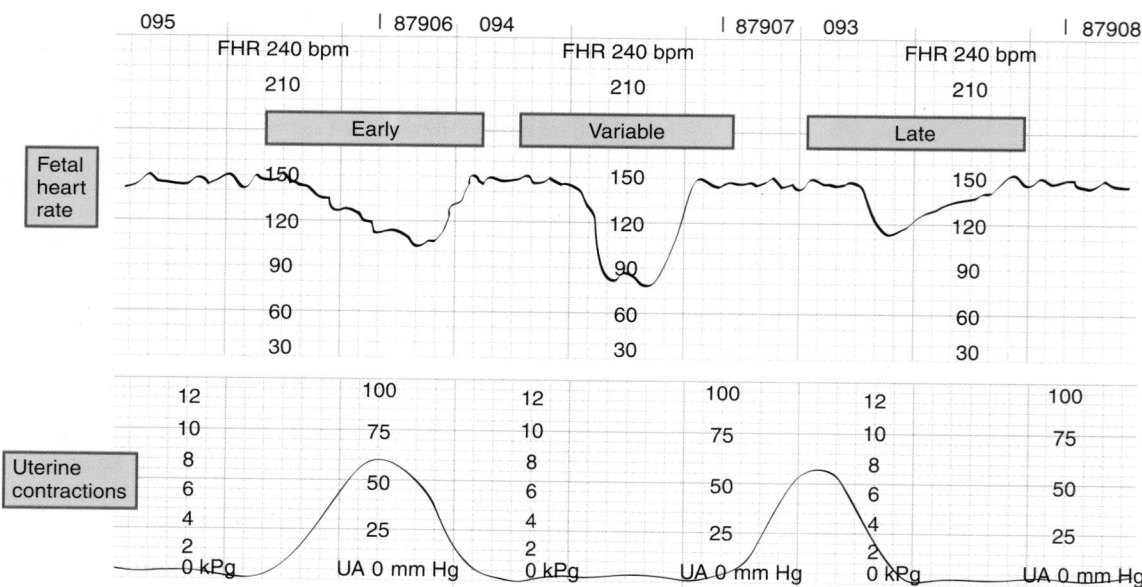

Fig. 177.5 Types of fetal heart rate decelerations. *bpm,* Beats per minute; *FHR,* fetal heart rate; *UA,* uterine activity.

typically from placental abruption. Therefore, once the traumatized mother is stabilized, the focus of care is directed toward the fetus. For the viable fetus (greater than 22 to 24 weeks' gestation), monitoring is the next step. Continuous monitoring maintained throughout all diagnostic and therapeutic actions is advisable. Because direct impact is not necessary for fetoplacental pathology to occur, the traumatized pregnant woman with no obvious abdominal injury still benefits from monitoring.

The recommended 4 hours of cardiotocographic observation of the viable fetus is extended to 24 hours if at any time during the first 4 hours there are more than three uterine contractions per hour, uterine tenderness persists, results on a fetal monitor strip are worrisome,

vaginal bleeding occurs, the membranes rupture, or any serious maternal injury is present. Most cases of placental abruption after maternal trauma are detected within the first 4 hours of monitoring.

On discharge from the hospital, the pregnant woman should be instructed to record fetal movements during the next week. If fewer than four movements per monitored hour are noted, the patient should see her obstetrician immediately and a nonstress test is warranted. The occurrence of preterm labor, membrane rupture, vaginal bleeding, or uterine pain also necessitates prompt reevaluation. Serial ultrasound and fetal heart rate tests on viable fetuses a few days after maternal trauma and periodically throughout the remaining portion of the pregnancy are helpful in monitoring fetal well-being.

Mother Stable, Fetus Unstable

Fetal death rates after maternal trauma are three to nine times higher than maternal death rates. If a viable fetus remains in distress despite optimization of maternal physiology, cesarean section should be considered.

Although fetal viability is first reached at 22 to 24 weeks, the ultimate determinant of the age of fetal viability is the level of neonatal care provided by the intensive care nursery unit in each hospital or accessible regional facility. Determining gestational age for fetuses of less than 29 weeks may be difficult. Emergency decisions on fetal viability are therefore made on the basis of the best ultrasonography and gestational age information available.

The presence of fetal heart tones is an important survival marker for fetuses about to undergo emergency cesarean section. The fetal survival rate is zero if there are no fetal heart tones present when emergency cesarean section commences. If fetal heart tones are present and the gestational age is 26 weeks or more, the infant survival rate may be as high as 75%.

Besides fetal distress, other reasons for a cesarean section include uterine rupture, placental rupture with significant vaginal bleeding, fetal malpresentation during preterm labor, and situations in which the uterus mechanically limits maternal repair. Fetal demise without any of the aforementioned conditions is not an indication for cesarean section, because most will pass spontaneously within 1 week.

Mother Unstable, Fetus Unstable

If the mother's condition is critical, primary repair of her wounds is the best course. This may apply even when the fetus is in distress, because a critically ill mother may not be able to withstand an additional operative procedure such as cesarean section, which prolongs laparotomy time and likely substantially increases blood loss. The best initial action on behalf of the fetus is early and rapid restoration of normal maternal physiology. If it is felt that the unstable mother can tolerate an emergency cesarean section, it should be considered for the distressed, viable fetus.

As with nonpregnant patients, operative intervention for blunt trauma and above-the-uterus stab wounds is dictated by clinical findings and diagnostic test results. Above-the-uterus intraperitoneal gunshot wounds require exploration. In situations of severe maternal hemorrhage, massive transfusion protocols should be initiated with fresh frozen plasma, platelets, and red blood cells in a 1:1:1 ratio to lower the rate of coagulopathy and improve survival. There is little evidence to support a definitive management strategy for penetrating trauma to the gravid uterus. In situations of a hemodynamically stable mother, expectant management has been recommended. However, no prospective study has verified this. Damage to the uterus alone can be quite devastating because of its increased circulation. Without exploration, it is impossible to know the occurrence, size, or depth of uterine penetration, and there are no guidelines indicating whether a uterine wound can be left unsutured without incurring an increased risk of infection or delayed uterine rupture. We recommend laparotomy or laparoscopy as the safest means of managing penetrating uterine wounds because missed maternal injuries can quickly compromise the fragile fetus.

Defibrillation

Electrical flow that bypasses the fetus has little effect on the pregnancy. Maternal elective and emergent cardioversion have been performed safely for cardiac dysrhythmias in all three stages of pregnancy. Energies up to 300 Joules on a monophasic defibrillator have been used without affecting the fetus or inducing preterm labor. Although the amount of energy reaching the fetal heart is thought to be small, it is advisable to monitor the fetal heart during maternal cardioversion.

Resuscitative Hysterotomy

Restoration of maternal and thus fetal circulation is the optimal goal with maternal hemodynamic instability. During maternal resuscitation, adequate oxygenation, fluid loading, and a 30-degree left tilting position or manual displacement of the gravid uterus is recommended to improve maternal circulation. If there is no response to advanced cardiac life support, a resuscitative hysterotomy, formerly known as a perimortem cesarean section, should be initiated by 4 minutes and completed by 5 minutes after the onset of maternal cardiac arrest with no return of spontaneous circulation (ROSC).[14-19]

In the event of maternal cardiopulmonary arrest, resuscitative hysterotomy is recommended to rapidly deliver the fetus to relieve aortocaval compression, improve hemodynamics, and optimize maternal and fetal survival.[20] A resuscitative hysterotomy is a rare but potentially lifesaving procedure for both the mother and neonate and is recommended only if uterine size exceeds the umbilicus (20 weeks' gestation or greater). Time since maternal circulation ceased is the critical factor in fetal outcome. Delivery increases venous return and cardiac output by 25% to 30% and leads to higher rates of ROSC and survival benefit for mother. Beyond 20 minutes, there is virtually never survival or favorable neurologic outcome for either mother or fetus.

The most experienced physician available should perform the procedure as cardiopulmonary resuscitation (CPR) is continuing. A midline vertical incision is made from the epigastrium to the symphysis pubis. The uterus is then entered with a midline vertical incision. If necessary, the placenta is incised to reach the fetus; once the fetus has been delivered, the cord is clamped and cut. Maternal revival after delivery of the fetus is reported due to relief of vena caval compression and improved hemodynamics.

DISPOSITION

The emergency clinician should consider the stability of the mother and the viability of the growing fetus when making management and disposition decisions. Any pregnant woman at 22 to 24 or more weeks of gestation who has sustained blunt trauma should undergo at least 4 hours of fetal monitoring, even if she appears well. In general, pregnant women who sustain minor trauma have a favorable pregnancy outcome. Other admission and operative criteria are similar for pregnant and nonpregnant trauma patients.

The references for this chapter can be found online at ExpertConsult. com.

Care of the Geriatric Patient

Denise Nassisi

FOUNDATIONS

Emergency department (ED) utilization for patients 65 and over is growing faster than for any other age group. The current growth in the population of older adults is unprecedented in the history of the world. In the United States approximately 10,000 of the "baby boomer" generation turn 65 years old each day, making those aged 65 years and older the fastest-growing segment of the population. By the year 2050, it is anticipated that they will comprise 21% of the population.

Older ED patients are a special population with unique needs and concerns. Altered homeostasis and decrease in physiologic reserve impacts their response to stressors and illness. Body composition changes predispose the older adult to dehydration and hypernatremia. Decreased subcutaneous fat places them at greater risk of hypothermia, and they are more at risk of developing hyperthermia when exposed to high ambient temperatures. The maximal heart rate achievable typically falls with age due to diminished responsiveness of the sympathetic nervous system, while resting heart rate may increase with age. Increases in heart rate may be blunted due to commonly prescribed medications. Reduced cardiac reserve predisposes to postural hypotension. Age-related decreases occur in hearing and vision that can markedly affect communication and functional status. Renal function, with creatinine clearance, declines with age. Changes in body composition and renal function result in pharmacokinetic and pharmacodynamic alterations that predispose older patients to medication adverse events. Polypharmacy is common in older patients, further increasing their risk of adverse drug reactions.

Emergency care should be approached in a holistic multidimensional manner with consideration for important confounding factors. Cognitive dysfunction, decreased functional reserve, frailty, mobility impairment, decreased hearing and decreased visual acuity can impact the ED evaluation and disposition decision making. The evaluation generally needs to be more comprehensive and extensive than those for younger patients. The average ED length of stay is longer for older adults who also have higher utilization of resources and rates of admission. They are more likely to have an emergent condition, higher morbidity and mortality, and are more likely to be misdiagnosed. Clinical presentations may be vague and nonspecific; "classic presentations" of disease are less likely in older patients. The differential diagnoses in the older adult are often expanded to included illnesses, such as mesenteric ischemia, aortic stenosis or giant cell (temporal) arteritis, that are not often seen in younger patients. Confounding chronic comorbidities, such as congestive heart failure, chronic obstructive pulmonary disease, and chronic kidney disease, add to the complexities of evaluation and treatment. Adverse effects of home medications should be considered as a possible cause of their ED visit, especially for presentations of falls or altered mental status.

Cognitive impairment may impact obtaining an accurate history, performing a diagnostic evaluation, and designing a treatment and disposition plan. Corroborating sources of information, especially from caregivers are often needed to obtain a full and accurate history. Cognitive impairment may make sending the patient home potentially more dangerous, particularly if the patient is in the ED unaccompanied. Attention to transitions of care with an evaluation of home and

BOX 178.1 Comprehensive Geriatric Assessment (CGA) Elements Important for ED Assessment

- Functional status
- Cognition
- Mood
- Comorbidities
- Polypharmacy and medications
- Fall risk
- Home situations and social supports

social supports is often needed. However, hospitalization poses its own risks in that it is associated with increased rates of delirium, nosocomial infections, iatrogenic complications, and adverse drug reactions. It is common for admitted older patients to have a loss of one or more of their basic activities of daily living (ADLs) with a permanent impairment occurring in up to 40% of these patients.

SPECIFIC ISSUES AND DISORDERS

Comprehensive Geriatric Assessment

The common multifactorial issues that affect older adults including chronic medical conditions, polypharmacy, cognitive problems, mobility and functional deficits, as well as psychosocial issues, are referred to as "geriatric syndromes." The Comprehensive Geriatric Assessment (CGA) (Box 178.1) is a multidisciplinary diagnostic and intervention process that identifies and addresses these issues that plague older adults.[1] This approach addresses the complex geriatric syndromes while keeping in mind the patient's goals of care, in an effort to improve the quality of life.

A complete CGA is time-consuming and not practical to be routinely performed for all older ED patients by busy emergency clinicians. However, identification of high-risk older adults may help target further evaluations and interventions and improve disposition planning. Widely disseminated geriatric ED guidelines recommend screening for high-risk patients.[2] CGA in the ED has been linked to reduced need for hospitalization without an increase in mortality, thus reducing exposure of the patient to the hazards of hospitalization. The use of CGA adapted to the ED is an active area of research that will facilitate safe and efficient care for the older adult.[3]

Cognitive Deficits: Delirium and Dementia

Older patients more often have cognitive, functional, and sensory impairments or depression that limit their ability to communicate. These conditions complicate the evaluation and management of older adults and may be underappreciated and underrecognized. Patients with cognitive dysfunction are less able to provide an accurate reason why they are in the ED and less able to comprehend discharge instructions. Patients and caregivers may have difficulties recalling all the details of a long and complex history or multiple medications; therefore, careful review of medical records and medication lists are important adjuncts to the history. Routine performance of a cognitive assessment in older patients is a geriatric quality indicator for EDs.

Delirium

Delirium, an acute confusional state with alterations in cognition and attention, occurs in 10% to 20% of older ED patients. Unfortunately, emergency clinicians miss recognizing delirium up to 75% of the time, especially with the hypoactive subtypes of delirium. There are several brief assessment tools available, including the well-established Confusion Assessment Method. The Delirium Triage Score with brief CAM (DTS and bCAM) is highly recommended for ED use (Fig. 178.1).

Delirium is generally caused by decreased neurologic reserve plus one or more acute precipitants, such as infection, metabolic abnormalities, and acute coronary syndromes. Delirium and dementia are sometimes difficult to distinguish from one another, but the distinction is important because the presence of delirium should lead to concern for a potentially life-threatening medical emergency. Inattention or the inability to sustain focus is a key feature of delirium. Patients with underlying dementia are at high risk for development of delirium and recognition of delirium is even more difficult in patients with dementia. Older ED patients with delirium have higher intensive care unit (ICU) admission, 30-day mortality and 30-day readmission rates.

Dementia

Studies that have universally screened older ED patients found rates of dementia of about 35%, mostly previously undiagnosed. *Dementia* is an umbrella term for chronic disorders causing impairment in two or more cognitive domains (i.e., memory loss, language, motor activity, object recognition, and disturbance of executive function). Although dementia would ideally be diagnosed by primary care physicians, this is not the norm. Detection of dementia by emergency clinicians allows a baseline cognitive status to be documented in the record and prompts patient and family to seek definitive evaluation for prognosis and planning. Most importantly, early recognition prompts additional history seeking from family and other collateral sources. Older adults with dementia are more likely to visit the ED and one recent study found that dementia is a predicator of 30-day ED revisits.[4]

Functional Decline, Vulnerability, and Frailty

Functional status is an important element in the evaluation of older ED patients and predicts short-term, repeat ED visits. Formal functional assessments, including ADLs and instrumental activities of daily living (IADLs), are important (Table 178.1) in that a sudden functional deterioration may be the only manifestation of an acute illness.

Vulnerability screening and risk assessment tools have been developed and utilized to sort out those elderly at highest risk in order to target them for further assessments and/or interventions. The Identification of Seniors at Risk (ISAR), Triage Risk Screening Tool (TRST) and the interRAI are vulnerability screening tools utilized in the ED setting. We recommend using the ISAR tool, which incorporates elements of cognitive impairment and functional decline together to estimate risk (Box 178.2). One study demonstrated that a high/positive ISAR score was associated with an increased risk of 30-day ED re-visits.[5]

Frailty

Older patients are a heterogeneous group and biologic age is not the same as chronologic age. Frailty is a geriatric syndrome or condition in which there is marked decrease in physiologic reserve and resilience. Frail patients have multidimensional failure involving several different organ systems. The stress of illness or injury places them at very high risk for adverse outcomes and mortality. Patients with frailty have higher resource utilization and are more likely to need placement in a skilled nursing facility. Frailty identification is used routinely in geriatric medicine and used for outcomes prediction in surgery and oncology. There is no gold standard for defining frailty, but several tools have been developed for clinical and research purposes.[6] The FRAIL Scale (Table 178.2) is a short 5-item screening instrument that requires no measurements. The Clinical Frailty Scale (Fig. 178.2) is a 9-point scale

Delirium Triage Screen (DTS)
Flow Sheet

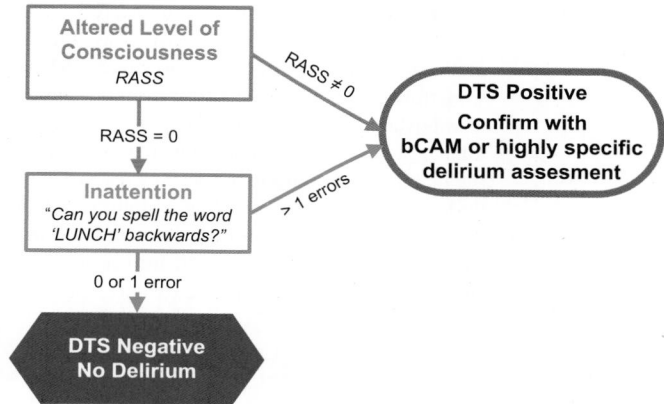

Instructions on using the Delirium Triage Screen

The Delirium Triage Screen (DTS) was developed to rapidly rule-out delirium and reduce the need for formal delirium assessments. It takes less than 20 seconds to perform and consists of two components:

1) Level of consciousness as measured by the Richmond Agitation Sedation Scale (RASS).
2) Inattention by spelling the word "LUNCH" backwards.

If the patient has a RASS of 0 (normal level of consciousness) and makes 0 or 1 errors on "LUNCH" backwards spelling test, then the DTS is considered negative. Because the DTS is 98% sensitive, delirium is ruled out in this case and no additional delirium testing is needed. If the patient has a RASS other than 0 (altered level of consciousness) or makes 2 or more errors on the "LUNCH" backwards spelling test, then the DTS is considered positive. Because the DTS is 55% specific, confirmatory testing is needed using the bCAM, 3D-CAM, CAM or 4AT to rule in delirium.

Han JH, Wilson A, Vasilevskis EE, Shintani A, Schnelle JF, Dittus RS, Graves AJ, Storrow AB, Shuster J, Ely EW. Diagnosing delirium in older emergency department patients: validity and reliability of the delirium triage screen and the brief confusion assessment method. *Ann Emerg Med.* 2013; 62(5):457-465.

A

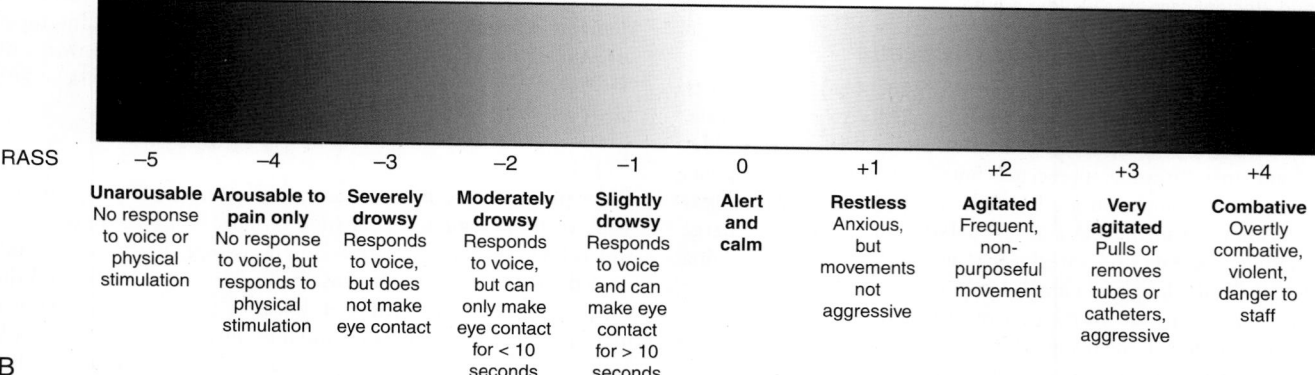

B

Figure 178.1 Delirium screen: combined (A) RASS, (B) DTS.

Continued

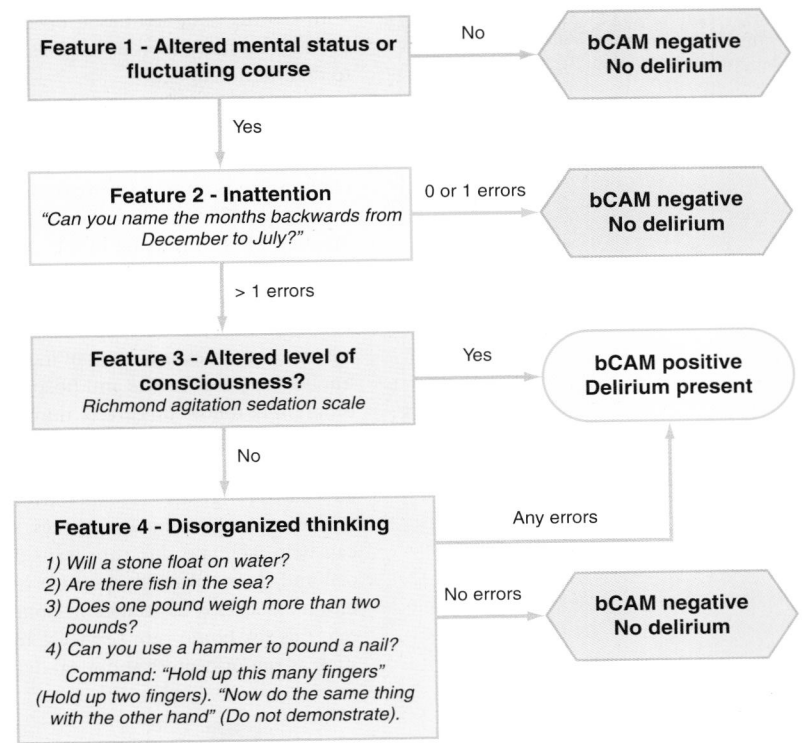

C

Figure 178.1 cont'd (C) bCAM. (A, From RASS, Richmond Agitation-Sedation Scale. Copyright 2012. Vanderbilt University; B, Han JH, Wilson A, Vasilevskis EE, et al. Diagnosing delirium in older emergency department patients: validity and reliability of the delirium triage screen and the brief confusion assessment method. *Ann Emerg Med.* 2013; 62(5):457-465. From Vanderbilt University, Nashville, TN. Copyright 2012; C, From Vanderbilt University, Nashville, TN. Copyright 2012; Adapted from: Ely EW, Inouye SK, Bernard GR, et al. Delirium in mechanically ventilated patients: validity and reliability of the confusion assessment method for the intensive care unit (CAM-ICU). *JAMA.* 2001;286(21):2703-2710; and Hospital Elder Life Program: Confusion assessment method (short CAM). https://help.agscocare.org/. © 2016. All rights reserved.)

TABLE 178.1	Functional Assessment	
Activities of Daily Living	**Instrumental Activities of Daily Living**
Bathing & grooming	Shopping
Getting dressed	Preparing meals
Transferring into/out of bed/chair	Housework
Maintaining continence	Laundry
Using the toilet	Using transportation
Eating	Using phone
	Managing medications
	Managing finances

Adapted from: Katz S, Ford AB, Moskowitz RW, Jackson BA, Jaffe MW. Studies of illness in the aged. The index of ADL: a standardized measure of biological and psychosocial function. *JAMA.* 21;185:914-9, 1963; Lawton MP, Brody EM. Assessment of older people: self-maintaining and instrumental activities of daily living. *Gerontologist.* 9(3):179-86,1969.

BOX 178.2 Identification of Seniors at Risk (ISAR) Tool

1. Before the illness or injury that brought you to the emergency department, did you need someone to help you on a regular basis? (yes)
2. Since the illness or injury that brought you to the emergency department, have you needed more help than usual to take care of yourself? (yes)
3. Have you been hospitalized for one or more nights during the past 6 months (excluding a stay in the emergency department)? (yes)
4. In general, do you see well? (no)
5. In general, do you have serious problems with your memory? (yes)
6. Do you take more than three different medications every day? (yes)
   Each "yes" response ("no" for question 4) counts as 1 point, for a total score ranging from 0 to 6. A patient is considered at high risk when the score is 2 or more.

Adapted from: McCusker J, Bellavance F, Cardin S, et al. Detection of older people at increased risk of adverse health outcomes after an emergency visit: the ISAR screening tool. *J Am Geriatr Soc.* 1999;47:1229-1237.

TABLE 178.2   FRAIL SCALE

F	Fatigue ("Have you felt fatigued? Most or all of the time over the past month?") Yes = 1, No = 0
R	Resistance ("Do you have difficulty climbing a flight of stairs?") Yes = 1, No = 0
A	Ambulation ("Do you have difficulty walking one block?") Yes = 1, No = 0
1	Illnesses ("Do you have any of these illnesses: hypertension, diabetes, cancer (other than a minor skin cancer), chronic lung disease, heart attack, congestive heart failure, angina, asthma, arthritis, stroke, and kidney disease?") Five or greater = 1, fewer than 5 = 0
L	Loss of weight ("Have you lost more than 5 percent of your weight in the past year?") Yes = 1, No ≠ 0
	Frail scale scores range from 0 to 5 (0 = best, 5 = worst) and represent frail (3 to 5), pre-frail (1 to 2), and robust (0) health status.

Data from: Morley JE, Malmstrom TK, Miller DK. A simple frailty questionnaire (FRAIL) predicts outcomes in middle aged African Americans. *J Nutr Health Aging.* 2012;16:601; and Woo J, Yu R, Wong M, et al. Frailty screening in the community using the FRAIL Scale. *J Am Med Dir Assoc.* 2015;16:412.

with scoring assigned based on clinical judgement. Both scales have been successfully used in the EDs, however further studies are needed to determine impact.

Goals of Care, Transitions of Care, and Palliative Care
Transitions in Care

Older patients undergo more transitions of care than younger patients. These transitions include home to ED, nursing home to ED, ED to inpatient, ED to nursing home, and ED to home. Transitions of care can be a risky period for patient safety; frail older patients are particularly vulnerable due to the complexity of their medical conditions and needs. Poor communication during transitions of care may result in adverse outcomes as a result of medication errors, adverse drug events, unnecessary treatments and hospitalizations, and lack of timely coordination of follow-up care. A number of groups, including the American College of Emergency Physicians, have identified management of transitions in care as a quality gap in emergency medicine and have advocated for greater vigilance around these transitions.

Depending on local resources, social work and/or case managers can help facilitate safe care transitions. They can identify psychosocial and financial needs, provide home safety assessments, transportation assistance, assistance in obtaining durable medical equipment, referrals for home care services, and access to community resources such as senior centers and meal delivery programs. Many transitional

CLINICAL FRAILTY SCALE

	1	VERY FIT	People who are robust, active, energetic and motivated. They tend to exercise regularly and are among the fittest for their age.
	2	FIT	People who have no active disease symptoms but are less fit than category 1. Often, they exercise or are very active occasionally, e.g., seasonally.
	3	MANAGING WELL	People whose medical problems are well controlled, even if occasionally symptomatic, but often are not regularly active beyond routine walking.
	4	LIVING WITH VERY MILD FRAILTY	Previously "vulnerable," this category marks early transition from complete independence. While not dependent on others for daily help, often symptoms limit activities. A common complaint is being "slowed up" and/or being tired during the day.
	5	LIVING WITH MILD FRAILTY	People who often have more evident slowing, and need help with high order instrumental activities of daily living (finances, transportation, heavy housework). Typically, mild frailty progressively impairs shopping and walking outside alone, meal preparation, medications and begins to restrict light housework.
	6	LIVING WITH MODERATE FRAILTY	People who need help with all outside activities and with keeping house. Inside, they often have problems with stairs and need help with bathing and might need minimal assistance (cuing, standby) with dressing.
	7	LIVING WITH SEVERE FRAILTY	Completely dependent for personal care, from whatever cause (physical or cognitive). Even so, they seem stable and not at high risk of dying (within ~6 months).
	8	LIVING WITH VERY SEVERE FRAILTY	Completely dependent for personal care and approaching end of life. Typically, they could not recover even from a minor illness.
	9	TERMINALLY ILL	Approaching the end of life. This category applies to people with a life expectancy <6 months, who are not otherwise living with severe frailty. (Many terminally ill people can still exercise until very close to death.)

SCORING FRAILTY IN PEOPLE WITH DEMENTIA

The degree of frailty generally corresponds to the degree of dementia. Common symptoms in mild dementia include forgetting the details of a recent event, though still remembering the event itself, repeating the same question/story and social withdrawal.

In moderate dementia, recent memory is very impaired, even though they seemingly can remember their past life events well. They can do personal care with prompting.

In severe dementia, they cannot do personal care without help.

In very severe dementia they are often bedfast. Many are virtually mute.

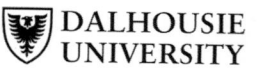

DALHOUSIE UNIVERSITY

Figure 178.2 The Clinical Frailty Scale. © 2007–2009. Version 1.2. All rights reserved. Geriatric Medicine Research, Dalhousie University, Halifax, Canada.

care models include rapid telephone follow-up post-ED discharge to reinforce adherence to instructions, identify needs, and assist with follow-up referrals. The use of a dedicated transitional care nurse was studied and found to be effective to reduce risk of inpatient admission and 30-day readmission.[7]

Goals of Care and Palliative Care

Older patients with advanced and end-stage disease frequently present to the ED with repeat visits. A patient-centered approach utilizing shared decision making to determine goals of care is especially important for older patients, with a balanced discussion on the benefits and harms of care.[8] Quality of life versus length of life preferences will vary by individual and also by the specifics of a particular situation.

For patients with advanced life-limiting disease, the role of the emergency clinician is a combination of curative care, such as infection management, and palliative care, with a focus on quality of life and symptom management. End-of-life frequent complaints include pain, dyspnea, anxiety, agitation and delirium, constipation, pruritus, excessive oral secretions, stomatitis and nausea, vomiting, and diarrhea. Prognostication in the ED setting is challenging, as is communication with patients and families regarding goals of care in an inherently fast-paced ED environment. However, these interventions are nonetheless necessary and the benefits of palliative care include improved patient satisfaction, reduced length of stay, cost savings, and improved outcomes.[9]

Nonspecific Complaints and Atypical Presentations

Unfortunately, the classic model of medical diagnosis, in which signs and symptoms are evaluated, tabulated, and formulated into a specific diagnosis, is not sufficient for older patients. Nonspecific complaints and atypical presentations are common in older patients, which makes arriving at a diagnosis challenging. Chief complaints such as generalized weakness, fatigue, or dizziness are consistently among the top presenting complaints for older ED patients. Sometimes patients complain that they "just don't feel well" and family or caregivers may complain that the patient "just isn't their normal self." Compounding the challenge is the fact that many patients who present with nonspecific complaints develop a serious condition within 30 days (e.g., infections, metabolic abnormalities, and malignancies.) One-third to one-half of older patients in the ED have atypical presentations of illness.[10]

Acute Coronary Syndrome

Cardiovascular heart disease is the leading cause of death in men and women older than 65 years. Older patients with acute coronary syndrome (ACS) have higher associated morbidity and mortality, and older age is an independent risk factor for mortality after both ST elevation myocardial infarction (STEMI) and non-STEMI. An accurate clinical assessment for older patients is needed, as well as an optimal therapeutic strategy, taking into consideration the patient's quality of life and goals of care.

The incidence of the "classic" symptoms of ACS diminishes with increasing age. Chest pain at presentation with STEMI occurs in only about 50% of patients who are 85 years or older. Atypical presentations of ACS occur more often in older patients who are more likely to present with dyspnea, syncope, diaphoresis, shoulder or back pain, abdominal pain, weakness, fatigue, and/or delirium. One-third of women older than 65 years with acute myocardial infarction present with abdominal pain alone. As a result, the diagnosis of ACS may be delayed, and older patients may present instead with delayed complications, such as acute congestive heart failure. Consideration should also be made to other conditions that are more prevalent in the elderly, including severe aortic stenosis, aortic dissection, and pulmonary embolism.

Acute heart failure at presentation occurs in nearly 50% of STEMI patients 85 years or older compared to only 1.7% of STEMI patients younger than 65 years. Myocardial ischemia impairs left ventricular relaxation, which leads to an increase in left ventricular end-diastolic pressure (LVEDP). This increased LVEDP, superimposed on age-related decreases in left ventricular compliance, frequently results in elevated pulmonary capillary wedge pressure and heart failure.

Current evidence supports an early invasive approach over conservative treatment for both non-STEMI and STEMI. American Heart Association (AHA) guidelines recommend no absolute age restrictions for revascularization therapy for non-STEMIs and STEMIs. However, older patients often do not receive as aggressive treatment, including early referral for cardiac catheterization, as their younger counterparts and are less likely to receive ACS care according to recommended guidelines.[11] The evidence to inform optimal care for elderly patients is limited. Despite the high prevalence of ACS and its higher morbidity and mortality in older patients, they were excluded and underrepresented in earlier randomized controlled trials of ACS. The After Eighty Study specifically targeted patients over 80 years of age with non-STEMI and unstable angina. The results demonstrated superior outcomes for an early invasive approach compared with conservative strategy for clinically stable octogenarians but were inconclusive for patients over 90 years of age.[12]

Syncope

Patients 65 and over with syncope are more likely to have a serious etiology than younger patients, with almost half of these patients ultimately being diagnosed with a cardiac condition, including dysrhythmias, valvular heart disease, acute coronary syndrome, and aortic dissection. Medication effect and results of polypharmacy (i.e., multiple drug interaction) is yet another concern.

In older patients, syncope should be considered as a possible etiology of any unexplained fall, and the elderly are more susceptible to serious injury. Amnesia may confound the evaluation. Vasovagal syncope in the elderly is less likely to have a prodrome. Orthostatic hypotension is more common in older patients due to reductions in baroreflex responsiveness, cardiac compliance, and attenuation of the vestibulosympathetic reflex.

Abdominal Pain

Older ED patients with acute abdominal pain are at increased risk of having a surgical condition and of dying. Presentations may be deceptively subtle, including the lack of rebound tenderness or guarding on abdominal palpation, despite serious intra-abdominal pathology. Etiologies of abdominal pain that are not intra-abdominal processes should also be considered in the differential diagnosis (e.g., myocardial ischemia or infarction, pneumonia, and herpes zoster).

Several factors in older patients that can complicate the ability to make a diagnosis based on the history and physical examination alone, include altered pain perception, aging effects on the immune system, medications that limit tachycardic response to stress, and decreased ability to mount a febrile response to infection. Additionally, sometimes older patients may present only with nonspecific generalized symptoms such as delirium, malaise, or dizziness when the cause is an acute abdominal condition. Laboratory values are frequently normal, despite the presence of surgical disease. There should be a low threshold for imaging, particularly computed tomography (CT).

Vascular disease increases with age and vascular emergencies remain some of the most time-sensitive and highly morbid causes of abdominal pain in the older patient. Abrupt onset symptoms are a red flag. Although the diagnosis of a ruptured abdominal aortic aneurysm

(AAA) may be fairly straightforward in the older patient who has abdominal pain, hypovolemic shock, and a pulsatile abdominal mass, most patients lack this triad at presentation. AAA is commonly misdiagnosed as acute renal colic, and any older patient presenting with symptoms of new-onset nephrolithiasis should have imaging to evaluate the aorta for AAA. Acute mesenteric ischemia is a disease of older adults and an important consideration in the differential diagnosis of abdominal pain. It is a more common etiology than appendicitis or AAA complications in patients over age 75.[13] Superior mesenteric artery occlusion is the most common cause of acute mesenteric ischemia. Risk factors for mesenteric ischemia include cardiac arrhythmias, atherosclerosis, and prothrombotic conditions such as infection.

Biliary tract disorders are the most common cause of abdominal pain in the older adult, with the incidence of gallstones increasing with age. Cholecystitis is the most common indication for abdominal surgery in the older patient. About one-third of older patients with cholecystitis have no fever or leukocytosis. Additionally, about one-third of older adults with acute cholecystitis will present with minimal abdominal pain and an absence of peritoneal signs. Due to the poor vascularity of the gallbladder, older patients are at increased risk of complications such as perforation and emphysematous cholecystitis. Additional complications seen more often in the elderly include bile stone ileus, pancreatitis and choledocholithiasis.

Appendicitis is the third most common indication for abdominal surgery in the older patient population. Older patients have a higher incidence of perforation and mortality due to much higher rates of delayed diagnoses and/or presentations. Appendicitis historically has been misdiagnosed half of the time in older adults because many patients lack fever, anorexia, or leukocytosis. One-quarter of older patients have no right lower quadrant pain at all.

Peptic ulcer disease (PUD) is more prevalent in older adults due to increased use of nonsteroidal antiinflammatory drugs and to increased *Helicobacter pylori* infections. Abdominal pain is lacking in approximately 30% of elderly patients with PUD. Complications of bleeding and perforation result in higher mortality rates in older patients. Diverticulitis and bowel obstructions are also more prevalent in older adults. Tumors are a cause of large bowel obstructions in older patients. Hernias should be considered in older patients with possible bowel obstruction, and they should be examined for hernias, especially those with significant cognitive deficits who may not realize or neglect to mention their presence.

Infections

As with other conditions, infections in the elderly often present atypically. Older patients with infection are less likely to have vital sign abnormalities of fever or tachycardia. Although fever of 38.0°C or higher is strongly associated with bacterial infection, the sensitivity is low with fever present in 12% to 25% with pneumonia and 20% with urinary tract infection (UTI).[14] Elevation in white blood cell count is similarly not a sensitive marker of infection with 20% to 45% of patients subsequently found to have bacteremia lacking leukocytosis. Older patients with pneumonia or UTI are less likely to have localizing symptoms. Further confounding the difficulty of diagnosing an

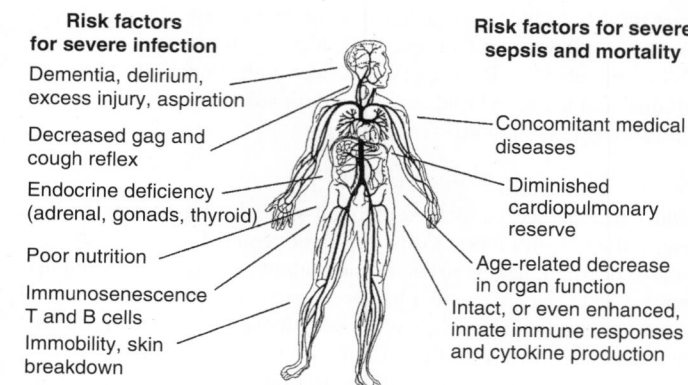

Risk factors for severe infection

Dementia, delirium, excess injury, aspiration

Decreased gag and cough reflex

Endocrine deficiency (adrenal, gonads, thyroid)

Poor nutrition

Immunosenescence T and B cells

Immobility, skin breakdown

Risk factors for severe sepsis and mortality

Concomitant medical diseases

Diminished cardiopulmonary reserve

Age-related decrease in organ function

Intact, or even enhanced, innate immune responses and cytokine production

Fig. 178.3 Predisposing factors for sepsis in older individuals. (From: Girard TD, Opal SM, Ely EW. Insights into sepsis in older patients: from epidemiology to evidence-based management. *Clin Infect Dis.* 2005;40:719-727.)

infection is that asymptomatic bacteriuria is common in older patients. Distinguishing asymptomatic bacteriuria from UTI is challenging especially in older cognitively impaired adults.

Older patients experience an increased incidence of severe infection and severe sepsis with advanced age. Mortality from sepsis approaches 40% for patients older than 85 years. Aging effects on immunity include a decline in cell-mediated immunity and antibody production. Older patients may also have multiple risk factors for sepsis (Fig. 178.3) including comorbid diseases, exposure to instrumentation, malnutrition, and institutionalization.

With aging, the ability to generate a fever in response to pyrogens is decreased. Because of this blunted fever response, and because medication use or cardiac disease may limit tachycardic response to infection, older patients may have systemic inflammatory response syndrome (SIRS)–negative sepsis. Abnormal triage vital signs in adults 75 years and older have poor sensitivity (73%) and specificity (50%) for predicting death or ICU admission. Emergency clinicians must look more broadly than just the typical SIRS criteria to suspect and diagnose sepsis accurately.

Management of suspected sepsis in older patients is similar to that for younger patients, with an emphasis on early identification of sepsis, fluid resuscitation, and early and appropriate antibiotics. Just as with younger adults, older patients with sepsis have improved mortality with comprehensive sepsis treatment. Older patients are more dependent on having an adequate preload to increase cardiac output in response to sepsis because the ability to raise the heart rate is blunted. However, aging-associated diastolic dysfunction is common, and fluid resuscitation goals may need adjustment if patients develop hypoxia or hypervolemia. In regard to the choice of empirical antibiotics, sepsis in older patients compared to younger patients is more likely to be due to respiratory or genitourinary infections, with pneumonia as the single most common cause of sepsis.

The references for this chapter can be found online at ExpertConsult.com.

179

Geriatric Trauma

Lauren T. Southerland and John J. Fath

KEY CONCEPTS

- Do not let a low-impact mechanism, patient cognitive impairment, or vital signs within the range of normal reduce your pretest probability of significant injury in an older patient.
- Age-specific trauma alert criteria improve the care of injured older adults.
- Vital signs, including tachycardia and hypotension, are unreliable to detect hemodynamic instability in older adults. Ultrasound is a helpful tool to assess volume status in the older trauma patient.
- Older patients are at high risk of hypothermia and develop pressure ulcers more rapidly than younger patients. Unnecessary spinal immobilization (cervical collars and backboards) causes pressure ulcers, respiratory distress, and delirium in this population.
- Clinical decision tools for radiographic imaging have generally excluded older patients. A low threshold for imaging should be used for older adults with trauma, and computed tomography (CT) should be used as the primary modality, except for extremity imaging.
- Falls are the leading cause of injury-related death in older adults, and ground-level falls can result in major injuries. Assessing the patient's future fall risk, home safety, and home resources is important prior to leaving the ED or hospital.
- Rib fractures and pulmonary contusions are associated with poor outcomes in older patients. ICU care should be considered for those with two or more rib fractures or pulmonary contusions.
- Older adults with hip fractures have improved survival on a dedicated orthogeriatric service. Consider transfer of patients to hospitals where these services are available.
- Routinely screen for elder abuse. A valid screening question is: "Has anyone close to you tried to hurt you or harm you recently?" Another query is: "Does anyone at home scare you or threaten you?"
- All older adults with fractures should be assessed for osteoporosis/osteopenia, and malnutrition as leaving this untreated reduces healing and increases morbidity and mortality.

FOUNDATIONS

Older adults make up a growing proportion of trauma patients in emergency departments (EDs). Although the general principles of trauma care for younger adults apply to older adults, there are special considerations for the older trauma patient from the initial decision to activate the trauma team through injury management and disposition.

Background and Importance

There is no standard definition of the term *geriatric trauma* in the literature; studies vary in their age criteria. In this chapter, unless noted, we are referring to patients 65 years and older. In 2016, older adults accounted for almost 13% of all injury-related ED visits in the United States, and this percentage is expected to increase with the aging of the population. Currently, unintentional injury is the sixth leading cause of death among older adults, and falls are the most common cause. Given the same mechanism of injury, older adults sustain more severe injuries than younger adults. Even low-energy mechanisms can cause morbidity and mortality. Managing these patients appropriately requires a holistic, multidisciplinary approach as recommended by the American College of Surgeons' Geriatric Trauma Management Guidelines, the Eastern Association for the Surgery of Trauma Practice Management Guidelines for Geriatric Trauma, and the Geriatric ED Guidelines. These guidelines incorporate geriatric principles into the care of the injured older adult from the trauma alert through the initial Advanced Trauma Life Support (ATLS) assessment, imaging decisions, and injury management.

SPECIFIC ISSUES

Age as a Trauma Triage Criterion

Trauma activation and/or transfer to a trauma center improves outcomes for older adults. Treatment at a trauma center reduces mortality in the first 7 days after injury (hazard ratio 0.62).[1] However, injured older adults are less likely to be transported to a trauma center either by emergency medical services (EMS) or by a referring hospital.[2] Traditional trauma triage criteria are less sensitive to the presenting signs and symptoms of older adults. For example, confusion could represent a baseline mental status or be a sign of acute traumatic brain injury (TBI). Medication effects such as anticoagulation must also be considered. Trauma triage criteria specific for older adults have been developed with age limits for triage criteria ranging from 55 years to 77 years. The most researched age-specific trauma criteria at this time is the Ohio Prehospital Geriatric Trauma Triage Criteria, which incorporates an age limit of 70 years old or older with additional mechanisms of fall and pedestrian struck by motor vehicle.[3] Pedestrians older than 50 years old who struck by a motor vehicle have a mean Injury Severity Score 9 points higher than younger adults, which is why this mechanism is part of geriatric trauma triage criteria. These criteria increase sensitivity from 61% to 93%, reducing the under-triage of older adults.

Mechanisms of Injury

Falls are the leading mechanism of injury and the leading cause of injury-related death in older adults. Most falls are from standing and occur at the place of residence; 12% of community-dwelling older adults fall each year. Traditional trauma criteria include a fall from a significant height or down a full flight of stairs, but for older adults a fall from standing or even out of a chair has an associated risk for injury. Mortality from a ground-level fall is only 0.1% for younger adults, but 4% to 5% for older adults.[4] The next most common injury mechanism is motor vehicle collisions. A detailed crash history is important, and single-vehicle crashes should raise the suspicion that a medical problem

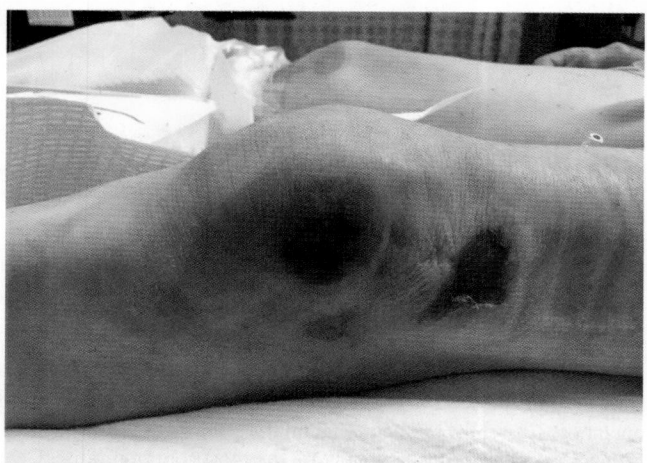

Fig. 179.1 Pressure damage to the skin occurs most frequently over bony prominences. This image shows pressure damage to the knee and thigh of an older man after being on the floor for several hours after a fall

caused the crash (e.g., syncope, myocardial infarction, stroke). An evaluation for coincident events leading to trauma should be undertaken during the ATLS trauma evaluation.

Thermal injuries, elder abuse/neglect, and self-injury are less common but are also important injury mechanisms. Burns can require significant wound care and recovery time which may be difficult for older adults to manage. In one multicenter study of older adults with a burned body surface area of 10% or greater, inpatient mortality was 25% and of the survivors, 15% required inpatient rehabilitation and 18% to 50% needed skilled nursing facility placement at discharge.[5] Burns, head and neck injuries, and delayed injury presentation are also all suspicious for elder abuse. Elder abuse is a complex problem (see Chapter 181). The secondary exam should include a full skin and genital exam and thorough documentation of any injuries. The Geri-IDT (Geriatric Injury Documentation Tool) can be helpful in guiding this assessment.[6]

A final concerning mechanism in geriatric trauma is self-injury. Older adults have a higher likelihood of completing suicide attempts than any other age group. Risk factors include recent bereavement, decreasing functional status, and increasing burden of disease. They are less likely to present with a chief complaint of depression/suicidality and less likely to receive mental health care in the ED.

Pathophysiology of Aging Affects Both the Injuries Sustained and the Recovery

Although older adults in a good state of health have sufficient reserves to accomplish activities of daily living, when they are stressed by acute trauma and the subsequent response to injury, the decrease in physiologic reserve can lead to rapid progression of tissue hypoperfusion and organ failure. In a trauma registry study out of Germany, 30% of older trauma patients experienced sepsis, 20% had multiple organ failure, and 45% had cardiovascular failure.[7] Renal function also decreases with age and can be misrepresented by assessing creatinine clearance. Serum creatinine is a muscle breakdown product; in an older adult creatinine clearance can appear artificially normal due to decreased overall muscle mass.

Skin changes predispose to skin tears, poor wound healing, and pressure ulcers (Fig. 179.1). Backboards and cervical collars placed during a trauma activation can lead to skin injury. In one study, trauma patients had a median time in a cervical collar of 117 minutes, 78%

developed pressure damage to the skin, and 28% developed severe indentations.[8] A final area of concern in older adults is age-related changes in the inflammatory and pain responses. Older adults have higher pain thresholds and reduced sensitivity to some types of painful stimuli. Decreases in the functionality of their white blood cells result in muted inflammatory responses and a lack of peritoneal abdominal signs on exam. In the older trauma patient, any abdominal tenderness is concerning for significant intra-abdominal injury.

Comorbidities

Older adults with polytrauma and a single comorbidity have 5.5 times higher risk of death than those without preexisting conditions. Comorbidities also increase the risk of injury by contributing to falls and impaired driving. Comorbidities complicate the evaluation process by impeding the ability to obtain an accurate history and interpret the physical exam. A patient with a blood pressure of 120/80 may be severely volume depleted if their normal systolic blood pressure is 150 due to hypertension. Table 179.1 provides examples of the effects various comorbidities can have on the evaluation and treatment of older adults following trauma.

Medications

A patient's daily medication regimen can increase the risk of a trauma and risk of death from an injury, obfuscate the clinical exam, and require changes in management and treatment of injuries. Medications also alter the response to resuscitative measures. A full medication review is essential for injured older adults with attention to specific drug classes (Table 179.2). Among older adults in a Canadian trauma registry, 30-day mortality increased by 24% for each medication a patient was taking. If the medication was potentially inappropriate based on the American Geriatrics Society Beers Criteria, the risk of death doubled.[9] Medication reconciliation in the setting of trauma is thus a matter of life and death. The most time-critical issue is the use of anticoagulation. Trauma patients on preexisting anticoagulation, regardless of type, have higher rates of complications and higher transfusion needs.[10] An "anticoagulation alert" system for older adult trauma activations may reduce mortality from injuries.

ATLS Assessment

A systematic trauma assessment per ATLS guidelines should be conducted in older adults (see Chapter 32). One change to the airway, breathing, circulation, disability mnemonic is to consider circulation alongside airway. Post intubation hypotension is more likely in older patients and 30% of these patients will die. Consideration should be given to resuscitation to restore perfusion prior to or concomitant with securing the airway.

Airway

Because older patients are likely to have multiple risk factors for a difficult airway, emergency clinicians should perform a systematic airway assessment. Early intubation is indicated for unstable patients, as defined by signs of shock, altered mental status, and significant chest trauma. However, this population is more likely to have advanced directives or other care planning documentation that should be consulted prior to intubation. Bilevel positive airway pressure (BIPAP) or high-flow oxygen may be used as temporizing measures while the goals of care are discussed.

If intubation is required, video laryngoscopy is recommended. Up to 30% of older trauma patients will require multiple intubation attempts. Consider sedation with ketamine to maintain the respiratory response and blood pressure (see Chapter 1). Etomidate is a second choice, as it is also not associated with significant hypotension, unlike propofol which may cause hypotension. We recommend rocuronium

TABLE 179.1 Comorbidities Common in Older Adults and Their Effects on the Evaluation and Management of the Patient After a Traumatic Injury

Comorbidity	Effect (*Contributing to Trauma, −Complicating the Trauma Exam, +Complicating Injury Management)
Cardiovascular disease	*Acute coronary syndrome may cause a fall or motor vehicle accident. −Higher risk of dissection with blunt chest trauma −Decreased peripheral perfusion from peripheral vascular disease +Risk of acute coronary syndrome from the catecholamine surge of trauma +Predisposed to pulmonary edema with large IV fluid boluses
Chronic kidney disease	+Need to decrease opioid and antibiotic doses and monitor for toxicity +More susceptible to volume depletion due to inability to concentrate the urine to conserve fluids +More susceptible to shock-induced acute on chronic kidney injury
Chronic lung disease	−Decreased pulmonary functional capacity can lead to significant respiratory compromise from cervical collars or lying flat. +Decreased tolerance of lung or chest wall injuries +Decreased ability to clear secretions from the lungs +Risk of encephalopathy from decreased ventilation and respiratory acidosis
Dementia	−Decreased ability to give a complete history −Agitation or behavioral disturbances from advanced dementia may complicate exam. +Increased risk of developing delirium from trauma or hospitalization +Decreased ability to express pain or request as needed (PRN) medications
Diabetes	−Results in peripheral neuropathy which can obscure injuries −Altered mental status with hyper- or hypoglycemia +Increased risk of wound infection and poor wound healing
Frailty	−Higher levels of mortality from even "minor" injuries +Higher risk of delirium +Need screening for nutritional deficits, home safety, and mobility issues. Consider early initiation of therapy (physical, occupational, speech) and geriatric consultations. +More likely to require skilled nursing facility placement, consider early case management and social work consultations
Joint replacements	−Periprosthetic or juxtahardware fractures may present with minimal deformity.
Neurovascular disease	*Neurologic deficits increase the risk of falls and injury. −Prior cerebrovascular accidents (CVA) or neurotrauma can obfuscate the neurologic exam. −Risk of recrudescence or another CVA with acute hypotension
Ophthalmologic	−Medications and prior surgeries (such as cataract repair) may change pupil exam for reactivity or symmetry.
Osteoporosis or Osteopenia	−Increased risk of fractures with minimal trauma −Prior atraumatic vertebral compression fractures complicating the evaluation of new injuries −X-rays have decreased sensitivity for detection of fractures. −Older adults will often still be able to ambulate despite pelvic or hip fractures; the ability to range a joint or ambulate cannot definitively rule out a fracture. +Osteopenia on CT scan is associated with a hazard ratio for death at 1 year of 12 times more than patients without osteopenia.
Rheumatoid Arthritis	*Associated cervical spine disease leads to fractures. −Joint deformities can be mistaken for acute fractures. Additional imaging may be needed to distinguish rheumatic disease from acute fracture.
Spinal diseases	*Degenerative disk disease of the spine increases the risk of endplate fractures. *Spinal stenosis can be associated with SCIWORET (Spinal Cord Injury without Radiographic Evidence of Trauma).

if a paralytic is required for an older trauma patient. Succinylcholine paralysis is contraindicated in the patient at risk for hyperkalemia from prolonged time on the floor after a fall. Limited mobility of the cervical spine and the temporal mandibular joint complicate visualization, making induction and paralysis key to successful airway management in the older adult. Dental changes such as bridges or lack of teeth can interfere with grip during scissoring and jaw thrust maneuvers. If dentures are securely in place, they do not need removal as they can improve the seal for bag mask ventilation.

Age is not a contraindication to performing a cricothyroidotomy, though this procedure can be more difficult in older patients. Flexion from cervical spine kyphosis compresses the anterior cervical anatomy which shortens and deepens the operative field, leading to a higher risk of failure of the procedure or injury to larger vessels.

Breathing

Older adults have more difficulty clearing secretions in the mouth and lungs and may require frequent suctioning. Lung disease and spinal kyphosis decrease functional lung volumes. A 45-degree incline can assist with oxygenation and ventilation. If there is concern for spinal injury, it is acceptable to ramp the entire bed (reverse Trendelenburg) to keep the head and chest elevated while the back is straight. Capnography

TABLE 179.2   Examples of Common Classes of Medications Taken by Older Adults and the Effects to Consider During Trauma Evaluation and Management of Injuries

Medication Class [Examples]	Medication Effects (*Contributing to Trauma –Complicating the Trauma Exam and Care)
Anticholinergics [Diphenhydramine, Meclizine, Promethazine, Hydroxyzine]	*Increase risk of falls, confusion, and delirium –Decrease urine output and cause constipation
Antihypertensives and Diuretics [Metoprolol, Carvedilol, Cardizem, Lisinopril, Furosemide]	*Increase risk of orthostatic hypotension and falls –AV nodal agents blunt the ability to mount a tachycardia response despite level of blood loss. –Baseline blood pressure may be hypertensive, so normotensive can signal relative blood loss.
Anticoagulants and Antiplatelets [Warfarin, Clopidogrel, direct oral anticoagulants (Apixaban, Rivaroxaban), aspirin, dabigatran, prasugrel, tigacrelor]	*Increase risk of spontaneous bleeding such as intracranial hemorrhage –Increase bleeding, bruising, and bleeding time –Increase mortality from intracranial hemorrhages
Corticosteroids [Prednisone, Dexamethasone]	*Chronic use increases risk of fractures. –Decrease wound healing –Decrease inflammatory response and may decrease sensitivity of exam for pain –Increase risk of wound infections –Increase risk of refractory hypotension
Hypoglycemic Agents [Metformin, Insulins, Sulfonylureas, Pioglitazone]	*Hypoglycemia can lead to falls or motor vehicle accidents. –Trauma patients are often placed on NPO (no oral intake) status causing iatrogenic hypoglycemia.
Opioids [Hydrocodone, Oxycodone, Codeine, illicit opioids]	*Sedative effects can lead to falls or motor vehicle collisions. –Blunt the pain response, increasing the risk of missed injury –Withdrawal may present with abdominal pain and tachycardia.
Sedatives [Benzodiazepines, Alcohol abuse, antipsychotic sedatives Mirtazapine and Trazodone]	*Increase risk of falls and motor vehicle accidents. –May affect Glasgow Coma Scale and cognitive assessments –Risk of respiratory sedation –Withdrawal may present as tachycardia and confusion.

is highly recommended if there is any concern for underlying lung disease, acute thoracic injury, or if analgesia or sedatives are given.

Circulation

As previously noted, older adults are particularly vulnerable to shock due to limited physiologic reserve. Adaptive responses to hypovolemia such as tachycardia and hypotension are reduced by physiologic changes and medications (see Tables 179.1 and 179.2). *Normal* initial vital signs are not reassuring, but *baseline* vital signs are helpful. Trends are more informative than specific cutoffs.

During resuscitation, the therapeutic window for cardiac preload is narrow, and inadequate monitoring of fluid status may lead to over- or under-resuscitation. Evaluation of the collapsibility of the inferior vena cava by ultrasound is recommended to assess overall fluid status and guide resuscitation. In patients in whom there is no obvious source of blood loss, incremental boluses (e.g., 500 mL) of warmed isotonic crystalloid can be used for resuscitation. Patients in shock with injuries that have a high likelihood of acute blood loss should be given blood early and empirically. The indicators for need of massive transfusion, such as the Assessment of Blood Consumption and the Trauma Associated Severe Hemorrhage scores, are not as sensitive in older adults. We recommend to start transfusing 1 unit packed red blood cells while obtaining imaging if there is any suspicion of significant blood loss. Frequent (every 30 minutes) reassessment of the hemodynamic status will avoid iatrogenic pulmonary edema and respiratory failure. Thoracic ultrasound is fast, available in most trauma bays, and with skilled operators is more sensitive for signs of pulmonary edema (B lines) than chest x-ray. Thoracic ultrasound for pulmonary edema or abdominal ultrasound of the inferior vena cava can be helpful in directing fluid resuscitation for the trauma patient.

Anticoagulation reversal is another method of improving circulation by reversing life-threatening bleeding. Considerations for reversing coagulation abnormalities in older trauma patients are the severity of injury, the volume of reversal agents required, the urgency for the reversal, the availability of various reversal agents and the corresponding risk of fluid overload (see Chapter 180).

Disability

Evaluation of older adults for disability includes examination for TBI, spinal cord trauma, vertebral fractures, and extremity injuries. In contrast to younger adults, older adults can have intracranial hemorrhages and yet maintain a Glasgow Coma Score (GCS) of 15. Any GCS less than 15 is concerning for TBI, and a GCS score below 8 is predictive of a poor outcome. Subtle changes in mental status such as confusion or decreased alertness or symptoms such as headache may be the only signs of TBI. Confirming baseline mental status with family or caregivers is essential. Ultimately, no combination of historical features and physical findings has been shown to reliably predict the absence of intracranial injuries in the older trauma population. Brain computed tomography (CT) is indicated for all older adults with head trauma, multisystem trauma, or symptoms or signs of TBI, because no clinical decision rule has been validated in older trauma patients.

The evaluation of the patient's cognitive status is critical to detecting delirium. A patient who is cognitively impaired or acutely delirious may not express pain or answer questions and therefore their physical examination may not be accurate. Delirium can be the cause of traumatic injury, such as falls, or can be the result of traumatic injuries. The Brief Delirium Triage Screen has high sensitivity in emergency department patients and is more rapid than the full CAM-ICU. Brief cognitive screening tests such as the Mini Cog or the 4AT Delirium Assessment tool are also helpful when probing for cognitive impairment. Delirium is common among all trauma patients, especially those in the ICU or intermediate care units, and is associated with worse outcomes. A quarter of older trauma patients with rib fractures will develop delirium. Missing delirium on the initial evaluation in the ED is associated with prolonged length of stay in the hospital and increased morbidity.

Exposure

Older trauma patients often have a combination of chronic, acute, and iatrogenic skin injuries. Because even minor wounds can cause serious complications in older patients, a thorough skin exam should be performed. Once exposed, older trauma patients are at risk of developing hypothermia because normal thermoregulatory mechanisms may no longer be intact, or are disrupted from the stress of trauma. Hypothermia on arrival should raise suspicion of infection leading to the fall and injury, or prolonged exposure or immobilization after the fall.

Secondary Assessment

A complete history should be obtained from the patient or a care provider, with particular emphasis on corroborating the accident history, past medical history, medications, allergies, and social history, including baseline functional status and living arrangements. Code status and confirmation of any advanced care planning documentation is essential. Baseline functional status includes the patient's ability to walk and any need for assistive devices prior to the injury. In addition to the basic history, a history of falls should be obtained and fall risk factors identified. Patients should be screened for alcohol abuse, substance abuse, and elder abuse. Home living situation, caregivers and caregiver availability, and home safety concerns need to be understood to ensure a safe discharge. Social workers often assist with this evaluation and early assistance from these teams can greatly speed care and disposition of the older trauma patient.

Laboratory Testing

In addition to the recommended trauma labs (see Chapter 32), we recommend a urine culture and a cardiac evaluation (ECG, troponin, and cardiac monitoring). A creatinine kinase level should be considered in every patient who has been immobilized by fall or injury. Electrocardiography (ECG) and cardiac monitoring are advised because of the risk of cardiac causes or complications of their traumatic event.

COMMON INJURIES IN OLDER ADULTS

Traumatic Brain Injury (TBI)

TBI can occur with minimal head trauma in older adults and can be initially asymptomatic. Physiologic changes of aging and the frequent use of anticoagulant medications increase the likelihood and severity of TBI in older adults. With aging, the size of the brain decreases by 10% on average, resulting in increased intracranial free space, stretching of bridging veins to the dura, and increased brain mobility within the calvarium. With this increased freedom of movement even minor trauma can lead to shearing of blood vessels and intracranial hemorrhage. These injuries can be devastating; a fifth of older adults admitted for TBI will die or enter a vegetative state.[11]

Clinical variables alone are insufficient to identify all cases of intracranial injury reliably in older patients; the New Orleans Criteria, NEXUS II CT Head Rule, and Canadian Head CT Rule all exclude older adults. Newer research into biomarkers of glial injury have shown some promise, but as of yet are not validated in older adults. A noncontrast head CT is the imaging of choice to diagnosis hemorrhagic TBI. The TBI spectrum in older adults also includes concussions, which as in sports related injury, may result in headaches, nausea, short-term memory deficits, and sleep disruption. We recommend the Center for Disease Control's Acute Concussion Evaluation.

Treatment of moderate to severe TBI includes supportive care, rapid reversal of anticoagulation, and early neurosurgical consultation (see Chapter 33). Patients with mild TBI (GCS 13 to 15) may be safe for monitoring and anticoagulation reversal (if required) on a regular hospital floor or observation unit. Physical therapy and occupational therapy consultations are recommended both to assess for subtle deficits and to address any home safety, safe mobility, or care needs. Older patients with head trauma who are not anticoagulated and have a normal head CT are generally safe for discharge if they have a safe environment, responsible care provider, and reliable follow-up. In patients on therapeutic anticoagulation, if the initial head CT does not show any injury, the risk of subsequent development of an intracranial hemorrhage is less than 2%.[12] Although this risk is low, we recommend that any patient with neurologic deficits, confusion, or who is without reliable monitoring at home should be observed for 12 to 24 hours to assess for concussion or evolving intracranial injury.

Vertebral Fractures and Spinal Cord Injuries

Changes in bone mineral density (BMD) and spinal kyphosis with aging contribute to several distinct fracture types in older adults: C1 to C2 cervical fractures and vertebral compression fractures. In contrast to younger patients, in older adults the most common cervical spine fractures are at the level of C1 and C2, with more than 50% of cervical fractures occurring at the level of C2. These fractures are usually the result of a fall with impact to the head, resulting in anterior or posterior displacement of the odontoid process. Mortality from these fractures is high (16% in the first month, up to 32% in the first year for nonoperatively treated C2 fractures).[13] Vertebral compression fractures are also common and can be asymptomatic other than the slight loss of height. In one series of hospitalized women, the prevalence of incidental thoracic vertebral fractures on chest x-ray was 2.4% in women aged 50 to 59 years, 8.9% in women aged 60 to 69 years, and 21.9% in women aged 70 years or older.[14] A lack of initial symptoms unfortunately does not mean that these fractures lack long-term morbidity.

Establishing a diagnosis of cervical spine fracture in older patients is complicated because 20% of adults older than 55 years with a cervical spinal fracture do not report neck pain. The Canadian C-Spine Rule classifies all patients 65 years or older as inherently high risk. The National Emergency X-Ray Utilization Study (NEXUS) criteria include all ages, but validation studies of NEXUS have shown lower sensitivity in older adults. In any blunt trauma to the older neck, lack of spinal tenderness or lack of pain on range of motion does not completely rule out spinal injury. We recommend CT imaging for any older adult with trauma and neurologic symptoms or cognitive impairment.

Older adults are also at increased risk of thoracic, lumbar, and sacral vertebral fractures. Per trauma guidelines, CT imaging should be used liberally for older adult trauma patients. Consider imaging the entire spine for those with altered mentation or dementia. Clinical exam can only rule out thoracolumbar injury in the awake, alert, older adult without cognitive impairment or other comorbidities/medications that limit the sensation or expression of pain.

Up to 20% of women over 70 years of age have suffered a vertebral compression fracture; magnetic resonance imaging (MRI) is helpful in determining acuity. Finally, if one acute spinal fracture is found, the rest of the spine should be imaged. In blunt trauma patients with a cervical fracture, 20% to 26% will have a noncontiguous thoracolumbar fracture. In the past, flexion/extension x-rays were used to evaluate for ligamentous injury, but this is controversial and no longer general practice.

Consultation with a spine surgeon is essential for all spinal injuries. Kyphoplasty or vertebroplasty can help control pain. Braces or collars can assist with pain and recovery, but these also limit an older adult's abilities to perform activities of daily living. Spinous process and other stable cervical fractures are sometimes managed without immobilization because of the respiratory effects and discomfort from cervical collars.

Thoracic Trauma

Older adults are at increased risk of rib and sternal fractures, pulmonary contusions, and their complications with low-force injuries. In-hospital mortality from thoracic trauma ranges from 3% to 15%.

Obtaining a chest x-ray combined with extended FAST exam has a sensitivity of only 64% for detecting clinically significant thoracic injuries; therefore, chest CT is recommended for the potentially multiply injured patient.

Management of the older adult with thoracic trauma is similar to management of younger adults, but a lower threshold for ICU monitoring is suggested. Although these patients may appear stable by vitals, admission to the ICU for older adults with multiple rib fractures significantly decreased complications, hospital length of stay, and need for discharge to a skilled nursing facility in one single-center study.[15] Alternatives to opioid analgesia such as epidural analgesia, paravertebral analgesia, and/or topical lidocaine can be considered for pain management.

Fragility Fractures

Fractures are common injuries in older adults with decreased BMD. Even nonoperative, distal extremity fractures can affect mobility and the ability to live independently. The most common upper extremity fractures sustained by older adults, in order of frequency, are distal radius fractures, proximal humerus fractures, and elbow fractures. The most common lower extremity fractures in older adults are ankle fractures, hip and pelvic fractures, and tibial plateau fractures. Pelvic fractures can occur with relatively little force in older adults and often patients continue to ambulate on a fractured pelvis. Although the majority of pelvic fractures are stable, these fractures can be associated with hemorrhage. In-hospital pelvic fracture mortality is 2.8%, and up to 21% in older patients with open pelvic fractures. The initial in-hospital mortality from hip fractures (intratrochanteric) is low, but due to debility the longer-term mortality in this population is high (45% at 1 year), with men twice as likely to die as women.

Hip fractures can be seen on plain x-ray films but occult fractures are a well-described phenomenon in older adults. Patients with the inability to ambulate or who have persistent pain after trauma require further evaluation; MRI is useful to delineate the pathology.

Older adults with hip fractures have better outcomes with early surgery (<72 hours) and care in a distinct orthogeriatric service. Emergency clinicians should consider transferring older adults with hip fractures to hospitals with such services. For pain management, consider ultrasound-guided blocks such as the fascia iliaca. For other fractures, management is similar to that of younger adults except that the emergency physician is uniquely poised to discuss the treatment and diagnosis of two common syndromes: low BMD and malnutrition.

A fragility fracture should be suspected in all women older than 50 years and men older than 70 years old presenting with a fracture. The classic fragility fractures are distal radius, hip, and spine, but in the setting of trauma low BMD can contribute to fractures anywhere. If osteopenia is seen on the trauma CTs, then low BMD can be presumed. Treatment includes testing calcium and vitamin D levels and starting

---

BOX 179.1   Suggestions to Limit the Side Effects and Complications of Analgesics for Injured Older Adults

- Limit NSAID (nonsteroidal antiinflammatory drug) use to 1 week or less to avoid renal and gastric injury. NSAIDs increase bleeding risk if patient is taking aspirin.
- Discuss total daily acetaminophen consumption limits and if any medications are combination pills with acetaminophen to avoid accidental overuse.
- Skeletal muscle relaxers such as cyclobenzaprine, methocarbamol, and benzodiazepines are discouraged for use by the American Geriatrics Society Beers Criteria.
- Tramadol lowers the seizure threshold, is renally metabolized, and can cause SIADH/hyponatremia and hypoglycemia in addition to the regular side effects of opioid medications. Use with caution.
- Tramadol, codeine, and morphine are not recommended for patients with renal insufficiency (GFR <30 mL/min).
- Discuss a bowel regimen that includes a promotility agent such as senna, docusate, bisacodyl, or prune juice.
- Consider topical agents such as lidocaine and topical NSAIDs.
- Consider early referral to physical therapy to assess mobility and pain, and reduce functional decline from injury.

Compiled from the American Geriatrics Society 2019 Beers Criteria and the American Geriatrics Society Geriatrics at Your Fingertips.

---

the patient on supplementation (if needed) pending full evaluation by their primary care doctor, orthopedist, or endocrinologist. The major contraindications to starting vitamin D and calcium supplementation from the ED include: end-stage renal disease, parathyroid disease, coronary atherosclerosis (currently debated), and renal stones.

Nutritional status also directly affects perioperative mortality and long-term healing from injuries. Malnutrition assessment in the older injured patient is endorsed by trauma guidelines. A study of older adults with hip fractures found that malnourishment was associated with increased in-hospital (27% versus 7%) and 1-year mortality (46% versus 17%).[16] Calcium levels, vitamin D levels, body mass index, and pre-albumin/albumin levels can all suggest malnourishment.

DISPOSITION, END-OF-LIFE CONSIDERATIONS, AND RECOVERY

Although age alone is not an indication to withhold aggressive treatment, comfort measures may be more appropriate than transferring patients to a trauma center in select cases (e.g., grave prognosis or when the patient's goals of care are known). Early referrals to palliative medicine and hospice from the ED help with pain and end-of-life care (see Chapter e5). The majority of older adults will recover from their injuries, but many will require additional help during recovery. Even minor decreases in range of motion of a joint can have a large impact on older adults' ability to care for themselves at home; additional help, equipment, or acute rehabilitation facility placement may be needed. An observation unit can be used to coordinate physical and occupational therapy consultations and home equipment prior to discharge from the ED. Lastly, prior to discharging an older adult to home, a safe and effective strategy for pain control is required (Box 179.1).

The references for this chapter can be found online at ExpertConsult.com.

180

Geriatric Drug Therapy

Christopher J. Edwards and Arthur B. Sanders

KEY CONCEPTS

- Those with a chronologic age of 65 years or older are commonly referred to as older adults (or the elderly), but physiologic age is more indicative of a drug's therapeutic or toxicologic effect. Besides age, overall patient assessment should include organ function, comorbidity, and functional status to guide drug dosing.
- Pharmacokinetic and pharmacodynamic changes that occur with age need to be considered to optimize drug dosing and minimize toxicity in older adults. In most cases, a "start low, go slow" approach is recommended. Multiple or repeated dosing is more likely to lead to drug accumulation compared to single doses in the emergency department (ED).
- Polypharmacy is common in older adults, predisposing them to adverse drug effects, drug interactions, and functional and cognitive impairment. Some of these medications do not have legitimate indications or may be inappropriate.
- Published lists of potentially inappropriate medications, such as the Beers list and the STOPP and START criteria, can help to identify potentially problematic medications; however, there are limited studies to enable extrapolation to the ED setting.
- Anticoagulation-related hemorrhagic complications are common in elderly patients, particularly if drug accumulation occurs in patients taking renally eliminated direct-acting oral anticoagulants.
- Older adults often present to the ED with altered mental status. Drug-related causes such as anticholinergic medication burden should be considered in the differential diagnosis.
- Geriatric patients with pain-related complaints are less likely to receive analgesics in the ED compared to younger adults, placing them at risk for poor pain control. Dosing of opioids should be cautious, with frequent monitoring and titration. Given the availability of alternative opioids, the use of meperidine should be avoided.
- A growing number of institutions have pharmacists practicing in the ED. In geriatric EDs, there is a great opportunity to integrate and consult with pharmacists, given the myriad drug therapy issues that can lead to suboptimal care.

FOUNDATIONS

There are approximately 23 million visits to United States (US) emergency departments (EDs) by adults over the age of 65 annually.[1] As the US population ages, the number of ED visits by older adults is expected to increase disproportionately compared to the general population based on estimates from the US census.[2] Drug therapy issues are particularly challenging in older adults because of altered pharmacokinetics and pharmacodynamics compared to younger adults. In addition, older patients take more medications, have more comorbidities, and are at increased risk for adverse drug effects because of the physiologic changes that occur with aging. Medication selection and dosing must be age-adapted for optimal patient outcomes. Also, given that advanced age is a commonly applied exclusion criterion in clinical trials, there is less high-quality evidence for many drug therapy interventions in older adults compared to younger adults. This can make extrapolating from studies and evaluating risks versus benefits for pharmacologic options more challenging, particularly for patients who are 80 years of age or older.

Most developed countries have adopted the chronologic age of 65 years to define the geriatric or older population.[3] The World Health Organization does not have a standard definition, but generally uses the age of 60 years or older to refer to older persons.[3] This categorization may be overly simplistic, and stratification, such as young old (60–69 years), middle old (70–79 years), and very old (≥80 years), is more suitable and medically useful. From a drug therapy perspective, physiologic age is more indicative of the anticipated therapeutic or toxicologic effect; however, there are no physiologic markers that define the aging process or that can be routinely used in clinical practice.[4] Most studies evaluating medication use in older adults have used a cut-off value of 65 years, and this serves as the basis for recommendations from the American Geriatrics Society.[5]

In this chapter, we refer to older adults as those with a chronologic age of 65 years or older; however, from the emergency clinicians' perspective, this is an arbitrary value for making drug therapy decisions. In addition to chronologic age alone, an overall assessment that incorporates organ function, comorbidity, functional status, and lifestyle is a better determinant of drug therapy selection and dosing. This should also be considered when interpreting recommendations for older adults, such as what is considered to be an inappropriate medication. This chapter reviews select aspects of pharmacology for older adults and the clinical implications in emergency medicine.

Pharmacokinetics

The time course of drug exposure is determined by pharmacokinetic parameters including absorption, distribution, metabolism, and elimination. The drug effect is primarily determined by this exposure, which can be quantified by serum drug concentrations over time. It is assumed that increased exposure is more likely to result in toxic medication effects. Thus, an understanding of pharmacokinetic changes in older adults is useful for determining risks of adverse drug reactions and can help guide medication selection and dosing.

The effect of physiologic changes on drug absorption is an important consideration for orally ingested medications. Changes in gastric pH, gastric emptying, splanchnic blood flow, bowel motility, and absorptive capacity all impact drug availability. For example, the increase in gastric pH seen in older adults can decrease the dissolution of medications that are weak bases, reducing absorption and resulting in lower serum drug levels. Conversely, decreased bowel motility can increase transit time, allowing more opportunity for absorption to occur, leading to increased serum drug levels. Clearly, age-related changes in the gastro-intestinal system can have a varied effect on drug absorption, leading to unpredictable effects on serum drug concentrations. As an example, decreased absorptive capacity coupled with decreased bowel motility can increase transit time, leading to a net neutral effect on drug exposure. Gastrointestinal and other comorbidities can have a greater effect on absorption than age alone. Given these considerations, it would be prudent in the ED to use the intravenous route for acute conditions, when rapid drug absorption is needed to achieve a therapeutic concentration.

Age-related changes in body composition have an effect on the distribution of drugs. There is an increase in total body fat and a decrease in relative skeletal muscle mass in older adults compared to young adults. This change in body composition accelerates between 60 to 75 years and then may start to decline. Lipophilic medications have a greater volume of distribution with increasing adiposity, whereas the opposite is true for hydrophilic medications. Opioid analgesics such as fentanyl and most sedatives (e.g., benzodiazepines, propofol) are very lipophilic, so there is distribution and accumulation of the drug within adipose tissue, and its metabolites are renally eliminated. With prolonged use, this can lead to an increased duration of effect due to redistribution of drug from tissue to serum and central nervous system. Conversely, hydrophilic medications such as digoxin would require lower loading doses in older adults to achieve similar serum concentrations due to a smaller volume of distribution. This has the potential for drug toxicity if not dosed appropriately for age.

Most drugs require biotransformation into polar metabolites before final elimination. This primarily occurs in the liver via phase 1 metabolism by cytochrome P450 enzymes (oxidation) or phase 2 (conjugation, acetylation, sulfation) reactions. With advanced age, hepatic mass and blood flow may decrease by up to 40%, which reduces the delivery of medications to the liver and their subsequent metabolism. This decrease in first-pass metabolism improves drug bioavailability resulting in increased serum levels and potentially increasing the risk of drug toxicity for certain agents. Drugs with a high hepatic extraction ratio are more dependent on hepatic blood flow for drug metabolism, and the slowing of hepatic metabolism seen with age has mainly been related to changes in phase 1 pathways. For example, morphine is a high–extraction ratio drug and would lead to greater drug exposure as hepatic blood flow is reduced. Commonly used benzodiazepines in the ED also vary in their metabolic pathways. Midazolam undergoes phase 1 metabolism, and hepatic impairment would lead to drug accumulation, especially with repeated or prolonged use. Conversely, lorazepam undergoes phase 2 conjugation and is preferred in patients with hepatic impairment because this metabolic pathway is less dependent on hepatic blood flow. The effect of aging on phase 1 metabolism via CYP3A4 is controversial. This enzyme represents the metabolic pathway for most medications, and studies have shown no significant differences between younger and older populations.

Renal blood blow, renal mass, and the number of nephrons decrease with age, leading to a decrease in renal function. In a longitudinal study, renal function decreased by approximately 10% for each decade between 30 and 80 years of age. This decrease was independent of comorbid conditions and was attributed to aging alone. Although this decline is likely to occur in most patients, up to one-third may have no decline, and some may have an increase in renal function. Kidney function is expressed as the glomerular filtration rate (GFR) and is routinely estimated by the Cockcroft-Gault equation. However, this equation may not accurately estimate the GFR, so the modification of diet and renal disease (MDRD) equation has been suggested as a more

BOX 180.1   Equations to Estimate Glomerular Filtration Rate (GFR, in mL/min)

Cockcroft-Gault Equation

Creatinine clearance (mL/min) = (140 − age) × (weight in kg) /72 × serum creatinine × (0.85 if female)

Use ideal body weight (IBW). If patient is obese, use adjusted body weight.

IBW (male) = 50 + [2.3× (height in inches − 60)]

IBW (female) = 45.5 + [2.3× (height in inches − 60)]

Adjusted body weight = IBW + [0.3 × (actual weight − IBM)]

Modification of Diet and Renal Disease Equation

GFR = 175 × serum creatinine^{-154} × age$^{-0.203}$
(× 1.212 if patient is black; × 0.742 if patient is female)

accurate estimation.[6] Common equations used to calculate creatinine clearance and estimate GFR are in Box 180.1. Discordance in drug doses selected may occur 10% to 40% of the time when comparing the two equations, and there has been considerable debate regarding the most appropriate equation to use in practice.[7,8]

Typically, drug dosing in manufacturers' labeling per the US Food and Drug Administration is based on creatinine clearance determined by the Cockcroft-Gault equation and, as such, most pharmacists continue to use this equation for drug dosing. The Cockcroft-Gault equation is also easier to calculate compared to the MDRD. While many electronic health records and laboratories use MDRD to calculate and report GFR, there is no universal industry standard approach, and it is important to know which equation is used to calculate the GFR reported in the medical record. Although cumbersome, one approach is to calculate estimated GFR based on both equations and evaluate if there is a discrepancy in dosing recommendations. This approach is useful if the initial estimate is close to a cut-off value that would alter the dosing regimen. If a discrepancy exists, the decision to use a more or less conservative dosing strategy will depend on the clinical scenario. In general, a low-dose approach should be used for medications with a narrow therapeutic index, particularly when the risk of toxicity is high and serum concentration monitoring is not available. In general, medication dosing should be higher in the ED when the implications for therapeutic failure warrant such an approach, assuming the medication has a broad safety margin. An example would be erring on the side of more aggressive dosing when using antibiotics in a patient with sepsis or febrile neutropenia. Thus, clinical circumstances may override drug dosing recommendations, especially when there is discordance between equations, and professional judgment is always required. These equations use the serum creatinine level to estimate creatinine clearance, which is affected by muscle mass. Therefore, although serum creatinine values may be normal, they may not accurately estimate renal function in some older adults, especially those with less musculature. For all older patients, some providers routinely round serum creatinine values less than 1 mg/dL up to 1 mg/dL to account for reduced muscle mass; however, this practice should be avoided because it has been shown to underestimate clearance.

Given the limited number of repeat doses typically administered in the ED, even in patients with hepatic or renal impairment, drug accumulation is unlikely to be clinically meaningful. If, however, several doses of a medication are administered in the ED, especially when patients are boarded, drug toxicity or prolonged effects may become

TABLE 180.1 Pharmacokinetic Changes in Older Adults

Parameter	Change	Comments
Absorption		
Gastric pH	↑	Net absorption may be increased or decreased.
Gastric emptying	↓	Peak effect will likely be delayed.
Splanchnic blood flow	↓	The intravenous route is preferred in the ED for rapid and predictable effect
Bowel motility	↓	
Absorptive capacity		
Distribution		
Adipose tissue	↑	Lipophilic medications will accumulate with repeated dosing, which increases duration of effect.
Total body water	↓	Hydrophilic medications will have a lower volume of distribution, requiring lower loading doses.
Metabolism		
Phase 1 metabolism	↓	Medications with phase 1 metabolism are more likely to accumulate than those metabolized via phase 2 pathways.
Phase 2 metabolism	↓	
Liver blood flow	↓	
Elimination		
Glomerular filtration rate	↓	This is the most important consideration for drug dosing. Calculate creatinine clearance using the equations in Box 180.1 and adjust dosing. First doses of antibiotics and most one-time doses do not require adjustment.

clinically relevant. In general, a "start low and go slow" approach is prudent in older patients. When this strategy is used, it is critical to reevaluate the patient after the anticipated onset of the administered medication to determine if additional doses are necessary because failure to do so could lead to undertreatment. The risks versus benefits of drug therapies generally increase with age, suggesting that a more conservative approach is warranted, particularly when using drugs with a narrow therapeutic index. Pharmacokinetic changes in older adults are listed in Table 180.1.

Pharmacodynamics

Even at similar plasma concentrations, drugs may have altered effects in older adults, perhaps because of changes in the number and sensitivity of receptors, signal transduction, and reduction in homeostatic processes that help maintain equilibrium. Thus, physiologic mechanisms that help restore function are attenuated, leading to an exaggerated or relatively unopposed pharmacologic effect. Pharmacodynamic changes in older adults that are most relevant to consider in the ED include those that pertain to the cardiovascular, central nervous, and coagulation systems. For example, there is a decreased response to both β-adrenergic receptor agonists and antagonists. Conversely, there is no age-related change in α_1-adrenergic receptor sensitivity. Calcium channel blockers cause a greater drop in blood pressure and heart rate in older adults compared to younger adults, so the risk for postural hypotension is higher in older adults. The diminished inotropic response to catecholamines contributes to this risk. In the ED, non-dihydropyridine calcium channel antagonists such as diltiazem or verapamil are commonly used for patients with supraventricular tachycardias. Lower doses are appropriate in older adults, especially when the patient has tenuous blood pressure.

There is increased sensitivity to benzodiazepines in older adults, and lower doses are needed to obtain similar sedative-hypnotic effects. This is because of changes in the structure, composition, and function of the γ-aminobutyric acid (GABA) receptor complex. Similarly, in one investigation, older patients required less propofol for the induction and maintenance of sedation during procedures in the ED.[9] The dose

required for induction was 0.5 mg/kg less than in the cohort of young adults. In older adults, it is more suitable to start propofol with a 0.5-mg/kg rather than the 1-mg/kg bolus that is typically recommended. Some studies have shown that older patients have increased sensitivity to opioids. Pharmacodynamic effects in these studies were measured in terms of electroencephalographic readings, which do not reliably indicate the presence of pain. However, the risk of adverse effects and interactions due to the use of concurrent medications is likely increased in older adults, suggesting that a cautious approach is appropriate when dosing opioids.

There is an age-related decrease in dopamine content in the central nervous system, which predisposes patients who are given neuroleptics and other dopamine antagonists to extrapyramidal symptoms. Similarly, there is a decrease in acetylcholine synthesis in older adults, which increases the risk for anticholinergic neurotoxicity with commonly used antihistamines, antispasmodics, and antiparkinsonian agents.

Bleeding is a potentially life-threatening consequence of anticoagulants. Historically, warfarin has been the most commonly used oral anticoagulant, although, more recently, newer oral agents such as direct thrombin and factor Xa inhibitors have become available. At similar warfarin plasma concentrations, there is greater vitamin K inhibition in older adults. Thus, it is recommended that warfarin should be initiated at a daily dose of 5 mg or less for older adults, when indicated. In the ED, this may occur for patients discharged after a venous thromboembolism in conjunction with low-molecular-weight heparin as bridge therapy. There is emerging evidence supporting the early use of direct-acting oral anticoagulants for certain patients presenting with a venous thromboembolism (VTE). While data regarding the use of direct-acting oral anticoagulants in older patients being discharged from the ED with VTE are sparse, when used, careful attention must be paid when selecting an agent and formulating a dosing regimen. Certain agents, such as dabigatran, should be avoided in advanced age (greater than 80 years of age), while others, such as apixaban, require an adjustment when renal dysfunction is present in patients above a certain age threshold (Table 180.2).[10,11] Dosing regimens and recommendations for adjustment also differ based on indication. In addition, therapeutic

TABLE 180.2   Harmful Drug Interactions From Studies in Older Patients

Object Drug	Adverse Event	Comments
ACE inhibitor or ARB	Hyperkalemia	Avoid potassium sparing diuretics or TMP-SMX Apixaban Subtherapeutic, increased VTE risk Interacts with carbamazepine
Benzodiazepines and sedative-hypnotics	Fractures, falls	Interacts with macrolides and has additive effect with other CNS depressants
Calcium channel blockers	Hypotension	Interacts with macrolides
Digoxin	Toxicity	Interacts with macrolides Haloperidol Toxicity Interacts with Parkinson's treatments
Lithium	Toxicity	Interacts with diuretics, ACE inhibitors, and NSAIDs
Phenytoin	Toxicity	Interacts with TMP-SMX
Sulfonylureas	Hypoglycemia	Interacts with TMP-SMX, fluconazole, macrolides, and fluoroquinolones
Theophylline	Toxicity	Interacts with ciprofloxacin
Warfarin	Bleeding	Interacts with most antibiotics and antifungal agents. Increased risk with NSAIDs

ACE, Angiotensin-converting enzyme; *ARB,* angiotensin receptor blocker; *CNS,* central nervous system; *NSAID,* nonsteroidal antiinflammatory drug; *TMP-SMX,* trimethoprim-sulfamethoxazole.

drug monitoring is not routinely available for these agents, making it difficult to assess the degree of anticoagulation, further enhancing the need for nuance and attention to detail to ensure they are being used appropriately. The other primary anticoagulant used in the ED is intravenous heparin for acute coronary syndrome or venous thromboembolism. Patient age does not correlate with heparin dose requirements, so heparin dose adjustments are not required.

SPECIFIC DISORDERS

Polypharmacy and Drug Interactions

The term *polypharmacy* is used to describe the use of multiple medications. There is no standard definition or consensus regarding the number of medications that serves as a cut point for this term; however, the American College of Emergency Physician's Geriatric Emergency Department Guidelines and other experts consider five or more medications to constitute polypharmacy.[12] Older patients are particularly prone to polypharmacy because they have a greater number of comorbidities and conditions requiring treatment for medications. In one national estimate of community-residing older adults, close to one-third of the population took five or more medications, and approximately half also took over-the-counter medications and dietary supplements. Polypharmacy may result in adverse drug effects, drug interactions, and functional and cognitive impairment, and can lead to falls, resulting in injury.[13,14] An estimated 10% of ED visits by older adults may be attributed to an adverse drug-related event.

An important consequence of polypharmacy is drug interactions, which occur more commonly in older adults. A drug interaction occurs when there is an alteration in the effect of a drug due to the coadministration of another. The alteration could be the increase in effect, leading to toxicity, or a decrease in effect, resulting in therapeutic failure. The mechanism of interaction could be pharmacokinetic, which is primarily due to the inhibition or induction of drug-metabolizing enzymes such as the cytochrome P450 system or alterations in drug transporter activity. Alternatively, the interaction could be pharmacodynamic, in which the change in effect is unrelated to pharmacokinetic mechanisms. This primarily occurs due to the pharmacologic effects of drugs, which may be additive or antagonistic. For example, the use of a benzodiazepine with an antibiotic that inhibits its metabolism leading to an increased or prolonged effect would be a pharmacokinetic interaction, whereas the use of a benzodiazepine with an opioid, leading to additive central nervous system depression, would be a pharmacodynamic interaction.

There are thousands of possible drug-drug interactions, which increase exponentially with the number of medications that a patient is taking. The use of ED pharmacists may help to identify clinically relevant drug-drug interactions, particularly in patients with complex medication regimens. Clinical decision support systems integrated with electronic medical records may also provide a useful mechanism to reduce this risk; however, there are several challenges that need to be overcome in the ED setting so that providers can make the best possible decisions. The identification of an interaction is dependent on an accurate medication history, which is often difficult to obtain. Clinical decision support systems identify many drug interactions that are not clinically meaningful, leading to alert fatigue. It is estimated that providers override more than 96% of alerts, even when the interactions are significant.[15] Furthermore, most interactions are based on preclinical studies during drug development, have a theoretical basis, and often lack high-level evidence. This leads to discrepancies in major drug information systems, and there is no standard classification to guide decisions.

A prudent approach is to focus on the most common drug interactions that have been known to result in patient harm and that may be most applicable to the emergency clinician. Single doses of drugs administered within the monitored setting of the ED are less likely to lead to harm than those prescribed on discharge and used for several days. Adverse events can be narrowed down to several interactions that resulted in hospitalization from hyperkalemia, hypotension, fractures, hypoglycemia, bleeding, and specific drug toxicities. The object drugs involved in these interactions should serve as important flags to alert prescribers when giving a new medication (Table 180.3). Most of these adverse events are seen to occur when new antibiotics are prescribed. Thus, antibiotics prescribed to patients need to be considered carefully for potential interactions, especially when patients are taking a medication such as one mentioned earlier. However, there are many other high-risk medications, such as antidepressants, neuroleptics, and antiepileptics, that are also known to have several drug-drug interactions. Ideally, consultation with a pharmacist is helpful in identifying and determining the risk of potential drug interactions and modifying the therapeutic plan, if necessary.

Potentially Inappropriate Medications
Beers Criteria

In 1991, Beers and colleagues developed explicit criteria defining inappropriate medication use in older adults. They are now known as the Beers criteria and are periodically updated by the American Geriatrics Society.[5] At that time, it was observed that residents of skilled nursing

TABLE 180.3 Dose Adjustments for Direct Oral Anticoagulants (DOACs)

Drug	Indication	Adult Regimen	Recommended Dose Adjustments
Apixaban	Venous Thromboembolism or Pulmonary Embolism	10 mg bid × 7 days followed by 5 mg bid	None
	Non-Valvular Atrial Fibrillation	5 mg bid	2.5 mg bid if 2 of the following: age > 80 y, weight ≤ 60 kg, sCr > 1.5 mg/dL
Dabigatran	Venous Thromboembolism or Pulmonary Embolism	150 mg bid after at least 5 days of parenteral therapy	Patients ≥ 75 y: Use extreme caution and consider other options[a] Patients > 65 y: Use with caution CrCl 30–50 mL/min and P-glycoprotein inhibitor use: 75 mg bid CrCl avoid use
	Non-Valvular Atrial Fibrillation	150 mg bid	Patients ≥ 75 y: Use extreme caution and consider other options[a] CrCl 50–80 mL/min: Use caution due to increased drug exposure CrCl 30–50 mL/min: Adjust if significant drug interactions, use with caution in advanced age CrCl ≤30 mL/min: Avoid use
Edoxaban	Venous Thromboembolism or Pulmonary Embolism	After at least 5 days of parenteral therapy and CrCl < 95 mL/min : 60 mg daily	CrCl 15–50 mL/min OR age >65 AND weight <60 kg OR use of concomitant P-glycoprotein inhibitors: 30 mg daily CrCl < 15 mL/min: Avoid use
	Non-Valvular Atrial Fibrillation	CrCl < 95 mL/min: 60 mg daily	CrCl 15–50 mL/min: 30 mg daily CrCl < 15 mL/min: Avoid use
Rivaroxaban	Venous Thromboembolism or Pulmonary Embolism	15 mg bid with food × 21 days followed by 20 mg daily with food	CrCl <30 mL/min: Avoid use
	Non-Valvular Atrial Fibrillation	20 mg daily with food	CrCl 15–50 mL/min: 15 mg once daily CrCl < 15 mL/min: Avoid use

[a]Dabigatran has shown an increased risk of excessive anticoagulation leading to hemorrhagic complications, including fatalities, with increased age. DOACs should be avoided in all patients with moderate to severe hepatic impairment and nursing mothers.

facilities were prescribed eight medications on average; more than 50% of them received a psychoactive medication. The Beers criteria were applied to the older residents in nursing homes, representing the frailest of the population. Inappropriate medications were defined by an expert panel as those that should be avoided, except under unusual clinical circumstances. This was because of the lack of effectiveness, risks outweighing the benefits, or safer alternatives that were available. The criteria were developed so that they could be assessed from easily identifiable pharmacy records using minimal clinical data. This made it feasible for use for the quality improvement initiatives in skilled nursing facilities. The Beers criteria were subsequently updated so that they could be applied to all older patients, regardless of the place of residence. The most recent version from the American Geriatrics Society was developed by a 13-member panel with expertise in geriatric medicine, nursing, pharmacy, research, and quality measures.[5] Each criterion for medication or class includes a quality of evidence rating and strength of recommendation, serving as a valuable resource for clinicians involved in the care of older adults.

However, important questions remain regarding the applicability of the Beers criteria to practice in the ED. For example, promethazine is considered to be an inappropriate medication for older adults because of its anticholinergic and central nervous system effects, and avoiding this agent was given a strong recommendation based on high-quality evidence by the expert panel. Although the chronic effects of promethazine, such as drug-related falls, constipation, and dry mouth, are not of particular concern in the ED, promethazine-induced confusion or

sedation may be problematic in patients presenting with altered mental status. A safer alternative for nausea or vomiting in this latter circumstance would be a 5-HT$_3$ receptor antagonist, such as ondansetron. However, ondansetron has been associated with QTc interval prolongation, which could be concerning in older patients who are already taking QTc-prolonging medications, leading to a potentially severe drug interaction. These nuanced therapeutic decisions require emergency clinicians to consider patient-specific parameters and realize that a "one size fits all" approach may not be appropriate.

Medications provided on discharge create another challenge. Although benzodiazepines appear on the Beers list, a single dose of a short-acting benzodiazepine used for procedural sedation in a controlled environment with monitoring and observation until the patient has returned to baseline is unlikely to cause long-term issues; however, medications prescribed on discharge must be more cautiously considered. Medications given to older patients on discharge should be prescribed for a limited duration until outpatient follow-up can be provided. In this setting, the Beers criteria may provide important guidance. For example, the Beers criteria expert panel has recommended that benzodiazepines should be avoided for the treatment of insomnia in older adults. This is because of the increased risk for cognitive impairment, delirium, falls, fractures, and motor vehicle collisions. Even short-term use of benzodiazepines after ED discharge could be associated with these adverse effects. In one randomized controlled trial, the use of a clinical decision support system in the ED was able to reduce the prescribing of potentially inappropriate medications in

TABLE 180.4 Most Common Beers List Medications Prescribed to Patients Discharged from the Emergency Department

Rank	Inappropriate Medication[a]
1	Promethazine
2	Diphenhydramine
3	Diazepam
4	Hydroxyzine
5	Amitriptyline
6	Cyclobenzaprine
7	Clonidine
8	Indomethacin

[a]Propoxyphene is not included because it is no longer available.

TABLE 180.5 Top 10 STOPP Criteria

Rank	Criteria
1	Long-term use of benzodiazepines
2	Duplicate prescriptions from the same drug class
3	Proton pump inhibitor for peptic ulcer disease at full dose for >8 wk
4	NSAIDs in patients with moderate to severe hypertension
5	Long-term use of opioids—first-line treatment for mild to moderate pain
6	Aspirin without adequate cardiovascular risk
7	Warfarin and NSAID used together
8	Beta blocker in patients with chronic obstructive pulmonary disease
9	Prolonged use of first-generation antihistamines
10	NSAID use in patients with chronic renal failure

NSAID, Nonsteroidal antiinflammatory drug; STOPP (Screening Tool of Older People's Potentially Inappropriate Prescriptions).

patients being discharged from the ED. Interestingly, the study targeted only a few medications, which accounted for 80% of the inappropriate medications prescribed on discharge. These medications, listed from the most to least commonly used, are in Table 180.4. Each institution should periodically evaluate trends in medications being prescribed and assessed for appropriateness because this can vary by center.

STOPP and START Criteria

In 2008, the STOPP (*S*creening *T*ool of *O*lder *P*eople's Potentially Inappropriate *P*rescriptions) and START (*S*creening *T*ool to *A*lert doctors to *R*ight *T*reatment) tools were developed and validated to build upon the Beers criteria and overcome some of their limitations. The Beers criteria account for only a small subset of medications that are prescribed inappropriately to older adults. In addition, many of the medications in the Beers criteria may not be available in European countries or are seldom prescribed. In the ED setting, these tools can be used to identify drug-related presentations, to determine if medications are suitable to be used in the ED during acute illness, and to guide medication prescribing on discharge. Even if a presentation is not drug-related, assessment in the ED is an opportunity to identify medications that may be problematic and lead to future admissions. In this regard, the STOPP screening tool was able to identify more elderly ED patients with potentially inappropriate medications than the Beers criteria (35% versus 25%). The STOPP-related medications also contributed to twice the number of admissions (12% versus 6%). The most recent version includes 80 STOPP and 34 START criteria.[16] The top 10 criteria that identified the most patients with inappropriate medications are listed in Table 180.5.

Anticoagulation and Bleeding

Oral anticoagulation use is common for age-related conditions such as atrial fibrillation. Warfarin has been used for several decades but is less than ideal because it has a narrow therapeutic range, routine laboratory monitoring is required, and numerous drug and food interactions lead to an unpredictable response, often resulting in hemorrhagic complications.

More recently, newer direct acting oral anticoagulants have become available that do not require routine laboratory monitoring and have fewer drug interactions and are not affected by diet. These include a direct thrombin inhibitor, dabigatran, and the factor Xa inhibitors rivaroxaban, apixaban, and edoxaban. High-quality randomized clinical trials of these direct oral anticoagulants (DOACs) have shown them to be equivalent or superior to warfarin with regard to stroke prevention and bleeding occurrence for patients in atrial fibrillation.

A recent meta-analysis of these agents found that when used for atrial fibrillation in elderly patients, DOACs were associated with a lower risk thromboembolic events when compared to warfarin.[17] This analysis also found no difference in the rate of major bleeding events, a decreased risk of intracranial bleeding, hemorrhagic stroke, and fatal bleeding compared to warfarin, but were associated with a higher risk of gastrointestinal bleeding compared to warfarin. Current prescribing trends indicate that warfarin use is declining and the use of DOACs is on the rise both in the general population and specifically in older adults.[18,19]

One drawback of these agents is that they undergo renal elimination, and patients with severe renal impairment were excluded from major trials. Although several of these agents provide recommendations for dosing adjustments based on creatinine clearance, the fluctuating course of renal function in older adults during an acute illness may contribute to accumulation and bleeding. Furthermore, routine laboratory testing does not quantify the level of anticoagulation. For warfarin-induced bleeding, reversal is achieved when the international normalized ratio (INR) is less than 1.5. The new oral anticoagulants increase prothrombin time (PT), activated partial thromboplastin time (aPTT), and thrombin time, but these measures do not reliably estimate the level of anticoagulation and thus have limited ability to guide therapy. Laboratory parameters such as ecarin clotting time, diluted thrombin time, and chromogenic antifactor Xa assay may be useful; however, these tests are not widely available.

The most common major hemorrhagic complication resulting from anticoagulation is intracranial hemorrhage (ICH) following traumatic brain injury. While high-quality prospective research is lacking, recent studies suggest that patients receiving DOACs have worse outcomes and increased risk for delayed ICH following TBI.[20,21] Prompt reversal of anticoagulation is recommended in the setting of a life-threatening hemorrhage after careful evaluation of the thromboembolic risk of reversal in relation to the anticipated benefit of achieving hemorrhage control. There is limited evidence to guide anticoagulation reversal specifically in elderly patients; however, in general, reversal strategies used in younger adults are reasonable to use in elderly patients.

Neurologic Conditions

Altered mental status and delirium are common chief complaints among older patients presenting to the ED. Although there are many factors that can influence mental status, medication-related adverse effects are a common cause of altered mental status and delirium. Evaluation of a patient presenting with altered mental status or delirium should include a thorough medication history, including prescription and nonprescription medications as well as over-the-counter nutritional supplements. Many of the medications are included on the Beers list are included due to their propensity for causing adverse neurologic effects. Medications with anticholinergic properties, benzodiazepines, sedatives, hypnotics, and opioids are commonly associated with delirium. Avoidance of anticholinergic agents in elderly patients was given a strong recommendation based on moderate- to high-quality evidence by the American Geriatrics Society.[5] There are numerous medications with anticholinergic effects, and toxicity is often due to a cumulative anticholinergic burden. Treatment begins with supportive care and nonpharmacologic measures, including discontinuation of the offending medications.

When nonpharmacologic measures have been unsuccessful and the patient is presenting a danger to themselves or others, pharmacologic management should be considered. Antipsychotic agents such as haloperidol or an atypical antipsychotic may be used. When used in older adults, lower starting doses are typically recommended (e.g., haloperidol doses of ≤5 mg IM [intramuscular] or IV) to reduce the risk of extrapyramidal symptoms.[22] Large doses of haloperidol given via the IV route have been associated with QTc interval prolongation, so monitoring of the electrocardiogram (ECG) is important, if feasible, especially if repeated doses are needed. Avoid haloperidol use in patients with Parkinson's due to increased risk of mortality. Use an intramuscular/intravenous atypical antipsychotic instead such as olanzapine or ziprasidone if one is needed.

There are certain, specific situations where short-term use of low-dose benzodiazepines may be considered for agitated delirium, including suspicion that the patient is withdrawing from alcohol or benzodiazepines or if the patient has comorbid conditions, such as Parkinson disease or QTc prolongation, that would preclude the use of an antipsychotic agent; however, there is weak to moderate-quality evidence that benzodiazepines may contribute to delirium, and they should generally be avoided in the elderly.[22]

There are also differences in the pharmacologic management of some key neurologic emergencies in older adults. In patients with community-acquired bacterial meningitis, the Infectious Disease Society of America has additional recommendations for older adults compared to young adults. In older adults, ampicillin is recommended in addition to the standard empirical regimen for coverage of *Listeria monocytogenes*. Thus, older patients should receive a triple regimen of vancomycin, ceftriaxone, and ampicillin. However, the cutoff value for age is 50 years rather than the traditional age definition. Similarly, there are differences in the eligibility criteria for thrombolytic therapy for ischemic stroke based on age. The American Heart Association guidelines on the management of ischemic stroke allow for extending the time window for the provision of thrombolysis from 3 to 4.5 hours after onset of symptoms in select patients.[23] This recommendation incorporates the exclusion criteria utilized in the primary trial showing benefit from this approach. The ECASS-3 trial excluded patients older than 80 years, and as a result, while extending the time window to 4.5 hours in patients over 80 years old is still recommended, it is given a lower level recommendation compared to younger patients.

Analgesia

In a national survey of US EDs, geriatric patients with pain-related complaints were less likely to receive any analgesics than young adults.[24] The risk for poor pain management in older adults is multifactorial and increases with logistic constraints, such as ED crowding. Pain perception and susceptibility to adverse drug effects of analgesics is also different in older patients. Dosing of opioids should be cautious and monitoring for respiratory depression needs to be vigilant. It is difficult to anticipate how much opioid would be required for pain control

in the ED. Instead of large single doses, a lower dose with titration consistent with pharmacokinetic and pharmacodynamic characteristics of the opioid is ideal. For example, morphine and hydromorphone have their peak analgesic effect at approximately 15 minutes. Thus, redosing every 1 to 2 hours is an unnecessarily long time and leads to suboptimal pain control. One strategy that has been successfully used in older patients for severe pain in the ED is a two-step hydromorphone protocol.[25] Patients are given 0.5 mg IV hydromorphone, which is repeated in 15 minutes if the patient desires another dose when asked, "Do you want more pain medication?" However, previous opioid exposure needs to be considered to determine appropriate dosing. For example, in some older cancer patients with chronic opioid consumption, doses will likely need to be escalated for pain control.

Meperidine use should be avoided in older patients. It has a neurotoxic metabolite that accumulates with renal impairment common in these patients. Given the availability of alternative opioids, there is little reason to use this medication in the ED, and it is also listed on the Beers criteria.

Regional anesthetics, such as fascia iliaca compartment blocks in patients with hip fractures, have been shown to reduce opioid requirements and should be considered, particularly in older patients, when feasible.[26] Other strategies, such as hematoma blocks and intra-articular steroid injections, should be considered to minimize systemic analgesics when appropriate.

Ketorolac is a valuable alternative to opioids in the ED, and single doses have been shown to be as effective as opioids for pain related to certain indications, such as renal or gallbladder stones. However, it is a potent nonsteroidal antiinflammatory drug (NSAID) with the possibility of causing renal failure or gastrointestinal hemorrhage. This is less likely to occur with isolated doses in the ED setting. Nonetheless, studies have demonstrated similar analgesic effects from ketorolac doses of 10 mg, 15 mg, and 30 mg, indicating a ceiling effect.[27] To minimize the possibility of adverse effects, doses over 10 mg are not recommended, particularly in older adults. Despite lacking antiinflammatory effects, IV acetaminophen has been shown to provide similar pain control compared to IV ketorolac in a heterogenous prehospital population that included older patients.[28] Acetaminophen is a reasonable alternative to NSAIDs in select patients; however, in most health systems, only oral and rectal acetaminophen are readily available. Studies in the perioperative and postoperative settings have failed to show a significant difference in pain reduction or opioid sparing effects between IV and oral acetaminophen leading many health systems to restrict the use of IV acetaminophen given the relatively high cost of the parenteral dosage form.[29]

Clinical Pharmacy Services

There are a growing number of institutions that have pharmacists who practice in the ED. The American College of Emergency Physicians (ACEP) has a policy statement advocating for dedicated pharmacy services to be provided to the ED to promote safe, efficient, and effective medication use in the emergency department.[30] In geriatric EDs, there is a great opportunity to integrate pharmacists, given the myriad drug therapy issues that can lead to suboptimal care.[12] Older adults have more medications prescribed, which increases the risk for medication errors.[31] Pharmacists are able to intercept these errors, preventing patient harm. Given the possibility of drug-induced admissions, pharmacy services can be used to identify medications that may have contributed to an ED presentation. However, resource constraints make it difficult for pharmacists to evaluate each geriatric patient, especially in EDs with large bed capacities.

Obtaining an accurate medication list is necessary for determining the cause of an adverse effect, but this often requires phone calls to multiple pharmacies and physicians' offices. One option is the use of pharmacy technicians who are also able to perform this function with similar accuracy.[32] Patients can also be referred to the pharmacist based on variables that have been associated with adverse drug events.[33] One clinical decision rule was able to identify 91.3% of patients with adverse drug events by limiting referral of less than half of patients to a pharmacist so that a full review could be conducted. This decision rule is shown in Fig. 180.1.

Even if the presentation is unrelated to an adverse drug event, clinical pharmacists can be used to identify potentially inappropriate therapies that the patient is taking to minimize the possibility for readmissions. For example, it is possible that a patient may be taking two medications from the same drug class prescribed by two different physicians. Applying the Beers, START, and STOPP criteria, the anticholinergic burden and other opportunities for drug therapy optimization can be assessed. Finally, pharmacists serve as an important safety net for drug therapy prescribed by ED clinicians, both within the ED and on discharge. Setting up a system whereby the pharmacist can be consulted and is available to review these medication orders for potential harm is a risk mitigation strategy that may help reduce readmissions by older adults.

Has the patient taken medications in the past 2 weeks?

☐ Yes ☐ No → **LOW RISK**

↓

Does the patient have any preexisting medical problems or has the patient taken antibiotics in the past 7 days?

☐ Yes ☐ No → **LOW RISK**

↓

Is the patient ≥ 80 years old *or* has the patient changed any medications in the past 28 days?

☐ Yes ☐ No → **LOW RISK**

↓

HIGH RISK

Fig. 180.1 Decision rule to identify adverse drug events. (Adapted from: Hohl CM, Badke K, Zhao A, et al. Prospective validation of clinical criteria to identify emergency department patients at high risk for adverse drug events. *Acad Emerg Med.* 2018;25(9):1015-1026.)

The references for this chapter can be found online at ExpertConsult.com.

181

Geriatric Abuse and Neglect

Tony Rosen

KEY CONCEPTS

- Elder mistreatment, which includes physical abuse, sexual abuse, neglect, emotional/psychological abuse, abandonment, financial/material exploitation, and self-neglect, is common and may have serious medical and social consequences.
- Elder mistreatment is under-recognized by emergency clinicians and under-reported to the authorities.
- Signs suggestive of potential elder abuse and neglect that should be recognized by emergency clinicians may exist in the medical history, physical examination, and medical/laboratory markers.
- Emergency clinicians should be vigilant in assessing for the possibility of elder abuse or neglect and routinely ask elderly patients about mistreatment, even in the absence of signs and symptoms. Screening protocols may be helpful.
- Using a team-based approach including social workers and other emergency department (ED)-based professionals may improve elder abuse detection, and Emergency Medical Services can play a critical role.
- ED management of elder abuse should include the following: treating acute medical and psychological issues, ensuring patient safety, and proper reporting to the authorities. Trauma-informed care should be provided.
- Emergency clinicians should hospitalize elderly patients who are in immediate danger or implement a care plan that prevents them from having any contact with the suspected abuser(s) but must respect the wishes of an older adult with decision-making capacity who refuses interventions and desires to return to an abusive situation. Trauma-informed care should be provided.
- Emergency clinicians should document completely and accurately the history and all physical findings in cases of suspected elder abuse or neglect, as this documentation may be critical to ensure justice for the victim.

FOUNDATIONS

Background

An ED encounter offers an important opportunity to identify and initiate intervention for elder abuse and neglect, a common but under-recognized phenomenon that may have serious medical and social consequences. Elder abuse and neglect includes: any actions or negligence that may cause harm or risk of harm committed by someone in a relationship of trust or when the victim is targeted due to age or disability, Table 181.1. Many victims may suffer concurrently from multiple types of abuse.

Epidemiology and Scope of the Problem

As many as 10% of older adults living in the community and more than 20% of nursing home residents experience some form of abuse, neglect, or exploitation each year. Psychological/emotional abuse, financial mistreatment, and neglect are most commonly reported, while physical and sexual abuse are less common. Elder abuse is strongly associated with adverse health outcomes, including depression, exacerbations of chronic illness, and dramatically increased mortality. Older adults suffering abuse are more likely to present to the ED, be hospitalized, and be placed in a nursing home. The direct medical costs of elder abuse and neglect, though challenging to quantify, are estimated to be many billions of dollars annually and growing as the geriatric population continues to increase.

Despite its frequency and potential for harm, elder abuse and neglect is under-recognized and under-reported, with many sufferers enduring it for years before discovery. Studies suggest that as few as 1 in 24 cases of elder abuse is reported to the authorities, and much of the associated morbidity and mortality is likely due to delay in identification and intervention.

Many factors contribute to elder abuse and neglect (Table 181.2), and researchers have attempted to identify risk factors for becoming a victim or perpetrator. Findings have been inconsistent and difficult to interpret, partly due to methodological limitations, and to the heterogeneity of elder mistreatment cases. Potential risk factors for becoming a victim or perpetrator based on existing evidence are described in Box 181.1. Cognitively impaired older adults are more likely to be victimized. Sub-populations including military veterans and lesbian/gay/bisexual/transgender older adults may be at particularly high risk. Many cases of elder mistreatment occur in the absence of risk factors, however, and the phenomenon crosses ethnic and socioeconomic boundaries.

Identifying Elder Abuse and Neglect in the Emergency Department

The ED visit provides an opportunity to identify elder abuse or neglect. For many older adults, assessment by health care providers is their only contact outside the family. Limited research suggests that elder abuse and neglect victims are less likely to see a primary care provider but receive ED care more frequently than other older adults,[1] often for management of acute illnesses or injuries. A recent study found that 7% of cognitively intact older ED patients reported a history of physical or psychological mistreatment during the previous year.[2] The actual prevalence is likely much higher, as abuse is more common among cognitively impaired older adults, and because neglect and financial exploitation were not included.

TABLE 181.1   Types of Elder Abuse and Neglect

Type	Definition	Examples
Physical abuse	Intentional use of physical force that may result in bodily injury, physical pain, or impairment	• Slapping, hitting, kicking, pushing, pulling hair • Use of physical restraints, force-feeding • Burning, use of household objects as weapons, use of firearms and knives
Sexual abuse	Any type of sexual contact with an elderly person that is non-consensual or sexual contact with any person incapable of giving consent	• Sexual assault or battery, such as rape, sodomy, coerced nudity, and sexually explicit photographing • Unwanted touching, verbal sexual advances • Indecent exposure
Neglect	Refusal or failure to fulfill any part of a person's obligations or duties to an elder, which may result in harm—may be intentional or unintentional	• Withholding of food, water, clothing, shelter, medications • Failure to ensure elder's personal hygiene or to provide physical aids, including walker, cane, glasses, hearing aids, dentures • Failure to ensure elder's personal safety and/or appropriate medical follow-up
Emotional/ psychological abuse	Intentional infliction of anguish, pain, or distress through verbal or nonverbal acts	• Verbal berating, harassment, or intimidation • Threats of punishment or deprivation • Treating the older person like an infant • Isolating the older person from others
Abandonment	Desertion of an elderly person by an individual who has assumed responsibility for providing care for an elder or by a person with physical custody	
Financial/material exploitation	Illegal or improper use of an older adult's money, property, or assets	• Stealing money or belongings • Cashing an older adult's checks without permission and/or forging his or her signature • Coercing an older adult into signing contracts, changing a will, or assigning durable power of attorney against his or her wishes or when the older adult does not possess the mental capacity to do so
Self-neglect	Behavior of an older adult that threatens his/her own health or safety—excluding when an older adult who understands the consequences of his or her actions makes a conscious and voluntary decision to engage in acts that threaten his/her health or safety	• Refusal or failure of an older adult to provide himself or herself with basic necessities such as food, water, shelter, medications, and appropriate personal hygiene • Disregard for maintenance of safe home environment and/or hoarding

Adapted from National Center on Elder Abuse: Types of abuse. Available at https://ncea.acl.gov/Suspect-Abuse/Abuse-Types.aspx.

TABLE 181.2   Selected Theories of the Underlying Causes of Elder Abuse and Neglect

Theory	Description
Transgenerational violence	Family violence is a learned behavior, and abused children grow up to potentially abuse not only their own children but also perhaps parents
Psychopathology of the abuser	Mental health issues of the abuser, including personality disorders, poorly treated mood disorders or schizophrenia, alcoholism, and other substance abuse problems, lead to abusive behavior
Dependency	Increasing frailty, including functional and cognitive disability, result in overwhelming care needs that leave an older adult vulnerable to abuse by an overburdened caregiver
Stressed caregiver	A caregiver who has become increasingly stressed (from caregiving or other causes) may be more likely to be abusive
Isolation	Greater social isolation due to disability, illness, and age increases an older adult's vulnerability to abuse or neglect

Adapted from: Jones JS, Holstege C, Holstege H. Elder abuse and neglect: understanding the causes and potential risk factors. *Am J Emerg Med.* 1997;15:579-583.

Additionally, the nature of an ED encounter increases the potential for detection, as an older adult is typically assessed over several hours by multiple providers.

Despite the opportunity, emergency clinicians seldom identify and report elder abuse and neglect. Several reasons exist for this missed opportunity, including inadequate training, difficulty distinguishing between intentional and unintentional injuries, lack of time to conduct a thorough evaluation for abuse, concern about involvement in the legal system, a victim's unwillingness to report, and a victim's inability to report due to cognitive impairment. For the health of our patients, it is critical that all emergency care providers embrace the challenge of identifying and initiating care for victims of elder abuse and neglect.

CLINICAL FEATURES

Observation and Medical History

When initially assessing an older adult with a caregiver present, carefully observe their interaction, identifying any clues of a strained relationship. Observations that increase suspicion for elder abuse or neglect are listed in Box 181.2.

History should be taken from the patient in as private a setting as possible, without caregivers or family present. The patient should be assured of privacy and confidentiality since victims may be reluctant to

BOX 181.1   Potential Risk Factors for Elder Abuse

For Becoming a Victim
Functional dependence or disability
Poor physical health
Cognitive impairment/dementia
Poor mental health
Low income/socioeconomic status
Social isolation/low social support
Previous history of family violence
Previous traumatic event exposure
Substance abuse

For Becoming a Perpetrator
Mental illness
Substance abuse
Caregiver stress
Previous history of family violence
Financial dependence on older adult

Acierno R, Hernandez MA, Amstadter AB, et al. Prevalence and correlates of emotional, physical, sexual, and financial abuse and potential neglect in the United States: the National Elder Mistreatment Study. *Am J Public Health.* 2010;100:292-297; Amstadter AB, Zajac K, Strachan M, et al. Prevalence and correlates of elder mistreatment in South Carolina: the South Carolina elder mistreatment study. *J Interpers Violence.* 2011;26:2947-2972; Pillemer K, Burnes D, Riffin C, et al. Elder abuse: background paper for the world report on ageing and health. *Gerontologist.* 2016;56(Suppl 2):S194-205; Gibbs LM. Understanding the medical markers of elder abuse and neglect: physical examination findings. *Clin Geriatr Med.* 2014;30:687-712.

BOX 181.2   Observations from Interaction Between Older Adult and Caregiver That Should Raise Concern for Elder Abuse or Neglect

Older adult and caregiver provide conflicting accounts of events
Caregiver interrupts/answers for the older adult
Older adult seems fearful of or hostile towards caregiver
Caregiver appears unengaged/inattentive in caring for the older adult
Caregiver appear frustrated, tired, angry, or burdened by the older adult
Caregiver appears overwhelmed by the older adult
Caregiver appears to lack knowledge of the patient's care needs
Evidence that the caregiver and/or older adult may be abusing alcohol or illicit drugs

BOX 181.3   Indicators from the Medical History of Possible Elder Mistreatment

Poor living conditions according to paramedics or others
Unexplained injuries
Past history of frequent injuries
Delay between onset of medical illness or injury and seeking of medical attention
Recurrent visits to the ED for similar injuries
Using multiple physicians and EDs for care rather than one primary care physician ("doctor hopping or shopping")
Noncompliance with medications, appointments, or physician directions
Patient or caregiver reluctant to answer questions
Strained patient/caregiver interaction
Inconsistent history of injury mechanism between the patient and caregiver
Elderly patient referred to as "accident prone"
Caregiver not able to give details of the patient's medical history or routine medications
Caregiver answers the questions regarding the patient
Abandonment of the patient in the ED by the caregiver

ED, Emergency department.

patient should be questioned about how the injury occurred, including directed questions regarding whether anyone has hit, punched, pushed, tripped, or kicked the patient. The evaluation should also include an assessment for behavioral signs and symptoms suggestive of potential elder mistreatment, including fear, anxiety, poor eye contact, low self-esteem, and helplessness.

Unfortunately, obtaining a reliable history from victims of elder abuse and neglect is often difficult. Many older adults have cognitive impairment that prevents them from providing an accurate medical history. Even in these cases, an attempt should be made to interview the patient, in that recent research suggests that older adults with cognitive impairment can reliably report abuse.[3] Whenever an older adult is unable to provide a history, information should be sought from others besides the caregiver such as other family members, the primary care physician, neighbors, or visiting nurses.

A separate interview of the caregiver or suspected abuser is often useful. It may reveal discrepancies from the patient's history. In addition, a caregiver who is unfamiliar with an older adult's routine medications and necessary medical care may be neglecting them. The interview should be conducted in a nonthreatening and nonjudgmental manner. Verbal expressions of sympathy, explicit recognition of the challenges, and demonstrations of support can be beneficial for the caregiver and also promote information sharing. Questions should also explore whether any important changes or recent stresses have occurred in the household, whether the caregiver feels that the patient is a burden, the caregiver's other dependents and responsibilities, and whether any respite services or other home help services have been made available.

Physical Examination

Physical examination should include a thorough exam for signs of injury and abuse, including identification of bruising peritoneal injury. Additional attention should be given to the skin and intra-oral exam. Geriatric patients with multiple suspicious physical findings may be more likely to be victims of elder abuse or neglect than those with isolated findings.

When an older adult presents with an acute injury (such as a fall), consider whether the reported mechanism is consistent with the injuries suffered. Research has begun to systematically explore

disclose due to a desire to protect the abuser (often a spouse or child), dependency on the caregiver, shame, cultural or ethnic beliefs, or a fear of reprisal or institutionalization. If a translator is needed, a professional translator or telephone/virtual translation service should be provided. A family member or the caregiver should not be used as an interpreter even if they are not suspected to be an abuser.

The assessment for elder mistreatment should be incorporated into the routine evaluation. Potential historical indicators of elder mistreatment are listed in Box 181.3. The emergency clinician may ask in detail about the reason for the visit and then inquire about the patient's health in general, focusing on the safety of the home environment, functional status, cognition, need for support or assistance, and any feelings of isolation and depression. Box 181.4 suggests potential questions to assess for abuse. If the older adult is presenting with an injury, the

BOX 181.4   Questions for Use in Asking Patients About Elder Abuse

Please explore any positive responses in more detail.
  In the last 6 months:

Physical Abuse	Has anyone tried to harm you? Have you been hit, slapped, pushed, grabbed, strangled, or kicked?
	Are there guns or other weapons in your home? Does anyone close to you have access to guns or other weapons?
Sexual Abuse	Has anyone touched you in ways or places you did not want to be touched?
Neglect/Functional Status	Have you relied on people for any of the following: bathing, dressing, shopping, banking, or meals?
	a. If yes, have you had someone who helps you with this?
	b. If yes, how often do you receive help? Is this help enough?
	c. Have they done a good job? Are they reliable?
	d. What happens if no one is available to help?
	Has anyone prevented you from getting food, clothes, medication, glasses, hearing aids, medical care, or anything else you need to stay healthy?

Psychological Abuse	Has anyone close to you called you names, put you down, or yelled at you?
	Has anyone close to you ever threatened to punish you or put you in an institution?
	Have you felt sad or lonely at home?
	Have you felt afraid of anyone close to you?
	Do you distrust anyone close to you?
	Does anyone close to you drink or use drugs?
Financial Exploitation	Has anyone tried to force you to sign papers against your will, or that you did not understand?
	a. Has anyone pressured you to give them money or property?
	Has anyone taken money or things that belong to you without asking?
	Does anyone close to you rely on you for housing and/or financial support?

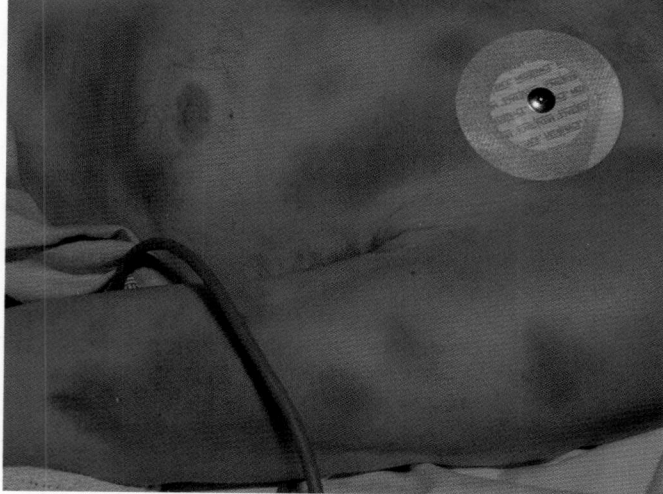

Fig. 181.1 Atypical bruising of the chest in a case of substantiated abuse. (From: Gibbs LM. Understanding the medical markers of elder abuse and neglect: physical examination findings. Clin Geriatr Med. 2014;30:687-712.)

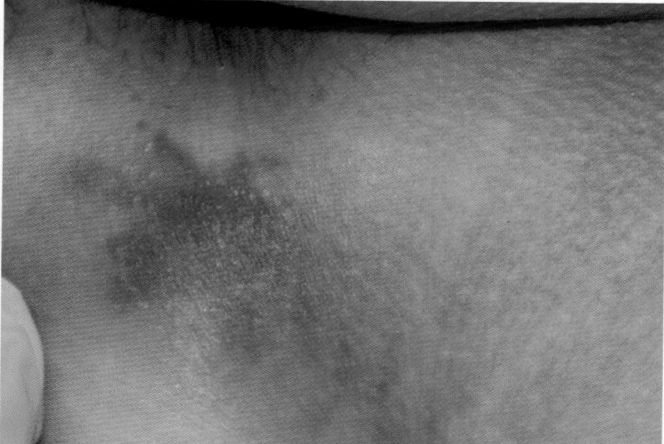

Fig. 181.2 Pattern bruise on the left buttock from unknown object. (From: Gibbs LM. Understanding the medical markers of elder abuse and neglect: physical examination findings. Clin Geriatr Med. 2014;30:687-712.)

whether injury patterns exist that are suggestive of, or specific for, elder mistreatment (analogous to findings in child abuse, such as shaken infant syndrome and bucket-handle metaphyseal fracture). Unfortunately, it can be difficult to distinguish between elder mistreatment and the sequelae of unintentional trauma or medical illness. This difficulty may be due to normal physiologic changes that occur with aging, such as osteopenia, thinning of the skin with easy bruising, as well as the impact of medications commonly used, including anticoagulants. Studies have found that abuse victims, in comparison to other older adults, have bruises that were more often large (>5 cm) and on the face, lateral right arm, or posterior torso.[1] Physical abuse and assault-related injuries most commonly occur on the head/face, neck, and upper extremities[4] (Fig. 181.1). Abuse victims are more likely than older adults presenting to the ED with a fall to have injuries to the left cheek/zygoma, with neck and ear

injuries occurring commonly in abuse victims but generally not after a fall. Additionally, physical elder abuse victims are more likely to have maxillofacial/dental/neck injuries combined with no upper and lower extremity injuries, suggesting that the simultaneous presence and absence of injuries may be helpful in differentiating intentional from unintentional injuries in older adults.[4] Patterned injuries, wrist or ankle lesions suggesting possible inappropriate restraint, burns suggesting immersion injury or cigarette burns, or fractures of different ages should suggest elder physical abuse (Figs. 181.2 to 181.5). These and other findings may be used to develop clinical prediction rules in the future to assist ED providers in identifying injury patterns suspicious for abuse.

Sexual assault of older adults occurs, is underrecognized, and should be considered. Perineal injury should illicit concern for sexual assault in the elderly and should prompt reporting (Figs. 181.6 to 181.7). If sexual abuse is suspected or reported, a complete sexual assault examination is recommended.

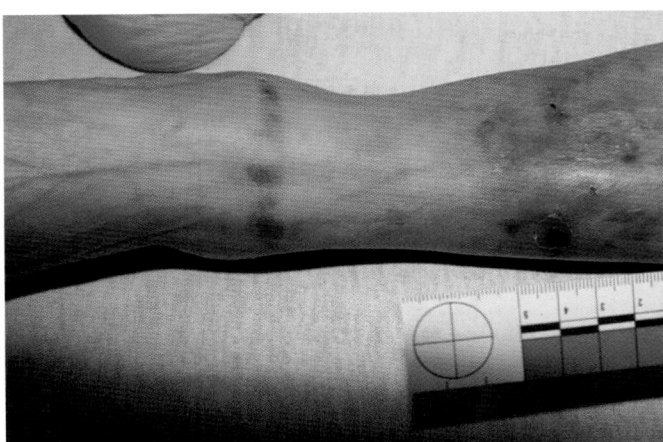

Fig. 181.3 Pattern bruising on lower leg from a ligature. (From: Gibbs LM. Understanding the medical markers of elder abuse and neglect: physical examination findings. Clin Geriatr Med. 2014;30:687-712.)

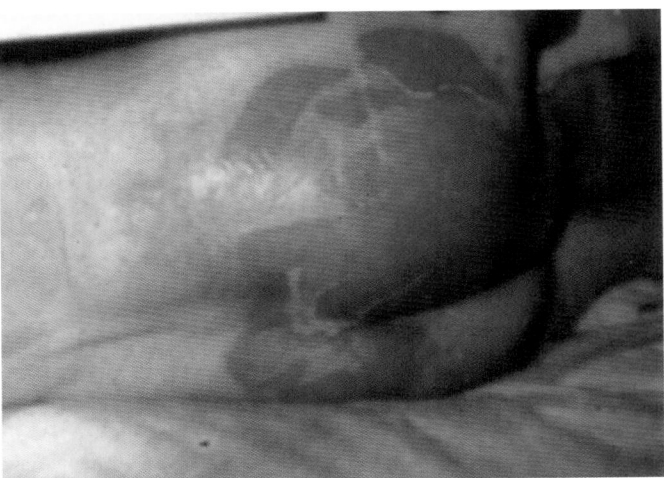

Fig. 181.4 Burn injuries on the back and buttocks from scalding water. (From: Gibbs LM. Understanding the medical markers of elder abuse and neglect: physical examination findings. Clin Geriatr Med. 2014;30:687-712.)

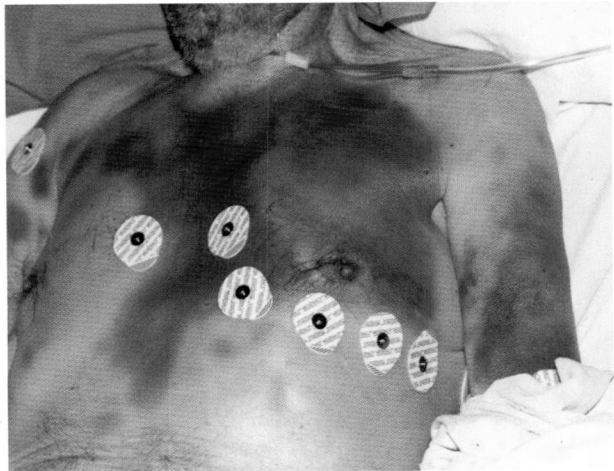

Fig. 181.5 A 70-year-old man was brought from his caregiver's home to the emergency department (ED) by police after his daughter found him severely bruised. He had multiple contusions at varying stages of healing on his chest and arms, as well as a linear patterned injury across his left anterior chest. The central and bilateral locations of the contusions, varying colors, and linear pattern of the bruise on the left side of his chest are highly suggestive of physical abuse. (Courtesy Dr. D.C. Homeier.)

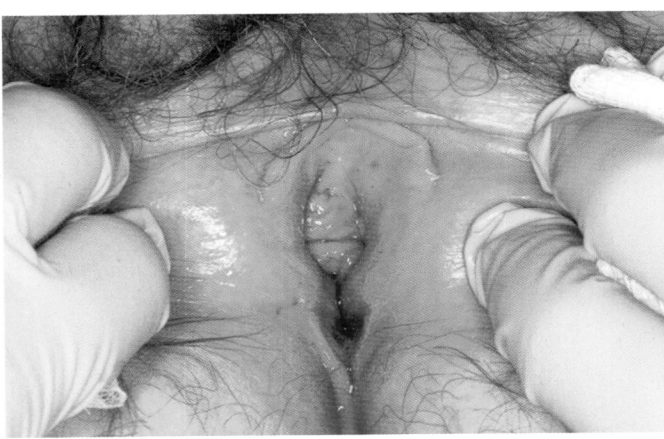

Fig. 181.6 A 65-year-old woman in a nursing home with posterior fourchette and perineum laceration from rape by resident. (From: Speck PM, Hartig MT, Likes W, et al. Case series of sexual assault in older persons. Clin Geriatr Med. 2014;30:779-806.)

Neglect needs to be considered when the elder in the care of others shows signs of poor care such as poor hygiene, advanced pressure ulcers, advanced medical disease that may have responded to early intervention, and neglected dental disease (Figs. 181.8 to 181.11).

DIAGNOSTIC TESTING

No laboratory tests exist to definitively detect abuse, but medical and laboratory findings may suggest elder mistreatment. These include biomarkers of malnutrition, dehydration, anemia, hypothermia/hyperthermia, and rhabdomyolysis. In addition, serum or urine drug levels may provide clues to medication by a caregiver. Perpetrators may divert controlled substances, such as narcotic pain medications, for their own use or to sell. Elevated serum levels of prescription medications may suggest intentional or unintentional overdose, and the presence of toxins or drugs that have not been prescribed may indicate poisoning. Platelet count and coagulation studies may be helpful in ruling out a medical etiology for unexplained or abnormal bruising. Evidence of sexually transmitted diseases in an older adult not known to be sexually active may suggest sexual abuse.

Diagnostic Imaging

Unlike child abuse, there is very limited literature on imaging correlates for elder abuse, and diagnostic radiologists typically receive no formal training in elder abuse detection. Findings suggestive of elder abuse or neglect include co-occurring old and new fractures, high-energy fractures despite low-energy mechanism, distal ulnar diaphyseal fractures, and small bowel hematomas. Any concern for elder abuse should be verbally communicated to the radiologist reading the images with a request that they consider whether the imaging findings are consistent with the purported history. They may also consider additional screening imaging tests, such as maxillofacial CT scan and chest x-ray, analogous to the skeletal survey used in child abuse to assess for occult acute and chronic fractures.

Screening

Though ED screening often consists of a single question about home safety, it is generally accepted that this is inadequate and represents a

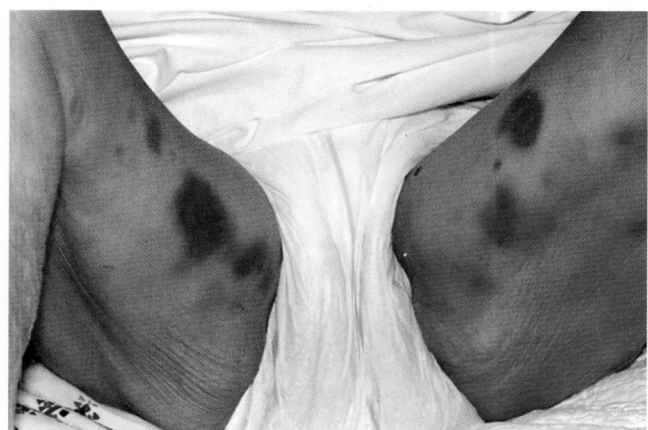

Fig. 181.7 A 69-year-old woman with severe dementia who resided in a skilled nursing facility was brought to the emergency department (ED) after her daughter noticed that the patient had bruises on her bilateral inner thighs. When the daughter inquired about the bruises, she was told by the facility staff that the patient had fallen. These bruises are in a location that raises suspicion for sexual abuse. The emergency clinician consulted the hospital's adult protection team, which contacted local law enforcement; the long-term care ombudsman was also notified for further investigation. The hospital's sexual assault response team was consulted and conducted a sexual assault forensic examination for evidence collection. (Courtesy Dr. D.C. Homeier.)

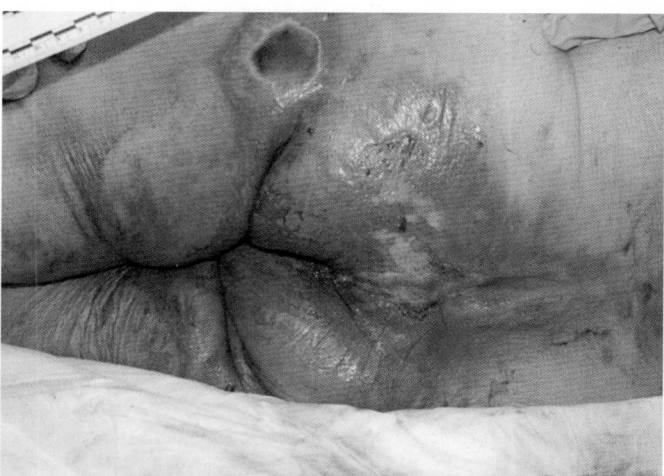

Fig. 181.8 Case of elder neglect showing moisture-associated skin damage (MASD) and ulcers in the sacrum, buttocks, and thighs. (From: Gibbs LM. Understanding the medical markers of elder abuse and neglect: physical examination findings. Clin Geriatr Med. 2014;30:687-712.)

missed opportunity. Multiple more robust screening tools have been developed, though none have yet been validated for use in the ED. The Elder Abuse Suspicion Index (EASI) is a short tool validated for cognitively intact patients in ambulatory care and may be appropriate for use in the ED. The ED Senior AID (Abuse Identification) tool is a promising recently developed ED-specific screening tool that is highly sensitive and specific and is currently undergoing multi-site validation.[5]

The American Medical Association, the American College of Emergency Physicians, and the Joint Commission have strongly supported routine assessment for all types of family violence, including elder mistreatment, but their choice of words has stopped short of recommending universal screening. Additionally, though screening for elder abuse has the potential to identify occult cases so that intervention may be

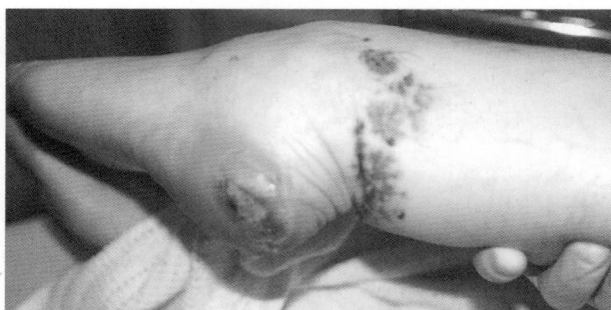

Fig. 181.9 A 65-year-old developmentally delayed but ambulatory woman was brought to the emergency department (ED) by her family on account of "unruly behavior." Examination of her left heel revealed a pressure ulcer, and her left ankle revealed an erythematous rash in a circumferential pattern. This may represent the use of a restraint, resulting in the pressure ulcer. (Courtesy Dr. D.C. Homeier.)

initiated, evidence of improved outcomes to support screening for elder mistreatment does not yet exist. The US Preventative Services Task has not recommended screening for elder abuse in health care settings.[6]

Targeted screening of only high-risk patients may be a desirable alternative to universal screening, reducing resources that need to be devoted to the screening process and increasing the proportion of patients who screen positive. High-yield demographic factors have yet to be identified. Future strategies may use data elements from the electronic health record or other health care utilization data combined with machine learning approaches to perform automated prescreening to identify high-risk patients.

MANAGEMENT

A multidisciplinary team-based approach is required to improve the recognition and management of elderly mistreatment. Key to success is empowering all members of the team to share observations and recommendations in a safe context. Large EDs typically have social workers or case managers in the department, while smaller EDs usually have access to them in the hospital or on-call. These professionals assess the patient's home situation, support system, financial resources, and social service needs, and also provide counseling. Their assessment may identify evidence or risks for mistreatment that is not detected by medical providers. If possible, dependent older adult ED patients being considered for discharge and any patient for whom a concern about elder abuse or neglect exists should be seen by a social worker or case manager. The Emergency Department Elder Mistreatment Assessment Tool for Social Workers (ED-EMATS), a structured assessment tool for ED social workers who have less experience evaluating patients for elder mistreatment, was recently developed.[7]

Nurses and patient care technologists (PCTs) are also instrumental members of the team since they have more face-to-face contact with patients, caregivers, and family than medical providers and may observe interactions that arouse suspicion requiring further investigation. Also, nurses and PCTs provide personal care (e.g., diaper changes) that may identify otherwise missed suspicious physical findings. Patient escort and radiology technicians are yet other personnel who may be confided in by the patient: Radiologic technicians may be particularly well-positioned to identify abuse, as they can privately assess and interview patients in the radiology suite while conducting imaging examinations.

Emergency Medical Services

Older adults are four times more likely than younger patients to use EMS, and these providers are the first clinicians to evaluate acutely

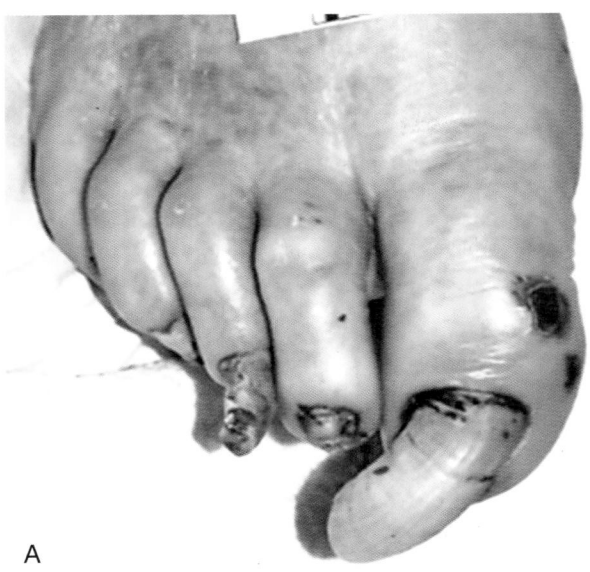 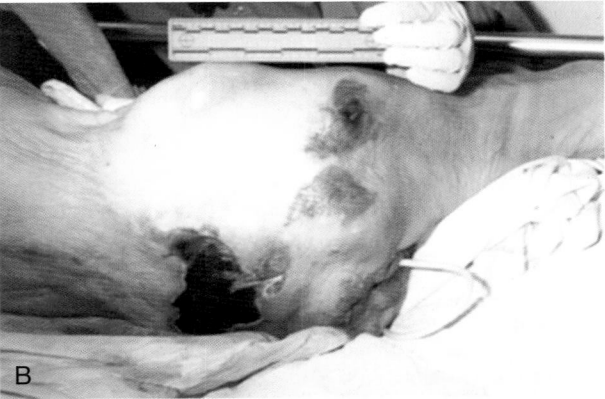

A

B

Fig. 181.10 A 72-year-old woman was brought to the emergency department (ED) by paramedics for "not eating for 5 days" according to her family. The paramedics noted she was covered in urine and feces. The following signs were of concern for neglect: elongated toenails (A), pressure sores (B), poor hygiene, and a delay in seeking medical care. (Courtesy Dr. D.C. Homeier.)

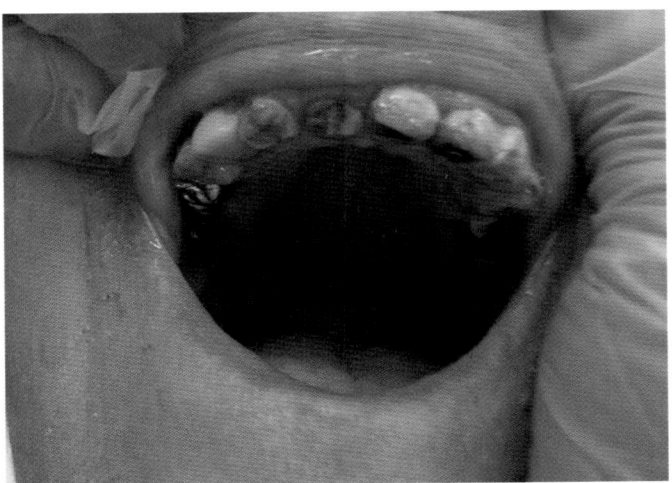

Fig. 181.11 Poor dentition in a substantiated case of dependent adult neglect. (From: Gibbs LM. Understanding the medical markers of elder abuse and neglect: physical examination findings. Clin Geriatr Med. 2014;30:687-712.)

injured or ill older adults, typically in the patient's home. EMS providers can identify unmarked medication bottles or expired medications, as well as multiple bottles of a single medication. They can check whether any food is available in the refrigerator or pantry. EMS providers have an opportunity to observe hazards including vermin infestation, extreme clutter/hoarding, inappropriately hot or cold temperature, or utilities that aren't working. Given that EMS activation is usually unplanned, an abusive or neglectful caregiver is often not able to clean up the patient or home before EMS arrives. EMS providers may observe unusual or inappropriate interpersonal dynamics between caregivers and older adults as well as evidence of drug or alcohol use. Further, EMS may provide care to older adult patients who decline ED transport.

The Detection of Elder Abuse Through Emergency Care Technicians (DETECT) screening tool has recently been developed and has been shown to be feasible for EMS providers to integrate into their practice.[8] As EMS practice is heavily protocolized, changes to improve elder abuse and neglect detection could be implemented broadly through changes at a system level. Hopefully, use of integrated electronic medical records and the development of standardized screening tools and protocols, will facilitate increased detection of elderly mistreatment by EMS and communication with hospital providers.

Management of suspected elder abuse or neglect includes treating acute medical and psychological issues, ensuring patient safety, and proper reporting to the authorities. Traumatic injuries and metabolic abnormalities including dehydration are common and should be stabilized and treated. Management of worsening chronic medical conditions may be required due to an abuser's failure to provide appropriate care. In some circumstances, hospitalization may be necessary to provide extended treatment and observation.

If a mistreatment victim is in immediate danger, the patient should be prevented from having any contact with the suspected abuser. In extreme cases, this may require a security watch for the patient and even having the abuser removed from the ED. In these cases, law enforcement, hospital social workers, and administrators should be alerted. Alternative living arrangements may need to be arranged for the patient, with a reliable family member or friend or in an appropriate emergency shelter. If none of these options are available, the patient may require hospital admission to ensure safety.

If the patient refuses intervention, a determination must be made whether the patient has the capacity to make this decision. A psychiatric consultation may be helpful. The wishes of an older adult with decision-making capacity who desires to return to an abusive situation must be respected, as in cases of intimate partner violence among younger adults. If possible, the patient should be educated about the potential for escalation in violence and abuse and provide appropriate referral materials for future use. If an older adult does not have decision-making capacity, treatments that are in the patient's best interest, including hospitalization, should be provided.

In some cases, a patient may not have decision-making capacity, and the suspected abuser may be the patient's official health care proxy or power of attorney. Under these circumstances, hospital administration, legal, and/or the ethics committee should be involved to assist with health care decision making and guardianship.

In suspected cases of elder mistreatment without an imminent threat to a patient's safety, interventions are individualized. If the patient wants to return home and may be safely discharged, follow-up should be coordinated with the patient's primary care physician. Social workers may be able to offer support resources to both the patient and the caregiver. Ideally, elder mistreatment cases are managed in the community by a case manager or a team and involve home visits and advocacy.

A multidisciplinary ED-based consultation team, modeled on child protection team interventions, may assist in optimizing the care and ensuring the safety of these vulnerable patients. This team coordinates medical, forensic, and social work evaluations, and assist with a safe disposition. The team's presence can lessen the burden on ED providers who are generally multitasking and caring for multiple patients. ED providers may be more willing to pursue suspicions about elder abuse and neglect because of the availability of a team to assist with care, which may lead to higher rates of identification. These multidisciplinary ED elder protection consultation teams have been developed and are undergoing impact evaluation.

Trauma-Informed Care

Trauma-informed care to older adult victims of abuse or neglect involves being sensitive to the profound impact of traumatic and stressful life experiences on a patient's mental and physical health. Ongoing abuse or neglect, which may occur daily for years, and also previous—even remote—traumatic experiences may cause depression, anxiety, or posttraumatic stress disorder. Trauma-informed care is particularly important for older adults, who have had a long life to experience stressful or traumatic events.

Providing trauma-informed care focuses on the patient's need for safety, respect, and acceptance. The victim's choice and control should be maximized while minimizing re-traumatization through treatment. Recommended bedside strategies include:

- Using language and grammar that is easily understood, neutral, and not intimidating
- Limiting the number of times a victim has to talk about the assault
- Avoiding words such as violence, abuse, or criminal behavior if the victim does not initially conceive of what has occurred as abusive or criminal
- Asking permission before touching a potential victim
- Maintaining the victim's privacy and confidentiality
- Offering the support of an advocate if available
- Being mindful of culturally specific expectations regarding interactions between older adult patients and younger care providers

ED clinicians should also use these trauma-informed strategies for cognitively impaired patients, as they may still be deeply affected by ongoing or previous traumatic exposures.

Documentation

The history should be documented in the patient's own words, and avoid using biased words such as "claims" or "alleged." Pertinent social history (e.g., patient's functional status, caregiver's relationship to patient, living arrangements) should be included. The patient's general appearance on initial arrival to the ED should be described including signs of potential neglect (e.g., soiled diaper, inappropriate or dirty clothing, or dirt under nails). Injuries of any type (e.g., fractures, lacerations, and contusions) should be described, including their number, size, location, and stage of healing, and comment about whether the injuries are consistent with the reported mechanism. Providers

should consider using a body diagram/traumagram to precisely document physical findings. The Geri-IDT, a practical tool to improve medical documentation of geriatric injuries for potential forensic use, was recently developed and may be helpful.[9] If possible, photographs of all injuries should be added to the medical record. The results of laboratory investigations and imaging studies should also be recorded. Careful documentation of interventions, follow-up plans, and referrals should be made. In cases of suspected elder abuse that result in legal action, thorough documentation may be critical to ensure justice for the victim.

Reporting

Suspected cases of elder abuse or neglect should be reported to the appropriate authorities. A reasonable cause to suspect abuse is all that is necessary. Health care providers are mandated reporters for elder abuse in most but not all US states and, in many states, elder abuse must be reported even if the victim does not want a report made. As laws differ, ED clinicians should be aware of their state's requirements. This information is available on a state's department of health website, and a summary is at: http://www.napsa-now.org/wp-content/uploads/2014/11/Mandatory-Reporting-Chart-Updated-FINAL.pdf.

Adult Protective Services (APS) is typically the agency that investigates these cases for community-dwelling older adults. Information on how to contact state or local APS in different areas is available at: http://www.napsa-now.org/get-help/help-in-your-area/. The scope of the APS response must be appreciated: in most US states, APS can only investigate cases where an older adult has cognitive or functional impairment, and the agency will not act on reports if they judge that the older adult does not meet these criteria. Additionally, APS functions differently than Child Protective Services and will not open their investigation while a patient is in the ED or hospital. They will only open an investigation after discharge, generally within 72 hours. Consequently, ED clinicians should consider reporting to the local police when concerned about a patient's immediate safety or that a crime has been committed.

Collaboration with the Community

EDs may benefit substantially from improving communication, connection, and collaboration with APS and other community-based service providers. In many communities, multidisciplinary teams (MDTs) have developed that meet regularly to manage complex elder abuse and neglect cases. Members of these MDTs include APS case workers, prosecutors, civil attorneys, law enforcement professionals, financial services professionals, and health care providers.

Resources

The Administration for Community Living's National Center on Elder Abuse website (https://ncea.acl.gov) is the most comprehensive online resource available on elder abuse and neglect. Also, http://www.elder-abuseemergency.org is a website designed for emergency clinicians that provides access to tools, information, and resources that may be useful for reference and when on shift.

SPECIFIC ISSUES

Elder Mistreatment in Institutions

Residents of skilled nursing facilities represent a large and growing percentage of older adults who present to the ED and are at particularly high risk for mistreatment. Over the last several decades, increased regulatory scrutiny has improved care and reduced staff mistreatment of older adults in skilled nursing facilities through the Long-Term Care

Ombudsman Program to investigate complaints, mandatory staff background checks, and minimizing the use of restraints.

In addition to staff abuse and neglect of nursing home residents, resident-to-resident elder mistreatment has been recently identified as an important problem.[10] Given that dementia and associated behavioral disturbance in long-term care facilities is high, aggressive behavior can occur between residents. Additional research is needed to improve understanding and recognition of this type of elder mistreatment. When abuse or neglect of any kind in patients from nursing homes is identified or suspected, it should be reported to the long-term care ombudsman in their state (https://theconsumervoice.org/get_help), the state's department of health, or APS for further investigation.

Self-Neglect

Self-neglect includes behaviors in which an older adult threatens his/her own health or safety by failing to perform or refusing assistance with essential self-care. This may include malnutrition due to not eating, failure to take necessary medications, inattention to personal hygiene, hoarding, and not maintaining a safe home environment.

Often, patients with self-neglect suffer from an underlying mental disorder, including mild cognitive impairment, depression, psychosis, or substance abuse disorders that prevents them from understanding that their health and safety are at risk and that they need to seek assistance. Self-neglect is associated with increased mortality. It is the most common form of elder mistreatment reported to social services, with reports rising. As with other types of elder mistreatment, recognition is critical because many of these older adults have virtually no other contact outside the home. EMS providers, who may note an empty refrigerator, expired pill bottles, or vermin infestation, may play a pivotal role in the patient's care. Although evidence-based strategies for intervention have not been established, a reasonable approach for an emergency clinician includes laboratory assessment for metabolic and nutritional abnormalities and social work evaluation to offer resources and services. Many of these patients will require hospital admission because it will be impossible to establish a safe discharge plan.

The references for this chapter can be found online at ExpertConsult.com.

182

The Immunocompromised Patient

Jack Perkins Jr. and Christopher P. Waasdorp Jr.

KEY CONCEPTS

- Immunocompromised patients who present with acute infections, especially those that are neutropenic, may appear deceptively benign initially. Their symptoms and signs often mimic noninfectious complications.
- Broad-spectrum antibiotics are indicated after obtaining appropriate cultures of all potential sites of infection, especially if the patient is neutropenic.
- Immunocompromised patients can have serious local or systemic infections without fever.
- Symptoms, signs, and findings of infection may include tachypnea, tachycardia, mental status change, metabolic acidosis, increased volume requirements, rapid changes in serum glucose or sodium concentration, or acute abdominal pain.
- The incidence and severity of febrile neutropenia are inversely proportional to the absolute neutrophil count and directly proportional to the duration of neutropenia.
- In neutropenic patients, the temperature should be measured orally or tympanically, not rectally, due to theoretical risk of bacterial translocation and subsequent bacteremia.
- Febrile neutropenia is more common in hematologic malignancy (compared with solid malignancy) and is most likely to occur 7 to 10 days after chemotherapy.
- Gram-positive organisms are responsible for most serious infections in neutropenic cancer patients, but infections due to gram-negative organisms are more rapidly lethal.
- Neutropenic cancer patients with chemotherapy-induced oral mucositis can develop rapid onset of fever with shock. Viridans streptococci is a common pathogen and requires Vancomycin.

- When pneumonia develops in patients with febrile neutropenia, purulent sputum may be absent, and the initial chest radiograph may not show an infiltrate.
- Some low-risk febrile neutropenic patients may not require admission to the hospital. After calculating a Multinational Association for Supportive Care in Cancer (MASCC) risk index score and consulting with their oncologist, discharge may be reasonable.
- Diabetic patients have a high incidence of MRSA infection, osteomyelitis, and wound infections and are at higher risk of bacteremia. Severe infections may be more insidious in presentation.
- Patients with cell-mediated immune deficiency, including those on high-dose corticosteroids, may develop life-threatening infections with intracellular bacteria (*Listeria*, *Salmonella*, tuberculosis), fungi (*Cryptococcus*, *Coccidioides*, *Histoplasma*), herpes simplex virus, and varicella-zoster virus.
- Guidelines no longer support empiric antibiotic treatment of aspiration in alcoholic patients.
- In patients with cirrhosis, empirical treatment of suspected spontaneous bacterial peritonitis (SBP) with antibiotics should be started regardless of ascitic cell count.
- Patients who require hemodialysis for end-stage renal disease have high mortality if they develop pneumonia, *C. difficile* disease, or infections of the dialysis access site.
- Functional or surgical asplenia predisposes to fulminant infection with pneumococci and other encapsulated organisms (*H. influenzae*, *N. meningitidis*, and *Capnocytophaga canimorsus* after dog bites) and, when seen early, may be misdiagnosed as a viral illness, gastroenteritis, or food poisoning.

FOUNDATIONS

Emergency clinicians must recognize and treat infectious complications of cancer, organ transplantation, diabetes, renal failure, cirrhosis, asplenism, human immunodeficiency virus (HIV) infection, and other immunosuppressive conditions. Infections are more common, progressive, and severe in immunocompromised patients, and a wider variety of microorganisms may lead to infection. Immunocompromised persons presenting with acute infections may initially appear deceptively benign. Additionally, they may present with symptoms and signs that mimic noninfectious conditions, only to deteriorate rapidly if they are not evaluated and treated urgently. Many factors result in immunocompromise and predispose patients to infections. These include disruption of the body's protective surfaces, such as skin and mucosal barriers (oral and respiratory mucosa and intestinal and genitourinary surfaces); disorders that directly impair the function of the body's immune system (e.g., lymphoma, asplenism, and myeloma); drugs and irradiation that suppress or alter immune function; alterations in body substances (hyperglycemia) or solid organ function (kidney and liver failure); and malnutrition, aging, and exposure to antimicrobial agents that inhibit the normal protective resident bacterial flora.

PHYSIOLOGY

Immunity and Immune Deficiency

The body's defense mechanisms consist of surface barriers, innate (natural) and acquired (adaptive) responses. Innate responses occur to the same extent regardless of how often the body encounters the infectious agent, whereas acquired responses improve with repeated exposure. Innate immunity is activated immediately on exposure to an infecting agent, rapidly controlling replication and allowing the requisite 3 to 5 days for the adaptive component to clone sufficient T and B cells to respond more specifically.

Non–Microbe-Specific Immunity

Physical Barriers. Physical barriers, the first line of defense against microorganisms, consist of intact skin, mucosa, cilia, biofilm, gastric acid, antimicrobial peptides and proteins on skin and mucous membranes, and resident microflora. Smoking and pulmonary disease impair physical barriers in the respiratory tract whereas mechanical ventilation or tracheostomy introduces large numbers of microbes that often overwhelm natural clearance. Gastric acid and pancreatic enzymes have antibacterial properties that prevent overgrowth in the upper gastrointestinal tract. Normal peristalsis and mucosal shedding help maintain normal gut flora. Alterations in these factors, such as broad-spectrum antibiotics, alter normal flora and permit overgrowth of pathogens such as *Candida*, multidrug-resistant organisms, and *Clostridium difficile.*

Initial Inflammatory Response and Innate Immunity. The initial inflammatory response to microbial invasion promotes phagocytosis and microbial killing while activating the immune system. This innate immune response is not dependent on prior exposure to the pathogen. The initial inflammatory response factors, mainly produced in the liver, activate many cell types to synthesize and release cytokines, chemokines, and "trigger molecules" that kill the invading organism. This response delivers humoral and cellular immune components to sites of inflammation and initiates antibody production. Cytokines, platelet-activating factor, and hormone-like proteins are secreted from various immune cells and play essential roles in mediation of this response. Cytokines cause migration and adhesion of polymorphonuclear leukocytes and monocytes to sites of bacterial invasion. These cells release granules of substances that mediate vasodilation and increased vascular permeability, leading to edema, warmth, and redness, and allow both phagocytic cells and humoral components to be concentrated at the site of infection.

Reticuloendothelial System. The reticuloendothelial system, composed of tissue macrophages and their blood-borne counterparts, monocytes, removes particulate matter, including microbes, from the lymph and blood. The tissue component is concentrated in the lymph nodes, spleen, liver, marrow, and lung and has particular affinity for encapsulated bacteria, such as pneumococci, meningococci, and *Haemophilus influenzae*. The overwhelming sepsis from encapsulated organisms that can occur in patients with asplenia demonstrates the vital importance of this non–microbe-specific system.

Adaptive (Microbe-Specific) Immunity

Humoral Immunity

Antibodies. Each B cell produces a single microbe-specific antibody type. Stimulation by an antigen (or microbe) causes proliferation of

this particular B cell so that large quantities of a specific circulating antibody can be produced. B cells are also active in presenting antigens to T lymphocytes, promoting cell-mediated immunity (CMI).

Immunoglobulins. Immunoglobulin M (IgM) is the first immunoglobulin to appear in response to a new antigen. Although it has less affinity at binding antigens than immunoglobulin G (IgG), IgM provides some recognition of antigens and begins B-cell proliferation before the subsequent development of IgG. IgM is detectable earlier in serum than IgG and serves as a marker for a patient's early response to acute infection.

Secretory immunoglobulin A (IgA) is the predominant immunoglobulin present in gastrointestinal fluids, nasal and oral secretions, tears, and other mucous fluids. IgA inhibits cell adherence of viral, bacterial, and protozoan pathogens and prevents invasion by organisms through the respiratory or gastrointestinal tract.

Immunoglobulin E (IgE), which is expressed in high concentration on the surface of mast cells and basophils, is responsible for immediate-type hypersensitivity responses. Mast cells and IgE are important in defense against helminthic pathogens.

IgG, widely distributed in tissues, accounts for 75% of the total immunoglobulin mass. It crosses the placenta and provides fetal immunity during the first 6 months of life. Congenital or acquired deficiencies of IgG lead to infection with encapsulated organisms because the predominant subtype (IgG2) has affinity for the dense polysaccharides of bacterial cell capsules, such as those of *Streptococcus pneumoniae* and *H. influenzae*.

Complement. The complement cascade, a complex interaction of 30 proteins, is another crucial component of humoral response. Complement is important in producing inflammation and leukocytosis and in recruiting leukocytes to sites of infection. Complement also neutralizes viruses, enhances bacterial binding of opsonin, and lyses bacterial cell walls and membranes.

IgG and IgM activate the classical complement pathway when they are in contact with an antigen, whereas molecules with repeating chemical structures (e.g., bacterial cell walls and capsules) activate the cascade through the alternative pathway. C3 is the merging point of the classical and alternative paths and modulates the response of lymphocytes (CMI). The terminal leg of the cascade, C5 through C9, forms the membrane attack complex, which inserts into cell walls and membranes and leads to cell death.

Individuals with inherited complement deficiencies are predisposed to frequent and recurrent infections with *S. pneumoniae*, *H. influenzae*, and especially *Neisseria meningitidis* and *Neisseria gonorrhoeae*. The risk of meningococcal infection is increased several thousand-fold, especially in people deficient in C3 and late complement components (C5 to C8). Paradoxically, the disease is usually milder with complement deficiency, and mortality is likewise reduced fivefold to tenfold. This suggests that the host response may be, in part, responsible for the severity of disease in normal individuals and is attenuated in complement deficiency. Acquired deficiencies of complement function may develop in people with rheumatologic diseases, especially systemic lupus erythematosus (SLE). Approximately 40% of patients with SLE have an inhibitor of C5a-derived chemotaxis in their serum, resulting in enhanced susceptibility to infection.

Cell-Mediated Immunity. Cell-mediated immunity (CMI) includes immune responses mediated by T lymphocytes, natural killer (NK) cells, and mononuclear phagocytes. CMI is crucial in controlling infections caused by microbes that survive and replicate intracellularly, including most viruses and some bacterial (obligate and facultative intracellular types), fungal, and protozoan pathogens.

Only 5% of lymphocytes are in circulating blood. Most mature and are active in the marrow, thymus, spleen, and lymph nodes. The last two sites expose T cells to circulating antigens from invading microbes. Specialized antigen-presenting cells in the lymphoid system sequester antigen and antigen-antibody complexes and present them to T cells via a cell surface molecule called the *major histocompatibility complex (MHC)*. Only with this specific presentation can a T lymphocyte become activated against a particular antigen.

Two major types of T lymphocytes are CD4 (helper cell) and CD8 (suppressor cell). CD4 lymphocytes provide help for other cells in the immune system, including enhanced B-cell antibody production and the production of cytokines. CD8 lymphocytes are generally cytotoxic and mediate the eradication of virally infected target cells and certain tumors. A decline in the number of CD4 cells, with predominance of CD8 cells, is responsible for the increased susceptibility to infection in patients with human immunodeficiency virus (HIV). Despite the cytotoxicity of CD8 cells, immunity is reduced without adequate numbers of CD4 cells.

Patients with defects in CMI are at increased risk for disseminated infection with intracellular bacteria, such as *Mycobacterium tuberculosis*, *Listeria monocytogenes*, and *Salmonella* species. The DNA viral infections, such as cytomegalovirus, herpes simplex, and varicella-zoster, also affect these patients more severely, as do fungal infections with *Candida*, *Cryptococcus*, *Mucor*, *Aspergillus*, and *Pneumocystis*. Finally, some protozoa are pathogenic in patients without intact CMI, such as *Toxoplasma gondii*. Some infections are seen only below a certain CD4 cell count. *Pneumocystis* pneumonia, for example, is seen almost exclusively in patients with CD4 counts below 200 cells/mL, whereas almost all patients with toxoplasmosis or cryptococcal meningitis have counts below 100 cells/mL. In settings where the CD4 count is not readily available, such as the ED, an absolute lymphocyte count of less than 1000 cells/mL is suggestive of a CD4 count of less than 200 cells/mL.

NK cells, closely related to lymphocytes, are important in the innate immune response and are found in high concentrations in blood and spleen. NK cells recognize infected cells and directly kill these cells while secreting cytokines that activate macrophages to destroy phagocytosed microbes. NK cells are important in defense against intracellular microbes, particularly viruses and intracellular bacteria such as *L. monocytogenes*.

Granulocytic Phagocytes. Granulocytic phagocytes are the cellular effectors of microbe killing, engulfing them and enzymatically lysing their cell membranes or walls. Two major types are polymorphonuclear leukocytes (neutrophils) and macrophages (the tissue version of circulating monocytes). Macrophages have surface receptors that recognize nonvertebrate carbohydrates, such as mannose, to identify and attack "invaders" rather than "self."

Two other types of granulocytes, eosinophils and basophils, are less involved in the ingestion of organisms. Eosinophils attack certain parasitic helminths through the release of toxic proteins. This cell type can increase from 3% to 20% during times of high parasite load. Basophils (rare in circulation) and their tissue counterparts, mast cells, have a high affinity for IgE. On exposure to bound IgE, they release granules with histamine, prostaglandins, leukotrienes, and endogenous heparin to promote blood flow and inflammatory response in combating arthropod ectoparasites or helminth endoparasites. Activation of basophils by IgE bound to pollen and other allergens may affect the allergic-inflammatory response with increased vascular permeability, bronchospasm, and vasodilation.

Half of all neutrophils that leave the bone marrow circulate in the plasma. The other half become marginated, adhering to endothelium, primarily in the lungs, liver, and spleen. During periods of stress or with endogenous or exogenous catecholamines or corticosteroids, these neutrophils demarginate and enter the circulation. If the patient

is not neutropenic, demargination causes an increased peripheral neutrophil count composed of mature cells. With bacterial infection, an increased proportion of immature (band) forms is more typically seen.

Neutrophils (and tissue macrophages) bind to and ingest bacteria through phagocytosis. This process is enhanced by proteins called *opsonins* that bind to bacterial surfaces, particularly important in defense against infection with *S. pneumoniae, Streptococcus pyogenes, H. influenzae,* and *Staphylococcus aureus.* C-reactive protein, one of the initial inflammatory response proteins, fulfills this function for certain bacteria, including *S. pneumoniae.* IgG and complement protein C3b also opsonize bacteria, again illustrating the interdependence of the immune system. Actual killing takes place within granulocytes when cytoplasmic granules enzymatically produce potent oxidants. Granulocytes further control bacterial proliferation at the site of infection by elaborating lactoferrin, which locally binds free iron necessary for bacterial replication.

In addition to phagocytosis, macrophages (located in the spleen, alveoli, liver, and lymph nodes) modulate the immune response by presenting antigens to lymphocytes and releasing cytokines and complement components. Activation of macrophages to ingest bacteria depends on interaction with interferon-γ, a cytokine manufactured by T cells, again bridging different components of the immune system.

SPECIFIC DISORDERS

Immune system defects in the immunocompromised patient and the most common pathogens associated with each defect are listed in Box 182.1.

Solid Organ Transplants

For specific issues regarding medication-induced immunocompromised states in solid organ transplant patients, refer to Chapter 183.

Cancer

Patients with cancer frequently suffer from neutropenia or impaired T and B cells function due to the cancer itself or chemotherapy. Defects in the physical barriers of the skin and mucous membranes, including the cytotoxic effects of chemotherapy on cells lining the gastrointestinal tract, predispose to infection. In addition, splenic dysfunction or splenectomy, use of long-term intravascular catheters, frequent use of complex invasive diagnostic and therapeutic procedures, toxic effects of radiation therapy, and frequent colonization with antimicrobial-resistant pathogens predispose to immune system compromise. Despite many advances in supportive care, infections continue to result in severe morbidity and mortality. Furthermore, increasing resistance to antimicrobials is occurring among common pathogens along with the emergence of new opportunistic infections.

Neutropenia
Background
Definitions of neutropenia vary, but the 2018 American Society of Clinical Oncology proposed the following based on absolute neutrophil count (ANC):[1]

Neutropenia: ANC less than 1000 cells/μL
Severe neutropenia: ANC less than 500 cells/μL
Profound neutropenia: ANC less than 100 cells/μL

The nadir of the ANC is usually 7 to 10 days after the conclusion of chemotherapy. Fever in the neutropenic patient is defined as a single oral temperature of 38.3°C (101°F) or greater or a temperature of 38.0°C (100.4°F) or greater sustained over 60 minutes.[1] Febrile neutropenia (FN) usually results from cytotoxic chemotherapy or the underlying malignancy. Risk of FN is largely determined by the

BOX 182.1   The Immunocompromised Patient: Immune System Defects Predisposing to Infection and the Most Common Pathogens Associated with Each

Neutropenia

Bacteria

Gram-negative bacilli

  Escherichia coli

  Klebsiella pneumoniae

  Pseudomonas aeruginosa

  Enterobacter sp.

  Serratia sp.

  Citrobacter sp.

  Proteus sp.

  Acinetobacter sp.

  Stenotrophomonas maltophilia

Gram-positive cocci

  Staphylococcus epidermidis

  Staphylococcus aureus including methicillin-resistant strains

  Viridans streptococci

  Streptococcus pneumoniae

  Streptococcus pyogenes

  Enterococcus sp., including vancomycin-resistant strains

Gram-positive rods

  Corynebacterium sp.

  Less common: *Bacillus* sp.

Fungi

  Candida sp.

  Aspergillus sp.

  Less common: *Mucor* sp., *Rhizopus* sp., *Trichosporon beigelii, Fusarium* sp., *Pseudallescheria boydii*

Cellular Immune Dysfunction

Bacteria

Listeria monocytogenes

Salmonella sp.

Mycobacterium tuberculosis

Mycobacterium avium-intracellulare

Legionella sp.

Nocardia sp.

Fungi

Cryptococcus neoformans

Histoplasma capsulatum

Coccidioides immitis

Candida sp.

Aspergillus sp.

Pneumocystis jiroveci (formerly *carinii*)

Viruses

Herpes simplex

Varicella zoster

Cytomegalovirus

Epstein-Barr

Less common: Measles, adenovirus

Parasites

Toxoplasma gondii

Cryptosporidium sp.

Strongyloides stercoralis

Humoral Immune Dysfunction (Antibody Deficiency)

Bacteria

S. pneumoniae

Haemophilus influenzae

Neisseria meningitidis

S. aureus

Splenectomy or Functional Asplenia

Bacteria

S. pneumoniae

H. influenzae

N. meningitidis

Capnocytophaga canimorsus

Bordetella holmesii

Parasites

Babesia sp.

Complement Deficiency

Bacteria

N. meningitidis

S. pneumoniae

H. influenzae

---

type of malignancy, with FN being far more common in hematologic malignancies. Additionally, other factors include the type of chemotherapy and where the patient is in relation to their chemotherapy regimen, with FN being much more common in the first or second cycle of chemotherapy. Mortality varies widely and is affected by comorbid illness, severity of neutropenia, presence of shock, and hematologic malignancy (worse outcomes), among other variables.[1] In a nationwide study in the United States of FN among patients with metastatic solid tumors, FN occurred in 13% to 20% during their chemotherapy course with a mortality of 4% to 10% per episode of neutropenia.[2]

The incidence and severity of infection in cancer patients with neutropenia is inversely proportional to the ANC and directly proportional to the duration of neutropenia.[3] Although the incidence begins to rise as the neutrophil count falls below 500 cells/μL, most severe infections and almost all bacteremias occur when the neutrophil count is less than 100 cells/μL.[3,4]

The most common sites of infection in neutropenic patients are the lung (25%); mouth and pharynx (25%); gastrointestinal tract (15%); skin, soft tissue, and intravascular catheters (15%); perineum and anorectal area (10%); urinary tract (5%); and nose and sinuses (5%).[3,4] Pneumonia and anorectal infection are more likely to be associated with bacteremia.[5,6] Bacteremia may occur without an obvious source despite intensive investigation. The most important bacteria infecting neutropenic patients are four gram-positive cocci—*Staphylococcus epidermidis,* viridans group *streptococci, Enterococcus* species, and *S. aureus*—and three gram-negative bacilli—*Escherichia coli, Klebsiella pneumoniae,* and *Pseudomonas aeruginosa.*[4,6] An increase in formerly uncommon gram-negative infections caused by *Enterobacter, Citrobacter,* and *Serratia* species has occurred, and infections caused by gram-negative organisms resistant to cephalosporins, extended-spectrum penicillins, and carbapenems are occurring more frequently. Anaerobes are uncommon but may be important in certain mixed infections (mouth, abdominal, and perianal).[3,4]

Infections caused by gram-positive organisms (coagulase-negative staphylococci, *S. aureus,* viridans streptococci, and *Enterococcus* species) are now the leading cause of bacterial infection (50% to 70% at some centers) in febrile neutropenic cancer patients in the United States, Canada, and western Europe.[4,6] Gram-negative organisms still predominate in developing countries. Most of these gram-positive organisms do not produce immediately life-threatening infections, in contrast to the rapid lethality of many gram-negative infections. However, bloodstream infections caused by viridans streptococci (especially *Streptococcus mitis*), may be life-threatening and result in rapid development of shock or acute respiratory distress syndrome (ARDS). These infections are common in many cancer centers and often respond poorly to penicillins and cephalosporins. Risk factors for serious viridans streptococcal infections include aggressive cytoreduction therapy for acute leukemia or allogeneic bone marrow transplantation, profound neutropenia, and severe oral mucositis. Other risk factors include prophylactic use of trimethoprim-sulfamethoxazole or fluoroquinolones, antacids or H$_2$ receptor antagonists, and pediatric age.[7]

Aspergillus and *Candida* species are the most common fungal pathogens in cancer patients with fever and neutropenia.[8-11] Infection is most likely to develop in neutropenic patients treated with broad-spectrum antimicrobials and in those whose fever persists for more than seven days.[8] *Aspergillus* species usually produce necrotizing infections in the lungs or sinuses. Pulmonary aspergillosis often manifests with pleuritic pain, hemoptysis, and localized wheezing. The chest radiograph demonstrates pleural effusions or focal infiltrates. Computed tomography (CT) is more sensitive in detecting pulmonary infiltrates compatible with aspergillosis and may demonstrate a distinct halo of low attenuation surrounding a pulmonary infiltrate. This pattern is highly suggestive of invasive aspergillosis, although zygomycosis (formerly mucormycosis) and other disorders may mimic the halo.

Invasive aspergillosis originating in the paranasal sinuses may extend to the surrounding bone and brain. Often, an initial red-purple lesion on the nasal turbinate or palate turns pale and then black as vascular invasion produces infarction of the mucosa and bone. The black eschar on the nose or palate can be misdiagnosed as dried blood. Patients presenting with headache, facial pain or swelling, or proptosis, should be rapidly evaluated for invasive aspergillosis and zygomycosis. *Candida* species produce infections of the skin, oral cavity, and esophagus, as well as fungemia. The sudden onset of generalized rash consisting of pink-purple, nontender subcutaneous nodules is characteristic of candidemia.

Mucositis involving the mouth and other mucous membranes is a painful and debilitating condition that commonly occurs in cancer patients receiving intense chemotherapy. It is a frequent prelude to viridans streptococcal bacteremia, which can produce sudden onset of acute respiratory distress syndrome, a toxic shock–like syndrome, rash, and pneumonia. Importantly, mucositis predisposes the patient to gram-positive infections, and vancomycin is appropriate in addition to a broad-spectrum gram-negative agent. History is helpful because mucositis tends to recur throughout the chemotherapy course.

Febrile Neutropenia Evaluation Pitfalls

- **Fever is the only sign of infection.** Fever is frequently the only sign of infection, partly because these patients are unable to mount a full inflammatory response.[4-6] Usual symptoms and signs of infection may not be present, especially when the neutrophil count is less than 100 cells/μL. Furthermore, aggressive education before and during chemotherapy makes these patients much more likely to present early in the course of an infectious illness when fever is the only symptom. Some patients may harbor a serious infection yet not be able to mount a febrile response (chronic prednisone

therapy, bone marrow transplant) or may present with hypothermia.
- **Assuming the patient does not harbor an infectious pathology if they are afebrile.** While most neutropenic patients are still able to mount a febrile response to infection, some patients will have serious infectious pathology and be afebrile.[4-6] Oral temperatures are unreliable, and rectal temperatures are contraindicated in FN, making it difficult to accurately identify patients who do not present with a complaint of fever at home.[12] Bone marrow transplant patients, patients on chronic corticosteroids, and elderly patients are all at higher risk of not mounting the expected febrile response to infection. Such infections may be manifested instead by unexplained tachypnea or tachycardia, mental status changes, metabolic acidosis, increased volume requirements, rapid changes in serum glucose or sodium concentration, or acute abdominal pain.
- **Physical examination that is misleading.** The FN patient with a localized infection may have shaking chills and a toxic appearance without localized findings. Areas of cellulitis may have minimal induration and redness and little or no purulent drainage. Tenderness may be the only finding in perineal and anal infections. Peritoneal signs may be absent even with surgical pathology due to a lack of the inflammatory response that results in the traditional peritoneal findings.
- **Failing to consider noninfectious causes of fever.** Noninfectious causes of fever need to be considered, including drug toxicity, drug allergy, transfusion reactions, and pulmonary emboli.
- **Overestimating sensitivity of diagnostic testing in febrile neutropenia.** When pneumonia develops, purulent sputum may be absent, and the initial chest radiograph may not show an infiltrate.[13,14] Pyuria may be absent in patients with a urinary tract infection.
- **Misinterpreting leukocytosis in a patient who has received a colony-stimulating factor.** Oncologic patients who are expected to become neutropenic after their course of chemotherapy may be administered colony-stimulating factor to boost their white blood cell production. Consequently, the emergency clinician may encounter a patient with a marked leukocytosis and fail to recognize that these patients should be evaluated and treated in the same manner as if they presented with neutropenia and fever.[3,6] Emergency clinicians should routinely inquire about the use of colony-stimulating factors during their initial history.
- **Obtaining a rectal temperature in neutropenic patients.** In neutropenic patients, the temperature should be measured orally, not rectally. Although no randomized controlled trials have ever been conducted, there is a theoretical risk of bacterial translocation with any rectal stimulation.[3]

Evaluation and Management

Box 182.2 describes a step-by-step approach to the evaluation and management of the adult patient with febrile neutropenia.

Unfortunately, only about 50% of FN episodes will have an identified focus of fever.[4-6] Up to 25% of patients have a microbiologically identified source of infection such as blood, urine, or wound cultures. Another 25% of patients have a clinically evident source of infection such as pneumonia but no microbiologic data confirms the precise pathogen. Consequently, many patients with FN are not able to have their antibiotics narrowed to minimize the risks of developing resistant bacteria or *Clostridium difficile.*

Antibiotic Therapy. The Infectious Disease Society of America and the American Society of Clinical Oncology recommend antibiotic therapy within 60 minutes of presentation to ED triage for patients with FN.[1] Afebrile neutropenic patients who have unstable vital signs (e.g.,

---

BOX 182.2   Evaluation and Management of the Adult Cancer Patient With Febrile Neutropenia in the Emergency Department

- Fever (or reported history of fever by patient) of single oral temperature ≥ 38.3°C (101°F) or temperature ≥ 38.0°C (100.4°F) sustained over 60 minutes. Some neutropenic patients will harbor serious infection without fever.
- Neutropenia = Absolute neutrophil count (ANC) < 1000 cells/μL
- If patient is septic, rapidly administer intravenous fluids and maintain mean arterial pressure ≥ 65 mm Hg.
- Contact oncologist early in ED course to assist in guiding evaluation and management especially regarding unique chemotherapy side effect considerations and unusual pathogens (e.g., fungal, viral).
- Query patient about previous episodes of neutropenic fever, recent travel, exposure to animals, vaccinations, and any current antimicrobial use.
- Obtain blood for measurement of electrolytes, renal and hepatic function, serum lactate.
- Obtain blood cultures from each lumen of any existing central venous catheters and from at least one peripheral site, or two blood cultures from separate venipunctures of peripheral veins if no central venous catheter is present.
- Review records for information pertaining to previous episodes of neutropenic fever, prior culture results and sensitivities, echocardiogram, and current chemotherapy regimen.
- Perform a careful physical examination to search for subtle symptoms or signs of infection, with particular attention to the mouth, nose and sinuses, lower esophagus, lung, and skin, including nails, perineum including anus, bone marrow aspiration sites, and vascular catheter sites.
- Understanding that peritoneal signs may be absent in neutropenia and that chest radiograph has marked limitations, consider CT of chest/abdomen/pelvis searching for a source if routine evaluation does not yield a likely source of fever.
- Obtain chest radiograph, understanding it is poorly sensitive for infiltrate with neutropenia.
- Obtain urinalysis with urine culture.
- Send influenza testing if appropriate (by season), understanding that rapid antigen testing has insufficient sensitivity to exclude influenza. Influenza PCR is a superior test to exclude influenza. Neutropenic patients are at high risk for morbidity and mortality from influenza and may present without fever. Empiric treatment (if PCR testing is unavailable) should be considered with oseltamivir based on clinical presentation.
- If diarrhea is present, send for culture, ova and parasites and *Clostridium difficile*.
- Lumbar puncture is not recommended as a routine procedure; however, classic findings such as meningismus may be absent in neutropenic patients.
- Evaluate joins for potential effusion and consideration of aspiration.

- Antibiotics (cefepime, a carbapenem, meropenem, imipenem, or piperacillin/tazobactam) should be initiated within 60 minutes of presentation. The specific agent will depend on institutional antibiogram for gram-negative pathogen sensitivities.
- For patients with a history of severe penicillin allergy, initiate empiric therapy with aztreonam and vancomycin. Avoid empirical use of a fluoroquinolone as coverage for gram-negative pathogens in penicillin-allergic patients.
- Once the initial antibiotic has been administered, consider additional antimicrobials based on suspected source.
  - Add coverage for atypical organisms in suspected community-acquired pneumonia.
  - Add metronidazole or clindamycin for suspected intra-abdominal infections (if broad-spectrum gram-negative agent does not have anaerobic activity such as cefepime).
- For patients with a minor penicillin allergy, empirical treatment with cefepime, meropenem or imipenem-cilastatin can usually be given safely.
- Empiric use of vancomycin is not routinely indicated for all febrile neutropenic patients. Vancomycin should be administered for: 1) suspected catheter-related infection; 2) known colonization with MRSA or penicillin-resistant pneumococci; 3) presence of shock; 4) severe mucositis; 5) prior fluoroquinolone prophylaxis; and 6) institutions in which MRSA, vancomycin-susceptible enterococci, and *Streptococcus mitis* (viridans streptococcus group) are frequent pathogens.
- Empirical antifungal therapy is only rarely indicated in the ED and should not be initiated by the emergency medicine provider without consultation with an infectious diseases specialist.
- Do not initiate outpatient therapy in low-risk patients without contacting the patient's oncologist or an infectious diseases specialist.
- Calculate the MASCC score if outpatient therapy is being considered in a stable patient.
- Patients being considered for early discharge and outpatient management should have a MASCC score ≥21 and have no other high-risk features. They should be observed for at least four hours after the initial antibiotic dose to monitor for stability.
- Low-risk patients may be monitored in an ED observation unit where they can be evaluated by an oncologist and/or infectious diseases specialist to determine whether early discharge to home is feasible.
- Avoiding an inpatient admission is advantageous for the stable low-risk patient because hospitalization exposes the patients to potential iatrogenic complications and antimicrobial-resistant nosocomial pathogens, and outpatient admission allows an improved quality of life.

CT, Computed tomography; *ED*, emergency department; *MASCC*, Multinational Association for Supportive Care in Cancer; *MRSA*, methicillin-resistant *Staphylococcus aureus*; *PCR*, polymerase chain reaction.

Data from: Taplitz RA, Kennedy EB, Bow EJ, et al. Outpatient management of fever and neutropenia in adults treated for malignancy: American Society of Clinical Oncology and Infectious Diseases Society of America clinical practice guideline update. *J Clin Oncol.* 2018;36(14):1443-1453. https://doi.org/10.1200/JCO.2017.77.6211; Baden LR, Swaminathan S, Angarone M, et al. Prevention and treatment of cancer-related infections, version 2.2016, NCCN clinical practice guidelines in oncology. *J Natl Compr Canc Netw.* 2016;14(7):882-913; Carmona-Bayonas A, Jiménez-Fonseca P, Virizuela Echaburu, J, et al. Prediction of serious complications in patients with seemingly stable febrile neutropenia: Validation of the clinical index of stable febrile neutropenia in a prospective cohort of patients from the FINITE study. J Clin Oncol. 2015;33(5):465-471. https://doi.org/10.1200/JCO.2014.57.2347; Rivas-Ruiz R, Villasis-Keever M, Miranda-Novales G, Castelán-Martínez OD, Rivas-Contreras S. Outpatient treatment for people with cancer who develop a low-risk febrile neutropaenic event. *Cochrane Database Syst Rev.* March 2019. https://doi.org/10.1002/14651858.CD009031.pub2.

hypotension), are ill-appearing, or have symptoms or signs of infection (e.g., abdominal tenderness) should be treated empirically regardless of the presence of fever.[1,7] The three most commonly used antibiotics are cefepime, piperacillin/tazobactam, or anti-Psuedomonal carbapenem. Use of a single antibiotic agent is preferred in most patients, because there is no conclusive evidence of benefit from multiple drugs.[1] Each hospital should have a preferred antibiotic agent based on the hospital antibiogram. The most common agents are cefepime, piperacillin/tazobactam, or an anti-Psuedomonal carbapenem, and they are typically used for empirical treatment of both sepsis and febrile neutropenia. Review of patient records for previous pathogens and sensitivities can help identify patients at higher risk of resistant organisms requiring adjustment in empiric therapy. It should be noted that monotherapy with cefepime, a carbapenem, or piperacillin-tazobactam will not be

TABLE 182.1   Selected Antimicrobial Agents Useful in the Immunocompromised Patient

Drug	DOSAGE Adult	DOSAGE Child (Age >28 Days)	Precautions and Comments[a]
Aminoglycosides			
Gentamicin or tobramycin	2 mg/kg loading dose, then 5 mg/kg/day IV every 8 to 12 hours, or 5 to 7 mg/kg IV once daily	Same as adult	Decrease maintenance dose in elderly or with renal dysfunction
Amikacin	Conventional: 10 mg/kg IV load then 5–7.5 mg/kg every 8 hours. High-dose extended interval: 15 mg/kg every 24 hours	Same as adult	Only active against aerobic gram-negative bacilli. Some gram-negative bacilli may be resistant to gentamicin and tobramycin
Extended-Spectrum Penicillins and β-Lactamase Inhibitors			
Piperacillin-tazobactam	4.5 g IV every 6 to 8 hours (depending on extended infusion)	240 to 400 mg/kg/day IV of piperacillin component every 6 hours	Broad activity against gram-positive organisms, *Pseudomonas aeruginosa*, and anaerobes
Cephalosporins			
Cefepime	1 to 2 g IV every 6 to 8 hours	150 mg/kg/day IV every 8 hours	Active against many gram-positive organisms, *P. aeruginosa* and many resistant gram-negative bacilli, but not anaerobes
Carbapenems			
Imipenem-cilastatin	0.5 to 1 g IV every 6 hours	60 to 100 mg/kg/day IV every 6 hours	Adjust dose in elderly or with renal dysfunction. Reduces VPA levels
Meropenem	1 g IV every 8 hours	60 to 120 mg/kg/day IV every 8 hours	Seizures are associated with imipenem. May be cross-allergenic with penicillin. Broad-spectrum activity against gram-positive and gram-negative organisms, including *P. aeruginosa* and anaerobes
Other			
Aztreonam	1 to 2 g IV every 8 hours	120 mg/kg/day IV every 6 hours	Active against gram-negative bacilli including *P. aeruginosa*. Not active against gram-positive organisms or anaerobes. Safe in penicillin-allergic patient
Vancomycin	15 mg/kg IV every 12 hours	40 mg/kg/day IV every 6 to 12 hours	Infuse during 2 hours (flushing, hypotension with rapid infusion). Rapid infusions associated with flushing and hypotension (red man syndrome)
Amphotericin B	0.5 to 1.5 mg/kg/day IV once daily	Same as adult	Refer to infectious disease or pharmacology text
Acyclovir			Infuse during 1 hour
• Herpes simplex, mucocutaneous[b]	5 mg/kg IV every 8 hours or 400 mg PO three times a day	250 mg/m² IV every 8 hours or 15 mg/kg/day PO every 4 hours	
• Herpes zoster			
• Not severe[c]	800 mg PO five times a day	20 mg/kg PO four times a day	
• Severe	10 mg/kg IV every 8 hours	500 mg/m² IV every 8 hours	
• Primary varicella	10 mg/kg IV every 8 hours	10 to 20 mg/kg IV every 8 hours	

[a]Antibiotics require renal/gestational age adjustments.
[b]Alternative for herpes simplex: valacyclovir 1 g two times a day PO.
[c]Alternative for herpes zoster: valacyclovir 1 g three times a day PO.
IV, Intravenous; *PO, per os* (by mouth).

active against vancomycin-resistant *Enterococcus* species or methicillin-resistant staphylococci.

For patients who are allergic to β-lactam antibiotics, coverage of gram-negative bacilli, including *P. aeruginosa,* can be provided by aztreonam. Because aztreonam is not active against gram-positive organisms, it should be combined with vancomycin. If anaerobes are suspected (oral, abdominal, or perianal infection) in the β-lactam–allergic patient or in the patient receiving cefepime monotherapy, an anti-anaerobic drug (clindamycin or metronidazole) should be administered. Empirical treatment with intravenous fluoroquinolones is not recommended in the febrile neutropenic cancer patient because of frequent prophylactic use of these agents in the cancer patient, risk for rapid emergence of resistance in gram-negative bacilli, and predisposition to *C. difficile* infection.[1]

When a focus of infection is identified, empirical therapy should cover the most likely pathogens causing infections at the site (Table 182.1). Patients with pneumonia may need coverage for *Legionella* (azithromycin or a fluoroquinolone), *Pneumocystis* (trimethoprim-sulfamethoxazole), or fungi (amphotericin B, micafungin, voriconazole), in addition to standard antibacterial coverage. Agents effective against anaerobes (clindamycin, metronidazole, meropenem, imipenem, or piperacillin-tazobactam) should be considered for patients with perianal or oral infection and those with abdominal pain, who may have appendicitis, diverticulitis, or typhlitis (neutropenic enterocolitis). Acyclovir should be considered for patients with ulcerative or vesicular lesions who may have herpes simplex or varicella-zoster virus infections. In patients with severe mucositis and FN, meropenem, imipenem, or piperacillin-tazobactam, often combined with vancomycin, are preferred for empirical treatment because of superior efficacy against viridans streptococci.[1]

"Routine" empirical use of vancomycin for all febrile neutropenic cancer patients is not recommended because of concern for the development of vancomycin-resistant organisms.[1,15] Indications for initial empirical vancomycin therapy include serious catheter-related infections (e.g., with hypotension), known colonization with penicillin-resistant pneumococci or methicillin-resistant *Staphylococcus aureus* (MRSA), and positive blood culture for gram-positive organisms before final identification and susceptibility testing.[1,15] Other indications include shock, severe mucositis, prior fluoroquinolone prophylaxis, and institutions in which MRSA, vancomycin-susceptible enterococci, and *S. mitis* are frequent pathogens.[1,15] Patients previously colonized or infected with MRSA, vancomycin-resistant enterococci, extended-spectrum β-lactamase–producing gram-negative bacteria, and carbapenemase-producing organisms may require modifications to initial empirical therapy.[1,7]

Amphotericin B (and its lipid formulations) is the drug of choice for treating invasive fungal infections in patients with neutropenia.[8-10] Due to amphotericin toxicity, micafungin or voriconazole may be considered for treatment of specific fungal infections. Up to one-third of febrile neutropenic patients not responding to one week of antibiotics have systemic fungal infections, usually *Candida* or *Aspergillus*.[8-11]

Risk Assessment and Disposition

Febrile neutropenic cancer patients can be classified into high-risk and low-risk groups. Some of the factors associated with high risk include the following: status as an inpatient when fever and neutropenia developed; presence of serious comorbid medical conditions; uncontrolled cancer; acute leukemia; hemodynamic instability; evidence of organ failure; presence of pneumonia, severe soft tissue infection, infection of a central line, abdominal pain, neurologic or mental status abnormalities; and neutropenia expected to last more than 10 days.[16-17] These patients should be treated in the hospital with intravenous antibiotics.

Outpatient empirical antibiotic therapy is safe and efficacious in carefully selected FN adults who are not at high risk for medical complications.[1,7,16-17] The Multinational Association for Supportive Care in Cancer (MASCC) risk index score (available at www.mascc.org/mascc-fn-risk-index-score) is an easy to use, validated clinical prediction rule for classification of low-risk adults (Table 182.2, Box 182.3). However, it should not be used as the sole factor to decide on low-risk status or outpatient management.[1,7,16-17] Three clinical practice guidelines, including the Infectious Diseases Society of America, the American Society of Clinical Oncology, and the National Comprehensive Cancer Network, support outpatient or short-stay oral antibiotic therapy in carefully selected low-risk patients with FN.[1,7,16] The only oral antibiotic regimen recommended is a fluoroquinolone *plus* amoxicillin-clavulanate (or *plus* clindamycin in penicillin-allergic patients).[1]

TABLE 182.2 Multinational Association for Supportive Care in Cancer Scoring System to Identify Patients With Cancer and Febrile Neutropenia at Low Risk of Medical Complications

Characteristic	Weight[a,b,c]
Burden of febrile neutropenia with mild or no symptoms	5
No hypotension (systolic blood pressure >90 mm Hg)	5
No chronic obstructive pulmonary disease	4
Solid tumor or hematologic malignancy with no previous fungal infection	4
No dehydration requiring parenteral fluids	3
Burden of febrile neutropenia with moderate symptoms	3
Outpatient status	3
Age younger than 60 years old	2

[a]Maximum score is 26. Higher score is better.
[b]Scores ≥21 indicate a low risk for medical complications.
[c]Burden of febrile neutropenia: The general clinical status of the patient as influenced by the febrile neutropenic episode is evaluated on the following scale: no or mild symptoms (score of 5); moderate symptoms (score of 3); and severe symptoms or moribund (score of 0). Choose only one score for burden of febrile neutropenia symptoms (5, 3, or 0). Adapted from: Taplitz RA, Kennedy EB, Bow EJ, et al. Outpatient management of fever and neutropenia in adults treated for malignancy: American Society of Clinical Oncology and Infectious Diseases Society of America clinical practice guideline update. *J Clin Oncol.* 2018;36(14):1443-1453. https://doi.org/10.1200/JCO.2017.77.6211. Available at: www.mascc.org/mascc-fn-risk-index-score.

BOX 182.3 Considerations for Outpatient Management of Cancer Patients With Febrile Neutropenia

Adult patients may be considered for outpatient therapy if:
- Patient has a MASCC score ≥21.
- Patient is medically stable without acute or chronic organ dysfunction or comorbid conditions and does not have acute leukemia.
- No focus of infection identified: Patient does not have pneumonia, infection of a central line or a severe soft tissue infection, and does not have acute abdominal pain or an intra-abdominal infection.
- Patient has access to a telephone and transportation to return to hospital available 24 hours a day and has a caregiver at home.
- Patient has a history of compliance with follow-up and treatment protocols.
- Patient is not on fluoroquinolone prophylaxis and there is a low prevalence of fluoroquinolone-resistance in the community.
- Patient's oncologist agrees to outpatient management.
- The emergency clinician should contact the patient's oncologist and/or an infectious diseases specialist before considering outpatient therapy.

Patients being considered for outpatient therapy should be observed for at least 4 hours in the ED (or in an ED observation unit) after the initial antibiotic dose, which should be administered intravenously as soon as possible after initial cultures are obtained.

The only recommended outpatient oral antimicrobial therapy for these patients is ciprofloxacin or levofloxacin *plus* amoxicillin/clavulanate (or *plus* clindamycin for those with penicillin allergy).

ED, Emergency department; *MASCC,* Multinational Association for Supportive Care in Cancer.

Recently, a second prognostic score has been developed and is termed the Clinical Index for Stable Febrile Neutropenia (CISNE). Importantly, it was derived and validated in patients with FN and solid tumor malignancy. Recent studies suggest that the CISNE and MASCC scores both perform well in FN patients with solid tumor malignancy.[1,18-19]

In the setting of a favorable MASCC score, the decision to pursue outpatient therapy for FN should be made in conjunction with the patient's oncologist when the patient lives within 60 minutes of a hospital, can seek care reliably, has the assistance of a caregiver at home, no barriers to obtaining antibiotics, and agrees to return for outpatient visits. While numerous criteria should be met for outpatient management, avoiding inpatient admission and exposure to nosocomial pathogens is advantageous for low-risk patients.[1]

Children With Cancer and Febrile Neutropenia

Box 182.4 lists unique considerations in the evaluation and management of children with cancer and febrile neutropenia.

Non-Neutropenic Conditions in the Cancer Patient

The Solid Organ Cancer Patient Without Neutropenia

Most solid organ cancer patients who have fever and infection are not neutropenic. Infections in these patients may occur after surgical procedures and can include wound infection, deep abscess, or perforated viscus. Infections may be associated with central venous or urinary catheters, stents, and prosthetic devices. In addition, solid tumor patients with large tumor lesions may have obstructive infections (e.g., bronchus, bile duct, or ureter). The spectrum of microorganisms includes a wide variety of community-acquired organisms (bacterial, fungal, and viral), as well as nosocomial multi-antibiotic–resistant pathogens.

Prompt initiation of antimicrobial therapy in the febrile non-neutropenic solid cancer patient is not always indicated. In febrile non-neutropenic cancer patients who are not ill-appearing and have no identified focus of infection, it may be appropriate to obtain culture specimens and to observe the patient. After consultation with an oncologist, some patients can be discharged home with close follow-up. Indications for urgent antibiotics include signs of sepsis, mental status

changes, lactic acidosis, shock, abdominal pain, history of splenectomy, and identification of a focal site of infection.[1,7]

Impaired Cell-Mediated Immunity

The T-cell defects resulting from impaired CMI in cancer patients usually result from cancer chemotherapy or corticosteroid treatment. The cancer itself impairs CMI in patients with Hodgkin disease, non-Hodgkin lymphoma, and hairy cell leukemia.

Bacterial Infections. *L. monocytogenes* is one of the more common bacterial organisms infecting cancer patients with impaired CMI. *Listeria* infection is also seen in patients with organ transplants, diabetes, cirrhosis, AIDS, late pregnancy, and those receiving high-dose corticosteroids or biologic therapies. No early characteristics distinguish *Listeria* infection from bacteremias caused by other organisms. Meningitis, which may be accompanied by cerebritis or brain abscess, is the most common focus of infection and may manifest with personality changes or focal neurologic signs. Cerebrospinal fluid examination frequently does not reveal the organism on Gram stain, but protein is elevated and pleocytosis is present. Ampicillin is the treatment. Trimethoprim-sulfamethoxazole is an alternative for patients with penicillin allergy. Vancomycin is not effective in the treatment of *Listeria* infections even when in vitro susceptibility is shown. Cephalosporins, such as ceftriaxone, are not active against *Listeria*. If meningitis is suspected, empiric ampicillin is recommended in any patient with impaired CMI regardless of age.

Infections caused by *Salmonella* species are common in patients with impaired CMI and usually are manifested with fever. Enteritis may or may not be present. Bacteremia can result in infection of bones, joints, central nervous system, and endovascular devices. Multidrug-resistant *Salmonella* species are increasing. Treatment usually includes a third-generation cephalosporin, like ceftriaxone, or a fluoroquinolone because many isolates are resistant to ampicillin and trimethoprim-sulfamethoxazole.

Patients with solid tumors, lymphoma, and leukemia (especially hairy cell leukemia) are at increased risk for pneumonia from *Legionella* species, with the highest risk in cancer patients receiving high-dose corticosteroids. Non-*pneumophila* species of *Legionella* (*Legionella micdadei* and *Legionella bozemanii*) are particularly common in these patients. Clinical and radiographic manifestations of *Legionella* infection in the immunocompromised patient often differ from those in the immunocompetent host. For example, pleuritic chest pain may be a prominent symptom in the immunocompromised patient and may mimic pulmonary embolism. These patients can have fever without any other symptoms of pneumonia despite the presence of radiographic pulmonary infiltrates. In addition, the chest radiograph may reveal an expanding pulmonary nodule or cavitation of a nodule or infiltrate rather than the usual lower lobe alveolar filling defects. Hyponatremia with a serum sodium less than 130 mEq/L [mmol/L] is particularly common.[20] Although gastrointestinal and neurologic findings are common in patients with *Legionella* infections, these are not more common in patients with *Legionella* than in other causes of pneumonia.[20] The treatment of choice for immunocompromised patients with suspected *Legionella* infection is a respiratory fluoroquinolone or azithromycin.

Nocardiosis is an uncommon but often severe bacterial infection caused by a weakly acid-fast gram-positive branching filamentous rod. It occurs in cancer patients, in those receiving high-dose corticosteroids, and in others with defective CMI. Subacute pneumonia with nodular infiltrates is the most common manifestation, usually without fever.[21] *Nocardia* may also produce cellulitis, subcutaneous abscesses, meningitis, and brain abscesses. Diagnosis requires biopsy, tissue stains, and culture. Treatment is with sulfonamides often combined with other agents.

Mycobacterial Infections. Tuberculosis and other mycobacterial diseases may produce severe disease in those with defective CMI and be manifested as fever of undetermined origin, pneumonia, lymphadenopathy, meningitis, or skin lesions. It is easily mistaken for signs caused by the patient's underlying disease or treatment. Disseminated nontuberculous mycobacterial infections are more common in patients with hairy cell leukemia or chronic myelogenous leukemia.

Fungal Infections. Infections with *Cryptococcus neoformans* and *Cryptococcus gattii* occur in patients with Hodgkin and non-Hodgkin lymphoma, chronic myelogenous leukemia, and chronic lymphocytic leukemia, especially those taking high-dose corticosteroids.[22] Patients with HIV infection, solid organ transplants, diabetes, renal insufficiency, and cirrhosis are also at risk, as are patients receiving prolonged high-dose corticosteroids for connective tissue diseases. Meningitis is the most common manifestation, often with the insidious onset of low-grade fever and subacute and often intermittent headache. Many other organ systems can become infected, including the lungs, skin, bones, and joints. Diagnosis is made by measuring cryptococcal antigen in the serum and cerebrospinal fluid, fungal cultures, and tissue biopsy. An opening pressure should be measured when obtaining cerebrospinal fluid in the evaluation of *Cryptococcal* meningitis as it is frequently elevated due to obstructive hydrocephalus by the *Cryptococcal* capsule.

Impaired CMI may result in reactivation of *Histoplasma capsulatum* and *Coccidioides immitis* with resultant disseminated disease. Infections with *Candida* species are also common in cancer patients with defective CMI, but disseminated disease is less likely than in patients with neutropenia. Invasive aspergillosis may develop in cancer patients receiving high-dose corticosteroids but not as commonly as in those with organ transplants or prolonged neutropenia.

Pneumocystis jirovecii (formerly *carinii*) pneumonia is most common in patients with AIDS, leukemia, lymphoma, and solid tumors taking high doses of corticosteroids. The presentation is often indolent and is characterized by progressive malaise, dyspnea on exertion, and a multitude of potential chest radiograph abnormalities.[23] Patients classically have hypoxia with ambulation which can raise clinical suspicion of pulmonary embolus.[23] High-risk patients (e.g., bone marrow transplant) may take antibiotic prophylaxis consisting of trimethoprim-sulfamethoxazole.

Parasitic Infections. Reactivation of central nervous system infection with the protozoan *T. gondii* occurs most often in patients with hematologic cancers and in patients with HIV. *Strongyloides stercoralis,* an intestinal nematode, is the only helminthic organism producing severe infection in patients with deficient CMI, almost exclusively in those receiving high-dose corticosteroids. Larvae of the parasite disseminate from the intestines to the lungs and other organs, including the central nervous system and skin, causing the *Strongyloides* hyperinfection syndrome, with very high mortality. Wheezing, cough, dyspnea, hemoptysis, and hemorrhagic rash are common. Chest radiographs may show focal or diffuse infiltrates. Dissemination is often accompanied by bacterial infection, usually caused by enteric gram-negative bacilli carried by the parasites from the intestinal tract. Diagnosis is made by examining stool, sputum, tissue or fluid obtained by bronchoscopy or endoscopy, or cerebrospinal fluid for larvae of the parasite. The treatment of choice is oral ivermectin.

Viral Infections. The most common viruses producing serious infections in cancer patients with defective CMI are varicella-zoster, herpes simplex, and cytomegalovirus. Visceral dissemination is common in primary varicella (chicken pox) in nonimmune immunocompromised children and adults, with development of pneumonia, encephalitis, hepatitis, and hemorrhagic lesions. When a nonimmune immunocompromised patient is exposed to varicella, varicella-zoster immune globulin (VariZIG in the United States) should be administered as soon as possible after exposure, up to 10 days postexposure, to ameliorate the disease.[24] Herpes zoster infection is common in cancer patients, particularly those with Hodgkin and non-Hodgkin lymphoma and leukemia. Disease usually remains localized to the primary dermatome, but dissemination occurs in approximately 11%

of patients.[25] Dissemination is usually limited to the skin, but visceral involvement (lung and liver) occasionally occurs. Skin lesions in primary varicella or zoster often become hemorrhagic in these patients.

Reactivation of herpes simplex virus is common, resulting in severe mucocutaneous infection in oral or genital areas. Spread may occur to the esophagus, lungs, or other organs. Herpetic lesions in cancer patients tend to be larger and deeper than those in the immunocompetent patient. Acyclovir given intravenously is the treatment of choice for varicella-zoster and herpes simplex infections in immunocompromised patients, but some stable patients may be treated with oral valacyclovir.[22]

Cytomegalovirus infection may occur in cancer patients treated with corticosteroids. Measles virus, although uncommon, may produce severe infection in those with defective CMI. Fever, rash, pneumonia, and encephalitis are common manifestations. Immune serum globulin may be given after exposure to ameliorate disease. Common community respiratory viruses, such as respiratory syncytial virus, influenza, and adenovirus, may produce severe or fatal pneumonia.

Influenza vaccination is indicated for all patients who are immunocompromised, and vaccination may attenuate symptoms and reduce mortality even if the patient develops influenza.[23] Influenza may mimic bacterial pneumonia, and patients with CMI who are diagnosed with influenza pneumonia should be concurrently treated for bacterial pneumonia due to the likelihood of coexisting disease.[26] Fever is not necessary to suspect or diagnose influenza. Recent Infectious Diseases Society of America (IDSA) guidelines recommend testing any patient who presents to the ED with influenza-related symptoms.[26] All patients with CMI would fall into the higher risk category for influenza-related morbidity and mortality, which warrants early treatment with oseltamivir.[26]

Humoral Immune (B-Cell) Defects

Hypogammaglobulinemia is common in patients with chronic lymphocytic leukemia and multiple myeloma. Low immunoglobulin levels predispose to infections with encapsulated bacteria, such as *S. pneumoniae, H. influenzae,* and *N. meningitides.*[24] Pneumonia is the most common manifestation, but sepsis, otitis media, cellulitis, and urinary tract infection may occur. After receiving cytotoxic agents and corticosteroids for treatment, these patients become susceptible to infections associated with impaired CMI, as well as bacterial infections caused by *S. aureus* and gram-negative bacilli, often with high mortality.[24] Regular infusions of intravenous immune globulin may decrease the incidence of infection but do not prolong survival. Patients should receive pneumococcal vaccine, but many do not respond.

Disruption of Natural Barriers

Disruption of natural anatomic barriers (mucous membranes and skin) by ulcerating tumors, chemotherapy, radiation therapy, diagnostic and therapeutic procedures, and catheters can lead to infection by gram-positive and gram-negative organisms, including anaerobes. Oral mucositis, a debilitating and intensely painful condition associated with radiation therapy and high-dose chemotherapy, frequently results in serious local and systemic infections, including life-threatening sepsis with viridans streptococci. Cancers may cause partial or total obstruction of body lumens and cavities, as may swelling and scarring from radiation therapy. Bronchial obstruction by tumor can lead to pneumonia. Obstruction of the urinary tract may result in infection. Gastrointestinal tract obstruction can lead to perforation and peritonitis.

Opportunistic Infections Mimicking Neoplasm

Infectious agents can produce laboratory, radiologic, or physical findings that resemble those caused by the spread of tumors. For example, mass lesions in the brain caused by *Nocardia* or *Toxoplasma* can be mistaken for cancer metastases. *Aspergillus, Mucor, Rhizopus,* and related fungi invade blood vessel walls and produce thrombosis, which may result in Budd-Chiari syndrome (hepatic vein obstruction), nephrotic syndrome, or oculomotor palsy that may be misattributed to the spread of tumor. Renal vein thrombosis can be caused by infection with gram-negative bacilli. *Candida* fungus balls may develop in one or both ureters, producing a picture of postrenal obstructive uropathy. *Histoplasma, Pneumocystis, Legionella, Aspergillus, Nocardia,* and other organisms can produce pulmonary nodules and be mistaken for pulmonary metastases.

Diabetes

Diabetic patients have increased susceptibility to infection because of defects in immune function, excess substrate for fungal and bacterial growth, vascular insufficiency related to microangiopathy and atherosclerosis, and sensory neuropathy that leads to wound neglect (see Chapter 115). Neutrophil and monocyte-macrophage functions are directly impaired in diabetic patients. These defects are exacerbated by hyperglycemia and improved by tight glucose control. Cellular immunity is affected by a decrease in proliferative response but otherwise remains primarily intact. As immunity is impaired, people with diabetes may present with infections but have atypical symptoms in their presentation. For example, they may present with malaise but lack fever, or may present with purulent wound discharge without pain.

Most diabetic wounds are appropriately managed with preventive techniques and outpatient wound care. Infectious complications include cellulitis, necrotizing skin and soft tissue infection (NSSTI), and osteomyelitis. The decision to treat with antibiotics should be based on signs and symptoms of infection such as purulent drainage, wound inflammation, pain, or systemic symptoms. Mild to moderate wound infections should target gram-positive cocci such as staphylococci and streptococci. These may be treated with oral agents such as cephalexin 500 mg every 6 hours or trimethoprim-sulfamethoxazole 160 mg/800 mg twice a day in the outpatient setting with close surgical follow-up.[25] More severe infections, deeper infections, or infections in patients with risks for multidrug-resistant organisms (MDRO) should be treated with broad-spectrum parenteral antibiotic agents and surgical consultation. X-ray can be specific for deeper infection, but CT is more sensitive for NSSTI and MRI is more sensitive for osteomyelitis. Biomarkers such as CRP and ESR may be elevated in infection but are not specific. Uninfected ulcers do not benefit from antibiotic therapy.[25] Wound swabs may assist in guiding antibiotic therapy in superficial wounds but become unreliable in deeper infection.[25] Procalcitonin testing has shown promise in differentiating infected from noninfected wounds in some small studies,[27] but its role in the ED is still to be determined.

Other infections often attributed to diabetes include: urinary tract infections including emphysematous cystitis and pyelonephritis; emphysematous cholecystitis; polymicrobial NSSTIs, especially involving the perineum (Fournier gangrene) and lower extremities; malignant otitis externa caused by *P. aeruginosa;* and the rare rhinocerebral zygomycosis caused by *Rhizopus* and *Mucor* species. The combination of organism risk, poor circulation, and impaired immune function often leads to an increased risk of tuberculosis. Patients with diabetes are at increased risk of candidiasis, including vulvovaginal candidiasis in women, psoas abscess, spinal epidural abscess, postoperative surgical site infections, and *S. aureus* and gram-negative pneumonia. Diabetic patients with pneumococcal pneumonia are more likely to become bacteremic and to have a higher mortality rate. With increased risk, diabetic patients often need broad-spectrum parental agents. Glycemic control is crucial in reestablishing proper immune function to promote healing.

Alcohol Use Disorder and Cirrhosis

Alcohol consumption predisposes to infection through direct suppression of the immune system, alterations in blood flow, depression of mental status, and delay in seeking medical care. Patients with alcohol use disorder also often have coexisting malnutrition, cigarette smoking, and chronic lung disease. Alcoholic cirrhosis results in deficient hepatic clearance and destruction of bacteria by reticuloendothelial cells, as well as splenic hypofunction. Complement deficiency occurs because the liver is the primary site of C3 synthesis. Neutrophils show impaired recruitment to infected sites and defective chemotaxis and phagocytosis. Cellular immune deficiency occurs and is often exacerbated by malnutrition. Bactericidal activity of IgM antibodies against gram-negative pathogens such as *E. coli* and *H. influenzae* is decreased.

Acute ethanol intoxication is associated with granulocytopenia and diminished leukocyte mobilization that is reversible with abstinence. Additionally, intoxication inhibits respiratory reflexes and mucous clearance leading to aspiration; concomitant withdrawal seizures or encephalopathy increase this risk. Prior data showed increased oropharyngeal colonization by gram-negative bacteria in alcoholics, but recent studies have demonstrated no increased risk of gram-negative infections in individuals with alcohol use disorder.[28] Recent guidelines from the American Thoracic Society and the IDSA include alcoholism as a comorbidity for combination antibiotic therapy in community-acquired pneumonia but recommend no deviation in routine inpatient therapy and no routine coverage of aspiration in the absence of empyema or lung abscess.[29]

Common infections in patients with cirrhosis include spontaneous bacteremia and sepsis caused by *E. coli, K. pneumoniae, Salmonella,* streptococci, *Vibrio vulnificus,* and *Aeromonas;* spontaneous bacterial peritonitis, usually caused by *E. coli, K. pneumoniae, S. pneumoniae,* or enterococci; pneumonia related to pneumococci, gram-negative bacilli (*E. coli, K. pneumoniae,* and *H. influenzae),* and anaerobes; tuberculosis; meningitis caused by *S. pneumoniae* and *L. monocytogenes;* and skin and soft tissue infections with *S. aureus,* streptococci, and gram-negative bacilli. Cirrhotic patients who present to the ED after a recent hospitalization often have health care–associated infections, including catheter-related and *C. difficile* infections, spontaneous bacteremia, urinary tract infections, and pneumonia, often with high mortality.

In cirrhotic patients with ascites and fever, abdominal pain, or concern for infectious encephalopathy, spontaneous bacterial peritonitis should be ruled out with ascitic fluid sampling and cell count. Patients with a PMN count of 250 cells/mm^3 or greater should be treated empirically with broad-spectrum coverage, such as ceftriaxone or ciprofloxacin, until cultures result. Additionally, patients receiving treatment for SBP have been shown to have increased survival and decreased incidence of hepatorenal syndrome when administered albumin 1.5 g/kg at presentation and 1 g/kg on day 3 of treatment.

Alcoholic patients with leukopenia may have delayed inflammatory responses; these patients should be watched more carefully and may warrant a higher level of care when infected. For example, leukopenic alcoholic patients with community-acquired pneumonia are more likely to have a delayed manifestation of septic shock or ARDS.

Renal Failure

Infections are a significant cause of death in patients with chronic renal failure and are the second most common cause of mortality after coronary artery disease. These patients often have diabetes, which increases their risk for severe morbidity and mortality from infections. Disruption of cutaneous barriers at vascular access sites and peritoneal dialysis catheter sites and numerous immune system defects are responsible for the increased incidence of infection. Uremic pruritus with excoriation, epidermal and sweat gland atrophy, dryness, and vesicular eruptions also compromise the cutaneous barrier. Reduced renal clearance of unknown toxins, nutritional deficiencies, and administration of immunosuppressive medications lead to aberrant immune regulation early in the course of renal failure.

Chronic kidney failure leads to a state of generalized immune hyporesponsiveness. Neutrophils show reduced mobility, chemotaxis, adherence, phagocytosis, and intracellular bactericidal activity. Leukopenia is common. CMI is severely impaired, with decreased activation and proliferation of T lymphocytes and reduced NK cell activity, which cannot be reversed by hemodialysis. Furthermore, humoral immunity is adversely affected, resulting in deficient production of specific IgG subclass antibodies. Inadequate response to vaccines is typical but can be improved by reinforced vaccination schedules, increased vaccine dosage, and adjunct immunomodulators. Additional predisposing factors to infection in uremic patients include low serum albumin, iron overload, increased intracellular calcium, circulating low-molecular-weight uremic toxins, metabolic acidosis, circulating inhibitors to chemotactic factors, decreased production of endogenous pyrogens, and invasive vascular procedures for dialysis access.

Severe infections with antibiotic-resistant bacteria are common, and empirical therapy for a suspected serious infection should include broad-spectrum antimicrobials active against MRSA and antibiotic-resistant gram-negative bacilli. Skin and soft tissue infections, especially those caused by *S. aureus,* are particularly severe in diabetics and in those with peripheral vascular disease or peripheral neuropathy. Vascular access site infections are usually caused by *S. aureus* but occasionally by gram-negative bacilli and enterococci. Patients using central venous catheters for dialysis have much higher rates of sepsis compared with fistulas or grafts. Infections of dialysis access sites, often due to *S. aureus,* are life-threatening and frequently associated with hematogenous seeding of infection to distant sites, including osteomyelitis (usually involving the ribs or thoracic vertebrae), endocarditis, meningitis, epidural abscess, and septic arthritis. Pneumonia may be severe, and there is an increased incidence of *Legionella* pneumonia. Pneumonia may be challenging to diagnose by chest radiograph in these patients due to changing pulmonary fluid dynamics. Because mortality is high, early antimicrobial treatment should be administered after appropriate cultures have been obtained if acute pneumonia is considered, considering antimicrobial coverage for health care–associated pathogens.

Tuberculosis and fungal infections caused by *Candida* species, *Cryptococcus, Histoplasma,* and *Coccidioides* occur with increased frequency. Diagnosis of tuberculosis may be difficult because of nonspecific symptoms and increased incidence of extrapulmonary disease. In addition, *C. difficile* infection occurs more frequently and is more severe with high mortality.

Infections of the urinary tract are more prevalent in patients who continue to produce urine, with urinary bladder catheterization being the most frequent predisposing factor. There is a poor correlation between the presence of pyuria and urinary tract infection in these patients. *Candida* infection of the urinary tract may develop in patients with chronic renal failure treated with broad-spectrum antibiotics.

Antibiotic selection and dosing should consider a kidney disease patient's lack of renal clearance. If a renally cleared regimen is selected, agents may often be dosed with dialysis treatments. In patients who are otherwise well and nontoxic but require parenteral agents due to drug resistance, this may be facilitated by outpatient dialysis if clinical stability and logistics allow.

Up to two-thirds of patients receiving chronic peritoneal dialysis have peritonitis in their first year, and one-third may be forced to discontinue dialysis because of recurrent infections. *S. aureus* and *S. epidermidis* predominate, followed by streptococci, gram-negative

bacilli, and *Candida* species. Fortunately, peritoneal dialysis patients have much lower rates of sepsis than those on hemodialysis. Patients presenting with fever, abdominal pain, or signs of local site infection should be evaluated for peritonitis including testing of effluent cell count and culture. Those with cell counts greater than 100 WBC/mL or PMNs greater than 50% for individuals using night-time dwells should be treated with renally dosed vancomycin and ciprofloxacin. Patients with recurrent infections or candidal infections will likely need to transition to hemodialysis.

Splenectomy, Hyposplenia, and Functional Asplenia

The spleen is the most crucial organ in the reticuloendothelial system and is the primary site for IgM synthesis, the first early immune response of the body. Opsonin production in the spleen facilitates phagocytosis of bacteria by intracellular macrophages. Patients without a spleen also have decreased production of neutrophils, NK cells, and immunomodulating cytokines.

The spleen is the principal site of clearance of *S. pneumoniae* from the blood. Splenectomy or functional asplenia predisposes to overwhelming pneumococcal infection and fulminant infection with other encapsulated organisms (*H. influenzae, N. meningitidis,* and *Capnocytophaga canimorsus* after dog bites) and gram-negative bacilli (*E. coli* and *P. aeruginosa*).[28,29] Asplenic patients who become infected with *Babesia microti,* a malaria-like protozoan transmitted by tick bite in the United States, may develop severe and often fatal hemolysis (see Chapter 123). Human granulocytic anaplasmosis (formerly ehrlichiosis), another tickborne infection, is severe and sometimes fatal in asplenic patients. In addition, the gram-negative coccobacillus *Bordetella holmesii* produces a non–life-threatening acute febrile illness with bacteremia in patients with asplenia. Pneumococcal sepsis represents 50% to 90% of cases. Most healthy adults who die after fulminating pneumococcal sepsis have had a splenectomy or have a congenitally small or abnormal spleen.

The incidence of overwhelming postsplenectomy sepsis in these patients is low; but when it occurs, the mortality rate is high—especially in children with hematologic disorders. The risk is more significant in children than in adults, with children younger than 2 years old at greatest risk. The risk is highest in the first few years after splenectomy but persists throughout life into old age. People undergoing splenectomy for a hematologic disorder or lymphoma are at much higher risk for overwhelming postsplenectomy infection than are those undergoing splenectomy for trauma. This is probably because of the occurrence of splenic implants (splenosis) or accessory spleens in traumatized patients. Patients with functional asplenia from sickle cell anemia or thalassemia major are at high risk for overwhelming bacterial infections.

Functional hyposplenism occurs in a variety of conditions besides sickle cell disease, including sickle cell–hemoglobin C disease, ulcerative colitis, celiac disease, sarcoidosis, amyloidosis, rheumatoid arthritis, and SLE. The presence of anatomic or functional hyposplenism may be recognized by the finding of Howell-Jolly bodies in red blood cells on a peripheral blood smear.

When overwhelming postsplenectomy infection occurs, often no obvious source of infection is found. Prodromal symptoms such as fever, rigors, malaise, myalgias, headache, vomiting, and diarrhea may be present for 1 or 2 days. Patients seen at this time may be misdiagnosed as having a viral illness, gastroenteritis, or food-borne illness. Abrupt deterioration then occurs over hours, with rapid progression to septic shock with disseminated intravascular coagulation, purpura, and multiorgan dysfunction. The mortality rate is high (50% to 70%), with younger children having the highest mortality rate. In addition, meningitis without overwhelming infection or shock is a common presentation of pneumococcal infection in asplenic patients. When fever develops in a person at risk for this disorder, treatment with an antimicrobial agent effective against *S. pneumoniae* should be initiated without delay. After a blood culture is performed, adults and children should receive ceftriaxone at meningitic doses, with the addition of vancomycin in areas where penicillin resistance is prevalent. Clindamycin, levofloxacin, or moxifloxacin are alternatives for patients with severe penicillin allergy. Children with a history of serious penicillin allergy should receive vancomycin plus levofloxacin.

Use of pneumococcal vaccine in patients at risk is especially important now that antimicrobial-resistant *S. pneumoniae* is prevalent, but the efficacy of this vaccine in these patients is unclear. Persons with functional hyposplenism related to severe underlying diseases often respond poorly to pneumococcal vaccination. Asplenic people should be immunized against pneumococcus, *H. influenzae* type b, *N. meningitidis,* and influenza virus. Although there is no evidence to support this, guidelines recommend that children should receive prophylaxis with oral penicillin or amoxicillin up to the age of 5 years and for at least 1 or 2 years after splenectomy, provided they have not had an invasive pneumococcal infection and have received pneumococcal immunizations. Long-term antimicrobial prophylaxis is generally not recommended in adults. These patients should have standby oral antibiotics at home (amoxicillin-clavulanate, levofloxacin, or moxifloxacin) with instructions to self-administer at the first sign of infection, and they should be provided with information and a medical alert bracelet. Fatal pneumococcal infection has occurred in patients immunized with pneumococcal vaccine who were also taking penicillin.

IMMUNOSUPPRESSIVE THERAPY

Corticosteroids

High doses of corticosteroids alter the distribution and function of neutrophils, monocytes, and lymphocytes. Corticosteroids suppress inflammation, impair mobilization of neutrophils and monocytes, inhibit neutrophil adherence, and decrease chemotaxis of neutrophils and monocytes. They also inhibit phagocytosis and intracellular killing, severely impair CMI, inhibit lymphocyte proliferation, inhibit complement activation, and cause hyperglycemia that contributes to infection.

Acute administration of corticosteroids produces marked alterations in circulating leukocyte numbers. Basophils, eosinophils, and monocytes decrease, whereas neutrophils increase. These changes occur within 4 to 6 hours and abate by 24 to 48 hours after a single steroid dose. Lymphocytes (predominantly T cells) redistribute out of the circulation, resulting in lymphocytopenia. Corticosteroid therapy has little effect on serum immunoglobulin levels.

The most common infections occurring in patients receiving high-dose corticosteroids are caused by pyogenic bacteria (*S. aureus,* streptococci, and gram-negative bacilli). Despite the profound depression of CMI in patients taking corticosteroids, these patients generally have few infections commonly recognized as associated with defective CMI. The most common are tuberculosis and severe or disseminated infections caused by varicella-zoster and herpes simplex viruses. Patients receiving moderate doses of corticosteroids for asthma and other disorders are at increased risk for lethal primary varicella infection. Other infections seen with corticosteroid use include those caused by *Listeria, Salmonella, Legionella, Nocardia, Candida, Aspergillus, Cryptococcus, Histoplasma, Coccidioides, Pneumocystis, Toxoplasma, Cryptosporidium,* and *Strongyloides.* Patients with neurologic diseases have much higher rates of infectious complications than do patients with intestinal, hepatic, or renal disease. The infectious complications related

to corticosteroid use increase with doses of prednisone equivalents of more than 20 mg/day in adults, with total doses of more than 700 mg, and with treatment longer than 30 days. The risk of adrenal suppression can be decreased by use of prednisone doses less than 7.5 mg/day, administration of doses early in the day, avoidance of split doses, and use of alternate-day dosing.

Corticosteroids decrease leukocyte accumulation at inflammatory sites, and the whole cascade of responses leading to local manifestations of infection is slowed. These effects result in delayed presentation of serious infections. In addition, prolonged administration of corticosteroids results in delayed wound healing. For example, skin sutures should be left 50% to 100% longer than in other patients. Short-term steroid treatment has little effect on wound healing.

Use of corticosteroids greatly increases the risk of hospital admission for complications of diverticular disease.[30] The diagnosis of peritonitis resulting from perforation of colonic diverticula, appendicitis, peptic ulcer, or another primary intra-abdominal condition is particularly challenging. These patients have abdominal discomfort, but they may have few abdominal findings and need rapid investigation for life-threatening abdominal disease. CT scan of the abdomen and pelvis and surgical consultation may be needed emergently in these patients, along with timely administration of broad-spectrum antimicrobials to cover for gram-negative enteric bacilli and anaerobes.

Other Immunosuppressive Medications

Commonly used immunosuppressives include cyclosporine, tacrolimus, sirolimus, mycophenolate, azathioprine, methotrexate, and cyclophosphamide. They treat a wide variety of conditions, including rheumatoid arthritis, psoriasis, nephrotic syndrome, and inflammatory bowel disease, and they are used in the prevention and treatment of organ transplant rejection. These drugs depress immune function, especially CMI. In addition, they have a narrow therapeutic window, wide-ranging toxic side effects, and many significant drug-drug and drug-food interactions. Patients may present for evaluation of symptoms caused by an adverse drug reaction or an infection. Before altering current medications or adding new ones, the emergency medicine clinician must check carefully for drug interactions.

Immunomodulating agents are available to treat a variety of immune-mediated inflammatory diseases, including rheumatoid arthritis, psoriasis, and psoriatic arthritis, ankylosing spondylitis, and inflammatory bowel disease. Some of these drugs include inhibitors of tumor necrosis factor alpha (infliximab, adalimumab, certolizumab, golimumab, etanercept), inhibitors of interleukins (tocilizumab, anakinra), inhibitor of pyrimidine synthesis (leflunomide), and inhibitor of T-cell activation (abatacept). These agents, particularly the tumor necrosis factor inhibitors, are associated with increased susceptibility to infection, particularly disseminated infection with various intracellular pathogens.[31] Reactivation of latent infection with *M. tuberculosis,* nontuberculous mycobacterial infection, histoplasmosis, and coccidioidomycosis is frequently disseminated and extrapulmonary at presentation. Additional infections seen at increased frequency include cryptococcosis, listeriosis, legionellosis, salmonellosis, aspergillosis, candidiasis, and pneumocystosis. The clinician should be alert to unusual manifestations of infection in patients taking these agents because misdiagnosis and delayed diagnosis increase mortality. These drugs may also cause impaired wound healing, so skin sutures should be left in place longer than usual.

The references for this chapter can be found online at ExpertConsult. com.

183

The Solid Organ Transplant Patient

Christine E. Koval and Michael P. Phelan

KEY CONCEPTS

- The solid organ transplant recipient's altered anatomy, denervated allograft, and immunosuppression frequently result in atypical disease presentations both related and unrelated to the transplanted organ.
- An understanding of the solid organ transplant recipient's altered anatomy, including vascular and nonvascular anastomoses, is critical to evaluating early post-transplantation complications.
- Rejection can manifest at any point post-transplantation with constitutional symptoms and signs of allograft insufficiency, requiring prompt recognition and augmented immunosuppression to salvage the transplanted organ.
- Timing post-transplantation, the net state of immunosuppression, and ongoing antimicrobial prophylaxis should be incorporated into the evaluation of a solid organ transplant recipient with fever and other concerns for infection.
- In addition to affecting a specific arm of the immune system, each antirejection agent is associated with unique toxicities which may be independently responsible for a solid organ transplant recipient's clinical condition.
- Cardiac allograft vasculopathy, a form of chronic rejection and similar to coronary artery disease in presentation, has emerged as a common complication of orthotopic heart transplantation as transplant recipients live longer.
- Especially in lung transplant recipients with underlying cystic fibrosis or bronchiectasis, prior imaging and culture data should help guide initial management of new respiratory symptoms.
- Recurrent allograft pyelonephritis post-transplantation merits thorough evaluation for ureteral stones and strictures, perinephric abscesses, and urinary retention to identify potentially actionable contributors to infection.
- Hepatic artery thrombosis is an uncommon but devastating early complication of liver transplantation resulting in allograft dysfunction, biliary necrosis, and sepsis if left undetected and untreated.
- Allograft rejection, bacterial or viral enteritis, and altered intestinal transit time can all contribute to diarrhea in the intestinal and multivisceral transplant recipient.
- As chronic corticosteroids are incorporated into immunosuppression regimens for the majority of solid organ transplant recipients, adrenal insufficiency should be considered in the differential of transplant recipients presenting with hypotension and fever.
- In addition to the organ-specific complications described in the sections above, solid organ transplant recipients experience graft-versus-host disease, malignancy, trauma, and psychosocial distress post-transplantation requiring heightened awareness and assembly of multidisciplinary teams.

INTRODUCTION

Solid organ transplantation has undergone significant advancement since the first successful kidney transplant in 1956. In 2019, over 39,000 solid organ transplants were performed in the United States (US).[1] As improvements in medical and surgical treatments allow more individuals to undergo transplantation and increase the life expectancy for transplant recipients, emergency clinicians should expect to encounter patients with illnesses complicated by their history of transplantation. This chapter provides a basic knowledge of organ transplant pathologies and their initial management as well as an appreciation for the utility of consultation with transplant surgeons and other subspecialists.

Pathophysiology

Altered anatomy and ongoing immunosuppression change how transplant recipients present with disease. Allografts are denervated, and thus pain is an unreliable sign of illness. Normal inflammatory and immunologic responses are impaired, limiting the recipient's ability to mount a fever or elevated leukocyte count.[2] Subtle signs and symptoms may be harbingers of serious complications. Transplant-related illness can generally be placed into one of four categories: anatomy, rejection, infection, and drug toxicity (Fig. 183.1). Rejection and infection may present similarly. Changes in baseline allograft function and time since transplantation guide the differential diagnosis. It is imperative to consider infectious risk and drug toxicity when recipients present with issues not directly involving the allograft.

Anatomy

Anatomic complications can involve vascular anastomoses, nonvascular anastomoses, or surgical wounds, and typically manifest within the first few months post-transplantation. Vascular anastomotic complications can include arterial or venous structures. Of these, arterial complications are more acutely devastating. Arterial stenosis or thrombosis may lead to fulminant organ failure. Pseudoaneurysms or mycotic aneurysms can precipitate hemorrhagic shock. Nonvascular organ anastomoses can develop leaks or obstructions from scarring or stent migration, which may provoke acute allograft dysfunction or infection. Early identification of these complications by laboratory investigation of allograft function, imaging, and prompt consultation of transplant specialists is vital to salvage the allograft.

Infection

Infection is the primary cause of mortality after transplantation. Timing since transplantation may predict the most likely pathogens and guide empirical antibiotic selection (Fig. 183.2).

Early Period: 0 to 4 Weeks Post-Transplantation. Infections within the first month of transplantation often relate to postoperative intensive care and surgical site complications.[2] Typical pathogens include nosocomial and multidrug-resistant organisms as well as the transplant recipient's colonizing bacteria identified pre-transplantation. Wound infections, pneumonias, urinary tract infections, and *Clostridioides difficile* colitis are encountered. Bloodstream infection may present without typical signs of sepsis syndrome.

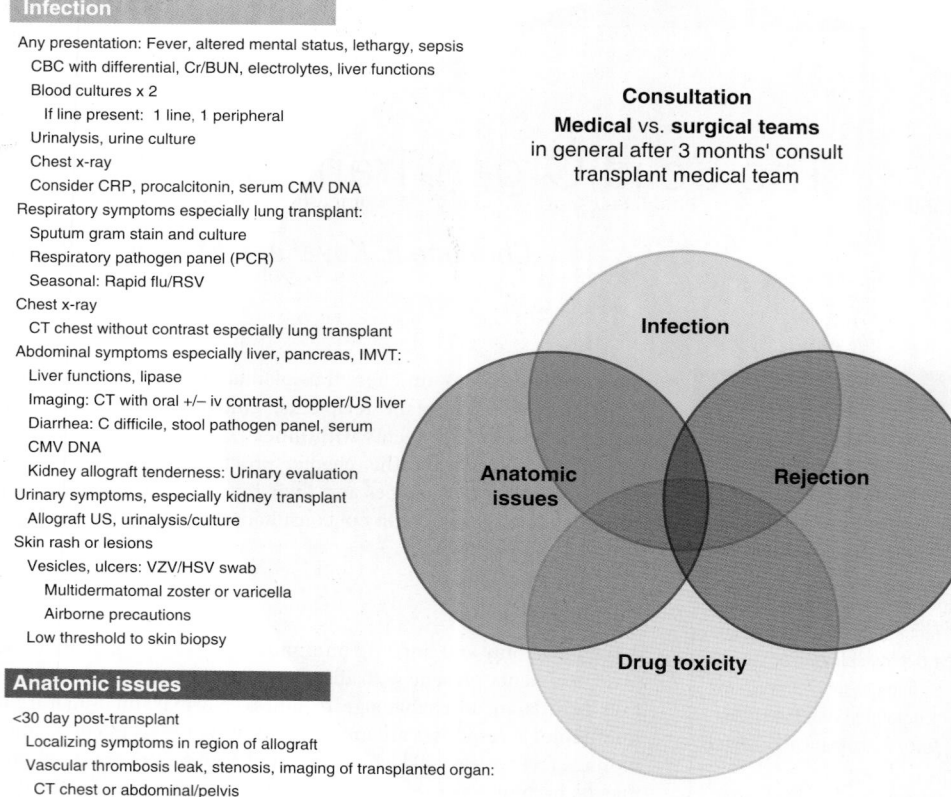

Infection

Any presentation: Fever, altered mental status, lethargy, sepsis
CBC with differential, Cr/BUN, electrolytes, liver functions
Blood cultures x 2
  If line present: 1 line, 1 peripheral
Urinalysis, urine culture
Chest x-ray
Consider CRP, procalcitonin, serum CMV DNA
Respiratory symptoms especially lung transplant:
  Sputum gram stain and culture
  Respiratory pathogen panel (PCR)
  Seasonal: Rapid flu/RSV
Chest x-ray
  CT chest without contrast especially lung transplant
Abdominal symptoms especially liver, pancreas, IMVT:
  Liver functions, lipase
  Imaging: CT with oral +/− iv contrast, doppler/US liver
  Diarrhea: C difficile, stool pathogen panel, serum
  CMV DNA
Kidney allograft tenderness: Urinary evaluation
Urinary symptoms, especially kidney transplant
  Allograft US, urinalysis/culture
Skin rash or lesions
  Vesicles, ulcers: VZV/HSV swab
    Multidermatomal zoster or varicella
    Airborne precautions
  Low threshold to skin biopsy

Anatomic issues

<30 day post-transplant
  Localizing symptoms in region of allograft
  Vascular thrombosis leak, stenosis, imaging of transplanted organ:
    CT chest or abdominal/pelvis
    Doppler/US of liver or kidney
  Transplant surgery consult
>30 day: Strictures, subacute thrombosis
  CT, doppler/US, need for in patient endoscopy (ERCP for biliary strictures)

Consultation
Medical vs. surgical teams
in general after 3 months' consult
transplant medical team

Rejection

General
Recent treatment for rejection increases
risk for infection
  Adherence to immunosuppressants
  New drugs that interact to lower drug levels
  Serum tacrolimus (trough ideal)
  Serum cyclosporine (trough ideal)
Organ specific testing
  Lung transplant: CXR, CT
  Liver transplant: LFTs, US
  Kidney: creatinine, US
  Heart: EKG, echocardiogram
  Pancreas: Lipase
  Intestine/MVT: CT
Tissue biopsy gold standard for all organs
Infection can mimic rejection

Drug toxicity

General: High levels of immunosuppression
increases risk for infection, decreases risk
for rejection and low levels of
immunosuppressant increases risk for
rejection, decreases risk for infection
  Assess for new drugs that may interact
  to raise drug levels
Look for worsening renal function
  Serum tacrolimus (trough ideal)
    High: Increased creatinine, tremor,
    headache, seizure/PRES
  Serum cyclosporine (trough ideal)
    High: Gingival hyperplasia
Mycophenolate: Diarrhea, leukopenia
Steroids: Hyperglycemia, psychosis

©CCF 2019

Fig. 183.1 Evaluation of the solid organ transplant recipient in the emergency department. (Reprinted with permission, The Cleveland Clinic Center for Medical Art & Photography © 2020. All Rights Reserved.)

Both donors and recipients undergo extensive serologic and nucleic acid testing pre-transplantation, but expected and unexpected pathogen transmissions from donor to recipient can occur.[2] Expected transmissions in some donor/recipient pairs include cytomegalovirus (CMV), Epstein-Barr virus (EBV), and hepatitis C virus (HCV). Transplant center–specific strategies to monitor and pre-emptively treat such infections effectively prevent end-organ disease. Unrecognized donor infection prior to transplantation can rarely result in unexpected transmissions and lead to tissue-based or systemic illness (e.g., rabies encephalitis, disseminated disease due to fungi, *Mycobacterium tuberculosis* [MTB], or *Strongyloides stercoralis*). While the focus should remain on addressing the more likely postoperative infections in this time period, consideration of donor-derived infections may be instrumental for diagnosis. Unexpected donor derived infections are reported to United Network for Organ Sharing (UNOS) for the safety of other transplant recipients.

Intermediate Period: 1 to 12 Months Post-Transplantation. Infections occurring within the first year of transplantation are generally divided into two categories: reactivation of latent infections and opportunistic infections.

Reactivation of CMV, the most prevalent viral infection observed during this time period, increases the risk of other infections, allograft rejection, and mortality due to CMV's immunomodulatory properties.[2,3] As all transplant centers provide valganciclovir prophylaxis or serum CMV deoxyribonucleic acid (DNA) monitoring, symptomatic CMV infection does not usually emerge until after prophylaxis is

stopped.[4] Duration of prophylaxis varies based on the type of allograft, donor/recipient serostatus, and transplant center, but typically ranges from 3 to 12 months post-transplantation. Common presentations of CMV reactivation include "CMV syndrome," characterized by fever, leukopenia, and viremia, and CMV gastrointestinal disease presenting with diarrhea, abdominal pain, or odynophagia with or without viremia. Other tissue-based infections (e.g., hepatitis, pneumonitis) involve their respective allografts, present with viremia, and are differentiated from alternative etiologies by allograft biopsy.

Reactivation of herpes simplex viruses (HSV) 1 and 2 and varicella zoster virus (VZV) can be prevented by valganciclovir or other acyclovir-derivatives. When these agents are stopped beyond the prophylaxis period, transplant recipients may present with localized or disseminated disease including multidermatomal zoster. Facial zoster involving the cornea and multidermatomal zoster require hospital admission. Multidermatomal zoster merits airborne and contact precautions. Timely treatment with acyclovir decreases post-herpetic neuralgia. Some adults may be VZV seronegative at the time of transplantation and are at risk for complications of primary varicella infection, including life-threatening pneumonia and encephalitis with or without classic skin lesions. Treatment includes intravenous acyclovir and sometimes varicella immune globulin.

Effective prophylaxis can also prevent many opportunistic infections post-transplantation. Thus, such infections merit particular consideration in transplant recipients who cannot tolerate prophylactic antimicrobials. For example, trimethoprim/sulfamethoxazole (TMP/

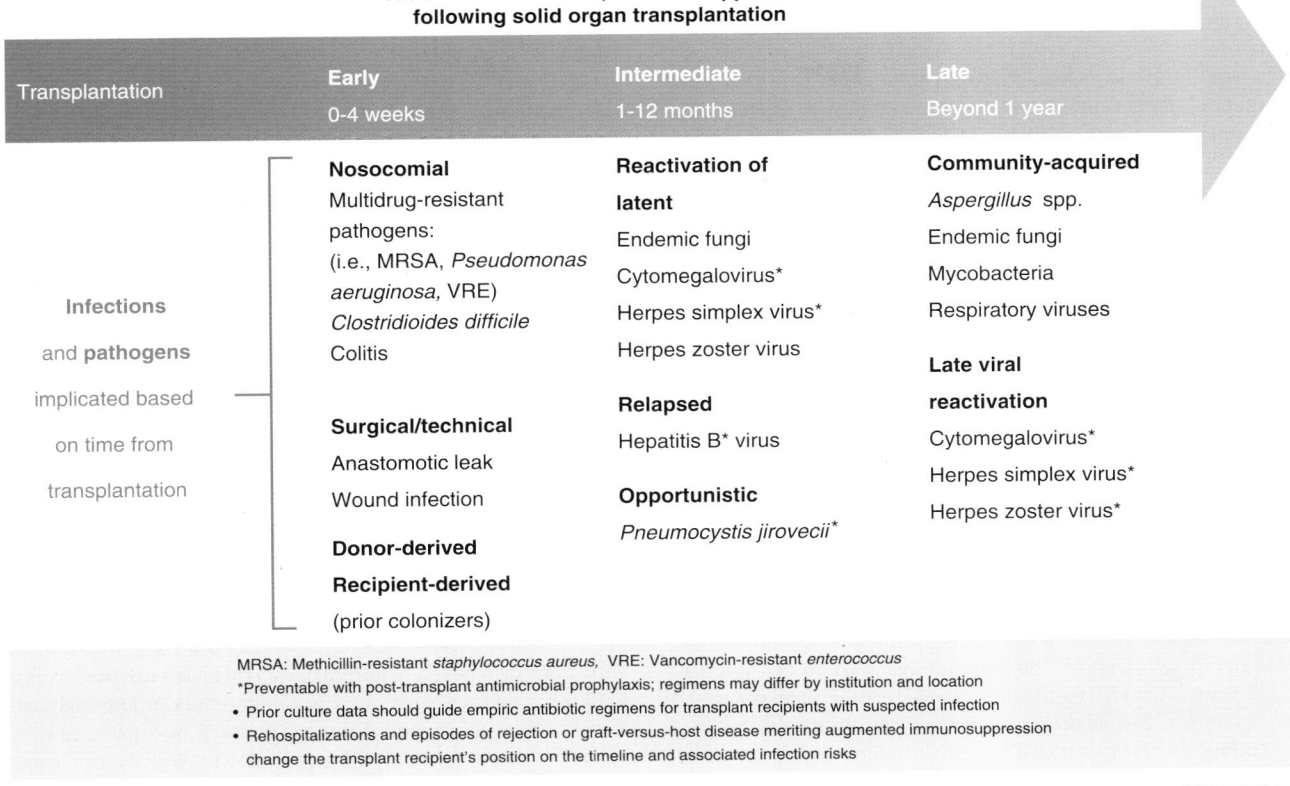

Timeline of infections, immunosuppression following solid organ transplantation

Transplantation	Early 0-4 weeks	Intermediate 1-12 months	Late Beyond 1 year
Infections and **pathogens** implicated based on time from transplantation	**Nosocomial** Multidrug-resistant pathogens: (i.e., MRSA, *Pseudomonas aeruginosa*, VRE) *Clostridioides difficile* Colitis **Surgical/technical** Anastomotic leak Wound infection **Donor-derived** **Recipient-derived** (prior colonizers)	**Reactivation of latent** Endemic fungi Cytomegalovirus* Herpes simplex virus* Herpes zoster virus **Relapsed** Hepatitis B* virus **Opportunistic** *Pneumocystis jirovecii**	**Community-acquired** *Aspergillus* spp. Endemic fungi Mycobacteria Respiratory viruses **Late viral reactivation** Cytomegalovirus* Herpes simplex virus* Herpes zoster virus*

MRSA: Methicillin-resistant *staphylococcus aureus*, VRE: Vancomycin-resistant *enterococcus*
*Preventable with post-transplant antimicrobial prophylaxis; regimens may differ by institution and location
• Prior culture data should guide empiric antibiotic regimens for transplant recipients with suspected infection
• Rehospitalizations and episodes of rejection or graft-versus-host disease meriting augmented immunosuppression
  change the transplant recipient's position on the timeline and associated infection risks

©CCF 2019

Fig. 183.2 Timeline for infectious complications after solid organ transplantation. (Adapted from: Fishman, J. Infection in organ transplantation. *Am J Transplant.* 2017;17:856-879. Reprinted with permission, The Cleveland Clinic Center for Medical Art & Photography © 2020. All Rights Reserved.)

SMX) is the drug of choice to prevent *Pneumocystis jirovecii* pneumonia (PCP) and concomitantly covers *Toxoplasma*, *Nocardia*, and *Listeria* species. Those with sulfa allergies or significant intolerance may be prescribed alternative agents (inhaled pentamidine, oral dapsone, or atovaquone) for PCP prophylaxis but these alternative agents do not sufficiently protect against these other pathogens.

Pneumocystis typically presents with a subacute, progressive, nonproductive cough and dyspnea and is accompanied by diffuse pulmonary infiltrates on imaging. Diagnosis is best made by molecular testing of induced sputum or bronchoalveolar lavage fluid. Optimal treatment is with 5 mg/kg of TMP/SMX every 6 to 8 hours, based on renal function. There is no proof that adjunctive steroid use is beneficial in patients with PCP but without human immunodeficiency virus (HIV), and high doses of steroids may be harmful, but data are extremely limited.[5]

Mycobacterial infections such as tuberculosis (TB) mostly represent reactivated disease, but can also represent primary disease from a new exposure. Transplant recipients may develop pulmonary TB or disseminated infection, presenting with nonspecific systemic symptoms or evident meningitis, peritonitis, or vertebral infection. Treatment is challenging due to public health concerns, serious drug-drug interactions with immunosuppression, and allograft toxicities.

Lung and liver transplant recipients are at highest risk for fungal infections post-transplantation.[6] Invasive aspergillosis frequently presents as pulmonary nodules but may disseminate to any organ system. Endemic mycoses (histoplasmosis, blastomycosis, and coccidiomycosis) manifesting with fever and respiratory symptoms should be considered based on geographic location and exposure history. These infections are uncommon but are more likely to disseminate from an original pulmonary source.[7] Amphotericin B may be appropriate for disseminated disease but newer azoles can be effective for pulmonary infection and are specifically indicated for certain fungi.

Toxoplasmosis is uncommon in solid organ transplantation. Risk is greatest in toxoplasma seronegative recipients who acquire an organ from a seropositive donor and do not receive TMP/SMX prophylaxis.[8] Toxoplasmosis presents as myocarditis in heart transplant recipients, resembling rejection, but can disseminate to cause pulmonary infiltrates, hepatosplenomegaly, and central nervous system (CNS) disease. Treatment involves intravenous sulfadiazine and pyrimethamine or TMP/SMX.

Cryptococcus neoformans presents as a meningoencephalitis with altered mental status. Serum cryptococcal antigen can diagnose disease. However, lumbar puncture for opening pressure and cryptococcal antigen is required to address CNS involvement. If the opening pressure is greater than 25 mm H_2O, relief of cerebrospinal fluid to reduce the opening pressure to less than 20 mm H_2O, or by 50% if the pressure is extremely high, is immediately warranted.[9] Repeated lumbar punctures or percutaneous drains may be required over subsequent days. Initial antimicrobial therapy for meningoencephalitis includes the lipid formulation of amphotericin and flucytosine.

Strongyloides stercoralis is an intestinal nematode that can present with hyperinfection syndrome, causing a necrotizing hemorrhagic enterocolitis and hemorrhagic pneumonia. Disseminated strongyloidiasis presents with severe abdominal pain, obstructive symptoms, hemorrhage and secondary peritonitis, sepsis from enteric pathogens, meningitis, and pneumonia. Diagnosis is by stool or bronchoalveolar lavage sample microscopy. Treatment of disseminated strongyloidiasis is with ivermectin and albendazole, although mortality is high if not detected early.[10]

Late Period: Beyond 1 Year Post-Transplantation. One year after transplantation, transplant recipients' susceptibility to infection is predominantly dependent on their net state of immunosuppression. Healthy transplant recipients have a functioning allograft and can generally be maintained on low doses of immunosuppression such that they achieve immunologic control of CMV and other herpes viruses. They face a mildly increased susceptibility to community-acquired infections, such as influenza and pneumococcal pneumonia, and still develop certain reactivated or opportunistic infections (i.e., VZV, TB, aspergillosis) with aging or environmental exposures. They remain at risk for more severe forms of community-acquired infections and endemic mycoses. In contrast, transplant recipients with chronic immune dysregulation require aggressive immunosuppression for rejection and are unable to develop adaptive immunity to CMV. They face high risk for life-threatening opportunistic infections, as well as standard community-acquired and nosocomial infections, and may require prolonged antimicrobial prophylaxis.

Rejection

Rejection is the process by which T cell receptor–mediated pathways lead to cytotoxic activity and B cell memory and antibody formation lead to allograft cell death.[11] This immune response to the allograft waxes and wanes, mandating lifelong surveillance. Hyperacute rejection occurs in the immediate postoperative period, caused by pre-formed antibodies against major histocompatibility complex or ABO blood type antigens. This complication is rare with careful donor-recipient matching or with aggressive desensitization strategies. Acute cellular rejection (ACR) and antibody mediated rejection (AMR) are both associated with constitutional symptoms and signs of allograft insufficiency occurring days to weeks after transplantation or any time immunosuppression is deliberately or accidentally decreased. ACR is mediated by T cells whereas AMR is due to circulating donor-specific antibodies, complement deposition, and neutrophilic inflammation of the allograft. Chronic rejection occurs over months to years and results in allograft failure.

Immunosuppressive therapy requires correctly timed drug combinations to establish a balance between rejection and infection. Regimens are transplant center–specific, but most include a calcineurin inhibitor (usually tacrolimus), an antimetabolite (usually mycophenolate mofetil), and steroids. Recognition of the side effects, toxicities, and potential drug-drug interactions of immunosuppressant medications is important for the care of any transplant recipient (Table 183.1). Consultation with a clinical pharmacist trained in transplant pharmacotherapy can help optimize the use of immunosuppressive and antibiotic agents.

Desensitization Regimens and Therapies for Antibody-Mediated Rejection. Desensitization regimens decrease circulating antibodies likely to react with donor antigens in patients sensitized to incompatible donors. These pretransplant regimens include plasmapheresis to remove antibodies, rituximab to deplete B cells, bortezomib to reduce antibody production, intravenous immune globulin (IVIG) to trigger antibody clearance, and eculizumab to target the complement cascade.[11]

Induction Agents. Induction immunosuppression is employed in the pre- or peri-transplantation period. Antithymocyte globulin (ATG) and alemtuzumab are both lymphocyte depleting agents, with ATG targeting T cells and alemtuzumab both T and B cells. ATG is also used to treat steroid-refractory acute cellular rejection. Lymphodepletion can last for 3 to 6 months, conferring increased risk of opportunistic

infections and post-transplantation lymphoproliferative disorder (PTLD). Non-lymphodepleting agents include basiliximab and daclizumab, anti-IL-2 monoclonal antibodies used in recipients at lower risk of rejection.[12]

Maintenance Immunosuppression

Calcineurin Inhibitors. The calcineurin inhibitors tacrolimus and cyclosporine have greatly improved patient- and allograft-related outcomes. However, calcineurin inhibitors (CNIs) have narrow therapeutic indices, variable pharmacokinetics, and adverse side effects.[12] Serum trough levels should be checked in patients with worsening renal function, because CNIs are cleared by the kidney and can cause kidney injury. Both CNIs have been associated with gout and pseudogout. CNI concentrations are altered by common post-transplantation medications including antibiotics; the initiation of such medications merits close communication with the transplant team to plan for CNI dose adjustments and prospective drug monitoring.

Tacrolimus is a macrolide compound that binds to lymphocyte proteins and inhibits cytokine synthesis. Adverse effects include dose-dependent nephrotoxicity as well as neurotoxicity, characterized by tremors, headache, and posterior reversible encephalopathy syndrome (PRES).[12] When combined with steroids, tacrolimus can lead to hyperglycemia and diabetes.

Cyclosporine inhibits both cellular and humoral immunity by binding to proteins which inhibit lymphocyte signal transduction between helper-inducer T cells and B cells. Cyclosporine is similarly associated with dose-dependent nephrotoxicity which is enhanced when used with other nephrotoxins, such as amphotericin or aminoglycosides.[12] Renal tubular injury and direct renal artery vasospasm can result in systemic hypertension. Rarely, cyclosporine toxicity can result in a neurologic syndrome of confusion, quadriplegia, and coma if left untreated.

Mammalian Target of Rapamycin Inhibitors. Sirolimus and everolimus are two drugs in the mammalian target of rapamycin (mTOR) class. mTOR is key in the pathway for T cell clonal activation. Adverse effects include delayed wound healing, hyperlipidemia, cytopenias, diarrhea, and sirolimus-induced lung injury.[12]

Antimetabolites. Azathioprine is an antimetabolite derivative of 6-mercaptopurine and inhibits both DNA and ribonucleic acid synthesis to suppress lymphocyte proliferation.[12] Transplant recipients may exhibit dose-dependent neutropenia, hepatic dysfunction, and gastrointestinal upset.

Mycophenolate mofetil (MMF) is an antimetabolite with more potent and selective inhibition of lymphocyte proliferation as well as a relatively low side effect profile.[12] The most common adverse effects are diarrhea and leukopenia. Because magnesium and aluminum antacids interfere with MMF absorption, care should be exercised in treatment of GI symptoms. MMF is usually switched to azathioprine in the setting of pregnancy to reduce risk of teratogenicity.

Corticosteroids. Corticosteroids have a wide range of effects on the immune system. Every effort is made to minimize corticosteroid use to prevent long-term consequences such as gastrointestinal bleeding, diabetes, and osteonecrosis. High-dose steroids to treat rejection may precipitate altered mental status. Acute withdrawal or severe illness may lead to Addisonian crisis, presenting with fevers, hypotension, and metabolic derangements and merit initiation of stress-dose steroids (e.g. hydrocortisone 100 mg IV).

Other Agents: Belatacept, Rituximab, Eculizumab. Belatacept is a fusion protein that blocks T cell co-stimulation at CD28 and is used primarily in kidney transplantation to avoid the nephrotoxicity of CNIs.[12] It is dosed on a monthly basis. It is associated with increased rates of PTLD and is contraindicated in EBV-seronegative recipients. Rituximab is a monoclonal antibody directed against the B-cell surface marker CD20 and

TABLE 183.1   Immunosuppression Agents Used in Solid Organ Transplantation

Agent	Mechanism	Metabolism	Drug-Drug Interactions	Toxicities and Other Considerations
Alemtuzumab	CD52 inhibitor	–	–	Lymphocyte depletion for 6–12 months
Antithymocyte globulin	Polyclonal T cell depletion	–	–	Lymphocyte depletion for 3–6 months Serum sickness, fevers with infusions
Azathioprine	Antimetabolite	Hepatic	↑ by allopurinol May ↓ anticoagulant effect of warfarin	Hepatotoxicity Bone marrow suppression, ↑ by valganciclovir
Basiliximab	IL-2Rα inhibitor	–	–	Duration of activity may last 4–6 weeks
Belatacept	CD80/86 inhibitor	–	–	Post-transplant lymphoproliferative disorder
Bortezomib	26S proteasome inhibitor	Hepatic CYP2C19, CYP3A4	↓ by phenytoin, carbamazepine, rifampin ↑ by azoles, CCBs, macrolides, PIs	Peripheral neuropathy
Cyclosporine A	Calcineurin inhibitor	Hepatic CYP3A4 and P-glycoprotein	↓ by phenytoin, carbamazepine, rifampin ↑ by azoles, CCBs, macrolides, PIs, letermovir	Nephrotoxicity, ↑ by AG, AMB, NSAIDs Hypertension Gingival hyperplasia
Eculizumab	Terminal complement inhibitor	–	–	*Neisseria meningitides* meningitis
Everolimus	Mammalian target of rapamycin inhibitor	Hepatic CYP3A4 and P-glycoprotein	↓ by phenytoin, carbamazepine, rifampin ↑ by azoles, CCBs, macrolides, PIs	Interstitial pneumonitis Nephrotoxicity Poor wound healing
Intravenous immunoglobulin	Antibody replacement	–	–	Serum sickness, fevers with infusions
Mycophenolate mofetil Mycophenolate sodium	Antimetabolite	Hepatic and gastrointestinal	↑ by antacids, cholestyramine	Hepatotoxicity Bone marrow suppression, ↑ by valganciclovir Gastrointestinal distress
Rituximab	CD20 inhibitor	–	–	Reactivation of hepatitis B, JC virus
Steroids	Variable	Hepatic cytochrome P450 (minor)	↑ by PIs	Weight gain and associated glucose intolerance, HLD Poor wound healing ↑ risk gastrointestinal bleeding with NSAIDs
Sirolimus	Mammalian target of rapamycin inhibitor	Hepatic CYP3A4 and P-glycoprotein	↓ by phenytoin, carbamazepine, rifampin ↑ by azoles, CCBs, macrolides, PIs	Interstitial pneumonitis Poor wound healing
Tacrolimus	Calcineurin inhibitor	Hepatic CYP3A4 and P-glycoprotein	↓ by some antiepileptics, caspofungin, rifampin ↑ by azoles, CCBs, macrolides, PIs, CBD	Nephrotoxicity, ↑ by AG, AMB, NSAIDs Neurotoxicity (PRES, Tremor)

CCB, Calcium channel blocker; *PI*, protease inhibitor; *AG*, aminoglycoside; *AMB*, amphotericin B; *NSAID*, nonsteroidal antiinflammatory; *HLD*, hyperlipidemia; *PRES*, posterior reversible encephalopathy syndrome.
Reprinted with permission, The Cleveland Clinic Center for Medical Art & Photography © 2020. All Rights Reserved.

results in B cell depletion. It is associated with cytopenias and hepatitis B reactivation. It also carries a black box warning for progressive multifocal leukoencephalopathy, although this is rare.[12] Eculizumab is a monoclonal antibody that acts as a terminal complement inhibitor and is associated with increased risk for meningococcemia.[13]

ORGAN-SPECIFIC CONSIDERATIONS

The following sections delineate organ-specific anatomic, rejection-related, infectious, and pharmacologic complications of transplantation with occasional reference to the general concepts of solid organ transplantation described previously.

Heart Transplantation

Heart transplantation is a curative option for patients with end-stage cardiomyopathy, recurrent ventricular arrhythmias, intractable angina, or primary tumors. In 2019, over 3500 heart transplants were performed in the United States.[1] Over 40% of candidates are bridged to transplantation with ventricular assist device (VAD) technologies. Current 1-, 3-, and 5-year patient and allograft survival rates are 90%, 85%, and 80%, respectively.[14] Main reasons for readmission early post-transplantation include cardiac dysrhythmias, allograft rejection, and infection; later causes include cerebrovascular and allograft vasculopathy. Renal dysfunction and diabetes are common comorbidities.[15]

Anatomic Considerations

Orthotopic heart transplants are usually bicaval, involving a single anastomosis between the donor and recipient left atria, aortic and pulmonary artery anastomoses, and two caval anastomoses. Alternatively, the biatrial method of orthotopic heart transplantation involves anastomoses between the aorta and pulmonary artery as well as both the right and left atria.[16] Leads from previous pacemakers or implantable cardioverter-defibrillators may be retained post-transplantation, limiting the transplant recipient's ability to undergo magnetic resonance imaging safely.

The transplanted heart is denervated of both parasympathetic and sympathetic nerve fibers, which causes clinically important physiologic changes.[17] Without parasympathetic tone, the transplant recipient's early resting heart rate varies from 95 to 110 beats/minute, but decreases by one year to a mean of 92 beats/minute.[18] Variation exists based on donor and recipient factors. Without sympathetic tone, transplant recipients may experience relative bradycardia during times of physical or mental stress. Transplant recipients presenting to the ED with brady- or tachyarrhythmias generally merit admission. For immediate intervention, beta-blockers, diltiazem, and amiodarone may be used to treat supraventricular tachyarrhythmias. The allograft is sensitive to adenosine with a risk of prolonged AV block, so the anticipated dose should be reduced by half prior to administration. Atropine and glycopyrrolate have no effect on the denervated heart and should not be used in the transplant recipient.

Denervation of the allograft also prevents heart transplant recipients from experiencing classic anginal symptoms.[17] Transplant recipients suffer silent myocardial infarctions and sudden cardiac death, compelling providers to remain aware of other signs and symptoms of cardiac ischemia. The most common electrocardiogram (ECG) abnormalities after heart transplantation, incomplete right bundle branch blocks and repolarization abnormalities, are not clinically meaningful.[19] Significant ECG abnormalities include consistent Q waves as well as ST segment elevations. Heart failure may present in an atypical fashion as well. Although a transthoracic echocardiogram may report normal left ventricular function and ejection fraction, microscopic scarring of the allograft can gradually lead to a restrictive cardiomyopathy.

Infection

In addition to the nosocomial infections described earlier in this chapter, infections related to the surgical site as well as the sites of prior device placement occur in the first month after heart transplantation. Mediastinitis may present with chest pain, sternal instability, wound breakdown, or with nonspecific symptoms of fever and tachycardia. Diagnosis requires computerized tomography (CT) scan of the chest, and treatment requires broad-spectrum antibiotics and surgical débridement. Infections of VAD components can be present at the time of transplantation and may impact post-transplantation infection risk. Prior VAD infection increases the risk for post-transplantation multidrug-resistant infections and can thus inform empirical antibiotic selection.[20]

Toxoplasmosis is a particular risk for heart transplant recipients, especially in those unable to take TMP/SMX prophylaxis, and presents with signs of myocarditis resembling rejection, pneumonia, or meningoencephalitis. Trypanosomiasis is rare in the United States but is a common indication for heart transplantation in endemic countries. Unmonitored, recurrent infection can cause myocarditis, subcutaneous nodules, or disseminated disease.[8]

Rejection

Hyperacute cellular or metabolic rejection is rare but can precipitate early allograft failure, requiring the temporary use of advanced heart therapies.[21] Acute cellular rejection occurs in 27% of recipients by one year post-transplantation and is diagnosed by allograft biopsy.[14] Many episodes are low-grade, asymptomatic, and left untreated. Severe rejection manifests with fever and signs of heart failure such as dyspnea, meriting admission for anti-rejection therapies.

Cardiac allograft vasculopathy is associated with chronic rejection and serves as a major determinant of morbidity and mortality for heart transplant recipients.[21] It is identified via angiography with diffuse, concentric narrowing of the coronary arteries. CAV may be asymptomatic or present with symptoms of heart failure, myocardial infarction, or sudden cardiac death. The definitive treatment for CAV is re-transplantation.

Drug Toxicity

Calcium channel blockers and amiodarone can increase cyclosporine, tacrolimus, and sirolimus levels. In contrast, cyclosporine can increase the drug levels of statin medications to result in muscle cramping and rhabdomyolysis. Sirolimus use in the early post-transplantation period can result in sternal wound dehiscence and is avoided early post-transplantation. Drug-drug interactions between antibiotics and warfarin require attention to ensure safe anticoagulation.

Kidney Transplantation

Kidney transplantation is a life-saving option for patients with end-stage renal disease compared to prolonged time on dialysis. Over 23,000 kidney transplants were performed in the United States in 2019.[1] One-, three-, and five-year patient survival post-deceased donor kidney transplantation is generally estimated at 97%, 94%, and 90%, respectively, with living donor outcomes exceeding these.[22] Up to 40% of transplant recipients present to the ED in the first year, usually due to allograft dysfunction, infection, or exacerbation of diabetes or hypertension.[23]

Anatomic Considerations

The renal allograft is usually transplanted in the right or left iliac fossa, with native kidneys and ureters left in situ. Allograft pyelonephritis presents with pain at the allograft in the lower abdomen rather than the flank pain observed with native pyelonephritis. However, denervation can prevent the development of pain altogether.[24] Rarely, nephrolithiasis and urinary tract infections still occur in the transplant recipient's retained native kidneys.[25]

Donor renal vessels are anastomosed to recipient iliac vessels. Although rare, vascular complications such as bleeding and thrombosis can occur up to a week post-transplantation.[23] Intra-abdominal hematomas can initially manifest with urinary obstruction and hydronephrosis. Renal artery and vein thromboses can also present with decreased urinary output and acute kidney injury. Vascular complications occurring months to years post-transplantation are typically due to arterial stricture or stenosis observed in the context of underlying peripheral vascular disease. Doppler ultrasound is the preferred method of evaluating vascular patency.

Nonvascular anastomoses are created between the donor ureter and either the recipient's ureter or bladder. Ureteral stents are endoscopically inserted during transplantation and remain in place for 6 weeks. Retention of the stent during episodes of infection may lead to recurrent urinary tract infections due to biofilm formation. Ureteric complications occur in up to 15% of transplants and include stent migration as well as ureteric leak or stricture. Unlike the native system, the transplanted ureter does not have a one-way valve at the insertion site in the native bladder to prevent reflux-associated injury to the allograft.

Delayed allograft function requires temporary dialysis until reasonable function is established. During dialysis, attention must be paid to central catheters, fistulas, and grafts, which may be potential sources of infection or thrombosis.

Infection

Urinary tract infections including allograft pyelonephritis are the most common infections post-transplantation. Classic presenting symptoms include fever, allograft tenderness, and pyuria, but symptoms may be nonspecific, including confusion, malaise, or weakness. Associated volume depletion can elevate creatinine, mirroring allograft rejection. If there is evidence of sepsis, obtain blood and urine cultures and initiate empirical antibiotic therapy until culture data are available.

Recurrent urinary tract infections can lead to allograft failure and merit a thorough investigation (including imaging) of potentially actionable contributors to disease such as perinephric abscesses, nephrolithiasis, residual ureteral stent, and urinary retention. Oral antibiotics may suffice to treat uncomplicated cystitis, though intravenous options are recommended in the setting of allograft pyelonephritis or urinary tract infections complicated by bacteremia or sepsis. Asymptomatic bacteriuria does not require routine treatment.[26]

Attention to remaining dialysis access sites may identify a source for bloodstream infections. BK virus infection results in chronic nephropathy in up to 10% of kidney transplant recipients but is rarely an emergent problem.[27] Reduction of immunosuppression is the only proven strategy for decreasing the risk of significant BK nephropathy and usually takes months to resolve.

Rejection

Acute rejection is a common complication of kidney transplantation, with an incidence of 10% at 1 year and associated reductions in allograft survival.[22] Renal allograft rejection manifests with fever, tenderness over the allograft, and signs and symptoms of allograft dysfunction including decreased urine output and elevated creatinine. Early consultation with the transplant nephrologist or urologist is prudent to pursue timely renal biopsy and empirical treatment.

Chronic transplant rejection occurs after long-term loss of adequate function due to nephrosclerosis or fibrosis of the blood vessels supplying the allograft. This process involves proliferation of the vascular intima of renal vessels with marked decrease in the lumen size. Findings include proteinuria, hypertension, and allograft dysfunction.

Drug Toxicity

Drug toxicities are a particular risk to the renal allograft. Supratherapeutic CNI concentrations can cause acute and chronic kidney injury.[12] Other nephrotoxic drugs can potentiate injury in the setting of CNIs or volume depletion. Nonsteroidal antiinflammatory drugs (NSAIDs) are not recommended in kidney transplant patients because even short courses for acute pain management have been demonstrated to result in acute allograft injury.[28] Amphotericin and foscarnet should be administered with caution.

Liver Transplantation

Over 8800 liver transplants were performed in the United States in 2019.[1] Since 2015, nonalcoholic steatohepatitis (NASH) has superseded hepatitis C as the primary indication for liver transplantation. One-, three-, and five-year patient survival is reported as 91%, 84%, and 76%, respectively.[29] Vascular and biliary complications, allograft dysfunction, and infection are common, with up to 45% of transplant recipients presenting to the ED in the first year post-transplantation and 78% of these requiring admission.[30]

Anatomic Considerations

Liver transplantation requires surgical anastomoses at biliary and vascular sites. Biliary anastomosis can be duct-to-duct or by choledochojejunostomy. Choledochojejunostomy (CDJ) is performed when donor or recipient ducts are not amenable to direct anastomosis, joining the allograft remnant bile duct directly into the roux limb of the recipient small bowel. CDJ increases the risk of intra-abdominal infections. The gallbladder is always removed during transplantation.

All vascular and biliary anastomoses can serve as sites of stenosis, obstruction, or leak. Hepatic artery rupture, caused by bacterial or fungal arteritis, can result in hemorrhagic shock. Portal vein thrombosis occurs in 1% to 2% of liver transplant recipients and presents with encephalopathy and refractory ascites characteristic of allograft failure.[31] Hepatic artery thrombosis (HAT) is the most common vascular complication and can result in immediate hepatic or biliary necrosis, manifesting with fever, jaundice, and right upper quadrant pain with or without elevated transaminases and hyperbilirubinemia.[31] Liver transplant recipients presenting to the ED in the first month post-transplantation should be screened for HAT with Doppler ultrasound. Treatment of acute HAT may require immediate thrombectomy or emergent re-transplantation.

Biliary complications including stricture, obstruction, leaks, and necrosis frequently manifest with fevers, abdominal pain, and relative hyperbilirubinemia.[31] Extrahepatic biliary leak presents with perihepatic collections or peritonitis. Intrahepatic biliary necrosis or stricture can present with intrahepatic bilomas and cholangitis. Biliary stricture typically manifests within 1 year post-transplantation.[31] Stents placed endoscopically may ameliorate the stricture but can themselves become obstructed and may require revision.

Living donor allografts are comprised of either the right or left lobe of the liver. Transplantation of these partial allografts may be complicated by small-for-size syndrome, or functional hepatic impairment occurring within one week postoperatively with coagulopathy, cholestasis, encephalopathy, and ascites.[32] Portal hypertension, a risk factor for small-for-size syndrome, is assessed intraoperatively and modulated with shunt formation or splenectomy. The vascular and biliary complications described in this section are more commonly observed in living donor liver transplant recipients due to complexities of both vessel and bile duct division during allograft donation and the creation of smaller anastomoses during transplantation.

Infection

Over 50% of bacterial infections causing sepsis in this population occur within the first two weeks of transplantation, usually due to pre-transplantation risk factors or surgical complications.[33] Later intra-abdominal infections are due to biliary strictures or preceding HAT. About 50% of living-donor liver transplant recipients experience infection within 1 year, usually due to biliary and vascular complications.[29] Fever, malaise, or abdominal pain should prompt laboratory evaluation with a complete blood count and differential and comprehensive metabolic panel, as well as blood cultures. Niduses of infection, including retained biliary stents, gallstones, and hepatic or intra-abdominal abscesses, should be identified via ultrasound and CT of the abdomen to coordinate surgical or procedural interventions as appropriate.

Enteric organisms, including *Enterococcus* species, gram-negative, and anaerobic organisms are typical pathogens meriting empirical coverage with beta-lactam/beta-lactamase inhibitor regimens. Pre-transplantation colonization with multidrug-resistant organisms may warrant even broader antibacterial coverage. Many recipients have received vaccinations against encapsulated organisms (*Streptococcus pneumoniae*, *Neisseria meningitidis*, and *Haemophilus influenzae*) in planning for possible splenectomy at the time of transplantation, but such infections should remain on the differential diagnosis. Overlying incisional wound infections may warrant coverage for *Staphylococcus aureus* (including methicillin-resistant strains). However, incisional infections and wound dehiscence often portend an underlying intra-abdominal source.

Liver transplant recipients are susceptible to some invasive fungal infections, mostly due to *Candida* species in the early post-transplantation period.[2,33] Risk is associated with biliary and operative bleeding complications and CDJ anastomosis. Invasive aspergillosis and endemic fungal infections usually emerge later but can occur within the first month in high-risk settings such as fulminant hepatic failure, re-transplantation, or severe renal failure post-transplantation. Empirical antifungal therapy is warranted for patients with these risk factors or with septic shock.

Rejection

Acute rejection occurs in up to 20% of liver transplant recipients within one year of transplantation.[29] Chronic rejection is more indolent and can be diagnosed years after initial presentation. Both acute and chronic allograft rejection may present with asymptomatic transaminase elevations or with fever, jaundice, and right upper quadrant pain. Eosinophilia may be noted. Anatomic complications, infections, and drug toxicities can mimic the clinical syndrome of acute rejection. Allograft biopsy is necessary to diagnose rejection but may be occasionally treated empirically in the setting of low tacrolimus concentrations and normal hepatic blood flow.

Drug Toxicity

Liver transplant recipients may be particularly vulnerable to hepatotoxic medications used in the post-transplantation period such as rifamycins or isoniazid used for TB treatment or azole antifungal agents. Up to 4 grams per day of acetaminophen is allowed, but NSAIDs are discouraged.[34]

Lung Transplantation

Over 2700 lung transplantations were performed in the United States in 2019 to treat patients with advanced lung diseases, including idiopathic pulmonary fibrosis, obstructive pulmonary disease, pulmonary hypertension, and cystic fibrosis.[1] Despite ongoing challenges with surgical complications, infections, and chronic allograft lung dysfunction, lung transplantation can significantly improve survival as well as quality of life. One-, three-, and five-year patient survival is estimated at 85%, 68%, and 56%, respectively.[35] Up to 45% of lung transplant recipients present to the ED and 67% face readmission in the first year.[36] Airway complications, infection, and atrial fibrillation are common causes for readmission.

Anatomic Considerations

Lung transplantation may involve a single lung transplant with bronchial anastomosis, bilateral lung transplant with tracheal anastomosis, sequential bilateral lung transplant with bronchial anastomoses, lobar transplant, or heart-lung transplant. Bilateral lung transplantation is indicated for patients with existing lung infection (i.e., cystic fibrosis and bronchiectasis) or significant pulmonary hypertension. Single lung transplantation is often pursued in older and more debilitated individuals as it is a shorter procedure associated with better early postoperative outcomes.

Single and sequential bilateral lung transplantation both require anastomoses of the main bronchi and pulmonary arteries as well as an anastomosis between the donor's pulmonary veins to the recipient's left atrium. Bronchial anastomotic complications such as stenosis, ischemia, tissue degeneration, and dehiscence can occur in up to 15% of transplant recipients, provoking prolonged air leak with pneumothorax or mediastinitis.[37] Vascular anastomotic complications can result in ischemia and allograft failure as well as hemothorax. Postoperative pleural complications such as pleural effusions and empyemas are most frequently observed within 1 week of transplantation.[38] In evaluating a lung transplant recipient with new respiratory symptoms, an initial chest radiograph may be helpful but a non-contrast CT scan of the chest will best evaluate the parenchyma, airways, and pleural spaces.[38]

Infection

Infection occurs in up to 60% of lung transplant recipients in the first year and remains a major cause of mortality.[33,35] Surgical denervation impairs the cough reflex and mucociliary clearance, disruption of vascularization and lymphatic channels results in stagnancy, and immunosuppression blunts appropriate responses to environmental pathogens. Gastroesophageal reflux affects a significant proportion of transplant recipients and contributes to aspiration-related infection events. Some patients such as those with cystic fibrosis also harbor bacteria in the sinuses which may infect the lower airways.

Infections are most commonly pulmonary in origin throughout the post-transplantation course. Early infections are typically hospital-acquired or ventilator-associated.[2] Native lung and allograft parenchyma alike can be affected by donor-derived and nosocomial organisms. Consideration should be given to previously grown pathogens to help guide empirical therapy of a lung transplant recipient with new fever, dyspnea, and cough. Community respiratory viruses are more likely to cause lower respiratory tract infections and inflammation, leading to chronic allograft dysfunction (CLAD).[39] Thus, available antivirals for influenza, respiratory syncytial, and even parainfluenza viruses are often used in conjunction with tapered courses of systemic steroids to control the immune response.[40]

Lung transplant recipients are prone to reactivation of CMV infection and manifest with CMV pneumonia. CT of the chest most often identifies ground-glass opacities and may resemble acute rejection or PJP. Definitive diagnosis requires lung biopsy, but detection of CMV viremia and clinical findings often warrants presumptive therapy, usually with intravenous ganciclovir. PJP is rare in the setting of prophylaxis, but invasive aspergillosis and other mold infections remain relevant throughout the post-transplantation course and should be considered in the setting of nodular or cavitary opacities on imaging or anastomotic wound infections.[41]

A final pair of donor-derived organisms affecting lung transplant recipients are *Mycoplasma hominis* and *Ureaplasma urealyticum*. These two urea-splitting bacteria alter the production and metabolism of ammonia in the allograft, resulting in hyperammonemia syndrome within 10 to 14 days post-transplantation.[42] This condition, characterized by altered mental status and elevated serum ammonia levels, can cause cerebral edema, coma, and eventual death over days to weeks if left unchecked.[43] Any lung transplant recipient, particularly early post-transplantation, with altered mental status should have a serum ammonia level checked. Treatment is multifaceted and includes direct measures to reduce ammonia as well as antibiotics.

Rejection

Approximately 18% of lung transplant recipients experience acute cellular or humoral rejection in the first year post-transplantation.[35] Surveillance spirometry is intended to detect early functional decline that directs further testing. Symptoms of acute rejection can present at any time point post-transplantation with fever, dyspnea, cough, and generalized malaise. While subtle findings of rejection may not be well-evaluated by chest x-ray, this imaging modality may demonstrate airspace disease, interlobular septal thickening, or pleural effusions.[38] Non-contrast CT of the chest reveals ground-glass opacities. Acute rejection is diagnosed by transbronchial biopsy.

CLAD is a manifestation of rejection characterized by airway scarring and fibrosis with resultant progressive deterioration of lung function.[44] Both restrictive and obstructive patterns of disease are described, with a variety of posited triggers, including infections and prior rejection. Clinically, CLAD presents with progressive cough, dyspnea, spirometry readings, and oxygen requirements over months to years. It is the leading cause of morbidity and mortality beyond the first year of transplantation.[35] Azithromycin can effectively prevent CLAD.[45]

Drug Toxicity

Sirolimus may be used in the setting of CLAD. It should not be used early post-transplantation due to its adverse effects on wound healing. Sirolimus itself can also cause pulmonary toxicity, presenting with a range of severity from ground-glass opacities to necrotizing consolidations.

In dosing empirical antibiotic therapy for lung transplant recipients with suspected infection, special attention must be paid to cystic fibrosis patients, who demonstrate elevated metabolic rates. Inhaled antibiotics can be used in addition to systemic antibiotics to provide directed therapy for suspected pneumonias or anastomotic infections.

Pancreas Transplantation

Pancreatic transplantation can provide complete insulin independence for patients with long-standing diabetes mellitus. It may be performed with simultaneous or sequential kidney transplantation in those with advanced renal disease due to diabetic glomerulonephritis. There were 143 pancreas-only and 872 kidney/pancreas transplants performed in the United States in 2019.[1]

The donor organ with its native duodenum is most often anastomosed to the recipient small intestine to allow for exocrine drainage.[46] Previous strategies to manage the exocrine secretions of the organ included anastomosis at the recipient bladder, but this led to non–anion gap acidosis, reflux pancreatitis, chronic pyuria, and recurrent urinary tract infections such that bladder anastomosis has largely been abandoned. Vascular anastomoses are at the right internal iliac vessels. Complications due to bleeding or thrombosis usually manifest in the first week post-transplantation. Fistulas and intra-abdominal abscesses may occur later with abdominal pain, hyperamylasemia, leukocytosis, and elevated serum creatinine.

Infections are usually bacterial but may contain *Candida* species. CMV infection risk warrants valganciclovir prophylaxis and monitoring. Rejection occurs in 11% to 19% of transplant recipients in the first year post-transplantation but long-term steroid use is avoided to prevent hyperglycemia, resulting in increased use of induction agents and higher CNI target troughs.[47] Assessment of allograft rejection includes laboratory evaluation of serum amylase and lipase as well as allograft function (glucose, insulin production) in addition to allograft biopsy.

Patients presenting with fever or allograft tenderness should be evaluated for intra-abdominal infections, CMV tissue-invasive disease of the gastrointestinal tract, and rejection. CT imaging may be particularly helpful. Most hospital readmissions post-transplantation, however, are due to dehydration and metabolic derangements.

Intestinal and Multivisceral Transplantation (IMVT)

IMVT is a life-saving option for patients with irreversible intestinal failure. There were 81 IMVTs performed in 2019 in the United States.[1] Transplant-related outcomes vary widely based on transplant recipient age as well as type of IMVT performed. One- and five-year patient survival range between 66% to 89% and 49% to 76%, respectively, while 1-, 3-, and 5-year allograft survival are reported as 72% to 78%, 57% to 61%, and 45% to 50%, respectively.[48] Over 90% of IMVT recipients require readmission in the first year post-transplantation due to allograft rejection, infection, and dehydration.[49]

Isolated intestinal transplantation is performed for patients with irreversible intestinal failure and is comprised of jejuno-ileum.[50] Combined intestine-liver transplantation is performed in the context of irreversible intestinal failure complicated by parenteral nutrition-associated liver failure. Multivisceral transplants are comprised of intestine, stomach, duodenum, and pancreas with or without the liver. The intestinal allograft is usually left as a stoma for several months post-transplantation to facilitate protocolized endoscopic evaluations for allograft rejection. Early post-IMVT complications are most often due to anastomotic leaks, organ ischemia, vascular thrombosis or bleeding. Attempts to manage pain or slow gut motility to increase absorptive time can result in ileus and vomiting.

Infection causes up to 50% of allograft failure and is most often bacterial.[50] Abdominal infection is the most likely, though bloodstream infections associated with catheters placed for fluid or nutritional support even after transplantation, pneumonia associated with reflux and aspiration, and urinary tract infections also occur. CMV and adenovirus enteritis, EBV-associated PTLD, and graft-versus-host disease (GVHD) are all of particular concern with IMVT recipients and require specialized care to identify and treat.

Rejection occurs in 25% of adults and 58% of children in the first year and can precipitate bacterial translocation and septicemia.[48] IMVT recipients presenting to the ED should be assessed for volume status, electrolytes, and liver and renal function. Any fever or subtle signs of infection, such as tachycardia or tachypnea, should be assessed with blood cultures, urinalysis and culture, chest radiograph, and consideration given to CT imaging of the abdomen. Prompt notification of the intestinal transplant team is imperative to directing further management strategies.

Of note, intestinal function may impact the use of enterically administered drugs and any essential therapies should be delivered by alternative means, such as sublingual or intravenous administration.

Vascularized Composite Allografts

Vascularized composite allografts including the uterus, limb, face, abdominal wall, trachea, and larynx are not essential to patient survival but rather designed to improve the patient's quality of life. Fourteen such transplants were performed in 2019 and are still under experimental status, requiring strict inclusion and exclusion criteria to guide transplantation eligibility and mandating timely adverse event reporting.[1]

OTHER CONSIDERATIONS

Post-Transplantation Malignancy

Solid organ transplant recipients face a two- to three-fold higher risk of malignancy compared to the general population, particularly for lung, colon, skin, and liver cancer as well as lymphoma. This has been attributed to underlying illnesses, long-term exposure to immunosuppression and antimicrobial agents, and chronic viral infections. Virus-associated malignancies including EBV-associated PTLD and HPV-associated cancers (cervical, anal, and oral) are important considerations.

Post-Transplantation Lymphoproliferative Disorder

PTLD affects up to 10% of solid organ transplant recipients.[51] It is a malignancy of T cell impairment that results in uninhibited monoclonal proliferation of EBV-infected B lymphocytes and their subsequent transformation into immortal lymphoblastoid B cells. Approximately 60% of cases occur within the first year post-transplantation, most often in EBV IgG donor-positive/recipient-negative pairs. Early disease may be asymptomatic and discovered on routine imaging or present with fever and weight loss. Cytopenias and EBV DNA may be detected with laboratory evaluation. Lymphadenopathy or hepatosplenomegaly concerning for PTLD detected on imaging in the emergency department merits discussion with the transplant team to arrange follow-up. Survival has improved since the availability of rituximab.[51]

Graft-versus-Host Disease in Solid Organ Transplantation

Graft-versus-host disease (GVHD) affects less than 10% of adult solid organ transplant recipients but is fatal in up to 70% of cases and thus requires recognition. GVHD occurs 2 to 6 weeks post-transplantation, usually in the context of immunogenic allografts such as the intestine and liver.[52,53] Donor T cells are transmitted with the organ and respond to recipient tissue-based antigens evoking apoptosis in skin, bowel, and bone marrow. Fever, rash, diarrhea, and cytopenias occur. Diagnosis is by skin or endoscopic biopsy and blood measures of donor T cell chimerism. If GVHD is confirmed, high-dose corticosteroids or T cell depleting agents are administered with antibiotic prophylaxis.

Viral Hepatitis in Solid Organ Transplantation

Patient- and allograft-related outcomes of transplant recipients with hepatitis B and hepatitis C infection have dramatically improved due to vaccination, screening practices, and antiviral therapies. Confidence in HBV and HCV management is reflected in the growing use of the organs from donors with known HBV or HCV infection and those at increased risk for such infections. Liver dysfunction in a transplant recipient with a history of pre-existing viral hepatitis, a known HBV- or HCV-positive donor, or an increased risk donor may prompt evaluation for active infection with serum HBsAg and HBV DNA as well as HCV RNA.

HBV infection can arise from a post-transplantation exposure, donor-derived transmission, or reactivation of latent disease.

Transplant recipients of hepatitis B surface antigen-positive or hepatitis B core antibody-positive organs (indicating active or occult HBV infection) merit potent nucleoside analog therapy (entecavir, tenofovir, or lamivudine) and monitoring for viremia suggestive of active infection.[54] Patients with underlying HBV-related liver disease prior to transplantation receive a potent nucleoside analog and possibly hepatitis B immunoglobulin with routine monitoring of HBsAg and HBV DNA. Transplant recipients should be continued on HBV-directed nucleoside analog therapy on presentation to avoid hepatitis B reactivation.

With direct-acting antiviral agents (DAAs) facilitating prompt sustained viral remissions, solid organ transplant recipients with HCV have experienced a marked decrease in morbidity and mortality.[54] HCV-positive organs have been successfully transplanted into HCV-negative recipients with subsequent cure of donor-derived HCV in most, allowing for expansion of the donor pool and reduced wait times to transplantation.

Human Immunodeficiency Virus in Solid Organ Transplantation

With effective antiretroviral therapy (ART) dramatically increasing life expectancy, more HIV-positive individuals survive to develop chronic end-stage renal, heart, lung and liver disease. Organ transplantation for kidney, liver, heart, or lung failure in this population has very good outcomes. HIV-positive solid organ transplant recipients face more allograft rejection but not more infection than HIV-negative recipients.[55] Evaluation of the HIV-positive transplant recipient should be similar to other transplant recipients, with additional attention provided to adherence to antiretroviral medications and possible drug-drug interactions. Although efforts are now made to choose ART that does not interact with immunosuppression, it is important to be aware that stopping certain drugs (ritonavir, cobicistat, and efavirenz) in the setting of acute illness can have important effects on CNI levels and allograft function. Assessing CD4 T cell count and HIV RNA viral loads helps to establish risk for opportunistic infection.

Trauma

The management of solid organ transplant trauma patients is generally no different from other trauma patients, except for a few considerations. Trauma may precipitate episodes of rejection. When possible, resuscitation with leuko-reduced and CMV-negative blood products is preferred for immunosuppressed transplant recipients to prevent transmission of viral infection. Heart transplant recipients may demonstrate clinical tamponade from scarring and adhesions, even in the absence of a pericardium. Pleural adhesions may complicate chest tube placement in a lung transplant patient. Traumatic injury of the transplanted kidney and pancreas is rare, despite their positioning in the anterior pelvis.

Eligible Organ Donors

Emergency clinicians caring for patients affected by devastating trauma or severe acute illness may address issues of organ donor eligibility of deceased individuals. Medical advancements and newer data on outcomes using organs previously considered ineligible have expanded the definition of a donor. Both donation after brain death and donation after cardiac death can yield successful outcomes for most organ types. Those dying of opioid overdose and those with known hepatitis B, hepatitis C, or HIV infection are now considered eligible donors. Immediate contraindications to organ donation include active malignancy and Creutzfeldt-Jakob disease. Questions regarding potential donor eligibility should be discussed with the local organ procurement organization.

Pregnancy and Solid Organ Transplantation

Women who undergo transplantation are able to pursue pregnancy and childbirth safely. However, pregnancy complications such as miscarriage, preeclampsia, preterm delivery, and need for caesarean section are more common in this population, affecting 1 in 2 pregnant transplant recipients.[56] Physiologic changes of pregnancy can affect allograft function (e.g., peripheral edema in a heart transplant recipient, shortness of breath in a lung transplant recipient, proteinuria in a renal transplant recipient), and should be assessed in consultation with the transplant team. Ideally, transplant recipients should attempt pregnancy with stable allograft function and no evidence of rejection in the previous year. Usual immunosuppression can be continued, though MMF will be stopped or changed to azathioprine to reduce risk of major fetal malformations.[57] Corticosteroids and tacrolimus increase risk of gestational diabetes. Most infections occurring in the pregnant transplant recipient are non-life-threatening urinary tract infections, but awareness of other infections discussed in prior sections (CMV, HSV, VZV, and toxoplasmosis) that can precipitate congenital disease is imperative.

Psychological Aspects

Transplant centers widely use psychosocial selection criteria aiming to optimize pre-transplantation mental health and psychosocial supports. While successful transplantation can improve the psychological well-being for many, the transplantation experience is challenging for most. The side effects of lifelong immunosuppression or steroid withdrawal can include anxiety, depression, delirium, and insomnia. Adherence to treatment recommendations may be markedly affected by depression and may be at issue in transplant recipients who present to the ED with allograft rejection or drug toxicities.[58] Triage to a psychiatrist with expertise in transplantation may be instrumental if depressive symptoms are identified.

DISPOSITION

Transplant recipients presenting to the ED are more likely to merit admission than members of the general population. The insidious nature of the diseases affecting this immunosuppressed population necessitates a thorough, structured approach to evaluation. If infection, rejection, or drug toxicity is suspected, transplant specialists should be consulted either in house or by phone. Transplant recipients who are deemed safe to discharge home require careful instructions, medication reconciliation, and close follow up with their transplant team.

Acknowledgements

The authors would like to acknowledge Anita Modi, MD, for her exceptional contributions to the writing and revising of this chapter, as well as the following individuals for their input: Leway Chen, MD; Koji Hashimoto, MD, PhD; Pavithra Srinivas, PharmD, BCPS; Shinya Unai, MD; and Alvin Wee, MD, MBA.

The references for this chapter can be found online at ExpertConsult. com.

The Morbidly Obese Patient

Matthew M. Hall

FOUNDATIONS

The last several decades have seen a dramatic increase in rates of obesity in children and adults in the United States and around the world.[1,2] In 2015 to 2016, it was estimated that 39.8% of adults and 18.5% of children in the United States were obese, with as many as 7.6% of Americans classified as severely obese.[1,3] Obesity is often defined as a body mass index (BMI, calculated as weight in kilograms divided by the square of the height in meters) greater than 30 (see Table 184.1). A range from 25 to 29 is considered overweight, and obesity can be further subdivided into grade I (BMI 30.1–34), grade II (BMI 35–39), and grade III or severe obesity (BMI ≥ 40).[4] The obese patient presents a host of management challenges including difficulties related to size and weight but also changes in physiology, procedural challenges, and drug pharmacokinetics.

PATHOPHYSIOLOGY

Changes to Respiratory Mechanics

Increased chest wall mass in conjunction with substantial abdominal fat mass leads to reduced lung compliance and collapse of small airways resulting in increased airway resistance (Table 184.2).[6] These changes in turn result in a decrease in functional residual capacity (FRC) leading to increased atelectasis.[6-8] Obese patients also preferentially aerate the upper portion of the lung and perfuse the more dependent portions leading to ventilation perfusion (V/Q) mismatch.[6] Each of these changes is exacerbated when the patient is supine and ameliorated when sitting upright.[6,7,9]

These physiologic perturbations lead to increases in work of breathing and oxygen consumption; obese patients consume 50% more oxygen than healthy-weight individuals.[6,7] Additionally, obese patients produce significantly more carbon dioxide than non-obese individuals, leading to an increased respiratory rate with a resting rate of 15 to 21 breaths per minute compared to 10 to 12 for those of a healthy weight.[6,7]

Obstructive Sleep Apnea and Obesity Hypoventilation Syndrome

Obstructive sleep apnea (OSA) is an obesity-related disorder characterized by upper airway collapse during sleep. Increases in adiposity of upper airway structures leads to reduced airway caliber and reduced pharyngeal muscle tone.[10,11] Symptoms include snoring and apneic episodes during sleep, daytime sleepiness, and morning headaches.[10] Diagnosis is usually confirmed with polysomnography. Treatment consists of continuous positive airway pressure (CPAP) at night and weight loss.[10,11]

Obesity hypoventilation syndrome (OHS), or Pickwickian syndrome, occurs when the physiologic changes described in the preceding paragraph lead to increased daytime hypercarbia. The Academy of Sleep Medicine defines OHS as daytime alveolar hypoventilation ($Paco_2 > 45$ when awake and at sea level) in individuals with a BMI greater than 30 when other etiologies of hypercarbia are excluded, such as chronic obstructive pulmonary disease, mechanical respiratory dysfunction such as severe kyphoscoliosis, and neuromuscular disease.[2,11,12] It is also prudent to screen for pharmaceutical and recreational substances that affect respiratory drive such as opioids, sedative-hypnotics, and alcohol.[12] While not all, or even most, patients with OSA will have OHS, 90% of those suffering from OHS also suffer from OSA with as many as 70% with severe OHS (characterized by more than 30 apnea-hypoxia events per hour during sleep).[2] Patients with OHS have increased rates of pulmonary hypertension, congestive heart failure (CHF), acute or chronic hypercapnic respiratory failure, and mortality compared to those with only OSA.[11] One recent study identified 600 patients in a 5-year period with OHS and noted 15% died on the index visit with another 16% dying in the approximately 3-year follow-up period.[13]

The American Thoracic Society recently issued a clinical practice guideline regarding evaluation and treatment of OHS. They suggest that patients with sleep disordered breathing but a low/moderate (<20%) pretest probability of OHS should undergo screening with serum bicarbonate levels. Patients with bicarbonate levels over 27 mmol/L or those with a high pretest probability of OHS should undergo confirmatory testing of arterial carbon dioxide levels. They also recommend immediate treatment with noninvasive ventilation and suggest evaluation for bariatric surgery.[2]

TABLE 184.1 Body Mass Index Classifications

BMI	WHO Classification
<18.4	Underweight
18.5–24.9	Normal Weight
25–29.9	Overweight
30–34.9	Grade I Obesity
35–39.9	Grade II Obesity
>40	Grade III Obesity[a]

[a]Alternative terms include Morbid Obesity and Extreme Obesity.[4,5]
BMI, Body mass index; WHO, World Health Organization.
Ogden CL, Carroll MD, Kit BK, Flegal KM. Prevalence of childhood and adult obesity in the United States, 2011-2012. *JAMA.* 2014;311(8):806-814; Anast N, Olejniczak M, Ingrande J, Brock-Utne J. The impact of blood pressure cuff location on the accuracy of noninvasive blood pressure measurements in obese patients: an observational study. *Can J Anaesth.* 2016;63(3):298-306.

TABLE 184.2 Changes to Pulmonary Physiology Observed in the Obese Patient

Parameter	Obesity-Related Change
Chest Wall/Abdominal Mass	Increased
Lung Compliance	Reduced
Airway Resistance	Increased
Functional Residual Capacity	Decreased
Atelectasis	Increased
V/Q Mismatch	Increased
Work of Breathing	Increased
Oxygen Consumption	Increased
CO_2 Production	Increased
Respiratory Rate	Increased
Safe Apnea Time	Decreased

Changes in Pharmacokinetics

The clinician faces several challenges regarding proper medication dosing in the obese patient. The volume of distribution (V_d) of a drug is the principal factor involved in the loading dose while subsequent maintenance dosing will primarily be governed by total body clearance (Cl).[14] The V_d is affected by many factors including drug lipophilicity, plasma binding, regional blood flow, body composition, molecular size, and degree of ionization.[9,14-18] Hydrophilic drugs will tend to not enter adipose tissue to a great extent resulting in lower V_d and will therefore tend to be dosed based upon ideal body weight (IBW). Lipophilic drugs will dissipate into fat tissue to a significant extent, leading to increases in the V_d and a situation where total body weight (TBW) may be appropriately used for dose calculations. Other drug loading doses will use an adjusted body weight (ABW) where a fraction of the adipose tissue, often 30% or 40%, is utilized in dose calculations (see Table 184.3 for scalers often used in medication dosage calculations).[14,15]

Drug maintenance doses are primarily determined by Cl, the sum of contributions from each organ involved in drug metabolism or excretion. As obese patients often have increased liver and kidney mass, as well as increased renal blood flow, obesity will often affect Cl.[14] Additionally, critically ill patients will have changes in vascular permeability, cardiac output, and hepatic and renal function that will impact both V_d and Cl.[16] Care in the emergency department (ED) will primarily involve the loading dose of a medication, but maintenance dosing may be required in departments faced with prolonged inpatient boarding where consultation with a pharmacist may be helpful.

Antibiotics

There is limited data on beta-lactam and cephalosporin use in obesity, but several trials have illustrated lower than normal drug concentrations and cure rates in obese patients when standard dosing is utilized. Until more data are available, we recommend initial dosing at the upper limit of the recommended dose and suggest extended infusion times (Table 184.4).[14-16]

Fluoroquinolones also have very limited pharmacokinetic data in the setting of obesity. There are insufficient data to provide clear recommendations for ciprofloxacin. Levofloxacin 750 mg/day has been shown to be effective against gram-negative infections in small studies of obese patients with preserved renal function, but further data is required before firm recommendations can be made for fluoroquinolones. Therefore, we recommend usual dosing.[14-16]

Vancomycin has both increased V_d and Cl in obese patients and obese patients have been found to have lower vancomycin troughs. The large V_d necessitates a loading dose recommended at 20 to 25 mg/kg TBW; doses >4 g/day are associated with vancomycin-induced nephrotoxicity. Variable Cl in conjunction with the large V_d makes maintenance dosing difficult and it is prudent to individualize subsequent doses to peak and trough levels so as to achieve therapeutic levels but avoid nephrotoxicity.[14,16]

Linezolid is noted to have subtherapeutic levels in obese patients, but data have not illustrated worse clinical outcomes. Expert recommendations are mixed at this time and there are insufficient data to give clear guidelines regarding linezolid dosing in obese patients; therefore, we recommend usual dosing.[14,15]

Aminoglycosides are hydrophilic but do have an increased V_d in obese patients, suggesting that the drug does distribute into fat tissue but not to nearly the same concentrations as other tissues. Limited evidence suggests dosing by ABW with a correction factor of 0.4 for the loading dose with maintenance dosing individualized for the patient.[14,15]

Sedatives and Induction Agents

Recent studies have demonstrated that both obese and non-obese children and adults often receive incorrect anesthetic and paralytic medications, with one investigation reporting only 75% of obese patients receiving an appropriate dose of etomidate and 60% being administered the correct dose of succinylcholine.[19,20] Propofol is highly lipophilic; in fact, one of the great advantages of this drug, its short duration of action, is not due to metabolism but rather to rapid redistribution into muscle and fat.[18] Historically there has been controversy regarding the appropriate scaler for propofol, but recent research has suggested that using ABW with a correction factor of 0.4 results in successful sedation (Table 184.5).[17,18,21-23] Although etomidate is ubiquitous in the ED, little research has been performed regarding optimal dosing in obese patients with some experts recommending TBW and others reduced doses.[6,17] One recent study did demonstrate IBW resulted in successful sedation, but currently there is insufficient evidence to give a strong recommendation regarding which scaler should be used.[24] At this time we suggest using TBW to dose etomidate. Similarly, there is a paucity of data for ketamine in the obese patient; however, given its large V_d, most experts suggest reducing from TBW with some suggesting IBW and others LBW. We suggest utilizing LBW.[6,17]

Neuromuscular Blocking Agents

Succinylcholine, a depolarizing neuromuscular blocking agent, is cleared via breakdown by plasma cholinesterase (PCE). Obese patients have increased levels of PCE proportional to total body weight and therefore succinylcholine (1.5 mg/kg IV) should be dosed

TABLE 184.3   Scalers for Various Body Weight Descriptors

Body Weight Descriptor		Formula	Example
IBW	Ideal Body Weight	Male: 50.0 + 2.3 (inches over 5 feet in height)	64 kg
		Female: 45.5 + 2.3 (inches over 5 feet in height)	59 kg
LBW	Lean Body Weight	Male: $(9270 \times TBW) / (6680 + 216 \times BMI)$	79 kg
		Female: $(9270 \times TBW) / (8780 + 244 \times BMI)$	65 kg
ABW	Adjusted Body Weight	$IBW + C^a \times (TBW–IBW)$	Male, C=0.3, 92 kg
			Male, C=0.4, 103 kg
			Female, C=0.3, 89 kg
			Female, C=0.4, 99 kg
TBW	Total Body Weight	Patients Actual Weight	159 kg
BMI	Body Mass Index	Weight × Height²	56 kg/m²

[a]C is correction factor, usually either 0.3 or 0.4. The example is for a 5 foot, 6 inch person (66 inches; 168 centimeters) weighing 350 pounds (159 kilograms).[14]

Meng L, Mui E, Holubar MK, Deresinski SC. Comprehensive guidance for antibiotic dosing in obese adults. *Pharmacotherapy*. 2017;37(11):1415-1431.

TABLE 184.4   Dosing Recommendations for Selected Antibiotic Classes

Drug Class	Dosing Recommendation
Beta-lactams/Cephalosporins	Limited data, upper limit of regular dose suggested
Fluoroquinolones	Limited data, upper limit of regular dose suggested
Vancomycin	Load with 20–25 mg/kg TBW; subsequent dose based on peak/trough levels
Linezolid	Limited data
Aminoglycosides	$ABW_{0.4}$

TABLE 184.5   Dosing Recommendations for Sedatives, Neuromuscular Blocking Agents, and Neuromuscular Blocking Reversal Agents

Drug	Dosing Recommendation
Propofol	Limited data, avoid TBW
Etomidate	Limited data, suggest TBW
Ketamine	Limited data, avoid TBW, suggest LBW
Succinylcholine	TBW
Rocuronium	TBW
Vecuronium	TBW
Sugammadex	TBW

by TBW.[6,17] The non-depolarizing neuromuscular blocking agents most commonly used in the ED, vecuronium and rocuronium, have both been shown to have prolonged duration of action when administered by total body weight.[6,17] One recent trial illustrated that using 0.6 mg/kg IBW of rocuronium did not result in slower time of onset than when using higher doses in obese patients.[25] However, given that the only complication of higher doses of non-depolarizing agents is prolonged duration of action and underdosing risks suboptimal intubating conditions, we recommend using TBW for these medications. Sugammadex rapidly reverses paralysis due to the non-depolarizing neuromuscular blocking agents (rocuronium and vecuronium). Recent research suggests the possibility of using IBW; however, as most trials investigating sugammadex are conducted in the operating room at the end of surgical cases as opposed to situations where it would likely be utilized in the ED, the end points of these trials allow for a time to onset that would be inappropriate in the emergency department.[17,26,27]

Anticoagulation

Unfractionated heparin remains a vital drug for the treatment of thromboembolic disease, acute coronary syndrome, and atrial fibrillation. Current recommendations suggest weight-based dosing for both an initial bolus and subsequent infusion, but are silent on dosing strategies in the obese patient.[28-30] Several studies have investigated various dosing methods in the obese, including reducing the initial bolus, capping the bolus, or using various weight scalers, but no clear superior dosing method has been described.[29] We suggest consultation with a pharmacist if local recommendations are not clear on dosing ceilings in the

obese patient because many institutions have specific local guidelines in this regard. It is clear that careful monitoring of heparin activity with either activated partial thromboplastin time (aPTT) or anti-Xa levels aids in titrating heparin infusions.[28] Low-molecular-weight heparin (LMWH) can be used in many cases, but activity should be monitored in those over 190 kg by following anti-Xa levels.

Direct oral anticoagulants (DOACs) have gained popularity over vitamin K antagonists such as warfarin in recent years. To date there have not been any large, prospective randomized trials investigating their efficacy and safety in the obese population. Both the Anticoagulation Forum VTE Treatment Guidance and the International Society on Thrombosis and Haemostasis have given recommendations to avoid DOACs in patients with a BMI greater than 40 and weights over 120 kg.[31,32] There have been several recent large retrospective chart review studies that suggest DOACs, and especially rivaroxaban, have reassuring efficacy and safety profiles in severely obese patients. These studies also remind the ED physician that there are large numbers of very obese patients taking these medications.[33-36] Given the paucity of prospective investigations, it would be prudent to avoid initiating DOACs in obese patients from the ED unless alternative medications are unavailable or follow-up care has been coordinated.

TRAUMA CONSIDERATIONS

Obese patients appear to display a change in injury pattern compared to healthy-weight patients with fewer head injuries but more lower abdominal and chest injuries.[37] Increasing BMI has been identified as a protective factor against intraperitoneal injury from stab wounds to

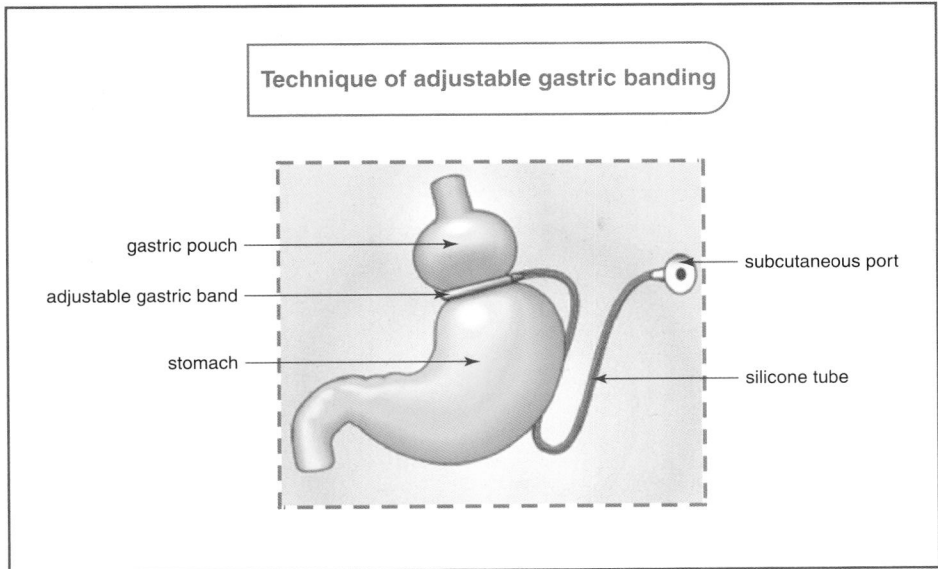

Fig. 184.1 Depiction of laparoscopic adjustable banding (LAB) procedure. (From: Contival N, Menahem B, Gautier T, Le Roux Y, Alves A. Guiding the non-bariatric surgeon through complications of bariatric surgery. *J Visc Surg.* 2018;155:27-40.)

the abdomen.[38] Morbidly obese patients have also been shown to have increased mortality and in-hospital complications as well as longer intensive care unit stays and increased time on mechanical ventilation when compared to non-obese patients.[37,39] We recommend following advanced trauma life support (ATLS) algorithms for the obese patient while paying particular attention to the respiratory status of obese patients laying supine during the primary and secondary surveys. Care should be taken when rolling the patient to protect both the patient and the staff from inadvertent injury.

BARIATRIC SURGERY

Overview

Bariatric surgery is the only intervention that has been demonstrated to produce sustained significant weight loss and treat comorbidities of obesity.[40-45] Severe postoperative complications such as pulmonary embolism (PE), acute coronary syndrome, and anastomotic leak are rare with an overall incidence of less than 1% in the first 30 days.[43] However, approximately 10% of postoperative patients will present to the ED in the first month and over one-third will do so in the first year after surgery.[41,44]

Bariatric surgery encourages weight loss through restrictive (reducing the amount of food that can be ingested at one time) or malabsorptive (reducing caloric absorption from a surgically altered small bowel) means.[45] The American Society for Metabolic and Bariatric Surgery recommends that surgery be offered to patients either with a BMI over 40 or with a BMI over 35 along with severe obesity-related comorbidities such as diabetes, OHS, and nonalcoholic fatty liver disease, among others. Although there are six different operations currently being performed in the United States, the vast majority of patients undergo laparoscopic adjustable banding (LAB), sleeve gastrectomy (SG), or the Roux-en-Y gastric bypass (RYGB). LAB (Fig. 184.1) is the insertion of an adjustable balloon circumferentially around the proximal stomach connected to a subcutaneous port allowing intermittent tightening or loosening of the band. In a SG (Fig. 184.2), the surgeon creates a small stomach remnant with a staple line excluding the greater curvature. In the RYGB (Fig. 184.3), the proximal stomach is separated with a staple line from the distal stomach, creating a small stomach pouch; the jejunum is transected and the distal portion (alimentary limb) is

anastomosed to the stomach pouch while the proximal biliopancreatic limb is anastomosed to the jejunum.

Gastric bypass via RYGB results in the greatest (reported at 62% of excess weight on average) and most sustained weight loss but tends to have the most complications. LAB results in less weight loss (about 40% of excess weight) with the fewest complications whereas SG offers intermediate weight loss and complication rates.[42,45] All three surgical options can present to the ED with short-term and long-term complications (Table 184.6).

Obese patients develop thromboembolic complications at a rate that is 2 to 3 times that of the non-obese population. Open surgical approaches have higher rates of PE than do laparoscopic procedures.[45] Given the previously described challenges regarding anticoagulation in the obese population, PE should be considered in postoperative patients presenting with suggestive signs and symptoms.

Laparoscopic Gastric Band

LGB has an exceedingly low mortality rate, but patients can still suffer from early and late complications. Early complications decrease dramatically with surgical experience and are most commonly related to esophageal or gastric perforation (usually but not always diagnosed intraoperatively) and acute gastric dilation. Dilation of the stomach pouch is rare, but because gastric distention can lead to local ischemia, it can result in gastric necrosis and necessitates operative repair. Patients suspected of having these complications should receive prompt resuscitation with IV fluids, pain control, IV antibiotics such as piperacillin-tazobactam targeting intra-abdominal pathogens along with emergent surgical consultation.[45]

Late complications are fairly common with LGB. It is not uncommon for the tubing connecting the subcutaneous port to the band to become kinked or to break. More ominous is a port infection. This may be related to instrumentation from adjustments to the gastric band, but as gastric mural erosion will often present as chronic purulent drainage at the port site, this more serious complication should be ruled out. Computed tomography (CT) or upper gastrointestinal series (UGIS) usually diagnoses this complication; however, upper endoscopy is the test of choice. Aside from purulence at the port site, patients may experience epigastric pain, fever, tachycardia, and

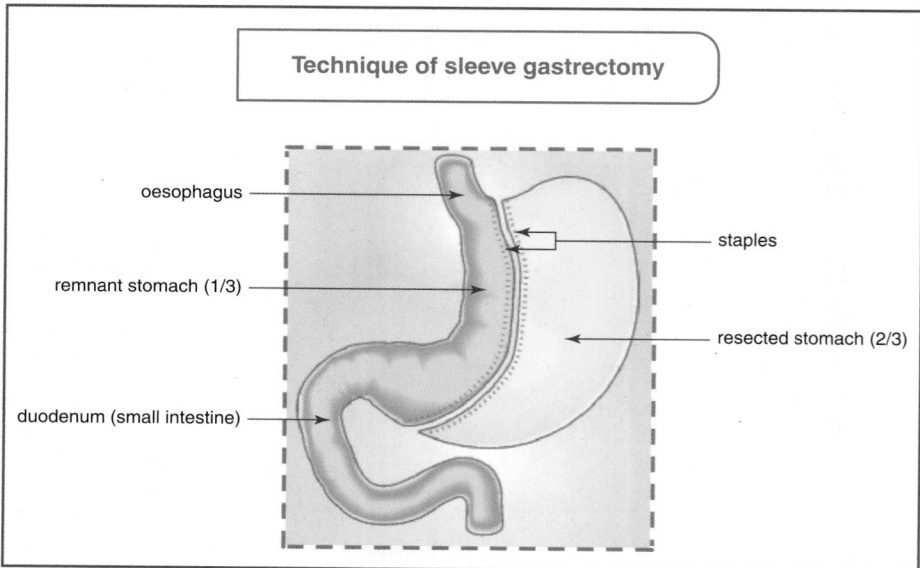

Fig. 184.2 Depiction of sleeve gastrectomy (SG) procedure. (From: Contival N, Menahem B, Gautier T, Le Roux Y, Alves A. Guiding the non-bariatric surgeon through complications of bariatric surgery. *J Visc Surg.* 2018;155:27-40.)

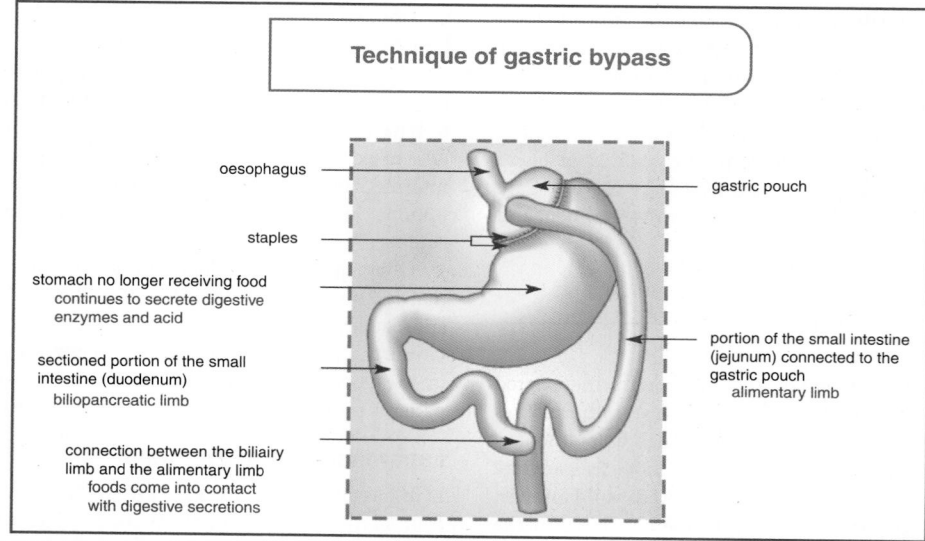

Fig. 184.3 Depiction of Roux-en-Y gastric bypass (RYGB) procedure. (From: Contival N, Menahem B, Gautier T, Le Roux Y, Alves A. Guiding the non-bariatric surgeon through complications of bariatric surgery. *J Visc Surg.* 2018;155:27-40.)

signs of GI bleeding. Pocket dilation and late slippage occurs when the band slowly and gradually slips distally, allowing for larger meals that in turn result in further slippage. Usually this is an insidious process resulting in a cessation of weight loss, but occasionally it can result in acute strangulation and gastric necrosis. It is best diagnosed via UGIS and is treated via prompt loosening of the gastric band by a surgeon. Esophageal dilation likely results from overly aggressive tightening of the band leading to accumulation of food in the esophagus. It is diagnosed via UGIS and treated by relaxation of the band.[45]

Sleeve Gastrectomy

The primary complication of SG centers on gastric leaks leading to fistula formation. It appears that leaks typically arise at the top of the staple line and occur in about 2% of patients undergoing SG. Repair of fistulas, once they appear, is a long and difficult process often requiring

multiple procedures and hospitalizations. Strictures will present with signs of obstruction and are resolved either surgically or endoscopically depending upon location. Gastroesophageal reflux disease (GERD) is the most common late complication.[45] As SG has gained significant popularity only since 2010, descriptions of its complications are not as thorough as with other common surgical procedures.

Roux-en-Y Gastric Bypass

The RYGB, the most common gastric bypass surgery in the United States, results in several early and late complications. Leaks can occur at each of the staple lines, which are located at the gastric pouch, the excluded stomach remnant, the jejuno-jejunostomy, and gastro-jejunostomy as well as small bowel division sites. Leaks and fistulas in the distal jejuno-jejunostomy are life-threatening and often present with abdominal pain, peritonitis, and signs of sepsis. However, possibly

TABLE 184.6   Common Early and Late Complications for Various Bariatric Surgeries

Procedure	Early Complications	Late Complications
Laparoscopic Gastric Band	Esophageal perforation	Tubing failure
	Gastric perforation	Port infection
	Gastric dilation	Gastric erosion
		Pocket dilation with late slippage
		Esophageal perforation
Sleeve Gastrectomy	Gastric leak	Gastroesophageal reflux disease
	Fistula formation	Dumping syndrome
Roux-en-Y Gastric Bypass	Staple line leak with or without fistula formation	Marginal ulcers
	Jejuno-jejunostomy obstruction	Internal herniation with or without obstruction
	Gastro-jejunostomy obstruction	Adhesions with obstruction
	Postoperative bleeding	Cholelithiasis
	Marginal ulcers	Dumping syndrome

related to the difficulties with physical examination of the morbidly obese patient, tachycardia may be the only presenting sign. Therefore, we advise urgent surgical evaluation for recent postoperative patients with unexplained heart rates over 120 beats/minute.[45] More proximal fistulas at the gastric pouch suture line or gastro-jejunostomy can be insidious and even asymptomatic and can therefore be managed conservatively with bowel rest. Those with pain or vital sign derangements often require operative intervention.[45]

Bowel obstruction due to anastomotic stricture of the jejuno-jejunostomy is another dangerous complication. Because the 70-cm biliopancreatic limb originates in the blind stomach remnant, it will fill with digestive secretions before the obstruction fills the gastric pouch through the longer alimentary limb (150 cm). Therefore, the excluded stomach may distend and subsequently perforate before the onset of vomiting. Prompt surgical consultation is advised when this diagnosis is considered. Epigastric pain, vomiting, and progressive dysphagia suggest stenosis of the more proximal gastro-jejunostomy and appear later (weeks after surgery) than jejuno-jejunostomy strictures (days after surgery). In contrast to more serious distal strictures, gastro-jejunostomy strictures are usually managed with endoscopy and dilation.[45]

Postoperative intraperitoneal bleeding most often occurs from staple lines, resulting in blood in abdominal drains. The diagnosis can be confirmed, if necessary, via laparoscopy and therefore prompt surgical consultation is recommended. As with all bleeding, unstable patients should be transfused early, while the diagnosis is confirmed. Intraluminal bleeding from a proximal source may be suggested by hematemesis or melena and is managed via endoscopy for both diagnosis and possible treatment. Distal bleeding from the jejuno-jejunostomy or the excluded portion of the stomach, suggested when patients present with melena, is usually managed supportively.[45] Marginal ulcers, or ulceration at the gastro-jejunostomy, tend to occur in those who smoke, suffer from *Helicobacter pylori* infection, or are on nonsteroidal antiinflammatory medication.[40] Patients often present with epigastric pain especially with eating, vomiting, and occasionally with signs of upper GI bleeding. Diagnosis is made by endoscopy. Medical treatment is usually sufficient with high-dose proton pump inhibitor and risk factor modification. Rarely, marginal ulcers can lead to strictures or even perforation.[45]

Patients who have undergone RYGB can suffer from several late complications. Marginal ulcers, although more common in the immediate postoperative period, are known to develop up to 2 years after surgery. Bowel obstruction may be related to postoperative adhesions but is due to internal herniation in 60% of cases. Weight loss will predispose patients to internal hernias as potential spaces open in the small bowel mesenteries. They can be particularly difficult to diagnose because they can be intermittent and CT scans are often falsely negative. Patients may complain of intermittent pain without clear etiology which may localize to the left flank. Exploratory laparoscopy may be required to confirm the diagnosis. Rapid weight loss associated with RYGB leads to formation of gallstones, particularly 6 to 18 months following surgery. Some surgeons will perform a prophylactic cholecystectomy during the gastric bypass procedure, but this is not a universal practice. Treatment of simple symptomatic cholecystitis and biliary colic is similar to patients without bariatric surgery, but clinicians should note that following RYGB the common bile duct is no longer accessible via routine endoscopic retrograde cholangiopancreatography (ERCP). Therefore, treatment of common duct stones requires a surgical approach rather than the typical endoscopic one.[40,45]

Anatomic changes associated with RYGB and SG can predispose patients to dumping syndrome. This occurs whereby a large bolus of partially digested food is rapidly released into the small bowel.[45,46] Early dumping syndrome is thought to be related to rapid fluid shifts as water is drawn into the hyperosmolar environment of the small bowel from the vascular compartment in the first hour after a meal. This leads to GI symptoms such as abdominal pain, bloating, nausea, borborygmi, and vomiting. Rapid fluid shifts can result in flushing, palpitations, fatigue, transient hypotension, tachycardia, diaphoresis, and rarely, syncope. Late dumping syndrome, typically 60 to 180 minutes following a meal, is thought to result from an incretin-driven hyperinsulinemic response leading to hypoglycemia. The patient will often experience typical symptoms of hypoglycemia such as fatigue, weakness, and hunger along with an adrenergic surge leading to tremor, tachycardia, and diaphoresis. First-line treatments for dumping syndrome focus on diet and include frequent small meals, elimination of refined sugar, and delaying fluid intake until 30 minutes after a meal.[46]

PROCEDURAL DIFFICULTIES

Lumbar Puncture

The lumbar puncture (LP) is typically performed using a landmark-based approach. However, this can be particularly challenging in the obese patient when familiar landmarks are obscured by adipose tissue.[47,48] Ultrasound can be of assistance in mapping out landmarks when they cannot be palpated.[49] Positioning the patient in a sitting position rather than lateral decubitus position may also make the procedure easier. Extra-long 5-inch (12.7 cm) needles may be necessary to reach the subarachnoid space. In cases where the LP cannot be successfully performed at the bedside, the patient may require a fluoroscopic-guided lumbar puncture.[47]

Venous Access

Excessive subcutaneous adipose tissue can lead to difficulties in establishing intravenous (IV) access. Ultrasound can successfully identify otherwise obscured veins in the obese population and aid in the establishment of IV access.[50] Central venous access may be required for access in general or in the case of an unstable patient. Care should be taken when placing obese patients in the Trendelenburg position as it can have severe negative consequences for pulmonary function in both the spontaneously breathing and the intubated obese patient. An assistant or tape may be required to position the panniculus out of the field when placing catheters in the femoral vessels. Intraosseous (IO) access can also be rapidly established when medications or blood needs to be given expeditiously. Recent research has suggested that so long as the tibial tuberosity can be palpated, a standard 25-mm IO needle can be placed in the proximal or distal tibia. A longer 45-mm needle should be placed in the proximal humerus in obese patients and in the tibia if the tibial tuberosity cannot be palpated.[51]

Cardiopulmonary Resuscitation

High-quality cardiopulmonary resuscitation (CPR) is critical in the chain of survival from cardiac arrest. Guidelines suggest placing the hands on "the lower half of the sternum" due to the common location of the maximal left ventricular outflow tract diameter.[52,53] Recent radiographic evidence suggests that the optimal compression location for CPR in obese patients is slightly more cranial than in healthy-weight individuals and that CPR is technically more difficult on obese patients than on healthy-sized individuals.[53,54] We encourage emergency providers to pay close attention to CPR quality in obese patients and use CPR quality feedback devices when available.

Endotracheal Intubation

Although controversial, obesity has been considered a risk factor for difficult intubation.[6,7,55,56] The pathophysiologic changes that occur in the lung due to obesity result in much shorter apnea times than in healthy-weight patients. Preoxygenation with noninvasive ventilation, when time and equipment allow, is recommended over non-rebreather mask use because it has been shown to increase safe apnea time by one minute in the obese patient, likely by reducing atelectasis.[7] Increases in safe apnea times may also be seen when the patient is maintained in an upright position during preoxygenation and intubation.[6,7,57] During intubation, we recommend placing obese patients in a head up or ramped position with the goal of aligning the external auditory meatus with the sternal notch. This will serve to both increase safe apnea times and improve the laryngoscopic view.[6,7,57] Intubation of the obese patient should be considered a difficult intubation and all airway adjuncts should be readily available. Clinicians should keep in mind that obesity is associated with difficult bag-valve-mask (BVM) ventilation and be prepared for two-person BVM ventilation with oral and/or nasal airways. Cricothyrotomy is likely to be technically difficult in the obese patient owing to difficulty palpating landmarks.[37]

Ventilator Management

Obese patients suffer from increased atelectasis and V/Q mismatch owing to changes in lung compliance and FRC. They also have increased respiratory rates, even at rest, compared to nonobese patients. After intubation, tidal volumes should typically be set to 6 to 8 mL/kg IBW rather than TBW to avoid pulmonary injury.[6,7] Respiratory rates should initially be set higher than for nonobese patients owing to the increased resting respiratory rate and can be titrated based on blood gas analysis. Patients who are known or predicted to be acidemic should usually have even higher respiratory rates. Positive end-expiratory pressure (PEEP) can be difficult to manage in the obese patient. Given their propensity for atelectasis, starting obese patients with PEEP of 10 cm H_2O is recommended. However, high levels of PEEP can lead to reduced venous return and therefore lower preload and can predispose patients to hypotension. Therefore, close attention should be paid to hemodynamics and ventilator settings adjusted as needed. Providers also are urged to monitor for auto-PEEP and change ventilator settings accordingly.[6,7] As with most patients, obese patients should be maintained in either a sitting position or reverse Trendelenburg to optimize pulmonary function.

Challenges with Hospital Equipment

Emergency departments should have equipment, including hospital beds, commodes, and wheelchairs, engineered to accommodate obese patients. This includes the ability to handle not only substantial weight but also the increased girth of these patients. Appropriate monitoring equipment such as blood pressure cuffs should also be readily available. Proper mechanical lifts and safe handling plans are also prudent; the National Institute for Occupational Safety and Health recommends that nurses lift no more than 35 pounds when providing patient care and currently workers in hospitals suffer from musculoskeletal injuries at twice the national rate.[9]

Imaging Challenges

Ultrasound has the advantage of portability and therefore table weight limits do not present a challenge. Adipose tissue will attenuate sound waves; however, with the proper settings and transducer, as well as by utilizing harmonic imaging, most obese patients can be evaluated with ultrasound. X-ray imaging is limited in the obese patient due to reductions in resolution and image contrast. Obese patients also will require increased exposure times which in turn lead to greater probability of motion artifact.[58]

CT imaging in the obese patient has both mechanical and radiographic challenges. Three different measurements must be taken into account when evaluating if an obese patient can be evaluated by a particular scanner. First is the table load limit, which not only protects against mechanical table failure and subsequent risk of patient injury, but also allows for smooth and predictable speed as the patient is passed through the scanner. Second is aperture size to ensure that the patient can physically pass through the CT machine. This is much more of a challenge when abdomen/pelvis CT is required than when a CT of the head is needed and may require measuring the girth of the patient. Third is the maximum reconstruction FOV (field of view). This denotes the area within the scanner where images will be captured. It is advised that the obese patient be positioned such that the area of interest lies within the FOV. Even when the obese patient is able to fit in the scanner, large amounts of adipose tissue will create artifacts that can limit the diagnostic utility of the image.[58] Additionally, patients must lie flat in the CT scanner, which can lead to respiratory complications in an obese patient. It is prudent to offer a trial of supine positioning in the safety of the ED with staff at the ready if there is a question regarding the ability of the patient to lie flat for the time required to obtain the desired images.

Obtaining useful MRI images often encounters problems similar to those outlined for CT imaging. The MRI table must be able to safely support and pass the patient into the scanner, and the patient must be able to fit into the scanner itself. Modern scanners are often 70 cm in diameter and slightly larger than previous generations of scanners (60 cm). Some radiology departments have "open MRI" machines that may accommodate larger patients.

The references for this chapter can be found online at ExpertConsult. com.

185

The Combative and Difficult Patient*

Malia J. Moore and Jason D. Heiner

THE COMBATIVE PATIENT

Foundations

Combative patients are among the most difficult patients encountered by emergency clinicians. Often brought in against their will, they can be agitated, confrontational, difficult to examine, and they may physically harm themselves or others. The emergency clinician should seek to control the patient and the situation, diagnose and treat reversible causes of violence, ensure that there is not an organic cause

---

*Disclaimer: The views expressed herein are solely those of the authors and do not represent the official views of the Department of Defense or Army Medical Department.

contributing to the behavior, and protect the patient, staff, and other patients from harm.

The emergency department (ED) is a volatile environment owing to high stress, illness, prolonged waiting times, and often perceived gaps in communication. Given that the ED is open 24 hours a day, 7 days a week, combined with the availability of potential hostages and accessibility to drugs or weapons, compound the potential for violent behavior. The assault-injury rate of health care occupations is nearly 10 times that of the general sector, and over half of all health care providers will be victims of violence of some form during their careers.

Emergency care providers throughout the world are more likely than other health care providers to experience violent events, such as verbal threats, physical assaults, or confrontations outside the workplace.[1-9] In 2018, The American College of Emergency Physicians (ACEP) conducted a poll of 3539 emergency physicians across the country in which nearly 50% reported having been assaulted while at work in the ED, with over 70% having witnessed an assault in the workplace.[7] In this survey, nearly all assaults were committed by the patient (97%), but in 28%, it was reported that family or friends acted as an accessory.[7] Similar rates of violence and aggression toward physician and nursing staff are typically observed, and both men and women generally appear to be at comparable risk.[1,4] Violent incidents are far more likely to be verbal threats or acts of intimidation than physical assaults and, in the ED, may be acted out by patients, as well as their family, friends, or other visitors.[1-7] The actions of combative patients have consequences that extend beyond the physical injury of ED caregivers, such as provider posttraumatic stress disorder symptoms or lost provider work productivity, and also serve as a major contributor to burnout.[1,6-8]

Clinical Presentation
Patient Characteristics

The pathogenesis of violent behavior is multifactorial, with potential contributing factors including environmental, historical, interpersonal, biochemical, genetic, hormonal, neurotransmitter, or substance abuse disorders.[10-12] Psychiatric illness is also a risk factor, with schizophrenia, personality disorders, mania, or psychotic depression most frequently associated with violence.[10-12] Delusional schizophrenic patients may become violent, believing that others are attempting to harm them. They may also have auditory hallucinations commanding harm to others. The patient with acute mania is unpredictably dangerous because of emotional lability, a situation in which pleasantness can quickly turn to aggression. Substance abuse disorders and drug-seeking behavior are consistently associated with violent behavior in both psychiatric and nonpsychiatric populations.

Biologically, the serotonin system largely controls aggression and inhibition, with a role of diminished serotonergic function in disinhibiting aggression against self and others.[11] Generalized brain

BOX 185.1   Selected Conditions Associated With Violence

Psychiatric
Schizophrenia
Paranoid ideation
Catatonic excitement
Mania
Personality disorders
    Borderline
    Antisocial
    Delusional depression
    Posttraumatic stress disorder
    Decompensating obsessive-compulsive disorders

Situational Frustration
Mutual hostility
Miscommunication
Fear of dependence or rejection
Fear of illness
Guilt about disease process

Antisocial Behavior
Violence with no associated medical or psychiatric explanation (these patients may be managed by the police or security)

Organic
Diseases
Delirium
Dementia
Trauma

Central nervous system infection
Seizure
Neoplasm
Cerebrovascular accident
Vascular malformation
Hypoglycemia
Hypoxia
Acquired immunodeficiency syndrome (AIDS)
Electrolyte abnormality
Hypothermia or hyperthermia
Anemia
Vitamin deficiency or toxicity (e.g., hypervitaminosis D)
Endocrine disorder

Drugs
Unanticipated reaction to prescribed medication (especially sedatives in brain-injured or elderly patients)
Alcohol (intoxication and withdrawal)
Amphetamines
Cocaine
Sedative-hypnotics (intoxication or withdrawal)
Phencyclidine (PCP)
Lysergic acid diethylamide (LSD)
Anticholinergics
Aromatic hydrocarbons (e.g., glue, paint, gasoline)
Steroids
Synthetic cannabinoids
Synthetic cathinones

dysfunction may predispose patients to violence by disruption of the regulation of aggression, particularly in the prefrontal or temporal cortex.[11] Cerebral imaging documents both functional and structural impairments in violent criminals and antisocial patients.

Violent behavior also occurs in association with head trauma, hypoxia, hypoglycemia, electrolyte imbalance, infections (particularly herpes encephalitis), drug intoxication or withdrawal or adverse reaction, or metabolic and endocrine derangements. Uncommon organic causes include seizures (e.g., temporal lobe), tumors (particularly those in the limbic system), limbic encephalitis, multiple sclerosis, porphyria, Wilson disease, Huntington disease, sleep disorders, hyperparathyroidism, or vitamin and mineral deficiencies (e.g., folate, vitamin B_{12}, niacin B_2, and pyridoxine vitamin B_6). Although drug or ethanol intoxication and withdrawal are the most common diagnoses in combative ED patients, the mnemonic FIND ME (functional [i.e., psychiatric], infectious, neurologic, drugs, metabolic, endocrine) helps in broadly categorizing many important causes of violence (Box 185.1).

Identification of *potentially* violent patients is more difficult; male gender, prior history of violence, and drug or ethanol abuse have historically been positive predictors, whereas ethnicity, diagnosis, age, marital status, and education have been unreliable identifiers. Overall, the most accurate tools for predicting acute violent behavior likely rely largely on current behavioral patterns and clinical observations in the context of prior patterns of violence of the patient when known or previously documented.[12]

Emergency Department Influences

An annual ED census over 50,000 patients, an average waiting time over 2 hours, and ED crowding are associated with an increased incidence of violence.[13] The risk of workplace assault in the ED, however, exists across hospitals of all sizes and reflects the rate of violence in the community. Despite these risks, health care providers have not been routinely trained in the identification and management of combative patients.[14]

Patients armed with lethal weapons pose a serious threat to staff and the potential risk posed by concealed weapons exists in all settings including pediatric EDs. In areas where community violence is prevalent, conflict may spill over into the ED when those involved in violent altercations are being treated for their injuries.[8] The carriage of weapons in the ED population has previously been estimated at approximately 4% to 8%, with up to 27% of major trauma patients; however, not all EDs screen for weapons or use metal detectors. Unfortunately, prediction of weapons carriage in any particular patient is challenging, and it is therefore prudent to assume that all violent patients are armed until it is proved otherwise, especially those presenting with major trauma.

The deleterious effects of violence in the ED can be minimized by employing certain preventive measures and by training staff in techniques to de-escalate and limit violent behavior when it occurs (Box 185.2).

Initial Patient Evaluation

Evaluation of the combative patient begins with attention to safety measures. All patients should be screened for weapons before the interview. The use of metal detection is ideal upon ED entry, and additional attention may be needed for patients brought to the ED by ambulance and thereby bypassing routine security screens. The practice of undressing patients and placing them in a gown is useful as a non-confrontational survey for potential weapons that also discourages fleeing in some circumstances or, conversely, aids in identification if a violent patient suddenly flees from the ED.

The ideal setting for the patient interview emphasizes privacy without isolation, such as a seclusion room specifically designed for the

BOX 185.2   Emergency Department Preparedness and Prevention of Violence

General Emergency Department Preparedness Considerations

Physical and system factors to minimize ED violence risk:

1. Prominently displayed warning signs prohibiting weapons and alerting all entering that they may be screened for weapons
2. Nondiscriminatory inquiry about weapon carriage and searches of individuals for weapons with clear local policies for staff about searches and contraband disposal
3. A panic or alarm system to activate hospital security or local police response
4. ED placement of dedicated telephone(s) with a direct line to police or security to request additional personnel if needed
5. Control flow into the ED by limiting access to one or two entrances and consider buzzer access systems, and protective bulletproof glass or metal bar barriers at front desks
6. A secure examination room with solid ceiling, shatterproof ceiling lights, heavy indestructible chairs, well-secured restraint bed, two outward swinging doors that can be locked from the outside, an emergency distress button that can be activated unobtrusively, and consideration of a video monitoring system

Primary Prevention

Control factors encouraging the development of frustration and aggression:

1. Minimize waiting times to the extent feasible
2. Optimize waiting room environment
3. The presence of visible surveillance cameras
4. The presence of a trained visible security force reflecting both hospital needs and anticipated violence based on local community prevalence

Secondary Prevention

Response to pre-violent agitation and aggression:

1. Recognition of risk (pre-violent patients and their companions)
2. Implementation of de-escalation techniques
3. Minimize treatment delays of pre-violent individuals
4. Ongoing staff training in violent management techniques to increase caregiver confidence and comfort while decreasing the rate of aggressive incidents

Tertiary Prevention

Limitation of the actual act of violence once it has occurred:

1. Use of physical and chemical restraints
2. Appropriate security and police intervention
3. Apply familiar protocols for dealing with the violent individual

ED, Emergency department.

BOX 185.3   Patient Behaviors Suggesting Impending Violence

Provocative behavior
Angry demeanor
Loud, aggressive speech
Tense posturing (e.g., gripping arm rails tightly, clenching fists)
Pacing or frequently changing body position
Aggressive acts (e.g., pounding walls, throwing objects, hitting oneself)

protection of the provider, earrings, necklaces, and neckties should be removed. Personal accessories that may be used against the caregiver, such as a stethoscope or scissors, should also be removed. The clinician should be aware of any objects within the room or on the patient's body that might be used as weapons, such as pens, watches, necklaces, key chains, cell phones, or belts.

Violence risk assessment of a potentially combative patient can be difficult. Violence often erupts after a period of mounting tension. The astute practitioner may identify verbal or nonverbal cues and may subsequently have the opportunity to defuse the situation. In a typical scenario, the patient first becomes angry, then resists authority, and finally becomes confrontational and violent. When clinicians have a "gut feeling" that a dangerous situation may be developing, they should take appropriate precautions. Violent behavior may also erupt without warning, especially in patients with an organic brain syndrome, so clinicians should not feel overly confident in their ability to sense impending danger. An obviously angry ED patient should be considered potentially violent. Patients with a history of violent behavior are more likely to inflict serious injury, and certain patient behaviors may suggest impending violence (Box 185.3).

To prevent escalation, the patient should be removed from contact with other agitated accomplices, as well as from other provocative patients. A quiet area enabling direct observation is optimal. Because increased waiting times correlate positively with violent behavior, consider evaluating the potentially violent patient accelerated to prevent escalation of aggression. When feasible, expeditious triage and evaluation of these patients may avoid the challenging consequences of violence for the patient at hand, the ED staff, and ultimately the care of other ED patients. Often, the perception of preferential treatment alone may serve to defuse the patient's anger.

Management

Verbal Management Techniques

Verbal de-escalation techniques should be considered in the setting of agitated or violent patients prior to implementation of physical restraints or chemical sedation. The agitated but cooperative patient may be amenable to verbal de-escalation techniques alone. This verbal interaction provides an opportunity to assess the patient's mental status and comprehension, as well as perception of the current situation. If the patient remains resistant or violent after verbal techniques, or incapable of interacting appropriately, then restraint is necessary. However, the uncooperative, actively violent or potentially violent patient may warrant immediate restraint to minimize risk to the patient and ED staff.

Successful verbal management techniques include an effort to make the patient as comfortable as possible, being honest and straightforward during the medical interview, adopting a non-confrontational demeanor, and being an attentive and receptive listener without conveying weakness or vulnerability (Box 185.4).[9,14] The interviewer should respond verbally in a calm and soothing tone of voice. It is also important to stand at least an arm's length away and to avoid prolonged

interview of potentially dangerous patients. Prior to the medical interview, security should be stationed strategically and the door left open to facilitate both intervention and escape for the provider. The patient and interviewer may be seated roughly equidistant from the door, or the interviewer may sit between the patient and the door. Blocking of the door, however, poses a risk of harm to the clinician if the patient feels the urge to escape. Ideally, examination room doors should swing out, and more than one exit should be available. The clinician should have unrestricted access to the door and avoid sitting behind a desk. The room should not contain heavy or potentially dangerous objects that may be thrown. There ideally should be a mechanism to alert others of danger, such as a panic button or a code word or phrase that summons security (e.g., "I need 'Dr. Armstrong' in here."). For personal

BOX 185.4 Ten Elements for Verbal De-Escalation

1. Respect personal space: Maintain a distance of two arm's lengths and provide space for easy exit for either party.
2. Purposefully avoid provocation: Keep your hands relaxed, maintain a non-confrontational body posture, and do not stare at the patient.
3. Establish verbal contact: The first person to successfully connect verbally should lead the effort.
4. Use concise, simple language: Elaborate and technical terms are hard for an impaired person to understand.
5. Identify feelings and desires: "What are you hoping for?"
6. Listen closely to what the patient is saying: After listening, restate what the patient said to improve mutual understanding (e.g., "Tell me if I have this right ...").
7. Agree, or agree to disagree: (a) Agree with clear specific truths; (b) agree in general (e.g., "Yes, everyone should be treated with respect."); (c) agree with minority situations (e.g., "There are others who would feel like you.").
8. Set clear limits: Inform the patient that violence or abuse cannot be tolerated.
9. Offer choices and optimism: Patients feel empowered if they have some choice in matters.
10. Debrief the patient and staff: Be sure to include an opportunity for the patient and staff to speak.

Adapted from the American Association for Emergency Psychiatry De-escalation Workgroup consensus statement: Richmond JS, Berlin JS, Fishkind AB, et al: Verbal de-escalation of the agitated patient: consensus statement of the American Association for Emergency Psychiatry Project BETA De-escalation Workgroup. *West J Emerg Med.* 2012;13:17-25.

direct eye contact, approaching the patient from behind, or sudden movements. In some cases, an agitated patient may be aware of the impulse control problem and welcome limit setting by the clinician (e.g., "I can help you with your problem, but I cannot allow you to continue threatening me, the emergency department staff, or other patients."). The interviewer should act as an advocate for the patient. Offering a soft chair, food, or beverage (though not a hot liquid, which may be used as a weapon) may help in establishing trust, and patients may de-escalate as a result of the attention to their basic human needs.

A key component of interviewing a potentially violent patient is addressing the issue of violence directly. The patient should be asked relevant questions about suicidal or homicidal ideations or plans, possession of weapons, history of violent behavior, and current use of intoxicants. Acknowledgment of the obvious (e.g., "You look angry.") may enable the patient to begin sharing emotions. If the patient becomes more agitated, it may be helpful to speak in a conciliatory manner and to offer supportive statements to guide and empower the patient in what you would like them to do (such as, "You seem to want to do the right thing. How can we come up with a solution together?") to help defuse the situation. If this is not successful, a respectful offer of medication or restraints to the patient may prevent further escalation.

Counterproductive approaches to the combative patient include arguing, threats, deception, or condescension, as they fail to build rapport and may challenge patients to "prove themselves," thereby further escalating the situation. An open threat to call security personnel also invites aggression. Clinicians should be aware of their own reactions to such patients and avoid transference of anger. Deliberate deception (e.g., "I am sure you will be out of here in no time.") may serve to invite violent consequences once the false promise is uncovered and an unsuspecting nurse or colleague who follows the initial interviewer

may be victimized. It is important to avoid denial or downplaying of threatening behavior, and if verbal techniques are unsuccessful and escalation occurs, the clinician should immediately seek refuge and summon help.

Physical Restraints

Physical restraints should be considered when verbal techniques prove unsuccessful. The use of restraints can be humane and effective in facilitating diagnosis and treatment while preventing injury to the patient or medical staff. Generally speaking, the liability one incurs for restraining a patient against his or her will is negligible compared with the potential liability for allowing a patient to lose control and cause physical harm to themselves or others. Restraints should not be applied for convenience or as a punitive response for disruptive behavior and should be removed as expeditiously as possible, usually once adequate chemical sedation is achieved.

Indications for emergency seclusion and restraint include the prevention of imminent harm to the patient, others, or the immediate environment, or as part of an effective ongoing behavior treatment program. Patients can typically be broadly classified into three categories: (1) those with an organic disorder for whom restraints facilitate evaluation, (2) those with functional psychosis for whom verbal techniques are less effective and restraints facilitate administration of neuroleptics, and (3) those with personality or other disorders prohibiting the utility of verbal techniques. Seclusion or restraint may be contraindicated because of the patient's clinical or medical condition. Seclusion should not be used in an unstable patient who requires close monitoring and should be avoided when the patient is suicidal (unless adequate continuous observation can occur), self-abusive or self-mutilating, or intentionally ingested drugs or poisons. The indications for the use of restraints should be documented. Specific statements (such as, "I restrained Mr. Smith because he told me he was going to beat me up and then took a swing at me.") are preferable to general statements (such as, "I restrained Mr. Smith because he was violent.").

The application of restraints should be systematic and ideally follow a predetermined ED protocol that is implemented when the examiner leaves the room after verbal techniques are unsuccessful. Whenever possible, the treating clinician should avoid active participation in restraint application to preserve the clinician-patient relationship. The restraint team ideally consists of at least five people, including a team leader. The leader, whether a physician, nurse, or security officer, should be experienced in implementing restraints and provide guidance and instruction for the restraint team. Before engaging with the patient, the leader outlines the restraint protocol and warns of anticipated danger, including the presence of objects that may be weaponized. All team members should remove personal objects that the patient could use against them. A mixed-gender restraint team should be considered to mitigate potential allegations such as sexual assault.

The team engages with the patient as a group and displays a professional rather than threatening attitude. Many violent individuals calm down at this point as a large show of force protects their ego (e.g., "I would have fought back but there were too many against me."). The leader speaks to the patient in a calm and organized manner, explaining why restraints are needed and how the course of events will transpire (e.g., "You require a medical and psychiatric examination, as well as treatment."). The patient is instructed to cooperate and to lie down on the gurney to have restraints applied. Some patients are relieved at the protection to self and others afforded by restraints when they feel themselves losing control. Even if the patient suddenly appears less dangerous once the decision to restrain is made, it is advisable to continue the process and avoid negotiation with the patient at this point.

If physical force becomes necessary, one team member restrains a preassigned extremity by controlling the major joint (knee or elbow). The team leader controls the head. If the patient is armed, two mattresses can be used to charge and immobilize (sandwich) the patient. Restraints are applied securely to each extremity and tied to the solid frame of the gurney (not side rails, as later repositioning of side rails also repositions the patient's extremities).

Leather is the optimal type of restraint, as it is a physically stronger material and less constricting than typical soft restraints. For this reason, gauze should not be used. Soft restraints may help restrict extremity use in the semi-cooperative patient, but are unlikely to be effective in the truly violent patient who is continuing to struggle and attempt escape. If chest restraints are used, it is vital that adequate chest expansion for ventilation is ensured. The application of a soft Philadelphia collar to the patient's neck may minimize head banging or biting. In this circumstance, ensuring continued adequacy of the patient's airway is similarly prudent. Although restraining patients on their sides helps prevent aspiration, we recommend the supine position with the head elevated, as it tends to be more comfortable and allows a more thorough medical examination while providing some protection against aspiration. Once the patient is immobilized, announcing "the patient is safe" may have a calming effect on the restraint team and the patient.

We recommend avoiding the prone restraint position when possible and employing chemical sedation when a patient continues to struggle against physical restraints. Sudden unexpected deaths have been reported in prone patients, particularly if left unattended during busy shifts or between multiple sign-outs with various treating clinicians. Although healthy volunteers, when restrained and undergoing physical exertion, do not appear to experience clinically significant positional asphyxia, combative ED patients often suffer from other conditions that may predispose to increased morbidity. Patients using cocaine or other stimulants who are restrained in the prone position appear to be uniquely at risk because increased sympathetic tone and altered pain sensation allow exertion beyond normal physiologic limits, and sympathetic-induced vasoconstriction may impede clearance of metabolic waste products and induce hyperthermia and rhabdomyolysis. Alteration of respiratory mechanics in an acidemic patient resulting from the position of restraint can be a contributing factor through impairment of respiratory compensation.

After restraints are successfully applied, the patient should be monitored frequently and positions changed to prevent neurovascular sequelae, such as circulatory obstruction, paresthesias, or rhabdomyolysis associated with continued combativeness. Standardized documentation is recommended for this monitoring to include the specific indication for restraint and, ideally, colleague agreement that restraints are necessary. Basic patient needs must be met (e.g., hydration, toileting needs) and physical restraints should be removed as soon as possible. Review of restraint team performance and critical discussion may reveal opportunities for improvement. Education and rehearsal by staff can improve and maintain restraint skill as well as improve comfort and confidence with this skill.

Chemical Restraints

Chemical sedation alone, or in conjunction with physical restraint, may assist in the safe management of an agitated or violent patient when verbal de-escalation techniques fail. Chemical restraints subdue patients who may otherwise harm themselves or others and serve to facilitate further medical evaluation and treatment. Clinical and administrative guidelines for their use are similar to those for physical restraints. The use of medication to calm a patient may obscure the mental status examination and clinical diagnosis. Caution should also be exercised because adverse events may result from sedation.

The most commonly observed adverse event is respiratory depression or hypoxia. In one study, the rate of adverse events was 16%, and the highest risk characteristics were found to be age greater than 65 years, alcohol intoxication, and more than one type of parenteral sedation administered within 60 minutes. The risk of adverse events should be weighed, however, against the increased risk to the patient and staff without medication administration.

The ideal agent for controlling combative patients is effective, safe, well tolerated, free of significant side effects or drug interactions, rapid in onset, titratable, and available through multiple routes of administration. Several pharmaceutical agents can quickly achieve safe behavioral control, or "rapid tranquilization," without oversedation. Medications should be used judiciously and with close patient monitoring, as there remains a paucity of rigorous clinical data regarding chemical sedation in certain settings such as acute delirium, the underlying comorbid or primary conditions of violent ED patients are often unknown, and a degree of individual variation in response to any medication should be anticipated.

The primary medications commonly used in the ED for chemical sedation include benzodiazepines, first-generation (typical) antipsychotics, second-generation (atypical) antipsychotics, or ketamine.[15-30] We suggest a patient-based approach to chemical sedative selection based on suspected or known clinical features (Box 185.5).

Benzodiazepines, antipsychotics (also known as *neuroleptics*), and ketamine are commonly used either alone or in combination for rapid tranquilization. Chemical restraints should ideally be offered to the patient for voluntary use, as the offer itself has potential to restore the patient's feeling of control and may lead to subsequent de-escalation. In the uncooperative or dangerous patient refusing an oral medication, the intramuscular (IM) route is preferred, with intravenous (IV) administration an alternative depending on IV catheter status. As with physical restraints, it is imperative that patients are frequently re-evaluated for changes in their clinical status.

Benzodiazepines. Benzodiazepines, particularly lorazepam (Ativan) and midazolam (Versed), are often used in the ED for rapid tranquilization of an agitated or violent patient. Benzodiazepines enhance the activity of the major inhibitory neurotransmitter gamma-aminobutyric acid to cause anxiolytic, anticonvulsant, and sedative effects. These agents are preferred for the management of agitation caused by ethanol withdrawal or sedative-hypnotic drug withdrawal, as well as cocaine, amphetamines, or sympathomimetic drug ingestions. Benzodiazepines may be more effective than antipsychotics in reducing delirium and mortality and are useful in patients at risk for seizure or when avoiding antipsychotic-associated akathisia and hyperthermia. For these reasons, we prefer the use of benzodiazepines when sedating the patient with agitation from an unknown cause. Although they are generally well tolerated, side effects of benzodiazepines include excessive sedation, ataxia, confusion, nausea, or respiratory depression, which may be amplified in the presence of concurrent alcohol and other depressant use.

Lorazepam is frequently preferred to other benzodiazepines because of its rapid onset of action, short half-life, hepatic and renal excretion, lack of active metabolites, and effectiveness by oral, IM, or IV routes of administration. Recommended initial oral, IM, or IV doses of lorazepam range from 0.5 mg to 2 mg. Typical doses for chemical restraint in the ED begin at 1 mg to 2 mg increments IM or IV with upward titration as needed. The onset of action after administration of lorazepam is generally 20 to 30 minutes if it is given IV or 15 to 30 minutes if it is given IM, with a duration of action of 6 to 8 hours. Caution should be employed when switching routes of administration; for example, synergy may be observed when doses are given IM followed by IV, and desired clinical effects coupled with undesirable side effects, such as respiratory depression, may be noted simultaneously.

BOX 185.5   Suggested Patient-Based Approach to Chemical Restraint

The Severely Violent Patient

Droperidol 2.5 to 5 mg IM/IV, titrate as needed

or

Midazolam 2.5 to 5 mg IM/IV, titrate as needed

or

Midazolam 2.5 to 5 mg IM/IV with droperidol 2.5 to 5 mg IM/IV, titrate either as needed

or

Haloperidol 2.5 to 5 mg IM/IV with lorazepam 1 to 2 mg IM/IV, titrate either as needed

or

Ketamine 1–2 mg IV/IM

The Undifferentiated Severely Agitated Patient or With Stimulant Intoxication

Lorazepam 1 to 2 mg IM/IV

or

Midazolam 2.5 to 5 mg IM/IV

or

Haloperidol 5 mg IM/IV with lorazepam 2 mg IM/IV

The Patient Intoxicated With a Central Nervous System Depressant (e.g., Alcohol)

Haloperidol 2.5 to 5 mg IM/IV

or

Droperidol 2.5 to 5 mg IM/IV

or

Ketamine 1–2 mg IV/IM

The Patient With a Known Psychotic/Psychiatric Disorder

Haloperidol 2.5 to 5 mg IM/IV

or

Droperidol 2.5 to 5 mg IM/IV

or

Haloperidol 2.5 to 5 mg IM/IV with lorazepam 2 mg IM/IV

or

Ziprasidone 10 to 20 mg IM[a]

or

Olanzapine 5 to 10 mg IM[a]

The Cooperative but Agitated Patient

Lorazepam 1 to 2 mg PO

or

Risperidone 2 mg PO [a]

or

Olanzapine 5 to 10 mg PO [a]

The Elderly Patient

Reduce above medication dose by half [a]

[a] The safety of atypical antipsychotics in geriatric patients remains somewhat uncertain.

IM, Intramuscular; *IV,* intravenous; *PO, per os* (by mouth).

Midazolam is another effective benzodiazepine for achievement of mild sedation and has a more rapid onset of action and a shorter duration of clinical effects than lorazepam. The IM route is used widely to calm the agitated patient with a typical initial dose of 2.5 mg to 5 mg IM. When it is administered IM, the medication usually takes effect in about 15 minutes with a mean duration of 2 hours. The choice of midazolam versus lorazepam may, in part, be guided by the duration of sedation desired and faster onset of action.

Antipsychotics. Antipsychotic medications play a prominent role in the chemical restraint of the violent ED patient. These medications include the older "typical" (or "classic") antipsychotics and the newer "atypical" antipsychotics. Typical antipsychotics appear to strongly block brain dopamine receptors, whereas the atypical antipsychotics less strongly and more specifically antagonize dopamine and serotonin receptors.[17] Both classes of antipsychotics have variable effects on other receptors, including adrenergic, cholinergic, or histaminergic receptors. The typical antipsychotics can be categorized in terms of their "potency," a description referring to the relative dosing of the medication and generally predictive of its side effect profile. The incidence of sedation, hypotension, and anticholinergic side effects is higher with the low-potency antipsychotics, whereas the incidence of extrapyramidal symptoms is greatest with the high-potency antipsychotics. Low-potency antipsychotics include chlorpromazine (Thorazine) and thioridazine (Mellaril), medium-potency antipsychotics include loxapine (Loxitane) and molindone (Moban), and high-potency antipsychotics include haloperidol (Haldol) and droperidol (Inapsine).

Of the older typical antipsychotics, the butyrophenones—haloperidol and droperidol—have been widely utilized in the emergency care setting. Haloperidol is the most frequently administered antipsychotic to control agitated ED patients.[17,24] It is available in oral, IM, and IV preparations, although the commonly used IV route of administration is not approved by the US Food and Drug Administration (FDA). Haloperidol is generally given in 2.5 mg to 10 mg IM doses (often 5 mg IM for the severely agitated, average sized adult), with half doses administered to elderly patients (e.g., 2.5 mg IM), followed by repeated dosing every 20 to 60 minutes as needed. Effects are usually seen within 30 minutes by the IM route, and the average patient typically requires fewer than three doses for the desired clinical effect.

Droperidol has been commonly used at doses of 2.5 to 10 mg IM or 2.5 to 5 mg IV to control the agitated or combative patient in a manner similar to haloperidol.[17,19,23] Compared with haloperidol, droperidol appears to more rapidly reduce agitation at equal IM dosing, has a shorter duration of effect, more sedation, a larger incidence of orthostatic hypotension, and a lesser incidence of extrapyramidal symptoms. When compared with midazolam 10 mg IM, droperidol 10 mg IM appears to have an equally rapid onset of action and requires fewer additional doses for sedation. The clinical use of droperidol decreased markedly after it was given a controversial black box warning in 2001 by the FDA for concern of QTc prolongation and torsades de pointes; however, subsequent studies have shown a low incidence of complications as well as superiority over other antipsychotics in its rapidity of action.[19,21] For instance, in a 2018 prehospital comparison of droperidol and midazolam, patients treated with droperidol had fewer adverse events and required fewer additional sedative doses.[20]

Haloperidol is also associated with QTc prolongation and torsades de pointes. Given the effectiveness and overall safety of these medications combined with the unclear risk association for QTc prolongation, we recommend the cautious use of both haloperidol and droperidol when administered to patients with other identified risk factors for, or the known presence of, QTc prolongation, such as in the setting of baseline antipsychotic or methadone use. We also recommend obtaining an electrocardiogram or placing the patient on a cardiac monitor before drug administration if feasible. If this is precluded by poor cooperation of a violent or agitated patient, we recommend obtaining an electrocardiogram once the patient becomes more cooperative.

Common side effects of haloperidol and droperidol include sedation, orthostatic hypotension, or extrapyramidal symptoms. Extrapyramidal symptoms are thought to be due to mesolimbic dopamine receptor blockade. They are not dose related and may occur immediately or days following medication administration. Patients can have akathisia (extreme restlessness) or uncoordinated involuntary movements known as dystonia, including of the muscles of the mouth (buccolingual), neck (torticollis), back (opisthotonos), eyes (oculogyric crisis), or trunk (abdominopelvic). Treatment includes diphenhydramine 25 mg to 50 mg IV or IM, or benztropine 1 mg to 2 mg IV or IM, acutely and extended for 3 days to minimize symptom recurrence. Both haloperidol and droperidol have some anticholinergic properties and are often co-administered with diphenhydramine or benztropine, and thus should not be used to control agitation in a patient with known or suspected anticholinergic intoxication. Haloperidol and droperidol should also be avoided in patients with alcohol, benzodiazepine, or other sedative withdrawal syndromes, patients with known seizure disorders, patients with phencyclidine overdose, and, when possible, in pregnant or lactating females.

Neuroleptic malignant syndrome is a rare and potentially lethal idiosyncratic reaction estimated to occur in 0.01% to 0.04% of patients receiving antipsychotic medications. Characteristic symptoms include autonomic instability, hyperthermia, "lead-pipe" muscle rigidity, and altered mental status. If neuroleptic malignant syndrome is suspected, further antipsychotics should be withheld, and we recommend initiation of supportive treatment and rapid external cooling (see Chapter 150).

Chemical restraint with newer atypical antipsychotics (such as olanzapine, ziprasidone, or aripiprazole) is generally safe and effective in the treatment of agitated patients.[17,22-24] Compared with the typical antipsychotics, these medications appear to provide more tranquilization than sedation and have fewer extrapyramidal side effects. Their use in the ED is facilitated by IM or oral dissolving tablet formulations that may assist in a smoother transition to oral dosing in those patients requiring ongoing antipsychotic therapy. Although the clinical significance is uncertain, atypical antipsychotics carry a black box warning for an increased risk of death in elders with dementia-related psychosis and they also cause QTc prolongation. As a result, we recommend employing the same precautions used with the typical antipsychotics. In a 2019 study comparing agitated patients with known alcohol intoxication who were treated with droperidol, haloperidol, or olanzapine, median ED length of stay was shortest for droperidol (499 minutes), which was significantly shorter than that of haloperidol (524 minutes) and olanzapine (533 minutes). No cases of sudden cardiac death occurred.[18]

Olanzapine (Zyprexa) is readily available in IM, oral, and oral-dissolving tablet formulations; and it has a reported distinct "calming" effect in clinical practice. It has FDA-approved indications for the treatment of agitation associated with bipolar I mania and schizophrenia. IM olanzapine has an onset of action of 15 to 45 minutes after initial administration and is typically administered as an initial dose of 2.5 mg to 10 mg IM followed by one or two subsequent doses every 2 to 4 hours for a total maximum dose of 30 mg IM. Although generally well tolerated, side effects include sedation (which may be compounded in the setting of concomitant benzodiazepine use), mild hypotension, and anticholinergic properties that can exacerbate existing anticholinergic intoxication. Mild hypoxia is common but critical hypoxia or serious airway compromise remains rare.[22] Olanzapine has minimal QTc-prolonging effects and a lesser occurrence of acute dystonia and akathisia compared with haloperidol. In a 2019 study comparing the need for an additional "rescue" sedation dose, both olanzapine and droperidol required lower rates of rescue sedation at one hour and overall when compared with haloperidol. There were no significant differences in major adverse events.[21]

Ziprasidone (Geodon) is FDA approved for treatment of the agitated schizophrenic and bipolar manic patient. Typical dosing is 10 mg IM every 2 hours or 20 mg IM every 4 hours (not to exceed 40 mg/day)

with an onset of action of 15 to 30 minutes. Ziprasidone is generally well tolerated, although side effects such as somnolence, dizziness, and headache are common, and it appears to have potentially notable QTc-prolonging effects.

Aripiprazole (Abilify) has FDA-approved indications for the treatment of agitation associated with the schizophrenia or bipolar disorders. Recommended doses for the acutely agitated patient are 5.25 to 15 mg IM (often 9.75 mg) every 2 hours as needed (to a maximum daily dose of 30 mg). Aripiprazole IM (9.75 and 15 mg) may have comparable efficacy to lorazepam 2 mg IM with a low risk of oversedation.

Risperidone (Risperdal) is typically used for schizophrenia and available in an oral or IM depot form with typical dosing of 1 mg to 2 mg. Given orally, risperidone appears to be as effective and tolerable as IM administration of haloperidol. The time to peak concentration is shorter than some oral second-generation antipsychotics and may be useful when rapid control of agitation by an oral medication is desired.

Combined Use of Benzodiazepines and Antipsychotics. Benzodiazepines and typical antipsychotics are commonly used in combination for chemical restraint. In a 2016 meta-analysis of chemical agents for sedation of agitated patients in the ED, combination therapy sedated a greater proportion of patients at 15 to 20 minutes than benzodiazepines alone.[17] Combination therapy was more effective and required fewer repeat doses for sedation, and the risk of adverse events was lower than for benzodiazepines alone.[17] A 2017 study of monotherapy with droperidol or olanzapine compared with combination therapy with midazolam and droperidol found significantly more patients in the midazolam-droperidol group were adequately sedated at 10 minutes.[23] The combination therapy was 6 minutes faster than either monotherapy.[23] Patients in the midazolam-droperidol group required fewer additional doses or alternative drugs to achieve adequate sedation, and the adverse event rate and length of stay did not differ between the three groups.[23] In a 2018 comparison of intramuscular midazolam, olanzapine, ziprasidone, or haloperidol for treating acute agitation in the emergency department, midazolam was found to work most rapidly and olanzapine appeared to have superior sedation without redosing, as well as less effect on QTc; however, no differences in adverse events in any treatment group were identified.[24]

Demonstrated effective combinations include midazolam (5 mg IV or IM) with droperidol (5 mg IV or IM) or lorazepam (2 mg IV or IM) with haloperidol (5 mg IV or IM). When given together, lorazepam and haloperidol appear to be more rapidly sedating than either medication alone, have fewer adverse effects, and are compatible within the same syringe. Half doses should be considered in carefully selected elders. If additional medication is immediately needed, we recommend consideration of IV midazolam every 3 to 5 minutes or IV lorazepam every 20 to 30 minutes. In summary, though antipsychotics and benzodiazepines are both safe and effective on their own, the combination is also safe, may have more rapid onset, with similar side effect profile to either medication alone.

Ketamine. Ketamine is a dissociative anesthetic with a good safety profile used to manage the violent and acutely agitated patient in the hospital or prehospital settings, including use following treatment failure with benzodiazepines or antipsychotics.[17,25-30] Although its use in agitated delirium in young adults is increasingly described, we recommend avoiding its use in elders with acute agitated delirium, patients at increased risk for heart disease, or patients with schizophrenia, given the possibility of exacerbating these conditions. For the treatment of acute violent agitation in the ED patient, we recommend an initial dose of 1 to 2 mg/kg IV or 4 to 5 mg/kg IM. The onset of drug action is typically 1 to 2 minutes after IV use and 4 minutes or longer after IM administration, with duration of action of approximately 20 minutes. It appears to be faster in onset via IM route

Clinical Feature	Delirium	Dementia	Functional
Onset	Acute	Gradual	Gradual
Age at onset	Any	>50 years old	<40 years old
Alertness	Altered	Normal	Normal or hyperalert
Orientation	Impaired	May be normal or impaired (depending on stage of dementia)	Normal
Hallucinations	Common; can be visual, auditory, or tactile	None	Auditory in schizophrenia, otherwise uncommon
Symptom picture	Fluctuating	Stable	Stable
Abnormal vital signs	Common	Uncommon	Uncommon
Psychiatric history	No	No	Yes

TABLE 185.1   Distinguishing Organic From Functional Causes of Violent Behavior (ORGANIC)

than other medications; however, due to its short duration of action, it frequently requires combination therapy or repeat doses.[26,27,28,30] Notable side effects include hypertension and tachycardia (usually mild and transient), drooling, laryngospasm or other respiratory complications (uncommon), emesis, or emergence reactions. In a 2016 comparison of prehospital administration of ketamine or haloperidol for severe agitation, ketamine worked faster but was associated with greater risk of complications or intubation.[30] Overall, studies reflect that patients receiving ketamine in the prehospital setting are more likely to require intubation than when ketamine is administered in the ED, though it is unclear whether this is caused by dosing differences, unfamiliarity with side effect profile, or increased severity of illness.

Post-Restraint Medical Evaluation

Once combative patients are controlled, evaluation is necessary to screen for organic causes of agitation. Separation of functional (psychiatric) from organic (medical) disease is a challenging task complicated by the fact that many patients with psychiatric disorders also suffer from organic medical disorders that may worsen symptoms. Patients who exhibit violent behavior that is caused or exacerbated by an organic problem may rapidly deteriorate if the medical issues are not addressed in a timely fashion.

Historical features may assist in distinguishing functional from organic illness (Table 185.1). Patients aged 40 years or older who exhibit new onset of psychiatric symptoms are more likely to have an organic cause. Elders are at higher risk for organic delirium from medical illness or adverse medication reactions. Patients with a history of drug or ethanol abuse may exhibit violent behavior as a manifestation of an intoxication or withdrawal syndrome. The acute onset of agitated behavior, as well as behavior that waxes and wanes over time, suggests an organic origin. Most psychiatric patients are alert and oriented and many have known psychiatric diagnoses.

The history includes medical, psychiatric, family, and social information, including suicidal or homicidal ideation, drug and alcohol use, medication use, and any recent changes to prescribed medications or dosages. The agitated patient may be unreliable; thus family or friends may provide valuable details. When family or friends are available, interview them independently from the patient.

The violent patient should be asked for permission to perform a thorough physical examination to search for an organic cause and to evaluate for resulting injury. Restraint of the patient may be necessary to accomplish even the most rudimentary physical examination, including accurate vital signs. Patients with persistently abnormal vital signs, a clouding of consciousness, or focal neurologic findings are more likely to suffer from organic disease and require further diagnostic evaluation. A careful examination of the agitated patient includes general appearance (e.g., hygiene, nourishment, tremors), vital signs, evidence of trauma or needle tracks, characteristic odors, neurologic and mental status, or signs of a possible toxidrome (Table 185.2).

We recommend tailoring diagnostic studies to clinical findings. An initial rapid blood glucose determination and pulse oximetry are prudent when they can be performed safely. Patients younger than 40 years of age with a prior psychiatric history, normal physical examination, calm demeanor, normal orientation, and no physical complaints are unlikely to require further diagnostic testing. Additional studies that may be useful in selected patients include serum electrolyte values, blood or urine toxicology screening, serum ethanol level, thyroid function panel, cranial imaging, or lumbar puncture. Diagnostic studies should be guided by the overall clinical scenario and are not required in most patients. Specific medication levels can be determined if toxic levels would impact treatment or disposition. An electrocardiogram may be useful in elders or in the setting of a suggested intentional ingestion. In the setting of intentional toxin ingestion, serum acetaminophen, and possibly aspirin, levels may be helpful.

Although serum ethanol or toxicology screening may not significantly influence the ED course, behavioral health or other consulting specialists may utilize the results in decision making. Ideally, an agreement on a diagnostic strategy is reached with the behavioral health specialist to assist in patient disposition. Unnecessary diagnostic testing may prolong ED length of stay and delay definitive psychiatric care.

Disposition and Medical Clearance

The emergency clinician often provides "medical clearance" for the psychiatric or combative patient brought to the ED in police custody or after being placed on a psychiatric hold in the prehospital setting. "Medical clearance" is a misnomer, as a patient is not "cleared" of all possible medical conditions during the ED evaluation; additionally, standard protocols for the provision of what is more accurately termed a "focused medical assessment" remain variable. A preferred phrase in this setting is "medically stable for psychiatric evaluation." Although few patients with primary psychiatric complaints are likely to have coexisting, emergent complications of chronic disease or medical problems contributing to their violent behavior, misattribution of aberrant organic behavior remains a pitfall in the evaluation of the combative patient.

Aspects of a focused medical assessment, including recommended laboratory tests, are often influenced or dictated by local policies or procedures. When feasible, we believe that patients with known psychiatric

TABLE 185.2 Vital Signs and Toxic Syndromes

Toxin	Blood Pressure	Pulse	Respiratory Rate	Temperature	Pupil Size	Skin	Example
Sympathomimetic	↑	↑	↑	↑	↑	Wet	Cocaine
Anticholinergic	↑/↓	↑	↑/↓	↑	↑	Dry	Diphenhydramine
Cholinergic	↑/↓	↑/↓	—	—	↓	Wet	Pesticides
Opioids	↓	↓	↓	↓	↓	—	Morphine
Sedatives	↓	↓	↓	↓	↑/↓	—	Lorazepam
Withdrawal (ethanol, sedative-hypnotics)	↑	↑	↑	↑	↑	Wet	Benzodiazepine withdrawal

disease who are deemed to be at low risk for active or significant, complicating organic medical conditions can be rapidly referred for psychiatric evaluation once they are calm and cooperative. Patients at higher risk for an acute organic illness typically require further diagnostic evaluation. Potential high-risk considerations in the prehospital or ED setting include altered mental status, ingestion, hanging, sexual assault, traumatic injury, or an unrelated medical complaint.[31] The findings of a focused medical assessment should ideally be both communicated to the mental health provider and documented in the medical record, reflecting consideration of an acute medical condition as a contributor or driver of the observed behavior. When the cause of the patient's violent behavior is drug or ethanol intoxication, further observation may reasonably be achieved in the ED or another facility where the patient can be safely monitored until the effects of the intoxicants have abated and further mental health evaluation can occur, as necessary.

Assault and Hostage Situations

Interventions to prevent assault and hostage situations, such as optimization of ED security and general preparedness (see Box 185.2), remain paramount because rates of extreme hospital and ED violence have increased over time.[32] Unfortunately, physical assault may occur despite appropriate precautions or interventions. The individual who is physically assaulted or threatened with harm with a weapon can take steps to protect both themselves and others in the ED setting (Box 185.6).

The frequency of hospital-based shootings has more than doubled in the early 21st century, with deadly incidents that may involve disgruntled, angry, desperate, or mentally ill patients, visitors, or even employees.[32] Weapons may be brought in from outside or appropriated from authorized carriers, such as police. Specific scenarios that should be considered are intimate partner violence, grudges or revenge against former health care providers or employers, mental illness leading to paranoid actions or suicide attempt, and prisoners attempting escape. Violence may be related to the setting (i.e., family member angry about a previous complication, or unrelated, such as an intimate partner seeking out their significant other at work). An emerging and concerning prompt for violence is ideologically or politically motivated. Hospitals should develop an action plan for cases of extreme violence. The plan should include prevention and safety measures, a means for rapid notification of security or police personnel, evacuation routing, medical treatment strategies, and crisis intervention. Scenario-based training drills for medical personnel and dedicated multidisciplinary hospital violence management teams may help optimize readiness and management of extreme patient aggression.[33]

THE DIFFICULT PATIENT

Foundations

The difficult patient is one who is perceived to interfere with the clinician's ability to establish a usual patient-clinician relationship. Difficult

BOX 185.6 Protective Responses to Physical Assault or Weapon Threat

If physically assaulted:
1. Immediately summon help (via panic button if possible).
2. Maintain a sideward posture and keep arms ready for self-protection.
3. Use an arm or leg to deflect a punch or kick.
4. If choked, tuck in the chin to protect the neck, carotid circulation, and ability to breathe.
5. If bitten, do not pull away—push toward the assailant's mouth and hold the assailant's nares shut.

If threatened with a weapon:
1. Appear calm, adopt a nonthreatening posture, and avoid sudden movements.
2. Do not reach for the weapon.
3. Comply with demands and avoid arguing, despair, or whining.
4. Do not bargain, make promises, or lie.
5. Attempt to establish a human connection with the hostage taker.
6. Appear less expendable by offering to administer aid to other hostages.
7. Reassure the hostage taker that a person of authority will arrive promptly to hear their complaints or demands.
8. If a weapon is put down, do not reach for it—instead attempt verbal resolution of the crisis while awaiting security.
9. Request a hostage negotiator from legal authorities if needed.

patients are encountered across medical specialties and may represent upwards of 15% to 30% of physician-patient encounters.[34] Difficult patients may carry a number of pejorative labels and can invoke feelings such as irritation, dread, anxiety, or dysphoria in their health care team, potentially leading to dissatisfying interactions for the patient and health care team alike. A high frequency of difficult patient encounters appears to be associated with clinician dissatisfaction and burnout.

The difficult patient-clinician relationship is a consequence of aspects of the ED environment, clinician characteristics, patient factors, and the complex dynamic interaction of these elements (Box 185.7).[33] These elements can act in concert to perpetuate a cycle of impaired patient-clinician interactions, which may dominate the clinical encounter with negative impacts on both the patient and clinician. This can be particularly problematic in the case of patients with maladaptive patterns of behavior. Clinicians may react negatively to perceived difficult or unreasonable patients, which may summon fear of abandonment in such patients. In response to this perceived threat, maladaptive responses of the patient may include an attempt to sustain the patient-clinician relationship through escalation of the actions that were originally perceived negatively by the clinician. The subsequent clinician reaction may be even greater in magnitude and result in even further escalation by the patient as the cycle continues. Ultimately,

BOX 185.7   Factors Impacting the Difficult Patient-Physician Interaction

Emergency Department Factors

Lack of patient choice of facility or physician

Time constraints, frequent interruptions, other priorities of care

Suboptimal patient privacy or comfort (e.g., hallway examinations)

Long waiting times, department crowding

Negative bias toward the patient from other members of the care team (e.g., by prehospital personnel, nursing)

Physician Factors

Poor communication

Difficulty expressing empathy or becoming easily frustrated

Personal negative bias and prejudices toward conditions and interactions

Limited knowledge of the patient's condition or psychosocial situation

Overly rigid medical agenda or interaction

Outside stressors affecting work

Emotional burnout or insecurity

Personal health issues

Situational stressors and perceived time pressure

Sleep deprivation or shift fatigue

Patient Factors

Behavioral issues (e.g., argumentative, manipulative, medical noncompliance)

Fear of abandonment

Psychiatric conditions

Low literacy

Financial constraints

Chronic pain syndromes

Multiple complaints

Beliefs or goals of care unknown to the physician

Unrealistic expectations or goals of care

Substance use disorder

Past or current physical, emotional, or mental abuse

Life stress or social disarray

Adapted from: Cannarella Lorenzetti R, Jacques CH, Donovan C, et al. Managing difficult encounters: understanding physician, patient, and situational factors. *Am Fam Physician*. 2013; 87:419-425; Breen KJ, Greenberg PB. Difficult physician-patient encounters. *Intern Med J*. 2010;40:682-688.

BOX 185.8   Tools for Managing Negative Reactions

Maintain Appropriate Emotional Distance

Avoid reciprocating hostile behaviors while maintaining a sense of empathy for the patient

Understand Negative Behavior as a Symptom

View the patient as a casualty of their own circumstances

Look for Cognitive Distortion

Be cautious not to overly stereotype or cloud clinical judgment and avoid perpetuating negative labels

View Negative Reactions in Context

Recognize when one feels overwhelmed by the expectations of the ED work environment to gain perspective on personal reactions

From: Cannarella Lorenzetti R, Jacques CH, Donovan C, et al. Managing difficult encounters: understanding physician, patient, and situational factors. *Am Fam Physician*. 2013;87:419-425.

the patient may feel dissatisfied with care, diagnoses may be missed or made incorrectly as a consequence of the dysfunctional interaction, and discharge from the ED may occur prematurely by either the patient or provider. Following such encounters, the clinician is prone to experience frustration, exhaustion, a sense of failure or defeat, or fear of litigation. Also, nonconstructive patient stereotypes or unrecognized prejudices may develop or perpetuate.

The clinician brings personal and professional experiences, biases, individual personality traits, and interpersonal skills to every patient encounter. Some clinicians appear to have more difficult encounters than others, and similar interactions or patients may not be perceived as "difficult" by other providers. Clinicians who are more likely to have difficult patient encounters include those with fewer years of experience, who are less comfortable with diagnostic uncertainty, and may be less adaptable in communication style or acceptance of alternative lifestyle choices. Within the complex difficult patient encounter, the clinician has the greatest opportunity to positively alter aspects of their contribution to the interaction. When recognized, strategies exist to help the clinician manage negative reactions to difficult patient experiences (Box 185.8). Communication is a critical aspect of the patient encounter affecting medical care, patient satisfaction, and overall patient perception of the experience—some general concepts of communication can aid the difficult patient interaction (Table 185.3).

Specific Disorders

The primary characteristic of a difficult patient is the ability to trigger a negative emotional response or frustration in the clinician. Difficult patients are more likely to be older, widowed or divorced, and have more acute or chronic medical problems. They are more likely to have notable psychiatric, substance or alcohol use disorders, or social issues such as homelessness. Rather than a diagnosis or demographic, it is typically the behaviors of these patients and subsequent therapeutic dynamic that characterize the difficult encounter. Categorizing potentially difficult patients based on four common dominant behavior types—attention seeking, demanding, repeat visitors, self-destructive—allows a structure for the clinician to approach and manage challenges that may arise (Table 185.4).

Attention-Seeking Patients

This patient may have associated personality disorders (dependent, borderline, or histrionic), be malingering, or possess somatoform disorders or other chronic psychiatric diagnoses. The patient is characterized in part by an excessive need for attention with an initial extreme delivery of gratitude, which the clinician may welcome. However, as the amount of care that the patient receives grows, so do their needs and demands. This cycle continues to often leave the clinician frustrated and exhausted and eager to discharge or refer the patient to another health care provider.

When such patients are identified, the clinician should carefully establish reasonable expectations and limits before the "cycle of need" has set into motion. Importantly, these patients are especially likely to seek care in the ED during times of personal crisis. Structuring the encounter to be particularly attentive to the underlying crisis may provide the opportunity to address the underlying problem rather than the patient's perceived needs. This scenario is often encountered with patients exhibiting drug-seeking behavior.

Demanding Patients

Demanding patients can include very important persons (VIPs) or other well-informed successful professionals, substance abusers, or people with personality disorders, such as narcissistic or paranoid.

TABLE 185.3   Communication Strategies for the Difficult Patient Encounter

Goal	Physician Action	Example
Structure the interview	Set time limits and expectation that interruptions may occur	"Thank you for your patience. I may have to excuse myself to care for another patient, but if we are interrupted, I will return to pick up where we left off and provide you with the care you need."
Set limits	Establish ground rules for behavior	"We want to help you and your language and behavior is offending other patients—making it difficult to care for you and other patients. Please be mindful of your remarks or you may need to be escorted out."
Active listening to improve understanding	Allow the patient to talk without interruption, summarize concerns, and recognize that anger is usually a secondary emotion	"Help me to understand what is upsetting you so much right now."
Understand the patient's agenda	Nonjudgmentally inquire about the patient's primary needs, concerns, and expectations	"What is the most important thing that we can do to help you right now?"
Validate emotion and empathize	Disarm intense emotion by attempting to name the patient's emotional state and express concern and empathy	"You seem upset." "You are right. It is frustrating to wait a long time to be seen."
Redirect the interview	Avoid pursuing trivial, chronic, or tangential complaints by redirecting focus	"I think I can help you most right now if we focus on your main concern first."
Take a time out	Leaving a patient's room and returning after both parties have regained composure is prudent if unable to contain one's frustration	"Thank you for your openness. I need to step out, and I will be back to see what we can do to help you."

Cannarella Lorenzetti R, Jacques CH, Donovan C, et al. Managing difficult encounters: understanding physician, patient, and situational factors. *Am Fam Physician*. 2013;87:419-425; Breuner CC, Moreno MA. Approaches to the difficult patient/parent encounter. *Pediatrics*. 2011;127:163-169.

TABLE 185.4   Approaches to Challenging Patient Behavior Types

Patient Type	Characteristic of Physician Response	Suggested Strategies
Attention Seeking • Excessive need for attention and reassurance • May use helplessness and seduction • Worried about abandonment • Escalating requests and demands	• Physician may initially feel special and welcome the patient's praise • As patient demands increase and physician time and energy commitment increases, feelings of frustration, exhaustion, and resentment may dominate	• Recognize the inflated positive self-esteem feeling that is being cultivated • Maintain a professional demeanor • Establish and maintain boundaries of care early • Crisis intervention may be needed • Involve the patient in decision making including appropriate follow-up
Demanding • Uses intimidation, hostility, name dropping, blame, or threats • May refuse necessary steps of assessment or treatment • Behavior caused by fear of loss of power or physician abandonment	• Initial desire may be to engage in the patient's conflict • Physician may feel intimidated, inadequate, or fear litigation	• Resist urge to enter into conflict and avoid power struggles • Reinforce concept that the patient is entitled to reasonable medical care while setting limits on unreasonable demands and behavior • Allow the patient to choose between reasonable treatment options • If a specific emotion is evident, recognize and address it with the patient
Repeat Visitor • Excessive need for attention through multiple visits or unsolvable problems • Rejects the possibility that any treatment will help	• Physician may feel frustrated and overlook significant illness, but also may share the patient's pessimism and fear that serious illness has been missed	• Be mindful of cognitive distortions that may obscure real illness • Set limits on expectations while being supportive
Self-Destructive • Disregard for own health with repeated self-destructive behaviors • Feels helpless or hopeless about changing the situation	• Physician may feel frustrated, helpless, or guilty for lack of empathy • Physician may avoid being available for the patient and unconsciously provide poor care	• Be mindful of one's own feelings and keep appropriate emotional distance • Set realistic expectations and provide appropriate care • Search for signs of mental health or social needs and consider referral or consultation as needed

From: Cannarella Lorenzetti R, Jacques CH, Donovan C, et al. Managing difficult encounters: understanding physician, patient, and situational factors. *Am Fam Physician*. 2013;87:419-425, 2013; Breuner CC, Moreno MA. Approaches to the difficult patient/parent encounter. *Pediatrics*. 2011;127:163-169.

Their behavior is often hostile, intimidating, or threatening, and they may have endless needs and unreasonable demands. These patients fear being helpless in the context of their medical needs, and behaviors that have promoted success in their professional lives become maladaptive behaviors of entitlement to protect themselves from their own insecurity.

The behavior of these patients can evoke feelings of anger or antagonism and a desire to engage in debate and conflict. These power struggles are often counterproductive and only escalate the maladaptive behavior. A clinician can address the underlying insecurity and fears by maintaining a supportive relationship. Limit setting is important to curb escalation of unreasonable demands. Clinicians may preserve the patients' sense of autonomy and control in situations where they otherwise feel helpless by engaging them to participate in the selection of reasonable recommended options of care.

Repeat Visitors

This category is largely characterized by desperate and numerous repeat ED and other medical visits despite expressed certainty that past visits have been failures. Behaviors may appear entitled, manipulative, and self-defeating. These patients may have borderline or antisocial personality disorders and may be malingering. Their complaints are often vague and defy diagnosis, and clinicians may feel a sense of futility or failure. The behavior of these patients often stems from a need for connection and relationship in the setting of a fear of rejection and such patients are also at risk for unrecognized depression.

The clinician is at risk of both prematurely dismissing the patient's complaint due to a pattern of frequent visits and medical noncompliance or prematurely beginning an extensive investigation from fear that a critical diagnosis has been missed. Awareness of one's own cognitive distortions and personal biases can aid in avoiding inappropriate premature discharge, and seeking collateral information from previous medical records may reveal additional information that can help limit the evaluation and coordinate ongoing consistent medical care. Although clarifying expectations and limit setting are important, support and empathy can be particularly valuable in these encounters, as expressed lack of concern and dismissal of the patient's fears may feed an underlying sense of rejection within the patient, thus fueling the maladaptive behavior.

Self-Destructive Patients

These patients may appear hopeless, helpless, and in profound denial of their self-destructive and neglectful behaviors. These patients may be violent, chronically suicidal, suffer from substance abuse issues, or have a borderline personality disorder. Untreated anxiety or depression may be present. These patients may not personally seek help but instead are referred for care by others. ED care may result in addressing immediate needs (such as food or shelter), but despite adequate medical intervention, it is likely that the patient's often serious problems will persist.

These self-destructive patients can be challenging to treat because ED staff may feel frustration or even loathing or disgust toward the patient and minimize contact with them. Consequently, the treating clinician and others may unconsciously provide substandard care. By recognizing one's own feelings and setting realistic expectations of care, the ED care team can avoid poor medical care and may discover patient needs, including mental health conditions or crises or unrecognized social needs.

The references for this chapter can be found online at ExpertConsult. com.

186

Multiculturalism, Diversity, and Care Delivery

Ava E. Pierce and Marquita S. Norman

FOUNDATIONS

Background and Importance

In recent years, many high-profile incidents have put the role of multiculturalism, diversity, inclusion, and health equity in the forefront of public discourse. To obtain high-quality care, patients must first enter a health care system where many have experienced barriers to access based on race, religion, ethnicity, socioeconomic status, age, sex, disability status, language, sexual orientation, gender identity, and residential location. These issues highlight both the progress and challenges in understanding equity in society. As a microcosm of larger society within health care, the practice of emergency medicine (EM) should embrace a greater understanding and awareness of the roles of multiculturalism and diversity in the delivery of health care.

The population of the United States (US) continues to become more diverse. Women now comprise over half of the US population. By 2030, one in five Americans is projected to be aged 65 years and over. Minority groups (any group other than non-Hispanic White alone) are projected to become the collective majority as early as 2044, and almost one in five of the nation's total population is expected to be foreign-born by 2060.[1] As a specialty, EM is in a unique position to serve this diverse population. In many emergency departments (EDs), the majority of visits are with patients from minority backgrounds.[2]

Emergency physicians routinely encounter patients from diverse cultural backgrounds representing various customs, practices or beliefs. All major national EM membership organizations now have policies and statements on diversity, inclusion, and equity. Policies on cultural awareness and emergency care focus on how emergency clinicians should consider the patient's culture, as it relates to history and presenting symptoms, in developing a treatment plan that is mutually agreed upon by the patient and physician. Statements also focus on beliefs and commitments to the goals of attaining equity, diversity, and inclusion in emergency medicine that reflects our multifaceted society. There is consensus around the development and promotion of education, research, and services that assist EDs in improving health for all, with a focus on eliminating health inequities.[3,4] To attain these goals, emergency clinicians must become culturally competent to meet the needs of diverse patient populations.

RATIONALE FOR CULTURAL COMPETENCE

Changing Demographics

Both the US population and the types of health problems seen by emergency clinicians are constantly changing.[5] According to US Census data from the 2018 American Community Survey, 14% of the US population identified as foreign-born.[6] Additionally, 28% of the population identified as other than "White alone" and 18% described themselves as Hispanic or Latino.[6] These changing demographics do not speak to the diversity within the various groups. The category Hispanic, for example, is an ethnic grouping counted in the race category of the census, but it fails to capture the significant range of diversity represented by Spanish speakers. Hispanics may share some cultural practices and speak similar versions of the Spanish language, but they have major differences in vocabulary and dialect, history, socioeconomic status, cultural identity, self-reference (Hispanic or Latino), levels of acculturation, health beliefs, habits, access to care, and health outcomes. The changing cultural landscape will challenge EM providers to recognize, account for, and address these differences when providing care for their patients.

Racial and Ethnic Disparities in Health Care Access and Outcomes

An overarching goal of the Healthy People 2030 Project is to "Eliminate health disparities, achieve health equity, and attain health literacy to improve the health and well-being of all."[7] Numerous studies find that we are not meeting that goal.[5] When compared to Whites, racial and ethnic minorities have a lower likelihood of having a usual source of care, fewer physician visits, and fewer health expenditures. Hispanics and Blacks are less likely to initiate or receive mental health services when compared to Whites. Hispanics have lower health care use, including ED visits and outpatient mental health services, when compared to Whites and Blacks. Hispanic, Asian, and Black patients are less likely to have a consistent primary care provider.[8] With respect to unmet needs from ED visits, Black women fared the worst compared to men and women from White, Hispanic, and Asian backgrounds. Black patients are among the most disadvantaged of the racial/ethnic groups with a greater proportion impoverished, unemployed but looking for work, or in poor to fair health.[8]

Factors resulting in racial/ethnic disparities in health care contribute to differences in access to care. While these differences in access to care may correlate with access to financial resources or health insurance, other factors such as culture, language, and discriminatory practices may also contribute to these variations. Studies indicate that "implicit bias against Black, Hispanic/Latino/Latina, and dark-skinned individuals is present among many health care providers of varying specialties, levels of training, and levels of experience."[9] Reproductive biology and conditions specific to gender may also result in differences in health service use as it relates to gender.[8]

Tests and Treatments

Disparities in ED pain treatment persist a decade after identification of racial and ethnic differences in analgesic administration.[10,11] Studies indicate that provider bias may contribute to a skewed assessment of pain and therefore inadequate treatment.[12] Lee et al. reviewed studies from 1990 to 2018 comparing racial and ethnic differences in the administration of analgesia for acute pain and found that Black and Hispanic patients were less likely than White patients to receive analgesia for acute pain.[13] Goyal et al. found that Black children with appendicitis are less likely to receive any pain medication for moderate pain and less likely to receive opioids for severe pain, suggesting a different threshold for treatment.[14]

Racial and ethnic differences in provision of medically appropriate procedures and therapies have been documented. Wilder et al. found that Blacks and Hispanics were significantly less likely to receive any antidote when presenting to the ED for acute drug overdose.[15] Miller et al. found that a protocol-driven care pathway eliminates the racial disparity among Black and White participants with chest pain in the acquisition of index-visit cardiovascular testing.[16] Despite decades-old identification of these differences and regardless of the setting, health care disparities remain a real and pervasive threat to patient care, but studies indicate that protocol-driven pathways may help to decrease racial disparities.

Health Outcomes

Even perceived discrimination has a significant effect on health.[17,18] Thames et al. performed a cross-sectional bioinformatic analysis relating perceived discrimination (measured by the Perceived Ethnic Discrimination Questionnaire [PED-Q]) to the activity of proinflammatory, neuroendocrine, and antiviral transcription control pathways relevant to the conserved transcriptional response to adversity (CTRA) in peripheral blood leukocytes. They found that differential exposure to racial discrimination may contribute to racial disparities in health outcomes in part by activating threat-related molecular programs that stimulate inflammation and contribute to increased risk of chronic illnesses.[19]

Lee et al. evaluated the association between discrimination and leukocyte telomere length (LTL), a biologic marker of systemic aging.

High discrimination was associated with shorter LTL after controlling for sociodemographic factors, health factors, depressive symptoms, and stress. Results suggest that discrimination experiences accelerate biologic aging in older African American males and females alike. This finding helps advance our understanding of how discrimination generates greater disease vulnerability and premature death in African Americans.[20]

Failure of Trust

Patients from minority communities have reason to be skeptical about the validity of medical research and appropriateness of medical recommendations. The legacy of Tuskegee, for example, has long been seen as the etiology of mistrust in the African American (AA) community. Lack of trust can result in failure to follow medical advice, arrange follow-up appointments, and obtain prescriptions.[21]

Higher levels of acculturation and lower levels of perceived discrimination are associated with higher levels of trust in health care providers. Patients often rate their physician interactions as longer, more participatory, and having more positive effects when their physician is of the same race.[22] For immigrants, shorter lengths of time spent in the United States and increased experiences with discrimination predicted increased distrust in the health care system. In one study, interventions aimed at the reduction of perceived discrimination reduced health care disparities in Korean Americans.[23]

SPECIFIC ISSUES

Communication and Use of Interpreters

Effective communication between patients and physicians is essential for improved health outcomes. There are over 300 languages other than English spoken in the United States. According to US Census data released in 2015, over 60 million Americans over the age of 5 years speak a language other than English at home, and 25 million speak English less than very well.[24] Patients with limited English proficiency are more likely to defer needed health services, leave against medical advice, miss appointments, fail to adhere to treatment regimens, lack a regular provider, and report poor health status.[25] Additional challenges faced by this diverse population with limited English proficiency include risk of increased medication errors, decreases in understanding medical conditions, and misdiagnosis resulting from the lack of physician understanding of complaints or patients' ability to effectively convey their symptoms.[26] The use of untrained nonprofessional interpreters (employees, family, friends, etc.) can result in patient confidentiality concerns and miscommunication due to oversimplification of medical problems or other interpretation errors, which potentially compromises quality, safety, and patient satisfaction.[27,28]

The National Standards for Culturally and Linguistically Appropriate Services in Health and Health Care (The National CLAS Standards), last modified in October 2018 and published by the US Department of Health and Human Services Office of Minority Health, aim to improve health care quality and advance health equity by establishing a framework for organizations to serve the nation's increasingly diverse communities. Institutions and practitioners are required to provide for medical needs in a patient's primary language and in a manner compatible with the patient's health beliefs and practices. The overarching goal of the CLAS standards is to "provide effective, equitable, understandable and respectful quality care and services that are responsive to diverse cultural health beliefs and practices, preferred languages, health literacy and other communication needs."[29] Health care institutions and providers are asked to collect data stratified by race, ethnicity, and language, and to institute quality improvement efforts when cross-cultural differences in outcomes of care, process indicators, or

BOX 186.1 Pitfalls in Language Communication Standards

- Use of family members, friends, or children
- Failure to translate documents such as consent forms and discharge instructions
- Lack of documentation of a patient's need for an interpreter or English language limitations
- Lack of documentation of the use of an interpreter and background and qualifications of the interpreter

patient satisfaction are detected. They are asked to develop culturally competent systems of care based on an assessment of the organization's mission, goals, policies, practices and services, staff training needs, and current diversity of the staff. After the assessment process, health care organizations must identify opportunities to improve the cultural competence of the organization and its delivery of health care services to a diverse population. At the top of the list is the improvement of interpreter services. Hospitals are asked to establish minimum performance standards for interpreters, which includes training in the culturally specific medical language and code of ethics.[29,30]

Standards and certification for medical interpreters are necessary to ensure consistency and quality.[31,32] As of 2019, every state and the District of Columbia had enacted multiple laws addressing language access.[33] The Joint Commission requires hospitals to provide professional interpretation services to every patient who needs it. The International Medical Interpreters Association recommends that standards cover interpretation, cultural interface, and ethical behavior.[34] Because the meaning inherent in the message is rooted in culturally specific beliefs, values, assumptions, customs, and norms, and language is itself an expression of culture, it may be necessary for a medical interpreter to go beyond a literal interpretation to explain unstated assumptions and find new ways of communicating untranslatable words or concepts. In addition to maintaining confidentiality, the medical interpreter has an ethical burden to uphold the trust of both parties and to assure them that the considerable power associated with the interpreter's role will not be abused, and that information will be faithfully conveyed without interjection of the subjective opinions and thoughts of the interpreter. Even with such qualified interpreters, the emergency clinician still needs to monitor the flow of the interview and, from time to time, clarify meaning and ensure understanding. This can be done by having the interpreter repeat what he or she thought the patient meant and asking the patient to repeat what the interpreter said. It is important to observe the interaction for phrase length as an indication of material not translated or added by the translator.

Finally, failure to meet language and communication standards in clinical scenarios can have financial implications. Professional interpreter usage has been demonstrated to have cost lowering effects resulting from decreased administration of intravenous fluids, unnecessary laboratory and radiologic testing, and admissions as a precaution.[27] In addition, the use of nonprofessional interpreters can yield medical malpractice claims resulting from harm caused because of language barriers. In a study of medical malpractice claims of a malpractice carrier that insures providers in four US states, researchers found that 2.5% of the carrier's total claims reviewed were related to language barriers resulting in patient death or irreparable harm. The study reported that the carrier paid $2.3 million in damages or settlements and $2.8 million in legal fees between 2005 and 2009. In 32 of the 35 cases, the health care providers did not use competent interpreters.[35] Box 186.1 lists common pitfalls in meeting language communication standards.

Disability and Accommodations

Overview

According to the World Health Organization (WHO), roughly 15% of the world's population (over a billion people) live with some form of a disability. Disability is defined as impairments, activity limitations, and participation restrictions of individuals with a health-related condition and their personal and environmental factors.[36,37] Increasing rates of disability are related to an aging population and increase in chronic conditions. All people with disabilities have basic health care needs requiring access to the mainstream health care services despite the diversity and complexities of the disability. According to the WHO, people with disabilities search for more health care options than people without disabilities and have greater unmet needs.[38] People with disabilities can be subject to prejudice and the resulting health disparities and poorer health care outcomes, similar to people from other stigmatized groups. They can experience many barriers in accessing health care, including factors such as prohibitive costs, limited availability of services, physical barriers to access facilities or treatment, and lack of knowledge and skills of health care workers.[38]

Patients living with disabilities present for a variety of reasons that may or may not result from their disability. The ED may be the first point of contact with the health care system and the visit may be the first presentation of a condition that could result in a disability or a complication arising from it.

The Hearing Impaired

Deaf and hard-of-hearing individuals over the age of 12 comprise 23% of the US population.[39] This group encompasses varying skills with spoken language, lip-reading, sign language, and written language. The level and type of skill usually depends on when in life the impairment occurred. For example, an individual with congenital hearing loss may be proficient in sign language, while someone with acquired deafness may be more proficient with written notes and may be less able to lip read.[40] Individuals whose language is American Sign Language (ASL) or another sign language face significant barriers to access to the health care system due to lack of health care sign language interpreters.[41] Although antidiscrimination legislation exists to protect the deaf community, persistent gaps in support and resources still exist that impacts accessibility for the hearing impaired. Communication barriers prevent deaf patients from being able to maintain strong patient-provider relationships with primary care. This can lead to overutilization of the ED and urgent care for routine health concerns.[41] Inadequate provision for sign language interpretive services can have legal, financial, and ethical implications. These consequences can include discrimination suits based on the American with Disabilities Act, breach of duty concerns in regard to patients' informed consent and their ability to participate in their health care, as well as professional conduct of health care providers as it relates to equitable patient-centered care.[40] The National Association of the Deaf (NAD) has outlined guidelines for health care providers to provide effective communication to deaf patients who communicate with sign language[41] (Box 186.2).

The Homeless

The homeless often encounter multiple barriers to accessing health care, yet they experience high levels of both chronic and acute medical problems. They are also disproportionately vulnerable to violence and injury and are at increased risk of premature death and disability.[42] Homeless individuals use the ED at higher rates, are more likely to have repeat ED visits, and are more likely to present via ambulance because of their lack of transportation than non-homeless persons.[43] Homeless individuals often use the ED for nonemergent medical needs because demands and costs for food, shelter, and safety supersede obtaining

BOX 186.2　National Association of the Deaf Communication Guidelines for Health Care Providers

- Clearly identify at-risk individuals for poor communication.
- Provide visual medical aids.
- Providers who know basic sign language can be beneficial but be aware of limitations.
- Establish an effective communication policy for the office or institution.
- Provide qualified sign language interpreters.
- Ineffective methods of communication are discouraged, including lip-reading or written notes.
- Be aware of effective communication approaches and resources.
- Make health care providers and staff aware of relevant laws and mandates that provide equal access and communication for deaf patients.

primary care. The high prevalence of concomitant substance abuse and psychiatric illness can make treating the homeless population more challenging. Homeless individuals have a significantly higher risk of opioid overdose and opioid-related ED visits and hospitalizations compared to low-income housed individuals.[44] This finding highlights the importance of recognizing the homeless population as high-risk for opioid overdose. Comprehensive discharge planning is required for homeless patients due to their comorbid psychiatric and substance abuse issues combined with their lack of consistent and safe shelter.

The ED presents a window of opportunity where early intervention strategies may be implemented to improve the health status of homeless patients. Intensive case management has been shown to reduce ED use and result in better health outcomes by connecting homeless patients with available community resources. Greater attention must be given to the hospital services that are provided to the homeless so that behavioral, environmental, and psychosocial needs are also addressed effectively and efficiently. Improved integration of health care facilities and shelters as overlapping systems of care may improve the quality of transitions of care and health care outcomes for homeless patients.[27] Caring for homeless patients in the ED requires attention to the social determinants of health[42] (see Chapter 189).

Prisoners

Prisoners have a higher incidence of physical and psychiatric disorders compared to the general population. The health disparity between prisoners and the general population has been attributed to socioeconomic and behavioral factors including increased rates of intravenous drug use, infectious diseases, alcohol abuse, and smoking, which have increased the risk of cardiovascular disease and some cancers. Approximately one in seven prisoners has a mental illness. Mental illness has been shown to increase the risk of crime and repeat offending. The disproportionate degree of physical and psychiatric disease in prisoners presents both unique public health challenges and opportunities for public health intervention. For many underserved individuals, prison provides an opportunity for diagnosis, disease management education, counseling, and treatment that they would not otherwise receive. Treating mental and physical illnesses of prisoners can improve public health.

Unfortunately, prisoners often have limited access to health care after release from prison.[27] Upon release from prison, the previously incarcerated return to their communities with their physical and psychiatric morbidity, occasionally untreated and sometimes worsened, creating additional societal burden within their communities. Psychiatric morbidity leads to increased suicide rates and contributes to repeat offending.

The Undocumented

Undocumented patients rely on the ED for a disproportionate degree of care due to barriers to health care access. For example, reliance on the ED for routine dialysis occurs because of ineligibility for Medicare and Medicaid, leading to increased mortality.[45-47]

Emergency clinicians should become familiar with strategies and resources that will impact the ED care of undocumented individuals. Also, strengthening ties with community-based organizations and medical legal partnerships can facilitate linking undocumented patients to social services and may help to facilitate successful discharge planning and follow up.

Understanding immigration status as a modifiable social determinant of health is a first step in improving the care and health of undocumented populations (see Chapter 189).

CULTURAL COMPETENCE

Appreciation of Different Beliefs, Values, and Experiences

The encounter between a clinician and patient is guided by perspectives dictated by cultural differences or similarities. Knowledge and awareness of those differences or similarities can often enhance satisfaction and health outcomes. A patient-centered approach to the clinical encounter requires the clinician to be carefully observant to sufficiently assess or even inquire about a patient's preexisting assumptions in order to provide culturally sensitive care.

Diagnosis of specific diseases can be interpreted differently depending upon differing cultural perspectives. For example, in African American and Puerto Rican communities, a cancer diagnosis may be perceived as fatal even if diagnosed at an early stage with a more favorable prognosis. As a result, patients may be more likely to avoid initial evaluation or choose no treatment when initially diagnosed. A health care provider who understands these health beliefs and concerns can work collaboratively with patients to provide health information in a format that the patient can accept.

Alternative healing systems have strong cultural roots. In the 2007 National Health Interview Survey (NHIS), approximately 38% of adults reported using complementary and alternative medicine (CAM) in the previous 12 months, with approximately 354 million visits to CAM practitioners and approximately 835 million purchases.[48] The National Center for Complementary and Integrated Health maintains an extensive database of literature on alternative healing methodologies in the United States.[49-52]

Folk medicine is too diverse for providers to know all possible practices, but emergency clinicians need to be aware of the more common folk therapies. For example, more than a few physicians have called social workers to investigate children with apparent bruises caused by coining, which involves vigorous rubbing of the skin with coins and warm oil (tiger balm) to release "bad wind" (reduce fever). These parents, who have attempted to help their children by using health care practices that are widely accepted in their communities of origin, feel accused, and the trust between the physician and family may be irrevocably lost. Similarly, herbal remedies can be effective or at least harmless, but they can occasionally be toxic, as in the case of clay ingestion by pregnant women, marijuana tea to treat asthma, and powders containing high concentrations of lead oxide to treat *empacho*, a condition in which it is believed that a substance (usually food or saliva) gets stuck to the walls of the stomach or intestines, causing an obstruction. Specific uses of folk medicine need to be elicited respectfully in a careful history and evaluated. Recommendations can then be presented nonjudgmentally, and alternative folk remedies that are benign can be prescribed along with needed allopathic medications.

The practitioner and patient will inevitably bring different beliefs and values to the medical encounter; the key to cultural competence is respectful negotiation of these differences without imposing the power of the physician's expertise, thereby protecting the patient's autonomy. If patients are satisfied, they will carry out follow-up recommendations and return to the ED in the future when they need emergency care.

Interpreting the Culture of Medicine for Patients From Diverse Backgrounds

There are inherent conflicts between the culture of western medical practice and the cultures of many patients. Physicians are experts in diagnosis and treatment of *disease*, the abnormal structures or functions of the human body (the pathophysiology of disease states). Patients, on the other hand, experience *illness*, a subjective feeling state that is interpreted through the lens of culture and has a personal and social meaning. The patient is an expert on his or her own illness and its effects on daily living, whereas a physician is expert on the effects of diseases on organ systems. Both ways of looking at the world have validity and a culturally competent approach recognizes both and works to integrate both perspectives for the best possible outcomes.

If patients with true disease remain asymptomatic or experience no alteration in functioning, they may be reluctant to accept a physician's diagnosis. On the other hand, a patient may be significantly, subjectively symptomatic in the absence of medical diagnosis, despite a thorough investigation. Concepts such as *susto* (fright), *coraje* (anger), and *fatalismo* (fatalism) are common cultural beliefs that manifest in physical symptoms. For example, *susto,* an illness recognized by Mexican Americans, causes listlessness, insomnia, depression, and anorexia, and is believed to be caused by exposure to a frightening experience. Treatment requires the patient to speak openly about the events that led to the susto, followed by bed rest and a ritual that includes prayers, incantations, and *barridas*—sweeping of the body with an egg, candle, or herbal tea. If these beliefs are not well understood by the health care provider, recommendations for treatment are likely to be discarded. As a result, the health care provider must develop trust with the patient. One useful approach is to engage a family member or *promotora* or *promotor* (community health worker) in the conversation.[53]

To be most effective, physicians need to investigate how patients view the causality of their illnesses and how they experience them to negotiate a therapeutic intervention. Exploration might take the form of comments and questions, such as, "Help me see through your eyes how you understand this problem," or "Have you or someone you know experienced it before?" The role of the physician is to accept the patient's experience as uniquely his or hers or, when possible, to reframe it in terms of medical knowledge. Then both physician and patient will be satisfied with the outcome of the encounter.

Every medical encounter is potentially a cross-cultural experience within this context and negotiation of the divide can be challenging for both patients and providers. Cultural competence involves reframing many of these unstated rules so that underlying circumstances and problems can be recognized and addressed. Circumstances may exist where patients may not feel comfortable sharing information with clinicians because of cultural, racial, sexual orientation, or language barriers. Vague complaints may be a sign of social stressors that result in mental health–related symptoms. These presentations may be further complicated by negative stimuli related to racial and ethnic discrimination.[54] People from minority cultures often experience significantly higher levels of daily stressors and there is mounting evidence that these types of negative encounters engender clinical depression and anxiety and contribute to hypertension and other medical sequelae.

Minority populations consume ED care at higher rates and are more likely to use the ED as a usual source of care.[55] Emergency clinicians must appreciate the context of their practice settings; recognize how rules, language, hierarchy and bias can potentially interfere with effective patient care; and work to provide care that is patient-centered and culturally sensitive. These actions can help create a safe environment for practitioners and patients who will experience higher levels of satisfaction with the care experience.

Combining Cultural Competence and Patient-Centered Care

Models for cultural competence and patient-centered care have evolved separately yet are closely aligned. The goal of both models is to improve the quality of the health care experience in a multicultural setting. Cultural competence involves providing equitable, evidence-based, high-quality care for diverse patient populations.[56] It requires the clinician to recognize and respect individual differences and the impact of individual interpretation on health, illness, and health care delivery. Patient and family–centered care is an approach to health care delivery that is a mutually beneficial partnership among the patient, family, and the health care team to address the planning, development, and assessment of the medical care.

Ideal health care systems incorporate the principles of both cultural competence and patient centeredness. A health care system built on patient-centered principles represents the heart of cultural competence—seeing the problem and solution from the point of view of the patient.[56] In 2015, the American Association of Pediatrics published a technical report which stated that "commitment to patient and family centered care ensures that the experiences and perspectives of patients and families guide the practice of coordinated and culturally sensitive care that promotes patient dignity, comfort, and autonomy."[57]

Medical education at the undergraduate, graduate, and professional levels about the impact of culture on health care encounters is a key component for the development of culturally appropriate health care and is a requirement for organizational accreditation. Students and residents in training consistently express greater levels of comfort in multicultural environments when they have had preparatory training. Training also helps students and residents understand that their own culture also affects clinical encounters and is equally participatory.

The Accreditation Council of Graduate Medicine Education (ACGME) and the Liaison Committee on Medical Education (LCME) have provided guidelines that graduate training programs and medical schools use to teach cultural competency through communication skills and professionalism.[27,58-59] The American Association of Medical Colleges (AAMC) also provides the Tool for Assessing Cultural Competency Training (TACCT) to assess cultural competency training in medical schools and provide medical schools and graduate medical education programs with a suggested rubric.[60]

According to the Emergency Medicine Milestones Project, patient-centered communication and professional values are assessed for every emergency medicine resident. This particular area addresses the learner's ability to elicit presenting symptoms from a diverse population of emergency department patients. Additionally, it assesses the learner's ability to communicate effectively with vulnerable populations. The professional values milestone requires learners to demonstrate cultural humility by providing compassion, integrity, and respect during patient care.[61]

RECOMMENDATIONS

Diversity among the ED patient population poses a challenge to emergency clinicians. Recognition of cultural differences, knowledge about diverse cultures, awareness of the health impact of cultural beliefs and practices, and sensitivity to patients' needs can reduce access barriers and improve clinical outcomes and hospital-community relationships while reducing the number of repeated visits and costs of health care. Diversity, inclusion, and health equity education also creates a rich environment for conceptualizing and researching health problems.

There are many opportunities for EDs and their institutions to improve their care of multicultural communities. These include plans to address problems related to lack of protocols for patient care and lack of resources for translation and cross-cultural interpretation. Cross-culture teaching guidelines and standards in medical education can correct false perceptions of culturally competent care such as negative impacts on flow and efficiency in the ED. Opportunities also exist to develop, recruit, and retain residents, faculty, and practitioners who are underrepresented in medicine in order to enhance multicultural patient care, opening the doors to community engagement.

Specific recommendations, based on the National Standards for Culturally and Linguistically Appropriate Services in Health and Health Care, have been proposed for pediatric emergency settings that can be applied universally. Institutions should use trained medical interpreters and should have a goal of employing a diverse workforce.

Pharmacies are encouraged to label prescriptions and provide medical instructions in the patient's primary language. Administrators should post multilingual signs and ensure that handouts and forms are translated. Quality improvement programs should collect and analyze data and provide information to monitor outcomes based on race and ethnicity. Efforts should be made to expand minority enrollment in research studies and clinical trials to improve the validity and applicability of discoveries and new therapies.

The process of change for the development of culturally competent medical systems has been slow, but progress is occurring. Evolution of culturally appropriate environments for patients and their families has begun on all levels and, with the development of new standards and performance monitoring systems, assurance of established culturally competent systems will be an expectation. These expectations are important and tightly linked to safety and quality. The linkage of cultural competence to social justice broadens the depth of comprehension for the learner and provides opportunities for enhanced engagement with consumers and greater quality of care.

The process of creating a successful plan to move cultural competency from a theoretical model to one of action and implementation has been outlined in six principles that incorporate key points recommended by the IOM report of 2003 for systems aligned with new cultural competence standards and expectations (Box 186.3).

Essential cultural competence tools for providers include recognition of cultural differences, respect for individual opinions and perspectives about health and illness and, most importantly, ability and willingness to negotiate differences to offer the best opportunity for good health care outcomes. Culturally appropriate health care systems should be incorporated into EDs, which serve as the gateway to our health care institutions.

The references for this chapter can be found online at ExpertConsult. com.

187

Human Trafficking

Wendy Macias-Konstantopoulos and Hanni Stoklosa

KEY CONCEPTS

- Labor and sex trafficking involve the exploitation of a person for labor or commercial sex, respectively, affecting up to 25 million persons worldwide.
- Human smuggling, a crime in which a person contracts a smuggler to facilitate their illegal entry into a country, can evolve into trafficking during transit or at the destination and under such circumstances the person is considered a victim of human trafficking.
- Child victims of sex trafficking are considered victims of child abuse and neglect under the law and thereby call into relevance state mandated reporting statutes.
- Populations at greater risk for trafficking include persons with histories of child abuse, family dysfunction, diverse sexual orientation or gender identity, intellectual disability, homelessness, financial insecurity, and migration.
- Human trafficking often involves the use of abusive and violent tactics, including forced substance use and psychological coercion to entrap and exert control over trafficked persons, with profound implications for survivors' physical, reproductive, and mental health.
- Trafficked persons seek health care services during their exploitation for a wide range of health conditions and the emergency department (ED) is the most common access point for this patient population where indicators of abuse, control, and the physical and psychosocial red flags of trafficking can assist in the recognition of trafficked victims.
- Inquiry about forms of interpersonal violence, including trafficking, is fundamentally different from screening for medical issues with the goal of providing a safe environment in which patients feel empowered to share as much or as little as they choose, and where strengths and resilience are recognized.
- Trafficked people may return to exploitative situations repeatedly before exiting permanently; therefore, safety planning is critical for the discharged trafficked patient.
- Trauma due to trafficking results in neurobiologic changes such that commonly occurring smells, sounds, sights, and procedures of the ED environment may be perceived as threats by those with trauma histories.
- The six principles of trauma-informed care include physical and psychological safety; trustworthiness and transparency; peer support; collaboration and mutuality; empowerment, voice, and choice; and cultural, historical, and gender acknowledgment.
- Law enforcement involvement should be limited to patient request, in state-specific mandated reporting scenarios, or when clinicians suspect imminent danger to staff or the patient.

FOUNDATIONS

Background and Importance

Human trafficking is an abusive and exploitative form of interpersonal violence. It is a global public health problem associated with a multitude of health problems. The United States (US) recognizes both labor trafficking and sex trafficking as "severe forms of trafficking in persons" punishable under federal and state laws. Under the US Trafficking Victims Protection Act (TVPA) of 2000 and its subsequent reauthorization acts, as amended (22 USC § 7102):

- *Labor trafficking* is "the recruitment, harboring, transportation, provision, or obtaining of a person for labor or services, through the use of force, fraud, or coercion for the purposes of subjection to involuntary servitude, peonage, debt bondage, or slavery," and
- *Sex trafficking* is "the recruitment, harboring, transportation, provision, obtaining, patronizing, or soliciting of a person for the purposes of a *commercial sex act*, in which the commercial sex act is induced by force, fraud, or coercion, or in which the person induced to perform such an act has not attained 18 years of age."[1,2]

Federal law assumes that persons under the age of 18 years performing commercial sex acts have been induced to engage in commercial sex and does not require that force, fraud, or coercion be proven for minors to be considered victims of sex trafficking. (Pursuant to Pub. L. 106-386, 114 Stat 1469 (2000), a commercial sex act refers to "any sex act on account of which anything of value is given to or received by any person.") Antitrafficking legislation since the TVPA of 2000 has focused further attention on prosecution, protection, and prevention of child trafficking. The Justice for Victims of Trafficking Act of 2015 authorized a range of provisions for combating trafficking and assisting victims, including an amendment to the Child Abuse Prevention and Treatment Act of 1988 by which the legal definition of *child abuse and neglect* was expanded to incorporate "sex trafficking" and "severe forms of trafficking in persons" involving minors.[3] Although mandated reporting statutes vary across jurisdictions, all states, the District of Columbia, and US territories mandate the report of suspected child abuse and neglect to the proper authorities.[4]

Finally, it is important for providers to understand that the law differentiates between human trafficking and human smuggling. Whereas human trafficking involves the exploitation of a victim for compelled labor or commercial sex, *human smuggling* involves a person contracting a smuggler to facilitate their voluntary and illegal entry into a country. Although human smuggling is a crime of migration committed against the state (not against a person), persons smuggled across international borders may be subjected to labor or sex trafficking during transit or upon arrival at their destination. Under these circumstances, their voluntary consent to smuggling does not render legal their subsequent entrapment in forced labor or commercial sex and such individuals are considered victims of the crime of human trafficking under federal law.[5] Understanding this distinction is important to educating victims about their legal rights and linking them to services where they can access the legal protections and redress to which they are entitled.

EPIDEMIOLOGY

Trafficking Typologies

The US Department of State has determined that human trafficking is an umbrella term that comprises a number of different forms of compelled service including forced labor, bonded labor (debt bondage), domestic servitude, sex trafficking, child sex trafficking, forced child labor, and child soldiering.[6] Exploitation of adults and children in the United States has been reported in typically formal labor markets (e.g., restaurant and hospitality, construction, agriculture, farming), informal labor sectors (e.g., domestic work, landscaping, traveling sales crew, peddling rings), and commercial sex industries.[7] In the United States, the illegal commercial sex economy may involve street-based commercial sex, brothels and cantinas, technology-facilitated rendezvousing, escort services, adult entertainment venues, child sex tourism abroad, live-streaming of child sexual abuse, and child and adult pornography.[7,8,9] Additionally, nail salons, massage parlors, health spas, and other unregulated bodywork businesses can serve as storefronts for both labor and sex trafficking.[7,9]

Global and US Prevalence

Prevalence estimates of human trafficking are historically wide-ranging and influenced by multiple factors. Data integrity and reliability are challenged by the clandestine nature of human trafficking, the failure to use a standardized definition of trafficking across organizations and countries, the focus of the data collecting agency (i.e., law enforcement versus social service agency, labor versus sex trafficking, adults versus minors), and the lack of centralization or even compatibility across databases. In 2016, the United Nation's International Labor Organization in collaboration with the Walk Free Foundation and International Organization for Migration (IOM) estimated that 24.9 million persons around the globe are trapped in forced labor, including sexual exploitation.[10] According to this study, women and girls account for 71% and children account for 25% of victims, and nonsexual forced labor comprises the majority of cases.[10] Centralized, reliable, high-quality data are needed to enhance our understanding of the scope of the problem globally and within individual countries.

Polaris, a US nongovernmental organization (NGO), has been monitoring human trafficking and operating the National Human Trafficking Hotline (NHTH) in the United States since 2000. Although reporting hotlines fail to capture all cases of trafficking, statistics from the national trafficking hotline offer relevant proxy data regarding the extent of the problem. According to published hotline statistics, nearly 52,000 *situations* of human trafficking involving one or more victims were identified across the US and US territories between December 2007 and December 2018.[11] In 2018 alone, the NHTH identified over 23,000 individual survivors of human trafficking, 64% of whom were survivors of sex trafficking, 24% labor trafficking, and 6% both forms of trafficking.[12]

Demographics of Trafficked Persons

Within the subset of tip calls received by the national hotline for which survivor demographic data are available, the majority of survivors are adults (≥18 years), female, and Latinx. Extrapolation from the limited data suggests that the average age (mode age range) at the onset of trafficking was 25 (15–17) years old for labor trafficking and 18 (15–17) years old for sex trafficking.[12,13] Given the challenges in collecting comprehensive and accurate information, demographic data from identified and reported cases in any local or national database may not accurately reflect the overall demographics of US trafficked persons.

Although human trafficking can affect persons of any age, gender identity, sexual orientation, ethnicity, race, citizenship, socioeconomic

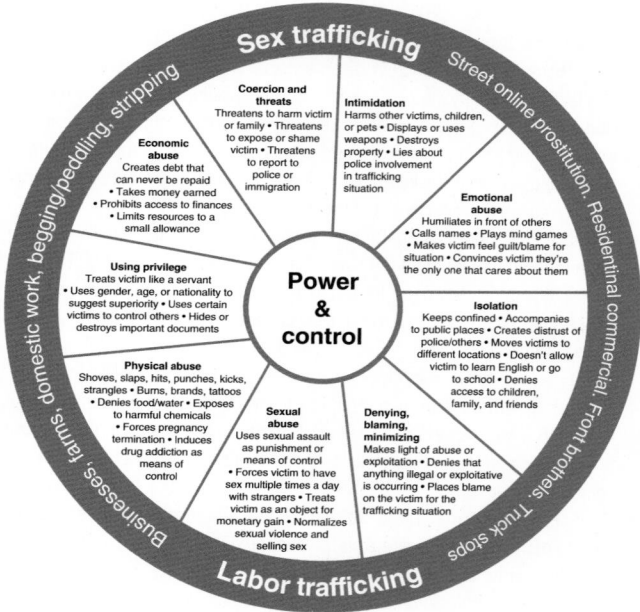

Fig. 187.1 Polaris Human Trafficking Power and Control Wheel. (Adapted from Polaris and available for download at https://human-traffickinghotline.org/resources/human-trafficking-power-and-control-wheel.)

standing, religion, and physical or intellectual ability, certain populations are at greater risk for trafficking. Circumstances that place individuals at risk for trafficking are those that increase their dependence on others to meet their basic needs or obtain something of value. Box 187.1 lists factors associated with increased vulnerability to human trafficking.[12,14-29]

Recruitment and Control Tactics

Traffickers entrap and maintain control over victims of human trafficking in multiple ways. Figure 187.1 summarizes the constellation of methods used, which often extends to financial disempowerment, debt bondage, coerced involvement in illegal activities, blackmail, and a host of other criminal tactics.[14,15,30]

According to 2018 NHTH data, the top *labor trafficking* recruitment methods used, in order of reported frequency, included false job offers or advertisements, false promises/fraud, smuggling-related initiation, coercion, and familial inducement.[12]

In nearly 12,000 cases of *child trafficking*, data from the Counter-Trafficking Data Collaborative suggest that children are most commonly trafficked by family members (41%), intimate partners (14%), and friends (11%) by means of psychological abuse (24%), physical force (16%), sexual violence (10%), and substance-related coercion (9%).[31]

IMPACT ON HEALTH

Traffickers often employ abusive and violent tactics to exert and maintain control over victims in order to effectuate the crime of human trafficking. These tactics have profound implications for the health of trafficked individuals, leading to physical, reproductive, and mental health problems. Accidental (occupational) and intentional (violence-related) traumatic injuries occur during trafficking as a result of the physical demands of manual labor, lack of personal protective equipment, hazardous working conditions, and physical and sexual violence.[17,32] Sex trafficking survivors and labor trafficking survivors experiencing sexual violence are at elevated risk for sexually transmitted infections (STIs) including human immunodeficiency virus (HIV) infection, pregnancies, and terminations.[17,33-36] In addition, trafficked persons may experience control through induced debilitation, specifically food and sleep deprivation, coerced substance use, and confiscation of needed medications or medical supplies.[30] The abuse and violence endured while trafficked can result in depression, anxiety, posttraumatic stress disorder (PTSD), dissociative states, psychosomatic pain syndromes, substance use, self-injurious behavior, and suicide attempts.[17,25,33-42]

Substance use, mental illness, and pregnancy merit special consideration given the unique degree of vulnerability conferred on victims. These health conditions can create or exacerbate relational imbalances of need and dependency that traffickers can exploit to subvert victims. When caring for patients with these conditions, providers must consider the possibility of the trafficker being a family member, intimate partner, or friend.

Substance Use

Research has established a correlation between substance use and human trafficking. A retrospective chart review of 12- to 18-year-old victims of sexual violence found that drug use rates were significantly higher among commercially sexually exploited and trafficked youth compared to sexually abused and assaulted youth.[19]

The complex relationship between substance use and human trafficking has been increasingly recognized and understood. Substances can play a key role throughout the various stages of trafficking, including in the recruitment, entrapment, and exploitation of victims. Highly addictive substances (e.g., opioids, stimulants) provide a relatively easy opportunity for traffickers to entrap experimenting adolescents and young adults by exploiting newly evolving addictions. In cases where the trafficker is someone close or known to the individual being targeted for recruitment, the trafficker may be the person who introduces the addictive substance and encourages its use with the intent of creating a vulnerability to exploit. Similarly, previously formed addictions offer traffickers a mechanism through which they can entrap individuals with addiction for the purpose of exploiting them.

In addition to facilitating recruitment and entrapment, victim accounts suggest substances may play a central role in maintaining control over trafficked persons. In some cases, traffickers force drug-naïve victims, particularly adolescents, to use substances as a means of weakening their defenses and creating an addiction that can be leveraged to exert control over them during their exploitation.[43] In other cases, the trafficker may simply ensure substances are available and trafficked persons may initiate use on their own as a way to cope with the physical and emotional trauma of their trafficking situation. Victims' reliance on substances to numb their pain and cope with the anxiety, depression, and PTSD related to their everyday experiences while trafficked creates high levels of dependence on the trafficker for access to the drug.[44] Traffickers are thus able to exert and maintain control over trafficked individuals by regulating the type (drug class), manner (route of administration), and extent (dosage and frequency) to which the substance is available to them.

Mental Illness

In addition to mental health disorders potentially heightening risk for trafficking, the traumatic experiences endured by victims while being trafficked may induce or unmask mental health disorders. Trafficking may exacerbate preexisting mental health disorders and lead to increased frequency or severity of psychiatric manifestations.[45] In a historical cohort study of trafficking survivors receiving mental health services in the United Kingdom, the most commonly encountered diagnoses in the adult sample included 34% affective disorders; 28% PTSD, severe stress, or adjustment disorder; 15% schizophrenia and related disorders; and 22% intentional self-injurious behaviors.[45] Similarly, 27% of the youth in the study were diagnosed with affective disorders and another 27% with PTSD, severe stress, or adjustment disorder. Among youth, 27% exhibited intentional self-harm while in care.[45] In a US study among court-involved commercially sexually exploited female youth, 88% endorsed substance use, 76% identified with having a mental health problem, 43% reported previous psychiatric admissions, and 14% reported suicidal ideation.[46]

Anecdotally, traffickers can use a victim's mental illness to remain undetected. A trafficked person who presents to an ED providing accounts of seemingly unrealistic events may be erroneously assumed to be suffering from acute paranoid delusions, persecutory delusions, or hallucinations. Any inconsistencies in their accounts might even raise suspicion among providers of malingering for secondary gain rather than memory gaps related to trauma.[47] Subsequent attempts to obtain assistance in the ED may be misdiagnosed as episodes of acutely decompensated psychiatric illness rather than real life events related to being trafficked. In this manner, traffickers can continue their abuse and control with less concern that the veracity of a victim's report will be investigated.

Pregnancy

Trafficked adolescent and adult women often experience decreased ability to negotiate condom use during transactional sexual encounters,[33,44] as well as decreased access to family planning services and prenatal care.[39,48] Decreased reproductive control and diminished access to family planning services theoretically increases the likelihood that trafficked women may present to an ED for such services (e.g., counseling about alternative discrete forms of contraception, STI screening and treatment, HIV counseling and testing, and emergency contraception). Moreover, lack of access to prenatal care is associated with adverse pregnancy outcomes, including insufficient gestational weight gain, premature rupture of membranes, and precipitous labor,[49] and these outcomes may be at play among trafficked women who present to the ED in the later stages of pregnancy seeking to either initiate prenatal care or deliver.

For trafficked adolescent and adult women, desires to carry or terminate a pregnancy are influenced by the circumstances of their trafficking situation, but such decisions may be unduly influenced by traffickers. As in intimate partner violence, pregnancy also carries an increased risk of trafficker-perpetrated abuse and violence,[44] which in turn is related to increased risk of preterm labor, small-for-gestational-age infants, postpartum depression, and decreased likelihood of breastfeeding.[50,51] Pregnant and postpartum women who present to an ED for violence-related injuries should be queried about other potentially exposed children. Limited evidence suggests that traffickers may use pregnancy and children (e.g., threats of forced abortion, threats to take away children, threats to cut off financial support) to exert and maintain control over their mothers.[14,18,48,52]

Little is known about the experiences of trafficked women's children in the United States. An exploratory study in 2016 found that children of sex workers or trafficked mothers experience significant health risks and outcomes, including behavioral and mental health problems, physical and sexual abuse, the use of cough medicine, alcohol, and other sedating substances to induce sleep, death from a wide range of causes including neglect (e.g., exposure after being left in a car, house fire after being left home), untreated HIV, poisoning, overdose, lethal physical abuse (e.g., abusive head trauma, previously *shaken baby syndrome*), and gang-related murder.[48]

SPECIFIC ISSUES

Recognition and Assessment

Indicators and Red Flags

While indicators and red flags of trafficking can assist in the recognition of possible trafficking, there is no single characteristic that is pathognomonic of human trafficking. Although there are certain segments of the population at higher risk for trafficking, the overall sociodemographic characteristics of trafficked persons are wide-ranging, and no two experiences of trafficking are exactly alike.

Currently there is no defined set of signs and symptoms that cuts across all forms of human trafficking with any sufficient degree of sensitivity and specificity to employ for the identification of victims in the ED. Familiarity with general indicators of abuse and control and the red flags of human trafficking can help elevate a suspicious situation into the level of awareness (Table 187.1).

Indicators of abuse and control can include the presence of an accompanying person who is reluctant to leave the examination room, insists on answering questions or providing language interpretation,

and attempts to control the encounter; combined with a patient who appears fearful or anxious, defers information sharing to the person accompanying them, and frequently glances at the accompanying person for evidence of approval after speaking.[35,36,53] Other potential indicators include patient communications that seem rehearsed or scripted, patient reluctance or inability to answer simple questions about their living or working situation, conflicting information, reported mechanism of injury inconsistent with the physical evidence, and evidence of psychological distress (e.g., limited eye contact, low trigger threshold, hypervigilance, hyperstartle reflex).[36,53]

Physical red flags of human trafficking include delayed presentation for care of injuries or infections; signs of abuse or neglect (e.g., malnourishment, poor oral health); work injuries or exposures that would be easily prevented by personal protective equipment (PPE); intravaginal foreign material to interrupt menstrual flow; delayed presentations for prenatal care; distinctive tattoos or other forms of branding; and multiple STIs, pregnancies, or abortions.[35,36]

Psychosocial red flags of human trafficking include a reluctance to expose or explain a tattoo or marking; unusually high numbers of sexual partners at an early age; truancy and absenteeism from school at certain hours of the day; chronic running away from home; multiple fake forms of identification; lack of identification or immigration documents; long work hours without breaks; limited access to PPE; living in overcrowded quarters; and weather-inappropriate clothing.[36,53]

Trafficking Inquiry

While it is routine in medical care for multiple providers to ask a patient their history, retelling of a traumatic event can be inherently retraumatizing. Concerted efforts to minimize the number of times a patient recounts their history can be conducive towards a feeling of safety. Furthermore, when there is concern for trafficking, the goal of a clinical encounter is not for the patient to disclose victimization, but for providers to treat, educate, and empower the patient.

Inquiry around forms of interpersonal violence, including trafficking, is fundamentally different from screening for medical issues. Rather than disclosure, the goal of inquiry is to provide a safe environment in which patients feel empowered to share as much or as little as they choose, and where their strengths and resilience are recognized. Inquiry-based assessment is an active process that includes open-ended questions and dialogue.[54] The context around which questions are asked, especially for issues where a trafficked patient may feel emotionally and physically unsafe (due to shame, judgment, threats of deportation, etc.) modulate how much a patient may feel comfortable

TABLE 187.1	Potential Trafficking Indicators and Red Flags	
Physical	**Relational**	**Other**
• Delayed presentations to care • Signs of physical, sexual, or dental trauma • Signs of neglect • Signs of malnourishment • Substance use • Multiple recurrent STIs • Foreign bodies to stop menstrual flow • Multiple previous pregnancies • Work injuries preventable with training and/or personal protective equipment • Tattoos or branding indicating ownership	• Accompanied by a person who attempts to control the encounter • Accompanied by a person who insists on translating • Scripted or restricted patient communications • Patient frequently glances to the accompanying person for approval after speaking • Patient avoids eye contact with accompanying person and/or provider • Other signs of submission, fear, or hypervigilance • Distrust of authority	• Difficulty answering simple questions (e.g., name, age, home address, work, current location) • Apparent vs. reported age discrepancy • Discrepancy between history and clinical presentation • Possession of multiple fake IDs or numerous hotel keys • Inappropriate clothing for weather • Truancy or absenteeism from school at certain times of day • Not in possession of identification or immigration documents • Excessive work hours • Possession of large sums of cash or payment in cash

Revised/adapted from Macias-Konstantopoulos W. Human trafficking: the role of medicine in interrupting the cycle of abuse and violence. *Annals of Internal Medicine*. 2016;165(8):582-8.

disclosing at a given point in time.[55] In contrast to inquiry, screening is a "process for evaluating the possible presence of a particular problem" and "the outcome is normally a simple yes or no."[56] Screening for trafficking through a checklist approach may unintentionally retraumatize the patient by triggering the patient's traumatic memories.[57] The only trafficking screening tool that has been validated for use in the pediatric ED is limited to English-speaking 13- to 17-year-olds who have been sex trafficked.[58] The Rapid Appraisal for Trafficking (RAFT) is a validated 4-item trafficking screening tool for labor and sex trafficking of adults in the ED.[58a]

Although evidence exists to support universal inquiry in domestic violence, the extant trafficking literature offers no evidence in support of this. Based on current evidence, trafficking inquiry may be focused on high-risk populations and patients exhibiting red flags. That inquiry may follow trauma-informed frameworks, such as the Privacy, Educate, Ask, Respect, Respond (PEARR) tool.[54] It should be noted that perception of red flags may be influenced by a provider's unconscious and conscious bias.[59] For example, if a clinician views trafficked persons as Caucasian, cis-gendered, and sex trafficked, they may miss an obvious case involving a labor trafficked Black transgender male patient who presents to their ED.[59a]

Use of Professional Interpreters

If the patient speaks a foreign language, emergency providers should use professional interpreter services. Accompanying persons (e.g., friends, relatives including children, or others) may unintentionally compromise confidentiality and even be a trafficker or trafficker's associate. Remote telephone interpretation services may be preferred in certain circumstances including if a potential trafficked person is from a small ethnic group where the interpreter's ties to the local community could pose a risk for a trafficked person.[60]

Evaluation and Treatment

The ED care of a trafficked person involves providing appropriate emergency medical care for the chief complaint, while respecting the patient's goals for the encounter. ED evaluation may include addressing acute medical issues, evaluation of possible untreated chronic medical problems, documentation of acute and remote injuries, STI testing and treatment, and consideration of a sexual assault medical forensic examination and evidence collection. For both labor and sex trafficking, empirical STI treatment and emergency contraception may be indicated.[60]

When a case of suspected human trafficking has been identified, a sexual assault medical forensic examination may be clinically appropriate. Research shows that the use of sexual assault or forensic nurse examiners results in better patient outcomes in legal and emotional support. To the extent that the resource is available, EDs may preferentially offer this service or consider transfer to a crisis center.[60]

Trauma-Informed Approach to Care

Studies of trafficked persons have demonstrated the critical importance of using trauma-informed approaches to care.[59,61] The Substance Abuse and Mental Health Services Administration (SAMHSA) defines trauma as "an event, series of events, or set of circumstances that is experienced by an individual as physically or emotionally harmful or life threatening and has lasting adverse effects on the individual's functioning and mental, physical, social, emotional, or spiritual well-being."[62] Trauma results in neurobiologic changes such that commonly occurring smells, sounds, sights, and procedures of the ED environment may be perceived as threats by those with trauma histories, including trafficked persons. For example, a patient who appears to be uncooperative, avoidant, jumpy, or agitated, may instead be manifesting a natural "fight," "flight," or "freeze" stress reaction.[63]

Sincere, empathetic, nonjudgmental communication is the foundation of trauma-informed care. This includes clinician awareness and mitigation of conscious and unconscious biases, including their manifestation in body language and word choice, in order to prevent retraumatization of trafficked persons.[59,63,64] Loss of control is a major part of the trafficking experience and the medical environment can exacerbate those feelings. Therefore, emergency clinicians should look for and offer choices when possible, helping the patient regain a sense of autonomy. Clear communication about the clinical team composition, the care plan, events to expect, and possible timeline, allows a trafficked patient to feel a sense of control.[59,63,64]

Helping a traumatized patient to feel safe and calm includes a mindfulness of a patient's stress reactions, including demeanor, speech, and even pulse rate. When these reactions are observed, clinicians may respond using psychological first-aid techniques of connectedness, calmness, safety, structure, self-efficacy, and hope (Fig. 187.2).[63] Potentially triggering environmental factors could include the visibility of security guards who may remind the patient of prior traumatizing law enforcement experiences. Trauma-informed approaches are especially important for the agitated patient with an experience of trauma. Beginning with de-escalation and psychological first-aid techniques can mitigate retraumatization and should be balanced with staff safety concerns. If restraints are necessary for the safety of the patient and staff, use of the least restrictive measures possible is recommended.[63]

The Privacy, Educate, Ask, Respect, and Respond (PEARR) tool provides a trauma-informed framework for the clinician assessing any form of interpersonal violence, including human trafficking.[54] The first step of the PEARR tool is to find a place to speak to a patient alone, explaining any limits to confidentiality with the patient before beginning this sensitive discussion. The clinician attempts to educate the patient regarding abuse, neglect, or violence in a nonjudgmental and normalized manner, and then asks about the patient's personal experience. The patient may or may not disclose their exploitation experience at this point in time. The final step involves ongoing respect of the patient's wishes and responding according to their goals. It is common for patients experiencing interpersonal violence, including trafficking, to choose to return to their exploiter. If a patient denies victimization or declines assistance, and there are persistent concerns about abuse, neglect, or violence, then the clinician may offer the patient information about resources that can assist in the event of an emergency (e.g., local service providers, crisis hotlines).

Multidisciplinary Response

Establishing multidisciplinary protocols inclusive of labor and sex trafficking and involving internal and external resources allows clinicians to respond to a trafficking disclosure in a safe, trauma-informed manner. In addition to a myriad of acute and chronic medical and mental health needs, trafficked persons may also require assistance with substance use treatment, housing, vocational, and legal needs. Response protocols will vary considerably based on a clinical practice setting. The majority of health care institutions already have protocols in place that address various forms of violence including intimate partner violence, child abuse, elder abuse, and sexual assault. Human trafficking responses may be incorporated into existing interpersonal violence protocols to streamline training, treatment, and referral processes.[60,65,66]

Breaches of privacy may harm the provider-patient relationship, compromise patient autonomy, and produce distrust among other trafficked persons. Therefore, EDs and health care institutions may consider establishing memorandums of understanding with external partners, including limitations of HIPAA, and need for patient consent for information sharing. If case management is not available, the patient may

Goals	Useful statements or actions
Connectedness	Assign a single team member to be the primary source of communication with the patient: "I am going to stay and help you with everything you go through here." For pediatric patients, if feasible, allow parental presence and support.
Calmness	Minimize presence of non-participatory members of the care team. Avoid excess noise/chatter. Encourage the patient to perform slow breathing exercises.
Safety	Provide patient a simple reminder that he or she has been removed from the site of injury: "You are in the safest place you could be right now."
Self-efficacy	Discuss care plan with patient to diminish sense of loss of control. Use language that acknowledges rather than undermines the patient's defense mechanisms; for example, "You are going through a tough situation" rather than "Tough it out." If feasible, allow patients to provide input into decisions about care. Identify resources (e.g., case management, community organizations) that can facilitate
Hope	Avoid statements that may exacerbate patient feelings of self-blame. Provide realistic statements of expected positive outcomes: "It will not be easy or fast, but I expect you will recover from your injuries."

Fig. 187.2 Statement or action examples grounded in psychological first-aid principles. (Adapted from: Fischer KR, Bakes KM, Corbin TJ, Fein JA, Harris EJ, James TL, Melzer-Lange MD. Trauma-informed care for violently injured patients in the emergency department. *Annals Emerg Med.* 2019 Feb 1;73(2):193-202.)

be encouraged to contact a local or statewide hotline or the National Human Trafficking Hotline to learn more about available resources.[60]

DISPOSITION

Admission versus Discharge

As with all admissions, the decision to admit a trafficked person should be made in a clinically grounded, patient-centered manner. The reason for admission may be medical; in some cases, health facilities may permit a "social" observation admission in order to carry out complex case management to facilitate a trafficked person's exit from exploitation. As with intimate partner violence, not all trafficked persons recognize or are ready to leave their exploitative situation. This happens for a variety of reasons, including fear of retribution, fear of endangering loved ones, threats of police or immigration involvement, blackmail, as well as trauma bonds. Clinicians may consider utilizing motivational interviewing techniques based on the Stages of Change model to engage the patient and provide support in the decision-making process (Box 187.2). Ultimately, trafficked persons are most knowledgeable about the potential risks involved with seeking help or beginning the process of leaving the trafficking situation and respecting their wishes aligns with trauma-informed care principles.[60]

Safety Planning

Trafficked persons may return to exploitative situations repeatedly before exiting permanently. Involving social workers, case managers, and advocates early in suspected cases of human trafficking helps facilitate safety planning for a patient who is not ready to commit to leaving. Safety planning involves assessing for potential future health risks and identifying strategies for avoiding or reducing the threat of harm when safety is threatened. Safety planning facilitates a sense of trust and safety with the health system and encourages patients to return when ready to access services or for further medical care.

Safety planning varies greatly depending on how the patient views their trafficking situation and whether the patient wants to stay in the situation, is in the process of leaving, or has left.

BOX 187.2   Stages of Change

Stage 1: Precontemplation—Feeling there is no control of your situation
Stage 2: Contemplation—Wondering if there might be a way of managing your situation
Stage 3: Preparation—Researching and planning ways to manage your situation
Stage 4: Action—Taking steps to manage your situation
Stage 5: Maintenance—Continuing positive steps and learning new strategies to maintain your new situation

---

Important determinants in assessing risk include the patient's level of fear and his or her own appraisal of both immediate and future safety needs. The following indicators of escalating lethality risk may be explored with the patient: an increase in the frequency or severity of threats or assaults; increasing or new threats of homicide or suicide by the trafficker if the patient discloses; the presence or availability of a firearm or other lethal weapon; and new or increasingly violent behavior by the perpetrator, including strangulation.[68]

Resources

A follow-up appointment can be a helpful component of safety planning for trafficked persons. This can take a variety of forms, depending on institutional resources, including arranging for an outreach worker (public health nurse or community health worker) to make a follow-up visit or returning to see the ED social worker. The means of conveying post-discharge resources will vary based on the patient's situation; clinicians may consider providing resources verbally to patients or through discrete messaging, while the patient is alone. Examples of discrete resource sharing include writing the human trafficking hotline number on a business card or on a sanitary napkin. Many patients will not be able to leave with written information because their belongings are monitored.

Resources to consider sharing with potential victims of trafficking include information about the National Human Trafficking Hotline which can be accessed 24/7 by texting "INFO" or "HELP" to BEFREE

(233733) or calling 1-888-373-7888 for information or help, though patients should be reminded that smartphones provided to them by the exploiter may be monitored. Other potentially helpful resources include a health system contact number to call or text if the patient wants further assistance; a referral and resource list from community partners for such needs as food, clothing, shelter, housing, social services, and legal services; and an address of local police departments should patients find themselves in imminent danger. Confirming with patients that it is safe for them to take such material with them can signal to patients that the clinician understands the potential gravity of their circumstances. The clinician may discuss with the patient the safest way to communicate with them and carefully consider whether it is safe to contact the patient for follow-up.

Some patients may be unwilling or unable to return for ongoing or follow-up care. For this reason, on discharge the clinician could consider explicitly reassuring patients that they deserve to be safe and free from abuse, that they are not to blame for their circumstance, and that the health care system is "always open" as a source of safe, confidential, and supportive care.[60]

SPECIAL CONSIDERATIONS

Mandatory Reporting

Notably, many human trafficking situations do not fall under mandated reporting requirements. Depending on the state, there may be components of a trafficked person's experience that fall under mandatory reporting laws for abuse of children, disabled adults, and elders; injuries resulting from burns, firearms, or knives; or threats of imminent harm to oneself or another. In certain states, mandatory reporting of sexual assault, domestic violence, or strangulation may come into play. These reporting requirements should be built into institutional human trafficking protocols. Mandated reporting can be executed in a trauma-informed manner, including explaining limits of confidentiality prior to a patient's disclosure, and if a disclosure is made, explaining why reporting is necessary, soliciting patient input into what information will be given to authorities and offering to have the patient present for the conveying of information.[60]

Medical Record Documentation

Because of the complexity of medical-legal issues around human trafficking cases, and great variation in state and local laws, institutions may consider consulting with local prosecutors, defense attorneys, and advocates, particularly those with expertise in privacy and rape shield laws when establishing documentation guidelines.

Depending on the legal climate, entering more or less information in the patient's chart can either be helpful or harmful. In some cases, accurate documentation can potentially substitute for, or supplement, the clinician's personal testimony in court. Alternatively, information in the medical record can potentially be harmful to the patient when the case goes to trial (e.g., if a trafficked person contracts HIV, in some states they could be criminalized for the transmission of HIV). In many jurisdictions, crimes committed by trafficked persons while under the control of their trafficker will be prosecuted (e.g., a patient coerced to sell sex may still be charged with prostitution). Sensitive information in the medical record may or may not be redacted during a court hearing or trial depending on whether the state has a rape shield law, and if that state has determined that the rape shield law applies to trafficking victims. It may be difficult to balance the need for inclusive information with medico-legal discretion. For example, obtaining information about prior injuries, consensual sex, number of partners, and STIs may influence the clinician's work-up, examination, and the anticipatory guidance, but documentation of these data may be used against the patient in certain legal circumstances.[60]

Inclusion of victim quotes in the medical record is often advised in cases of injury or sexual assault, but such details about a victim's story may not be helpful should they change their account later, which is a common phenomenon when someone has experienced trauma. Keeping the documentation of history simple can prevent insignificant points from becoming a disputed fact in a legal case. Similar to cases of sexual assault, careful documentation of the physical examination includes signs of abuse such as old scars, surgical incisions, birthmarks, skin lesions, tattoos, and piercings.[60]

Diagnostic Codification

The International Classification of Diseases, 10th Revision, Clinical Modification (ICD-10-CM) released the first ever trafficking-specific abuse codes in October 2018 developed through a partnership between the American Hospital Association, Catholic Health Initiatives, and Massachusetts General Hospital.[69] Inclusion of one of these 29 ICD-10 abuse codes for forced labor and sexual exploitation, when appropriate and relevant as a finding, diagnosis, or problem, may help strengthen data collection on human trafficking in the health care system and inform the allocation of resources and future development of services equipped to respond to the needs of trafficking victims and survivors. Care must be taken to ensure that the use of these codes does not stigmatize or cause harm to already traumatized survivors.[69a]

Law Enforcement Considerations

Many trafficked persons have a negative or fearful perception of law enforcement (LE) officials because of previous arrests, fear of arrest or deportation, or abuses imposed by authority figures, so a thoughtful approach to law enforcement engagement with suspected human trafficking cases is advised. Law enforcement involvement should be limited to patient request, in state-specific mandated reporting scenarios that require LE involvement, or when clinicians appreciate imminent danger to staff or the patient.[60] In cases where LE involvement is mandated by law, trust and rapport can be safeguarded by ensuring a transparent, predictable, and non-retraumatizing process. It is not advisable, however, for providers to promise safety.

Barriers to Identification and Care

Trafficked persons generally do not self-identify as victims of human trafficking. In some cases, trafficked persons may not recognize their victimization, especially when cultural practices or beliefs cast a sense of normalcy on their circumstances (e.g., gender inequality, domestic violence, sex work).[14,25,70] In other cases, the victim narrative may not resonate with trafficked persons due to its failure to accurately capture their experience of and relationship to their trafficker, particularly when emotional or romantic bonds exist (e.g., parent, family member, boyfriend).[70] Still, in other cases, a trafficked person may outright reject the label of victim, opting instead for more empowering interpretations of their trafficking experiences.[70] Nevertheless, even when the trafficked person is acutely aware of their victimization and desires assistance, disclosure and engagement in care is hampered by shame, fear of physical retaliation, fear of harm to loved ones, fear of immigration authorities, and fear of police if compelled to commit crimes as part of their exploitation (e.g., shoplifting, drug selling, peer recruitment into trafficking).[14,17,53,71]

A recent systematic review on health care access barriers found that extrinsic, intrinsic, and structural barriers contribute to the reluctance among trafficked youth to access care.[72] Barriers identified included trafficker control, physical confinement, diminished trust in health care providers, concerns over discrimination, lack of confidentiality, language barriers, and complex registration process.[72] Similarly, a mixed-methods study identified three distinct profiles of survivor

Key element	Preparedness actions
Multidisciplinary teams	Identify champions among the key stakeholders whose discipline, expertise, local knowledge of the problem, and community partnership will enhance preparedness and response (e.g., medical, nursing, mental health, social work, child protection, forensic examiners, legal counsel, security, risk management).
Institutional policy	Adopt an institutional policy that is survivor-centered, based on available evidence or "promising practices," and in accordance with applicable state mandatory reporting laws.
Resources compendium	Create and maintain an up-to-date database of hospital and community resources available to address the varying needs of trafficking survivors.
Network partnerships	Partner with law enforcement, government agencies, social service organizations, hospital-based services, and other community stakeholders to determine best practices for collaboration and referrals, and more effectively serve survivors.
Response protocol	Develop a stepwise algorithm that leverages interdisciplinary teams, promotes a trauma-informed care approach, and accounts for the unique needs of adults and children when responding to the disclosure or identification of a trafficked patient.
Knowledge, training, and quality & safety	Establish mechanisms for knowledge dissemination (i.e., human trafficking and trauma-informed care education), response protocol implementation training, monitoring and evaluation of response incidents, evaluation of quality and safety gaps and opportunities, and protocol revisions when needed and appropriate.

Fig. 187.3 Health care preparedness: framework for developing human trafficking response protocols. (Adapted from: Macias-Konstantopoulos W. Human trafficking: the role of medicine in interrupting the cycle of abuse and violence. *Annals Internal Med.* 2016;165(8):582-588.)

experiences and engagement with health care: avoidant, distrustful, and constrained. Common across the three profiles was a feeling of disenfranchisement that contributed to decreased care access behaviors.[73] Trauma-informed, culturally sensitive, and survivor-centered care practices may mitigate this sense of disenfranchisement by minimizing retraumatization, fostering psycho emotional safety and well-being, and empowering survivors in their recovery.[73]

Studies have established that the ED is a significant health care access point for trafficked persons.[74] Identification is central to a more comprehensive and effective health care response for this patient population. One of the most consequential barriers to identification and care is the lack of formal human trafficking curricula in education and training which reinforces an underappreciation of its relevance to clinical practice, perpetuates a gap in knowledge and skill, and leads to preconceived biases about who victims are and what they look like. Other barriers include failure to establish trust, interview the patient alone, use professional interpreters, recognize red flags, and carry out more in-depth assessments.[17,53] This gap in knowledge and skill not only places the emergency practitioner at a disadvantage in caring for trafficking survivors, but also may place the trafficked patient at greater risk of harm if the provider proceeds with the evaluation and response in a manner that is unsafe, no matter how well-intentioned. A focus on education and training has been growing in the last decade.[36,75-80]

Similarly, there has been increased advocacy for clinical guidelines and protocols that guide a safe, effective, and comprehensive response, including the need for trauma-informed care, patient privacy, professional interpreters, mandatory reporting when appropriate (e.g., children), and referrals to national and local community resources for unmet needs.[53,80] Existing protocols for identifying and assisting trafficking patients in hospitals across the United States vary widely.[62] A "health care preparedness" framework for the development of response protocols proposes six main elements: interdisciplinary teams, survivor-centered institutional policy based on evidence or promising practices, collaborations and partnerships with community resources and cross-sector agencies, a stepwise trauma-informed response algorithm, and a plan for provider education/training and quality assurance of response protocols (Fig. 187.3).[53]

The ED visit represents a critical opportunity for trafficked persons to receive assistance and a potentially life-altering intervention. Through universal adoption of trauma-informed principles, labor and sex trafficking education, and development of multidisciplinary policies and procedures, emergency clinicians can positively impact the lives and health of trafficked patients.

The references for this chapter can be found online at ExpertConsult. com.

188

Sexual Minority Populations (LGBTQ)

Joel Moll and Carolyn Kluwe Holland

KEY CONCEPTS

- Sexual orientation, gender identity, and gender expression occur along a continuum and may be completely separate and discordant from one another.
- Multiple health disparities exist in sexual minority populations, but many of the contributing factors are likely unknown due to lack of studies.
- ED provider education about sexual minorities is often inadequate, limited, or absent.
- Transgender individuals may utilize a variety of medical and surgical interventions in their transition to affirm their gender identity. Emergency clinicians should be aware of complications related to these practices that may require treatment in the ED.
- Sexual minority patients at extremes of age, or who share another minority identity, have additional disparities that require consideration to deliver equitable and safe care.
- Open, inclusive, and nonjudgmental patient-centered communication using appropriate terminology is fundamental to fostering provider trust and minimizing health disparities in sexual minorities.

FOUNDATIONS

Background and Importance

Sexual minority individuals cross every demographic, and multiple cultural and societal influences can affect their visibility and disclosure of sexual and gender identity. They represent a diverse continuum of individuals without a strict heterosexual identity (lesbian, gay, bisexual. queer, or questioning [LGBTQ]) and include those whose gender identity is different or fluid from their sex-based gender assigned at birth. Although sexual minorities share many similarities, there are also key differences. There is a wide range of perceptions on the prevalence of sexual minorities in the United States (US). This reflects societal bias, lack of research, and barriers to disclosing or collecting data regarding an individual's sexual and gender identities. One recent estimate is that 4.5% or 11 million Americans identify as a sexual minority,[1] and at least 0.6% or 1.4 million identify as transgender.[2,3] Importantly, sexual and gender identities should be considered separate from sexual behavior. It is estimated that 8.7% of women and 8.2% of men have had same-sex sexual behavior.[4]

Terminology and Concepts

To create a welcome and inclusive environment for sexual minorities, health care providers should be familiar with culturally competent terminology to better communicate and avoid unintentional offense (Table 188.1). Providers should avoid terms associated with bias or prejudice. Terms like "homosexual" or "sexual preference" may be common in language, but have stigma when used in the sexual minority community. The use of the word "homosexual" is associated with past bias and discrimination; therefore preferred terms include lesbian, gay, or bisexual. Similarly, because there is no legitimate evidence that sexual orientation is a choice, the term "sexual preference" should not be used. Patients should be asked about their partner(s) in gender neutral terms without assuming that they are in a heterosexual relationship. Asking open-ended questions will signal being receptive to patients not in traditional heterosexual relationships or gender identities. When in doubt, ask the patient for their preferred terms, or allow them to define their relationships.

Historical Context

Same-sex relationships and transgender identity have existed throughout recorded history, although societal acceptance and tolerance has varied over time. Laws and attitudes against same-sex sexual behavior were common in the United States, which adversely influenced attitudes of health care providers and isolated sexual minorities from medical care. Despite recent increased acceptance of sexual minorities, past actions and discrimination can still be a powerful barrier to equitable care. Although the majority of Americans support sexual minority rights,[5] it is far from universal, and continued implicit and explicit bias along with outright discrimination and refusal of care still exist. Basic health care rights and choices assumed by the majority are often not afforded to sexual minorities, or are incomplete. Some forms of discrimination, including employment discrimination, are still legal in many states, making patient-provider trust and confidentiality of substantial importance to the sexual minority patient. Emergency care providers should be prepared to assure LGBTQ patients of laws protecting their medical records from disclosure.

Identity

Sexual minorities undergo a deeply personal process of accepting their sexual orientation or gender identity and then disclosing it to the outside world, known as "coming out." This process should occur on the patient's own terms and timeline. Since many individuals who engage in same-sex behaviors may never identify themselves as a sexual minority for a variety of reasons, clinicians should inquire about specific sexual activity and not just sexual orientation or identity when it is pertinent to their clinical presentation.

Legal identity and the patient's gender identity may be discordant for transgender patients, leading to confusion and discomfort. If the patient's insurance uses their gender assigned at birth, their preferred name and gender may not appear in many electronic health records (EHRs), and services and prescriptions using their preferred name and gender may not be covered. Few transgender people have all of their identification materials with their preferred name and gender, and for 68% none of their identification reflects their preferred name and gender, financial costs being one of the largest barriers to acquiring updated identification.[6] Creating an inclusive environment

TABLE 188.1   Terms and Definitions for Sexual Minorities

	Term	Definition
General Terms	Sexual Minority	Term for the diverse group of people whose sexual orientation and gender identity fall on a spectrum outside of strictly heterosexual and/or their gender identity of sex at birth
	Sex	Biologically male or female
	Gender	Psychological, behavioral, and cultural characteristics of being male or female
	Queer	Overarching term for sexual minorities
	Questioning	Person unsure of sexual and/or gender identities
Sexual Attraction	Gay	Man or woman who identifies as someone with sexual attraction to the same sex
	Lesbian	Woman who identifies as someone with sexual attraction to the same sex
	Bisexual	Man or woman who identifies as someone with sexual attraction to both men and women. This attraction may be more female or male.
	Sexually Fluid	Identity is not fixed as purely opposite or same-sex attraction
Gender	Gender Identity	Identity along a spectrum from female to male
	Gender Expression	Expressions and behavior of traits traditionally associated with women or men
	Cisgender	Gender identity is similar to identity associated with sex at birth
	Transgender, Trans, or Gender Nonconforming	Gender identity is different or opposite of identity associated with sex at birth
	Gender Affirming	Behaviors or interventions to affirm gender identity
	Transitioning	Undergoing interventions to affirm gender identity different from gender associated with sex at birth

without assumptions or judgment about identity will best promote an honest and trusting dialogue that will enhance health decisions and care.

SPECIFIC ISSUES

Factors Affecting Equitable Care

Legal Barriers

Legal issues can affect sexual minority patients' care in unique ways. Prior to marriage equality, many same-sex couples completed legal documents to provide some of the rights automatically provided by marriage. These issues include medical decision making and hospital visitation rights. Despite these documents, the wishes of patients were not always respected by hospitals, courts, or families. In 2010, the Department of Health and Human Services prohibited hospitals that participate in Medicare or Medicaid from denying visitation on the basis of race, color, national origin, religion, sex, sexual orientation, gender identity, or disability.[7] Marriage equality in 2015 provided the opportunity for stronger and automatic protections previously denied to same-sex couples; however, only 50% of same-sex couples' households are legally married compared to over 90% of heterosexual households[8,9] Same-sex spouses in the ED should be given the same level of access to health care information, decision making, and visitation as married heterosexual couples without having to provide a marriage certificate to prove their relationship status. Additionally, unmarried same-sex couples who have completed legally structured powers-of-attorney for health care and finance should have those documents respected and followed to the fullest extent of local and state laws.

Sexual Minority Parental Barriers

Up to 3.7 million children under 18 years old have an LGBTQ parent, with 200,000 being raised by same-sex couples. This represents approximately 16% of all same-sex couples (8% of male and 24% of female same-sex couples), while almost 40% of heterosexual coupled households have children.[10] These same-sex couples with children are far more likely to have an adopted child (20%) or foster child (3%) than majority couples (3%, 0.4% respectively).[8]

Legal recognition of parenthood is currently derived from marriage, adoption, or biology. Even with marriage equality, not all states recognize the same rights of parenthood to nonbiological parents. The legal recognition of nonbiological married same-sex parents varies state by state, and there are no requirements for a different state to recognize a legal tie between parent and child granted elsewhere. Additionally, some states will allow a single LGBTQ person to adopt a child, but will not allow the second parent to also be named as a legal guardian. This can leave same-sex parents in a precarious position when trying to access health care for their children.[11] Until there are consistent standards that provide clear legal status to nonbiological same-sex parents, health care providers need to be aware of and follow their local laws as they relate to consent for procedures and treatments.

In additional to lack of standardized legal recognition of nonbiological parents of children born to same-sex couples, there are other barriers to obtaining health care for these families. On arrival to the emergency department (ED), registration forms and the EHR often are not structured to accommodate same-sex couples. Typically, there are data fields to document a mother or father, but not two mothers or two fathers. This may keep providers from having accurate information about a child's family structure, and may put one parent in the position of not having decision-making authority concerning the child's medical care.[12] Heteronormative assumptions about adults accompanying a child in the ED may cause a provider to not recognize that a full family is present by assuming that the second adult is a nonparent relative or family friend.[12] Nonbiological parents may fear their lack of genetic ties to the child could cause them to be inappropriately ineligible to make health decisions for their child.[13] By focusing on a child's genetic parentage and not the legal and emotional relationships that make a family, nonbiological parents from same-sex couples feel a lack of respect for their family which can act as a barrier to full and candid communication between providers and parents.

Remedies to these described barriers include the development of cultural competency in the health care team and adaptation of the EHR and paper forms to accommodate all family structures and parent roles. Cuing from the EHR about unique family structures can alert providers to be mindful of how and to whom questions are asked about the child, and assist in the collection of relevant information without inadvertently offending parents.

Barriers to Health Care Access

Sexual minority patients have less access to health care than their majority counterparts. They are less likely to have health insurance and more likely to live in poverty. Patients may fear sensitive information being disclosed to their employer, and if they have insurance, it may not cover gender affirming treatment. These factors can lead to delays in medical diagnosis and treatment. A quarter of transgender patients experience health insurance–related problems, including being denied coverage for nonemergent care due to their transgender status.[6] One in ten transgender people report having access to a bathroom denied to them, and may experience verbal harassment and even physical or sexual assault when accessing a restroom.[6] A third of transgender people have limited their fluid intake to avoid public restrooms, resulting in 8% reporting urinary tract infections due to avoidance and holding urine.[6]

Health Care Experience

Many sexual minorities report negative experiences in navigating the health care system, especially among the transgender population, leading to avoidance and delay of care.[14,15] In a small survey of transgender individuals in Ontario, Canada, half felt that presenting as their stated gender had prompted negative experiences in the ED, leading 21% to avoid visiting an ED in the future.[15] This was also demonstrated in the 2015 US Transgender Survey where 33% had at least one negative experience related to their transgender status, and 23% reported avoiding needed health care.[6,16] Issues include: being "misgendered" even after disclosing their gender identity; lack of provider knowledge about transgender health, including hormone effects; unnecessary questions about gender-related surgeries for unrelated chief complaints; and a persistent focus on genital examinations.[17,18] In the San Francisco area, where LGBTQ individuals are more visible than in many other regions, most practicing nurses had very little understanding of gender-related terminology, and many health care organizations did not have inclusive forms or standard language to discuss transgender patient issues.[2] However, despite these experiences, for some sexual minorities the anonymity of the ED may be preferred over their primary care physician, who may not be aware of their sexual behaviors or gender identity. Limited research suggests increased ED utilization among some sexual minorities compared to their majority counterparts.[19,20] Because the majority of these patients are in relationships, partners should be included in health discussions if desired by the patient.

Provider Education

A significant number of sexual minority patients do not disclose their sexual orientation, same-sex sexual behavior, or gender identity to their physician. A mix of societal, patient, and provider factors account for this nondisclosure. Prior to 2019, the Model of the Clinical Practice of Emergency Medicine (EM) jointly developed by the major EM organizations and published by the American Board of Emergency Medicine did not specifically include sexual minority health, and medical school and EM residency training often offers limited, if any, sexual minority education. Recent initiatives have been undertaken to determine needs and knowledge gaps. One study of EM residents found that 43% felt obtaining history and physical examinations from transgender patients was more challenging, and 25% felt similarly about LGB patients.[21] Most EM residents did not ask patients about sexual orientation or sexual behaviors even when pertinent to the chief complaint (e.g., abdominal or genitourinary concerns). Another survey of emergency physicians found that although most cared for transgender patients,

few had formal training regarding their health needs or care. More than half asked patients about gender affirming surgeries, regardless of the chief complaint. Only 9% could identify the most commonly used non-hormonal medication used by female transgender patients (spironolactone), and only 26% could identify the most commonly used surgery by male transgender patients (mastectomy with thoracoplasty).[22] One should take an organ and hormone inventory only when relevant to the complaint. Similarly, when related to the presenting condition, one should inquire about sexual partners, specific sexual practices, and sexually transmitted infections (STIs; past diagnoses, use of protection) to improve health care to sexual minority patients.[23]

All emergency health care providers should receive training on LGBTQ inclusion and cultural competency. Education on terminology, sex differentiation, hormone therapy, mitigation of personal bias, and creating a safe environment has been shown to improve knowledge of, comfort with, and attitudes toward sexual minorities.[24,25] Creating an atmosphere of inclusion is fundamental to candid health care conversations and providing equitable and competent care.[26]

Health Disparities

Sexual minorities have the same basic health care requirements as others, but also have specific health needs intrinsic to their sexual orientation, gender identity, and behavior. Obstacles to equitable health can lead to health care disparities. The Minority Stress Model, described by Meyer, explains that minority groups, including sexual minorities, experience chronically high levels of stress from societal stigmatization. Sexual minority health disparities adversely affect both physical and mental health (Table 188.2). Higher prevalence of mood and substance abuse disorders result from increased stress caused by discrimination, rejection, and the adoption of societies' negative attitudes toward oneself. Research on disparities is limited, due in part to infrequent collection of sexual orientation or gender identity data, so many disparities are likely currently unidentified.

When considering health disparities among sexual minorities, HIV infection is often the focus despite the fact that the vast majority are HIV negative. However, in 2017, 70% of new cases of HIV were among men who have sex with men (MSM), making treatment and prevention important considerations.[27] One in six MSM who are HIV positive are unaware of their status.[27] Intimate partner violence among MSM has been associated with riskier sexual practices and increased risk of sexually transmitted infections, including HIV.[28] Men who have receptive anal sex are 13 times more at risk for HIV transmission than those who have insertive anal sex.[27] Sexually active MSM should be tested for HIV at least annually, or more frequently based on individual risk.[29] HIV treatment is paramount since an undetectable viral load markedly decreases the risk of transmission to seronegative partners, and treatment can significantly prolong life. Unfortunately, only 62% of HIV-positive MSM are receiving treatment, and only 52% have achieved viral suppression at levels that decrease transmission.[30] ED HIV testing and referral can provide an impactful opportunity on sexual minority health care. Additionally, pre and postexposure prophylaxis against HIV can provide further risk reduction, and has been shown to be effective and well tolerated.[31] Tenofovir disoproxil fumarate and emtricitabine (Truvada) is the only FDA-approved regimen for preexposure prophylaxis (PrEP).[32] Emergency care providers should be trained and prepared to prescribe these treatments for at-risk individuals.

Transgender Health

Health care delivery to a transgender patient can be challenging for providers due to lack of education and familiarity with transgender health (Table 188.3). Transgender individuals who are "out" or are

TABLE 188.2 Known Health Disparities for Sexual Minorities

	Gay Men	Lesbians	Bisexual	Transgender
Cardiovascular	↑Heart Disease[58] ↑Hypertension[58]	↑Heart Disease[20] ↑Hyperlipidemia[20] ↑Stroke[58]		↑Heart Disease (trans♀) ↑Hyperlipidemia[38] ↑Hypertension[38] ↑Thromboembolic Disease[33] (trans♀)
Endocrine		↑Diabetes[20] ↑Obesity/BMI[58,59]		↑Diabetes[38] ↑Obesity/ BMI[33,38]
Gastro Intestinal	↑Hepatitis[60]	↑Hepatitis[60]		↑Gallstones[33] (trans♀)
Hematology Oncology	↑Anal Cancer[61] ↑Kaposi Sarcoma	↑Breast Cancer[62] ↑Lung Cancer[62]		Polycythemia (trans♂)[38]
Infectious Disease	↑HIV ↑Rectal GC[63] ↑Hepatitis A, B, C[62] ↑HPV[64]		↑Hepatitis A, B, C♂[62]	
Mental Health	↑Mood Disorders[20,62] ↑Suicidality and Suicide Attempts[62] ↑Eating Disorders[65]	↑Mood Disorders[62,66] ↑Suicidality and Suicide Attempts[62,67] ↑Eating Disorders[65]	↑Mood Disorder[62,66] ↑Suicidality and Suicide Attempts ♀[67] ↑Eating Disorders[65]	↑Suicidality and Suicide[6]
Pulmonary		↑Asthma[20]	↑COPD[60]	↑COPD[68]
Safety	↑Sexual assault[69] ↑IPV-↓reporting[70] ↑Homelessness[71]	↑Sexual assault[69] ↑IPV[70] ↑Homelessness[71]	↑Sexual assault[69] ↑IPV[70] ↑Homelessness[71]	↑Sexual assault[6] ↑IPV[6] ↑Homelessness[6]
Substance Use	↑Heavy Drinking[72] ↑Moderate Smoking[72] ↑Lifetime Pain Reliever Misuse[73]	↑Heavy Drinking[58] ↑Heavy Smoking[72] ↑Lifetime Pain Reliever Misuse[73] ↑Lifetime Heroin Misuse[73] ↑Lifetime IV Heroin Misuse[73]	↑Heavy Drinking[72] ↑Heavy Smoking[72] ↑Moderate Smoking ♀[72] ↑Lifetime Pain Reliever Misuse[73] ↑Lifetime Heroin Misuse[73] ↑Lifetime IV Heroin Misuse[73]	↑Heavy Drinking[74] ↑Heavy Smoking[74] ↑Lifetime Pain Reliever Misuse[74]
Other	↑Arthritis[60] ↑Sleep Disturbances[75]	↑Arthritis[72] ↑Sleep Disturbances[75] ↑Pregnant Unmet Health Needs[76]	↑Sleep Disturbances[75]	↑Acne (trans♂)[38] ↑Sleep Disturbances[68] Osteoporosis[77] (trans♀)

TABLE 188.3 Best Practices in Caring for Transgender Patients

Area	Best Practice
Registration	Collect sexual orientation and gender identity so health needs can be identified early. Include preferred pronouns and name to be utilized during their ED visit.[17]
Identification	Call for patients by their last name only without the use of gender prefixes when in group settings such as waiting rooms.[17]
Scripting	Use standardized scripts to facilitate cultural sensitivity for sexual and gender minorities.[78]
Health Records	EHRs should have the ability to record and display preferred name and pronouns of patients for all users in all views. Once a patient has legal documents that reflect their gender identity and chosen name, indicators of transgender status should be removed from the view of casual users.
Organ and Hormone Inventory	Information about a patient's transition history, including an inventory of organs and hormone use information, are best stored in the medical/surgical history of the EHR.[79,34]
Accommodation	Restrooms should be defined as gender-neutral, or have specific signage and policies that patients may choose either the women's or men's room based on their own preference and identity. If patients have to choose a gendered bathroom, making at least one gender-neutral/all-gendered bathroom available will be helpful and supportive to nonbinary patients as well as those patients who are in transition.[34,17]
Patient Room	Patients should have single-occupancy rooms.

perceived as transgender experience verbal harassment (54%), physical assault (24%), and sexual assault (13%) because of their gender identity. Forty percent of transgender individuals have attempted suicide, almost nine times the rate of the general population.[6] Many transgender people have challenges with their families or religious communities and experience psychological stress due to rejection from previous sources of nurturing and support. Ten percent of transgender people report violence from an immediate family member, 8% have been kicked out of their homes, and 20% leave their spiritual or religious community due to rejection based on their gender identity.[6] Nearly a third of transgender people live in poverty, compared to 12% of the general US population.

Medical Gender Affirming Therapy and Complications

Transgender Female. For the transgender female, medical gender affirmation therapy commonly includes hormone supplementation with androgen blocking medication, in conjunction with estrogen in physiologic doses. The most commonly used androgen blocker in the United States is spironolactone, with alternative androgen blocking medications including 5-alpha reductase inhibitors (finasteride, dutasteride). Outside the United States, cyproterone acetate, a synthetic progestogen commonly used in the treatment for prostate cancer, is used as an androgen blocker. Options for estradiol administration include daily oral or sublingual, weekly transdermal, or biweekly intramuscular (IM) dosing. Use of feminizing hormone therapy for transgender women is considered off-label, and may need to be administered in higher doses than normally used in postmenopausal cisgender women.[33] Additionally, some transgender women may also take progestogens to enhance breast development, mood, or libido. Common changes seen with the implementation of hormone therapy include breast development, facial and body subcutaneous fat redistribution, muscle mass reduction, body hair reduction, and slowing or reversal of scalp hair loss. Erectile dysfunction, decreased or absent sperm count, and reduced testicular size also occur.[33] Some transgender women still produce sperm even in the setting of androgen blockade and estrogen use, and are at risk for causing an unplanned pregnancy if they are engaging in sexual activity that could cause fertilization.[33] Transgender women who went through puberty and had exposure to testosterone will not have complete elimination of male patterned facial or body hair, change in skeletal bone structure, or change in pitch of their voice with hormone therapy alone. These individuals require specific interventions such as plastic surgery, laser hair removal or electrolysis, and voice therapy.

Although the use of estrogen and progesterone are associated with mental health conditions among cisgender women, such as premenstrual dysphoric disorder, this does not appear to occur in transgender women. The use of feminizing hormones does likely lead to increased risk for cardiovascular disease and diabetes when other risk factors are present. Additionally, venous thromboembolism (VTE), gall stones, elevated liver enzymes, and weight gain are exacerbated in individuals taking supraphysiologic doses of estrogen feminizing hormones. Estrogen should be discontinued during the acute treatment of VTE.[34] While the use of progestogens in combination with estrogens is associated with increased cardiovascular events and breast cancer in postmenopausal cisgender women, there are no specific studies defining this risk in transgender women.[33] There is also no conclusive increased risk for breast cancer.[33,35] There is a theoretical pro-growth impact of estrogen on human testicular cells; however, there is no specific link between exogenous estrogen and testicular cancer risk.[36]

"Tucking" of testicles and the penis provides a more feminine appearing contour of the genital area and involves manually displacing the testes into the inguinal canal followed by positioning of the penis and scrotal skin between the legs directed rearward toward the anus. The position is maintained with tight underwear, tape, or a special garment known as a gaff, with some transgender women staying "tucked" up to 24 hours per day. Prolonged tucking is associated with increased risk of urinary tract infections.[34]

Injection of very small amounts of medical-grade free silicone with the intent of causing local reaction of fibroblasts and collagen growth is often used in the management of HIV-related lipodystrophy. In the transgender community, "silicone injections" may involve the injection of up to 3 liters of a variety of non–medical grade substances such as aircraft lubricant, tire sealant, window caulk, mineral oil, methyl acrylates, or petroleum jelly.[37] An estimated 20% to 50% of transgender women may have received these injections from nonmedical providers in their efforts to relieve their gender dysphoria and have immediate body changes that conform to their gender identity. Unfortunately, this practice often leads to significant immediate, early, and late-term health consequences (Table 188.4). Patients may not be forthcoming with information about having received filler injections in a nonmedical setting, so health care providers must be diligent in determining if injections might be a possible cause of patients' symptoms.

Transgender Male. The most common gender affirming medical treatment utilized by transgender men is testosterone. It can be administered IM, subcutaneously, or topically. With topical use, there is a modest risk of exposure to other people from skin to skin contact, and caution should be taken around patients with more sensitivity to testosterone such as pregnant women and small children.[38] Adjuvant therapies include progestogens, 5-alpha reductase inhibitors, aromatase inhibitors, gonadotropin-releasing hormone antagonists, and direct application of topical testosterone to the clitoris.[38] Use of hormone replacement therapy mimics male puberty, taking 4 to 5 years for full

TABLE 188.4	Silicone Injection Adverse Effects and Complications
Immediate	• Bleeding, pain, focal tissue necrosis, hypersensitivity reactions • Silicone embolization causing ARDS, multisystem organ failure, or loss of limbs
Early Onset *days to weeks*	All of the immediate adverse events, PLUS • Infected inflammatory nodules that may be fluctuant • Angioedema • Non-inflamed nodules that are painful, pruritic, and cause hypopigmentation
Long Term *weeks to years*	All of the immediate and early adverse events, PLUS • Nodules (inflamed and non-inflamed) may form sterile abscesses or fistulae • Migration of silicone causing pain or deformity • Silicone granulomas • Hypercalcemia • Sepsis, hypersensitivity pneumonitis, immune reconstitution inflammatory syndrome (IRIS) • Organ failure from direct mass effects

effect. Clitoral growth starts in as soon as 3 months and peaks at 1 to 2 years. Some may also try off label use of dihydrotesterone (DHT) to enhance clitoromegaly. Menses usually stop after 3 to 6 months of testosterone treatment, but this is dose dependent.

Transmen who were amenorrhoeic from testosterone may also present with new vaginal bleeding. This may be due to inadequate suppression of menses by the testosterone, but evaluation for pregnancy, infection, or malignancy, and gynecologic consultation may be necessary.[38] Testosterone provides ineffective birth control. In transgender men who became pregnant, 60% used testosterone prior to pregnancy, 20% conceived while amenorrhoeic from testosterone, and 32% of the pregnancies were unplanned.[39] If transgender men engage in vaginal receptive intercourse, they should use contraception such as condoms, progesterone-only birth control, or a hormonal IUD.[38] Testosterone is contraindicated in pregnancy and should be discontinued immediately if the pregnancy is desired.

Transgender men may also experience vaginal atrophy similar to that which occurs in postmenopausal women.[38] Atrophic vaginal tissue with decreased tissue resiliency and an altered microbial environment can be present due to relative estrogen deficiency. This can lead to bacterial vaginosis, cystitis, or cervicitis. Treatment with vaginal estrogen for symptom relief and comfort is appropriate, and should be accompanied by reassurance that the minimal systemic absorption of estrogen should not interfere with masculinization effects of testosterone. If patients are uncomfortable with intravaginal administration, they can just apply the estrogen cream on their external genitalia.

Transgender men on masculinizing hormones should have their labs interpreted based on standard male values, except for hemoglobin values. If the patient is still having menses, their hemoglobin should be interpreted relative to female values. Use of masculinizing hormones leads to an increased risk for polycythemia, weight gain, acne, androgenic alopecia, and sleep apnea. Additionally, there are possible increased risks for elevated liver enzymes, hypercholesterolemia, cardiovascular disease, hypertension, and diabetes if additional factors are present. Psychiatric disorders that include manic or psychotic symptoms may have an increased risk of destabilization from masculinizing hormones. There is no conclusive increased risk for bone density loss, breast cancer, cervical cancer, ovarian cancer, or uterine cancer.[35,38]

Masculinizing hormone treatment may not shrink breasts, and thus transmen may bind their breasts with tight-fitting sports bras, shirts, ace bandages or specially made binders to flatten the contour of the chest. Larger-breasted people may use multiple garments at the same time, which can lead to pain, diminished respiratory capacity, skin breakdown, or fungal infections.[40] Sensitive and appropriate history taking and physical examination of patients who may be reluctant to remove bindings is key to providing culturally competent care and allowing a discussion about safe binding.[34]

Surgical Gender Affirming Therapy and Complications

Transgender Women. Gender affirming surgeries for transgender women included genital procedures such as orchiectomy, vaginoplasty involving the creation of a neovagina, clitoris, urethral rerouting, and labiaplasty, most commonly using the penile inversion technique. Nongenital procedures commonly seen include breast augmentation, facial feminization with plastic surgery, and reduction thyroid chondroplasty to decrease prominence of the "Adam's apple."[33] Of note, the prostate is generally not removed with any of these procedures, so health maintenance including screening for prostate cancer is still required.

Transgender Men. Mastectomy is one of the most commonly requested surgery by transgender men. They experience the same rate and type of complications as cisgender women who have mastectomies.[41] Genital surgical procedures include metoidioplasty

(movement of the hypertrophied clitoris anteriorly to a normal penile position) and phalloplasty (construction of a neophallus using free and/or pedicled flaps). Complications of both procedures include spraying or dribbling of urine, urethral strictures or fistulas, and, with phalloplasty, the additional risk of vascular compromise of the flap and necrosis.[38]

Physical Examination

Examination of a neovagina in a transgender woman involves looking at a blind cuff that lacks a cervix or surrounding fornices. It may be more posteriorly oriented than expected. Using an anoscope instead of a vaginal speculum may provide a more anatomic approach. Once inserted, the trocar can be removed from the anoscope, and direct visualization of the walls of the neovagina can occur as it is withdrawn and the walls collapse around the end of the anoscope.[34]

Physicians evaluating transgender men who present with complaints of pelvic pain should take the same general anatomic based approach as a non-transgender woman, considering urologic, gynecologic, gastrointestinal, musculoskeletal, and psychiatric causes. Recognizing that transgender men may engage in receptive vaginal sex, a comprehensive sexual history including specific behaviors (vaginal-vaginal contact, vaginal or anal or receptive penile sex) should be collected.[42] Pregnancy should also be considered in any patient who still has a uterus and ovaries. Explaining that pregnancy testing is part of a standard protocol may ameliorate any offense taken by patients who deny any sexual activity with a partner capable of insemination.[34]

Even when medically necessary, having a pelvic examination can be traumatic and anxiety provoking for transgender men. It may have been a long time since their last exam, and they may not be up to date on screening for cervical cancer or STIs. Techniques for decreasing discomfort with pelvic exam include: discussing the procedure beforehand; allowing the patient to have a support person in the room; directly explaining each step before performing it; using the patient's terms for their body parts instead of medical terms. Some transgender men may decline speculum exam, transvaginal ultrasound, or bimanual exams as it may exacerbate their gender dysphoria. If the patient requires a transvaginal ultrasound, a low-dose benzodiazepine may be considered in conjunction with the application of lidocaine ointment to the vulva and vagina prior to the procedure. Having the patient insert the intravaginal ultrasound themselves may also facilitate a transvaginal ultrasound.[34]

Special Populations
Youth

Sexual minority youth have similar health disparities as adults; however, they also face challenges unique to their developmental stage and vulnerable position. In addition to typical formative milestones, LGBTQ adolescents are challenged by the realization that their sexual attraction and/or gender identity may be different than what is expected of them by their parents, peers, or society. Parents, peers, and medical providers may lack insight or knowledge into the complexities of their situation, and heteronormative assumptions may cause unintended harm. Youth can become disconnected from support and social networks by self-isolation or rejection. In 2017, the Youth Risk Behavior Surveillance study found that sexual minority youth reported much higher rates of mistreatment than their heterosexual counterparts.[43] One-third of LGBTQ teens were bullied at school, 27% were bullied electronically, 30% were victims of physical violence, and 22% experienced sexual violence.[43] Ten percent of LGBTQ students had missed school due to safety concerns.[43] Sexual minority adolescents also have an increased rate of mental health disorders, substance abuse, STIs, and self-harm or risky behaviors compared to majority adolescents.[44]

While 13% of heterosexual students contemplate suicide, the number rises to 48% of sexual minority youth.[43] Up to 40% of homeless youth identify as LGBTQ.[44]

For transgender youth, puberty-suppressing medications may be prescribed. The purpose is to allow more time to explore their gender identity and other developmental issues, and potentially facilitate future transition by preventing the development of secondary sex characteristics, such as facial hair, breasts, or deepened voice. These secondary sex characteristics are otherwise difficult to impossible to reverse if the person later chooses to pursue gender confirming procedures. Adolescent patients with male genitalia may be taking gonadotropin-releasing hormone analogues to stop luteinizing hormone secretion, or medications that block secretion or action of testosterone, such as progestins. Adolescent patients with female genitalia may also be treated with gonadotropin-releasing hormone analogues to stop production of estrogen and progesterone. Surgical interventions should not be carried out until the patients reach the legal age to consent for medical procedures and have met other criteria for gender affirming surgeries.[35]

Elders

There are approximately 3 million Americans over the age of 55 years who identify as LGBTQ, and by 2030 it is estimated there will be 6 million.[45] Significant health disparities also disproportionately affect older sexual minorities (see Table 188.2). Physical disparities may result in significant disability later in life. Mental health concerns are staggering with over half of sexual minority individuals over age 65 experiencing depression, almost 40% have contemplated suicide, and over 50% feel isolated.[46] Like other sexual minorities, they are less likely to have medical insurance and more likely to live in poverty.[46]

Although LGBTQ individuals and couples are increasingly parents through surrogacy, adoption, or other means, most do not have children who may assist them in advanced age compared to heterosexuals. Elder sexual minorities are twice as likely to live alone and may be estranged from biological family.[46] Sexual minorities commonly rely more on friends and community, but may become separated from social support by declining independence and health.[47] As a result, sexual minority individuals anticipate more use of institutional long-term care.[48] Among elder transgender individuals, 35% are concerned about being judged by their health care providers and believe that their health care will be limited (65%) or denied (55%) as they age.[49] Sexual minorities dependent on others have a high rate of abuse from caregivers. In one study, 22% of sexual minorities over 60 years of age reported that they had been harmed or neglected by a caregiver, and 26% reported knowing someone else who had been mistreated.[50] These factors are essential in consideration of a safe discharge from the ED.

People of Color

Although sexual minorities face many barriers in the obtainment of equitable health care, those of color have additional burdens. African American and Latino sexual minorities experience greater stigma relative to white counterparts.[51] Even within the sexual minority community, African Americans have the highest levels of racial/ethnic stigma, Caucasians the least, and Latinos and Asians in between.[52] Being LGBTQ and an underrepresented minority due to race, creed, ethnicity, or religion can potentially cause direct conflict with strongly held community values. As a cohort, African Americans and Hispanics have higher spirituality,[53] and religious institutions can therefore have an important role in helping or exacerbating their double minority stress.[54] Providers should be aware of how different cultural expectations that form identity can conflict and have an impact on the overall mental and physical health of these patients, and potentially magnify preexisting disparities.

African American and Latino sexual minorities are disproportionately affected by HIV compared to other racial groups, accounting for 37% and 29% respectively of new HIV infections among MSM.[27] Black MSM have a one in two chance of acquiring HIV during their lifetime,[55] and Latino MSM have a one in four lifetime risk.[30] Both are also are less likely to use PrEP, but this alone does not account for the difference between racial groups.[56] Although overall rates of HIV have been stable in the last decade, rates rose 52% among Asian and 18% among Latino MSM.[27] The HIV infection rate was stable among Black MSM, and the rate among white MSM rate decreased by 16%.[27] Intimate partner violence has been shown to be independently associated with HIV risk in Latino MSM.[57]

The references for this chapter can be found online at ExpertConsult. com.

Social Determinants

Dennis Hsieh

TABLE 189.1   Patient and Provider Factors

Patient and Provider Factors	Rosen's Chapter
Race, ethnicity, and diversity	Chapter 186
Cultural humility	Chapter 186
Implicit bias	Chapter 186
Sexual orientation and gender identity	Chapter 188
Mental health	Chapters 96-101
Disability	N/A
Language and literacy	Chapter 189 (this chapter)

FOUNDATIONS

The emergency department (ED) serves as the interface between health care and the community in a nexus where health care delivery can become a complex integration of significant physical and mental health crises intertwined with other life emergencies such as homelessness, poverty, and hunger.[1] These social and economic factors are collectively known as the social determinants of health (SDOH).

SDOH create barriers to health care access and result in nonadherence to medical interventions. It is estimated that 20% of a patient's health outcome is influenced by medical care, whereas social and economic factors account for 50% of such outcomes, highlighting the importance of concurrent medical and social interventions to advance patient health outcomes.[2]

Furthermore, left unaddressed, SDOH drive both health care cost and utilization. Even for those with access to care, many competing social needs impede the ability of the individual to adhere to treatment plans. These factors have a significant effect on health. For many of these concerns, providers can connect patients to concrete resources regardless of whether or not social work is available.

SPECIFIC ISSUES

Patient and Provider Factors

A large number of patient and provider factors affect the care of patients (Table 189.1).[2a]

Language

Many ED patients do not speak English as a first language. Title VI of the Civil Rights Law requires all recipients of federal funding to provide interpretation for patients with limited English proficiency. With time pressure in the emergency department and lack of proper training, providers do not always use a certified interpreter and instead use their limited knowledge of a second language or a patient family member. Failure to use a certified interpreter leads to poorer health outcomes and persistent health disparities.[3] Given this, emergency clinicians should use certified interpreters for patients with limited English proficiency.

Health Literacy

Even patients who speak English as a first language may have limited health literacy, which is defined as limited capacity to obtain, process, and understand basic health information and services needed to make appropriate health decisions. Those who have low health literacy may have trouble with tasks including reading appointment slips, understanding medication labels, and comprehending information from their providers, all of which are associated with poorer adherence to care plans and poorer health outcomes.[4] To address this, ED providers can use techniques such as "teach back" by providers and engaging with family members and friends to support patients.

Insurance and Access to Care

Uninsured and underinsured patients are often unable to access care prior to an ED visit.[5] This leads to delayed presentations of serious health conditions, poor health outcomes, and higher mortality.[6] For those who have poor access to care, two of the main drivers are the lack of ability to afford care and low health literacy regarding how to utilize care once coverage is obtained.[7]

For emergency clinicians, insurance and access to care are crucial to ensure proper follow up for patients. Rapid follow up reduces both return ED visits[8] and avoidable hospital admissions.[9] Thus, making sure patients have a practical and accessible follow-up plan is key. For those patients who have trouble navigating the system, case management can reduce ED recidivism.[10]

Employment, Income, and Financial Strain

The United States (US) has an extremely high rate of income inequality that has continued to grow in recent years.[11,12] As income inequality has grown, so have health care disparities: lower-income Americans have higher rates of chronic disease, anxiety, and depression, as well as lower life expectancy.[13,14] Low income, financial strain, and resulting poverty lead to increased stress, poor access to healthy foods, unsafe housing, and challenges with other SDOH.

Medical debt is related to income, employment, and financial security and is estimated to contribute to 67.5% of all bankruptcies, even after passage of the Affordable Care Act.[15] Hospitalization itself leads to decreased employment and income with a rise in out-of-pocket spending on medical care.[16] This highlights the importance of ensuring patients are connected to health care coverage and other programs to minimize the impact that an ED visit and/or hospitalization has on their lives.

Food Insecurity

Food insecurity, defined as a condition in which individuals do not have access to nutritionally adequate and safe food because of limited financial or other resources, is a leading health issue in the United States.[17] Lack of access to healthy foods leads to increased rates of low birth weight, hypertension, diabetes, and mental health disorders, particularly depression.[18] Not surprisingly, this is associated with increased emergency department visits and acute care utilization[19] and therefore increased costs within the health care system. Food insecurity led to an estimated $53 billion dollars of excess health care spending in the United States in 2016.[20]

Food insecurity leads to poor health by forcing individuals to choose between eating and medications, medical care, housing, education, utilities, and transportation.[21] Furthermore, food insecurity makes it difficult for individuals to follow a healthy diet and reduces the cognitive bandwidth available to manage chronic illnesses.[21]

Poverty, lack of education, and unemployment lead to individuals and households not having enough to eat and substituting cheaper, less nutritious items for healthy foods[22] or choosing not to eat to meet other basic needs. Low-income individuals often live in areas that have been historically underdeveloped with poor public transit and lack access to healthy foods. These areas, known as food deserts, lead to poor outcomes for those with chronic disease, including cardiovascular disease[23] and diabetes.[24]

Homelessness and Housing

Lack of access to safe, habitable housing is an important social determinant of health for many patients. These individuals have worse health outcomes and mortality compared with those who are housed.[25] Unhoused individuals may be unable to properly store certain medications, which can affect their efficacy (e.g., refrigeration of insulin or other antidiabetic agents may not be possible). Additionally, patients with housing insecurity may take irregularly or avoid taking certain medications based on expected side effects and potential legal implications. An example includes the use of diuretics, which cause increased need for urination; due to lack of access to bathroom, patients may be unable to reliably relieve themselves or be charged with indecent exposure or public urination. Housing First programs that provide housing and supportive case management decrease the use of nonroutine health care services, including ED visits, while improving self-perceived health.[26,27] However, compared to other federal, state, and local means-tested programs such as Medicaid and SNAP, housing programs have a limited supply and long waitlists.

For those with housing, utility payments can be challenging. Utility assistance programs are available for low-income patients and have been shown to improve health.[28,29]

Transportation

Lack of access to transportation leads to missed appointments, poor adherence to medications, and delayed access to care, resulting in increased costs and poorer health outcomes.[30] Lack of transportation also impacts access to services, healthy foods, jobs, and other social determinants of health.

Barriers to transportation include poor infrastructure, costs, lack of access to vehicles, distance and time burden, and policy-related issues.[31]

Elders, veterans, children, women, minorities, and those with lower incomes and chronic conditions face more transportation barriers.[32] Rural settings are especially challenging, given the great distances and lack of public transportation.[33] Providing transportation improves adherence to care, thereby decreasing costs and improving outcomes.[34]

Immigration Status

The immigration experience has profound effects on individuals and their health.[35] Immigration status is linked to ability to work and access public benefits, including health care.[36] The lack of proper immigrant status causes stress and poorer health.[37] Immigration law and policy are complicated and continuously changing. Important interventions that can be initiated in the ED include identifying vulnerable patients and educating them about potential opportunities to adjust their immigration status through mechanisms such as the T-Visa, U-Visa, and Violence Against Women Act (VAWA), as well as providing education and dispelling fear regarding accessing medical and social services.

Education

Youth behavioral issues in school can be related to mental health or developmental delay, resulting in the youth being brought to the ED. Parents or guardians may express concerns regarding the issues of truancy, suspension, expulsion, and reasonable accommodation, challenges that appropriate social services can help them address. For adults, educational needs are more subtle and tied to employment opportunities and income. Lower educational attainment is correlated with lower health literacy and poor health outcomes. More years of education are directly linked to a lower risk of mortality, a lower risk of obesity, and a lower risk of smoking.[38]

Legal Concerns

Health-harming legal needs is a term used to describe the legal avenues that exist to address many SDOH. For example, if an individual has mold, pests, or other housing issues that a landlord refuses to address, or an individual is improperly denied Medicaid coverage for durable medical equipment, a lawyer can help advocate and enforce housing and Medicaid regulations, respectively. Addressing SDOH through the law diminishes stress, decreases ED visits, and improves adherence to care and health outcomes.[39]

Justice Involvement

The United States has the largest population of incarcerated individuals in the world.[40] Individuals in custody or otherwise justice-involved are often seen in the ED. Many of these individuals experience comorbid psychiatric and substance use disorders, chronic health conditions, or homelessness, making these populations extremely vulnerable.[41] Furthermore, individuals in custody lose their rights and privacy. Being justice-involved is associated with higher mortality, morbidity, and poorer health outcomes.[42]

The Built Environment

Emergency clinicians must view and treat patients within the context of their lives and their communities. As such, the built environment, the surrounding physical environment, and conditions that are constructed by human activity affect patients' ability to follow up for care, exercise, access transportation, eat healthy food, and address other social determinants of health.[43] Improvement in the built environment is associated with better health outcomes in areas such as increased physical activity, better mental health, and improved dietary behaviors.[44] Emergency clinicians often see patients who reside in poorer areas, where following common preventative measures such as healthy eating and exercise is often challenging. Providers can address specific barriers, such as food insecurity and challenges with transportation, as previously discussed. Beyond this, however, changing the built environment requires gathering evidence from the bedside and engaging with health systems, local and state government, and the community to help bring about systematic change.

MANAGEMENT

Overview

Most EDs do not currently screen for social needs. Instead, social needs arise during the course of the patient encounter. Options for systematic screening exist but require implementing a framework for both identifying and addressing social needs.[45] After identifying concerns with the social determinants of health, patients can be linked to resources. Social workers or ED staff can help assess and provide emotional support prior to providing patients with a list of resources. Some systems have adopted electronic platforms such as One Degree (www.1deg.org), 211 (www.211.org), or Aunt Bertha (www.findhelp.org), which are accessible for patients to use themselves.[46] Some systems also use patient navigators to help more actively connect patients to resources.[47,48]

EDs, hospitals, and health systems cannot address SDOH and poverty alone. In addition to working across specialties, health systems must look outside of health care to meet patients' social needs. There are many community groups, nonprofit organizations, and government agencies working on factors affecting SDOH. Together, these partnerships not only provide an opportunity to invite service organizations into the health care setting to connect with patients, but also ensure closed-loop communication that ensures that patients actually receive help.

Apart from connecting patients to resources, community engagement can lead to building capacity within the community through infrastructure changes such as offering low-cost day care and early childhood education opportunities, introducing violence prevention programs in schools, increasing the number of parks and green spaces, reducing unhealthy food options, creating bike lanes, or introducing farmer's markets to combat food deserts. Even with these types of changes, other challenges such as the lack of affordable housing and low wages require further advocacy in partnership with the community at the local, state, and federal levels.

Health Care Access and Literacy

Even for those who have health care coverage, access to follow-up care from the ED can be challenging. There are no federal standards requiring that appointments be available within a certain number of days, or how many providers there must be for a certain number of enrollees. However, most states do require that Medicaid and managed care plans provide adequate networks and timely access.[49] Patients having trouble accessing care can call their insurance plan to find out who their doctor is, what specialists are available, and how quickly they should be able to get an appointment. If, despite contacting their doctor and their insurance plan, they are still unable to access care in a timely manner, patients can contact their state's department of insurance for further assistance.

Health Care Coverage

When a patient does not have health care coverage, there are a number of options to consider.

Medicaid was created by the Title XIX of the Social Security Act in 1965 and is a means-tested program, meaning that eligibility depends in part on income. The program is administered by states and jointly funded by federal and state dollars. At a minimum, coverage must be provided to individuals who are pregnant, blind, disabled, over 65 years of age, and parents or caretakers of a dependent child whose household income falls below a certain amount. Beyond this, states have the option to cover additional populations. Income levels are set by the state.[50] Patients can look to their state government website for more information and to sign up for Medicaid.

Medicare was established in 1965 under Title XVIII of the Social Security Act for individuals age 65 (currently) and older, those less than 65 who receive Social Security Disability Insurance, and those who suffer from end-stage renal disease. People who fall into one of these three categories must have worked or be linked to an individual who has worked at least 40 quarters (10 years) during their lifetime. Medicare is administered and funded by the federal government and contains several parts including inpatient hospital coverage (Part A), outpatient medical coverage (Part B), and alternative coverage options—Medicare Advantage (Part C), and prescription drug coverage (Part D). To sign up for Medicare, one must go through the Social Security Administration by either visiting a Social Security Office or registering online: https://www.ssa.gov/benefits/medicare/.

In addition, all states have a health care marketplace (healthcare.gov) under the Affordable Care Act (ACA) where individuals can see plan options and sign up for health care. Generally, the exchanges have a period of open enrollment during which an individual must sign up for insurance. However, instances such as a job loss or relocation will permit signing up for insurance outside of open enrollment periods. If an individual is not eligible for Medicaid or Medicare, signing up for insurance via the exchanges is the most appropriate option.

There are specific programs focused on providing access to care for children under the age of 18, including the Children's Health Insurance Program (CHIP). However, transitional age youth between the ages of 18 to 25 years face special challenges because they become ineligible for many benefits, including health care, during this age range and can also lose access to their pediatrician. The Affordable Care Act requires plans and issuers that offer dependent child coverage to make coverage available until the child reaches the age of 26.

Individuals who are not eligible for these options will receive a bill of charges that is higher than the negotiated rates that insurance companies pay. These individuals should be advised to call the health care provider or hospital to discuss options that include free care, a reduced rate, or a payment plan. A reduced rate or free care (collectively also known as charity care) is available at the discretion of the provider and is generally based on income. A payment plan is a plan where the amount due after negotiations can be paid in installments, much like credit card payments. Note that facilities built with assistance from the Hill-Burton Act of 1946 (usually hospitals) have legally mandated charity care obligations.

Patients who have trouble navigating these options, feel that they have been wrongly denied benefits, or have been sent to collections can contact the patient advocate at the hospital and a local free legal services organization for assistance. Those sent to collections can call the original provider to ask that the bill be taken back from collections to work out a payment plan as the provider receives substantially less reimbursement when a medical bill is sold to a collection agency. Additionally, patients may be unable to afford some or all of their medications, leading to repeated presentations to the ED. Determining alternative strategies from different medication options (e.g., transitioning from SGLT-2 inhibitor or GLP-1 inhibitor for treatment of diabetes mellitus to a sulfonylurea) or different mechanisms for payment may be crucial to prevent additional visits.

Disability and Loss of Employment

Emergency clinicians often care for individuals who have suffered an injury that affects their ability to work. Depending on the nature of the injury, the patient may qualify for either short-term or long-term disability insurance that will pay them a portion of their wages while they are unable to work. States administer short-term disability, which is anticipated to last less than one year. For long-term or permanent disability, people must apply through the Social Security Administration for either Social Security Disability Insurance (SSDI) or Supplemental Security Insurance (SSI).

The Family and Medical Leave Act of 1983 (FMLA) protects individuals who have to take leave from their jobs due to the birth of a new child, caring for a sick family member, or recovering from a serious illness, allowing for unpaid leave for up to one year without the risk of job loss. Those taking time off for pregnancy and childbirth also qualify for short-term disability insurance.

Challenges with Employers

Clinicians will also encounter patients who feel that they have been wronged by their employer. Complaints may include employment discrimination, denial of meals and breaks, improper termination, unpaid overtime, and unpaid wages. For these concerns, referral to a legal services attorney or an employment law attorney is the appropriate next step.

Finding Employment

Patients who need assistance in finding employment can contact local workforce development agencies and nonprofits that help individuals find and retain employment. For those who have misdemeanors or felonies on their records, referral to legal services for record expungement may help these individuals obtain jobs.

Income Support

Patients who are employed but earn very little may qualify for earned income tax credit (EITC). Those who are able to work but have lost their jobs can apply for unemployment insurance, which is administered on a state-by-state basis. Those who have minor children may qualify for Temporary Assistance for Needy Families (TANF), which is funded by the federal government and administered by states. For those without minor children, local jurisdictions may have limited cash aid, such as General Assistance or General Relief. These programs are generally administered by the local department of social services. Those who are older may also qualify for Social Security retirement benefits, which is administered by the Social Security Agency. Individuals who have a history of military service may be eligible for income assistance from the Department of Veterans Affairs. Providers should also make sure that these patients are linked with other programs that assist with basic needs, such as programs that help with food and housing.

Management of Food Insecurity

Health Care Based Resources

Some hospitals and health systems have partnered with local food recovery organizations, food banks, and farmers to set up food pharmacies that provide healthy produce for free to patients who are food insecure and/or have chronic disease.[51] These food pharmacies are often supplemented with cooking classes and nutrition education for patients. Many hospitals and health systems also partner with local growers to host on-site farmers markets to make healthy food accessible to patients and some institute a 1-to-1 match for supplemental nutrition assistance program (SNAP match) purchasers.[52]

Community-Based Resources

Patients can also be referred to community resources that provide food ready for consumption, such as churches, soup kitchens, and shelters, as well as those that provide groceries, such as food banks and pantries.[53] Other sources include farmers markets that provide a SNAP match, food delivery services such as Meals on Wheels, and medically tailored meals, such as those provided by Project Open Hand in the San Francisco Bay Area.

Public Programs

Public programs are generally limited to those who have legal status in the country. The supplemental nutrition assistance program (SNAP), formerly known as food stamps, is a federally funded program through the United States Department of Agriculture (USDA) that is based on financial need. Local offices can be found on the USDA website.[54]

The Special Supplemental Nutrition Program for Women, Infants, and Children (WIC) is a program open to postpartum women and children up to the age of five. This program is also administered by the USDA and local offices can be found on the USDA website.[55]

Housing and Homelessness

Clinicians also care for many patients who are experiencing challenges with housing, including the imminent risk of homelessness. Given already substantial challenges in obtain housing, any pending eviction or loss of a Section 8 voucher should be treated as a legal emergency with an immediate referral to a legal services provider given often strict timelines (days) to respond to any pending legal action.

For those who have concerns with the habitability of their housing due to pests, mold, rodents or other health hazards, or have nonfunctioning heating or appliances, a request can be made of the landlord to adhere to codes of habitability to resolve the concerns. Patients may also require reasonable accommodation because of a disability or feel that they have been discriminated against in violation of the Fair Housing Act. For patients who own their homes and are at risk of foreclosure, working with a lawyer who specializes in housing may allow individuals to negotiate a modification on their mortgage or a payment plan in order to keep their housing. All of these patients can be connected to their local legal services organizations for additional support.

Challenges may also exist with utilities. Many regions or states have heating assistance programs for low-income individuals. There are also other utility assistance programs for electricity, gas, telephone, and even internet services. Patients with limited income should inquire with their utility companies about any available assistance.

Those experiencing homelessness can apply for Section 8, the federal housing assistance voucher program that pays a portion of an individual's rent. Section 8 is extremely limited in supply, and in many jurisdictions the waitlist for Section 8 is only open a few days each year for new individuals to sign up. Once an individual registers, the wait can be as long as 5 to 10 years.

Health care organizations may support funding for housing through a Housing First model, which has been shown to improve health while reducing costs.[55a] For those with medical needs and insurance, skilled nursing facilities, congregate living, medical respite, and recuperative care are options. For those with limited income, board and care facilities or renting a room may be an option. Individuals with immediate housing needs can access available shelter systems. Shelters often offer little privacy, do not allow individuals to stay during the day, and require people to line up for a bed on a daily basis. Shelters often also have restrictions based on age and gender, making it challenging for families or couples to stay together. Given these restrictions and limited availability, many individuals opt to live under less stable conditions—in their vehicles, with friends or family, or on the streets.

Transportation Challenges

Most EDs offer a range of transportation options for patients at the time of discharge, including public transit assistance, taxi, rideshare, shuttle service, and medical transportation. This is the perfect time to make sure that patients understand their transportation options to obtain follow-up appointments.

Health plans often have transportation benefits included. Medicaid is legally required to provide nonemergency transportation for patients. Ensuring patients understand how to use this service can decrease barriers to transportation, improve adherence to follow-up, result in improved health outcomes, and lead to significant savings.[56] Those who are having trouble accessing required benefits should contact legal services.

Health facilities either provide patients with transportation vouchers in partnership with local providers or let providers know that the patient would benefit from transportation assistance. The vouchers can be for public transportation, taxis, or rideshare programs such as Lyft. Some health facilities have taken on this approach[57] while others have created shuttle services or used volunteer drivers to address the challenge of transportation.[58]

Immigration Status

Adjustment of Status

For those who are without legal status, there are several options for adjusting status. A family-based petition process is available if there is a family member who is a US citizen to adjust their status and become a legal permanent resident (green card holder). However, initial entry to the United States without permission may require the petitioner to leave the United States for up to 10 years prior to reentering even if they qualify for a green card. Petitioning for and support by an employer for a green card is also an option.[59] A number of other special categories that qualify a petitioner for legal status can be found on the US Citizenship and Immigration Services (USCIS) website (https://www.uscis.gov/citizenship). Immigration is a complex issue, and individuals with immigration questions should be connected to the local bar association to work with a qualified attorney.

Victims of Violence and Crime

Interpersonal violence is an important cause of morbidity and mortality. For further discussion of this issue, please see the chapters on community violence and intimate partner violence and abuse (see Chapters 190 and 192). Clinicians can work with social services to help victims in reporting their crime to law enforcement and to ensure a safe ED discharge plan. Furthermore, victims of interpersonal violence may be eligible for a temporary or permanent restraining order as part of their safety plan. Courthouse self-help centers and legal aid organizations can help victims apply for a restraining order. Regarding financial assistance for victims of violence, any victim (and their families) are eligible for the Crime Victims Fund established by the Victims of Crime Act of 1984. This fund is managed by the Office for Victims of Crime and administered by each state.[60] For those victims who are without legal status, cooperating with law enforcement to investigate and/or prosecute the crime may allow the individual to apply for a special visa or to become a legal permanent resident (green card holder)

Victims of violence and crime are especially vulnerable when they are without legal immigration status because their abusers may threaten to report them to immigration officials as a deterrent to reporting the crime and seeking help. Victims of intimate partner violence can adjust their status and apply to become legal permanent residents (green card holder) through either the federal Violence Against Women Act (VAWA)[61] or the Victims of Criminal Activity U Nonimmigrant Status (U Visa),[62] as long as the victims make a police report and cooperate

with law enforcement to investigate and prosecute the crime. Those who are the victims or witness to other crimes, including but not limited to assault, rape, kidnapping, and blackmail, are also eligible for the U Visa.[63]

Those who are victims of sex or labor trafficking and/or who are certain family members of these victims are eligible to apply for the T nonimmigrant status as long as they cooperate with law enforcement to investigate and/or prosecute the crime[64] (see Chapter 187).

Although complicated, a path to legalization and citizenship for these vulnerable patients is possible. Ensuring appropriate documentation such as police reports, discussing options with social work, and ensuring connection to a local legal services provider are all important next steps of which the emergency clinician should be aware.

Refugees and Asylees

Refugees are individuals who have been persecuted or fear that they will be persecuted based on their race, religion, nationality, political opinions, or membership in a particular social group who seek refugee status from outside of the United States. Asylees are individuals who are already in the United States, or those who are actively seeking to enter the United States and meet the definition of a refugee. If asylees do not have legal status, they can apply for adjustment of status through USCIS (recommended to do so with an attorney's help).[65]

Asylees under 21 years of age who are seen in the ED may qualify for Special Immigrant Juvenile Status. To qualify to apply through USCIS (recommended to do so with an attorney's help), the individual must be currently unmarried, cannot be reunited with parents because of abuse, abandonment, neglect or other similar reasons, and cannot in their best interest return to the country of nationality.[66]

Hospital Safe Spaces Initiatives

Immigrants often fear seeking medical care because of confusion caused by complicated and ever-changing immigration policies.[67] Educating patients that the ED and hospital are safe spaces where providers are focused on treating health and will not report patients to the USCIS is crucial to ensuring that patients seek care in a timely manner. Providers should respect patient privacy and not disclose patient information unless served with a valid warrant. Any questions that arise should be deferred to the hospital's legal counsel and the administrator on duty.

Immigration Status and Public Charge

The idea of becoming a "public charge" or one who is reliant on public benefits, has caused fear and hesitation among immigrant communities to seek care.[68] Although applying for and receiving certain public benefit programs *may* make one a public charge, seeking and receiving health care services never does. However, for the undocumented individual, eligibility to receive public benefits is impermissible unless the specific exceptions are met. Individuals should be reassured that obtaining health care never makes them a public charge and providers should refer them to a legal services attorney to evaluate their individual case and public benefits.

Education-Related Challenges

For youth with school-related concerns regarding truancy, suspension and expulsion, or with respect to reasonable accommodation with an Individualized Education Plan (IEP), clinicians can connect the youth and their parents or guardians to an attorney specializing in education law. Connecting with the local bar association is one way to find low-cost or no-cost attorneys who specialize in education law.

For adults, connection to the local community college or other special adult education programs allows for exploration of affordable educational options.

TABLE 189.2	Health Harming Legal Needs	
Health Harming Legal Needs Categories	**Specific Needs**
Housing	Eviction, Section 8 voucher termination/denial, habitability, discrimination, reasonable accommodation
Employment	Improper termination, discrimination, unpaid wages, unpaid overtime, lack of breaks/meals/accommodation
Family	Divorce, custody, child support, restraining orders, guardianship, adoption
Immigration	Adjustment of status (family-based, employment based, U-Visa, T-Visa, VAWA, SJIS, asylee/refugee), naturalization, deportation defense
Healthcare Benefits	Denial/termination of coverage (Medicaid, Medicare, other insurance), denial of specific benefits, lack of timely access, medical debt/charity care/negotiating a payment plan
Other Public Benefits	Denial/termination of TANF, VA benefits, SSI, SSDI, SNAP, IHS, unemployment, short term disability, other cash aid; overpayments; improper amount of benefit
Consumer	Debt, fraud
Elder	Advanced directives, conservatorship, wills and trusts
Justice-Involved	Expungement, tickets, warrants,
Miscellaneous	Name change, gender change

Domestic Concerns and Social Isolation

Troubled family dynamics and relationships can be a source of stress and lead to ED visits and poor health.[69] In most jurisdictions, emergency providers are required to report cases of suspected child or elder abuse. Patients may face challenges with marriage and children. If there is no intimate partner violence, then a referral to the local legal services agency, courthouse, and/or bar association can help patients access resources to resolve these concerns.

Patients are sometimes dropped off in the ED because family members are unable to care for them. Medicaid offers in-home support services (IHSS) as part of its benefit to help individuals remain in the least restrictive environment. This is often an option for elders or disabled patients. The local social service agency may provide some assistance with childcare as part of its Temporary Assistance for Needy Families (TANF) benefit.

Elders and their families may request assistance with creating an advanced directive. In addition to assisting patients and their families fill out the portable medical order (POLST) form, caregivers can refer patients to the local bar association for assistance. Providers may see patients who feel socially isolated. Working with social work and local agencies can provide options such as day programs for elders and support groups for individuals with special needs.

Legal Concerns

Legal Assistance

Reduced cost or free legal services are available to help low-income individuals with issues such as public benefits, housing, and family law (Table 189.2). Many of the nonprofit legal services providers who offer low-cost or free legal services programs are federally funded.[70] For issues that legal aid providers do not assist with, clinicians can refer patients to the local bar association for help.

Medical legal partnerships are arrangements that place attorneys into the health care setting to work as part of the health care team.[71] These attorneys can be hired by the health care team directly or come from local nonprofit legal services organizations. They work with the health care team to address health-harming legal needs. The co-location and communication allows the provider to make the legal team part of the treatment plan while the legal team works with the provider to demonstrate the health harm that patients are suffering.

Patients in Police Custody

Clinicians often care for patients who are in police custody, where there is a significant power imbalance between the patient and law enforcement. It is often difficult for patients in custody to obtain health care, so providers should ensure thorough medical assessments are performed in this vulnerable patient population where routine care is limited.[72] Best practices support patient interviews in private, clear communication of results, and follow-up instructions clearly documented in discharge instructions confidentially communicated to the correctional facility's health care staff. Any physical or medical limitations for the patient should be communicated to accompanying officers.

To avoid conflict between the emergency clinician and law enforcement officials when the question of blood draws for legal purposes arises, policies should be in place to allow providers to respect patient autonomy. This will help the clinician avoid the difficult legal circumstance of having to choose between either defying a request from law enforcement or being potentially liable for assault.

Tickets and Outstanding Warrants

Patients who are not in custody may have concerns about unpaid tickets and outstanding warrants. These public records may make it difficult for them to access housing or jobs. Such concerns are becoming more prevalent as jurisdictions criminalize homelessness and poverty with laws such as the sit-lie laws that prohibit sitting or lying on the sidewalk or in other public spaces. Referral to local legal services providers can allow patients to receive an evaluation and potentially address these concerns.

The references for this chapter can be found online at ExpertConsult. com.

190

Community Violence

Theodore Corbin and Thea James

FOUNDATIONS

Population Characteristics and Violence

Young adults and adolescents in the United States (US) are exposed to crime and violence at much higher rates than those in other developed nations.[1] Rates of violence in the United States also vary by location, with higher homicide rates in metropolitan communities compared to suburban or rural areas.[2] Over 80% of the 12,979 firearm homicides in the United States in 2015 occurred in urban areas,[3] and disparities are larger in certain areas of large cities (e.g., racially and ethnically diverse neighborhoods). For instance, in Philadelphia's safest police district, which is approximately 85% white, there were no reports of anyone being killed by gun violence. Conversely, the most violent district, with a roughly 90% African American population, had over 180 shooting victims and 40 deaths.[4] African American youth in the United States disproportionately carry the largest burden of violent experiences. The homicide rate for African Americans in the United States is eight times higher than that of their white counterparts,[3] and African Americans are 500 times more likely to die this way.[5] While African American young adults and adolescents only make up about 2.4% of the US population, they are disproportionately victims of injuries from assault (26%) and homicide (20.7%).[3,6]

Contributing factors to these differences in rates of violence by location are rooted in historical, present day, and persistent structural racism (e.g., racial segregation), inequality, and poverty.[7] Structural barriers that impact present day rates of violence were established decades ago.[8-11] In the 1930s, President Franklin D. Roosevelt (FDR) created opportunities for wealth-building to help Americans recover from their financial losses in the 1929 Great Depression, securing home ownership through access to guaranteed financial services. In the same decade, FDR's administration established redlining, a practice with long-lasting effects that segregated America both racially and socioeconomically. Redlining policies drew red lines through cities across America, and residents living behind red lines were denied access to financial services (i.e., mortgages, loans, insurance companies) needed for wealth-building through home ownership and the benefits of home equity. A majority of people living behind red lines were people of color and low income. Redlining policies established two distinct socioeconomic populations that still exist today.[8-11] Communities located behind historic red lines have lower rates of education attainment, income, and life expectancy, and higher rates of homicide.[9,12,13] In general, populations in these communities have lower rates of health, as do their children[12] as beneficiaries of their parents' limited resources.[14]

Community Violence

Community violence is a complex and persistent health issue that disproportionately affects low-income neighborhoods and communities of color in the United States. Community violence occurs primarily in public settings, occurs between individuals or groups who may or may not know each other, and is often an impulsive or loosely planned act.[15] The effects of community violence are severe and often result in injuries or death. Both those who contribute to and are survivors of community violence are disproportionately young men and adolescent males from historically disadvantaged backgrounds and communities.[15] Analysis of 2017 data from the National Vital Statistics System, National Crime Victimization Survey, and the Youth Risk Behavior Surveillance System concluded that African American young adults and adolescents are at a much greater risk of violence (e.g., homicides, fights with injuries, aggravated assaults) compared to their white counterparts.[16] Furthermore, the frequency of exposure to community violence is higher in large urban cities and within impoverished communities. There is an overrepresentation of racial minorities, especially African American males, among youth who live in these communities and are disproportionately exposed to violence.[17]

Further exacerbating community violence is the lack of economic growth in an area, further contributing to the cycle of urban flight. For instance, there is slower growth in businesses, new retail, and a depreciation of home values in communities with higher rates of violence.[18] Families of victims and survivors of gun violence often experience financial stress, such as having challenges in paying rent, bills, and phone services because of the loss in earnings from employment and medical costs.[19] Exposure to community violence can be very traumatic for individuals and contributes to poor health among African American young adults and adolescents. Community violence exposure has been found to be associated with an increase in psychological health problems, including posttraumatic stress disorder, depression or anxiety, and aggression.[17] Alarmingly, the disproportionate impact of violence on young African Americans comes from forms of violence having the greatest immediate negative consequences on physical and mental health, such as aggravated assault and homicide.

SPECIFIC ISSUES

Root Causes of Community Violence

Since the first Africans were brought to the United States, African Americans were forced to live in poor physical and social conditions. For over 250 years, enslaved African Americans suffered social, physical, and mental abuse and brutalization. Although slavery has ended, African Americans still live in a country that is unjust, and one that has systemically discriminated against and oppressed them. Slavery and present day structural and institutionalized racism have contributed to the poor health among African Americans.[20] African Americans in the United States are exposed to constant racism that is systemic (organized socially and culturally) through exclusion, prejudice, and discrimination.[21] Racism is also correlated with second-rate employment, housing, education, income, and access to health services. Racism is a factor in health disparities and inequities that is not explained by other demographic factors such as age, gender, and educational attainment.[21] Due to their lower socioeconomic status, racial or ethnic minorities suffer disproportionate risks for poor health outcomes: occupational hazards, exposures to toxic substances and allergens in the home, low-quality schooling, and lack of availability of healthy foods.[20] While these risk factors are not clinical in nature, they make up the social determinants of health which includes factors such as race/racism, poverty, education, housing, access to healthy food, environmental exposures, violence, and gender. Compared to their white counterparts, proportionately fewer African Americans in the United States graduate from high school or earn a college degree,[22] and they are more than two times as likely to be unemployed.[23,24] The social determinants of health predict the health needs of a population, and the health risks, much more than clinical care.[20]

African Americans, through poverty and residential segregation, live in some of the poorest neighborhoods throughout the United States, areas with high rates of homicide.[20] Violence influences health greatly and can cause injury, disability, and preventable death. African American youth are more than four times more likely to die from a gunshot wound than their white counterparts.[20] African American children are much more likely to witness violence and 20 times more likely to witness a murder than their white counterparts.[25]

Race or ethnicity alone are not risk factors for violence, but rather are associated with socioeconomic risk factors for violence.[26] Therefore, it is important for prevention efforts, including those in hospitals and emergency departments, to consider unjust social conditions that are disproportionately experienced by minorities, and especially African Americans, including generational poverty, residential segregation, and other forms of racism that limit opportunities to grow up in healthy and violence-free environments. Addressing these conditions is critical to lessening and eliminating violence exposure among African American and other minority and vulnerable communities.[16]

Psychological and Mental Health

Trauma has been defined as an emotional response to a distressing event, such as an accident, rape, violent attack, or natural disaster.[27] Trauma can invoke long-term reactions and adverse effects such as flashbacks to the traumatic event, unpredictable emotions, poor mental, physical, social, emotional, or spiritual well-being.[27,28] Experiencing traumatic events or chronic traumatic events, such as exposure to community violence, is also associated with traumatic stress reactions that include fear, anger, sadness, shame, guilt, aggression, and behavioral health issues.[29-33]

The physical and mental health consequences of experiencing violence over time can lead to the development of preventable chronic conditions and can result in considerable health burdens and costs, lower quality of life, and lost productivity.[34] Racial and ethnic minorities, particularly African American young adults and adolescents in urban areas, are experiencing trauma from community violence at levels that impede their ability to cope in healthful ways.[35] The stressful and traumatic events from community violence contribute negatively to mental health and overall quality of life through emotional changes, and this is also passed on through generations. With poverty and high exposure to racism and discrimination, African Americans suffer from more frequent and intense poor mental and behavioral health compared to their white counterparts.[36]

Disparities in Access to Mental Health Care Services and Treatment

Community violence disproportionately persists in communities of color. Also disproportionately impacting African American young men and adolescents, exposure to community violence is negatively associated with psychological and behavioral health issues. Disparities in access to and utilization of mental health care services among African Americans and Latinos stem from limited access, mistrust, stigma, misdiagnosis, little understanding about mental illness, and feeling culturally misunderstood.[37-38] Shame, ridicule from peers, mistrust of health care service providers, and mental health stigma can deter African American young men and adolescents from receiving mental health treatment.[39] One study observed that African American parents were much less likely to seek mental health care services for their children if they themselves held high levels of stigma towards mental health.[40] Furthermore, uninsured African Americans with depression are less likely to be prescribed antidepressants compared to those who are insured, and those who are insured are still less likely to be prescribed medications compared to their white counterparts.[41]

PHYSICAL TRAUMA FROM VIOLENT INJURY AND THE ROLE OF HOSPITALS, EMERGENCY DEPARTMENTS, AND TRAUMA CENTERS

Victims of interpersonal violence may experience traumatic physical injuries and seek treatment from hospitals, emergency departments (EDs), and trauma centers. The vast majority of these centers focus almost exclusively on stabilizing patients, and clinicians in these settings may not recognize the importance of assessing psychological and mental health issues that victims may experience post-injury. Most trauma centers are not equipped with the resources, staff, and systematic approach to identify and address the social factors that contribute to persistent community violence among the patient populations they serve.[42] Individuals who are victims of interpersonal violence and have exposure to community violence are more at risk for recurrent trauma.[43] Health care providers that care for victims of physical injury have an opportunity to incorporate violence prevention into their care. With emerging acceptance that violence is structural in the United States, emergency and trauma physicians have been inspired to participate in the reduction of violence through prevention and intervention efforts.[44-47]

Hospital-Based Violence Intervention Programs

The first hospital-based violence intervention programs (HVIPs) in the United States were developed in the 1990s: the "Caught in the Crossfire" program in Oakland, California, and Project Ujima in Milwaukee, Wisconsin.[42] Since then, several HVIPs have been developed and implemented in the United States with the National Network of Hospital-Based

Violence Intervention Programs, now known as the Health Alliance for Violence Intervention (HAVI).[48] According to Rosenblatt et al., several fundamental principles of HVIPs include the following:

"1) Violence is preventable,

2) Hospitals should use public health-based principles to approach violence prevention, including working to address the following in the patients and communities they serve: poor education, lack of job opportunities, injury and criminal recidivism, socioeconomically deprived neighborhoods, substance abuse, complex post-traumatic stress disorder, lack of positive role models,

3) There is a 'teachable' moment during which a patient may be more receptive to psychological first aid and prevention principles following a traumatic injury, and

4) Intervention will begin in the hospital but must follow the patient and family into their community. Case management principles are implemented, ideally including professionals with therapeutic skill sets and 'credible messengers' with knowledge of the patient population."[42]

Several studies have suggested that HVIPs are beneficial for patients who are exposed to community violence and who are survivors of interpersonal violence. A recent review found that HVIP programs that incorporate case management and at least some brief intervention observed decreases in recidivism, and that HVIPs are cost-effective. Furthermore, it must be emphasized that social determinants such as health, stable housing, and increase in income are important components to include in HVIPs.[49,50,51] Several studies have shown that HIVPs can decrease the reinjury rates of participants by up to 50% and that even applying a brief intervention to reduce violence among youth (ages 14 to 20) was associated with increased self-efficacy for avoiding fighting and a decrease in aggression frequency.[52,53]

It is feasible to integrate health data on violence and other patient characteristics (e.g., social determinants of health information) into ED electronic medical records across institutions, with minimal impact on workflow and triage times, to collectively gather data on violence and aid in public health surveillance of community violence data trends.[54] Organizations such as the Centers for Disease Control and Prevention could then use this data to fund HVIPs where they are needed the most.[55]

HVIPs can also incorporate digital health tools. One study of a technology-augmented violence and depression intervention tool for high-risk adolescents found a high level of acceptance among participants, who experienced less depression and less subsequent violence compared to the control group.[56]

Peers and community members with similar lived experiences as victims of violence should be included in the process of operating an HVIP. This approach has been effective for EDs trying to understand how their HVIP can improve the lives of individuals experiencing violence in their communities.[57,58] An HVIP housed at Drexel University in Philadelphia has an ongoing evaluation that assesses delivery of services and trauma symptom reduction. Preliminarily, the HVIP demonstrates that the services provided by the team decrease trauma symptoms. Using a focus on structural determinants of health to mitigate and eliminate gaps to thriving, HVIPs have served as models for health care systems aiming to sustainably reduce costs and improve health outcomes in the communities they serve.[59,60]

Boston University HVIP Model

A Boston University emergency medicine–based HVIP began with a "no assumptions" approach to building its program. The program engaged survivors of violence to help understand the root causes of the city's disproportionate geographic prevalence of community violence. Knowledge of the structural barriers in communities, and in their patients' lived experiences, shaped expectations of what was possible for them to achieve.[8] The program learned that its patients who were survivors of violence were coming from communities that had been disinvested in for decades and predictably experienced low income, education attainment, economic mobility, and opportunities to build wealth. These communities were among those negatively affected historically by redlining policies.[10] The Boston HVIP survivors of violence expressed overwhelming themes of hopelessness.

Guided by intervention models of the network of HVIPs nationally,[11] the Boston HVIP program made a conscious decision to set high bars to alter the quality of life course for their patients through intentional disruption of structural barriers. The program encouraged survivors of violence to identify their goals and then partnered with them to achieve those goals. Common goals were education, steady employment, stable housing, and safety. The program hired and embedded a career specialist for workforce development, hired a housing advocate, and expanded its multisector community partnerships in workforce development, financial literacy, education, and housing.

The Boston HVIP's hospital health care system is now using the same model expanded to all patients. This occurred in large part to a charge by its largest payer, Massachusetts Medicaid or Mass Health, in 2018. Its hospital health care system is the largest recipient of Medicaid payments in Massachusetts. Mass Health addressed its decade-long upward trajectory of rising costs and poor health outcomes by changing from a fee-for-service to value-based care reimbursement. It charged Boston health care systems, who are Medicaid payees, to lower cost and improve outcomes prescriptively by focusing on social determinants of health. HVIPs have years of experience in this area.

The Boston HVIP's hospital health care system is now using an HVIP model to alter life course for all patients. Examples of how the Boston HVIP hospital has targeted structural barriers to health to alter the quality of life course of its patients and communities where they live include the following:

1. Development and operationalization of a screening tool in ambulatory clinics that identifies gaps people have, and connects them to resources to mitigate and eliminate the gaps; the tool is embedded in their electronic medical record for providers to see. A built analytics platform evaluates and monitors results monthly.
2. The hospital joined the Healthcare Anchor Network, a national collaboration of 45 health care systems. Their goal is to build more inclusive local economies through hospitals being intentional about how they make daily decisions in three pillars; hiring, investment, and procurement.[12]
3. Invested in a private equity fund that explicitly funds developments that provide access to affordable housing, employment, green walking space, transit, and healthy affordable food.[13,14]
a. The investment contributed to what is becoming 323 units of new mixed-income housing to own and to rent.
b. Seventy percent of laborers at the construction site come from the community.
c. The hospital was able to help a grocery store mitigate expansion costs of moving to the site by giving it a no interest loan.
4. The hospital invested to support a local organization that invests in local small business development.
5. The hospital health care system expanded its procurement operations to include more local vendors. It built an analytics platform to monitor and evaluate progress.
6. The Affordable Care Act requires hospitals to conduct a community health needs assessment with an improvement plan every

three years. In 2019, the Boston hospitals conducted an assessment together. Prioritized improvement plan areas that emerged from the assessment are housing, finance and economic mobility, access, and behavioral health. The hospitals will collectively address the first two domains in communities with goals to have measurable impact.[60]

7. The Boston HVIP hospital created an innovative Stable Housing Initiative.[59] Subsequently, two other Boston academic medical centers joined them and together they have partnered and invested in innovative solutions to housing instability.

The HVIP model of altering quality of life course has served as a proof of concept for all patients who face perpetual life and health instability due to structural barriers.

The references for this chapter can be found online at ExpertConsult. com.

191

Sexual Assault

Jennie Alison Buchanan and Sarah Tolford Selby

KEY CONCEPTS

- Sexual assault is most common in women but can happen to gay and heterosexual men and to lesbian, gay, bisexual, transgender, and gender-nonconforming individuals.
- Sexual assault often results in no physical signs of injury.
- Optimal care includes creating a safe confidential environment while incorporating the principles of trauma-informed care. The patient should be included in decision making and ultimately decide treatment. Options include injury evaluation, treatment to prevent pregnancy and sexually transmitted infections (STIs), support and trauma counseling, evidence collection, and comprehensive toxicology testing if appropriate.
- The sexual assault evidence collection examination is an intensive, protocol-driven, multistep process, best performed by a certified sexual assault examiner.
- Adult sexual assault patients should be treated empirically according to Center for Disease Control (CDC) guidelines to prevent STIs (e.g., gonorrhea, syphilis, chlamydia, trichomonas, human immunodeficiency virus [HIV], human papillomavirus [HPV], and hepatitis B). Children and adolescents should be tested and, if symptoms develop, treated for STIs.
- All adolescent and adult female sexual assault patients should be offered pregnancy prophylaxis.
- HIV postexposure prophylaxis should be offered if the assailant is known to be HIV-positive, multiple assailants are involved, or if the HIV status of the assailant is unknown.
- Alcohol and drugs may have been ingested voluntarily or involuntarily by the patient. If the patient consents, comprehensive toxicology testing may be performed.
- A strangulation attempt with loss of consciousness, bowel and bladder incontinence, persistent voice changes, difficulty swallowing, or shortness of breath should be comprehensively evaluated in the emergency department (ED). Evaluation options include a chest x-ray, flexible laryngoscopy, and CTA or MRI of the neck. We recommend prolonged observation or hospital admission for persistent symptoms.
- Many victims will not have obvious physical injuries; this does not imply consent or refute a sexual assault.
- The emergency clinician should record observations, statements, and findings that were gathered during the course of ED treatment objectively.

FOUNDATIONS

Sexual assault is the deliberate act of sexual contact or behavior towards another person without that person's explicit consent. Rape is a form of *sexual assault* and is defined by the Federal Bureau of Investigation (FBI) as "penetration, no matter how slight, of the vagina or anus with any body part or object, or oral penetration by a sex organ of another person, without the consent of the victim."[1] *Sexual assault* is a form of *sexual violence*. The term *sexual violence* is defined by the World Health Organization (WHO) as "any sexual act, attempt to obtain a sexual act, unwanted sexual comments or advances, or acts to traffic, or otherwise directed, against a person's sexuality using coercion, by any person regardless of relationship to the victim, in any setting, including but not limited to home and work."[2] Sexual assault is never the victim's fault and can lead to chronic physical and psychological adverse health effects.

According to the 2015 Centers for Disease Control and Prevention (CDC) National Intimate Partner and Sexual Violence Survey (NISVS), 43.6% of women and 24.8% of men have experienced some form of contact sexual violence in their lifetime.[3] During their lifetime, 1 in 5 women have been victims of completed or attempted rape and 1 in 14 men have been made (i.e., forced or threatened) to penetrate someone else (completed or attempted).[3]

National database estimates on nonfatal injuries treated in emergency departments (EDs) have revealed that 5.4% of all assault-related visits to the ED were for sexual assault.[4] Most of these victims were women. The lifetime prevalence of sexual assault for women and men respectively is 43.6% and 24.8%.[3] Male victims are often younger than their female counterparts with 26% of victimization occurring in males 10 years old or younger and 12.7% in females 10 or younger.[3] Given the prevalence and role in the evaluation and treatment of survivors of sexual assault, emergency clinicians should be comfortable evaluating, treating, and coordinating their care. In many areas, dedicated sexual assault teams or forensic examiners are available to assist with specialized care, detailed evidence collection, and thorough documentation. The team often includes a specialty-trained registered nurse, victims advocate, or social worker, and may involve local police or sexual assault detective(s). The emergency clinician's responsibilities include providing compassionate nonjudgmental care, diagnosing and treating acute injuries, administering medications to prevent pregnancy and sexually transmitted infections (STIs), offering forensic evidence collection and comprehensive toxicology testing when appropriate, and providing linkage to support and follow-up services.[4]

The ED evaluation and treatment can take hours and requires the coordination of multiple resources. Evaluation and treatment of the patient are nuanced, with intertwined medical, legal, and forensic components. Medical stabilization and evaluation take priority over forensic evaluation. The role of the emergency clinician is to objectively record information heard, observed, examined, or photographed. In many cases, a trained forensic examiner will be available to complete the formal forensic evidence collection process. The emergency clinician may be called to testify, sometimes years after the event, necessitating thorough and accurate documentation.

CLINICAL FEATURES

Many sexual assaults are never reported to police or health care providers. Victims who report to the police and who sustain injuries are more likely to present to the ED for evaluation. Many victims present with concerns about injuries, risk of pregnancy, or contracting STIs (including human immunodeficiency virus [HIV] and hepatitis). Victims may present with mental health concerns, including depression, acute stress reaction, posttraumatic stress disorder (PTSD), and suicidal ideation. Acquaintance and intimate partner rape are less commonly reported to police and health care providers.[1,3] When these victims do present to the ED, they are more likely to present in a delayed manner, when medications to decrease pregnancy rates and STI transmission are less likely to be effective. Most patients who present to the ED with the complaint of sexual assault are women.[2,3] Although some studies have reported a similar age distribution for males and females, others have noted males are assaulted at a younger age (<9 years).[3] Populations at increased risk for sexual assault include the homeless, those with severe disabilities (e.g., serious injury, chronic disease, chronic mental health problems), incarcerated men and women, and the young.[1,5] Other populations at increased risk include college-aged women, non-heterosexuals, those who use illicit drugs and ethanol, and sex workers.[1,5]

Patients who come to the ED with the complaint of sexual assault or rape may present with injuries related to the assault, with general body injuries in up to 67%. It is not uncommon to have minimal or no genital injury from a rape. Genital findings depend on time to presentation, victim's age, parity, and methods used to evaluate for genital injury. Nonfatal strangulation, associated with rape, carries a risk of immediate and delayed psychological and medical sequelae, including airway obstruction, pulmonary edema, and vascular dissection leading to stroke. Nonfatal strangulation has also been associated with an increased risk of future lethality.

Rape can occur in the context of force or coercion or in the context of drug or alcohol ingestion. About 50% of all rapes are in the context of alcohol or drug ingestion, especially in the adolescent or college-aged population. Alcohol or drugs may have been ingested voluntarily by the victim or administered surreptitiously by the assailant. Comprehensive toxicology testing can be considered in those presenting within the specific jurisdiction's time limits (approximately 72–96 hours) but should be approached cautiously as false negatives are common.

Acute reactions to sexual assault vary and are influenced by prior sexual assault or trauma, events surrounding the assault, and preexisting mental health conditions. Victims may appear calm and collected, detached, agitated, angry, depressed, tearful, or anxious. Anger may be directed outwardly toward health care providers, making interactions between the patient and provider challenging. Victim advocates are helpful in supporting the patient and their reactions.

The neurochemical changes in the brain that occur in response to trauma can make recalling details difficult. Recall may be sporadic and disorganized but may become clearer with time and should not be construed as fabrication. Recent research has focused on the concept of tonic immobility, whereby the victim experiences paralysis, increased muscular rigidity, eye closing, and suppressed vocal cord activity in response to an extremely traumatic event. Increasing evidence has suggested that humans may respond this way to a life-threatening event when coupled with inescapability. Although tonic immobility may occur in any traumatic event, it is more common in victims of childhood sexual assault. Victims who report tonic immobility often experience increased feelings of guilt, are at increased risk of developing PTSD, and are much less likely to respond to pharmacologic mental health therapy.

DIFFERENTIAL DIAGNOSES

The purpose of the medical forensic sexual assault examination is to document history and physical findings and collect evidentiary material, not to determine whether or not a rape occurred. Final diagnosis and discharge instructions should avoid the words "rule out" and

---

BOX 191.1 Indications for Comprehensive Toxicology Screening[a]

- Period of unconsciousness
- Period of loss of motor control
- Amnesia or confused state with suspicion of sexual assault
- Patient suspicion or belief that she or he was drugged prior to or during sexual assault *and*
- Less than 72–96 hours since assault (depending on jurisdictional protocol)

[a]Toxicology screening should be approached with caution as false negatives are common.

"alleged." Alternative medicolegal options may include "evaluation following sexual assault," or "sexual assault." As many as 71% of sexual assault victims sustain nongenital injuries. Fortunately, most injuries are minor and rarely require emergent medical or operative intervention. A majority of injuries are from blunt trauma and include contusions, lacerations, incised wounds, bruises, hematomas, sprains or strains, fractures, closed head injuries, intracranial injuries, and intra-abdominal injuries. Treatment of life-threatening injuries should follow advanced trauma life support (ATLS) protocol and take precedence over evidence collection.

DIAGNOSTIC TESTING

There are no specific diagnostic tests for sexual assault. Traumatic injuries should be evaluated per standard protocols. There is no test that can determine if a rape occurred; even visualization of sperm on wet mount by emergency clinicians is often inaccurate.

Sexually Transmitted Infections

Testing for STIs is controversial in adult sexual assault patients. Despite rape shield laws prohibiting the use of a victim's past sexual behavior in court cases, there remains concern that the presence of a preexisting STI may be used to discredit the victim's claim. Furthermore, STI prophylaxis is provided to sexual assault victims and, therefore, will treat any preexisting STIs. Proponents for testing cite public health concerns; identifying preexisting disease allows for notification of previous contacts.[1,2,3] In children, the presence of an STI can be conclusive proof of a sexual assault, and STI testing is uniformly recommended. We recommend testing adults for STIs if the patient complains of signs or symptoms of STIs or when the patient requests testing, along with routine testing of children and young adolescents.

Drug-Facilitated Sexual Assault

Drug-facilitated sexual assault (DFSA) occurs when alcohol or drugs are used to compromise a victim's ability to consent to sexual activity, inhibit the victim's ability to resist, and impair memory of the event. Alcohol is the most common drug used, but many other "drugs" are utilized including illicit agents, prescription medications, and over-the-counter substances. Comprehensive toxicology testing, often performed in specialized forensic laboratories, is recommended in cases of suspected DFSA and can test for multiple illicit, prescription, and over-the-counter substances. The most commonly detected substances include ethanol, cannabinoids, cocaine, amphetamines, and benzodiazepines.[6] Box 191.1 lists symptoms and conditions suspicious for DFSA. Because many substances have a short half-life, toxicology testing should be performed expeditiously; most protocols obtain specimens up to 72 to 96 hours post-assault or after ingestion. Many jurisdictions have specific collection requirements and kits that are sent to comprehensive crime laboratories. At least 100 mL of urine and 12 mL of blood (sodium fluoride tube) should be collected, and specimens refrigerated, with the chain of custod carefully maintained (Fig. 191.1).

Evaluating the Victim of Attempted Strangulation

Strangulation is a serious and potentially life-threatening injury. Intimate partner violence (IPV) survivors with nonfatal strangulation have a sevenfold increased risk of future completed homicide. Hypoxia is the final common pathway in strangulation and can occur by three main mechanisms—jugular vein occlusion, carotid artery occlusion, or laryngeal occlusion. Symptoms of dysphagia, odynophagia, and dysphonia may accompany physical findings, including facial, periorbital, auricular, intraoral, and neck petechiae (Fig. 191.2) and subconjunctival

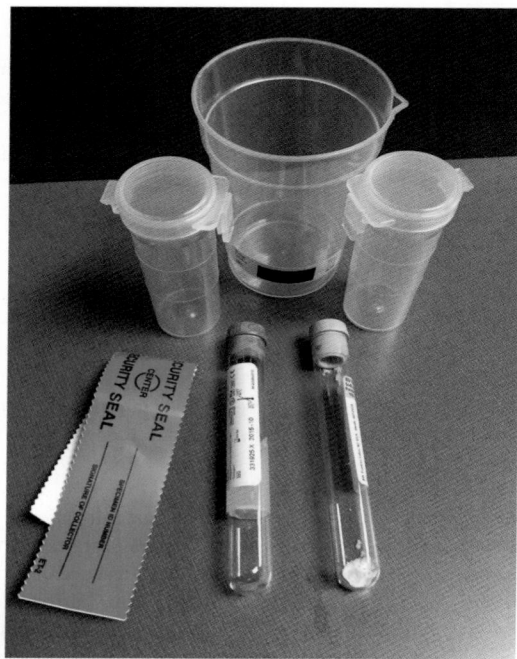

Fig. 191.1 Example of a forensic toxicology test kit for urine and serum specimens.

hemorrhages, the result of venous occlusion causing increased intravessel pressure and rupture. Other possible findings include bruising in the shape of fingerprints on the neck (Fig. 191.3), and defensive scratch marks on the neck from the victim attempting to pry off the assailant's fingers (Fig. 191.4). Alteration in consciousness, neurologic complaints, and urinary or fecal incontinence may result from restricted blood flow to the brain. Direct laryngeal injury may lead to vocal cord injury and laryngeal or hyoid fractures. Carotid artery injury, dissection, or intraluminal thrombosis may cause stroke symptoms, which may not present until months or years after the assault.[7]

We recommend imaging for patients with facial petechiae, loss of consciousness, incontinence, stroke-like symptoms, or voice changes. Imaging modalities and strategies for patient evaluation are listed in Tables 191.1 and 191.2.[7] Consider chest x-ray to evaluate for early pulmonary edema or aspiration pneumonitis, fiberoptic imaging to assess upper airway patency, and computed tomography angiography (CTA) or magnetic resonance imaging (MRI) to evaluate for arterial dissection (most commonly, carotid).[7] Patients with persistent altered levels of consciousness, laryngeal fractures, carotid injuries, or neurologic symptoms should be admitted for close airway monitoring. We recommend that patients with reported loss of consciousness, incontinence, facial or conjunctival petechiae, or signs and symptoms of soft tissue neck injury, or who are under the influence of drugs or alcohol, be observed and monitored for delayed sequelae of injury. Patients with no loss of consciousness, minimal or no physical findings, no intoxication, and a safe discharge environment can be discharged with precautions relating to signs of delayed neurologic, pulmonary or laryngeal sequelae from strangulation.

MANAGEMENT

Management of the sexually assaulted patient requires an organized victim-centered and trauma-informed approach, defined by institutional protocols and available support resources. In most cases, a sexual assault nurse examiner (SANE) or sexual assault forensic examiner (SAFE) will perform the evidentiary examination. Most hospitals should have a protocol concerning the activation of a sexual assault response team (SART), which includes a SANE/SAFE, social worker, and victim's advocate. If there is no SART available at the hospital,

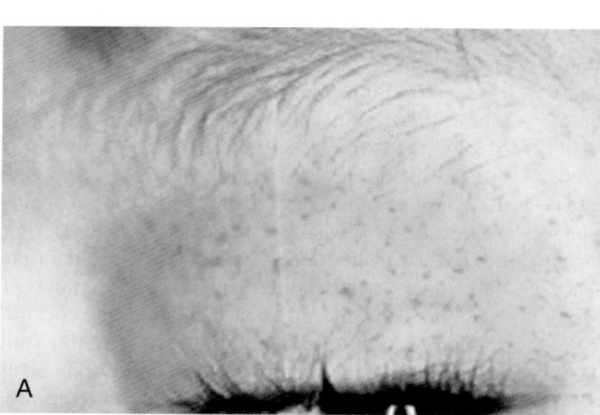
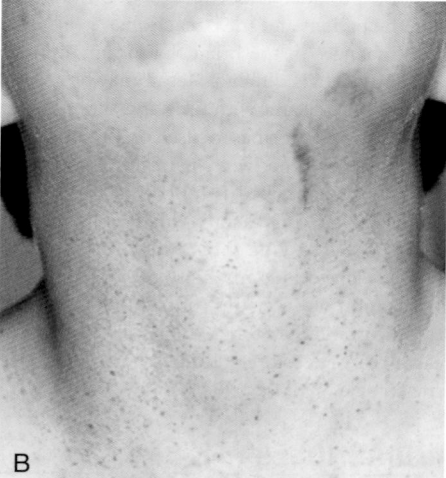

Fig. 191.2 Petechiae in nonfatal strangulation. (A) Eyelid petechiae following the nonfatal strangulation of a child. (B) Neck petechiae seen in the same patient. There is also an abrasion present on the left side of the neck and ecchymosis of the left and right mandibles. (Courtesy Training Institute on Strangulation Prevention, San Diego, CA; used with permission.)

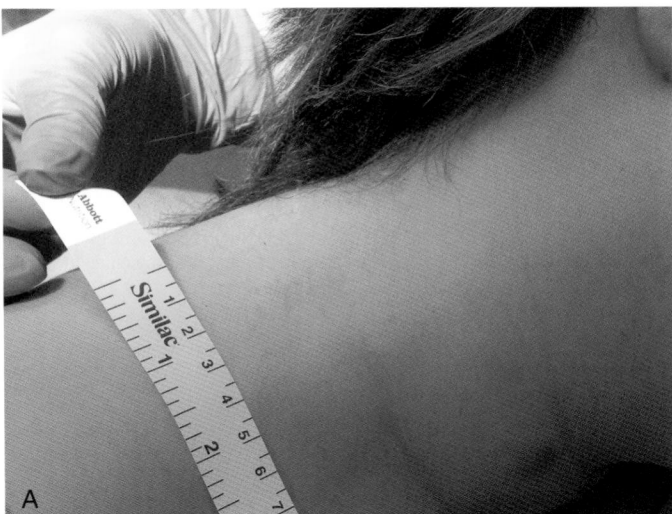

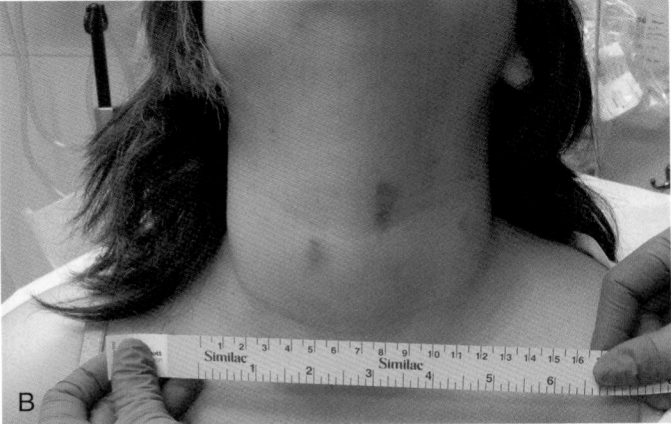

Fig. 191.3 Neck bruising in nonfatal strangulation. (A) Circular neck bruising following manual strangulation. This injury is referred to as a fingertip bruise. (B) Other bruises of the neck on the same patient, most likely made by the assailant's fingers.

the American College of Emergency Physicians supports the triage of medically stable sexual assault victims to designated examination facilities for evidence collection by specially educated and clinically trained personnel.[7-9]

On arrival to the ED, the sexual assault patient should be triaged and placed in a private area or examination room. The SART should be mobilized, and depending on department protocol and patient complaints, the patient may or may not be evaluated by the emergency clinician immediately. The goal of the history is to rule out potentially serious injury, determine which medications are needed for prophylaxis, and decipher if the patient is in the time range for evidence collection; however, if there is a question, we recommend contacting the SART team. Some questions include the following:

- When did it happen?
- What types of assault occurred?
- Where did penetration occur?
- Were any objects used during the assault?
- Have there been symptoms since the assault?
- Was there loss of memory, incoordination, or suspicion for drug-facilitated sexual assault?

As with any ED patient, providers should elicit the patient's medical complaints, past medical history, current medications, allergies, and last menstrual period.

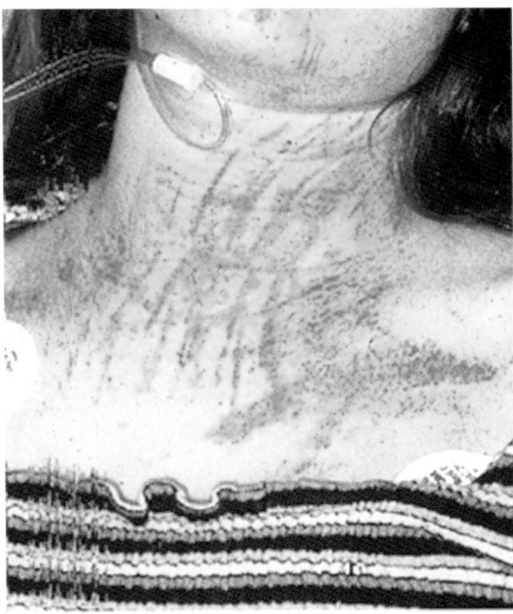

Fig. 191.4 Claw marks in nonfatal strangulation. The patient caused these injuries as she attempted to pry the assailant's hands off of her neck. (Courtesy Training Institute on Strangulation Prevention, San Diego, CA; used with permission.)

Medical Forensic Examination

The medical forensic examination should be organized, coordinated, and the patient should be informed of all steps during the exam. The examination can be conducted up to 7 days following assault, depending on jurisdiction policy, with most using 5 days as an evidentiary cutoff.[8-9] In cases of oral and anal assault, evidence is usually not collected more than 24 hours after the assault. In vaginal assaults, DNA and sperm may be recovered from the cervix up to 120 hours (5 days) later. Evidence is collected using a jurisdictionally specific sexual assault evidence kit or physical evidence recovery kit (rape kit). This kit contains all the supplies necessary to collect and properly store recovered evidence (Fig. 191.5).

The patient should consent to the examination and collection of evidence, forensic photography, and their decision on reporting to law enforcement (Fig. 191.6). The consent process begins with the forensic examiner explaining the purpose of the examination, steps, and process involved. The forensic examination process should proceed only after the patient has a thorough understanding of the examination process and has consented. The patient has the right to decline any or all parts of the examination and can revoke or change that consent at any time during the process—this is their decision and right and should be reinforced to the patient who may feel vulnerable after a sexual assault. The Violence Against Women Act (VAWA) creates and supports comprehensive, cost-effective responses to sexual assault, intimate partner violence, dating violence, and stalking. VAWA also allows for sexual assault examination without requiring law enforcement involvement. Many jurisdictions have policies that allow the patient to have evidence collected and stored for a given amount of time, leaving the patient the option to report to the police at a later date. The VAWA program also ensures patients are not required to pay for the services provided. VAWA's recent reauthorization in 2019 improved services for all victims, especially immigrants, lesbian, gay, bisexual, and transgender victims, Native American women, college students and youth, and public housing residents.

TABLE 191.1   Imaging Modalities in Nonfatal Strangulation

Modality	Indications	Advantages	Disadvantages
Plain radiograph (bone technique)	Visualize cervical vertebral fracture	Readily available in the emergency department (ED)	Limited information provided because C-spine fractures are rare
Plain radiograph (soft tissue technique)	Tracheal injury (subcutaneous emphysema, edema, tracheal deviation) Hyoid fractures	Readily available in the ED	Low sensitivity in detecting rare signs of deep soft tissue and laryngeal injury, and hyoid bone fracture is rare
Computed tomography (CT)	Soft tissue and laryngeal injuries Neuroimaging (brain)	Readily available in the ED High sensitivity Easy to perform	May need IV contrast, and screening for renal dysfunction
CT angiography (CTA)	Carotid artery injury, dissection, or thrombosis	Readily available in the ED High sensitivity	Requires IV contrast, and screening for renal dysfunction
Magnetic resonance imaging (MRI)	Soft tissue injuries of the neck and airway	Highest sensitivity	Not readily available Expensive
Doppler ultrasound	Visualize intimal injury (dissection) or thrombosis of carotid artery	Available in the ED Portable for unstable patients	Less sensitive for carotid injury or thrombosis
Fiberoptic laryngoscopy	Visualize vocal cords and adjacent structures	Sensitive for vocal cord and laryngeal injury	Availability depends on institution and expertise

TABLE 191.2   Imaging Strategy for Nonfatal Strangulation[a]

Scenario and Findings	Recommended Modality	Alternative Modality
No loss of consciousness, no physical complaints	None	None
No loss of consciousness, but voice changes	Four-vessel cervicocranial CT angiography with fiberoptic laryngoscopy	Magnetic resonance imaging (MRI) with and without contrast
Loss of consciousness and physical findings of force to the neck (e.g., bruising, petechiae)	Four-vessel cervicocranial CT angiography	MRI without contrast
Persistent unconsciousness	Four-vessel cervicocranial CT angiography	MRI without contrast
Intact consciousness with unilateral neurologic findings	Four-vessel cervicocranial CT angiography	Doppler ultrasound of the carotid artery—four-vessel angiography

[a]Imaging modality chosen will vary based on institution-specific protocols and availability of imaging modalities.

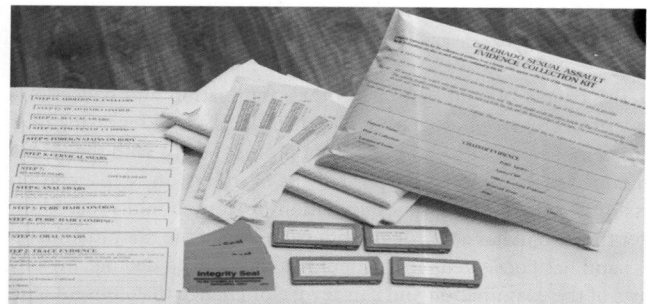

Fig. 191.5 Sexual assault evidence collection kit. Contents of kits vary by state and jurisdiction. This is an example of a customized jurisdictional evidence kit including envelopes, swabs, and microscope slides used to collect, package, and store evidence. This kit shows how the chain of evidence must be followed with signatures, seals, and appropriate transfer of property to establish integrity of the evidence. (Courtesy of the University of Colorado Forensic Nursing Program)

Questions regarding consent are often complex, especially when the victim is a minor, intellectually disabled, or incapacitated by drugs or alcohol. In the case of the minor who is unable to legally consent (due to age), the doctrine of the mature minor (one who has been supporting himself or herself, is a parent, or is in the armed forces, depending on state statutes) may allow the minor to consent without guardian notification. In many states, the minor who is in danger of having been exposed to pregnancy or an STI can also consent. If the minor does not assent to examination, the SANE/SAFE should not force the patient to undergo the examination—the minor also has the right to determine what happens to her or his body. An examination cannot be forced per the request of police or a parent or guardian. For the person unable to give consent due to mental health, psychological, or neurologic conditions, consent should be obtained from a guardian or legally authorized representative. In the case of the patient who is temporarily incapacitated due to drugs or alcohol, the examination can be delayed until the effects of the intoxicants have worn off and the patient is able to consent. In patients unable to give consent for a prolonged period of time (e.g., severe head injury or requiring intubation), the decision to proceed with a medical forensic examination is complicated, as lack of patient consent may be perceived as a further violation. Because many patients would desire evidence collection if incapacitated, and because there is a limited window of time for collection, institutional protocols should be crafted to address these specific scenarios.[8-9] At some institutions, a family member or guardian can consent to evidence collection on behalf of the patient. In these situations, evidence is collected (as an anonymous kit) and held until the patient is able to make the decision. Institutional legal counsel and ethics consults should be used when protocols have not been established.

The medical forensic examination begins with the detailed forensic history, followed by thorough physical examination, documentation of injuries with diagrams, and evidence collection, including photographs. Medical record documentation should be securely protected from nonclinical personnel. Evidence collection kits often require their own supporting documentation. Key features of the forensic history are detailed in Box 191.2. The examination should proceed in a head-to-toe fashion, with the more intrusive parts (e.g., pelvic and rectal areas) examined at the end. Each part of the body is uncovered, one area at a time, to maintain as much modesty as possible. Each jurisdiction has a standard protocol for the sequence of evidentiary collection, modified by elements of the history. Table 191.3 highlights potential steps during the forensic examination and describes the technique for each step. Some jurisdictions may require additional steps (e.g., a wet mount to look for motile sperm and for slides to be made in addition to swabs). For victims who were unconscious or cannot remember

specifics of the assault, oral, external genital, vaginal, cervical, anal and rectal, neck, and breast swabs should be obtained because these areas have a high likelihood of DNA recovery.

A recent study of over 2000 victims found that 27% sustained an anogenital injury; historically, the literature reports a variable rate of such injuries.[10] Anogenital injuries are usually seen at the posterior fourchette, fossa navicularis, and hymen (see Fig. 191.7 for diagrams and terminology of female genitalia). Injuries are documented using the face of a clock, with 12:00 representing anterior and 6:00 representing posterior injuries. Although genital injury can occur in up to 52% of women after consensual intercourse, sexual assault victims are more likely to have multiple injuries, abrasions, and a higher frequency of lesions beyond the posterior genital area.[10] The mnemonic TEARS (*t*ears/cuts, *e*cchymosis,

COLORADO SEXUAL ASSAULT CONSENT and INFORMATION FORM

Collection, Analysis/Release, and Consent Withdrawal of Sexual Assault Evidence/Information

▶ **You have the right to have this form explained and all of your questions answered. Please initial and sign where appropriate. You will receive a copy of this form after it is completed.**

Law Enforcement Agency:	Case No:
Officer Name:	Phone No:

Medical Forensic Exam

▶ _____ **I consent to a medical forensic exam**. I understand I can stop the exam at any time and can decline any portion of the exam or collection of any sample.

Reporting Decision (initial only one)

▶ _____ **I am choosing to make a report to law enforcement**. I give permission for evidence collected and information gathered during my sexual assault exam to be released to law enforcement for use in investigation(s) and potential prosecution(s). I understand the investigating law enforcement agency will be given my name and contact information.

▶ _____ At this time, **I am choosing NOT TO REPORT TO LAW ENFORCEMENT OR PARTICIPATE** in any investigation. I understand I can change my mind and later report to law enforcement. I understand law enforcement may be given my name. I understand law enforcement may choose to investigate but I do not have to participate.

Evidence Analysis/Release of Results (initial only one)

▶ _____ **I consent for law enforcement to release the collected evidence to a forensic lab for analysis**. I understand law enforcement **may** submit the evidence to a lab no later than 21 days after receiving it. I understand if the evidence is analyzed, law enforcement **will** receive the results for the purposes of investigation(s) and potential prosecution(s).

▶ _____ **I consent only to the collection and storage of evidence** at a law enforcement agency. I understand this means the evidence will **NOT** be submitted to a forensic lab for analysis. I understand I can change my mind, make a report to law enforcement and possibly have the evidence analyzed at a forensic lab. I understand law enforcement is only required to hold the evidence for a minimum of 2 years.

Withdrawal of Consent for Evidence Analysis/Release of Results (only patients 18 years & older)

▶ _____ **I understand I may withdraw my consent for evidence analysis/release of results** by contacting the law enforcement agency listed on this form. I understand the withdrawal of consent becomes effective when law enforcement verifies my identity, but will not apply to any actions already taken. I understand that once analysis has begun, consent cannot be withdrawn.

_____   _____   _____
Printed Patient Name   Patient Signature   Date

_____   _____   _____
Printed Witness Name/Title   Witness Signature   Date

White Copy – Enclose with Kit   Yellow Copy – Law Enforcement   Pink Copy – Medical Records   Green Copy – Patient

A

Fig. 191.6 Sample consent forms for a medical forensic examination. (A) General consent form.

Fig. 191.6, cont'd (B) Anonymous form. (https://www.colorado.gov/pacific/sites/default/files/ECP-v6.pdf.)

abrasions, redness, and swelling) can be used to describe specific findings (Figs. 191.8 to 191.11). The Genital Injury Severity Scale (GISS) is another available instrument that uses gross visualization, colposcopy, and toluidine blue staining. Variables include five types of injuries—swelling, color change, tissue break, hymen and introitus injury, toluidine blue dye uptake—and two classes of severity—tissue integrity intact and disrupted. The GISS can help distinguish sexual assault patients from consensual intercourse subjects based on type and class of injury. In a cohort of sexual assault victims, 40% had class B or tissue-disrupted injuries versus 10% in the consensual group. Although not commonly used in clinical practice by emergency clinicians, the GISS has been validated in defining and measuring external genital injury after sexual intercourse and is most commonly used by sexual assault experts.

General Principles of Evidence Collection

Gloves should be worn during collection, processing, and packaging of evidence and should be changed in between each step of evidence collection to avoid cross-contamination of evidence. Clothing should be collected, especially if it has been ripped or torn, taking care not to cut through existing holes or tears. Areas of clothing with possible DNA (including underwear not worn at the time of assault but put on later) should also be collected. Clothing and other evidence should be placed in paper bags because plastic promotes mold and bacteria growth and can destroy DNA evidence. If a piece of evidence is wet when collected, the package should be labeled as such, and the police or crime laboratory be made aware of this so that they can dry and repackage the evidence. A minimum of two swabs should be taken when swabbing an area, allowing the crime laboratory to save one swab for future analysis

BOX 191.2   Important Historical Information for the Medical Forensic Examination[a]

Patient History
- Pertinent past medical history
- Last consensual intercourse[b]—when? with whom? areas penetrated? ejaculation?
- Voluntary drug or alcohol use

Assault History
- Date
- Time
- Surroundings
- Assailant(s)
- Involuntary drug or alcohol ingestion
- Genital and nongenital injury, pain, bleeding
- Loss of memory
- Loss of consciousness
- Vomiting
- Injury inflicted on assailant? consumption?

Methods Used by Assailant
- Weapons—type? use? injury?
- Physical blows—slapping? hitting? punching?
- Grabbing, holding, pinching
- Threats of harm
- Physical restraints
- Choking/strangulation
- Burns
- Targets of threat

Victim Post-Assault Hygiene, Activity
- Urinated
- Defecated
- Genital, body wipes
- Douched
- Removed, inserted tampon
- Removed, inserted diaphragm
- Ate
- Drank
- Gargled
- Brushed teeth
- Changed clothes
- Washed clothes

Assault Acts[c]
- Vaginal penetration—penis? object? finger?
- Oral penetration—penis? object? finger?
- Anal penetration—penis? object? finger?
- Oral copulation of genitals—of patient by assailant? of assailant by patient?
- Oral copulation of anus—of patient by assailant? of assailant by patient?
- Nongenital acts—biting? sucking? licking? kissing? locations?
- Did ejaculation occur? location?
- Contraception or lubricant used—foam? jelly? lubricant? condom?

[a] These questions should only be asked by emergency clinician if they are performing the entire medical forensic examination, including evidence collection.
[b] This information is needed for uploading the DNA profile into CODIS to prevent confusion with DNA from a consensual partner.
[c] Yes, no, attempted, or unsure answer choices.

TABLE 191.3   Steps in Sexual Assault Evidence Collection Kit

Step	Technique
Clothing collection	Collect clothing the patient wore during the assault. • Have the patient disrobe on a sheet laid on the floor. Keep clothing articles separate. • Place each item of clothing in a paper bag; label and seal. • Fold the sheet and package the same way.
Debris collection	Scan the body from head to toe looking for potential evidentiary materials. • Document findings and collect objects using tweezers, tape, or lint roller. • Package each piece separately in an envelope; label and seal.
Biologic evidence	Scan the body for potential biologic material and fluids and bite or suck marks. • Use an alternative light source, location guided by patient history. • Use swab to collect evidence, air-dry, package, label, and seal.
Fingernail evidence	Obtain evidence from the fingernails if applicable. • Use rosewood stick, broken tongue blade, or moistened swab to scrape beneath the nails. • Nail clippers can be used to cut the nails. • Package, label, and seal.
Pubic hair combings	Obtain foreign material from pubic hair. • Place collection sheet under the buttocks. • Use plastic comb to comb through hair toward the sheet. • If pubic hair is absent or trimmed, a lint roller may be used. • Package sheet and comb, label, and seal.
Pubic hair pulling (painful, typically not collected unless requested by police)	To obtain reference DNA on patient: • Pull ≈25 pubic hairs, without cutting or using tweezers, trying to obtain the root. • Package, label, and seal.

TABLE 191.3   Steps in Sexual Assault Evidence Collection Kit—cont'd

Step	Technique
Head hair pulling (painful, typically not collected unless requested by police)	To obtain patient reference DNA: • Pull ≈25 head hair strands from different parts of the scalp to try to obtain the root. • Package, label, and seal.
External genital examination and swabs	Obtain biologic evidence from the external GU sites—vulva and perineum—while inspecting for injury. • Use retraction and separation technique to look for evidence of genital injury. • Use moistened swabs to swab the areas. • If matted pubic hair is present, use scissors to cut the matted section. • Package, label, and seal.
Internal genital swabs	Obtain biologic evidence from internal GU sites—vagina and cervix—to assess for genital injury. • Use swabs to collect fluid and evidence from the posterior fornices. • Collect any foreign object, such as a tampon or condom. • Insert swab into cervix and gently twirl. • Obtaining STI cultures is done at this time. • Package, label, and seal.
Anal examination and swabs	Obtain biologic evidence from the anus/rectum and assess for injury. • Gently retract the anus with slow steady pressure to allow natural dilation, and inspect for injury. • Gently insert swabs and twirl. • An anoscope can be used to assess for injury. • Package, label, and seal.
DNA reference sample	Obtain a DNA reference sample. • As per protocol, collect a blood or buccal swab sample.
General principles	• Two sterile cotton-tipped swabs are used simultaneously to collect samples. One will be used for the crime laboratory, and one is available for the defense, if requested. • Dry swabs are used to collect evidence from moist areas; swabs moistened with control sterile water are used to collect evidence from dry areas. • Swabs are air-dried, placed back in the sleeves, and then placed in an envelope. • All evidence is placed in paper (not plastic) because moisture may cause mold growth and destroy DNA.

GU, Genitourinary; *STI*, sexually transmitted infection.

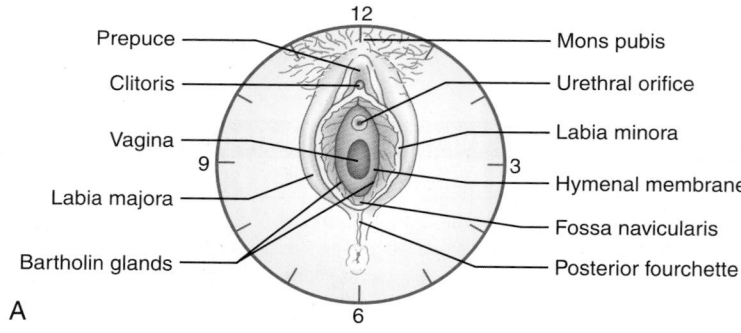

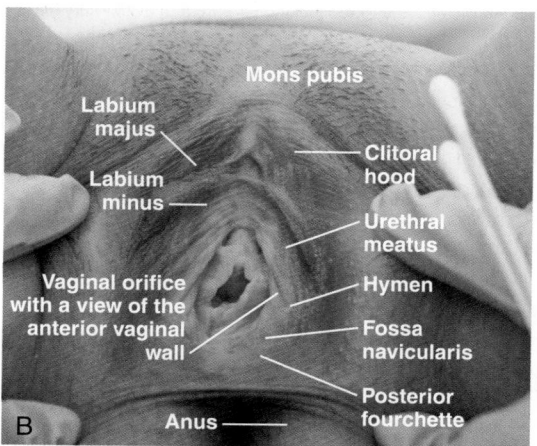

Fig. 191.7 Female genitalia. (A) Anatomy of the female external genitalia with the clock positions used in documentation. (B) Actual photograph highlighting the relative anatomy of the female external genitalia important in a medical forensic examination. (From: Roberts JR, Custalow CB, Thompsen TW. *Roberts and Hedges' Clinical Procedures in Emergency Medicine*, ed 6. Philadelphia: Elsevier Saunders; 2013.)

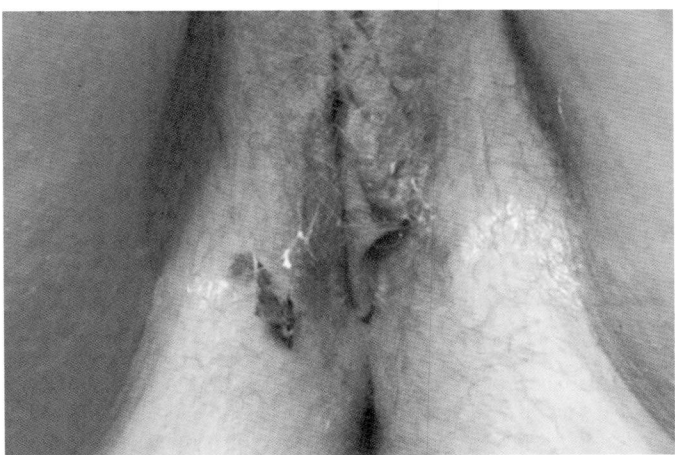

Fig. 191.8 Examination of the external genitalia. This illustrates foreign debris (presumed semen and piece of paper) on the external genitalia of a rape victim.

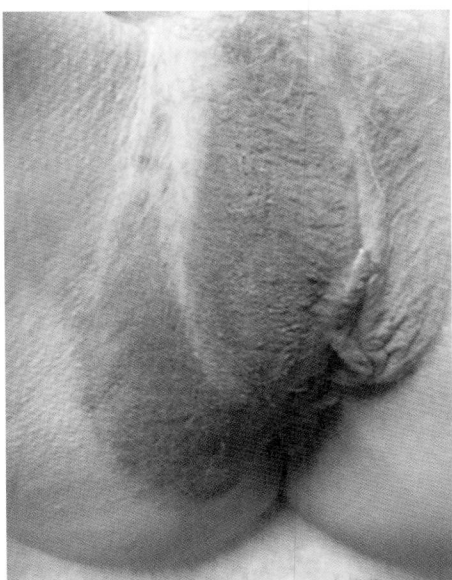

Fig. 191.9 External genitalia injury. Shown are marked swelling and ecchymosis of the right labia major, inguinal area, and buttocks in a middle-aged woman following sexual assault by a single perpetrator.

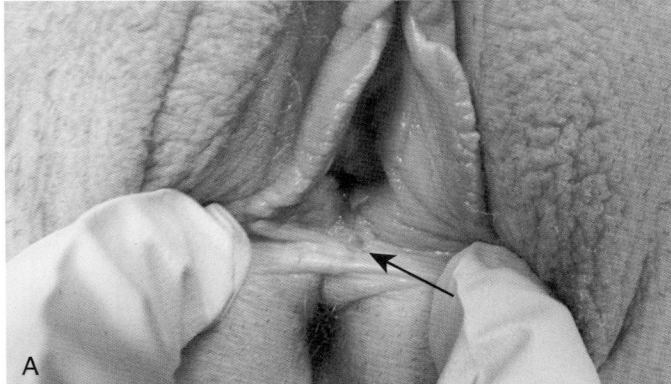

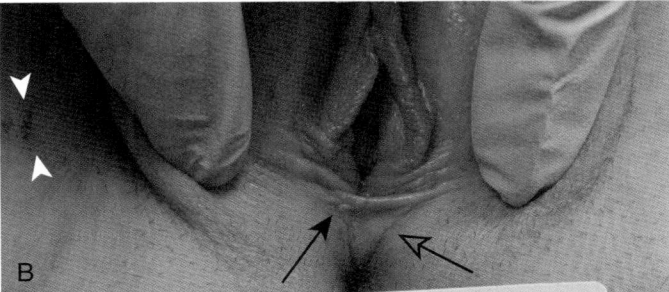

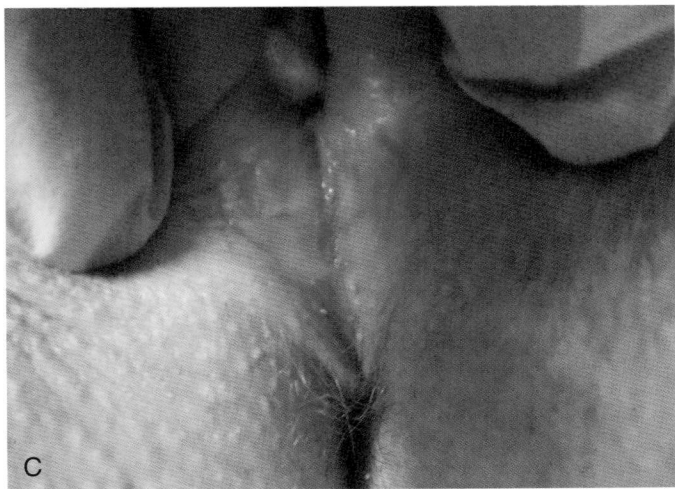

Fig. 191.10 External genitalia injury. (A) Tear and abrasion at the 6 o'clock position of the fossa navicularis. (B) *Closed arrow* is abrasion to the posterior fourchette at 6:30. *Open arrow* is abrasion of the perineum (anterior to the rectum). *Arrowheads* are abrasion and ecchymosis of right medial thigh. (C) The patient in this picture sustained multiple tears and abrasions. There is a large linear tear extending from the fossa navicularis through the posterior fourchette and onto the perineum all in the midline. There are also tears bilaterally on the labia minora, three at the 7 o'clock position and two at the 5 o'clock position.

by the defense's laboratory. In general, wet stains should be collected with a dry swab or cotton-tipped applicator; dry stains are collected with a swab moistened with sterile or distilled water. For dried specimens and bite marks, a double-swab technique is performed. First, the area is swabbed in a rolling fashion with a moistened swab, and then a dry one is rolled over the area. All swabs should be allowed to dry by air, using a desiccant pack, or in a swab dryer. The evidence is packaged into envelopes once the examination is completed, and all swabs have dried. The completed evidentiary collection kit is labeled and sealed. While maintaining a chain of custody, the kit should be stored according to departmental policy or turned over to law enforcement.

The chain of custody describes the path evidence takes once it is collected from the body and ensures the evidence was not tampered with or mishandled. Failure to maintain the chain of custody calls into question the validity of the evidence and may make it inadmissible in court. Chain of custody documentation should describe how the evidence was handled and include a log of those who have had contact

with it. The medical forensic examination kit will typically contain chain of custody forms (Fig. 191.12.)

Special Techniques

Colposcopy. Colposcopy is a diagnostic procedure to illuminate, magnify, photograph, or digitally record external and internal genital structures. Having widespread application in gynecology, the colposcope microscopically improves gross visualization. The colposcope has a magnification of 4× to 30× and can be equipped with a still or video camera. Colposcopy is superior to gross visualization

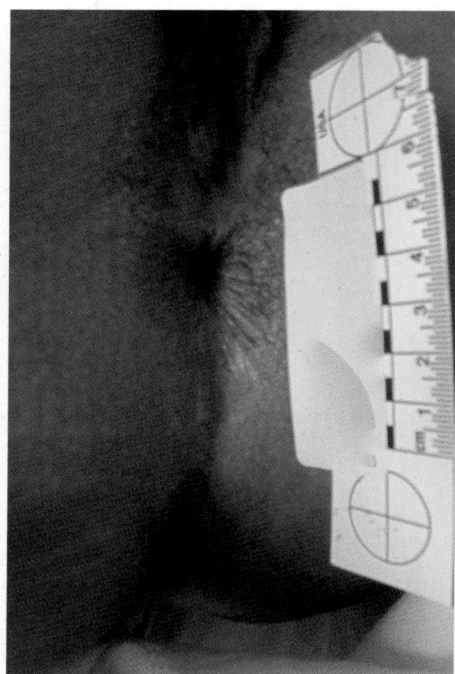

Fig. 191.11 Anal injury. There is a linear anal abrasion and tear at the 6 o'clock position with the patient in the lithotomy position.

EVIDENCE

INITIAL HERE:
WARNING! SECURITY SEAL - DO NOT REMOVE

STEP 16	Chain of Custody Form

Patient Name, Label or ID

Items

☐ Sexual Assault Evidence Collection Kit   ☐ Clothing Bag _____

☐ Clothing Bag _____   ☐ Other _____

☐ Clothing Bag _____   ☐ DFSA _____

Items Sealed by:

Nurse/Physician—sign   Hospital and City

Print   Date and Time

Items Released by:

Nurse/Physician—signature

Print   Date and Time

Items Released to:

Law Enforcement—sign   Badge/Agency

Print   Date and Time

EVIDENCE

INITIAL HERE:
WARNING! SECURITY SEAL - DO NOT REMOVE

Fig. 191.12 Sample chain of custody form which includes inventory of items collected as well as names and signatures of the persons collecting, releasing, and law enforcement receiving the evidence. Evidence seals shown in image as well. (From the Ohio Commercial Kit.)

for detecting anogenital injuries. Most SANEs/SAFEs routinely use colposcopy in their evaluations. Limitations of colposcopy include the cost and size of the instrument, as well as the technical training required. Because of this, several programs use digital photography alone to detect and document genital injury. Although no study has directly compared colposcopy to digital photography for detecting injury, we recommend colposcopy when available; however, some studies have questioned the use of colposcopy due to the psychological trauma of examination with magnification.[11]

Toluidine Blue Dye. Toluidine blue dye (TBD) is a stain that adheres to nuclei in damaged epithelial cells and has not been shown to interfere with DNA testing. More tears were identified with TBD enhancement by direct visualization and colposcopy. The dye should be applied prior to speculum insertion since the speculum may introduce genital injury. The dye is applied to the external genitalia and then gently wiped with surgical lubricant, 1% acetic acid solution, or baby wipes to remove excess solution (Figs. 191.13 and 191.14) which can lead to false-positive findings of injury.

Alternate Light Source. An alternative light source (ALS) uses ultraviolet light to fluoresce biologic material. In sexual assault examinations, the ALS is used to scan the body and genitalia for areas of fluorescence that can be swabbed and submitted for potential DNA identification. Semen and saliva fluoresce under an ultraviolet (UV) light wavelength of 450 nm (range, 390–500 nm). Although the ALS is sensitive to semen, it is not specific. False-positive ALS results may be seen with hand cream, powder, body gel, laundry detergent, fabric softeners, soaps, and other ointments and creams. However, physician training can improve the ability to distinguish semen from other substances (e.g., hand cream, soap, and bacitracin). A Wood's lamp, which emits UV light at wavelengths less than 390 nm, is a poor substitute for an ALS device, and thus not recommended for detecting biologic evidence.

SPECIAL POPULATIONS

Older Adult Sexual Assault

From 2003 to 2013, the National Crime Victimization Survey reported 0.2/1000 cases of rape or sexual assault to elderly victims aged 65 years or older. Older persons may be at risk for sexual assault due to neurologic or cognitive disease, physical disabilities, frailty, and institutionalized living arrangements. In one study, older victims reported verbal threats more frequently.[12] Postmenopausal women are thought to be at particular risk for genital injury due to atrophy of connective tissue, loss of tissue elasticity, and atrophy of vaginal epithelium.

Studies have shown mixed results regarding the severity of genital injury. A recent study of 122 postmenopausal women found that 37% suffered a genital injury compared to 17% of premenopausal women. Although postmenopausal women had similar rates of extragenital injury, they were more likely to have sustained large bruises.[12] The locations of the genital injuries are similar to those of younger victims, but older victims tend to have more anogenital lacerations and abrasions.[12] The medical forensic examination of the older patient should proceed in the same manner as for other patients. The history may be difficult due to neurologic or cognitive impairment in the victim. Patient positioning may be more challenging due to physical disabilities; the typical dorsal lithotomy position may not be possible, and other positions (e.g., left lateral Sims, lateral recumbent, and dorsal recumbent) may be needed for a patient's comfort (Fig. 191.15). Prophylaxis against STIs and HIV infection should be offered while considering potential medication interactions or side effects. Older victims can also suffer major psychological trauma, including PTSD and rape trauma syndrome, and should be referred to rape crisis center services.

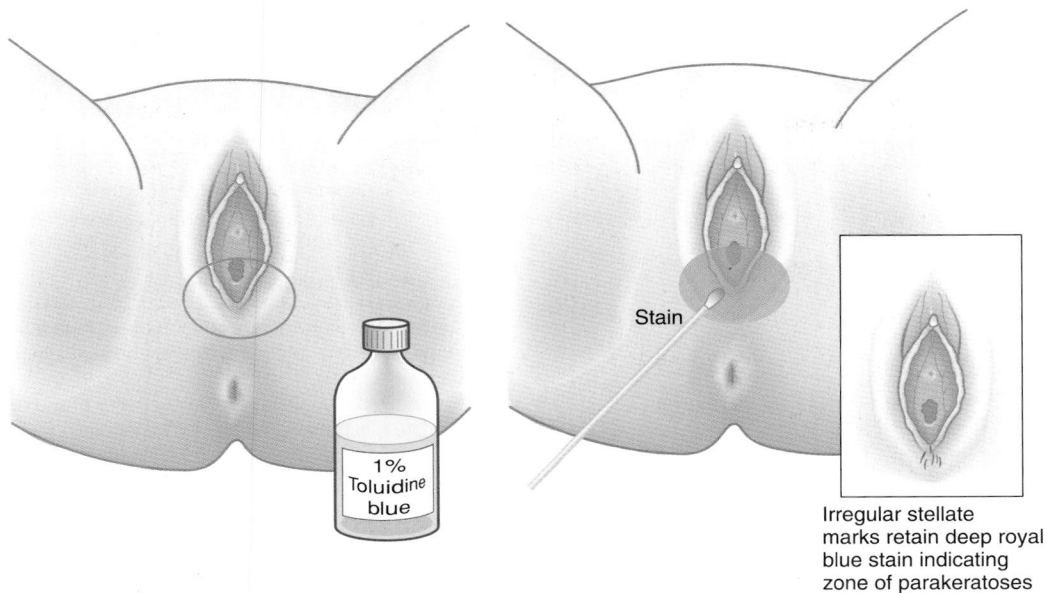

Fig. 191.13 Toluidine blue dye (TBD) application. This figure illustrates the application and removal of TBD during a forensic medical examination.

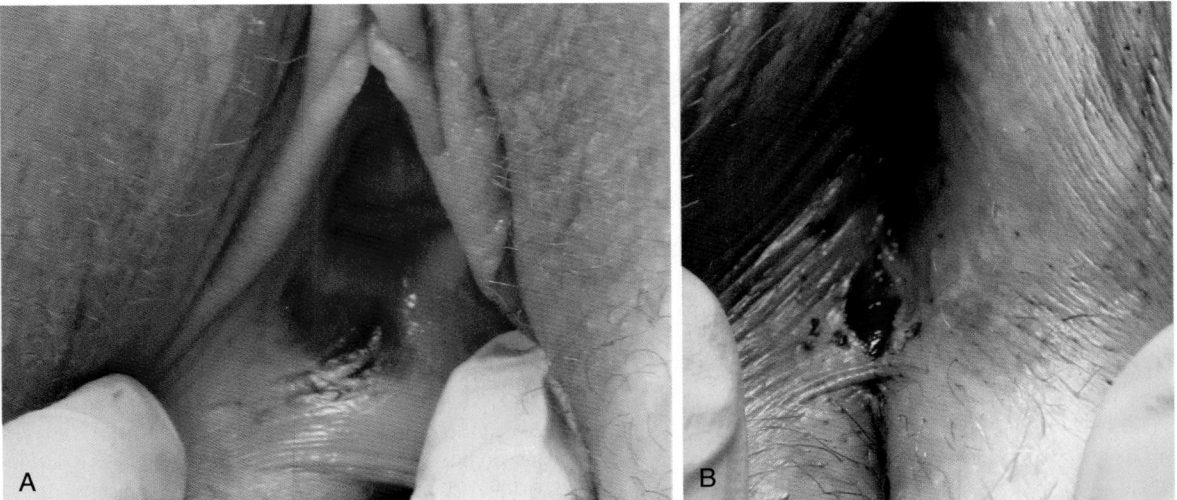

Fig. 191.14 External genitalia examination after toluidine blue dye (TBD) application. (A) After the TBD was applied, two tears of the fossa navicularis were seen between the 6 and 7 o'clock positions. (B) TBD application highlighting a large tear and abrasion of the fossa navicularis at the 6 o'clock position. There are also other scattered, smaller injuries present.

Male Sexual Assault

Male sexual assaults occur in straight, homosexual, and bisexual individuals, college students, prisoners, military personnel, gang members, and institutionalized individuals. According to the 2015 NISVS, nearly one-quarter of men (24.8%) in the United States. have experienced some form of contact sexual violence at some point in their lives, with about 2.6% experiencing completed or attempted rape victimization in their lifetime.[3] Males are raped by men or women, tend to underreport their rape, and seek medical services much less frequently than females.[3] Compared to women, males tend to be of a similar age (20–30 years), report more forcible penetration (52% anal, 15% oral, and 33% both), have more anal trauma and injury, suffer more object and digital penetration, have multiple assailants, have more weapons used, and know their assailant(s) less often. Male sexual assault includes forced oral copulation or vaginal and anal penetration of the victim or assailant. Male victims may ejaculate during the assault due to fear and physical stimulation.[3] This can cause increased feelings of guilt and shame and can be used to argue in a court of law that the victim was a willing participant.

The forensic history and physical examination proceed in a similar fashion to that for a female patient. During the physical examination, attention is paid to the oral cavity, penis and scrotum, and anus and rectum. See Fig. 191.16 for a diagram of the terminology for male genitalia. Swabs should be taken from the oral cavity, external genitals, and anus. When swabbing the genitals, all parts of the penis should be assessed, including the base of the penis and anterior scrotum. The anal and rectal examination should include visualization to look for potential foreign bodies and gross injury such as tears, abrasions, bleeding,

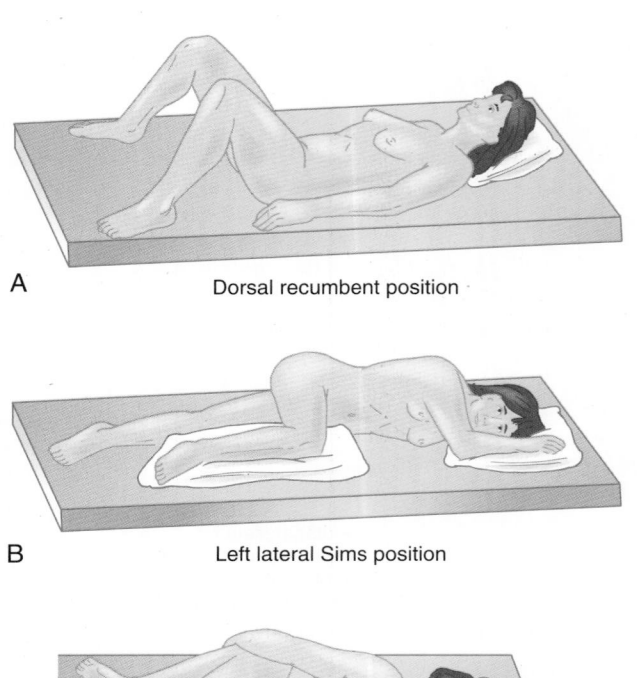

A Dorsal recumbent position

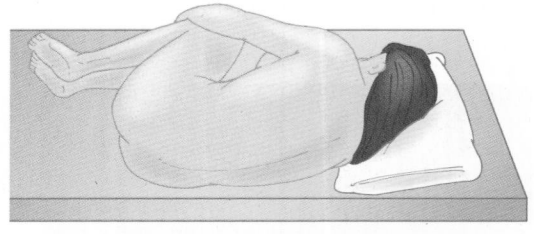

B Left lateral Sims position

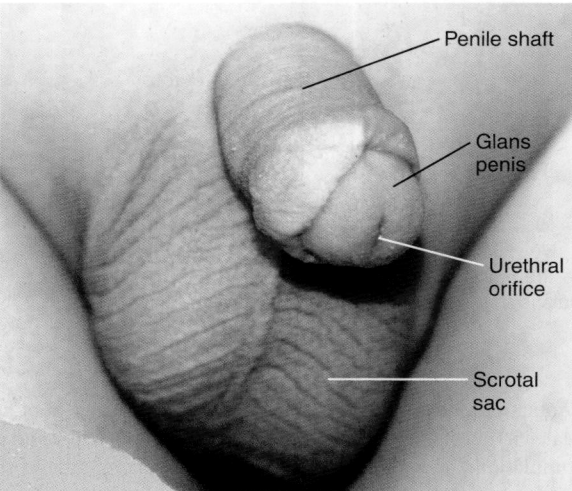

C Left lateral recumbent position

Fig. 191.15 (A) Dorsal recumbent position. (B) Left lateral Sims position. (C) Left lateral recumbent position.

Fig. 191.16 Male genitalia. This picture highlights the relative anatomy of the male genitalia important in a medical forensic examination. (From: Roberts JR, Custalow CB, Thompsen TW. *Roberts and Hedges' Clinical Procedures in Emergency Medicine*, ed. 6, Philadelphia: Elsevier Saunders; 2013.)

Labels: Penile shaft; Glans penis; Urethral orifice; Scrotal sac

erythema, hematoma, fissures, engorgement, and friability. Anal swabs should be inserted approximately 2 cm into the rectum. Visualization can be enhanced using TBD and anoscopy. Anoscopy has been shown to detect more injuries than colposcopy or an unassisted examination. Significant pain and an inability to tolerate anoscopy may warrant an

TABLE 191.4 Calculated Risks of Acquiring HIV from Isolated Sexual Contact With Known HIV-Positive Individual

Type of Contact	Risk[a]
Oral	Negligible
Anal	0.5%–3.0%
Vaginal	0.08%–0.3%
Health care worker percutaneous needlestick	0.3%

[a]Risk is higher in early or late HIV infection, higher viral load in assailant, presence of trauma or genital ulcers, and sexually transmitted infection in victim.
Data from: Dosekun O, Fox J. An overview of the relative risks of different sexual behaviours on HIV transmission. *Curr Opin HIV AIDS*. 2010;5:291-297; and Boily MC, Baggaley RF, Wang L, et al. Heterosexual risk of HIV-1 infection per sexual act: systematic review and meta-analysis of observational studies. *Lancet Infect Dis*. 2009;9:118-129.

examination under anesthesia, with some victims requiring surgical evaluation and treatment.

Male victims should be offered similar STI prophylaxis. HIV prophylaxis should be considered given the high risk of transmission from anal receptive and anal insertive intercourse. Victims should also be given (or referred for) rape crisis counseling services.

Definitive Treatment to Prevent Sexually Transmitted Infections and Pregnancy

One of the most common concerns of survivors who present to the ED is that of becoming pregnant and acquiring STIs, including HIV. The risk of becoming pregnant after rape has been estimated at 5%, but depends on the age of the patient, use of birth control by the patient, condoms in the assailant, and timing in the menstrual cycle. The risk of acquiring STIs after a rape depends on the local prevalence of the infections. Prior research has shown the risk is greatest for acquiring bacterial vaginosis (19%), trichomonas (12%), *Neisseria gonorrhea* (4%), and chlamydia (2%).[1,3,13] The risk of acquiring HIV is very low, estimated to be 0.1% to 0.3% for receptive vaginal intercourse and 0.5% to 3.0% for receptive anal intercourse (Table 191.4).[1,3,13] However, estimates do not take into account the increased risks associated with sexual violence and injuries. The risk of HIV transmission is also related to viral load in the assailant (highest in very early and very late HIV infection), route of assault, and presence of STIs in the victim.

According to CDC recommendations, all sexual assault victims presenting to the ED should be offered treatments for STIs (i.e., gonorrhea, chlamydia, and trichomonas), emergency contraception, postexposure hepatitis B vaccination, human papillomavirus (HPV) vaccination, and HIV postexposure prophylaxis (PEP) (Table 191.5). Many states mandate that emergency clinicians offer pregnancy prevention to sexual assault victims (www.ncsl.org/research/health/emergency-contraception-state-laws.aspx). Emergency contraceptives prevent pregnancy by inhibiting ovulation, fertilization, or implantation, and do not disrupt an existing pregnancy. Emergency contraception may be taken up to 5 days after sexual contact, but ideally within 72 hours. See Table 191.6 for emergency contraception options. All victims should also be given a tetanus booster if indicated. HIV PEP should be offered to sexual assault patients who have been assaulted by multiple assailants, a known HIV-positive assailant, or high-risk exposure. Unfortunately, because the HIV status of the assailant is usually unknown, the CDC recommends offering prophylaxis

TABLE 191.5 Recommended Treatment to Prevent Sexually Transmitted Infection and Pregnancy

Infection or Condition	Medication
Gonorrhea[a]	Ceftriaxone, ≤150 kg 500 mg IM; >150 kg ≥ 1 gm. Alternative treatment, cefixime 800 mg PO daily; not preferred due to treatment failure risk. For moderate to severe penicillin allergy gentamicin 240 mg IM daily and azithromycin 2 gm PO daily (note: poor efficacy in OP, do not use this regimen in pregnancy)
Chlamydia	Doxycycline, 100 mg PO bid × 7 days *or* Azithromycin, 1 g PO *or* Amoxicillin 500 mg PO TID × 7 days; toc in 21 to 28 days
Trichomoniasis	Metronidazole, 2 g PO (recommended to take at home later)
HIV	See most recent CDC guidelines[b] and Fig. 191.17 for decision to treat
Hepatitis B	First dose of 3-dose vaccination series if not vaccinated or unsure if vaccinated
HPV	First dose of 2- or 3-dose vaccination series, approved for ages 9 to 45 years old
Tetanus	Tdap, 0.5 mL IM
Pregnancy	Levonorgestrel, 1.5 g PO within 72 hours *or* Ulipristal acetate, 30 mg PO within 120 hours
Antiemetic	Practitioner's discretion

[a]If patient reports a severe penicillin allergy (anaphylaxis, TEN, or Stephens-Johnson syndrome), treat with gentamicin 240 mg IM once plus azithromycin 2 gm PO once. There has been an increase in *N. gonorrhea* resistance to azithromycin, so follow-up testing is recommended in this scenario.
[b]Centers for Disease Control and Prevention. 2015 sexually transmitted diseases treatment guidelines. https://www.cdc.gov/std/tg2015/default.htm.

on a case-by-case basis, taking into account patient preferences and ability to comply with the 1-month course of medications and follow up. See Fig. 191.17 for the CDC algorithm on the decision to treat possible nonoccupational HIV exposures. When HIV PEP is recommended, the emergency clinician should refer to hospital guidelines or infectious disease consultation for the recommended triple-drug regimens and provide the victim at least a 3-to-7-day starter pack with prompt infectious disease follow up. The National HIV Clinician's Consultation Center offers online information and telephone consultation for providers who do not have access to a local HIV expert (nccc.ucsf.edu/clinician-consultation/pep-post-exposure-prophylaxis/).[3,13]

DISPOSITION

Most sexual assault patients will be discharged from the ED. There are websites that can assist the emergency clinician who is caring for the sexual assault patient (Box 191.3). If available in the ED, social services and a victim's advocate can help formulate a safe discharge plan. Victims of attempted strangulation, especially those with loss of consciousness, bowel or bladder incontinence, or persistent shortness of breath or voice changes, should be admitted for observation. If safe house resources or respite are unavailable, consider admitting patients who do not have a safe place to go. The discharge instructions should include the number of the forensic kit collected. Patients should be encouraged to follow up with their local rape crisis center, primary care provider (or another medical provider), and mental health provider, as needed. Medical follow up should include any needed completion of the hepatitis B series, repeat pregnancy testing, vaccines, STI testing (if they did not get treated), and repeat HIV testing (at 6 weeks). If they received HIV prophylaxis, they should follow up with local HIV experts or clinics to have follow-up laboratory testing, assess for medication compliance, and be monitored for side effects.

Patients may experience subsequent symptoms of PTSD or rape trauma syndrome (RTS). Symptoms may include depression, anxiety, flashbacks, and difficulty sleeping and interacting with friends and

TABLE 191.6 Emergency Contraception

Method	Brand Name	Dose	Timing After Intercourse	Efficacy	Adverse Effects	Relative Contraindications[a]	Notes
Copper IUD	Paragard	Single IUD	0–120 h	>99%	Pain, bleeding	Infection, copper allergy, uterine anomalies	Consider in IPV where recurrent assault more likely (effective up to 10 yr) Most effective, but often not feasible or desirable from the ED after assault
Levonorgestrel[b]	Plan B, Plan B One-Step, Next Choice	1.5 mg	0–72 h (may be used with decreased efficacy up to 120 h)	85%	Nausea, vomiting, headache, menstrual changes		Less effective if >72 h or BMI >26
Ulipristal acetate[c]	Ella, Ella One	30 mg	0–120 h	85%	Nausea, vomiting, headache, menstrual changes	Renal, hepatic impairment, uncontrolled asthma, breast-feeding	More effective than LNG at 72–120 h More effective for BMI 26–35 (less effective in BMI >35)

BMI, Body mass index; *ED*, emergency department; *IUD*, intrauterine device; *IPV*, intimate partner violence; *LNG*, levonorgestrel.
[a]There are no absolute contraindications to EC, except for an established pregnancy, because they will not be effective.
[b]Levonorgestrel is not an abortifacient and is not teratogenic.
[c]Ulipristal acetate is not an abortifacient. It has not been tested adequately in human studies in pregnancy or breast-feeding; animal studies showed increased pregnancy loss.
Adapted from. Glasier AF, Cameron ST, Fine PM, et al. Ulipristal acetate versus levonorgestrel for emergency contraception: a randomised non-inferiority trial and meta-analysis. *Lancet.* 2010;375:555-562; and Glasier A, Cameron ST, Blithe D, et al. Can we identify women at risk of pregnancy despite using emergency contraception? Data from randomized trials of ulipristal acetate and levonorgestrel. *Contraception, 84,* 363-367.

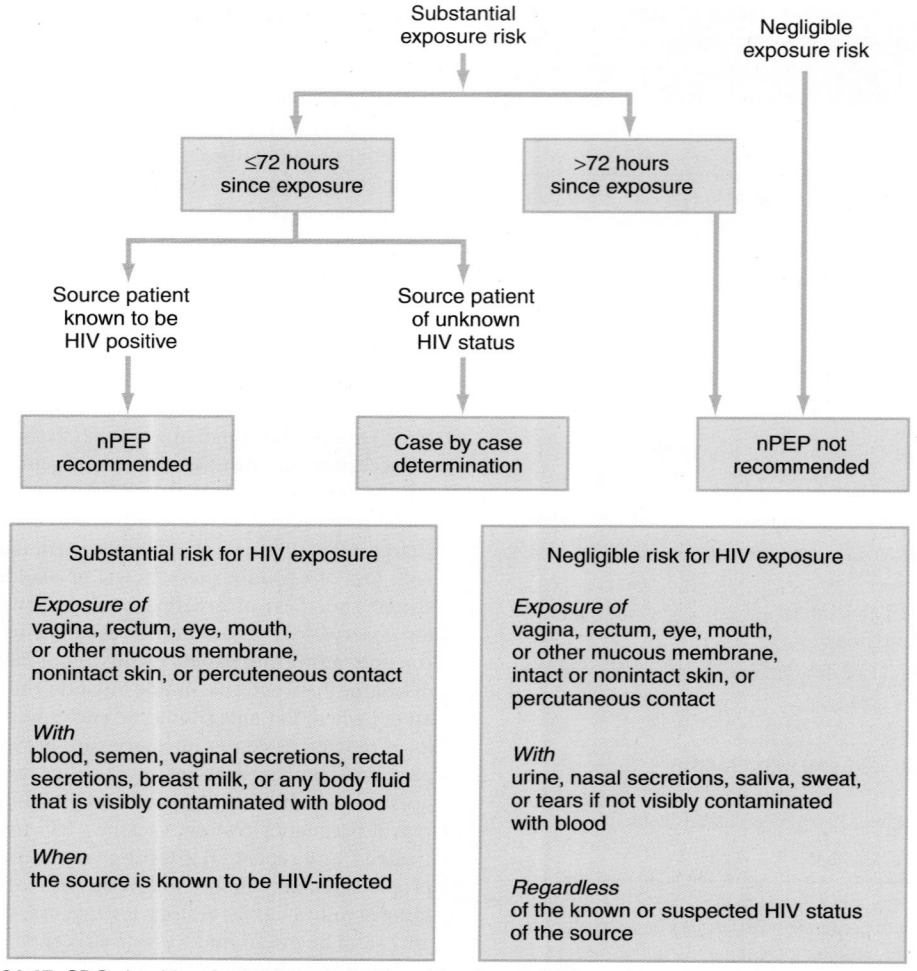

Fig. 191.17 CDC algorithm for HIV prophylaxis and for the evaluation and treatment of possible nonoccupational HIV exposure. *nPEP,* Nonoccupational postexposure prophylaxis.

loved ones. Acute pain after sexual assault is common and often undertreated, sometimes involving areas that were not traumatized. Delayed or worsening pain in many regions of the body has been shown to occur in up to 60% of sexual assault survivors at 6 weeks and 3 months post-assault.

TESTIFYING IN COURT

Although good medical care is the primary goal of ED treatment, the emergency clinician may at times be responsible for collecting sexual assault evidence. In this case, the emergency clinician may be asked to testify in court. The key to competent testimony is preparation and knowledge of the court process.

In most cases, the emergency clinician will be called on as a fact witness or as someone who testifies to what the patient said or did, as well as findings on physical examination. Occasionally, the emergency clinician may be called as an expert witness. An expert witness has specific training and may be called on to provide an explanation or educate the jury, even if he or she did not actually care for the patient. Box 191.4 outlines the steps in court testimony and includes some helpful suggestions for the emergency clinician in preparation for trial.

BOX 191.4 Steps in Court Testimony

Preparation for Trial

1. Respond to the subpoena in a timely fashion; a delay can result in criminal charges for you.
2. Notify and consult with the institutional legal counsel.
3. Update your CV and be able to recite dates of education and certification.
4. Ask to meet with the prosecutor to review the medical records, evidence collection kit, and a list of questions the prosecutor plans to ask the emergency clinician.

Day of the Trial

1. The day of the trial may change due to motions and order of witnesses.
2. Arrive early and dress in professional attire—a suit is preferred rather than a white coat.
3. Before testifying, the emergency clinician will be sworn in and seated in the witness box. There are three parts to the testimony—questioning by the prosecution (testimony), cross-examination by the defense attorney, and redirect by the prosecution.
4. In general, the emergency clinician should look at the prosecution or defense attorney when being questioned, and the jury when answering questions; this is the provider's opportunity to educate the judge and jury.
5. Responses to questions should be brief and answer only the question; do not add information and explanations unless asked, and resist using medical jargon such as *ecchymosis* in favor of clearly understood terms such as *bruising*.
6. All answers should be verbal, taking care not to nod in response. The line of questioning will often start with asking the provider to state her or his name and then describe training and certification, including how long he or she has been practicing emergency medicine.
7. Do not refer to the patient as the "victim."
8. If an answer cannot be recalled, then just simply state, "I cannot recall."
9. Documents can be reviewed in court (e.g., medical or evidentiary kit records) on request.
10. If the question is not understood, the emergency clinician can ask the attorney to repeat the question or clarify it prior to answering.

ACKNOWLEDGMENT

We would like to thank Judith A. Linden and Ralph J. Riviello for their significant contribution to the prior edition of this chapter.

The references for this chapter can be found online at ExpertConsult.com.

192

Intimate Partner Violence and Abuse

Carolyn Joy Sachs

KEY CONCEPTS

- Intimate partner violence encompasses a pattern of controlling behaviors, including intentional physical assault, sexual assault, psychological violence, and financial control.
- Intimate partner violence (IPV) patients are best served by a coordinated system response plan that includes staff training, social work, victim advocates, and a close relationship with area IPV service provider groups and law enforcement.
- The emergency clinician's role in caring for patients affected by intimate partner violence involves 4 basic steps.
  1. Identification (asking the patient)
  2. Treatment (supporting messages and medical issues)
  3. Documentation (regarding violent actions and threats)
  4. Referral (e.g., community, social services, legal)
- Sequelae of IPV include chronic pain, mental health issues (e.g., depression, posttraumatic stress syndrome [PTSD], substance abuse), sexually transmitted infections (STIs) and unintended pregnancy, and worsening of medical illnesses.

FOUNDATIONS

Background

Intimate partner violence (IPV) consists of acts or threats of physical, psychological, or sexual violence between intimate (or formerly intimate) partners. Physical violence includes any behavior with the potential to cause death, disability, injury, or other harm: pushing, hitting, slapping, punching, kicking, biting, burning, strangulation, and aggressive use of objects or weapons. Exact legal definitions of criminal IPV acts vary by country and even within countries by local and state laws. Each state in the United States (US) maintains separate penal codes for IPV crimes, with differing legal definitions of IPV. Definitions and crimes also differ under federal law, military law, and tribal law, among others. Psychological or emotional violence also fulfills the medical and sociologic definitions of IPV: words and behaviors meant to intimidate, degrade, humiliate, or isolate the victim from family and friends; threats; controlling access to clothing, transportation, money, and other basic needs; and limiting professional and social activities. Sexual violence involves threats or physical force to attempt or complete sexual contact and includes any physical contact with a sexual organ with a person unable to consent. Sexual violence within a current or former dating or intimate relationship most often fulfills criteria for a separate crime, in addition to IPV. Reproductive coercion, a relatively recently described subset of sexual IPV, involves prevention of (or interference with) the use of birth control and refusal to use condoms to prevent the transmission of sexually transmitted infections (STIs) and human immunodeficiency virus (HIV).

The Centers for Disease Control (CDC) periodically performs a National Intimate Partner and Sexual Violence Survey (NISVS) which assesses sexual violence, stalking, and intimate partner violence victimization among adults in the United States. According to the 2015 NISVS, 36.4% of US women experience physical violence, rape, or stalking during their lives. One in three of those reporting IPV experienced multiple forms of IPV.[1]

Emergency department (ED) patients suffering from injuries due to IPV may present with a clear history of the IPV but may also fail to disclose the true nature of the injuries due to shame or fear of retaliation. Thus, national estimates of IPV injuries among ED patients likely underestimate the true prevalence. In ED studies, observed IPV prevalence among women ranges from 12% to 19%. Though the majority of injured IPV patients are females injured by a male partner, men may also be victims; IPV is at least as common in same-sex relationships as in heterosexual relationships.[2,3] Eleven percent of US men self-report IPV during their lifetime, including contact sexual violence, physical violence, or stalking by an intimate partner.

The high prevalence of IPV reported by men may be partly understood by the frequently bidirectional nature of partner conflict and violence. In a simplified model, IPV falls into two distinct forms: intimate terrorism and situational couple violence. Intimate terrorism is defined as "the attempt to dominate one's partner and to exert general control over the relationship," whereas situational couple violence is "violence that is not connected to a general pattern of control." Situational couple violence is usually less physically severe and more likely to be engaged in by either member of the couple. Intimate terrorism characteristically involves more severe injury, occurs more frequently, and is perpetrated more often by men against women. The type of IPV is unlikely to change the role of the ED clinician, which remains identification, treatment, documentation, and referral (Box 192.1). Overall, women continue to be the primary targets of violence, and to experience high rates of health sequelae. Therefore, health care responses to IPV, as well as community resources for survivors, are largely directed toward women. This may translate to decreased community resources available for male victims who also deserve our compassionate and complete care. Although this chapter often assumes the more common female victim and male perpetrator, principles herein apply to all IPV victims, irrespective of gender identity.

IPV affects many aspects of health and is associated with risky health behaviors, such as cigarette smoking, heavy alcohol and drug use, and physical inactivity, as well as mental illness (e.g., depression, anxiety, posttraumatic stress disorder [PTSD], suicidality).[3,4,5,6] IPV patients often have poor maintenance of chronic medical conditions, such as asthma, diabetes, and chronic pain syndromes. Pregnant IPV victims tend to seek prenatal care late and are at risk for termination of pregnancy, placental abruption, preterm delivery, and low infant birth weight.[7,8,9]

BOX 192.1 Emergency Department Role in IPV

Identification (Ask)

- Injured patients may self-present or be transported by prehospital care with trauma known to be IPV or they may require additional physician queries to uncover the true cause of injuries.
- Directed screening involves questioning those with risk factors about IPV
- Routine screening involves asking all patients about IPV

Treatment

- Medical
- Support: This most often involves giving support and information and does not mean a victimized patient will always leave her/his perpetrator. Emergency clinicians should accept that intervention in intimate partner violence may be an ongoing process and most often not resolved in one ED visit.
- Danger assessment (often with social work or IPV advocate)

Documentation

- Medical record
- Reporting forms in applicable
- Photography if applicable and available

Referral (Will be patient specific)

- Minimum: IPV community resources
- Hospital social work
- IPV community/legal advocate
- Law enforcement (depending on patient preference or mandatory reporting)
- Reporting is mandated by state law in certain cases
  - Patients with certain injuries/weapon use
  - When children are involved (to child protective services)
  - When the victim is also a dependent adult or elder (to adult protective services)
  - The mandate reporting supersedes the patient's right to privacy under HIPPA

The majority of all assaults on women worldwide and in the US are by intimate partners. Approximately half of all female homicides with a known perpetrator are committed by a former or current partner.[10] Partner violence is a precursor in 75% of IPV homicide cases, and many IPV homicide victims see a health care provider within the year before their death. ED visits provide an opportunity to identify IPV and those at high risk for future severe injury or death.

The morbidity and mortality associated with IPV translates to an economic burden of 3.6 trillion US dollars over the lifetime of those suffering. Both victims and perpetrators generate some of these costs with lost productivity and criminal justice activities, however, more than half of the estimated costs have been attributed to medical care.[11] Encouragingly, survivor health care use has been observed to return to normal rates several years after the cessation of IPV, suggesting that interventions against IPV may have a positive overall effect on health.

Causes and Natural History of Intimate Partner Violence

Clinicians may find it difficult to comprehend why humans choose to physically, sexually, or psychologically hurt someone whom they purport to love. Potential answers to this paradox involve multiple societal, community, relationship, and individual factors. Individual-level risk factors for both perpetration and victimization include childhood exposure to IPV or other abuse, presence of a physical or mental disability, and use of alcohol or drugs.[12] Though prevalent in all socioeconomic groups, IPV occurs at increased rates among those with lower

income, job or housing instability, and male unemployment. Housing instability also increases the risk of sequelae, such as PTSD, depression, and increased ED use in IPV victims. Lack of social support for women, and delinquent peer associations for men, have been associated with victimization and perpetration, respectively.

Finally, human beings are not uniform and reflect different cultures with their own laws, attitudes, norms, and biases, including degrees of societal tolerance toward violence. Historically and worldwide, increased violence against women can be seen in societies with greater gender inequity. All aspects of our community, including law enforcement agencies, schools, the media, social services, and medical professionals play a role in changing dangerous attitudes that ignore IPV and helping those who are already affected find refuge. The literature overwhelmingly supports the concept that IPV victims want help from their doctors, and that they frequently seek help in the medical setting. Though medical resources alone cannot solve the societal problems that lead to IPV, through a collaborative community response and the four principles of identification, documentation, treatment, and referral, emergency clinicians can give their patients a chance to live without the excess burden of IPV.

Identification

Optimal medical intervention for IPV requires systematic screening for identification, and multidisciplinary care for treatment and referral. In addition to providing acute medical care, emergency clinicians need resources to secure that patients with positive IPV screens have access to primary care physicians and IPV community agencies for what is often a long-term, recurring problem, requiring long-term physical and mental health care, counseling and advocacy, legal aid, and long-term strategies for financial and social independence. Due to the human suffering and potential efficacy of treatment, the US Preventive Services Taskforce (USPSTF) recommends routine screening for IPV in women of childbearing age, even in the absence of overt injuries.[13]

Emergency clinicians may perceive barriers to identification, treatment, documentation, and referral of patients suffering from IPV. For the last few decades, medical schools have included some education on the identification and treatment of victimized patients, but many current emergency clinicians lack comprehensive training. In busy clinical settings such as the ED, the high volume of patients and acuity of disease may preclude private screening and more in-depth discussions of partner abuse. Given the complex psychosocial issues that may accompany IPV, emergency clinicians may also fear opening a Pandora's box, uncovering additional interventional needs that may be impossible to effectively address during an ED visit.[14]

Furthermore, ED providers may harbor their own prejudices and misunderstandings that can interfere with identifying and treating IPV victims. Despite obstacles, the majority of EDs endorse screening patients for IPV, and most EDs provide universal screening during triage nurse evaluations. Though nurses most often verbally query patients and record the screening information in the patient's chart, paper or computer self-administered private surveys may provide improved disclosure rates.

Screening

Asking all patients about partner violence (past or present) is called IPV screening. The USPSTF recommends routine screening of asymptomatic women of childbearing age for IPV in the health care setting, with referral to intervention services. Directed screening for IPV involves questioning patients presenting with illnesses and conditions associated with IPV (e.g., chronic pain, multiple ED visits, STIs, unintended pregnancy, mental health issues such as depression, anxiety, PTSD, and suicide, alcohol and drug presentations).

BOX 192.2 Screening Question Options for Intimate Partner Violence

Partner Violence Screen

- Have you been hit, kicked, punched, or otherwise hurt by someone within the past year? If so, by whom?
- Do you feel safe in your current relationship?
- Is there a partner from a previous relationship who is making you feel unsafe now?

Modified Abuse Assessment Screen

- Has your partner or someone important to you ever emotionally or physically hurt you?
- Within the last year, have you been hit, slapped, kicked, or otherwise physically hurt by someone?
- Within the last year, has anyone forced you to participate in sexual activity?
- Are you afraid of your partner or anyone listed above?

Indirect Questioning

- Because relationship conflict and violence are problems in many of my patients' lives, I ask all my patients about this: Is violence at home occurring in your life?
- You seem bothered by something today. Often relationship problems are a source of concern in my patients' lives. Do you have concerns about your relationship?
- All couples argue sometimes. What happens when you and your partner argue? Do the arguments ever become physical?
- Often when I have seen this type of injury, it is due to a punch or a slap. Is this how your injury happened? (This may be used for a patient with a suspicious injury.)
- Often when I have seen patients with these symptoms, it is due to stress or fighting at home (or with a partner). Is this going on in your life? (This is an approach to a patient with complaints potentially related to anxiety/mental health/pain syndrome.)
- What happens when your partner wants to have sex but you don't?

Although studies have shown an increase in identification, proving a decrease in violence and increase in quality of life for ED screening has remained a challenge.[15] The USPSTF screening recommendation does not name a specific medical site, but given that IPV survivors use the ED at high rates, the ED provides a safe place for intervention. When surveyed in the ED, 26% of women in a past-year relationship screened positive for IPV; at 1 week and 3 months follow-up, there was no report of increased violence or harm as a result of screening.

Despite the organizational recommendations and institutional protocols to screen for IPV, practical implementations of screening cast doubt on the efficacy of the protocols. Challenges to ED protocol implementation include time constraints, privacy issues, and continued provider discomfort or indifference. Documentation of screening is often included in the triage section of the medical record and tasked to the triage nurse in a hectic and sometimes public area. This approach puts privacy and security at risk, because IPV survivors may be accompanied by their abusive partner. Additionally, other companions with the patient may not be aware of the situation and patients will rarely disclose without privacy.

Some well-studied IPV screening tools—the Partner Violence Screen (PVS) and Modified Abuse Assessment Screen (AAS)—are presented in Box 192.2. Studies that investigate the incidence and prevalence of IPV most often use a second longer survey, the Conflict Tactics Scale (CTS), as a gold standard to determine sensitivity and specificity of the tool. However, the CTS was developed for purposes

of research rather than detecting IPV in the acute medical setting and may not be the most applicable gold standard for ED use. Emergency clinicians should ask about specific actions and avoid using the terms "victim" and "abuse," as patients may not yet see the actions as abuse or themselves as victims. Paper and electronic screening, an underutilized method, are at least as effective as face-to-face screening and more likely to be universally applied with less bias introduced by interprovider variability.[16] Patients should be informed about state-specific reporting requirements that may accompany disclosure of IPV. Triage screening should be followed up privately, after all visitors have been asked to step out of the room. Initial framing statements can normalize and destigmatize IPV and may improve victims' disclosure to providers (Box 192.2). Patients are more likely to disclose abuse if the provider asks at least one additional related question.

We recommend asking open-ended questions to give patients a chance to tell their story. Questioning about IPV should be done in a nonthreatening manner, devoid of blame and judgment. An atmosphere of support and understanding will facilitate patient disclosure. We recommend inclusive terms, such as *partner*, for those in same-sex or gender nonconforming relationships. Those in same-sex relationships may feel added challenges to disclosing abuse. Abusive partners may use the threat of outing a victim's sexuality to intimidate them into silence.[2,17]

Partners should be asked to leave the room before the patient is asked about IPV. Patients will rarely admit to abusive acts unless they are guaranteed privacy. Moreover, when asked in the presence of an abusive partner, questions about IPV can put the patient in future danger. Usually, a patient's companion will agree to leave cooperatively before the physical examination. If a companion is resistant to leaving, the patient may be taken to the restroom (e.g., for a urine sample) or taken to the radiology area and privately asked about IPV.

CLINICAL FEATURES

Injuries and Comorbidities

Classic injury patterns (e.g., facial injuries, multiple injuries, extremity fractures) have demonstrated limited predictive value in screening for IPV. Most IPV victims present to the ED for non-injury visits, including gynecology-related complaints, mental health and substance abuse complaints, pain syndromes, and uncontrolled medical illnesses. Historical elements that may suggest an abuser is preventing the patient's access to care include a delay in seeking medical care, noncompliance with medications, or missed medical appointments. Unless probed about IPV, these patients may not be identified. If an injury is a result of IPV, the patient may be reluctant to divulge the information. Additional historical clues of IPV are a vague or changing history, a history that is inconsistent with the injuries, a statement by the patient that he or she is accident-prone, and a past history of injuries.

IPV is often considered in women who present with injuries or assault but should also be considered in men and teenage boys with injuries. Presenting injuries in male patients are commonly less severe (e.g., abrasions) and the mechanism is often scratching, punching, or being hit with a blunt object. Though rarely discussed, emergency clinicians treat perpetrators who might be suffering from mental illness or substance abuse. These patients may want help with their violent behavior but lack assistance to accomplish a change. While making known the obligations of mandatory reporting (see later), clinicians should give patients a chance to disclose perpetration of IPV, providing treatment resources and helping attenuate abuse.[18]

Questioning Injury Presentations

Emergency clinicians should inquire about abuse in an open-ended and non-accusatory way, asking how injuries occurred and if another

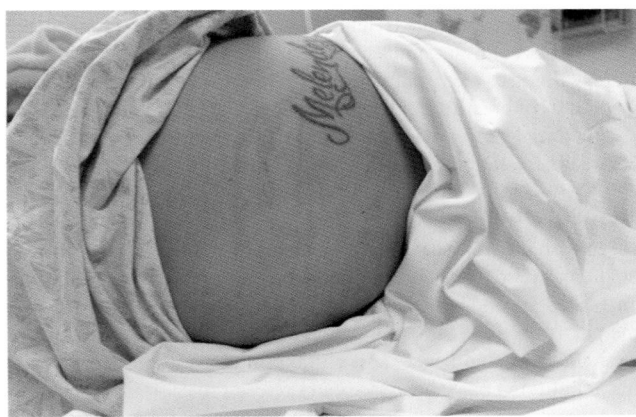

Fig. 192.1 Central location of injury common in IPV. (Image copyright of Malinda Wheeler RN, NP, SANE.)

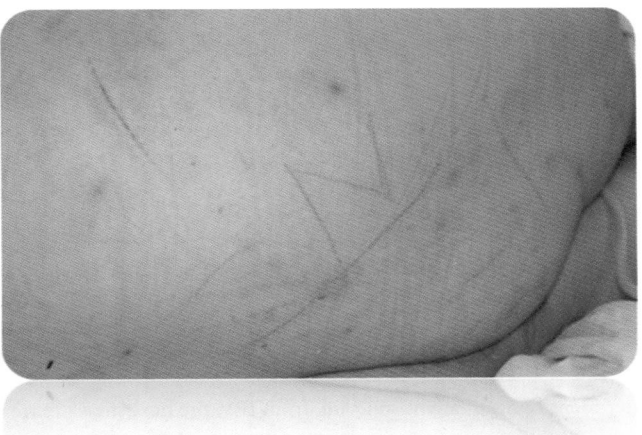

Fig. 192.2 Pattern injury: perpetrator carved his initials on the patients back and buttock. (Image copyright of Malinda Wheeler RN, NP, SANE.)

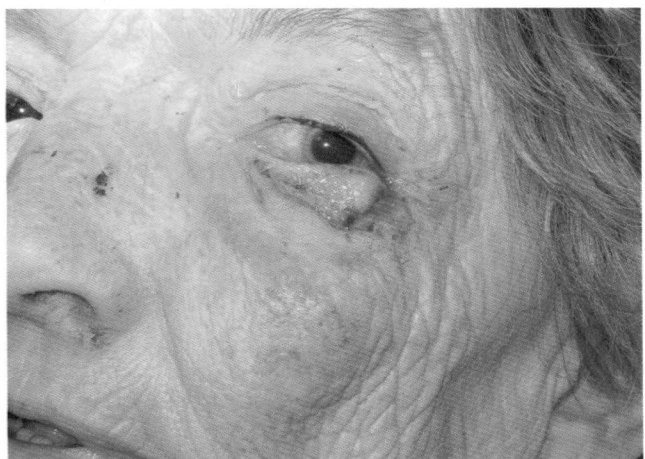

Fig. 192.3 Facial injury from blunt force assault. (Image copyright of Malinda Wheeler RN, NP, SANE.)

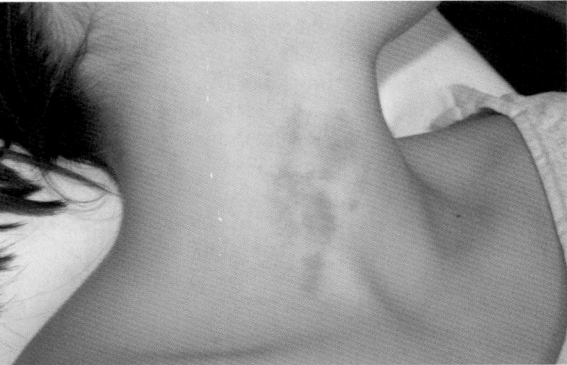

Fig. 192.4 Neck abrasions from strangulation injury. (Image copyright of Malinda Wheeler RN, NP, SANE.)

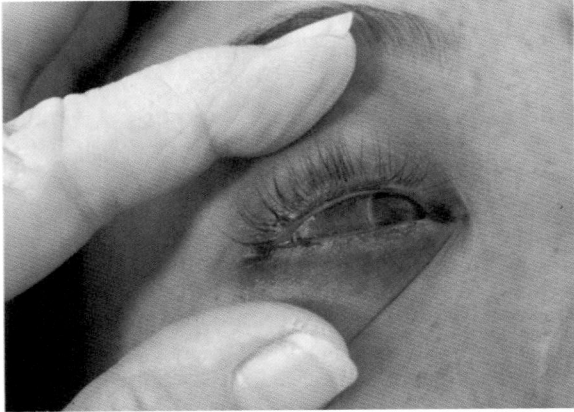

Fig. 192.5 Subconjunctival hemorrhages from strangulation injury and jugular venous obstruction. (Image copyright of Malinda Wheeler RN, NP, SANE.)

person played a role. Victimized patients may come to the ED with acute injuries, or injuries may be an incidental finding discovered during the physical examination. The emergency clinician should look for clues that an injury may be intentional. Injuries more likely to be intentional include: a central location (e.g., trunk, breasts Fig. 192.1); bilateral injuries (i.e., both arms or both legs); defensive injuries (e.g., ecchymoses on the ulnar aspect of the forearm or back of the hand); and patterned injuries (i.e., markings of an object—sole of a shoe, a cigarette or imprint pattern burn, or knife tip carving Fig. 192.2). Common locations for IPV injuries are the head, face, mouth, and neck (Fig. 192.3). Common ED head injuries from IPV include: facial contusions, lacerations, or fractures; alopecia from the perpetrator chronically pulling the victim by the hair; or acute scalp lacerations from pulling injuries. Strangulation can cause neck abrasions and contusions, facial and conjunctival petechiae, or subconjunctival hemorrhages (Figs. 192.4 and 192.5). Strangled patients may report a loss of consciousness or difficulty swallowing, speaking, or breathing. Patterned fingertip-shaped contusions (i.e., grab marks) to the upper arms suggest a violent relationship (Fig. 192.6). Emergency clinicians should document injury location, size, swelling, tenderness, coloration, evidence of healing, and presence of a pattern. The electronic medical record often provides a format to upload photographic images with patient consent.

SPECIFIC ISSUES

Gynecologic-Related Presentations

IPV victims commonly present to the ED with obstetric and gynecologic complaints.[19] Presentations related to IPV include unintended pregnancy-related complications, requests for emergency

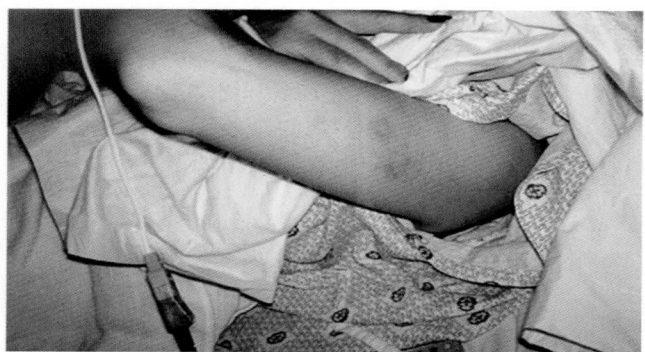

Fig. 192.6 Contusions suggestive of fingertip marks from forceful grabbing by perpetrator. (Image copyright of Malinda Wheeler RN, NP, SANE.)

contraception or termination of pregnancy, and frequent sexually transmitted infections. Unintended pregnancy and STIs may be a consequence of loss of reproductive control or sexual assault. Sexual violence is a common tactic used for intimidation and control in IPV; approximately half of abused women admit to sexual assault in the context of abuse. Similarly, approximately half of sexual assault patients name an intimate or formerly intimate partner as the perpetrator. If the sexual assault occurred within 3 to 5 days (depending on state law) of the ED visit, a forensic sexual assault examination should be offered to the patient (see Chapter 191).[20]

The sequelae of intimate partner sexual abuse are at least as serious as those of stranger sexual assault and those who disclose and submit to examination display more nongenital injuries than victims of stranger assault. IPV screening tools should include questions about sexual abuse or reproductive coercion but often fail to do so. Emergency clinicians should ask all patients reporting sexual assault about IPV and safety at home, including what happens when the patient does not want to have sex. Patients may not label forced sex from a partner as sexual assault, a message given by the perpetrator or incorrect societal views. Providers can inform patients that, as of 1993, forced or incapacitated sex with a spouse carries the same legal felony charges as stranger assault in all states with specific state laws available at the RAINN website.[21]

Mental Health Presentations

Repeated physical, sexual, and psychological assaults often carry serious mental health consequences for those living with IPV. Patients presenting to the ED with depression, suicidal ideation, homicidal ideation, PTSD, eating disorders, and alcohol and drug misuse are more likely to have a history of IPV.

Alcohol and Drug Use and Intimate Partner Violence

Substance abuse in either or both parties in an IPV relationship places women at greater risk for physical and sexual intimate partner victimization. Alcohol and drug use may be used to cope with the emotional and physical sequelae of IPV, but can also increase perpetrator violence and leave impaired victims more vulnerable. Victims with substance abuse issues often face negative social and provider bias, reducing the likelihood of accessing medical and community intervention resources. Despite the added difficulties, emergency clinicians play a key role in identifying IPV victims and connecting them with needed help.

Chronic Medical Conditions

IPV patients commonly seek care for chronic medical conditions from previous injuries or those associated with abuse, including mental

health disorders, musculoskeletal disorders, and gynecological complaints. Other common medical presentations of IPV include cardiorespiratory illnesses (e.g., palpitations, chest pain, asthma exacerbations, or shortness of breath), gastrointestinal disorders (e.g., abdominal pain and functional bowel disease), and general constitutional complaints (e.g., weakness, fatigue, dizziness, and pain syndromes).

Pain Syndromes

As seen with other posttraumatic syndromes, patients recovering from IPV often suffer from chronic pain, including headache, abdominal pain, back pain, and bone and joint pain, with disability and pain symptoms persisting for years after leaving the violence. Those with more severe abuse, sexual abuse, and childhood abuse report more symptoms. Identifying past abuse facilitates referral to critical resources and decreases use of ineffective medical interventions.

Human Trafficking

Because a trafficker often maintains a sexually intimate relationship with the victim, a victim of human trafficking (HT) can be mistaken for an IPV victim. Human trafficking perpetrators often use physical, emotional, and sexual violence to control victims, frequently forcing the use of drugs or alcohol. Human trafficking entails unique dynamics, challenges, and approaches to intervention and resources (see Chapters 187 and 172).

DIAGNOSTIC TESTING

Diagnostic testing for specific injuries and illnesses related to IPV follows general medical, trauma, and injury guidelines.

MANAGEMENT

After identifying a patient suffering from IPV, the next steps are treatment and documentation. To ensure safety for staff and patients, we recommend notifying hospital security of high-risk situations, such as a victim presenting immediately after leaving their perpetrator.

ED screening for IPV should be determined by a coordinated institutional response: ED staff training; development of institution-wide easily accessible policies and protocols; and in-person resources that include an advocate with IPV expertise (e.g., social worker). Hospitals often partner with local IPV shelters to provide real-time responses to a patient in crisis and safety planning. The US Veteran's Affairs (VA) coordinated and comprehensive program is one example of an effective multifaceted institutional response. Every VA medical facility implements and maintains an IPV Assistance Program for veterans and their intimate partners. Those impacted by IPV have access to resources, assessment intervention, and referrals, and some interventions have demonstrated successful primary prevention outcomes.[22] For institutions that lack a hospital-based IPV program, partnering with a local domestic violence agency or shelter increases resources and can facilitate coordination of care.

IPV victims should receive a trauma-informed approach that recognizes the effect of past and present trauma on the individual and their community, as well as how this trauma is impacted by treatment in the health care system. Emergency clinicians should sympathize with the victim's situation, while emphasizing the strengths of the survivor. Victims should be recognized as the experts in their situation, allowing them to use their unique insights to determine needed interventions.

Physician-Delivered Messages

IPV patients with traumatic injuries or medical conditions should be treated appropriately, and physical symptoms should not be

BOX 192.3 Simple Steps for Discussing IPV Post Disclosure

1. Give supportive messages, for example:
   - "Thank you for sharing this with me. I know it took courage."
   - "No one deserves to be treated this way. It doesn't matter what you did or what your partner said you did, you do not deserve to be hit."
   - "You are not the only one who has suffered this kind of abuse. IPV is a common problem."
   - "You don't have to deal with this alone. We have people here (or in the community) who can help you."
2. Explain that you would like to help them today. Ask permission to get an advocate or social worker involved. Ask how else staff can help today.
3. Safety and danger assessment—assess immediate safety concerns; have further discussion and planning with the social worker or advocate.
4. Make a plan for follow-up. Reinforce that IPV is a health care problem and that the patient can return for assistance.

minimized or ascribed solely to IPV. Psychological treatment and support are essential; supportive counseling from an emergency clinician can facilitate catharsis for a victim who has been suffering in silence. Victims universally feel they deserve the abuse, because abusers introduce and reinforce this notion throughout the relationship. Emergency clinicians should unequivocally tell IPV victims that the abuse is *not* their fault, emphasizing that no one deserves to suffer physical, psychological, or sexual abuse. Use compassionate and supportive statements that acknowledge the abuse experience, commend the patient for disclosing, and explain how information will facilitate good care. A few kind and supportive words from a provider can help alleviate the guilt and shame felt when revealing the abuse. Box 192.3 provides examples of comforting phrases and dialogue.

Documentation

Physicians should document the identity of the other person involved in the injury, including that person's relationship to the patient. A victim living with their assailant will need unique resources, and the nature of the relationship is also needed for appropriate diagnostic coding. Medical record documentation can help future health care providers deliver optimal care. Medical records may also be used in court to help victims seeking legal recourse, child custody, or restraining orders. Patient statements should be documented in quotes or preceded with "patient states." Injuries should be described, recording the size or length, type of injury (e.g., bruise, incised wound, abrasion), and location. Injuries should be digitally photographed (usually by law enforcement or forensic specialist) with adequate quality for legal use. We recommend at least 4 photographs of every injury:

- 1 long-range picture, including the face for identification,
- 1 medium range,
- 1 close range without ruler, and
- 1 close range with ruler.

Many electronic medical records incorporate a way to upload photographs directly into the medical record with the time and date recorded. Patients who decline photography in the ED should be encouraged to privately document their injuries with their own cameras or phones, as self-obtained images have been used successfully in prosecution of IPV. Referral agencies, social work, and law enforcement involvement, follow-up, and referrals should be recorded in the medical record. The diagnosis of IPV or suspected IPV should be documented for possible use in legal proceedings.

Immigration Issues

Due to cultural norms that embrace husband-to-wife marital violence and control, immigrant women are less likely to reveal abuse. Many cultures blame the woman for any type of marital discord, including violence. A victim's own family may desert her if she leaves her partner for any reason, even fear of homicide. As abuse draws the attention of law enforcement agencies, undocumented immigrant women may fear deportation of themselves or their partners. Additionally, a citizen perpetrator may use the victim's immigration status to force the victim to remain in the violent relationship (including marriage). Language barriers may further impede a victim's ability to obtain help. In recent years, federal and state governments have attempted to correct some of the legal problems that plague immigrant IPV victims. According to the federal Violence Against Women Act (VAWA), victims who depend on their perpetrator to legally stay in the United States may self-petition for legal permanent residence as they attempt to separate.[20,23] Programs and protocols for treating IPV victims should include information on local resources for ethnic minorities and immigrants.

Referral

Referral services can help assess the risk of acute danger to the patient or their children, determine readiness to separate from the perpetrator, and provide specific means to increase safety. Protocols should include intervention (e.g., from IPV advocates or social workers) and referral resources, including safe housing. If separating from the violent partner, patients may need legal advice (e.g., orders for protection, custody, or other official charges), shelter placement, and ongoing support groups. A discussion about past strategies, what has or has not been successful, can help guide management. Discussing the scope and consequences of the violence (e.g., on the patient or their children) may help the patient make the safest decisions. Orders for protection have been shown to be effective in decreasing future violence, but cannot guarantee safety, and perpetrators with past criminal records may be less likely to respect law enforcement directives. Although survivors may not be ready to leave an abusive situation, the provider should support the survivor and encourage disclosure to future health care providers or IPV agencies.

If children are present in the home, have experienced violence, or are at risk for becoming targets of violence, the emergency clinician may be mandated by law to report the situation to child protective services. Emergency clinicians should explain that reporting helps keep the children safe, demonstrates the victim's desire to protect the children, and is more likely to reflect positively on the victim in the event of future custody hearings. A brief discussion about the long-term health effects of violence on children may be helpful, as victims are often more focused on the immediate consequences to children.[24] Individualized safety planning may be complex and time consuming and is best accomplished by an experienced social worker or IPV advocate.

If the patient has not disclosed, but the emergency clinician suspects IPV, a disclosure should not be forced. It is more important to express concern for the patient, explain how the condition may be related to stress, and offer support, community domestic violence resources, and the opportunity to return for assistance. "My Plan" is a valuable smart phone or computer resource to assess danger and plan for safety (available at https://www.myplanapp.org/home) (Fig. 192.7). In the absence of an advocate, social worker, or law enforcement specialist, victims can use My Plan to learn more about IPV and develop a detailed safety plan. Clinicians can also consult or advocate using the national 24-hour IPV hotline (1-800-799-SAFE).

Danger Assessment

Campbell and colleagues have developed a 20-item danger assessment tool (Fig. 192.8) that was developed and validated based on reviews

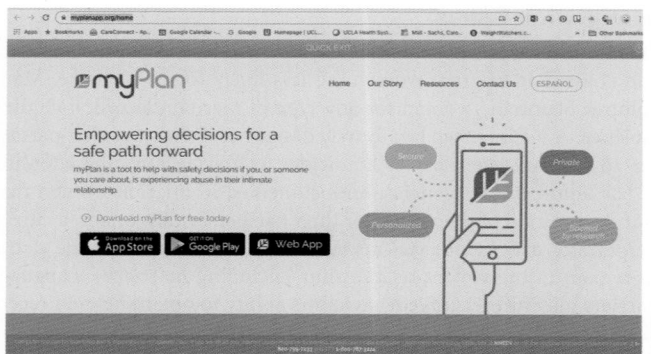

Fig. 192.7 Downloadable My Plan for smart phone and computer application with danger assessment.

of IPV-related homicides across 11 cities. This study identified factors more often correlated with IPV leading to homicide or attempted homicide and can assess immediate risk for future severe violence and lethality, however, the tool is somewhat complex to score and requires familiarity. A self-administered version of this tool is available through the MyPlan application for IOS and Android (see Fig. 192.7). A brief, five-item version of this tool (Box 192.4) can identify ED patients at high risk; a threshold of three "yes" answers has shown an 83% sensitivity for predicting future severe or potentially lethal assault. This information should be shared with the patient, ideally in conjunction with social work and an advocate to help the patient in planning for safety and the desired course of action upon discharge. The MyPlan app also contains specific recommendations for safety planning.

DANGER ASSESSMENT

Jacquelyn C. Campbell, Ph.D., R.N. Copyright, 2003; update 2019; www.dangerassessment.com

Several risk factors have been associated with increased risk of homicides (murders) of women and men in violent relationships. We cannot predict what will happen in your case, but we would like you to be aware of the danger of homicide in situations of abuse and for you to see how many of the risk factors apply to your situation.

Using the calendar, please mark the approximate dates during the past year when you were abused by your partner or ex-partner. Write on that date how bad the incident was according to the following scale:

1. Slapping, pushing; no injuries and/or lasting pain
2. Punching, kicking; bruises, cuts, and/or continuing pain
3. "Beating up"; severe contusions, burns, broken bones
4. Threat to use weapon; head injury, internal injury, permanent injury, miscarriage or choking" (use a © in the date to indicate choking/strangulation/cut off your breathing- example 4©)
5. Use of weapon; wounds from weapon
   (If any of the descriptions for the higher number apply, use the higher number.)

Mark **Yes** or **No** for each of the following. ("He" refers to your husband, partner, ex-husband, ex-partner, or whoever is currently physically hurting you.)

_____ 1. Has the physical violence increased in severity or frequency over the past year?
_____ 2. Does he own a gun?
_____ 3. Have you left him after living together during the past year?
            3a. (If you have *never* lived with him, check here: ___)
_____ 4. Is he unemployed?
_____ 5. Has he ever used a weapon against you or threatened you with a lethal weapon?(If yes, was the weapon a gun? check here: ___)
_____ 6. Does he threaten to kill you?
_____ 7. Has he avoided being arrested for domestic violence?
_____ 8. Do you have a child that is not his?
_____ 9. Has he ever forced you to have sex when you did not wish to do so?
_____ 10. Does he ever try to choke/strangle you or cut off your breathing?
            10a. (If yes, has he done it more than once, or did it make you pass out or black out or make you dizzy? check here: ___)
_____ 11. Does he use illegal drugs? By drugs, I mean "uppers" or amphetamines, "meth", speed, angel dust, cocaine, "crack", street drugs or mixtures.
_____ 12. Is he an alcoholic or problem drinker?
_____ 13. Does he control most or all of your daily activities? For instance, does he tell you who you can be friends with, when you can see your family, how much money you can use, or when you can take the car? (If he tries, but you do not let him, check here: ___)
_____ 14. Is he violently and constantly jealous of you? (For instance, does he say: "If I can't have you, no one can.")
_____ 15. Have you ever been beaten by him while you were pregnant? (If you have never been pregnant by him, check here: ___)
_____ 16. Has he ever threatened or tried to commit suicide?
_____ 17. Does he threaten to harm your children?
_____ 18. Do you believe he is capable of killing you?
_____ 19. Does he follow or spy on you, leave threatening notes or messages, destroy your property, or call you when you don't want him to?
_____ 20. Have you ever threatened or tried to commit suicide?

_____ Total "Yes" answers

Thank you. Please talk to your nurse, advocate, or counselor about what the Danger Assessment means in your situation.

Fig. 192.8 Danger assessment tool.

BOX 192.4   Brief Danger Assessment

1. Has the physical violence increased in frequency or severity over the past 6 months?
2. Has [he/she] ever used a weapon or threatened you with a weapon?
3. Do you believe [he/she] is capable of killing you?
4. Have you ever been beaten by [him/her] while you were pregnant?
5. Is [he/she] violently and constantly jealous of you?

Mental Health Screening

Given the increased prevalence of mental health disorders in IPV survivors, including depression, anxiety, and suicide, providers should refer for supportive counseling and treatment.

Privacy and Confidentiality Considerations

Privacy is a concern for many IPV survivors. Any referrals or records should only be released with permission of the survivor. IPV should not be reported to police without the consent of the survivor, unless mandated by law in cases of coexisting child, elder, or disabled abuse or based on state-specific reporting statutes (e.g., burns or injuries inflicted by weapons). Links to state legislation governing the reporting of injuries due to assault may be found at the victim rights website.[25] If reporting is mandated, the emergency clinician should make every effort to involve the patient. Health Insurance Portability and Accountability Act (HIPAA) violations do not apply in this circumstance; the privacy rule contains a provision allowing disclosure of protected health information to law enforcement in the case of reporting required by law.

Involvement of Law Enforcement Agencies

Unless required by mandatory reporting laws, patients should be given the choice of whether or not to involve law enforcement. Consultation with law enforcement personnel may enhance victim safety through immediate access to restraining orders (in some states). Additionally, acute injuries to the victim can lead to the immediate arrest of the perpetrator, thus temporary victim safety. Almost all states have laws that require medical personnel to notify law enforcement agencies in special circumstances, such as when a patient presents with injuries caused by a firearm or other deadly weapon. Many states also require that emergency clinicians report any victim of aggravated assault or a violent crime. In the last few decades, many states, counties, and cities have implemented IPV training for law enforcement officers. Courses can provide the sensitivity-training and knowledge needed to appropriately interview and counsel victims. However, this training is not universal, and clinicians should be aware of the limitations of their local law enforcement agencies.

Intimate Partner Violence Coding and Diagnosis

International Classification of Diseases (ICD)-10 coding provides increased specificity for the coding of IPV (Table 192.1). New codes added to the primary category allow the provider to include adult

TABLE 192.1   ICD-10 Coding Categories Used for Intimate Partner Violence

ICD-10 Code	Description
995.8_	Maltreatment (abuse)
995.81	Physically abused adult
995.82	Adult emotional and psychological
995.83	Adult sexual
995.84	Adult neglect
995.85	Other, multiple forms
E	Who, intentionality, nature of abuse
T4	Suspected abuse
T7	Confirmed abuse
V	Past history of abuse

ICD, International Classification of Diseases.

maltreatment and neglect. Other codes added include suspected IPV (T codes) and past IPV and counseling (V codes). Similar to ICD-9, ICD-10 also includes E codes, which are used to describe the nature of the cause of the injury—for example, "Who committed the act of violence" (E967.0–E967.9), the nature of the abuse (E960–E968), the intent of the abuse or neglect (E904.0–E968.4), and the intentionality of the abuse (E980–E989).

DISPOSITION

Patients with potentially life-threatening injuries, particularly attempted strangulation, are at high risk of future violence and should have safe plans for discharge or be offered temporary admission. Although shelters are one option, they may not be available in all locations. Patients who qualify and choose to go to an IPV shelter are typically required to disengage from their lives to protect the location and safety of the shelter. They cannot contact family or friends, nor can they contact their job or their children's schools. Even when present, local shelters may lack enough space to take a victim with children, or may not accept patients with substance abuse issues, teenage male children of survivors, or male or transgender survivors.

All survivors who are being discharged should receive patient-appropriate resources for IPV, mental health, substance abuse, and social services. The emergency clinician may not agree with the choices made by the survivor but should always respect these decisions and offer encouragement and validation. This approach will increase the chances of a positive interaction and increase the likelihood of further help-seeking behavior.

The references for this chapter can be found online at ExpertConsult.com.

Global Emergency Medicine

Sean M. Kivlehan and Stephanie Kayden

OUTLINE

For the complete chapter text, go to ExpertConsult.com. To access your account, look for your activation instructions on the inside front cover of this book.

Humanitarian Aid in Disaster and Conflict

Shawn D'Andrea and Stephanie Kayden

OUTLINE

For the complete chapter text, go to ExpertConsult.com. To access your account, look for your activation instructions on the inside front cover of this book.

Emergency Ultrasound

L. Connor Nickels and Petra Duran-Gehring

OUTLINE

For the complete chapter text, go to ExpertConsult.com. To access your account, look for your activation instructions on the inside front cover of this book.

The Geriatric Emergency Department

Kevin Biese and Ula Hwang

For the complete chapter text, go to ExpertConsult.com. To access your account, look for your activation instructions on the inside front cover of this book.

e5

End of Life

Ashley Shreves and Tammie E. Quest

OUTLINE

For the complete chapter text, go to ExpertConsult.com. To access your account, look for your activation instructions on the inside front cover of this book.

Bioethics

Kenneth V. Iserson and Carlton E. Heine

OUTLINE

For the complete chapter text, go to ExpertConsult.com. To access your account, look for your activation instructions on the inside front cover of this book.

Emergency Medical Treatment and Labor Act and Medicolegal Issues

Robert A. Bitterman

OUTLINE

For the complete chapter text, go to ExpertConsult.com. To access your account, look for your activation instructions on the inside front cover of this book.

Quality Improvement and Patient Safety

Bryan A. Stenson and Shamai A. Grossman

OUTLINE

For the complete chapter text, go to ExpertConsult.com. To access your account, look for your activation instructions on the inside front cover of this book.

e9

Patient Experience in the Emergency Department

Emily L. Aaronson and Benjamin White

OUTLINE

For the complete chapter text, go to ExpertConsult.com. To access your account, look for your activation instructions on the inside front cover of this book.

Wellness, Stress, and the Impaired Physician

Lori Weichenthal and Julius (Jay) A. Kaplan

OUTLINE

For the complete chapter text, go to ExpertConsult.com. To access your account, look for your activation instructions on the inside front cover of this book.

e11

Forensic Emergency Medicine

Adedamola A. Ogunniyi and Andrea W. Wu

OUTLINE

For the complete chapter text, go to the ExpertConsult.website. To access your account, look for your activation instructions on the inside front cover of this book.

Emergency Medical Services: Overview and Ground Transport

Thomas H. Blackwell

OUTLINE

For the complete chapter text, go to ExpertConsult.com. To access your account, look for your activation instructions on the inside front cover of this book.

e13

Air Medical Transport

Ira J. Blumen and Howard Rodenberg

OUTLINE

For the complete chapter text, go to ExpertConsult.com. To access your account, look for your activation instructions on the inside front cover of this book.

Disaster Preparedness

Carl H. Schultz and Romeo Fairley

OUTLINE

For the complete chapter text, go to ExpertConsult.com. To access your account, look for your activation instructions on the inside front cover of this book.

Weapons of Mass Destruction

Kristi L. Koenig and Romeo Fairley

OUTLINE

For the complete chapter text, go to ExpertConsult.com. To access your account, look for your activation instructions on the inside front cover of this book.

Tactical Emergency Medical Support and Urban Search and Rescue

Nelson Tang and Matthew J. Levy

OUTLINE

For the complete chapter text, go to ExpertConsult.com. To access your account, look for your activation instructions on the inside front cover of this book.

INDEX

Note: Page numbers followed by "f" indicate figures "t" indicate tables and "b" indicate boxes.

Myocardial infarction (MI)
  acute, 851
    anatomic location of, 858–862
    anterior, 858–860, 859f
    anterolateral, 858–860, 859f, 861f
    classification of, 851
    early complications of, 854–855
    electrocardiography in, 856f
    inferior, 860–861, 860f
    lateral, 859f, 860, 861f
    in left bundle branch block, 864, 866f
    posterior, 861–862, 862f, 867, 869f
    regional ST segment changes in, 858–860,
      859t
    ST segment-T wave morphology
      in, 855, 857f
    ventricular paced pattern with,
      865, 868f
  anterior, 858–860, 859f
  chest pain and, 208t–209t
  in diabetes, 1549
  fibrinolytic therapy and, 886
  heart failure and, 939–940, 943t
  inferior, 860–861, 860f, 862f
  non-Q wave, 851, 867
  non-ST segment elevation, 867
  nontransmural, 851
  posterior, 861–862, 862f
  post-MI syndrome, 854
  post-myocardial infarction, 965
  Q wave, 851
  reperfusion therapy for, 887
  right ventricular, 862, 863f
  rule-out MI protocol and, 873
  STEMI alert responses, 879–880
  transmural, 851
  types of, 851
  vomiting in, 229t–230t
Myocardial ischemia, 939–940
Myocardial rupture, 388–389
  anatomy of, 388
  clinical features of, 388
  diagnostic testing for, 388–389, 389f
  importance of, 388
  management of, 389
  pathophysiology of, 388
  physiology of, 388
Myocardial scintigraphy, 874
Myocardial stunning, 852, 935
Myocarditis, 960–962
  in children, 2127
    clinical features of, 2127
    diagnostic testing for, 2127
    foundations of, 2127
    management of, 2127
  clinical features of, 961
  diagnostic testing for, 961
  differential diagnosis of, 961
  foundations of, 960–961
  infectious causes of, 961b
  key concepts, 955b
  management of, 961–962
  patient disposition in, 962
Myoglobin, 1562
  in acute coronary syndrome, 871t,
    872f, 873
  normal physiology of, 1559
  serum, 1562
  urine, 1562
Myoglobin-induced acute kidney injury, in
  rhabdomyolysis, 1561–1562
Myopathies, 1317
Myositis ossificans, 583–584, 584f
MyPlan application, 2443–2444,
  2444f
Myristica fragrans, 1923

Myxedema coma, 1576, 1577t
  factors, 1577b
  management of, 1578
  patient disposition, 1578
  recognition of, 1577t
  treatment of, 1578b

N

Nadolol, 1891t
Naegleria, 1667
  drug regimens for, 1658t–1663t
Naftifine, for tinea corporis, 1439
Nail, 459–460, 460f
Nail bed injuries, lacerations, 488–490,
  491f
Nalbuphine, 70t
Naldemedine (Symproic), 255t–256t
Nalmefene, 1961
Naloxegol (Movantik), 255t–256t
Naloxone, 73–74, 1961
  for opioid overdose, 1960
  in pregnancy, 2281
  for PSA reversal and rescue, 88, 2029
  safety, 1960–1961
Nanocrystalline silver, for burns, 716t
Napoleonic Wars, e112
Naproxen
  for gouty arthritis, 1378
  for vaginal bleeding, 267t
Naproxen sodium, for migraine
  attacks, 1257t
Narcolepsy, 2187
Narcotics, 2025
Narrow-complex tachycardia, 901–903
Nasal bleeding, 788
Nasal flaring, 2000, 2001f
Nasal fractures, 331
Nasal packing, 789
NASEMSO. *See* National Association of State
  Emergency Medical Service Officials
Nasopharynx, 183, 184f
Nasotracheal intubation, in neck, 374
Nateglinide, 1546t
National Academy of Sciences-National Re-
  search Council, e112
National Association of State Emergency Medi-
  cal Service Officials (NASEMSO), e115
National Button Battery Ingestion
  Hotline, 1047
National Capital Poison Center, 2146
National Emergency X-Radiography Utilization
  Study (NEXUS), 340b–361b, 357–358
  for cervical spine injury, 2329
National Highway Traffic Safety Administration
  (NHTSA), e112
National Incident Management System (NIMS),
  2459.e139, 2459.e143
National Institutes of Health Stroke Scale (NI-
  HSS), 1228, 1229t
National Intimate Partner and Sexual Violence
  Survey (NISVS), 2438
National Response Center, 1823t
National Response Framework, 2459.e135t,
  2459.e139, 2459.e143
National Response Plan, 2459.e143
Natriuretic peptide
  hemodynamic effects, 984t
  for hypertension, 984t
Natural barriers, disruption of, 2357
Natural disasters, e10–e11, e11t
Natural killer (NK) cells, 2350
Natural rubber latex, as triggers for anaphylaxis,
  1420
Nausea and vomiting, 227–239
  ancillary studies for, 232–233
  associated symptoms with, 231

Nausea and vomiting (Continued)
  cannabinoid hyperemesis syndrome,
    229t–230t, 238
  causes of, 231t
  in chemotherapy, 238
  cyclical vomiting and, 238
  diagnostic algorithm for, 233
  diagnostic approach to, 227–233, 234f–235f
  differential diagnosis considerations for,
    227–228
  differential diagnosis of, 231t
  epidemiology of, 227
  in gastroparesis, 239
  headache in, 238
  history of similar episodes of, 231–232
  key concepts, 227b
  management of, empirical, 233–239, 237f
    adults, 233–236
    pediatrics, 238
  medications for treatment of, 236t
  opioid-induced vomiting and, 238
  past medical history of, 231
  pathophysiology of, 227, 228f
  patient disposition in, 239
  physical examination of, 232, 232t
  pivotal findings for, 228–233
  in pregnancy, 238
  signs of, 232
  social history of, 231
  symptoms of, 228–232
  in vertigo, 239
Navicular anatomy, 642
Navicular dislocations, 643
Navicular fractures, 642–643
  body fractures, 642
  clinical features of, 642
  diagnostic testing for, 642
  dorsal avulsion fractures, 642
  management of, 642–643
  pathophysiology of, 642
  patient disposition for, 643
  radiology in, 642
  tuberosity fractures, 642
NCSE. *See* Nonconvulsive status epilepticus
NDMS. *See* National Disaster Medical System
Near drowning, 1815
Near-fatal asthma, 803–804
Near field, definition of, e20b
Near-infrared spectroscopy, in peripheral vascular injury, 434
Nebulizers, for asthma in children, 2092
Necator americanus, drug regimens for,
  1658t–1663t
Neck
  anatomy of, 368–369, 369f, 737–739
  deep infection in, 737–741
  fascial planes of, 737
  mobility, 4–5
Neck bruising, in nonfatal strangulation, 2425f
Neck injury, 143
  electrical, 1784–1785
Neck masses, 791–793
  clinical features of, 791–792
  diagnostic testing for, 792
  differential diagnosis of, 792, 792b
  management and patient disposition in,
    792–793
  rule of 80 or 80% rule for, 791
Neck trauma, 368–375, 368b
  airway management in, 374
  blunt trauma
    diagnostic testing for, 372
    management of, 374, 374t
  clinical features of, 370–371
  diagnostic testing for, 371–373
  differential diagnosis of, 371, 372t

Vesicant (blistering agents), 2460.e156–2460. e157, 728–729, 728t
Vestibular neuritis, 144t–145t
  diagnosis of, 143t
  differentiating benign paroxysmal positional vertigo, 148t
Vestibular schwannoma, 1288
  clinical features of, 1288
  diagnostic testing for, 1288
  differential diagnosis of, 1288
  foundations of, 1288
  key concepts, 1281b
  management of, 1288
  patient disposition in, 1288
Vestibulocochlear nerve (CN VIII), 1285t–1286t
Vibrio cholera infection, treatment of, 2157t–2158t
Vibrio cholerae infection enteritis, 1115t, 1123–1124
Vibrio gastroenteritis, 1115t, 1123–1124
  clinical features of, 1123
  diagnostic testing for, 1123
  epidemiology of, 1123
  management of, 1123–1124
  pathophysiology of, 1123
Vibrio parahaemolyticus infection
  gastroenteritis, 1120–1121, 1123
    clinical features of, 1120–1121
    diagnostic testing for, 1121
    epidemiology of, 1114t, 1120
    management of, 1121
    pathophysiology of, 1120
    treatment of, 1115t, 2157t–2158t
Vibrio vulnificus infection
  in enteritis, 1123
  in skin, 1730
Videolaryngoscopes, 18–20, 20f
Videolaryngoscopy, 2013–2014
  devices, 2014t
  direct laryngoscopy *versus*, 18
  for trauma patients, 290
Vincent angina, 734
Violence
  community, 2418–2421, 2418b
    Boston University HVIP Model, 2420–2421
    disparities in access to mental health care services and treatment, 2419
    hospital-based violence intervention programs, 2419–2421
    physical trauma from, 2419–2421
    population characteristics and, 2418
    psychological and mental health, 2419
    root causes of, 2419
  conditions associated with, 2380b
  emergency department preparedness and prevention of, 2381b
  interpersonal, in pregnancy, 2311
  patient behaviors suggesting impending, 2381b
  risk assessment of, 2381
Violence Against Women Act (VAWA), 2425
Violent behavior, 2380
  organic from functional causes of, 2386t
  pathogenesis of, 2379
Viperidae snakes, 691
Viral arthritis, 1376t
Viral conjunctivitis, 763–764, 763f
Viral croup, 2084–2085
Viral disease, dyspnea and, 197t
Viral encephalitis, 1323–1324
  management of, 1331
Viral exanthems, 1437–1438, 1438f
Viral gastroenteritis, 1125–1126, 1125t
  diagnosis and treatment of, 1116t
Viral hepatitis, 1059–1065
  in solid organ transplantation, 2370

Viral infections
  causing nonspecific febrile illness, 1617–1620
  impaired cell-mediated immunity, 2357
  with neurologic manifestations, 1623–1630
  skin and, 1435–1438
  with vesicular rash, 1614–1617
Viral meningitis, 1323
  management of, 1331
Viral pharyngitis, 816
Viral pneumonia, 2102
  radiographic findings of, 2103f
  syndromes, 2102t
Viral vaccines, 1612t
Viruses, 1610–1634, 1610b
  associated with diarrheal illness, 1623
  classification of, 1611t
  foundations of, 1610
  in infectious diarrhea, 2152–2161, 2154t
Viscera
  electrical injury to, 1785
  peripheral arterial aneurysms, 1016–1017
Visceral larva migrans, drug regimens for, 1658t–1663t
Visceral leishmaniasis, in HIV infection and AIDS, 1673
Visceral pain, 64, 211
Viscosity, 1935
Vision, primary disorders of, 769–776, 769f
Vision loss
  chiasmal, 770
  functional, 775–776
  neuro-ophthalmologic, 770
  post-chiasmal, 770
  prechiasmal, 770
Visual acuity, 167, 170
Visual analogue scale (VAS), 2022
Visual field deficits, 772–774
Visual field testing, 170
Vital signs
  in children, 2032b
  in dizziness, 144
  pediatric, 1997t, 2111–2112, 2112t
  predicting toxicity from, 1831b
  toxic syndromes and, 2387t
Vitamin A, for rubeola, 1438
Vitamin B$_6$ (pyridoxine), in pregnancy, 2288
Vitamin B$_{12}$, 1470t
Vitamin B$_{12}$ deficiency, 1468–1469, 1469b
Vitamin K, 1497–1498
Vitreous detachment, 772
Vitreous hemorrhage, 772, 773f
Vocal cord paralysis, 2083–2084
Volar plate, 461
Volatility, 1935
Volcanic activity, 2459.e134
Voltage, 1781
Volume, resuscitation, for thyroid storm, 1570b
Volume-controlled ventilation (VCV), 25, 25t
Volume expanders, for neonatal resuscitation, 2050, 2050t
Volume expansion, in anaphylaxis, 1425
Volume of distribution (V$_d$), of drug, 2373
Volume overload, heart failure and, 938
Volume regulation, in acute kidney injury, 1171
Volume replacement, 39–40
Volume resuscitation, for hypothermia, 1758
Volvulus, 1138–1140
  bird's beak sign of, 1139f
  cecal, 1138
    clinical features of, 1138
    diagnostic testing for, 1139, 1139f–1140f
    management of, 1140
  clinical features of, 1138
  diagnostic testing for, 1138–1139
  differential diagnosis of, 1138

Volvulus (*Continued*)
  foundations of, 1138
  gastric, 1056–1057
  key concepts, 1132b
  management of, 1139–1140
  patient disposition in, 1140
  sigmoid, 1138
    bird's beak sign of, 1139f
    clinical features of, 1138
    diagnostic testing for, 1138–1139, 1139f
    management of, 1139–1140
  small bowel, 1095
Vomiting, 227
  acute, 227–228
  in children, 2162, 2163t
  cyclical, 238
  differential considerations for, 2137t
  disorders associated with, 229t–230t
  duration of, 231
  opioid-induced, 238
  in pediatric after head injury, 2056–2057
  process of, 228f
  sequelae of, 236t
  timing of, 231
Vomiting center, 227
Vomitus, differential diagnosis based on content of, 232t
von Willebrand disease, 1497
V/Q mismatch, 102
V/Q ratios
  high, 102
  low, 102
VTE-BLEED score, 1029b
Vulnerable triage populations, 2459.e138
Vulvovaginal candidiasis, 1191, 1441
VVEEPP, mnemonic, 169–170
VX, 2460.e155–2460.e156, 2460.e156b, 728, 728t
V-Y wound closure, 658, 662f

W

Wait times, patient experience and, 2454.e85
Wallenberg syndrome, 144t–145t
Warfarin
  excessive anticoagulation from, 1497–1498
  older patients and, 2334t
  in pregnancy, 2279
Warm ischemia, 431
Warts, genital, 1191–1192, 1191f
WASH regimen, 1154, 1154b
Washed RBCs, 1455
Wasp, 699
Wasp stings, 699
Water, humanitarian response and, e13
Water-borne infections, 1730
Water hammer, or Corrigan's, pulse, 975–976
Water-soluble contrast enema
  in complicated diverticulitis, 1136
  in large bowel obstruction, 1138
Water-soluble ingestants, 1835
Waterhouse-Friderichsen syndrome, 1324
Watson-Jones classification, 619, 619f
Watson scaphoid shift test, 511
WBC count, abdominal pain and, 214
WBI. *See* Whole bowel irrigation
Weakness, 96–101, 1316
  bilateral, 99–100
    all four extremities without facial involvement, 99
    distal portions of extremities only, 100
    lower extremities only, 99
    proximal portions of extremities only, 99–100
    upper extremities only, 99
  common clinical patterns of, 98f
  critical diagnoses of, 97, 99t